AMERICAN COLLEGE OF SURGEONS

ACS SURGERY

Principles & Practice

AMERICAN COLLEGE OF SURGEONS

ACS SURGERY

Principles & Practice

Formerly known as Scientific American® Surgery

DOUGLAS W. WILMORE, M.D., F.A.C.S.
Frank Sawyer Professor of Surgery,
Harvard Medical School
EDITORIAL CHAIRMAN

LAURENCE Y. CHEUNG, M.D., F.A.C.S.
Professor and Chairman, Department of Surgery,
University of Kansas School of Medicine
EDITOR

ALDEN H. HARKEN, M.D., F.A.C.S.
Professor and Chairman, Department of Surgery,
University of Colorado Health Sciences Center
EDITOR

JAMES W. HOLCROFT, M.D., F.A.C.S.
Professor, Department of Surgery,
University of California, Davis,
School of Medicine
EDITOR

JONATHAN L. MEAKINS, M.D., D.Sc., F.A.C.S.
Edward W. Archibald Professor and Chairman,
Department of Surgery,
McGill University Faculty of Medicine
EDITOR

NATHANIEL J. SOPER, M.D., F.A.C.S.
Professor, Department of Surgery,
Washington University School of Medicine
EDITOR

WebMD®
www.webmd.com

Library of Congress Cataloging-in-Publication Data

ACS surgery: principles and practice / Douglas W. Wilmore ... [et al.], editor.
   p. ; cm.
  Includes bibliographical references and index.
  ISBN 0-9703902-1-1 (alk. paper)
   1. Therapeutics, Surgical. 2. Surgery. I. Wilmore, Douglas W. (Douglas Wayne), date.
 II. American College of Surgeons.
  [DNLM: 1. Surgical Procedures, Operative—methods. 2. Perioperative Care—methods.
WA 300 G775c 2000]
  RD49 .A275 2001
  617'.9—dc21

2001026575

Content Development Manager	Richard P. Lindsey
Senior Producer	John J. Anello
Production Editor	Dave Terry
Art and Design Editor	Elizabeth Klarfeld
Electronic Composition	Carol Hansen, Diane Joiner, and Jennifer Smith
Manufacturing Coordinator	Kelly Mercado
Indexer	Julia Brooks Figures

© 2002 WebMD Corporation. All rights reserved.

No part of this book may be reproduced in any form by any means, including photocopying, or translated, transmitted, framed, or stored in a retrieval system for public or private use without the written permission of the publisher, WebMD Corporation. Scientific American® and Scientific American® Surgery are trademarks of Scientific American, Inc., and are used by WebMD Corporation under license from Scientific American, Inc.

Printed in the United States of America.

Published by WebMD Corporation.

WebMD Reference
WebMD Corporation
825 Third Avenue, 15th Floor
New York, NY 10022

ACS Surgery: Principles and Practice is sponsored by the American College of Surgeons and written by individuals who are recognized experts. The text represents the authors' approaches to clinical problems and to other important issues in surgical practice. It should be used as a general reference with other sources in the formation of an integrated care plan.

The authors, editors, and publisher have conscientiously and carefully tried to ensure that recommended measures and drug dosages in these pages are accurate and conform to the standards that prevailed at the time of publication. The reader is advised, however, to check the product information sheet accompanying each drug to be familiar with any changes in the dosage schedule or in the contraindications. This advice should be taken with particular seriousness if the agent to be administered is a new one or one that is infrequently used. *ACS Surgery: Principles and Practice* describes basic principles of diagnosis and therapy. Because of the uniqueness of each patient and the need to take into account a number of concurrent considerations, however, this information should be used by physicians only as a general guide to clinical decision making.

A Message from the American College of Surgeons

The American College of Surgeons was founded in 1913 to improve the quality of care for the surgical patient by setting high standards for surgical education and practice. As part of the College's continuing medical education (CME) efforts, it traditionally has produced a variety of publications on topics of interest to practicing surgeons. From the early 1960s until the late 1970s, the College published a variety of surgical manuals that covered specific areas, including trauma, infection, nutrition, and perioperative care. When interest in those publications decreased in the early 1980s, the Pre- and Postoperative Care Committee of the College decided to revitalize the manuals by creating a complete surgical reference for practicing surgeons that could be updated regularly. That surgical reference—*Scientific American® Surgery* (which began as *Care of the Surgical Patient*)—was launched in the late 1980s, and the College has sponsored it since its inception.

Last year, WebMD acquired *Scientific American® Surgery,* and this new publisher used this work to create the first online comprehensive surgical reference for the 21st century. The relationship between WebMD and the American College of Surgeons is strong. When the publisher approached us with the idea of renaming this CME resource *ACS Surgery: Principles and Practice,* we agreed that this new title is an appropriate acknowledgment of the College's commitment to providing CME for its members as well as a fitting recognition of the outstanding work done by the Editorial Board and the authors, who are superb representatives of the American College of Surgeons.

We hope that all our members, current and future, in the United States and abroad, will find *ACS Surgery: Principles and Practice* a useful tool in their ongoing efforts to improve patient care.

Thomas R. Russell, M.D., F.A.C.S.
Executive Director, American College of Surgeons
Chicago, Illinois
August 2001

To better care for all surgical patients

CONTENTS

Contributors	xv
Foreword, by Claude H. Organ, Jr., M.D., F.A.C.S.	xxiii
Preface	xxv

I RESUSCITATION

1	**Initial Emergency Management of Noninjured Patients: Cardiopulmonary Resuscitation and Correction of Acute Dysrhythmias** Steven R. Lowenstein, M.D., M.P.H., and Alden H. Harken, M.D.	3
2	**Trauma Resuscitation** Frederick A. Moore, M.D., and Ernest E. Moore, M.D.	31
3	**Burn Care in the Immediate Resuscitation Period** Robert H. Demling, M.D.	49
4	**Shock** James W. Holcroft, M.D.	63
5	**Bleeding and Transfusion** John T. Owings, M.D., and Robert C. Gosselin, M.T.	77
6	**Life-Threatening Electrolyte Abnormalities** Kimberly J. Van Zee, M.D., and Stephen F. Lowry, M.D.	91
7	**Life-Threatening Acid-Base Disorders** Lena M. Napolitano, M.D., and Anthony A. Meyer, M.D., Ph.D.	107
8	**Acute Wound Care** W. Thomas Lawrence, M.D., A. Griswold Bevin, M.D., and George F. Sheldon, M.D.	121
9	**Coma, Seizures, Cognitive Impairment, and Brain Death** Marike Zwienenberg, M.D., and J. Paul Muizelaar, M.D., Ph.D.	143
10	**Substance Abuse** John A. Marx, M.D., and Mark Kirk, M.D.	169

II COMMON PRESENTING PROBLEMS

11	**Neck Mass** Barry J. Roseman, M.D., and Orlo H. Clark, M.D.	183
12	**Asymptomatic Carotid Bruit** Claudio S. Cinà, M.D., Sp. Chir. (It.), M.Sc., Catherine M. Clase, M.B., B.Chir., M.Sc., and Aleksandar Radan, M.D., B.Sc., B.F.A.	195
13	**Breast Complaints** Barbara L. Smith, M.D., Ph.D., and Wiley W. Souba, M.D., Sc.D.	207

14	**Acute Abdominal Pain** *Romano Delcore, M.D., and Laurence Y. Cheung, M.D.*	225
15	**Abdominal Mass** *Romano Delcore, M.D., and Laurence Y. Cheung, M.D.*	241
16	**Jaundice** *Jeffrey S. Barkun, M.D., and Alan N. Barkun, M.D.*	251
17	**Intestinal Obstruction** *W. Scott Helton, M.D.*	263
18	**Upper Gastrointestinal Bleeding** *Richard T. Schlinkert, M.D., and Keith A. Kelly, M.D.*	283
19	**Lower Gastrointestinal Bleeding** *Margaret Schnitzler, M.B.B.S., and Robin S. McLeod, M.D.*	293
20	**Skin Lesions** *Alan E. Seyfer, M.D.*	301
21	**Soft Tissue Infection** *Ronald T. Lewis, M.B.B.S., M.Sc.*	313

III TRAUMA AND THERMAL INJURY

22	**Emergency Department Evaluation of the Patient with Multiple Injuries** *Felix D. Battistella, M.D.*	337
23	**Injuries to the Central Nervous System** *Marike Zwienenberg, M.D., and J. Paul Muizelaar, M.D., Ph.D.*	355
24	**Injuries to the Face and Jaw** *Seth Thaller, M.D., and F. William Blaisdell, M.D.*	369
25	**Injuries to the Neck** *David Wisner, M.D., and F. William Blaisdell, M.D.*	379
26	**Injuries to the Chest** *Kenneth L. Mattox, M.D., and Asher Hirshberg, M.D.*	395
27	**Operative Exposure of Abdominal Injuries and Closure of the Abdomen** *Erwin R. Thal, M.D., Brian J. Eastridge, M.D., and Rusty Milhoan, M.D.*	405
28	**Injuries to the Liver, Biliary Tract, Spleen, and Diaphragm** *Jon M. Burch, M.D., and Ernest E. Moore, M.D.*	413
29	**Injuries to the Stomach, Duodenum, Pancreas, Small Bowel, Colon, and Rectum** *Charles E. Lucas, M.D., and Anna M. Ledgerwood, M.D.*	425
30	**Injuries to the Great Vessels of the Abdomen** *David V. Feliciano, M.D.*	437
31	**Injuries to the Urogenital Tract** *Hunter Wessells, M.D., and Jack W. McAninch, M.D.*	449
32	**Injuries to the Extremities** *John T. Owings, M.D., James P. Kennedy, M.D., and F. William Blaisdell, M.D.*	463
33	**Burn Care in the Early Postresuscitation Period** *Robert H. Demling, M.D.*	479
34	**Burn Care after the First Postburn Week** *Robert H. Demling, M.D.*	491
35	**Miscellaneous Thermal Injuries** *Robert H. Demling, M.D.*	505

IV PREOPERATIVE PREPARATION

36	**Elements of Cost-Effective Nonemergency Surgical Care** Robert S. Rhodes, M.D., and Charles L. Rice, M.D.	519
37	**Nonemergency Surgery: Initial Evaluation, Preoperative Planning, Perioperative Issues, and Postoperative Care** Nicolas V. Christou, M.D., Ph.D., and Richard B. Reiling, M.D.	535
38	**Evaluation of Cardiac Risk** David A. Fullerton, M.D., Alden H. Harken, M.D., and Keith A. Horvath, M.D.	559
39	**Prevention of Postoperative Infection** Jonathan L. Meakins, M.D., D.Sc., Byron J. Masterson, M.D., and Ronald Lee Nichols, M.D., M.S.	567
40	**Preparing the Operating Room** Ramon Berguer, M.D., Denise Joffe, M.D., Rene Lafreniere, M.D., C.M., James T. Lee, M.D., Ph.D., Joseph LoCicero III, M.D., Edward J. Quebbeman, M.D., Ph.D., H. David Reines, M.D., Cynthia Spry, R.N., M.S.N., and Karen Stanley Williams, M.D.	591
41	**Perioperative Effects of Anesthesia** William C. Tullock, M.D., Charles D. Boucek, M.D., Wilbert A. Cusano, D.O., and W. David Watkins, M.D., Ph.D.	605

V OPERATIVE MANAGEMENT

42	**Thyroid and Parathyroid Procedures** Gregg H. Jossart, M.D., and Orlo H. Clark, M.D.	621
43	**Breast Procedures** Barbara L. Smith, M.D., Ph.D., and Wiley W. Souba, M.D., Sc.D.	629
44	**Lymphatic Mapping and Sentinel Lymph Node Biopsy** Douglas Reintgen, M.D., Fadi Haddad, M.D., Solange Pendas, M.D., Ni Ni Ku, M.D., Claudia Berman, M.D., Frank Glass, M.D., Jane Messina, M.D., and Charles Cox, M.D.	643
45	**Ultrasonography: Surgical Applications** Grace S. Rozycki, M.D.	659
46	**Thoracoscopy** Valerie W. Rusch, M.D.	673
47	**Gastrointestinal Endoscopy** Jeffrey L. Ponsky, M.D.	687
48	**Esophageal Procedures: Minimally Invasive Approaches** Marco G. Patti, M.D., and Carlos A. Pellegrini, M.D.	697
49	**Gastric Procedures** John L. Sawyers, M.D.	707
50	**Gastric Procedures for Morbid Obesity** Eric J. DeMaria, M.D., and Harvey J. Sugerman, M.D.	721
51	**Biliary Tract Procedures** Bernard Langer, M.D., and Bryce R. Taylor, M.D.	735
52	**Laparoscopic Cholecystectomy** Gerald M. Fried, M.D., and Liane S. Feldman, M.D.	753
53	**Pancreatic Procedures** John L. Cameron, M.D.	773
54	**Laparoscopic Splenectomy** Eric C. Poulin, M.D., M.Sc., Christopher M. Schlachta, M.D., and Joseph Mamazza, M.D.	787

55	**Intestinal Anastomosis** Zane Cohen, M.D., and Barry Sullivan, M.D.	803
56	**Appendectomy** Hung S. Ho, M.D.	815
57	**Colorectal Procedures** Theodore R. Schrock, M.D.	825
58	**Laparoscopic Colectomy** Babak N. Rad, M.D., and Robert W. Beart, Jr., M.D.	837
59	**Anal Procedures** Ira J. Kodner, M.D.	843
60	**Open Repair of Hernias of the Abdominal Wall** George E. Wantz, M.D.	857
61	**Laparoscopic Hernia Repair** Liane S. Feldman, M.D., and Marvin J. Wexler, M.D.	877
62	**Vascular and Peritoneal Access** Bernard Montreuil, M.D., Laurie Morrison, M.D., Lawrence Rosenberg, M.D., Ph.D., and Carl Nohr, M.D., Ph.D.	897
63	**Carotid Arterial Procedures** Wesley S. Moore, M.D.	921
64	**Repair of Infrarenal Abdominal Aortic Aneurysms** Frank R. Arko, M.D., and Christopher K. Zarins, M.D.	937
65	**Lower-Extremity Amputation for Ischemia** William C. Pevec, M.D.	949
66	**Organ Procurement** Charles M. Miller, M.D., Felix T. Rapaport, M.D., and Thomas E. Starzl, M.D., Ph.D.	959
67	**Plastic Surgical Reconstruction** David A. Hidalgo, M.D., and Joseph J. Disa, M.D.	973

VI SPECIAL PERIOPERATIVE PROBLEMS

68	**Diabetes Mellitus** Maha F. Ansara, M.D., Philip E. Cryer, M.D., and David W. Scharp, M.D.	993
69	**Obesity** Harvey J. Sugerman, M.D.	1003
70	**Thromboembolic Problems** F. William Blaisdell, M.D., and John T. Owings, M.D.	1013
71	**Pulmonary Insufficiency** Robert H. Bartlett, M.D.	1039
72	**Renal Dysfunction** Nicholas L. Tilney, M.D., Julian L. Seifter, M.D., and Robert J. Rizzo, M.D.	1051
73	**Adrenal Insufficiency** Valerie J. Halpin, M.D., and Jeffrey A. Norton, M.D.	1063
74	**Non-AIDS Immunosuppression** Carl Nohr, M.D., Ph.D.	1071
75	**The Elderly Surgical Patient** James M. Watters, M.D., and Jacqueline C. McClaran, M.D.	1091
76	**The Pediatric Surgical Patient** Arnold G. Coran, M.D.	1121
77	**The Pregnant Surgical Patient** David C. Brooks, M.D., and Laura A. Sznyter, M.D.	1145

78	**Clinical and Laboratory Diagnosis of Infection** *David C. Evans, M.D., and Jonathan L. Meakins, M.D., D.Sc.*	1163
79	**Blood Cultures and Infection in the Patient with the Septic Response** *Donald E. Fry, M.D.*	1175
80	**Antibiotics** *Nicolas V. Christou, M.D., Ph.D.*	1191
81	**Nosocomial Infection** *E. Patchen Dellinger, M.D.*	1221
82	**Peritonitis and Intra-abdominal Abscesses** *Ori D. Rotstein, M.D., M.Sc., and Avery B. Nathens, M.D., Ph.D., M.P.H.*	1239
83	**Infections in the Upper Abdomen: Biliary Tract, Pancreas, Liver, and Spleen** *Jeffrey S. Barkun, M.D., and Ronald T. Lewis, M.B.B.S., M.Sc.*	1263
84	**Hand Infection** *Thomas M. Sinclair, M.D., C.M., and H. Bruce Williams, M.D.*	1279
85	**Fungal Infection** *Elias J. Anaissie, M.D., Bishara B. Albair, M.D., and Joseph S. Solomkin, M.D.*	1289
86	**Viral Infection** *Jennifer W. Janelle, M.D., and Richard J. Howard, M.D., Ph.D.*	1309
87	**Acquired Immunodeficiency Syndrome** *John Mihran Davis, M.D.*	1333
88	**Immunomodulation** *David L. Dunn, M.D., Ph.D.*	1347

VII CARE IN THE ICU

89	**Cardiopulmonary Monitoring** *Jerome H. Abrams, M.D., Frank Cerra, M.D., and James W. Holcroft, M.D.*	1365
90	**Support of the Failing Heart** *Charles L. Rice, M.D., and R. John Solaro, Ph.D.*	1391
91	**Pulmonary Dysfunction** *Robert H. Demling, M.D.*	1401
92	**Use of the Mechanical Ventilator** *Robert H. Bartlett, M.D.*	1423
93	**Acute Renal Failure** *Anthony A. Meyer, M.D., Ph.D.*	1441
94	**Hepatic Failure** *Walid S. Arnaout, M.D., and Achilles A. Demetriou, M.D., Ph.D.*	1455
95	**Multiple Organ Dysfunction Syndrome** *John C. Marshall, M.D., and Avery B. Nathens, M.D., Ph.D., M.P.H.*	1473
96	**Metabolic Response to Critical Illness** *Palmer Q. Bessey, M.D.*	1495
97	**Nutritional Support** *John L. Rombeau, M.D., Rolando H. Rolandelli, M.D., Douglas W. Wilmore, M.D., and John M. Daly, M.D.*	1521
98	**Fever, Hyperpyrexia, and Hypothermia** *Douglas W. Wilmore, M.D.*	1549
99	**Reactive Oxygen Metabolites** *Patrick M. Reilly, M.D., Susan A. Kelly, M.D., Henry J. Schiller, M.D., and Gregory B. Bulkley, M.D.*	1559

100	**Eicosanoids in Surgery** Martin R. Weiser, M.D., James Hill, M.B., Ch.B., Thomas Lindsay, M.D., and Herbert B. Hechtman, M.D.	1591
101	**Cytokines and the Cellular Response to Injury and Infection** Yuman Fong, M.D., and Stephen F. Lowry, M.D.	1603

VIII POSTOPERATIVE MANAGEMENT

102	**Postoperative Management** Samir M. Fakhry, M.D., Edmund J. Rutherford, M.D., and George F. Sheldon, M.D.	1625
103	**Early Postoperative Pneumonia** David W. Chang, M.D., and Robert H. Demling, M.D.	1647
104	**Postoperative Pain** Henrik Kehlet, Prof. M.D., Ph.D., and F. Michael Ferrante, M.D.	1659
105	**Stomal Care** M. Joyce Rosenthal, R.N., M.S., C.E.T.N., and Daniel Rosenthal, M.D.	1675
106	**Rehabilitation of the Burn Patient** Robert H. Demling, M.D.	1691

IX MISCELLANEOUS CONCERNS

107	**Pharmacokinetics in Surgical Practice** C. Edward Hartford, M.D., and G. Patrick Kealey, M.D., M.S.	1697
108	**Infection Control in Surgical Practice** A. Peter McLean, M.D., and Catherine M. Dixon, R.N., B.A.	1717
109	**The Impaired Physician** David B. Hoyt, M.D., Martha C. Martell, M.S., and Peter Rosen, M.D.	1729
	Index	1741

CONTRIBUTORS

JEROME H. ABRAMS, M.D., F.A.C.S. Associate Professor, Department of Surgery, University of Minnesota Medical School—Minneapolis, and Chief, Surgical Critical Care, Veterans Affairs Medical Center, Minneapolis

BISHARA B. ALBAIR, M.D. Postdoctoral Fellow, Department of Surgery, University of Arkansas College of Medicine, Little Rock

ELIAS J. ANAISSIE, M.D. Professor of Medicine, Department of Medicine, Myeloma and Transplantation Research Center, University of Arkansas College of Medicine, and Director, Department of Clinical Affairs, University Hospital of Arkansas, Little Rock

MAHA F. ANSARA, M.D. Fellow, Endocrinology and Metabolism, Division of Endocrinology, Diabetes and Metabolism, New Hanover Regional Medical Center, Wilmington, North Carolina

FRANK R. ARKO, M.D. Postdoctoral Fellow/Endovascular Fellow, Division of Vascular Surgery, Department of Surgery, Stanford University School of Medicine

WALID S. ARNAOUT, M.D., F.A.C.S. Associate Director, Center for Liver Diseases and Transplantation, Cedars-Sinai Medical Center, Los Angeles

ALAN N. BARKUN, M.D. Associate Professor and Director, Division of Gastroenterology, Department of Medicine, McGill University Faculty of Medicine, and Director, Division of Gastroenterology, McGill University Health Centre

JEFFREY S. BARKUN, M.D. Associate Professor, Department of Surgery, McGill University Faculty of Medicine

ROBERT H. BARTLETT, M.D., F.A.C.S. Professor, Division of General and Thoracic Surgery, Department of Surgery, University of Michigan Medical School

FELIX D. BATTISTELLA, M.D., F.A.C.S. Associate Professor, Division of Trauma, Department of Surgery, University of California, Davis, School of Medicine, and Attending Physician, Department of Surgery, University of California, Davis, Medical Center

ROBERT W. BEART, JR., M.D., F.A.C.S. Chairman of Colon and Rectal Surgery and Costello Professor of Surgery, Division of Colorectal Surgery, Department of Surgery, Keck School of Medicine, University of Southern California

RAMON BERGUER, M.D., F.A.C.S. Professor of Surgery, Wayne State University School of Medicine, and Chief, Division of Vascular Surgery, Detroit Medical Center

CLAUDIA BERMAN, M.D. Professor, Department of Radiology, University of South Florida College of Medicine, and Attending Radiologist, H. Lee Moffitt Cancer Center and Research Institute

PALMER Q. BESSEY, M.D., F.A.C.S. Professor, Department of Surgery, Weill Medical College of Cornell University, and Associate Director, William Randolf Hearst Burn Center, New York Presbyterian Hospital-Cornell Medical Center

A. GRISWOLD BEVIN, M.D. Professor Emeritus, Division of Plastic Surgery, Department of Surgery, University of North Carolina at Chapel Hill School of Medicine

F. WILLIAM BLAISDELL, M.D., F.A.C.S. Professor and Chairman, Department of Surgery, University of California, Davis, School of Medicine, and Chief of Surgical Services, Department of Surgery, Mather Veterans Affairs Hospital, Mather, California

CHARLES D. BOUCEK, M.D. Associate Professor of Clinical Anesthesiology and Staff, Anesthesiology, University of Pittsburgh Medical Center

DAVID C. BROOKS, M.D., F.A.C.S. Associate Professor, Department of Surgery, Harvard Medical School, and Senior Surgeon, Department of Surgery, Brigham and Women's Hospital

GREGORY B. BULKLEY, M.D., F.A.C.S. Mark M. Ravitch Professor, Department of Surgery, Johns Hopkins University School of Medicine, and Director, Department of Surgical Research, Johns Hopkins Hospital

JON M. BURCH, M.D., F.A.C.S. Professor, Department of Surgery, University of Colorado Health Sciences Center, and Chief, Department of General and Vascular Surgery, Denver Health Medical Center

JOHN L. CAMERON, M.D., F.A.C.S. Professor and Chairman, Department of Surgery, Johns Hopkins University School of Medicine, and Surgeon-in-Chief, Johns Hopkins Hospital

Frank Cerra, M.D., F.A.C.S. Professor, Department of Surgery, and Senior Vice President for Health Sciences, Academic Health Center, University of Minnesota; and Attending Surgeon, Department of Surgery, Fairview University Medical Center

David W. Chang, M.D. Fellow in Critical Care, Brigham and Women's Hospital

Laurence Y. Cheung, M.D., F.A.C.S. Professor and Chairman, Department of Surgery, University of Kansas School of Medicine, and Chief of Surgery, Department of Surgical Services, University of Kansas Hospital, Kansas City

Nicolas V. Christou, M.D., Ph.D., F.A.C.S. Professor, Department of Surgery, McGill University Faculty of Medicine, and Head, Division of General Surgery, McGill University Health Centre

Claudio S. Cinà, M.D., Sp. Chir. (It.), M.Sc., F.R.S.C.(C) Assistant Clinical Professor, Department of Surgery, McMaster University Faculty of Health Sciences, Hamilton, Ontario, Canada

Orlo H. Clark, M.D., F.A.C.S. Professor and Vice Chair, Department of Surgery, University of California, San Francisco, School of Medicine, and Chief, Department of Surgery, Mount Zion Medical Center of UC-San Francisco

Catherine M. Clase, M.B., B.Chir., M.Sc., F.R.C.P.(C) Assistant Professor, Department of Medicine, Dalhousie University Faculty of Medicine, and Nephrologist, Department of Medicine, QE 2 Health Sciences Center

Zane Cohen, M.D., F.A.C.S. Professor, Department of Surgery, University of Toronto Faculty of Medicine, and Surgeon-in-Chief, Mount Sinai Hospital, Toronto

Arnold G. Coran, M.D., F.A.C.S. Professor, Division of Pediatric Surgery, Department of Surgery, University of Michigan Medical School, and Surgeon-in-Chief, Section of Pediatric Surgery, Department of Surgery, C. S. Mott Children's Hospital

Charles Cox, M.D., F.A.C.S. Professor, Department of Surgery, University of South Florida College of Medicine, and Breast Cancer Program Leader, H. Lee Moffitt Cancer Center and Research Institute

Philip E. Cryer, M.D. Irene E. and Michael M. Karl Professor of Endocrinology, Diabetes, and Metabolism, Professor of Medicine, and Director, Division of Endocrinology, Diabetes, and Metabolism, and Director of General Clinical Research Center, Washington University School of Medicine; and Physician, Department of Medicine, Barnes Jewish Hospital of St. Louis

Wilbert A. Cusano, D.O. Assistant Professor of Anesthesiology, Department of Anesthesiology/CCM, Montefiore University Hospital, University of Pittsburgh School of Medicine

John M. Daly, M.D., F.A.C.S. Lewis Atterbury Stimson Professor and Chairman, Department of Surgery, Weill Medical College of Cornell University, and Surgeon-in-Chief, New York Presbyterian Hospital-Cornell Medical Center

John Mihran Davis, M.D., F.A.C.S. Professor, Department of Surgery, University of Medicine and Dentistry of New Jersey Robert Wood Johnson Medical School, and Surgery Program Director, Jersey Shore Medical Center

Romano Delcore, M.D., F.A.C.S. Professor, Department of Surgery, University of Kansas School of Medicine, and Medical Director, Department of Surgery, University of Kansas Medical Center

E. Patchen Dellinger, M.D., F.A.C.S. Professor and Vice Chairman, Department of Surgery, University of Washington School of Medicine, and Chief and Associate Medical Director, Department of Surgery, University of Washington Medical Center

Eric J. DeMaria, M.D., F.A.C.S. Professor, Division of General/Trauma Surgery, Virginia Commonwealth University Medical College of Virginia, and Section Chief, General and Endoscopic Surgery, and Director, Medical College of Virginia's Hospital for Minimally Invasive Surgery

Achilles A. Demetriou, M.D., Ph.D., F.A.C.S. Chairman, Department of Surgery, Cedars-Sinai Medical Center, Los Angeles

Robert H. Demling, M.D., F.A.C.S. Professor, Department of Surgery, Harvard Medical School, and Director, Burn Center, Brigham and Women's Hospital

Joseph J. Disa, M.D. Assistant Attending Surgeon, Department of Plastic and Reconstructive Surgery, Memorial Sloan-Kettering Cancer Center

Catherine M. Dixon, R.N., B.A. Infection Control Coordinator (Retired), Royal Victoria Hospital, Montreal

David L. Dunn, M.D., Ph.D., F.A.C.S. Jay Phillips Professor and Chairman, Department of Surgery, and Head, Division of Surgical Infectious Diseases, University of Minnesota Medical School

Brian J. Eastridge, M.D., F.A.C.S. Assistant Professor, Department of Surgery, University of Texas Southwestern Medical School

David C. Evans, M.D. Assistant Professor, Department of Surgery, McGill University Faculty of Medicine, and Director, Trauma Unit, Montreal General Hospital

Samir M. Fakhry, M.D., F.A.C.S. Clinical Professor, Department of Surgery, Georgetown University School of Medicine, and Director, Trauma Services/Trauma Intensive Care Unit, Inova Fairfax Hospital, Falls Church, Virginia

Liane S. Feldman, M.D. Assistant Professor, Department of Surgery, McGill University Faculty of Medicine, and Staff, Departments of Videoendoscopic Surgery and Surgery, McGill University Hospital Centre

David V. Feliciano, M.D., F.A.C.S. Professor, Department of Surgery, Emory University School of Medicine, and Chief of Surgery, Grady Memorial Hospital, Atlanta

F. Michael Ferrante, M.D. Professor, Departments of Anesthesiology and Medicine, University of Pennsylvania School of Medicine, and Director, Anesthesia Pain Medicine Program and Cancer Pain and Symptom Management Program, University of Pennsylvania Health Systems

Yuman Fong, M.D., F.A.C.S. Associate Professor of Cell Biology and Anatomy, Cornell University Medical College, and Associate Professor of Surgery, Memorial Sloan-Kettering Cancer Center

Gerald M. Fried, M.D., F.A.C.S. Professor of Surgery, Division of General Surgery, McGill University Faculty of Medicine, and Senior Surgeon, McGill University Health Centre

Donald E. Fry, M.D., F.A.C.S. Professor and Chairman, Department of Surgery, University of New Mexico School of Medicine

David A. Fullerton, M.D., F.A.C.S. Professor of Surgery and Chief, Division of Cardiothoracic Surgery, Northwestern University Medical School

Frank Glass, M.D. Associate Professor, Departments of Medicine and Pathology, H. Lee Moffitt Cancer Center and Research Institute, University of South Florida College of Medicine

Robert C. Gosselin, M.T. Senior Specialist, Hematology/Hemostasis, University of California, Davis, Medical Center

Fadi Haddad, M.D., F.A.C.S. Clinical Research Fellow, Department of Surgery, H. Lee Moffitt Cancer Center and Research Institute, University of South Florida College of Medicine

Valerie J. Halpin, M.D. Resident, Department of Surgery, Washington University School of Medicine

Alden H. Harken, M.D., F.A.C.S. Professor and Chairman, Department of Surgery, University of Colorado Health Sciences Center

C. Edward Hartford, M.D., F.A.C.S. Professor of Surgery, University of Colorado Health Sciences Center

Herbert B. Hechtman, M.D., F.A.C.S. Professor, Department of Surgery, Harvard Medical School, and Surgeon Emeritus, Brigham and Women's Hospital

W. Scott Helton, M.D., F.A.C.S. Professor and Chief, Division of General Surgery, Department of Surgery, University of Illinois College of Medicine

David A. Hidalgo, M.D., F.A.C.S. Associate Professor, Department of Surgery, Weill Medical College of Cornell University, and Associate Professor, Division of Plastic and Reconstructive Surgery, Manhattan Eye, Ear, and Throat Hospital

James Hill, M.B., Ch.B., F.R.C.S. Senior Registrar, Manchester Royal Infirmary, England

Asher Hirshberg, M.D. Lecturer in Surgery, Shackler School of Medicine, and Staff Surgeon, Department of General and Vascular Surgery, and Co-Director, Trauma Service, B. Chaim Sheba Medical Center, Tel Hashomer, Israel

Hung S. Ho, M.D., F.A.C.S. Associate Professor, Division of Gastrointestinal and Laparoscopic Surgery, Department of Surgery, University of California, Davis, School of Medicine, and Medical Director and Attending Staff, Section of Gastrointestinal and Laparoscopic Surgery, Department of Surgery, University of California, Davis, Medical Center

James W. Holcroft, M.D., F.A.C.S. Professor, Department of Surgery, University of California, Davis, School of Medicine

Keith A. Horvath, M.D., F.A.C.S. Assistant Professor, Department of Surgery, Northwestern University Medical School, and Attending Surgeon, Northwestern Memorial Hospital

Richard J. Howard, M.D., Ph.D., F.A.C.S. Robert H. and Kathleen M. Axline Professor of Surgery, Division of General Surgery and Transplantation, Department of Surgery, University of Florida College of Medicine

David B. Hoyt, M.D., F.A.C.S. Professor, Department of Surgery, University of California, San Diego, School of Medicine, and Chief, Division of Trauma, Burns, and Surgical Intensive Care, University of California, San Diego, Medical Center

Jennifer W. Janelle, M.D. Clinical Professor of Medicine, Division of Infectious Diseases, Department of Medicine, University of Florida College of Medicine

Denise Joffe, M.D. Associate Professor, Department of Anesthesiology, University of Medicine and Dentistry of New Jersey Robert Wood Johnson Medical School

Gregg H. Jossart, M.D. Director of Minimal Invasive Surgery, California Pacific Medical Center, San Francisco

G. Patrick Kealey, MD., M.S., F.A.C.S., F.C.C.M. Professor, Department of Surgery, University of Iowa College of Medicine, and Director, Trauma, Burn, and Surgical Critical Care Services, University of Iowa Hospitals and Clinics

Henrik Kehlet, Prof. M.D., Ph.D. Professor, Department of Surgery, University of Copenhagen School of Medicine, and Chief Surgeon, Section of Surgical Gastroenterology, Department of Surgery, Københavns Kommunes Hvidovre Hospital, Hvidovre, Denmark

Keith A. Kelly, M.D., F.A.C.S. Professor, Department of Surgery, Mayo Medical School, and Consultant, Department of Surgery, Mayo Clinic Arizona

Susan A. Kelly, M.D. Private practice, Obstetrics and Gynecology, Wilmington, Delaware

James P. Kennedy, M.D. Assistant Professor, Division of Clinical Orthopedic Surgery, Department of Surgery, Northeastern Ohio Universities College of Medicine

Mark Kirk, M.D. Medical Toxicology Fellowship Director, Indiana Poison Control Center and the Emergency Medicine and Trauma Center at Methodist Hospital, Indiana University School of Medicine

Ira J. Kodner, M.D., F.A.C.S. Solon and Bettie Gershman Professor, Division of Colon and Rectal Surgery, Department of Surgery, Washington University School of Medicine

Ni Ni Ku, M.D. Clinical Associate Professor of Pathology, University of South Florida College of Medicine, and Director of Anatomic Pathology, Department of Pathology, Bayfront Medical Center, St. Petersburg, Florida

Rene Lafreniere, M.D., C.M., F.A.C.S. Professor and Head, Department of Surgery, University of Calgary Faculty of Medicine, and Regional Clinical Department Head of Surgery, Calgary Regional Health Authority, Calgary, Alberta, Canada

Bernard Langer, M.D., F.R.C.S.(C), F.A.C.S. Professor, Department of Surgery, University of Toronto Faculty of Medicine, and Senior Staff Surgeon, Toronto General Hospital

W. Thomas Lawrence, M.D., F.A.C.S. Professor and Chief, Division of Plastic Surgery, Department of Surgery, University of Kansas School of Medicine

Anna M. Ledgerwood, M.D., F.A.C.S. Professor, Department of Surgery, Wayne State University School of Medicine, and General Surgeon, Detroit Receiving Hospital

James T. Lee, M.D., Ph.D., F.A.C.S. Professor, Department of Surgery, University of Minnesota Medical School

Ronald T. Lewis, M.B.B.S., M.Sc., F.R.C.S.(C), F.A.C.S. Associate Professor, Department of Surgery, McGill University Faculty of Medicine, and Chief, Vascular Surgery, Department of Surgery, McGill University Health Centre

Thomas Lindsay, M.D., F.R.C.S.(C) Associate Professor of Vascular Surgery, Department of Surgery, University of Toronto Faculty of Medicine, and Staff Surgeon, Vascular Surgery, Toronto General Hospital

Joseph LoCicero III, M.D., F.A.C.S. Associate Professor of Surgery, Harvard Medical School, and Chief, General Thoracic Surgery, Department of Surgery, Beth Israel Deaconess Medical Center

Steven R. Lowenstein, M.D., M.P.H. Associate Professor of Surgery, Medicine, and Preventive Medicine and Biometrics, University of Colorado School of Medicine, and Associate Director, Emergency Department, University of Colorado Hospital

Stephen F. Lowry, M.D., F.A.C.S. Professor and Chairman, Department of Surgery, University of Medicine and Dentistry of New Jersey Robert Wood Johnson Medical School

Charles E. Lucas, M.D., F.A.C.S. Professor, Department of Surgery, Wayne State University School of Medicine, and Surgeon, Detroit Receiving Hospital

Joseph Mamazza, M.D. Assistant Professor, Department of Surgery, University of Toronto Faculty of Medicine, and Medical Director of Minimal Access Therapeutics and Diseases of Digestive Systems and Director of Minimally Invasive Surgery, St. Michael's Hospital

John C. Marshall, M.D., F.R.C.S.(C), F.A.C.S. Professor, Department of Surgery, University of Toronto Faculty of Medicine, and Director of Research, Medical and Surgical Intensive Care Unit, and Staff Surgeon, Toronto General Hospital University Health Network

Martha C. Martell, M.S. Managing Editor, *Journal of Emergency Medicine*, Department of Emergency Medicine, University of California, San Diego, Medical Center

John A. Marx, M.D. Clinical Professor, Department of Emergency Medicine, University of North Carolina at Chapel Hill School of Medicine, and Chairman, Department of Emergency Medicine, Carolinas Medical Center, Charlotte, North Carolina

Byron J. Masterson, M.D., F.A.C.S. J. Wayne Reitz Professor of Gynecologic Surgery and Chairman Emeritus, University of Florida College of Medicine, Gainesville, and Professor, School of Public Health, University of South Florida (courtesy), Tampa

Kenneth L. Mattox, M.D., F.A.C.S. Professor and Vice Chairman, Division of Thoracic Surgery, Department of Surgery, Baylor College of Medicine, and Chief of Staff and Chief of Surgery, Ben Taub General Hospital, Houston

Jack W. McAninch, M.D., F.A.C.S. Professor, Department of Urology, University of California, San Francisco, School of Medicine, and Chief, Department of Urology, San Francisco General Hospital

Jacqueline C. McClaran, M.D. Associate Professor, Departments of Family Medicine and Medicine, McGill University Faculty of Medicine, and Director, Department of Discharge Planning, McGill University Health Centre

A. Peter McLean, M.D., F.A.C.S. Associate Professor, Department of Surgery, McGill University Faculty of Medicine, and Senior Surgeon, McGill University Health Centre

Robin S. McLeod, M.D., F.A.C.S. Professor, Department of Surgery, University of Toronto Faculty of Medicine, and Head, Division of General Surgery, Mount Sinai Hospital, Toronto

Jonathan L. Meakins, M.D., D.Sc., F.A.C.S. Edward W. Archibald Professor and Chairman, Department of Surgery, McGill University Faculty of Medicine, and Surgeon-in-Chief, McGill University Health Centre

Jane Messina, M.D. Associate Professor, Department of Pathology, H. Lee Moffitt Cancer Center and Research Institute, University of South Florida College of Medicine

Anthony Meyer, M.D., Ph.D., F.A.C.S. Professor, Vice Chairman, and Chief, Division of General Surgery, Department of Surgery, University of North Carolina at Chapel Hill School of Medicine, and Chief of General Surgery, North Carolina Jaycee Burn Center, University of North Carolina Hospitals and Clinics

Rusty Milhoan, M.D., F.A.C.S. Trauma Surgeon, Department of Trauma Services, Christus St. Elizabeth Hospital, Beaumont, Texas

Charles M. Miller, M.D., F.A.C.S. Alfred and Florence Gross Professor of Surgery, Mt. Sinai School of Medicine of the City University of New York, and Director, Recanati-Miller Transplantation Institute, Mount Sinai Medical Center, New York City

Bernard Montreuil, M.D. Assistant Professor, Division of Vascular Surgery, Department of Surgery, Royal Victoria Hospital, Montreal, Quebec, Canada

Ernest E. Moore, M.D., F.A.C.S. Professor and Vice Chairman, Department of Surgery, University of Colorado Health Sciences Center, and Chief, Department of Surgery, Denver Health Medical Center

Frederick A. Moore, M.D., F.A.C.S. Professor and Vice Chairman, Department of Surgery, University of Texas Medical School at Houston, and Chief, Department of General Surgery, Trauma, and Critical Care, Memorial Hermann Hospital

Wesley S. Moore, M.D., F.A.C.S. Professor, Division of Vascular Surgery, Department of Surgery, University of California, Los Angeles, UCLA School of Medicine

Laurie Morrison, M.D. Fellow, Division of Vascular Surgery, Department of Surgery, McGill University Faculty of Medicine

J. Paul Muizelaar, M.D., Ph.D. Professor and Chairman, Department of Neurological Surgery, University of California, Davis, School of Medicine

Lena M. Napolitano, M.D., F.A.C.S. Associate Professor, Department of Surgery, University of Maryland Medical System, and Director of Surgical Critical Care, Surgical Care Center, VA Maryland Health Care System, Baltimore

Avery B. Nathens, M.D., Ph.D., M.P.H., F.A.C.S. Assistant Professor of Surgery, Harborview Medical Center, Seattle

Ronald Lee Nichols, M.D., M.S., F.A.C.S. William Henderson Professor, Department of Surgery and Microbiology, Tulane University School of Medicine, and Attending Surgeon, Department of Surgery, Tulane University Hospital and Clinic

Carl Nohr, M.D., Ph.D., F.R.C.S.(C), F.A.C.S. Chief, Department of Surgery, Palliser Health Region, Alberta, Canada

Jeffrey A. Norton, M.D., F.A.C.S. Professor and Vice Chair, Department of Surgery, University of California, San Francisco, School of Medicine, and Chief of Surgical Service, San Francisco VA Medical Center

John T. Owings, M.D., F.A.C.S. Associate Professor, Division of Trauma, Department of Surgery, University of California, Davis, School of Medicine, and Attending Physician, Department of Surgery, University of California, Davis, Medical Center

Marco G. Patti, M.D., F.A.C.S. Associate Professor, Department of Surgery, University of California, San Francisco, School of Medicine, and Director, Center for the Study of GI Motility and Secretion, University of California, San Francisco, Medical Center

Carlos A. Pellegrini, M.D., F.A.C.S. Henry N. Harkins Professor and Chair, Department of Surgery, University of Washington School of Medicine, and Attending Surgeon, Department of Surgery, University of Washington Medical Center

Solange Pendas, M.D. Surgical Resident, Department of Surgery, Maimonides Medical Center

William C. Pevec, M.D., F.A.C.S. Associate Professor of Vascular Surgery, Department of Surgery, University of California, Davis, School of Medicine, and Chief of Vascular Surgery, Department of Surgery, University of California, Davis, Medical Center

Jeffrey L. Ponsky, M.D., F.A.C.S. Professor of Surgery, Cleveland Clinic Health Sciences Center of the Ohio State University, and Director, Section of Endoscopic Surgery, Department of General Surgery, Cleveland Clinic Foundation

Eric C. Poulin, M.D., M.Sc. Professor, Department of Surgery, University of Toronto Faculty of Medicine, and Surgeon-in-Chief, St. Michael's Hospital

Edward J. Quebbeman, M.D., Ph.D., F.A.C.S. Professor of Trauma and Emergency Surgery, Department of Surgery, Medical College of Wisconsin

Babak N. Rad, M.D. Fellow in Colorectal Surgery, Keck School of Medicine, University of Southern California

Aleksandar Radan, M.D., B.Sc., B.F.A. General Surgery Resident, Department of Surgery, McMaster University Faculty of Health Sciences

Felix T. Rapaport, M.D. Distinguished Professor, Department of Surgery, State University of New York at Stony Brook School of Medicine (deceased)

Richard B. Reiling, M.D., F.A.C.S. Clinical Professor of Surgery, Wright State University School of Medicine, and Vice President for Cancer Services, Grant/Riverside Methodist Hospitals, Columbus, Ohio

Patrick M. Reilly, M.D., F.A.C.S. Assistant Professor and Trauma Program Director, Division of Traumatology and Surgical Critical Care, Department of Surgery, University of Pennsylvania Medical Center

H. David Reines, M.D., F.A.C.S. Professor of Surgery, Tufts University School of Medicine, and Chairman of Surgery, Newton-Wellesley Hospital, Newton, Massachusetts

Douglas Reintgen, M.D., F.A.C.S. Professor, Department of Surgery, University of South Florida College of Medicine, and Program Leader, Department of Cutaneous Oncology, H. Lee Moffitt Cancer Center and Research Institute

Robert S. Rhodes, M.D., F.A.C.S. Adjunct Professor, Department of Surgery, University of Pennsylvania School of Medicine, and Associate Executive Director and Director of Evaluation, American Board of Surgery, Philadelphia

Charles L. Rice, M.D., F.A.C.S. Professor, Departments of Surgery and Physiology and Biophysics, and Vice Chancellor for Health Affairs, University of Illinois at Chicago Medical Center

Robert J. Rizzo, M.D., F.A.C.S. Assistant Professor, Division of Cardiac Surgery, Department of Surgery, Harvard Medical School, and Associate Surgeon, Division of Cardiac Surgery, Brigham and Women's Hospital

Rolando H. Rolandelli, M.D., F.A.C.S. Professor, Department of Surgery, and Chief, Section of General Surgery, Temple University Hospital

John L. Rombeau, M.D., F.A.C.S. Professor, Division of Colorectal Surgery, Department of Surgery, University of Pennsylvania School of Medicine, and Staff Colorectal Surgeon, Division of Gastrointestinal Surgery, Department of Surgery, Hospital of the University of Pennsylvania

Barry J. Roseman, M.D. Roseman and Budayr, M.D., P.C., Maryville, Tennessee

Peter Rosen, M.D., F.A.C.S. Professor, Department of Clinical Medicine and Surgery, University of California, San Diego, School of Medicine

Lawrence Rosenberg, M.D., Ph.D., F.A.C.S. Professor of Surgery and Medicine and Director, Division of Surgical Research, McGill University Faculty of Medicine, and Senior Surgeon, McGill University Health Centre

Daniel Rosenthal, M.D., F.A.C.S. Clinical Professor, Department of Surgery, University of Texas Medical School at San Antonio, and Uniformed Services University of the Health Sciences School of Medicine, Bethesda

M. Joyce Rosenthal, R.N., M.S., C.E.T.N. Gastrointestinal Nurse, Baptist Medical Center, San Antonio

Ori D. Rotstein, M.D., M.Sc., F.R.C.S.(C), F.A.C.S. Professor, Department of Surgery, University of Toronto Faculty of Medicine, and Staff Surgeon, Toronto General Hospital

GRACE S. ROZYCKI, M.D., F.A.C.S. Associate Professor, Department of Surgery, Emory University School of Medicine, and Director of Trauma/Surgical Critical Care, Grady Memorial Hospital

VALERIE W. RUSCH, M.D., F.A.C.S. Professor, Department of Surgery, Weill Medical College of Cornell University, and William G. Cahan Chair of Surgery and Chief of Thoracic Surgery, Memorial Sloan-Kettering Cancer Center

EDMUND J. RUTHERFORD, M.D., F.A.C.S. Associate Professor, Department of Surgery, University of North Carolina at Chapel Hill School of Medicine, and Chief of Surgical Critical Care, UNC Hospitals

JOHN L. SAWYERS, M.D., F.A.C.S. John Clinton Foshee Distinguished Professor (Emeritus), Department of Surgery, Vanderbilt University School of Medicine

DAVID W. SCHARP, M.D., F.A.C.S. Chief Scientific Officer, Novocell, Inc., Irvine, California

HENRY J. SCHILLER, M.D. Associate Professor of Surgery and Director, Clark Burn Center, State University of New York Health Science Center at Syracuse

CHRISTOPHER M. SCHLACHTA, M.D. Lecturer and General Surgeon, Department of Surgery, University of Toronto Faculty of Medicine

RICHARD T. SCHLINKERT, M.D., F.A.C.S. Professor, Department of Surgery, Mayo Graduate School of Medicine, and General Surgeon, Department of Surgery, Mayo Clinic Scottsdale

MARGARET SCHNITZLER, M.B.B.S. Associate Professor, Department of Surgery, University of Sydney Faculty of Medicine, Australia

THEODORE R. SCHROCK, M.D., F.A.C.S. Chairman, Associate Dean for Clinical Services, and J. Englebert Dunphy Professor, Department of Surgery, University of California, San Francisco, School of Medicine

JULIAN L. SEIFTER, M.D. Associate Professor, Department of Medicine, Harvard Medical School, and Director of Training Programs and Associate Director, Nephrology and Renal Division, Brigham and Women's Hospital

ALAN E. SEYFER, M.D., F.A.C.S. Professor of Surgery, Anatomy, and Cell/Developmental Biology, Division of Plastic and Reconstructive Surgery, Oregon Health Sciences University, and Staff Surgeon, Department of Plastic Surgery, Doernbecher Children's Hospital

GEORGE F. SHELDON, M.D., F.A.C.S. Zack D. Owens Professor and Chairman, Department of Surgery, University of North Carolina at Chapel Hill School of Medicine

THOMAS M. SINCLAIR, M.D., C.M., F.R.C.S. Attending Plastic Surgeon, Department of Surgery, Mineral Springs Hospital, Banff, Alberta, Canada

BARBARA L. SMITH, M.D., Ph.D., F.A.C.S. Assistant Professor, Department of Surgery, Harvard Medical School; Director, Comprehensive Breast Health Center, Massachusetts General Hospital; Co-Director, Women's Cancers Program, Dana Farber/Partner's Cancer Care; and Chief of Breast Surgical Services, Gillette Center at the Dana Farber Cancer Institute

R. JOHN SOLARO, Ph.D. Professor and Head, Department of Physiology and Biophysics, University of Illinois at Chicago College of Medicine

JOSEPH S. SOLOMKIN, M.D., F.A.C.S. Professor, Department of Surgery, and Director, Surgical Infectious Diseases Division, University of Cincinnati College of Medicine

WILEY W. SOUBA, M.D., Sc.D., F.A.C.S. John A. and Marian T. Waldhaun Professor of Surgery, and Chair, Department of Surgery, Penn State College of Medicine, and Surgeon-in-Chief, Milton S. Hershey Medical Center

CYNTHIA SPRY, R.N., M.S.N. International Clinical Consultant, Johnson & Johnson

THOMAS E. STARZL, M.D., Ph.D., F.A.C.S. Professor, Department of Surgery, and Director, Thomas E. Starzl Transplantation Institute, University of Pittsburgh School of Medicine

HARVEY J. SUGERMAN, M.D., F.A.C.S. David M. Hume Professor and Head, Division of General and Trauma Surgery, Department of Surgery, Virginia Commonwealth University, Medical College of Virginia

BARRY SULLIVAN, M.D. Assistant Professor, Department of Surgery, University of British Columbia, and Surgeon, St. Paul's Hospital, Vancouver, British Columbia

LAURA A. SZNYTER, M.D. Instructor of Surgery, Harvard Medical School, and Assistant to the Surgeon-in-Chief, Brigham and Women's Hospital

BRYCE R. TAYLOR, M.D., F.A.C.S. Professor and Associate Chair, Division of General Surgery, Department of Surgery, University of Toronto Faculty of Medicine, and McCutcheon Chair in Surgery, Surgeon-in-Chief, and Director of Surgical Services, University Health Network

ERWIN R. THAL, M.D., F.A.C.S. Professor, Department of Surgery, University of Texas Southwestern Medical Center, Dallas

SETH THALLER, M.D., F.A.C.S. Professor and Chief, Department of Plastic Surgery, University of Miami School of Medicine

NICHOLAS L. TILNEY, M.D., F.A.C.S. Francis D. Moore Professor, Department of Surgery, and Director, Surgical Research Laboratory, Harvard Medical School, and Director, Center for Transplant Research, Brigham and Women's Hospital

WILLIAM C. TULLOCK, M.D. Assistant Professor of Anesthesiology, Department of Anesthesiology/CCM, University of Pittsburgh Medical Center

KIMBERLY J. VAN ZEE, M.D., F.A.C.S. Assistant Professor, Department of Surgery, Weill Medical College of Cornell University, and Assistant Attending Surgeon, Breast Service, Memorial Sloan-Kettering Cancer Center

GEORGE E. WANTZ, M.D. Clinical Professor of Surgery, Cornell University Medical College (deceased)

W. DAVID WATKINS, M.D., Ph.D. Professor, Department of Anesthesiology/CCM, and Medical Director, Pittsburgh Clinical Research Network, University of Pittsburgh Medical Center

JAMES M. WATTERS, M.D., F.A.C.S. Professor, Department of Surgery, University of Ottawa Faculty of Medicine, and Attending Surgeon, Department of Surgery, Ottawa Hospital-Civic Campus

MARTIN R. WEISER, M.D. Fellow, Memorial Sloan-Kettering Cancer Center

HUNTER WESSELLS, M.D., F.A.C.S. Associate Professor, Department of Urology, University of Washington School of Medicine

MARVIN J. WEXLER, M.D., F.A.C.S. Professor, Departments of Surgery and Oncology, McGill University Faculty of Medicine, and Senior Surgeon, Department of Surgery, Royal Victoria Hospital, Montreal

H. BRUCE WILLIAMS, M.D. Professor, Department of Surgery, McGill University Faculty of Medicine, and Surgeon-in-Chief, Department of Surgery, Montreal Children's Hospital

KAREN STANLEY WILLIAMS, M.D. Chief, Anesthesia and Surgical Services, Warren G. Magnuson Clinical Center, National Institutes of Health

DOUGLAS W. WILMORE, M.D., F.A.C.S. Frank Sawyer Professor of Surgery, Harvard Medical School, and Senior Staff Surgeon, Department of Surgery, Brigham and Women's Hospital

DAVID WISNER, M.D., F.A.C.S. Professor and Chief, Division of Trauma Surgery, Department of Surgery, University of California, Davis, School of Medicine

CHRISTOPHER K. ZARINS, M.D., F.A.C.S. Chidester Professor of Surgery, Stanford University School of Medicine, and Chief, Division of Vascular Surgery, Stanford University Medical Center

MARIKE ZWIENENBERG, M.D. Research Fellow, Department of Neurological Surgery, University of California, Davis, School of Medicine

FOREWORD

> The amount of writings of a profession is a measure of its vitality and activity whilst their quality is vindication of its intellectual state.
> Sir Robert Hutchinson, Lancet 2:1059, 1939

The art and science of surgery have perennially depended on both empirical and experimental learning—that is, on both intuition and evidence. Contemporary textbooks increasingly focus on the acquisition, evaluation, and application of evidence in caring for the individual patient. *ACS Surgery: Principles and Practice* is an excellent practical example of the modern focus. Under the sponsorship of the American College of Surgeons, this seminal compilation has been guided and directed by a highly distinguished Editorial Board, comprising Douglas W. Wilmore, M.D., F.A.C.S. (Harvard Medical School), Editorial Chairman; Laurence Y. Cheung, M.D., F.A.C.S. (University of Kansas); Alden H. Harken, M.D., F.A.C.S. (University of Colorado); James W. Holcroft, M.D., F.A.C.S. (University of California, Davis); Jonathan L. Meakins, M.D., D.Sc., F.A.C.S. (McGill University); and Nathaniel J. Soper, M.D., F.A.C.S. (Washington University). These surgeons represent the best of North American surgery and constitute a sui generis group. Within the surgical community, they exemplify the highest ideals of patient care, creative research, and education, and they have brought these ideals, along with their considerable experience and skills, to the present volume.

ACS Surgery: Principles and Practice is divided into nine major sections comprising 109 chapters from nearly 200 contributors. In its current form, it is the latest step in a strategic planning process that has been ongoing for more than 15 years. Through this process, Dr. Wilmore and his colleagues have developed a highly functional reference that not only is textually superb but also is liberally augmented with interpretive pictures, diagrams, and algorithms. What is more, they have skillfully and with admirable consistency outlined rational approaches to decision making for common problems presenting to the general surgeon and have supplemented these decision-making approaches with excellent correlative narrations and reference lists.

In particular, the Editors have clearly been concerned to address issues of informational access. Throughout, they have been at pains to ensure that surgeons can readily obtain the concepts and data they need to know most urgently. By way of illustration, most of the chapters (other than those specifically concerned with operative technique) exhibit a three-part structure specifically designed to facilitate informational access. This structure typically includes (1) an algorithm that graphically depicts the basic approach to the problem, (2) an initial decision-making section that reverses the usual textbook structure by placing the critical diagnostic and therapeutic decision-making information at the beginning of the chapter rather than the end, and (3) a correlative discussion section at the end that addresses less urgent issues, such as basic science, investigational diagnostic and therapeutic alternatives, and peripheral concerns. As further illustration, the procedures described in the section on operative management are broken down into discrete and easily comprehensible steps, and practical troubleshooting tips are provided along the way. This welcome attention to the prioritization of information, in my view, can only benefit readers, who continue to have less and less time to pore over textbooks and journals.

ACS Surgery: Principles and Practice is not an ordinary textbook of surgery, nor is it just another edition. It can perhaps be best described as a panorama of surgical care from the inception of a disease or injury phase through therapeutic options and complications. As such, it is the culmination of a development phase that began with the original loose-leaf from which this volume derives—*Care of the Surgical Patient*, later renamed *Scientific American® Surgery*—as well as a harbinger of further growth to come as the field of surgery continues to develop and change.

Readers already familiar with *Scientific American® Surgery* will find in *ACS Surgery: Principles and Practice* all the same strengths they have been accustomed to expect, including (but by no means limited to) the expert coverage of trauma and critical care, the concise and thoughtful approaches to the workup of common clinical presenting problems, and the beautifully illustrated technique chapters. However, they will also find a number of new chapters, and they will encounter an all-new organizational structure aimed at more closely reflecting the flow of modern surgical care—yet another instance of the Editors' concern with the appropriate presentation of information.

Drs. Wilmore, Cheung, Harken, Holcroft, Meakins, and Soper are all sedulous students of surgery. In this text, they have successfully achieved their strategic goal of creating a book that is simul-

sible without the ongoing efforts of an outstanding Editorial Board, which currently includes Laurence Y. Cheung, M.D., F.A.C.S.; Alden H. Harken, M.D., F.A.C.S.; James W. Holcroft, M.D., F.A.C.S.; Jonathan L. Meakins, M.D., D.Sc., F.A.C.S.; and Nathaniel J. Soper, M.D., F.A.C.S. Acknowledgment is also due here to Murray F. Brennan, M.D., F.A.C.S., who contributed a great deal to the early development of the book and was a founding member of the Editorial Board. The Editors have been and continue to be both active and committed, and they are constantly writing, editing, and reworking text for this book and seeking new contributions. They have devoted considerable time and effort to this project in order to provide a contemporary information base for the practicing surgeon. We are deeply grateful for their long-standing commitment.

In addition, the Editors and I are indebted to the authors for their participation and to the publishers for their enthusiastic support. Special thanks go to WebMD staff members Richard Lindsey, Content Development Manager, Bill Day, Editorial Director, and Nancy Chorpenning, Vice President and Publisher for Professional Content, for their signal contributions. Acknowledgment is also due to Nancy Ehrlich, who served as the original Managing Editor of *Care of the Surgical Patient,* and to Aileen McHugh, who shepherded the transition to *Scientific American® Surgery.*

Finally, we are also greatly appreciative of the support given this project by the staff of the ACS and, in particular, of the specific help provided by Linn Meyer, Director of Communications, and Thomas R. Russell, M.D., F.A.C.S., Executive Director.

It is our hope that *ACS Surgery: Principles and Practice* provides useful practical information, adds new knowledge to the field, and advances the art and practice of surgery.

Douglas W. Wilmore, M.D., F.A.C.S.

1 INITIAL EMERGENCY MANAGEMENT OF NONINJURED PATIENTS: CARDIOPULMONARY RESUSCITATION AND CORRECTION OF ACUTE DYSRHYTHMIAS

Steven R. Lowenstein, M.D., M.P.H., and Alden H. Harken, M.D.

Management of Cardiac Arrest and Acute Dysrhythmia

Cardiopulmonary arrest is the sudden cessation of breathing and circulation in a patient who is not expected to die. Victims are unresponsive, and their skin is ashen and mottled. Respirations are agonal or absent, and no pulses are present in the large arteries. The success of cardiopulmonary resuscitation (CPR) is directly related to how soon it is begun.

The approach to the patient in cardiac arrest must be organized, vigorous, and bold. First, verify the patency of the airway. Second, assure adequacy of the breathing effort. Third, restore the circulatory bed. The ABCs—*A*irway, *B*reathing, and *C*irculation—apply not only to resuscitation of victims of full cardiopulmonary arrest but also to resuscitation of all sick or injured patients. The ABCs have stood the test of time as the most basic mnemonic in all of medicine.

There are two important exceptions to the orderly rule of the ABCs. The first applies to the patient in a monitored setting who experiences sudden ventricular fibrillation (VF). On discovery of VF, immediate electrical defibrillation takes precedence over airway management, pharmacologic therapy, and CPR.

The second exception applies to the trauma patient in cardiac arrest [*see 2 Trauma Resuscitation*]. In these patients, the cause of cardiac arrest is usually exsanguination or a critical thoracic injury (e.g., cardiac tamponade, tension pneumothorax, or flail chest). In trauma patients, the head tilt [*see Basic Life Support, below*] should not be used to open the airway if there is suspicion of cervical spine injury. There is also no evidence that external chest compressions are effective in traumatic (hypovolemic) cardiac arrest[1]; instead, restoration of circulating blood volume and a resuscitative thoracotomy are urgently needed. In what follows, we consider only the resuscitation of noninjured patients.

Basic Life Support

Basic life support (BLS) consists of placing the victim on his or her back, opening the airway, performing mouth-to-mouth breathing, and initiating rhythmic chest compressions. Each of these sequential BLS steps has been delineated in the guidelines of the American Heart Association (AHA).[2] Each of the ABC steps should begin with an assessment phase—verify unresponsiveness, evaluate airway patency, assess breathing—before active intervention. Unfortunately, BLS provides suboptimal blood flow to the heart, brain, and other vital tissues, and it cannot reverse cardiac arrhythmias. BLS only buys time. Advanced life support (ALS) provides the definitive treatment [*see Advanced Life Support, below*]. ALS includes defibrillation, tracheal intubation, drug and fluid therapy, and various procedures (e.g., external or internal pacemaker placement, pericardiocentesis, tube thoracostomy, and open thoracotomy).

INITIAL STEPS

Verify cardiopulmonary arrest Shout at or gently shake the victim to determine unresponsiveness. Next, to establish the absence of functional ventilation, listen and feel for airway movement at the nose and mouth, and look for movement of the thoracic cage. If the patient is unresponsive and if breathing is absent or agonal, CPR must be initiated. It is not necessary to check pupils, pulses, or heart sounds.

Call for help and position the patient If the patient is outside the hospital, activate the emergency medical services (EMS) system. Place the victim supine on a hard surface (floor or backboard). If trauma is likely, take precautions to minimize motion of the cervical spine: hold the head in a neutral position, and then logroll the victim to the supine position, conveying the head, the neck, and the torso as a single unit [*see 2 Trauma Resuscitation*].

THE ABCS

Airway

Basic life support begins with relief of airway obstruction. The most common cause of airway obstruction in unconscious humans is the tongue, which falls backward against the posterior pharyngeal wall. In addition, during labored breathing, negative pressure is generated in the hypopharynx; the tongue and

Management of Cardiac Arrest

Verify cardiac arrest

Position patient. Call for help. Diagnose rhythm with quick-look paddles.

Rhythm is ventricular fibrillation or pulseless ventricular tachycardia

Deliver countershock of 200 joules

Ventricular fibrillation persists: deliver countershock of 300 joules

Ventricular fibrillation persists: deliver countershock of 360 joules

Successful defibrillation

Start I.V. Administer O₂. Infuse lidocaine in a 1.5 mg/kg bolus; continue at 1–4 mg/min. Continue ECG monitoring.

Ventricular fibrillation persists

Initiate CPR: open airway (use head tilt–chin lift). Insert oropharyngeal airway. Begin mouth-to-mask or bag-mask ventilation. Suction and clear debris. Begin chest compressions, 80–100/min.

Intubate trachea; administer 100% O₂. Initiate continuous ECG monitoring. Start I.V.

Give epinephrine (1:10,000) I.V. in escalating doses (1 mg, 3 mg, and 5 mg, 3 min apart) during arrest. High doses (0.1 mg/kg q. 3–5 min) are an option if ventricular fibrillation is refractory. ET epinephrine is acceptable. Repeat countershock of 300–360 joules.

Give lidocaine, 1.5 mg/kg I.V. Repeat countershock of 300–360 joules. Repeat lidocaine in 5 min to total loading dose of 3 mg/kg.

Give bretylium, 5 mg/kg I.V. Repeat countershock of 300–360 joules. If necessary, repeat bretylium in 5 min at 10 mg/kg.

Give magnesium sulfate, 4 g slow I.V., especially in case of torsade de pointes. Repeat countershock of 300–360 joules.

Consider beta blocker or procainamide. Consider emergency cardiac bypass or thoracotomy, open-chest massage, and defibrillation.

Rhythm is not ventricular fibrillation

Initiate CPR: open airway (use head tilt–chin lift). Insert oropharyngeal airway. Begin mouth-to-mask or bag-mask ventilation. Suction and clear debris. Begin chest compressions, 80–100/min.

Intubate trachea; administer 100% O_2. Initiate continuous ECG monitoring. Start I.V. Recheck rhythm.

Ventricular fibrillation

Deliver countershock of 200 joules.

Asystole

Verify asystole

Verify that patient is attached to monitor. Rotate leads 90°; rule out fine or null-plane ventricular fibrillation.

Give epinephrine (1:10,000) I.V. in escalating doses (1 mg, 3 mg, and 5 mg, 3 min apart) during arrest. High doses (0.1 mg/kg q. 3–5 min) are an option. ET epinephrine is acceptable.

Give atropine, 1 mg I.V.; repeat twice q. 5 min to maximum of 3 mg. ET atropine is acceptable.

Attempt defibrillatory countershock of 300–360 joules if ventricular fibrillation is suspected.

Consider cardiac pacing if early in arrest.

Pulseless electrical activity

Diagnose and reverse underlying causes

Consider: tension pneumothorax, cardiac tamponade, hypovolemia, ruptured abdominal aortic aneurysm, GI bleeding, anaphylaxis, acidosis, drug overdose, and hyperkalemia.

Give epinephrine (1:10,000) I.V. in escalating doses (1 mg, 3 mg, and 5 mg, 3 min apart), during arrest. High doses (0.1 mg/kg q. 3–5 min) are an option. ET epinephrine is acceptable.

Give atropine, 1 mg I.V., if electrical activity is slow; repeat twice q. 5 min to maximum of 3 mg.

Consider calcium chloride, 500 mg I.V., especially in presence of hyperkalemia, hypocalcemia, or use of calcium channel blockers or if arrest is protracted.

In presence of hyperkalemia or tricyclic antidepressant overdose, administer sodium bicarbonate.

Consider cardiac pacing, thoracotomy, and open-chest cardiac massage.

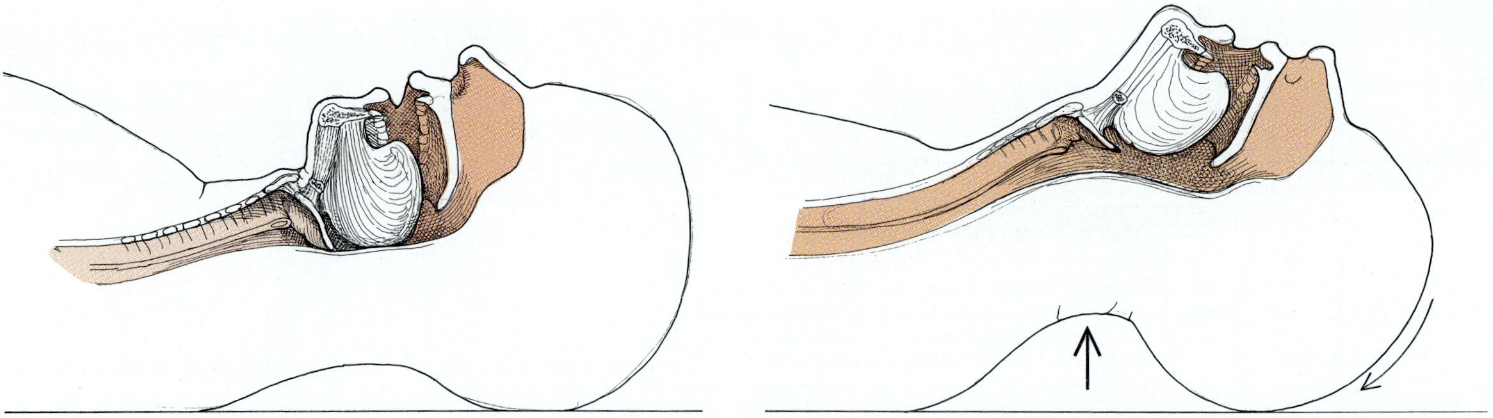

Figure 1 In unconscious, apneic patients, the patency of the airway may be improved by maneuvers that cause anterior displacement of the mandible. The tongue, which is the most frequent cause of airway obstruction, is attached to the lower mandible. The epiglottis also attaches to the mandible via the hyoid bone and the mylohyoid and digastric muscles. Therefore, when the mandible is raised, the tongue and epiglottis move anteriorly, widening the glottic opening.

epiglottis are drawn back over the entrance to the trachea [see Figure 1], thereby exacerbating obstruction.[3]

Glottal obstruction may also be caused by blood, teeth, vomitus, secretions, and other foreign debris. Obstructive asphyxia may also be precipitated by swelling of laryngeal tissues, as occurs in smoke inhalation, epiglottitis, and anaphylaxis.

Verify airway patency To assess the patency of the airway, listen to and feel for the exchange of air at the nose and mouth. Partial airflow obstruction produces inspiratory stridor. Gurgling, choking, hoarseness, and difficulty with speech also signify upper airway obstruction. Another cardinal sign of airway obstruction is extreme respiratory effort, manifested by gasping breaths, the use of accessory respiratory muscles, or a strained, weak cough. An inability to deliver air by mouth-to-mouth or bag-valve-mask ventilation (see below) also signifies airway obstruction.

Open the airway In most patients with apnea or obstructive asphyxia, the airway can be improved with manual maneuvers aimed at providing forward displacement of the mandible: when the mandible is raised, the tongue and epiglottis, which are attached to the mandible, move anteriorly, thus widening the glottic opening [see Figure 1].[3]

The simplest technique for opening the airway is the head tilt maneuver. (The head tilt maneuver is contraindicated in victims of blunt trauma.) To perform this maneuver, place the palm of one hand on the victim's forehead and apply firm backward pressure to tip the head posteriorly [see Figure 2]. Place the other hand behind the victim's neck. The head tilt maneuver alone can relieve glottal obstruction in many unconscious victims.[2]

A second maneuver, the chin lift, is accomplished by hooking the index and third finger of one hand beneath the bony chin and lifting the chin upward to bring the teeth almost to occlusion [see

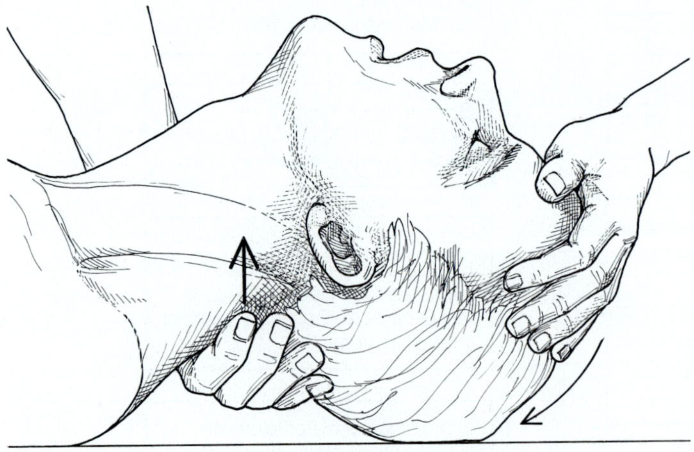

Figure 2 The head tilt maneuver, which provides anterior displacement of the mandible, is easy to perform but usually provides only partial airway opening. To perform the head tilt, place the palm of one hand on the victim's forehead and apply firm backward pressure to tip the head posteriorly. Place the other hand behind the victim's neck.

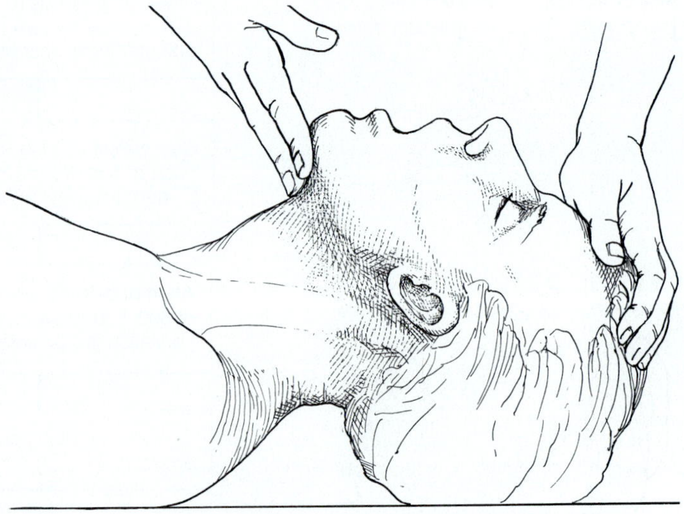

Figure 3 The head tilt–chin lift is the procedure of choice for opening the airway in nontrauma victims. This maneuver is the easiest to perform and provides the greatest glottal opening. To perform the chin lift, place the index and third fingers (not the thumb) under the bony chin. Then, lift the chin upward to bring the teeth almost to occlusion.

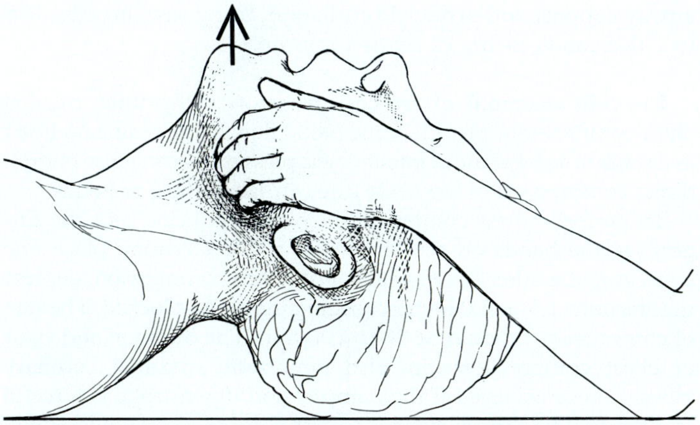

Figure 4 The jaw thrust is an effective, although technically difficult, airway opening procedure. To perform it, grasp the angles of the lower jaw and lift, using both hands, to bring the mandible anteriorly to the maximal prognathic position. The jaw thrust without a head tilt is the procedure of choice in trauma victims.

Figure 3].[2] The combined head tilt–chin lift maneuver is the easiest, least fatiguing airway maneuver to perform. It also provides the greatest forward displacement of the mandible, the greatest relief of glottal obstruction, and the largest tidal volumes during rescue breathing.

The jaw thrust is also an effective technique for improving patency of the airway. To perform the jaw thrust, grasp the angles of the lower jaw and lift, using both hands, to bring the mandible anteriorly to the maximal prognathic position [*see Figure 4*]. The combined head tilt–jaw thrust maneuver provides satisfactory airway patency, although it is more difficult and tiring to perform.

Check for resumption of spontaneous respirations Once the head, neck, and jaw are optimally positioned, check for spontaneous ventilation. Some patients who have suffered obstructive asphyxia may resume breathing.

Improving airway patency The oropharyngeal tube is a useful adjunct to improve airway patency in unconscious patients [*see Figure 5*]. It is a plastic, semicircular device that lifts the base of the tongue off the posterior pharynx. When the tube is well into the patient's mouth, rotate it 180° into its proper position. The oropharyngeal tube should not be inserted in conscious patients, because it provokes laryngospasm, gagging, vomiting, and aspiration. Patients with intact gag reflexes will better tolerate a rubber nasopharyngeal (trumpet) airway [*see Figure 6*].

Breathing

Perform mouth-to-mouth breathing To perform rescue breathing, gently pinch the victim's nose closed, inhale deeply, seal your lips around and over the victim's mouth, and deliver two slow rescue breaths. Each inflation should last 1.5 to 2.0 seconds, and there should be time for full deflation after each breath. An adequate tidal volume is about 800 ml, or just enough to make the chest rise visibly. The mouth-to-nose technique is preferable if trismus precludes mouth-to-mouth ventilation.

The fraction of inspired oxygen (F_IO_2) in a rescuer's exhaled air is 0.16, a value sufficient to meet a victim's needs.[4] Still, mouth-to-mouth breathing is not a perfect form of airway management. Air leaks at the victim's face often lead to inadequate lung inflation, atelectasis, arteriovenous shunting, and hypoxemia. The chief hazard of artificial ventilation is gastric insufflation followed by regurgitation and aspiration. Gastric insufflation is more likely if quick breaths are delivered at a high peak inspiratory pressure (PIP).[5] An excessive PIP overcomes the opening pressure of the lower esophageal sphincter. In simulated models of CPR, as much as 75% of each mouth-to-mouth breath enters the stomach, not the lungs.[5] Furthermore, as lung compliance declines during cardiopulmonary arrest, the chance of inflating the stomach instead of the lungs increases.

Three strategies are available to reduce the risk of gastric inflation and regurgitation.[5] First, maintain proper head position and airway patency. Second, perform rescue breathing slowly, allowing full exhalation between breaths. Third, employ the Sellick maneuver: pressure applied to the cricoid cartilage reduces the risk of gastric inflation and emesis during CPR [*see Figure 7*].[5]

Performing direct mouth-to-mouth resuscitation may expose rescuers to saliva, blood, and other body fluids, increasing the risk that rescuers will acquire hepatitis, tuberculosis, herpes simplex virus, HIV infection. The probability that a rescuer will acquire an infection after CPR is minimal. Although cases of tuberculosis and

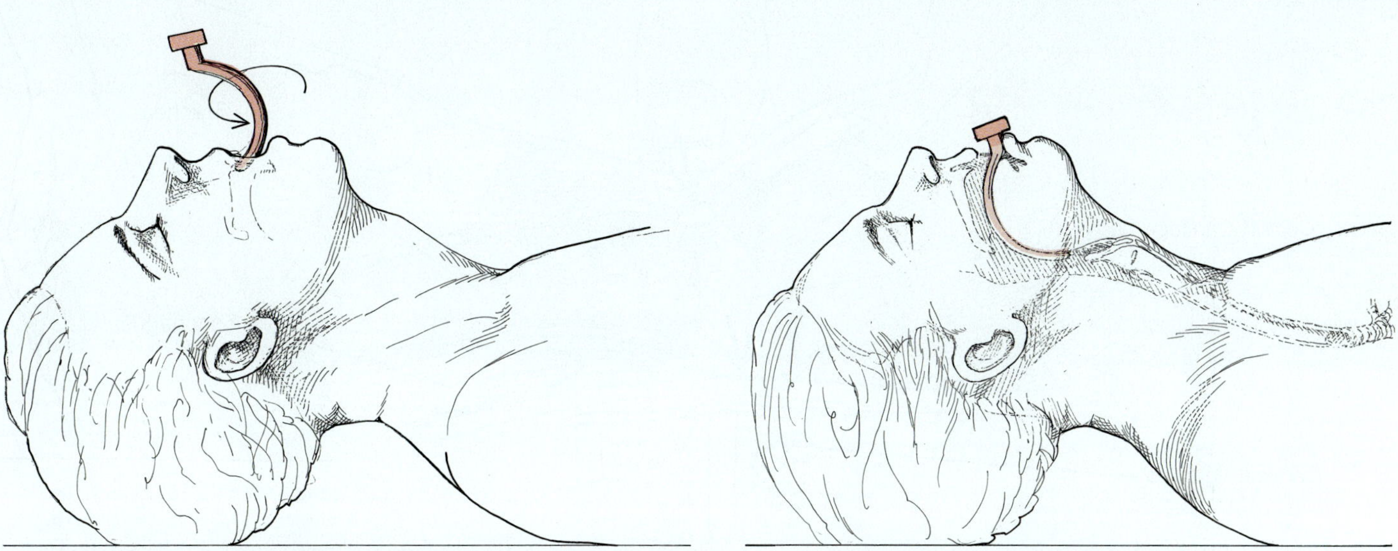

Figure 5 The oropharyngeal airway is inserted into the posterior pharynx in unconscious patients to relieve obstruction of the airway. This plastic device is inserted in an inverted position and then rotated 180°. Once properly positioned, the oropharyngeal airway lifts the base of the tongue, thus improving airway patency.

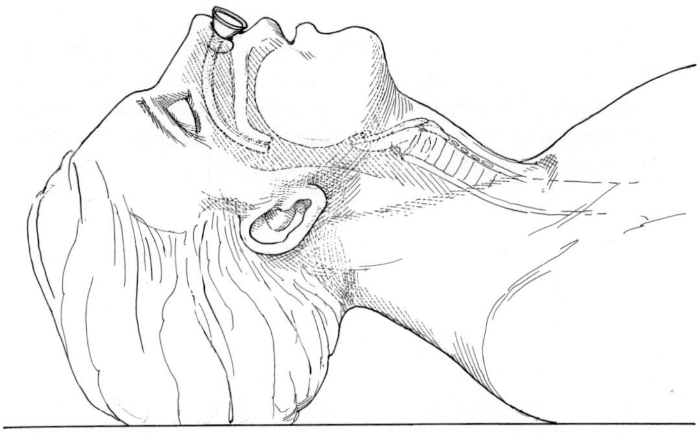

Figure 6 In conscious patients, the oropharyngeal airway is often poorly tolerated and frequently produces laryngospasm, coughing, vomiting, and aspiration. The rubber nasopharyngeal (trumpet) airway (shown here) is a better choice for conscious patients with an intact gag reflex.

herpesvirus transmission have been reported, cases of HIV and hepatitis transmission have not.[2] Nevertheless, universal blood and body fluid precautions [see 86 *Viral Infection* and 108 *Infection Control in Surgical Practice*] should be observed during all phases of CPR. Goggles, gowns, and latex gloves should be worn. Rescuers should perform mouth-to-mouth breathing with the assistance of a protective face shield or mask, preferably one that has a one-way valve to divert expired air away from the rescuer.[2]

Circulation

Verify pulselessness After opening the airway and delivering the first two rescue breaths, check for a carotid arterial pulse. If none is present, circulatory arrest is confirmed, and chest compressions must begin at once. If pulses are present, continue airway support and artificial ventilation, using slow breaths (1.5 to 2.0 seconds each), 12 times a minute.[5]

Provide external chest compression Rhythmic, manual chest compressions provide some blood flow to the brain and heart as a result of a global rise in intrathoracic pressure (the thoracic pump), direct compression of the heart (the cardiac pump), or both.[6]

To perform chest compressions, place the heels (not the fingers) of the hands on the lower half of the sternum; place one hand atop the other [see *Figure 8*]. With each compression, depress the sternum 1.5 to 2.0 inches, keeping the elbows locked. The rate of compressions should be 80 to 100/min. The duration and vigor of chest compressions are also important; maximal coronary blood flow is achieved if the compression downstroke is forceful and brief.[7] The time allowed for chest compression should equal, but not exceed, the time allowed for release.

Avoid the ribs and the xiphoid process during chest compressions. Errant or overvigorous chest thrusts increase the incidence of abdominal visceral trauma, rib fractures, mediastinal bleeding, hemopericardium, hemopneumothorax, and other complications. About 40% of CPR recipients suffer at least one CPR-related complication.[8,9]

Advanced Life Support

Under the best circumstances, CPR provides only 25% of the prearrest cardiac output. Although peak systolic blood pressures of 60 mm Hg are often achieved, diastolic pressures seldom exceed 20 mm Hg. Blood flow to the brain is only 15% of normal, and coronary arterial blood flow is essentially zero.[6,10]

ADJUNCTS TO ASSIST VENTILATION

Bag-Valve-Mask Devices

The resuscitation bag is self-inflating and attaches via a nonrebreathing valve to a clear mask [see *Figure 9*]. This device can

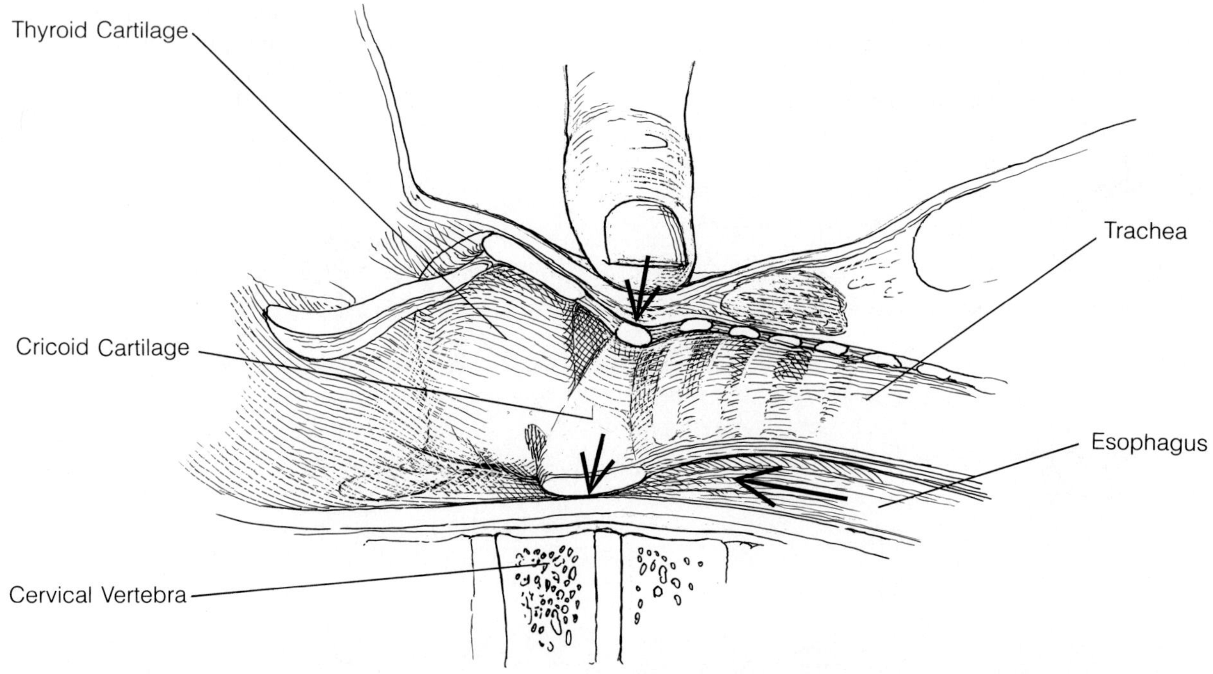

Figure 7 During assisted ventilation in unintubated patients, gastric insufflation, vomiting, and aspiration are constant hazards. The risk of aspiration is reduced if digital pressure is applied to the cricoid cartilage. This simple procedure (the Sellick maneuver) should be employed during bag-valve-mask and mouth-to-mask ventilation.

deliver adequate oxygenation and tidal volume if properly used. An oropharyngeal airway must be in place, the victim's head extended, and the jaw elevated to support the airway. The bag is compressed evenly and forcefully while a patent airway and a leakproof seal are maintained. The bag is attached to a long-tubing reservoir with a capacity that equals or exceeds the tidal volume of the bag. High-flow oxygen is delivered to the reservoir at a flow rate that meets or exceeds the patient's minute ventilation. With proper technique, adequate tidal volumes and an F_IO_2 of at least 0.75 can be achieved.

TRACHEAL INTUBATION

Intubation provides better tidal volumes and better oxygenation than mouth-to-mouth or mouth-to-mask breathing and is the only reliable protection against aspiration of gastric contents. A secure endotracheal tube also provides a conduit to evacuate secretions and a route to administer first-line resuscitation drugs.

The decision to secure an airway can be made by rapid evaluation of five parameters: (1) airway patency, (2) adequacy of ventilation, (3) adequacy of oxygenation, (4) level of consciousness, and (5) overall patient condition. Virtually all patients with cardiopulmonary arrest who cannot be immediately resuscitated by an electrical countershock [see Treatment of Ventricular Fibrillation, Electrical Defibrillation, below] will require intubation. The trachea can be intubated by the oral, the nasal, or the transcricoid route, but with the exception of patients who have suffered foreign-body aspiration and upper airway obstruction, all noninjured cardiac arrest victims should be intubated by the oral route.

Orotracheal Intubation

Preparation Success in intubation is dependent on steps taken before the endotracheal tube is touched. First, assemble all essential equipment: suction apparatus, a working laryngoscope blade and handle, and an endotracheal tube of the correct size (for adults, 7.5 to 8.5 mm in internal diameter or, more roughly, about the diameter of the patient's thumbnail). Second, preoxygenate the patient by mouth-to-mask or bag-valve-mask ventilation. Third, place the patient in the so-called sniffing position. Hyperextension of the neck is not desirable. Instead, flex the lower cervical vertebral segments in relation to the trunk and extend the head only at the atlanto-occipital joint. More simply, (1) keep the plane of the patient's face parallel to the floor, (2) leave the shoulders on the stretcher, (3) elevate the occiput anteriorly to shoulder level on a pillow or towel, and then (4) extend the head at the atlanto-occipital joint. This pose brings the trachea, larynx, pharynx, and mouth (as well as the eye of the rescuer) into alignment.

Intubation Intubation requires a good view of the larynx. Begin the intubation process with the laryngoscope in the left hand and a suction catheter, not an endotracheal tube, in the right hand. Clear away secretions, vomitus, and blood. Only then, after the larynx is clearly visualized, exchange the suction tube for the ET tube and insert the ET tube.

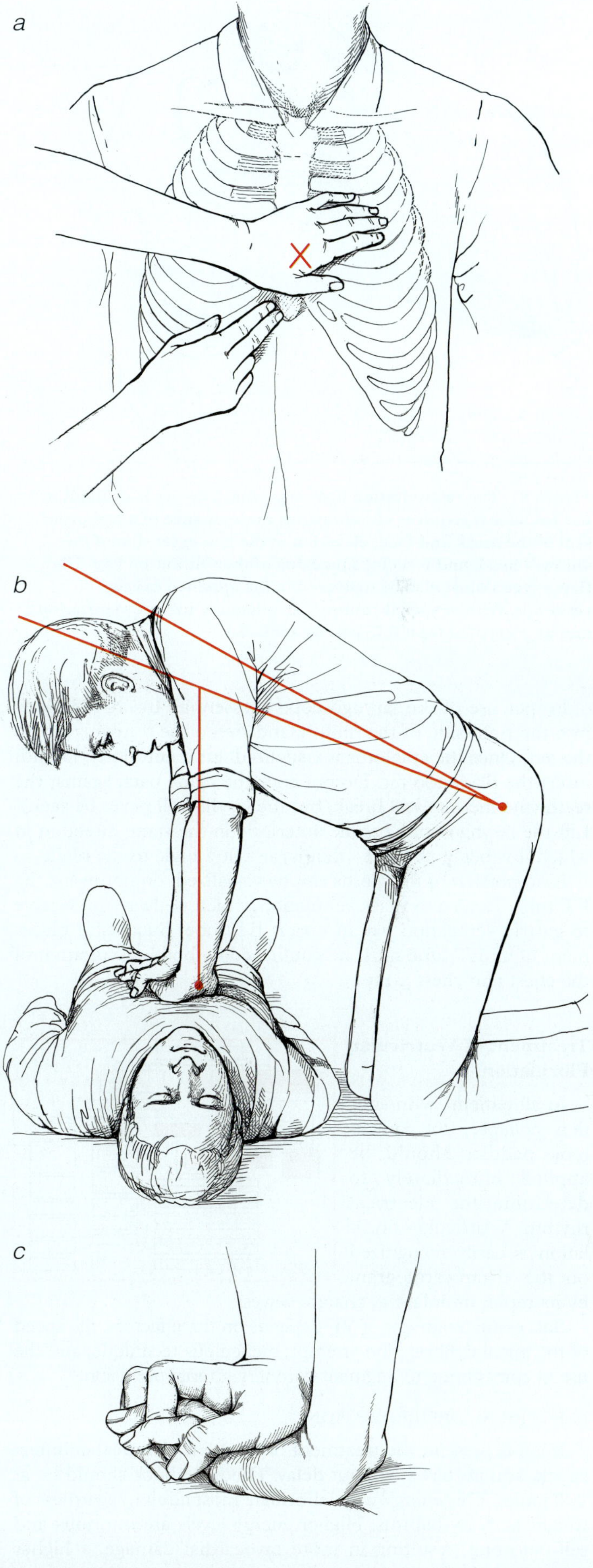

Figure 8 The proper hand position for external chest compression is the lower end of the sternum (*a*). Avoid the ribs and the xiphoid process to reduce the risk of thoracic or abdominal visceral injury. To perform chest compressions, place the heel of one hand on the lower half of the sternum, with the long axis of the hand along the long axis of the victim's sternum (*b*). Place the second hand on top of the first (*c*). With the elbows locked, begin forceful, rhythmic chest compressions at a rate of 80 to 100/min.

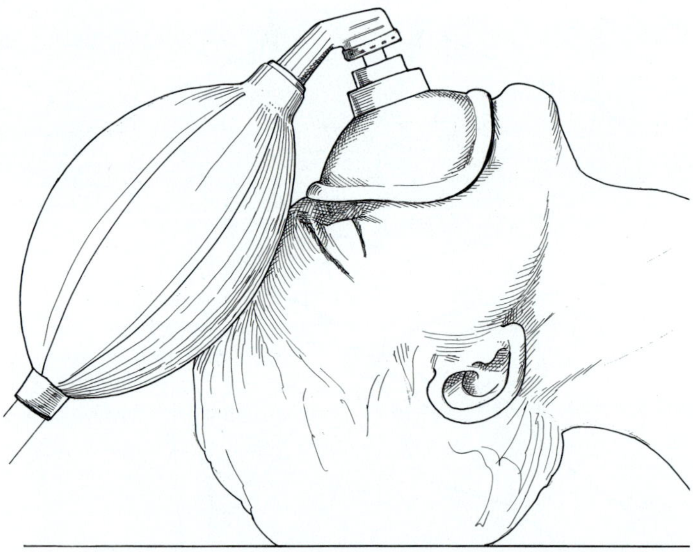

Figure 9 The resuscitation bag-valve-mask device is difficult to use because it requires simultaneous maintenance of a leakproof seal of the mask and face, elevation of the jaw, extension of the victim's head, and forceful squeezing of the ventilation bag. High-flow oxygen must also be delivered to the attached oxygen reservoir. With proper technique, an adequate minute ventilation and an F_IO_2 of at least 0.75 can be achieved.

Proper use of the laryngoscope is essential. Insert the blade into the right side of the mouth, and sweep the tongue away to the left. Once the epiglottis is visualized, lift it anteriorly. Do not insert the blade too far. Do not cock the blade back against the teeth (the incisors will break, but the larynx will never be seen). Lift the laryngoscope handle anteriorly in the same direction in which it is being pointed—that is, at a 90° angle to the blade.

If no portion of the glottis can be visualized, do not insert the ET tube. Return to mask ventilation, which is always preferable to gastric ventilation via an errant ET tube. Successful placement of an ET tube must be confirmed by both auscultation of the chest and chest x-ray.

Treatment of Ventricular Fibrillation

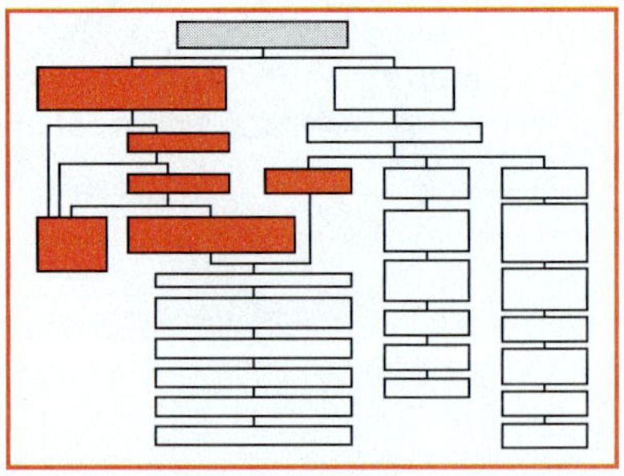

In all patients with sudden collapse, the quick-look paddles should be applied immediately to determine the electrical rhythm. Ventricular fibrillation is easily recognized on the electrocardiogram by its rapid, undulating, chaotic waves.

Successful treatment of VF depends on three factors: the speed of the initial defibrillation attempt, meticulous technique, and the use of epinephrine to augment coronary arterial perfusion.

ELECTRICAL DEFIBRILLATION

If VF is present, the treatment of choice is electrical countershock, administered without delay. The first shock should be at 200 joules. This energy will defibrillate most adults, regardless of weight or body habitus. Higher energy levels are injurious and self-defeating, resulting in more myocardial damage, a higher incidence of postshock arrhythmias, and a lower rate of survival.[11] If the initial shock fails, a second should be administered immediately at 300 joules. The third attempt, if needed, should be at 360 joules. The first three defibrillatory shocks must be performed expeditiously, without any pause for BLS, airway management, or drugs.[12] Mortality increases by 10% for each minute that the first countershock is delayed.[13]

Although time is the most critical determinant of the success of defibrillation, technique is also important. Success depends on correct paddle placement, firm paddle pressure, and the use of a low-resistance conducting gel [*see Figure 10*]. Defibrillation during the exhalation phase of ventilation and delivery of two or three countershocks in rapid succession will lower transthoracic impedance and facilitate defibrillation.[11,14]

If the initial three defibrillatory shocks fail, CPR must be initiated. The airway and an intravenous line should be secured, and pharmacologic therapy should be started.

EPINEPHRINE

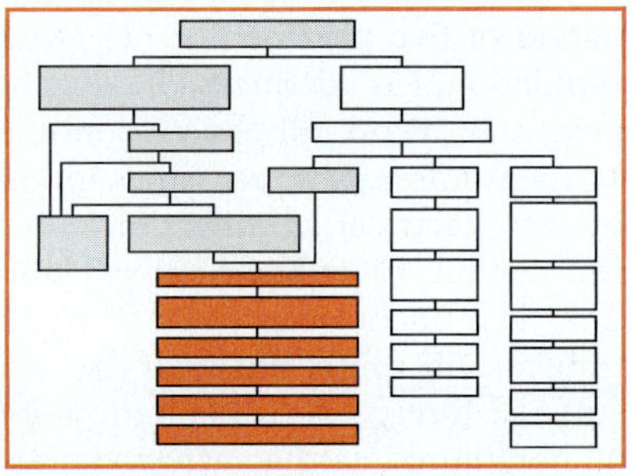

If the first three attempts at defibrillation fail, the first drug administered should be epinephrine (1 mg I.V. or 3 mg endotracheally in a 1:10,000 dilution). By means of its alpha-adrenergic (pressor) properties, epinephrine augments aortic diastolic blood pressure and increases perfusion to the heart.[15] It may not coarsen the fibrillatory waves or enhance electrical defibrillation per se, but it is critical to restoring a pulsatile rhythm, especially after a delayed defibrillation.[6,16]

After administration of epinephrine, defibrillation (at a maximal output of 360 joules) should be attempted. If VF persists, check paddle placement and technique, and verify the placement of the endotracheal tube and the adequacy of ventilation. Epinephrine administration must be repeated every 3 to 5 minutes. Epinephrine has proven merit in resuscitation. One acceptable regimen is to administer escalating doses of epinephrine (1 mg, 3 mg, and 5 mg) 3 minutes apart, continued at 5 mg every 5 minutes thereafter [*see Table 1 and* Discussion, Drug Therapy, *below*].

ANTIDYSRHYTHMIC DRUGS

If VF is resistant to electrical countershock and epinephrine, a loading dose of lidocaine (1.5 mg/kg) should be administered. This lidocaine dose should be repeated in 5 minutes to a total loading dose of 3 mg/kg. Only bolus therapy is indicated in cardiac arrest. A single endotracheal dose (3 mg/kg) may also be effective.

Bretylium should be given if lidocaine fails (earlier use of bretylium has been recommended if VF is caused by hypothermia). The combination of lidocaine and bretylium may act synergistically to prevent the recurrence of VF.[17] Initiate treatment with 5 mg/kg by intravenous push. An additional bolus (10 mg/kg) may be given in 5 minutes.

Lidocaine, bretylium, and procainamide are recommended in refractory VF because they are familiar, fast-acting drugs. All three agents have proven efficacy in suppressing ventricular ectopic activity in ischemic hearts. However, no clinical study has demonstrated that these agents are helpful in VF patients. In fact, lidocaine may increase the energy requirement for electrical defibrillation.[17,18] In one randomized prehospital trial of VF

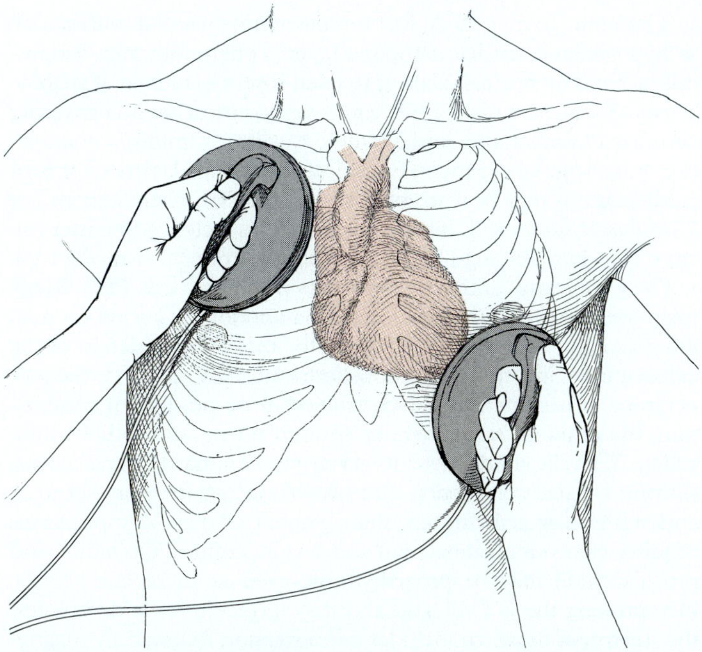

Figure 10 Proper electrode placement is essential to promote defibrillation. The apical paddle should be placed just lateral to the left nipple in the midaxillary line; the other paddle should be placed beneath the right clavicle, just to the right of the upper sternum. The two paddles should be well separated. Myocardial current flow and defibrillation are enhanced if firm paddle pressure and a conducting gel are used and if defibrillation is performed during the exhalation phase of the respiratory cycle.

patients, administration of lidocaine resulted in an increase in the incidence of postcountershock bradyasystolic rhythms.[19]

After successful defibrillation, the myocardium remains electrically unstable and prone to refibrillation. Therefore, all patients should be treated with full loading doses and an I.V. infusion of lidocaine. If the patient proves refractory to lidocaine during the resuscitation, an infusion of procainamide or bretylium is indicated.

OTHER ANTIFIBRILLATORY AGENTS

In cases of refractory VF, it may also be helpful to administer magnesium sulfate, 4 g over a period of 1 minute, particularly to patients receiving digitalis or diuretics. In one retrospective report, amiodarone was administered intravenously to 14 patients who were in prolonged arrest from ventricular tachycardia (VT) or VF. Eleven of the 14 were successfully resuscitated, and eight survived to hospital discharge.[20]

Table 1 Epinephrine Dosing

Standard first dose
 1 mg I.V. push every 3–5 min
Escalating dose*
 1 mg, then 3 mg, then 5 mg I.V. push, administered 3 min apart
 5 mg every 3–5 min thereafter
High dose†
 0.1 mg/kg every 5 min

*Use if standard first dose fails.
†Optional—recommended before countershock when ventricular fibrillation is prolonged or refractory.

Treatment of Asystole

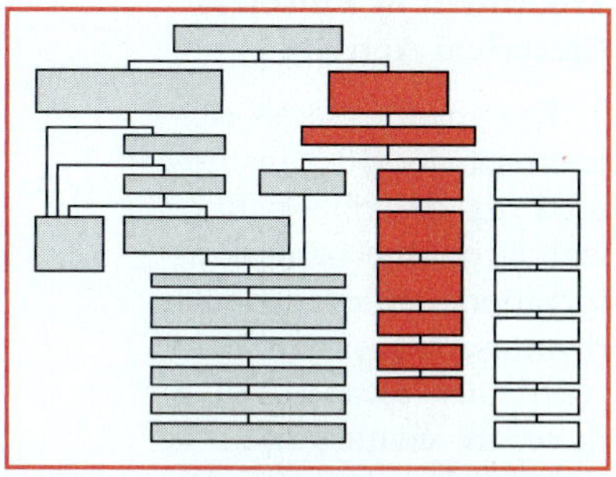

Whenever a flat-line or low-amplitude electrocardiogram is recorded, it is important to confirm the absence of cardiac activity. First, verify the absence of pulses; then, check for technical failures, such as a low battery or loose or disconnected monitor leads.[21] Third, rotate the monitoring leads 90° to detect a null-plane episode of VF. Defibrillation should be attempted only if the rhythm is unclear or if it appears to be fine VF.[14,21] In fine VF, pretreatment with a high dose of epinephrine (5 mg) is indicated before a countershock is administered [see Table 1]. Fine VF usually signals a long elapsed arrest time and a poorly perfused heart.

PHARMACOLOGIC THERAPY

Asystole is an ominous condition. The pharmacologic management of asystole consists of a two-pronged attack. First, administer epinephrine. Epinephrine acts via its vasoconstrictive action, not its inotropic action, to increase diastolic blood pressure (thus enhancing coronary perfusion), increase venous return, augment cardiac output during chest compression, and increase perfusion to the heart and brain.[6,22,23] The goal is to evoke good, coarse VF that should be responsive to cardioversion.

Epinephrine should be administered by the intravenous route in rapidly escalating or high doses [see Table 1]. Endotracheal administration is acceptable, but intracardiac injections should be utilized only if no other route of drug administration is available.

The second prong of antiasystole therapy is atropine, a parasympatholytic drug. Administer 1 mg intravenously (or 2 mg intratracheally), and repeat every 5 minutes to a maximum dosage of 3 mg. In theory, high levels of parasympathetic tone may accompany or cause cardiopulmonary arrest. Acidosis, hypoxia, and manipulation of the oropharynx during assisted ventilation or endotracheal intubation may add to parasympathetic overactivity.

Some patients with bradyasystole may respond favorably to intravenous administration of aminophylline, even after oxygenation, epinephrine, and atropine therapies have failed.[24] Aminophylline may act by blocking the effects of adenosine, an endogenous nucleoside that inhibits supraventricular activity, pacemaker activity, and atrioventricular conduction.

ELECTRICAL THERAPY

Electrical defibrillation is often employed to treat asystole. Occasionally, fine VF may masquerade as asystole, especially if it is of low amplitude or if the polarity of the fibrillatory waves is at right angles to the monitoring lead.[25] According to careful studies of prehospital cardiac arrest, however, the frequency with which VF masquerades as a flat-line electrocardiogram is low. More commonly, so-called reversible asystole is actually caused by technical failures, such as a faulty battery, a loose lead, or a disconnected monitor; these technical problems must always be addressed before defibrillation is attempted.[21]

Pacemaker therapy, when applied late in the resuscitation effort, is seldom effective. Electrical capture is common, but mechanical activity is rare and survival is nil. Transcutaneous (external) pacing may be slightly more efficacious if initiated early for postdefibrillation asystole and heart block,[26] and it is considerably more expeditious than internal pacing.

Treatment of Pulseless Electrical Activity

The term pulseless electrical activity (PEA) is now used to describe patients with electromechanical dissociation, idioventricular rhythms, bradyasystole, or ventricular escapes. All of these are characterized by organized electrocardiographic activity without effective myocardial contractions. In PEA, although some synchronous myocardial contractions (demonstrable only by central aortic pressure measurements or by echocardiography) may occur,[26,27] peripheral perfusion and effective cardiac output have ceased. PEA is the proximate cause of death in the majority of delayed or difficult resuscitations.

To manage PEA, first search for reversible causes [see Table 2]. PEA may signal absolute or relative hypovolemia. Causes include gastrointestinal hemorrhage, rupture of an abdominal aortic aneurysm, the septic response, and anaphylaxis. These disorders are characterized by flat jugular veins and a rapid, narrow-complex ECG rhythm (sinus tachycardia). Tension pneumothorax, pulmonary embolus, cardiac tamponade, and acute prosthetic valve dysfunction, which present mechanical barriers to ventricular filling, are also important reversible causes of PEA. In these disorders, cardiac filling is reduced but jugular venous pressure is paradoxically elevated because intrathoracic pressure is high. One robust clue to the presence of a treatable form of PEA is the finding of a rapid, narrow-complex rhythm (sinus tachycardia) on the ECG.[28]

Therefore, to treat PEA, first reverse nonmyocardial causes, such as hypovolemia, cardiac tamponade, and pneumothorax. Empirically administer normal saline or lactated Ringer's solution. If anaphylaxis is a likely cause of the PEA (e.g., if cardiac arrest has occurred after contrast administration in the radiology suite), administer epinephrine and a volume expander. Empirical chest tube placement or pericardiocentesis may be warranted in difficult PEA resuscitations [see 2 Trauma Resuscitation]. If hyperkalemia is suspected, administer calcium chloride (500 mg I.V.) and sodium bicarbonate (1 mg/kg I.V.).

Drug overdoses and toxic exposures may also incite PEA. Many toxic overdoses have specific, lifesaving antidotes. Carbon monoxide poisoning occurs with exposure to smoke or inhalation of the exhaust from incomplete combustion; high-flow oxygen is the cornerstone of treatment. Cyanide is another by-product of combustion; the antidote is intravenous sodium nitrite and sodium thiosulfate. Tricyclic antidepressants act as type Ia antiarrhythmic agents, slowing cardiac conduction and provoking hypotension, seizures, and ventricular arrhythmias; management of these complications requires vigorous alkalinization and seizure control. Quinidine and procainamide may be proarrhythmic even at therapeutic levels; they prolong the QT interval and may induce torsade de pointes, the treatment of which includes cardioversion followed by magnesium and ventricular pacing. Other common drug overdoses that cause PEA include overdose of beta blockers, calcium channel blockers, and digitalis. Calcium channel blocker and beta-blocker overdoses necessitate atropine, pressor agents, intravenous calcium, glucagon, pacing, or, in desperate cases, cardiopulmonary bypass. Digitalis overdose is treated with digoxin-specific antibodies.

The only hope in refractory PEA is to restore coronary perfusion; therefore, the treatment of choice is epinephrine in rapidly escalating or high doses [see Table 1]. Other alpha-adrenergic drugs

Table 2 Reversible Causes of Pulseless Electromechanical Activity

Etiology	History and Physical Findings	Jugular Venous Pressure	ECG Findings	Treatment
Tension pneumothorax	History of asthma, mechanical ventilation, or trauma Decreased breath sounds Cyanosis Deviated trachea Resistance to ventilation Rib fractures Subcutaneous emphysema	Elevated	Narrow complex Rapid heart rate Right axis deviation	Chest tube
Pulmonary embolus	Acute pulmonary hypertension Risk factor for thromboembolism	Elevated	Narrow complex Rapid heart rate Right axis deviation	Thoracotomy or thrombolytic therapy
Cardiac tamponade	History of malignancy or recent myocardial infarction Aortic dissection Trauma	Elevated	Narrow or wide complex Reduced voltage Electrical alternans	Pericardiocentesis
GI bleeding	Evidence of bleeding	Nonelevated	Narrow complex Rapid heart rate	Blood and volume expansion
Ruptured abdominal aneurysm	Back or abdominal pain Abdominal pulsatile mass or distention	Nonelevated	Narrow complex Rapid heart rate	Volume expansion, MAST suit, operation
Anaphylaxis	Arrest after drug or contrast administration Urticaria, thick tongue, angioedema Stridor or wheezing	Nonelevated	Narrow complex Rapid heart rate	Epinephrine Volume expansion
Hyperkalemia	Renal failure, dialysis fistula Diabetes or severe acidosis Chemotherapy (cell lysis)	Nonelevated	Wide, slow complex Absent P waves	Calcium and sodium bicarbonate Insulin and glucose

(e.g., methoxamine) may also exert a salutary effect; in canine models of PEA, epinephrine and other alpha-adrenergic catecholamines augment diastolic blood pressure, coronary arterial blood flow, and myocardial contractility and lead to improved survival.[29]

There is no other pharmacologic antidote for PEA. Oxygenation and ventilation should be optimized. Atropine should be administered if the rate is slow. Sodium bicarbonate should be used with restraint, if at all, because it generates new CO_2 and leads to intracellular acidosis. In the heart, intracellular acidosis worsens the contractile state and may contribute to refractory PEA.

Prevention of In-Hospital Cardiac Arrest

Even expeditious treatment of cardiopulmonary arrest is not always successful, and for all patients, an ounce of prevention may offer more hope than a pound of cure. Although the incidence of preventable or iatrogenic cardiac arrest cannot be known, it is certain that errors of omission and commission occur.

Anesthetic and sedating agents are responsible for a small number of inpatient cardiac arrests.[30] Suppressive drugs and iatrogenic hypoventilation—especially in emergency cases—are usually responsible. In almost every case, progressive bradycardia is a harbinger of trouble, and its significance must be appreciated. Dyspnea, tachypnea, and sudden changes in mental status (acute confusion) are the most frequent signals.[31,32]

Resuscitation: Summary

In addition to time, only four ingredients are critical to resuscitation: (1) prompt, proper BLS, (2) rapid defibrillation, (3) airway management, and (4) epinephrine, if needed. Epinephrine is the vasopressor agent of choice in cardiopulmonary resuscitation. Epinephrine augments peripheral vascular tone, increases stroke volume during CPR, optimizes arteriovenous pressure gradients, and improves regional blood flow to the heart and brain. Epinephrine and other alpha agonists have proved efficacious in resuscitation, regardless of the electrocardiographic pattern.

Management of Acute Dysrhythmia Arising after Resuscitation

After successful CPR, the most common hemodynamically destabilizing problem is an abnormal heart rhythm. In what follows, we outline the approach to a resuscitated patient with an apparent acute cardiac dysrhythmia [see Figure 11].

The purpose of the heart's electrical activity is to induce mechanical activity. Abnormal electrical activity (arrhythmia or dysrhythmia) that occurs in the absence of hemodynamic compromise should be examined and treated with forbearance because therapy itself poses some hazards: all antidysrhythmic agents except oxygen are negatively inotropic. Thus, there are four questions that should be asked in the evaluation of a patient who appears to exhibit an acute cardiac dysrhythmia:

1. Does the patient actually have a cardiac dysrhythmia?
2. Does the patient require therapy (i.e., is the patient sufficiently stable that treatment is NOT indicated)?
3. How soon should therapy be started?
4. Which therapy is the safest and most effective?

PATIENT IS HEMODYNAMICALLY UNSTABLE

The choice of therapy is determined by the stability of the patient and the origin of the dysrhythmia. An electrocardiogram is required. All hemodynamically unstable patients who have a dysrhythmia other than asystole should be treated immediately by cardioversion (see below); treatment of asystole has already been examined [see Treatment of Asystole, above].

The two primary goals in the management of an acute dysrhythmia are to control the ventricular rate and to maintain a normal sinus rhythm. However, hemodynamic instability in a patient who has a ventricular rate between 60 and 100 beats/min is almost certainly not the result of a cardiac rhythm disturbance. Furthermore, heart rates in excess of 100 beats/min do not necessarily require therapy. Most patients can remain hemodynamically stable—and, in fact, increase their cardiac output—while increasing their heart rate up to 220 beats/min minus their age. In addition, it is not critical to reestablish normal sinus rhythm in all cases.[33] In a young, healthy patient with a normal heart, the so-called atrial kick adds almost nothing to cardiac output.[34] If normal sinus rhythm is abolished and atrial fibrillation is electrically induced in such patients, the ventricles and the rest of the cardiovascular system compensate almost immediately to prevent a fall in cardiac output.[35] On the other hand, loss of synchronous atrial activity in patients with end-stage cardiac decompensation may decrease cardiac output by as much as 40%[36]; such a degree of end-stage cardiac compromise, however, is rare.

Cardioversion

Cardioversion delivers sufficient electrical energy to the precordium (or directly to the heart) to depolarize cells, even those in a relatively refractory state. Cardioversion attempts to impose an electrical organization on the heart, the theory being that after depolarization, all the myocardial cells will repolarize simultaneously and continue to beat synchronously thereafter [see Sidebar The Intracardiac Cardioverter Defibrillator].

Certain precautions are necessary with cardioversion. It is of no use in patients who are in asystole or who have fine VF, because there is no cardiac activity to organize. Supraventricular dysrhythmias such as atrial flutter can be converted by using extremely low energies (e.g., ≤ 5 joules), but such low energies should not be employed in emergency situations. When an unstable patient is treated, it is critical to use an energy level that will work. For a hemodynamically unstable patient, the initial cardioverting energy should be 100 joules; if the dysrhythmia is not abolished, the voltage should be increased rapidly (to a maximum of 360 joules).

PATIENT IS HEMODYNAMICALLY STABLE

Ventricular Rate Is Slow

If the patient is bradycardic before or after cardioversion, atropine should be administered in a 0.5 mg I.V. push. This dose may be repeated at 2-minute intervals. Because the effects of atropine are transient, a temporary internal or external pacemaker should be used to maintain the heart rate [see Sidebar Troubleshooting a Pacemaker].

Ventricular Rate Is Fast

If a patient is hemodynamically stable, a full 12-lead electrocardiogram should be obtained; a long rhythm strip should be obtained as well. The best ECG lead to use for evaluating acute dysrhythmias is one that has good-voltage QRS complexes and maximal P waves, if the latter are present.

Electrocardiography A cardiac impulse produces a positive, or upward, deflection on the monitor or oscilloscope as it

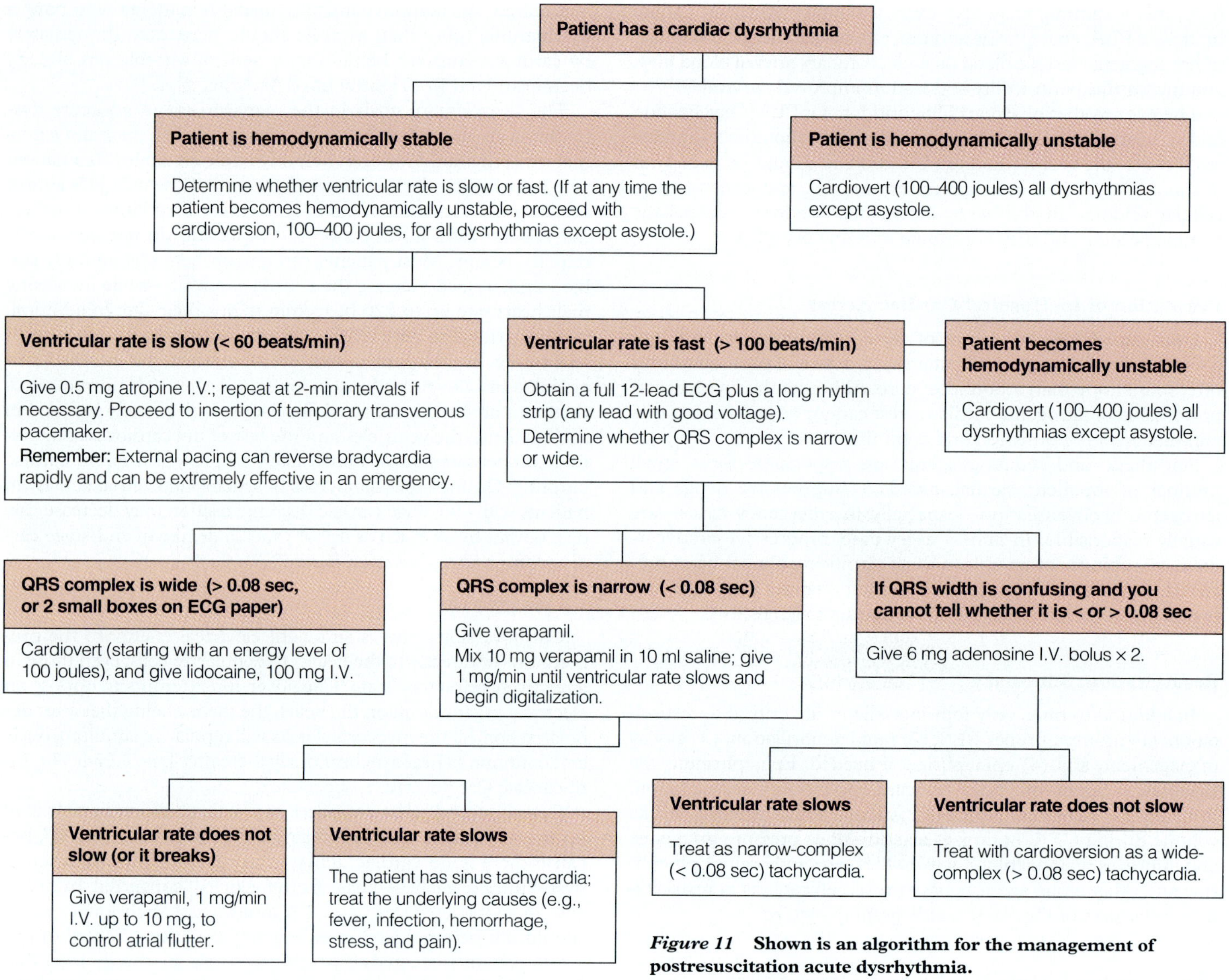

```
                        ┌─────────────────────────────────┐
                        │ Patient has a cardiac dysrhythmia│
                        └─────────────────────────────────┘
```

Patient is hemodynamically stable
Determine whether ventricular rate is slow or fast. (If at any time the patient becomes hemodynamically unstable, proceed with cardioversion, 100–400 joules, for all dysrhythmias except asystole.)

Patient is hemodynamically unstable
Cardiovert (100–400 joules) all dysrhythmias except asystole.

Ventricular rate is slow (< 60 beats/min)
Give 0.5 mg atropine I.V.; repeat at 2-min intervals if necessary. Proceed to insertion of temporary transvenous pacemaker.
Remember: External pacing can reverse bradycardia rapidly and can be extremely effective in an emergency.

Ventricular rate is fast (> 100 beats/min)
Obtain a full 12-lead ECG plus a long rhythm strip (any lead with good voltage). Determine whether QRS complex is narrow or wide.

Patient becomes hemodynamically unstable
Cardiovert (100–400 joules) all dysrhythmias except asystole.

QRS complex is wide (> 0.08 sec, or 2 small boxes on ECG paper)
Cardiovert (starting with an energy level of 100 joules), and give lidocaine, 100 mg I.V.

QRS complex is narrow (< 0.08 sec)
Give verapamil.
Mix 10 mg verapamil in 10 ml saline; give 1 mg/min until ventricular rate slows and begin digitalization.

If QRS width is confusing and you cannot tell whether it is < or > 0.08 sec
Give 6 mg adenosine I.V. bolus × 2.

Ventricular rate does not slow (or it breaks)
Give verapamil, 1 mg/min I.V. up to 10 mg, to control atrial flutter.

Ventricular rate slows
The patient has sinus tachycardia; treat the underlying causes (e.g., fever, infection, hemorrhage, stress, and pain).

Ventricular rate slows
Treat as narrow-complex (< 0.08 sec) tachycardia.

Ventricular rate does not slow
Treat with cardioversion as a wide-complex (> 0.08 sec) tachycardia.

Figure 11 Shown is an algorithm for the management of postresuscitation acute dysrhythmia.

approaches an ECG electrode and a negative, or downward, deflection as it moves away from the electrode. The important factor in dysrhythmia recognition, however, is not the direction of the impulse but its duration. Normal conduction velocity is fast: an impulse is transmitted by healthy Purkinje fibers at a rate of 2 to 3 m/sec.[35] Hence, when an impulse that arises in the atrium (supraventricular) is transmitted via the atrioventricular (AV) node to the high-velocity Purkinje system, the entire ventricle is electrically activated in 0.08 second. An impulse that is generated at an ectopic ventricular site, however, cannot access the high-velocity Purkinje fibers as rapidly as a normal impulse, and ventricular activation is delayed. The QRS complex arising from an ectopic ventricular focus is therefore wider, signifying aberrant ventricular conduction.

Because dysrhythmias of supraventricular origin typically display a narrow QRS complex, the width of the QRS can generally be used to distinguish dysrhythmias of ventricular origin from those of supraventricular origin [see Figure 12]. A wide QRS, however, may also be produced by an impulse that originates in the atrium and is aberrantly conducted to or through the ventricles (supraventricular rhythm with aberrancy). Such rhythms do not pose a serious problem, however, because they are relatively uncommon (the incidence is approximately 10%); more important, the patient will never suffer if all dysrhythmias with a wide QRS [see Figure 13] are treated as if they were of ventricular origin.

When the ventricular rate is fast and the QRS is narrow, the 12-lead ECG should be searched for P waves, which indicate the presence of atrial activity. If P waves are absent and the QRS complexes are irregular [see Figure 14], the patient probably has atrial fibrillation. It is not, however, crucial to know this; the focus again should be on the width of the QRS complex. Verapamil should be administered to control the ventricular rate (mix 10 mg of verapamil in 10 ml of saline; give 1 mg/min until the ventricular rate slows). A patient with a wide-complex tachycardia is treated by cardioversion (see above) accompanied by administration of lidocaine, 100 mg I.V., whereas a patient with a narrow-complex tachycardia is treated with verapamil.[35,37] Therefore, it is not necessary to identify the specific type of dysrhythmia to treat it effectively.

Verapamil acts by producing profound AV nodal blockade (see below); however, it is also a peripheral vasodilator. Moderate to profound systemic hypotension can be anticipated until the patient converts to sinus rhythm.

Much has been written about the risks of using verapamil in patients who are already receiving beta blockers. Abrupt and com-

> ### The Intracardiac Cardioverter Defibrillator
>
> Over 30 years ago, Michel Mirowski developed the first automatic intracardiac cardioverter defibrillator (ICD), a device that detects dangerous tachyarrhythmias and delivers a cardioverting shock.[130] In the intervening time, it has become abundantly clear that some of the 400,000 Americans who die "suddenly" of tachyarrhythmias each year could have been identified as high risk, although they could not have been saved by pharmacologic or surgical treatment. For these patients, an ICD can be lifesaving.[131]
>
> The ICD identifies dangerous rhythm patterns by means of two algorithms. The first of these algorithms analyzes the patient's heart rate. The patient's maximum attainable sinus rate must be determined by exercise testing before the device is implanted; the ICD is then programmed to detect heart rates above this value. (The ICD can be externally programmed to detect rates between 155 and 200 beats/min.[132])
>
> Using rate criteria alone, however, the ICD cannot discriminate between sinus tachycardia and ventricular or supraventricular tachycardia. Inappropriate shocks are the Achilles heel of the ICD: almost one third of patients experience at least one inappropriate shock annually, when the device detects an episode of sinus tachycardia in which the rate exceeds the threshold programmed earlier. The ICD misinterprets the event as ventricular tachycardia and delivers a shock to the hemodynamically stable patient.[133] Patients liken this to being punched hard in the chest. Although rarely of electrophysiologic significance, an inappropriate shock can be psychologically crippling.[134]
>
> Although computer circuitry is facile and rapid, an ICD recognizes patterns poorly. Fine (or even coarse) VF may not exhibit enough positive spikes to be recognized as a tachyarrhythmia by the ICD. A second algorithm (the probability density function algorithm) was developed to analyze electrophysiologic data and improve the specificity of the ICD's sensing circuitry. A unique feature of ventricular fibrillation is the virtual absence of isoelectric time. Conversely, during sinus tachycardia and supraventricular tachycardia, the ECG is at the isoelectric baseline much of the time. The probability density function algorithm enables the ICD to determine the proportion of time that the ECG is spending at the isoelectric baseline and thereby to detect ventricular fibrillation.
>
> The ICD typically requires more than 5 seconds to appreciate ventricular tachycardia or fibrillation. It then charges its energy storage capacitors for 15 seconds and delivers a 30-joule cardioverting shock. If necessary, the device will deliver a second, third, fourth, and fifth countershock. If the rhythm disorder persists after the fifth countershock, the device will not recycle.
>
> ICD systems are not complex. The device consists of a battery, which is heavy (though newer batteries are becoming lighter), and circuitry, which is light, with a total weight of less than 100 g. Most implanted defibrillators are currently placed without a thoracotomy. A sensing and defibrillating lead system (14 French) is inserted percutaneously via the subclavian vein into right ventricular–right atrial position. The distal electrode tip senses ventricular fibrillation and tachycardia. The cardioverting energy is then discharged between a coil electrode on the diaphragmatic surface of the right ventricle and another coil electrode positioned in the superior vena cava.
>
> It is now clear that ICDs really do work and are capable of extending life. The most effective predictor of outcome in patients with ICDs is the severity of heart failure.[135] The ICD does not prevent malignant arrhythmias: it is, in essence, a safety net that cardioverts ventricular tachycardia or VF when it occurs. Therefore, it must still be used in conjunction with antidysrhythmic drugs.[136,137]
>
> It is easy for a surgeon to become spooked by an ICD. The most effective strategy for managing a patient with an ICD is simply to ignore the ICD. If such a patient is being transported to the OR, however, the device should be inactivated before the electrocautery is used: the ICD will misinterpret the cautery current as VF and respond by delivering a shock to the patient.
>
> The aura of mystery surrounding the ICD may be instantly eliminated by turning off the device (see below). Once the ICD is inactivated, the patient can be treated as any other patient would be. If external cardioversion is indicated, the ICD can be disregarded; external cardioversion will not harm or activate it.
>
> #### How to Turn the ICD Off
>
> 1. If you can find the industry representative to program the device to remain off, do so. Then treat the patient exactly as you would if the ICD were not present.
> 2. If you cannot find the representative or the situation is urgent:
>   a. Palpate the ICD generator, which is typically implanted in the left subcostal region.
>   b. Place a heavy pacemaker (or, better yet, an ICD magnet) over the upper corner of the device, toward the patient's left shoulder. Older devices used to emit a soft beep (synchronous with the heartbeat) in response to a magnet when they were active. Unfortunately, that feature has since been engineered out, and newer ICDs are silent.
>   c. Tape the magnet in place over the upper border of the device. As long as the magnet is in place, the ICD is off and the electrocautery can be used safely.

plete AV block rarely occurs. In the vast majority of patients, however, the risk of persistent supraventricular tachycardia is greater than the risk of third-degree heart block. Previous beta blockade should not be considered a contraindication to the use of verapamil. Some clinicians may prefer to use adenosine.

Adenosine (see below) produces conduction delay in the AV node and deserves recognition as a second very good (albeit transiently effective) option for treatment of paroxysmal narrow-complex tachycardia or for diagnosis of supraventricular tachycardia with aberrancy (including Wolff-Parkinson-White syndrome). Adenosine is given in a 6 mg I.V. push, followed 2 minutes later by a 12 mg I.V. push and, after another 2 minutes, by a final 12 mg I.V. push over 2 seconds.[34,38]

Patients receiving adenosine complain of a frightening feeling of breathlessness and pressure that is not angina or dyspnea. This feeling typically resolves within 30 seconds. Facial flushing is also common. Unlike verapamil, adenosine is associated with hypotension in fewer than 1% of patients. Transient atrial or ventricular ectopy, with varying degrees of AV block, occurs in more than half of patients. None of the side effects of adenosine necessitate therapy. Compared with verapamil, adenosine has certain advantages. Adenosine's rapid onset and short-duration AV nodal blockade permit diagnostic probing of questionable wide-complex tachycardias, and its side effects are trivial and self-limited. On the other hand, the profound neuroendocrine and electrolyte perturbations that provoked the dysrhythmias in the first place—perturbations that are very common in the surgical intensive care unit—are likely to persist, and the rhythm disorder typically recurs. If adenosine works, the longer-acting verapamil should also work.

Verapamil Both the sinoatrial (SA) node and the AV node are activated by the movement of calcium through the so-called slow calcium channels.[39] Verapamil, a calcium channel blocker, is the most powerful agent currently available for blocking the transmission of impulses across the AV node. A supraventricular dysrhythmia produces an acceleration in the ventricular rate because impulses generated by an ectopic source above the AV node are transmitted too rapidly to the ventricle [see Figure 15]. Verapamil produces a pharmacologic blockade of the AV node, reducing the number of impulses reaching the ventricles and thereby controlling the ventricular rate.

Adenosine Adenosine is an endogenous nucleoside that has differential antidysrhythmic effects in both supraventricular and ventricular tissue. The real appeal of adenosine as a therapeutic

Troubleshooting a Pacemaker

Patient with pacemaker experiences palpitations or presyncope
Obtain 30-second rhythm strip to assess pacing and sensing functions.

- **All wide (paced) QRS complexes are preceded by pacemaker artifacts**
  Pacing function is normal.

- **Heart rate is adequate, and no pacemaker artifacts are visible**
  Place magnet over pacemaker to inactivate sensing circuit and convert to fixed-rate mode.
  - **No pacemaker artifacts are visible with magnet**
    Pacemaker battery is dead.
  - **Pacemaker artifacts that appear at appropriate distances from prior QRS complexes (i.e., outside refractory period) provoke paced QRS**
    Sensing and pacing functions are normal.
  - **Pacemaker artifacts that appear at appropriate distances from prior QRS complexes (i.e., outside refractory period) do not provoke paced QRS**
    Consider two possibilities:
    - Adequate pacemaker output may not be reaching an excitable portion of the ventricle, or
    - Ventricular pacing threshold is higher than pacemaker output.

- **Some or all pacemaker artifacts are not followed by wide (paced) QRS complexes**
  Ventricular pacing threshold is higher than pacemaker output.

Obtain drug history to rule out an increase in ventricular threshold caused by antidysrhythmic agents.
Obtain chest x-ray to determine whether endocardial lead has been fractured or dislodged.

Endocardial lead is intact and in good anatomic position
Reprogram pacemaker to higher output.

- **All pacemaker artifacts are followed by a paced beat**
- **Intermittent capture persists**
  Relocate endocardial lead to lower threshold site.

Troubleshooting a Pacemaker

Few industries have benefited more from the United States space program than has the cardiac pacemaker industry. Much of the microcircuitry developed for the space shuttle is directly applicable to pacemakers. Yet the array of programmable parameters that has become standard in most implanted pacemakers, while providing therapeutic flexibility to electrophysiologists, can be intimidating to the mere mortal surgeon. The purpose of this discussion is to delineate simple methods for identifying problems with the two dominant pacemaker functions: pacing and sensing (see above and right).

Any of the following situations might prompt evaluation of pacemaker function: (1) the patient informs you that he or she has a pacemaker, (2) you note a pacemaker bulge in the pectoral area, (3) a chest x-ray reveals a pacemaker with a wire descending onto the diaphragmatic surface of the right ventricle, or (4) a patient with an implanted pacemaker notes symptoms of palpitations or presyncope. At this point, you need to obtain a 30-second rhythm strip to determine whether the pacemaker can capture the patient's ventricle—that is, whether the pacemaker emits an impulse that stimulates the ventricle to depolarize.

(continued)

---

and diagnostic tool is that it depresses automaticity and conduction within the SA and AV nodes.[40] Two clinically relevant types of adenosine receptors are present in cardiac tissue: (1) A_1 receptors, which are present on AV nodal tissue and cardiomyocytes and promote AV block and bradycardia, and (2) A_2 receptors, which reside on vascular endothelial and smooth muscle cells and mediate coronary vasodilatation. A_3 receptors are present in the myocardium, and selective activation of these has a cardioprotective effect; however, these receptors are not important in antidysrhythmic therapy.[41]

Adenosine and acetylcholine exhibit identical cardiac effects and share similar receptor-effector coupling systems. Adenosine and acetylcholine provide an opposing balance to the sympathetic neurotransmitters norepinephrine and epinephrine. Thus, predictably, the adenosine antagonists caffeine, theophylline, and aminophylline provoke tachycardia and ectopy.

Because of the rapid intravascular metabolism of adenosine (half-life, 6 seconds), an intravenous bolus of adenosine (6 mg or 100 μg/kg) produces a negligible effect on systemic blood pressure, as confirmed by multiple clinical studies. Thus, adenosine is safe, but its effects are transient.

Adenosine is useful in blocking AV nodal conduction. Intracardiac recordings exhibit prolongation of the A-H interval with no alteration in conduction distal to the His bundle and on into the ventricular myocardium (the His-Purkinje system is unaffected).

In more than 90% of cases, adenosine is effective in terminating supraventricular tachycardia. Interestingly, adenosine was as

Troubleshooting a Pacemaker (continued)

Ventricular Capture

a

Note the pacemaker artifact (↑) that precedes each wide QRS complex in rhythm strip *a*, above. The QRS complex is wide because ventricular activation does not originate from the AV node, and ventricular conduction is therefore aberrant. At this point, you know that your patient is pacing, and you can determine the pacing rate. You do not, however, know the pacing threshold (i.e., the minimum voltage required for ventricular capture) or the safety margin between pacemaker output and pacing threshold. At this moment (and presumably yesterday and tomorrow), this pacemaker is appropriately discharging its most important function—pacing the heart and maintaining an adequate rate.

Ventricular Sensing

b

In rhythm strip *b,* above, normal P waves are followed by regular QRS complexes, and no pacemaker artifacts are evident. It is most likely that this patient's pacemaker has been programmed to fire at a paced rate that is slower than this patient's intrinsic heart rate, and the pacemaker is thus appropriately sensing each QRS complex. It is unlikely but possible, however, that the pacemaker is not sensing appropriately. Instead, one of the following problems may be occurring: (1) the pacemaker battery is dead, which is unlikely unless the battery was implanted more than 5 years ago, (2) the intracardiac electrode has been fractured, which is also unlikely, because current leads are remarkably durable, (3) the intracardiac electrode has been dislodged (this is an uncommon late problem that typically results in pacemaker artifacts unrelated to each QRS complex), or (4) the patient is taking an antidysrhythmic drug that has profoundly depressed ventricular excitability below threshold level for capture (this problem is very rare and can be excluded by taking a drug history). It is overwhelmingly likely, therefore, that rhythm strip *b* simply demonstrates that the pacemaker is sensing appropriately.

Assessing Ventricular Capture When the Spontaneous Heart Rate Is High

Typically, by the time you see the syncopal patient in the emergency department or recovery room, the patient is sufficiently excited that his or her heart rate has recovered, and the rhythm strip will look like rhythm strip *b*. In a patient in whom heart rate is adequate and no pacemaker artifacts are visible, it is necessary to override the pacemaker's sensing circuit to determine whether the pacemaker is capable of emitting a pacing impulse that will capture the ventricle. The pacemaker's sensing circuit may be inactivated by placing a magnet over the pacemaker. Alternatively, the pacemaker may be reprogrammed to a paced rate that is faster than the patient's intrinsic heart rate. In this fashion, capture may easily be assessed. (Unfortunately, the programmers are expensive and are therefore often locked in some inaccessible closet. Programmers have great theoretical value but very little practical value to the surgeon.)

c

|←———— Magnet ————→|

In rhythm strip *c*, above, a magnet has converted the patient's pacemaker from the demand mode to the fixed-rate mode. The pacemaker artifacts that precede the wide (paced) QRS complexes in this rhythm strip (black arrows) show that the pacing function of this pacemaker is intact. Occasionally, a pacemaker artifact occurs during the electrical refractory period that immediately follows the QRS complex (red arrows). Pacing during the refractory period will not result in ventricular capture. Pacing during the refractory period should not result in ventricular capture and must not be interpreted as intermittent capture. In a patient whose pacemaker seems to be sensing appropriately (as in rhythm strip *b*), the magnet permits assessment of ventricular capture. Rhythm strip *c* demonstrates normal ventricular capture in the presence of a magnet.

Some or All Pacemaker Artifacts Are Not Followed by Wide QRS Complexes

If a pacemaker impulse that occurs outside the refractory period is not followed by a wide QRS complex, two possibilities should be considered. First, an adequate pacemaker impulse may not be reaching an excitable portion of the ventricle because of fracture or dislodgment of the endocardial lead. This problem can usually be identified by a chest x-ray. Second, if the chest x-ray shows that the lead is intact and in good anatomic position, the pacemaker output is not sufficient to reach the pacing threshold. Occasionally, this problem is caused by fibrosis at the endocardial electrode tip. If the pacemaker can be reprogrammed to a higher output, the capture problem should resolve. Otherwise, the lead must be repositioned to a site at which the pacing threshold is lower.

Occasional Pacemaker Artifacts Closely Follow a Spontaneous QRS Complex

If the patient's rhythm strip looks like rhythm strip *c, in the absence of a magnet,* the pacemaker is not sensing properly. In the demand mode, most pacemakers require at least a 2.5 mV signal to suppress output. Thus, if the pacemaker emits stimuli in spite of a normal spontaneous heart rate, an adequate QRS signal either is not being sensed (the lead tip may be lodged at the site of a prior myocardial infarction or scar) or is not being transmitted to the pacemaker (because of lead fracture or dislodgment).

---

effective at terminating atrioventricular reentry (85%) as at terminating atrioventricular node reentry (86%).[40] Because of adenosine's short half-life, however, the supraventricular dysrhythmia is likely to recur within 2 minutes in up to one third of patients. Thus, adenosine is diagnostically valuable in discriminating supraventricular from ventricular dysrhythmias. Continuous (therapeutic) infusion of adenosine (150 to 300 μg/kg/min) is rational from a physiologic standpoint but is frighteningly expensive. The transient (and safe) characteristics of adenosine permit its diagnostic use [*see Figure 11*]. If the QRS width is confusing and it is therefore uncertain whether the rhythm disorder is supraventricular (QRS < 0.08 second) or ventricular (QRS > 0.08 second),

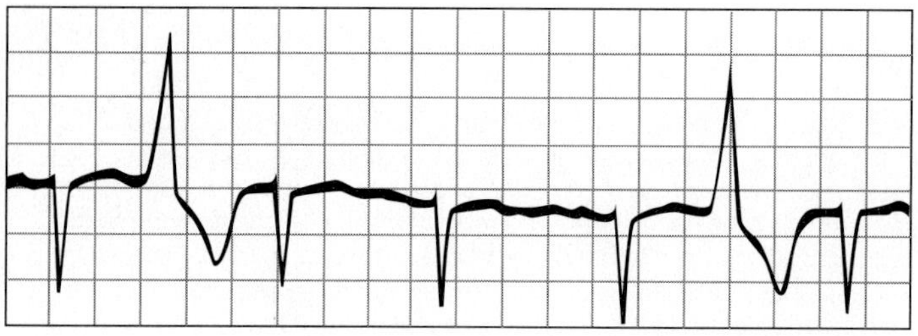

Figure 12 This tracing depicts frequent ventricular ectopic depolarizations interspersed among depolarizations from a supraventricular source. Note that the QRS depolarizations of supraventricular origin are narrow, whereas the QRS complexes of ectopic ventricular origin are wide.

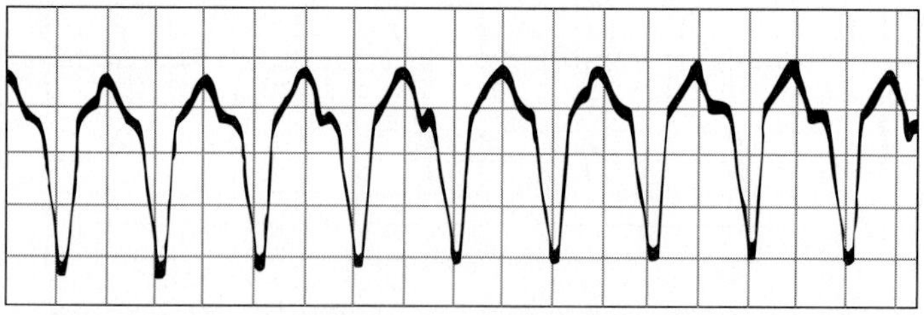

Figure 13 In a wide-complex tachycardia, each impulse is conducted aberrantly through the ventricles. The QRS complex is therefore prolonged to more than 0.08 second and occupies more than two small boxes on the ECG tracing.

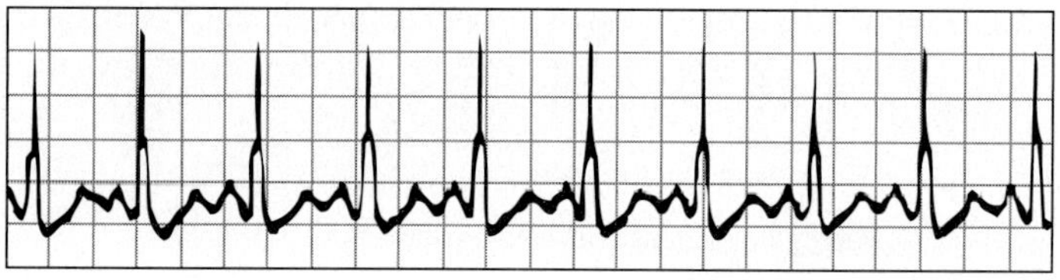

Figure 14 P waves are absent and the QRS complexes are narrow and irregular in this ECG tracing from a patient with atrial fibrillation.

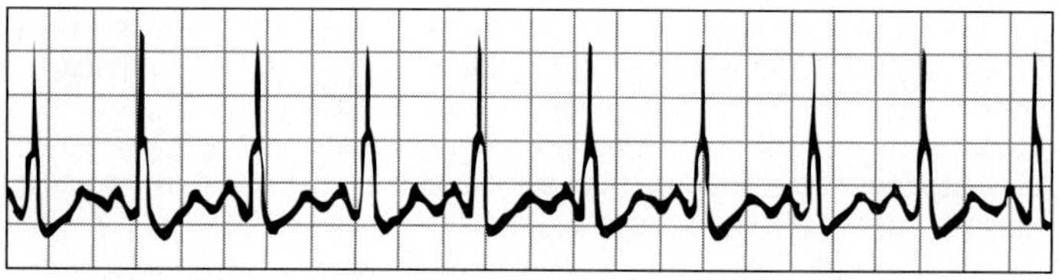

Figure 15 In a narrow-complex tachycardia, the entire ventricle is activated in less than 0.08 second. Presumably, the impulse originated at a supraventricular source and accessed the ventricle via the high-velocity Purkinje system.

adenosine (6 mg I.V. bolus) may be infused and repeated if necessary. If the dysrhythmia breaks, that means it was supraventricular. If it does not break, proceed to cardioversion (see above).

Several clinical studies have compared adenosine with verapamil for therapeutic AV nodal blockade, with predictable results. Both agents block the AV node and control the ventricular rate: cumulative efficacy with either agent is more than 90%. Postconversion dysrhythmias in the two groups were similar. Spontaneous reinitiation of supraventricular dysrhythmias occurs more frequently with adenosine, whereas systemic hypotension is more commonly associated with verapamil (at least until the dysrhythmia breaks). Thus, for help in seconds (approximately 20 seconds), use adenosine (6 mg I.V. bolus, may be repeated); for help in minutes (3 to 5 minutes), use verapamil (1 mg/min I.V. up to 10 mg); and for help in hours, infuse digoxin, 0.5 mg I.V. Although digitalis effectively blocks the AV node, it should be remembered that digitalis actually increases automaticity and excitability in both the atrium and the ventricle. The calcium channel blockers are superior to digoxin in controlling the ventricular rate.[39]

The adverse effects of adenosine, like the beneficial effects, are transient.[40] Facial flushing, chest pressure (adenosine has been implicated in the sensation of angina), and transient third-degree heart block are very common. Significant side effects are rare. Nebulized adenosine can cause bronchoconstriction, especially in asthmatic patients. Bronchoconstriction has not been reported after intravenous administration of adenosine.

Magnesium Magnesium is the second most abundant cation in man. It is involved in many enzymatic reactions that influence the production and utilization of cellular energy. Abnormalities in electrolyte homeostasis (potassium and calcium in particular) are associated with a robust increase in cardiac myocellular excitability and automaticity, especially when these abnormalities are concurrent with myocardial ischemia.[42] Multiple clinical studies confirm the efficacy of intravenous magnesium infusion even in the absence of objective hypomagnesemia.[43,44] Magnesium appears to be uniquely beneficial in the setting of digitalis toxicity and acute myocardial ischemia. Intravenous magnesium appears to help even when the measured serum values are normal. No one knows the mechanism. When confronted with a patient exhibiting either supraventricular or ventricular ectopy, it is safe (and often effective) to administer magnesium chloride at a dosage of 7 g or 100 mg/kg I.V. over 1 to 3 hours. It is not necessary to measure the serum magnesium concentration first; the serum value will not influence therapy.

Amiodarone Amiodarone is a potent inhibitor of alpha- and beta-adrenergic stimulation with a half-life of 1 month. It prolongs the myocardial action potential and refractory period and delays both sinus node function and AV conduction.

Although the primary effect of amiodarone is to slow down cardiac activity (actually, amiodarone exhibits electrophysiologic characteristics of all four antiarrhythmic classes [*see* Discussion, Drug Therapy, *below*]),[45] it must have additional therapeutic efficacy. It reduces transmural proarrhythmic heterogeneity (which predisposes to arrhythmias) in the human heart[46] [*see* Discussion, Reentrant Dysrhythmias, *below*]. Intravenous amiodarone has also proved effective against refractory ventricular tachycardia and VF. In one randomized trial,[44] I.V. amiodarone brought about a significant improvement in survival compared with placebo in patients suffering out-of-hospital cardiac arrest.

Intravenous amiodarone was approved in the United States for use against malignant ventricular tachyarrhythmias in 1995. Rates of effective suppression for ventricular arrhythmias have been reported to be as high as 91% in uncontrolled trials.[47] Although this gratifyingly effective agent is available and works well, it has significant side effects. In trials of low-dose amiodarone (200 mg/day), thyroid, neurologic, cutaneous, ocular, bradycardic, and hypotensive problems were statistically more frequent; interestingly, pulmonary fibrosis was not.[48] The recommended dosages for adults are as follows: loading dose, 150 mg I.V. over 10 minutes; maintenance infusion, 0.5 mg/min; and oral dose, 200 to 400 mg/day (after loading).

Cardiac Dysrhythmias during Pregnancy

Fortunately, cardiac dysrhythmias are not frequent in young women of childbearing age. When rhythm problems do occur, they tend not to be hemodynamically destabilizing. The most commonly used obstetric drug with electrophysiologic side effects is magnesium.[49] When magnesium is infused intravenously into the mother, the fetus may exhibit a dose-dependent bradycardia and a progressive decrease in healthy heart rate variability.[50,51] Antidysrhythmic (indeed, any) drugs should be avoided during the first trimester of pregnancy, although most antidysrhythmic agents carry relatively little risk.[49] Quinidine, procainamide, lidocaine, digoxin, adenosine, and beta blockers all have a long record of safety during pregnancy. Flecainide has proved to be effective in treating fetal supraventricular tachycardia complicated by hydrops. Phenytoin and amiodarone have been associated with congenital abnormalities.[49]

The important point is that if the mother is unstable, direct current cardioversion is safe and effective.

Proarrhythmia with Antidysrhythmic Drugs

Proarrhythmic manifestations have been linked primarily to agents that prolong repolarization. Early afterdepolarizations (see below) associated with agents that retard repolarization or an increase in spatial and temporal dispersion of repolarization are the putative mechanisms of proarrhythmia.[52]

The class III antidysrhythmic agents have traditionally been the agents most likely to cause dysrhythmias.[52] The best way of preventing dysrhythmias, however, is to follow the general policy of not using drugs at all if they are not needed.[53]

Discussion

In the fifth century B.C., the Greek poet Pindar admonished all physicians: "Thou shall treat and thou shall not kill, but do not attempt to return a dead soul to life."[54] Fortunately, no one listened to the poet then, and no one is listening now. Since Biblical times, humans have sought to reanimate the dead, mixing science, prayer, alchemy, and the magic arts. Today, CPR is the cornerstone of resuscitation and is practiced by millions of health professionals and laypersons in communities throughout the world.

In recent years, investigators have made fundamental new discoveries in CPR. A mechanism of blood flow that contradicts the conventional notion of cardiac massage has been identified. Some apocryphal drugs, including calcium and isoproterenol (and, in some circles, sodium bicarbonate), have finally been abandoned. One old technique, open-chest cardiac massage, has resurfaced and appears promising. Controversies have arisen at every turn.

What has prompted the renaissance of interest and research in resuscitation? Primarily, it has been the observation that the majority of cardiac arrest victims do not survive. Only 15% of patients with prehospital cardiopulmonary arrest survive to hospital discharge.[55] Much higher survival rates (30% to 50%) have been reported in some urban communities, but only if (1) the arrest is witnessed, (2) a bystander administers CPR, (3) the initial rhythm is ventricular fibrillation, (4) BLS is provided within 4 minutes, and (5) definitive ALS is provided within 8 minutes of arrest.[55]

Among long-term survivors of prehospital arrest, permanent neurologic impairment is all too common. At least 20% of prehospital victims who are resuscitated and admitted to hospitals never regain consciousness. Permanent brain dysfunction occurs in one half of all long-term survivors.[56] To promote resuscitation with preservation of intellect and independence, the new field of cardiopulmonary-cerebral resuscitation (CPCR) has evolved.

Sudden, unexpected cardiac arrests are also common in the hospital setting. In fact, in teaching hospitals, resuscitation is attempted on 1% of patients admitted and on 30% of patients who die.[57] Although response times are short, resuscitation equipment is at hand, and the bystanders are physicians and nurses, success rates for resuscitation in general hospitals are low: 50% of patients remain alive for 1 hour or longer, but only 10% survive to discharge.[57] For those patients who do survive cardiac arrest and resuscitation efforts, however, the long-term outcome is favorable. Most survivors walk out of the hospital and return to their homes,[58] and 6 months later, 80% of those who returned home are still alive and well. When longevity, independence, and mental fitness are considered, the majority of patients who survive resuscitation have an excellent prognosis. In one study, 21 (55%) of 38 patients who survived for 6 months or longer said that they would choose to undergo cardiopulmonary resuscitation again.[55,58]

Most patients who experience in-hospital cardiac arrest have critical circulatory, respiratory, malignant, or neurologic disorders, which may explain their poor survival rate. Indeed, azotemia, cancer, sepsis, hypotension, and a homebound lifestyle have all been shown to predict a poor outcome. In the absence of a witness[57] or in the presence of a rhythm other than VF or VT,[59] resuscitation is likely to be unsuccessful. Advanced age does not appear to be an independent predictor of poor outcome when comorbidity and illness severity are controlled for[58,60]; thus, CPR is not precluded in elderly patients. Nevertheless, most chronically ill elderly patients will not survive resuscitation in the hospital.[57,61] When a patient is both elderly and irreversibly ill, the physician and the patient or family should give careful consideration to the hazards (and the probable futility) of CPR.[62]

Circulatory Physiology during CPR

CARDIAC PUMP

Kouwenhoven and coworkers first suggested that during CPR the heart is squeezed like a pump between the sternum and the spine.[63] According to this theory, each downstroke on the chest results in a systole, during which the left ventricle is compressed and blood is propelled into the arterial circulation. Because the cardiac valves operate in only one direction, anterograde blood flow is assured. The relaxation phase of CPR (diastole) also mimics the natural circulation. As the sternum recoils to its normal position, intracardiac pressures fall, the atrioventricular valves open, and blood is drawn into the heart from the lungs and the venae cavae.

During the intercompression interval, a small inflow of air occurs from the trachea. However, because this flow is insufficient for ventilation, positive pressure ventilation must be applied. The cardiac pump concept is the basis for the current standards of CPR: ventilation and compression are alternated so that inflation of the lungs will not impede direct massage of the heart.

THORACIC PUMP

Many physiologists now favor a different mechanism of blood flow during CPR: the thoracic pump. According to this theory, external chest compression does not massage the heart; instead, each deflection of the sternum generates an abrupt increase in intrathoracic pressure, which in turn propels blood into the arterial tree.[6] The increase in pressure is uniform in all hollow viscera of the thorax, including the four chambers of the heart, the intrathoracic aorta, and the great veins. The mitral and tricuspid valves are rendered incompetent, and no atrioventricular or ventriculoaortic pressure gradients are established. While the extrathoracic jugular veins collapse during thoracic compression, the thick-walled carotid arteries remain patent and receive the forward spurt of blood. Thus, in contrast to the cardiac pump, the thoracic pump generates forward blood flow because of an arteriovenous pressure gradient established outside, not within, the chest. According to the thoracic pump concept, the heart is a passive conduit, not a pump, during CPR.

The relative contributions of the cardiac and thoracic pumps remain unsettled.[64] Each mechanism probably contributes to systemic perfusion, depending on the configuration and stiffness of the chest wall, the presence or absence of cardiac enlargement, and the method of CPR.[6] In an individual patient, there may even be variations in the mechanism of blood flow. Cardiac compressions may predominate early in the resuscitation effort, especially at the points of maximal sternal deflection and minimal lung inflation. In any case, whether the cardiac or thoracic pump is operative, the blood flow generated increases with the depth, force, and rate of chest compressions.

LIMITED VITAL ORGAN PERFUSION DURING CPR

Blood flow during CPR can barely sustain life. When standard CPR is applied to the patient in cardiac arrest, the cardiac output is only 25% of normal.[6,10,16] Although the peak systolic blood pressure at the downstroke of the chest compression may reach 60 mm Hg, the diastolic blood pressure is less than 20 mm Hg.

Cerebral cortical flow seldom exceeds 15% of prearrest values. Standard CPR does not sustain cerebral oxygenation, pupillary reactivity, or electroencephalographic activity during prolonged resuscitation.[10]

The situation in the coronary circulation is even more precarious. During conventional CPR, blood flow in the coronary vascular bed falls to 5% of normal.[10] In fact, reverse coronary flow has been observed. Indeed, the thoracic pump provides no mechanism at all for blood flow to the heart. In the cardiac arrest victim, the sole determinant of coronary blood flow is the coronary perfusion pressure (i.e., aortic diastolic pressure minus right atrial diastolic pressure). Both components of this equation lie within the thorax and increase and decrease together during CPR. In addition, unlike the cerebral vascular bed, the coronary venous circulation has no one-way valves to protect it from pressure increases. Therefore, the essential problem with CPR is that it raises arterial pressure and venous pressure to virtually the same degree, generating no gradient for coronary blood flow at all.

MEASURES OF EFFECTIVE CPR

Traditionally, clinicians have judged the effectiveness of CPR by the strength of the victim's pulses and the size of the pupils. Near-normal blood gas levels have also been considered a favorable sign. However, none of these parameters actually correlates with vital organ perfusion or with success of resuscitation.[65] Instead, the best predictors of outcome are hemodynamic measures: the success of resuscitation correlates most closely with the coronary perfusion gradient (i.e., aortic blood pressure minus right atrial pressure) during the release phase (diastole) of CPR.[6,16] In prolonged CPR, neurologic recovery and long-term survival are possible only if certain critical hemodynamic thresholds are met or exceeded: aortic diastolic (coronary perfusion) blood pressure must equal 30 mm Hg; calculated coronary perfusion gradient, 20 mm Hg; and myocardial blood flow, 20 ml/min/100 g (about 30% of baseline). These requisite hemodynamic parameters are highly correlated with one another and with survival. A cerebrocortical blood flow of 20 ml/min/100 g (20% of the prearrest level) is essential for neurologic recovery. None of these critical indices can be achieved by conventional CPR alone.

NEW CPR TECHNIQUES

Volume Loading during CPR

For many years, dextrose and water at a keep-open rate has been considered the appropriate fluid for CPR. Now, however, volume expansion may be more appropriate. Volume infusion is helpful in some cases of PEA, especially those caused by blood loss, systemic inflammatory response syndrome, anaphylaxis, pericardial tamponade, pulmonary embolus, and tension pneumothorax. In one porcine model of PEA, prearrest volume expansion with a crystalloid-hydroxyethyl starch mixture improved survival.[66] Expansion of the central circulatory volume is a logical adjunct to improve cardiac output and vital organ perfusion during CPR.

Interposed Abdominal Compression CPR

A more promising modification of CPR is the technique of manual interposed abdominal compression (IAC-CPR). In IAC-CPR, a third rescuer is recruited whose role is to apply pressure to the midabdomen during the release phase (i.e., diastole) of the chest compression-relaxation cycle. Otherwise, standard CPR is administered by using alternating ventilation and compression. Like an intra-aortic balloon pump, IAC-CPR augments aortic diastolic blood pressure and improves cerebral and myocardial perfusion. As noted earlier, coronary flow and survival are closely related to the central arteriovenous pressure difference during the release phase of CPR.

Active Compression-Decompression CPR

Early clinical studies suggested that active compression-decompression CPR (ACD-CPR) might outperform standard CPR. In one study of 10 patients in whom standard advanced life-support interventions had failed, institution of ACD-CPR resulted in immediate augmentation of cardiac output and coronary arterial perfusion.[67] A randomized clinical trial of 62 patients on a hospital ward demonstrated the superiority of ACD-CPR over standard CPR.[68] Short-term survival (24 hours) was 45% in the ACD-CPR group, compared with only 9% in the standard-CPR group. Neurologic recovery was higher in the ACD-CPR group as well. ACD-CPR may also improve ventilation. In contrast, Schwab and colleagues found no improvement in outcome with ACD-CPR in a large out-of-hospital trial.[69]

CURRENT-BASED DEFIBRILLATION

Rapid electrical defibrillation is the key to resuscitation success. One promising new technique is current-based defibrillation, which imposes an electrical current on the heart that is strong enough to interrupt the VF reentry circuit. The optimal current for successful defibrillation is about 30 to 40 amperes. Today, operators of defibrillators do not select the current needed; rather, they select the total energy dose, measured in joules.

However, selection of a standard energy dose fails to take into account that the flow of current is determined not only by the energy dose but also by the patient's transthoracic impedance (measured in ohms).[70] Transthoracic impedance varies from case to case because of differences in paddle pressure, patient size, chest wall configuration, conducting gels, lung inflation, and previous countershocks. The average transthoracic impedance in humans is about 70 ohms; however, impedance varies widely among cardiac arrest patients—from 15 to 150 ohms. If a patient's transthoracic impedance is high, the standard energy dose of 200 joules may deliver insufficient current. In a patient with low transthoracic resistance, this energy dose may be too high, provoking postcountershock bradyasystole.

Drug Therapy

AGENTS USED IN RESUSCITATION

Physicians have traditionally practiced resuscitation with "the empiricism of a grandmother's cooking,"[71] mixing sodium bicarbonate, calcium, and inotropes "according to taste." In truth, only one class of drugs—the alpha-adrenergic agonists—has proved effective in CPR.

Epinephrine and Other Alpha Agonists

In 1906, Crile and Dolley recognized that "the basic problem in resuscitation is to secure by means of some infusion a coronary [perfusion] pressure amounting to 30 to 40 mm Hg."[72] Of course, the aortic diastolic blood pressure is the driving force for coronary perfusion; indeed, in 1963, Redding and Pearson demonstrated experimentally that an aortic diastolic blood pressure of 40 mm Hg was a prerequisite for resuscitability.[73] Subsequent investigations have indicated that it is virtually impossible to attain this level of aortic blood pressure by external chest compression alone. Epinephrine is an essential adjunct.[15]

Alpha-adrenergic (pressor) agents cause venoconstriction, thus augmenting stroke volume during chest compression. Alpha-adrenergic agents also improve regional blood flow during CPR by inducing a selective increase in noncerebral and noncoronary vascular tone.[22] For example, epinephrine augments cerebrocortical blood flow by vasoconstricting peripheral arterial beds, by preventing or reversing carotid artery collapse at the thoracic outlet, and by constricting the extracerebral carotid artery,[22] thereby reducing blood flow to the tongue and facial musculature. Epinephrine and phenylephrine administration leads to improved cerebral cortical blood flow and neurologic recovery after CPR.[22,74]

Epinephrine also has a positive effect on the aortic diastolic (coronary perfusion) blood pressure. The myocardial perfusion pressure increases after epinephrine infusion because this drug augments aortic diastolic blood pressure without substantially increasing the right atrial pressure.[10]

Resuscitation is critically dependent on alpha-adrenergic tone no matter what the arrest rhythm. In prolonged ventricular fibrillation, successful electrical reversion to a pulsatile rhythm is enhanced by administration of epinephrine. This enhances defibrillation not by coarsening the fibrillatory waves (a beta-adrenergic effect) but by augmenting myocardial perfusion. Isoproterenol, a pure beta-adrenergic agonist, increases the frequency and amplitude of the fibrillatory waves; there is no proof that this coarser fibrillatory pattern is more easily cardioverted, but it certainly seems to suggest a more favorable outcome. Isoproterenol may even be detrimental: its unopposed beta-adrenergic activity causes peripheral vasodilatation, increases intraventricular pressures, reduces subendocardial blood flow, increases oxygen demand, and is detrimental to the CPR effect. Indeed, isoproterenol is no longer recommended in any cardiac arrest situation.

Alpha agonists are also critical in the treatment of asystole. When epinephrine is administered to asystolic animals, it is the alpha-adrenergic (pressor) action, not the beta-adrenergic (inotropic-chronotropic) action, that facilitates the return of a spontaneous rhythm.[73] In asphyxiated dogs, asystole may be reverted with equal success by using epinephrine, phenylephrine, metaraminol, or methoxamine.

Although the catecholamine of choice for resuscitation in all forms of cardiac arrest is epinephrine (a balanced alpha- and beta-adrenergic drug), preliminary studies suggested that the use of pure alpha-adrenergic agonists, such as methoxamine or phenylephrine, might be preferable. The standard dose of epinephrine in cardiac resuscitation has long been 1 mg, but this dose has no clinical or experimental basis. In fact, in the landmark animal studies of epinephrine performed over 90 years ago, 1 mg was a homeopathic dose.[29,72] Adequate coronary perfusion pressure is achieved in dogs only with the administration of 0.05 to 0.20 mg/kg—the equivalent of 3.5 to 14.0 mg every 5 minutes in a 70 kg human. Recent experimental and clinical studies have demonstrated that only these larger doses of epinephrine will consistently produce coronary perfusion pressures that exceed the threshold required for return of spontaneous circulation.[16]

Investigators have attempted to determine whether high-dose epinephrine is beneficial in cardiac arrest patients. In one large prehospital trial, patients who received a high dose (15 mg) of epinephrine had a higher return of spontaneous pulse and a higher hospital admission rate than patients who received a standard dose (1 mg).[75] However, survival to hospital discharge was not improved. In a large out-of-hospital study, high-dose epinephrine (0.2 mg/kg) did not increase the return of spontaneous pulse, number of hospital admissions, consciousness at hospital discharge, or overall survival.[76] A randomized trial comparing epinephrine doses of 1 mg and 7 mg for both in-hospital and out-of-hospital cardiac arrests found that the use of high-dose epinephrine did not improve 1-hour survival, survival to discharge, or neurologic recovery.[77]

Human and animal studies of epinephrine have consistently demonstrated that a moderate dose (5 mg) of epinephrine is superior to the standard dose (1 mg) in augmenting myocardial perfusion.[16] However, it remains unclear whether moderate-dose and high-dose epinephrine enhance long-term survival or neurologic recovery. In addition, high doses of epinephrine may increase cardiac metabolic demand during VF and may even cause recurrent or refractory VF. Therefore, an escalating dosing regimen is advised [*see Table 1*]. The first dose of epinephrine should be 1 mg, but if this is ineffective, the dose should be increased after 3 minutes to 3 mg, and then, after 3 additional minutes, to 5 mg; a dose of 5 mg should then be repeated every 3 to 5 minutes.

Calcium

Calcium excites the myocardium and has long been advocated as a first-line panacea in all forms of cardiac arrest. Indeed, in the spontaneously beating heart, calcium augments contractile force, facilitates excitation-contraction coupling, and stimulates impulse formation and conduction.[78,79] Unfortunately, the arrested heart, unlike the beating heart, does not respond to infusions of calcium. In clinical trials, calcium has not been effective in patients with PEA, asystole, or VF.[79]

Calcium can also have pernicious effects. After injection of standard doses of calcium, dangerously high serum levels of calcium are frequently observed.[80] Rapid boluses can cause sinus arrest, suppression of normal automaticity, provocation of ventricular ectopy, and cerebrovascular spasm.[80] Hypercalcemia is particularly dangerous in patients receiving digitalis.

Calcium should not be administered routinely in cardiac arrest. With delayed or prolonged resuscitation, however, administration of calcium chloride may be helpful. Investigators have documented a time-dependent state of ionized hypocalcemia that may impede resuscitation.[81,82] Calcium should be administered if hyperkalemia is suspected (e.g., when cardiac arrest occurs in renal failure), if hypocalcemia is suspected, or if patients are receiving calcium channel blockers. Today, there is greater interest in treatment with calcium blockers than in treatment with calcium to promote tissue salvage and to aid in resuscitation.[79,83]

Sodium Bicarbonate

Acidemia is inevitable during prolonged cardiopulmonary arrest. Inadequate ventilation leads to carbon dioxide accumulation. CO_2 then passes readily across biologic membranes into cells. The result is a fall in pH in the cytosol, as predicted by the Henderson-Hasselbalch equation [see 7 Life-Threatening Acid-Base Disorders]. Metabolic acidosis also occurs during protracted arrest, even if CPR is effective. The critical reduction in delivery of oxygen to tissues leads to anaerobic metabolism and lactic acidosis [see 7 Life-Threatening Acid-Base Disorders].

Unmitigated acidosis exerts noxious effects on circulation.[84] Acidosis increases pulmonary vascular resistance but causes a loss of vasomotor tone in the peripheral arterial circulation. It causes arteriolar dilatation but venous constriction, leading to capillary stasis. Acidosis attenuates both the vascular and the cardiac responses to circulating adrenergic amines while enhancing the effects of vagal stimulation. Thus, acidosis leads to reduced chronotropy, inotropy, and vascular tone and predisposes to cardiovascular collapse. In addition, a fall in pH is associated with ventricular irritability and a lower threshold for VF.

It is actually the intracellular pH that matters. Therefore, respiratory acidosis is the more critical cause of myocardial dysfunction during cardiopulmonary arrest.[85] Myocardial contractile function is exquisitely sensitive to increases and decreases in arterial carbon dioxide tension because CO_2 enters cells so readily. As intracellular pH falls, myocardial contractile function declines. Thus, hypercapnia and intracellular acidosis are potent negative inotropes that can cause refractory PEA.[64]

The primary treatment of the acidemia that results from cardiac arrest is adequate ventilation, which ensures removal of CO_2. In clinical and animal studies, survival and correction of the pH correlate most closely with adequacy of ventilation.[86]

Traditionally, bicarbonate has also been administered to cardiac arrest victims to correct the base deficit associated with metabolic acidosis. In the myocardium, intracellular hypercapnia is a powerful negative inotrope (see above). In the globally ischemic heart, excessive sodium bicarbonate administration may cause contractile failure, refractory PEA, and a failed resuscitation effort (but only in the absence of adequate ventilation).[85] The second hazard of sodium bicarbonate administration is its hypertonicity. Each 50 mEq ampule of sodium bicarbonate contains 2,000 mOsm of the agent. This hypertonicity reduces aortic vasomotor tone, which, in turn, lowers the coronary arterial perfusion pressure. When coronary perfusion falls, a successful return of a perfusing rhythm is unlikely regardless of the pH achieved. Coronary blood flow—not arterial pH—is the critical factor that determines the success or failure of CPR.[87] No clinical or animal studies have documented that sodium bicarbonate helps in resuscitation except in cases of hyperkalemia and of tricyclic antidepressant overdose.[88] There is no evidence that administration of sodium bicarbonate helps manage the pH, improves the rate of defibrillation, or aids resuscitation.

Monitoring pH and Cardiac Output during Resuscitation

Measurements of arterial blood gases are usually considered the best guides for managing acid-base disturbances, and in most clinical circumstances, arterial and venous measurements of pH and carbon dioxide tension (P_{CO_2}) are roughly equivalent.[89] However, cardiopulmonary arrest may be an exception: a striking discordance between venous and arterial blood gas measurements has been uncovered.[85,90] During the initial minutes of cardiac resuscitation, marked mixed venous hypercapnia and acidosis occur routinely. Venous hypercapnia and acidosis probably reflect the production of lactic acid in underperfused tissues and the subsequent generation of new CO_2 as the anaerobically produced lactic acid is buffered by sodium bicarbonate. Venous hypercapnia also reflects venous pooling and impaired pulmonary excretion of CO_2, as a consequence of the drastic fall in cardiac output.

It is interesting to note that the mixed venous hypercapnia and acidosis are selective; that is, they are usually not reflected in the arterial blood. Arterial blood gases often reveal a low P_{CO_2} and alkalosis if lung ventilation is adequate. Researchers have found venous-arterial P_{CO_2} gradients of greater than 60 mm Hg.[85]

Arteriovenous differences in pH and P_{CO_2} may have clinical importance in CPR. Mixed venous blood, with its high P_{CO_2} and low pH, may reflect tissue hypoperfusion more accurately. Venous pH is also more predictive of the outcome of CPR because it is a marker of both circulatory and ventilatory adequacy. Administration of sodium bicarbonate in an effort to maintain normal arterial blood gases may exacerbate the disparity between arterial and venous pH and P_{CO_2} in the absence of adequate ventilation.[90]

End-tidal CO_2 monitoring The best and least invasive monitor of the efficacy of CPR is the expired CO_2 concentration because it is an indicator of circulatory delivery of CO_2 to the lung. The end-tidal CO_2 concentration rises and falls with pulmonary blood flow and therefore with cardiac output. End-tidal CO_2 monitoring (also known as capnography) provides continuous measurements of the blood flow generated during CPR, and its utilization correlates directly with increased coronary perfusion and survival.[91] Because end-tidal CO_2 varies not only with pulmonary perfusion but also with alveolar ventilation, sodium bicarbonate load, and carbon dioxide production,[92] it may provide a superb minute-by-minute window on the arrest victim's circulatory function, ventilation, and metabolism. Monitoring the end-tidal CO_2 at the bedside is almost as easy as palpating the carotid pulse; furthermore, the end-tidal CO_2 is a far more accurate measure of blood flow and the efficacy of CPR.

Median-frequency analysis of VF During prolonged VF, myocardial work and oxygen demand continue at nearly the same level as they do during sinus rhythm. Because myocardial blood flow is nil, myocardial oxygen, glucose, and high-energy phosphate stores are rapidly depleted and intracellular lactic acidosis becomes pronounced.[93,94] After a long period of VF, the fibrillatory waveform becomes less coarse. This pattern, often called fine VF, has long been recognized as a marker of a long arrest time[95] and a predictor of a poor outcome. The amplitude of the fibrillatory waves declines linearly as time elapses and signals that the heart is desperately underperfused.

Computer-assisted analyses of the fibrillatory waves have led to useful insights regarding VF. The median frequency of the ECG signals during VF is now recognized as a better marker of downtime and the adequacy of myocardial perfusion.[96] The median frequency of VF correlates with myocardial perfusion and appears to predict accurately the success or failure of electrical defibrillation. The median frequency of the VF tracing can be measured in seconds and may therefore serve as a valuable guide to the timing of defibrillation and the optimal dosing of epinephrine.[97]

Drug Administration: Peripheral, Central, Tracheal, or Cardiac?

A lifeline is essential in CPR. The safest and most expedient access to the circulation is generally considered to be a peripheral antecubital vein. However, medications reach the arterial circulation faster if injected into the internal jugular or subclavian vein. Central venous injections also result in higher peak arterial concentrations.[98] Therefore, central drug administration is recommended. A supradiaphragmatic (subclavian or internal jugular) vein should be cannulated because perfusion to, and drug absorption from, the lower extremities and subdiaphragmatic torso are markedly impaired during CPR.[99] After delivery of each drug, a 20 to 30 ml bolus of fluid should be given to speed delivery to the central circulation.[2]

If vascular access is not feasible, an endotracheal tube provides a satisfactory route for administration of some first-line resuscitation drugs. Most lipophilic drugs, including epinephrine, atropine, lidocaine, diazepam, and naloxone, can be administered by this route. Sodium bicarbonate, calcium, and vasopressors should not be administered intratracheally, because excessive volumes, tissue necrosis, and inactivation of surfactant result. Drug administration by endotracheal (ET) tube takes advantage of the relatively high blood flow to the lungs and the vast (70 m^2) absorptive area of the alveolar-capillary membrane.[100,101]

The pharmacokinetics of endotracheal drugs is best understood in the case of epinephrine. Its absorption is very rapid: peak drug levels and physiologic responses are detected 15 and 120 seconds after injection. Administration into the lungs also provides a beneficial depot effect: 5 minutes after injection of epinephrine, 80% of the initial blood level is still present in circulation. However, the peak blood concentration of epinephrine after ET administration is only 10% of that achieved with an equal I.V. dose.[100,101]

The method of ET drug injection is simple. About 2.5 times the standard I.V. dose (epinephrine, 2 to 5 mg; atropine, 3 mg; lidocaine, 3 mg/kg) should be administered after dilution in 10 ml of distilled water or saline. Shallow instillation is ineffective; the drug must be injected forcibly into a catheter that is placed beyond the distal end of the endotracheal tube and disseminated into the alveolar space by forced manual hyperventilation.[102] The efficacy and risks of endotracheal administration of drugs in patients with parenchymal lung disease are not known.

An alternative route to venous access, used primarily for children, is the tibial bone marrow. A large-bore needle can be inserted directly into the medullary cavity of the tibia in a matter of seconds.[103,104]

ANTIDYSRHYTHMIC AGENTS

Verapamil, lidocaine, and adenosine are the only drugs of value for the acute treatment of cardiac dysrhythmias. Because patients may already be taking oral agents for chronic dysrhythmias, however, it is important to be aware of the actions and side effects of these drugs when treating an individual with an acute dysrhythmia. Antidysrhythmic drugs have been classified on the basis of their dominant electrophysiologic effect[105]; this classification has been reviewed and placed in a clinical context.[37] Adenosine has a unique receptor that modulates cyclic adenosine monophosphate (cAMP), resulting in cholinergic activity. It is not similar to other antidysrhythmic agents and is therefore unclassified.

Class I Agents (Membrane Active)

Class I agents are fast sodium channel blockers. All class I agents—which include lidocaine, procainamide, quinidine, and disopyramide—are local anesthetics. These agents block the fast inward sodium current and thereby decrease both the amplitude of the action potential, or phase 0 depolarization (see below), and conduction velocity. These agents also depress the rate of spontaneous phase 4 depolarization, or automaticity, and thus are useful for abolishing premature ventricular contractions (PVCs); class I agents are sometimes termed PVC killers.

Because these agents slow the conduction velocity, they can predispose to reentrant cardiac dysrhythmias in some patients.[52,53]

Class II Agents (Beta Blockers)

Class II agents are beta blockers and include such drugs as propranolol. Sympathetic hyperactivity, marked by increased release of catecholamines, is one of the major causes of cardiac dysrhythmias that result from increased automaticity.[52,53,106] Beta-adrenergic blockade has produced a decrease in such automatic dysrhythmias under both clinical and experimental conditions.[106]

Class III Agents (to Prolong Repolarization)

Class III agents, such as bretylium, act directly on the myocardial cell membrane to delay phases 2 and 3 of repolarization and thereby prolong refractoriness. Bretylium is effective in terminating reentrant dysrhythmias because it prolongs the refractory period of the ectopic focus to the point where this region is still unexcitable when an impulse returns to reenter the circuit.[33,34] Bretylium apparently has no effect on either automaticity or conduction velocity.[107]

Class IV Agents (Calcium Channel Blockers)

Class IV agents, of which verapamil is the most effective, block the movement of calcium across the slow calcium channels but have virtually no effect on the so-called fast sodium channels.[105] Because both the SA node and the AV node are composed of slow-response fibers that are activated by the movement of calcium ions across the slow channels, the class IV agents are particularly effective in preventing unwanted supraventricular impulses from reaching the ventricles. Verapamil decreases the conduction velocity through the AV node and increases the refractory period of the AV node.

Class V Agents (Unclassified)

The vagus nerve innervates the SA node, the atria, and the AV node, but it has almost no influence over the His-Purkinje system or ventricular muscle. At therapeutic levels, digitalis has an antidysrhythmic action that is mediated almost exclusively via the vagus nerve. Toxic doses of digitalis, however, may produce an increased automaticity characterized by multifocal premature ventricular depolarizations [see Pathophysiology of Cardiac Dysrhythmias, *below*]. Caution must be observed in digitalizing a patient who is prone to atrial dysrhythmias, because digitalis increases atrial excitability and hence increases the risk of atrial ectopy. Because digitalis also induces AV nodal blockade mediated by the vagus nerve, however, any atrial dysrhythmias produced by digitalization will be less clinically significant.[108,109]

Cellular Electrophysiology

Electromechanical activity of all muscle, including the heart, is determined by the concentration and flow of ions, particularly calcium, potassium, and sodium. Knowledge of cardiac electrophysiology can serve as a conceptual framework on which to build a rational therapeutic program. Direct observation of cellular electrical activity using a glass microelectrode reveals that the cell membrane is semipermeable: it permits easy passage of cations such as sodium, potassium, and calcium but provides a barrier to anions such as proteins. Negatively charged intracellular proteins that cannot cross the cell membrane create a transmembrane potential in which the interior of the cell is negatively charged relative to the exterior. The membrane potential of a cell, E_K, is proportional to the difference between the logarithms of the intracellular potassium concentration, $[K]_i$, and the extracellular potassium concentration, $[K]_o$:

$$E_K = c(\log [K]_i - \log [K]_o)$$

The proportionality constant, c, varies with temperature, but at 37° C it is –60 mV. Thus, under physiologic conditions,

$$E_K = -60 \text{ mV} \times \log \frac{[K]_i}{[K]_o}$$

This relation, termed the Nernst equation, can be used to calculate the myocardial cell membrane potential if the potassium concentrations are known. For example, if the potassium concentration is normal—that is, 150 mEq/L intracellularly and 3.8 mEq/L extracellularly—then the membrane potential is

$$E_K = -60 \text{ mV} \times \log \frac{150}{3.8}$$

$$E_K = -90 \text{ mV}$$

If, however, the serum potassium concentration rises to 6.0 mEq/L, then the membrane potential also changes:

$$E_K = -60 \text{ mV} \times \log \frac{150}{6.0}$$

$$E_K = -80 \text{ mV}$$

Thus, the resting membrane potential is determined primarily by the concentration gradient for potassium across the cell membrane. The transmembrane potential can be calculated if the transmembrane potassium concentrations are measured with a glass microelectrode. Under clinical conditions, however, only the serum potassium level can be measured. This value does not provide an adequate guide to the transmembrane electrical voltage, because many physiologic factors are capable of altering the intracellular potassium concentration.[43] Such factors include electrolyte and acid-base balance, the level of osmotic and metabolic activity, and the serum levels of glucose and insulin.

Any factor that causes osmotic movement of water into the cell will produce a decrease in the intracellular potassium concentration. The transmembrane gradients of sodium and calcium are maintained by energy-requiring pumps in the cell membrane. When these pumps are inactivated, as during myocardial ischemia,[42] sodium and calcium can leak into the cell. If, as often occurs, sodium leaks into the cell faster than potassium leaks out, water will be drawn in, producing myocardial edema. Tissue acidosis can also alter the transmembrane potassium gradient. In acidosis, hydrogen ions can leak into the cell in exchange for potassium, thereby decreasing the intracellular potassium concentration and increasing the membrane potential. Variations in glucose transport can also affect the potassium gradient. Under the influence of insulin and epinephrine, glucose may move across the membrane into the myocardial cell, drawing in water by osmosis. The decline in intracellular potassium concentrations stimulates the sodium pump to exchange extracellular potassium for intracellular sodium. Concurrent administration of glucose and insulin is the standard method for treating hyperkalemia because it shifts potassium from the extracellular fluid into the cells.

ACTION POTENTIAL GENERATION

Stimulation of either cardiac muscle or skeletal muscle produces an action potential. Unlike a skeletal muscle action potential, which lasts only several milliseconds, a cardiac action potential may persist for as long as several hundred milliseconds.[110] The standard Purkinje, or ventricular muscle, action potential has five discernible phases [see Figure 16].

Phase 4

In phase 4, the resting membrane potential, or the diastolic potential, of the cell is generated by active metabolic processes that produce substantial transmembrane potassium and sodium gradients. An energy-dependent sodium-potassium pump counteracts a significant influx of sodium and efflux of potassium in the resting cell to maintain this resting membrane potential. As noted, when the extracellular potassium concentration rises from a typical value of 3.8 mEq/L to 6.0 mEq/L, the resting membrane potential increases from –90 mV to –80 mV. This effect would tend to increase automaticity, but it is superseded by the effect of hyperkalemia on the sodium current. A rise in the extracellular potassium level progressively impairs the flux of sodium through sodium-specific channels, leading to an overall decrease in myocardial excitability.

Phase 0

During phase 0, an electrical stimulus causes the sodium-specific fast channels and the calcium-specific slow channels to open, usually for no longer than one millisecond. As positive ions rush in, depolarization occurs as the membrane potential rises to threshold, or –60 mV, and an action potential is generated [see Figure 16]. Under normal physiologic conditions, the stimulus that produces an action potential is electrical, but any stimulus—electrical, physical (such as a precordial thump), or chemical—that depolarizes a membrane to threshold can generate an action potential. There are various abnormalities that can cause the resting membrane potential to move toward threshold. For example, conditions that produce a decrease in energy supply (or, alternatively, an increase in energy demand) will have this effect because energy is required to maintain the potassium and sodium gradients across the resting membrane. Under such conditions, automaticity is enhanced because lesser stimuli can achieve the threshold potential, and the cardiac muscle is said to be hyperexcitable, or irritable.

Phases 1 and 2

Phase 1 is characterized by repolarization to the plateau phase, or phase 2. During phase 2, the slow calcium channels as well as the fast sodium channels are activated, and the membrane potential remains relatively constant for as long as 100 milliseconds.[80] The long duration of this plateau phase is the most dramatic difference that is observed between an action potential in cardiac

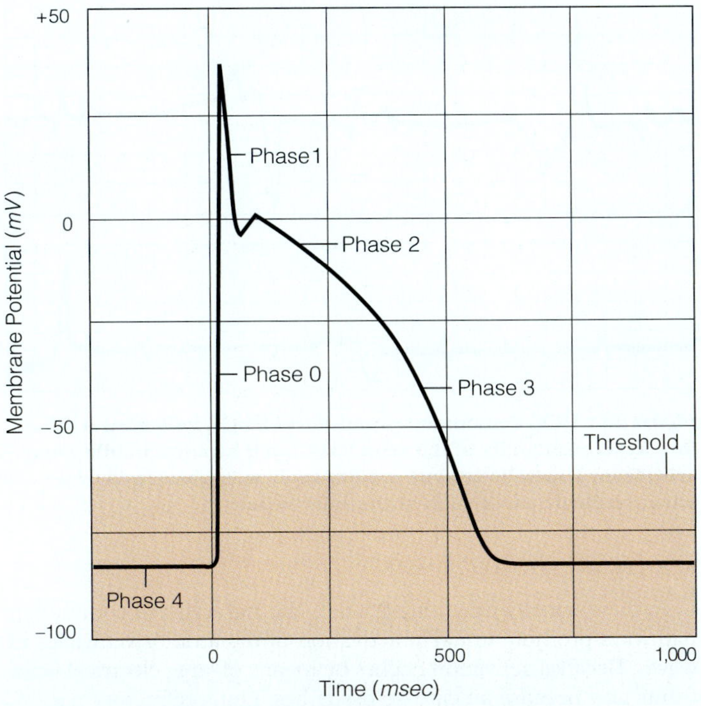

Figure 16 The standard Purkinje (or ventricular muscle) action potential has five distinct phases: phase 0, rapid depolarization; phase 1, early repolarization; phase 2, plateau; phase 3, rapid repolarization; and phase 4, diastole.

Pathophysiology of Cardiac Dysrhythmias

All dysrhythmias are caused by enhanced automaticity, reentry, or a combination of these two mechanisms.

AUTOMATIC DYSRHYTHMIAS

Any area of myocardial tissue that independently depolarizes, reaches threshold, and fires is termed automatic, and the electrical impulse that activates the adjacent myocardium generates an automatic rhythm. Acute dysrhythmias tend to be automatic; such automatic dysrhythmias are frequently seen in patients in emergency rooms and coronary care units and in patients undergoing operation. Five major clinical phenomena that tend to increase automaticity have been identified: local myocardial hypoxia, hypokalemia, hypercalcemia, increased catecholamine levels, and digitalis administration.

Local Myocardial Hypoxia

Energy-dependent cell membrane pumps maintain the resting membrane potential, and when oxygen supply to myocardial tissue is inadequate because of ischemia, the pumps fail to function properly. Consequently, the potassium gradient declines, and the membrane potential drifts closer toward threshold. Small membrane potential fluctuations or stimuli of less than normal magnitude are then sufficient to bump the membrane potential up to threshold and initiate an action potential. Ventricular muscle cells, not only those cells in specialized conduction tissue, can spontaneously generate electrical fluctuations, or oscillations, in membrane potential [*see* Slow Afterdepolarizations, *below*]. If the resting membrane potential is initially closer to normal because of local myocardial hypoxia, then these spontaneous oscillations are more likely to achieve threshold and fire an action potential.[112]

Hypokalemia

Extracellular hypokalemia increases the resting membrane potential, drawing it further away from threshold and producing hyperpolarization. This effect tends to decrease tissue excitability or automaticity.[112,113] Hypokalemia, however, also increases the size of the sodium channels, thereby promoting more rapid influx of sodium during phase 0. Because the net result of hypokalemia is increased automaticity, the effect of hypokalemia on sodium influx appears to override its effect on membrane hyperpolarization. Hypokalemia is one of the most easily treated (and overtreated) forms of hyperexcitability.

Hypercalcemia

Calcium is a potent inotropic agent, mediating the interaction between actin and myosin that produces muscle contraction.[80]

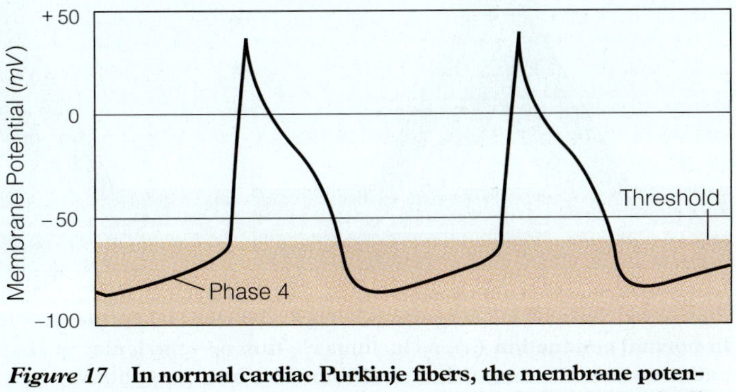

muscle and one in skeletal muscle. During this interval, termed the effective refractory period, the myocardium is relatively refractory to excitation.

Phase 3

During phase 3, potassium channels reopen to promote efflux of potassium from the cell. Rapid repolarization ensues, and the resting membrane potential is reestablished at –90 mV.

Spontaneous Phase 4 Depolarization

Unlike ordinary atrial and ventricular muscle, the Purkinje fibers do not have a stable phase 4 diastolic potential [*see Figure 17*]. Instead, these fibers undergo continuous depolarization during diastole as a result of deactivation of the potassium efflux current.[80,111] If the Purkinje fibers reach the threshold voltage, they will fire an action potential. Under normal conditions, however, the SA and AV nodes exhibit faster diastolic depolarization and reach threshold sooner than the Purkinje fibers. Because the cardiac impulse in the SA node normally reaches threshold first, the SA node typically assumes the pacemaker function of the heart. Premature ventricular contractions develop when a hyperexcitable cell or fiber in ventricular myocardium undergoes rapid diastolic depolarization and reaches threshold before the cells in the SA node. This cell or fiber then assumes the pacemaker function of the heart for that beat. The PVCs that result from such ventricular ectopy can be abolished by overdrive pacing. In this manner, a mechanical pacemaker is used to pace the heart at a rate faster than that of the PVC (i.e., the RR interval is shorter). The artificial device thereby assumes the pacemaker function and regularizes the heart rate, producing a beneficial cosmetic effect on the ECG without altering the hyperexcitability of the diseased cell.

Figure 17 In normal cardiac Purkinje fibers, the membrane potential does not remain flat during phase 4 but instead rises gradually. This spontaneous phase 4 depolarization is the result of a resting potassium current.

High extracellular calcium levels may cause myocardial work to exceed the energy supply and thus impair the function of the membrane pump. As a result, the resting membrane potential drifts up toward threshold, enhancing automaticity. Excess calcium also appears to promote spontaneous oscillations in membrane potential [see Slow Afterdepolarizations, below].[114] Because of calcium's inotropic effect, such oscillations are accompanied by muscle activity.

Elevated Catecholamine Levels

Increased catecholamine levels also appear to predispose to automaticity, as evidenced by a significant increase in the incidence of multiple premature ventricular contractions reported in patients who have been infused with high doses of catecholamines, such as epinephrine or dopamine. Catecholamines increase both heart rate and contractility. As with hypercalcemia, elevated catecholamine levels may increase cardiac work beyond the limits of energy supply and cause the membrane potential to move closer to threshold. This effect on the energy-dependent membrane pumps has been observed in isolated preparations of Purkinje muscle fibers. The addition of catecholamines to preparations of Purkinje muscle fibers has decreased the outward potassium current to the point that the resting membrane potential was shifted as much as 25 mV toward depolarization, enhancing automaticity.[80,111] In addition to affecting the operation of the membrane pumps, catecholamines can also produce large spontaneous oscillations in membrane voltage.[80,114] Catecholamines are elaborated endogenously; a patient who is in pain, for example, may be releasing large amounts of epinephrine into his or her own circulation. In such cases, morphine can be used effectively as an antidysrhythmic agent.[115]

Drugs

Digitalis is the prototypical cardiac stimulant. Typically, any agent other than oxygen that causes the heart to pump harder and faster also increases cardiac excitability. Digitalis toxicity can produce diffuse myocardial hyperexcitability, manifested by automatic ventricular ectopy. In this condition, the cardiac impulse originates from multiple sites in the ventricle. In patients with ventricular ectopy caused by digitalis intoxication, the QRS complex has an altered morphology, and multifocal PVCs are apparent on the ECG—the classic multifocal ectopy of digitalis toxicity [see Figure 18].[116-118]

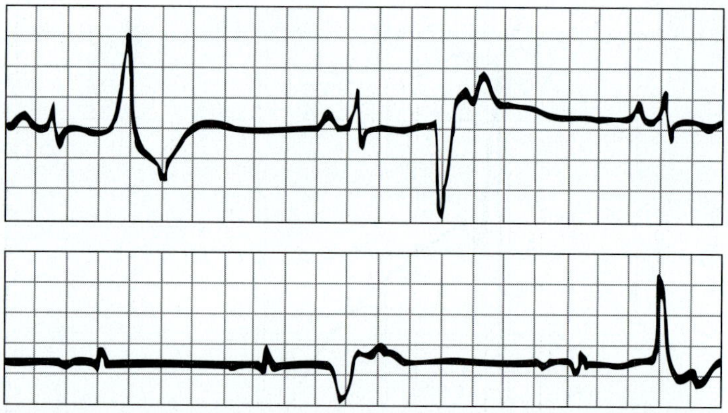

Figure 18 ECG demonstrates multifocal PVCs, indicating a diffuse hyperexcitability of the ventricles. Such hyperexcitability may arise from a metabolic abnormality such as hypokalemia or a pharmacologic cause such as digitalis toxicity.

REENTRANT DYSRHYTHMIAS

In the normally functioning heart, the rich cell-cell conduction pathways promote uniform activation of the atria or ventricles in waves. Because activation occurs by means of large electrical wave fronts and because all cardiac tissue has a long refractory period, it is highly unlikely that any cells remain excitable at the completion of each beat. However, disorders such as myocardial ischemia, fibrosis, and necrosis slow electrical conduction and also produce nonconductive areas that interrupt the normal electrical wavefront.[119] These conditions set up one of the requirements for reentry: areas of differential myocardial repolarization.[120]

A circuit whose length exceeds the length of the reentrant impulse circuit is required for the initiation of reentry of continuous conduction; such a circuit may develop because of anatomic or physiologic heterogeneity in myocardial tissue.[119,120] Slow conduction, a shortened refractory period, and anatomic heterogeneity all favor reentry [see Figure 19]. The circuit wavelength of an impulse is the product of the conduction velocity and the duration of the longest refractory period in the circuit.[121] For example, for normal myocardium, the conduction velocity is 200 cm/sec and the refractory period is 0.4 second; therefore, the circuit length for a normally conducted myocardial impulse would have to be 80 cm. Because the reentrant circuit would have to be extraordinarily tortuous to encompass 80 cm, it

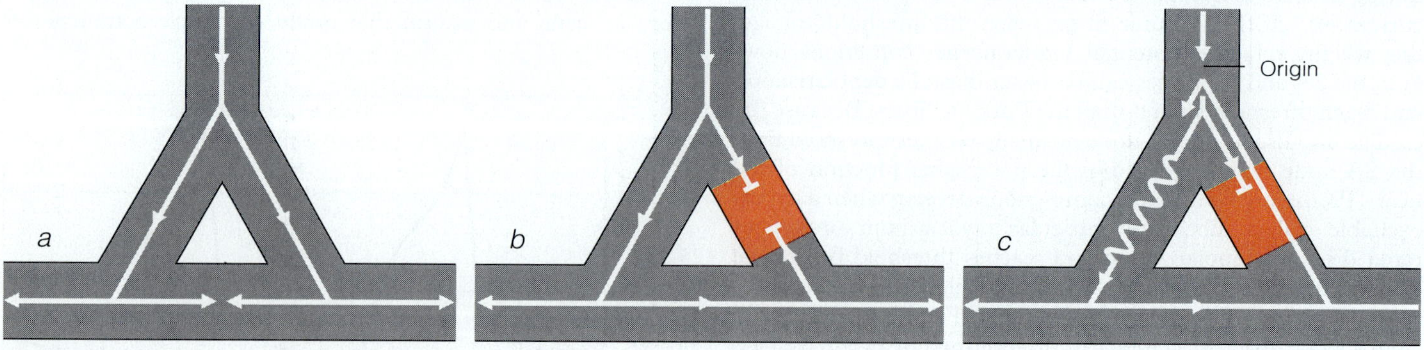

Figure 19 Schematic diagram portrays a conceptual framework for understanding the generation of reentrant dysrhythmias. In normal conduction (*a*), as in sinus rhythm or ventricular pacing, an impulse is propagated along two different anatomic pathways and is extinguished at the bottom. In *b*, one pathway has a region of slow conduction (red area), which results in a rate-dependent block. In *c*, the impulse is also blocked in the right limb (red area), but it travels over the alternative pathway sufficiently slowly (zigzag line) for the origin to be able to repolarize before the initial impulse returns; the conducted impulse then depolarizes the origin and reenters the circuit.

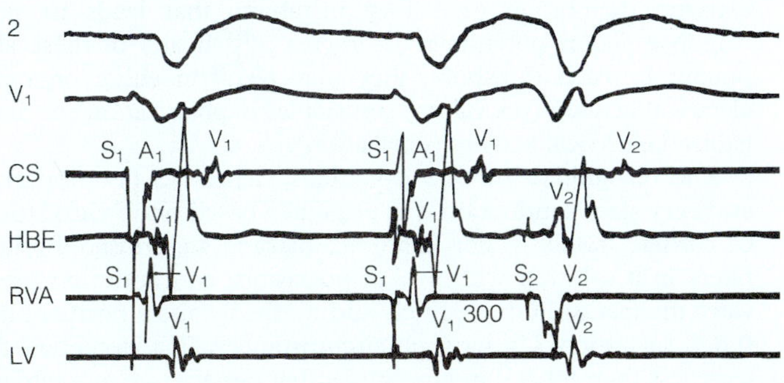

Figure 20 In electrophysiologic testing, the electrical complexes are spread out to facilitate the recognition of ventricular electrical morphology. In panel *a,* critically timed paced stimuli capture one ventricle, but when pacing is stopped, the rhythm reverts to sinus rhythm. In panel *b,* critically timed paced stimuli achieve rate-dependent block in one arm of a reentrant circuit. When the activation wave front returns to the origin, this tissue is no longer refractory and undergoes depolarization. With reexcitation, the conditions for reentry are met, and the impulse continues after pacing stops.

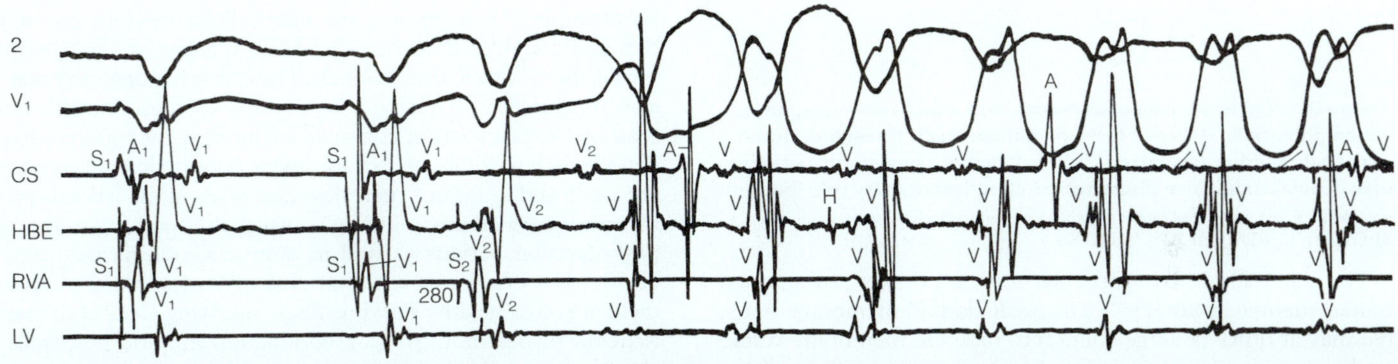

would appear that concomitant slow conduction is essentially mandatory to shorten the circuit wavelength and permit initiation of a reentrant dysrhythmia. Regions such as the AV and SA nodes normally exhibit slow conduction, and therefore, any disturbance that produces minor additional slowing in these areas predisposes to reentry. It has also been suggested that extreme anatomic heterogeneity might permit microreentry.[120] For example, a tortuous path over stunned, slowly conducting ventricular muscle in an individual with heterogeneous myocardial infarction might achieve the prerequisites for reentry.

In vitro studies have investigated physiologic factors that might produce changes in conduction and excitability that predispose to reentrant dysrhythmias. For example, abnormal conduction has been observed in a Purkinje network subjected to local changes in potassium concentration.[110,115] The decrease in conduction velocity can vary in different areas of the Purkinje network, leading to functional conduction block.[112,113] In T- or X-shaped Purkinje preparations, the impulses were observed either to summate electrically or, conversely, to inhibit each other when they arrived at the same junction simultaneously. It is difficult to study the cardiac microenvironment in living animals or humans, but in these studies,[122] the Purkinje network was subjected to potassium fluctuations that certainly occur during induced cardioplegia and that may well exist in cases of myocardial ischemia that lead to the formation of necrotic areas adjacent to healthy cells.

Electrophysiologic testing with programmed stimulation in a patient with a history of cardiac dysrhythmias can reveal whether latent substrates of reentry are present. Because organized ventricular reentry does not occur in normal myocardium, all reentrant dysrhythmias, whether they are induced or spontaneous, are pathologic. Rapidly paced stimuli may provoke a decrease in action potential duration and shorten refractoriness in myocardium in which the conduction velocity has already been reduced. Critically timed premature paced stimuli may then penetrate selective zones of myocardium, leading to a reentrant dysrhythmia [see Figure 20].[123] A ventricular tachydysrhythmia that can be induced by programmed stimulation carries an ominous prognosis unless it can be abolished by pharmacotherapy or operation.[123]

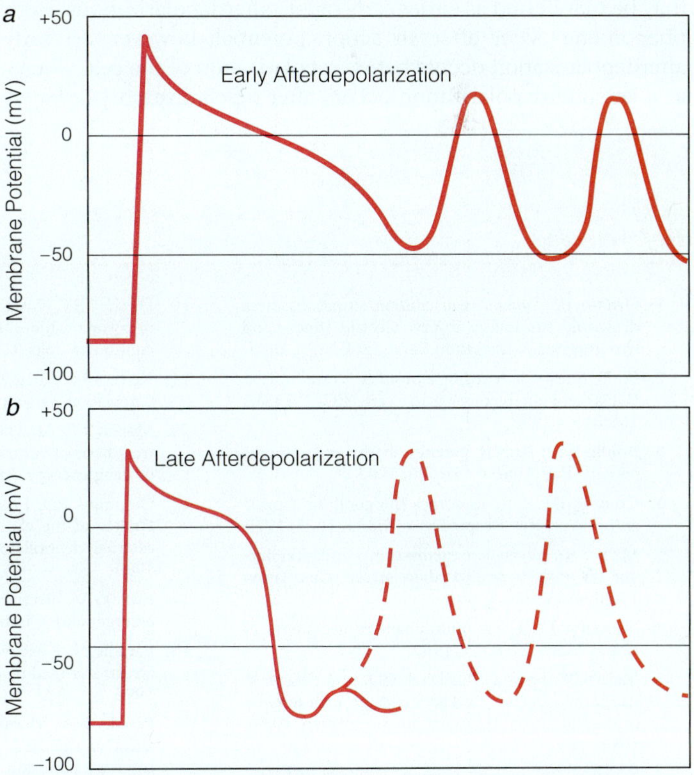

Figure 21 Membrane oscillatory instability may be manifested by either (*a*) early afterdepolarizations or (*b*) late afterdepolarizations. If the late afterdepolarizations achieve the threshold voltage, they can fire an action potential (dotted lines).

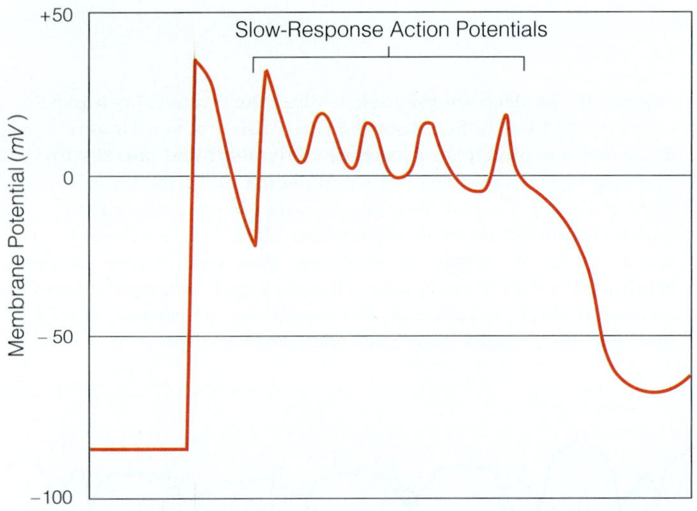

Figure 22 Early afterdepolarizations may lead to slow-response action potentials. If any of these potentials reach threshold, they may lead to either organized electrical activity (premature ventricular depolarization) or disorganized electrical activity (fibrillation).

SLOW AFTERDEPOLARIZATIONS

Damaged atrial and ventricular muscle exhibits resting membrane potential instability.[124] The oscillations in membrane potential may at times be large enough to raise the membrane voltage to threshold level and fire. The phenomenon of oscillatory instability, which was first recognized in the 1940s,[125] is now thought to play an important role in the genesis of cardiac dysrhythmias. Injury,[124] elevated calcium levels,[110] digitalis,[116,117] and catecholamines all promote membrane oscillatory instability, which may be manifested as either early or late afterdepolarizations. Both phenomena occur after an action potential; however, an early afterdepolarization occurs before repolarization of the cell, whereas a late afterdepolarization occurs after repolarization [see Figure 21]. Both early and late afterdepolarizations may be followed by extreme membrane oscillatory instability that leads to slow-response action potentials [see Figure 22]. If any of these slow potentials reach threshold, they may result in either organized electrical activity (premature ventricular depolarization) or disorganized electrical activity (fibrillation).

The recognition of slow potentials, depressed fast responses, and very slow conduction was originally based on in vitro studies of cardiac tissue.[126] For example, bathing superfused Purkinje fibers in a solution with a high potassium concentration inactivates the fast sodium channels and markedly alters normal phase 0 depolarization. Under such circumstances, slow potentials that were less than 80 mV in amplitude, that depolarized at a rate of 1 to 2 V/sec, and that lasted for up to 1 second were observed.[115,126] The amplitude and the overshoot of these slow potentials could be magnified by increasing the extracellular calcium concentration and could be abolished by adding manganese, an agent that blocks the slow calcium channels. These results suggested that the slow potentials were mediated by the slow calcium channels rather than by the fast sodium channels responsible for routine phase 0 depolarization. Although extraordinary nonphysiologic conditions are employed to induce such slow potentials in the laboratory, the myocardial microenvironment during the peri-infarction and postinfarction periods as well as after cardioplegia may well be bizarre. For example, even after extensive myocardial infarction, there are often healthy Purkinje fibers overlying areas of damaged, ischemic myocardium.[127] Slow conduction and slow potentials are characteristic of stunned myocardium.[128,129]

Slow potentials have been incriminated in the generation of reentrant dysrhythmias for three reasons: (1) because they are caused by an active calcium influx that produces 40 to 80 mV depolarizations, they may be conducted long distances; (2) because the conduction velocity may be 1,000 times slower than normal, the circuit wavelength is reduced accordingly; and (3) because slow potentials leave a long refractory wake, they set up zones of functional conduction block.[128,129]

References

1. Ornato JP: Special resuscitation situations: near drowning, traumatic injury, electric shock, and hypothermia. Circulation 74(suppl IV):23, 1986
2. Guidelines for cardiopulmonary resuscitation (CPR) and emergency cardiac care (ECC). JAMA 268:2171, 1992
3. Boidin MP: Airway patency in the unconscious patient. Br J Anaesth 57:306, 1985
4. Comroe JH: ". . . In comes the good air" (pts 1 and 2). Am Rev Respir Dis 119:803, 1025, 1979
5. Melker RJ: Alternative methods of ventilation during respiratory and cardiac arrest. Circulation 74(suppl IV):63, 1986
6. Niemann JT: Cardiopulmonary resuscitation. N Engl J Med 327:1075, 1992
7. Maier GW, Tyson GS Jr, Olsen CO, et al: The physiology of external cardiac massage: high-impulse cardiopulmonary resuscitation. Circulation 70:86, 1984
8. Bedell SE, Fulton EJ: Unexpected findings and complications at autopsy after cardiopulmonary resuscitation (CPR). Arch Intern Med 146:1725, 1986
9. Powner DJ, Holcombe PA, Mello LA: Cardiopulmonary resuscitation–related injuries. Crit Care Med 12:54, 1984
10. Ditchey RV, Winkler JV, Rhodes CA: Relative lack of coronary blood flow during closed-chest resuscitation in dogs. Circulation 66:297, 1982
11. Kerber RE: Energy requirements for defibrillation. Circulation 74(suppl IV):117, 1986
12. Martin TG, Hawkins NS, Weigel JA, et al: Initial treatment of ventricular fibrillation: defibrillation or drug therapy. Am J Emerg Med 6:113, 1988
13. Cummins RO: From concept to standard-of-care? Review of the clinical experience with automated external defibrillators. Ann Emerg Med 18:1269, 1989
14. Ewy GA: Electrical therapy for cardiovascular emergencies. Circulation 74(suppl IV):111, 1986
15. Paradis N, Koscove EM: Epinephrine in cardiac arrest: a critical review. Ann Emerg Med 19:1288, 1990
16. Paradis NA, Martin GB, Rosenberg J, et al: The effect of standard- and high-dose epinephrine on coronary perfusion pressure during prolonged cardiopulmonary resuscitation. JAMA 265:1139, 1991
17. Jaffe AS: The use of antiarrhythmics in advanced cardiac life support. Ann Emerg Med 22:307, 1991
18. Wesely RC, Resh W, Zimmerman D: Reconsiderations of the routine and preferential use of lidocaine in the emergent treatment of ventricular arrhythmias. Crit Care Med 19:1439, 1991
19. Weaver WD, Fahrenbruch CE, Johnson DD, et al: Effect of epinephrine and lidocaine therapy on outcome after cardiac arrest due to ventricular fibrillation. Circulation 82:2027, 1990
20. Williams ML, Woelfel A, Cascio WE, et al: Intravenous amiodarone during prolonged resuscitation from cardiac arrest. Ann Intern Med 110:839, 1989
21. Cummins RO, Austin D Jr: The frequency of 'occult' ventricular fibrillation masquerading as a flat line in prehospital cardiac arrest. Ann Emerg Med 17:813, 1988
22. Koehler RC, Michael JR, Guerci AD, et al: Beneficial effect of epinephrine infusion on cerebral and myocardial blood flows during CPR. Ann Emerg Med 14:744, 1985
23. Paradis NA, Martin GB, Rivers EP, et al: Coronary perfusion pressure and the return of spontaneous circulation in human cardiopulmonary resuscitation. JAMA 263:1106, 1990
24. Bertolet BD, McMurtrie EB, Hill JA, et al: Theophylline for the treatment of atrioventricular block after myocardial infarction. Ann Intern Med 123:509, 1995

25. Ewy GA: Ventricular fibrillation masquerading as asystole. Ann Emerg Med 13:811, 1984
26. Cummins RO, Graves JR, Larsen MP, et al: Out-of-hospital transcutaneous pacing by emergency medical technicians in patients with asystolic cardiac arrest. N Engl J Med 328:1377, 1993
27. Bocka JJ, Overton DT, Hauser A: Electromechanical dissociation in human beings: an echocardiographic evaluation. Ann Emerg Med 17:450, 1988
28. Paradis NA, Martin GB, Goetting MG, et al: Aortic pressure during human cardiac arrest: identification of pseudo-electromechanical dissociation. Chest 101:123, 1992
29. Brown CG, Werman HA: Adrenergic agonists during cardiopulmonary resuscitation. Resuscitation 19:1, 1990
30. Keenan RL, Boyan CP: Cardiac arrest due to anesthesia: a study of incidence and causes. JAMA 253:2373, 1985
31. Bedell SE, Deitz DC, Leeman D, et al: Incidence and characteristics of preventable iatrogenic cardiac arrests. JAMA 265:2815, 1991
32. Franklin C, Mathew J: Developing strategies to prevent inhospital cardiac arrest: analyzing responses of physicians and nurses in the hours before the event. Crit Care Med 22:244, 1994
33. Cannom DS, Prystowsky EN: Management of ventricular arrhythmias: detection, drugs and devices. JAMA 281:172, 1999
34. Reiffel JA: Selecting an antiarrhythmic agent for atrial fibrillation should be a patient-specific, data-driven decision. Am J Cardiol 82:72N, 1998
35. Harken AH, Honigman B, VanWay CW III: Cardiac dysrhythmias in the acute setting: recognition and treatment or anyone can treat cardiac dysrhythmias. J Emerg Med 5:129, 1987
36. Raichlen JS, Campbell FW, Edie RN, et al: Effect of the site of placement of temporary epicardial pacemakers on ventricular function in patients undergoing cardiac surgery. Circulation 70:I, 1984
37. Sarubbi B, Ducceschi V, D'Andrea A, et al: Atrial fibrillation: what are the effects of drug therapy on the effectiveness and complications of electrical cardioversion? Can J Cardiol 14:1267, 1998
38. Bigger JT Jr: Epidemiological and mechanistic studies of atrial fibrillation as a basis for treatment strategies. Circulation 98:943, 1998
39. Botto GL, Bonini W, Broffoni T: Modulation of ventricular rate in permanent atrial fibrillation: randomized, crossover study of the effects of slow-release formulations of gallopamil, diltiazem, or verapamil. Clin Cardiol 11:837, 1998
40. Glatter KA, Cheng J, Dorostkar P, et al: Electrophysiologic effects of adenosine in patients with supraventricular tachycardia. Circulation 99:1034, 1999
41. Tracy WR, Magee W, Masamune H, et al: Selective activation of adenosine A3 receptors with N6-(C3-chlorobenzyl)-5′-N-methylcarboxamideoadenosine (CB-MECA) provides cardioprotection via KATP channel activation. Cardiovasc Res 40:138, 1998
42. Zumino AP, Baiardi G, Schanne OF, et al: Differential electrophysiologic effects of global and regional ischemia and reperfusion in perfused rat hearts. Effects of Mg^{2+} concentration. Mol Cell Biochem 186:79, 1998
43. Siddiqui MN, Zafar H, Alvi R, et al: Hypomagnesaemia in postoperative patients: an important contributing factor in postoperative mortality. Int J Clin Pract 52:265, 1998
44. Hobbs WJ, Fitchet A, Cotter L: Atrial arrhythmias after cardiac surgery. N Engl J Med 337:860, 1997
45. Gonzalez ER, Kannewurf BS, Ornato JP: Intravenous amiodarone for ventricular arrhythmias: overview and clinical use. Resuscitation 39:33, 1998
46. Drouin E, Lande G, Charpentier F: Amiodarone reduces transmural heterogeneity of repolarization in the human heart. J Am Coll Cardiol 32:1063, 1998
47. Kowey PR, Marinchak RA, Rials SJ, et al: Intravenous amiodarone. J Am Coll Cardiol 29:1190, 1997
48. Vorperian VR, Havighurst TC, Miller S, et al: Adverse effects of low-dose amiodarone: a meta-analysis. J Am Coll Cardiol 30:791, 1997
49. Joglar JA, Page RL: Treatment of cardiac arrhythmias during pregnancy: safety considerations. Drug Saf 20:85, 1999
50. Cardosi RJ, Chez RA: Magnesium sulfate, maternal hypothermia, and fetal bradycardia with loss of heart rate variability. Obstet Gynecol 92:691, 1998
51. Hamersley SL, Landy HJ, O'Sullivan MJ: Fetal bradycardia secondary to magnesium sulfate therapy for preterm labor. A case report. J Reprod Med 43:206, 1998
52. Hohnloser SH: Proarrhythmia with class III antiarrhythmic drugs: types, risks, and management. Am J Cardiol 80:82G, 1997
53. Sager PT: New advances in class III antiarrhythmic drug therapy. Curr Opin Cardiol 14:15, 1999
54. Negovsky VA: Reanimatology today: some scientific and philosophic considerations. Crit Care Med 10:130, 1982
55. Cummins RO, Eisenberg MS: Prehospital cardiopulmonary resuscitation: is it effective? JAMA 253:2408, 1985
56. Eisenberg MS, Bergner L, Hallstrom A: Survivors of out-of-hospital cardiac arrest: morbidity and long-term survival. Am J Emerg Med 2:189, 1984
57. Taffet GE, Teasdale TA, Luchi RJ: In-hospital cardiopulmonary resuscitation. JAMA 260:2069, 1988
58. Lowenstein SR, Sabyan EM, Lassen CF, et al: Benefits of training physicians in advanced cardiac life support. Chest 89:512, 1986
59. Skovron ML, Goldberg E, Suljaga-Petchel K: Factors predicting survival for six months after cardiopulmonary resuscitation: multivariate analysis of a prospective study. Mt Sinai J Med 52:271, 1985
60. Office of Technology Assessment: Life-sustaining technologies in the elderly. OTA-BA-306. US Congress, 1987, p 167
61. Murphy DJ, Murray AM, Robinson BE, et al: Outcomes of cardiopulmonary resuscitation in the elderly. Ann Intern Med 111:199, 1989
62. Schiedermayer DL: The decision to forgo CPR in the elderly patient. JAMA 260:2096, 1988
63. Kouwenhoven WB, Jude JR, Knickerbocker GG: Closed-chest cardiac massage. JAMA 173:1064, 1960
64. Chandra NC: Mechanisms of blood flow during CPR. Ann Emerg Med 22:281, 1993
65. Steen-Hansen JE, Hansen NN, Vaagenes P, et al: Pupil size and light reactivity during cardiopulmonary resuscitation: a clinical study. Crit Care Med 16:69, 1988
66. Grundler W, Weil MH, Rackow EC: Effects of volume expansion on reversal of electromechanical dissociation. Chest 86:282, 1984
67. Cohen TJ, Tucker KJ, Lurie KG, et al: Active compression-decompression: a new method of cardiopulmonary resuscitation. Cardiopulmonary Resuscitation Working Group. JAMA 267:2916, 1992
68. Cohen TJ, Goldner BG, Maccaro PC, et al: A comparison of active compression-decompression cardiopulmonary resuscitation with standard cardiopulmonary resuscitation for cardiac arrests occurring in the hospital. N Engl J Med 329:1918, 1993
69. Schwab TM, Callaham ML, Madsen CD, et al: A randomized clinical trial of active compression-decompression CPR vs standard CPR in out-of-hospital cardiac arrest in two cities. JAMA 273:1261, 1995
70. Kerber RE: Electrical treatment of cardiac arrhythmias: defibrillation and cardioversion. Ann Emerg Med 22:296, 1993
71. Greenberg MI: Drug selection and delivery in cardiopulmonary resuscitation. Am J Emerg Med 2:457, 1984
72. Crile G, Dolley DH: Experimental resuscitation of dogs killed by anesthetics and asphyxia. J Exp Med 6:713, 1906
73. Redding JS, Pearson JW: Evaluation of drugs for cardiac resuscitation. Anesthesiology 24:203, 1963
74. Brown CG, Werman HA, Davis EA, et al: The effect of high-dose phenylephrine versus epinephrine on regional cerebral blood flow during CPR. Ann Emerg Med 16:743, 1987
75. Callaham M, Madsen CD, Barton CW, et al: A randomized clinical trial of high-dose epinephrine and norepinephrine vs standard-dose epinephrine in prehospital cardiac arrest. JAMA 268:2667, 1992
76. Brown CG, Martin DR, Pepe PE, et al: A comparison of standard-dose and high-dose epinephrine in cardiac arrest outside the hospital. Multicenter High-Dose Epinephrine Study Group. N Engl J Med 327:1051, 1992
77. Stiell IG, Hebert PC, Weitzman BN, et al: High-dose epinephrine in adult cardiac arrest. N Engl J Med 327:1045, 1992
78. Hughes WG, Ruedy JR: Should calcium be used in cardiac arrest? Am J Med 81:285, 1986
79. Thompson BM, Steuven HS, Tonsfeldt DJ, et al: Calcium: limited indications, some danger. Circulation 74(suppl IV):90, 1986
80. Meldrum DR, Cleveland JC Jr, Rowland RT, et al: Cardiac surgical implications of calcium dyshomeostasis in the heart. Ann Thorac Surg 61:1273, 1996
81. Urban P, Scheidegger D, Buchmann B, et al: Cardiac arrest and blood ionized calcium levels. Ann Intern Med 109:110, 1988
82. Katz AM: Is calcium beneficial or deleterious in patients with cardiac arrest? Ann Intern Med 109:91, 1988
83. White BC, Winegar CD, Wilson RF, et al: Possible role of calcium blockers in cerebral resuscitation: a review of the literature and synthesis for future studies. Crit Care Med 11:202, 1983
84. Narins RG, Cohen JJ: Bicarbonate therapy for organic acidosis: the case for its continued use. Ann Intern Med 106:615, 1987
85. Weil MH, Rackow EC, Trevino R, et al: Difference in acid-base state between venous and arterial blood during cardiopulmonary resuscitation. N Engl J Med 315:153, 1986
86. Bishop RL, Weisfeldt ML: Sodium bicarbonate administration during cardiac arrest: effect on arterial pH, Pco_2 and osmolality. JAMA 235:506, 1976
87. Weisfeldt ML, Guerci AD: Sodium bicarbonate in CPR. JAMA 266:2129, 1991
88. Planta M, Bar-Joseph G, Wiklund L, et al: Pathophysiologic and therapeutic implications of acid-base changes during CPR. Ann Emerg Med 22:404, 1993
89. Relman AS: "Blood gases": arterial or venous? (editorial). N Engl J Med 315:188, 1986
90. Adrogue HJ, Rashad MN, Gorin AB, et al: Assessing acid-base status in circulatory failure: differences between arterial and central venous blood. N Engl J Med 320:1312, 1989
91. Gudipati CV, Weil MH, Bisera J, et al: Expired carbon dioxide: a noninvasive monitor of cardiopulmonary resuscitation. Circulation 77:234, 1988
92. Falk JL, Rackow EC, Weil MH: End-tidal carbon dioxide concentration during cardiopulmonary resuscitation. N Engl J Med 318:607, 1988

93. Kern KB, Garewal HS, Sanders AB, et al: Depletion of myocardial adenosine triphosphate during prolonged untreated ventricular fibrillation: effect on defibrillation success. Resuscitation 20:221, 1990
94. Neumar RW, Brown CG, Van Ligten P, et al: Estimation of myocardial ischemic injury during ventricular fibrillation with total circulatory arrest using high-energy phosphates and lactate as metabolic markers. Ann Emerg Med 20:222, 1991
95. Weaver WD, Cobb LA, Dennis D, et al: Amplitude of ventricular fibrillation waveform and outcome after cardiac arrest. Ann Intern Med 102:53, 1985
96. Brown CG, Griffith RF, Van Ligten P, et al: Median frequency—a new parameter for predicting defibrillation success rate. Ann Emerg Med 20:787, 1991
97. Brown CG, Dzwonczyk R, Martin DR: Physiologic measurement of the ventricular fibrillation ECG signal: estimating the duration of ventricular fibrillation. Ann Emerg Med 22:70, 1993
98. Talit U, Braun S, Halkin H, et al: Pharmacokinetic differences between peripheral and central drug administration during cardiopulmonary resuscitation. J Am Coll Cardiol 6:1073, 1985
99. Emerman CL, Bellon EM, Lukens TW, et al: A prospective study of femoral versus subclavian vein catheterization during cardiac arrest. Ann Emerg Med 19:26, 1990
100. Greenberg MI, Roberts JR, Baskin SI, et al: The use of endotracheal medication in cardiac emergencies. Emergency Medicine Annual 2:91, 1983
101. Hasegawa EA: The endotracheal use of emergency drugs. Heart Lung 15:60, 1986
102. Gonzalez ER: Pharmacologic controversies in CPR. Ann Emerg Med 22:317, 1993
103. Rosetti VA, Thompson BM, Miller J, et al: Intraosseous infusion: an alternative route of pediatric intravascular access. Ann Emerg Med 14:885, 1985
104. Iserson KV, Criss E: Intraosseous infusions: a usable technique. Am J Emerg Med 4:540, 1986
105. The Sicilian gambit: a new approach to the classification of antiarrhythmic drugs based on their actions on arrhythmogenic mechanisms. Task Force of the Working Group on Arrhythmias of the European Society of Cardiology. Circulation 84:1831, 1991
106. Brodsky MA, Orlov MV, Allen BJ, et al: Clinical assessment of adrenergic tone and responsiveness to beta-blocker therapy in patients with symptomatic ventricular tachycardia and no apparent structural heart disease. Am Heart J 131:51, 1996
107. Kowey PR, Marinchak RA, Rials SJ, et al: Pharmacologic and pharmacokinetic profile of class III antiarrhythmic drugs. Am J Cardiol 80:16G, 1997
108. Stafford RS, Robson DC, Misra B, et al: Rate controls and sinus rhythm maintenance in atrial fibrillation: national trends in medication use, 1980-1996. Arch Intern Med 158:2144, 1998
109. Van Gelder IC, Brugemann J, Crijns HJ: Current treatment recommendations in antiarrhythmic therapy. Drugs 55:331, 1998
110. Uchida T, Yashima M, Gotoh M, et al: Mechanism of acceleration of functional reentry in the ventricle: effects of ATP-sensitive potassium channel opener. Circulation 99:704, 1999
111. Cleveland JC Jr, Meldrum DR, Rowland RT, et al: Optimal myocardial preservation: cooling, cardioplegia, and conditioning. Ann Thorac Surg 61:760, 1996
112. Janse MJ: Why does atrial fibrillation occur? Eur Heart J 18(suppl C):C12, 1997
113. Yue L, Feng J, Gaspo R, et al: Ionic remodeling underlying action potential changes in a canine model of atrial fibrillation. Circ Res 81:512, 1997
114. Priebe L, Beuckelmann DJ: Simulation study of cellular electric properties in heart failure. Circ Res 82:1206, 1998
115. Levi AJ, Dalton GR, Hancox JC, et al: Role of intracellular sodium overload in the genesis of cardiac arrhythmias. J Cardiovasc Electrophysiol 8:700, 1997
116. Riaz K, Forker AD: Digoxin use in congestive heart failure. Current status. Drugs 55:747, 1998
117. Reddy S, Benatar D, Gheorghiade M: Update on digoxin and other oral positive inotropic agents for chronic heart failure. Curr Opin Cardiol 12:233, 1997
118. Umans VA, Cornel JH, Hic C: Digoxin in patients with heart failure. N Engl J Med 337:129, 1997
119. Patterson E, Kalcich M, Scherlag BJ: Phase 1B ventricular arrhythmia in the dog: localized reentry with the mid-myocardium. J Interv Card Electrophysiol 2:145, 1998
120. Boineau JP, Cox JL: Slow ventricular activation in acute myocardial infarction: source of reentrant premature ventricular contractions. Circulation 48:702, 1973
121. Swynghedaauw B: Molecular mechanisms of myocardial remodeling. Physiol Rev 79:215, 1999
122. Koning MMG, Gho BCG, Klaarwater EV, et al: Rapid ventricular pacing produces myocardial protection by nonischemic activation of K$^+$-ATP channels. Circulation 93:178, 1996
123. Kastor JA, Horowitz LN, Harken AH, et al: Clinical electrophysiology of ventricular tachycardia. N Engl J Med 304:1004, 1981
124. Yamabe H, Okumura K, Misumi I, et al: Role of bipolar electrogram polarity mapping in localizing recurrent conduction in the isthmus early and late after ablation of atrial flutter. J Am Coll Cardiol 33:39, 1999
125. Bozler E: The initiation of the cardiac impulse. Am J Physiol 138:273, 1943
126. Carmeliet EE, Vereecke J: Adrenaline and the plateau phase of the cardiac action potential. Pflugers Arch 313:303, 1969
127. Friedman P, Stewarts J, Fenoglio J: Survival of subendocardial Purkinje fibers after extensive myocardial infarction in dogs. Circ Res 33:597, 1973
128. Masui A, Tamura K, Tarumi N, et al: Resolution of late potentials with improvement of left ventricular systolic pressure in patients with first myocardial infarction. Clin Cardiol 20:466, 1997
129. Ferrari R, Pepi P, Ferrari F, et al: Metabolic derangement in ischemic heart disease and its therapeutic control. Am J Cardiol 82:2K, 1998
130. Pires LA, Lehmann MH, Steinman RT, et al: Sudden death in implantable cardioverter-defibrillator recipients: clinical context, arrhythmic events and device responses. J Am Coll Cardiol 33:24, 1999
131. Yee R, Connolly SJ, Gillis AM: Appropriate use of the implantable cardioverter defibrillator: a Canadian perspective. Canadian Working Group on Cardiac Pacing. Pacing Clin Electrophysiol 22:1, 1999
132. Swygman CA, Homoud MK, Link MS, et al: Technologic advances in implantable cardioverter defibrillators. Curr Opin Cardiol 14:9, 1999
133. Grimm W, Menz V, Hoffmann J, et al: Complications of third generation implantable cardioverter defibrillator therapy. Pacing Clin Electrophysiol 22:201, 1999
134. Pauli P, Wiedemann G, Dengler W, et al: Anxiety in patients with an automatic implantable cardioverter defibrillator: what differentiates them from panic patients? Psychosom Med 61:69, 1999
135. Anvari A, Gottsauner-Wolf M, Turel Z, et al: Predictors of outcome in patients with implantable cardioverter defibrillators. Cardiology 90:180, 1998
136. Movsowitz C, Marchlinski FE: Interactions between implantable cardioverter-defibrillators and class III agents. Am J Cardiol 82:41I, 1998
137. Dorian P, Newman D, Greene M: Implantable defibrillators and/or amiodarone: alternatives or complementary therapies. Int J Clin Pract 52:425, 1998

Acknowledgment

Figures 1 through 10   Carol Donner.

2 TRAUMA RESUSCITATION

Frederick A. Moore, M.D., and Ernest E. Moore, M.D.

Initial Approach to the Critically Injured Patient

Salvage of the critically injured is optimized by a coordinated team effort in an organized trauma system. Management of life-threatening injuries must be decided according to physiologic necessity for survival; that is, active efforts to support airway, breathing, and circulation (the ABCs) are usually initiated before specific diagnosis. This chapter presents a systematic approach to severely injured patients within the so-called golden hour. The discussion is divided into prehospital care and emergency department management; the ED component is further divided into (1) primary survey and initial resuscitation, (2) evaluation, with continuation of resuscitation, and (3) secondary survey and definitive diagnosis.

Prehospital Care

Resuscitation and evaluation of trauma patients begin at the injury site. Prehospital care and hospital destination are much different from those of the medical arrest victim. Whereas provision of advanced cardiac life support (ACLS) at the scene clearly improves survival for the medical patient,[1] the goal in trauma is to get the *right patient to the right hospital at the right time*. First responders (typically, firefighters and police) provide rapid basic trauma life support (BTLS) and are followed by paramedics and flight nurses with advanced skills. Medical control is ensured by preestablished field protocols, radio communication with a base hospital physician, and subsequent trip audits. Management priorities of BTLS on the scene are to (1) assess and control the scene for the safety of the patient and the prehospital care provider, (2) tamponade external hemorrhage with direct pressure, (3) protect the spine after blunt trauma, (4) supplement inspired oxygen, (5) extricate the patient, and (6) stabilize long bone fractures. Active airway support is a major asset of advanced trauma life support (ATLS) in prehospital systems, achieved with skilled paramedics under close medical control.[2] However, the value of intravenous fluid administration in such systems remains controversial.[3-5] The heart of the controversy is whether it is preferable (1) to give fluids until a normal blood pressure is reached, thus causing hemodilution and disruption of early hemostatic clots, or (2) to withhold resuscitation, thus prolonging cellular shock, which may become irreversible by the time operative control is accomplished. The compromise between these two approaches is moderate volume loading.[5-8]

Application of the pneumatic antishock garment (PASG) is warranted for active hemorrhage caused by major pelvic fractures and may be appropriate for profound shock if transport time is expected to exceed 30 minutes.[6,9,10] In any situation, implementation of ATLS depends on the expertise of field personnel, the patient's condition, and the distance to the hospital.[11-13]

Prehospital trauma scores have been devised to identify critically injured trauma victims, who represent about 10% to 15% of all injured patients. When it is geographically and logistically feasible, critically injured patients should be taken directly to a designated level I facility (i.e., an Urban Regional Trauma Center) or to a level II facility (i.e., a Rural Regional Trauma Center). The currently available field trauma scores, however, are imperfect for identifying critically injured patients.[14] A 25% over-triage is probably necessary to capture most of the patients with life-threatening injury. Advance transmission of key patient information to the receiving trauma center facilitates organization of the trauma team and ensures availability of ancillary services.

Emergency Department Management

Initial ED management of seriously injured patients requires simultaneous treatment and evaluation. Rapid assessment of vital function is done while an empirical sequence of lifesaving therapeutic and diagnostic procedures is initiated.[15] The ultimate goal is to establish adequate oxygen delivery to the vital organs. This is accomplished by first progressing through the ABCs: airway control with cervical spine precautions—along with assisted breathing, ventilation, and occasional empirical tube thoracostomy to relieve a pneumothorax—maximizes oxygen delivery to the alveoli. Support of circulation (tamponade of external bleeding and fluid administration via large-bore I.V. catheters) is required to restore effective blood volume, thus enhancing myocardial performance and oxygen delivery to the tissues.

PRIMARY SURVEY AND INITIAL RESUSCITATION

Airway/Breathing

After blunt trauma, airway control should proceed on the assumption that an unstable cervical spine fracture exists; thus, hyperextension of the neck must be avoided. Airway management in the seriously injured victim can usually be accomplished with simple techniques, but occasionally, it can be extremely challenging. Evaluation begins by asking the patient a question such as "How are you?" A response given in a normal voice indicates that the airway is not in immediate jeopardy; a breathless, hoarse response or no response at all indicates that the airway may be compromised.

Initial Approach to the Critically Injured Patient

Communicate with base hospital

Field triage: Level I, II, or III facility
Assemble trauma team:
- Trauma surgeon
- ED physician
- Surgical specialist
- Radiology technicians
- Nurses
- Respiratory technicians

Ensure ancillary services:
- OR
- CT scanning
- Blood bank
- Interventional radiology

Hemodynamic stability is restored

Cardiogenic shock

Tension pneumothorax
Place chest tube.

Myocardial contusion
Monitor with ECG. Prevent hypoxia. Provide pharmacologic cardiac support.

Pericardial tamponade

Air embolism

Chest trauma

Hemodynamic stability is restored

Arrest is not imminent
Perform pericardiocentesis.

Impending cardiac arrest

Arrest is not imminent
Place chest tube.
Criteria for operation:
- Continued shock
- Continued bleeding (250 ml/hr for 3 hr)

Patient stabilizes

Shock persists

Perform ED thoracotomy.

Secondary survey (perform systematic assessment)

Question EMT/flight nurse. Obtain medical history. Conduct rapid, systematic physical exam. Assess potential sites of ongoing blood loss by means of DPL, abdominal ultrasonography, chest x-ray, and pelvic x-ray. Initiate flow sheet and treatment:
- Ensure adequate ventilation.
- Insert NG tube and Foley catheter. • Monitor core T°.
- Give tetanus prophylaxis. • Splint long bone fractures.
- Give systemic antibiotics for specific indications only.
- Obtain CBC, urinalysis, and ECG. • Type and crossmatch.
- Measure arterial blood gases for significant chest injuries.

Obtain radiologic studies as needed to assess occult injuries and clarify indications for operation.

Transport to SICU.

Urban: < 15 minutes
(Rural: > 30 minutes)

Initiate resuscitation and evaluation of trauma patients at the injury scene; communicate with base hospital

Management priorities of basic trauma life support are the following:
- Assess and control the accident scene
- Tamponade external hemorrhage with direct pressure
- Protect the spine after blunt trauma
- Extricate the patient
- Supplement inspired O_2
- Stabilize long bone fractures

Advanced trauma life support may include the following:
- Active airway support
- I.V. fluid administration
- Decompression of thorax for suspected pneumothorax
- Application of pneumatic antishock garment (PASG) for pelvic crush injuries

3 Minutes

Primary survey (evaluate and initiate management of airway, breathing, and circulation)

Listen to prehospital report. **Airway:** Clear airway and establish patency; obtain cervical spine x-ray. **Breathing:** Assist ventilation; vent suspected hemopneumothoraces with chest tubes. **Circulation:** Establish I.V. access; infuse fluid (crystalloid); draw blood samples.

5 Minutes

Evaluate response to initial resuscitation

Assess response to crystalloid infusion (i.e., BP, heart rate, respiratory rate, mental status). Identify easily reversible causes of shock.
Assess chest and abdomen with ultrasonography.
Blunt trauma: obtain x-rays of cervical spine, chest, and pelvis.

Shock persists

Reassess physical signs. Monitor CVP.
Repeat ultrasonography; perform DPL if ultrasonography is equivocal.

Secondary survey:
Unstable patients: 5 minutes
(Stable patients: up to 30 minutes)

Hypovolemic shock

Neurogenic shock

[*See 4 Shock.*]

Abdominal trauma

Pelvic fracture

Compress with sheet or C-clamp; administer blood.

Impending cardiac arrest

Multisystem trauma

Isolated injury

Hemodynamic stability is restored

Consider pelvic fixation (consult orthopedic surgeon).

Shock persists

Perform open DPL.

Abdominal ultrasonography is positive

Abdominal ultrasonography is equivocal

Perform DPL.

DPL is grossly positive

DPL is positive by red cell count or negative

Perform angiography and percutaneous embolization, depending on fracture geography. If DPL was negative, transport to ICU. If DPL was positive, evaluate by CT scan.

Perform ED thoracotomy.

Transport to OR.

< 60 Minutes

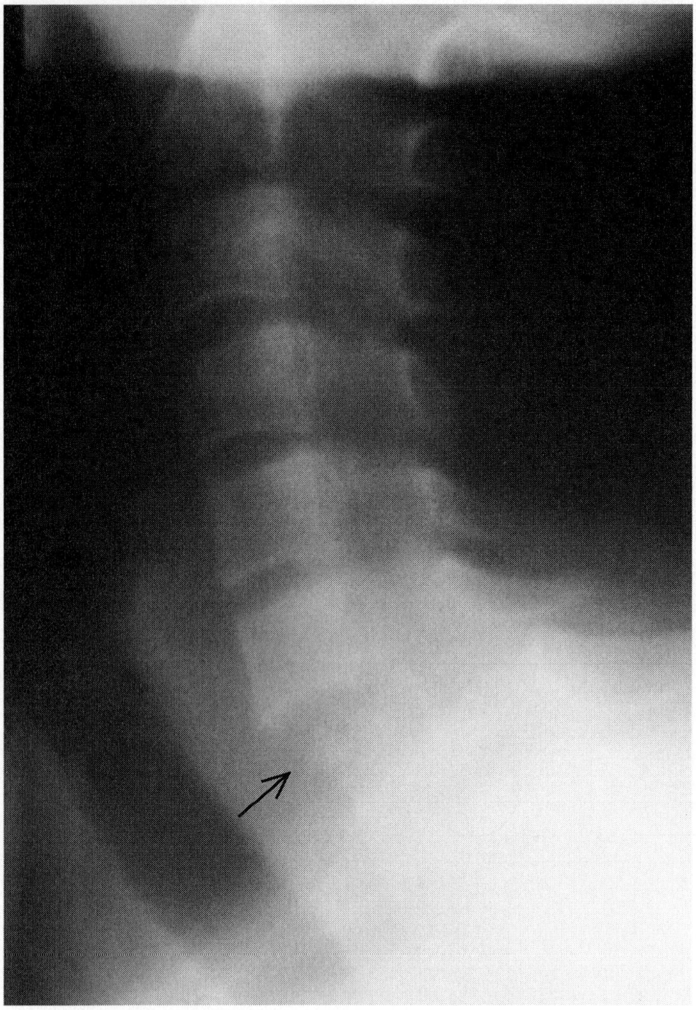

Figure 1 The cross-table lateral cervical spine x-ray is integral to acute airway management decisions. The most frequent mistake is inadequate visualization of the seventh cervical vertebra (arrow).

Airway obstruction and hypoventilation are the most likely causes of respiratory failure. The critical decision is whether active airway intervention is needed. The first maneuver is to clear the airway of debris and to suction secretions. In the obtunded patient, this procedure is followed by elevation of the angle of the mandible to alleviate pharyngeal obstruction and placement of an oropharyngeal or nasopharyngeal tube to maintain airway patency. Supplemental oxygen is given via a nasal cannula (6 L/min) or a non-rebreathing oxygen mask (12 L/min). Airway patency does not ensure adequate ventilation. Clinical evidence of hypoventilation includes poor air exchange at the nose and mouth, diminished breath sounds, and decreased chest wall excursion; the most likely causes are head injury, spinal cord transection, hemopneumothorax, flail chest, and profound shock. Suspected hemopneumothoraces should be vented with large-bore chest tubes inserted via the midlateral thorax.

Early cervical spine assessment is integral to airway management. The timing of active airway control is pivotal. The majority of significant spinal injuries in adults arriving alive at the emergency department are at the C5 to C7 levels.[16] In children 8 years old or younger, the most frequent site of spinal injury is between the occiput and C3 level.[17] Moreover, children experience a higher incidence of significant spinal cord injury without radiographic abnormalities (i.e., the SCIWORA syndrome).[18] A fractured cervical spine is usually tender to direct palpation in alert patients, but pain may be masked by distracting injuries.[19] A good-quality cross-table lateral cervical spine (CTLCS) x-ray will delineate 98% of unstable fractures [*see Figure 1*]. In high-risk patients, initial airway management is based on the CTLCS film and clinical judgment,[20] although a cervical collar is left in place until the cervical spine has been radiologically evaluated for bony integrity.

Ideally, after blunt trauma or transcervical gunshot wounds, intubation should be deferred until CTLCS films are available, although neurologic injury from a gunshot wound to the neck is virtually always complete at the time of injury. Bag-mask ventilation is an effective temporizing measure, but it consumes the attention of a skilled trauma team member, it may insufflate air into the stomach, it is resisted by spontaneously breathing patients, and it is ineffective in the presence of severe maxillofacial trauma. The decision for urgent airway control is clinical; there is no time to obtain a confirmatory arterial blood gas (ABG) analysis.[21] Persistent airway obstruction or signs of inadequate ventilation mandate prompt intervention. Patients with expanding neck hematomas, deteriorating vital signs, or severe head trauma are also best managed with an aggressive airway approach. On the other hand, in equivocal situations (e.g., increased P_aCO_2 or base deficit despite a satisfactory S_aO_2), an ABG analysis may be decisive.

The best method of airway control depends on (1) the presence of maxillofacial trauma, (2) suspected cervical spine injury, (3) overall patient condition, and (4) the experience of the physician. Patients in respiratory distress with severe maxillofacial trauma warrant operative intervention. Cricothyrotomy is the preferred approach in adults and has virtually replaced tracheostomy in the ED [*see Figure 2*]; the rare exceptions are in patients with direct laryngeal trauma or complete tracheal disruption. Percutaneous transtracheal ventilation may be safer than both of these surgical procedures for temporary airway management, particularly in children.[22] Nasotracheal intubation is the airway route of choice in nonapneic patients with potential cervical injury in the field but is rarely employed in the ED. The current standard approach is rapid sequence intubation (RSI) of the trachea orally with inline immobilization.[23,24] Our RSI guidelines include nine steps: (1) preparation of equipment and supplies; (2) preoxygenation; (3) sedation to decrease anxiety; (4) premedication to mitigate the negative effects of intubation (e.g., a defasciculating dose of pancuronium or lidocaine for patients with head injuries to prevent increased intracranial pressure); (5) cricoid pressure; (6) paralysis with either succinylcholine, 1.0 to 1.5 mg/kg, or rocuronium, 0.5 to 1.2 mg/kg; (7) intubation with visualization of the vocal cords to permit confident airway access; (8) confirmation of tube position by auscultation and capnography; and (9) securing of the airway. In adults, a large (8 mm internal diameter) cuffed endotracheal tube should be inserted to a distance of 23 cm from the incisors. In children, tube size is gauged to equal the diameter of the little finger or may be estimated by the following formula:

$$\frac{age + 16}{4} = \text{internal diameter (mm) of endotracheal tube}$$

The proper depth (in centimeters) to which the tube should be inserted can be estimated by multiplying the tube's internal diameter (in millimeters) by 3. A chest x-ray should be obtained as soon as possible to rule out the common problem of right mainstem intubation.

Circulation

Once alveolar ventilation is ensured, the next priority is to optimize oxygen delivery by maximizing cardiovascular performance. Hypovolemia is the most likely cause of shock that occurs after the patient receives an injury [*see 4 Shock*]; therefore, treatment is

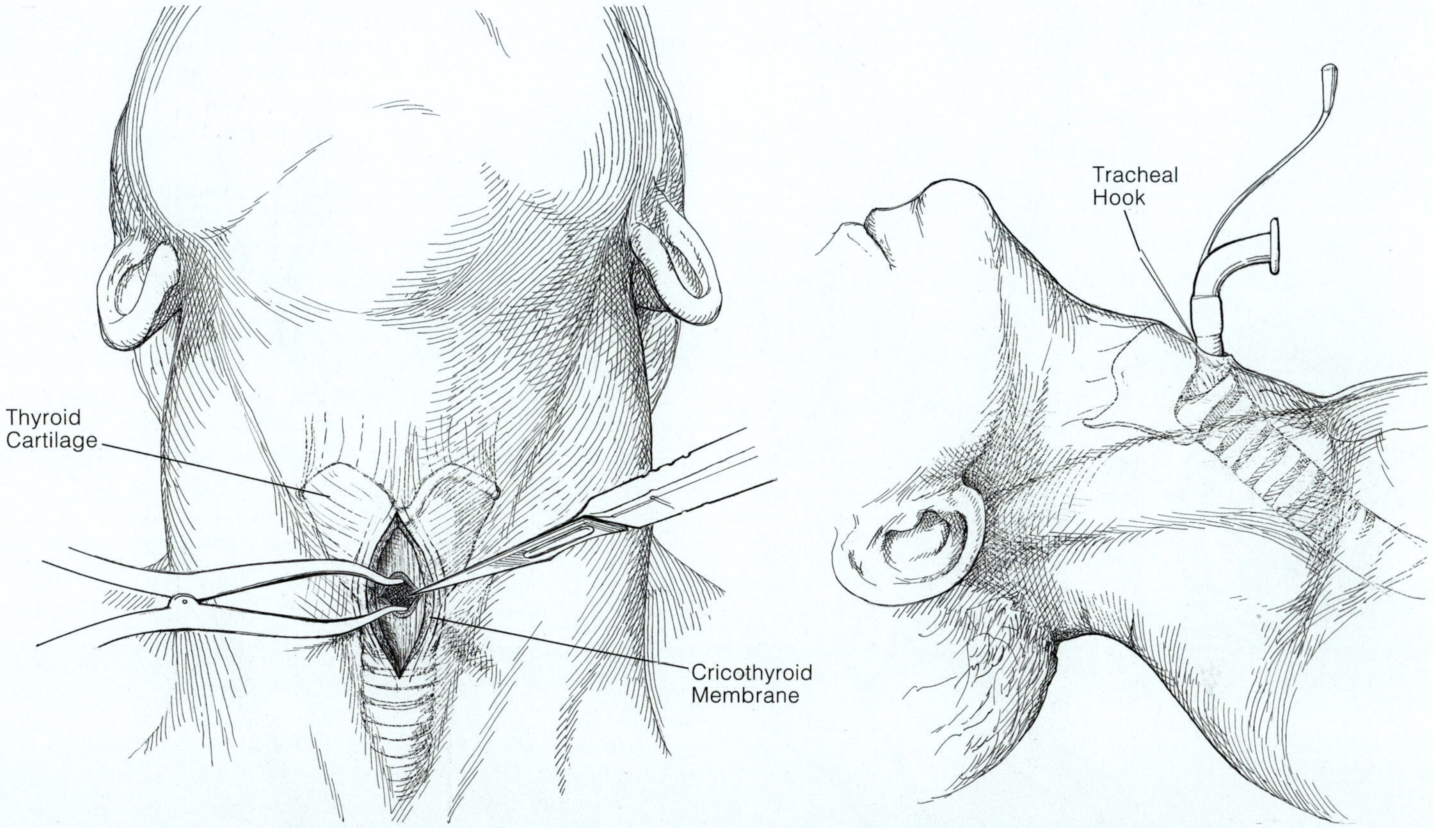

Figure 2 Technique for cricothyrotomy is illustrated here. The larynx is stabilized with one hand, and a 2 cm vertical incision is made over the cricothyroid space. The cricothyroid membrane is palpated and incised horizontally. A Trosseau dilator is inserted and spread vertically for visualization of the subglottic space (left). A tracheal hook is used to retract the inferior border of the thyroid cartilage as a tracheostomy tube with a 6 mm internal diameter is inserted into the trachea (right).

initiated with crystalloid infusion via large-bore I.V. cannulas, and external hemorrhage is controlled by manual compression. If the PASG has been applied in the field, it should not be removed until effective volume restitution has been achieved. Of special concern are cases in which the PASG has been applied to manage otherwise uncontrollable lower-extremity hemorrhage. In such cases, with effective volume loading, bleeding may become profuse. Application of the PASG in the ED should be reserved for the control of bleeding from major pelvic fractures—if used at all. In fact, wrapping the pelvis with a sheet in the ED is now preferred for initial mechanical stabilization of major pelvic fractures.

The size, number, and sites of I.V. catheters depend on the degree of shock and on estimates of the severity of the injury. If the patient arrives in shock or has obvious multiple injuries, a short 14 French catheter should be placed in each antecubital vein. When vascular collapse precludes peripheral percutaneous access, saphenous vein cutdown at the ankle is preferred [*see Figure 3*] because the site is distant from sites of other resuscitative efforts, the vein will easily accept a large catheter, and the only adjacent structure is a trivial branch of the saphenous nerve. An acceptable alternative is intubation of the femoral vein at the groin by means of the Seldinger technique. Intraosseous infusion through a cannula placed in the medullary cavity of a long bone is a safe and efficacious method for emergency vascular access in infants and children 6 years old or younger. This procedure is typically performed in the anteromedial aspect of the tibial plateau in an uninjured extremity; the distal femur, the distal tibia, and the sternum are other potential sites. Intraosseous infusion generally allows administration of sufficient fluid to facilitate subsequent cannulation of the venous circulation.[25] With establishment of the first intravenous line, blood should be drawn for hematocrit, white blood cell count, amylase level, electrolyte concentrations, blood-group typing, coagulation profile, and toxicology screen as indicated.

EVALUATION AND CONTINUED RESUSCITATION

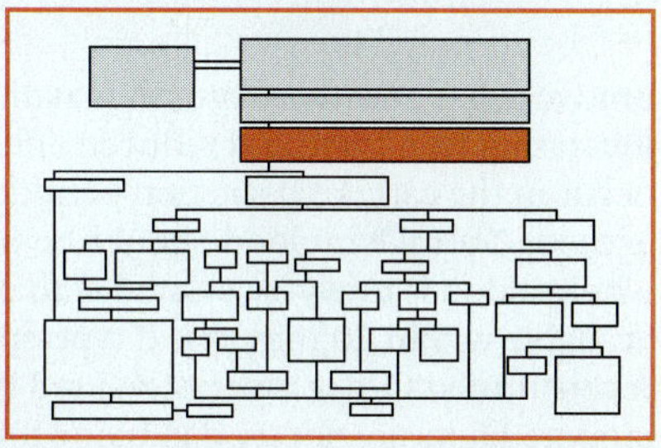

Systemic blood pressure, heart rate, respiratory rate, and the patient's general appearance are most helpful in judging the degree of acute blood loss and in assessing the response to initial crystalloid resuscitation. As a general rule, the carotid pulse is palpable at a systolic blood pressure of 60 mm Hg, the femoral pulse at 70 mm Hg, and the radial pulse at 80 mm Hg. In patients with hypovolemic shock, crystalloid loading is initiated with ongoing monitoring of vital signs. Studies from Houston, however, emphasize that in patients with free intraperitoneal or intrathoracic bleeding, overzealous fluid administration before definitive vascular control is achieved may increase blood loss.[3] Consequently, such patients should be promptly transported to the operating room without aggressive efforts to normalize vital signs. It is important to note that acute massive blood loss may paradoxically trigger a vagal-mediated

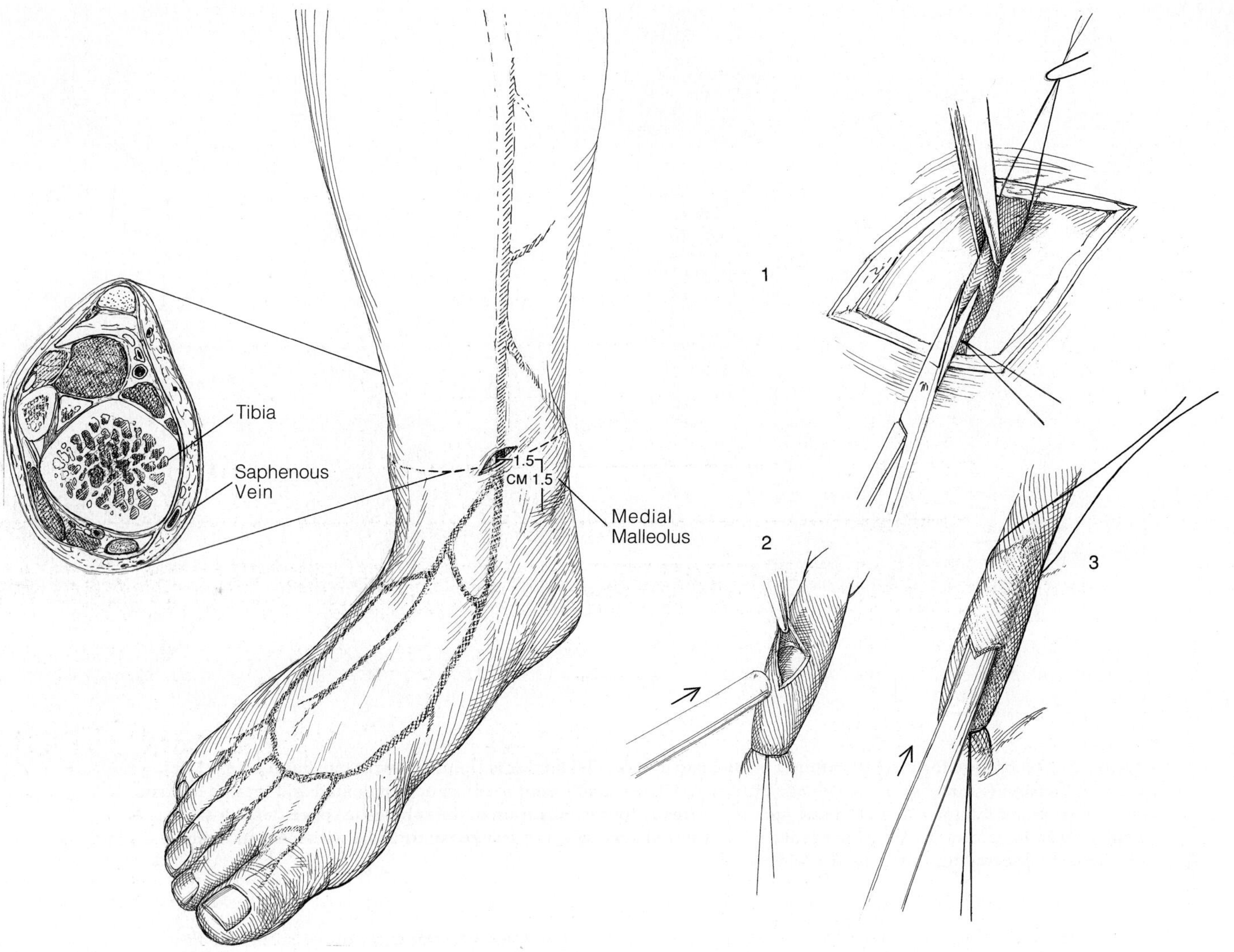

Figure 3 Saphenous vein cutdown is indicated when vascular collapse precludes peripheral access. The greater saphenous vein lies superficial to the anterior periosteum at the medial malleolus. A transverse skin incision is made one fingerbreadth superior and anterior to the malleolus. A hemostat is inserted and brought across the anteromedial aspect of the tibia. The only structures that should be included under the hemostat are the saphenous vein and a trivial branch of the saphenous nerve.

bradycardia, and therefore, the traditional inverse correlation of increasing heart rate and reduced effective blood volume may not occur in the early resuscitation period.[26] When crystalloid infusion exceeds 50 ml/kg, blood should be administered[27]; type-specific whole blood is rarely associated with complications and should be available within 20 minutes. If type-specific blood is not available, reconstituted O-negative packed red blood cells may be used. Micropore filters are not used in blood infusion lines in hemodynamically unstable patients, because they impede infusion capabilities.[28] In the future, hemoglobin-based blood substitutes may become available that would obviate the need for crossmatching and filtration. Electrocardiographic monitoring, serial measurement of vital signs, rapid physical examination, rectal temperature reading, and initiation of a flow sheet complete the initial assessment of the patient.

The next step is to evaluate the response to resuscitation. In patients with persistent shock, chest x-rays [*see Figure 4*], pelvic x-rays, and thoracic and abdominal ultrasonography are performed early in the resuscitation to identify occult sources of hemorrhage.[29,30]

Persistent shock may be hypovolemic, cardiogenic, or neurogenic [*see 4 Shock*]. Measurement of central venous pressure (CVP) may aid in differentiating between these types of shock. With hypovolemic shock, the CVP is generally less than 5 mm Hg, whereas in clinically significant cardiogenic shock, the CVP usually exceeds 20 mm Hg. Unfortunately, the CVP may be falsely elevated because of rapid volume infusion, hyperventilation, patient straining, a malfunctioning catheter, or improper location of the catheter tip.

The differential diagnosis of traumatic cardiogenic shock consists basically of (1) tension pneumothorax, (2) pericardial tamponade, (3) myocardial contusion, and (4) air embolism. Except for refractory shock, telltale physical signs are frequently hard to discern in a noisy ED, especially when compounded by persistent hypovolemia. Timely diagnosis requires a high index of suspicion. Tension pneumothorax, the most common etiology, is often confirmed with emergency chest tube placement [*see Figure 5*]. In traumatic pericardial tamponade, the classic signs of tamponade, termed Beck's triad (hypotension, muffled heart sounds, and jugular venous distention), are frequently absent, and pulsus paradoxus is rarely detectable. With

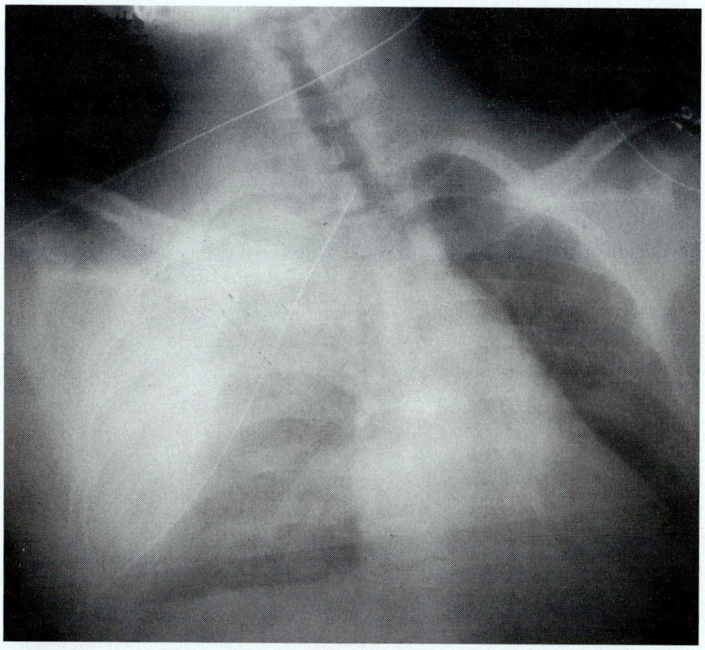

Figure 4 ED chest x-ray shows a massive hemothorax. If the chest tube fails to evacuate the blood, this is a so-called caked hemothorax, which is an indication for emergency thoracostomy in the OR.

the wider use of ultrasonography by trauma surgeons, ED echocardiography should be the first test employed in patients with a high-risk penetrating wound, clinical signs of tamponade, and persistent central venous hypertension.[31,32] With documented pericardial blood on echocardiography and persistent tachycardia, pericardiocentesis should be performed even in the presence of normal systolic blood pressure to relieve any ongoing subendocardial ischemia [*see Figure 6*]. Patients who have persistent signs of pericardial tamponade despite a negative echocardiogram or pericardiocentesis should be transported to the OR for a subxiphoid pericardial window. It is important to remember that results of pericardial aspiration for acute hemopericardium are falsely negative in 15% of patients because the blood in the pericardial sac is clotted and cannot be aspirated. If the patient is in extremis, ED thoracotomy should be performed promptly [*see Figure 7*].[33] Myocardial contusion should be suspected in a patient with unexplained cardiogenic shock or arrhythmia. ECG changes are usually nonspecific.[34,35] Fundamental measures include correction of acidosis, hypoxia, and electrolyte abnormalities; judicious administration of fluid; and pharmacologic suppression of life-threatening arrhythmias. Air embolism into the left atrium from a pulmonary laceration is probably more common than is recognized[36]; typically, hemodynamic instability occurs after positive pressure ventilation is initiated, forcing

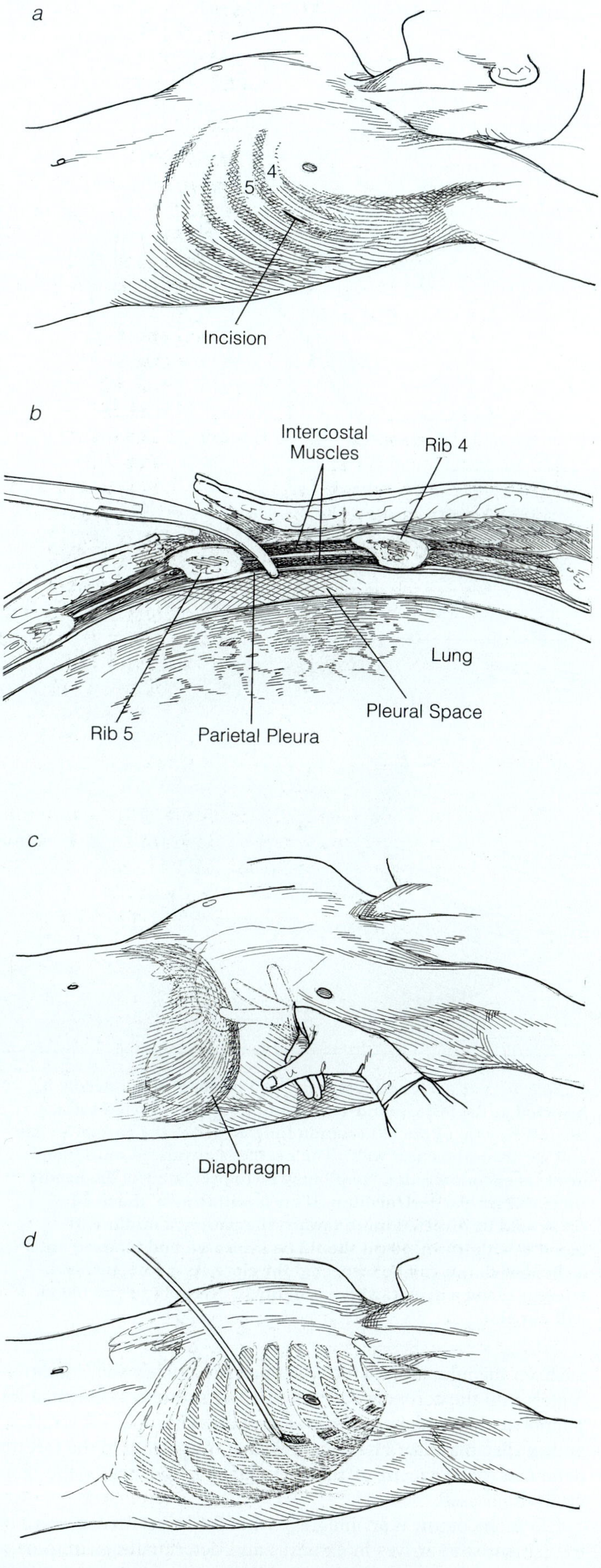

Figure 5 In acute trauma, a tube thoracostomy is performed through the fourth or fifth interspace at the midaxillary line, well above the diaphragm (*a*). A short subcutaneous tunnel is fashioned over the superior edge of the rib, and the overlying fascia and intercostal muscle are divided sharply. The pleural space is entered by bluntly perforating the pleura with a Kelly clamp (*b*). A gloved finger is then inserted to confirm penetration of the thoracic cavity and to free up intrapleural adhesions (*c*). A large-bore tube (36 French) is directed posteriorly toward the pleural apex; the proximal port must be well inside the chest (*d*). The tube is then secured to the chest wall with No. 5 braided polyethylene suture and connected to a standard collection apparatus.

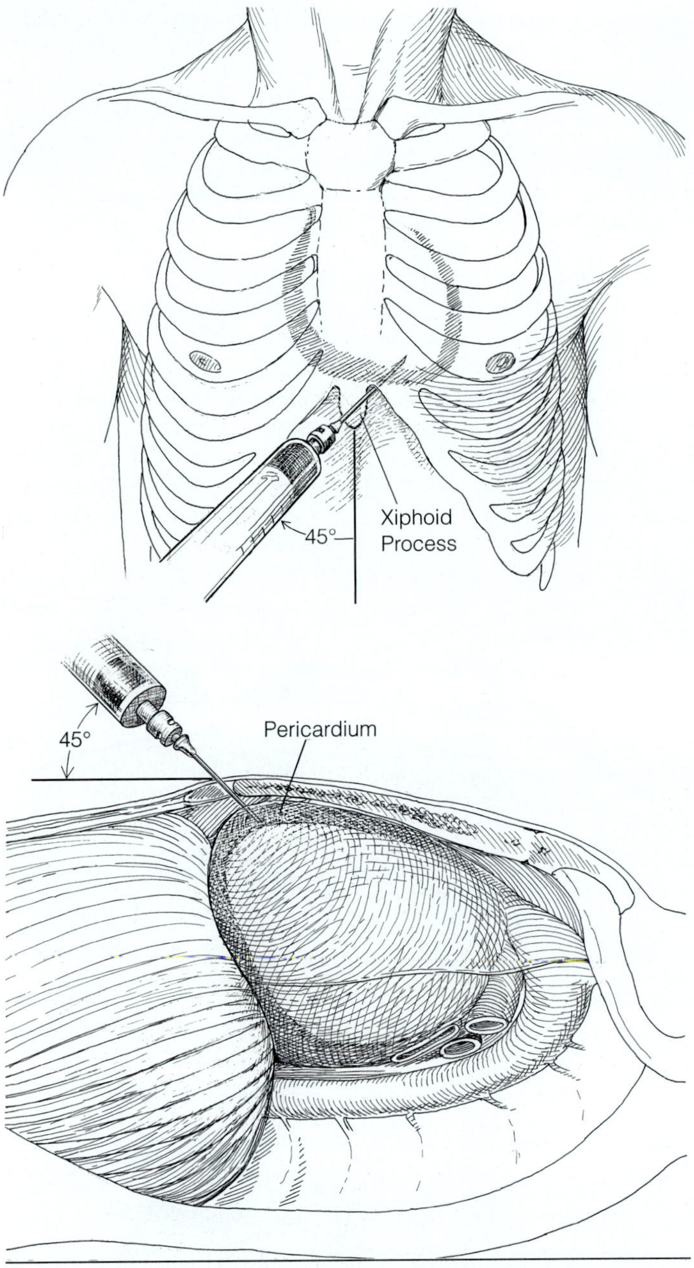

cardiac arrest [see Figures 7 and 8].[33] The physiologic rationale is to minimize the time of profound shock; ED thoracotomy permits (1) release of pericardial tamponade, (2) control of intrathoracic blood loss, (3) internal cardiac massage, and (4) cross-clamping of the descending thoracic aorta to enhance coronary and cerebral perfusion as well as to reduce subdiaphragmatic bleeding. Internal cardiac massage should be done bimanually; otherwise, a forceful thumb may rupture the relatively thin right ventricle as it becomes distended. Simple ventricular lacerations are repaired with pledgeted horizontal mattress sutures, whereas atrial injuries are controlled with a partially occluding vascular clamp and repaired with a running suture [see Figure 8].

SECONDARY SURVEY AND DEFINITIVE DIAGNOSIS

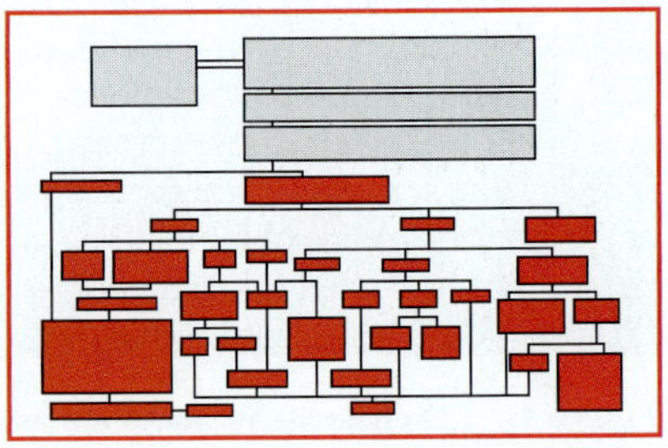

After immediate physiologic demands have been addressed, acutely injured patients can usually be rendered hemodynamically stable, and the secondary survey phase can begin. In this phase, the goal is to complete a systematic assessment to identify all potentially life-threatening injuries. Such assessment is crucial to allow proper triage from the ED to the OR, the CT scanning suite, the interventional suite, or the ICU. Mechanism of injury, severity of shock, and response to resuscitation will dictate the time expended. Details of the patient's medical history as well as those related to the injury are critical. The prehospital emergency medical technicians can provide important details and should be questioned before they leave the ED. A minimal review of the patient's medical history should include preexisting medical illness, current medications and when they were most recently ingested, allergies, tetanus immunization, and time of last meal. A rapid but systematic physical examination is done, literally from head to toe. Patients must be completely disrobed and, once spinal injury is excluded, rolled side to side so that the back and flanks can be inspected. Rectal examination for blood and sphincter tone, inspection of the perineum and axillae, and assessment of neurologic function and peripheral pulses are essential.

A good-quality lateral cervical spine x-ray should be obtained as soon as possible after blunt trauma. Until the x-ray is available and all seven cervical vertebral bodies are clearly visualized, the neck is rigidly immobilized. Splinting of long bone fractures minimizes pain, blood loss, and soft tissue damage. Insertion of a nasogastric tube serves to decompress the stomach and reduce the risk of pulmonary aspiration, but because maxillofacial injury may provide a pathway into the cranial vault,[37] the tube should be placed orally when there are midfacial fractures. Blood in the gastric aspirate may be the only sign of an otherwise occult injury of the stomach and duodenum. A Foley catheter empties the bladder, may disclose hematuria, and permits the physician to monitor urinary output, but it should not be inserted until abdominal ultrasonography is completed. Urine volume is a sensitive index of tissue perfusion. The trauma victim is uniquely susceptible to hypothermia; a rectal temperature probe is therefore essential in patients who have been exposed to a cold environment or who require massive volume replacement. A core temperature reading lower than 32° C (89.6° F) should be confirmed with an esophageal probe, and rewarming measures appropriate for the degree of hypothermia should be initiated [see 98 Fever, Hyperpyrexia, and Hypothermia].[38-40] Tetanus prophylaxis is routine. Systemic antibiotics should be withheld until a

Figure 6 For pericardiocentesis, an 18-gauge spinal needle is inserted at the left xiphoid-costal junction and inserted toward the inferior tip of the left scapula (angled 45° to the patient's right and 45° from the chest wall). The needle is advanced until blood or air is encountered; a "pop" may be appreciated as the needle tip traverses the pericardium. If air is withdrawn, the needle tip should be directed more toward the patient's midline. If blood is withdrawn, 50 ml should be aspirated and injected onto a sheet so that it can be inspected for clots. As a rule, intraventricular blood will clot, whereas defibrinated pericardial blood will not clot.

air from the injured lung into the open pulmonary veins and ultimately into the coronary arteries. ED thoracotomy is essential for pulmonary hilar cross-clamping, air aspiration from the left ventricle, and cardiac massage. The patient is then transferred to the OR for definitive management of the pulmonary lesion before the hilar clamp is released.

ED thoracotomy is an integral part of the initial management of the patient who arrives in extremis and deteriorates to imminent

specific indication arises. Minimal laboratory tests for trauma include a complete blood count and urinalysis. An electrocardiogram is obtained after blunt chest trauma, and an ABG analysis is done in select patients to confirm adequate ventilation and metabolic balance. The size of the base deficit can be a useful measure of the depth of hemorrhagic shock.[41] In any patient with evidence of hypovolemia, a blood sample should be sent for blood-group typing.

All potential sites of ongoing blood loss should be evaluated in the hypovolemic patient. A chest x-ray is the most reliable screening test for intrathoracic bleeding; it also confirms the location of endotracheal, nasogastric, and thoracostomy tubes as well as the central venous catheter. Pleural fluid can be difficult to appreciate on a supine chest x-ray; 1 L of blood may produce only a hazy appearance in a hemithorax. Hemothoraces should be drained promptly by tube thoracostomy [see Figure 5]. Continued bleeding must be monitored carefully by means of chest tube output, serial chest films to detect retained intrapleural blood, and vital signs. Abrupt cessation of chest tube output may be deceptive; if hypotension persists or recurs, a second chest tube should be inserted and another chest x-ray should be obtained. The inability to clear the thorax with chest tubes (so-called caked hemothorax [see Figure 4]) is an indication for prompt thoracotomy.

Abdominal examination is notoriously misleading in detecting acute hemoperitoneum.[42] The peritoneal cavity may sequester up to 3,000 ml of blood with only minimal abdominal distention. Laparotomy is clearly indicated for gunshot wounds with violation of the peritoneum[43] or in patients with overt peritonitis after a stab wound or blunt trauma. After blunt trauma, however, head injury or intoxication frequently alters the patient's response to acute injury, and pain from associated fractures may overshadow peritoneal irritation secondary to bleeding. Ultrasonography is the most rapid method of identifying free blood, but it may yield false negative results in as many as 5% to 10% of patients on initial examination. Diagnostic peritoneal lavage (DPL) [see Figure 9] is the most expedient and reliable method of identifying significant intraperitoneal hemorrhage; in patients with life-threatening bleeding, sensitivity approaches 100%. Paradoxically, because of its extreme sensitivity in identifying blood, DPL lacks specificity for determining the need for laparotomy in stable patients.[44,45] A grossly positive aspirate (> 10 ml of blood) mandates emergency laparotomy in cases of penetrating wounds and in cases of blunt trauma with hemodynamic instability. A red blood cell count higher than 100,000/mm³ in a patient with penetrating trauma is an indication for semiemergent celiotomy, whereas a red blood cell count exceeding 50,000/mm³ in a patient with blunt trauma

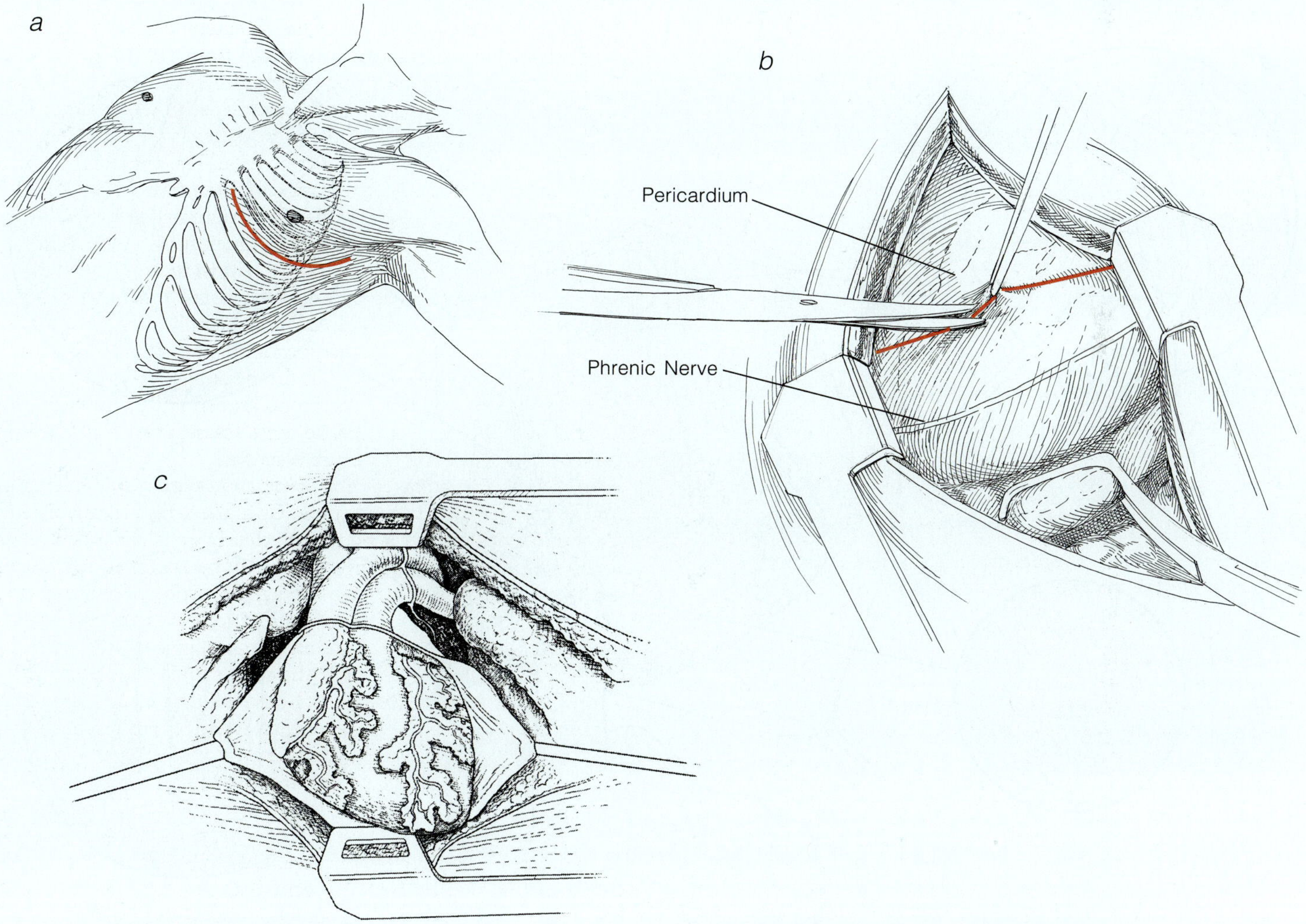

Figure 7 (*a*) **A left anterolateral thoracotomy is performed through the fifth intercostal space. (*b*) The lung is reflected superomedially, and a Satinsky vascular clamp is placed on the descending thoracic aorta. A pericardiotomy is performed with scissors anterior to the phrenic nerve. (*c*) A so-called butterfly extension across the sternum creates a bilateral anterolateral thoracotomy, providing access to both thoracic cavities and to the pulmonary hila, heart, and proximal great vessels.**

warrants further evaluation by computed tomography of the abdomen. Furthermore, in the setting of both blunt trauma and penetrating trauma, elevation in the peritoneal lavage white blood cell count, the amylase level, and the alkaline phosphatase concentration may identify hollow viscus injury; threshold levels, however, have not been determined.[46-48] In penetrating wounds to the lower chest, the red blood cell count threshold for abdominal exploration is lowered to 10,000/mm^3 because isolated diaphragmatic perforations may not bleed.[49] An intermediate red blood cell count of 1,000 to 10,000/mm^3 warrants further definitive evaluation by thoracoscopy.[49,50] Because DPL does not sample the retroperitoneum, triple-contrast CT scanning may be of help in cases of high-risk penetrating wounds to the back or the flank.[51,52] Most injuries to retroperitoneal hollow viscera, however, are identified on the basis of extraluminal gas or fluid rather than contrast extravasation.

Assessment of bony stability by physical examination and plain films of the pelvis is crucial for the early identification of major pelvic fractures. Life-threatening hemorrhage occurs most commonly with fracture patterns involving the posterior columns [see Figure 10].[53,54] Appropriate initial management includes vigorous blood volume replacement and mechanical support of the pelvis [see Figure 11]. Most patients can be rendered hemodynamically stable and are potential candidates for external skeletal fixation if the fracture geography is appropriate.[55,56] The unstable patient with a clearly positive ultrasonogram should undergo laparotomy because of a high probability of major hepatic, splenic, or mesenteric bleeding.[57] Conversely, the hemodynamically unstable patient in whom the ultrasonogram is normal and DPL yields confirmatory negative results should undergo prompt pelvic arteriography for selective embolization.[58]

The length of time expended in the ED, the decision for urgent operation, and the need for special radiologic studies are critical triage decisions that must take into account the mechanism of injury, the response to resuscitation, and the availability of a staffed OR. A patient in refractory shock with a central abdominal gunshot wound, for example, should be assigned by triage to the OR in a matter of minutes, whereas a far more complex decision is required in the case of a motor vehicle accident victim with altered mental status, a widened mediastinum on chest x-ray, and a positive ultrasonogram. If the latter patient is hemodynamically unstable, laparotomy should be performed first because intraperitoneal bleeding is the most likely cause of persistent shock. If this patient is hemodynamically stable, however, CT scanning and aortography should be performed first because the results of these procedures facilitate a multiteam approach and allow prioritizing of operative needs.[59,60]

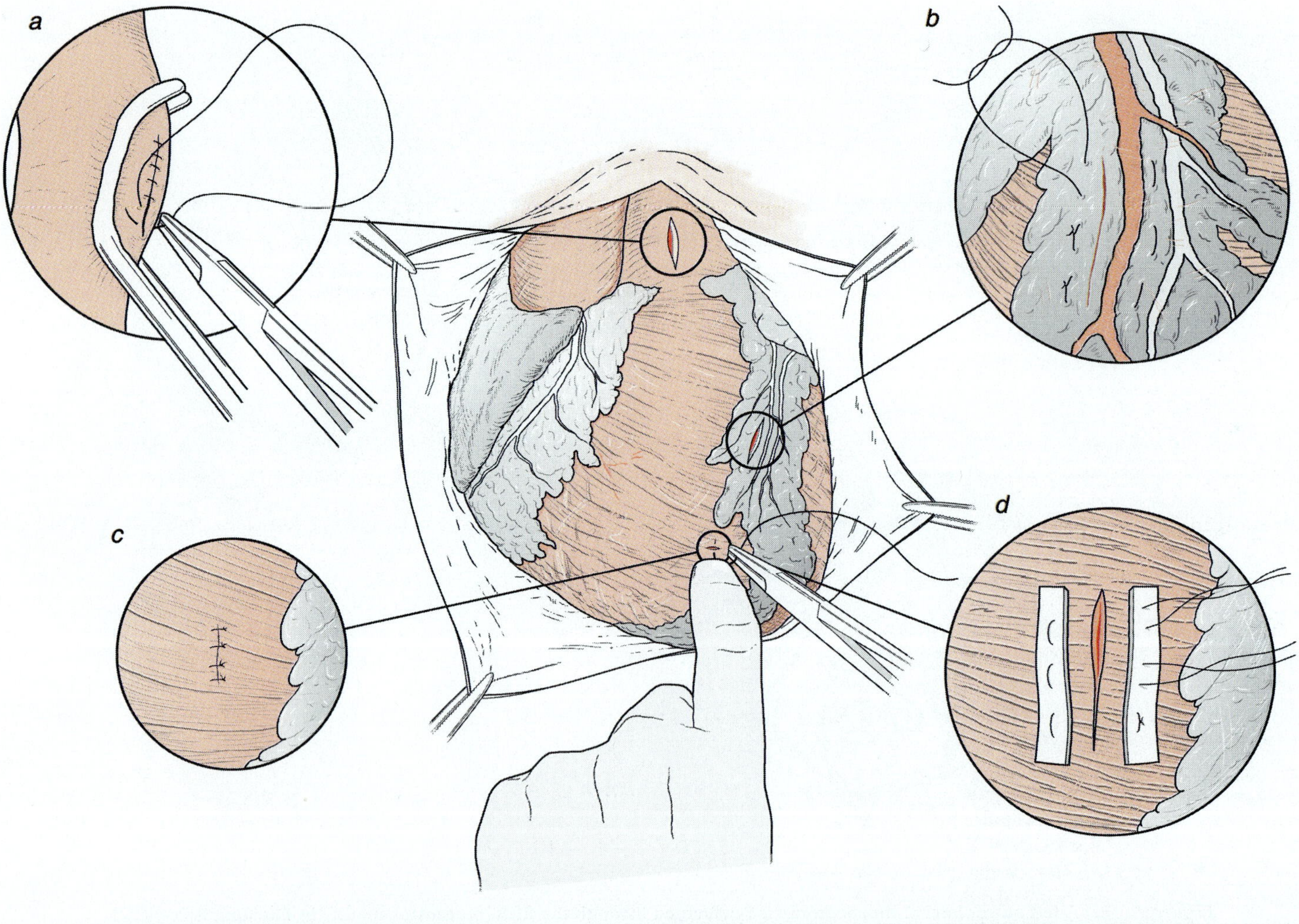

Figure 8 (a) A Satinsky vascular clamp is used to control arterial and major vessel injuries while they are closed with a running suture. (b) For wounds close to coronary arteries, horizontal mattress sutures should be used to exclude the arteries. (c) Small wounds to the thick left ventricle can be closed with interrupted simple sutures. (d) Larger wounds should be closed using pledgets.

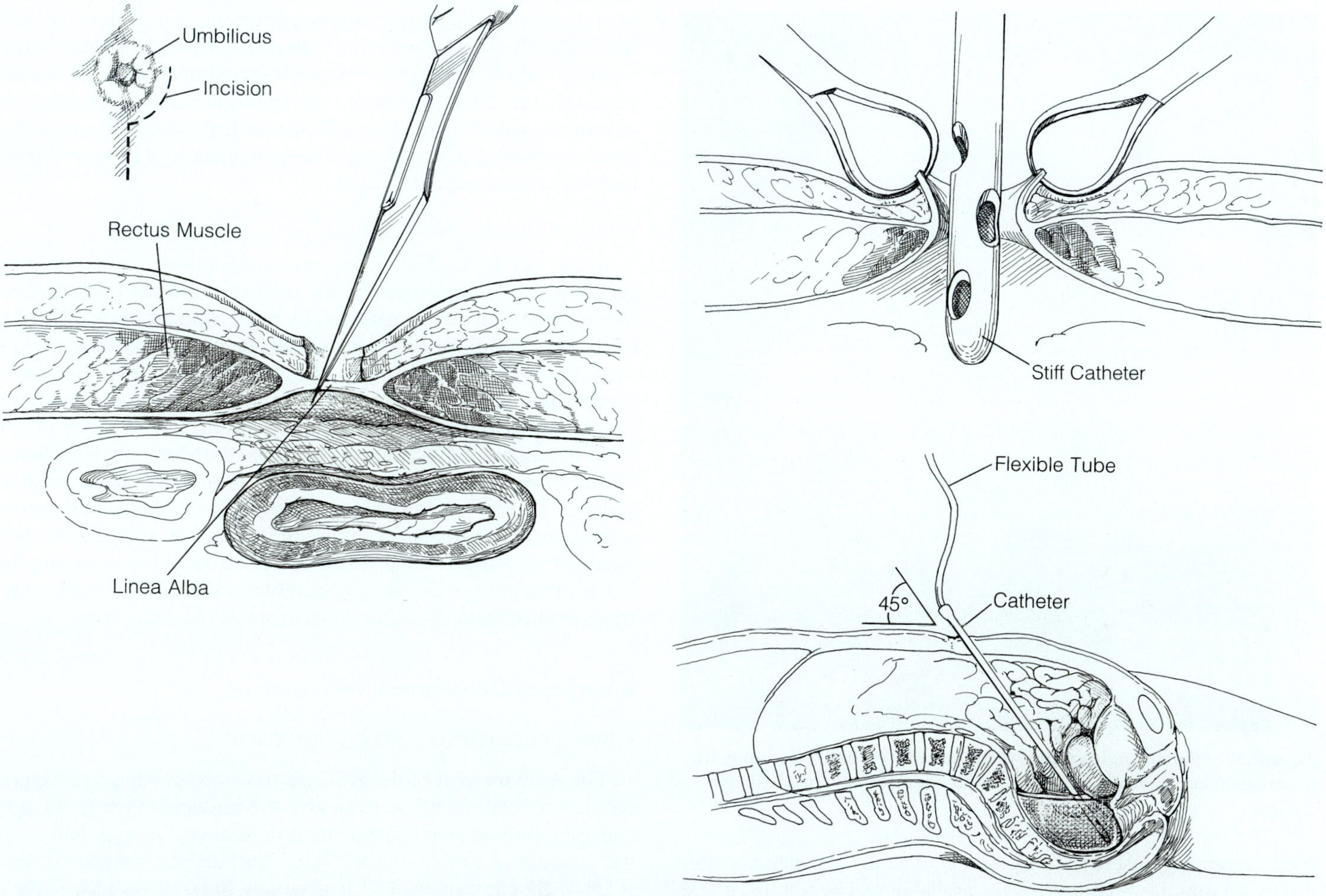

Figure 9 Illustrated here is the semiopen technique for peritoneal lavage. A 3 to 4 cm incision is made over the infraumbilical ring, and the linea alba is incised vertically for 1 cm. The fascial edges are grasped with towel clips and elevated. A standard peritoneal dialysis catheter is introduced into the peritoneum at a 45° angle and then advanced into the pelvis without use of the trocar. If 10 ml of gross blood is aspirated, the study is considered to be positive. Otherwise, 1 L of normal saline (10 ml/kg for children) is infused. The lavage fluid is retrieved by gravity siphonage; the empty saline bag is dropped to the floor. A 50 ml sample of the fluid is submitted for laboratory analysis.

Discussion

Prehospital Care

ADVANCED TRAUMA LIFE SUPPORT

The principles of initial assessment and management in ACLS and ATLS are based on the ABCs—airway maintenance, breathing, and circulation. In both settings, upper airway control and assisted ventilation are imperative for optimizing alveolar oxygen tension. With respect to circulation, however, the protocols diverge markedly because of differing pathophysiology.

It is estimated that 60% of deaths caused by coronary artery disease occur within 1 hour of initial symptoms, usually before the patient can receive medical care.[61] Rhythm disturbance is the most frequent cause of death after cardiac arrest; there is only a 6-minute period until irreversible cerebral damage occurs.[62] Temporary artificial circulation in these normovolemic patients can be achieved by closed-chest compression. The technique is simple and effective and requires no special equipment. However, arrhythmias, the most common cause of preventable death, become refractory if pharmacologic or electrical treatment is delayed.[63] ECG monitoring and venous access allow the necessary interventions to be initiated effectively in the field, and indeed, ACLS results in a fivefold reduction in the incidence of cardiac arrest en route to the hospital. In contrast, the major reversible threat to life for the severely injured patient is persistent hemorrhage, which requires hospital facilities for effective treatment.

Sophistication of emergency medical services has dramatically expanded the scope of prehospital care. Qualified paramedics using ACLS skills have produced dramatic improvement in survival of acute myocardial infarction by treating arrhythmias in the field.[64] Unquestionably, these efforts also improve trauma resuscitation, but the extent of prehospital ATLS remains a highly controversial issue. Advocates of the so-called scope-and-run philosophy argue that field stabilization is detrimental because it delays definitive care. However, in systems with rigorous medical control, the addition of advanced techniques (e.g., endotracheal intubation, I.V. access, and fluid administration) adds less than 10 minutes to the on-scene time.[2] In the Denver Emergency Medical Service system, para-

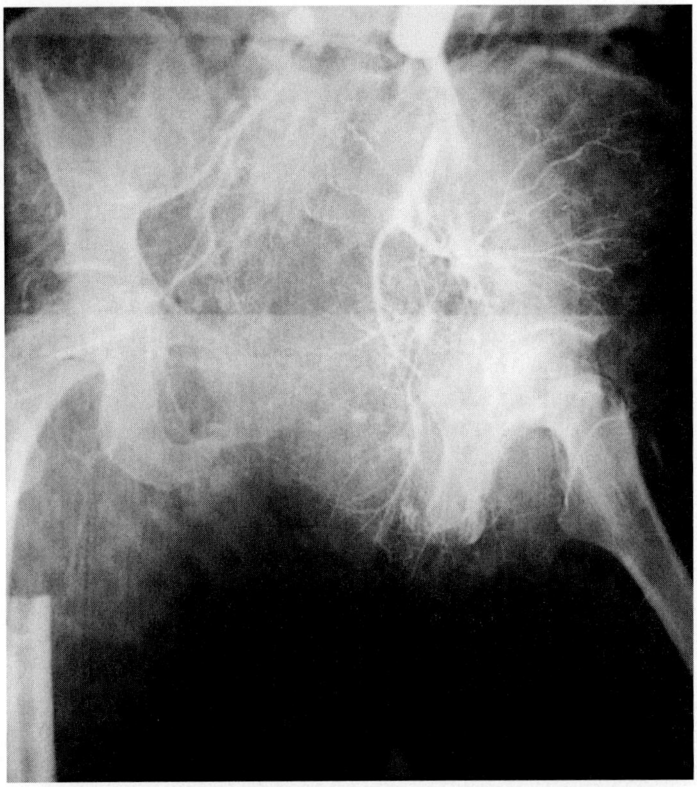

Figure 10 Pelvic angiography with selective embolization may be an integral component in the early management of a pelvic crush injury.

medics routinely insert I.V. catheters in critically ill patients within 1.0 to 1.5 minutes.[65] Moreover, the availability of hypertonic saline solution and human polymerized hemoglobin for prehospital fluid resuscitation may provide an undisputed physiologic rationale for establishing I.V. access at the scene.[66-71] Clearly, the relative benefits of paramedic intervention depend on mechanism of injury, patient status, and availability of a trauma center. An efficient prehospital care system should be tailored to the community's needs, providing well-thought-out protocols, appropriate field personnel, and active medical control. Unfortunately, a paradox exists: ATLS skills are needed most in sparsely populated rural areas where transport time exceeds 30 minutes, but the limited volume of trauma precludes the experience necessary to maintain this expertise.

AIRWAY MANAGEMENT

The principles of initial resuscitation are governed by physiologic rationale. The goal is to reestablish adequate oxygen delivery to vital organs. Efforts to improve tissue perfusion will be unproductive unless the oxygen content of the circulating blood is sufficient. Airway patency and maintenance of adequate ventilation are thus the initial priorities. Current policy dictates that emergency airway control after blunt vehicular trauma be performed with the assumption that an unstable cervical spine fracture exists until such injuries are excluded radiologically; however, this policy does not preclude RSI.[72] Cervical neck injury has been documented in 25% of accidental fatalities[73] and in 60% of fatalities in which the patient had sustained head trauma,[74] but the incidence of truly occult unstable cervical fractures in neurologically intact survivors of vehicular trauma is unknown. The current recommendation of orotracheal intubation with in-line manual stabilization of the head and neck has proved safe in clinical series to date. For patients with extensive maxillofacial trauma that precludes oral intubation, the traditional alternative has been to do a cricothyrotomy, but this surgical procedure has definite risks. The success achieved with percutaneous dilatational tracheostomy in ICU patients[75] suggests that similar approaches with percutaneous cricothyrotomy may be easier and would pose less risk to the patient. Finally, we believe that percutaneous transtracheal ventilation is a viable option in challenging airway problems and that it remains underutilized.[22]

PNEUMATIC ANTISHOCK GARMENT

In the 1970s, the PASG was mandated as essential prehospital equipment for ambulances on the basis of the assumption that inflation produced autotransfusion by redistributing blood from the lower extremities into the central circulation. Subsequent experimental work challenged this concept and showed that the rise in mean arterial pressure is merely the result of an elevated systemic vascular resistance.[76] Randomized prospective evaluations of the PASG in urban prehospital care have failed to demonstrate a benefit and in fact suggest that PASG inflation may be detrimental in cases of thoracic trauma.[6] However, the role of PASGs in the rural setting, in which transport times are longer, has not been studied adequately. In the hospital setting, we consider either wrapping the pelvis or use of the C clamp preferable to the PASG for management of unrelenting bleeding from unstable pelvic fractures.

Emergency Department Management

AIRWAY, BREATHING, AND CIRCULATION

The primary goal of the ABCs is to establish adequate oxygen delivery to vital organs so as to give the physician time to identify and treat immediately life-threatening injuries. Oxygen delivery is the product of cardiac output (CO) and arterial oxygen content (C_aO_2). By convention, CO is generally indexed to body surface area and expressed as cardiac index (CI), which when multiplied by C_aO_2 yields an oxygen delivery index (D_{O_2}). Normal D_{O_2} is roughly 500 ml/min/m²; it will increase by as much as 30% in response to injury. C_aO_2 and D_{O_2} are calculated as follows:

$$C_aO_2 \text{ (ml/dl)} = [Hb] \text{ (g/dl)} \times 1.38 \times S_aO_2 \text{ (\%)} + [P_aO_2 \text{ (mm Hg)}] \times 0.003$$
$$D_{O_2} \text{ (ml/min/m}^2\text{)} = CI \text{ (L/min/m)} \times C_aO_2 \text{ (ml/dl)} \times 10$$

where [Hb] is the hemoglobin concentration, S_aO_2 is oxyhemoglobin saturation, P_aO_2 is arterial oxygen tension, and 0.003 is the solubility of O_2 in blood.

S_aO_2 is the first important variable to consider. Given the low solubility of oxygen in plasma, the level of P_aO_2 is only important insofar as it relates to S_aO_2. A review of the oxyhemoglobin dissociation curve [*see 7 Life-Threatening Acid-Base Disorders*] makes it clear why pushing P_aO_2 to levels higher than 100 mm Hg will not affect S_aO_2 appreciably and thus will have little impact on D_{O_2}. During initial resuscitation, a high fraction of inspired oxygen (F_IO_2) is administered, and pulse oximetry is used to assess S_aO_2. As a rule, a low S_aO_2 is easily treated by increasing the F_IO_2 further. Intubated patients who do not respond when the F_IO_2 is increased to 100% can be treated with low levels of positive end-expiratory pressure (PEEP) once adequate volume status is ensured.

The second important variable is the hemoglobin concentration. The initial hemoglobin level is notoriously misleading because the patients have not yet been volume loaded and because there has not been sufficient time for substantial flux of interstitial fluid into the intravascular space. The initial hemoglobin level is also problematic because of the lag time before the results come back from the laborato-

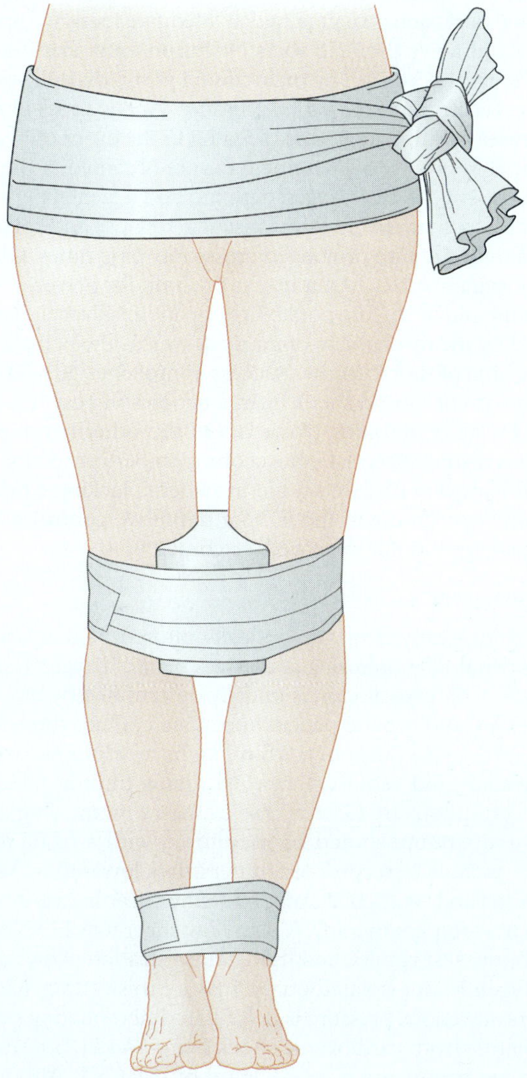

Figure 11 Shown is the wrapping technique currently used for mechanical support of the pelvis.

ry. Once recognized, a low hemoglobin level is easily treated with blood transfusion. Given the concerns just mentioned, however, early blood transfusion should be empirically administered in patients who arrive in severe class IV hemorrhagic shock or who have injuries associated with significant bleeding (e.g., vertical shear pelvic fracture or bilateral femur fractures), especially if they are elderly.

CO is the third important variable to consider. Unfortunately, it is difficult to monitor CO in the ED. Decreased preload is by far the most likely problem; consequently, empirical volume loading is recommended. When the patient is unresponsive, a central venous pressure reading can be helpful in differentiating persistent hypovolemia from cardiogenic shock. There is evidence to suggest that noninvasive monitoring of subcutaneous tissue perfusion status may be a valuable adjunct in assessing the adequacy of DO_2.[77]

BLOOD VOLUME RESTITUTION

During profound shock, fluid is lost from the intravascular as well as interstitial space because of sodium flux into the cellular compartment.[78] Crystalloid solutions, which rapidly equilibrate with the total extracellular space, are preferred.[79] Most authorities agree that albumin or artificial plasma expanders are no more effective in restoring tissue perfusion when adequate sodium is provided.[80,81] Moreover, they are costly and may aggravate posttraumatic complications. The type of crystalloid fluid used for initial volume replacement is of less importance. Lactated Ringer solution is theoretically preferred to normal saline because it provides a better buffer for metabolic acidosis of protracted shock.[82,83] The role of hypertonic saline continues to be investigated. There is some evidence to suggest that hypertonic saline may attenuate neutrophil-mediated injury.[84,85] Acute whole blood loss can be replaced initially with crystalloid because (1) this solution repletes the total extracellular space, (2) hemodilution enhances perfusion by means of reduced blood viscosity, and (3) increased CO and peripheral oxygen extraction provide adequate tissue oxygenation.[86] There is, of course, a limit to these compensatory mechanisms. With massive hemorrhage, the crystalloid replacement for blood may approach a ratio of 8:1 because of a progressive fall in plasma oncotic pressure and intracellular sequestration of sodium.[87] In general, blood should be added to fluid resuscitation when crystalloid infusion exceeds 50 ml/kg.[27,88] Diagnosis and management of shock, as well as the pathophysiology of the various shock states, is discussed in detail elsewhere [*see 4 Shock*].

Fully crossmatched blood is rarely available for emergency trauma resuscitation. Uncrossmatched type-specific whole blood or packed red blood cells can be safely administered[89,90] and are available in most hospitals within 20 minutes. If type-specific blood is unavailable, reconstituted O-negative packed red blood cells should be used. Type O-negative blood has no cellular antigens; therefore, the risk of major hemolytic reactions caused by patient antibodies attacking donor antigens is minimal. However, O-negative whole blood, the universal donor, is not considered safe, because its plasma contains anti-A and anti-B antibodies.[91] When O-negative packed cells are unavailable, the O-positive packed red blood cells may be used. The patient will become sensitized to the Rh factor, but this is significant only in women of childbearing age.

A 1994 clinical trial found that for hypotensive patients with penetrating torso injuries, survival improved when fluid resuscitation was delayed until surgical intervention had controlled the source of hemorrhage.[3] A subsequent subset analysis revealed that survival was improved only in patients who had sustained cardiac injuries and not in patients who had sustained major vascular, abdominal solid organ, and noncardiac thoracic injuries.[92] Although this clinical trial had some methodologic flaws, it is important for the appropriate emphasis it placed on source control of hemorrhage as an imperative priority. Whether resuscitation should be totally withheld until control of hemorrhage is achieved is doubtful; such an approach is clearly not the current standard of care.[15]

Animal studies using the traditional controlled hemorrhagic shock models have shown that if shock is allowed to persist for several hours, an irreversible shock state occurs from which the animals cannot be resuscitated.[93] On the other hand, more recent animal studies using uncontrolled hemorrhagic shock models with graded resuscitation have found that moderately resuscitated animals survive better than animals who receive either less aggressive or more aggressive resuscitation. A systolic pressure of 90 mm Hg may be acceptable, but the overriding priority must be timely surgical intervention. What this means in blunt trauma is not clear. If a non–head-injured patient arrives in class IV shock with a positive abdominal ultrasonogram, operative control of bleeding is the overriding priority. However, the possibility of a serious associated head injury frequently exists. The surgeon cannot determine whether the low Glasgow Coma Scale score is attributable to cerebral hypoperfusion or to intracranial pathology. If the brain is indeed injured, decreased perfusion pressure can produce secondary brain injury and worsen outcome.[94] Moreover, prehospital extrication and initial ED assessment times are longer with blunt trauma, and definitive con-

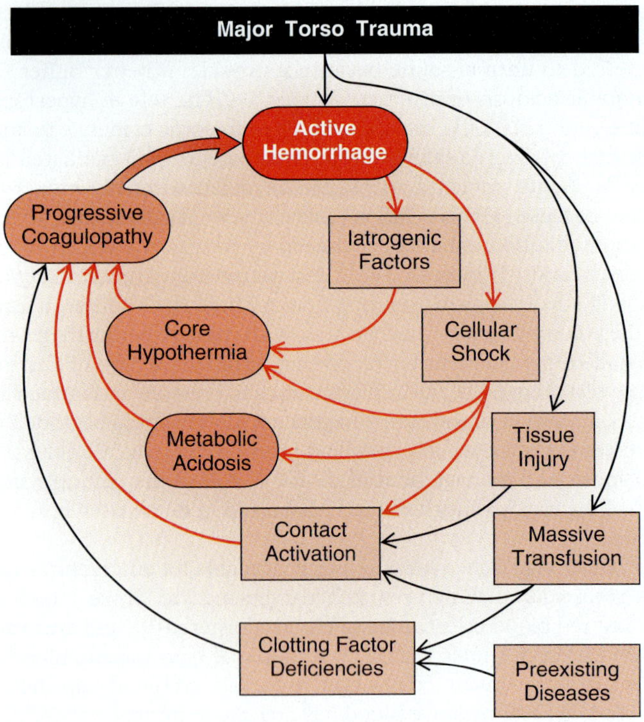

Figure 12 Illustrated is the so-called bloody vicious cycle. This syndrome has a multifactorial pathogenesis, with the usual manifestations including coagulopathy, hypothermia, and metabolic acidosis.[118]

trol of bleeding may take hours to orchestrate. Finally, for blunt trauma patients who survive early prolonged hypoperfusion, soft tissue injury combined with severe shock contributes to a high incidence of late multiple organ failure.[95]

Diverse clinical experience has substantiated the feasibility of autotransfusion, and in trauma, there has been increasing enthusiasm for its use in the ED as well as in the OR.[96] Autotransfusion clearly eliminates the infectious, allergic, and incompatibility problems of stored blood, an important concern because of the acquired immunodeficiency syndrome (AIDS). However, when large amounts of unprocessed collected blood are reinfused, a consumptive coagulopathy and platelet dysfunction occur.[97] These risks may outweigh the benefits of autotransfusion in the critically injured patient who has multiple potential bleeding sites.

Much attention has been directed toward production of a red blood cell substitute. Fluosol-DA, a perfluorocarbon, appeared promising,[98] but clinical trials failed to demonstrate an advantage over standard lactated Ringer solution, and animal studies clearly established an immunologic penalty.[99] Consequently, Fluosol-DA failed to receive the approval of the Food and Drug Administration. In contrast, progress has been made with hemoglobin-based blood substitutes, although tetrameric hemoglobin has been problematic.[71,100] Experience with human polymerized hemoglobin as a blood substitute after major surgical procedures suggests that this agent may be available for trauma resuscitation in the near future. Transfusion considerations are discussed in detail elsewhere [*see 5 Bleeding and Transfusion*].

EMERGENCY DEPARTMENT THORACOTOMY

ED thoracotomy is an integral part of the initial management of trauma patients who arrive in extremis.[33,101] With insufficient blood volume, open cardiac massage is superior to closed-chest compression in maintaining systemic blood flow[102]; coronary and cerebral perfusion is maintained at adequate levels for up to 30 minutes. Adjunctive thoracic aorta occlusion enhances both coronary and cerebral perfusion by maintaining aortic diastolic pressure and by increasing carotid systolic pressure. Aortic cross-clamping also decreases subdiaphragmatic bleeding in the event of associated abdominal injury.[103,104] These benefits are obtained at the expense of increased myocardial oxygen demand and a lack of perfusion to the lower torso. Irreversible cardiovascular collapse and splanchnic dysfunction occur with prolonged cross-clamping times. Clinical experience suggests that 30 minutes is the limit for prevention of serious ischemic sequelae. The possibility of patient salvage is largely determined by the mechanism of injury as well as the patient's condition at the time of thoracotomy. Success approaches 50% in patients arriving with profound shock from a penetrating cardiac wound and 20% for all penetrating wounds. On the other hand, patient outcome is dismal when ED thoracotomy is performed for blunt trauma; it is now considered futile in patients lacking cardiac activity. Adding laparotomy in the ED for definitive control of abdominal hemorrhage has not improved outcome.[105]

PHYSIOLOGIC MONITORING

It is imperative that the critically injured patient undergo early hemodynamic monitoring and assessment of oxygen transport. The adequacy of resuscitation is initially determined by blood pressure, pulse rate, and general patient appearance. Once these factors have stabilized, urine output (> 0.5 ml/kg/hr in adults) is used to gauge additional fluid requirements. All major trauma patients should have continuous ECG and pulse oximetry monitoring. In addition, core temperature should be monitored with a rectal temperature probe capable of recording temperatures lower than 32° C (89.6° F). Atrial and ventricular arrhythmias from cardiac contusion or ischemia may require therapy. A data flow sheet for physiologic indices, laboratory test results, and fluid administration allows quick analysis of trends, but isolated points may be misleading. Measurement of central venous pressure is helpful in differentiating persistent hypovolemia from cardiogenic shock [*see 4 Shock*], but several conditions can produce a false elevation of the CVP. Although arterial lines and pulmonary arterial catheters are of limited use in ED trauma management, they are important in the radiology suite, particularly if the patient requires beta blockade for a suspected torn aorta.[60] End-tidal CO_2 monitoring should be available for patients undergoing emergency endotracheal intubation.

COAGULOPATHY

The most devastating complication of massive blood and fluid resuscitation is a bleeding diathesis. Paradoxically, although clotting is accelerated at the capillary level because of shock and tissue damage,[106] the circulating blood becomes hypocoagulable.[107,108] The pathogenesis of bloody vicious cycle is complex [*see Figure 12*]. Factors predictive of a severe coagulopathic state (i.e., prothrombin time [PT] > 2 times normal and partial thromboplastin time [PTT] > 2 times normal) include (1) massive rapid blood transfusion (10 units/4 hr), (2) persistent cellular shock (oxygen consumption index < 110 ml/min/m², lactate concentration > 5 mmol/L), (3) progressive metabolic acidosis (pH < 7.20, base deficit > 14 mEq/L), and (4) refractory core hypothermia (< 34° C).[109] The extent of tissue disruption (as quantitated by the Injury Severity Score) is not a strong independent risk factor; however, it clearly is a facilitating event.

Stored blood is deficient in factors V and VIII and platelets and replete with fibrin split products and vasoactive substances. Timely administration of fresh frozen plasma and platelets will minimize the risk of coagulopathy after massive transfusion [*see 5 Bleeding and*

Transfusion]. Although blood components are not usually indicated in the early resuscitation phase, they may be appropriate in patients with massive hemorrhage caused by pelvic fracture.

Germane to the initial period of massive blood transfusion are the potential complications of hypocalcemia, acidosis, and hypothermia. Hypocalcemia caused by citrate binding of ionized calcium does not occur until the blood transfusion rate exceeds 100 ml/min (1 U/5 min). Decreased serum levels of ionized calcium depress myocardial function before impairing coagulation.[110,111] Calcium gluconate (10 mg/kg I.V.) should be reserved for cases in which there is ECG evidence of ST interval prolongation or, rarely, for cases of unexplained hypotension during massive transfusion. Moderate hypothermia (< 32° C) causes platelet sequestration and inhibits the release of platelet factors that are important in the intrinsic clotting pathway.[39] In addition, moderate hypothermia has consistently been associated with poor outcome in trauma patients.[112] Core temperature often falls insidiously because of exposure at the scene and in the ED and because of administration of resuscitation fluids stored at ambient temperature. The first step is to prevent further heat loss by covering the body (including the head) and infusing warm blood and fluid. Another simple technique is to heat and aerosolize ventilator gases. Active external rewarming with heating blankets and increased room temperature should also be used. However, it is important to note that the above techniques are not very effective in reversing established hypothermia. In this setting, lavage of the abdominal or chest cavities can increase core temperature at a rate of 1° to 2° C an hour. Recently, Gentilello and others have introduced relatively simple extracorporeal techniques that can increase core temperature at a rate of 2° to 5° C an hour.[113] Whether these rapid rewarming techniques improve patient outcome is currently being investigated.

The use of bicarbonate in the treatment of systemic acidosis remains controversial. Moderate acidosis (pH < 7.20) impairs coagulation,[114] myocardial contractility,[115] and oxidative metabolism.[116] Acidosis in the trauma patient is caused primarily by a rise in lactic acid production secondary to tissue hypoxia and will usually resolve when the volume deficit has been corrected [*see 7 Life-Threatening Acid-Base Disorders*]. Administration of sodium bicarbonate may cause a leftward shift of the oxyhemoglobin dissociation curve, reducing tissue oxygen extraction, and it may worsen intracellular acidosis caused by carbon dioxide production.[117] Bicarbonate infusion, therefore, should be limited to persons with protracted shock. Patients in shock should be ventilated on 100% oxygen; thus, blood gases obtained from a central venous line are clinically useful in the assessment of acid-base status. Blood gases should be corrected for core body temperature; pH should be increased by 0.15 for every 1° C drop below normal.

References

1. Eisenberg MS, Bergner L, Hallstrom A: Cardiac resuscitation in the community: importance of rapid provision and implications for program planning. JAMA 241:1905, 1979
2. Copass MK, Oreskovich MR, Baldergroen MR, et al: Prehospital cardiopulmonary resuscitation of the critically injured patient. Am J Surg 148:20, 1984
3. Bickell WH, Wall MJ Jr, Pepe PE, et al: Immediate versus delayed fluid resuscitation for hypotensive patients with penetrating torso injuries. N Engl J Med 331:1105, 1994
4. Soucy DM, Rude M, Hsrg WC, et al: The effects of varying fluid volume and rate of resuscitation during uncontrolled hemorrhage. J Trauma 46:209, 1999
5. Burris D, Rhee P, Kaufman C, et al: Controlled resuscitation for uncontrolled hemorrhagic shock. J Trauma 46:216, 1999
6. Mattox KL, Bickell WH, Pepe PE, et al: Prospective randomized evaluation of antishock MAST in posttraumatic hypotension. J Trauma 26:779, 1986
7. Capone AC, Safar P, Stezoski W, et al: Improved outcome with fluid restriction in treatment of uncontrolled hemorrhagic shock. J Am Coll Surg 180:49, 1995
8. Kowalenko T, Stern S, Dronen S, et al: Improved outcome with hypotensive resuscitation of uncontrolled hemorrhagic shock in a swine model. J Trauma 33:349, 1992
9. Cayten CG, Berendt BM, Byrne DW, et al: A study of pneumatic antishock garments in severely hypotensive trauma patients. J Trauma 34:728, 1993
10. Domerer RM, O'Conner, Delbridge TR, et al: National Association of EMS Physicians, Position Paper: Use of the pneumatic anti-shock garment (PASG). Prehosp Emerg Care 1:32, 1997
11. Aprahamian C, Thompson BM, Towne JB, et al: The effects of a paramedic system on mortality of major open intra-abdominal vascular trauma. J Trauma 23:687, 1983
12. Jacobs LM, Sinclair A, Beiser A, et al: Prehospital advanced life support: benefits in trauma. J Trauma 24:8, 1984
13. Pons PT, Honigman B, Moore EE, et al: Prehospital advanced trauma life support for critical penetrating wounds to the thorax and abdomen. J Trauma 25:828, 1985
14. Hoyt DB, Mikulaschek AW, Winchel RJ: Trauma triage and interhospital transfer. Trauma, 4th ed. Mattox KL, Feliciano DV, Moore EE, Eds. McGraw-Hill, New York, 2000
15. Committee on Trauma, American College of Surgeons: Advanced Trauma Life Support Manual. American College of Surgeons, Chicago, 1981
16. Ducker TB, Russo GL, Bellegarrique R, et al: Complete sensorimotor paralysis after cord injury: mortality, recovery, and therapeutic implications. J Trauma 19:837, 1979
17. Bohn D, Armstrong D, Becker L, et al: Cervical spine injuries in children. J Trauma 30:463, 1990
18. Pang D, Pollack IF: Spinal cord injury without radiographic abnormality in children—the SCIWORA syndrome. J Trauma 29:654, 1989
19. Roth BJ, Martin RR: Roentgenographic evaluation of the cervical spine: a selective approach. Arch Surg 129:643, 1994
20. Shaffer MA, Doris PE: Limitation of the cross table lateral view in detecting cervical spine injuries: a retrospective analysis. Ann Emerg Med 10:508, 1981
21. Robinson RJS, Mulder DS: Airway control. Trauma, 4th ed. Mattox KL, Feliciano DV, Moore EE, Eds. McGraw-Hill, New York, 2000
22. Jorden RC, Moore EE, Marx JA, et al: A comparison of PTV and endotracheal ventilation in an acute trauma model. J Trauma 25:978, 1985
23. Norwood S, Myers MB, Butler TJ: The safety of emergency neuromuscular blockade and orotracheal intubation in the acutely injured trauma patient. J Am Coll Surg 179:646, 1994
24. Vijayakumar E, Bosscher H: The use of neuromuscular blocking agents in the Emergency Department to facilitate tracheal intubation in the trauma patient: help or hindrance? J Crit Care 13:1, 1998
25. Sawyer RW, Bodai BI, Blaisdell FW, et al: The current status of intraosseous infusion. J Am Coll Surg 179:353, 1994
26. Vayer JS, Henderson JV, Bellamy RF, et al: Absence of a tachycardic response to shock in penetrating intraperitoneal injury. Ann Emerg Med 17:227, 1988
27. Rush BF Jr, Richardson JD, Bosomworth P, et al: Limitations of blood replacement with electrolyte solutions: a controlled clinical study. Arch Surg 98:49, 1969
28. Durtschi MB, Haisch CE, Reynolds L, et al: Effect of micropore filtration on pulmonary function after massive transfusion. Am J Surg 138:8, 1979
29. Rozycki GS, Ochsner MG, Jaffin JH, et al: Prospective evaluation of surgeon's use of ultrasound in the evaluation of trauma patients. J Trauma 34:516, 1993
30. Rozycki GS, Feliciano DV, Ochsner MG, et al: The role of ultrasound in patients with possible penetrating cardiac wounds: a prospective multicenter study. J Trauma 46:543, 1999
31. Breaux EP, Dupont JB Jr, Albert HM, et al: Cardiac tamponade following penetrating mediastinal injuries: improved survival with early pericardiocentesis. J Trauma 19:361, 1979
32. Plummer D, Brunette D, Asinger R, et al: Emergency department echocardiography improves outcome in penetrating cardiac injury. Ann Emerg Med 21:709, 1992
33. Biffl WL, Moore EE, Harken AH: Emergency department thoracotomy. Trauma, 4th ed. Mattox KL, Feliciano DV, Moore EE, Eds. McGraw-Hill, New York, 2000
34. Biffl WL, Moore FA, Moore EE, et al: Cardiac enzymes are irrelevant in the patient with suspected myocardial contusion. Am J Surg 169:523, 1994
35. Illig KA, Swierzewski MJ, Feliciano DV, et al: A rational screening and treatment strategy based on the electrocardiogram alone for suspected cardiac contusion. Am J Surg 162:537, 1991
36. King MW, Aitchison JM, Nel JP: Fatal air embolism following penetrating lung trauma: an autopsy study. J Trauma 24:753, 1984
37. Fremstad JD, Martin SH: Lethal complication from insertion of nasogastric tube after severe basilar skull fracture. J Trauma 18:820, 1978

38. Gentilello LM: Temperature-associated injuries and syndromes. Trauma, 4th ed. Mattox KL, Feliciano DV, Moore EE, Eds. McGraw-Hill, New York, 2000
39. Patt A, McCroskey BL, Moore EE: Hypothermia induced coagulopathies in trauma. Surg Clin North Am 68:775, 1988
40. Reed RL II, Bracey AW Jr, Hudson JD, et al: Hypothermia and blood coagulation: dissociation between enzyme activity and clotting factor levels. Circ Shock 32:141, 1990
41. Davis JW, Kaups KL: Base deficit in the elderly: a marker of severe injury and death. J Trauma 45:873, 1998
42. Thompson JS, Moore EE, Van Duzer-Moore S, et al: The evolution of abdominal stab wound management. J Trauma 20:478, 1980
43. Moore EE, Moore JB, Van Duzer-Moore S, et al: Mandatory laparotomy for gunshot wounds penetrating the abdomen. Am J Surg 140:847, 1980
44. Marx JA, Moore EE, Jorden RC, et al: Limitations of computed tomography in the evaluation of acute abdominal trauma: a prospective comparison with diagnostic peritoneal lavage. J Trauma 25:933, 1985
45. Fabian TC, Mangiante EC, White TJ, et al: A prospective study of 91 patients undergoing both computed tomography and peritoneal lavage following blunt abdominal trauma. J Trauma 26:602, 1986
46. Feliciano DV, Bitondo-Dyer CG: Vagaries of the lavage white blood cell count in evaluating abdominal stab wounds. Am J Surg 168:680, 1994
47. Jacobs DG, Angus A, Rodriguez A, et al: Peritoneal lavage white count: a reassessment. J Trauma 30:607, 1990
48. McAnena OJ, Marx JA, Moore EE: Peritoneal lavage enzyme determinations following blunt and penetrating abdominal trauma. J Trauma 31:1161, 1991
49. Moore JB, Moore EE, Thompson JS: Abdominal injuries associated with penetrating trauma in the lower chest. Am J Surg 140:724, 1980
50. Uribe RA, Pachon CE, Frame SB, et al: A prospective evaluation of thoracoscopy for the diagnosis of penetrating thoracoabdominal trauma. J Trauma 37:650, 1994
51. McAllister E, Perez M, Albrink MH, et al: Is triple contrast computed tomographic scanning useful in the selective management of stab wounds to the back? J Trauma 37:401, 1994
52. Easter DW, Shackford SR, Mattrey RF: A prospective, randomized comparison of computed tomography with conventional diagnostic methods in the evaluation of penetrating injuries to the back and flank. Arch Surg 126:1115, 1991
53. Burgess AR, Eastridge BJ, Young JWR, et al: Pelvic ring disruptions: effective classification system and treatment protocols. J Trauma 30:848, 1990
54. Cryer HM, Miller FB, Evers BM, et al: Pelvic fracture classification: correlation with hemorrhage. J Trauma 28:973, 1988
55. Latenser BA, Gentilello LM, Tarver AA, et al: Improved outcome with early fixation of skeletally unstable pelvic fractures. J Trauma 31:28, 1991
56. Riemer BL, Butterfield SL, Diamond DL, et al: Acute mortality associated with injuries to the pelvic ring: the role of early patient mobilization and external fixation. J Trauma 35:671, 1993
57. Moreno C, Moore EE, Rosenberger A, et al: Hemorrhage associated with major pelvic fracture: a multispecialty challenge. J Trauma 26:987, 1986
58. Panetta T, Sclafani SJA, Goldstein AS, et al: Percutaneous transcatheter embolization for massive bleeding from pelvic fractures. J Trauma 25:1021, 1985
59. Harris JH, Horowitz DR, Zelitt DL: Unenhanced dynamic mediastinal computed tomography in the selection of patients requiring aortography for detection of acute traumatic aortic injury. Emerg Radiol 2:67, 1995
60. Fabian TC, Davis KA, Gavant ML, et al: Prospective study of blunt aortic injury: helical CT is diagnostic and antihypertensive therapy reduces rupture. Ann Surg 227:666, 1998
61. Lombardi G, Gallagher EJ, Gennis P: Outcome of out-of-hospital cardiac arrest in New York City. JAMA 271:678, 1994
62. Messer JV: Management of emergencies: XIV. Cardiac arrest. N Engl J Med 275:35, 1966
63. Roth R, Stewart RD, Rogers K, et al: Out-of-hospital cardiac arrest: factors associated with survival. Ann Emerg Med 13:237, 1984
64. DeBard ML: Cardiopulmonary resuscitation: analysis of six years' experience and review of the literature. Ann Emerg Med 10:408, 1981
65. Pons PT, Moore EE, Cusick JM, et al: Prehospital venous access in an urban paramedic system: a prospective on-scene analysis. J Trauma 28:1460, 1988
66. Kramer GC, Perron PR, Lindsey DC, et al: Small-volume resuscitation with hypertonic saline dextran solution. Surgery 100:239, 1986
67. Mattox KL, Maningas PA, Moore EE, et al: Prehospital hypertonic saline/dextran infusion for post-traumatic hypotension. Ann Surg 213:482, 1991
68. Younes RN, Aun F, Accioly CQ, et al: Hypertonic solutions in the treatment of hypovolemic shock: a prospective, randomized study in patients admitted to the emergency room. Surgery 111:380, 1992
69. Vassar MJ, Fischer RP, O'Brien PE, et al: A multicenter trial for resuscitation of injured patients with 7.5% sodium chloride. Arch Surg 128:1003, 1993
70. Shackford SR, Schmoker JD, Zhuang J: The effect of hypertonic resuscitation on pial arteriolar tone after brain injury and shock. J Trauma 37:899, 1994
71. Gould SA, Moore EE, Holt D, et al: The first randomized trial of human polymerized hemoglobin as a blood substitute in acute trauma and emergency surgery. J Am Coll Surg 187:113, 1998
72. Aprahamian C, Thompson BM, Finger WA, et al: Experimental cervical spine injury model: evaluation of airway management and splinting techniques. Ann Emerg Med 13:584, 1984
73. Bucholz RW, Burkhead WZ, Graham W, et al: Occult cervical spine injuries in fatal traffic accidents. J Trauma 19:768, 1979
74. Davis D, Bohlman H, Walker AE, et al: The pathological findings in fatal craniospinal injuries. J Neurosurg 34:603, 1971
75. Moore FA, Haenel JB, Moore EE, et al: Percutaneous tracheostomy/gastrostomy in brain-injured patients: a minimally invasive alternative. J Trauma 33:435, 1992
76. Gaffney FA, Thal ER, Taylor WF, et al: Hemodynamic effects of medical anti-shock trousers (MAST garment). J Trauma 21:931, 1981
77. McKinley BA, Marvin RG, Cocanour CS, et al: Tissue hemoglobin O_2 saturation during resuscitation of traumatic shock monitored using near infrared spectometry. J Trauma 48:637, 2000
78. Shires GT, Cunningham JN, Backer CR, et al: Alterations in cellular membrane function during hemorrhagic shock in primates. Ann Surg 176:288, 1972
79. Shires GT, Canizaro PC: Fluid resuscitation in the severely injured. Surg Clin North Am 53:1341, 1973
80. Cochrane Injuries Group Albumin Reviewers: Human albumin administration in critically ill patients: systematic review of randomised controlled trials. BMJ 317:235, 1998
81. Choi PT-L, Yip G, Quinonez LF, et al: Crystalloids vs. colloids in fluid resuscitation: a systematic review. Crit Care Med 27:200, 1999
82. Trinkle JK, Rush BF, Eiseman B: Metabolism of lactate following major blood loss. Surgery 63:782, 1968
83. Healey MA, Davis RE, Liu FC, et al: Lactated Ringer's is superior to normal saline in a model of massive hemorrhage and resuscitation. J Trauma 45:894, 1998
84. Ciesla DJ, Moore EE, Gonzalez R, et al: Hypertonic saline inhibits neutrophil (PMN) priming via attenuation of p38 MAPK signaling. Shock 14:265, 2000
85. Rhee P, Wang D, Ruff P, et al: Human neutrophil activation and increased adhesion by various resuscitation fluids. Crit Care Med 28:74, 2000
86. Moore FD, Dagher FJ, Boyden CM, et al: Hemorrhage in normal man: I. Distribution and dispersal of saline infusions following acute blood loss: clinical kinetics of blood volume support. Ann Surg 163:485, 1966
87. Cervera AL, Moss G: Progressive hypovolemia leading to shock after continuous hemorrhage and 3:1 crystalloid replacement. Am J Surg 129:670, 1975
88. Mann DV, Robinson MK, Rounds JD, et al: Superiority of blood over saline resuscitation from hemorrhagic shock: a ^{31}P magnetic resonance spectroscopy study. Ann Surg 226:653, 1997
89. Blumberg N, Bove JR: Un–cross-matched blood for emergency transfusion: one year's experience in a civilian setting. JAMA 240:2057, 1978
90. Gervin AS, Fischer RP: Resuscitation of trauma patients with type-specific uncrossmatched blood. J Trauma 24:327, 1984
91. Barnes A Jr, Allen TE: Transfusions subsequent to administration of universal donor blood in Vietnam. JAMA 203:695, 1968
92. Wall MJ, Granchi T, Liscum K, et al: Delayed versus immediate resuscitation in patients with penetrating trauma: subgroup analysis. J Trauma 39:173, 1995
93. Wiggers CJ: Physiology of Shock. Commonwealth Publications, New York, 1950
94. Rosner MJ, Daughton S: Cerebral perfusion pressure management in head injury. J Trauma 30:933, 1990
95. Sauaia AJ, Moore FA, Moore EE, et al: Multiple organ failure can be predicted as early as 12 hrs postinjury. J Trauma 45:291, 1998
96. Jurkovich GJ, Moore EE, Medina G: Auto-transfusion in trauma: a pragmatic analysis. Am J Surg 148:782, 1984
97. Silva R, Moore EE, Bar-Or D, et al: The risk:benefit of autotransfusion—comparison to banked blood in a canine model. J Trauma 24:557, 1984
98. Tremper KK, Friedman AE, Levine EM, et al: The preoperative treatment of severely anemic patients with a perfluorochemical oxygen-transport fluid, Fluosol-DA. N Engl J Med 314:1653, 1986
99. Gould SA, Rosen AL, Lakshman RS, et al: Fluosol-DA as a red-cell substitute in acute anemia. N Engl J Med 314:1653, 1986
100. Sloan EP, Koenigsberg M, et al: Diaspirin cross-linked hemoglobin (DCLHb) in the treatment of severe traumatic hemorrhagic shock: a randomized controlled efficacy trial. JAMA 282:1857, 1999
101. Rhee PM, Acosta J, Bridgeman A, et al: Survival after emergency department thoracotomy: review of published data from the past 25 years. J Am Coll Surg 190:288, 2000
102. Sanders AB, Kern KB, Ewy GA, et al: Improved resuscitation from cardiac arrest with open-chest massage. Ann Emerg Med 13:672, 1984
103. Ledgerwood AM, Kazmers M, Lucas CE: The role of thoracic aortic occlusion for massive hemoperitoneum. J Trauma 16:610, 1976
104. Millikan JS, Moore EE: Outcome of resuscitative thoracotomy and descending aortic occlusion performed in the operating room. J Trauma 24:387, 1984
105. Mattox KL, Allen MK, Feliciano DV: Laparotomy in the emergency department. JACEP 8:180, 1979
106. Hardaway RM, Chun B, Rutherford RB: Coagulation in shock in various species including man. Acta Chir Scand 130:157, 1965
107. Collins JA: Problems associated with the massive transfusion of stored blood. Surgery 75:274, 1974
108. Miller RD, Robbins TO, Tong MJ, et al: Coagulation defects associated with massive blood transfusions. Ann Surg 174:794, 1971
109. Cosgriff N, Moore EE, Sauaia A, et al: Predicting life-threatening coagulopathy in the massively transfused trauma patient: hypothermia and acidoses revisited. J Trauma 42:857, 1997

110. Stulz PM, Scheidegger D, Drop LJ, et al: Ventricular pump performance during hypocalcemia: clinical and experimental studies. J Thorac Cardiovasc Surg 78:185, 1979
111. Trunkey D, Carpenter MA, Holcroft J: Calcium flux during hemorrhagic shock in baboons. J Trauma 16:633, 1976
112. Jurkovich GJ, Greiser WB, Luterman A, et al: Hypothermia in trauma victims: an ominous predictor of survival. J Trauma 27:1019, 1987
113. Gentilello LM, Jurkovich GJ, Maier R, et al: Is hypothermia in the victim of major trauma protective or harmful? a randomized prospective study. Ann Surg 226:439, 1997
114. Dunn EL, Moore EE, Breslich DJ, et al: Acidosis-induced coagulopathy. Forum on Fundamental Surgical Problems 30:471, 1979
115. Clowes GHA Jr, Sabga GH, Konitaxis A, et al: Effects of acidosis on cardiovascular function in surgical patients. Ann Surg 154:524, 1961
116. Fry DE, Ratcliffe DJ, Yates JR: The effects of acidosis on canine hepatic and renal oxidative phosphorylation. Surgery 88:269, 1980
117. Douglas ME, Downs JB, Mantini EL, et al: Alteration of oxygen tension and oxyhemoglobin saturation: a hazard of sodium bicarbonate administration. Arch Surg 114:326, 1979
118. Moore EE: Thomas G. Orr Memorial Lecture. Staged laparotomy for the hypothermia, acidosis, and coagulopathy syndrome. Am J Surg 172:405, 1996

Acknowledgments

Figures 2 and 6   Carol Donner, revised by Tom Moore.
Figures 3, 5, 7a, 7b, and 9   Carol Donner.
Figures 7c, 8, and 11   Tom Moore.
Figure 12   Seward Hung.

3 BURN CARE IN THE IMMEDIATE RESUSCITATION PERIOD

Robert H. Demling, M.D.

Approach to the Burn Patient in the First 24 Hours

Neutralization of the Source of the Burn

CLOTHING

The first objective is to stop the burning process because the deeper the burn, the greater the potential for mortality and morbidity. With chemical burns, chemicals can remain in fabric and on skin for long periods. With a flame or scald burn, clothing can retain heat for a considerable time. Rapid removal of clothing is thus essential. Clothes are often still smoldering when the patient arrives at the emergency room. If clothing is burned or melted into the tissues, the surrounding fabric can be cut off. Adherent clothing can be removed after admission, when further wound cleaning and debridement are performed.

CHEMICAL BURNS

Removal of the chemical is urgent. Acid burns should be irrigated for up to 60 minutes with warm tap water. For burns resulting from alkali contact, lavage for at least 60 minutes may be beneficial [*see Table 1*]. If necessary, particles of corrosive powders should be surgically removed before the wound is irrigated. The skin burn itself is not the only concern, because the absorption of certain chemicals can lead to systemic toxicities such as neurologic dysfunction, red cell hemolysis, and liver and kidney failure.

It is important to avoid severe hypothermia during irrigation because hypothermia results in significant morbidity. Therefore, once the burn source is removed, the patient should be covered with clean, dry dressings or sheets.

Establishment of Airway and Adequate Ventilation

DIAGNOSIS AND TREATMENT OF CARBON MONOXIDE TOXICITY

Carbon monoxide toxicity is one of the leading causes of death associated with fires. As oxygen is being consumed in the process of combustion, CO is being released. Carbon monoxide is rapidly transported across the alveolar membrane and preferentially binds to hemoglobin in place of oxygen to form carboxyhemoglobin (COHb). In addition, CO causes the oxyhemoglobin dissociation curve to shift to the left, thereby impairing oxygen unloading at the tissue level; this shift results in a substantial reduction in oxygen delivery, given that 98% of the oxygen supplied to the tissues comes bound to hemoglobin. With prolonged exposure, CO can saturate the cell, binding to cytochrome oxidase and thereby further impairing mitochondrial function and adenosine triphosphate (ATP) production.

Patients who were injured in a closed space or who have inhalation injuries should be suspected of inhaling CO [*see Table 2*]. CO toxicity is determined by a high index of suspicion and by measuring the COHb level. Persistent metabolic acidosis in a patient with adequate volume resuscitation and adequate cardiac output indicates persistent impairment of oxygen utilization and delivery by CO or hydrocyanide. The chemical alteration of hemoglobin or of the cytochrome system by CO will not affect the amount of oxygen dissolved in plasma, and arterial oxygen tension (P_aO_2) will thus remain relatively normal. However, the measured oxygen saturation of hemoglobin will be markedly decreased relative to the oxygen tension.

Treatment of CO toxicity consists of promptly displacing CO from hemoglobin by administering 90% to 100% oxygen until the COHb level is less than 7%. If 20% oxygen is administered, the half-life of COHb is about 90 minutes; if concentrated high-flow oxygen is administered, the half-life is 20 to 30 minutes. The concentration of COHb is thus reduced by approximately 50% every 20 to 30 minutes if an oxygen concentration of 90% to 100% is used. Hyperbaric oxygen (2 to 3 atm) yields even more rapid displacement, particularly from the cell cytochrome system, and can be used to treat severe CO toxicity (i.e., a CO level > 50% or an elevated CO level that does not respond to standard oxygen therapy).

DIAGNOSIS AND TREATMENT OF CYANIDE TOXICITY

Hydrocyanide, the gaseous form of cyanide, is a well-recognized cause of fire-associated morbidity and mortality, particularly when synthetics such as

```
┌─────────────────────────────────────────┐
│ Patient presents with burn              │
├─────────────────────────────────────────┤
│ Neutralize the burn source: remove      │
│ clothing and chemicals.                 │
│ Irrigate acid and alkali burns.         │
│ Continue wet dressings only in 2° burns │
│ < 15% TBS.                              │
│ Avoid hypothermia at all times.         │
└─────────────────────────────────────────┘
```

1. Establish and maintain airway and adequate ventilation

- Patient is conscious,
- No airway or ventilation problems, *and*
- No deep facial burn

Give 100% O_2 by mask.
Obtain blood gases, COHb levels, cyanide levels.

COHb is normal

Give O_2 to maintain O_2 sat. > 90%.
Monitor for pulmonary problems.

COHb ↑

Give O_2 until COHb < 7%.
If COHb > 40%, intubate and use PEEP.
Reserve hyperbaria for most severe cases.

Cyanide ↑

Give sodium nitrite, followed by sodium thiosulfate.

One of the following is present:
- Unconsciousness
- Deep facial burn
- Hypoventilation
- Hypoxia on mask O_2

Secure airway (use tube ≥ 7 mm).
Diagnose and treat ↑ COHb.
Begin CPAP or PEEP at 5 cm H_2O; ↑ to maintain O_2 sat. > 90%.
Assess lower airways.
Obtain baseline chest x-ray.

Ventilation is inadequate

Consider bronchodilators for airway spasm.
Chest wall burn present?
- Circumferential 3°: perform escharotomy
- Noncircumferential: monitor closely; perform escharotomy on symptoms of restriction

Begin standard Rx for smoke exposure

Maintain
- Aggressive pulmonary toilet
- Close monitoring of gas exchange
- Controlled fluid Rx
- Airway assessment

Do not use prophylactic corticosteroids.

Approach to the Burn Patient in the First 24 Hours

2. Establish and maintain adequate circulation

Burns > 20% TBS

Begin administration of lactated Ringer solution
Estimate initial rate according to % TBS burned and weight.

Maintain
- BP > 90 mm Hg systolic
- Urine output 0.5–1.0 ml/kg/hr
- Pulse < 130 beats/min
- T° ≥ 37° C

Modify protocol in the presence of massive burns, inhalation injury, or shock and in elderly patients

Include hypertonic lactated saline (first 8–10 hr) or colloid.
Consider inotrope if fluid alone is inadequate (low-dose dopamine is first choice).
Use pulse oximeter (ideal for measuring O_2 sat.).
Add arterial line to monitor BP and blood gases.
Monitor cardiac output, PAWP, mixed venous P_{O_2} with pulmonary arterial line in the presence of
- heart disease, or
- persistent hemodynamic instability, or
- inotrope administration.

3. Initiate wound management

Determine extent of injury

Estimate depth.
Estimate area, using Rule of Nines.
Consider risk factors: age, inhalation injury, trauma, concomitant illness.

Follow ACS guidelines for tetanus prophylaxis

Maintain perfusion

Elevate burned extremities.
Remove constricting items.
Monitor distal perfusion; perform escharotomy if necessary.

Control pain with frequent small doses of I.V. narcotics

Clean the wound

Use chlorhexidine in warm solution.
Avoid body immersion.
Debride loose tissue and dirt; spare large blisters, hands, and feet.

Dress the wound

Superficial 2° burn

Face or neck: Apply bacitracin t.i.d. No dressing.
Extremities or flat surfaces: Temporary skin substitute or grease gauze dressing. Second choice: topical antibiotics.
Perineum or buttocks; gross contamination anywhere: Silver sulfadiazine b.i.d. with or without dressings.

Medium to deep 2° burn

Apply silver sulfadiazine, with dressings in most areas.
Change b.i.d. or t.i.d.

3° burn

Dressings preferred in most areas.
Uninfected wound: Use silver sulfadiazine b.i.d.
Infected wound: Use mafenide b.i.d.

polyurethane are burned. Although cyanide can be absorbed through the GI tract or through skin, it is most dangerous when aerosolized and inhaled because it is absorbed especially rapidly through the respiratory tract. Once absorbed, cyanide binds to the cytochrome system, thereby inhibiting cell metabolism and ATP production. All cells, and hepatocytes in particular, have a detoxifying system in which the enzyme rhodenase converts hydrocyanide to thiocyanate, which is then excreted in the urine. If, however, a large amount of cyanide is absorbed, this protective system can be overwhelmed, especially in the face of hypovolemia, which hinders metabolism and clearance of cyanide.

The diagnosis of cyanide toxicity is made on the basis of the history and a high index of suspicion and is confirmed by the presence of elevated blood cyanide levels (normal, < 0.1 mg/L; values higher than 1 mg/L are usually lethal). Treatment begins with volume replenishment. From 10 to 20 ml of a 3% sodium nitrite solution is then given over a period of 10 minutes; methemoglobin is produced as the cyanide is detoxified. Finally, 50 ml of a 25% solution of sodium thiosulfate is given; this converts the cyanide to sodium thiocyanate, which is excreted in the urine.

DIAGNOSIS OF THE PRESENCE AND EXTENT OF INHALATION INJURY

Inhalation injury, a complex and deadly disease process, occurs when the heat and toxins in smoke make contact with airway mucosa and alveoli. The degree of injury depends on the composition of the smoke, which varies according to its source. Heat affects primarily the supraglottic area and causes edema and upper airway obstruction, whereas the gas and particle components of the smoke affect primarily the airway mucosa and cause the actual chemical burn. The initial smoke injury occurs shortly after exposure, but the ensuing intense inflammatory reaction evolves over a period of hours to days [see Figure 1]. The degree of mucosal damage can range from simple erythema and irritation to complete mucosal sloughing that leads to distal airway obstruction and subsequently to atelectasis and increased shunting. Alveolar instability can also occur as a result of direct surfactant denaturation. Alveolar edema is a late finding.

Table 1 Chemical Burns

Agent	Pathophysiology	Treatment
Acids	Acids cause deep skin burns through tissue desiccation and protein denaturation; with concentrated acids, injury may extend well below skin. Acids such as H_2SO_4, HCl, and HNO_3 cause local damage. Burned area is tan to gray in appearance; extreme pain is a common finding. *Hydrofluoric acid:* Hydrofluoric acid causes a deep skin burn that may be extensive. It also exerts systemic effects, which are attributable to hypocalcemia resulting from the formation of a Ca^{2+}-F^- complex.	Perform vigorous water lavage for as long as 60 min after injury; use warm water with extensive exposure to prevent hypothermia. Assume that the burn will be much deeper than initial appearance indicates. Apply standard fluid resuscitation principles. *Hydrofluoric acid:* Perform vigorous water lavage. Inject calcium gluconate locally, and apply 2.5% calcium gluconate gel topically; end point of calcium gluconate administration is relief of pain. Monitor plasma calcium levels, and replace calcium deficits if necessary.
Alkalies	Alkalies cause deep skin burns through tissue desiccation and protein denaturation resulting from chemical reaction with hydrated tissue. Alkali burns tend to be worse than acid burns, but alkalies tend not to be absorbed systemically and thus rarely exert systemic effects. The burned area is tan to gray; extreme pain is a characteristic finding.	Perform vigorous water lavage for at least 60 min after injury—longer for lye burns—and take pains to prevent hypothermia. Assume that the burn will increase in depth. Apply standard fluid resuscitation principles.
Gasoline	Gasoline immersion produces both superficial skin injury and systemic injury (resulting from absorption of hydrocarbons). The systemic injury comprises the following: *Renal injury:* lipid degenerative changes to proximal tubules *Pulmonary injury:* surfactant denaturation, atelectasis, lipoid pneumonia *CNS injury:* edema producing seizures or coma *Hepatic injury:* lipid degenerative changes, hepatitis Burned area is erythematous in appearance.	Immerse injured area in water. Aggressively maintain hydration and pulmonary support, and provide general critical care support.
Phenol	Phenol produces both a partial-thickness burn and systemic injury (resulting from absorption), which is directly proportional to amount of skin exposed. The systemic injury comprises the following: *Renal injury:* direct glomerular and tubular damage as well as indirect damage from precipitated hemoglobin *Hematologic injury:* red cell hemolysis *CNS injury:* seizures or coma *Hepatic injury:* centrolobular necrosis Burned area is dull tan to gray in appearance.	Spray or pour large amounts of water on burned surface. Do not swab or use small amounts of water; these actions serve only to increase surface area of exposure. After lavage, quickly wipe skin with polyethylene or propylene glycol. To minimize hemoglobin precipitation, keep urine alkaline by administering bicarbonate. Maintain optimal hydration and blood volume to support injured kidney and any other injured organs.
Tar	Hot tar causes a superficial to deep skin burn, depending on the temperature of the tar when it contacts the skin. As a rule, there is no systemic absorption.	Remove tar to allow burn wound management. Bacitracin ointment and Neosporin (polymyxin B–bacitracin–neomycin) ointment contain the emulsifier Tween-80, which is very useful for dissolving tar. Apply the ointment and wash it off several times a day until tar is removed. Avoid hydrocarbon solvents. Perform general mechanical debridement if desired.

Table 2 Symptoms of Carbon Monoxide Intoxication

Carboxyhemoglobin Level (%)	Symptoms
0–15	None
15–20	Headache, confusion
20–40	Disorientation, fatigue, nausea, visual impairment
40–60	Hallucination, combativeness, coma, shock
60+	Death

Inhalation injury should be suspected in (1) individuals who were injured in a closed space; (2) patients with extensive burns or with burns of the face; (3) patients who were unconscious at the time of injury; (4) patients with singed nasal hairs, hoarseness, or wheezing; and (5) patients who are coughing up carbonaceous sputum.

Pulmonary injury is known to result in substantially increased late burn mortality and morbidity as well as increased early fluid requirements and metabolic demands. Early intubation and positive pressure ventilation have been reported to improve outcome. The mode of ventilation used depends on the specific physiologic problem present; different modes may become necessary as the disease changes over time.

Pulmonary changes can be classified according to cause: thermal injury (heat) or chemical injury (incomplete products of combustion).

Thermal Injury

A number of techniques have been used to assess the degree of supraglottic injury and to determine the need for endotracheal intubation. Fiberoptic bronchoscopy or laryngoscopy will reveal physical evidence of mucosal injury. Spirometry detects early obstructive patterns in the airways, but reliable data can be obtained only in a cooperative patient without severe facial burns. Because the injury process is progressive during the first 18 to 24 hours, none of these tests accurately predicts the severity of subsequent airway compromise; serial studies must be performed.

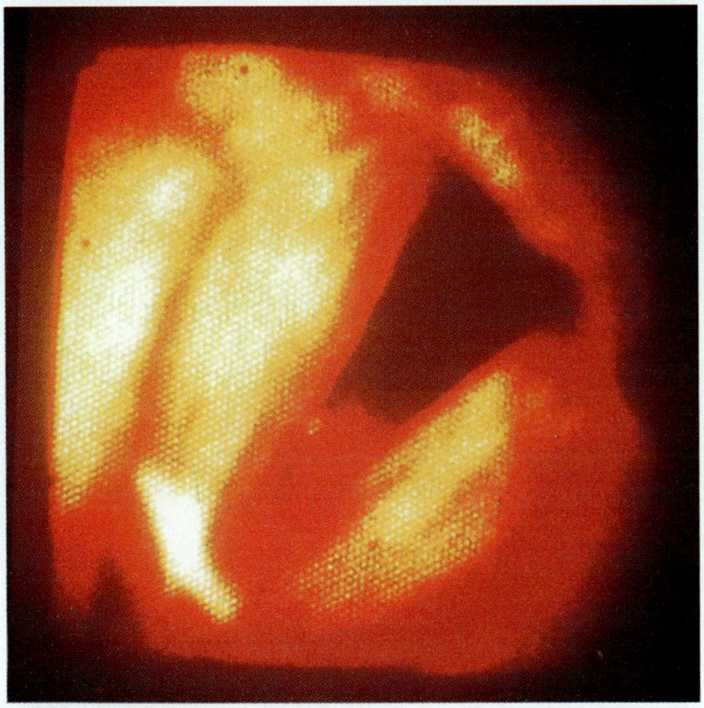

Chemical Injury

Diagnosis of chemical injury is complicated by the fact that facial burns or other signs evident in heat injury may be absent; indeed, the patient may not have been exposed to heat. Fiberoptic bronchoscopy detects the reddened, sometimes ulcerated mucosa that indicates the presence—but not the severity—of chemical injury. Ventilation-perfusion lung scans using xenon-133 reportedly detect early changes in the small airways, as do analyses of flow-volume curves and a simple 1-second forced expiratory volume (FEV_1). Preexisting lung disease, however, will alter the interpretation of findings. Measurement of lung water is of minimal benefit because major changes in water content usually occur only in an alveolar injury in which early respiratory failure is prominent. Initial chest x-ray, blood gas levels, and physical examination results are frequently normal.

INTUBATION

Endotracheal intubation is indicated for (1) deep facial burns—especially of the lips, the mouth, the neck, or the oropharynx—because subsequent edema will impair airway patency; (2) cases of smoke inhalation in which heat or chemical burns to the airway have been demonstrated by laryngoscopy or bronchoscopy; and (3) massive body burns, especially in the presence of circumferential chest burns, because ventilatory support is needed.

With deep burns of the face, the mouth, or the neck, the airway can be compromised by anatomic distortion and compression from the burn-edema process. Edema-induced distortion peaks at 18 to 24 hours after a burn; both airway patency and the ability to clear secretions are impaired. As edema increases, it becomes much more difficult to secure an airway. Endotracheal intubation is thus preferably performed on admission, before severe edema develops. A patient with inhalation injury can be closely monitored for upper airway obstruction without a tube, preferably with the head elevated at 30°, only if intubation will be technically possible later. However, if anatomic distortion from face and neck burns is increasing to a point where safe intubation might soon be precluded, the procedure is carried out immediately. Tracheostomy through burned tissue is contraindicated because the risk of infection, both in the wound and in the airway, is substantially increased.

Heat injury usually heals in a matter of a few days to a week, as the mucosal edema resolves and the relatively superficial mucosal injury heals.

Positive end-expiratory pressure (PEEP) is frequently necessary to keep the edematous airways open and to maintain an adequate functional residual capacity; it is also often used in the early management of severe CO toxicity (COHb > 40%). Prophylactic endotracheal intubation and PEEP have been reported to decrease deaths from early pulmonary complications after severe burns and smoke inhalation. A large enough tube (i.e., approximately 7.5 mm internal diameter in adults) should be used because very thick secretions develop as the lung injury becomes manifest, and changing tubes in the presence of edema is very dangerous. Therefore, although the nasotracheal route may be more comfortable for the patient, the choice of a route of placement must be based on the tube size required.

Figure 1 The view through a fiberoptic bronchoscope shows erythema and edema of the larynx 18 hours after a burn.

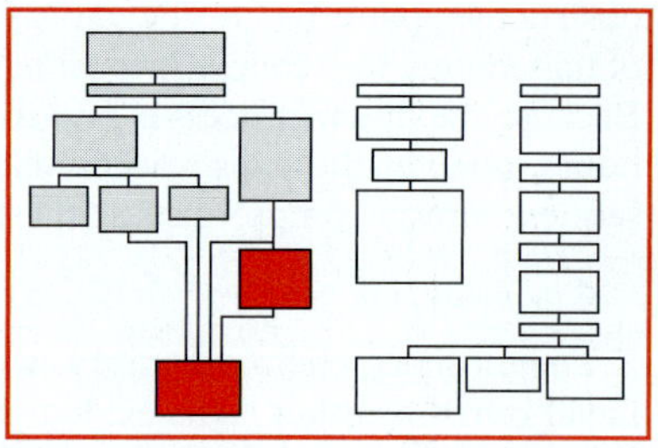

INITIATION OF AGGRESSIVE PULMONARY SUPPORT

Continuous administration of humidified oxygen is indicated to maintain adequate oxygen delivery as well as to assist in the clearance of secretions. If the patient's hemodynamic condition will tolerate it, elevation of the head and chest by 20° to 30° is helpful in reducing neck and chest wall edema. The early addition of bronchodilators, usually by aerosol, is especially advantageous in managing the bronchospasm seen after chemical injury. The beta$_2$-adrenergic agent metaproterenol (via nebulizer) is an effective bronchodilator. Intravenous aminophylline, although helpful, is frequently limited in its use because of the tachycardia seen in the early postburn period. Intravenous steroids have not been found to decrease the degree of injury; however, aerosolized steroid preparations identical to those used in asthma patients can decrease airway hyperreactivity, which is often a major problem in patients with smoke inhalation injury and which may not be responsive to aerosolized beta agonists. On the other hand, intravenous steroids have been successful in attenuating obliterative bronchiolitis, an uncommon but uniformly fatal late complication of severe smoke inhalation injury. Prophylactic antibiotics are not indicated to prevent a lung infection after smoke injury.

Close monitoring of the adequacy of gas exchange by serial blood gas determination is necessary, particularly during the early evolution of complications from the inhalation injury. An indwelling arterial line is indicated in the presence of severe injuries. When placement of such a line is not possible, a pulse oximeter is very useful if an unburned finger or earlobe is available. The pulse oximeter reads arterial oxygen saturation by means of a photosensor, which detects the color of the blood flowing beneath the probe.

Chest Wall Escharotomy

A full-thickness burn of the anterior and lateral chest wall can lead to severe restriction of chest wall motion as edema develops beneath the nonviable tissue (eschar), even in the absence of a completely circumferential burn. Chest wall escharotomy is required to relieve the restriction; the incision must penetrate completely through the eschar so that the subeschar space can expand and decrease tissue pressure. In a full-thickness burn, nerve endings are destroyed along with the entire epidermis and dermis. Analgesics are thus usually not necessary for escharotomy. The escharotomy incisions are placed along the anterior axillary lines, with bilateral incisions connected by a subcostal incision [see Figure 2 and Initiation of Wound Management, Subeschar Edema in Extremities, below]. Occasionally, another incision from the suprasternal notch to the xiphoid process is needed. Bleeding can usually be managed by pressure and occasional use of the electrocautery unit.

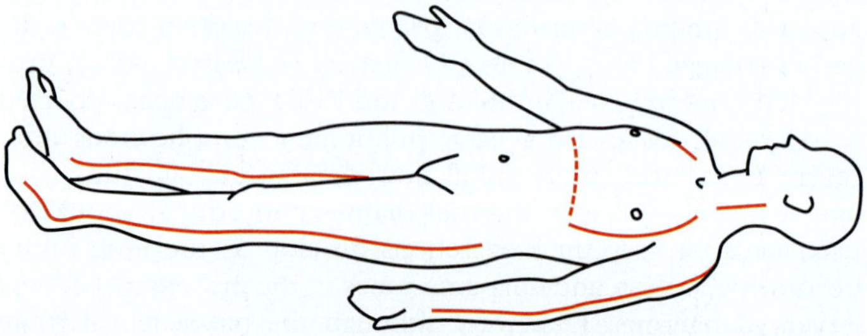

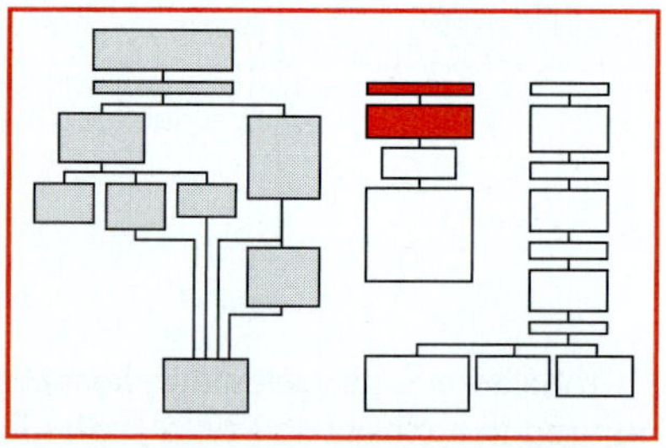

Restoration and Maintenance of Hemodynamic Stability

ESTIMATION OF BURN SIZE

Fluid requirements depend on the size of the burn. A simple determination of the burn surface area can be made using the Rule of Nines: each arm is considered to be 9% of total body surface (TBS), each leg 18%, the anterior trunk 18%, the posterior trunk 18%, and the head 9% [see Figure 3]. In small children, the determination must be modified because the head approaches 18% of TBS.

INTRAVENOUS ACCESS

A peripheral venous catheter through unburned tissue is the preferred route for fluid administration. A central venous line or pulmonary arterial line is only occasionally needed to monitor the patient during the initial resuscitation period and is removed as soon as it is no longer needed. These lines are usually required only in elderly patients or in patients who have severe heart disease. An extremely high complication rate reportedly accompanies the use of central catheters in burn patients because of infection and embolic episodes related to a hypercoagulable state. Because of the high infection rate, an intravenous catheter should not be placed through burn tissue unless every other possible route has been ruled out. A line that is dedicated to total parenteral nutrition should be completely isolated from the burn wound and cared for by covering the entrance site with an occlusive dressing [see 34 Burn Care after the First Postburn Week].

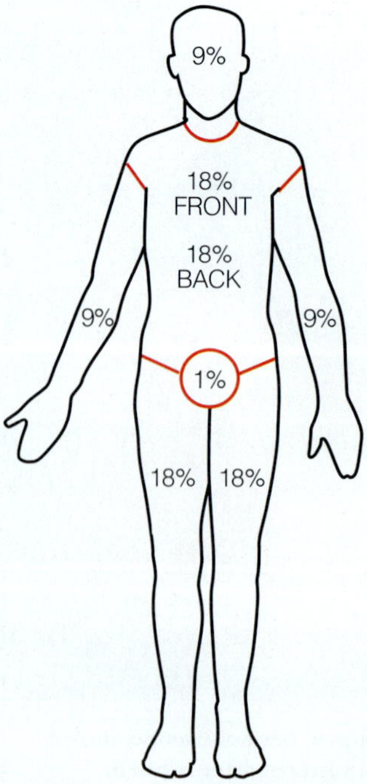

Figure 2 The red lines on the illustrated human figure represent guidelines for the placement of escharotomy incisions.

Figure 3 The size of a burn can be estimated by means of the Rule of Nines, which assigns percentages of total body surface to the head, the extremities, and the front and back of the torso.

RESUSCITATION FLUIDS

In general, fluids containing salt in quantities at least isotonic with plasma are appropriate for use in resuscitation after burn injury if given in sufficient amounts. These fluids should be free of glucose because burn patients exhibit early glucose intolerance as a result of the early release of catecholamines and other stress hormones. The oral route can be used in the case of smaller burns, but intestinal ileus frequently occurs after deep burns in excess of 20% of total body surface. A number of intravenous fluids, including colloids, are used to decrease edema in unburned tissues and to maintain a higher blood volume.

Crystalloid

Crystalloid—in particular, lactated Ringer solution, with a sodium concentration of 130 mEq/L—is the most popular resuscitation fluid in the United States. The loss of large quantities of sodium and water from the vascular space into the burn wound is well described. Isotonic crystalloid, if given in sufficient amounts, can restore cardiac output toward normal in most patients, the exceptions being patients who are extremely young or extremely old, those whose burns are massive, and those with superimposed inhalation injury. Lactated Ringer solution is preferred to normal saline because of its physiologic pH of 6.5 versus saline's pH of 5.0. Because isotonic salt solutions generate no differential in osmotic pressure between plasma and interstitial spaces, the entire extracellular space must be expanded to replace intravascular losses.

The amount of isotonic crystalloid required in the first 24 hours is based primarily on the calculated deficit of sodium from the extracellular space. This amount has been estimated to be 0.5 to 0.6 mEq sodium/kg/% TBS burned, which is equal to 4 ml/kg/% TBS burned of lactated Ringer solution. The quantity of crystalloid needed is also determined by measuring the parameters used to monitor resuscitation. In most burn centers, a urine output of 0.5 ml/kg/hr is considered an indication of adequate perfusion. The patient will require about 3 to 5 ml/kg/% TBS burned in the first 24 hours; about half of this amount is given in the first 8 hours [see Table 3].

Sodium is apparently the key element in crystalloid infusion; water is primarily the solvent. Solutions with increased sodium concentration therefore have a theoretical advantage because less water is infused. The hypertonic salt solutions used clinically have an osmolarity of 400 to 600 mOsm/L (isotonic solutions have an osmolarity of 280 to 300 mOsm/L); these solutions thereby transiently generate potential osmotic pressures of several thousand mm Hg relative to the normal isosmolar state. Hypertonic salt solutions have been known for many years to be effective in treating shock states, including burns. Essentially, they induce the body to borrow intracellular water to fill the extracellular space deficit. Infusion of hypertonic solutions thereby limits edema, compared with treatment by infusion of isotonic solutions.

Hypertonic solutions have also been reported to increase myocardial contractility, produce precapillary dilatation, and decrease vascular resistance by exerting a direct effect on the capillary smooth muscle. Current practice is to use a solution with a sodium concentration of approximately 240 mEq/L, which is prepared by adding two ampules of sodium lactate to each liter of normal saline. It is recommended that serum sodium levels not be allowed to exceed 160 mEq/L during infusion of the solution. Complications of hypertonic saline administration relate primarily to hyperosmolarity. A more isotonic solution should be given if an excessive hyperosmolar state develops. Free water cannot be given during infusion, because such action will simply lead to a more isotonic solution and in turn no decrease in total administered fluid. Increased water retention is likely to occur with the institution of hypotonic solutions beginning on postburn day 2, at least until isotonicity results.

Colloids

Unburned tissue appears to regain normal permeability very soon after injury. Because hypoproteinemia may accentuate edema in uninjured tissues, protein restoration should begin 8 to 12 hours after a burn if nonburn edema and total fluid requirements are to be minimized. This method is particularly advantageous in patients who have massive burns and in elderly patients.

The amount of protein to be infused remains undefined. Many investigators have arbitrarily used between 0.5 and 1.0 ml/kg/% TBS burned during the first 24 hours. The amount depends on the magnitude of the injury and on the degree of hemodynamic instability. The protein should be infused at a constant rate [see Adjustment of Infusion Rate, below]; pulsed infusion will transiently increase pressure and increase the rate of edema formation.

If early administration of colloids is required because hemodynamic instability persists despite the infusion of large quantities of crystalloid (about 4 ml/kg/% TBS burned), nonprotein colloids are more economical. Although the weight of dextran 70 (70 kd) is almost identical to that of albumin, dextran's molecular size is considerably larger because of its branched configuration. A standard 6% solution of dextran 70 exerts an oncotic pressure more than twice that generated by a 6% albumin solution. This property makes the compound advantageous as a volume expander. Dextran 40 (40 kd) in a 10% solution, infused at about 2 ml/kg/hr, is an even more potent volume expander because it generates a colloid osmotic pressure six to eight times that of a protein of comparable weight. To prevent platelet deficits, the total dose of dextran 70 during any 24-hour period should not exceed 33 ml/kg; the total

---

Table 3 Calculations to Determine Resuscitation Requirements in a Young Patient without an Inhalation Injury

The patient is a 35-year-old male. His weight is 70 kg. His burns cover 50% TBS, most of which are second degree.

Recommendations:
 3–4 ml lactated Ringer solution/kg body weight/% TBS burned
 Administer 1/2 the required volume in the first 8 hr after the burn.
 Administer 1/2 the required volume during the next 16 hr.

Calculation:
 4 ml × 70 kg × 50% TBS burned = 14,000 ml/24 hr

Give
 7,000 ml during the first 8 hr (875 ml/hr)
 7,000 ml during the next 16 hr (435 ml/hr)

Monitor
 Blood pressure (systolic > 90 mm Hg; mean > 80 mm Hg)
 Pulse (< 120 beats/min)
 Urine output (30–50 ml/hr)
 Arterial blood gases (P_{O_2} > 90 mm Hg)
 pH (> 7.35)

Adjust fluid administration in response to circulatory requirements:
 Diminish fluid administration if hemodynamic stability is achieved at these infusion rates

  or

 Add colloid if adequate hemodynamic stability is not achieved at 4 ml/kg/% TBS burned.

dose of dextran 40 should not exceed 15 ml/kg during any 24-hour period. Therefore, these preparations are usually used in the early resuscitation period and are replaced by protein in the later resuscitation period. The use of the hapten PROMIT—a 1 kd dextran—before the administration of the dextran solution essentially precludes allergic reactions to the dextran molecule.

Hetastarch, a 6% starch solution, has colloid properties very similar to those of a 6% protein solution and generates a comparable oncotic pressure. Hetastarch molecules are much larger than those of most dextrans, and vascular clearance is therefore much slower. This solution is being used with increasing frequency as a volume expander.

Blood

Because there is no actual early red cell deficit with a burn alone, blood replacement is usually not needed during this period unless severe hemolysis occurs. Occasionally, however, blood can be a very useful volume expander to restore cardiac output if perfusion is not adequately maintained by other resuscitation fluids.

ADJUSTMENT OF INFUSION RATE

Fluids should be infused at a constant rate because rapid fluid challenge transiently increases pressure above the level required for adequate perfusion and contributes to edema formation. Fluid requirements in the first 6 to 8 hours after a burn will clearly exceed those in the subsequent 18 hours because the largest fluid shifts occur early. Approximately half of the total amount of fluid required in the first 24 hours will be given in the first 8 hours. During those first 8 hours, once a fluid infusion rate is reached at which adequate perfusion is maintained, only minor changes should be made so as to avoid large hemodynamic fluctuations. Beginning 8 to 10 hours after a burn, when fluid requirements begin to diminish, an attempt should be made to decrease the infusion rate gradually and to determine the smallest amount of fluid or fluids necessary to maintain adequate perfusion. The rate required in the 12- to 24-hour period must usually deliver around 50% to 60% of the initial requirements. Fluid requirements during the first 24 hours usually range from 3 to 4 ml/kg/% TBS burned, depending on the type of fluid, the patient's age, and the presence of other injuries [see Table 3].

HEMODYNAMIC PARAMETERS TO MONITOR

Perfusion-Related Parameters

The adequacy of perfusion is difficult to assess after major burns. Burn injury leads to increased tissue demand for oxygen, but at the same time, the body's ability to increase oxygen delivery is impaired by capillary leakage into the burn. Inhalation injury places additional fluid requirements and metabolic demands on burn patients. The increased hemodynamic instability seen in burn patients is probably attributable to activation of systemic inflammation by the burn as well as to airway injury. Infusion of larger amounts of resuscitation fluid may be necessary; however, this may lead to additional edema, which also results in complications. The best approach is to rely on repeated clinical assessments based on sound physiologic principles. Monitoring the following parameters can facilitate the assessment and improvement of perfusion.

Mean arterial pressure The increased sympathetic tone characteristic of the early postburn period makes arterial pressure an insensitive measure of volume status; however, minimal perfusion pressure (mean, > 90 mm Hg) must be maintained, which means that blood pressure must be monitored. In each patient, however, the precise blood pressure required to maintain adequate organ perfusion and tissue oxygenation becomes evident only in the process of observing the patient's response to fluid infusion.

If the patient is hemodynamically unstable, if the extremities are burned to such an extent that a sphygmomanometer cannot be used, or if frequent measurement of not only P_aO_2 but also pH and arterial carbon dioxide tension (P_aCO_2) is required, insertion of an arterial catheter may be necessary. The catheter should be placed through unburned skin and should be removed as soon as possible. A pulse oximeter can provide continuous readings of oxygen saturation and has the additional benefit of being noninvasive.

Pulse rate Tachycardia is inevitable in the early postburn period, given the development of hypovolemia and the release of catecholamines as a result of tissue trauma and pain. The degree of tachycardia can be a useful indicator of the adequacy of volume replacement, except in elderly patients or in patients with preexisting heart disease, whose heart rate cannot increase in proportion to the stimulus. In most patients, a pulse rate lower than 120 beats/min usually indicates adequate volume, whereas a pulse rate higher than 130 beats/min usually indicates that more fluid is needed. This guideline assumes that the pulse rate response corresponds to the other monitors of perfusion being used. Sometimes, the pulse rate does not follow the other indicators of impaired perfusion, in which case it becomes less useful for monitoring purposes. A case in point is a burn patient who is taking a beta blocker.

Pulmonary arterial wedge pressure In most young patients, even those with massive burns, it is not necessary to measure pulmonary arterial wedge pressure (PAWP) in the course of initial resuscitation: the risks associated with inserting a pulmonary arterial catheter may well exceed any benefits to be gained with respect to assessing adequacy of perfusion. Like central venous pressure, PAWP is usually normal to low (6 to 10 mm Hg) in the early postburn period, even when perfusion is adequate. Hypoperfusion is almost always attributable to hypovolemia; other well-recognized causes are (1) impaired left ventricular function resulting from impaired left ventricular filling (as with high mean airway pressure or pneumothorax) and (2) a marked increase in afterload resulting from high levels of circulating vasoconstrictors. There are three main patient groups in whom measurement of PAWP may be beneficial: (1) elderly patients who have deep burns covering more than 30% of TBS or who have suffered substantial smoke inhalation injury, (2) patients with preexisting heart disease who have massive burns or substantial smoke inhalation injury, and (3) young patients with massive burns who are not maintaining adequate perfusion despite fluid intake well in excess of predicted requirements.

Cardiac output and mixed venous oxygen tension The primary objective of fluid management is maintenance of adequate delivery of oxygen to tissues. Direct measurement of cardiac output (usually expressed as cardiac index) facilitates this task. In an uninjured person, a cardiac index of 2.5 L/min/m² or higher would be considered normal. In an injured person, however, such a value would not necessarily be indicative of adequate oxygen delivery, because injured tissue requires more oxygen than normal tissue does. Monitoring of mixed venous oxygen tension ($P_{mv}O_2$) can be of great assistance in this situation. A $P_{mv}O_2$ higher than 35 mm Hg indicates that oxygen delivery is adequate, a $P_{mv}O_2$ between 30 and 35 mm Hg indicates that oxygen delivery is marginal, and a $P_{mv}O_2$ lower than 30 mm Hg indicates that oxygen delivery is inadequate.

Arterial blood gas values Whether P_aO_2 and P_aCO_2 must be monitored depends on the percentage of TBS burned and on the risk of respiratory abnormalities (particularly in patients with a history of smoke exposure). Pulse oximetry is useful for measuring P_aO_2. Measurement of pH and evaluation of acid-base balance are also extremely useful in the assessment of tissue oxygenation. A base deficit during the early postburn phase usually reflects impaired tissue oxygenation caused by hypovolemia or by carbon monoxide or hydrocyanide toxicity [*see 7 Life-Threatening Acid-Base Abnormalities*].

Blood lactate concentration A normal blood lactate concentration does not indicate that perfusion is optimal; it only indicates that anaerobic metabolism is not taking place. A high lactate concentration, on the other hand, reflects severe hypoperfusion.

Urine output Urine output via a Foley catheter is a valuable indicator of adequate renal blood flow if the urine is nonglycosuric and if output has not been increased by administration of solutes (e.g., mannitol or dextran). An output of 0.5 ml/kg/hr in adults or 1.0 ml/kg/hr in children is adequate. Antidiuretic hormone and aldosterone are automatically released in response to the burn stress; therefore, a urine output greater than 0.5 to 1.0 ml/kg/hr may necessitate a rate of fluid infusion far higher than that necessary to maintain perfusion, and excess edema will result.

Other Parameters

Serum creatinine and blood urea nitrogen concentration Baseline values for serum creatinine and blood urea nitrogen may help rule out intrinsic renal disease, which impairs the reliability of urine output as an index of perfusion.

Body weight and temperature Obtaining a baseline body weight as early as possible after the burn will facilitate assessment of fluid balance. The preburn weight should be used to determine nutrition needs and drug dosages.

Body temperature should be obtained as well. Hypothermia is a major complication of burns; it is controlled by warming the environment. Hyperthermia can also occur as a result of early pyrogen release and can alter vital signs to be misleadingly suggestive of profound hypovolemia; it should be treated with antipyrogens.

Electrocardiographic status Arrhythmias are not common in young patients with burns as long as oxygenation is adequate, but they become a major concern in patients older than 45 years as a result of the stress response to the burn. Because arrhythmias may be the first clues to the presence of hypoxia and electrolyte or acid-base abnormalities, continuous electrocardiographic monitoring is required during the early postburn period.

Intake and output What goes in and what comes out should be carefully tabulated. Intake will far exceed output during the early postburn period as edema develops.

Hematocrit and hemoglobin concentration Although it is helpful to monitor the hematocrit and the hemoglobin concentration, changes in these values may not accurately reflect changes in blood volume. The rate of plasma loss often exceeds the rate of whole blood loss, which means that the hematocrit may be normal even in the face of severe volume depletion; consequently, blood loss (e.g., from escharotomies, line placement, internal bleeding, or fractures) can easily be underestimated. If, however, the hematocrit declines in the absence of hemolysis, this is a clear indication that there is a significant source of blood loss somewhere. After large burns, normalization of blood volume is almost impossible until 24 to 48 hours after the burn.

White blood cell count The initial white blood cell count may be high, normal, or low, depending on the magnitude of the stress response and the degree of white cell sequestration into the burn. The absolute value is not a particularly useful parameter during the early postburn period.

Blood glucose level The increased release of catecholamines in burn patients often leads to hyperglycemia. In elderly and diabetic patients, insulin may be required; some glucose should be infused at this time as well. Infants are prone to hypoglycemia as a result of decreased glucose stores.

Electrolyte status Because most of the fluid lost initially is plasma rather than whole blood, concentrations of sodium, chloride, and potassium remain relatively constant despite hypovolemia; variations in these values are mainly a function of the type of resuscitation fluid used. The potassium concentration will rise if severe hemolysis has occurred or if renal impairment is present. The HCO_3^- concentration varies according to perfusion status and acid-base balance.

Plasma protein and myoglobin levels A marked decrease in the plasma protein level occurs soon after a burn, with the greater part of the decrease coming in the first 4 to 6 hours. Not much can be done about this change until about 10 to 12 hours after the burn, given the rapid fluid and protein shifts. The plasma albumin level should be maintained above 2.5 g/dl.

In patients with very deep burns, especially if the burns are electrical in origin, the plasma myoglobin level should be measured. Myoglobin released from deeply injured muscles will affect renal function. This problem can be largely prevented by maintaining a higher than normal urine output.

Prothrombin time, partial thromboplastin time, and platelet count Initial values for prothrombin time and partial thromboplastin time and an initial platelet count are useful for determining whether administration of coagulation factors will be necessary. In the first 36 hours after the burn, coagulation factors and platelets are rarely needed unless a prolonged shock state has initiated disseminated intravascular coagulation or unless the patient has preexisting hepatic or hematologic disease.

INOTROPIC SUPPORT

Inotropic support in the first 24 hours is indicated if inadequate perfusion persists despite vigorous fluid resuscitation. This situation is most common in the elderly burn patient. If improved renal blood flow is the major goal, low-dose dopamine (1 to 4 µg/kg/min) is preferred. Moderate-dose dopamine (5 to 10 µg/kg/min) or dobutamine will increase contractility and improve cardiac output. Dobutamine results in less tachycardia. Digoxin is not recommended in the immediate postburn period, because the rapid fluid shifts during this period can lead to digitalis toxicity; in addition, digoxin is generally a less potent inotropic agent than dopamine or dobutamine.

DIURETICS

Diuretics are rarely indicated in the first 24 hours of resuscitation. The exceptions are when hemoglobinuria or myoglobinuria is present, as may occur after electrical injuries.

Initiation of Wound Management

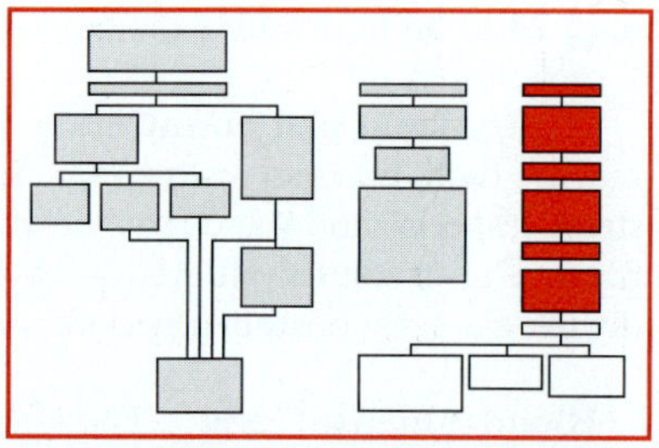

COOLING THE WOUND

Cooling will increase heat loss, and neutralizing the heat source is a primary goal of initial management. Immediate cooling of the burn also decreases edema, apparently by stabilizing skin mast cells and thereby preventing histamine release. This effect, however, is short-lived. After the first 30 minutes, the benefit of cooling with water at a temperature of approximately 20° C is principally that of pain relief in superficially burned tissues. Prolonged cooling for pain relief is indicated only in second-degree burns covering less than 15% of TBS. Ice should never be used directly on the skin, because a freezing injury can result.

After a deep burn, the normal protective mechanism of skin vasoconstriction is absent. The barrier to water loss by evaporation—and hence the barrier to heat loss—is markedly impaired, an extremely important problem to recognize in the resuscitation period. Body heat is lost 25 times more quickly in water (wet dressings or hydrotherapy) than in air because of increased heat conductivity in water. Once hypothermia develops, rewarming is extremely slow, and decreased body temperature may affect cardiac output and perfusion of vital organs.

ASSESSMENT OF BURN DEPTH

At this point, more precise assessments of burn size and depth are needed to determine the manner of burn care and the need for transfer to a burn facility [see Figure 4 and Table 4]. The size of second- and third-degree burns must be determined in relation to total body surface [see Figure 3].

Burn depth is classified by degree of injury. Unfortunately, clinical assessment of the depth of anything more serious than a superficial second-degree burn is difficult at admission. Moreover, deeper burns tend to increase in depth over a period of hours to days as the injured but viable tissue eventually becomes nonviable, usually as a result of a low-flow state (initially) or inflammation (in the later stages). A number of techniques for clinical determination of burn depth have been employed; all have met with some success, but none have been widely adopted.

First-Degree Burns

A first-degree burn involves only the thinner outer epidermis layer and is characterized by erythema and mild discomfort. Tissue damage is minimal, and protective functions of the skin are intact. Pain, the chief symptom, usually resolves in 48 to 72 hours, and healing takes place uneventfully. The pain is probably caused by local vasodilator prostaglandin production. In 5 to 10 days, the damaged epithelium peels off in small scales, leaving no residual scarring. The most common causes of first-degree burns are overexposure to sunlight and brief scalding by hot liquids.

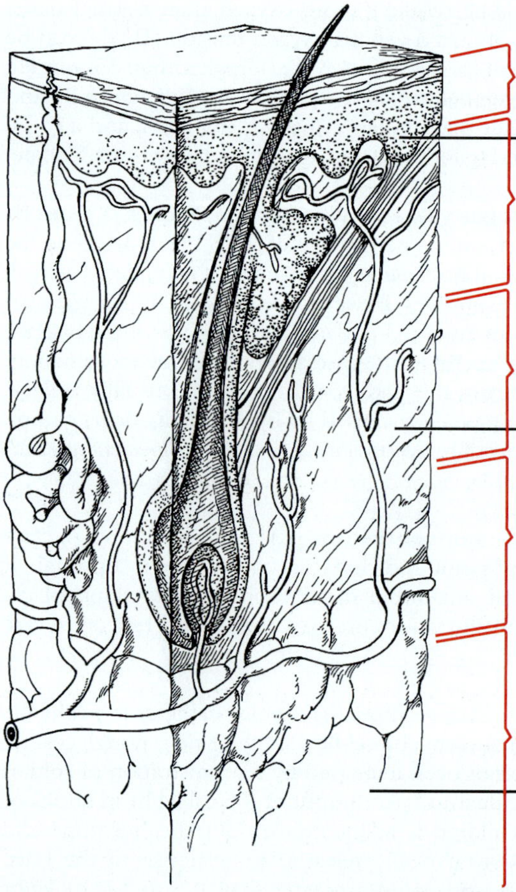

Second-Degree Burns

Second-degree burns [see Figure 5] are those in which the entire epidermis and variable portions of the dermis have been destroyed by heat. A superficial second-degree burn involves heat injury to the upper third of the dermis. The microvessels perfusing this area are injured, and permeability is increased, with the result that large amounts of plasma leak into the interstitium. This fluid in turn lifts the thin, heat-destroyed epidermis, forming blisters. Despite the

Figure 4 Illustrated here are the depths to which skin damage extends with burns of varying degrees.

Table 4 Physical Characteristics of Burns

Cause	Appearance	Depth	Pain
Hot liquids			
Short exposure	Wet; pink; blisters	2°	Severe
Long exposure	Wet; dark red	2°–3°	Minimal
Flames			
Flash exposure	Wet; pink; blisters	2°	Severe
Direct contact	Dry, white, and waxy; leathery brown or black	3°	Minimal
Chemicals			
Acid, alkalies	Light brown to light gray	2° (converts to 3°)	Severe

loss of the entire basal layer of the epidermis, a superficial second-degree burn will heal in 7 to 14 days owing to repopulation by the epithelial cells that line the hair follicles, sweat glands, and other skin appendages anchored deep in the dermis. Minimal scarring occurs because the wound closes rapidly; consequently, inflammation, which stimulates excessive collagen deposition, is short-lived. A deep dermal second-degree burn extends well into the dermal layer; fewer viable epidermal cells remain. Epithelialization is extremely slow, sometimes requiring months. Blister formation is not characteristically seen: because the layer of dead tissue is thick and adherent to underlying dermal collagen, it cannot be readily lifted off the surface. Exceptions occur in very young or very old patients, who have a very thin dermis. The surface of the wound is usually red, with some evidence of plasma leakage from remaining intact blood vessels. Blood supply to the burned tissue is marginal; thus, there is a high probability that tissue damage will deepen with time. Pain is present but to a lesser degree than in more superficial burns. Fluid losses and the metabolic effects of deep dermal burns are basically the same as those seen with third-degree burns. Dense scarring usually results if skin grafts are not performed.

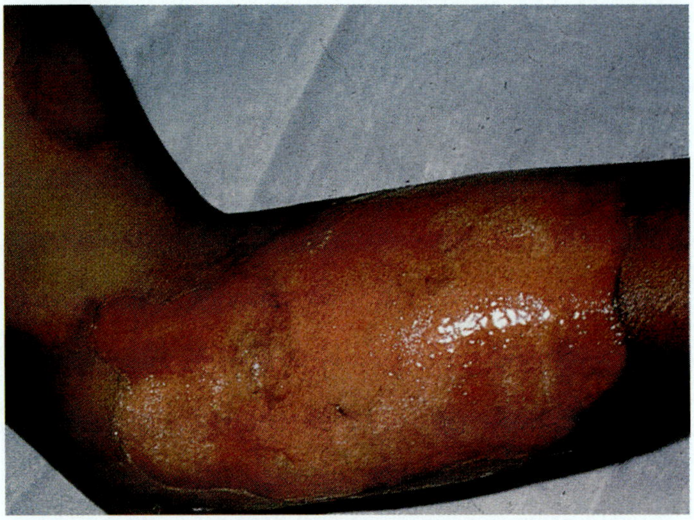

Figure 5 Immediately after injury, a second-degree burn typically has a wet, reddish appearance.

Third-Degree Burns

In a full or third-degree burn [*see Figure 6*], the entire epidermis and dermis are destroyed; no residual epidermal cells remain to repopulate or epithelialize. Areas of the wound not closed by wound contraction will require skin grafting. Characteristically, avascular burned tissue has the waxy white color typical of any avascular tissue. If the burn extends into the fat or if contact with a flame source has been prolonged, the leathery brown or black color typical of charred tissue is seen. The most common cause of third-degree burns is a short exposure to a very high temperature, such as direct contact with a flame. However, prolonged contact with only moderately hot liquids (e.g., water at 125° F), as seen with intentional scalding, can result in a third-degree burn. Prolonged contact with hot liquid that leads to a third-degree burn will also lead to red cell hemolysis and release of myoglobin from underlying muscle, resulting in a red pigment deposition in the wound. The red-pigmented wound can be mistaken for viable dermis; the same appearance in a flame burn would represent only a deep second-degree injury. Therefore, a dark-red appearance in a scald burn may actually represent a full-thickness injury. The microvessels are not immediately thrombosed in second-degree injury and therefore continue to leak plasma for days. In full-thickness flame burns, however, injured capillaries are usually immediately occluded by thrombosis. The absence of pain sensation in full-thickness burns is the result of heat destruction of nerve endings. This sensory deficit distinguishes a third-degree burn from a partial-thickness injury.

Full-thickness chemical burns are light gray to brown in appearance. Pain is usually extreme because retained chemicals prolong the burning process; these retained chemicals commonly convert partial burns to full-thickness burns.

In the early postburn period (24 to 72 hours after the burn), a zone of ischemia is usually present below the dead tissue and above the deeper living tissue. The vasculature to this area has been injured. Some vessels are thrombosed; others are patent but have endothelial cell damage. The marginally viable tissue can readily convert to eschar if blood flow is further decreased because of local mediator release or infection. A deep second-degree burn—in which healing is still possible—can therefore progress to a third-degree burn. Wound conversion is prevented or minimized with prompt, adequate resuscitation.

PAIN MEDICATION

Pain medication is necessary for partial-thickness burns, particularly when the wounds are cleaned. Pain control should be initiated before aggressive wound manipulation because it is important to minimize the subsequent stress response. With minor burns, oral or intramuscular narcotics may be adequate if given about 30 minutes before wound care. For major burns [*see Table 5*], intravenous narcotics in small doses are appropriate; erratic absorption from the gastrointestinal tract, skin, and muscles makes these routes of administration both ineffective and dangerous.

REMOVAL OF FOREIGN BODIES AND LOOSE NONVIABLE TISSUE

When a patent airway, breathing, and circulation are ensured, the wound can be debrided and cleaned. Soot and dirt are best removed with a mild dilute detergent such as a chlorhexidine product. Gross debris, loose sloughed skin, or skin overlying broken blisters should be gently removed with forceps and scissors. Rough scrubbing should be avoided to prevent further harm to the injured tissues. Ground-in dirt will gradually work its way to the surface with daily dressing changes. The surrounding skin should be

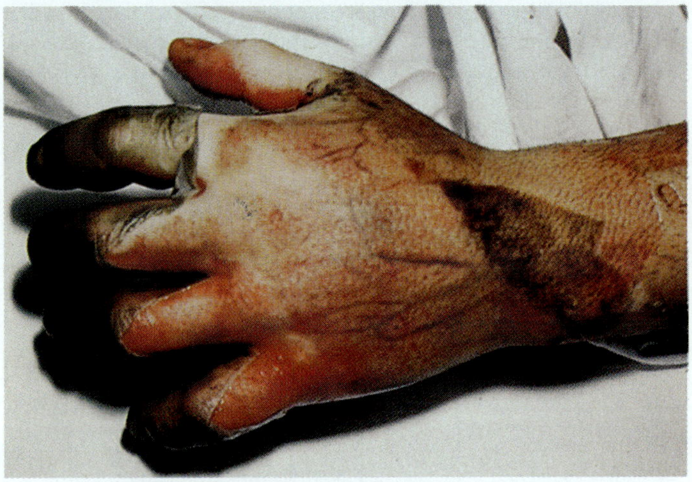

Figure 6 Shown is a full-thickness burn of the hand that actually extends below the dermis into subdermal tissue.

Table 5 **Classification of Severity of Burn Injury**

Critical burns
- 2° burns involving > 30% TBS
- 3° burns involving > 10% TBS
- Any burns complicated by respiratory tract injury, fractures, or involvement of critical areas (i.e., face, hands, feet, perineum)
- High-voltage electrical burns
- Lesser burns in patients with significant preexisting disease

Moderate burns
- 2° burns involving 15%–20% TBS (if critical areas are not involved)
- 3° burns involving 2%–10% TBS (if critical areas are not involved)

Minor burns
- 2° burns involving < 15% TBS (if critical areas are not involved)
- 3° burns involving < 2% TBS (if critical areas are not involved)

shaved to facilitate local wound care. Large intact blisters can be left in place for 48 hours, reducing discomfort and the risk of underlying dermal desiccation.

If a hydrotherapy tank is to be used at this time for wound cleaning, the patient must be hemodynamically stable because good hemodynamic monitoring will be impossible during the procedure. Sequential cleaning of the various burned areas at bedside allows continuous monitoring and minimizes hypothermia and is thus a safer approach. A warm environment during burn care, preferably 30° to 35° C (86° to 95° F), is necessary to avoid heat loss.

Tar burns present unique problems. Tar removal is particularly difficult because the heat of the tar (150° to 200° C) usually results in a deep burn, and the rapid cooling leads to adherence to the skin. Tar can be gently removed without further tissue damage by means of repeated applications of petroleum-based ointments (such as Neosporin), which also contain surface-active emulsifying agents that dissolve the tar and make it easier to remove.

TETANUS PROPHYLAXIS

As with any large wound, the risk of tetanus must be minimized by using standard measures [see 8 Acute Wound Care].

PROPHYLACTIC ANTIBIOTICS

Numerous studies have demonstrated that prophylactic systemic antibiotics do not decrease wound infection rates in either minor or major burns. The blood supply to the relatively avascular deep burn is insufficient to provide adequate tissue antibiotic levels. In addition, any open wound will become colonized with bacteria. The only exception to the dictum against prophylactic systemic antibiotics would be prophylaxis against β-hemolytic streptococcus with low-dose penicillin, particularly if the patient is at high risk for infection with this organism (i.e., if the patient is a carrier or was recently exposed).

EARLY INFECTION CONTROL: TOPICAL ANTIBIOTICS AND SKIN SUBSTITUTES

Topical Antibiotics

Because topical antibiotics decrease the rate of wound healing (in particular, the rate of epithelialization) as compared with biologic dressings or other forms of temporary skin substitutes, these agents are most useful for deep burns with eschar present and are less useful for most superficial burns or clean, healing burns. Topical agents are applied to the wound, which is then covered with dressings or left open to the environment. Both techniques are used, but the closed dressing technique is employed more because pain, heat, and fluid loss are decreased if dressings are applied. In addition, residual dermis is less likely to desiccate under a dressing.

The deep burn must be protected from early bacterial invasion, which can rapidly convert the wound to a still deeper injury. Topical antibiotics that are sufficiently water soluble to penetrate the burn eschar will temporarily control bacterial growth in the wound [see Table 6]. The half-life of the currently available topical agents is only a few hours; therefore, the agent must be applied at least twice daily to achieve a reasonable level of antibacterial protection.

Silver sulfadiazine (Silvadene) is the most commonly used topical agent because it has good antibacterial properties and because fewer complications are associated with its use. This agent, however, penetrates thick eschar less readily than some other agents and is therefore better used to prevent infection than to treat an established infection. Antibacterial properties are primarily directed against gram-negative organisms, with some antifungal effects. The primary complication of silver sulfadiazine is leukopenia as a result of transient bone marrow suppression. A white blood cell count of 2,000 to 3,000/mm³ can be seen after application is begun. The effect is transient; the white cell count returns toward normal after several days, even if the agent is continued.

Mafenide (Sulfamylon) is the most effective agent in its ability to penetrate burn eschar. It also has the most potent antibacterial

Table 6 **Topical Antibiotic Agents**

Agent	Antimicrobial Spectrum	Eschar Penetration	Local Tissue Toxicity	Systemic Toxicity	Pain on Application	Occlusive Dressings
10% Mafenide (Sulfamylon)	Broad*	Excellent	Moderate	Acidosis; carbonic anhydrase inhibition	Yes	Unnecessary
1% Silver sulfadiazine (Silvadene)	Broad	Good	Low	Transient leukopenia	Minimal	Preferred
0.1% Gentamicin sulfate ointment	Broad†	Fair	Low	? Renal toxicity; ? ototoxicity	Minimal	Preferred
0.5% Povidone-iodine (Betadine)	Broad	Fair	Low	Renal, CNS, and iodine toxicity	Yes	Preferred
Bacitracin ointment	Gram-positive organisms	Surface only	Low	Renal toxicity	No	Optional

*Most potent of the topical agents. †Has no antifungal properties.

properties and is particularly effective against gram-negative organisms. The agent has some antifungal properties as well. However, mafenide, as a carbonic anhydrase inhibitor, can potentiate pulmonary insufficiency and metabolic acidosis; hence, it also produces the most significant complications. In addition, application is painful in many cases. This agent is used primarily as a second line of defense or as a primary treatment for small, infected wounds.

Povidone-iodine (Betadine) ointment is usually used only on relatively thin eschar because its tissue penetration is not very good. The active agent is iodine, which is quite effective against both bacteria and fungi. Agents such as gentamicin and bacitracin can be used for more selective infections [see Table 6], but systemic toxicity can occur if these agents are used over large open wounds. Bacitracin is reasonably effective against wound colonization with gram-positive organisms. Bacitracin and gentamicin, however, have no antifungal properties, and prolonged use on an open wound can precipitate fungal growth.

Temporary Skin Substitutes

A number of temporary skin substitutes have been developed to improve healing of partial-thickness wounds as well as to protect clean, excised wounds when autografts are not performed immediately. Skin substitutes allow excision of burned tissue even if insufficient skin is available for autograft, permitting more rapid removal of devitalized tissue. The properties required of a temporary skin substitute have been well defined. Most important, it must adhere to the wound to maximize the epithelialization rate and minimize inflammation and fibrosis.

There are two types of temporary skin: biologic and synthetic. Biologic dressings are from previously living tissue, including amniotic membranes, xenografts, and allografts (or cadaver skin), although the last is only of limited availability and is used primarily to cover excised wounds. A number of synthetic skin substitutes have been developed that have the advantages of ready availability, long shelf life, and minimal risk of disease transmission.

SUBESCHAR EDEMA IN EXTREMITIES

The increased pressure that accompanies the development of subeschar edema is of particular concern in extremities with circumferential burns. In such cases, if the increasing pressure cannot be dissipated, a decrease in venous outflow results; this effect speeds the rate of edema formation and further elevates tissue pressure until there is marked impairment of arterial blood flow to the tissues distal to the obstruction.

Immediate elevation of the burned extremity decreases the magnitude of tissue edema. Perfusion is best monitored by the Doppler flowmeter or by assessment of capillary refill. Immediate escharotomy is indicated [see Figure 2] if there is a decrease in pulsatile flow beyond the burn.

Transfer to Specialized Burn Facility

Patients whose burns are critical [see Table 5] should be transferred to specialized burn facilities as early as possible after their injury, once the initial assessment and resuscitation have begun. Moderate burns necessitate hospitalization but may be manageable outside a burn facility if a local surgeon with an interest or expertise in burns will accept responsibility for the patient's care. Minor burns may be manageable on an outpatient basis.

A major reason for the impressive progress made in the field of burn therapy has been the expansion of the concept of specialized centers for burns. There are now more than 150 burn units in the United States as compared with a mere dozen 30 years ago. About 21,000 burn patients—approximately one third of all hospitalized burn patients—are treated yearly in these 1,700 specialized burn care beds. The centralization of patients has made possible not only improved care but also multidisciplinary research.

Recommended Reading

Barillo D, Goode R, Esch V: Cyanide poisoning in victims of fire: analysis of 364 cases and review of the literature. J Burn Care Rehabil 15:46, 1994

Crapo R: Causes of respiratory injury. Respiratory Injury: Smoke Inhalation and Burns. Haponik E, Munster A, Eds. McGraw-Hill Book Co, New York, 1990, p 47

Crum RL: Cardiovascular and neurohumoral responses following burn injury. Arch Surg 125:1065, 1990

Deitch E: The management of burns. N Engl J Med 323:1249, 1990

Demling R: Fluid resuscitation. The Art and Science of Burn Care. Boswick J, Ed. Aspen, Rockville, Maryland, 1982, p 189

Demling R: Smoke inhalation injury. New Horizons in Critical Care. Demling R, Ed. Williams & Wilkins, Baltimore, 1993, p 422

Demling R, Knox J, Youn Y, et al: Oxygen consumption early post burn becomes oxygen dependent with the addition of smoke inhalation injury. J Trauma 32:593, 1992

Fitzpatrick J, Cioffi W: Diagnosis and treatment of inhalation injury. Total Burn Care. Herndon D, Ed. WB Saunders Co, Philadelphia, 1996, p 174

Fratianno R, Brandt C: Improved survival of adults with extensive burns. J Burn Care Rehabil 18:347, 1997

Heimbach D: Burn depth. World J Surg 16:10, 1992

Jeng J, Lee K, Jordan M: Serum lactate and base deficit suggest inadequate resuscitation of patients with burn injury. J Burn Care Rehabil 18:402, 1997

Masanes M, Legendre C: Fiberoptic bronchoscopy for the early diagnosis of subglottal inhalation injury: comparative value in the assessment of prognosis. J Trauma 36:59, 1994

Pruitt B: The evolutionary development of biologic dressings and skin substitutes. J Burn Care Rehabil 18:52, 1997

Scheulen JJ, Munster AM: The Parkland formula in patients with burns and inhalation injury. J Trauma 22:869, 1982

Silverman S, Purdue G, Hunt J, et al: Cyanide toxicity in burned patients. J Trauma 28:171, 1988

Vinus B, Matsuda T, Coprizo JB, et al: Prophylactic intubation and continuous positive airway pressure in the management of inhalation injury in burn victims. Crit Care Med 9:519, 1981

Youn Y, LaLonde C, Demling R: Oxidants and pathophysiology of burn and smoke inhalation injury. Free Radic Biol Med 12:409, 1992

Acknowledgment

Figures 2 through 4 Carol Donner.

4 SHOCK

James W. Holcroft, M.D.

Approach to the Treatment of Shock

Classification of Shock

Shock may be defined as a state in which either (1) the cardiovascular system lacks adequate power for perfusion of the peripheral tissues or (2) there is adequate power for perfusion, but only at the cost of excessive and inefficient use of oxygen by the heart, which renders the heart vulnerable to ischemia. The first type of shock is commonly termed decompensated shock; the second, compensated shock.

Shock, whether decompensated or compensated, can be classified into five categories according to the physiologic derangement that is the primary cause of the shock state: (1) extracardiac compressive/obstructive shock, (2) hypovolemic shock, (3) inflammatory shock, (4) neurogenic shock, and (5) cardiogenic shock [*see Tables 1 and 2*]. Frequently, this classification is a non-exclusive one—that is, a given clinical condition (e.g., tension pneumothorax) might cause shock by several mechanisms. Nonetheless, a physiologic classification of shock that emphasizes a single primary cause is frequently helpful in the initial stages of treatment.

In extracardiac compressive shock, forces external to the heart compress the thin-walled chambers of the heart (the atria and right ventricle) and the great veins (both systemic and pulmonary) as they enter the heart, thus decreasing ventricular end-diastolic volumes. In extracardiac obstructive shock, the heart fails because it encounters excessive hindrance during contraction or because the extrapericardial veins returning blood to the heart become compressed. Many of the conditions associated with excessive hindrance to contraction also compress the great systemic and pulmonary veins.

In hypovolemic shock, small ventricular end-diastolic volumes lead to inefficient or inadequate cardiac production of power.

Inflammatory shock arises from the release of inflammatory and coagulatory mediators. It can be caused by ischemia-reperfusion injuries, trauma, or infection (in which case it is sometimes referred to as septic shock). Inflammatory shock is also known as distributive shock because the abnormalities in some cases derive partly from increased blood flow to the skin or stagnation of blood in dilated peripheral venules and small veins.

Inflammatory and coagulatory mediators cause inflammatory shock via three main mechanisms: (1) disruption of the microvascular endothelium, both at the inflammatory site and distally, (2) dilation of the microvasculature, both locally and distally, and (3) depression of the myocardium. The result is plasma loss into the interstitium, which produces a hypovolemic state, distant organ failure, and cardiac insufficiency or inadequacy. If the predominant feature of the shock state is loss of plasma volume into the interstitium through a permeable microvasculature, the patient's skin will be cool and clammy (hence the terms cold septic shock and cold inflammatory shock). If blood volume has been restored or the predominant feature of the shock state is cutaneous vasodilatation, the skin will be flushed and warm (hence the term warm inflammatory shock).

The causes of inflammatory shock are all associated with the presence of large amounts of infected or traumatized tissue in proximity to a robust blood supply and drainage. An avascular infection (e.g., a contained abscess) will not cause inflammatory shock, because the inflammatory mediators do not have access to the circulation; however, an uncontained abscess (e.g., a ruptured appendiceal abscess or a surgically drained subphrenic abscess) can cause inflammatory shock because the mediators that spill out of the abscess are picked up by the vasculature in the surrounding tissue. In like manner, dry gangrene, because of its poor vascular supply, will not cause inflammatory shock, whereas wet gangrene can.

Neurogenic shock arises from loss of autonomic innervation of the vasculature and, in some cases, of the heart. Causes include spinal cord injury, regional anesthesia, administration of drugs that block the adrenergic nervous system (including some systemically administered anesthetic agents), certain neurologic disorders, and fainting. Loss of arteriolar tone leads to hypotension; loss of venular and small venous tone leads to pooling of blood in the denervated parts of the body. If the blockade is generalized or at a high enough level, the denervation can also decrease myocardial contractility and heart rate.

In cardiogenic shock, the heart itself, through an intrinsic abnormality, is incapable of efficiently pushing its contained blood into the vasculature with adequate power.

Recognition of Shock

The presence of a shock state is typically signaled by one or more characteristic clinical markers [*see Table 3*].

HYPOTENSION

A low blood pressure is a specific sign of shock but not a sensitive one. A very low blood pressure (≤ 89 mm Hg) almost always indicates some form of shock. Postural falls in blood pressure can also be a helpful signal: a sustained (> 30 seconds) systolic pressure drop greater than 10 mm Hg in a patient who has arisen from a supine position to an upright one is abnormal and frequently is an indication of underlying shock.

The absence of hypotension does not, however, rule out shock. Adrenergic discharge and the release of circulating and locally produced vasoconstrictors during shock often sustain blood pressure despite volume depletion or depressed myocardial contractility. Furthermore, how hypotension should be defined in a particular case depends on the patient's usual blood pressure, which may not be known to the physician. For instance, in a patient with severe preexisting hypertension, a systolic pressure of 120 mm Hg might reflect shock. Thus, hypotension—either supine or postural—can strongly suggest the diagnosis of shock, but normotension in a patient suspected of being in shock means nothing.

Approach to the Treatment of Shock

Patient shows signs of possible shock

Characteristic signs include
- Hypotension
- Tachycardia or bradycardia
- Tachypnea
- Cutaneous hypoperfusion
- Mental abnormalities
- Oliguria
- Myocardial ischemia
- Metabolic acidemia
- Hypoxemia

Shock resolves

Extracardiac compressive/obstructive shock

Compression or obstruction of the heart or great vessels, as an immediately life-threatening condition (see above), should already have been treated. However, periodic reassessment during workup is appropriate because this type of shock can develop secondary to another process.

Hypovolemic shock

Control bleeding.
Obtain vascular access, and infuse NS or lactated Ringer solution (to 60 ml/kg or more).
If [Hb] ≤ 9 g/dl, consider giving RBCs. [Hb] should be ≥ 7 g/dl in young healthy patients with controlled bleeding, up to ≥ 11 g/dl in other patients.
Treat pain, hypothermia, acidemia, and coagulopathy.

Inflammatory shock

Obtain vascular access, and infuse fluids as necessary to replenish volume.
Give RBCs as for hypovolemic shock.
Treat pain, hypothermia, and acidemia.
Once resuscitation is well under way, search for and treat underlying inflammatory cause of shock.

Shock resolves

Periphery is priority

Goals: SV 60–100 ml, MAP 90 mm Hg, HR 60–100/min, filling pressures in midteens.

Treatment measures:
- Infuse fluids to ensure generous end-diastolic volumes.
- Increase contractility as needed with dobutamine (5–15 µg/kg/min) and milrinone (50 µg, then 0.375–0.75 µg/kg/min).
- If absolutely necessary to increase BP, give a vasoconstrictor—dopamine (2–20 µg/kg/min) if HR ≤ 90/min, norepinephrine (4–12 µg/kg/min) if HR > 90/min.

Periphery and heart are equal priorities

Goals: SV 55–85 ml, MAP 80 mm Hg, HR 60–90/min, filling pressures in low teens.

Treatment measures:
- Give fluids or initiate diuresis so that the smaller of the two end-diastolic volumes is slightly greater than normal.
- Cautiously increase contractility as necessary with dobutamine (5–15 µg/kg/min) and milrinone (50 µg, then 0.375–0.75 µg/kg/min).
- If absolutely necessary, give a vasoconstrictor—dopamine (2–20 µg/kg/min) if HR ≤ 70/min, norepinephrine (4–12 µg/kg/min) if HR > 70/min.
- For HR ≥ 110/min, initiate beta blockade with esmolol (500 µg/kg, then 50 µg/kg/min), followed by metoprolol (5–10 mg q. 6 hr).

```
Search for and treat any immediately life-threatening
conditions:
  • Dysrhythmias              • Bleeding
  • Loss of airway or         • Anaphylaxis
    inadequate ventilation    • Electrolyte or glucose
  • Compression or obstruction  abnormalities
    of heart or great vessels
```

Shock persists

Secure airway, and ensure adequate ventilation.
Treat on basis of underlying physiologic abnormality.

Neurogenic shock

Place patient in Trendelenburg position.
Obtain vascular access, and infuse fluids as necessary.
Give vasoconstrictors if required, provided that shock state has no hypovolemic component.

Cardiogenic shock

If ventricular end-diastolic volumes seem large, initiate diuresis (e.g., with furosemide, 10–40 mg).
Control hypertension, if present.
Initiate beta blockade to keep HR ≤ 90/min, unless patient is hypotensive or periphery is underperfused.
If [Hb] ≤ 11g/dl, give RBCs.
Search for and treat cardiac cause of shock.

Shock persists

Insert systemic and pulmonary arterial catheters.
Overall goal is to reverse clinical abnormalities. Failing that, temporary goals can be formulated on the basis of measurements from catheters. Goals for SV, HR, MAP, and filling pressures should be based on relative priorities of heart and periphery.

Heart is priority

Goals: SV 50–70 ml, MAP 80 mm Hg, HR 60–80/min, filling pressures in low teens.

Treatment measures:
• Initiate diuresis so that smaller end-diastolic volume is normal or (if necessary for adequate SV and filling pressures) slightly larger.
• Control BP with nitroprusside (0.5–10 µg/kg/min), nitroglycerin (5–200 µg/min), or ACE inhibitors (e.g., enalaprilat, 1.25–5 mg q. 6 hr). as needed.
• Initiate beta blockade to keep HR ≤ 90/min.
• Obtain coronary arteriogram and initiate cardiac catheterization as needed.
• Intervene with coronary angioplasty, balloon pump, or cardiac surgery as indicated.

Table 1 Pathophysiologic Classification of Shock

Type of Shock	Abnormality	Causes
Extracardiac Compressive	Compression of the thin-walled chambers of the heart—the atria and the right ventricle—and compression of the great veins entering the heart	Pericardial tamponade, elevated diaphragm from pregnancy or abdominal bleeding or intestinal distention or ascites, ruptured diaphragm, tension pneumothorax, positive pressure ventilation with large tidal volumes
Obstructive	Excessive hindrance to ventricular emptying imposed by cardiac valvular stenosis or excessive vascular stiffness or resistance	Pulmonary embolism, air embolism, systemic hypertension, tension pneumothorax, hemothorax, ruptured diaphragm, positive pressure ventilation, aortic or pulmonary valvular stenosis
Hypovolemic	Depletion of vascular volume	Bleeding, protracted vomiting or diarrhea, fluid sequestration in obstructed gut or injured tissue, excessive use of diuretics, adrenal insufficiency, diabetes insipidus, dehydration, anaphylaxis
Inflammatory (formerly known as septic or traumatic shock)	Complex response associated with the systemic inflammatory and coagulative reaction to infected or injured tissues	Pneumonia, peritonitis, cholangitis, pyelonephritis, soft tissue infection, meningitis, mediastinitis, crush injuries, major fractures, high-velocity penetrating wounds, major burns, retained necrotic tissue, pancreatitis, anaphylaxis
Neurogenic	Pooling of blood in autonomically denervated venules and small veins; hypotension arising from denervated arterioles and sometimes from a denervated heart	Spinal cord injury, regional anesthetic, administration of drugs that produce autonomic blockade
Cardiogenic	Decreased myocardial contractility	Bradyarrhythmias, tachyarrhythmias, cardiac valvular insufficiency, papillary muscle rupture, myocardiopathy, myocarditis, myocardial ischemia, myocardial contusion (rare), septal defects

Table 2 Clinical Features of Compensated and Decompensated Shock

Parameter	Hypovolemic Shock		Inflammatory Shock		Neurogenic Shock		Left-Sided Cardiogenic Shock	
	Compensated	Decompensated	Compensated	Decompensated	Compensated	Decompensated	Compensated	Decompensated
Cardiovascular								
Heart rate	Increased	Variable	Increased	Increased	Increased	Decreased	Normal	Normal
BP	Normal	Decreased	Decreased	Decreased	Decreased	Decreased	Normal	Decreased
Cardiac output	Normal	Decreased	Increased	Normal	Increased	Decreased	Normal	Decreased
Power	Normal	Decreased	Normal	Decreased	Normal	Decreased	Normal	Decreased
Cardiac efficiency*	Decreased	Decreased	Decreased	Decreased	Decreased	Decreased	Decreased	Decreased
Metabolic								
Acid-base status	Normal	Metabolic acidemia	Metabolic acidemia	Metabolic acidemia	Normal	Metabolic acidemia	Normal	Metabolic acidemia
O_2 consumption	Normal	Decreased	Normal	Decreased	Normal	Decreased	Normal	Decreased
Glucose concentration	Moderately increased	Moderately increased	Increased	Variable	Normal	Normal	Normal	Normal
Clinical								
Temperature	Normal	Normal to decreased	Increased	Variable	Normal	Normal to decreased	Normal	Normal
Respiratory rate	Increased	Increased	Increased	Increased	Normal	Variable	Normal	Increased
Skin	Pale, cool	Pale, cool, clammy	Pink, warm	Pale, cool, clammy	Pink, warm in denervated areas	Pink, warm in denervated areas	Normal	Pale, cool, clammy
Neurologic state	Anxious	Anxious, confused, combative, obtunded	Anxious	Obtunded	Anxious; lower body paralyzed	Anxious; upper and lower body paralyzed	Normal	Anxious
Urine output	Decreased	Minimal	Decreased	Minimal	Decreased	Minimal	Decreased	Minimal

*Cardiovascular power divided by myocardial O_2 requirements.

TACHYCARDIA OR BRADYCARDIA

The pulse rate—perhaps the most evident of all the physical findings in clinical medicine—can increase in shock; such an increase is frequently cited as a cardinal feature of shock. When tachycardia is present, the possibility of shock should be considered; however, the absence of tachycardia should not be taken as a sign that the patient is not in shock. In extreme cases of shock, the pulse rate eventually falls to 0/min. Even in less extreme cases, the pulse rate may slow down, presumably to allow added time both for ventricular filling and for coronary perfusion of the myocardium as well as to reduce myocardial oxygen requirements. Thus, a normal or even a slow heart rate does not rule out shock and may even be an indication of a decompensated shock state.[1-3]

TACHYPNEA

A rapid respiratory rate may be a response to a metabolic acidemia, which is a typical finding with decompensated shock of any cause.

CUTANEOUS HYPOPERFUSION

Poor skin perfusion is often the first sign of shock. In all types of shock other than warm inflammatory shock and neurogenic shock, adrenergic discharge and the release of vasopressin and angiotensin II constrict the arterioles, venules, and small veins throughout the body. This constriction compensates for what otherwise could be profound hypotension. Cutaneous vasoconstriction produces the most sensitive sign of shock: the pale, cool, and clammy skin of someone exhibiting the fight-or-flight reaction. This sign is not specific for shock—it can also be the result of hypothermia, for example—but when it is seen in conjunction with collapsed and constricted subcutaneous veins in a patient with suspected hypovolemic or decompensated inflammatory shock, it establishes the diagnosis.

MENTAL ABNORMALITIES

Patients in severe decompensated shock frequently exhibit mental abnormalities, which can range from anxiousness to agitation to indifference to obtundation. These findings are not sensitive—indeed, they develop only in the late stages of shock—nor are they specific. They are, however, a strong warning to the physician that something must be done quickly. The body protects the brain at all costs; if blood supply to the brain is becoming inadequate, there usually is little time left.

OLIGURIA

Whenever the diagnosis of shock is being entertained, a Foley catheter should be placed. In many cases of compensated shock and in all cases of decompensated shock (except those in which shock results from inappropriate diuresis involving either a previously administered drug or ingestion of ethanol), urine output falls off. Oliguria is one of the most sensitive and specific of all the signs of shock.

MYOCARDIAL ISCHEMIA

An electrocardiogram, which should be obtained promptly whenever a patient is suspected of being in shock, may show signs of ischemia. The ischemia may be caused either by a primary myocardial problem or by a secondary extracardiac problem (e.g., hypotension resulting from hemorrhage or excess hindrance to ventricular contraction resulting from pulmonary embolism). In either case, the presence of myocardial ischemia, like the presence of mental abnormalities, should prompt quick action.

METABOLIC ACIDEMIA

Metabolic acidemia, as a sign of shock, may be manifested by an increased respiratory rate, but analysis of blood gases is usually re-

Table 3 Clinical Markers of Possible Shock State

Clinical Marker	Value or Findings Indicative of Shock
Systolic blood pressure	
Adult	≤ 110 mm Hg
Schoolchild	≤ 100 mm Hg
Preschool child	≤ 90 mm Hg
Infant	≤ 80 mm Hg
Sinus tachycardia	
Adult	≥ 90 beats/min
Schoolchild	≥ 120 beats/min
Preschool child	≥ 140 beats/min
Infant	≥ 160 beats/min
Cutaneous vasoconstriction	Pale, cool, clammy skin with constricted subcutaneous veins
Mental changes	Anxiousness, agitation, indifference, lethargy, obtundation
Urine output	
Adult	≤ 0.5 ml·kg^{-1}·hr^{-1}
Child	≤ 1.0 ml·kg^{-1}·hr^{-1}
Infant	≤ 2.0 ml·kg^{-1}·hr^{-1}
Myocardial ischemia or failure	Chest pain, third heart sound, pulmonary edema, abnormal ECG
Metabolic acidemia	[HCO$_3^-$] ≤ 21 mEq/L Base deficit ≥ 3 mEq/L
Hypoxemia (on room air)	
0–50 yr	≤ 90 mm Hg
51–70 yr	≤ 80 mm Hg
≥ 71 yr	≤ 70 mm Hg

quired for confirmation. The acidemia may take the form of either a low calculated bicarbonate level or a base deficit.[4] Some patients in the early stages of shock—even severe shock—are not acidemic. If flow is sufficiently reduced, the anaerobic products of metabolism will be confined to the periphery; they may not be washed into the central circulation until some degree of resuscitation has taken place. Systemic arterial acidemia may become evident only after the diagnosis has been made and treatment initiated.

HYPOXEMIA

Systemic arterial hypoxemia is a common sign of shock. Low flow results in marked desaturation of blood leaving the metabolizing peripheral tissues and entering the pulmonary artery. If pulmonary function is compromised to any significant degree, as is often the case with shock, the markedly desaturated pulmonary arterial blood becomes only partially saturated as it passes through the lungs.

Identification and Treatment of Immediately Life-Threatening Conditions

If the patient shows signs of possible shock, the next step is to search for and treat any conditions that could kill the patient immediately. Such conditions include dysrhythmias, loss of airway or inadequate ventilation, extracardiac compression of the heart or obstruction of the vasculature, bleeding, and certain life-threatening medical conditions (e.g., anaphylaxis and highly abnormal electrolyte concentrations).

DYSRHYTHMIAS

Given that an electrocardiogram should be obtained promptly in any patient suspected of being in shock, any dysrhythmias present will usually be recognized at an early point. An agonal patient with a dysrhythmia should undergo cardioversion, ideally even before the airway is secured and before I.V. access is obtained. Cardioversion, when successful, can restore a moribund patient with ventricular fibrillation, ventricular tachycardia, or atrial fibrillation to life with full neurologic recovery. It is of no value for a patient in asystole; however, the possibility of fully resuscitating a patient in ventricular standstill is so remote that it usually makes little difference what mode of therapy is attempted or whether therapy is attempted at all.

A nonagonal patient should be treated in accordance with standard resuscitation routines [see 1 Initial Emergency Management of Noninjured Patients: Cardiopulmonary Resuscitation and Correction of Acute Dysrhythmias].

LOSS OF AIRWAY OR INADEQUATE VENTILATION

If a patient can talk in a full voice without undue effort, the airway can be assumed to be intact; if not, the possibility of airway compromise must be considered. Airway compromise has a number of possible causes, ranging from loss of protective reflexes to mechanical obstruction. Sometimes, a jaw thrust is all that is needed for the physician to make the diagnosis and treat the problem.[5] In cases of profound shock, however, a definitive airway, such as that gained by inserting an oral endotracheal tube, becomes necessary. A definitive airway allows the physician to proceed with other lifesaving measures. If, after initial resuscitation, shock resolves and the patient regains consciousness and begins to struggle against intubation, the tube may be removed.

Of all the conditions that can render ventilation inadequate, tension pneumothorax is the most deadly. The most common causes of tension pneumothorax are trauma and therapeutic interventions by medical personnel (e.g., central venous punctures and positive pressure ventilation). Characteristic signs include decreased or absent breath sounds on the involved side, a hyperresonant hemithorax, and, if the patient is normovolemic, distended neck veins. (A tracheal shift—a commonly described feature in patients with tension pneumothoraces—is hard to detect and, in my experience, rarely helpful in making the diagnosis.) Treatment consists of needle decompression or tube thoracostomy.

Institution of mechanical ventilation does not guarantee that the patient will be adequately ventilated. The ventilator may malfunction, or the endotracheal tube may be misplaced or obstructed. If the chest wall does not rise with inspiration, mechanical ventilation should be promptly discontinued, and ventilation with an Ambu bag should be initiated at an inspired oxygen fraction (F_IO_2) of 1.0. If increasing abdominal distention is apparent, the possibility of esophageal intubation or displacement of the endotracheal tube into the hypopharynx should be considered. Treatment consists of reintubation. If breath sounds are absent on the left, right mainstem bronchial intubation should be considered. Treatment consists of partial withdrawal of the tube. Endotracheal tubes can become obstructed with clotted blood or inspissated secretions. Treatment consists of suctioning. Bleeding in the tracheobronchial tree (from injuries or from friable bronchial mucosa or tumor tissue) can eliminate ventilation from the lung segment supplied by the injured or obstructed bronchus and flood the initially uninjured lung with blood. If the bleeding is thought to be coming from the left lung, the endotracheal tube should be advanced into the right mainstem bronchus. Bleeding from the right lung can be more problematic because selective left mainstem intubation may be impossible. Prompt control of bleeding can sometimes be obtained via endobronchial or open surgical intervention; both interventions also may be needed either for acute control or for definitive management of bleeding from the left lung.

Massive hemothoraces with collapse and compression of the lung should be treated with tube thoracostomy and, if necessary, surgical intervention. A massive left-side air leak from trauma or a ruptured bleb can be treated by advancing the endotracheal tube into the right mainstem bronchus. A massive right-side air leak usually necessitates surgical intervention, as does any leak that does not close quickly.

COMPRESSION OR OBSTRUCTION OF THE HEART OR THE GREAT VESSELS

Acute pericardial tamponade is usually manifested by muffled heart tones and occasionally by an exaggerated (> 10 mm Hg) decrease in systolic blood pressure on spontaneous breathing. If the patient is not hypovolemic, the neck veins are typically distended. Treatment consists of needle decompression or surgical creation of a pericardial window. Chronic tamponade can also produce shock but often does not give rise to the findings characteristic of acute tamponade; it is treated in the same way.

Diaphragmatic rupture and the ensuing intrusion of abdominal viscera into the chest can compress the heart, the great veins, and the extracardiac pulmonary vasculature, as can an intact but elevated diaphragm. Such compression can become a major problem if the patient is also hypovolemic. Treatment of a ruptured hemidiaphragm consists of operative reduction and repair; treatment of gut distention, decompression; treatment of bleeding, vascular control; and treatment of ascites, paracentesis of small amounts of fluid (just enough to lower intra-abdominal pressure).[6] Late-term pregnant women should be turned onto the left side so as to relieve compression of the right common iliac vein and the inferior vena cava.

Positive pressure ventilation can compress the heart, the great veins, and the vasculature in the pulmonary parenchyma.[7-11] In cases of suspected shock, tidal volumes should be kept small (≤ 7 ml/kg ideal body weight); inspiratory times should be short (≤ 1 second); end-expiratory pressure should be set at 0; and the initial respiratory rate should be kept low to minimize the total time spent in inspiration. Oxygenation can be maintained by using a high F_IO_2 (initially, 1.0). When blood gas analysis becomes available, the respiratory rate should be adjusted to prevent respiratory acidemia, and the inspired oxygen concentration should be decreased, provided that arterial saturation remains above 95%. When the patient is more stable, arterial saturation can be kept at a slightly lower level (≥ 92%); however, in the acute setting, it should be kept higher to buffer unanticipated decreases in oxygenation.

Besides compromising ventilation, tension pneumothoraces can compress the heart, the great systemic and pulmonary veins as they enter the atria, and the extracardiac pulmonary vasculature. Massive hemothoraces can exert similar effects. These conditions are treated as previously described [see Loss of Airway or Inadequate Ventilation, above].

Intravascular obstruction from a pulmonary thromboembolism or air embolism can kill quickly. Treatment of massive thromboembolism consists of prompt administration of fibrinolytics or heparin [see 70 Thromboembolic Problems], followed, in many cases, by pulmonary arteriography and further lytic therapy. Right-side air embolism can arise from penetrating injuries to large veins in the upper part of the body or from a percutaneous puncture with a large-bore needle if air is allowed access to the venous system while the patient takes a deep breath, especially if the patient is upright. Right-side air embolism can also arise as a complication of insufflation of gas into the peritoneal cavity during laparoscopy. Initial treatment consists of elimination of the source of air. Air that forms an air trap in the outflow tract of the right ventricle can sometimes be translocated to the apex of the ventricle by placing the patient in the Trendelenburg position with the left side down. Treatment consists of administration of 100% oxygen to wash out any residual nitrogen, followed by attempts to aspirate the air with a long central venous catheter. Coronary air embolism can occur whenever a patient with a penetrating injury to the lung parenchyma, either from trauma or from a needle puncture, is placed on positive pressure ventilation. The positive airway pressure can push air from an injured bronchus into an adjacent injured pulmonary vein, thereby allowing the air access to the left ventricle, the coronary arteries, and the brain. The diagnosis is usually made when a patient at risk goes into arrest shortly after initiation of positive pressure ventilation. Coronary air embolism is treated by giving 100% oxygen, opening the chest on the side with the suspected pulmonary penetration, and cross-clamping the hilum of the lung. The heart is then massaged while the descending thoracic aorta is compressed, and vasoconstrictors are administered.

BLEEDING

Bleeding should be controlled by any means necessary. Bleeding from an easily accessible site in an extremity, for instance, may be readily controlled with compression, whereas bleeding from an injury to the suprarenal aorta calls for meticulous exposure and control. Fracture-dislocations should be reduced if possible or, if not immediately reduced, immobilized.

ACUTE MEDICAL CONDITIONS

Anaphylaxis and life-threatening abnormalities in electrolyte or glucose concentrations usually are not recognized in the initial stages of shock management, but once they come to light, they should be treated promptly.

Treatment of Shock on the Basis of the Underlying Physiologic Abnormality

If shock persists after immediately life-threatening conditions have been treated, the next step in management is to categorize the shock state on the basis of the underlying physiologic abnormality and to initiate treatment accordingly.

As a rule, all that is needed to make this preliminary classification is the history, the physical examination, a chest x-ray, an electrocardiogram, and, in some cases, a complete blood count, electrolyte concentrations, a glucose level, and an arterial blood gas analysis. The classification is seldom neat: more than one cause of cardiovascular inadequacy is usually present, as when a patient with a myocardial infarction (MI) requires ventilation or when a patient with a ruptured abdominal aortic aneurysm has a distended abdomen. Nevertheless, such categorization is useful, in that it focuses the physician's attention on the primary problem, the cause of the persistent shock state.

First, the airway should be secured (if it has not been secured already), and supplemental oxygen should be given via a mask or a nasal cannula. The patient should be intubated, and ventilatory support should be provided if needed. The F_IO_2 should be 1.0 initially. Tidal volumes should be kept small (approximately 7 ml/kg ideal body weight) to minimize overdistention of alveoli and compression of the pulmonary vasculature and the heart. No end-expiratory pressure should be used initially. Inspiratory times should be kept short (≤ 1 second), and the respiratory rate should be kept as slow as possible. These measures will minimize ventilation-induced obstruction of the pulmonary vasculature and compression of the vena cavae and the heart—hemodynamic consequences that can be fatal, especially when superimposed on preexisting shock.

EXTRACARDIAC COMPRESSIVE/OBSTRUCTIVE SHOCK

As a condition that can kill quickly, extracardiac compressive/obstructive shock should already have been treated [see Compression or Obstruction of the Heart or the Great Vessels, above]. It is wise, however, to keep these two causes of shock in mind as workup proceeds: they often develop secondarily, as when tension pneumothorax develops in a mechanically ventilated patient who is being worked up or treated for some nonpulmonary problem.

HYPOVOLEMIC SHOCK

Treatment of Underlying Cause

At first glance, it might seem obvious that treatment of the underlying causes of shock should have the highest of priorities. This is indeed the case for hypovolemic shock caused by hemorrhage: it makes no sense to pour fluid and blood into a patient while controllable bleeding continues unchecked. For other types of shock, however, it is better to postpone treatment of the underlying causes until after the patient has been adequately resuscitated [see Inflammatory Shock, below].

Vascular Access

Simultaneously with efforts to control the underlying cause of hypovolemic shock, vascular access should be obtained, if it has not been already. If possible, superficial veins in the upper extremities should be cannulated with two large-bore catheters. If this is impossible, cutdowns may be performed on an antecubital or a basilic vein in the upper extremity, a cephalic vein at the shoulder, an external jugular vein at the base of the neck, or a saphenous vein at the ankle or in the groin.

Cutdowns in the upper extremity cause little morbidity but can take time to perform because upper-extremity veins are most likely to be thrombosed from earlier use. Morbidity is also low with the cephalic veins and the external jugular veins; however, exposure is sometimes difficult because of either the overlying fascia (in the case of the cephalic veins) or the overlying muscle (in the case of the external jugular veins). The saphenous vein at the ankle is readily exposed, large, and easy to cannulate. It cannot be used if there is extensive trauma to the extremity: if the cannula is left in place at the ankle for more than 24 hours, it is likely to cause superficial thrombophlebitis. The saphenous vein in the groin is harder to expose, but it too is large and easy to cannulate. If the cannula is left in place in the groin for more than 24 hours, there is a substantial chance that it will cause iliofemoral thrombophlebitis, which can lead to massive and possibly disabling edema in the involved extremity. Therapeutic anticoagulation is required in patients who may be at high risk for bleeding.

Percutaneous cannulation of the internal jugular vein provides not only access for infusion of fluids and drugs but also a port for central venous monitoring. In hypovolemic patients, this vein is usually collapsed, and puncture of the adjacent common carotid artery becomes a possibility; if puncture does occur, it may be difficult to recognize. The pulsatility of blood drawn from an arterial catheter may not be apparent; desaturated arterial blood may take on the appearance of a venous aspirate.

Percutaneous puncture of the subclavian vein provides large-bore access and monitoring capability; however, it may be difficult to accomplish in a hypovolemic patient. Pneumothorax may result, but it is usually easy to treat if recognized early. Puncture of the subclavian artery with decompression into the pleural cavity (a nontamponading space) can be fatal, especially in a patient made vulnerable by coexisting shock.

Percutaneous puncture of the common femoral vein is among the easiest of all techniques for venous access and provides large-bore monitoring capability. Because the femoral artery is immediately adjacent to the vein, unintentional puncture of the artery is common under urgent conditions. If the patient is in extremis, the artery should be cannulated. Intra-arterial infusion of fluids is as effective as I.V. infusion. Great care must be taken to ensure that no air gains entry to the system, and the catheter should be removed as soon as other access is gained. A femoral venous catheter should be removed as soon as possible as well. Percutaneous puncture of the common femoral vein is usually a fallback approach. If it is used in the resuscitation of a hypercoagulable shock patient (the usual scenario) and if the catheter is left in place for more than even a few hours, there is a substantial risk of iliofemoral deep vein thrombosis or even septic deep vein thrombosis—a potentially fatal complication in a critically ill patient.

In pediatric patients, intraosseous access has become a useful means of gaining vascular access under difficult conditions. On rare occasions, this approach may be used in young adults.[12,13]

The first attempts at obtaining vascular access should be made in the upper extremities with a percutaneous technique. If these attempts fail, the physician should fall back on a technique with which he or she is comfortable. There is no single best approach.

Fluid Administration

Once vascular access is obtained, a 20 ml/kg bolus of normal saline should be infused. If the patient is in profound shock, the fluid bolus should be given within 5 minutes if possible; if the situation is less urgent, it may be given over a period of 15 minutes or so. If shock does not resolve, two more boluses should be given.

I consider normal saline the fluid of choice for initial resuscitation in most patients. Its sodium concentration (154 mmol/L) is close to that of normal serum. Its chloride concentration (also 154 mmol/L) can induce hyperchloremic metabolic acidemia, but this state seems not to be harmful to the patient; if it is not severe, it may even augment myocardial contractility. The slight hyperosmolality of the solution may yield a modest increase in contractility as well. If the patient has severe metabolic acidemia with a chloride concentration exceeding 115 mmol/L, lactated or acetated Ringer solution is used. Both the lactate and the acetate accept a proton to form an organic acid, which is converted in the liver to carbon dioxide and water. As long as hepatic function and pulmonary function are adequate, which is usually the case, the result of this process is buffering of the acidemia that can accompany the shock state. Both of these solutions, however, are hyponatremic and hypoosmotic; the latter is a potential problem in patients at risk for increased intracranial pressure.

Solutions containing glucose should not be used in the initial resuscitation of a patient in shock unless the patient is known to be hypoglycemic. Most patients in shock, in fact, are hyperglycemic as a result of high plasma levels of epinephrine and cortisol.[14] Excessively high plasma glucose concentrations can induce an inappropriate diuresis.

Hypertonic saline solutions containing up to 7.5% sodium chloride (compared with 0.9% for normal saline) show promise for resuscitating patients in situations where large-volume resuscitation with isotonic solutions is impossible (e.g., battle, events involving mass casualties, and prehospital trauma care). Hypertonic solutions provide far more blood volume expansion than isotonic solutions do. They also have advantages in treating hypotensive patients with head injuries. These solutions are approved for use and are commercially available in Brazil (the country where the idea originated), Chile, Argentina, and Europe; they are not currently approved for use in the United States.[15-21]

Albumin-containing solutions should not be given in the acute phase of shock resuscitation except perhaps in unusual circumstances—for example, when only small amounts of resuscitative fluids can be given because of logistical problems, such as those encountered with mass casualties or under battlefield conditions. Initially, protein- or colloid-containing solutions achieve greater plasma volume expansion than crystalloid solutions, but the data from randomized trials with albumin convincingly demonstrate that long-term survival is no better and possibly worse if albumin is used in a setting where large-volume crystalloid can be given instead.[22] The reasons for the poorer survival rates are not entirely clear, but it may be that administration of albumin under conditions of increased microvascular permeability results in accumulation of excessive amounts of albumin in the interstitium. Once in the interstitium, albumin, unlike water and other smaller molecules, can regain access to the plasma space only via lymphatic drainage. If lymphatic drainage capacity is exceeded, persistent postoperative edema may result.

Blood should be given to ensure that the hemoglobin concentration is at least 7 g/dl, if not substantially higher. Certain patients require higher concentrations, as reflected in the following guidelines:

1. A hemoglobin concentration of 7 g/dl is adequate in a young patient who has good coronary arteries and whose bleeding is known to be completely under control.[23]
2. A hemoglobin concentration of 8 g/dl is adequate in a young patient who is at slight risk for further bleeding.
3. A hemoglobin concentration of 9 g/dl is required if the risk of bleeding is substantial.
4. A hemoglobin concentration of 10 g/dl should be the goal if there is any possibility of coronary artery disease, even in the absence of ongoing myocardial ischemia. (The heart is a working muscle, even when the body is at rest, and uses much of the oxygen delivered to it by the coronary arteries. Obstruction of the arteries proximal to the working muscle can lead to usage of all the oxygen carried in the blood. Accordingly, it is crucial to maintain an adequate hemoglobin concentration in this setting. Provided that the arteries are not obstructed, the other organs in the resting body are not susceptible, because they use only a fraction of the oxygen delivered to them.)
5. A hemoglobin concentration of 11 g/dl should be maintained if the heart shows any signs of ongoing myocardial ischemia.

In an emergency, O-negative red blood cells reconstituted with normal saline may be given. If the patient can wait a few more minutes, type-specific blood may be given so as to conserve the blood bank's supply of O-negative blood. Whole blood can be administered more quickly than packed red blood cells, but use of packed cells has the advantage of conserving the blood bank's supply of fresh frozen plasma. Filtering reduces the amount of particulate material administered with the blood but may also reduce the rate at which blood can be administered.

The use of blood substitutes for resuscitation is an attractive option from a conceptual perspective. To date, however, clinical trials using these agents in this setting have yielded disappointing results.[24,25]

Treatment of Pain, Hypothermia, Acidemia, and Coagulopathy

Once blood volume has been at least partially replenished, pain may be treated with small I.V. doses of narcotics. Pain relief can decrease the stress response associated with shock and perhaps diminish the severity of its late sequelae; however, narcotics can also decrease tone in the venules and small veins, thereby exacerbating the shock state. Accordingly, it is vital to keep doses small, to titrate the dosage carefully, and to be ready to reverse the effect with a narcotic antagonist if necessary. Sometimes, a drop in blood pressure after administration of a narcotic can even be a good thing if it alerts the physician to an underlying hypovolemia that should be treated more aggressively.

If hypothermia is present initially, it should be corrected; if it is not present initially, it should not be allowed to develop. Hypothermia slows metabolic processes. In some situations (e.g., cold-water drowning), this may be beneficial to a degree. In the majority of cases, however, it is better for the patient to have a normal body temperature, normal myocardial contractility, and intact coagulatory and immune function. The patient must be unclothed during the initial evaluation, but after that, he or she should be covered, especially the head (a potential source of major heat loss). The room should be kept warm, and any fluids administered should be prewarmed either in an oven or with heating devices.

A low arterial pH should be brought up to a 7.20 by means of either modest degrees of hyperventilation or administration of bicarbonate. Attempts to achieve higher values, at least in the initial shock setting, are probably counterproductive. As noted [*see* Fluid Administration, *above*], moderate acidemia may enhance myocardial contractility and immune function. Ideally, acidemia is corrected by treating the underlying cause of shock. Administration of bicarbonate should be kept to a minimum.

Coagulopathy should be treated with fresh frozen plasma and platelets [*see* 5 Bleeding and Transfusion]. The decision to use these components should be based on observation of bleeding and clotting in the patient, not on laboratory measurements of coagulation or platelet counts, which can be normal even during exsanguination.

INFLAMMATORY SHOCK

For the most part, initial treatment of inflammatory shock is similar to that of hypovolemic shock because the most pronounced feature of inflammatory shock is loss of plasma into the interstitium through a permeable microvasculature, leading to depletion of vascular volume. The main difference between treatment of hypovolemic shock and treatment of inflammatory shock has to do with when the underlying cause of the shock state should be treated. With hemorrhagic shock, the first priority is control of bleeding. With inflammatory shock, the first priority is replenishment of vascular volume, and definitive treatment (e.g., debridement of dead tissue, drainage of pus, or diversion of the GI tract) should be postponed until the patient is at least partially resuscitated. Such definitive procedures can impose a major physiologic burden on the patient; thus, it is usually best to wait until the patient can withstand the operative insult.

Other potential differences between treatment of inflammatory shock and treatment of hypovolemic shock have to do with the replenishment of depleted compensatory factors and with the use of blockers of inflammatory mediators. A 2001 study suggested that infusion of activated protein C might well be lifesaving for some patients with the septic response.[26] To date, however, studies using blockers of inflammatory mediators to treat inflammatory shock have yielded disappointing results.[27,28]

NEUROGENIC SHOCK

Initial management of neurogenic shock is similar to that of hypovolemic shock, with two exceptions. First, patients in neurogenic shock often benefit from being placed in the Trendelenburg position. Autonomic denervation of the systemic venules and small veins leads to pooling of blood in these capacitance vessels. The Trendelenburg position causes this blood to be translocated to the vascular structures in the chest, including the heart, thereby helping to restore ventricular end-diastolic volumes. Patients with other forms of shock, however, derive no benefit from the Trendelenburg position. In hypovolemic shock, for example, the systemic venules and small veins are already depleted of their blood, as a consequence of both volume loss and adrenergic constriction of the vessel walls. Thus, no blood can be translocated. Furthermore, the left ventricle must pump its blood uphill to perfuse the abdominal viscera and the lower extremities, and the increased work can exhaust an overworked heart.[29]

Second, patients in neurogenic shock often benefit from the use of vasoconstrictors. Vasoconstrictors play no role in the initial management of hypovolemic or inflammatory shock. In these forms of shock, fluid replenishment is a crucial initial measure, and constrictors can be deadly in these settings because they can shut off residual flow to organs already rendered ischemic by depletion of the vascular volume. In neurogenic shock, however, the arterioles are fully dilated in the denervated parts of the body, and this dilatation can lead to central hypotension and inadequate perfusion of the brain and heart. Vasoconstrictors constrict the denervated arterioles, thereby helping to restore central pressures. They also constrict denervated systemic venules and small veins, thereby helping to restore ventricular end-diastolic volumes.

If the heart rate is slow, as it may be if denervation extends high enough to block the sympathetic nerves going to the heart, dopamine (2 to 20 μg/kg/min) may be used. If the heart rate is rapid, norepinephrine or phenylephrine is a good choice. Norepinephrine is given by continuous infusion at a dosage of 4 to 12 μg/min; phenylephrine is initially given at a dosage of 100 to 180 μg/min, which is then decreased to 40 to 60 μg/min.

The danger in giving a vasoconstrictor to a patient in neurogenic shock is that the underlying cause of shock may also have caused occult bleeding. Thus, the vasoconstrictor may maintain the blood pressure, reassuring the physician while the patient bleeds to death. Vasoconstrictors should be used in patients in neurogenic shock only after it has been established that the shock state has no hypovolemic component.

CARDIOGENIC SHOCK

In most cases of cardiogenic shock, management begins with diuresis rather than fluid administration. Furosemide (10 to 40 mg I.V. over a period of 2 to 5 minutes) is a good first choice. If the patient has been receiving furosemide for an extended period, high dosages may be necessary, or spironolactone (25 to 200 mg orally) may have to be added.

Hypertension, if present, may be treated in several ways, depending on the conditions observed. Morphine sulfate (1 to 6 mg I.V. every 1 to 4 hours) is a good first choice if the patient is in pain from an MI and if the physical examination and the chest x-ray indicate pulmonary edema. Nitroglycerine is a good choice if the patient is experiencing angina. It should initially be given I.V. at a dosage of 5 µg/min, which may then be raised in increments of 5 µg/min every 5 minutes. When the dosage reaches 20 µg/min, it may then be raised in increments of 10 µg/min to a maximum dosage of 200 µg/min. Nitroprusside is effective under any conditions. It should initially be given at a dosage of 0.5 µg/kg/min, which may then be raised in increments of 0.5 µg/kg/min to a maximum dosage of 3 µg/kg/min. An angiotensin-converting enzyme (ACE) inhibitor (e.g., enalaprilat, 1.25 to 5.0 mg every 6 hours) is a good choice if the patient's renal function is not compromised and if time is not critical. Sometimes, all of these drugs can be used.

As a rule, hydralazine should not be used; it can increase the heart rate and can markedly increase myocardial oxygen requirements. Calcium channel blockers should be given only after other approaches have failed; they can reduce myocardial oxygen requirements but at the cost of a substantially decreased cardiac output. Nitroprusside and ACE inhibitors generally do not reduce cardiac output, nor, in patients with large ventricular end-diastolic volumes, do morphine and nitroglycerine.

Beta blockade can be extremely effective in controlling blood pressure in a hypertensive patient and heart rate in any patient. Esmolol, a short-acting agent, is the best first choice. A loading dose of 500 µg/kg is given, followed by infusion at a rate of 50 µg/kg/min. If it proves necessary to increase the dosage, another 500 µg/kg loading dose is given, and the infusion rate is raised to 100 µg/kg/min. If the patient responds well to this regimen, he or she should be switched from esmolol to the long-acting agent metoprolol (5 to 15 mg every 6 hours).

Beta blockers can reduce cardiac output, but they also markedly reduce myocardial oxygen requirements by decreasing heart rate, blood pressure, stroke volume, and myocardial contractility. These agents should not be given to patients who are hypotensive or show signs of marked peripheral hypoperfusion, but they should be given to all other patients in whom myocardial ischemia is a possibility.

In many patients with acute myocardial ischemia and shock, all of the aforementioned treatments should be employed, with the addition of heparin anticoagulation and emergency coronary angiography. The mortality associated with cardiogenic shock in a patient with an acute MI is extremely high. Accordingly, every effort should be made to find a correctable lesion and treat it with coronary angioplasty, stenting, or surgical revascularization. If necessary, an intra-aortic balloon pump may be placed once angiography, angioplasty, and stenting have been completed or in preparation for surgical correction of ischemia.

The hemoglobin concentration in patients with cardiogenic shock should be maintained at a generous level (i.e., about 11 g/dl).

Treatment of Shock That Persists Despite Initial Management

INVASIVE MONITORING

In most cases of shock, regardless of category, the initial approach just described leads to resolution of all the clinical abnormalities. Some patients, however, do not respond to these treament measures. In my view, invasive monitoring is warranted for these unresponsive patients.

Invasive monitoring permits direct assessment of patients' thermodynamic needs, thus allowing the physician to deal with the most difficult problem in managing unresponsive shock patients—namely, how to balance the metabolic needs of the noncardiac tissues against the demands made on a potentially ischemic myocardium. Almost all interventions that increase perfusion of the peripheral tissues also increase myocardial oxygen requirements, and almost all interventions that decrease myocardial oxygen requirements also decrease perfusion of noncardiac tissues [see Sidebar Thermodynamic Concepts of Clinical Relevance to Shock].[30,31]

GOALS OF RESUSCITATION

The primary goal of shock management is to correct the clinical abnormalities that led to the diagnosis in the first place. The secondary goal is to enable the patient to generate adequate blood pressure and cardiac output—that is, adequate power [see Table 4]—for perfusion of the tissues without overburdening the heart.

Determining what constitutes adequate blood pressure can be difficult at times. The pressure must be, at the very least, high enough to perfuse the brain, an organ that has a very active metabolic rate and very little vascular tone. Drops in blood pressure put the brain at risk because, unlike all the other organs in the body, it is unable to vasodilate in response to falling perfusion pressure. In an alert patient, determining adequate blood pressure is not difficult. In an obtunded patient, an arbitrary value must be assigned; a reasonable systolic pressure might be 90 mm Hg in a younger patient and somewhat higher in an older patient. Carotid stenosis necessitates a higher pressure, and stenoses in any of the arteries supplying actively metabolizing organs call for higher central pressures.

Although, under ordinary circumstances, all noncerebral organs have some tonic contracture of the arterioles that allows vasodilatation if pressure falls, the arterioles in an organ made ischemic by proximal obstruction and active metabolism are maximally dilated; the organ therefore becomes vulnerable to hypotension. The classic example of this phenomenon is the heart in a patient with coronary disease, but the same mechanism comes into play in the gut in a patient with mesenteric arterial occlusive disease, in the kidney in a patient with renal artery stenosis, in the spinal cord in a patient with obstructed intercostal arteries, and in the extremities in a patient with peripheral arterial disease.

In sum, the only way of setting the goal for adequate blood pressure is to combine clinical judgment with assessment of the patient's response to treatment. If a given blood pressure is associated with an altered level of consciousness, myocardial ischemia, oliguria, or any other sign suggesting inadequate flow, it must be increased.

Although there is general agreement on how to set goals for adequate blood pressure, there is little agreement on how to set goals for optimum cardiac output. One approach is to attempt to determine whether the patient's oxygen consumption (measured with a pulmonary arterial catheter and based in part on measurements of cardiac output) is dependent on oxygen delivery (the product of cardiac output, hemoglobin concentration, and arterial oxygen saturation). At very low levels of oxygen delivery, there is no question that oxygen consumption must decrease.[32] At excessively high levels, however, oxygen consumption may continue to rise if oxygen delivery is increased by the administration of inotropes. These agents usually have beta-adrenergic effects and can increase peripheral oxygen metabolism; they also increase myocardial oxygen requirements. Thus, the act of increasing delivery can increase peripheral consumption.

Another approach is to maintain all patients at very high levels of oxygen delivery without making any attempt to see if there is a correlation between delivery and peripheral consumption. This proposed approach was examined in randomized trials in critically ill patients, which found that maintaining supranormal levels of oxygen delivery was of no benefit.[33-36]

A third approach is to use mixed venous oxygen saturation (also measured with a pulmonary arterial catheter) as a primary end point in resuscitation. This approach has the advantage of simplicity and is certainly useful with some forms of shock (e.g., hypovolemic

Table 4 Different Forms of Power Generated in the Cardiovascular System

Form of Power	Formula
Power delivered into aortic root each minute	SV · HR · LVESP
Power generated by left atrium	SV · HR · LAP
Power generated by left ventricle	SV · HR · (LVESP−LAP)
Mean power delivered into aortic root	SV · HR · MAP
Oscillatory power delivered into aortic root	SV · HR · (LVESP−MAP)
Power used to perfuse peripheral tissues	SV · HR · (MAP−RAP)
Power used to fill right atrium	SV · HR · RAP

Note: see 89 Cardiopulmonary Monitoring.
HR—heart rate   LAP— mean left atrial pressure   LVESP—left ventricular end-systolic pressure   MAP—mean arterial pressure (equivalent to mean aortic root pressure)   RAP—mean right atrial pressure   SV—stroke volume

shock). Many patients in inflammatory shock, however, have quite high mixed venous oxygen saturations, partly because of peripheral shunting through the cutaneous vasculature and partly because of functional shunting by cells that cannot metabolize the oxygen presented to them. In these patients, a high mixed venous oxygen saturation might even indicate a severe metabolic derangement rather than resolution of shock.[34]

Yet another resuscitation approach is to avoid using any direct measurement of cardiovascular adequacy and to use other end points of resuscitation instead. Perhaps the most attractive such end point is gastric mucosal pH. In many forms of shock, the gut is quickly made ischemic; conceivably, if the gut mucosa can be shown to be well perfused, one can assume that the rest of the body is also well perfused. Further trials are necessary to ascertain whether gastric mucosal pH can be used in lieu of detailed measurements of cardiac performance.[37]

Thermodynamic principles may also be employed to set resuscitation end points. Such an approach implies that cardiac output itself should be used in conjunction with blood pressure to assess adequacy of resuscitation. Recent work by Chang and associates suggests that a normal cardiac output is probably an adequate one.[38,39] One might wish to aim for slightly supranormal values in patients with major injuries or overwhelming infections, but excessively high values should rarely be necessary.

To define what a normal cardiac output is, one must take some account of patient size, expressed in terms either of body weight (ideal, current, or premorbid) or of body surface area (which in turn is calculated in part on the basis of weight). I prefer to use ideal body weight in the calculations rather than current body weight or premorbid weight. Ideal body weight is calculated on the basis of the patient's height, with adjustments made for age, on the assumption that ideal weight in an unconditioned older individual decreases by 10% each decade after 50 years of age. The age adjustment can have a substantial effect on the calculation. For example, a patient who is 80 years old—not an uncommon age for an ICU patient today—might have had an ideal body weight of 70 kg at age 50. At 80 years of age, if the patient is not in good condition, ideal body weight will have fallen to 51 kg. This makes a significant difference in terms of target cardiac output: whereas a cardiac output of 7 L/min might have been required when the patient was 50 years old, an output of 5 L/min is probably more than adequate 30 years later. Finally, the choice of a goal for cardiac output is sometimes facilitated by trial and error. For example, if a supranormal cardiac output causes an abnormality (e.g., metabolic acidemia) to resolve when a normal output did not, then an effort should be made to keep the output high for a while.

Thermodynamic Concepts of Clinical Relevance to Shock

In my view, treatment of shock is best approached with an eye to the thermodynamics of cardiovascular function. Thermodynamics is the scientific discipline developed in the 19th century to explain the generation and transfer of energy, including power and heat, between systems. For the purposes of this chapter, an exhaustive familiarity with thermodynamic principles is unnecessary; however, there are a few thermodynamic concepts of direct clinical relevance that are worth outlining here. These concepts become increasingly pertinent as one moves from easily managed patients to more challenging ones.

A key concept is that of power. Power, in thermodynamic terms, is flow multiplied by pressure [see Table 4]. In the case of the heart, the power generated by the left atrium and the left ventricle (and consequently the power delivered into the aortic root) is approximately equal to cardiac output multiplied by left ventricular end-systolic pressure (LVESP):

Power into aortic root = SV · HR · LVESP

where cardiac output is expressed as the product of stroke volume (SV) and heart rate (HR).

The main challenge in treating the patient in shock is to balance the needs of the peripheral circulation against the demands made on the heart. Left ventricular oxygen requirements are directly proportional to left ventricular power: doubling power doubles oxygen requirements. The significance of this relation in the management of shock will be apparent from an examination of the formulas for left ventricular power and power for peripheral tissue perfusion:

Left ventricular power = SV · HR · (LVESP−LAP)
Power for peripheral perfusion = SV · HR · (MAP−RAP)

where LAP is mean left atrial pressure, MAP is mean arterial pressure (which is equivalent to mean aortic root pressure), and RAP is mean right atrial pressure.

From these formulas, it is clear that any therapy that increases SV or HR will increase both power for peripheral perfusion and left ventricular power (and thus left ventricular oxygen requirements). Any therapy that increases MAP will increase power for peripheral perfusion and usually will increase ventricular oxygen requirements because LVESP generally rises when MAP rises. Finally, any therapy that decreases RAP will increase power for peripheral perfusion and usually will increase left ventricular oxygen requirements because LAP generally falls when RAP falls. Thus, in increasing power for perfusion of the peripheral tissues, one almost always increases left ventricular oxygen requirements as well. In other words, there is no thermodynamic free lunch.

Thus, the end points of shock management are for the most part clinical end points—namely, reversal of cutaneous signs of shock, hypotension, mental abnormalities, myocardial ischemia, metabolic acidemia, hypoxemia, and heart rate abnormalities. If these end points cannot be reached initially, the goal should then be to reach thermodynamic end points—that is, adequate pressures and adequate flow (power [see Table 4])—while trying to minimize myocardial oxygen requirements. This is the main challenge in resuscitating a patient from shock. As a rule, increasing the heart rate, end-diastolic volumes, contractility, and the hindrance against which the ventricles contract (up to a limit) all increase the power output of the heart; they also all increase myocardial oxygen requirements. Incorporating a thermodynamic perspective into management brings this problem into the open.

Depending on the resuscitative priorities in a given patient, one of the following three hemodynamic goals is generally appropriate:

1. Increased provision of nutrients to noncardiac tissues along with robust amounts of energy, even though production of that energy by the heart puts a strain on the myocardium.
2. Decreased demands on the heart, even though, as a consequence, less energy will be available for perfusion of noncardiac tissues.
3. A balance between (1) and (2), aimed at achieving the most efficient possible production of energy by the heart while admitting the possibility that a compromise between the two might end up achieving neither.

An example of a patient for whom the first goal might be appropriate is a young trauma patient with a robust myocardium but extensive noncardiac injuries. The second goal might be appropriate for a patient with an uncomplicated MI. The third goal might be appropriate for a patient with known coronary artery disease who has just undergone resection of a ruptured abdominal aortic aneurysm.

ASSESSMENT OF RELATIVE PRIORITIES OF PERIPHERY AND HEART

The next task in the management of unresponsive shock states is to determine whether priority should be given to the needs of the periphery or to those of the heart. The difficulty here is that many of the patients who have reached this stage of treatment—that is, in whom initial therapeutic measures have been unsuccessful—have both cardiac and noncardiac problems. Management of these patients is a challenge.

Periphery Is Priority

Fluid administration and assessment of ventricular end-diastolic volumes If priority is given to the periphery, the patient will probably require fluids. As a starting point, the goal should be to achieve a pulmonary arterial wedge pressure in the midteens (assuming that the patient is being mechanically ventilated). As therapy progresses and as more measurements are made, this goal may have to be modified. The ultimate goal, however, is not to produce any specific wedge pressure but rather to produce generous right and left ventricular end-diastolic volumes.[40] To estimate these volumes, it is necessary to synthesize several pieces of information.

Intracavitary right atrial pressure (a commonly measured value obtained via the proximal port of a pulmonary arterial catheter) yields a good estimate of intracavitary right ventricular end-diastolic pressure. Pulmonary arterial wedge pressure is equivalent to intracavitary left atrial pressure (which, in the absence of mitral valvular stenosis, is the same as left ventricular end-diastolic pressure) if there is an open column of blood when the balloon is inflated between the end of the catheter and the left atrium. This open communication between the catheter tip and the atrium is usually present because the catheter, once inserted, is directed by flow into the well-perfused parts of the pulmonary vasculature. On occasion, however, the catheter ends up in a poorly perfused part of the lung (zone I), in which case it measures intra-alveolar pressure instead of left atrial pressure. This malpositioning is usually signaled by excessive swings in wedge pressure that coincide with the cycling of the ventilator. In theory, inaccuracies can creep into pressure measurements if there is robust collateral flow around the vasculature occluded by the balloon, as with the bronchial circulation. In practice, however, this is seldom a problem.

Given acceptably accurate intracavitary end-diastolic pressure values, the challenge is to extrapolate from these values to reasonably good estimates of ventricular end-diastolic volume. There is not a simple proportional correspondence between pressure and volume, because volume depends not only on pressure but also on the stiffness of the ventricle during diastole and on the stiffness of the structures surrounding the heart.[41-43]

In a patient breathing spontaneously, a right atrial pressure of 2 to 5 mm Hg measured with respect to atmosphere with the transducer zeroed at the midaxillary line is generally sufficient to generate an adequate right ventricular end-diastolic volume. For the left ventricle, a wedge pressure of 5 to 8 mm Hg usually suffices. In a patient with compression of the heart as a result of inflation of the lungs by positive pressure ventilation, an intracavitary right atrial (or right ventricular end-diastolic) pressure of 9 to 12 mm Hg is usually necessary for a normal right ventricular end-diastolic volume; a wedge pressure of 12 to 15 mm Hg is usually necessary for a normal left ventricular end-diastolic volume.

These values work for patients with essentially normal lungs; however, most patients on mechanical ventilators do not have normal lungs. In such patients, the lungs can form a stiff compartment around the heart that does not give when the heart is pushed into the compartment by an elevated diaphragm. To complicate matters further, the diastolic stiffness of the ventricular musculature is increased in many critically ill patients, and the intracavitary pressures must overcome this added stiffness as well. On occasion, right and left intracavitary ventricular end-diastolic pressures exceeding 20 mm Hg are necessary to produce normal end-diastolic volumes.

The estimates of end-diastolic pressure can sometimes be confirmed by increasing the filling pressures of the heart with a fluid bolus and assessing the cardiovascular response. Increases in stroke volume, especially if associated with increases in pulmonary and systemic arterial pressures, suggest that the initial end-diastolic volumes were too small and that more fluid is needed. In other cases, initial end-diastolic volumes might have been unnecessarily large. If so, a diuretic can be given. If stroke volumes and blood pressures do not decrease, further diuresis is indicated.

Right ventricular end-diastolic volume can be measured directly by means of a pulmonary arterial catheter equipped with a fast-response thermistor. These catheters are more expensive than those not so equipped, but they can be helpful in complicated cases.[44] Left ventricular end-diastolic volume can be measured directly with transesophageal echocardiography in difficult cases (e.g., a patient with an elevated diaphragm).

If measurements are available from only one ventricle, the physician can cautiously use this information to estimate the corresponding values from the other, keeping in mind that in many critically ill patients, there is a marked discrepancy between right and left ventricular end-diastolic volumes. The general finding from studies comparing right ventricular end-diastolic volumes (measured with a fast thermistor) and left ventricular end-diastolic volumes (measured with transesophageal echocardiography) is that right ventricular values are frequently larger than left ventricular values in patients in inflammatory shock, sometimes by a factor of 3.[45] In patients with left-sided congestive heart failure, however, left ventricular end-diastolic volumes can be substantially larger than right. Thus, knowing the volume of one chamber does not necessarily mean that one knows the volume of the other, but the clinical scenario can provide some guidance.

Inotropes Inotropes such as dobutamine (5 to 15 µg/kg/min) and milrinone (50 µg, then 0.375 to 0.75 µg/kg/min) can be given freely. They will increase myocardial oxygen requirements, but this is not a problem in a patient with a strong heart. The only limitation on use of the inotropes is the development of a tachycardia. If the heart rate begins to exceed 100 beats/min, the dosage should be reduced.

Vasoconstrictors There are only three indications for administration of vasoconstrictors to patients in whom the primary concern is perfusion of the periphery: (1) profound hypotension in a patient who is in neurogenic shock; (2) hypotension so severe that cerebral or spinal cord perfusion is thought to be inadequate on the basis of either neurologic symptoms (if the patient is neurologically intact) or cerebral perfusion pressure (if the patient is not neurologically intact); and (3) hypotension in a patient who has critical stenosis in the cerebral, coronary, mesenteric, or renal arteries or in the arteries supplying the spinal cord or who has a severely ischemic extremity. For virtually all other patients whose main problem is inadequate perfusion of the periphery, fluids and, occasionally, inotropes are enough.

If a vasoconstrictor is indicated, dopamine may be given if the initial heart rate is 90 beats/min or slower. The heart rate should not be driven above 100 beat/min. Norepinephrine may be given if the initial heart rate exceeds 90 beats/min.

Periphery and Heart Are Equal Priorities

Fluid management in patients who have both inadequate peripheral perfusion and marginal myocardial reserve must be finely tuned. Every effort should be made to estimate the ventricular end-diastolic volumes accurately. Excessively large end-diastolic volumes will increase myocardial oxygen requirements unnecessarily, and inadequate end-diastolic volumes will make it impossible for the ventricles to produce adequate pressure and stroke volumes. In some patients, diuresis is indicated; in others, administration of fluids. Frequently, trial and error will be necessary.

If pressures and stroke volumes are still inadequate after fluids have been replenished, inotropes should be tried. These agents must be used with some caution because they will increase myocardial oxygen requirements.

Vasoconstrictors should be used only as previously discussed [*see* Periphery Is Priority, *above*]. Dopamine may be given if the initial heart rate is 70 beats/min or slower. The heart rate should not be driven above 90 beats/min. Norepinephrine may be given if the heart rate exceeds 70 beats/min.

Beta blockade is frequently necessary when the heart rate exceeds 90 beats/min. Maintenance of a slow heart rate is the single most important factor in minimizing myocardial oxygen requirements, but it usually can be achieved only at the cost of decreasing pressures and stroke volumes. Esmolol is a good first choice because it is quickly reversible; metoprolol may be given later if it is clear that beta blockade was needed and the patient is stable.

Heart Is Priority

If the priority is the heart and there is comparatively little reason for concern about noncardiac tissues, treatment is usually straightforward, though the results may be less than might be hoped for. The treatment approach should be patterned on that for cardiogenic shock (see above). Invasive monitoring allows precise measurements that can be useful, particularly during diuresis. The goal of diuresis is to produce normal ventricular end-diastolic volumes so as to minimize myocardial oxygen requirements. Often, this proves impossible. Larger end-diastolic volumes are necessary to make up for poor contractility. Invasive monitoring helps the physician strike the necessary balance. Vasoconstrictors and inotropes should not be used, because they will increase myocardial oxygen requirements. If blood pressure or stroke volumes become inadequate, the therapeutic approach should be changed to take the needs of the periphery into account as described earlier [*see* Periphery and Heart Are Equal Priorities, *above*].

References

1. Demetriades D, Chan LS, Bhasin P, et al: Relative bradycardia in patients with traumatic hypotension. J Trauma 45:534, 1998
2. Little RA: 1988 Fitts Lecture: heart rate changes after haemorrhage and injury—a reappraisal. J Trauma 29:903, 1989
3. Shenkin HA, Cheney RH, Govons SR, et al: On the diagnosis of hemorrhage in man: a study of volunteers bled large amounts. Am J Med Sci 208:421, 1944
4. Gore DC, Ferrando A, Barnett J, et al: Influence of glucose kinetics on plasma lactate concentration and energy expenditure in severely burned patients. J Trauma 49:673, 2000
5. Gausche M, Lewis RJ, Stratton SJ, et al: Effect of out-of-hospital pediatric endotracheal intubation on survival and neurological outcome: a controlled clinical trial. JAMA 283:783, 2000
6. Chang MC, Miller PR, D'Agostino R, et al: Effects of abdominal decompression on cardiopulmonary function and visceral perfusion in patients with intra-abdominal hypertension. J Trauma 44:440, 1998
7. Ventilation with lower tidal volumes as compared with traditional tidal volumes for acute lung injury and the acute respiratory distress syndrome. Acute Respiratory Distress Syndrome Network. N Engl J Med 342:1301, 2000
8. Amato MBP, Barbas CSV, Medeiros DM, et al: Effect of a protective-ventilation strategy on mortality in the acute respiratory distress syndrome. N Engl J Med 338:347, 1998
9. Bulger EM, Jurkovich GJ, Gentilello LM, et al: Current clinical options for the treatment and management of acute respiratory distress syndrome. J Trauma 48:562, 2000
10. Ranieri VM, Suter PM, Tortorella C, et al: Effect of mechanical ventilation on inflammatory mediators in patients with acute respiratory distress syndrome: a randomized controlled trial. JAMA 282:54, 1999
11. Rankin JS, Olsen CO, Arentzen CE, et al: The effects

of airway pressure on cardiac function in intact dogs and man. Circulation 66:108, 1982
12. Sawyer RW, Bodai BI, Blaisdell FW, et al: The current status of intraosseous infusion. J Am Coll Surg 179:353, 1994
13. Waisman M, Waisman D: Bone marrow infusion in adults. J Trauma 42:288, 1997
14. Wilmore DW: Metabolic response to severe surgical illness: overview. World J Surg 24:705, 2000
15. Angle N, Hoyt DB, Coimbra R, et al: Hypertonic saline resuscitation diminishes lung injury by suppressing neutrophil activation after hemorrhagic shock. Shock 9:164, 1998
16. Ciesla DJ, Moore EE, Zallen G, et al: Hypertonic saline attenuation of polymorphonuclear neutrophil cytotoxicity: timing is everything. J Trauma 48:388, 2000
17. Ho HS, Liu H, Cala PM, et al: Hypertonic perfusion inhibits intracellular Na and Ca accumulation in hypoxic myocardium. Am J Physiol Cell Physiol 278:C953, 2000
18. Rotstein OD: Novel strategies for immunomodulation after trauma: revisiting hypertonic saline as a resuscitation strategy for hemorrhagic shock. J Trauma 49:580, 2000
19. Vassar MJ, Fischer RP, O'Brien PE, et al: A multicenter trial for resuscitation of injured patients with 7.5% sodium chloride. Arch Surg 128:1003, 1993
20. Velasco IT, Pontieri V, Rocha e Silva M, et al: Hyperosmotic NaCl and severe hemorrhagic shock. Am J Physiol 239:H664, 1980
21. Wade CE, Grady JJ, Kramer GC, et al: Individual patient cohort analysis of the efficacy of hypertonic saline/dextran in patients with traumatic brain injury and hypotension. J Trauma 42:S61, 1997
22. Human albumin administration in critically ill patients: systematic review of randomised controlled trials. Cochrane Injuries Group Albumin Reviewers. BMJ 317:235, 1998
23. Hébert PC, Wells G, Blajchman MA, et al: A multicenter, randomized, controlled clinical trial of transfusion requirements in critical care. N Engl J Med 340:409, 1999
24. Cohn SM: Surgical research review: blood substitutes in surgery. Surgery 127:599, 2000
25. Sloan EP, Koenigsberg M, Gens D, et al: Diaspirin cross-linked hemoglobin (DCLHb) in the treatment of severe traumatic hemorrhagic shock: a randomized controlled efficacy trial. JAMA 282:1857, 1999
26. Bernard GR, Vincent JL, Laterre PF, et al: Efficacy and safety of recombinant human activated protein C for severe sepsis. N Engl J Med 344:699, 2001
27. Angus DC, Birmingham MC, Balk RA, et al: E5 murine monoclonal antiendotoxin antibody in gram-negative sepsis: a randomized controlled trial. JAMA 283:1723, 2000
28. Ketoconazole for early treatment of acute lung injury and acute respiratory distress syndrome: a randomized controlled trial. ARDS Network Authors. JAMA 283:1995, 2000
29. Sibbald WJ, Paterson NAM, Holliday RL, et al: The Trendelenburg position: hemodynamic effects in hypotensive and normotensive patients. Crit Care Med 7:218, 1979
30. McDonald's Blood Flow in Arteries: Theoretical, Experimental and Clinical Principles, 4th ed. Nichols WW, O'Rourke MF, Eds. Arnold and Oxford University Press, London and New York, 1998
31. Suga H: Ventricular energetics. Physiol Rev 70:247, 1990
32. Cain SM: Oxygen delivery and uptake in dogs during anemic and hypoxic hypoxia. J Appl Physiol 42:228, 1977
33. Durham RM, Neunaber K, Mazuski JE, et al: The use of oxygen consumption and delivery as endpoints for resuscitation in critically ill patients. J Trauma 41:32, 1996
34. Gattinoni L, Brazzi L, Pelosi P, et al: A trial of goal-oriented hemodynamic therapy in critically ill patients. N Engl J Med 333:1025, 1995
35. Hayes MA, Timmins AC, Yau EHS, et al: Elevation of systemic oxygen delivery in the treatment of critically ill patients. N Engl J Med 330:1717, 1994
36. Velmahos GC, Demetriades D, Shoemaker WC, et al: Endpoints of resuscitation of critically injured patients: normal or supranormal? A prospective randomized trial. Ann Surg 232:409, 2000
37. Ivatury RR, Simon RJ, Islam S, et al: A prospective randomized study of end points of resuscitation after major trauma: global oxygen transport indices versus organ-specific gastric mucosal pH. J Am Coll Surg 183:145, 1996
38. Chang MC, Meredith JW, Kincaid EH, et al: Maintaining survivors' values of left ventricular power output during shock resuscitation: a prospective pilot study. J Trauma 49:26, 2000
39. Chang MC, Mondy JS, Meredith JW, et al: Redefining cardiovascular performance during resuscitation: ventricular stroke work, power, and the pressure-volume diagram. J Trauma 45:470, 1998
40. Miller PR, Meredith JW, Chang MC: Randomized, prospective comparison of increased preload versus inotropes in the resuscitation of trauma patients: effects on cardiopulmonary function and visceral perfusion. J Trauma 44:107, 1998
41. Grossman W: Diastolic dysfunction in congestive heart failure. N Engl J Med 325:1557, 1991
42. Hess OM, Osakada G, Lavelle JF, et al: Diastolic myocardial wall stiffness and ventricular relaxation during partial and complete coronary occlusions in the conscious dog. Circ Res 52:387, 1983
43. Isoyama S, Apstein CS, Wexler LF, et al: Acute decrease in left ventricular diastolic chamber distensibility during simulated angina in isolated hearts. Circ Res 61:925, 1987
44. Chang MC, Blinman TA, Rutherford EJ, et al: Preload assessment in trauma patients during large volume shock resuscitation. Arch Surg 131:728, 1996
45. Kraut EJ, Owings JT, Anderson JT, et al: Right ventricular volumes overestimate left ventricular preload in critically ill patients. J Trauma 42:839, 1997
46. Perdue PW, Balser JR, Lipsett PA, et al: "Renal dose" dopamine in surgical patients: dogma or science? Ann Surg 227:470, 1998

5 BLEEDING AND TRANSFUSION

John T. Owings, M.D., and Robert C. Gosselin, M.T.

Approach to the Patient with Ongoing Bleeding

A surgeon is often the first person to be called when a patient experiences ongoing bleeding. To treat such a patient appropriately, the surgeon must identify the cause or source of the bleeding. Causes fall into two main categories: (1) conditions leading to loss of vascular integrity, as in a postoperative patient with an unligated vessel that is bleeding or a trauma patient with a ruptured spleen, and (2) conditions leading to derangement of the hemostatic process. In this chapter, we focus on the latter category, which includes a broad spectrum of conditions ranging from aspirin-induced platelet dysfunction to von Willebrand disease (vWD) to disseminated intravascular coagulation (DIC) and even to hemophilia.

Coagulopathies are varied in their causes, treatments, and prognoses. Our aim is not to obviate the hematologic tests required for identification of rare congenital or acquired clotting abnormalities but to outline effective management approaches to the coagulopathies surgeons see most frequently. The vast majority of these coagulopathies can be diagnosed by means of a brief patient and family history, a review of medications, physical examination, and laboratory studies—in particular, activated partial thromboplastin time (aPTT), prothrombin time (PT, commonly expressed as an international normalized ratio [INR]), complete blood count (CBC), and D-dimer assay.

Exclusion of Technical Causes of Bleeding

It is critical for the surgeon to recognize that the most common causes of postoperative bleeding are technical: an unligated vessel or an unrecognized injury is much more likely to be the cause of a falling hematocrit than either a drug effect or an endogenous hemostatic defect. Furthermore, if an unligated vessel is treated as though it were an endogenous hemostatic defect (i.e., with transfusions), the outcome is likely to be disastrous. For these reasons, in all cases of ongoing bleeding, the first consideration must always be to exclude a surgically correctable cause.

Ongoing bleeding may be surprisingly difficult to diagnose. Healthy young patients can usually maintain a normal blood pressure until their blood loss exceeds 40% of their blood volume (roughly 2 L). If the bleeding is from a laceration to an extremity, it will be obvious; however, if the bleeding is occurring internally (e.g., from a ruptured spleen or an intraluminal GI source), there may be few physiologic signs [*see 4 Shock*]. For the purposes of the ensuing discussion, we assume that bleeding is known to have occurred or to be occurring.

Even when a technical cause of bleeding has seemingly been excluded, the possibility often must be reconsidered periodically throughout assessment. Patients who are either unresuscitated or underresuscitated undergo vasospasm, which may cause tamponade of the bleeding point.[1] As resuscitation proceeds, the catecholamine-induced vasospasm subsides and the bleeding may recur. For this reason, constant reassessment of the possibility of a technical cause of bleeding is appropriate. Only when the surgeon is confident that a missed injury or unligated vessel is not the cause of the bleeding should other potential causes be investigated.

Initial Assessment of Potential Coagulopathy

The first step in assessment of a patient with a potential coagulopathy is to draw a blood sample. The blood should be distributed into a tube containing ethylenediaminetetraacetic acid (EDTA) (for a CBC) and a citrated tube (for coagulation analysis).

At the same time, the patient's temperature should be noted. Because coagulation is a chemical reaction, it slows with increasing cold.[2] Thus, a patient with a temperature lower than 35° C (95° F) clots more slowly and less efficiently than one with a temperature of 37° C (98.6° F).[3] The resulting coagulatory abnormality is what is known as a hypothermic coagulopathy. Upon receipt of the drawn specimen, the laboratory warms the sample to 37° C to run the coagulation assays (aPTT and INR). In a patient with a purely hypothermic coagulopathy, this step results in normal coagulation parameters. Hypothermic patients should be actively rewarmed.[4] Typically, such patients cease to bleed after rewarming, and no further treatment is required. If the patient is normothermic and exhibits normal coagulation values but bleeding continues, attention should again be focused on the possibility of an unligated bleeding vessel or an uncontrolled occult bleeding source (e.g., the GI tract).

Ongoing bleeding in conjunction with abnormal coagulation parameters may have any of several underlying causes. In this setting, one of the most useful pieces of information to obtain is a personal and family history. A patient who has had dental extractions without major problems or who had a normal adolescence without any history of bleeding dyscrasias is very unlikely to have a congenital or hereditary bleeding disorder.[5] If there is a personal or family history of a specific bleeding disorder, appropriate steps should be taken to diagnose and treat the disorder [*see* Discussion, Bleeding Disorders, *below*].

Approach to Patient with Ongoing Bleeding

Patient experiences ongoing bleeding

First, consider possible technical cause (unligated vessel after operation or unrecognized injury).

Patient has unligated vessel or unrecognized injury

Control bleeding vessel.

Patient has family history of bleeding disorder

Initiate directed testing and therapy.

Patient has normal INR and aPTT

Consider platelet dysfunction.
Give platelets and initiate directed therapy.

Patient has normal INR and prolonged aPTT

Consider drug effects (heparin, lepirudin), acquired factor deficiency, and vWD.
Give protamine (to reverse heprin), replace factors, or initiate directed therapy for vWD.

```
┌─────────────────────────────────────────────────┐
│ **No technical cause of bleeding is apparent**  │
│ Draw blood for laboratory tests.                │
│ Check T°.                                        │
└─────────────────────────────────────────────────┘
```

T° is normal

T° is low
Warm patient.

Bleeding continues

Bleeding stops

Assess platelet status and coagulation parameters.

Platelet status or coagulation parameters are abnormal
Look for family history of specific bleeding disorder.

Platelet status and coagulation parameters are normal
DIC is not present.
Reconsider possibility of unligated vessel [see above, left].

Patient has no family history of bleeding disorder
Continue evaluation guided by laboratory test results.

Patient has increased INR and normal aPTT
Consider drug effects (warfarin), hepatic failure, and malnutrition.
Give I.V. vitamin K or FFP as appropriate; treat cirrhosis-related variceal bleeding surgically.

Patient has increased INR and prolonged aPTT
If D-dimer level is elevated, assume DIC and treat accordingly.
If D-dimer level is normal, consider end-stage renal disease and multifactor deficiency.
Give FFP, and initiate directed therapy.

Measurement of Coagulation Parameters

NORMAL INR, NORMAL aPTT

Patients with a normal INR and aPTT who exhibit ongoing bleeding may have impaired platelet activity. Inadequate platelet activity is frequently manifested as persistent oozing from wound edges or as low-volume bleeding. Such bleeding is rarely the cause of exsanguinating hemorrhage, though it may be life-threatening on occasion, depending on its location (e.g., the head or the pericardium). Inadequate platelet activity may be attributable either to an insufficient number of platelets or to platelet dysfunction. In the absence of a major surgical insult, a platelet count of 20,000/mm^3 or higher is usually adequate for normal coagulation.[6,7] There is some disagreement regarding the absolute level to which the platelet count must fall before platelet transfusion is justified in the absence of active bleeding. Patients undergoing procedures in which even capillary oozing is potentially life-threatening (e.g., craniotomy) should be maintained at a higher platelet count (i.e., > 20,000/mm^3). Patients without ongoing bleeding who are not specifically at increased risk for major complications from low-volume bleeding may be safely watched with platelet counts lower than 20,000/mm^3.

Oozing in a patient who has an adequate platelet count and normal coagulation parameters may be a signal of platelet dysfunction. The now-routine administration of aspirin to reduce the risk of myocardial infarction and stroke has led to a rise in the incidence of aspirin-induced platelet dysfunction. Aspirin causes irreversible platelet dysfunction through the cyclo-oxygenase pathway; the effect of aspirin can thus be expected to last for approximately 10 days. The platelet dysfunction caused by other nonsteroidal anti-inflammatory drugs (e.g., ibuprofen) is reversible and consequently does not last as long as that caused by aspirin. Newer platelet-blocking agents have been found to be effective in improving outcome after coronary angioplasty.[8] These drugs function predominantly by blocking the platelet surface receptor glycoprotein (GP) IIb-IIIa, which binds platelets to fibrinogen.

In patients with platelet dysfunction caused by an inhibitor of platelet function, such as an elevated blood urea nitrogen (BUN) level, 1-desamino-8-D-arginine vasopressin (DDAVP) is capable of partially reversing the dysfunction.[9] DDAVP has also been successful in partially reversing aspirin-induced platelet dysfunction.

Less common causes of bleeding in patients with a normal INR and a normal aPTT include factor XIII deficiency, hypofibrinogenemia or dysfibrinogenemia, and derangements in the fibrinolytic pathway [see Discussion, Mechanics of Hemostasis, below].

NORMAL INR, PROLONGED aPTT

Patients with a normal INR and an abnormal aPTT are likely to have a drug-induced coagulation defect. The agent most commonly responsible is unfractionated heparin. Reversal of the heparin effect, if desired, can be accomplished by administering protamine sulfate. Protamine should be given with caution, however, because it has been reported to induce a hypercoagulable state.[10] It is likely that many of the thrombotic complications are related to simple reversal of a needed anticoagulant state. Protamine should also be used with caution in diabetic patients. These persons sometimes become sensitized to impurities in protamine through their exposure to similar impurities in insulin, and this sensitization may result in an anaphylactic reaction.

It should be remembered that the aPTT does not accurately measure the anticoagulant activity of low-molecular-weight heparins. Because such heparins exert the greater proportion of their anticoagulant effect by potentiating antithrombin to inactivate factor Xa rather than factor IIa, an assay that measures anti-Xa activity is needed to measure the anticoagulant effect. This effect, however, like that of unfractionated heparin, is reversible by protamine. A crucial point is that the administration of fresh frozen plasma (FFP) will not correct the anticoagulant effect of either unfractionated heparin or low-molecular-weight heparins. In fact, given that plasma contains antithrombin and that both unfractionated heparin and low-molecular-weight heparins act by potentiating antithrombin, administration of FFP could actually enhance the heparins' anticoagulant effect.

A variety of direct thrombin inhibitors (e.g., hirulog and lepirudin) are currently available in Europe, Asia, and North America.[11] Many of them cause prolongation of the aPTT. One disadvantage shared by most of the direct thrombin inhibitors is that the effects are not reversible; if thrombin inhibition is no longer wanted, FFP must be given to correct the aPTT. Because the inhibitor that is circulating but not bound at the time of FFP administration will bind the prothrombin in the FFP, the amount of FFP required to correct the aPTT may be greater than would be needed with a simple factor deficiency.

von Willebrand disease is frequently, though not always, associated with a slight prolongation of the aPTT. Its clinical expression is variable. Confirmation of the diagnosis can be obtained by testing for circulating factor levels. Platelet function analysis will also show abnormal function. Correction is accomplished by administering directed therapy (von Willebrand factor [vWF]) [see Discussion, Bleeding Disorders, below], DDAVP, or cryoprecipitate.

Hemophilia may either cause spontaneous bleeding or lead to prolonged bleeding after a surgical or traumatic insult. As noted, hemophilia is rare in the absence of a personal or family history of the disorder. The most common forms of hemophilia involve deficiencies of factors VIII, IX, and XI (hemophilia A, hemophilia B, and hemophilia C, respectively). In contrast to depletion of natural anticoagulants such as antithrombin and protein C [see 70 Thromboembolic Problems], depletion of procoagulant factors rarely gives rise to significant manifestations until it is relatively severe. Typically, no laboratory abnormalities result from depletion of procoagulant factors until factor activity levels fall below 40% of normal, and clinical abnormalities are frequently absent even when factor activity levels fall to only 10% of normal. This tolerance for subcritical degrees of depletion is a reflection of the built-in redundancies in the procoagulant pathways.

If hemophilia is suspected, specific factor analysis is indicated. Appropriate therapy involves administering the deficient factor or factors [see Table 1]. Hemophiliac patients who have undergone extensive transfusion therapy may pose a particular challenge: massive transfusions frequently lead to the development of antibodies that make subsequent transfusion or even directed therapy impossible. Accordingly, several alternatives to transfusion or directed factor therapy (e.g., recombinant activated factor VII) have been developed for use in this population.

Table 1 Preparations Used in Directed Therapy for Hemophilia

Product (Manufacturer)	Origin	Factors Contained		
		Factor VIII	Factor IX	vWF
Alphanate (Alpha Therapeutic)	Plasma	Yes	—	Yes
Monarc-M (American Red Cross)	Plasma	Yes	—	Yes
Hemofil M (Baxter Healthcare)	Plasma	Yes	—	Yes
Humate-P (Centeon)	Plasma	Yes	—	Yes
Koāte-HP (Bayer)	Plasma	Yes	—	Yes
Monoclate-P (Centeon)	Plasma	Yes	—	Yes
Recombinate (Baxter Healthcare)	Recombinant	Yes	—	—
Kogenate (Bayer)	Recombinant	Yes	—	—
Bioclate (Baxter Healthcare), Helixate (Centeon)	Recombinant	Yes	—	—
Hyate:C (Speywood)	Porcine plasma	Yes	—	—
Autoplex T (prothrombin complex concentrate) (NABI)	Plasma	—	Yes	—
Feiba VH Immuno (prothrombin complex concentrate) (Immuno-US)	Plasma	—	Yes	—
Mononine (Centeon)	Plasma	—	Yes	—
AlphaNine-SD (Alpha Therapeutic)	Plasma	—	Yes	—
Bebulin VH Immuno (Immuno-US)	Plasma	—	Yes	—
Proplex T (Baxter Healthcare)	Plasma	—	Yes	—
Konȳne 80 (Bayer)	Plasma	—	Yes	—
Profilnine SD (Alpha Therapeutic)	Plasma	—	Yes	—
BeneFix (Genetics Institute)	Recombinant	—	Yes	—
Novo Seven (Novo Nordisk)	Recombinant	Yes	Yes	—

INCREASED INR, NORMAL aPTT

An increased INR in association with a normal aPTT is a more ominous finding in a patient with a coagulopathy. Any of a number of causes, all centering on factor deficiency, may be responsible.

Cirrhosis is arguably the most serious of the causes of an elevated INR. It is a major problem not so much because of the coagulopathy itself but because of the associated deficits in wound healing and immune function that result from the synthetic dysfunction and the loss of reticuloendothelial function. In all cases, factor replacement should be instituted with FFP. If the bleeding is a manifestation of the cirrhosis (as in variceal bleeding), emergency portal decompression should be accomplished before the coagulopathy worsens. Management of cirrhotic patients who have sustained injuries is particularly troublesome because such patients are at disproportionately high risk for subdural hematoma. The reason this risk is so high is that in addition to their pathologic autoanticoagulation, these patients often have some degree of cerebral atrophy as a result of one of the more frequent causes of cirrhosis—namely, alcoholism. As a result, the bridging intracranial veins are more vulnerable to tears and more likely to bleed. Modest elevations of the INR in patients who are not actively bleeding, have not recently undergone operation, and are not specifically at increased risk for life-threatening hemorrhage may be observed without correction.

An elevated INR with a normal aPTT may also be a consequence of warfarin administration. Such a coagulopathy is the result of a pure factor deficiency, and its degree is proportional to the prolongation of the INR. Because warfarin acts by disrupting vitamin K metabolism, the coagulopathy may be corrected by giving vitamin K [see Table 2].[12] If the patient is actively bleeding, vitamin K should still be given, but the primary corrective measure should be to administer FFP in an amount proportional to the patient's size and the relative increase in the INR. The INR should subsequently be rechecked to ensure that replacement therapy is adequate. Vitamin K replacement therapy has two main potential drawbacks: (1) if the patient is to be reanticoagulated with warfarin in the near future, dosing will be difficult because the patient will exhibit resistance to warfarin for a variable period; and (2) anaphylactic reactions have been reported when vitamin K is given I.V.

Table 2 Management of the Patient with an Increased INR[12]

Indication	Recommended Treatment
INR above therapeutic range but < 5.0	If no bleeding is present or surgery is indicated, lower or hold next dose
INR > 5.0 but < 9.0	
Patient has no significant bleeding	In the absence of additional risk factors for bleeding, withhold next 1–2 doses; alternatively, withhold next dose and give vitamin K, 1.0–2.5 mg (oral route is acceptable)
Rapid reduction of INR is required	Give vitamin K, 2.0–4.0 mg p.o.; expected reduction of INR should occur within 24 hr
INR > 9.0	
Patient has no significant bleeding	Give vitamin K, 3.0–5.0 mg p.o.; expected reduction of INR should occur within 24 hr
Patient has serious bleeding or is overly anticoagulated (INR > 20.0)	Give vitamin K, 10 mg I.V., and FFP; further vitamin K supplementation may be required every 12 hr
Patient has life-threatening bleeding or is seriously overanticoagulated	Prothrombin complexes may be indicated, along with vitamin K, 10 mg I.V.

INCREASED INR, PROLONGED aPTT

Increases in both the INR and the aPTT may be the most problematic finding of all. When both assays show increases, the patient is likely to have multiple factor deficiencies; possible causes include DIC, severe hemodilution, and renal failure with severe nephrotic syndrome. However, when dramatic elevations of the aPTT and the INR are observed in a seemingly asymptomatic patient, the problem may lie not in the patient's condition but in the laboratory analysis. If the tube in which the blood sample was placed for these tests was not adequately filled, the results of the coagulation assays may be inaccurate. In such cases, the blood sample should be redrawn and the tests repeated.

Hemodilution and nephrotic syndrome result in a coagulopathy that is attributable to decreased concentration of coagulation proteins. Dilutional coagulopathy may occur when a patient who is given a large volume of packed red blood cell (RBC) units is not also given coagulation factors.[13] Because of the tremendous redundancy of the hemostatic process, pure dilutional coagulopathy is rare. It is considered an unlikely diagnosis until after one full blood volume has been replaced (as when a patient requires 10 units of packed RBCs to maintain a stable hematocrit). Nephrotic syndrome is associated with loss of protein (coagulation proteins as well as other body proteins) from the kidneys.

Both hemodilution and nephrotic syndrome should be distinguished from DIC (which is a consumptive rather than a dilutional process[14]), though on occasion this distinction is a difficult one to make. A blood sample should be sent for D-dimer assay. If the D-dimer level is low (< 1,000 ng/ml), DIC is unlikely; if it is very high (> 2,000 ng/ml) and there is no other clear explanation (e.g., a complex unstable pelvic fracture), the diagnosis of DIC rather than dilution should be made. Treatment of dilutional coagulopathy should be directed at replacement of lost factors. FFP should be given first, followed by cryoprecipitate, calcium, and platelets. Transfusion should be continued until the coagulation parameters are corrected and the bleeding stops.

DIC is a diffuse, disorganized activation of the clotting cascade within the vascular space. It may result either from intravascular presentation of an overwhelming clotting stimulus (e.g., massive crush injury or transfusion reaction) or from presentation of a moderate clotting stimulus in the context of shock. Different degrees of severity have been described. In the mildest form of DIC, acceleration of the clotting cascade is seen, and microthrombi are formed in the vascular space but are cleared effectively. Thus, mild DIC may be little more than an acceleration of the clotting cascade that escapes recognition. In the moderate form of DIC, the microthrombi are ineffectively lysed and cause occlusion of the microcirculation. This process is clinically manifested in the lungs as the acute respiratory distress syndrome (ARDS), in the kidneys as renal failure, and in the liver as hepatic failure.

Neither mild DIC nor moderate DIC is what surgeons traditionally think of as DIC. Severe DIC arises when congestion of the microvasculature with thrombi occurs, resulting in large-scale activation of the fibrinolytic system to restore circulation. This fibrinolytic activity results in breakdown of clot at previously hemostatic sites of microscopic injury (e.g., endothelial damage) and macroscopic injury (e.g., I.V. catheter sites, fractures, or surgical wounds). Bleeding and reexposure to tissue factor stimulate activation of factor VII with increased coagulation activity; thus, microthrombi are formed, and the vicious circle continues. The ultimate manifestation of severe DIC is bleeding from (1) fibrinolysis and (2) depletion (consumption) of coagulation factors.

Several scoring systems have been devised to assess the severity of DIC. These scoring systems are most useful for distinguishing DIC from other causes of coagulopathy (e.g., hypothermia, dilution, or drug effects) [see Table 3].[15]

DIC is a diagnosis of exclusion, largely because none of the various treatment strategies tried to date have been particularly successful. Heparin has been given in large doses in an attempt to break the cycle by stopping the clotting, thus allowing clotting factor levels to return to normal. Antifibrinolytic agents (e.g., ε-aminocaproic acid) have also been tried in an attempt to reduce fibrinolytic activity and thus slow the bleeding that stimulates subsequent clot formation. Antithrombotics (e.g., antithrombin and protein C) have been used as well; improvements have been noted in laboratory measures of DIC but not in survival.

Currently, the most appropriate way of treating a patient with severe DIC is to follow a multifaceted approach. First, the clotting stimulus, if still present, should be removed: dead or devitalized tissue should be amputated, abscesses drained, and suspect transfusions discontinued. Second, hypothermia, of any degree of severity, should be corrected. Third, both blood loss (as measured by the hematocrit) and clotting factor deficits (as measured by the INR) should be aggressively corrected (with blood and plasma, respec-

Table 3 Coagulopathy (DIC) Score

Score	INR (sec)	aPTT (sec)	Platelets (1,000/mm³)	Fibrinogen (mg/dl)	D-dimer (ng/ml)
0	< 1.2	< 34	> 150	> 200	< 1,000
1	> 1.2	> 34	< 150	< 200	< 2,000
2	> 1.4	> 39	< 100	< 150	< 4,000
3	> 1.6	> 54	< 60	< 100	> 4,000

DIC—disseminated intravascular coagulopathy   INR—international normalized ratio   aPTT—activated partial thromboplastin

tively). This supportive approach is only modestly successful. For certain groups of patients in whom DIC develops (e.g., those who have sustained head injuries), mortality approaches 100%. This alarmingly high death rate is probably related more to the underlying pathology than to the hematologic derangement.

An increased INR with a prolonged aPTT may also be caused by various isolated factor deficiencies of the common pathway. Congenital deficiencies of factors X, V, and prothrombin are very rare. Acquired factor V deficiencies have been observed in patients with autoimmune disorders. Acquired hypoprothrombinemia has been documented in a small percentage of patients with lupus anticoagulants who exhibit abnormal bleeding. Factor X deficiencies have been noted in patients with amyloidosis.

Stabilized warfarin therapy will increase both the INR and the aPTT. Several current rodenticides (e.g., brodifacoum) exert the same effect on these parameters that warfarin does; however, because they have a considerably longer half-life than warfarin, the reversal of the anticoagulation effect with vitamin K or FFP may be correspondingly longer.[16] Animal venoms may also increase the INR and the aPTT.

Management of Anemia and Indications for Transfusion

Treatment of anemia has changed substantially since the early 1990s. Blood cell transfusions have been shown to have significant immunosuppressive potential, and transmission of fatal diseases through the blood supply has been extensively documented. Moreover, at least one large trial found that using a restrictive RBC transfusion protocol in place of a more traditional one improved survival.[17] These findings have led to a paradigm shift with respect to RBC transfusion: whereas the traditional view was that anemia by itself was a sufficient indication for transfusion, the current consensus is that a second indication must be present in addition to a decreased hemoglobin concentration.

The decision whether to transfuse should be based on the patient's current or predicted need for additional oxygen-carrying capacity [see Figure 1]. A major component of this decision is to determine as promptly as possible whether the patient is in a steady state with respect to hemoglobin supply (in which case transfusions are less likely to be needed) or not (in which case transfusions are usually indicated). Thus, there is no specific hemoglobin concentration or hematocrit (i.e., transfusion trigger) at which all patients should receive transfusions.

There are two large groups of patients who should be managed more aggressively than the general patient population with respect to RBC transfusion. Patients who are either actively bleeding or at high risk for active bleeding and patients who have significant coronary artery disease (CAD) should receive transfusions according to a more liberal protocol than that applied to other patients.

ACTIVE BLEEDING

Patients who are actively bleeding (e.g., those with GI hemorrhage) should receive transfusions up to a level sufficient to keep up with blood loss. Coagulation factors must also be replaced as necessary [see Measurement of Coagulation Parameters, Increased INR, Prolonged aPTT, above]. Patients at high risk for active bleeding (e.g., from massive liver injury) should receive transfusions up to a level at which, if bleeding occurs or recurs, enough reserve oxygen-carrying capacity is afforded to allow diagnosis and correction of the hemorrhage without significant compromise of oxygen delivery. In cases of major injury, we advocate a target hematocrit of 30%; however, this is not a fixed value but a rule-of-thumb figure that may be increased or decreased as appropriate, depending on the individual patient's reserves and the individual surgical team's ability to diagnose and correct the underlying problem.

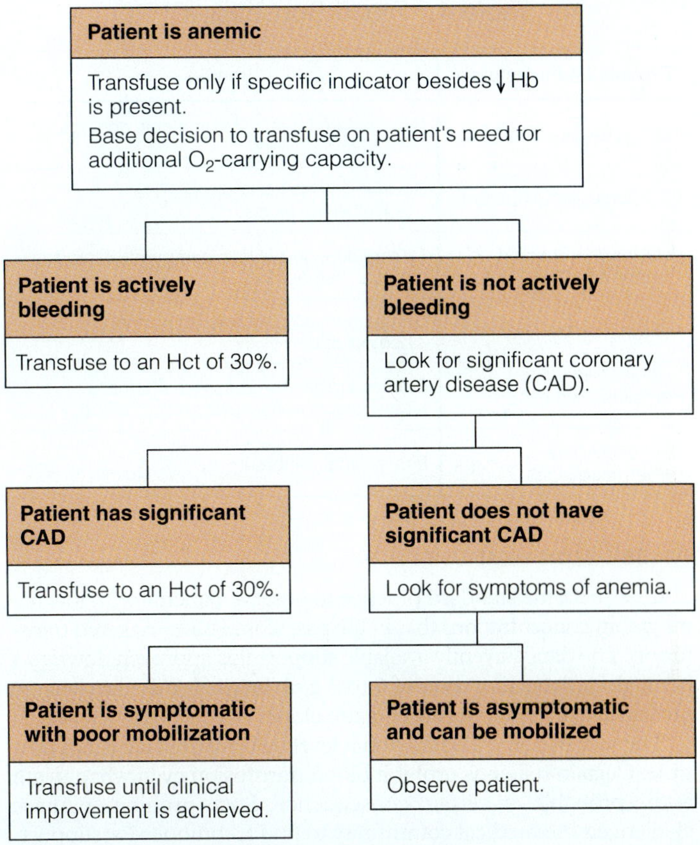

Figure 1 Algorithm depicts decision-making process for transfusion in anemic patients.

SIGNIFICANT CORONARY ARTERY DISEASE

Although no studies have conclusively shown that patients with significant CAD benefit from increased RBC mass, there is also no published evidence to support a restrictive transfusion policy.[17] The major trials that found most patients to benefit from a restrictive transfusion policy specifically excluded CAD patients out of concern that adverse cardiovascular events (e.g., myocardial infarction and cerebrovascular accidents) might increase in frequency at lower hematocrits. Studies evaluating the potential benefit of a more aggressive transfusion policy (i.e., to hematocrits > 30%) failed to show any benefit. Consequently, a target hematocrit of 30% is generally considered appropriate for patients with significant CAD.

SYMPTOMATIC ANEMIA

An additional indication for transfusion is oxygen-carrying capacity that is insufficient to support necessary activities (e.g., wound healing, mobilization, and physical therapy). Typical manifestations are light-headedness, tachycardia, and tachypnea either during the activity in question or at rest. Clearly, some degree of tachycardia is to be expected in any patient who has undergone a major operation or sustained a serious injury. The key point with respect to symptomatic anemia is that patients who have physiologically compensated for anemia must be distinguished from those whose health or recovery is compromised by anemia, and only the latter group should receive transfusions.

Table 4 Blood Substitutes[76]

Product (Manufacturer)	Source
PHP (Apex Bioscience)	Pyridoxylated human hemoglobin conjugated to polyoxyethylene
PEG-hemoglobin (Enzon)	Bovine hemoglobin conjugated to polyethylene glycol
PolyHeme (Northfield Laboratories)	Glutaraldehyde-polymerized pyridoxylated human hemoglobin
Hemopure (Biopure)	Glutaraldehyde-polymerized bovine hemoglobin
Hemolink (Hemosol)	Oxidized raffinose–crosslinked human hemoglobin from expired stored blood
Oxygent (Alliance Pharmaceutical)	Emulsified perflubron

OBSERVATION OF ANEMIA

It has become standard practice to observe patients with low hemoglobin concentrations that in the past would have triggered transfusion. The data currently available support this approach down to a hemoglobin concentration of 6 to 7 g/dl; below 6 g/dl, the data are not sufficient to support observation alone.

There does come a hemoglobin level below which life is not possible. Certain religions prohibit blood transfusion even when death is the probable or certain consequence. Such prohibitions have challenged the medical community to find techniques for supporting life at lower and lower hemoglobin concentrations. In addition, they have helped to define the limits beyond which a restrictive transfusion protocol may be fatal.

When RBC transfusion is not possible (whether for cultural reasons or because compatible blood is unavailable), there are a number of temporizing measures that can be used to support life. If oxygen-carrying capacity cannot be increased, one option is simply to decrease oxygen demand. Oxygen demand is directly proportional to metabolic activity; that is, as metabolic rate increases, so too does oxygen demand. Once unnecessary activity (e.g., assuming an upright posture or walking) has been eliminated, respiration becomes an activity that requires a significant amount of energy. Mechanical ventilation reduces the work of breathing and with it the oxygen requirements of the respiratory muscles. Even with full mechanical ventilation, however, most patients continue to initiate breaths on their own. This energy-requiring activity can be eliminated by administering a neuromuscular blocking agent, which dramatically reduces oxygen demand in essentially all skeletal muscle. The metabolic rate can be further reduced by inducing hypothermia. This measure should be used with caution, however, because hypothermia in the absence of neuromuscular blockade results in uncontrollable shivering, which actually increases the metabolic rate. In addition, trials addressing the use of hypothermia in head injury patients to reduce cerebral oxygen demand reported increased infection rates in the hypothermic groups.

A completely different approach to the issue of the unacceptability or unavailability of RBC transfusion involves the use of RBC substitutes to augment oxygen-carrying capacity. A variety of different substitutes are currently under investigation [see Table 4].[18] None have been approved for routine use by the United States Food and Drug Administration, but several have demonstrated promise in clinical trials. Without modification, the hemoglobin molecule is nephrotoxic. Accordingly, virtually all of the products now being studied depend on techniques for making an acellular hemoglobin molecule nontoxic for I.V. administration.

Acellular blood substitutes clearly possess a number of advantages, including greatly increased shelf life, reduced risk of viral transmission, availability that is not limited by donor supply, reduced or eliminated risk of incompatibility reactions, and—potentially, at least—reduced cultural and religious objections.[19] To what extent this approach is suited to the treatment of anemia in surgical patients should be clarified when the results of the trials now under way are published.[18]

Discussion

Mechanics of Hemostasis

Hemostasis is the term for the process by which cellular and plasma components interact in response to vessel injury in order to maintain vascular integrity and promote wound healing. The initial response to vascular injury (primary hemostasis) involves the recruitment and activation of platelets, which then adhere to the site of injury. Subsequently, plasma proteins, in concert with cellular components, begin to generate thrombin, which causes further activation of platelets and converts fibrinogen to fibrin monomers that polymerize into a fibrin clot. The final step is the release of plasminogen activators that induce clot lysis and tissue repair.

The cellular components of hemostasis include endothelium, white blood cells (WBCs), RBCs, and platelets. The plasma components include a number of procoagulant and regulatory proteins that, once activated, can accelerate or downregulate thrombin formation or clot lysis to facilitate wound healing. In normal individuals, these hemostatic components are in a regulatory balance; thus, any abnormality involving one or more of these components can result in a pathologic state, whether of uncontrolled clot formation (thrombosis) or of excessive bleeding (hemorrhage). These pathologies can result from either hereditary defects of protein synthesis or acquired deficiencies attributable to metabolic causes.

CELLULAR COMPONENTS

Endothelium

The endothelium has both procoagulant and anticoagulant properties. When vascular injury occurs, the endothelium serves as a nidus for recruitment of platelets, adhesion of platelets to the endothelial surface, platelet aggregation, migration of platelets across the endothelial surface, generation of fibrin, and expression of adhesion molecule receptors (E-selectin and P-selectin). Exposure of collagen fibrils and release of vWF from the Weibel-Palade bodies cause platelets to adhere to the cellular surface of the endothelium. The presence of interleukin-1β (IL-1β), tissue necrosis factor (TNF), interferon-8 (IFN-8), and thrombin promotes expression of tissue factor (TF) on the endothelium.[20,21] TF activates factors X and VII, and these activated factors generate additional thrombin, which increases both fibrin formation and platelet aggregation.

The endothelium also acts in numerous ways to downregulate coagulation.[22] Heparan sulfate and thrombomodulin are both downregulators of thrombin formation. In the presence of thrombin, the endothelium responds by (1) releasing thrombomodulin, which forms a complex with thrombin to activate protein C; (2) producing endothelium-derived relaxing factor (i.e., nitric oxide[23]) and prostacyclin, which have vasodilating and platelet aggregation–inhibiting effects, respectively; and (3) releasing tissue plasminogen activator (t-PA) or urokinase-type plasminogen activator (u-PA), either of which converts the zymogen plasminogen to an active form (i.e., plasmin) that degrades fibrin and fibrinogen.[20,24] Heparan sulfate, on the endothelium wall, forms a complex with plasma antithrombin to neutralize thrombin. The endothelium is also the source of tissue factor pathway inhibitor (TFPI), which downregulates TF-VIIa-Xa complexes.

Erythrocytes and Leukocytes

The nonplatelet cellular components of blood play indirect roles in hemostasis. RBCs contain thromboplastins that are potent stimulators of various procoagulant proteins. In addition, the concentration of RBCs within the bloodstream (expressed as the hematocrit) assists in primary hemostasis by physically forcing the platelets toward the endothelial surfaces. When the RBC count is low enough, the absence of this force results in inadequate endothelium-platelet interaction and a bleeding diathesis.

Leukocytes have several functions in the hemostatic process. The interaction between the adhesion molecules expressed on both leukocytes and endothelium results in cytokine production, initiation of inflammatory responses, and degradation of extracellular matrix to facilitate tissue healing. In the presence of thrombin, monocytes express TF, which is an integral procoagulant for thrombin generation. Neutrophils and activated monocytes bind to stimulated platelets and endothelial cells that express P-selectin. Adhesion and rolling of neutrophils, mediated by fibrinogen and selectins on the endothelium, appear to facilitate vessel integrity but may also lead to inflammatory responses.[25,26] Lymphocytes also adhere to endothelium via adhesion molecule receptors and appear to be responsible for cytokine production and inflammatory responses.

Platelets

The roles platelets play in hemostasis and subsequent fibrin formation rest on providing a phospholipid surface for localizing procoagulant activation. Activation of platelets by agonists such as adenosine triphosphate (ATP), adenosine diphosphate (ADP), epinephrine, thromboxane A_2, collagen, and thrombin causes platelets to undergo morphologic changes and degranulation. Degranulation of platelets results in the release of procoagulants that promote further platelet adhesion and aggregation (e.g., thrombospondin, vWF, fibrinogen, ADP, and ATP), vasodilation (e.g., serotonin), and surface expression of P-selectin, which induces cellular adhesion. Platelet degranulation also results in the release of β-thromboglobulin, platelet factor 4 (which has antiheparin properties), various growth factors, coagulation procoagulants, and calcium as well as the formation of platelet microparticles. Plasminogen activator inhibitor–I (PAI-I) released from degranulated platelets neutralizes the fibrinolytic pathway by forming a complex with t-PA.

Upon exposure to vascular injury, platelets adhere to the exposed endothelium via binding of vWF to the GPIb-IX-V complex.[27] Conformational changes in the GPIIb-IIIa complex on the activated platelet surface enhance fibrinogen binding, which results in platelet-to-platelet interaction (i.e., aggregation). The phospholipid surface of the platelet membranes anchors activated IXa-VIIIa and Xa-Va complexes, thereby localizing thrombin generation.[28]

PLASMA COMPONENTS

Procoagulants

Traditional diagrams of the coagulation cascade depict two distinct pathways for thrombin generation: the intrinsic pathway and the extrinsic pathway. The premise for the distinction between the two is that the intrinsic pathway requires no extravascular source for initiation, whereas the extrinsic pathway requires an extravascular component (i.e., TF). This traditional depiction is useful in interpreting coagulation tests, but it is not an accurate reflection of the hemostatic process in vivo. Accordingly, our focus is not on this standard view but rather on the roles contact factors (within the intrinsic cascade) and TF play in coagulation. As noted, circulating plasma vWF is necessary for normal adhesion of platelets to the endothelium. Plasma vWF also serves as the carrier protein for factor VIII, preventing its neutralization by the protein C regulatory pathway.

Even in patients in whom laboratory tests strongly suggest a severe clotting abnormality (i.e., the aPTT is markedly prolonged), contact factors do not play a significant role in the generation of thrombin. However, contact factor activation does appear to play secondary roles that are essential to normal hemostasis and tissue repair. Factor XII, prekallikrein, and high-molecular-weight kininogen are bound to the endothelium to activate the bradykinin (BK) pathway. The BK pathway exerts profibrinolytic effects by stimulating endothelial release of plasminogen activators. It also stimulates endothelial production of nitric oxide and prostacyclin, which play vital regulatory roles in vasodilation and regulation of platelet activation.[29]

The key initiator of plasma procoagulant formation is the expression of TF on cell surfaces.[21,30] TF activates factor VII and binds with it to form the TF-VIIa complex, which activates factors X and IX. Factor Xa also enhances its own production by activating factor IX, which in turn activates factor X to form factor Xa. Factor Xa also produces minimal amounts of thrombin by cleaving the prothrombin molecule. The thrombin generated from this process cleaves the coagulation cofactors V and VIII to enhance production of the factor complexes IXa-VIIIa (intrinsic tenase) and Xa-Va (prothrombinase), which catalyze conversion of prothrombin to thrombin [see Figure 2].[31]

Thrombin has numerous functions, including prothrombotic and regulatory functions. Its procoagulant properties include cleaving fibrinogen, activating the coagulation cofactors V and VIII, inducing platelet aggregation, inducing expression of TF on cell surfaces, and activating factor XIII. In cleaving fibrinogen, thrombin causes the release of fibrinopeptides A and B (fibrin monomer). The fibrin monomer undergoes conformational changes that expose the α and β chains of the molecule, which then polymerize with other fibrin monomers to form a fibrin mesh. Activated factor XIII cross-links the polymerized fibrin (between the α chains and the γ chains) to stabilize the fibrin clot and delay fibrinolysis.

Fibrin(ogen)olysis

Plasminogen is the primary fibrinolytic zymogen that circulates in plasma. In the presence of t-PA or u-PA (released from the endothelium), plasminogen is converted to the active form, plasmin. Plasmin cleaves fibrin (or fibrinogen) between the molecule's D and E domains, causing the formation of X, Y, D, and E fragments. The secondary function of the fibrinolytic pathway is the activation by u-PA of matrix metalloproteinases that degrade the extracellular matrix.[32]

Regulatory Factors

In persons with normal coagulation status, downregulation of hemostasis occurs simultaneously with the production of procoagulants (e.g., activated plasma factors, stimulated endothelium, and stimulated platelets). In addition to their procoagulant activity, both thrombin and contact factors stimulate downregulation of the coagulation process. Thrombin forms a complex with endothelium-bound thrombomodulin to activate protein C, which inhibits factors Va and VIIIa. The thrombin-thrombomodulin complex also regu-

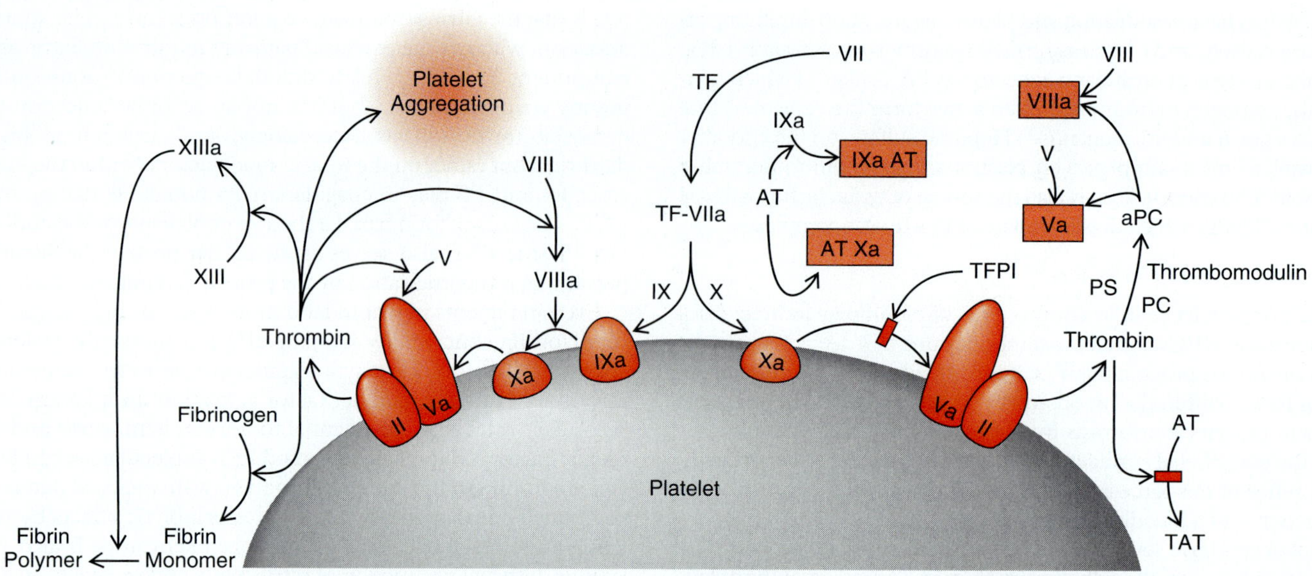

Figure 2 Shown is a schematic representation of the procoagulant pathways.

lates the fibrinolytic pathway by activating a circulating plasma protein known as thrombin-activatable fibrinolysis inhibitor (TAFI), which appears to suppress conversion of plasminogen to plasmin.[33] Contact factors are known to be required for normal surface-dependent fibrinolysis, and there is some evidence that contact factor deficiencies can lead to thromboembolism. Another plasma protein responsible for regulation of fibrinolysis is α_2-antiplasmin, which binds to circulating and bound plasmin to limit breakdown of fibrin.

Circulating downregulating proteins include antithrombin (a serine protease inhibitor of activated factors—especially factors IXa, Xa, and XIa—and thrombin[31]), proteins C and S (regulators of factors VIIIa and Va[34]), C1 inhibitor (a regulator of factor XIa), TFPI (a regulator of the TF-VIIa-Xa complex[35]), and α_2-macroglobulin (a thrombin inhibitor—the primary thrombin inhibitor in neonates[36]). Limitation of platelet activation occurs secondarily as a result of decreased levels of circulating agonists and endothelial release of prostacyclin [see Figure 2].

Bleeding Disorders

INHERITED COAGULOPATHIES

Numerous congenital abnormalities of the coagulation system have been identified. In particular, various abnormalities involving plasma proteins (e.g., hemophilia and vWD), platelet receptors (e.g., Glanzmann thrombasthenia and Bernard-Soulier syndrome), and endothelium (e.g., telangiectasia) have been described in detail. For the sake of brevity, we will refer to abnormal protein synthesis resulting in a dysfunctional coagulation protein as a defect and to abnormal protein synthesis resulting in decreased protein production as a deficiency.

Most of the coagulation defects associated with endothelium are closely related to thrombosis or atherosclerosis. Defects or deficiencies of thrombomodulin, TFPI, and t-PA, albeit rare, are associated with thrombosis.[37,38] Vascular defects (e.g., hemorrhagic telangiectasias) may carry an increased risk of bleeding as a consequence of dysfunctional fibrinolysis, concomitant platelet dysfunction, or coagulation factor deficiencies.[39]

Defects or deficiencies of RBCs and WBCs have other primary clinical manifestations that are not related to hemostasis. Alterations in the physical properties of blood (e.g., decreased blood flow from increased viscosity, polycythemia vera, leukocytosis, and sickle-cell anemia) have been reported to lead to thrombosis, but usually not to major bleeding.

Inherited platelet membrane receptor defects are relatively common. Of these, vWD is the one that most frequently causes bleeding.[40] The condition is characterized by vWF abnormalities, which may take three forms: vWF may be present in a reduced concentration (type I vWD), dysfunctional (type II vWD), or absent altogether (type III). Diagnosis of vWD is based on a combination of the patient history (e.g., previous mucosal bleeding) and laboratory parameters [see Laboratory Assessment of Bleeding, below]. It is necessary to identify the correct type or subtype of vWD: some treatments (e.g., DDAVP) are contraindicated in patients with type IIb vWD.[41]

Less common receptor defects include Glanzmann thrombasthenia (a defect in the GPIIb-IIIa complex), Bernard-Soulier syndrome (a defect in the GPIb-IX complex), and Scott syndrome (a defect in the platelet's activated surface that promotes thrombin formation); other agonist receptors on the platelet membrane may be affected as well.[42,43] Intracellular platelet defects are relatively rare but do occur; examples are gray platelet syndromes (e.g., alpha granule defects), Hermansky-Pudlak syndrome, dense granule defects, Wiskott-Aldrich syndrome, and various defects in intracellular production and signaling (involving defects of cyclooxygenase synthase and phospholipase C, respectively).[43]

Numerous pathologic states are also associated with deficiencies or defects of plasma procoagulants. Inherited sex-linked deficiencies of factor VIII (i.e., hemophilia A) and factor IX (i.e., hemophilia B and Christmas disease) are relatively common.[44-46] The clinical presentations of hemophilia A and hemophilia B are similar: hemarthroses are the most common clinical manifestations, ultimately leading to degenerative joint deformities. Spontaneous bleeding may also occur, resulting in intracranial hemorrhage, large hematomas in the muscles of extremities, hematuria, and GI bleeding. Factor XI deficiency is relatively common in Jewish persons but rarely results in spontaneous bleeding.[47,48] Such deficiency may result in bleeding after oral operations and trauma; however, there are a number of major procedures (e.g., cardiac bypass surgery) that do not result in postoperative bleeding in this population.[49]

Inherited deficiencies of the other coagulation factors are very rare. Factor XIII deficiencies result in delayed postoperative or posttraumatic bleeding. Congenital deficiencies of factor V, factor VII, factor X, prothrombin, and fibrinogen may become apparent in the neonatal period (presenting, for example, as umbilical stump bleeding); later in life, they result in clinical presentations such as epistaxis, intracranial bleeding, GI bleeding, deep and superficial bruising, and menorrhagia.

Defects or deficiencies in the fibrinolytic pathway are also rare and are most commonly associated with thromboembolic events. α_2-Antiplasmin deficiencies and primary fibrin(ogen)olysis are rare congenital coagulopathies with clinical presentations similar to those of factor deficiencies. In primary fibrin(ogen)olysis, failure of regulation of t-PA and u-PA leads to increases in circulating plasmin levels, which result in rapid degradation of clot and fibrinogen.[50,51]

ACQUIRED COAGULOPATHIES

A wide range of clinical conditions may cause deficiencies of the primary, secondary, or fibrinolytic pathways. Acquired coagulopathies are very common, and most do not result in spontaneous bleeding. (DIC is an exception [see below].)

As noted, coagulopathies related to the endothelium are primarily associated with thrombosis rather than bleeding. There are a number of disorders that may cause vascular injury, including sickle-cell anemia, hemolytic-uremic syndrome, and thrombotic thrombocytopenic purpura.

Acquired platelet abnormalities, both qualitative (i.e., dysfunction) and quantitative (i.e., decreases in absolute numbers), are common occurrences. Many acquired thrombocytopathies are attributable to either foods (e.g., fish oils, chocolate, red wine, garlic, and herbs) or drugs (e.g., aspirin, ibuprofen, other nonsteroidal anti-inflammatory drugs, ticlopidine, various antibiotics, certain antihistamines, and phenytoin).[52-56] Direct anti–platelet receptor drugs (e.g., abciximab and eptifibatide) block the GPIIb-IIIa complex, thereby preventing platelet aggregation.[57] Thrombocytopenia can be primary or secondary to a number of clinical conditions. Primary bone disorders (e.g., myelodysplastic or myelophthisic syndromes) and spontaneous bleeding may arise when platelet counts fall below 10,000/mm³. Thrombocytopenia can be associated with immune causes (e.g., immune thrombocytopenic purpura or thrombotic thrombocytopenic purpura) or can occur secondary to administration of drugs (e.g., heparin). Acquired platelet dysfunction (e.g., acquired vWD) that is not related to dietary or pharmacologic causes has been observed in patients with immune disorders or cancer.

Acquired plasma factor deficiencies are common as well. Patients with severe renal disease typically exhibit platelet dysfunction (from excessive amounts of uremic metabolites), factor deficiencies associated with impaired synthesis or protein loss (as with increased urinary excretion), or thrombocytopenia (from diminished thrombopoietin production).[58,59] Patients with severe hepatic disease commonly have impairment of coagulation factor synthesis, increases in circulating levels of paraproteins, and splenic sequestration of platelets.

Hemodilution from massive RBC transfusions can occur if more than 10 packed RBC units are given within a short period without plasma supplementation. Immunologic reactions to ABO/Rh mismatches can induce immune-mediated hypercoagulation. Acquired multifactorial deficiencies associated with extracorporeal circuits (e.g., cardiopulmonary bypass, hemodialysis, and continuous venovenous dialysis) can arise as a consequence of hemodilution of circuit priming fluid or activation of procoagulants after exposure to thrombogenic surfaces.[60-62] Thrombocytopenia can result from platelet destruction and activation caused by circuit membrane exposure, or it can be secondary to the presence of heparin antibody.

Animal venoms can be either procoagulant or prothrombotic. The majority of the poisonous snakes in the United States (rattlesnakes in particular) have venom that works by activating prothrombin, but cross-breeding has produced a number of new venoms with different hemostatic consequences. The clinical presentation of coagulopathies associated with snakebites generally mimics that of consumptive coagulopathies.[63]

Drug-induced factor deficiencies are common, particularly as a result of anticoagulant therapy. The most commonly used anticoagulants are heparin and warfarin. Heparin does not cause a factor deficiency; rather, it accelerates production of antithrombin, which inhibits factor IXa, factor Xa, and thrombin, thereby prolonging clot formation. Warfarin reduces procoagulant potential by inhibiting vitamin K synthesis, thereby reducing carboxylation of factor VII, factor IX, factor X, prothrombin, and proteins C and S. Newer drugs that may also cause factor deficiencies include direct thrombin inhibitors (e.g., lepirudin and hirulog[64]) and fibrinogen-degrading drugs (e.g., ancrod[65]).

Isolated acquired factor deficiencies are relatively rare. Clinically, they present in exactly the same way as inherited factor deficiencies, except that there is no history of earlier bleeding. In most cases, there is a secondary disease (e.g., lymphoma or an autoimmune disorder) that results in the development of antibody to a procoagulant (e.g., factor V, factor VIII, factor IX, vWF, prothrombin, or fibrinogen).[66-68]

Disseminated Intravascular Coagulation

DIC is a complex coagulation process that involves activation of the coagulation system with resultant activation of the fibrinolytic pathway and deposition of fibrin; the eventual consequence is the multiple organ dysfunction syndrome (MODS).[69] The activation occurs at all levels (platelets, endothelium, and procoagulants), but it is not known whether this process is initiated by a local stimulus or a systemic one. It is crucial to emphasize that DIC is an acquired disorder that occurs secondary to an underlying clinical event (e.g., a complicated birth, severe gram-negative infection, shock, major head injury, polytrauma, severe burns, or cancer. As noted [see Measurement of Coagulation Parameters, Increased INR, Prolonged aPTT, *above*], there is some controversy regarding the best approach to therapy, but there is no doubt that treating the underlying cause of DIC is paramount to patient recovery.

DIC is not always clinically evident: low-grade DIC may lack clinical symptoms altogether and manifest itself only through laboratory abnormalities, even when thrombin generation and fibrin deposition are occurring. In an attempt to facilitate recognition of DIC, the disorder has been divided into three phases, distinguished on the basis of clinical and laboratory evidence. In phase I DIC, there are no clinical symptoms, and the routine screening tests (i.e., INR, aPTT, fibrinogen level, and platelet count) are within normal limits.[70] Secondary testing (i.e., measurement of antithrombin, prothrombin fragment, thrombin-antithrombin complex, and soluble fibrin levels) may reveal subtle changes indicative of thrombin generation. In phase II DIC, there are usually clinical signs of bleeding around wounds, suture sites, I.V. sites, or venous puncture sites, and decreased function is noted in specific organs (e.g., lung, liver, and kidneys). The INR is increased, the aPTT is prolonged, and the fibrinogen level and platelet count are decreased or decreasing. Other markers of thrombin generation and fibrinolysis (e.g., D-dimer level) show sizable elevations. In phase III DIC, MODS is observed, the INR and the aPTT are markedly increased, and fibrinogen and D-dimer levels are markedly depressed. A peripheral blood smear would show large numbers of schistocytes, indicating RBC shearing resulting from fibrin deposition.

The activation of the coagulation system seen in DIC appears to be primarily caused by TF. The brain, the placenta, and solid tumors are all rich sources of TF. Gram-negative endotoxins also in-

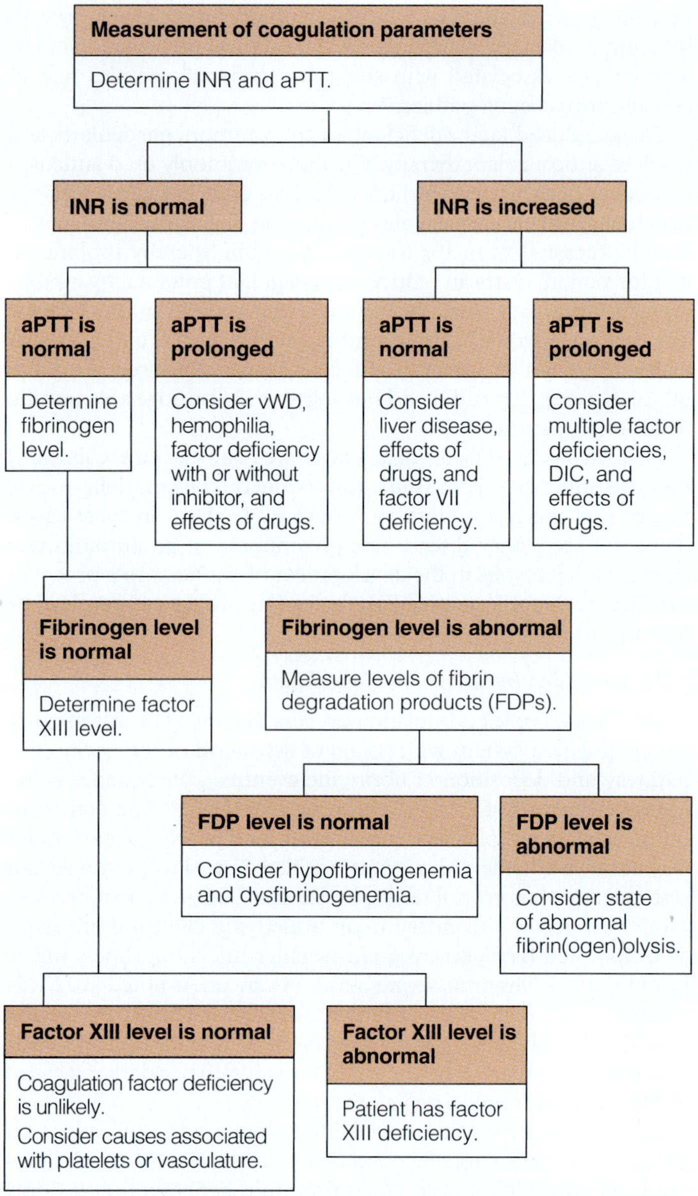

Figure 3 Algorithm depicts use of coagulation parameters in assessment of coagulopathies.

duce TF expression. The exposure of TF on cellular surfaces causes activation of factors VII and IX, which ultimately leads to thrombin generation. Circulating thrombin is rapidly cleared by antithrombin. Moreover, the coagulation pathway is downregulated by activated protein C and protein S. However, constant exposure of TF (as a result of underlying disorders) results in constant generation of thrombin, and these regulator proteins are rapidly consumed. TAFI and PAI also contribute to fibrin deposition by restricting fibrinolysis and subsequent fibrin degradation and clearance. Finally, it is likely that release of cytokines (e.g., IL-6, IL-10, and TNF) may play some role in causing the sequelae of DIC by modulating or activating the coagulation pathway.

Laboratory Assessment of Bleeding

Laboratory testing is an integral part of the diagnostic algorithm used in assessing the bleeding patient. It may not be prudent to wait for laboratory values before beginning treatment of acute bleeding, but it is imperative that blood samples for coagulation testing be drawn before therapy. The development of microprocessor technology has made it possible to perform diagnostic laboratory testing outside the confines of the clinical laboratory (so-called near-care testing). Whether near-care testing or clinical laboratory testing is employed, it is important to recognize that valuable as such testing is, it does not provide all of the needed diagnostic information.

In particular, the value of a careful patient history must not be underestimated. Previous bleeding events and a familial history of bleeding are both suggestive of a congenital coagulopathy. A thorough medication inventory is necessary to assess the possible impact of drugs on laboratory and clinical presentations. In the patient history query, it is advisable to ask explicitly about nonprescription drugs—using expressions such as "over-the-counter drugs," "cold medicines," and "Pepto-Bismol"—because unless specifically reminded, patients tend to equate the term medications with prescription drugs. If this is not done, many drugs that are capable of influencing hemostasis in vivo and in vitro (e.g., salicylates, cold and allergy medicines, and herbal supplements) may be missed. Mucosal and superficial bleeding is suggestive of platelet abnormalities, and deep bleeding is suggestive of factor deficiency.

It is important to be clear on the limitations of coagulation testing. At present, there are no laboratory or ex vivo methods capable of directly measuring the physiologic properties of the endothelium. Indirect assessments of endothelial damage can be obtained by

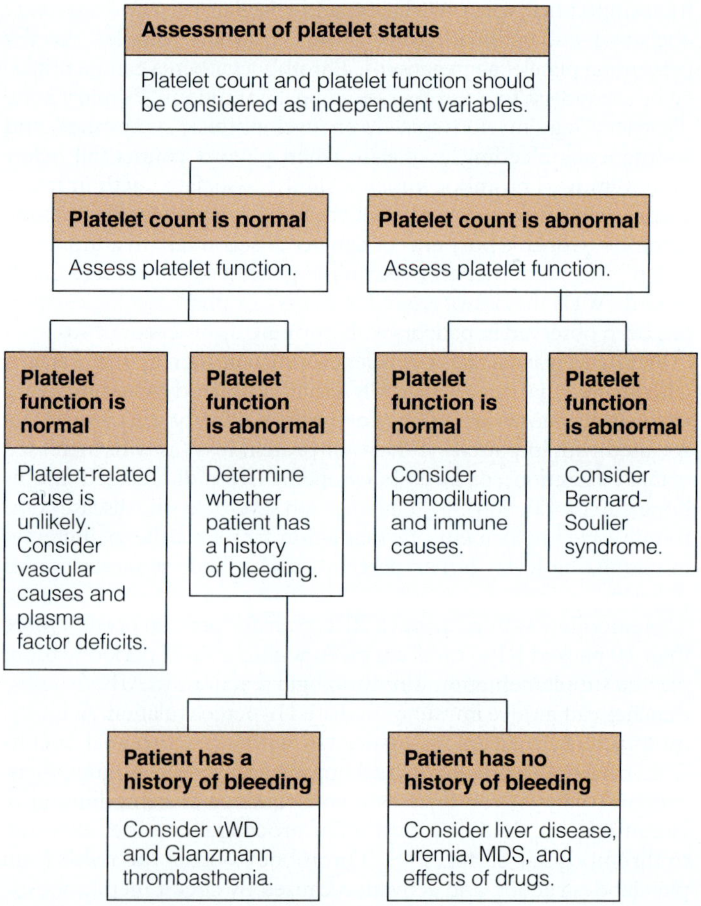

Figure 4 Algorithm depicts use of platelet count and platelet functional status in assessment of coagulopathies.

Table 5 Tests of Platelet Function

Product (Manufacturer)	Method
PFA-100 (Dade Behring)	Measures time required to occlude aperture after exposure to platelet agonists at shear rates
hemoSTATUS (Medtronic)	Measures activated clotting time; platelet-activating factor is the platelet agonist
AggreStat (Centocor)	Measures changes in voltage (impedance) after addition of platelet agonist
Thromboelastograph (Haemascope)	Measures changes in the viscoelastic properties of clotting blood induced by a rotating piston
Sonoclot Analyzer (Sienco)	Measures changes in the viscoelastic properties of clotting blood induced by a vibrating probe
Clot Signature Analyzer (Xylum)	Measures changes in platelet function at shear rates
Ultegra Analyzer (Accumetrics)	Used primarily for measuring the effect of platelet glycoprotein blockers (e.g., abciximab and eptifibatide); thrombin receptor activator peptide is the agonist

measuring levels of several laboratory parameters (e.g., vWF, the soluble cytokines endothelian-1 and E-selectin, and thrombomodulin), but such measurements have no clinical utility in the assessment of a bleeding patient.

Another issue is that of bias resulting from technical factors. PT (i.e., INR) and aPTT testing involves adding activators, phospholipids, and calcium to plasma in a test tube (or the equivalent) and determining the time to clot formation. Time to clot formation is a relative value, in that it is compared with the time in a normal population. A perturbation within the coagulation cascade, an excess of calcium, or poor sampling techniques (e.g., inadequately filled coagulation tubes, excessive tourniquet time, and clotted or activated samples) can bias the results. Hemolysis from the drawing of blood can also bias results via the effects of thromboplastins released from RBC membranes to initiate the coagulation process. In addition, many coagulation factors are highly labile, and failure to process and run coagulation samples immediately can bias test results.

Finally, not all coagulation tests are functionally equivalent: different laboratory methods may yield differing results.[71] Coagulation reagents have been manufactured in such a way as to ensure that the coagulation screening tests are sensitive to factor VIII and IX deficiencies and the effects of anticoagulation with warfarin or heparin. Thus, a normal aPTT in a patient with an abnormal INR may not exclude the possibility of common pathway deficiencies (e.g., deficiencies of factors X, V, and II), and most current methods of determining the INR and the aPTT do not detect low fibrinogen levels. The approach we use assumes that the methods used to assess INR and aPTT can discriminate normal factor activity levels from abnormal levels (< 0.4 IU/ml).

The CBC (including platelet count and differential count), the INR, and the aPTT tests should be the primary laboratory tests for differentiating coagulopathies [see Figure 3].

Platelet count and platelet function should be considered as independent values [see Figure 4]. Patients with congenital thrombocytopathies often have normal platelet counts; therefore, assessment of platelet function is required as well. Historically, the bleeding time has been used to assess platelet function. This test is grossly inadequate, in that it may yield normal results in as many as 50% of patients with congenital thrombocytopathies.[72,73] Numerous rapid tests of platelet function are currently available that can be used to screen for platelet defects; these tests can and should be included in the diagnostic approach to the bleeding patient [see Table 5].[73-75]

References

1. Bickell WH, Wall MJ Jr, Pepe PE, et al: Immediate versus delayed fluid resuscitation for hypotensive patients with penetrating torso injuries. N Engl J Med 331:1105, 1994
2. Gubler KD, Gentilello LM, Hassantash SA, et al: The impact of hypothermia on dilutional coagulopathy. J Trauma 36:847, 1994
3. Watts DD, Trask A, Soeken K, et al: Hypothermic coagulopathy in trauma: effect of varying levels of hypothermia on enzyme speed, platelet function, and fibrinolytic activity. J Trauma 44:846, 1998
4. Gentilello LM, Jurkovich GJ, Stark MS, et al: Is hypothermia in the victim of major trauma protective or harmful? A randomized, prospective study. Ann Surg 226:439, 1997
5. Rapaport SI: Blood coagulation and its alterations in hemorrhagic and thrombotic disorders. West J Med 158:153, 1993
6. Practice guidelines for blood component therapy: a report by the American Society of Anesthesiologists Task Force on Blood Component Therapy. Anesthesiology 84:732, 1996
7. Heckman KD, Weiner GJ, Davis CS, et al: Randomized study of prophylactic platelet transfusion threshold during induction therapy for adult acute leukemia: 10,000/μL versus 20,000/μL. J Clin Oncol 15:1143, 1997
8. Dyke CM, Bhatia D, Lorenz TJ, et al: Immediate coronary artery bypass surgery after platelet inhibition with eptifibatide: results from PURSUIT. Platelet Glycoprotein IIb/IIIa in Unstable Angina: Receptor Suppression Using Integrelin Therapy. Ann Thorac Surg 70:866, 2000
9. Despotis GJ, Levine V, Saleem R, et al: Use of point-of-care test in identification of patients who can benefit from desmopressin during cardiac surgery: a randomised controlled trial. Lancet 354:106, 1999
10. Levy JH, Schwieger IM, Zaidan JR, et al: Evaluation of patients at risk for protamine reactions. J Thorac Cardiovasc Surg 98:200, 1989
11. Fenton JW 2nd, Ofosu FA, Brezniak DV, et al: Thrombin and antithrombotics. Semin Thromb Hemost 24:87, 1998
12. Hirsh J, Dalen JE, Anderson DR, et al: Oral anticoagulants: mechanism of action, clinical effectiveness, and optimal therapeutic range. Chest 114(5 suppl):445S, 1998
13. Murray DJ, Pennell BJ, Weinstein SL, et al: Packed red cells in acute blood loss: dilutional coagulopathy as a cause of surgical bleeding. Anesth Analg 80:336, 1995
14. Holcroft JW, Blaisdell FW, Trunkey DD, et al: Intravascular coagulation and pulmonary edema in the septic baboon. J Surg Res 22:209, 1977
15. Owings JT, Bagley M, Gosselin R, et al: Effect of critical injury on plasma antithrombin activity: low antithrombin levels are associated with thromboembolic complications. J Trauma 41:396, 1996
16. Weitzel JN, Sadowski JA, Furie BC, et al: Surreptitious ingestion of a long-acting vitamin K antagonist/rodenticide, brodifacoum: clinical and metabolic studies of three cases. Blood 76:2555, 1990
17. Hébert PC, Wells G, Blajchman MA, et al: A multicenter, randomized, controlled clinical trial of transfusion requirements in critical care. Transfusion Requirements in Critical Care Investigators, Canadian Critical Care Trials Group. N Engl J Med 340:409, 1999
18. Maxwell RA, Gibson JB, Fabian TC, et al: Resuscitation of severe chest trauma with four different hemoglobin-based oxygen-carrying solutions. J Trauma 49:200, 2000
19. Creteur J, Sibbald W, Vincent JL: Hemoglobin solutions—not just red blood cell substitutes. Crit Care Med 28:3025, 2000
20. Mantovani A, Sozzani S, Vecchi A, et al: Cytokine activation of endothelial cells: new molecules for an old paradigm. Thromb Haemost 78:406, 1997
21. Edington TS, Mackman N, Brand K, et al: The structural biology of expression and function of tissue factor. Thromb Haemost 66:67, 1991
22. Vane JR, Anggard EE, Botting RM: Regulatory function of the vascular endothelium. N Engl J Med 323:27, 1990
23. Ignarro LJ, Buga GM, Wood KS, et al: Endothelium-derived relaxing factor produced and released from artery and vein is nitric oxide. Proc Natl Acad Sci 84:9265, 1987
24. ten Cate JW, van der Poll T, Levi M, et al: Cytokines:

triggers of clinical thrombotic disease. Thromb Haemost 78:415, 1997

25. Cerletti C, Evangelista V, de Gaetano G: P-selectin-β2-integrin crosstalk: a molecular mechanism for polymorphonuclear leukocyte recruitment at the site of vascular damage. Thromb Haemost 82:787, 1999
26. Brunetti M, Martelli N, Manarini S, et al: Polymorphonuclear apoptosis is inhibited by platelet mediated-released mediators, role of TGFβ-1. Thromb Haemost 84:478, 2000
27. Stel HV, Sakariassen KS, de Groot PG, et al: Von-Willebrand factor in the vessel wall mediates platelet adherence. Blood 65:85, 1985
28. Michelson AD, Barnard MR: Thrombin-induced changes in platelet membrane glycoproteins Ib, IX, and IIb-IIIa complex. Blood 70:1673, 1987
29. Motta G, Rojkjaer R, Hasan AA, et al: High molecular weight kininogen regulates prekallikrein assembly and activation on endothelial cells: a novel mechanism for contact activation. Blood 91:516, 1998
30. Osterud B, Rappaport SI: Activation of factor IX by the reaction product of tissue factor and factor VII: additional pathway for initiating blood coagulation. Proc Natl Acad Sci USA 74:5260, 1997
31. Mann KG: Biochemistry and physiology of blood coagulation. Thromb Haemost 82:165, 1999
32. Collen D, Lijnen HR: Basic and clinical aspects of fibrinolysis and thrombolysis. Blood 78:3114, 1991
33. Chetaille P, Alessi MC, Kouassi D, et al: Plasma TAFI antigen variations in healthy subjects. Thromb Haemost 83:902, 2000
34. Esmon CT, Owen WG: Identification of an endothelial cell cofactor for thrombin-catalyzed activation of protein C. Proc Natl Acad Sci USA 78:2249, 1981
35. Broze GJ, Warren LA, Novotny WF, et al: The lipoprotein-associated coagulation inhibitor that inhibits factor Xa: insight into its possible mechanism of action. Blood 71:335, 1988
36. Schmidt B, Mitchell L, Ofosu FA, et al: Alpha-2-macroglobulin is an important progressive inhibitor of thrombin in neonatal and infant plasma. Thromb Haemost 62:1074, 1989
37. Juhan-Vague I, Valadier J, Alessi MC, et al: Deficient tPA release and elevated PA inhibitor levels on patients with spontaneous recurrent DVT. Thromb Haemost 57:67, 1987
38. Korninger C, Lechner K, Niessner H, et al: Impaired fibrinolytic capacity predisposes for recurrence of venous thrombosis. Thromb Haemost 52:127, 1984
39. Shovlin CL: Molecular defects in rare bleeding disorders: hereditary hemorrhagic telangiectasia. Thromb Haemost 78:145, 1997
40. Sadler JE, Mannucci PM, Berntop E, et al: Impact, diagnosis, and treatment of von Willebrand's disease. Thromb Haemost 84:160, 2000
41. Mannucci PM: Desmopressin: a nontransfusional form of treatment for congenital and acquired bleeding disorders. Blood 72:1449, 1988
42. Weiss HJ: Congenital disorders of platelet function. Semin Thromb Hemost 17:228, 1980
43. Nurden AT: Inherited abnormalities of platelets. Thromb Haemost 82:468, 1999
44. Ljung RC: Prenatal diagnosis of haemophilia. Haemophilia 5:84, 1999
45. Lillicrap D: Molecular diagnosis of inherited bleeding disorders and thrombophilia. Semin Hematol 36:340, 1999
46. Cawthern KM, van't Veer C, Lock JB, et al: Blood coagulation in hemophilia A and hemophilia C. Blood 91:4581, 1998
47. Rodriguez-Merchan EC: Common orthopaedic problems in haemophilia. Haemophilia 5[suppl 1]:53, 1999
48. Mannucci PM, Tuddenbam EG: The hemophilias: progress and problems. Semin Hematol 36[4 suppl 7]:104, 1999
49. Bolton-Maggs PH: The management of factor XI deficiency. Haemophilia 4:683, 1998
50. Minowa H, Takahashi Y, Tanaka T, et al: Four cases of bleeding diathesis in children due to congenital plasminogen activator inhibitor-1 deficiency. Haemostasis 29:286, 1999
51. Lind B, Thorsen S: A novel missense mutation in the human plasmin inhibitor (alpha2-antiplasmin) gene associated with a bleeding tendency. Br J Haematol 107:317, 1999
52. Turpeinen AM, Mutanen M: Similar effects of diets high in oleic or linoleic acids on coagulation and fibrinolytic factors in healthy humans. Nutr Metab Cardiovasc Dis 9(2):65, 1999
53. Li D, Sinclair A, Mann N, et al: The association of diet and thrombotic risk factors in healthy male vegetarians and meat-eaters. Eur J Clin Nutr 53:612, 1999
54. Temme EH, Mensink RP, Hornstra G: Effects of diets enriched in lauric, palmitic or oleic acids on blood coagulation and fibrinolysis. Thromb Haemost 81:259, 1999
55. Rein D, Paglieroni T, Wun T, et al: Cocoa inhibits platelet activation and function. Am J Clin Nutr 72:30, 2000
56. Rein D, Paglieroni T, Wun T, et al: Cocoa and wine polyphenols modulate platelet activation and function. J Nutr 130:2120S, 2000
57. Bhatt DL, Topol EJ: Current role of platelet glycoprotein IIb/IIIa inhibitors in acute coronary syndromes. JAMA 284:1549, 2000
58. Humphries JE: Transfusion therapy in acquired coagulopathies. Hematol Oncol Clin North Am 8:1181, 1994
59. Zachee P, Vermylen J, Boogaerts MA: Hematologic aspects of end-stage renal failure. Ann Hematol 69:33, 1994
60. Peek GJ, Firmin RK: The inflammatory and coagulative response to prolonged extracorporeal membrane oxygenation. ASAIO J 45:250, 1999
61. Hobisch-Hagen P, Wirleitner B, Mair J, et al: Consequences of acute normovolaemic haemodilution on haemostasis during major orthopaedic surgery. Br J Anaesth 82:503, 1999
62. Konrad C, Markl T, Schuepfer G, et al: The effects of in vitro hemodilution with gelatin, hydroxyethyl starch, and lactated Ringer's solution on markers of coagulation: an analysis using SONOCLOT. Anesth Analg 88:483, 1999
63. Boyer LV, Seifert SA, Clark RF, et al: Recurrent and persistent coagulopathy following pit viper envenomation. Arch Intern Med 159:706, 1999
64. Eriksson BI, Kalebo P, Ekman S, et al: Direct thrombin inhibition with rec-hirudin CGP 39393 as prophylaxis of thromboembolic complications after total hip replacement. Thromb Haemost 72:227, 1994
65. Sherman DG, Atkinson RP, Chippendale T, et al: Intravenous ancrod for treatment of acute ischemic stroke: the STAT study: a randomized controlled trial. Stroke Treatment with Ancrod Trial. JAMA 282:2395, 2000
66. Oleksowicz L, Bhagwati N, DeLeon-Fernandez M: Deficient activity of von Willebrand's factor-cleaving protease in patients with disseminated malignancies. Cancer Res 59:2244, 1999
67. Francis JL, Biggerstaff J, Amirkhosravi A: Hemostasis and malignancy. Semin Thromb Hemost 24:93, 1998
68. Amirkhosravi M, Francis JL: Coagulation activation by MC28 fibrosarcoma cells facilitates lung tumor formation. Thromb Haemost 73:59, 1995
69. Williams EC, Moshen DF: Disseminated intravascular coagulation. Hematology: Basic Principles and Practice. Hoffman R, Benz EJ Sr, Shattil SJ, et al, Eds. Churchill-Livingstone, New York, 1995, p 1758
70. Muller-Berghaus G, ten Cate H, Levi M: Disseminated intravascular coagulation: clinical spectrum and established as well as new diagnostic approaches. Thromb Haemost 82:706, 1999
71. Lawrie AS, Kitchen S, Purdy G, et al: Assessment of Actin FS and Actin FSL sensitivity to specific clotting factor deficiencies. Clin Lab Haematol 20:179, 1998
72. Lind SE: The bleeding time does not predict surgical bleeding. Blood 77:2547, 1991
73. Mammen EF, Comp PC, Gosselin R, et al: PFA-100™ System: A new method for assessment of platelet dysfunction. Semin Thromb Hemost 24:195, 1998
74. Speiss BD: Coagulation function in the operating room. Anesth Clin North Am 8:481, 1990
75. LeForce WR, Bruno DS, Kanot WP, et al: Evaluation of the Sonoclot analyzer for the measurement of platelet function in whole blood. Am Clin Lab Sci 22:30, 1992
76. Winslow RM: Blood substitutes. Adv Drug Deliv Rev 40:131, 2000

Acknowledgments

Figures 1, 3, and 4   Marcia Kammerer.
Figure 2   Seward Hung.

6 LIFE-THREATENING ELECTROLYTE ABNORMALITIES

Kimberly J. Van Zee, M.D., and Stephen F. Lowry, M.D.

Evaluation and Treatment of Electrolyte Emergencies

Assessment of Volume Status

Proper management of any life-threatening electrolyte abnormality must include the clinical assessment of extracellular fluid (ECF) volume status. Because no simple specific laboratory test is sufficient for accurate determination of intravascular and interstitial fluid volume, clinical assessment aimed at detecting signs and symptoms of deficits or excesses of body fluid is necessary. Such assessment should include historical information that might bear on the pathogenesis of these volume changes.

EVALUATION AND TREATMENT OF
EXTRACELLULAR FLUID VOLUME DEFICITS

Deficits in ECF volume may adversely affect cardiovascular function, central nervous system function, and metabolic and temperature regulation, as well as induce more subtle changes in peripheral muscle function. Moderate decreases in ECF volume lead to orthostatic hypotension and associated tachycardia with evidence of reduced venous filling; drowsiness and a mild decrease in body temperature may result as well. Such decreases in ECF volume are also associated with a small, soft tongue and reduced skin turgor. More severe volume deficits eventually lead to stupor or coma, with reduced deep tendon reflexes and muscle atony. These deficits also result in hypotension and reduced pulse pressure with cutaneous lividity. A marked decrease in body temperature to 34° to 36° C (93° to 97° F) may also be observed.

ECF volume depletion results from loss of both sodium and water, not necessarily in the same proportion. In surgical patients, sodium is often lost in acute or chronic losses of gastrointestinal fluids. Postoperatively or after injury, fluid sequestration, or so-called third spacing, often causes subtle deficits in isotonic fluid volume.[1,2] In addition, preexisting renal or adrenal disease or previous administration of diuretics may lead to excess sodium loss in urine and thereby cause volume deficiencies.

Severe ECF volume deficits must be corrected as quickly as possible. Initially, until further abnormalities of electrolyte or acid-base status are identified, fluid should be replaced through the administration of a physiologic salt solution. In some patients, except for those with symptomatic hypernatremia, it may be preferable to begin fluid volume resuscitation with normal saline until adequate renal function and urine output can be established. Hemodynamically stable patients should initially receive 100 to 200 ml. Unstable patients can receive initial boluses of up to 500 ml according to need. There is no standard formula for calculating the amount of saline required to correct ECF volume depletion. Consequently, the adequacy of repletion must be clinically assessed. Blood pressure, pulse, urine output, and hematocrit should be monitored during the initial phases of this resuscitation. If further abnormalities of electrolyte status are discovered, management should be continued (see below).

EVALUATION AND TREATMENT OF
EXTRACELLULAR FLUID VOLUME EXCESS

Extracellular fluid volume excess may be associated with both systemic and organ-specific findings. Unless ECF excess is associated with other problems related to oxygen transport, however, it does not give rise to specific central nervous system signs of fluid volume excess. On the other hand, moderate ECF excess yields several significant cardiovascular findings, including higher pulse pressure, evidence of venous distention, and, possibly, congestive heart failure. More severe ECF excess results in pulmonary edema. Pitting edema may occur even with moderate ECF excess, and in more extreme cases, there is associated vomiting and diarrhea as intestinal edema progresses.

Acute volume excess usually results from acute or chronic renal or cardiovascular failure and occasionally from underlying liver disease. In surgical patients, volume excess from organ failure may be compounded by administration of too much fluid or failure to recognize fluid mobilization postoperatively.

Whatever the underlying cause, water intake should be restricted in patients with evidence of ECF volume excess. Fluid replacement should be the minimal daily requirement of approximately 500 ml, with additions to replace significant extraneous losses or to maintain hemodynamic stability. Further measures, such as administration of diuretics or inotropic cardiac agents or, in extreme cases, the use of dialysis, may be necessary to reduce fluid volume successfully. In such circumstances, serial determinations of electrolytes, particularly potassium, should be performed because changes in electrolyte status will inevitably influence subsequent therapeutic efforts.

Evaluation and Treatment of Electrolyte Emergencies

Patient presents with undefined change in neurologic, cardiovascular, renal, or volume status

Suspect abnormality of electrolyte status. Obtain history, and perform physical examination; assess fluid volume, blood glucose, liver function, and acid-base status; rule out organ-specific causes. Assess serum electrolysis.

Patient is hyponatremic

Rule out artifacts (e.g., from presence of glucose, mannitol, or glycine). Suspect renal dysfunction and acid-base disorders. Initiate continuous cardiovascular, renal, and neurologic monitoring. Assess volume status.

- **Volume is low**
  Correct volume deficit:
  - Administer isotonic saline if patient is alkalotic.
  - Administer lactated Ringer's solution if patient is acidotic.

- **Volume is normal**

- **Volume is increased**
  Consider administration of a loop diuretic.

Evaluate severity of symptoms including CNS alterations hypotension, and oliguria.

- **Symptoms are mild**
  Restrict water intake.

- **Symptoms are severe**
  Infuse hyperpertonic (3%) saline. Do not raise serum sodium by more than 12 mEq/L in first 24 hr. Discontinue infusion when symptoms improve.

Patient is hypernatremic

Assess volume status. Monitor cardiovascular, renal, and neurologic function.

- **Volume is low**
  Replace volume deficit with isotonic saline or lactated Ringer's solution.

- **Volume is normal**

- **Volume is increased**
  Give diuretics.

Replace water deficit (no more than half in first 24 hr; remainder over 1–2 days). Discontinue infusion when symptoms improve. If neurogenic diabetes insipidus is present, administer vasopressin.

Serum potassium < 3.0 mEq/L

Assess immediate risk. Watch for any ECG changes or neuromuscular changes. Ensure adequare urine output.

ECG or neuromuscular changes are present

Initiate immediate I.V. therapy and monitoring. Give up to 40 mEq K$^+$/hr in normal saline with 60 mEq K$^+$/L. Recheck serum level after 40–50 mEq has been given.

Serum potassium < 2.5 mEq/L

Repeat 50 mEq infusion; recheck serum level afterward.

```
                                                    ┌─────────────────────────────┐
                                                    │ Patient is hyperkalemic     │
┌──────────────────────────┐                        │                             │
│ Patient is hypokalemic   │                        │ Assess immediate risk.      │
└──────────────────────────┘                        │ Evaluate renal function.    │
              │                                     │ Monitor ECG continuously.   │
              ▼                                     └─────────────────────────────┘
┌──────────────────────────┐                                    │
│ Serum potassium          │                    ┌───────────────┴────────────────┐
│ > 3.0 mEq/L              │                    ▼                                ▼
│                          │       ┌────────────────────────┐      ┌────────────────────────┐
│ Administer oral          │       │ Kidneys are functioning│      │ Patient is in renal    │
│ supplements or slow I.V. │       └────────────────────────┘      │ failure                │
│ supplementation.         │                    │                  │                        │
└──────────────────────────┘                    │                  │ Initiate dialysis.     │
                                                │                  └────────────────────────┘
```

Patient is hypokalemic

Serum potassium > 3.0 mEq/L → Administer oral supplements or slow I.V. supplementation.

- **No ECG or neuromuscular changes are present**
- **Patient is receiving digitalis or is acidotic**

Serum potassium > 2.5 mEq/L and no ECG changes are present → Give 10 mEq K$^+$/hr I.V. in normal saline with 30 mEq K$^+$/L.

Patient is hyperkalemic

Assess immediate risk. Evaluate renal function. Monitor ECG continuously.

- **Kidneys are functioning**
- **Patient is in renal failure** → Initiate dialysis.

Serum potassium < 6.0 mEq/L; no ECG changes
Administer cation exchange resins. Give orally, if tolerated. If not, give rectally.

Serum potassium > 6.0 mEq/L, or ECG changes present
Administer cation exchange resins. Give orally, if tolerated. If not, give rectally.

- **Patient is not receiving digitalis**
  Give 10% calcium gluconate 10 ml I.V. over 2 min. If ECG changes persist, repeat over 15 min.

- **Patient is receiving digitalis**
  Give sodium bicarbonate, 45 mEq I.V. over 5 min.

ECG changes resolve | ECG changes persist
Give sodium bicarbonate, 45 mEq I.V. over 5 min. If ECG changes persist, repeat over 15 min.

ECG changes resolve | ECG changes persist
Give 1 ampule D50W with 10 U regular insulin I.V. over 15 min. If patient is well hydrated, consider furosemide, 20–40 mg I.V.

ECG changes resolve | ECG changes persist
Initiate dialysis.

Table 1 Approximate Values for Serum and Total Body Electrolytes

Electrolyte	Serum Level (mEq/L)	Total Body Level (mEq)
Sodium	136–145	3,000
Potassium	3.5–5.0	3,400
Calcium	4.4–5.2	50,000
Magnesium	1.5–2.5	2,000

Assessment of Sodium Status

Serum sodium concentration cannot be assumed to be related to ECF volume status. Marked changes in sodium concentration result in specific clinical signs and symptoms. Altered levels of circulating sodium should be sought and assessed in the light of historical and clinical evidence indicating the status of the total body sodium balance [see Table 1]. The initial evaluation should include a search for organ-specific and generalized findings that can be useful in determining the extent of tonicity derangement and in guiding initial therapeutic interventions.

EVALUATION AND TREATMENT OF HYPONATREMIA

Artifactual hyponatremia may be induced by other circulating osmotic substances, such as mannitol or glycine (absorbed from the irrigant used during prostate procedures) or, most commonly, glucose. In hyperglycemic patients, the serum sodium concentration is reduced by 1.6 mEq/L for every 100 mg/dl (5.5 mmol/L) rise in glucose above normal. Evaluation of hyponatremia should begin with an attempt to rule out artifacts, along with assessment of renal function and acid-base status. Volume status should also be assessed. Volume deficits in alkalotic patients should be replaced with isotonic saline. In the presence of acidosis, deficits should be replaced with lactated Ringer's solution.

Acute symptomatic hyponatremia is characterized by alterations of CNS function, such as increased deep tendon reflexes and muscle twitching, as well as the more specific signs of excessive intracellular fluid, such as increased blood pressure and reduced pulse rate. As hyponatremia becomes more severe, convulsions occur, deep tendon reflexes are reduced, hypothermia becomes evident, and oliguria and watery diarrhea may appear. In hyponatremia associated with decreased total body sodium, hypotension and oliguria may occur; these conditions must be corrected immediately if irreversible renal failure is to be prevented. Hyponatremia with increased total body sodium is often associated with renal failure and with cirrhosis. In these circumstances, there will be evidence of pitting edema.[3]

Hyponatremia may also occur in the presence of relatively normal total body sodium levels. This situation is less common in surgical patients, but it may occur, for example, when hypotonic or sodium-free solutions have been administered in excess to patients who are unable to modulate their sodium and fluid intake; it may also be associated with the syndrome of inappropriate secretion of antidiuretic hormone (SIADH), which is characterized by impaired excretion of renal free water. In patients with this syndrome, urine is excessively concentrated (osmolarity > 100 mOsm/L), and high urinary sodium concentrations occur.[4] Hyponatremia caused by SIADH or administration of excess free water is treated by free water restriction.

If hyponatremia gives rise to serious side effects that warrant emergency treatment (e.g., coma, seizures, myoclonus, or focal neurologic deficits), infusion of hypertonic saline may be initiated. The estimated sodium deficit [see Sidebar Calculation of Sodium Deficit and Replacement] can serve as the initial guide for sodium replacement. To avoid neurologic complications, the serum sodium concentration should not be raised by more than 12 mEq/L during the first 24 hours. Once the serum sodium level is 120 mEq/L or higher or symptoms have resolved, further correction generally is not required. Rapid extracellular volume expansion and pulmonary edema are potential problems during hypertonic volume infusions; however, they may be anticipated and avoided through careful monitoring. If treatment is required, loop diuretics are effective.

EVALUATION AND TREATMENT OF HYPERNATREMIA

Hypernatremia is always associated with hypertonicity. Cellular dehydration resulting from the movement of free water out of the cell down the concentration gradient into the ECF is a universal feature of hypernatremia and is responsible for the characteristic signs: thirst, agitation, lethargy, tachycardia, reduced blood pressure, and core temperature elevation.[5,6] Oliguria and dry, sticky mucous membranes are often found, and a swollen, red tongue and flushed skin may also be evident. As this state of cellular dehydration progresses, delirium and cardiovascular collapse may occur. Consequently, the first step in management is to monitor cardiovascular, renal, and neurologic function to assess fluid volume status.

Calculation of Sodium Deficit and Replacement

Normal serum Na$^+$ (mEq/L) − actual serum Na$^+$ (mEq/L) = sodium deficit (mEq/L)

Example: 140 − 110 = 30

0.6 × body weight (kg) = normal body water volume (L)

Example: 0.6 × 60 = 36

Normal body water volume (L) × sodium deficit (mEq/L) = estimated body Na$^+$ deficit (mEq)

Example: 36 × 30 = 1,080

Because a 3.0 percent hypertonic saline solution contains 0.5 mEq sodium/ml, the volume of solution needed for sodium replacement can be calculated as follows:

$$\frac{\text{Estimated body Na}^+ \text{ deficit (mEq)}}{0.5} = \text{necessary volume of 3.0 percent saline (ml)}$$

Example: 1,080/0.5 = 2,160

Hypernatremia may occur in conjunction with hypovolemia, isovolemia, or hypervolemia. Careful clinical evaluation of ECF volume is therefore essential. In hypernatremia associated with hypovolemia, there is generally a total body sodium deficit. This condition may occur in patients with excessive GI losses (from nasogastric suction, severe diarrhea, or vomiting), renal losses (from osmotic diuresis caused by hyperglycemia, hyperalimentation, or diuretic administration), cutaneous losses (from burns, hyperthermia, or excessive sweating), or peritoneal losses (from peritonitis or peritoneal dialysis). It should be treated by administering isotonic saline or lactated Ringer's solution.

Hypernatremia may also result from the administration of hypertonic saline (e.g., solutions containing sodium bicarbonate), hyperaldosteronism, or Cushing's syndrome. In hypernatremic patients who are hypervolemic, diuretics and water replacement are indicated.

Neurogenic diabetes insipidus (DI) is a not uncommon cause of hypernatremia in the ICU. In this condition, total body sodium is often normal, but a relative state of pure water deficit exists. The diagnosis of DI is suggested by polyuria and a urine osmolarity lower than 200 mOsm/L. Treatment comprises administration of vasopressin and replacement of free water.

Water deficits can be calculated as follows:

$$\text{Normal body water (L)} = 0.6 \times \text{body weight (kg)}$$

$$\text{Current body water (L)} = \frac{\text{normal serum Na}^+ \text{ (mEq/L)} \times \text{normal body water (L)}}{\text{measured serum Na}^+ \text{ (mEq/L)}}$$

$$\text{Body water deficit (L)} = \text{normal body water (L)} - \text{current body water (L)}$$

An amount equal to one half of the calculated water deficit should be administered over the first 24 hours; the remaining deficit should be corrected over the next one to two days. More rapid correction of the hypernatremia may result in lethargy or convulsions secondary to cerebral edema.

Assessment of Potassium Status

Because 98 percent of potassium is intracellular and only two percent is extracellular, a shift of a small amount of potassium into or out of the intracellular compartment can result in a dramatic change in the serum potassium concentration. The resultant alteration of the potassium gradient across the cell membrane causes neuromuscular dysfunction, especially in cardiac tissue, with potentially grave consequences. The distribution of potassium is affected by a number of factors, including acid-base balance, hormone levels, body fluid tonicity, the actions of pharmacological agents, and changes in body cell mass.[7]

EVALUATION AND TREATMENT OF HYPOKALEMIA

Hypokalemia may result from inadequate intake of potassium, excessive renal or GI losses, or redistribution of normal body stores.[8] Management of hypokalemia includes an assessment of immediate risk and is based on monitoring changes in neuromuscular activity (e.g., weakness or hyporeflexia) as well as on monitoring electrocardiographic changes. Evidence of neuromuscular changes or of progressive ECG changes (frequent premature ventricular contractions → flat or inverted T waves → U waves → depressed ST segments → prolonged PR intervals → tall P waves → widened QRS complexes) is an indication for immediate intravenous therapy.[5] In patients with severe hypokalemia, cautious administration of up to 40 mEq/hr of potassium may be undertaken but only with continuous electrocardiographic monitoring and close physician supervision. Any potassium infusion at rates greater than 10 mEq/hr should be administered into a central vein to avoid inadvertent formation of a potassium bolus, which could result in myocardial depression. Even in the absence of clinical and electrocardiographic evidence of impending severe hypokalemic complications, patients who are receiving digitalis or who have concurrent metabolic acidosis should also receive immediate intravenous potassium supplementation. In the latter cases, administration of up to 10 mEq/hr may be cautiously undertaken. For patients whose serum potassium level is 3 mEq/L or greater, either oral supplementation or slow intravenous potassium supplementation is appropriate. Patients who present with simultaneous hypokalemia and hypomagnesemia will require magnesium replacement before abnormalities in potassium levels can be fully corrected.

EVALUATION AND TREATMENT OF HYPERKALEMIA

The classic signs of hyperkalemia are progressive electrocardiographic changes: tall peaked T waves → widened QRS complexes → depressed ST segments → decreased amplitude of R waves → prolonged PR interval → diminished P waves → widened QRS complex with prolongation of the QT interval, resulting in a sine wave pattern → diastolic arrest.[5] These changes are usually seen when the potassium level is 6.0 to 6.5 mEq/L or higher but may also occur with potassium levels between 5.0 and 6.0 mEq/L.

Treatment of hyperkalemia consists of taking immediate measures to reduce the serum potassium level, withholding any exogenous potassium, limiting severe catabolism, and correcting renal failure. As with hypokalemia, the immediate risk must be assessed; in addition, the adequacy of renal function must be established, and continuous ECG monitoring must be initiated. If the kidneys are functioning but the serum potassium level is higher than 6 mEq/L or electrocardiographic changes are present, patients not receiving digitalis therapy may undergo intravenous calcium gluconate infusion (90 mg of elemental calcium in a 10 ml ampule, given over two minutes). The calcium antagonizes the membrane effects of hyperkalemia in a matter of minutes and has a duration of action of about one hour. The next step is sodium bicarbonate (45 mEq I.V. over five minutes). Bicarbonate causes potassium to shift into the intracellular space within 15 to 30 minutes and has a duration of action of about one to two hours. Patients who are taking digitalis should not receive intravenous calcium. Instead, they should initially receive sodium bicarbonate (45 mEq over five minutes).

If ECG changes persist, the following additional approaches may be tried: (1) administration of glucose and insulin (one ampule of 50 percent dextrose in water and 10 units of regular insulin), which also shifts potassium into cells within 15 to 30 minutes and has a duration of action of two to four hours, and (2) administration of furosemide (20 to 40 mg I.V.), which increases renal excretion of potassium within about 15 to 30 minutes in well-hydrated patients with functioning kidneys. Cation exchange resins, given by either the oral or the rectal route, should be administered simultaneously with this immediate intravenous therapy in patients with life-threatening hyperkalemia or as a means of primary therapy in patients with less severe hyperkalemia. Patients who show evidence of impaired renal function or who respond inadequately to the measures just described should be prepared to undergo dialysis immediately.

Assessment of Calcium Status

Calcium is present in the plasma in two forms: either bound to protein or as a positively charged ion. The degree to which calcium is bound is influenced by the amount of protein present in the plasma. Several corrective calculations have been suggested to determine the true total calcium in the presence of low levels of serum proteins. The following is one such calculation:

$$\text{Corrected calcium (mg/dl)} = \text{measured calcium} + [(4 - \text{albumin [g/dl]}) \times 0.8]$$

A simpler way of determining true total calcium is to assume that every 1 g/dl decrease in serum albumin falsely lowers the serum calcium by 1 mg/dl. Serum calcium can also be markedly altered by the degree of acid-base abnormality. In severe alkalosis, the ionic calcium level can be lowered and hypocalcemic symptoms precipitated, even if the patient has a normal or low normal total calcium. Similarly, hyperventilation alkalosis can lower the ionic calcium and precipitate symptoms. In much the same way, renal tubular acidosis can lead to elevated serum calcium levels.

EVALUATION AND TREATMENT OF HYPERCALCEMIA

Because calcium is ubiquitous in the body, symptoms and signs of hypercalcemia are widespread and often nonspecific, and their etiology is frequently unclear [see Table 2]. The common gastrointestinal symptoms are early, nonspecific, and often vague. Increased gastric acid secretion and pancreatitis are much more often noted in patients whose elevated calcium levels result from primary hyperparathyroidism. There is considerable controversy regarding this point, however, and the true prevalence of hyperparathyroidism as an etiology is still unknown. The neuromuscular symptoms are widespread and, like the GI symptoms, nonspecific; they usually consist of depression, fatigue, lethargy, and clouding of consciousness. Profound muscle weakness, usually of proximal muscle type, may be followed by stupor and even by irreversible coma in late or unrecognized states. Characteristic electroencephalographic abnormalities have been described.[9,10]

The major renal symptom of hypercalcemia is a reversible renal tubular defect in the ability to concentrate urine that mimics the manifestations of diabetes insipidus, resulting in some degree of total body water deficit and sodium deficit in most patients. Dehydration decreases the glomerular filtration rate, thereby exacerbating the renal damage and bringing about a progressive increase in hypercalcemia, which leads to further renal failure.

In patients with primary hyperparathyroidism and prolonged urinary loss of calcium, nephrocalcinosis or renal stones are common; however, renal stones are relatively rare in patients with primary hypercalcemia of malignancy.

The cardiovascular symptoms of hypercalcemia are related to the major role calcium plays in neurotransmission. Acute hypercalcemia can actually slow the heart rate and shorten the ventricular systole. In moderate hypercalcemia, the QT interval is shortened, whereas in severe hypercalcemia (calcium levels > 16 mg/dl), the QT interval lengthens. Digitalis must be used cautiously in patients with hypercalcemia.

Severe hypercalcemia is a medical emergency and requires hospitalization and aggressive treatment. Although the definitive treatment of acute hypercalcemic crisis in patients with primary hyperparathyroidism is surgical, calcium levels should, if possible, be reduced before exploration is begun. The patient must be monitored so that fluid balance and central venous pressure may be accurately determined. Foley catheterization is usually required to assess renal function and volume status. As acute treatment progresses, the etiology of the hypercalcemia should be actively investigated [see Figure 1].

The first step is rehydration with normal saline solution. In mild to moderate cases, the usual amount infused is 3 to 5 L/day, but in severe cases, as much as 10 L/day may be required. These larger amounts should be accompanied by administration of furosemide, beginning with a dose of 40 mg, followed by dosages of 40 to 80 mg every two to four hours. Ethacrynic acid is acceptable as an alternative diuretic, but the thiazides are not. In addition to serum calcium levels, serum sodium, potassium,

---

Table 2 Causes of Hypercalcemia

Primary hyperparathyroidism

Malignancy
- With bone metastasis
- Without bone metastasis

Drugs
- Thiazide or other diuretics
- Vitamins A and D
- Calcium carbonate

Granulomatous diseases
- Wegener's granulomatosis
- Sarcoid

Metabolic disorders
- Paget's disease
- Osteoporosis
- Familial hypercalcemic hypocalciuria
- Thyrotoxicosis
- Renal tubular acidosis

Other
- Pheochromocytoma

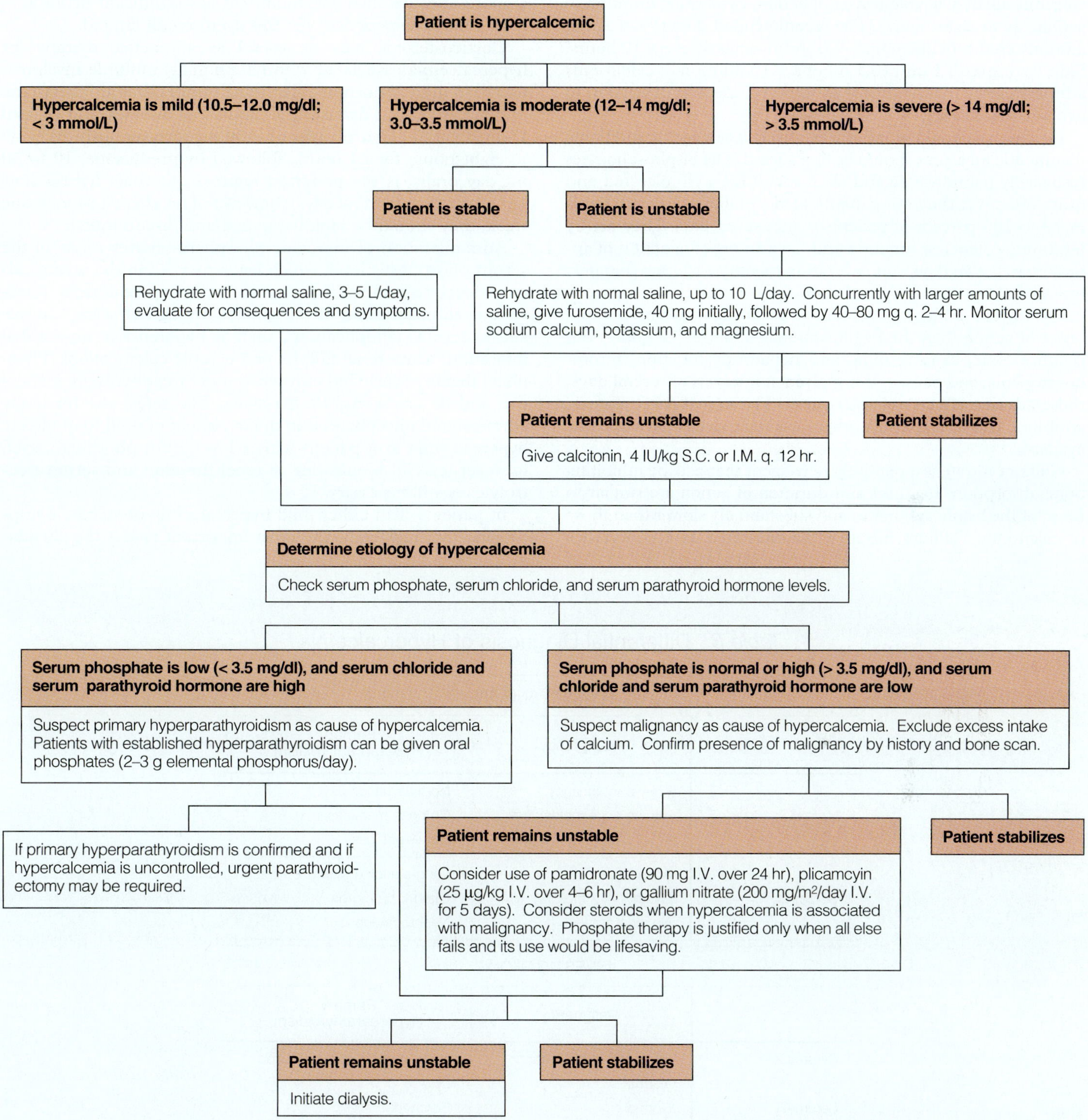

```
                        ┌─────────────────────────┐
                        │ Patient is hypercalcemic│
                        └─────────────────────────┘
```

Figure 1 Illustrated is an algorithm for management of hypercalcemia.

and magnesium levels must be monitored constantly to ensure that major deficits of these electrolytes do not result in a parallel metabolic derangement.

If hydration in conjunction with furosemide fails, or if hypercalcemia is life threatening, calcitonin should be used. Calcitonin acts by inhibiting bone resorption and increasing renal excretion of calcium and is the most rapidly acting anticalcemic agent available (onset of action, two hours; duration of action, six to eight hours). The recommended dosage is 4 IU/kg administered subcutaneously or intramuscularly every 12 hours. Skin testing with 1 unit (0.1 ml of a 1:10 dilution of calcitonin) administered subcutaneously should precede administration to exclude any allergy.

Because calcitonin alone is a relatively weak agent, additional therapeutic measures should be considered. The bisphosphonates (especially pamidronate and clodronate) are well tolerated and quite effective: they are capable of normalizing calcium levels in 70 to 100 percent of patients within seven days. They act by inhibiting osteoclast function and have an onset of action of approximately two days and a duration of action of approximately one week.[11]

Plicamycin (25 µg/kg over four to six hours) has a more rapid onset of action than the bisphosphonates (about 12 hours) but is more toxic, causing renal and hepatic dysfunction, thrombocytopenia, and nausea. If it is given at intervals of several days, these adverse effects are infrequent. The use of this cytotoxic antibiotic has decreased as other, less toxic drugs have become available.

Gallium nitrate is a relatively new agent that acts by inhibiting bone absorption. Its onset and duration of action are similar to those of the bisphosphonates and substantially slower than those of calcitonin. Gallium nitrate is administered as a continuous intravenous infusion (200 mg/m^2/day for five days). Although it is more effective than calcitonin,[12] it has significant nephrotoxicity. Clinical experience with this agent is still limited.

Corticosteroids may be useful as adjunctive therapy for hypercalcemia associated with lymphomas, multiple myeloma, non–parathyroid hormone–secreting tumors that are metastatic to bone, Addison's disease, granulomatous diseases, and vitamin D intoxication. Hydrocortisone, 100 mg intravenously every six to eight hours for 24 hours, followed by prednisone, 10 to 30 mg/day orally, is the preferred regimen. Steroids have a slow onset of action (several days); however, if no effect is seen in one week, they should be rapidly tapered and discontinued.

Administration of inorganic phosphates causes a rise in the serum phosphorus level, which leads to a fall in the serum calcium level, regardless of the cause of the hypercalcemia. Intravenous administration of phosphates, though effective, can result in serious complications, such as hypotension, myocardial infarction, acute renal failure, and ectopic calcifications. Phosphate therapy is justified only when other treatments are ineffective and its use would be lifesaving. The safest use for orally administered phosphates is in the treatment of mild to moderate hypercalcemia in a patient with a low serum phosphate level; however, careful monitoring of renal function and serum electrolytes is still necessary.

In patients with either mild hypercalcemia or stable, asymptomatic hypercalcemia, the most important task is the elucida-

Table 3 Differential Diagnosis of Hypercalcemia

	SYMPTOMS AND SIGNS	
	Malignancy	Primary Hyperparathyroidism
History	Known malignancy Known bone metastases Weight loss	No malignancy No bone metastases No weight loss
Serum Ca^{2+}	Abrupt rise Usually > 12 mg/dl No renal stones	Long-standing slow rise Often < 12 mg/dl Nephrocalcinosis
	INVESTIGATIONS	
	Malignancy	Primary Hyperparathyroidism
Serum Ca^{2+}	Recent abrupt elevation	Long-standing slow elevation
Serum PO$_4$*	Normal	Low
Serum Cl$^-$	Normal	Elevated
Cl$^-$ to PO$_4$ ratio	> 33	< 33
Serum parathyroid hormone	Normal	Elevated
Urinary Ca^{2+}	Normal or elevated	Elevated
Urinary cAMP	Normal	Elevated
Serum bicarbonate	Normal	Low
Alkaline PO$_4$*	Normal or elevated	Normal or elevated
Bone scan	Isolated sites of increased uptake; metastatic disease	Diffuse, increased uptake

*PO$_4$ stands for H$_2$PO$_4^-$, HPO$_4^{2-}$, and PO$_4^{3-}$.

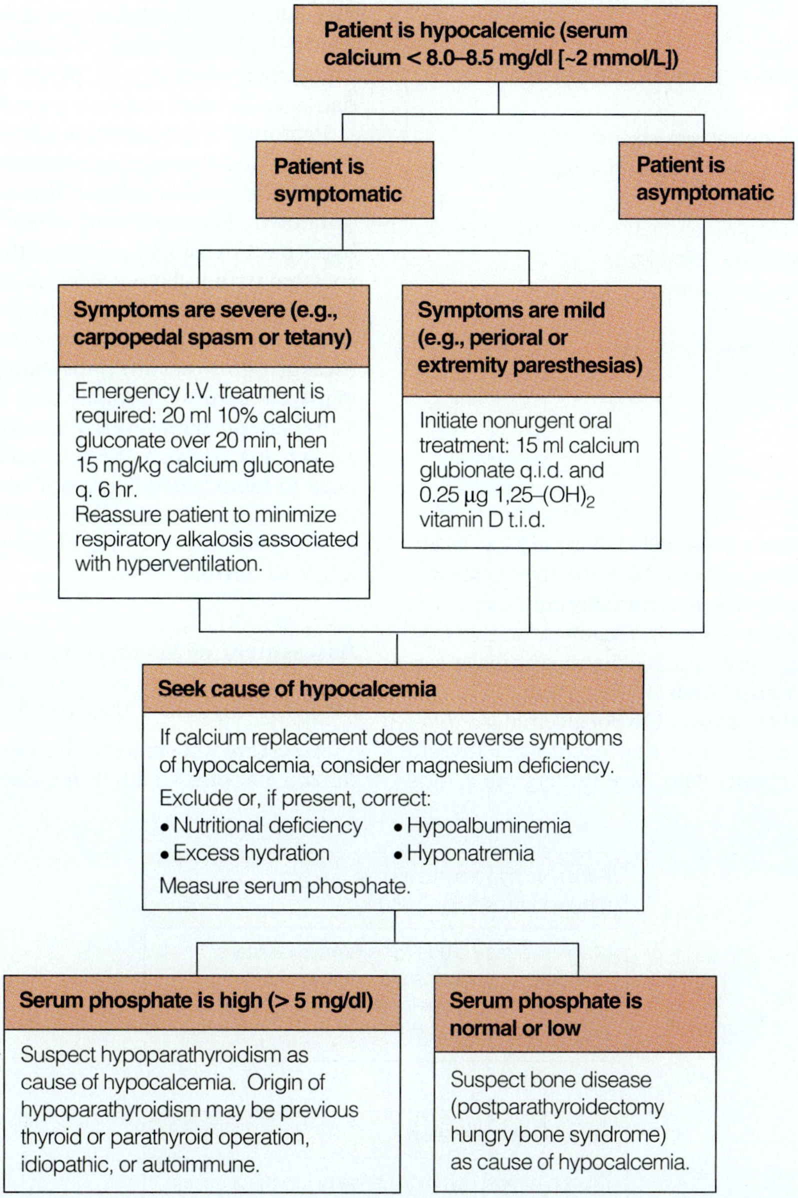

Figure 2 Illustrated is an algorithm for management of hypocalcemia.

tion of the etiology. The essential distinction that must be made is between hypercalcemia of parathyroid origin and hypercalcemia that is caused by malignant disease [see Table 3]. Other conditions rarely progress to major life-threatening hypercalcemia.

EVALUATION AND TREATMENT OF HYPOCALCEMIA

Biochemical hypocalcemia is usually defined as a serum calcium level below the lower limit of normal in the laboratory—usually 8.0 to 8.5 mg/dl (2.0 to 2.1 mmol/L). In asymptomatic patients, no immediate therapy is required other than a search for the cause of the hypocalcemia. In symptomatic patients who have perioral or extremity paresthesias, treatment can be initiated on a nonurgent basis with oral medication. In patients with more severe symptoms, particularly those of carpopedal spasm and tetany, emergency intravenous treatment is required. Not the least important part of this urgent treatment is reassurance of the patient; reassurance serves to diminish hyperventilation and the accompanying respiratory alkalosis, which merely compounds the hypocalcemia [see Figure 2].

Ten milliliters of a 10 percent calcium gluconate solution contains 93 mg (4.6 mEq) of elemental calcium. Ten milliliters of a 10 percent calcium chloride solution contains 273 mg of elemental calcium (14 mEq). The calcium chloride solution thus has a greater osmolarity (2.04 mOsm/ml) than the calcium gluconate solution (0.7 mOsm/ml), which makes it potentially more irritating to the vein on infusion. The 15 mg/kg of calcium gluconate can be given as five ampules in 1,000 ml at 100 ml/hr. In oral replacement, 5 ml of a calcium glubionate preparation has 115 mg of elemental calcium, which is equivalent to 1.2 g of calcium gluconate. Calciferol, which contains 1,25-dihydroxy-vitamin D, has a brief half-life of three to six hours and can be given in a dosage of 0.25 μg three or four times a day.

Mild biochemical hypocalcemia is more common in hospitalized patients who are severely malnourished and have been rigorously treated with intravenous fluids. It is rarely symptomatic,

Table 4 Causes of Hypocalcemia

- Thyroidectomy or parathyroidectomy
- Idiopathic autoimmune hypoparathyroidism
- Pseudohypoparathyroidism
- Acute pancreatitis
- Dilutional or nutritional deficiency
- Severe magnesium depletion
- Drugs
- Chronic vitamin D deficiency
- Multiple transfusions
- Chronic renal failure

although the serum calcium can occasionally fall to very low levels. Low levels of serum albumin may exacerbate the hypocalcemia. For practical purposes, a 1 g/dl fall in serum albumin can cause the total serum calcium to fall by 1 mg/dl. Treatment in this case should be directed at restoring the overall biochemical imbalances, along with meeting the nutritional needs of the patient.

There are numerous possible causes of hypocalcemia [see Table 4]. The more acute problems are those that occur after thyroid or parathyroid operations. Patients who have undergone a total thyroidectomy have postoperative hypocalcemic symptoms that can be highly dramatic. Similarly, patients who have undergone a parathyroidectomy, in which all parathyroid tissue has been damaged or removed, can experience profound hypocalcemia.

Profound hypocalcemia is more commonly seen in patients who are undergoing a reoperation for parathyroid disease and in whom the amount of parathyroid tissue previously removed is unknown. These patients often have severe and long-standing hyperparathyroidism, along with the significant bone disease associated with it. Hypocalcemia can be compounded by two conditions: (1) hypoparathyroidism and (2) so-called hungry bones. Differentiation between these two entities is best achieved by measuring the serum phosphate levels. In hypoparathyroid patients, the serum phosphate level will rise, often to 6 mg/dl, whereas in patients with severe bone disease, the serum phosphate will remain low, despite the low calcium level. If symptoms attributed to hypocalcemia are not reversed by calcium replacement, magnesium deficiency should always be considered because it is a not uncommon cause of inability to restore serum calcium levels to normal.

Assessment of Magnesium Status

EVALUATION AND TREATMENT OF HYPOMAGNESEMIA

An estimated six to twelve percent of ambulatory and hospitalized patients are hypomagnesemic [see Figure 3]. Because

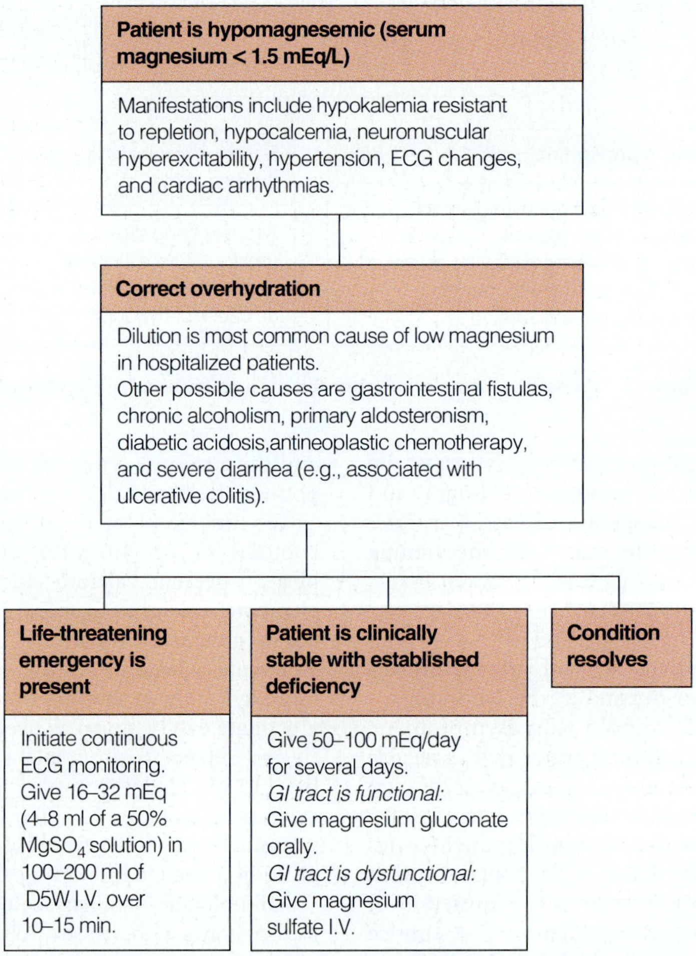

Figure 3 Presented here are guidelines for management of hypomagnesemia.

magnesium is not included in the usual panel of electrolytes, disorders of magnesium are often overlooked. The daily requirement for magnesium is about 10 to 30 mEq, and inadequate magnesium intake for as short a period as one week can result in hypomagnesemia. Vigilance and appropriate replacement can decrease the incidence of complications.

Common causes of hypomagnesemia in hospitalized patients include dilution, GI fistulas, diarrhea, prolonged bowel rest, alcoholism, diabetic ketoacidosis, primary aldosteronism, and excessive urinary losses resulting from chemotherapy (especially with cisplatin). Manifestations of magnesium deficiency include hypokalemia that is resistant to repletion, hypocalcemia, neuromuscular hyperexcitability, hypertension, ECG changes, and cardiac arrhythmias.[13]

In a life-threatening emergency, such as severe hypomagnesemia that is causing seizures, cardiac arrhythmias, or neuromuscular excitability, large doses of magnesium should be administered. In conjunction with continuous ECG monitoring, 16 to 32 mEq (4 to 8 ml of a 50 percent $MgSO_4$ solution) in 100 to 200 ml of five percent dextrose in water should be infused intravenously over 10 to 15 minutes.

In clinically stable patients with an established magnesium deficiency, it may be necessary to give 50 to 100 mEq/day for several days to replenish body stores. Patients at high risk for magnesium deficiency include those who are on bowel rest, those who are receiving total parenteral nutrition, and those who have chronic diarrhea or fistulas. Magnesium should be given intravenously (in a dose of 10 to 50 mEq) to patients with dysfunctional GI tracts; patients with functional GI tracts can receive magnesium orally. Although a 500 mg magnesium gluconate tablet supplies only 2.4 mEq of elemental magnesium (compared with 122.4 mEq from 15 g of $MgSO_4$ powder), it is much better tolerated than magnesium sulfate, which commonly causes diarrhea and abdominal cramps.

EVALUATION AND TREATMENT OF HYPERMAGNESEMIA

Hypermagnesemia is much less common than hypomagnesemia: it is seen only in renal insufficiency. In patients with renal failure who are on a normal diet and are taking no magnesium-containing supplements, serum magnesium levels will stabilize at about 2.5 mEq/L. If, however, magnesium-containing supplements (e.g., antacids) are being administered, plasma concentrations can reach 4 to 6 mEq/L, a level at which signs and symptoms of toxicity often begin to appear. At a serum magnesium level of 4 mEq/L, the most common symptoms are drowsiness, lethargy, diaphoresis, nausea, and vomiting. At higher levels, hyporeflexia and abnormal cardiac conduction are seen. As serum magnesium levels approach 10 mEq/L, respiratory paralysis, narcosis, hypotension, and even complete heart block may occur.[14]

Treatment consists of immediate withholding of all exogenous magnesium, hydration, and intravenous administration of calcium, starting with 90 to 180 mg (10 to 20 ml of a 10 percent calcium gluconate solution) over five to 10 minutes. The calcium will immediately reverse the effects of magnesium toxicity, but the effect is transient. Dialysis may be required to sustain a decrease in magnesium levels in patients with severe hypermagnesemia.

Discussion

Physiology of Body Fluids

Knowledge of the extent and composition of various body fluid compartments is a necessary basis for rational treatment of pathophysiological changes in electrolyte and water balance. Total body water generally constitutes between 50 and 70 percent of total body weight; however, it can be radically altered by a number of variables, including age, sex, and organ-specific or systemic disease. For example, in young men, total body water accounts for 60 percent of body weight, whereas in young women, it accounts for 50 percent. As a percentage of total body weight, total body water decreases steadily and significantly with age, eventually reaching a low of approximately 52 percent in men and 47 percent women. The percentage of total body weight accounted for by water is also higher in thin subjects than in obese ones and higher in infants than in adults.

The body water is divided into three functional compartments. The first, the intracellular compartment, accounts for 30 to 40 percent of body weight. Extracellular fluid represents approximately 20 percent of body weight; it can be further subdivided into intravascular fluid, or plasma (accounting for five percent of body weight), which makes up the second compartment, and interstitial, or extravascular, extracellular fluid (accounting for 15 percent of body weight), which makes up the third compartment.

INTRACELLULAR AND EXTRACELLULAR FLUID

Isotopic and biopsy studies of the intracellular compartment have yielded accurate measurements of the composition of intracellular fluid [see Figure 4]. In addition to water, its major constituents are potassium and magnesium, which are the principal cations, and phosphates and proteins, which are the principal anions.

The interstitial fluid has two main components, one of which equilibrates rather rapidly (functional) and the other relatively slowly (nonfunctional). The second component includes connective tissue water as well as what is termed transcellular water, which includes cerebrospinal fluid and joint fluids. This nonfunctional component of the interstitial fluid represents only a minor portion (10 percent) of the interstitial fluid volume and is not the same as the additional nonfunctional extracellular fluid, commonly referred to as third space, that is found after burns, soft tissue injuries, or surgery. In normal extracellular fluid, sodium is the predominant cation, and chloride and bicarbonate are the principal anions [see Figure 4]. The plasma compartment has a higher protein content; consequently, the total concentration of cations is higher and the concentration of inorganic anions somewhat lower than in the interstitial compartment. For clinical purposes, however, the concentration and composition of the plasma and the interstitial compartment can be considered to be equivalent.

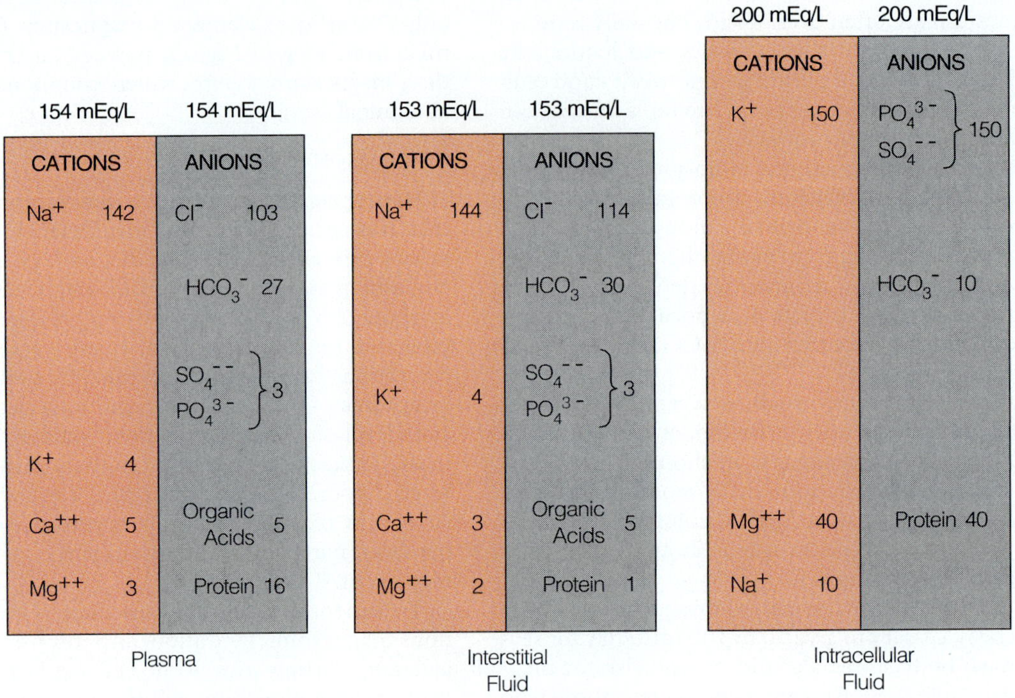

Figure 4 This schematic diagram represents the composition of plasma, interstitial fluid, and intracellular fluid.[17]

OSMOTIC PRESSURE

The activity of electrolytes within a compartment depends on (1) the number of particles present per unit volume (mmol/L), (2) the number of electric charges per unit volume (mEq/L), and (3) the number of osmotically active particles or ions per unit volume (mOsm/L). The molar expression of a substance is commonly encountered, but this definition gives no information about the number of osmotically active particles in solution or about the electric charge present in solution. The electrolytes of the body are customarily expressed in terms of their chemical combining power or equivalents. Within any compartment, the number of equivalents of anions must balance the number of equivalents of cations.

The number of osmotically active particles within any given compartment is between 290 and 310 mOsm/L. Protein dissolved in the plasma compartment is responsible for the effective osmotic pressure between the plasma and the interstitial compartment, commonly referred to as the colloid oncotic pressure. Differences in ionic composition between the intracellular and extracellular fluid compartments are maintained by the cell wall, which functions as a semipermeable membrane. The effective osmotic pressure between the extracellular and intracellular fluid compartments is altered in proportion to the levels of substances that do not freely traverse the cell membrane. Sodium, which is the principal cation of the extracellular fluid, accounts for most of the osmotic pressure of the interstitial fluid. Other substances that do not penetrate the cell membrane freely, such as glucose, can also increase the effective osmotic pressure.

The effective osmotic pressure in the two compartments must be maintained. Because the cell membrane is completely permeable to water, any condition that alters the effective osmotic pressure in either the intracellular or the extracellular compartment will result in redistribution of water. For example, an increase in serum sodium concentration will result in increased extracellular fluid volume, with a net transfer of water from intracellular to extracellular fluid. This transfer of water continues until the osmotic pressure between the two compartments is equalized. On the other hand, a reduction in serum sodium will result in a net transfer of water from the extracellular to the intracellular fluid compartment, whereas isosmotic depletion of the extracellular fluid, which does not change the concentration of ions, causes no transfer of water between compartments. Thus, the intracellular fluid is affected by losses that involve a change in the concentration or composition of the extracellular fluid, but it is affected little, if at all, by losses involving isotonic volume.

Pathophysiological Body Fluid Changes

Disorders of fluid and electrolyte balance may be generally classified into three categories: volume disturbances, concentration disturbances, and composition disturbances. Although these disturbances may be interrelated, and any or all of them may occur in clinically complex patterns, for purposes of management and interpretation of data, each one should be analyzed as a separate entity. Changes in volume are most readily identified as loss of isotonic saline solution from the extracellular fluid space. If the osmolarity in the intracellular and extracellular spaces remains unchanged, net transfer of fluid from the intracellular space to the depleted extracellular space is unlikely. If, however, water alone is added to or lost from the extracellular

Table 5 Normal Volume and Composition of Gastrointestinal Secretions

Secretion	Volume (L/day)	Concentration (mEq/L)			
		Na^+	K^+	Cl^-	HCO_3^-
Saliva	≈1	20–80	10–20	20–40	20–160
Gastric juice	1–2	20–100	5–10	120–160	—
Bile	≈1	150–250	5–10	40–60	20–60
Pancreatic juice	1–2	120	5–10	10–60	80–120
Succus entericus	1–2	140	5	variable	variable

fluid or the concentration of osmotically active particles changes, water will pass between the intracellular and extracellular spaces and so return the osmolarity to normal. The extracellular concentration of most ions—except for sodium, which is the dominant extracellular ion—can change without significantly affecting the total osmolarity. Such changes, commonly referred to as compositional changes, are infrequent when the kidneys are functioning normally.

VOLUME DISTURBANCES

Extracellular Fluid Volume Depletion

ECF volume depletion results from loss of both sodium and water, but the two constituents may be lost in differing proportions. For instance, the sodium content of gastrointestinal secretions varies widely throughout the GI tract; the precise amounts of sodium and water lost are governed by the source of the loss [see Table 5]. If the loss is isonatremic, the tonicity of the ECF is relatively unaffected and the intracellular volume will not change. If, however, as is common, water loss exceeds sodium loss (as in sweating, hyperventilation, nasogastric suction, and severe diarrhea), hypernatremia results, leading to increased ECF osmolarity and shifting of intracellular water to the extracellular compartment. By contrast, hyponatremia may result if excessive administration of fluid lowers the ECF sodium concentration below the normal level. Measurement of serum sodium only determines the concentration of sodium with respect to water: it provides no information about the absolute quantities of either substance present in the body.

Among the extrarenal causes of extracellular fluid volume depletion is volume depletion caused by losses of gastrointestinal fluid. Sequestration of fluid after injury may also result in significant extracellular fluid volume depletion if not enough of the lost fluid is replaced or if inappropriately concentrated solutions are administered. Preexisting renal or adrenal disease or previous administration of diuretics may lead to excess sodium loss in urine.

The aim of management is to restore reduced ECF volume by administering solutions designed to replace both the lost fluid and the lost electrolytes. Several different saline solutions can be used [see Table 6]. There is no standard formula for calculating the amount of saline required to correct ECF volume depletion. Consequently, the adequacy of repletion must be assessed clinically through physical signs, renal function, and hematocrit.

Extracellular Fluid Volume Excess

In surgical patients, ECF volume excess is usually iatrogenic or secondary to renal disease. It can be aggravated by coexisting conditions, such as congestive heart failure, nephrosis, cirrhosis, and conditions associated with hypoalbuminemia. These latter conditions are thought to result in a reduction of the effective arterial volume, leading to renal salt and water retention.

Table 6 Electrolyte Content of Parenteral Fluids (mEq/L)

Solution	Cations					Anions		
	Na^+	K^+	Ca^{2+}	Mg^{2+}	NH_4^+	Cl^-	HCO_3^-	HPO_4^-
Extracellular fluid	142	4	5	3	0.3	103	27	3
Lactated Ringer's solution	130	4	2.7			109	28*	
0.9% sodium chloride (saline)	154					154		
M/6 sodium lactate	167						167*	
M (molar) sodium lactate	1,000						1,000*	
3% sodium chloride	513					513		
5% sodium chloride	855					855		
0.9% ammonium chloride					168	168		

*Present in solution as lactate, which is converted to bicarbonate.

ABNORMALITIES OF SODIUM CONCENTRATION

Hyponatremia

Hyponatremia may be defined as a lower than normal concentration of sodium in the serum. Serum osmolarity is reduced. Because concentration is a measure not of total sodium but of the ratio of sodium to water, the presence of hyponatremia does not necessarily imply a deficit of body sodium; in fact, hyponatremia is often associated with an excess of total body salt (as in the edema-forming state). Consequently, an estimate of the total body sodium balance is necessary for the proper interpretation of an abnormality of serum sodium.

When there is no loss of sodium without water, hyponatremia is the net result of loss of isotonic or hypotonic fluid that is replaced by water without salt. In such circumstances, the administration of an isotonic saline solution is the treatment of choice because volume depletion is more threatening than hypotonicity, and water diuresis may be restored when volume depletion is corrected.

Water intoxication, which is usually caused by administration of water to patients unable to manifest a water diuresis (e.g., those who have just undergone operation or who have renal insufficiency), is usually managed by restriction of water intake. Administration of hypertonic saline may be indicated in those rare cases in which hyponatremia is severe and symptomatic. In such circumstances, administration of hypertonic saline solution should be used only to increase the serum sodium concentration to the point where clinical symptoms are resolved; it should not be used to restore serum sodium concentration to normal. This potentially dangerous mode of therapy can result in severe circulatory overload and therefore should be performed only in certain rare situations in which severe symptoms, such as delirium, exist. Careful physiologic monitoring is essential.

A state of severe hyponatremia that has been associated with SIADH may occur in a variety of disorders, most often in lesions of the pulmonary or central nervous system. The hyponatremia initially is a result of water retention but then is complicated by urinary loss of sodium. The essential criteria for diagnosis of this syndrome are (1) hyponatremia, (2) urine that is hypertonic to plasma at all times, even during water administration, (3) inappropriately large amounts of urinary sodium, even after water loading, (4) no renal or adrenal cause for this constellation of abnormalities, and (5) disappearance of all abnormalities after adequate restriction of water intake.

Both hyperglycemia and hyperlipidemia may increase extracellular osmolarity, thereby causing water to move from the intracellular to the extracellular compartment. As a result, the tonicity of extracellular fluid is underestimated; in general, however, no immediate therapy is required other than that aimed at rectifying the underlying metabolic disorder.

Hypernatremia

Hypernatremia leads to increased tonicity (osmolarity) and may result from either loss of water or gain of sodium. When hypernatremia is from loss of water, both intracellular and extracellular fluid compartments are diminished in volume; when it is from gain of sodium, extracellular fluid volume is increased, and intracellular fluid volume is decreased.

Hypernatremia most often occurs in patients unable to obtain free water. This inability may be the result of insufficient water intake, as in coma, vomiting, hypothalamic lesions, excessive sweating, hyperpnea, diarrhea, and polyuria of renal or extrarenal origin (e.g., diabetes insipidus or mellitus or administration of osmotic diuretics). Hypernatremia caused by pure salt gain is uncommon and usually iatrogenic but may be chronic in hyperaldosteronism and Cushing's syndrome.

Although urine volume is usually diminished and specific gravity increased during hypernatremia, the hematocrit may not be increased because of proportionate loss of plasma and red blood cell water. The change in ECF volume may be small unless water depletion is severe. The resulting loss of intracellular fluid volume leads to diminished skin turgor as well as to changes in pressure and in pressure regulation.

The usual treatment for hypernatremia is administration of solute-free water. The amount of water required is calculated according to the equation supplied earlier [see Assessment of Sodium Status, above].

Mixed Volume and Concentration Changes

The clinical picture associated with combined fluid and concentration abnormalities tends to be a composite of the signs and symptoms associated with each state. One of the more common mixed abnormalities is the combination of extracellular fluid deficit and hyponatremia. In surgical patients, this problem frequently occurs during the postoperative period, when lost gastrointestinal fluids are replaced with hypotonic or solute-free solutions. Extracellular fluid excess combined with hypernatremia is also seen in surgical patients, typically as a result of prolonged administration of excessive quantities of sodium salts and restricted water intake, as when pure water losses (such as insensible loss of water from skin and lungs) are replaced with sodium-containing solutions only. In patients with renal insufficiency and an associated inability to generate a water diuresis, excessive administration of water or hypotonic salt solutions may

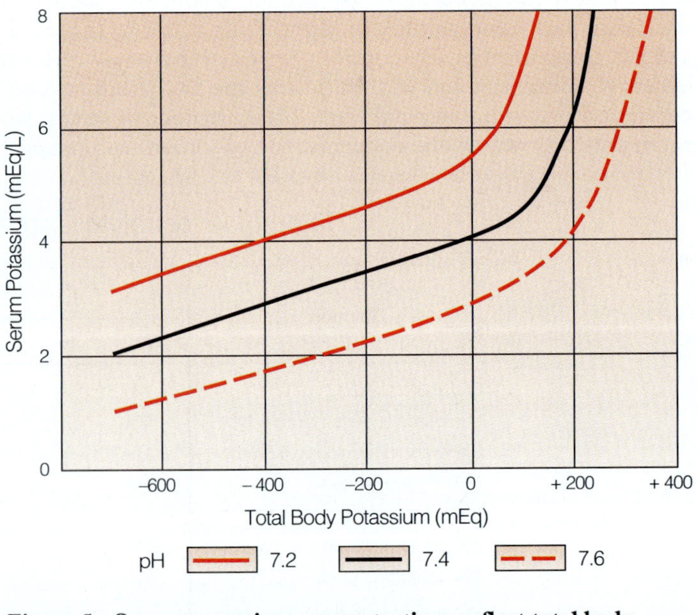

Figure 5 Serum potassium concentrations reflect total body potassium concentrations, as illustrated here. The effect of arterial pH on their relation is also shown.[18]

induce extracellular fluid volume excess in combination with hyponatremia.

ABNORMALITIES OF POTASSIUM CONCENTRATION

Body Balance

Urinary correction accounts for the majority of potassium lost from the body. The kidneys, which are responsible for regulating body potassium balance, are able to increase excretion in response to high potassium intake; however, they are less able to adjust to very low levels of potassium intake. There are no major renal conservation mechanisms for potassium, as there are for sodium; consequently, 5 to 10 mEq of potassium continues to appear in the urine even after a prolonged period of potassium-free intake.

On the whole, even though ECF contains only about two percent of total body potassium, the serum potassium concentration reflects the total body potassium content. Therefore, when total body potassium is elevated, serum concentration is high as well; when total body potassium is low, serum levels are also reduced [see Figure 5].

The distribution of potassium between intracellular and extracellular compartments can be influenced by many pathophysiological conditions. Large quantities of intracellular potassium may be released into the extracellular space as a consequence of severe injury, surgical stress, or acidosis or during catabolic states. In these conditions, there may be a significant rise in serum potassium if oliguric or anuric renal failure is present, but life-threatening hyperkalemia is rarely encountered when renal function is normal.

Hypokalemia

Reductions in serum potassium may result either from loss of potassium from the body or from a shift of potassium in the cells. Potassium deficiency in the surgical patient is commonly the result of excess losses; for practical purposes, the only potassium deficiencies caused by movement from serum to cells result from insulin use, respiratory alkalosis, or athletic training. Diarrhea, intestinal or biliary fistulas, ureteroenterostomy, vomiting, and nasogastric suction can all cause significant potassium losses from the gastrointestinal tract. Losses associated with vomiting or nasogastric suction may induce a potassium deficit greater than can be explained by the loss of potassium in fluids; such a deficit usually results from the enhanced urinary excretion of potassium that is associated with alkalosis and ECF volume contraction. Common causes of urinary loss of potassium include renal tubular disorders, osmotic diuresis, diuretic or corticosteroid therapies, Cushing's syndrome, hyperaldosteronism, and Bartter's syndrome. Reductions in circulating potassium level may also result from intracellular potassium shift resulting from administration of alkali or from parenteral administration of glucose or insulin without adequate potassium supplementation.

Although a mild depression in serum potassium may not be a life-threatening emergency, a risk assessment is essential in any patient with a serum potassium level of less than 3 mEq/L. A variety of oral supplementations providing potassium are available, including potassium chloride, which may be administered diluted in juice. Other potassium formulations, including potassium gluconate and potassium bicarbonate, are also available for oral administration and can be administered to patients whose serum chloride is normal. When hypokalemic alkalosis is present, however, potassium chloride is preferable because the chloride component is necessary for correction of the alkalosis and the associated chloride deficit.

Intravenous administration of potassium must always be undertaken with great caution and in conjunction with intensive monitoring. Rates of administration higher than 10 mEq/hr are seldom indicated except when signs of impending neuromuscular or cardiovascular collapse are present.

When there is evidence of potassium loss through gastrointestinal fluids, fluid replacement can be initiated, with the composition of the fluid to be determined by the level of the loss [see Table 5]. In such conditions, it is safe to replace the entire amount that it is anticipated will be lost because patients with normal renal function can easily handle any excess.

Hyperkalemia

Hyperkalemia invariably results from decreased renal excretion of potassium caused by intrinsic dysfunction or secondary to rapid release of potassium from cells after massive cellular injury or transcellular shifts related to a fall in blood pH. Artifactual elevations of serum potassium concentration may occur in association with an elevated platelet count or in conjunction with hemolysis or prolonged refrigeration of blood samples.

Hyperkalemia may be treated by measures that counteract the effects of potassium, those that force cellular entry of potassium, or those that actually remove potassium from the body. The urgency of the situation should be assessed on the basis both of the serum potassium concentration and of any ECG changes that are observed.

CALCIUM METABOLISM

Calcium is a key electrolyte in numerous body functions. The normal daily dietary intake of calcium is about 1,000 mg, and the overall net absorption is about 100 mg. Secretion into the intestine is variable but usually is about 300 mg; about 40 percent of what is ingested is absorbed [see Table 7].

Table 7 Calcium Metabolism

Total Body Calcium	
Exchangeable bone pool	4 g
Stable bone pool	1,000 g
Intracellular fluid	11 g
Extracellular fluid	0.9 g
GI tract	1.5 g
Calcium Lost Daily	
Feces	1 g
Urine	100 mg
Skin	30–100 mg
Calcium Exchanged Daily	
Bone	500 mg
GI tract	1 g
Glomerular filtrate	10 g

The greater part of the roughly 1,000 mg of calcium distributed throughout the extracellular fluid is exchanged with bone. This exchange is both rapid and slow. The exchangeable bone pool is approximately 4 g, and the stable bone pool is approximately 1,000 g. From 300 to 500 mg of calcium is exchanged with bone each day; accretion depends on the age of the patient. About 10,000 mg of calcium is exchanged daily by glomerular filtration, which means that the entire supply of extracellular fluid is exchanged 40 to 50 times every 24 hours. Virtually all excreted calcium is reabsorbed in the kidney; only 100 mg is excreted daily in the urine, and only 900 to 1,000 mg in the feces. Even in severe hypercalcemia, urinary excretion of calcium barely reaches 500 mg/day. This fact partially explains why in hypercalcemic states urinary excretion of calcium cannot compensate for the excess mobilization of bone calcium.

Plasma and blood levels remain stable within narrow limits, and disturbances of these levels can cause numerous abnormalities of function. The primary causes of disturbed calcium metabolism resulting in hypercalcemia are primary hyperparathyroidism and malignancy. In five to 10 percent of all cases of malignancy, elevated calcium levels will develop at some time in the course of the illness. Hypercalcemia is linked with a number of different neoplasms, the most common of which are breast cancer, renal cell cancer, lung cancer, and multiple myeloma. Primary hyperparathyroidism is common, occurring in up to 1,000 to 2,000 of the general population. There are numerous other causes of hypercalcemia, but they neither are as common as hyperparathyroidism or malignancy nor cause such severe hypercalcemia. Hyperparathyroidism and malignancy can coexist: of 100 patients with proven primary hyperparathyroidism in a cancer hospital, 34 (34 percent) also had a malignant disorder, whereas of 180 patients with proven primary hyperparathyroidism at an adjacent general hospital, 17 (nine percent) had a malignant disorder within a similar interval.[15] One review of patients with breast malignancy suggests that the prevalence of hyperparathyroidism in these patients is similar to that in the general population.[16]

MAGNESIUM METABOLISM

The total body content of magnesium is approximately 2,000 mEq. More than half of this amount is contained in bone; the remainder is distributed intracellularly. Only one percent is in the ECF, which means that the rate of magnesium loss must be slow because the exchangeable pool is turning over slowly. Normal intake is approximately 20 mEq/day; the majority is excreted in feces, and a lesser amount is excreted in urine. Virtually all absorbed magnesium is excreted by the kidneys. Magnesium plays a major role in intracellular enzyme function. The homeostatic mechanism by which it is controlled is not well understood, but it is known to involve parathyroid hormone. Urine has a strong tendency to retain magnesium, and normally functioning kidneys protect against excessive losses by this route.

References

1. Shires GT, Williams J, Brown F: Acute changes in extracellular fluids associated with major surgical procedures. Ann Surg 154:803, 1961
2. Wright HK, Gann DS: Correction of defect in free water excretion in postoperative patients by extracellular fluid volume expansion. Ann Surg 158:70, 1963
3. Schrier RW, Anderson RJ: Renal sodium excretion, edematous disorders, and diuretic use. Renal and Electrolyte Disorders, 2nd ed. Schrier RW, Ed. Little, Brown & Co, Boston, 1980
4. Goldberg M: Hyponatremia. Med Clin North Am 65:251, 1981
5. Van Zee KJ, Barie PS, Lowry SF: Electrolyte disorders. Current Surgical Therapy, 4th ed. Cameron JL, Ed. Mosby-Year Book, St Louis, 1992, p 1005
6. Feig PU, McCurdy DK: The hypertonic state. N Engl J Med 297:1444, 1977
7. Cox M: Potassium homeostasis. Med Clin North Am 65:363, 1981
8. Knochel JP: Etiologies and management of potassium deficiency. Hosp Pract 22:153, 1987
9. Allen EM, Singer FR, Melamed D: Electroencephalographic abnormalities in hypercalcemia. Neurology 20:15, 1970
10. Moure JMB: The electroencephalogram in hypercalcemia. Arch Neurol 17:34, 1967
11. Bilezikian JP: Management of acute hypercalcemia. N Engl J Med 326:1196, 1992
12. Warrell RP, Israel R, Frisone M, et al: Gallium nitrate for acute treatment of cancer-related hypercalcemia: a randomized, double-blind comparison to calcitonin. Ann Intern Med 108:669, 1988
13. England MR, Gordon G, Salem M, et al: Magnesium administration and dysrhythmias after cardiac surgery: a placebo-controlled, double-blind, randomized trial. JAMA 268:2395, 1992
14. Agus ZS, Massry SG: Hypomagnesemia and hypermagnesemia. Maxwell & Kleeman's Clinical Disorders of Fluid and Electrolyte Metabolism, 5th ed. Narins RG, Ed. McGraw-Hill, New York, 1994, p 1099
15. Farr HW: Hyperparathyroidism and cancer. CA Cancer J Clin 26:66, 1976
16. Axelrod DM, Bockman RS, Wong GY, et al: Distinguishing features of primary hyperparathyroidism in breast cancer patients. Cancer 60:1620, 1987
17. Shires GT, Canizaro PC, Lowry SF: Fluid, electrolyte, and nutritional management of the surgical patient. Principles of Surgery, 4th ed. Schwartz SI, Shires GT, Spencer FC, et al, Eds. McGraw-Hill Book Co, New York, 1984, p 45
18. Taggart DD: Fluid and electrolyte disturbances. Manual of Medical Therapeutics, 20th ed. Rosenfeld MG, Ed. Little, Brown & Co, Boston, 1971

Acknowledgments

Figures 1 through 3   Talar Agasyan.
Figures 4 and 5   Al Miller.

7 LIFE-THREATENING ACID-BASE DISORDERS

Lena M. Napolitano, M.D., and Anthony A. Meyer, M.D., Ph.D.

Evaluation of Acid-Base Imbalance

Normal acid-base balance is maintained via complex interactions among the cardiovascular, renal, pulmonary, gastrointestinal, and hepatic systems. Perturbations in one or more of these systems result in the many different disorders of acid-base metabolism. These disorders vary with respect to cause, severity of presentation, and management. For all of them, however, the fundamental goal of management is to reestablish acid-base homeostasis.

Given that acid-base disorders are very common in critically ill patients, a working knowledge of these conditions is essential for any physician who treats such patients. Early diagnosis and early therapeutic intervention may prevent serious complications. In what follows, we place special emphasis on those acid-base disorders that are common in surgical patients and on those that are potentially life-threatening.

Definitions and Measurement Issues

Arterial pH is very tightly regulated and is normally maintained between 7.35 and 7.45. Because mixed venous carbon dioxide tension ($P_{mv}CO_2$) is higher than arterial carbon dioxide tension (P_aCO_2) as a result of production of CO_2 by tissues, venous pH is usually slightly lower than arterial pH. Consequently, acid-base balance can be more accurately determined by using arterial blood samples, which is therefore highly recommended.

The following definitions will be used throughout the chapter:

- Acidemia: a blood pH value lower than 7.35.
- Alkalemia: a blood pH value higher than 7.45.
- Acidosis: a physiologic process that causes acidemia if not compensated.
- Alkalosis: a physiologic process that causes alkalemia if not compensated.

TEMPERATURE CORRECTION FOR ARTERIAL BLOOD SAMPLES

It is known that temperature variation alters measured blood gas values in vitro, thereby changing measured pH in a linear fashion.[1] Although arterial blood samples are drawn at the patient's body temperature, which may be lower or higher than normal, they are always warmed or cooled to 37° C before undergoing analysis for measurement of pH, P_aCO_2, and arterial oxygen tension (P_aO_2). The numbers obtained, therefore, reflect what pH, P_aCO_2, and P_aO_2 would be if the patient's temperature were 37° C, not necessarily what they are at the patient's actual body temperature.

Temperature correction is the process by which mathematical adjustments based on the patient's true body temperature at the time of blood sampling are applied to the arterial blood gas values obtained at 37° C to make these values a more accurate reflection of the true in vivo values. There is considerable controversy regarding whether such temperature correction is necessary; it is not clear whether it has any real impact on either clinical interpretation or the choice of therapeutic intervention.[2,3] In our view, uncorrected arterial blood gas values provide the most useful information for assessment and management of acid-base disturbances in hypothermic patients; corrected values have little clinical relevance. In most cases, therefore, temperature correction of arterial blood samples for acid-base analysis is unnecessary.[4]

MEASURED VERSUS CALCULATED BICARBONATE CONCENTRATION

In the evaluation of acid-base balance, it is extremely important to consider the bicarbonate concentration. The bicarbonate concentration in serum or arterial blood can be either measured directly or calculated by means of the Henderson-Hasselbalch equation:

$$pH = pK_a + \log \frac{[HCO_3^-]}{[H_2CO_3]}$$

As a rule, the carbonic acid (H_2CO_3) concentration is not measured directly in clinical laboratories, but it can be approximated by multiplying P_aCO_2 by the CO_2 solubility coefficient, for which the generally accepted value is 0.0301 at physiologic pH.

In most cases, calculated values for the bicarbonate concentration are roughly equivalent to measured values. Sometimes, however, they differ by as much as 7 to 8 mEq/L. When this occurs, the measured bicarbonate concentration is considered correct: the CO_2 solubility coefficients used in the Henderson-Hasselbalch equation may change in patients with acute acid-base disorders, and such change renders calculated bicarbonate concentrations less accurate. For this reason, assessment of acid-base homeostasis should make use of the bicarbonate value that is directly measured in the serum electrolyte panel, not the calculated value that is derived from arterial blood gas analysis.

Primary versus Mixed Acid-Base Disturbances

The primary acid-base disturbances are metabolic acidosis, respiratory acidosis, metabolic alkalosis, and respiratory alkalosis. When one of these primary acid-base disturbances is present and chemical buffering is unable to prevent a change in pH, the body initiates compensatory responses in an attempt to maintain electrical neutrality. These compensatory responses are dependent on the renal sys-

```
                        ┌─────────────────────────────┐
                        │ Patient has acid-base imbalance │
                        └─────────────────────────────┘
                                    │
            ┌───────────────────────┴───────────────────────┐
            │                                               │
┌───────────────────────────────────────┐   ┌───────────────────────────────────────┐
│ Metabolic acidosis (pH < 7.35, $P_aco_2$ < 40 mm Hg) │   │ Respiratory acidosis (pH < 7.35, $P_aco_2$ < 40 mm Hg) │
└───────────────────────────────────────┘   └───────────────────────────────────────┘
```

Metabolic acidosis branch

Condition is life-threatening (pH < 7.2)

Correct hypoxemia, hypovolemia, and hypoperfusion.

Initiate fluid resuscitation.

Consider placing a central venous or pulmonary arterial catheter.

Consider HCO_3^- therapy to raise pH to ≥ 7.2.

Condition is not life-threatening

Identify and treat cause of acidosis

Calculate anion gap:
Anion gap = $[Na^+] - ([Cl^-] + [HCO_3^-])$

Anion gap is increased

Possible causes include
- Lactic acidosis
- Diabetic ketoacidosis
- Alcoholic ketoacidosis
- Renal failure
- Ingestion of toxins
- Rhabdomyolysis

Anion gap is normal

Possible causes include
- Excessive HCO_3^- loss
  Diarrhea
  Enteric fistulas
  Ureterosigmoidostomy
  Renal tubular acidosis
  Carbonic anhydrase inhibitors (e.g., acetazolamide)
- Hypoaldosteronism
- Addison's disease
- Excessive acid administration

Respiratory acidosis branch

Condition is life-threatening (pH < 7.2, P_aco_2 > 60 mm Hg, or patient has respiratory distress or is unresponsive)

Perform emergency endotracheal intubation and institute mechanical ventilation.

Condition is not life-threatening

Determine whether there is a history of pulmonary disease or chronic hypercapnia.

Identify and treat cause of acidosis

Airway obstruction

Possible causes include
- Laryngospasm
- Foreign body
- External compression
- Sleep apnea

For laryngospasm, correct the cause and give racemic epinephrine.

For external compression, correct problem surgically.

Pulmonary disease

Conditions that may be present include
- Asthma exacerbation
- COPD
- Pneumonia
- Empyema
- Pulmonary edema
- ARDS
- Pneumothorax
- Hemothorax

For asthma, give bronchodilators and consider high-dose steroid therapy if pulmonary inflammation is present

Respiratory muscle weakness

Possible causes include
- Hypokalemia
- Hypophosphatemia
- Neuromuscular blockade
- Aminoglycosides
- Muscular and neurologic disorders

Correct electrolyte abnormalities and provide nutritional support.

Reverse neuromuscular blockade.

Depressed respiratory drive

Possible causes include
- Drugs
- CNS pathology
- Primary idiopathic alveolar hypoventilation

Reverse effects of narcotics or sedatives. Avoid excessive O_2 therapy.

Metabolic alkalosis (pH > 7.45, P_aco_2 > 35 mm Hg)

Condition is life-threatening (pH > 7.6, [HCO_3^-] > 40 mEq/L)

Consider administering acetazolamide, 250–500 mg I.V.

If this is ineffective, calculate chloride deficit: Cl^- deficit = 0.2 L/kg × weight (kg) × (103 − [Cl^-] [mEq/L]).

Administer exogenous acid (0.1N HCl solution) at a rate no faster than 2 mEq/kg/hr or 125 ml/hr.

Condition is not life-threatening

Identify and treat cause of alkalosis

Obtain spot measurement of urine [Cl^-].

[Cl^-] > 10 mEq/L

Alkalosis is saline-responsive. Possible causes include
- Gastric drainage
- GI loss of HCl via vomiting
- Diuretic therapy
- Overshoot from alkalinizing therapy
- Excess acetate in parenteral nutrition solutions

Restore fluid volume with normal saline.

Correct hypokalemia with KCl.

Give H_2 receptor blockers to decrease H^+ secretion.

Consider discontinuing diuretics.

[Cl^-] > 20 mEq/L

Alkalosis is saline-unresponsive. Possible causes include
- Mineralocorticoid excess
- Primary aldosteronism
- Cushing's syndrome
- Hypokalemia
- Hypomagnesemia
- Hypophosphatemia

Correct electrolyte abnormalities.

Remove mineralocorticoid source or block action of mineralocorticoid with spironolactone or amiloride.

Respiratory alkalosis (pH > 7.45, P_aco_2 < 35 mm Hg)

Condition is life-threatening (pH > 7.6, P_aco_2 < 20 mm Hg, or cardiac arrhythmias are present)

Consider emergency intubation and mechanical ventilation.

Condition is not life-threatening

Identify and treat cause of alkalosis

Central causes

Possible causes include
- Anxiety
- Pain
- Hypoxemia
- Sepsis
- Intracranial pathology
- Hepatic encephalopathy

Consider anxiolytic therapy, supplemental O_2, pain medication, and treatment of infection.

For possible intracranial pathology, perform CT scan of the head.

Pulmonary causes

Possible causes include
- Asthma
- Pneumonia
- Pulmonary embolism
- Congestive heart failure
- Atelectasis
- Pneumothorax

Treat underlying pulmonary disorder.

Iatrogenic causes

Possible causes include
- Inappropriate ventilator management
- Drugs

Adjust mechanical ventilation.

Discontinue drug responsible for alkalosis; if this is not possible, adjust dose.

Evaluation of Acid-Base Imbalance

Table 1 Expected Compensation for Primary Acid-Base Disorders[31,32]

Disorder	Primary Event*	Compensation	Rate of Compensation
Metabolic acidosis	↓ [HCO_3^-]	↓ P_aCO_2	For 1 mEq/L ↓ [HCO_3^-], P_aCO_2 ↓ 1–1.5 mm Hg
Metabolic alkalosis	↑ [HCO_3^-]	↑ P_aCO_2	For 1 mEq/L ↑ [HCO_3^-], P_aCO_2 ↑ 0.5–1 mm Hg
Respiratory acidosis Acute (< 12–24 hr) Chronic (3–5 days)	 ↑ P_aCO_2 ↑ P_aCO_2	 ↑ [HCO_3^-] ↑ ↑ [HCO_3^-]	 For 10 mm Hg ↑ P_aCO_2, [HCO_3^-] ↑ 1 mEq/L For 10 mm Hg ↑ P_aCO_2, [HCO_3^-] ↑ 4 mEq/L
Respiratory alkalosis Acute (< 12 hr) Chronic (1–2 days)	 ↓ P_aCO_2 ↓ P_aCO_2	 ↓ [HCO_3^-] ↓ ↓ [HCO_3^-]	 For 10 mm Hg ↓ P_aCO_2, [HCO_3^-] ↓ 1–3 mEq/L For 10 mm Hg ↓ P_aCO_2, [HCO_3^-] ↓ 2–5 mEq/L

*Normal serum [HCO_3^-] is 24 mEq/L; normal P_aCO_2 is 40 mm Hg.

tem and the pulmonary system. Primary metabolic disorders evoke compensatory respiratory changes, whereas primary respiratory disorders evoke compensatory metabolic changes. For instance, metabolic acidosis, which is characterized by a decreased blood bicarbonate concentration, initiates compensatory hyperventilation, which decreases P_aCO_2. Similarly, respiratory acidosis, which is characterized by increased P_aCO_2, initiates a renal compensatory change that raises the blood bicarbonate concentration. Whether renal or respiratory, these compensatory responses act in essentially the same way: they attempt to counteract the change in pH by reversing the change in the ratio of P_aCO_2 to [HCO_3^-].

The compensatory metabolic and respiratory changes that occur in response to primary acid-base disorders are quite predictable. When the individual patient's compensatory responses fall outside the usual range [see Table 1], there are two main possibilities: either not enough time has passed for compensation to occur or the patient has a mixed acid-base disorder—that is, a combination of primary acid-base disorders (e.g., respiratory acidosis and metabolic alkalosis in a patient with chronic obstructive pulmonary disease [COPD] who is receiving diuretics).

Metabolic Acidosis

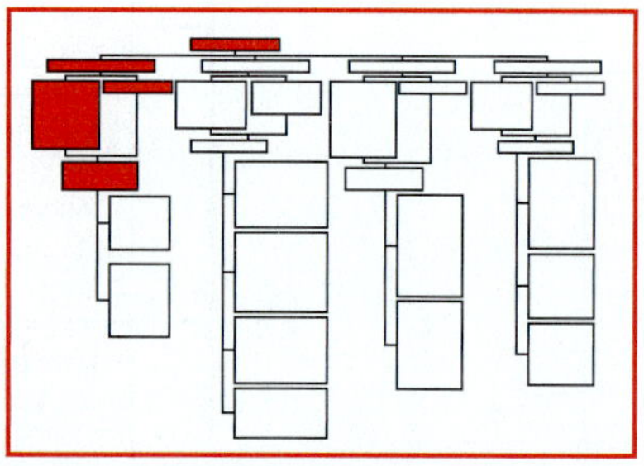

Of the primary acid-base disorders, metabolic acidosis is the one that is most often life-threatening in surgical patients. It is characterized by a loss of bicarbonate or an accumulation of fixed acids, either of which can lead to a decrease in pH.

In surgical patients, life-threatening metabolic acidosis is most often the result of inadequate oxygen delivery as a consequence of inadequate perfusion from hypovolemia or blood loss. Treatment must therefore be directed at restoration of perfusion and correction of the underlying disorder whenever possible. Restoration of perfusion is accomplished by means of fluid resuscitation with crystalloid, colloid, or blood products, depending on the patient's clinical condition. If the patient is healthy, intravascular volume resuscitation can be guided by simple measures of urine output. If, however, the patient has cardiac disease or other medical problems, such as respiratory insufficiency or renal insufficiency, placement of a pulmonary artery catheter to guide resuscitation should be considered. Severe metabolic acidosis can also be caused by inadequate oxygen delivery resulting from hypoxemia, anemia, or inadequate cardiac output, especially in critically ill patients.

It is rarely necessary to administer sodium bicarbonate to patients with acute metabolic acidosis, provided that aggressive fluid resuscitation and treatment of underlying disorders are initiated promptly. Experimental studies have documented that cardiac function and catecholamine responsiveness are unaffected as long as pH remains at or above 7.2. In addition, metabolic acidosis causes the oxyhemoglobin dissociation curve to shift to the right, thereby augmenting oxygen delivery [see Figure 1]. Consequently, we do not recommend bicarbonate treatment for clinically stable patients with metabolic acidosis and a pH of 7.2 or higher.

Once blood pH falls below 7.2, however, the risk of cardiac dysfunction and arrhythmias is increased, and life-threatening problems may occur suddenly. When metabolic acidosis is life-threatening secondary to impairment of cardiac function, judicious administration of sodium bicarbonate may be required. It is important, however, to titrate bicarbonate therapy very carefully to prevent iatrogenic metabolic alkalosis. Iatrogenic metabolic alkalosis may be difficult to correct and may impair oxygen delivery to the tissues by decreasing cardiac contractility and shifting the oxyhemoglobin dissociation curve to the left [see Figure 1], thereby causing hemoglobin to bind oxygen more avidly. In addition, the bicarbonate ad-

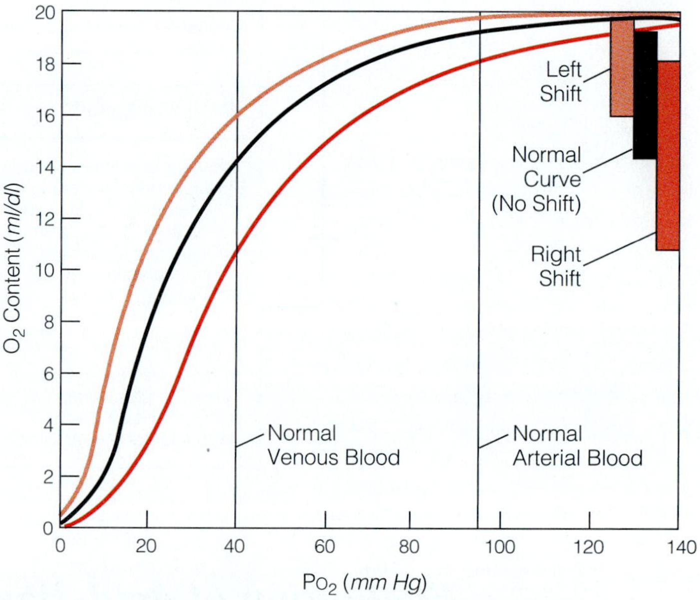

Figure 1 Depicted is the oxyhemoglobin dissociation curve. Shifting this curve to the left (light-red line and bar) or the right (dark-red line and bar) affects the amount of oxygen available for extraction by tissues.

ministered constitutes an excess alkali load that must be excreted by the body.

Metabolic acidosis can be divided into two broad categories on the basis of whether the anion gap is increased or normal. The anion gap is the difference between measured cations and measured anions in serum. This difference does not reflect a true disparity between positive and negative charges, given that serum actually is electrically neutral when all serum cations and anions are measured. Rather, the anion gap is a measurement artifact resulting from the fact that only certain cations and anions (Na^+, K^+, Cl^-, and HCO_3^-) are routinely measured. The anion gap is usually calculated by subtracting the serum chloride and bicarbonate concentrations from the serum sodium concentration:

$$\text{Anion gap} = [Na^+] - ([Cl^-] + [HCO_3^-])$$

The normal range for the anion gap is 8 to 12 mEq/L.

INCREASED ANION GAP

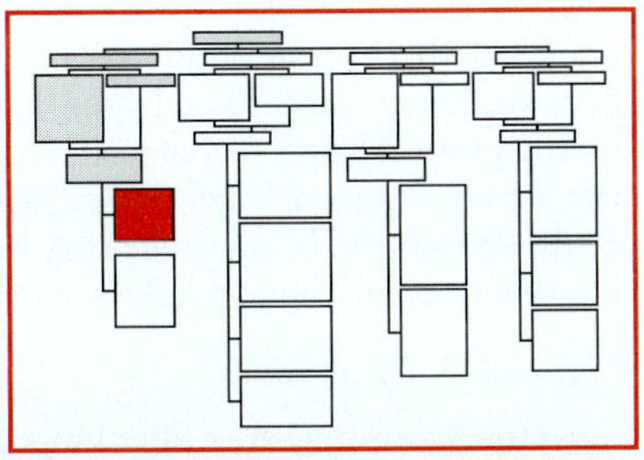

Metabolic acidosis with an increased anion gap is secondary to the addition of endogenous or exogenous acid. There are numerous possible causes. When it has been determined that an increased anion gap metabolic acidosis is present, there are specific laboratory values the surgeon should consider obtaining: arterial or mixed venous lactate concentrations, serum and urine ketone levels, blood glucose levels, serum potassium concentrations, blood urea nitrogen (BUN) and serum creatinine concentrations, and blood alcohol levels. Serum and urine toxic drug screens should be considered as well. Blood creatine kinase levels and urine myoglobin concentrations should be measured if rhabdomyolysis is a possibility. Other values that are useful in the assessment of increased anion gap metabolic acidosis are methanol and ethylene glycol levels and serum osmolality. The results of these laboratory tests should help determine the cause of the acidosis. If, however, a patient appears underperfused and the increased anion gap metabolic acidosis improves with therapy, further workup usually is not necessary.

Lactic Acidosis

Inadequate tissue perfusion leads to inadequate aerobic metabolism at the cellular level and triggers anaerobic metabolism, which results in the production of lactic acid and an increased anion gap metabolic acidosis [see Discussion, below]. The right shift in the oxyhemoglobin dissociation curve facilitates the release of oxygen to the tissues as a protective mechanism. When tissue oxygenation is restored to normal through resuscitation and improvement of oxygen delivery, the lactic acid that has accumulated as a result of anaerobic metabolism is rapidly metabolized to bicarbonate by the liver and the kidneys, and the metabolic acidosis resolves.

Tissue hypoperfusion is the most common cause of lactic acidosis in critically ill patients. Prolonged hypoperfusion leads to tissue hypoxia and cellular acidosis and can trigger a cascade of events that leads to irreversible damage and cell death unless oxygen delivery is promptly reestablished [see Figure 2]. Consequently, the most important treatment priority in these patients is to restore tissue perfusion rapidly by improving oxygen delivery and limiting oxygen consumption as much as possible. Oxygen delivery may be improved by increasing cardiac output (through volume resuscitation or inotropic support), increasing the hemoglobin concentration (through trans-

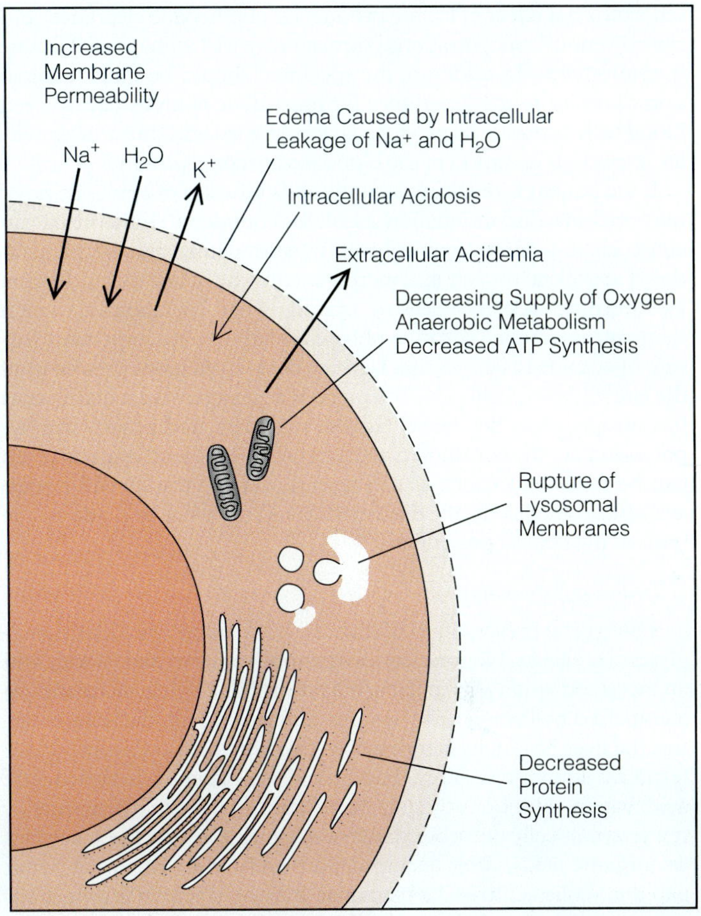

Figure 2 Energy pathways are affected by cellular changes that are associated with hypoxia. Decreased production of adenosine triphosphate (ATP) and loss of cellular integrity result.[29]

fusion of red blood cells), or increasing arterial oxygen saturation. Oxygen consumption may be decreased by administering sedatives judiciously, eliminating fever and shivering, or instituting mechanical ventilation in patients with increased work of breathing [see 89 Cardiopulmonary Monitoring].

The morbidity and mortality associated with lactic acidosis are related to the severity of the acidosis and the response of the underlying disorder to treatment. Severe, acute lactic acidosis is associated with a low survival rate; the survival rate is inversely correlated with the blood lactate concentration. Bicarbonate therapy may actually increase morbidity and mortality in patients with severe, life-threatening acidosis; however, judicious use of such therapy to raise pH to 7.2 or higher may still be prudent, especially in patients with myocardial dysfunction. Administration of dichloroacetate (DCA), which enhances cardiac output and promotes oxidation of pyruvate and lactate by stimulating pyruvate dehydrogenase activity, may eventually prove to be an important therapeutic modality for patients with severe, unremitting lactic acidosis.[5,6]

In the absence of renal or hepatic insufficiency, blood lactate concentrations can help quantitate the degree of tissue hypoxia present or the extent to which perfusion is inadequate. They can also be useful in monitoring the patient's response to therapeutic interventions, such as fluid resuscitation, transfusion, or augmentation of cardiac output. Only values obtained from arterial or mixed venous blood samples should be relied on, however. Peripheral venous lactate concentrations reflect regional, rather than systemic, perfusion and lactate metabolism; arterial lactate concentrations, on the other hand, reflect the net effect of lactate production and hepatic clearance, and mixed venous concentrations correlate very well with arterial lactate measurements. In addition, the specimen should be quickly transported on ice to the laboratory for immediate analysis because red blood cells continue to produce lactate in vitro and thus may generate a spurious elevation in the blood lactate concentration.

If the patient is receiving a continuous infusion of epinephrine or nitroprusside, discontinuation should be considered. Either drug can cause lactic acidosis, epinephrine by stimulating glycogen breakdown in skeletal muscle and increasing the rate of lactate production and nitroprusside by releasing cyanide when metabolized, which then can uncouple oxidative phosphorylation. One important feature of cyanide toxicity is that lactic acidosis is often not present until the late stages of the illness. Tolerance of and increasing requirements for nitroprusside, headache, nausea, weakness, and progressive hypotension are the common clinical signs. Whole blood cyanide levels can be measured (normal < 5 µg/ml), but the results will not be available immediately; the diagnosis should therefore be made on the basis of the clinical presentation.

Diabetic Ketoacidosis

The typical presentation of diabetic ketoacidosis includes hyperglycemia, elevated ketone concentrations in urine and blood, and an increased anion gap metabolic acidosis. When glucose utilization is impaired by fasting or by insulin deficiency, as in diabetes mellitus, the liver produces ketones from free fatty acids to supply an alternative source of energy. The first ketone formed is acetoacetic acid, which subsequently may be reduced to β-hydroxybutyrate or nonenzymatically decarboxylated to acetone. Because these ketones are organic acids, their accumulation leads to an increased anion gap metabolic acidosis. Ketoacidosis may be severe in insulin-deficient patients with diabetes mellitus; insulin deficiency impairs ketone utilization as well as glucose utilization, and it promotes lipolysis, which causes more free fatty acids to be delivered to the liver and converted into keto acids.

The test that is used to measure keto acids in blood and urine—the nitroprusside test—is not entirely accurate: it may underestimate the degree of ketoacidosis or even fail to detect it in severe cases. The reason is that the nitroprusside test detects only acetoacetate and acetone, not β-hydroxybutyrate, which is the most prevalent keto acid in all types of ketoacidosis. A simple way of compensating for this flaw is to add a few drops of hydrogen peroxide to a urine sample. The hydrogen peroxide nonenzymatically converts the β-hydroxybutyrate to acetoacetate, which is detectable by the nitroprusside test.[7]

The aim of therapy for diabetic ketoacidosis is to correct hypovolemia, hyperglycemia, ketoacidosis, and potassium and phosphorus depletion. Because insulin deficiency is responsible for many of these abnormalities, insulin administration is extremely important. Exogenous insulin administration helps correct the hyperglycemia, reduces ketoacidosis by increasing peripheral ketone utilization, and limits further ketone production by decreasing the rate of lipolysis and decreasing glucagon secretion. Initially, regular insulin is administered as an intravenous bolus; it has a half-life of only 4 to 5 minutes and is completely cleared from plasma within 30 minutes. Subsequently, regular insulin is administered by continuous intravenous infusion so that the amount of insulin required to lower the plasma glucose concentration into the normal range can be accurately determined. Regular insulin should not be administered to critically ill patients by the subcutaneous route. Absorption may be erratic if this is done, especially in patients who require vigorous volume resuscitation and in whom anasarca may develop.

Fluid resuscitation corrects the hypovolemia present in diabetic ketoacidosis. Fluid resuscitation also helps correct hyperglycemia and ketoacidosis by virtue of its dilutional effect, and it leads to improved renal function and thus improved renal glucose clearance. Serum creatinine concentrations are often falsely elevated in patients with diabetic ketoacidosis because acetoacetate can be mismeasured as creatinine.

Potassium replacement is necessary in all patients with diabetic ketoacidosis, even though serum potassium concentrations may be normal or high initially. These deceptive findings reflect the movement of potassium from the cells into the extracellular space secondary to insulin deficiency and hyperglycemia. Continuous ECG monitoring is necessary in all cases as well: the acid-base and potassium imbalances place these patients at risk for severe cardiac dysrhythmias.

Phosphate depletion is also a common finding in patients with diabetic ketoacidosis. Routine phosphate replacement is not recommended, however: two clinical studies have documented that it has no effect on morbidity or outcome, does not accelerate correction of electrolyte abnormalities, and may induce hyperphosphatemia or hypocalcemia.[8-10] Phosphate therapy is therefore reserved for patients with severe (serum phosphate < 1.0 mEq/dl) or symptomatic hypophosphatemia. Administration of bicarbonate should also be avoided because it may exacerbate hyperosmolality and hypokalemia, prolong hyperventilation so that respiratory alkalosis develops, and cause iatrogenic metabolic alkalosis as the keto acids are metabolized. Small amounts of bicarbonate may be indicated when arterial pH is less than 7.2 [*see* Lactic Acidosis, *above*].

Alcoholic Ketoacidosis

Ketoacidosis may arise after binge drinking or sudden abstinence on the part of an alcoholic, usually in association with low food intake or vomiting. Alcoholic ketoacidosis results from the interplay among the effects of ethanol, starvation, and volume depletion. Alcoholic ketoacidosis can be differentiated from diabetic ketoacidosis by the absence of significant hyperglycemia. Perhaps surprisingly, serum ethanol concentrations may be low in patients with alcoholic ketoacidosis; this condition usually occurs with abstinence or 1 to 3 days after heavy drinking, by which time the ethanol has undergone oxidation by the liver. Serum ketone levels may be low as well. The ratio of β-hydroxybutyrate to acetoacetate is higher in patients with alcoholic ketoacidosis than in those with diabetic ketoacidosis because of the NADH production consequent to the oxidation of alcohol. As a result, the nitroprusside test, being unable to measure β-hydroxybutyrate [*see* Diabetic Ketoacidosis, *above*], typically yields a weakly positive or even a negative reaction. Patients who have alcoholic ketoacidosis often respond dramatically to fluid resuscitation and usually do not require bicarbonate therapy. Infusion of glucose decreases keto acid formation in the liver, and infusion of saline promotes renal clearance of keto acids.

Acute and Chronic Renal Failure

Increased anion gap metabolic acidosis occurs in renal failure as a consequence of decreased renal ammoniagenesis and decreased excretion of titratable acids. Patients with advanced renal failure cannot excrete the fixed acids (phosphate, sulfates, and other organic acids) generated as by-products of the body's normal metabolic processes, and the accumulation of these acids leads to the increased anion gap metabolic acidosis. For metabolic acidosis caused by chronic renal failure, treatment is rarely required; for severe metabolic acidosis caused by acute renal failure, supplemental bicarbonate therapy may be necessary.

Ingestion of Toxins

Salicylate Salicylate intoxication may give rise to an increased anion gap metabolic acidosis as a result of the accumulation of salicylate anion and other organic anions, such as lactate and keto anions. Salicylates also uncouple oxidative phosphorylation, thereby increasing the production of organic acids and CO_2. The diagnosis of salicylate intoxication should be considered in any patient who has an increased anion gap metabolic acidosis of unknown origin. Chemical determination of blood salicylate levels establishes the diagnosis: levels higher than 30 mg/dl are considered above the therapeutic limit. Therapy is instituted immediately. The first step is to ensure that the airway is open and that oxygenation and ventilation are adequate. Correction of fluid deficits is mandatory. Gastric lavage and administration of charcoal are then undertaken to prevent further absorption of salicylates from the GI tract.

In systemic acidemia, the nonionized form of salicylate (the form that enters the cells) becomes more prevalent, which means that tissue uptake is increased. In addition, the nonionized species is reabsorbed in the renal tubules, whereas the ionized form is not, which means that renal excretion of salicylates is lower than normal. Immediate correction of systemic acidemia is therefore of utmost importance. Respiratory acidosis (which may also be present in salicylate intoxication as a result of hypoventilation) is corrected by mechanical ventilation, and metabolic acidosis is corrected by the administration of bicarbonate until a mild systemic alkalemia (pH = 7.46 to 7.49) is achieved. Urinary alkalinization also prevents tubular reabsorption and promotes effective renal excretion of the salicylates. Dialysis is reserved for patients who have renal dysfunction or life-threatening complications.

Methanol and ethylene glycol Ketoacidosis may occur in adult alcoholics as a result of methanol or ethylene glycol ingestion. Both drugs are consumed as cheap alternatives to ethanol. Methanol is used in industry and is being studied as an energy source; ethylene glycol is found in antifreeze solutions. Methanol and ethylene glycol are rapidly converted to toxic metabolites (formic acid and glycolic acid, respectively) in the liver, and even small amounts of these metabolites may be lethal. In determining whether ethanol, methanol, or ethylene glycol is responsible for an increased anion gap metabolic acidosis, it may be helpful to calculate the serum osmolal gap, which is the difference between measured serum osmolality and calculated serum osmolality. Calculated serum osmolality is derived by using three variables: sodium ion concentration, BUN, and glucose concentration. If ethanol is present and the blood ethanol concentration is available, a fourth expression (ethanol [mg/dl]/4.6) should be added to the calculation.

$$\text{Calculated serum osmolality (mOsm/L)} = 2[Na^+] \text{ (mEq/L)} + \frac{BUN \text{ (mg/dl)}}{2.8} + \frac{\text{glucose (mg/dl)}}{18}$$

Normally, the serum osmolal gap is less than 10 mOsm/L. An increased osmolal gap indicates the presence in plasma of an osmotically active substance that normally is absent. The substances that most frequently cause an increased osmolal gap are ethanol, ketones, lactate, mannitol, methanol, and ethylene glycol.

Therapy for methanol or ethylene glycol ingestion should be instituted immediately and should include gastric lavage, administration of activated charcoal (to remove unabsorbed toxin), intravenous infusion of ethanol (to competitively inhibit metabolism of methanol or ethylene glycol to their toxic metabolites), and, in life-threatening situations, hemodialysis.

Paraldehyde Paraldehyde has been used clinically as a sedative and an anticonvulsant; currently, however, it is rarely given. Paraldehyde intoxication is associated with an increased anion gap metabolic acidosis, hyperkalemia, and leukocytosis. The increased anion gap acidosis is likely to be secondary to increased concentrations of β-hydroxybutyrate, which means that the nitroprusside test commonly yields negative results in these patients. Treatment should include intravenous hydration to correct fluid deficits, correction of systemic acidemia with bicarbonate administration, and emergency dialysis if acute renal failure is present or other life-threatening complications exist.

Rhabdomyolysis

Rhabdomyolysis—extensive muscle breakdown caused by myonecrosis—may also cause an increased anion gap metabolic acidosis. The acidosis results from the accumulation of organic acids and may worsen if acute myoglobinuric renal failure develops. Measurement of serum concentrations of creatine kinase or aldolase (an enzyme confined to skeletal muscle) and urine concentrations of myoglobin may facilitate diagnosis. Fluid resuscitation should be begun immediately; early aggressive management may prevent acute renal failure and ensure a favorable prognosis.

NORMAL ANION GAP

When a surgical patient has a metabolic acidosis but the calculated anion gap is within normal limits (8 to 12 mEq/L), the most likely cause is the loss of excess bicarbonate via the GI tract. Other possible causes must also be considered, however.

Excessive Bicarbonate Loss

Metabolic acidosis associated with a normal anion gap is characterized by impairment of bicarbonate buffering. In surgical patients, this is commonly secondary to loss of bicarbonate from the GI tract. Intestinal fluids, including pancreatic and biliary secretions, are relatively alkaline. Consequently, any process that causes the loss of such fluids (e.g., diarrhea, a villous adenoma, or the removal of pancreatic, biliary, or intestinal secretions via tube drainage or fistulas) can lead to a normal anion gap metabolic acidosis. When bicarbonate is lost in urine or stool, there is a compensatory increase in chloride, so that the anion gap remains normal. Another possible initiating process is occult laxative use, which should be considered in any patient with a hyperchloremic metabolic acidosis of unknown etiology.

Ureterosigmoidostomy can also lead to a hyperchloremic metabolic acidosis through two mechanisms: (1) chloride entering the colon from the urine is exchanged with bicarbonate, so that an increased amount of bicarbonate is lost, and (2) the colon reabsorbs NH_4^+, which is derived from urine and from colonic bacteria, and NH_4^+ is metabolized in the liver to NH_3 and H^+. The development of the ureteroileostomy procedure has minimized these complications.

Renal tubular acidosis is another possible cause of normal anion gap acidosis in surgical patients. Normally, about 50 to 100 mEq of acid is generated each day by tissue catabolism; in critically ill patients, this value may be significantly higher. Renal tubular cells excrete H^+ into the urine, thereby triggering the production of bicarbonate, which is then secreted back into the blood. Failure of this normal mechanism leads to renal tubular acidosis. There are several different forms of renal tubular acidosis, depending on which part of the nephron is abnormal. The urinary anion gap is useful in the assessment of renal tubular acidosis. It is calculated by subtracting the urine chloride concentration from the sum of the urine sodium concentration and the urine potassium concentration:

$$\text{Urinary anion gap} = ([Na^+] + [K^+]) - [Cl^-]$$

The urinary anion gap can be used to identify defects in renal tubular acidification in patients with normal anion gap metabolic acidosis. When this value is considered in tandem with urinary pH, it is possible to determine whether the likely cause of the acidosis is excessive gastrointestinal bicarbonate losses or defective renal tubular acidification [see Table 2]. Basically, the urinary anion gap serves as a crude index of urinary ammonium excretion, thereby reflecting, in part, net acid excretion.

The antifungal agent amphotericin B has also been reported to result in renal tubular acidosis, probably by altering the extent to which the membrane of the distal nephron is permeable to hydrogen and potassium ions. In general, the renal tubular acidosis tends to be mild and does not necessitate withdrawal of amphotericin B. Enteral potassium and bicarbonate supplements are useful for maintaining normal serum electrolyte concentrations.

The administration of carbonic anhydrase inhibitors (such as acetazolamide) can also lead to the development of hyperchloremic normal anion gap acidosis in critically ill patients by impairing proximal bicarbonate reabsorption. The clinical presentation of this acidosis can be indistinguishable from that of renal tubular acidosis. Patients should be asked if they routinely take carbonic anhydrase inhibitors (e.g., for glaucoma), and these agents should be used with caution in the ICU.

Hypoaldosteronism and Addison's Disease

Hypoaldosteronism may be an important pathogenetic factor in the acidification defect noted in patients with hyperkalemic distal renal tubular acidosis, which is also known as type IV renal tubular acidosis. Aldosterone deficiency causes a reduction in net acid secretion in the distal nephron. Other disorders that are associated with mineralocorticoid deficiency, including Addison's disease, may also lead to the development of renal tubular acidosis.

Excessive Acid Administration

The administration of ammonium chloride, the transfusion of massive amounts of blood preserved with citrate, and high-volume resuscitation with normal saline can all present the body with an excessively large acid load. Excessive acid administration can lead to the accumulation of inorganic acids and consequently to the development of a hyperchloremic normal anion gap metabolic acidosis. When high-volume crystalloid resuscitation is required in a surgical patient (e.g., after trauma), lactated Ringer's solution is preferred to normal saline for resuscitation: the higher chloride content of normal saline may contribute to the development of a hyperchloremic normal anion gap metabolic acidosis.

Table 2 Use of Urinary Anion Gap and Urinary pH in Differential Diagnosis of Normal Anion Gap Metabolic Acidosis[33,34]

Urinary Anion Gap	Urinary pH	Diagnosis
Negative	< 5.5	Normal
Positive	> 5.5	Renal tubular acidosis
Negative	> 5.5	Diarrhea or enteric fistula

Respiratory Acidosis

ACUTE

Acute respiratory acidosis is caused by alveolar hypoventilation, which results in retention of CO_2 and an acute increase in P_aCO_2 (hypercapnia) and ultimately may lead to acute respiratory failure. The body's compensatory response to acute respiratory acidosis is renal retention of bicarbonate: the plasma bicarbonate concentration rises by an average of 1 mEq/L for every 10 mm Hg increase in P_aCO_2. Because the renal response takes time to develop, the cell buffers, particularly hemoglobin and proteins, constitute the only protection against acute hypercapnia.

Acute respiratory acidosis also depresses myocardial function. Many studies have documented that increased P_aCO_2 (as in respiratory acidosis) impairs myocardial contractility to a greater degree than decreased bicarbonate concentration (as in metabolic acidosis).[11,12] This finding is related to the observation that intracellular pH changes more quickly in response to extracellular respiratory acidosis than in response to metabolic acidosis.[13,14]

Respiratory acidosis should be considered potentially life-threatening in patients who appear to be in respiratory distress, are unresponsive or have altered mental status (CO_2 narcosis), or exhibit acute changes in arterial pH (to < 7.2) or P_aCO_2 (to > 60 mm Hg). Emergency endotracheal intubation and mechanical ventilatory support are indicated for these patients. Once this treatment has been implemented, it is imperative to determine the underlying cause of the acute respiratory acidosis and to initiate appropriate treatment.

If acute respiratory acidosis is identified, the patient is stable, and emergency intubation is not indicated, it is important to identify the cause, institute appropriate treatment, and determine whether there is any history of pulmonary disease (e.g., COPD or asthma) or chronic hypercapnia. The major objectives in the treatment of acute respiratory acidosis, regardless of the specific cause, are correction of hypoxia and correction of hypercapnia. Initial treatment involves administering supplemental oxygen, correcting anemia, attempting to correct reversible problems such as sedative or narcotic overdose, improving pulmonary function and tissue oxygenation, and, if other treatments fail, initiating mechanical ventilation. Bicarbonate therapy should not be administered to patients who have a pure respiratory acidosis: it will only increase the body's carbon dioxide load.

There are four main causes of the alveolar hypoventilation that underlies acute respiratory acidosis: (1) airway obstruction, (2) pulmonary diseases that affect alveolar-capillary gas exchange, (3) weakened respiratory muscles, and (4) depressed respiratory drive.

Airway Obstruction

Airway obstruction can lead to acute severe respiratory acidosis. If the obstruction is caused by laryngospasm, the preferred treatment is correction of the specific cause of the laryngospasm (e.g., removal of a foreign body) or administration of racemic epinephrine. Slight positive pressure bag-valve-mask ventilation and steroid administration may also be helpful in some instances. Airway obstruction may also be caused by external compression (for example, from head and neck tumors, a large thyroid gland, or excess pharyngeal tissue, as in the sleep apnea syndrome). In most cases, external causes of airway obstruction leading to respiratory acidosis must be corrected surgically.

Pulmonary Diseases

A variety of pulmonary diseases, including asthma, pneumonia, pulmonary edema, acute respiratory distress syndrome (ARDS), acute lung injury, and aspiration pneumonia, can lead to acute respiratory acidosis. All of them induce some degree of ventilation-perfusion mismatch. Structural causes of acute CO_2 retention leading to respiratory acidosis include pneumothorax, hemothorax, empyema, and severe chest wall injury with underlying pulmonary contusions.

Asthma exacerbation and COPD are the two most common causes of acute respiratory acidosis. In the initial stages of an asthma exacerbation, respiratory alkalosis is often present because bronchospasm-induced hypoxia causes patients to hyperventilate. During more sustained episodes of bronchospasm, respiratory muscle fatigue eventually develops, and patients are unable to sustain hyperventilation. A normocapnic state ensues, followed by hypercapnic respiratory acidosis, which is a harbinger of impending respiratory failure in patients who have severe reactive small airway disease. The presence of acute respiratory acidosis in patients who have asthma is therefore indicative of a poor prognosis and suggests that intubation and mechanical ventilation are likely to be necessary.

In addition to general treatment measures for acute respiratory acidosis (see above), aggressive treatment of respiratory acidosis caused by asthma includes administering inhaled and parenteral bronchodilators (e.g., beta-adrenergic agents, theophylline, and, in children and young adults, epinephrine). Inhaled steroids and high-dose parenteral steroids should be considered in patients with associated pulmonary inflammation. Magnesium sulfate (a smooth muscle relaxant) may be helpful in the treatment of severe asthma.

Respiratory Muscle Weakness

Various disorders that affect the respiratory muscles and the chest wall can also cause acute respiratory acidosis. Both hypokalemia and hypophosphatemia are known to weaken respiratory muscles; aggressive replacement therapy should be instituted if either abnormality is identified. The administration of aminoglycosides is associated with renal potassium and magnesium wasting and may lead to severe hypokalemia. Myopathy secondary to hypokalemia can be rapidly reversed by the administration of large quantities of potassium. Serum potassium and phosphate levels should be monitored in critically ill patients, especially when active weaning from mechanical ventilatory support is being considered.

Neuromuscular blockade induces respiratory muscle weakness, especially when it is prolonged. There have been numerous reports of persistent paralysis in critically ill patients after the administration of neuromuscular blocking agents.[15] Consequently, these agents should not be used unless absolutely required. If they are required, the patient should be monitored with a peripheral nerve stimulator to ensure that the dosage is appropriate.

Certain muscular and neurologic disorders (e.g., myasthenia gravis, multiple sclerosis, Guillain-Barré syndrome, amyotrophic lateral sclerosis, and muscular dystrophy) can affect respiratory muscles and thus lead to acute respiratory acidosis, as can some spinal column abnormalities (e.g., kyphoscoliosis). In patients with these disorders, treatment centers on preventing any electrolyte abnormalities that might further impair respiratory muscle function, providing ongoing medical therapy for the underlying disorders, attempting to prevent pulmonary infection, and providing nutritional support to keep muscle function from degenerating further.

Depressed Respiratory Drive

The central nervous system controls the rate of pulmonary CO_2 excretion (and thus whole body CO_2 balance) through both voluntary and involuntary modulations of the frequency and depth of respiration. Accordingly, drugs that inhibit the medullary respiratory centers (e.g., sedatives, general anesthetics, and narcotics) may induce acute respiratory acidosis by causing primary failure in the drive to ventilation; care should be taken when these drugs are given to critically ill patients. Depressed respiratory drive can also be a long-term sequela of a cerebrovascular accident or cerebral trauma, and patients with respiratory acidosis should be evaluated for possible intracranial pathology.

Primary idiopathic alveolar hypoventilation is another possible cause of acute respiratory acidosis secondary to depressed respiratory drive. In this disorder, the respiratory centers lack normal responsiveness to hypercapnia, and this lack results in hypoventilation. Primary idiopathic alveolar hypoventilation can also occur in patients with chronic respiratory acidosis who have pulmonary diseases that cause CO_2 retention, and excessive oxygen therapy may exacerbate respiratory failure in patients with COPD. Hypnotic or sedative drugs should be administered with great caution to these patients, who are particularly susceptible to further respiratory depression.

CHRONIC

Chronic respiratory acidosis differs from acute respiratory acidosis primarily with respect to the duration of CO_2 retention. Chronic CO_2 retention can occur secondary to the same mechanisms that produce the initial hypercapnia that results in acute respiratory acidosis: chronic airway obstruction, depression of respiratory drive, respiratory muscle weakness, and pulmonary diseases that interfere with the efficient exchange of CO_2 or cause persistent ventilation-perfusion mismatch.

The body's compensatory response to chronic respiratory acidosis differs from its response to acute respiratory acidosis: the plasma bicarbonate concentration rises by approximately 4 mEq/L for every 10 mm Hg increase in P_aCO_2 [see Table 1]. The persistent elevation in P_aCO_2 stimulates renal secretion of H^+ over a period of 3 to 5 days, resulting in the addition of bicarbonate to the extracellular fluid. The efficiency of this renal compensation is such that the associated changes in arterial pH are relatively small; this means that P_aCO_2 can rise to much higher levels in patients with chronic respiratory acidosis than in those with acute hypercapnia.

Treatment of chronic respiratory acidosis also differs from that of acute respiratory acidosis. Extensive efforts should be made to avoid having to institute intubation and mechanical ventilation because patients with chronic respiratory acidosis are often difficult to wean. Excessive supplemental oxygen therapy should be avoided because it may suppress spontaneous respiratory efforts. Aggressive supportive therapy is indicated, including treatment of any underlying pulmonary infections, treatment of associated congestive heart failure, administration of oral or inhaled bronchodilators, prevention of associated acid-base abnormalities (e.g., metabolic alkalosis resulting from diuretic therapy), and, possibly, pharmacologic stimulation of respiration.

Metabolic Alkalosis

Metabolic alkalosis results from any pathophysiologic process that causes the loss of H^+, the addition of bicarbonate, or the loss of extracellular fluid (which leads to alkalemia because this fluid contains more chloride than bicarbonate). When metabolic alkalosis is potentially life-threatening (pH > 7.6 or [HCO_3^-] > 40 mEq/L), administration of the carbonic anhydrase inhibitor acetazolamide should be considered; however, this agent is associated with renal loss of potassium, which must be anticipated and managed appropriately. If acetazolamide is not effective or the metabolic alkalosis worsens, exogenous acid, in the form of a 0.1N solution of hydrochloric acid (100 mEq/L), should be administered through a central venous catheter. The amount of exogenous acid to be given should be determined on the basis of the calculated chloride deficit, which is derived as follows:

$$\text{Calculated Cl}^- \text{ deficit} = 0.2 \text{ L/kg} \times \text{weight (kg)} \times (103 - [\text{Cl}^-] \text{ [mEq/L]})$$

Arterial blood gases must be monitored frequently to ensure that only the amount necessary is given; overshoot can cause metabolic acidosis.

A number of complications are commonly associated with metabolic alkalosis. In critically ill patients, metabolic alkalosis may lead to supraventricular or ventricular arrhythmias that are refractory to medical therapy until the metabolic alkalosis has been corrected and normal acid-base balance restored. Moreover, metabolic alkalosis can induce a reduction in cardiac output and cause the oxyhemoglobin dissociation curve to shift to the left, thereby diminishing oxygen delivery to the tissues. Alkalosis may also stimulate glycolysis, thereby increasing oxygen consumption at a time when oxygen delivery is already impaired. Furthermore, the respiratory compensation for metabolic alkalosis is hypoventilation with CO_2 retention (secondary hypercapnia), which may lead to hypoxemia; these conditions may produce further impairment of tissue oxygenation. An additional problem is that this respiratory compensation may hinder weaning from mechanical ventilation. Aggressive efforts must be made to correct the underlying disorder that caused the metabolic alkalosis before weaning from mechanical ventilation can be resumed.

Severe alkalemia (pH > 7.6) may cause neuromuscular abnormalities in critically ill patients, including mental confusion, stupor, lethargy, muscle weakness and cramping, and, possibly, seizures. The mechanism by which alkalemia causes these neuromuscular abnormalities is not fully understood; it may be related to reduced plasma ionized calcium concentrations resulting from increased binding of calcium to plasma proteins.

A useful first step in determining the cause of metabolic alkalosis is a spot measurement of the urine chloride concentration. If the urine chloride concentration is lower than 10 mEq/L, the metabolic alkalosis is likely to be saline-responsive; if it is higher than 20 mEq/L, the metabolic alkalosis is saline-unresponsive and may be more difficult to treat.

SALINE-RESPONSIVE

Two of the most common causes of saline-responsive metabolic alkalosis in surgical patients are continuous gastric aspiration and gastrointestinal loss of hydrochloric acid secondary to vomiting. The severity of the alkalosis depends on the magnitude and duration of the acid losses, the extent of volume depletion, and the severity of potassium depletion.

Initial therapy involves restoring extracellular fluid volume by infusing normal saline, correcting hypokalemia by administering potassium chloride, and monitoring the patient closely for possible associated complications. Because the serum potassium concentrations may not reflect the full extent of total body potassium deficiency, potassium replacement should be aggressive; the goal should be to achieve serum levels of 4.5 to 5.5 mEq/L. The administration of an H_2 receptor antagonist (e.g., cimetidine or ranitidine) may help attenuate further loss of H^+ from the GI tract.

Long-term administration of thiazide or loop diuretics is also a common cause of saline-responsive metabolic alkalosis in surgical patients. The degree of metabolic alkalosis caused by diuretic administration is directly correlated with the degree of volume depletion. Ideally, diuretic therapy should be discontinued and the lost potassium and chloride should be replaced; however, this is not always possible. If diuretic therapy must be continued, the potassium and chloride deficits must be corrected. The use of potassium-sparing diuretics may also be considered for patients who require long-term diuretic therapy.

Iatrogenic causes of metabolic alkalosis include the overenthusiastic application of exogenous alkali therapy [see Metabolic Acidosis, above] and the provision of excess acetate in parenteral nutrition solutions.

SALINE-UNRESPONSIVE

Saline-unresponsive metabolic alkalosis is a persistent condition characterized by normal or increased extracellular fluid volume and an elevated urinary chloride concentration. It is most often observed in association with mineralocorticoid excess, and it is resistant to sodium chloride therapy.

Primary aldosteronism is a common cause of saline-unresponsive metabolic alkalosis: the aldosterone excess enhances acid secretion in the distal nephron and results in a metabolic alkalosis. The clinical presentation includes arterial hypertension and hypokalemia as well as metabolic alkalosis. Cushing's syndrome may also be associated with metabolic alkalosis: cortisol possesses some intrinsic mineralocorticoid activity, and consequently, cortisol excess mimics some of the physiologic effects of aldosterone excess.

Treatment of saline-unresponsive metabolic alkalosis involves correcting the electrolyte deficiencies and removing the source of the mineralocorticoid excess. If surgical removal of the mineralocorticoid source is not possible, the action of the mineralocorticoid can be blocked by means of spironolactone or amiloride.

Respiratory Alkalosis

Care must be taken at all times in surgical patients to avoid hyperventilation and respiratory alkalosis so as not to impair tissue oxygenation. In this patient population, respiratory alkalosis is most often attributable to early sepsis or early ARDS. Mild respiratory alkalosis may result from pain or anxiety and subsequent hyperventilation. In addition, iatrogenic respiratory alkalosis secondary to excessive ventilation is quite common and is often overlooked. Overventilation can lead to decreased oxygen delivery by shifting the oxyhemoglobin dissociation curve to the left.

If respiratory alkalosis is potentially life-threatening (pH > 7.6, P_aCO_2 < 20 mm Hg, or cardiac arrhythmias are present), emergency intubation and mechanical ventilation must be considered. If respiratory alkalosis is not life-threatening, management should focus on identifying and correcting the underlying disorder that caused it.

Central causes of respiratory alkalosis include hyperventilation resulting from anxiety, hypoxemia, pain, or sepsis. Anxiolytic therapy, supplemental oxygen, pain medication, and treatment of infections, respectively, are appropriate for this group of patients. Intracranial pathology (e.g., CNS infection, tumor, or trauma) can also cause hyperventilation and thus respiratory alkalosis. A computed tomography scan of the head is the most reliable diagnostic test for determining whether such pathology is a possible cause of the respiratory alkalosis.

Pulmonary causes of respiratory alkalosis include those diseases that affect the alveolar-capillary membrane, hindering gas exchange, creating a ventilation-perfusion mismatch, and eventually leading to hypoxia. The body's response to hypoxia is hyperventilation, which results in respiratory alkalosis. The pulmonary diseases that are most often responsible for respiratory alkalosis in surgical patients are asthma, pneumonia, pulmonary embolism, congestive heart failure, atelectasis, and pneumothorax.

Iatrogenic causes of respiratory alkalosis are mainly related to inappropriate management of mechanical ventilation. Various drugs can also cause iatrogenic respiratory alkalosis. Discontinuation of the medication is the optimal therapy. If the medication is necessary, adjustment of the dose may be helpful.

Mixed Acid-Base Disorders

The mixed acid-base disorders fall into two main categories [see Table 3]. In additive combinations, the pH deviations are in the same direction, whereas in counterbalancing combinations, the pH deviations are in opposite directions. Depending on the precise combination present, a mixed acid-base disorder can result in normal arterial pH, acidemia, or alkalemia [see Figure 3].

The patients at highest risk for life-threatening complications associated with mixed acid-base disorders are those who have additive combinations. For example, a patient who has severe diabetic ketoacidosis (primary metabolic acidosis) and who subsequently experiences acute respiratory failure (primary respiratory acidosis) may have life-threatening acidemia, which would necessitate emergency intubation and mechanical ventilation for immediate correction of the primary respiratory acidosis as well as continued treatment for diabetic ketoacidosis. Similarly, a patient who has a contraction alkalosis resulting from excessive diuretic therapy (primary metabolic alkalosis) and who subsequently requires mechanical ventilation for respiratory failure and is erroneously overventilated (primary respiratory alkalosis) may have life-threatening alkalemia.

Interpretation and diagnosis of complex mixed acid-base disorders can be quite difficult, often involving numerous calculations.

Table 3 Classification of Mixed Acid-Base Disorders[35]

Additive Combinations	Causes	Counterbalancing Combinations	Causes
Respiratory acidosis and metabolic acidosis	Cardiopulmonary arrest Pulmonary edema Chronic lung disease with hypoxia Hypokalemic myopathy plus metabolic acidosis Severe phosphorus depletion Poisoning—drug toxicity (ethanol, methanol, or ethylene glycol)	Respiratory acidosis and metabolic alkalosis	Excess diuresis in chronic lung disease Severe potassium depletion
Respiratory alkalosis and metabolic alkalosis	Severe trauma Blood transfusion Pregnancy Respirator-induced	Respiratory alkalosis and metabolic acidosis	Aspirin intoxication Advanced liver disease Pulmonary-renal syndromes

Mixed elevated anion gap and normal anion gap metabolic acidosis (high anion gap metabolic acidosis with excessive decrease in [HCO_3^-]: change in [HCO_3^-] > change in anion gap)	Renal-related causes
	  Early chronic renal failure
	  Uremic acidosis with proximal or distal renal tubular acidosis
	Diabetes mellitus
	Diarrhea
	Hypoaldosteronism
	Repair phase of diabetic ketoacidosis
	Lactic acidosis complicating diarrhea or other causes of normal anion gap metabolic acidosis
		Metabolic acidosis and metabolic alkalosis (high anion gap with less than equimolar reduction in serum [HCO_3^-]: change in [HCO_3^-] < change in anion gap)	Renal-related causes
			  Uremic vomiting
			  Alkali therapy in uremia
			  Transfusion alkalosis
			  Aluminum hydroxide (Amphojel) plus sodium polystyrene sulfonate (Kayexalate)
			  Diuretic administration
			Diabetes mellitus
			  Diabetic ketoacidosis and vomiting
			  $NaHCO_3^-$ therapy for diabetic ketoacidosis
			Lactic acidosis when complicated by various causes of metabolic alkalosis

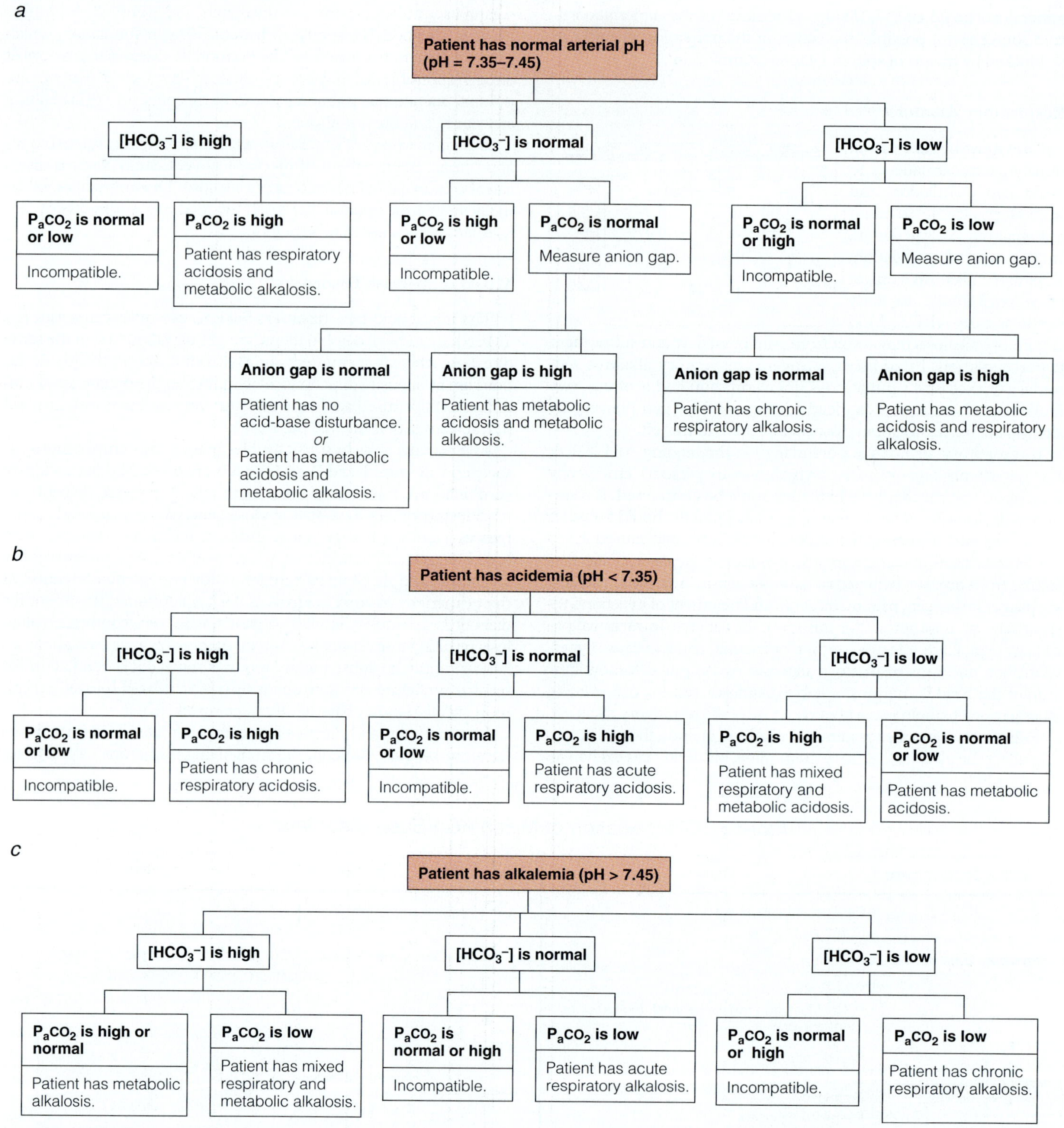

Figure 3 Patients with mixed acid-base disorders can have normal arterial pH (*a*), acidemia (*b*), or alkalemia (*c*), depending on the precise combination of disorders present.[30] Shown are algorithms that may facilitate the evaluation of such disorders.

Automatic computer interpretation of acid-base disturbances was initiated in the late 1960s; however, the systems that were developed were highly complex, and few were implemented in clinical practice.[16-18] In the early 1990s, a computer system was designed to help clinicians interpret complex acid-base disturbances on the basis of numerical laboratory measurements.[19] In accuracy, versatility, and clinical utility, this system compared favorably with a medical expert; moreover, it saved time by performing all necessary calculations. Similar computer programs have been put into routine practice in a number of ICUs and are now commercially available. It is of the utmost importance that the data and conclusions generated by computer systems such as this be used in tandem with the clinical findings obtained by examining the patient. The integration of computer system analysis with clinical examination may result in the timely diagnosis of complex mixed acid-base disturbances and allow earlier initiation of appropriate therapy, especially in life-threatening situations.

Discussion

Biochemical Basis of Lactic Acidosis

Lactic acidosis results from excessive production or impaired degradation of lactic acid or from a combination of the two. In virtually all cells, the formation of pyruvate in the cytosol by anaerobic glycolysis is the first step in glucose metabolism. Pyruvate then enters the cellular mitochondria, where it is metabolized to NADH via the citric acid (Krebs) cycle:

$$\text{Pyruvate} + \text{coenzyme A} + \text{NAD}^+ \rightarrow \text{acetyl coenzyme A} + CO_2 + \text{NADH}$$

Oxidative phosphorylation then results in the production of adenosine triphosphate (ATP). This aerobic metabolism is a highly efficient process: 36 mol of ATP is produced for each 1 mol of glucose consumed.

When oxygen is not available at the cellular level, pyruvate is metabolized to lactate by the enzyme lactate dehydrogenase (LDH):

$$\text{Pyruvate} + \text{NADH} + H^+ \xrightarrow{\text{LDH}} \text{lactate} + \text{NAD}^+$$

Compared with the aerobic pathway, the anaerobic pathway is very inefficient, producing only 2 mol of ATP for every 1 mol of glucose that is converted to lactate.

Most of the lactate produced by the body is cleared by the liver; a lesser amount is cleared by the kidney. The heart, the liver, and the kidneys are capable of converting lactate to pyruvate and then converting pyruvate to CO_2 and ATP via aerobic metabolism. In addition, the liver and the kidneys are able to produce glucose from lactate via gluconeogenesis. From a quantitative viewpoint, gluconeogenesis is the most important process for removing lactate from the blood. The continuous cyclic flow of lactate from peripheral tissues (e.g., skeletal muscle, which is the main source of lactate) to the liver, where it is converted to glucose, and back to the peripheral tissues is known as the Cori cycle. The Cori cycle ensures a continuous supply of glucose to the tissues that have an absolute requirement for glucose, namely, the brain, erythrocytes, and the medullae of the kidneys. When hepatic or renal insufficiency develops in critically ill patients, lactate clearance is altered as a result, and blood lactate concentrations thus become a less accurate indicator of the extent of tissue hypoxia present.

Patients with lactic acidosis were initially classified by Huckabee[20] into two groups on the basis of whether the ratio of lactate to pyruvate was normal (10:1) or increased. A revised classification formulated by Cohen and Woods[21] divided patients into two categories on the basis of whether tissue hypoxia was apparent (type A) or not (type B); these categories were then broken down into subcategories [see Table 4]. The fundamental point made by this classification is that the determination of whether lactic acidosis is caused by tissue hypoxia or not is important for initiating appropriate treatment. The various causes of lactic acidosis have been reviewed more extensively elsewhere.[22]

Therapy for Lactic Acidosis: Alkalinizing Agents and Dichloroacetate

Alkalinizing agents have been given to patients who have lactic acidosis with the aim of reducing the excess acid load and treating its associated adverse effects. In 1992, the National Conference on Cardiopulmonary Resuscitation established current guidelines, according to which the routine use of sodium bicarbonate is no longer recommended.[23] Occasionally, however, patients with severe lactic acidosis still require alkalinizing agents; accordingly, clinicians must be familiar with the indications for the use of these agents and knowledgeable about potential complications.

Parenteral bicarbonate therapy can induce a hyperosmolar state and may further increase lactate production by increasing phosphofructokinase activity and accelerating glycolysis. In addition, it can lead to so-called overshoot alkalosis. The increase in arterial pH associated with bicarbonate administration may increase the affinity of hemoglobin for oxygen, thereby impairing tissue oxygen delivery and worsening tissue hypoxia. Experimental studies have shown that mortality after bicarbonate therapy is not significantly lower than mortality after saline administration, and clinical studies have confirmed these findings. Therefore, bicarbonate administration may have no real advantages as a treatment modality.

Other alkalinizing agents, such as Carbicarb (an equimolar solution of sodium bicarbonate and sodium carbonate) and tris-hydroxymethyl aminomethane (THAM), have been studied. Because of the substitution of carbonate for bicarbonate, Carbicarb tends to cause less production of CO_2, and it is better than bicarbonate at raising serum pH without increasing the serum lactate concentration.[24] THAM has vasodilatory properties that lead to decreased peripheral vascular resistance, an effect that is potentially detrimental in many patients. At present, there is little clinical experience with these agents; further study is required.

DCA is receiving increased attention as a potential adjunctive treatment of lactic acidosis.[25] By inhibiting the action of a protein kinase that inactivates the enzyme pyruvate dehydrogenase, DCA brings about enhanced metabolism of pyruvate and hence lactate. DCA may also have a direct inotropic effect on myocardium: studies have demonstrated improvements in cardiac output and blood pressure that do not appear to be related to changes in extracellular pH. These effects may result in improved oxygen delivery, thereby decreasing lactate production. Clinical trials using DCA have demonstrated overall improvements in blood lactate concentration, pH, cardiac output, and blood pressure; however, follow-up studies have documented no improvement in clinical outcome.[5,26] It has also been documented that DCA alleviates lactic acidosis during liver transplantation. Two clinical studies concluded that DCA, 40 to 80 mg/kg, safely and effectively attenuated lactic acid accumulation, moderated acidosis, decreased

Table 4 Classification of Lactic Acidosis[21]

Tissue Hypoxia	Type	Cause
Apparent	A	Severe hypoxia, asthma, or CO poisoning; severe anemia; hypovolemic shock, hemorrhage, hypotension, or cardiac arrest; congestive heart failure or pulmonary edema; cardiogenic shock
Not apparent	B1	Acquired disease: diabetes mellitus, hepatic failure, Reye's syndrome, sepsis, malignancies, alcoholic ketoacidosis, renal failure, pancreatitis, systemic inflammatory response syndrome
Not apparent	B2	Drugs or toxins: ethanol, ethylene glycol, methanol, sodium nitroprusside, acetaminophen, salicylates, epinephrine, norepinephrine, isoniazid, streptozocin, nalidixic acid
Not apparent	B3	Congenital disorders: glucose-6-phosphatase deficiency, fructose-1,6-diphosphatase deficiency, pyruvate dehydrogenase deficiency, pyruvate carboxylase deficiency

NaHCO₃ requirements, and reduced the incidence of hypernatremia during orthotopic liver transplantation.[27,28]

Although the findings from preliminary clinical study of DCA are promising, it appears that for the time being, use of this agent should be reserved for patients with type B lactic acidosis (i.e., lactic acidosis associated with adequate oxygen delivery). Primary therapy for type A lactic acidosis involves attempting to restore tissue oxygen delivery by administering appropriate fluid resuscitation therapy, providing inotropic support, and, if necessary, transfusing blood or giving supplemental oxygen.

References

1. Rosenthal TB: The effects of temperature on the pH of the blood and plasma in vitro. J Biol Chem 173:25, 1948
2. Ream AK, Reitz BA, Silverberg G: Temperature correction of pCO₂ and pH in estimating acid-base status: an example of the emperor's new clothes? Anesthesiology 56:41, 1982
3. Hansen JE, Sue DY: Should blood gas measurements be corrected for the patient's temperature? N Engl J Med 303:341, 1980
4. Delaney KA, Howland MA, Vassallo S, et al: Assessment of acid-base disturbances in hypothermia and their physiologic consequences. Ann Emerg Med 18:72, 1989
5. Narins RG, Cohen JJ: Bicarbonate therapy for organic acidosis: the case for its continued use. Ann Intern Med 106:615, 1987
6. Stacpoole PW, Lorenz AC, Thomas RG, et al: Dichloroacetate in the treatment of lactic acidosis. Ann Intern Med 108:58, 1988
7. Narins RG, Jones ER, Stom MC, et al: Diagnostic strategies in disorders of fluid, electrolyte and acid-base homeostasis. Am J Med 72:496, 1982
8. Keller U, Berger W: Prevention of hypophosphatemia by phosphate infusion during treatment of diabetic ketoacidosis and hyperosmolar coma. Diabetes 29:87, 1980
9. Wilson HK, Kever SP, Lea AS, et al: Phosphate therapy in diabetic ketoacidosis. Arch Intern Med 142:527, 1982
10. Winter RJ, Harris CJ, Phillips LS, et al: Diabetic ketoacidosis: induction of hypocalcemia and hypomagnesemia by phosphate therapy. Am J Med 67:897, 1979
11. Cingolani HE, Mattiaze AR, Blesa ES, et al: Contractility in isolated mammalian heart muscle after acid-base changes. Circ Res 26:269, 1970
12. Pannier JL, Leusen I: Contraction characteristics of papillary muscle during changes in acid-base composition of the bathing fluid. Arch Intern Physiol Biochim 76:624, 1968
13. Cingolani HE, Blesa ES, Gonzalez NC, et al: Extracellular vs. intracellular pH as a determinant of myocardial contractility. Life Sci 8:775, 1969
14. Poole-Wilson PA, Cameron IR: A comparison of the control of intracellular pH in cardiac and skeletal muscle. Clin Sci 44:15P, 1973
15. Hoyt JW: Neuromuscular blockade in critical care. New Horizons 2:1, 1994
16. Cohen ML: A computer program for the interpretation of blood gas analysis. Comp Biomed Res 2:549, 1969
17. Bleich HL: The computer as a consultant. N Engl J Med 284:141, 1971
18. Bleich HL: Computer-based consultation: electrolyte and acid-base disorders. Am J Med 53:285, 1972
19. Pince H, Verberckmoes R, Willems JL: Computer aided interpretation of acid-base disorders. Int J Biomed Comput 25:177, 1990
20. Huckabee WE: Abnormal resting blood lactate: II. Lactic acidosis. Am J Med 30:840, 1961
21. Cohen RD, Woods HF: Clinical and Biochemical Aspects of Lactic Acidosis. Blackwell, Oxford, 1976
22. Vary TC, Siegel JH, Rivkind A: Clinical and therapeutic significance of metabolic patterns of lactic acidosis. Perspectives in Critical Care 1:85, 1988
23. Emergency Cardiac Care Committee and Subcommittees, American Heart Association: Standards and guidelines for cardiopulmonary resuscitation and emergency cardiac care. JAMA 268:2171, 1992
24. Sun JH, Filley GF, Hord K, et al: Carbicarb: an effective substitute for NaHCO⁻ for the treatment of acidosis. Surgery 102:835, 1987
25. Stacpoole PW, Henderson GN, Yan Z, et al: Clinical pharmacology and toxicology of dichloroacetate. Environ Health Perspect 106(suppl 4):989, 1998
26. Stacpoole PW, Harman EM, Curry SH, et al: Treatment of lactic acidosis with dichloroacetate. N Engl J Med 309:390, 1983
27. Shangraw RE, Rabkin JM, Lopaschuk GD: Hepatic pyruvate dehydrogenase activity in humans: effect of cirrhosis, transplantation and dichloroacetate. Am J Physiol 274:G569, 1998
28. Shangraw RE, Winter R, Hromco J, et al: Amelioration of lactic acidosis with dichloroacetate during liver transplantation in humans. Anesthesiology 81:1127, 1994
29. Arturson G, de Verdier C-H: Respiratory functions of blood. Surgical Physiology. Burke JF, Ed. WB Saunders Co, Philadelphia, 1983, p 451
30. Walmsley RN, White GH: A Guide to Diagnostic Clinical Chemistry. Blackwell Scientific, Melbourne, 1983, p 114
31. Brewer ED: Disorders of acid-base balance. Pediatr Clin North Am 37:429, 1990
32. Bernards WC, Kirby RR: Acid-base chemistry and physiology. Critical Care, 2nd ed. Civetta JM, Taylor RW, Kirby RR, Eds. JB Lippincott Co, Philadelphia, 1992, p 343
33. Battle DC, Hizon M, Cohen E, et al: The use of the urinary anion gap in the diagnosis of hyperchloremic metabolic acidosis. N Engl J Med 318:594, 1988
34. Marino PL: The ICU Book. Williams & Wilkins, Baltimore, 1998
35. Riley LJ, Ilson BE, Narins RG: Acute metabolic acid-base disorders. Crit Care Clin 5:699, 1987

Reviews

Brenner M, Welliver J: Pulmonary and acid-base assessment. Nurs Clin North Am 25:761, 1990

Clinical Disorders of Fluid and Electrolyte Metabolism, 4th ed. Maxwell MH, Kleeman CR, Narins RG, Eds. McGraw-Hill Book Co, New York, 1987

Fluids and Electrolytes, 2nd ed. Kokko JP, Tannen RL, Eds. WB Saunders Co, Philadelphia, 1990

Kruse JA, Carlson RW: Lactate metabolism. Crit Care Clin 5:725, 1987

Rose BD: Clinical Physiology of Acid-Base and Electrolyte Disorders, 2nd ed. McGraw-Hill Book Co, New York, 1984

Walmsley RN, Guerin MD: Disorders of Fluid and Electrolyte Balance. John Wright & Sons Ltd, Bristol, 1984

Acknowledgments

Figure 1 Albert Miller.
Figure 2 Seward Hung.
Figure 3 Talar Agasyan.

8 ACUTE WOUND CARE

W. Thomas Lawrence, M.D., A. Griswold Bevin, M.D., and George F. Sheldon, M.D.

Approach to Acute Wound Management

When a patient presents with an acute wound, the priorities are a careful, complete history and a thorough physical examination. Most cutaneous wounds are obvious and easily diagnosed but are not life threatening. However, the wounded patient may also have less apparent problems that are potentially lethal and demand immediate attention. The management of such potentially life-endangering problems takes precedence over wound management.

After more urgent problems have been ruled out or corrected, wound management can be addressed. Information about the time and mechanism of injury must be obtained. The patient should be asked about a coagulopathy and about conditions (e.g., diabetes, immune disorders, renal disease, hepatic dysfunction, and malignancies), practices (e.g., smoking), and medications (e.g., corticosteroids or chemotherapeutic agents) that could interfere with healing. The patient's nutritional status must be assessed, and the patient must be checked for signs of arterial or venous insufficiency in the wounded area.

The wound must then be carefully examined. Active hemorrhage must be noted. Wounded tissue must be assessed for viability, and foreign bodies must be sought. The possibility of damage to nerves, ducts, muscles, or bones in proximity to the injury must be assessed. X-rays and a careful motor and sensory examination may be required to rule out such coexistent injuries. It may be necessary to probe such ducts as the parotid or the lacrimal duct to assess them for injury. The patient's tetanus immunization status should be considered [see Tetanus Prophylaxis, below]. Antirabies treatment should be considered for patients who have been bitten by wild animals such as skunks, raccoons, foxes, and bats [see 21 Soft Tissue Infection and 86 Viral Infection].

Tetanus Prophylaxis

With any wound, it is important to consider the status of the patient's tetanus immunization.[1] The effectiveness of antibiotics for the prophylaxis of tetanus is uncertain.[2] Large, deep wounds with devitalized tissue are especially prone to tetanus infection and are defined as tetanus prone[3] [see Tables 1 and 2]. There is no one characteristic that defines a wound as tetanus prone: instead, wounds are considered tetanus prone if they have a significant number of the characteristics considered to define this state.

For non–tetanus-prone wounds, tetanus immune globulin (human) (TIG) is never indicated. If a patient with a non–tetanus-prone wound was never completely immunized or has not received a tetanus booster dose within the past 10 years, a booster dose of tetanus and diphtheria toxoids adsorbed (Td) is required. For a patient who has been previously immunized and has received a tetanus booster within the past 10 years, no further treatment is required.

For a patient with a tetanus-prone wound who has been completely immunized and has received a booster dose within the past 5 years, no treatment is indicated. If a previously immunized patient with a tetanus-prone wound has not been immunized within the past 5 years, a booster Td dose is administered. If a patient with a tetanus-prone wound either was not immunized or was incompletely immunized, TIG is given along with a dose of Td.

Antibiotic Prophylaxis

Antibiotics are indicated for cellulitis in the tissues surrounding the wounded area and for contaminated wounds in immunocompromised individuals. They are also indicated for patients with extensive injuries to the central area of the face, to prevent spread of infection through the venous system to the meninges; for patients with valvular disease, to prevent endocarditis; and for patients with prostheses, to limit the chance of bacterial seeding of the prosthesis. Lymphedematous extremities are particularly prone to cellulitis, and antibiotics are indicated when such extremities are wounded. Stool-contaminated wounds and human-bite wounds are considered infected from the moment of infliction and must be treated with antibiotics [see 21 Soft Tissue Infection].[4,5] In all these

Table 1 Wound Classification[3]

Clinical Features	Tetanus-Prone Wounds	Non–Tetanus-Prone Wounds
Age of wound	> 6 hr	≤ 6 hr
Configuration	Stellate wound, avulsion, abrasion	Linear wound
Depth	> 1 cm	≤ 1 cm
Mechanism of injury	Missile, crush, burn, frostbite	Sharp surface (e.g., knife or glass)
Signs of infection	Present	Absent
Devitalized tissue	Present	Absent
Contaminants (e.g., dirt, feces, soil, or saliva)	Present	Absent

```
┌─────────────────────────────────────────────────────┐
│ Obtain history and perform physical examination     │
├─────────────────────────────────────────────────────┤
│ Life-threatening conditions take priority over      │
│ wound care.                                         │
└─────────────────────────────────────────────────────┘
                          │
┌─────────────────────────────────────────────────────┐
│ Consider prophylaxis against tetanus or rabies, or both │
└─────────────────────────────────────────────────────┘
                          │
┌─────────────────────────────────────────────────────┐
│ Consider antibiotic therapy for contaminated wounds in immunocompromised │
│ patients for cellulitis around the wound, for human-bite wounds, for abscesses of │
│ the central area of the face, for patients with valvular heart disease or prostheses, │
│ for stool-contaminated wounds, and for wounds in lymphedematous extremities │
└─────────────────────────────────────────────────────┘
                          │
┌─────────────────────────────────────────────────────┐
│ Determine timing of wound closure                   │
└─────────────────────────────────────────────────────┘
```

Small or superficial wound that will heal secondarily within 2 weeks

Example:
  Puncture wounds
  Superficial abrasions

Secondary healing:
Clean and dress the wound and allow it to heal.

Fresh, acute wound with viable wound margins, limited bacterial contamination, and no unusual problems with foreign bodies or hemorrhage

Examples:
  Dog-bite wounds
  Kitchen-knife wounds
  Surgical wounds

Primary closure:
Proceed immediately to consideration of method of wound closure.

Determine method of wound closure

Choices:
  Direct approximation
  Skin graft
  Flap (local or distant)

Simplest method possible in a given situation is preferred.

Provide general or local anesthesia as needed; prepare wound for closure.

Wound with edges in proximity

Close wound by direct approximation.
Consider use of drains.

Wound edges cannot be approximated; wound contains no denuded bones, cartilage, nerve, or tendon; and a skin graft is cosmetically and functionally acceptable

Apply a skin graft.

Wound edges cannot be approximated, and a skin graft is not possible or desirable

Utilize a flap for wound closure.
Consider use of drains.

Approach to Acute Wound Management

Acute wound with uncontrollable hemorrhage	**Acute wound with questionably viable tissue or extreme contamination with foreign bodies**	**Acute or neglected wound with excessive bacterial contamination**

Example:
   Wound in a hemophiliac
 	
Tertiary closure:
Pack or wrap wound tightly until bleeding is controlled; then proceed with closure.
	Examples:
	   Wounds with embedded road tar
	   Wounds with severely contused tissue
	
	Tertiary closure:
	Proceed with debridement of foreign bodies and necrotic tissue, and initiate dressing changes until wound is clean; then proceed with closure.
		Example:
		   Human-bite wounds
		
		Tertiary closure:
		Debride and irrigate wound and initiate dressing changes with antibacterial cream until bacterial count is $< 10^5$/g tissue; then proceed with closure.

cases, the choice of antibiotics depends on the species of bacteria present within the wound. Gram's stain often provides an early clue to the type of bacteria present. The mechanism of injury also provides useful clues. Human bites should be treated with broad-spectrum antibiotics or combinations of antibiotics to ensure coverage of the various species present in human saliva; penicillin plus a penicillinase-resistant penicillin or a cephalosporin is a common choice. Animal-bite wounds generally may be treated with penicillin alone, although the need for prophylactic antibiotics is not as great.[6] Routine soft tissue infections are usually caused by staphylococci or streptococci, and gram-positive coverage is generally indicated. The presence of crepitus or a foul smell suggests a possible anaerobic infection. Initial antibiotic choices are made empirically; more specific antibiotic treatment can be instituted when the results of bacterial culture and sensitivity studies become available.

Timing of Wound Closure

The goal of acute wound management should be a closed, healing wound. The first issue to address is the timing of closure. The choices are (1) primary closure, that is, to close the wound at the time of initial presentation; (2) secondary closure, that is, to allow the wound to heal on its own; and (3) tertiary closure, that is, to close the wound after a period of secondary healing. The proper choice depends on how the following questions are answered:

1. Must the wound be closed, or will secondary healing produce an acceptable result?
2. If closure is required,
   a. Can hemorrhage be easily controlled?
   b. Can all necrotic material and foreign bodies be clearly identified and excised?
   c. Is excessive bacterial contamination present?

Table 2 Immunization Schedule[3]*

History of Tetanus Immunization (Doses)	Tetanus-Prone Wounds		Non–Tetanus-Prone Wounds	
	Td†	TIG	Td†	TIG‡
Uncertain	Yes	Yes	Yes	No
0 or 1	Yes	Yes	Yes	No
2	Yes	No§	Yes	No
3 or more	No‖	No	No¶	No

Note: The only contraindication to tetanus and diphtheria toxoids for the wounded patient is a history of neurologic or severe hypersensitivity reaction to a previous dose. Local side effects alone do not preclude continued use. If a systemic reaction is suspected to represent allergic hypersensitivity, postpone immunization until appropriate skin testing is performed. If a contraindication to a tetanus toxoid–containing preparation exists, consider passive immunization against tetanus for a tetanus-prone wound.
*Verify a history of tetanus immunization from medical records so that appropriate tetanus prophylaxis can be accomplished.
†For children younger than 7 years, diphtheria and tetanus toxoids and pertussis vaccine adsorbed (or diphtheria and tetanus toxoids adsorbed, if pertussis vaccine is contraindicated) is preferable to tetanus toxoid alone. For persons 7 years of age and older, Td is preferable to tetanus toxoid alone.
‡When administering TIG and Td concurrently, use separate syringes and separate sites.
§Yes, if wound is more than 24 hours old.
‖Yes, if more than 5 years since last dose. (More frequent boosters are not needed and can accentuate side effects.)
¶Yes, if more than 10 years since last dose.
Td—tetanus and diphtheria toxoids adsorbed (for adult use)
TIG—tetanus immune globulin (human)

Normal healing can proceed only if tissues are viable, the wound contains no foreign bodies, and tissues are free of excessive bacterial contamination.

SMALL OR SUPERFICIAL WOUNDS

Superficial wounds involving only the epidermis and a portion of the dermis will frequently heal secondarily within 1 to 2 weeks. In such wounds, the functional and aesthetic results of secondary healing are generally as good as or better than those obtained by primary or tertiary closure. For puncture wounds, secondary healing is preferred because it diminishes the likelihood of infection and produces an aesthetically acceptable scar. For wounds on concave surfaces such as the medial canthal region and the nasolabial region, secondary healing generally yields excellent aesthetic results.[7]

ACUTE WOUNDS WITHOUT BACTERIAL CONTAMINATION, FOREIGN BODIES, OR NECROTIC TISSUE

If wound closure is required, primary closure is preferred if it is feasible: it eliminates the need for extensive wound care; the wound reaches its final, healed state more quickly; and it minimizes patient discomfort. However, a wound with foreign bodies or necrotic tissue that cannot be removed by irrigation or debridement, or a wound with excessive bacterial contamination, should not be closed primarily (see below), nor should wounds in which hemostasis is incomplete. Hematomas,[8] necrotic tissue,[9] and foreign bodies[10] promote the growth of bacteria and provide a mechanical barrier between healing tissues.

ACUTE WOUNDS WITH EXCESSIVE BLEEDING

Hemorrhage can be readily controlled in most wounds with pressure, cautery, or ligatures. Occasionally, as with a patient with a bleeding diathesis, primary wound closure is precluded by inadequate hemostasis. In such cases, the wound should be packed or wrapped tightly and elevated if the anatomic site of the wound allows. The wound should then be re-examined within 24 hours to determine whether hemostasis is sufficient to allow safe closure. If bleeding within a wound occurs after closure, the course of action depends on the size of the resulting hematoma. Small hematomas, which will be resorbed, can be ignored. Larger hematomas, which provide a significant barrier to healing, require drainage.

ACUTE WOUNDS WITH FOREIGN BODIES OR NECROTIC TISSUE

Foreign Bodies

Most foreign bodies can be easily removed from wounds manually or debrided surgically. Patients injured in motorcycle accidents, however, frequently slide along asphalt pavements for long distances at high speeds, with the result that many small fragments of asphalt become embedded in and beneath the skin. Exploding gunpowder also causes many small pieces of foreign material to be embedded within the skin. These foreign bodies are often difficult to extract, but they should be removed as soon as possible after the injury. High-pressure irrigation with saline will remove many foreign bodies. Surgical debridement or vigorous scrubbing with a wire brush may be required for the removal of more firmly embedded foreign material. If too much time elapses between injury and treatment, the embedded material is gradually covered and encapsulated by advancing epithelium and thereby becomes sealed within the dermis. In such instances, surgical dermabrasion is necessary for the removal of the foreign material.[11,12]

Foreign materials such as paint, oil, and grease are sometimes inadvertently injected subcutaneously under pressure (600 to 12,000 psi) by the spray guns used for painting, automotive body work, or industrial purposes.[13,14] On initial examination, the injury may appear deceptively benign in that a punctate entry wound draining foreign material is often the only sign of injury other than edema. Nevertheless, these wounds must be treated aggressively if extensive tissue loss is to be avoided. With some injected materials, radiographs are useful for demonstrating the extent of distribution. The involved area, which is frequently the hand, should be incised, and as much of the foreign material as possible should be surgically debrided (preferably, if the hand is involved, by a surgeon who specializes in hand injuries). Because the foreign material is often widely distributed in the soft tissues, extensive incisions may be necessary. Antibiotics and tetanus prophylaxis are also recommended. The ultimate prognosis is at least partially determined by the type of material injected: paint is associated with a particularly poor prognosis, whereas water is associated with a good one.[15] Early aggressive therapy does not rule out the possibility of amputation, especially if the injected material is notably caustic.

High-velocity missiles such as bullets are rendered sterile by the explosion required for their propulsion; therefore, deeply embedded bullets can often be left safely where they have lodged. Center-fire rifle bullets and .44 magnum pistol bullets carry a large amount of kinetic energy and can produce extensive tissue damage. Wounds created by such high-velocity missiles may have to be debrided to permit excision of necrotic tissue. The mechanism of injury may suggest the possibility of a foreign body within the wound that is not immediately apparent. If a radiopaque material, such as metal or leaded glass, is being looked for, radiographs may detect its presence. For less opaque materials, xeroradiography, magnified radiographs, and computed tomography scans are sometimes diagnostically useful.[16]

Identification and Debridement of Necrotic Tissue

The necrotic tissue in most wounds can be identified and surgically debrided at initial presentation. In some wounds, there may be a significant amount of tissue of questionable viability. If the amount of questionable material precludes acute debridement, dressing changes may be initiated. When all tissue has been identified as viable or necrotic, and when the necrotic tissue has been debrided surgically or by means of dressing changes, the wound can be closed.

Sometimes, a flap of tissue may be of questionable viability. Signs that suggest whether tissue is viable include color, bright-red arteriolar bleeding, and blanching on pressure followed by capillary refill. A flap can also be evaluated acutely by administering up to 15 mg/kg of fluorescein intravenously and observing the flap for fluorescence under an ultraviolet lamp after 10 to 15 minutes have elapsed.[17] Viable tissue fluoresces. Flap tissue that is thought to be devascularized, on the basis of physical examination or fluorescein examination, should be debrided. If the viability of a segment of tissue is in doubt, it may be sewn back in its anatomic location and allowed to define itself as viable or nonviable over time.

In burn wounds, it is impossible to assess the extent of final tissue damage at presentation because the injury can worsen during the first few days after the burn.[18] Closure of the burn wound is often delayed until all of the necrotic tissue can be defined and removed [*see 34 Burn Care after the First Postburn Week*].

Another type of wound in which the severity of the injury may not be readily apparent is the crush injury. With a crush injury, there may not be an external laceration, even though tissue damage may be extensive. The primary concern is whether muscle damage in the fascial compartments is severe enough to induce swelling sufficient to compromise the vascularity of the muscle. If pulses are diminished or paresthesias are developing, the pressure within the fascial compartment is clearly excessive, and fasciotomies are indicated. In less clear-cut cases, intracompartmental pressures may be assessed by percutaneous placement of catheters or wicks into the fascial compartments. The catheters or wicks are attached to pressure monitors or transducers. An intracompartmental pressure greater than 40 mm Hg indicates that capillary filling pressure has been exceeded and muscle perfusion is compromised. The fascial compartment must then be released to prevent ischemic muscle damage; the fasciotomies must be performed on an emergent basis. If the degree of damage is not severe enough to necessitate fasciotomy, the injured part should be elevated and dressed in a mildly compressive dressing to limit edema formation. If there is muscle damage, the possibility of crush syndrome with renal damage caused by rhabdomyolysis must be considered. If myoglobin is found in the urine, diuresis should be induced, and the urine should be alkalinized.

ACUTE OR NEGLECTED WOUNDS WITH BACTERIAL CONTAMINATION

An infected wound is defined as one with bacterial concentrations greater than 10^5 organisms/g tissue.[19,20] β-Hemolytic streptococci are an exception to this rule and can produce clinical infections in lower concentrations.[21] It is often difficult to assess the degree of bacterial contamination of a wound solely by visual inspection. The age of the wound is one factor correlated with the degree of bacterial contamination. The initial 6 to 8 hours after wounding have been referred to as the golden period because closure can usually be accomplished safely during this period. In a clinical study in a civilian setting, most wounds less than 5 to 6 hours old were contaminated with fewer than 10^5 bacteria/g tissue and therefore could be safely closed primarily.[22] Experimental data suggest that bacteria trapped within the fibrinous exudate that forms over a wound's surface cause the infections seen in wounds closed after 6 to 8 hours.[23,24] The bacteria proliferate after wounding and generally take 6 to 8 hours to reach levels of 10^5/g tissue. The longer wounds remain open, the greater the likelihood that they will become infected.[25]

The location of the injury is also significant. Lacerations of the face, which has an abundant blood supply, are more likely to resist bacterial proliferation (and to do so for a longer time) than injuries to less adequately perfused areas, such as the lower extremities.[26] Immune status is also important. A wound is less likely to become infected in a young, healthy person than in an elderly, debilitated patient or a person receiving immunosuppressive medication.[27]

The mechanism of injury can suggest whether a wound may become infected and what species of bacteria are most likely to be present in the wound. Human saliva contains up to 10^8 bacteria/ml; it contains a mixture of aerobic and anaerobic gram-positive and gram-negative species. Human-bite wounds should be considered infected from the moment they occur.[4] *Staphylococcus aureus*, α-hemolytic streptococci, *Eikenella corrodens*, *Hemophilus* species, and anaerobes are often cultured from human-bite wounds.[6,28] Animal-bite wounds are generally less contaminated than human-bite wounds; infection is more likely when bites and scratches are seen late [see 21 Soft Tissue Infection]. *Pasteurella multocida* is the most common infecting organism in cat-bite wounds; it is also common in dog-bite wounds, although α-hemolytic streptococci and *S. aureus* also are frequently seen.[6,28] Mutilating injuries caused by farm equipment are often contaminated with a mixture of gram-positive and gram-negative organisms, although they are not always excessively contaminated from inception.[29]

An infected wound can sometimes be excised to produce a fresh, less contaminated wound. However, in situations in which the nature of the injury precludes complete wound excision or in which there is cellulitis of surrounding tissues, dressing changes should be initiated. The use of certain topical agents will lead to a decreased bacterial count. Silver sulfadiazine (Silvadene) is used frequently because its antibacterial spectrum is broad, it is comfortable for the patient, and it does not commonly lead to metabolic problems such as those seen with other agents, such as mafenide (Sulfamylon) or silver nitrate.[30,31] Silver sulfadiazine may also speed the rate of epithelialization.[32] Parenteral antibiotics are not useful for killing bacteria in the wound itself, because they do not penetrate the wound directly.[33] In experiments on animals, parenteral antibiotics have proved useful for controlling bacteria within wounds when used in conjunction with proteolytic enzymes such as Travase.[23,34] This combination of treatments has not been widely used clinically.

Once bacterial control has been accomplished, the wound can be closed. In one series, tertiary closure was successful in more than 90% of cases when bacterial counts in tissue had diminished to less than $10^5/g$.[35]

In many cases, the degree of bacterial contamination is uncertain. Ideally, quantitative cultures can be obtained to provide precise information about the type and numbers of bacteria present. With the rapid slide technique, information about bacterial counts can be obtained within an hour.[36] If this information cannot be obtained, the clinician can initiate dressing changes or, alternatively, close the wounds over drains and administer topical and systemic antibiotics. The latter approach has yielded low infection rates in some series.[37,38]

An alternative to either primary closure or dressing changes in these patients is delayed primary closure, a technique developed empirically during wartime. Saline-soaked gauze is packed into the wound at the time of injury, and the wound is reexamined after several days. If the wound appears clean, the wound edges are then approximated. If the wound appears to be contaminated at follow-up, dressing changes are instituted. This approach limits the infection rate in potentially contaminated wounds.

When infection develops after closure of a wound, treatment involves removal of some or all of the sutures and initiation of dressing changes, often with use of topical antibacterials [see Dressings, below]. Any cellulitis surrounding the wound is treated with systemic antibiotics [see 21 Soft Tissue Infection].

Surgical Wounds

The American College of Surgeons has divided operative wounds into four major categories [see Table 3]. The likelihood of infection after any surgical procedure is correlated with the category of wound.[39] Wounds in classes I and II have low infection rates, whereas wounds in class IV have infection rates as high as 40%.

Wounds Resulting from Wild-Animal Bites: Special Considerations

Rabies prophylaxis must be considered for bite wounds from high-risk wild animals such as skunks, raccoons, foxes, coyotes, and bats.[40] Rabies is generally not a risk in bite wounds from rodents, rabbits, pets, and domestic animals unless the animal is acting unusually aggressive and is salivating excessively. If there is any possibility that the biting animal has rabies and the animal is available, it should be watched for symptoms of rabies for 10 days. If the biting animal can be killed and examined, rabies can be confirmed or excluded by means of an immunofluorescent antibody study of its brain. If rabies is confirmed or if the biting animal is not available for examination and rabies is suspected, the patient should be treated with both rabies immune globulin and human diploid cell vaccine. Specific schedules for administration appear elsewhere [see 21 Soft Tissue Infection].

With snakebite wounds, the possibility of envenomation must be considered. The poisonous snakes native to the United States are coral snakes and three species of pit vipers—namely, rattlesnakes, copperheads, and water moccasins.[41-43] The pit vipers can be identified by the pit between the eye and nostril on each side of the head, the vertical elliptic pupils, the triangular shape of the head, the single row of caudal plates, and the characteristic fang marks they inflict when they bite. Coral snakes have rounder heads and eyes and lack fangs; they are identified by their characteristic color pattern, consisting of red, yellow, and black vertical bands. Patients bitten by any of the pit vipers must be examined for massive swelling and pain, which, along with fang marks, suggest envenomation. The pain and swelling generally develop within 30 minutes of the bite, although it may take up to 4 hours to become manifest. Secondary local signs, such as erythema, petechiae, ecchymoses, and bullae, sometimes appear; if envenomation is extensive, systemic signs, such as disseminated intravascular coagulation, bleeding, shock, acute respiratory distress syndrome, and renal failure, may also be seen. Patients bitten by coral snakes, on the other hand, show no obvious local signs when envenomation has occurred. Consequently, the physician must look for systemic signs, such as paresthesias, increased salivation, fasciculations of the tongue, dysphagia, difficulty in speaking, visual disturbances, respiratory distress, convulsions, and shock. These symptoms may not develop until several hours after the bite.

No local care is necessary for coral snake bite wounds; however, a variety of techniques have been used for local care of pit viper bite wounds. Some groups have advocated surgical approaches, such as early incision with suction and wound excision, whereas others have suggested topical application of ice or use of tourniquets to limit the

Table 3 Classification and Infection Rates of Operative Wounds

Classification	Infection Rate (%)	Wound Characteristics
Clean (class I)	1.5–5.1	Atraumatic, uninfected; no entry of GU, GI, or respiratory tract
Clean-contaminated (class II)	7.7–10.8	Minor breaks in sterile technique; entry of GU, GI, or respiratory tract without significant spillage
Contaminated (class III)	15.2–16.3	Traumatic wounds; gross spillage from GI tract; entry into infected tissue, bone, urine, or bile
Dirty (class IV)	28.0–40.0	Drainage of abscess; debridement of soft tissue infection

spread of venom. None of these treatments have been shown to provide a definite benefit. At present, topical application of ice is discouraged because it is more likely to lead to secondary injuries than to benefit the patient. Tight tourniquets cannot be left in place for long periods without risking damage to the extremity; however, loose tourniquets that slow lymphatic drainage may be of some value. Excision of the bite wound may be effective if it is performed within 1 to 2 hours of injury. To reduce the incidence of unintentional injuries, excision should be performed only by persons with medical training.

Antivenin is indicated if pain and swelling are substantial enough to suggest extensive envenomation. It should be administered only if it is clearly necessary because it is of equine origin and frequently produces serum sickness. Antivenin is almost never required for copperhead bites but is more commonly needed for rattlesnake bites.[44] When indicated, it should be administered as soon as possible because it is less effective when given after signs of envenomation have become severe.

Whenever there is any suggestion of envenomation, a battery of tests, including hematocrit, fibrinogen level, coagulation studies, platelet count, urinalysis, and serum chemistry values, should be performed. These tests should be repeated every 8 to 24 hours to evaluate any venom-induced changes. With severe envenomation, decreased fibrinogen levels, coagulopathies, and bleeding may be seen, as may myoglobinuria.

Envenomation is also a consideration with the bites of brown recluse spiders and black widow spiders.[43] The brown recluse spider has a violin-shaped mark on its dorsum; is found in dark, dry places; and is nocturnal. The symptoms of the bite may range from minor irritation to extreme tenderness associated with edema and erythema; the tenderness, erythema, and edema generally do not develop until 2 to 8 hours after the bite. In more severe cases, tissue necrosis can develop in as little as 12 hours, although more often the area of necrosis does not demarcate itself for weeks. Severe systemic reactions, including hemolysis and disseminated intravascular coagulation, have been reported. The tissue necrosis resulting from the bite of the brown recluse can be minimized by the use of dapsone.[45] The black widow often has a red hourglass mark on its abdomen and lives in dark, dry, protected areas.[43] The venom is a neurotoxin that produces severe local pain. Neurologic signs usually develop within 15 minutes and consist of muscle pain and cramps starting in the vicinity of the bite. The abdominal muscles frequently become involved. Other symptoms that may develop are vomiting, tremors, increased salivation, paresthesias, hyperreflexia, and, with severe envenomation, shock. In sensitive individuals, paralysis, hemolysis, renal failure, or coma may be seen. Treatment of black widow envenomation includes parenteral 10% calcium gluconate, parenteral methocarbamol, and one dose of parenteral antivenin.

Method of Wound Closure

When a wound is ready to be closed, the appropriate type of wound closure must be chosen. The types of wound closure are (1) direct approximation, (2) skin graft (autograft), (3) local flap, and (4) distant flap. In general, the simplest method possible in a given situation is preferred.

DIRECT WOUND APPROXIMATION

The most common surgical problem is the deep, relatively acute traumatic or surgical wound that is suitable for primary closure by direct approximation of the edges of the wound. In this setting, the goal is to provide the best possible chance for uncomplicated healing.

Adequate general or local anesthesia is an extremely important first step. If local anesthesia is indicated, as for small traumatic injuries, 0.5% or 1.0% lidocaine (Xylocaine) is generally injected directly into the wounded tissues. Although other local anesthetic agents can be used, lidocaine is the most popular choice because it acts quickly, it rarely provokes allergic reactions, and it provides local anesthesia for the 1 to 2 hours required for most wound closures. Epinephrine in a dilution of 1:100,000 or 1:200,000 is used in combination with the lidocaine in most areas except the fingers and toes, where it can induce vasospasm, leading to digital loss. Epinephrine prolongs the effectiveness of the anesthetic, increases the anesthetic dose that can be safely used, and aids hemostasis.[46] Lower concentrations of epinephrine can be effective, but it becomes unstable if stored for long periods at low concentrations. However, one experimental study, as yet unsubstantiated clinically, has suggested that the use of epinephrine is associated with an increased incidence of infection.[47] The maximum safe doses of lidocaine traditionally cited are 4 mg/kg without epinephrine and 7 mg/kg with epinephrine. The upper limit of the maximum safe dose has been questioned. During liposuction procedures, up to 35 mg/kg of lidocaine has been administered in a 0.1% solution containing epinephrine in a 1:1,000,000 dilution without reaching toxic drug levels.[48,49] The pain involved in injecting the local anesthetic can be minimized by using a small-caliber needle, warming the drug, injecting the drug slowly, using the subcutaneous rather than the intradermal route (even though the rate of onset is thereby slowed),[50] and buffering the agent with sodium bicarbonate to limit its acidity.[51]

Topical local anesthetics have been gaining in popularity as adjuncts to injectable local anesthetics. TAC (a solution of 0.5% tetracaine, 1:2,000 adrenaline [epinephrine], and 11.8% cocaine) and other topical agents have been demonstrated to induce local anesthesia when applied topically to an open wound, especially in the face or scalp.[52,53] EMLA, a eutectic mixture of lidocaine and prilocaine, induces anesthesia in intact skin, but it must be in contact with the skin for 1 to 2 hours to be effective.[54]

Hair may be clipped to facilitate exposure and wound closure, if necessary. Close shaving should be avoided, however, because it potentiates wound infections.[55] Clipping of eyebrows should also be avoided because they may not grow back.

The next step is to irrigate the wound with a high-pressure (≥ 8 psi) spray to decrease the number of bacteria in the wound.[56-58] A pressurized irrigation device is preferred, but if none is available, high-pressure irrigation may be performed by using (1) a 30 to 50 ml syringe and a 19-gauge needle or catheter or (2) a flexible bag of intravenous 0.9% saline attached to tubing and a 19-gauge catheter with a pressure device.[56] Low-pressure irrigation and scrubbing of the wound with a saline-soaked sponge have not been demonstrated to decrease the incidence of wound infections.[58,59] The only irrigants that have been demonstrated to be nontoxic to tissues are 0.9% saline[60] and Pluronic F-68,[61,62] though lactated Ringer's solution is also acceptable. Pluronic F-68 has surfactant properties that improve wound cleansing without damaging tissues. Antibiotics are sometimes added to irrigation solutions to increase their effectiveness at killing bacteria. Solutions of 1% neomycin sulfate and 2% kanamycin sulfate, which do not kill fibroblasts in culture,[60] have limited toxicity to tissues. There is some evidence[63] that antibiotic supplements are more effective than saline solution in decreasing bacterial counts in contaminated wounds.

There are a number of solutions that should never be placed on a wound. Povidone-iodine scrub and soaps containing hexachlorophene are especially damaging to normal tissues.[60,64,65] Chlorhexidine, which is found in various brands of soaps, has also been demonstrated to impede the healing process.[66,67] Alcohol is toxic to tissues and should not be placed in wounds.[68] A 0.5% solution of sodium hypochlorite (Dakin's solution) has been demonstrated to be toxic to fibroblasts, to impair neutrophil function, and to slow epithelialization in open wounds.[69,70] A 0.25% solution of acetic acid has been demonstrated to kill fibroblasts in culture and to slow epithelialization in open wounds.[70] Hydrogen peroxide has been shown to kill fibroblasts in culture and to cause histologic damage to tissues.[60,70] Even standard hand soap can induce some tissue damage that is visible on histologic examination.[60,68] The dictum "Don't put in a wound what you wouldn't put in your eye" is a valid guideline.[71]

After adequate anesthesia has been achieved, hair has been clipped, and the wound has been irrigated, the tissue surrounding the wound is prepared with an antibacterial solution such as povidone-iodine,[72,73] and a sterile field is created by using sterile drapes. Skin preparation limits contamination of the wound by bacteria from adjacent skin. The wound is surgically debrided of any foreign bodies or necrotic material to limit the chances of postoperative infection.[74] If the wound edges are beveled and adequate local tissue is available, the wound edges should be excised by means of incisions perpendicular to the skin.

Although wound closure can usually proceed in a straightforward manner, special caution is necessary in certain situations. When a wound crosses tissues with different characteristics, such as at the vermilion border of the lip, at the eyebrow, or at the hairline of the scalp, great care must be taken to align the damaged structures accurately. Injured nerves or ducts should generally be repaired at the time of wound closure. In acute wounds, it is generally best to avoid more complex tissue rearrangements such as a Z-plasty or W-plasty. Actual reconstructive surgery in the face of trauma is rarely indicated [see 67 Plastic Surgical Reconstruction]. Direct approximation of wounds does not always produce a uniform or aesthetically desirable result, particularly in extensive wounds, wounds lying outside normal skin folds or creases, wounds in children older than 2 years, wounds in the sternal and deltoid regions, U-shaped wounds, wounds with beveled edges, or wounds in regions of thick oily skin, such as the tip of the nose, where scars are often less acceptable. Wounds heal optimally when two perpendicular, well-vascularized wound edges are approximated in a tension-free manner.

An ideal method of wound closure would support the wound until it had nearly reached full strength (i.e., about 6 weeks), would not induce inflammation, would not induce ischemia, would not penetrate the epidermis and predispose to additional scars, and would not interfere with the healing process in any way. No existing method of wound closure accomplishes all of these goals: some sort of compromise is virtually always necessary.

Materials for Wound Closure

Materials available for wound closure are sutures, staples, tapes, and tissue adhesives. Of these, sutures are most commonly used. Absorbable sutures, such as those made of plain or chromic catgut, polyglactin 910 (Vicryl), polyglycolic acid (Dexon), polyglyconate (Maxon), or polydioxanone (PDS), are generally used for dermis, fat, muscle, or superficial fascia. Nonabsorbable sutures, such as those made of nylon, Ethibond, or polypropylene (Prolene), are most commonly used either for the skin (in which case they are removed) or for deeper structures that require prolonged wound support, such as the fascia of the abdominal wall or tendons.

The suture should be as small in diameter as possible while still being able to maintain approximation. The decision to remove skin sutures or staples involves balancing of optimal cosmesis with the need for wound support. Optimal cosmesis demands early removal of sutures, before inflammation can develop and before epithelialization can occur along the suture tracts. An epithelialized tract will develop around a suture or staple that remains in the skin for more than 7 to 10 days; after removal of the stitch, the tract will be replaced by an unwanted scar.[75] On the other hand, it takes a number of weeks for the wound to gain significant tensile strength, and early removal of wound support can lead to dehiscence of wounds subject to substantial tension. Wounds on the face and wounds along skin tension lines (e.g., incisions for thyroidectomy) are subject to limited tension, and sutures can be removed from these areas relatively early. Sutures are generally removed at day 4 or 5 from the face and generally by day 7 from other areas where skin tension is limited.

Sutures should remain longer in wounds subject to a greater amount of stress, such as wounds in the lower extremities and wounds closed under tension. Sutures also remain longer in wounds in persons with healing limitations, such as malnutrition. Less aesthetically pleasing consequences may have to be accepted in these cases.

One way of sustaining skin wound support while avoiding unwanted scars from skin sutures is to use buried dermal sutures. Synthetic materials, such as Vicryl, Dexon, PDS, or Maxon, are preferable to chromic or plain catgut because the former are absorbed by simple hydrolysis with little inflammatory response, whereas the latter provoke an active cellular inflammatory response that slows the healing process. Buried dermal sutures are often used in conjunction with either tapes (e.g., SteriStrips) or fine epidermal sutures to aid in precise epidermal alignment.

Closure with staples is more rapid than suture closure, although approximation may not be as precise.[76] Tape is easy to apply, is comfortable for the patient, and leaves no marks on the skin.[77-79] However, patients may inadvertently remove tapes, and approximation is less precise with tapes alone than with sutures. Furthermore, wound edema tends to cause inversion of taped wound edges.

Cyanoacrylate tissue adhesives, used by surgeons for over 30 years, are strong, reasonably flexible, and biocompatible. When these compounds first became available, isobutyl cyanoacrylate and trifluoropropyl cyanoacrylate were placed between wound edges to hold them together. Adhesives used in this way created a mechanical barrier to healing and increased wound inflammation and infection rates. This use of cyanoacrylate tissue adhesives was abandoned relatively quickly.[80]

More recently, cyanoacrylates have been applied topically to intact skin at the edge of wounds to hold injured surfaces together. Contact with open wounds is carefully avoided to limit toxicity. Hystoacryl Blue (n-butyl-2-cyanoacrylate) has been used extensively with good clinical results.[81] It creates limited wound strength during the first day after injury and should not be used in wounds subject to stress.[82]

A new octylcyanoacrylate is stronger than Hystoacryl Blue. A prospective, randomized trial in Canada[83] compared octylcyanoacrylate to sutures for wound closure. There were few cases of dehiscence, and the aesthetic results of wounds assessed 3 months after closure were similar to those obtained with sutures. As would be expected, octylcyanoacrylate closures were faster for the surgeon and less painful to the patient. Octylcyanoacrylate was not used in deep wounds that penetrated fascia, and the authors also specifically recommended against its use on the hands and over joints where either washing or repetitive motion might lead to premature removal of the adhesive.[83]

Fibrin glue has been utilized to improve the adherence and take of skin grafts[84,85]; it has also been used with a limited number of sutures to close wounds subjected to limited tension (e.g., blepharoplasty incisions[86]) and to curtail seroma formation under flaps.[87]

Although fibrin glue is helpful in these settings, it is not strong enough to be usable alone for the closure of wounds subject to even limited tension. It is more widely employed in Europe, where multi-donor glue is commercially available. In the United States, only autologous material is used (to avoid the risk of AIDS), which means that fibrin glue is an option only where blood banks have glue-producing capability.

The old surgical principle that dead space should be closed or obliterated seems to call for the closure of subcutaneous tissues. However, studies in both laboratory animals and humans have demonstrated that multiple layers of closure contribute to an increased incidence of infection.[88,89] Therefore, sutures should be avoided whenever possible in subcutaneous fat, which cannot hold them. Deeper fascial layers that contribute to the structural integrity of areas such as the abdomen or the chest should be closed as a separate layer to prevent hernias or other structural deformities.

If there appears to be a potential risk of fluid collecting in an unclosed subcutaneous space, drains are a more suitable alternative than subcutaneous stitches. In addition to preventing the accumulation of blood or serum in the wound, suction drains also aid in the approximation of tissues. They are particularly useful in aiding tissue approximation under flaps. Most drains—especially those made of silicone rubber—are relatively inert. However, all drains tend to potentiate bacterial infections and should be removed from a wound as soon as possible.[90]

Drains can usually be safely removed when drainage reaches levels of 25 to 50 ml/day. If a seroma develops after drain removal, intermittent sterile aspirations followed by application of a compressive dressing are indicated. In the unusual case in which drainage is persistent and refractory to intermittent aspirations, a drain may be reintroduced. In unusual cases with prolonged drainage, drains have been left in place for weeks to avoid the development of a seroma.[91]

Occasionally, despite a surgeon's best efforts, a closed wound will dehisce. Dehiscence usually results from tension combined with local and systemic factors. Local factors include poor surgical technique and tissue damage by trauma, prior surgery, or radiation—or, in the case of the abdomen, increased intra-abdominal pressure. Systemic factors include malnutrition, obesity, and concurrent use of medications such as steroids or chemotherapeutic agents. If the dehiscence is noted within 6 to 8 hours and it involves only skin and superficial tissues, the wound can be reclosed or, alternatively, be allowed to heal secondarily with dressing changes. Dehiscence of deeper structures such as the abdominal fascia can be a more serious problem. Fascial dehiscence in the abdomen is often heralded by serosanguineous discharge between sutures on days 5 to 8. Fascial separation of less than a few centimeters can be treated expectantly; if the dehiscence is larger, reoperation for fascial reclosure should be performed if the patient's condition permits.

SKIN GRAFTS

If a wound can be directly approximated without excessive tension or distortion of normal structures, that is almost always the method of choice. If a wound is so extensive that direct approximation is impossible, skin grafts should be considered [see 67 Plastic Surgical Reconstruction]. However, skin grafts cannot be used to close injuries that involve bone denuded of periosteum, cartilage denuded of perichondrium, tendon denuded of paratenon, and nerve denuded of perineurium. Skin grafts will not heal over large areas (> 1.0 to 1.5 cm^2) of denuded bone, cartilage, nerve, or tendon, because these structures are relatively, if not totally, avascular, and blood vessels are not present to revascularize the graft. For such wounds, flaps must be considered (see below).

Skin grafting produces a second wound at the donor site. Skin grafts vary in thickness, from very thin split-thickness grafts that incorporate the epidermis and only a small portion of the dermis to full-thickness grafts that incorporate the entire dermis. (There are further variations within these two classifications.) Thin full-thickness skin grafts from areas such as the eyelid, the retroauricular region, or the medial surface of the upper arm heal more reliably than thicker ones taken from other areas. Thin split-thickness grafts heal readily, as do their donor sites. Thick skin grafts that incorporate most or all of the dermis maximally inhibit wound contraction. The ability to inhibit wound contraction is not dependent on the absolute thickness of the graft but instead is related to the amount of the deeper dermis the graft contains.[92] Donor sites for thick skin grafts heal more slowly and in some cases may have to be closed separately.

Skin grafts can be meshed and expanded like a pantograph. This technique increases the area that can be covered and facilitates drainage of fluid through the resulting interstices. Meshed grafts conform well to irregular surfaces. However, the aesthetic result of a meshed graft is usually less satisfactory than that of an intact, unmeshed skin graft, especially if the meshed graft is expanded widely. Wound contraction is increased with an expanded meshed skin graft, which can be a problem around flexion and extension creases near joints.

A suitable donor site should provide a good color match for the wounded tissue and be as inconspicuous as possible.[93] Because humans are relatively symmetrical, the ideal graft tissue in terms of color and texture match is tissue from the contralateral structure. However, this type of graft is often impractical because the donor site is frequently too conspicuous. In general, skin anywhere above the clavicles resembles facial skin; the retroauricular and supraclavicular regions and the scalp are relatively inconspicuous donor sites for facial wounds. The buttocks and upper thighs are preferred donor sites for wounds of the trunk or the extremities.

Grafts will not take if bacterial contamination is excessive,[94] if a seroma or hematoma develops between the graft and the wound site, or if shearing occurs between the graft and the wound site. Infected wounds and wounds in which bleeding is inadequately controlled should not be grafted. Compressive, immobilizing dressing techniques and elevation can help prevent shearing and limit seroma formation. A graft must be protected to some extent until it reaches maturity, usually 6 months after placement.[95] Such measures are especially important for lower-extremity grafts, which may be more susceptible to trauma and dependent edema.

The color of grafted skin generally changes after transfer and is usually darker than it appeared in situ.[96] Hair is transferred only with full-thickness or very thick split-thickness skin grafts. In thicker split-thickness skin grafts, sebaceous activity is lost initially but resumes within 3 months. In the interim, the graft must be lubricated with skin creams. Sensibility in skin grafts is more like that of the recipient site than that of the area from which the graft was taken.[97] Perspiration returns with sensibility, and its pattern also is determined by that of the recipient site.[97] Full-thickness skin grafts have normal growth potential when they are placed during the early years of life, but the growth of split-thickness skin grafts is limited.[98] Skin grafts can be remarkably durable after complete healing and can be used effectively even on the soles of the feet.

FLAPS

Like skin grafts, flaps allow coverage of a wound that cannot be satisfactorily closed primarily; again, the cost is a secondary wound at the donor site. Flaps can be used to close any uninfected wound. They do not require as vascular a wound bed as grafts do, because they maintain their blood supply after transfer and do not depend on revascularization for survival. Flaps are indicated for wounds containing denuded bone, cartilage, tendon, or nerve that cannot be closed by direct approximation. Flaps may be used in some situations in which skin grafts are also a possible choice because they may provide tissue with desirable characteristics such as bulk or a more natural appearance. Flaps that include bone or muscle may also be indicated for functional purposes. Any flap creates at least some functional or aesthetic deficit, a consideration when deciding what type of flap should be used. When feasible, use of local flaps is generally preferred because they usually require a less complex operation and because local tissue is generally the most natural-looking substitute for the wounded tissue. Sometimes, however, specific tissue requirements mandate use of distant flaps.

A flap can be classified as either random or axial. A random flap is supplied with blood from the subdermal plexus but has no specific blood vessel supplying it. An axial flap must be supplied by a specific, predictable blood vessel. Generally, a flap that includes large amounts of tissue or specialized tissue such as muscle or bone is constructed as an axial flap. The most complex distant flap is an axial one that requires microvascular anastomoses of the primary blood vessels of the flap to appropriate recipient vessels in surrounding tissue [see 67 Plastic Surgical Reconstruction].

The blood supply to the flap must not be impaired by poor design, kinking of the vascular pedicle, pressure from an ill-placed dressing, poor patient positioning, or hematoma formation. Drains are frequently placed under flaps both to encourage tissue approximation and to prevent collection of blood and serum under the flap. Flaps will retain their color, texture, hair-bearing characteristics, and sebaceous activity regardless of the recipient site. Sensibility and perspiration return to some extent between 6 weeks and 3 months after flap transfer. With certain axial flaps, sensibility and other neural functions are preserved from the outset. In children, flaps are also durable and have normal growth potential.

Dressings

Different types of dressings perform different functions. Therefore, for any wound, the purpose a dressing is to serve must be carefully considered before the dressing is applied.

Partial-thickness injuries, such as abrasions and skin graft donor sites, heal primarily by epithelialization and are best treated with dressings that maintain a warm, moist environment.[99,100] A variety of dressings can accomplish this goal, including biologic dressings (e.g., allograft,[101] amnion,[102] or xenograft[103]), synthetic biologic dressings (e.g., Biobrane[104]), hydrogel dressings, and dressings of semipermeable or nonpermeable membranes (e.g., Op-Site or Duoderm).[100] These dressings need not be changed as long as they remain adherent. Small, superficial wounds also heal readily when dressed with Xeroform or Scarlet Red; these dressings are often changed with greater regularity.[105] The traditional approach to these partial-thickness injuries has been to apply gauze, often impregnated with a petrolatum-based antimicrobial such as bismuth tribromophenate (Xeroform), and to allow it to dry. Heat lamps have been used to accelerate the drying process. With this method, the gauze provides a matrix that facilitates scab formation.

A scab, which consists of dried fibrin, blood cells, and wound exudate, will protect a wound and limit desiccation and bacterial invasion. Epithelial cells advancing beneath a scab, however, must debride the scab-wound interface enzymatically to migrate across the wound surface beneath the scab.[106] Epithelialization is therefore slower under a scab than it would be under an occlusive dressing. Thus, wounds covered with a scab tend to be more painful than wounds covered with occlusive dressings as well.

For wounds containing necrotic tissue, foreign bodies, or other debris, wet-to-dry dressings are preferred. In this approach, saline-soaked, wide-meshed gauze dressings are applied, allowed to dry, and then changed every 4 to 6 hours. Granulation tissue (including necrotic tissue and other debris) and wound exudate become incorporated within the wide-meshed gauze; thus, a debriding effect is produced when the gauze is removed.[107,108] The disadvantage of this type of dressing is that some viable cells are damaged by the debridement process. Wet-to-wet dressing changes, in which the saline is not allowed to dry, minimize tissue damage but do not produce as much debridement. Enzymatic agents (e.g., Travase ointment) have been used for debridement and may have some advantages over plain dressings.[109]

Virtually any type of dressing change will lower the bacterial count in infected wounds[36]; however, application of antibacterial agents, which directly affect the infecting bacteria, generally decrease the bacterial count more quickly than other dressing-change regimens. Silver sulfadiazine is frequently used because in addition to its broad antibacterial spectrum and low incidence of side effects, it has the secondary benefits of maintaining the wound in a moist state and speeding epithelialization.[31]

For wounds with exposed tendons or nerves, it is particularly important to maintain a moist environment to prevent desiccation of the exposed vital structures. Although the biologic and membrane dressings mentioned accomplish this, they are difficult to use on deep or irregular wounds and wounds with a great deal of drainage. Consequently, wet-to-wet dressings or dressings including creams that contain agents such as silver sulfadiazine are often used.

For sutured wounds, the purpose of a dressing is to prevent bacterial contamination, protect the wound from trauma, manage any drainage, and facilitate epithelialization. One approach is to use a dressing with multiple layers, each of which serves a different purpose. The contact layer immediately adjacent to the wound must be sterile and nontoxic. An ideal contact layer does not stick to the wound or absorb fluid but instead facilitates drainage through itself to the overlying layers of the dressing. Materials with these characteristics include Xeroflo, a fine-meshed gauze impregnated with a hydrophilic substance, and N-terface, a synthetic fine-meshed gauze. The dressing layer directly over the contact layer should be absorptive and capable of conveying exudate or transudate away from the wound surface. Wide-meshed gauze facilitates capillary action and drainage.[110] Such absorptive layers must not be allowed to become soaked, because if they do, exudate collects on the wound surface, and maceration and bacterial contamination may occur. The outermost dressing layer is a binding layer, the purpose of which is to fix the dressing in place. Tape is most commonly used as a binding layer, though elastic wraps or other materials may sometimes be used instead. With sutured wounds, dressings are required only until drainage from the wound ceases. With nondraining wounds, dressings may be removed after 48 hours, by which time epithelial cells will have sealed the superficial layers of the wound. An alternative method of treating minimally draining incisional wounds is to apply an antibacterial ointment. Such ointments are occlusive and maintain a sterile, moist environment for the 48 hours required for epithelialization.

Some physicians use occlusive dressings for incisional wounds. These dressings, as mentioned, create a warm, moist, sterile environment that is optimal for epithelialization. Some of these are transparent, allowing observation of the wound. The disadvantage of most of these dressings is their limited absorptive capacity, allowing drainage from the wound to collect under the dressing.

In certain small wounds in areas that are difficult to dress, such as the scalp, it may be reasonable to forgo a synthetic dressing and simply allow a scab to form on the wound surface.

Discussion

Physiology of Wound Healing

Phylogenetically, humans have lost the ability of many lower animals, such as planaria and salamanders, to regenerate specialized structures in most of their tissues. Although the wound-healing process differs slightly from tissue to tissue, the process is similar throughout the body. The result in almost all tissues is scar, the so-called glue that repairs injuries. The goal of acute wound management is to facilitate the body's innate tendency to heal so that a strong but minimally apparent scar results. Generally, however, the normal wound-healing process cannot be accelerated.

The physiology of wound healing is usually described in phases [see Figure 1]. Although each of these phases will be discussed as a separate entity, the phases blend without distinct boundaries.

HEMOSTASIS

Most wounds extend into the dermis, injuring blood vessels and resulting in bleeding. Platelets adhere to the collagen exposed by damage to the blood vessel endothelium and form a plug. Platelet aggregation during the hemostatic process results in the release of cytokines and other proteins from the alpha granules of the cytoplasm of platelet cells. These cytokines include platelet-derived growth factor (PDGF), transforming growth factor–β (TGF-β), transforming growth factor–α (TGF-α), basic fibroblast growth factor or fibroblast growth factor 2 (bFGF or FGF2), platelet-derived epidermal growth factor (PD-EGF), and platelet-derived endothelial cell growth factor (PD-ECGF). Some of these cytokines have direct effects early in the healing process, and others are bound locally and play critical roles in later aspects of healing.

Activation of factor XII, which occurs when blood is exposed to foreign surfaces, stimulates the intrinsic coagulation cascade. The extrinsic coagulation cascade is stimulated by a tissue factor released from the injured tissues. Both coagulation cascades generate fibrin, which acts with platelets to form a clot in the injured area [see 5 Bleeding and Transfusion]. In a large wound, the superficial portion of this clot may dehydrate over time to produce a scab.

In addition to contributing to hemostasis, fibrin is the primary component of the provisional matrix that forms in the wound during early healing. Fibrin becomes coated with vitronectin from the serum and fibronectin derived from both serum and aggregating platelets. Fibronectins are a class of glycoproteins that facilitate the attachment of migrating fibroblasts as well as other cell types to the fibrin lattice.[111] By influencing cellular attachment, fibronectin is a key modulator of the migration of various cell types in the wound.[112,113] In addition, the fibrin-fibronectin lattice binds various cytokines released at the time of injury and serves as a reservoir for these factors in the later stages of healing.[114]

INFLAMMATION

Tissue damage at the site of injury stimulates the inflammatory response. This response is most prominent during the first 24 hours after a wound is sustained. In clean wounds, signs of inflammation dissipate relatively quickly, and few if any inflammatory cells are seen after 5 to 7 days. In contaminated wounds, inflammation may persist for a prolonged period. The signs of inflammation, originally described by Hunter in 1794, include erythema, edema, heat, and pain.

The signs of inflammation are generated primarily by changes in the 20 to 30 µm diameter venules on the distal side of the capillary bed. In the first 5 to 10 minutes after wounding, the skin blanches as a result of vasoconstriction mediated by prostaglandins such as PGF_{2a}, by thromboxane A_2, and by catecholamines. The initial vasoconstriction is followed by vasodilatation, which generates the characteristic erythema. The vasodilatation is mediated by (1) vasodilator prostaglandins such as PGE_2 and prostacyclin, released by injured cells, (2) histamine, released by mast cells and possibly by platelets to a lesser degree, (3) serotonin, also released by mast cells, (4) kinins, the release of which is stimulated by the coagulation cascade, and possibly by other factors as well. The endothelial cells lining the microvenules tend to contract and separate from one another, resulting in increased vascular permeability.

Serum migrates into the extravascular space, giving rise to edema. Inflammatory cells initially adhere loosely to endothelial cells lining the capillaries and roll along the endothelial surface of the vessels. The inflammatory cells eventually adhere to the vessel wall, in a process mediated by the β2 class of integrins, and subsequently transmigrate into the extravascular space.[115] Chemoattractants stimulate the migration of inflammatory cells to the injured area. As monocytes migrate from the capillaries into the extravascular space, they transform into macrophages in a process mediated by serum factors and fibronectin.[116-118] Neutrophils are the predominant inflammatory cell in the wound during the 2 to 3 days after wounding, but macrophages eventually become the predominant inflammatory cell in the wound.

Because monocytes are present in the serum in much lower numbers than neutrophils, it is not unexpected that they are rarely seen in the wound area initially. The shift in predominance is at least partly caused by the fact that macrophages live longer than neutrophils. There may also be macrophage-specific chemotactic factors that selectively attract macrophages into the wound.

Neutrophils and macrophages engulf damaged tissue and bacteria, digesting them in lysosomes. Macrophages, which secrete metalloproteinases (MMPs) that break down damaged tissue, survive after phagocytosing bacteria or necrotic material; neutrophils die, releasing lysosomal contents that can contribute to tissue damage and prolong the inflammatory response. The dying cells and liquefied tissue are the constituents of pus, which may or may not be sterile, depending on whether bacteria are present. Experimental studies have demonstrated that neutrophils are not essential to normal healing,[119] whereas macrophages are necessary.[120] In addition to performing other functions, macrophages are a primary source of cytokines that mediate other aspects of the healing process; this role is probably what makes macrophages essential for healing.

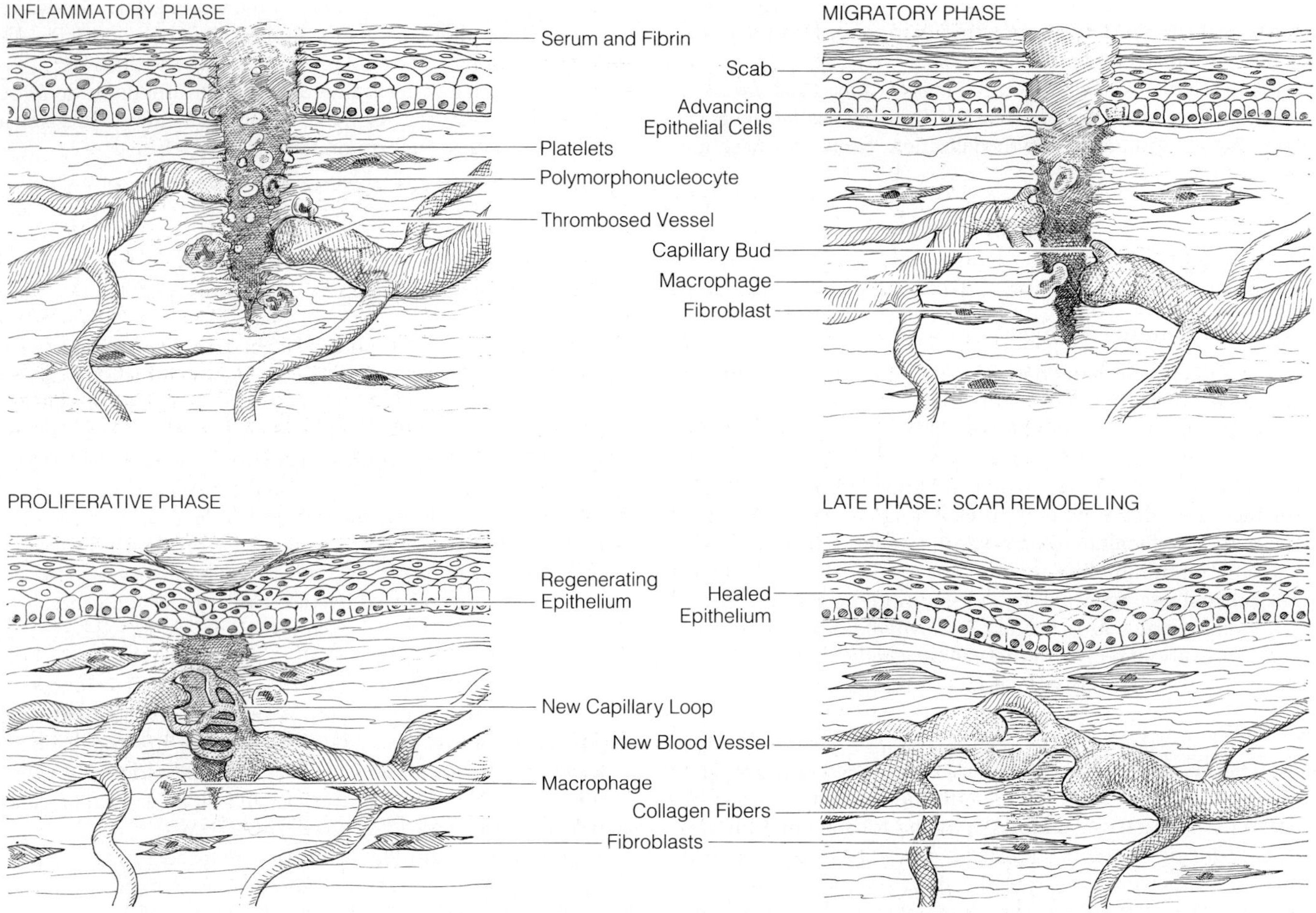

Figure 1 Depicted are the phases of wound healing. In the early phases (top, left), platelets adhere to collagen exposed by damage to blood vessels to form a plug. The intrinsic and extrinsic coagulation cascades generate fibrin, which combines with platelets to form a clot in the injured area. Initial local vasoconstriction is followed by vasodilatation mediated by histamine, PGE_2, PGI_2, serotonin, and kinins. Neutrophils are the predominant inflammatory cells (a polymorphonucleocyte is shown here). In the migratory phase (top, right), additional inflammatory cells, as well as fibroblasts and other mesenchymal cells, migrate into the wound area. Gradually, macrophages replace neutrophils as the predominant inflammatory cells. Angiogenic factors induce the development of new blood vessels as capillaries. Epithelial cells advance across the wound area from the basal layer of the epidermis. The fibrin-platelet clot may dehydrate to form a scab. In the proliferative phase (bottom, left), the advancing epithelial cells have covered the wound area. New capillaries form. The wound's strength grows as a result of steadily increasing production of collagen and glycosaminoglycans by fibroblasts. Myofibroblasts induce wound contraction. In the late phase (bottom, right), scar remodeling occurs. The overall level of collagen in the wound plateaus; old collagen is broken down as new collagen is produced. The number of cross-links between collagen molecules increases, and the new collagen fibers are aligned so as to provide a gradual increase in wound tensile strength. New capillaries combine to form larger vessels. The epithelium is healed, although it never quite regains its normal architecture.

MIGRATORY PHASE

Many substances attract fibroblasts and other mesenchymal cells into the wound during the migratory phase, including many of the cytokines[111,121,122] [see Table 4]. It is not known which of them are most active biologically at different points after wounding. The fibroblasts migrate along the scaffold of fibrin and fibronectin, as mentioned. Additional cytokines stimulate the proliferation of mesenchymal cells important in the wound-healing process once these cells have been attracted into the wound area[123-125] [see Table 4].

Angiogenesis

Angiogenesis is also initiated in the migratory phase during the first 2 or 3 days after wounding. Before revascularization of the injured area, the wound microenvironment is hypoxic and is characterized by high lactic acid levels and a low pH. Angiogenic factors stimulate the process of neovascularization. Some of the more potent angiogenic factors are derived from platelets and macrophages[126,127] [see Tables 4 and 5]. New vessels develop from existing vessels as capillaries. They produce fibrinolysin, which allows them to progress through areas of fibrin clot. The capillaries grow from the edges of the wound toward areas of inadequate perfusion, where lactate levels are increased and tissue oxygen tension is low. When they meet other developing capillaries, they join and establish new blood vessels. Initially, the capillaries advance in a brushlike configuration, but as they begin to function, they consolidate to form larger blood vessels.

Epithelialization

Epithelialization of skin involves the migration of cells from the basal layer of the epidermis across the denuded wound area.[128] This migratory process begins approximately 24 hours after wounding. The migrating cells develop bands 40 to 80 Å wide that can be seen with electron microscopy and stained with antiactin antibodies.

Table 4 Involvement of Cytokines in Wound-Healing Functions

Wound-Healing Function	Cytokines Involved
Neutrophil chemotaxis	PDGF IL-1
Macrophage chemotaxis	PDGF TGF-β IL-1
Fibroblast chemotaxis	EGF PDGF TGF-β
Fibroblast mitogenesis	EGF PDGF IGF TGF-β TGF-α IL-1 TNF-α
Angiogenesis, endothelial cell chemotaxis, mitogenesis	EGF Acidic and basic FGF (FGF1 and FGF2) TGF-β TGF-α TNF-α VEGF PD-ECGF
Epithelialization	EGF Basic FGF (FGF2) TGF-β TGF-α KGF IGF
Collagen synthesis	EGF Basic FGF (FGF2) PDGF TGF-β IL-1 TNF-α
Fibronectin synthesis	Basic FGF (FGF2) PDGF TGF-β EGF
Proteoglycan synthesis	Basic FGF (FGF2) PDGF TGF-β IL-1
Wound contraction	Basic FGF (FGF2) TGF-β
Scar remodeling, collagenase stimulation	EGF PDGF TGF-β IL-1 TNF-α

PDGF—platelet-derived growth factor IL-1—interleukin-1 TGF—transforming growth factor EGF—epidermal growth factor IGF—insulinlike growth factor TNF—tumor necrosis factor FGF—fibroblast growth factor VEGF—vascular endothelial growth factor PD-ECGF—platelet-derived endothelial cell growth factor KGF—keratinocyte growth factor

Forty-eight hours after wounding, the basal epidermal cells at the wound edge enlarge and begin to proliferate, producing more migratory cells. When epithelial cells migrating from two areas meet, contact inhibition prevents further migration. The cells making up the epithelial monolayer then differentiate into basal cells and divide, eventually yielding a neoepidermis consisting of multiple cell layers. Epithelialization progresses both from wound edges and from epithelial appendages. Epithelial advancement is facilitated by adequate debridement and decreased bacterial counts, as well as by the flattening of rete pegs in the dermis adjacent to the wound area. The epithelium never returns to its previous state. The new epidermis at the edge of the wound remains somewhat hyperplastic and thickened, whereas the epidermis over the remainder of the wound is thinner and more fragile than normal. True rete pegs do not form in the healed area.

PROLIFERATIVE PHASE AND COLLAGEN SYNTHESIS

The proliferative phase of wound healing usually begins approximately five days after wounding. During this phase, the fibroblasts that have migrated into the wound begin to synthesize proteoglycans and collagen, and the wound gains strength. Until this point, fibrin has provided most of the wound's strength. Although a small amount of collagen is synthesized during the first 5 days of the healing process,[129] the rate of collagen synthesis increases greatly after the fifth day. Wound collagen content continually increases for 3 weeks, at which point it begins to plateau.[130]

Although there are at least 18 types of collagen, the ones of primary importance in skin are type I, which makes up 80% to 90% of the collagen in skin, and type III, which makes up the remaining 10% to 20%. A higher percentage of type III collagen is seen in embryologic skin and in early wound healing. A critical aspect of collagen synthesis is the hydroxylation of lysine and proline moieties within the collagen molecule. This process requires specific enzymes as well as oxygen, vitamin C, α-ketoglutarate, and ferrous iron, which function as cofactors. Hydroxyproline, which is found almost exclusively in collagen, serves as a marker of the quantity of collagen in tissue. Hydroxylysine is required for covalent cross-link

Table 5 Cell Sources of Cytokines

Cell Type	Cytokines
Platelet	EGF PDGF TGF-β TGF-α
Macrophage	FGF PDGF TFG-β TGF-α IL-1 TNF-α IGF-1
Lymphocyte	TGF-β IL-2
Endothelial cell	FGF PDGF
Epithelial cell	TGF-α PDGF TGF-β
Smooth muscle cell	PDGF

formation between collagen molecules, which contributes greatly to wound strength. Deficiencies in oxygen or vitamin C or the suppression of enzymatic activity by corticosteroids may lead to underhydroxylated collagen incapable of generating strong crosslinks. Underhydroxylated collagen is easily broken down. After collagen molecules are synthesized by fibroblasts, they are released into the extracellular space. There, after enzymatic modification, they align themselves into fibrils and fibers that give the wound strength.

Proteoglycans, also synthesized during the proliferative phase of healing, consist of a protein core linked to one or more glycosaminoglycans. Dermatan sulfate, heparin, heparin sulfate, keratan sulfate, and hyaluronic acid are the more common proteoglycans. The biologic effects of proteoglycans are less well understood than those of collagen. They generally anchor specific proteins in certain locations and affect the biologic activity of target proteins. Heparin is an important cofactor of bFGF (FGF2) during angiogenesis. Other proteoglycans most likely facilitate the alignment of collagen molecules into fibrils and fibers.

Wound Contraction

Collagen has no contractile properties, and its synthesis is not required for wound contraction. During the proliferative phase, myofibroblasts appear in the wound and probably contribute to its contraction.[131] Myofibroblasts are unique cells that resemble normal fibroblasts and may be derived from them. They have convoluted nuclei, vigorous rough endoplasmic reticula, and microfilament bundles 60 to 80 Å in diameter. These microfilaments can be stained with antiactin and antimyosin antibodies. The wound edges are pulled together at a rate of 0.60 to 0.75 mm/day. The rate of contraction varies with tissue laxity. Contraction is greatest in anatomic sites where there is redundant tissue. Wound contraction generally continues most actively for 12 to 15 days or until wound edges meet.

LATE PHASE: SCAR REMODELING

Approximately 3 weeks after wounding, scar remodeling becomes the predominant feature of the healing process. Collagen synthesis is down-regulated, and the wound becomes less cellular as apoptosis occurs. During this phase, there is continual turnover of collagen molecules as old collagen is broken down and new collagen is synthesized along lines of stress.[132,133] Collagen breakdown is mediated by several MMPs, found in scar tissue as well as in normal connective tissues.[134] MMP-1 is interstitial collagenase, MMP-2 is elastase, and MMP-3 is stromelysin. The activity of these collagenolytic enzymes is modulated by several tissue inhibitors of metalloproteinases (TIMPs). During this phase, there is little net change in total wound collagen,[132] but the number of crosslinks between collagen strands increases.

The realigned, highly cross-linked collagen is much stronger than the collagen produced during the earlier phases of healing. The result is a steady, gradual growth in wound tensile strength that continues for 6 to 12 months after wounding [see Figure 2]. Scar tissue never reaches the tensile strength of unwounded tissue, however. The rate of gain in tensile strength begins to plateau at 6 weeks after injury. The common clinical recommendation that patients avoid heavy lifting or straining for 6 weeks after laparotomy, hernia repair, or many orthopedic procedures is based on the time required for increased tensile strength.

Role of Cytokines in Wound Healing

Wounding stimulates specific cellular activities in a consistent manner that is reproducible from wound to wound. It is becoming increasingly apparent that many, if not all, of these cellular activities are mediated by cytokines. The predictability with which cellular activities start and stop after wounding suggests that the cytokines mediating them are released in a closely regulated fashion; however, the details of this process have not yet been elucidated.

Numerous cytokines are known to be capable of mediating the major biologic activities involved in wound healing [see Table 4]. Most of these activities can be mediated by more than one factor, and researchers have not yet been able to determine which factors are the most important stimulants of wound-healing functions in vivo. One possible explanation for the duplication in mediating functions is that factors with similar activities may act at different times in the course of the wound-healing process.

Cytokines are produced by platelets, macrophages, lymphocytes, endothelial cells, epithelial cells, and smooth muscle cells [see Table 5]. Some cytokines, such as PDGF, are produced by several cell types,[135-138] whereas others, such as interleukin-2 (IL-2), are produced by only one cell type.[139,140] The cell of origin is a key variable that determines the time at which a factor will be present after wounding. Platelets, for example, release PDGF,[135] TGF-β,[141] and epidermal growth factor (EGF),[142] and it would be expected that these cytokines would be found in a wound soon after injury. Factors produced by several different cell types may be released by individual cell types at different times. For example, PDGF[136,137] and TGF-β,[143] which are produced by both platelets and macrophages, might be released by platelets soon after wounding and by macrophages at a later stage in the healing process.

The names of cytokines are frequently misleading. In many cases, they derive from the first known cell of origin or from the first function discovered (or hypothesized) for the factor. As a result, a polyfunctional factor may have a name implying that it has only one function, a factor produced by multiple cell types may have a name suggesting that it is produced by a single cell type, or a factor's name may lay claim to a capability that the factor does not have. For example, TGF-β received its name because it was originally believed to be capable of transforming normal cells into malignant ones. Although it is now known that TGF-β does not have this capability, the name has not been altered.

Cytokines are also a promising tool in the biologic modification of the wound-healing process. Early experimental work was done with small quantities of factors extracted from biologic sources

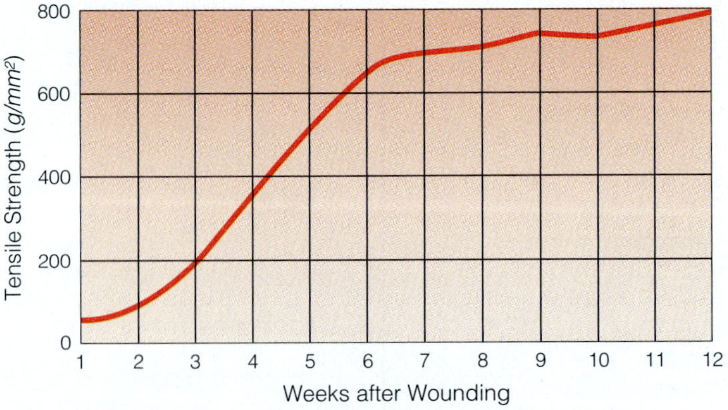

Figure 2 The tensile strength of skin wounds begins to increase gradually about 3 weeks after wounding. The collagen elaborated early in the healing process is replaced by stronger collagen that is aligned along the lines of stress in the tissue. Closer bonding and a greater number of cross-links between fibers augment the wound's tensile strength. The process of collagen replacement and scar remodeling continues for years.[236]

(e.g., platelets). More recently, recombinant technology has provided large quantities of highly purified material that can be used clinically. It has been experimentally demonstrated that many of the cytokines are capable of accelerating wound healing in normal and healing-impaired models. TGF-β has markedly increased wound-breaking strength in incisional wounds in rats soon after wounding.[144] bFGF or FGF2 has increased the strength of incisional wounds when injected on day 3 after wounding.[145] EGF has accelerated the closure of partial-thickness wounds in pigs when applied topically,[146] and it has accelerated collagen accumulation in a wound chamber model.[147] PDGF has accelerated healing in incisional wounds in rats when administered in a slow-release vehicle at the time of wounding.[148] Cytokines have also been observed to reverse healing deficits produced by diabetes,[149] steroids,[150] doxorubicin,[151] and radiation[152] in experimental models.

The positive results of these experimental studies encouraged the use of cytokines in clinical trials in humans. In an early human study, EGF accelerated the healing of skin graft donor sites.[153] In another study, it was applied topically to chronic nonhealing wounds in an uncontrolled group of patients and was considered to contribute to improved healing in the majority.[154] Autogenous platelet extracts have been used on chronic nonhealing wounds as well, with good results.[155] In a better-controlled study, recombinant human PDGF-bb accelerated healing when applied topically to pressure sores in a randomized, double-blind, placebo-controlled fashion.[156] In another carefully controlled, randomized, prospective study, bFGF was also demonstrated to be efficacious as a topical wound-healing supplement for pressure sores.[157] PDGF-bb has been demonstrated to be efficacious and has been approved for use on diabetic ulcers.[158] It is being marketed as Regranex.

It is not known which factors will be most effective as healing adjuvants in either normal or impaired healing states. It would seem logical that addition of a combination of factors in a sequence mimicking that characteristic of normal healing would produce optimal effects when healing is unimpaired. When healing is impaired, it would seem logical to augment the quantity of whatever factors are lacking or present at reduced levels. However, much work remains to be done—first, to determine which factors are most critical in normal states and, second, to determine which factors are lacking in impaired states so that the best use can be made of the recombinant factors now available.

Physiology of Skin Graft Healing

Although the physiology of skin graft healing is similar to that of open wound healing, differences arise because the wound is covered by the graft and because the graft has its own intrinsic architectural nature. Initially, fibrin holds the graft on the recipient site. The strength of attachment increases rapidly for the first 8 hours after graft placement, after which the rate of increase tapers off slightly.[159] For the first 48 hours, the graft survives by serum imbibition[160]: plasmalike fluid is absorbed by the graft, which increases in weight by up to 30% during this period. The absorbed fluid supports only minimal metabolic activities and maintains cellular viability until revascularization occurs. After approximately 48 hours, new blood vessels begin to grow into the graft from the recipient site.[161] It is not known whether a new vascular network grows within the graft or whether vessels from the recipient site simply connect with existing vessels in the graft. Skin graft revascularization probably involves a combination of these two processes.[162] Blood flow in the graft reaches nearly normal levels approximately 7 days after grafting. The vascular system continues to mature, with smaller vessels merging into larger ones. By 21 days after grafting, the graft's vascular supply appears nearly normal on dye injection studies.[161]

Lymphatic channels begin to develop 4 to 5 days after grafting, and the lymphatic system gradually matures until it, too, is nearly normal after 21 days.[163] Epithelial cells and fibroblasts remain dormant for 3 days after placement of a skin graft and subsequently proliferate.[164] The epithelium remains hyperplastic for 6 weeks.[165] By 7 to 8 days after grafting, fibroblasts are more plentiful in the graft than in the surrounding skin, and new collagen is being synthesized.[164,165] Collagenolytic activity develops simultaneously and actually exceeds collagen synthesis for 2 weeks, leading to a net loss in graft collagen. However, during the third week after grafting, the net amount of collagen starts to increase as the rate of collagen synthesis begins to exceed the rate of collagenolysis. Active collagen synthesis continues for at least 20 weeks.[95]

Disturbances of Wound Healing

Healing does not always occur in a straightforward, undisturbed fashion. Both local and systemic factors can interfere with healing. Local factors include infection, foreign bodies, tissue hypoxia, venous insufficiency, local toxins, mechanical trauma, irradiation, and cigarette smoking. Systemic factors include malnutrition, cancer, diabetes mellitus, uremia, jaundice, old age, corticosteroids, chemotherapeutic agents, and alcoholism. Several of these local and systemic factors [see Table 6] will be discussed in more detail.

LOCAL FACTORS

Infection

The body maintains a symbiotic relationship with bacteria. Normal dry skin contains up to 1,000 bacteria/g,[4] and saliva contains 100 million bacteria/ml.[166] The bacterial population is kept in control by several mechanisms. Invasion is mechanically limited by an intact stratum corneum in the skin and intact oral mucosa.[5] Sebaceous secretions contain bactericidal and fungicidal fatty acids that modulate bacterial proliferation.[167] Edema dilutes these fatty acids, making edematous areas more infection prone. Lysozymes in skin hydrolyze bacterial cell membranes, further limiting bacterial proliferation.[168] The immune system augments local barriers to infection.

Infection occurs when the number or virulence of bacteria exceeds the ability of local tissue defenses to control them. Generally, as mentioned, infection exists when bacteria have proliferated to levels beyond 10^5 organisms/g tissue. At this level, bacteria overwhelm host defenses and proliferate in an uncontrolled fashion. This number has been defined by studies performed at the United States Army Institute of Surgical Research and elsewhere.[19,169-171] Local factors such as impaired circulation or radiation injury increase the

Table 6 Factors Impairing Wound Healing

Local	Systemic
Infection	Malnutrition
Foreign bodies	Cancer
Ischemia/hypoxia	Diabetes mellitus
Venous insufficiency	Uremia
Toxins (e.g., spider venom)	Jaundice
Previous trauma	Old age
Radiation	Systemic corticosteroids
Cigarette smoking	Chemotherapeutic agents
	Alcoholism

risk of infection. Systemic diseases such as diabetes, AIDS, uremia, and cancer also increase the susceptibility to wound infection.

Hypoxia and Smoking

Delivery of oxygen to healing tissues is critical for prompt wound repair. Oxygen is necessary for cellular respiration as well as for hydroxylation of proline and lysine residues. Adequate tissue oxygenation requires an adequate circulating blood volume,[172] adequate cardiac function, and adequate local vasculature. Vascular disorders may be systemic, as in peripheral vascular disease, or localized, caused by scarring from trauma or prior surgery. Wound healing in ischemic extremities is directly correlated with transcutaneous oxygen tension.[173] Hyperbaric oxygen has been used in the treatment of many types of wounds in which tissue hypoxia may impair healing. Anemia, however, is not associated with impaired healing unless the anemia is severe enough to limit circulating blood volume.[174]

Smoking can impair tissue oxygenation. Smoking stimulates vasoconstriction acutely and contributes to the development of atherosclerosis and vascular disease over time.[175-177] Approximately 3% to 6% of cigarette smoke is carbon monoxide, which binds to hemoglobin, producing carboxyhemoglobin. Smokers have carboxyhemoglobin levels between 1% and 20%.[178] Carboxyhemoglobin limits the oxygen-carrying capacity of the blood, increases platelet adhesives,[179] and produces endothelial changes.[180,181]

Irradiation

Irradiation damages the DNA of cells in exposed areas. Some cells die, while others are rendered incapable of undergoing mitosis. When radiation is administered therapeutically, doses are fractionated and tangential fields are used to limit damage to normal cells while maximizing damage to tumor cells. Despite such techniques, normal cells are damaged by irradiation.

Radiation therapy initially produces inflammation and desquamation in a dose-dependent fashion.[182] After a course of irradiation, healing ensues if surrounding normal tissues have not been irreparably damaged. Additional cells must migrate into the treated area for adequate healing to occur. Fibroblasts migrating into irradiated tissue are often abnormal because of irradiation. These cells are characterized by multiple vacuoles, irregular rough endoplasmic reticulum, degenerating mitochondria, and cytoplasmic crystalline inclusion bodies. Increased levels of inflammatory mediators contribute to an abnormal healing response. Collagen is synthesized to an abnormal degree in irradiated tissue, causing characteristic fibrosis. The media of dermal blood vessels in irradiated areas thickens and some blood vessels become occluded, resulting in a decrease in the total number of blood vessels. Superficial telangiectasias may be seen. The epidermis becomes thinned, and changes in pigmentation often develop. Irradiated skin is dry because of damage to sebaceous and sweat glands, and it has little hair. The epidermal basement membrane is abnormal, and nuclear atypia is common in keratinocytes.

Abnormal healing is predictable after wounding of previously irradiated tissue. Decreased vascularity and increased fibrosis limit the ability of platelets and inflammatory cells to gain access to wounds in the area. The quantity of cytokines released is therefore limited in wounds in irradiated tissue. This relative cytokine deficiency causes impairment of virtually all cellular aspects of healing. Damaged fibroblasts and keratinocytes in the area may not respond normally to wound-healing stimulants. In addition, irradiated tissue is predisposed to infection, which can further slow the healing process.

Clinically, impaired healing is manifest by a higher rate of complications when an operation is performed on irradiated tissue.[183] Vitamin A has been used to reverse the healing impairment caused by radiation therapy.[184] Difficult wounds in irradiated tissue can often be managed surgically by bringing a new blood supply to the area with flaps from nonirradiated areas.

SYSTEMIC FACTORS

Malnutrition

Adequate amounts of protein, carbohydrates, fatty acids, vitamins, and other nutrients are required for wounds to heal. Malnutrition frequently contributes to suboptimal healing.[185] In experimental studies,[186] a loss of 15% to 20% of lean body mass has been associated with a decrease in wound-breaking strength and a decrease in colonic bursting pressure. Hypoproteinemia inhibits proper wound healing by limiting the supply of critical amino acids required for synthesis of collagen and other proteins. Collagen synthesis essentially stops in the absence of protein intake,[187] resulting in impaired healing.[188,189] Arginine and glutamine appear to be particularly important amino acids. Cystine residues are found along the nonhelical peptide chain associated with procollagen; in the absence of these cystine residues, proper alignment of peptide chains into a triple helix is inhibited.[190]

Carbohydrates and fats provide energy for healing, and wound healing slows when carbohydrate or fat stores are limited. As an alternative energy source, protein is broken down instead of contributing primarily to tissue growth.[191] Fatty acids are also vital components of cell membranes.

Several vitamins are essential for normal healing. As mentioned, vitamin C is a necessary cofactor for hydroxylation of lysine and proline during collagen synthesis. The ability of fibroblasts to produce new, strongly cross-linked collagen is diminished if vitamin C is deficient. Clinically, existing scars dissolve because collagenolytic activity continues without adequate compensatory collagen synthesis, and new wounds fail to heal. Vitamin C deficiency is also associated with impaired resistance to infection.[192] Because vitamin A is essential for normal epithelialization, proteoglycan synthesis, and normal immune function,[192-194] healing is impaired when vitamin A is deficient. Thiamine deficiency has also been associated with impaired healing.[195] Vitamin D, required for normal calcium metabolism, is needed for bone healing. Exogenous vitamin E impairs wound healing in rats, most likely by influencing the inflammatory response in a corticosteroid-like manner.[196]

The minerals necessary for normal healing include the trace element zinc, a necessary cofactor for DNA polymerase and reverse transcriptase. Because zinc deficiency can result in an inhibition of cellular proliferation and deficient granulation tissue formation[197] and healing,[198] zinc replacement should be given if a deficiency is diagnosed. Pharmacologic overdosing with zinc does not accelerate wound healing and can have detrimental effects.[198]

Correction of generalized malnutrition requires refeeding. The amount of food ingested in the immediate preoperative period may have a greater influence than the overall degree of malnutrition, possibly by inducing positive nitrogen balance.[199] A prospective, randomized study of patients undergoing total parenteral nutrition prior to surgery demonstrated a significant reduction in postoperative morbidity and mortality.[200]

Cancer

Impaired wound healing associated with cancer has been demonstrated experimentally[201] and is often noted clinically. Cancer-bearing hosts may have impaired healing for a variety of reasons. Cancer-induced cachexia, manifest as weight loss, anorexia, and asthenia, significantly limits healing. Cachexia is a result of either decreased caloric intake, increased energy expenditure, or both.

Decreased oral intake may be due to anorexia or mechanical factors. Anorexia is mediated through as yet imperfectly defined circulating factors. Changes in taste perception, hypothalamic function, and tryptophan metabolism may contribute to anorexia. Tumors in the gastrointestinal tract can produce obstruction and generate fistulae that limit nutrient absorption. Other cancers generate peptides such as gastrin and vasoactive intestinal polypeptide (VIP) that alter transit times and interfere with absorption of nutrients.

Cancers alter host metabolism in dysfunctional ways as well. Glucose turnover may be increased, sometimes leading to glucose intolerance. The effect of increased glucose use is higher energy needs.[202] Protein catabolism may be accelerated. Protein breakdown in muscle is increased, as is hepatic utilization of amino acids. Such changes in protein metabolism produce a net loss of plasma protein. Unlike malnourished patients, cancer patients may not be able to alter their metabolism to rely on fat for most energy needs. In tumor-bearing animals, fat accumulates, while other, more vital tissues are broken down for energy. In addition, vitamin C may be taken up preferentially by some tumors, limiting availability of the vitamin for hydroxylation of proline and lysine moieties in collagen. All of these metabolic changes contribute to a negative energy balance and inefficient energy use.

Cancer patients may be relatively anergic, most likely because of abnormal inflammatory cell activity. Macrophages do not migrate or function normally in cancer patients. Inflammatory cell dysfunction may limit the availability of cytokines required for healing and may also predispose to infection.

Impaired healing must be anticipated in cancer patients because of the many alterations in metabolism and immune function. It has been suggested that vitamin A can improve healing in tumor-bearing mice,[203] but this effect has not been demonstrated in humans.

Old Age

The elderly heal less efficiently than younger persons. DuNuoy and Carrell,[204] who studied patients injured during World War I, demonstrated that wounds in 20-year-old patients contracted more rapidly than those in 30-year-old patients. In a blister epithelialization model,[205] younger patients also healed more rapidly than older patients. Another study[206] found that wound disruption occurred with less force in the elderly.

Diabetes

Diabetes mellitus is also associated with impaired healing. In a prospective study of 23,649 surgical wounds,[207] the risk of infection was five times greater in diabetic patients than in nondiabetic patients. This impairment has been demonstrated experimentally in several models.[208-210] A major contributor to this phenomenon is the impaired inflammatory response associated with hyperglycemia. Diabetes is associated with impaired granulocyte chemotaxis,[211] phagocytic function,[212-214] and humoral and cellular immunity. In addition, diabetes is associated with a microangiopathy that can limit blood supply to the healing wound, particularly in older diabetic patients.[215] Diabetic neuropathy impairs sensation, classically in a stocking or glove nerve distribution in extremities. Although this neuropathy does not limit healing directly, it can diminish an individual's ability to protect himself or herself from trauma. The diabetes-induced impairment in healing may be reduced by tight control of blood sugar levels with insulin.[216-218]

Uremia

Uremia has been associated with impaired healing, partially as a direct effect of urea and partially as the result of coexisting malnutrition. This healing impairment has been demonstrated experimentally in both incisional skin wounds and intestinal anastomoses in rats[219] and in an implantable Gore-Tex wound-healing model in humans.[220] This impairment may be ameliorated by regular dialysis.

Alcoholism

In mice chronically fed alcohol, cellular ingrowth and collagen accumulation were diminished in a sponge model.[221]

Steroids and Immunosuppression

Adrenocortical steroids inhibit all aspects of healing. In incisional wounds, steroids slow the development of breaking strength[222]; in open wounds healing secondarily, they impede wound contraction[223,224] and epithelialization.

This impaired healing results from derangements in cellular function induced by steroids. A primary feature of wounds in steroid-treated individuals is a deficiency in inflammatory cell function. As discussed, inflammatory cells, particularly macrophages, mediate essentially all aspects of healing through cytokines. By diminishing the supply of cytokines, steroids and other immunosuppressive agents profoundly impair all aspects of healing. Macrophage migration, fibroblast proliferation, collagen accumulation, and angiogenesis are among the processes diminished by steroid administration. Sandberg[225] demonstrated that the effects of steroids on healing are most pronounced when the drug is administered several days before or after wounding.

All aspects of steroid-induced healing impairment other than wound contraction can be reversed by supplemental vitamin A. The recommended dose is 25,000 IU/day. Topical vitamin A has also been found effective for open wounds.[226] Anabolic steroids and growth hormone–releasing factor have also reversed steroid-induced healing impairments.

Chemotherapeutic Agents

Chemotherapeutic agents impair healing primarily through inhibition of cellular proliferation. Many agents have been examined in experimental models, and virtually all agents impair healing.[227] Nitrogen mustard, cyclophosphamide, methotrexate, BCNU (carmustine), and doxorubicin are the most damaging to the healing process. Most chemotherapeutic regimens use a combination of agents, compounding their deleterious effects. Clinical trials with chemotherapeutic agents have not been associated with as high an incidence of complications as might be anticipated from experimental evidence. The timing of drug administration as well as the doses utilized may explain this apparent contradiction. Doxorubicin, for example, is a more potent inhibitor of wound healing when delivered preoperatively than postoperatively.[228]

Jaundice and Liver Failure

Liver dysfunction most likely impairs healing through the direct effect of hyperbilirubinemia and through metabolic impairments, such as hypoalbuminemia and hypoprothrombinemia, that develop when the synthetic functions of the liver are impaired. The effect of obstructive jaundice on wound healing has been examined experimentally by several investigators. Bayer and Ellis[229] demonstrated decreased wound-breaking strength in abdominal wounds in rats with obstructive jaundice. In jaundiced animals with gastric wounds, angiogenesis was subjectively diminished, but wound-breaking strength was normal. Arnaud and coworkers[230] demonstrated impaired healing with obstructive jaundice,[230] but Greaney and associates[231] could not duplicate their results in a similar model. Greaney did show diminished collagen accumulation, however, in the wounds of jaundiced animals. In humans, Ellis and Heddle[232] noted an increased incidence of wound dehiscence and hernias in patients undergoing surgery for relief of obstructive jaundice,[232] although others have disagreed.

Clinicians must be aware of both local and systemic factors that can influence healing in an individual patient and take appropriate measures, whenever possible, to improve chances for optimal healing.

HYPERTROPHIC SCARS AND KELOIDS

The events involved in normal healing begin and end in a controlled fashion, producing flat, unobtrusive scars. Healing is a biologic process, and as with all biologic processes, it may occur to a greater or lesser degree. Disturbances that diminish healing have already been discussed. Excessive healing can result in a raised, thickened scar with both functional and cosmetic complications. If the scar is confined to the margins of the original wound, it is called a hypertrophic scar.[233] Keloids extend beyond the confines of the original injury, so that the original wound often can no longer be distinguished.

Certain patients and certain wounds are at higher risk for abnormal scarring. Dark-skinned persons and patients between the ages of 2 and 40 are at higher risk for the development of hypertrophic scars or keloids. Wounds in the presternal or deltoid area, wounds that cross skin tension lines, and wounds in thicker skin have a greater tendency to heal with a thickened scar. Some parts of the body, such as the genitalia, the eyelids, the palms of the hands, and the soles of the feet, almost never develop abnormal scars.

Certain patient and wound characteristics increase the relative likelihood of developing a hypertrophic scar as opposed to a keloid.[234] Keloids are more likely than hypertrophic scars to be familial. Hypertrophic scars are more likely to be seen in light-skinned people, though both occur more frequently in dark-skinned people. Hypertrophic scars generally develop soon after injury, whereas keloids may develop up to a year after an injury. Hypertrophic scars may subside in time, whereas keloids rarely do. Hypertrophic scars are more likely to be associated with a contracture across a joint surface.

Keloids and hypertrophic scars result from a net increase in the quantity of collagen synthesized by fibroblasts in the wound area. Recent evidence has suggested that the fibroblasts within keloids are different in terms of their biologic responsiveness from those within normal dermis. Although many theories have been suggested, the etiology of keloids and hypertrophic scars is unknown. Treatment of hypertrophic scars and keloids has included surgical excision, steroid injection, pressure garments, topical Silastic gel, radiation therapy, and combinations of these approaches. The absence of a uniform treatment program accurately suggests that no specific treatment is predictably effective for these lesions.[235]

Conclusion

Acute wound care is organized to achieve a closed wound that heals without complications. The first decision to make about an acute wound is when to close it. A wound should be closed as soon as necrotic tissue and foreign material have been debrided, hemorrhage has ceased, and bacterial contamination has been controlled. Less severe wounds may be allowed to heal secondarily without formal closure. The next decision to make about the wound is how to close it. Direct wound approximation is preferred whenever it can be accomplished without excessive tension or distortion of surrounding tissues. If direct wound approximation is not possible, a skin graft may be used unless there is significant denuded bone, cartilage, tendon, or nerve or unless the wound requires closure with tissue that has specific characteristics available only with a flap. When a flap is indicated, local flaps are preferred if possible. In certain cases, distant flaps are necessary to obtain appropriate functional or aesthetic results [see 67 Plastic Surgical Reconstruction]. Regardless of the method chosen for closure, careful consideration must be given to the biology of wound healing to produce a durable, healed wound with the least possible apparent scar formation.

References

1. Committee on Trauma, American College of Surgeons: Early Care of the Injured Patient, 3rd ed. Walt AJ, Peltier LF, Pruitt BA Jr, et al, Eds. WB Saunders Co, Philadelphia, 1982, p 69
2. Grossman JAI, Adams JP, Kunec J: Prophylactic antibiotics in simple hand lacerations. JAMA 245: 1055, 1981
3. Committee on Trauma, American College of Surgeons: A Guide to Prophylaxis against Tetanus in Wound Management, 1984 Revision. The American College of Surgeons, Chicago, 1984
4. Peeples C, Bowick JA Jr, Scott FA: Wounds of the hand contaminated by human or animal saliva. J Trauma 20:383, 1980
5. Edlich RF, Rodeheaver GT, Morgan RF, et al: Principles of emergency wound management. Ann Emerg Med 17:1284, 1988
6. Cummings P: Antibodies to prevent infection in patients with dog bite wounds: a meta-analysis of randomized trials. Ann Emerg Med 23:536, 1994
7. Zitelli JA: Wound healing by secondary intention: a cosmetic appraisal. J Am Acad Dermatol 9:407, 1983
8. Krizek TJ, Davis JH: The role of the red cell in subcutaneous infection. J Trauma 5:85, 1965
9. Howe CW: Experimental studies on determinants of wound infection. Surg Gynecol Obstet 123:507, 1966
10. Elek SD: Experimental staphylococcal infections in the skin of man. Ann NY Acad Sci 65:85, 1956
11. Iverson PC: Surgical removal of traumatic tattoos of the face. Plast Reconstr Surg 2:427, 1947
12. Agris J: Traumatic tattooing. J Trauma 16:798, 1976
13. Gelberman RH, Posch JL, Jurist JM: High-pressure injection injuries of the hand. J Bone Joint Surg [Am] 57:935, 1975
14. Mrvos RM, Dean BS, Krenzelok EP: High pressure injection injuries: a serious occupational hazard. J Toxicol Clin Toxicol 25:297, 1987
15. Weltmer JB Jr, Pack LL: High-pressure water-gun injection injuries to the extremities: a report of six cases. J Bone Joint Surg [Am] 70:1221, 1988
16. Lammers RL: Soft tissue foreign bodies. Ann Emerg Med 17:1336, 1988
17. Myers MB: Prediction of skin sloughs at the time of operation with the use of fluorescein dye. Surgery 51:158, 1962
18. Hinshaw JR: Progressive changes in the depth of burns. Arch Surg 87:993, 1963
19. Teplitz C, Davis D, Mason AD, et al: Pseudomonas burn wound sepsis: I. Pathogenesis of experimental burn wound sepsis. J Surg Res 4:200, 1964
20. Shuck JM, Moncreif JA: The management of burns: I. General considerations and the Sulfamylon method. Current Problems in Surgery. Year Book Medical Publishers, Inc, Chicago, 1969
21. Robson MC, Heggers JP: Surgical infection: II. The beta-hemolytic streptococcus. J Surg Res 9:289, 1969
22. Hepburn HH: Delayed primary suture of wounds. Br Med J 1:181, 1919
23. Rodeheaver GT, Rye DR, Rust R, et al: Mechanisms by which proteolytic enzymes prolong the golden period of antibiotic action. Am J Surg 136: 379, 1978
24. Edlich RF, Smith OT, Edgerton MT: Resistance of the surgical wound to antimicrobial prophylaxis and its mechanism of development. Am J Surg 126:583, 1973
25. Robson MC, Duke WF, Krizek TJ: Rapid bacterial screening in the treatment of civilian wounds. J Surg Res 14:426, 1973
26. Kanthak FF, Dubrul EL: The immediate repair of war wound of the face. Plast Reconstr Surg 2:110, 1947
27. Ad Hoc Committee of the Committee on Trauma, Division of Medical Sciences, National Academy of Sciences–National Research Council: Postoperative wound infections: the influence of ultraviolet radiation of the operating room and of various other features. Ann Surg 160(suppl 1):1, 1964
28. Brook I: Human and animal bite infections. J Fam Pract 28:713, 1989
29. Fitzgerald RH Jr, Cooney WP III, Washington JA II, et al: Bacterial colonization of mutilating hand injuries and its treatment. J Hand Surg [Am] 2:85, 1977
30. Kucan JO, Robson MC, Heggers JP, et al: Comparison of silver sulfadiazine, povidone-iodine and

physiologic saline in the treatment of chronic pressure ulcers. J Am Geriatr Soc 24:232, 1981

31. Moncrief JA: Topical therapy for control of bacteria in the burn wound. World J Surg 2:151, 1978

32. Geronemus RG, Mertz PM, Eaglstein WH: Wound healing: the effects of topical antimicrobial agents. Arch Dermatol 115:1311, 1979

33. Robson MC, Edstrom LE, Krizek TJ, et al: The efficacy of systemic antibiotics in the treatment of granulating wounds. J Surg Res 16:299, 1974

34. Rodeheaver G, Edgerton MT, Elliott MB, et al: Proteolytic enzymes as adjuncts to antibiotic prophylaxis of surgical wounds. Am J Surg 127:564, 1974

35. Robson MC, Heggers JP: Delayed wound closure based on bacterial counts. J Surg Oncol 2:379, 1970

36. Heggers JP, Robson MC, Ristroph JD: A rapid method of performing quantitative wound cultures. Milit Med 134:666, 1969

37. McIlrath DC, van Heerden JA, Edis AJ, et al: Closure of abdominal incisions with subcutaneous catheters. Surgery 60:411, 1976

38. Zelko JR, Moore EE: Primary closure of the contaminated wound: closed suction wound catheter. Am J Surg 142:704, 1981

39. Cruise PJE, Foord R: The epidemiology of wound infection: a 10-year prospective study of 62,939 wounds. Surg Clin North Am 60:27, 1980

40. Klein M: Nondomestic mammalian bites. Am Fam Physician 32:137, 1985

41. Kurecki BA 3rd, Brownlee HJ Jr: Venomous snakebites in the United States. J Fam Pract 25:386, 1987

42. Sprenger TR, Bailey WJ: Snakebite treatment in the United States. Int J Dermatol 25:479, 1986

43. Pennell TC, Babu S-S, Meredith JW: The management of snake and spider bites in the southeastern United States. Am Surg 53:198, 1987

44. Lawrence WT, Giannopoulos A, Hansen A: Pit viper bites: rational management in locales in which copperheads and cottonmouths predominate. Ann Plast Surg 36:276, 1996

45. Rees RS, Altenbern P, Lynch JB, et al: Brown recluse spider bites: a comparison of early surgical excision versus dapsone and delayed surgical excision. Ann Surg 202:659, 1985

46. Siegel RJ, Vistnes LM, Iverson RE: Effective hemostasis with less epinephrine: an experimental and clinical study. Plast Reconstr Surg 51:129, 1973

47. Tran D-T, Miller SH, Buck DS, et al: Potentiation of infection by epinephrine. Plast Reconstr Surg 76:933, 1985

48. Klein JA: Tumescent technique for local anesthesia improves safety in large-volume liposuction. Plast Reconstr Surg 92:1085, 1993

49. Samdal F, Amland PF, Bugge JF: Plasma lidocaine levels during suction-assisted lipectomy using large doses of dilute lidocaine with epinephrine. Plast Reconstr Surg 93:1217, 1994

50. Arndt KA, Burton C, Noe JM: Minimizing the pain of local anesthesia. Plast Reconstr Surg 72:676, 1983

51. Christoph RA, Buchanan L, Begalla K, et al: Pain reduction in local anesthesia administration through pH buffering. Ann Emerg Med 17:117, 1988

52. Anderson AB, Colecchi C, Baronoski R, et al: Local anesthesia in pediatric patients: topical TAC versus lidocaine. Ann Emerg Med 19:519, 1990

53. Schilling CG, Bank DE, Borchert BA, et al: Tetracaine, epinephrine (adrenalin) and cocaine (TAC) versus lidocaine, epinephrine and tetracaine (LET) for anesthesia of lacerations in children. Ann Emerg Med 25:203, 1995

54. Lander J, Hodgins M, Nazarali S, et al: Determinants of success and failure of EMLA. Pain 64:89, 1996

55. Alexander JW, Fischer JE, Boyajian M, et al: The influence of hair-removal methods on wound infections. Arch Surg 118:347, 1983

56. Madden H, Edlich RF, Schauerhamer R, et al: Application of principles of fluid dynamics to surgical wound irrigation. Current Topics in Surgical Research 3:85, 1971

57. Gross A, Cutright DE, Bhaskar SN: Effectiveness of pulsating water jet lavage in treatment of contaminated crushed wounds. Am J Surg 124:373, 1972

58. Hamer ML, Robson MC, Krizek TJ, et al: Quantitative bacterial analysis of comparative wound irrigations. Ann Surg 181:819, 1975

59. Schauerhamer RA, Edlich RF, Panek P, et al: Studies in the management of the contaminated wound: VII. Susceptibility of surgical wounds to postoperative surface contamination. Am J Surg 122:74, 1971

60. Branemark PI, Albrektsson B, Lindstrom J, et al: Local tissue effects of wound disinfectants. Acta Chir Scand 357(suppl):166, 1966

61. Rodeheaver GT, Smith SL, Thacker JG, et al: Mechanical cleansing of contaminated wounds with a surfactant. Am J Surg 129:241, 1975

62. Rodeheaver G, Turnbull V, Edgerton MT, et al: Pharmacokinetics of a new skin cleanser. Am J Surg 132:67, 1976

63. Dirschl DR, Wilson FC: Topical antibiotic irrigation in the prophylaxis of operative wound infections in orthopedic surgery. Ortho Clin North Am 22:419, 1991

64. Rodeheaver G, Bellamy W, Kody M, et al: Bactericidal activity and toxicity of iodine-containing solutions in wounds. Arch Surg 117:181, 1982

65. Custer J, Edlich RF, Prusak M, et al: Studies in the management of the contaminated wound: V. An assessment of the effectiveness of pHisoHex and betadine surgical scrub solutions. Am J Surg 121:572, 1971

66. Mobacken H, Wengstrom C: Interference with healing of rat skin incisions treated with chlorhexidine. Acta Derm Venereol (Stockh) 54:29, 1974

67. Saatman RA, Carlton WW, Hubben K, et al: A wound healing study of chlorhexidine digluconate in guinea pigs. Fundam Appl Toxicol 6:1, 1986

68. Branemark PI, Ekholm R: Tissue injury caused by wound disinfectants. J Bone Joint Surg [Am] 49:48, 1967

69. Kozol RA, Gillies C, Elgebaly SA: Effects of sodium hypochlorite (Dakin's solution) on cells of the wound module. Arch Surg 123:420, 1988

70. Lineaweaver W, Howard R, Soucy D, et al: Topical antimicrobial toxicity. Arch Surg 120:267, 1985

71. Rodeheaver G: Controversies in wound management. Wounds 1:19, 1989

72. Lowbury EJL, Lilly HA, Bull JP: Methods for disinfection of hands and operation sites. Br Med J 2:531, 1964

73. Saggers BA, Stewart GT: Polyvinyl-pyrrolidone-iodine: an assessment of antibacterial activity. J Hyg (Camb) 62:509, 1964

74. Haury B, Rodeheaver G, Vensko J, et al: Debridement: an essential component of traumatic wound care. Am J Surg 135:238, 1978

75. Ordman LJ, Gillman T: Studies in the healing of cutaneous wounds: II. The healing of epidermal, appendageal, and dermal injuries inflicted by suture needles and by suture material in the skin of pigs. Arch Surg 93:883, 1966

76. George TK, Simpson DC: Skin wound closure with staples in the accident and emergency department. J R Coll Surg Edinb 30:54, 1985

77. Golden T: Non-irritating, multipurpose surgical adhesive tape. Am J Surg 100:789, 1960

78. Golden T, Levy AH, O'Connor WT: Primary healing of skin wounds and incisions with a threadless suture. Am J Surg 104:603, 1962

79. Conolly WB, Hunt TK, Zederfeldt B, et al: Clinical comparison of surgical wounds closed by suture and adhesive tapes. Am J Surg 117:318, 1969

80. Edlich RF, Prusak M, Panek P, et al: Studies in the management of the contaminated wound: VIII. Assessment of tissue adhesives for repair of contaminated tissue. Am J Surg 122:394, 1971

81. Mizrahi S, Bicke A, Ben-Layisfh E: Use of tissue adhesives in the repair of lacerations in children. J Ped Surg 23:312, 1988

82. Yaron M, Halperin M, Huffler W, et al: Efficacy of tissue glue for laceration repair in an animal model. Acad Emerg Med 2:259, 1995

83. Quinn J, Wells G, Sutcliffe T, et al: A randomized trial comparing octylcyanoacrylate tissue adhesive and sutures in the management of lacerations. JAMA 277:1527, 1997

84. Saltz R, Sierra D, Feldman D, et al: Experimental and clinical applications of fibrin glue. Plast Reconstr Surg 88:1005, 1991

85. Jabs AD Jr, Wider TM, DeBellis J, et al: The effect of fibrin glue on skin grafts in infected sites. Plast Reconstr Surg 89:268, 1992

86. Mandel MA: Minimal suture blepharoplasty: closure of incisions with autologous fibrin glue. Aesthetic Plast Surg 16:269, 1992

87. Ersek RA, Schade K: Subcutaneous pseudobursa secondary to suction and surgery. Plast Reconstr Surg 85:442, 1991

88. Ferguson DJ: Clinical application of experimental relations between technique and wound infection. Surgery 63:377, 1968

89. DeHoll D, Rodeheaver G, Edgerton MT, et al: Potentiation of infection by suture closure of dead space. Am J Surg 127:716, 1974

90. Magee C, Rodeheaver GT, Golden GT, et al: Potentiation of wound infection by surgical drains. Am J Surg 131:547, 1976

91. Taldych L, Donegan WL: Postmastectomy seroma and wound drainage. Surg Gynecol Obstet 165:483, 1987

92. Rudolph R: The effect of skin graft preparation on wound contraction. Surg Gynecol Obstet 142:49, 1976

93. Edgerton MT, Hansen FC: Matching facial color with split thickness skin grafts from adjacent areas. Plast Reconstr Surg 25:455, 1960

94. Krizek TJ, Robson MC, Kho E: Bacterial growth and skin graft survival. Forum on Fundamental Surgical Problems 18:518, 1967

95. Klein L, Rudolph R: 3 H-Collagen turnover in skin grafts. Surg Gynecol Obstet 135:49, 1972

96. Mir y Mir L: The problem of pigmentation in the cutaneous graft. Br J Plast Surg 14:303, 1961

97. Ponten B: Grafted skin—observations on innervation and other qualities. Acta Chir Scand 257(suppl):1, 1960

98. Baran NK, Horton CE: Growth of skin grafts, flaps, and scars in young minipigs. Plast Reconstr Surg 50:487, 1972

99. Gimbel NS, Farris W: Skin grafting: the influence of surface temperature on the epithelialization rate of split thickness skin donor sites. Arch Surg 92:554, 1966

100. Alvarez OM, Mertz PM, Eaglstein WH: The effect of occlusive dressings on collagen synthesis and re-epithelialization in superficial wounds. J Surg Res 35:142, 1983

101. Shuck JM, Pruitt BA, Moncrief JA: Homograft skin for wound coverage: a study of versatility. Arch Surg 98:472, 1969

102. Robson MC, Krizek TJ, Koss N, et al: Amniotic membranes as a temporary wound dressing. Surg Gynecol Obstet 136:904, 1973

103. Bromberg BE, Song IC, Mohn MP: The use of pig skin as a temporary biologic dressing. Plast Reconstr Surg 36:80, 1965

104. Woodruff EA: Biobrane, a biosynthetic skin prosthesis. Burn Wound Coverings. Wise DL, Ed. CRC Press, New York, 1984

105. Salomon JC, Diegelman RF, Cohen IK: Effect of dressings on donor site epithelialization. Forum on Fundamental Surgical Problems 25:516, 1974
106. Winter GD, Scales JT: Effect of air drying and dressings on the surface of a wound. Nature 197:91, 1963
107. Noe JM, Kalish S: The problem of adherence in dressed wounds. Surg Gynecol Obstet 147:185, 1978
108. Noe JM, Kalish S: Wound Care. Chesebrough Pond's, Greenwich, Connecticut, 1976
109. Varma AO, Bugatch E, German FM: Debridement of dermal ulcers with collagenase. Surg Gynecol Obstet 136:281, 1973
110. Noe JM, Kalish S: The mechanism of capillarity in surgical dressings. Surg Gynecol Obstet 143:454, 1976
111. Grinnell F, Billingham RE, Burgess L: Distribution of fibronectin during wound healing in vivo. J Invest Dermatol 76:181, 1981
112. Clark RAF, Folkvord JM, Wertz RL: Fibronectin as well as other extracellular matrix proteins mediate human keratinocyte adherence. J Invest Dermatol 84:378, 1985
113. Grinnell F: Fibronectin and wound healing. J Cell Biochem 25:107, 1984
114. Wysocki AB, Grinnell F: Fibronectin profiles in normal and chronic wound fluid. Lab Invest 63:825, 1990
115. Ley K: Leukocyte adhesion to vascular endothelium. J Reconstr Microsurg 8:495, 1992
116. Newman SL, Henson JE, Henson PM: Phagocytosis of senescent neutrophils by human monocyte-derived macrophages and rabbit inflammatory macrophages. J Exp Med 156:430, 1982
117. Proveddini DM, Deftos LJ, Manolagas SC: 1,25-Dihydroxyvitamin D3 promotes in vitro morphologic and enzymatic changes in normal human monocytes consistent with their differentiation into macrophages. Bone 7:23, 1986
118. Wright SD, Meyer BC: Fibronectin receptor of human macrophages recognizes sequence Arg-Gly-Asp-Ser. J Exp Med 162:762, 1985
119. Simpson DM, Ross R: Effects of heterologous antineutrophil serum in guinea pigs: hematologic and ultrastructural observations. Am J Pathol 65:79, 1971
120. Leibovich SJ, Ross R: The role of the macrophage in wound repair: a study with hydrocortisone and antimacrophage serum. Am J Pathol 78:71, 1975
121. Seppa H, Grotendorst G, Seppa S, et al: Platelet-derived growth factor is chemotactic for fibroblasts. J Cell Biol 92:584, 1982
122. Gauss-Miller V, Kleinman H, Martin GR, et al: Role of attachment factors and attractants in fibroblast chemotaxis. J Lab Clin Med 96:1071, 1980
123. Grotendorst GR, Chang T, Seppa HEJ, et al: Platelet-derived growth factor is a chemoattractant for vascular smooth muscle cells. J Cell Physiol 113:261, 1982
124. Stiles CF, Capone GT, Scher CD, et al: Dual control of cell growth by somatomedins and platelet-derived growth factor. Proc Natl Acad Sci USA 76:1279, 1979
125. Leibovich SJ, Ross R: A macrophage-dependent factor that stimulates the proliferation of fibroblasts in vitro. Am J Pathol 84:501, 1976
126. Thakral KK, Goodson WH III, Hunt TK: Stimulation of wound blood vessel growth by wound macrophages. J Surg Res 26:430, 1979
127. Knighton DR, Hunt TK, Thakral KK, et al: Role of platelets and fibrin in the healing sequence: an in vivo study of angiogenesis and collagen synthesis. Ann Surg 196:379, 1982
128. Van Winkle W Jr: The epithelium in wound healing. Surg Gynecol Obstet 127:1089, 1968
129. Cohen IK, Moore CD, Diegelman RF: Onset and localization of collagen synthesis during wound healing in open rat skin wounds. Proc Soc Exp Biol Med 160:458, 1979
130. Peacock EE Jr: Wound Repair, 3rd ed. WB Saunders Co, Philadelphia, 1984
131. Rudolph R, Guber S, Suzuki M, et al: The life cycle of the myofibroblast. Surg Gynecol Obstet 145:389, 1977
132. Madden JW, Peacock EE Jr: Studies on the biology of collagen during wound healing: III. Dynamic metabolism of scar collagen and remodelling of dermal wounds. Ann Surg 174:511, 1971
133. Forrester JC, Zederfeldt BH, Hayes TL, et al: Wolff's law in relation to the healing skin wound. J Trauma 10:770, 1970
134. Riley WB Jr, Peacock EE Jr: Identification, distribution and significance of a collagenolytic enzyme in human tissue. Proc Soc Biol Med 214:207, 1967
135. Witte LD, Kaplan KL, Nossel HL, et al: Studies of the release from human platelets of the growth factor for cultured human arterial smooth muscle cells. Circ Res 42:402, 1978
136. Martinet Y, Bitterman PB, Mornex JF, et al: Activated human monocytes express the c-sis proto-oncogene and release a mediator showing PDGF-like activity. Nature 319:158, 1986
137. Shimokado K, Raines EW, Madtes DK, et al: A significant part of macrophage-derived growth factor consists of at least two forms of PDGF. Cell 43:277, 1985
138. Walker LN, Bowen-Pope DF, Ross R, et al: Production of platelet-derived growth factor-like molecules by cultured arterial smooth muscle cells accompanies proliferation after arterial injury. Proc Natl Acad Sci USA 83:7311, 1986
139. Barbul A, Knud-Hansen J, Wasserkrug HL, et al: Interleukin 2 enhances wound healing in rats. J Surg Res 40:315, 1986
140. DeCunzo LP, MacKenzie JW, Marafino BJ Jr, et al: The effect of interleukin-2 administration on wound healing in Adriamycin-treated rats. J Surg Res 49:419, 1990
141. Assoian RK, Komoriya A, Meyers CA, et al: Transforming growth factor-β in human platelets: identification of a major storage site, purification, and characterization. J Biol Chem 258:7155, 1983
142. Pesonen K, Viinikka L, Myllyla G, et al: Characterization of material with epidermal growth factor immunoreactivity in human serum and platelets. J Clin Endocrinol Metab 68:486, 1989
143. Assoian RK, Fleurdelys BE, Stevenson HC, et al: Expression and secretion of type β transforming growth factor by activated human macrophages. Proc Natl Acad Sci USA 84:6020, 1987
144. Mustoe TA, Pierce GF, Thomason A, et al: Accelerated healing of incisional wounds in rats induced by transforming growth factor-β. Science 237:1333, 1987
145. McGee GS, Davidson JM, Buckley A, et al: Recombinant basic fibroblast growth factor accelerates wound healing. J Surg Res 45:145, 1988
146. Brown GL, Curtsinger L III, Brightwell JR, et al: Enhancement of epidermal regeneration by biosynthetic epidermal growth factor. J Exp Med 163:1319, 1986
147. Laato M, Niinikoski J, Lebel L, et al: Stimulation of wound healing by epidermal growth factor: a dose-dependent effect. Ann Surg 203:379, 1986
148. Pierce GF, Mustoe TA, Senior RM, et al: In vivo incisional wound healing augmented by platelet-derived growth factor and recombinant c-sis gene homodimeric proteins. J Exp Med 167:974, 1988
149. Tsuboi R, Rifkin DB: Recombinant basic fibroblast growth factor stimulates wound healing in healing-impaired db/db mice. J Exp Med 172:245, 1990
150. Pierce GF, Mustoe TA, Lingelbach J, et al: Transforming growth factor-β reverses the glucocorticoid-induced wound-healing deficit in rats: possible regulation in macrophages by platelet-derived growth factor. Proc Natl Acad Sci USA 86:2229, 1989
151. Curtsinger LJ, Pietsch JD, Brown GL, et al: Reversal of Adriamycin-impaired wound healing by transforming growth factor-beta. Surg Gynecol Obstet 168:517, 1989
152. Mustoe TA, Purdy J, Gramates P, et al: Reversal of impaired wound healing in irradiated rats by platelet-derived growth factor-BB. Am J Surg 158:345, 1989
153. Brown GL, Nanney LB, Griffen J, et al: Enhancement of wound healing by topical treatment with epidermal growth factor. N Engl J Med 321:76, 1989
154. Brown GL, Curtsinger L, Jurkiewicz MJ, et al: Stimulation of healing of chronic wounds by epidermal growth factor. Plast Reconstr Surg 88:189, 1991
155. Knighton DR, Ciresi K, Fiegel VD, et al: Stimulation of repair in chronic, nonhealing, cutaneous ulcers using platelet-derived wound healing formula. Surg Gynecol Obstet 170:56, 1990
156. Robson MC, Phillips LG, Thomason A, et al: Recombinant human platelet-derived growth factor-BB for the treatment of chronic pressure ulcers. Ann Plast Surg 29:193, 1992
157. Robson MC, Phillips LG, Lawrence WT, et al: The safety and effect of topically applied recombinant basic fibroblast growth factor on the healing of chronic pressure sores. Ann Surg 216:401, 1992
158. Steed DL, Diabetic Ulcer Study Group: Clinical evaluation of recombinant human platelet derived growth factor for the treatment of lower extremity diabetic ulcers. J Vasc Surg 21:71, 1995
159. Polk HC: Adherence of thin skin grafts. Forum on Fundamental Surgical Problems 17:487, 1966
160. Converse JM, Uhlschmid GK, Ballantyne DL Jr: "Plasmatic circulation" in skin grafts: the phase of serum imbibition. Plast Reconstr Surg 43:495, 1969
161. Marckmann A: Autologous skin grafts in the rat: vital microscopic studies of the microcirculation. Angiology 17:475, 1966
162. Smahel J: The healing of skin grafts. Clin Plast Surg 4:409, 1977
163. Psillakis JM: Lymphatic vascularization of skin grafts. Plast Reconstr Surg 43:287, 1969
164. Converse JM, Ballantyne DL: Distribution of diphosphopyridine nucleotide diaphorase in rat skin autografts and homografts. Plast Reconstr Surg 30:415, 1962
165. Hinshaw JR, Miller ER: Histology of healing split-thickness, full-thickness autogenous skin grafts and donor sites. Arch Surg 91:658, 1965
166. Kligman AM: The bacteriology of normal skin. Skin Bacteria and Their Role in Infection. Wolcott BW, Rund DA, Eds. McGraw-Hill, New York, 1965, p 13
167. Ricketts CR, Squire JR, Topley E: Human skin lipids with particular reference to the self sterilising power of the skin. Clin Sci 10:89, 1951
168. Heggers JP: Natural host defense mechanisms. Clin Plast Surg 6:505, 1979
169. Lindberg RB, Moncrief JA, Switzer WE, et al: The successful control of burn wound sepsis. J Trauma 5:601, 1965
170. Kass EH: Asymptomatic infections of the urinary tract. Trans Assoc Am Physicians 69:56, 1956
171. Bendy RH, Nuccio PA, Wolfe E, et al: Relationship of quantitative bacterial counts to healing of decubiti: effect of gentamycin. Antimicrob Agents Chemother 4:147, 1964
172. Hunt TK, Zederfeldt BH, Goldstick TK, et al: Tissue oxygen tensions during controlled hemorrhage. Surg Forum 18:3, 1967
173. Hauser CJ: Tissue salvage by mapping of skin transcutaneous oxygen tension index. Arch Surg 122:1128, 1987
174. Heughan C, Grislis G, Hunt TK: The effect of anemia on wound healing. Ann Surg 179:163, 1974

175. Roth GJ, McDonald JB, Sheard C: The effect of cigarettes and of intravenous injections of nicotine on the electrocardiogram, basal metabolic rate, cutaneous temperature, blood pressure, and pulse rate of normal persons. JAMA 125:761, 1944

176. Bruce JW, Miller JR, Hooker DR: The effect of smoking upon the blood pressures and upon the volume of the hand. Am J Physiol 24:104, 1909

177. Wright IS, Moffat D: The effects of tobacco on the peripheral vascular system. JAMA 103:315, 1934

178. Sackett DL, Gibson RW, Bross IDJ, et al: Relation between aortic atherosclerosis and the use of cigarettes and alcohol: an autopsy study. N Engl J Med 279:1413, 1968

179. Birnstingl MA, Brinson K, Chakrabarti R: The effect of short-term exposure to carbon monoxide on platelet stickiness. Br J Surg 58:837, 1971

180. Astrup P, Kjeldsen K: Carbon monoxide, smoking and atherosclerosis. Med Clin North Am 58:323, 1973

181. Kjeldsen K, Astrup P, Wanstrup J: Ultra-structural intimal changes in the rabbit aorta after a moderate carbon monoxide exposure. Atherosclerosis 16:67, 1972

182. Fajardo LF, Berthong M: Radiation injury in surgical pathology. Part III. Salivary glands, pancreas and skin. Am J Surg Pathol 5:279, 1981

183. Rudolph R: Complications of surgery for radiotherapy skin damage. Plast Reconstr Surg 70:179, 1982

184. Levenson SM, Gruber CA, Rettura G, et al: Supplemental vitamin A prevents the acute radiation-induced defect in wound healing. Ann Surg 200:494, 1984

185. Howes EL, Briggs H, Shea R, et al: Effect of complete and partial starvation on the rate of fibroplasia in the healing wound. Arch Surg 27:846, 1933

186. Ward MW, Danzi M, Lewin MR, et al: The effects of subclinical malnutrition and refeeding on the healing of experimental colonic anastomoses. Br J Surg 69:308, 1982

187. Haydock DA, Hill GL: Impaired wound healing in surgical patients with varying degrees of malnutrition. JPEN J Parenter Enteral Nutr 10:550, 1986

188. Thompson WD, Ravdin IS, Frank IL: Effect of hypoproteinemia on wound disruption. Arch Surg 36:500, 1938

189. Devereux DF, Thistlewaite PA, Thibault LF, et al: Effect of tumor bearing and protein depletion on wound breaking strength in the rat. J Surg Res 27:233, 1979

190. Williamson MB, Fromm HJ: Effect of cystine and methionine on healing of experimental wounds. Proc Soc Exp Biol Med 80:623, 1957

191. Levenson SM, Seifter E: Dysnutrition, wound healing, and resistance to infection. Clin Plast Surg 4:375, 1977

192. Freiman M, Seifter E, Connerton C, et al: Vitamin A deficiency and surgical stress. Surg Forum 21:81, 1970

193. Shapiro SS, Mott DJ: Modulation of glycosaminoglycan synthesis by retinoids. Ann NY Acad Sci 359:306, 1981

194. Cohen BE, Till G, Cullen PR, et al: Reversal of postoperative immunosuppression in man by vitamin A. Surg Gynecol Obstet 149:658, 1979

195. Alvarez OM, Gilbreath RL: Effect of dietary thiamine on intermolecular collagen crosslinking during wound repair: a mechanical and biochemical assessment. J Trauma 22:20, 1982

196. Ehrlich HP, Tarver H, Hunt TK: Inhibitory effects of vitamin E on collagen synthesis and wound repair. Ann Surg 175:235, 1972

197. Fernandez-Madrid F, Prasad AS, Oberleas D: Effect of zinc deficiency on nucleic acids, collagen, and noncollagenous protein of the connective tissue. J Lab Clin Med 82:951, 1973

198. Haley JV: Zinc sulfate and wound healing. J Surg Res 27:168, 1979

199. Windsor JA, Knight GS, Hill GL: Wound healing response in surgical patients: recent food intake is more important than nutritional status. Br J Surg 75:135, 1988

200. Muller JM, Brenner U, Dienst C, et al: Preoperative parenteral nutrition in patients with gastrointestinal carcinomas. Lancet 1:68, 1982

201. Lawrence WT, Norton JA, Harvey AK, et al: Wound healing in sarcoma-bearing rats: tumor effects on cutaneous and deep wounds. J Surg Oncol 35:7, 1987

202. Chlebowski RT, Heber D: Metabolic abnormalities in cancer patients: carbohydrate metabolism. Surg Clin North Am 66:957, 1986

203. Weingweg J, Levenson SM, Rettura G, et al: Supplemental vitamin A prevents the tumor-induced defect in wound healing. Ann Surg 211:269, 1990

204. DuNuoy P, Carrell A: Cicatrization of wounds. J Exp Biol 34:339, 1921

205. Grove GL: Age-related differences in healing of superficial skin wounds in humans. Arch Dermatol Res 272:381, 1982

206. Sandblom P, Peterson P, Muren A: Determination of the tensile strength of the healing wound as a clinical test. Acta Chir Scand 105:252, 1953

207. Cruse PJE, Foord RA: A prospective study of 23,649 surgical wounds. Arch Surg 107:206, 1973

208. Goodson WH, Hunt TK: Studies of wound healing in experimental diabetes mellitus. J Surg Res 22:221, 1977

209. Prakash A, Pandit PN, Sharma LK: Studies in wound healing in experimental diabetes. Int Surg 59:25, 1974

210. Arquilla ER, Weringer EJ, Nakajo M: Wound healing: a model for the study of diabetic microangiopathy. Diabetes 25(suppl 2):811, 1976

211. Mowat AG, Baum J: Chemotaxis of polymorphonuclear leukocytes from patients with diabetes mellitus. N Engl J Med 284:621, 1971

212. Bybee JD, Rogers DE: The phagocytic activity of polymorphonuclear leukocytes obtained from patients with diabetes mellitus. J Lab Clin Med 64:1, 1964

213. Nolan CM, Beaty HN, Bagdade JD: Further characterization of the impaired bactericidal function of granulocytes in patients with poorly controlled diabetes. Diabetes 27:889, 1978

214. Bagdade JD, Root RK, Bugler RJ: Impaired leukocyte function in patients with poorly controlled diabetes. Diabetes 23:9, 1974

215. Duncan HJ, Faris IB: Skin vascular resistance and skin perfusion pressure as predictors of healing of ischemic lesions of the lower limb: influences of diabetes mellitus, hypertension, and age. Surgery 99:432, 1986

216. Gottrup F, Andreassen TT: Healing of incisional wounds in stomach and duodenum: the influence of experimental diabetes. J Surg Res 31:61, 1981

217. Weringer EJ, Kelso JM, Tamai IY, et al: Effects of insulin on wound healing in diabetic mice. Acta Endocrinol 99:101, 1982

218. Yue DK, McLennan S, Marsh M, et al: Effects of experimental diabetes, uremia, and malnutrition on wound healing. Diabetes 36:295, 1987

219. Colin JF, Elliot P, Ellis H: The effect of uremia upon wound healing: an experimental study. Br J Surg 66:793, 1979

220. Goodson WH III, Lindenfield SM, Omachi RS, et al: Chronic uremia causes poor healing. Surg Forum 33:54, 1982

221. Benveniste K, Thut P: The effect of chronic alcoholism on wound healing. Proc Soc Exp Biol Med 166:568, 1981

222. Howes EL, Plotz CM, Blunt JW, et al: Retardation of wound healing by cortisone. Surgery 28:177, 1950

223. Hunt TK, Ehrlich HP, Garcia JA, et al: The effect of vitamin A on reversing the inhibitory effect of cortisone on the healing of open wounds in animals. Ann Surg 170:633, 1969

224. Stephens FO, Dunphy JE, Hunt TK: Effect of delayed administration of corticosteroids on wound contraction. Ann Surg 173:214, 1971

225. Sandberg N: Time relationship between administration of cortisone and wound healing in rats. Acta Clin Scand 127:446, 1964

226. Hunt TK, Ehrlich HP, Garcia JA, et al: Effects of vitamin A on reversing the inhibitory effects of cortisone on healing of open wounds in animals and man. Ann Surg 170:633, 1969

227. Shamberger RC, Devereux DF, Brennan MF: The effect of chemotherapeutic agents on wound healing. Int Adv Surg Oncol 4:15, 1981

228. Lawrence WT, Talbot TL, Norton JA: Preoperative or postoperative doxorubicin hydrochloride (Adriamycin): which is better for wound healing? Surgery 100:9, 1986

229. Bayer I, Ellis HL: Jaundice and wound healing: an experimental study. Br J Surg 63:392, 1976

230. Arnaud J-P, Humbert W, Eloy M-R, et al: Effect of obstructive jaundice on wound healing. Am J Surg 141:593, 1981

231. Greaney MG, Van Noort R, Smythe A, et al: Does obstructive jaundice adversely affect wound healing? Br J Surg 66:478, 1979

232. Ellis H, Heddle R: Does the peritoneum need to be closed at laparotomy? Br J Surg 64:733, 1977

233. Peacock EE Jr, Madden JW, Trier WC: Biologic basis for the treatment of keloids and hypertrophic scars. South Med J 63:755, 1970

234. Brody GS, Peng STJ, Landel RF: The etiology of hypertrophic scar contracture: another view. Plast Reconstr Surg 67:673, 1981

235. Lawrence WT: In search of the optimal treatment of keloids: report of a series and a review of the literature. Ann Plast Surg 27:164, 1991

236. Levenson SM, Greever EF, Crowley IV, et al: The healing of rat skin wounds. Ann Surg 161:293, 1965

Acknowledgments

Figure 1 Carol Donner.
Figure 2 Janet Betries.

9 COMA, SEIZURES, COGNITIVE IMPAIRMENT, AND BRAIN DEATH

Marike Zwienenberg, M.D., and J. Paul Muizelaar, M.D., Ph.D.

Management of the Patient with Altered Consciousness

Every clinician will at some point encounter a patient who is in an altered state of consciousness. Altered consciousness is not a disease per se but rather a symptom of some underlying process. It is variable in degree, ranging from mere confusion to deep coma.

Consciousness depends on both the reticular activating system (RAS), which is responsible for general alertness, and the cerebral cortex, which is responsible for the quality of behavior. The integrity of the cerebral hemispheres, the RAS, and the connections between them is essential for the maintenance of conscious behavior.

Coma is thought to result from a lesion to the hemispheres, the RAS, or both and may be caused by structural or toxic metabolic abnormalities. Specific causes of coma are numerous and include alcohol and drug intoxication, epilepsy, infection, uremia and other metabolic disorders, head injury, cerebral tumors, hypothermia, psychiatric disorders, and stroke and other vascular diseases. Accordingly, the management of coma is complex. In what follows, we discuss the various underlying causes of coma and provide general and specific guidelines.

Loss of consciousness associated with seizure activity is thought to result from a global disturbance of electrochemical activity that involves both hemispheres. Brain death represents the extreme end of the spectrum of altered consciousness and results when the loss of cerebral and brain-stem function is irreversible. Management of seizures and determination of brain death are discussed separately from management of coma.

Cognitive impairment is common in surgical patients, particularly in those who undergo major surgical procedures. The degree and nature of impairment are dependent on the underlying disease and the presence of precipitating factors, which may range from communication deficits, anxiety, and sleep deprivation to drug withdrawal, metabolic disturbances, and infection. Cornerstones of management include identification and alleviation of risk factors as well as recognition of frequent causes of cognitive impairment, such as delirium, depression, and dementia.

Often, little information is available about the circumstances leading to the disturbance in consciousness or about the patient's medical history. It is therefore essential that the surgeon follow a systematic management approach that quickly establishes the etiology and prevents unnecessary delay in initiating appropriate treatment.

Initial Management of the Comatose Patient

Initial management of the comatose patient is aimed at stabilization of the patient's condition and prevention of further central nervous system damage. The immediately occurring damage that is preventable results from cerebral hypoxia, ischemia, and low blood glucose levels. Therefore, initial evaluation and treatment of the comatose patient must be carried out simultaneously: the airway (A), breathing (B), and circulation (C) must be assessed and controlled, and hypoglycemia must be excluded or corrected. Attention should then be directed toward treatment of specific causes of coma, such as seizures, drug or alcohol overdose, head injury, or infection. Specific questions regarding medical history, recent changes in behavior, use of medications or drugs, recent trauma, and history of seizures must be asked so that the events leading to coma can be reconstructed. If the cause of coma remains elusive, the physical and neurologic examinations may yield clues that clarify the underlying etiology. In addition, laboratory tests and diagnostic imaging methods, such as computed tomography and magnetic resonance imaging, can provide important information for establishing a diagnosis and instituting proper treatment.

AIRWAY

To ensure adequate oxygenation and ventilation, the patient's airway must be cleared of all foreign material, the patency of the airway must be verified, and oxygen must be administered. The spontaneous rate and rhythm of respiration should be noted before they are obscured by therapeutic measures. The respiratory pattern is a good indicator of the depth of depression and the etiology of the coma [*see* Physical and Neurologic Examinations, *below*].

BREATHING

An oropharyngeal or nasopharyngeal airway may suffice in unresponsive patients who are breathing normally; however, endotracheal intubation is indicated in patients who are dyspneic, hypoventilating, or vomiting uncontrollably. Hyperventilation with a bag

Patient is in state of altered consciousness

Patient is in coma

Coma is defined as a sleeplike state of continuous unarousable unresponsiveness in which there is no spontaneous activity.

Ensure adequate ventilation and circulatory support. Obtain specimens for laboratory screening:
- CBC
- Serum electrolytes
- BUN
- Creatinine
- Glucose
- Liver function tests
- Osmolarity
- Toxic screen

Patient has seizure

Seizure is self-limited

Emergency treatment is not required.

Tonic-clonic seizure persists

Treat status epilepticus:
- Obtain quick history and perform physical examination while assistant draws blood and inserts venous line.
- Perform bedside blood glucose determination. If glucose < 60 mg/dl or not immediately available, infuse dextrose (50 ml of 50% solution for adults and 1–2 ml/kg of 25% solution for children).
- Give adult patients 100 mg thiamine I.V.
- Correct hyponatremia with 3% NaCl solution in slow I.V. infusion.
- Give calcium (1–2 ampules of calcium gluconate for 5–10 min) if necessary.

Administer anticonvulsants in the following sequence:
- Phenytoin
- Benzodiazepines
- Phenobarbital

Last resort: general anesthesia or pentobarbital-induced coma

Administer glucose and thiamine

Assess glucose level by bedside technique. If level is low or not immediately obtainable, give 50 mg of 50% glucose solution I.V. immediately. Before glucose administration, give 50–100 mg of thiamine I.V., followed by 100 mg I.M. daily for 3 days.

Manage intoxication

Provide early intubation and respiratory support; maintain normal BP. Perform gastric lavage if
- Ingestion occurred within 4 hr (or within 10 hr for salicylates), or
- Patient has been in shock, or
- Time of ingestion is not known.

Excretion of toxins can be facilitated with catharsis, diuresis, dialysis, or charcoal hemoperfusion. Give antidotes (if known).

Perform basic physical and neurologic examinations

Physical: Search for signs of trauma, systemic illness, infection, or drug ingestion.
Neurologic: Ascertain cause of coma and site of impairment. Differentiate between anatomic and structural lesions:
- Presence of lateralizing signs suggests structural lesion.
- Presence of pupillary light response is an important feature of metabolic coma, except in cases of drug ingestion or prolonged anoxia.
- Absence of pulillary response to light suggests structural lesion.
- Decorticate posturing suggests structural lesion; decerebrate rigidity may be caused by structural or metabolic coma (posturing has little diagnostic value after the acute phase of the coma).

If structural coma is suspected, the clinical diagnosis may be confirmed by appropriate imaging studies (CT or MRI).

Metabolic coma

Restore acid-base balance.
Restore electrolyte balance.
Restore normal body temperature.

Treat underlying conditions:
- Hypoxia
- Hypoglycemia or hyperglycemia
- Infection
- Overdose
- Specific disease process

Structural coma

Treat structural lesions. Determine severity of symptoms and rapidity of their evolution as soon as possible.
If patient is stable, obtain CT scan or MRI urgently: perform contrast study (CT or MRI) if structural lesion is suspected on the basis of noncontrast studies. If patient is deeply comatose or symptoms are evolving rapidly, treat elevated ICP urgently:
- Hyperventilate patient to P_aco_2 of 25–30 mm Hg.
- Give osmotic diuretics (e.g., 0.25–1.5 g/kg of 20% mannitol solution I.V.).
- If patient does not have severe intracranial hypertension, consider elevating head of bed 30°–50°.
- If patient does not respond to hyperventilation or mannitol, consider barbiturate administration or, if possible, ventriculostomy.

Other causes of coma and similar syndromes

Alternative causes of coma and coma-resembling states include hypothermia, psychiatric disorders, persistant vegetative states, and locked-in syndrome.
Treat causative conditions as appropriate.

Patient is cognitively impaired

Eliminate or mitigate known risk factors for cognitive impairment.

Institute general supportive measures and perioperative precautions.

Treat causative conditions:
- Delirium
- Dementia
- Depression
- Head injury
- Side effects of drugs

Patient is suspected of being brain-dead

Document the presence of a potential cause of brain death. CT suffices in most cases; perform CSF examination if a definite diagnosis cannot be made.

Rule out complicating medical conditions and drug intoxication or poisoning.

Ensure that core T° ≥ is 32° C.

Initial conditions for brain death are met

Test for three cardinal features of brain death.
- Coma or unresponsiveness
- Absence of brain-stem reflexes
- Apnea (via apnea test)

Order confirmatory tests if (1) clinical criteria cannot be evaluated reliably or (2) the country, locality, or institution requires such confirmation.

Initial conditions for brain death are not met

Reevaluate patient.

Management of the Patient with Altered Consciousness

and mask and 100% oxygen should be performed before intubation to ensure adequate oxygenation during the procedure. If there is any possibility of a cervical spine injury, intubation should be delayed until fracture can be ruled out radiographically. If, however, the patient's condition is such that delay is inadvisable, intubation should be done without manipulation of the spine. In patients with head injury who are at risk for basilar skull fractures, the oropharyngeal route is preferred for intubation. In these patients, an aggressive approach to early intubation is usually indicated because hypoxia aggravates brain injury. In the Traumatic Coma Data Bank study, mortality was almost twice as high among hypoxic patients as among nonhypoxic patients (50% versus 27%).[1] It should be noted, however, that hypoxia alone adds little to mortality; it is the combination of ischemia and hypoxia that appears to be responsible for the increase in mortality.

CIRCULATION

Because substrate delivery to the brain is dependent on the cardiovascular system, circulation must be vigorously supported. A large-bore I.V. or central venous catheter is inserted, and blood volume is replenished with fluids or volume expanders. Solutions that contain free water (e.g., 5% dextrose in water) should be avoided, particularly in patients with head injury, because they may exacerbate brain edema. Vasoactive agents are infused if necessary. An electrocardiographic monitor is placed, and cardiac rate and rhythm are recorded. When vasopressor therapy is instituted, insertion of a pulmonary catheter is recommended in elderly patients or in patients with current or past cardiopulmonary disease. In patients suffering from head injury, hypotension and shock rarely result from a cerebral lesion; their presence should alert the physician to seek a source of extracorporeal or intracorporeal hemorrhage. However, when hypertension is present in these patients, it should be left untreated because it is likely to be an adaptive response (i.e., part of the Cushing response) of the brain to the increase in intracranial pressure (ICP) [see 23 Injuries to the Central Nervous System].

LABORATORY SCREENING

As soon as the venous line is in place, blood specimens are obtained for laboratory screening. The following tests and measurements should be performed:

1. Complete blood count.
2. Serum electrolyte (Na, K, Cl, CO_2, Ca, PO_4) levels.
3. Blood urea nitrogen level.
4. Creatinine level.
5. Glucose level.
6. Liver function tests.
7. Osmolarity.
8. Toxic screen (including drugs and alcohol).

GLUCOSE ADMINISTRATION

Glucose is the basic substrate for cerebral metabolism. Even a transient decrease in oxidative metabolism of glucose may lead to an abrupt disruption of brain function. Blood glucose levels should be assessed by means of a rapid bedside technique and verified in the laboratory. If the bedside determination yields a low value (< 40 to 60 mg/dl) or cannot be done immediately, 50 mg of a 50% glucose solution is administered I.V., even if laboratory verification of the blood glucose level is not yet available. The risk of hypoglycemic cerebral damage outweighs the risk of temporary worsening of the rare case of hyperosmolar coma. Many patients admitted to the emergency ward while in coma are chronic alcoholics or malnourished and thus are prone to Wernicke encephalopathy, which is caused by thiamine deficiency and can be precipitated by a large glucose load. To prevent acute symptomatic thiamine deficiency, 50 to 100 mg of thiamine should be given I.V. to all patients before glucose is administered. Afterward, 100 mg is given I.M. every day for 3 days.

Physical and Neurologic Examinations

When the necessary resuscitative measures have been initiated, the next step is to perform basic physical and neurologic examinations. These examinations should be brief yet sufficiently thorough to yield the key information required for further evaluation and treatment. The physical examination should focus on signs of trauma, chronic disease (e.g., alcoholism or renal failure), infection, or self-administration of drugs. The neurologic examination should focus on diagnosing those conditions that call for rapid treatment, such as the following:

1. Lateralizing signs in trauma patients.
2. Signs of an increase in ICP.
3. Meningism.
4. Seizures.

LEVEL OF CONSCIOUSNESS

The patient's level of consciousness is assessed by means of the Glasgow Coma Scale (GCS), which is widely accepted as the standard method [see 23 Injuries to the Central Nervous System]. The GCS consists of three components: eye opening (E), motor function (M), and verbal response (V) [see Table 1]. The score on each component is assessed by recording the response of the patient to verbal or noxious stimuli, such as pressure on the supraorbital notch or compression of the distal interphalangeal joints; the total GCS score is the sum of the scores of these three components [see Table 1]. The maximum GCS score is 15, and the minimum score is 3. Coma is usually defined as a GCS score of 9 or less.

A persistent misconception about the GCS, which results from equating abnormal flexion with so-called decorticate rigidity and extensor response with so-called decerebrate rigidity, is that the type of motor response corresponds to the level of the lesion. In this view, decorticate rigidity would indicate a lesion affecting the hemispheres or the diencephalon, and decerebrate rigidity would suggest a lesion affecting the midbrain or the brain stem, as shown in the Sherrington preparations.[2,3] It is now clear, however, that in patients with head injury, decerebrate motor posturing and prolonged coma are not associated with brain-stem dysfunction but rather with dysfunction of the hemispheres.[4] Therefore, we prefer to use the terms abnormal flexion and extension or flexor and extensor posturing instead of the terms decorticate and decerebrate rigidity.

LOCALIZING OR LATERALIZING SIGNS

The presence of localizing or lateralizing signs suggests that the underlying abnormality of coma is structural (i.e., caused by a focal lesion) rather than metabolic. Rapid radiologic evaluation (CT scan) is essential in these cases, particularly in patients with head injuries who may harbor an expanding intracranial hematoma, for which

Table 1 Glasgow Coma Scale[80]

Test	Response	Score
Eye opening (E)	Spontaneous	4
	To verbal command	3
	To pain	2
	None	1
Best motor response (arm) (M)	Obedience to verbal command	6
	Localization of painful stimulus	5
	Flexion withdrawal response to pain	4
	Abnormal flexion response to pain (decorticate rigidity)	3
	Extension response to pain (decerebrate rigidity)	2
	None	1
Best verbal response (V)	Oriented conversation	5
	Disoriented conversation	4
	Inappropriate words	3
	Incomprehensible sounds	2
	None	1
	Total (E + M + V)	3–15

rapid surgical intervention is indicated. Patients are observed for asymmetrical movements of the extremities, which may occur spontaneously or in response to noxious stimuli. They are also evaluated for asymmetry of tone and reflexes, with special attention paid to such signs as unilateral flaccidity, spasticity, clonus, or Babinski signs. Most comatose patients, however, will have bilateral Babinski signs regardless of the cause of their condition.

PUPILLARY SIZE AND RESPONSE

The pathways involved in the pupillary response to light are relatively resistant to most metabolic causes of coma; unless the patient is under the influence of certain drugs, this response is preserved until the near-terminal stages of metabolic coma. Consequently, the presence or absence of the pupillary light reflex is the most useful single sign for distinguishing metabolic causes of coma from structural causes. Both the size of the pupil and its direct and consensual response to light should be noted.

Bilateral reactive constricted pupils are most often seen in patients in metabolic coma. Pinpoint pupils are indicative of either a pontine lesion or an overdose of narcotics; the latter is more likely if the pupillary constriction is reversed when naloxone is administered. Fixed dilated pupils can be the result of an intrinsic midbrain lesion or, more commonly, damage to the parasympathetic fibers accompanying the third nerve in its intracranial course. Unilateral pupillary dilatation usually indicates an ipsilateral mass and is typically a sign of uncal herniation when associated with contralateral hemiplegia. Rarely, unilateral pupillary dilatation is associated with ipsilateral hemiplegia as a result of a mass that compresses the cerebral peduncle of the midbrain against the opposite tentorial margin (Kernohan's notch). Bilateral fixed dilated pupils indicate severe midbrain damage, usually from transtentorial herniation. Fixed midposition pupils are the result of injury at the midbrain level, which impairs both sympathetic (dilatation) and parasympathetic (constriction) outflow.

It has been suggested that a decrease in brain-stem blood flow, rather than direct mechanical compression of the third cranial nerve, may be a cause of mydriasis after severe head injury.[5] The investigators measured cerebral blood flow (CBF) in the brain stems of 162 patients with severe head injury and correlated these findings with pupillary response. Brain-stem blood flow was significantly lower in patients with bilateral nonreactive pupils than in patients with responsive pupils, indicating that decreased pupillary reactivity may be the result of brain-stem ischemia. This hypothesis is supported by a subsequent study documenting significantly decreased brain-stem CBF and absent pupillary response in the presence of transtentorial herniation, both of which findings were reversed after administration of hypertonic saline.[6]

EYE MOVEMENTS

Eye movements are of major importance in the physical diagnosis of coma because they involve pathways that stretch through a large part of the brain and the brain stem. In conscious patients, eye movements are either voluntary—that is, controlled by the hemispheres—or dictated by superimposed involuntary brain-stem reflexes (which in turn are influenced by afferent impulses from the labyrinth and the vestibular nuclei). In deeply comatose patients, spontaneous eye movements are usually absent; however, they may occur even in the absence of functioning frontal or occipital cortices, in which case they generally take the form of conjugate horizontal roving. This movement indicates that the midbrain and the pontine tegmentum are spared. Ocular bobbing, a brisk downward and slow upward conjugate motion of the globes, is an indication of bilateral pontine damage. Conjugate lateral deviation of the eyes suggests the presence of either an ipsilateral hemispheric lesion or a contralateral pontine lesion. Seizures may cause sustained eye deviation, in which the eyes look away from the seizure focus and exhibit rhythmic, jerky movements in the direction of the deviation.

In drowsy patients, divergence of eye positions in the horizontal plane is normal; it disappears when consciousness returns or the coma deepens. An adducted eye signals sixth-nerve palsy or pontine damage. Unilateral or bilateral sixth-nerve palsy may be associated with increased ICP. An abducted eye signals third-nerve palsy. Skew deviation, in which the eyes are not in the same horizontal plane, is usually the result of pontine or cerebellar damage.

BRAIN-STEM REFLEXES

If spontaneous eye movements are absent, the integrity of the brain stem can be assessed by means of the so-called doll's-eyes maneuver or the caloric test. These tests are based on the observation that brain-stem reflexes become hyperactive when they are released from hemispheric inhibitory influences, as in coma or sleep. The anatomic pathways involved in these brain-stem reflexes arise from the upper cervical spinal cord and the medulla (the sources of vestibular and proprioceptive input from head turning) and from the inner ear via the vestibular and sixth nerves. The fibers then pass through the contralateral medial longitudinal fasciculus to the level of the third nerve in the midbrain.

The doll's-eyes maneuver tests the oculocephalic reflex. When coma is caused by hemispheric disease and the brain stem is intact, the doll's-eyes maneuver yields horizontal conjugate deviation of the eye in the direction opposite the direction of rotation, flexion, or extension; thus, the gaze remains stationary as the head is turned. When the brain stem is dysfunctional, there is no such deviation of the eyes; thus, the gaze does not remain stationary but moves as the head is turned. The connection between the vestibular nuclei and the third, fourth, and sixth cranial nerves, which is termed the medial longitudinal fasciculus, is interrupted. As a result, the oculocephalic reflexes are impaired, so that patients with bilateral lesions are unable to maintain a stationary gaze as the head is turned and those with unilateral lesions are unable to turn their gaze toward the side on which the lesion is located.

The caloric test is used to evaluate the oculovestibular reflex. It yields much the same information as the doll's-eyes maneuver; however, it is a stronger stimulus to reflex eye movements and therefore should be performed only if the doll's-eyes maneuver yields negative results. The patient's head is elevated 30°, and the external auditory canal is irrigated with 20 to 50 ml of ice water. The ice-water injection generates convection currents in the endolymph of the labyrinth that inhibit the normal spontaneous firing of the vestibular nerve. If the coma is caused by hemispheric disease and the brain stem is intact, the normal response is sustained conjugate deviation of the eyes toward the side of the irrigated ear. Structural brain-stem lesions may abolish these responses, as may an overdose of a sedative, a hypnotic, or phenytoin. Disconjugate ocular deviation suggests the presence of either a unilateral brain-stem lesion or a metabolic depression of the brain-stem pathways. Failure of one or both eyes to adduct indicates that the lesion is located in the medial longitudinal fasciculus or the third cranial nerve. Failure to abduct signals a sixth-nerve lesion.

Other brain-stem reflexes are the corneal reflex and the gag reflex. The corneal reflex is mediated by the fifth and seventh cranial nerves and is elicited by briefly striking the corneal surface with a piece of cotton wool twisted to a point. Both eyes should blink quickly in response to this stimulus. Bilateral absence of the corneal reflex usually suggests a deep coma, and unilateral absence of the reflex indicates an ipsilateral lesion. The gag reflex is elicited by stimulating the back of the throat or by passing a suction tube down the endotracheal tube while the patient is intubated. In unconscious patients who are at risk for aspiration, this reflex should be elicited only when the airway is protected (i.e., when the endotracheal cuff is inflated). The sensory stimulus is relayed via the ninth cranial nerve, but the 10th cranial nerve mediates the resulting palatal movement. A depressed or absent gag reflex usually indicates significant brain-stem pathology.

RESPIRATION

Respiration is dependent on neural influences arising from nearly every level of the brain, from the forebrain to the upper cervical spinal cord. Oxygenation and acid-base balance are primarily regulated in the lower brain stem. If the function of the hemispheres or the thalamus is structurally or metabolically impaired, the respiratory response to carbon dioxide is reset, so that a higher level of carbon dioxide is required to trigger the respiratory drive. The resulting respiratory pattern, known as Cheyne-Stokes respiration, is characterized by periods of increasing hyperventilation alternating with apnea in a crescendo-decrescendo fashion. If more caudal regions at the level of the midbrain and the upper pons are injured, central neurogenic hyperventilation may result. This pattern of respiration, characterized by hyperventilation with forced and prolonged inspiration and expiration, is commonly seen in metabolic disorders such as hypoxia. In the lower brain stem, if the lower pons or the medulla is injured, any of several respiratory patterns may occur. Apneusis, a pattern in which long inspiration is followed by a pause lasting a few seconds and then by normal expiration, results from pontine lesions and occasionally from metabolic suppression. Cluster breathing, a pattern in which breaths are irregular and fall into groups, is associated with lower pontine lesions. Atactic breathing, characterized by irregular respiratory rate and amplitude, with gasps held in inspiration intermingling with periods of apnea, is associated with lower medullary lesions and may be indicative of a terminal respiratory pattern in severely brain-damaged patients.

Other patterns of respiration, such as slow and shallow but regular breathing, are suggestive of metabolic or drug-induced depression. Kussmaul respiration, a pattern of rapid, deep breathing that is also known as air hunger, occurs with metabolic acidosis.

ELEVATED INTRACRANIAL PRESSURE

An increase in ICP occurs when an increase in the volume of one of the three components of the intracranial cavity (i.e., blood, cerebrospinal fluid, and brain parenchyma) cannot be compensated for by a similar decrease in the volume of one of the other components.[7,8] Causes of increased intracranial volume include intracranial hematoma, hydrocephalus, tumor, vascular congestion, and cerebral edema. Cerebral edema is a nonspecific accompaniment of many disorders, such as head injury, tumor, stroke, and infection. Cerebral edema and increased ICP are particularly common after severe head injury and are important determinants of the prognosis of these patients[9-11] [see 23 Injuries to the Central Nervous System]. Signs and symptoms of rising ICP include increasing arterial blood pressure, slowing of the pulse rate, and slowing or periodic respiration. This so-called Cushing response has been related to brain-stem ischemia; however, brain-stem blood flow is not always decreased in the presence of a Cushing response.[12] Papilledema caused by raised ICP takes several weeks to develop and is usually not a presenting symptom in patients with rapidly rising ICP.

MENINGISM

Meningism, or neck stiffness, occurs when the meninges are irritated by inflammation (as in meningitis) or the presence of blood (as in subarachnoid hemorrhage). In addition to nuchal rigidity, signs of meningeal irritation include a positive Kernig sign (elicited by flexing the thigh to 90° with the knee bent and then straightening the knee; the sign is positive when this maneuver causes pain in the hamstrings) and a positive Brudzinski sign (elicited by flexing the neck in a supine patient, which results in involuntary flexion of the hip).

Differential Diagnosis of Coma: Metabolic, Structural, and Other Causes

The differential diagnosis of coma is complex. It is essential to differentiate coma of metabolic origin from coma caused by structural lesions. In addition, both of these varieties of coma must be distinguished from psychogenic and other causes of coma and similar states, such as a persistent vegetative state and locked-in syndrome. Each of these types of coma has a characteristic clinical presentation and evolution [see Table 2].

TOXIC METABOLIC COMA

General Considerations

Toxic metabolic coma results from derangement of metabolism, alteration in resting membrane potentials, or suppression of neurotransmission in the cerebral cortex or the brain stem. Both exogenous toxins, such as sedatives and alcohol, and endogenous toxins, such as those produced in the course of uremia and hepatic failure, may suppress metabolic and electrical processing in the brain. Hypoxia and hypoglycemia lead to acute deficiencies of metabolic substrates. Acid-base and electrolyte imbalance suppress neuronal excitability, as do osmolarity abnormalities. Metabolic causes of coma usually cannot be demonstrated by means of radiography; however, signs of cerebral edema or increased ICP may be apparent on CT scan.

The hallmark of metabolic coma is that it is difficult to attribute neurologic signs to a restricted region because not all levels of the CNS are depressed concurrently and equally; for example, pupillary responses may be normal, and consciousness and respiration may be suppressed. The preservation of the pupillary light reflex even in the presence of signs of lower brain injury is an important feature distinguishing metabolic from structural coma. This rule does not, however, hold true for patients who have ingested drugs or sustained anoxic damage. The ingestion of narcotics results in reactive pinpoint pupils; the ingestion of the anticholinergic agents atropine and scopolamine gives rise to fixed fully dilated pupils; and the ingestion of glutethimide yields moderately dilated pupils that are unequal in size and frequently fixed. Severe anoxia may lead to bilateral fixed dilated pupils. Profound barbiturate poisoning or hypothermia may cause pupils to be both fixed and dilated. Although asymmetry of motor function is rare in metabolic coma, it does occur, often fluctuating from side to side. Abnormal motor signs such as tremor, myoclonus, and asterixis are characteristic of a metabolic derangement.

Specific Causes

Hypoglycemic coma Hypoglycemic coma is a serious complication of long-term insulin use, with a single episode occurring in at least one third of these patients at some point in their lives.[13] Tremor, tachycardia, sweating, blurring of vision, confusion, irritability, and abnormal behavior may precede the loss of consciousness, but in patients who are long-term insulin users, the premonitory symptoms may be absent and these patients may slip into a coma without any warning.

Diabetic ketoacidosis Diabetic ketoacidosis is a metabolic acidosis that develops in diabetic patients as a result of raised levels of circulating ketone bodies.[13] It is a severe complication of uncontrolled diabetes that requires emergency treatment. Initially, these patients present with severe dehydration, compensatory hyperventilation (Kussmaul respiration), vomiting, depression of consciousness, and sometimes abdominal pain. Coma is not common.

Uncontrolled hyperglycemia Nonketotic hyperosmolar coma results when uncontrolled hyperglycemia leads to dehydration and increased osmolality.[13] In this type of uncontrolled hyperglycemia, endogenous insulin secretion is still sufficient (and thus peripheral lipolysis and hepatic ketogenesis are inhibited), but hepatic glucose production, which is less sensitive to insulin control, is unrestrained. Patients with this disorder typically are in middle or later life and have been previously diagnosed with mild diabetes or have undiagnosed diabetes. Initial symptoms are profound dehydration and a decreased level of consciousness. The condition may be precipitated by an underlying infection or, in older patients, by vascular disease.

Hepatic and renal failure Hepatic encephalopathy may occur in the setting of acute fulminant hepatitis, in which there is no history of liver disease, or after rapidly progressive chronic liver disease.[14] The exact cause of the encephalopathy is not known, but possible factors include the release of toxins from the damaged liver, failure to detoxify metabolic products, and alterations in cerebral neurotransmitters caused by amino acid imbalances. Initial symptoms include slowness of mentation and affect, fluctuant mild confusion, reversed sleep rhythm, slurred speech, alternating euphoria and depression, and untidiness. Additional clues to underlying liver disease include fetor hepaticus, flapping tremor (asterixis), and constructional apraxia. A progressive deterioration in mental status and behavior usually follows, leading eventually to coma. In the early stages of coma, patients hyperventilate and their pupils react sluggishly to light. There is a general muscle hypertonia, and a grasp reflex may be elicited. Deeper coma develops rapidly if no treatment is instituted, and extensor posturing, loss of oculovestibular reflexes, hypotension, cardiac arrhythmias, and respiratory arrest occur.

Untreated acute and chronic renal failure may lead to uremic encephalopathy, which is associated with a progressive decrease in the level of consciousness, hyperventilation, asterixis, myoclonic jerking, tetany, and convulsions.[15] Higher mental functions are affected first, followed by motor symptoms. The onset of uremic encephalopathy depends on both the severity of the uremia and its rate of onset; rapid onset is associated with early CNS manifestations.

Table 2 Etiology of Coma

Causes of structural coma	Tumor
	Vascular
	   Cerebrovascular accident
	   Subarachnoid hemorrhage
	   Arteriovenous malformation
	   Global ischemia (vasospasm)
	Trauma
	   Intracranial hematoma
	   Multiple contusions
	   Diffuse axonal injury
	Infection
	   Cerebral abscess
	   Meningoencephalitis

Causes of toxic metabolic coma	Hypoxia Hypercarbia Hypoglycemia Hepatic failure Renal failure Electrolyte disorders Endocrine abnormalities Poisons Drugs
Other causes of coma	Hypothermia Hypotension and shock Psychiatric disorders

Electrolyte disturbances Coma can result from disturbances in sodium, potassium, and magnesium homeostasis.[16] Hyponatremia (e.g., from renal or GI sodium loss) may cause coma when the plasma sodium concentration falls below 110 to 115 mmol/L, particularly when the fall is rapid. Hypernatremia occurs in a hyperosmolar nonketotic coma. The level of consciousness falls and convulsions develop when the plasma sodium concentration rises above 155 to 160 mmol/L. Hypokalemia usually does not produce a frank coma, but rather a decrease in the level of consciousness. Death in these patients is caused by ventricular tachycardia. Both hypomagnesemia (e.g., from severe vomiting and diarrhea) and hypermagnesemia (e.g., from renal failure) can produce coma. Increased irritability, hallucinations, convulsions, myoclonus, and chorea usually precede hypomagnesemia, whereas hypermagnesemia is preceded by increased lethargy and generalized weakness. Death in patients with hypermagnesemia results from respiratory paralysis.

STRUCTURAL COMA

General Considerations

Structural brain lesions produce coma either by destroying the brain parenchyma or by causing shifting or herniation of the brain within the rigid confines of the tentorium and skull [*see* Discussion, Pathophysiology of Coma, Herniation Syndromes, *below*]. Supratentorial lesions produce coma by causing a caudal shift of the cerebral contents beyond the confines of the tentorium, which results in compression of the brain stem and dysfunction of the ascending RAS. Infratentorial lesions produce coma by compressing the brain stem from either inside (i.e., intrinsic brain-stem lesions) or outside (i.e., cerebellar lesions).

As mentioned previously, the hallmark of a structural lesion underlying coma is the presence of localizing signs. In addition, unilateral pupillary abnormalities and unilaterally absent brain-stem reflexes are highly suggestive of an anatomic lesion. Some structural lesions (e.g., aneurysmal subarachnoid hemorrhage) often have a typical clinical presentation, and this may aid in the differential diagnosis. Specific structural causes of coma and their clinical presentation are discussed below.

Specific Causes

Cerebral tumor Coma is usually not the presenting symptom in patients with brain tumors. In most patients with cerebral tumors, a progressive neurologic deficit or focal seizure activity precedes the onset of coma, and their presence is an important clue in the differential diagnosis. Headache is also a common presenting symptom and is present in approximately 50% of patients with primary brain tumors or metastatic lesions. The classic headache associated with a brain tumor is described as being worse in the morning; exacerbated by coughing, straining, or bending forward; and accompanied by nausea and vomiting, which often afford relief for the patient. However, this classic pattern occurs only in a subset of patients. In a study of 111 patients with brain tumors, investigators showed that 77% of the patients had headaches that were similar to tension headaches, 9% had headaches that were migrainelike, and only 8% had the typical headache symptoms of a brain tumor.[17]

Signs and symptoms of supratentorial tumors include those caused by raised ICP (e.g., mass effect of the tumor or blockage of CSF drainage), focal deficits (e.g., destruction of the brain parenchyma; compression of the parenchyma by edema, mass, or hemorrhage; and compression of the cranial nerves), headache, seizures, mental status changes, transient ischemic attack symptoms (caused by vessel occlusion or hemorrhage into the tumor), and, in the case of pituitary tumors, endocrine symptoms and visual impairment. Patients with infratentorial tumors usually do not present with seizures, because such seizures are thought to arise from irritation of the cerebral cortex. Signs and symptoms of these lesions include headache, nausea, vomiting, papilledema, gait disturbances, vertigo, diplopia, and cranial nerve abnormalities and nystagmus when there is brain-stem involvement.

Stroke Stroke is categorized as cerebral infarction (thromboembolic or ischemic stroke), which signifies ischemic brain damage, or cerebral hemorrhage (hemorrhagic stroke), in which damage to the brain mainly consists of vascular rupture and extravasation of blood into the brain parenchyma. The hallmark of both types of stroke is the abrupt onset of a focal neurologic deficit. Whereas brain-stem infarcts can result in an immediate coma, ischemic stroke usually does not produce coma as a predominant symptom. In most cases, coma develops later, when edema develops in and around the infarct or when hemorrhagic conversion of the infarct results in the development of a massive hematoma that produces brain herniation.

In intracerebral hemorrhage (ICH), loss of consciousness is a prominent feature. The hallmarks of ICH are a rapidly developing neurologic deficit, vomiting, and a fluctuating level of consciousness. Coma usually indicates a large lobar or ganglionic hemorrhage (> 60 ml),[18] and coma is thought to result either from direct destruction or from herniation caused by the mass effect of the hemorrhage.

Both hemorrhagic and thromboembolic stroke predominantly affect the elderly. Diabetes, atherosclerosis, cardiac disease, hypertension, vasculitis, and hematologic disorders are important risk factors for ischemic stroke. The main causes of ICH include hypertension, arteriovenous (AV) malformations, ruptured aneurysms, arteriopathies, tumors, coagulation or clotting disorders, venous or dural sinus thrombosis, abuse of drugs (e.g., cocaine or amphetamines), eclampsia, postsurgical complications (e.g., repair of congenital heart defects in children, hyperemia after carotid endarterectomy, or repair of AV malformation), and infection. Whether hypertension actually causes ICH is still subject to debate because 66% of patients older than 65 years are hypertensive, and the observed hypertension associated with ICH may in fact be part of the physiologic Cushing response and not a preexisting condition.[19]

Aneurysmal subarachnoid hemorrhage Subarachnoid hemorrhage (SAH) refers to bleeding within the subarachnoid space rather than the brain parenchyma and is the result of either a ruptured aneurysm (aneurysmal SAH) or a severe head injury (traumatic SAH). Aneurysmal SAH occurs most frequently in the fourth to sixth decades of life. The classic manifestations of aneurysmal SAH are headache of sudden onset (commonly described as the most severe headache ever experienced), a variable period of consciousness, meningism, photophobia, vomiting, and focal signs. The clinical severity of SAH is graded by using the Hunt and Hess Scale [*see Table 3*][20] or the World Federation of Neurological Surgeons Scale [*see Table 4*].[21]

Delayed cerebral ischemia or vasospasm is responsible for considerable morbidity and mortality and is an important cause of impaired consciousness and coma in patients with aneurysmal SAH. Vasospasm has a typical pattern of development. It generally occurs between day 5 and day 14 after aneurysmal SAH, with a peak incidence between day 7 and day 10. Clinical signs and symptoms include an insidious decrease in the level of consciousness and fluctuating neurologic signs. The diagnosis is confirmed by means of transcranial Doppler ultrasonography or cerebral angiography.

Table 3 Hunt and Hess Classification of Subarachnoid Hemorrhage[20]

Score*	Definition
0	Unruptured aneurysm
1	Asymptomatic; or mild headache and slight nuchal rigidity
1a	No acute meningeal/brain reaction, but with fixed neurologic deficit
2	Moderate to severe headache and nuchal rigidity; or CNS palsy (e.g., III, IV)
3	Lethargy or confusion; mild focal deficit
4	Stupor; moderate to severe hemiparesis
5	Deep coma, extensor posturing, moribund appearance

*Add one grade for serious systemic disease (e.g., hypertension, diabetes mellitus, severe atherosclerosis, chronic obstructive pulmonary disease) or severe vasospasm on arteriography.

Table 4 World Federation of Neurological Surgeons Committee on Universal Subarachnoid Hemorrhage Grading Scale[21]

Grade	GCS Score	Motor Deficit
I	15	Absent
II	13–14	Absent
III	13–14	Present
IV	7–12	Present or absent
V	3–6	Present or absent

GCS—Glasgow Coma Scale

Traumatic SAH is a common phenomenon in patients with severe head injuries. The diagnosis is made by means of CT. In a study from the National Institutes of Health Traumatic Coma Data Bank, traumatic SAH was identified in 39% of 753 patients with severe head injury.[22] Clinically, traumatic SAH is associated with signs and symptoms of vasospasm that are similar to those occurring with aneurysmal SAH. Vasospasm affects between 25% and 40% of patients with severe head injuries,[23] and the presence of traumatic SAH appears to be related to an unfavorable outcome.

Meningoencephalitis and cerebral abscess Bacteria, viruses, spirochetes, and fungi may infect the meninges and the subarachnoid space. In most cases, infection of the CNS results from an infection that originates somewhere else. For example, meningococcal meningitis is often a complication of meningococcal bacteremia; tuberculous meningitis is the result of breakdown of a tuberculous lesion or miliary tuberculosis; and herpes zoster, listeriosis, and cryptococcal meningitis are opportunistic CNS infections that typically occur with debilitating disease or altered immune status. After neurosurgery, gram-negative aerobic bacilli usually cause meningitis. Signs and symptoms of meningoencephalitis include fever, headache, raised ICP, meningism, photophobia, seizures, and focal signs. A depressed level of consciousness, sometimes progressing to a frank coma, is a relatively common clinical manifestation of CNS infection. About 50% of patients with acute meningitis have a depressed level of consciousness.[24] The exact mechanism behind depressed levels of consciousness in CNS infection is unknown. A direct effect of the organism or its toxins on the brain parenchyma has been suggested, but disturbance of the cerebral microcirculation and occlusion of the larger vessels through either vessel wall thickening or vasospasm have also been suggested.[25]

Cerebral abscesses commonly produce focal signs or seizures but may lead to brain herniation and coma when they expand. In the classic case, the presentation is acute, with fever followed by confusion and the development of focal signs over the course of days; however, a cerebral abscess may also develop gradually, without overt disease. Cerebral abscesses may be associated with sinusitis, otitis, cranial trauma, or disseminated infection.

Head injury Head injury is discussed in more detail elsewhere [see 23 Injuries to the Central Nervous System].

OTHER CAUSES OF COMA AND COMA-RESEMBLING SYNDROMES

Hypothermia

Hypothermia occurs when the body's core temperature is 35° C or lower. It can result from exposure (i.e., from cold stress exceeding the body's maximum heat production), exhaustion (i.e., from depletion of the body's available energy sources), or failure of central temperature regulation (mainly in elderly patients and newborns). Loss of consciousness by itself may result in hypothermia. Consciousness decreases when the core body temperature is at or below 32° C and progresses to coma with further temperature decline. Metabolic processes slow, and for each 1° C decrease in body temperature, CBF diminishes by about 6%. At 28° C, the metabolic rate is 50% of normal, and below 25° C, asystole and death occur. At this point, cerebral autoregulation fails, and CBF follows the systemic blood pressure in a pressure-passive manner.[26]

Psychiatric Disorders

Psychogenic coma is an uncommon cause of unresponsiveness. It may be observed in patients with psychiatric disorders such as conversion reactions, catatonic schizophrenia, severe psychotic depression, or frank malingering. In most cases, the physical examination reveals normal tone and reflexes, as well as normal oculocephalic and oculovestibular reflexes. Occasionally, EEG is necessary to demonstrate a normal waking pattern.

Persistent Vegetative State

A vegetative state is a syndrome of diffuse cortical damage in which brain-stem activity is preserved. Consequently, eye opening and muscle movements are observed, but there is no voluntary control of the movements. A vegetative state is usually a long-term and often a permanent state associated with injuries such as head trauma and global ischemia.

Locked-in Syndrome

The locked-in syndrome is a state in which quadriplegia and paralysis of the lower cranial nerves are present but the level of consciousness is normal. This syndrome is rare and usually results from thrombosis of the basilar artery, which is attributed to a variety of causes. Patients can communicate only by eye movements (e.g., blinking). Long-term survival is uncommon but has been reported.[27]

Radiologic Imaging

Radiologic imaging modalities depict the anatomic configuration of intracranial structures and play a crucial role in the evaluation of comatose patients, particularly when an adequate history cannot be obtained and the physical examination is inconclusive. They can be used to confirm or exclude the presence of clinically suspected abnormalities or, in some instances, to make a specific diagnosis, thereby greatly expediting treatment or intervention.

TYPES OF IMAGING MODALITIES

Plain Skull Radiography

Plain skull radiography is particularly useful in the evaluation of patients with head injuries. Bullets and bullet fragments can be easily detected, and the points of entry and exit can generally be determined with this method. In patients with closed head injuries, plain skull radiography is used to detect fractures of the cranial vault and base. It is important to obtain a skull radiograph in patients with head injuries because the presence of a fracture is related to intracranial hematoma and thus is an indication of the severity of head injury [see Table 5].

Computed Tomography and Magnetic Resonance Imaging

Both CT and MRI provide detailed information on brain anatomy, including the configuration and size of the ventricular chambers; the presence of midline displacements; the presence of subfalcial, transtentorial, or uncal herniations; and the position of vascular structures. CT is usually the first investigation performed in comatose patients. Compared with MRI, CT takes less time for a complete investigation, and the CT unit is much easier to access. These are significant advantages of CT in comatose patients, who are usually monitored with multiple electronic devices—a practice that, by itself, limits the use of MRI because of the effect of the magnetic field on these devices. In addition, CT is better at imaging bony structures than MRI is, it is an excellent method of demonstrating ICH, and it offers the best resolution for demonstrating SAH. MRI, however, offers the advantage of imaging in multiple planes, which allows accurate anatomic visualization of the lesion. Furthermore, it is more sensitive than CT in detecting intracranial abnormalities and thus is better able to find small lesions. In addition, the absence of bony artifacts makes MRI more useful for imaging lesions in the

Table 5 Relation between Presence of Skull Fracture and Intracranial Hematoma in Patients with Severe, Moderate, and Minor Head Injury[124]

Severity	Hematoma on CT	No Hematoma on CT	Total
Severe (GCS 8)			
Fracture	74 (44%)	94 (56%)	168
No fracture	43 (32%)*	91 (68%)	134
Moderate (GCS 9–12)			
Fracture	49 (29%)	118 (71%)	167
No fracture	25 (8%)†	299 (92%)	324
Minor (GCS 13–15)			
Fracture	42 (10%)	391 (90%)	433
No fracture	27 (1%)‡	2,549 (99%)	2,576
Total	260	3,542	3,802

*$P < 0.05$. †$P < 0.001$. ‡$P < 0.0001$.
GCS—Glasgow Coma Scale

posterior and temporal fossae. Overall, CT is preferred for initial evaluation of comatose patients. MRI should be reserved for patients who require less monitoring, who are able to remain still for prolonged examination, and in whom CT has not been beneficial or is inconclusive.

RADIOLOGIC DIAGNOSIS OF SPECIFIC CAUSES OF COMA

Cerebral Tumor

CT (with and without injection of contrast) is a useful and quick first investigation for detecting a tumor. It demonstrates mass effect, edema, calcifications, and accompanying disorders that may necessitate rapid intervention (e.g., hydrocephalus). Low-grade gliomas show a decreased density on CT scans that does not enhance with contrast. The surrounding edema is minimal. Calcifications may be present, particularly in certain subtypes (e.g., oligodendrogliomas). High-grade gliomas are usually large and enhance intensely after contrast administration [*see Figure 1*]. In most cases, the enhancement is irregular. A central area of low density may also be present, indicating necrosis. High-grade gliomas are usually surrounded by marked cerebral edema and compression of the ipsilateral ventricle by a hemispheric mass; alternatively, the surrounding edema may result in obstructive hydrocephalus with dilatation of the contralateral ventricle.

On MRI, low-grade gliomas may present as abnormal areas of decreased T_1 signal (spin-lattice or longitudinal relaxation time) and increased T_2 signal (spin-spin or transverse relaxation time), even in the absence of CT evidence of a tumor. High-grade gliomas characteristically have a low signal intensity on T_1-weighted images and a high signal on T_2-weighted images. Gadolinium enhancement is more likely to occur in high-grade gliomas. Metastatic lesions have a variable intensity on T_2-weighted images, and they commonly enhance with gadolinium. Meningiomas are hypointense to isointense on T_1 and hyperintense to isointense on T_2, and they enhance strongly with contrast. Nerve sheath tumors are isointense or hypointense on T_1 and hyperintense on T_2 and enhance intensely with contrast. Pituitary tumors are best visualized on T_1-weighted imaging. They are hypointense lesions within the intermediate intensity of the anterior lobe. Lymphomas are usually hypointense to isointense on T_1-weighted images and isointense to hyperintense on T_2-weighted images. These tumors enhance after I.V. injection of gadolinium.

Stroke

CT abnormalities can be detected a few hours after an ischemic stroke. In patients with a middle cerebral artery (MCA) stroke, CT findings include effacement of the sulci, loss of distinction of the caudate nucleus and lentiform nucleus, and loss of the insular ribbon. The hyperdense MCA sign, which is caused by the clot in the artery, is present in almost 50% of patients when a CT scan is performed within the first 2 hours.[28,29] The characteristic triangle-shaped hypodensity usually develops fully within 3 days, and the mass effect, caused by cerebral swelling as well as petechial hemorrhages and indicating hemorrhagic conversion, may be seen at this time. The likelihood of edema increases with the size of MCA infarcts; if the infarct size, as determined on CT scan within 5 hours after the insult, is larger than 50% of the MCA territory, significant edema develops in 85% of patients.[30]

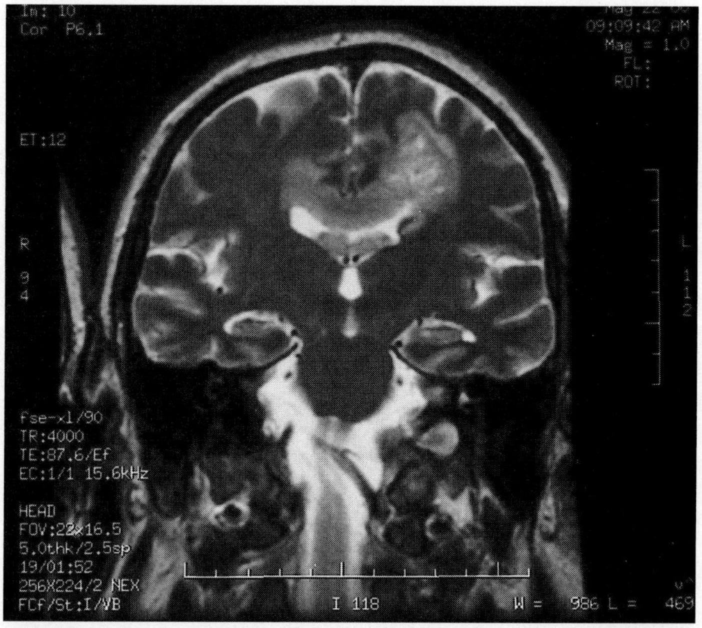

Figure 1 Characteristic appearance of butterfly glioma is apparent on coronal T_1-weighted MRI. The tumor mass extends to the contralateral side across the corpus callosum.

Table 6 Fisher CT Classification of Subarachnoid Hemorrhage[31]

Grade	Amount of Blood on CT	No. of Patients	Angiographic Vasospasm		DIND
			Slight	Severe	
1	No SAH detected	11	2	2	0
2	Diffuse or vertical layers* < 1 mm	7	3	0	0
3	Localized clot and/or vertical layer > 1 mm	24	1	23	23
4	Intracerebral or intraventricular clot with diffuse or no SAH	5	2	0	0

*Vertical layers refer to blood within the vertical subarachnoid spaces, including the interhemispheric fissure, insular cistern, and ambient cistern.
DIND—delayed ischemic neurologic deficit   SAH—subarachnoid hemorrhage

Supratentorial, cerebellar, and brain-stem hemorrhages appear as hyperdense lesions on CT scan. Putaminal hemorrhages may extend into the thalamus and enter the ventricular system. Caudate hemorrhage may be difficult to detect because the ventricular extension may predominate. Lobar hematomas on CT scan may show compression of the sulci, midline shift, and compression of the lateral ventricle. MRI is a useful test for excluding metastasis, occult vascular malformations, previous hemorrhages associated with amyloid angiopathy, or cerebral venous thrombosis that is not detected with CT.

Cerebellar hematomas may cause significant compression and obliteration of the basal cisterns, resulting in CSF obstruction and hydrocephalus; these signs, together with the size of the hematoma, are important determinants of further management. In patients with pontine hemorrhage, massive hemorrhages are most frequent, but small ones occur as well.

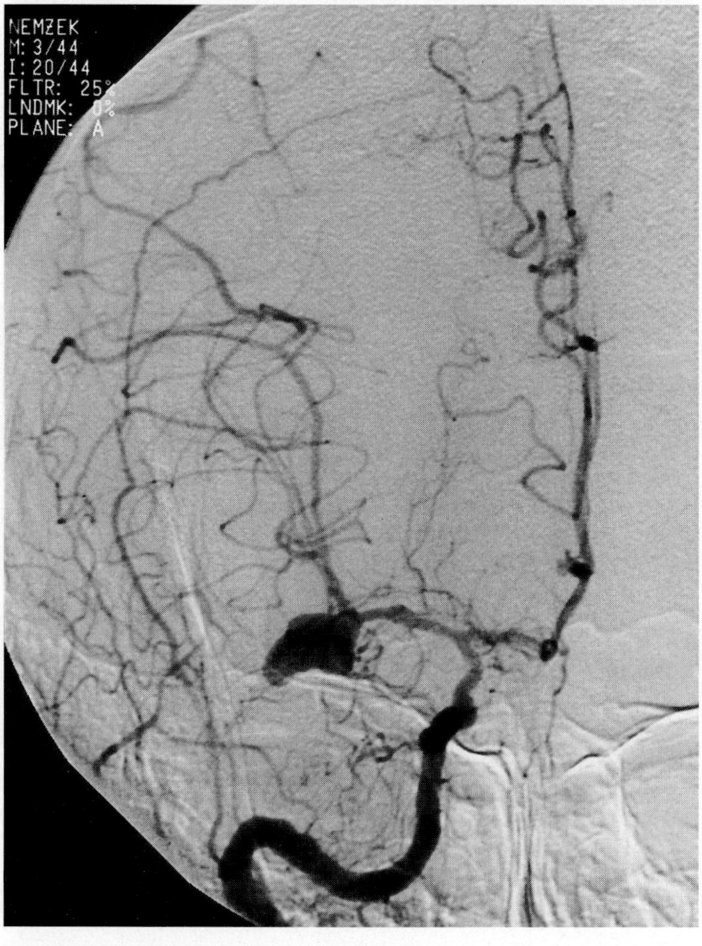

Subarachnoid Hemorrhage

Aneurysmal SAH is classified according to the Fisher CT classification, which relates severity of bleeding to prognosis [see Table 6].[31] The sensitivity of CT scanning for detecting SAH is very high, approximately 95%.[32,33] In many cases, there is a slight preponderance of blood deposited in the area of the ruptured aneurysm, which may aid in determining the location of the aneurysm or the location of multiple intracranial aneurysms. Cerebral angiography [see Figure 2] is the gold standard for evaluating the size and location of the aneurysm, though newer methods (e.g., MR angiography and CT angiography) are being used increasingly.[34-38]

Lumbar puncture is never the first choice of investigation for confirming a diagnosis of SAH. As noted, a mass lesion in the posterior fossa may closely mimic the signs and symptoms of SAH, and patients are at considerable risk for herniation if a lumbar puncture is performed. A CT scan usually yields the diagnosis, and a lumbar puncture is rarely necessary. If SAH is suspected and CT is not available, it is safer to transport the patient to a facility where CT scanning is available, particularly when the patient is rapidly deteriorating.[33] Lumbar puncture, however, must be used when the CT scan is negative and there is even a slight suspicion of aneurysmal SAH.

Meningoencephalitis and Cerebral Abscess

Other than diffuse basal dural enhancement on MRI, meningoencephalitis usually does not produce specific signs on CT or MRI. A CT scan is indicated in comatose patients, however, to rule out complications of meningitis such as hydrocephalus, subdural empyema, and abscess. On CT, a cerebral abscess appears as a smooth thin-walled lesion with a low-density center that enhances brightly after administration of contrast. In some cases, it is difficult to distinguish between a tumor and an abscess on CT, and stereotactic biopsy is essential to confirm the diagnosis [see Figure 3]. Diffusion-weighed MRI also may be useful in these cases.[39] MRI can show intracranial abscesses with a much greater resolution than CT scanning can, and it is excellent for detecting cerebritis and abscesses that are undetectable or uncertain on CT.[40]

Head Injury

Fractures of the cranial vault and base are sometimes difficult to detect, particularly by the inexperienced investigator. Depressed and linear fractures are the most common types [see Figure 4]. Types of ICH that are often seen after head injury and that can be detected with CT include contusions and epidural, subdural, subarachnoid, and intraparenchymal hemorrhages. An epidural hematoma

Figure 2 Cerebral angiography shows a large right middle cerebral artery aneurysm.

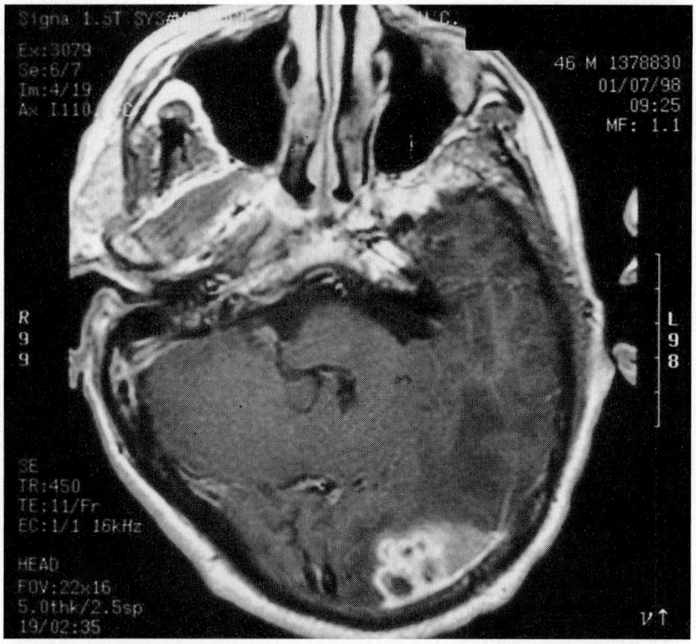

respect to the adjacent brain, subacute hematomas are hyperdense to isodense, and chronic hematomas [see Figure 6c] are hypodense.

Intraparenchymal lesions appear as an area of increased density on CT scans [see Figure 7]. The hematomas are usually associated with extensive lobar contusions, from which they are indistinguishable in many cases.[43,44] The amount of blood in a lesion determines whether the lesion is classified as a hematoma or a contusion. If blood accounts for at least two thirds of the lesion, the lesion is classified as an intracerebral hematoma. The remaining lesions are described as disrupted tissue with areas of microscopic hemorrhage.[45] A hemorrhagic mass should be considered an intracerebral hematoma when there is a homogeneous collection of blood with relatively well-defined margins. Multiple intracerebral hematomas are found in approximately 20% of cases.[46]

Contusions, appearing as small hyperdense lesions on CT, usually have a characteristic distribution, affecting the frontal poles, the orbital gyri, the cortex above and below the sylvian fissures, the temporal poles, and the lateral and inferior aspects of the temporal lobes. Over time, significant swelling may accompany these lesions, appearing as hypodense areas around the contusion.

Diffuse axonal injury is characterized by the presence of punctate hemorrhages or so-called Strich hemorrhages and indicates severe head injury.[47] Strich hemorrhages are most commonly found in the corpus callosum, the walls of the third ventricle (hypothalamus, columns of the fornix, and anterior commissure), the internal capsule, the basal ganglia, the dorsolateral brain stem, and the superior cerebellar peduncles.

Midline shift and compression of the subarachnoid space are parameters indicating the extent of mass expansion or cerebral swelling. The National Institutes of Health Traumatic Coma Data Bank introduced a classification of head injury based on initial CT findings [see Table 7].[48] This classification is commonly used in clinical trials investigating new treatments for severe head injury. Eisenberg and colleagues have shown a correlation between some of the CT scan characteristics after severe head injury (i.e., compression of the basal cisterns, the presence of SAH, and midline shift) and the frequency of raised ICP, mortality, and other outcomes.[22]

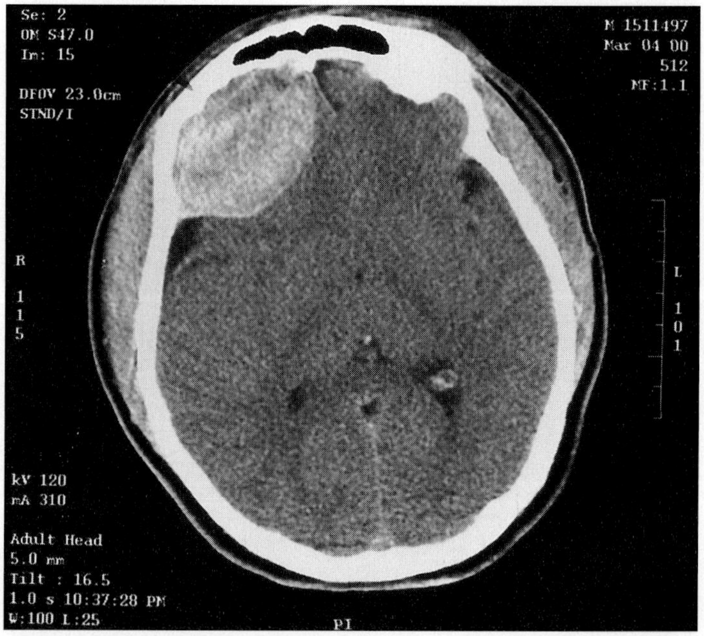

Figure 3 MRI reveals a cerebral abscess. Axial T_1-weighted image with gadolinium contrast medium shows multiloculated, brightly enhancing mass. Signal intensity is low at the abscess wall. There is significant surrounding edema and mass effect, which results in effacement of the ipsilateral occipital horn of the left lateral ventricle. Local involvement of the meninges is indicated by enhancement of the overlying meninges.

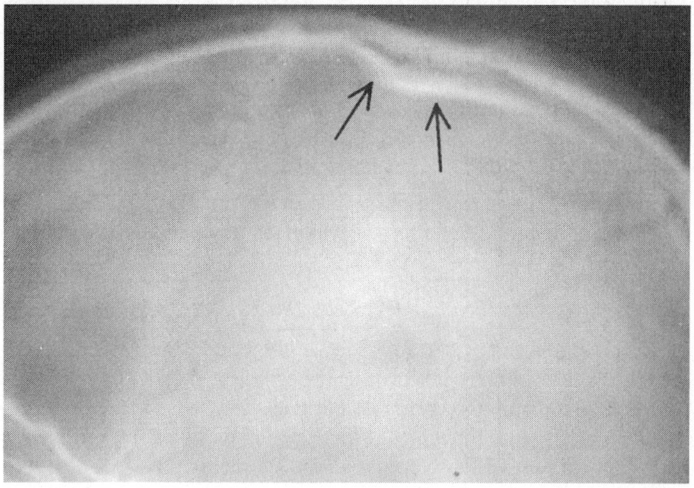

Figure 4 Conventional lateral radiograph shows a skull fracture.

characteristically appears as a biconvex hyperdense lesion [see Figure 5]. Epidural hematomas have been classified into three types on the basis of CT scan criteria.[41] Type I (acute) hematomas are characterized by a lucent swirl (unclotted blood) in a dense hematoma. Some investigators call these hematomas hyperacute extradural hematomas. Type II (subacute) hematomas appear as solid clots. Type III (chronic) hematomas appear as mixed-density or lucent hematomas with a contrast-enhanced membrane.

Subdural hematomas appear as convex-concave lesions on CT [see Figure 6a, b]. In many cases, subdural hemorrhage is accompanied by SAH, indicating severe injury.[42] The complex of subdural hematoma and adjacent contusion in the brain is sometimes referred to as a burst lobe. Acute subdural hematomas are hyperdense with

Figure 5 CT scan shows acute epidural hematoma. Note the characteristic biconvex hyperdense lesion.

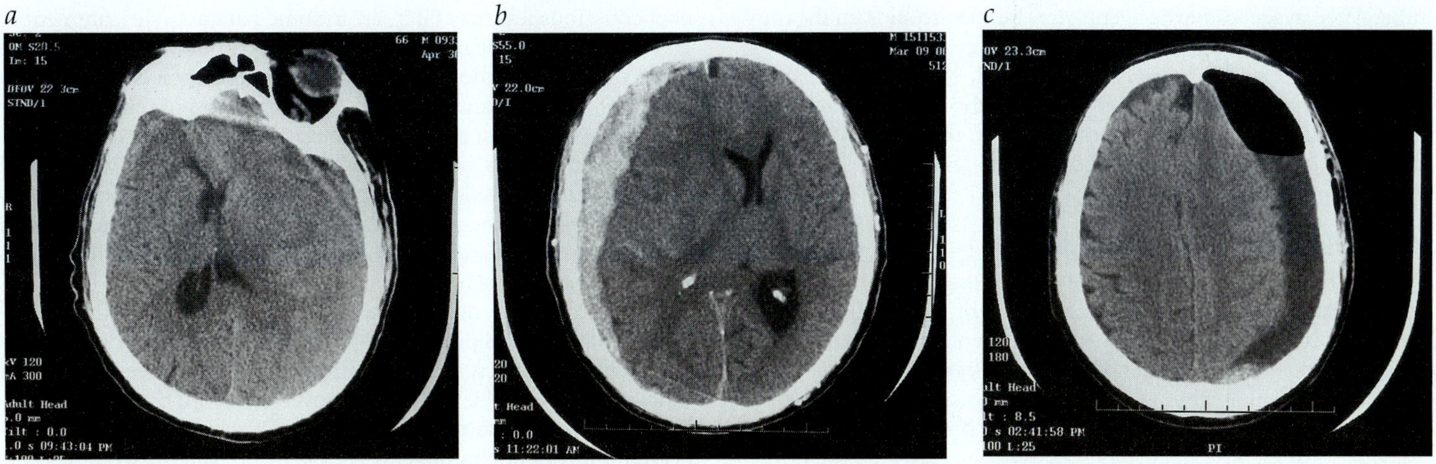

Figure 6 Shown are three examples of subdural hematoma: (*a*) hyperacute subdural hematoma (note that there is only a slight difference in density between the convex-concave hematoma and the brain parenchyma; the hematoma causes significant midline shift and ipsilateral brain compression), (*b*) acute subdural hematoma, and (*c*) chronic subdural hematoma after surgical evacuation.

Treatment of Coma

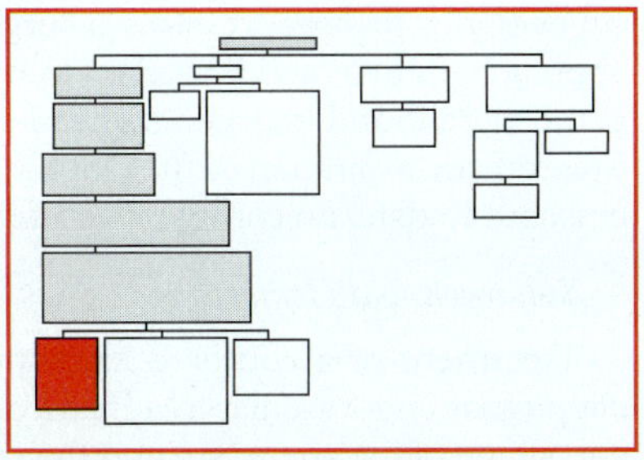

METABOLIC COMA

Management of Intoxication

Many comatose patients who are seen in the emergency ward are suffering from an overdose of alcohol, narcotics, sedatives, or a combination thereof. Most of these drugs induce respiratory and cardiovascular depression, which is a major cause of mortality in comatose patients. Anticipation and early treatment of these complications may alleviate their effects.

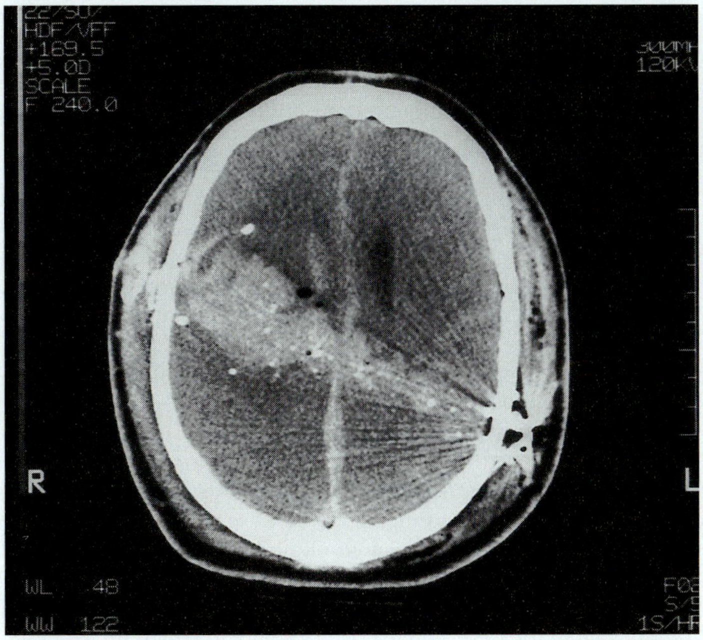

Early intubation, respiratory support, and maintenance of normal blood pressure are essential. Gastric lavage is effective when ingestion of a drug is discovered no more than 4 hours after the event, except in the case of salicylates, which may be removed in substantial amounts as long as 10 hours after ingestion. As a rule, little is gained by performing gastric lavage more than 4 hours after ingestion, unless the patient has been in shock and consequently manifests delayed gastric emptying and slowed absorption. In comatose or uncooperative patients, however, it is rarely possible to determine the exact time of ingestion; thus, gastric lavage is almost always indicated.

Patients are intubated with a cuffed endotracheal tube (to protect the airway from aspirated gastric contents) and then positioned on their left side (to allow pooling of the gastric contents) with the head down. Lavage is then performed with copious amounts of fluid until the return is clear. After evacuation, a slurry of 10 g of activated charcoal in 30 to 50 ml is instilled in the stomach via a nasogastric

Figure 7 CT scan shows intracerebral hematoma resulting from a cranial gunshot wound.

Table 7 Classification of Head Injury Based on Initial CT Findings

Category	Definition
Diffuse injury I	No visible intracranial pathology on CT scan

Diffuse injury II	Cisterns present with midline shift of 0–5 mm and/or the following:
	    Lesion densities present
	    No high- or mixed-density lesion > 25 ml
	    May include bone fragments and foreign bodies

Diffuse injury III (swelling)	Cisterns compressed or absent, with midline shift of 0–5 mm; no high- or mixed-density lesion > 25 ml
Diffuse injury IV	Midline shift > 5 mm; no high- or mixed-density lesion > 25 ml
Evacuated mass lesion	Any lesion surgically evacuated
Nonevacuated mass lesion	High- or mixed-density lesion > 25 ml, not surgically evacuated

tube. After lavage, cathartic agents may be used to shorten the transit time through the GI tract and thus to decrease absorption of the ingested material. Diuresis (saline, ionized, or osmotic), dialysis, and charcoal hemoperfusion all facilitate the excretion of toxins. Specific antidotes exist for several common intoxicants; however, these antidotes are beyond the scope of the present discussion [see 12 Substance Abuse].

Hypoglycemic Coma

Initial treatment of hypoglycemic coma is discussed elsewhere [see Initial Management of the Comatose Patient, above]. In addition, treatment consists of prevention, in the form of education in the use of insulin and encouragement of patients to carry glucose tablets or sweets with them at all times. A supply of glucagon (1 g I.M.) that can be administered by relatives may also be stored at home.

Diabetic Ketotic Coma

Treatment must be initiated as soon as possible because these patients often present with profound dehydration. Key points in the management of diabetic ketoacidosis include the following:

1. Replace fluid losses (the average fluid loss is approximately 7 L).
2. Replace electrolytes and monitor potassium carefully.
3. Restore acid-base balance (with bicarbonate infusion only in severe cases).
4. Replace insulin deficiency (4 to 6 U/hr).
5. Replace energy losses (dextrose infusion with insulin cover until the patient can eat).
6. Look for an underlying cause (infection is common).

Hyperglycemic Hyperosmolar Nonketotic Coma

Management of hyperosmolar nonketotic coma does not differ from that of diabetic ketotic coma; however, meticulous rehydration should be performed, particularly because many patients with this condition are elderly.

STRUCTURAL COMA

Cerebral Tumor

Management of brain tumors consists of surgery, radiotherapy, and other adjuvant treatments (e.g., chemotherapy). Ultimately, treatment of these lesions depends on both tumor characteristics (e.g., localization, malignancy, tumor spread, and associated edema) and patient characteristics (e.g., age, medical history, and personal beliefs). An in-depth discussion of the diverse treatment strategies, however, is beyond the scope of this chapter.

In the comatose patient, two interventions deserve particular consideration. First, to reduce cerebral edema, patients should be started on glucocorticosteroid therapy (e.g., dexamethasone), particularly when signs of elevated ICP are present. Second, coexisting hydrocephalus may be alleviated by the insertion of a ventricular catheter.

Stroke

In patients with thromboembolic stroke, coma is usually caused by brain swelling. Cerebral edema occurs in approximately 10% to 20% of patients with MCA stroke and in almost 100% of those with complete MCA occlusion.[49,50] It typically occurs after 2 to 7 days and is characterized by a gradual deterioration, though the level of consciousness may fluctuate in some patients. Measurement of ICP is indicated because it has been shown that ICP may predict the ultimate outcome of these patients[49] and thus can serve as a guide for patient management.[51] Administration of mannitol is initially selected to treat an increase in ICP. Acute episodes of impending herniation may be treated with hyperventilation if mannitol fails, and further clinical deterioration can be followed by decompressive surgery if the patient has no other significant disease and is relatively young. In addition, a ventriculostomy can be placed if significant contralateral hydrocephalus is present.

In patients with nondominant ischemic stroke, including comatose patients and patients with a fixed dilated pupil, decompressive surgery has been successful, though it has not been tested in a randomized clinical trial.[52-57] Moreover, it should be noted that although mortality may decrease substantially with decompressive surgery, it may not be desirable to salvage those patients who may end up with a severe disability or in a vegetative state. In a recent study of 32 surgically treated patients, mortality decreased by 35% in comparison with historic controls, but one in four patients experienced severe disability.[55]

Treatment of so-called supratentorial hypertensive intraparenchymal hemorrhage is still subject to considerable debate. No uniform treatment guidelines are available, and there is very little clinical evidence to support either a surgical or a conservative medical approach. In two randomized trials, no significant differences in outcome were found between surgical and medical management.[58,59] Stereotactic aspiration of the clot has achieved some degree of success, but to date, no comparative studies have been published.[60,61]

Subarachnoid Hemorrhage

Treatment of a ruptured aneurysm consists of either surgical clipping or endovascular treatment, depending on the location, size, and shape of the aneurysm and the age, clinical condition, and past medical history of the patient. Ideally, patients are treated within 48 hours of hemorrhage because the risk of rebleeding is highest early after the initial bleeding episode. The estimated frequency of repeat bleeding in untreated patients is 4% on day 1 and 1.5% from day 2 to day 14. Overall, 15% to 20% of patients experience repeat bleeding within 14 days, and 50% within 6 months; thereafter, the risk is 3% per year, with an annual mortality of 2%.[62,63] An advantage of clipping or coiling the aneurysm is that it allows the institution of so-called triple-H therapy (i.e., therapy for hypertension, hypervolemia, and hemodilution) and transluminal balloon angioplasty in the case of vasospasm. In a subset of patients (i.e., those with poor neurologic condition or those who present with symptomatic vasospasm), surgical treatment may be postponed, or the aneurysm may be treated by means of endovascular techniques.

Cerebral vasospasm is initially treated with ample fluid replacement and discontinuance of any antihypertensive or diuretic agents. When necessary, triple-H therapy and transluminal balloon angioplasty to dilate the vasospastic vessels are instituted.[64,65] Prevention of vasospasm by means of prophylactic transluminal balloon angioplasty is currently under investigation.[66]

Meningoencephalitis and Cerebral Abscess

If there is a strong suspicion of bacterial meningitis, I.V. antibiotics should be started immediately because this condition can be rapidly fatal. If there is a delay in obtaining the CSF, one should start treatment blind. Antibiotic selection depends on the initial expectation of the organism most likely to be involved, the results of Gram stain of the CSF, and the drug's ability to penetrate the CNS. Neurosurgical consultation is obtained in the case of a suspected cerebral abscess or hydrocephalus, both of which may require emergency drainage. Subdural empyema is a rare complication of meningitis that usually requires drainage. In the case of diffuse cerebral edema, management and monitoring of ICP are indicated.

Treatment of a cerebral abscess consists of identification of the bacterial organisms, institution of antibiotic therapy, and drainage or excision of the abscess through a craniotomy or bur hole.[67-70] Repeated aspiration of the abscess may be necessary. Surgical excision is considered if there is persistent reaccumulation of the abscess, if the abscess is in an accessible site or is located in the cerebellum, or if there is a well-formed fibrous capsule that fails to collapse despite repeated aspiration.

Head Injury

The main goal in the management of head injury is the prevention of secondary injury. Treatment of such injuries is addressed more fully elsewhere [see 23 Injuries to the Central Nervous System].

OTHER CAUSES OF COMA

Hypothermia

Early intubation and respiratory support facilitate oxygenation and rewarming. In the case of circulatory arrest, for every decrease of 1° C in body temperature, the time during which there is hope for recovery without cardiopulmonary resuscitation can be doubled (this applies only to patients with primary hypothermia, not to those who are hypothermic because of cardiac arrest). Hypothermia can cause considerable coagulation disturbances, which predispose the patient to bleeding. To detect these abnormalities, the physician should perform clotting tests at the patient's core body temperature rather than at 37° C.

External or surface rewarming by covering the patient, by conducting treatment in a warm room, and by giving warmed I.V. fluids and warmed humidified oxygen is indicated in patients with a core body temperature higher than 30° C. In patients with a core body temperature below 30° C, surface rewarming is contraindicated. In these patients, surface rewarming could cause shunting of the blood to the dilated skin vessels, thereby exacerbating hypotension and further decreasing the core temperature, both of which predispose these patients to ventricular fibrillation. Active core rewarming is therefore instituted in these patients, which consists of delivering warmed humidified gases and parenteral fluids, performing peritoneal dialysis (4 to 8 L/hr at a temperature of 37° to 42° C), circulating water at 42° C through a closed irrigation system inserted into the esophagus or stomach (3 L/hr), or performing hemodialysis with the blood flowing past a dialysis solution warmed to 40° C. Considerations in the management of hypothermia are discussed more fully elsewhere [see 98 Fever, Hyperpyrexia, and Hypothermia].[71-77]

Seizures

Seizures or epileptic attacks are episodes of transient disturbance of electrochemical activity within the brain, expressed as abnormal motor, sensory, or psychological behavior. Epilepsy is defined as a condition characterized by recurrent unprovoked seizures. Traditionally, epileptic attacks are classified into three main groups [see Table 8]. Partial (focal) seizures are often associated with a structural abnormality, such as a scar, a tumor, or an AV malformation. Generalized seizures are a result of diffuse neuronal hyperactivity; there is usually no identifiable structural abnormality. Seizures that induce loss of consciousness may involve both cerebral hemispheres and may either be generalized from onset (primary generalized seizures) or begin focally and then spread to involve both hemispheres (secondary generalized seizures).

Table 8 **Classification of Epilepsy**

Generalized: bilaterally symmetrical; no local onset; loss of consciousness from onset
  Generalized tonic-clonic: idiopathic, no anatomic abnormality
  Absence (petit mal seizure): impaired consciousness with mild or no motor involvement
  Bilateral myoclonus: syndrome of three seizure types, including myoclonic jerks, generalized tonic-clonic seizures, and absence
  Infants and children: infantile spasms, atonic seizures, and tonic seizures

Partial: focal from onset
  Simple (usually no loss of consciousness)
  Complex (any alteration of consciousness, automatisms)
  Partial with secondary generalization

Unclassified epileptic seizures

Several systemic and neurologic diseases can give rise to seizures. Head trauma, cerebrovascular disease, and CNS infections are common causes, as are metabolic imbalances such as hypoglycemia, hypoxia, hyponatremia, hypernatremia, hypocalcemia, and hypomagnesemia. In addition, hypothermia can induce seizures. Drugs and toxins, such as methylxanthines, tricyclic antidepressants, phenothiazine, cocaine, and local anesthetics (e.g., lidocaine), can lead to seizures. Withdrawal of a drug—particularly of a barbiturate, alcohol, or a hypnotic—can cause seizures if too abrupt.

Generalized tonic-clonic seizures are characterized by sudden loss of consciousness associated with tonic-clonic movements. There is no preceding aura, but occasionally, there may be preictal irritability or a rising epigastric sensation. During the seizure, the patient falls to the ground, sometimes with a cry; tongue biting and loss of sphincter control are often noted. After an initial period of tonic rigidity and short-lived apnea, clonic jerking of the neck, trunk, and extremities ensues. The clonic jerking gives way to flaccid relaxation accompanied by labored breathing, pallor, and hypersalivation. Consciousness, lost at the beginning of the seizure, is gradually regained, but postictal confusion and drowsiness may last for hours. Grand mal seizures may predispose the patient to serious bodily injuries, such as vertebral compression fractures, cerebral trauma, and drowning.

Status epilepticus occurs when the seizures follow one another without recovery of consciousness between episodes. Specifically, it is defined as more than 30 minutes of convulsive activity or repeated convulsions over the course of 30 minutes without return of consciousness in between. This arbitrary definition is related to the onset of cerebral metabolic and systemic consequences of prolonged seizure activity [see Discussion, Cellular, Metabolic, and Systemic Effects of Status Epilepticus, below]. Withdrawal of antiepileptic drugs is the most common cause of status epilepticus among patients with epilepsy. Status epilepticus can be classified into convulsive status epilepticus and nonconvulsive status epilepticus. Tonic-clonic status epilepticus is the most feared complication of epilepsy and is potentially lethal. The death rate approaches 60% in untreated patients; even with skilled management, the death rate is 10%.[78] In what follows, we focus on management of tonic-clonic status epilepticus.

MANAGEMENT OF STATUS EPILEPTICUS

General Management of Seizures

Most seizures are self-limited and therefore rarely require emergency treatment. When a seizure does not resolve quickly and spontaneously, treatment must be rapid and efficient. The primary goals of treatment are (1) to ensure adequate ventilation so as to prevent hypoxia and (2) to prevent complications such as aspiration and physical injuries. A quick history and physical examination are performed in an attempt to determine the underlying cause of the seizure, while an assistant begins drawing blood and inserting a venous line. Blood specimens are obtained for measurement of anticonvulsant drug levels, biochemical tests, a hemogram, and assessment of arterial blood gas pressures. Blood glucose level is determined by means of rapid bedside techniques; if it cannot be estimated immediately or is estimated to be lower than 60 mg/dl, dextrose is infused (50 ml of a 50% solution for adults and 1 to 2 ml/kg of a 25% solution for children). Adult patients are also given 100 mg of thiamine I.V. as a safeguard against an exacerbation of Wernicke encephalopathy, which is a relatively common disease among patients with status epilepticus. Thiamine is always given before dextrose is administered.

Patients with hyponatremia, whose condition may be associated with compulsive water drinking, fluid overload, or the syndrome of inappropriate antidiuretic hormone secretion, are given a hypertonic (3%) solution of sodium chloride by slow I.V. infusion. Half the calculated sodium deficit is administered, which is usually sufficient to stop seizures; the remaining deficit can be corrected by fluid restriction and diuresis. Excessively rapid correction of hyponatremia may result in cardiovascular overload or central pontine myelinosis. Patients with a recent history of thyroid or parathyroid surgery as well as a prolonged QT interval on the ECG should immediately be given I.V. calcium—1 to 2 ampules of calcium gluconate for 5 to 10 minutes—even if confirmatory laboratory results are not yet available. Because oxygenation, blood pressure, acid-base balance, and blood glucose may all be disturbed by prolonged convulsions, supportive medical care is just as important as anticonvulsant drug therapy.

Pharmacotherapy for Status Epilepticus

The three main drugs or drug classes used in the treatment of status epilepticus are the benzodiazepines, phenytoin, and the barbiturates. Usually a benzodiazepine is administered first, followed immediately by a loading dose of phenytoin. Benzodiazepines exert their effect by enhancing γ-aminobutyric acid (GABA) inhibition, whereas phenytoin interferes with sodium entry into the cell [*see* Discussion, *below*]. Among the benzodiazepines, lorazepam is the preferred drug. Because diazepam is redistributed rapidly in fatty tissue, seizures may recur within 10 to 20 minutes. Furthermore, diazepam appears to be less effective in aborting status epilepticus. A 1995 study showed that lorazepam aborted status epilepticus in 97% of cases and diazepam in only 68%.[79] A side effect of benzodiazepines is respiratory depression, which occurs in approximately 12% of patients. Lorazepam appears to cause less respiratory depression than diazepam. In adults, lorazepam is given I.V. in a dosage of 4 mg over 2 minutes; the dose may be repeated after 5 minutes. In pediatric patients, a dose of 0.1 mg/kg is used, up to a maximum of 5 to 6 mg.

In adult patients who are not already taking phenytoin, the loading dose is 20 mg/kg, infused at a maximum rate of 50 mg/min. In patients taking phenytoin, 0.74 mg/kg is given to raise the level by 1 μg/ml. If the phenytoin level is unknown, a loading dose of 500 mg is given. In pediatric patients, the loading dose is 20 mg/kg infused at a rate of 1 to 3 mg/kg/min.

If the seizures continue, the initial strategy is to give additional doses of phenytoin (5 mg/kg each, to a maximum of 30 mg/kg). Thereafter, phenobarbital is loaded (20 mg/kg in adults, to a maximum of 100 mg/minute; 5 to 10 mg/kg in pediatric patients every 20 to 30 minutes, to a maximum of 30 to 40 mg/kg), or diazepam is given (100 mg/500 ml drip at 40 ml/min). As a last resort, general anesthesia is instituted, usually with pentobarbital. EEG monitoring should be performed in these patients, and pentobarbital should be titrated until burst-suppression occurs. In addition, blood pressure should be monitored closely because hypotension may occur.

Cognitive Impairment

Cognitive functions include consciousness; attention; orientation to time, place, and person; immediate, recent, and remote memory; abstraction; language; praxis; and visuomotor ability. Cognitive impairment is a common consequence of coma, particularly in patients with structural lesions. It may also follow status epilepticus, though more likely as a result of underlying brain abnormalities than of status epilepticus itself.[80]

In surgical settings, however, cognitive impairment is most common in patients who undergo major operations. It is often the result of delirium but may also be associated with dementia, amnestic disorders, depression, and various other mental disorders. In addition, several drugs may cause cognitive impairment, especially when administered in combination. Early detection is important because patients with cognitive deficits have higher rates of perioperative morbidity and mortality, longer hospital stays, and higher rates of institutionalization than patients with normal cognitive function do.

PERIOPERATIVE CARE: RISK FACTORS AND PREVENTIVE MEASURES

Certain factors increase the risk that cognitive impairment will develop in a surgical patient [*see* Table 9].[81,82] It is important to iden-

Table 9 Risk Factors and Exacerbating Factors for Cognitive Impairment

Risk factors	Exacerbating factors
Age > 60 yr	Unfamiliar environment
Addiction to alcohol, narcotics, or both	Communication deficits
Cerebral damage or disease	Sensory deprivation or overload
Cardiac, renal, or hepatic disease	Sleep deprivation
Visual or auditory impairment	Immobilization
Preoperative depression	Anxiety
History of delirium or functional psychosis	Pain
Family history of psychosis	

Table 10 **Precipitating Medical and Surgical Causes of Delirium**

Drug intoxication
  Alcohol, anesthesia, antianxiety agents, anticholinergics, anticonvulsants, antidepressants, antihistamines, antihypertensives, antiparkinsonian agents, cimetidine, clonidine, digitalis, insulin, lithium, neuroleptics, opiates, salicylates, sedative-hypnotics

Drug withdrawal
  Alcohol, antianxiety agents, sedative-hypnotics

Metabolic disturbances
  Electrolyte, fluid, or acid-base imbalance; endocrine disorders; hepatic or renal failure; hypoglycemia; hypothermia; hypoxia; paraneoplasm

Acute cerebral disorders
  Edema, encephalitis, epilepsy, fat emboli, primary or metastatic neoplasm, stroke, transient ischemic attack, vasculitis

Infections
  Bacterial endocarditis, meningitis, pneumonia, septicemia, urinary tract infection

Hemodynamic disturbances
  Anemia, arrhythmia, congestive heart failure, hypertensive encephalopathy, hypotension, hypovolemia, myocardial infarction, orthostatic hypotension

Respiratory disorders
  Pulmonary embolus

Nutritional and vitamin deficiency

Trauma
  Burns, fractures, head injury

tify and, when possible, reduce these risk factors by adopting the following measures:

1. Simplify drug regimens.
2. Taper and discontinue unnecessary medications. Obtain psychiatric consultation for patients receiving monoamine oxidase (MAO) inhibitors to determine whether the drug can be discontinued 2 weeks before operation.
3. Ensure therapeutic blood levels of drugs such as digitalis, anticonvulsants, and lithium. Lithium should be discontinued 1 to 2 days before operation.
4. For patients dependent on alcohol, analgesics, or anxiolytic-sedatives, stabilize drug intake, make proper substitutions, or, if time permits, gradually withdraw the agent.
5. Ensure nutritional, thiamine, and multivitamin supplementation in alcoholic patients and in malnourished elderly patients.
6. Review the management of the patient's existing medical and psychiatric disorders and obtain early consultation to provide optimal preoperative management.
7. Correct visual and auditory deficits if possible.

In addition, general supportive measures should be instituted as early as possible, and factors that exacerbate cognitive impairment should be mitigated [see Table 9]. Patients with cognitive impairment should be further evaluated for suicidal intent and behavior. If the patient is at risk of suicide or exhibits dangerous behavior (e.g., wandering, falling, or acting aggressively), psychiatric consultation should be obtained immediately, the physical environment should be secured, and a sitter should be present when family and staff are absent. Pharmacologic management may be necessary and is usually preferable to physical restraints, which can increase agitation, decrease mobility, and damage soft tissue.

Meticulous intraoperative care can prevent or diminish postoperative delirium in high-risk and cognitively impaired patients. The following precautionary measures are recommended:

1. If the patient has received an MAO inhibitor within 2 weeks of operation, monitor blood pressure levels carefully. If hypotension develops, treat with a direct-acting sympathomimetic such as phenylephrine.[83]
2. Plan anesthesia and surgical interventions so as to minimize operative time, hypotension, tissue damage, and the use of psychoactive drugs.
3. Avoid premedication with highly anticholinergic drugs (e.g., scopolamine or atropine).
4. Schedule the operation to minimize waiting time, anxiety, and fasting.
5. Maintain normal body temperature, especially in an elderly patient.
6. Carefully monitor hemodynamic, cardiac, and metabolic functions.
7. Ensure that orienting procedures and the use of glasses and hearing aids are resumed in the recovery room.

In the postoperative period, measures to prevent medical and surgical causes of delirium include the following:

1. Administer essential medications, sufficient calories, and detoxification agents parenterally until oral intake can be resumed.
2. Avoid excessive analgesic administration or routine use of long-acting benzodiazepines (e.g., diazepam or flurazepam).
3. Initiate early and vigorous treatment of metabolic imbalances, infection, hemodynamic disturbances, respiratory failure, and trauma (e.g., from falls or bedsores).
4. Reduce factors that contribute to cognitive impairment by continuing the supportive measures that were initiated before the operation.
5. Preserve maximum possible visual input in eye-surgery patients; enhance tactile and auditory clues.
6. Encourage all patients to become mobile and to resume autonomous functioning as soon as physical and cognitive abilities permit.

DIAGNOSIS AND MANAGEMENT OF FREQUENT CAUSES OF COGNITIVE IMPAIRMENT

The Mini-Mental State Examination and the Confusion Assessment Method are useful, rapid tests for evaluating cognitive functions,[84-87] though their sensitivity largely depends on the experience and background of the investigator.[88] These tests should be repeated daily in patients with cognitive impairment and in high-risk patients. The most frequent causes of cognitive impairment are delirium, dementia, depression, head injury, and pharmacotherapy.

Delirium

An obvious deterioration in cognitive ability, behavior, or mood during the first week after operation is usually caused by delirium and signals the presence of potentially life-threatening disorders [see Table 10]. Delirium is a transient mental disorder characterized by acute onset of global impairment of cognitive functions and widespread disturbance of cerebral metabolism. Delirium may arise immediately after the operation but typically follows after an interval of several days. Early manifestations include restlessness, irritability, insomnia, lethargy, kinesthetic sensations, vivid and frightening dreams, illusions, difficulty in thinking, and thickening or slurring of speech. As

Table 11 **DSM-IV Diagnostic Criteria for Delirium**

Disturbance of consciousness (i.e., reduced clarity of awareness of environment) with reduced ability to focus or sustain or shift attention

Change in cognition (e.g., memory deficit, disorientation, language disturbance) or the development of a perceptual disturbance that is not better accounted for by a preexisting, established, or evolving dementia

Development of the disturbance over a short time (usually hours to days) and fluctuation during the course of the day

Evidence from the history, physical examination, or laboratory findings that the disturbance is caused by a general medical condition, substance intoxication, substance withdrawal, or more than one such cause

DSM-IV—Diagnostic and Statistical Manual of Mental Disorders, 4th edition.

Table 12 **Laboratory Studies to Investigate Delirium**

Routine procedures
  Complete blood count
  Blood chemistry tests for electrolytes; calcium, phosphate, and glucose; blood urea nitrogen; liver enzymes
  Urinalysis
  Erythrocyte sedimentation rate
  Serologic test for syphilis
  Chest x-ray
  Electrocardiogram

Special procedures
  Blood chemistry tests for creatinine, magnesium, vitamin B_{12}, folate, thyroxine, ammonia, serum proteins, osmolality, arterial blood gases, cortisol
  Test for levels of medications in the blood
  Blood and urine toxicology screens
  Blood cultures
  HIV antibody test
  Lupus erythematosus preparation and antinuclear antibody test
  Urine tests for osmolality, porphobilinogen, 5-hydroxyindoleacetic acid
  CSF examination for cells, protein, glucose, culture, viral serology, pressure
  Cranial CT scan or MRI
  Electroencephalogram

the syndrome progresses, fluctuations in attention, perception, orientation, language, and intellectual functioning may become apparent. Sleep becomes fragmented, and day and night cycles may be reversed. Urinary incontinence, loss of motor coordination, focal neurologic signs, nystagmus, and various types of tremor may also be noted. Bilateral asterixis and multifocal myoclonus are highly suggestive of delirium. Current diagnostic criteria for delirium are given in the fourth edition of the *Diagnostic and Statistical Manual of Mental Disorders (DSM-IV)* [see Table 11].

When delirium is suspected on clinical grounds, appropriate laboratory studies should be performed to help identify precipitating organic causes [see Table 12]. Management of delirium includes treatment of precipitating factors [see Table 9], control of exacerbating factors [see Table 9], continuation of prophylactic measures, and management of agitation (see below).

Dementia

Dementia is a clinical syndrome that usually occurs in the elderly [see 75 The Elderly Surgical Patient]. Dementia has a protracted course that is characterized by loss of cognitive abilities, disorganization of personality, and decreased ability to perform activities of daily living. Consciousness is usually not disturbed, unless delirium is present. Dementia can be totally reversed in 10% to 15% of patients if detected early and treated appropriately, and it can be arrested or at least partially improved in 25% to 30%.[89,90] Of the many disorders that cause dementia [see Table 13], Alzheimer disease and vascular diseases (multi-infarct dementia) are most commonly implicated, accounting for, respectively, 40% to 60% and 10% to 25% of all cases.[89,90] The diagnosis of Alzheimer disease is based on the presence of a progressive dementia of insidious onset with prominent aphasia, apraxia, and cognitive impairment, but with relatively intact motor functions until the final stages of the disease.[91] A family history of the disease may be present. The diagnosis of vascular dementia is suggested by a sudden onset, a stepwise deteriorating course, focal neurologic signs and symptoms, and evidence of significant cerebrovascular disease from the history, clinical examination, or laboratory tests. Other causes of dementia are excluded by the history, clinical examination, and laboratory results.[90,92] *DSM-IV* also lists criteria for dementia [see Table 14], and recommended investigations for suspected dementia are similar to those outlined previously [see Table 12]. In addition, psychological tests may be helpful in certain cases.[89,93,94]

Management of dementia includes treating underlying causes and superimposed delirium or coexisting depression, minimizing exacerbating factors for cognitive impairment [see Table 9], and alleviating common manifestations of dementia (e.g., intellectual impairment, depression, insomnia, wandering, agitation, immobility, motor instability, incontinence, iatrogenic conditions, and family

Table 13 **Causes of Dementia**

Degenerative
  Senile dementia, Alzheimer disease, Pick disease, Huntington chorea, Parkinson disease, Creutzfeldt-Jakob disease, normal-pressure hydrocephalus, multiple sclerosis

Intracranial space-occupying lesions
  Tumor, subdural hematoma

Trauma
  Single severe head injury, repeated head injury (e.g., in boxers, football players)

Infections and related conditions
  Encephalitis, neurosyphilis, cerebral sarcoidosis

Vascular
  Multi-infarct dementia, occlusion of the carotid artery, cranial arteritis

Metabolic
  Sustained uremia, liver failure, remote effects of carcinoma or lymphoma, renal dialysis

Toxic
  Alcohol, poisoning with heavy metals (e.g., lead, arsenic, thallium)

Anoxia
  Anemia, postanesthesia, carbon monoxide, cardiac arrest, chronic respiratory failure

Vitamin deficiency
  Sustained lack of vitamin B_{12}, folic acid, thiamine

> **Table 14 DSM-IV Diagnostic Criteria for Dementia**
>
> Development of multiple cognitive deficits
> Impaired memory (new and previously learned information)
> One or more of the following: aphasia, apraxia, agnosia, and disturbed executive functioning (planning, organizing, sequencing, abstracting)
> Each of the above cognitive deficits must cause significant social or occupational impairment and represent a significant decline from previous functioning
> Deficits do not occur exclusively during the course of delirium
> *Additional criteria* are required for diagnosis of one of the following dementia types
> *Dementia of Alzheimer type*
>   Gradual onset and continuing cognitive decline; cognitive deficits resulting from other CNS conditions, systemic conditions, or substance-induced conditions not better accounted for by other axis I disorders
> *Vascular dementia*
>   Focal signs and symptoms or laboratory evidence of cerebrovascular disases that are judged to be etiologically related
> *Dementia resulting from other general medical conditions*
>   Evidence that the disturbance is a direct physiologic consequence of a general medical disorder (to be coded on axis III)
> *Substance-induced persistent dementia*
>   Deficits present beyond the usual duration of substance intoxication or withdrawal. Evidence that deficits are etiologically related to the persisting effects of substance use.
> *Dementia resulting from multiple etiologies*
>   Evidence that the disturbance has more than one cause
>
> DSM–IV—*Diagnostic and Statistical Manual of Mental Disorders*, 4th edition.

burden). Specific patient management and pharmacologic interventions are discussed elsewhere.[95-102]

Depression

Features that suggest a depressive disorder underlying cognitive impairment include a history of affective disorder in the patient or the family, a clearly depressed mood, and an atypical recent history of cognitive deficit.[103-105] Depression may also be the result of a general medical condition or an underlying organic cause; in addition, medications, substance abuse, endocrinopathies, malignant disorders, head injury, infectious disorders, and metabolic disorders should always be considered. Furthermore, the depressive episode may continue even after the precipitating organic factor has been removed and may require the same treatment as a major depressive episode. *DSM-IV* outlines the criteria for a major depressive episode [see Table 15].

If the patient is currently depressed and is already receiving a maintenance regimen of antidepressants, the dose should be increased every 2 to 5 days until the maximum daily dose is reached, intolerable side effects occur, or a clinical response is achieved. If the patient is starting antidepressant therapy and there is no history of a good response to any particular drug in either the patient or the family, the treatment of choice should be a tricyclic antidepressant (TCA) with minimal anticholinergic properties (e.g., desipramine) or a selective serotonin reuptake inhibitor (SSRI) (e.g., fluoxetine or sertraline). In elderly patients, it is wise to initiate therapy with a low dose and to increase the dose gradually while watching for adverse effects, such as delirium or orthostatic hypotension with a TCA and nausea, anxiety, insomnia, or headache with an SSRI.[106-108]

A combined antidepressant-neuroleptic regimen or electroconvulsive therapy may be indicated in delusional patients. Electroconvulsive therapy is also indicated for severely depressed patients at risk of suicide or rapid physical decline. Depressed patients with a personal or family history of hypomania may need additional medication with lithium or anticonvulsant agents (i.e., carbamazepine or valproate). In these last three groups of patients, psychiatric consultation is advisable.

Head Injury

Cognitive impairment is common after severe head injury. The extent of cognitive impairment is not always clearly reflected in the Glasgow Outcome Scale (GOS) [see Table 16], however, which is one of the most popular scales used to assess outcome after head injury.[109,110] Many patients cannot function normally months or years after severe traumatic brain injury; common cognitive deficits include memory and behavior disturbances. In the group of patients with so-called GOS good recovery, a substantial number of patients undergo personality changes that interfere with their personal lives and careers.[111-113] In a study of 82 patients with severe head injury, the investigators monitored GOS scores and psychosocial reintegration (defined in terms of employment, interpersonal relationships, social contacts, and leisure interests) for 6 years after injury.[114] Of the 82 patients, 76% were classified as having poor or substantially limited reintegration; among the patients with favorable GOS scores (i.e., good recovery or moderate disability), only 50% were found to have good reintegration.

The severity of cognitive impairment is related to the severity of the initial injury (as reflected in the GCS), the time between injury and hospital admission, the type of brain lesion, the duration of coma, and the extent of posttraumatic amnesia.[115,116] In a study of 117 patients with severe head injuries, neuropsychological sequelae were ascertained from two examinations in 30 of the conscious survivors within the first year after injury and were related to CT examinations. CT findings included diffuse axonal injury, diffuse swelling,

> **Table 15 DSM-IV Diagnostic Criteria for Major Depressive Episodes**
>
> At least five of the following symptoms have been present during the same 2-week period and represent a change from previous functioning
>
> *and*
>
> either symptom 1 or 2 is present
>
> *and*
>
> symptoms are not caused by a general medical condition or by mood-incongruent delusions or hallucinations.
>
> 1. Depressed mood
> 2. Markedly diminished interest or pleasure
> 3. Significant gain or loss of weight or appetite
> 4. Insomnia or hypersomnia
> 5. Psychomotor agitation or retardation
> 6. Fatigue or loss of energy
> 7. Feelings of worthlessness or excessive or inappropriate guilt
> 8. Diminished ability to think, concentrate, or make decisions
> 9. Recurrent thoughts of death or suicide, suicide attempt, or suicide plan
>
> Symptoms do not meet criteria for a mixed (with manic features) episode.
> Symptoms cause clinically significant distress or impairment of functioning.
> Symptoms do not result from a substance (e.g., drug or abuse of medication) or a general medical condition.
> Symptoms are not explained by bereavement.
>
> DSM–IV—*Diagnostic and Statistical Manual of Mental Disorders*, 4th edition.

Table 16 Glasgow Outcome Scale[110]

Description	Score
Good recovery	5
Moderate disability	4
Severe disability	3
Vegetative state	2
Death	1

and focal injuries. Neuropsychological outcome varied with the type of CT lesion and the function measured. Overall differences in memory and learning were found among the three categories of CT lesions, whereas differences in intelligence and visuomotor functions were not significant. Levels of memory, learning, and visuomotor speed were higher after diffuse swelling injuries, but less improvement was noted. Greater improvements in memory, learning, and visuomotor speed occurred after diffuse axonal injury. After focal injuries, visuomotor speed improved, but recall and learning did not.[117]

Cognitive Side Effects of Pharmacologic Therapy

Cognitive side effects may be produced by a variety of medications from multiple drug classes. As noted, multidrug pharmacotherapy is an important cause of cognitive impairment, and drug regimens should be carefully evaluated, particularly in elderly patients. Impaired renal and hepatic function and the use of medications that interfere with hepatic and renal drug excretion may predispose patients to untoward effects. Elderly patients are more susceptible to cognitive side effects because of age-related alterations in pharmacokinetics, increased use of medications, and an increased incidence of premorbid cognitive impairment. Cognitive impairment in demented patients may be exacerbated by medications, and dementia increases the risk of delirium by twofold to threefold.[118] A comprehensive review of the cognitive side effects of pharmacotherapy together with an excellent source of references is available elsewhere.[119]

MANAGEMENT OF AGITATION

Agitation is frequently seen in patients with cognitive impairment and may present as increased psychomotor activity, often accompanied by wandering, shouting, and verbal or physical aggression. Management includes treatment of underlying disorders and intervention to reduce symptoms. The first steps in management consist of removing any obvious causes of the behavior, orienting the patient, increasing levels of safe activity, and improving pain control, any or all of which may suffice. If these measures are inadequate or the situation becomes life-threatening, psychopharmacologic management is indicated.

In several delirium syndromes, an antipsychotic drug is not the treatment of choice. In anticholinergic delirium, anticholinergic drugs are discontinued and supportive care is provided. If the delirium is life-threatening (i.e., associated with coma, seizures, or cardiac arrhythmias), parenteral physostigmine may reverse the danger. Because of its side effects, however, this drug should be used with caution.[120] For hepatic encephalopathy, a short-acting benzodiazepine that requires little hepatic degradation is preferred (e.g., oral oxazepam 15 to 30 mg every 6 hours as required). For delirium caused by alcohol or benzodiazepine withdrawal, benzodiazepines are preferred to antipsychotics, which are epileptogenic and may cause akathisia (motor restlessness). For alcohol withdrawal, 50 to 100 mg of thiamine should also be administered.[121] In emergency situations, 50 mg of chlordiazepoxide, 10 mg of diazepam, or 2 mg of lorazepam may be given slowly I.V. every 1 or 2 hours until control is established. Alternatively, 4 mg of lorazepam may be given I.M. In less urgent situations, 25 to 50 mg of chlordiazepoxide given I.M. or orally four times a day will suffice. As soon as the patient's condition is stable, the dosage can be tapered at a daily rate of about one tenth to one quarter of the initial dose. Fuller descriptions of the management of alcohol, benzodiazepine, barbiturate, and other sedative-hypnotic withdrawal syndromes are available elsewhere [*see 10 Substance Abuse*].

Haloperidol is the drug of choice for most other causes of agitation, particularly if patients display psychosis, aggression, or both. Haloperidol is relatively free from anticholinergic, autonomic, and drug-interaction effects. Side effects of the drug include extrapyramidal syndromes (i.e., Parkinson-like symptoms, akathisia, dyskinesia, or dystonia) and neuroleptic malignant syndrome, which is a rare but life-threatening complication. Brief treatment, however, does not usually cause severe side effects.

Mild forms of agitation are managed with haloperidol dosages of 2 to 15 mg orally twice a day. In elderly patients, 0.5 to 3 mg/day is usually sufficient. In emergency situations, haloperidol should be administered I.V. in a dose of 1 to 5 mg, and the dose should be increased by 5 to 10 mg/hour until an effective dose is achieved. Use of single doses of 30 mg and maximum daily doses of 100 mg has been reported.[121] For refractory cases, 1 to 4 mg of I.V. lorazepam may be added. Once improvement occurs, the regimen may be continued via the I.M. or oral route. In less urgent situations, severely agitated patients will usually respond to haloperidol, 2 to 10 mg/hr I.M., up to a daily dose of 10 to 60 mg (one third of this dose in the elderly). Supplementary parenteral dosages of 2 to 10 mg/hr may be administered. When the patient's behavior is controlled, haloperidol should be continued orally; if no supplementary doses are necessary, the dosage should be decreased by one quarter each day until discontinuance.

For delirium, the total duration of treatment with haloperidol is usually 3 to 5 days. For agitation associated with psychoses, longer

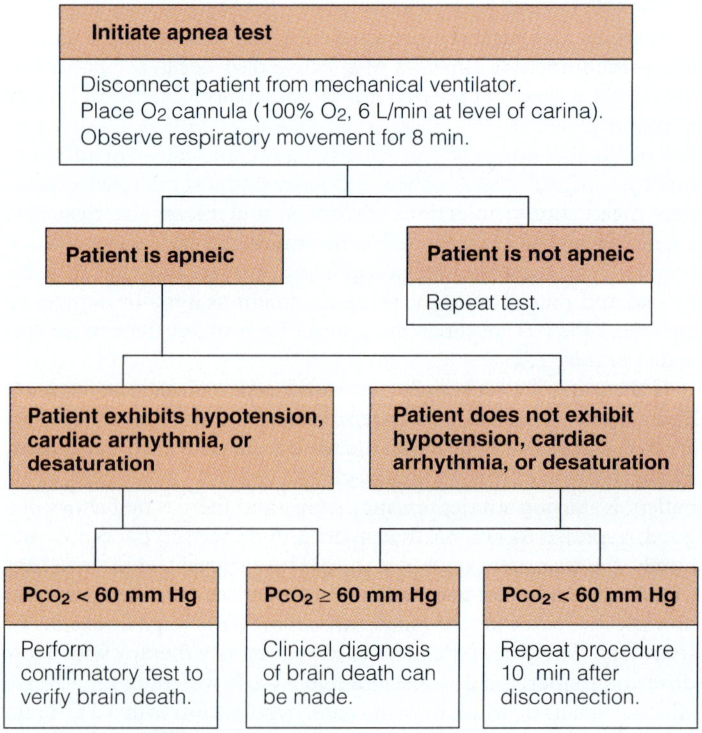

```
┌─────────────────────────────────────────┐
│ Initiate apnea test                     │
├─────────────────────────────────────────┤
│ Disconnect patient from mechanical ventilator. │
│ Place O₂ cannula (100% O₂, 6 L/min at level of carina). │
│ Observe respiratory movement for 8 min. │
└─────────────────────────────────────────┘
```

Patient is apneic / Patient is not apneic (Repeat test.)

Patient exhibits hypotension, cardiac arrhythmia, or desaturation / Patient does not exhibit hypotension, cardiac arrhythmia, or desaturation

P_{CO_2} < 60 mm Hg — Perform confirmatory test to verify brain death.
P_{CO_2} ≥ 60 mm Hg — Clinical diagnosis of brain death can be made.
P_{CO_2} < 60 mm Hg — Repeat procedure 10 min after disconnection.

Figure 8 Algorithm depicts the procedure for the apnea test in brain death.[124]

treatment is usually required and psychiatric follow-up is advisable. Patients who cannot tolerate or fail to respond to haloperidol may respond to a phenothiazine antipsychotic such as chlorpromazine (25 to 50 mg I.M. every hour, followed by 25 to 100 mg orally every 4 to 6 hours). Side effects of chlorpromazine include hypotension, drowsiness, cardiac arrhythmias, seizures, respiratory depression, and coma.

Brain Death

The term brain death implies irreversible cessation of activity in the cerebrum and brain stem. Brain death is frequently a consequence of severe head injury, (re)rupture of a cerebral aneurysm, or ICH[122,123]; less commonly, it is a consequence of fulminant encephalitis, bacterial meningitis, or anoxic-ischemic encephalopathy. A qualified physician should determine the occurrence of brain death, but legal requirements are different in various states and countries. Areas of concern include recognition of conditions that may mimic brain death, the procedure for the apnea test, indications for confirmatory tests, and management of physiologic changes associated with brain death. In addition, early identification of potential donor candidates is important, though selection of these candidates can proceed only after the clinical diagnosis of brain death has been established and family members have given their consent.

GUIDELINES FOR THE DETERMINATION OF BRAIN DEATH

The guidelines for determining brain death in adults and children have been published elsewhere[124]; accordingly, we provide here only a brief summary of the procedures involved. In most cases, the differences in the criteria for brain death from one state or country to another have to do with the type and number of confirmatory tests (see below) that are needed. The clinical diagnosis of brain death requires the following:

1. The presence of a cause that is compatible with brain death.
2. The absence of complicating medical conditions that may confound clinical assessment.
3. The absence of drug intoxication or poisoning.
4. A core temperature of at least 32° C.

In most patients, a CT scan will document an abnormality that is compatible with brain death. In patients with normal CT scans, the diagnosis should be reconsidered, unless there is a high certainty about the mechanism that has led to brain death (e.g., ischemic-anoxic brain death caused by cardiac arrest or asphyxia). CSF examination is indicated if a definite diagnosis cannot be made. Severe electrolyte, acid-base, and endocrine disturbances should be excluded, and a drug screen may be helpful to detect a specific drug or poison. In the presence of barbiturates, the diagnosis of brain death can likely be made when the levels are subtherapeutic; however, supportive data for this approach are available only for pediatric patients.[125] The core temperature should be at least 32° C because brain-stem reflexes are absent below 27° C.

If these conditions are met, clinical testing should follow. Three cardinal features of brain death are evaluated, as follows:

1. Coma or unresponsiveness.
2. Absence of brain-stem reflexes.
3. Apnea.

Coma or unresponsiveness is evaluated by assessing the motor response to painful stimuli, such as either supraorbital pressure or nail-bed pressure; this response should be absent. Pitfalls include the observation of spontaneous spinal motor responses (Lazarus sign), which may occur during pain stimuli, during the apnea test, and after recent administration of neuromuscular blocking agents. In the latter case, examination with a bedside nerve stimulator is required (so-called train-of-four monitoring). In a brain-dead patient, the pupils are typically in the middle position (4 to 6 mm) and fixed, although dilated pupils may be observed as well. Many drugs affect pupil size, but the light reflex usually remains intact. Topical ocular instillation of drugs, trauma to the cornea or the bulbus oculi, preexisting anatomic abnormalities, and previous surgical procedures should all be considered in the evaluation of the pupils and the pupillary response. The oculocephalic and caloric responses are then tested; these too should be absent. The caloric response can be diminished or abolished by a variety of drugs, including sedatives, TCAs, anticholinergics, antiepileptics, and chemotherapeutics. In addition, clotted blood or cerumen may occlude the external auditory canal, and fracture of the petrous bone may result in unilateral absence of a response. Finally, the corneal, pharyngeal, and tracheal reflexes are tested, all of which should be absent.

If all brain-stem reflexes are absent, the apnea test is performed [see Figure 8].[126] To minimize confounding factors, such as marked hypotension, severe cardiac dysrhythmias, and desaturations, the following precautions are taken[125]:

1. Core temperature must be 36° C or higher (rewarm the patient if temperature is lower).
2. Systolic BP must be 90 mm Hg or higher (use dopamine if BP is lower).
3. Fluid balance must be positive for 6 hours or longer (use vasopressin if this cannot be accomplished).
4. Arterial PCO_2 must be 40 mm Hg or higher (decrease minute ventilation if PCO_2 is lower).

Table 17 **Guidelines for the Determination of Brain Death in Children**

Historical criteria
  Determination of the proximate cause of coma
  Absence of remediable or reversible conditions such as toxins, drugs (sedatives, hypnotics, paralytics), metabolic disorders, surgically correctable conditions, hypotension, and hypothermia

Physical examination criteria
  Coexisting coma and apnea (standardized apnea test)
  Absence of brain-stem function
  Absence of hypothermia or hypotension
  Flaccid tone or absence of spontaneous or induced movements (except spinal cord events)
  Consistent examination findings throughout observation and testing periods

Observation periods and laboratory testing
  7 days to 2 months: two clinical examinations and apnea tests and two EEGs at least 48 hr apart
  2 to 12 months: two clinical examinations and apnea tests and two EEGs at least 24 hr apart*
  > 12 months: two clinical examinations and apnea tests at least 12 hr apart†

*Repeat examination and EEG are obviated by the absence of flow on cerebral angiogram.
†If hypoxic-ischemic encephalopathy is suspected, the observation period should be extended to 24 hr. Laboratory testing is not required if there is absence of a remediable or reversible condition.

5. Arterial PO_2 must be 200 mm Hg or higher (inspired oxygen fraction = 1.0 for 10 minutes).

CONFIRMATORY TESTS

Brain death is essentially a clinical diagnosis; it may be repeated after 6 hours to establish the final diagnosis. In most cases, this clinical diagnosis is sufficient; however, in cases in which the specific components of clinical testing cannot be evaluated reliably (e.g., as a result of drug intoxication, altered metabolic status, shock, or hypothermia), confirmatory tests may be indicated. Moreover, some countries require such confirmation by law, and many hospitals have their own policies for determining brain death. Generally accepted tests include EEG, cerebral angiography, single-photon emission CT, and, more recently, transcranial Doppler ultrasonography. In our experience, angiography not only is the most reliable and rapid way of establishing brain death but also occasionally shows that the cerebral circulation is normal and that further therapeutic efforts (such as hemicraniectomy) are justified. The tests are particularly important when organ and tissue donation are under consideration.

DETERMINATION OF BRAIN DEATH IN CHILDREN

Finally, a word is reserved for the determination of brain death in children. In children younger than 5 years, caution is indicated in applying the neurologic criteria for brain death. In comparison with adult brains, the brains of infants and young children have an increased resistance to cerebral damage that makes it easier for them to recover substantial functions, even after exhibiting unresponsiveness for longer than is possible in adults. Guidelines for the determination of brain death in children are available [see Table 17], but clear recommendations are lacking.[124,127,128]

Discussion

Pathophysiology of Coma

The pathophysiologic basis of coma is either a structural disruption of crucial areas in the cerebral hemispheres or brain stem (structural coma) or a diffuse depression of cerebral metabolism (metabolic coma). Cerebral metabolism is described in greater detail elsewhere [see 23 Injuries to the Central Nervous Sysytem]. Key variables for understanding the pathophysiology of coma include ICP, mean arterial pressure (MAP), cerebral perfusion pressure (CPP) (defined as MAP minus ICP), CBF (derived from CPP via the Poiseuille equation), the global arterial–jugular venous oxygen difference (A-VDO_2), and the cerebral metabolic rate of oxygen ($CMRO_2$) (derived via the Fick equation, CBF times A-VDO_2).

Because 95% of the energy in the normal brain is generated by oxidative metabolism, $CMRO_2$ is considered a sensitive measure of cerebral metabolism. Metabolic causes of coma predominantly interfere with $CMRO_2$, whereas structural causes of coma may interfere with both $CMRO_2$ and the supply of substrates. In patients with head injury, the observed depression in $CMRO_2$ has been related to impairment of mitochondrial function and consequently to depression of oxidative ATP generation.[129]

The resting CBF is approximately 55 ml/100 g/min, which is adequate for meeting normal metabolic demands and includes a modest safety margin to accommodate most physiologic changes. Between a CBF of 55 ml/100g/min and one of 25 ml/100 g/min, increased oxygen extraction compensates for the decrease in CBF, and $CMRO_2$ can be maintained. When the mean CBF drops below 25 ml/100 g/min, slowing of brain electrical activity is apparent on EEG, and a progressive depression of consciousness occurs clinically. This represents a stage of reversible brain dysfunction. Below a CBF of 18 ml/100 g/min, however, ATP generation is insufficient to support $CMRO_2$. Consequently, arrest of the sodium-potassium pump occurs, leading to membrane failure, cell swelling, and irreversible brain dysfunction. The resulting cell damage depends on both the duration and the amount of CBF depression.[130] In most circumstances, structural lesions affect CBF by their effect on the CPP.

Because CPP is defined as MAP minus ICP, it follows that CPP can be decreased by severe hypotension, which is a common complication in structural lesions such as head injuries, or by raised ICP, which may accompany any type of intracranial lesion.

As mentioned before, ICP is the product of a constantly changing interplay between CSF volume, brain tissue volume, and cerebral blood volume (CBV). These three compartments are enclosed within a rigid cranium, which implies that if ICP is to remain constant, any volume gained (e.g., from tumor, hematoma, or abscess) must be balanced by volume lost. In the presence of a cerebral mass, ICP can be maintained initially because CSF is displaced to the spinal compartment. At a certain volume, however, this compensatory mechanism is exhausted, and ICP rises rapidly [see Figure 9]. The resulting pressure-volume curve is exponential in shape; in other words, a relatively small increase in volume may cause only a small rise in ICP at the flat portion of the curve but a large increase in ICP at the steep portion. A small increase in volume (such as results from CO_2 retention [see below] or obstruction of venous outflow) can prove fatal to a patient with an elevated ICP.

Manipulation of CBV is an artificial method of compensating for raised ICP. CBV is determined by the total diameter of the vascular bed, and changes in diameter thus affect CBV. The cerebral vessels are sensitive to changes in the pH of the CSF and thus respond to changes in the partial pressure of CO_2 with caliber adjustments. CO_2 can be regulated by adjusting ventilatory settings, and hyperventilation (i.e., induction of hypocapnia) to induce vasoconstriction is a useful method to manage acute episodes of raised ICP. For long-term treatment of ICP, however, hyperventilation is not recommended [see 23 Injuries to the Central Nervous System].

Translocation of different parts of the brain produces specific herniation syndromes that have characteristic clinical presentations and temporal profiles. Brain herniation occurs in five major patterns.[1]

HERNIATION SYNDROMES

Subfalcial (Cingulate) Herniation

Mass lesions in the anterior or middle fossa may result in herniation of the cingulate gyrus under the free edge of the falx cerebri. Usually, patients with this condition are asymptomatic. If the herniation is severe, however, the pericallosal arteries may be compressed, resulting in unilateral or bilateral frontal infarcts in their region of distribution. Clinically, this may result in paresis of one or both legs.

Lateral (Uncal) Tentorial Herniation

Uncal herniation is caused by mass lesions in the lateral middle fossa or temporal lobe, which displace the medial edge of the uncus and hippocampal gyrus medially over the ipsilateral edge of the tentorium cerebelli. The uncus and the hippocampus thus herniate in the space between the midbrain and the tentorial edge, resulting in compression of the midbrain from side to side and elongation of its anteroposterior diameter. The ipsilateral cerebral peduncle and the

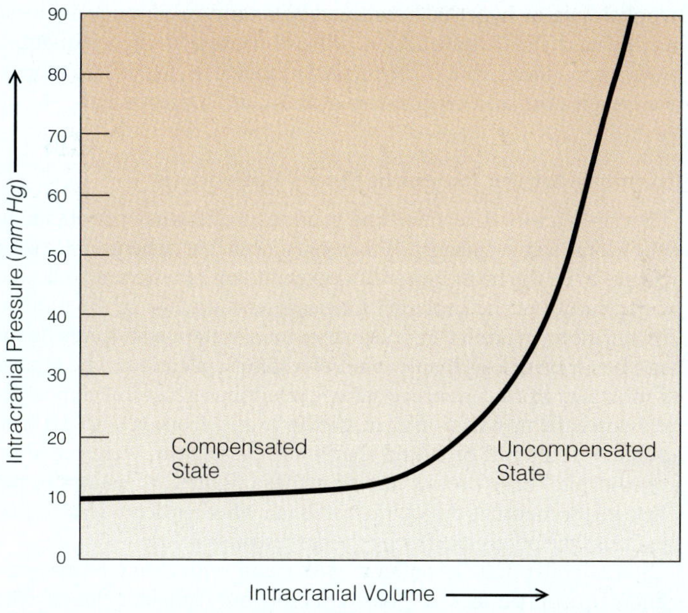

Figure 9 Depicted is the relation between ICP and intracranial volume.

oculomotor nerve are compressed, resulting in the classic syndrome of uncal herniation, which consists of contralateral hemiparesis, decreased consciousness (possibly caused by distortion or deafferentiation of the upper part of the RAS), and ipsilateral pupillary dilatation. In some cases, the herniation may cause compression of the contralateral cerebral peduncle against the tentorium, resulting in ipsilateral hemiparesis (Kernohan's notch). In these cases, the contralateral oculomotor nerve may also be stretched.

As uncal herniation progresses, it becomes clinically indistinguishable from central herniation. Early recognition of uncal herniation is important because deterioration may proceed rapidly once signs of herniation and brain-stem compression appear. In its initial stages, uncal herniation is fully reversible; however, as it evolves, neurologic recovery becomes progressively less likely.

Posterior (Tectal) Herniation

Posterior or tectal herniation may occur in patients who have purely frontal or occipital lesions or have bilateral lesions such as a bilateral chronic subdural hematoma. Under these circumstances, the medial temporal structures do not herniate between the tentorium and midbrain; instead, they herniate posteriorly or on both sides, thereby compressing the quadrigeminal plate at the level of the superior colliculi. Clinically, this results in findings resembling Parinaud syndrome. The patient has bilateral ptosis and an upward gaze paralysis in the presence of initially preserved pupillary response.

Central (Axial) Herniation

Central or axial herniation is defined as a downward shift of the entire brain stem toward the foramen magnum. Because of the downward herniation, the brain stem is elongated in its anteroposterior diameter, and stretching may occur in the central perforating branches of the basilar artery. This stretching is thought to produce ischemia and hemorrhage, although hemorrhage occasionally results from reversal of the displacement by operative decompression. Impaired consciousness has been related to this axial displacement. The Cushing response (arterial hypertension, bradycardia, and respiratory irregularity) has also been related to brain-stem ischemia.

Brain-stem blood flow is not always decreased in the presence of a Cushing response, however, and variant Cushing responses (e.g., hypotension) exist.[12,131]

The first clinical signs are reduced consciousness; symmetrical, small, reactive pupils; paresis of the upward gaze; signs of bilateral corticospinal tract dysfunction; and periodic breathing (Cheyne-Stokes respiration). As herniation progresses, flexor and eventually extensor posturing occurs, the pupils become fixed and dilated or remain in midposition, and hyperpnea results. At later stages, the lower pons and upper medulla are affected; this is characterized by fixed midposition pupils, limb flaccidity, bilateral Babinski responses, abolished oculovestibular reflexes, and shallow, regular breathing, often at an increased rate. Finally, medullary dysfunction occurs; patients display slow, irregular respiration interrupted by deep sighs and gasps. All reflexes disappear and the pupils become widely dilated.

Tonsillar Herniation

Prolapse of the cerebral tonsils through the foramen magnum can occur with either supratentorial or infratentorial masses or with a generalized increase in ICP. Tonsillar herniation causes obliteration of the cisterna magna and compression of the medulla oblongata, the latter resulting in apnea. The shape and size of the tentorial opening determine whether signs of tentorial or tonsillar herniation predominate with supratentorial mass lesions. When the opening is small, major symptoms are usually tentorial in nature; however, when the opening is large, tonsillar herniation may follow without any preceding signs of tentorial herniation.

Prognosis for the Comatose Patient

Even when optimal treatment is provided, the overall prognosis for the comatose patient is poor. Only about 40% of patients who are unconscious as a result of head trauma make a satisfactory recovery. In nontraumatic coma, the outcome is worse. In a study of 596 patients who were admitted for cardiac arrest (31%), cerebral infarction (36%), or ICH (36%), follow-up at 2 months showed that 69% had died, 20% survived with severe disability, 8% survived without severe disability, and 3% survived with unknown functional status.[132]

Outcome depends primarily on the etiology and the duration of coma, the initial clinical signs of neurologic damage, and the general medical condition and age of the patient. In patients with head injury, a motor score of 3 on admission, episodes of hypoxia (PO_2 < 60 mm Hg), hypotension (systolic blood pressure < 90 mm Hg), and raised ICP are important prognosticators of poor outcome.[133] Coma caused by depressant drug poisoning carries the most favorable prognosis if treated early: overall mortality is 1% to 5%.[134,135] Hypoxic-ischemic coma carries the worst prognosis: overall mortality is as high as 54%.[135,136] Most patients who recover from drug overdose suffer no residual brain damage, even after prolonged coma, whereas in one study, more than 50% of patients with hypoxic-ischemic coma who survived for at least 2 weeks remained comatose and suffered permanent brain damage.[135]

Cellular, Metabolic, and Systemic Effects of Status Epilepticus

The events that initiate status epilepticus are not known. The presence of an abnormally prolonged seizure has been attributed to excessive excitation, a failure of inhibition, or a combination of the two. However, relatively little is known about the cellular and molecular changes within a neuronal network that are responsible for persistent seizure activity. Excitation is a glutamate-dependent process and is initiated when the neurotransmitter glutamate binds to postsynaptic N-methyl-D-aspartate (NMDA) and non-NMDA glutamate receptors.[137] Initially, only non-NMDA channels are activated, resulting in the influx of sodium and depolarization. Ion flow through NMDA channels is blocked because of the presence of magnesium in the ion channel and because of GABA-mediated inhibitory mechanisms. In status epilepticus, however, GABA-mediated inhibition is suppressed, resulting in depolarization of the NMDA receptor, removal of magnesium from the ion channel, and influx of calcium, followed by further depolarization and intracellular calcium accumulation. Cell death after status epilepticus has been attributed to increased calcium accumulation, initiation of cell swelling, and calcium-mediated cell destruction.[138]

The effects of status epilepticus on cerebral metabolism and circulation can be divided into two phases, whereby the transition from phase 1 to phase 2 typically occurs at 30 to 60 minutes of continuous seizure activity.[138] In phase 1, an increase in CBF compensates for the increase in cerebral metabolic activity caused by the seizures, and the delivery of oxygen and glucose is maintained. In phase 2, the physiologic compensation mechanism (i.e., cerebral autoregulation) begins to fail because CBF is no longer sufficient to support the high metabolic demands of the epileptic tissue, and ischemia ensues.[139-141] Ischemia is further precipitated by systemic hypotension, which almost invariably occurs in phase 2 and which is in turn greatly exacerbated by I.V. antiepileptic drug therapy, particularly when these drugs are infused quickly. ICP can rise exponentially in late status epilepticus, and this rise, combined with hypotension, results in a decrease in CPP, which further compromises the cerebral circulation.

Other general metabolic and systemic effects of status epilepticus occurring in phase 1 include autonomic changes such as tachycardia, cardiac dysrhythmias, hypertension, apnea, pupillary enlargement, hypersecretion, sweating, incontinence, hyperglycemia, and lactic acidosis. In phase 2, changes include hypoglycemia, hyponatremia, hypokalemia or hyperkalemia, metabolic and respiratory acidosis, hepatic and renal dysfunction, diffuse intravascular coagulation, multiorgan failure, rhabdomyolysis, leukocytosis, hypoxia, hypotension, respiratory and cardiac impairment, and hyperpyrexia.[138]

Prognosis for the Patient in Status Epilepticus

Several factors determine the prognosis of status epilepticus. In tonic-clonic status epilepticus, the actual time that patients are seizing appears to be the most important determinant of outcome, followed by the nature of the underlying disease and the age of the patient. Furthermore, in adults it appears that intermittent status epilepticus has a better prognosis than continuous status epilepticus. The reported mortality from convulsive status epilepticus in several clinical series varied from 0% to 6% in children and from 0% to 10% in adults.[142] It should be noted that all of these cases were retrieved from hospital-based series and that these figures are estimates because it is sometimes difficult to establish whether death was caused by status epilepticus itself or by the underlying disease.

Status epilepticus in patients with head injury may represent a significant contribution to poor outcome, but sufficient clinical data are unavailable. Seizure prophylaxis is recommended in patients with head injuries, but no guidelines are currently available to indicate who should receive it (i.e., patients with severe head injuries only or those with moderate head injuries as well). In a recent study of 94 patients with moderate to severe head injuries who underwent continuous EEG monitoring, seizure activity was demonstrated in 22% of patients despite phenytoin prophylaxis. Six of them displayed status epilepticus, all of whom subsequently died; these results indicate that continuous evaluation for seizures or status epilepticus should be seriously considered in these patients, together with aggressive intervention.[143]

References

1. Miller J, Becker D: Pathophysiology of head injury. Neurological Surgery, 2nd ed. Youmans J, Ed. WB Saunders Co, Philadelphia, 1982, p 1896
2. Denny-Brown D: Selected Writings of Sir Charles Sherrington. Oxford University Press, Oxford, 1979
3. Eccles J, Gibson W: Sherrington, His Life and Thought. Springer International, Berlin, 1979
4. Greenberg RP, Stablein DM, Becker DP: Noninvasive localization of brain-stem lesions in the cat with multimodality evoked potentials: correlation with human head-injury data. J Neurosurg 54:740, 1981
5. Ritter AM, Muizelaar JP, Barnes T, et al: Brain stem blood flow, pupillary response, and outcome in patients with severe head injuries. Neurosurgery 44:941, 1999
6. Qureshi A, Wilson D, Traystman R: Treatment of elevated intracranial pressure in experimental intracerebral hemorrhage: comparison between mannitol and hypertonic saline. Neurosurgery 44:1055, 1999
7. Kellie G: On death from cold, and on congestions of the brain. An account of the appearances observed in the dissection of two of three individuals presumed to have perished in the storm of 3rd November 1821; with some reflections on the pathology of the brain. Trans Med Chir Soc Edinburgh 1:84, 1824
8. Monro A: Observations on the Structure and Function of the Nervous System. Creech and Johnson, Edinburgh, 1783
9. Chesnut RM, Marshall LF: Management of head injury. Treatment of abnormal intracranial pressure. Neurosurg Clin N Am 2:267, 1991
10. Eisenberg HM, Frankowski RF, Contant CF, et al: High-dose barbiturate control of elevated intracranial pressure in patients with severe head injury. J Neurosurg 69:15, 1988
11. Miller JD, Becker DP, Ward JD, et al: Significance of intracranial hypertension in severe head injury. J Neurosurg 47:503, 1977
12. Rowan JO, Teasdale G: Brain stem blood flow during raised intracranial pressure. Acta Neurol Scand Suppl 64:520, 1977
13. Souhami R, Moxham J: Textbook of Medicine. Churchill Livingstone, Edinburgh, 1990, p 747
14. Souhami R, Moxham J: Textbook of Medicine. Churchill Livingstone, Edinburgh, 1990, p 971
15. Souhami R, Moxham J: Textbook of Medicine. Churchill Livingstone, Edinburgh, 1990, p 806
16. Souhami R, Moxham J: Textbook of Medicine. Churchill Livingstone, Edinburgh, 1990, p 968
17. Forsyth PA, Posner JB: Headaches in patients with brain tumors: a study of 111 patients. Neurology 43:1678, 1993
18. Ropper A, Gress D: Computerized tomography and clinical features of large cerebral hemorrhages. Cerebrovasc Dis 1:38, 1991
19. Brott T, Thalinger K, Hertzberg V: Hypertension as a risk factor for spontaneous intracerebral hemorrhage. Stroke 17:1078, 1986
20. Hunt WE, Hess RM: Surgical risk as related to time of intervention in the repair of intracranial aneurysms. J Neurosurg 28:14, 1968
21. Drake C: Report of World Federation of Neurological Surgeons Committee on a universal subarachnoid hemorrhage grading scale. J Neurosurg 68:985, 1988
22. Eisenberg HM, Gary HE Jr, Aldrich EF, et al: Initial CT findings in 753 patients with severe head injury. A report from the NIH Traumatic Coma Data Bank. J Neurosurg 73:688, 1990
23. Martin NA, Doberstein C, Alexander M, et al: Post-traumatic cerebral arterial spasm. J Neurotrauma 12:897, 1995
24. Romer F: Difficulties in the diagnosis of acute bacterial meningitis: evaluation of antibiotic pretreatment and causes of admission to the hospital. Lancet 2:345, 1977
25. Bolton C: Infections of the central nervous system. Coma and Impaired Consciousness. Young G, Ropper A, Bolton C, Eds. McGraw-Hill Book Co, New York, 1998, p 228
26. Young G: Impaired consciousness and disorders of temperature. Coma and Impaired Consciousness. Young G, Ropper A, Bolton C, Eds. McGraw-Hill Book Co, New York, 1998, p 213
27. Katz RT, Haig AJ, Clark BB, et al: Long-term survival, prognosis, and life-care planning for 29 patients with chronic locked-in syndrome. Arch Phys Med Rehabil 73:403, 1992
28. Tomsick TA, Brott TG, Chambers AA, et al: Hyperdense middle cerebral artery sign on CT: efficacy in detecting middle cerebral artery thrombosis. AJNR Am J Neuroradiol 11:473, 1990
29. Tomsick T, Brott T, Barsan W, et al: Thrombus localization with emergency cerebral CT. AJNR Am J Neuroradiol 13:257, 1992
30. Wijdicks E: The Clinical Practice of Critical Care Neurology. Lippincott-Raven, Philadelphia, 1997, p 193

31. Fisher CM, Kistler JP, Davis JM: Relation of cerebral vasospasm to subarachnoid hemorrhage visualized by computerized tomographic scanning. Neurosurgery 6:1, 1980
32. Brouwers PJ, Wijdicks EF, Van Gijn J: Infarction after aneurysm rupture does not depend on distribution or clearance rate of blood. Stroke 23:374, 1992
33. Hillman J: Should computed tomography scanning replace lumbar puncture in the diagnostic process in suspected subarachnoid hemorrhage? Surg Neurol 26:547, 1986
34. Hashimoto H, Iida J, Hironaka Y, et al: Use of spiral computerized tomography angiography in patients with subarachnoid hemorrhage in whom subtraction angiography did not reveal cerebral aneurysms. J Neurosurg 92:278, 2000
35. Strayle-Batra M, Skalej M, Wakhloo AK, et al: Three-dimensional spiral CT angiography in the detection of cerebral aneurysm. Acta Radiol 39:233, 1998
36. Velthuis BK, Rinkel GJ, Ramos LM, et al: Subarachnoid hemorrhage: aneurysm detection and preoperative evaluation with CT angiography. Radiology 208:423, 1998
37. Harrison MJ, Johnson BA, Gardner GM, et al: Preliminary results on the management of unruptured intracranial aneurysms with magnetic resonance angiography and computed tomographic angiography. Neurosurgery 40:947, discussion 955, 1997
38. Wardlaw JM, White PM: The detection and management of unruptured intracranial aneurysms. Brain 123:205, 2000
39. Desprechins B, Stadnik T, Koerts G, et al: Use of diffusion-weighted MR imaging in differential diagnosis between intracerebral necrotic tumors and cerebral abscesses [see comments]. AJNR Am J Neuroradiol 20:1252, 1999
40. Miller ES, Dias PS, Uttley D: CT scanning in the management of intracranial abscess: a review of 100 cases. Br J Neurosurg 2:439, 1988
41. Zimmerman RA, Bilaniuk LT: Computed tomographic staging of traumatic epidural bleeding. Radiology 144:809, 1982
42. Gennarelli TA, Thibault LE: Biomechanics of acute subdural hematoma. J Trauma 22:680, 1982
43. Gudeman SK, Kishore PR, Miller JD, et al: The genesis and significance of delayed traumatic intracerebral hematoma. Neurosurgery 5:309, 1979
44. Ribas G, Jane J: Traumatic contusions and intracerebral hematomas. Central Nervous System Trauma Status Report 1991. J Neurotrauma 9[suppl 1]:S265, 1992
45. Becker D, Doberstein C, Hovda D: Craniocerebral Trauma: Mechanisms, Management, and the Cellular Response to Injury. Current Concepts. The Upjohn Co, Kalamazoo, Michigan, 1994
46. Chesnut R, Servadei F: Surgical treatment of post-traumatic mass lesions. Traumatic Brain Injury. Marion D, Ed. Thieme Medical Publishers, New York, 1999, p 81
47. Strich S: Shearing of nerve fibers as a cause of brain damage due to head injury: a pathological study of twenty cases. Lancet 2:443, 1961
48. Marshall LF, Marshall SB, Klauber MR, et al: The diagnosis of head injury requires a classification based on computed axial tomography. J Neurotrauma 9(suppl 1):S287, 1992
49. Ropper AH, Shafran B: Brain edema after stroke. Clinical syndrome and intracranial pressure. Arch Neurol 41:26, 1984
50. Shaw C, Alvord E, Berry R: Swelling of the brain following ischemic infarction with arterial occlusion. Arch Neurol 1:161, 1959
51. Schwab S, Aschoff A, Spranger M, et al: The value of intracranial pressure monitoring in acute hemispheric stroke. Neurology 47:393, 1996
52. Doerfler A, Forsting M, Reith W, et al: Decompressive craniectomy in a rat model of "malignant" cerebral hemispheric stroke: experimental support for an aggressive therapeutic approach. J Neurosurg 85:853, 1996
53. Forsting M, Reith W, Scheabitz WR, et al: Decompressive craniectomy for cerebral infarction: an experimental study in rats. Stroke 26:259, 1995
54. Rabb CH: Surgical treatment strategies in ischemic stroke. Neuroimaging Clin N Am 9:527, 1999
55. Rieke K, Schwab S, Krieger D, et al: Decompressive surgery in space-occupying hemispheric infarction: results of an open, prospective trial. Crit Care Med 23:1576, 1995
56. Sakai K, Iwahashi K, Terada K, et al: Outcome after external decompression for massive cerebral infarction. Neurol Med Chir (Tokyo) 38:131, 1998
57. Schwab S, Steiner T, Aschoff A, et al: Early hemicraniectomy in patients with complete middle cerebral artery infarction. Stroke 29:1888, 1998
58. McKissock W, Richardson A, Taylor J: Primary intracerebral hemorrhage: a controlled trial of surgical and conservative treatment in 180 unselected cases. Lancet 2:221, 1961
59. Juvela S, Heiskanen O, Poranen A, et al: The treatment of spontaneous intracerebral hemorrhage: a prospective randomized trial of surgical and conservative treatment. J Neurosurg 70:755, 1989
60. Kandel EI, Peresedov VV: Stereotaxic evacuation of spontaneous intracerebral hematomas. J Neurosurg 62:206, 1985
61. Kanno T, Nagata J, Nonomura K, et al: New approaches in the treatment of hypertensive intracerebral hemorrhage. Stroke 24(12 suppl):I96, 1993
62. Winn HR, Richardson AE, Jane JA: The long-term prognosis in untreated cerebral aneurysms: I. The incidence of late hemorrhage in cerebral aneurysm: a 10-year evaluation of 364 patients. Ann Neurol 1:358, 1977
63. Winn HR, Richardson AE, O'Brien W, et al: The long-term prognosis in untreated cerebral aneurysms: II. Late morbidity and mortality. Ann Neurol 4:418, 1978
64. Dorsch NW: Cerebral arterial spasm—a clinical review. Br J Neurosurg 9:403, 1995
65. Levy ML, Giannotta SL: Induced hypertension and hypervolemia for treatment of cerebral vasospasm. Neurosurg Clin North Am 1:357, 1990
66. Muizelaar JP, Zwienenberg M, Rudisill NA, et al: The prophylactic use of transluminal balloon angioplasty in patients with Fisher grade 3 subarachnoid hemorrhage: a pilot study. J Neurosurg 91:51, 1999
67. Dyste GN, Hitchon PW, Menezes AH, et al: Stereotaxic surgery in the treatment of multiple brain abscesses. J Neurosurg 69:188, 1988
68. Kala M: Aspiration or extirpation in cerebral abscess surgery? Neurosurg Rev 16:121, 1993
69. Mampalam TJ, Rosenblum ML: Trends in the management of bacterial brain abscesses: a review of 102 cases over 17 years. Neurosurgery 23:451, 1988
70. Tekkeok IH, Erbengi A: Management of brain abscess in children: review of 130 cases over a period of 21 years. Childs Nerv Syst 8:411, 1992
71. Ballester JM, Harchelroad FP: Hypothermia: an easy-to-miss, dangerous disorder in winter weather. Geriatrics 54:51, 1999
72. Gentilello LM: Advances in the management of hypothermia. Surg Clin N Am 75:243, 1995
73. Goodlock JL: Methods of rewarming the hypothermic patient in the accident and emergency department. Accid Emerg Nurs 3:114, 1995
74. Haskell RM, Boruta B, Rotondo MF, et al: Hypothermia. AACN Clinical Issues 8:368, 1997
75. Kofstad J: Blood gases and hypothermia: some theoretical and practical considerations. Scand J Clin Lab Invest Suppl 224:21, 1996
76. Lloyd EL: Accidental hypothermia. Resuscitation 32:111, 1996
77. McGowan J: Management of hypothermia in adults. Nursing Crit Care 4:59, 1999
78. Patten J: Attacks of Altered Consciousness, 2nd ed. Springer-Verlag, Berlin, 1996
79. Appleton R, Sweeney A, Choonara I, et al: Lorazepam versus diazepam in the acute treatment of epileptic seizures and status epilepticus. Dev Med Child Neurol 37:682, 1995
80. Dodrill CB, Wilensky AJ: Intellectual impairment as an outcome of status epilepticus. Neurology 40 (suppl 2):23, 1990
81. Lipowski Z: Delirium in surgery: historical introduction. Delirium: Acute Brain Failure in Man. Charles C Thomas, Springfield, Illinois, 1980, p 213
82. Fisher B, Gilchrist D: Postoperative delirium in the elderly. Ann R Coll Phys Surg Canada 26:358, 1993
83. El-Ganzouri A, Ivankovich A, Braverman B, et al: Monoamine oxidase inhibitors: should they be discontinued preoperatively? Anesth Analg 64:592, 1985
84. Grigoletto F, Zappalaa G, Anderson DW, et al: Norms for the Mini-Mental State Examination in a healthy population. Neurology 53:315, 1999
85. McDowell I, Kristjansson B, Hill GB, et al: Community screening for dementia: the Mini-Mental State Exam (MMSE) and Modified Mini-Mental State Exam (3MS) compared. J Clin Epidemiol 50:377, 1997
86. Rapp CG, Wakefield B, Kundrat M, et al: Acute confusion assessment instruments: clinical versus research usability. Appl Nurs Res 13:37, 2000
87. Wind AW, Schellevis FG, Van Staveren G, et al: Limitations of the Mini-Mental State Examination in diagnosing dementia in general practice. Int J Geriatr Psychiatry 12:101, 1997
88. Rolfson DB, McElhaney JE, Jhangri GS, et al: Validity of the confusion assessment method in detecting postoperative delirium in the elderly. Int Psychogeriatrics 11:431, 1999
89. Spar JE: Dementia in the aged. Psychiatr Clin N Am 5:67, 1982
90. Kaplan H, Sadock B, Grebb J: Dementia. Synopsis of Psychiatry. Williams & Wilkins, Baltimore, 1994, p 345
91. McKhann G, Drachman D, Folstein M, et al: Clinical diagnosis of Alzheimer's disease: report of the NINCDS-ADRDA Work Group under the auspices of Department of Health and Human Services Task Force on Alzheimer's Disease. Neurology 34:939, 1984
92. Cummings J: Neuropsychiatric aspects of Alzheimer's disease and other dementing illnesses. Textbook of Neuropsychiatry. Yudofsky S, Hales R, Eds. American Psychiatric Association, Washington, DC, 1992, p 605
93. McEvoy J: Organic brain syndromes. Ann Intern Med 95:212, 1981
94. Wells C: Organic syndromes: dementia. Comprehensive Textbook of Psychiatry. Kaplan H, Sadock B, Eds. William & Wilkins, Baltimore, 1985, p 851
95. Daly MP: Diagnosis and management of Alzheimer disease. J Am Board Fam Pract 12:375, 1999
96. Davis RE, Emmerling MR, Jaen JC, et al: Therapeutic intervention in dementia. Crit Rev Neurobiol 7:41, 1993
97. Diaz Brinton R, Yamazaki RS: Advances and challenges in the prevention and treatment of Alzheimer's disease. Pharm Res 15:386, 1998
98. Flint AJ, van Reekum R: The pharmacologic treatment of Alzheimer's disease: a guide for the general psychiatrist. Can J Psychiatry 43:689, 1998
99. Foy JM, Starr JM: Assessment and treatment of dementia in medical patients. Psychother Psychosom 69:59, 2000
100. Nyenhuis DL, Gorelick PB: Vascular dementia: a contemporary review of epidemiology, diagnosis, prevention, and treatment. J Am Geriatr Soc 46:1437, 1998
101. Rabins PV: Developing treatment guidelines for Alz-

heimer's disease and other dementias. J Clin Psychiatry 59(suppl 11):17, 1998

102. Scheltens P, van Gool WA: Emerging treatments in dementia. Eur Neurol 38:184, 1997

103. Sadavoy J: A review of pseudodementia. Mod Med Canada 39:319, 1984

104. Wells C: Pseudodementia. Am J Psychiatry 136:895, 1979

105. Yesavage J: Differential diagnosis between depression and dementia. Am J Med 94(suppl 5a):23s, 1993

106. Touringny-Rivard M: Treatment of depression in the elderly. Med North Am 1:56, 1986

107. Jenike M: Treatment of affective illness in the elderly with drugs and electroconvulsive therapy. Geriatr Psychiatry Neurol 22:77, 1989

108. Rosenberg D, Wright B, Gerson S: Depression in the elderly. Dementia 3:157, 1992

109. Jennett B, Snoek J, Bond MR, et al: Disability after severe head injury: observations on the use of the Glasgow Outcome Scale. J Neurol Neurosurg Psychiatry 44:285, 1981

110. Teasdale GM, Pettigrew LE, Wilson JT, et al: Analyzing outcome of treatment of severe head injury: a review and update on advancing the use of the Glasgow Outcome Scale. J Neurotrauma 15:587, 1998

111. Blyth B: The outcome of severe head injuries. N Z Med J 93:267, 1981

112. Gensemer IB, McMurry FG, Walker JC, et al: Behavioral consequences of trauma. J Trauma 28:44, 1988

113. Gensemer IB, Smith JL, Walker JC, et al: Psychological consequences of blunt head trauma and relation to other indices of severity of injury. Ann Emerg Med 18:9, 1989

114. Tate RL, Broe GA, Lulham JM: Impairment after severe blunt head injury: the results from a consecutive series of 100 patients. Acta Neurol Scand 79:97, 1989

115. Dikmen S, Temkin N, McLean A, et al: Memory and head injury severity. J Neurol Neurosurg Psychiatry 50:1613, 1987

116. Paniak CE, Shore DL, Rourke BP: Recovery of memory after severe closed head injury: dissociations in recovery of memory parameters and predictors of outcome. J Clin Exp Neuropsychol 11:631, 1989

117. Uzzell BP, Dolinskas CA, Wiser RF, et al: Influence of lesions detected by computed tomography on outcome and neuropsychological recovery after severe head injury. Neurosurgery 20:396, 1987

118. Francis J: Delirium in older patients. J Am Geriatr Soc 40:829, 1992

119. Meador KJ: Cognitive side effects of medications. Neurol Clin 16:141, 1998

120. Burns MJ, Linden CU, Grandins A, et al: A comparison of physostigmine and benzodiazepines for the treatment of anticholinergic poisoning. Ann Emerg Med 35:374, 2000

121. Tesar GE, Murray GB, Cassem NH: Use of high-dose intravenous haloperidol in the treatment of agitated cardiac patients. J Clin Psychopharmacol 5:344, 1985

122. Black PM: Brain death (pt 1). N Engl J Med 299:338, 1978

123. Black PM: Brain death (pt 2). N Engl J Med 299:393, 1978

124. Report of Special Task Force: Guidelines for the determination of brain death in children. Pediatrics 80:298, 1987

125. LaMancusa J, Cooper R, Vieth R, et al: The effects of the falling therapeutic and subtherapeutic barbiturate blood levels on electrocerebral silence in clinically brain-dead children. Clin Electroencephalogr 22:112, 1991

126. Wijdicks E: Precautions for the apnea test in brain death. Neurology of Critical Illness. FA Davis Co, Philadelphia, 1995, p 329

127. Lynch J, Eldadah MK: Brain-death criteria currently used by pediatric intensivists. Clin Pediatr 31:457, 1992

128. Mejia RE, Pollack MM: Variability in brain death determination practices in children [see comments]. JAMA 274:550, 1995

129. Verweij BH, Muizelaar JP, Vinas FC, et al: Mitochondrial dysfunction after experimental and human brain injury and its possible reversal with a selective N-type calcium channel antagonist (SNX-111). Neurol Res 19:334, 1997

130. Jones T: Thresholds of focal cerebral ischemia in awake monkeys. J Neurosurg 54:773, 1981

131. Marshiman L: Cushing's variant response (acute hypotension) after subarachnoid hemorrhage. Association with moderate intracranial hypertension and subacute cardiovascular collapse. Stroke 28:1445, 1997

132. Hamel MB, Goldman L, Teno J, et al: Identification of comatose patients at high risk for death or severe disability. SUPPORT Investigators. Understand Prognoses and Preferences for Outcomes and Risks of Treatments. JAMA 273:1842, 1995

133. Combes P, Fauvage B, Colonna M, et al: Severe head injuries: an outcome prediction and survival analysis. Intensive Care Med 22:1391, 1996

134. Ghodse A: Deliberate self-poisoning: a study in London casualty departments. Br Med J 1:805, 1977

135. Sacco RL, VanGool R, Mohr JP, et al: Nontraumatic coma. Glasgow Coma Score and coma etiology as predictors of 2-week outcome. Arch Neurol 47:1181, 1990

136. Bertini G, Margheri M, Giglioli C, et al: Prognostic significance of early clinical manifestations in postanoxic coma: a retrospective study of 58 patients resuscitated after prehospital cardiac arrest. Crit Care Med 17:627, 1989

137. Fountain N, Bleck T: Mechanism of action of drugs for status epilepticus. Epilepsy Quarterly, winter 1996

138. Shorvon S: Status Epilepticus: Its Clinical Features and Treatment in Children and Adults. Cambridge University Press, Cambridge, 1994, p 54

139. Meldrum B: Metabolic factors during prolonged seizures and their relation to cell death. Status Epilepticus. Mechanisms of Brain Damage and Treatment, Vol 34. Delgado-Escueta A, Wasterlain C, Treiman D, et al, Eds. Raven Press, New York, 1986, p 261

140. Franck G, Sadzot B, Salmon F, et al: Regional cerebral blood flow and metabolic rates in human focal epilepsy and status epilepticus. Basic Mechanisms of the Epilepsies: Molecular and Cellular Approaches, Vol 44. Delgado-Escueta A Jr., Woodbury D, Porter R, Eds. Raven Press, New York, 1986, p 935

141. Siesjo B, Wieloch T: Epileptic brain damage: pathophysiology and neurochemical pathology. Basic Mechanisms of the Epilepsies: Molecular and Cellular Approaches, Vol 44. Delgado-Escueta A Jr., Woodbury D, Porter R, Eds. Raven Press, New York, 1986, p 813

142. Shorvon S: Status Epilepticus: Its Clinical Features and Treatment in Children and Adults. Cambridge University Press, Cambridge, 1994, p 296

143. Vespa P, Prins M, Ronne-Engstrom E, et al: Increase in extracellular glutamate caused by reduced cerebral perfusion pressure and seizures after human traumatic brain injury: a microdialysis study. J Neurosurg 89:971, 1998

Acknowledgments

Portions of this chapter are adapted from material contained in two chapters previously published in *Scientific American® Surgery*: "Coma, Seizures, and Brain Death," by Ehud Arbit, M.D., and George Krol, M.D., and "Cognitive and Sensory Deficits," by Richard Monks, M.D.

10 SUBSTANCE ABUSE

John A. Marx, M.D., and Mark Kirk, M.D.

The Substance Abuser in the Emergency Department

Substance abuse may take the form of acute toxic exposure, chronic use, withdrawal, or a combination thereof; each form in itself poses a significant threat. Furthermore, substance abuse and abstinence may mask or masquerade as clinical features of surgical disease, thereby greatly complicating management. Four classes of abused substances will be considered in some detail: narcotics, stimulants, hallucinogens, and alcohols. Other classes of substances (e.g., sedative-hypnotics) are abused as well, but we consider these four classes to comprise the substances of greatest concern for practicing surgeons. Acute exposure, chronic use, and withdrawal will be separately addressed.

Resuscitation

The first priority is establishment of a patent airway. Because drug toxicity produces obtundation and loss of airway-protective reflexes, aspiration is a common complication. Aspiration pneumonitis carries increased risks of prolonged ventilatory support, pneumonia, prolonged hypoxic states, and progression to acute respiratory distress syndrome. Left lateral decubitus positioning helps prevent aspiration in patients who are obtunded and do not have a protective endotracheal tube in position. Vomitus in the airway should be suctioned. Proper head positioning and use of oral airway equipment may be sufficient to keep the upper airway unobstructed. The need for endotracheal intubation is determined clinically. Indications include inability to protect the airway, hypoxemia despite supplemental oxygen administration, significant hypercapnia, and severe respiratory distress. The presence or absence of the gag reflex is not a reliable indicator of need.

Any abnormality in one or more vital signs warrants insertion of an intravenous catheter. In acute overdose, even if vital signs do not appear abnormal, intravenous access should routinely be obtained and maintained, together with cardiac monitoring (see below), until it is clear that the responsible substance or substances are benign or that the patient's clinical course has progressed to the point where intravenous access is no longer needed. Standard routes for intravenous access may not exist in the chronic intravenous drug abuser. These patients can often direct the clinician to the most viable venous alternative. Central venous lines and extremity cutdowns may be necessary.

Continuous cardiac monitoring and pulse oximetry are appropriate in patients with or at risk for alterations in vital signs, respiratory failure, seizures, or acidosis. Appropriate measures should be taken to manage hypoxemia, hypotension, hypertension, and acid-base abnormalities, as well as their precipitating factors.

Urgent Syndromes

There are three common urgent syndromes associated with substance abuse that warrant discussion. These three syndromes are coma or altered mental status, seizures, and severe agitation [*see 9 Coma, Seizures, Cognitive Impairment, and Brain Death*]. For each of these three syndromes, there is a wide spectrum of possible causes to be identified and managed, both within and outside the category of toxic exposure.

COMA AND ALTERED MENTAL STATUS

Depressed mental status, including coma, can result from high doses of ethanol, narcotics, or sedative-hypnotics. It is an unusual presentation for Wernicke-Korsakoff syndrome, a nutritional complication of chronic ethanol abuse and poor diet. Complications of poisoning, as opposed to direct toxic effects causing altered mental status, include the following: anoxic brain injury, cerebral hemorrhage, cerebral infarction, central nervous system infections, and septic emboli. The depth of coma can be appraised with brain stem reflex testing. Prolonged coma or waxing-and-waning states of consciousness are seen with some toxins. Coma with fixed, dilated pupils and an isoelectric electroencephalogram can mimic brain death.[1]

Antidotes

Dextrose One ampule (50 ml = 25 g dextrose) of 50 percent dextrose in water (D50W) should immediately be given intravenously when delirium, obtundation, or coma is present and when hypoglycemia (blood glucose < 60 mg/dl) is confirmed by rapid bedside testing (e.g., Dextrostix). If rapid bedside testing is unavailable, patients with altered mentation or coma but without focal neurologic findings should be treat-

The Substance Abuser in the Emergency Department

Patient presents with symptoms and signs of substance abuse

Symptoms and signs include
- Unusual or bizarre behavior
- Lethargy, confusion
- Pressure-dependent ecchymoses, bullae, necrotic areas
- Cyanosis
- Hypotension
- Altered respiration
- Track marks
- ↑ or ↓ T°
- Mydriasis, miosis, horizontal or vertical nystagmus
- Peculiar odors
- Tachyarrhythmias

Suggestive clinical scenarios include
- Trauma
- Near-drownings, fires
- Domestic violence, suicide attempts, homicide
- Reckless driving, single-car accidents

↓

Assess airway and ventilatory status and vital signs

If airway is inadequate: place obtunded patients in left lateral decubitus position; suction vomitus; place ET tube if necessary.

↓

Vital signs are abnormal, or acute overdose is present

Establish I.V. access.
Monitor via continuous ECG or pulse oximetry.
Correct hypoxemia, hypotension, hypertension, and acid-base abnormalities.
Manage any urgent syndromes present.

Vital signs are normal, and acute overdose is absent

Patient is comatose, delirious, or obtunded

Administer appropriate antidotes:
- D50W, 50 ml
- Naloxone, 2 mg I.V., repeated q. 2–3 min to total of 10 mg as necessary (ineffective against ethanol-induced coma)
- Thiamine, 50–100 mg by I.V. bolus, for suspected chronic alcoholism, poor diet, or Wernicke-Korsakoff syndrome

Patient has seizures

Protect patient from injury.
Administer anticonvulsants:
- Diazepam, 5 mg I.V. q. 5 min as needed, or lorazepam, 1–2 mg I.V. q. 5 min as needed to total of 10–12 mg
- Phenobarbital, 10–20 mg/kg for status epilepticus

Patient is severely agitated

Rule out hypoxemia, closed head injury, pain, and respiratory distress.
Use physical restraints as necessary. If patient is violent, sedate with haloperidol, 5–10 mg I.V. q. 10 min as needed. Give benzodiazepines for stimulant- or withdrawal-induced agitation once patient's violent behavior is controlled.

↓

Continue evaluation and consider perioperative needs

If possible, obtain history, focusing on
- Course of symptoms and signs
- Amount, route, and time of exposure
- Bizarre or violent behavior
- Trauma
- Accidents
- Other medications or drugs

Perform detailed physical exam to rule out traumatic, metabolic, and endocrine causes.
Order lab tests (serum electrolytes, blood gases, skeletal muscle enzymes, renal function, x-rays, ECG) as necessary on the basis of clinical findings. Qualitative and quantitative toxicologic analyses are often of limited utility.
Consider gut decontamination (lavage or charcoal therapy).
Preoperative considerations: need for and risks of anesthesia; universal HIV precautions
Postoperative considerations: pain control (narcotic addicts may require large doses); possible withdrawal syndromes

↓

Initiate specific management

ed empirically. Hemiplegia is present in most patients with cerebral ischemia but in only 2.5 percent of patients with hypoglycemia. If empirical glucose administration is withheld from this subset of patients until glucose levels can be measured, the adverse effects of hyperglycemia after cerebral ischemia can be prevented.[2] Substance abuse–related causes of hypoglycemia include poor nutrition, liver failure, and alcohol-induced hypoglycemia in chronic alcoholics, as well as systemic infection in intravenous drug abusers.

Naloxone Naloxone is a pure opioid antagonist with a therapeutic half-life of 30 to 60 minutes for reversal of respiratory depression. It is indicated in any patient with depressed mentation or coma and is effective against both natural and synthetic opioids. The standard dose of naloxone is 2 mg I.V. for adults and for children weighing more than 20 kg, with onset of action in one to three minutes. For children weighing less than 20 kg, 0.1 to 0.2 mg/kg should be given. These doses can be repeated up to a total dose of 10 mg when the response is only partial or when opioids known to be less susceptible to naloxone (e.g., propoxyphene, diphenoxylate, pentazocine, or butorphanol) are suspected.[2] If necessary, naloxone can be administered via subcutaneous, intramuscular, or intralingual routes or via an endotracheal tube. There are no well-documented adverse consequences of naloxone administration, with the exception of opioid withdrawal in narcotic-dependent patients. If narcotic addiction is known or suspected, a lower dose (0.1 to 0.2 mg) may be used to prevent violent withdrawal and can be titrated to the cessation of respiratory and CNS depression. The need to protect the airway with suction or endotracheal intubation should be anticipated because withdrawal may precipitate vomiting without arousal. A patient suspected of narcotic overdose who responds to naloxone must be observed for at least two hours after the last dose of naloxone has been administered.

Flumazenil Flumazenil is a pure competitive benzodiazepine antagonist. It is safe and effective for the reversal of benzodiazepine-induced sedation in short diagnostic or surgical procedures. However, securing the airway should take precedence over the reversal of benzodiazepine-induced respiratory and CNS depression. Because the half-life of this agent is 30 to 80 minutes (much shorter than that of virtually all benzodiazepines currently used), resedation is likely after its administration. Because flumazenil can precipitate severe benzodiazepine withdrawal or seizures and dysrhythmias from co-ingestants (e.g., cyclic antidepressants),[3] it should not be used in patients with mixed or unknown overdoses.

Thiamine Thiamine is a water-soluble vitamin whose absence causes Wernicke-Korsakoff syndrome. It should be administered to patients who are chronic ethanol abusers, have a poor diet, or are suspected of having Wernicke-Korsakoff syndrome. Specific indications include lethargy, confusion, bradycardia, hypotension, and hypothermia of unknown cause. Thiamine can be safely administered in doses of 50 to 100 mg by I.V. bolus.[4] A 50 mg dose of thiamine is frequently part of intravenous multivitamin preparations.

SEIZURES

Toxin-caused seizures are grand mal unless there is preexisting focal CNS pathology. They can be direct sequelae of acute narcotic and stimulant use or hyperadrenergic events attributed to ethanol and sedative-hypnotic withdrawal. Hypoxemia caused by airway compromise, hypoventilation, or respiratory complications should be considered.

Management of seizures includes avoidance of physical injury to the patient and, when required, intervention to protect the airway. Because most grand mal seizures are brief and self-limited, immediate pharmacological intervention is rarely necessary. For persistent seizures, the first-line medication is a benzodiazepine administered intravenously (e.g., diazepam, 5 mg every five minutes in adults and 0.1 to 0.3 mg/kg every five minutes in children, or lorazepam, 1 to 2 mg every five minutes up to 10 to 12 mg in adults and 0.05 to 0.10 mg/kg in children). If there is an ongoing risk of seizure, phenobarbital, 10 to 20 mg/kg I.V., should be administered. Phenytoin has no role in emergent treatment of toxin-induced seizures. Elimination of the substance or condition that precipitated the seizure (e.g., a toxin or hypoxemia) should be undertaken simultaneously with these measures.

SEVERE AGITATION

Causes of combativeness should be sought, including respiratory distress, closed head injury, and significant pain. Irritability and agitation should be interpreted as hypoxemia until this is ruled out. When violent behavior endangers the patient and staff or hinders urgent management, application of physical restraints and judicious sedation are indicated. To gain control of agitated patients who could harm the staff or themselves, intravenous haloperidol or droperidol (5 to 10 mg I.V. initially, then every 10 minutes as needed) is effective within 10 minutes.[5] These agents do not cause cardiorespiratory deterioration, lower the seizure threshold, or interfere with neurosurgical assessment. Use of opioids, barbiturates, or benzodiazepines to sedate combative patients can lead to depressed circulatory and respiratory function and can exacerbate acute toxic effects if the abused substance is from the same pharmaceutical class. Once the patient is under control, however, benzodiazepines are the most beneficial agents for treatment of agitation, seizures, hyperthermia, and hyperdynamic states caused by stimulants (e.g., cocaine) and by sedative-hypnotic withdrawal.

Patient Evaluation

HISTORY

The patient, the family, friends, and paramedics can all provide useful data regarding the current presentation, patterns of substance abuse, and associated medical complications. It is helpful to determine when, in what quantity, and by what route the patient was exposed to the substance; whether additional substances were involved; what symptoms occurred and how they developed over time; and what medications the patient is taking. In addition, certain clinical scenarios should prompt concern. Unexpected or bizarre patterns of behavior suggest drug toxicity. Substance abuse is frequently involved in domestic violence, suicide, and homicide and

common, an endotracheal tube should usually be inserted and well secured before naloxone is administered. Naloxone is a pure competitive antagonist at the opioid receptors.[18] The onset of action of naloxone occurs one to three minutes after administration, with maximum effect in five to 10 minutes [see Urgent Syndromes, above]. With some opioids, higher doses (up to 10 mg) are required for a reversal response. Gut decontamination may be helpful if the ingestion is recent, but no form of elimination enhancement is indicated. Noncardiogenic pulmonary edema is treated by optimizing oxygen delivery. Positive end-expiratory pressure may be necessary.

Prescription analgesic medications are often opioids in combination with other drugs, such as acetaminophen or salicylates. In an overdose, the toxic effects of the coingestant must be taken into account. Abusers may use combinations, such as heroin and cocaine (a so-called speedball). Reversal of the opioid effect may allow the coingestant to have predominant toxic effects.

CHRONIC USE

A variety of infectious complications ensue from contaminated drugs or unsterile intravenous injection practices.[19] These include bacterial endocarditis, extremity abscesses and cellulitis, wound botulism, diskitis, and septic emboli. Acute and chronic forms of hepatitis, especially hepatitis B, and HIV infection are extremely prevalent in this population.[20]

The clinical presentation (e.g., fever or signs of endocarditis) dictates the cultures and serologic analyses that should be requested. Empirical laboratory studies are not indicated.

Management

Management of infectious and other complications is directed by clinical need and the laboratory results.

WITHDRAWAL

The time course of abstinence withdrawal depends on the particular narcotic abused.[21] With short-acting drugs (e.g., meperidine and hydromorphone), the syndrome begins within three to six hours and lasts four to five days. With less potent drugs (e.g., codeine and propoxyphene) or longer-acting drugs (e.g., methadone), it begins within 24 hours and lasts two to four days. Manifestations include yawning, lacrimation, rhinorrhea, restlessness, gooseflesh, aching, cramps, nausea, vomiting, and diarrhea. Fever and hypertension may be present. These symptoms and signs progress to a peak and then subside over a period of hours to days.

Naloxone administration can provoke intense withdrawal that begins within five minutes, peaks in 30 minutes, and lasts one to two hours, regardless of the opioid involved. Longer-acting opioid antagonists (e.g., nalmefene and naltrexone) can precipitate withdrawal that will persist for many hours.

Attention to electrolyte levels may be necessary if gastrointestinal losses are marked.

Management

The opiate abstinence syndrome may be ameliorated with clonidine, a central alpha$_2$ agonist. A 0.2 mg oral dose is given initially, followed by 0.1 to 0.2 mg every eight hours.[22] Methadone, a long-acting opioid, is an alternative treatment for detoxification. The administration of other drugs for reducing anxiety (e.g., benzodiazepines), abdominal cramps (e.g., anticholinergics), or nausea (e.g., prochlorperazine) may be considered.

Stimulants

The stimulants commonly abused include cocaine, amphetamines, and amphetamine-like drugs. Stimulants cause catecholamine excess, both within the CNS and peripherally. Clinically, all stimulant intoxications are similar. CNS excitation causes agitation and seizures; cardiovascular provocation causes tachycardia and hypertension. Hyperthermia can be severe.

COCAINE

Users snort cocaine as a powder; smoke it as an alkaloid (crack) or, less frequently, as a coca paste; and administer it intravenously. Recently, much attention has focused on the combination of cocaine and ethanol. A metabolite of this combination (cocaethylene) can be more toxic to the heart than cocaine alone.

Acute Exposure

Cocaine is a sympathomimetic agent and a CNS stimulant. Mild intoxication produces minimal alteration of vital signs. Changes in mental status include euphoria, excitement, and irritability. Mydriasis may be seen. Hypertension, hyperthermia, tachycardia, and agitation predominate in overdose. A single generalized seizure or status epilepticus can occur. Cerebral hemorrhage and ischemic strokes have been reported.[23] In extreme cases, coma, hypotension, severe metabolic acidosis, hyperkalemia, hyperthermia, and wide QRS complex dysrhythmias can lead to rapid death. Chest pain after cocaine use is a particular clinical dilemma. The pronounced Valsalva maneuver associated with smoking cocaine can result in pneumothorax or pneumomediastinum.[24] CNS stimulation produces severe anxiety, which may contribute to atypical chest pain. Myocardial infarction has been reported in patients with and without preexisting coronary artery disease. The myocardium becomes ischemic because cocaine constricts coronary arteries, forms thrombi, and accelerates atherosclerosis.[25,26] Acute aortic dissection can also occur. Ischemic infarction of the skin, bowel, kidneys, and muscle have all resulted from intense vasoconstriction attributable to cocaine.

Cocaine can be detected in the blood for a very short time after exposure, but a metabolite (benzoylecgonine) can be detected in urine for 48 to 72 hours. Adrenergic excess from cocaine causes leukocytosis, hypokalemia, metabolic acidosis, and hyperglycemia. Serum creatine kinase levels should be monitored because cocaine-induced muscle injury can result in acute renal failure from myoglobinuria.

Management Beyond good supportive care, therapy to inhibit excess adrenergic stimulation may be necessary. Benzodiazepines are most effective in inhibiting CNS stimulation and can attenuate cardiovascular stimulation both centrally and peripherally. Beta blockers, which have been associated with worsening clinical outcome, should be avoided. Wide QRS complex arrhythmias should be treated with intravenous sodium bicarbonate. Severe hypertension is managed with benzodiazepines and, if necessary, nitroprusside, phentolamine, or nifedipine. A patient who is seizing should receive benzodiazepines and, if necessary, phenobarbital. If hyperthermia is present, benzodiazepines and aggressive external cooling are indicated. For myocardial ischemia and myocardial infarction, generous benzodiazepine therapy is necessary in addition to the usual measures. Thrombolytics have been used successfully in patients with acute myocardial infarction caused by cocaine.[26]

Decontamination should be considered only in cases of recent exposure to large doses, such as those that result from packet breakage inside the body. Emesis, lavage, and attempts at endoscopic removal can result in the sudden release of large amounts of cocaine, with severe consequences, including death.

Chronic Use

Chronic insufflation of cocaine can lead to rhinitis and nasal erosions and perforations. A variety of psychiatric disorders may be present, including euphoria, dysphoria, and psychosis. Complications of parenteral drug abuse should be anticipated.

Withdrawal

During withdrawal, chronic cocaine users may experience depression, tiredness, nausea, and vomiting with abstinence. A severe withdrawal syndrome is highly unusual.

AMPHETAMINES

Acute Exposure

Amphetamine, its isomers (dextroamphetamine and methamphetamine), and numerous analogues are all available for misuse (for weight loss, prolonged wakefulness, and enhanced athletic performance) and abuse. Patients may be exposed by the oral, inhalational, subcutaneous, or intravenous route. The duration of clinical effect, regardless of the route of exposure, is typically long, ranging from six hours to several days.

Acute amphetamine overdose manifests itself via stimulation of the cardiovascular and central nervous systems. Mild toxic effects include restlessness, insomnia, irritability, nausea and vomiting, flushing, diaphoresis, mydriasis, and combativeness. Moderate toxic effects include chest pain, vomiting and abdominal pain with hypertension, tachycardia, tachypnea, mild temperature elevation, profuse diaphoresis, and hallucinations. Indicators of severe overdose include more marked alterations in vital signs, such as hyperpyrexia and severe hypotension or hypertension, cardiac arrhythmias, seizures, focal neurologic signs, and coma.

Acute complications are cardiovascular (myocardial infarction and dysrhythmias), cerebrovascular (intracranial hemorrhage and vasospasm), hyperthermic (hypermetabolic state and status epilepticus), renal (myoglobinuric renal failure), neurologic (amphetamine psychosis, with paranoia and hallucinations), and peripheral vascular (infectious and vasospastic complications of injection).

Qualitative analysis can confirm amphetamine exposure; quantitative analysis is not clinically useful. Leukocytosis with no other apparent cause is frequent after amphetamine use. Hypokalemia, hyperglycemia, and a mild metabolic acidosis may be seen. It may be necessary to evaluate cardiac and skeletal muscle enzyme activity as well as the effect of rhabdomyolysis on electrolyte concentrations, renal function, and coagulation. CT of the head, which is indicated for severe headache, meningismus, or localizing CNS findings, may reveal intracerebral, subdural, or subarachnoid hemorrhage. Cerebral angiography may demonstrate characteristic beading of small-caliber arteries.[27]

Management Management should focus on life-threatening cardiovascular and cerebrovascular complications of acute amphetamine overdose. Benzodiazepines are the treatment of choice to decrease CNS stimulation and centrally mediated cardiovascular stimulation. Acute severe hypertension that is unresponsive to benzodiazepines can be treated with nitroprusside, phentolamine, or calcium channel blockers. Seizures should be managed with parenteral benzodiazepines and phenobarbital. Patients in status epilepticus who do not respond to these measures may have to be intubated and paralyzed to prevent hyperthermia, profound acidemia, and rhabdomyolysis. Agitation and combativeness can be treated with either benzodiazepines or haloperidol. Haloperidol and appropriate physical restraints are indicated for patients with amphetamine psychosis. Activated charcoal therapy is indicated for acute ingestions. Alteration of pH to enhance elimination is contraindicated, and hemodialysis and hemoperfusion are not useful.

Chronic Use

Chronic amphetamine abusers may present with complaints of insomnia, weight loss, depression, hypertension, or toxic psychosis. Patients who use these drugs by parenteral means are subject to infectious and extremity complications similar to those found in narcotic abusers.

Toxicologic analysis can reveal the source of the patient's concerns. Other laboratory studies are generally unhelpful.

Management Clinical need is sufficient to guide management of chronic abusers; therapy is directed at the clinical signs and symptoms.

Withdrawal

Abstinence after chronic use of amphetamines is characterized by depression, anxiety, sleep disturbance, abdominal pain, myalgia, and voracious appetite. These manifestations typically last three to six days and are not life threatening. Seizures should not be anticipated.

Hallucinogens

The hallucinogens include the psychedelics (lysergic acid diethylamide [LSD], mescaline, and psilocybin), phencyclidine (PCP), and marijuana. Of these, the first two are the most germane to surgical practice.

LSD

Acute Exposure

LSD is the prototypical psychedelic. It occurs naturally as an ergot alkaloid, but far more of it is manufactured than is found in nature. LSD has no medical uses in the United States. It is ingested as capsules, tablets, or a solution on blotting paper, sugar cubes, or gelatin; it is rarely taken intravenously or by insufflation. Unlike opioids, amphetamines, and cocaine, which are associated with repetitive, sustained patterns of abuse, LSD is used only intermittently. It is well absorbed from the gastrointestinal tract; the clinical effect begins to be noticeable 30 to 90 minutes after ingestion, peaks in three to five hours, and lasts eight to 12 hours.

Typical physiologic alterations include mild increases in pulse, temperature, respiratory rate, and pupil size. Nausea, vomiting, weakness, ataxia, and modest increases in salivation and lacrimation may occur. CNS manifestations predominate among the clinical effects.[28] Behavior is unpredictable and ranges from passive and reserved to hostile and threatening. Although LSD experiences are intended to be pleasurable, they often are not. Acute panic reactions are the most commonly seen complications. Acute toxic psychosis with distorted perceptions and hallucinations is also common. Orientation is usually preserved, but judgment is grossly impaired. Impaired judgment, coupled with depressive reactions, may prompt unintentional self-destructive behavior, such as attempting to fly.

Flashbacks involving visual, time, and body image distortion can follow LSD use. These may be precipitated by physiologic or emotional stresses. Flashbacks occurring more than six months after use of the drug are seen predominantly in patients with obsessive and schizoid personalities.

Rare but severe complications of LSD use include seizures and coma. Vasospasm and angiitis may cause focal neurologic deficits. Massive overdoses and violent hyperactivity may result in pronounced temperature elevations, rhabdomyolysis, and metabolic acidosis.[29]

LSD can be detected in urine to verify exposure. Urine should be routinely screened for myoglobin in patients with a history of seizures or prolonged hyperactivity.

Management Seizure, coma, and rhabdomyolysis are rare with LSD use. If these life-threatening manifestations occur, the usual measures are indicated. Gut decontamination is usually futile. Panic attacks respond best to reduction of sensory stimuli and constant reassurance. Physical restraints or administration of benzodiazepines or haloperidol may be required for panic and psychotic reactions. Use of phenothiazines as neuroleptics may be unsafe and should be avoided.

Withdrawal

No abstinence syndrome for LSD has been reported.

PCP

Acute Exposure

PCP was discovered in 1957 and was briefly used for anesthesia in humans and animals. Currently, it is classified as a dissociative anesthetic, but it has no medical uses. PCP is well absorbed by all routes. Most users either sprinkle PCP powder onto a marijuana or tobacco cigarette or dip the cigarette into a liquid form of the drug. Some snort or ingest PCP, but the development of clinical toxicity is more difficult to predict when these methods are adopted.

Symptoms and signs of PCP intoxication include increased heart rate and blood pressure, nystagmus (horizontal, vertical, or rotatory), miosis, markedly diminished ability to feel pain and temperature, ataxia, increased muscle tone, and slurred speech.[30] The patient's behavior can be lethargic, bizarre, agitated, euphoric, or violent. These changes usually last six hours after exposure but occasionally last as long as 24 hours. Toxic psychosis is heralded by delusions, hallucinations, depersonalization, and disorganized thoughts and can last four hours to seven days (average, one to two days). The combination of psychosis and lack of pain sensation can lead to violent and combative acts of extraordinary proportions.

Medical complications include acute hypertension, hyperpyrexia, seizures, and rhabdomyolysis with renal failure.[31] Severe trauma is common. Drowning and other types of accidental death, violent suicide, and homicide are well known to occur in this population.

Toxicology screens can detect the presence of PCP in urine. Quantitative blood analysis is poorly correlated with toxic patterns.

Management Respiratory depression, seizures, and coma are treated in the standard fashion. Gut decontamination is usually ineffective; in addition, it is generally difficult to perform, given the patient's pattern of behavior. Urinary acidification is dangerous in patients with PCP intoxication. Although urinary acidification enhances urinary excretion of PCP, its effect on clinical outcome is unclear, and it may exacerbate renal injury resulting from rhabdomyolysis.[31]

Supportive care and pharmacological therapy may be required for patients with hypertension, hyperthermia, and rhabdomyolysis. Typically, the greatest problem encountered by medical staff is control of the violent patient. Outbreaks are unpredictable, and the patient's strength can be superhuman. A coordinated effort must be made by all available personnel to ensure the safety of the patient and the staff. Liberal use of benzodiazepines, butyrophenones (haloperidol or droperidol), or both may be necessary.

Chronic Use

Chronic use of PCP is associated with memory deficits, emotional lability, social isolation, and, in rare instances, organic brain syndrome.

Withdrawal

No severe physical reactions occur in withdrawal, but depression, anxiety, and fatigue may be seen for weeks to months after the initiation of abstinence.

Alcohols

Alcohol exists in many forms and remains an immensely popular and exceedingly prevalent drug throughout the world. The pathology it creates or contributes to is exceptionally varied and frequently serious, and no organ system is unaffected. Moreover, alcohol is the leading cause of morbidity and mortality as well as the principal risk factor for unintentional and intentional injuries in the United States.[6]

ACUTE EXPOSURE

Clinical Findings

Ethanol is rapidly absorbed in the stomach and the proximal small bowel. Blood concentration peaks 30 to 120 minutes after ingestion. Alcohol is primarily metabolized in the liver by alcohol dehydrogenase; chronic alcoholics have auxiliary degradative enzyme systems. The hourly rate of metabolism ranges from 15 to 20 mg/dl in the nonalcoholic to 40 mg/dl in chronic alcoholics.

At low concentrations, ethanol impairs higher cortical function, and at high concentrations, it can inhibit brain stem function. The primary manifestations of ethanol intoxication reflect its cerebellar effects; thus, dysarthria, nystagmus, and gait disturbance are prominent. Prediction of serum ethanol levels according to clinical presentation demands careful scrutiny of the patient's history, his or her experience with drinking, and the examination findings. Whereas inexperienced drinkers may be grossly ataxic and stuporous at blood ethanol levels of 100 mg/dl, chronic alcoholics are often alert and conversant at levels in excess of 500 mg/dl.

Acute ethanol intoxication may cause delayed or erroneous diagnosis in patients with concomitant disorders.[7] It is imperative to perform a careful initial examination and serial evaluations in acutely intoxicated patients. The differential diagnosis of altered mentation in cases of suspected ethanol intoxication is broad. Closed head injury is exceedingly common in intoxicated patients. Metabolic conditions, including alcohol-induced hypoglycemia, hepatic encephalopathy, the presence of other alcohols or drugs, the presence of disulfiram alone or in combination with ethanol, and hypothermia are frequently seen as well. Infections are more common in chronic alcoholics, and particular attention should be given to the possibility of CNS infections and aspiration or bacterial pneumonia. Most alcohol-related causes of abnormal mentation are neurologic; these include the postictal state that follows an alcohol withdrawal seizure, alcohol withdrawal itself, and Wernicke-Korsakoff syndrome.

Alcohol-induced hypoglycemia is a common disorder ascribed to impaired gluconeogenesis and inadequate glycogen stores. Chronic alcoholics, binge drinkers, and children (because of their marginal glycogen stores) are at the greatest risk.[32] Hypoglycemia may occur during intoxication or as much as six to 20 hours after the last drink. Its onset is insidious, and the clinical picture is dominated by neuroglycopenia rather than catecholamine response. Lethargy and obtundation proceed to seizures and coma. Focal neurologic signs are frequently seen in adults, and seizures are common in children.[33]

Nonethanol alcohols (e.g., methanol, ethylene glycol, and isopropyl alcohol) are consumed either accidentally or deliberately and are both common and readily available.[34] Methanol is found in windshield-washer cleaner, gas-line antifreeze, and shellacs. Symptoms appear 40 minutes to 72 hours after ingestion. Nausea, vomiting, abdominal pain, and tenderness may be accompanied by gastrointestinal bleeding. Ophthalmologic abnormalities include blurred vision and "spots" or "snow" before the eyes, optic disk hyperemia, and retinal edema; permanent blindness may result. Methanol may also cause lethargy, confusion, and, in severe cases, seizures and coma. High anion gap metabolic acidosis occurs as a result of the toxic metabolic product formic acid. Ethylene glycol is most often used in radiator antifreeze and windshield deicer. Its clinical course proceeds through three stages: stage 1—metabolic acidosis and CNS depression, including seizures and coma, are seen in the first 30 minutes to 12 hours after ingestion; stage 2—in severe cases, cardiopulmonary findings, including pulmonary edema, cardiomegaly, and cardiovascular collapse, occur 12 to 36 hours after ingestion; and stage 3—acute renal failure becomes apparent 48 to 72 hours after exposure. Isopropyl alcohol (also termed rubbing alcohol) is found in numerous home products. The manifestations of isopropyl alcohol intoxication are very similar to those of acute ethanol intoxication; however, at the same dosage, isopropyl alcohol produces more profound clinical intoxication than ethanol. Isopropyl alcohol is metabolized partly to acetone, resulting in ketosis without acidosis.[35]

Disulfiram, a drug that is widely prescribed for the treatment of chronic alcoholism, can itself cause psychosis, delirium, and seizures in rare cases. Ingestion of alcohol by a patient on long-term disulfiram therapy can cause the disulfiram-ethanol reaction (DER), which can be severe and sometimes fatal.[36] Chronic disulfiram users who ingest alcohol will experience clinical symptoms that appear within five to 15 minutes, peak within 20 to 30 minutes, and usually dissipate within two to four hours. Because disulfiram has a long elimination half-life, the DER can occur in patients who stopped taking disulfiram as long as two weeks before ingesting alcohol. Patients who have taken their first dose of disulfiram and then ingest alcohol may not show symptoms for eight to 12 hours. Characteristic features of the DER include facial and truncal skin flushing, headache, nausea, and vomiting; more serious reactions include severe dyspnea, chest pain, and shock.

Laboratory Studies

Quantitative assessment of ethanol can be accomplished by analysis of blood or alveolar air. Most laboratories test for ethanol only, although some routinely screen for ethanol, methanol, and isopropyl alcohol. Ethylene glycol is analyzed by different methods and should be requested separately when indicated. The Breathalyzer provides reasonably accurate measurements of ethanol in the blood, but it has two drawbacks: first, inadequate ventilation can render levels falsely low, and second, the device measures all alcohols but cannot distinguish one from another. Saliva test strips show good correlation with serum measurements but only at low concentrations of ethanol.[37]

Mandatory serum glucose analysis in the intoxicated patient is unnecessarily expensive. Alcohol-induced hypoglycemia can be easily and rapidly detected by bedside determinations.

Obtaining quantitative measurements of nonethanol alcohols facilitates management. When serum levels are not available, they can be estimated on the basis of the osmolar gap (measured osmolality minus calculated osmolality). Ancillary tests in poisonings by nonethanol alcohols include serum electrolyte concentrations, arterial blood gas values, assessment of renal function, and urinalysis.

Management

Patients with suspected ethanol intoxication in whom other causes for altered mentation have been excluded by clinical or laboratory means should be observed and examined repeatedly. Airway patency and ventilation should be assured. Extremely obtunded patients should be placed in the left lateral decubitus position to prevent aspiration. In the presence of craniofacial trauma, cervical spine immobilization and appropriate x-rays are indicated. Intravenous access is helpful and allows administration of 50 mg of thiamine as prophylaxis against Wernicke-Korsakoff syndrome. The welfare of the patient should be safeguarded with physical restraints and haloperidol when necessary. Intoxicated patients should remain under close observation until clinical sobriety has been attained. Gut decontamination is rarely effective.[38] Hemodialysis has rarely been used and is not clinically useful.

Patients with alcohol-induced hypoglycemia should immediately be given one or two ampules of D50W, followed by 1 to 2 L of D5W or D10W over a period of six to 10 hours. Their return to a normal diet should be assured before they are discharged.

Treatment for nonethanol alcohol poisoning is determined by the substance ingested, the time of ingestion, and the clinical and laboratory findings. Isopropyl alcohol intoxication can be handled in much the same way as ethanol intoxication. Methanol and ethylene glycol are relatively nontoxic in themselves; it is their by-products that are dangerous. Prevention of metabolism to harmful by-products is accomplished by means of intravenous ethanol administration and, when required, hemodialysis.[39]

Patients with severe DER must be monitored. Hypotension is managed by infusing crystalloid. Pressors are rarely required.

CHRONIC USE

Clinical Findings

The effects of chronic ethanol abuse are myriad. Physical findings include spider telangiectasis, jaundice, caput medusae, palmar erythema, ascites, and generalized wasting. Acute, subacute, and chronic myopathies of cardiac and skeletal muscle occur. Atrial dysrhythmias are common during intoxication and withdrawal. Numerous diseases of the gastrointestinal and biliary systems follow prolonged use. The incidence of gastrointestinal hemorrhage caused by gastritis, peptic ulcer, Mallory-Weiss tears, and esophageal varices is increased in patients with cirrhosis. Abdominal pain and tenderness can be caused by alcoholic hepatitis and acute or chronic pancreatitis.

The hematologic manifestations of alcoholism are caused by the direct actions of alcohol, nutritional deficiency, and liver involvement. Each of the three major hematopoietic cell lines is affected.[40] Megaloblastic anemia is extremely common. Hypersplenism, sideroblastic changes, and iron deficiency contribute to the development of anemia. Leukopenia occurs in three to eight percent of alcoholics, most often affecting the granulocytic line. Thrombocytopenia is found in as many as 40 percent of alcoholics and is caused by decreased production, folate deficiency, and hypersplenism. Levels below 20,000/mm^3 are rarely seen. Because the liver is the site of production of all coagulation factors except factor VIII, alcohol-related liver disease leads to synthetic incompetence of these factors and resultant abnormalities in prothrombin time, partial thromboplastin time, and thrombin time.[41]

The neurologic consequences of chronic alcoholism are the most frequently seen and the most devastating.[42] Peripheral neuropathy is frequent. Cerebellar dysfunction is common and can be profound. Cortical atrophy and loss of higher function are well documented. Wernicke-Korsakoff syndrome is caused by thiamine deficiency and, in the United States, is seen almost exclusively in chronic alcoholics with poor diet. In this syndrome, ophthalmoplegia, gait disturbance, and mental status changes tend to develop over a period of several days to weeks.[43] Generally, all three are found, although the mental changes may lag behind the others by days to weeks. Ocular changes include horizontal and vertical nystagmus and ophthalmoplegia. Bilateral abducens nerve palsy is virtually pathognomonic of the disease. Gait and stance ataxia are nonspecific findings and generally are not accompanied by tremor, appendicular ataxia, or a cerebellar speech pattern. Abnormal mentation usually presents as mild delirium, disorientation, and apathy. Full Korsakoff's syndrome, characterized by anterograde and retrograde amnesia with the former dominating, often follows. Unusual presentations of Wernicke-Korsakoff syndrome include coma, hypothermia, and hypotension.

Laboratory Studies

Hematologic, chemical, and radiographic examinations are based on the clinical presentation. Diagnosis of Wernicke-Korsakoff syndrome is entirely clinical. Specialized assays to detect chronic alcoholism exist, but they are never available without delay and are no substitute for clinical judgment.

Management

Abstinence stabilizes and improves most chronic-use conditions. If Wernicke-Korsakoff syndrome is suspected, 100 mg of thiamine should be given intravenously at the outset and each day until the patient returns to a normal diet.[44] Magnesium, a necessary cofactor for thiamine, is frequently depleted in chronic alcoholics and must be replenished if thiamine therapy is to be effective.

WITHDRAWAL

Clinical Findings

The manifestations of abstinence from ethanol typically depend on the habitual dose and chronicity of use, but there is wide interindividual variation. Patients with a history of withdrawal are likely to experience similar manifestations with subsequent periods of abstinence. Generally, four to five weeks of daily and significant ethanol ingestion is required to produce significant withdrawal, although as little as five days may be sufficient. Alcohol withdrawal can be divided into five syndromes: (1) minor withdrawal, (2) alcoholic hallucinosis, (3) alcohol withdrawal seizures, (4) delirium tremens, and (5) alcoholic ketoacidosis, a frequent metabolic complication of the withdrawal period. These syndromes frequently merge and share features. They do not necessarily progress in any particular order.

Minor withdrawal The minor withdrawal syndrome begins six to eight hours after the cessation of alcohol use, peaks in 24 to 36 hours, and may persist as long as 10 to 14 days. Patients with the minor withdrawal syndrome are hyperalert and anorectic, with nausea and vomiting, and may show mild tachycardia, hypertension, hyperreflexia, and tremor on examination.

Alcoholic hallucinosis Alcoholic hallucinations occur six to 96 hours after the beginning of abstinence and usually peak at 12 to 48 hours. Hallucinations are typically visual (as opposed to the auditory hallucinations associated with schizophrenia), and the images tend to be frightening to the patient. The duration of illness is generally two to three days.

Alcohol withdrawal seizures The majority of alcohol withdrawal seizures occur between six and 48 hours after discontinuance of ethanol, with the peak incidence coming between 13 and 24 hours; virtually all seizures occur within 96 hours.[45] Withdrawal seizures occur singly in about 50 percent of patients and in groups of two to six in the remainder. Status epilepticus is rare. When multiple seizures do occur, they tend to cluster within a 12-hour period in 95 percent of patients. Alcohol withdrawal seizure tends to be grand mal and self-limited; however, the high prevalence of prior closed head injury in chronic alcoholics explains why focal seizures are seen in as many as 40 percent of cases. Other features of withdrawal, including autonomic hyperactivity, hallucinosis, and tremor, may or may not be seen.

Delirium tremens Delirium tremens usually appears 72 to 96 hours after cessation of drinking and lasts one to three days. It is the most dramatic and serious form of alcohol withdrawal and is characterized by profound confusion, disorientation, delusions, vivid hallucinations, tremor, agitation, insomnia, and psychomotor, speech, and autonomic hyperactivity.[46] The most distinguishing features are hypersympathetic symptoms with tachycardia, hypertension, fever, mydriasis, and profuse diaphoresis. Cardiovascular collapse may occur. Associated illnesses (particularly pneumonia, pancreatitis, and hepatitis) are common and often contribute to the cause of death.

Alcoholic ketoacidosis Alcoholic ketoacidosis is typically seen after a long drinking binge followed by several days of abstinence, anorexia, nausea, and vomiting.[47] Examination may reveal signs of hypovolemia, tachycardia, and Kussmaul's respiration if acidemia is severe. Abdominal pain is a typical symptom, and tenderness is common. In extreme cases, rebound and guarding can be severe enough to mimic the signs of an acute abdomen. Sensorium is usually normal.

Laboratory Studies

Patients with alcoholic ketoacidosis exhibit a high anion gap metabolic acidosis caused by the production of ketoacids.[48] Because metabolic alkalosis secondary to vomiting and respiratory alkalosis secondary to alcohol withdrawal often coexist, the pH in these patients is extremely variable. Serum glucose levels should be normal or low (the opposite of the situation with diabetic ketoacidosis). Hypokalemia and hypophosphatemia are frequent. Ketoacids are detectable in the serum or urine; however, it must be remembered that routine ketoacid measurements are not sensitive to β-hydroxybutyric acid, the predominant ketoacid species in this disorder.

For the other alcohol withdrawal syndromes, laboratory studies are of negligible diagnostic value. Fluid and electrolyte deficits may be severe in patients with delirium tremens or alcoholic ketoacidosis.

Management

The goals of treatment are to prevent progression of withdrawal, to alleviate symptoms, and to recognize and treat underlying disorders.[49] A variety of drugs may be administered, of which the benzodiazepines are the most widely used.[50] In mild cases of withdrawal, oral delivery may suffice. In severe cases, intravenous administration permits immediate loading and titration of the sedative. Intramuscular administration is contraindicated because of poor and variable absorption and the risk of hematoma or abscess formation in compromised alcoholics. None of the benzodiazepines has demonstrated clear superiority in the treatment of alcohol withdrawal; however, oxazepam and lorazepam are less dependent on hepatic function and may be preferred when severe hepatic dysfunction exists. The dosages required are widely variable and should be governed by the clinical presentation and the response to therapy. Continued observation for persistent or worsening manifestations is required in all patients.[51] Deterioration despite benzodiazepine therapy may necessitate careful management in an ICU.

Antipsychotics may be required for management of hallucinosis or combativeness. Beta blockers, barbiturates, paraldehyde, and chloral hydrate have no advantages over the benzodiazepines for treatment of withdrawal.

Patients who respond to pharmacological intervention and who do not require admission for alcohol withdrawal or other illnesses are best referred to a detoxification facility, where their withdrawal can be carefully observed until it is complete and symptoms have abated entirely.

Minor withdrawal Supportive therapy, including two days of oral administration of benzodiazepines or beta blockers, is sufficient.

Alcoholic hallucinosis Alcoholic hallucinosis is distinguished from delirium tremens by the absence of autonomic hyperactivity. Haloperidol is appropriate.

Alcohol withdrawal seizures The first time a patient presents with alcohol withdrawal seizure, a diagnostic workup, including serum chemistries, computed tomography of the head, and electroencephalography, should be performed.[52] As many as 10 percent of patients with alcohol withdrawal seizures have focal CNS pathology that necessitates additional diagnostic or therapeutic efforts. Repeat presentations for suspected alcohol withdrawal seizure call for careful examination and exclusion of traumatic, infectious, and metabolic causes, but further workup is not necessary. Because withdrawal seizures are usually self-limited, there is no need for acute pharmacotherapy (e.g., with diazepam). Long-term outpatient antiepileptic therapy should not be initiated unless a structural focus has been identified.[53] Prophylaxis against withdrawal seizures (e.g., clorazepate, 15 mg, or lorazepam, 1 to 2 mg, twice daily for three days) during abstinence is probably warranted, particularly in patients who have a history of withdrawal seizures.[54]

Delirium tremens Patients with delirium tremens require continuous intensive care monitoring, crystalloid therapy for volume deficits, cooling measures for hypothermia, physical restraints, and parenteral benzodiazepines. Benzodiazepines should be administered intravenously to produce a state of calm; tremendous dosages, titrated over five- to 15-minute intervals, may be necessary. These patients have vivid and threatening hallucinations, and their behavior is unpredictable. Thus, physical restraints must be maintained until calm is ensured. Serious coexisting medical conditions are common.

Alcoholic ketoacidosis I.V. fluids with dextrose should be given at a minimum rate of 125 ml/hr. Potassium and phosphate are often required. Sodium bicarbonate administration is rarely necessary, and insulin is not indicated. The condition generally resolves within eight to 12 hours.

Consultation and Referral

Early consultation with a toxicologist or regional poison center is appropriate. Patients with acute or chronic conditions related to substance abuse should ultimately be referred to counselors, psychiatrists, and centers expert in the medical and psychosocial complications of alcoholism. Family members and friends are often unwitting codependents and can benefit from similar referrals.

References

1. Powner D: Drug-associated isoelectric EEGs: a hazard in brain death certification. JAMA 236:1123, 1976
2. Hoffman RS, Goldfrank LR: The poisoned patient with altered consciousness: controversies in the use of a 'coma cocktail.' JAMA 274:562, 1995
3. Spivey WH, Roberts JR, Derlet RW: A clinical trial of escalating doses of flumazenil for reversal of suspected benzodiazepine overdose in the emergency department. Ann Emerg Med 22:1813, 1993
4. Frommer DA, Marx J: Wernicke's encephalopathy (letter). N Engl J Med 313:638, 1985
5. Silverstein SC, Frommer DA, Marx JA, et al: The safety and efficacy of parenteral haloperidol for the combative patient: a prospective study (abstr). Ann Emerg Med 15:636, 1986
6. Seventh Special Report to Congress on Alcohol and Health. National Institute on Alcohol Abuse and Alcoholism. US Department of Health and Human Services. Rockville, Maryland, 1990
7. Marx JA: Alcohol and trauma. Emerg Med Clin North Am 8:929, 1990
8. Alcohol as a risk factor for injuries—United States. MMWR 32:61, 1983
9. Kulig K: Initial management of ingestions of toxic substances. N Engl J Med 326:1677, 1992
10. Wiltbank TB, Sine HE, Brody BB: Are emergency toxicology measurements really used? Clin Chem 20:116, 1974
11. Brett AS: Implications of discordance between clinical impression and toxicology analysis in drug overdose. Arch Intern Med 148:437, 1988
12. Kulig K, Bar-Or D, Cantrill SV, et al: Management of acutely poisoned patients without gastric emptying. Ann Emerg Med 14:562, 1985
13. Pond SM, Olson KR, Osterloh JD, et al: Randomized study of the treatment of phenobarbital overdose with repeated doses of activated charcoal. JAMA 251:3104, 1984
14. Utecht MJ, Stone AF, McCarron MM: Heroin body packers. J Emerg Med 11:33, 1983
15. Marc B, Baud FJ, Maison P, et al: Cardiac monitoring during medical management of cocaine body packers. Clin Tox 30:387, 1992
16. Eneanya DI, Bianchine JR, Duran DO, et al: The actions of metabolic rate of disulfiram. Annu Rev Pharmacol Toxicol 21:575, 1981
17. Duberstein JL, Kaufman DM: A clinical study of an epidemic of heroin intoxication and heroin-induced pulmonary edema. Am J Med 51:704, 1971
18. Ford M, Hoffman R, Goldfrank L: Opioids and designer drugs. Emerg Med Clin North Am 8:495, 1990
19. Cherubin CE, Sapira JD: The medical complications of drug addiction and the medical assessment of the intravenous drug user: 25 years later. Ann Intern Med 119:1017, 1993
20. Friedland GH, Harris C, Butkus-Small C, et al: Intravenous drug abusers and the acquired immunodeficiency syndrome (AIDS). Arch Intern Med 145:1413, 1985
21. Freitas PM: Narcotic withdrawal in the emergency department. Am J Emerg Med 3:456, 1985
22. Holman PW: Clonidine and naloxone in ultrashort opiate detoxification. Clin Pharm 4:100, 1985
23. Brody SL, Slovis CM, Wrenn KD: Cocaine-related medical problems: consecutive series of 233 patients. Am J Med 88:325, 1990
24. Shesser R, Davis C, Edelstein S: Pneumomediastinum and pneumothorax after inhaling alkaloidal cocaine. Ann Emerg Med 10:213, 1981
25. Hollander JE, Hoffman RS, Gennis P, et al: Prospective multicenter evaluation of cocaine-associated chest pain. Acad Emerg Med 1:330, 1994
26. Hollander JE: The management of cocaine-associated myocardial ischemia. N Engl J Med 333:1267, 1995
27. Rumbaugh CL, Bergeron RT, Fang HC, et al: Cerebral angiographic changes in the drug abuse patient. Radiology 101:335, 1971
28. Kulig K: Emergency aspects of drug abuse. Emerg Med Clin North Am 8:551, 1990
29. Klock JC, Boerner U, Becker CE: Coma, hyperthermia and bleeding associated with massive LSD overdose: a report of eight cases. West J Med 120:183, 1974
30. Baldridge EB, Bessen HA: Phencyclidine. Emerg Med Clin North Am 8:541, 1990
31. McCarron MM, Schulze BW, Thompson GA, et al: Acute phencyclidine intoxication: clinical patterns, complications, and treatment. Ann Emerg Med 10:290, 1981
32. Sporer KA, Ernst AA, Conte R, et al: The incidence of ethanol-induced hypoglycemia. Am J Emerg Med 10:403, 1992
33. Madison LL: Ethanol-induced hypoglycemia. Advances in Metabolic Disorders 3:85, 1968
34. Kulig K, Duffy JP, Lenden CH, et al: Toxic effects of methanol, ethylene glycol and isopropyl alcohol. Topics in Emergency Medicine 6:14, 1984
35. Marx JA, Duffens K: Response to E. Otten's letter (ketoacidosis and isopropyl alcohol). J Emerg Med 6:342, 1988
36. Brewer C: Recent developments in disulfiram treatment. Alcohol 28:383, 1993
37. Bates ME, Brick J, White HR: The correspondence between saliva and breath estimates of blood alcohol concentration: advantages and limitations of the saliva method. J Stud Alcohol 54:17, 1993
38. Pollack CV Jr, Jorden RC, Carlton FB, et al: Gastric emptying in the acutely inebriated patient. J Emerg Med 10:1, 1992
39. Christiansson LK, Kaspersson KE, Kulling PE: Treatment of severe ethylene glycol intoxication with continuous arteriovenous hemofiltration dialysis. J Toxicol Clin Toxicol 33:267, 1995
40. Eichner ER, Hillman RS: The evolution of anemia in alcoholic patients. Am J Med 50:218, 1971
41. Cowan DH: Effect of alcoholism on hemostasis. Semin Hematol 17:137, 1980
42. Diamond I, Messing RO: Neurologic effects of alcoholism. West J Med 161:279, 1994
43. Victor M, Adams RD, Collins GH: The Wernicke-Korsakoff Syndrome. FA Davis Co, Philadelphia, 1971
44. Frommer D, Kulig K, Marx J, et al: Tricyclic antidepressant overdose patients managed in an emergency department observation unit. Presented to the III World Congress of the World Federation of Associations of Clinical Toxicology and Poison Control Centres and the XII International Congress of the European Association of Poison Control Centres, Brussels, Belgium, August 1986
45. Victor M, Brausch C: The role of abstinence in the genesis of alcoholic epilepsy. Epilepsia 8:1, 1967
46. Schuckit MA, Tipp JE, Reich T, et al: The histories of withdrawal convulsions and delirium tremens in 1648 alcohol dependent subjects. Addiction 90:1335, 1995
47. Duffens K, Marx JA: Alcohol ketoacidosis—a review. J Emerg Med 5:399, 1987
48. Wrenn KD, Slovis CM, Minion GE, et al: The syndrome of alcoholic ketoacidosis. Am J Med 91:119, 1991
49. Saitz R, Mayo-Smith MF, Roberts MS, et al: Individualized treatment for alcohol withdrawal: a randomized double-blind controlled trial. JAMA 272:519, 1994
50. Hoey LL, Nahum A, Vance-Bryan K: A retrospective review and assessment of benzodiazepines in the treatment of alcohol withdrawal in hospitalized patients. Ann Med 26:101, 1994
51. Lohr RH: Treatment of alcohol withdrawal in hospitalized patients. Mayo Clin Proc 70:777, 1995
52. Earnest MP, Feldman H, Marx JA, et al: Intracranial lesions shown by CT scans in 259 cases of first alcohol-related seizures. Neurology 38:1561, 1988
53. Chance JF: Emergency department treatment of alcohol withdrawal seizures with phenytoin. Ann Emerg Med 20:520, 1991
54. Marx JA, Berner J, Bar-Or D, et al: Prophylaxis of alcohol withdrawal seizures: a prospective study (abstr). Ann Emerg Med 15:637, 1986

II COMMON PRESENTING PROBLEMS

11 NECK MASS

Barry J. Roseman, M.D., and Orlo H. Clark, M.D.

Assessment of a Neck Mass

History

The evaluation of any neck mass begins with a careful history. The history should be taken with the differential diagnosis in mind [see Table 1] because directed questions can narrow down the diagnostic possibilities and focus subsequent investigations. For example, in younger patients, one would tend to look for congenital lesions, whereas in older adults, the first concern would always be neoplasia.

The duration and growth rate of the mass should be determined: malignant lesions are far more likely to exhibit rapid growth than benign ones, which may grow and shrink. Next, the location of the mass in the neck should be determined. This is particularly important for differentiating congenital masses from developmental ones because each type usually occurs consistently in particular locations. In addition, the location of a neoplasm is both diagnostically and prognostically significant. The possibility that the mass reflects an infectious or inflammatory process should also be assessed. One should check for evidence of infection or inflammation (e.g., fever, pain, or tenderness); a recent history of tuberculosis, sarcoidosis, or fungal infection; the presence of dental problems; and a history of trauma to the head and neck. Masses that appear inflamed or infected are far more likely to be benign.

Finally, factors suggestive of cancer should be sought: a previous malignancy elsewhere in the head and neck (e.g., a skin lesion or a head and neck tumor); night sweats (suggestive of lymphoma); excessive exposure to the sun (a risk factor for skin cancer); smoking or excessive alcohol consumption (risk factors for squamous cell carcinoma of the head and neck); nasal obstruction or bleeding, otalgia, odynophagia, dysphagia, or hoarseness (suggestive of a malignancy in the upper aerodigestive tract); or exposure to low-dose therapeutic radiation (a risk factor for thyroid cancer).

Physical Examination

Examination of the head and neck is challenging in that much of the area to be examined is not easily visualized. Patience and practice are necessary to master the special instruments and techniques of examination. A head and neck examination is usually performed with the patient sitting in front of the physician. Constant repositioning of the head is

Table 1 Etiology of Neck Mass

Inflammatory and infectious disorders	Acute lymphadenitis (bacterial or viral infection)
	Subcutaneous abscess (carbuncle)
	Infectious mononucleosis
	Cat-scratch fever
	Acquired immunodeficiency syndrome
	Tuberculous lymphadenitis (scrofula)
	Fungal lymphadenitis (actinomycosis)
	Sarcoidosis
Congenital cystic lesions	Thyroglossal duct cyst
	Branchial cleft cyst
	Cystic hygroma (lymphangioma)
	Vascular malformation (hemangioma)
	Laryngocele
Benign neoplasms	Salivary gland tumor
	Thyroid nodules or goiter
	Soft tissue tumor (lipoma, sebaceous cyst)
	Chemodectoma (carotid body tumor)
	Neurogenic tumor (neurofibroma, neurilemoma)
	Laryngeal tumor (chondroma)
Malignant neoplasms	*Primary*
	Salivary gland tumor
	Thyroid cancer
	Upper aerodigestive tract cancer
	Soft tissue sarcoma
	Skin cancer (melanoma, squamous cell carcinoma, and basal cell carcinoma)
	Lymphoma
	Metastatic
	Upper aerodigestive tract cancer
	Skin cancer (melanoma, squamous cell carcinoma)
	Salivary gland tumor
	Thyroid cancer
	Adenocarcinoma (breast, GI tract, GU tract, lung)
	Unknown primary

Assessment of a Neck Mass

Patient presents with a neck mass

Obtain clinical history

Determine
- Duration and growth rate of mass
- Location of mass

Ask about
- Factors suggestive of infection or inflammatory disorder
- Factors suggestive of cancer

Perform physical examination of head and neck

Look for
- Asymmetry • Signs of trauma • Skin changes
- Movement of mass on deglutition • Bruit
- Vocal changes

Attempt to determine source of mass, and assess its physical characteristics. Examine the following areas in detail:
- Cervical lymph nodes • Skin • Thyroid
- Salivary glands • Oral cavity and oropharynx
- Larynx and hypopharynx • Nasal cavity and nasopharynx

Formulate initial diagnostic impressions

Diagnosis is probable, and further diagnostic investigation is unnecessary

Diagnosis is uncertain, or further information is needed or desired

Consider investigative studies:
Biopsy: Fine-needle aspiration (FNA) is preferred method.
Imaging studies: Not routinely called for, but ultrasonography, CT, MRI, arteriography, angiography, and plain x-rays are sometimes helpful. Consultation with a head and neck radiologist is desirable.

FNA is diagnostic or confirmatory

FNA yields negative or inconclusive results

Repeat FNA or perform open biopsy.

Inflammatory or infectious disorder

Treat medically.
Drain abscesses.

Congenital cystic lesion

These include
- Thyroglossal duct cysts and branchial cleft cysts (treated surgically)
- Cystic hygromas and hemangiomas (treated expectantly)

Benign neoplasm

These include
- Salivary gland tumors
- Thyroid nodules and goiters
- Soft tissue tumors
- Chemodectomas
- Neurogenic tumors
- Laryngeal tumors

Treat surgically. (Observation is appropriate in some cases.)

Malignant neoplasm

Determine whether cancer is primary or metastatic.

Primary neoplasm

These include
- Lymphoma • Thyroid cancer • Upper aerodigestive tract cancer • Soft tissue sarcoma
- Skin cancer

Treat with surgery, radiation therapy, and/or chemotherapy, as appropriate.

Metastatic tumor

Primary is known

Metastatic squamous cell carcinoma: Perform selective neck dissection, and consider adjuvant radiation therapy.
Metastatic adenocarcinoma: Perform neck dissection (selective or other), and consider adjuvant radiation therapy.
Metastatic melanoma: Perform full-thickness excision, then modified neck dissection, depending on tumor thickness.

Primary is unknown

Evaluate nasopharynx, larynx, esophagus, hypopharynx, and tracheobronchial tree endoscopically.
Biopsy nasopharynx, tonsils, and hypopharynx.
Perform unilateral neck dissection followed by irradiation of neck, entire pharynx, and nasopharynx.

necessary to obtain adequate visualization of the various areas. Gloves must be worn during the examination, particularly if the mucous membranes are to be examined. Good illumination is essential. The time-honored but cumbersome head mirror has been largely supplanted by the headlight (usually a high-intensity halogen lamp). Fiberoptic endoscopy with a flexible laryngoscope and a nasopharyngoscope has become a common component of the physical examination for evaluating the larynx, the nasopharynx, and the paranasal sinuses, especially when these areas cannot be adequately visualized with more standard techniques.

The examination should begin with inspection for asymmetry, signs of trauma, and skin changes. One should ask the patient to swallow to see if the mass moves with deglutition. Palpation should be done both from the front and from behind. Auscultation is performed to detect audible bruits. One should also ask about the patient's voice, changes in which may suggest either a laryngeal tumor or recurrent nerve dysfunction from locally invasive thyroid cancer.

During the physical examination, one should be thinking about the following questions: What structure is the neck mass arising from? Is it a lymph node? Is the mass arising from a normally occurring structure, such as the thyroid gland, a nerve, a blood vessel, or a muscle? Or is it arising from an abnormal structure, such as a laryngocele, a branchial cleft cyst, or a cystic hygroma? Is the mass soft, fluctuant, easily mobile, well-encapsulated, and smooth? Or is it firm, poorly mobile, and fixed to surrounding structures? Does it pulsate? Is there a bruit? Does it appear to be superficial, or is it deeper in the neck? Is it attached to the skin? Is it tender?

The following areas of the head and neck are examined in some detail.

CERVICAL LYMPH NODES

Enlarged lymph nodes are by far the most common neck masses encountered. The cervical lymphatic system consists of interconnected groups or chains of nodes that parallel the major neurovascular structures in the head and neck. The skin and mucosal surfaces of the head and neck all have specific and predictable nodes associated with them. The classification of cervical lymph nodes has been standardized to comprise six levels [see Table 2 and Figure 1]. Accurate determination of lymph node level on physical examination and in surgical specimens not only helps establish a common language among clinicians but also permits comparison of data among different institutions.

The location, size, and consistency of lymph nodes furnish valuable clues to the nature of the primary disease. Other physical characteristics of the adenopathy should be noted as well, including the number of lymph nodes affected, their mobility, their degree of fixation, and their relation to surrounding anatomic structures. One can often establish a tentative diagnosis on the basis of these findings alone. For example, soft or tender nodes are more likely to derive from an inflammatory or infectious condition, whereas hard, fixed, painless nodes are more likely to represent metastatic cancer. Multiple regions of enlarged lymph nodes are usually a sign of systemic disease (e.g., lymphoma, tuberculosis, or infectious mononucleosis), whereas solitary nodes are more often due to malignancy. Firm, rubbery nodes are typical of lymphoma. Low cervical nodes are more likely to contain metastases from a primary source other than the head and neck, whereas upper cervical nodes are more likely to contain metastases from the head and neck.

The submental and submandibular nodes (level I) are palpated bimanually. Metastases to level I are commonly from the lips, the oral cavity, or the facial skin. The three levels of internal jugular chain nodes (levels II, III, and IV) are best examined by gently rolling the sternocleidomastoid muscle between the thumb and the index finger. Level II and level III lymph nodes are common sites for lymph node metastases from primary cancers of the oropharynx, the larynx, and the hypopharynx. Metastases in level IV lymph nodes can arise from cancers of the upper aerodigestive tract, from cancers of the thyroid gland, or from cancers arising below the clavicle (Virchow's node). The nodes in the posterior triangle (level V) are all palpated. Nodal metastases in this region can arise from nasopharyngeal and thyroid cancers as well as from squamous cell carcinoma or melanoma of the posterior scalp and the pinna of the ear. The tracheoesophageal groove nodes (level VI) are then palpated.

SKIN

Careful examination of the scalp, the ears, the face, and the neck will identify potentially malignant skin lesions, which may give rise to lymph node metastases.

THYROID GLAND

The thyroid gland is palpated, and its size and consistency are assessed. One determines whether it is smooth, diffusely enlarged, or nodular and whether one nodule or several are present. If it is unclear whether the mass is truly thyroid, one should ask the patient to swallow and watch to see whether the mass moves. Signs of superior mediastinal syndrome (e.g., cervical venous engorgement and facial edema) suggest retrosternal extension of a thyroid goiter. The larynx and trachea are examined, with special attention to the cricothyroid membrane, over which Delphian nodes can be palpated. These nodes can be a harbinger of thyroid or laryngeal cancer.

MAJOR SALIVARY GLANDS

Examination of the paired parotid and submandibular glands involves not only palpation of the neck but also an intraoral examination to inspect the duct openings. The submandibular

Table 2 Classification of Cervical Lymph Nodes

Level	Nodes
I	Submental nodes Submandibular nodes
II	Upper internal jugular chain nodes
III	Middle internal jugular chain nodes
IV	Lower internal jugular chain nodes
V	Spinal accessory nodes Transverse cervical nodes
VI	Tracheoesophageal groove nodes

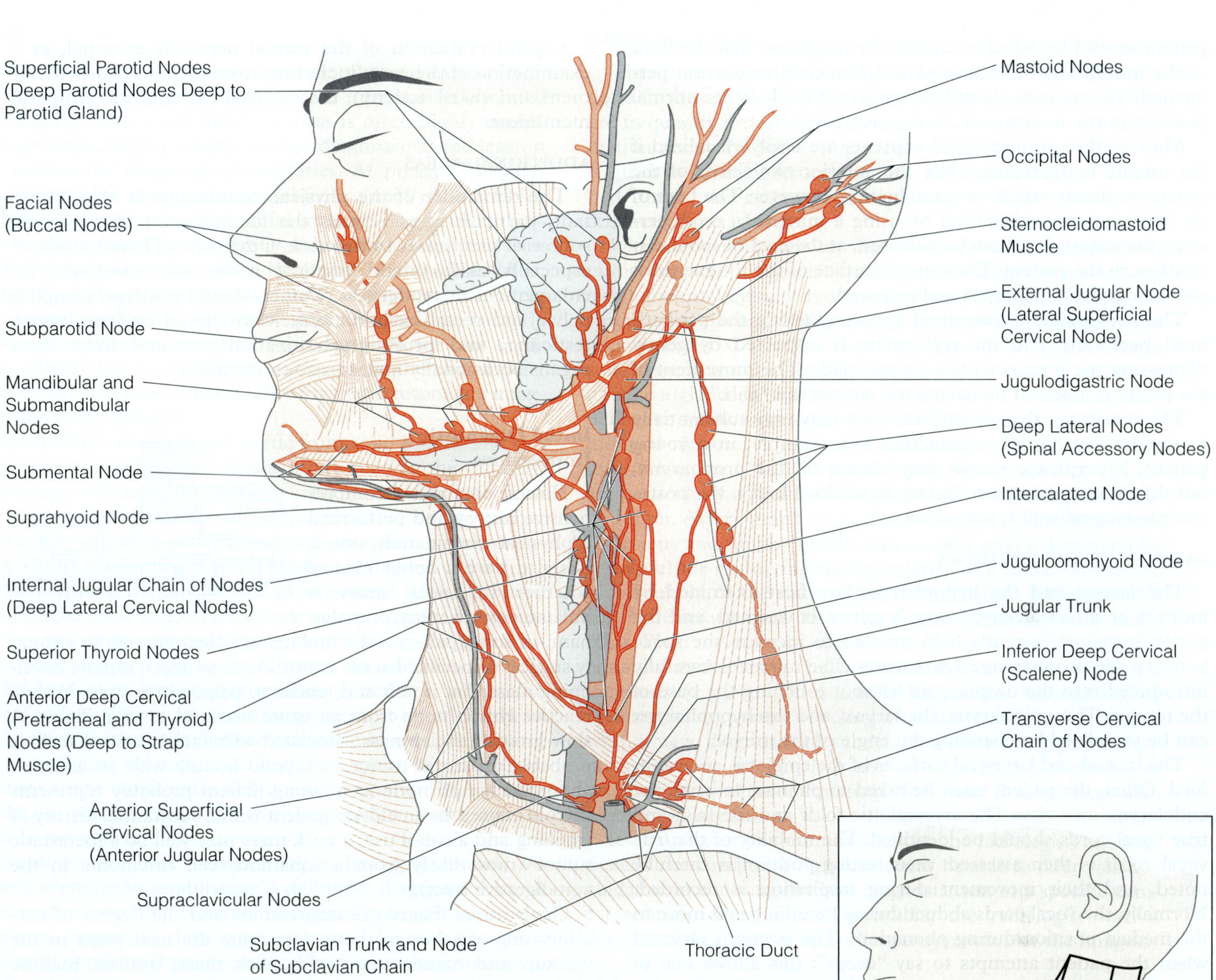

Figure 1 Cervical lymph nodes can be classified into six levels (inset) on the basis of their location in the neck.

glands are best assessed by bimanual palpation, with one finger in the mouth and one in the neck. They are normally lower and more prominent in older patients. The parotid glands are often palpable in the neck, though the deep lobe cannot always be assessed. A mass in the region of the tail of the parotid must be distinguished from enlarged level II jugular nodes. The oropharynx is inspected for distortion of the lateral walls. The parotid (Stensen's) duct may be found opening into the buccal mucosa, opposite the second upper molar.

ORAL CAVITY AND OROPHARYNX

The lips should be inspected and palpated. Dentures should be removed before the mouth is examined. The buccal mucosa, the teeth, and the gingiva are then inspected. The

buncles (most often occurring in the back of the neck in a patient with diabetes mellitus). The physical characteristics of abscesses make recognition of these problems relatively straightforward.

On occasion, primary head and neck bacterial infections can lead to infection of the fascial spaces of the neck. A high index of suspicion is required: such infections are sometimes difficult to diagnose. Aggressive treatment with antibiotics and drainage of closed spaces is indicated to prevent overwhelming fasciitis.

Various chronic infections (e.g., tuberculosis, fungal lymphadenitis, syphilis, cat-scratch fever, and acquired immunodeficiency syndrome [AIDS]) may also involve cervical lymph nodes. Certain chronic inflammatory disorders (e.g., sarcoidosis) may present with cervical lymphadenopathy as well. Because of the chronic lymph node involvement, these conditions are easily confused with neoplasms, especially lymphomas. Biopsy is occasionally necessary; however, skin tests and serologic studies are often more useful for establishing a diagnosis. Treatment of these conditions is primarily medical; surgery is reserved for complications.

CONGENITAL CYSTIC LESIONS

Thyroglossal Duct Cysts

Thyroglossal duct cysts are remnants of the tract along which the thyroid gland descended into the neck from the foramen cecum [*see Figure 2*]. They account for about 70 percent of all congenital abnormalities of the neck. Thyroglossal duct cysts may be found in patients of any age but are most common in the first decade of life. They may take the form of a lone cyst, a cyst with a sinus tract, or a solid core of thyroid tissue. They may be so small as to be barely perceptible, as large as a grapefruit, or anything in between. Thyroglossal duct cysts are almost always found in the midline, at or below the level of the hyoid bone; however, they may be situated anywhere from the base of the tongue to the suprasternal notch. They occasionally present slightly lateral to the midline and are sometimes associated with an external fistula to the skin of the anterior neck. They are often ballotable and can usually be moved slightly from side to side but not up or down; however, they do move up and down when patients swallow or protrude the tongue.

Thyroglossal duct cysts must be differentiated from dermoid cysts, lymphadenomegaly in the anterior jugular chain, and cutaneous lesions (e.g., lipomas and sebaceous cysts). Operative treatment is almost always required, not only because of cosmetic considerations but also because of the high incidence of recurrent infection, including abscess formation. About one percent of thyroglossal duct cysts contain cancer; papillary cancer is the neoplasm most commonly encountered, followed by squamous cell carcinoma.

Branchial Cleft Cysts

Branchial cleft cysts are vestigial remnants of the fetal branchial apparatus from which all neck structures are derived. Early in embryonic development, there are five branchial arches and four grooves (or clefts) between them. The internal tract or opening of a branchial cleft cyst is situated at the embryologic derivative of the corresponding pharyngeal groove, such as the tonsil (second arch) or the piriform sinus (third and fourth arches). The second arch is the most common area of origin for such cysts. The position of the cyst tract is also determined by the embryologic relation of its arch to the derivatives of the arches on either side of it.

The majority of branchial cleft cysts (those that develop from the second, third, and fourth arches) tend to present as a bulge along the anterior border of the sternocleidomastoid muscle, with or without a sinus tract. Branchial cleft cysts may become symptomatic at any age, but most are diagnosed in the first two decades of life. They often present as a smooth, painless, slowly enlarging mass in the lateral neck. Frequently, there is a history of fluctuating size and intermittent tenderness. The diagnosis is more obvious when there is an external fistulous tract and there is a history of intermittent discharge. Infection of the cyst may be the reason for the first symptoms.

Treatment consists of complete surgical removal of the cyst and the sinus tract. Any infection or inflammation should be treated and allowed to resolve before the cyst and the tract are removed.

Cystic Hygromas (Lymphangiomas)

A cystic hygroma is a lymphangioma that arises from vestigial lymph channels in the neck. Almost always, this condition is first noted by the second year of life; on rare occasions, it is first diagnosed in adulthood. A cystic hygroma may present as a relatively simple thin-walled cyst in the floor of the mouth or may involve all the tissues from the floor of the mouth to the mediastinum. About 80 percent of the time, there is only a painless cyst in the posterior cervical triangle or in the supraclavicular area. A cystic hygroma can also occur, however, at the root of the neck, in the angle of the jaw (where it may involve the parotid gland), and in the midline (where it may involve the tongue, the floor of the mouth, or the larynx).

The typical clinical picture is of a diffuse, soft, doughy, irregular mass that is readily transilluminated. Cystic hygromas look and feel somewhat like lipomas but have less well defined margins. Aspiration of cystic hygromas yields straw-colored fluid. They may be confused with angiomas (which are compressible), pneumatoceles from the apex of the lung, or aneurysms. They can be distinguished from vascular lesions by means of arteriography. On occasion, a cystic hygroma grows suddenly as a result of an upper respiratory tract infection, infection of the hygroma itself, or hemorrhage into the tissues. If the mass becomes large enough, it can compress the trachea or hinder swallowing.

In the absence of pressure symptoms (i.e., obstruction of the airway or interference with swallowing) or gross deformity, cystic hygromas may be treated expectantly. They tend to regress spontaneously; if they do not, complete surgical excision is indicated. Excision can be difficult because of the numerous satellite extensions that often surround the main mass and because of the association of the tumor with vital structures such as the cranial nerves. Recurrences are common; staged resections for complete excision are often necessary.

Vascular Malformation (Hemangiomas)

Hemangiomas are usually considered congenital because they either are present at birth or appear within the first year

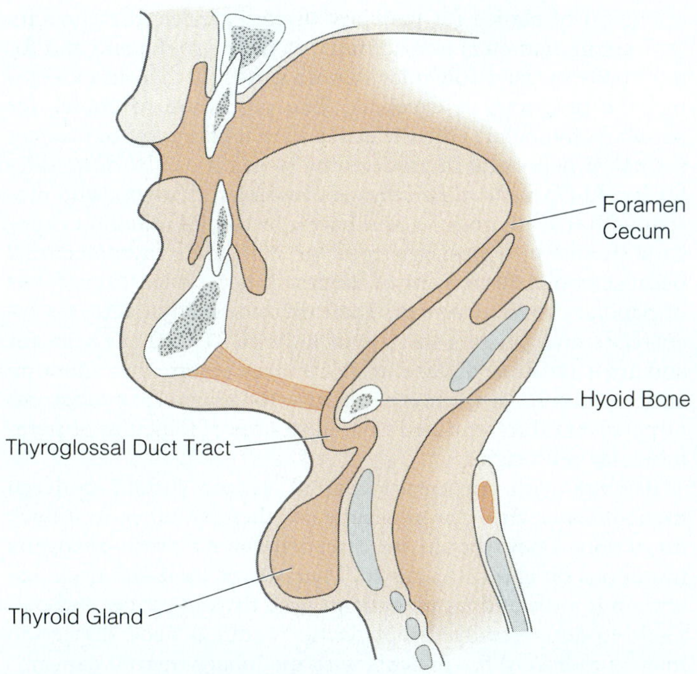

Figure 2 Shown is the course of the thyroglossal duct tract from its origin in the area of the foramen cecum to the pyramidal lobe of the thyroid gland. In the operative treatment of a thyroglossal duct cyst, the central portion of the hyoid bone must be removed to ensure complete removal of the tract and to prevent recurrence.

of life. A number of characteristic findings—bluish-purple coloration, increased warmth, compressibility followed by refilling, bruit, and thrill—distinguish them from other head and neck masses. Angiography is diagnostic but is rarely indicated.

Given that most of these congenital lesions resolve spontaneously, the treatment approach of choice is observation alone unless there is rapid growth, thrombocytopenia, or involvement of vital structures.

BENIGN NEOPLASMS

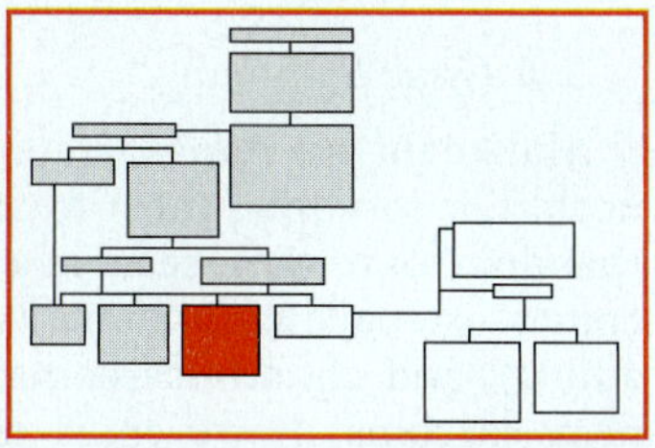

Salivary Gland Tumors

The possibility of a salivary gland neoplasm must be considered whenever an enlarging solid mass lies in front of and below the ear, at the angle of the mandible, or in the submandibular triangle. Benign salivary gland lesions are often asymptomatic; malignant ones are often associated with seventh cranial nerve symptoms or skin fixation. Diagnostic radiographic studies (CT or MRI) indicate whether the mass is salivary in origin but do not help classify it histologically. The diagnostic test of preference is open biopsy in the form of complete submandibular gland removal or superficial parotidectomy.

With any mass in or around the ear, one should be prepared to remove the superficial lobes of the parotid, the deep lobes, or both and to perform a careful facial nerve dissection. Any less complete approach reduces the chances of a cure: there is a high risk of implantation and seeding of malignant tumors. Benign mixed tumors make up two thirds of all salivary tumors; these must also be completely removed because recurrence is common after incomplete resection.

Benign Thyroid Nodules and Nodular Goiters

Thyroid disease is a relatively common cause of neck masses: in the United States, about four percent of women and two percent of men have a palpable nodular goiter. Patients should be questioned about local symptoms (pain, dysphagia, pressure, hoarseness, or a change in the voice), about the duration of the nodule, and about systemic symptoms (from hyperthyroidism, hypothyroidism, or any other illness). Although most nodules are benign, malignancy is a significant concern. Nodules in children, young men, pregnant women, or persons with a history of radiation exposure or a family history of thyroid cancer are more likely to be malignant. Nodules that are truly solitary, feel firm or hard on examination, are growing rapidly, or are nonfunctional on scans are more likely to be malignant.

If physical examination suggests a discrete thyroid nodule, FNA should be done to ascertain whether malignancy is present within the nodule. If malignancy is confirmed or suspected, surgery is indicated. If the nodule is histologically benign or disappears with aspiration, thyroid suppression and observation are often sufficient. FNA often yields unrepresentative results in patients with a history of radiation exposure, in whom there is approximately a 40 percent chance that one of the nodules present contains cancer.

Surgery for thyroid nodules involves excisional biopsy consisting of at least total lobectomy; enucleation is almost never indicated. The surgical approach of choice for most patients with Graves' disease or multinodular goiter is subtotal thyroidectomy or total lobectomy on one side and subtotal lobectomy on the other (Dunhill's operation). Treatment of thyroid cancer is discussed elsewhere [see Primary Malignant Neoplasms, Thyroid Cancer, *below*].

Soft Tissue Tumors (Lipomas, Sebaceous Cysts)

Superficial intracutaneous or subcutaneous masses may be sebaceous (or epidermal inclusion) cysts or lipomas. Final diagnosis and treatment usually involve simple surgical excision, often done as an office procedure with local anesthesia.

Chemodectomas (Carotid Body Tumors)

Carotid body tumors belong to a group of tumors known as chemodectomas (or, alternatively, as glomus tumors or nonchromaffin paragangliomas), which derive from the chemoreceptive tissue of the head and neck. In the head and neck, chemodectomas most often arise from the tympanic bodies in the middle ear, the glomus jugulare at the skull base, the vagal body near the skull base along the inferior ganglion of the vagus, and the carotid body at the carotid bifurcation. They are occasionally familial and sometimes occur bilaterally.

A carotid body tumor presents as a firm, round, slowly growing mass at the carotid bifurcation. Occasionally, a bruit is present. The tumor cannot be separated from the carotid artery by palpation and can usually be moved laterally and medially but not in a cephalocaudal plane. The differential diagnosis includes a carotid aneurysm, a branchial cleft cyst, a neurogenic tumor, and nodal metastases fixed to the carotid sheath. The diagnosis is made by means of CT scanning or arteriography, which demonstrates a characteristic highly vascular mass at the carotid bifurcation. Neurofibromas tend to displace, encircle, or compress a portion of the carotid artery system, events that are readily demonstrated by carotid angiography. Given the low incidence of multiple chemodectomas, carotid angiography should be done via a transfemoral route if a chemodectoma is suspected.

Biopsy should be avoided. Chemodectomas are sometimes malignant and should therefore be removed in most cases to prevent subsequent growth and pressure symptoms. Fortunately, even malignant chemodectomas are usually low grade; long-term results after removal are excellent on the whole. Some experience with vascular surgery is desirable: bleeding may occur, and clamping of the carotid artery may result in a stroke. Expectant treatment may be indicated in older or debilitated individuals. Radiotherapy may be appropriate for patients with unresectable tumors.

Neurogenic Tumors (Neurofibromas, Neurilemomas)

The large number of nerves in the head and neck renders the area susceptible to neurogenic tumors. The most common of such tumors, neurilemomas (schwannomas) and neurofibromas, arise from the neurilemma and usually present as painless, slowly growing masses in the lateral neck. Neurilemomas can be differentiated from neurofibromas only by means of histologic examination.

Given the potential these tumors possess for malignant degeneration and slow but progressive growth, surgical resection is indicated. This may include resection of the involved nerves, particularly with neurofibromas, which tend to be more invasive and less encapsulated than neurilemomas.

Laryngeal Tumors

In rare cases, a chondroma may arise from the thyroid cartilage or the cricoid cartilage. It is firmly fixed to the cartilage and may present as a mass in the neck or as the cause of a progressively compromised airway. Surgical excision is indicated.

PRIMARY MALIGNANT NEOPLASMS

Lymphomas

Cervical adenopathy is one of the most common presenting symptoms in patients with Hodgkin's and non-Hodgkin's lymphoma. The nodes tend to be softer, smoother, more elastic, and more mobile than nodes containing metastatic carcinoma would be. Rapid growth is not unusual, particularly in non-Hodgkin's lymphoma. Involvement of extranodal sites, particularly Waldeyer's tonsillar ring, is often seen in patients with non-Hodgkin's lymphoma; enlargement of these sites may provide a clue to the diagnosis. The diagnosis is confirmed via excisional biopsy of an intact lymph node. As noted, the precise histologic subtype usually cannot be determined by FNA alone; open biopsy must be done, and fresh tissue must be submitted for surface marker and electron microscopic studies.

Lymphoma is treated by means of radiation therapy, chemotherapy, or both, depending on the disease's pathological type and clinical stage.

Thyroid Cancer

The approach to suspected thyroid cancer differs in some respects from the approach to benign thyroid disease. The operation of choice for papillary thyroid cancer that is occult (< 1 cm in diameter) and confined to the thyroid gland and for minimally invasive follicular thyroid cancer is thyroid lobectomy; the prognosis is excellent. The procedure of choice for papillary, follicular, Hürthle cell, and medullary thyroid cancer is total or near-total thyroidectomy (when it can be done safely) [see 42 Thyroid and Parathyroid Procedures]. Patients who present with thyroid nodules and have a history of radiation exposure should also undergo total or near-total thyroidectomy because about 40 percent of them will have at least one focus of papillary thyroid cancer. Total thyroidectomy decreases recurrence and permits the use of iodine-131 (^{131}I) to scan for and treat residual disease; it also makes serum thyroglobulin and calcitonin assays more sensitive for diagnosing recurrent or persistent differentiated thyroid tumors of follicular or parafollicular cell origin.

Patients with medullary thyroid cancer should undergo meticulous elective (prophylactic) or therapeutic central neck dissection. They should be screened for *ret* proto-oncogene mutations on chromosome 10. Therapeutic modified neck dissection is indicated for all patients with thyroid cancer and palpable nodes laterally. Prophylactic modified neck dissection may be indicated for patients with medullary thyroid cancer.

Patients with anaplastic thyroid cancer are probably best treated with a combination of chemotherapy and radiation therapy, in conjunction with the removal of as much of the neoplasm as can safely be excised. Chemotherapy and radiation therapy are indicated for most patients with thyroid lymphoma, a much less common entity.

Upper Aerodigestive Tract Cancer

Deciding on the optimal therapeutic approach to tumors of the aerodigestive tract (i.e., surgery, radiation therapy, or some combination of the two) generally requires expertise beyond that of most general surgeons. Therefore, cancers involving the nose, the paranasal sinuses, the nasopharynx, the floor of the mouth, the tongue, the palate, the tonsils, the piriform sinus, the hypopharynx, or the larynx are best managed by an experienced head and neck oncological surgeon in conjunction with a radiation therapist and a medical oncologist.

Soft Tissue Sarcomas

Malignant sarcomas are not common in the head and neck. The sarcomas most frequently encountered include the rhabdomyosarcoma seen in children, fibrosarcoma, liposarcoma, osteogenic sarcoma (which usually arises in young adults), and chondrosarcoma. The most common head and neck sarcoma, however, is malignant fibrous histiocytoma (MFH). MFH is seen most frequently in the elderly and extremely rarely in children, but it can arise at any age. It is often difficult to differentiate pathologically from other entities (e.g., fibrosarcoma). MFH can occur in the soft tissues of the neck or involve the bone of the maxilla or the mandible. The preferred treatment is wide surgical resection; adjuvant radiation therapy and chemotherapy are currently being studied in clinical trials.

Rhabdomyosarcoma, usually of the embryonic form, is the most common form of sarcoma in children. It generally occurs near the orbit, the nasopharynx, or the paranasal sinuses. The diagnosis is confirmed by biopsy. A thorough search for distal metastases is made before treatment—consisting of a combination of surgical resection, radiation therapy, and chemotherapy—is begun.

Skin Cancer

Basal cell carcinoma is the most common of the skin malignancies [see 20 Skin Lesions]. It arises in areas that have been extensively exposed to sunlight (e.g., the nose, the forehead, the cheeks, and the ears). Metastases are rare (< one percent of cases), and the prognosis is excellent. If treatment is inadequate, however, basal cell carcinomas can cause extensive local destruction. Basal cell carcinoma of the medial canthus may invade the orbit, the ethmoid sinus, and even the brain. Periauricular basal cell carcinoma can spread across the cartilage of the ear canal or into the parotid gland. Treatment consists of local resection with adequate clear margins.

Squamous cell carcinoma also arises in areas associated with extensive sunlight exposure; the lower lip and the pinna are the most common sites. Unlike basal cell carcinoma, however, squamous cell carcinoma tends to metastasize regionally and distally. This tumor must also be excised with an adequate margin.

Melanoma is classified on the basis of size, location, depth of invasion, and histologic subtype, although the prognosis is closely related to the thickness of the tumor [see Metastatic Tumors, Metastatic Melanomas, below]. In addition to the typical pigmented, irregularly shaped skin lesions [see 20 Skin Lesions], malignant melanoma may also arise on the mucous membranes of the nose or the throat, on the hard palate, or on the buccal mucosa. The treatment of choice is wide surgical resection. Radiation therapy, chemotherapy, and immunotherapy may also be considered.

METASTATIC TUMORS

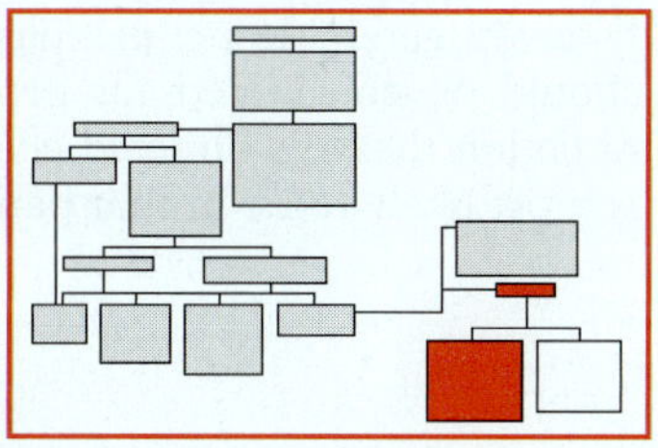

Any surgeon who is managing patients with head and neck cancers must have a thorough understanding of neck dissections and should have sufficient training and experience to perform these operations in the appropriate clinical circumstances.

Types of Neck Dissections

There are two classification systems for neck dissections. The first is based on the indications and goals of surgery. An *elective* (or *prophylactic*) neck dissection is done when the neck is clinically negative (that is, when no abnormal lymph nodes are palpable or visible on radiographic imaging). A *therapeutic* neck dissection is done to remove all palpable and occult disease in patients with suspicious lymph nodes discovered via physical examination or CT scanning.

The second system is based on the extent and type of dissection. *Comprehensive* neck dissections include the classic radical neck dissection as well as the modified radical (or functional) neck dissection [see Figure 3]. In a radical neck dissection, the sternocleidomastoid muscle, the internal and external jugular veins, the spinal accessory nerve, and the submaxillary gland are removed, along with all lymph node–bearing tissues. The modified radical or functional neck dissection is a modification of the radical neck dissection in which the lymphatic tissue from these areas is removed but the functional structures are preserved. *Selective* neck dissections involve the removal of specific levels of lymph nodes [see Figure 1]. The rationale for selective dissections is that several head and neck cancers consistently metastasize to specific localized lymph node regions. The following are examples of selective neck dissections: suprahyoid neck dissection (levels I and II); supraomohyoid neck dissection (levels I, II, and III); lateral neck dissection (levels II, III, and IV); and posterolateral neck dissection (levels II, III, IV, and V).

Metastatic Squamous Cell Carcinomas

The basic principle in the management of metastatic squamous cell carcinoma is to treat all regional lymph node groups at highest risk for metastases by means of surgery or radiation therapy, depending on the clinical circumstances. Selective lymph node dissection can be performed along with wide excision of the primary tumor at the time of initial operation. For example, carcinomas of the oral cavity are treated with supraomohyoid neck dissection, and carcinomas of the oropharynx, the hypopharynx, and the larynx are treated with lateral neck dissection. If extranodal extension or the presence of multiple levels of positive nodes is confirmed by the pathological findings, the patient should receive adjuvant bilateral neck radiation for four to six weeks after operation.

Metastatic Adenocarcinomas

Adenocarcinoma in a cervical node most frequently represents a metastasis from the thyroid gland, the salivary glands, or the GI tract. The primary tumor must therefore be sought through endoscopic and radiologic study of the bronchopulmonary tract, the GI tract, the genitourinary tract, the salivary glands, and the thyroid gland. Other possible primary malignancies to be considered include breast and pelvic tumors in women and prostate cancer in men.

If the primary site is controlled and the patient is potentially curable or if the primary site is not found and the neck dis-

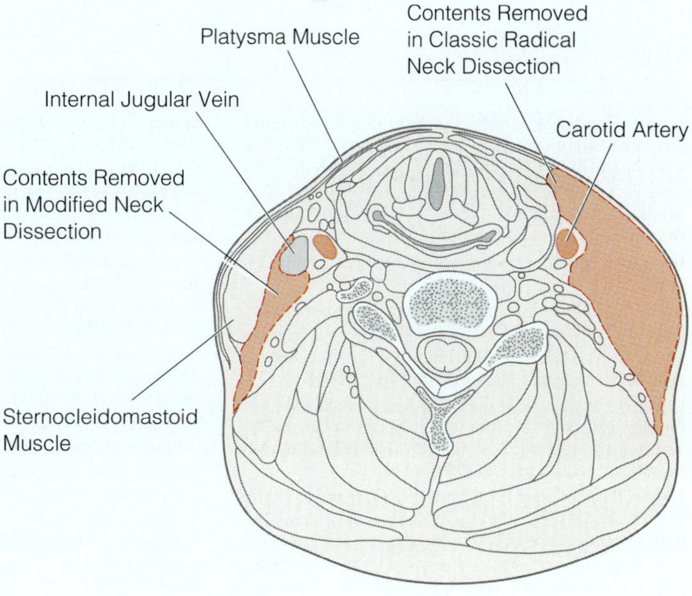

Figure 3 Cross section of the neck shows the structures removed in a classic radical neck dissection (right) and in a modified radical neck dissection (left).

ease is the only established site of malignancy, neck dissection is the appropriate treatment. Postoperative adjuvant radiation may also be considered. If the patient has thyroid cancer and palpable nodes, lateral neck dissection and ipsilateral central neck dissection are recommended.

Overall survival is low—about 20 percent at two years and nine percent at five years—except for patients with papillary or follicular thyroid cancer, who have a good prognosis. Two factors associated with a better prognosis are unilateral neck involvement and limitation of disease to lymph nodes above the cricoid cartilage.

Metastatic Melanomas

Ten to 15 percent of cutaneous malignant melanomas occur in the head and neck. These tumors commonly metastasize to lymph nodes in the parotid region and in the ipsilateral neck. If the patient has a thin melanoma (< 1.0 mm), full-thickness excision with 1 cm margins should be done. If the patient has palpable nodal metastases or a tumor of intermediate thickness (1.0 to 4.0 mm), modified neck dissection is indicated. Parotidectomy should be included if there are lesions on the upper face or the anterior scalp. The technique of sentinel lymph node biopsy with selective neck dissection has been used to identify patients with clinically negative but microscopically positive nodes and may help identify those patients with intermediate-thickness melanomas who will benefit from neck dissection.

Metastases from an Unknown Primary Malignancy

Management of patients with an unknown primary malignancy is challenging for the surgeon. It is helpful to know that when cervical lymph nodes are found to contain metastatic squamous cell carcinoma, the primary tumor is in the head and neck about 90 percent of the time. Typically, such patients are found to have squamous cell carcinoma on the basis of FNA of an abnormal cervical lymph node; this finding calls for an exhaustive review of systems as well as a detailed physical examination of the head and neck.

If no primary tumor is identified, the patient should undergo endoscopic evaluation of the nasopharynx, the hypopharynx, the esophagus, the larynx, and the tracheobronchial tree under general anesthesia. Biopsies of the nasopharynx, the tonsils, and the hypopharynx often identify the site of origin (although there is some debate on this point). If the biopsies do not reveal a primary source of cancer, the preferred treatment is unilateral neck dissection, followed by radiation therapy directed toward the neck, the entire pharynx, and the nasopharynx. In 15 to 20 percent of cases, the primary cancer is ultimately detected. Overall five-year survival in such cases ranges from 25 to 50 percent.

If a malignant melanoma is found in a cervical lymph node but no primary tumor is evident, the patient should be asked about previous skin lesions, and a thorough repeat head and neck examination should be done, with particular attention to the scalp, the nose, the oral cavities, and the sinuses. An ophthalmologic examination is also required. If physical examination and radiographic studies find no evidence of metastases, modified neck dissection should be performed on the involved side.

Metastatic adenocarcinoma in a cervical lymph node with no known primary tumor is discussed elsewhere [*see* Metastatic Adenocarcinomas, *above*]. The most common primary sites in the head and neck are the salivary glands and the thyroid gland. The possibility of an isolated metastasis from the breast, the GI tract, or the genitourinary tract must also be rigorously investigated. If no primary site is identified, the patient should be considered for protocol-based chemotherapy and radiation therapy, directed according to what the primary site is most likely to be in that patient.

Recommended Reading

Adams GL: Malignant tumors of the head and neck. Boie's Fundamentals of Otolaryngology: A Textbook of Ear, Nose and Throat Disease, 6th ed. Adams GL, Boie LR Jr, Hilger PA, Eds. WB Saunders Co, Philadelphia, 1989, p 443

Beenken SW, Maddox WA, Urist MM: Workup of a patient with a mass in the neck. Adv Surg 28:371, 1995

Byers RM: Modified neck dissection. Am J Surg 150:414, 1985

Byers RM: Neck dissection: concepts, controversies and technique. Semin Surg Oncol 7:9, 1991

Chandler JR, Mitchell B: Branchial cleft cysts, sinuses and fistulas. Otolaryngol Clin North Am 14:175, 1981

Cohen JI: Benign neck masses. Boie's Fundamentals of Otolaryngology: A Textbook of Ear, Nose and Throat Disease, 6th ed. Adams GL, Boie LR Jr, Hilger PA, Eds. WB Saunders Co, Philadelphia, 1989, p 429

Coker DD, Casterline PF, Chambers RG, et al: Metastases to lymph nodes of the head and neck from an unknown primary site. Am J Surg 134:517, 1977

Coleman JJ III, Sultan MR: Tumors of the head and neck. Principles of Surgery, 6th ed. Schwartz SI, Shires GT, Spencer FC, Eds. McGraw-Hill Book Co., New York, 1994, p 595.

Fabian RL: Benign and malignant diseases of the head and neck. Current Practice of Surgery, Vol. 2. Levine BA, Copeland EM III, Howard RJ, et al, Eds. Churchill Livingstone, New York, 1993, Ch. 1.

Gluckman JL, Waner M: Physical examination of the head and neck. Otolaryngology Volume II: Diagnosis of Disorders of the Head and Neck, 3rd ed. Paparella MM, Shumrick DA, Eds. WB Saunders Co, Philadelphia, 1991, p 1811

Hainsworth JD: Poorly differentiated carcinoma and poorly differentiated adenocarcinoma of unknown primary tumor site of the neck. Semin Oncol 20:279, 1993

Jesse RH, Perez CA, Fletcher GH: Cervical lymph node metastasis: unknown primary cause. Cancer 31:854, 1973

Lee NK, Byers RM, Abbruzzese JL, et al: Metastatic adenocarcinoma to the neck from an unknown primary source. Am J Surg 162:306, 1991

Lefebvre JL, Coche-Dequeant B, Van JT, et al: Cervical lymph nodes from an unknown primary tumor. Am J Surg 160:443, 1990

McGuirt WF: The unknown primary in metastatic head and neck cancer: a clinical approach. N C Med J 39:299, 1978

McGuirt WF: Diagnosis and management of masses in the neck, with special emphasis on metastatic disease. Oncology 4:85, 1990

Medina JE, Byers RM: Supraomohyoid neck dissection: rationale, indications, and surgical technique. Head Neck 11:111, 1989

Montgomery WW: Surgery of the neck. Surgery of the Upper Respiratory System, 2nd ed. Lea & Febiger, Philadelphia, 1989, p 83

Nadol JB: Evaluation of neck masses. Quick Reference to Ear, Nose, and Throat Disorders. Wilson WR, Nadol JB, Eds. JB Lippincott Co, Philadelphia, 1983

Shah JP, Medina JE, Shaha AR, et al: Cervical lymph node metastasis. Curr Probl Surg 30:1, 1993

Acknowledgment

Figures 1 through 3   Tom Moore.

12 ASYMPTOMATIC CAROTID BRUIT

Claudio S. Cinà, M.D., Sp.Chir. (It.), M.Sc., Catherine M. Clase, M.B., B.Chir., M.Sc., and Aleksandar Radan, M.D., B.Sc., B.F.A.

Assessment of Asymptomatic Carotid Bruit

The term bruit refers to any noise detected on auscultation in the neck. The conventional method of auscultation is to use the bell of the stethoscope and listen over an area extending from the upper end of the thyroid cartilage to just below the angle of the jaw.[1-3] The principal reason why bruits in the neck are matters of some concern is that they may reflect underlying occlusive carotid artery disease, which carries an increased risk of stroke.

In what follows, we outline a problem-oriented approach to the workup of patients found to have cervical bruits at the time of routine or focused vascular examination.

Clinical Assessment

CAROTID BRUITS VERSUS OTHER CERVICAL SOUNDS

Clinical assessment begins with evaluation of the character of the bruit and examination of the precordium and the cervical structures. Carotid bruits must be distinguished from other sounds heard in the neck. Venous hums are relatively common, being reported in 27% of young adults.[4] They tend to have a diastolic component, are louder when the patient sits or turns the head away from the side of auscultation, and disappear when the patient lies down or when the Valsalva maneuver is performed.[4] Ejection systolic murmurs of cardiac origin may radiate into the neck, but generally, they are bilateral, are louder within the chest, and are less audible distally in the neck[5]; the same is true of bruits arising in other intrathoracic vessels.[6,7] No definitive clinical sign has yet been identified that clearly differentiates bruits from transmitted cardiac murmurs. On occasion, a bruit may be heard over the thyroid gland; however, this finding is extremely rare and is usually accompanied by thyromegaly and other features of autoimmune thyroid disease.[5] In dialysis patients, a bruit may be generated by the increased flow resulting from the creation of an arteriovenous fistula in the forearm.[8]

SYMPTOMATIC VERSUS ASYMPTOMATIC CAROTID BRUITS

Transient ischemic attacks (TIAs) are defined as brief episodes of focal loss of brain function that can usually be localized to a specific portion of the brain supplied by a single vascular system.[9] By arbitrary convention, such an ischemic episode is considered a TIA if it lasts less than 24 hours; a similar episode, in the absence of evidence of trauma or hemorrhage, is considered an ischemic stroke if it lasts more than 24 hours or causes death.[9] Amaurosis fugax is a transient (< 24 hours) loss of vision in one eye or a portion of the visual field.[9] If a patient with a carotid bruit has a history of any of these conditions in the ipsilateral eye or brain, then the bruit is regarded as neurologically symptomatic, and the relevant question at that point is whether the patient has significant carotid stenosis and may be a candidate for carotid endarterectomy on that basis. Given the substantial differences between the management of patients with symptomatic bruits and those with asymptomatic bruits, the distinction between these two patient groups is crucial.

The history is of critical importance in the diagnosis of TIA because most TIAs last less than 4 hours,[10] which means that patients typically are not seen by physicians during the period of neurologic deficit.[11] Patients should be specifically asked about transient focal problems with vision, language, facial paresis, dysarthria, and arm or leg numbness or weakness. A 1984 study reported good interobserver agreement ($\kappa = 0.65$) [see Table 1] between clinicians diagnosing previous ischemic episodes.[12] Assigning a probable neurologic territory to a TIA or stroke, however, proved more difficult: for TIAs, the interobserver agreement between two independent neurologists asked to distinguish between carotid and vertebrobasilar events was relatively poor ($\kappa = 0.31$).[12] There is some evidence that using a standardized protocol for the diagnosis of previous ischemic episodes might improve this low interobserver agreement (e.g., to $\kappa = 0.65$[12] or $\kappa = 0.77$[13]). Similar difficulties attend diagnosis of stroke by means of history and physical examination.[14]

Many patients with a possible TIA or stroke will have undergone neurologic imaging. Such imaging is unhelpful if it yields negative results; however, in some cases, it reveals the presence of an infarct, thereby confirming the ischemic nature of the event and establish-

Table 1 Quantification of Interobserver Agreement*

κ†	Strength of Agreement
≤ 0.2	Poor
$> 0.2, \leq 0.4$	Fair
$> 0.4, \leq 0.6$	Moderate
$> 0.6, \leq 0.8$	Good
$> 0.8, \leq 1$	Very good

*Reliability (how closely an assessment agrees with another similar assessment on a second occasion or by a second observer) and validity (how closely the assessment agrees with another criterion or a gold standard) are the key properties of any assessment. When agreement between two observers is poor, the assessment in question, whether it is a physical finding, a clinical diagnosis, or an interpretation of a diagnostic test, is lacking in reliability; if more reliable methods are available, they should be considered instead. In clinical medicine, however, more reliable methods are not always available. When this is the case, the physician must use a relatively unreliable assessment as the best available alternative, while remaining aware of its limitations.[118]

†κ is a statistical measure used to quantify agreement between two or more observers. It takes a value between 0 and 1, where 0 represents agreement no better than that expected by chance alone and 1 represents perfect agreement.[118]

Approach to the Patient with an Asymptomatic Carotid Bruit

Noise is detected on auscultation of neck
Determine nature of cervical sound.

Sound is carotid bruit
Distinguish symptomatic bruits from asymptomatic bruits; the decision affects treatment.

Bruit is symptomatic

Bruit is asymptomatic
Perform vascular risk assessment, looking for vascular risk factors (e.g., ↑BP, ↑lipids, diabetes, smoking) and vascular disease (e.g., ischemic cardiac disease, peripheral vascular disease).
Initiate modification of vascular risk. Determine subsequent management approach.

Risk associated with CE is low (Goldman class I or II)
Assess risk of carotid stenosis.

Risk of carotid stenosis is high
Risk factors include ↑age, ↑BP, smoking, peripheral vascular disease.
Assess risk of stroke.

Risk of carotid stenosis is low

Risk of stroke is high
Risk factors include age > 70, male sex, ↑BP, ↑lipids, diabetes, smoking, ischemic cardiac disease, peripheral vascular disease.
Consult patient preferences regarding surgical treatment.

Risk of stroke is low

Patient prefers surgical management
Determine presence and degree of carotid stenosis with duplex ultrasonography and carotid angiography.

Patient prefers medical management

Severe stenosis is present
Perform prophylactic CE.

Moderate stenosis is present
Reevaluate with duplex ultrasonography every 1– 2 yr unless patient status changes.

Minimal or no stenosis is present

Sound is venous hum, radiating cardiac murmur or intrathoracic bruit, or thyroid bruit

Patient is to be assessed as candidate for carotid endarterectomy (CE)

Determine level of risk associated with procedure.

Risk associated with CE is high (Goldman class ≥ III)

Patient is to be managed conservatively

Continue modification of vascular risk.
Educate patient regarding symptoms and signs of stroke.
Carry out nonsurgical follow-up.
Re-refer patient promptly if he or she ever becomes symptomatic.

ing its location. For a bruit to be regarded as symptomatic on the basis of imaging studies, at least one infarct must be seen in the appropriate ipsilateral anterior vasculature.

It is evident that distinguishing between symptomatic and asymptomatic bruits on clinical grounds may be difficult; nonetheless, it is worthwhile to make the effort because the risk of stroke in the asymptomatic population is quite different from that in the symptomatic population. For example, whereas the Asymptomatic Carotid Atherosclerosis Study (ACAS), which included patients believed on clinical grounds to be neurologically asymptomatic, reported an overall stroke rate of 6.2% at 2.7 years in its medically managed group,[15] the North American Symptomatic Carotid Endarterectomy Trial (NASCET), which included patients assessed as neurologically symptomatic (i.e., with a history of amaurosis fugax, TIA, or minor stroke), reported a stroke rate of 26% at 3 years in its medically managed group.[16]

In determining whether a unilateral bruit is symptomatic or asymptomatic, the physician should concentrate primarily on ischemic deficits in the ipsilateral hemisphere (i.e., those causing focal contralateral motor or sensory deficits) and ipsilateral amaurosis fugax. However, symptoms referable to the contralateral carotid artery, even if no bruit is heard on that side, might prompt evaluation of the patient for symptomatic carotid stenosis on the contralateral side. The absence of a bruit by no means excludes the diagnosis: carotid bruits are absent in 20% to 35% of patients with high-grade stenosis of the internal carotid artery.[17] In the NASCET subgroup in which the physical finding of a carotid bruit was compared with angiographic imaging of the carotid system, the presence of a focal ipsilateral carotid bruit had a sensitivity of 63% and a specificity of 61% for high-grade (70% to 99%) stenosis; the absence of a bruit did not significantly change the probability of significant stenosis in this population (pretest 52%, posttest 40%).[18]

Workup of patients with symptomatic bruits is beyond the scope of this chapter. Accordingly, the ensuing discussion focuses on assessment of patients with asymptomatic bruits.

VASCULAR RISK ASSESSMENT

Vascular diseases and other vascular risk factors are common in patients with asymptomatic carotid bruits. Hypertension is twice as common in patients who have bruits as in those who do not[19]; smoking, ischemic heart disease, and peripheral vascular disease are also more prevalent.[20,21] Consequently, detection of a bruit should prompt a thorough vascular risk assessment. Standard vascular risk factors—hypertension, hyperlipidemia, diabetes, and smoking—can be integrated into risk profiles for particular patients by using either the New Zealand risk tables (http://www.nzgg.org.nz/library/gl_complete/bloodpressure/appendix.cfm) or the formula and spreadsheets provided by Anderson et al.[22,23] The probability of stroke for various follow-up periods may be quantified by using the Framingham stroke-risk profile.[24] From age, systolic blood pressure, diabetes, smoking, cardiovascular disease, atrial fibrillation, and left ventricular hypertrophy, probability of stroke may be calculated for men and women according to a point system.[24]

Smoking cessation should be recommended to all patients,[25-27] and hypertension should be controlled (BP < 140/90).[28-31] Depending on a patient's individual risk profile, dietary and pharmacologic management of hyperlipidemia may also be warranted.[32-34] Diabetic control should be optimized.[35,36]

Patients should be asked specifically about any concurrent vascular disease—in particular, symptoms suggestive of ischemic heart disease or of claudication or rest pain. In patients with established vascular disease, the risk that future vascular events (e.g., coronary-related death, myocardial infarction [MI], new angina, stroke, TIA, new congestive heart failure, or peripheral vascular syndrome) will occur in the next 5 years is greater than 20%.[22,37] In such patients, consultation of formulas or tables is unnecessary, and all modifiable risk factors should be aggressively managed (target BP < 140/90; target ratio of total cholesterol to high-density lipoprotein [HDL] cholesterol < 4).[22]

A meta-analysis of randomized, controlled trials showed that aspirin reduced the risk of subsequent stroke, MI, and death from vascular events for patients who had previously experienced a cerebrovascular event, MI, or unstable angina.[38] Other meta-analyses of randomized, controlled trials[39,40] were unable to confirm the effectiveness of aspirin in preventing cerebrovascular events in asymptomatic patients or in patients with TIAs or strokes of noncardiac (and presumably vascular) origin[41]; however, one randomized, controlled trial involving hypertensive patients at modest vascular risk found that aspirin reduced the risk of vascular events, if not the risk of stroke.[42] In the absence of contraindications, we recommend that aspirin be considered for all patients who have established vascular disease elsewhere and for all patients who have a bruit in association with any vascular risk factors.

INDICATIONS FOR SURGICAL INTERVENTION

The absolute risk of stroke is increased in the presence of a carotid bruit. In population-based studies, the annual risk of stroke was 2.1% (95% confidence interval [CI], 0.6 to 8.5)[19,20,43,44] for persons who had a carotid bruit and 0.86% (95% CI, 0.8 to 0.9) for those who did not.[19,43,44] These figures represent an absolute risk increase for stroke of 1.24% a year and a relative risk for stroke of 2.4. The mean patient age in these studies was approximately 65 years, and sex distribution and prevalence of risk factors for atherosclerotic disease were similar in patients with bruits and those without bruits. Even after adjustment for age, sex, and the presence of hypertension, the presence of a carotid bruit remained an independently significant variable, with a relative risk of 2.0.[19]

Table 2 Annual Risk of Stroke

Patient Population	Annual Risk of Stroke
Population without bruits, age > 60 yr[19,43,44]	0.86% (95% CI, 0.8–0.9)
Population with bruits, age > 60 yr[19,20,43]	2.1% (95% CI, 0.6–8.5)
Male population without bruits, age > 60 yr[19,24]	0.9% (95% CI, 0.1–3.0)
Male population with bruits, age > 60 yr[19]	8.0% (95% CI, 0.2–38.0)
Female population without bruits, age > 60 yr[24]	2.0% (95% CI, 0.8–4.2)
Female population with bruits, age > 60 yr[19]	2.4% (95% CI, 0.7–5.5)

Table 3 Prevalence of Carotid Stenosis in Patients with Bruits and in Healthy Volunteers

Patient Population	Prevalence of Carotid Stenosis
Overall population with cervical bruits	
> 35% stenosis[20,56-58,119]	58% (95% CI, 55–60)
> 60%–75% stenosis[56-58]	21% (95% CI, 18–24)
Healthy volunteers*	
Age > 70 yr[89]	5.1% (95% CI, 2.6–9.0)
Age ≤ 70 yr[89]	1.5% (95% CI, 0.2–5.3)

*In healthy volunteers, the incidence of asymptomatic carotid stenosis is significantly correlated with age ($P < 0.01$) and with the presence of hypertension ($P < 0.005$).

Table 4 Necessary Criteria for Offering an Interventional Approach to Selected Patients with Carotid Bruits

Center-specific criteria
 Either
  DUS is documented to have a > 90% PPV for stenosis > 50% on angiography and is used alone
 or
  DUS has a lower PPV and is used as a screening test only, and angiography in patients with cerebrovascular disease has a documented complication (stroke or death) rate of around 1%
Surgeon-specific criterion
 Perioperative rate of stroke or death is < 3% for carotid endarterectomy

DUS—duplex ultrasonography PPV—positive predictive value

Given the low absolute risk of stroke in asymptomatic patients with bruits [see Table 2], the low prevalence of surgically relevant stenosis in patients with bruits [see Table 3], and the small (and only marginally statistically significant) absolute benefit of carotid endarterectomy in patients with asymptomatic stenosis,[45,46] we and others[47-51] do not believe that further investigation with a view to carotid endarterectomy is mandatory in the asymptomatic population. Many surgeons may prefer to manage these patients conservatively, reevaluating them promptly if they become symptomatic [see Discussion, below]. Other surgeons may wish to pursue a more interventional strategy with selected patients, in which case further evaluation with an eye to surgical treatment depends on the presence of the following key findings in a given patient: (1) low risk associated with carotid endarterectomy, (2) relatively high risk of carotid stenosis, and (3) high risk of stroke if carotid stenosis is documented. In addition, the patient's preferences should be consulted: no patient should be subjected to further evaluation who is not prepared to undergo surgical treatment if such management is recommended. Patients who, on the basis of any of these criteria, are not suitable candidates for intervention will not benefit from imaging studies and should be managed medically.

Finally, surgeons and centers who are contemplating offering prophylactic carotid endarterectomy for asymptomatic stenosis should be able to document that their rates of stroke or perioperative death for this procedure are lower than 3% [see Table 4]. When complication rates exceed this threshold, the value of carotid endarterectomy becomes negligible, and surgeons may find themselves doing more harm than good.[45,46]

Low Risk Associated with Carotid Endarterectomy

In NASCET and ACAS, patients were excluded if they had coexisting medical disease likely to produce significant mortality and morbidity (e.g., cardiac valvular or rhythm disorders, uncontrolled hypertension or diabetes, unstable angina pectoris, or MI in the previous 4 months)[16]; accordingly, the results of these trials are not generalizable to patients who have such conditions. Further evidence for the impact of operative risk on outcomes is provided by a retrospective review of 562 patients who underwent carotid endarterectomy for symptomatic and asymptomatic disease in a large community hospital.[52] For patients in Goldman class I or II,[53] the overall rate of death or nonfatal MI was 2% (95% CI, 1.1 to 3.9), whereas for patients in class III or IV, the corresponding figure was 21% (95% CI, 9.2 to 39.9) [see Table 5]. Given that 50 prophylactic carotid endarterectomies would have to be performed to prevent one stroke over the subsequent 3-year period (i.e., the number needed to treat [NNT] is 50), it is clearly unacceptable to perform this procedure in a population facing a 21% incidence of MI or death, in which for every 5 patients undergoing the operation, one would experience an MI or die (i.e., the number needed to harm [NNH] is only 5). Further consideration of prophylactic carotid endarterectomy in patients for whom the procedure carries a high risk is not warranted.

High Risk of Carotid Stenosis

Cohort[45,54-60] and population-based[19,61,62] studies suggest that patients with asymptomatic carotid bruits are more likely to have significant carotid stenosis if they are older, are hypertensive, smoke, or have advanced peripheral vascular disease. In one study, hemodynamically significant stenosis (i.e., > 50%) was found by means of ultrasonography in 32% of patients scheduled to undergo peripheral vascular procedures but in only 6.8% of those scheduled to undergo coronary artery bypass grafting (CABG).[63] (All figures for degree of stenosis in this chapter are determined according to the formula used in NASCET [see Table 6 and Figure 1].)

Further consideration of carotid endarterectomy may be warranted in patients with vascular risk factors or known peripheral vascular disease; in the absence of these findings, the risk of significant carotid stenosis is low. Further evaluation is unnecessary for patients who are younger, do not smoke, are not hypertensive or diabetic, and are not known to have peripheral vascular disease.

High Risk of Stroke

Within the group of patients with asymptomatic carotid stenosis, there is only limited direct evidence for the existence of subgroups of patients at higher risk for stroke. Men seem to be at higher risk for stroke than women are: in the medical arm of ACAS, the incidence of stroke or death at 2.7 years was 7.0% (95% CI, 4.9 to 9.4) for men and 4.9% (95% CI, 2.7 to 8.0) for women. Gender-related differences aside, however, identification of other subgroups at higher risk relies on extrapolation of data from other populations at risk for artery-to-artery embolism. Data from NASCET indicate that for symptomatic patients with greater than 70% carotid stenosis, the presence of a higher number of identifiable clinical risk factors (age > 70 years; male sex; systolic or diastolic hypertension; the occurrence of a cerebrovascular event within the preceding 31 days; the occurrence of a more serious cerebrovascular event, namely, stroke rather than a TIA or amaurosis fugax; smoking; MI; congestive heart failure; diabetes; intermittent claudication; or hyperlipidemia) was associated with a higher annual stroke risk. For patients with zero to three risk factors, the annual stroke risk was 6.6%; for those with four or five, 9.2%; and for those with six or more, 15.8%. Data from the same study indicate that among patients with a contralateral asymptomatic stenosed carotid artery, patients with zero to three risk factors have an annual stroke risk of 1.4% in the territory of the asymptomatic stenosis; those with four or five, 2.8%; and those with six or more, 3.8%.[64]

Obesity is another risk factor for stroke.[49,50] Some 60% of patients who experience a stroke before 65 years of age have a body mass index greater than 24 kg/m².[49] This finding, in conjunction with a history of smoking, was found to predict 60% of strokes in men in this age group.[50]

Patients with carotid bruits who do not have significant systemic risk factors or other vascular disease are at low absolute risk for stroke and are unlikely to benefit from carotid endarterectomy; hence, further investigation is not warranted.[5,18,49] Patients with numerous (i.e., six or more) clinical risk factors [see Table 7] are at relatively high risk for stroke, and it is in this population that most of the benefit from carotid endarterectomy is likely to be concentrated.

Patient Preference for Surgical Intervention

Before pursuing the diagnosis of carotid stenosis with imaging techniques, the surgeon must discuss prophylactic surgical intervention with the patient. The essential question is, if significant stenosis is documented, will the patient wish to undergo carotid endarterectomy? It should be remembered that at this point in the workup, we are considering only those patients (1) for whom the cardiac risk associated with the procedure is acceptably low and (2) who are considered to be at relatively high risk for stroke if carotid stenosis is demonstrated.

Patients should be informed that if they are found to have significant carotid stenosis, their risk of stroke is 6.3% over the ensuing 2.7 years if they do not undergo operation and 4.0% over the same period if they do.[15] They should also be informed that these figures take into account a 3% risk of perioperative stroke or death (2.7% risk of stroke and 0.3% risk of death).[15] The 2.3% absolute risk reduction associated with surgical treatment translates into an NNT of 43, meaning that 43 patients would have to undergo endarterectomy to prevent one stroke over the next 2.7 years.

Given the front-loaded risks of surgery, some patients will prefer a simple risk-modification strategy to a strategy including both risk modification and surgical intervention. In such cases, carotid imaging is not necessary, because knowledge of the degree of stenosis will not affect subsequent management.

Diagnosis of Asymptomatic Carotid Stenosis

The purpose of investigation of asymptomatic neck bruits is to identify persons with significant carotid stenosis who are at increased risk for cerebrovascular disease[65,66] and who are likely to benefit from carotid endarterectomy. In the absence of other significant findings, cervical bruits are not sufficiently predictive of significant carotid stenosis or ischemic stroke to be useful in selecting candidates for noninvasive imaging.[51] Noninvasive testing is a reasonable step in patients with the characteristics listed above, but routine screening of all patients with asymptomatic carotid bruits is not warranted.[51]

DUPLEX ULTRASONOGRAPHY

Duplex ultrasonography (DUS) should be performed bilaterally. A meta-analysis conducted in 1995 found that for detecting greater

Table 5 Cardiac Risk Assessment*

Parameter	Weighted Score on Cardiac Risk Index		
	Goldman	Detsky	Eagle
Age > 70 yr	5	5	1
MI			1
< 6 mo	10	10	
> 6 mo		5	
Angina			1
Class III		10	
Class IV		20	
Unstable		10	
Diabetes			1
Operation			
Emergency	4	10	
Aortic, abdominal, or thoracic	3		
CHF	11		1
< 1 wk		10	
> 1 wk		5	
ECG			
Rhythm other than sinus	7	5	
> 5 PVCs/min	7	5	
Poor medical status†	3	5	

Risk of Perioperative Cardiac Events

Low	0–12 (class I, II)	0–15	0
Intermediate	13–25 (class III)	16–30	1–2
High	> 25 (class IV)	> 30	≥ 3

*The Goldman cardiac risk index[53] is a multifactorial index of cardiac risk in patients undergoing noncardiac surgery. Modifications have been proposed by Detsky,[121-123] who included angina and institution-specific perioperative cardiac event rates in the model. The Eagle index[124-126] is another risk index based on five clinical variables. Despite the lack of consensus regarding the relative merits of these tools for preoperative cardiac risk assessment, stratification of patients into risk categories is helpful in assessing the risk and benefits of a procedure such as carotid endarterectomy.
†P_{aO_2} < 60 mm Hg; P_{aCO_2} > 50 mm Hg; K^+ < 3 mmol/L; serum HCO_3 < 20 mmol/L; serum urea > 18 mmol/L; creatinine > 260 μmol/L; abnormal ALT; signs of chronic liver disease; bedridden from cardiac causes.
CHF—congestive heart failure   MI—myocardial infarction   PVC—premature ventricular contraction

than 50% stenosis (determined by means of angiography, the gold standard), DUS had a sensitivity of 91% (95% CI, 89 to 94) and a specificity of 93% (95% CI, 88 to 95).[67] Given a disease prevalence of approximately 41% in patients referred for DUS, these findings translate into a positive predictive value of 90% and an accuracy of 92%.[67] A subsequent prospective study of patients (both symptomatic and asymptomatic) in whom carotid endarterectomy was being considered reported a sensitivity of 100% and a specificity of 98% for greater than 60% stenosis, with a positive predictive value of 99%.[68]

At centers where DUS has been internally validated in comparison with angiography and where this level of performance has been documented, the surgeons may choose to proceed to surgery without angiography.[68-70] At centers where DUS is less reliable, however, it should be regarded as a screening test, and angiography should be performed when DUS suggests greater than 50% stenosis.

CAROTID ANGIOGRAPHY

As an invasive procedure, carotid angiography carries a significant risk of morbidity and mortality. All centers performing carotid angiography for cerebrovascular disease should audit their stroke rates

Table 6 Conversion between Different Methods of Measuring Degree of Carotid Stenosis

Method	Severity of Disease				
	Minimal	Moderate		Severe	Occlusion
ECST*	24%–57%	58%–69%	70%–81%	82%–99%	100%
NASCET	0%–29%	30%–49%	50%–69%	70%–99%	100%
CC method†	35%–56%	57%–61%	62%–80%	81%–99%	100%

*Conversion from ECST to NASCET was done according to the following formula: ECST % stenosis = 0.6(NASCET % stenosis) + 40.[127]
†The relation of the NASCET method to the CC method is linear, with a ratio of 0.62 between the distal internal carotid diameter and the common carotid diameter.[117]

periodically. Since 1990, four prospective studies[71-74] have addressed the question of the risks associated with angiography in patients with atherosclerotic cerebrovascular disease. When the data from these studies were pooled, the risk of permanent neurologic deficit or death was 1.1% (95% CI, 0.6 to 2.0).[75] In ACAS, the 1.2% of patients in the intervention arm who experienced stroke or died after angiography accounted for 40% of the strokes and deaths attributable to surgical intervention.[15] Angiographic complication rates significantly worse than these will adversely impact the risk-benefit ratio associated with surgical intervention. Centers that consistently record relatively high angiographic complication rates should not offer evaluation for and surgical treatment of asymptomatic carotid disease.

Carotid Endarterectomy

At this point in management, it is reasonable to offer surgical treatment of asymptomatic disease to patients with greater than 50% stenosis. ACAS[15] and two meta-analyses[45,46] that included other trials of surgical therapy for asymptomatic carotid stenosis documented a small and marginally statistically significant benefit from prophylactic carotid endarterectomy in asymptomatic patients with greater than 50% to 60% carotid stenosis. Because the absolute benefit is small, we do not consider it obligatory to pursue the diagnosis or to follow an invasive strategy in patients identified solely on the basis of an asymptomatic bruit; however, patients possessing all the characteristics listed earlier [see Indications for Surgical Intervention, *above*] probably constitute a group that is particularly able to benefit from surgical intervention. Patients with higher degrees of stenosis are at higher risk for stroke and are therefore most likely to benefit.[76-79]

The degree of stenosis and the presence or absence of plaque ulceration may modify the final decision for or against operative management [see Discussion, Subgroup Analyses for Potential High-Risk Factors, *below*].

Technical details of carotid endarterectomy are discussed elsewhere [see 63 *Carotid Arterial Procedures*].

Patient Education

All patients with asymptomatic carotid bruits, whether they are undergoing prophylactic endarterectomy or not, should be carefully advised regarding the symptoms and signs of stroke, TIAs, and amaurosis fugax and should be strongly encouraged to seek urgent medical attention if such problems arise. Patients who experience one of these untoward events should undergo full reevaluation for stroke risk factors (e.g., hypertension, hyperlipidemia, diabetes, smoking, and atrial fibrillation); in the absence of atrial fibrillation (which should prompt consideration of prophylactic anticoagulation[80-82]), a change in antiplatelet therapy should be considered. Both ticlopidine[83] and clopidogrel[84,85] are more effective than aspirin in preventing stroke. (Ticlopidine is associated with reversible but severe neutropenia in fewer than 1% of cases; accordingly, monitoring for this complication is indicated.)

If a patient who is a surgical candidate experiences a TIA or stroke as a result of an ischemic event in the carotid region in the absence of atrial fibrillation, he or she must be promptly referred back to the vascular surgeon. This possibility should be clearly explained to patients once the initial evaluation is complete and they have been referred back to their primary care physicians. Patients referred back to a vascular surgeon under these circumstances should then be regarded as having symptomatic carotid disease. A subgroup analysis of patients with symptomatic stenosis reported that carotid endarterectomy performed soon after a nondisabling stroke was not associated with a significantly higher operative complication rate than endarterectomy performed 30 days or longer after a stroke.[75,86] Performing endarterectomy early reduces the risk period for recurrent stroke and may therefore increase the potential benefit of the intervention; the usual approach is to perform the procedure within a week or two of a patient's first neurologic event.[86]

Management of cardiovascular risk factors and concurrent vascular disease should continue. In the absence of concurrent vascular disease, patients may be referred back to the family practitioner, internist, or cardiologist in place of specific surgical follow-up.

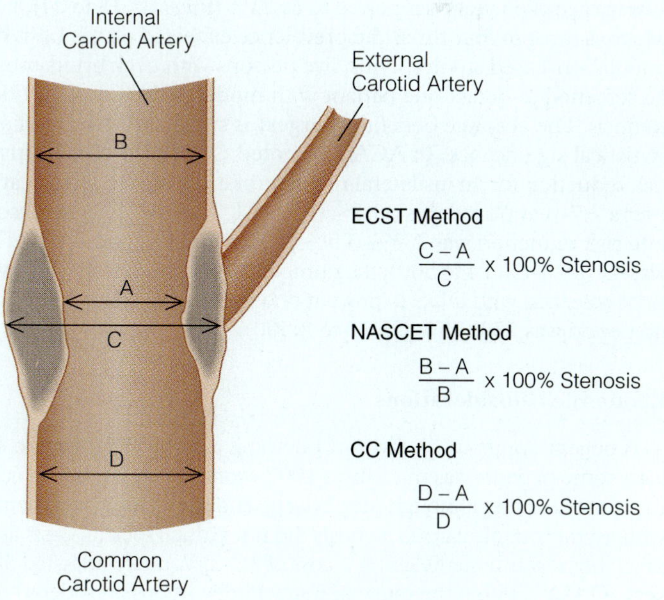

ECST Method

$$\frac{C - A}{C} \times 100\% \text{ Stenosis}$$

NASCET Method

$$\frac{B - A}{B} \times 100\% \text{ Stenosis}$$

CC Method

$$\frac{D - A}{D} \times 100\% \text{ Stenosis}$$

Figure 1 Carotid angiography remains the gold standard for determining the extent of carotid arterial disease. Several methods of reporting angiographically defined stenosis have been described in the literature.[115] The most commonly used methods are those adopted by the NASCET and ECST investigators, though the so-called common carotid (CC) method has its advocates as well.[116,117]

Table 7	Risk Factors for Stroke[128,129]
Age > 70 yr	Smoking (or history of smoking)
Male sex	> 80% carotid stenosis
Hypertension*	Presence of ulceration
Hyperlipidemia	Ischemic heart disease†
Diabetes	Peripheral vascular disease

*Defined as systolic BP > 160 mm Hg or diastolic BP > 90 mm Hg.
†MI or CHF.

Follow-up of Patients with Lower-Grade Stenosis

Carotid stenosis progresses in about one quarter of patients with asymptomatic carotid stenosis monitored with DUS over a 2-year period.[87] In a population of asymptomatic patients with bruits who were referred to a vascular laboratory, 282 stenotic carotid arteries (average stenosis, 50%) were followed for 38 ± 18 months. Progression of stenosis, defined as an increase in degree of stenosis to 80% or beyond, occurred in 17% of arteries, and 2% became completely occluded. Progression was associated with an increase in stroke risk of 4.9% at 1 year, 16.7% at 3 years, and 26.5% at 5 years. In comparison, the estimated stroke risk in an asymptomatic population of patients with 50% to 79% stenosis was 0.85%, 3.6%, and 5.4% for the same three periods ($P = 0.001$).[76]

Although carotid stenosis, once identified, tends to progress over time,[20,54,76,88] the data are currently insufficient to permit recommendation of routine ultrasonographic or other surveillance for all patients with neck bruits outside a research setting. In our view, reevaluation every 1 to 2 years with noninvasive diagnostic tests is a reasonable approach to patients (1) who are already known to have greater than 50% stenosis, (2) who do not undergo surgery, and (3) who are at high risk for stroke, are surgical candidates, and are not averse to surgery.

Discussion

Epidemiology

In cross-sectional and population-based studies, the overall prevalence of greater than 75% carotid stenosis has been low. A 1992 study reported a 2.3% prevalence in men and a 1.1% prevalence in women; there was a significant ($P < 0.0001$) increase with age with each decade from 65 years to beyond 85 years, but there were no significant differences between men and women.[62] In the Framingham study population, the incidence of greater than 50% stenosis was 8% (95% CI, 6.5 to 9.8).[61] In a study of healthy volunteers, the incidence of greater than 50% stenosis was 5.1% (95% CI, 2.6 to 9.0) in patients 70 years of age or older and 1.5% (95% CI, 0.2 to 5.3) in younger patients.[89]

The pooled risk of greater than 60% to 75% stenosis in patients with carotid bruits referred for noninvasive vascular evaluation at an average age of 65 years is reported to be 21% (95% CI, 18 to 24),[56-58] which is three to four times the prevalence expected on the basis of population-based studies. Thus, five persons with neck bruits must be screened to detect one patient with moderate to severe carotid stenosis. The absolute benefit of surgery is small and of borderline statistical significance. In ACAS, as noted (see above), the relative risk reduction for an ipsilateral major stroke or perioperative death over a 2.7-year period was 36.5% (95% CI, 27.5 to 47.1), the absolute risk reduction was 2.3% (95% CI, 0.2 to 7.0), and the NNT was 43 (95% CI, 14 to 500); the number of patients that would have to be screened with DUS to prevent one stroke over a 3-year follow-up period was 250 (95% CI, 70 to 2,500).

Economic Considerations

A cogent argument in favor of pursuing a surgical strategy in at least some patients was made by a 1997 economic analysis,[90] which demonstrated that although prophylactic endarterectomy in patients with asymptomatic carotid stenosis did not reduce societal costs appreciably, it was nonetheless, at a cost of $8,000/quality-adjusted life year (QALY), within the range of many interventions considered by society to be cost-effective. It should be pointed out, however, that this economic analysis addressed only carotid endarterectomy in patients with identified carotid stenosis, not screening strategies for patients with bruits, and consequently did not consider costs associated with investigation and follow-up to the point of recommendation for or against carotid endarterectomy in the broader group of patients with bruits. These costs would alter the economic analysis substantially, and if they are included, it is far from clear whether the resulting overall cost/QALY would still be acceptable. To date, no trial or economic analysis of a screening strategy has been published.

Screening Issues

For the reasons previously discussed, we do not feel justified in recommending routine screening for patients with asymptomatic carotid bruits. Given the available evidence, we believe that such patients may reasonably be managed in either of two ways. One choice is simply to conclude that screening patients with carotid bruits as possible candidates for carotid endarterectomy has not been proved to be a useful intervention and to concentrate instead on general vascular risk reduction. The other, which is appropriate in centers where noninvasive or invasive diagnostic tests reach acceptable standards with an acceptable degree of risk and where the procedure is done by surgeons whose documented perioperative stroke and death rates are less than 3%, is to take a selective approach that addresses various issues related to stroke risk, cardiac risk, and patient preferences before noninvasive tests are ordered.

Subgroup Analyses for Potential High-Risk Factors

Given the small absolute risk reduction reported by ACAS[15] and by the two meta-analyses of all asymptomatic carotid stenosis trials,[45,46] it would be useful to be able to identify one or more high-risk groups within the broader group of patients identified as having stenosis.

SEX

ACAS included a subgroup analysis addressing the effect of sex on ability to benefit from surgery: the absolute reduction in the risk of perioperative stroke or death or ipsilateral stroke at 2.7 years was 3.6% (95% CI, 1.1 to 9.9) for men and 0.5% (95% CI, 0.01 to 2.7) for women.

DEGREE OF STENOSIS

In asymptomatic patients stratified according to their ultrasonographically determined degree of stenosis, the risk of stroke is low both for patients with less than 30% stenosis (4% cumulative event rate at 3 years) and for those with 30% to 74% stenosis (9% cumulative event rate at 3 years); it is highest for those with greater than 75% stenosis (21% cumulative event rate at 3 years).[20] The European Carotid Surgery Trialists (ECST) study,[47] using angiographic data from the asymptomatic carotid arteries of 2,295 patients, reported that the Kaplan-Meyer estimate of stroke risk at 3 years was only 2% and remained low (< 2%) when patients with less than 79% stenosis were considered; stroke risk increased to 9.8% for patients with 70% to 79% stenosis and to 14.4% for those with 80% to 99% stenosis. In a population of patients referred to a vascular laboratory with asymptomatic carotid stenosis on DUS who were followed for a mean of 38 months, the incidence of stroke was 2.1% in patients with 50% to 79% stenosis and 10.4% in those with greater than 80% stenosis.[76]

In ACAS, there were too few strokes to permit subgroup analysis of the effect of degree of stenosis on ability to benefit from carotid endarterectomy. In both ECST[79] and NASCET,[75,77,78,91] however, higher degrees of stenosis in symptomatic patients were consistently observed to be associated with higher stroke risk as well as with greater ability to benefit from surgical treatment [see Table 8].

PLAQUE ULCERATION AND PLAQUE STRUCTURE

At present, there are no subgroup analyses examining the effect of plaque ulceration on the ability of asymptomatic patients to benefit from surgical treatment. In NASCET, however, when symptomatic patients with 70% to 99% stenosis were considered, those with angiographic evidence of plaque ulceration were at higher risk for stroke than those without ulceration[92] and derived greater benefit from surgery.[75] Angiography had a sensitivity of 46% and a specificity of 74% in the detection of ulcerated plaques, with a positive predictive value of 72%.[93] A 1994 study reported that when ulceration was detected with B-mode imaging in patients with asymptomatic carotid stenosis, the incidence of silent cerebral infarction detected by magnetic resonance imaging was 75%, compared with an incidence of 25% when ulceration was absent.[94]

It has also been suggested that carotid plaques of differing structures may have differing embolic potentials.[95] DUS can distinguish between fibrous plaques (which are highly echogenic) and plaques with high concentrations of lipid and necrotic material (which are echolucent). Echolucent plaques are more frequently associated with neurologic symptoms and computed tomography–proven cerebral infarction.[95-97] Interobserver reliability for plaque echostructure, however, seems to be highly variable, ranging from good ($\kappa = 0.79$) for greater than 70% stenosis[95] to average ($\kappa = 0.51$) for greater than 40% stenosis[98] to poor ($\kappa = 0.29$) for greater than 80% stenosis.[99] A 1994 report found no correlation between the presence or type of symptoms and plaque structure as determined by DUS.[100] The true importance of carotid plaque echomorphology and surface characteristics as predictors of cerebrovascular events remains to be defined.

CONTRALATERAL DISEASE

It has been suggested that the presence of contralateral carotid disease is a risk factor for future cerebrovascular events. In NASCET patients with greater than 70% stenosis,[101] contralateral occlusion significantly increased the benefit of surgery with respect to the incidence of stroke or death, but contralateral high-grade stenosis did not.[75]

ASYMPTOMATIC CEREBRAL INFARCTION

The presence of areas of asymptomatic cerebral infarction ipsilateral to the area of carotid stenosis on head CT may identify patients who would benefit from surgery.[102] In asymptomatic patients with carotid stenosis, the incidence of silent strokes demonstrated by CT has been reported to be 10% in patients with 35% to 50% stenosis on DUS, 17% in those with 50% to 75% stenosis, and 30% in those with greater than 75% stenosis.[103] The incidence of silent cerebral infarctions demonstrated by MRI in the same type of population has been reported to be 42%, increasing to 75% for greater than 50% stenosis.[94] Use of CT and MRI of the brain in risk stratification of patients with asymptomatic carotid stenosis is controversial and currently is not advised.

CONCLUSIONS

Although only limited data on patients with asymptomatic stenosis are available, we believe that consideration of sex, degree of stenosis, and possibly the presence of plaque ulceration may be helpful in making the final decision on whether to offer carotid endarterectomy to these patients; at present, plaque morphology is insufficiently reliable to be a useful guide to clinical management.

Special Situations

RESTENOSIS OR PREVIOUS CAROTID SURGERY

Patients who have previously undergone carotid surgery have been excluded from most studies of asymptomatic patients; when they have been included in trials addressing symptomatic stenosis, they have experienced increased rates of perioperative complications.[16,50] Patients in whom restenosis occurs after an earlier carotid endarterectomy should be advised against surgery while they remain asymptomatic.[15] It is therefore unnecessary to follow patients with ultrasonography after carotid endarterectomy if no symptoms develop.

PREOPERATIVE ASSESSMENT FOR CORONARY ARTERY BYPASS GRAFTING

Some 20% to 30% of patients undergoing assessment for CABG are found to have carotid bruits,[49,104] and 5% to 20% have greater than 50% stenosis on DUS[105-107] or ocular plethysmography.[108] In asymptomatic patients with carotid stenosis who are undergoing CABG, there is no direct evidence favoring prophylactic carotid endarterectomy either before or in conjunction with CABG. Cohort studies including symptomatic and asymptomatic carotid ste-

Table 8 Effectiveness of Surgery by Degree of Stenosis in Patients with Symptomatic Carotid Stenosis[75]

Degree of Stenosis	Relative Risk Reduction or Increase	Absolute Risk Reduction or Increase	Number Needed to Treat or Harm
70%–99%	RRR, 48% (95% CI, 27–63)	ARR, 6.7% (95% CI, 3.2–10)	NNT, 15 (95% CI, 10–31)
50%–69%	RRR, 27% (95% CI, 5–44)	ARR, 4.7% (95% CI, 0.8–8.7)	NNT, 21 (95% CI, 11–125)
≤ 49%	RRI, 20% (95% CI, 0–44)	ARI, 2.2% (95% CI, 0–4.4)	NNH, 45 (95% CI, 22–∞)

ARI—absolute risk increase   ARR—absolute risk reduction   NNH—number needed to harm   NNT—number needed to treat
RRI—relative risk increase   RRR—relative risk reduction

nosis indicate that patients undergoing CABG and carotid endarterectomy in the same operation have a stroke rate of 6% (95% CI, 4.6 to 7.8), an MI rate of 4.6% (95% CI, 3.1 to 6.5), and a mortality of 4.7% (95% CI, 3.4 to 6.4).[109] For cohorts in which carotid endarterectomy was performed before CABG, the stroke rate is 3.2% (95% CI, 2.1 to 4.5), the MI rate is 5.2% (95% CI, 3.6 to 6.9)—a nonsignificant increase—and the mortality is 4.7% (95% CI, 3.4 to 6.4).[109] For cohorts in which CABG was done first and carotid stenosis was treated on its own after the cardiac procedure, the stroke rate is 3.5% (95% CI, 1.0 to 9.0), the MI rate is 2% (95% CI, 0.2 to 6.0), and the mortality is 0.8% (95% CI, 0.02 to 4.8).[110-112]

We recommend against a combined surgical approach in patients with asymptomatic carotid stenosis. Given the equivalent stroke rate and the lower MI rate and mortality, we believe that the preferred strategy in patients with bruits is first to proceed with CABG if indicated and then to determine whether the patient should be further evaluated as a candidate for carotid endarterectomy in the same manner as other elective patients would be.

Effect of Center-Specific Variations on Risk-to-Benefit Ratio

In ACAS, 1.2% of the overall 2.7% perioperative stroke rate was accounted for by strokes occurring after angiography. Centers where ultrasonography has been documented to have high predictive values may avoid this risk by proceeding directly from ultrasonography to surgery. If these complications had been avoided in ACAS, the absolute risk reduction would have been more substantial: 3.43% (95% CI, 1.1 to 9.9), corresponding to an NNT of 29 (95% CI, 1 to 80). The true perioperative combined stroke and death rate achieved in this study was 1.5%, a result that is definitive of excellence in the surgical management of carotid endarterectomy and that constitutes a useful quality assurance measure for centers and individual surgeons.

Issues for the Future

It is possible, perhaps likely, that in the future, magnetic resonance angiography[67] and three-dimensional CT angiography,[113,114] together with DUS, will replace angiography as preferred imaging methods for diagnosing internal carotid artery stenosis. As for surgical treatment and screening, further data on patients with asymptomatic carotid stenosis are necessary before definitive recommendations can be made. The Asymptomatic Carotid Surgery Trial (ACST), a large study currently under way in Europe, will be completed in the next few years; it is to be hoped that this trial will provide these additional data.

References

1. Chambers BR, Norris JW: Clinical significance of asymptomatic neck bruits. Neurology 35:742, 1985
2. Harrison MJ: Cervical bruits and asymptomatic carotid stenosis. Br J Hosp Med 32:80, 1984
3. Ratcheson RA: Clinical diagnosis of atherosclerotic carotid artery disease. Clin Neurosurg 29:464, 1982
4. Jones FL: Frequency, characteristics and importance of the cervical venous hum in adults. N Engl J Med 267:658, 1962
5. Sauve JS, Laupacis A, Ostbye T, et al: Does this patient have a clinically important carotid bruit? JAMA 270:2843, 1993
6. Caplan LR: Carotid artery disease. N Engl J Med 315:886, 1986
7. Thompson JE, Patman RD, Talkington CM: Asymptomatic carotid bruit: long term outcome of patients having endarterectomy compared with unoperated controls. Ann Surg 188:308, 1978
8. Messert B, Marra TR, Zerofsky RA: Supraclavicular and carotid bruits in hemodialysis patients. Ann Neurol 2:535, 1977
9. National Institute of Neurological Disorders and Stroke: Special Report from the National Institute of Neurological Disorders and Stroke. Classification of Cerebrovascular Diseases III. Stroke 21:637, 1990
10. Werdelin L, Juhler M: The course of transient ischemic attacks. Neurology 38:677, 1988
11. Albers GW, Hart RG, Lutsep HL, et al: AHA Scientific Statement. Supplement to the guidelines for the management of transient ischemic attacks: a statement from the Ad Hoc Committee on Guidelines for the Management of Transient Ischemic Attacks, Stroke Council, American Heart Association. Stroke 30:2502, 1999
12. Kraaijeveld CL, van Gijn J, Schouten HJ, et al: Interobserver agreement for the diagnosis of transient ischemic attacks. Stroke 15:723, 1984
13. Koudstaal PJ, van Gijn J, Staal A, et al: Diagnosis of transient ischemic attacks: improvement of interobserver agreement by a check-list in ordinary language. Stroke 17:723, 1986
14. von Arbin M, Britton M, de Faire U, et al: Validation of admission criteria to a stroke unit. J Chronic Dis 33:215, 1980
15. Toole JF, Baker WH, Castaldo JE, et al: Endarterectomy for asymptomatic carotid artery stenosis. JAMA 273:1421, 1995
16. North American Symptomatic Carotid Endarterectomy Trial Collaborators (NASCET): Beneficial effect of carotid endarterectomy in symptomatic patients with high-grade carotid stenosis. N Engl J Med 325:445, 1991
17. Davies KN, Humphrey PRD: Do carotid bruits predict disease of the internal carotid arteries? Postgrad Med J 70:433, 1994
18. Sauve JS, Thorpe KE, Sackett DL, et al: Can bruits distinguish high-grade from moderate symptomatic carotid stenosis? The North American Symptomatic Carotid Endarterectomy Trial. Ann Intern Med 120:633, 1994
19. Heyman A, Wilkinson WE, Heyden S, et al: Risk of stroke in asymptomatic persons with cervical arterial bruits: a population study in Evans County, Georgia. N Engl J Med 302:838, 1980
20. Chambers BR, Norris JW: Outcome in patients with asymptomatic neck bruits. N Engl J Med 315:860, 1986
21. Meissner I, Wiebers DO, Whisnant JP, et al: The natural history of asymptomatic carotid artery occlusive lesions. JAMA 258:2704, 1987
22. Anderson KM, Odell PM, Wilson PW, et al: Cardiovascular disease risk profiles. Am Heart J 121(1 pt 2):293, 1991
23. Anderson KM, Wilson PW, Odell PM, et al: An updated coronary risk profile: a statement for health professionals. Circulation 83:356, 1991
24. Wolf PA, D'Agostino RB, Belanger AJ, et al: Probability of stroke: a risk profile from the Framingham Study. Stroke 22:312, 1991
25. Wolf PA, D'Agostino RB, Kannel WB, et al: Cigarette smoking as a risk factor for stroke. The Framingham Study. JAMA 259:1025, 1988
26. Wannamethee SG, Shaper AG, Whincup PH, et al: Smoking cessation and the risk of stroke in middle-aged men. JAMA 274:155, 1995
27. Shinton R, Beevers G: Meta-analysis of relation between cigarette smoking and stroke. BMJ 298:789, 1989
28. Prevention of stroke by antihypertensive drug treatment in older persons with isolated systolic hypertension: final results of the Systolic Hypertension in the Elderly Program (SHEP). SHEP Cooperative Research Group. JAMA 265:3255, 1991
29. Sutton-Tyrrell K, Alcorn HG, Herzog H, et al: Morbidity, mortality, and antihypertensive treatment effects by extent of atherosclerosis in older adults with isolated systolic hypertension. Stroke 26:1319, 1995
30. Sutton-Tyrrell K, Wolfson SK Jr, Kuller LH: Blood pressure treatment slows the progression of carotid stenosis in patients with isolated systolic hypertension. Stroke 25:44, 1994
31. Collins R, Peto R, MacMahon S, et al: Blood pressure, stroke, and coronary heart disease. Part 2, Short-term reductions in blood pressure: overview of randomised drug trials in their epidemiological context. Lancet 335:827, 1990
32. Randomised trial of cholesterol lowering in 4444 patients with coronary heart disease: the Scandinavian Simvastatin Survival Study (4S). Lancet 344:1383, 1994
33. Furberg CD: Lipid-lowering trials: results and limitations. Am Heart J 128(6 pt 2):1304, 1994
34. Furberg CD, Adams HP Jr, Applegate WB, et al: Effect of lovastatin on early carotid atherosclerosis and cardiovascular events. Asymptomatic Carotid Artery Progression Study (ACAPS) Research Group. Circulation 90:1679, 1994
35. The effect of intensive treatment of diabetes on the development and progression of long-term complications in insulin-dependent diabetes mellitus. The Diabetes Control and Complications Trial Research Group. N Engl J Med 329:977, 1993
36. Intensive blood-glucose control with sulphonyl-ureas or insulin compared with conventional treatment and risk of complications in patients with type 2 diabetes (UKPDS 33). UK Prospective Diabetes Study (UKPDS) Group [published erratum appears in Lancet 354:602, 1999]. Lancet 352:837, 1998

37. Anderson KM, Wilson PW, Odell PM, et al: An updated coronary risk profile: a statement for health professionals. Circulation 83:356, 1991
38. Collaborative overview of randomised trials of antiplatelet therapy—I. Prevention of death, myocardial infarction, and stroke by prolonged antiplatelet therapy in various categories of patients. Antiplatelet Trialists' Collaboration [published erratum appears in BMJ 308:1540, 1994]. BMJ 308:81, 1994
39. Hart RG, Halperin JL, McBride R, et al: Aspirin for the primary prevention of stroke and other major vascular events: meta-analysis and hypotheses. Arch Neurol 57:326, 2000
40. Kronmal RA, Hart RG, Manolio TA, et al: Aspirin use and incident stroke in the cardiovascular health study. CHS Collaborative Research Group. Stroke 29:887, 1998
41. Barnett HJM, Eliasziw M, Meldrum HE: Drugs and surgery in the prevention of ischemic stroke. N Engl J Med 332:238, 1995
42. Hansson L, Zanchetti A, Carruthers SG, et al: Effects of intensive blood-pressure lowering and low-dose aspirin in patients with hypertension: principal results of the Hypertension Optimal Treatment (HOT) randomised trial. HOT Study Group. Lancet 351:1755, 1988
43. Wiebers DO, Whisnant JP, Sandok BA, et al: Prospective comparison of a cohort with asymptomatic carotid bruit and a population-based cohort without carotid bruit. Stroke 21:984, 1990
44. Shorr RI, Johnson KC, Wan JY, et al: The prognostic significance of asymptomatic carotid bruits in the elderly. J Gen Intern Med 13:86, 1998
45. Benavente OR, Moher D, Pham B: Carotid endarterectomy for asymptomatic carotid stenosis: a meta-analysis. BMJ 317:1477, 1998
46. Chambers BR, You RX, Donnan GA: Carotid endarterectomy for asymptomatic carotid stenosis. Cochrane Database Syst Rev (2):CD001923, 2000
47. European Carotid Surgery Trialists' Collaborative Group: Risk of stroke in the distribution of an asymptomatic carotid artery. Lancet 345:209, 1995
48. Gorelick PB: Carotid endarterectomy: where do we draw the line? (editorial) Stroke 30:1745, 1999
49. Gorelick PB, Sacco RL, Smith DB, et al: Prevention of a first stroke: a review of guidelines and a multidisciplinary consensus statement from the National Stroke Association. JAMA 281:1112, 1999
50. Feinberg RW: Primary and secondary stroke prevention. Curr Opin Neurol 9:46, 1996
51. Lee TT, Solomon NA, Heidenreich PA, et al: Cost-effectiveness of screening for carotid stenosis in asymptomatic persons. Ann Intern Med 126:337, 1997
52. Musser DJ, Nicholas GG, Reed JF III: Death and adverse cardiac events after carotid endarterectomy. J Vasc Surg 19:615, 1994
53. Goldman L, Caldera DL, Nussbaum SR, et al: Multifactorial index of cardiac risk in noncardiac surgical procedures. N Engl J Med 297:845, 1977
54. Roederer GO, Langlois YE, Jager KA, et al: The natural history of carotid arterial disease in asymptomatic patients with cervical bruits. Stroke 15:605, 1984
55. Fowl RJ, Marsh JG, Love M, et al: Prevalence of hemodynamically significant stenosis of the carotid artery in an asymptomatic veteran population. Surg Gynecol Obstet 172:13, 1991
56. Zhu CZ, Norris JW: Role of carotid stenosis in ischemic stroke. Stroke 21:1131, 1990
57. AbuRahma AF, Robinson PA: Prospective clinicopathophysiologic follow-up study of asymptomatic neck bruit. Am Surg 56:108, 1990
58. Lusiani L, Visonà A, Castellani V, et al: Prevalence of atherosclerotic lesions at the carotid bifurcation in patients with asymptomatic bruits: an echo-Doppler (duplex) study. Angiology 36:235, 1985
59. Kartchner MM, McRae LP: Noninvasive evaluation and management of the "asymptomatic" carotid bruit. Surgery 82:840, 1977
60. Clagett GP, Youkey JR, Brigham RA, et al: Asymptomatic cervical bruit and abnormal ocular pneumoplethysmography: a prospective study comparing two approaches to management. Surgery 96:823, 1984
61. Wilson PWF, Hoeg JM, D'Agostino RB, et al: Cumulative effects of high cholesterol levels, high blood pressure, and cigarette smoking on carotid stenosis. N Engl J Med 337:516, 1997
62. O'Leary DH, Polak JF, Kronmal RA, et al: Distribution and correlates of sonographically detected carotid artery disease in the Cardiovascular Health Study. The CHS Collaborative Research Group. Stroke 23:1752, 1992
63. Hennerici M, Aulich A, Sandmann W, et al: Incidence of asymptomatic extracranial arterial disease. Stroke 12:750, 1981
64. Barnett HJ, Eliasziw M, Meldrum HE, et al: Do the facts and figures warrant a 10-fold increase in the performance of carotid endarterectomy on asymptomatic patients? Neurology 46:603, 1996
65. Warlow C: Endarterectomy for asymptomatic carotid stenosis? Lancet 345:1254, 1995
66. Amarenco P, Cohen A, Tzourio C, et al: Atherosclerotic disease of the aortic arch and the risk of ischemic stroke. N Engl J Med 331:1474, 1994
67. Blakeley DD, Oddone EZ, Hasselblad V, et al: Noninvasive carotid artery testing: a meta-analytic review. Ann Intern Med 122:360, 1997
68. Ballotta E, DaGiau G, Abbruzzese E, et al: Carotid endarterectomy without angiography: can clinical evaluation and duplex ultrasonographic scanning alone replace traditional arteriography for carotid surgery workup? A prospective study. Surgery 126:20, 1999
69. Wolf RK, Williams EL II, Kistler PC: Transbrachial balloon catheter tamponade of ruptured abdominal aortic aneurysms without fluoroscopic control. Surg Gynecol Obstet 164:463, 1987
70. Baird RN: Should carotid endarterectomy be purchased? treatment avoids much morbidity. BMJ 310:316, 1995
71. Hankey GJ, Warlow CP, Molyneux AJ: Complications of cerebral angiography for patients with mild carotid territory ischaemia being considered for carotid endarterectomy. J Neurol Neurosurg Psychiatry 53:542, 1990
72. Heiserman JE, Dean BL, Hodak JA, et al: Neurologic complications of cerebral angiography. AJNR Am J Neuroradiol 15:1401, 1994
73. Davies KN, Humphrey PR: Complications of cerebral angiography in patients with symptomatic carotid territory ischaemia screened by carotid ultrasound. J Neurol Neurosurg Psychiatry 56:967, 1993
74. Grzyska J, Freitag Z, Zeumer H: Selective cerebral intraarterial DSA. Complication rate and control of risk factors. Neuroradiology 32:296, 1990
75. Cinà CS, Clase CM, Haynes RB: Refining indications for carotid endarterectomy in patients with symptomatic carotid stenosis: a systematic review. J Vasc Surg 30:606, 1999
76. Rockman CB, Riles TS, Lamparello PJ, et al: Natural history and management of the asymptomatic, moderately stenotic internal carotid artery. J Vasc Surg 25:423, 1997
77. Cina CS, Clase CM, Haynes RB: Carotid endarterectomy for symptomatic carotid stenosis. Cochrane Database Syst Rev (2):CD001081, 2000
78. Rothwell PM, Slattery J, Warlow CP: Clinical and angiographic predictors of stroke and death from carotid endarterectomy: systematic review. BMJ 315:1571, 1997
79. European Carotid Surgery Trialists' Collaborative Group: Randomized trial of endarterectomy for recently symptomatic carotid stenosis: final results of the MRC European Carotid Surgery Trial. Lancet 351:1379, 1998
80. Stroke Prevention in Atrial Fibrillation Study: Final results. Circulation 84:527, 1991
81. Warfarin versus aspirin for prevention of thromboembolism in atrial fibrillation: Stroke Prevention in Atrial Fibrillation II Study. Lancet 343:687, 1994
82. Go AS, Hylek EM, Phillips KA, et al: Implications of stroke risk criteria on the anticoagulation decision in nonvalvular atrial fibrillation: the Anticoagulation and Risk Factors in Atrial Fibrillation (ATRIA) study. Circulation 102:11, 2000
83. Hass WK, Easton JD, Adams HP Jr, et al: A randomized trial comparing ticlopidine hydrochloride with aspirin for the prevention of stroke in high-risk patients. Ticlopidine Aspirin Stroke Study Group. N Engl J Med 321:501, 1989
84. Creager MA: Results of the CAPRIE trial: efficacy and safety of clopidogrel. Clopidogrel versus aspirin in patients at risk of ischaemic events. Vasc Med 3:257, 1998
85. A randomised, blinded trial of clopidogrel versus aspirin in patients at risk of ischaemic events (CAPRIE). CAPRIE Steering Committee. Lancet 348:1329, 1996
86. Gasecki AP, Ferguson GG, Eliasziw M, et al: Early endarterectomy for severe carotid artery stenosis after a nondisabling stroke: results from the North American Symptomatic Carotid Endarterectomy Trial. J Vasc Surg 20:288, 1994
87. Bornstein NM, Chadwick LG, Norris JW: The value of carotid Doppler ultrasound in asymptomatic extracranial arterial disease. Can J Neurol Sci 15:378, 1988
88. Bornstein NM, Norris JW: Management of patients with asymptomatic neck bruits and carotid stenosis. Neurol Clin 10:269, 1992
89. Colgan MP, Strode GR, Sommer JD, et al: Prevalence of asymptomatic carotid disease: results of duplex scanning in 348 unselected volunteers. J Vasc Surg 8:674, 1988
90. Cronenwett JL, Birkmeyer JD, Nackman GB, et al: Cost-effectiveness of carotid endarterectomy in asymptomatic patients. J Vasc Surg 25:298, 1997
91. Barnett HJ, Taylor DW, Eliasziw M, et al: Benefit of carotid endarterectomy in patients with symptomatic moderate or severe stenosis. North American Symptomatic Carotid Endarterectomy Trial Collaborators (NASCET). N Engl J Med 339:1415, 1998
92. Eliasziw M, Streifler JY, Fox AJ, et al: Significance of plaque ulceration in symptomatic patients with high-grade carotid stenosis. North American Symptomatic Carotid Endarterectomy Trial. Stroke 25:304, 1994
93. Streifler JY, Eliasziw M, Fox AJ, et al: Angiographic detection of carotid plaque ulceration. comparison with surgical observations in a multicenter study. North American Symptomatic Carotid Endarterectomy Trial. Stroke 25:1130, 1994
94. Hougaku H, Matsumoto M, Handa N, et al: Asymptomatic carotid lesions and silent cerebral infarction. Stroke 25:566, 1994
95. Sabetai MM, Tegos TJ, Nicolaides AN, et al: Hemispheric symptoms and carotid plaque echomorphology. J Vasc Surg 31(1 pt 1):39, 2000
96. Meairs S, Hennerici M: Four-dimensional ultrasonographic characterization of plaque surface motion in patients with symptomatic and asymptomatic carotid artery stenosis. Stroke 30:1807, 1999
97. Kessler C, von Maravic M, Bruckmann H, et al: Ultrasound for the assessment of the embolic risk of carotid plaques. Acta Neurol Scand 92:231, 1995
98. de Bray JM, Baud JM, Delanoy P, et al: Reproducibility in ultrasonic characterization of carotid plaques. Cerebrovasc Dis 8:273, 1998
99. Albers GW: Expanding the window for thrombolytic therapy in acute stroke: the potential role of acute MRI for patient selection. Stroke 30:2230, 1999
100. Hill SL, Donato AT: Ability of the carotid duplex scan to predict stenosis, symptoms, and plaque structure. Surgery 116:914, 1994
101. Gasecki AP, Eliasziw M, Ferguson GG, et al: Long-term prognosis and effect of endarterectomy in pa-

tients with symptomatic severe carotid stenosis and contralateral carotid stenosis or occlusion: results from nascet. North American Symptomatic Carotid Endarterectomy Trial (NASCET) group. J Neurosurg 83:778, 1995

102. Findlay JM, Tucker WS, Ferguson GG, et al: Guidelines for the use of carotid endarterectomy: current recommendations from the Canadian Neurosurgical Society. Can Med Assoc J 157:653, 1997

103. Norris JW, Zhu CZ: Silent stroke and carotid stenosis. Stroke 23:483, 1992

104. Halliday AW, Thomas D, Mansfield A: The Asymptomatic Carotid Surgery Trial (ACST): rationale and design. Steering Committee. Eur J Vasc Surg 8:703, 1994

105. Ricotta JJ, O'Brien MS, DeWeese JA: Carotid endarterectomy for non-hemispheric ischaemia: long-term follow-up. Cardiovasc Surg 2:561, 1994

106. Faggioli GL, Curl GR, Ricotta JJ: The role of carotid screening before coronary artery bypass. J Vasc Surg 12:724, 1990

107. Courbier R, Jausseran JM, Poyen V: Current status of vascular grafting in supraaortic trunks. Personal experience. Int Surgery 73:210, 1988

108. Pillai L, Gutierrez IZ, Curl GR, et al: Evaluation and treatment of carotid stenosis in open-heart surgery patients. J Surg Res 57:312, 1994

109. Borger MA, Fremes SE, Weisel RD, et al: Coronary bypass and carotid endarterectomy: does a combined approach increase risk? A metaanalysis. Ann Thorac Surg 68:14, 1999

110. Rosenthal D, Caudill DR, Lamis PA, et al: Carotid and coronary arterial disease: a rational approach. Am Surg 50:233, 1984

111. Newman DC, Hicks RG, Horton DA: Coexistent carotid and coronary arterial disease. Outcome in 50 cases and method of management. J Cardiovasc Surg (Torino) 28:599, 1987

112. Ennix CL Jr, Lawrie GM, Morris GC Jr, et al: Improved results of carotid endarterectomy in patients with symptomatic coronary disease: an analysis of 1,546 consecutive carotid operations. Stroke 10:122, 1979

113. Sameshima T, Miyao J, Oda T, et al: [Effects of allopurinol on renal damage following renal ischemia.] Masui—Japan J Anesthesiol 44:349, 1995

114. Cinat ME, Pham H, Vo D, et al: Improved imaging of carotid artery bifurcation using helical computed tomographic angiography. Ann Vasc Surg 13:178, 1999

115. Fox AJ: How to measure carotid stenosis (editorial). Radiology 186:316, 1993

116. Rothwell PM, Gibson RJ, Slattery J, et al: Equivalence of measurements of carotid stenosis: a comparison of three methods on 1001 angiograms. European Carotid Surgery Trialists' collaborative group. Stroke 25:2435, 1994

117. Eliasziw M, Smith RF, Singh N, et al: Further comments on the measurement of carotid stenosis from angiograms. North American Symptomatic Carotid Endarterectomy Trial (NASCET) group. Stroke 25:2445, 1994

118. Landis R, Koch G: The measurement of observer agreement for categorical data. Biometrics 33:159, 1997

119. Floriani M, Giulini SM, Anzola GP, et al: Predictive value of cervical bruit for the detection of obstructive lesions of the internal carotid artery: data from 2000 patients. Ital J Neurol Sci 10:321, 1989

120. Thiele BL, Jones AM, Hobson RW, et al: Standards in noninvasive cerebrovascular testing. Report from the Committee on Standards for Noninvasive Vascular Testing of the Joint Council of the Society for Vascular Surgery and the North American Chapter of the International Society for Cardiovascular Surgery. J Vasc Surg 15:495, 1992

121. Detsky AS, Abrams HB, Forbath N, et al: Cardiac assessment for patients undergoing noncardiac surgery. Arch Intern Med 146:2131, 1986

122. Detsky AS, Abrams HB, McLaughlin JR, et al: Predicting cardiac complications in patients undergoing non-cardiac surgery. J Gen Intern Med 1(July–August):211, 1986

123. Wong T, Detsky AS: Preoperative cardiac risk assessment for patients having peripheral vascular srugery. Ann Intern Med 116:743, 1992

124. Eagle K, Brundage B, Chaitman B, et al: Guidelines for perioperative cardiovascular evaluation for noncardiac surgery: report of the American College of Cardiology/American Heart Association Task Force on Practice Guidelines (Committee on Perioperative Cardiovascular Evaluation for Noncardiac Surgery). J Am Coll Cardiol 27:910, 1996

125. Eagle K, Froelich J: Reducing cardiovascular risk in patients undergoing noncardiac surgery (editorial). N Engl J Med 335:1761, 1996

126. Eagle KA, Coley CM, Newell JB, et al: Combining clinical and thallium data optimizes preoperative assessment of cardiac risk before major vascular surgery. Ann Intern Med 110:859, 1989

127. Rothwell PM, Gibson RJ, Slattery J, et al: Prognostic value and reproducibility of measurements of carotid stenosis: a comparison of three methods on 1001 angiograms. European Carotid Surgery Trialists' collaborative group. Stroke 25:2440, 1994

128. NASCET: Clinical alert: benefit of carotid endarterectomy for patients with high-grade stenosis of the internal carotid artery. national institute of neurological disorders and stroke stroke and trauma division. North American Symptomatic Carotid Endarterectomy Trial (NASCET) investigators. Stroke 22:816, 1991

129. NASCET: North American Symptomatic Carotid Endarterectomy Trial. Methods, patient characteristics, and progress. Stroke 22:711, 1991

Acknowledgment

Figure 1   Laurie Grace.

13 BREAST COMPLAINTS

Barbara L. Smith, M.D., Ph.D., and Wiley W. Souba, M.D., Sc.D.

Assessment and Management of Breast Complaints

One of every two women will consult her physician about a breast disorder at some point in her life. Although breast cancer is the most common malignancy of women in the United States, most breast disorders are nonmalignant: it is estimated that 80% to 90% of clinical presentations related to the breast are caused by benign disease. (The true incidence of benign diseases of the breast is difficult to estimate because of the blurred distinction between true breast disease and physiologic breast symptoms such as nodularity, lumpiness, and tenderness.) Because breast disorders are so common, it is important for the practicing general surgeon to be knowledgeable about the workup, diagnosis, and management of breast complaints.

Common Presenting Symptoms of Breast Disease

Most of the breast problems surgeons encounter in routine practice fall into six general categories, which are associated with varying degrees of risk for breast cancer [see Table 1]. Some presentations, such as a dominant mass in a postmenopausal woman, are clearly suggestive of malignancy, and their workup is relatively straightforward. Others, such as a tender thickening in a premenopausal woman, usually reflect benign disease. It is important to recognize, however, that any of these presenting symptoms can be associated with a malignancy, and thus all of them warrant a complete evaluation. In fact, it is the evaluation of the usually benign symptoms that places the greatest demands on the physician's clinical judgment. When such symptoms are the main presenting complaint of a breast cancer, their apparently benign nature may be misleadingly reassuring and delay the diagnosis of malignancy.

Risk Factors for Breast Cancer

The central task facing a physician examining a patient with a breast complaint is to determine whether the abnormality is benign or malignant. To this end, knowledge of the main risk factors for breast cancer is essential: prompt identification of the patients at highest risk for malignancy allows the physician to take an appropriately vigorous approach from the beginning of the diagnostic workup.

Various factors that place women at increased risk for breast carcinoma have been identified[1] [see Table 2]. These risk factors include increasing age; mutations in breast cancer risk genes (including *BRCA1* and *BRCA2, PTEN*, and *p53*) and other factors related to a family history of breast cancer[2]; hormonal and reproductive factors, including early menarche, late menopause, nulliparity, the absence of lactation, and the use of exogenous hormones[1,3-9]; environmental factors, including diet and the lifestyle characteristic of developed Western nations[10-12]; certain pathologic findings within breast tissue, including previous breast cancer and various premalignant lesions[13-15]; and certain nonbreast malignancies, including ovarian and endometrial carcinomas. There are also a number of molecular markers that can be correlated with prognosis.

Recognition of risk factors facilitates appropriate screening and clinical management of the individual patient. It is important to recognize, however, that in many women in whom breast cancer develops, known risk factors for breast carcinoma are entirely absent. The absence of these risk factors should not prevent full evaluation or biopsy of a suspicious breast lesion.

Workup of the Patient with a Breast Complaint

Evaluation of any breast problem should include a detailed history of the presenting complaint, previous breast problems, and any risk factors for breast carcinoma; a thorough physical examination of the breasts; appropriate imaging studies; and evaluation of the patient's general medical condition. Particular attention must be paid to any findings that increase the suspicion of malignancy.

HISTORY

The patient should be asked to describe when and how the problem was first identified. Changes in the size or tenderness of any palpable abnormalities since their initial discovery should be recorded, with particular attention paid to any changes that occurred during the menstrual cycle. Previous breast problems or breast operations should be documented, and pathology reports from any such operations should be obtained. All imaging studies or medical evaluations that have already been performed should be reviewed.

Next, those portions of the medical history that bear on the risk of breast cancer should be explored in detail. Age at menarche and either the date of the last menstrual period or, if applicable, age at menopause should be recorded. Parity, age at the first term pregnancy, and duration of lactation should be determined. Any use of exogenous hormones should be recorded, including use of oral contraceptives (with years of use before the first term pregnancy recorded separately), use of postmenopausal estrogen replacement therapy, and use of any other hormones as part of a fertility program or for other purposes.

In addition, any history of breast cancer in family members, up to and including third-degree relatives, should be detailed, and age

Assessment and Management of Breast Complaints

Patient presents with breast complaint

The most common presenting problems are
- Palpable mass
- Normal physical examination with abnormal mammogram
- Vague thickening or nodularity
- Nipple discharge
- Breast pain
- Breast infection or inflammation

Evaluate likelihood that lesion reflects cancer [see Table 1], and be aware of patient risk factors for cancer [see Table 2].

Palpable mass

Factors increasing suspicion of malignancy:
- Skin dimpling
- Palpable axillary nodes
- Mass with irregular borders
- Increasing age

Determine whether mass is cystic or solid.

Mass is cystic

If fluid is bloody or mass remains after aspiration, obtain tissue diagnosis. If not, follow up as for a simple cyst.

Mass is solid

Obtain tissue diagnosis by means of fine-needle aspiration, core-needle, or open surgical biopsy.

Abnormal mammogram after normal breast examination

Factors increasing suspicion of malignancy:
- Previous normal mammogram
- Localized soft tissue mass
- Stellate-appearing lesion
- Clustered microcalcifications

Mammogram is suspicious

Perform biopsy (open or stereotactic or ultrasound-guided core-needle).

Mammogram is not suspicious

Follow up with mammograms every 6 mo for 2 yr.

Vague thickening or nodularity

Factors increasing suspicion of malignancy:
- Skin changes
- Asymmetry between right and left breast
- No generic hormonal changes (e.g., pregnancy, beginning or ceasing contraception)
- Palpable axillary nodes

Order mammogram if patient is > 35 yr or > 30 yr with a family history of breast cancer.

Thickening is suspicious

Perform open biopsy (FNA is not appropriate).

Thickening is not suspicious

Reexamine patient after 2 menstrual cycles. If area resolves, provide routine follow-up. If lesion persists or worsens, perform open biopsy.

Malignancy is present

Perform clinical staging.
Consider treatment options.
Initiate definitive therapy for breast cancer.

No malignancy is present

Continue routine screening, as appropriate for patient's age.

Work up patient:
- History, with particular attention to risk factors for breast cancer
- Physical examination
- Imaging studies (e.g., mammography)

Initiate evaluation of specific breast problem.

Nipple discharge

Factors increasing suspicion of malignancy:
- Bloody discharge
- Unilateral discharge
- Palpable mass (see facing page)
- Abnormal mammogram (see facing page)

Breast pain

Factors increasing suspicion of malignancy:
- Abnormal skin changes
- Noncyclic pain

Order mammogram if pain is noncyclic and patient is > 35 yr or > 30 yr with a family history of breast cancer.

Breast infection or inflammation

Factors increasing suspicion of malignancy:
- No elevation of white blood cell count
- No response to antibiotics
- Symptoms not associated with lactation

Mammogram is abnormal, or palpable mass is detected

Work up as indicated for palpable mass or abnormal mammogram.

Mammogram is normal, and physical examination yields normal results

Offer comfort, reassure, and perform follow-up examination in 2 mo. If pain resolves or there is still no palpable abnormality, reassure further and follow up routinely. If there is a palpable abnormality, obtain tissue diagnosis.

High-risk patients without symptons

Perform risk assessment (e.g., using Gail or Claus model).

Consider genetic testing for risk gene mutations.

Discuss risk with patient.

Select treatment option:
1. Close surveillance
2. Prophylactic mastectomy
3. Chemoprevention with tamoxifen or participation in chemoprevention trial

---

Discharge is suspicious

Order mammogram. Perform biopsy of any lesions found. If a single duct is the source of the pathologic discharge, excise duct. If source of discharge can only be localized to a quadrant, excise ducts in that quadrant.

Discharge is not suspicious (physiologic discharge or galactorrhea)

If discharge is physiologic, reassure patient; no further treatment is needed. If galactorrhea is present, initiate appropriate workup (serum prolactin levels, thyroid function tests, and MRI if necessary).

Patient is lactating

Give oral antibiotics to cover gram-positive cocci, use warm soaks, and attempt to keep breast emptied. If abscess forms, incise and drain.

Patient is not lactating

Incise and drain any abscesses, and give antibiotics to cover skin organisms (including anaerobes).

If there is no response to short course of antibiotics, rule out inflammatory carcinoma; perform biopsy, including skin. If infection is chronic, excise subareolar duct complex.

Table 1 Common Presenting Symptoms of Breast Disease

Symptom	Likelihood of Malignancy	Risk of Missed Malignancy
Palpable mass	Highest ↑	Lowest ↑
Abnormal mammogram with normal breast examination		
Vague thickening or nodularity		
Nipple discharge		
Breast pain		
Breast infection	Lowest ↓	Highest ↓

at diagnosis should be recorded. Similarly, any family history of ovarian cancer or other cancers (particularly those that developed when the relative was young) should be recorded, along with age at diagnosis. Any personal history of cancer should be recorded, with particular attention paid to breast, ovarian, and endometrial cancers. Previous exposure to radiation, especially in the area of the chest wall, should be noted.

Finally, as with any surgical patient, an overview of the general medical history should be obtained that includes current medications, allergies, tobacco and alcohol use, previous surgical procedures, medical problems, and a brief social history.

PHYSICAL EXAMINATION

First, as the patient sits with her hands behind her head and her elbows back, the breasts should be inspected for asymmetry, dimpling of the skin, erythema, or edema. Each breast should then be carefully palpated from the clavicle to below the inframammary fold and from the sternum to the posterior axillary line, with pains taken to include the subareolar area. This is done with the patient both supine and sitting. If an abnormal area is identified, its size, contour, texture, tenderness, and position should be described; a diagram of the lesion is extremely useful for future reference.

Table 2 Risk Factors for Breast Cancer

Increasing age
Caucasian race
Age at menarche ≤ 11 years
Age at menopause ≥ 55 years
Nulliparity
Age at first pregnancy ≥ 30 years
Absence of history of lactation
? Prolonged use of oral contraceptives before first pregnancy
Use of postmenopausal estrogen replacement, especially if prolonged
Use of other hormones, fertility regimens, or diethylstilbestrol
Mutations in breast cancer risk genes, including *BRCA1* and *BRCA2*, *PTEN*, and *p53*
Family history of breast cancer: multiple affected relatives, early onset, bilaterality
Family history of ovarian cancer: multiple affected relatives, early onset
Pathologic findings that indicate increased risk (e.g., atypical hyperplasia, lobular carcinoma in situ, proliferative fibrocystic disease)
Previous breast cancer
Previous breast problems
Previous breast operations
Previous exposure to radiation

Next, the nipples and areolae are inspected for skin breakdown and squeezed gently to check for discharge. The number and position of any ducts from which discharge is obtained should be recorded, and the color of the discharge (milky, green, yellow, clear, brown, or bloody) and its consistency (watery, sticky, or thick) should be noted. Discharge on one side calls for a careful search for discharge on the other side because unilateral, single-duct discharge is much more suspicious than bilateral, multiple-duct discharge. Any discharge obtained should be tested for occult blood. Cytologic study of nipple discharge generally is not indicated: it adds expense and rarely contributes significantly to the decision whether biopsy is needed.

Finally, the axillary and supraclavicular nodes are examined bilaterally. If enlarged nodes are discovered, their size, mobility, and number should be recorded. Any matting of nodes or fixation of nodes to the chest walls should also be recorded. Tenderness of enlarged nodes may suggest a reactive process and should therefore be recorded as well.

IMAGING STUDIES

Mammography

According to current recommendations, a baseline screening mammogram need not be performed until 40 (or possibly, as some suggest, until 50[16]) years of age; however, it is reasonable to perform a mammogram to rule out synchronous, nonpalpable lesions whenever a woman older than 35 years presents with a palpable breast mass or other specific symptoms. Approximately 4% to 5% of breast cancers occur in women younger than 40 years, and about 25% occur in women younger than 50 years.[17,18] On the other hand, mammography fails to detect 10% to 15% of all palpable malignant lesions, and its sensitivity is particularly decreased in women with lobular carcinoma or radiographically dense breast tissue. It must therefore be emphasized that a negative mammogram should not influence the decision to perform a biopsy of a clinically palpable lesion. The purpose of mammography is to look for synchronous lesions or nonpalpable calcifications surrounding the palpable abnormality, not to determine whether to perform a biopsy of the palpable lesion.

Ultrasonography

The main value of ultrasonography is in distinguishing cystic from solid lesions. If the lesion is palpable, this distinction is best made by direct needle aspiration, which is both diagnostic and therapeutic; if the lesion is not palpable, ultrasonography can determine whether the lesion is cystic and thus potentially eliminate the need for additional workup or treatment. Ultrasonography has not proved useful for screening: it fails to detect calcifications, misses a large number of malignancies, and identifies a great deal of normal breast texture as potential nodules. It is useful, however, for directing fine-needle or core-needle biopsy of the lesions that it does visualize: it permits real-time manipulation of the needle and direct confirmation of the position of the needle within the lesion. The use of advanced ultrasound technology for diagnostic purposes in the breast is currently being explored.

Magnetic Resonance Imaging

A promising addition to breast imaging options is magnetic resonance imaging. MRI after injection of gadolinium contrast enhances many malignant lesions in relation to normal breast parenchyma. Although some benign lesions (e.g., fibroadenomas) are also enhanced by gadolinium, the contrast agent appears to enhance malignant lesions more rapidly and often to a greater extent.

The sensitivity and specificity of MRI in distinguishing benign from malignant lesions are still being assessed. The main approved use of MRI in breast disease is for identification of leaks in silicone breast implants, because MRI can detect the ruptured silicone membrane within the silicone gel. MRI is also useful in identifying occult primary tumors in women who have palpable axillary nodes but no palpable or mammographically identified primary breast lesion. MRI appears to be effective for assessing the extent of vaguely defined tumors, identifying unsuspected multifocal disease, and helping identify patients who are not eligible for breast-conserving surgery. In addition, it appears that MRI can distinguish between a locally recurrent tumor and surgical scarring or radiation change after lumpectomy and radiation, although the technology may not provide reliable readings until 18 months or more after surgery or the completion of radiation therapy. The utility of MRI for screening of young high-risk women with mammographically dense breast tissue is being explored.

Nuclear medicine studies such as sestamibi scintimammography and positron emission tomography (PET) scanning remain primarily investigational tools. There is currently no role for thermography or xerography in the evaluation of breast problems.

Management of Specific Breast Problems

PALPABLE MASS

The workup and management of a discrete breast mass are governed by the age of the patient, the physical characteristics of the palpable lesion, and the patient's medical history.[19] The likelihood of malignancy is greater when the patient is 40 years of age or older, when the mass has irregular borders, or when skin dimpling or enlarged axillary nodes are present. A prebiopsy mammogram is indicated for women older than 35 years and for those younger than 35 years who have a strong family history of premenopausal breast cancer.

It is important to determine whether the mass is solid or cystic. Cysts are almost always benign; usually, aspiration is all that is required. Solid masses are more likely to be cancerous; a tissue diagnosis must be obtained to rule out malignancy. Clinical examination is not accurate in distinguishing cysts from a solid mass. In one study, only 58% of 66 palpable cysts were correctly identified on physical examination.[20]

Cystic Masses

If it is suspected that a palpable mass is a cyst, the suspicion should generally be confirmed by aspiration, even if ultrasound examination has already shown the mass to be a simple cyst. Aspiration verifies that the palpable mass corresponds to the lesion seen on ultrasonography; it also permits more thorough examination of the surrounding breast tissue. If the cyst fluid is bloody or a mass remains after aspiration, there is a significant chance of malignancy, and the aspirate should be sent for cytologic analysis.[21] At this point, excisional biopsy is generally indicated, even if the cytologic analysis reveals no malignancy. If the cyst fluid is not bloody and no mass remains after aspiration, there is little chance of malignancy, and the aspirate need not be sent for cytologic analysis.[22,23] In one study, there were no malignancies in 6,747 nonbloody cyst aspirates.[24]

If a cyst is aspirated without having been demonstrated to be a simple cyst by ultrasonography, the patient should be reexamined in 4 to 8 weeks. Fewer than 20% of simple cysts recur after a single aspiration, and fewer than 9% recur after two or three aspirations.[25] If a cyst recurs rapidly after aspiration, it should be reaspirated and its contents sent for cytologic analysis. If the results of the analysis are suspicious or if the cyst recurs yet again, an excisional biopsy should be performed. If, however, a new cyst appears in a different area of breast tissue, this additional workup is not required, and the new cyst should be evaluated as a new problem. Additional cysts may be expected to occur in more than 50% of patients.[26]

Solid Masses

If a discrete mass in the breast is believed to be solid, either on the basis of ultrasonographic findings or because attempts at aspiration yield no fluid, a tissue diagnosis is necessary to rule out malignancy. Physical examination alone is insufficient: it correctly identifies masses as malignant in only 60% to 85% of cases.[27,28] Furthermore, experienced examiners often disagree on whether biopsy is needed for a particular lesion: in one study, four surgeons unanimously agreed on the necessity of biopsy for only 11 (73%) of 15 palpable masses that were later shown by biopsy to be malignant. Tissue diagnosis may be accomplished by fine-needle aspiration (FNA) biopsy, core-needle biopsy, or open surgical biopsy [see Sidebar Breast Biopsy].

Phyllodes tumors The phyllodes tumor, a mesenchymal tumor limited to mammary tissue, is a rare condition. The tumor is typically smooth, round, firm, well defined, and mobile and causes no pain. It has no pathognomonic mammographic or ultrasonographic features and is difficult, if not impossible, to distinguish from a fibroadenoma on physical examination or radiologic evaluation unless it is quite large. Palpable axillary lymph nodes are encountered in 20% of patients with phyllodes tumors, but histologic evidence of malignancy is encountered in fewer than 5% of axillary lymph node dissections for clinically positive nodes. The remainder of the nodes are enlarged as a result of necrosis of the primary tumor.

Tumors are classified as low, intermediate, or high grade on the basis of five criteria: stromal cellularity, stromal atypia, the microscopic appearance of the tumor margin (infiltrating, effacing, or bulging), mitoses per 10 high-power fields, and the macroscopic size of the tumor. Structural[29] and cytogenetic[30] studies of constituent cells have demonstrated similarities between fibroadenomas and phyllodes tumors, and there is evidence[31] that certain fibroadenomas develop into phyllodes tumors. FNA is usually nondiagnostic, primarily because of the difficulty of obtaining adequate numbers of stromal cells for cytogenic analysis.[32] Although phyllodes tumors have minimal metastatic potential, they have a proclivity for local recurrence and should be excised with a 1 cm margin. Local recurrence has been correlated with excision margins but not with tumor grade or size.[33]

The diagnosis of phyllodes tumor should be considered in all patients with a history of a firm, rounded, well-circumscribed, solid (i.e., noncystic) lesion in the breast. Simple excisional biopsy should be performed if aspiration fails to return cyst fluid or if ultrasonography demonstrates a solid lesion. Because phyllodes tumors mimic fibroadenomas, they are often enucleated or excised with a close margin. If a 1 cm margin is not obtained after examination of the permanent section, the patient should undergo reexcision to obtain wider margins. Otherwise, a recurrence rate of 15% to 20% can be expected. If a simple excision cannot be accomplished without gross cosmetic deformity or if the tumor burden is too large, a simple mastectomy may be performed. Axillary lymph node dissection should be reserved for clinically palpable nodes. Radiation therapy may have a role in patients with chest wall invasion. Chemotherapy, which is reserved for patients with metastatic disease, is based on guidelines for the treatment of sarcomas, rather than breast adenocarcinomas.

talgia.[46,47] Pharmacotherapy for mastalgia is contraindicated in patients who are trying to become pregnant.

BREAST INFECTION OR INFLAMMATION

Infections of the breast fall into two general categories: (1) lactational infections and (2) chronic subareolar infections associated with duct ectasia. These benign infections must be distinguished from inflammatory carcinoma.

Both cellulitis and abscesses may occur in lactating women, often during weaning or at other times when engorgement occurs. In the early stages, infections are treated by giving oral antibiotics that cover gram-positive cocci, applying warm packs to the breast, and actively attempting to keep the breast emptied. Weaning is not necessary: the infant is not adversely affected by nursing from the infected breast.[48,49]

Once a breast abscess forms, however, surgical drainage is necessary, and the infant generally must be weaned. Because of the network of fibrous septa within the breast, breast abscesses in lactating women rarely form fluctuant masses.[48] The diagnosis is established by the clinical picture of fever, leukocytosis, and exquisite point tenderness in the breast. General anesthesia is almost always required for drainage of these abscesses, because of the tenderness of the affected area and the amount of manipulation necessary to break up the loculated abscess cavity adequately. The cavity should be packed open, as with any abscess.

Nonlactational infections of the breast often present as chronic relapsing infections of the subareolar ducts associated with periductal mastitis or duct ectasia. These infections usually involve multiple organisms, including skin anaerobes.[50,51] Retraction or inversion of the nipple, subareolar masses, recurrent periareolar abscesses, or a chronic fistula to the periareolar skin may result,[41,52] as may palpable masses and mammographic changes that mimic carcinoma. In the acute phase of infection, treatment entails incision, drainage, and administration of antibiotics that cover skin organisms, including anaerobes. In cases of repeated infection, the entire subareolar duct complex should be excised after the acute infection has completely resolved, with antibiotic coverage provided during the perioperative period. The necessity of drain placement is debated. Even after wide excision of the subareolar duct complex and intravenous antibiotic coverage, infections recur in some patients; these can be treated by excising the nipple and the areola.[40,53]

HIGH-RISK PATIENTS PRESENTING FOR SCREENING

On the basis of established risk factors [see Risk Factors for Breast Cancer, above, and Table 2], certain asymptomatic women can be determined to be at increased risk for the development of breast cancer. The risk can be assessed by genetic testing for mutations in breast cancer risk genes or by the use of mathematical models to estimate risk. The Gail model,[54] which relies on data from the Breast Cancer Detection Demonstration Project, and the Claus model,[55] which relies on data from the Cancer and Steroid Hormone Project, are two of the tools that have been used to make this determination. At present, there are three treatment options for women at high risk for breast cancer: (1) close surveillance, (2) prophylactic mastectomy, and (3) chemoprevention with tamoxifen or other agents in the setting of a clinical trial. Although most women at high risk choose the option of close surveillance, recent data on chemoprevention with tamoxifen or other selective estrogen receptor modulators (SERMs), as well as new data on the efficacy of prophylactic mastectomy, may increase selection of the other two options.

Studies have reported that tamoxifen, 20 mg/day, reduces the risk of developing breast cancer. A meta-analysis[56] of trials in which tamoxifen was used to treat women with breast cancer demonstrated a 47% reduction in contralateral breast cancers in women taking tamoxifen for 5 years compared with those taking placebo. The National Surgical Adjuvant Breast and Bowel Project (NSABP) P-1 trial of tamoxifen, 20 mg/day, versus placebo in high-risk women reported a 44% reduction in new breast cancers in the tamoxifen group.[57] Two other trials in high-risk women[58,59] failed to show that tamoxifen reduced the rate of new breast cancers, but eligibility criteria and trial designs were different from those used in the NSABP trial.[60]

Other SERMs, such as raloxifene, show promise as chemoprevention agents and may have fewer side effects than tamoxifen.[61] The NSABP P-2 trial will compare tamoxifen and raloxifene with respect to their efficacy in preventing breast cancer and their side effects.

Long-term results of prophylactic mastectomy in high-risk women[62] indicate that breast cancer risk was reduced by at least 90% in women at high or very high risk who underwent this procedure compared with women who did not, with risk predicted by the Gail model.[54] Mathematical modeling suggests that prophylactic mastectomy could translate into improved survival for women at very high risk if it confers a 90% reduction in risk.[63]

For women with a previous diagnosis of breast cancer, surveillance protocols are described elsewhere [see Management of the Patient with Breast Cancer, Follow-up after Treatment, below]. For women with lobular carcinoma in situ (LCIS) or a family history of breast carcinoma, surveillance should include twice-yearly physical examinations. Mammography should be performed annually after the diagnosis of LCIS or atypical hyperplasia. For women with a family history of breast cancer, mammography should be performed annually, beginning at least 5 years before the earliest age at which cancer was diagnosed in a relative and in any case no later than the age of 35 years.[64] For women who carry BRCA1 or BRCA2 mutations and other women from families with an autosomal dominant pattern of breast cancer transmission, annual mammographic screening should begin at least 10 years before the earliest age at which the cancer was diagnosed in a relative and no later than 25 years of age.[64]

Management of the Patient with Breast Cancer

STAGING

In patients with newly diagnosed breast cancer, it is important to determine the overall extent of disease before embarking on definitive therapy. This process, referred to as clinical staging, includes (1) physical examination to identify any areas of palpable disease in the breasts or the axillary and supraclavicular nodes, along with a detailed clinical history to identify symptoms that may suggest metastatic disease; (2) imaging studies, including mammography, chest x-ray, and, sometimes, bone scans or CT scans of the chest, the abdomen, or the head; and (3) laboratory studies, including a complete blood

Table 3 **TNM Clinical Classification of Breast Cancer**[116]

Tumor (T)
- TX Primary tumor cannot be assessed
- T0 No evidence of primary tumor
- Tis Carcinoma in situ: intraductal carcinoma, lobular carcinoma in situ, or Paget's disease of the nipple with no invasive tumor
- T1 Tumor ≤ 2 cm in greatest dimension
    - T1mic: Microinvasion ≤ 0.1 cm
        - T1a: Tumor > 0.1 cm and ≤ 0.5 cm
        - T1b: Tumor > 0.5 cm and ≤ 1.0 cm
        - T1c: Tumor > 1 cm and ≤ 2 cm
- T2 Tumor > 2 cm and ≤ 5 cm in greatest dimension
- T3 Tumor > 5 cm in greatest dimension
- T4 Tumor of any size; direct extension to chest wall or skin
    - T4a Extension to chest wall
    - T4b Edema (including *peau d'orange*) or ulceration of the skin of the breast or satellite skin nodules confined to the same breast
    - T4c Both T4a and T4b
    - T4d Inflammatory carcinoma

Nodes (N)
- NX Regional lymph nodes cannot be assessed (e.g., previously removed)
- N0 No regional lymph node metastases
- N1 Metastasis to movable ipsilateral axillary node(s)
- N2 Metastasis to ipsilateral axillary node(s) fixed to one another or other structures
- N3 Metastasis to ipsilateral internal mammary lymph node(s)

Metastasis (M)
- MX Presence of distant metastasis cannot be assessed
- M0 No distant metastases
- M1 Distant metastasis, including metastasis to ipsilateral supraclavicular lymph node(s)

Table 4 **Staging of Breast Cancer**[116]

Stage	T	N	M
Stage 0	Tis	N0	M0
Stage I	T1	N0	M0
Stage IIA	T0	N1	M0
	T1	N1	M0
	T2	N0	M0
Stage IIB	T2	N1	M0
	T3	N0	M0
Stage IIIA	T0	N2	M0
	T1	N2	M0
	T2	N2	M0
	T3	N1, N2	M0
Stage IIIB	T4	Any N	M0
	Any T	N3	M0
Stage IV	Any T	Any N	M1

count (CBC) and liver function tests. Several clinical staging systems for breast cancer are currently in use [*see Tables 3 and 4*].

The extent of preoperative staging should be guided by the size and other characteristics of the primary tumor and by the patient's history and physical examination. For patients with early-stage cancer and a low probability of metastatic disease, extensive testing adds cost without offering much benefit and should therefore be discouraged. For patients with stage I or II disease, a CBC, liver function tests, and a chest x-ray should be performed before definitive surgical therapy is initiated, and imaging studies should be reserved for patients who have abnormal test results or clinical symptoms that suggest metastatic disease (e.g., bone pain). For patients with higher-stage disease at presentation, the use of additional staging studies should be guided by the patient's clinical situation.

TREATMENT OPTIONS

Mastectomy versus Limited Surgery

Clinical trials in the 1970s and 1980s clearly demonstrated that in eligible women with stage I and II breast carcinoma, limited surgery—consisting of lumpectomy or quadrantectomy, axillary dissection, and radiation—yielded overall survival rates that were equivalent to those achieved with radical or modified radical mastectomy.[65-68] Certain categories of patients are now widely considered to be eligible for breast conservation and radiation therapy [*see Table 5*]: not only are long-term survival rates after breast conservation with limited surgery identical to those achieved with mastectomy in these groups, but local recurrence rates are low as well (5% to 10%). Approximately two thirds of all women with breast cancer are eligible for breast conservation. Nevertheless, many eligible women in the United States are still treated with mastectomy.[69-73] When a patient is eligible for limited surgery, the decision between mastectomy and breast conservation with radiation therapy is made on the basis of patient and physician preference, access or lack of access to radiation therapy, and the presence or absence of contraindications to breast conservation.

Contraindications to breast conservation There remain patients for whom mastectomy is still clearly the treatment of choice. These patients fall into four broad categories: (1) those in whom radiation therapy is contraindicated, (2) those in whom lumpectomy would have an unacceptable cosmetic result, (3) those for whom local recurrence is a concern, and (4) those high-risk patients in whom surgical prophylaxis is appropriate [*see Management of Specific Breast Problems, High-Risk Patients Presenting for Screening, above*].

Radiation therapy may be contraindicated for any of several reasons. Some patients choose not to undergo radiation therapy, either because it is inconvenient or because they are concerned about potential complications (including the induction of second malignancies). Some patients simply do not have access to radiation therapy, either because they live in a rural area or because they have physical conditions that make daily trips for therapy cumbersome. Other patients have medical or psychiatric disorders that would make it ex-

Table 5 **Determinants of Patient Eligibility for Lumpectomy and Radiation Therapy**

Primary tumor ≤ 5 cm (may be larger in selected cases)
Tumor of lobular or ductal histology
Any location of primary within breast if lumpectomy to clean margins (including central lesions) will yield acceptable cosmetic results
Clinically suspicious but mobile axillary nodes
Tumor either positive or negative for estrogen and progesterone receptors
Any patient age

tremely difficult for them to comply with the daily treatment schedule. Still others have specific medical contraindications to radiation therapy, including pregnancy, collagen vascular disease, or previous irradiation of the chest wall (as in a woman with a local recurrence of a breast carcinoma that was treated with radiation therapy). Although there are some clinical data supporting the use of repeat local excision without further irradiation to treat local recurrence after radiation therapy, most authorities favor mastectomy.[74,75]

When resection of the primary tumor to clean margins would render the appearance of the remaining breast tissue cosmetically unacceptable, mastectomy with immediate reconstruction may be preferable. This is likely to be the case, for example, in patients with large primary tumors relative to their breast size: resection of the primary tumor would remove a substantial portion of the breast tissue. Another example is patients with multiple primary tumors, who would have not only an increased risk of local recurrence but also poor cosmetic results after multiple wide excisions. Patients with superficial central lesions, including Paget's disease, are eligible for wide excision (including the nipple and areola) followed by radiation therapy, provided that clean margins are obtained. The survival and local recurrence rates in these patients are equivalent to those in other groups of patients undergoing lumpectomy and radiation.[76-78] In many cases, the cosmetic results of this procedure are preferable to those of immediate reconstruction, and there is always the option to reconstruct the nipple and areola later.

Patients who are at high risk for local recurrence often choose mastectomy as primary therapy. Features of primary tumors that are associated with higher local recurrence rates after limited surgery and radiation include gross residual disease after lumpectomy, multiple primary tumors within the breast, an extensive intraductal component, large tumor size, lymphatic vessel invasion, and lobular histologic findings.

In practice, obtaining clean margins is probably the most critical factor in decreasing the risk of local recurrence. The difficulty of obtaining microscopically clean margins in tumors with an extensive intraductal component and in lobular carcinomas may account for the higher local recurrence rates sometimes seen with these tumors. Histologic analysis of mastectomy specimens from patients with tumors with an extensive intraductal component has shown a high rate of multifocality within ipsilateral breast tissue; this residual disease is thought to be the nidus for local recurrence.[79]

The long-term benefits of choosing mastectomy to reduce local recurrences are not clear. Whereas the appearance of distant metastases typically heralds incurable and ultimately fatal disease, local recurrence after breast conservation appears to have little, if any, impact on overall survival. Prospective, randomized trials have had difficulty showing a statistically significant reduction in survival in women who have had a local recurrence after limited surgery and radiation. It has been suggested that additional follow-up may eventually confirm reduced survival in some patients with local recurrences.[80] Still, most of the evidence suggests that local recurrences are not the source of subsequent distant metastases. It is worthwhile to keep in mind, however, that even if mastectomy to prevent local recurrence does not actually improve survival, it may nevertheless provide significant benefit by reducing patient anxiety, the amount of follow-up testing required, and the need for subsequent treatment.

Options for axillary staging Axillary node status is one of the most powerful predictors of prognosis in breast cancer. Staging of the axilla, generally via a level I or II axillary dissection, has been a standard component of breast cancer surgery. Decisions about systemic and radiation therapy are often made on the basis of the number of axillary nodes involved by metastatic disease. The value of axillary dissection has been questioned, however, because of the increased use of systemic therapy even for many node-negative breast cancers as well as the morbidity associated with axillary dissection, including pain, reduced arm mobility, and the risk of lymphedema.

As an alternative to axillary dissection, sentinel lymph node (SLN) biopsy [see 44 Lymphatic Mapping and Sentinel Lymph Node Biopsy] has become increasingly popular as a way of assessing axillary node status with less morbidity.[81,82] The technique is technically demanding, however, and discussion continues as to the most appropriate way of implementing this approach in general practice.[83] SLN biopsy identifies an increased number of patients with micrometastases, with some identified by immunohistochemical staining alone. Treatment of patients with only micrometastases to axillary nodes remains a topic of debate, to be addressed in a planned clinical trial of SLN biopsy by the American College of Surgeons Oncology Group.

Breast reconstruction after mastectomy Breast reconstruction after mastectomy may provide both cosmetic and psychological benefits. In the past, reconstruction was generally delayed for 1 to 2 years after mastectomy; now, it is most often performed immediately after mastectomy.[17] This change has not been shown to have any serious adverse effects: it has not significantly increased recurrence or shortened survival, nor has it significantly delayed the detection of local recurrence or the administration of adjuvant chemotherapy.[84] Reconstruction options [see 43 Breast Procedures] include the placement of subpectoral saline implants (either immediately or after tissue expansion), latissimus dorsi myocutaneous flap reconstruction, and transverse rectus abdominis muscle myocutaneous flap reconstruction. Free flaps may also be employed under special circumstances.

Radiation Therapy

Current radiation therapy regimens consist of the delivery of approximately 5,000 cGy to the whole breast at a dosage of approximately 200 cGy/day, along with, in most cases, the delivery of an additional 1,000 to 1,500 cGy to the tumor bed, again at a dosage of 200 cGy/day. Axillary node fields are not irradiated unless there is evidence that the patient is at high risk for axillary relapse—namely, multiple (generally more than four) positive lymph nodes, extranodal extension of tumor, or bulky axillary disease (i.e., palpable nodes several centimeters in diameter). Because the combination of surgical therapy and radiation therapy increases the risk of lymphedema of the arm, it is appropriate only when there is sufficient risk of axillary relapse to justify the increased complication rate. As a rule, supraclavicular node fields are irradiated only in patients with multiple positive axillary nodes, who are at increased risk for supraclavicular disease. The internal mammary nodes are seldom irradiated prophylactically.

Postmastectomy radiation therapy involves the delivery of radiation to the chest wall after mastectomy; it is mainly reserved for patients with T3 or T4 primary tumors or multiple positive lymph nodes. Such therapy is recommended particularly when there are multiple positive axillary lymph nodes: significant axillary disease predicts higher rates of chest wall recurrence after mastectomy. Two series[85,86] have suggested that postmastectomy radiation therapy significantly improves survival in premenopausal women with any positive axillary nodes.

Irradiation of the breast or chest wall is generally well tolerated: most women experience only minor side effects, such as transient skin erythema, mild skin desquamation, and mild fatigue. Because a small amount of lung volume is included in the irradiated fields, there is usually a clinically insignificant but measurable reduction in pulmonary function. In addition, because the heart receives some radiation when the left breast or left chest wall is treated, there may be a slightly increased risk of future myocardial infarction. There is also a 1% to 2% chance that the radiation will induce a second malignancy (sarcoma, leukemia, or a second breast carcinoma). These radiation-induced malignancies appear after a long lag time, generally 7 to 15 years or longer.

Systemic Drug and Hormone Therapy

Despite the success of surgical treatment and radiation therapy in achieving local control of breast cancer, distant metastases still develop in many patients. Various drugs and hormones have therefore been used to treat both measurable and occult metastatic disease. It became clear in early trials that multiple-agent (or combination) chemotherapy was superior to single-agent chemotherapy.[87,88] It also became clear that chemotherapy and hormone therapy were limited in their ability to control large tumor masses, although on occasion, patients with large tumor masses showed dramatic partial responses or even complete responses to therapy.

With the goal of eradicating breast cancer metastases while they are still microscopic, systemic therapy is now administered in a so-called adjuvant setting—that is, when there is no evidence of distant metastases but there is sufficient suspicion that metastasis may have occurred. Until the late 1980s, adjuvant chemotherapy was given primarily to women who had axillary node metastases but no other evidence of disease.[87,89,90] In node-positive premenopausal women, adjuvant chemotherapy appeared to be significantly more beneficial than adjuvant hormone therapy. In node-positive postmenopausal women, on the other hand, hormone therapy appeared to be as beneficial as chemotherapy and less toxic.[89]

This approach to adjuvant systemic therapy changed in 1988, when the National Cancer Institute issued a clinical alert stating that there was sufficient evidence of benefit to allow recommendation of adjuvant chemotherapy or hormone therapy for even node-negative breast cancer patients.[91] By that time, a number of studies had shown that adjuvant chemotherapy could improve survival in node-negative breast cancer patients.[90-93] A consensus conference of experts in the field suggested that such therapy be reserved for node-negative women with primary tumors larger than 1 cm in diameter.[94] In 1992, a meta-analysis that reviewed the treatment of 75,000 women in 133 randomized clinical trials of adjuvant therapy for breast cancer concluded that overall long-term survival was increased by 20% to 30% in node-negative premenopausal women who received chemotherapy in comparison with those who did not.[95] This benefit also appeared to extend to postmenopausal women between 50 and 60 years of age. A 1998 overview of the use of adjuvant tamoxifen in randomized trials[56] demonstrated a 47% reduction in recurrence and a 26% reduction in mortality with 5 years of the use of tamoxifen rather than placebo in women with estrogen receptor (ER)–positive tumors. In this analysis, the effects of tamoxifen on recurrence and survival were independent of age and menopausal status. Tamoxifen did not appear to improve survival, however, in women with ER-negative tumors. These results, together with recent data on the efficacy of tamoxifen for chemoprevention, have led to increased use of tamoxifen for premenopausal women and for women with small tumors.

TREATMENT OF NONINVASIVE CANCER

Ductal Carcinoma in Situ

Before mammographic screening was widely practiced, ductal carcinoma in situ (DCIS) was generally identified either as a palpable lesion (usually with comedo histology) or as an incidental finding on a biopsy performed for another lesion. With the increasing use of mammography, DCIS is accounting for a growing proportion of breast cancer cases. The diagnosis of DCIS is now made in 6.6% of all needle-localized breast biopsies and 1.4% of breast biopsies for palpable lesions. About 30% of all mammographically detected malignancies are DCIS.[14]

It was recognized early on that DCIS had a very favorable prognosis compared with other forms of breast cancer: long-term survival approached 100% after treatment with mastectomy. Axillary lymph nodes were positive in only 1% to 2% of patients, most of whom had large or palpable lesions or comedo histology. The prognosis for DCIS continues to be very favorable in relation to that for invasive breast cancers. In theory, there is no potential for metastatic disease with a purely in situ lesion. In practice, however, axillary node metastases continue to be found in 1% to 2% of patients thought to have pure DCIS, presumably arising from a small area of invasion that was missed on pathologic evaluation.

DCIS is believed to be a true anatomic precursor of invasive breast cancer. There are at least two lines of evidence that support this conclusion. First, when DCIS is treated with biopsy alone (usually because it was missed on the initial biopsy and not found until subsequent review), invasive carcinoma develops in 25% to 50% of patients at the site of the initial biopsy; all these tumors appear within 10 years and are of ductal histology. Second, when DCIS recurs locally after breast conservation, invasive ductal carcinoma appears in about 50% of patients. The true relationship between DCIS and invasive ductal carcinoma awaits a better understanding of the molecular biology of breast cancer development.

The consequence of the view that DCIS is a precursor of invasive cancer is that treatment is required once the diagnosis is made. Treatment options for DCIS are similar to those for invasive breast cancer [*see Figure 1*]; however, it should be remembered that although the risk of local recurrence is greater after breast conservation for DCIS than after mastectomy, the likelihood of metastatic disease is very small. Wide excision to microscopically clean margins followed by radiation therapy has become an accepted alternative to mastectomy. Smaller areas of DCIS, particularly of low to intermediate nuclear grade, are increasingly treated with wide excision without radiation.[96] If clean margins cannot be obtained or if the cosmetic result is expected to be poor after excision to clean margins, mastectomy should be performed. The NSABP B-17 study,[97] which examined the role of radiation in the treatment of DCIS, found that the addition of radiation therapy to wide excision reduced the recurrence rate at 43 months after operation by approximately half, from 16.4% with wide excision alone to 7.0% with wide excision and radiation. The report also suggested that the addition of radiation therapy may reduce the incidence of invasive recurrences.

Most patients in whom DCIS is identified mammographically can choose between mastectomy and wide excision with or without radiation, either of which yields excellent long-term survival. Given the lack of any significant difference in survival between the two options, the patient must weigh her feelings about the risk of a local, possibly invasive, recurrence after breast conservation against her feelings about the cosmetic and psychological effects of mastectomy. Mastectomy remains a reasonable treatment even for patients with very small DCIS lesions if the primary concern is to maximize local control of the cancer. Breast reconstruction after mastectomy for DCIS is an option that is open to most such patients.

Axillary dissection is not usually performed in conjunction with lumpectomy for DCIS, because the probability of positive nodes is low: it increases morbidity and expense while providing little prognostic information. On the other hand, low axillary dissection is often included in mastectomy for DCIS: a level I axillary dissection adds little morbidity to a mastectomy, and many surgeons believe

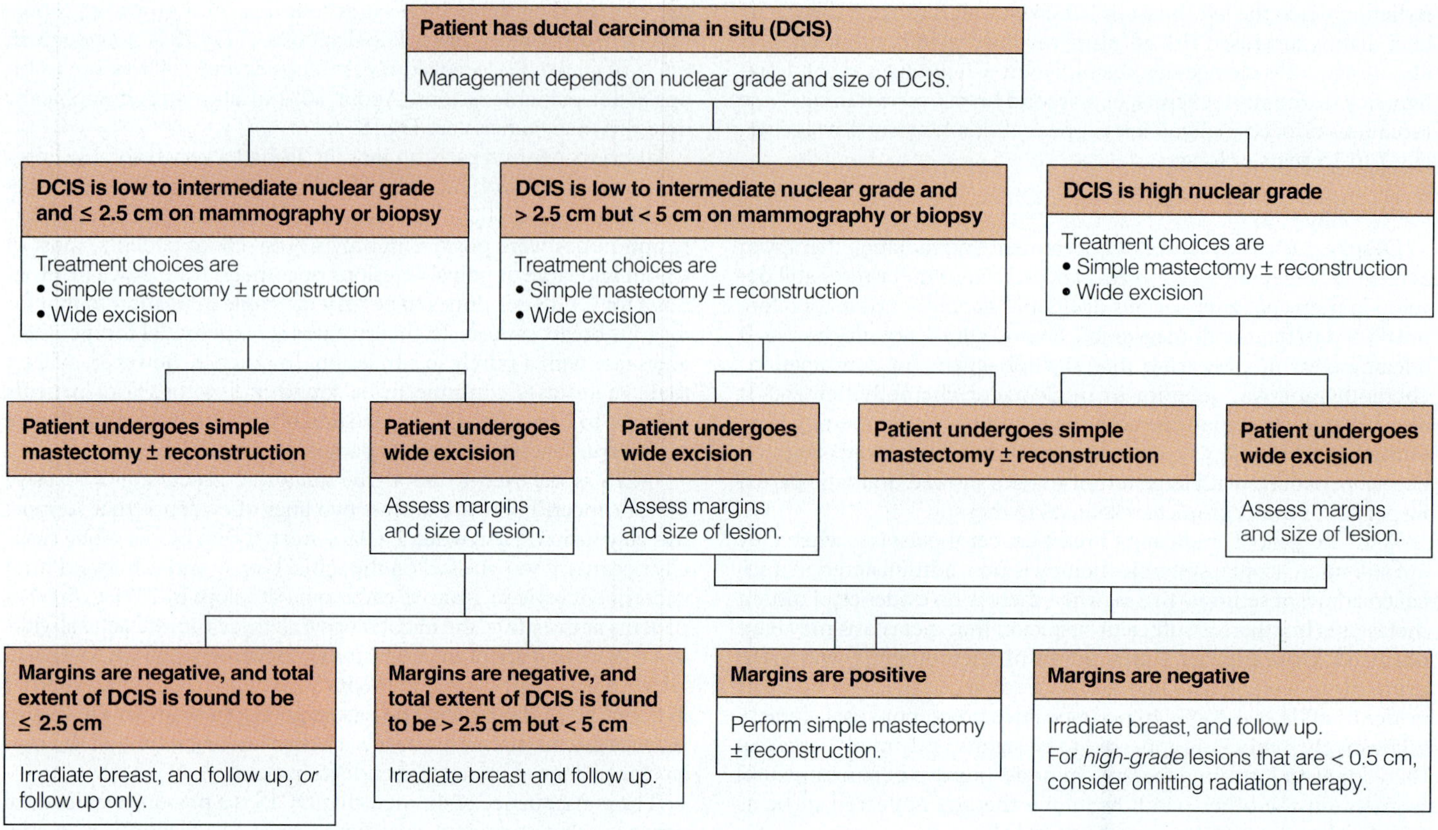

```
┌─────────────────────────────────────────────────┐
│  Patient has ductal carcinoma in situ (DCIS)    │
│  Management depends on nuclear grade and size of DCIS. │
└─────────────────────────────────────────────────┘
```

DCIS is low to intermediate nuclear grade and ≤ 2.5 cm on mammography or biopsy	DCIS is low to intermediate nuclear grade and > 2.5 cm but < 5 cm on mammography or biopsy	DCIS is high nuclear grade
Treatment choices are • Simple mastectomy ± reconstruction • Wide excision	Treatment choices are • Simple mastectomy ± reconstruction • Wide excision	Treatment choices are • Simple mastectomy ± reconstruction • Wide excision

Patient undergoes simple mastectomy ± reconstruction	Patient undergoes wide excision	Patient undergoes wide excision	Patient undergoes simple mastectomy ± reconstruction	Patient undergoes wide excision
	Assess margins and size of lesion.	Assess margins and size of lesion.		Assess margins and size of lesion.

Margins are negative, and total extent of DCIS is found to be ≤ 2.5 cm	Margins are negative, and total extent of DCIS is found to be > 2.5 cm but < 5 cm	Margins are positive	Margins are negative
Irradiate breast, and follow up, *or* follow up only.	Irradiate breast and follow up.	Perform simple mastectomy ± reconstruction.	Irradiate breast, and follow up. For *high-grade* lesions that are < 0.5 cm, consider omitting radiation therapy.

Figure 1 Algorithm illustrates the approach to managing ductal carcinoma in situ.

that dissection must be carried into the low axilla to ensure that the entire axillary tail of the breast is removed.

In some patients with areas of mammographically detected DCIS lesions measuring less than 2.5 cm in diameter, it may be possible to omit radiation therapy, particularly if the lesions do not have comedo histology. Omission of radiation therapy is a complex decision that should be based on the individual patient's histology, the presence or absence of other risk factors, the presence or absence of contraindications to radiation therapy, and the degree to which the patient is willing to accept a higher local recurrence rate. This option is probably best pursued in the context of a clinical trial.

There are certain patients with DCIS for whom mastectomy remains the preferred treatment, such as those who have lesions larger than 5 cm in diameter. Some surgeons would also include those who have comedo lesions larger than 2.5 cm and those who present with palpable DCIS in this category. In these patients, the local recurrence rate after breast conservation, even in conjunction with radiation therapy, remains high. As many as half of these recurrences will contain invasive cancer with metastatic potential. These also are the DCIS patients who are at highest risk for positive axillary nodes. For this reason, an axillary node sampling is often performed in conjunction with the mastectomy.

Lobular Carcinoma in Situ

LCIS, also referred to as lobular neoplasia,[98] does not have the same clinical implications as DCIS, invasive ductal carcinoma, or invasive lobular carcinoma. It is now generally accepted that LCIS is a predictor of increased risk of subsequent invasive breast carcinoma rather than a marker of the site at which the subsequent carcinoma will arise.[13,14] Most of the carcinomas that develop after a biopsy showing LCIS are of ductal histology.[99-101] The increased risk of subsequent carcinoma is equally distributed between the biopsied breast and the contralateral breast and is thought to be between 20% and 25% in patients with LCIS and no other risk factors; it may be additive with other risk factors [*see* Risk Factors for Breast Cancer, *above*]. Because the two breasts are at equal risk for future carcinoma, unilateral mastectomy is inappropriate. Appropriate treatment options include (1) careful observation coupled with physical examination two or three times annually and mammograms annually, (2) prophylactic bilateral simple mastectomies with or without reconstruction, and (3) chemoprevention with tamoxifen or participation in chemoprevention trials with other agents. Most patients choose the first option, but there are some patients for whom prophylactic mastectomy is still preferable, either because of patient anxiety or because of concurrent risk factors.[102]

Management of tumors that contain LCIS mixed with invasive carcinoma of either lobular or ductal histology is dictated primarily by the features of the invasive carcinoma. Staging is not affected by the presence of LCIS.

TREATMENT OF INVASIVE CANCER

Although the optimal treatment regimen for breast cancer continues to be the subject of active investigation, there is at least a partial consensus regarding current treatment options for the various stages of breast cancer.

Early-Stage Invasive Cancer

Local treatment   In patients with stage I or II breast cancer, lumpectomy to microscopically clean margins combined with axillary dissection and radiation therapy [*see Figure 2*] appears to yield approximately the same long-term survival rates as mastectomy. Patients undergoing lumpectomy and radiation are, however, at risk for local recurrence in the treated breast as well as for the development of a new primary tumor in the remaining breast tissue. Local recurrences can generally be managed with mastectomy; overall survival is equivalent to that of women who underwent mastectomy at the time of initial diagnosis. There may, however, be a significant cost to the patient in terms of anxiety about recurrence, as well as the morbidity and potential mortality associated with undergoing a second surgical procedure.

On the other hand, patients who choose mastectomy as their initial surgical treatment face the psychological consequences of losing a breast. Although they are at lower risk for local recurrence than patients who choose lumpectomy, axillary node dissection, and radiation, their overall survival does not seem to be significantly improved. Each physician and each patient must weigh the inconvenience and potential complications of radiation therapy and the risk of local recurrence against the value of breast preservation, keeping in mind that the choice between procedures appears to have no significant effect on survival.

Adjuvant therapy It is generally agreed that adjuvant chemotherapy, adjuvant hormone therapy, or both should be considered for all women with tumors larger than 1 cm in diameter, even those with negative axillary lymph nodes.[94,95] For patients with tumors that have a very favorable prognosis (i.e., that are smaller than 1 cm or have a favorable histology), the potential benefits of adjuvant therapy are probably outweighed by its risks. Tamoxifen therapy is now being reconsidered for women with such low-risk tumors, given recent data[56] on the efficacy of this agent for both treatment and prevention of breast cancers. In premenopausal women, adjuvant therapy should consist of combination chemotherapy, with hormone therapy reserved for clinical trials; in postmenopausal women, hormone therapy (generally consisting of tamoxifen, 10 mg twice daily) is the first-line treatment. Currently, however, the idea that menopause should be an absolute cutoff point for consideration of chemotherapy is being reassessed. For healthy postmenopausal women, particularly those between 50 and 60 years of age, the decision between hormone therapy and chemotherapy plus hormone therapy is made on an individual basis and takes into account the woman's overall health and the specifics of her tumor.

In cases of node-positive disease, combination chemotherapy is used for premenopausal women and for healthy postmenopausal women up to 60 years of age or even older. Hormone therapy is generally the treatment of choice in postmenopausal women who are older than 60 years and in poor health, particularly those with ER-positive tumors. There is currently renewed interest in other hormonal manipulations, such as oophorectomy and chemical castration, for premenopausal women who are at high risk for metastatic disease.[103]

Locally Advanced Cancer

Patients with locally advanced breast cancer include those with primary tumors larger than 5 cm (particularly those with palpable axillary lymph nodes), those with fixed or matted N2 axillary nodes, and those with inflammatory breast carcinoma. These patients are

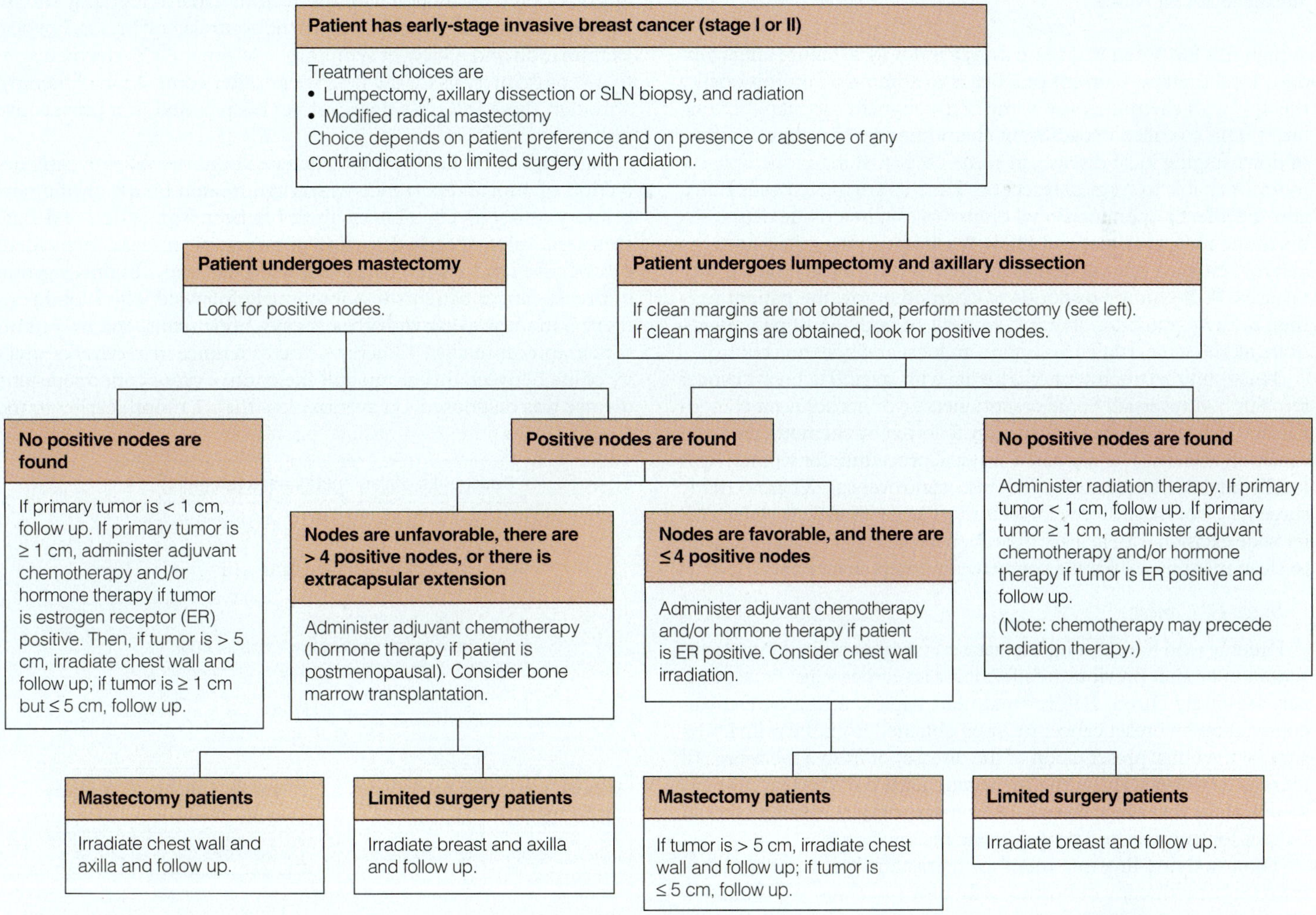

Figure 2 Algorithm illustrates the approach to managing early-stage invasive breast cancer.

```
┌─────────────────────────────────────────┐
│ Patient has locally advanced breast cancer (stage │
│ III or inflammatory carcinoma)          │
├─────────────────────────────────────────┤
│ Perform needle or incisional biopsy to obtain tissue │
│ diagnosis and hormone receptor data.    │
│ Administer "neoadjuvant" chemotherapy.  │
│ Restage to identify distant metastases. │
└─────────────────────────────────────────┘
        │
   ┌────┴────┐
   ▼         ▼
┌──────────────────────┐  ┌──────────────────────┐
│ Metastases are       │  │ No metastases are    │
│ identified on        │  │ identified on        │
│ restaging            │  │ restaging            │
├──────────────────────┤  ├──────────────────────┤
│ Initiate appropriate │  │ Determine whether    │
│ management [see      │  │ tumor is operable.   │
│ Figure 4].           │  │                      │
└──────────────────────┘  └──────────────────────┘
                              │
                         ┌────┴────┐
                         ▼         ▼
                 ┌──────────────────┐  ┌──────────────────────┐
                 │ Tumor is         │  │ Tumor is operable    │
                 │ inoperable       │  ├──────────────────────┤
                 ├──────────────────┤  │ Perform modified     │
                 │ Administer a     │  │ radical mastectomy.  │
                 │ different        │  │ Lumpectomy with      │
                 │ chemotherapy or  │  │ axillary dissection  │
                 │ hormone therapy  │  │ is an option for     │
                 │ regimen.         │  │ some patients.       │
                 │ Restage to       │  │ Consider radiation   │
                 │ assess           │  │ to the chest wall    │
                 │ operability.     │  │ and axilla. (Most    │
                 │                  │  │ patients require     │
                 │                  │  │ both surgery and     │
                 │                  │  │ radiation in         │
                 │                  │  │ addition to          │
                 │                  │  │ chemotherapy.)       │
                 │                  │  │ Follow up.           │
                 └──────────────────┘  └──────────────────────┘
```

Figure 3 Algorithm illustrates the approach to managing locally advanced breast cancer.

at high risk for systemic disease as well as for local failure after standard local therapy. Current practice is to administer multimodality therapy, with chemotherapy as the first treatment modality [*see Figure 3*]. This so-called neoadjuvant chemotherapy often has the effect of downstaging local disease, in some cases making inoperable tumors amenable to surgical resection. Patients are treated with FNA, core-needle, or open incisional biopsy to obtain a tissue diagnosis, hormone receptor data, and HER-2/*neu* status; they then undergo careful restaging after systemic therapy to identify any distant metastases. If the tumor responds to chemotherapy, the patient may then undergo radiation therapy, surgery, or both. Most patients require all three modalities for optimum local and systemic control.

The optimum treatment of patients with stage IIIa breast cancer remains controversial. Some practitioners favor neoadjuvant chemotherapy, whereas others favor surgery followed by chemotherapy and radiation therapy. The choice of surgical procedure for women with locally advanced breast cancer is also controversial. Whereas many surgeons favor mastectomy for all tumors larger than 5 cm, others offer wide excision with axillary dissection to patients in whom excision to clean margins will leave a cosmetically acceptable breast.

Stage IV Cancer

Patients who have distant metastases, whether at their initial presentation or after previous treatment for an earlier-stage breast cancer, are rarely cured. Before treatment begins, a tissue diagnosis consistent with breast cancer must be obtained from the primary lesion (at the initial presentation of the disease) or from a metastasis (if there is any doubt about the metastatic nature of the lesion or the source of the metastatic disease). Any tissue samples obtained should be sent for estrogen and progesterone receptor assays.

The usual first-line treatment for metastatic breast cancer is cytotoxic chemotherapy or hormone therapy [*see Figure 4*]. Radiation therapy may be used to relieve pain from bone metastases or to avert a pathologic fracture at a site of metastatic disease. There is also oc-

casionally a role for so-called toilet mastectomy for patients who have metastatic disease and a locally advanced and ulcerated primary tumor if the condition of the primary tumor prevents the administration of needed chemotherapy.

Treatment for stage IV breast cancer should be on protocol whenever possible. For patients who are ineligible for therapy on protocol, palliative chemotherapy or hormone therapy may be the best treatment option.

FOLLOW-UP AFTER TREATMENT

Patients who have been treated for breast cancer remain at risk for both the recurrence of their original tumor and the development of a new primary breast cancer. The rate of recurrence of breast cancer is nearly linear over the first 10 years after treatment. After the first decade, recurrence becomes less likely, but it continues at a significant rate through the second decade and beyond. In patients who have undergone limited surgery and radiation therapy, radiation-induced breast and chest wall malignancies begin to appear 7 or more years after treatment and continue to appear for at least 20 years after treatment.

Follow-up of breast cancer patients thus includes screening of the breasts and nodal areas for locoregional recurrence or a new primary tumor by means of physical examination and mammography. There is no general agreement on the optimum intervals for follow-up. For patients treated with breast conservation, annual mammography is appropriate, beginning after any acute radiation reaction has resolved (generally 6 to 9 months after completion of radiation therapy). For patients treated with mastectomy, mammography should be continued on an annual basis for the contralateral breast. Physical examination and review of symptoms are generally performed at 3- to 6-month intervals for the first 5 years after completion of therapy, although these intervals have not yet been tested in a prospective fashion.

Although there has been little debate about the value of early detection of a local recurrence within the treated breast or of a new primary tumor in either breast, there has been a great deal of debate about the value of early detection of metastatic disease. Two recent prospective randomized trials addressed this issue. In one, a group of breast cancer patients was intensively followed with blood tests every 3 months along with chest x-rays, bone scans, and liver ultrasonography annually.[104] There was no difference in survival or quality of life between this group and the control group, and metastatic disease was diagnosed, on average, less than 1 month earlier in the

```
┌─────────────────────────────────────────┐
│ Patient has distant metastases (stage IV)│
├─────────────────────────────────────────┤
│ Determine whether patient is eligible for│
│ therapy on protocol.                    │
│ Consider radiation therapy to relieve   │
│ pain from bone marrow metastases or     │
│ avert pathologic fracture at metastatic │
│ site.                                   │
│ Consider "toilet mastectomy" if patient │
│ has locally advanced and ulcerated      │
│ primary tumor that hinders              │
│ administration of chemotherapy.         │
└─────────────────────────────────────────┘
              │
         ┌────┴────┐
         ▼         ▼
┌──────────────────────┐  ┌──────────────────────┐
│ Patient is ineligible│  │ Patient is eligible  │
│ for therapy on       │  │ for therapy on       │
│ protocol             │  │ protocol             │
├──────────────────────┤  ├──────────────────────┤
│ Initiate palliative  │  │ Initiate therapy on  │
│ chemotherapy or      │  │ protocol.            │
│ hormone therapy.     │  │                      │
└──────────────────────┘  └──────────────────────┘
```

Figure 4 Algorithm illustrates the approach to managing stage IV breast cancer.

intensively followed group than in the control group. In the second study, a group of breast cancer patients received chest x-rays and bone scans every 6 months for 5 years.[105] Pulmonary and bone metastases were detected significantly earlier in this group than in the control group, but there was no improvement in survival. This study demonstrated that early detection of metastatic disease could be achieved with short-interval screening, but given current therapeutic options, early detection had no beneficial effect on survival. Both studies concluded that at present, there is no role for routine imaging studies in the follow-up of breast cancer patients and that imaging studies should be ordered only as prompted by clinical findings.

FUTURE DIRECTIONS IN TREATMENT

Efforts continue to be made to minimize the number and extent of invasive treatments for breast cancer without compromising survival or local control. Trials are now under way whose aim is to explore the need for radiation therapy for tumors in elderly women or tumors consisting of pure DCIS. The need for axillary dissection has been questioned, and the idea that features of the primary tumor rather than axillary node status should be used to determine the prognosis and the need for adjuvant therapy is being discussed. Trials of SLN biopsy are under way.

Many current trials of chemotherapy for breast cancer focus on increasing the efficacy of treatment through dose intensification. Very high dose chemotherapy in conjunction with administration of growth factor or autologous bone marrow transplantation is being assessed in the hope that higher doses of chemotherapy will improve response rates and duration of response.

The early results from studies of bone marrow transplantation have been somewhat disappointing: median survival is prolonged by only 7 to 10 months beyond what is achievable with more standard chemotherapy.[106] There is, however, a small but significant group of long-term survivors who remain free of disease for more than 5 years after undergoing bone marrow transplantation to treat breast cancer with 10 or more positive lymph nodes at initial presentation.[105] Trials of improved bone marrow transplantation regimens continue in the hope that the toxicity and cost of the treatment can be reduced and the number of long-term survivors increased.

Immune therapy using antibodies to HER-2/*neu* protein, alone or in conjunction with chemotherapy, is being evaluated for tumors that overexpress the oncogene HER-2/*neu*. At present, there is no definitive evidence that the biologic therapies and immune therapies now available are of significant value in the treatment of breast cancer. These types of therapy continue to be actively explored.

Even more exciting than the prospect of improved therapy is the concept of chemoprevention—that is, the use of pharmacologic, hormonal, or other interventions to prevent the development or progression of a malignancy. Positive results of trials using tamoxifen for chemoprevention have raised hopes that many breast cancers can be prevented and have increased interest in identifying additional agents that can reduce breast cancer risk with minimal side effects. These results underscore the importance of understanding risk factors for breast cancer, including gene mutations, to better identify women who might benefit from chemoprevention.

MULTIDISCIPLINARY BREAST CANCER CARE

Care of even the earliest breast cancers now routinely entails consultation with and treatment by several specialists, including surgeons, radiation oncologists, medical oncologists, radiologists, and pathologists. The selection and timing of individual treatments are determined by this team of physicians in consultation with the patient. This process is greatly simplified when the physicians concerned are able to coordinate their visits with the patient, thereby both saving time for the patient and facilitating decision making among the various specialists. A number of centers have established multidisciplinary breast centers that allow a patient to see all the specialists in a single visit while also allowing the physicians to consult with each other in reviewing the clinical data, imaging studies, and pathology and determining treatment options.

Patient education is also becoming more and more critical in the management of breast cancer. Patients are increasingly being asked to participate in decision making, and as hospital stays for breast cancer treatments become shorter, they are also being asked to participate more actively in their own care. To participate effectively, patients must be educated about the advantages and disadvantages of the various aspects of cancer management. The shifting of a larger proportion of cancer care to the outpatient setting also necessitates the use of other support services, such as visiting nurses, social workers, and outpatient infusion services. How best to coordinate these complex services while maintaining a focus on the problems and needs of the individual patient remains one of the major challenges faced by physicians caring for patients with breast cancer.

References

1. Henderson IC: Risk factors for breast cancer development. Cancer 71(suppl):2127, 1993
2. Slattery ML, Kerber RA: A comprehensive evaluation of family history and breast cancer risk. JAMA 270:1563, 1993
3. Newcomb PA, Storer BE, Longnecker MP, et al: Lactation and a reduced risk of premenopausal breast cancer. N Engl J Med 330:81, 1994
4. Marchant DJ: Estrogen-replacement therapy after breast cancer: risk versus benefits. Cancer 71(suppl):2169, 1993
5. Squitieri R, Tartter PI, Ahmed S, et al: Carcinoma of the breast in postmenopausal hormone user and nonuser control groups. J Am Coll Surg 178:167, 1994
6. Steinberg KK, Thacker SB, Smith SJ, et al: A meta-analysis of the effect of estrogen replacement therapy. JAMA 265:1985, 1991
7. Wingo PA, Lee NC, Ory H, et al: Age specific differences in the relationship between oral contraceptive use and breast cancer. Obstet Gynecol 78:161, 1991
8. Colditz GA, Stampfer MJ, Willett WC: Prospective study of estrogen replacement therapy and risk of breast cancer in post-menopausal women. JAMA 264:2648, 1990
9. Dupont WD, Page DL: Menopausal estrogen-replacement therapy and breast cancer. Arch Intern Med 151:67, 1991
10. Hunter DJ, Manson JE, Colditz GA, et al: A prospective study of the intake of vitamins C, E, and A and the risk of breast cancer. N Engl J Med 329:234, 1993
11. Willett WC, Hunter DJ, Stampfer MJ, et al: Dietary fat and fiber in relation to risk of breast cancer: an 8-year follow-up. JAMA 268:2037, 1992
12. Armstrong B, Doll R: Environmental factors and cancer incidence and mortality in different countries, with special reference to dietary practices. Int J Cancer 15:617, 1975
13. Page DL, Jensen RA: Evaluation and management of high risk and premalignant lesions of the breast. World J Surg 18:32, 1994
14. Frykberg ER, Bland KI: Management of in situ and minimally invasive breast carcinoma. World J Surg 18:45, 1994
15. Jacobs TJ, Byrne C, Colditz G, et al: Radial scars in benign breast-biopsy specimens and the risk of breast cancer. N Engl J Med 340:430, 1999
16. Fletcher SW, Black W, Harris R, et al: Report of the International Workshop on Screening for Breast Cancer. J Natl Cancer Inst 85:1644, 1989
17. Osteen RT, Cady B, Chmiel JS, et al: 1991 national survey of carcinoma of the breast by the Commission on Cancer. J Am Coll Surg 178:213, 1994
18. Surveillance, Epidemiology, and End Results: Incidence and Mortality Data, 1973-1977. DHEW Publ No. (NIH)81-2330. Public Health Service, Bethesda, Maryland, 1981
19. Donegan WL: Evaluation of a palpable breast mass. N Engl J Med 327:937, 1992
20. Rosner D, Blaird D: What ultrasonography can tell in breast masses that mammography and physical examination cannot. J Surg Oncol 28:308, 1985
21. Hamed H, Coady A, Chaudary MA, et al: Follow-up

22. Cowen PN, Benson GA: Cytological study of fluid from benign breast cysts. Br J Surg 66:209, 1979
23. Sartorius O, Smith H, Morris P, et al: Cytologic evaluation of breast fluid in the detection of breast disease. J Natl Cancer Inst 59:1073, 1977
24. Ciatto S, Cariaggi P, Bulgaresi P: The value of routine cytologic examination of breast cyst fluids. Acta Cytol 31:301, 1987
25. Leis HP Jr: Gross breast cysts: significance and management. Contemp Surg 39(2):13, 1991
26. Hughes LE, Bundred NJ: Breast macrocysts. World J Surg 13:711, 1989
27. Boyd NF, Sutherland HJ, Fish EB, et al: Prospective evaluation of physical examination of the breast. Am J Surg 142:331, 1981
28. Layfield LJ, Glasgow BJ, Cramer H: Fine-needle aspiration in the management of breast masses. Pathol Annu 24:23, 1989
29. Silverman JS, Tameness A: Mammary fibroadenoma and some phyllodes tumor stroma are composed of CD34+ fibroblasts and factor XIIIa+ dendrophages. Histopathology 29:411, 1996
30. Dietrich CU: Karyotypic changes in phyllodes tumors of the breast. Cancer Genet Cytogenet 78:200, 1994
31. Noguchi S, Yokouchi H, Aihara T, et al: Progression of fibroadenoma to phyllodes tumor demonstrated by clonal analysis. Cancer 76:1779, 1995
32. Shimizu K: Cytologic evaluation of phyllodes tumors as compared to fibroadenomas of breast. Acta Cytol 38:891, 1994
33. Mangi AA, Smith BL, Gadd MA, et al: Surgical management of phyllodes tumors. Arch Surg 134:487, 1999
34. Hall FM, Storella JM, Silverstone DZ, et al: Nonpalpable breast lesions: recommendations for biopsy based on suspicion of carcinoma at mammography. Radiology 167:353, 1988
35. Sickles EA: Periodic mammographic follow-up of probably benign lesions: results in 3,184 consecutive cases. Radiology 179:463, 1991
36. Wolfe JN, Buck KA, Salane M, et al: Xeroradiography of the breast: overview of 21,057 consecutive cases. Radiology 165:305, 1987
37. Helvie MA, Pennes DR, Rebner M, et al: Mammographic follow-up of low-suspicion lesions: compliance rate and diagnostic yield. Radiology 178:155, 1991
38. Takeda T, Suzuki M, Sato Y, et al: Cytologic studies of nipple discharge. Acta Cytol 26:35, 1982
39. Chaudary M, Millis R, Davies G, et al: Nipple discharge: the diagnostic value of testing for occult blood. Ann Surg 196:651, 1982
40. Urban JA: Excision of the major duct system of the breast. Cancer 16:516, 1963
41. Passaro ME, Broughan TA, Sebek BA, et al: Lactiferous fistula. J Am Coll Surg 178:29, 1994
42. Watt-Boolsen S, Eskildsen P, Blaehr H: Release of prolactin, thyrotropin and growth hormone in women with cyclical mastalgia and fibrocystic disease of the breast. Cancer 56:500, 1985
43. Pashby NL, Mansel RE, Hughes LE, et al: A clinical trial of evening primrose oil in mastalgia. Br J Surg 68:801, 1981
44. Baker H, Snedecor P: Clinical trial of danazol for benign breast disease. Am Surg 45:727, 1979
45. Lauersen N, Wilson K: The effect of danazol in the treatment of chronic cystic mastitis. Obstet Gynecol 48:93, 1976
46. Mansel R, Preece P, Hughes L: A double blind trial of the prolactin inhibitor bromocriptine in painful benign breast disease. Br J Surg 65:724, 1978
47. Fentiman I, Caleffi M, Brame K, et al: Double-blind controlled trial of tamoxifen therapy for mastalgia. Lancet 1:287, 1986
48. Benson EA: Management of breast abscesses. World J Surg 13:753, 1989
49. Niebyl JR, Spence MR, Parmley TH: Sporadic (nonepidemic) puerperal mastitis. J Reprod Med 20:97, 1978
50. Brook I: Microbiology of non-puerperal breast abscesses. J Infect Dis 157:377, 1988
51. Walker AP, Edmiston CE, Krepel CJ, et al: A prospective study of the microflora of nonpuerperal breast abscess. Arch Surg 123:908, 1988
52. Smith BL: Duct ectasia, periductal mastitis, and breast infections. Breast Diseases. Harris JR, Hellman S, Henderson IC, et al, Eds. JB Lippincott Co, Philadelphia, 1991, p 38
53. Hadfield J: Excision of the major duct system for benign disease of the breast. Br J Surg 47:472, 1960
54. Gail MG, Brinton LA, Byar DP, et al: Projecting individualized probabilities of developing breast cancer for white females who are being examined annually. J Natl Cancer Inst 81:1879, 1989
55. Claus EB, Risch N, Thompson WD: Autosomal dominant inheritance of early-onset breast cancer: implications for risk prediction. Cancer 73:643, 1994
56. Tamoxifen for early breast cancer: an overview of the randomised trials. Early Breast Cancer Trialists' Collaborative Group. Lancet 351:1451, 1998
57. Fisher B, Costantino JP, Wickerham DL, et al: Tamoxifen for prevention of breast cancer: report of the National Surgical Adjuvant Breast and Bowel Project P-1 Study. J Natl Cancer Inst 90:1371, 1998
58. Powles T, Eeles R, Ashley S, et al: Interim analysis of the incidence of breast cancer in the Royal Marsden Hospital tamoxifen randomised chemoprevention trial. Lancet 352:98, 1998
59. Veronesi U, Maisonneuve P, Costs A, et al: Prevention of breast cancer with tamoxifen: preliminary findings from the Italian randomised trial among hysterectomised women. Lancet 352:93, 1998
60. Pritchard KI: Is tamoxifen effective in prevention of breast cancer? Lancet 352:80, 1998
61. Jordan VC: Antiestrogenic action of tamoxifen and raloxifene: today and tomorrow. J Natl Cancer Inst 90:967, 1998
62. Hartmann LC, Schaid DJ, Woods JE, et al: Efficacy of bilateral prophylactic mastectomy in women with a family history of breast cancer. N Engl J Med 340:77, 1999
63. Schrag D, Kuntz KM, Garber JE, et al: Decision analysis—effects of prophylactic mastectomy and oophorectomy on life expectancy among women with BRCA1 or BRCA2 mutations. N Engl J Med 336:1465, 1997
64. Lynch HT, Marcus JN, Watson P, et al: Familial breast cancer, family cancer syndromes and predisposition to breast neoplasia. The Breast: Comprehensive Management of Benign and Malignant Diseases. Bland KI, Copeland EM, Eds. WB Saunders Co, Philadelphia, 1991, p 262
65. Veronesi U, Banfi A, DelVecchio M, et al: Comparison of Halstead mastectomy with quadrantectomy, axillary dissection and radiotherapy in early breast cancer: long term results. Eur J Cancer Clin Oncol 22:1085, 1986
66. Sarrazin D, Le M, Rouesse J, et al: Conservative treatment versus mastectomy in breast cancer tumors with macroscopic diameter of 20 millimeters or less: the experience of the Institut Gustave Roussy. Cancer 53:1209, 1984
67. Fisher B, Bauer M, Margolese R, et al: Five-year results of a randomized clinical trial comparing total mastectomy and segmental mastectomy with or without radiation in the treatment of breast cancer. N Engl J Med 312:665, 1985
68. Fisher B, Redmond C, Poisson R, et al: Eight year results of a randomized clinical trial comparing total mastectomy and lumpectomy with or without irradiation in the treatment of breast cancer. N Engl J Med 320:822, 1989
69. Farrow DC, Hunt WC, Samot JM: Geographic variation in the treatment of localized breast cancer. N Engl J Med 326:1097, 1992
70. Nattinger AB, Gottlieb MS, Veum J, et al: Geographic variation in the use of breast-conserving treatment for breast cancer. N Engl J Med 326:1102, 1992
71. Osteen RT, Steele GD, Menck HR, et al: Regional differences in surgical management of breast cancer. Cancer 42:39, 1992
72. Lazovich D, White E, Thomas DB, et al: Underutilization of breast conserving surgery and radiation therapy among women with stage I or II breast cancer. JAMA 266:3433, 1991
73. Lee-Feldstein A, Anton-Culver H, Feldstein PJ: Treatment differences and other prognostic factors related to breast cancer survival: delivery systems and medical outcomes. JAMA 271:1163, 1994
74. Kurtz JM, Spitalier JM, Almaric R, et al: Results of wide excision for local recurrence after breast-conserving therapy. Cancer 61:1969, 1989
75. Haffty GB, Goldberg NB, Rose M, et al: Conservative surgery with radiation therapy in clinical stage I and II breast cancer: results of a 20 year experience. Arch Surg 124:1266, 1989
76. Harris JR, Hellman S, Kinne DW: Limited surgery and radiotherapy for early breast cancer. N Engl J Med 313:1365, 1985
77. Clarke DH, Le M, Sarrazin D, et al: Analysis of local regional relapses in patients with early breast cancers treated by excision and radiotherapy: experience of the Institut Gustave Roussy. Int J Radiat Oncol Biol Phys 11:137, 1985
78. Fisher B, Wolmark N: Limited surgical management for primary breast cancer: a commentary on the NSABP reports. World J Surg 9:682, 1985
79. Holland R, Connolly JL, Gelman R, et al: The presence of an extensive intraductal component following a limited excision correlates with prominent residual disease in the remainder of the breast. J Clin Oncol 8:113, 1990
80. Harris JR, Osteen RT: Patients with early breast cancer benefit from effective axillary treatment. Breast Cancer Res Treat 5:17, 1985
81. Krag D, Weaver D, Ashikaga T, et al: The sentinel node in breast cancer: a multicenter validation study. N Engl J Med 339:941, 1998
82. Giuliano AE, Jones RC, Brennan MM, et al: Sentinel lymphadenectomy in breast cancer. J Clin Oncol 15:2345, 1997
83. McMasters KM, Giuliano AE, Ross MI, et al: Sentinel-lymph node biopsy for breast cancer—not yet the standard of care. N Engl J Med 339:990, 1998
84. Eberlein TJ, Crespo LD, Smith BL, et al: Prospective evaluation of immediate reconstruction following mastectomy. Ann Surg 218:29, 1993
85. Overgaard M, Hansen PS, Overgaard J, et al: Postoperative radiotherapy in high-risk premenopausal women with breast cancer who receive adjuvant chemotherapy. N Engl J Med 337:949, 1997
86. Ragaz J, Jackson SM, Le N, et al: Adjuvant radiotherapy and chemotherapy in node-positive premenopausal women with breast cancer. N Engl J Med 337:956, 1997
87. Bonadonna G, Valagussa P, Tancini G, et al: Current status of Milan adjuvant chemotherapy trials for node-positive and node-negative breast cancer. J Natl Cancer Inst Monogr 1:45, 1986
88. Fisher B, Redmond C, Fisher E, et al: Systemic adjuvant therapy in treatment of primary operable breast cancer: NSABP experience. J Natl Cancer Inst Monogr 1:35, 1986
89. Consensus Conference: Adjuvant chemotherapy for breast cancer. JAMA 254:3461, 1985
90. Fisher B, Costantino J, Redmond C, et al: A randomized trial evaluating tamoxifen in the treatment of patients with node-negative breast cancer who have estrogen-receptor-positive tumors. N Engl J Med 320:479, 1989
91. Clinical Alert from the National Cancer Institute. Department of Human Services, National Cancer Institute, National Institutes of Health, May 16, 1988
92. Fisher B, Redmond C, Dimitrov NV, et al: A ran-

domized clinical trial evaluating sequential methotrexate and fluorouracil in the treatment of patients with node-negative breast cancer who have estrogen-receptor-negative tumors. N Engl J Med 320:473, 1989
93. Mansour EG, Gray R, Shatila NH, et al: Efficacy of adjuvant chemotherapy in high-risk node-negative breast cancer. N Engl J Med 320:485, 1989
94. NIH Consensus Conference: Treatment of early-stage breast cancer. JAMA 265:391, 1991
95. Early Breast Cancer Trialists' Collaborative Group: Systemic treatment of early breast cancer by hormonal, cytotoxic, or immune therapy: 133 randomised trials involving 31,000 recurrences and 24,000 deaths among 75,000 women. Lancet 339:71, 1992
96. Silverstein MJ, Lagios MD, Groshen S, et al: The influence of margin width on local control of ductal carcinoma in situ of the breast. N Engl J Med 340:1455, 1999
97. Fisher B, Costantino J, Redmond C, et al: Lumpectomy compared with lumpectomy and radiation therapy for the treatment of intraductal breast cancer. N Engl J Med 328:1581, 1993
98. Haagensen CD, Lane N, Lattes R, et al: Lobular neoplasia (so-called lobular carcinoma in situ) of the breast. Cancer 42:737, 1978
99. Rosen PP: Lobular carcinoma in situ and intraductal carcinoma of the breast. Monogr Pathol 25:59, 1984
100. Rosen PP, Kosloff C, Lieberman PH, et al: Lobular carcinoma in situ of the breast: detailed analysis of 99 patients with average follow-up of 24 years. Am J Surg Pathol 2:225, 1978
101. Fisher ER, Fisher B: Lobular carcinoma of the breast: an overview. Ann Surg 185:377, 1977
102. Kinne D: Clinical management of lobular carcinoma in situ. Breast Diseases. Harris JR, Hellman S, Henderson IC, et al, Eds. JB Lippincott Co, Philadelphia, 1991, p 239
103. Scottish Cancer Trials Breast Group: Adjuvant ovarian ablation versus CMF chemotherapy in premenopausal women with pathological stage II breast carcinoma: the Scottish trial. Lancet 341:1293, 1993
104. GIVIO Investigators: Impact of follow-up testing on survival and health-related quality of life in breast cancer patients. JAMA 271:1587, 1994
105. Del Turco MR, Palli D, Cariddi A, et al: National Research Council Project on Breast Cancer Follow-up. Intensive diagnostic follow-up after treatment of primary breast cancer: a randomized trial. JAMA 271:1593, 1994
106. Peters WP: High-dose chemotherapy and autologous bone marrow support for breast cancer. Important Advances in Oncology. DeVita VT Jr, Hellman S, Rosenberg SA, Eds. JB Lippincott Co, Philadelphia, 1991, p 135
107. Hammond S, Keyhani-Rofagha S, O'Toole RV: Statistical analysis of fine needle aspiration cytology of the breast: a review of 678 cases plus 4,265 cases from the literature. Acta Cytol 31:276, 1987
108. Dowlatshahi KD, Yaremko ML, Kluskens LF, et al: Nonpalpable breast lesions: findings of stereotaxic needle-core biopsy and fine-needle aspiration cytology. Radiology 181:745, 1991
109. Ballo MS, Sneige N: Can core needle biopsy replace fine needle aspiration cytology in the diagnosis of palpable breast carcinoma: a comparative study of 124 women. Cancer 78:773, 1996
110. Smith DN, Christian R, Meyer JE: Large-core needle biopsy of nonpalpable breast cancers: the impact on subsequent surgical excisions. Arch Surg 132:256, 1997
111. El-Ashry D, Lippman ME: Molecular biology of breast carcinoma. World J Surg 18:12, 1994
112. Slamon DJ, Godolphin W, Jones LA, et al: Studies of the HER-2/neu proto-oncogene in human breast and ovarian cancer. Science 244:707, 1989
113. Gusterson BA, Gelber RD, Goldhirsch A, et al: Prognostic importance of c-erbB-2 expression in breast cancer: International (Ludwig) Breast Cancer Study Group. J Clin Oncol 10:1049, 1992
114. Perren TJ: C-erbB-2 oncogene as a prognostic marker in breast cancer (editorial). Br J Cancer 63:328, 1991
115. Gullick WJ, Love SB, Wright C, et al: C-erbB-2 protein overexpression in breast cancer is a risk factor in patients with involved and uninvolved lymph nodes. Br J Cancer 63:434, 1991
116. American Joint Committee on Cancer: AJCC Cancer Staging Manual, 5th ed. Lippincott-Raven Publishers, Philadelphia, 1997, p 171

Acknowledgments

Figure 1   Marcia Kammerer.
Figures 2 through 4   Talar Agasyan.

ABDOMINAL PAIN CHART

NAME _____ REG. NUMBER _____

MALE _____ FEMALE _____ AGE _____ FORM FILLED BY _____

MODE OF ARRIVAL _____ DATE _____ TIME _____

PAIN

Site of Pain
- At Onset
- At Present

Radiation

Aggravating Factors
- movement
- coughing
- respiration
- food
- other
- none

Relieving Factors
- lying still
- vomiting
- antacids
- food
- other
- none

Progression of Pain
- better
- same
- worse

Duration

Type
- intermittent
- steady
- colicky

Severity
- moderate
- severe

HISTORY

Nausea yes no

Vomiting yes no

Anorexia yes no

Indigestion yes no

Jaundice yes no

Bowels
- normal
- constipation
- diarrhea
- blood
- mucus

Micturition
- normal
- frequency
- dysuria
- dark
- hematuria

Previous Similar Pain yes no

Previous Abdominal Surgery yes no

Drugs for Abdominal Pain yes no

Female-LMP
- pregnant
- vaginal discharge
- dizzy/faint

EXAMINATION

Temp. Pulse
BP

Mood
- normal
- upset
- anxious

Color
- normal
- pale
- flushed
- jaundiced
- cyanotic

Intestinal Movement
- normal
- poor/nil
- peristalsis

Scars yes no

Distention yes no

Location of Tenderness

Rebound yes no

Guarding yes no

Rigidity yes no

Mass yes no

Murphy's Sign Present yes no

Bowel Sounds
- normal
- absent
- increased

Rectal-Vaginal Tenderness
- left
- right
- general
- mass
- none

Initial Diagnosis & Plan

Results
- amylase
- blood count (WBC)
- urine
- x-ray

other

Diagnosis & Plan after Investigation

(time   )

Discharge Diagnosis

History and examination of other systems on separate case notes.

information for the Research Committee of the OMGE and other groups studying acute abdominal pain.[12,13] Given that the data sheet is by no means exhaustive, individual surgeons may want to add to it; however, they would be well advised not to omit any of the symptoms and signs on the data sheet from their routine examination of patients with acute abdominal pain.[14]

When the surgeon obtains a complete clinical history with an open mind, the patient often provides important clues to the correct diagnosis. Patients should be allowed to relate the history in their own words, and examiners should refrain from suggesting specific symptoms, except as a last resort. Any questions that must be asked should be open-ended—for example, "What happens when you eat?" rather than "Does eating make the pain worse?" Leading questions should be avoided. When a leading question must be asked, it should be posed first as a negative question (i.e., one that calls for an answer in the negative), since a negative answer to a question is more likely to be honest and accurate. For example, if peritoneal inflammation is suspected, the question asked should be "Does coughing make the pain better?" rather than "Does coughing make the pain worse?"

The mode of onset of abdominal pain may help the examiner determine the severity of the underlying disease. Pain that has a sudden onset suggests an intra-abdominal catastrophe, such as a ruptured abdominal aortic aneurysm, a perforated viscus, or a ruptured ectopic pregnancy. Rapidly progressive pain that becomes intensely centered in a well-defined area within a period of a few minutes to an hour or two suggests a condition such as acute cholecystitis or pancreatitis. Pain that has a gradual onset over several hours, usually beginning as slight or vague discomfort and slowly progressing to steady and more localized pain, suggests a subacute process and is characteristic of peritoneal inflammation. Numerous disorders may be associated with this mode of onset, including acute appendicitis, diverticulitis, pelvic inflammatory disease (PID), and intestinal obstruction.

Pain can be either intermittent or continuous. Intermittent or cramping pain (colic) is pain that occurs for a short period (a few minutes), followed by longer periods (a few minutes to one-half hour) of complete remission during which there is no pain at all. Intermittent pain is characteristic of obstruction of a hollow viscus and results from vigorous peristalsis in the wall of the viscus proximal to the site of obstruction. This pain is perceived as deep in the abdomen and is poorly localized. The patient is restless, may writhe about incessantly in an effort to find a comfortable position, and often presses on the abdominal wall in an attempt to alleviate the pain. Whereas the intermittent pain associated with intestinal obstruction (typically described as gripping and mounting) is usually severe but bearable, the pain associated with obstruction of small conduits (e.g., the biliary tract, the ureters, and the uterine tubes) often becomes unbearable. Obstruction of the gallbladder or bile ducts gives rise to a type of pain often referred to as biliary colic; however, this term is a misnomer, in that biliary pain is usually constant because of the lack of a strong muscular coat in the biliary tree and the absence of regular peristalsis.

Continuous or constant pain is pain that is present for hours or days without any period of complete relief; it is more common than intermittent pain. Continuous pain is usually indicative of peritoneal inflammation or ischemia. It may be of steady intensity throughout, or it may be associated with intermittent pain. For example, the typical colicky pain associated with simple intestinal obstruction changes when strangulation occurs, becoming continuous pain that persists between episodes or waves of cramping pain.

Certain types of pain are generally held to be typical of certain pathologic states—for example, the general burning pain of a perforated gastric ulcer, the tearing pain of a dissecting aneurysm, and the gripping pain of intestinal obstruction. However, the character of the pain is not always a reliable clue to its cause.

For several reasons—atypical pain patterns, dual innervation by visceral and somatic afferents, normal variations in organ position, and widely diverse underlying pathologic states—the location of abdominal pain is only a rough guide to diagnosis. It is nevertheless true that in most disorders, the pain tends to occur in characteristic locations, such as the right upper quadrant (cholecystitis), the right lower quadrant (appendicitis), the epigastrium (pancreatitis), or the left lower quadrant (sigmoid diverticulitis) [see Figure 2]. It is important to determine the location of the pain at onset because this may differ from the location at the time of presentation (so-called shifting pain). In fact, the chronological sequence of events in the patient's history is often more important for diagnosis than the location of the pain alone. For example, the classic pain of appendicitis begins in the periumbilical region and settles in the right lower quadrant. A similar shift in location can occur when escaping gastroduodenal contents from a perforated ulcer pool in the right lower quadrant.

It is also important to take into account radiation or referral of the pain, which tends to occur in characteristic patterns [see Figure 3]. For example, biliary pain is referred to the right subscapular area, and the boring pain of pancreatitis typically radiates straight through to the back. The more severe the pain is, the more likely it is to be referred.

The intensity or severity of the pain is related to the magnitude of the underlying insult. It is important to distinguish between the intensity of the pain and the patient's reaction to it because there appear to be significant individual differences with respect to tolerance of and reaction to pain. Pain that is intense enough to awaken the patient from sleep usually indicates a significant underlying organic cause. Past episodes of pain and factors that aggravate or relieve the pain often provide useful diagnostic clues. For example, pain caused by peritonitis tends to be exacerbated by motion, deep breathing, coughing, or sneezing, and patients with peritonitis tend to lie quietly in bed and avoid any movement. The typical pain of acute pancreatitis is exacerbated by lying down and relieved by sitting up. Pain that is relieved by eating or taking antacids suggests duodenal ulcer disease, whereas diffuse abdominal pain that appears 30 minutes to 1 hour after meals suggests intestinal angina.

Associated gastrointestinal symptoms, such as nausea, vomiting, anorexia, diarrhea, and constipation, often accompany abdominal pain; however, these symptoms are nonspecific and therefore may not be of great value in the differential diagnosis. Vomiting in particular is common: when sufficiently stimulated by pain impulses traveling via secondary visceral afferent fibers, the medullary vomiting centers activate efferent fibers and cause reflex vomiting. Once again, the chronology of events is important, in that pain often precedes vomiting in patients with conditions necessitating operation, whereas the opposite is usually the case in patients with medical (i.e., nonsurgical) conditions.[4,6] This is particularly true for patients with acute appendicitis, in whom pain almost always precedes vomiting by several hours. Similarly, constipation may result from a reflex paralytic ileus when sufficiently stimulated visceral afferent fibers activate efferent sympathetic fibers (splanchnic nerves) to

Figure 1 Shown on facing page is a data sheet modified from the abdominal pain chart developed by the OMGE.[13]

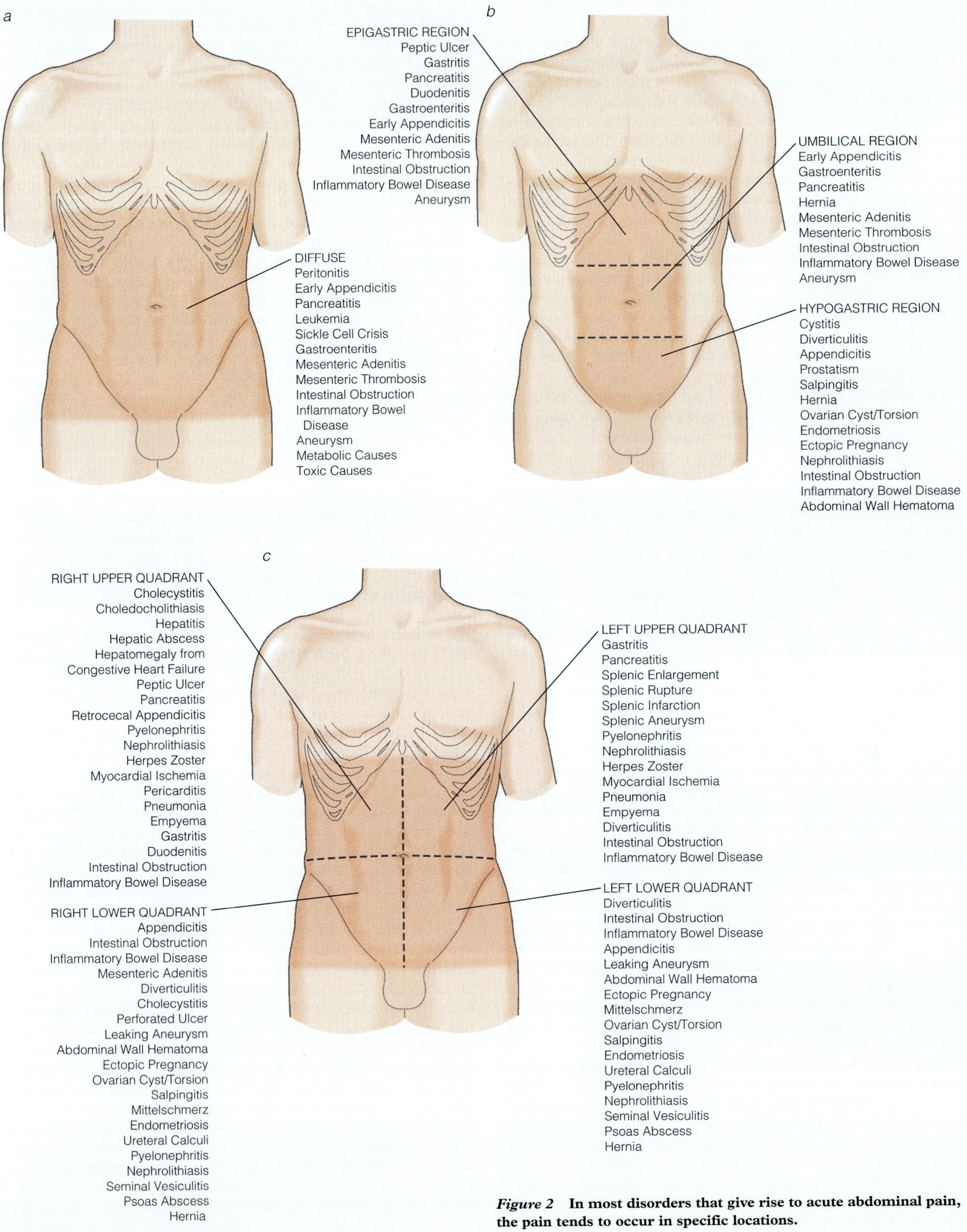

a

DIFFUSE
Peritonitis
Early Appendicitis
Pancreatitis
Leukemia
Sickle Cell Crisis
Gastroenteritis
Mesenteric Adenitis
Mesenteric Thrombosis
Intestinal Obstruction
Inflammatory Bowel Disease
Aneurysm
Metabolic Causes
Toxic Causes

b

EPIGASTRIC REGION
Peptic Ulcer
Gastritis
Pancreatitis
Duodenitis
Gastroenteritis
Early Appendicitis
Mesenteric Adenitis
Mesenteric Thrombosis
Intestinal Obstruction
Inflammatory Bowel Disease
Aneurysm

UMBILICAL REGION
Early Appendicitis
Gastroenteritis
Pancreatitis
Hernia
Mesenteric Adenitis
Mesenteric Thrombosis
Intestinal Obstruction
Inflammatory Bowel Disease
Aneurysm

HYPOGASTRIC REGION
Cystitis
Diverticulitis
Appendicitis
Prostatism
Salpingitis
Hernia
Ovarian Cyst/Torsion
Endometriosis
Ectopic Pregnancy
Nephrolithiasis
Intestinal Obstruction
Inflammatory Bowel Disease
Abdominal Wall Hematoma

c

RIGHT UPPER QUADRANT
Cholecystitis
Choledocholithiasis
Hepatitis
Hepatic Abscess
Hepatomegaly from
 Congestive Heart Failure
Peptic Ulcer
Pancreatitis
Retrocecal Appendicitis
Pyelonephritis
Nephrolithiasis
Herpes Zoster
Myocardial Ischemia
Pericarditis
Pneumonia
Empyema
Gastritis
Duodenitis
Intestinal Obstruction
Inflammatory Bowel Disease

RIGHT LOWER QUADRANT
Appendicitis
Intestinal Obstruction
Inflammatory Bowel Disease
Mesenteric Adenitis
Diverticulitis
Cholecystitis
Perforated Ulcer
Leaking Aneurysm
Abdominal Wall Hematoma
Ectopic Pregnancy
Ovarian Cyst/Torsion
Salpingitis
Mittelschmerz
Endometriosis
Ureteral Calculi
Pyelonephritis
Nephrolithiasis
Seminal Vesiculitis
Psoas Abscess
Hernia

LEFT UPPER QUADRANT
Gastritis
Pancreatitis
Splenic Enlargement
Splenic Rupture
Splenic Infarction
Splenic Aneurysm
Pyelonephritis
Nephrolithiasis
Herpes Zoster
Myocardial Ischemia
Pneumonia
Empyema
Diverticulitis
Intestinal Obstruction
Inflammatory Bowel Disease

LEFT LOWER QUADRANT
Diverticulitis
Intestinal Obstruction
Inflammatory Bowel Disease
Appendicitis
Leaking Aneurysm
Abdominal Wall Hematoma
Ectopic Pregnancy
Mittelschmerz
Ovarian Cyst/Torsion
Salpingitis
Endometriosis
Ureteral Calculi
Pyelonephritis
Nephrolithiasis
Seminal Vesiculitis
Psoas Abscess
Hernia

Figure 2 In most disorders that give rise to acute abdominal pain, the pain tends to occur in specific locations.

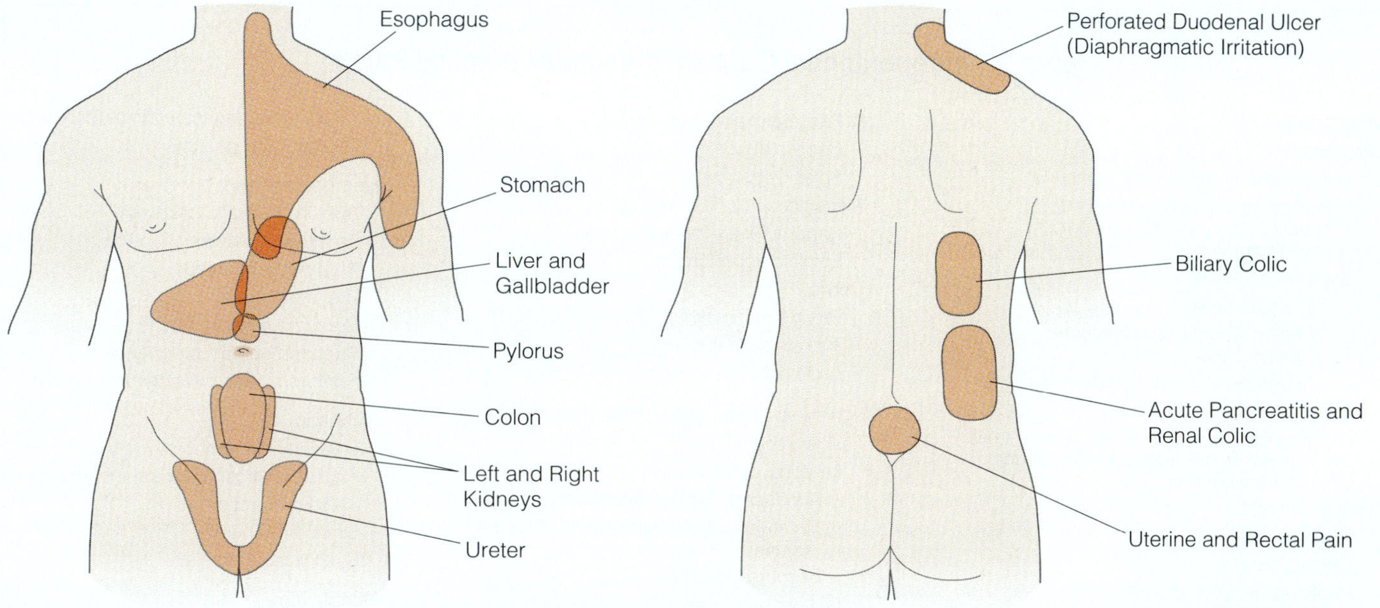

Figure 3 **Pain of abdominal origin tends to be referred in characteristic patterns.[43] The more severe the pain is, the more likely it is to be referred. Shown are anterior (left) and posterior (right) areas of referred pain.**

reduce intestinal peristalsis. Diarrhea is characteristic of gastroenteritis but may also accompany incomplete intestinal obstruction. More significant is a history of obstipation, because if it can be definitely established that a patient with acute abdominal pain has not passed gas or stool for 24 to 48 hours, it is certain that some degree of intestinal obstruction is present. Other associated symptoms that should be noted include jaundice, melena, hematochezia, hematemesis, and hematuria. These symptoms are much more specific than the ones just discussed and can be extremely valuable in the differential diagnosis. Most conditions that cause acute abdominal pain of surgical significance are associated with some degree of fever. Fever suggests an inflammatory process; however, it is usually low grade and often absent altogether, particularly in elderly and immunocompromised patients. The combination of a high fever with chills and rigors indicates bacteremia, and concomitant changes in mental status (e.g., agitation, disorientation, and lethargy) suggest impending septic shock.

A history of trauma (even if the patient considers the traumatic event trivial) should be actively sought in all cases of unexplained acute abdominal pain; such a history may not be readily volunteered (as is often the case with trauma resulting from domestic violence). With female patients, it is essential to obtain a detailed gynecologic history that includes the timing of symptoms within the menstrual cycle, the date of the last menses, previous and current use of contraception, any abnormal vaginal bleeding or discharge, an obstetric history, and any risk factors for ectopic pregnancy (e.g., PID, use of an intrauterine device, or previous ectopic or tubal surgery).

A complete history of previous medical conditions must be obtained because associated diseases of the cardiac, pulmonary, and renal systems may give rise to acute abdominal symptoms and may also significantly affect the morbidity and mortality associated with surgical intervention. Weight changes, past illnesses, recent travel, environmental exposure to toxins or infectious agents, and medications used should also be investigated. A history of previous abdominal operations should be obtained but should not be relied on too heavily in the absence of operative reports. A careful family history is important for detection of hereditary disorders that may cause acute abdominal pain. A detailed social history should also be obtained that includes tobacco, alcohol, or illicit drug use as well as a sexual history.

Tentative Differential Diagnosis

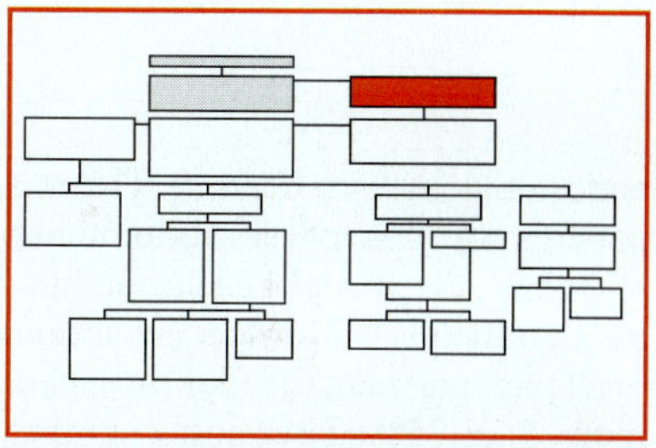

Once the patient's history has been obtained, the examiner should generate a tentative differential diagnosis and carry out the physical examination in search of specific signs or findings that either rule out or confirm the diagnostic possibilities. Given that the list of conditions that can cause acute abdominal pain is almost endless [see Tables 1 and 2], there is no substitute for some general knowledge of what the most common causes of acute abdominal pain are and how age, gender, and geography may affect the likelihood that any of these potential causes is present.

Ambulatory patients with acute abdominal pain as a chief complaint constitute 2% to 3% of all patients in an office practice and 5% to 10% of all patients seen in the emergency department.[4,13,15] At least two thirds of these patients have disorders that do not call for surgical intervention.[2,4,5] Although acute abdominal pain is the most common surgical emergency and most non–trauma-related surgical admissions (and 1% of all hospital admissions) are accounted for by patients complaining of abdominal pain, little information is available regarding the clinical spectrum of disease in these patients.[16] Nevertheless, detailed epidemiologic information can be an invaluable asset in the diagnosis and treatment of acute abdominal pain.

The most extensive information available comes from the ongoing survey begun in 1977 by the Research Committee of the OMGE. As of the last progress report on this survey, which was published in 1988,[12] more than 200 physicians at 26 centers in 17 countries had accumulated data on 10,320 patients with acute

Table 1 Intraperitoneal Causes of Acute Abdominal Pain[44]

Inflammatory
  Peritoneal
    Chemical and nonbacterial peritonitis
      Perforated peptic ulcer/biliary tree, pancreatitis, ruptured ovarian cyst, mittelschmerz
    Bacterial peritonitis
      Primary peritonitis
        Pneumococcal, streptococcal, tuberculous
        Spontaneous bacterial peritonitis
      Perforated hollow viscus
        Esophagus, stomach, duodenum, small intestine, bile duct, gallbladder, colon, urinary bladder
  Hollow visceral
    Appendicitis
    Cholecystitis
    Peptic ulcer
    Gastroenteritis
    Gastritis
    Duodenitis
    Inflammatory bowel disease
    Meckel diverticulitis
    Colitis (bacterial, amebic)
    Diverticulitis
  Solid visceral
    Pancreatitis
    Hepatitis
    Pancreatic abscess
    Hepatic abscess
    Splenic abscess
  Mesenteric
    Lymphadenitis (bacterial, viral)
    Epiploic appendagitis
  Pelvic
    Pelvic inflammatory disease (salpingitis)
    Tubo-ovarian abscess
    Endometritis

Mechanical (obstruction, acute distention)
  Hollow visceral
    Intestinal obstruction
      Adhesions, hernias, neoplasms, volvulus
      Intussusception, gallstone ileus, foreign bodies
      Bezoars, parasites
    Biliary obstruction
      Calculi, neoplasms, choledochal cyst, hemobilia
  Solid visceral
    Acute splenomegaly
    Acute hepatomegaly (congestive heart failure, Budd-Chiari syndrome)
  Mesenteric
    Omental torsion
  Pelvic
    Ovarian cyst
    Torsion or degeneration of fibroid
    Ectopic pregnancy

Hemoperitoneum
  Ruptured hepatic neoplasm
  Spontaneous splenic rupture
  Ruptured mesentery
  Ruptured uterus
  Ruptured graafian follicle
  Ruptured ectopic pregnancy
  Ruptured aortic or visceral aneurysm

Ischemic
  Mesenteric thrombosis
  Hepatic infarction (toxemia, purpura)
  Splenic infarction
  Omental ischemia
  Strangulated hernia

Neoplastic
  Primary or metastatic intraperitoneal neoplasms

Traumatic
  Blunt trauma
  Penetrating trauma
  Iatrogenic trauma
  Domestic violence

Miscellaneous
  Endometriosis

---

abdominal pain [*see Table 3*]. The most common diagnosis in these patients was nonspecific abdominal pain (NSAP)—that is, the retrospective diagnosis of exclusion in which no cause for the pain can be identified.[17,18] Nonspecific abdominal pain accounted for 34% of all patients seen; the four most common diagnoses accounted for more than 75%. The most common surgical diagnosis was acute appendicitis, followed by acute cholecystitis, small bowel obstruction, and gynecologic disorders. Relatively few patients had perforated peptic ulcer, a finding that confirms the recent downward trend in the incidence of this condition. Cancer was found to be a significant cause of acute abdominal pain. There was little variation in the geographic distribution of surgical causes of acute abdominal pain (i.e., conditions necessitating operation) among developed countries. In patients who required operation, the most common causes were acute appendicitis (42.6%), acute cholecystitis (14.7%), small bowel obstruction (6.2%), perforated peptic ulcer (3.7%), and acute pancreatitis (4.5%).[12]

The finding that NSAP is the most common diagnosis in patients with acute abdominal pain has been confirmed by several other clinical studies[4,5,16,19]; the finding that acute appendicitis, cholecystitis, and intestinal obstruction are the three most common diagnoses in patients with acute abdominal pain who require operation has also been amply confirmed[1,4,5,16,19] [*see Table 3*].

The data described so far provide a comprehensive picture of the most likely diagnoses for patients with acute abdominal pain in many centers around the world; however, this picture does not take into account the effect of age on the relative likelihood of the various potential diagnoses. It is well known that the disease spectrum of acute abdominal pain is different in different age groups, especially in the very old and the very young.[20] This variation is apparent when the 10,320 patients from the OMGE study are segregated by age[21] [*see Table 4*]. In patients 50 years of age or older, cholecystitis was more common than either NSAP or acute appendicitis, and small bowel obstruction, diverticular disease, and pancreatitis were all approximately five times more common than in patients younger than 50 years. Hernias were also a much more common problem in older patients. In the entire group of patients, only one of every 10 instances of intestinal obstruction was attributable to a hernia, whereas in patients 50 years of age or older, one of every three instances was caused by an undiagnosed hernia. Cancer was 40 times more likely to be the cause of acute abdominal pain in patients 50 years of age or older; vascular diseases (including myocardial infarction, mesenteric ischemia, and ruptured abdominal aortic aneurysm) were 25 times more common in patients 50 years of age or older and 100 times more common in patients older than 70 years. What is more, outcome was clearly related to age: mortality was significantly higher in patients older than 70 years (5%) than in those younger than 50 years (less than 1%). Whereas the peak incidence of acute abdominal pain occurred in patients in their teens and 20s, the great majority of deaths occurred in patients older than 70 years.[22]

Further analysis of the data from the OMGE survey also makes it clear that the disease spectrum in children is different from that in adults: well over 90% of cases of acute abdominal pain in children are diagnosed as either acute appendicitis (32%) or nonspecific abdominal pain (62%).[22] Similar age-related differences in the spectrum of disease have been confirmed by other studies,[16] as have various gender-related differences.

Knowledge of the most common causes of acute abdominal pain and familiarity with the special circumstances that make particular causes more likely than others allow the surgeon to play the odds.[14] As has often been said, common things are common—or, to put it another way, most people get what most people get.

Physical Examination

In physical examination, as in history taking, there is no substitute for organization and patience; the amount of information that can be obtained is directly proportional to the gentleness and thoroughness of the examiner. The physical examination begins with a brief but thorough evaluation of the patient's general appearance and ability to answer questions. The degree of obvious pain should be estimated. The patient's position in bed should be noted: as an example, a patient who lies motionless with flexed hips and knees is more likely to have generalized peritonitis, whereas a restless patient who writhes about in bed is more likely to have colicky pain, which suggests different diagnoses. The area of maximal pain should be identified before the physical examination is begun. The examiner can easily do this by simply asking the patient to cough and then to point with one finger to the area of maximal pain. This allows the examiner to avoid the area in the early stages of the examination and to confirm it at a later stage without causing the patient unnecessary discomfort in the meantime.

A complete physical examination should be performed and extra-abdominal causes of pain and signs of systemic illness should be sought before attention is directed to the patient's abdomen. Systemic signs of shock, such as diaphoresis, pallor, hypothermia, tachypnea, tachycardia with orthostasis, and frank hypotension, usually accompany a rapidly progressive or advanced intra-abdominal condition and, in the absence of extra-abdominal causes, are an indication for immediate laparotomy. The absence of any alteration in vital signs, however, does not necessarily exclude a serious intra-abdominal process.

The surgeon then begins the abdominal examination. This is done with the patient resting in a comfortable supine position. The examination should include inspection, auscultation, percussion, and palpation of all areas of the abdomen, the flanks, and the groin (including all hernia orifices) in addition to rectal and genital examinations (and, in female patients, a full gynecologic examination). A systematic approach is crucial: an examiner who methodically follows a set pattern of abdominal examination every time will be rewarded more frequently than one who improvises haphazardly with each patient.

Table 2 **Extraperitoneal Causes of Acute Abdominal Pain**

Genitourinary
- Pyelonephritis
- Perinephric abscess
- Renal infarct
- Nephrolithiasis
- Ureteral obstruction (lithiasis, tumor)
- Acute cystitis
- Prostatitis
- Seminal vesiculitis
- Epididymitis
- Orchitis
- Testicular torsion
- Dysmenorrhea
- Threatened abortion

Pulmonary
- Pneumonia
- Empyema
- Pulmonary embolus
- Pulmonary infarction
- Pneumothorax

Cardiac
- Myocardial ischemia
- Myocardial infarction
- Acute rheumatic fever
- Acute pericarditis

Metabolic
- Acute intermittent porphyria
- Familial Mediterranean fever
- Hypolipoproteinemia
- Hemochromatosis
- Hereditary angioneurotic edema

Endocrine
- Diabetic ketoacidosis
- Hyperparathyroidism (hypercalcemia)
- Acute adrenal insufficiency (Addisonian crisis)
- Hyperthyroidism or hypothyroidism

Musculoskeletal
- Rectus sheath hematoma
- Arthritis/diskitis of thoracolumbar spine

Neurogenic
- Herpes zoster
- Tabes dorsalis
- Nerve root compression
- Spinal cord tumors
- Osteomyelitis of the spine
- Abdominal epilepsy
- Abdominal migraine
- Multiple sclerosis

Inflammatory
- Schönlein-Henoch purpura
- Systemic lupus erythematosus
- Polyarteritis nodosa
- Dermatomyositis
- Scleroderma

Infectious
- Bacterial
- Parasitic (malaria)
- Viral (measles, mumps, infectious mononucleosis)
- Rickettsial (Rocky Mountain spotted fever)

Hematologic
- Sickle cell crisis
- Acute leukemia
- Acute hemolytic states
- Coagulopathies
- Pernicious anemia
- Other dyscrasias

Vascular
- Vasculitis
- Periarteritis

Toxins
- Bacterial toxins (tetanus, staphylococcus)
- Insect venom (black widow spider)
- Animal venom
- Heavy metals (lead, arsenic, mercury)
- Poisonous mushrooms
- Drugs
- Withdrawal from narcotics

Retroperitoneal
- Retroperitoneal hemorrhage (spontaneous adrenal hemorrhage)
- Psoas abscess

Psychogenic
- Hypochondriasis
- Somatization disorders

Factitious
- Munchausen syndrome
- Malingering

Table 3 Frequency of Specific Diagnoses in Patients with Acute Abdominal Pain

Diagnosis	Frequency in Individual Studies (% of Patients)					
	OMGE[12] (N = 10,320)	Wilson[19] (N = 1,196)	Irvin[16] (N = 1,190)	Brewer[4] (N = 1,000)	de Dombal[1] (N = 552)	Hawthorn[5] (N = 496)
Nonspecific abdominal pain	34.0	45.6	34.9	41.3	50.5	36.0
Acute appendicitis	28.1	15.6	16.8	4.3	26.3	14.9
Acute cholecystitis	9.7	5.8	5.1	2.5	7.6	5.9
Small bowel obstruction	4.1	2.6	14.8	2.5	3.6	8.6
Acute gynecologic disease	4.0	4.0	1.1	8.5	—	—
Acute pancreatitis	2.9	1.3	2.4	—	2.9	2.1
Urologic disorders	2.9	4.7	5.9	11.4	—	12.8
Perforated peptic ulcer	2.5	2.3	2.5	2.0	3.1	—
Cancer	1.5	—	3.0	—	—	—
Diverticular disease	1.5	1.1	3.9	—	2.0	3.0
Dyspepsia	1.4	7.6	1.4	1.4	—	—
Gastroenteritis	—	—	0.3	6.9	—	5.1
Inflammatory bowel disease	—	—	0.8	—	—	2.1
Mesenteric adenitis	—	3.6	—	—	—	1.5
Gastritis	—	2.1	—	1.4	—	—
Constipation	—	2.4	—	2.3	—	—
Amebic hepatic abscess	1.2	—	1.9	—	—	—
Miscellaneous	6.3	1.3	5.2	15.5	4.0	8.0

The first step in the abdominal examination is careful inspection of the anterior and posterior abdominal walls, the flanks, the perineum, and the genitalia for previous surgical scars (possible adhesions), hernias (incarceration or strangulation), distention (intestinal obstruction), obvious masses (distended gallbladder, abscesses, or tumors), ecchymosis or abrasions (trauma), striae (pregnancy or ascites), everted umbilicus (increased intra-abdominal pressure), visible pulsations (aneurysm), visible peristalsis (obstruction), limitation of movement of the abdominal wall with ventilatory movements (peritonitis), or engorged veins (portal hypertension).

The next step in the abdominal examination is auscultation. Although it is important to note the presence (or absence) of bowel sounds and their quality, auscultation is probably the least rewarding aspect of the physical examination. Severe intra-abdominal conditions, even intra-abdominal catastrophes, may occur in patients with normal bowel sounds, and patients with silent abdomens may have no significant intra-abdominal pathology at all. In general, however, the absence of bowel sounds indicates a paralytic ileus; hyperactive or hypoactive bowel sounds often are variations of normal activity; and high-pitched bowel sounds with splashes, tinkles (echoing as in a large cavern), or rushes (prolonged, loud gurgles) indicate mechanical bowel obstruction.

The third step is percussion to search for any areas of dullness, fluid collections, sections of gas-filled bowel, or pockets of free air under the abdominal wall. Tympany may be present in patients with bowel obstruction or hollow viscus perforation. Percussion can be useful as a way of estimating organ size and of determining the presence of ascites (signaled by a fluid wave or shifting dullness). It is most useful, however, as a means of demonstrating peritoneal irritation (rebound tenderness). The customary technique is to dig the fingers deep into the patient's abdomen and then let go abruptly. This technique is a time-honored one, but it is painful and often misleads the examiner into assuming that an acute process is present when none exists. Gentle percussion over the four quadrants of the abdomen is much better tolerated by the patient; in addition, it is much more accurate in demonstrating rebound tenderness.

The last step, palpation, is the most informative aspect of the physical examination. Palpation of the abdomen must be done very gently to avoid causing additional pain early in the examination. It should begin as far as possible from the area of maximal pain and then should gradually advance toward this area, which should be the last to be palpated. The examiner should place the entire hand on the patient's abdomen with the fingers together and extended, applying pressure with the pulps (not the tips) of the fingers by flexing the wrists and the metacarpophalangeal joints. It is essential to determine whether true involuntary muscle guarding (muscle spasm) is present. This determination is made by means of gentle palpation over the abdominal wall while the patient takes a long, deep breath. If guarding is voluntary, the underlying muscle immediately relaxes under the gentle pressure of the palpating hand. If, however, the patient has true involuntary guarding, the muscle remains in spasm (i.e., taut and rigid) throughout the respiratory cycle (so-called boardlike abdomen). True involuntary guarding is indicative of localized or generalized peritonitis. It must be remembered that muscle rigidity is relative: for example, muscle guarding may be less pronounced or absent in debilitated and elderly patients who have poor abdominal musculature. In addition, the evaluation of muscle guarding is dependent on the patient's cooperation.

Palpation is also useful for determining the extent and severity of the patient's tenderness. Diffuse tenderness indicates generalized peritoneal inflammation. Mild diffuse tenderness without guarding usually indicates gastroenteritis or some other inflammatory intestinal process without peritoneal inflammation. Localized tenderness suggests an early stage of disease with limited peritoneal inflammation.

Careful palpation can elicit several specific signs [see Table 5]—such as the Rovsing sign (associated with acute appendicitis) and the Murphy sign (acute cholecystitis)—that are indicative of localized peritoneal inflammation. Similarly, specific maneuvers can elicit signs of localized peritoneal irritation, such as the psoas sign (associated with retrocecal appendicitis), the obturator sign (pelvic appendicitis), and the Kehr sign (diaphragmatic irritation). One very important maneuver is the Carnett test, in which the patient elevates his or her head off the bed, thus tensing the abdominal muscles. Tenderness to palpation persists when the pain is caused by abdominal wall conditions (e.g., rectal sheath hematoma) but decreases or disappears when the pain is caused by intraperitoneal conditions (the Carnett sign).

Rectal, genital, and (in women) pelvic examinations are an essential part of the evaluation in all patients with acute abdominal pain. The rectal examination should include evaluation of sphincter tone, tenderness (localized versus diffuse), and prostate size and tenderness, as well as a search for the presence of hemorrhoids, masses, fecal impaction, foreign bodies, and gross or occult blood. The genital examination should search for adenopathy, masses, discoloration, edema, and crepitus. The pelvic examination in women should check for vaginal discharge or bleeding, cervical discharge or bleeding, cervical mobility and tenderness, uterine tenderness, uterine size, and adnexal tenderness or masses. Although a carefully performed pelvic examination can be invaluable in differentiating nonsurgical conditions (e.g., PID) from conditions necessitating prompt operation (e.g., acute appendicitis), the possibility that a surgical condition is present should not be prematurely dismissed solely on the basis of a finding of tenderness on pelvic or rectal examination.

Basic Investigative Studies

Although laboratory and radiologic studies rarely, if ever, establish a definitive diagnosis by themselves, they are often useful for confirming the diagnosis suggested by the history and the physical examination.

LABORATORY STUDIES

In all except extremely hemodynamically unstable patients, a complete blood count, blood chemistries, and a urinalysis are routinely obtained. The hematocrit is important in that it allows the surgeon to detect significant changes in plasma volume (e.g., dehydration caused by vomiting, diarrhea, or fluid loss into the peritoneum or the intestinal lumen), preexisting anemia, or bleeding. An elevated white blood cell count is indicative of an inflammatory process and is a particularly helpful finding if associated with a marked left shift; however, the presence or absence of leukocytosis should never be the single deciding factor as to whether the patient should undergo an operation. A low white blood cell count may be a feature of viral infections, gastroenteritis, or NSAP.

Serum electrolyte, blood urea nitrogen, and creatinine concentrations are useful in determining the nature and extent of fluid losses. Blood glucose and other blood chemistries may also be helpful. Liver function tests (serum bilirubin, alkaline phosphatase, and transaminase levels) are mandatory when abdominal pain is suspected to be hepatobiliary in origin. Similarly, amylase and lipase determinations are mandatory when pancreatitis is suspected, although it must be remembered that amylase levels may be low or normal in patients with pancreatitis and may be markedly elevated in patients with other conditions (e.g., intestinal obstruction, mesenteric thrombosis, and perforated ulcer).

Urinalysis may reveal red blood cells (suggestive of renal or ureteral calculi), white blood cells (urinary tract infection or inflammatory processes adjacent to the ureters, such as retrocecal appendicitis), increased specific gravity (dehydration), glucose, ketones (diabetes), or bilirubin (hepatitis). A pregnancy test should be considered in any woman of childbearing age with acute abdominal pain.

An electrocardiogram is mandatory in elderly patients and in patients with a history of atherosclerotic heart disease. Abdominal pain may be a manifestation of myocardial disease, and the physiologic stress of acute abdominal pain can increase myocardial oxygen demands and induce ischemia in patients with coronary artery disease.

RADIOLOGIC STUDIES

In most patients with acute abdominal pain, initial radiologic evaluation should include plain films of the abdomen in the

Table 4 Frequency of Specific Diagnoses in Younger and Older Patients with Acute Abdominal Pain in the OMGE Study[12,21]

Diagnosis	Frequency (% of Patients)	
	Age < 50 Yr (N = 6,317)	Age ≥ 50 Yr (N = 2,406)
Nonspecific abdominal pain	39.5	15.7
Appendicitis	32.0	15.2
Cholecystitis	6.3	20.9
Obstruction	2.5	12.3
Pancreatitis	1.6	7.3
Diverticular disease	< 0.1	5.5
Cancer	< 0.1	4.1
Hernia	< 0.1	3.1
Vascular disease	< 0.1	2.3

Table 5 Common Abdominal Signs and Findings Noted on Physical Examination[7]

Sign or Finding	Description	Associated Clinical Condition(s)
Aaron sign	Referred pain or feeling of distress in epigastrium or precordial region on continued firm pressure over the McBurney point	Acute appendicitis
Ballance sign	Presence of dull percussion note in both flanks, constant on left side but shifting with change of position on right side	Ruptured spleen
Bassler sign	Sharp pain elicited by pinching appendix between thumb of examiner and iliacus muscle	Chronic appendicitis
Beevor sign	Upward movement of umbilicus	Paralysis of lower portions of rectus abdominis muscles
Blumberg sign	Transient abdominal wall rebound tenderness	Peritoneal inflammation
Carnett sign	Disappearance of abdominal tenderness when anterior abdominal muscles are contracted	Abdominal pain of intra-abdominal origin
Chandelier sign	Intense lower abdominal and pelvic pain on manipulation of cervix	Pelvic inflammatory disease
Charcot sign	Intermittent right upper quadrant abdominal pain, jaundice, and fever	Choledocholithiasis
Chaussier sign	Severe epigastric pain in gravid female	Prodrome of eclampsia
Claybrook sign	Transmission of breath and heart sounds through abdominal wall	Ruptured abdominal viscus
Courvoisier sign	Palpable, nontender gallbladder in presence of clinical jaundice	Periampullary neoplasm
Cruveilhier sign	Varicose veins radiating from umbilicus (*caput medusae*)	Portal hypertension
Cullen sign	Periumbilical darkening of skin from blood	Hemoperitoneum (especially in ruptured ectopic pregnancy)
Cutaneous hyperesthesia	Increased abdominal wall sensation to light touch	Parietal peritoneal inflammation secondary to inflammatory intra-abdominal pathology
Dance sign	Slight retraction in area of right iliac fossa	Intussusception
Danforth sign	Shoulder pain on inspiration	Hemoperitoneum (especially in ruptured ectopic pregnancy)
Direct abdominal wall tenderness	—	Localized inflammation of abdominal wall, peritoneum, or an intra-abdominal viscus
Fothergill sign	Abdominal wall mass that does not cross midline and remains palpable when rectus muscle is tense	Rectus muscle hematoma

supine and standing positions and chest radiographs.[23] If the patient is unable to stand, a left lateral decubitus radiograph should be obtained. Like the basic laboratory studies (see above), these plain radiographs may help confirm diagnoses suggested by the history and the physical examination, such as pneumonia (signaled by pulmonary infiltrates); intestinal obstruction (air-fluid levels and dilated loops of bowel); intestinal perforation (pneumoperitoneum); biliary, renal, or ureteral calculi (abnormal calcifications); appendicitis (fecalith); incarcerated hernia (bowel protruding beyond the confines of the peritoneal cavity); mesenteric infarction (air in the portal vein); chronic pancreatitis (pancreatic calcifications); acute pancreatitis (the so-called colon cutoff sign); visceral aneurysms (calcified rim); retroperitoneal hematoma or abscess (obliteration of the psoas shadow); and ischemic colitis (so-called thumbprinting on the colonic wall).

A prospective study published in 1999 evaluated the utility of routine plain abdominal radiographs in the management of adult patients with acute right lower quadrant abdominal pain.[24] The results seem to demonstrate that indiscriminate use of such radiographs in this patient subset is not helpful but that discriminating use in selected patients with clinically suspected small bowel obstruction or urinary symptoms may be worthwhile. Admittedly, plain abdominal radiographs cost relatively little; still, refraining from routinely obtaining them in all patients with suspected acute appendicitis would help reduce the cost of medical care appreciably.

Working Diagnosis

Ideally, the tentative differential diagnosis list generated after the clinical history was obtained should be narrowed down to a working diagnosis by the physical examination and the information provided by the basic laboratory and radiologic studies. Once this working diagnosis has been established, subsequent management depends on the accepted treatment for the particular condition believed to be present. In general, the course of management follows four basic pathways (see below), depending on whether the patient (1) is in need of immediate laparotomy, (2) is believed to have an underlying surgical condition, (3) has an uncertain diagnosis, or (4) is believed to have an underlying nonsurgical condition.

It must be emphasized that the patient must be constantly reevaluated (preferably by the same examiner) even after the working diagnosis has been established. If the patient does not

Table 5 (continued)

Sign or Finding	Description	Associated Clinical Condition(s)
Grey Turner sign	Local areas of discoloration around umbilicus and flanks	Acute hemorrhagic pancreatitis
Iliopsoas sign	Elevation and extension of leg against pressure of examiner's hand causes pain	Appendicitis (retrocecal) or an inflammatory mass in contact with psoas
Kehr sign	Left shoulder pain when patient is supine or in the Trendelenburg position (pain may occur spontaneously or after application of pressure to left subcostal region)	Hemoperitoneum (especially ruptured spleen)
Kustner sign	Palpable mass anterior to uterus	Dermoid cyst of ovary
Mannkopf sign	Acceleration of pulse when a painful point is pressed on by examiner	Absent in factitious abdominal pain
McClintock sign	Heart rate > 100 beats/min 1 hr post partum	Postpartum hemorrhage
Murphy sign	Palpation of right upper abdominal quadrant during deep inspiration results in right upper quadrant abdominal pain	Acute cholecystitis
Obturator sign	Flexion of right thigh at right angles to trunk and external rotation of same leg in supine position result in hypogastric pain	Appendicitis (pelvic appendix); pelvic abscess; an inflammatory mass in contact with muscle
Puddle sign	Alteration in intensity of transmitted sound in intra-abdominal cavity secondary to percussion when patient is positioned on all fours and stethoscope is gradually moved toward flank opposite percussion	Free peritoneal fluid
Ransohoff sign	Yellow pigmentation in umbilical region	Ruptured common bile duct
Rovsing sign	Pain referred to the McBurney point on application of pressure to descending colon	Acute appendicitis
Subcutaneous crepitance	Palpable crepitus in abdominal wall	Subcutaneous emphysema or gas gangrene
Summer sign	Increased abdominal muscle tone on exceedingly gentle palpation of right or left iliac fossa	Early appendicitis; nephrolithiasis; ureterolithiasis; ovarian torsion
Ten Horn sign	Pain caused by gentle traction on right spermatic cord	Acute appendicitis
Toma sign	Right-sided tympany and left-sided dullness in supine position as a result of peritoneal inflammation and subsequent mesenteric contraction of intestine to right side of abdominal cavity	Inflammatory ascites

respond to treatment as expected, the working diagnosis must be reassessed and the possibility that another condition exists must be immediately entertained and investigated by returning to the differential diagnosis list.

Indications for Immediate Laparotomy

A systematic approach to patients with acute abdominal pain is essential because in some patients, action must be taken immediately and there is not enough time for an exhaustive evaluation. As outlined (see above), such an approach should include a brief initial assessment, a complete clinical history, a thorough physical examination, and basic laboratory and radiologic studies. These steps can usually be completed in less than 1 hour and should be insisted on in the evaluation of most patients.

There are, in fact, very few abdominal crises that mandate immediate operation, and even with these conditions, it is still necessary to spend a few minutes on assessing the seriousness of the problem and establishing a probable diagnosis. Among the most common of the abdominal catastrophes that necessitate immediate operation are ruptured abdominal aortic or visceral aneurysms, ruptured ectopic pregnancies, and spontaneous hepatic or splenic ruptures. The relative rarity of such conditions notwithstanding, it must always be remembered that patients with acute abdominal pain may have a progressive underlying intra-abdominal disorder causing the acute pain and that unnecessary delays in diagnosis and treatment can adversely affect outcome, often with catastrophic consequences.

When immediate operation is not called for, the physician must decide whether urgent or nonurgent but early operation is necessary, whether additional tests are required before a decision can be made, whether the patient should be admitted to the hospital for careful observation, or whether nonsurgical treatment is indicated [see Suspected Surgical Abdomen, Uncertain Diagnosis, and Suspected Nonsurgical Abdomen, below].

Suspected Surgical Abdomen

INDICATIONS FOR URGENT LAPAROTOMY OR LAPAROSCOPY

Once a definitive diagnosis has been made, it is easy to decide whether a patient should undergo operation. On occasion, however, a patient must be operated on before a precise diagnosis is reached. In contemporary clinical practice, the misuse or abuse of available technology frequently undermines the importance of sound surgical judgment at the bedside: in particular, too many patients with obvious surgical abdomens are subjected to time-consuming imaging studies before surgical consultation is obtained. *It cannot be emphasized too strongly that although diagnostic accuracy is intellectually satisfying and undoubtedly important, the primary goal in the management of patients with acute abdominal pain is not to arrive at an exact clinicopathologic diagnosis but rather to determine which patients require immediate or urgent surgical intervention.* Indications for immediate laparotomy (see above) are essentially limited to severe hemodynamic instability. Indications for urgent laparotomy are somewhat more numerous.

Urgent laparotomy implies operation within 1 to 2 hours of the patient's arrival; thus, there is usually sufficient time for adequate resuscitation, with proper rehydration and restoration of vital organ function, before the procedure. Indications for urgent laparotomy may be encountered during the physical examination, may be revealed by the basic laboratory and radiologic studies, or may not become apparent until other investigative studies are performed. Involuntary guarding or rigidity during the physical examination, particularly if spreading, is a strong indication for urgent laparotomy. Other indications include increasing severe localized tenderness, progressive tense distention, physical signs of sepsis (e.g., high fever, tachycardia, hypotension, and mental status changes), and physical signs of ischemia (e.g., fever and tachycardia). Basic laboratory and radiologic indications for urgent laparotomy include pneumoperitoneum, massive or progressive intestinal distention, signs of sepsis (e.g., marked or rising leukocytosis, increasing glucose intolerance, and acidosis), and signs of continued hemorrhage (e.g., a falling hematocrit). Additional findings that constitute indications for urgent laparotomy include free extravasation of radiologic contrast material, mesenteric occlusion on angiography, endoscopically uncontrollable bleeding, and positive results from peritoneal lavage (i.e., the presence of blood, pus, bile, urine, or gastrointestinal contents). Acute appendicitis, perforated hollow viscera, and strangulated hernias are examples of common conditions that necessitate urgent laparotomy.

Several studies from the 1990s suggest that laparoscopy is the procedure of choice when the primary clinical diagnosis is acute appendicitis or perforated peptic ulcer.[25-30] In a prospective, randomized trial,[26] Hansen and associates reported that laparoscopic appendectomy is as safe as open appendectomy. Although laparoscopic appendectomy requires a longer operating time (63 minutes versus 40 minutes), it has two advantages: the surgical site infection rate is lower, and patients return to normal activities earlier. Accordingly, we recommend laparoscopic appendectomy as a worthwhile alternative for patients with a clinical diagnosis of acute appendicitis. It has also been shown that diagnostic laparoscopy through the right lower abdominal incision is very helpful in establishing the correct diagnosis in patients who are operated on for suspected acute appendicitis but in whom the appendix is grossly normal.[27]

Laparoscopic treatment of perforated peptic ulcers—either with an omental patch or with sutures[28-30]—is becoming more popular as surgeons gain experience and competence with the technique. Compared with open approaches, laparoscopic repair results in reduced wound pain and respiratory complications as well as earlier return to normal activities.

HOSPITALIZATION AND ACTIVE OBSERVATION

Numerous studies have shown that of all patients admitted for acute abdominal pain, only a minority require immediate or urgent operation.[2,4,5] It is therefore cost-effective as well as prudent to adopt a system of evaluation that allows for thought and investigation before definitive treatment in all patients with acute abdominal pain except those identified early on as needing immediate or urgent laparotomy. The traditional wisdom is that spending time on observation opens the door for complications (e.g., perforating appendicitis, intestinal perforation associated with bowel obstruction, or strangulation of an incarcerated hernia); however, careful clinical trials evaluating active in-hospital observation of patients with acute abdominal pain of uncertain origin have demonstrated that such observation is safe, is not accompanied by an increased incidence of complications, and results in fewer negative laparotomies.[31]

After the initial assessment has been completed, narcotic analgesia for pain relief should not be withheld.[32,33] In appropriately titrated doses, analgesics neither obscure important physical findings nor mask their subsequent development. In fact, some physical signs may be more easily identified after adequate pain relief.[34,35] Severe pain that persists in spite of adequate doses of narcotics suggests a serious condition that is likely to call for operative intervention.[33]

Active observation allows the surgeon to identify most of the patients whose acute abdominal pain is caused by NSAP or various specific nonsurgical conditions. It must be emphasized that active observation means something more than simply admitting the patient to the hospital: it implies an active process of thoughtful, discriminating, and meticulous reevaluation of the patient (preferably by the same examiner) at intervals ranging from minutes to a few hours, to be complemented by appropriately timed additional investigative studies.

Additional investigative studies beyond the basic ones already mentioned should be obtained only if the results are likely to alter or improve patient management significantly. Furthermore, the invasiveness, morbidity, and cost-effectiveness of each additional test must be carefully weighed. More liberal use of supplemental studies is justified in those patients in whom the history and physical findings tend to be less reliable (e.g., the very young, the elderly, the critically ill, or the immunocompromised).

Supplemental studies that may be considered include computed tomography, ultrasonography, diagnostic peritoneal lavage, radionuclide imaging, angiography, magnetic resonance imaging, gastrointestinal endoscopy [*see 47 Gastrointestinal Endoscopy*], and diagnostic laparoscopy. Diagnostic laparoscopy has been recommended when surgical disease is suspected but its probability is not high enough to warrant open laparotomy.[36] It is particularly valuable in young women of childbearing age, in whom gynecologic disorders frequently mimic acute appendicitis.[37] A report by Chung and coworkers showed that diagnostic laparoscopy had the same diagnostic yield as open laparotomy in 55 patients with acute abdomen[38]; 34 (62%) of these patients were safely managed with laparoscopy alone, with no increase in morbidity and with a shorter average hospital stay. Diagnostic laparoscopy has also been shown to be useful in the assessment of acute abdominal pain in ICU patients[39] and patients with AIDS.[40]

Indications for Early or Elective Laparotomy or Laparoscopy

Early laparotomy or laparoscopy (within 24 to 48 hours of the initial evaluation) is reserved for patients whose conditions are not likely to become life threatening if operation is delayed to permit further resuscitation or additional investigative studies. It is often possible to perform early laparotomy or laparoscopy in patients with uncomplicated acute cholecystitis or diverticulitis and those with nonstrangulated incarcerated hernias, thereby preventing the increased patient risk that always accompanies unplanned emergency operations as well as avoiding the logistical impediments to unscheduled surgical procedures in the middle of the night or on weekends or holidays. Similarly, patients with simple uncomplicated intestinal obstructions often benefit from several hours of nasogastric tube decompression and fluid and electrolyte resuscitation.

Elective laparotomy or laparoscopy is reserved for patients whose condition is highly likely to respond to conservative medical management or highly unlikely to become life threatening during prolonged periods (several days or even weeks) of diagnostic evaluation.

Uncertain Diagnosis

Hospitalization and Active Observation

If the diagnosis is unclear, the surgeon's task is to determine whether hospitalization and active observation are necessary or whether outpatient evaluation is an option. All patients with acute abdominal pain and evidence of extracellular fluid deficits, electrolyte imbalances, or sepsis must be hospitalized. Furthermore, any patient with unexplained abdominal symptoms whose condition has not improved within 24 hours of the initial evaluation should be hospitalized.[41]

Supplemental studies are often required for further evaluation and complete workup of patients with uncertain diagnoses and for the exclusion of many medical conditions that do not call for operation. When the diagnosis is not obvious from the history and the physical examination, apparent on the plain radiographs, or suggested by the basic laboratory studies, ultrasonography and CT, both of which are now widely available, should be considered. CT is more useful in the early evaluation of patients with acute abdominal pain because it is not operator dependent, is not hampered by the presence of overlying gas (which transmits sound waves poorly and interferes with ultrasonography), and can be performed rapidly (a complete scan of the abdomen and pelvis takes less than 15 minutes). Although watchful observation with ongoing reexamination is a time-honored approach to the patient with acute abdominal pain of uncertain origin, excessive reliance on this practice or on esoteric physical diagnosis maneuvers (which most medical students have witnessed in awe at one time or another) suggests that the surgeon is unaware of how valuable, rapid, and accurate a CT scan can be in the early diagnosis of these patients.

Diagnostic peritoneal lavage, although most useful in the evaluation of blunt abdominal trauma, may be particularly helpful in obtunded or critically ill patients, whose condition is difficult to assess by means of history taking and physical examination.[42]

Outpatient Evaluation

The epidemiology of acute abdominal pain is such that for every patient who requires hospitalization, there are at least two or three others who have self-limiting conditions for which neither operation nor hospitalization is necessary. Much or all of the evaluation of such patients, as well as any treatment that may be needed, can now be completed in the outpatient department. To treat acute abdominal pain cost-effectively and efficiently, the surgeon must be able not only to identify patients who need immediate or urgent laparotomy or laparoscopy but also to reliably identify those whose condition does not present a serious risk and who therefore can be managed without hospitalization. The reliability and intelligence of the patient, the proximity and availability of medical facilities, and the availability of responsible adults to observe and assist the patient at home are factors that should be carefully considered before the decision is made to evaluate or treat individuals with acute abdominal pain as outpatients.

Suspected Nonsurgical Abdomen

There are numerous disorders that cause acute abdominal pain but do not call for surgical intervention. These nonsurgical conditions are often extremely difficult to differentiate from surgical conditions that present with almost indistinguishable characteristics.[2] For example, the acute abdominal pain of lead poisoning or acute porphyria is difficult to differentiate from the intermittent pain of intestinal obstruction, in that marked hyperperistalsis is the hallmark of both. The pain of acute hypolipoproteinemia may be accompanied by pancreatitis, which, if not recognized, can lead to unnecessary laparotomy. Similarly, acute and prostrating abdominal pain accompanied by rigidity of the abdominal wall and a low hematocrit may lead to unnecessary urgent laparotomy in patients with sickle cell anemia crises. To further complicate the clinical picture, cholelithiasis is also often found in patients with sickle cell anemia.

In addition to numerous extraperitoneal disorders [see Table 2], nonsurgical causes of acute abdominal pain include a wide variety of intraperitoneal disorders, such as acute gastroenteritis (from enteric bacterial, viral, parasitic, or fungal infection), acute gastritis, acute duodenitis, hepatitis, mesenteric adenitis, salpingitis, Fitz-Hugh–Curtis syndrome, mittelschmerz, ovarian cyst, endometritis, endometriosis, threatened abortion, spontaneous bacterial peritonitis, and tuberculous peritonitis. Acute abdominal pain in immunosuppressed patients or patients with AIDS is now encountered with increasing frequency and can be caused by a number of unusual conditions (e.g., cytomegalovirus enterocolitis, opportunistic infections, lymphoma, and Kaposi sarcoma) as well as by the more usual ones.

As noted [see Tentative Differential Diagnosis, *above*], most patients with acute abdominal pain presenting to the office or the emergency department have an underlying nonsurgical condition and do not require operation.[2,4,5] Again, the single most common diagnosis in these patients is NSAP.[5,12,16-19] Although the natural history of NSAP has been well documented (harmless abdominal pain that is relieved in a few days without any treatment), there have been no prospective studies detailing the symptomatology and physical findings associated with this disorder. Furthermore, it remains unclear whether NSAP is in fact a single disease entity or is simply the presenting symptom complex for many different minor and self-limited conditions.[18] A complete clinical history and physical examination, coupled with careful in-hospital observation and a high index of suspicion, will in most cases prevent unnecessary laparotomy in patients with nonsurgical causes of acute abdominal pain. On rare occasions, diagnostic laparoscopy may be employed to prevent unnecessary laparotomy.

Conclusion

In the management of patients with acute abdominal pain, it occasionally happens that even with the aid of considerable clinical acumen and liberal use of diagnostic tests, the surgeon cannot readily determine whether a patient requires operation. In such cases, laparotomy or diagnostic laparoscopy may constitute the definitive, as well as the safest, approach to the evaluation of acute abdominal pain.

References

1. de Dombal FT: Diagnosis of Acute Abdominal Pain, 2nd ed. Churchill Livingstone, London, 1991
2. Purcell TB: Nonsurgical and extraperitoneal causes of abdominal pain. Emerg Med Clin North Am 7:721, 1989
3. Silen W: Cope's Early Diagnosis of the Acute Abdomen, 17th ed. Oxford University Press, New York, 1990
4. Brewer RJ, Golden GT, Hitch DC, et al: Abdominal pain: an analysis of 1,000 consecutive cases in a university hospital emergency room. Am J Surg 131:219, 1976
5. Hawthorn IE: Abdominal pain as a cause of acute admission to hospital. J R Coll Surg Edinb 37:389, 1992
6. Staniland JR, Ditchburn J, de Dombal FT: Clinical presentation of acute abdomen: study of 600 patients. Br Med J 3:393, 1972
7. Hickey MS, Kiernan GJ, Weaver KE: Evaluation of abdominal pain. Emerg Med Clin North Am 7:437, 1989
8. Adams ID, Chan M, Clifford PC, et al: Computer aided diagnosis of acute abdominal pain: a multicentre study. Br Med J 293:800, 1986
9. Paterson-Brown S, Vipond MN: Modern aids to clinical decision-making in the acute abdomen. Br J Surg 77:13, 1990
10. Wellwood J, Johannessen S, Spiegelhalter DJ: How does computer-aided diagnosis improve the management of acute abdominal pain? Ann R Coll Surg Engl 74:40, 1992
11. de Dombal FT: Computers, diagnoses and patients with acute abdominal pain. Arch Emerg Med 9:267, 1992
12. de Dombal FT: The OMGE acute abdominal pain survey. Progress Report, 1986. Scand J Gastroenterol 144(suppl):35, 1988
13. American College of Emergency Physicians: Clinical policy for the initial approach to patients presenting with a chief complaint of nontraumatic acute abdominal pain. Ann Emerg Med 23:906, 1994
14. de Dombal FT: Surgical Decision Making in Practice: Acute Abdominal Pain. Butterworth-Heinemann Ltd, Oxford, 1993, p 65
15. Walters DT, Wendel HF: Abdominal pain. Prim Care 13:3, 1986
16. Irvin TT: Abdominal pain: a surgical audit of 1190 emergency admissions. Br J Surg 76:1121, 1989
17. Jess P, Bjerregaard B, Brynitz S, et al: Prognosis of acute nonspecific abdominal pain: a prospective study. Am J Surg 144:338, 1982
18. Gray DW, Collin J: Non-specific abdominal pain as a cause of acute admission to hospital. Br J Surg 74:239, 1987
19. Wilson DH, Wilson PD, Walmsley RG, et al: Diagnosis of acute abdominal pain in the accident and emergency department. Br J Surg 64:249, 1977
20. Bender JS: Approach to the acute abdomen. Med Clin North Am 73:1413, 1989
21. Telfer S, Fenyo G, Holt PR, et al: Acute abdominal pain in patients over 50 years of age. Scand J Gastroenterol. Suppl 144:47, 1988
22. Dickson JAS, Jones A, Telfer S, et al: Acute abdominal pain in children. Progress Report, 1986. Scand J Gastroenterol. Suppl 144:43, 1988
23. Plewa MC: Emergency abdominal radiography. Emerg Med Clin North Am 9:827, 1991
24. Boleslawski E, Panis Y, Benoist S, et al: Plain abdominal radiography as a routine procedure for acute abdominal pain of the right lower quadrant: prospective evaluation. World J Surg 23:262, 1999
25. Fritts LL, Orlando R: Laparoscopic appendectomy: a safety and cost analysis. Arch Surg 128:521, 1993
26. Hansen JB, Smithers BM, Schache D, et al: Laparoscopic versus open appendectomy: prospective randomized trial. World J Surg 20:17, 1996
27. Schrenk P, Rieger R, Shamiyeh A, et al: Diagnostic laparoscopy through the right lower abdominal incision following open appendectomy. Surg Endosc 13:133, 1999
28. Matsuda M, Nishiyama M, Hanai T, et al: Laparoscopic omental patch repair for the perforated peptic ulcer. Ann Surg 221:236, 1995
29. Tate JJ, Dawson JW, Lau WY, et al: Sutureless laparoscopic treatment of perforated duodenal ulcer. Br J Surg 80:235, 1993
30. Darzi A, Cheshire NJ, Somers SS, et al: Laparoscopic omental patch repair of perforated duodenal ulcer with an automated stapler. Br J Surg 80:1552, 1993
31. Thomson HJ, Jones PF: Active observation in acute abdominal pain. Am J Surg 152:522, 1986
32. Zoltie N, Cust MP: Analgesia in the acute abdomen. Ann R Coll Surg Engl 68:209, 1986
33. Boey JH: The acute abdomen. Current Surgical Diagnosis and Treatment, 10th ed. Way LW, Ed. Appleton & Lange, Norwalk, Connecticut, 1994, p 441
34. Cuschieri A: The acute abdomen and disorders of the peritoneal cavity. Essential Surgical Practice. Cuschieri A, Giles GT, Moosa AR, Eds. Wright PSG, Bristol, 1982, p 885
35. Attard AR, Corlett MJ, Kidner NJ, et al: Safety of early pain relief for acute abdominal pain. BMJ 305:554, 1992
36. Salky BA, Edye MB: The role of laparoscopy in the diagnosis and treatment of abdominal pain syndromes. Surg Endosc 12: 911, 1998
37. Borgstein PJ, Gordijn RV, Eijsbouts QA, et al: Acute appendicitis—a clear-cut case in men, a guessing game in young women: a prospective study on the role of laparoscopy. Surg Endosc 11:923, 1997
38. Chung RS, Diaz JJ, Chari V: Efficacy of routine laparoscopy for the acute abdomen. Surg Endosc 12:219, 1998
39. Orlando R, Crowell KL: Laparoscopy in the critically ill. Surg Endosc 11:1072, 1997
40. Box JC, Duncan T, Ramshaw B, et al: Laparoscopy in the evaluation and treatment of patients with AIDS and acute abdominal complaints. Surg Endosc 11:1026, 1997
41. Hobsley M: An approach to the acute abdomen. Pathways in Surgical Management, 2nd ed. Edward Arnold Ltd, London, 1986
42. Larson FA, Haller CC, Delcore R, et al: Diagnostic peritoneal lavage in acute peritonitis. Am J Surg 164:449, 1992
43. Cheung LY, Ballinger WF: Manifestations and diagnosis of gastrointestinal diseases. Hardy's Textbook of Surgery. Hardy JD, Ed. JB Lippincott Co, Philadelphia, 1983, p 445
44. McFadden DW, Zinner MJ: Manifestations of gastrointestinal disease. Principles of Surgery, 6th ed. Schwartz SI, Shires GT, Spencer FC, Eds. McGraw-Hill, New York, 1994, p 1015

Acknowledgment

Figures 2 and 3   Tom Moore.

15 ABDOMINAL MASS

Romano Delcore, M.D., and Laurence Y. Cheung, M.D.

Evaluation of Abdominal Masses

Abdominal masses are mentioned in some of the earliest known medical writings. The Papyrus Ebers (ca. 1500 B.C.) discusses the differential diagnosis of abdominal masses and describes methods of abdominal examination by palpation.[1] In his *Book of Prognostics* (ca. 400 B.C.), Hippocrates discussed the prognostic significance of abdominal masses:

> That state of the hypochondrium is best when it is free from pain, soft, and of equal size on the right side and the left. But if inflamed, or painful, or distended; or when the right and left sides are of disproportionate sizes; all these appearances are to be dreaded.... Such swellings as are soft, free from pain, and yield to the finger, occasion more protracted crises, and are less dangerous than the others.... Such, then, as are painful, hard, and large, indicate danger of speedy death.[2]

The term abdominal mass generally refers to a palpable mass that is anterior to the paraspinous muscles and is located anywhere between the costal margins, the iliac crests, and the pubic symphysis. An abdominal mass may be noticed initially by the patient or may be discovered by the surgeon as a new finding. In either case, the mass may have been present for days, months, or even years and may be caused by any of a great variety of intra-abdominal, pelvic, or retroperitoneal disorders as well as by any of numerous different abdominal wall lesions.

Occasionally, after examining a patient with an abdominal mass, the surgeon is so certain about the diagnosis that no further investigation is necessary and appropriate management for the condition can be instituted immediately. Conditions that often can be readily diagnosed in this fashion include obesity, ascites, pregnancy, abdominal wall hernias, sebaceous cysts, and lipomas. It must be remembered, however, that even when an experienced clinician is convinced of the presence of a mass, it is still possible that no abnormality exists. In one study, 22% of patients thought to have a palpable mass on the basis of physical examination proved not to have any abnormalities on further investigation.[3]

Most often, the surgeon is confronted with a diagnostic challenge, in which assessing the origin and character of the abdominal mass proves difficult, time consuming, and expensive. This challenge involves not only establishing the correct diagnosis but also determining whether this can be accomplished without operative intervention. Making the correct decision regarding whether to operate on a patient with an abdominal mass requires sound surgical judgment. The decision must be based on a detailed medical and surgical history as well as on a meticulous physical examination. These, in turn, must be guided by experience; a thorough knowledge of the anatomy and physiology of the abdominal wall, abdominal cavity, and retroperitoneum; and a clear understanding of the physiologic and pathologic processes within and around the abdomen. The arrival of new diseases, coupled with the continuous development of new diagnostic technologies, calls for constant broadening of the differential diagnosis and periodic revision of established approaches to the evaluation of abdominal masses.

Clinical History

A careful and methodical clinical history should be obtained that includes the mode of onset, duration, character, location, and chronology of the abdominal mass as well as the presence or absence of any associated symptoms. When the surgeon obtains an unhurried and complete clinical history, the patient often provides all the information needed for making the correct diagnosis. In addition, such a history is often more valuable than any single laboratory or radiologic finding and determines the course of subsequent evaluation and management. Patients should be allowed to relate the history in their own words, and examiners should refrain from suggesting specific chronologies or symptoms except as a last resort. Any questions that must be asked should be open-ended—for example, "When did you first notice a mass?" rather than "Did you just notice the mass?" Leading questions should be avoided. When a leading question must be asked, it should be posed first as a negative question (i.e., one that calls for an answer in the negative), since a negative answer to a question is more likely to be honest and accurate.

Various GI symptoms (e.g., nausea, vomiting, anorexia, diarrhea, constipation, and a decrease in stool caliber) often accompany an abdominal mass. These symptoms are nonspecific but may still be of some value in the differential diagnosis. Other associated symptoms that should be noted are jaundice, melena, hematochezia, hematemesis, hematuria, and menorrhagia. These symptoms are more specific and can be very valuable in the differential diagnosis. Urinary hesitancy or urgency in the presence of a lower abdominal mass may suggest bladder distention secondary to urethral obstruction or urinary retention caused by anticholinergic medications (e.g., phenothiazines). A female patient with a pelvic mass should be asked for a detailed gynecologic history that includes the timing of symptoms within the menstrual cycle, the date of the last menses, previous and current use of contraception, any abnormal vaginal bleeding or discharge, and a complete obstetric history. All patients with abdominal masses should also be asked about previous injuries, however minor: even a traumatic event the patient considers trivial can be diagnostically significant.

Evaluation of Abdominal Masses

Patient presents with abdominal mass

Obtain clinical history

Assess mode of onset, duration, character, location, and chronology.
Look for associated symptoms.
Ask about previous injuries and medical conditions and recent suggestive events (e.g., weight changes, foreign travel).
Obtain family history and (if relevant) gynecologic history.

Generate tentative differential diagnosis

Perform physical examination

Evaluate general appearance; note any pain or discomfort; look for extra-abdominal causes of the mass and signs of systemic illness.
Perform systematic abdominal examination: (1) inspection, (2) auscultation, (3) percussion, (4) palpation.
Determine whether patient has generalized swelling or discrete mass(es).

Patient has generalized abdominal swelling

The most common causes are the six Fs: fat, fluid, flatus, fetus, feces, and fatal growths. Of these, the most common is gaseous distention

Diagnosis is obvious

Working diagnosis guides subsequent evaluation and management.

Diagnosis is unknown

Perform investigative studies

Laboratory: occult blood in stool, electrolytes, creatinine, blood urea nitrogen, liver function tests, urinalysis, complete blood count with differential.
Radiologic: Ultrasonography or CT.

Diagnosis is not established

Perform image-guided percutaneous biopsy.

Biopsy is nondiagnostic

Perform exploratory laparotomy.

Diagnosis is established

Evaluate and treat as appropriate for diagnosis.

```
                    ┌──────────────────────────────┐
                    │  Patient has discrete mass   │
                    └──────────────┬───────────────┘
                                   │
                    ┌──────────────┴───────────────┐
                    │     Diagnosis is obvious     │
                    └──────────────┬───────────────┘
                                   │
        ┌──────────────────────────┴──────────────────────────────┐
┌───────┴──────────────────────────────────┐  ┌───────────────────┴──────────────────────────────┐
│ Patient appears to have distended bladder│  │ Patient does not have distended bladder or stomach│
│ or stomach                               │  │                                                  │
│ Decompress with Foley catheter or NG tube.│ │ Working diagnosis guides subsequent evaluation   │
│                                          │  │ and management.                                  │
└───────┬──────────────────────┬───────────┘  └──────────────────────────────────────────────────┘
        │                      │
┌───────┴───────┐      ┌───────┴────────┐
│ Mass persists │      │ Mass disappears│
└───────────────┘      └────────────────┘
```

243

A complete history of previous medical conditions must be obtained because associated diseases may give rise to abdominal masses and may also significantly affect morbidity and mortality from subsequent surgical intervention. Weight changes suggesting carcinoma, past illnesses, previous abdominal operations, and recent travel (raising the possibility of amebic abscess or parasitic cyst) should also be investigated. A careful family history is important for detection of hereditary disorders that may cause abdominal masses.

Tentative Differential Diagnosis

Once the history has been obtained, the examiner should generate a tentative differential diagnosis and carry out the physical examination in search of specific signs or findings that either confirm or rule out the diagnostic possibilities. Failure to include a broad array of possibilities in the tentative differential diagnosis is a common and often costly mistake. For example, when urinary retention is not considered as part of the early differential diagnosis of a large lower abdominal mass, the patient may undergo needlessly extensive and expensive evaluations.

In the light of the large number of conditions that can give rise to an abdominal mass, the task of arriving at a specific diagnosis can appear overwhelming. To lessen the difficulty of this task, it would be invaluable to have some general knowledge of what the most common causes of abdominal masses are as well as how age, gender, associated symptoms, and geography may affect the likelihood that any of these potential causes is present. Unfortunately, abdominal masses as such usually are not coded in the medical record; rather, specific diseases or definitive diagnoses are coded. Consequently, the true incidence of abdominal mass remains unknown, nor is there much information in the literature regarding the relative frequency with which specific diseases present with an abdominal mass.[4] As of early 1999, only two series had been published that provided a differential diagnosis of abdominal masses based on statistical analysis and relative frequency.[1,5] These two series have now been rendered hopelessly outdated by modern medical practice and the advent of newer diagnostic and therapeutic modalities. Nevertheless, knowledge of the most common disease processes associated with abdominal masses and familiarity with the characteristic signs and symptoms that accompany the most common causes of this presenting symptom can greatly facilitate and shorten the evaluation of patients presenting with abdominal masses.

Physical Examination

In physical examination, as in history taking, there is no substitute for organization and patience; the amount of information that can be obtained is directly proportional to the gentleness and thoroughness of the examiner. As in the evaluation of the acute abdomen [see 14 Acute Abdominal Pain], the physical examination begins with a brief but thorough evaluation of the patient's general appearance. Any obvious pain or associated discomfort should be noted. A complete physical examination should be performed, and possible extra-abdominal causes of the mass as well as signs of systemic illness should be sought before attention is directed to the mass. Systemic signs of shock, such as tachycardia, tachypnea, diaphoresis, pallor, orthostasis, and frank hypotension, usually accompany a rapidly progressive or advanced condition and are an indication for immediate resuscitation and laparotomy. Abdominal masses that may occur in association with systemic signs of shock and that must be recognized as soon as possible include abdominal aortic and other visceral aneurysms, hepatic and splenic subcapsular hematomas, blood-filled pancreatic pseudocysts, and empyema of the gallbladder with associated ascending cholangitis. The abdominal examination should include inspection, auscultation, palpation, and percussion, generally in that order; these maneuvers are described in more detail elsewhere [see 14 Acute Abdominal Pain].

Inspection of the abdomen may reveal either generalized enlargement or distention of the entire abdomen or the presence of one or more discrete masses of varying sizes. Conditions that may give rise to generalized abdominal distention include obesity, tympanites or meteorism (swelling of the abdomen caused by gas within the intestine or peritoneal cavity), ascites, pregnancy, fecal impaction, and neoplasm. An easy way of remembering these conditions is to use the so-called six Fs mnemonic device: Fat, Fluid, Flatus, Fetus, Feces, and Fatal growths.[6-8]

The most common cause of transient generalized enlargement of the abdomen is intestinal gas or bloating. Gaseous distention may appear or disappear in minutes to hours and is usually accompanied by discomfort. Percussion of the abdomen elicits tympany. Because aerophagia and certain foods are common causes of gaseous distention, the differential diagnosis necessitates a detailed dietary history. Intestinal ileus and intestinal obstruction (in particular, distal obstruction) can present with generalized abdominal enlargement resulting from gaseous distention.

The most common cause of chronic abdominal enlargement is obesity. This condition is usually readily apparent on inspection and is confirmed on examination by the greatly increased skinfold thickness of the abdominal wall. When obesity results from adipose tissue in the mesentery, the omentum, and the extraperitoneal layer, the diagnosis may not be so readily apparent. In general, obesity makes evaluation of discrete abdominal masses by means of physical examination much more difficult, to the point where masses of remarkable size can be missed by even the most careful examiner. Massive enlargement of a single organ (e.g., the liver, the spleen, or the kidneys) or a large fluid-filled cyst can also cause generalized abdominal enlargement, as can accumulation of ascitic fluid in the peritoneal cavity. A common and often overlooked cause of an abdominal mass, particularly in elderly or institutionalized patients, is fecal impaction. Removal of the impaction causes the mass to disappear.

A distended urinary bladder may extend up to the level of the umbilicus; it is usually in the midline, and because of its extreme size, it is commonly mistaken for an abdominal mass. The swelling is fluctuant and resolves with catheterization. In cases of acute gastric dilatation, the distended stomach may also occasionally be large enough to all but fill the abdomen. Decompression with a nasogastric tube leads to complete resolution.

When the mass is discrete rather than generalized, the examiner should note whether it moves with respiration; such movement suggests that the mass is associated with a mobile organ in the abdominal cavity rather than located in the retroperitoneum or attached to the abdominal wall. Inspection should be followed by auscultation, before percussion and palpation stimulate the abdominal viscera to abnormal activity that may obscure vascular bruits.

The examination begins with light palpation of the entire abdomen, which may reveal regions of tenderness and increased resistance that should be examined later in detail. Light palpation can determine only the presence of a mass and its location; further information must be sought through deep palpation, which is done to confirm the findings from inspection and light palpation and to search for previously unsuspected masses. Frequently, a mass that is not visible on inspection is easily felt on palpation. Normal structures felt during palpation must not be confused with abdominal masses. Prominent segments of the abdominal wall musculature, the abdominal aorta, and the sacral promontory may be mistaken for abdominal masses on a cursory examination. Masses must also be distinguished from muscle spasms.

During palpation of the mass, every effort should be made to determine as many of the following characteristics as possible: location, size, shape, consistency, surface (smooth or nodular), presence or absence of tenderness, temperature, the color of the overlying skin, degree of mobility, any fixation or attachments, pulsatility, fluctuation, response to ballottement, and appearance on transillumination. Clearly, it is not possible to determine all of these characteristics in every case. Knowing the location of the mass in the abdomen limits the number of possible organs to be considered and may give an insight into the nature and extent of the pathologic process.

Whether the mass is located within the abdominal cavity or in the wall of the abdomen is also an important diagnostic factor. A rectus sheath hematoma is an example of an abdominal wall lesion that is frequently mistaken for an intra-abdominal mass. Masses situated in the abdominal wall itself can be recognized on the basis of their superficial location; their adherence to skin, subcutaneous fascia, or muscles; or their failure to follow the movements of the viscera immediately underlying the abdominal wall. It may, however, be impossible to differentiate an intra-abdominal mass that has become attached to the abdominal wall (as either an inflammatory or a neoplastic process) from an abdominal wall lesion. A simple test that should be done with any patient who has an abdominal mass is to direct the patient to raise the head and shoulders or the legs from the examining table. This maneuver produces tightening of the abdominal muscles. If the mass is in the abdominal wall itself, it remains palpable, but if it is within or behind the abdominal cavity, it is obscured.

Some pathologic processes are suggested by the consistency of the mass and its resistance to pressure: for instance, carcinoma may be rock-hard, whereas an abscess may be soft and fluctuant. A smooth surface implies diffuse involvement, and a nodular surface suggests neoplastic metastases or granulomas. Tenderness may be caused by an acute inflammatory process or by distention of the capsule of a viscus. As noted, mobility with respiration tends to distinguish a peritoneal mass from an extraperitoneal one. Pulsatility should alert the examiner to the possibility that the mass is of vascular origin. Pulsation in the epigastrium of a thin patient is apparent almost routinely on palpation and usually results from the normal pulsation of the aorta lying over the vertebral bodies. In most cases, pulsation associated with an epigastric mass represents a pulsation transmitted through a pancreatic tumor or cyst or a gastric tumor. If, however, pulsation is associated with an expanding mass, it quite possibly represents an abdominal aortic aneurysm. Fluctuation may indicate a cyst, a pseudocyst, a hematoma, or an abscess.

Working Diagnosis

The tentative differential diagnosis list that is generated after the clinical history has been obtained can often be narrowed down to a working diagnosis on the basis of the physical examination. Once a working diagnosis has been established, subsequent management depends on the accepted methods of evaluation and treatment for the particular condition believed to be present. In a number of cases, however, the diagnosis remains unknown even after the physical examination. When this is the case, investigative studies are required. Often, basic investigative studies (e.g., laboratory testing, ultrasonography, or CT) are sufficient to establish the diagnosis. Occasionally, they are not, and further investigative studies are needed.

Investigative Studies

Integrating the information provided by one investigative test with that provided by preceding and subsequent tests yields a higher degree of diagnostic accuracy. Clearly, not every available mode of investigation should be used in each patient. The best evaluative approach in a given case depends somewhat on the preferences of the patient, the physician, and the institution as well as on consideration of relative costs. Most patients with abdominal masses can be evaluated as outpatients, but in making this decision, the examiner must be sure that the patient is both available and reliable. Investigative studies must be individualized so that the examiner can reach an accurate diagnosis in the shortest possible time using the fewest, least invasive, and (ideally) least expensive diagnostic tests possible.

LABORATORY STUDIES

If the cause of the mass can be determined without question on the basis of the history and the physical examination, laboratory evaluation may be unnecessary. If the cause of the abdominal mass remains unknown, the patient should undergo testing for occult blood in the stool, a chemistry profile (which should include at least electrolytes, blood urea nitrogen [BUN], creatinine, and liver function tests), a urinalysis, and a complete blood count with differential. An unexpected abnormal laboratory value may be the only finding that steers the surgeon toward the correct diagnosis. For example, an elevated alkaline phosphatase concentration may suggest metastasis to the liver, and an elevated serum amylase concentration may lead to the diagnosis of a pancreatic pseudocyst.

RADIOGRAPHIC STUDIES

Advances in cross-sectional imaging modalities, such as ultrasonography, CT, and magnetic resonance imaging, have made characterization of abdominal masses relatively simple and direct. The exquisite resolution of these imaging modalities permits accurate diagnosis, and when they are used to guide percutaneous biopsy, they make exploratory laparotomy solely for the purpose of diagnosis unnecessary in almost all instances.[9]

Each imaging modality has its unique strengths and weaknesses. The surgeon must correlate the clinical location of the mass with the history and the laboratory findings to determine which imaging modality is the most expeditious and cost-effective in a given instance. Of the currently available imaging procedures, ultrasonography [see 45 Ultrasonography: Surgical

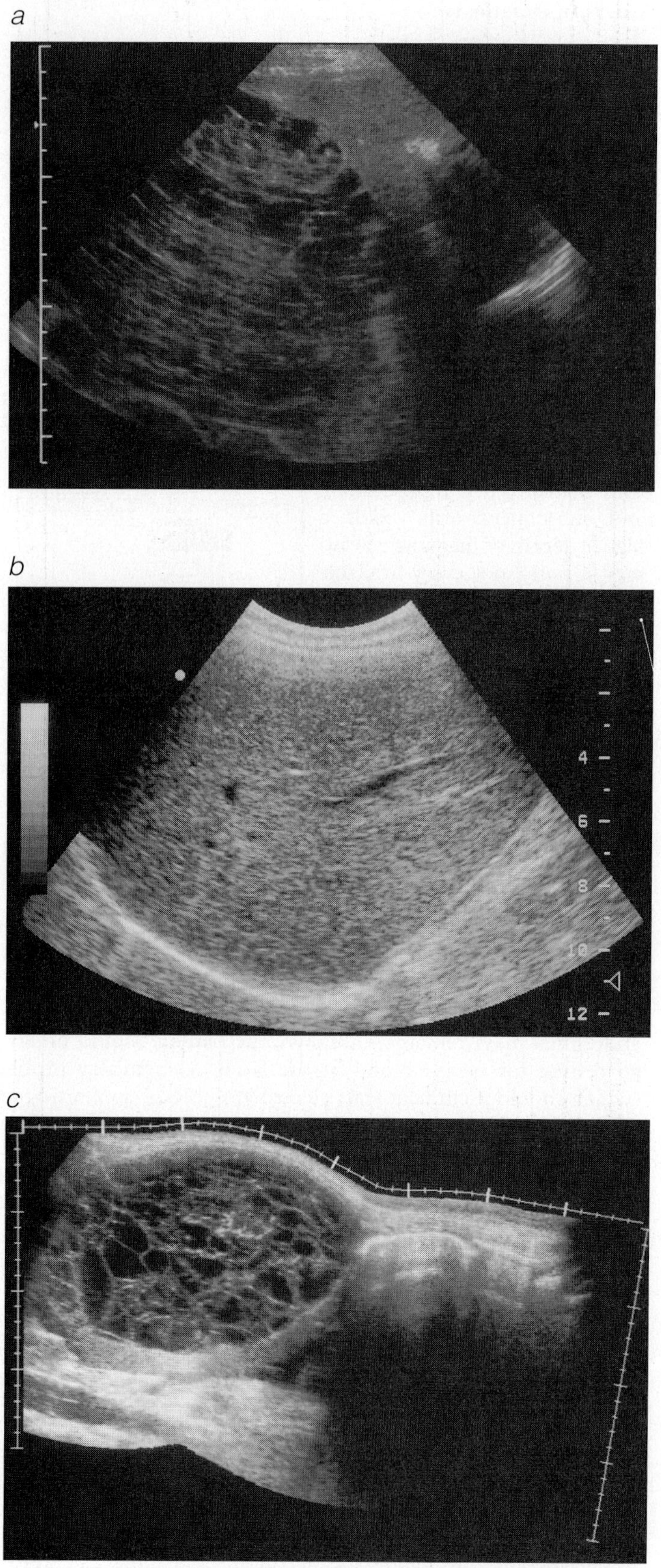

Figure 1 A 51-year-old patient presented with a palpable abdominal mass. (*a*) A transverse ultrasonogram showed a complex, multiply septated peritoneal cyst. A normal transverse ultrasonogram of the same region (*b*) is provided for purposes of comparison. (*c*) A longitudinal ultrasonogram of the same patient shows the cyst from a different viewpoint.

Applications] is the least expensive, the least invasive, and the most readily available. Proper interpretation of ultrasonograms is highly dependent on the skill and experience of the ultrasonographer; however, even examiners who lack great expertise with this modality generally are still able to obtain most of the information they need to evaluate an abdominal mass. The essential information available from the ultrasonogram includes where the mass is anatomically located, whether it is solid or cystic, and on what surrounding structures it impinges [*see Figure 1*]. Once this information is obtained, further imaging procedures are often unnecessary.

Plain Abdominal Radiographs

The plain abdominal radiograph (kidneys-ureters-bladder [KUB]) usually reveals only nonspecific and indirect evidence of a mass, such as alteration in the size or density of an organ or displacement of normal structures or fat planes. Occasionally, however, this low-cost technique can make specific diagnoses, such as a calcified aortic aneurysm, acute gastric distention, fecal impaction, or an enlarged porcelain gallbladder.

Conventional Barium Studies

At one time, barium studies were the best noninvasive method for evaluating abdominal masses. The advent of cross-sectional imaging has relegated barium studies to an adjunctive role in the evaluation of upper abdominal and midabdominal masses because unless a mass arises directly from the alimentary tract, barium studies yield only indirect signs of its presence. Barium studies still play an important role in the evaluation of adult patients with lower abdominal masses whose history suggests GI pathology (e.g., anemia and weight loss, suggesting a colonic neoplasm, or fever and leukocytosis, suggesting a diverticular inflammatory mass).

Excretory Urography

Excretory urography is not recommended as an initial examination in the evaluation of abdominal masses, because unless the mass originates directly from the kidney or bladder, this technique yields only indirect signs, such as displacement or obstruction of the kidney, the ureter, or the bladder.

Angiography

Cross-sectional imaging modalities have relegated arteriography and venography to secondary roles in the evaluation of abdominal masses. The major role of these techniques is to provide a vascular road map for the surgeon before operation.

Radionucleotide Scanning

Cross-sectional imaging has essentially eliminated the use of radionucleotide studies in the evaluation of abdominal masses.

Magnetic Resonance Imaging

MRI can display abdominal masses directly and is excellent at discriminating varying degrees of density in soft tissue. Because MRI is not as widely available as ultrasonography or CT and because its cost-effectiveness in relation to these modalities has not been demonstrated, MRI is not used as a primary imaging modality for abdominal masses.

Ultrasonography

Ultrasonography has several advantages in the evaluation of abdominal masses: widespread availability, speed, absence of ionizing radiation, portability, low cost, and the ability to document a

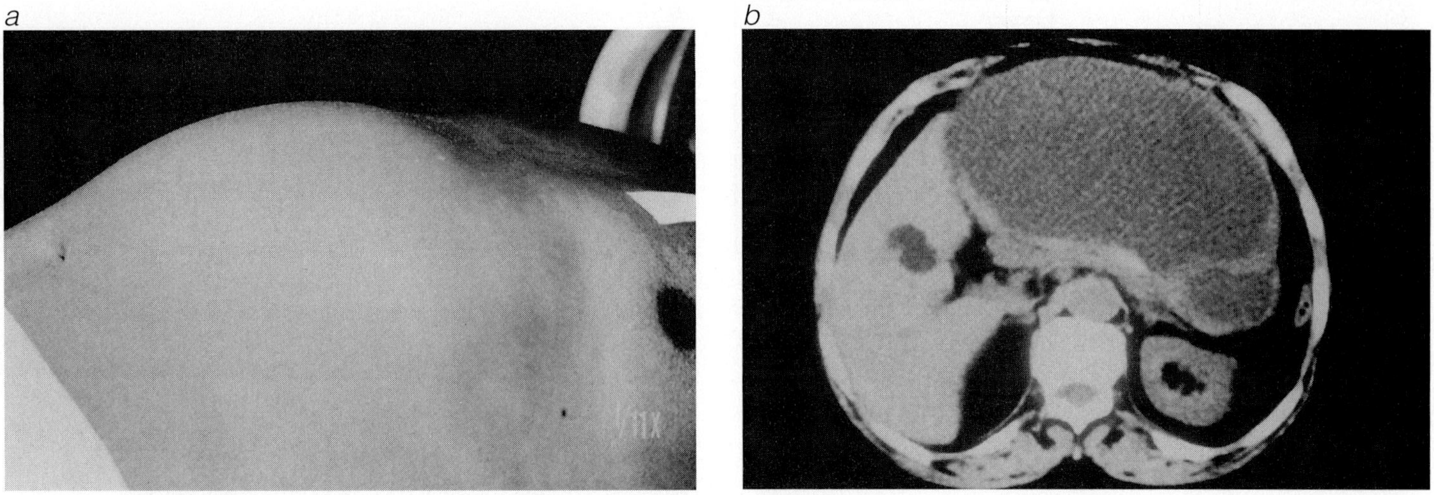

Figure 2 A 58-year-old male patient presented with a palpable, visible (*a*) abdominal mass. (*b*) A CT scan showed a mass arising from the omentum. An omental leiomyosarcoma was surgically resected.

mass's size, consistency, and (usually) origin in real time.[10,11] In addition, the necessary equipment can be transported to the patient's bedside, and the test requires no patient preparation and only minimal patient cooperation.

Ultrasonography can readily differentiate solid from cystic masses, but its ability to visualize the abdominal cavity is limited by the acoustic barriers presented by intestinal gas and bone, which prevent the evaluation of underlying structures. Another limitation is that spatial resolution decreases as depth of penetration increases [*see 45 Ultrasonography: Surgical Applications*]. For these reasons, ultrasonography is most effective in regions where an acoustic window exists, such as the right upper quadrant, the pelvis, and the left upper quadrant.

The principal disadvantage of ultrasonography is its dependence on the technical proficiency of the operator. Because ultrasonography is so operator dependent, it is quite possible that in the hands of an inexperienced ultrasonographer, it can contribute to misdiagnosis. The experience level of the ultrasonographer must always be taken into account when ultrasonography is used in the evaluation of an abdominal mass.

Computed Tomography

Currently, CT is the most efficient imaging modality available for the evaluation of abdominal masses[3,9,12]: it has excellent spatial resolution and exquisite density discrimination, and it provides cross-sectional images that are unaffected by bowel gas, bone, excessive abdominal fat, or unusually large body size [*see Figures 2 and 3*]. CT yields excellent visualization of vascular structures and can assess the vascularity of an abdominal mass after intravenous administration of contrast material. It routinely visualizes retroperitoneal and abdominal wall structures and perfectly displays the peritoneal compartments, clearly defining tissue planes and illustrating relations between masses and adjacent organs and structures.[13-15] If, however, the bowel is not opacified, the accuracy of CT in evaluating abdominal masses is significantly reduced because unopacified intestinal loops can simulate a mass or an abscess.

When the examiner suspects that an abdominal mass is neoplastic, CT is the initial imaging procedure of choice because in addition to imaging the mass itself directly, CT provides invaluable information for staging purposes (e.g., evidence of contiguous spread or the presence of distant metastases).

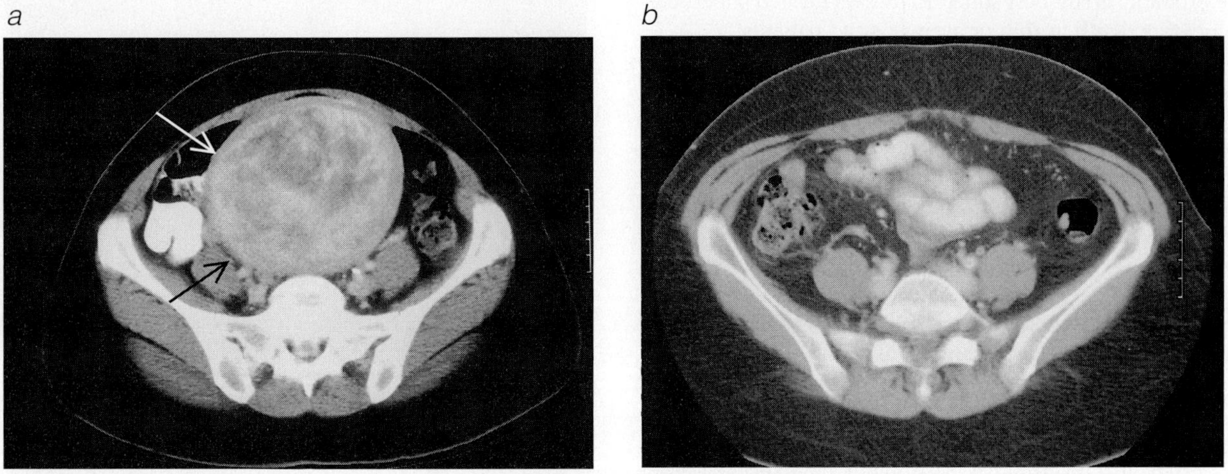

Figure 3 A 49-year-old female patient presented with an abdominal mass. (*a*) A CT scan reveals a uterine fibroid presenting as a pelvic mass. A normal CT of the same region (*b*) is provided for purposes of comparison.

BIOPSY

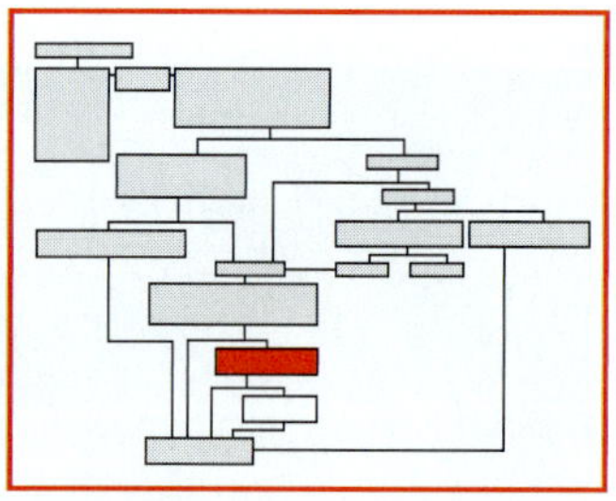

Image-Guided Percutaneous Biopsy

The value of image-guided percutaneous biopsy in the evaluation of abdominal masses is now firmly established.[16,17] Recent improvements in imaging techniques (in particular, developments in high-resolution cross-sectional imaging), advances in cytologic methods (in terms of both performance technique and interpretation of findings) that permit accurate evaluation of minute quantities of aspirated material, and the availability of fine flexible needles for obtaining tissue specimens have all contributed to the rapid growth in the use of this diagnostic method.[18]

Both ultrasonography and CT can be used to guide percutaneous needle insertion.[19-23] The choice between the two depends on several factors, including how large the mass is, where it is, whether it is better visualized with one imaging modality than with the other, and which modality is more readily available. With many masses, either ultrasound guidance or CT guidance will yield good results; in these cases, the choice depends largely on the personal preference and experience of the radiologist performing the biopsy. MRI can also be used to guide needle biopsy, but it has not yet been thoroughly evaluated against ultrasonography and CT in this role.

Traditionally, ultrasound guidance has been used for biopsy of large, superficial, and cystic masses. Currently, however, because of improvements in instrumentation and biopsy techniques, ultrasonography can also accurately guide biopsy of small, deep, and solid masses. The greatest advantage ultrasonography possesses as a guidance modality is that it enables real-time visualization of the needle tip as it passes through tissue planes into the mass. This real-time visualization allows the examiner to place the needle with considerable precision and to avoid important intervening structures. Another advantage ultrasonography has is that it facilitates angled approaches to the mass, in that it is capable of providing guidance in multiple transverse, longitudinal, or oblique planes. In addition, color flow Doppler imaging can identify blood vessels in and around a mass and can prevent complications by helping the examiner to avoid any vascular structures lying in the path of the needle. Theoretically, any mass that is well visualized on an ultrasonogram is amenable to ultrasound-guided biopsy; in practice, however, this technique probably is still best suited to masses located superficially or at moderate depth in thin or average-sized patients.

CT is well established as an accurate guidance method for percutaneous biopsy of most regions of the body. In the abdomen, CT provides excellent spatial resolution of all structures between the skin and the lesion, regardless of how large the patient is or how deep the mass is. Its only limitation is that it does not provide continuous visualization of the needle during insertion and biopsy. In most cases, however, the direction and depth of the needle can be established reliably with CT guidance [*see Figure 4*]; substantial repositioning of the needle is rarely necessary.

Numerous different needles of varying caliber, length, and tip design have been used for percutaneous image-guided biopsy. They can be grouped into two general categories: small caliber (20 to 25 gauge) and large caliber (14 to 19 gauge). Small-caliber needles are employed primarily to obtain specimens for cytologic analysis but may also be employed to obtain small pieces of tissue for histologic examination. Their flexible shafts permit movement of the needle during respiration and minimize the risk of tissue or

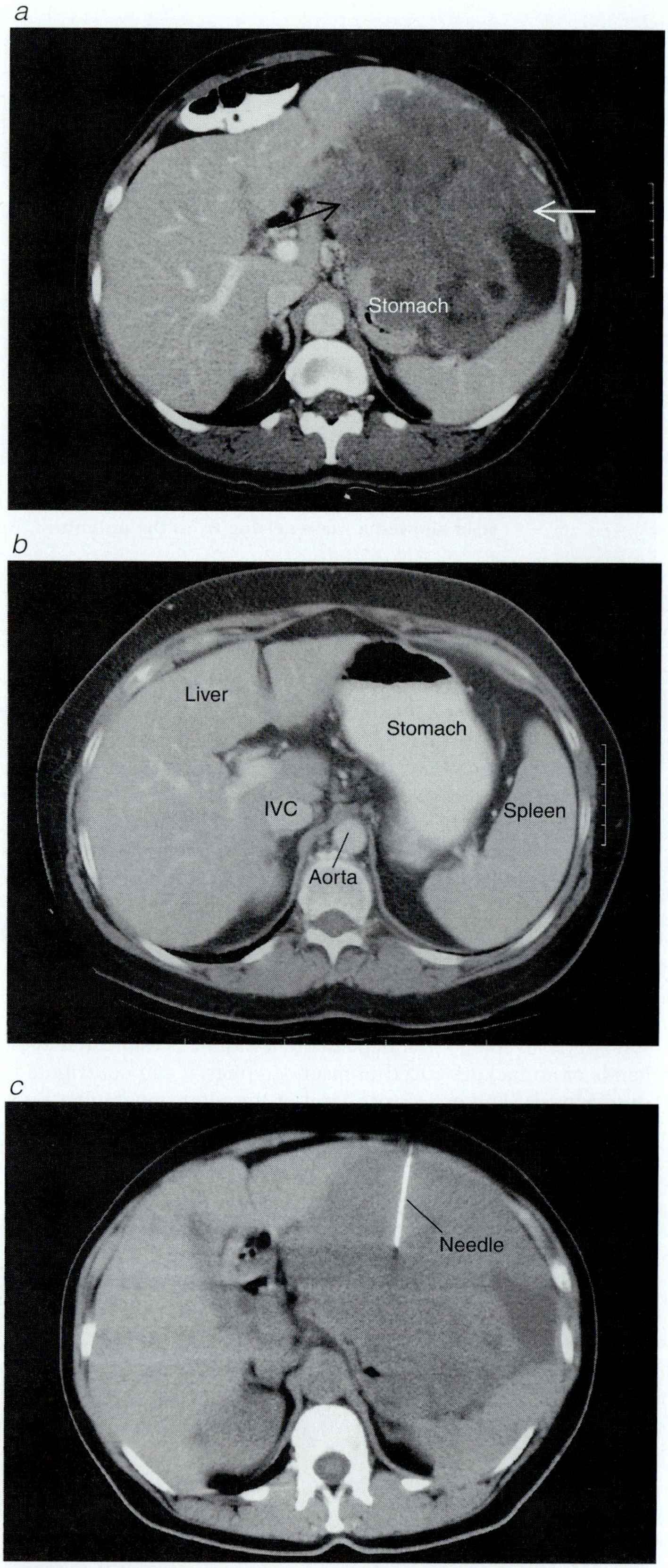

Figure 4 A 51-year-old female patient presented with a palpable abdominal mass. (*a*) A CT scan located a suspicious lesion. A normal CT scan of the same region (*b*) is provided for purposes of comparison. (IVC—inferior vena cava) (*c*) A CT-guided needle biopsy was performed, and the results indicated that the lesion was a gastric leiomyosarcoma.

organ laceration and damage from tearing. The main advantage of these smaller needles is that biopsies of masses situated behind loops of bowel can be done with minimal risk of infection. Large-caliber needles are employed to obtain greater amounts of material for histologic as well as cytologic analysis.

The following three events are relative contraindications to percutaneous biopsy:

1. Uncorrectable coagulopathy. Although postbiopsy embolization of the needle tract is capable of controlling hemorrhage in patients with uncorrectable coagulopathy, special expertise and equipment are required.
2. Absence of a safe biopsy route. When the location of the mass necessitates that the biopsy path extend through a large blood vessel, the stomach, or an intestinal loop, the potential for hemorrhage or infection increases; however, neither potential complication is a contraindication if a small-caliber needle is used. Biopsies done through collections of ascitic fluid have also proved safe.
3. Lack of cooperation on the part of the patient. An uncooperative patient's uncontrolled motion during needle placement can substantially increase the risk of tissue laceration and hemorrhage; in such cases, sedation or anesthesia may be necessary.

The safety of image-guided percutaneous biopsy is well attested.[18,24] Several large multi-institutional reviews have reported mortalities ranging from 0.008% to 0.031% and major complication rates ranging from 0.05% to 0.18%.[25-27] A review of 11,700 patients who underwent percutaneous abdominal biopsy with 20- to 23-gauge needles between 1969 and 1982 found a total complication rate of only 0.05% and a mortality of only 0.008%.[25] Another study, involving 63,180 patients, demonstrated a complication rate of 0.16%.[28] A single-institution review of 8,000 ultrasound-guided needle biopsies done with both large- and small-caliber needles reported similar results: a mortality of 0.038% and a major complication rate of 0.187%.[29] A prospective study of 3,393 biopsies (1,825 ultrasound-guided and 1,568 CT-guided) showed a mortality of 0.06% and a complication rate of 0.34% (0.3% for ultrasound-guided biopsies and 0.5% for CT-guided biopsies).[24]

Of the major complications, hemorrhage is the most commonly reported. Other major complications reported are pneumothorax, pancreatitis, bile leakage, peritonitis, and needle-track seeding. Although needle-track seeding is an important theoretical consideration when a mass seems likely to be of malignant neoplastic origin, it remains an exceedingly rare complication: fewer than 100 cases have been reported in the literature, for an estimated frequency of only 0.005%.[28,30,31] Because seeding is so rare, it should affect the decision to perform percutaneous biopsy only when the surgeon is convinced the lesion is amenable to curative surgical resection. Most cases of needle-track seeding have occurred after biopsy of a pancreatic carcinoma; however, it has also been reported after biopsy of hepatic and retroperitoneal lesions. There is some evidence to suggest that with masses in solid organs, using large-caliber needles or cutting needles does not lead to a significantly higher complication rate than fine-needle aspiration biopsy does, provided that there is a direct path to the mass.[24,32,33]

The reported accuracy of ultrasound-guided biopsy ranges from 66% to 97%, depending on the location, size, and histologic origin of the mass.[24] In one series of ultrasound-guided biopsies of 126 consecutive small (< 3 cm) solid masses in various anatomic locations and of various histologic types, the overall accuracy of biopsy was 91%.[34] Results improved as the size of the mass increased, rising from 79% in masses 1 cm or less in diameter to 98% in masses 2 to 3 cm in diameter. The accuracy of biopsy for hepatic masses of any size was 96%.[34] Another report found ultrasound-guided biopsy to be 91% accurate for small (< 2.5 cm) abdominal masses.[35] Two organ-specific reviews demonstrated 94% accuracy for ultrasound-guided liver biopsy[36] and 95% accuracy for ultrasound-guided biopsy of pancreatic masses.[37]

The reported accuracy of CT-guided biopsy ranges from 80% to 100%, depending on the location, size, and histologic origin of the mass.[21,22,33] In a study of 200 consecutive CT-guided needle biopsies, the overall accuracy for all sites was 95%. Accuracy of diagnosis was very high for hepatic (99%) and renal (100%) biopsies and for characterization of fluid collections (100%) but somewhat lower for retroperitoneal (87.5%) and pancreatic (82%) biopsies.[21] In a prospective study of 1,000 consecutive CT-guided biopsies, the procedure was 91.8% sensitive and 98.9% specific.[33]

Laparoscopic Biopsy

Even though laparoscopy provides excellent visualization of the inside of the abdominal cavity and now plays an important role in the staging of some abdominal neoplasms, its role in the evaluation of abdominal masses is limited.[38] Laparoscopic biopsy specimens are best obtained under direct vision with a biopsy needle introduced at an independent site rather than with a biopsy forceps: forceps biopsy usually produces superficial, small, squeezed, and distorted specimens. Although percutaneous biopsies of this type can be especially useful when bleeding from the biopsy site is a concern, image-guided percutaneous biopsy usually offers a more expedient, less invasive, cheaper, and often safer means of obtaining the diagnosis. More important, in the presence of adhesions, laparoscopic biopsy is much less effective and typically fails to make a diagnosis altogether unless the mass is clearly visible on the anterior surface of the viscera.

Exploratory Laparotomy

Despite recent advances in diagnostic imaging and laparoscopic procedures, it still occasionally proves necessary to perform an exploratory laparotomy for the sole purpose of establishing a diagnosis in the patient with an abdominal mass. It is essential to keep in mind, however, that many patients with abdominal masses have disorders for which operative intervention is not required. In addition, although exploratory laparotomy can yield crucial information and may be, in a sense, the "ultimate diagnostic test" (as some have referred to it), it is not infallible. Errors in the intra-abdominal surgical diagnosis of abdominal masses can and do occur. For example, in six instances observed during an 18-month period at a single institution, exploratory laparotomy failed to reveal abdominal masses that had already been demonstrated by preoperative evaluation and were subsequently confirmed during the postoperative period.[39]

Conclusion

Management of the patient with an abdominal mass ultimately depends on the accurate tissue diagnosis established by microscopic examination of histologic specimens obtained from the mass. To obtain an adequate tissue sample safely, without subjecting the patient to an otherwise unnecessary laparotomy, remains the surgeon's primary responsibility.

References

1. Butler DB, Bargen JA: Abdominal masses. Gastroenterology 19:1, 1951
2. Hippocrates: The Book of Prognostics, part 7. The Internet Classics Archives, http://classics.mit.edu/Hippocrates/prognost.7.7.html
3. Dixon AK, Kingham JGC, Fry IK, et al: Computed tomography in patients with an abdominal mass: effective and efficient? A controlled trial. Lancet 1:1199, 1981
4. Cassidy D: Abdominal mass. The Clinical Practice of Emergency Medicine, 2nd ed. Harwood-Nuss AL, Linden CH, Luten RC, et al, Eds. Lippincott-Raven, Philadelphia, 1996, p 133
5. Cabot RC: Differential Diagnosis, Presented Through an Analysis of 317 Cases, 2nd ed. WB Saunders Co, Philadelphia, 1915, vol 2, p 709
6. Schaffner F: Abdominal enlargement and masses. Gastroenterology. Haubrich WS, Schaffner F, Berk JE, Eds. WB Saunders Co, Philadelphia, 1998, p 138
7. Morales TG, Fennerty MB: Abdominal distention. Clinical Medicine, 2nd ed. Greene HL, Fincher RME, Johnson WP, et al, Eds. Mosby–Year Book, St. Louis, 1996, p 290
8. DeGowin EL, DeGowin RL: Bedside Diagnostic Examination. Macmillan Publishing Co, New York, 1976, p 471
9. Gore RM: Palpable abdominal masses. Diagnostic Imaging: An Algorithmic Approach. Eisenberg RL, Ed. JB Lippincott Co, Philadelphia, 1988, p 214
10. Aspelin P, Hildell J, Karlsson S, et al: Ultrasonic evaluation of palpable abdominal masses. Acta Chir Scand 156:501, 1980
11. Barker CS, Lindsell DRM: Ultrasound of the palpable abdominal mass. Clin Radiol 41:98, 1990
12. Williams MP, Scott IHK, Dixon AK: Computed tomography in 101 patients with a palpable abdominal mass. Clin Radiol 35:293, 1984
13. Engel IA, Auh YH, Rubenstein WA, et al: Large posterior abdominal masses: computed tomographic localization. Radiology 149:203, 1983
14. Pistolesi GF, Procacci C, Caudana R, et al: C.T. criteria of the differential diagnosis in primary retroperitoneal masses. Eur J Radiol 4:127, 1984
15. Pandolfo I, Blandino A, Gaeta M, et al: CT findings in palpable lesions of the anterior abdominal wall. J Comput Assist Tomogr 10:629, 1986
16. Gazelle GS, Haaga JR: Guided percutaneous biopsy of intraabdominal lesions. AJR Am J Radiol 153:929, 1989
17. Welch TJ, Reading CC: Imaging-guided biopsy. Mayo Clin Proc 64:1295, 1989
18. Grainger RG, Allison D: Interventional radiology. Diagnostic Radiology: A Textbook of Medical Imaging. Grainger RG, Allison D, Eds. Churchill Livingstone, New York, 1997, p 2485
19. Staab EV, Jaques PF, Partain CL: Percutaneous biopsy in the management of solid intra-abdominal masses of unknown etiology. Radiol Clin North Am 17:435, 1979
20. Ennis MG, MacErlean DP: Percutaneous aspiration biopsy of abdomen and retroperitoneum. Clin Radiol 31:611, 1980
21. Sundaram M, Wolverson MK, Heiberg E, et al: Utility of CT-guided abdominal aspiration procedures. AJR Am J Radiol 139:1111, 1982
22. Smith C, Butler JA: Efficacy of directed percutaneous fine-needle aspiration cytology in the diagnosis of intra-abdominal masses. Arch Surg 123:820, 1988
23. Jaeger HJ, MacFie J, Mitchell CJ, et al: Diagnosis of abdominal masses with percutaneous biopsy guided by ultrasound. Br Med J 301:1188, 1990
24. Rumack CM, Wilson SR, Charboneau JW: Ultrasound-guided biopsy and drainage of the abdomen and pelvis. Diagnostic Ultrasound. Rumack CM, Wilson SR, Charboneau JW, Eds. Mosby–Year Book, New York, 1998, p 600
25. Livraghi R, Damascelli B, Lombardi C, et al: Risk in fine needle abdominal biopsy. J Clin Ultrasound 11:77, 1983
26. Fornari F, Civardi G, Cavanna L, et al: Complications of ultrasonically guided fine needle abdominal biopsy: results of a multi-centre Italian study and a review of the literature (The Cooperative Italian Study Group). Scand J Gastroenterol 24:949, 1989
27. Smith EH: Complications of percutaneous abdominal fine needle biopsy. Review Radiology 178:253, 1991
28. Smith EH: The hazards of fine needle aspiration biopsy. Ultrasound Med Biol 10:629, 1984
29. Nolsoe C, Nielsen L, Torp-Pedersen S, et al: Major complications and deaths due to interventional ultrasonography: a review of 8000 cases. J Clin Ultrasound 18:179, 1990
30. Engzell U, Esposti PL, Rubio C, et al: Investigation on tumour spread in connection with aspiration biopsy. Acta Radiol Ther Phys Biol 10:385, 1971
31. Smith FP, Macdonald JS, Schein PS, et al: Cutaneous seeding of pancreatic cancer by skinny-needle aspiration biopsy. Arch Intern Med 140:855, 1980
32. Martino CR, Haaga JR, Bryan PJ, et al: CT-guided liver biopsies: eight years' experience. Radiology 152:755, 1984
33. Welch TJ, Sheedy PF, Johnson CD, et al: CT-guided biopsy: prospective analysis of 1,000 procedures. Radiology 171:493, 1989
34. Reading CC, Charboneau JW, James EM, et al: Sonographically guided percutaneous biopsy of small (3 cm or less) masses. AJR Am J Radiol 151:189, 1988
35. Downey DB, Wilson SR: Ultrasonographically guided biopsy of small intra-abdominal masses. Can Assoc Radiol J 44:350, 1993
36. Buscarini L, Fornari F, Bolondi L, et al: Ultrasound-guided fine-needle biopsy of focal liver lesions: technique, diagnostic accuracy and complications: a retrospective study on 2091 biopsies. J Hepatol 11:344, 1990
37. Brandt KR, Charboneau JW, Stephens DH, et al: CT- and US-guided biopsy of the pancreas. Radiology 187:99, 1993
38. Sackier JM, Berci G, Paz-Partlow M: Elective diagnostic laparoscopy. Am J Surg 161:326, 1991
39. Harbin WP, Wittenberg J, Ferrucci JT, et al: Fallibility of exploratory laparotomy in detection of hepatic and retroperitoneal masses. AJR Am J Roentgenol 135:115, 1980

16 JAUNDICE

Jeffrey S. Barkun, M.D., and Alan N. Barkun, M.D.

Approach to the Jaundiced Patient

The term jaundice refers to the yellowish discoloration of skin, sclerae, and mucous membranes that results from excessive deposition of bilirubin in tissues. It usually is unmistakable but on occasion may manifest itself subtly. It is generally held that jaundice develops when serum bilirubin levels rise above 42 μmol/L (2 mg/dl)[1]; however, the appearance of jaundice also depends on whether it is conjugated or unconjugated bilirubin that is elevated and on how long the episode of jaundice lasts.

In what follows, we outline a problem-based approach to the jaundiced patient that involves assessing the incremental information provided by successive clinical and laboratory investigations as well as the information obtained by means of modern imaging modalities. We also propose a classification of jaundice that stresses the therapeutic options most pertinent to surgeons. We have not attempted a detailed review of bilirubin metabolism and the various pediatric disorders that cause jaundice; such issues are beyond the scope of this chapter. Finally, we emphasize that modern decision making in the approach to the jaundiced patient includes not only careful evaluation of anatomic issues but also close attention to patient morbidity and quality-of-life concerns, as well as a focus on working up the patient in a cost-effective fashion. For optimal treatment, in our view, an integrated approach that involves the surgeon, the gastroenterologist, and the radiologist is essential.

Clinical Assessment

When a patient presents with a skin discoloration suggestive of jaundice, the first step is to confirm that icterus is indeed present. To this end, the mucous membranes of the mouth, the palms, the soles, and the sclerae should be examined in natural light. Because such areas are protected from the sun, photodegradation of bile is minimized; thus, the yellowish discoloration of elastic tissues may be more easily detected. Occasionally, deposition of a yellowish pigment on skin may mimic jaundice but may in fact be related to the consumption of large quantities of food containing lycopene or carotene or drugs such as rifampin or quinacrine. In these cases, the skin is usually the only site of coloration, and careful inspection of sclerae and mucous membranes generally reveals no icteric pigmentation. In certain cultures, long-term application of tea bags to the eyes may lead to a brownish discoloration of the sclerae that can mimic jaundice.[2]

DIRECT VERSUS INDIRECT HYPERBILIRUBINEMIA

Once the presence of jaundice has been confirmed, further clinical assessment determines whether the hyperbilirubinemia is predominantly direct or indirect. This distinction is based on the division of bilirubin into conjugated and unconjugated fractions, which are also known, respectively, as direct and indirect fractions on the basis of their behavior in the van den Bergh (diazo) reaction.[3] If the patient has normal-colored urine and stools, unconjugated bilirubin [see Sidebar Unconjugated (Indirect) Bilirubin] is predominant [see Table 1]. If the patient has dark urine, pale stools, or any other signs or symptoms of a cholestatic syndrome (see below), the serum bilirubin fractionation usually indicates that conjugated biliru-

---

Unconjugated (Indirect) Bilirubin

The breakdown of heme leads to the production of unconjugated bilirubin, which is water insoluble, is tightly bound to albumin, and does not pass into the urine. Excessive production of unconjugated bilirubin typically follows an episode of hemolysis. In the absence of concomitant liver disease or biliary obstruction, the liver can usually handle the extra bilirubin, and only a modest rise in serum levels is observed. There is a substantial increase in bile pigment excretion, leading to large quantities of stercobilinogen in the stool. A patient with hemolysis may therefore be slightly jaundiced with normal-colored urine and stools. Blood tests reveal that 60 to 85 percent of bilirubin is indirect.[67]

Possible causes of indirect hyperbilirubinemia include a variety of disorders that result in significant hemolysis or ineffective erythropoiesis. The diagnosis of indirect hyperbilirubinemia attributable to hemolysis is confirmed by an elevated serum lactate dehydrogenase (LDH) level, a decreased serum haptoglobin level, and evidence of hemolysis on microscopic examination of the blood smear.

Disorders associated with defects in hepatic bilirubin uptake or conjugation can also produce unconjugated hyperbilirubinemia. The most common of these, Gilbert syndrome, is a benign condition affecting up to seven percent of the general population.[68,69] It is not a single disease but a heterogeneous group of disorders, all of which are characterized by a homozygosity for a defect in the promoter controlling the transcription of the UDP glucuronyl transferase I gene.[70] The consequent impairment of bilirubin glucuronidation presents as a mild unconjugated hyperbilirubinemia. The elevated bilirubin level is usually detected on routine blood testing, and affected patients may report that their skin turns yellow when they are fatigued or at stressful times (e.g., after missing meals, after vomiting, or in the presence of an infection). Other causes of an unconjugated hyperbilirubinemia are beyond the scope of this chapter.

Approach to the Jaundiced Patient

Patient has confirmed hepatic jaundice

[*See Sidebar* Hepatic Jaundice.]

Patient has presumed posthepatic jaundice

Obtain ultrasonogram to confirm posthepatic jaundice and identify level of biliary obstruction.

In some unusual clinical situations, ultrasonography may not detect the posthepatic cause of jaundice, and hepato-iminodiacetic acid (HIDA) scanning, endoscopic retrograde cholangiopancreatography (ERCP), percutaneous transhepatic cholangiography (PTC), or repeat ultrasonography may be necessary.
If all these situations are ruled out, seek a hepatic cause and consider liver biopsy.

Patient has confirmed posthepatic jaundice

Proceed according to clinical scenario present.

Suspected cholangitis

Choledocholithiasis is the most likely diagnosis.

Resuscitate, correct any coagulopathy, and give appropriate antibiotics.

Perform ERCP for definitive diagnosis and treatment. If ERCP cannot be done, consider transhepatic drainage or surgery.

Suspected choledocholithiasis

Perform preoperative ERCP and laparoscopic cholecystectomy.

Alternatively, perform laparoscopic cholecystectomy with intraoperative cholangiography.

Patient presents with skin discoloration suggestive of jaundice	→	**Perform clinical assessment**

Perform clinical assessment

Perform physical exam and obtain history.

Confirm icterus by examining oral mucous membranes, palms, soles, and sclerae in natural light.

Distinguish indirect (unconjugated) from direct (conjugated) hyperbilirubinemia:
- Normal-colored urine and stools suggest indirect hyperbilirubinemia
- Dark urine, pale stools, and signs or symptoms of a cholestatic syndrome suggest direct hyperbilirubinemia

Measure total serum bilirubin and percentage of conjugated bilirubin.

Patient has indirect hyperbilirubinemia

[See Sidebar Unconjugated (Indirect) Bilirubin.]

Patient has direct hyperbilirubinemia

Distinguish hepatic ("medical") jaundice from posthepatic ("surgical") jaundice.
- Acute hepatitis, alcohol abuse, and physical evidence of cirrhosis or portal hypertension suggest hepatic jaundice
- Abdominal pain, rigors, itching, and a palpable liver > 2 cm below costal margin suggest posthepatic jaundice

Patient has presumed hepatic jaundice

[See Sidebar Hepatic Jaundice.]

Suspected lesion other than choledocholithiasis

The most common single cause is pancreatic cancer; many of the other possible causes also involve malignancy.

Perform dynamic CT to diagnose lesion and assess resectability.

Consider Doppler ultrasonography to stage lesion further.

Perform ERCP to assess intrahepatic biliary system in patients with middle-third or upper-third obstruction.

Lesion appears unresectable, and surgical palliation is not indicated

Treat with ERCP or PTC and drainage. For advanced malignant disease, supportive care alone may be indicated.

Lesion appears resectable, or surgical palliation is indicated

Treat with surgical bypass or resection as appropriate for level of obstruction.

Perform laparoscopy to confirm resectability before laparotomy.

Upper-third obstruction

Palliation: bypass with left (segment III) hepaticojejunostomy.

Resection for cure: resection of tumor, possibly with hepatectomy or segmentectomy, and reconstruction with hepaticojejunostomy or cholangiojejunostomy.

Middle-third obstruction

Palliation: bypass with hepaticojejunostomy.

Resection for cure: resection of tumor and reconstruction with hepaticojejunostomy.

Lower-third obstruction

Palliation: bypass with Roux-en-Y choledochojejunostomy.

Resection for cure: resection of tumor with pancreaticoduodenectomy or local ampullary excision.

Table 1 Causes of Unconjugated Hyperbilirubinemia

Increased RBC breakdown
  Acute hemolysis
  Chronic hemolytic disorders
  Large hematoma resorption, multiple blood transfusions
  Gilbert syndrome
Decreased hepatic bilirubin conjugation
  Gilbert syndrome
  Crigler-Najjar syndrome types I and II
  Familial unconjugated hyperbilirubinemia

bin is predominant. Rarely, the clinical picture may be secondary to a massive increase in both direct and indirect bilirubin production after the latter has overcome the ability of the hepatocytes to secrete conjugated bilirubin.

It is nearly always possible to distinguish between direct and indirect hyperbilirubinemia on clinical grounds alone.[4] Our emphasis here is on direct hyperbilirubinemia, which is the type that is more relevant to general surgeons.

Cholestatic Syndrome

The term cholestasis refers to decreased delivery of bilirubin into the intestine (and subsequent accumulation in the hepatocytes and in blood), irrespective of the underlying cause. When cholestasis is mild, it may not be associated with clinical jaundice. As it worsens, a conjugated hyperbilirubinemia develops that presents as jaundice. The conjugated hyperbilirubinemia may derive either from a defect in hepatocellular function (hepatic jaundice, also referred to as nonobstructive or medical jaundice) or from a blockage somewhere in the biliary tree (posthepatic jaundice, also referred to as obstructive or surgical jaundice). In this chapter, we refer to hepatic and posthepatic causes of jaundice, reserving the term cholestasis for the specific clinical syndrome that is attributable to a chronic lack of delivery of bile into the intestine. This syndrome is characterized by signs and symptoms that are related either to the conjugated hyperbilirubinemia or to chronic malabsorption of fat-soluble vitamins: jaundice, dark urine, pale stools, pruritus, bruising, steatorrhea, night blindness, osteomalacia, and neuromuscular weakness.[5]

HEPATIC VERSUS POSTHEPATIC JAUNDICE

Once the presence of direct hyperbilirubinemia is confirmed, the next step is to determine whether the jaundice is hepatic or posthepatic. A number of authors have studied the reliability of clinical assessment for making this determination.[6-17] The sensitivities of history, physical examination, and blood tests alone range from 70 to 95 percent,[6-11] whereas the specificities are approximately 75 percent.[10,11] The overall accuracy of clinical assessment of hepatic and posthepatic causes of jaundice ranges from 87 to 97 percent.[8,12] Clinically, hepatic jaundice is most often signaled by acute hepatitis, a history of alcohol abuse, or physical findings reflecting cirrhosis or portal hypertension[13]; posthepatic jaundice is most often signaled by abdominal pain, rigors, itching, or a palpable liver more than 2 cm below the costal margin.[14]

By using discriminant analysis in a pediatric patient population, two investigators[15] were able to isolate three biochemical tests that differentiated between biliary atresia and intrahepatic cholestasis with an accuracy of 95 percent: total serum bilirubin concentration, alkaline phosphatase level, and γ-glutamyltranspeptidase level. Serum transaminase levels added no independent information of significance to the model. Another multivariate analysis model[16] demonstrated that patients with posthepatic jaundice were younger, had a longer history of jaundice, were more likely to present with fever, and had greater elevations of serum protein concentrations and shorter coagulation times than patients with hepatic jaundice. This model, however, despite its 96 percent sensitivity (greater than that of any single radiologic diagnostic modality), could not accurately predict the level of a biliary obstruction. Other investigators[8,12,13] have reported similar findings.

In one study,[17] clinical and laboratory assessments alone were sufficient to identify not only the level of obstruction but also the exact source of jaundice in 78 percent of patients; however, the authors concluded that an approach that omitted ultrasonography altogether was clearly inferior to a combined strategy.

In summary, a clinical approach supported by simple biochemical evaluation displays good predictive ability to distinguish hepatic from posthepatic jaundice; however, a clinical approach alone does not accurately identify the level of biliary obstruction in a patient with posthepatic jaundice.

The remainder of this chapter focuses primarily on management of posthepatic jaundice; hepatic jaundice is less often seen and dealt with by general surgeons [see *Table 2* and *Sidebar Hepatic Jaundice*].

Imaging

Once the history has been obtained and bedside and laboratory assessments have been completed, the next step is imaging, the goals of which are (1) to confirm the presence of an extrahepatic obstruction (i.e., to verify that the jaundice is indeed posthepatic rather than hepatic), (2) to determine the level of the obstruction, (3) to identify the specific cause of the obstruction, and (4) to provide complementary information relating to the underlying diagnosis (e.g., staging information in cases of malignancy).

Of the many imaging methods available today, the gold standard for defining the level of a biliary obstruction before operation in a jaundiced patient remains direct cholangiography, which can be performed either via endoscopic retrograde cholangiopancreatography (ERCP) or via percutaneous transhepatic cholangiography (PTC). Unlike other imaging modalities, direct cholangiography poses significant risks to the patient: there is a four to six percent incidence of pancreatitis or cholangitis after ERCP[18] and a four percent incidence of

Table 2 — Causes of Hepatic Jaundice

Hepatitis
   Viral
   Autoimmune
   Alcoholic
Drugs and hormones
Diseases of intrahepatic bile ducts
Liver infiltration and storage disorders
Systemic infections
Total parenteral nutrition
Postoperative intrahepatic cholestasis
Cholestasis of pregnancy
Benign recurrent intrahepatic cholestasis
Infantile cholestatic syndromes
Inherited metabolic defects
No identifiable cause (idiopathic hepatic jaundice)

---

bile leakage, cholangitis, or bleeding after PTC.[19] There are also several risks that are particular to the manipulation of an obstructed biliary system (see below). For these reasons and because both modalities have therapeutic capability, it is important to gather as much imaging information as possible on the likely cause of the jaundice before performing ERCP or PTC. We have found the following approach to be an efficacious, cost-effective,[20] and safe way of obtaining such information in a patient with presumed posthepatic jaundice.

The presence of ductal dilatation of the intrahepatic or extrahepatic biliary system confirms that a posthepatic cause is responsible for the jaundice. Ultrasonography detects ductal dilatation with an accuracy of 95 percent, although results are to some extent operator-dependent.[21] If ultrasonography does not reveal bile duct dilatation, it is very unlikely that an obstructing lesion is present. Even in the absence of ductal dilatation, other ultrasonographic findings may still point to a specific hepatic cause of jaundice (e.g., multiple liver metastases, cirrhosis, or infiltration of the liver by tumor).

There are a few instances in which ultrasonography may fail to detect a posthepatic cause of jaundice. For instance, very early in the course of an obstructive process, not enough time may have elapsed for biliary dilatation to occur. In this setting, a hepato-iminodiacetic acid (HIDA) scan may help identify bile duct blockage.[22] The yield from this test is highest when the serum bilirubin level is lower than 100 μmol/L, and it diminishes as the serum bilirubin level rises.[1] Occasionally, the intrahepatic biliary tree is unable to dilate; possible causes of such inability include extensive hepatic fibrosis, cirrhosis, sclerosing cholangitis, and recent liver transplantation. If one of these diagnoses is suspected, either ERCP or PTC will eventually be required to confirm the diagnosis of biliary obstruction. Occasionally, the biliary tree dilatation may be intermittent; possible causes of this condition include choledocholithiasis and some biliary tumors. If one of these diagnoses is suspected, ultrasonography may be repeated after a short period of observation (when clinically applicable); biliary

---

Hepatic Jaundice

Hepatic jaundice may be either acute or chronic and may be caused by a variety of conditions [see Table 2].

Acute hepatic jaundice may arise de novo or in the setting of ongoing liver disease. Historical clues may suggest a particular cause, such as medications or viral hepatitis. Physical examination usually reveals little; however, an enlarged liver is sometimes palpated. In the presence of preexisting chronic liver disease, bedside stigmata (e.g., ascites, spider nevi, caput medusae, palmar erythema, gynecomastia, or Dupuytren's contractures) may be present. Although specific therapies exist for certain clinical problems (e.g., acetylcysteine for acetaminophen ingestion and penicillin plus silibinin for *Amanita phalloides* poisoning), treatment in most cases remains supportive. Patients in whom encephalopathy develops within two to eight weeks of the onset of jaundice are usually classified as having fulminant hepatic failure. Evidence of encephalopathy, renal failure, or a severe coagulopathy is predictive of poor outcome in this setting.[71] The most common causes of fulminant hepatic failure are viral hepatitis and drug toxicity. The mortality from fulminant hepatic failure remains high even though liver transplantation has favorably affected the prognosis.[72]

In cases of chronic hepatic jaundice, the patient may have chronic hepatitis or cholestasis, with or without cirrhosis. The cause usually is determined on the basis of the history in conjunction with the results of serology, biochemistry, and, occasionally, histology. Causes include viral infection, drug-induced chronic hepatitis, autoimmune liver disease, genetic disorders (e.g., Wilson's disease and α_1-antitrypsin deficiency), chronic cholestatic disorders, alcoholic liver disease, and steatohepatitis.[73] Physical examination reveals the stigmata of chronic liver disease and occasionally suggests a specific cause (e.g., Kayser-Fleischer rings on slit-lamp examination in Wilson's disease). Treatment, once again, is usually supportive, depending on the clinical presentation; whether more specific therapy is needed and what form it takes depend on the cause of liver disease. Although physiologic tests have been developed to quantify hepatic reserve, the most widely used and best-validated prognostic index remains the Child-Pugh classification (see below), which correlates with individual survival and has been shown to predict operative risk.[74] Liver transplantation is the treatment of choice in most cases of end-stage liver disease.

The Child-Pugh Classification
Numerical Score (*points*)

Variable	1	2	3
Encephalopathy	Nil (0)	Slight to moderate (1, 2)	Moderate to severe (3–5)
Ascites	Nil	Slight	Moderate to severe
Bilirubin, mg/dl (umol/L*)	< 2 (< 34)	2–3 (34–51)	> 3 (> 51)
Albumin, g/dl (g/L*)	> 3.5 (> 35)	2.8–3.5 (28–35)	< 2.8 (< 28)
Prothrombin index	> 70%	40–70%	< 40%

Modified Child's risk grade (depending on total score): 5 or 6 points, grade A: 7 to 9 points, grade B: 10 to 15 points, grade C.
*Système International d'Unités, or SI units.

ductal dilatation will often be apparent on the subsequent ultrasonogram. If all of these unusual clinical situations have been ruled out, a hepatic cause for the jaundice should be sought [see Table 2] and a liver biopsy considered.[23]

Besides being able to identify the presence of extrahepatic ductal obstruction with a high degree of reliability, ultrasonography can accurately determine the level of the obstruction in 90 percent of cases.[24] For example, a dilated gallbladder suggests that the obstruction is probably located in the middle third or the distal third of the common bile duct (CBD).

Some centers prefer CT to ultrasonography as the initial imaging modality,[25] but we, like a number of other authors,[26] find ultrasonography to be the most expedient, most readily available, least invasive, and most economical imaging method for differentiating between hepatic and posthepatic causes of jaundice as well as for suggesting the level of obstruction. Traditional imaging techniques, such as oral or intravenous cholangiography, have a negligible role to play in this setting because of their very poor accuracy and safety, especially in jaundiced patients.

Magnetic resonance cholangiopancreatography (MRCP) [see Figure 1], three-dimensional CT (3D-CT) scanning, and endoscopic ultrasonography have been used to visualize the biliary and pancreatic trees in a variety of patient populations, including patients with CBD stones; the results are encouraging but not conclusive.[27-31]

Workup and Management of Posthepatic Jaundice

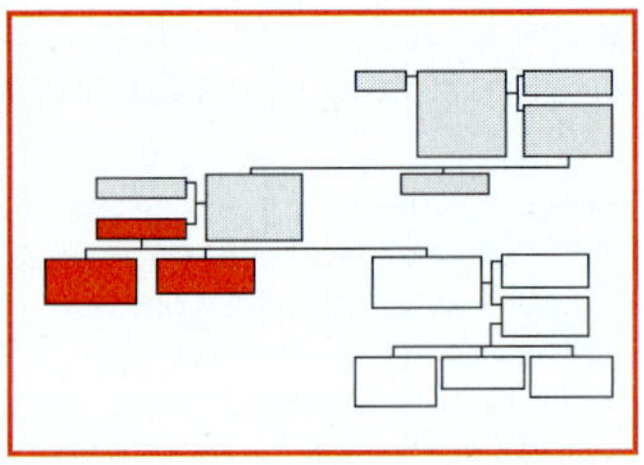

Once ultrasonography has confirmed that ductal obstruction is present, there are three possible clinical scenarios: suspected cholangitis, suspected choledocholithiasis without cholangitis, and a suspected lesion other than choledocholithiasis.

SUSPECTED CHOLANGITIS

If a jaundiced patient exhibits a clinical picture compatible with acute suppurative cholangitis (Charcot's triad or Raynaud's pentad), the most likely diagnosis is choledocholithiasis. After appropriate resuscitation, correction of any coagulopathies present, and administration of antibiotics, ERCP is indicated for diagnosis and treatment.[32] If ERCP is unavailable or is not feasible (e.g., because of previous Roux-en-Y reconstruction), transhepatic drainage or surgery may be necessary. It is important to emphasize here that the mainstay of treatment of severe cholangitis is not just the administration of appropriate antibiotics but rather the establishment of adequate biliary drainage.

SUSPECTED CHOLEDOCHOLITHIASIS WITHOUT CHOLANGITIS

Choledocholithiasis is the most common cause of biliary obstruction[13,14] and should be strongly suspected if the jaundice is episodic or painful or if ultrasonography has demonstrated the presence of gallstones or bile duct stones. Patients with suspected choledocholithiasis should be referred for laparoscopic cholecystectomy with either preoperative ERCP or intraoperative cholangiography. We favor preoperative ERCP in this setting because its diagnostic yield is high,[33] it

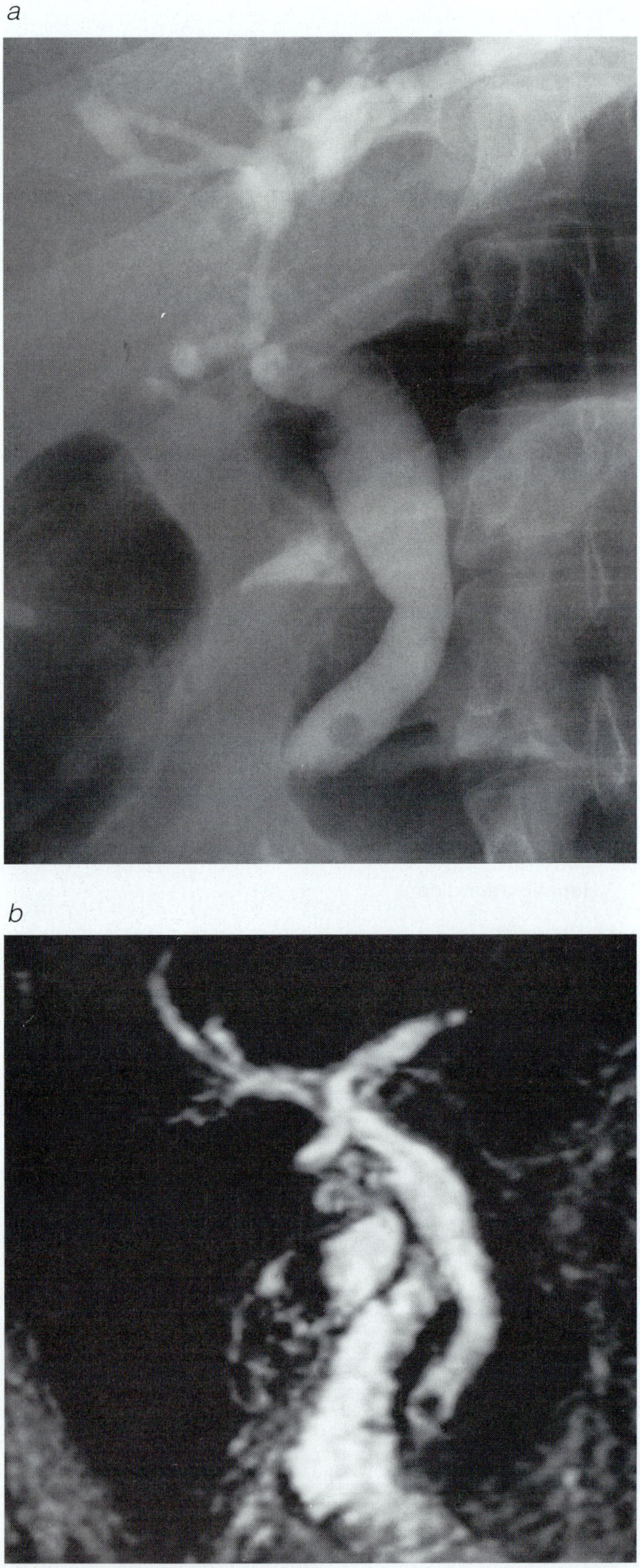

Figure 1 ERCP (*a*) and corresponding MRCP (*b*) demonstrate the presence of a stone in the distal CBD.

allows confirmation of the diagnosis preoperatively (thus obviating intraoperative surprises), and it is capable of clearing the CBD of stones in 95 percent of cases.

SUSPECTED LESION OTHER THAN CHOLEDOCHOLITHIASIS

If no gallstones are identified, if the clinical presentation is less acute (e.g., constant abdominal or back pain), or if there are associated constitutional symptoms (e.g., weight loss, fatigue, and long-standing anorexia), the presence of a lesion other than choledocholithiasis should be suspected. In such cases, another imaging modality besides the ultrasonography already performed must be considered before the decision is made to proceed to cholangiography or operation.

Possible causes of posthepatic obstruction (other than choledocholithiasis) may be classified into three categories depending on the location of the obstructing lesion (as suggested by the earlier ultrasonogram): the upper third of the biliary tree, the middle third, or the lower (distal) third [see Table 3]. After choledocholithiasis, the most common cause of such obstruction is pancreatic cancer.[13,14] In adults, many of the other possible causes also involve malignant processes. Consequently, the next step in the workup of the patient is typically the assessment of resectability and operability [see 51 Biliary Tract Procedures].

Diagnosis and Assessment of Resectability

Because surgery is the only chance for definitive treatment of a biliary or pancreatic malignancy, it is important not to deny a patient this chance. Assessment of the resectability of a tumor usually hinges on whether the superior mesenteric vein, the portal vein, and the superior mesenteric artery are free of tumor and on whether there is evidence of significant local adenopathy or extrapancreatic extension of tumor. A number of lesions will be clearly unresectable, either because of tumor extension or because of the presence of liver metastases.

Many imaging modalities are currently being used to determine resectability, and several of these are also being investigated as possible alternatives to direct cholangiography because they involve little if any morbidity. Their accuracy varies according to the underlying pathology and the expertise of the user. They have been studied mostly with respect to the staging and diagnosis of pancreatic or biliary hilar cancers.

For determining resectability and staging lesions before operation, we rely mainly on high-resolution incremental dynamic contrast-enhanced CT (so-called dynamic CT), which allows good definition of the nature and extent of the lesion. At present, this modality is thought to be superior for the diagnosis and staging of lesions such as pancreatic cancer, especially if a spiral CT scanner is used.[34-36] Dynamic CT exhibits a high negative predictive value and has a false positive rate of less than 10 percent; its sensitivity is optimal for pancreatic lesions larger than 1.5 cm in diameter. The presence of ascites, liver metastases, lymph nodes larger than 2 cm in diameter, and invasion into adjacent organs are all signs of advanced disease.[37] On the basis of these criteria, dynamic CT can predict that a lesion will not be resectable with an accuracy approaching 95 percent; however, as many as 33 percent of tumors that appear to be resectable on dynamic CT are found to be unresectable at operation.[35,36] Occasionally, dynamic CT does not yield sufficient information, and as a result, supplementary imaging studies are required. The accuracy of these ancillary modalities varies.

As yet, only preliminary data on the use of MRI in this context are available; however, the initial results appear promising.[37] MRI may be particularly useful for following up patients in whom clip artifacts interfere with a CT image.[37]

Only in a few selected cases is angiography used to assess resectability or stage a hepatobiliary or pancreatic neoplasm: increasingly, it is being replaced by duplex Doppler ultrasonography, which can confirm the presence of flow in the hepatic arterial or portal venous systems and occasionally can demonstrate invasion of these vessels by tumor.[38]

Endoscopic ultrasonography probably has a role to play in assessing the resectability of pancreatic tumors.[39,40] In a large study comprising 232 patients,[41] this modality was found to be superior to CT and standard ultrasonography in detecting venous and gastric invasion by cancers measuring 3 cm or less

Table 3 Causes of Posthepatic Jaundice

Upper-third obstruction
  Polycystic liver disease
  Caroli's disease
  Hepatocellular carcinoma
  Oriental cholangiohepatitis
  Hepatic arterial thrombosis (e.g., after liver transplantation or chemotherapy)
  Hemobilia (e.g., after biliary manipulation)
  Iatrogenic bile duct injury (e.g., after laparoscopic cholecystectomy)
  Cholangiocarcinoma (Klatskin's tumor)
  Sclerosing cholangitis
  Papillomas of the bile duct

Middle-third obstruction
  Cholangiocarcinoma
  Sclerosing cholangitis
  Papillomas of the bile duct
  Gallbladder cancer
  Choledochal cyst
  Intrabiliary parasites
  Mirizzi syndrome
  Extrinsic nodal compression (e.g., from breast cancer or lymphoma)
  Iatrogenic bile duct injury (e.g., after open cholecystectomy)
  Cystic fibrosis
  Benign idiopathic bile duct stricture

Lower-third obstruction
  Cholangiocarcinoma
  Sclerosing cholangitis
  Papillomas of the bile duct
  Pancreatic tumors
  Periampullary tumors
  Chronic pancreatitis
  Sphincter of Oddi dysfunction
  Papillary stenosis
  Duodenal diverticula
  Penetrating duodenal ulcer
  Retroduodenal adenopathy (e.g., lymphoma, carcinoid)

in diameter. In another large series,[42] it was reported to be more accurate than CT in the comparative staging of pancreatic and ampullary cancers. Occasionally, the presence of a small (< 2 cm) pancreatic tumor may be suspected in a patient with an obstruction of the distal third of the bile duct and a normal CT scan; endoscopic ultrasonography may be particularly helpful in this setting.[40]

At this point in the evaluation, patients with an upper-third or middle-third lesion are referred for cholangiography to delineate the proximal biliary anatomy; patients with a distal-third obstruction for which the diagnosis is still unclear are also referred for cholangiography.

If a biliary stricture is detected at cholangiography, brush cytology or biopsy is mandatory. Biliary cytology, however, has been disappointing, particularly at ERCP: diagnostic accuracy ranges from 40 to 85 percent,[43,44] mostly because the negative predictive value is poor. Accuracy improves with multiple sampling and when a biliary rather than a pancreatic malignancy is detected. In addition, biopsy tends to be more accurate than brush cytology.[43]

If a pancreatic tumor is suspected, percutaneous fine-needle aspiration (FNA) cytology may be helpful; the yield is best for larger tumors. In the case of potentially resectable lesions, however, this modality adds very little to the decision-making process. The limited data currently available suggest that assays of tumor markers in serum and pancreatic fluid are useful, particularly for cystic lesions of the pancreas.[45]

Nonoperative Management: Drainage and Cholangiography

In the majority of patients with malignant obstructions, treatment is palliative rather than curative. It is therefore especially important to recognize and minimize the iatrogenic risks related to the manipulation of an obstructed biliary system.

Cholangiography and decompression of obstructed biliary system As a rule, we favor ERCP, although PTC may be preferable for obstructions near the hepatic duct bifurcation. Whichever imaging modality is used, the following four principles apply.

1. In the absence of preexisting or concomitant hepatocellular dysfunction, drainage of one half of the liver is sufficient for resolution of jaundice.
2. Because of its external diameter, a transhepatic drain, once inserted, does not necessarily permit equal drainage of all segments of the liver, particularly if there are a number of intrahepatic ductal stenoses. Accordingly, some patients with conditions such as sclerosing cholangitis or a growing tumor may experience persistent sepsis from an infected excluded liver segment even when the prosthesis is patent [*see Figure 2*]. An excluded segment may even be responsible for severe persistent pruritus.
3. Any attempt at opacifying an obstructed biliary tree introduces a significant risk of subsequent cholangitis, even when appropriate antibiotic prophylaxis is provided. The referring surgeon should therefore plan for biliary drainage either at the time of cholangiography (ERCP or PTC) or soon thereafter.
4. Routine preoperative drainage of an obstructed biliary system does not benefit patients who will soon undergo operative correction.[46,47] This is true even though jaundice is associated with multiple adverse systemic effects (e.g., renal failure, sepsis, and impaired wound healing).[48,49]

Cholangiography is more than just a diagnostic test: it is the ideal setting for cytology, biopsy, or even drainage of the obstructed bile duct via a sphincterotomy, a nasobiliary tube, or a catheter or stent. Accordingly, it is essential that the surgeon, the gastroenterologist, and the radiologist discuss the possible need for drainage well before it is required. Early, open communication among all the members of the treating team is a hallmark of the modern management of biliary obstruction.

Palliation in patients with advanced malignant disease
When a patient has advanced malignant disease, drainage of the biliary system for palliation is not routinely indicated, because the risk of complications related to the procedure may outweigh the potential benefit. Indeed, the best treatment for a patient with asymptomatic obstructive jaundice and liver metastases may be supportive care alone. Biliary decompression is indicated if cholangitis or severe pruritus that interferes with quality of life is present.

We, like others,[20] consider a stent placed with ERCP to be the palliative modality of choice for advanced disease, although upper-third lesions may be managed most easily through the initial placement of an internal/external catheter at the time of PTC. Metal expandable stents remain patent longer than large conventional plastic stents,[50,51] but the high price of the metal stents has kept them from being widely used, and their overall cost-effectiveness has yet to be clearly demonstrated.

Randomized controlled trials suggest that surgical bypass should be reserved for patients who are expected to survive for prolonged periods because bypass is associated with more prolonged palliation at the cost of greater initial morbidity.[52]

The role of prophylactic gastric drainage at the time of operative biliary drainage remains controversial.[53] Jaundiced patients with unresectable lesions who also present with duodenal or jejunal obstruction should be referred for gastrojejunostomy and biliary bypass surgery.

Operative Management at Specific Sites: Bypass and Resection

Surgical treatment of tumors causing biliary obstruction is determined primarily by the level of the biliary obstruction. There is a growing body of evidence indicating that modern surgical approaches are resulting in lower postoperative morbidity and, possibly, improved five-year survival[54]; however, the prognosis is still uniformly poor, except for patients with periampullary tumors. In fact, the surgical procedure rarely proves curative, even after meticulous preoperative patient selection.

The first step in any operation to resect a potential jaundice-causing cancer should be laparoscopy to determine resectability before laparotomy and to prevent the hospital stay and pro-

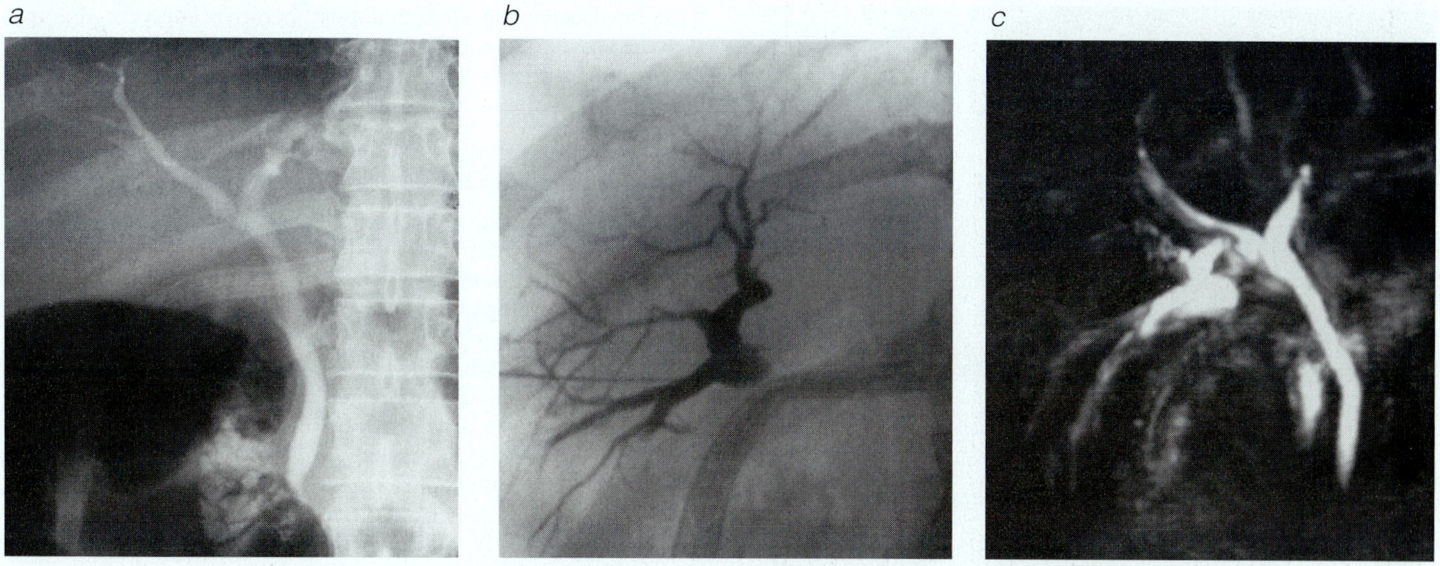

Figure 2 ERCP (*a*) demonstrates missing liver segments. Transhepatic cholangiography (*b*) of segment VI reveals excluded liver ductal system. MRCP (*c*)[75] shows the excluded liver segments as well as the biliary system, which still communicates with the common hepatic duct.

longed convalescence associated with an unnecessary laparotomy. Laparoscopy is used to detect peritoneal carcinomatosis, liver metastases, malignant ascites, and gross hilar adenopathy.[55,56] In a 1996 trial involving 115 patients with potentially resectable peripancreatic tumors, full laparoscopic staging could be performed in 94 percent, and the overall resectability rate was 76 percent. The hospital stay for patients who underwent staging laparoscopy alone was five days shorter than that for patients who underwent open staging.[55] In a preliminary study that examined laparoscopic ultrasonography in 38 patients,[56] this modality appeared to be superior to simple laparoscopy in 30 percent of cases, and its specificity and accuracy were approximately 88 percent.[56,57]

Once laparoscopy confirms that there is no obvious advanced disease, the patient should undergo a full laparotomy, usually in the same setting.

In what follows, only the general principles of resection or bypass at each level of obstruction are discussed: operative technical details are addressed elsewhere [*see 51 Biliary Tract Procedures*]. Our preferred method of biliary anastomosis, for either reconstruction or bypass, involves the fashioning of a Roux-en-Y loop, followed by a mucosa-to-mucosa anastomosis. In all cases, a cholecystectomy is performed to facilitate access to the biliary tree.

Upper-third obstruction

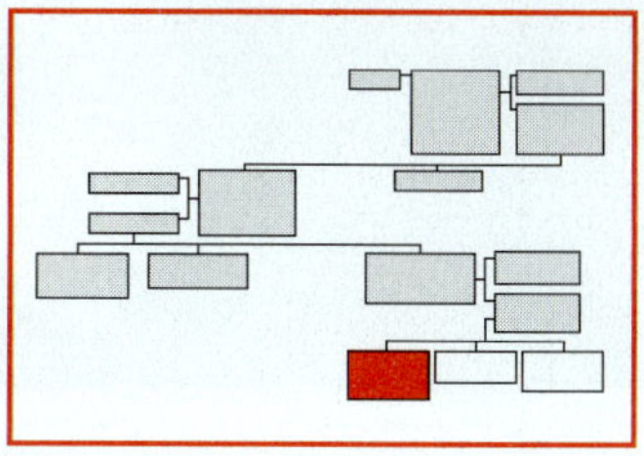

Palliation. In the absence of liver compromise, drainage of one half of the liver usually leads to clearance of jaundice.[58] Because the left hepatic duct has a long extrahepatic segment that makes it more accessible, the preferred bypass technique for an obstructing upper-third lesion is a left (or segment III) hepaticojejunostomy. This operation has superseded the Longmire procedure because it does not involve formal resection of liver parenchyma. More recently, laparoscopic bypass techniques that make use of segment III have been developed, but their performance has yet to be assessed.[59]

Resection for cure. The hilar plate is taken down to lengthen the hepatic duct segment available for subsequent anastomosis. Often, a formal hepatectomy or segmentectomy is required to ensure an adequate margin of resection. If the resection must be carried out proximal to the hepatic duct bifurcation, several cholangiojejunostomies will have to be done to anastomose individual hepatic biliary branches. Frozen section examination of the proximal and distal resection margins is important because of the propensity of tumors such as cholangiocarcinoma to spread in a submucosal or perineural plane.

Middle-third obstruction

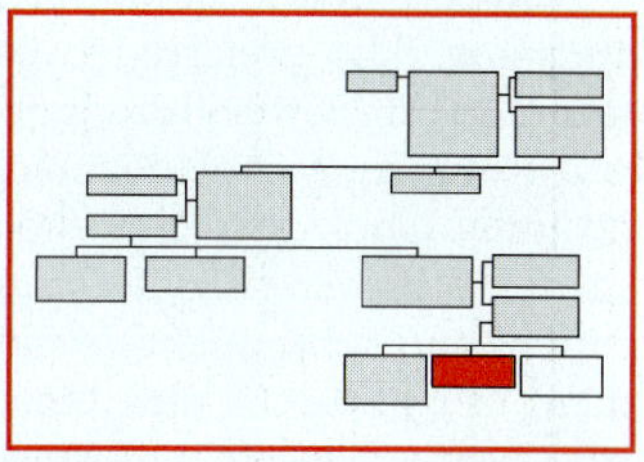

Palliation. Surgical bypass of middle-third lesions is technically simpler because a hepaticojejunostomy can often be performed distal to the hepatic duct bifurcation, which means that exposure of the hilar plate or the intrahepatic ducts is unnecessary.

Resection for cure. Discrete tumors in this part of the bile duct are usually quite amenable to resection along with the lymphatic chains in the porta hepatis. Resection of an early gallbladder cancer may, on occasion, necessitate the concomitant resection of segment V, although the value of resecting this segment prophylactically has not been conclusively demonstrated. Sometimes, jaundice from a suspected middle-third lesion is in fact caused by a case of Mirizzi syndrome [*see Figure 3*]. In such cases, a gallstone is responsible for extrinsic obstruction of the CBD, either by causing inflammation of the gallbladder wall or via direct impingement. Proper treatment of this syndrome may involve hepaticojejunostomy in addition to chole-

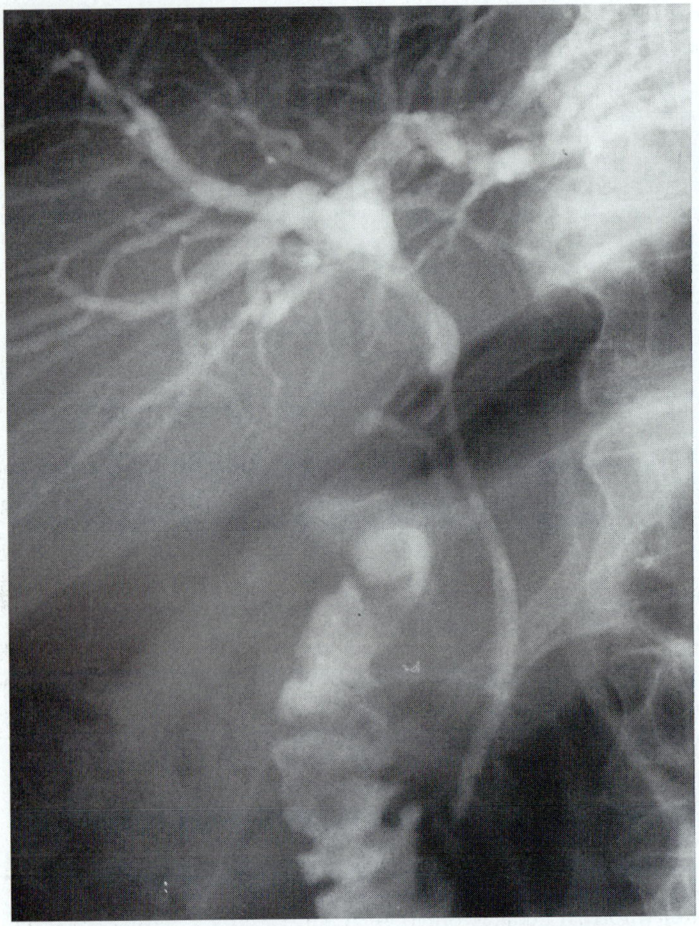

Figure 3 ERCP demonstrates extrinsic compression of the common hepatic duct by a stone in Hartmann's pouch. A biliary stent has been inserted for drainage.

cystectomy if a cholecystocholedochal fistula is present.[60]

Lower-third obstruction 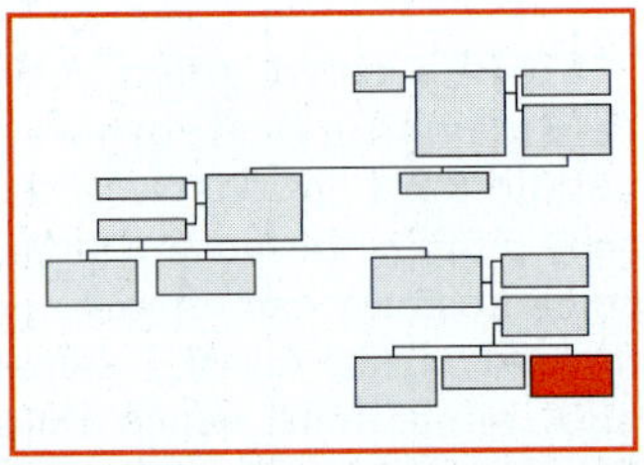
Palliation. The preferred bypass technique for lower-third lesions is a Roux-en-Y choledochojejunostomy. Cholecystojejunostomy carries a higher risk of complications and subsequent development of jaundice[61]; this remains true even when it is performed laparoscopically.[59] Occasionally, it may be done as a temporizing measure before a more definitive procedure in the context of an upcoming transfer to a specialized center.

Resection for cure. Occasionally, an impacted CBD stone at the duodenal ampulla mimics a tumor and is not clearly identified preoperatively. In this situation, intraoperative choledochoscopy before resection helps confirm the diagnosis and may even permit removal of the stone. Resection of a lower-third lesion usually involves a pancreaticoduodenectomy [*see 53 Pancreatic Procedures*], although local ampullary resection may be an acceptable alternative for a small adenoma of the ampulla. For optimal results, pancreaticoduodenectomy probably is best performed in specialized centers.[62]

It has been suggested that postoperative adjuvant therapy may improve the prognosis after resection, or even simply palliation, of a pancreatic adenocarcinoma,[54] but this debate falls outside the scope of our discussion.

Postoperative Jaundice

A clinical scenario of particular pertinence to surgeons that we have not yet addressed is the development of jaundice in the postoperative setting.

Jaundice develops in approximately one percent of all surgical patients after operation.[63] When jaundice occurs after a hepatobiliary procedure, it may be attributable to specific biliary causes, such as retained CBD stones, postoperative biliary leakage (through reabsorption of bile leaking into the peritoneum) [*see Figure 4*], injury to the CBD, and the subsequent development of biliary strictures. In most instances, however, the jaundice derives from a combination of disease processes, and only rarely is invasive testing or active treatment required.[64]

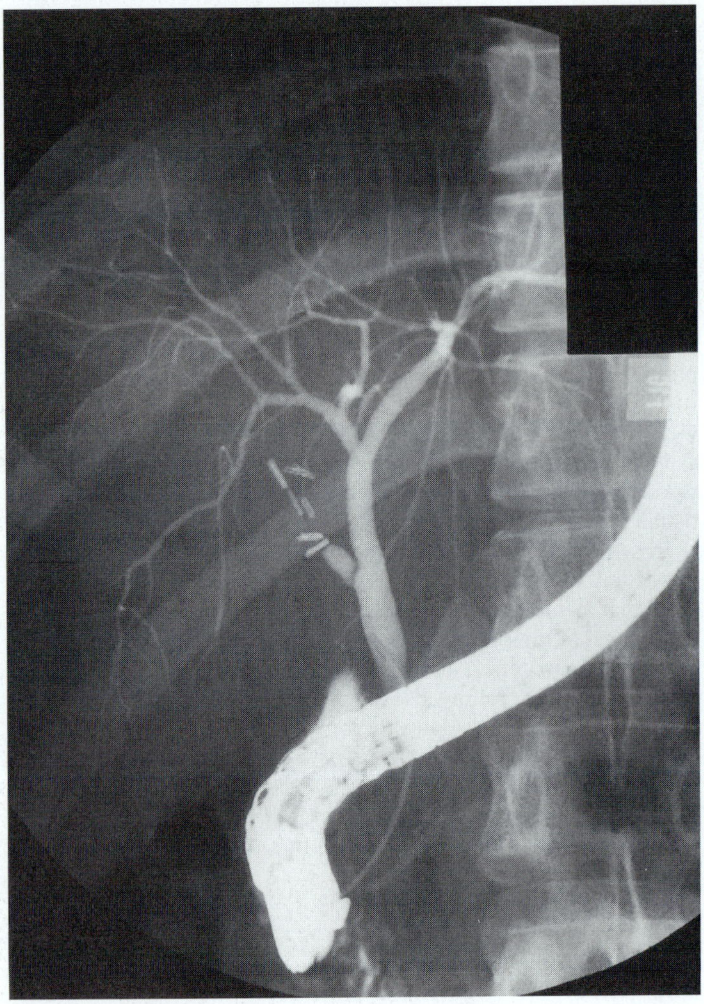

Figure 4 Jaundice has occurred after laparoscopic cholecystectomy as a result of bile leakage from a distal biliary tributary. A stent has been inserted to decrease bile duct luminal pressure and foster spontaneous resolution.

A diagnostic approach similar to the one outlined earlier (see above) is applicable to postoperative jaundice; however, another useful approach is to consider the possible causes in the light of the time interval between the operation and the subsequent development of jaundice.

- Jaundice may develop within 48 hours of the operation; this is most often the result of the breakdown of red blood cells, occurring in the context of multiple blood transfusions (particularly with stored blood), the resorption of a large hematoma, or a transfusion reaction. Hemolysis may also develop in a patient with a known underlying hemolytic anemia and may be precipitated by the administration of specific drugs (e.g., sulfa drugs in a patient who has glucose-6-phosphate dehydrogenase deficiency).[65] Cardiopulmonary bypass or the insertion of a prosthetic valve may be associated with the development of early postoperative jaundice as well. Gilbert syndrome [see Sidebar Hepatic Jaundice] may first manifest itself early in the postoperative period. Occasionally, a mild conjugated hyperbilirubinemia may be related to Dubin-Johnson syndrome, which is an inherited disorder of bilirubin metabolism. This condition is usually self-limited and is characterized by the presence of a melaninlike pigment in the liver.

- Intraoperative hypotension or hypoxemia or the early development of heart failure can lead to conjugated hyperbilirubinemia within five to 10 days after operation. The hyperbilirubinemia may be associated with other end-organ damage (e.g., acute tubular necrosis). In fact, any impairment of renal function causes a decrease in bilirubin excretion and can be responsible for a mild hyperbilirubinemia.

- Jaundice may develop seven to 10 days after operation in association with a medication-induced hepatitis attributable to an anesthetic agent. This syndrome has an estimated incidence of one in 10,000 after an initial exposure.[65] More commonly, the jaundice is related to the administration of antibiotics or other medications used in the perioperative setting.[65]

- After the first week, jaundice associated with intrahepatic cholestasis is often a manifestation of a septic response and usually presents in the setting of overt infection, particularly in patients with multiple organ dysfunction syndrome. Gram-negative sepsis from an intra-abdominal source is typical; if it persists, the outcome is likely to be poor. Jaundice may occur in as many as 30 percent of patients receiving total parenteral nutrition (TPN). It may be attributable to steatosis, particularly with formulas containing large amounts of carbohydrates. In addition, decreased export of bilirubin from the hepatocytes may lead to cholestasis, the severity of which appears to be related to the duration of TPN administration. Acalculous cholecystitis or even ductal obstruction may develop as a result of sludge in the gallbladder and the CBD. An elevated postoperative bilirubin level at any time may also result from unsuspected hepatic or posthepatic causes (e.g., occult cirrhosis, choledocholithiasis, or cholecystitis). A rare cause of postoperative jaundice is the development of thyrotoxicosis. Another entity to consider (as a diagnosis of exclusion) is so-called benign postoperative cholestasis, a primarily cholestatic, self-limited process with no clearly demonstrable cause that typically arises within two to 10 days after operation. Benign postoperative cholestasis may be attributable to a combination of mechanisms, including an increased pigment load, impaired liver function resulting from hypoxemia and hypotension, and decreased renal bilirubin excretion caused by varying degrees of tubular necrosis.[66] The predominantly conjugated hyperbilirubinemia may reach 40 mg/dl and remain elevated for as long as three weeks.[65] This is a diagnosis of exclusion.

- In the late postoperative period, the development of non-A, non-B, non-C viral hepatitis after transfusion of blood products will usually occur within five to 12 weeks of operation.

References

1. Schiff L: Jaundice: a clinical approach. Diseases of the Liver, 7th ed. Schiff L, Schiff ER, Eds. JB Lippincott Co, Philadelphia, 1993, p 334
2. Jabbari M: Personal communication
3. Scharschmidt BF, Gollan JL: Current concepts of bilirubin metabolism and hereditary hyperbilirubinemia. Progress in Liver Diseases. Popper H, Schaffner F, Eds. Grune & Stratton, New York, 1979, p 187
4. Frank BB: Clinical evaluation of jaundice: a guideline of the Patient Care Committee of the American Gastroenterological Association. JAMA 262:3031, 1989
5. Sherlock S: Cholestasis. Diseases of the Liver and Biliary System, 8th ed. Sherlock S, Ed. Blackwell Scientific Publications, Oxford, 1989, p 257
6. Lindberg G, Björkman A, Helmers C: A description of diagnostic strategies in jaundice. Scand J Gastroenterol 18:257, 1983
7. Lumeng L, Snodgrass PJ, Swonder JW: Final report of a blinded prospective study comparing current non-invasive approaches in the differential diagnosis of medical and surgical jaundice. Gastroenterology 78:1312, 1980
8. Martin W, Apostolakos PC, Roazen H: Clinical versus actuarial prediction in the differential diagnosis of jaundice. Am J Med Sci 240:571, 1960
9. Matzen P, Malchow-Möller A, Hilden J, et al: Differential diagnosis of jaundice: a pocket diagnostic chart. Liver 4:360, 1984
10. O'Connor K, Snodgrass PJ, Swonder JE, et al: A blinded prospective study comparing four current non-invasive approaches in the differential diagnosis of medical versus surgical jaundice. Gastroenterology 84:1498, 1983
11. Schenker S, Balint J, Schiff L: Differential diagnosis of jaundice: report of a prospective study of 61 proved cases. Am J Dig Dis 7:449, 1962
12. Theodossi A, Spiegelhalter D, Portmann B, et al: The value of clinical, biochemical, ultrasound and liver biopsy data in assessing patients with liver disease. Liver 3:315, 1983
13. Pasanen PA, Pikkarainen P, Alhava E, et al: The value of clinical assessment in the diagnosis of icterus and cholestasis. Ital J Gastroenterol 24:313, 1992
14. Theodossi A: The value of symptoms and signs in the assessment of jaundiced patients. Clin Gastroenterol 14:545, 1985
15. Fung KP, Lau SP: Differentiation between extrahepatic and intrahepatic cholestasis by discriminant analysis. J Paediatr Child Health 26:132, 1990
16. Pasanen PA, Pikkarainen P, Alhava E, et al: Evaluation of a computer-based diagnostic score system in the diagnosis of jaundice and cholestasis. Scand J Gastroenterol 28:732, 1993
17. Malchow-Möller A, Gronvall S, Hilden J, et al: Ultrasound examination in jaundiced patients: is computer-assisted preclassification helpful? J Hepatol 12:321, 1991
18. Cotton PB, Lehman G, Vennes J, et al: Endoscopic sphincterotomy complications and their management: an attempt at consensus. Gastrointest Endoscopy 37:383, 1991
19. Gibson RN: Percutaneous transhepatic cholangiography. Surgery of the Liver and Biliary Tract, 2nd ed, Vol 1. Blumgart LH, Ed. Churchill Livingstone, New York, 1994, p 294
20. Rossi LR, Traverso W, Pimentel F: Malignant obstructive jaundice: evaluation and management. Surg Clin North Am 76:63, 1996
21. Taylor KJW, Rosenfield A: Grey-scale ultrasonog-

22. Kaplun L, Weissman HS, Rosenblatt RR, et al: The early diagnosis of common bile duct obstruction using cholescintigraphy. JAMA 254:2431, 1985
23. Richter JM, Silverstein MD, Schapiro R: Suspected obstructive jaundice: a decision analysis of diagnostic strategies. Ann Intern Med 99:46, 1983
24. Blackbourne LH, Earnhardt RC, Sistrom CL, et al: The sensitivity and role of ultrasound in the evaluation of biliary obstruction. Am Surg 60:683, 1994
25. Sherlock S: Ultrasound (US), computerized axial tomography (CT) and magnetic resonance imaging (MRI). Diseases of the Liver and Biliary System 5:70, 1989
26. Cosgrove DO: Ultrasound in surgery of the liver and biliary tract. Surgery of the Liver and Biliary Tract, 2nd ed, Vol 1. Blumgart LH, Ed. New York, Churchill Livingstone, 1994, p 189
27. Gillams A, Gardener J, Richards R, et al: Three-dimensional computed tomography cholangiography: a new technique for biliary tract imaging. Br J Radiol 67:445, 1994
28. Low RN, Sigeti JS, Francis IR, et al: Evaluation of malignant biliary obstruction: efficacy of fast multiplanar spoiled gradient-recalled MR imaging vs spin-echo MR imaging, CT, and cholangiography. AJR Am J Roentgenol 162:315, 1994
29. Amouyal P, Amouyal G, Levy P, et al: Diagnosis of choledocholithiasis by endoscopic ultrasonography. Gastroenterology 106:1062, 1994
30. Guibaud L, Bret PM, Reinhold C, et al: Bile duct obstruction and choledocholithiasis: diagnosis with MR cholangiography. Radiology 197:109, 1995
31. Ishizaki Y, Wakayama T, Okada Y, et al: MR cholangiography for evaluation of obstructed jaundice. Am J Gastroenterol 88:2072, 1993
32. Lai EC, Mok FP, Tan ES, et al: Endoscopic biliary drainage for severe acute cholangitis. N Engl J Med 326:1582, 1992
33. Barkun JS, Fried GM, Barkun AN, et al: Cholecystectomy without operative cholangiography: implications for bile duct injury and common bile duct stones. Ann Surg 218:371, 1993
34. Freeny PC, Traverso LW, Ryan JA: Diagnosis and staging of pancreatic adenocarcinoma with dynamic computed tomography. Am J Surg 165:600, 1993
35. Freeny PC, Marks WM, Ryan JA, et al: Pancreatic ductal adenocarcinoma: diagnosis and staging with dynamic CT. Radiology 166:125, 1988
36. Moosa AR, Gamagami RA: Diagnosis and staging of pancreatic neoplasms. Surg Clin North Am 75:871, 1995
37. Megibow AJ, Zhou XH, Rotterdam H, et al: Pancreatic carcinoma: CT vs MR imaging in the evaluation of resectability. Radiology 195:327, 1995
38. Smits NJ, Reeders JW: Current applicability of duplex doppler ultrasonography in pancreatic head and biliary malignancies. Bailliere's Clin Gastroenterol 9:153, 1995
39. Giovannini M, Seitz JF: Endoscopic ultrasonography with a linear-type echoendoscope in the evaluation of 94 patients with pancreatobiliary disease. Endoscopy 26:579, 1994
40. Snady H, Cooperman A, Siegel J: Endoscopic ultrasonography compared with computed tomography and E.R.C.P. in patients with obstructive jaundice or small peri-pancreatic mass. Gastrointest Endoscopy 38:27, 1992
41. Nakaizumi A, Uehara H, Iishi H, et al: Endoscopic ultrasonography in diagnosis and staging of pancreatic cancer. Dig Dis Sci 40:696, 1995
42. Bakkevold KE, Arnesjo B, Kambestad B: Carcinoma of the pancreas and papilla of Vater—assessment of resectability and factors influencing resectability in stage I carcinoma: a prospective multicentre trial in 472 patients. Eur J Surg Oncol 18:494, 1992
43. Davidson BR: Progress in determining the nature of biliary strictures. Gut 34:725, 1993
44. Hawes RH: Endoscopy and non-calculus biliary obstruction. Annuals of Gastrointestinal Endoscopy, 8th ed. Cotton PB, Tytgat GNJ, Williams CB, Eds. Current Science, England, 1995, p 101
45. Fernandez Del Castillo C, Warshaw AL: Cystic tumors of the pancreas. Surg Clin North Am 75:1001, 1995
46. Pitt HA, Gomes AS, Lois JF: Does preoperative percutaneous biliary drainage reduce operative risk or increase hospital cost? Ann Surg 201:545, 1985
47. McPherson GA, Benjamin IS, Hodgson HJ, et al: Preoperative percutaneous transhepatic biliary drainage: results of a controlled trial. Br J Surg 71:371, 1984
48. Rege RV: Adverse effects of biliary obstruction: implications for treatment of patients with obstructive jaundice. AJR Am J Roentgenol 164:287, 1995
49. Grande L, Garcia-Valdecasas JC, Fuster J, et al: Obstructive jaundice and wound healing. Br J Surg 77:440, 1990
50. Knyrim K, Wagner HJ, Pausch J, et al: A prospective, randomized controlled trial of metal stents for malignant obstruction of the common bile duct. Endoscopy 25:207, 1993
51. Davids P, Groen A, Rauws E, et al: Randomized trial of self-expanding metal stents versus polyethylene stents for distal malignant biliary obstruction. Lancet 340:1488, 1992
52. Smith AC, Dowsett JF, Russell RC, et al: Randomized trial of endoscopic stenting vs surgical bypass in malignant low bile duct obstruction. Lancet 344:1655, 1994
53. Lillemoe KD, Sauter P, Pitt HA, et al: Current status of surgical palliation of periampullary carcinoma. Surg Gynecol Obstet 176:1, 1993
54. Lillemoe KD, Cameron JL, Yeo CJ, et al: Pancreaticoduodenectomy: does it have a role in the palliation of pancreatic cancer? Ann Surg 22:718, 1996
55. Conlon KC, Dougherty E, Klimstra DS, et al: The value of minimal access surgery in the staging of patients with potentially resectable pancreatic malignancy. Ann Surg 223:134, 1996
56. John TG, Greig JD, Carter DC, et al: Carcinoma of the pancreatic head and periampullary region. Tumor staging with laparoscopy and laparoscopic ultrasonography. Ann Surg 221:156, 1995
57. Hunerbein M, Rau B, Schlag PM: Laparoscopic ultrasound for staging of upper gastrointestinal tumours. Eur J Surg Oncol 21:50, 1995
58. Baer HU, Rhyner M, Stain SC, et al: The effect of communication between the right and left liver on the outcome of surgical drainage for jaundice due to malignant obstruction at the hilus of the liver. HPG Surg 8:27, 1994
59. Gagner M: Personal communication
60. Baer HU, Matthews JB, Schweizer WP, et al: Management of the Mirizzi syndrome and the surgical implications of cholecystocholedochal fistula. Br J Surg 77:743, 1990
61. Sarfeh MG, Rypins EB, Jakowatz JG, et al: A prospective, randomized clinical investigation of cholecystoenterostomy and choledochoenterostomy. Am J Surg 155:411, 1988
62. Lieberman MD, Kilburn H, Lindsey M, et al: Relation of perioperative deaths to hospital volume among patients undergoing pancreatic resection for malignancy. Ann Surg 222:638, 1995
63. Lamont JT, Isselbacher KJ: Current concepts of postoperative hepatic dysfunction. Conn Med 39:461, 1975
64. Matlof DS, Kaplan MM: Postoperative jaundice. Orthop Clin North Am 9:799, 1978
65. Moody FG, Potts JR III: Postoperative jaundice. Diseases of the Liver, 7th ed. Schiff L, Schiff ER, Eds. JB Lippincott Co, Philadelphia, 1993, p 370
66. Isselbacher KJ: Bilirubin metabolism and hyperbilirubinemia. Harrison's Principles of Internal Medicine, 12th ed. Wilson JD, Braunwald E, Isselbacher KJ, et al, Eds. McGraw-Hill, New York, 1991, p 1320
67. Watson CJ: Prognosis and treatment of hepatic insufficiency. Ann Intern Med 31:405, 1959
68. Sherlock S: Jaundice. Diseases of the Liver and Biliary System, 8th ed. Sherlock S, Ed. Blackwell Scientific Publications, Oxford, 1989, p 230
69. Gollan JL, Keefe EB, Scharschmidt BF: Cholestasis and hyperbilirubinemia. Current Hepatology, Vol I. Gitnick G, Ed. Houghton Mifflin, Boston, 1980, p 277
70. Bosma PJ, Chowdhury JR, Bakker C, et al: The genetic basis of the reduced expression of bilirubin UCP-glucuronosyltransferase 1 in Gilbert's syndrome. N Engl J Med 333:1171, 1995
71. O'Grady JG, Portmann B, Williams R: Fulminant hepatic failure. Diseases of the Liver, 7th ed. Schiff L, Schiff ER, Eds. JB Lippincott Co, Philadelphia, 1993, p 1077
72. Bismuth H, Samuel D, Castaing D, et al: Orthotopic liver transplantation in fulminant and subfulminant hepatitis. Ann Surg 222:109, 1995
73. Boyer JL, Reuben A: Chronic hepatitis. Diseases of the Liver, 7th ed. Schiff L, Schiff ER, Eds. JB Lippincott Co, Philadelphia, 1993, p 586
74. Pugh RN, Murray-Lyon IM, Dawson JL, et al: Transection of the esophagus for bleeding esophageal varices. Br J Surg 60:646, 1973
75. Semelka RC, Asher SM, Reinhold C: MRI of the Abdomen and Pelvis: A Text-Atlas. John Wiley and Sons, New York, 1997

17 INTESTINAL OBSTRUCTION

W. Scott Helton, M.D.

Assessment of Intestinal Obstruction

Intestinal obstruction is a common medical problem and accounts for a large percentage of surgical admissions for acute abdominal pain [*see 14 Acute Abdominal Pain*].[1] It develops when air and secretions are prevented from passing aborally as a result of either intrinsic or extrinsic compression (i.e., mechanical obstruction) or gastrointestinal paralysis (i.e., nonmechanical obstruction in the form of ileus or pseudo-obstruction). Small intestinal ileus is the most common form of intestinal obstruction; it occurs after most abdominal operations and is a common response to acute extra-abdominal medical conditions and intra-abdominal inflammatory conditions [*see Table 1*]. Mechanical small bowel obstruction is somewhat less common; such obstruction is secondary to intra-abdominal adhesions, hernias, or cancer in about 90 percent of cases [*see Table 2*]. Mechanical colonic obstruction accounts for only 10 to 15 percent of all cases of mechanical obstruction and most often develops in response to obstructing carcinoma, diverticulitis, or volvulus [*see Table 3*]. Acute colonic pseudo-obstruction occurs most frequently in the postoperative period or in response to another acute medical illness.

In what follows, several different methods of classifying mechanical obstruction are used: acute versus chronic, partial versus complete, simple versus closed-loop, and gangrenous versus nongangrenous. The importance of these classifications is that the natural history of the condition, its response to treatment, and the associated morbidity and mortality all vary according to which type of obstruction is present.

When chyme and gas can traverse the point of obstruction, obstruction is partial; when this is not the case, obstruction is complete. When the bowel is occluded at a single point along the intestinal tract, leading to intestinal dilatation, hypersecretion, and bacterial overgrowth proximal to the obstruction and decompression distal to the obstruction, simple obstruction is present. When a segment of bowel is occluded at two points along its course by a single constrictive lesion that occludes both the proximal and the distal end of the intestinal loop as well as traps the bowel's mesentery, closed-loop obstruction is present. When the blood supply to a closed-loop segment of bowel becomes compromised, leading to ischemia and eventually to bowel wall necrosis and perforation, strangulation is present. The most common causes of simple obstruction are intra-abdominal adhesions, tumors, and strictures; the most common causes of closed-loop obstruction are hernias, adhesions, and volvulus.

One of the most difficult tasks in general surgery is deciding when to operate on a patient with intestinal obstruction. The purpose of the following discussion is to outline a safe and efficient stepwise approach to making this often difficult decision and to optimizing the management of patients with this problem. Absolutes are few and far between: treatment must always be highly individualized. Consequently, the following recommendations are intended only as guidelines, not as surgical dicta.

History and Clinical Setting

When a patient complains of acute obstipation, abdominal pain and distention, nausea, and vomiting, the probability that either mechanical bowel obstruction or ileus is present is very high.[2] Mechanical obstruction can often be distinguished from ileus or pseudo-obstruction on the basis of the location, character, and severity of abdominal pain. Pain from mechanical obstruction is usually located in the middle of the abdomen, whereas pain from ileus and pseudo-obstruction is diffuse. Pain from ileus is usually mild, and pain from obstruction is typically more severe. In general, pain increases in severity and depth over time as obstruction progresses; however, in mechanical obstruction, pain severity may decrease over time as a result of bowel fatigue and atony. The periodicity of pain can help localize the level of obstruction: pain from proximal intestinal obstruction has a short periodicity (three to four minutes), and distal small bowel or colonic pain has longer intervals (15 to 20 minutes) between episodes of nausea, cramping, and vomiting.

Abdominal distention, nausea, and vomiting usually develop after pain has already been felt for some time. The patient should be asked what degree of abdominal distention is present and whether there has been a sudden or rapid change. Distention developing over many weeks suggests a chronic process or progressive partial obstruction. Massive abdominal distention coupled with minimal crampy pain, nausea, and vomiting suggests long-standing intermittent mechanical obstruction or some form of chronic intestinal pseudo-obstruction. The combination of a gradual change in bowel habits, progressive abdominal distention, early satiety, mild crampy pain after meals, and weight loss also suggests chronic partial mechanical bowel obstruction. If the patient has undergone evaluation for similar symptoms before, any previous

Assessment of Intestinal Obstruction

Patient presents with signs and symptoms of intestinal obstruction (abdominal pain or distention, nausea, vomiting, obstipation)

Obtain clinical history

Assess character, severity, location, and periodicity of pain.

Assess degree of abdominal distention, and ask about any sudden or rapid changes.

Ask about changes in bowel habits, weight loss, and last passage of flatus.

Ask about (1) previous obstruction, (2) previous abdominal or pelvic procedures, (3) abdominal cancer, (4) intra-abdominal inflammation.

Consider clinical setting: ask about medical conditions or metabolic derangements, exposure to radiation, all medications. Immediate postoperative state is special situation.

Mechanical obstruction

Determine whether obstruction is complete or partial.

Nonmechanical obstruction

Ileus

[See Figure 12.]

Pseudo-obstruction

[See Figure 13.]

Classify obstruction

The most useful distinction is mechanical vs. nonmechanical.

If nature of obstruction is still unclear, perform additional diagnostic tests: sigmoidoscopy, ultrasonography, CT, or contrast studies.

Terminally ill patients: consider no treatment other than comfort measures and hospice care.

Complete obstruction

Immediate operation

Perform physical examination and resuscitate as necessary

Develop gestalt of patient's illness, and assess patient's vital signs, hydration, and cardiopulmonary system.

Place NG tube, Foley catheter, and I.V. line immediately. Assess volume and character of NG aspirate, and measure urine output.

Replace lost fluid with isotonic saline or lactated Ringer's solution. Look for signs of abscess, pneumonia, or myocardial infarction, and be alert for dyspnea, labored breathing, or jaundice.

Perform systematic abdominal examination: observation → auscultation → palpation and percussion. Look for abdominal masses, tenderness, incisions, and hernias; assess bowel sounds; examine rectum for masses, fecal impaction, and occult blood.

Perform investigative studies

Obtain chest x-rays and abdominal films.

If uncertainty about presence or nature of colonic obstruction remains, perform sigmoidoscopy and barium enema examination.

Measure serum electrolytes and creatinine, determine hematocrit, and order coagulation profile. If ileus is suspected, measure serum magnesium and calcium and order urinalysis.

Partial obstruction

Look for associated factors that may necessitate immediate operation.

Patient has peritonitis, incarcerated hernia, suspected or confirmed strangulation, pneumatosis cystoides intestinalis, sigmoid volvulus with systemic toxicity or peritoneal irritation, small bowel volvulus, colonic volvulus above sigmoid, or fecal impaction

No indications for immediate operation are present

Manage initially with nonoperative measures.

Reassess patient frequently.

Look for changes in pain, abdominal findings, and volume and character of NG aspirate.

Repeat abdominal x-rays, and look for changes in gas distribution, pneumatosis cystoides intestinalis, and free intraperitoneal air.

Classify patient's condition as improved, unchanged, or worse.

Decide whether operative treatment is necessary and, if so, whether it should be done on urgent or elective basis.

Urgent operation

Indications include
- Lack of response to 24–48 hr of nonoperative therapy (increasing abdominal pain, distention, or tenderness; NG aspirate changing from nonfeculent to feculent; ↑ proximal small bowel distention with ↓ distal gas).
- Early technical complications of operation (abscess, phlegmon, hematoma, hernia, intussusception, anastomotic obstruction).

No operation

Conditions that typically resolve with nonoperative therapy include adhesive obstruction (unless it does not improve in 12 hr), early postoperative obstruction (unless it does not improve in 2 wk), and various inflammatory conditions (IBD, radiation enteritis, diverticulitis, acute Crohn's disease).

Elective operation

Indications include nontoxic, nontender sigmoid volvulus with sigmoidoscopically managed obstruction; recurrent adhesive or stricture-related small bowel obstruction; partial colonic obstruction unresponsive to 24 hr of nonoperative therapy; development and resolution of small bowel obstruction in patient who has never undergone abdominal operation.

266 — II COMMON PRESENTING PROBLEMS

Table 1 Causes of Ileus

Intra-abdominal causes
  Intraperitoneal problems
    Peritonitis or abscess
    Inflammatory condition
      Mechanical: operation, foreign body
      Chemical: gastric juice, bile, blood
      Autoimmune: serositis, vasculitis
    Intestinal ischemia: arterial or venous, sickle-cell disease
  Retroperitoneal problems
    Pancreatitis
    Retroperitoneal hematoma
    Spine fracture
    Aortic operation
    Renal colic
    Pyelonephritis
    Metastasis

Extra-abdominal causes
  Thoracic problems
    Myocardial infarction
    Pneumonia
    Congestive heart failure
    Rib fractures
  Metabolic abnormalities
    Electrolyte imbalance (e.g., hypokalemia)
    Sepsis
    Lead poisoning
    Porphyria
    Hypothyroidism
    Hypoparathyroidism
    Uremia
  Medicines
    Opiates
    Anticholinergics
    Alpha agonists
    Antihistamines
    Catecholamines
  Spinal cord injury or operations
  Head, thoracic, or retroperitoneal trauma
  Chemotherapy, radiation therapy

---

recurrent cancer. Obstructive symptoms that come and go suddenly over several days in a patient older than 65 years should increase the index of suspicion for gallstone ileus.[3] If the patient has experienced episodes of obstruction before, one should ask about the etiology and the response to treatment. If the patient has ever undergone an abdominal operation, one should try to obtain and read the operative report, which can provide a great deal of helpful information (e.g., description of adhesions, assessment of their severity, and evaluation of intra-abdominal pathology and anatomy). If abdominal cancer was present, one should find out what operation was performed and attempt to determine the likelihood of intra-abdominal recurrence.

The clinical setting often provides clues to the cause and type of bowel obstruction. In hospitalized patients, there is likely to be an associated medical condition or metabolic derangement that led to obstruction. A thorough review of the patient's medical history and hospital course should be undertaken to identify precipitating events that could have led to intestinal obstipation. One should ask the patient about any previous abdominal irradiation and should note and take into account all medications the patient is taking, especially anticoagulants and agents with anticholinergic side effects. Patients who are receiving chemotherapy or have undergone abdominal radiation therapy are prone to ileus. Severe infection, fluid and electrolyte imbalances, narcotic and anticholinergic medications, and intra-abdominal inflammation of any origin may be implicated. Acute

abdominal radiographs or contrast studies should be reviewed. The patient should be asked when flatus was last passed: failure to pass flatus may signal a transition from partial to complete bowel obstruction. Patients with an intestinal stoma (ileostomy or colostomy) who present with signs and symptoms of obstruction often report abdominal distention and pain after a sudden change in stomal output of stool, liquid, or air.

The patient should also be asked about (1) previous episodes of bowel obstruction, (2) previous abdominal or pelvic operations, (3) a history of abdominal cancer, and (4) a history of intra-abdominal inflammation (e.g., inflammatory bowel disease, cholecystitis, pancreatitis, pelvic inflammatory disease, or abdominal trauma). Any of these factors increases the chance that the obstruction is secondary to an adhesion or

Table 2 Causes of Small Bowel Obstruction in Adults

Extrinsic causes
  Adhesions*
  Hernias (external, internal, incisional)*
  Metastatic cancer*
  Volvulus
  Intra-abdominal abscess
  Intra-abdominal hematoma
  Pancreatic pseudocyst
  Intra-abdominal drains
  Tight fascial opening at stoma

Intraluminal causes
  Tumors*
  Gallstones
  Foreign body
  Worms
  Bezoars

Intramural abnormalities
  Tumors
  Strictures
  Hematoma
  Intussusception
  Regional enteritis
  Radiation enteritis

*Approximately 85% of all small bowel obstructions are secondary to adhesions, hernias, or tumors.

Table 3 Causes of Colonic Obstruction

Common causes
- Cancer (primary, anastomotic, metastatic)
- Volvulus
- Diverticulitis
- Pseudo-obstruction
- Hernia
- Anastomotic stricture

Unusual causes
- Intussusception
- Fecal impaction
- Strictures (from one of the following)
  - Inflammatory bowel disease
  - Endometriosis
  - Radiation therapy
  - Ischemia
- Foreign body
- Extrinsic compression by a mass
  - Pancreatic pseudocyst
  - Hematoma
  - Metastasis
  - Primary tumors

massive abdominal distention in a hospitalized patient usually results from acute gastric distention, small bowel ileus, or acute colonic pseudo-obstruction. Excessive anticoagulation can lead to retroperitoneal, intra-abdominal, or intramural hematoma that can cause mechanical obstruction or ileus. Finally, there are specific problems that tend to arise in the postoperative period; these are discussed more fully elsewhere [*see* Urgent Operation, Early Postoperative Technical Complications, *and* No Operation, Early Postoperative Obstruction].

Physical Examination and Resuscitation

The initial steps in the physical examination are (1) developing a gestalt of the patient's illness and (2) assessing the patient's vital signs, hydration status, and cardiopulmonary system. A nasogastric tube, a Foley catheter, and an I.V. line are placed immediately while the physical examination is in progress. The volume and character of the gastric aspirate and urine are noted. A clear, gastric effluent is suggestive of gastric outlet obstruction. A bilious, nonfeculent aspirate is a typical sign of medial to proximal small bowel obstruction or colonic obstruction with a competent ileocecal valve. A feculent aspirate is a typical sign of distal small bowel obstruction. Volume replacement, if necessary, is initiated with isotonic saline solution or lactated Ringer's solution. Urine output must be adequate (at least 0.5 ml/kg/hr) before the patient can be taken to the OR; supplemental potassium chloride (40 mEq/L) is administered once this is achieved.

Fever may be present, suggesting that the obstruction may be a manifestation of an intra-abdominal abscess. Signs of pneumonia or myocardial infarction should be sought: these conditions, like intestinal obstruction, can have upper abdominal pain, distention, nausea, and vomiting as presenting symptoms. Dyspnea and labored breathing may occur secondary to severe abdominal distention or pain, in which case immediate relief should be provided by placing the patient in the lateral decubitus position and offering narcotics as soon as the initial physical examination is performed. Jaundice raises the possibility of gallstone ileus or metastatic cancer.

Examination of the abdomen proceeds in an orderly manner from observation to auscultation to palpation and percussion. The patient is placed in the supine position with the legs flexed at the hip to decrease tension on the rectus muscles. The degree of abdominal distention observed varies, depending on the level of obstruction: proximal obstructions may cause little or no distention. Abdominal scars should be noted. Abdominal asymmetry or a protruding mass suggests an underlying malignancy, an abscess, or closed-loop obstruction. The abdominal wall should be observed for evidence of peristaltic waves, which are indicative of acute small bowel obstruction.

Auscultation should be performed for at least three to four minutes to determine the presence and quality of bowel sounds. High-pitched bowel tones, tingles, and rushes are suggestive of an obstructive process, especially when temporally associated with waves of crampy pain, nausea, or vomiting. The absence of bowel tones is typical of intestinal paralysis but may also indicate intestinal fatigue from long-standing obstruction, closed-loop obstruction, or pseudo-obstruction.

Approximately 70 percent of patients with bowel obstruction have symmetric tenderness, whereas fewer than half have rebound tenderness, guarding, or rigidity.[2] The traditional teaching is that localized tenderness and guarding indicate underlying strangulated bowel; however, prospective studies have demonstrated that these physical findings are neither specific nor sensitive for detecting underlying strangulation[4] or even obstruction.[2] Nevertheless, most surgeons still believe that guarding, rebound tenderness, and localized tenderness reflect underlying strangulation and therefore are indications for operation. Patients with ileus tend to have generalized abdominal tenderness that cannot be distinguished from the tenderness of mechanical obstruction. Gentle percussion is performed over all quadrants of the abdomen to search for areas of dullness (suggestive of an underlying mass), tympany (suggestive of underlying distended bowel), and peritoneal irritation.

A thorough search is made for inguinal, femoral, umbilical, and incisional hernias. The rectum is examined for masses, fecal impaction, and occult blood. If the patient has an ileostomy or a colostomy, the stoma is examined digitally to make sure that there is no obstruction at the level of the fascia.

Investigative Studies

IMAGING STUDIES

One should obtain a chest x-ray in all patients with bowel obstruction to exclude a pneumonic process and to look for subdiaphragmatic air. In most

patients into those with mechanical obstruction and those with nonmechanical obstruction. In patients with mechanical bowel obstruction, an effort should be made to determine whether the obstruction is complete or partial. Except for a few clinical situations, patients with complete bowel obstruction require immediate operation; conversely, patients with partial bowel obstruction rarely do. Finally, an effort should be made to establish the level and cause of obstruction because these factors often help guide therapy and affect the probability of success in response to specific therapeutic intervention. Patients with nonmechanical obstruction, which derives from ileus or pseudo-obstruction [see Ileus and Pseudo-obstruction, below], do not require immediate operation.

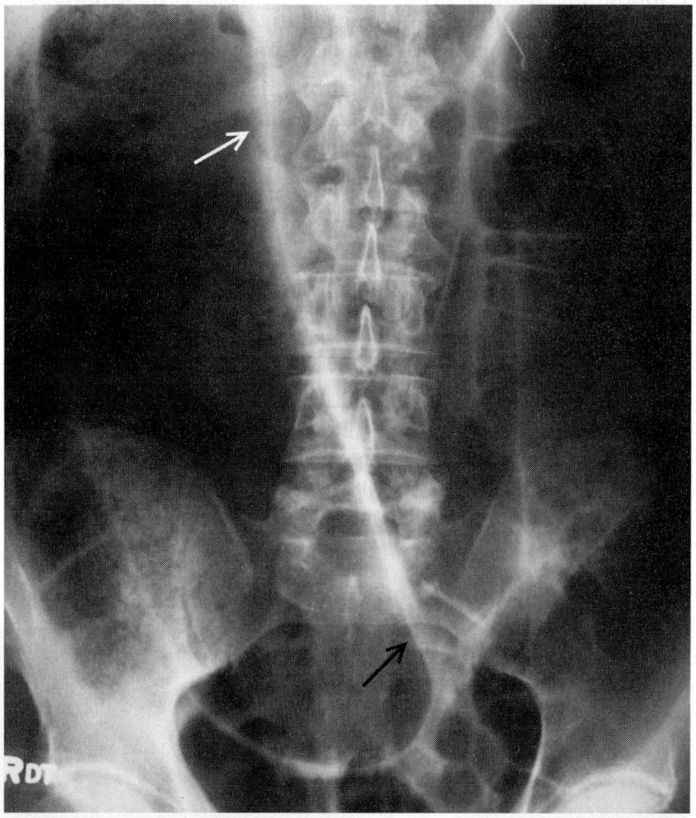

ADJUNCTIVE TESTS FOR EQUIVOCAL SITUATIONS

Sigmoidoscopy

When one is uncertain whether the obstruction is mechanical or not on the basis of the information in hand, additional diagnostic measures are immediately indicated. When large amounts of colonic air extend down to the rectum, flexible or rigid sigmoidoscopy will readily exclude a rectal or distal sigmoid obstruction. If sigmoidoscopy yields normal findings and partial colonic obstruction is the most likely diagnosis, a barium enema with water-soluble contrast material should immediately be performed.[6] Abdominal ultrasonography, though not as definitive as a contrast examination, is also able to diagnose suspected colonic obstruction in 85 percent of patients.[7]

Ultrasonography and CT Scanning

Abdominal radiographs can be entirely normal in patients with complete, closed-loop, or strangulation obstruction.[8] Therefore, if the patient's clinical profile and the results of physical examination are consistent with intestinal obstruction despite normal abdominal radiographs, abdominal ultrasonography, followed by CT scanning if necessary, should be performed immediately.[8-10] Both of these imaging modalities are highly sensitive and specific for intestinal obstruction when performed properly and interpreted by experienced clinicians. In addition, both are capable of detecting the cause of the obstruction as well as the presence of closed-loop or strangulation obstruction.[7,9,11-14] Sonographic criteria have been established for small bowel and colonic obstruction[7,11,12]: (1) simultaneous observation of distended and collapsed bowel segments, (2) free peritoneal fluid, (3) inspissated intestinal contents, (4) paradoxical pendulating peristalsis, (5) highly reflecting fluid within the bowel lumen, (6) bowel wall edema between serosa and mucosa, and (7) a fixed mass of aperistaltic, fluid-filled, dilated intestinal loops. One group of authors[7] has recommended that when abdominal radiographs are inconclusive or normal in patients with suspected colonic

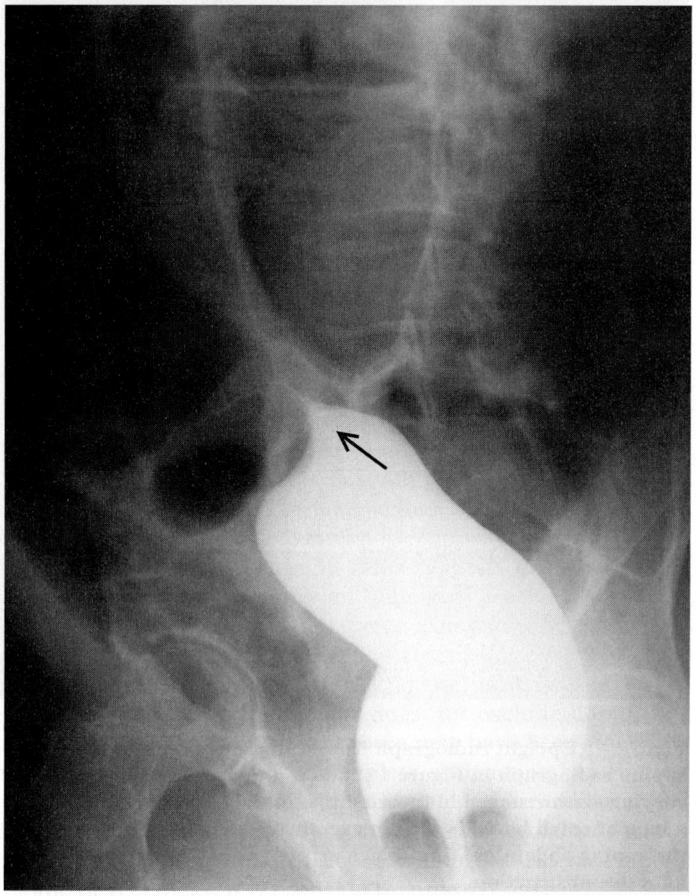

Figure 5 (*a*) Radiograph from a patient with massive sigmoid volvulus shows a distended ahaustral sigmoid loop (white arrow), inferior convergence of the walls of the sigmoid loop to the left of the midline, and approximation of the medial walls of the sigmoid loop as a summation line (black arrow). (*b*) Barium enema of the colon shows a tapered obstruction at the rectosigmoid junction with a typical bird's-beak deformity (black arrow).

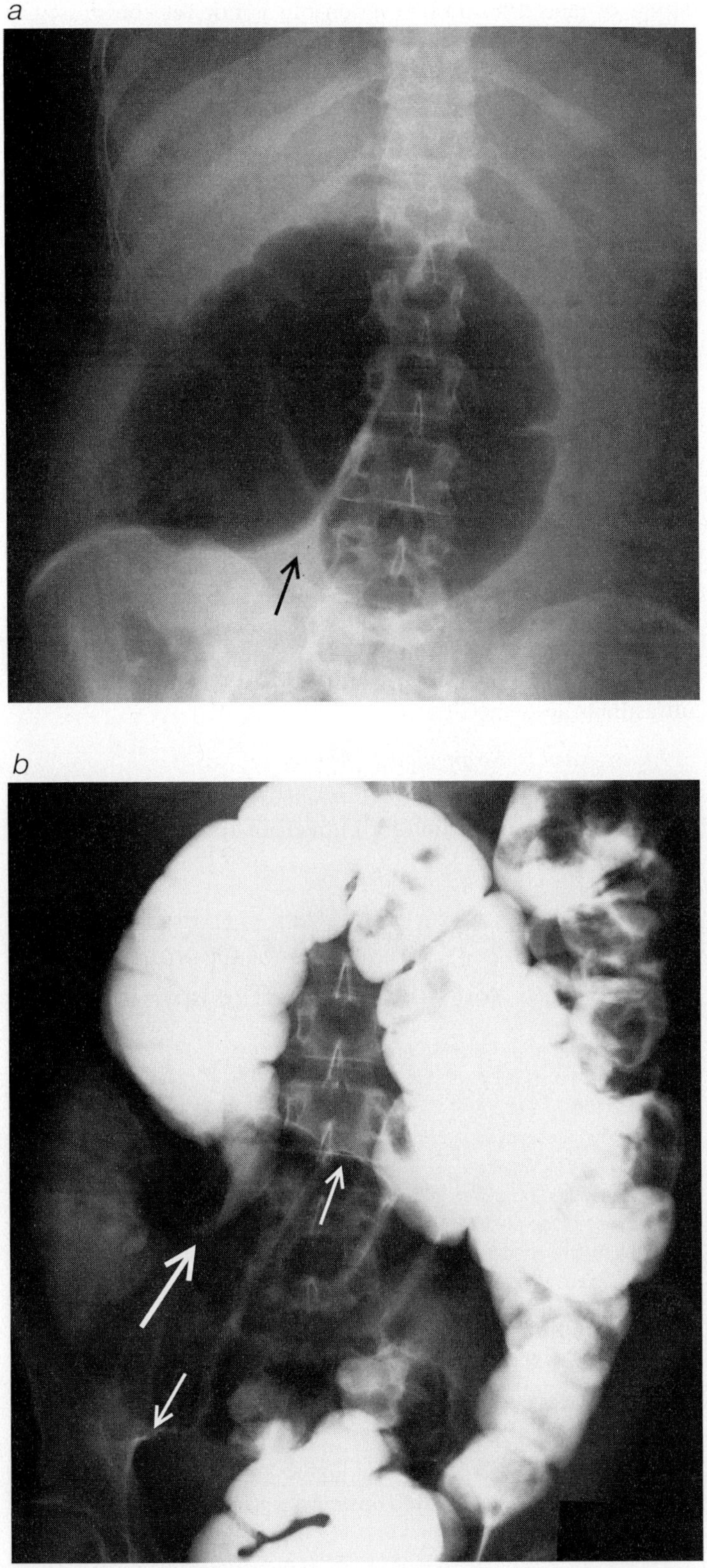

Figure 6 (*a*) Radiograph from a patient with cecal volvulus shows a dilated cecum with no air distally in the colorectum. Convergence of the medial walls of the loop (black arrow) points to the right, a typical finding in cecal volvulus. (*b*) Barium examination demonstrates a bird's-beak deformity tapering at the point of volvulus (large white arrow). Note walls of dilated cecum (small white arrows).

obstruction, ultrasonography, rather than CT or barium enema, should be the next diagnostic step. Ultrasonography is well suited to critically ill patients: because it can be performed at the bedside, the risk associated with transport to the radiology suite is avoided. Given that ultrasonography is relatively inexpensive, is easy and quick to perform, and often can provide a great deal of information about the location, nature, and severity of the obstruction, it should be employed early on in the evaluation of all patients with intestinal obstruction.

Another author[10] has recommended that patients with suspected small bowel obstruction and equivocal plain abdominal films undergo CT scanning before a small bowel contrast series is ordered. CT scanning has several advantages over a small bowel contrast examination in this setting: (1) it can ascertain the level of obstruction, (2) it can assess the severity of the obstruction and determine its cause, and (3) it can detect closed-loop obstruction and early strangulation [*see Figures 8, 9, 10, and 11*]. CT can also detect inflammatory or neoplastic processes both outside and inside the peritoneal cavity and can visualize small amounts of intraperitoneal air or pneumatosis cystoides intestinalis not seen on conventional films [*see Figure 10*]. Prospective studies have demonstrated that the accuracy of CT in diagnosing bowel obstruction is higher than 95 percent and its sensitivity and specificity are each higher than 94 percent.[13,14] It has been argued that only after a nondiagnostic CT scan or ultrasonogram should patients be evaluated with a barium contrast study; however, the sensitivity and specificity of this recommended approach have yet to be established by prospective trials.

Contrast Studies

Enteroclysis (direct injection of $BaSO_4$ into the small bowel) is generally considered the most sensitive method of distinguishing between ileus and partial mechanical small bowel obstruction: it has a diagnostic sensitivity of 87 percent for adhesive obstruction.[15,16] Many surgeons are concerned that injection of barium might cause partial obstruction to progress to complete obstruction; however, there is no evidence that this ever occurs, and one therefore should not refrain from using enteroclysis to diagnose partial small bowel obstruction.[17,18] If complete obstruction is identified, the patient should undergo immediate operation. If partial obstruction is identified in either the small or the large bowel, the patient is treated accordingly. If mechanical obstruction is not identified and abdominal ultrasonography yields normal findings, the diagnosis is almost certainly ileus, in which case one's attention is directed toward identifying and correcting the underlying precipitating cause [*see Table 1*].

Mechanical Obstruction

TERMINAL ILLNESS

Patients with a terminal illness (e.g., acquired immunodeficiency syndrome [AIDS] or advanced carcinomatosis) to whom surgical treatment offers little hope of improved quality or duration of life may choose not to undergo operative intervention for acute bowel obstruction. These patients should be offered comfort measures, including continuous morphine infusion and an octreotide drip. Patients who do not wish to die of malignant bowel obstruction in a hospital should be offered hospice care or home visiting nurse services with continuous octreotide infusion, intravenous rehydration or total parenteral nutrition (TPN), and gastrostomy decompression.[19,20] It is essential to always pay attention to quality-of-life issues and to the patient's potential interest in pursuing nonoperative forms of palliation. For many terminally ill or incurable patients with bowel obstruction, the most humane and sensible treatment comprises nothing more than gastric decompression, intravenous rehydration, and morphine.

IMMEDIATE OPERATION

All patients with complete bowel obstruction, whether of the small intestine or the large, should undergo immediate operation unless extraordinary circumstances (e.g., diffuse carcinomatosis, terminal illness, or sigmoid volvulus that responds to sigmoidoscopic decompression) are present. If one attempts to manage complete intestinal obstruction nonoperatively, one risks delaying definitive treatment of patients with intestinal ischemia and subjecting them to significantly increased morbidity and mortality should perforation or severe infection develop.[4,21]

Immediate operation is also indicated when bowel obstruction is associated with peritonitis; incarcerated strangulated hernias; suspected or confirmed strangulation; pneumatosis cystoides intestinalis; sigmoid volvulus accompanied by systemic toxicity or peritoneal irritation; colonic volvulus above the sigmoid colon; or fecal impaction. These conditions will not resolve without operation and are associated with increased morbidity, mortality, and cost if diagnosis and treatment are delayed. The only time one would not operate immediately on any patient with one of these diagnoses is when the patient requires cardiopulmonary stabilization, additional resuscitation, or both. Whenever there is any doubt as to the presence of any of these conditions, additional diagnostic tests (e.g., ultrasonography, CT, or contrast studies) are indicated to confirm or exclude them.

Strangulation and Closed-Loop Obstruction

Morbidity and mortality from intestinal obstruction vary significantly and depend primarily on the presence of strangulation and subsequent infection. Strangulation obstruction occurs in approximately 10 percent of all patients with small intestinal obstruction. It carries a mortality of 10 to 37 percent, whereas simple obstruction carries a mortality of less than five percent.[4,17,22,23] Early recognition and immediate operative treatment of strangulation obstruction are the only current means of decreasing this mortality. Strangulation obstruction occurs most frequently in patients with incarcerated hernias, closed-loop obstruction, volvulus, or complete bowel obstruction; hence, identification of any of these specific causes of obstruction is an important and clear indication for immediate operation. Radiographic evidence of pneumatosis cystoides intestinalis or free intraperitoneal air in a patient with a clinical picture of bowel obstruction is indicative of strangulation, perforation, or both and constitutes an indication for operation. High-quality abdominal CT with intravenous contrast can detect advanced strangulation as well as identify early, reversible strangulation [*see Figure 11*]. Abdominal ultrasonography can also identify edematous, hemorrhagic loops of intestine. Accordingly, whenever one is concerned about possible strangulation or closed-loop obstruction but is not yet committed to taking the patient immediately to the OR, an ultrasonogram or a CT scan should be obtained. In fact, given that ultrasonography and CT are the only well-established means of diagnosing strangulation obstruction short of exploratory laparotomy or laparoscopy, an argument can be made that one or the other should be performed in all patients who have been admitted to the hospital with bowel obstruction and are initially being treated nonoperatively.

Many surgeons base the decision whether to operate on patients with bowel obstruction on the presence or absence of the so-called classic signs of strangulation obstruction—continuous abdominal pain, fever, tachycardia, peritoneal signs, and leukocytosis—and on their clinical experience. Unfortunately, these classically taught signs, even in conjunction with abdominal x-rays and clinical judgment, are incapable of reliably detecting closed-loop or gangrenous bowel obstruction.[4,17,21-24] In fact, one prospective clinical trial concluded that the five classic signs of strangulation obstruction and experienced clinical judgment were not sensitive for, specific for, or predictive of strangulation[4]: in more than 50 percent of the patients who had intestinal strangulation, the condition was not recognized preoperatively. Such findings suggest that early nonoperative recognition of intestinal strangulation is not feasible without ultrasonography or CT.

Incarcerated or Strangulated Hernias

A hernia that is incarcerated, tender, erythematous, warm, or edematous is an indication for immediate operation. Primary or

Table 4 **Guidelines for Operative and Nonoperative Therapy**

Situations necessitating emergent operation
- Incarcerated, strangulated hernias
- Peritonitis
- Pneumatosis cystoides intestinalis
- Pneumoperitoneum
- Suspected or proven intestinal strangulation
- Closed-loop obstruction
- Nonsigmoid colonic volvulus
- Sigmoid volvulus associated with toxicity or peritoneal signs
- Complete bowel obstruction

Situations necessitating urgent operation
- Progressive bowel obstruction at any time after nonoperative measures are started
- Failure to improve with conservative therapy within 24–48 hr
- Early postoperative technical complications

Situations in which delayed operation is usually safe
- Immediate postoperative obstruction
- Sigmoid volvulus successfully decompressed by sigmoidoscopy
- Acute exacerbation of Crohn's disease, diverticulitis, or radiation enteritis
- Chronic, recurrent partial obstruction
- Gastric outlet obstruction
- Postoperative adhesions
- Resolved partial colonic obstruction

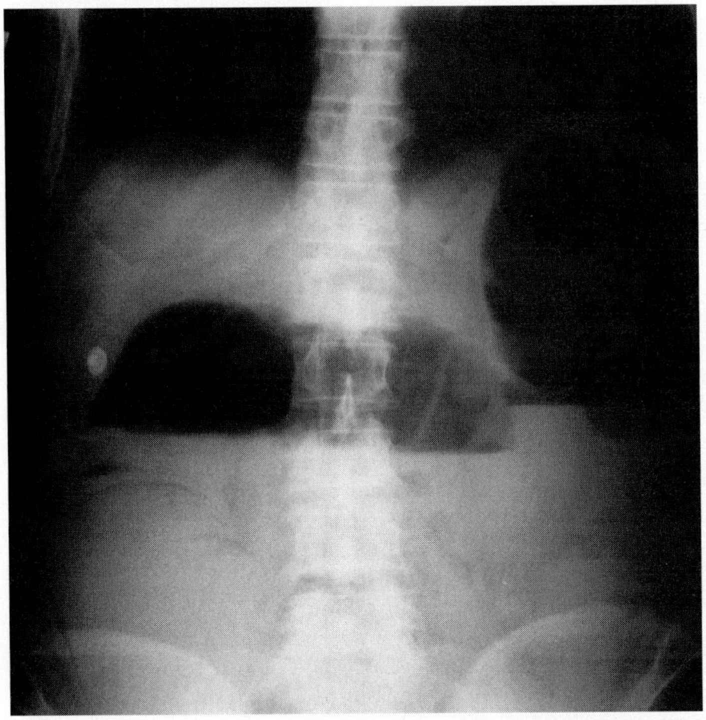

Figure 7 Shown is a radiograph from a patient with complete colonic obstruction from an obstructing carcinoma in the descending left colon with proximal air-fluid levels. The absence of air distally in the rectum or the sigmoid is suggestive of complete obstruction. The ileocecal valve is competent, and thus, there is no small bowel air.

incisional hernias may not be palpable in obese patients, in which case ultrasonography or CT scanning should be performed.

Nonsigmoid Volvulus and Sigmoid Volvulus with Systemic Toxicity or Peritoneal Signs

All intestinal volvuli are closed-loop obstructions and thus carry a high risk of intestinal strangulation, infarction, and perforation. Patients typically present with acute, colicky abdominal pain, massive distention, nausea, and vomiting. Sigmoid volvulus is the most common form of colonic volvulus, followed by cecal volvulus. Abdominal radiographs are fairly diagnostic for colonic volvulus [*see Figures 5 and 6*]. In contrast, small bowel volvulus may not be visualized on plain radiographs, because the closed loop fills completely with fluid and no air-fluid level can be seen. Small bowel volvulus is readily detected by ultrasonography or CT scanning; one or both of these procedures should be performed in patients presenting with signs and symptoms of bowel obstruction and normal abdominal radiographs. Small bowel volvulus is an indication for immediate operation.

If one observes signs of systemic toxicity, a bloody rectal discharge, fever, leukocytosis, or peritoneal irritation in a patient with sigmoid volvulus, the patient should undergo immediate operation; if all of these signs are absent, the patient should undergo sigmoidoscopy. When there are no signs of peritonitis or generalized toxicity, sigmoidoscopic decompression is safe and effective in more than 95 percent of patients with sigmoid volvulus.[25] If mucosal gangrene or a bloody effluent is noted at the time of sigmoidoscopy, immediate operative intervention is necessary even in the absence of any clinical signs or symptoms of strangulation. After sigmoidoscopy, the patient can undergo elective bowel preparation and a single-stage sigmoid resection before being discharged from the hospital. If, howev-

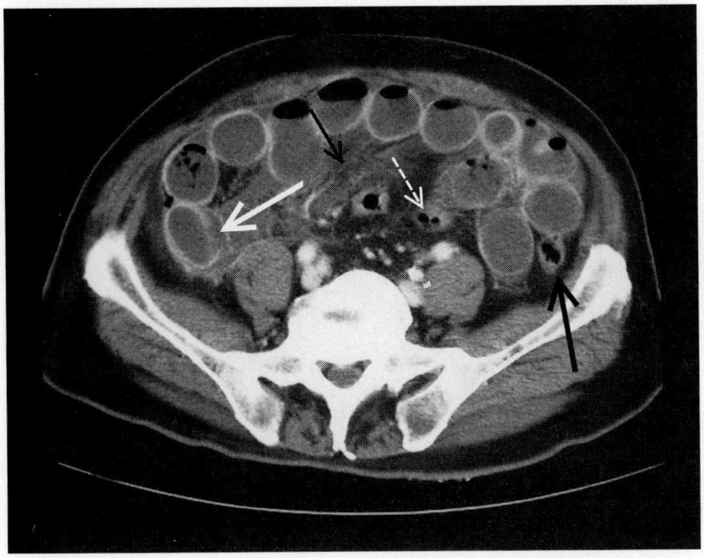

Figure 8 CT scan from a patient with partial small bowel obstruction shows distended, fluid-filled loops of small bowel with air-fluid levels, hyperemia, and bowel wall thickening (large white arrow). Note the discrepancy in caliber between dilated small bowel and decompressed small bowel (dashed white arrow) and the stranding (small black arrow) in the small bowel mesentery. Air in a decompressed descending colon (large black arrow) is indicative of partial obstruction.

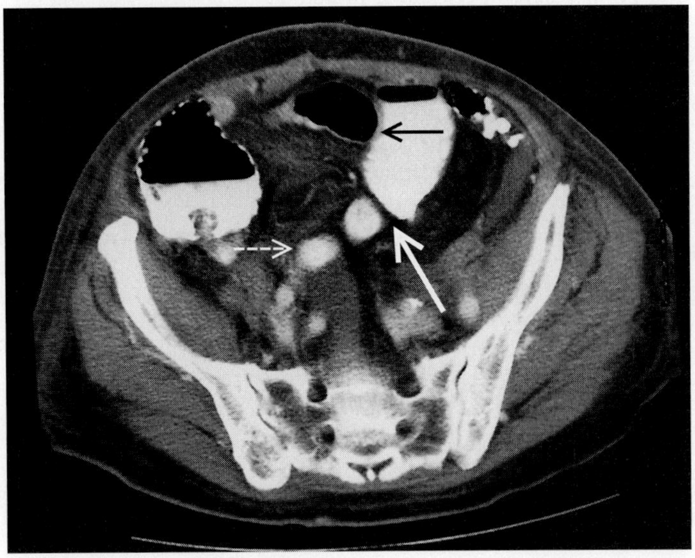

Figure 9 CT scan from a patient with adhesive partial small bowel obstruction shows massively dilated small intestine (black arrow) proximal to a thick adhesive band (large white arrow) and decompressed small bowel distal to the adhesion (dashed white arrow). The patient was operated on because of the low probability that this obstruction would resolve with conservative management.

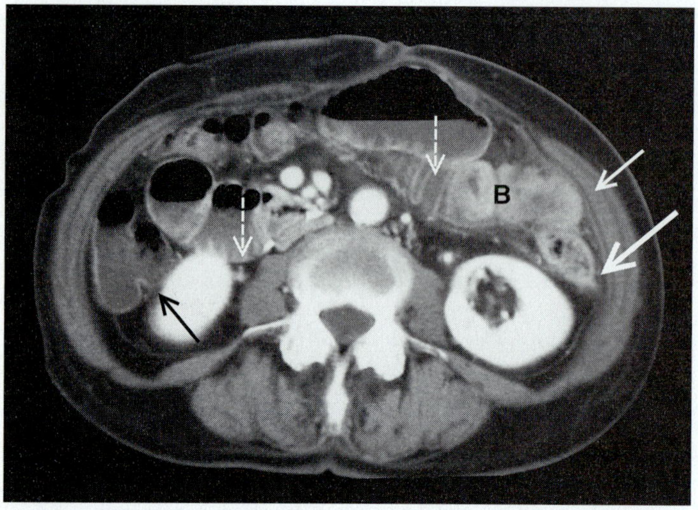

Figure 10 CT scan from a patient with partial small bowel obstruction from cancer shows distended small bowel (dashed white arrows) proximal to a mass (small white arrow). There is air in the cecum (black arrow), the transverse colon, and the descending colon (large white arrow). The small bowel is maximally dilated, with hyperemic, edematous bowel wall (B) just proximal to an obstructing recurrent colon carcinoma. Even though plain radiographs showed partial small bowel obstruction, this CT scan led to early operation because continued nonoperative management would not resolve the problem.

but is undetected. Furthermore, there is the risk that while the patient is being observed, partial obstruction will progress to complete obstruction or strangulation and perforation will develop. It is therefore crucial to be alert to changes in the patient's condition.

Repeated examination of the abdomen by the same clinician is the most sensitive way of detecting progressive obstruction. Examinations should be performed every three hours. If abdominal pain, tenderness, or distention increases or the gastric aspirate changes from nonfeculent to feculent, abdominal exploration is indicated. Abdominal radiographs should be repeated six to 12 hours after nasogastric decompression. If proximal small bowel distention increases or distal intestinal gas decreases, nonoperative therapy is considered to have failed, and operative intervention is indicated. Conversely, if the patient's condition appears stable or improved and x-rays indicate that the obstruction either has resolved somewhat or at least is no worse, it is generally safe to continue nonoperative care for another 12 to 24 hours. If the clinical picture is stable after 24 hours of observation, one must decide whether to operate or to continue nonoperative therapy. One's clinical judgment and experience, coupled with a thorough and accurate assessment of the patient's underlying diagnosis and clinical condition, are the most reliable guides for making this decision. Even in stable patients who are not in a toxic state, continued observation carries certain risks (e.g., progressive bowel ischemia with possible bowel infarction and perforation).

Early Postoperative Technical Complications

When normal bowel function initially returns after an abdominal operation but then is replaced by a clinical picture

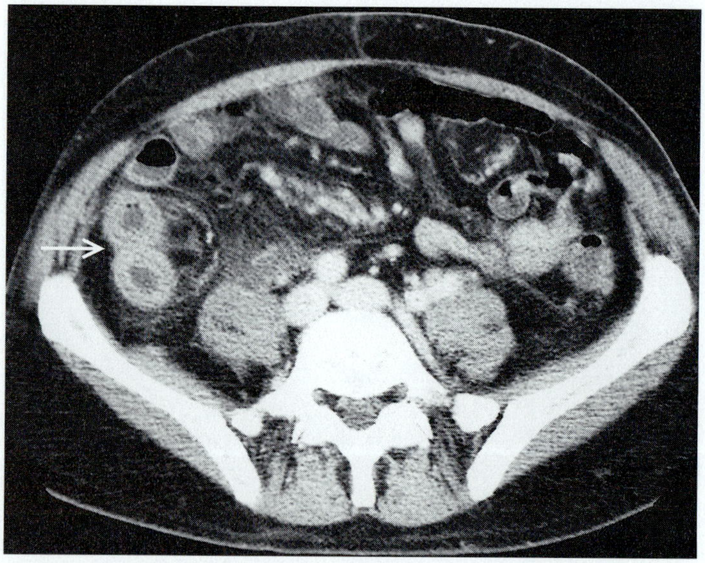

er, clinical toxicity, a bloody rectal discharge, fever, or peritoneal irritation arise at any time after sigmoidoscopic decompression while the patient is being prepared for elective operation, immediate operation is indicated.

Patients with volvulus proximal to the sigmoid colon should undergo immediate operation regardless of whether peritoneal irritation is present. The incidence of strangulation infarction is high in such patients, and nonoperative therapy often fails. If the diagnosis of nonsigmoid colonic volvulus is in doubt, a barium enema is indicated to exclude colonic pseudo-obstruction.

Fecal Impaction

Complete colonic obstruction secondary to fecal impaction in the rectum can sometimes be successfully relieved through disimpaction at the bedside; however, this can be difficult and extremely uncomfortable for the patient. The most expeditious and successful method of relieving the obstruction is to disimpact the patient while he or she is under general or spinal anesthesia.

URGENT OPERATION

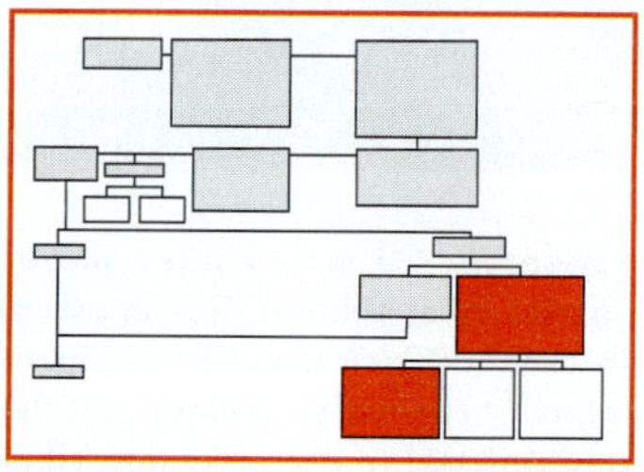

Lack of Response to Nonoperative Therapy within 24 to 48 Hours

It is usually safe to manage partial bowel obstruction initially by nonoperative means: a nihil per os (NPO) regimen, nasogastric decompression, analgesics, and octreotide. Such therapy is successful in many cases, but there is always the risk that complete bowel obstruction or strangulation already exists

Figure 11 CT scan from a patient with early closed-loop obstruction of the small intestine shows markedly edematous, hyperemic small bowel, a finding indicative of early strangulation (white arrow). The patient had minimal symptoms, and there was air in the transverse colon and the descending colon (a finding indicative of partial small bowel obstruction); however, the finding of gangrenous, nonperforated small bowel on this CT scan led to early operation.

suggestive of early postoperative mechanical obstruction, the explanation may be a technical complication of the operation (e.g., phlegmon, abscess, intussusception, a narrow anastomosis, an internal hernia, or obstruction at the level of a stoma). An early, aggressive diagnostic workup should be performed to identify or exclude these problems because they are unlikely to respond to nasogastric decompression or other forms of conservative management. It is critical to know exactly what was done within the abdomen in the course of the operation. To this end, one should try to speak directly with the operating surgeon rather than attempt to deduce the needed information from the operative report.

If the patient had peritonitis or a colonic anastomosis at the initial operation, one should order a CT scan to look for an intra-abdominal abscess. An abscess or a phlegmon at the site of an anastomosis is usually secondary to anastomotic leakage and is an indication for reoperation. CT scanning can also identify intra-abdominal hematomas, which should be evacuated through early reoperation. In patients recovering from a proctectomy, herniation of the small bowel through a defect in the pelvic floor is a common cause of intestinal obstruction. Oral contrast studies can help identify patients with an internal hernia, intussusception, or anastomotic obstruction and should be performed after the CT scan. A retrograde barium examination should be performed in patients thought to have a problem related to a stoma or an intestinal anastomosis. When none of the above factors appear to be the cause of the postoperative obstruction, it is reasonable for the surgeon to assume that the obstruction is secondary to postoperative adhesions, which are best treated conservatively (see below).

NO OPERATION

In selected patients, nonoperative management of partial small bowel obstruction is highly successful and carries an acceptably low mortality. Such patients include those whose partial obstruction is secondary to intra-abdominal adhesions, occurs in the immediate postoperative period, or derives from an inflammatory condition (e.g., inflammatory bowel disease, radiation enteritis, or diverticulitis).

Adhesive Partial Small Bowel Obstruction

Adhesive partial small bowel obstruction is treated initially with nasogastric decompression, intravenous rehydration, and analgesia. Parenteral nutrition should be begun if one believes that oral or enteral nutrition will not be adequate within five days. Nonoperative therapy leads to resolution of adhesive partial obstruction in as many as 90 percent of patients.[26] Some studies suggest that the nature of the previous abdominal operation may influence the probability that the obstruction will not respond to medical therapy. Operations associated with intestinal obstruction that is not likely to respond to medical therapy include procedures involving the aorta, the pelvic adnexa, or the appendix and those done to relieve carcinomatous obstruction. In a patient with this kind of operative history, strong consideration should be given to surgical intervention unless comorbid medical conditions tip the risk-benefit balance in the direction of nonoperative therapy.

There is constant debate regarding how long patients with partial adhesive obstruction should be treated conservatively. After 48 hours of nonoperative management, the risk of complications increases substantially, and the probability that the obstruction will resolve diminishes.[23] Generally, if the obstruction is going to resolve with nonoperative therapy, there will be a fairly prompt response within the first eight to 12 hours. Therefore, if a patient's condition has deteriorated or has not significantly improved by 12 hours after the operation, exploratory laparotomy is advisable. During this observation period, the patient must be constantly reevaluated, ideally by the same examiner. Analgesics can be safely administered, and repeat abdominal examinations should be performed at three-hour intervals when the influence of narcotics has waned. Repeat abdominal x-rays should be obtained no later than six hours after nasogastric decompression, and the pattern of gas distribution should be compared with that seen on the admission films. A decrease in intestinal gas distal to a point of obstruction coupled with an increase in proximal dilatation suggests that the obstruction is worsening; conversely, a decrease in intestinal distention coupled with the appearance of more gas distally in the colon suggests that the obstruction is being reduced. The degree of abdominal distention, the passage of flatus, and the nature of the nasogastric aspirate should be evaluated periodically. If abdominal distention does not decrease or the gastric aspirate changes from bilious to feculent, the patient should be operated on.

Experimental and clinical studies suggest that patients undergoing nonoperative treatment for bowel obstruction may benefit from the administration of somatostatin analogues as a result of the potent effects these substances exert on intestinal sodium, chloride, and water absorption.[27] In one study, animals with either complete or closed-loop partial small bowel obstruction were given either long-acting somatostatin or saline; the treatment group had significantly less intestinal distention, less infarction, and longer survival than the control group.[27,28] In a prospective, randomized clinical trial evaluating the use of somatostatin in patients who had complete small bowel obstruction without clinical or radiologic evidence of strangulation, the treatment group was less likely to need operation, had less proximal intestinal distention, and exhibited decreased mucosal necrosis proximal to the point of obstruction.[29] Long-acting somatostatin analogues also significantly decrease the amount of gastric aspirate and reduce the symptoms of intestinal obstruction in terminally ill patients with malignant disease.[19,20] Prospective, randomized trials are needed to determine whether somatostatin analogues can significantly benefit patients with adhesive partial small bowel obstruction.

Some clinicians have advocated routine intragastric administration of water-soluble contrast agents to patients with partial small bowel obstruction[30-32] on the grounds that this practice not only permits the identification of patients who are likely to respond to nonoperative therapy but also is capable of relieving adhesive partial small bowel obstruction. Two prospective, randomized clinical trials independently reported that intragastric administration of 100 ml of diatrizoate meglumine or iohexol significantly enhanced the resolution of adhesive partial small bowel obstruction and significantly reduced the length of hospital stay.[31,32] In one of these studies,[32] 10 percent of patients receiving diatrizoate meglumine required operation (compared with 21 percent of control subjects), and the mean length of hospital stay for these patients was 2.2 days (compared with 4.4 days for the control subjects). Furthermore, when intestinal function did not return within 12 hours of the administration of the contrast agent, there was an increased probability that operation would eventually be necessary to correct the underlying cause of obstruction. In another study,[30] administration of diatrizoate meglumine did not lead to resolution of partial intestinal obstruction in any of the patients with carcinomatous obstruction.

By accelerating the resolution of partial small bowel obstruction and ileus, administration of water-soluble contrast agents shortens the expected hospital stay and thereby also reduces the cost of care. Thus, it is reasonable that the first step in managing suspected partial small bowel obstruction from adhesions or postoperative ileus is to administer water-soluble contrast material intragastrically. If bowel function does not return within 24 hours, then the obstruction is less likely to resolve with nonoperative therapy, and early operation may be the best option for shortening hospital stay. If ileus persists after intragastric administration of the contrast material and mechanical obstruction is excluded, then continued observation is warranted, with close attention paid to factors that may be causing the ileus. Prospective trials will be necessary to assess this potentially cost-effective strategy.

Early Postoperative Obstruction

Early postoperative mechanical small bowel obstruction is often difficult to diagnose because it gives rise to many of the same signs and symptoms as postoperative ileus: obstipation, distention, nausea, vomiting, abdominal pain, and altered bowel sounds. In most cases, there are roentgenographic signs indicative of small bowel obstruction rather than ileus; however, in some cases, abdominal x-rays fail to diagnose the obstruction.[33] Traditionally, when plain radiographs are equivocal, an upper GI barium study with follow-through views is the next test performed to distinguish ileus from partial or complete small bowel obstruction[34]; however, such studies may yield the wrong diagnosis in as many as 30 percent of cases.[15,33,35] A number of authorities believe that abdominal ultrasonography is excellent at distinguishing postoperative ileus from mechanical obstruction and recommend that it be done before any contrast study.[12]

Early postoperative obstruction is caused by adhesions in about 90 percent of patients.[33,36] When there are no signs of toxicity and no acute abdominal signs, such obstruction can usually be managed safely with nasogastric decompression.[33,35,36] As many as 75 percent of patients respond to nasogastric suction within two weeks. About 70 percent of the patients who respond to nonoperative treatment do so within one week, and an additional 25 percent respond during the following seven days. If postoperative obstruction does not resolve in the first two weeks, it is unlikely to do so with continued nonoperative therapy, and reoperation is probably indicated[33,36]; about 25 percent of patients whose postoperative obstruction was initially treated nonoperatively eventually require reoperation. An exception to this guideline arises in patients known to have severe dense adhesions (sometimes referred to as obliterative peritonitis) in response to multiple sequential laparotomies. These patients may have a combination of mechanical obstruction and diffuse small bowel and colonic ileus. The risk of closed-loop obstruction, volvulus, or strangulation in this group of patients is low. Repeat laparotomies and attempts to lyse adhesions may lead to complications, the development of enterocutaneous fistulae, or exacerbation of the adhesions. Often, the best approach to managing these patients is observation for prolonged periods (i.e., months). Parenteral nutritional support is necessary in these patients. The addition of octreotide to the TPN solution may be helpful.

Long intestinal tubes have no role to play in the management of postoperative bowel obstruction[17]; in fact, some authorities have reported that the use of such tubes increases morbidity.[17,23,34] Because the risk of intestinal strangulation in patients with postoperative adhesive obstruction is extremely small (less than one percent),[33,37] one can generally treat these patients nonoperatively for longer periods. In fact, the conservative approach is often the wise one: reoperation may do more harm than good (e.g., by causing enterotomies and inducing denser adhesions).

The traditional indications for operation in patients with early postoperative obstruction include (1) deteriorating clinical status, (2) worsening obstructive symptoms, and (3) failure to respond to nonoperative management within two weeks. With the rising cost of hospitalization, it might in fact be more cost-effective to reoperate on patients who have persistent obstruction after seven days. This speculation would have to be tested by a well-organized cost-benefit study conducted in a prospective fashion.

Inflammatory Conditions

Partial bowel obstruction secondary to inflammatory bowel disease, radiation enteritis, or diverticulitis usually resolves with nonoperative therapy. Bowel obstruction accompanying an acute exacerbation of Crohn's disease usually resolves with nasogastric suction, intravenous antibiotics, and anti-inflammatory agents. If, however, CT scanning detects intra-abdominal abscess, there is evidence of a chronic stricture, or the patient exhibits persistent obstructive symptoms, operation may be necessary. Similarly, bowel obstruction arising from acute enteritis caused by radiation exposure or chemotherapy usually resolves with supportive care. Chronic radiation-induced strictures are problematic; astute clinical judgment must be exercised to determine when operative treatment is the best option.

Patients with acute diverticulitis typically present with a history of altered bowel movements, fever, leukocytosis, localized pain, tenderness, and guarding in the left lower quadrant of the abdomen. Twenty percent of patients with colonic diverticulitis also present with signs and symptoms of partial colonic obstruction. A CT scan should be obtained early in all patients with diverticulitis to ascertain whether there is a pericolic abscess that could be drained percutaneously.[38] Partial colonic obstruction in these patients usually resolves with antibiotic therapy, an NPO regimen, and nasogastric decompression. If obstructive symptoms persist for more than seven days or if obstructive symptoms from a documented stricture recur, operation is indicated.

ELECTIVE OPERATION

Nontoxic, Nontender Sigmoid Volvulus

Patients with nontoxic, nontender sigmoid volvulus whose bowel obstruction is initially treated successfully with sigmoidoscopic decompression are at risk for recurrent colonic obstruction. Accordingly, these patients should undergo elective sigmoid resection after complete bowel preparation.

Recurrent Adhesive or Stricture-Related Partial Small Bowel Obstruction

Many patients whose adhesive bowel obstruction resolves experience no further obstructive episodes. If a patient does present with recurrent obstruction from presumed adhesions, one should perform a contrast examination of the bowel to look for a point of stenosis that can be surgically corrected. A strong argument can be made that non–high-risk patients should undergo elective operation after presenting with their second episode of mechanical obstruction. Similarly, patients with recurrent obstruction from strictures of any sort should undergo elective operation, given that these lesions are unlikely to resolve.

Partial Colonic Obstruction

The most common causes of partial colonic obstruction are colon cancer, strictures, and diverticulitis. Cancer and strictures usually must be managed surgically because they generally go on to cause obstruction later. Strictures from ischemia or endometriosis usually call for elective colonic resection. Inflammatory strictures from diverticulitis may resolve; however, if obstructive symptoms persist or if barium enema examination continues to yield evidence of colonic narrowing, elective resection is warranted.

When abdominal x-rays suggest distal colonic obstruction, digital examination and rigid sigmoidoscopy are performed to exclude fecal impaction, tumors, strictures, and sigmoid volvulus. If obstruction is proximal to the sigmoidoscope, barium contrast examination is indicated. If barium examination does not demonstrate mechanical obstruction, a presumptive diagnosis of colonic pseudo-obstruction is made.

The morbidity and mortality associated with elective colorectal procedures are significantly lower than those associated with emergent colonic surgery. Furthermore, immediate operation for left-side colonic obstruction almost always necessitates the creation of a diverting colostomy. If a colostomy takedown subsequently proves necessary, the overall cost of caring for the patient will be significantly higher than it would have been had a single-stage procedure been performed. For these reasons, one should initially treat patients with partial colonic obstruction with nasogastric suction, enemas, and intravenous rehydration in the hope that the obstruction will resolve and that the patient thus can undergo mechanical and antibiotic bowel preparation and a single-stage procedure comprising resection and primary anastomosis. Patients who do not respond to nonoperative measures within 24 hours should undergo operation within 12 hours with the aim of preventing perforation.

In patients with partially obstructing rectal or distal sigmoid tumors or strictures that can be traversed with a radiologic guide wire, balloon dilatation should be performed and a self-expanding stent deployed.[39,40] With restoration of the bowel lumen, patients can be prepared for elective surgery, can be spared the creation of a diverting colostomy, and can avoid the extra expense and morbidity associated with the performance of two operations. In patients with large, fixed rectal masses, one should obtain CT scans of the pelvis to assess the extent of the tumor. Transrectal laser fulguration and endoluminal stenting are palliative treatment options for restoring bowel lumen patency that may be considered for patients with nonresectable recurrent rectal cancer or radiation strictures in whom operative risk is prohibitively high.

Bowel Obstruction without Previous Abdominal Operation

When partial small bowel obstruction develops and resolves in a patient who has not previously undergone an abdominal operation, one should perform a diagnostic workup to identify the cause of the obstruction; there may be an underlying condition that is likely to cause recurrent obstruction (e.g., an internal hernia, a tumor, malrotation, or metastatic cancer). The first diagnostic test to be ordered should be a CT scan, followed by an upper GI barium study with follow-through views and a barium enema.[41] If a pathological lesion is identified, elective operation is indicated. An argument can be made that no additional diagnostic tests should be performed in these patients and that diagnostic laparoscopy should be performed instead to enable laparoscopic surgery in case a cause of obstruction is identified that can be treated with a minimally invasive procedure. If no cause of obstruction is found at laparoscopy, open laparotomy is performed.

Nonmechanical Obstruction

ILEUS

Ileus, or intestinal paralysis, is most common after abdominal operations but can also occur in response to any acute medical condition or metabolic derangement [*see Table 1*]. The pathophysiological mechanisms that cause ileus are incompletely understood but appear to involve disruption of normal neurohumoral responses.[42] Ileus may be classified into two broad categories: postoperative ileus and ileus without antecedent abdominal operation. Postoperative ileus is manifested by atony of the stomach, the small intestine, and the colon and usually resolves spontaneously within a few days as normal bowel motility returns. Typically, the small bowel regains its motility within 24 hours of operation, followed three to four days later by the stomach and the colon. Initial therapy of ileus is directed at identifying and correcting the presumed cause [*see Figure 12*]. If the patient experiences abdominal distention, abdominal pain, nausea, or vomiting, then nasogastric decompression, placement of a Foley catheter, and intravenous rehydration are indicated. In postoperative patients, it is best not to use strong narcotics for analgesia and instead to rely on epidural anesthesia and nonsteroidal anti-inflammatory drugs. When ileus develops in patients who have not recently undergone an operation, a thorough history, a careful physical examination, and well-chosen laboratory tests are necessary to identify the possible causes.

When ileus persists for what is, in one's best clinical judgment, an inordinate length of time for the operation performed (typically, longer than three to four days), the possibility of partial mechanical obstruction, possibly associated with an intra-abdominal abscess or another source of infection, must be considered. If an abscess is suspected, an abdominal CT scan should be obtained. Abdominal ultrasonography has been

treatment of—small bowel obstruction at eight days a person is about $1.8 billion annually in the United States. Accordingly, reducing the average hospital stay by one day would save about $225 million annually. Given the escalating cost of delivering hospital-based care, it would be wise and prudent to implement strategies designed to reduce the length of hospital stay for patients with small bowel obstruction.

Strategies for accomplishing this (as well as for reducing costs overall) may take several forms: the development of diagnostic and therapeutic methods that lead to more rapid diagnosis and resolution of ileus and partial small bowel obstruction; the development of techniques for rapid identification of patients with complete or closed-loop obstruction and early reversible strangulation, which would permit earlier operative intervention and thereby reduce the incidence of complications; the development of therapeutic approaches that prevent postoperative ileus; and the development of methods for preventing intra-abdominal adhesions, which would significantly reduce the overall incidence of bowel obstruction.

If a specific diagnostic test or medication costs less than $500 and saves one day of hospitalization, it immediately becomes cost-effective from a management viewpoint. Intragastric administration of a water-soluble contrast agent to relieve small bowel ileus or partial adhesive obstruction is an example of an innovative cost-effective therapeutic strategy. Diagnostic laparoscopy with local anesthesia, abdominal ultrasonography, and CT scanning have all been used successfully to diagnose early closed-loop or strangulation obstruction. When complete or closed-loop obstruction is present, administration of long-acting somatostatin analogues, such as octreotide, may decrease the magnitude of intestinal injury and thereby decrease morbidity and cost. Prospective, randomized trials are needed to establish the cost-effectiveness of these approaches in managing patients with intestinal obstruction or ileus.

Most patients are not discharged until they can eat and drink satisfactorily; thus, when ileus develops, the result usually is a significantly prolonged hospital stay, along with an increased overall cost of care. Laparoscopic abdominal procedures, by decreasing the magnitude and duration of postoperative ileus, may lead to earlier hospital discharge than would similar operative procedures performed through an open approach. Jejunal feeding immediately after a major abdominal operation or injury may prevent the development of intestinal ileus and permit quicker resumption of a complete oral diet. If prospective, randomized trials substantiate these findings, a strong argument can be made for immediate postoperative jejunal feeding in all patients undergoing major abdominal operations as well as operations associated with a high incidence of postoperative ileus.

References

1. Irvin T: Abdominal pain: a surgical audit of 1190 emergency admissions. Br J Surg 76:1121, 1989
2. Eskelinen M, Ikonen J, Lipponen P: Contributions of history-taking, physical examination, and computer assistance to diagnosis of acute small-bowel obstruction: a prospective study of 1333 patients with acute abdominal pain. Scand J Gastroenterol 29:715, 1994
3. Reisner R, Cohen J: Gallstone ileus: a review of 1001 reported cases. Am Surg 60:441, 1994
4. Sarr M, Bulkley G, Zuidema G: Preoperative recognition of intestinal strangulation obstruction: prospective evaluation of diagnostic capability. Am J Surg 145:176, 1983
5. Burrell H, Baker D, Wardrop P, et al: Significant plain film findings in sigmoid volvulus. Clin Radiol 49:317, 1994
6. Fatarr S, Schulman A: Small bowel obstruction masking synchronous large bowel obstruction: a need for emergency barium enema. AJR Am J Roentgenol 140:1159, 1983
7. Lim J, Ko Y, Lee D, et al: Determining the site and causes of colonic obstruction with sonography. AJR Am J Roentgenol 163:113, 1994
8. Gough I: Strangulating adhesive small bowel obstruction with normal radiographs. Br J Surg 65:431, 1978
9. Ko Y, Lim J, Le D, et al: Small bowel obstruction: sonographic evaluation. Radiology 188:649, 1993
10. Balthazar E: For suspected small-bowel obstruction and an equivocal plain film, should we perform CT or a small-bowel series? AJR Am J Roentgenol 163:1260, 1994
11. Meiser G, Meissner K: Intermittent incomplete intestinal obstruction: a frequently mistaken identity. Ultrasonographic diagnosis and management. Surg Endosc 3:46, 1989
12. Meiser G, Meissner K: Ileus and intestinal obstruction—ultrasonographic findings as a guideline to therapy. Hepatogastroenterology 34:194, 1987
13. Megibow A: Bowel obstruction: evaluation with CT. Radiol Clin North Am 32:861, 1994
14. Balthazar E: CT of small-bowel obstruction. AJR Am J Roentgenol 162:255, 1994
15. Dunn JT, Halls JM, Berne TV: Roentgenographic contrast studies in acute small-bowel obstruction. Arch Surg 119:1305, 1984
16. Caroline DF, Herlinger H, Laufer I, et al: Small bowel enema in the diagnosis of adhesive obstructions. AJR Am J Roentgenol 142:1133, 1984
17. Brolin R: Partial small bowel obstruction. Surgery 95:145, 1984
18. Maglinte D, Peterson D, Vahey T, et al: Enteroclysis in partial small bowel obstruction. Am J Surg 147:325, 1984
19. Khoo D, Hall E, Motson R, et al: Palliation of malignant intestinal obstruction using octreotide. Eur J Cancer 30A:28, 1994
20. Stiefel F, Morant R: Vapreotide, a new somatostatin analogue in the palliative management of obstructive ileus in advanced cancer. Support-Care-Cancer 1:57, 1993
21. Silen W, Hein MF, Goldman L: Strangulation obstruction of the small intestine. Arch Surg 85:137, 1962
22. Laws H, Aldrete J: Small bowel obstruction: a review of 465 cases. South Med J 69:733, 1976
23. Sosa J, Gardner B: Management of patients diagnosed as acute intestinal obstruction secondary to adhesions. Am Surg 59:125, 1993
24. Snyder EN, McCranie D: Closed loop obstruction of the small bowel. Am J Surg 111:398, 1966
25. Mangiante E, Croce M, Fabian T, et al: Sigmoid volvulus: a four-decade experience. Am Surg 55:41, 1989
26. Bizer L, Liebling R, Delany H, et al: Small bowel obstruction: the role of non-operative treatment in simple intestinal obstruction and predictive criteria for strangulation obstruction. Surgery 89:407, 1981
27. Mulvihill S, Pappas T, Fonkalsrud Z, et al: The effect of somatostatin on experimental intestinal obstruction. Ann Surg 207:169, 1988
28. Gittes G, Nelson M, Debas H, et al: Improvement in survival of mice with proximal small bowel obstruction treated with octreotide. Am J Surg 163:231, 1992
29. Bastounis E, Hadjinikolaou L, Ioannou N, et al: Somatostatin as adjuvant therapy in the management of obstructive ileus. Hepatogastroenterology 36:538, 1989
30. Stordahl A, Laerum F, Gjolberg T, et al: Water-soluble contrast media in radiography of small bowel obstruction. Acta Radiol 29:53, 1988
31. Stordahl A: Water-soluble contrast media in obstructed ischemic small intestine: a clinical and experimental study. Journal of the City Hospitals of Oslo 39(1-2):3, 1989
32. Assalia A, Schein M, Kopelman D, et al: Therapeutic effect of oral Gastrografin in adhesive, partial small-bowel obstruction: a prospective randomized trial. Surgery 115:433, 1994
33. Pickleman J, Lee R: The management of patients with suspected early postoperative small bowel obstruction. Ann Surg 212:216, 1989
34. Brolin R: The role of gastrointestinal tube decompression in the treatment of mechanical intestinal obstruction. Am Surg 49:131, 1983
35. Quatromoni J, Rosoff L, Halls J, et al: Early postoperative small bowel obstruction. Ann Surg 191:72, 1980
36. Stewart R, Page C, Brender J, et al: The incidence

and risk of early postoperative small bowel obstruction. Am J Surg 154:643, 1987
37. Spears H, Petrelli N, Herrera L, et al: Treatment of small bowel obstruction after colorectal carcinoma. Am J Surg 155:383, 1988
38. Hulnick D, Megibow A, Balthazar E, et al: Computed tomography in the evaluation of diverticulitis. Radiology 152:491, 1984
39. Tejero E, Mainar A, Fernández L, et al: New procedure for the treatment of colorectal neoplastic obstructions. Dis Colon Rectum 37:1158, 1994
40. Itabashi M, Hamano K, Kameoka S, et al: Self-expanding stainless steel stent application in rectosigmoid stricture. Dis Colon Rectum 36:508, 1993
41. Stelmach W, Cass A: Small bowel obstructions: the case for investigation for occult large bowel carcinoma. Aust NZ J Surg 59:181, 1989
42. Fromm D: Ileus and obstruction. Surgery: Scientific Principles and Practice. Greenfield LJ, Mulholland MW, Oldham KT, et al, Eds. JB Lippincott Co, Philadelphia, 1993, p 731
43. Watkins D, Robertson C: Water-soluble radiocontrast material in the treatment of the postoperative ileus. Am J Obstet Gynecol 152:450, 1985
44. Zer M, Kanzenelson D, Feigenberg Z, et al: The value of Gastrografin in the differential diagnosis of paralytic ileus and mechanical obstruction. Dis Colon Rectum 20:573, 1977
45. Vanek V, Al-Salti M: Acute pseudo-obstruction of the colon (Ogilvie's syndrome): an analysis of 400 cases. Dis Colon Rectum 29:203, 1986
46. Sloyer A, Panella V, Demas B: Ogilvie's syndrome: successful management with colonoscopy. Dig Dis Sci 33:1391, 1988
47. Nakhgevany KB: Colonoscopic decompression of the colon in patients with Ogilvie's syndrome. Am J Surg 148:317, 1984
48. Hutchinson R, Griffiths C: Acute colonic pseudo-obstruction: a pharmacological approach. Ann R Coll Surg Engl 74:364, 1992
49. Faulk D, Anuras S, Christensen J: Chronic intestinal pseudo-obstruction. Gastroenterology 74:922, 1978
50. Schuffler M, Deitch E: Chronic idiopathic intestinal pseudo-obstruction: a surgical approach. Ann Surg 192:752, 1980
51. Knoll RF Jr, Schuffler MD, Helton WS: Small bowel resection for relief of chronic intestinal pseudo-obstruction. Am J Gastroenterol 90:1142, 1995

Acknowledgment

Figures 12 and 13   Marcia Kammerer.

18 UPPER GASTROINTESTINAL BLEEDING

Richard T. Schlinkert, M.D., and Keith A. Kelly, M.D.

Assessment and Management of Upper Gastrointestinal Bleeding

The most common causes of upper gastrointestinal bleeding are chronic duodenal ulcers, chronic gastric ulcers, esophageal varices, gastric varices, Mallory-Weiss tears, acute hemorrhagic gastritis, and gastric neoplasms [*see* Management of Specific Sources of Upper GI Bleeding, *below*]. Less common causes include various other gastrointestinal conditions as well as certain hepatobiliary and pancreatic disorders.

Presentation and Initial Management

INITIAL ASSESSMENT AND MANAGEMENT

Upper gastrointestinal hemorrhage may present as severe bleeding with hematemesis, hematochezia, and hypotension; as gradual bleeding with melena; or as occult bleeding detected by positive tests for blood in the stool. The initial steps in the evaluation of patients with upper gastrointestinal bleeding are based on the perceived rate of bleeding and the degree of hemodynamic stability. Whereas patients with hematochezia or hematemesis should be hospitalized, stable patients with melenic stools may be treated as outpatients.

The airway, breathing, and circulation should be rapidly assessed, and the examiner should note whether the patient has a history of or currently exhibits hematemesis, melena, or hematochezia. Blood should be drawn for a complete blood count, blood chemistries (including tests of liver function and renal function), and measurement of the prothrombin time (PT) and the partial thromboplastin time (PTT). Blood should be sent to the blood bank for typing and crossmatching.

If the patient is stable and shows no evidence of recent or active hemorrhage, the surgeon may proceed with the workup.

If, however, the patient is stable but shows evidence of recent or active bleeding, a large-bore intravenous line should be placed before workup is begun; the presence of the line ensures immediate I.V. access should the patient subsequently become unstable.

If the patient is unstable, resuscitation should be begun immediately.

RESUSCITATION

Resuscitation of an unstable patient is begun by establishing a secure airway and ensuring adequate ventilation. Oxygen should be given as necessary, either by mask or by endotracheal tube and ventilator. A large-bore I.V. line should then be placed, through which lactated Ringer's solution should be infused at a rate high enough to maintain tissue perfusion. A urinary catheter should be inserted and urine output monitored. Blood should be given as necessary, and any coagulopathies should be corrected if possible. It is all too easy to forget these basic steps in a desire to evaluate and manage massive GI hemorrhage.

If the patient remains unstable and continues to bleed despite supportive measures, he or she should be taken to the operating room for intraoperative diagnosis. The abdomen should be opened through an upper midline incision. A 7 cm anterior gastroduodenotomy that is centered on the pylorus should be made. If no bleeding lesion is discovered, a proximal corporeal gastrotomy should be done and a bleeding site in the proximal stomach sought.

Workup

HISTORY

Only after the initial measures to protect the airway and stabilize the patient have been completed should an attempt be made to establish the cause of the bleeding. The history should focus on known causes of upper GI bleeding (e.g., ulcers, recent trauma or stress, liver disease, varices, alcoholism, and vomiting) and on the possible use of medications that interfere with coagulation (e.g., aspirin, nonsteroidal anti-inflammatory drugs [NSAIDs], and dipyridamole) or alter hemodynamics (e.g., beta blockers and antihypertensive agents). The cardiac history is particularly important for assessing the patient's ability to withstand varying degrees of anemia.

PHYSICAL EXAMINATION

The physical examination is seldom of much help in determining the exact site of bleeding, but it may reveal jaundice, ascites, or other signs of hepatic disease; a tumor mass; or a bruit from an abdominal vascular lesion.

NASOGASTRIC ASPIRATION

The next step is nasogastric aspiration. A bloody aspirate is an indication for esophagogastroduodenoscopy (EGD), as is a clear, nonbilious aspirate if a bleeding site distal to the pylorus has not been excluded. If the aspirate is clear and bile-stained, the source of the bleeding is unlikely to be the stomach, the duodenum, the liver, the biliary tree, or the pancreas. Nonetheless, if subsequent evaluation of the lower GI tract for the source of the bleeding is unrewarding, an upper GI site that had stopped bleeding when the nasogastric tube was passed or that was distal to the ligament of Treitz should still be considered.

UPPER GI ENDOSCOPY (ESOPHAGOGASTRODUODENOSCOPY)

EGD [see 47 Gastrointestinal Endoscopy] almost always reveals the source of upper GI bleeding; its utility and accuracy have been well documented in the literature. This procedure requires considerable skill: identification of bleeding sites in a blood-filled stomach is far from easy. Hematemesis is an indication for emergent EGD, usually within one hour of presentation. If the rate of bleeding is high, saline lavage may be performed to clear the stomach of blood and clots. If the rate of bleeding is moderate or low, as is often the case in patients with melena, urgent EGD is indicated.

EGD is not only an excellent diagnostic tool but also a valuable therapeutic modality. Indeed, most upper GI hemorrhages may be controlled endoscopically, though the degree of success to be expected in individual cases varies according to the expertise of the endoscopist and the specific cause of the bleeding. Therapeutic endoscopic maneuvers include injection sclerotherapy, rubber banding of varices, electrocoagulation, the use of the heater probe, the injection of ethanol or epinephrine, and laser coagulation; the choice of therapy depends on the cause, the site, and the rate of bleeding.

OTHER TESTS

If endoscopic examination reveals no lesions in the stomach or the duodenum, enteroclysis (direct introduction of $BaSO_4$ into the small bowel) and roentgenography of the duodenum and the jejunum should be done next. This is probably a more sensitive radiologic test than a standard small bowel roentgenogram. Nonetheless, the absence of a lesion on this test does not rule out the small bowel as the source of the hemorrhage; not uncommonly, the x-ray is negative when a bleeding small bowel lesion is present.

Tagged red cell scans may confirm the presence of an active bleeding site; however, scans are fairly nonspecific with respect to determining the anatomic location of the bleeding. Arteriography may demonstrate that a lesion is present, but it cannot reliably identify a bleeding site unless the bleeding is brisk (> 1 ml/min). Occasionally, arteriography reveals a vascular malformation that is the cause of the bleeding.

When a patient has recurrent bleeding that is believed to originate in the small bowel, intraoperative endoscopic exploration may prove useful. Before the small bowel is manipulated, a pediatric colonoscope is introduced either orally or through a distal jejunal enterotomy; the latter method allows easier viewing of the entire small bowel. The mucosal detail is examined as the surgeon guides the scope through the small bowel. The bowel must be handled gently to avoid a mucosal injury, which could mimic a significant lesion.

These tests, in conjunction with EGD, should allow the surgeon to establish the cause of upper GI bleeding at least 90 percent of the time.

Management of Specific Sources of Upper GI Bleeding

CHRONIC DUODENAL ULCER

The development of effective medical regimens for controlling uncomplicated duodenal ulcers has led to a drastic reduction in the number of elective surgical procedures performed for this purpose. Nevertheless, the incidence of bleeding from duodenal ulcers that is severe enough to necessitate emergent operative intervention has not decreased.

Once EGD has demonstrated that a duodenal ulcer is the source of the bleeding, the first question that must be addressed is whether active bleeding is present. If it is, an attempt should be made to control the hemorrhage endoscopically through use of the heater probe, electrocoagulation, or injection sclerotherapy [see Figure 1]. Because ongoing blood loss eventually leads to coagulopathies, the surgeon must exercise good judgment in deciding how long to pursue endoscopic treatment before concluding that such treatment has failed and that surgical treatment is necessary. In general, substantial bleeding (four to six units or more) that is not easily controlled endoscopically is an indication for immediate surgical intervention. Likewise, ongoing hemorrhage in a hemodynamically unstable patient (especially an elderly one) calls for immediate surgical therapy.

If bleeding is controlled endoscopically, then an H_2-receptor blocker should be given intravenously. In addition, antibiotic therapy directed against Helicobacter pylori should be considered if the organism is present; such therapy has been shown to decrease rebleeding rates after antacid medication has been stopped. Food need not be withheld unless the likelihood of rebleeding is high, in which case operation or repeat endoscopy would be necessary. Resumption of oral feeding does not appear to affect rebleeding rates. Early oral intake also allows earlier initiation of omeprazole therapy.

If bleeding continues despite medical and endoscopic therapy, it should be managed surgically. In addition, certain patients whose bleeding was controlled endoscopically—such as those with a visible gastroduodenal artery and a clot in the base of the ulcer, those who experience rebleeding despite medical and endoscopic therapy, those who will require long-term use of NSAIDs, and those with giant ulcers—should be strongly considered for surgical therapy.

At operation, an upper midline incision is made. The duodenum is kocherized and an anterior longitudinal duodenotomy performed over the site of the ulcer. The bleeding vessel, which is usually on the posterior wall of the first portion of the

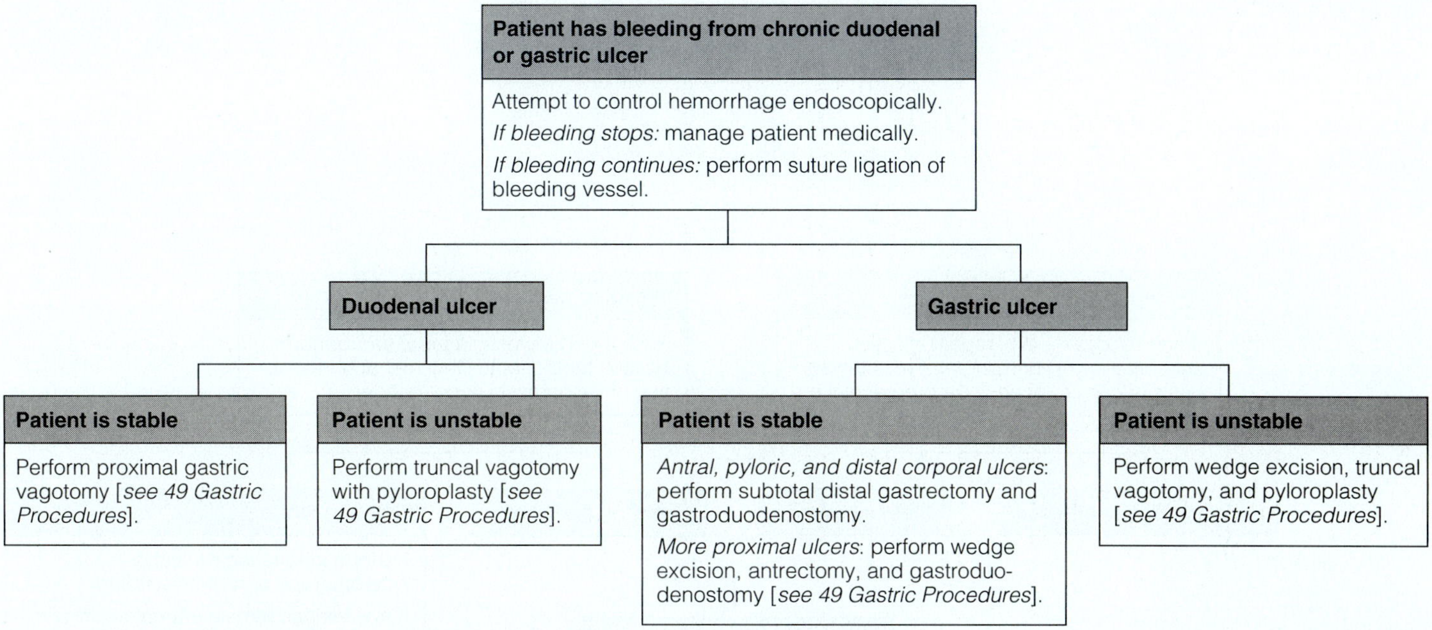

```
┌─────────────────────────────────────┐
│ Patient has bleeding from chronic   │
│ duodenal or gastric ulcer           │
├─────────────────────────────────────┤
│ Attempt to control hemorrhage       │
│ endoscopically.                     │
│ If bleeding stops: manage patient   │
│ medically.                          │
│ If bleeding continues: perform      │
│ suture ligation of bleeding vessel. │
└─────────────────────────────────────┘
```

Duodenal ulcer
- *Patient is stable*: Perform proximal gastric vagotomy [see 49 Gastric Procedures].
- *Patient is unstable*: Perform truncal vagotomy with pyloroplasty [see 49 Gastric Procedures].

Gastric ulcer
- *Patient is stable*:
  - *Antral, pyloric, and distal corporal ulcers*: perform subtotal distal gastrectomy and gastroduodenostomy.
  - *More proximal ulcers*: perform wedge excision, antrectomy, and gastroduodenostomy [see 49 Gastric Procedures].
- *Patient is unstable*: Perform wedge excision, truncal vagotomy, and pyloroplasty [see 49 Gastric Procedures].

Figure 1 Shown is an algorithm for management of bleeding from chronic duodenal or gastric ulcers.

duodenum, is oversewn with nonabsorbable sutures at sites proximal and distal to the bleeding point. A third stitch is placed posterior to the bleeding vessel. Pains must be taken to avoid injury to the common bile duct during the placement of these sutures. The duodenotomy is then closed.

If the patient is stable, the next step is to perform a proximal gastric vagotomy [see 49 Gastric Procedures]; the safety of this procedure in stable patients has been well documented. Proximal gastric vagotogmy is preferable to truncal vagotomy because it is less likely to result in gastric atony, alkaline reflux gastritis, dumping, and diarrhea. If the patient is unstable, a truncal vagotomy should be performed in conjunction with pyloroplasty [see 49 Gastric Procedures]. Frozen section to confirm the presence of nerve tissue is helpful for ensuring that the vagotomy is complete.

This recommendation of vagotomy is based on data from studies done before omeprazole and anti–*H. pylori* therapy came into use, in which in-hospital rebleeding rates of approximately 15 percent were recorded when a vagotomy was not performed. Subsequent studies that evaluated rebleeding rates with current medical regimens, however, have demonstrated much lower rebleeding rates. Furthermore, it seems probable that long-term omeprazole, being the medical equivalent of vagotomy, should decrease rebleeding rates significantly. Therefore, one may consider an alternative treatment approach in patients who had not been receiving ulcer therapy before the bleeding began—namely, ligation of the bleeding vessel, postoperative administration of H_2-receptor blockers, and anti–*H. pylori* therapy. Whether omeprazole would confer any additional benefit is unknown. This approach could alleviate the complications associated with truncal vagotomy.

CHRONIC GASTRIC ULCER

Initially, bleeding from a chronic gastric ulcer is managed in much the same way as that from a chronic duodenal ulcer (i.e., endoscopically) [see Figure 1]. To prevent aggravation of the bleeding, early biopsy generally is not recommended; repeat endoscopy and biopsy are done at a later date. Emergent surgical indications for gastric ulcers are the same as those for duodenal ulcers. In addition, if bleeding from a gastric ulcer does not resolve after six weeks of medical therapy, surgical excision is often indicated.

In stable patients, surgical management of a nonhealing chronic gastric ulcer generally consists of a hemigastrectomy that includes the ulcer site; if the ulcer is located more proximally, wedge excision of the ulcer, antrectomy, and gastroduodenostomy are done [see 49 Gastric Procedures]. Excision of the ulcer should be immediately followed by frozen section to rule out cancer. There is no need for a vagotomy in these instances. In unstable patients, hemigastrectomy should probably be avoided because of the increased morbidity and mortality that can follow it; wedge excision, truncal vagotomy, and pyloroplasty are preferred.

ESOPHAGEAL VARICES

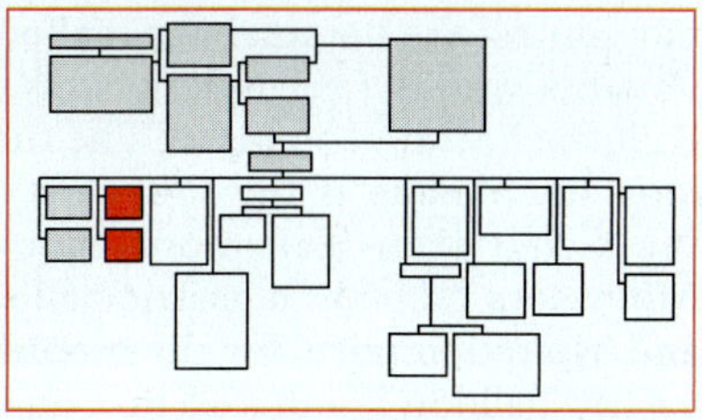

The value of endoscopy in the diagnosis and management of variceal bleeding cannot be overemphasized. Even in patients with known varices, the site of bleeding is frequently nonvariceal; endoscopy is therefore essential. If bleeding varices are identified, rubber banding or

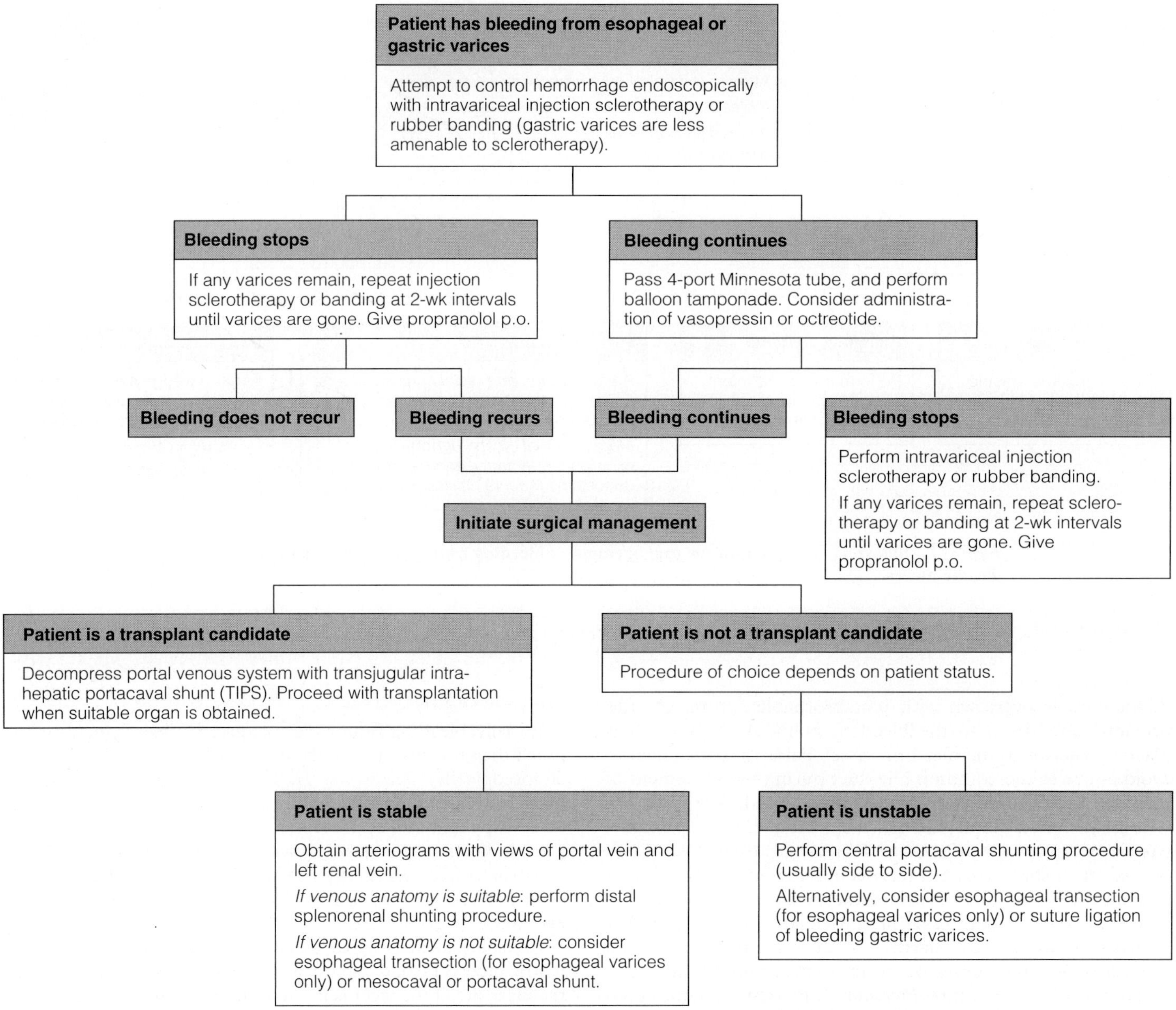

```
┌─────────────────────────────────────┐
│ Patient has bleeding from esophageal │
│ or gastric varices                   │
├─────────────────────────────────────┤
│ Attempt to control hemorrhage        │
│ endoscopically with intravariceal    │
│ injection sclerotherapy or rubber    │
│ banding (gastric varices are less    │
│ amenable to sclerotherapy).          │
└─────────────────────────────────────┘
```

Bleeding stops
If any varices remain, repeat injection sclerotherapy or banding at 2-wk intervals until varices are gone. Give propranolol p.o.

- **Bleeding does not recur**
- **Bleeding recurs**

Bleeding continues
Pass 4-port Minnesota tube, and perform balloon tamponade. Consider administration of vasopressin or octreotide.

- **Bleeding continues**
- **Bleeding stops**: Perform intravariceal injection sclerotherapy or rubber banding. If any varices remain, repeat sclerotherapy or banding at 2-wk intervals until varices are gone. Give propranolol p.o.

Initiate surgical management

Patient is a transplant candidate
Decompress portal venous system with transjugular intrahepatic portacaval shunt (TIPS). Proceed with transplantation when suitable organ is obtained.

Patient is not a transplant candidate
Procedure of choice depends on patient status.

Patient is stable
Obtain arteriograms with views of portal vein and left renal vein.
If venous anatomy is suitable: perform distal splenorenal shunting procedure.
If venous anatomy is not suitable: consider esophageal transection (for esophageal varices only) or mesocaval or portacaval shunt.

Patient is unstable
Perform central portacaval shunting procedure (usually side to side).
Alternatively, consider esophageal transection (for esophageal varices only) or suture ligation of bleeding gastric varices.

Figure 2 Shown is an algorithm for management of bleeding from esophageal or gastric varices.

intravariceal sclerotherapy with 1.5 percent sodium tetradecyl sulfate is performed [*see Figure 2*]. If these measures do not control the hemorrhage, balloon tamponade is indicated. Patients who are to undergo this procedure should have an endotracheal tube in place. The tube we prefer to use for balloon tamponade is the four-port Minnesota tube, although the Sengstaken-Blakemore tube is also acceptable. The Minnesota tube has a gastric balloon, an esophageal balloon, and aspiration ports for the esophagus and the stomach. The gastric balloon is inflated first and placed on traction. If the bleeding is not controlled, the esophageal balloon is then inflated. The pressure in the balloons should be released in 24 to 48 hours to prevent necrosis of the esophageal or the gastric wall. Successful balloon tamponade is followed by endoscopic variceal injection or variceal banding.

Systemically administered vasopressin (10 units/hr I.V.) or octreotide (100 μg q.i.d., s.c.) may also be used in conjunction with the above-mentioned steps. Vasopressin causes diffuse vasoconstriction; a nitroglycerin patch may be required to alleviate cardiac side effects. Octreotide has few side effects; when administered as an intravenous drip, it appears to be as effective as vasopressin in controlling variceal hemorrhage. Some authors question the effectiveness of vasopressin and octreotide, but these agents are still commonly used in the treatment of variceal hemorrhage.

Multiple prospective, randomized trials have shown that propranolol (40 mg b.i.d., p.o.) decreases the incidence of first-time variceal bleeding as well as the incidence of recurrent variceal bleeding. Propranolol should not be used during active bleeding but should be started once bleeding stops.

After the acute variceal bleeding has been controlled, any remaining varices should be subjected to injection sclerotherapy or banding at two-week intervals until they too are obliterated.

The main indications for surgical intervention in patients with bleeding esophageal varices are uncontrolled hemorrhage and persistent rebleeding despite endoscopic and medical therapy. When surgical intervention is planned, it is essential to determine whether the patient is a transplant candidate. If so, operation should be avoided and bleeding managed by decompressing the portal venous system with a transjugular intrahepatic portacaval shunt (TIPS). TIPS yields excellent short-term results with respect to stopping bleeding and providing time to locate a liver suitable for transplantation; however, it has not been shown to have the capacity to control hemorrhage by itself over the long term. Thus, its use in patients who are not transplant candidates is questionable.

If the patient is not a transplant candidate and is not actively bleeding, a distal splenorenal shunt is preferable. Arteriograms with views of the portal vein and the left renal vein are obtained. If the venous anatomy is suitable—that is, if the diameter of the splenic vein is greater than 0.75 cm (preferably greater than 1.0 cm) and the vein is within one vertebral body of the renal vein on venography—a distal splenorenal shunting procedure should be feasible. If the venous anatomy is not suitable, then esophageal transection, a mesocaval venous graft, or a portacaval shunt is required.

In the emergency setting, we prefer a central portacaval shunt, usually in a side-to-side fashion. Esophageal transection is also a reasonable choice. This procedure is associated with a lower incidence of encephalopathy than a portacaval shunting procedure; however, it is associated with higher rates of rebleeding (particularly late rebleeding), and it can be difficult to perform when active bleeding is present. Suture ligation of the bleeding varices (the Segura procedure) should also be considered.

In general, prognosis is related to the underlying liver disease. For example, patients with varices that are secondary to chronic extrahepatic portal venous or splenic venous occlusion generally have a much better prognosis than those whose portal hypertension is secondary to hepatic parenchymal causes. The severity of the cirrhosis also determines short-term and long-term survival and may influence the decision whether to perform a shunting procedure.

Varices in children are generally secondary to portal vein thrombosis. A conservative, nonoperative approach is preferred. If operation is required, either a portacaval shunt, a distal splenorenal shunt, or a devascularization procedure is performed. In children or adults with varices that are secondary to splenic vein thrombosis (sinistral portal hypertension), a splenectomy is usually curative.

GASTRIC VARICES

Gastric varices are managed in much the same way as esophageal varices [see Figure 2], though they are less amenable to sclerotherapy. The surgical options are the same, except that esophageal transection is not a good choice. If bleeding from gastric varices is not controlled by sclerotherapy, suture ligation is indicated.

MALLORY-WEISS TEARS

Mallory-Weiss tears are linear tears at the esophagogastric junction that are usually caused by vomiting. Any patient who presents with vomiting that initially was not bloody but later turns so should be suspected of having a Mallory-Weiss tear. As a rule, these lesions stop bleeding without therapy. If bleeding is substantial or persistent, however, endoscopic coagulation may be necessary. In rare instances, the tear will have to be oversewn at operation. This is accomplished via an anterior gastrotomy and direct suture ligation of the tear.

ACUTE HEMORRHAGIC GASTRITIS

Bleeding from gastritis is virtually always managed medically with H_2-receptor blockers, omeprazole, sucralfate, or antacids (either alone or in combination), along with antibiotics if *H. pylori* is present. Sometimes, administration of vasopressin via the left gastric artery is needed to control bleeding. In rare cases, total or near-total gastrectomy [see 49 Gastric Procedures] is required; however, the mortality associated with this operation in this setting is high. Stress ulcer prophylaxis in severely ill or traumatized patients is essential to prevent this problem. The gastric pH should be kept as close to neutral as possible. If the gastritis is relatively mild, a biopsy specimen should be obtained and tested for *H. pylori*. Treatment consists of acid reduction and anti–*H. pylori* therapy.

NEOPLASMS

Benign tumors of the upper GI tract (e.g., leiomyomas, hamartomas, and hemangiomas) bleed at times. Wedge excision of the offending lesion is the procedure of choice.

Bleeding from malignant neoplasms, whether early-stage or late-stage, generally can be controlled initially by endoscopic means; however, rebleeding rates are high. If the lesion is resectable, it should be excised promptly once the patient is stable and any coagulopathies have been corrected. If disease is advanced, however, surgical options are limited, and thus a nonoperative approach, though necessarily imperfect, is preferable.

ESOPHAGEAL HIATAL HERNIA

Not infrequently, the source of chronic enteric blood loss is an esophageal hiatal hernia. Major bleeding is rare in this condition but may occur as a result of linear erosions at the level of the diaphragm (Cameron's lesions), gastritis within the hernia, or torsion of a paraesophageal hernia. Endoscopy is generally diagnostic, though the sources of chronic blood loss are not always obvious. Recognition that the bleeding derives from a Cameron's lesion should incline the surgeon toward operative intervention: this lesion is usually mechanically induced and therefore tends to be less responsive to antacid therapy.

Chronic bleeding from a sliding esophageal hiatal hernia should be treated initially with antacids; anti–*H. pylori* therapy should be added if biopsy shows this organism to be present. Operation (i.e., Nissen fundoplication [see 48 *Esophageal Procedures: Minimally Invasive Approaches*]) is reserved for patients who do not respond to medical therapy. A paraesophageal hernia should be repaired surgically. This has generally been done via open laparotomy; however, given the growing favorable experience with laparoscopic repair, it is likely that minimally invasive approaches will soon supplant repair by open laparotomy.

DIEULAFOY'S LESION

Dieulafoy's lesion (also referred to as exulceratio simplex) is the rupturing of a 1 to 3 mm bleeding vessel through the gastric mucosa (usually in the proximal stomach) without surrounding ulceration. This lesion tends to be found high on the lesser curvature, but it can also occur in other locations. Histologic studies have not revealed any intrinsic abnormalities either of the mucosa or of the vessel.

Initial treatment consists of coagulation of the bleeding vessel with a heater probe; local injection of epinephrine may help control acute hemorrhage while this is being done. If endoscopic therapy fails, surgical options, including ligation or excision of the vessel involved, come into play.

HEMOBILIA

Hemobilia should be suspected in all patients who present with the classic triad of epigastric and right upper quadrant pain, GI bleeding, and jaundice; however, only about 40 percent of patients with hemobilia present with the entire triad. Endoscopy demonstrating blood coming from the ampulla of Vater points to a source in the biliary tree or the pancreas (hemosuccus pancreaticus).

Arteriography may provide the definitive diagnosis: a bleeding tumor, a ruptured artery from trauma, or another cause. Arteriographic embolization of the affected portion of the liver is the preferred treatment option; hepatic artery ligation (selective if possible) or hepatic resection may be required.

HEMOSUCCUS PANCREATICUS

Bleeding into the pancreatic duct, generally from erosion of a pancreatic pseudocyst into the splenic artery, is signaled by upper abdominal pain followed by hematochezia. If endoscopy is performed when hematochezia is present, the bleeding site may not be seen; however, if endoscopy is performed when pain is first noted, blood may be seen coming from the ampulla of Vater. Distal pancreatectomy [see 53 *Pancreatic Procedures*], including excision of the pseudocyst and ligation of the splenic artery, is the preferred treatment and generally leads to cure.

AORTOENTERIC FISTULA

Aortoenteric fistulas may occur spontaneously as a result of rupture of an aortic aneurysm or perforation of a duodenal lesion; more often, they arise after aortic surgery. A common initial manifestation of an aortoenteric fistula is a small herald bleed that is followed a few days later by a massive hemorrhage. A high index of suspicion facilitates diagnosis. Endoscopy may show an aortic graft eroding into the enteric lumen, but this is an uncommon finding. CT scanning is the procedure of choice for diagnosis. The finding of air around the aorta or the aortic graft is diagnostic and is an indication for emergency exploration. The preferred surgical treatment is resection of the graft with extra-abdominal bypass.

ARTERIOVENOUS MALFORMATIONS

Arteriovenous malformations may bleed briskly. As a rule, the lesions are readily identified and the bleeding controlled by endoscopic means. Lesions that continue to bleed, either acutely or chronically, despite endoscopic measures should be excised. Some patients have multiple and extensive arteriovenous malformations that necessitate resection of large portions of the stomach or the small intestine.

DUODENAL AND JEJUNAL DIVERTICULA

Duodenal and jejunal diverticula are rare causes of upper GI bleeding. Accurate identification of a bleeding site within a given diverticulum is difficult, but an attempt should be made to accomplish this by means of peroral enteroscopy. Excision is the preferred treatment. Great care must be taken in the treatment of duodenal diverticula in the region of the ampulla of Vater to ensure that the pancreatic duct and the bile ducts are not injured during excision.

JEJUNAL ULCER

Ulcerations of the jejunum are also rare. They may be secondary to medication, infection, a gastrinoma, or idiopathic causes. Offending medications should be stopped, infections should be treated, and gastrinomas should be excised. If these measures do not control the hemorrhage, the bleeding segment of the jejunum should be excised.

Recommended Reading

PROSPECTIVE, RANDOMIZED, CONTROLLED TRIALS

Cello JP, Grendell JH, Crass RA, et al: Endoscopic sclerotherapy versus portacaval shunt in patients with severe cirrhosis and variceal hemorrhage. N Engl J Med 311:1589, 1984

Clark AW, Westaby D, Silk DBA, et al: Prospective controlled trial of injection sclerotherapy in patients with cirrhosis and recent variceal hemorrhage. Lancet 2:552, 1980

Conn HO, Grace ND, Bosch J, et al: Propranolol in the prevention of the first hemorrhage from esophagogastric varices: a multicenter, randomized clinical trial. Hepatology 13:902, 1991

Garcia-Pagan JC, Feu F, Bosch J, et al: Propranolol compared with propranolol plus isosorbide-5-mononitrate for portal hypertension in cirrhosis: a randomized controlled study. Ann Intern Med 114:869, 1991

Graham DY, Hepps KS, Ramirez FC, et al: Treatment of *Helicobacter pylori* reduces the rate of rebleeding in peptic ulcer disease. Scand J Gastroenterol 28:939, 1993

Gregory PB: Prophylactic sclerotherapy for esophageal varices in men with alcoholic liver disease: a randomized, single-blind, multicenter trial. N Engl J Med 324:1779, 1991

Groszmann RJ, Bosch J, Grace ND, et al: Hemodynamic events in a prospective randomized trial of propranolol versus placebo in the prevention of a first variceal hemorrhage. Gastroenterology 99:1401, 1990

Krejs GJ, Little KH, Westergaard H, et al: Laser photocoagulation for the treatment of acute peptic-ulcer bleeding: a randomized controlled clinical trial. N Engl J Med 316:1618, 1987

Laine L: Multipolar electrocoagulation versus injection therapy in the treatment of bleeding peptic ulcers: a prospective, randomized trial. Gastroenterology 99:1303, 1990

Laine L, Cohen H, Brodhead J, et al: Prospective evaluation of immediate versus delayed refeeding and prognostic value of endoscopy in patients with upper gastrointestinal hemorrhage. Gastroenterology 102:314, 1992

Metz CA, Livingston DH, Smith JS, et al: Impact of multiple risk factors and ranitidine prophylaxis on the development of stress-related upper gastrointestinal bleeding: a prospective, multicenter, double-blind, randomized trial. Crit Care Med 21:1844, 1993

Pascal JP, Cales P: Propranolol in the prevention of first upper gastrointestinal tract hemorrhage in patients with cirrhosis of the liver and esophageal varices. N Engl J Med 317:856, 1987

Saeed ZA, Winchester CB, Michaletz PA, et al: A scoring system to predict rebleeding after endoscopic therapy of nonvariceal upper gastrointestinal hemorrhage, with a comparison of heat probe and ethanol injection. Am J Gastroenterol 88:1842, 1993

Vinel JP, Lamouliatte H, Cales P, et al: Propranolol reduces the rebleeding rate during endoscopic sclerotherapy before variceal obliteration. Gastroenterology 102:1760, 1992

Warren WD, Henderson JM, Millikan WJ, et al: Distal splenorenal shunt versus endoscopic sclerotherapy for long-term management of variceal bleeding: preliminary report of a prospective, randomized trial. Ann Surg 203:454, 1986

META-ANALYSES

Cook DJ, Guyatt GH, Salena BJ, et al: Endoscopic therapy for acute nonvariceal upper gastrointestinal hemorrhage: a meta-analysis. Gastroenterology 102:139, 1992

Poynard T, Cales P, Pasta L, et al: Beta-adrenergic-antagonist drugs in the prevention of gastrointestinal bleeding in patients with cirrhosis and esophageal varices. N Engl J Med 324:1532, 1991

Tryba M: Prophylaxis of stress ulcer bleeding: a meta-analysis. J Clin Gastroenterol 13(suppl 2):S44, 1991

PROSPECTIVE STUDIES

Branicki FJ, Coleman SY, Pritchett CJ, et al: Emergency surgical treatment for nonvariceal bleeding of the upper part of the gastrointestinal tract. Surg Gynecol Obstet 172:113, 1991

Gostout CJ, Wang KK, Ahlquist DA, et al: Acute gastrointestinal bleeding: experience of a specialized management team. J Clin Gastroenterol 14:260, 1992

Hunt PS, Fracs MS, Korman MG, et al: An 8-year prospective experience with balloon tamponade in emergency control of bleeding esophageal varices. Dig Dis Sci 27:413, 1982

Loftus EV, Alexander GL, Ahlquist DA, et al: Endoscopic treatment of major bleeding from advanced gastroduodenal malignant lesions. Mayo Clin Proc 69:736, 1994

Rockey DC, Cello JP: Evaluation of the gastrointestinal tract in patients with iron-deficiency anemia. N Engl J Med 329:1691, 1993

Terblanche J, Northoever JMA, Bornman P, et al: A prospective evaluation of injection sclerotherapy in the treatment of acute bleeding from esophageal varices. Surgery 85:239, 1979

Zuckerman G, Benitez J: A prospective study of bidirectional endoscopy (colonoscopy and upper endoscopy) in the evaluation of patients with occult gastrointestinal bleeding. Am J Gastroenterol 87:62, 1992

RETROSPECTIVE STUDIES

Arora A, Mehrotra R, Patnaik PK, et al: Dieulafoy's lesion: a rare cause of massive upper gastrointestinal haemorrhage. Trop Gastroenterol 12:25, 1991

Cotton PB, Rosenberg MT, Waldram RPL, et al: Early endoscopy of oesophagus, stomach, and duodenal bulb in patients with haematemesis and melaena. Br Med J 2:505, 1973

Dempsey DT, Burke DR, Reilly RS, et al: Angiography in poor-risk patients with massive nonvariceal upper gastrointestinal bleeding. Am J Surg 159:282, 1990

Fox JG, Hunt PS: Management of acute bleeding gastric malignancy. Aust NZ J Surg 63:462, 1993

Gaisford WD: Endoscopic electrohemostasis of active upper gastrointestinal bleeding. Am J Surg 137:47, 1979

Henriksson AE, Svensson J-O: Upper gastrointestinal bleeding (with special reference to blood transfusion). Eur J Surg 157:193, 1991

Himal HS, Perrault C, Mzabi R: Upper gastrointestinal hemorrhage: aggressive management decreases mortality. Surgery 84:448, 1978

Jacobson AR, Cerqueira MD: Prognostic significance of late imaging results in technetium-99m-labeled red blood cell gastrointestinal bleeding studies with early negative images. J Nucl Med 33:202, 1992

Jim G, Rikkers LF: Cause and management of upper gastrointestinal bleeding after distal splenorenal shunt. Surgery 112:719, 1992

Kaye GL, McCormick A, Siringo S, et al: Bleeding from staple line erosion after esophageal transection: effect of omeprazole. Hepatology 15:1031, 1992

Liebler JM, Benner K, Putnam T, et al: Respiratory complications in critically ill medical patients with acute upper gastrointestinal bleeding. Crit Care Med 19:1152, 1991

Lipper B, Simon D, Cerrone F: Pulmonary aspiration during emergency endoscopy in patients with upper gastrointestinal hemorrhage. Crit Care Med 19:330, 1991

Miller AR, Farnell MB, Kelly KA, et al: The impact of therapeutic endoscopy on the treatment of bleeding duodenal ulcers, 1980–90. World J Surg 19:89, 1995

Sugawa C, Benishek D, Walt AJ: Mallory-Weiss syndrome: a study of 224 patients. Am J Surg 145:30, 1983

Sugawa C, Steffes CP, Nakamura R, et al: Upper gastrointestinal bleeding in an urban hospital: etiology, recurrence, and prognosis. Ann Surg 212:521, 1990

Sugawa C, Werner MH, Hayes DF, et al: Early endoscopy: a guide to therapy for acute hemorrhage in the upper gastrointestinal tract. Arch Surg 107:133, 1973

Wilairatana S, Sriussadaporn S, Tanphaiphat C: A review of 1338 patients with acute upper gastrointestinal bleeding at Chulalongkorn University Hospital, Bangkok. Gastroenterologia Japonica 26:58, 1991

Reviews

Groszmann RJ, Grace ND: Complications of portal hypertension: esophagogastric varices and ascites. Gastroenterol Clin North Am 21:103, 1992

Kankaria AG, Fleischer DE: The critical care management of nonvariceal upper gastrointestinal bleeding. Crit Care Clin 11:347, 1995

Katz PO, Salas L: Less frequent causes of upper gastrointestinal bleeding. Gastroenterol Clin North Am 22:875, 1993

Kleber G, Ansari H, Sauerbruch T: Prophylaxis of first variceal bleeding. Bailliere's Clinical Gastroenterology 6:563, 1992

Sugawa C: Endoscopic diagnosis and treatment of upper gastrointestinal bleeding. Surg Clin North Am 69:1167, 1989

19 LOWER GASTROINTESTINAL BLEEDING

Margaret Schnitzler, M.B.B.S., and Robin S. McLeod, M.D.

Assessment and Management of Lower Gastrointestinal Bleeding

Many pathological conditions of the colon and rectum can cause lower gastrointestinal bleeding, which may be major or minor in nature. Major bleeding is most often caused by diverticular disease or vascular malformations of the colon but can also be caused by neoplasms, mucosal inflammation, ischemic colitis, aortoduodenal fistula, and a variety of other lesions. Minor bleeding may be related to anal conditions, such as hemorrhoids and anal fissures, or to colonic or rectal lesions, including neoplasms and inflammatory bowel disease. This chapter will consider only patients who present with overt bleeding and will not discuss the management of occult GI blood loss that is detected only by stool examination.

Presentation and Initial Assessment

The initial approach to the patient who presents with lower GI bleeding involves a rapid assessment of the extent of the bleeding. Minor bleeding often has an anorectal cause and, in most cases, can be investigated and managed on a nonurgent basis [*see* Investigation and Management of Minor Bleeding, *below*]. By contrast, major lower GI hemorrhage can be a life-threatening emergency and requires immediate attention. The airway, respiratory system, and circulation should be rapidly assessed, and the extent of blood loss should be estimated. A history of passage of a large amount of rectal blood—particularly of bright-red blood—or the presence of any symptoms or signs of hemodynamic compromise indicate the need for resuscitation and urgent investigation.

RESUSCITATION

In hemodynamically compromised patients or patients with a history of major bleeding, resuscitative therapy with I.V. crystalloid or colloid fluids should be instituted via a large-bore cannula. Oxygen should be administered by mask or, if the airway is compromised, by endotracheal tube and ventilator. A urinary catheter should be inserted, and urine output should be monitored hourly. Blood should be drawn for baseline measurements of complete blood count, coagulation studies, and blood chemistry, as well as for typing and cross-matching. If the patient continues to bleed or is unstable, blood transfusion should be commenced.

Because massive rectal bleeding is caused by a lesion proximal to the ligament of Treitz in up to 10 percent of cases, a nasogastric tube should be inserted in patients with significant rectal bleeding to exclude an upper GI source. If a bloody aspirate is returned or if an upper GI lesion seems likely on the basis of the history, esophagogastroduodenoscopy should be carried out [*see* 18 Upper Gastrointestinal Bleeding and 47 Gastrointestinal Endoscopy].

Investigation and Management of Major Bleeding

Patients who have significant lower GI bleeding, as indicated by blood loss of more than 100 ml, or who have bleeding and hemodynamic instability should be admitted to the hospital for observation and monitoring. If major bleeding continues in a stable patient, he or she must be closely observed and monitored for signs of hemodynamic instability. Resuscitation with I.V. fluids and blood, if necessary, should be continued, and urgent investigations should be performed to identify the source of the bleeding. It should be emphasized that in these circumstances, there is no role for exploratory laparotomy as a means of localizing the site of bleeding; it is usually not possible to identify any obvious colonic lesions, and blind segmental resection has a high rate of rebleeding.

UNSTABLE PATIENTS WHO CONTINUE TO BLEED

In a minority of patients presenting with lower GI hemorrhage, the bleeding is massive and continuous, leading to hemodynamic instability. Such bleeding is most likely a result of diverticular disease, but it may also be associated with other colonic lesions or with an

Assessment and Management of Lower Gastrointestinal Bleeding

Patient presents with lower GI bleeding

Perform initial assessment:
- Evaluate airway, breathing, and circulation.
- Establish extent of blood loss.

Patient has major bleeding or exhibits signs and symptoms of hemodynamic compromise

Resuscitate with I.V. crystalloid or colloid fluids administered via large-bore cannula.
Give oxygen by mask or by ET tube and ventilator.
Insert urinary catheter and monitor urine output.
Give blood as needed.
Draw blood for CBC, coagulation studies, blood chemistry analysis, typing, and crossmatching.
Perform nasogastric aspiration.

Bloody aspirate is returned

Upper GI bleeding suspected. Proceed with esophagogastroduodenoscopy [see 47 Gastrointestinal Endoscopy]. Treat appropriately [see 18 Upper Gastrointestinal Bleeding].

No bloody aspirate is returned

Lower GI bleeding suspected.

Patient continues to bleed

Assess hemodynamic stability.

Patient is hemodynamically stable

Obtain history of bleeding, bowel habit, medications, and concomitant illnesses.
Perform physical examination and rigid sigmoidoscopy.

Patient is hemodynamically unstable

Attempt to localize site of bleeding.
Perform urgent angiography or radionuclide scanning.
Perform rigid sigmoidoscopy.

Bleeding site localized

Undertake endoscopic therapy [see 47 Gastrointestinal Endoscopy] or surgical therapy, as appropriate.

Bleeding site not localized

Patient continues to bleed

Observe and monitor for signs of hemodynamic instability.
Perform urgent investigations to identify source of bleeding:
- Emergency colonoscopy
- Radionuclide scanning
- Selective angiography

Cause of bleeding is identified

Treat cause (e.g., angiodysplasia, neoplasia, diverticular disease, inflammatory bowel disease) appropriately.

Bleeding site localized

Perform segmental resection.

Bleeding site not localized

Examine entire colon and small bowel during laparotomy.
If localization remains unsuccessful and patient continues to bleed, perform urgent colectomy and ileorectal anastomosis [see 57 Colorectal Procedures].

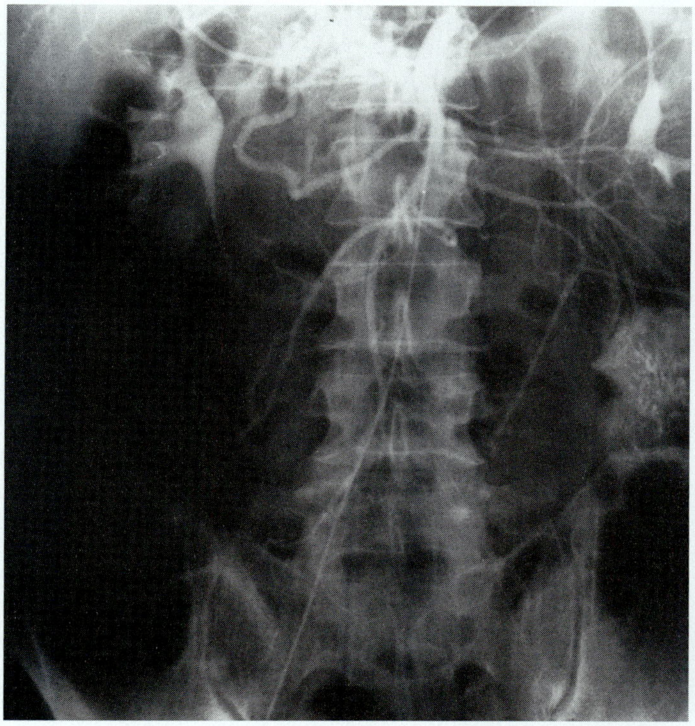

Figure 4 Angiography was performed in a young patient who presented with recurrent episodes of rectal bleeding despite normal results on previous repeated colonoscopy and gastroduodenoscopy. The angiogram reveals an abnormal vascular lesion in the left lower quadrant. Histology of the resected specimen revealed it to be a leiomyoma of the jejunum.

for 12 to 24 hours; if bleeding has ceased on cessation of treatment, the catheter is withdrawn. Intra-arterial vasopressin infusion has been reported to be successful in controlling bleeding in up to 90 percent of patients, but there is a high rate of recurrent bleeding on cessation of therapy and a significant incidence of complications—particularly abdominal pain, cardiac arrhythmias, and decreased cardiac output. Nonetheless, intra-arterial vasopressin infusion may be useful as a temporizing measure in massively bleeding patients before operation and in those who are unsuitable for operation. An angiographically localized bleeding source—particularly vascular malformations—may also be amenable to colonoscopic therapy (see above).

Therapy Once the bleeding site has been successfully localized, endoscopic or surgical therapy can be undertaken. In the case of patients with angiodysplastic lesions of the right colon, nonoperative treatment should be attempted, as it is highly likely that control of the bleeding will be achieved by endoscopic therapy with sclerosing or vasoconstricting agents, electrocoagulation, or laser therapy. Bleeding that is associated with diverticular disease is unlikely to be controlled by endoscopic therapy and may require segmental resection of the affected portion of the colon if the bleeding continues [*see 57 Colorectal Procedures*]. After resection, the decision to perform a primary anastomosis or to create a stoma will depend on the general condition of the patient and the state of the colon.

Management of Stable Patients in Whom Bleeding Stops

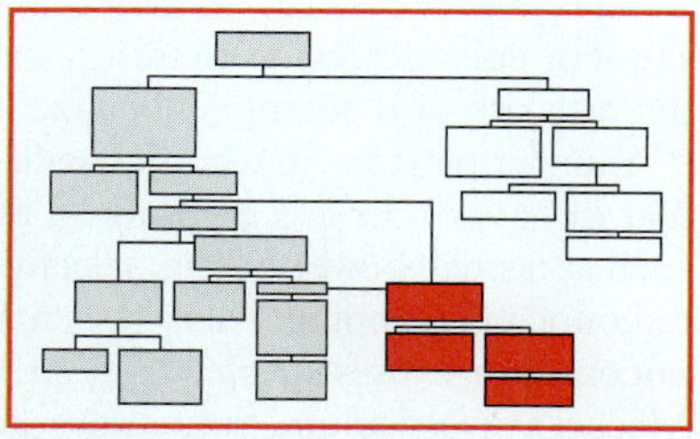

If bleeding stops and the patient remains hemodynamically stable, urgent investigation is not required, but colonoscopy should be performed within 24 hours or as soon as is feasible [*see 47 Gastrointestinal Endoscopy*]. Blood within the colon acts as a cathartic agent, and adequate preparation of the bowel may be achieved by the administration of enemas without the need for oral preparation. This may identify a specific source of bleeding, such as a vascular malformation or a colonic neoplasm. If no obvious source of blood loss is identified, a repeat colonoscopy after full preparation should be performed electively.

Barium enema should not be performed in the acutely bleeding patient, as it is of limited use in the identification of vascular malformations; although diverticula may be seen, they will not necessarily be the source of the bleeding. In addition, the presence of barium in the colon precludes the subsequent performance of angiography or colonoscopy and is undesirable if operation is required. If colonoscopy cannot be carried out or is contraindicated, a barium enema may be performed electively after discharge from the hospital.

Despite a careful endoscopic or radiologic examination of the colon, it may not be possible to identify an obvious source of hemorrhage. In older patients, it is likely that the bleeding has originated from diverticular disease or from an angiodysplastic lesion that was not visualized. In these patients, no further investigation is needed unless the bleeding is recurrent. If bleeding is recurrent, repeated colonoscopy, angiography, or radionuclide scanning should be carried out at the time of sub-

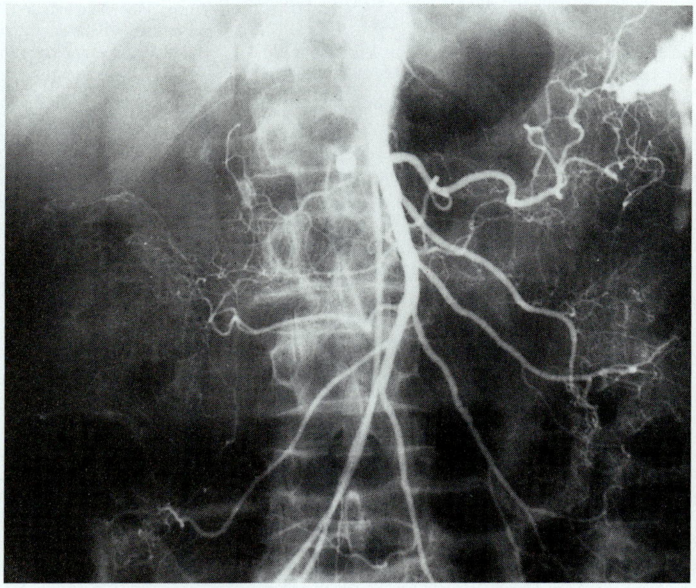

Figure 5 This angiogram of an elderly woman who presented with massive rectal bleeding reveals extravasation of contrast in the left upper quadrant. At operation, the patient was found to have an ulcerated carcinoma of the splenic flexure of the colon.

sequent episodes, and operation should be performed only if a definite site of bleeding is localized.

Younger patients, in whom vascular abnormalities and diverticular disease occur less commonly, require further investigations, such as a small bowel enema, selective mesenteric angiography, or radionuclide scanning. These tests may lead to the identification of uncommon causes of bleeding, such as small bowel tumors or Meckel's diverticulum. Sometimes, laparotomy and intraoperative endoscopy are necessary for the management of recurrent GI bleeding of unknown cause.

Investigation and Management of Minor Bleeding

Many patients describe the passage of small amounts of red blood, either mixed with or on the surface of the stool. When the bleeding is obvious and bright red in color, it can be assumed that the site of blood loss is within or distal to the left colon. If the bleeding has been of small volume (i.e., < 20 ml) and the patient is in stable condition, further investigation can be performed on an outpatient basis. In a young and otherwise healthy person with an obvious anorectal cause of bleeding, no further investigation is required. Treatment of the cause—which may include rubber band ligation or surgical hemorrhoidectomy for bleeding hemorrhoids or lateral internal sphincterectomy for a symptomatic anal fissure—is all that is required [see 59 Anal Procedures].

In patients older than 40 years, patients with a family history of colon cancer, and patients in whom no obvious bleeding source can be identified by means of anoscopy and sigmoidoscopy, further investigation is necessary. The preferred investigation is elective colonoscopy after bowel preparation [see 47 Gastrointestinal Endoscopy] because this is the most sensitive and specific test for the detection of neoplasms and mucosal abnormalities of the colon. If colonoscopic examination cannot be performed, a barium enema and sigmoidoscopy can be substituted. Subsequent management, such as surgical resection of a neoplasm or treatment of inflammatory bowel disease, will depend on the findings of these investigations. If no abnormality is identified after a complete colonoscopic investigation, a policy of observation can be adopted.

Recommended Reading

Alavi A, Dann R, Baum S, et al: Scintigraphic detection of acute gastrointestinal bleeding. Radiology 124:753, 1977

Alavi A, Ring EJ: Localization of gastrointestinal bleeding: superiority of 99 technetium sulfur colloid compared with angiography. AJR Am J Roentgenol 137:741, 1981

Bender JS, Wiencek RG, Bouwman DL: Morbidity and mortality following total abdominal colectomy for massive lower gastrointestinal bleeding. Am Surg 57:536, 1991

Boley SJ, Sprayregen S, Sammartano RJ, et al: The pathophysiologic basis of the angiographic signs of vascular ectasias of the colon. Radiology 125:615, 1977

Boley SJ, Dibiase A, Brandt LJ, et al: Lower intestinal bleeding in the elderly. Am J Surg 137:56, 1979

Boley SJ, Brandt LJ: Vascular ectasias of the colon. Dig Dis Sci 31(suppl):265, 1986

Browder W, Cerise EJ, Litwin MS: Impact of emergency angiography in massive lower gastrointestinal bleeding. Ann Surg 204:530, 1986

Davis GB, Bookstein JJ, Coel MN: Advantage of intraarterial over intravenous vasopressin infusion in gastrointestinal hemorrhage. AJR Am J Roentgenol 128:733, 1977

Flickinger EG, Stanforth AC, Sinar DR, et al: Intraoperative video panendoscopy for diagnosing sites of chronic intestinal bleeding. Am J Surg 157:137, 1989

Foutch PG: Angiodysplasia of the gastrointestinal tract. Am J Gastroenterol 88:807, 1993

Guy GE, Shetty PC, Sharma RP, et al: Acute lower gastrointestinal hemorrhage: treatment by superselective embolization with polyvinyl alcohol particles. AJR Am J Roentgenol 159:521, 1992

Hunter JM, Pezim ME: Limited value of technetium 99m–labeled red cell scintigraphy in localization of lower gastrointestinal bleeding. Am J Surg 159:504, 1990

Jensen DM, Machicado GA: Diagnosis and treatment of severe hematochezia: the role of urgent colonoscopy after purge. Gastroenterology 95:1569, 1988

Naveau S, Aubert A, Poynard T, et al: Long-term results of treatment of vascular malformations of the gastrointestinal tract by neodymium Yag laser photocoagulation. Dig Dis Sci 35:821, 1990

Nussbaum M, Baum S: Radiographic demonstration of unknown sites of gastrointestinal bleeding. Surg Forum 14:374, 1963

Potter GD, Sellin JH: Lower gastrointestinal bleeding. Gastroenterol Clin North Am 17:341, 1988

Richter JM, Christensen MR, Colditz GA, et al: Angiodysplasia: natural history and efficacy of therapeutic interventions. Dig Dis Sci 34:1542, 1989

Roberts PL, Schoetz DJ, Coller JA: Vascular ectasia: diagnosis and treatment by colonoscopy. Am Surg 54:56, 1988

Rosen RJ, Sanchez G: Angiographic diagnosis and management of gastrointestinal hemorrhage. Radiol Clin North Am 32:951, 1994

Rutgeerts R, Van Gompel F, Gebos K, et al: Long-term results of treatment of vascular malformations of the gastrointestinal tract by Neodymium-Yag laser photocoagulation. Gut 26:586, 1985

Santos JCM, Aprilli F, Guimarais AS, et al: Angiodysplasia of the colon: endoscopic diagnosis and treatment. Br J Surg 75:256, 1988

Sharma R: Angiodysplasia and lower gastrointestinal tract bleeding in elderly patients. Arch Intern Med 155:807, 1995

Welch CE, Athanasoulis CA, Galbadini JJ: Hemorrhage from the large bowel with special reference to angiodysplasia and diverticular disease. World J Surg 2:73, 1978

Zuckerman DA, Bocchini TP, Birnbaum EH: Massive hemorrhage in the lower gastrointestinal tract in adults: diagnostic imaging and intervention. AJR Am J Roentgenol 161:703, 1993

20 SKIN LESIONS

Alan E. Seyfer, M.D.

Assessment and Management of Skin Lesions

The clinical assessment and treatment of skin lesions can be challenging, since some skin lesions are capricious in their biologic behavior. History is of great importance. Recent changes in the appearance of a lesion usually indicate active growth, which increases the chance that the lesion is malignant. Likewise, a history of chronic sun exposure—particularly in a patient who has a fair complexion—multiplies the patient's risk of malignancy. Certain congenital lesions must also be viewed with suspicion, even though the incidence of malignancy in such lesions can be extremely variable. Any history that departs from the natural history of a simple nevus should raise suspicion of malignancy. In general, nevus tissue becomes apparent at four or five years of age. Nevi often darken with puberty and pregnancy and fade in the seventh to eighth decades of life. Malignancies usually differ from the characteristic clinical pattern of a simple nevus.

Nonsuspicious Lesions

In general, lesions are nonsuspicious if they remain stable and uniform in their physical characteristics (e.g., size, shape, color, profile, texture). Nonsuspicious lesions may be safely monitored conservatively, especially if they are located in regions easily visible to the patient. Excisional biopsy is warranted if the lesions change in size, shape, color, profile, or texture. Cosmesis is always a subjective and relative indication for excision.

Suspicious Lesions

Changes and irregularities in the physical characteristics of a skin lesion (e.g., size, shape, color, profile, and texture) are important in helping determine whether the lesion is suspicious. For example, an irregular physical pattern, large size (1 to 2 cm or larger), or unfavorable location (e.g., on skin that is unprotected from sun exposure) places the lesion in the suspicious category and is a relative indication for performing an excisional biopsy.

BIOPSY

If the lesion is suspicious, a biopsy is warranted. If the suspicious area is small, it should be completely excised with a 1 to 4 mm margin, depending on the clinical characteristics. The important principle is to include a margin of normal skin around the lesion. This helps the pathologist and may include occult areas of importance. Shave biopsies should *never* be performed, because the depth of the lesion is of great diagnostic importance, and lesion depth is destroyed by this technique. To provide a complete specimen for study, my preference is to include a full thickness of the dermis with subcutaneous fat. As noted above, a small margin of normal skin is helpful to the pathologist [*see* Surgical Technique, Excisional Biopsy, *below*].

If the lesion is found to be benign, further treatment is unwarranted. If the lesion proves to be malignant, further excision with an appropriate margin is usually necessary, and staging of the tumor becomes important (see below). Presentation of the biopsy to the tumor board is of great value both clinically and medicolegally. In cases of melanoma or other so-called liquid tumors that shed their cells readily in all tissue, ancillary treatment (e.g., with perfusion therapy, radiation therapy, or chemotherapy) may be reasonable before reexcision with wider margins.

CLINICAL STAGING OF MALIGNANCY

If a malignancy is suspected, regional node status is important, and the nodes that drain the region should be thoroughly examined. If nodes are palpable and the lesion proves to be a malignancy, a regional node dissection, or sampling, is necessary to stage the patient's tumor and plan for further treatment. Likewise, a node dissection may be therapeutic and may contribute to local control of the lesion. If the nodes are positive, it is reasonable to consider adjuvant therapy or ancillary treatment. If the nodes are negative microscopically, it is reasonable to follow the patient with serial examinations. Again, an interdisciplinary tumor board will assist in making the appropriate management decision once a malignancy is confirmed by biopsy.

Assessment and Management of Skin Lesions

Determine whether skin lesion is suspicious for malignancy

Obtain history and examine the patient's skin lesion.

Lesion is suspicious

Changes and irregularities in physical characteristics, history of chronic sun exposure, unfavorable location, and presence of certain congenital lesions (e.g., dysplastic nevi) all raise suspicion of malignancy.

Lesion is nonsuspicious

The lesion is stable and uniform in its physical characteristics (e.g., size, shape, color, profile, texture). Monitor conservatively. Patient may choose elective excision for cosmesis.

Perform excisional biopsy

Suspicious lesion should be completely excised with a 1–4 mm margin (depending on clinical characteristics), including the full thickness of the dermis with subcutaneous fat. Shave biopsies should *never* be performed on suspicious lesions.

Lesion is benign

No further treatment is necessary.

Lesion is malignant

Present biopsy to tumor board. If tumor is melanoma or other so-called liquid tumor, consider ancillary treatment (e.g., perfusion therapy, radiation therapy, chemotherapy) before reexcision.

Perform reexcision with appropriate margin and assess regional node status

---

Nodes are nonpalpable

Follow clinically.

Nodes are palpable

Perform appropriate regional node dissection.

Nodes are negative

Follow clinically.

Nodes are positive

Consider ancillary treatment (e.g., perfusion therapy, radiation therapy, chemotherapy).

Discussion

Nonmelanoma skin cancers are the most common cancers in the United States, making up approximately 35 percent of all cancers diagnosed every year.[1,2] Nonmelanoma skin cancers can be capricious, and it may be difficult to assess their biologic behavior from their appearance alone. Certainly, it is possible for a benign-looking papule to exhibit aggressive biologic behavior. Melanomas, at the more malignant end of the spectrum, can metastasize early and even present initially with cerebral metastasis.

Sun exposure with actinic changes in the skin is a predisposing factor for skin cancers of all types.[3-5] Fair-skinned persons lacking protective pigmentation are at a much higher risk for the development of skin cancers.[6] Recent evidence also implicates failure of the immunologic surveillance system, decreased cell-mediated immunity, and use of immunosuppressive agents as factors that may influence a patient's predisposition for malignant skin lesions.[7,8]

Basal Cell Carcinoma

Basal cell carcinomas originate in the pluripotential epithelial cells of the epidermis and skin adnexa.[1] These tumors tend to be characterized by slow growth and progressive morbidity by local extension. Their viability seems to depend on attachment to the dermis, and systemic metastases are therefore rare. However, certain types of basal cell carcinoma may be extremely aggressive, resulting in morbidity, mutilation, and death by local extension. This is particularly true of midface and sclerosing basal cell cancers.

Clinically, there are several types of basal cell carcinomas [see Figure 1]. The most common is the nodular type, which begins as a flesh-colored, raised, telangiectatic lesion that may be difficult to distinguish from a common nevus.[9] The nodular lesion is rounded in appearance during its early phase and characteristically assumes a raised rim with a craterlike central region, often with scaling of superficial skin cells at its center [see Figure 1a]. Perhaps the most dangerous type is the sclerosing, or morpheaform, basal cell carcinoma—a light, plaquelike lesion that can resemble a stellate scar [see Figure 1b]. Morpheaform basal cell carcinomas tend to be locally invasive, with multiple cancer projections, resembling tentacles, that penetrate toward the deep portions of the tissue. Therefore, it is possible—even likely—to perform an excisional biopsy of the lesion and inadvertently leave tumor behind.[10] Such tumors can also ulcerate and resemble pigmented melanomas [see Figure 1c].

The distribution of basal cell cancers has a strong predilection for the midface, cheek, and ear regions.[11] Treatment is usually surgical, with removal of a rim of normal skin around the lesion. Morpheaform basal cell cancers should be treated with a wider margin of excision, and careful attention should be paid to the margins to ascertain clearance of tumor cells. In most cases, closure can be accomplished by wide undermining of the skin and fat and direct closure. Otherwise, a skin graft is a useful alternative.

Radiation therapy for basal cell carcinomas claims an overall cure rate of over 90 percent.[12] This therapy can be offered to each patient, but the repeated treatments require multiple visits. Radiation therapy is a safe, noninvasive form of treatment that can be an attractive alternative for patients who are, for whatever reasons, considered bad candidates for surgical extirpation. Radiation is a particularly attractive alternative for the treatment of lesions in areas that are difficult to reconstruct, such as the medial canthal margin of the eyelids, certain external ear lesions, and the nostril rim.

Another therapeutic option is Mohs' micrographic surgical operation. Frederic Mohs, a general surgeon, developed the technique for lesions like basal cell carcinomas without metastatic potential that were of full thickness and involved the skin and mucous membranes of the nose.[13] Perhaps the best indication

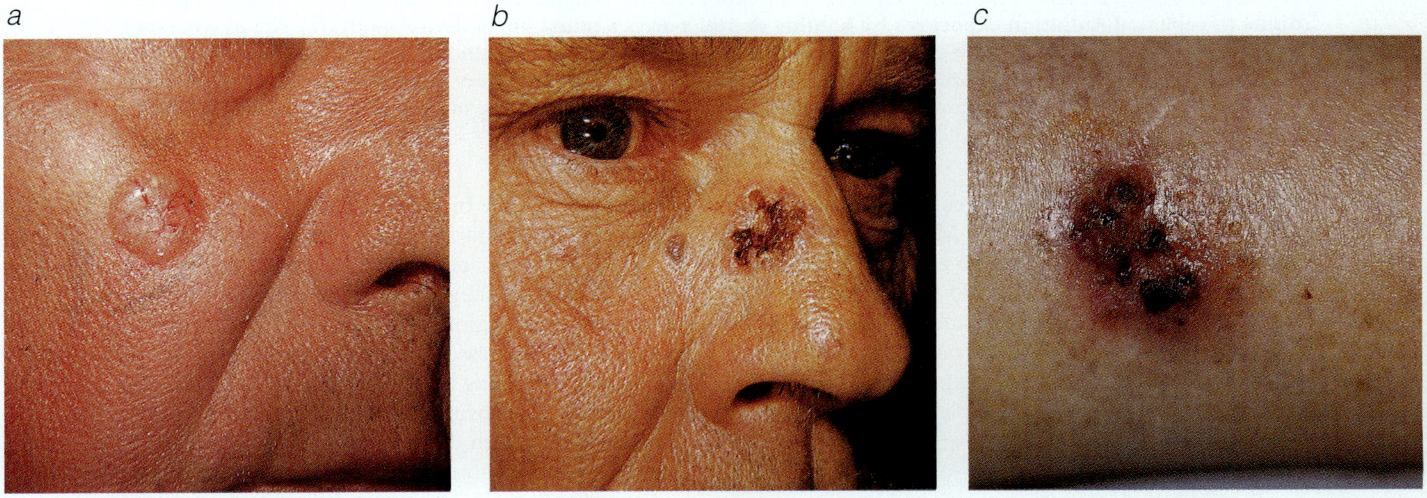

Figure 1 (*a*) A pearly luster and telangiectasias are evident in this typical basal cell carcinoma on the cheek of a 43-year-old man. (*b*) This sclerosing (morpheaform) basal cell carcinoma on the nose of a 55-year-old man was found to be deeply invasive and exhibited multidirectional growth. (*c*) This basal cell carcinoma on the lower leg of a 91-year-old woman showed ulceration and pigmentation similar to that of a melanoma.

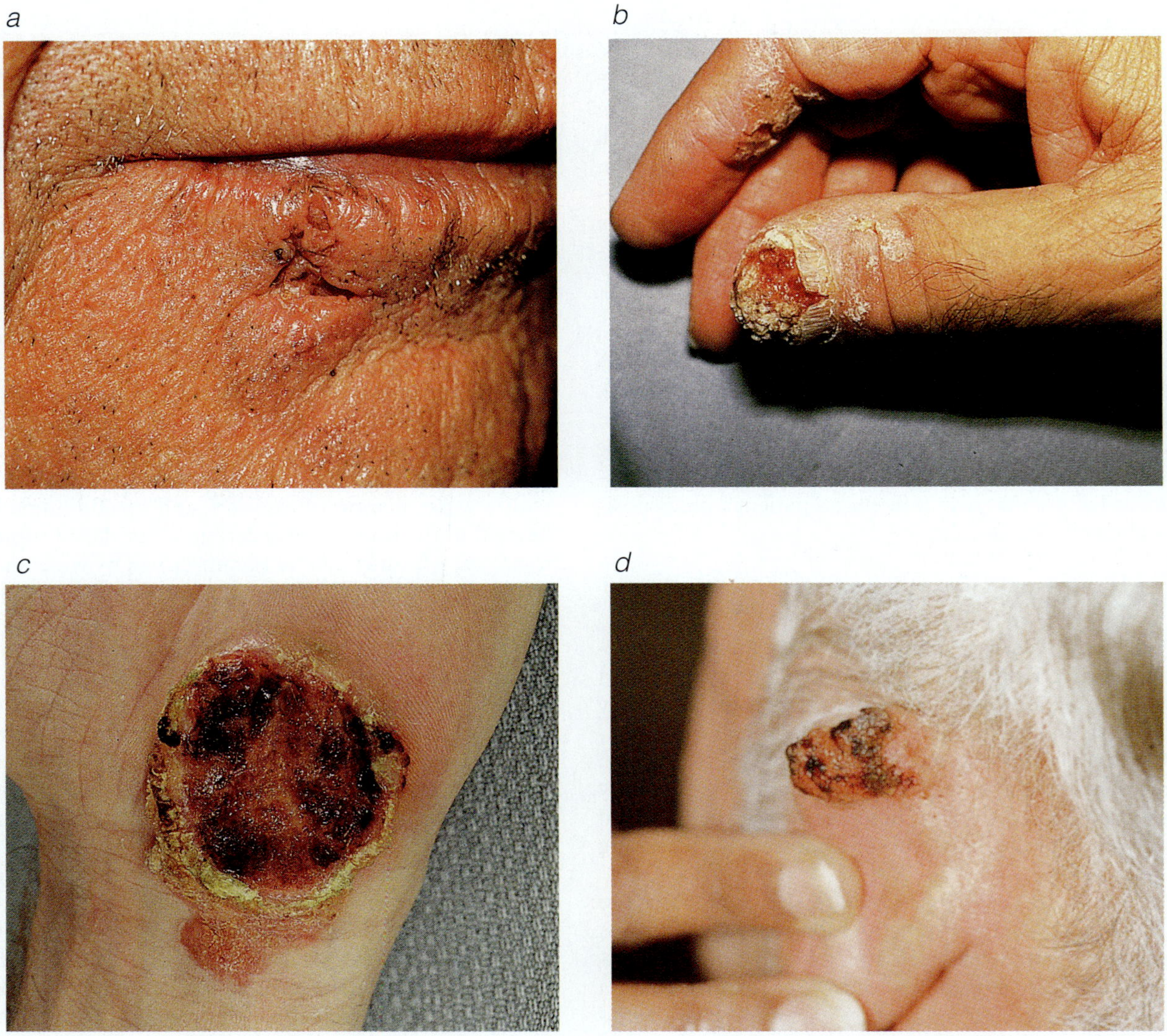

Figure 2 (*a*) This squamous cell carcinoma on the lip of a 70-year-old man was related to sun exposure; the patient was a nonsmoker. (*b*) This squamous cell carcinoma involving the thumb and index finger of a 72-year-old man, a retired dentist, was related to exposure to occupational hazards; he had subjected these digits to repeated radiation exposures by holding dental x-rays against his patients' teeth. (*c*) The 61-year-old man who had this indolent, slow-growing squamous cell carcinoma on the hand also had a synchronous penile erythroplasia of Queyrat (localized)—a squamous cell carcinoma in situ; there was no evidence of metastasis from either lesion. (*d*) This squamous cell carcinoma on the helix of the external ear in a 73-year-old man can be seen extending to the scalp.

for the Mohs procedure is recurrent basal cell carcinomas, especially those of the morpheaform type. The Mohs technique usually incorporates wide enough margins to ensure a reasonable cure rate. The Mohs technique may also be appropriate for microcystic adnexal carcinoma and dermatofibrosarcoma protuberans.[14] The drawbacks to the Mohs procedure are that it requires a considerable amount of time, exposure, and expense but has a cure rate similar to that of simple surgical excision.

Squamous Cell Carcinoma

Like basal cell cancers, squamous cell cancers are associated with actinic solar damage but may also arise out of old scars, radiation-damaged skin, or chronic, open wounds[15] [*see Figures 2*]. Chronic inflammation and irritation appear to be the common denominators. The biologic activity of squamous cell cancers is aggressive in comparison with that of basal cell cancers; fortunately, they are less common. Persons of fair complexion are at increased risk; all skin cancers have a predilection for developing in sun-exposed regions[16] [*see Figure 2a*]. Certain occupational hazards have been associated with an increased risk for squamous cell cancer, including those experienced by dental personnel who habitually expose their hands to x-ray energy and technicians who paint radium watch dials [*see Figure 2b*].

Histologically, squamous cell lesions are characterized by masses of squamous epithelium that invade downward through the dermis in a palisade arrangement. The degree of epithelial differentiation determines the grade of the tumor. This grade is measured as a ratio of atypical cells to normal cells. In higher grades of tumor (i.e., those with a high degree of biologic aggressiveness), differentiation and keratinization are greatly diminished.[1] Anaplastic (i.e., undifferentiated) tumors may require further characterization. The presence of cytokeratin antibodies (indicative of squamous cells) or antibody to S100 protein (which may identify melanocytes, indicative of melanoma) may also help in assessing the more anaplastic tumors. Immunoperoxidase staining may help distinguish between the desmoplastic variety of melanoma and certain squamous cell cancers.[1,17] Differentiation of a squamous cell cancer, depth of invasion, and the presence of perineural invasion correlate with biologic aggressiveness.[1]

Clinically, the lesion may appear as a gradually enlarging, nonhealing, nontender sore [see Figure 2c], or it may present as an actinic patch—typically on the cheek or external ear [see Figure 2d]. Tumors that arise in old scars or open wounds are characteristically aggressive. Squamous cell carcinomas that develop from Marjolin's ulcer (which arises in burn scars and open wounds such as osteomyelitis drainage sites) are characterized by extreme aggressiveness after surgical resection; this aggressive behavior may be attributable to the relatively immunologically privileged status of the tumors before extirpation. Surgical excision seems to activate certain lesions. Although the lesion may have remained indolent for many years, tumor recurrence and metastasis are common after treatment.[18,19]

Certain areas of the body are especially prone to early metastases and have a higher risk of regional nodal metastases. For example, squamous cell cancers of the scalp, nose, and extremities seem to metastasize early. Regional metastases are associated with a poorer prognosis.[1,20]

Bowen's disease, a carcinoma in situ, presents as a red patch or plaque with small areas of crusting. The recommended treatment is wide-margin (0.5 to 1.0 cm) surgical excision.[16]

Malignant Melanoma

Recent advances in the understanding of the biologic activity of melanoma have provided insight into the therapy and prognosis of this dangerous lesion. Although the clinical course of the disease is characteristically unpredictable, treatment strategies for primary lesions and nodal drainage systems can be developed with the assistance of some important prognostic markers: the thickness of the lesion (Breslow's level) and the depth of tissue invasion (Clark's level)[21] [see Melanoma Staging, below]. Melanomas tend to grow both vertically and radially; those that have a rapid onset in the vertical phase present as thicker lesions and have a worse prognosis.[22]

Over the past 35 years, the incidence of melanoma has increased; it is now the most rapidly increasing cancer among white males and the fourth most rapidly increasing cancer among white females.[23] Despite the poor prognosis associated with melanoma, survival after therapy has improved over the past 50 years. Some innovative and exciting immunotherapeutic strategies have been attempted, but the viable treatment options remain exclusively surgical.

As with other dermal neoplasms, a positive correlation is seen between sun exposure and the incidence of malignant melanoma. Ninety-eight percent of melanomas occur in whites, and within this population, the lighter-skinned persons are most at risk. Painful, blistering sunburns, early childhood exposure,[24] and sun-induced freckling are associated with a two to three times higher risk of cutaneous melanoma.[25]

DIFFERENTIAL CHARACTERISTICS OF BENIGN NEVI AND MALIGNANT MELANOMA

Unfortunately, the clinical presentation of malignant and benign pigmented lesions can be quite similar [see Figures 3]. However, certain differences do exist that can be helpful in making the distinction. For example, benign lesions tend to be less than 1 cm in diameter and have regular borders, a homogeneous color, and a smooth texture. Malignant lesions, on the other hand, are often larger, exhibit variable pigmentation and irregular borders, and are less orderly in their presentation.

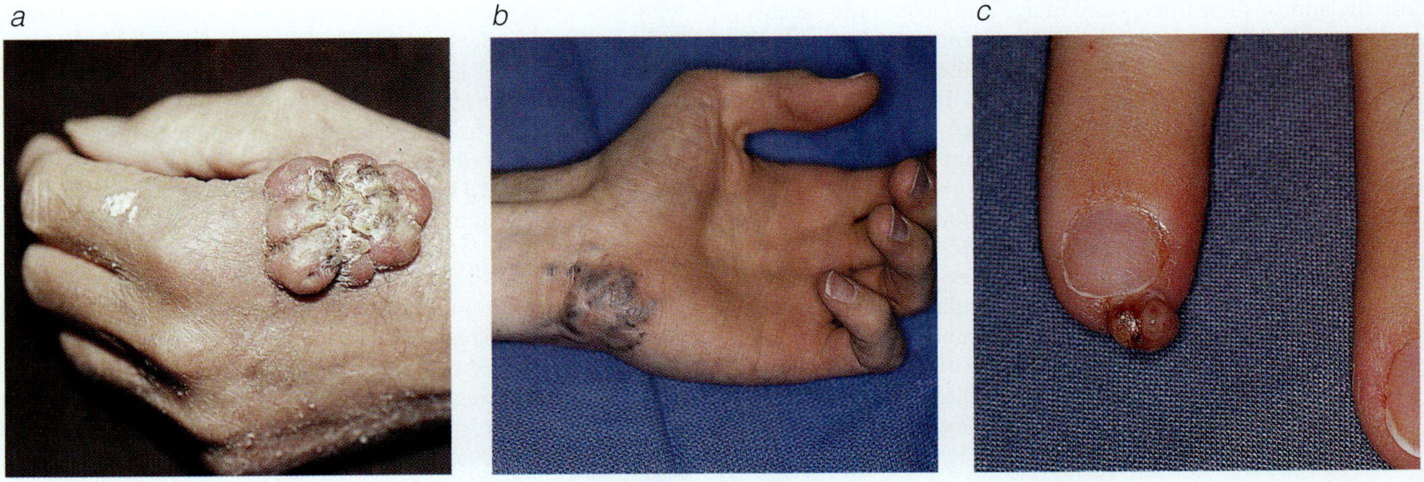

Figure 3 (a) Benign keratoacanthoma, such as this one on the hand of a 67-year-old man, is a rapidly growing lesion that can be mistaken for a malignancy. (b) This dark lesion on the distal ulnar area of a 31-year-old man, a posttraumatic arteriovenous fistula, is similar in appearance to a pigmented dermal lesion. (c) This rapidly growing pyogenic granuloma on the index finger of a 24-year-old woman developed after a small skin wound; microscopically, the lesion represents granulation tissue.

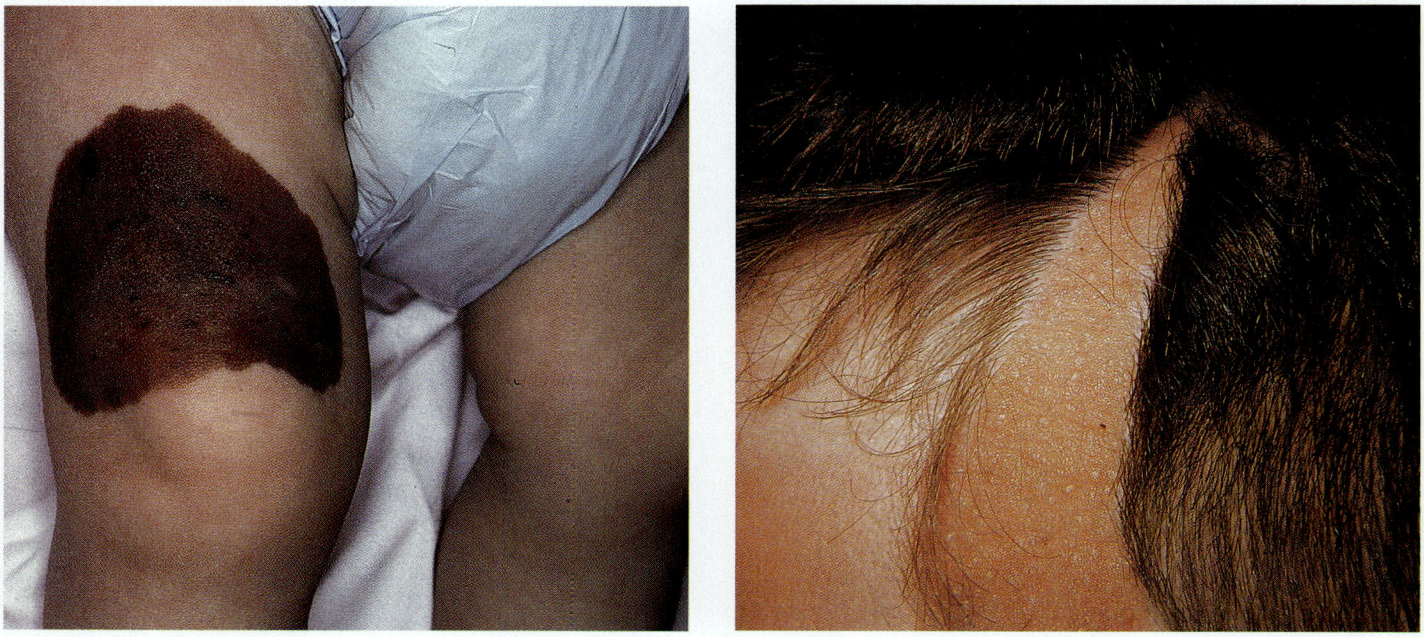

Figure 4 (*a*) This nevus on the thigh of an infant is problematic because of its congenital nature. (*b*) This sebaceous nevus, or Jadassohn-Tièche nevus, involving the temporal scalp in a 19-year-old white man may undergo malignant change.

Benign Nevi

Benign nevi, the most common pigmented lesions, are divided into three major histologic groups: (1) junctional, (2) compound, and (3) dermal. This classification, though arbitrary, refers to characteristic features of acquired melanocytic nevi.

Junctional nevi are the earliest stage of intraepidermal proliferation, the stage in which cells form nests along the dermal-epidermal junction. These lesions are relatively sessile and have a homogeneous, brownish pigmentation. Junctional nevi are characteristically smooth and have round or oval borders. They usually appear after three years of age and before adolescence, darken with the onset of puberty or pregnancy, and gradually fade in color and decrease in height in the later years of life. *Compound nevi* have junctional as well as dermal components. *Dermal nevi* are slightly raised, homogeneous in pigmentation, and well circumscribed, but they are confined to the dermis histologically.[26] Any lesion that tends to drift from this natural history should be regarded with suspicion, especially in the years after adolescence [*see Figures 4a and 4b*].

Certain lesions, including dysplastic nevi, have a higher risk for malignant transformation.[27] The familial dysplastic nevus syndrome is characterized by an autosomal dominant pattern and a unique histologic appearance. Dysplastic nevi are typically larger than ordinary nevi, and significantly, their borders and color are irregular. Over time, dysplastic nevi progress to melanoma.

Malignant Melanoma

Malignant melanoma is characterized by radial and vertical growth phases.[21,22,26] During the radial growth phase, melanocytes within the epidermis and papillary dermis grow in all directions. The result is slow radial enlargement of the lesion. Vertical growth, which usually follows the radial growth phase, consists of growth perpendicular to the direction of growth that occurred in the radial phase. This pattern is characterized by deep invasion and subsequent development of metastases.

Three types of melanoma are clinically distinguishable [*see Figures 5*]. *Superficial spreading melanoma* is the most common type of melanoma, and it may arise in a preexisting nevus. The less common *nodular melanoma* usually exhibits more rapid and aggressive growth. Nodular melanoma is not usually associated with preexisting nevi, is more common in males, has a higher incidence in middle age, and typically presents over the trunk, head, and neck.[26] *Lentigo malignant melanoma* represents only seven to eight percent of all melanomas.[28,29] It presents in older patients and tends to be indolent. Lentigo malignant melanoma was originally described by Hutchinson in 1894, and although it has been termed Hutchinson's freckle—a name that implies benignity—the lesion does have clear malignant potential.

MELANOMA STAGING

The most common criteria for the staging of melanomas are Clark's level and Breslow's level.

Clark categorized tumors according to their level of invasion into five separate regions [*see Figure 6*]. Level I, in which the tumor involves the epidermis, is essentially carcinoma in situ. Level II indicates extension of the tumor into the papillary dermis. Level III signifies a spreading of tumor cells along the papillary-reticular dermal interface. Level IV indicates invasion into the reticular dermis. Level V indicates extension into the subcutaneous tissue. According to Clark's criteria, survival decreases as the depth of invasion increases.[30]

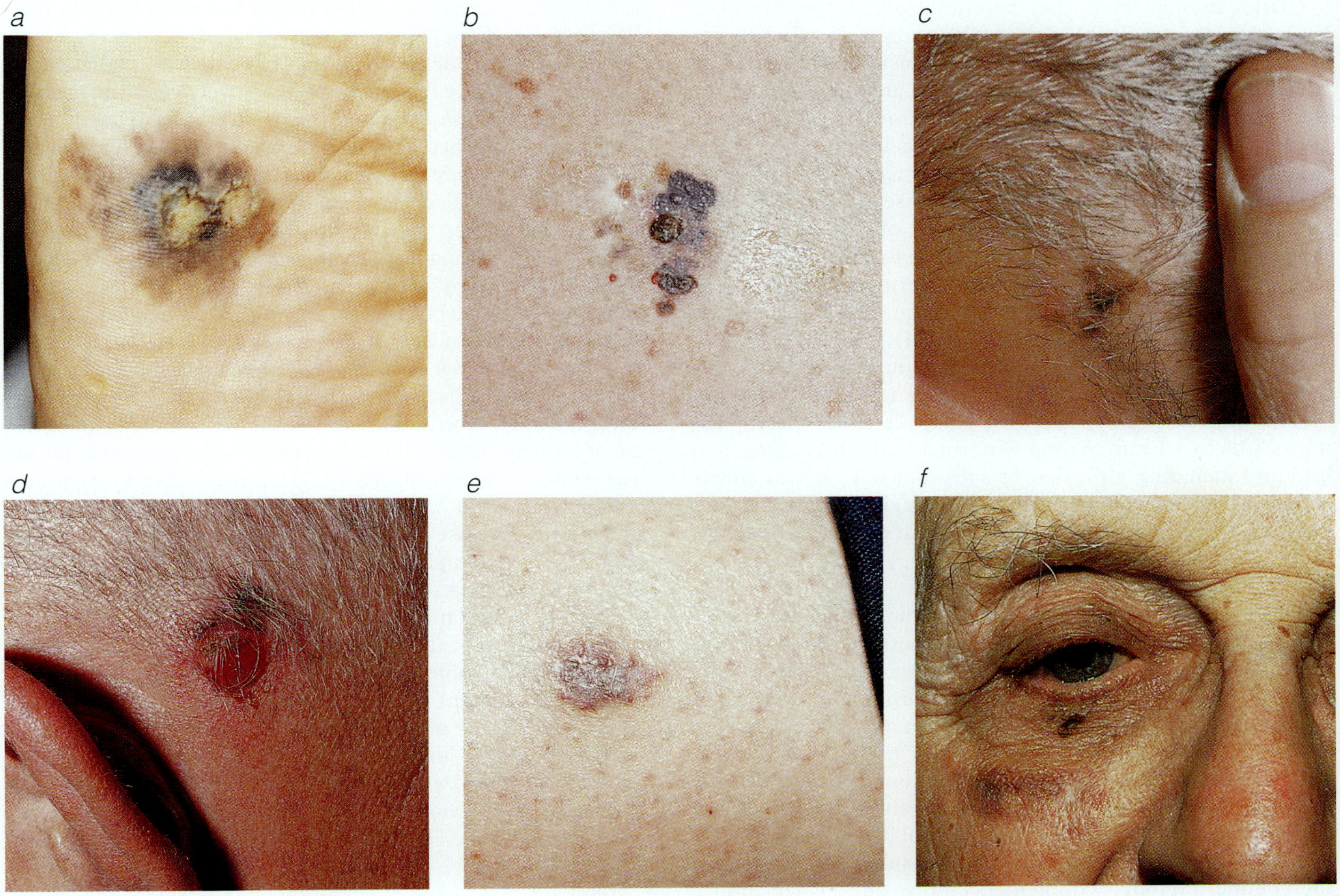

Figure 5 (*a*) This melanoma, on the sole of the foot of a 47-year-old black woman, shows irregularities in shape, contour, and pigmentation. (*b*) A so-called halo effect is visible along the left margin of this melanoma on the upper back of a 33-year-old white woman; irregularities in shape, contour, and pigmentation are also evident. (*c*) This melanoma of the postauricular scalp in a 56-year-old man exhibited ulceration and new growth (*d*) over the lower portion of the lesion two weeks later. (*e*) This melanoma on the thigh of a 31-year-old woman shows a slightly umbilicated center, irregular shape, and nonhomogeneous coloration. (*f*) This melanoma of the lower eyelid in another patient is visible as the darkly pigmented area just below the eyelashes.

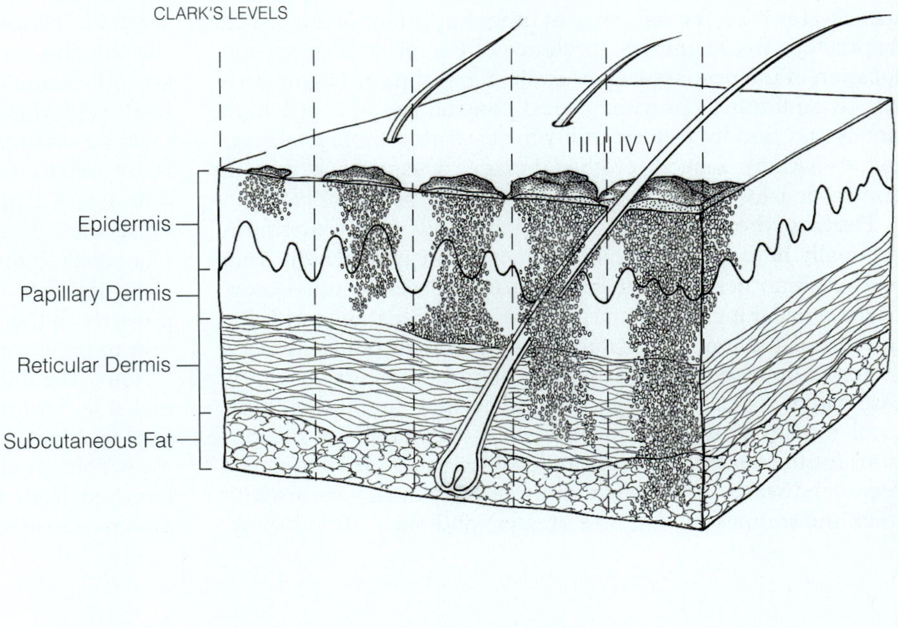

Figure 6 Clark categorized skin tumors according to their level of invasion. Tumors of level I involve the epidermis and are essentially carcinoma in situ. In level II, the tumor has extended into the papillary dermis. Tumor cells at level III are spread along the papillary-reticular dermal interface. Invasion into the reticular dermis occurs at level IV. Level V tumors extend into the subcutaneous tissue. In general, survival decreases as the depth of invasion increases.

Clark's dermal layers may be cumbersome, but Breslow's levels provide comparable therapeutic and prognostic discrimination. Breslow classified the level of invasion by use of an ocular micrometer to measure from the granular layer in the epidermis to the deepest point of invasion in the dermis. Under Breslow's criteria, thin melanomas invade 0.75 mm or less into the dermis (stage IA, T1). Intermediate-thickness melanomas invade 0.76 to 3.99 mm; these are further subdivided into thin intermediate melanomas of 0.76 to 1.49 mm (stage IB, T2), intermediate intermediate melanomas of 1.5 to 2.49 mm (stage IIA, T3a), and thick intermediate melanomas of 2.5 mm to 3.99 mm (stage IIA, T3b). Thick melanomas invade 4.0 mm and deeper (stage IIB, T4).[31]

It is important to note that *any* suspicious lesion should initially be removed by means of a full-thickness excisional biopsy. This diagnostic excisional biopsy may be close, encompassing as little as a 1 mm margin of normal skin. Sharp dissection into and including a portion of subcutaneous fat will enable accurate histologic (depth and levels) staging. Shave biopsies must always be condemned because depth cannot be assessed.

TREATMENT

Effective treatment of melanoma remains exclusively surgical. Initial complete excision is the therapeutic goal. Thin melanomas can be safely excised with surgical margins of only 1 cm.[32,33] However, the appropriate margins for excision of intermediate-thickness lesions remain a matter of controversy.

The benefit of prophylactic regional node dissections in patients with intermediate-thickness lesions and nonpalpable nodes is also controversial. Prospective, randomized trials and a mathematical model indicate no survival benefit with elective lymph node dissection compared with subsequent so-called therapeutic regional lymphadenectomy only when nodes become palpable.[34,35] Intraoperative lymphatic mapping and selective lymphadenectomy may be warranted in a case-specific approach.[36]

Patients with intermediate-thickness tumors (between 0.76 and 3.99 mm) may benefit if an elective regional lymph node dissection (of nonpalpable nodes) is included in their initial surgical management. Benefit has also been shown with the use of elective regional lymph node dissection for the treatment of thick melanomas (4 mm and greater) and thin intermediate melanomas (between 0.76 mm and 1.49 mm) in men.[37] However, the influence of other important factors, such as previous treatment, age, presence of comorbid disease, and location of the primary lesion, awaits the results of ongoing trials. In addition to providing local control, removal of lymph nodes may find its greatest utility in accurate pathological staging.[38-40] Many aspects of this therapeutic approach remain controversial.[41]

Patients who have N1 or N2 regional node involvement traditionally have an unfavorable outcome but may benefit from isolated limb perfusion or limb infusion. Several investigators have reported increased survival rates in such patients with the use of isolated limb perfusion.[42] Perfusion with tumor necrosis factor–α appears to yield high local response rates, but the associated toxicity is high.[43] Intralesional immunotherapy, local radiation therapy, and systemic chemotherapy are options for the control of recurrent local lesions.[21] Unfortunately, regional disease develops within three years in all patients with thick melanomas (4 mm and greater) and stage IIIA disease, and distant metastases develop within five years in more than 60 percent of these patients.[30,31,37]

Although one might expect that patients with malignancies that have a high incidence of systemic involvement might benefit from adjuvant therapy, none has been proved to be uniformly effective. Allogeneic tumor vaccines (comprising a mixture of different tumor antigens) and other immunostimulation strategies are being studied in clinical trials.[21]

Trials of newer agents for the treatment of stage IV melanoma (involving distant metastases) continue to be disappointing. Studies of interleukin-2 (IL-2) immunotherapy for metastatic disease, both alone and with lymphokine-activated killer cells (LAK cells, or lymphocytes grown in IL-2), continue to show potential rewards. IL-2 appears to have a 10 to 25 percent response rate in metastatic melanoma. Unfortunately, fewer than 50 percent of the responses are complete, and most are of limited duration. IL-2 is currently approved only for the treatment of renal cell cancer. IL-2 and other cytokines in combination with chemotherapeutic agents have generally shown little increase in benefit at the expense of higher toxicity. IL-12, a macrophage-derived cytokine, enhances cellular immunity and may soon enter clinical trials.[21,44,45]

Certain melanoma surface antigens may be common to other tumors and may be recognized in an HLA class I molecule–restricted fashion. Melanoma patients who are HLA-A1 positive (26 percent of all whites) and whose tumors contain *MAGE-1* (a tumor gene found in melanoma and other human tumors) could be immunized against their tumors with cytotoxic T cells sensitized to the melanoma cell surface antigen or against *MAGE-1* alone. Vaccinia recognizance (viral) vectors incorporating this *MAGE-1* gene are already being prepared for clinical trials.[21]

Surgical Technique

EXCISIONAL BIOPSY

The biopsy can often be performed in the clinic operating room under local anesthesia. Care should be taken to avoid injecting the lesion itself because the resulting bleeding may distort the histologic fixation of the specimen. A field block is usually sufficient.

Attention to proper surgical technique will prevent the spread of cancer cells and allow the pathologist sufficient tissue to make an accurate diagnosis. For the histologic diagnosis and staging of all skin lesions, the surgeon should submit at least a full-thickness portion of the lesion and preferably perform an excisional biopsy. When dealing with a larger tumor, it is important to incorporate a representative portion of the lesion with 1 mm of normal skin at the margin so the pathologist can examine the skin adjacent to the neoplasm. Diagnostic biopsies should not be allowed to be damaged by electrocautery. It is important to orient and mark the specimen properly so the adequacy of the margins can be studied in relation to the overall anatomy.

Thus, the initial biopsy should include at least 1 mm of normal skin, and the surgeon should take care to perform a full-thickness excision into the fat. The tissue is gently retracted as the incision is continued around the lesion. Before the lesion is removed from the field, an orientation suture is placed. My preference is to make a small drawing on the pathology sheet, indicating where the suture is located in relation to the site on the body from which the lesion came. For example, a suture is placed at 12 o'clock, a small drawing is made of the patient's hand or face, and the specimen is sketched on the drawing itself. This allows the pathologist to identify and localize any margin that exhibits microscopic involvement with tumor cells. Similarly, excision of a segment of subcutaneous fat allows the pathologist to assess depth of invasion.

SUPERFICIAL AND RADICAL GROIN DISSECTIONS

The inguinal nodes drain the anterior and inferior abdominal wall, perineum, genitalia, hips, buttocks, and thighs. A superficial groin dissection removes the inguinal nodes, whereas a radical dissection additionally incorporates the iliac and obturator nodes. Palpable nodes can be marked on the patient before operation. Photography can be very helpful for both orientation and documentation.

In cases of skin lesions overlying the anteromedial portion of the thigh, the primary excision can often incorporate an incontinuity groin dissection that is designed to eradicate the primary tumor along with the lymphatic drainage system.[46] As a general principle, the skin lesion, subcutaneous fat, lymphatic tissue, and investing fascia are removed as a unit.

Technique

The patient is usually placed in a supine position on the operating table, with the hip slightly abducted and supported by a pillow, the hip and knee slightly flexed. A Foley catheter is inserted, the patient is prepared and draped, and the drapes are stapled in position.

A wide ellipse (4 cm margin) incorporating the skin lesion is marked. The femoral artery is palpated and marked, and a diagonally oriented skin incision is planned. The incision will course from the region of the anterosuperior iliac spine, caudally over the central groin region, through the femoral trigone, and terminate at midthigh level on the anteromedial surface of the thigh. This incision interferes least with the musculocutaneous and cutaneous vascular territories of the skin, usually avoids ischemia to the skin, and promotes subsequent healing. The incision is made with a scalpel, and electrocautery is employed sparingly. The initial incision should include the skin and subcutaneous fat and continue down through the deep investing fascia overlying the muscle. The dissection proceeds downward in a caudal direction, incorporating the fascia and exposing the inguinal ligament, deep fascia, and femoral vessels. Fat and nodal tissue are dissected off the external oblique aponeurosis, spermatic cord,

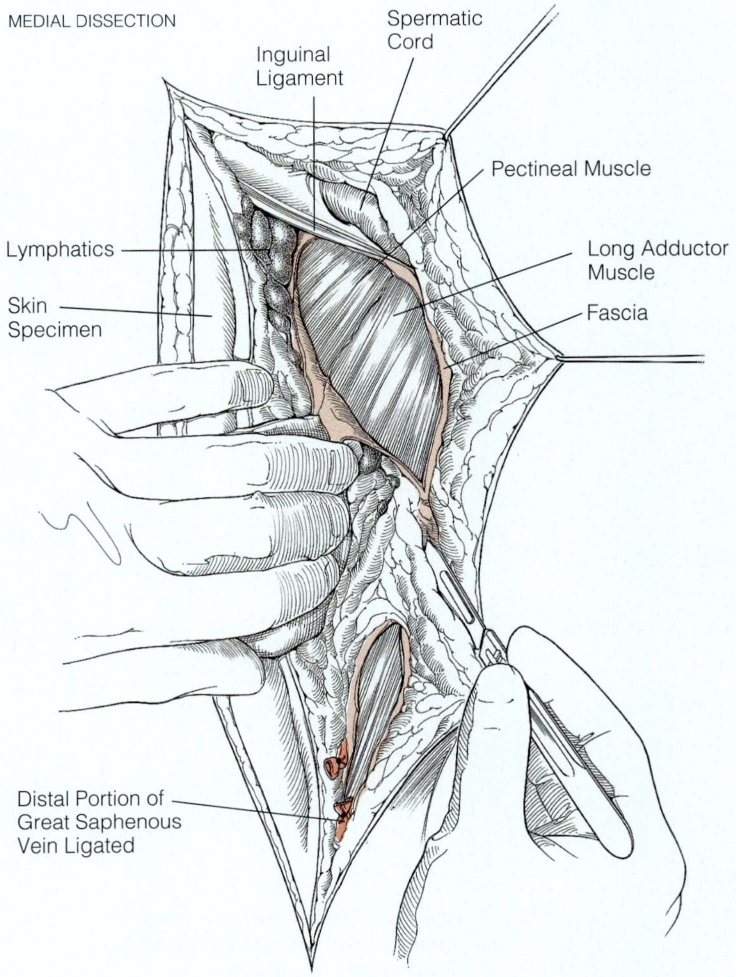

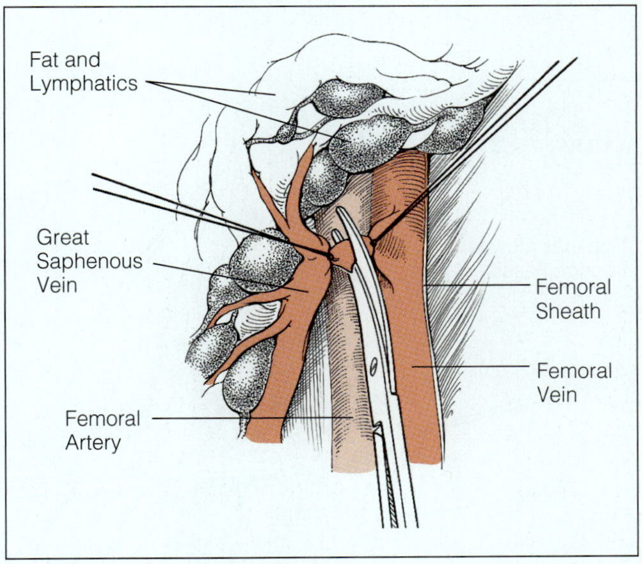

Figure 7 In a superficial groin dissection, the incision is deepened to include the deep muscular fascia. The great saphenous vein is ligated and divided (inset).

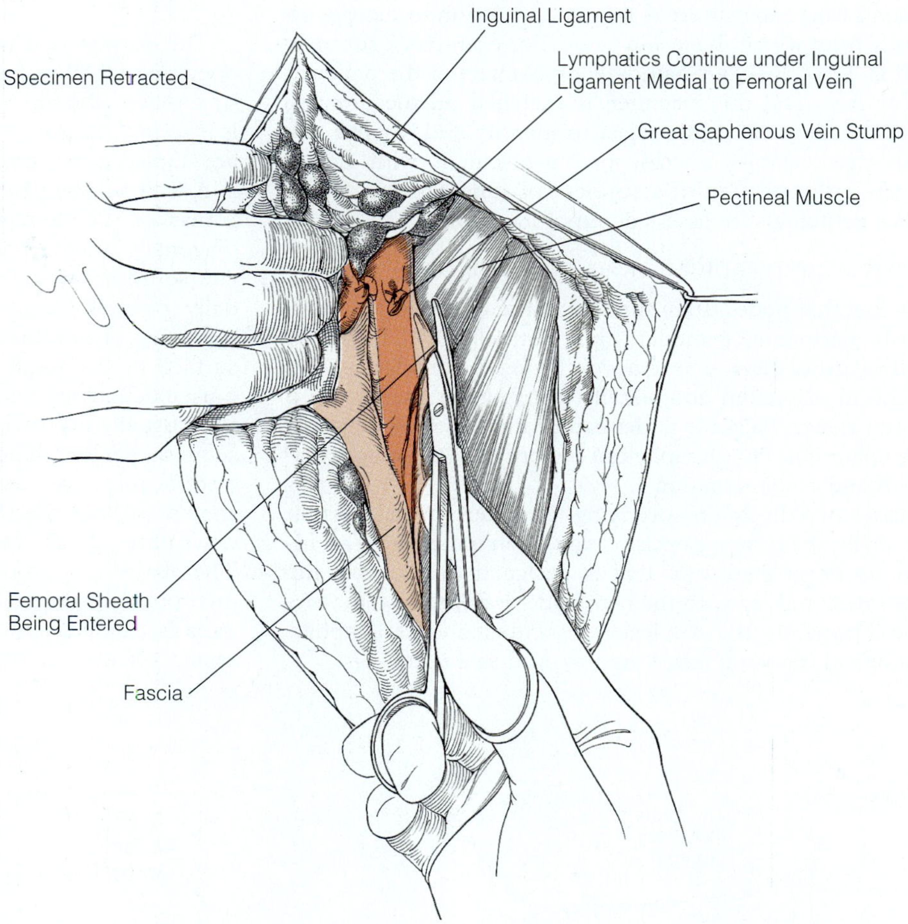

310 — II COMMON PRESENTING PROBLEMS

Figure 8 As the superficial groin dissection proceeds, the investing fascia overlying the femoral nerve and vessels is removed.

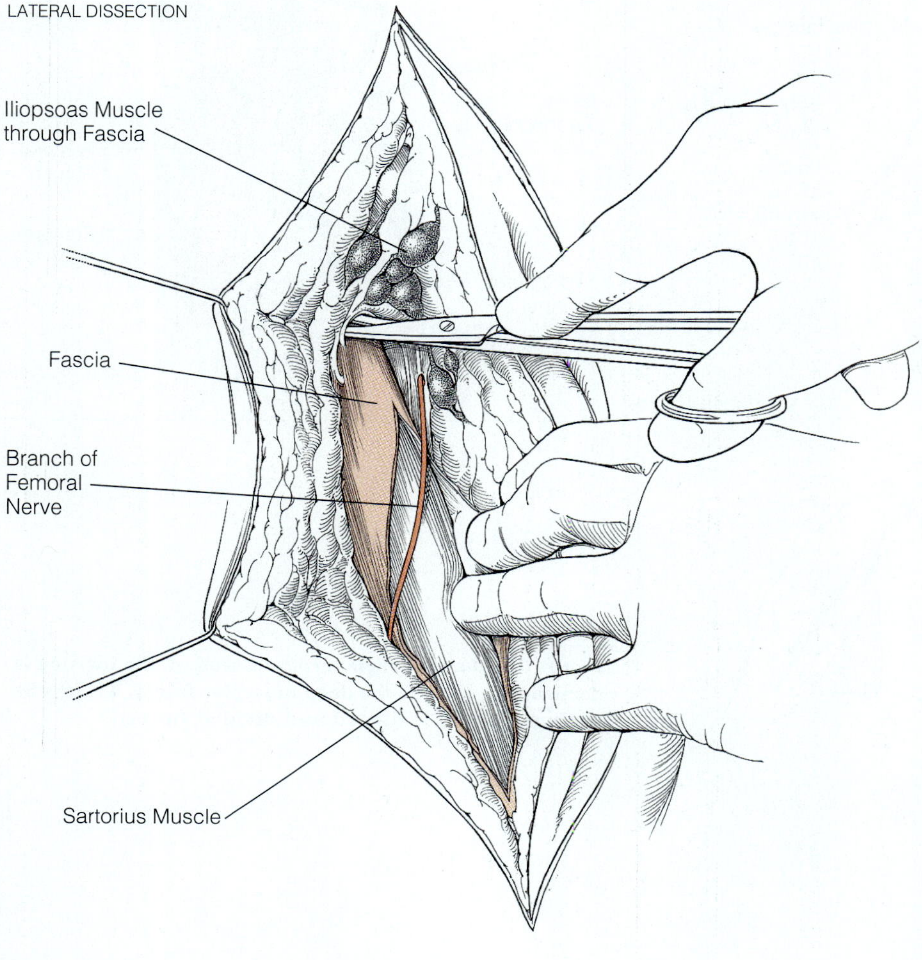

Figure 9 The superficial groin dissection is continued at the same level on the lateral side.

and inguinal ligament [see Figure 7a]. The superficial fascia over the vessels is removed, together with the fat and contents of the femoral trigone, proceeding from lateral to medial. The femoral vessels and femoral nerve are left undisturbed, and the dissection proceeds to the fossa ovalis femoris. The great saphenous vein is incorporated into the specimen, ligated by a suture at its junction with the femoral vein [see Figure 7b]. The fascia is removed from the sartorius muscle, adductor muscle group, and rectus femoris, including all lymphatic tissue in the surgical specimen [see Figures 8 and 9]. The dissection proceeds medially to the medial aspect of the femoral trigone. This completes the superficial portion of the groin dissection.

If the surgeon decides to perform a radical (ilioinguinal) node dissection, the incision is extended through the inguinal ligament, beginning medial to the anterosuperior iliac spine and continuing to a point approximately 2 cm lateral to the femoral artery. The inguinal canal is further exposed by releasing the internal oblique abdominal muscle, transversus abdominus, and the fascia transversalis and dissecting into the retroperitoneal space. The deep circumflex iliac vessels are ligated, and blunt finger dissection separates the peritoneum from the preperitoneal fat and nodes.

Retractors are inserted to widen the retroperitoneal space, and the peritoneum and abdominal viscera are retracted medially. The chain of lymph nodes, areolar tissue, and adventitial tissues along the external iliac vessels is dissected, proceeding proximally to the origins of the internal iliac vessels and incorporating the nodes overlying the obturator foramen by removing the internal obturator fascia. The deep epigastric vessels are usually ligated at their origins from the external iliac artery and vein. The lymph node–bearing specimen is then removed as a unit, oriented, and labeled appropriately with sutures. The inguinal canal is reconstructed to prevent a hernia, and the sartorius muscle is mobilized to the midportion of the wound to cover the femoral vessels. The skin and subcutaneous tissues are then closed in layers over a soft suction drain.

References

1. Cottel WI: Skin tumors: basal cell and squamous cell carcinoma. Selected Readings in Plastic Surgery 7(6):1, 1992
2. Silverberg E, Lubera J: Cancer statistics. CA Cancer J Clin 39:3, 1989
3. Cancer of the Skin. Friedman RJ, Rigel DS, Kopf AW, et al, Eds. WB Saunders Co, Philadelphia, 1991
4. Koh HK, Kligler BE, Lew RA: Sunlight and cutaneous malignant melanoma: evidence for and against causation. Photochem Photobiol 51:765, 1990
5. Green HA, Drake L: Aging, sun damage, and sunscreens. Clin Plast Surg 20:1, 1993
6. Urbach F: Geographic distribution of skin cancer. J Surg Oncol 3:219, 1971
7. Dellon AL: Host-tumor relationship in basal cell and squamous cell cancer of the skin. Plast Reconstr Surg 62:37, 1978
8. Marshall V: Premalignant and malignant skin tumors in immunosuppressed patients. Transplantation 17:272, 1974
9. Wade TR, Ackerman AB: The many faces of basal cell carcinoma. J Dermatol Surg Oncol 4:23, 1978
10. Salasche SJ, Amonette RA: Morpheaform basal cell epitheliomas: a study of subclinical extension in a series of 51 cases. J Dermatol Surg Oncol 7:387, 1981
11. Shanoff LB, Spira M, Hardy SB: Basal cell carcinoma: a statistical approach to rational management. Plast Reconstr Surg 39:619, 1967
12. Bart RS, Kopf AW, Peratos MA: X-ray therapy of skin cancer: evaluation of a "standardized" method for treating basal cell carcinoma. Fifth National Cancer Conference. JB Lippincott, Philadelphia, 1970, p 559
13. Mohs FE: Chemosurgery: microscopically controlled methods of cancer excision. Arch Surg 42:279, 1941
14. Robinson JK: Mohs micrographic surgery. Clin Plast Surg 20:149, 1993
15. Brownstein MH, Rabinowitz AD: The precursors of cutaneous squamous cell carcinoma. Int J Dermatol 18:1, 1979
16. Albricht SM: Treatment of malignant cutaneous tumors. Clin Plast Surg 20:167, 1993
17. Kohn H, Baumal R, From L: Role of immunohistochemistry in the diagnosis of undifferentiated tumors involving the skin. J Am Acad Dermatol 14:1063, 1986
18. Bostwick J, Pendergrast J, Vasconez L: Marjolin's ulcer: an immunologically privileged tumor? Plast Reconstr Surg 57:66, 1976
19. Traves N, Pack GT: The development of cancer in burn scars: analysis and report of 34 cases. Surg Gynecol Obstet 51:749, 1930
20. Ames FC, Hickey RC: Mestastasis from squamous cell skin cancer of the extremities. South Med J 75:920, 1982
21. Vetto J: Advances in the Therapy of Malignant Melanoma (monograph). Department of Surgery, Oregon Health Sciences University, Portland, Oregon, 1994
22. Morton DL, Dartyan DG, Wanek LA, et al: Multivariate analysis of the relationship between survival and the microstage of primary melanoma by Clark level and Breslow thickness. Cancer 71:3737, 1993
23. Koh HK: Cutaneous melanoma. N Engl J Med 325:171, 1991
24. Armstrong BK: Epidemiology of malignant melanoma: intermittent or total accumulated exposure to the sun. J Dermatol Surg Oncol 14:835, 1988
25. Lew RA, Saber AJ, Cook N, et al: Sun exposure habits in patients with cutaneous melanoma: a case control study. J Dermatol Surg Oncol 9:981, 1983
26. Evans GR, Manson PN: Review and current perspectives of cutaneous malignant melanoma. J Am Coll Surg 178:523, 1994
27. Anderson RG: Skin tumors II: melanoma. Selected Readings in Plastic Surgery 7(7):1, 1992
28. Mihm MC, Clark WH, From L: The clinical diagnosis, classification, and histogenic concepts of the early stages of cutaneous melanoma. N Engl J Med 284:1078, 1971
29. Friedman RJ, Rigel DS, Silverman MK, et al: Malignant melanoma in the 1990's: the continued importance of early detection and the role of physician examinations and self-examination of the skin. CA Cancer J Clin 41:201, 1991
30. Clark WH, From L, Bernardino EA, et al: The histogenesis and biologic behavior of primary human malignant melanomas of the skin. Cancer Res 29:705, 1969
31. Breslow A: Thickness, cross-sectional areas and depth of invasion in the prognosis of cutaneous melanoma. Ann Surg 172:902, 1970
32. Balch CM, Murad TM, Soong S, et al: Tumor thickness as a guide to surgical management of clinical stage I melanoma patients. Cancer 43:883, 1979
33. Veronisi U, Cascinelli N, Adamus J, et al: Thin stage I primary cutaneous malignant melanoma: comparison of excision with margins of 1 or 3 cm. N Engl J Med 318:1159, 1988
34. Sim FH, Taylor WF, Prichard DC, et al: Lymphadenectomy in the management of stage I malignant melanoma: a prospective randomized study. Mayo Clin Proc 61:697, 1986
35. Veronesi U, Adamus J, Bandiera DC, et al: Delayed regional lymph node dissection in stage I melanoma of the skin and lower extremities. Cancer 49:2420, 1982
36. Morton DL, Wen DR, Wong JH, et al: Technical details of intraoperative lymphatic mapping for early stage melanoma. Arch Surg 127:392, 1992
37. Balch CM, Soong SJ, Milton GW, et al: A comparison of prognostic factors and surgical results in 1,786 patients with localized (stage I) melanoma treated in Alabama, USA, and New South Wales, Australia. Ann Surg 196:677, 1982
38. Crowley NJ: The case against elective lymphadenectomy. Surg Oncol Clin North Am 1:223, 1992
39. Coates AS, Ingvar CI, Petersen-Schaefer K, et al: Elective lymph node dissection in patients with primary melanoma of the trunk and limbs treated at the

Sydney melanoma unit from 1960 to 1991. J Am Coll Surg 180:402, 1995
40. Krag DN, Meijer SJ, Weaver DL, et al: Minimal-access surgery for staging of malignant melanoma. Arch Surg 130:654, 1995
41. Vetto J: Elective lymph node dissection for intermediate thickness melanoma: does it have a future? Clin Oncol Alert 11:6, 1996
42. Hartley JW, Fletcher WS: Improved survival of patients with stage II melanoma of the extremity using hyperthermic isolation perfusion with 1-phenylalanine mustard. J Surg Oncol 36:170, 1987
43. Lienard D, Lejeune FJ, Ewalenko P: In transit metastases of malignant melanoma treated by high dose rTNF-α in combination with interferon-gamma and melphalan isolation perfusion. World J Surg 16:234, 1992
44. Rosenberg SA, Lotze MT, Yang JC, et al: Prospective trial of high-dose interleukin-2 alone or in conjunction with lymphokine-activated killer cells for the treatment of patients with advanced cancer. J Natl Cancer Inst 85:622, 1993
45. Nastala CL, Edington HD, Storkus WJ, et al: Recombinant interleukin-12 (r-mil-12) mediates regression of both subcutaneous and metastatic murine tumors. Surg Forum 44:518, 1993
46. Karakousis CP: Technique of lymphadenectomy for melanoma. Surg Oncol Clin North Am 1:157, 1992

Acknowledgments

Figures 7 through 9   Susan E. Brust, C.M.I.

The author is grateful to John Vetto, M.D., and Paul Manson, M.D., for their suggestions in the preparation of this chapter.

21 SOFT TISSUE INFECTION

Ronald T. Lewis, M.B.B.S., M.Sc.

Approach to the Patient with Soft Tissue Infection

The key to successful treatment of soft tissue infection is early recognition of infections that require prompt surgical drainage and debridement. It is convenient to classify lesions into those that are focal, such as cutaneous abscesses and pyoderma gangrenosum, and those that are diffuse and often require emergency treatment, such as cellulitis and necrotizing cellulitic infections. (There are also certain miscellaneous conditions, such as bite wound infections and purpura fulminans, that do not fit neatly into either category; these conditions are considered separately.) Many lesions appear deceptively innocent at first and are mistaken for nonspecific inflammation. To prompt recognition and effective treatment of any lesion, the answers to five questions should be sought:

1. Is infection present?
2. Is there an underlying systemic condition present that favors infection?
3. Should antibiotics be given?
4. Which antibiotics are most appropriate?
5. Is surgical treatment required?

Focal Inflammation

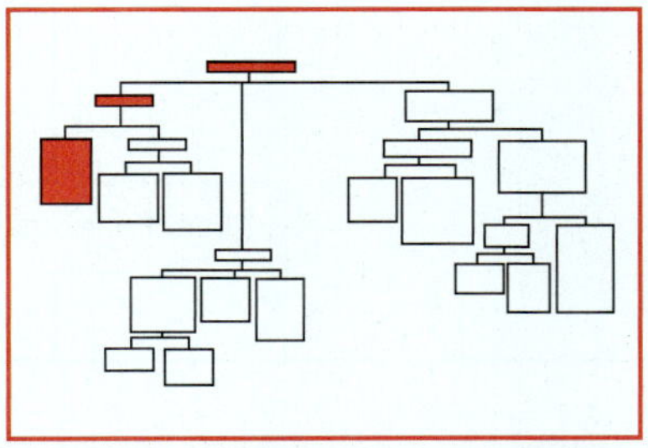

The history together with the clinical appearance of a focal lesion will indicate whether it is a minor, confined cutaneous abscess or a more serious, spreading focal lesion such as pyoderma gangrenosum. Cutaneous abscesses are very common and are readily recognized. Pyoderma gangrenosum, on the other hand, is a rare condition.

CONFINED CUTANEOUS ABSCESS

A cutaneous abscess is a walled-off collection of pus that presents as a painful fluctuant mass, usually with surrounding erythema and firm granulation tissue. It is treated by incision and drainage. Gram stain and culture of the pus are not done routinely, because antibiotics are not generally given. Antibiotics may be helpful, however, in immunocompromised patients and in patients with abscesses of the central area of the face. In such cases, the findings on Gram stain suggest appropriate antibiotic therapy. Gram-positive cocci in clusters indicate *Staphylococcus aureus*, which may be treated with an oral semisynthetic penicillin (e.g., cloxacillin, 0.5 to 1.0 g every 6 hours for 5 to 7 days). Mixed gram-positive and gram-negative bacilli represent an infection by aerobic and anaerobic organisms that can be treated with an oral cephalosporin (e.g., cephalexin, 0.5 g every 6 hours for 5 to 7 days). Occasionally, white blood cells but no organisms are seen. This finding confirms a sterile abscess, for which antibiotics are not needed.

SPREADING FOCAL LESION

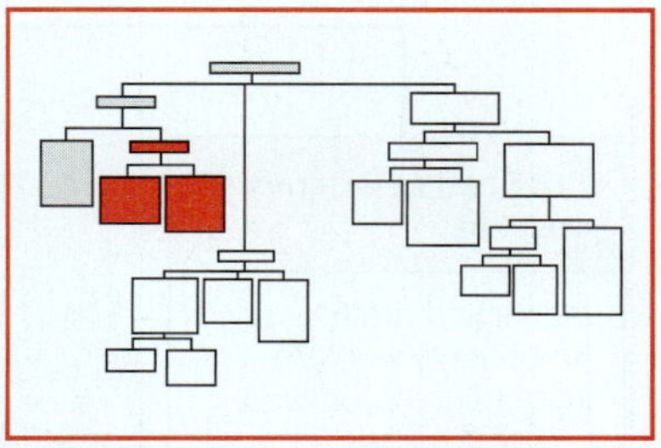

Classic Pyoderma Gangrenosum

Classic pyoderma gangrenosum is characterized by a painful, raised pustular lesion that progresses to spreading ulceration with a typical necrotic center, bluish undermined edges, and surrounding erythema [see Figure 1].[1] It occurs either singly or in groups, most often on the legs. The lesions may localize at sites of minor trauma (so-called pathergy). Fever, malaise, myalgias, and arthralgias are common. A biopsy is usually performed to rule out disorders that produce similar lesions: ischemic ulceration, vasculitis of periarteritis nodosa, and chronic bacterial, mycobacterial, or fungal disorders. Massive neutrophil infiltration and necrosis of the epidermis are typical. In contrast with vasculitis, only minor vessel wall infiltration is present with pyoderma gangrenosum. Underlying disease, often parainflammatory or hemoproliferative, is present in 60% to 80% of cases.[2] The most common concomitant conditions are inflammatory bowel disease (especially ulcerative colitis),[1] polyarthritis,[3] monoclonal gammopathy,[4] and malignant hematologic neoplasms (especially leukemia).[5] Four variants have been identified: peristomal (seen, for example, in Crohn disease); vulvar or penoscrotal, simulating the lesions of Behçet disease; oral (peristomatitis vegetans); and bullous. The skin le-

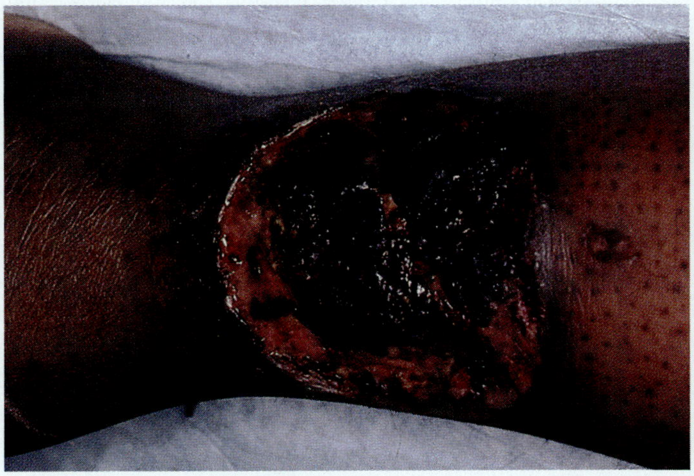

Figure 1 In this photograph of an advanced pyoderma gangrenosum lesion, the darker area surrounding the necrotic center corresponds to the violaceous zone of intense erythema.

```
Patient has soft tissue infection
```

Focal inflammation

Confined cutaneous abscess
Incise and drain. (In patients who are immunocompromised or who have an abscess of the central area of the face, identify the pathogen and administer antibiotics.)

Spreading focal lesion

Postoperative progressive bacterial gangrene
Identify the pathogen. Give I.V. penicillin (or cloxacillin) and gentamicin. Perform wide excision. Consider nutritional Rx.

Classic pyoderma gangrenosum
Identify and treat underlying disease. Obtain Gram stain and culture of biopsy specimen. Give sulfasalazine, clofazimine, or glucocorticoids and cyclosporin.

Miscellaneous infections

Animal bites and scratches
All bites:
- Give tetanus prophylaxis.
- Irrigate and debride.
- Suture dog bites; *do not close other bites primarily.*
- Begin antibiotics.
- Consider rabies prophylaxis.

Early infection
Give oral amoxicillin-clavulanate.

Late infection
Give broad-spectrum I.V. antibiotics (e.g., ticarcillin-clavulanate). Elevate and soak affected part; debride.

Human bites
Give tetanus prophylaxis. Irrigate and debride. Give broad-spectrum antibiotics. Do not close primarily.

Purpura fulminans
Resuscitate. Give I.V. antibiotics, I.V. heparin, protein C concentrates, and standard coagulation support. Survivors may require debridement, topical silver sulfadiazine, and grafting.

Diffuse inflammation

Recognize necrotizing infection that requires operation, on the basis of clinical signs and ancillary tests.

Nonoperative cellulitis

Identification of pathogen may be helpful.

Cellulitis caused by streptococci or *Staphylococcus aureus*

Give oral or I.V. antibiotics (e.g., cloxacillin). Provide rest, heat, and elevation.

Cellulitis from other causes

Gram-negative cellulitis: Give I.V. or oral cephalosporins or ciprofloxacin.

High-risk cellulitis:
Facial—give I.V. cloxacillin or cefuroxime.
Postadenectomy/postvenectomy—give I.V. cloxacillin.
Bites—see "Miscellaneous Infections" (left).

Necrotizing infection requiring operation

Review Gram stain and culture; study biopsy and frozen section.
(Clinical indications include edema beyond erythema, crepitus, skin vesicles, cutaneous anesthesia or focal gangrene, shock, abnormal coagulation, and elevated creatine kinase and lactic dehydrogenase.)

No inflammatory response

Infection is clostridial.

Nontoxic cellulitis

Debride and drain wound; inspect muscle. Give I.V. penicillin.

Toxic myonecrosis

Resuscitate. Perform radical debridement. Give I.V. penicillin. Consider hyperbaric oxygen.

Inflammation is present

Infection is nonclostridial.
- Treat hypovolemia with rapid resuscitation; correct electrolyte abnormalities.
- Give broad-spectrum combination therapy (penicillin plus gentamicin plus clindamycin or ciprofloxacin plus metronidazole) or monotherapy (imipenem-cilastatin or ticarcillin-clavulante).
- Debride extensively.

Approach to the Patient with Soft Tissue Infection

sion seen in leukemia is typically the bullous variant: it remains superficial and exhibits more subdued colors than the classic lesion. About 30% of cases are idiopathic and remain so on follow-up of more than 2 years.[6]

Investigations should include Gram stain and culture of a biopsy specimen. Pyogenic organisms commonly grow from swabs of the central ulcer, but it is unlikely that these organisms are significant. Studies that should be performed to rule out underlying diseases include a complete blood count; blood chemistry studies; and immunologic tests, including assays for antinuclear antibody, rheumatoid factor, and serum protein as well as immunoglobulin electrophoresis. A chest x-ray, upper gastrointestinal series, and barium enema should also be done.

Treatment is controversial but should always include *specific therapy for the underlying disorder*. Thus, in patients with inflammatory bowel disease, colon resection may produce lasting remission of the skin lesions,[2] and in some patients with leukemia, pyoderma gangrenosum has improved or cleared completely after chemotherapy.[5]

Various antimicrobials have been used with success. They include sulfasalazine (4 g/day) and the antimycobacterial agent clofazimine (300 mg/day), as well as minocycline and rifampin. These agents, particularly sulfasalazine and clofazimine, may act not as antibiotics but by enhancing neutrophil phagocytosis and intracellular bacterial killing and by stimulating macrophage activity. Prednisone, 40 to 120 mg/day, and cyclosporin A, 5 mg/day, produce long-term remission in almost half of cases; however, 3 to 6 months of glucocorticoid treatment may be required before lesions heal, and fatal complications have been reported after such treatment.[3] Current theories suggest that the lesions of pyoderma gangrenosum may be caused by serum immune complexes or by defects in cellular or humoral immunity. Overexpression of interleukin-8 (IL-8) has been identified in subepidermal neutrophils. Cyclosporin A acts on T cells to limit production of interleukins, thereby reversing the ratio of T helper to T suppressor cells.[7] Resistant cases may respond to oral tacrolimus, 0.1 to 0.3 mg/kg/day, and topical tacrolimus, 0.1% in paraffin or beeswax.[8] This new immunosuppressive drug inhibits T-cell activation by blocking receptor-mediated signal transduction pathways. Intravenous immunoglobulin therapy may be helpful in cases of resistant disease.[9] Immunosuppressive therapy with azathioprine, cyclophosphamide, or dapsone is less effective[10] but is useful for maintenance purposes in patients with inflammatory bowel disease.

Topical measures include wet-to-dry dressings and intralesional injection or surface application of antibacterials and immune agents. Saline compresses provide some debridement. Aggressive debridement and skin grafting have been condemned,[2] but some workers[11] have reported dramatic improvement with surgical debridement. Heng has observed abundant formation of granulation tissue and arrest of extension of ulceration by a simplified topical application of hyperbaric oxygen (HBO).[12]

Superficial Atypical Mycobacterial Lesions

In cases of nonhealing extremity ulcers unresponsive to conventional surgical and antibiotic treatment, the possibility of an atypical

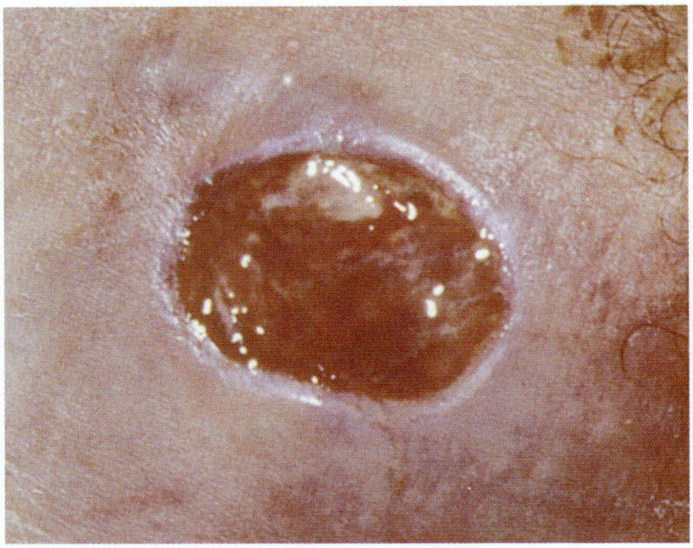

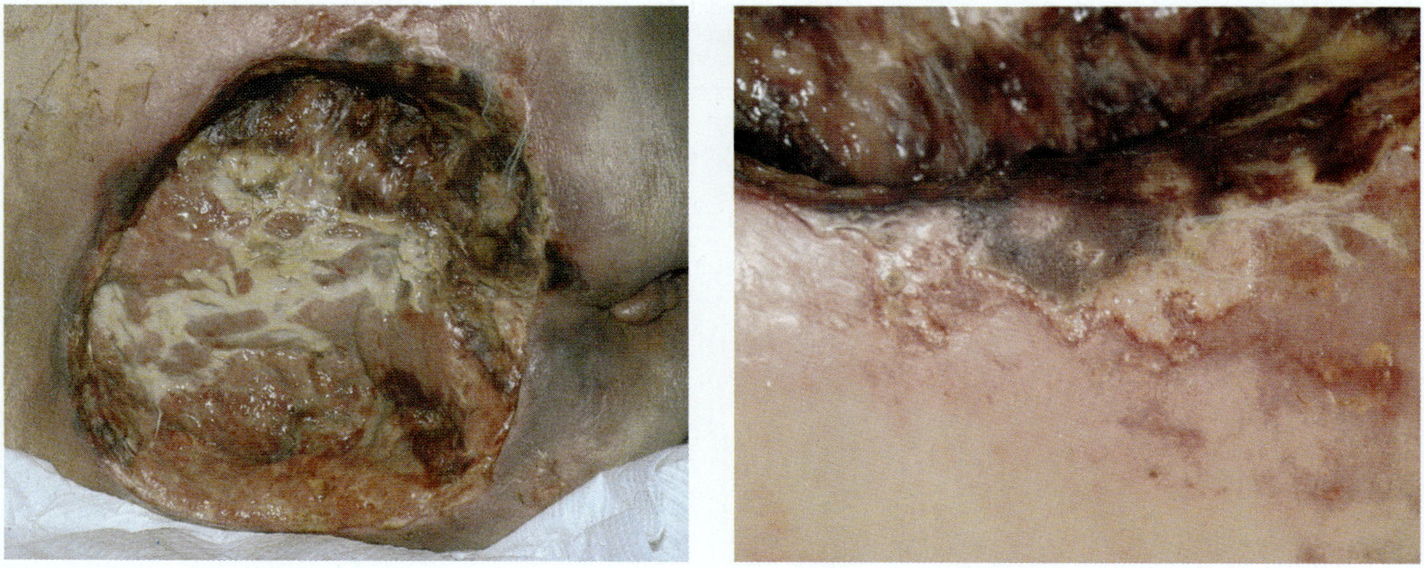

Figure 2 This chronic ulcer of the lateral malleolus shows the violaceous discoloration, rolled edges, nongranulating base, and watery discharge characteristic of an atypical mycobacterial lesion.

Figure 3 Progressive bacterial gangrene has developed in the decubitus ulcer shown at left. The edge of the necrotic lesion shows the three characteristic zones of necrosis, discoloration, and erythema (right).

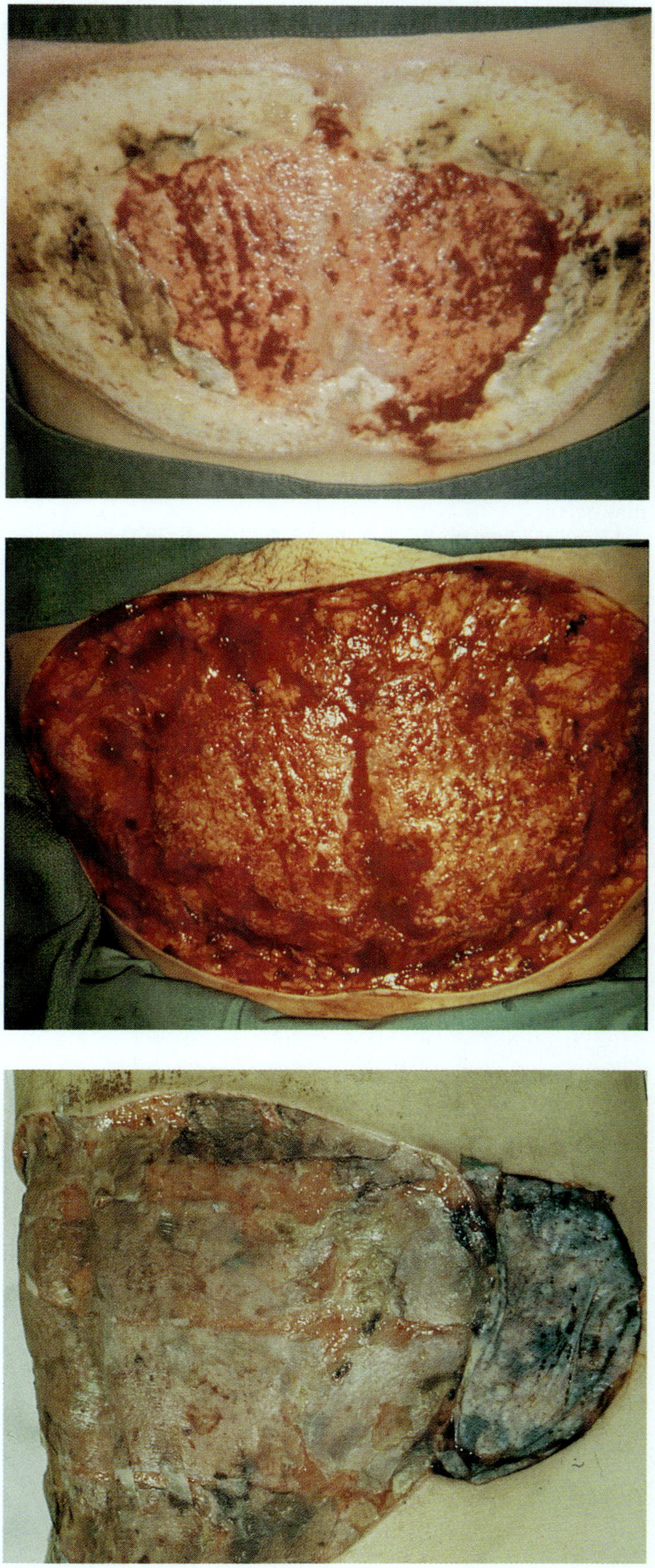

mycobacterial infection should be considered. Although rare, indolent mycobacterial lesions that closely resemble pyoderma gangrenosum have been observed. In one study, infected ulcers in four steroid-dependent patients yielded atypical mycobacteria upon culture of the excised tissue. Two ulcers contained *Mycobacterium smegmatis*, which rarely causes disease in humans; the third, *M. kansasii;* and the fourth, *M. chelonei*.[13] The lesions presented as chronic ulcerations with violaceous edges, rolled margins, a nongranulating base, and watery discharge [see Figure 2]. In three of the four patients, wide local excision and intravenous antibiotic therapy followed by oral antibiotic therapy were required for successful treatment. One patient was treated successfully with debridement and oral antibiotic therapy.

Because experience in treating these ulcers has been limited, the best antibiotic therapy is uncertain. *M. kansasii* is usually sensitive to rifampin, isoniazid, and ethambutol; and *M. chelonei* is sensitive to amikacin, cefoxitin, tetracycline, and erythromycin. All three species respond well to cefoxitin (1 g every 6 hours) or to quinolones (e.g., ciprofloxacin, 0.4 g every 12 hours); accordingly, these agents should be prescribed.

Postoperative Progressive Bacterial Gangrene

The postoperative progressive bacterial gangrene of Meleney[14] is considered to be a variant of classic pyoderma gangrenosum.[11] The lesion appears 2 weeks or more after accidental trauma or after operative management of purulent peritoneal or pleural infection; it is characterized by wound edema, redness, and tenderness that progress to the three characteristic zones of pyoderma gangrenosum: a necrotic center, bluish undermined edges, and surrounding erythema [see Figure 3]. Fever, muscle wasting, and toxicity are often present. A swab taken from the central necrotic area usually yields hemolytic *S. aureus* on culture; later in the course of the illness, it may show gram-negative bacilli. Needle aspirate from the outer zone may grow microaerophilic nonhemolytic streptococci.

Broad-spectrum parenteral antibiotics should be started promptly and are useful in reducing systemic toxicity. Penicillin, 1 to 2 million units I.V. every 6 hours, along with gentamicin, 1.5 mg/kg every 8 hours, may be given, but if *S. aureus* is found on Gram stain, cloxacillin, 1 to 2 g every 6 hours, is substituted for penicillin. Antibiotic therapy is followed by wide excision of the skin lesion [see Figure 4]. The wound is left open to granulate, and skin grafts are applied later. Researchers found that HBO reduced the extent of excision required,[15,16] but the value of HBO therapy is controversial in this and other necrotizing soft tissue infections [see Diffuse Inflammation, Inflammatory Response Is Absent (Clostridial Infection), *below*]. Because these patients have marked systemic manifestations and significant muscle wasting, supportive nutritional therapy may be of benefit [see 97 Nutritional Support].

Diffuse Inflammation

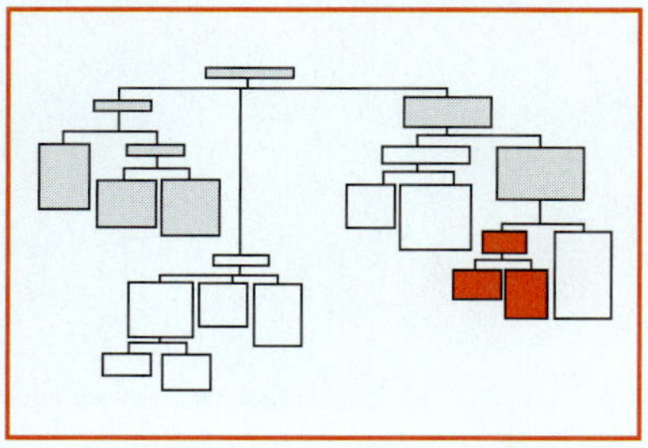

NECROTIZING INFECTION REQUIRING OPERATION

In managing diffuse inflammatory lesions, it is crucial to recognize necrotizing infections promptly because they require surgical debridement. To spot a necrotizing infection, one must know the clinical setting in which it often occurs and must identify cer-

Figure 4 Progressive bacterial gangrene developed in this patient's abdominal wall after cesarean section. In photograph at top, the lesion has been partially excised; extension of necrosis is evident. The lesion was widely excised (center). Extension of necrosis into the flank necessitated further excision and skin grafting (bottom); skin grafts done earlier on the central lesion are healing.

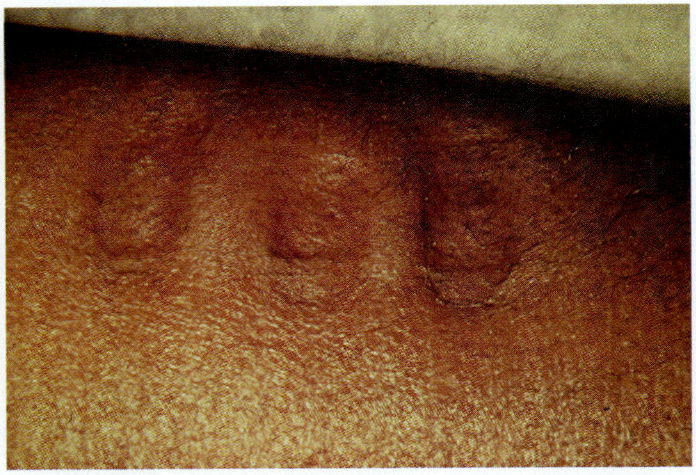

318 — II COMMON PRESENTING PROBLEMS

Figure 5 Edema extending beyond the area of erythema is a marker of necrotizing soft tissue infection.

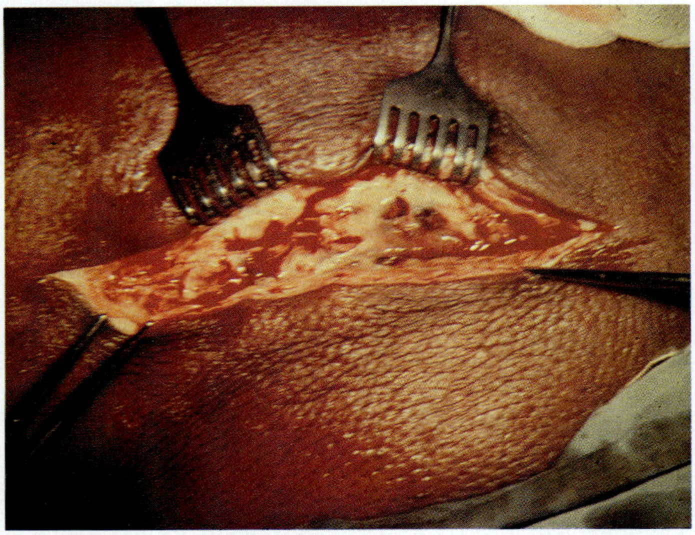

Figure 6 In this patient with necrotizing fasciitis, edema is present without skin vesicles, and there is necrosis of the deep layer of the superficial fascia.

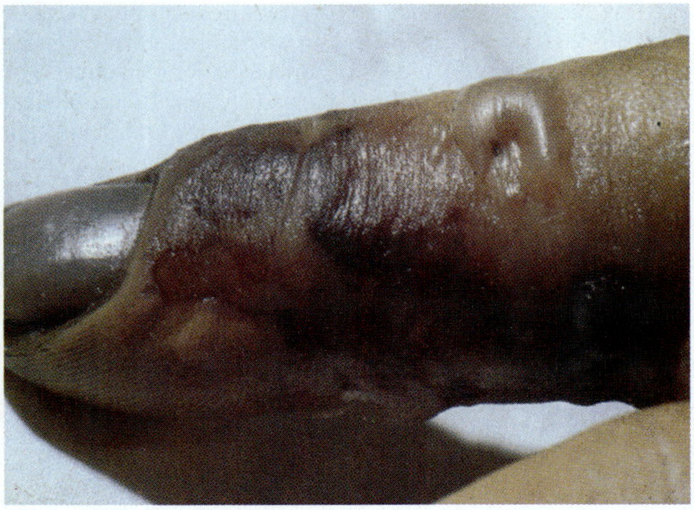

Figure 7 Skin vesicles such as those on this patient's finger are seen early in streptococcal gangrene.

tain clinical clues. In some cases, ancillary studies may help finalize the diagnosis. Necrotizing infections usually occur in patients with impaired host defense mechanisms, such as the elderly, those receiving immunosuppressive therapy, or those with an underlying systemic illness, such as cancer, chronic renal failure, chronic alcoholism, diabetes mellitus, or peripheral vascular disease. When cellulitis occurs in these patients, a necrotizing infection should be suspected. The initiating factor for necrotizing infections is often surprisingly minor, perhaps because of the poor host resistance. For example, necrotizing infections can occur in areas of blunt soft tissue contusion associated with a distant focus of infection.[17]

Important early clinical markers of necrotizing soft tissue infection include edema beyond the area of erythema, crepitus, and skin vesicles [see Figures 5 through 7]. The lymphangitis and lymphadenitis commonly seen in patients with nonoperative cellulitis are absent. In later stages of infection, cutaneous anesthesia, focal skin gangrene, shock, and impaired blood coagulation may occur.

Useful ancillary studies include soft tissue x-rays and blood chemistry studies. X-ray examination of the affected area may disclose soft tissue gas in patients in whom crepitus is not present on palpation [see Figure 8].[18] In addition, elevated blood levels of the muscle proteins creatine kinase and lactate dehydrogenase may suggest skeletal muscle breakdown.[19] Isoenzyme analysis may confirm the origin of these elevated enzymes.

Even in the initial absence of such clinical markers, a necrotizing infection should be suspected when cellulitis is refractory to appropriate antibiotic treatment. This is a signal to explore the wound.[20-23] On exploration, the diagnosis is almost always confirmed by the presence of gray necrotic fascia with little free pus and by easy dissection and undermining of the wound. Thrombosed blood vessels may also be seen. Incisional biopsies and frozen sections are favored for rapid diagnosis of necrotizing fasciitis.[24] The histologic criteria for diagnosis are the following:

1. Necrosis of the superficial fascia.
2. Infiltration of the dermis and of the fascia by polymorphic neutrophils.
3. Thrombosis of subcutaneous arteries and veins.
4. Angiitis and fibrinoid necrosis of arterial and venous walls.
5. Presence of microorganisms in the fascia and dermis on Gram stain.
6. Absence of muscle involvement.

In practice, the diagnosis of necrotizing infection is usually confirmed by the gross findings on surgical exploration. Histologic studies are not required for the initial diagnosis, although they are helpful in defining the cause of the infection [see Inflammatory Response Is Absent (Clostridial Infection), *below*].

Serial measurements of muscle compartment pressure have been used to confirm the need for operation.[19] Normal recumbent muscle compartment pressures are 0 to 8 mm Hg; pressures above 30 mm Hg are abnormal.[25]

Inflammatory Response Is Absent (Clostridial Infection)

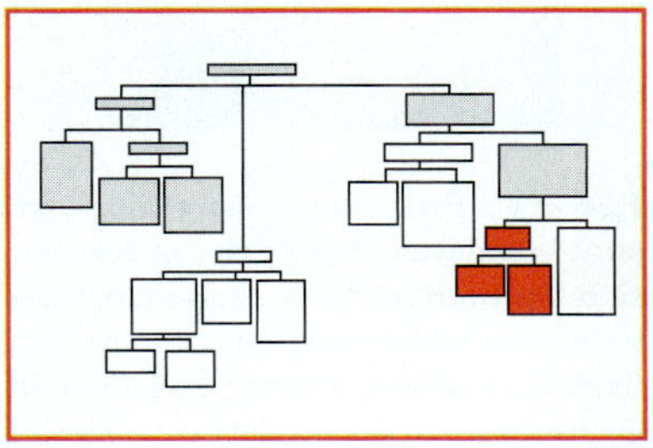

On Gram stain or frozen section, histotoxic clostridial infection yields gram-positive rods without white blood cells [see Figure 9], whereas nonclostridial soft

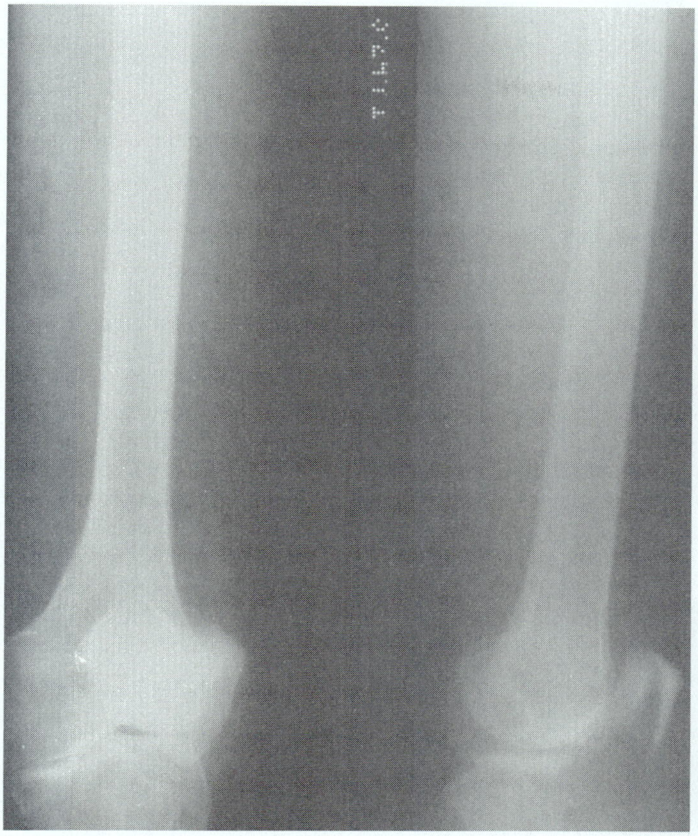

Figure 8 In some patients with necrotizing soft tissue infection, air may be seen in the soft tissues on x-ray even in the absence of crepitus.

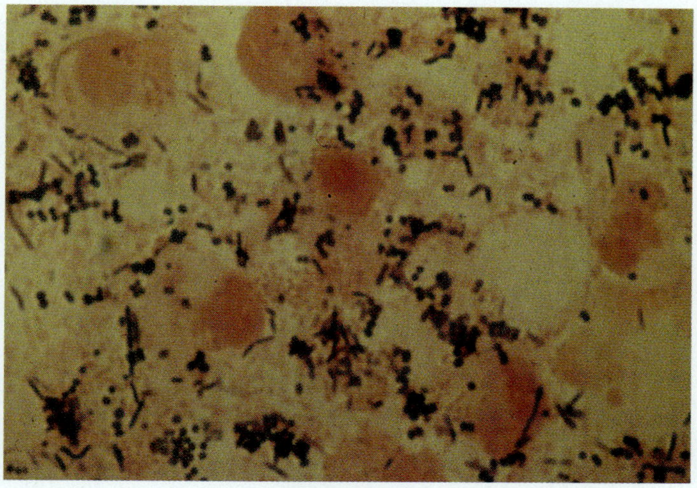

Figure 10 In necrotizing fasciitis, an inflammatory response is present.

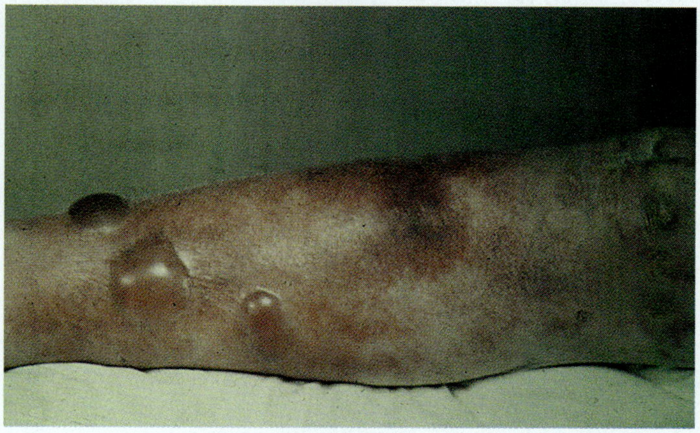

Figure 11 Bronzing of the skin occurs early in gas gangrene. Skin vesicles, as seen on this patient with advanced gas gangrene, occur later.

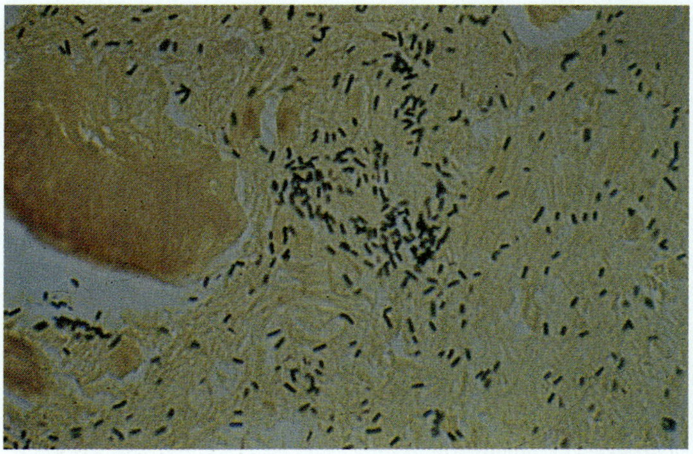

Figure 9 In clostridial myonecrosis, there is no inflammatory response.

tissue infection is associated with a significant number of white blood cells in the wound [see Figure 10].[26] Clostridial infection may present as a nontoxic cellulitis or toxic myonecrosis. Clostridial cellulitis develops 3 to 5 days after a wound is sustained. It is characterized by pain, a foul-smelling seropurulent discharge, skin vesicles that are small and flat, and limited systemic toxicity. Although pain may be severe, it does not compare to that experienced by patients with clostridial myonecrosis. Crepitus may be present. Effective treatment includes debridement and drainage of the wound and inspection of muscle to ensure that it is intact. Intravenous penicillin (6 to 12 million U/day for 7 to 10 days) decreases toxemia and limits the spread of infection.

Clostridial myonecrosis, also known as gas gangrene, occurs most commonly in the extremities of injured young men, in the abdominal wall of older men, and in the extremities of elderly patients with diabetes and peripheral arterial occlusive disease. The hallmarks of this infection are severe wound pain, marked swelling, and systemic toxicity. Hemolysis and coagulopathies are common. There may be a watery wound discharge with a musty odor, and a bronzing of the skin may occur. Skin vesicles, cutaneous gangrene, and crepitus, which may occur early in clostridial cellulitis, are late signs in myonecrosis [see Figure 11]. Resuscitation with I.V. fluids is required [see 4 Shock], and administration of I.V. penicillin (12 million U/day) is helpful, but radical surgical debridement is the mainstay of treatment.

The use of HBO in clostridial myonecrosis remains controversial; it inhibits production of exotoxins but does not neutralize those already present. However, edema is reduced, progression of necrosis may be halted,[27] and tissue may be spared.[28,29] It has been suggested that mortality may be decreased by HBO,[28,30] but no comparative controlled studies exist. HBO may be a useful adjunct, but it is not a substitute for surgical treatment and must not be allowed to delay surgical debridement.

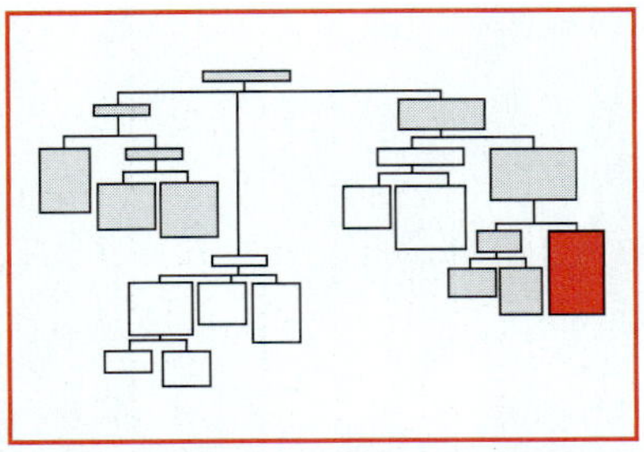

Inflammatory Response Is Present (Nonclostridial Infection)

The nonclostridial diffuse necrotizing soft tissue infections seen most often are hemolytic streptococcal gangrene [see Figure 7], necrotizing fasciitis with or without streptococcal toxic-shock syndrome (TSS), gram-negative synergistic necrotizing cellulitis, and idiopathic scrotal gangrene. Much confusion has arisen from reports that merge these syndromes under the single name of necrotizing fasciitis; in fact, they are multiple entities requiring a common initial approach.[26] The specific final diagnosis can be made only in retrospect. Although this diagnosis is valuable for fine-tuning therapy, it is not required for effective empirical initial treatment. Factors that increase mortality include delay in making the diagnosis, immunocompromise, shock and organ failure, a polymicrobial flora, and disease of the trunk rather than of the extremities. The principles of treatment are rapid resuscitation of the hypovolemia and correction of the electrolyte abnormalities [see 4 Shock and 6 Life-Threatening Electrolyte Abnormalities], administration of broad-spectrum antibiotics, extensive surgical debridement of all necrotic tissue, and supportive care.

Broad-spectrum antibiotics are usually given initially to cover the variety of organisms that may cause similar syndromes. Combination therapy may be used, such as penicillin (6 to 12 million U/day) with gentamicin (1.5 mg/kg every 8 hours) and clindamycin (600 mg every 6 hours) or ciprofloxacin (400 mg every 12 hours) with metronidazole (500 mg every 8 hours). Alternatively, monotherapy that is effective against gram-negative bacilli, streptococci, and anaerobes may be given, such as imipenem-cilastatin (0.5 to 1.0 g I.V. every 6 hours) or ticarcillin-clavulanate (3.1 g I.V. every 6 hours). Later, when pathogens are identified in blood or tissue, antibiotic therapy should be tailored to the organisms identified.

The initial surgical debridement of the wound should be aggressive. The wound should be incised, and the necrotic tissue should be excised. Wherever possible, however, viable skin should be preserved, and skin incisions should be placed so as to minimize devascularization. The deep fascia should be incised to allow inspection of the muscle. Finally, the wound should be packed open. Further debridement of the wound is the rule and should be performed 24 to 48 hours after the initial debridement. The extent of further debridement depends on the findings during operation and on the evolving clinical syndrome.

Adjunctive fasciotomy has been recommended.[19] Temporary dressings with amniotic membrane[31] or porcine xenografts[32] may be helpful in minimizing colonization of debrided wounds and may promote the growth of granulation tissue, allowing early initiation of split-thickness skin grafts. In immunocompromised patients with perineal gangrene, a diverting colostomy[33] established early in treatment minimizes further contamination of the wound.

Supportive care includes nutritional therapy[21,34] [see 97 Nutritional Support] and the use of low-dose subcutaneous heparin in order to reduce the risk of venous thrombosis.[35] HBO is the approach favored by some researchers[19,36] but not by others.[21,37,38]

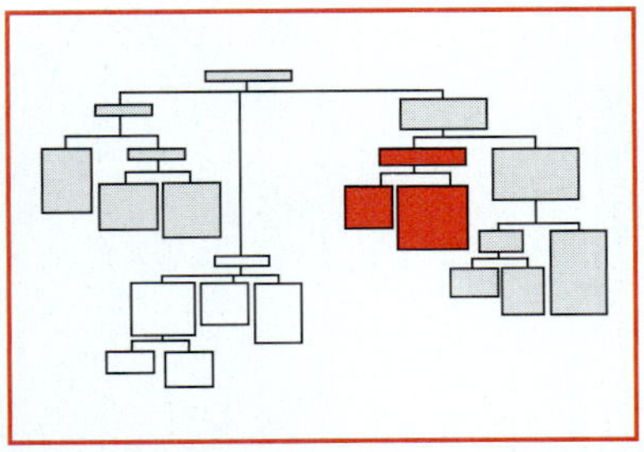

NONOPERATIVE CELLULITIS

In the absence of clinical clues or histologic findings indicating necrotizing infection, diffuse inflammation is probably simple nonoperative cellulitis. The classic lesion is a warm, erythematous, edematous, painful spreading inflammation of the skin with nonelevated, poorly defined, advancing margins. Lymphangitis and lymphadenitis are often present in nonoperative cellulitis but not in necrotizing infection requiring operation [see Figure 12].

The identification of pathogens involved is not essential but may be helpful. If a primary lesion is found, swabs taken from it give the highest yields of positive cultures.[39] Needle aspiration of the advancing edge of cellulitis,[40] preferably without preliminary saline injection, yields positive cultures in only 20% to 40% of cases.[39,41,42] Blood cultures are positive in only 2% of cases, and false positive results are twice as common. Therefore, routine blood cultures are not cost-effective; however, blood cultures may be of value in cases where cellulitis of abrupt onset occurs in conjunction with high fever (> 38.4° C [101.1° F]), leukocytosis (> 13,500/mm³), or immunodeficiency.[43] Serologic tests are of limited value.[44]

Most cellulitis is caused by group A streptococci (occasionally by groups B, C, D, and G) or by *S. aureus*. Oral or intravenous antibiotics are the primary treatment. Because streptococcal and staphylococcal cellulitis often cannot be differentiated clinically, a semisynthetic penicillin is commonly used, such as cloxacillin (4 to 6 g/day). Nonspecific measures such as rest, elevation, and warm compresses are also helpful.

Although cellulitis in adults is rarely caused by organisms other than streptococci or *S. aureus*, gram-negative cellulitis and high-risk cellulitis are nonetheless important variants. Gram-negative bacilli, particularly *Proteus mirabilis* and *Klebsiella* species, may cause cellulitis in immunocompromised patients and in patients with underlying disease (e.g., cirrhosis and congestive heart failure). Fever is often absent, but the white blood cell count is typically higher than 13,500/mm³, and severe edema of the dermal papillae produces characteristic subepidermal vesicles or hemorrhagic bullae.[45] Similarly, cellulitis may develop in a laceration that has been exposed to soil or to water infested with *Aeromonas* species. These conditions all require broad-spectrum antibiotic therapy,[44] such as cefazolin or ce-

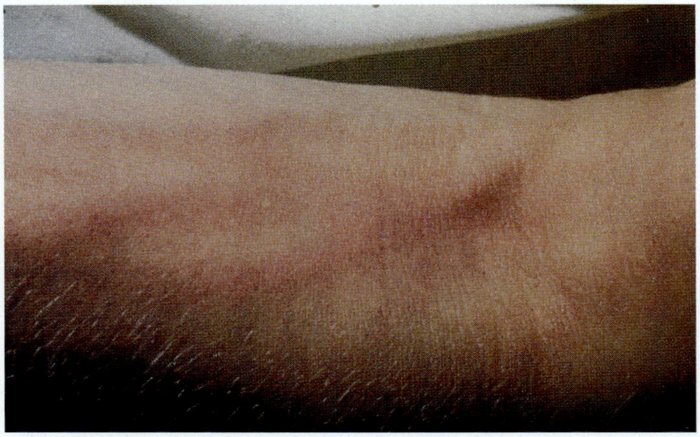

Figure 12 Lymphangitis, as illustrated here, is commonly associated with nonoperative cellulitis but not with necrotizing infection requiring operation.

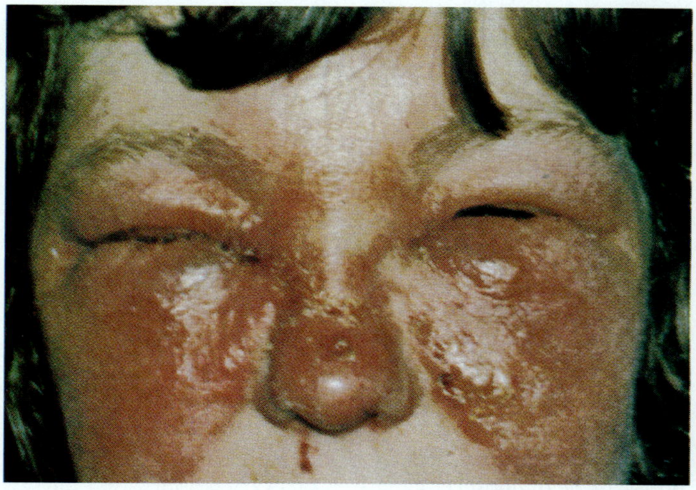

Figure 13 In this patient with late-stage erysipelas, bullae and induration of the cheeks are present along with well-demarcated erythema on the forehead.

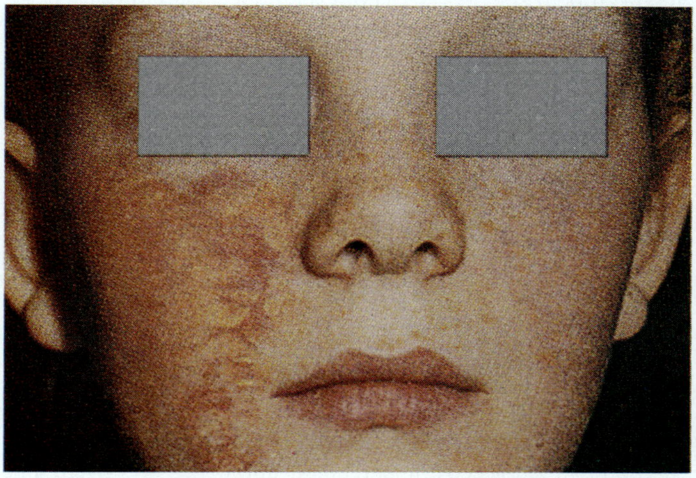

Figure 14 This child has *Haemophilus influenzae* type b cellulitis of the right cheek.

foxitin, 4 to 6 g/day in divided doses; oral ciprofloxacin, 500 mg twice daily; or oral cephalexin, 2 to 4 g/day.

High-risk cellulitis is often caused by unusual organisms. It occurs in critical locations, such as the face and the extremities (especially the hand), that are particularly vulnerable to serious complications. The term high-risk cellulitis includes several distinct conditions, namely, facial cellulitis, postadenectomy and postvenectomy cellulitis, and cellulitis after animal or human bites.

Facial cellulitis may be odontogenic, originating from the teeth and gums in older children, but most cases are nonodontogenic and occur in the upper face of infants and younger children. The best examples of facial cellulitis are erysipelas, *Haemophilus influenzae* type b (Hib) cellulitis, and orbital cellulitis. In erysipelas, a streptococcal upper respiratory infection invades the dermis and epidermis and produces a *peau d'orange* of the cheek [see Figure 13]. It responds to penicillin G, 1 million units I.V. four times daily. Hib cellulitis (now uncommon with the widespread use of *H. influenzae* vaccine) gives the cheek a bluish, bruised appearance [see Figure 14]. It is accompanied by severe respiratory infection, fever, leukocytosis, and Hib bacteremia.[46] A similar disorder occasionally occurs in adults.[47] Traditionally, ampicillin, 2 to 3 g/day I.V. in divided doses, has been used for treatment, but currently, cefuroxime, 125 mg I.V. twice daily, is preferred. Orbital and periorbital cellulitis are characterized by pain, erythema, and swelling of the eyelids. Periorbital infections are common in children after minor trauma. Orbital cellulitis is a rare complication of acute sinusitis. The Chandler classification describes five stages of orbital cellulitis, determined on the basis of clinical findings and CT scanning: preseptal, postseptal, subperiosteal abscess, orbital abscess, and meningitis or brain abscess.[48] *S. aureus,* streptococci, and, occasionally, gram-negative aerobes are the usual causative organisms; accordingly, broad-spectrum antibiotics are the preferred agents. When an abscess is present, prompt orbital exploration and decompression are indicated if 36 hours of I.V. antibiotic therapy yields no improvement or if visual acuity or globe motion becomes impaired.[49]

Recurrent cellulitis may develop after adenectomy and in lymphedematous limbs after venectomy. Fever, toxic reactions, and chills are common. Non–group A streptococci (especially groups B, C, and G) are the usual causative organisms[50]; cloxacillin, 1 g I.V. every 4 to 6 hours, is the standard treatment. Similar syndromes related to lymphatic insufficiency have been reported in the breast after breast conservation therapy for carcinoma[51] and in the buttock after hip surgery.[52] In the former instance, *S. epidermidis, Streptococcus agalactiae,* and group B streptococci were incriminated. Initial treatment consists of oral cloxacillin or cephalexin, 500 mg to 1 g every 6 to 8 hours; if the infection does not respond to this regimen, specific therapy based on Gram staining or culture may be required. Patients with cellulitis of the buttock after hip surgery have been followed for several years, and no evidence of infection of the prosthetic implant has been found.

Animal and human bites may be complicated by severe infection, especially when they occur on the hands; they are discussed in more detail elsewhere (see below). Another high-risk infection of the hand is erysipeloid, in which cellulitis caused by a gram-positive rod, *Erysipelothrix rhusiopathae,* produces a purple-red infection of the finger or hand in fishers or butchers[53] [see Figure 15]. On rare occasions, erysipeloid is complicated by bacteremia or endocarditis. If the lesion is not recognized, diagnosis can be difficult, in that the organism lies deep in the skin and is hard to culture. A new PCR assay developed for diagnosis of swine erysipeloid has now been successfully applied in a human.[53] Erysipeloid responds to oral or parenteral penicillins (e.g., cloxacillin, 1 g every 6 hours).

Miscellaneous Infections

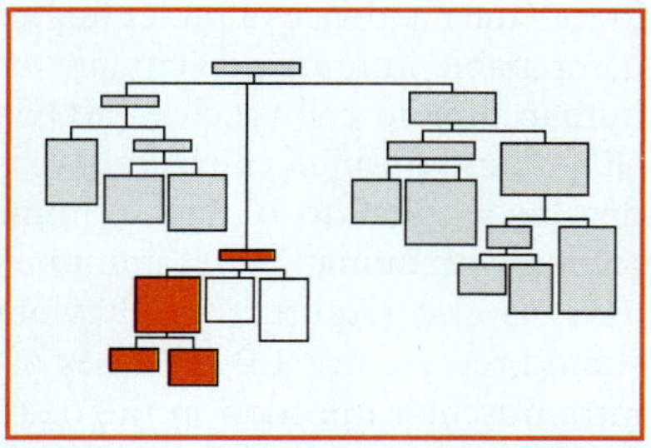

Of the miscellaneous soft tissue infections, only the common wound infections that occur after human and animal bites as well as the rare condition purpura fulminans are considered here. Established infection is more likely to occur when animal bites and scratches are seen late. When bites are seen early, infection is usually mild and responds well to treatment, which includes cleansing, tetanus prophylaxis [see 8 Acute Wound Care], rabies prophylaxis (see below), administration of antibiotics (see below), and surgical debridement.

INFECTION AFTER ANIMAL BITES

From 80% to 90% of reported animal bites are caused by dogs, 10% to 20% by cats, and 1% to 2% by nondomestic animals. About 50% of animal bites are trivial; 1% to 2% necessitate hospitaliza-

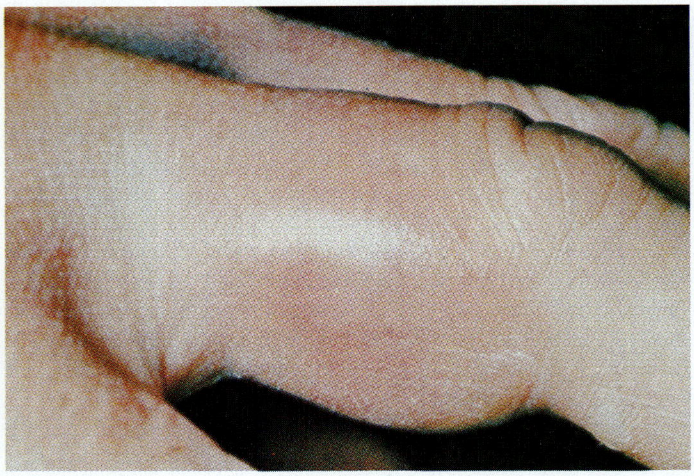

Figure 15 Characteristic of erysipeloid is an indolent, purple, nonpurulent swelling of the finger.

tion.[54] Washing with soap and water is effective immediately after a bite; later, high-pressure jet irrigation with saline is best. Fresh puncture wounds should be cleansed but not irrigated, because irrigation may compound tissue injury. Older puncture wounds should be opened to allow irrigation. Local anesthetics should be infiltrated to facilitate cleansing and debridement. When seen early, dog bites may be debrided and closed; infection is unlikely provided that appropriate antibiotics are also given. Cat bites and monkey bites are better debrided and left open, except when they occur on the face. Infected wounds and wounds that are older than 24 hours should be left open. Tetanus prophylaxis is given by intramuscular injection [see 8 Acute Wound Care].

Another important consideration is rabies prophylaxis. Rabies is a viral infection transmitted in the saliva of infected animals. The virus enters the central nervous system of the host and results in encephalomyelitis that is nearly always fatal. Rabies prophylaxis is always indicated for bites by carnivorous wild animals (in particular, skunks, raccoons, foxes, and coyotes) and by bats but not for bites by a domestic animal unless the animal is thought to be rabid or unless it becomes rabid while confined. Prophylaxis is almost never indicated after bites by rodents such as mice, rats, or squirrels. In animal studies, wound cleansing and irrigation with virucidal agents such as povidone-iodine lowers the incidence of rabies markedly. Three rabies vaccines of comparable immunogenicity are available for commercial use: human diploid cell vaccine (HDCV); rabies vaccine adsorbed (RVA), and purified chick embryo vaccine (PCEC). Antibodies develop within 7 to 10 days of immunization; thus, passive protection with human rabies immune globulin (RIG) (half-life, 21 days) is also required.[54,55] Previously nonimmunized persons should receive five 1.0 ml doses of HDCV, RVA, or PCEC by intramuscular injection in the deltoid on days 0, 3, 7, 14, and 28. The recommended dose of human RIG is 20 IU/kg on day 0 or up to day 8; half of the dose should be infiltrated in the area of the wound, and the remainder should be given by intramuscular injection. The animal involved must be observed for rabies. A domestic animal should be confined for 10 days and killed only if it becomes rabid. A wild, stray, or unwanted animal—especially one that is behaving erratically—should be killed immediately, and its brain should be tested for evidence of rabies by means of immunofluorescence techniques.

About 85% of reported animal bites harbor pathogens, and about 15% to 20% of dog bites and 50% to 60% of cat bites become infected. The most common pathogens in animal bites are *Pasteurella multocida, S. aureus,* and viridans streptococci.[54] Infections that occur within 24 hours of a bite are usually caused by *P. multocida* and deserve special attention. This gram-negative coccobacillus occurs in the mouths of up to 54% of dogs and 70% of cats and is the most common source of infection in wounds from domestic animal bites and scratches.[56] Typically, it causes infection within 12 to 18 hours, with marked local pain and tenderness. A serosanguineous discharge, low-grade fever, and regional adenopathy are less common. Infections that develop later are most often caused by *S. aureus* and viridans streptococci.

The ideal antibiotic for outpatient treatment of domestic animal bites is amoxicillin-clavulanate, 500 mg amoxicillin with 125 mg potassium clavulanate, given for 5 to 7 days. For inpatient treatment of infected bites, ampicillin-sulbactam, 3 g I.V. every 6 hours, or ticarcillin-clavulanate, 3.1 g every 6 hours for 7 days, is best. For patients allergic to penicillin, either (1) trimethoprim-sulfamethoxazole plus clindamycin or (2) cefuroxime axetil or cefuroxime sodium plus metronidazole is recommended. Elevation of the affected part is also helpful. Obvious pus must be drained and necrotic tissue debrided; however, unnecessary surgical treatment can cause marked disability.

INFECTION AFTER HUMAN BITES

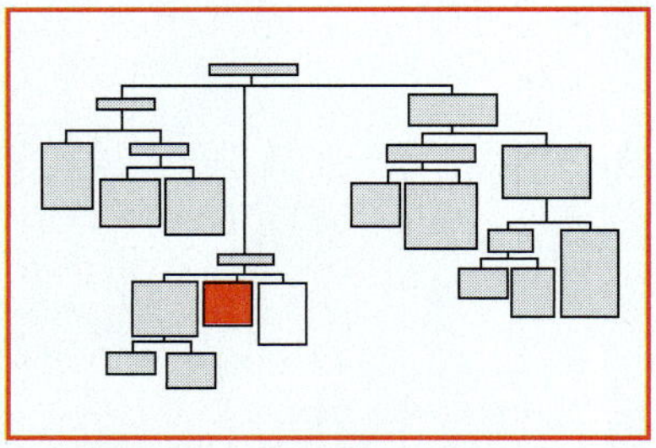

Human bites are rarely seen before infection is established,[54] and they therefore require more vigorous treatment than do animal bites. The minimum treatment of those presenting early includes tetanus prophylaxis [see 8 Acute Wound Care], high-pressure saline irrigation, broad-spectrum antibiotics, and local debridement without closure of the wounds. The severely infected wound must be treated in the hospital. Wide debridement is necessary, and broad-spectrum parenteral antibiotics are given. The largest percentage of human bite wound infections are attributable to anaerobic bacteria (50%), including *Bacteroides* species (40%); however, viridans streptococci (25%), *S. aureus* (25%), *Eikenella corrodens* (15%), and others are also common pathogens. Appropriate antibiotic therapy consists of cefoxitin, 2 g every 8 hours, ceftriaxone, 2 g every 24 hours, or ticarcillin-clavulanate, 3.1 g every 6 hours for 7 to 10 days. Bites to a clenched fist in which tendon sheaths and joint spaces are entered typically are seen late and often are severely infected at presentation. *E. corrodens* is often isolated from these wounds. Since *E. corrodens* is not sensitive to erythromycin, patients who are allergic to penicillin should receive a cephalosporin instead.

Transmission of HIV and hepatitis B is an additional concern. Transmission of HIV through a human bite is extremely unlikely because proteolytic enzymes in the saliva usually inactivate the virus; consequently, postexposure HIV prophylaxis is not recommended. Hepatitis B, on the other hand, may be transmitted through mucosal contact with blood or saliva from actively infected subjects. A hepatitis B surface antigen (HbsAg)–positive person who bites another person and breaks the skin may transmit the virus; likewise, a seronegative person who bites an HBsAg-positive subject and breaks the skin may acquire the virus. Accordingly, hepatitis B immunoglobulin should be given to all nonimmunized exposed persons.

PURPURA FULMINANS

Purpura fulminans is a rare, life-threatening condition associated with meningococcal or pneumococcal bacteremia. The clinical picture consists of bacteremia, shock, and disseminated intravascular coagulation (DIC) causing symmetrical purpura in the skin and subcutaneous tissues of the distal extremities or the face.[57] Treatment includes immediate resuscitation for shock and sepsis and correction of the coagulation defects.[57] Complete volume replacement to establish a normal urine output, cardiotonic drugs, and specific antibiotic therapy are required. Heparin is advised for DIC. The heparin is given by continuous drip in sufficient dosage to maintain the activated partial thromboplastin time at twice the normal value; standard coagulation support is provided to keep the platelet count above 50,000/mm³ and the serum fibrinogen level above 2.0 g/L. DIC is known to be associated with a profound decrease in protein C levels; consequently, administration of protein C concentrates early in the course of DIC plays a central role in current therapy. Protein C concentrates are given first in a 10 IU/kg test dose, then in a 100 IU/kg bolus, and finally in a continuous infusion at a rate of 10 to 15 IU/kg/hour to keep the protein C level between 80 and 120 IU/ml. Antithrombin III is administered when the plasma level falls to 35 IU/ml, below which point heparin is ineffective as an anticoagulant. A 25 IU/kg bolus is given every 6 hours while plasma levels are being monitored. Usually, this approach leads to reversal of DIC within 5 days. Protein C therapy is then withdrawn gradually over a period of 2 days while heparin infusion is maintained at 5 to 10 IU/kg/hour.

If the patient survives the first few days, organ failure is the main problem. Surgical treatment is seldom required early in the course of the disease. The initial mortality is 40%, but some patients who survive may need amputation; others require debridement, topical silver sulfadiazine dressing, and skin grafts.

Discussion

Recognizing the Disorder

In the management of soft tissue infection, success depends on early recognition and prompt treatment of the disorder. The primary treatment is often surgical operation, chosen empirically. When antibiotics are indicated, the initial selection of an antibiotic is also largely empirical. The first goal, then, is not to find the precise diagnosis but to decide whether the condition requires operation. This approach holds for focal lesions, for which diagnosis is easy and treatment of the usual cutaneous abscess is simple. It also holds for diffuse lesions, but the diagnosis of necrotizing infection is often difficult, and the management is challenging.

Value of Classification Systems

Although several classification systems for necrotizing soft tissue infections have been proposed, most are impractical, and some contribute to the confusion that surrounds these disorders. A practical classification system for diffuse necrotizing soft tissue infection is based on the clinical presentation, the anatomic site of primary tissue involvement, and the microbiology of the causative organisms [see Table 1]. These factors determine the course of the various clinical syndromes and are sufficiently predictable to influence the plan of treatment after the initial empirical approach.

Role of Operation

Operation is often the main treatment of soft tissue infection. Furthermore, in necrotizing infection, operation must be performed early to limit tissue damage. The extent of surgical debridement depends on operative findings and cannot be predicted before operation. Therefore, it is more important to recognize that operation is required than to identify exactly which procedure will be done. Incision and drainage suffice for cutaneous abscesses. Various modifications, such as primary closure,[58] excision, and marsupialization, have been shown to be effective and are well known to most surgeons, although they are practiced infrequently. These methods, compared with incision and drainage, result in shorter healing times but are associated with a higher rate of recurrence.[59,60] The role of operation in pyoderma gangrenosum is controversial,[2,10] but wide excision is generally required in the postoperative progressive bacterial gangrene of Meleney. In diffuse necrotizing infection, the wound is explored, by incision if necessary, to confirm the diagnosis. In necrotizing fasciitis, debridement of necrotic superficial fascia may create large, randomly based skin flaps that are poorly perfused. Some researchers have advocated preoperative planning of incisions by means of digital dermofluorometry.[61] Incision along a line joining the points of least fluorescence produces skin flaps with well-perfused bases. Thus, mutilation and disability are minimized.

In treating diffuse necrotizing soft tissue infections, reoperation is almost always required to inspect and debride the wound. The extent of debridement depends on the specific clinical syndrome,

Table 1 Classification and Characteristics of Diffuse Necrotizing Infections

Type	Characteristics
Clostridial	
Necrotizing cellulitis	Early local signs, moderate pain, and involvement of superficial tissue (skin and subcutaneous tissue)
Myonecrosis	Early systemic signs, severe pain, and involvement of deeper layers of tissue (primarily muscle)
Nonclostridial	
Monomicrobial necrotizing cellulitis Streptococcal gangrene *Vibrio* necrotizing infections	Rapid onset (1 to 3 days), single causative organism, and involvement of superficial tissue (skin and subcutaneous tissue)
Necrotizing fasciitis Classic bacteria Phycomycotic	Slower onset (4 to 7 days), bacterial synergy, some anaerobic activity, and involvement of deeper layers of tissue (Scarpa's fascia)
Synergistic necrotizing cellulitis caused by gram-negative bacteria	Slowest onset (5 to 10 days), bacterial synergy, greatest anaerobic activity, and involvement of deepest layers of tissue (deep fascia and possibly muscle)

which should be identifiable 24 to 48 hours after initial treatment on the basis of clinical, operative, and microbiological findings. Thus, in monomicrobial necrotizing cellulitis, only focal patchy areas of necrotic skin and subcutaneous tissue need to be excised. In necrotizing fasciitis, the superficial fascia requires further excision, whereas in synergistic necrotizing cellulitis and in clostridial myonecrosis, further debridement of muscle is required, and amputation of part or all of an extremity may be necessary.

Roles of Antibiotics and Pathogen Identification

Antibiotics play a limited role in treating focal soft tissue infection. They are not indicated in otherwise healthy patients with cutaneous abscesses.[62] In about 25% of patients,[63] however, systemic antibiotics are required because of the severity of associated systemic infection, because the patient is immunodeficient, or because a significant infection occurs in the central area of the face and carries a risk of cavernous sinus infection and thrombosis. The choice of antibiotics depends on the bacteria present. The anatomic site of the lesion, the duration of illness, the findings on Gram staining of specimens obtained by drainage or tissue aspiration, the odor of the pus, and the previous medical condition of the patient all provide clues to the likely pathogens.

Anaerobes are dominant in the perineum and rare on the hand. Swabs from cutaneous abscesses often initially yield *S. epidermidis* and streptococci; later, *S. aureus* may appear.[64] Pus that is foul smelling suggests anaerobic bacteria; *Clostridium* species, when present, cause a mousy odor. An abdominal wall abscess after bowel surgery may originate from an intestinal fistula. Gram stains obtained in these situations closely reflect the results of subsequent cultures.[63]

Only 4% of cutaneous abscesses are sterile. One third yield single isolates, usually *S. aureus* or occasionally *P. mirabilis;* the remainder yield a polymicrobial flora that includes many anaerobes.[63] *Bacteroides* species are the most common anaerobes. *B. melaninogenicus* and *B. ureolyticus* occur more frequently than *B. fragilis;* anaerobic gram-positive cocci occur less often, and *Clostridium* species are rare.

In patients with pyoderma gangrenosum, the significance of the pathogens obtained on primary lesion culture and needle aspirate culture is uncertain. A link between the pyogenic organisms found in the central lesion and the progressive destructive process of the skin has been proposed,[1] but this suggestion has not been substantiated, and the organisms are widely regarded as being merely opportunistic. The choice of antibiotics in classic pyoderma gangrenosum is not dictated by the pathogens identified. In his review of the postoperative variant of pyoderma gangrenosum, Meleney reported that when microaerophilic *Streptococcus* organisms and *S. aureus* were injected together into an experimental animal, cutaneous gangrene developed.[14] Injection of a pure culture of either organism failed to produce the skin lesion. These experiments confirmed the role of bacterial synergy in causing the clinical lesion. Gram-negative bacilli are sometimes found in the central area. Although the lesion must be excised for cure, broad-spectrum antibiotics are usually given empirically before surgery.

In diffuse necrotizing fasciitis, the initial antibiotic therapy is given empirically to manage the usual causative organisms. The best approaches are (1) combination therapy with I.V. penicillin, gentamicin, and clindamycin or with ciprofloxacin and metronidazole or (2) monotherapy with I.V. imipenem-cilastatin or ticarcillin-clavulanate [see Diffuse Inflammation, Inflammatory Response Is Present (Nonclostridial Infection), *above*]. Within 48 hours, the precise syndrome, whether clostridial or nonclostridial, may be defined by the results of Gram stain and culture of the tissue from the wound, by the clinical findings and course, and by the anatomic and pathologic findings at operation. For monomicrobial necrotizing cellulitis or clostridial myonecrosis, treatment with penicillin (6 to 12 million U/day I.V.) is sufficient. In necrotizing fasciitis, use of antibiotics directed against *B. fragilis* may be eliminated if this organism is not found on culture. In necrotizing fasciitis with streptococcal TSS, penicillin (18 million U/day), clindamycin (2.7 g/day), and human immunoglobulin (400 mg/kg/day for 5 days) are recommended. Intravenous amphotericin B may be added if hyphae on Gram stain or histologic section suggest necrotizing fasciitis of phycomycotic origin. The initial broad-spectrum antibiotic therapy should be maintained if muscle necrosis and the presence of aerobic and anaerobic gram-negative bacilli, including *B. fragilis*, suggest synergistic necrotizing cellulitis caused by gram-negative bacteria.

In patients with nonoperative cellulitis, systemic antibiotics are the main mode of therapy. There is no indication for autogenous vaccine therapy or for operation, both of which were popular many years ago.[65] The choice of antibiotic is based on the knowledge that cellulitis is usually caused by group A streptococci or by *S. aureus*. A semisynthetic penicillin covers both organisms adequately. Significant improvement can be observed within 48 hours.

The causative bacteria in the usual case of cellulitis are not as predictable as in specifically identified conditions such as erysipelas, but there are three lines of evidence that suggest the role of streptococci and staphylococci. First, the role of streptococci in spontaneous cellulitis occurring in the lymphedematous extremity of the dog has been documented.[66] Second, a rising titer of antistreptolysins and antifibrinolysins has been demonstrated in patients recovering from acute attacks of recurrent tropical lymphangitis[67]; these titers fall again over time. Third, in the few cases in which pus is present, streptococci and staphylococci are often cultured from patients with cellulitis.[41,68] Thus, the usual case of cellulitis may be treated without identification of the pathogen. Moreover, attempts to find bacteria by means of needle aspiration culture, blood culture, or even tissue biopsy culture are often unrewarding.[39]

Although clinical evaluation for the presence of infection is fairly accurate in most instances, it lacks specificity for a variety of disorders within the spectrum of extremity infection. Accordingly, to identify necrosis of soft tissue or infections in bone—complications that may jeopardize the integrity of the limb—further evaluation is useful. For years, plain roentgenograms and scintigrams have been used to define musculoskeletal infection. Currently, however, magnetic resonance imaging with I.V. gadolinium contrast is becoming the preferred modality for evaluating and diagnosing complicated extremity infections because it accurately depicts the degree to which bone and soft tissue are involved and identifies areas of necrosis.[68] Thus, MRI yields superior anatomic delineation of the extent of infection; furthermore, visualization of the bone marrow and definition of bony changes such as cortical destruction allow sensitive detection of osteomyelitis. These findings may be the stimulus for prolonged antibiotic therapy or for surgical intervention.

Traditionally, severe and high-risk cellulitis have been treated in the hospital setting, both to ensure access to surgical debridement when necessary and to facilitate I.V. administration of antibiotics. Often, such treatment has necessitated prolonged hospital stays. With the technology and the antibiotics currently available, however, it is usually possible to discharge patients early and to offer them outpatient parenteral antibiotic therapy (OPAT) or conversion to oral antibiotic therapy. This change in practice derives from (1) the evolution of safe techniques of central venous access for outpatient use, (2) the development of effective antibiotics with long half-lives for daily or twice-daily administration, and (3) the development of antibiotics of such high bioavailability when taken orally that oral regimens match the effectiveness of parenteral regimens. In the United States, skin and soft tissue infection is now the most common indication for referral for outpatient antibiotic therapy.

The vascular access modalities currently in use include peripherally inserted central catheters (PICCs), tunneled central catheters, and implanted ports. Of these, implanted ports are the least likely to become infected, but PICCs are now the most widely used because they are safe and easy to insert and use and because they have proved dependable and durable for prolonged antibiotic administration both in and outside the hospital setting.[69] The delivery systems used with these catheters include (1) slow I.V. injection (so-called I.V. push), which is suitable for time-dependent antibiotics (e.g., cephalosporins) but not for antibiotics that must be given over longer periods of time for reasons of safety and that depend on peak levels or prolonged persistent effects for efficacy (e.g., aminoglycosides and antifungals); (2) minibag and tubing systems that are used with rate-controlling roller clamps to generate a premixed diluted drip; and (3) a variety of portable electronic pumps and specialized tubing that are simple to use but expensive.

A number of antibiotics with long half-lives (e.g., ceftriaxone) have been developed that may be given once daily and are ideal for OPAT. One study of children with preseptal orbital cellulitis concluded that the maximum time for resolution of inflammatory signs was 36 hours, after which time transition to oral antibiotic therapy was appropriate.[70] Other antibiotics (e.g., cefazolin) that are given twice daily, either alone or with probenecid, have also been shown to be effective for home parenteral treatment of moderate and severe cellulitis. In one prospective trial of 61 such episodes of cellulitis, 88% of patients were cured, all peak antibiotic concentrations were higher than 40 μg/ml, and all trough concentrations were above the minimum inhibitory concentration for the expected pathogens.[71]

Antibiotics that possess high bioavailability after oral administration (e.g., quinolones) have greatly facilitated oral therapy for moderate to severe cellulitis. Quinolones are effective against moderate wound infections[72]; combined with single-dose or short-term parenteral antibiotics, they may also be used to treat more severe infections. Oral semisynthetic penicillins and first- or second-generation cephalosporins have long been used alone to treat mild infections or to complete the treatment of moderate cellulitis. Current data suggest that compared with other antibiotics, cephalexin may have a relatively high failure rate (40%) in treating uncomplicated cellulitis and that concomitant acid-suppressive therapy may explain this failure in part.[73]

Pathogenesis of Necrotizing Infections

The pathogenesis of the necrotizing soft tissue infections has been well discussed in the literature,[37,74,75] particularly the pathogenesis of clostridial infections. However, what causes a necrotizing infection rather than nonoperative cellulitis to develop is poorly understood, and even less is known about why a particular type of necrotizing infection occurs. The following are the four known pathogenetic factors in necrotizing soft tissue infections:

1. An anaerobic wound environment.
2. The presence of toxic lytic enzymes.
3. Bacterial synergy.
4. Thrombosis of nutrient blood vessels to skin and subcutaneous tissue.

CLOSTRIDIAL NECROTIZING INFECTIONS

The role of clostridia in producing gas gangrene has been well studied. Six species of clostridia have been reported to cause gas gangrene in humans: *C. perfringens*, *C. novyi*, *C. septicum*, *C. histolyticum*, *C. bifermentans*, and *C. fallax*. *C. perfringens* accounts for more than 80% of cases, *C. novyi* for 30% to 60%, and *C. septicum* for 5% to 20%. About 30% of trauma wounds are contaminated by *C. perfringens*,[74] but in only a few does gas gangrene develop. A fall in redox potential in contaminated puncture wounds or in limbs with ischemic muscle allows the spores to be converted to the vegetative, toxic form. The isolation of clostridia from the wound does not, however, establish the diagnosis of gas gangrene. Simple contamination and clostridial cellulitis must be differentiated from gas gangrene. The diagnosis is clinical.[75] Acceptable criteria for the diagnosis of gas gangrene are the presence of necrotic tissue with seropurulent exudate, gas bubbling from the wound or wound crepitus, and recovery of *C. perfringens* or gram-positive bacilli without spores from a symptomatic patient. In clostridial cellulitis, local signs of infection, including pus formation, predominate over systemic findings.

The hallmarks of gas gangrene—liquefaction of muscle fiber and systemic toxicity—are caused by the exotoxins of clostridia. *C. perfringens* produces at least 12 well-described exotoxins in infected wounds; *C. novyi*, eight; and *C. septicum*, four. The best known of these exotoxins is the α-toxin, lecithinase. It destroys cell membranes, alters capillary permeability, causes hemolysis, and is highly lethal. The θ-toxin causes hemolysis and necrosis and is cardiotoxic; the κ-toxin, a collagenase, lyses protein; the ν-toxin, a hyaluronidase, acts as a spreading factor; the μ-toxin affects cell DNA; and neuraminidase destroys immunologic receptors on erythrocytes. Prominent systemic signs of gas gangrene are apathy, tachycardia out of proportion to increased body temperature, and cardiovascular collapse. Renal failure resulting from the combined effects of cardiovascular collapse and hemolysis is the most common complication.

NONCLOSTRIDIAL NECROTIZING INFECTIONS

The four pathogenetic factors in necrotizing infections (i.e., an anaerobic wound environment, the presence of toxic lytic enzymes, bacterial synergy, and thrombosis of nutrient blood vessels supplying skin and subcutaneous tissue) are less well understood in nonclostridial than in clostridial infections. However, although the mechanisms of action of these factors are not well understood, their roles in infection are known. An anaerobic wound environment facilitates bacterial synergy, especially between aerobic and anaerobic bacteria, and may also explain why radiographs show subcutaneous gas in the wound in 90% of cases [*see* Gas in the Wound, *below*].[34] Local findings in the wound, such as skin necrosis, are caused by the action of lytic enzymes and by the thrombosis of nutrient blood vessels to the skin.

The range of clinical presentations of the nonclostridial necrotizing infections has changed since the original description of streptococcal gangrene by Meleney in 1924[76] and now includes necrotizing fasciitis and necrotizing fasciitis with TSS. These changes may be related to differences in pathogenesis.

Streptococcal Gangrene

Meleney emphasized the rapid development of streptococcal gangrene: the initial erythema appears within 24 hours and is associated with fever and toxicity; in 48 hours, blue-purple discoloration, blisters, and bullae appear; and by day 4 or 5, the purple patches become gangrenous[76] [*see Table 2*]. McCafferty attributed this rapid spread to proteolytic enzymes activated by streptokinase or staphylokinase. Skin necrosis appears early because of thrombosis of subcutaneous blood vessels [*see Figure 7*].[77]

Necrotizing Fasciitis

Necrotizing fasciitis was recognized in the 1950s.[78] It differs from

Table 2 Changes in Characteristics of Nonclostridial Necrotizing Soft Tissue Infections

Factor	Streptococcal Gangrene	Necrotizing Fasciitis	Necrotizing Fasciitis with Group A Streptococcal Toxic-Shock Syndrome
Historical description	Meleney (1924)[76]	Wilson (1952)[78]	Greenberg (1983)[87]
Patients	Healthy, minor trauma	Multiple medical problems	Healthy, minor trauma Elderly with diabetes
Bacteria	Hemolytic streptococci	Mixed organisms	Group A streptococci
Pathogenesis	Lytic toxins	Bacterial synergy plus lytic toxins	Toxins Virulence (because of superantigens, M proteins, or susceptibility)
Symptoms	Erythema within 24 hr Blisters Gangrene within 4–5 days	Pain Erythema Blisters in the second week	Pain Edema Fever Shock Organ failure
Mortality	20% (preantibiotic era)	20%	20%–60%

streptococcal gangrene in the preponderance of systemic over local findings and in the slower onset of symptoms [*see Table 2*]. No clear explanation is available for these differences. Although few toxic lytic enzymes have been identified during pathogenesis, clinical and experimental evidence of their role in necrotizing fasciitis is available. Meade and Mueller found in 1968 that a collagenase elaborated by *Pseudomonas* species causes the rapid progression of necrosis in the subcutaneous tissue and along the superficial fascia.[79] More recently, Talkington and coworkers found that necrotizing tissue lesions in streptococcal necrotizing fasciitis are associated with a protease elaborated by the bacteria.[80] Thrombosis of nutrient blood vessels occurs late and may also cause skin necrosis. Barker and coworkers reported that the incidence of thrombosis of nutrient blood vessels is higher in patients with acute skin necrosis than in those with subacute cases.[81]

There are two main bacteriologic types of necrotizing fasciitis.[82] Most cases are type I, in which synergy occurs between Enterobacteriaceae or non–group A β-hemolytic streptococci and anaerobic cocci or penicillin-sensitive *Bacteroides* organisms. Type II cases are far less frequent and include group A streptococci either alone or with staphylococci. The clinical features in patients with type I or type II bacteriologies are indistinguishable. The hemolytic streptococcus seen in necrotizing fasciitis may be a different strain from that which produces hemolytic streptococcal gangrene: Meleney noted that different strains of hemolytic streptococcus injected under the skin of rabbits caused different outcomes.[76]

Bacterial synergy is the rule in the pathogenesis of necrotizing fasciitis. Using an animal model, Seal and Kingston[83] studied the role of bacterial synergy and lytic toxin in promoting both local progression and systemic toxicity in necrotizing fasciitis. Intradermal injection of group A β-hemolytic streptococci produced spreading infection and toxicity in 12% of animals. However, when cultures of *S. aureus* were coinjected with β-hemolytic streptococci, spreading infection occurred in 50% of cases; and when the α-lysin of *S. aureus* was coinjected with β-hemolytic streptococci, spreading lesions occurred in 75%. The predominantly anaerobic wound environment in necrotizing fasciitis and gram-negative synergistic necrotizing cellulitis facilitates the bacterial synergy between aerobic and anaerobic bacteria that is important in the pathogenesis of these syndromes.

Necrotizing soft tissue infection caused by halophilic noncholera marine *Vibrio* bacteria has been described.[84] Such infection occurs in minor wounds that have been exposed to seawater or in puncture wounds or small lacerations sustained when the patient is cleaning seafood. The clinical presentation is similar to the presentations of other types of monomicrobial necrotizing cellulitis and is more like that of hemolytic streptococcal gangrene than that of necrotizing fasciitis, which has a slower course. The onset is abrupt and is marked by swelling, erythema, and toxemia. *V. vulnificus, V. parahaemolyticus,* and *V. alginolyticus* are the usual bacteria. The mechanism of pathogenicity is not well understood, but *V. vulnificus* can cause transmural acute necrotizing vasculitis, which leads to thrombosis of subcutaneous blood vessels.

A variant form of necrotizing fasciitis caused by phycomyces has been described.[85,86] As in other forms of necrotizing fasciitis, the clinical presentation of this form is insidious. The main causative organisms are *Rhizopus arrhizus, Mucor* species, and *Absidia* species. Phycomycotic necrotizing fasciitis can be identified promptly only by histologic examination of the infected tissue. The recommended therapeutic measures are urgent radical excision and I.V. amphotericin B.

Necrotizing Fasciitis with Streptococcal Toxic-Shock Syndrome

Since the 1980s, a marked increase in cases of streptococcal TSS—highly invasive group A streptococcal soft tissue infections largely associated with shock and organ failure—has been noted.[87] Streptococcal TSS is still uncommon (approximately 10 to 20 cases per 100,000 persons), but the increase may be accurately described as epidemic. However, this does not mean that widespread dissemination of infection by these so-called flesh-eating bacteria is imminent. The characteristics of streptococcal gangrene, necrotizing fasciitis, and necrotizing fasciitis with streptococcal TSS differ [*see Table 2*].

The pathogenesis of group A streptococcal TSS is particularly interesting—especially the roles exotoxins play in producing shock and in enhancing virulence of the bacteria. Streptococcal pyrogenic exotoxins (SPEs), produced by specific strains of *S. pyogenes,* are responsible for the characteristic fever, shock, and tissue injury of streptococcal TSS. SPE-A is associated with most cases of streptococcal TSS in the United States, whereas SPE-B and SPE-C are more prevalent causes in Europe and Canada. Some workers have shown that SPE-A and SPE-B cause monocytes to produce monokines, especially tumor necrosis factor–α (TNF-α), a prominent mediator of fever, shock, and tissue injury; IL-1β; and IL-6. Other

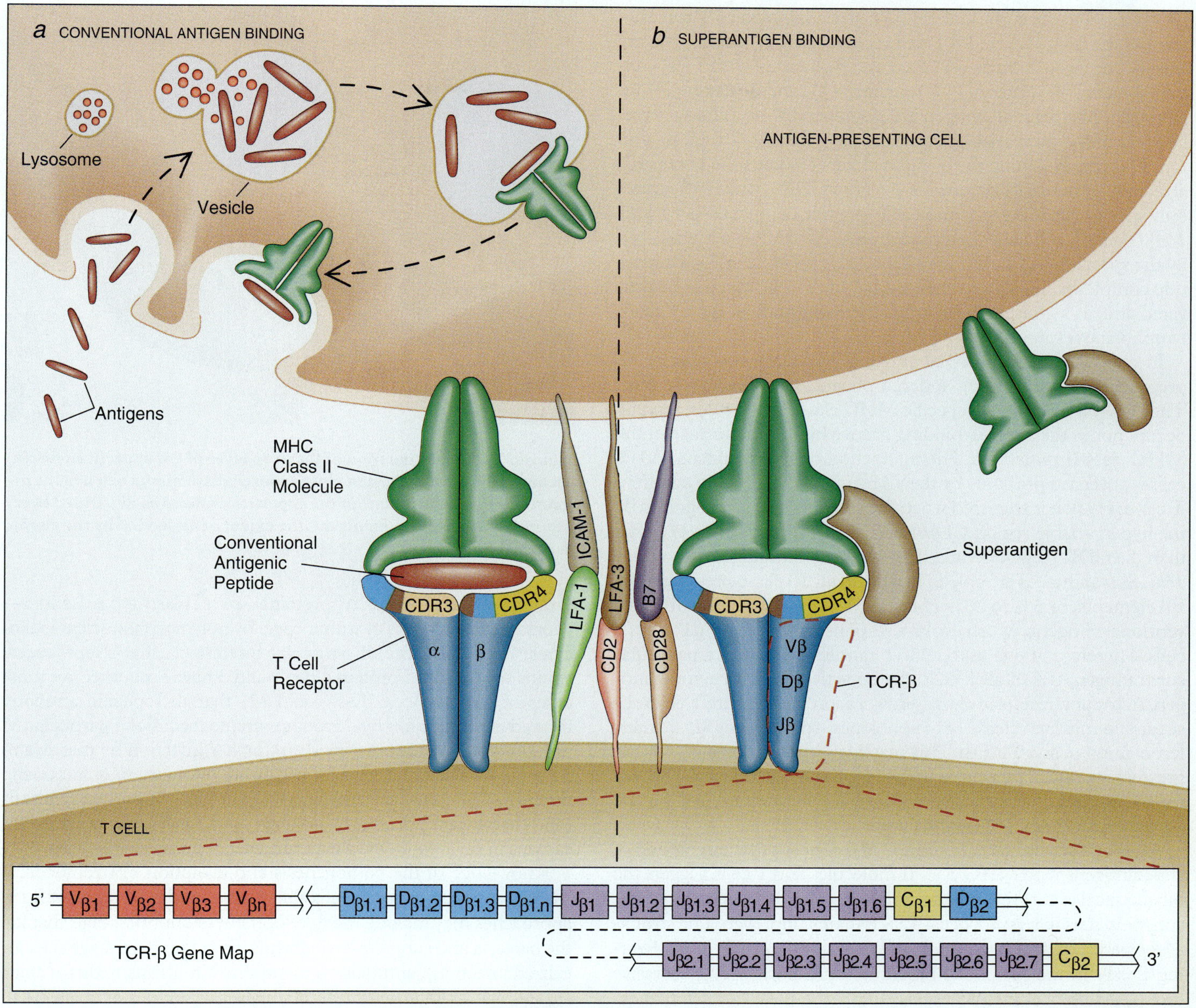

Figure 16 Superantigens differ from conventional antigens in how they bind to and interact with T cells. A conventional antigen (*a*) is phagocytosed by an antigen-presenting cell (APC) and processed into an antigenic peptide in a lysosomal compartment. The processed peptide passes to a vesicle, where it binds to a major histocompatibility complex (MHC) class II molecule at the molecule's peptide-binding groove. The resultant MHC class II molecule–peptide complex travels to the surface of the APC to be sampled by T cells, whose specificity for the peptide is determined by the amino acid sequences of the five variable regions of the T cell receptor (TCR): the $V\beta$, $V\alpha$, $J\beta$, $J\alpha$, and $D\beta$ segments. As a result, a conventional antigen is likely to be recognized by approximately 0.01% of T cells.

Superantigens (*b*), by contrast, are not phagocytosed and are far less restricted to specific molecules. For example, binding occurs not in the peptide-binding groove of the MHC class II molecule but on the molecule's surface. Interaction between the MHC class II molecule–superantigen complex and the T cell is governed primarily by a single variable region of the TCR—the $V\beta$ segment. The T cell is activated when the superantigen is recognized by the hypervariable complementarity-determining region CDR4 on the side of the $V\beta$ chain rather than the CDR3 region employed by conventional antigens. Thus, superantigens are able to react with all T cells that have the same TCR-β chain, or between 5% and 20% of resting T cells.

exotoxins, such as streptolysin O, are also potent inducers of TNF-α and IL-1β. Peptidoglycan and lipotechoic acid also cause TNF-α release by monocytes. These mechanisms, added to the effects of the SPEs, result in shock.

Some investigators have tried to account for the increased virulence of group A streptococci in streptococcal TSS and for the dramatic morbidity of the syndrome by proposing that the SPEs also act as superantigens, which differ from conventional antigens in their interactions with T cells.

Conventional antigens interact with T cells in three phases: internalization and preprocessing (i.e., phagocytosis), binding, and T cell activation [*see Figure 16a*]. In phase 1—phagocytosis—antigens are internalized by monocytes and other antigen-presenting cells (APCs) and are processed into small peptide antigen determinants in the lysosomes. In phase 2, binding occurs: the peptides pass into special vesicles, where they form complexes with major histocompatibility complex (MHC) class II molecules at the molecules' peptide-binding groove. In phase 3, the MHC class II molecule–peptide complexes travel to the surface of the APC to be sampled by T cells that express the unique α and β T cell receptor (TCR) chains that are specific for those complexes. The α and β chains of each TCR contain constant (C), variable (V), joining (J), and diversity (D) regions. Specificity for an antigen is determined by the amino acid sequences of the five variable regions of the TCR: Vβ, Vα, Jβ, Jα, and Dβ. The region joining the α and β chains contains the hypervariable complementarity-determining region CDR3, which recognizes only specific MHC class II molecule–peptide complexes [see Figure 16a]. Thus, T cell activation by conventional antigens is restricted by the specificity of the TCR and the MHC class II molecule–peptide complexes. This limits the number of T cells that can be activated and, as a consequence, limits the magnitude of the resultant lymphokine response.

In contrast to conventional antigens, superantigens require no preprocessing and do not undergo phagocytosis [see Figure 16b]. They are less restricted to specific MHC class II molecules; binding occurs not in the peptide-binding groove but on the surface of the MHC class II molecules. The interaction of superantigens with T cells is governed primarily by the Vβ region of the TCR. In addition, T cell activation is triggered when the superantigen is recognized by the hypervariable region CDR4 on the side of the Vβ chain rather than the CDR3 region required by conventional antigens [see Figure 16b]. Superantigens are able to react with all T cells expressing those Vβ elements, or 5% to 20% of resting T cells, compared with conventional antigens, which evoke a response from only 0.01% of T cells. Therefore, if two of the 25 Vβ families recognize a particular superantigen, 8% of all T cells can be activated by that superantigen. Activation results in clonal proliferation of the entire T cell subset and in massive release of lymphokines—particularly IL-2, interferon gamma, and TNF-β. This massive response accounts for the greater virulence of group A streptococci in streptococcal TSS, for the extent and severity of the systemic manifestations, and for the increased mortality of the syndrome.

Although several studies support the concept that interaction of superantigens with MHC class II molecules and T cells triggers the biochemical events that initiate clonal expansion, the role of specific superantigens in streptococcal TSS remains unproven. The strongest evidence to date is the finding of selective depletion of Vβ-bearing T cells in the peripheral blood of patients with severe invasive group A streptococcal infection and TSS.[88] It is well known that exposure of T cells to superantigens can result either in proliferation or in deletion of target T cell subsets. When a superantigen, such as staphylococcal enterotoxin A (SEA), is injected into mice, an initial marked increase is seen in the number of circulating SEA-specific Vβ-bearing T cells for 4 days, after which a second phase ensues in which those T cells are deleted by the induction of anergy and programmed cell death, or apoptosis, and their numbers fall to very low levels for 1 to 4 months.[89] Other studies suggest that the amount of superantigen may determine whether T cell expansion or deletion occurs.[90] The activation of T cells by superantigens is facilitated by APC costimulatory molecules, such as B7 and intracellular adhesion molecule–1, and their respective ligands on the T cell, CD28 and leukocyte function–associated antigen–1. T cell–superantigen interaction may bring the costimulatory molecules and ligands closer together, allowing better transduction of the signals that direct T cell activation and proliferation. In the absence of costimulatory molecules, interaction of the TCR and superantigen may induce T cell anergy. On the other hand, when the interaction is primed by TNF-α or interferon gamma, preactivated T cells may undergo apoptosis and selective deletion when reexposed to a superantigen.

A further mechanism contributing to the syndrome of streptococcal TSS is an increased susceptibility to infection induced by M proteins on streptococci. M proteins—particularly types 1 and 3—decrease phagocytosis of streptococci by polymorphonuclear leukocytes.[91] It is therefore of particular interest (1) that streptococcal strains that carry M protein types 1 and 3 have accounted for most cases of streptococcal TSS[92] and (2) that the specific antibody formed after infection by a group A streptococcus of a particular M protein type provides resistance to further infection by that strain. M proteins also enhance exotoxin production, thereby increasing tissue destruction. Clindamycin, which impairs M protein synthesis (and therefore suppresses exotoxin production), is particularly efficacious in the treatment of experimental S. pyogenes infections.

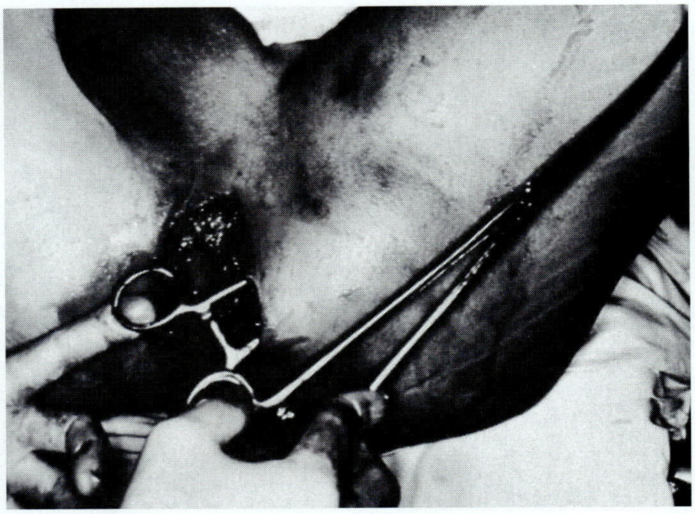

Knowledge of the pathogenesis and evolution of streptococcal TSS may suggest specific possible future modes of therapy. Such approaches may include the development of antimicrobials that kill the bacteria and suppress toxin formation at the initial stage (i.e., localized infection), antitoxins to neutralize circulating toxins at stage II, and agents that neutralize circulating cytokines at stage III to control the syndrome and prevent progression to the multiple organ dysfunction syndrome of stage IV. Takei and coworkers have shown that human immunoglobulin contains antibodies that inhibit activation of T cells by staphylococcal toxin superantigens in cases of staphylococcal TSS.[93]

Figure 17 The destruction of the deep layer of the superficial fascia accounts for the classic sign of unopposed dissection when a blunt instrument probes the plane of the superficial fascia, as illustrated here. The right-hand clamp points out the extent of dissection by the clamp in the left hand.

Streptococcal Myositis

Neither muscle nor deep fascia is involved in hemolytic streptococcal gangrene or in necrotizing fasciitis. The term fasciitis refers to the constant involvement of the deep layer of superficial fascia.[78] The destruction of this layer accounts for the classic sign of unopposed dissection when a blunt instrument probes the plane of the superficial fascia [see Figure 17].[23] An interesting variant with muscle involvement is streptococcal myositis, which has been differentiated from gas gangrene.[94] Most patients present with bacteremia and severe pain, but crepitus or gas in the tissues is unusual.[95] In streptococcal myositis, a group A hemolytic streptococcus is associated with anaerobic streptococci, S. aureus, or gram-negative bacilli. The muscle is inflamed but shows no evidence of the necrosis typical of gas gangrene.

Myositis may also occur as one element of necrotizing fasciitis with streptococcal TSS.[95] This so-called gangrenous streptococcal

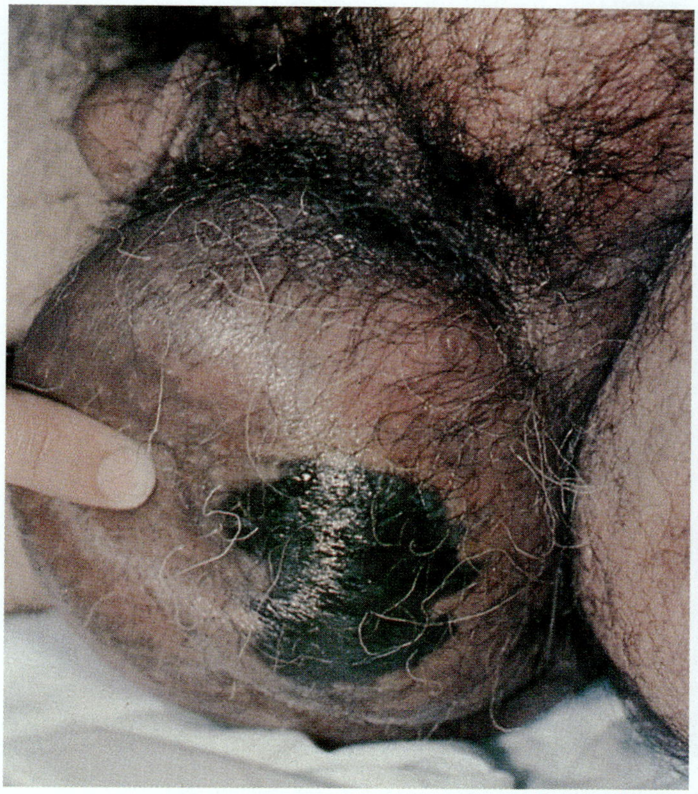

Gram-Negative Synergistic Necrotizing Cellulitis

True muscle necrosis also occurs in synergistic cellulitis caused by gram-negative bacteria. In this condition, the slow onset of disease, the deep anatomic location, and the anaerobic environment favoring bacterial synergy produce more extensive tissue necrosis than is generally seen in monomicrobial necrotizing cellulitis or in necrotizing fasciitis.[96] Although the perineal form of synergistic necrotizing cellulitis caused by gram-negative bacteria has been called Fournier's gangrene,[97] it is quite different from the idiopathic scrotal gangrene described by Fournier [see Figure 18].[98,99] Indeed, the parallel between idiopathic scrotal gangrene and so-called Fournier's gangrene is similar to the parallel between hemolytic streptococcal gangrene and necrotizing fasciitis. Synergistic necrotizing cellulitis is caused by synergy between anaerobic and aerobic gram-negative bacteria—usually *B. fragilis* or peptostreptococci and Enterobacteriaceae. Thus, it is polymicrobial from the outset. In addition, unlike idiopathic scrotal gangrene, perineal synergistic necrotizing cellulitis caused by gram-negative bacteria may extend onto the abdominal wall, necessitating extensive and repeated debridement [see Figures 19 and 20].

Idiopathic Scrotal Gangrene

Idiopathic scrotal gangrene[98,99] is characterized by sudden onset of fever, rapid progressive gangrene of the scrotal skin within 24 to 30 hours, and quick separation of the slough from the testes. The main causative organisms are anaerobic streptococci,[100] but secondary overgrowth of gram-negative bacilli may occur later.[101] The tissue loss is more superficial than that which occurs in Fournier's gangrene. Prompt and repeated surgical debridement reduces mortality. The wound granulates rapidly, and skin grafting may be performed later.

Gas in the Wound

Gas in the wound is an ominous sign to most physicians, perhaps because of its association with gas gangrene.[102,103] The significance of gas in the wound, however, depends on its source.

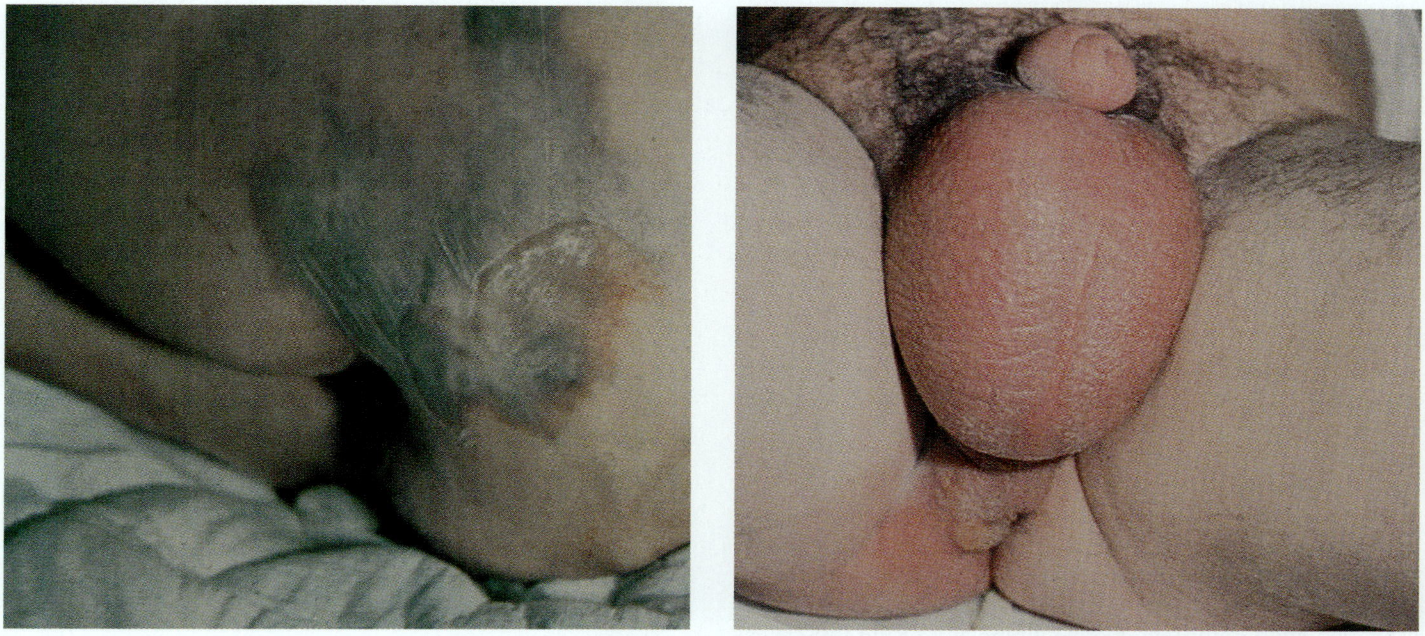

Figure 18 Fournier's gangrene of the scrotum is shown in this photograph.

myositis is similar to clostridial myonecrosis in abruptness of onset, severity of pain, and high mortality, but it differs in the absence of underlying disease or of recent trauma and in the lack of crepitus or gas in the tissues. It has been suggested that the bacteria reach the muscle by hematogenous dissemination; a prodromal viral myositis may predispose the involved muscle to localization of coincident streptococcal infection.

Figure 19 Patients with synergistic necrotizing cellulitis caused by gram-negative bacteria may have necrotizing infection of the buttock (left). A perineal form is also seen (right).

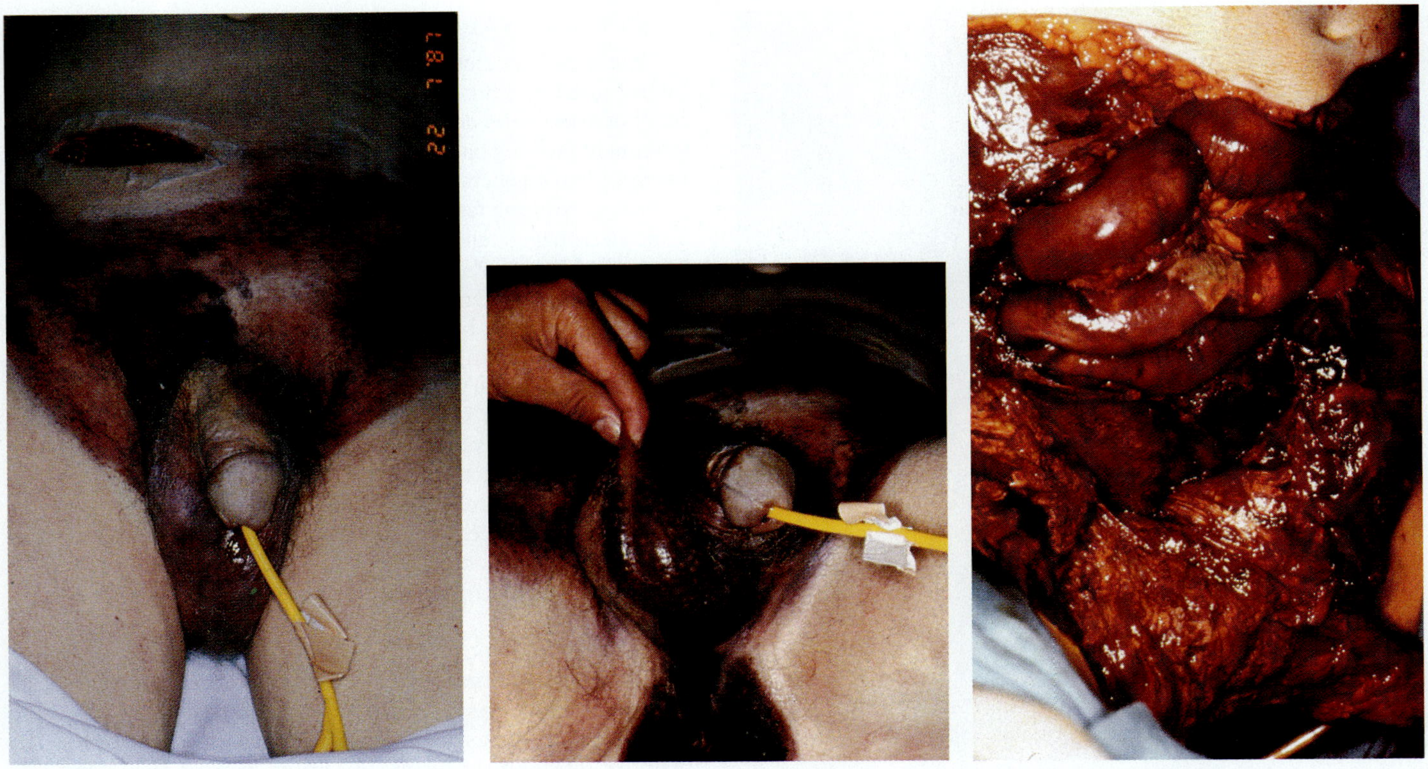

Figure 20 Synergistic necrotizing cellulitis caused by gram-negative bacteria on the anterior abdominal wall followed laparotomy for perforated carcinoma of the cecum in this patient. Ecchymosis and vesicles were present in the groin and anterior abdominal wall (left). Retroperitoneal dissection of infection and ecchymosis of the perianal region and scrotum are evident (center). Wide excision of the anterior abdominal wall revealed normal muscle in the flank but necrotic rectus abdominis and inguinal muscles in the lower abdomen (right).

Gas found in the wound may result from installation, leakage, or formation de novo. Installed gas is that left in the tissues in the course of tissue manipulation. It is characterized by the absence of other symptoms or signs and by gradual decrease in quantity over time.

Gas leakage into the tissues is characterized by a history of a predisposing event. It may occur after trauma—surgical or accidental—or after the violent retching and vomiting associated with spontaneous rupture of the esophagus. Air leakage from the esophagus, trachea, or lungs may follow blunt or penetrating trauma, and subcutaneous emphysema may follow tracheostomy or the insertion of a chest tube into the pleural space.

Gas formed in the tissues is truly spontaneous. It implies an anaerobic environment in which aerobic bacteria such as *E. coli, Klebsiella, Enterobacter,* or *Pseudomonas* or anaerobic bacteria such as peptostreptococci or *Bacteroides* species can produce gas. Usually, hydrogen and nitrogen are formed by processes of denitrification, fermentation, and deamination.[104] The volume of gas formed is quite variable. In some conditions, particularly synergistic necrotizing cellulitis caused by gram-negative bacteria, large volumes of gas may form, which dissect well beyond the area of infection. This occurrence, however, does not imply the need to excise or debride tissues beyond the area of infection. Simple incision will confirm that these tissues are not infected [see Figure 21].

Diagnosis and management of the patient with formed gas in the tissues is the same as that of the patient with a diffuse soft tissue infection. A search for telltale clinical features of necrotizing infection is combined with ancillary investigation—soft tissue x-ray, needle aspiration and Gram stain, blood culture, and serum muscle enzyme assay. The finding of gas within the muscle on x-ray is a telling sign of myonecrosis [see Figure 22].

Bite Wounds

Interesting differences between animal- and human-bite wounds should be noted because they affect management. Domestic animal bites and scratches occur far more often than human bites, but they are less serious. Only about half of all dog bites even receive medical attention. Human bites are more serious, in part because they usually present later, when infection is well established. In addition, the human oral cavity has a huge diversity of aerobic and anaerobic bac-

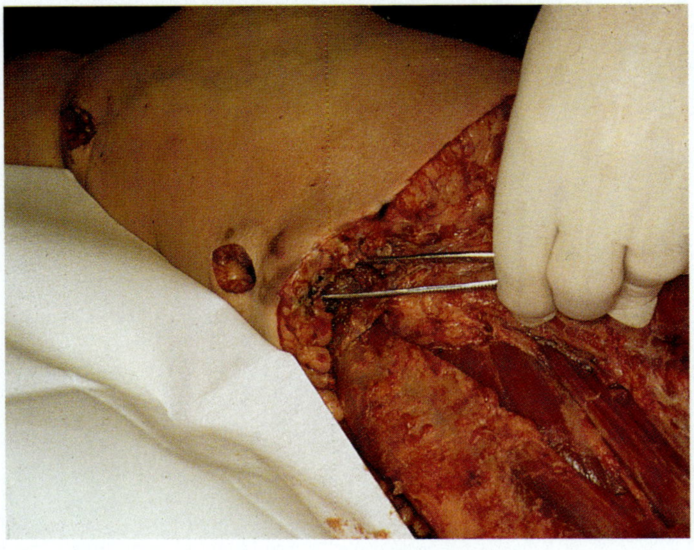

Figure 21 Exploratory incision must often be made to detect the presence of gas in the tissues beyond the area of necrosis.

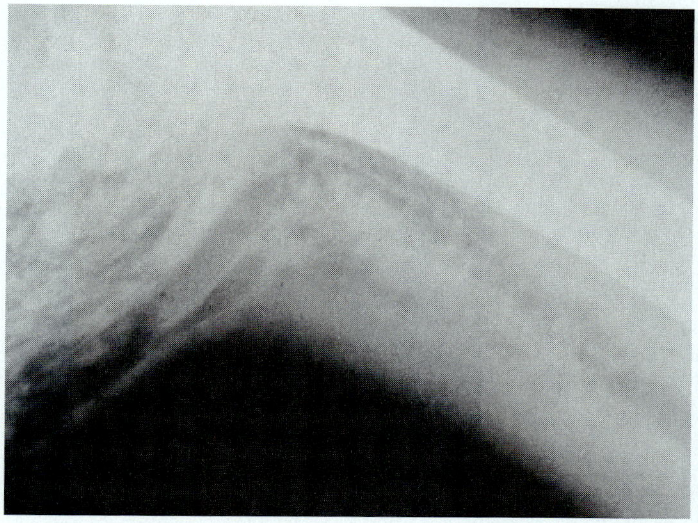

Figure 22 Gas seen within the muscle on x-ray is a telling sign of myonecrosis.

teria. All human-bite wounds should be considered infected; therefore, they call for a broader spectrum of antibiotic coverage and wider debridement than animal bites. Above all, the wounds must not be closed primarily. Of all animal wounds, dog bites have the lowest risk of infection. They may be debrided and closed primarily, provided antibiotics are given.[105]

Finally, the special risk of rabies after animal bites often raises questions about the need for prophylaxis. The risk of rabies depends on the species of animal involved, the circumstances of the bite, and the type of exposure. Bites by wild carnivorous animals involved in unprovoked attacks carry the highest risk. The HDCV is more immunogenic and better tolerated than the duck embryo vaccine used formerly. Pregnancy is not a contraindication to the use of HDCV. Patients with a history of hypersensitivity, however, should be given HDCV with caution: antihistamines may be used, epinephrine should be close at hand, and the patient should be observed carefully.

Pathogenesis of Purpura Fulminans

The pathogenesis of purpura fulminans is interesting but controversial. The earmarks of acute purpura fulminans, typically associated with meningococcemia, are purpuric skin and severe acute DIC. The skin changes differ from those characteristic of simple hemorrhage in that the lesions are raised, indurated, and circumferential and tend to coalesce, blister, and break. These changes are due to rapidly progressive microvascular thrombosis in the dermis, resulting in perivascular hemorrhage and necrosis with minimal inflammation. Acute purpura fulminans closely resembles the Shwartzman reaction, induced in experimental animals by two I.V. injections of endotoxin 12 to 24 hours apart.[106] Endotoxin damages endothelial cells and activates the Hageman factor (factor XII), thereby initiating intravascular thrombosis and causing ischemia, vessel wall damage, and bleeding.[107]

Endotoxin-induced microvascular thrombosis is also associated with severe DIC, which is particularly interesting because of the related profound and disproportionate fall in plasma concentration of protein C and the recently defined central role of protein C administration in therapy. Protein C is a vitamin K–dependent glycoprotein that acts as a natural anticoagulant. It combines with thrombomodulin and small amounts of thrombin on the endothelial surface to form activated protein C (APC), which with cofactor protein S blocks further generation of thrombin by inhibiting factors Va and VIIIa. Factor VIIIa normally activates factor X and acts in conjunction with factors Va and Xa in the prothrombinase complex that generates thrombin from prothrombin. By limiting thrombin generation, APC limits fibrin formation; moreover, by promoting fibrinolysis, it limits fibrin accumulation.

In meningococcemia, induced microvascular thrombosis initiates a vicious circle that triggers disproportionate consumption of protein C and produces severe DIC. The endotoxemia also promotes release of TNF-α and IL-1, resulting in elevated levels of plasminogen activator inhibitor–1, which blocks fibrinolysis. In addition, TNF-α increases vascular permeability and white blood cell trapping.[108] Through its anticoagulant and fibrinolytic actions, administered protein C decreases microvascular thrombosis. This effect is critical in preventing organ failure and digital gangrene.[108] Administered protein C is also anti-inflammatory because APC blocks release of TNF-α and IL-1. Steroid therapy has also been suggested for this condition but should not be used because the Shwartzman reaction can be primed with cortisone.[109]

Chronic purpura fulminans is seen only in children. It presents many days after a febrile illness, usually a viral upper respiratory tract infection. Antigen-antibody complexes are deposited in the skin and lead to patches of skin necrosis.

References

1. Brunsting LA, Goeckerm WH, O'Leary PA: Pyoderma (echthyma) gangrenosum: clinical and experimental observations in five cases occurring in adults. Archives of Dermatology and Syphilology 22:655, 1930
2. Newell LM, Malkinson FD: Commentary: pyoderma gangrenosum. Arch Dermatol 118:769, 1982
3. Holt PJA, Davies MG, Saunders KC, et al: Pyoderma gangrenosum. Medicine (Baltimore) 59:114, 1980
4. van der Sluis I: Two cases of pyoderma (ecthyma) gangraenosum associated with the presence of an abnormal serum protein (β₂ A-paraprotein). Dermatologica 132:409, 1966
5. Perry HO, Winkelmann RK: Bullous pyoderma gangrenosum and leukemia. Arch Dermatol 106:901, 1972
6. von den Driesch P: Pyoderma gangrenosum: a report of 44 cases with follow-up. Br J Dermatol 137:1000, 1997
7. Hughes JR, Smith E, Berry H, et al: Pyoderma gangrenosum in a patient with rheumatoid arthritis responding to treatment with cyclosporin A. Br J Rheumatol 33:680, 1994
8. Jolles S, Niclasse S, Benson E: Combination of oral and topical tacrolimus in therapy-resistant pyoderma gangrenosum. Br J Dermatol 140:564, 1999
9. Dirschka T, Kastner U, Behrens S, et al: Successful treatment of pyoderma gangrenosum with intravenous human immunoglobulin. J Am Acad Dermatol 39:789, 1998
10. Read AE: Pyoderma gangrenosum (editorial). Q J Med 55:99, 1985
11. Lewis SJ, Poh-Fitzpatrick MB, Walther RR: Atypical pyoderma gangrenosum with leukemia. JAMA 239:935, 1978
12. Heng MCY: Hyperbaric oxygen therapy for pyoderma gangrenosum. Aust NZ J Med 14:618, 1984
13. Plaus WJ, Hermann G: The surgical management of superficial infections caused by atypical mycobacteria. Surgery 110:99, 1991
14. Brewer GE, Meleney FL: Progressive gangrenous infection of the skin and subcutaneous tissues, following operation for acute perforative appendicitis. Ann Surg 84:438, 1926
15. Grainger RW, MacKenzie DA, McLachlin AD: Progressive bacterial synergistic gangrene: chronic undermining ulcer of Meleney. Can J Surg 10:439, 1967
16. Ledingham IMcA, Tehrani MA: Diagnosis, clinical course and treatment of acute dermal gangrene. Br J Surg 62:364, 1975
17. Svensson LG, Brookstone AJ, Wellsted M: Necrotizing fasciitis in contused areas. J Trauma 25:260, 1985

18. Fisher JR, Conway MJ, Takeshita RT, et al: Necrotizing fasciitis: importance of roentgenographic studies for soft-tissue gas. JAMA 241:803, 1979
19. Aitken DR, Mackett MCT, Smith LL: The changing pattern of hemolytic streptococcal gangrene. Arch Surg 117:561, 1982
20. Baxter CR: Surgical management of soft tissue infections. Surg Clin North Am 52:1483, 1972
21. Kaiser RE, Cerra FB: Progressive necrotizing surgical infections—a unified approach. J Trauma 21:349, 1981
22. Freischlag JA, Ajalat G, Busuttil RW: Treatment of necrotizing soft tissue infections: the need for a new approach. Am J Surg 149:751, 1985
23. Miller JD: The importance of early diagnosis and surgical treatment of necrotizing fasciitis. Surg Gynecol Obstet 157:197, 1983
24. Stamenkovic I, Lew PD: Early recognition of potentially fatal necrotizing fasciitis: the use of frozen-section biopsy. N Engl J Med 310:1689, 1984
25. Mubarak SJ, Hargens AR, Owen CA, et al: The wick catheter technique for measurement of intramuscular pressure: a new research and clinical tool. J Bone Joint Surg [Am] 58A:1016, 1976
26. Dellinger EP: Severe necrotizing soft-tissue infections: multiple disease entities requiring a common approach. JAMA 246:1717, 1981
27. Shupak A, Halpern P, Ziser A, et al: Hyperbaric oxygen therapy for gas gangrene casualties in the Lebanon War, 1982. Isr J Med Sci 20:323, 1984
28. Hitchcock CR, Demello FJ, Haglin JJ: Gangrene infection: new approaches to an old disease. Surg Clin North Am 55:1403, 1975
29. Hill GB, Osterhout S: Experimental effects of hyperbaric oxygen on selected clostridial species: II. In-vivo studies in mice. J Infect Dis 125:26, 1972
30. Heimbach RD, Boerema I, Brummelkamp WH, et al: Current therapy of gas gangrene. Hyperbaric Oxygen Therapy. Davis JC, Hunt TK, Eds. Undersea Medical Society, Inc, Bethesda, Maryland, 1977, p 153
31. Zarutskie P, Silverberg F: Amniotic membranes as a temporary wound dressing in necrotizing fasciitis. Obstet Gynecol 64:284, 1984
32. Sutton GP, Smirz LR, Clark DH, et al: Group B streptococcal necrotizing fasciitis arising from an episiotomy. Obstet Gynecol 66:733, 1985
33. Hiatt JR, Kuchenbecker SL, Winston DJ: Perineal gangrene in the patient with granulocytopenia: the importance of early diverting colostomy. Surgery 100:912, 1986
34. Majeski JA, Alexander JW: Early diagnosis, nutritional support, and immediate extensive debridement improve survival in necrotizing fasciitis. Am J Surg 145:784, 1983
35. Hammar H, Wanger L: Erysipelas and necrotizing fasciitis. Br J Dermatol 96:409, 1977
36. Gozal D, Ziser A, Shupak A, et al: Necrotizing fasciitis. Arch Surg 121:233, 1986
37. Tehrani MA, Ledingham IMcA: Necrotizing fasciitis. Postgrad Med J 53:237, 1977
38. Barzilai A, Zaaroor M, Toledano C: Necrotizing fasciitis: early awareness and principles of treatment. Isr J Med Sci 21:127, 1985
39. Hook EW III, Hooton TM, Horton CA, et al: Microbiologic evaluation of cutaneous cellulitis in adults. Arch Intern Med 146:295, 1986
40. Uman SJ, Kunin CM: Needle aspiration in the diagnosis of soft tissue infections. Arch Intern Med 135:959, 1975
41. Ginsberg MB: Cellulitis: analysis of 101 cases and review of the literature. South Med J 74:530, 1981
42. Leppard BJ, Seal DV, Colman G, et al: The value of bacteriology and serology in the diagnosis of cellulitis and erysipelas. Br J Dermatol 112:559, 1985
43. Perl B, Gottehrer NP, Schlesinger Y, et al: Cost-effectiveness of blood cultures for adult patients with cellulitis. Clin Infect Dis 29:1483, 1999
44. Slutkin G, Marzouk J, Dall L, et al: Comparison of cefonicid and cefazolin for treatment of soft-tissue infections. Rev Infect Dis 6(suppl 4):S853, 1984
45. Yoon TY, Jung SK, Chang SH: Cellulitis due to *Escherichia coli* in three immunocompromised subjects. Br J Dermatol 139:885, 1998
46. Fleisher G, Heeger P, Topf P: *Hemophilus influenzae* cellulitis. Am J Emerg Med 3:274, 1983
47. Drapkin MS, Wilson ME, Shrager SM, et al: Bacteremic *Hemophilus influenzae* type B cellulitis in the adult. Am J Med 63:449, 1977
48. Chandler JR, Langenbrunner DJ, Stevens ER: The pathogenesis of orbital complications in acute sinusitis. Laryngoscope 80:1414, 1970
49. Goodwin WJ Jr, Weinshall M, Chandler JR: The role of high resolution computerized tomography and standardized ultrasound in the evaluation of orbital cellulitis. Laryngoscope 92:729, 1982
50. Baddour LM, Bisno AL: Non-group A beta-hemolytic streptococcal cellulitis: association with venous and lymphatic compromise. Am J Med 79:155, 1985
51. Mertz KB, Baddour LM, Bell JL: Breast cellulitis following breast conservation therapy: a novel complication of medical progress. Clin Infect Dis 26:481, 1998
52. Studer-Sachsenberg EM, Ruffieux PH, Saurat J-H: Cellulitis after hip surgery: long term follow-up of seven cases. Br J Dermatol 137:133, 1997
53. Brooke CJ, Riley TV: Erysipelothrix rhusiopathiae: bacteriology, epidemiology and clinical manifestations of an occupational pathogen. J Med Microbiol 48:789, 1999
54. Fleisher GR: The management of bite wounds. N Engl J Med 340:138, 1999
55. Advisory Committee on Immunization Practices: Human rabies prevention—United States 1999. Recommendations of the Advisory Committee on Immunization Practices. MMWR 48:1, 1999
56. Francis DP, Holmes MA, Brandon G: *Pasteurella multocida*: infections after domestic animal bites and scratches. JAMA 233:42, 1975
57. Smith OP, White B: Infectious purpura fulminans: diagnosis and treatment. Br J Haematol 104:202, 1999
58. Ellis M: Incision and primary suture of abscesses of the anal region. Proc R Soc Med 53:652, 1960
59. Macfie J, Harvey J: The treatment of acute superficial abscesses: a prospective clinical trial. Br J Surg 64:264, 1977
60. Sorensen C, Hjortrup A, Moesgaard F, et al: Linear incision and curettage vs deroofing and drainage in subcutaneous abscess: a randomized clinical trial. Acta Chir Scand 153:659, 1987
61. Bongard FS, Elings VB, Markison RE: New uses of fluorescence in the surgical management of necrotizing soft tissue infection. Am J Surg 150:281, 1985
62. Llera JL, Levy RC: Treatment of cutaneous abscess: a double-blind clinical study. Ann Emerg Med 14:15, 1985
63. Becker LE, Tschen E: Common bacterial infections of the skin. Primary Care 10:397, 1983
64. Meislin HW, Lerner SA, Graves MH, et al: Cutaneous abscesses: anaerobic and aerobic bacteriology and outpatient management. Ann Intern Med 87:145, 1977
65. Hughes B: The treatment of cellulitis with special reference to the hand and arm. Practitioner 89:142, 1912
66. Drinker CK, Field ME, Ward HK, et al: Increased susceptibility to local infection following blockage of lymph drainage. Am J Physiol 112:74, 1935
67. Morales-Otero P, Pomales-Lebrón A: The development of antistreptolysins and antifibrinolysins following acute attacks of recurrent tropical lymphangitis. Trans R Soc Trop Med Hyg 30:191, 1936
68. Towers JD: The use of intravenous contrast in MRI of extremity infection. Semin Ultrasound CT MR 18:269, 1997
69. Brown JM: An overview of vascular access for the alternate care setting. Infusion 1:11, 1995
70. Blumer J, O'Brien C, Lemon E, et al: Skin and soft tissue infections: pharmacologic approaches. Pediatr Infect Dis 4:336, 1985
71. Leder K, Turnidge JD, Grayson ML: Home-based treatment of cellulitis with twice-daily cefazolin. Med J Australia 169:519, 1998
72. Lipsky BA, Miller B, Schwartz R, et al: Sparfloxacin versus ciprofloxacin for the treatment of community-acquired complicated skin and skin-structure infections. Clin Therapeutics 21:675, 1999
73. Madaras-Kelly KJ, Arbogast R, Jue S: Increased therapeutic failure for cephalexin versus comparator antibiotics in the treatment of uncomplicated outpatient cellulitis. Pharmacotherapy 20:199, 2000
74. Altemeier WA, Fullen WD: Prevention and treatment of gas gangrene. JAMA 217:806, 1971
75. MacLennan JD: The histotoxic clostridial infections of man. Bact Review 26:177, 1962
76. Meleney FL: Hemolytic streptococcus gangrene. Arch Surg 9:317, 1924
77. McCafferty EL, Lyons C: Suppurative fasciitis as the essential feature of hemolytic streptococcus gangrene. Surgery 24:438, 1948
78. Wilson B: Necrotizing fasciitis. Am Surg 18:416, 1952
79. Meade JW, Mueller CB: Necrotizing infections of subcutaneous tissue and fascia. Ann Surg 168:274, 1968
80. Talkington DF, Schwartz B, Black CM, et al: Association of phenotypic and genotypic characteristics of invasive *Streptococcus pyogenes* isolates with clinical components of streptococcal toxic shock syndrome. Infect Immun 61:3369, 1993
81. Barker FG, Leppard BJ, Seal DV: Streptococcal necrotizing fasciitis: comparison between histological and clinical features. J Clin Pathol 40:335, 1987
82. Giuliano A, Lewis F, Hadley K, et al: Bacteriology of necrotizing fasciitis. Am J Surg 134:52, 1977
83. Seal DV, Kingston D: Streptococcal necrotizing fasciitis: development of an animal model to study its pathogenesis. Br J Exp Pathol 69:813, 1988
84. Howard RJ, Pesa ME, Brennaman BH, et al: Necrotizing soft tissue infections caused by marine vibrios. Surgery 98:126, 1985
85. Wilson CB, Siber GR, O'Brien TF, et al: Phycomycotic gangrenous cellulitis. Arch Surg 111:532, 1976
86. Patino JF, Castro D, Valencia A, et al: Necrotizing soft-tissue lesions after a volcanic cataclysm. World J Surg 15:240, 1991
87. Greenberg RN, Willoughby BG, Kennedy DJ, et al: Hypocalcemia and "toxic" syndrome associated with streptococcal fasciitis. South Med J 76:916, 1983
88. Watanabe-Ohnishi R, Low DE, McGeer A, et al: Selective depletion of Vβ-bearing T cells in patients with severe invasive group A streptococcal disease and streptococcal toxic shock syndrome: implications for a novel superantigen. J Infect Dis 171:74, 1995
89. Kawabe Y, Ochi A: Selective anergy of Vβ8+, CD4+ T cells in *Staphylococcus* enterotoxin B–primed mice. J Exp Med 172:1065, 1990
90. McCormack JE, Callahan JE, Kappler J, et al: Profound depletion of mature T cells in vivo by chronic exposure to exogenous superantigen. J Immunol 150:3785, 1993
91. Lancefield RC: Current knowledge of type-specific M antigens of group A streptococci. J Immunol 89:307, 1962
92. Schwartz B, Facklam RR, Brieman RF: Changing epidemiology of group A streptococcal infection in the USA. Lancet 336:1167, 1990
93. Takei S, Arora YK, Walker SM: Intravenous immunoglobulin contains specific antibodies inhibitory to activation of T cells by staphylococcal toxin superantigens. J Clin Invest 91:602, 1993
94. MacLennan JD: Streptococcal infection of muscle. Lancet 1:582, 1943

95. Yoder EL, Mendez J, Khatib R: Spontaneous gangrenous myositis induced by *Streptococcus pyogenes*: case report and review of the literature. Rev Infect Dis 9:382, 1987
96. Stone HH, Martin JD Jr: Synergistic necrotizing cellulitis. Ann Surg 129:702, 1972
97. Rouse TM, Malangoni MA, Schulte WJ: Necrotizing fasciitis: a preventable disaster. Surgery 92:765, 1982
98. Fournier JA: Gangrène foudroyante de la verge. La Semaine Médicale 3:345, 1883
99. Rudolf R, Soloway M, DePalma RG, et al: Fournier's syndrome: synergistic gangrene of the scrotum. Am J Surg 129:591, 1975
100. Coenen H, Przedborski J: Die gangrän des penis und scrotums. Beitrage zur Klinischen Chirurgie 75:136, 1911
101. Slater DN, Smith GT, Mundy K: Diabetes mellitus with ketoacidosis presenting as Fournier's gangrene. J R Soc Med 75:530, 1982
102. MacLennan JD: Anaerobic infections of war wounds in the Middle East. Lancet 2:63, 1943
103. Altemeier WA, Culbertson WR: Acute non-clostridial crepitant cellulitis. Surg Gynecol Obstet 87:207, 1948
104. Van Beek A, Zook E, Yaw P, et al: Nonclostridial gas-forming infections: a collective review and report of seven cases. Arch Surg 108:552, 1974
105. Zook EG, Miller M, Van Beek AL, et al: Successful treatment protocol for canine fang injuries. J Trauma 20:243, 1980
106. Good RA, Thomas L: Studies on the generalized Shwartzman reaction: IV. Prevention of the local and generalized Shwartzman reactions with heparin. J Exp Med 97:871, 1953
107. Silbart S, Oppenheim W: Purpura fulminans: medical, surgical and rehabilitative considerations. Clin Orthop 193:206, 1985
108. Smith OP, White B, Vaughan D, et al: Use of protein C concentrate, heparin and haemofiltration in meningococcus induced purpura fulminans. Lancet 350:1590, 1997
109. Thomas L, Good RA: The effect of cortisone on the Shwartzman reaction: the production of lesions resembling the dermal and generalized Shwartzman reactions by a single injection of bacterial toxin in cortisone-treated rabbits. J Exp Med 95:409, 1952

Acknowledgments

Figure 1   Wolfin/Medichrome.

Figure 2   From "The Surgical Management of Superficial Infection Caused by Atypical Mycobacteria," by W. J. Plaus and G. Hermann, in *Surgery* 110:99, 1991.

Figures 5 through 8, 21, and 22   Courtesy of Jonathan L. Meakins, M.D., Royal Victoria Hospital, Montreal.

Figures 9 and 10   Courtesy of E. Patchen Dellinger, M.D., Harborview Medical Center, Seattle.

Figures 13 and 15   From *Infectious Diseases Illustrated*, by Harold Lambert and W. Edmund Farrar. Gower Medical Publishing Ltd., London, 1981.

Figure 14   From *Color Atlas of Paediatric Dermatology*, by Julian Verbow and Neil Morley. MTP Press, Lancaster, England, 1983.

Figure 16   Dimitry Schidlovsky.

Figure 17   Courtesy of Charles R. Baxter, M.D., University of Texas Health Science Center at Dallas.

Figures 18 and 19   From *A Visual Exploration of Anaerobic Infections*, by Charles A. Kallick. Merck-Frosst Canada, Inc., Kirkland, Quebec, 1978.

III TRAUMA AND THERMAL INJURY

22 EMERGENCY DEPARTMENT EVALUATION OF THE PATIENT WITH MULTIPLE INJURIES

Felix D. Battistella, M.D.

Approach to the Multiply Injured Patient in the Emergency Department

Morbidity and mortality resulting from trauma can be minimized if evaluation of the acutely injured patient proceeds logically and efficiently. Given the rapid deterioration that can occur as injuries progress, trauma systems should be geared to expedite the initial evaluation, resuscitation, and treatment of multiply injured patients. Preestablished management strategies and protocols can be useful in organizing and coordinating the efforts of the trauma team.

The algorithms presented in the discussion that follows suggest strategies for the early management of trauma victims. They may not anticipate all possible scenarios, but they should at least provide a framework that facilitates the rapid decision making needed to get patients from the emergency department to the operating suite. These algorithms may have to be modified to some extent to take account of differences in local resources and expertise or the introduction of new technologies; however, the basic principles they embody are unlikely to be superseded for some time yet.

The approaches outlined in this chapter were developed according to two main premises:

1. The goal of trauma care should be to minimize preventable morbidity and mortality for all trauma victims. To this end, trauma care providers should place the same emphasis on identifying occult injuries in minimally injured patients as on treating patients with catastrophic injury.
2. Prioritization of diagnostic and therapeutic maneuvers is crucial for optimizing outcome after critical injury. Treatment priority is determined by the severity of the injury, its rate of progression, and its complexity. Easily correctable, rapidly progressive, life-threatening injuries should be addressed first; complex or slowly progressive injuries should receive a lower priority. Once a correctable life-threatening injury is identified, the trauma team should focus its efforts on stabilizing this condition before looking for additional life-threatening injuries that may not be apparent.

Initial evaluation and treatment of trauma victims are governed by the mechanism of injury (i.e., penetrating or blunt) and by the patient's hemodynamic status. Evaluation and treatment priorities for penetrating injury differ from those for blunt trauma because the two mechanisms give rise to different patterns of injury: penetrating trauma typically results in a localized injury, whereas blunt trauma frequently results in multiple injuries that involve several body regions. Furthermore, within each class of injury, evaluation and treatment priorities for hypotensive patients differ from those for hemodynamically stable patients. Whenever hemodynamic instability is present, its cause must be identified and corrected promptly to increase the patient's chance for survival. At my institution, hemodynamic instability is defined as either a systolic blood pressure lower than 90 mm Hg or a documented decrease of more than 30 mm Hg in systolic blood pressure. Admittedly, hemodynamic stability is a relative term, in that most patients, especially young ones, can compensate for hypovolemia and maintain a normal blood pressure even in the face of significant ongoing hemorrhage; nevertheless, even though blood pressure is not a sensitive detector of early shock, it is still a useful guide in the emergency department because it can be obtained promptly and frequently. Regardless of the patient's blood pressure, the evaluation and treatment of all injured patients should proceed without undue delay because ongoing bleeding can be occult.

I begin with guidelines for managing trauma patients who present in cardiac arrest. The subsequent guidelines for penetrating and blunt trauma patients who are not in cardiac arrest are based on the assumption that the ABCs of trauma and the primary survey have been completed [*see 2 Trauma Resuscitation*]. Penetrating injuries are addressed according to their primary location—neck, chest, thoracoabdominal region, or extremities.

The neck is defined as the region below the mastoid process and above the clavicles; the chest, as the area below the clavicles but above the mamillary line; the thoracoabdominal region, as the area between the mamillary line and the inguinal ligaments; and the extremities, as the area distal to the deltopectoral groove or distal to the inguinal ligaments. Penetrating injuries that span more than one of these body regions require the surgeon to prioritize initial evaluation and treatment on the basis of the physical findings. Because blunt injuries typically involve more than one body region, they are addressed according to the patient's hemodynamic status. Finally, specific injuries or findings that are associated with blunt injury (e.g., potential cervical spine injury, wide mediastinum, and hematuria) are discussed.

Approach to the Multiply Injured Patient in the Emergency Department

```
                    Multiply injured patient presents to ED
                                    │
                ┌───────────────────┴───────────────────┐
    Patient is in cardiopulmonary arrest     Patient is not in cardiopulmonary arrest
    Determine mechanism of injury.           Determine mechanism of injury.
            │                                           │
      ┌─────┴─────┐                             ┌───────┴───────┐
 Penetrating   Blunt injury                Penetrating         Blunt injury
   injury                                    injury
 [See Figure 1.] [See Figure 2.]          Determine primary    Assess hemodynamic
                                          location of injury.  status.
```

- **Injury is primarily to neck** [See Figure 3.]
- **Injury is primarily thoracoabdominal**
  - Patient is unstable [See Figure 6.]
  - Patient is stable [See Figure 7.]
- **Injury is primarily to chest**
  - Patient is unstable [See Figure 4.]
  - Patient is stable [See Figure 5.]
- **Injury is primarily to extremity** [See Figure 8.]

Penetrating injury branch (not in arrest):
- Patient is unstable [See Figure 9.]
- Patient is stable — Obtain chest x-ray.
  - Patient has evidence of acute injury on chest x-ray [See Figure 10.]
  - Patient has no evidence of acute injury on chest x-ray [See Figure 11.]

Traumatic Cardiopulmonary Arrest

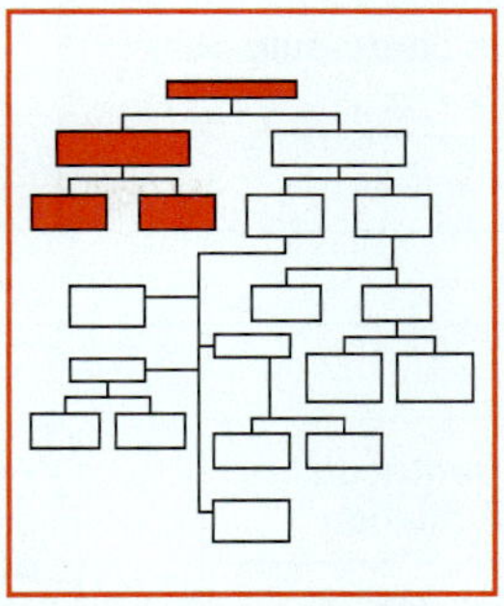

Survival after traumatic cardiopulmonary arrest is substantially influenced by mechanism of injury: the prognosis is dismal when cardiopulmonary arrest is attributable to blunt trauma and somewhat better when it is attributable to penetrating trauma.[1,2] The main reason for this divergence in outcomes is that cardiopulmonary arrest in a blunt trauma patient may be secondary to any of a number of causes, most of which are quite difficult to reverse rapidly (e.g., brain injury, high spinal cord injury, proximal aortic disruption, and exsanguination from a variety of injuries). The best survival rates after traumatic cardiopulmonary arrest are reported in patients with stab wounds to the heart, in whom the cardiac arrest is attributable to cardiac tamponade. In patients with cardiac tamponade, the heart often can be resuscitated simply by decompressing the pericardium [see 2 Trauma Resuscitation].

It follows, then, that management of a patient in traumatic cardiac arrest after penetrating injury should be much more aggressive than that of a patient in cardiac arrest after blunt injury.

PENETRATING TRAUMA

Even given the generally better prognosis associated with cardiac arrest after penetrating trauma, resuscitation is futile if cardiopulmonary arrest has persisted for a prolonged period [see Figure 1]. If no signs of life (e.g., spontaneous respirations, a pulse, or spontaneous movement) are observed by medical personnel at the scene or in transport and the ECG in the emergency department shows anything but a narrow complex sinus rhythm, the victim should be pronounced dead on arrival. If the history is unclear or signs of life are observed, the patient should undergo an emergency room thoracotomy without delay. If the wound is to the chest, the injured side should be opened first. The incision can be extended across the sternum if necessary.

The pericardium should be opened and the heart inspected. Any pericardial blood should be evacuated and the heart massaged. When a central pulmonary injury is present, the hilum should be cross-clamped to control hemorrhage and prevent air embolization. If the surgeon believes the central pulmonary injury to be correctable, resuscitation should proceed and the patient should be taken to the operating room for definitive repair.

If no intrathoracic injury is identified, efforts should be focused on reestablishing spontaneous cardiac activity. If this cannot be accomplished by giving intravenous fluids and providing cardiac support, resuscitation may be terminated and the patient pronounced dead. If spontaneous cardiac activity is restored, the patient should be taken to the OR, where the injuries should be dealt with as expeditiously as possible. Bleeding vessels should be ligated rather than reconstructed, and treatment of intra-abdominal injuries should be limited to control of hemorrhage. Reoperation for definitive treatment of abdominal injuries should be scheduled in the next 24 to 48 hours once the coagulopathy is reversed and the patient is hemodynamically stable.

BLUNT TRAUMA

Given the extremely poor survival rate for patients in cardiac arrest as a result of blunt trauma, resuscitative efforts should focus on the relatively few patients in this group whose arrest was witnessed in the ED or who present with a normal sinus rhythm [see Figure 2]. The electrical activity of the heart is a useful guide to the potential benefit to be derived from continued resuscitative efforts.[3] If the victim has no cardiac activity or exhibits an agonal rhythm or a wide-complex rhythm, no further resuscitative efforts are warranted, and the patient

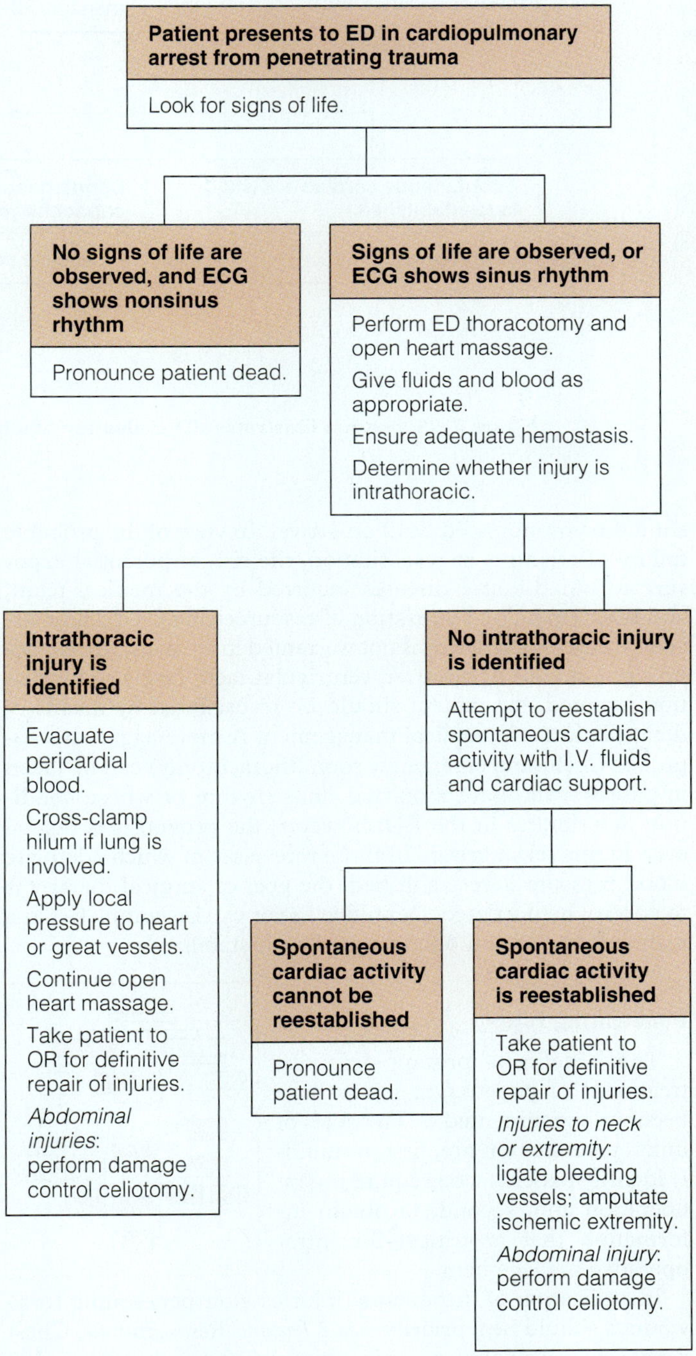

Figure 1 Algorithm illustrates ED evaluation of a penetrating trauma victim in cardiopulmonary arrest.

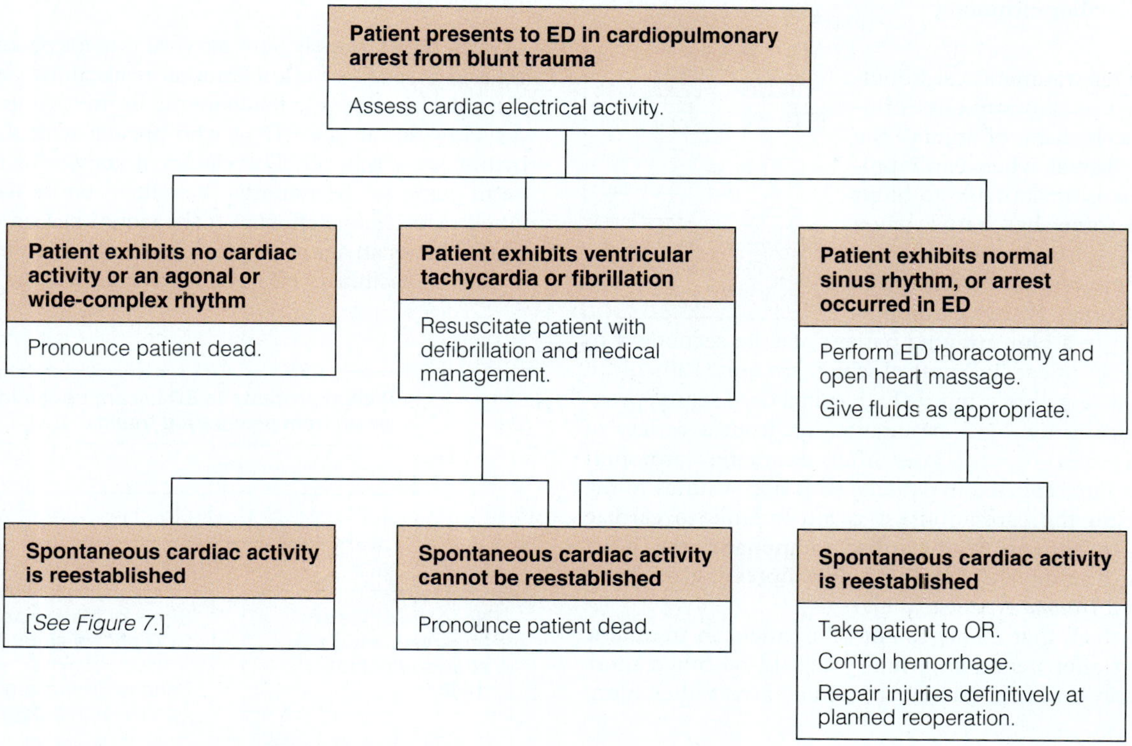

```
┌─────────────────────────────────┐
│ Patient presents to ED in       │
│ cardiopulmonary arrest from     │
│ blunt trauma                    │
│ Assess cardiac electrical       │
│ activity.                       │
└─────────────────────────────────┘
```

Patient exhibits no cardiac activity or an agonal or wide-complex rhythm
Pronounce patient dead.

Patient exhibits ventricular tachycardia or fibrillation
Resuscitate patient with defibrillation and medical management.

Patient exhibits normal sinus rhythm, or arrest occurred in ED
Perform ED thoracotomy and open heart massage.
Give fluids as appropriate.

Spontaneous cardiac activity is reestablished
[See Figure 7.]

Spontaneous cardiac activity cannot be reestablished
Pronounce patient dead.

Spontaneous cardiac activity is reestablished
Take patient to OR.
Control hemorrhage.
Repair injuries definitively at planned reoperation.

Figure 2 Algorithm illustrates ED evaluation of a blunt trauma victim in cardiopulmonary arrest.

should be pronounced dead on arrival. In view of the probable failure of attempts at resuscitation, the risk of potential exposure to blood-borne diseases incurred by the medical team, and the tremendous utilization of resources involved, an emergency room thoracotomy is not warranted in a patient who shows no signs of life.[4] If, however, ventricular tachycardia or fibrillation is noted, the patient should be resuscitated by means of defibrillation and medical management A more aggressive approach (including emergency room thoracotomy) can be taken in patients who have a normal sinus rhythm or whose condition deteriorates in the ED; however, the prognosis is dismal even in this select group. In those rare cases in which adequate blood pressure is reestablished, the goal of surgical therapy is to control hemorrhage. Definitive repair can be completed in a planned reoperation once the patient is stabilized.

Penetrating Injury

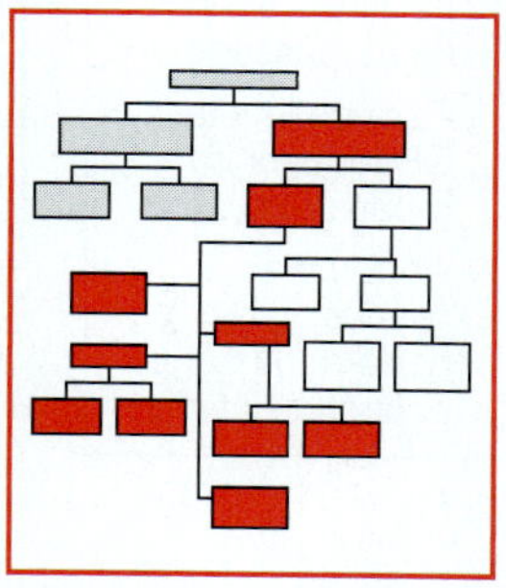

The benefits of prompt definitive treatment of penetrating injury have been well documented.[5-7] The goals of initial resuscitation are, first, to rapidly identify patients who require urgent operation and, second, to obtain information that is critical for intraoperative management.

Identification of intrapleural injuries after penetrating torso wounds should be a priority [see *2 Trauma Resuscitation*]. Chest x-ray is an invaluable screening modality for such injuries. If a hemothorax or a pneumothorax is clinically obvious, a thoracostomy tube should be inserted before a chest x-ray is obtained, especially if the patient is hemodynamically unstable. In all other patients, a chest x-ray should be obtained immediately. Chest x-rays are helpful in most gunshot wound victims, even if the wound site is some distance from the thorax, because the path of the bullet is often unknown.

Factors affecting the management of penetrating injuries include the hemodynamic stability of the patient, the location of the wound, and the weapon used. Which diagnostic tests are performed and how quickly evaluation proceeds are determined primarily by the hemodynamic stability of the patient.

NECK

Although the airway is always a priority in critically injured patients, it is a particular concern in a patient with a penetrating neck wound because of the potential for compromise resulting from an expanding hematoma or edema associated with the injury. Accordingly, the airway should be monitored frequently during diagnostic procedures. A chest x-ray should be obtained early in the course of resuscitation to rule out intrathoracic injury [*see Figure 3*]. If an intrathoracic injury is identified, it should be evaluated and treated as outlined elsewhere [see *Chest, below*].

ED management of a hemodynamically unstable patient with a penetrating neck injury should be limited to applying local pressure, establishing intravenous access, and obtaining a chest x-ray. Exploration and definitive management of the injury in the operating suite should follow as soon as possible. The results of the neurologic examination done at the time of presentation should be documented because asymmetric neurologic findings may influence whether a carotid artery injury is repaired or ligated.[8]

In the past, evaluation and management of stable patients with neck injuries that penetrated the platysma depended on the location of the injury: injuries to zones I and III were evaluated roentgenographically, whereas injuries to zone II were an indication for mandatory exploration. Currently, however, thanks to the increased availability and improved safety of arteriography, the selective exploration strategy is favored for evaluating stable patients with penetrating neck injuries. Patients who have an obvious injury to a vascular or visceral structure (manifested by hypovolemic shock, pulsatile bleeding, airway compromise, or subcutaneous air in the neck) should undergo prompt exploration and treatment. Stable patients who do not have an obvious injury can be evaluated by means of urgent arteriography to exclude vascular injury. If arteriography identifies an injury, the patient should undergo exploration and treatment in the OR without further delay; if the arteriogram is normal, the airway and the esophagus should be evaluated endoscopically and roentgenographically.

Whenever a neck injury penetrates the platysma, evaluation of the carotid arteries is indicated; however, whether evaluation of the larynx and the trachea or of the pharynx and the esophagus is also indicated depends on the patient's symptoms and physical findings. Patients with difficulty in swallowing, voice changes, stridor, difficulty in breathing, or anterior neck pain should undergo both laryngotracheal and pharyngoesophageal evaluation. Direct laryngoscopy is the best means of evaluating the larynx and the trachea, and esophagography is the best means of evaluating the pharynx and the esophagus. Esophagoscopy can be performed either as an alternative or as an adjunct to esophagography. Individually, both esophagoscopy and esophagography have false negative rates of 10 to 15 percent, but when the two are combined, their sensitivity for detecting esophageal injuries rises to nearly 100 percent.[9,10] Delayed recognition and treatment of pharyngoesophageal injuries can lead to significant increases in morbidity and mortality; a high index of suspicion and early evaluation allow prompt identification of injuries and minimize morbidity.

If the platysma is intact or diagnostic tests yield negative results, the patient can simply be given local wound care and then discharged.

CHEST

Insertion of a therapeutic and diagnostic thoracostomy tube should be a priority in a hemodynamically unstable patient with a penetrating chest injury [see Figure 4]. This should be done before a chest x-ray is obtained so that adequate lung reexpansion can be ensured and any hemothorax present drained.

Urgent thoracotomy is indicated when the initial chest tube output is greater than 20 ml/kg or when subsequent chest tube output is greater than 2 ml/kg/hr for two consecutive hours. Patients with large undrained hemothoraces should also undergo early thoracotomy, especially if they are hemodynamically compromised. Thoracotomy is best done through an anterolateral incision with the patient supine; this approach permits simultaneous abdominal exploration if a diaphragmatic or intra-abdominal injury is found. Injuries to the esophagus, the descending thoracic aorta, and the distal airway are difficult to treat through an anterolateral exposure; if these structures are injured, a temporary closure can be performed once the bleeding is controlled, and the patient can then be repositioned for a formal posterolateral thoracotomy to treat the injuries.

An unstable patient who remains hypotensive but whose chest tube output and x-ray findings do not meet the criteria for urgent thoracotomy should undergo urgent celiotomy to exclude an intra-abdominal source of bleeding. If the injury is close to the heart, a pericardial window should be created at

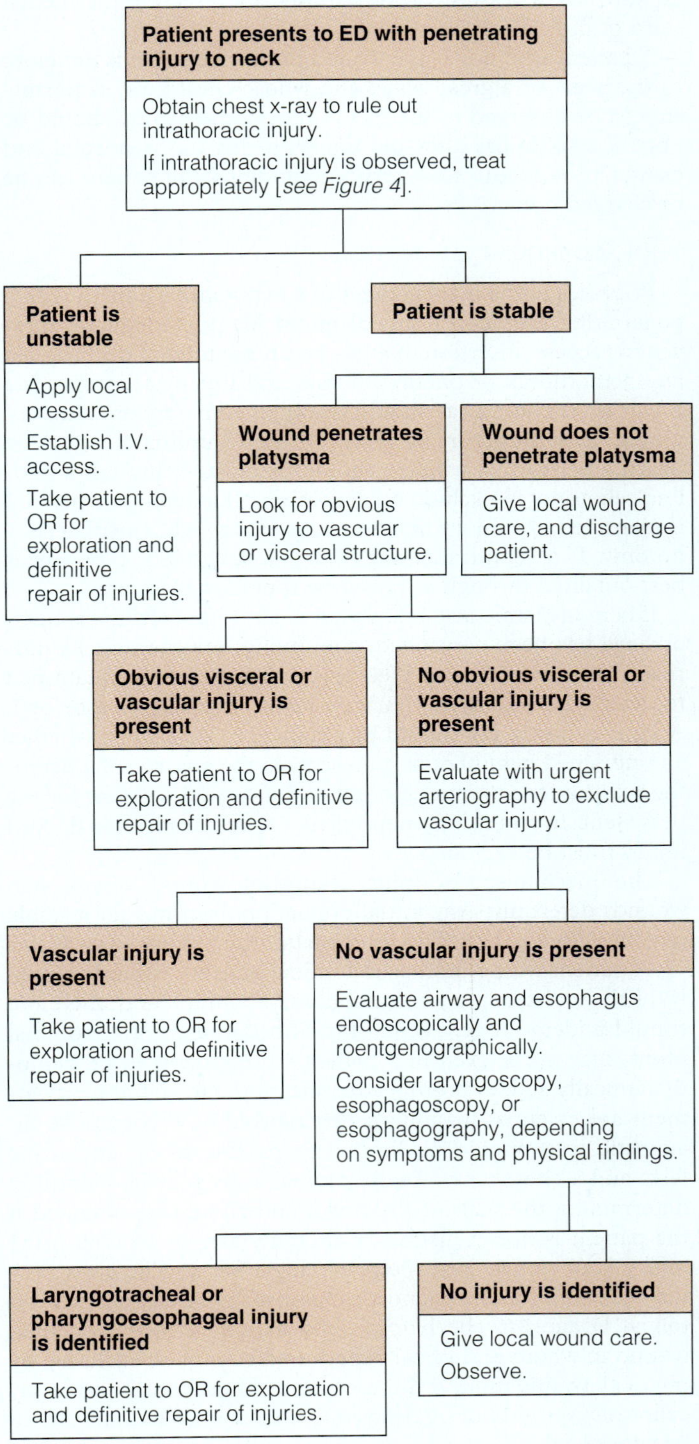

Figure 3 Algorithm illustrates ED evaluation of a patient with penetrating injury to the neck.

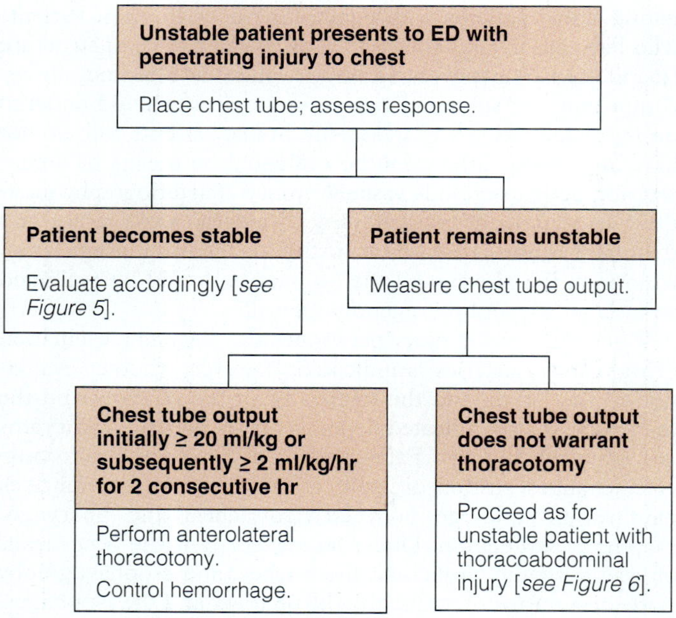

Figure 4

Unstable patient presents to ED with penetrating injury to chest
Place chest tube; assess response.

- **Patient becomes stable**
  Evaluate accordingly [see Figure 5].
- **Patient remains unstable**
  Measure chest tube output.
  - **Chest tube output initially ≥ 20 ml/kg or subsequently ≥ 2 ml/kg/hr for 2 consecutive hr**
    Perform anterolateral thoracotomy.
    Control hemorrhage.
  - **Chest tube output does not warrant thoracotomy**
    Proceed as for unstable patient with thoracoabdominal injury [see Figure 6].

Figure 4 Algorithm illustrates ED evaluation of an unstable patient with penetrating injury to the chest.

---

the time of laparotomy to rule out cardiac injury. A spinal cord injury should be suspected in a persistently hypotensive patient who exhibits no evidence of significant intra-abdominal or intrapericardial injury.

Most penetrating injuries to the chest can be managed simply by placing a chest tube in the affected hemithorax [see Figure 5]. Thoracotomy is indicated in a hemodynamically stable patient if there is evidence of significant bleeding (i.e., substantial chest tube output or a large clotted hemothorax), a tracheobronchial injury, a cardiovascular injury, or an esophageal injury. Exploration of the chest for a large hemothorax (evidenced by an initial chest tube output greater than 20 ml/kg, a subsequent chest tube output greater than 2 ml/kg/hr for two consecutive hours, or a cumulative 12-hour chest tube output greater than 30 ml/kg) can be performed through a posterolateral thoracotomy once intra-abdominal injury has been excluded.

A patient with a large air leak, massive subcutaneous or mediastinal emphysema, or a persistent pneumothorax should be evaluated via bronchoscopy to rule out tracheobronchial injury. Injuries to the intrathoracic trachea, the carina tracheae, or the right mainstem bronchus are best approached through a right anterolateral thoracotomy; injuries to the left mainstem bronchus are best approached through a left posterolateral thoracotomy.

A patient who is hemodynamically stable and does not require thoracotomy for hemorrhage or tracheobronchial injury should be evaluated for possible cardiac or vascular injury via echocardiography and arteriography if the injury is close to the heart or a great vessel. Most such injuries are associated with significant hemodynamic instability as a result of hemorrhage or pericardial tamponade; however, in rare cases, injuries to the heart or the great vessels may be occult. Echocardiographic evidence of pericardial fluid in a patient with a penetrating injury close to the heart is an indication for further evaluation via a subxiphoid pericardial window.[11] If a hemopericardium is confirmed, the pericardial blood may be evacuated and the cardiac injury treated through a median sternotomy. Arteriography may reveal pseudoaneurysms, arteriovenous fistulas, or intimal flaps in stable patients with wounds close to great vessels. Injuries to the innominate artery or the common carotid arteries may be exposed via a median sternotomy; injuries to the proximal left subclavian artery should be exposed via an anterolateral thoracotomy for proximal control. The distal subclavian vessels can be exposed by resecting the medial third of the clavicle.

A patient who has a stab wound to the chest that is not close to the heart or a great vessel and whose chest x-ray is normal should be observed in the ED. A repeat chest x-ray should be obtained six hours after the injury; if this too is normal and examination reveals no worrisome findings, the patient can be discharged home.[12,13]

THORACOABDOMINAL REGION

Priorities in the management of a hypotensive patient with a penetrating thoracoabdominal injury include adequate intravenous access, insertion of a thoracostomy tube to decompress any hemothorax or pneumothorax, and urgent celiotomy [see Figure 6]. A chest x-ray should be obtained before operation to identify any intrathoracic injury. If the wound is close to the heart, a pericardial window should be created through a midline celiotomy to exclude cardiac injury. If a hemopericardium is identified, the injury may be exposed through a median sternotomy. If a significant lung injury is suspected, exposure is best obtained through a transverse thoracosternotomy.

If hemodynamic instability persists after intraperitoneal hemorrhage has been controlled, continuing intrathoracic hemorrhage must be excluded. Pleural bleeding should be quantified to determine whether a thoracotomy is necessary (see below). A repeat chest x-ray should be obtained to determine whether an undrained hemothorax is present. In the absence of a hemothorax or a tension pneumothorax that would account for the persistent hypotension, neurogenic shock from spinal cord injury must be excluded.

The mechanism of injury (gunshot wound versus stab wound) determines the initial evaluation priorities for a stable patient with a penetrating thoracoabdominal injury [see Figure 7]. A patient with a thoracoabdominal gunshot wound is highly likely to harbor an intra-abdominal injury and therefore should undergo urgent celiotomy. Substantial intra-abdominal injury may occur even in a patient who appears to be hemodynamically stable; prompt identification and definitive treatment are essential for minimizing morbidity. Preoperative diagnostic tests should be limited to routine blood and urine tests and a chest x-ray. An abdominal x-ray may be helpful in determining the path of the bullet and should be obtained if the patient is not in distress. Celiotomy can be avoided if the injury is obviously superficial or tangential and involves only the abdominal wall. Diagnostic laparoscopy or diagnostic peritoneal lavage may be helpful in a patient with a tangential wound in whom peritoneal penetration cannot be excluded by physical examination. If there are signs of peritonitis, however, celiotomy should not be delayed, even if the wound appears to be superficial.

Management of a thoracoabdominal stab wound in a stable patient varies according to the location of the wound and the

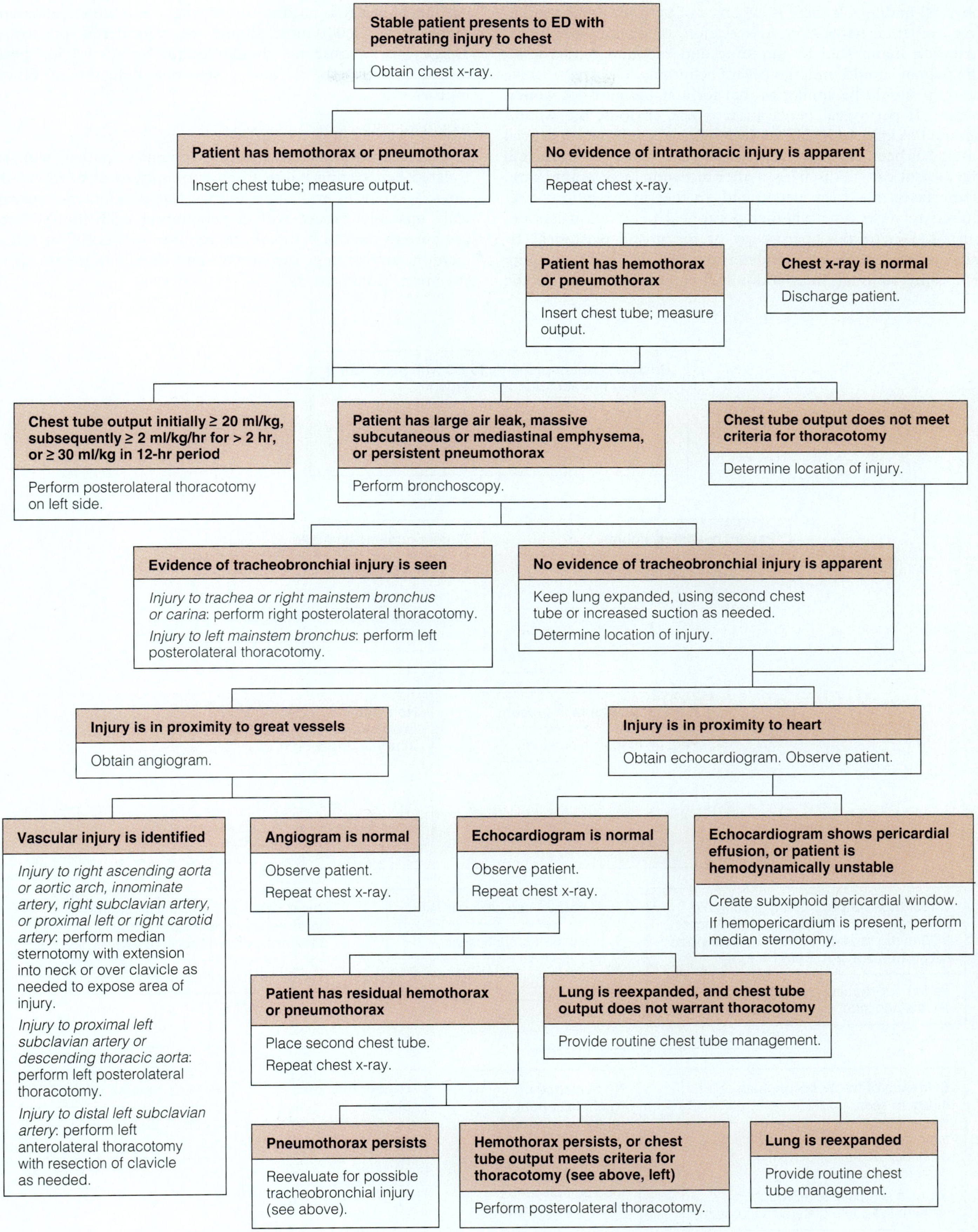

22 ED EVALUATION OF MULTIPLE INJURIES — 343

```
                    ┌─────────────────────────────────────┐
                    │ Stable patient presents to ED with  │
                    │ penetrating injury to chest         │
                    ├─────────────────────────────────────┤
                    │ Obtain chest x-ray.                 │
                    └─────────────────────────────────────┘
```

Patient has hemothorax or pneumothorax
Insert chest tube; measure output.

No evidence of intrathoracic injury is apparent
Repeat chest x-ray.

Patient has hemothorax or pneumothorax
Insert chest tube; measure output.

Chest x-ray is normal
Discharge patient.

Chest tube output initially ≥ 20 ml/kg, subsequently ≥ 2 ml/kg/hr for > 2 hr, or ≥ 30 ml/kg in 12-hr period
Perform posterolateral thoracotomy on left side.

Patient has large air leak, massive subcutaneous or mediastinal emphysema, or persistent pneumothorax
Perform bronchoscopy.

Chest tube output does not meet criteria for thoracotomy
Determine location of injury.

Evidence of tracheobronchial injury is seen
Injury to trachea or right mainstem bronchus or carina: perform right posterolateral thoracotomy.
Injury to left mainstem bronchus: perform left posterolateral thoracotomy.

No evidence of tracheobronchial injury is apparent
Keep lung expanded, using second chest tube or increased suction as needed.
Determine location of injury.

Injury is in proximity to great vessels
Obtain angiogram.

Injury is in proximity to heart
Obtain echocardiogram. Observe patient.

Vascular injury is identified
Injury to right ascending aorta or aortic arch, innominate artery, right subclavian artery, or proximal left or right carotid artery: perform median sternotomy with extension into neck or over clavicle as needed to expose area of injury.
Injury to proximal left subclavian artery or descending thoracic aorta: perform left posterolateral thoracotomy.
Injury to distal left subclavian artery: perform left anterolateral thoracotomy with resection of clavicle as needed.

Angiogram is normal
Observe patient.
Repeat chest x-ray.

Echocardiogram is normal
Observe patient.
Repeat chest x-ray.

Echocardiogram shows pericardial effusion, or patient is hemodynamically unstable
Create subxiphoid pericardial window.
If hemopericardium is present, perform median sternotomy.

Patient has residual hemothorax or pneumothorax
Place second chest tube.
Repeat chest x-ray.

Lung is reexpanded, and chest tube output does not warrant thoracotomy
Provide routine chest tube management.

Pneumothorax persists
Reevaluate for possible tracheobronchial injury (see above).

Hemothorax persists, or chest tube output meets criteria for thoracotomy (see above, left)
Perform posterolateral thoracotomy.

Lung is reexpanded
Provide routine chest tube management.

Figure 5 Algorithm illustrates ED evaluation of a stable patient with penetrating injury to the chest.

physical findings. If there is evidence of peritoneal penetration (e.g., omental herniation, evisceration, or obvious peritoneal irritation manifested by guarding and rebound tenderness), the patient should undergo urgent celiotomy. The preoperative workup should be similar to that for a stable gunshot wound victim. If peritoneal penetration is not obvious, the wound should be explored locally to determine whether the superficial fascia has been violated. If no fascial penetration has occurred, the patient can be discharged after receiving local wound care; if the fascia has been penetrated, further investigation is required to determine whether peritoneal penetration has occurred. Diagnostic laparoscopy or diagnostic peritoneal lavage can be performed to determine which patients require celiotomy to treat intra-abdominal injury. When diagnostic peritoneal lavage is used in this setting, a red blood cell count higher than $1,000/mm^3$ should be considered positive.[14] Diagnostic laparoscopy, though useful for identifying peritoneal penetration, is not a sensitive detector of bowel injuries.[15-18]

EXTREMITIES

Evaluation and treatment of a hypotensive patient with an isolated penetrating injury to an extremity involve essentially the same steps as evaluation and treatment of a hemodynamically unstable patient with a penetrating neck injury: local pressure to control hemorrhage, intravenous access for resuscitation, and prompt exploration and definitive treatment of the injury [see Figure 8].

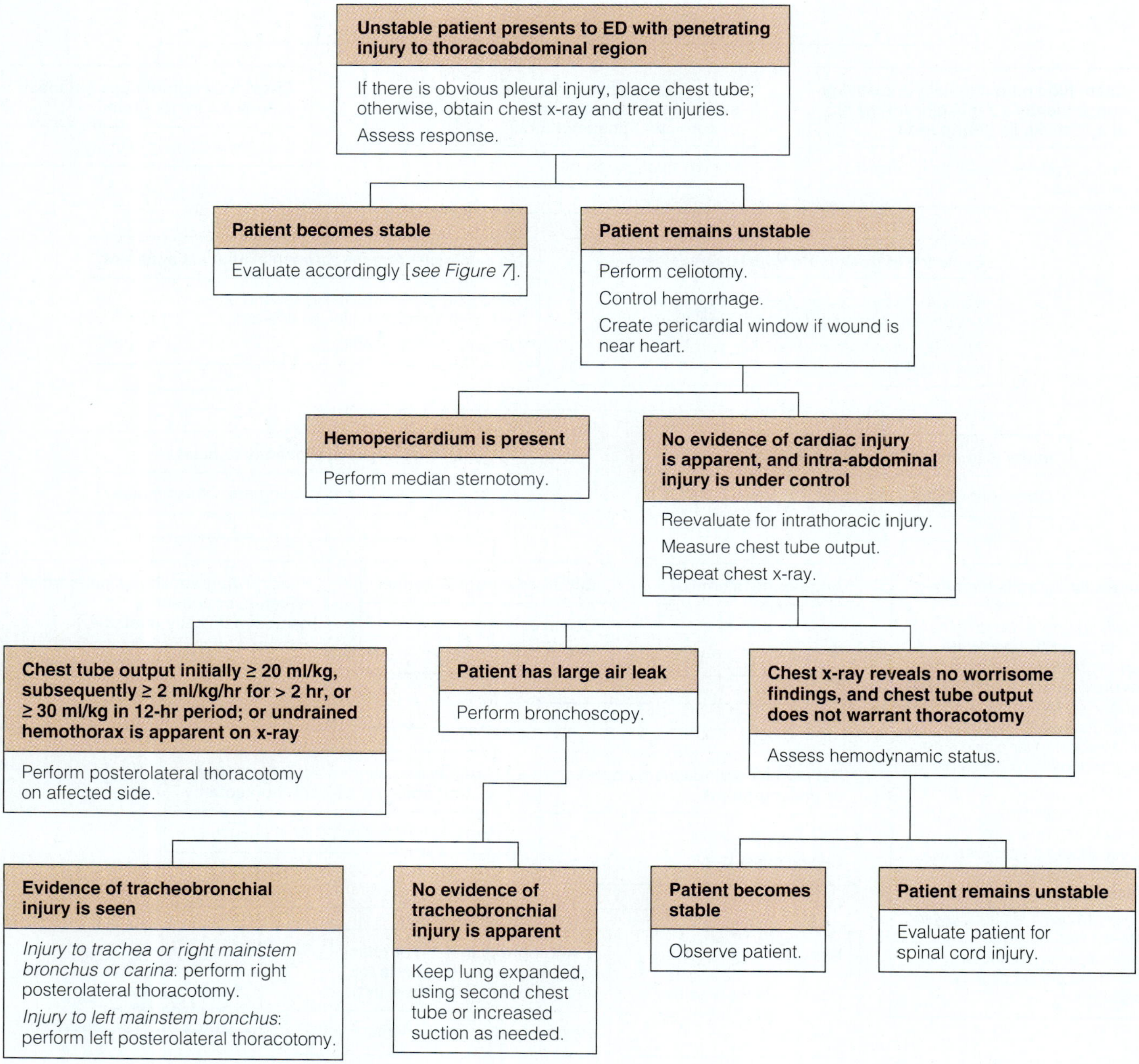

Figure 6 Algorithm illustrates ED evaluation of an unstable patient with penetrating injury to the thoracoabdominal region.

Management of a stable patient with a penetrating injury to an extremity depends on the pulses distal to the injury. If distal pulses are absent, the patient should undergo exploration in the OR to identify any arterial injury present. Early exploration and repair of an arterial injury minimize ischemic time and subsequent reperfusion injury. If an arterial injury is not readily identified at exploration, an intraoperative arteriogram may be obtained to exclude thrombosis.

If distal pulses are normal and there is a penetrating injury close to an artery, the patient should undergo arterial duplex evaluation to exclude vascular injury.[19-21] I recommend duplex evaluation of all extremity gunshot wounds because of the possibility of stretch injuries to the artery as a result of the tremendous energy dispersed in the tissues. If the vascular examination is not suggestive of arterial injury, duplex evaluation is not urgent; instead, the patient can be observed and duplex evaluation performed once the resources are available (within 12 to 24 hours).

Distal vascular pulses should be monitored during the observation period; if distal pulses are lost, the patient should undergo prompt exploration of the affected artery. Any arterial injury identified by duplex evaluation should be confirmed and further defined by arteriography unless there is evidence of arterial occlusion, in which case the affected artery should be explored and repaired.

X-rays of the injured extremity should be obtained to exclude associated fractures and to localize any retained foreign bodies. If not all of the bullets can be accounted for, intravascular embolization should be suspected and the patient evaluated via multiple x-rays or fluoroscopy.

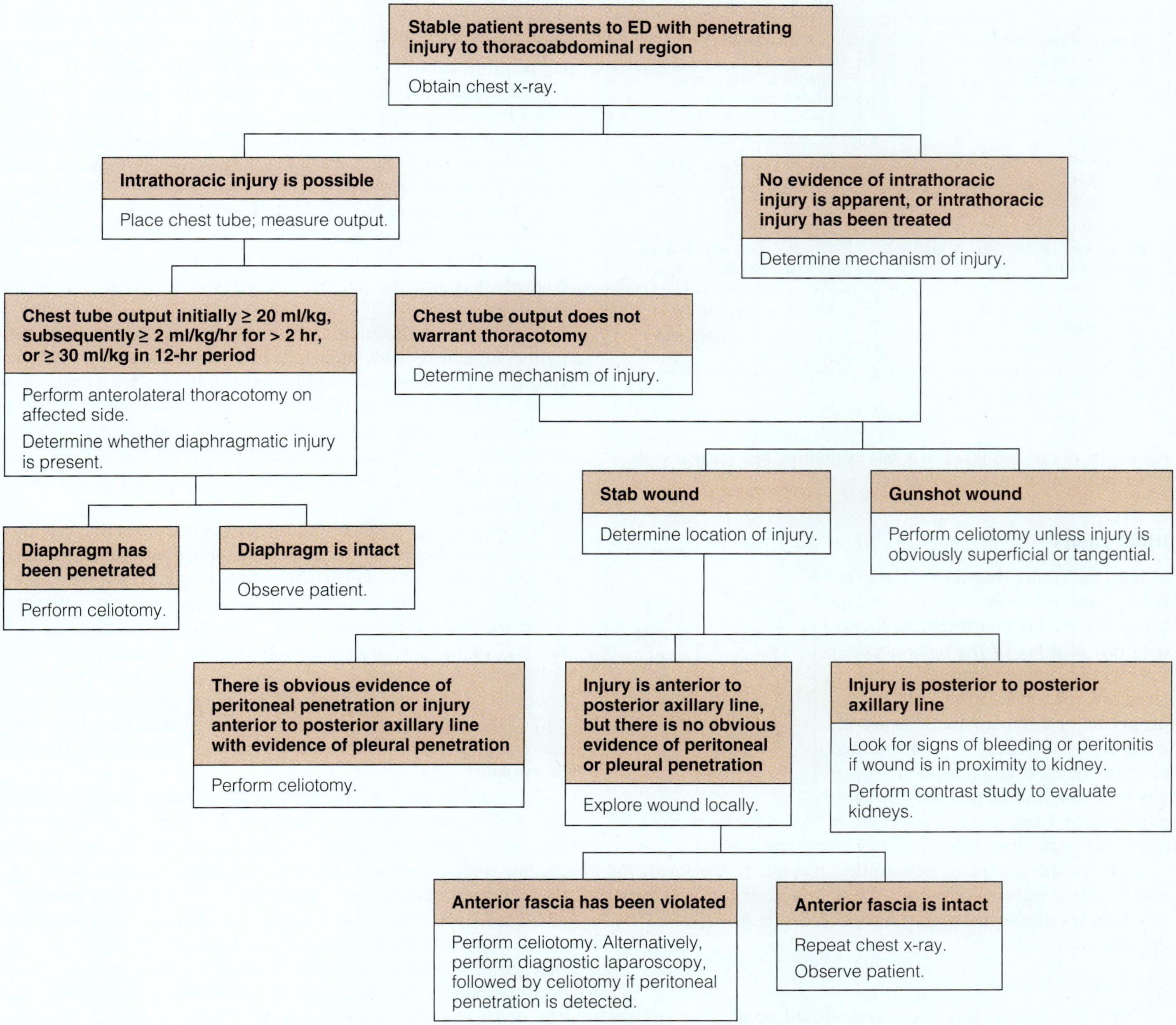

Figure 7 Algorithm illustrates ED evaluation of a stable patient with penetrating injury to the thoracoabdominal region.

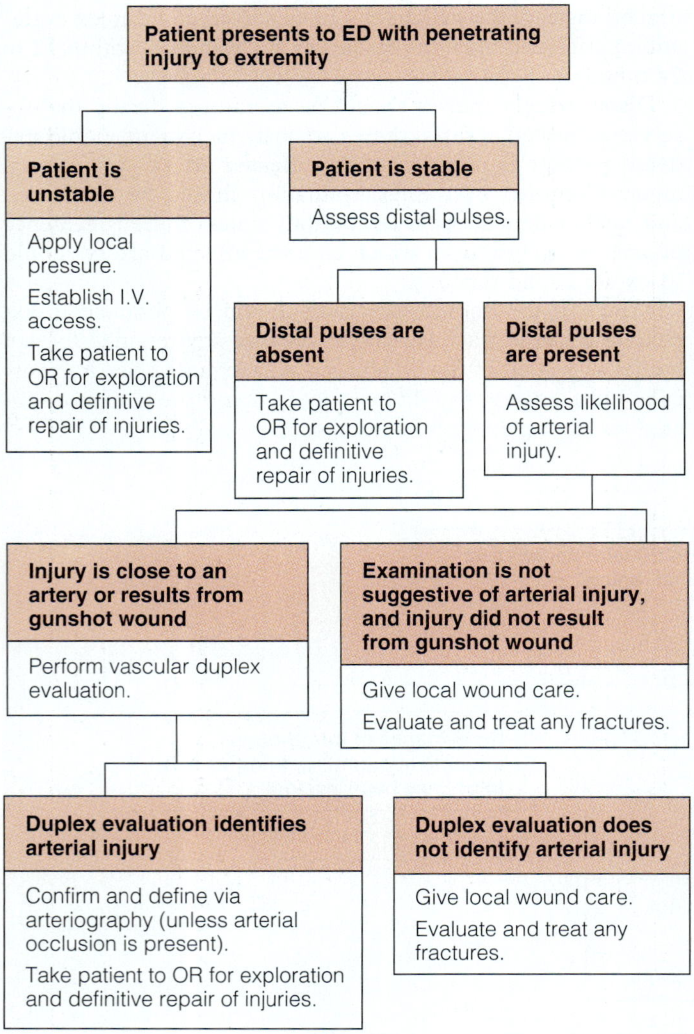

Figure 8 Algorithm

Patient presents to ED with penetrating injury to extremity

- **Patient is unstable**
  - Apply local pressure.
  - Establish I.V. access.
  - Take patient to OR for exploration and definitive repair of injuries.

- **Patient is stable**
  - Assess distal pulses.
    - **Distal pulses are absent**
      - Take patient to OR for exploration and definitive repair of injuries.
    - **Distal pulses are present**
      - Assess likelihood of arterial injury.
        - **Injury is close to an artery or results from gunshot wound**
          - Perform vascular duplex evaluation.
            - **Duplex evaluation identifies arterial injury**
              - Confirm and define via arteriography (unless arterial occlusion is present).
              - Take patient to OR for exploration and definitive repair of injuries.
            - **Duplex evaluation does not identify arterial injury**
              - Give local wound care.
              - Evaluate and treat any fractures.
        - **Examination is not suggestive of arterial injury, and injury did not result from gunshot wound**
          - Give local wound care.
          - Evaluate and treat any fractures.

Figure 8 Algorithm illustrates ED evaluation of a patient with penetrating injury to an extremity.

Blunt Injury

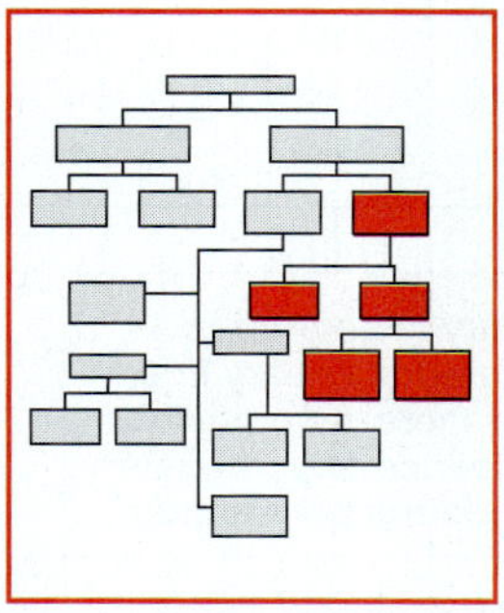

Because blunt trauma typically involves multiple body regions, evaluation is directed primarily by the hemodynamic stability of the patient rather than by the location of the main injury. Extensive ED evaluation may be appropriate for a stable patient; however, a hypotensive patient should undergo an abbreviated evaluation, rapid resuscitation, and, if indicated, urgent operative intervention, with assessment of non–life-threatening injuries left until after the patient has been stabilized.

Like the discussion of penetrating trauma (see above), the ensuing discussion is based on the assumption that the initial ABCs of trauma resuscitation have been addressed [see 2 Trauma Resuscitation].

UNSTABLE PATIENT

Once the airway has been established, evaluation of the chest and prompt decompression of any hemothorax or pneumothorax are priorities in a hypotensive blunt trauma victim [see Figure 9]. A chest tube should be inserted if breath sounds are diminished, the chest wall is grossly unstable, or subcutaneous emphysema is present. A chest x-ray should be obtained after the chest tube has been inserted to ensure proper placement and adequate decompression. In a patient without clinical signs of a hemothorax or a pneumothorax, a chest film should be obtained early in the initial evaluation period to detect occult thoracic injuries. If the patient's vital signs normalize after tube thoracoscopy, evaluation proceeds according to the specific injuries identified [see Stable Patient, below]. If the patient remains hemodynamically compromised, an urgent celiotomy should be performed to diagnose and treat any intra-abdominal injury.

When an urgent celiotomy is indicated, further evaluation is directed by the operative findings and the patient's response to the resuscitative efforts. If the intra-abdominal findings account for the patient's hemodynamic instability and the patient stabilizes after treatment, evaluation proceeds as dictated by the physical and laboratory findings. A damage control laparotomy should be performed in patients with continued hemodynamic instability and ongoing coagulopathy.[22] Non–life-threatening intra-abdominal injuries can be treated definitively at the time of reoperation. If the abdominal exploration reveals uncontrolled hemorrhage from a massive liver injury, the bleeding should be controlled and the patient transferred to the intensive care unit [see 28 Injuries to the Liver, Biliary Tract, Spleen, and Diaphragm]. Further workup for associated injuries should proceed only after the coagulopathy has resolved and the patient's hemodynamic status has been stabilized.

If the intra-abdominal findings do not account for the patient's persistent hypotension, both chest cavities should be vented (if this has not already been done) and a pericardial window created. The presence of a hemopericardium signals a cardiac injury. Blunt cardiac rupture is associated with a high mortality; however, prompt identification and treatment can increase the chances that the patient will survive this devastating injury.[23]

If laparotomy reveals a large pelvic hematoma, the stability of the pelvis should be reassessed. If the pelvic ring is disrupted and unstable, the pelvis should be stabilized by rigid fixation. This will control bleeding in most patients with unstable pelvic fractures. If pelvic bleeding continues after reduction and fixation of the fracture, it can be treated with angiographic embolization; however, in my experience, this is rarely required once the bones are stabilized. The hemodynamic instability and coagulopathy associated with massive blood loss should be corrected in the ICU before the patient is subjected to further diagnostic tests.

The indications for thoracotomy after blunt trauma are similar to those for penetrating injuries: an initial chest tube output greater than 20 ml/kg or a subsequent chest tube output greater than 2 ml/kg/hr for two consecutive hours. Although thoracic exploration can be performed through an anterolateral incision with the patient supine, pulmonary and posterior mediastinal injuries are best exposed through a posterolateral thoracotomy. Thus, once the intra-abdominal injuries have been corrected and the patient's condition is sufficiently stable, he or she can be moved to the lateral decubitus position for a posterolateral thoracotomy.

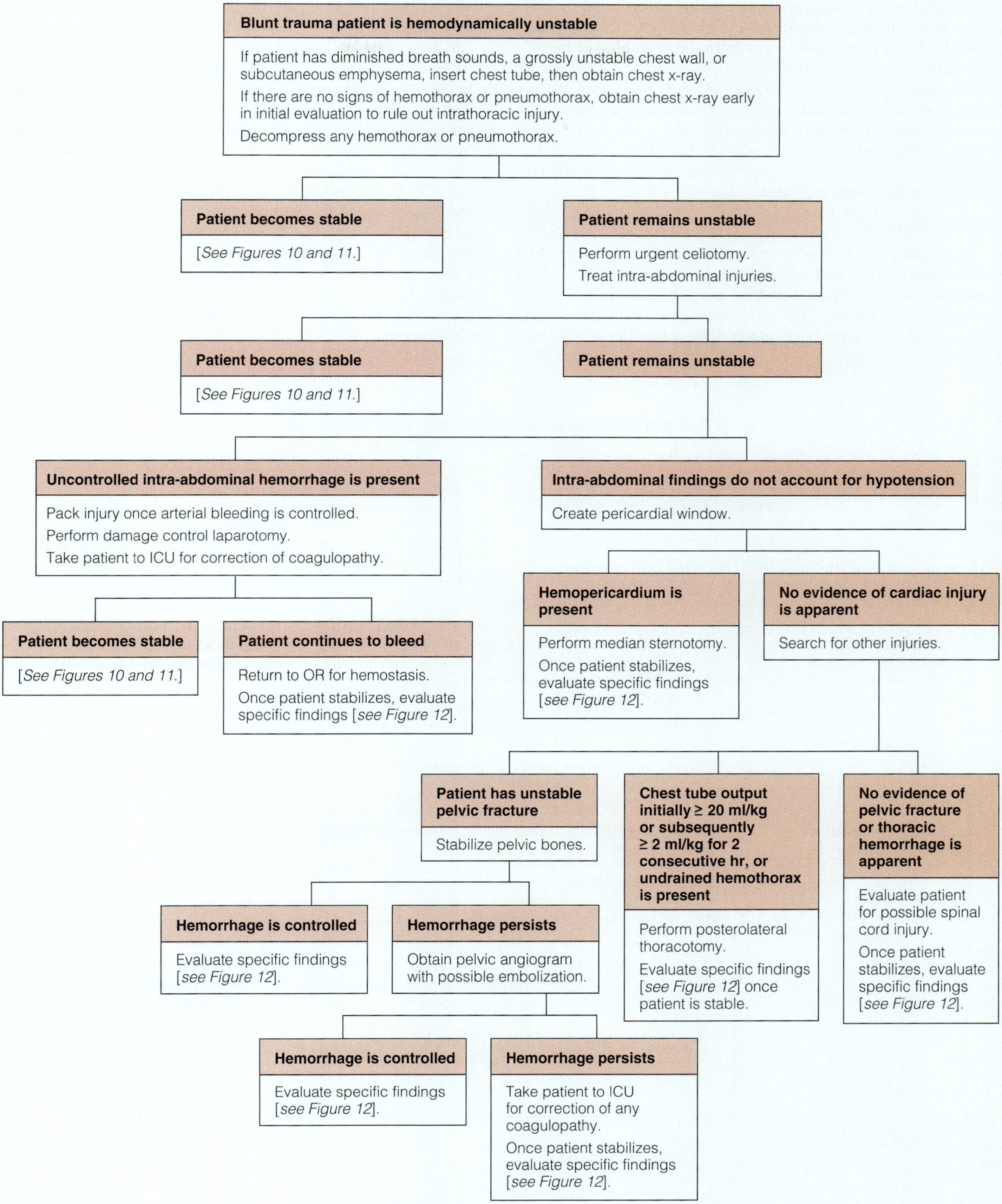

```
┌─────────────────────────────────────────────┐
│ Blunt trauma patient is hemodynamically unstable │
├─────────────────────────────────────────────┤
│ If patient has diminished breath sounds, a grossly unstable chest wall, or │
│ subcutaneous emphysema, insert chest tube, then obtain chest x-ray. │
│ If there are no signs of hemothorax or pneumothorax, obtain chest x-ray early │
│ in initial evaluation to rule out intrathoracic injury. │
│ Decompress any hemothorax or pneumothorax. │
└─────────────────────────────────────────────┘
```

Patient becomes stable
[See Figures 10 and 11.]

Patient remains unstable
Perform urgent celiotomy.
Treat intra-abdominal injuries.

Patient becomes stable
[See Figures 10 and 11.]

Patient remains unstable

Uncontrolled intra-abdominal hemorrhage is present
Pack injury once arterial bleeding is controlled.
Perform damage control laparotomy.
Take patient to ICU for correction of coagulopathy.

Intra-abdominal findings do not account for hypotension
Create pericardial window.

Patient becomes stable
[See Figures 10 and 11.]

Patient continues to bleed
Return to OR for hemostasis.
Once patient stabilizes, evaluate specific findings [see Figure 12].

Hemopericardium is present
Perform median sternotomy.
Once patient stabilizes, evaluate specific findings [see Figure 12].

No evidence of cardiac injury is apparent
Search for other injuries.

Patient has unstable pelvic fracture
Stabilize pelvic bones.

Chest tube output initially ≥ 20 ml/kg or subsequently ≥ 2 ml/kg for 2 consecutive hr, or undrained hemothorax is present
Perform posterolateral thoracotomy.
Evaluate specific findings [see Figure 12] once patient is stable.

No evidence of pelvic fracture or thoracic hemorrhage is apparent
Evaluate patient for possible spinal cord injury.
Once patient stabilizes, evaluate specific findings [see Figure 12].

Hemorrhage is controlled
Evaluate specific findings [see Figure 12].

Hemorrhage persists
Obtain pelvic angiogram with possible embolization.

Hemorrhage is controlled
Evaluate specific findings [see Figure 12].

Hemorrhage persists
Take patient to ICU for correction of any coagulopathy.
Once patient stabilizes, evaluate specific findings [see Figure 12].

Figure 9 Algorithm illustrates ED evaluation of an unstable blunt trauma patient.

Hypotension after blunt trauma should not be automatically ascribed to a head injury; instead, it should be assumed to result from hemorrhage. Hypotension associated with a head injury indicates brain stem involvement from direct trauma or herniation, either of which portends a hopeless prognosis. To assume that hypotension is the result of a head injury may delay prompt identification and treatment of hemorrhagic shock caused by a condition that may be easily manageable (e.g., a ruptured spleen). Thus, central nervous system injuries should be considered as causes of hypotension only after intra-abdominal and intrathoracic bleeding have been excluded.

STABLE PATIENT

Evaluation of a stable blunt trauma patient should proceed in the same rapid and efficient manner as evaluation of an unstable patient. Clearly, obvious peritonitis is an indication for prompt celiotomy. The real challenge in managing stable blunt trauma patients, particularly those who appear minimally injured, is to identify occult injuries, especially intra-abdominal injuries that may not be obvious at the time of initial presentation.

A chest x-ray early in the course of resuscitation provides information that is critical to the decision-making process [see Figure 10]. If a diaphragmatic hernia is identified, urgent celiotomy is indicated and further evaluation for intra-abdominal injury is unnecessary. If, however, a hemothorax large enough to warrant immediate thoracic exploration is identified [see Unstable Patient, above], diagnostic peritoneal lavage should be performed in the OR before thoracotomy. If the lavage fluid contains gross blood, celiotomy should precede thoracotomy. Once the abdominal bleeding is controlled, thoracic exploration can be performed through an anterolateral thoracotomy with the patient supine, or the patient can be repositioned for a posterolateral thoracotomy. If the lavage fluid is not bloody, the patient should be placed in the lateral decubitus position for a posterolateral thoracotomy.

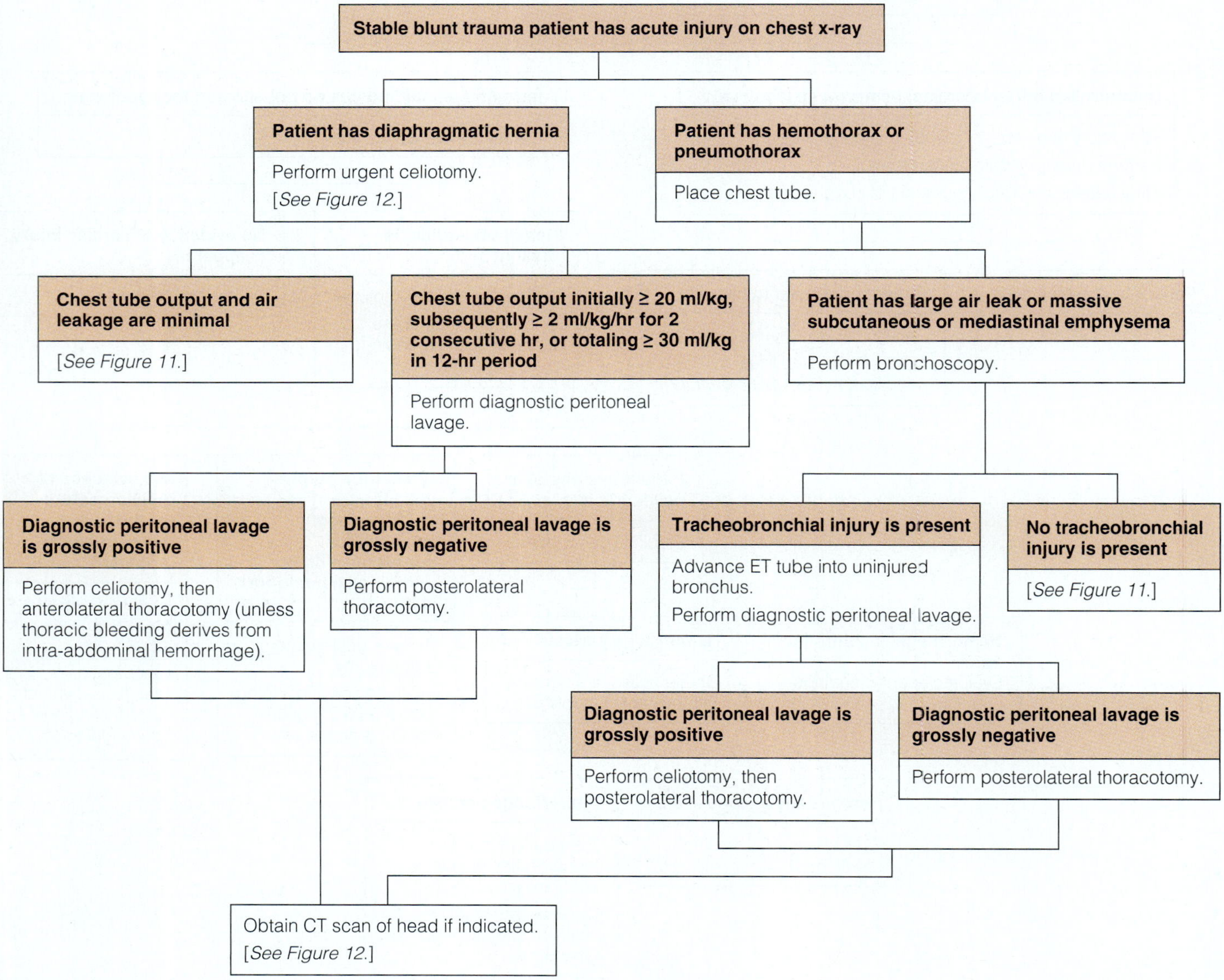

Figure 10 Algorithm illustrates ED evaluation of a stable blunt trauma patient with obvious injury.

A patient with a large air leak in the chest tube or massive subcutaneous or mediastinal emphysema should undergo bronchoscopy so that the tracheobronchial tree can be evaluated. If there is evidence of a tracheobronchial injury, the patient should undergo diagnostic peritoneal lavage before thoracotomy. Again, if the aspirate is bloody, abdominal exploration and control of bleeding should precede thoracotomy. In a patient with a large air leak caused by a tracheobronchial injury, ventilation can often be facilitated by advancing the endotracheal tube into the unaffected bronchus at the time of diagnostic bronchoscopy. The evaluation for other non–life-threatening injuries can be completed once thoracic and abdominal hemorrhage are controlled and major airway injuries are repaired.

Evaluation of the abdomen in a stable patient without intrathoracic injury or in a patient whose thoracic injury has been treated depends on the patient's neurologic status [see Figure 11]. If the patient is awake and alert, observation with serial abdominal examinations and serial blood counts is appropriate. If there is a significant associated injury (i.e., one with an abdominal injury severity [AIS] score >2),[24] such as an extremity fracture, a rib fracture, a pelvic fracture, or a head injury, the patient should be admitted to the hospital for observation.

If peritonitis develops during the observation period, celiotomy is indicated for evaluation and treatment of the intra-abdominal injury. If the patient will require prolonged surgery for associated injuries, the abdomen should be assessed preoperatively by means of CT scanning, ultrasonography, or diagnostic peritoneal lavage. If abdominal examinations yield normal results but blood counts drop significantly (i.e., the hematocrit falls by more than six percent), either CT scanning or ultrasonography is indicated to rule out occult intra-abdominal hemorrhage. If abdominal examinations continue to reveal no significant abnormalities and blood counts remain stable, the patient can be discharged after 24 hours of observation.

Evaluation of the abdomen in an obtunded or comatose patient is complicated by the unreliability of the abdominal examination. The combination of an abdominal injury that necessitates therapeutic laparotomy with a head injury that necessitates craniotomy is a rare occurrence; however, a small number of patients who have both intracranial and intra-abdominal injuries may benefit from simultaneous abdominal and cranial procedures.[25] A comatose patient should be evaluated with early diagnostic peritoneal lavage or abdominal ultrasonography in the ED to facilitate triage.[26-28] If the lavage fluid is not grossly bloody or there is no free abdominal fluid on ultrasonography, an urgent CT scan of the head should be performed. If there is gross blood in the aspirate or free abdominal fluid is apparent on ultrasonography, further steps are determined by the results of the neurologic examination. Because of the strong correlation between lateralizing motor deficits and intracranial hemorrhage that necessitates craniotomy, patients with asymmetric motor deficits should undergo a CT scan of the head before celiotomy even if there is evidence of intra-abdominal injury, provided that the patient remains hemodynamically stable. If the patient becomes hemodynamically unstable during evaluation, CT scanning should be omitted and an urgent celiotomy performed to control hemorrhage; evaluation of the brain can proceed once bleeding is controlled. The celiotomy may lead to short delays in the evaluation of the head injury; however, because hemorrhagic shock is detrimental to the injured brain as well as the rest of the patient, control of bleeding benefits both peripheral and central nervous perfusion. A patient with a nonfocal neurologic examination and evidence of intra-abdominal hemorrhage should undergo celiotomy, followed by an urgent CT scan of the head. Mannitol infusion can be used empirically to treat suspected high intracranial pressure in patients requiring urgent laparotomy or thoracotomy for hemostasis.

Evaluation of Specific Findings after Blunt Trauma

Physical examination and roentgenography will identify specific worrisome findings that call for further evaluation [see Figure 12]. When and how these findings are investigated depends on the stability of the patient, the need for surgical intervention to treat abdominal or thoracic hemorrhage, and the combination of injuries present. The trauma surgeon must prioritize the evaluation of specific findings according to the relative likelihood that a poor outcome will ensue if diagnosis is delayed. In what follows, these findings are addressed in decreasing order of urgency.

Loss of consciousness Once hemodynamic stability has been established, assessment for neurologic injury should be a priority. Whenever there has been a loss of consciousness or the neurologic examination reveals abnormalities, a CT scan of the head should be obtained.[29,30] The incidence of significant intracranial injury in patients with minor neurologic abnormalities is low; however, if an injury is missed, the potential for a poor clinical outcome is great.

A high index of suspicion is required for the diagnosis of blunt carotid artery injuries. Any patient who exhibits evidence of major cervical trauma or transient neurologic findings (e.g., hemiplegia or hemiparesis) may have a blunt carotid artery injury and should be evaluated with carotid artery duplex evaluation or arteriography.[31]

Wide mediastinum Traumatic pseudoaneurysms of the aorta should be suspected in victims of accidents involving rapid deceleration. Although x-ray findings (e.g., a depressed left mainstem bronchus, apical capping, a deviated trachea, or a deviated esophagus visualized with a nasogastric tube) may be suggestive, the mechanism of injury and the mediastinal silhouette are the two most sensitive markers for an injured thoracic aorta.[32] Evaluation of a wide mediastinum should proceed promptly once intra-abdominal hemorrhage has been controlled.

Aortography remains the gold standard for evaluating the aorta. Transesophageal echocardiography has been proposed as a screening tool; however, its sensitivity in identifying aortic injuries remains to be established.[33] Computed tomography of the chest is neither specific nor sensitive for traumatic aortic pseudoaneurysms and should not be relied on to exclude the diagnosis.[34]

Pulseless extremity The absence of distal pulses in a fractured or dislocated extremity demands urgent attention once life-threatening thoracoabdominal and head injuries have been addressed. Fractures and dislocations should be reduced promptly. If pulses return and are symmetric, no further eval-

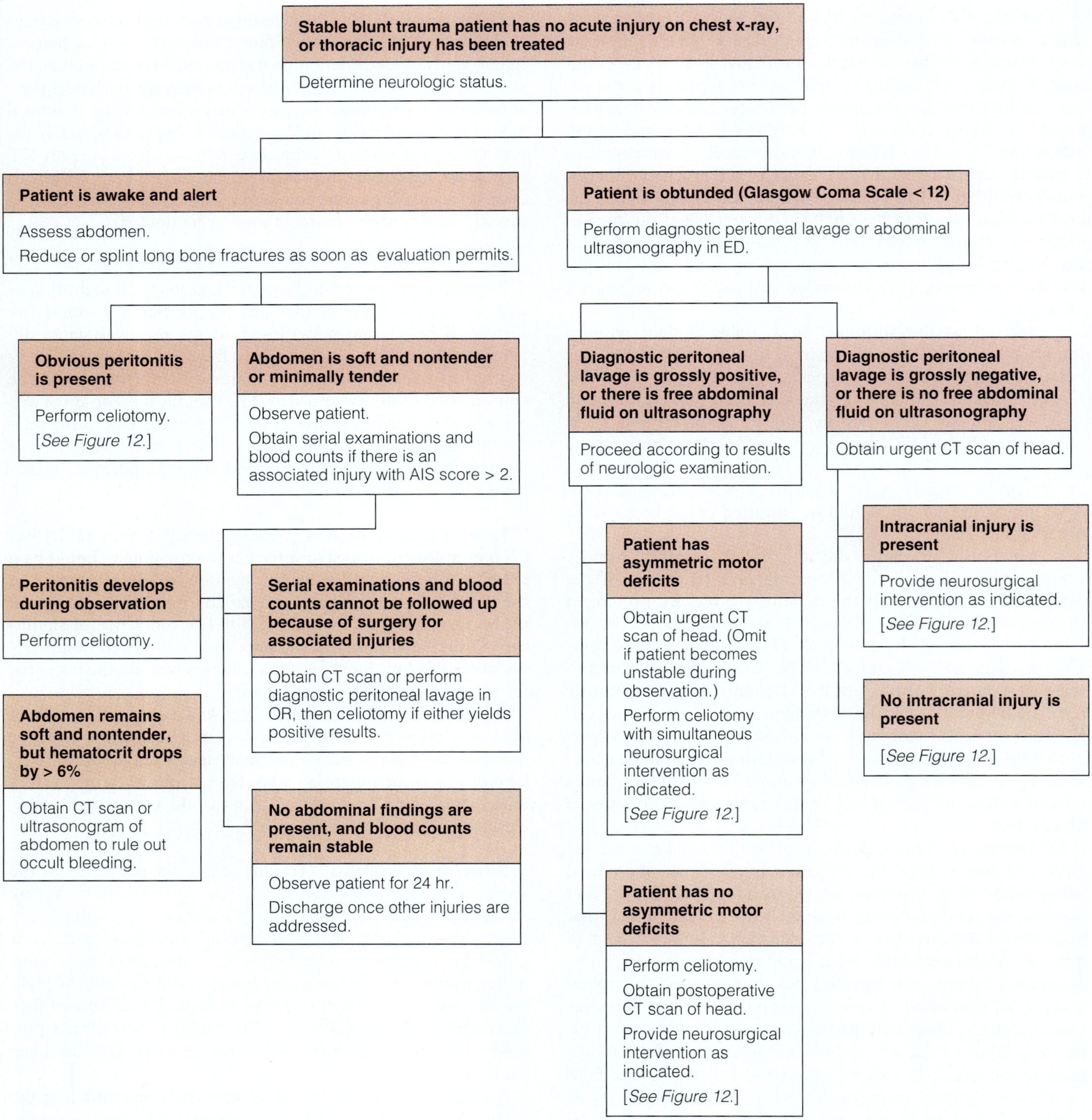

```
┌─────────────────────────────────────────────────────────┐
│ Stable blunt trauma patient has no acute injury on      │
│ chest x-ray, or thoracic injury has been treated        │
├─────────────────────────────────────────────────────────┤
│ Determine neurologic status.                            │
└─────────────────────────────────────────────────────────┘
```

Patient is awake and alert
Assess abdomen.
Reduce or splint long bone fractures as soon as evaluation permits.

Patient is obtunded (Glasgow Coma Scale < 12)
Perform diagnostic peritoneal lavage or abdominal ultrasonography in ED.

Obvious peritonitis is present
Perform celiotomy. [See Figure 12.]

Abdomen is soft and nontender or minimally tender
Observe patient.
Obtain serial examinations and blood counts if there is an associated injury with AIS score > 2.

Diagnostic peritoneal lavage is grossly positive, or there is free abdominal fluid on ultrasonography
Proceed according to results of neurologic examination.

Diagnostic peritoneal lavage is grossly negative, or there is no free abdominal fluid on ultrasonography
Obtain urgent CT scan of head.

Peritonitis develops during observation
Perform celiotomy.

Abdomen remains soft and nontender, but hematocrit drops by > 6%
Obtain CT scan or ultrasonogram of abdomen to rule out occult bleeding.

Serial examinations and blood counts cannot be followed up because of surgery for associated injuries
Obtain CT scan or perform diagnostic peritoneal lavage in OR, then celiotomy if either yields positive results.

No abdominal findings are present, and blood counts remain stable
Observe patient for 24 hr.
Discharge once other injuries are addressed.

Patient has asymmetric motor deficits
Obtain urgent CT scan of head. (Omit if patient becomes unstable during observation.)
Perform celiotomy with simultaneous neurosurgical intervention as indicated.
[See Figure 12.]

Patient has no asymmetric motor deficits
Perform celiotomy.
Obtain postoperative CT scan of head.
Provide neurosurgical intervention as indicated.
[See Figure 12.]

Intracranial injury is present
Provide neurosurgical intervention as indicated.
[See Figure 12.]

No intracranial injury is present
[See Figure 12.]

Figure 11 Algorithm illustrates ED evaluation of a stable blunt trauma patient without obvious injury.

uation is necessary; however, the patient should be monitored for the development of compartment syndrome. If vascular injury is suspected because of a weak, asymmetric pulse or if a knee dislocation is present, the artery in question should be examined with either vascular duplex evaluation or arteriography. The pulseless extremity is best evaluated in the OR. An on-table arteriogram should suffice to localize the area of injury. The vessels can then be explored and repaired promptly, and the time to reperfusion of the extremity can thereby be minimized.

Cervical spine injury Cervical spine injury is present in fewer than five percent of cases of blunt trauma.[35] Nevertheless, all patients should be screened for cervical spine injury because of the potentially devastating consequences if an injury is missed. Every patient with known or suspected

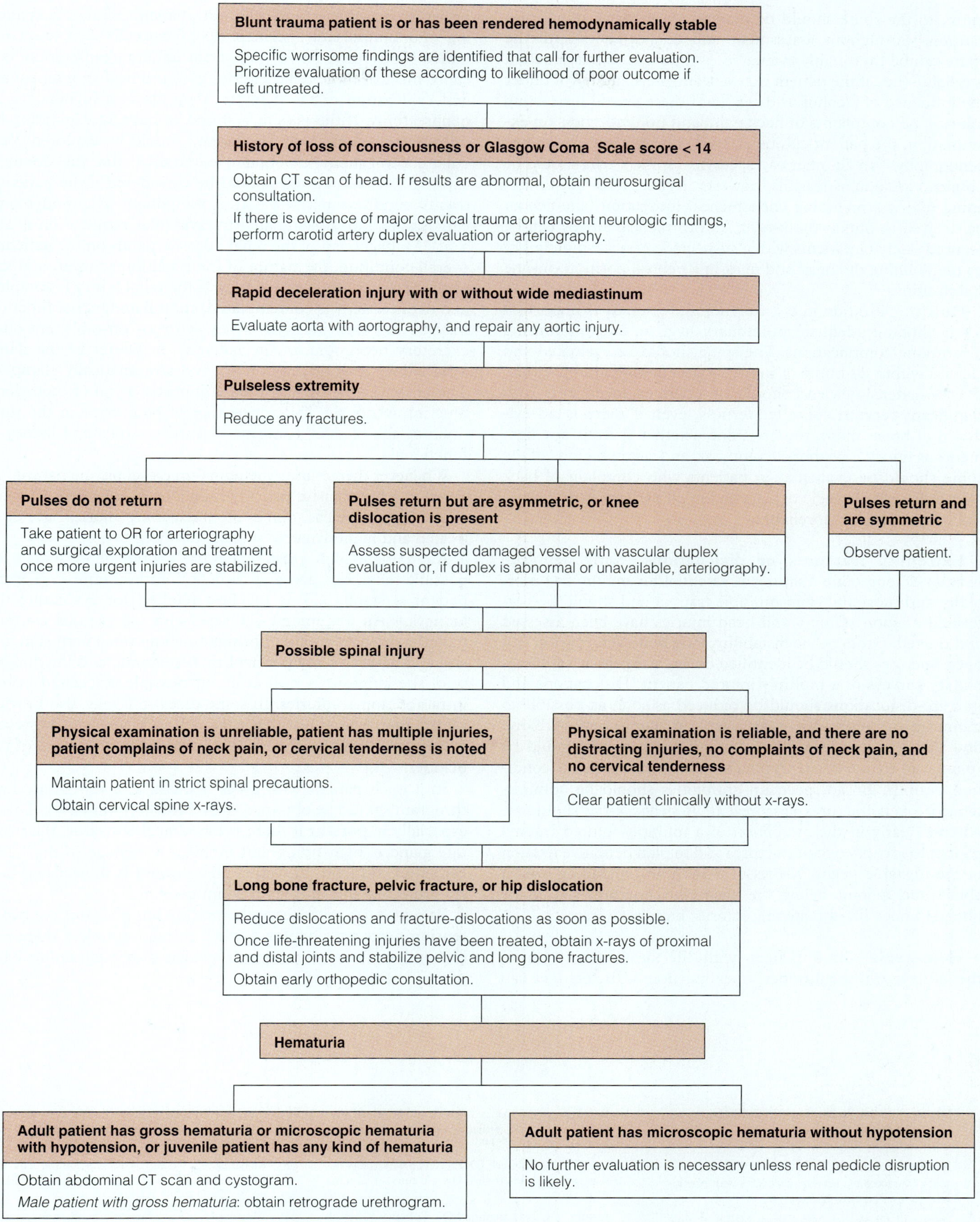

Blunt trauma patient is or has been rendered hemodynamically stable

Specific worrisome findings are identified that call for further evaluation. Prioritize evaluation of these according to likelihood of poor outcome if left untreated.

History of loss of consciousness or Glasgow Coma Scale score < 14

Obtain CT scan of head. If results are abnormal, obtain neurosurgical consultation.

If there is evidence of major cervical trauma or transient neurologic findings, perform carotid artery duplex evaluation or arteriography.

Rapid deceleration injury with or without wide mediastinum

Evaluate aorta with aortography, and repair any aortic injury.

Pulseless extremity

Reduce any fractures.

Pulses do not return

Take patient to OR for arteriography and surgical exploration and treatment once more urgent injuries are stabilized.

Pulses return but are asymmetric, or knee dislocation is present

Assess suspected damaged vessel with vascular duplex evaluation or, if duplex is abnormal or unavailable, arteriography.

Pulses return and are symmetric

Observe patient.

Possible spinal injury

Physical examination is unreliable, patient has multiple injuries, patient complains of neck pain, or cervical tenderness is noted

Maintain patient in strict spinal precautions.
Obtain cervical spine x-rays.

Physical examination is reliable, and there are no distracting injuries, no complaints of neck pain, and no cervical tenderness

Clear patient clinically without x-rays.

Long bone fracture, pelvic fracture, or hip dislocation

Reduce dislocations and fracture-dislocations as soon as possible.
Once life-threatening injuries have been treated, obtain x-rays of proximal and distal joints and stabilize pelvic and long bone fractures.
Obtain early orthopedic consultation.

Hematuria

Adult patient has gross hematuria or microscopic hematuria with hypotension, or juvenile patient has any kind of hematuria

Obtain abdominal CT scan and cystogram.
Male patient with gross hematuria: obtain retrograde urethrogram.

Adult patient has microscopic hematuria without hypotension

No further evaluation is necessary unless renal pedicle disruption is likely.

Figure 12 Algorithm illustrates evaluation of specific findings associated with blunt trauma after hemodynamic stability has been established.

injury to the spine should be maintained in strict spinal precautions throughout assessment and resuscitation until the spine can be thoroughly evaluated. If the physical examination is reliable (i.e., if the patient is awake and alert and is not under the influence of alcohol or drugs) and there are no distracting injuries, no complaints of neck pain, and no tenderness on examination, the patient can be cleared clinically without roentgenography.[36] In all other cases, cervical spine x-rays should be obtained as soon as feasible; however, treatment of life-threatening injuries (including endotracheal intubation) should not be delayed to obtain the x-rays. An orotracheal airway can be secured safely in patients with a suspected cervical spine injury by maintaining the head and neck in a neutral position (in-line stabilization).[37]

Early mobilization in critically injured patients is important for facilitating adequate pulmonary hygiene and minimizing thrombotic complications. The spine should be evaluated and cleared within 24 hours of injury to permit early mobilization. Flexion-extension views should be obtained in patients with significant cervical spine tenderness, even if there is no evidence of bone injury, to determine whether there is any ligamentous injury. The thoracic, lumbar, and sacral regions of the spine should be evaluated in patients who complain of back pain or have neurologic deficits and in all patients whose physical examination is unreliable.

Extremity fractures or dislocations Early definitive fixation of long bone fractures is essential for minimizing morbidity and mortality from multiple trauma and should be performed as soon as torso and head injuries have been assessed and treated. Gross pelvic instability, long bone deformities, and open fractures should be identified during the primary and secondary surveys of a multiply injured patient. Dislocations and fracture-dislocations should be reduced as soon as possible to minimize the morbidity associated with compromised blood flow distal to the dislocation. Long bone fractures should be splinted to reduce tissue trauma as soon as the patient's condition permits. Broad-spectrum antibiotics should be administered if open fractures are present. A pelvic x-ray should be obtained early in the evaluation of a multiply injured trauma patient to identify occult fractures and to plan definitive fixation of the unstable pelvis. X-rays of extremities, including a joint above and a joint below the suspected fracture, should be obtained once life-threatening injuries have been treated.

Hematuria In a patient with life-threatening injuries, the kidneys and the intraperitoneal portion of the bladder can be assessed at the time of celiotomy. Patients with nonexpanding and nonpulsatile perinephric hematomas that are contained by Gerota's fascia should not undergo exploration, because most of these renal injuries go on to heal spontaneously and exploration of the hematoma results in a higher rate of nephrectomy. If the patient is found to have an expanding or uncontained hematoma, the kidney should be explored. Vascular control should be obtained centrally before the kidney is exposed.[38] Renal salvage should be considered if the patient's overall condition permits (i.e., if the patient is hemodynamically stable and disseminated intravascular coagulation is absent). Management of the renal injury depends on the patient's overall condition, the nature of the renal injury itself, and the status of the contralateral kidney. If the renal injury is complex and nephrectomy is contemplated, contralateral renal function may be assessed intraoperatively with an on-table one-shot excretory nephrogram. Alternatively, the ureter of the damaged kidney may be temporarily and atraumatically clamped. The anesthesiologist may then administer a vial of methylene blue intravenously. The appearance of blue urine in the tube draining the bladder confirms that the contralateral kidney is functional.

Whenever hematuria, including microscopic hematuria, is noted in a hypotensive patient, evaluation is indicated.[39] Evaluation may proceed as soon as life-threatening injuries have been treated and hemodynamic stability has been restored.

Any patient with gross hematuria should be evaluated for possible renal, bladder, and (if male) urethral injuries.[39] If the patient is stable, CT is the best method for evaluating the kidneys.[40] An abdominal CT scan with intravenous contrast material provides useful information about renal perfusion, the size and nature of any perinephric hematoma, and the integrity of the kidneys, as well as about possible associated occult intra-abdominal injuries. In some cases, CT may also provide information about bladder injuries.[41,42] At present, however, cystography remains the study of choice for evaluation of the bladder.

In a male patient with gross hematuria, a retrograde urethrogram should be obtained to exclude urethral injury. This is especially important if there is blood at the meatus, the prostate gland is high-riding and mobile, or passage of the Foley catheter is difficult. In women, the urethra is shorter and better protected and thus is rarely injured.

Patients with microscopic hematuria but no history of hypotension need not undergo further evaluation unless there is a high index of suspicion for renal pedicle disruption on the basis of the mechanism of injury.

References

1. Durham LA 3d, Richardson RJ, Wall MJ Jr, et al: Emergency center thoracotomy: impact of prehospital resuscitation. J Trauma 32:775, 1992
2. Lorenz HP, Steinmetz B, Lieberman J, et al: Emergency thoracotomy: survival correlates with physiologic status. J Trauma 32:780, 1992
3. Harnar TJ, Oreskovich MR, Copass MK, et al: Role of emergency thoracotomy in the resuscitation of moribund trauma victims: 100 consecutive cases. Am J Surg 142:96, 1981
4. Rosemurgy AS, Norris PA, Olson SM, et al: Prehospital traumatic cardiac arrest: the cost of futility. J Trauma 35:468, 1993
5. Lerer LB, Knottenbelt JD: Preventable mortality following sharp penetrating chest trauma. J Trauma 37:9, 1994
6. Ivatury RR, Nallathambi MN, Roberge RJ, et al: Penetrating thoracic injuries: in-field stabilization vs. prompt transport. J Trauma 27:1066, 1987
7. Pepe PE, Wyatt CH, Bickell WH, et al: The relationship between total prehospital time and outcome in hypotensive victims of penetrating injuries. Ann Emerg Med 16:293, 1987
8. Richardson R, Obeid FN, Richardson JD, et al: Neurologic consequences of cerebrovascular injury. J Trauma 32:755, 1992
9. Weigelt JA, Thal ER, Snyder WH 3d, et al: Diagnosis of penetrating cervical esophageal injuries. Am J Surg 154:619, 1987
10. Noyes LD, McSwain NE Jr, Markowitz IP: Pan-

endoscopy with arteriography versus mandatory exploration of penetrating wounds of the neck. Ann Surg 204:21, 1986
11. Meyer DM, Jessen ME, Grayburn PA: Use of echocardiography to detect occult cardiac injury after penetrating thoracic trauma: a prospective study. J Trauma 39:902, 1995
12. Ordog GJ, Balasubramanium S, Wasserberger J: Outpatient management of 357 gunshot wounds to the chest. J Trauma 23:832, 1983
13. Weigelt JA, Aurbakken CM, Meier DE, et al: Management of asymptomatic patients following stab wounds to the chest. J Trauma 22:291, 1982
14. Oreskovich MR, Carrico CJ: Stab wounds of the anterior abdomen: analysis of a management plan using local wound exploration and quantitative peritoneal lavage. Ann Surg 198:411, 1993
15. Fabian TC, Croce MA, Stewart RM, et al: A prospective analysis of diagnostic laparoscopy in trauma. Ann Surg 217:557 (discussion, 564), 1993
16. Rossi P, Mullins D, Thal E: Role of laparoscopy in the evaluation of abdominal trauma. Am J Surg 166:707, 1993
17. Ivatury RR, Simon RJ, Stahl WM: A critical evaluation of laparoscopy in penetrating abdominal trauma. J Trauma 34:822, 1993
18. Fabian TC, Croce MA, Stewart RM, et al: A prospective analysis of diagnostic laparoscopy in trauma. Ann Surg 217:557, 1993
19. Bynoe RP, Miles WS, Bell RM, et al: Noninvasive diagnosis of vascular trauma by duplex ultrasonography. J Vasc Surg 14:346, 1991
20. Fry WR, Smith RS, Sayers DV, et al: The success of duplex ultrasonographic scanning in diagnosis of extremity vascular proximity trauma. Arch Surg 128:1368, 1993
21. Knudson MM, Lewis FR, Atkinson K, et al: The role of duplex ultrasound arterial imaging in patients with penetrating extremity trauma. Arch Surg 128:1033, 1993
22. Rotondo MF, Schwab CW, McGonigal MD, et al: "Damage control": an approach for improved survival in exsanguinating penetrating abdominal injury. J Trauma 35:375, 1993
23. Leavitt BJ, Meyer JA, Morton JR, et al: Survival following nonpenetrating traumatic rupture of cardiac chambers. Ann Thorac Surg 44:532, 1987
24. Association for the Advancement of Automotive Medicine: The abbreviated injury scale. Association for the Advancement of Automotive Medicine, Des Plaines, Illinois, 1990
25. Wisner DH, Victor NS, Holcroft J: Priorities in the management of multiple trauma: intracranial versus intra-abdominal injury. J Trauma 35:271, 1993
26. Rozycki GS, Ochsner MG, Schmidt JA, et al: A prospective study of surgeon-performed ultrasound as the primary adjuvant modality for injured patient assessment. J Trauma 39:492, 1995
27. Bolton JW, Bynoe RP, Lazar HL, et al: Two-dimensional echocardiography in the evaluation of penetrating intrapericardial injuries. Ann Thorac Surg 56:506, 1993
28. Rozycki GS, Ochsner MG, Jaffin JH, et al: Prospective evaluation of surgeons' use of ultrasound in the evaluation of trauma patients. J Trauma 34:516, 1993
29. Moran SG, McCarthy MC, Uddin DE, et al: Predictors of positive CT scans in the trauma patient with minor head injury. Am Surg 60:533, 1994
30. Shackford SR, Wald SL, Ross SE, et al: The clinical utility of computed tomographic scanning and neurologic examination in the management of patients with minor head injuries. J Trauma 33:385, 1992
31. Cogbill TH, Moore EE, Meissner M, et al: The spectrum of blunt injury to the carotid artery: a multicenter perspective. J Trauma 37:473, 1994
32. Kirsh MM, Behrendt DM, Orringer MB, et al: The treatment of acute traumatic rupture of the aorta: a 10-year experience. Ann Surg 184:308, 1976
33. Smith MD, Cassidy JM, Souther S, et al: Transesophageal echocardiography in the diagnosis of traumatic rupture of the aorta. N Engl J Med 332:356, 1995
34. Durham RM, Zuckerman D, Wolverson M, et al: Computed tomography as a screening exam in patients with suspected blunt aortic injury. Ann Surg 220:699, 1994
35. Soicher E, Demetriades D: Cervical spine injuries in patients with head injuries. Br J Surg 78:1013, 1991
36. Roberge RJ, Wears RC, Kelly M, et al: Selective application of cervical spine radiography in alert victims of blunt trauma: a prospective study. J Trauma 28:784, 1988
37. Rhee KJ, Green W, Holcroft JW, et al: Oral intubation in the multiply injured patient: the risk of exacerbating spinal cord damage. Ann Emerg Med 19:511, 1990
38. Carroll PR, Klosterman P, McAninch JW: Early vascular control for renal trauma: a critical review. J Urol 141:826, 1989
39. Nicolaisen GS, McAninch JW, Marshall GA, et al: Renal trauma: re-evaluation of the indications for radiographic assessment. J Urol 133:183, 1985
40. Herschorn S, Radomski SB, Shoskes DA, et al: Evaluation and treatment of blunt renal trauma. J Urol 146:274, 1991
41. Kane NM, Francis IR, Ellis JH: The value of CT in the detection of bladder and posterior urethral injuries. Am J Roentgenology 153:1243, 1989
42. Horstman WG, McClennan BL, Heiken JP: Comparison of computed tomography and conventional cystography for detection of traumatic bladder rupture. Urol Radiol 12:188, 1991

Acknowledgment

Figures 1 through 12   Marcia Kammerer.

23 INJURIES TO THE CENTRAL NERVOUS SYSTEM

Marike Zwienenberg, M.D., and J. Paul Muizelaar, M.D., Ph.D.

Approach to Injuries to the Head and Spinal Cord

It is estimated that each year, two million patients present to physicians with a primary or secondary diagnosis of head injury. Of these patients, approximately 400,000 are admitted and 70,000 die, most of traumatic brain injury. Thus, brain injury can be considered epidemic. Neurosurgeons, who number 4,000 in the United States, are probably best trained to manage patients with severe head injuries, but the initial resuscitation and stabilization is usually performed by emergency department physicians, general surgeons, and trauma surgeons. These professionals are the ones who can make a difference for patients: recent insights into the pathophysiology of traumatic brain injury indicate that treatment during the first few hours is critical and often determines outcome.

Nonetheless, the role of surgeons immediately after resuscitation and in the ensuing days is not to be underestimated. Patients with multiple system injuries often receive care in surgical intensive care units under the supervision of a general surgeon. Less than optimal management at an early stage will have a greater impact because of the larger number of patients involved, but less than optimal management at a later stage, even in a mildly injured patient, will have a much more dramatic impact. Initial recovery, followed by relentless decline attributable to insufficient cerebral perfusion, is not an expected outcome. Although we cannot promote healing of the brain with pharmacologic means, we can prevent secondary injury to the brain by ensuring adequate cerebral circulation and oxygenation.

The reported incidence of spinal cord injury in the United States ranges from 29 to 53 per million.[1-3] About 50% of the injuries are related to motor vehicle accidents, 15% to 20% to falls, 15% to 20% to interpersonal violence, and the remaining 15% to 20% to sports and recreational activity. In general, the group at highest risk is between 16 and 30 years of age, not unlike the group at highest risk for head injuries. Most of those injured are males: several studies report that the percentage is approximately 75%.[4] Between 45% and 50% of patients with spinal cord injury have associated injuries that seriously affect their prognosis.[5]

The cervical spine is most often involved in spinal cord injury. The major study of trauma outcome, conducted from 1982 to 1989, revealed that the cervical spinal cord was involved in 55% of cases, the thoracic spinal cord in 30% of cases, and the lumbar spinal cord in 15% of cases of acute injury.[6] In an analysis of 358 patients with spinal cord injury, 78% of the 71 cases of thoracic injury were accompanied by complete neurologic injury; 60% of the 202 cases of cervical injury and 65% of the 85 cases of thoracolumbar injury were accompanied by complete neurologic injury.[7] Average direct costs of spinal cord injury (including hospitalization, rehabilitation, residence modification, and long-term care) are tremendous. In 1992, it was estimated that lifetime costs (in 1989 dollars) were $210,379 for a paraplegic and $571,854 for a quadriplegic.[8]

Initial resuscitation and evaluation of injured patients are discussed more fully elsewhere [*see* 2 Trauma Resuscitation and 22 Emergency Department Evaluation of the Patient with Multiple Injuries]. In this chapter, we outline approaches to the management of severe head injury and acute spinal cord injury. In addition, we address the pathophysiology of such injuries to provide the reader with the understanding required for making appropriate decisions about diagnosis and treatment of injured patients [*see* Discussion, *below*].

Head Injury

EMERGENCY DEPARTMENT MANAGEMENT

Because hypoxia and hypotension interfere with cerebral oxygenation, complete and rapid physiologic resuscitation is the first priority for patients with head injuries. A large study from the Traumatic Coma Data Bank demonstrated that a single observation of systolic blood pressure below 90 mm Hg in the field or hypoxia (arterial oxygen tension [P_aO_2] below 60 mm Hg) was a major predictor of poor outcome.[9] A multidisciplinary team should provide the patient with an adequate airway and ventilation (intubation, ventilation, and detection of hemothorax or pneumothorax) and restore and maintain hemodynamic stability (with adequate fluid replacement and detection and treatment of any bleeding), all according to the principles developed by the Advanced Trauma Life Support system.[10] The ABCs of emergency care (airway, breathing, and circulation) take precedence, irrespective of neurologic injuries. The initial neurologic assessment, which does not take more than 10 seconds, consists of rating the patient on the Glasgow Coma Scale (GCS) [*see Table 1*] and assessing the width and reactivity of the pupils. Although the same assessment is made after resuscitation as a guide for prognosis and therapy, it should also be made (and recorded) before resuscitation to permit evaluation of the effect of resuscitative measures and differentiation between primary and secondary neurologic injury.

Early orotracheal intubation and ventilation, if not performed in the field, is recommended for patients with a GCS score of 8 or lower or a motor score of 4 or lower. Other indications for immediate intubation are loss of protective laryngeal reflexes and ventilatory insufficiency (indicated by measurement of blood gases), including hypoxemia ($P_aO_2 < 60$ mm Hg), hypercarbia (arterial carbon dioxide tension [P_aCO_2] > 45 mm Hg), spontaneous hyperventilation (causing $P_aCO_2 < 26$ mm Hg), and respiratory arrhythmia. Indications for intubation before transport are deteriorating consciousness (even if the patient is not in a coma), bilateral fractured mandible, copious bleeding into the mouth (as occurs with fracture of the base of the skull), and seizures. An intubated patient must also be ventilated ($P_aCO_2 \approx 35$ mm Hg).

Table 1 Glasgow Coma Scale

Test	Response	Score
Eye opening (E)	Spontaneous	4
	To verbal command	3
	To pain	2
	None	1
Best motor response (arm) (M)	Obedience to verbal command	6
	Localization of painful stimulus	5
	Flexion withdrawal response to pain	4
	Abnormal flexion response to pain (decorticate rigidity)	3
	Extension response to pain (decerebrate rigidity)	2
	None	1
Best verbal response (V)	Oriented conversation	5
	Disoriented conversation	4
	Inappropriate words	3
	Incomprehensible sounds	2
	None	1
	Total (E + M + V)	3–15

Fluid replacement should be performed with isotonic solutions such as lactated Ringer's solution, normal saline, or packed red blood cells when appropriate. The patient should be examined rapidly and thoroughly for any concomitant life-threatening injuries.

Patients with spinal cord injury above T5 and vasogenic spinal shock may have severe hypotension, which should be treated vigorously; induction of mild hypertension or application of pneumatic antishock trousers may be necessary. Intracranial hypertension should be suspected if there is rapid neurologic deterioration. Clinical evidence of intracranial hypertension, manifest by signs of herniation, includes unilateral or bilateral dilatation of the pupils, asymmetrical pupillary reactivity, and motor posturing.

Intracranial hypertension should be treated aggressively. Hyperventilation, which does not interfere with volume resuscitation and results in rapid reduction of intracranial pressure (ICP), should be established immediately in cases of pupillary abnormalities. Recent research has shown that unilateral or bilateral pupillary abnormalities do not result from compression of the third cranial nerves, as previously thought, but from compression of the brain stem, with resulting brain stem ischemia.[11] Therefore, administration of mannitol is effective because it not only decreases ICP but also increases cerebral blood flow (CBF) through modulation of viscosity. Because mannitol is not used to dehydrate the body, all fluid losses through diuresis must be replaced immediately or even preventively, especially in patients suffering shock as a result of blood loss. Although arterial hypertension occurring after a severe head injury may reflect intracranial hypertension (Cushing's phenomenon), especially when accompanied by bradycardia, it should not be treated, because it may be the sole mechanism permitting the brain to maintain perfusion despite increasing intracranial pressure.

In the absence of signs of herniation, sedation should be used when indicated for safe and efficient transport of the patient. Transport of the patient should be kept to a minimum because it is often accompanied by secondary insults (e.g., hypoxia or hypotension). Pharmacologic paralysis, which interferes with neurologic examination, should be used only if sedation alone is inadequate for safe and effective transport and resuscitation of the patient. When pharmacologic paralysis is used, short-acting agents are preferred. Prophylactic hyperventilation, which may exacerbate early ischemia, is not recommended for these patients. A guide to the resuscitation and initial treatment of patients with severe head injuries will assist in management [see Figure 1].

Minimal radiologic evaluation consists of a lateral cervical spine film or a swimmer's view [see Spinal Cord Injury, below]. After hemodynamic stability is achieved, unenhanced CT of the head should be used for all patients with persistent impairment of consciousness.

Operative Management

Rapid evacuation of mass lesions decreases intracranial pressure and consequently improves cerebral perfusion pressure (CPP) and CBF. Schroder and colleagues[12] have demonstrated reversal of ischemia soon after removal of a subdural hematoma. Subdural hematomas require emergent evacuation by a neurosurgeon; evacuation performed within 4 hours of injury has been shown to result in a better outcome.

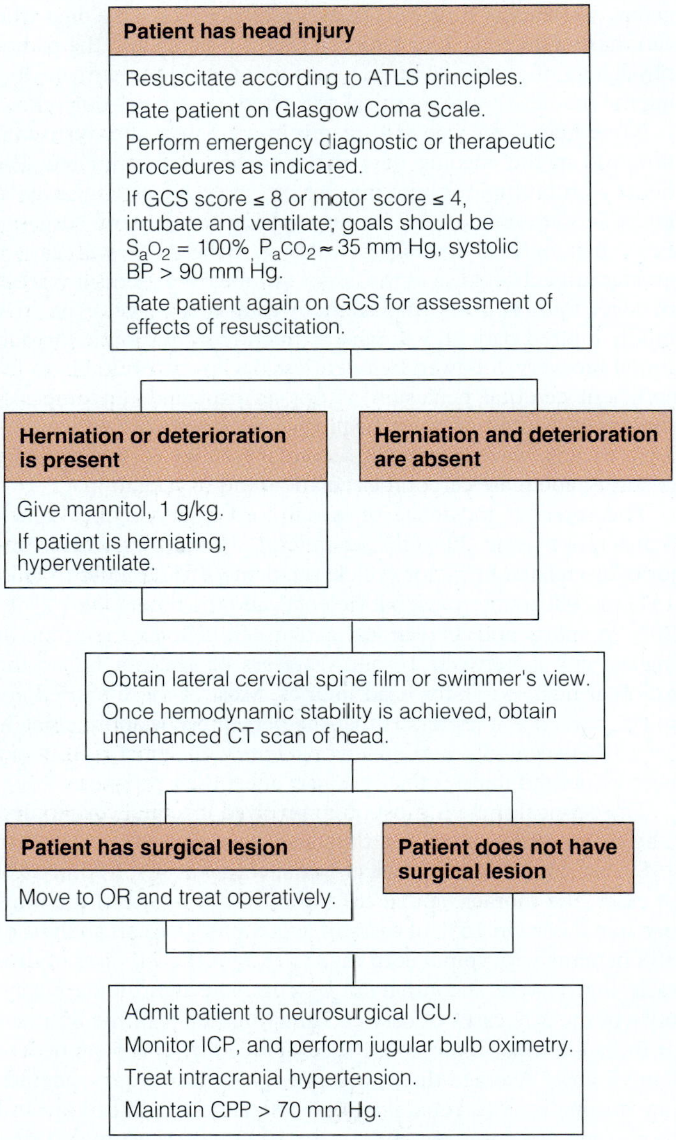

Patient has head injury

Resuscitate according to ATLS principles.
Rate patient on Glasgow Coma Scale.
Perform emergency diagnostic or therapeutic procedures as indicated.
If GCS score ≤ 8 or motor score ≤ 4, intubate and ventilate; goals should be S_aO_2 = 100% P_aCO_2 ≈ 35 mm Hg, systolic BP > 90 mm Hg.
Rate patient again on GCS for assessment of effects of resuscitation.

Herniation or deterioration is present

Give mannitol, 1 g/kg.
If patient is herniating, hyperventilate.

Herniation and deterioration are absent

Obtain lateral cervical spine film or swimmer's view.
Once hemodynamic stability is achieved, obtain unenhanced CT scan of head.

Patient has surgical lesion

Move to OR and treat operatively.

Patient does not have surgical lesion

Admit patient to neurosurgical ICU.
Monitor ICP, and perform jugular bulb oximetry.
Treat intracranial hypertension.
Maintain CPP > 70 mm Hg.

Figure 1 Shown is an algorithm for initial management of the patient with a severe head injury.

An epidural hematoma, which is a life-threatening neurosurgical emergency, should be evacuated urgently. In cases of temporal fracture and rapid clinical deterioration, a temporal craniectomy can be performed. If there is no temporal fracture, an unenhanced CT scan should be obtained to avoid searching for a lesion with multiple bur holes. In cases of progressive deterioration, moderate hyperventilation ($P_aCO_2 \approx 30$) should be initiated and mannitol (1 g/kg) given while the patient is being readied for surgery.

Posterior fossa hematomas, which are rare, also require urgent evacuation, because obstructive hydrocephalus and brain stem compression can result in rapid neurologic deterioration. An intracerebral hematoma causing a midline shift larger than 5 mm is an indication for operative treatment, but surgery can usually be delayed for a few hours.

ICU MANAGEMENT

A GCS score of 8 or lower after resuscitation is an indication for admission to a neurosurgical ICU. Although the focus of ICU management is prevention of secondary injury and maintenance of adequate cerebral oxygenation, admission to an ICU does not eliminate the occurrence of secondary insults.[13] In a series of 124 patients admitted to a neurosurgical ICU, more than one episode of hypotension occurred in 73% of all patients, and more than one episode of hypoxia occurred in 40%.[14] Kirkpatrick and coworkers[15] performed online monitoring of CPP, jugular venous saturation, local CBF, and local tissue oxygenation in 14 patients who had sustained a severe head injury; 37% of the episodes involving decreased CBF, CPP, and saturation were related to clinical and nursing procedures.

Monitoring

A variety of bedside devices are available for monitoring of ICP, local CBF, and local and global cerebral oxygenation.[13,15,16] Aside from monitors for ICP and jugular venous oxygen saturation, most of these devices are experimental.

Intracranial pressure Monitoring of ICP has never been subjected to a prospective, randomized clinical trial designed to assess its efficacy in improving patient outcome. Nevertheless, many clinical studies indicate that ICP monitoring is useful for early detection of intracranial mass lesions; that it allows calculation of CPP, an important clinical indicator of CBF; that it limits the indiscriminate use of potentially harmful therapies for control of ICP; that it helps determine prognosis; and that it may improve outcome. ICP monitoring is indicated in patients with a GCS score of 3 to 7 after resuscitation or a GCS score of 8 to 12 and an abnormal CT scan at the time of admission. In patients with a GCS score of 8 to 9 and a normal CT scan, ICP monitoring is indicated if the patient is older than 40 years, has a systolic BP below 90 mm Hg, and exhibits unilateral or bilateral motor posturing.[16]

Jugular bulb oximetry CBF is an important determinant of neurologic outcome, and the arterial–jugular venous oxygen difference (A-VDO$_2$) is an important parameter of the adequacy of CBF. Monitoring of therapy by measuring CBF and A-VDO$_2$ would be ideal, but there is no practical way of doing this directly and continuously.

An estimate of global A-VDO$_2$ can be obtained from simultaneous monitoring of arterial oxygen saturation (S_aO_2) and jugular venous oxygen saturation ($S_{jv}O_2$). Jugular venous oxygen saturation is monitored by percutaneous retrograde insertion of a fiberoptic catheter in the internal jugular vein, with the tip of the catheter located in the jugular bulb. The catheter is usually inserted into the jugular vein with the dominant cerebral venous drainage (the right jugular vein in 80% to 90% of the population), but some prefer to insert the catheter at the site of most significant brain damage.

A-VDO$_2$ is calculated according to the following formula:

$$A\text{-}VDO_2 = (S_aO_2 - S_{jv}O_2) \times 1.34 \times Hb + [(P_aO_2 - P_{jv}O_2) \times 0.0031]$$

The contribution of the variables within the brackets, which is small, is usually ignored for practical purposes. Because calculation of A-VDO$_2$ requires the drawing of blood samples, it can be done only intermittently.

For continuous monitoring, $S_{jv}O_2$, the result of arterial oxygen input and cerebral extraction, is used. In normal individuals, $S_{jv}O_2$ ranges from 50% to 70%.[17] If $S_{jv}O_2$ values below 50% last for more than 15 minutes, they are considered desaturations, resulting either from insufficient arterial oxygenation (S_aO_2) or oxygen-carrying capacity (Hb concentration) or, when arterial saturation and oxygen-carrying capacity are normal, from inadequate CBF. Gopinath and colleagues[18] [see Table 2] described a relation between the occurrence of desaturations and neurologic outcome in patients with severe head injuries. Without desaturation, mortality was 16%; with one documented desaturation, 42%; and with multiple desaturations, 70%. High $S_{jv}O_2$ values indicate low oxygen extraction, which is the case when the cerebral metabolic rate of oxygen (CMRO$_2$) is low.

The limitations of jugular bulb oximetry should be kept in mind when $S_{jv}O_2$ values are interpreted.[19,20] Because $S_{jv}O_2$ represents global oxygenation, regional ischemia may go undetected if the ischemic region is too small to be represented in the total hemispheric $S_{jv}O_2$ value. Ischemia may also occur in a part of the brain being drained by the opposite jugular vein. In addition, extracerebral veins drain into the internal jugular vein approximately 2 cm below the jugular bulb. With low flow values, significant extracerebral contamination may occur, resulting in deceptively high $S_{jv}O_2$ values. Finally, artifactual readings are often encountered as a result of reduced light intensity when the catheter lodges against the vessel wall. With a new type of catheter, however, the number of artifacts appears to be much lower.

Management of Cerebral Perfusion Pressure

The rationale behind CPP therapy is expressed in Poiseuille's law [see Discussion, Pathophysiology, below]. Although the effect of CPP therapy has not been investigated in a randomized, controlled clinical trial, several studies suggest that a CPP of 70 to 80 mm Hg may be the clinical threshold below which mortality and morbidity increase.[21,22] CPP therapy involves manipulation of both arterial BP and ICP, but its objective is the reduction of ICP. If ICP reduction does not achieve a CPP of 70 mm Hg, arterial

Table 2 Jugular Desaturation* and Outcome in 116 Patients with Severe Head Injuries[18]

Jugular Desaturations (No.)	Outcome		
	Good Recovery/ Moderate Disability (%)	Severe Disability/ Vegetative (%)	Deceased (%)
0	45	39	16
1	26	32	42
>1	10	20	70

*Defined as jugular venous oxygen saturation < 50% for longer than 15 min.

hypertension is instituted. Mean arterial BP should be raised first by achieving good volume status: ample fluids, including albumin (25 to 30 ml/hr), are administered to maintain central venous pressure at 5 to 10 mm Hg. A pulmonary arterial catheter is suggested for patients older than 50 years and for individuals with known cardiac disease, multiple trauma (particularly chest or abdominal injuries), or a need for vasopressors or high-dose barbiturates. Pulmonary arterial wedge pressure (PAWP) should be maintained between 10 and 14 mm Hg. If necessary, an alpha-adrenergic drug (e.g., phenylephrine, 80 mg in 250 or 500 ml of normal saline) can be combined with the fluids.

Management of Intracranial Pressure

Because ICP is a determinant of CPP, treatment of ICP inevitably affects CPP. Because the goal is maintenance or improvement of CBF, measures for treating ICP should be evaluated in the light of their effect on CBF. It is not possible to establish an arbitrary threshold for treatment of elevated ICP that would be applicable in all situations. Any interpretation of ICP must be combined with assessment of clinical features and evaluation of CT scan findings because it is possible to have transtentorial herniation with an ICP of 20 mm Hg in the presence of a mass lesion. Conversely, with diffuse brain swelling, adequate CPP can be maintained despite an ICP as high as 30 mm Hg. As a general rule, ICP values between 20 and 25 mm Hg indicate that therapy should be initiated.

The recommended regimen for treatment of ICP starts with drainage of CSF through a ventriculostomy-ICP catheter and continues with sedation of the patient with morphine sulfate or propofol, administration of mannitol, paralysis of the patient with pancuronium or vecuronium, initiation of hyperventilation, and induction of a coma with pentobarbital or etomidate.

Although drainage of CSF has no documented deleterious side effects, concern is occasionally expressed that it may aggravate brain shift. Therefore, only a minimal amount should be drained to decrease the ICP below 20 mm Hg. Sedation with morphine sulfate, 4 mg I.V., is standard treatment. Muscular paralysis, which is used by many clinicians, has been shown to increase the risk of respiratory complications.

Mannitol is usually administered in I.V. boluses of 0.25 to 1 g/kg over 10 to 15 minutes until ICP is controlled or serum osmolality reaches 320 mOsm/L. Because volume depletion is an important side effect of mannitol therapy, urine losses should be replaced.

As mentioned, hyperventilation reduces ICP (by vasoconstriction) and CBF, which may be at ischemic levels in certain parts of the brain. Therefore, hyperventilation ($P_aCO_2 < 30$) should not be instituted prophylactically. If P_aCO_2 must be reduced to extremely low levels, hyperventilation can be combined with mannitol, improving CBF by reducing blood viscosity. Jugular bulb oximetry is recommended in these situations because it will determine how much the cerebral blood flow can be constricted.

Hemoglobin, Hematocrit, and Blood Viscosity

To ensure optimal cerebral oxygenation, CPP, hemoglobin concentration, and oxygen saturation should be optimized; vessel diameter should be maximized; and viscosity should be in the low range. The hematocrit and viscosity are inversely related, and a balance must be established to ensure optimal oxygenation. If the hematocrit is too high, viscosity increases; if the hematocrit is too low, the oxygen-carrying capacity of blood decreases. Maintaining the hematocrit between 0.30 and 0.35 is recommended: below 0.30, the oxygen-carrying capacity falls without a significant change in viscosity, and above 0.35, the viscosity increases out of proportion to the oxygen-carrying capacity.

Brain Protection

When oxygen delivery cannot be sufficiently improved, the brain can be protected by decreasing $CMRO_2$. Barbiturates appear to protect the brain and lower ICP through several mechanisms, including alteration of vascular tone, suppression of metabolism, and inhibition of free radical lipid peroxidation. The most important effect may involve coupling of CBF to regional metabolic demands, so that the lower the metabolic requirements, the lower the CBF and the related cerebral blood volume (CBV), with subsequent beneficial effects on ICP and global cerebral perfusion. Barbiturate therapy (usually pentobarbital to a blood level of 4 mg/L) is instituted when other measures to control ICP fail. Marshall and associates,[23] in a series of 25 patients with an ICP higher than 40 mm Hg, reported that barbiturates not only controlled ICP but also improved outcome. Of the patients whose ICP was controlled, 50% had a good recovery; in the patients whose ICP was not controlled by barbiturates, 83% died. Prophylactic barbiturate therapy failed to improve neurologic outcome.[24] Of the barbiturate-treated patients, 54% were hypotensive, compared with 7% of the control subjects,[24] but this trial was conducted before the present emphasis on maintaining CPP was recognized.

Etomidate, a rapidly acting agent with hypnotic properties similar to those of barbiturates, has fewer adverse effects on systemic BP or ICP. However, it suppresses adrenocortical function, and its solvent, propylene glycol, can cause renal insufficiency.[25]

Propofol is a sedative hypnotic with a rapid onset and a short duration of action.[26,27] It depresses $CMRO_2$, but not as effectively as barbiturates and etomidate. Studies of patients with head injuries have demonstrated that ICP decreases with administration of propofol, but systemic BP usually decreases as well, resulting in a net decrease in CPP. Blood lactate levels do not increase when propofol is administered, indicating that cerebral oxygenation is adequate. Propofol is being used with increasing frequency in neurosurgical ICUs, mainly because its short half-life allows accurate neurologic examination minutes after discontinuance of its use. If propofol is used, correction of hypovolemia is recommended to prevent hypotension associated with bolus injection. Finally, because of its preservative-free, lipid-base vehicle, there is an increased risk of bacterial or fungal infection, and the high caloric content (1 kcal/ml) may be problematic during a prolonged infusion.

Hypothermia produces a balanced reduction in energy production and utilization, decreasing $CMRO_2$ and CBF proportionally. Current protocols for hypothermia include cooling to 32° to 33° C (89.6° to 91.4° F) within 6 hours of injury and maintenance of this temperature for 24 to 48 hours. Two pilot clinical trials have shown an improvement in neurologic outcome, and the results of a multicenter trial are expected in December 1998.[28,29] Hypothermia to 33° C has also been shown to be effective for refractory high intracranial pressure and for improved outcome under those conditions. Side effects of hypothermia are cardiac arrhythmias and coagulation disorders, reported after cooling to 32° to 33° C. Another drawback of hypothermia is that it is difficult to detect infection because of the lack of warning signs (e.g, spiking and elevated temperature). Finally, hypothermia requires specialized equipment (rotor beds with cooling control) as well as personnel to induce and maintain the condition.

Spinal Cord Injury

DIAGNOSIS AND INITIAL MANAGEMENT

In the field, all patients with significant trauma, any trauma patients who lose consciousness, and any patients suffering minor trauma who have complaints referable to the spine or spinal cord should be treated as if they had a spinal cord injury until proven otherwise [see Figure 2]. If cardiopulmonary resuscitation is necessary, it takes precedence. The objectives are to maintain adequate oxygenation and maintain blood pressure by administering fluids and vasopressors (avoiding phenylephrine) and placing the patient in military antishock trousers (MAST). The main concerns of management in the field are immobilization before and during extrication from a vehicle (or removal from the scene of another type of accident) and immobilization during transport to prevent active or passive movement of the spine. Subsequently, the patient may require a rigid Philadelphia collar, support from sandbags and straps, a spine board, or a log-roll for turning. A brief motor examination may detect possible deficits.

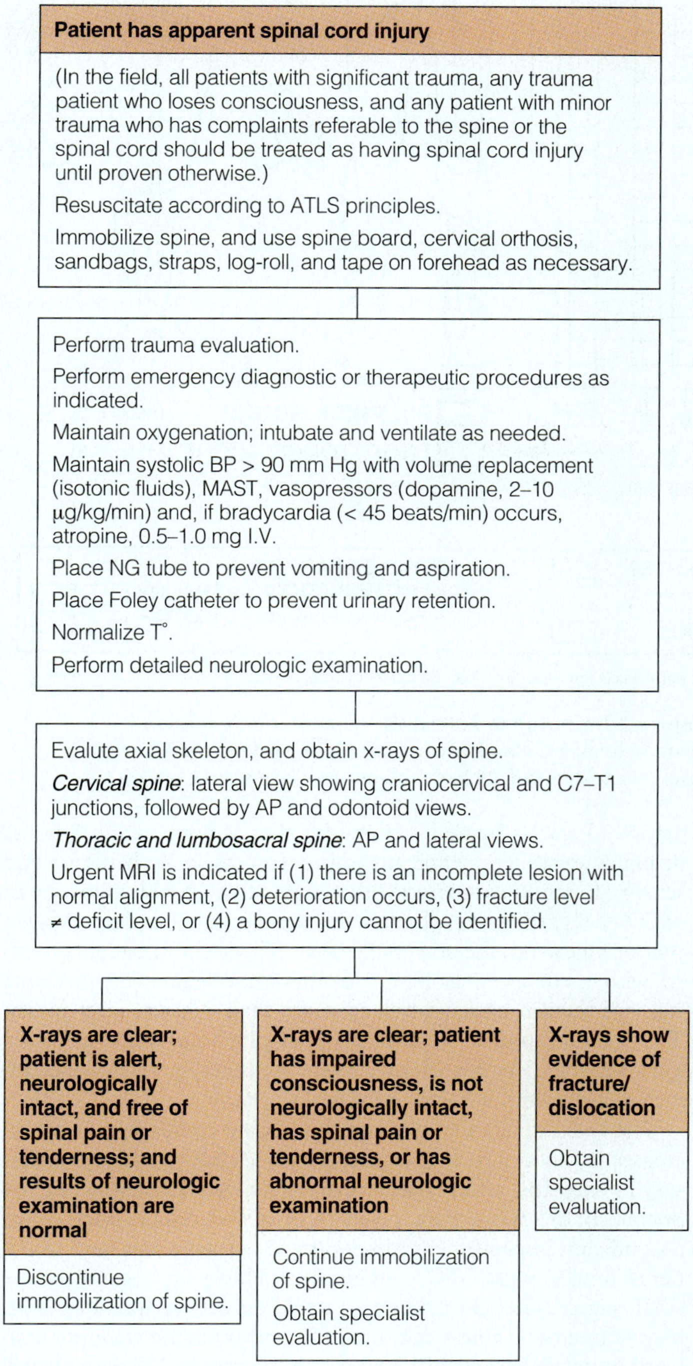

Patient has apparent spinal cord injury
(In the field, all patients with significant trauma, any trauma patient who loses consciousness, and any patient with minor trauma who has complaints referable to the spine or the spinal cord should be treated as having spinal cord injury until proven otherwise.) Resuscitate according to ATLS principles. Immobilize spine, and use spine board, cervical orthosis, sandbags, straps, log-roll, and tape on forehead as necessary.

Perform trauma evaluation.
Perform emergency diagnostic or therapeutic procedures as indicated.
Maintain oxygenation; intubate and ventilate as needed.
Maintain systolic BP > 90 mm Hg with volume replacement (isotonic fluids), MAST, vasopressors (dopamine, 2–10 μg/kg/min) and, if bradycardia (< 45 beats/min) occurs, atropine, 0.5–1.0 mg I.V.
Place NG tube to prevent vomiting and aspiration.
Place Foley catheter to prevent urinary retention.
Normalize T°.
Perform detailed neurologic examination.

Evalute axial skeleton, and obtain x-rays of spine.
Cervical spine: lateral view showing craniocervical and C7–T1 junctions, followed by AP and odontoid views.
Thoracic and lumbosacral spine: AP and lateral views.
Urgent MRI is indicated if (1) there is an incomplete lesion with normal alignment, (2) deterioration occurs, (3) fracture level ≠ deficit level, or (4) a bony injury cannot be identified.

X-rays are clear; patient is alert, neurologically intact, and free of spinal pain or tenderness; and results of neurologic examination are normal	X-rays are clear; patient has impaired consciousness, is not neurologically intact, has spinal pain or tenderness, or has abnormal neurologic examination	X-rays show evidence of fracture/dislocation
Discontinue immobilization of spine.	Continue immobilization of spine. Obtain specialist evaluation.	Obtain specialist evaluation.

Figure 2 Shown is an algorithm for management of the patient with an acute spinal cord injury.

When the patient arrives at the hospital, care should be taken to provide adequate oxygenation, prevent hypotension, and maintain immobilization. Patients with an injury above C4, who may have respiratory paralysis, may need ventilatory assistance. Lesions above T5 may be accompanied by loss of sympathetic tone and consequently by significant venous pooling and arterial hypotension. Because paralytic ileus is common, usually lasting several days, a nasogastric tube should be placed to prevent vomiting and aspiration. Because urinary retention is common, a Foley catheter should be inserted. Vasomotor paralysis may cause poikilothermy (uncontrolled temperature regulation), which should be treated with cooling blankets when necessary.

A detailed neurologic examination should ascertain whether the injury is complete or incomplete and at what level of the spinal cord the injury has occurred. If possible, a history should be taken to determine the mechanism of injury (e.g., hyperflexion, extension, axial loading, or rotation). There exists a protocol for sensory and motor examination of patients with spinal cord injuries, developed by the American Spinal Injury Association, that is precise and relatively easy to follow [see Figure 3].

Spinal shock, which occurs during major injury to the spinal cord, consists of loss of motor, sensory, and autonomic function. The motor component may consist of paralysis, flaccidity, and areflexia. The sensory component may involve both spinothalamic and dorsal column sensory function, and the autonomic component may include systemic hypotension, bradycardia, skin hyperemia, and warmth. Although the cause of spinal shock is unknown, it may be related to a disturbance in impulse conduction caused by a reversible imbalance of electrolytes or neurotransmitters. Usually, motor and sensory symptoms of spinal shock last 1 hour or less; longer-lasting deficits should be attributed to pathologic changes in the cord. Autonomic symptoms, however, may persist for days to months.

All patients with possible spine injuries should be examined radiologically. Roentgenography of the cervical spine, while the patient is in a rigid collar, should include a lateral view showing both the craniocervical and the C7-T1 junction. If the lateral view is obtained and the patient is coherent and has no neck tenderness or neurologic deficit, the collar can be removed for anteroposterior and odontoid views. If the lower cervical spine or the cervical-thoracic junction (or both) are not well visualized, a lateral view with caudal traction on the arms, or a swimmer's view, should be obtained. If the spine is still not visualized or if there is neurologic deficit, a CT scan should be obtained through the poorly visualized levels.

Anteroposterior and lateral views of thoracic and lumbosacral vertebrae should be obtained for all trauma patients who were thrown from a vehicle or fell more than 6 ft to the ground, complain of back pain, are unconscious, cannot reliably describe back pain or have altered mental status preventing adequate examination, or have an unknown mechanism of injury or other injuries that suggest the possibility of spinal injury.

Indications for an urgent MRI include the following: an incomplete lesion with normal alignment (to rule out the possibility that soft tissue is compressing the spinal cord); deterioration (worsening deficit or rising level); a fracture level different from the level of deficit; and the inability to identify a bony injury (to rule out the possibilities of soft tissue compression, disk herniation, or hematoma that would necessitate surgery).

In approximately 10% to 15% of adults and 40% of children with injury to the cervical spinal cord, no radiologic abnormalities are evident in plain, flexion, and extension films. Many patients have reversible incomplete cord lesions, but more severe lesions

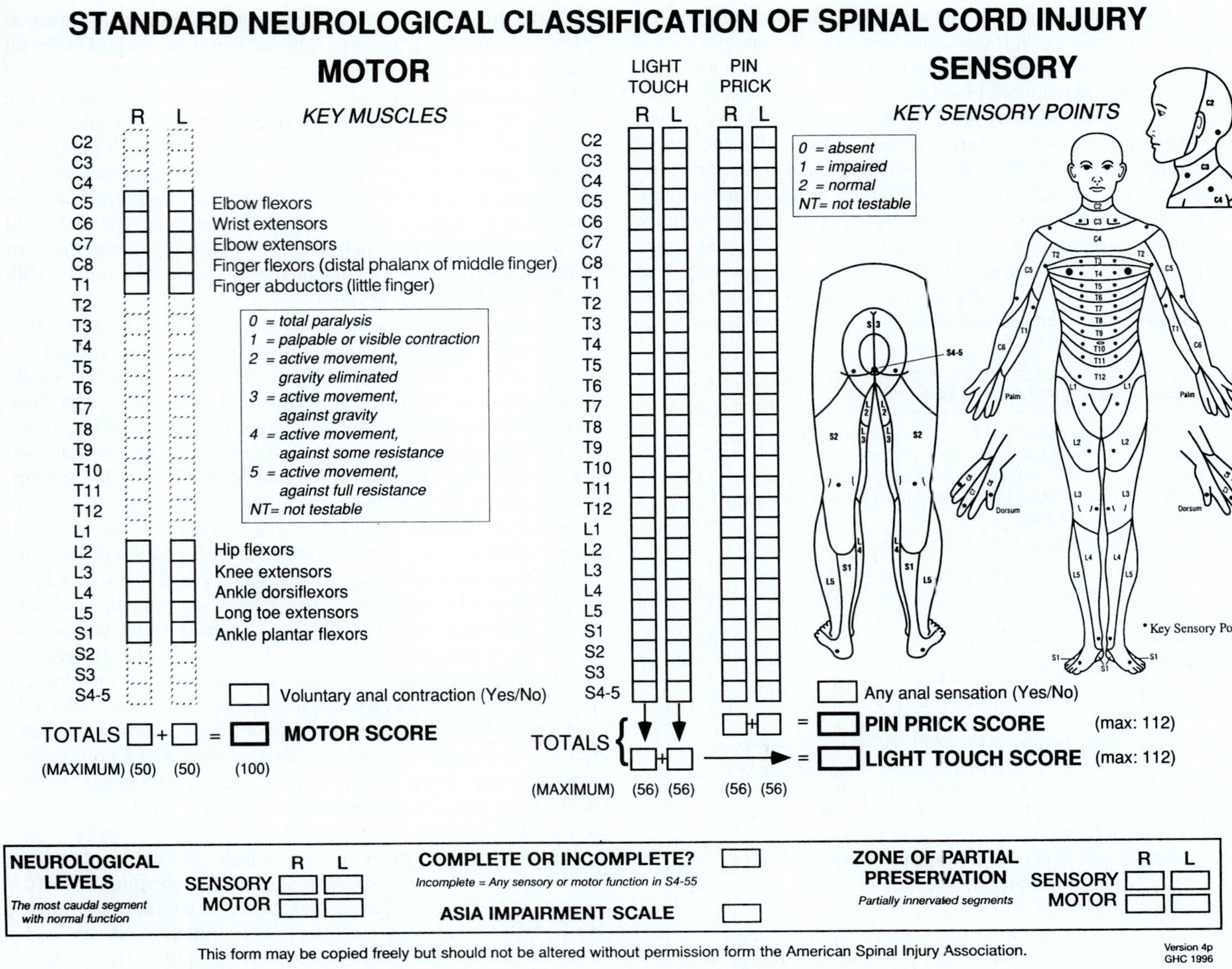

STANDARD NEUROLOGICAL CLASSIFICATION OF SPINAL CORD INJURY

MOTOR

KEY MUSCLES

	R	L	
C2			
C3			
C4			
C5			Elbow flexors
C6			Wrist extensors
C7			Elbow extensors
C8			Finger flexors (distal phalanx of middle finger)
T1			Finger abductors (little finger)
T2			
T3			
T4			
T5			
T6			
T7			
T8			
T9			
T10			
T11			
T12			
L1			
L2			Hip flexors
L3			Knee extensors
L4			Ankle dorsiflexors
L5			Long toe extensors
S1			Ankle plantar flexors
S2			
S3			
S4-5			Voluntary anal contraction (Yes/No)

0 = total paralysis
1 = palpable or visible contraction
2 = active movement, gravity eliminated
3 = active movement, against gravity
4 = active movement, against some resistance
5 = active movement, against full resistance
NT= not testable

TOTALS ☐+☐ = ☐ MOTOR SCORE
(MAXIMUM) (50) (50) (100)

SENSORY

KEY SENSORY POINTS

LIGHT TOUCH R L — PIN PRICK R L: C2, C3, C4, C5, C6, C7, C8, T1, T2, T3, T4, T5, T6, T7, T8, T9, T10, T11, T12, L1, L2, L3, L4, L5, S1, S2, S3, S4-5

0 = absent
1 = impaired
2 = normal
NT= not testable

Any anal sensation (Yes/No)

TOTALS ☐+☐ = PIN PRICK SCORE (max: 112)
☐+☐ = LIGHT TOUCH SCORE (max: 112)
(MAXIMUM) (56) (56) (56) (56)

• Key Sensory Points

NEUROLOGICAL LEVELS The most caudal segment with normal function		R	L	COMPLETE OR INCOMPLETE? Incomplete = Any sensory or motor function in S4-55	☐	ZONE OF PARTIAL PRESERVATION Partially innervated segments		R	L
	SENSORY	☐	☐				SENSORY	☐	☐
	MOTOR	☐	☐	ASIA IMPAIRMENT SCALE	☐		MOTOR	☐	☐

This form may be copied freely but should not be altered without permission form the American Spinal Injury Association.

Version 4p GHC 1996

Figure 3 **Shown is a form developed by the American Spinal Injury Association to record the principal information about motor, sensory, and sphincter function required for accurate neurologic classification of spinal cord injury. For the motor examination, 10 key muscles are tested (left). For the sensory examination, 28 key dermatomes are tested (right).**

are observed in elderly people. Explanations for this phenomenon include spontaneous reduction of a subluxation, hyperextension injury, and disk prolapse. With MRI, T_2 (spin-spin)-weighted images may show increased signal within the spinal cord parenchyma.

TREATMENT

Traction

The objectives of craniocervical traction are to reduce fracture-dislocations, to maintain normal alignment or immobility of the cervical spine, to prevent further injury, to decompress the spinal cord and roots, and to facilitate bone healing. A common technique is placement of Gardner-Wells tongs.

Pharmacologic Treatment

A variety of drugs are known to interfere with the processes of secondary injury. The challenge is to identify the most effective treatment or combination of treatments with the fewest severe side effects, a challenge requiring many experiments for each treatment tested. Methylprednisolone, thought to act by scavenging free radicals, has been reported to be neuroprotective in spinal cord injury.[30,31] Patients treated with methylprednisolone within 8 hours of injury exhibited significant improvements in both motor and sensory function compared with patients treated with naloxone or placebo, regardless of whether the injury was complete. After 1 year of follow-up, the advantage was still evident in patients treated with methylprednisolone, but this improvement in outcome was not seen in patients treated more than 8 hours after injury. The regimen studied comprised a 30 mg/kg bolus followed by 5.4 mg/kg/hr for 23 hours. Many centers use methylprednisolone, administered within 8 hours of injury.

The calcium channel blocker nimodipine causes significant increases in blood flow in the spinal cord,[32,33] but the dosage necessary to exert this effect is accompanied by significant systemic hypotension. In a prospective, placebo-controlled, double-blind study, a significant improvement in neurologic outcome was seen in patients treated with GM_1 ganglioside.[34] However, because of the small sample size (34 patients), certain aspects of spinal cord injury or treatment that might have affected outcome were not analyzed in detail. Results of a large phase III trial in 800 patients will be available in November 1998. The third National Acute Spinal Cord Injury Study (NASCIS), initiated in 1991, compared methylprednisolone given for either 24 or 48 hours with tirilazad mesylate (an oxygen and lipid radical scavenger).[35] Methylprednisolone was administered in a bolus of 30 mg/kg within 8 hours of injury. Patients receiving methylprednisolone for 48 hours exhibited significant improvement in motor function compared with patients treated with the same agent for 24 hours after injury; however, the patients treated for 48 hours suffered from more severe sepsis and pneumonia. Overall, mortality was identical in the two groups receiving methylprednisolone. Motor function after 6 months in patients treated with tirilazad was similar to that of patients treated with methylprednisolone for 24 hours. On the basis of these findings, the authors suggested that methylprednisolone therapy started within 3 hours of injury should be continued for 24 hours, whereas methylprednisolone treatment started 3 to 8 hours after injury should be continued for 48 hours.

Surgical Treatment

The role of neurosurgery in the treatment of spinal fractures and spinal cord injury is controversial. There is considerable disagreement as to whether surgery should be performed, what type of surgery should be done, and when should it be done. The primary goal of treatment is to restore spinal stability, provide for early mobilization and rehabilitation, and maximize neurologic recovery.

There is general agreement among physicians that early immobilization and early stabilization of fractures and dislocations of the spine are necessary. The single widely accepted indication for early surgical treatment is ongoing neurologic deterioration in the presence of spinal canal compromise from bone and disk fragments, hematoma, or unreduced subluxation. Surgical indications still under debate include incomplete spinal cord injury (with persistent spinal cord deformity) and complete spinal cord injury with the possibility of some neurologic recovery.

Early surgical intervention has been associated with an increased risk of systemic complications (especially pulmonary) and neurologic deterioration. Marshall and coworkers[36] found that one third of all cases of neurologic deterioration could be attributed directly to surgical intervention; 4 of 26 patients who underwent spinal surgery within 5 days deteriorated, while none of the patients treated after 5 days had any neurologic sequelae.

Other studies, however, have not found an increased risk of deterioration with early intervention. Wilberger[37] studied 110 patients with cervical spinal cord injury, of whom 88 underwent surgery for spinal stabilization; in the 39 patients treated within 24 hours, the incidence of systemic complications was reduced by 50% compared with the incidence in the 49 patients treated 24 hours to 3 weeks after injury. In addition, the incidence of neurologic deterioration was 0% in the early-stabilization group versus 2.5% in the late-stabilization group. Data from the NASCIS II study showed improved outcome in patients undergoing surgery within 24 hours of injury compared with patients treated after 200 hours, but the difference was not statistically significant.[38] To date, there is no clear evidence that early surgical intervention improves outcome.

Diagnosis and Treatment of Specific Fractures and Dislocations

Cervical spine Injuries to the cervical spine include atlas fractures, axis fractures, fractures of the lower cervical spine, and atlanto-occipital and atlantoaxial dislocations. Atlanto-occipital dislocations are rare, occurring in approximately 1% of the patients with injury to the cervical spine. Most of these patients die immediately after trauma because of brain stem injury and respiratory arrest. Treatment, which is controversial, consists of either operative fusion or 4 to 6 months of immobilization in a Halo brace. Atlantoaxial dislocations, which are often fatal and therefore seldom encountered in clinical practice, are usually associated with an odontoid fracture. Because of severe ligamentous injury, these lesions are unstable.

Atlas (Jefferson) fractures, which represent 5% to 10% of all cervical spine fractures, result from axial load. Because of the large diameter of the spinal canal and the tendency of fragments to move outward, these fractures usually are not accompanied by significant neurologic injury, but 40% of patients with an atlas fracture have another cervical fracture (e.g., a fracture through both C1 arches). Treatment requires rigid immobilization in a Halo vest.

Axis fractures account for 10% to 20% of all cervical spine fractures in adults and 70% of cervical fractures in children. Odontoid fractures are the most common (60%). Fractures of the tip of the odontoid process (avulsion fracture, type I) are uncommon and unstable and may require surgical fusion. Fractures of the neck (type II) or at the junction of the odontoid process and the axis (type III) are more common (65% to 80% and 20% to 35%, respectively); they call for Halo-vest immobilization when the dislocation is less than 6 mm and open reduction and internal fixation when the dislocation is greater than 6 mm. Traumatic spondylolisthesis, or hangman's fracture, accounts for approximately 20% of C2 fractures. Injury usually results from axial compression in combination with hyperextension of the occipito-atlanto-axial complex on the lower spine, resulting in bilateral fracture of the pars interarticularis. Fractures affecting the ring of the axis without C2-C3 angulation are stable and can be treated with immobilization in a Philadelphia collar or a sterno-occipito-mandibular immobilizer (SOMI) brace. Halo-vest immobilization is recommended in unreliable patients or patients with both C1 and C2 fractures. The average healing time is 11.5 weeks.

Approximately 80% of all fractures of the lower cervical spine are produced by indirect forces. The vertebra most commonly involved is C5, and dislocations are most frequent at the C5-C6 level. The following injury mechanisms are observed: flexion and distraction (approximately 40% of cases), flexion and compression (22%), vertical compression (8%), extension and compression (24%), extension and distraction (6%), and lateral flexion (3%).

Flexion and distraction injuries usually result from a blow to the occiput from below. The initial disruption is within the posterior ligamentous complex, leading to facet dislocation and abnormally large divergence of the spinous processes. Unilateral facet dislocation and facet interlocking result when a rotatory component is involved. Bilateral facet dislocation with anterior translation of the superior vertebra results from severe hyperflexion. Cord and root involvement vary with the degree of luxation and translation: 50% of patients with unilateral facet dislocation present with moderate cord and root injury, and 90% of patients with bilateral facet dislocation and a full translation of the vertebral body have neurologic deficits, predominantly a complete cord lesion. Teardrop fractures (a bone chip just beyond the anterior inferior edge of the vertebral body) result from severe hyperflexion injury, and the fractured vertebra is usually displaced posteriorly on the vertebra below; these patients are often quadriplegic. Flexion and extension x-rays should be obtained to evaluate ligamentous injury.

Flexion and compression injuries, usually observed at C4-C5 and C5-C6 levels, usually result from a blow to the back of the head. The effect on the anterior vertebral body varies from a moderate rounding or loss of anterior height to a wedge shape with an oblique fracture from the anterior surface to the inferior subchondral plate. Approximately 50% of patients with the latter type of injury have a neurologic deficit. More severe injuries are accompanied by translation of the inferior posterior margin of the vertebral body into the neural canal. About 75% of pa-

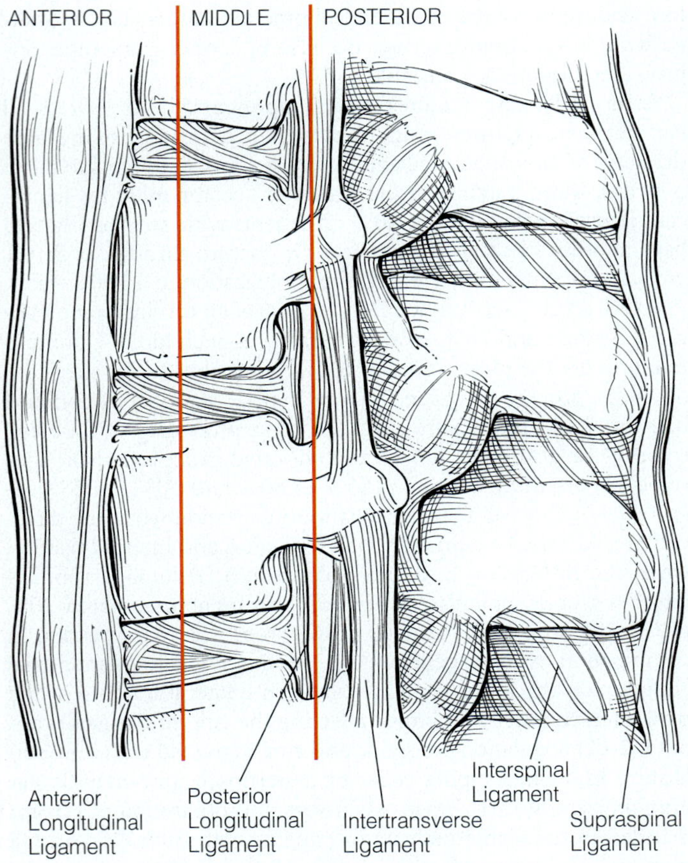

Figure 4 **Illustrated is the three-column concept for assessment of spinal stability. If two or more columns are destroyed or nonfunctional, instability is likely.**

tients have neurologic involvement. Translations of more than 3 mm result in a complete spinal cord lesion in most cases.

Extension and compression injuries are usually caused by a blow to the forehead and result in fractures of the posterior complex. About 40% of patients with unilateral vertebral arch fractures (articular process, pedicle, or lamina) have a neurologic deficit, predominantly a radiculopathy. Bilaminar fractures are accompanied by a complete cord lesion in 40% of cases. Bilateral vertebral arch fractures with complete anterior translation of the vertebral body present with radiculopathy (30%), central cord syndrome (30%), or incomplete cord lesion (30%). In Allen's series,[39] no complete cord lesions were observed with this type of injury.

Treatment of injuries to the lower cervical spine has not been standardized. As a general rule, severe ligament involvement and severe vertical compression require surgical intervention. Severely comminuted vertebral body fractures may also require surgery because of the high risk of progressive kyphosis. In the series reported by Lind and Nordwall,[40] 87% of patients with distractive flexion injury and 88% of those with compressive flexion injury healed with Halo-vest immobilization.

Thoracolumbar spine Approximately 64% of fractures of the spine occur at the T12-L1 junction, and 70% of these fractures are unaccompanied by immediate neurologic injury. Evaluation according to Denis' three-column principle[41] [see Figure 4] is useful for determining whether a fracture is stable, although the precise definition of stability remains controversial. Fractures of the thoracic spine (T1–T10) are more stable because of support from the surrounding rib cage and the strong costovertebral ligaments. When two of the three columns are affected, the fracture is considered unstable and generally requires surgical intervention. If there is no neurologic deficit, surgery can be performed by an orthopedic surgeon or a general surgeon, but if there is a neurologic deficit, a neurosurgeon should perform the operation. In general, the following conditions require surgical intervention: open lesions and dural lacerations, progressive neurologic deficit, marked and progressive angulation, and spinal instability.

The four major types of thoracolumbar spine injuries are compression fractures, burst fractures, seat belt fractures, and fracture-dislocations. These four types of fracture involve the anterior, middle, and posterior columns of the spine in different ways [see Table 3].

Minimal to moderate compression fractures with an intact posterior column can be treated with analgesics and bed rest. Ambulation should be started early, and depending on the degree of kyphosis, external immobilization (from a corset or a Boston brace) may or may not be indicated.

Severe compression injuries and seat-belt injuries should be treated with external immobilization in extension. If the loss of anterior height of the vertebral body exceeds 75%, there is an increased risk of progressive kyphosis. Occasionally, surgical intervention is required. An anterior injury is considered unstable if more than three elements in a row, or more than 50% of the height in a single element with angulation, is present.

Burst fractures are considered unstable even if there is no initial neurologic deficit. Early ambulation should be avoided because the axial loading may result in progressive collapse or angulation, with concomitant neurologic damage. Severe burst fractures with neurodeficit should be treated with surgical decompression and stabilization. L5 burst fractures are usually managed conservatively, because it is difficult for spinal instrumentation to maintain alignment at this level; if progressive deformity occurs, L4-S1 fixation is indicated.

Fracture-dislocations require surgical decompression and stabilization.

Table 3 Column Failure in the Four Types of Major Thoracolumbar Spinal Injury[41]

Fracture Type	Anterior Column	Middle Column	Posterior Column
Compression	Compression	Intact	Intact, or distraction if severe
Burst	Compression	Compression	Intact
Seat belt	Intact or mild compression of 10%–20% of anterior vertebral body	Distraction	Distraction
Fracture-dislocation	Compression, rotation, shear	Distraction, rotation, shear	Distraction, rotation, shear

Discussion

Pathophysiology

HEAD INJURY

Cerebral Metabolism

At 1,200 to 1,400 g, the brain accounts for only 2% to 3% of total body weight and does not do any mechanical work; yet it receives 15% to 20% of all cardiac output to meet its high metabolic demands. Of the total energy generated, 50% is used for interneuronal communication and the generation, release, and reuptake of neurotransmitters (synaptic activity), 25% is used for maintenance and restoration of ion gradients across the cell membrane, and the remaining 25% is used for molecular transport, biosynthesis, and other, as yet unidentified, processes.

Cell metabolism involves the consumption of adenosine triphosphate (ATP) during work and the ensuing consumption of metabolic substrates to resynthesize ATP from adenosine diphosphate (ADP). ATP is generated both in the cytosol (via glycolysis) and in the mitochondria (via oxidative phosphorylation). Glucose is the sole energy substrate, unless there is ketosis, and 95% of the energy requirement of the normal brain comes from aerobic conversion of glucose to water and CO_2. ATP generation is highly efficient. Glycolysis and subsequent oxidative phosphorylation result in the generation of 38 molecules of ATP for each molecule of glucose:

$$1 \text{ glucose} + 6\, O_2 + 38\, ADP + 38\, P_i \rightarrow 6\, CO_2 + 44\, H_2O + 38\, ATP$$

In the absence of oxygen, anaerobic glycolysis can proceed, but energy production is much less efficient. Two molecules of ATP and two molecules of lactate are generated for each molecule of glucose:

$$1 \text{ glucose} + 2\, ADP + 2\, P_i \rightarrow 2 \text{ lactate} + 2\, ATP$$

Regulation of Blood Flow

Because the reserves of glucose and glycogen within the astrocytes of the brain are limited and there is no significant storage capacity for oxygen, the brain depends on blood to supply the oxygen and glucose it requires. More specifically, substrate availability is determined by its concentration in blood, flow volume, and the rate of passage across the blood-brain barrier.

Under normal circumstances and with certain physiologic alterations, an adequate supply of substrates can be maintained by regulation of CBF. CBF increases with vasodilatation and decreases with vasoconstriction. Caliber changes take place mainly in cerebral resistance vessels (i.e., arterioles with a diameter of 300 μm down to 15 μm).[42,43] Control of CBF by influencing vessel caliber is commonly referred to as autoregulation of blood flow.

Metabolic autoregulation CBF is functionally coupled to cerebral metabolism, changing proportionally with increasing or decreasing regional or global metabolic demand. Thus, the brain precisely matches local CBF to local metabolic needs. Because 95% of the energy in the normal brain is generated by oxidative metabolism of glucose, $CMRO_2$ is considered to be a sensitive measure of cerebral metabolism. The relation between CBF and metabolism is expressed in the Fick equation:

$$CMRO_2 = CBF \times A\text{-}VDO_2$$

$CMRO_2$, expressed in milliliters per 100 g of brain tissue, is normally about 3.2 ml/100 g/min in awake adults.[17] The average CBF value for mixed cortical flow is 53 ml/100 g/min in a healthy adult. $A\text{-}VDO_2$, a measure of cerebral oxygen extraction, can be calculated by subtracting the oxygen content of jugular venous blood (6.7 ml/dl) from that of arterial blood (13 ml/dl), resulting in a value of 6.3 ml/dl; this value can then be corrected for hemoglobin content according to the formula discussed earlier [see Head Injury, ICU Management, above]. Under conditions of increasing metabolic demand (increased $CMRO_2$), such as seizures or fever, CBF increases proportionally, thus keeping $A\text{-}VDO_2$ constant. With decreasing metabolism (anesthesia, deep coma), CBF decreases.

Pressure autoregulation Another important physiologic property of the cerebral circulation is maintenance of a constant supply of substrates at the level set by metabolism. According to Poiseuille's equation,

$$CBF = k\, \frac{CPP \times d^4}{8 \times l \times v}$$

in which d represents vessel diameter, l represents vessel length, and v represents blood viscosity, changes in CPP (e.g., arterial hypotension or increases in ICP) would be followed by changes in CBF, unless diameter regulation (so-called pressure autoregulation) takes place.[44] In humans, the limits of pressure autoregulation range from 40 to 150 mm Hg of perfusion pressure.

Viscosity autoregulation In accordance with Poiseuille's equation, CBF can vary with changes in the viscosity of blood. Blood viscosity changes with variations in hematocrit, γ-globulin, and fibrinogen components of plasma protein. Increased viscosity would increase cerebrovascular resistance ($8 \times l \times v/d^4$). By means of diameter adjustment (viscosity autoregulation), cerebrovascular resistance is decreased and CBF can be kept constant.[45]

CO_2 reactivity Vascular caliber and cerebral blood flow are also responsive to changes in arterial P_aCO_2. Cerebral blood flow changes 2% to 3% for each mm Hg in P_aCO_2 within the range of 20 to 60 mm Hg. Hypercarbia (hypoventilation) results in vasodilatation and higher CBF, and hypocarbia (hyperventilation) results in vasoconstriction and lower CBF. Autoregulation is a compensatory or adaptive response adjusting cerebral blood flow to metabolism; with CO_2 variation, vessel caliber changes and CBF follow passively. The vessels respond not to changes in P_aCO_2 but to the pH in the perivascular space. CO_2 can cross the blood-brain barrier freely, thus changing the pH, but over 20 to 24 hours, with a constant new level of P_aCO_2, the pH in blood and in the perivascular space returns to baseline, and the diameter of cerebral blood vessels also returns to baseline.[46] With CO_2 reactivity, changes in CBF are compensated for by changes in $A\text{-}VDO_2$, so that a constant supply of substrates is maintained at the level set by metabolism ($CMRO_2$). A constant $A\text{-}VDO_2$ is a common feature of metabolic, pressure, and viscosity autoregulation; because CBF is tuned to metabolism ($CBF \approx CMRO_2$), $A\text{-}VDO_2$ can be kept constant.

Cerebral Circulation and Metabolism after Severe Head Injury

Arterial hypoxia and hypotension It is known from eyewitness reports of head injury and experimental studies immediately after the impact that arterial hypotension and interruption of normal respiration, sometimes with a period of prolonged apnea, are common findings. In the days after a head injury, there are many occasions and opportunities for hypoxic and hypotensive insults. Studies have identified hypotension (systolic BP below 90 mm Hg) and hypoxia (P_aO_2 below 60 mm Hg) as major determinants of poor outcome.[9,14,47]

The effect of hypotension on the brain depends on the status of autoregulation. If autoregulation is defective, decreased blood pressure leads directly and linearly to a decrease in CBF. If autoregulation is intact, arterial hypotension can lead to a considerable increase in ICP, which interferes with CBF by decreasing perfusion pressure.

Raised intracranial pressure According to the Monro-Kellie doctrine,[48,49] ICP is governed by three factors within the confines of the skull: brain parenchyma plus cytotoxic edema; CSF plus vasogenic edema; and CBV. When the volume in one compartment increases, ICP increases unless there is a compensatory decrease in volume in the other compartments. The relation between intracranial volume and ICP is expressed in the pressure-volume index (PVI).[50] PVI is defined by the volume that must be added to or withdrawn from the craniospinal axis to raise or decrease ICP 10-fold:

$$PVI = \frac{\Delta V}{\log ICP_i / ICP_o}$$

where ΔV represents the change in volume, ICP_o represents ICP before the volume change, and ICP_i represents ICP after the volume change. PVI is thus a measure for the compliance ($\Delta V/\Delta P$) or tightness of the brain. Under normal circumstances, PVI is 26 ± 4 ml; 26 ml of volume will raise ICP from 1 to 10 mm Hg, but the same volume will also raise ICP from 10 to 100 mm Hg. Conversely, a change in volume of only 6.4 ml is necessary to increase intracranial pressure from 10 mm Hg (normal) to the treatment threshold of 20 mm Hg. Thus, small changes in volume have a relatively large effect on ICP.

Apart from mass lesions, intracranial pressure typically increases after severe head injury because of cerebral edema. Initial compensation is by displacement of CSF from the cranium, which is visualized in a CT scan of the head as small ventricles and basal cisterns. Subsequent compensation would be by a decrease in CBV, which can be accomplished by means of vasoconstriction.

Relation between vessel diameter, cerebral blood volume, and intracranial pressure The total diameter of the cerebrovascular bed determines CBV. Cerebral veins contain most of the total blood volume, but their diameter and, thus, their volume are relatively constant. Approximately 20 ml of blood (i.e., one third of total CBV) is located in the cerebral resistance vessels (which range in diameter from 300 μm down to 15 μm).[51] Because most autoregulatory and CO_2-dependent variations in diameter take place in these vessels, cerebral blood volume is determined mainly by their diameter. Typically, the diameter ranges from 80% to 160% of baseline, resulting in volume changes between 64% and 256% of baseline. With a baseline value of 20 ml in the resistance vessels, CBV will range from 13 ml (maximal vasoconstriction) to 51 ml (maximal vasodilatation). Given a pressure-volume index of 26, change from maximal vasoconstriction to maximal vasodilatation will be accompanied by an almost 29-fold change in ICP.

Cerebral blood volume, intracranial pressure, and cerebral blood flow CBF and CBV are governed by vascular diameter. Thus, depending on other parameters influencing CBF (such as mean arterial BP, ICP, and blood viscosity), changes in vascular caliber also affect CBF.

Hypocarbia reduces ICP by means of vasoconstriction, consequently improving CPP. However, net CBF is decreased because in Poiseuille's equation, vessel diameter is carried to the fourth power. A randomized clinical trial has shown that preventive hyperventilation retards clinical improvement after severe head injury, perhaps through reduction of CBF to ischemic levels.[52] However, its rapid effect on ICP is of great advantage in cases of acute neurologic deterioration (e.g., in the presence of an expanding mass lesion before evacuation can take place) and should be reserved for these situations.

There are two methods of reducing ICP by means of vasoconstriction without affecting CBF. The first is to reduce blood viscosity. As can be deduced from Poiseuille's equation, decreasing the blood viscosity will, by itself, lead to vasoconstriction, provided that viscosity autoregulation is intact. With impaired autoregulation, decreased viscosity will result in an increase in CBF but no decrease in ICP. However, this effect can be used to maintain CBF under vasoconstriction with hypocarbia. The effect of mannitol on ICP is thought to be mediated in part by lowering blood viscosity.[53,54]

The second method of reducing ICP without affecting CBF is to increase CPP, which can be done by raising blood pressure. Again, with intact autoregulation, an increase in CPP will lead to vasoconstriction, with net CBF remaining constant. With impaired autoregulation, CBF will follow CPP passively, and maintenance of normal blood pressure may be indicated in these cases. More important, however, is the avoidance of hypotension under these circumstances; the effect of CPP therapy may be attributable in part simply to prevention of hypotension.[21,55]

Cerebral ischemia Cerebral ischemia, defined as CBF that is inadequate to meet the metabolic demands of the brain, is an important mechanism of secondary injury in patients with severe head injury, and the adequacy of CBF has been associated with neurologic outcome. In autopsy findings from patients dying after severe head injury, histologic damage indicative of cerebral ischemia was seen in 80% of cases.[56] Bouma and associates[57] found ischemia (CBF < 18 ml/dl with abnormally high A-VDO_2 values) in 20% to 33% of patients with severe head injuries within 4 to 12 hours of injury, and the ischemia was associated with a poor prognosis. Of the intracranial lesions, acute subdural hematoma and diffuse cerebral swelling were most often associated with ischemia.

The relation between cerebral metabolism and CBF is expressed in the Fick equation [see Metabolic Autoregulation, above]. The normal brain tends to keep A-VDO_2 constant and to react to changes in metabolism with adjustments in blood flow. When CBF decreases in response to metabolism (as with hyperventilation or decreasing CPP with impaired autoregulation), oxygen supply is maintained by increasing oxygen extraction (i.e., A-VDO_2 increases). Increasing A-VDO_2 is thus a sensitive marker of insufficient cerebral perfusion. However, oxygen extraction is limited, and this limit is reached when A-VDO_2 is doubled (13.2 ml/dl). Consequently, any further reduction in CBF results in neuronal dysfunction (i.e., $CMRO_2$ decreases). Because 50% of the energy is used for synaptic activity, a reversible and functional loss is usually observed first. Further decline, however, will result in ion pump failure, loss of membrane integrity, consequent cell swelling (cytotoxic edema), and cell death (irreversible infarction). The occurrence of irreversible infarction depends on both the level and the duration of ischemia. When cerebral blood flow decreases to approximately 18 ml/100 g/min for more than 4 hours, it reaches the threshold for irreversible infarction.[58]

Maintenance or improvement of CBF is thus essential to the treatment of severe head injury, and A-VDO$_2$ is a sensitive marker of the adequacy of therapy. When therapeutic measures fail to sustain CBF, CMRo$_2$ can be decreased to reinstate the match between CBF and metabolism. CNS suppression can be obtained with the administration of hypnotic agents (e.g., barbiturates or propofol) or the induction of hypothermia. Decreasing cell metabolism will result in reduced production of CO$_2$, lactic acid, or both and (with blood vessels almost always remaining responsive to perivascular pH changes) in vasoconstriction accompanied by reductions in both CBF and ICP. The relations between CMRo$_2$, CBF, CBV, CPP, and A-VDO$_2$ are complicated. An overview is available elsewhere[59] [see Table 4].

Altered cerebral metabolism Anaerobic metabolism of glucose to the end product lactate is characteristic of cerebral hypoxia/ischemia.[60] Increased lactate production, hyperglycolysis, and low tissue glucose levels have been observed after severe head injury, suggesting an increased turnover of glucose by the anaerobic glycolytic pathway. Increased lactate levels have also been found in the presence of preserved CBF,[61,62] suggesting impairment not only of oxygen delivery but also of oxidative metabolism (i.e., of mitochondrial function). Recent findings in animals and humans indicate that mitochondrial function is impaired after severe head injury, which may explain poor outcomes despite adequate CBF levels; ATP generation by anaerobic glycolysis is usually insufficient to maintain the metabolic activity of the brain.[63,64] In part, however, such poor outcomes may be attributable to the effects of lactate production (acidosis), because high lactate and hydrogen ion levels interfere with the functional recovery of tissue.

SPINAL CORD INJURY

Spinal cord injury is often viewed as an all-or-nothing event that is irreversible from the moment of injury. By this view, spinal cord injury is classified as either incomplete or complete. This dichotomy is not absolute, however, because some functional recovery occurs even after severe spinal cord injury. The Second National Acute Spinal Cord Injury Study revealed that patients with so-called complete loss of neurologic function recovered on average 8% of the function they had lost, and patients with an incomplete injury recovered 59% of what they had lost.[65] An injury classified as complete does not necessarily involve loss of all connections. Several studies have demonstrated that many patients with a clinically complete lesion show evidence of residual connection.[66] A certain number of intact connections is probably necessary for functional recovery. The determinants of functional outcome are complex, however, and probably include not only the extent of axonal loss but also the level of dysfunction of the surviving axons and the plasticity of the spinal cord.

Animal studies have found that a small number of axons may be sufficient to support functional recovery.[67-69] Animals recover evoked potentials and the ability to walk with as few as 10% of their spinal axons. Nerve sprouting, one of the mechanisms of plasticity, allows a few nerves to carry out the function of many. Finally, animal studies have also shown that many of the axons surviving traumatic injury are dysfunctional and that many of the axons had lost part or all of their myelin sheath, which is the structural component that improves the reliability and speed of conduction. 4-Aminopyridine, an axon-excitatory drug used for the treatment of multiple sclerosis, has significantly improved conduction in animals and humans with spinal cord injury.[70-72] Unfortunately, the drug must be given continuously to support axon function, and this is not feasible in humans because of its side effects (seizures, tachycardia, and hyperthermia).

Injury initiates complex responses in the body and the spinal cord. Ischemia is a prominent feature of events occurring after spinal cord injury.[73,74] Within 2 hours of a spinal cord injury, there is a significant reduction in spinal cord blood flow. It is unclear whether this is mechanically or biochemically induced. Like the brain, the spinal cord possesses autoregulatory capacity (pressure autoregulation). When this autoregulation is impaired, blood flow becomes dependent on systemic blood pressure. In a patient with multiple injuries or vasogenic spinal shock (a lesion above T5) complicating the spinal cord injury, severe systemic hypotension may exacerbate the effects of spinal cord injury.

Edema, another prominent feature of spinal cord injury, tends to develop first at the injured site, subsequently spreading to adjacent and sometimes distant segments. The relation between spreading edema and potential worsening of neurologic function is poorly understood. The inflammatory response to injury ideally cleans up cellular debris and repairs tissue. This response is accompanied, however, by the release of toxic substances, which cause further tissue damage, or secondary injury. Processes resulting in secondary injury involve generation of free radicals, excessive calcium influx and excitotoxicity, the release of eicosanoids and cytokines, and programmed cell death.

Conclusion

Mortality has decreased considerably in patients with severe head injury. In the patients we have studied, mortality has decreased from approximately 40% to 45% in the decade between 1975 and 1984 to 25% to 30% at present, with a further downward trend evident. Increased recognition of the mechanism of secondary brain injury as well as avoidance of secondary insults by optimizing cerebral perfusion and oxygenation are probably responsible for most of the improvement in outcome. Pharmacologic brain protection and attempts to intervene in the damaging cascade of biochemical events occurring after injury have shown some beneficial effects in phase II trials, but no compound has clearly shown efficacy when tested in multicenter phase II clinical trials. Targeted strategies or combinations of drugs, based on

Table 4 Changes in CBF, CBV, ICP, and A-VDO$_2$ Associated with Primary Reduction of Selected Variables[59]

Variable Reduced	CBF	CBV (ICP)	A-VDO$_2$
CMRO$_2$	↓	↓	—
CPP (autoregulation intact)	—	↑	—
CPP (autoregulation defective)	↓	↓	↑
Blood viscosity (autoregulation intact)	—	↓	—
Blood viscosity (autoregulation defective)	↑	—	↓
P$_a$CO$_2$	↓	↓	↑
Conductance vessel diameter (vasospasm above ischemia threshold)	↓	↑	↑

A-VDO$_2$—arteriovenous oxygen content difference CBF—cerebral blood flow CBV—cerebral blood volume CMRO$_2$—cerebral metabolic rate of oxygen CPP—cerebral perfusion pressure ICP—intracranial pressure P$_a$CO$_2$—arterial carbon dioxide tension

pathophysiologic concepts, are expected to provide the major breakthrough in research on treatment of head injury.

The results in patients with acute spinal cord injury are not spectacular. Methylprednisolone has provided a modest improvement in outcome, suggesting that pharmacologic intervention can curtail damage from ongoing biochemical cascades in central nervous system injuries. As in research on head injuries, better insight into pathophysiology is a major focus. Early stabilization and multidisciplinary care, which can prevent some of the systemic and neurologic complications of spinal cord injury, can improve outcome.

References

1. Fine P, Kuhlemeier K, DeVivo M, et al: Spinal cord injury: an epidemiological perspective. Paraplegia 17:237, 1979
2. Kalsbeek W, McLaurin R, Harris B, et al: The National Head and Spinal Cord Injury Survey: major findings. J Neurosurg 53:S19, 1982
3. Kraus J, Franti C, Riggins R, et al: Incidence of traumatic spinal cord lesions. J Chron Dis 28:471, 1975
4. Kraus J: Epidemiological aspects of acute spinal cord injury: review of incidence, prevalence, causes and outcome. Central Nervous System Trauma Status Report, 1985. Becker D, Poulishock J, Eds. National Institute of Neurological and Communicative Disorders and Stroke, Bethesda, Maryland, 1985, p 313
5. Factsheet No. 2: Spinal cord injury statistical information. National Spinal Cord Injury Association, Woburn, Massachusetts, 1992
6. Burney R, Maio R, Maynard F, et al: Incidence, characteristics, and outcome of spinal cord injury at trauma centers in North America. Arch Surg 128:596, 1992
7. Tator C: Spine-spinal cord relationships in spinal cord trauma. Clin Neurosurg 30:479, 1983
8. Gibson C: An overview of spinal cord injury. Phys Med Rehab Clin North Am 3:699, 1992
9. Chesnut RM, Marshall SB, Piek J, et al: Early and late systemic hypotension as a frequent and fundamental source of cerebral ischemia following severe brain injury in the Traumatic Coma Data Bank. Acta Neurochir Suppl (Wien) 59:121, 1993
10. American College of Surgeons Committee on Trauma: Advanced Life Support Course for Physicians, Instructor Manual, 2nd ed. American College of Surgeons, Chicago, 1985
11. Ritter AM, Muizelaar J, Barnes T, et al: Brain stem blood flow, pupillary response and outcome in patients with severe head injures. Neurosurgery 44:941, 1999
12. Schroder M, Muizelaar J, Kuta A: Documented reversal of global ischemia immediately after removal of a subdural hematoma: report of two cases. J Neurosurg 80:324, 1994
13. Andrews P, Piper I, Dearden N, et al: Secondary insults during intrahospital transport of head injured patients. Lancet 335:327, 1990
14. Jones P, Andrews P, Midgley S: Measuring the burden of secondary insults in head-injured patients during intensive care. J Neurosurg Anesthesiol 6:4, 1994
15. Kirkpatrick P, Smielewski P, Czosnyka M, et al: Near-infrared spectroscopy use in patients with severe head injury. J Neurosurg 83:963, 1995
16. Kanter M, Narayan R: Management of head injury: intracranial pressure monitoring. Neurosurg Clin North Am 2:257, 1991
17. Gibbs E, Lennox W, Nims L, et al: Arterial and cerebral venous blood: arteriovenous differences in man. J Biol Chem 144:325, 1942
18. Gopinath S, Robertson C, Contant C, et al: Jugular venous desaturation and outcome after severe head injury. J Neurol Neurosurg Psychiatry 57:171, 1994
19. Robertson C, Gopinath SP, Goodman J, et al: $S_{jv}O_2$ monitoring in head-injured patients. J Neurotrauma 12:891, 1995
20. Stochetti N, Paparella A, Bridelli F, et al: Cerebral venous oxygen saturation studied with bilateral samples in the internal jugular veins. Neurosurgery 34:38, 1994
21. Rosner M, Rosner S, Johnson A: Cerebral perfusion pressure: management protocol and clinical results. J Neurosurg 83:949, 1995
22. McGraw C: A cerebral perfusion pressure greater than 80 mm Hg is more beneficial. Springer-Verlag, Berlin, 1989
23. Marshall L, Smith R, Shapiro H: The outcome with aggressive treatment in severe head injuries, part II: acute and chronic barbiturate administration in the management of head injury. J Neurosurg 50:26, 1979
24. Ward J, Becker D, Miller JD, et al: Failure of prophylactic barbiturate coma in the treatment of severe head injury. J Neurosurg 62:383, 1985
25. Levy M, Aranda M, Zelman V, et al: Propylene glycol toxicity following continuous etomidate infusion for the control of refractory cerebral edema. Neurosurgery 37:363, 1995
26. Pinaud M, Lelasque J, Chetanneau A, et al: Effects of Diprivan on cerebral blood flow, intracranial pressure and cerebral metabolism in head-injured patients. Annales Françaises d'Anesthésie et de Réanimation 10:2, 1991
27. Bullock R, Stewart L, Rafferty C, et al: Continuous monitoring of jugular bulb oxygen saturation and the effect of drugs acting on cerebral metabolism. Acta Neurochir (Wien) 59:113, 1993
28. Clifton G, Allen S, Barrodale P, et al: A phase II study of moderate hypothermia in severe brain injury. J Neurotrauma 10:263, 1993
29. Marion D, Obrist W, Carlier P, et al: The use of moderate therapeutic hypothermia for patients with severe head injuries: a preliminary report. J Neurosurg 79:354, 1993
30. Bracken M, Shepard M, Collins W, et al: A randomized controlled trial of methylprednisolone or naloxone in the treatment of acute spinal cord injury. N Engl J Med 322:1405, 1990
31. Bracken M, Shepard M, Collins W, et al: Methylprednisolone or naloxone treatment after acute spinal cord injury: 1-year follow-up data. J Neurosurg 76:23, 1992
32. Guha A, Tator C, Piper I, et al: Increase in rat spinal cord blood flow with the calcium channel blocker nimodipine. J Neurosurg 63:250, 1985
33. Guha A, Tator C, Smith C, et al: Improvement in posttraumatic spinal cord blood flow with a combination of a calcium channel blocker and a vasopressor. J Trauma 29:1440, 1989
34. Geisler F: GM-1 ganglioside and motor recovery following human spinal cord injury. J Emerg Med 11(SII):49, 1993
35. Bracken M, Shepard M, Holford T, et al: Administration of methylprednisolone for 24 or 48 hours or tirilazad mesylate for 48 hours in the treatment of acute spinal cord injury: results of the Third National Acute Spinal Cord Injury Randomized Controlled Trial. National Acute Spinal Cord Injury Study. JAMA 227:1597, 1997
36. Marshall L, Knowlton S, Garfan S, et al: Deterioration following spinal cord injury: a multi-center study. J Neurosurg 66:400, 1987
37. Wilberger J: Advances in the diagnosis and management of spinal cord trauma. J Neurotrauma 8:75, 1992
38. Wilberger J, Duh M: Surgical treatment of spinal cord injury—the NASCIS II experience. Presented at the annual meeting of the AANS, Boston, Massachusetts, April 1993
39. Allen BL Jr: Recognition of injuries to the lower cervical spine. The Cervical Spine, 2nd ed. The Cervical Spine Research Society, Ed. JB Lippincott Co, Philadelphia, 1989, p 286
40. Lind BL, Nordwall A: Halo-vest treatment of unstable traumatic cervical spine injuries. Spine 13:425, 1988
41. Denis F: The three column spine and its significance in the classification of acute thoracolumbar spinal injuries. Spine 8:817, 1983
42. Kontos H, Raper A, Patterson J: Analysis of vasoreactivity of local pH, pCO_2, and bicarbonate on pial vessels. Stroke 8:358, 1977
43. Kontos H, Wei E, Navari R, et al: Responses of cerebral arteries and arterioles to acute hypotension and hypertension. Am J Physiol 234:H371, 1978
44. McHenry LC Jr, West JW, Cooper ES: Cerebral autoregulation in man. Stroke 5:695, 1974
45. Muizelaar J, Wei E, Kontos H, et al: Cerebral blood flow is regulated by changes in blood pressure and in blood viscosity alike. Stroke 17:44, 1986
46. Muizelaar J, Poel H, Li Z, et al: Pial arteriolar vessel diameter and CO_2 reactivity during prolonged hyperventilation in the rabbit. J Neurosurg 69:923, 1988
47. Chesnut R, Marshall L, Klauber MR, et al: The role of secondary brain injury in determining outcome after severe head injury. J Trauma 34:216, 1993
48. Monro A: Observations on the structure and function of the nervous system. Creech and Johnson, Edinburgh, 1783
49. Kellie G: On death from cold, and on congestions of the brain: an account of the appearances observed in the dissection of two of three individuals presumed to have perished in the storm of 3rd November 1821; with some reflections on the pathology of the brain. Trans Med Chir Soc Edinburgh 84-169, 1824
50. Marmarou A, Shulman K, Rosende R: A nonlinear analysis of the cerebral spinal fluid system and intracranial pressure dynamics. J Neurosurg 48:332, 1978
51. Muizelaar JP: Cerebral Blood Flow, Cerebral Blood Volume, and Cerebral Metabolism after Severe Head Injury. WB Saunders Co, Philadelphia, 1989
52. Muizelaar JP, Marmarou A, Ward JD, et al: Adverse effects of prolonged hyperventilation in patients with severe head injury: a randomized clinical trial. J Neurosurg 75:731, 1991
53. Muizelaar JP, Wei EP, Kontos H, et al: Mannitol causes compensatory cerebral vasoconstriction and vasodilation in response to blood viscosity changes. J Neurosurg 59:822, 1983
54. Muizelaar JP, Lutz HI, Becker D: Effect of mannitol on ICP and CBF and correlation with pressure autoregulation in severely head-injured patients. J Neurosurg 61:700, 1984
55. Rosner M, Daughton S: Cerebral perfusion management in head injury. J Trauma 30:933, 1990
56. Adams J, D: G: The Pathology of Blunt Head Injury. Heinemann, London, 1972
57. Bouma G, Muizelaar JP, Choi S, et al: Cerebral circulation and metabolism after severe traumatic brain injury: the elusive role of ischemia. J Neurosurg 75:685, 1991
58. Jones T, Morawetz R, Crowell R, et al: Thresholds of

focal cerebral ischemia in awake monkeys. J Neurosurg 54:773, 1981
59. Muizelaar JP, Schroder M: Overview of monitoring of cerebral blood flow and metabolism after severe head injury. Can J Neurol Sci 21:S6, 1994
60. Hochachka P, Mommsen T: Protons and anaerobiosis. Science 219:1391, 1983
61. Andersen B, Marmarou A: Functional compartmentalization of energy production in neural tissue. Brain Res 585:190, 1992
62. Inao S, Marmarou A, Clarke G, et al: Production and clearance of lactate from brain tissue, CSF and serum following experimental brain injury. J Neurosurg 69:736, 1988
63. Verweij B, Muizelaar J: Mitochondrial dysfunction after experimental and human brain injury and its possible reversal with a selective N-type calcium channel antagonist (SNX-111). Neurol Res 19:334, 1997
64. Xiong Y, Gu Q, Peterson P, et al: Mitochondrial dysfunction and calcium perturbation induced by traumatic brain injury. J Neurotrauma 14:23, 1997
65. Young W, Bracken M: The second National Acute Spinal Cord Injury Study. J Neurotrauma 9:S429, 1992
66. Dimitrijevic M, Dimitrijevic M, Faganel J, et al: Residual Motor Functions in Spinal Cord Injury. Raven Press, New York, 1988
67. Blight A, Young W: Central axons in injured cat spinal cord recover electrophysiological function following remyelination by Schwann cells. J Neurol Sci 91:15, 1989
68. Blight A, Decrescito V: Morphometric analysis of experimental spinal cord injury in the cat: the relation of injury intensity to survival of myelinated axons. Neuroscience 19:321, 1986
69. Blight A, Young W: Axonal morphometric correlates of evoked potentials in experimental spinal cord injury. Humana Press, New York, 1990
70. Blight A, Gruner J: Augmentation by 4-aminopyridine of vestibulospinal free fall responses in chronic phases of traumatic spinal cord injury in dogs: a phase I clinical trial. J Neurol Sci 82:155, 1987
71. Hayes K, Blight A, Potter P, et al: Preclinical trial of 4-aminopyridine in patients with chronic spinal cord injury. Paraplegia 31:216, 1993
72. Hayes K, Potter P, Wolfe D, et al: 4-aminopyridine-sensitive neurologic deficits in patients with spinal cord injury. J Neurotrauma 11:433, 1994
73. Sandler A, Tator C: Review of the effects of spinal trauma on vessels and blood flow in the spinal cord. J Neurosurg 45:638, 1972
74. Young W: Blood flow, metabolic and neurophysiologic mechanisms in spinal cord injury. Central Nervous System Trauma Status Report, 1985. Becker D, Poulishock J, Eds. National Institute of Neurological and Communicative Disorders and Stroke, Bethesda, Maryland, 1985

Acknowledgments

Figure 3 Reprinted courtesy of the American Spinal Injury Association, Chicago, Illinois.
Figure 4 Susan Brust, C.M.I.

24 INJURIES TO THE FACE AND JAW

Seth Thaller, M.D., and F. William Blaisdell, M.D.

Assessment and Management of Maxillofacial Injuries

Tremendous progress has been made in the management of patients with facial injuries. Reconstructive surgeons are treating an increasing number of challenging facial injuries because of excellent advances in the transportation of trauma victims and the regionalization of care in trauma centers. Although severe facial injuries are often associated with devastating cosmetic and functional defects, reconstructive surgeons are achieving better long-term surgical results and are able to repair certain injuries that were once considered nonreconstructible by employing craniofacial surgical techniques developed through the pioneering efforts of Dr. Paul Tessier, of Paris. These techniques include widespread subperiosteal exposure, rigid internal fixation with miniature plates and screws, and widespread primary bone grafting.

Initial Survey

Maxillofacial injuries are secondary to either blunt or penetrating trauma. Motor vehicle accidents remain the most common cause of facial injuries characterized by bony comminution and distraction. However, penetrating injuries, such as knife wounds, can cause extensive soft tissue injuries to skin and underlying nerves, blood vessels, parotid structures, and other structures of the upper aerodigestive system. Gunshot wounds can cause devastating injuries that necessitate extensive flap reconstruction to provide satisfactory soft tissue coverage of the underlying bone.

On initial assessment, the physician must always pay special attention to correcting the most life-threatening problems, including an obstructed airway, bleeding, and shock [see 2 Trauma Resuscitation, 4 Shock, and 5 Bleeding and Transfusion]. Patients with facial injuries often have multisystem involvement; priorities in the evaluation and treatment of associated significant injuries are discussed elsewhere [see 22 Emergency Department Evaluation of the Patient with Multiple Injuries]. After establishing that the patient is stable, the examiner should quickly make note of lacerations and contusions, extensive bony disruptions, loss of vision, malocclusion, trismus, and bleeding.

When evaluating facial injuries, a quick analysis of occlusion provides extremely important diagnostic information that serves as the foundation for future fracture repair. Angle's classification of malocclusion, which is more than 100 years old, remains one of the most commonly used systems. The maxillomandibular relation is determined by the position of the mesiobuccal cusp of the maxillary first molar in relation to the buccal groove of the mandibular first molar. Angle's class I, or neutroclusion, exists when the permanent maxillary first molar is ideally positioned—that is, the buccal cusp of the maxillary first molar and the mesiobuccal groove of the mandibular first molar occlude, resulting in a normal anteroposterior relation of the maxillary and mandibular dentition. Angle's class II, or distoclusion, exists when the maxillary first molar is mesial (i.e., toward the midline) to the corresponding mandibular first molar. Angle's class III, or mesioclusion, exists when the mandibular first molar is mesial to the maxillary first molar.

AIRWAY ASSESSMENT

Facial bone fractures, bleeding, loose dentition, debris, and laryngeal injuries can contribute to airway compromise. Accordingly, whenever there is any evidence of maxillofacial injuries, it is essential to monitor the airway status carefully. If the patient is conscious, alert, and breathing at a rate of less than 20 respirations/min, without excessive airway secretions or excessive hemorrhage, it can be assumed that the patient has an adequate airway.

In a comatose patient with compromised vital reflexes (i.e., gag, cough, and swallow), an endotracheal tube must be inserted immediately to prevent aspiration. In the presence of nasopharyngeal bleeding, major maxillofacial injuries, or cerebrospinal fluid leakage, nasal intubation should be avoided because of the potential for intracranial contamination. If there is a possible fracture of the cribriform plate, either an orotracheal tube should be placed or a cricothyrotomy should be performed. In an agitated or restless patient, only a single attempt should be made at inserting an endotracheal or nasotracheal tube; if the attempt is unsuccessful, an emergency cricothyrotomy should be performed [see 2 Trauma Resuscitation]. In slightly more elective circumstances, a deliberate tracheotomy may be the optimal means of ensuring an adequate airway. Cricothyrotomy and tracheotomy must never be taken lightly, because they can lead to significant complications. In addition, because newer treatment modalities using rigid fixation decrease the time required for extensive maxillomandibular fixation, more conservative methods of airway control are often indicated.

Assessment and Management of Maxillofacial Injuries

```
┌─────────────────────────────────────┐
│ Known or suspected facial injury    │
├─────────────────────────────────────┤
│ Assess airway, breathing, and       │
│ circulation.                        │
└─────────────────────────────────────┘
             │
      ┌──────┴──────┐
      │             │
┌─────────────┐  ┌─────────────────┐
│ Airway      │  │ No airway       │
│ compromise  │  │ compromise      │
├─────────────┤  ├─────────────────┤
│ Perform     │  │ Assess for major│
│ orotracheal │  │ nasopharyngeal  │
│ intubation, │  │ bleeding.       │
│ cricothyro- │  └─────────────────┘
│ tomy, or              │
│ tracheotomy.          │
└─────────────┘  ┌──────┴──────┐
                 │             │
        ┌──────────────┐  ┌──────────────┐
        │ Major        │  │ No major     │
        │ nasopharyn-  │  │ bleeding     │
        │ geal bleeding│  └──────────────┘
        ├──────────────┤
        │ Attempt      │
        │ control...   │
        └──────────────┘
```

Known or suspected facial injury
Assess airway, breathing, and circulation.

Airway compromise
Perform orotracheal intubation, cricothyrotomy, or tracheotomy.

No airway compromise
Assess for major nasopharyngeal bleeding.

Major nasopharyngeal bleeding
Attempt control of bleeding by packing oropharynx or nasopharynx with anterior or posterior nasal packing.

No major bleeding

Bleeding is not controlled
Transport patient to operating room for fracture reduction, ligation of external carotid artery, or both.

Bleeding is controlled →

Treat truncal and central nervous system injuries
- Evaluate facial injuries.
- Suture facial lacerations.
- Perform routine and specialized x-ray evaluations.

Treat specific facial injuries
- Eye and orbital injuries.
- Maxillary injuries.
- Mandibular injuries.
- Soft tissue injuries.

If the respiratory rate is higher than 25/min or if there is evidence that the airway is obstructed or compromised, the patient should be carefully monitored. When the respiratory rate increases to 30/min or higher, an immediate assessment of arterial blood gases should be made under close observation. A respiratory rate of higher than 35/min is an indication for both intubation and respiratory support unless the cause of the rapid rate can be identified and immediately reversed.

MAXILLOFACIAL BLEEDING

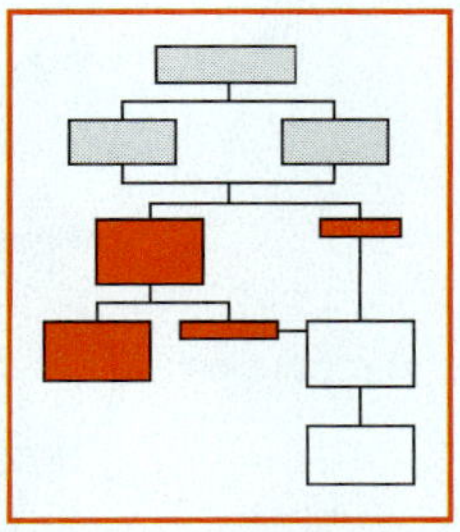

Once the airway has been satisfactorily stabilized, the next priority is to manage maxillofacial bleeding. There is a misconception that patients do not bleed profusely from facial injuries and that facial bleeding can be controlled easily.[1] Unfortunately, this is not necessarily always the case. In addition, because facial injuries themselves can be so striking, associated significant hemorrhage can often be overlooked or underestimated. Firm compression with moist sponges will temporarily stop most arterial and venous bleeding. Careful application of digital pressure or definitive ligation of the bleeding point can often control external bleeding. These procedures are best performed in the operating room, with the patient under general anesthesia.

If the source of hemorrhage is in the depths of a narrow laceration, bleeding can be controlled temporarily by packing. Blind clamping or suture ligation can damage important underlying facial structures, particularly branches of the facial nerve; therefore, such procedures must be avoided. Insertion of an anterior pack moistened with 1:10,000 epinephrine may be used to control nasal bleeding. However, persistent nasopharyngeal hemorrhage will necessitate either placement of a posterior pack or ligation of the internal maxillary artery or the external carotid artery.

In major maxillofacial injuries with extensive pharyngeal bleeding, immediate airway access is mandatory, either with an endotracheal tube or by cricothyrotomy. Once airway control has been achieved, the patient should be brought to the operating room for reduction of gross bony injuries, which will often stop uncontrollable hemorrhage. In those rare instances when maxillofacial injuries are associated with serious and uncontrollable hemorrhage, it may be necessary to obtain access to the external carotid artery for ligation of the major trunk or a branch if either is the source of bleeding [see 25 Injuries to the Neck].

Definitive Evaluation

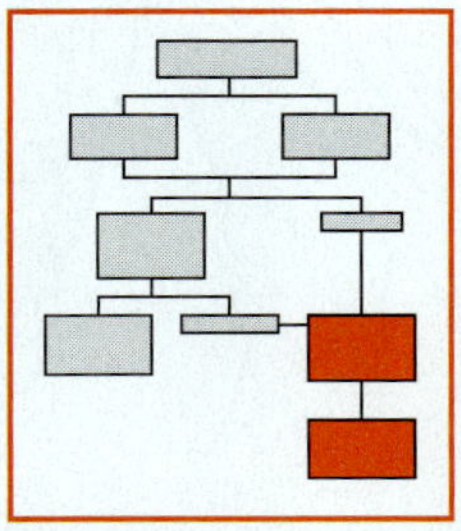

When there is no associated airway compromise, facial injuries are a lower priority than potential thoracic, abdominal, or head injuries [see 22 Emergency Department Evaluation of the Patient with Multiple Injuries]. In fact, in the absence of airway compromise and severe hemorrhage, definitive diagnostic evaluation and management of maxillofacial injuries can be delayed until the more life-threatening injuries have been stabilized and treated.

EXAMINATION

Like any other anatomic region, the face must be examined in an orderly fashion, with careful attention paid to gross asymmetry, paralysis, weakness, eye movements, occlusal discrepancies, and ecchymosis. Areas of hypesthesia or anesthesia should be noted. Special attention should be directed toward bimanual palpation of bony prominences within the craniofacial region to look for crepitus, tenderness, irregularities, and step-offs. Palpation should start with the frontal bones and lateral and inferior orbital rims.

The zygomatic arch should be palpated for evidence of depression, and the region of the malar eminence should be evaluated for recession [see Figures 1 through 4]. Fracture of the zygomatic complex is often identified with an inferiorly dis-

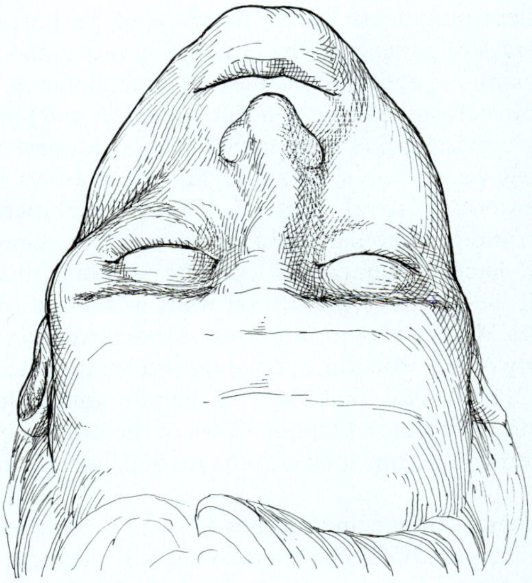

Figure 1 Broken nose.

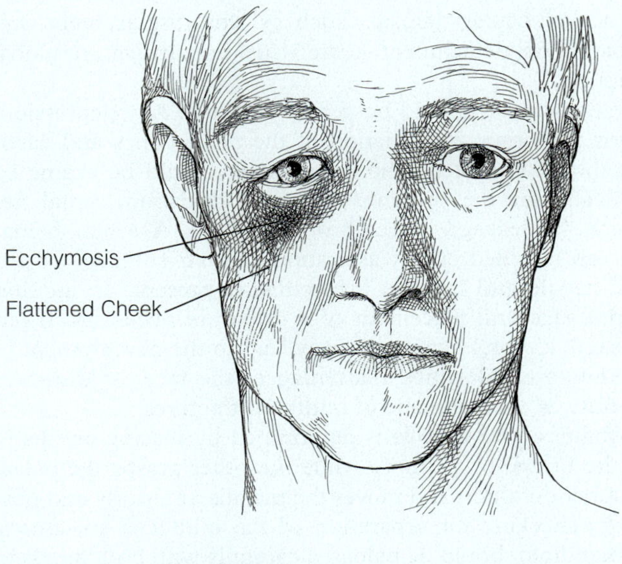

Figure 2 Fractured zygoma.

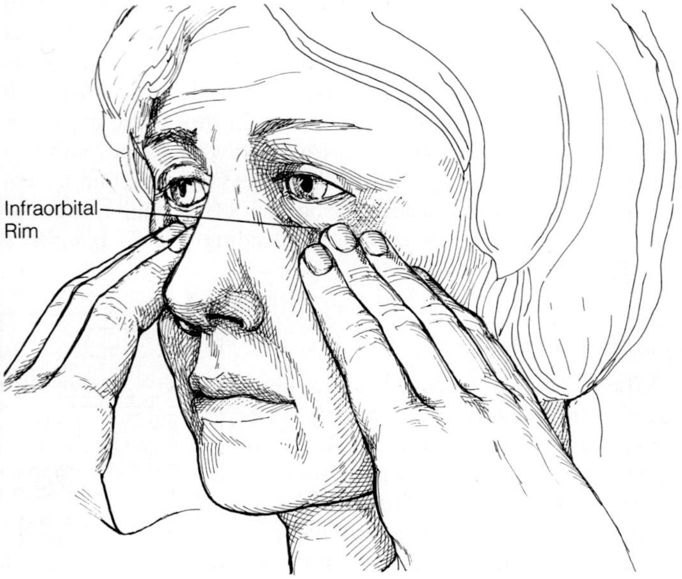

Figure 3 **Infraorbital fracture.**

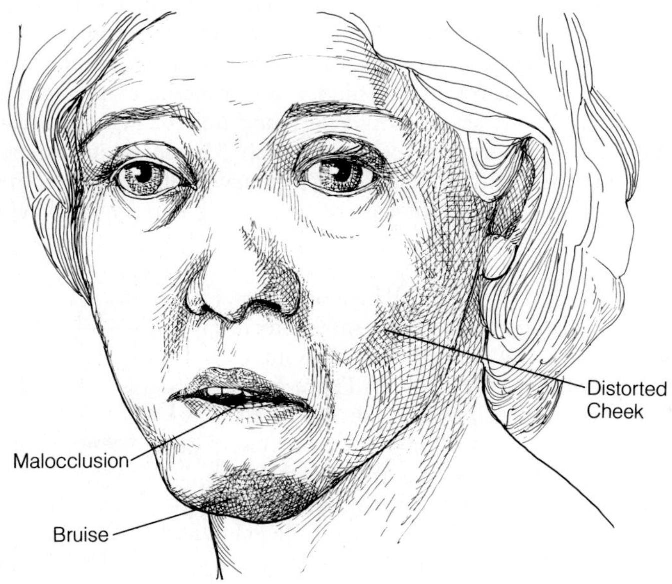

Figure 4 **Fractured mandible.**

placed lateral canthus, paresthesias of the infraorbital nerve, visual impairment, displacement of the globe, or trismus secondary to impingement of the zygomatic arch on the coronoid process or temporal muscle.

Orbital evaluation is key to the assessment of facial injuries. The nasolacrimal duct should be inspected, and the distance between the medial canthi should be measured for the presence of telecanthus. (The normal intercanthal distance in the average adult is less than 35 mm.) Pupils should be checked for reactivity, and extraocular muscle motion should be assessed. Diplopia secondary to extraocular muscle entrapment should be determined. The position of the globe should also be assessed; orbital floor fractures may cause enophthalmos and severe swelling, and a blow-in type fracture may result in exophthalmos. A visual acuity test must be performed before any surgical intervention for correction of facial fractures. An ophthalmologic consultation is essential if there is any evidence of ocular damage, such as lens displacement, hyphema, retinal detachment, acute visual impairment, or global disruption.

Next, the nose should be gently palpated. Any depression, abnormal motion, or deviation of the nasal bones and cartilages should be noted. The nasal cavity should be examined specifically for the presence of septal deviation, septal hematoma, or leakage of cerebrospinal fluid. A septal hematoma can be ruled out by aspiration with an 18-gauge or 20-gauge needle and syringe; if bleeding is present, an incision and drainage and placement of a drain are necessary. If left untreated, a septal hematoma may lead to the development of a saddle-nose deformity. Flattening of the face, or dish-face deformity, is characteristic of midfacial fractures.

Mobility of the maxilla is determined by placing one hand over the bridge of the nose while the other grasps the palate and upper dentition and moves the maxilla anteriorly and posteriorly, checking for separation of the midfacial structures. The mandible should be palpated carefully with both hands to locate any intraoral mucosal lacerations or lesions. Bimanual palpation of the mandible is accomplished by placing the thumbs over the molar occlusal surfaces and the index fingers externally over the inferior border of the mandible and torquing the bone to check for movement. Any missing or mobile teeth must be recorded. The floor of the mouth should also be examined with bimanual palpation.

The ears should be examined for evidence of lacerations or contusions of the external auditory canal that may be caused by condylar neck fractures. A simple diagnostic method is to insert the fingertip into the external auditory canal on one side; if no movement can be determined with mandibular excursion, a diagnosis of condylar fracture can be made.

FACIAL X-RAYS

A spectrum of available radiologic modalities plays a significant role in the diagnosis and treatment of facial injuries. Appropriate studies are mandatory. In addition, x-rays provide an excellent permanent record for medicolegal purposes. The initial x-rays of patients in the emergency room (the first level for assessment and clarification of maxillofacial injuries) should be performed using conventional films and should consist of a cervical spine series (with all the cervical vertebrae adequately visualized), skull x-rays, and facial x-rays, including anteroposterior, lateral, Waters', Towne's, submentovertex, panorex, and mandibular views. More definitive x-rays can be obtained later to completely evaluate specific injuries. The Caldwell view defines the orbital walls and the frontal sinus structures. Waters' view is important for determining the bony continuity of the orbit, nose, zygoma, and lateral portion of the maxilla. The lateral skull view is helpful for evaluation of frontal sinus fractures. Oblique views of the orbit are excellent for demonstrating the apex and the medial, lateral, and orbital walls.

The lateral oblique and modified Towne's views are used to evaluate the mandible. The lateral oblique is the most common and useful view and provides evaluation of the body, angle of the body, and the ascending ramus. A posteroanterior view is helpful in assessing the symphyseal and body regions as well as the condylar and coronoid processes. Panoramic x-rays are the best screening views for assessing mandibular fractures, especially within the condyles. Associated injuries to the dentition and supporting structures may necessitate dental spot films for more specific information.

OTHER STUDIES

Computed tomographic scanning can be of great value in diagnosing the more complex traumatic injuries, such as craniomaxillofacial injuries and associated central nervous system injuries. Computed tomography is used to evaluate most critically injured patients with craniocerebral trauma, and the studies can easily be extended to include the patient's facial skeleton with little additional risk. Both 3 mm axial and coronal computed tomographic cuts of the facial skeletal should be obtained, especially for examination of the orbit. A lateral oblique scan through the midportion of the globe provides additional information regarding the bony architecture of the orbit. This information can be reformatted, and three-dimensional reconstructions can be made for further evaluation. Magnetic resonance imaging is proving to be of benefit in assessing both bony and soft tissue injuries. Arteriography may be needed to evaluate the source of a hemorrhage or to rule out major vascular injuries.

Treatment of Soft Tissue Injuries

Soft tissue injuries are most often the result of penetrating trauma but can also be the result of blunt trauma [see Treatment of Maxillofacial Fractures, below]. Any patients who need general anesthesia, such as a child or a patient with extensive complex lacerations involving deeper structures, should be treated in the operating room after appropriate evaluation of their overall status. Soft tissue injuries can involve nerves, parotid ducts, lacrimal ducts, and other critical facial structures. Abrasions must be thoroughly cleaned, and lacerations should be irrigated with normal saline and conservatively debrided as necessary. With deeply embedded foreign material, debridement and irrigation must be particularly meticulous and extensive to prevent residual cosmetic deformities. Dermabrasion is especially good for large involved areas. Most facial lacerations can be closed primarily with standard suturing procedures [see 8 Acute Wound Care]. Antibiotic coverage is left to individual preferences; however, 24 hours of prophylactic perioperative antibiotic coverage with a cephalosporin is strongly recommended. The examiner must always consider the possibility of underlying injuries, and careful palpation and visualization of important underlying structures should be part of the definitive wound evaluation and treatment.

Local anesthetic agents used in the head and neck region should always contain epinephrine for hemostasis. To decrease pain and discomfort, the local anesthetic should be administered through the margins of the wound rather than through the surrounding skin. Regional nerve blocks are preferred for suture closure of lacerations involving the forehead, cheeks, lips, and chin. The forehead can be blocked by local infiltration of the supraorbital nerve, which is located just superior to the eyebrow. The upper lip, side of the nose, and adjacent skin can be blocked by anesthetizing the infraorbital nerve. Injection of the mental nerve, located between the first and second bicuspids, will anesthetize the lower lip and surrounding chin. Regional blocks also provide the advantage of minimizing tissue damage to already traumatized skin and lead to less scar formation.

NERVE INJURIES

The facial nerve is the nerve most vulnerable to maxillofacial trauma, and its function must be thoroughly evaluated before the administration of any local anesthetic. In addition, facial nerve injuries result in the most serious functional disabilities and aesthetic defects. Sensory nerves, such as the infraorbital and supraorbital nerves, can also be involved in traumatic injuries; however, the associated hypesthesia causes only minimal long-term disability.

Whenever the posterior half of the parotid gland suffers a deep laceration, it should be assumed that a major branch of the facial nerve has been divided, and the face should be carefully examined. If there is a clean, sharp division of one of the five major trunks or of the proximal main nerve trunk, it can be repaired immediately with microanastomotic techniques. If there is substantial nerve loss, the nerve ends should be identified and appropriately tagged for future nerve grafting. If a nerve laceration occurs anterior to the region of the lateral canthus, nerve repair is generally unnecessary because there is sufficient crossover from the opposite side. Peripheral branch injury is manifest by inability to raise the eyebrow (frontal branch), inability to close the eyelids (malar), smoothness of the cheek (infraorbital), inability to smile (buccal), and inability to frown (marginal mandibular).

PAROTID DUCT INJURIES

The parotid duct is located between the parotid gland and the oral mucosa, opening opposite the second upper molar. Any deep laceration of the anterior parotid gland can damage this duct. If there is a possibility that the parotid duct is injured, the orifice of Stensen's duct should be probed. Should the probe enter the wound, division of the duct is verified. The proximal cut end of the duct can be located by expressing saliva from the gland. A catheter should then be passed through Stensen's duct and through the area of laceration, and the duct should be repaired over the catheter [see Figure 5].

LACRIMAL DUCT INJURIES

Whenever there is a laceration involving the medial canthal region, a lacrimal duct injury should be assumed. Acute reconstruction of the lacrimal duct is controversial. If both ends of the duct can be easily discerned, the severed ends should be realigned, splinted internally, and repaired. This procedure is best accomplished over a fine Silastic rod. Dissection to locate the residual parts of the duct should be delicate and meticulous, because traumatic dissection can aggravate the injury and result in further permanent damage.

SCALP INJURIES

When scalp injuries are repaired, extensive shaving is unnecessary. Scalp injuries can be associated with profuse bleeding because of the scalp's extensive vascular supply. To obtain adequate control of hemorrhage from the wound margins, closure can be achieved in a single layer with a running, locking 3-0

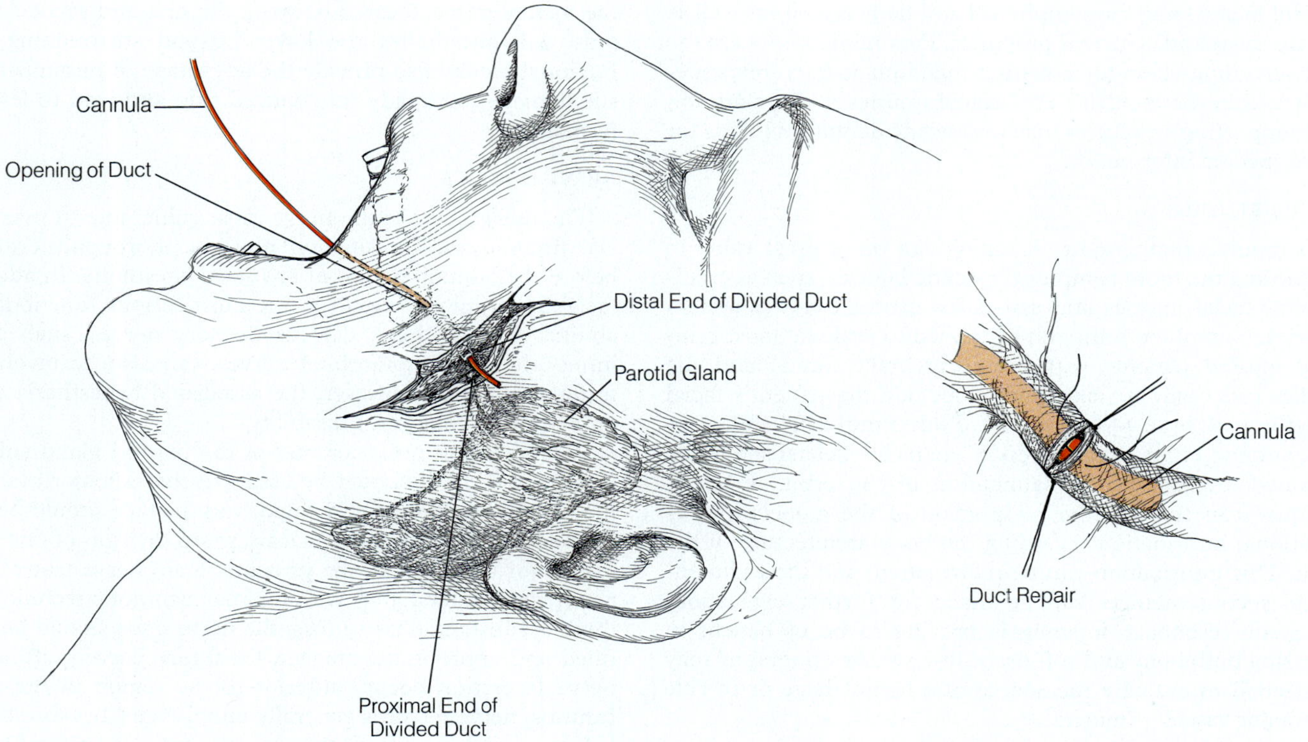

Figure 5 Injuries to the parotid duct are repaired by passing a catheter through Stensen's duct and through the area of laceration and then repairing the parotid duct over the catheter.

chromic suture on a large cutting needle. Associated underlying skull fractures are always a possibility, and the skull should be palpated and inspected through any full-thickness scalp wound.

EYELID INJURIES

If the patient reports excessive eye pain, the initial examiner must always first rule out an associated ocular injury. In addition, when faced with through-and-through lid lacerations, the examiner must perform a very careful eye examination. Lacerations of the eyelid should be meticulously repaired by approximation of the margins of the lid defect, followed by closure of the laceration in three layers. The conjunctiva may be left unsutured if good apposition can be obtained by closing the tarsal plate and the pretarsal muscles that occupy the middle layer, which is preferably closed with fine absorbable sutures. Fine nonabsorbable skin sutures are employed to close the final layer. All skin sutures should be removed within 48 hours. When there is extensive tissue loss, it may be necessary to use plastic techniques to mobilize sufficient conjunctiva for closure.

EYEBROW INJURIES

For optimal cosmetic results, the eyebrows should be closed meticulously in layers with careful alignment of the eyebrow margins. Lacerations passing through the eyebrow should not be shaved; leaving them intact facilitates good plastic closure. Because the hairs of the eyebrow run obliquely to the surface of the skin, any incision for debridement should follow the line of the eyebrows to avoid further loss of hair.

EXTERNAL-EAR INJURIES

If avulsions of the ear are properly repaired, the chances are good that they will heal because of the highly vascular pedicle. Circulation is maintained if even a small pedicle is present. Repair of ear wounds should be done in three layers by using fine nonabsorbable sutures to approximate the cartilage and the skin. If the ear is completely detached, the cartilage should be preserved within a subcutaneous pocket in the mastoid region for future reconstruction.

Hematomas can occur secondary to the shearing of the vascular mucoperichondrium from the underlying cartilage. These must be evacuated early, and a conforming pressure dressing should be placed to maintain the normal ear contour.

NASAL INJURIES

Through-and-through lacerations of the nose and near-avulsion injuries are cosmetic problems. Because the nose is extremely vascular, repair of these injuries should be especially meticulous and done in layers. The cartilage and skin should be aligned with fine nonabsorbable interrupted sutures. Absorbable sutures should be employed for repair of the mucosa. Key cosmetic points (i.e., epidermal-mucosal junctions, nasal fold junctions, or critical angles in jagged lacerations) should be sutured first to ensure that no deformity results.

LIP INJURIES

If the margin of the lip has been divided, the vermilion border should be carefully identified and tattooed, and the first sutures should be placed to approximate this critical margin. A common problem in the treatment of lip injuries is that it may become more difficult to identify landmarks when they are obliterated by local anesthetic injections or associated edema.

Treatment of Maxillofacial Fractures

Management of maxillofacial fractures can be extremely challenging. The common maxillofacial fractures include nasal, mandibular, orbital, zygomatic complex, sinus (e.g., maxillary, sphenoid, ethmoid, and frontal), and maxillary fractures (e.g., Le Fort I, II, or III). Management of these fractures often requires sophisticated specialty treatment involving plastic surgeons, ophthalmologists, neurosurgeons, otolaryngologists, or a combination of these.

FRONTAL SINUS FRACTURES

The frontal sinus region is prone to injury because of its prominent location and relatively thin anterior bony wall.[2,3] Injuries to the frontal sinus area require comprehensive treatment, often with a team approach. The key to treatment lies in determining the status of the nasofrontal ducts.[4,5] Patients with such injuries also require careful, regular, long-term follow-up care because potentially life-threatening complications, such as meningitis, osteomyelitis, and mucopyocele, may develop.[6-9]

NASAL AND NASO-ORBITO-ETHMOIDAL FRACTURES

The nasal bone is the most commonly fractured facial bone.[10] Before any treatment is embarked on, it is always helpful to have the patient provide a preinjury photo of himself or herself so that it can be determined whether the nasal deformity is from the acute episode. If a patient is seen almost immediately after injury and the associated swelling and ecchymosis are minimal, closed reduction can be performed at once. Nasal bone fractures can be reduced simply by inserting a scalpel handle or large hemostat into the nostril; the fracture segments can then be elevated and relocated. Usually, the nasal cavity is packed with petroleum jelly gauze to maintain alignment of the fracture and nasal septum, and a malleable splint is taped over the nose to provide counterpressure and assist in maintaining alignment. Packing is removed within 48 hours. However, treatment is generally not urgent and, depending on the individual situation, may be delayed for seven to 10 days.

Naso-orbito-ethmoidal fractures generally occur secondary to direct force applied over the nasal bridge, resulting in posterior displacement of bony structures and involvement of the medial canthus, lacrimal duct, canaliculi, and sac.[11] Repair of naso-orbito-ethmoidal fractures can be extremely challenging because of the number of important structures involved and their extensive comminution.[12] Satisfactory surgical management should be conducted through a coronal approach, thereby permitting precise three-dimensional reduction and stabilization and extensive primary bone grafting for replacement augmentation.[13] If there is associated CSF rhinorrhea, neurosurgical assistance should be obtained and early fracture reduction done.

ORBITAL FRACTURES

Orbital fractures can occur as isolated events or as a component of more extensive injuries. Orbital fractures, such as lacrimal duct lacerations and injuries to the globe, require highly specialized management with the aid of an ophthalmologist. Naso-orbital fractures with telecanthus should be treated with open reduction and fixation, as should all displaced fractures of the orbital rim and floor.[14,15]

ZYGOMATIC FRACTURES

The zygoma is a tetrapod structure that forms the malar prominence and the inferior and lateral aspects of the orbit. Fractures of the zygomatic complex should be repaired to prevent the development of serious aesthetic and functional deformities. Satisfactory stabilization requires three-point fixation achieved through incisions placed within the regions of the upper and lower lids and the upper buccal sulcus.

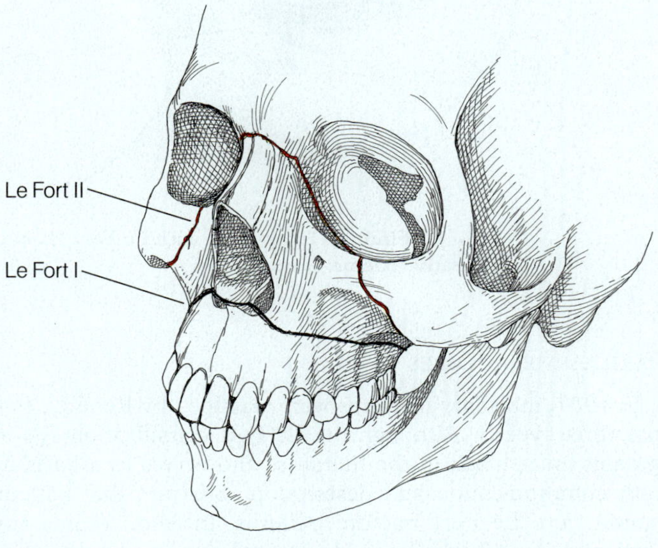

Figure 6 Le Fort I fractures (black line) affect the upper jaw alone. In Le Fort II fractures (red line), the upper jaw and the central portion of the face are separated from the skull.

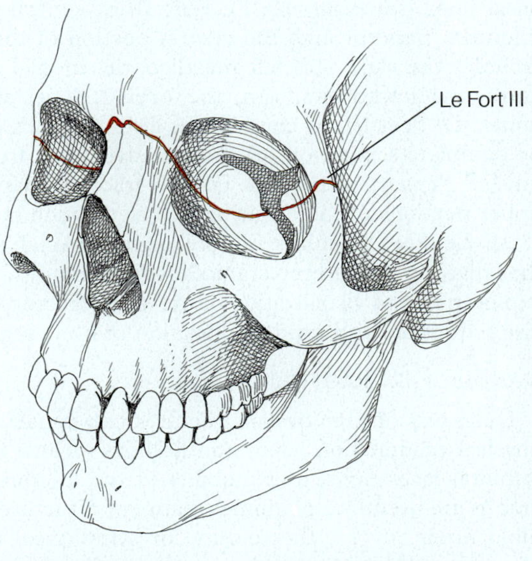

Figure 7 In Le Fort III fractures, all of the facial bones are separated from the skull.

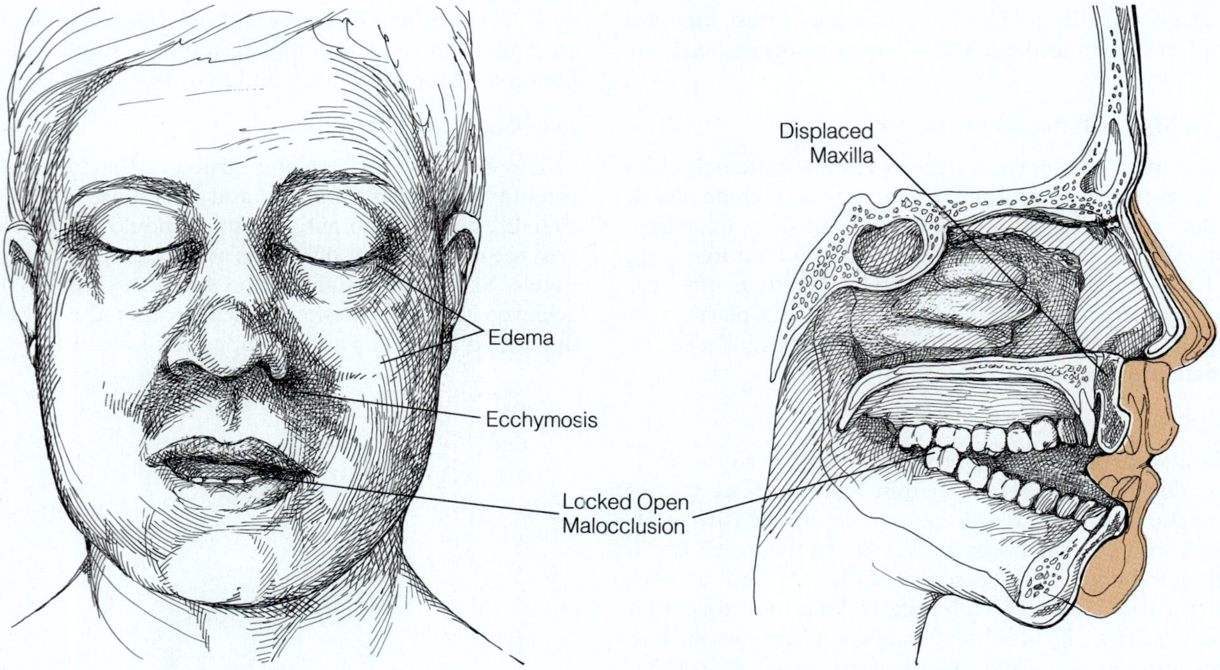

Figure 8 Findings in patients with Le Fort III maxillary fractures immediately after injury, before obliterative edema develops.

MAXILLARY FRACTURES

In 1901, maxillary fractures were classified by René Le Fort into three types.[16] Although the Le Fort classification system remains entrenched in the literature and serves as a basis for both communication and description, it is rare that patients exhibit pure Le Fort fracture patterns. Instead, trauma surgeons are generally challenged by severe bony comminution and distraction.

Le Fort I, or lower maxillary fractures, are the simplest type of maxillary fracture, consisting of horizontal detachment of the tooth-bearing segment of the maxilla at the level of the nasal floor [see Figure 6]. Le Fort II, or central or pyramidal fractures, pass through the central portion of the face, which includes the right and left maxillae, the medial aspect of the antra, the infraorbital rim, the orbital floor, and the nasal bones. Le Fort III, or craniofacial disjunction, is characterized by complete separation of all facial structures from the cranium [see Figures 7 and 8]. Le Fort III fractures pass through the upper portions of the orbits as well as through both zygomas.

All Le Fort fractures require highly specialized treatment that involves the use of craniofacial techniques, consisting of exploration and visualization of the entire fracture pattern, precise reduction, and rigid stabilization of bony segments.

MANDIBULAR FRACTURES

Diagnosis of mandibular fractures can usually be made on physical examination. Common findings include malocclusion, intraoral lacerations, and mobility at the fracture site. Radiographs are useful for planning treatment. Fractures of the mandible rarely involve the midline or symphyseal region. Most often, fractures will pass through areas of weakness, including the parasymphyseal region and the angle or neck of the condyle [see Figure 9]. The fracture pattern is usually determined by the site and mechanism of injury. Because of the mandible's architectural arrangement, more than one half of mandibular fractures involve multiple sites.

Mandibular fractures are not an emergency, but early definitive treatment results in a decreased number of complications. Preinjury occlusal relations remain the keystone to treatment. Mandibular fractures can be repaired by closed reduction with maxillomandibular fixation or by open reduction and fixation with wire osteosynthesis. However, newer techniques with rigid internal fixation with miniature plates and screws have

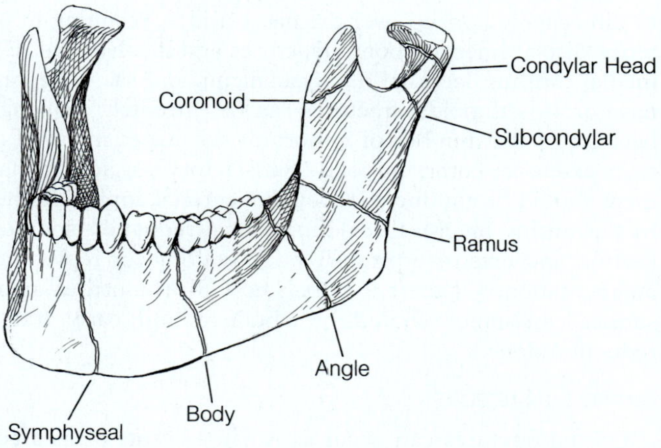

Figure 9 Mandibular fractures.

attained widespread popularity because of increased patient comfort.[17-20] In cooperative patients, a nondisplaced fracture can sometimes be handled conservatively with a dental soft diet and serial x-rays.

Discussion

Because the face is so thoroughly exposed, it is one of the most frequently injured areas of the body. Facial injuries can occur under a variety of circumstances, such as automobile accidents, altercations, or falls; more specifically, these injuries can be the results of bites, fires, explosions, lacerations, and contact with sharp or blunt objects. In automobile accidents, shards of glass may penetrate the wound, and these shards may not be radiopaque. If abrasions are present, note should be made of the abrading agent, whether it be grease, particles of dirt, gravel from a highway, or other contaminants. Underlying bony injury may or may not be obvious near the wounds. Because such injuries can expose the patient to tetanus or other anaerobic infections, antitetanic agents should be administered as part of the treatment regimen [see 8 Acute Wound Care]. If treatment is delayed for any reason, a systemic prophylactic antibiotic should be administered. Minor lacerations of the face caused by domestic assaults or household accidents can be adequately treated in the emergency department under local anesthesia [see 8 Acute Wound Care]. Lacerations that are contaminated are often best treated in the operating room with the patient under general anesthesia.

Only as much hair should be removed as is necessary for adequate assessment of the wound or for effective suturing. Eyebrows are best left unshaved to facilitate cosmetic repair. Local anesthesia should be induced, and abrasions should be scrubbed with a stiff brush until every particle of dirt is removed. If the dirt is deeply embedded, some tissue may have to be excised; this step can often be accomplished through the use of a fine curette or the point of a No. 11 blade. If dirt is not removed initially, it may be extremely difficult to remove later, and permanent tattooing may result.

Any dead or devitalized tissue should be excised, but there is no place for radical debridement of facial wounds. Tissue can survive on small pedicles. Full-thickness skin loss can be replaced with a free graft, which provides a better cosmetic match than a split-thickness skin graft [see 67 Plastic Surgical Reconstruction]. If the wound is so ragged that it cannot be approximated, careful squaring of the edges may be advisable to facilitate a cosmetic closure. Dead or devitalized subcutaneous tissue should be removed conservatively.

Most facial wounds can be closed by simple suturing. Although the deadline for closure of wounds to other sites is usually six to eight hours, facial wounds, unless heavily contaminated, can be closed as long as 24 hours after injury, particularly if meticulous attention is paid to procedural details. Such details include irrigation of the wound, removal of all foreign bodies, excision of devitalized tissue, and accurate approximation of tissue, with minimal dead space and no tension.

If the wound cannot be closed within the first 24 hours, delayed primary closure may be undertaken after 48 hours. In this event, the patient should be given systemic antibiotics, and the wound should be kept moist and protected as much as possible in the interval before closure. For best cosmetic results, the wound should be closed in multiple layers.

Sutures made of fine monofilament nylon, such as 6-0, are ideal for approximating the skin, because they are nonreactive. The sutures should be applied loosely so that they do not strangulate tissue.

Key anatomic points should be identified and tattooed, mucosal edges should be approximated, and irregular margins of the skin should be excised and squared to provide the best possible fit. Margins of damaged structures, such as the nose or the ear, should be defined, and the critical margins should be determined and approximated initially. While the wound is being closed, all dead space in the wound should be obliterated and the edges everted. If the needle is passed through the skin at right angles, the edges of the skin will abut and eversion will occur. If, however, the needle is passed through the skin edge obliquely, inversion will result, and healing will be compromised. Subcutaneous or subcuticular sutures should be placed in such a way as to allow the skin edges to be approximated with minimal tension. If this procedure is done, through-and-through sutures can be removed in three days, and no marks will be left on the skin.

Any skin defects that require closure should be closed by grafting. No facial wound should be allowed to heal by granulation, because this would lead to excessive scarring. Instead, a temporary cover in the form of a skin graft should be provided to minimize scar formation; any deformity that results from the graft can be repaired at a later date [see 67 Plastic Surgical Reconstruction].

The more complex of the maxillofacial fractures, such as major maxillary fractures, orbital fractures, malar fractures, and mandibular fractures [see Treatment of Maxillofacial Fractures, above], must be treated with specialty techniques; therefore, corresponding specialty consultation must be sought. However, in treating these fractures and soft tissue injuries [see Treatment of Soft Tissue Injuries, above], the priorities are to ensure adequacy of the airway and to control immediate bleeding. Once these aims have been achieved, none of the defects described, except for facial lacerations, require emergency treatment; they can be repaired days to even months later, if necessary, without jeopardizing a good cosmetic result.

References

1. Thaller S, Beal S: Maxillofacial trauma: a potentially fatal injury. Ann Plast Surg 27:281, 1991
2. Stanley R: Management of frontal sinus fractures. Facial Plast Surg 5:231, 1988
3. Stanley R: Fractures of the frontal sinus. Clin Plast Surg 16:115, 1989
4. Wolfe SA, Johnson P: Frontal sinus injuries: primary care and management of late complications. Plast Reconstr Surg 82:781, 1988
5. Luce E: Frontal sinus fractures: guidelines to management. Plast Reconstr Surg 80:500, 1987
6. Wilson B, Davidson B, Corey J, et al: Comparison of complications following frontal sinus fractures managed with exploration with or without obliteration over 10 years. Laryngoscope 98:516, 1988
7. Shockley W, Stucker F, White L, et al: Frontal sinus fractures: some problems and some solutions. Laryngoscope 98:18, 1988
8. Wallis A, Donald P: Frontal sinus fractures: a review of 72 cases. Laryngoscope 98:593, 1988
9. Rohrich R, Hollier L: Management of frontal sinus fractures. Clin Plast Surg 19:219, 1992
10. Spira M, Hardy S: Management of the injured nose. Tex Med 67:72, 1971
11. Gruss J: Naso-ethmoid-orbital fractures: classification and role of primary bone grafting. Plast Reconstr Surg 75:303, 1985
12. Gruss J, Pollock R, Phillips J, et al: Combined injuries of the cranium and face. Br J Plast Surg 42:385, 1989
13. Manson P, Crawley W, Yaremchuk M, et al: Midface fractures: advantages of immediate extended open reduction and bone grafting. Plast Reconstr Surg 76:1, 1985
14. Koutroupas S, Meyerhoff W: Surgical treatment of orbital floor fractures. Arch Otolaryngol 108:184, 1982
15. Antonyshyn O, Gruss J, Galbraith D, et al: Complex orbital fractures: a critical analysis of immediate bone reconstruction. Ann Plast Surg 22:220, 1989
16. Le Fort R: Etude expérimentale sur les fractures de la mâchoire supérieure. Rev Chir 23:208, 1901
17. Pogrel M: Compression osteosynthesis in mandibular fractures. Int J Oral Maxillofac Surg 15:521, 1986
18. El-Degwi A, Mathog R: Mandible fractures: economic considerations. Otolaryngol Head Neck Surg 108:213, 1993
19. Eid K, Lynch D, Whitaker L: Mandibular fractures: the problem patient. J Trauma 16:658, 1976
20. Thaller S, Reavie D, Daniller A: Rigid internal fixation with miniplates and screws: a cost-effective technique for treating mandible fractures? Ann Plast Surg 24:469, 1990

Acknowledgment

Figures 1 through 9   Carol Donner.

25 INJURIES TO THE NECK

David Wisner, M.D., and F. William Blaisdell, M.D.

Assessment and Management of Neck Injuries

Injuries to the neck can be secondary to both blunt and penetrating trauma. Most blunt injuries to the neck are managed nonoperatively; the initial diagnosis and treatment of these injuries in the emergency department setting are discussed elsewhere [*see* 22 Emergency Department Evaluation of the Patient with Multiple Injuries]. Occasionally, blunt trauma to the neck causes injury to the airway, the carotid artery system, or the vertebral artery system. Blunt airway injuries are sometimes surgical emergencies; the approach to these injuries is similar to that of penetrating injuries [*see* Airway Compromise *and* Isolated Laryngotracheal Injuries, *below*]. Blunt arterial injuries are almost always discovered by angiography and are usually treated nonoperatively. In the rare instance of a patient who undergoes operative treatment for a blunt injury to carotid or vertebral arteries, the operative and postoperative principles for penetrating arterial injuries should be applied [*see* Injuries to the Carotid Arteries, Jugular Veins, Pharynx, and Esophagus, *below*].

Patients with penetrating wounds of the neck can be loosely categorized into the following six groups according to the location and nature of the wound:

1. Patients with emergency or impending airway compromise.
2. Patients with an isolated injury to the larynx or trachea.
3. Patients with suspected or known injuries to the carotid arteries, jugular veins, pharynx, or esophagus.
4. Patients with wounds at the base of the neck (particularly when intrathoracic injury is suspected).
5. Patients with known injury to the vertebral arteries.
6. Patients with obviously superficial wounds of the neck.

Division of patients into these groups, though somewhat arbitrary, helps in choosing an incision and the initial operative priorities at exploration.

Airway Compromise

Some patients will present with emergency or impending airway compromise. The initial priority should be to ensure an adequate airway. In some patients, this requires orotracheal intubation. In other patients, the creation of a surgical airway is necessary by cricothyrotomy (in emergency cases) or tracheotomy (in less extreme cases).

CRICOTHYROTOMY

In true emergency situations, a cricothyrotomy should be done. The landmarks of the superior (notched) and inferior borders of the thyroid and the cricoid cartilage should be palpated. For this, it is helpful to stand on the patient's right side (for a right-handed surgeon) and to stabilize the cartilaginous framework by holding the thyroid cartilage in place with the left hand. A transverse incision should be made at the level of the cricothyroid membrane and developed rapidly through the subcutaneous tissue [*see 2 Trauma Resuscitation*]. As with any transversely oriented incision of the anterior neck, the anterior jugular veins are at risk for injury. If such injury occurs, the damaged veins are best controlled with suture ligation after an airway is obtained. In true emergency circumstances when the exact site of injury is unknown, a vertical rather than transverse incision should be used to allow access to as much of the anterior surface of the airway as possible and to decrease the chance of injury to the anterior jugular veins.

After the skin and subcutaneous tissue have been divided, an incision should be made through the cricothyroid membrane. This is most rapidly done with a No. 11 knife blade. It is important to avoid pushing the knife blade too far and causing injury to the posterior wall of the airway or to the posteriorly located hypopharynx and esophagus. After the incision has been made, the opening should be enlarged by placing the knife handle in the incision and twisting it 90°. At this point, an indwelling endotracheal airway should be placed and secured. In most adults, a No. 6 airway is the largest that can be inserted; a No. 4 or larger airway is adequate for initial placement. Any incisional bleeding from the anterior jugular vein or other vessels should be controlled. Cricothyrotomies should be converted to tracheotomies within 48 to 72 hours as long as the patient's general condition permits [*see* Discussion, Conversion of Cricothyrotomy to Tracheotomy, *below*].

TRACHEOTOMY

In some instances, airway compromise may not be extreme but a surgical airway may still be necessary for safety or subsequent management of a laryngeal injury. In such circumstances, a tracheotomy rather than a cricothyrotomy should be done, because cricothyrotomy is more likely than tracheotomy to make definitive treatment more difficult.

Assessment and Management of Neck Injuries

Patient has penetrating neck injury

Determine the location and nature of the injury.

Airway compromise

Ensure an adequate airway by orotracheal intubation or by creating a surgical airway.

- **Emergency airway compromise**

  Perform cricothyrotomy.

- **Nonemergency or potential airway compromise**

  Perform tracheotomy.

Isolated laryngotracheal injuries

Perform collar incision.

- **Small injuries to trachea**

  Close primarily, without tracheotomy.

- **Large injuries to trachea**
  - Anterior injuries: convert to tracheotomy.
  - Lateral and posterior injuries: close primarily and protect with tracheotomy.

- **Injuries to larynx**

  Perform tracheotomy and minimal debridement of laryngeal structures. Defer definitive treatment.

Known or suspected injuries to carotid arteries, jugular veins, pharynx, and esophagus

Perform anterior sternocleidomastoid incision for exposure and exploration of sites of injury [see Figure 1].

Wounds to the base of the neck

Assess known or suspected injuries to innominate or right subclavian artery [see Figure 5] and to left subclavian artery [see Figure 6].

Known vertebral artery injuries

Assess injuries [see Figure 7].

Superficial wounds

Achieve vascular control and debride the wound.

The initial approach for emergency tracheotomy is similar to that for cricothyrotomy, the difference being that a so-called collar incision is made at a point one to two fingerbreadths inferior to the level of the cricothyroid membrane. The incision should be wide enough to provide rapid exposure and should extend as far as the anterior border of the sternocleidomastoid bilaterally. Anteriorly located injuries at the level of the cricoid or trachea may already have a hole in the airway. In such cases, if the need for a surgical airway is immediate, the wound should be enlarged and used as a route of access to the airway.

On rare occasions, the injury is in the distal cervical or proximal intrathoracic trachea. In such circumstances, access to the trachea may not be possible through a cervical incision alone. Median sternotomy and lateral retraction of the innominate artery and left internal carotid artery allow exposure of the anterior surface of the trachea at the thoracic inlet. Right thoracotomy provides access to the more distal intrathoracic trachea.

Isolated Laryngotracheal Injuries

Most commonly, the presence of an isolated laryngotracheal injury is not known preoperatively. On occasion, however, isolated injuries to the larynx and trachea are known preoperatively on the basis of a suspicious history and the results of diagnostic studies, such as laryngoscopy and bronchoscopy.

Injuries to the larynx should be treated initially with a collar incision for the creation of a surgical airway [see Airway Compromise, Tracheotomy, *above*]; however, definitive treatment should be deferred. Minimal debridement of laryngeal structures should be carried out during the initial operative procedure. Injuries to the larynx should be handled on a semielective basis by otolaryngologists with expertise in laryngeal repair and reconstruction. Further investigation of the larynx, including laryngeal x-rays, laryngoscopy, and computed tomographic scanning, may be necessary.

Small injuries of the trachea can be repaired primarily without tracheotomy. Absorbable 3-0 or 4-0 sutures should be placed transversely, if possible, and should include tracheal rings above and below the site of injury. Large anterior defects should be converted to a tracheotomy, whereas defects to the lateral or posterior aspects of the trachea should be closed primarily and protected with a tracheotomy. Tension can be relieved from a repair by mobilizing the trachea proximally and distally. During this mobilization, the recurrent laryngeal nerves are subject to injury if the dissection is carried into the tracheoesophageal groove. Laryngotracheal injuries do not require routine drainage unless there is an associated injury to the pharynx or esophagus [see Injuries to the Carotid Arteries, Jugular Veins, Pharynx, and Esophagus, *below*].

If a large segment of trachea has been destroyed, primary anastomosis can be accomplished for defects up to five or six tracheal rings in length. Anastomosis requires mobilization of the intrathoracic trachea inferiorly and the laryngeal complex superiorly and is best done electively.[1,2]

Patients with laryngeal injuries should be watched carefully in the postoperative period for signs of mediastinitis, which may be from persistent airway leak or a missed pharyngoesophageal injury. The chest x-ray should also be checked for pneumomediastinum as a sign of continued airway leakage, particularly in patients who remain on positive pressure ventilation.

Injuries to the Carotid Arteries, Jugular Veins, Pharynx, and Esophagus

Probably the most common situation in penetrating cervical trauma is the patient with underlying structural injuries, the precise location and nature of which are unknown. Patients with known injuries to the carotid arteries, jugular veins, pharynx, and esophagus are also common. An anterior sternocleidomastoid incision provides good access to these areas and should be employed because of its relative ease and versatility.

STERNOCLEIDOMASTOID INCISION

If the location of underlying neck injuries is either unknown or confirmed by preoperative studies to be in the carotid arteries, the jugular veins, the pharynx, or the esophagus, an incision along the anterior border of the sternocleidomastoid muscle should be used [see Figure 1]. The sternocleidomastoid incision is particularly important in patients with true emergency conditions, such as external bleeding, focal neurologic deficits, coma, and an expanding neck hematoma. When bilateral exploration is necessary, separate sternocleidomastoid incisions should be done.

The use of an incision along the anterior border of the sternocleidomastoid muscle has several important advantages [see Figure 2]. For example, the incision can be lengthened to provide more extensive proximal or distal exposure. If a superior extension to below the earlobe is necessary, the incision should be curved posteriorly to avoid injury to the marginal mandibular branch of the facial nerve. Another advantage of the sternocleidomastoid incision is that it provides exposure of the carotid sheath, the pharynx, and the cervical esophagus.

Operative Technique

The patient should be supine with the head turned away from the side of exploration and the neck extended. In this regard, it is helpful to clear the cervical spine before operation. If both sides of the neck require exploration, the head should be left in the midposition, facing up. The entire neck and the appropriate side of the face and head should be prepped. The anterior chest should also be included in the preparation in case a median sternotomy is necessary for proximal control [see Exploration and Exposure, Arteries and Veins, *below*]. The patient should be draped in such a way as to leave the lateral neck as the primary field while the chest is kept easily accessible. The lateral chin and tip of the earlobe should also be kept in the field to provide landmarks. If the possibility exists that the injury is to the distal subclavian artery or the axillary artery, the patient's arm should be draped in a way that allows it to be manipulated.

The skin incision should be carried through the dermis and the platysma. After the platysma is divided in the direction of the incision, the investing fascia overlying the anterior border of the sternocleidomastoid muscle is incised, and the muscle is

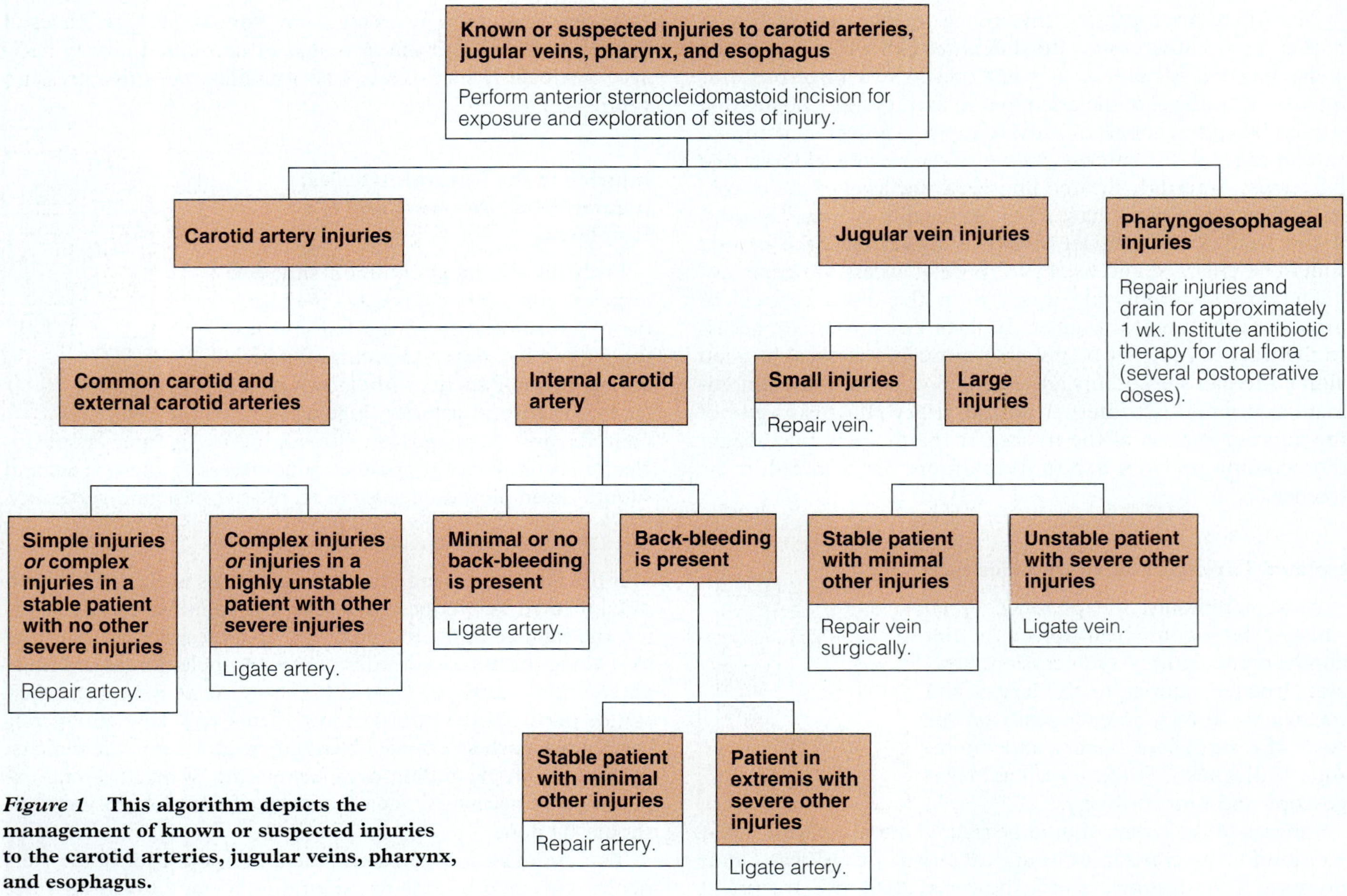

Figure 1 This algorithm depicts the management of known or suspected injuries to the carotid arteries, jugular veins, pharynx, and esophagus.

Known or suspected injuries to carotid arteries, jugular veins, pharynx, and esophagus
Perform anterior sternocleidomastoid incision for exposure and exploration of sites of injury.

- **Carotid artery injuries**
  - **Common carotid and external carotid arteries**
    - Simple injuries *or* complex injuries in a stable patient with no other severe injuries — Repair artery.
    - Complex injuries *or* injuries in a highly unstable patient with other severe injuries — Ligate artery.
  - **Internal carotid artery**
    - Minimal or no back-bleeding is present — Ligate artery.
    - Back-bleeding is present
      - Stable patient with minimal other injuries — Repair artery.
      - Patient in extremis with severe other injuries — Ligate artery.
- **Jugular vein injuries**
  - Small injuries — Repair vein.
  - Large injuries
    - Stable patient with minimal other injuries — Repair vein surgically.
    - Unstable patient with severe other injuries — Ligate vein.
- **Pharyngoesophageal injuries** — Repair injuries and drain for approximately 1 wk. Institute antibiotic therapy for oral flora (several postoperative doses).

---

retracted laterally and posteriorly to expose the carotid sheath. It is often necessary to divide a venous branch that connects the external jugular vein posterolaterally to the anterior jugular vein anteromedially. This vein lies in a plane immediately deep to the platysma.

Exploration and Exposure

When possible, proximal and distal control should be obtained before exploration of a carotid artery injury. In practice, obtaining proximal control before entering a perivascular hematoma is all that is absolutely necessary. Distal bleeding can be controlled with digital pressure while the dissection of the injured vessel is completed. Although it is often difficult to obtain control before addressing the area of injury, proximal and distal control of the vessel should be obtained at some point before any attempts at definitive repair. For injuries near the carotid bifurcation, it is necessary to control the common, internal, and external carotid arteries as well as the proximal branches of the external carotid artery.

Arteries and veins The initial exploration should attempt to rule out arterial or venous injury, unless an overt airway injury is present and requires immediate attention [*see* Airway Compromise, *above*]. If the airway is patent, the location of the carotid artery can then be confirmed by the presence of a pulse. It is often necessary to retract the jugular vein posterolaterally to provide adequate arterial exposure [*see*

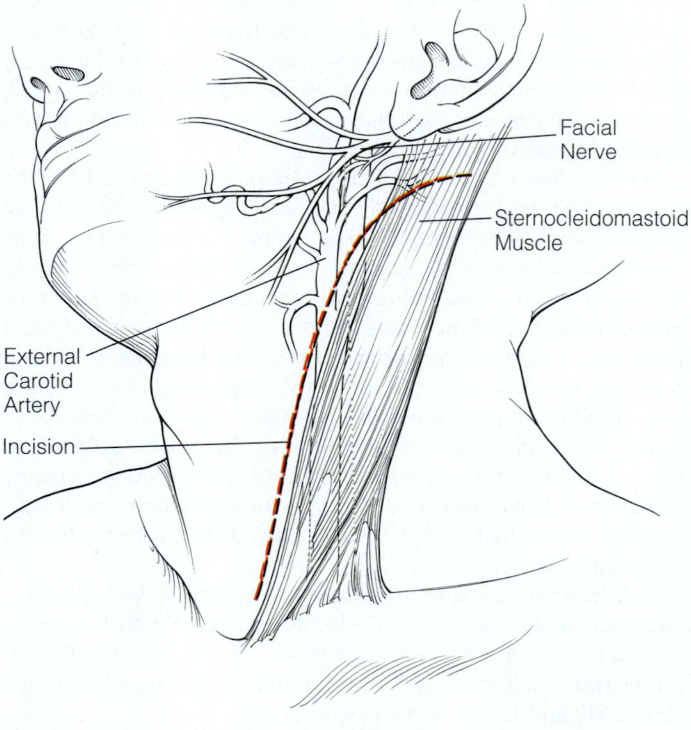

Figure 2 In general, exposure of structures in the anterior areas of the neck is best done through an incision oriented along the anterior border of the sternocleidomastoid muscle.

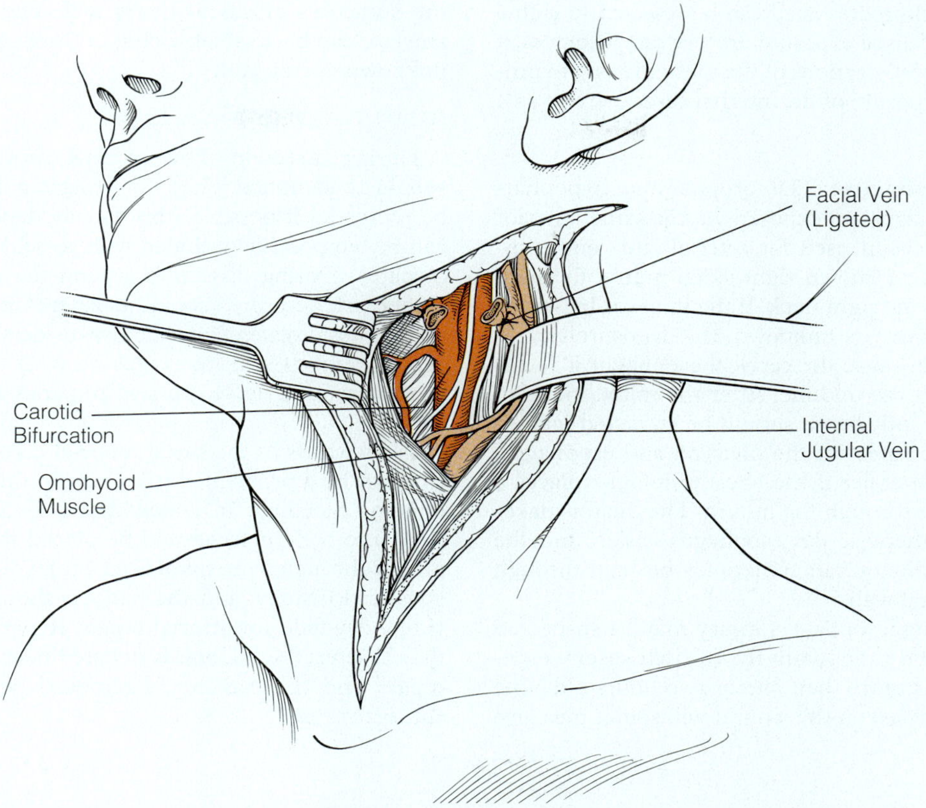

Figure 3 After a plane along the anterior border of the sternocleidomastoid muscle has been developed, dissection is carried down to the level of the carotid sheath. Suture ligation of the facial vein facilitates this dissection. Lateral retraction of the internal jugular vein improves exposure of the carotid bifurcation.

Figure 3]. Jugular vein retraction is facilitated by division of the facial vein, which is superficial to the carotid bifurcation. The severed ends of the facial vein should be suture-ligated to ensure that the ties will not come off with increased intravenous pressure in the postoperative period—for example, secondary to a cough or a Valsalva maneuver.

Exposure of the proximal common carotid artery at the base of the neck is easier after division of the omohyoid muscle at the point where its superior and inferior bellies are joined. Division of the omohyoid muscle results in minimal functional deficit postoperatively. For proximal control of the common carotid artery, it may be necessary to enter the chest via median sternotomy. To minimize blood loss, the decision to do a sternotomy should be made without undue delay. Control of the proximal right common carotid artery via this route is relatively easy and is accomplished by first obtaining control of the innominate artery and then dissecting distally. Proximal control of the left common carotid artery via median sternotomy is more difficult, because its origin from the aortic arch is more posterior than the origin of the innominate artery.

Exposure of the distal internal carotid artery can be very difficult, particularly if there is an injury in that location. As dissection is carried distally on the internal carotid artery, a number of important structures should be identified and protected [see Figure 4]. The hypoglossal nerve is usually encountered within several centimeters of the carotid bifurcation and should be dissected free of the internal carotid and retracted upward. This is facilitated by division of the occipital artery, which crosses superficial to the hypoglossal nerve on its course from the external carotid artery toward the occiput. It is also helpful to divide the ansa cervicalis branches that run inferiorly from the hypoglossal nerve to supply the muscles of the neck. Injury to the hypoglossal nerve results in impaired motor function of the tongue and can lead to dysarthria and dysphagia. Injury to or sectioning of the ansa cervicalis causes little or no morbidity.

Further distal exposure of the internal carotid artery may require unilateral mandibular subluxation or division of the ascending ramus of the mandible.[3,4] Such maneuvers are somewhat easier when the patient is nasotracheally intubated. They increase the size of the small area immediately behind the condyle and allow for easier division of the stylohyoid ligament and the styloglossus and stylopharyngeus muscles. These three structures can be divided together adjacent to their common origin at the styloid process. If this is done, care should be taken to preserve the facial nerve, which lies superficial to these muscles. The underlying glossopharyngeal nerve, which lies deep to these muscles and superficial to the internal carotid artery, should also be protected. Injury to the facial nerve results in loss of function of the muscles of facial expression. If the glossopharyngeal nerve is injured, loss of motor and sensory supply to parts of the tongue and pharynx increases the risk of aspiration.

Once the muscles originating from the styloid process have

been divided, the styloid process itself can be resected to gain a further short distance of distal exposure. In very rare instances, it may prove useful to remove portions of the mastoid bone to provide even more distal exposure of the internal carotid artery as it enters the carotid canal.

Pharynx and esophagus The oropharynx, hypopharynx, and cervical esophagus are exposed via the same anterior sternocleidomastoid incision used for arterial and venous injuries. If the patient has a known right-sided injury, the incision should be made in the right neck. If the injury is left-sided or if the exact site of injury is unknown, the exposure should be made from the left because the cervical esophagus is located slightly to the left of the midline. After the initial incision, the contents of the carotid sheath should be retracted laterally, exposing the lateral aspect of the pharynx and esophagus. This maneuver is made easier if the anesthesiologist places a large esophageal dilator through the mouth. The dilator makes identification of the otherwise flat esophagus easier, and the colored tubing of the dilator can sometimes be seen through defects in the esophageal wall.[5]

Sometimes, a pharyngoesophageal injury may be suspected but cannot be confirmed preoperatively. In such cases—especially when the injury is more than one or two hours old—the presence of salivary amylase in the wound will sometimes give the surgeon's gloves a greasy feel. The presence of salivary amylase can be a valuable clue to the existence of an otherwise unknown occult injury.

CAROTID ARTERY INJURIES

During dissection of the external carotid artery, the branches should be identified. They can be ligated if necessary but should be preserved if possible (this usually depends on whether they can be temporarily occluded with vessel loops, a looped suture, or clips). During dissection around the common and internal carotid arteries, care should be taken to avoid cutting or clamping the posterolaterally located vagus nerve; the recurrent laryngeal nerve runs with the vagus nerve at this level, and damage to the laryngeal nerve can lead to paralysis of the ipsilateral vocal cord.

For wounds of the distal internal carotid artery, distal control may be a problem, particularly in the presence of vigorous ongoing bleeding, in which case a Fogarty balloon catheter (size 3 to 5 French) should be placed through the area of injury or through a proximal arteriotomy. The catheter should be advanced distally, and the balloon should be inflated to provide a dry field for arterial repair. Repair can be done around the catheter; the balloon is deflated near the conclusion of the repair, and the catheter is removed before the final several sutures are tied.

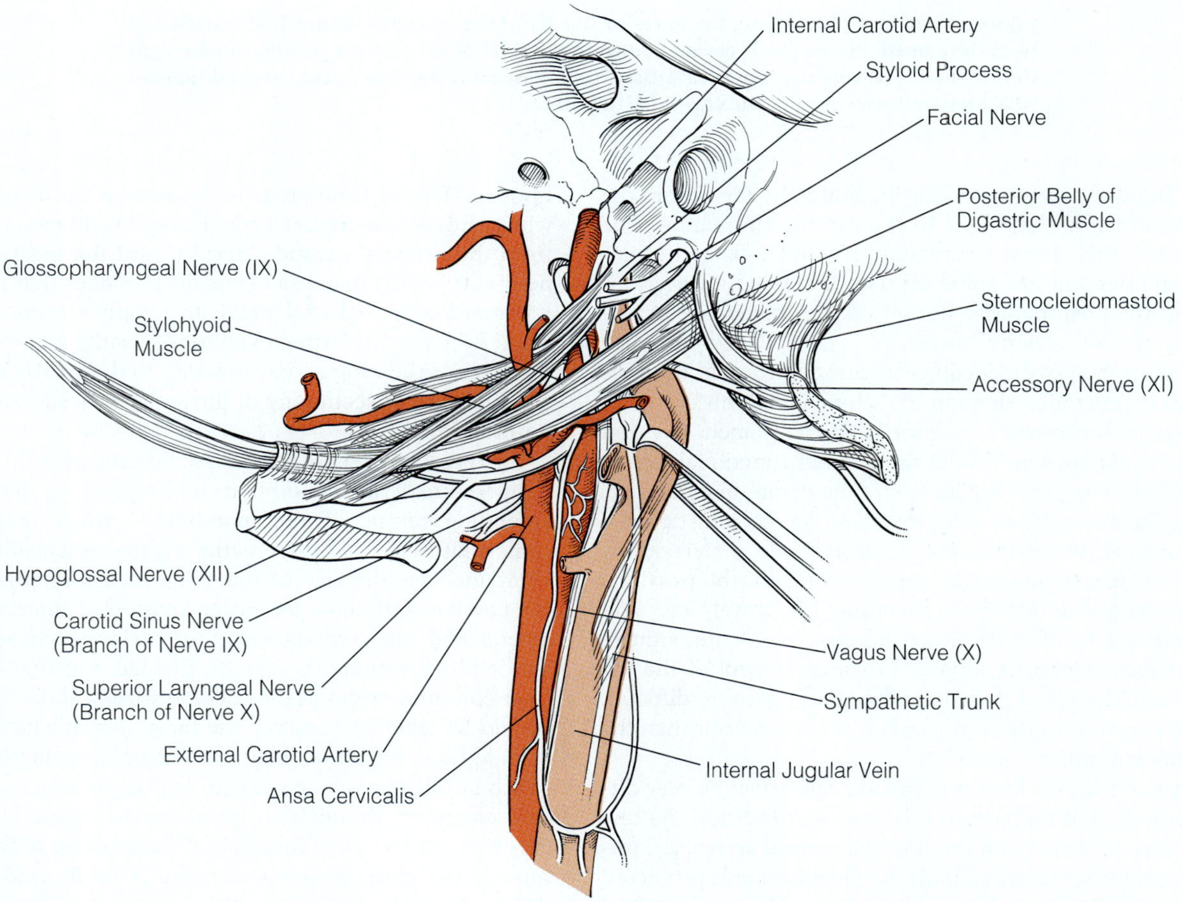

Figure 4 During distal dissection of the internal and external carotid arteries, a number of important structures are encountered, including the hypoglossal nerve and the occipital artery.

If associated injuries allow, a bolus of 5,000 to 10,000 units of heparin should be given before occluding any of the arteries in the neck. Because they have no branches, the common and internal carotid arteries can be safely mobilized for some distance from the injury to ensure a tension-free repair.

Management of injuries to the carotid arterial system is determined by the location of the injury, whereas management of common or external carotid artery injuries is governed by the extent of injury and the overall status of the patient. Small, simple injuries should be repaired. Complex injuries should be repaired in stable patients and treated with ligation in patients with severe hemodynamic instability or major associated injuries.

Initial management of injuries to the internal carotid artery depends on a determination of the amount of back-bleeding from the artery distal to the site of injury.[6,7] If back-bleeding is minimal or absent, the artery should be ligated. If significant back-bleeding is present, the overall status of the patient and the nature of the associated injuries should be taken into account [see Discussion, Repair versus Ligation of Carotid Arteries, below]. If the patient is hemodynamically stable and has minimal or moderate associated injuries, the internal carotid artery should be repaired. If the patient is hemodynamically unstable or has devastating associated injuries, the internal carotid artery should be ligated even when back-bleeding is present.

If a carotid artery injury involves minimal loss of vascular wall, primary repair is straightforward and can be done with either a running or interrupted technique; interrupted sutures will not purse-string the vessel. In younger patients who are still growing, interrupted sutures should be used to prevent later stenosis. As in elective vascular surgery, nonabsorbable sutures should be used; the carotid arteries generally require a 5-0, 6-0, or 7-0 monofilament suture, depending on the location of the injury and the type of suture material employed.

Defects greater than 1 to 2 cm in length should not be repaired primarily, because this will place excessive tension on the repair. For large defects limited to one surface of the vessel, a patch repair should be done. Either a venous patch or a synthetic patch can be used; when available, a venous patch is preferred for better long-term patency and to avoid placing a foreign body in a potentially contaminated wound.[8] Saphenous vein from the groin is preferable for patches because of its durability; a saphenous vein from the ankle is easiest to harvest when time is of the essence.[9] Although the jugular vein is in the operative field and can be easily harvested, it is better not to interfere with venous outflow in a neck in which the arterial inflow is to undergo repair; in addition, the jugular vein is very thin and difficult to handle.

For repairs near the carotid bifurcation, an alternative to venous patches and synthetic patches is the use of the proximal external carotid artery. This approach is especially appropriate when the origin of the external carotid artery is itself involved in the area of injury. If the injury is to the proximal internal carotid artery and the origin of the external carotid artery is free of injury, it is better to leave the external carotid artery patent and to use a venous patch or a synthetic patch instead; if the repair fails, the external carotid artery provides collateral distribution to the internal carotid artery via the ophthalmic artery.

Repair of circumferential loss of the common or internal carotid arteries is difficult. In this circumstance, if the defect is too long for primary anastomosis and the patient's general and neurologic condition permits, an interposition graft should be done. As with patch grafts, either venous or synthetic material can be used. As for patch grafts, saphenous vein from the groin is generally the donor material of first choice because of its strength. The saphenous vein from the groin is also well suited for reconstruction of the common carotid artery.

Completion angiography should be done after interposition graft placements and complex repairs of the common or internal carotid arteries. In general, patients with carotid artery injuries should be admitted postoperatively to an intensive care unit. ICU observation does not need to be prolonged but should be continued for at least 12 to 24 hours postoperatively. In the early postoperative period, the patient should be observed for bleeding or for the development of a neck hematoma; large postoperative hematomas may compromise the airway. If the patient develops a tense hematoma postoperatively, the neck should be reexplored.

Labile blood pressure—particularly in patients with extensive dissection around the carotid bifurcation—is another potential postoperative problem. It is related to manipulation of the carotid body, and control may require pharmacological intervention. Labile blood pressure is usually self-limiting and disappears over the first one to three days after operation, but it is another reason why patients with carotid artery repairs should be monitored initially in the ICU.

Antibiotics should be administered to cover common skin flora and should generally be continued only for one or two postoperative doses.

JUGULAR VEIN INJURIES

Any of the veins in the neck can be ligated when necessary. An exception to this rule is the rare instance when both internal jugular veins have been injured, in which case an attempt should be made to repair one of the veins, if possible. However, even in such cases, bilateral internal jugular ligation, if necessary, is usually tolerated. It is particularly important to use suture ligatures rather than simple ligatures on the cut ends of the internal jugular vein.

If the injury to the internal jugular is simple, the vein should be repaired. Large jugular vein injuries should be repaired only if the patient's general condition and associated injuries allow; if the patient is hemodynamically unstable or has severe associated injuries, large jugular vein injuries should be treated with ligation.

It is not always necessary to completely encircle the jugular vein proximal and distal to the site of injury; pressure with a finger or sponge stick will sometimes control bleeding while simple lateral venorrhaphy is done. In the case of more elaborate repairs, it is better either to encircle and occlude the proximal and distal vein or to place a side-biting vascular clamp for control during repair. Nonabsorbable 4-0 or 5-0 sutures should be used.

PHARYNGOESOPHAGEAL INJURIES

Either one- or two-layer repair of the pharynx and esophagus is acceptable, for which 3-0 or 4-0 absorbable sutures should be used. Attempts should be made to repair nearly all injuries, even when they are severe or are found on a delayed basis. In extreme cases of very large injuries or very delayed operative intervention, it may be necessary simply to drain the neck widely and turn the injury into a cervical esophagostomy. Esophageal diversion with distal esophageal ligation is rarely necessary in patients with isolated cervical esophageal injuries, except in cases when the injury is very low in the neck or in the thoracic esophagus.

Pharyngoesophageal injuries should be drained; either closed or Penrose drainage can be used. The drains should be left in place for approximately one week, at which time a radiographic contrast study should be obtained to determine whether the repair is competent. If the contrast study is negative for extravasation and the patient's general status permits, feeding can begin. If the feedings are well tolerated, the drains can be removed.[10]

Patients with pharyngoesophageal injuries should receive antibiotics appropriate for oral flora for several postoperative doses. If the repair is inadequate or breaks down, the resultant fistula will often heal with nonoperative management, provided that drainage is adequate. A high index of suspicion for mediastinitis should be maintained; the prevertebral space provides a ready route of access from the pharynx and cervical esophagus into the mediastinum. Therefore, missed or inadequately drained injuries may result in profound infection and a septic response.

Wounds at the Base of the Neck

Patients with wounds at the base of the neck should be identified early—particularly when an intrathoracic injury is suspected—so that the appropriate incision and operative approach can be undertaken.

A median sternotomy should be done for (1) patients with injuries at the base of the right neck and (2) patients in whom the superior mediastinum is the most likely site of injury and the most likely arterial injuries are to either the innominate artery or right subclavian artery[11,12] [see Figure 5]. Exposure of injuries to the proximal left subclavian artery is extremely difficult via sternotomy because of the artery's posterior location; in patients with such injuries, a left thoracotomy is needed [see Figure 6]. If a left thoracotomy is necessary, it is helpful to bump up the patient's left hip and shoulder to position the left chest 20° to 30° anteriorly. The head should be turned to the right, and the left arm should be prepped to the elbow and draped in such a way as to allow it free movement. Moving the arm is helpful in cases in which proximal exposure and control are done through the chest and distal exposure and control are done through a supraclavicular incision. It also allows for improved exposure of the axillary artery if necessary.

In stable patients with angiographically diagnosed injuries to either subclavian artery, a supraclavicular approach alone can be used, thereby avoiding initial entry into the chest. Because proximal control may not be feasible via this limited incision, the patient should still be positioned, prepped, and draped so that sternotomy or thoracotomy is possible. If the injury is on the right side of the neck and proximal control is not possible, a median sternotomy should be done. If the injury is on the left side of the neck and proximal control is not possible, a left thoracotomy should be performed.

If a median sternotomy has been done for exposure of an innominate artery or right subclavian artery injury, it may prove necessary to extend the incision into the right neck to obtain adequate distal control and exposure. Either a right supraclavicular or anterior sternocleidomastoid extension can be used. Although both are easily accomplished, the anterior sternocleidomastoid extension is the more versatile of the two. If a left thoracotomy is done for proximal control and exposure of the left subclavian artery, the distal subclavian artery should be exposed via a left supraclavicular incision. Improved exposure of the left subclavian artery at the thoracic outlet can be obtained either by resection of the medial one third to one half of the left clavicle or by a so-called trapdoor incision.[13] The trapdoor incision consists of a superior sternotomy and connection of the medial aspects of the thoracotomy and supraclavicular incisions. We find the trapdoor approach somewhat limited and cumbersome and prefer clavicular resection. Medial clavicular resection is accomplished by encircling the midclavicle in the subperiosteal plane via the supraclavicular incision. A Gigli's wire saw is then passed around the clavicle, and the clavicle is divided. The medial aspect of the divided bone is then grasped with a bone hook or Kocher clamp, and the dissection is carried medially in the subperiosteal plane to the sternoclavicular joint, which is disarticulated. If necessary, this dissection and resection can be accomplished in a matter of a few minutes.

After adequate exposure and control of innominate or subclavian artery injuries has been obtained, further management is determined by the nature of the injury and the status of the patient. Small injuries should always be repaired. Large injuries are not often seen, because they are usually incompatible with survival to medical attention. Nonetheless, they do occur, and their management is influenced by the status of the patient. Attempts at repair should be made for most such injuries, but in highly unstable patients, the artery should be ligated. However, there is sometimes severe morbidity associated with artery ligation, and it should be avoided if possible.

The wall of the subclavian artery is thin, and extra care should be taken when dissecting around it. Primary repair should be done with either interrupted or running nonabsorbable 4-0 or 5-0 sutures, laterally placed. Because of its location and the large number of branches, the subclavian artery is difficult to mobilize extensively. None of the branches are vital, however, and all can be divided as necessary to gain mobility. The vertebral artery should be preserved if possible, because in rare instances, ligation of the artery can lead to cerebral ischemia. Even with division of arterial branches, only short segments of the artery can be removed without the need for an interposition graft to avoid an anastomosis under tension. Saphenous vein is usually too small to be used as a graft, even when it is harvested from the groin. Accordingly, a synthetic graft is usually the better choice. Infections in this location are rare, even when the graft is placed in a contaminated field.[14]

Complex injuries of the innominate and subclavian veins should be treated with suture ligation, particularly when the patient has severe associated injuries. Simple injuries can be treated with lateral venorrhaphy. Depending on the circumstances, formal control of the proximal and distal vein can first be obtained, or pressure can be applied proximally and distally to provide for a bloodless field during repair. Another alternative for control of bleeding during venous repair is the use of a side-biting vascular clamp.

Some patients with injuries to the subclavian artery or subclavian vein require dissection of the supraclavicular area. The supraclavicular fat pad contains a large number of lymph nodes and lymphatic channels, and dissection of the fat pad can result in considerable weeping of lymphatic fluid; these wounds should therefore be drained. Either a closed or open drain can be used, and the drain should be brought out through a separate stab wound near the incision. After a left-sided procedure, persistent milky drainage via either drains or the wound suggests injury to the thoracic duct and may necessitate repeat operative intervention if it persists.

Elevation or paralysis of the hemidiaphragm ipsilateral to the side of dissection can indicate injury to the phrenic nerve, which courses in the field of dissection on the anterior surface of the anterior scalene muscle.

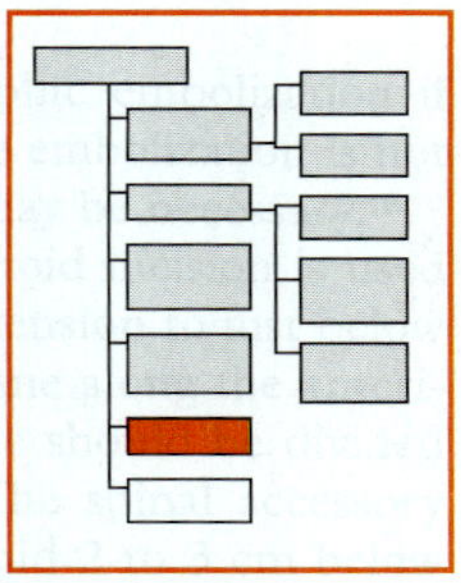

Known Vertebral Artery Injuries

On occasion, patients who present with penetrating cervical wounds and are hemodynamically and neurologically stable are demonstrated on angiographic workup to have an injury to the vertebral artery. In rarer instances, the location of an injury in the posterior triangle of the neck and the presence of ongoing hemorrhage may also indicate the high likelihood of an injury to the distal vertebral artery [see Figure 7].

Most vertebral artery injuries occur in stable patients and are discovered on angiography. Because operative attempts at ligation are associated with blood loss that can be problematic, an alternative approach utilizing angiographic embolization has been developed.[15] In most cases of injury to the distal vertebral artery, the angiographic approach is preferred if available [see Discussion, Angiographic Embolization of Distal

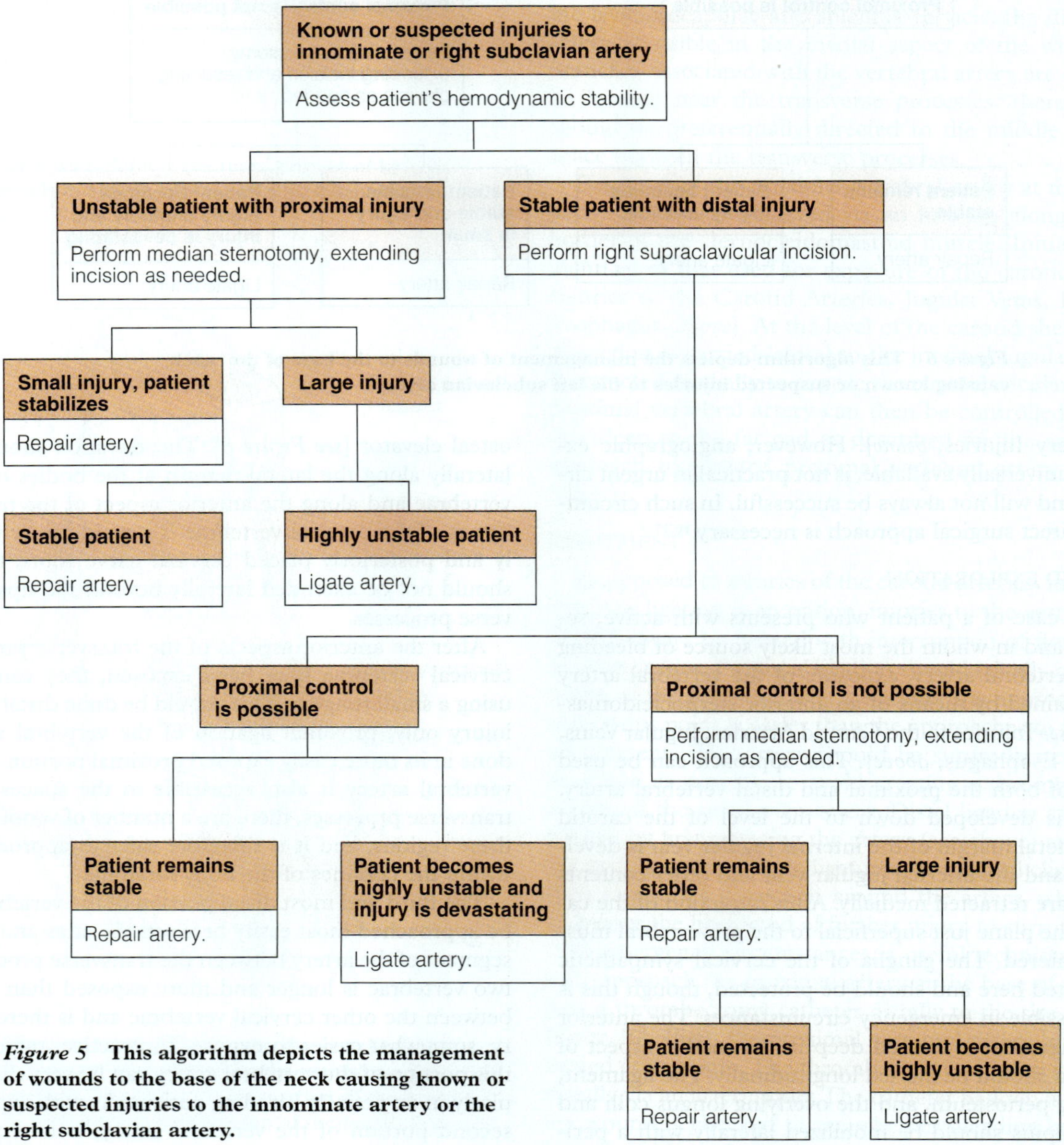

Figure 5 This algorithm depicts the management of wounds to the base of the neck causing known or suspected injuries to the innominate artery or the right subclavian artery.

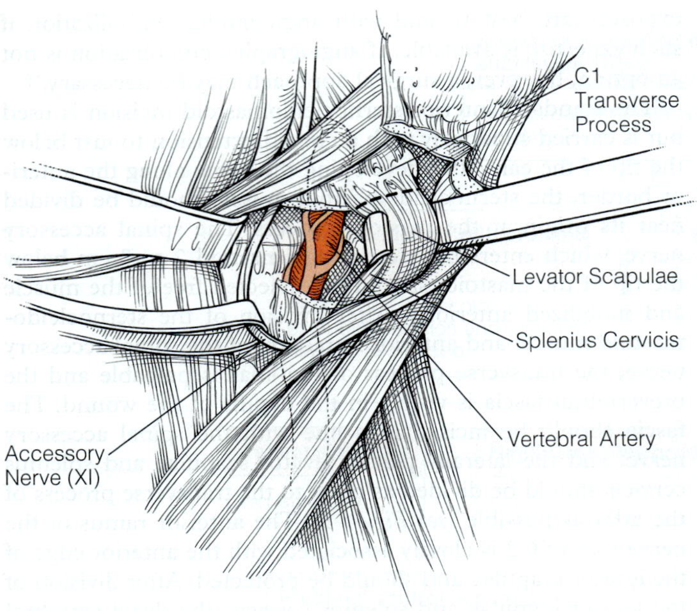

Figure 9 Exposure of the distal vertebral artery is done via an incision along the anterior border of the sternocleidomastoid muscle. The sternocleidomastoid muscle is then divided near its origin at the mastoid process. The spinal accessory nerve is mobilized anteriorly. The vertebral artery is accessible after division of the levator scapulae and splenius cervicis.

should be divided with the electrocautery at its insertion on the clavicle. The muscle is then retracted superiorly and medially. In the plane deep to the sternocleidomastoid muscle, the omohyoid muscle should be divided in its middle tendinous portion with the electrocautery.

At a level just deep to the sternocleidomastoid and omohyoid muscles, the carotid sheath is encountered in the medial aspect of the wound. The lateral border of the internal jugular vein should be dissected free of adjacent tissue and retracted medially. If the operation is on the left, the thoracic duct may be found in the medial portion of the wound. The thoracic duct is easily injured with retraction and should be divided and ligated if it is in the way.

Just lateral to the internal jugular vein at the same depth is the supraclavicular fat pad, which should be dissected from the supraclavicular fossa in which it lies. Exposure is further enhanced by dissection and division of the laterally located anterior scalene muscle. The phrenic nerve is closely applied to the anterior surface of the anterior scalene muscle and should be dissected free from the underlying muscle and retracted out of the field with a vessel loop. The anterior scalene muscle can then be divided with the electrocautery. During dissection of the supraclavicular fat pad, it may be necessary to divide branches of the thyrocervical and costocervical trunks. The most prominent of these branches is the inferior thyroid artery,

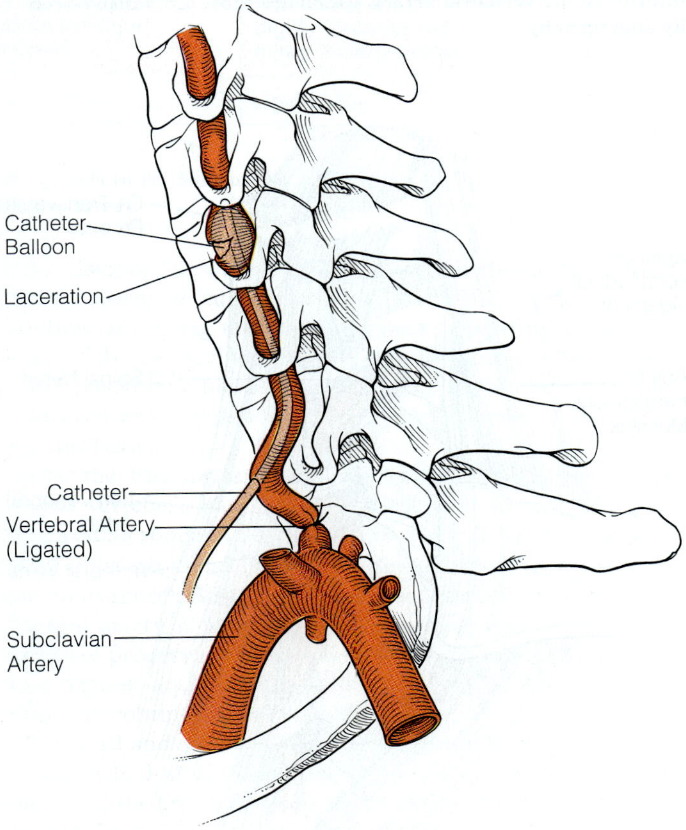

catheter is left in place, and the proximal end is brought out through the wound. The catheter is left in situ for approximately 48 hours, at which time the balloon is deflated and the wound is again checked for bleeding. If there is no bleeding for four to six hours, the catheter can be withdrawn. If the use of a thrombectomy catheter is unsuccessful, a direct surgical approach to the second or third portion of the artery is necessary. However, one of the potential disadvantages of adopting a surgical approach is that proximal ligation of the vertebral artery precludes angiographic embolization except via the contralateral vertebral artery. Embolization via the contralateral vertebral artery is extremely difficult and may result in ischemia or uncontrolled embolization.

If the injury is known by preoperative angiography to be isolated to the first portion of the vertebral artery, both proximal and distal ligation may be possible via a supraclavicular incision [see Figure 11]. The patient is positioned with the head turned away from the side of injury, and the chest and ipsilateral neck are prepared and draped. Preparation and draping include the chest so that a left thoracotomy can be done later if necessary for proximal control of the left subclavian artery. In such cases, it is helpful to bump the patient up on the left so that an anterolateral thoracotomy incision can be carried further posteriorly.

The supraclavicular incision should be made approximately one fingerbreadth superior to the clavicle and should extend medially to the midpoint of the sternocleidomastoid insertion and laterally to the juncture of the middle and lateral thirds of the clavicle. The skin, subcutaneous tissue, and platysma should be incised. The external jugular vein, if in the operating field, should be suture-ligated. The clavicular head of the sternocleidomastoid muscle is encountered next, and its lateral aspect

Figure 10 Bleeding from vertebral artery injuries located within the transverse process of the cervical vertebrae can sometimes be controlled by exposing the proximal vertebral artery at the base of the neck, passing a thrombectomy catheter distally, and inflating the balloon at the site of injury.

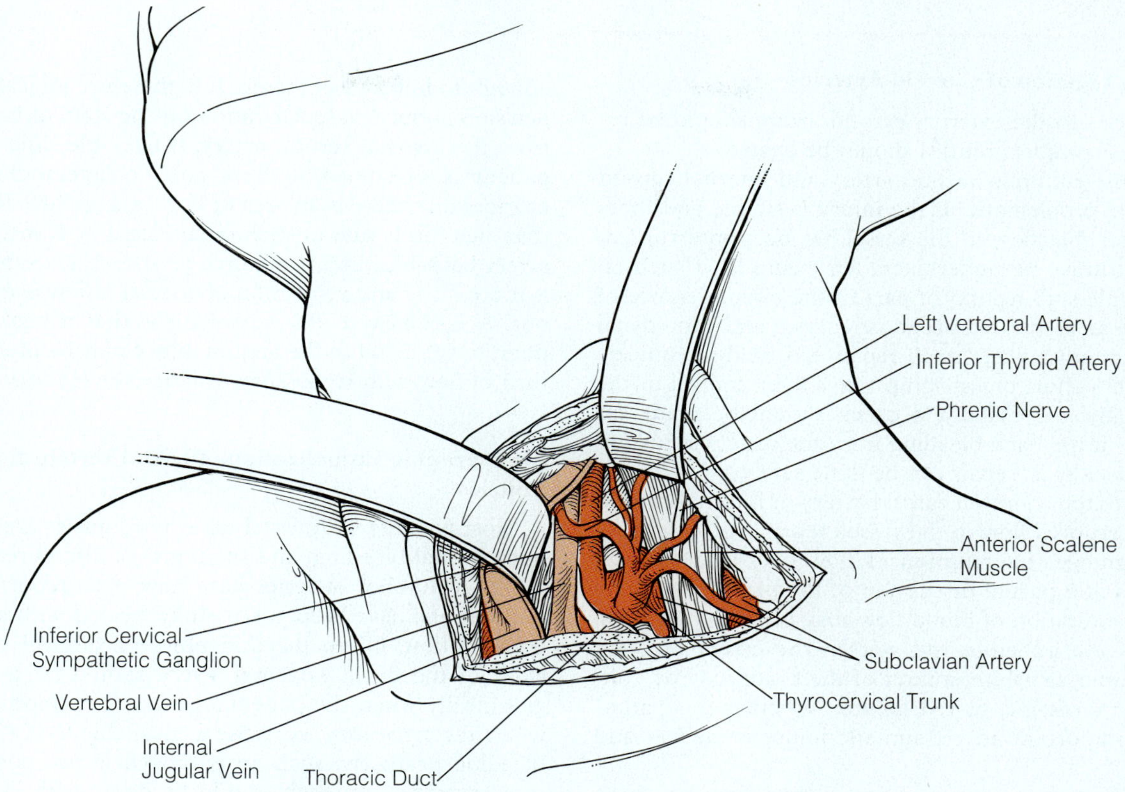

Figure 11 The proximal vertebral artery can be approached via a supraclavicular incision. Dissection of the supraclavicular fat pad reveals the underlying vertebral artery where it diverges from the subclavian artery. During dissection, care should be taken to avoid injuring the phrenic nerve.

which stems from the thyrocervical trunk and courses medially toward the thyroid.

After the supraclavicular fat pad has been dissected, the proximal portion of the vertebral artery is reached. The vertebral vein usually lies slightly superficial and medial to the vertebral artery. It should be divided and suture-ligated for better exposure. Care should be taken not to retract too vigorously on the vertebral vein before suture ligation to avoid its avulsion from the subclavian vein. At the depth of the vertebral artery, the white, cordlike elements of the brachial plexus are often visible in the superolateral aspect of the wound. If possible, traction should not be placed on the brachial plexus, and use of the electrocautery around the plexus should be minimized. After exposure, the proximal vertebral artery should be ligated both proximal and distal to the site of injury. No attempts at repair should be made.

Angiographic embolization, the preferred treatment of angiographically diagnosed injuries of the distal vertebral artery, depends on the availability of equipment and expertise with the procedure [*see* Discussion, Angiographic Embolization of Distal Vertebral Artery Injuries, *below*]. If angiographic embolization is not available, exposure and ligation should be carried out as described above.

In cases where angiographic embolization of the vertebral artery has been employed, a postprocedure angiogram should be done several days to weeks after the procedure to ensure that the artery remains occluded and that no arteriovenous fistula between the injured vertebral artery and the surrounding venous plexus has developed. Duplex scanning has also been used to a limited extent for follow-up screening. It can be used as an alternative to angiography, but its sensitivity relative to angiography is not yet proved.

Superficial Wounds

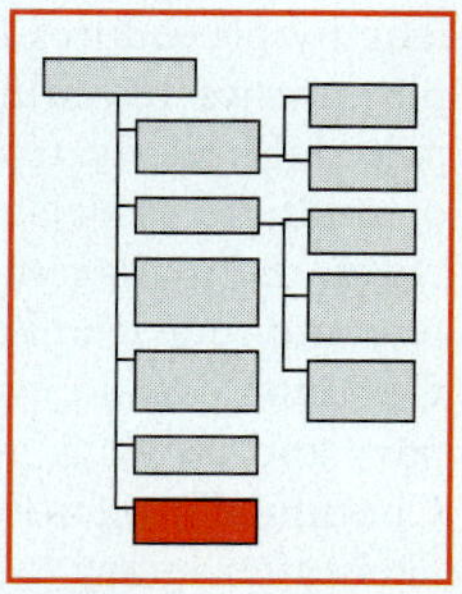

Some wounds are obviously superficial on the initial physical examination. Most commonly, these wounds are slash wounds caused by a knife or other sharp object as opposed to being true stab wounds. Rapid exposure and vascular control are sometimes easily accomplished through these wounds. In such circumstances, the surgical procedure consists of debridement of the neck wound, and deep dissection is not necessary. If greater access and control are needed to rule out further injuries or for definitive repair, a standard anterior sternocleidomastoid incision should be done [*see* Injuries to the Carotid Arteries, Jugular Veins, Pharynx, and Esophagus, *above*].

Discussion

Repair versus Ligation of Carotid Arteries

Simple injuries to the external carotid artery should be repaired, whereas complex injuries should be ligated.

Injuries to the common carotid artery and internal carotid artery are more problematic. If the injury is simple and there is no suggestion that flow in the vessel has been interrupted, repair should always be undertaken. An example of such an injury is a simple stab wound of part of the circumference of the artery with an associated pseudoaneurysm and good distal flow. In this circumstance, lateral repair can be done quickly and easily with a short cross-clamp time. After control of the vessel proximally and distally, a check should be made for back-bleeding. If the back-bleeding from the distal circulation is brisk, as it usually is, repair can be done safely.

If an injury to the common carotid artery or internal carotid artery has interrupted flow in the vessel, repair creates a theoretical disadvantage. Interruption of flow may lead to focal brain ischemia and partial disruption of the blood-brain barrier. Sudden restoration of blood flow may cause hemorrhage in the area of the ischemia and worsen the extent of brain injury; an anemic, or white, infarct of the brain may be converted to a hemorrhagic, or red, infarct. Whether this pathophysiology is important after traumatic injury is unclear and controversial.

Deciding whether to repair or ligate when flow has been interrupted is often difficult.[6,7] One approach is to base the decision on the patient's preoperative neurologic status. If there is no neurologic deficit, it is presumed that there are no areas of brain ischemia and that repair is safe. Conversely, a focal neurologic deficit is presumed to be related to ischemia, and in such cases, the risk of worsening the patient's neurologic status with restoration of blood flow is increased. Even though this approach is rational, it is not applicable in cases in which a detailed neurologic examination before surgery is not possible. Furthermore, this approach may be applicable only to patients in coma or with severe neurologic deficits. There are indications that milder neurologic deficits respond favorably to revascularization.

Yet another approach is to gauge the appropriateness of repair according to the nature of the injury itself. In this approach, large, complicated injuries requiring involved and lengthy procedures for repair should be ligated, whereas simple injuries requiring only simple and quick repairs are repaired. Similarly, repair is not indicated in patients with severe or multiple associated injuries. There is also a difference between the management of injuries of the common carotid artery and management of injuries of the internal carotid artery. Common carotid injuries are more accessible and easier to repair, and repair is generally associated with a good outcome. Continued prograde flow in the internal carotid artery is more likely after injury to the common carotid artery than to the internal carotid artery because of the possibility of collateral flow via the external carotid artery.

A reasonable way to deal with repair dilemmas is to make the decision on the basis of distal back-bleeding. Interruption of blood flow to the brain is tolerated only for a short time, and restoration of flow is unlikely to be accomplished quickly enough to improve outcome. It is therefore logical to base the decision about revascularization on the state of back-bleeding from the internal carotid artery. If back-bleeding is brisk, the patient is presumed to have good collateral flow, and the chances that there is an area of ischemia are low. Repair rather than ligation is safe in such circumstances. If internal carotid artery back-bleeding is minimal or absent, an ischemic infarct is more likely and restitution of arterial inflow is more dangerous. A corollary to this reasoning is that if back-bleeding is poor, a clot distal to the area of injury may be present, and return of flow with repair may dislodge the clot distally.

Angiographic Embolization of Distal Vertebral Artery Injuries

Most patients with vertebral artery injuries are stable without external bleeding, and the injury is discovered by angiography. A number of series have now been reported in which such lesions have been successfully treated with angiographic embolization. Given the difficulties of surgical exposure, lesions of the distal vertebral artery should be treated angiographically when the patient's general condition permits and when the necessary expertise is available.[15] If the patient is bleeding profusely, such an approach is not possible, and a rapid surgical approach should be done, with ligation of the proximal vertebral artery and an attempt at thrombectomy catheter control or packing of the wound until an angiographic approach can be attempted. If this is unsuccessful, the lesion should be approached directly [see Known Vertebral Artery Injuries, above].

If a patient with a distal vertebral artery lesion is stable—particularly when the lesion is otherwise silent and has been detected angiographically—an attempt should be made at angiographic embolization if the necessary expertise is available. Embolization is done via the ipsilateral proximal vertebral artery. Detachable balloons or coils can be used.

Conversion of Cricothyrotomy to Tracheotomy

Cricothyrotomy is typically reserved for life-threatening airway compromise when the need for a rapid surgical airway is paramount [see Airway Compromise, above, and 2 Trauma Resuscitation]. Tracheotomy is preferred if time and a lesser degree of urgency permit. Similarly, in the postoperative period, tracheotomy is preferred to cricothyrotomy. Traditional thinking, initially promulgated by Chevalier Jackson in 1921, is that cricothyrotomy is more likely than tracheotomy to result in airway stricture or damage to more proximal structures in the larynx. On the basis of this rationale, cricothyrotomies are converted to tracheotomies on a semielective basis within 24 to 48 hours of admission if the patient's general condition permits.[19,20]

Evidence to support a policy of routine conversion is mixed. Several series document a low but increased incidence of complications to the larynx and trachea from prolonged maintenance of cricothyrotomies. Even though incidence is low, the complications can be severe and may require extensive reconstructive procedures. Conversely, studies of cardiac patients undergoing routine cricothyrotomy do not demonstrate a significant increase in the incidence of airway complications. Cricothyrotomy is sometimes favored over tracheotomy in these patients because of concerns about the proximity of tracheotomy wounds to the patient's sternotomy incision. The results of studies of routine cardiac patients may be different from results of studies showing an increase in complications after cricothyrotomy, in that cardiac patients were intubated for shorter periods.

There have been no studies documenting a high incidence of complications in trauma patients who have undergone emergency cricothyrotomy and have remained intubated via the cricothyrotomy for longer than two or three days. Because complications are potentially so devastating, however, emergency cricothyrotomies should be converted to tracheotomy within one to two days of admission in stable patients. Assuming a stable patient, the risks of conversion are minimal, and conversion is justified to avoid the possibility of future complications.

References

1. Fuhrman GM, Steig FH III, Buerk CA: Blunt laryngeal trauma: classification and management protocol. J Trauma 30:87, 1990
2. Symbas IN, Hatcher CR Jr, Boehm GAW: Acute penetrating tracheal trauma. Ann Thorac Surg 22:473, 1976
3. Dossa C, Shepard AD, Wolford DG, et al: Distal internal carotid exposure: a simplified technique for temporary mandibular subluxation. J Vasc Surg 12:319, 1990
4. Fisher DF Jr, Clagett GP, Parker JI, et al: Mandibular subluxation for high carotid exposure. J Vasc Surg 1:727, 1984
5. Beal SL, Pottmeyer EW, Spisso JM: Esophageal perforation following external blunt trauma. J Trauma 28:1425, 1988
6. Fabian TC, George SM Jr, Croce MA, et al: Carotid artery trauma: management based on mechanism of injury. J Trauma 30:953, 1990
7. Richardson R, Obeid FN, Richardson JD, et al: Neurologic consequences of cerebrovascular injury. J Trauma 32:755, 1992
8. Feliciano DV, Mattox KL, Graham JM, et al: Five-year experience with PTFE grafts in vascular wounds. J Trauma 25:71, 1985
9. Archie JP Jr, Green JJ Jr: Saphenous vein rupture pressure, rupture stress, and carotid endarterectomy vein patch reconstruction. Surgery 107:389, 1990
10. Winter RP, Weigelt JA: Cervical esophageal trauma: incidence and cause of esophageal fistulas. Arch Surg 125:849, 1990
11. Abouljoud MS, Obeid FN, Horst HM, et al: Arterial injuries of the thoracic outlet: a ten-year experience. Am Surg 59:590, 1993
12. Rich NM, Baugh JH, Hughes CW: Acute arterial injuries in Vietnam: 1,000 cases. J Trauma 10:359, 1970
13. Wood VE: The results of total claviculectomy. Clin Orthop 207:186, 1986
14. McCready RA, Procter CD, Hyde GL: Subclavian-axillary vascular trauma. J Vasc Surg 3:24, 1986
15. Higashida RT, Halbach VV, Tsai FY, et al: Interventional neurovascular treatment of traumatic carotid and vertebral artery lesions: results in 234 cases. AJR Am J Roentgenol 153:577, 1989
16. Hatzitheofilou C, Demetriades D, Melissas J, et al: Surgical approaches to vertebral artery injuries. Br J Surg 75:234, 1988
17. Reid JD, Weigelt JA: Forty-three cases of vertebral artery trauma. J Trauma 28:1007, 1988
18. Blickenstaff KL, Weaver FA, Yellin AE, et al: Trends in the management of traumatic vertebral artery injuries. Am J Surg 158:101, 1989
19. Esses BA, Jafek BW: Cricothyroidotomy: a decade of experience in Denver. Ann Otol Rhinol Laryngol 96:519, 1987
20. Milner SM, Bennett JDC: Review article: emergency cricothyrotomy. J Laryngol Otol 105:883, 1991

Reviews

Surgical Anatomy, 6th ed. Anson B, McVay CB, Eds. WB Saunders Co, Philadelphia, 1984

Anatomic Exposures in Vascular Surgery. Wind G, Valentine R, Eds. Williams & Wilkins, Baltimore, 1991

Acknowledgments

Figure 1   Marcia Kammerer.
Figures 2 through 4   Susan E. Brust, C.M.I.
Figures 5 through 7   Marcia Kammerer.
Figures 8 through 11   Susan E. Brust, C.M.I.

26 INJURIES TO THE CHEST

Kenneth L. Mattox, M.D., and Asher Hirshberg, M.D.

Choice of Incision

The operative approach to thoracic trauma is determined primarily by the hemodynamic stability of the injured patient. As a general rule, anterolateral thoracotomy is the incision of choice in the unstable patient. This incision allows rapid access to the visceral content of the hemithorax, does not require special positioning, and does not interfere with access to other visceral compartments. The incision may also be rapidly extended across the sternum to the contralateral hemithorax. In the stable patient, thoracotomy follows a diagnostic workup with precise delineation of the injury, and thus, the incision can be targeted on the injured structure. The choice of thoracotomy incision in stable patients with bleeding into the pleural cavity or the airway is determined by the location of the injury. In patients with blunt or penetrating trauma to the right lower chest, bleeding is usually from an injured liver, and therefore, the initial approach is via a midline laparotomy. The right chest is entered only if laparotomy fails to reveal the source of bleeding. Injuries above the right nipple line and to any part of the left chest are approached through an anterolateral thoracotomy on the injured side.

Penetrating wounds to the base of the neck present special access problems. Injuries to the base of the right neck or those bleeding into the right pleural cavity are approached by median sternotomy. However, the first part of the left subclavian artery is intrapleural and posterior, and the appropriate incision for proximal control of this vessel is a left anterolateral thoracotomy in the third or fourth intercostal space. This incision is used for thoracic inlet injuries bleeding into the left pleura or for presumed left subclavian artery laceration. The more lateral parts of both subclavian arteries are approached through a supraclavicular incision, and exposure can be facilitated by removal of the medial third of the clavicle. An important operative adjunct is the insertion of a Foley balloon catheter into the missile tract to achieve temporary hemostasis by inflating the balloon while access and direct control are obtained.

The initial incision chosen for access to an actively bleeding thoracic inlet injury may prove inadequate and is immediately extended if necessary. A median sternotomy can be extended along the border of the sternocleidomastoid muscle or along the clavicle to improve access to the carotid or subclavian arteries. A so-called trapdoor incision is created by extending the median sternotomy into an anterolateral thoracotomy in conjunction with a supraclavicular incision. This incision is useful for proximal left carotid injuries and for obtaining control of the proximal left subclavian artery if the initial incision was a median sternotomy.

The choice of thoracotomy incision in stable patients hinges on precise delineation of the injured structures. The heart, ascending aorta, arch, and thoracic inlet vessels are approached via a median sternotomy. A posterolateral thoracotomy is indicated for injuries to the descending aorta, esophagus, lung, and bronchus.

Resuscitative Thoracotomy

The incision for resuscitative thoracotomy is made immediately beneath the nipple in men or beneath the manually retracted breast in women. It extends from the sternum medially as far lateral as possible. The incision is rapidly performed with a knife, and heavy scissors are used to cut the intercostal muscles. Time is not wasted on skin preparation, wound hemostasis, or identification of the severed internal mammary artery. A chest wall retractor is inserted with the handle away from the sternum and facing the axilla.

The subsequent operative maneuvers depend on the clinical circumstances. If a tamponade is suspected, the pericardial sac is opened longitudinally—anterior and parallel to the phrenic nerve—up to the aortic root superiorly and the diaphragm inferiorly. The heart is manually delivered into the left hemithorax and carefully examined for injuries. External visualization of the intact pericardium is misleading and should never be relied upon to exclude a tamponade. Attempts to repair cardiac lacerations in the suboptimal technical circumstances of the emergency room are frequently futile. Evacuation of blood and temporary control of the lacerations by digital pressure, a Foley catheter, or a skin stapler will allow transfer of the patient to the operating room for definitive repair under optimal conditions.

The descending thoracic aorta should be clamped to maintain cerebral and coronary perfusion in the agonal patient; clamping is also an important adjunct to open cardiac massage. This maneuver involves manual upward traction of the left lung, division of the inferior pulmonary ligament, incision of the mediastinal pleura, and just enough blunt finger dissection around the aorta to accommodate an aortic clamp. Digital aortic occlusion may be a safer and less traumatic alternative when visualization of the area is not optimal. When hemorrhage arises from the pulmonary hilum or parenchyma and when coronary air embolism is suspected, the pulmonary hilum is clamped. This maneuver also requires mobilization of the inferior pulmonary ligament.

As a general rule, the injured hemithorax is entered first. However, when it becomes apparent that the patient's agonal state is not explained by the findings in the open hemithorax, the incision should rapidly be extended across the sternum into the other hemithorax. This is particularly true for a right-sided thoracotomy, which does not provide access to the heart and the descending thoracic aorta. Extension of a left thoracotomy to the right hemithorax is done in the fourth intercostal space to facilitate access to the innominate artery. The resulting clam shell incision provides excellent access to all thoracic viscera (except the posterior mediastinal structures), albeit at the price of increased morbidity.

The technical keys to resuscitative thoracotomy are speed in entering the chest and avoiding complex repairs or maneuvers until the patient is in the operating room, where definitive repair of injuries is accomplished. The major pitfalls are iatrogenic injuries to the phrenic nerve or heart during pericardiotomy, avulsion of an intercostal artery, or esophageal perforation during attempted aortic clamping. Care should be taken to avoid laceration of the inferior pulmonary vein during division of the inferior pulmonary ligament. The transected internal mammary artery should be identified and ligated before closure.

Cardiac Trauma

SIMPLE INJURIES

Repair of simple anterolateral cardiac lacerations is a straightforward matter. The major determinants of a successful outcome in these cases are timely diagnosis and swift thoracotomy. The laceration itself is repaired either by simple or pledgeted monofilament suture. The most common site of myocardial disruption from blunt trauma is the right atrium, usually at the atriocaval junction. Atrial lacerations can sometimes be controlled with a partially occluding clamp to facilitate the repair.

COMPLEX INJURIES

Several factors may complicate the cardiorrhaphy [see Figure 1]. Injuries to the right side of the heart may not be accessible via a left thoracotomy and, thus, may require transsternal extension. Multiple holes or lacerations may require temporary control using digital pressure, an occluding balloon catheter, or a skin stapler. Lacerations involving a coronary artery present a special problem. Ligation of a distal coronary artery is rarely associated with significant arrhythmias or infarction, whereas proximal coronary lacerations should be repaired. When the cardiac perforation is in close proximity to a coronary artery, horizontal mattress sutures passed beneath the artery help avoid inadvertent interruption of the vessel [see Figure 2].

Temporary inflow occlusion is a key maneuver in difficult situations, such as posterior lacerations or injuries to the intrapericardial great vessels. Both venae cavae are rapidly clamped, and the heart is allowed to empty. This results in a temporarily dry operative field, which may be just enough for several quick critical stitches. Large posterior atrial lacerations can sometimes be repaired from within the heart by atriotomy combined with inflow occlusion. Cardiopulmonary bypass is always a theoretical possibility but rarely a practical option in the acute situation.

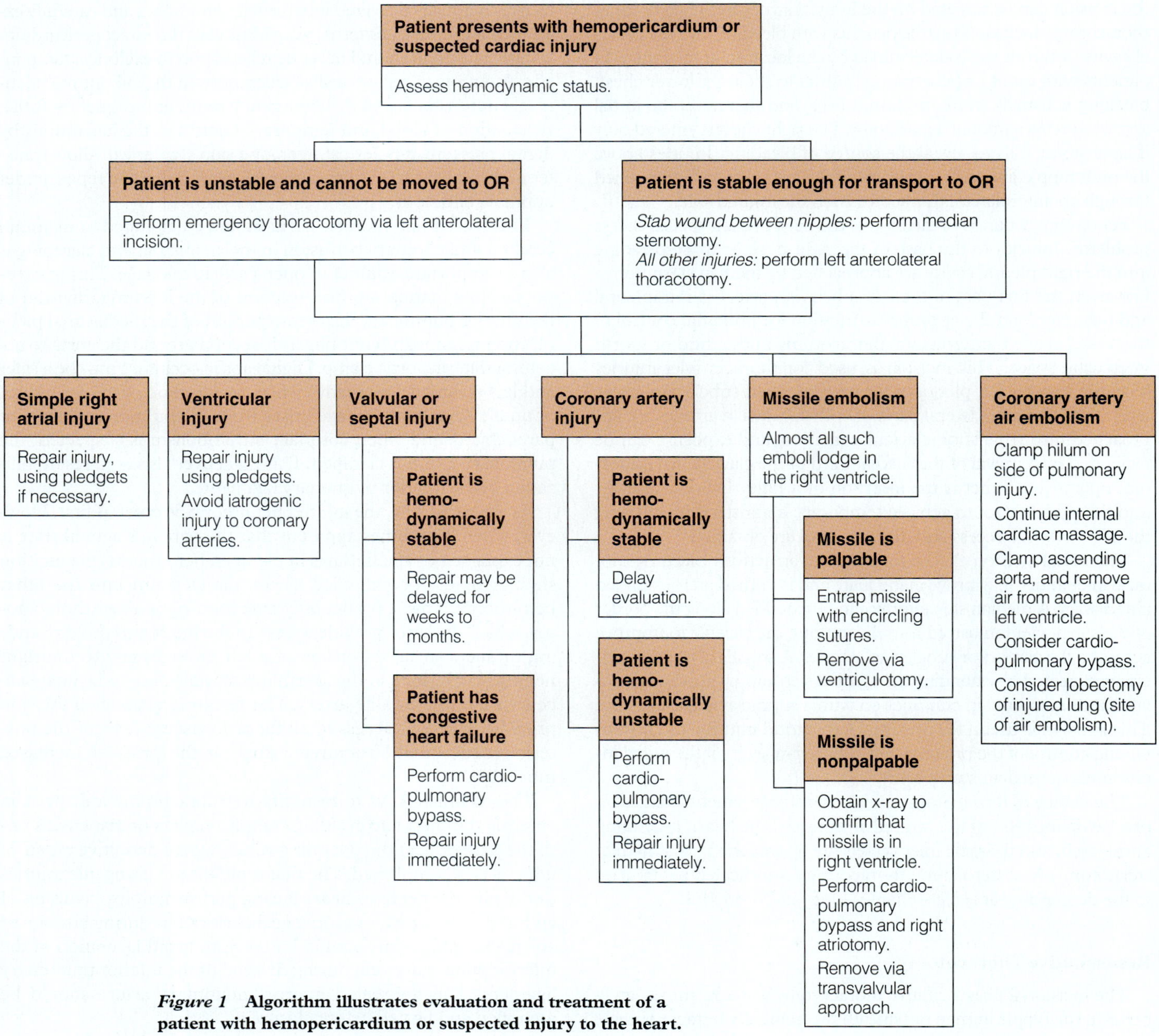

Figure 1 Algorithm illustrates evaluation and treatment of a patient with hemopericardium or suspected injury to the heart.

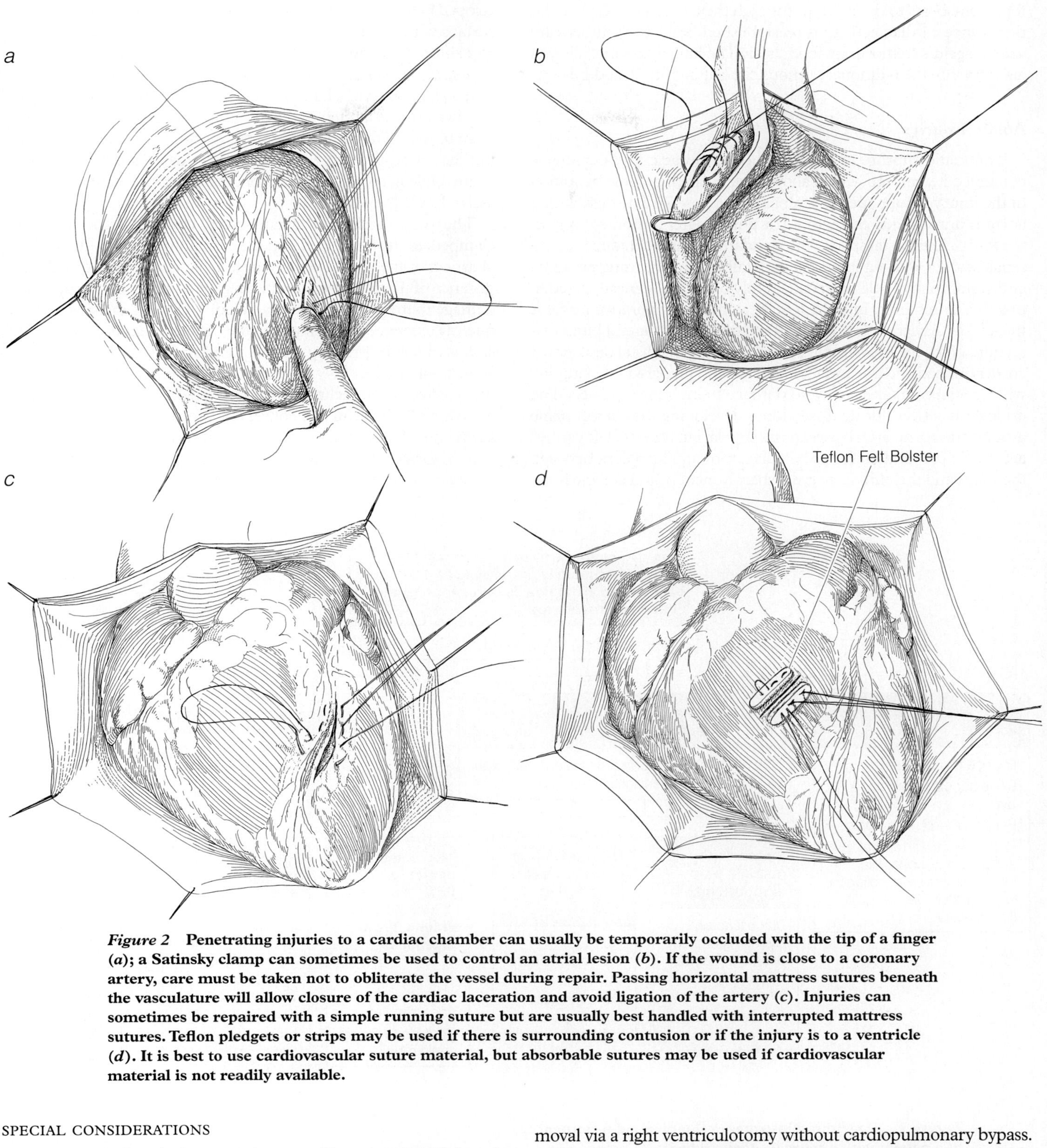

Figure 2 Penetrating injuries to a cardiac chamber can usually be temporarily occluded with the tip of a finger (*a*); a Satinsky clamp can sometimes be used to control an atrial lesion (*b*). If the wound is close to a coronary artery, care must be taken not to obliterate the vessel during repair. Passing horizontal mattress sutures beneath the vasculature will allow closure of the cardiac laceration and avoid ligation of the artery (*c*). Injuries can sometimes be repaired with a simple running suture but are usually best handled with interrupted mattress sutures. Teflon pledgets or strips may be used if there is surrounding contusion or if the injury is to a ventricle (*d*). It is best to use cardiovascular suture material, but absorbable sutures may be used if cardiovascular material is not readily available.

SPECIAL CONSIDERATIONS

Missile emboli to the heart can be caused by migration of air and particles from the peripheral venous injury site. Almost all such bullets will become embedded within the right ventricular trabeculations. Left in place, such a missile embolism can cause arrhythmias, further embolization to pulmonary arteries, endocarditis, and interference with tricuspid valve function. Such emboli have been removed by use of interventional radiologic techniques, cardiopulmonary bypass and right atriotomy, and entrapment and simple removal via a right ventriculotomy without cardiopulmonary bypass.

The diagnosis of coronary air embolism is made intraoperatively when air bubbles are noted in the coronary arteries. This calls for immediate hilar clamping of the injured lung in conjunction with venting of air from the left side of the heart and ascending aorta by a needle inserted into the most ventral aspect of these structures. Manual occlusion of the aortic root is then accomplished by placing the fingers of the left hand into the transverse sinus and compressing the aorta between the thumb and the forefinger. The heart is massaged for several beats to drive the air through the coronary microcirculation. Once cardiac activity is reestablished, the left chambers are vented again to remove any residual air. The lung injury that allowed air entry into the pulmonary venous circulation must be addressed.

Aortic Injuries

Traumatic rupture of the descending thoracic aorta creates a contained hematoma, which allows precise angiographic definition of the injury before operative repair [see Figure 3]. The descending aorta is approached through a left posterolateral thoracotomy in the fourth intercostal space. The standard repair technique is direct repair with or without interposition graft placement using proximal and distal control (clamp repair). Only one lung is anesthetized, if possible. After entry into the left chest, the first operative target is the left subclavian artery, which is encircled using careful blunt dissection. Next, the mediastinal pleura overlying the distal descending aorta is incised and the aorta is encircled and prepared for clamping with special care taken to avoid damage to intercostal vessels. The critical maneuver during dissection is developing the correct plane around the aortic arch between the subclavian and the left carotid arteries in preparation for proximal clamping. The pleura between the vagus and the phrenic nerve is sharply incised, and a plane is developed between the left (or main) pulmonary artery and the undersurface of the aortic arch. This is done with a combination of blunt and sharp dissection and may be especially difficult in elderly patients, who often have tough fibrous periaortic tissue at this location. A large curved clamp is used to encircle the aortic arch, and the dissection is limited to the minimum necessary for safe passage of an umbilical tape and subsequent cross-clamping. Before clamping the aorta, the surgeon may elect to use a temporary passive shunt, pharmacological control of central hypertension, or a pump-assist device [see Figure 4].

The aortic arch, subclavian artery, and distal aorta are then clamped, in this sequence, and the hematoma is entered. The lateral aspect of the aortic wall is carefully incised longitudinally for a distance of no more than 2 cm, a vein retractor is inserted, and the damage to the aortic wall is evaluated. This small incision is subsequently extended, as dictated by the operative findings, and a decision is made for primary repair or graft insertion. The aortic incision should be carefully tailored to both the extent of damage and the selected repair technique. Similarly, debridement of the injured wall should be careful and conservative, especially if primary repair seems possible. Direct repair is accomplished with a 4-0 Prolene suture. Graft interposition is accomplished in a standard end-to-end fashion by using a soft woven graft and taking care not to enter

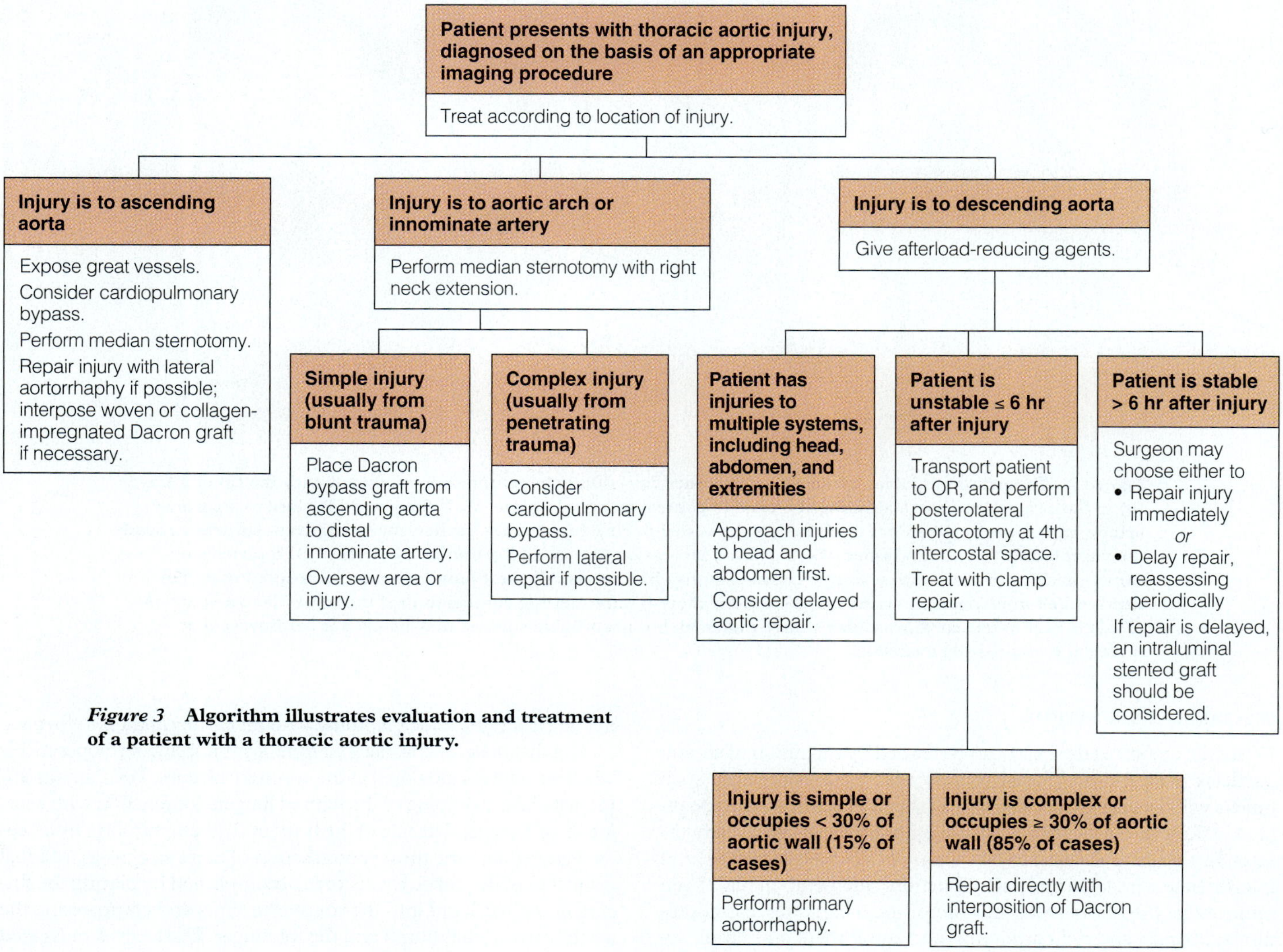

Figure 3 Algorithm illustrates evaluation and treatment of a patient with a thoracic aortic injury.

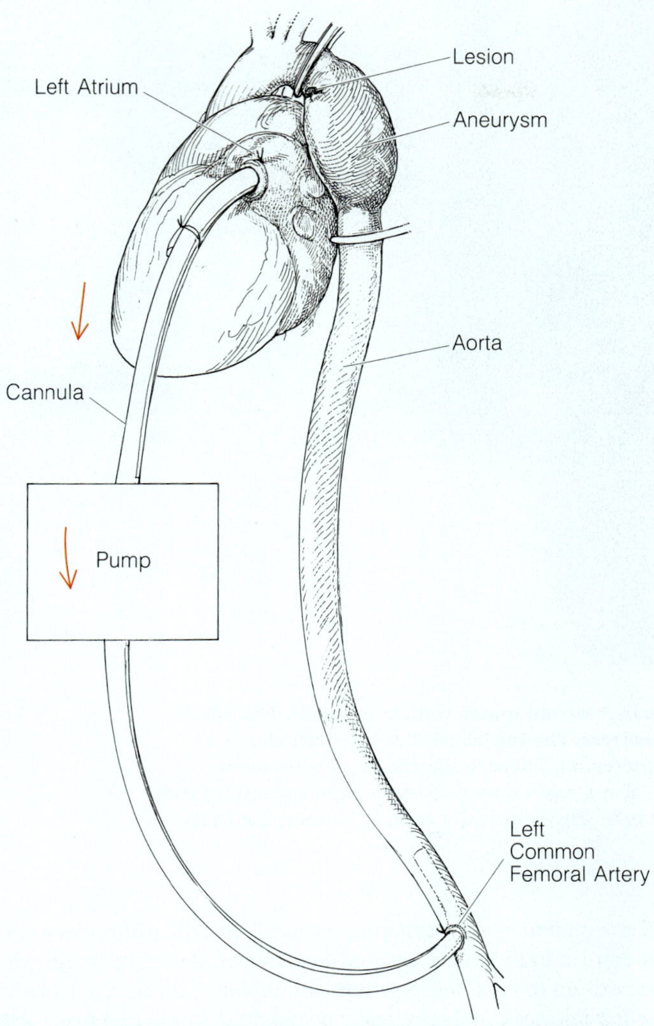

Figure 4 Illustrated is a bypass from the left atrium to the left common femoral artery during operation for a transected descending thoracic aorta. This maneuver permits decompression of upper body hypertension, complete perfusion of the viscera, and some perfusion of the spinal cord. Once the transected area has been dissected out, the clamps should be placed as close as possible to the damaged area to allow maximal perfusion of the collateral circulation.

the esophagus with the posterior bites. After completion of the proximal anastomosis, the clamp should not be moved to the graft, particularly in young adults, because the aorta of young persons is relatively friable and should not be subjected to excessive tension. Aortic declamping is a critical maneuver that should be accomplished slowly and only after the nitroprusside infusion used to control central hypertension has been discontinued.

Thoracic Outlet Injuries

The second most common blunt thoracic vascular injury is a tear at the origin of the innominate artery off the aortic arch. This injury is repaired by following the bypass and exclusion principle, thus avoiding the need for cardiopulmonary bypass, shunts, or heparinization. After precise angiographic definition of the injury, access is obtained via a median sternotomy. The ascending aorta is exposed inside the pericardium. The distal innominate, right subclavian, and right carotid arteries are dissected out and encircled preparatory to clamping, with care taken to avoid the hematoma itself. With a partially occluding (Satinsky) clamp on the ascending aorta, a 12 mm knitted Dacron graft is sewn to the normal ascending aorta in an end-to-side fashion, away from the injury. Occasionally, the innominate vein is ligated to optimize exposure. A second, partially occluding clamp is placed on the aortic arch at the origin of the innominate artery, with special care taken not to accidentally occlude the left carotid artery origin. The distal innominate artery or its branches are then clamped, and the distal anastomosis is completed. Only then is the hematoma entered and the injury oversewn by placing a row of pledgeted sutures on the aortic arch.

Penetrating injuries to the innominate vessels and proximal carotid arteries produce a mediastinal hematoma and, sometimes, torrential hemorrhage, which can be temporarily controlled either digitally or by placing a balloon catheter in the missile tract before obtaining access. The cardinal technical principle in the management of these injuries is never to enter a contained or partially contained mediastinal hematoma without prior proximal and distal control. Proximal control of these vessels can be obtained from within the pericardium, where the anatomy is not obscured by the hematoma. During dissection within the hematoma, the technical key is identification of the innominate vein, which may be ligated and divided with impunity if needed.

Injuries to the distal subclavian vessels can often be approached via a limited supraclavicular incision, but the safest approach, especially in the presence of active bleeding, is a more extensive incision. The medial third of the clavicle is rapidly resected by early subperiosteal division of the bone, grasping it with a towel clip and lifting it out of its bed. The subclavian artery is a very friable vessel, and limited resection of the injured segment with interposition of a graft (preferably one made of knitted Dacron) is a safer option than extensive mobilization and attempted end-to-end anastomosis.

Major Airway Disruption

The precise location of major airway injury is determined by bronchoscopy, and the operative approach is planned accordingly. Use of a double-lumen endotracheal tube is an important adjunct. The thoracic trachea and the right mainstem bronchus are approached via a right posterolateral thoracotomy, and the left mainstem bronchus is approached through a similar incision on the left. The anterior and left lateral aspects of the mediastinal trachea can also be approached through a median sternotomy. More than 80 percent of blunt tracheobronchial disruptions occur within 2 cm from the carina [*see Figure 5*].

The underlying technical principle in the management of airway injuries is to achieve primary repair with precise mucosa-to-mucosa apposition of the lacerated edges using interrupted absorbable sutures. Small tracheal wounds with well-opposed edges and no tissue loss can be managed conservatively by tracheal intubation and inflation of the balloon distal to the laceration. Large tracheobronchial wounds are managed by conservative debridement and airtight single-layer closure of the defect. Lacerations of the distal airways resulting in a large air leak or bleeding into the airway are managed by resection of the injured lung parenchyma.

Pulmonary Lacerations

Bleeding pulmonary lacerations can be either oversewn or resected [*see Figure 6*]. A continuous over-and-over Prolene suture

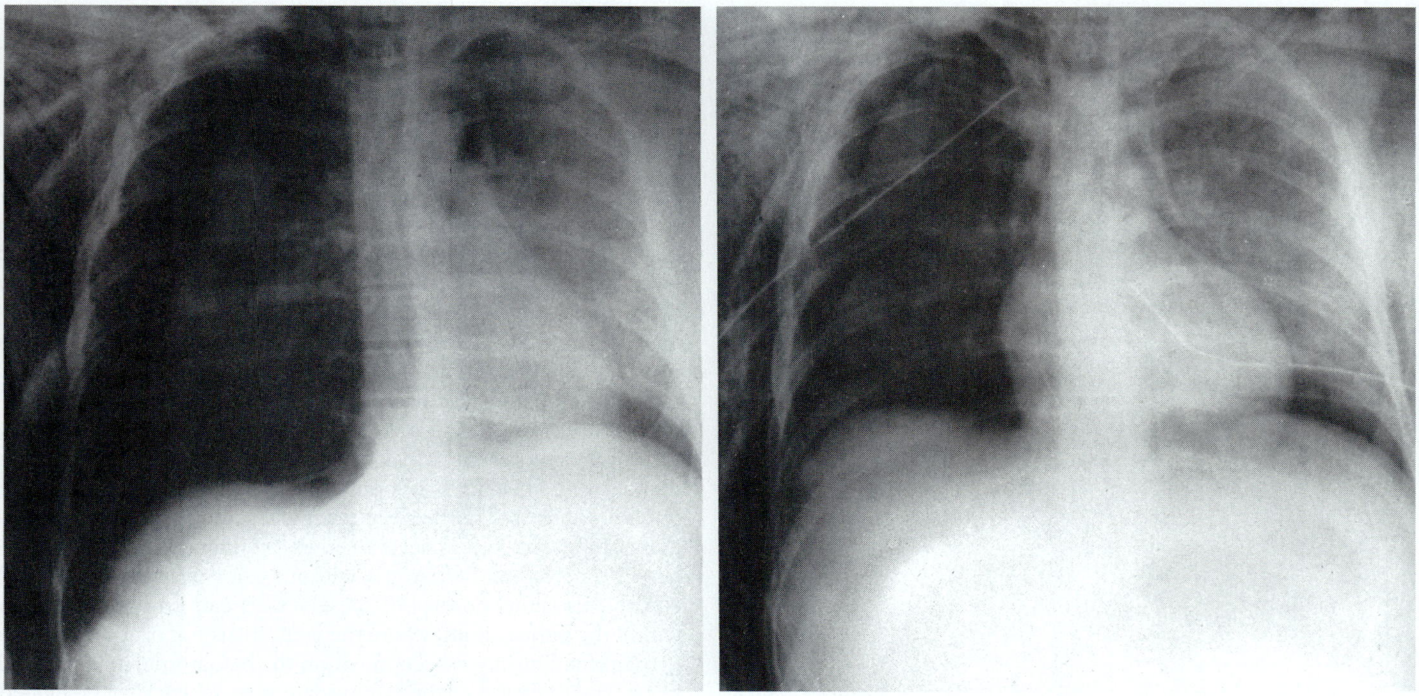

Figure 5 These x-rays are of a patient who was involved in a high-speed motor vehicle accident. His initial blood pressure was 90/60 mm Hg, and he was in respiratory distress. The initial chest x-ray (left) shows a right pneumothorax and a left hemothorax with pulmonary contusion. There is significant subcutaneous and mediastinal air. After bilateral tube thoracostomies, the chest x-ray shows persistent right pneumothorax (right); there was also a significant air leak through the chest tube. Bronchoscopy revealed disruption of the right mainstem bronchus, which was repaired.

controls bleeding from small or shallow lacerations, whereas deeper wounds require resection of the injured parenchyma. As a general rule, parenchymal resections for trauma are not anatomic. Rapid and simple resection of the injured lung tissue is usually accomplished using a wide linear stapler (TA-90), which is positioned just proximal to the injured segment, closed, and fired across. The tissue distal to the stapled line is then amputated, and the stapler is opened. Any residual bleeding or air leak from the stapled line is then oversewn with a Prolene suture.

Deep through-and-through injuries to the lung that do not involve hilar structures present a special technical problem because simple closure of the entry and exit wounds is inadequate. These injuries are managed by pulmonary tractotomy between two aortic clamps. The bridge of tissue between the clamps is cut, thus opening the tract and allowing selective suture-ligation of bleeders and air leaks. The tract is carefully inspected to ensure that no major vascular or bronchial injury is present that would require a formal resection. The lung tissue held by the aortic clamps is then oversewn with continuous Prolene suture, and the tractotomy is left open.

Central lung injuries are the source of exsanguinating hemorrhage, as well as air embolism. The key operative maneuver in the management of these injuries is early hilar clamping. The inferior pulmonary ligament is rapidly divided, and the entire hilum is clamped with a large vascular clamp, incorporating the pulmonary artery, both pulmonary veins, and the mainstem bronchus. The next step is a meticulous evaluation of the injuries to determine the method of definitive repair (i.e., vascular repair or pulmonary resection). If the vascular injury is immediately below the hilar clamp and the patient's hemodynamic status allows, the pulmonary vessels can be individually isolated and controlled from within the pericardium to facilitate exposure and repair of the injury. Isolated vascular injuries can theoretically be repaired, but in practice, these wounds are often associated with extensive parenchymal destruc-

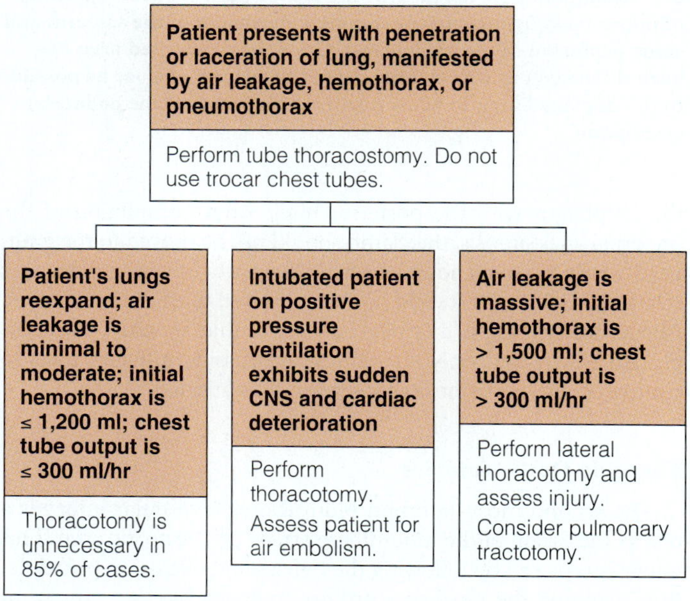

Figure 6 Algorithm illustrates evaluation and treatment of a patient with penetrations or lacerations of the lung.

tion and massive blood loss. Under these circumstances, rapid resection of the lobe or the entire lung is the only practical option.

Esophageal Injuries

Injuries to the upper and middle thoracic esophagus are approached via a right posterolateral thoracotomy, and similar injuries to the lower esophagus are best approached through the same incision on the left side. Anterolateral thoracotomy provides suboptimal exposure of these injuries. The thoracic esophagus is totally inaccessible when the chest is entered through a median sternotomy.

The key consideration in esophageal repair is timing. An early perforation (less than 12 hours old) is associated with minimal spillage into the adjacent mediastinum and is, therefore, amenable to primary repair. Late perforations are associated with a marked inflammatory response in the esophageal wall and surrounding mediastinum, thus making primary repair unsafe or technically impossible. Under these circumstances, excision and diversion are the only options. While a 12- to 16-hour delay usually serves as the dividing line between early and late injuries, the final decision depends more on the amount of local inflammation and the feasibility of a sound closure than on arbitrary time limits.

Repair of an esophageal perforation is done in one or two layers, with the aim of obtaining a tension-free, watertight closure. It is important to maintain the suture line in a transverse orientation to avoid narrowing the repaired segment. The repair is buttressed with nontraumatized adjacent tissue, such as a small intercostal muscle flap, a tongue of parietal pleura, or the fundus of the stomach (by means of a Thal patch or a Nissen fundoplication). Wide mediastinal drainage with a large Argyle tube completes the repair.

Delayed operation for esophageal perforation employs the principles of proximal diversion and wide drainage to effectively control an inflamed and friable esophageal wall that does not hold sutures [see Figure 7]. The noninflamed intact esophagus above and below the injured segment is mobilized, encircled, and stapled with a linear stapler, and the area is widely drained. This step is then followed by laparotomy with construction of a gastrostomy and a feeding jejunostomy. The final step is the creation of a loop cervical esophagostomy into the left neck. Total exclusion and diversion as described above will later require esophageal resection and reconstruction using colon interposition. Thus, when the local situation allows and repair of the perforation is technically feasible, a less radical technical solution should be considered. The perforation may be repaired and temporarily excluded in continuity by means of Teflon band closure of the gastroesophageal junction in conjunction with a lateral cervical esophagostomy. The decision to repair or exclude an esophageal injury is not based solely on the length of delay and the local inflammatory response. Even with early perforations, it is safer to exclude the esophageal injury when it is extensive or in the presence of other serious associated injuries.

Chest Wall Injuries

The source of bleeding in the patient with ongoing hemorrhage into the pleural cavity is usually a lacerated intercostal artery. The keys to successful control of chest wall bleeders are adequate exposure and ligation of the bleeding intercostal vessel on both sides of the injury; each intercostal artery has a bidirectional blood supply. Occasionally, the bleeding vessel cannot be directly controlled because of extensive surrounding soft tissue destruction. Temporary effective packing of the area may be the only feasible technical so-

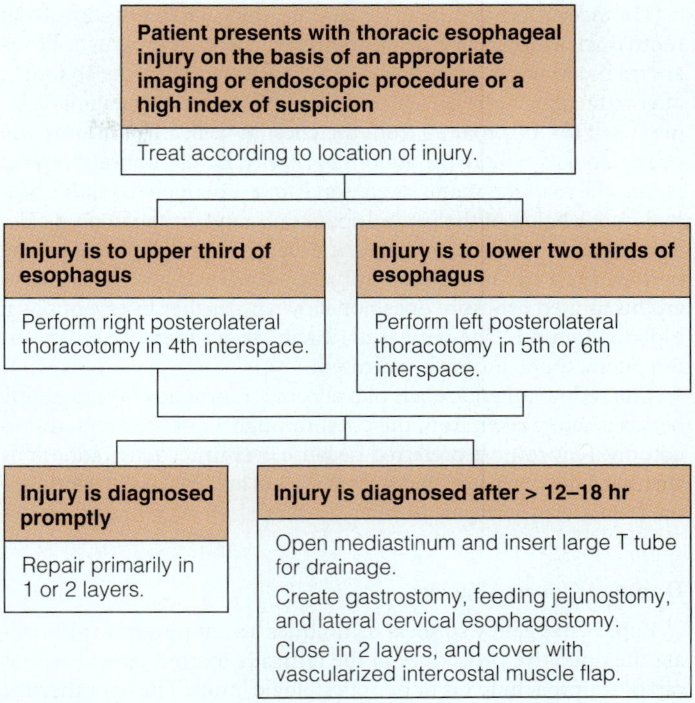

Figure 7 Algorithm illustrates evaluation and treatment of a patient with thoracic esophageal injury.

lution, especially in the presence of other life-threatening visceral injuries that demand immediate attention.

Massive chest wall defects are uncommon and are usually associated with extensive underlying visceral damage. Chest wall reconstruction is a low priority under these circumstances and is accomplished after the patient is stabilized. A myocutaneous flap based on the latissimus dorsi or on the pectoralis major muscle is the surgical solution for these wounds.

Surgical reduction and stabilization of the fractured sternum is indicated only when the fracture interferes with cardiac or pulmonary function or when the fractured segments override and may produce a painful pseudoarthrosis. It is important to remember that a sternal fracture is often a marker of underlying visceral damage, which is the first priority.

Special Operative Considerations

Thoracic injuries involving more than one truncal visceral compartment present unique operative problems. Transmediastinal penetrations are serious injuries for which the diagnostic and operative approaches have to be individualized. Whenever a transmediastinal penetration is suspected on the basis of the chest x-ray, the missile trajectory, or the clinical circumstances, injury to all three mediastinal components (i.e., heart, great vessels, and esophagus) must be ruled out. In hemodynamically unstable patients, this is done during operative exploration, but it should be remembered that an esophageal injury cannot be ruled out through a median sternotomy and thus requires either a different incision or esophagoscopy. Penetrating great vessel injuries cause massive hemorrhage and immediately become the focus of clinical attention. On the other hand, cardiac wounds do not always present with a dramatic clinical picture and may be missed even during surgical exploration if the pericardium is not opened.

Thoracoabdominal injury is another type of trauma involving more than one truncal visceral compartment. Diaphragmatic lacerations discovered at celiotomy are repaired from within the abdomen after reduction of any herniated viscera. While the diaphragmatic injury itself can be repaired from the chest as well, a laparotomy will be required to explore the abdominal cavity. Before transabdominal repair, the diaphragmatic laceration can be enlarged to enable limited visualization of the pleural space and lung on the injured side. The presence of blood in the pericardial space can be ruled out by performing a transabdominal subxiphoid pericardiotomy. However, this limited exposure does not allow any further interventions if blood is found in the pericardial cavity, so an immediate left anterolateral thoracotomy is indicated.

The reduction and repair of a chronic traumatic diaphragmatic hernia is undertaken from the chest through a posterolateral thoracotomy. This route is preferred because over time, dense adhesions surround the herniated abdominal viscera and make transabdominal reduction and repair technically difficult or even impossible.

Damage Control Tactics

Rapid emergency surgical techniques are employed to abbreviate the operative procedure in the critically injured patient who is rapidly approaching his or her physiologic limits. The hypothermic and coagulopathic patient is a poor candidate for lengthy formal procedures, and temporary or unorthodox technical solutions to control bleeding, air leak, and spillage are often employed in these patients. Formal anatomic repair either is postponed until after restitution of the patient's physiologic reserves postoperatively or is not performed at all.

Stapled lobectomy and pneumonectomy provide a rapid technical solution to exsanguinating hemorrhage from central lung injuries. The technique involves firing a wide linear stapler across the entire bronchovascular pedicle and subsequently oversewing any residual bleeding from the stump with a continuous Prolene suture. Pulmonary tractotomy and selective ligation is another useful damage-control technique. Pulmonary tractotomy is accomplished by placing two vascular clamps completely through a penetrating injury (ignoring anatomic lobar planes) and cutting between the clamps. Vascular control is achieved at the base of the tract, and a running suture line or linear staples are placed beneath each clamp for rapid control of bleeding and air leaks. Patients tolerate such techniques with virtually no postoperative sequelae.

Under emergency conditions, the subclavian and innominate arteries are sometimes ligated and not reconstructed. Rather, coagulopathic bleeding from soft tissue damage to the chest wall is packed, and the perforated esophagus is excluded by ligation of the esophagus above and below the injured segment with cotton tapes.

If reoperation is planned for definitive repair of the injuries, formal chest closure is not undertaken, because it is time consuming and unnecessary. Only the skin is closed, with a row of towel clips 1 to 2 cm apart or a running heavy nylon suture.

General Postoperative Concerns

The three major concerns in the immediate postoperative management of the critical patient with thoracic trauma are oxygenation, hypothermia, and bleeding. The combination of pulmonary trauma, massive bleeding, and aggressive preoperative and intraoperative fluid administration translates into compromised oxygen delivery. Early insertion of a pulmonary artery catheter is the key to maintaining adequate oxygenation under these circumstances. The physiologic insight provided by the pulmonary artery catheter allows tailored support of the preload, cardiac contractility, and afterload, as well as optimization of positive end-expiratory pressure (PEEP) and fraction of inspired oxygen (F_IO_2). Every attempt is made to avoid fluid overload, because the posttraumatic lung exhibits a marked degree of capillary leakage, and thus, fluid overload is immediately translated into interstitial pulmonary congestion and adversely affects oxygenation.

All critically injured patients are hypothermic, and rapid reversal of hypothermia is an urgent concern in an injured patient. Heat loss is especially severe in patients who underwent thoracotomy in conjunction with laparotomy and in patients who underwent prolonged operative procedures. In the intensive care unit, the patient is meticulously protected from additional conductive heat loss and undergoes aggressive active external rewarming. All intravenous fluids and blood components are warmed before they are administered. Extracorporeal rewarming may be indicated in selected patients.

Bleeding is the third urgent concern in the immediate postoperative period. Massive transfusion and hypothermia contribute to the development of coagulopathy, which is clinically apparent by continuous oozing of blood into the chest tubes and from the surgical incisions. This coagulopathy is managed by rewarming the patient and by empirical administration of fresh frozen plasma and platelets, because coagulation studies are unreliable in hypothermic patients. Continuous bleeding from the operated hemithorax raises the question of reoperation. As a general rule, the first priority is always to correct hypothermia and coagulopathy, and reoperation can be considered later.

A specific consideration in the postoperative patient operated on for a chest injury is that the cause of a sudden deterioration in oxygenation or hemodynamic collapse can often be found in the operated hemithorax. Tension pneumothorax, cardiac tamponade, and systemic air embolism are three mechanisms of sudden cardiovascular collapse that require immediate surgical action. If the patient has also had a laparotomy, a sudden deterioration in oxygenation, coupled with excessive inspiratory pressures, decreasing urinary output, and increased intra-abdominal pressure, should lead the surgeon to suspect the presence of the abdominal compartment syndrome, and immediate decompression should be performed.

Misleading chest tube output is a major pitfall in the postoperative patient. Chest tubes often become clogged, are misplaced, or are incorrectly connected to the underwater seal and suction system. Whenever the chest tube output becomes a cause for concern, the tube and its connections should be examined closely for evidence of clogging, kinking, and misplacement. A chest x-ray should be obtained and the tube exchanged if it is felt that the tube is not functioning properly. A chest tube is removed when it is no longer functioning for the purpose of its insertion. In the ventilated postoperative patient, a functioning chest tube is retained until the patient is weaned from positive pressure ventilation.

The possibility of a missed injury should be considered when there is any deviation from the expected course of recovery in the postoperative patient. Unexplained bleeding and unexpected sepsis are the two most common manifestations that should prompt a diligent search for a missed injury. The two most common sites for missed thoracic injuries are the chest wall vessels (intercostal and internal mammary arteries) and the heart. Both require urgent reoperation. Missed esophageal perforations are uncommon but devastating, and management is by proximal diversion, drainage of the perforation, distal drainage of GI contents via a large tube gastrostomy, and feeding tube jejunostomy. Total esophageal diversion is no longer considered an option.

Reoperation for thoracic trauma may be either planned or unplanned. Planned reoperation is performed in patients who underwent a damage control procedure and subsequent stabilization in the intensive care unit. The aim of this reoperation is to perform definitive repairs and formal chest closure. It is undertaken only after correction of hypothermia and coagulopathy and after oxygen delivery has been optimized. Unplanned procedures are usually performed for bleeding and may need to be undertaken in the surgical intensive care unit in a rapidly deteriorating patient. There are no firm quantitative guidelines to urgent reoperation, but reoperation should be considered in any patient whose postoperative bleeding markedly exceeds the surgeon's expectations. This decision should always be made by the surgeon who performed the initial thoracotomy.

Specific Postoperative Problems

PULMONARY COMPLICATIONS

Persistent Air Leak

Patients on sustained PEEP or with elevated ventilatory pressures may have a persistent and at times large-volume air leak. Often, increasing the negative pressure on the pleural space produces parietal and visceral pleura apposition that results in a decreased air leak. However, increased negative pressure may sometimes increase the air leak and create hypoxemia. On rare occasions, operative repair of a large torn lung or of a missed injury to a major bronchus is required. Operative repair should be undertaken only after the patient is off PEEP and has normal ventilatory pressures.

Retained Clotted Hemothorax

Unevacuated or retained clotted hemothorax is an indication for early evacuation, often by thoracoscopy and occasionally by thoracotomy. Use of thrombolytics and conservative treatment results in prolonged hospitalization and increased infectious complications.

Effusion and Empyema

Effusion and empyema may occur because of undrained pleural fluid, undetected esophageal or pulmonary leakage, or sympathetic reaction to subdiaphragmatic conditions. Both effusion and empyema require early detection and drainage.

Systemic Air Embolism

Systemic air embolism can occur with pulmonary parenchymal injury and increased intrabronchial pressure, creating a bronchopulmonary venous fistula. Sudden cerebral or cardiac insufficiency may be the initial sentinel clue that air has embolized to the coronary or cerebral vessels. Immediate prevention of further embolization of air with possible removal of the intravascular air is a therapeutic goal. Mortality associated with this complication is high.

CARDIAC COMPLICATIONS

Intracardiac Shunts

Left-to-right intracardiac shunts, which are manifested by continuous murmurs, are often found postoperatively. Detection may be aided by color Doppler imaging. Depending on the size of the fistula, closure of the fistula may be required by operative or transvascular interventional techniques.

Cardiac Herniation

Cardiac herniation can occur postoperatively in patients with a pericardium that has been only partially incised or incompletely repaired. It usually occurs when a patient is lying on the left side, and it is manifested by sudden hypotension and distended neck veins. Cardiac herniation is often reversible if the patient lies with the right side down. Such cases require either pericardiorrhaphy or wider pericardectomy.

Pericardial Effusion

Pericardial effusion is a rare but real entity that occurs after pericardiotomy or cardiorrhaphy. Such effusion may be sympathetic, chylous, reactive, or infectious. Diagnosis is made via echocardiography or a pericardial window. Such effusion may be part of a postpericardiotomy syndrome in some patients.

COMPLICATIONS OF THE GREAT VESSELS

Paraplegia

The dreaded complication of thoracic aortic surgery, paraplegia is the result of spinal cord ischemia, and there is currently no universally recognized preventive measure to reduce its incidence. Although ischemic myelopathy is most often apparent immediately after operation, it may occur as long as five days after surgery, suggesting other etiologies, such as spinal compartment syndrome and reperfusion injury.

False Aneurysms

False aneurysms occur at the site of undetected arterial injury or at vascular anastomotic sites. Some surgeons have recommended postoperative arteriograms in thoracic vascular reconstructions to establish a baseline study, whereas others obtain vascular images only when routine radiographs or symptoms suggest a posttraumatic false aneurysm. Delayed thoracic posttraumatic aneurysms frequently appear weeks or months after the injury rather than in the intensive care unit. Depending on the location of the aneurysm, direct surgical repair is indicated. Stenting of both arteriovenous fistulae and traumatic false aneurysms with intraluminal stents is a modern therapeutic option.

Arteriovenous Fistula

Arteriovenous fistula can occur in many thoracic locations, including the intercostal vessels, aorta to pulmonary artery, or pulmonary artery to pulmonary vein. The location of the last fistula listed may be the pulmonary parenchyma. Diagnosis is by arteriography, and treatment is by vascular reconstruction, occasionally after pulmonary resection.

ESOPHAGEAL, TRACHEAL, AND DIAPHRAGMATIC COMPLICATIONS

Esophageal Repair Breakdown

Penetrating injury to the thoracic esophagus repaired via an anterior thoracic incision has a 50 percent breakdown rate. Thus, it is recommended that a contrast esophagogram be performed in every patient who underwent an esophageal repair before resumption of oral food intake. When esophageal injury is discovered, it is best repaired via a posterior approach. Late esophageal leaks are handled as outlined earlier in this chapter.

Stenosis

Tracheal or bronchial stenosis can occur either from a missed injury, a constricted repair, or a buildup of granulation tissue around suture material at the site of a bronchial or tracheal repair. Suture line granuloma is less common when absorbable suture material is used. When braided or polypropylene suture materials are used, the externally placed knots are often discovered to be intraluminal at later bronchoscopy.

Posttraumatic Diaphragmatic Hernia

Acute diaphragmatic herniation is rare, because the appearance of this condition is usually delayed for months or years. Diagnosis is aided by gastric or colonic contrast studies. A posttraumatic diaphragmatic hernia is repaired via a thoracic incision, as opposed to acute herniations, which are approached via a laparotomy incision.

COMPLICATIONS OF THE CHEST WALL

Chylothorax

An uncommon but real occurrence, chylothorax usually becomes manifest on postinjury days 3 to 7. Conservative therapy involves either intravenous alimentation or enteral feedings with medium-chain triglycerides. To assist in the localization of persistent chylous leaks, preoperative or intraoperative gastrointestinal olive oil can be administered.

Causalgia

Posttraumatic causalgia, or reflex sympathetic dystrophy, may be caused by a partial injury to a peripheral nerve. Causalgia is also common after a so-called trap-door thoracotomy and is occasionally seen when a median sternotomy is opened very widely. Management is conservative and is based on response to physical therapy and stellate ganglion blocks. Occasionally, dorsal sympathectomy is required.

Radicular Pain

Intercostal radicular pain is common after a lateral thoracotomy. Frequently controlled by analgesics and intercostal nerve blocks initially, chronic pain of this etiology can be disabling. Use of permanent suture material for pericostal sutures during rib reapproximation contributes to radicular pain as the intercostal nerve becomes entrapped. Symptoms may be lessened by permanent intercostal nerve ablation.

Costal Chondritis

Thoracoabdominal incisions across the chondral border in trauma patients lead to a significant rate of chronic chondritis. This painful condition may be due to devascularization of the cartilaginous structures as a result of necrosis or infection. Such conditions are best treated by placement of a muscle flap into the adequately debrided area.

Recommended Reading

CHOICE OF INCISION

Mattox KL: Thoracic injury requiring surgery. World J Surg 7:47, 1982

Mattox KL: Indications for thoracotomy: deciding to operate. Surg Clin North Am 69:47, 1989

Pickard LR, Mattox KL: Thoracic trauma and indications for thoracotomy. Trauma. Mattox KL, Moore EE, Feliciano DV, Eds. Appleton & Lange, Norwalk, Connecticut, 1988, p 315

RESUSCITATIVE THORACOTOMY

Champion HR, Sykes L: Emergency room thoracotomy. Trauma Surgery, Part 1, 4th ed. Champion HR, Robbs JV, Trunkey DD, Eds. Butterworth & Co, London, 1989, p 70

Feliciano DV, Bitondo CG, Cruse PA, et al: Liberal use of emergency center thoracotomy. Am J Surg 152:654, 1986

Shannon FL, Moore EE, Moore JB: Emergency department thoracotomy. Trauma. Mattox KL, Moore EE, Feliciano DV, Eds. Appleton & Lange, Norwalk, Connecticut, 1988, p 175

CARDIAC INJURIES

Mattox KL, Beal AC Jr, Jordan GL Jr, et al: Cardiorrhaphy in the emergency center. J Thorac Cardiovasc Surg 68:886, 1974

Mitchell ME, Muakkassa FF, Poole GV, et al: Surgical approach of choice for penetrating cardiac wounds. J Trauma 34:17, 1993

Symbas PN: Cardiothoracic trauma. WB Saunders Co, Philadelphia, 1989, p 300

AORTIC INJURIES

Mattox KL, Holzman M, Pickard LR, et al: Clamp-repair: a safe technique for treatment of blunt injury to the descending thoracic aorta. Ann Thorac Surg 40:456, 1985

Mattox KL, Wall MJ Jr, Hirshberg A: Traumatic aneurysm of the thoracic aorta. Aneurysms—New Findings and Treatments. Yao JST, Pearce WH, Eds. Appleton & Lange, Norwalk, Connecticut, 1994, p 207

Mattox KL: Red River Anthology. J Trauma 42:353, 1997

von Oppell UO, Dunne TT, De Groot MK, et al: Traumatic aortic rupture: twenty-year metaanalysis of mortality and risk of paraplegia. Ann Thorac Surg 58:585, 1994

THE EXTRAPERICARDIAL VESSELS

Brawley RK, Murray GF, Crisler C, et al: Management of wounds of the innominate, subclavian and axillary blood vessels. Surg Gynecol Obstet 148:1130, 1970

Graham JM, Feliciano DV, Mattox KL: Management of subclavian vascular injuries. J Trauma 20:537, 1980

Johnston RH, Wall MJ Jr, Mattox KL: Innominate artery trauma: a thirty year experience. J Vasc Surg 17:134, 1993

MAJOR AIRWAY DISRUPTION

Symbas PN: Cardiothoracic trauma. Curr Probl Surg 28:747, 1991

Urschel HC, Razzuk MA: Management of acute traumatic injuries of tracheobronchial tree. Surg Gynecol Obstet 136:113, 1973

PULMONARY LACERATIONS

Wall MJ Jr, Hirshberg A, Mattox KL: Pulmonary tractotomy with selective vascular ligation for penetrating injuries to the lung. Am J Surg 168:665, 1994

Weincek RG Jr, Wilson RF: Central lung injuries: a need for early vascular control. J Trauma 28:1418, 1988

ESOPHAGEAL INJURIES

Cheadle W, Richardson JD: Options in management of trauma to the esophagus. Surg Gynecol Obstet 155:380, 1982

Defore WW Jr, Mattox KL, Hansen HA, et al: Surgical management of penetrating injuries of the esophagus. Am J Surg 134:734, 1977

CHEST WALL

Pate JW: Chest wall injuries. Surg Clin North Am 69:59, 1989

DAMAGE CONTROL TACTICS

Hirshberg A, Wall MJ Jr, Mattox KL: Planned reoperation for trauma: a two year experience with 124 consecutive patients. J Trauma 37:365, 1994

GENERAL POSTOPERATIVE CONCERNS

Hirshberg A, Wall MJ Jr, Ramchandani MK, et al: Reoperation for bleeding in trauma. Arch Surg 128:1163, 1993

Acknowledgments

Figures 1, 3, 6, and 7   Marcia Kammerer.
Figures 2 and 4   Carol Donner.

27 OPERATIVE EXPOSURE OF ABDOMINAL INJURIES AND CLOSURE OF THE ABDOMEN

Erwin R. Thal, M.D., Brian J. Eastridge, M.D., and Rusty Milhoan, M.D.

Management of abdominal trauma has changed significantly since the beginning of the 1990s. In part, the change is attributable to improvements in the available diagnostic studies and to the advent of nonoperative therapeutic approaches. Those patients who require operative intervention for treatment of abdominal injuries often present a major challenge to the surgical team. Although each such patient is unique, we believe that the application of a standard operative approach is nonetheless necessary to optimize patient care and to minimize the risk of missing injuries. The primary objective of this operative approach is the expeditious prioritization and treatment of injuries. To this end, all surgeons treating injured patients should have a general routine to follow and should be familiar with a variety of exposures and techniques that may be used to carry out this routine. Adequate exposure, rapid assessment, and sound clinical judgment are essential ingredients of the care of patients with abdominal injuries.

Patient Preparation

Before the celiotomy is begun, the patient must be adequately prepared. All contingencies must be planned for in advance. A nasogastric tube and a Foley catheter should be inserted, and a single dose of a broad-spectrum antibiotic should be given before the initial incision is made. With the patient positioned on the operating table, skin preparation is performed in such a way as to include the anterior chest as well as the abdomen; one thus has virtually immediate access to the chest in the event that a thoracic injury is discovered or thoracic vascular control is required. In addition, skin preparation should be extended over the anterior thighs in case distal vascular control is warranted or a vascular reconstruction conduit is needed. All exposed areas of the body that were not prepared must be covered to optimize thermoregulation. Drapes should be placed widely to allow easy access to all potential injuries.

Resuscitation, including the use of blood and blood products, should be continued as the patient is prepared. Both rapid volume infusion systems and cell saver systems are useful adjuncts in this setting. Room temperature must be controlled to minimize loss of heat from the patient during the operation.

Incision and Initial Exploration

CHOICE OF INCISION

A midline incision is the most expedient choice for opening the abdomen. It has several key advantages: it allows the abdominal cavity to be accessed easily and quickly, it provides good exposure (including exposure of the pelvis), and it can be extended into a median sternotomy or into either thoracic cavity if necessary. Its main disadvantage is the occasional difficulty that may be encountered in exploring the deep recesses of the upper quadrants.

Patients who have had previous midline incisions may be more challenging to operate on, depending on the extent to which intraperitoneal adhesions are present. Accordingly, alternative incisions may be considered. For example, a chevron incision or a transverse incision might allow better visualization of viscera adhering to a previous midline wound and thus might tend to protect them better from iatrogenic injury; however, these incisions are associated with certain disadvantages, in particular the need to divide the large rectus abdominis muscle, the restricted exposure provided, the additional time needed to close the incision, and the inherent limitations on extension of the incision if the need arises. Consequently, chevron and transverse incisions are rarely used and seldom recommended in this setting.

There are additional alternative incisions, such as paramedian, subcostal, retroperitoneal, and flank incisions, but they are not recommended, because they generally do not provide adequate exposure for assessment and treatment of abdominal injuries.

INITIAL EXPLORATION

Once the peritoneal cavity has been entered, initial exploration should proceed in an orderly manner so as to minimize hemorrhage and contamination and facilitate the identification of injuries. There may be an incipient drop in blood pressure when the abdomen is opened. The abdominal organs are eviscerated, and any gross blood, clotted or nonclotted, is evacuated. Laparotomy pads are then used for rapid packing of all four quadrants of the abdomen. When bleeding is under control, anesthesia is allowed to catch up with the resuscitation efforts before abdominal exploration is continued.

Once hemodynamic stability has been achieved, the peritoneal portion of the initial exploration is begun. If there is no discrete site of hemorrhage, the temporary packs are carefully removed, except for those around the solid viscera. The enteric viscera are inspected in an orderly fashion. The anterior aspect of the stomach is inspected from the esophagogastric junction to the pylorus. If there is a high index of suspicion, on the basis of the mechanism of injury or the presence of hematoma or soilage in the lesser sac, the gastrocolic omentum is opened to permit inspection of the posterior aspect of the stomach; this exposure also facilitates examination of the body of the pancreas. Exploration then continues distally. If duodenal or pancreatic injury is suspected, the Kocher maneuver is performed to mobilize the duodenum and the head of the pancreas fully. Once the duodenum has been visualized, the small bowel is inspected from the ligament of Treitz to the ileocecal valve. Careful consideration should be given to the possibility of mesenteric vascular injury, which is often manifested as a mesenteric hematoma. Next, the colon is inspected from the cecum to the peritoneal reflection over the rectum. If there are injuries or missile tracts in proximity to a portion of the ascending or descending colon, the colon must be mobilized by incising the peritoneal reflection (the white line of Toldt) so as to permit inspection of the posterior wall of the bowel as well. Finally, attention is turned toward evaluation of the solid viscera. The laparotomy pads are removed, and the liver and the spleen are visualized to ascertain whether any injury is present.

Once the peritoneal survey has been completed, the retroperitoneum is inspected for potential injury. Retroperitoneal hematomas are classified according to their location: zone 1 is the central portion of the retroperitoneum, zone 2 comprises the two lateral portions, and zone 3 is the pelvic portion [*see Figure 1*]. The decision whether to explore a retroperitoneal hematoma is based on its location and on the mechanism of injury [*see Priorities in Management, Repair of Retroperitoneal Injuries, below*]. The retroperitoneum is also evaluated with an eye to identifying any occult injuries to organs such as the pancreas, the duodenum, the posterior colon, the kidneys, and vascular structures. The initial exploration concludes with a brief pelvic survey undertaken to exclude injury to the rectum or the distal genitourinary tract (including the urinary bladder).

Operative Exposure

In what follows, we focus on exposure of specific organs and vessels in patients with abdominal injuries. Definitive repair of such injuries is addressed in more detail elsewhere [*see 28 Injuries to the Liver, Biliary Tract, Spleen, and Diaphragm; 29 Injuries to the Stomach, Duodenum, Pancreas, Small Bowel, Colon, and Rectum; and 30 Injuries to the Great Vessels of the Abdomen*].

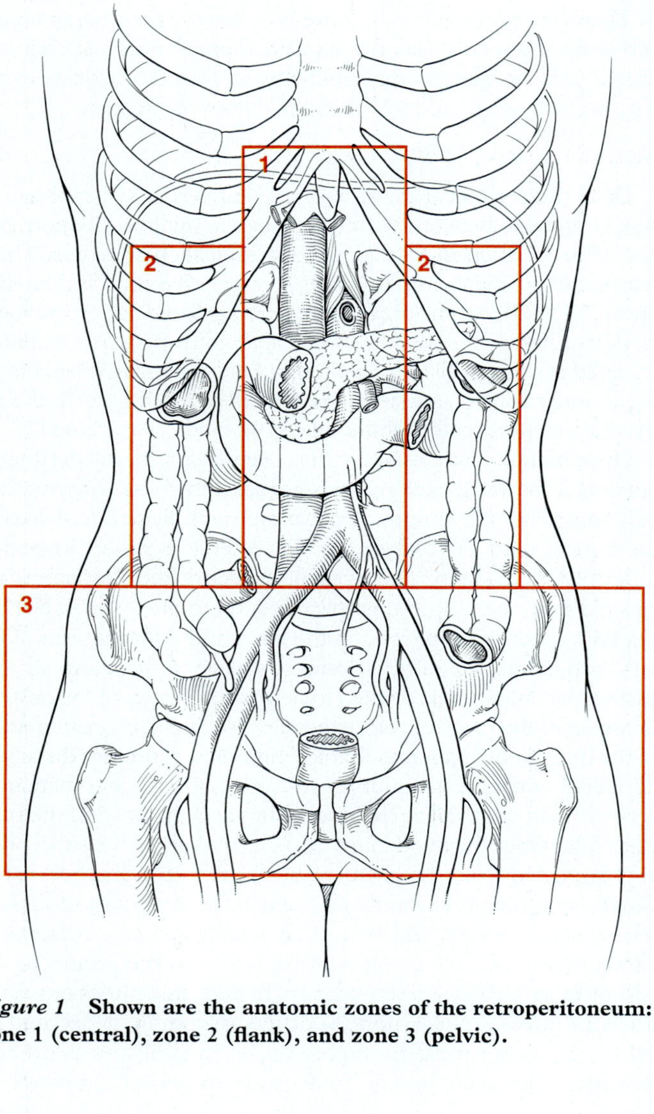

AORTA

Control of the aorta can be achieved at several different levels, depending on the site of injury. The supraceliac aorta can be exposed by incising the gastrohepatic ligament, retracting the left lobe of the liver cephalad, and retracting the stomach caudad. The esophagus and the periesophageal soft tissue are then mobilized laterally to permit identification of the abdominal aorta at the diaphragmatic hiatus, at which point the vessel can be clamped or compressed. The exposure this method gives is limited with respect to vascular access for definitive repair. Better exposure of the supraceliac aorta can be obtained by means of left medial visceral rotation [*see Figure 2*]. To reflect the left-sided viscera, the splenorenal ligament is mobilized with a combination of blunt and sharp dissection. The peritoneal reflection is incised, and the incision is extended down the left paracolic gutter to the level of the distal sigmoid colon. With the aid of blunt dissection, the left-sided viscera are gently mobilized to the right in a plane anterior to Gerota's fascia. This technique permits exploration of the entire length of the abdominal aorta as well as the origin of the celiac axis, the origin of the superior mesenteric artery, the left iliac system, and the origin of the right common iliac artery. In addition, it facilitates control of the left renal pedicle before exploration of a left-sided hematoma within Gerota's fascia.

If only distal access to the aorta is necessary, the vessel can be approached transperitoneally. The small bowel is retracted to the right, the transverse colon is retracted cephalad, and the descending colon is retracted to the left. The peritoneum is incised over the aorta, and the third and fourth portions of the duodenum are mobilized cephalad. The proximal limit of this dissection extends to the level of the left renal vein, which can, if necessary, be divided to provide access to the suprarenal aorta. If the left renal vein is ligated, care should be taken to place the ligature close to the vena cava so as to spare important venous collaterals. A somewhat more limited dissection may suffice to expose the distal infrarenal aorta; the exposure can subsequently be extended distally to expose both iliac vessels.

VENA CAVA

Access to the suprahepatic vena cava can be gained by incising the central tendon of the diaphragm or by performing a median sternotomy and opening the pericardium. The infrahepatic inferior vena cava can be exposed by means of right medial visceral rotation [*see Figure 3*] in much the same way as the aorta is exposed by means of left medial visceral rotation [*see Aorta, above*]. The right colon is mobilized by taking down the hepatic flexure and incising the peritoneal reflection within the right paracolic gutter. The colon, again, is reflected medially toward the aorta in a plane anterior to Gerota's fascia with the aid of blunt dissection. If additional exposure is necessary, the inferior margin of the peritoneal incision can be extended to the root of the mesentery and even beyond by sacrificing the inferior mesenteric vein. This exposure allows visualization of both the aorta below the origin of the superior mesenteric artery and the vena cava below the third portion of the duodenum. The portion of the inferior vena cava immediately below the liver can be exposed by performing the Kocher maneuver [*see Figure 4*] with subsequent medial mobilization of the duodenum and head of the pancreas.

Figure 1 Shown are the anatomic zones of the retroperitoneum: zone 1 (central), zone 2 (flank), and zone 3 (pelvic).

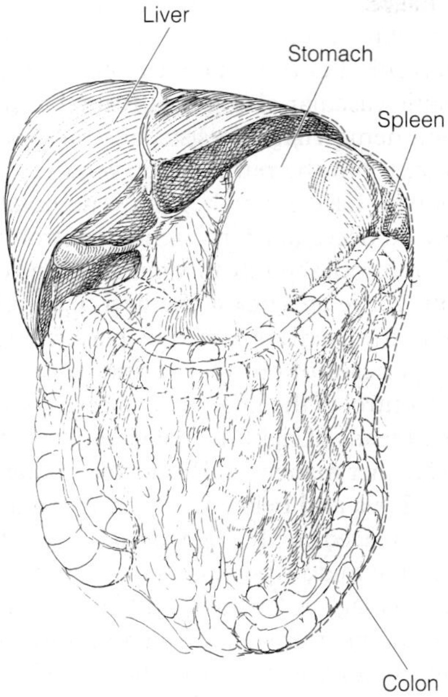

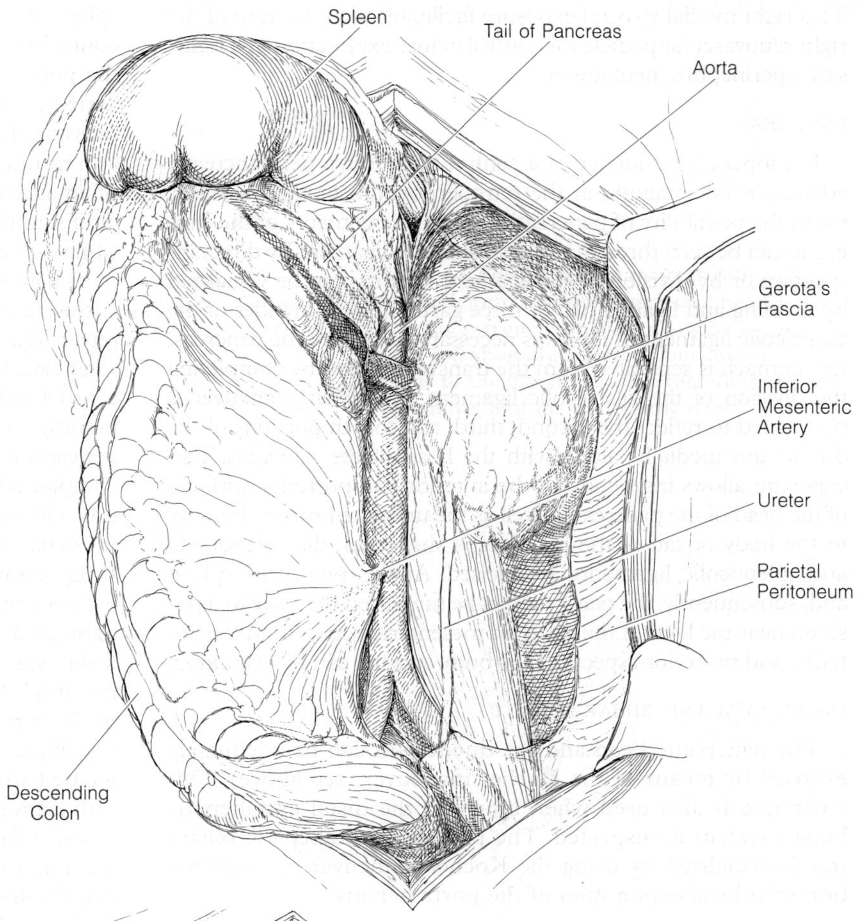

Figure 2 Left medial visceral rotation is performed to provide exposure of the entire length of the abdominal aorta, the left renal vasculature, the origins of the mesenteric arteries, and the common iliac bifurcation.

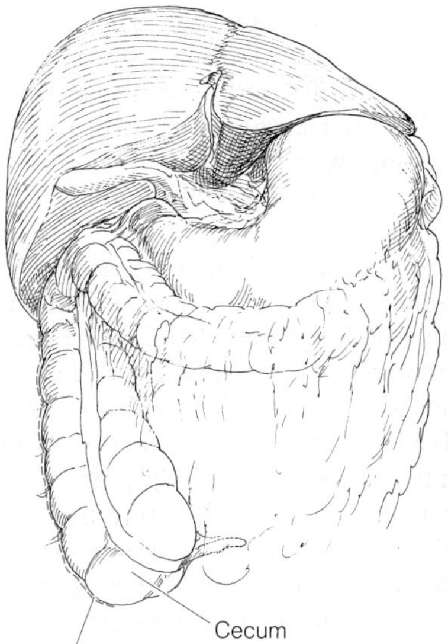

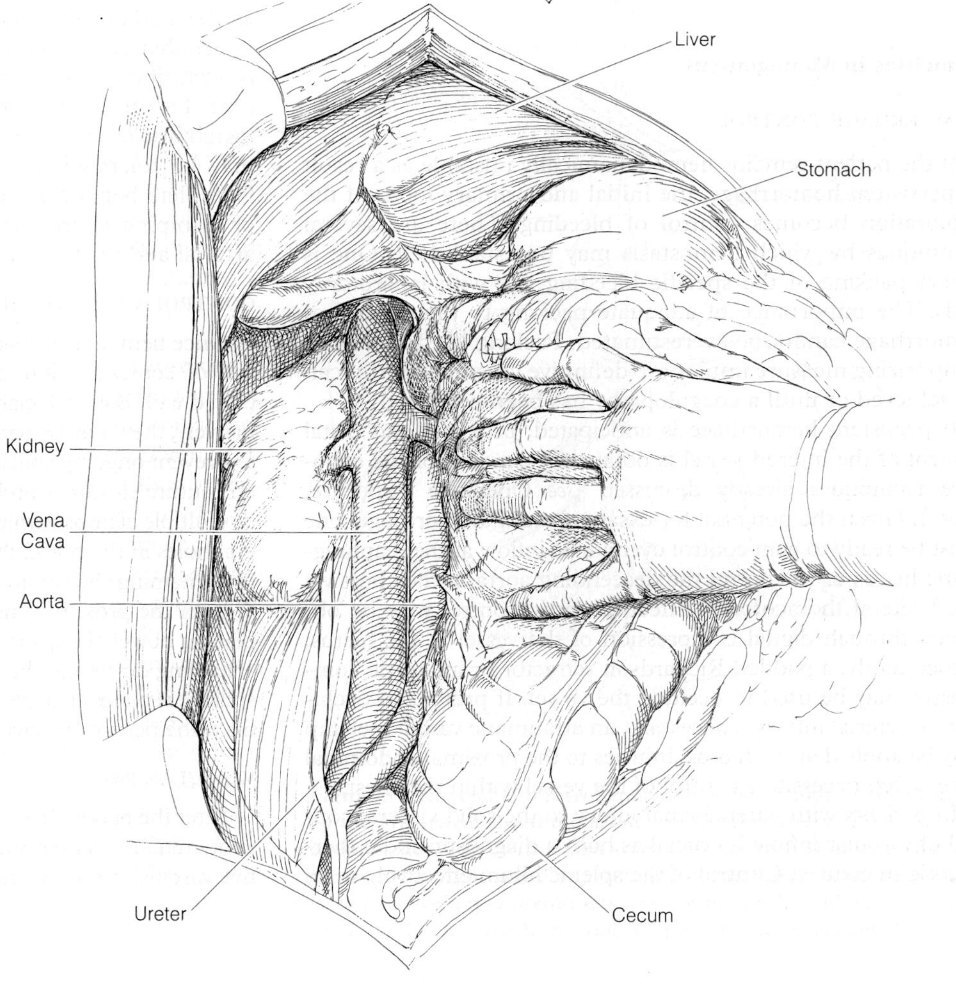

Figure 3 Right medial visceral rotation is performed to provide exposure of the inferior vena cava, the infrarenal abdominal aorta and iliac vessels, and the right renovascular pedicle.

length, a Hartmann procedure can be performed. When significant left colon injury occurs in association with shock or gross contamination, proximal diversion should be considered.

REPAIR OF RETROPERITONEAL INJURIES

Once injuries within the peritoneal cavity have been addressed, the retroperitoneum should be inspected again, with particular attention paid to the possibility of hematoma expansion. Zonal distribution and mechanism of injury are the two important determinants governing the decision whether to explore a retroperitoneal hematoma. All zone 1 hematomas should be explored regardless of the mechanism: they signal possible aortic, vena caval, duodenal, or pancreatic injury. Zone 2 and 3 hematomas should be explored if the patient sustained a penetrating injury. Generally, except for expanding zone 2 hematomas, zone 2 and 3 hematomas need not be explored in cases of blunt trauma. Even in blunt trauma patients with pelvic fractures, zone 3 hematomas are not explored if one is certain that there is no injury to the distal aorta or the iliac vessels. Before exploration of retroperitoneal hematomas, it is important to gain proximal vascular control to minimize hemorrhage once the retroperitoneal tamponade effect is lost. Vascular injuries discovered at this juncture should be repaired as discussed earlier (see above). Injuries to retroperitoneal organs (e.g., kidneys, pancreas, or adrenals) may be treated with debridement or resection with drainage as indicated.

Closure

GENERAL TECHNIQUE

Once the abdominal exploration has been completed, the abdomen should be copiously irrigated with a balanced salt solution. Generally, the optimal closure technique is chosen on the basis of five main considerations: the amount of blood lost, the volume of fluid received, the degree of contamination present, the patient's nutritional status, and the patient's overall stability. In some cases, the speed with which a closure can be performed may be the determining factor. Every effort should be made to close the fascia primarily. There are several methods that can be used to accomplish this. The most commonly used technique involves placement of a continuous monofilament suture. The major benefit of this type of closure is that it can be done relatively quickly. Alternatively, the fascia can be closed with interrupted sutures. There is no difference between the two techniques with respect to the rate of fascial dehiscence; however, the extent of the dehiscence is generally more limited with the interrupted suture method. Whichever method is used, the most important technical point is the necessity of avoiding excessive tension on the tissue.

Large monofilament sutures placed at intervals within the standard closure can serve as retention sutures [see Figure 6]. These sutures are used to support standard closure methods in patients who are at increased risk for fascial dehiscence and wound breakdown. They can be tied over bolsters fashioned from a red rubber catheter or tied over plastic skin bridges. When time is of the essence, the abdomen can be rapidly closed with four or five retention sutures of this type that are placed through and through all layers of the abdominal wall. These sutures should be checked daily and loosened if edema creates tension on the wound.

SKIN CLOSURE

The skin is closed primarily in patients who have minimal

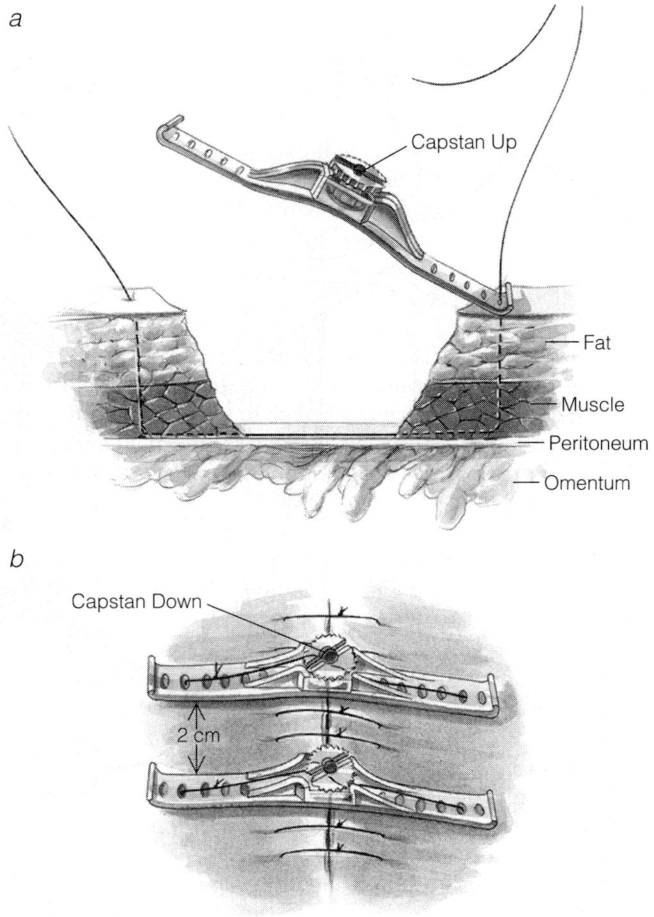

Figure 6 Retention sutures may be used to bolster fascial closure in wounds at high risk for breakdown. (*a*) Sutures are placed in the subfascial plane. (*b*) The defect is approximated over skin bridges.

injuries and show no evidence of enteric contamination. Either a stapled closure or a sewn closure is acceptable. A degree of clinical judgment is required in dealing with clean-contaminated wounds. In some cases, the skin may be closed primarily; however, one should stand ready to open the wound again without undue delay if subsequent infection is suspected. Alternatively, the wound may be left open for three to five days and then loosely approximated with Steri-Strips if there is no evidence of contamination or infection. When gross intraperitoneal contamination was noted at the time of celiotomy, the patient is best served by leaving the wound open to heal by either secondary intention or delayed primary closure.

OPEN FASCIAL CLOSURE

On occasion, a multiply injured patient must undergo a protracted procedure or must receive massive volume resuscitation to maintain hemodynamic stability. Extensive interstitial edema may occur, precluding primary fascial closure. Closure of the abdomen in these circumstances may result in compromise of respiratory function or increased intra-abdominal pressure and its attendant sequelae. Consequently, a number of materials have been developed for use in both temporary and permanent abdominal closure in such conditions. Several absorbable meshes are available [see Figure 7]. Their main advantages are their inherent porosity and their ability to be easily incorporated into tissue. Subsequent abdominal wounds can be left open to heal by secondary intention; ventral hernias may be expected to form at a later date. Abdominal fascial defects may also be closed with sheets of nonincorporable synthetics, such as Gore-Tex. The advantages of these nonabsorbable materials are their innate lack of reactivity with tissue and the decreased rate of complications (e.g., enterocutaneous fistula). On the other hand, they are expensive and must ultimately be removed unless the skin is closed over them to protect the graft from contamination. If a temporary closure that lasts only a few days is all that is needed, then materials such as sterile I.V. bags can be used to close the fascial defect.

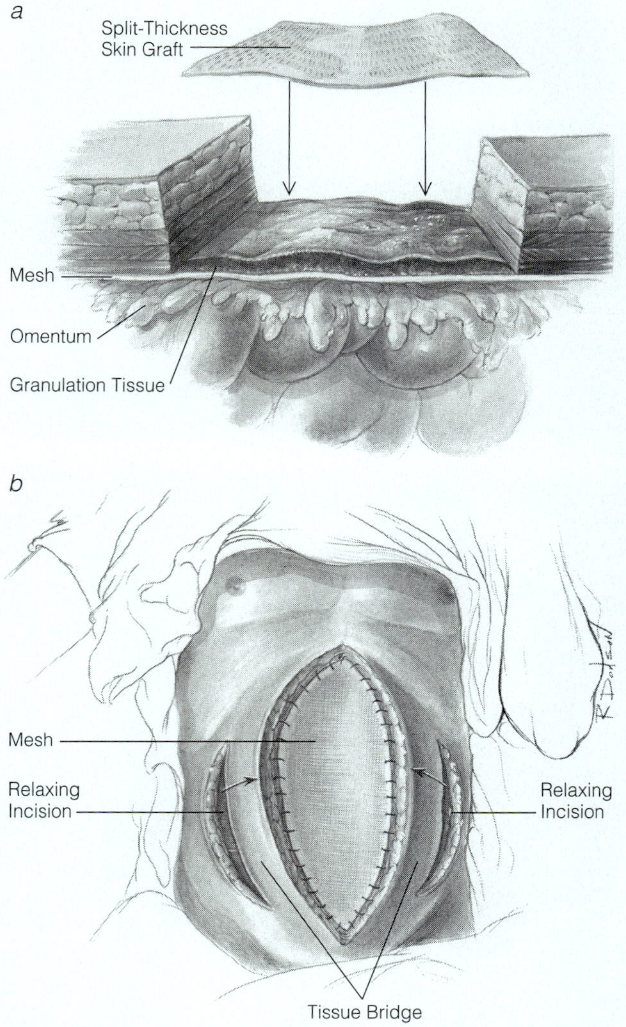

Figure 7 Mesh may be used for temporary or permanent abdominal closure in patients at risk for increased abdominal pressure. (*a*) Mesh is sutured into the fascial plane. (*b*) The abdominal defect is closed with mesh.

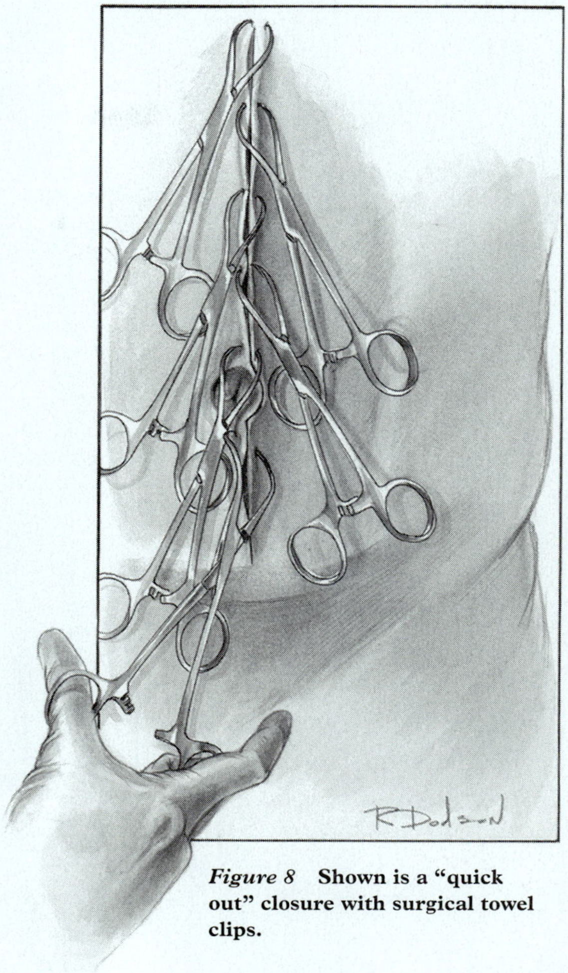

Figure 8 Shown is a "quick out" closure with surgical towel clips.

"QUICK OUTS" AND DAMAGE CONTROL

In grossly unstable or coagulopathic patients in whom surgical bleeding and contamination have been controlled, rapid abdominal closure may be necessary with the proviso that further exploration will be required. The basic objectives of the closure techniques used in these situations are control of peritoneal contamination and maintenance of intra-abdominal tamponade. One example of such a "quick out" is the use of towel clips to approximate skin [*see Figure 8*] in conjunction with a biooclusive dressing for control of contamination. Another technique involves placement of a sterile plastic barrier within the fascial defect, followed by insertion of several closed suction drains over which open laparotomy pads are placed. Subsequently, an adherent biooclusive sheet is draped over the abdominal wall to minimize thermal and insensible water losses.

Recommended Reading

Blaisdell FW, Trunkey DD: Abdominal Trauma. Thieme Medical Publishers, New York, 1993

Donovan AJ: Trauma Surgery. Mosby–Year Book Co, St Louis, 1994

Feliciano DV, Moore EE, Mattox KL: Trauma. Appleton & Lange, Stamford, Connecticut, 1996

Greenfield LJ: Complications in Surgery and Trauma. JB Lippincott Co, Grand Rapids, Michigan, 1990

Ivatury RR, Cayten CG: The Textbook of Penetrating Trauma. Williams & Wilkins, Baltimore, 1996

Mattox KL: Complications of Trauma. Churchill Livingstone, New York, 1994

Maull KI, Rodriguez A, Wiles CE: Complications in Trauma and Critical Care. WB Saunders Co, Philadelphia, 1996

Acknowledgments

Figures 1, 4, and 5   Susan Brust, C.M.I.
Figures 2 and 3   Carol Donner.
Figures 6 through 8   R. Dodson. Adapted from *Management of Operative Trauma: An Atlas,* by C. J. Carrico, E. R. Thal, and J. A. Weigelt. Appleton & Lange, Stamford, Connecticut, 1998.

28 INJURIES TO THE LIVER, BILIARY TRACT, SPLEEN, AND DIAPHRAGM

Jon M. Burch, M.D., and Ernest E. Moore, M.D.

Assessment and Management of Injuries to the Liver, Biliary Tract, Spleen, and Diaphragm

Injuries to the Liver

ASSESSMENT

The initial step in the management of penetrating abdominal injuries and of blunt abdominal injuries in cases when nonoperative treatment is contraindicated or has failed is exploratory laparotomy.

Visualization of the right lobe of the liver is hindered by the lobe's posterior attachments and by the right lower costal margin. Exposure of the right lobe is facilitated by elevating the right costal margin with a large Richardson retractor. Further exposure can be achieved with mobilization, which requires division of the right triangular and coronary ligaments. In dividing the superior coronary ligament, care must be taken not to injure the lateral wall of the right hepatic vein; in dividing the inferior coronary ligament, care must be taken not to injure the right adrenal gland (which is vulnerable because it lies directly beneath the peritoneal reflection) or the retrohepatic vena cava. When the ligaments have been divided, the right lobe of the liver can be rotated medially into the surgical field. Mobilization of the left lobe poses no unusual problems other than the risk of injury to the left hepatic vein, the left inferior phrenic vein, and the retrohepatic vena cava.

If optimal exposure of the junction of the hepatic veins and the retrohepatic vena cava is necessary, the midline abdominal incision can be extended by means of a median sternotomy. The pericardium and the diaphragm can then be divided toward the center of the inferior vena cava. This combination of incisions provides superb exposure of the hepatic veins and the retrohepatic vena cava while avoiding injury to the phrenic nerves.

The American Association for the Surgery of Trauma's Committee on Organ Injury Scaling has developed a grading system for classifying injuries to the liver [see Table 1 and Figure 1].[1] Hepatic injuries are graded on a scale of I to VI, with I representing superficial lacerations and small subcapsular hematomas and VI representing avulsion of the liver from the vena cava. Isolated injuries that are not extensive (grades I to III) often require little or no treatment; however, extensive parenchymal injuries and those involving the juxtahepatic veins (grades IV and V) may require complex maneuvers for successful treatment, and hepatic avulsion (grade VI) is lethal.

Clamping of the hepatic pedicle—the Pringle maneuver—is a helpful technique for evaluating grade IV and V hepatic injuries [see Figure 2]. This maneuver allows one to distinguish between hemorrhage from branches of the hepatic artery or the portal vein, which ceases when the clamp is applied, and hemorrhage from the hepatic veins or the retrohepatic vena cava, which does not. When performing the Pringle maneuver, we prefer to tear the lesser omentum manually and place the clamp from the left side while guiding the posterior blade of the clamp through the foramen of Winslow with the aid of the left index finger. The advantages of this approach are the avoidance of injury to the structures within the hepatic pedicle, the assurance that the clamp will be properly placed the first time, and the inclusion of a replacing or accessory left hepatic artery between the blades of the clamp.

MANAGEMENT OF INJURIES

Techniques for Temporary Control of Hemorrhage

Temporary control of hemorrhage is essential for two reasons. First, during treatment of a major hepatic injury, ongoing hem-

Table 1 AAST Liver Injury Scale (1994 Revision)[1]

Grade*	Injury Description
I	Hematoma: subcapsular, nonexpanding, < 10% surface area Laceration: capsular tear, nonbleeding, < 1 cm parenchymal depth
II	Hematoma: subcapsular, nonexpanding, 10%–50% surface area; intraparenchymal, nonexpanding, < 10 cm in diameter Laceration: capsular tear, active bleeding, 1–3 cm parenchymal depth, < 10 cm in length
III	Hematoma: subcapsular, > 50% surface area, expanding; ruptured subcapsular hematoma with active bleeding; intraparenchymal, > 10 cm or expanding Laceration: > 3 cm parenchymal depth
IV	Hematoma: ruptured intraparenchymal hematoma with active bleeding Laceration: parenchymal disruption involving 25%–75% of hepatic lobe or 1–3 Couinaud's segments within a single lobe
V	Laceration: parenchymal disruption involving > 75% of hepatic lobe or > 3 Couinaud's segments within a single lobe Vascular: juxtahepatic venous injuries (i.e., injuries to retrohepatic vena cava or central major hepatic veins)
VI	Vascular: hepatic avulsion

*Advance one grade for multiple injuries, up to grade III.
AAST—American Association for the Surgery of Trauma

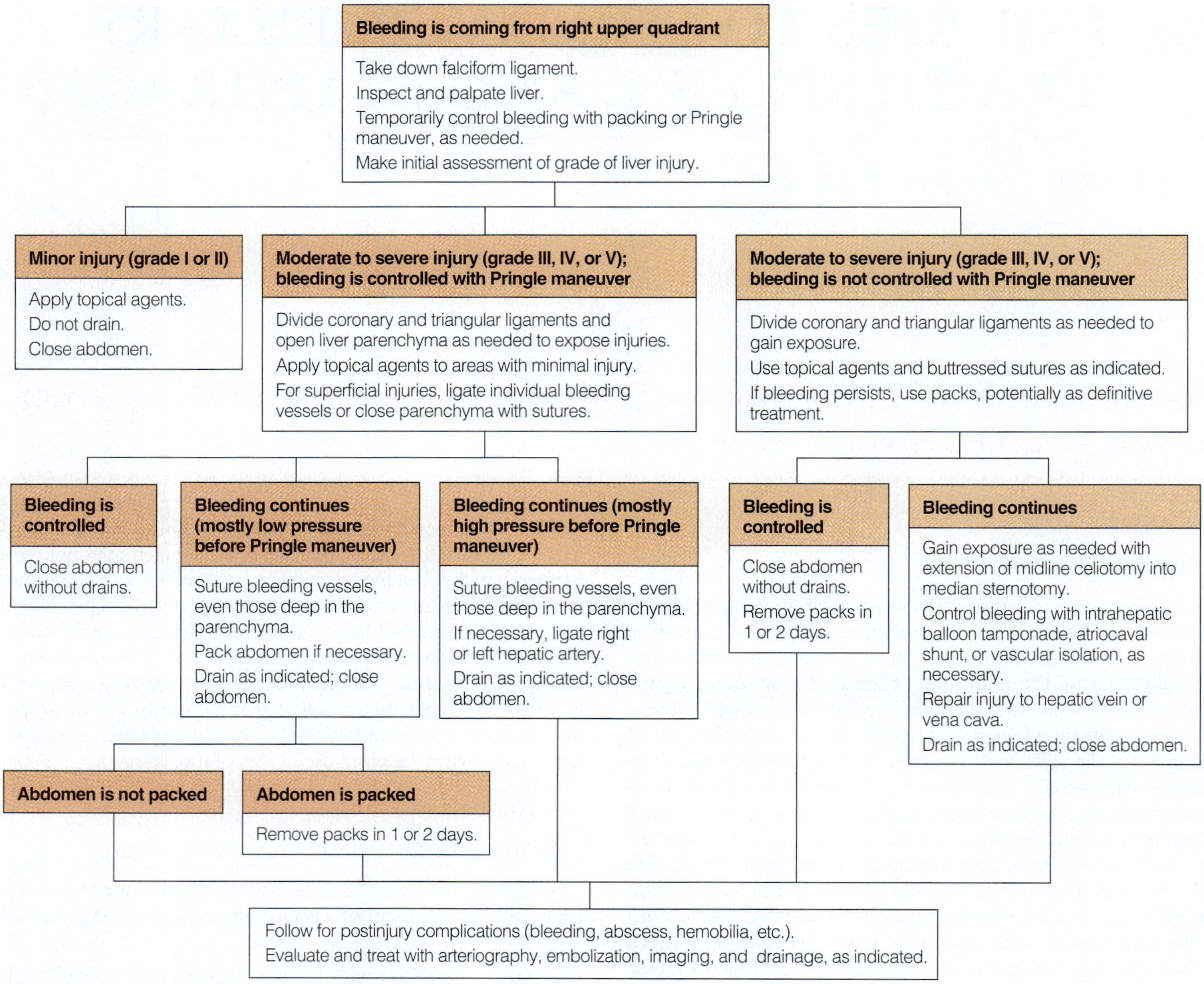

```
┌─────────────────────────────────────────┐
│ Bleeding is coming from right upper quadrant │
│ Take down falciform ligament.           │
│ Inspect and palpate liver.              │
│ Temporarily control bleeding with packing or Pringle │
│ maneuver, as needed.                    │
│ Make initial assessment of grade of liver injury. │
└─────────────────────────────────────────┘
```

Minor injury (grade I or II)
Apply topical agents.
Do not drain.
Close abdomen.

Moderate to severe injury (grade III, IV, or V); bleeding is controlled with Pringle maneuver
Divide coronary and triangular ligaments and open liver parenchyma as needed to expose injuries.
Apply topical agents to areas with minimal injury.
For superficial injuries, ligate individual bleeding vessels or close parenchyma with sutures.

Moderate to severe injury (grade III, IV, or V); bleeding is not controlled with Pringle maneuver
Divide coronary and triangular ligaments as needed to gain exposure.
Use topical agents and buttressed sutures as indicated.
If bleeding persists, use packs, potentially as definitive treatment.

Bleeding is controlled
Close abdomen without drains.

Bleeding continues (mostly low pressure before Pringle maneuver)
Suture bleeding vessels, even those deep in the parenchyma.
Pack abdomen if necessary.
Drain as indicated; close abdomen.

Bleeding continues (mostly high pressure before Pringle maneuver)
Suture bleeding vessels, even those deep in the parenchyma.
If necessary, ligate right or left hepatic artery.
Drain as indicated; close abdomen.

Bleeding is controlled
Close abdomen without drains.
Remove packs in 1 or 2 days.

Bleeding continues
Gain exposure as needed with extension of midline celiotomy into median sternotomy.
Control bleeding with intrahepatic balloon tamponade, atriocaval shunt, or vascular isolation, as necessary.
Repair injury to hepatic vein or vena cava.
Drain as indicated; close abdomen.

Abdomen is not packed

Abdomen is packed
Remove packs in 1 or 2 days.

Follow for postinjury complications (bleeding, abscess, hemobilia, etc.).
Evaluate and treat with arteriography, embolization, imaging, and drainage, as indicated.

Figure 1 Shown is an algorithm for the treatment of hepatic injuries.

orrhage may pose an immediate threat to the patient's life, and temporary control gives the anesthesiologist time to restore the circulating volume before further blood loss occurs. Second, multiple bleeding sites are common with both blunt and penetrating trauma, and if the liver is not the highest priority, temporary control of hepatic bleeding allows repair of other injuries without unnecessary blood loss. The most useful techniques for the temporary control of hepatic hemorrhage are manual compression, perihepatic packing, and the Pringle maneuver.

Periodic manual compression with the addition of laparotomy pads is useful in the treatment of complex hepatic injuries to provide time for resuscitation [see Figure 3].[2-4]

Perihepatic packing with carefully placed laparotomy pads is capable of controlling hemorrhage from almost all hepatic injuries.[5-9] The right costal margin is elevated, and the pads are strategically placed over and around the bleeding site [see Figure 4]. Additional pads may be placed between the liver and the diaphragm and between the liver and the anterior chest wall until the bleeding has been controlled. Ten to 15 pads may be required to control the hemorrhage from an extensive right lobar injury. Packing is not as effective for injuries of the left lobe, because with the abdomen open, there is insufficient abdominal and thoracic wall anterior to the left lobe to provide adequate compression. Fortunately, hemorrhage from the left lobe can be controlled by dividing the left triangular and coronary ligaments and compressing the lobe between the hands. Two complications may be encountered with the packing of hepatic injuries. First, tight packing compresses the inferior vena cava, decreases venous return, and reduces left ventricular filling; hypovolemic patients may not tolerate the resultant decrease in cardiac output. Second, perihepatic packing forces the right diaphragm superiorly and impairs its motion; this may lead to increased airway pressures and decreased tidal volume. Careful consideration of the patient's condition is necessary to determine whether the risk of these complications outweighs the risk of additional blood loss.

The Pringle maneuver is often used as an adjunct to packing for the temporary control of hemorrhage.[3] Over the years, the length of time for which surgeons believe a Pringle maneuver can be maintained without causing irreversible ischemic damage to the liver has increased. Several authors have documented the maintenance of a Pringle maneuver for longer than 1 hour in patients with complex injuries, without appreciable hepatic damage.[4,10] When a life-threatening hepatic injury is encountered on entry into the abdomen, the Pringle maneuver should

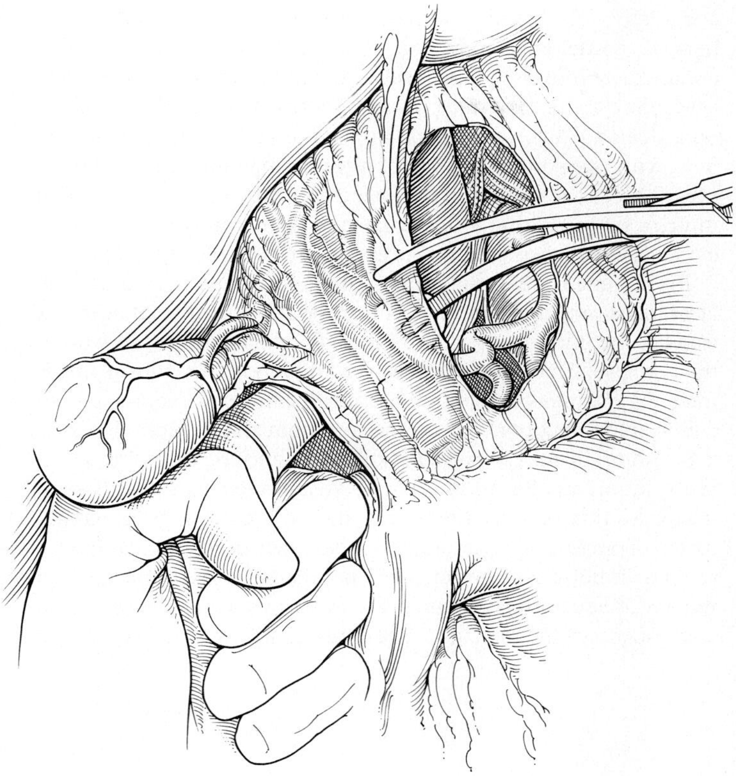

Figure 2 The Pringle maneuver controls arterial and portal vein hemorrhage from the liver. Any hemorrhage that continues must come from the hepatic veins.

be performed immediately and perihepatic packs placed. This combination of techniques should eliminate all hepatopetal blood flow and control retrograde venous bleeding.

Another technique for temporary control of hepatic hemorrhage is the application of a tourniquet or a liver clamp.[11] Once the bleeding lobe is mobilized, a 1 in. Penrose drain is wrapped around the liver near the anatomic division between the left lobe and the right. The drain is stretched until hemorrhage ceases, and tension is maintained by clamping the drain. Unfortunately, tourniquets are difficult to use: they tend to slip off or tear through the parenchyma if placed over an injured area. An alternative is the use of a liver clamp; however, the application of such devices is hindered by the variability in the size and shape of the liver.

Juxtahepatic venous injuries are technically challenging and often lethal. Complex procedures may be required for temporary control of these large veins. Of these procedures, the most important are hepatic vascular isolation with clamps, placement of the atriocaval shunt, and use of the Moore-Pilcher balloon.

Hepatic vascular isolation is accomplished by executing a Pringle maneuver, clamping the aorta at the diaphragm, and clamping the suprarenal and suprahepatic vena cava.[12] In patients scheduled for elective procedures, this technique has enjoyed nearly uniform success, but in trauma patients, the results have been disappointing. The relative ineffectiveness of hepatic vascular isolation with clamps in this setting is presumably due to the inability of a patient in shock to tolerate an acute reduction in left ventricular filling pressure; on occasion, sudden death has occurred on placement of the venous clamps.[13] If, however, a trauma patient requiring hepatic vascular isolation has been maintained in a relatively normal physiologic condition, it is reasonable to consider this method.

A new approach to exposure of complex injuries to the retrohepatic vena cava and the hepatic veins has recently been developed.[14] Vascular isolation of the liver is achieved by means of the clamping technique, and the suprahepatic vena cava is divided between vascular clamps. The liver and the suprahepatic vena cava are then rotated anteriorly to provide direct access to the posterior aspect of the retrohepatic vena cava. Anterior injuries of the large veins are repaired through an incision in the posterior aspect of the retrohepatic vena cava.

The atriocaval shunt was designed to achieve hepatic vascular isolation while still permitting some venous blood from below the diaphragm to flow through the shunt into the right atrium.[4] After a few early successes, the initial enthusiasm for the atriocaval shunt declined as high mortalities associated with its use began to be reported.[15-20] Surgeons' lack of familiarity with the technique; manipulation of a cold, acidotic heart; and poor patient selection have all contributed to the poor overall results.[13] A variation on the original atriocaval shunt has been described in which a 9 mm endotracheal tube is substituted for the usual large chest tube [see Figure 5].[21] The balloon of the endotracheal tube makes it unnecessary to surround the suprarenal vena cava with an umbilical tape. This minor change eliminates one of the most difficult maneuvers required for the original shunt procedure: because hemorrhage must be controlled by posterior pressure on the liver during the insertion of the shunt, access to the suprarenal vena cava is severely restricted, and thus, surrounding this vessel with an umbilical tape is almost impossible. A side hole must be cut in the tube to allow blood to enter the right atrium. Care must be taken to avoid damage to the integral inflation channel for the balloon.

An alternative to the atriocaval shunt is the Moore-Pilcher balloon.[22] This device is inserted through the femoral vein and advanced into the retrohepatic vena cava. When the balloon is properly positioned and inflated, it occludes the hepatic veins and the vena cava, thus achieving vascular isolation. The catheter itself is hollow, and appropriately placed holes below the balloon permit blood to flow into the right atrium, in much the same way as the atriocaval shunt. At present, the survival rate for patients with juxtahepatic venous injuries who are

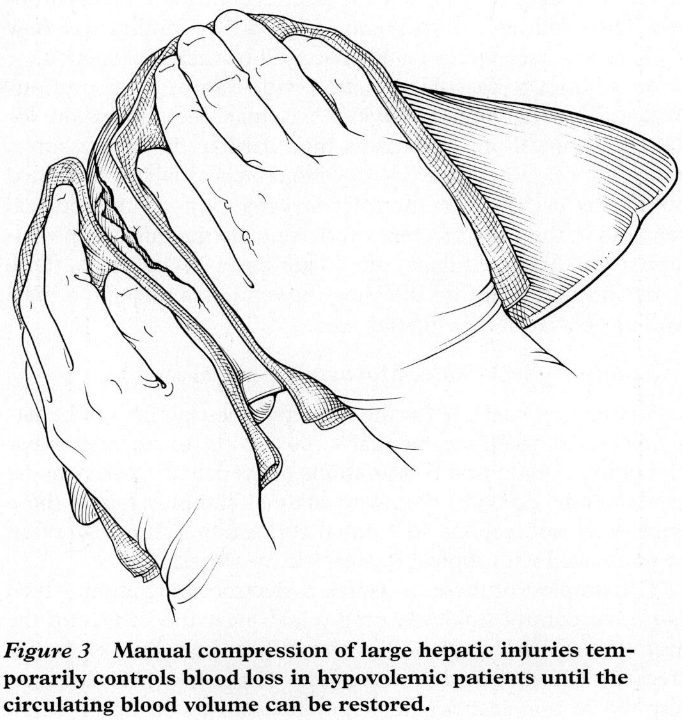

Figure 3 Manual compression of large hepatic injuries temporarily controls blood loss in hypovolemic patients until the circulating blood volume can be restored.

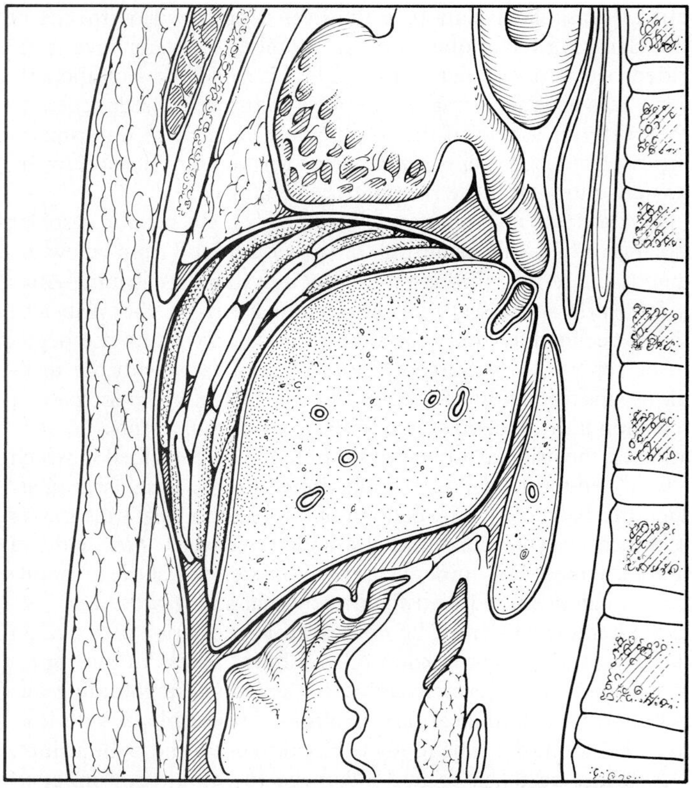

Figure 4 **Perihepatic packing is often effective in managing extensive parenchymal injuries. It has also been successfully employed for grade V juxtahepatic venous injuries.**

coagulator. This device imparts less heat to the surrounding hepatic tissue and creates a more consistent eschar, which enhances hemostasis. Also useful in similar situations is microcrystalline collagen in the powdered form. The powder is placed on a clean 4 × 4 in. sponge and applied directly to the oozing surface, with pressure maintained on the sponge for five to 10 minutes. Thrombin can also be applied topically to minor bleeding injuries by saturating either a gelatin foam sponge or a microcrystalline collagen pad and pressing it to the bleeding site.

Fibrin glue has been used in treating both superficial and deep lacerations and appears to be the most effective topical agent. It can also be injected deep into bleeding gunshot and stab wound tracts to prevent extensive dissection and blood loss. Fibrin glue is made by mixing concentrated human fibrinogen (cryoprecipitate) with a solution containing bovine thrombin and calcium. Because a coagulum forms quickly, the fibrinogen and the thrombin-calcium solution are placed in separate syringes joined with a Y connector, so that they are not mixed until immediately before application. Spray-on applicators have also been used. Topical hemostasis with fibrin glue became very popular after the publication of reports of large series of patients with serious hepatic injuries that were successfully managed with this material.[2,23,24] The initial

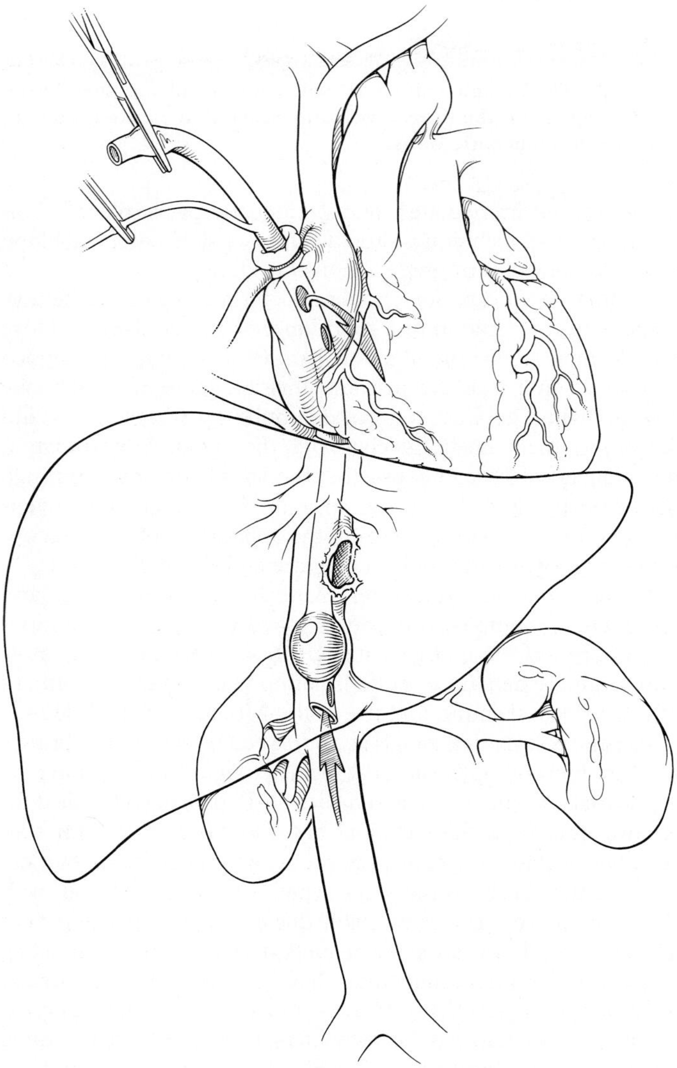

treated with this device is similar to that for patients treated with the atriocaval shunt.[18]

Surgeons who attempt hepatic vascular isolation should be aware that none of these techniques provide complete hemostasis. Drainage from the right adrenal vein and the inferior phrenic veins and persistent hepatopetal flow resulting from unrecognized replacing or accessory left hepatic arteries contribute to this problem. The relatively small volume of blood that continues to flow after vascular isolation is readily removed by means of suction.

An adjunct to vascular isolation with clamps is venovenous bypass. This technique provides vascular decompression for the small bowel and maintains high cardiac filling pressures, which are often necessary. Venovenous bypass is accomplished by placing catheters in the inferior vena cava via the femoral vein and in the superior mesenteric vein via the inferior mesenteric vein. A centrifugal pump withdraws blood from these veins and pumps it into the superior vena cava through a third catheter placed in the jugular vein.

Techniques for Definitive Management of Injuries

Techniques available for the definitive management of hepatic injuries range from manual compression to hepatic transplantation. Grade I or II lacerations of the hepatic parenchyma can generally be controlled with manual compression. If these injuries do not respond to manual compression, they can often be controlled with topical hemostatic measures.

The simplest of these measures is electrocauterization, which can often control small bleeding vessels near the surface of the liver (though the machine's power output may have to be increased). Bleeding from raw surfaces of the liver that does not respond to the electrocautery may respond to the argon beam

Figure 5 **Shown is a method of achieving hepatic vascular isolation with a 9 mm endotracheal tube.**

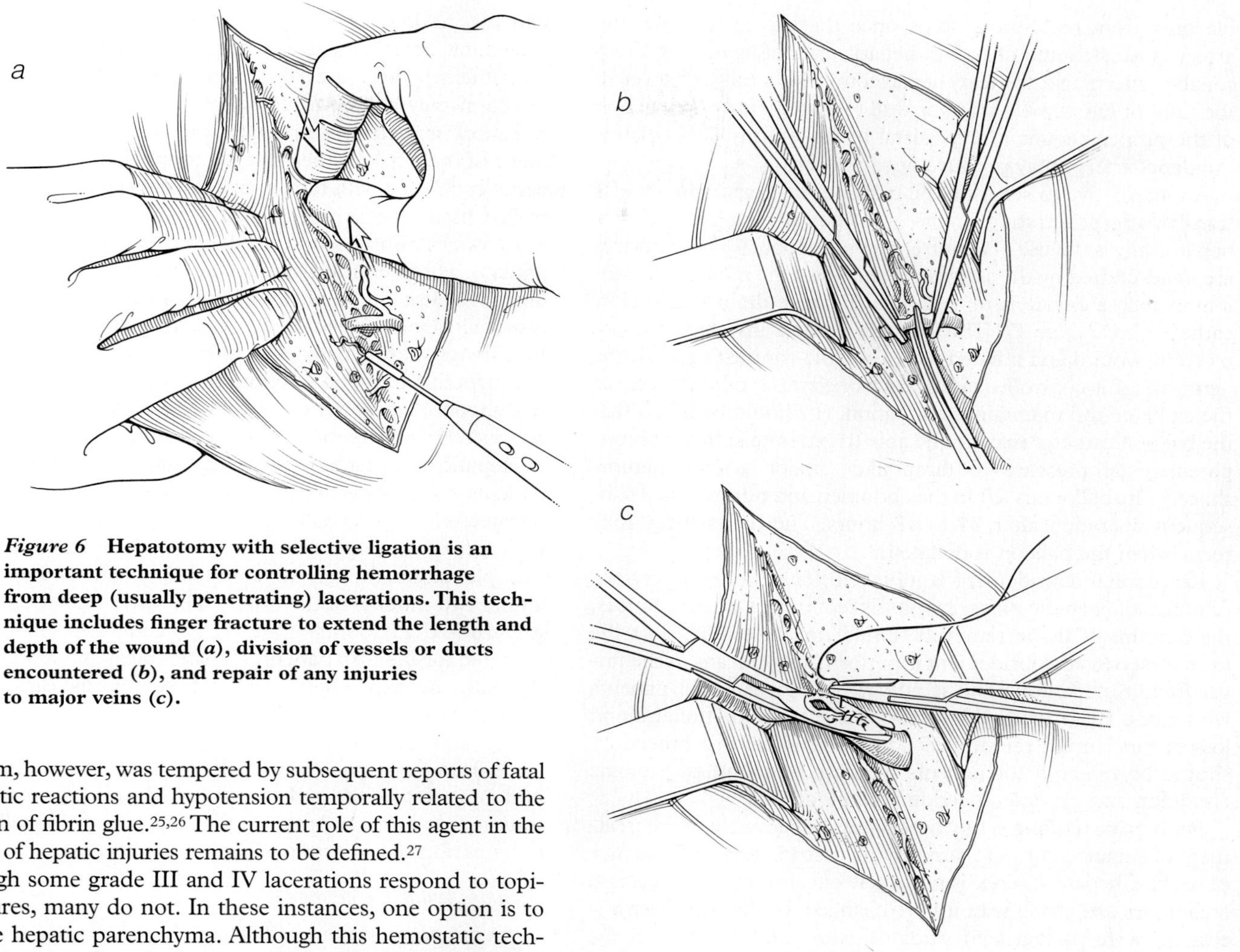

Figure 6 Hepatotomy with selective ligation is an important technique for controlling hemorrhage from deep (usually penetrating) lacerations. This technique includes finger fracture to extend the length and depth of the wound (*a*), division of vessels or ducts encountered (*b*), and repair of any injuries to major veins (*c*).

enthusiasm, however, was tempered by subsequent reports of fatal anaphylactic reactions and hypotension temporally related to the application of fibrin glue.[25,26] The current role of this agent in the treatment of hepatic injuries remains to be defined.[27]

Although some grade III and IV lacerations respond to topical measures, many do not. In these instances, one option is to suture the hepatic parenchyma. Although this hemostatic technique has been maligned as a cause of hepatic necrosis, it still is frequently used.[3,4,10,17,28,29] Suturing of the hepatic parenchyma is often employed to control persistently bleeding lacerations less than 3 cm in depth; it is also an appropriate alternative for deeper lacerations if the patient cannot tolerate the further hemorrhage associated with hepatotomy and selective ligation. If, however, the capsule of the liver has been stripped away by the injury, this technique is far less effective.

The preferred suture material is 0 or 2-0 chromic catgut attached to a large, blunt-tipped, curved needle; the large diameter prevents the suture from pulling through Glisson's capsule. For shallow lacerations, a simple continuous suture may be used to approximate the edges of the laceration. For deeper lacerations, interrupted horizontal mattress sutures may be placed parallel to the edges. When tying sutures, one may be sure that adequate tension has been achieved when hemorrhage ceases or the liver blanches around the suture.

Most sources of venous hemorrhage can be managed with parenchymal sutures. Even injuries to the retrohepatic vena cava and the hepatic veins have been successfully tamponaded by closing the hepatic parenchyma over the bleeding vessels.[13,30] Venous hemorrhage caused by penetrating wounds traversing the central portion of the liver may be managed by closing the entrance and exit wounds with interrupted horizontal mattress sutures. Although this measure may lead to the formation of intrahepatic hematomas that may then become infected, the risk is reasonable compared with the risks posed by an intracaval shunt or a deep hepatotomy. Still, suturing of the hepatic parenchyma is not always successful in controlling hemorrhage, particularly hemorrhage from the larger branches of the hepatic artery. If it fails, one must acknowledge the failure promptly and remove the sutures so that the wound can be explored.

Hepatotomy with selective ligation of bleeding vessels is an important technique that is usually reserved for deep or transhepatic penetrating wounds. Most authorities prefer it to parenchymal suturing[3,4,10,31,32]; some even favor it over placement of an atriocaval shunt for exposure and repair of juxtahepatic venous injuries.[20] The finger-fracture technique is used to extend the length and depth of a laceration or a missile tract until the bleeding vessels can be identified and controlled [*see Figure 6*]. It should be remembered that considerable blood loss may be incurred with the division of viable hepatic tissue in the pursuit of bleeding from deep penetrating wounds.

An adjunct to parenchymal suturing or hepatotomy is the use of the omentum to fill large defects in the liver and to buttress hepatic sutures. The rationale for this use of the omentum is that it provides an excellent source for macrophages and fills a potential dead space with viable tissue.[33] In addition, the omentum can provide a little extra support for parenchymal sutures, often enough to prevent them from cutting through Glisson's capsule.

Hepatic arterial ligation may be appropriate for patients with arterial hemorrhage from deep within the liver[34]; however, it plays only a limited role in the overall treatment of hepatic injuries, because it does not stop hemorrhage from the portal and hepatic venous systems.[35] Its primary role is in the management of deep lobar injuries when application of the Pringle maneuver results in the cessation of arterial hemorrhage. If the bleeding from the wound stops once the left or right hepatic artery is isolated and clamped, hepatic arterial ligation is a reasonable alternative to deep hepatotomy. Generally, ligation of the right or left hepatic artery is well tolerated; however, ligation of the proper hepatic artery (distal to the origin of the gastroduodenal artery) may produce hepatic necrosis.[36]

An alternative to suturing the entrance and exit wounds of a transhepatic penetrating injury or to performing an extensive hepatotomy is the use of an intrahepatic balloon.[37] These devices are hand-crafted by the surgeon in the OR. One method of fashioning such a device is to tie a 1 in. Penrose drain to a hollow catheter [see Figure 7]. The balloon is then inserted into the bleeding wound and inflated with a soluble contrast agent. If the hemorrhage is controlled, a stopcock or clamp is used to occlude the catheter and maintain the inflation. (It should be noted that the balloon catheter may not be able to generate sufficient intraparenchymal pressure to tamponade major arterial hemorrhage.) The balloon is left in the abdomen and removed at a subsequent operation after 24 to 48 hours. The hemorrhage may recur when the balloon is deflated.

Resectional debridement is indicated for peripheral portions of nonviable hepatic parenchyma. Except in rare circumstances, the amount of tissue removed should not exceed 25% of the liver. Resectional debridement is performed by means of the finger-fracture technique and is appropriate for selected patients with grade III to grade V lacerations. Because additional blood loss occurs during removal of nonviable tissue, this procedure should be reserved for patients who are in sound physiologic condition and can tolerate additional blood loss.

Perihepatic packing is the most significant advance in the treatment of hepatic injuries to occur in the past 15 years. The practice of packing hepatic injuries is not a new one, but the concepts and techniques associated with it have changed. In the past, liver lacerations were packed with yards of gauze, and one end of the gauze strip was brought out of the abdomen through a separate stab wound[38]; the remainder of the gauze was then teased out of the wound over a period of days. Unfortunately, this approach often led to abdominal infection and failed to control the hemorrhage, and as a result, it eventually fell from favor. The current approach is not to place packing material in the laceration itself but rather to place it over and around the injury to compress the wound by compressing the liver between the anterior chest wall, the diaphragm, and the retroperitoneum.[5-9] The abdomen is closed, and the patient is taken to the SICU for resuscitation and correction of metabolic derangements. Within 24 hours, the patient is returned to the OR for removal of the packs. Perihepatic packing is indicated for grade IV and V lacerations and for less severe injuries in patients who have a coagulopathy caused by associated injuries.

A technique that may be attempted if packing fails is to wrap the injured portion of the liver with a fine porous material (e.g., polyglycolic acid mesh) after the injured lobe has been mobilized.[39,40] Using a continuous suture or a linear stapler, the surgeon constructs a tight-fitting stocking that encloses the injured lobe. Blood clots beneath the mesh, which results in tamponade of the hepatic injury. Although this technique is intuitively attractive, to date it has achieved only limited success.

The final alternative for patients with extensive unilobar injuries is anatomic hepatic resection. In elective circumstances, anatomic lobectomies can be performed with excellent results; however, in the setting of trauma, the mortality associated with this procedure exceeds 50% in most series.[28,29,31,41-43] Consequently, hepatic resection is rarely performed in trauma patients, having been largely replaced by perihepatic packing, resectional debridement, and hepatotomy with selective ligation. Nonetheless, there are two circumstances in which anatomic resection may still be a reasonable choice. The first is prompt resection in patients with extensive injuries of the lateral segment of the left lobe; because hemorrhage from the left lobe is easily controlled with bimanual compression, the risk of uncontrolled blood loss is not as high as with left or right anatomic lobectomies. The second is delayed anatomic lobectomy in patients whose hemorrhage has been controlled but whose left or right lobe is nonviable as a result of ligation or thrombosis of essential blood vessels. Because of the large mass of necrotic liver tissue, there is a high risk of subsequent infection or persistent hyperinflammation, setting the stage for the multiple organ dysfunction syndrome (MODS). The necrotic lobe should be removed as soon as the patient's condition permits.

Hepatic transplantation has been successful in several trauma patients with devastating hepatic injuries who required total hepatectomy.[44-47] In each of these five patients, the mean anhepatic period was approximately 24 hours. All five survived the transplantation, though two died of disseminated viral infections within two months of the procedure. Two others were alive and well 16 and 17 months after the procedure; no follow-up was reported for the fifth patient. Hepatic transplantation represents the ultimate expression of aggressive trauma care. All other injuries must be well delineated (particularly injuries to the CNS), and the patient must have an excellent chance of survival aside from the hepatic injury. High cost and limited availability of donors restrict the performance of hepatic transplantation for trauma, but it seems probable that this procedure will continue to be performed in extraordinary circumstances.

Subcapsular Hematoma

An uncommon but troublesome hepatic injury is subcapsular hematoma, which arises when the parenchyma of the liver

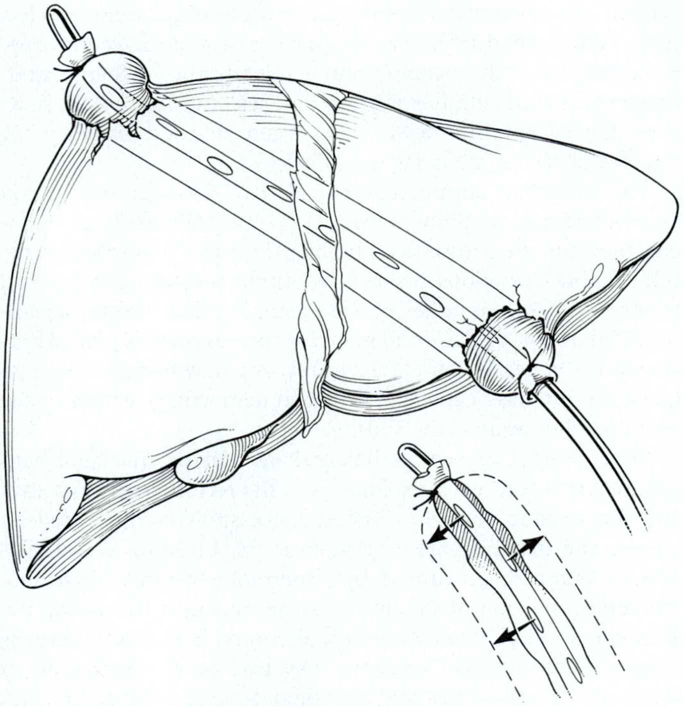

Figure 7 A hand-made balloon from a Robinson catheter and a Penrose drain may effectively control hemorrhage from a transhepatic penetrating wound.

is disrupted by blunt trauma but Glisson's capsule remains intact. Subcapsular hematomas range in severity from minor blisters on the surface of the liver to ruptured central hematomas accompanied by severe hemorrhage [see Table 1]. They may be recognized either at the time of the operation or in the course of CT scanning.

Regardless of how the lesion is diagnosed, subsequent decision making is often difficult. If a grade I or II subcapsular hematoma—that is, a hematoma involving less than 50% of the surface of the liver that is not expanding and is not ruptured—is discovered during an exploratory laparotomy, it should be left alone. If the hematoma is explored, hepatotomy with selective ligation may be required to control bleeding vessels. Even if hepatotomy with ligation is effective, one must still contend with diffuse hemorrhage from the large denuded surface, and packing may also be required. A hematoma that is expanding during operation (grade III) may have to be explored. Such lesions are often the result of uncontrolled arterial hemorrhage, and packing alone may not be successful. An alternative strategy is to pack the liver to control venous hemorrhage, close the abdomen, and transport the patient to the interventional radiology suite for hepatic arteriography and embolization of the bleeding vessels. Ruptured grades III and IV hematomas are treated with exploration and selective ligation, with or without packing.

Perihepatic Drainage

For years, all hepatic injuries were drained via Penrose drains brought out laterally or through the bed of the resected 12th rib; recently, the use of large sump drains and closed suction drains has become increasingly popular. Several prospective and retrospective studies have demonstrated that the use of either Penrose or sump drains carries a higher risk of intra-abdominal infection than the use of either closed suction drains or no drains at all.[48-51] It is clear that if drains are to be used, closed suction devices are preferred. What is not clear, however, is whether closed suction drains are better or worse than no drains, particularly in view of the advent of percutaneous catheter drainage. Patients who are initially treated with perihepatic packing may also require drainage; however, drainage is not indicated at the initial procedure, given that the patient will be returned to the OR within the next 48 hours.

MORTALITY AND COMPLICATIONS

Overall mortality for patients with hepatic injuries is approximately 10%. The most common cause of death is exsanguination, followed by MODS and intracranial injury. Three generalizations may be made regarding the risk of death and complications: (1) both increase in proportion to the injury grade and to the complexity of repair; (2) hepatic injuries caused by blunt trauma carry a higher mortality than those caused by penetrating trauma; and (3) infectious complications occur more often with penetrating trauma.

Postoperative hemorrhage occurs in a small percentage of patients with hepatic injuries. The source may be either a coagulopathy or a missed vascular injury (usually to an artery). In most instances of persistent postoperative hemorrhage, the patient is best served by being returned to the OR. Arteriography with embolization may be considered in selected patients. If coagulation studies indicate that a coagulopathy is the likely cause of postoperative hemorrhage, there is little to be gained by reoperation until the coagulopathy is corrected.

Perihepatic infections occur in fewer than 5% of patients with significant hepatic injuries. They develop more often in patients with penetrating injuries than in patients with blunt injuries, presumably because of the greater frequency of enteric contamination. An elevated temperature and a higher than normal white blood cell count after postoperative day 3 or 4 should prompt a search for intra-abdominal infection. In the absence of pneumonia, an infected line, or urinary tract infection, an abdominal CT scan with intravenous and upper gastrointestinal contrast should be obtained. Many perihepatic infections can be treated with CT-guided drainage; however, infected hematomas and infected necrotic liver tissue cannot be expected to respond to percutaneous drainage. Right 12th rib resection remains an excellent approach for posterior infections and provides superior drainage in refractory cases.

Bilomas are loculated collections of bile that may or may not be infected. If a biloma is infected, it is essentially an abscess and should be treated as such; if it is sterile, it will eventually be resorbed. Biliary ascites is caused by disruption of a major bile duct. Reoperation after the establishment of appropriate drainage is the prudent course. Even if the source of the leaking bile can be identified, primary repair of the injured duct is unlikely to be successful. It is best to wait until a firm fistulous communication is established with adequate drainage.

Biliary fistulas occur in approximately 3% of patients with major hepatic injuries.[42] They are usually of little consequence and generally close without specific treatment. In rare instances, a fistulous communication with intrathoracic structures forms in patients with associated diaphragmatic injuries, resulting in a bronchobiliary or pleurobiliary fistula. Because of the pressure differential between the biliary tract and the thoracic cavity, most of these fistulas must be closed operatively; however, we know of one pleurobiliary fistula that closed spontaneously after endoscopic sphincterotomy and stent placement.

Hemorrhage from hepatic injuries is often treated without identifying and controlling each bleeding vessel individually, and arterial pseudoaneurysms may develop as a consequence. As the pseudoaneurysm enlarges, it may rupture into the parenchyma of the liver, into a bile duct, or into an adjacent branch of the portal vein. Rupture into a bile duct results in hemobilia, which is characterized by intermittent episodes of right upper quadrant pain, upper gastrointestinal hemorrhage, and jaundice; rupture into a portal vein may result in portal vein hypertension with bleeding varices. Both of these complications are exceedingly rare and are best managed with hepatic arteriography and embolization.

Injuries to the Bile Ducts and Gallbladder

Injuries to the extrahepatic bile ducts can be caused by either penetrating or blunt trauma; however, they are rare in either case.[52-55] The diagnosis is usually made by noting the accumulation of bile in the upper quadrant during laparotomy for treatment of associated injuries. Treatment of common bile duct (CBD) injuries after external trauma is complicated by the small size and thin wall of the normal duct, which render primary repair almost impossible except when the laceration is small and there is no tissue loss. When there is tissue loss or the laceration is larger than 25% to 50% of the diameter of the duct, the best treatment option is a Roux-en-Y choledochojejunostomy [*51 Biliary Tract Procedures*].[56,57] Treatment of injuries to the left or right hepatic duct is even more difficult—so much so that we question whether repair should even be attempted under emergency conditions. If only one hepatic duct is injured, a reasonable approach is to ligate it and deal with any infections or atrophy of the lobe rather than to attempt repair.[58] If both ducts are injured, each should be intubated with a small catheter brought through the abdominal wall. Once the patient has recovered sufficiently, delayed repair is performed under elective conditions. Injuries to the intrapancreatic portion of the CBD are treated by dividing the duct at the superior border of the pancreas, ligating the distal portion, and performing a Roux-en-Y choledochojejunostomy.

The Roux-en-Y choledochojejunostomy is done in a single layer with interrupted 5-0 absorbable monofilament sutures. To prevent ischemia and possible stricture, no circumferential dissection of the duct is performed. A round patch of approximately the same diameter as the CBD is removed from the seromuscular layer of the small bowel, but the mucosa and submucosa are only perforated, not resected. The posterior row of sutures is placed first, with full-thickness bites taken through both the duct and the small bowel. The anterior row is then completed. Finally, three or four 3-0 polypropylene sutures are placed to secure the small bowel around the anastomosis to the connective tissue of the porta hepatis. The only purpose for these sutures is to spare the fragile anastomosis any potential tension. No T tubes or stents are employed. Closed suction drainage is added in the case of injuries to the intrapancreatic portion of the duct or at the surgeon's discretion.

Injuries to the gallbladder are treated by means of either lateral repair with absorbable sutures or cholecystectomy; the decision between the two approaches depends on which is easier in a given situation. Cholecystostomy is rarely, if ever, indicated.

Injuries to the Spleen

Splenic injuries are treated operatively by means of splenic repair (splenorrhaphy), partial splenectomy, or resection, depending on the extent of the injury [see Table 2] and the condition of the patient.[59-63] Currently, there is considerable enthusiasm for splenic salvage as a consequence of the evolving trend toward nonoperative management of solid organ injuries and the growing concern about the rare but often fatal complication known as overwhelming postsplenectomy infection (OPSI). OPSI is caused by encapsulated bacteria (e.g., *Streptococcus pneumoniae*, *Hemophilus influenzae*, and *Neisseria meningitidis*) and is very resistant to treatment: mortality may exceed 50%.[59] OPSI occurs most often in young children and immunocompromised adults and is uncommon in otherwise healthy adults. For this reason, splenic salvage is attempted more vigorously in pediatric patients than in adult ones.

To ensure safe removal or repair, the spleen should be mobilized to the point where it can be brought to the surface of the abdominal wall without tension. To this end, the soft tissue attachments between the spleen and the splenic flexure of the colon must be divided. Next, an incision is made in the peritoneum and the endoabdominal fascia, beginning at the inferior pole, 1 to 2 cm lateral to the posterior peritoneal reflection of the spleen, and continuing posteriorly and superiorly until the esophagus is encountered [see Figure 8a]. Care must be taken not to pull on the spleen, so that it will not tear at the posterior peritoneal reflection, causing significant hemorrhage. Instead, the spleen should be rotated counterclockwise, with posterior pressure applied to expose the peritoneal reflection. It is often helpful to rotate the operating table 20° to the patient's right so that the weight of the abdominal viscera facilitates their retraction. A plane is thus established between the spleen and pancreas and Gerota's fascia that can be extended to the aorta [see Figure 8b]. With this step, mobilization is complete, and the spleen can be repaired or removed without any need to struggle to achieve adequate exposure.

Splenectomy is the usual treatment for hilar injuries or a pulverized splenic parenchyma. It is also indicated for lesser splenic injuries in patients who have multiple abdominal injuries and a coagulopathy, and it is frequently necessary in patients in whom splenic salvage attempts have failed. Partial splenectomy is suitable for patients in whom only a portion of the spleen (usually the superior or inferior half) has been destroyed. Once the damaged portion has been removed, the same methods used to control hemorrhage from hepatic parenchyma can be used to control hemorrhage from splenic parenchyma [see Figure 9]. When horizontal mattress sutures are placed across a raw edge, gentle compression of the parenchyma by an assistant facilitates hemostasis; when the sutures are tied and compression is released, the spleen will expand slightly and tighten the sutures further. Drains are never used after completion of the repair or resection.

If splenectomy is performed, vaccines effective against the encapsulated bacteria are administered. The pneumococcal vaccine is routinely given, and vaccines effective against *H. influenzae* and *N. meningitidis* should also be given if available.

Injuries to the Diaphragm

In cases of blunt trauma to the diaphragm, the injury is on the left side 75% of the time, presumably because the liver diffuses some of the energy on the right side. With both blunt and penetrating injuries, the diagnosis is suggested by an abnormality of the diaphragmatic shadow on chest x-ray. Many of these abnormalities are subtle, particularly with penetrating injuries, and further diagnostic evaluation may be warranted. The typical injury from blunt trauma is a tear in the central tendon; often, the tear is quite large. Regardless of the cause, acute injuries are repaired through an abdominal incision. Because of the concave shape of the diaphragm and the overlying anterior ribs, anterior diaphragmatic injuries may be difficult to suture. Repair is greatly facilitated by using a long Allis clamp to grasp part of the injury and evert the diaphragm. Lacerations are repaired with continuous No. 1 monofilament nonabsorbable sutures. Occasionally, with large avulsions or gunshot wounds accompanied by extensive tissue loss, polypropylene mesh is required to bridge the defect.

Table 2 AAST Spleen Injury Scale (1994 Revision)[1]

Grade*	Injury Description
I	Hematoma: subcapsular, nonexpanding, < 10% surface area Laceration: capsular tear, nonbleeding, < 1 cm parenchymal depth
II	Hematoma: subcapsular, nonexpanding, 10%–50% surface area; intraparenchymal, nonexpanding, < 5 cm in diameter Laceration: capsular tear, active bleeding, 1–3 cm parenchymal depth, not involving a trabecular vessel
III	Hematoma: subcapsular, > 50% surface area or expanding; ruptured subcapsular hematoma with active bleeding; intraparenchymal, > 5 cm or expanding Laceration: > 3 cm parenchymal depth or involving trabecular vessels
IV	Hematoma: ruptured intraparenchymal hematoma with active bleeding Laceration: laceration involving segmental or hilar vessels producing major devascularization (> 25% of spleen)
V	Laceration: completely shattered spleen Vascular: hilar vascular injury that devascularizes spleen

*Advance one grade for multiple injuries, up to grade III.

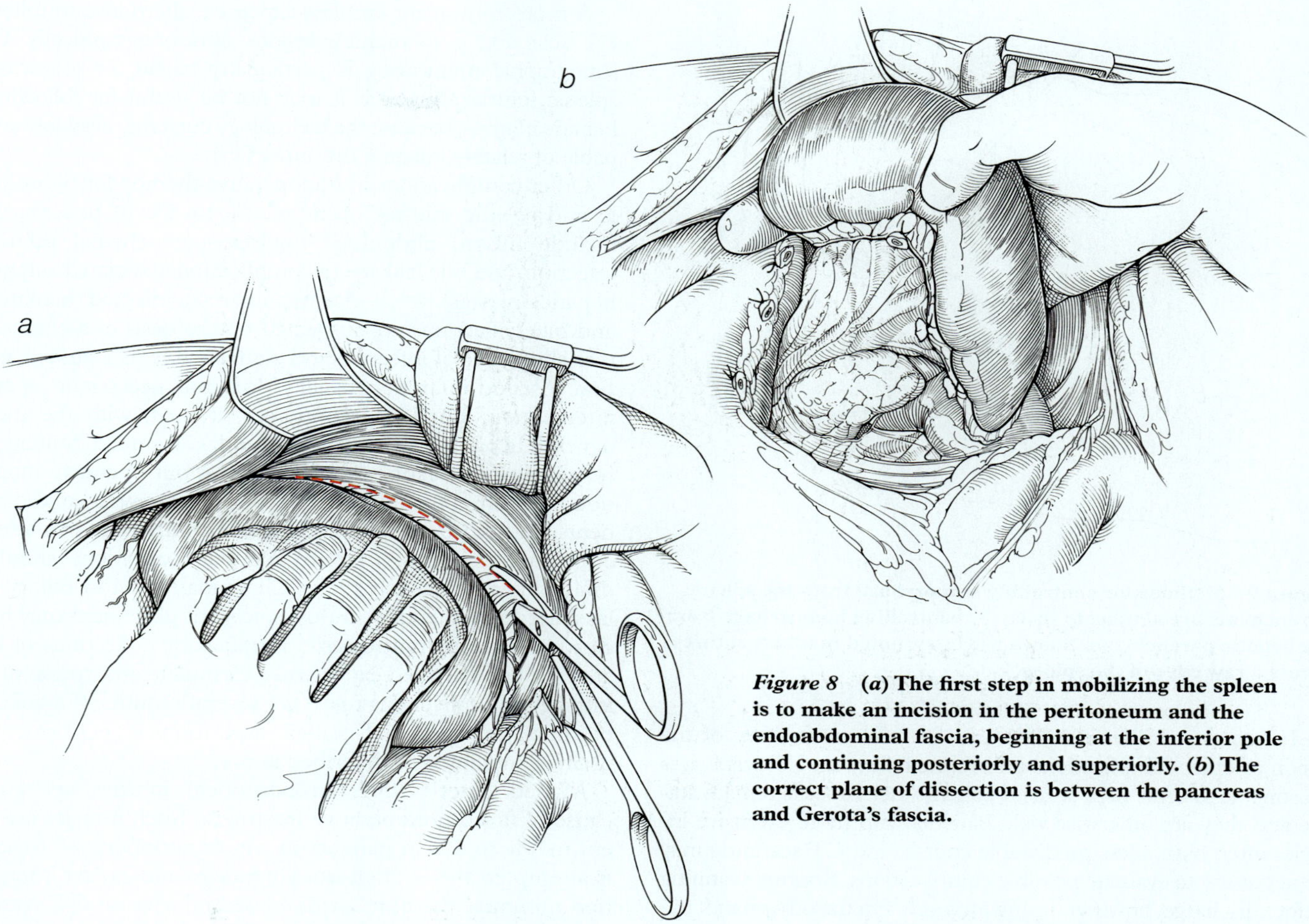

Figure 8 (*a*) The first step in mobilizing the spleen is to make an incision in the peritoneum and the endoabdominal fascia, beginning at the inferior pole and continuing posteriorly and superiorly. (*b*) The correct plane of dissection is between the pancreas and Gerota's fascia.

The explosive growth of laparoscopic procedures has led to the application of this technology for both diagnostic and therapeutic purposes in trauma patients. In a number of patients with low anterior thoracic stab wounds who otherwise were not candidates for a laparotomy, small diaphragmatic lacerations have been identified and repaired with laparoscopy and stapling.

Discussion

Nonoperative Treatment of Blunt Hepatic and Splenic Injury

Only a few years ago, blunt and penetrating hepatic and splenic injuries were managed in a similar fashion on the basis of a positive diagnostic peritoneal lavage or the probability of peritoneal penetration: a laparotomy was performed, and the injured organs were identified and treated. Currently, although penetrating abdominal injuries are still treated in the same way, nearly all children and 50% to 80% of adults with blunt hepatic and splenic injuries are treated without laparotomy.[64-74] This remarkable change was made possible by the development of the high-speed helical CT scanner, the replacement of diagnostic peritoneal lavage by ultrasonography, and the growth of interventional radiology.

The diagnosis of blunt abdominal trauma is suspected on the basis of the mechanism of injury and the presence of associated injuries (e.g., right or left lower rib fractures). In contemporary urban trauma centers, ultrasonographic examination of the abdomen may reveal a fluid stripe in Morrison's pouch, the left upper quadrant, or the pelvis, which suggests a hemoperitoneum. This observation prompts a CT scan of the abdomen, which delineates injuries of the liver or spleen. CT scanning is a less than optimal means of grading hepatic and splenic injuries; however, patients may be observed either in the SICU or on the ward, depending on the apparent severity of the parenchymal injury on the CT scan and the presence and extent of any associated injuries.[75,76]

The primary requirement for nonoperative therapy is hemodynamic stability.[63-72] To confirm stability, frequent assessment of vital signs and monitoring of the hematocrit are necessary. Continued hemorrhage occurs in 1% to 4% of patients.[65,66,68-73] Hypotension may develop, usually within the first 24 hours after hepatic injury but sometimes several days later, especially when splenic injury is present.[77,78] It is often an indication that operative intervention is necessary. A persistently falling hematocrit should be treated with packed red blood cell (PRBC) transfusions. If the hematocrit continues to fall after two or three units of PRBCs, embolization in the interventional radiology suite should be considered.[74] Overall, nonoperative treatment obviates laparotomy in more than 95% of cases.[65,66,68-73]

Out of concern over the risk of delayed hemorrhage or other complications, follow-up CT scans have often been recommended; unfortunately, there is no consensus as to when or even whether they should be obtained. Given that patients with grade I

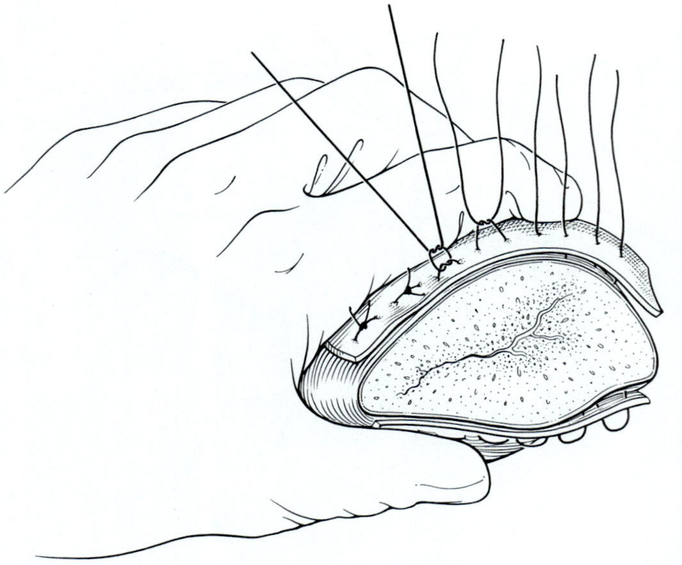

Figure 9 Methods for controlling hemorrhage from the splenic parenchyma are similar to those for controlling hemorrhage from the hepatic parenchyma. Shown are interrupted mattress sutures across a raw edge of the spleen.

A more convenient and less expensive alternative to follow-up CT scanning is to monitor lesions ultrasonographically. Ultrasonographic monitoring is particularly useful for following up splenic injuries; however, it may not be useful for following up hepatic injuries, because the technology currently available is incapable of reliably imaging the entire liver.

Other complications of nonoperative therapy for blunt hepatic and splenic injuries occur in 2% to 5% of patients; these include missed abdominal injuries, parenchymal infarction, infection, and bile leakage (a complication associated solely with hepatic injuries).[65,68-71] Aseptic infarcts, infected hematomas, and bile collections are suspected on the basis of a clinical picture suggestive of infection and confirmed by CT-guided aspiration. Aseptic infarction usually does not necessitate operative intervention. Fluid collections are drained, with the method depending on the viscosity of the fluid: CT-guided drainage may be effective in treating thin collections, but operative intervention is required for thicker collections, those with solid components, and those for which percutaneous drainage was attempted without success. Extrahepatic bile collections should be drained percutaneously under CT guidance. Most biliary fistulas close spontaneously; endoscopic stent placement may hasten closure in recalcitrant cases.[79] Intrahepatic collections of blood and bile are managed expectantly. Complete absorption of large intrahepatic collections may take several months. If a collection becomes infected, CT-guided aspiration is performed and drainage obtained as described above.

Missed enteric and retroperitoneal injuries are another cause of failed nonoperative treatment. Such injuries are present in 1% to 4% of patients in whom nonoperative treatment is attempted.[65,68-71] High-quality images and expert interpretation minimize the number of missed injuries on CT scans but cannot eliminate them entirely. Therefore, patients must be watched carefully for the development of peritoneal irritation and other signs of intra-abdominal pathology.

or II hepatic or splenic injuries rarely show progression of the lesion or other complications on routine follow-up CT scans, it is reasonable to omit such scans if patients' hematocrits remain stable and they are otherwise well. Patients with more extensive injuries often have a less predictable course, and CT scanning may be necessary to evaluate possible complications. Routine scanning before discharge, however, is unwarranted. On the other hand, patients who participate in vigorous or contact sports should have CT documentation of virtually complete healing before resuming those activities.

References

1. Moore EE, Cogbill TH, Jurkovich GJ, et al: Organ injury scaling: spleen and liver (1994 revision). J Trauma 38:323, 1995
2. Hepatic trauma revisited. Feliciano DV, Pachter HL, Eds. Curr Probl Surg 26, 1986
3. Moore EE: Critical decisions in the management of hepatic trauma. Am J Surg 148:712, 1984
4. Feliciano DV, Mattox KL, Jordan GL, et al: Management of 1000 consecutive cases of hepatic trauma (1979–1984). Ann Surg 204:438, 1986
5. Feliciano DV, Mattox KL, Burch JM, et al: Packing for control of hepatic hemorrhage. J Trauma 26:738, 1986
6. Ivantury RR, Nallathambi M, Gunduz Y, et al: Liver packing for uncontrolled hemorrhage: a reappraisal. J Trauma 26:744, 1986
7. Carmona RH, Peck DZ, Lim RC: The role of packing and planned reoperation in severe hepatic trauma. J Trauma 24:779, 1984
8. Cue JI, Cryer HG, Miller FB, et al: Packing and planned reexploration for hepatic and retroperitoneal hemorrhage: critical refinements of a useful technique. J Trauma 30:1007, 1990
9. Beal SL: Fatal hepatic hemorrhage: an unresolved problem in the management of complex liver injuries. J Trauma 30:163, 1990
10. Pachter HL, Spencer FC, Hofstetter SR, et al: Significant trends in the treatment of hepatic trauma: experience with 411 injuries. Ann Surg 215:492, 1992
11. Murray DH Jr, Borge JD, Pouteau GG: Tourniquet control of liver bleeding. J Trauma 18:771, 1978
12. Heaney JP, Stanton WR, Halbert DS, et al: An improved technic for vascular isolation of the liver. Ann Surg 163:237, 1966
13. Burch JM, Feliciano DV, Mattox KL: The atriocaval shunt: facts and fiction. Ann Surg 207:555, 1988
14. Buechter KJ, Gomez GA, Zeppa R: A new technique for exposure of injuries at the confluence of the retrohepatic veins and the retrohepatic vena cava. J Trauma 30:328, 1990
15. Schrock T, Blaisdell FW, Matthewson C Jr: Management of blunt trauma to the liver and hepatic veins. Arch Surg 96:698, 1968
16. Bricker DL, Morton JR, Okies JE, et al: Surgical management of injuries to the vena cava: changing patterns of injury and newer techniques of repair. J Trauma 11:725, 1971
17. Yellin AE, Chaffee CB, Donovan AJ: Vascular isolation in treatment of juxtahepatic venous injuries. Arch Surg 102:566, 1971
18. Walt AJ: The mythology of hepatic trauma: or Babel revisited. Am J Surg 125:12, 1978
19. Millikan JS, Moore EE, Cogbill TH, et al: Inferior vena cava injuries: a continuing challenge. J Trauma 23:207, 1983
20. Pachter HL, Spencer FC, Hofstetter SR, et al: The management of juxtahepatic venous injuries without an atriocaval shunt. Surgery 99:569, 1986
21. Rovito PF: Atrial caval shunting in blunt hepatic vascular injury. Ann Surg 205:318, 1987
22. Pilcher DB, Harman PK, Moore EE: Retrohepatic vena cava balloon shunt introduced via the saphenofemoral junction. J Trauma 17:837, 1977
23. Kram HB, Reuben BI, Flemming AW: Use of fibrin glue in hepatic trauma. J Trauma 28:1195, 1988
24. Kram HB, Nathan RC, Stafford FJ, et al: Fibrin glue achieves hemostasis in patients with coagulation disorders. Arch Surg 124:385, 1989
25. Berguer R, Staerkel RL, Moore EE, et al: Warning: fatal reaction to the use of fibrin glue in deep hepatic wounds: case reports. J Trauma 31:408, 1991
26. Ochsner MG, Maniscalco-Theberge ME, Champion HR: Fibrin glue as a hemostatic agent in hepatic and splenic trauma. J Trauma 30:884, 1990
27. Feliciano DV: Continuing evolution in the approach to severe liver trauma (editorial). Ann Surg 216:521, 1992
28. Trunkey DD, Shires GT, McClelland R: Manage-

28. ment of liver trauma in 811 consecutive patients. Ann Surg 179:722, 1974
29. Levin A, Gover P, Nance FC: Surgical restraint in the management of hepatic injury: a review of Charity Hospital experience. J Trauma 18:399, 1978
30. Lucas CE, Ledgerwood AM: Prospective evaluation of hemostatic techniques for liver injuries. J Trauma 16:442, 1976
31. Camona RH, Lim RC Jr, Clark GC: Morbidity and mortality in hepatic trauma: a 5 year study. Am J Surg 144:88, 1982
32. Moore FA, Moore EE, Seagrave A: Nonresectional management of major hepatic trauma: an evolving concept. Am J Surg 150:725, 1985
33. Stone HH, Lamb JM: Use of pedicled omentum as an autogenous pack for control of hemorrhage in major injuries of the liver. Surg Gynecol Obstet 141:92, 1975
34. Mays ET: Lobar dearterialization for exsanguinating wounds of the liver. J Trauma 12:397, 1972
35. Flint LM, Polk HC: Selective hepatic artery ligation: limitations and failures. J Trauma 19:319, 1979
36. Lucas CE: Discussion of: Flint LM, Polk HC. Selective hepatic artery ligation: limitations and failures. J Trauma 19:319, 1979
37. Poggetti RS, Moore EE, Moore FA, et al: Balloon tamponade for bilobar transfixing hepatic gunshot wounds. J Trauma 33:694, 1992
38. Madding GF, Lawrence KB, Kennedy PA: War wounds of the liver. Tex State J Med 42:267, 1946
39. Reed RL, Merrell RC, Meyers WC, et al: Continuing evolution in the approach to severe liver trauma. Ann Surg 216:524, 1992
40. Jacobson LE, Kirton OC, Gomez GA: The use of an absorbable mesh wrap in the management of major liver injuries. Surgery 111:455, 1992
41. Lim RC Jr, Knudson J, Steele M: Liver trauma: current method of management. Arch Surg 104:544, 1972
42. Donovan AJ, Michaelian MJ, Yellin AE: Anatomical hepatic lobectomy in trauma to the liver. Surgery 73:833, 1973
43. Defore WW, Mattox KL, Jordan GL, et al: Management of 1590 consecutive cases of liver trauma. Arch Surg 111:493, 1976
44. Esquivel CO, Bernardos A, Makowka L, et al: Liver replacement after massive hepatic trauma. J Trauma 27:800, 1987
45. Angstadt J, Jarrell B, Moritz M, et al: Surgical management of severe liver trauma: a role for liver transplantation. J Trauma 29:606, 1989
46. Ringe B, Pichlmayr R, Ziegler H, et al: Management of severe hepatic trauma by two-stage total hepatectomy and subsequent liver transplantation. Surgery 109:792, 1991
47. Jeng LB, Hsu C, Wang C, et al: Emergent liver transplantation to salvage a hepatic avulsion injury with a disrupted suprahepatic vena cava. Arch Surg 128:1075, 1993
48. Fischer RP, O'Farrell KA, Perry JF Jr: The value of peritoneal drains in the treatment of liver injuries. J Trauma 18:393, 1978
49. Gillmore D, McSwain NE, Browder IW: Hepatic trauma: to drain or not to drain? J Trauma 27:989, 1987
50. Noyes LD, Doyle DJ, McSwain NE: Septic complications associated with the use of peritoneal drains in liver trauma. J Trauma 28:337, 1988
51. Fabian TC, Croce MA, Stanford GG, et al: Factors affecting morbidity after hepatic trauma. Ann Surg 213:540, 1991
52. Posner MC, Moore EE: Extrahepatic biliary tract injury: operative management plan. J Trauma 25:833, 1985
53. Ivatury RR, Rohman M, Nallathami M, et al: The morbidity of injuries of the extra-hepatic biliary system. J Trauma 25:967, 1985
54. Sheldon GF, Lim RC, Yee ES, et al: Management of injuries to the porta hepatis. Ann Surg 202:539, 1985
55. Feliciano DV, Bitondo CG, Burch JM, et al: Management of traumatic injuries to the extrahepatic biliary ducts. Am J Surg 150:705, 1985
56. Bade PG, Thomson SR, Hirshberg A, et al: Surgical options in traumatic injury to the extrahepatic biliary tract. Br J Surg 76:256, 1989
57. Csendes A, Diaz JC, Burdiles P, et al: Late results of immediate primary end to end repair in accidental section of the common bile duct. Surg Gynecol Obstet 168:125, 1989
58. Howdieshell TR, Hawkins ML, Osler TM, et al: Management of blunt hepatic duct transection by ligation. South Med J 83:579, 1990
59. Sherman R: Perspective in management of trauma to the spleen: 1979 presidential address, American Association for the Surgery of Trauma. J Trauma 20:1, 1980
60. Barrett J, Sheaff C, Abuabara S, et al: Splenic preservation in adults after blunt and penetrating trauma. Am J Surg 145:313, 1983
61. Delany HM, Rudavsky AZ, Lan S: Preliminary clinical experience with the use of absorbable mesh splenorrhaphy. J Trauma 25:909, 1985
62. Beal SL, Spisso JM: The risk of splenorrhaphy. Arch Surg 123:1158, 1988
63. Feliciano DV, Spjut-Patrinely V, Burch JM, et al: Splenorrhaphy: the alternative. Ann Surg 211:569 1990
64. Schiffman MA: Nonoperative management of blunt abdominal trauma in pediatrics. Emerg Med Clin North Am 7:519, 1989
65. Cogbill TH, Moore EE, Jurkovich JJ, et al: Nonoperative management of blunt septic trauma: a multicenter experience. J Trauma 29, 1312, 1989
66. Meredith JW, Young JS, Bowling J, et al: Nonoperative management of blunt hepatic trauma: the exception or the rule? J Trauma 36:529, 1994
67. Morrell DG, Chang FC, Helmer SD: Changing trends in the management of splenic injury. Am J Surg 170:686, 1995
68. Pachter HL, Hofstetter ST: The current status of nonoperative management of adult blunt hepatic injuries. Am J Surg 169:442, 1995
69. Croce MA, Fabian TC, Menke PG, et al: Nonoperative management of blunt hepatic trauma is the treatment of choice for hemodynamically stable patients. Ann Surg 221:744, 1995
70. Boone DC, Federle M, Billiar TR, et al: Evolution of management of major hepatic trauma: identification of patterns of injury. J Trauma 39:344, 1995
71. Pachter HL, Knudson MM, Esrig B, et al: Status of nonoperative management of blunt hepatic injuries in 1995: a multicenter experience with 404 patients. J Trauma 40:31, 1996
72. Smith JS, Cooney RN, Mucha P: Nonoperative management of the ruptured spleen: a revalidation of criteria. Surgery 120:745, 1996
73. Powell M, Courcoulas A, Gardner M, et al: Management of blunt splenic trauma: significant differences between adults and children. Surgery 122:654, 1997
74. Sclafani SJA, Shaftan GW, Scalea TM, et al: Nonoperative salvage of computed tomography–diagnosed splenic injuries: utilization of angiography for triage and embolization for hemostasis. J Trauma 39:818, 1995
75. Sutyak JP, Chiu WC, D'Amelio LF, et al: Computed tomography is inaccurate in estimating the severity of adult splenic injury. J Trauma 39:514, 1995
76. Croce MA, Fabian TC, Kudsk KA, et al: AAST organ injury scale: correlation of CT-graded liver injuries and operative findings. J Trauma 31:806, 1991
77. Gates JD: Delayed hemorrhage with free rupture complicating the nonsurgical management of blunt hepatic trauma: a case report and review of the literature. J Trauma 36:572, 1994
78. MacGillivray DC, Valentine RJ: Nonoperative management of blunt pediatric liver injury—late complications: case report. J Trauma 29:251, 1989
79. Sugimoto K, Asari Y, Sakaguchi T, et al: Endoscopic retrograde cholangiography in the nonsurgical management of blunt liver injury. J Trauma 35:192, 1993

Acknowledgments

Figure 1   Marcia Kammerer.
Figures 2 through 9   Susan Brust, C.M.I.

29 INJURIES TO THE STOMACH, DUODENUM, PANCREAS, SMALL BOWEL, COLON, AND RECTUM

Charles E. Lucas, M.D., and Anna M. Ledgerwood, M.D.

Injuries to the stomach, duodenum, pancreas, small bowel, colon, and rectum present a broad spectrum of challenges necessitating widely different solutions. The first priorities are recognizing injury and making the decision to operate. Initial evaluation of injured patients is addressed more fully elsewhere [see 22 Emergency Department Evaluation of the Patient with Multiple Injuries]. In what follows, we assume that the patient has been stabilized and injuries have been localized to one or more of the organs just mentioned.

Injuries to the Stomach

The treatment of gastric injuries varies according to their severity [see Figure 1 and Table 1]. Most intramural hematomas (grades 1 and 2) are treated by careful evacuation, hemostasis, and seromuscular closure. Perforations from stabs and bullets are usually small in grade 1 and grade 2 injuries and can be closed primarily in two layers.[1,2] Because the stomach is quite vascular, even small perforations may bleed profusely, especially along the greater curvature. Consequently, the recommended closure is an inner layer of locked hemostatic sutures followed by an outer inverting layer of sutures.

Large (grade 3) injuries near the greater curvature can be closed by the same technique or by excising the injury with a long gastrointestinal anastomosis (GIA) stapler. Careful hemostasis and inversion of the staple line provide extra security when the lumen is not compromised. Extensive (grade 4) injuries may necessitate proximal or distal gastrectomy. The type of resection depends on the presence of associated injuries to the duodenum, pancreas, or esophagus. Patients with associated duodenal injuries or pancreatic injuries, or both, are best treated with gastrojejunal reconstruction after distal gastrectomy. In patients who survive extensive injury to the cardioesophageal region, an end-to-side esophagogastrostomy can be performed after proximal gastrectomy; a pyloroplasty is added. When total gastrectomy is performed for grade 5 injury, Roux-en-Y esophagojejunostomy is advocated [see 49 Gastric Procedures].

Injuries to the Duodenum

The diagnosis of penetrating duodenal injury is usually made during laparotomy performed for hypotension or peritoneal irritation. The decision to explore for isolated blunt duodenal injury is based on the physical examination and roentgenographic findings. Duodenal injury may be present

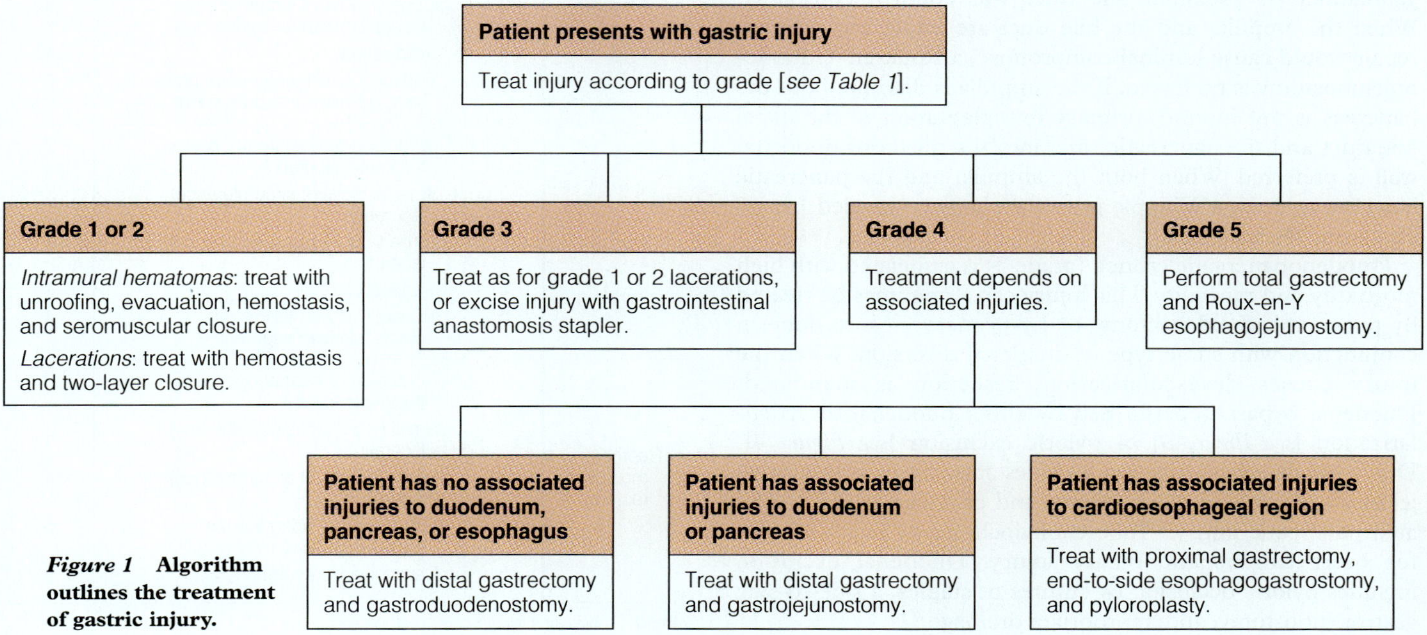

Figure 1 Algorithm outlines the treatment of gastric injury.

despite negative findings from diagnostic peritoneal lavage (DPL), and the symptoms of duodenal injury are often slow to evolve.[3] Roentgenograms made within two hours of injury typically show scoliosis and partial obliteration of the right psoas shadow. Retroperitoneal gas along the right psoas margin, over the right pole of the kidney, or in the lower mediastinum is seen within six hours in most patients. Computed tomography performed with a contrast agent will identify the site of perforation.

Treatment varies according to the location (segments D1 through D4) and severity of injury [see Figure 2 and Table 1].[4,5] Single-segment (grade 1) intramural hematoma usually occurs in segment D1 or D2, seldom leads to obstruction, and can be treated expectantly. Partial-thickness (grade 1) lacerations are best treated by simple seromuscular closure. Multisegment hematomas (grade 2) often require operative evacuation, especially when the obstruction lasts for more than 10 days and there is CT documentation that the hematoma persists. A generous longitudinal serosal incision along the antimesenteric border permits gentle evacuation without inadvertent injury to the underlying muscular and mucosal layers. The serosa with attached muscle is carefully reapproximated. Drainage is not necessary. Perforations involving less than 50 percent of the circumference of the duodenum, whether caused by penetrating wounds or blunt injury, are best treated by simple two-layer closure, preferably in a transverse manner.

Grade 3 perforations, which involve more than 50 percent of the circumference, require careful suture placement along the mesentery border to prevent inadvertent vascular compromise.[6] Near D3 and D4 injuries, careful suture placement and gentle duodenal mobilization help prevent iatrogenic injury to the superior mesenteric vessels. If a transected duodenum is ragged, the distal end may be oversewn and the proximal end anastomosed to a jejunal loop.[7] Alternatively, if primary closure would compromise lumen patency, a retrocolic Roux-en-Y jejunal limb can be used to close large defects.

Grade 4 ruptures at D2 can be closed primarily if the adjacent ampulla and mesentery are spared.[8] If the condition of the distal bile duct is unknown, choledochography through the gallbladder or proximal bile duct will confirm continuity. When the ampulla and the bile duct are intact but primary repair would cause luminal compromise, a Roux-en-Y duodenojejunostomy is preferred. If the ampulla is disrupted but the pancreas is not injured, primary reimplantation of the distal bile duct and the pancreatic duct into the posterior duodenal wall is preferred. When both the ampulla and the pancreatic head are injured, a Whipple procedure may be needed [see 53 Pancreatic Procedures].

Duodenopancreatic crunch (grade 5) is associated with high morbidity and mortality. This injury can sometimes be treated by pancreaticoduodenectomy or by primary closure done in conjunction with some type of duodenal diversion. When the injury causes devascularization, resection is mandated. Duodenal bypass is performed by either duodenal diverticularization [see Figure 3] or pyloric exclusion [see Figure 4]. Duodenal diverticularization includes antrectomy with gastrojejunostomy, tube duodenostomy, and drainage of the associated pancreatic injury.[6] Tube choledochostomy is added only for overt extrahepatic biliary injury. Duodenal exclusion includes pyloric occlusion by sutures or staples, a side-to-side gastrojejunostomy, and appropriate drainage.[9,10]

Table 1 Gradation of Injuries to Stomach, Duodenum, Pancreas, Small Bowel, Colon, and Rectum

Injured Structure	Grade	Characteristics of Injury	AIS-90 Score
Stomach	1	Intramural hematoma < 3 cm; partial-thickness laceration	2
	2	Intramural hematoma ≥ 3 cm; small (< 3 cm) laceration	2
	3	Large (> 3 cm) laceration	3
	4	Large laceration involving vessels on greater or lesser curvature	3
	5	Extensive (> 50%) rupture; stomach devascularized	4
Duodenum	1	Single-segment hematoma; partial-thickness laceration	2; 3
	2	Multiple-segment hematoma; small (< 50% of circumference) laceration	2; 4
	3	Large laceration (50%–75% of circumference of segment D2 or 50%–100% of circumference of segment D1, D3, or D4)	4
	4	Very large (75%–100%) laceration of segment D2; rupture of ampullary or distal bile duct	5
	5	Massive duodenopancreatic injury; devascularization	5
Pancreas	1	Small hematoma without duct injury; superficial laceration without duct injury	2
	2	Large hematoma without duct injury or tissue loss; major laceration without duct injury or tissue loss	2; 3
	3	Distal transection or parenchymal laceration with duct injury	4
	4	Proximal transection or parenchymal laceration involving ampulla	4
	5	Massive disruption of pancreatic head	5
Small bowel	1	Contusion or hematoma without devascularization; partial-thickness laceration	2
	2	Small (< 50% of circumference) laceration	3
	3	Large (≥ 50% of circumference) laceration without transection	3
	4	Transection	4
	5	Transection with segmental tissue loss; devascularized segment	4
Colon	1	Contusion or hematoma; partial-thickness laceration	2
	2	Small (< 50% of circumference) laceration	3
	3	Large (≥ 50% of circumference) laceration	3
	4	Transection	4
	5	Transection with tissue loss; devascularized segment	4
Rectosigmoid and rectum	1	Contusion or hematoma; partial-thickness laceration	2
	2	Small (< 50% of circumference) laceration	3
	3	Large (≥ 50% of circumference) laceration	4
	4	Full-thickness laceration with perineal extension	5
	5	Devascularized segment	5

AIS-90—Abbreviated Injury Score, 1990 version

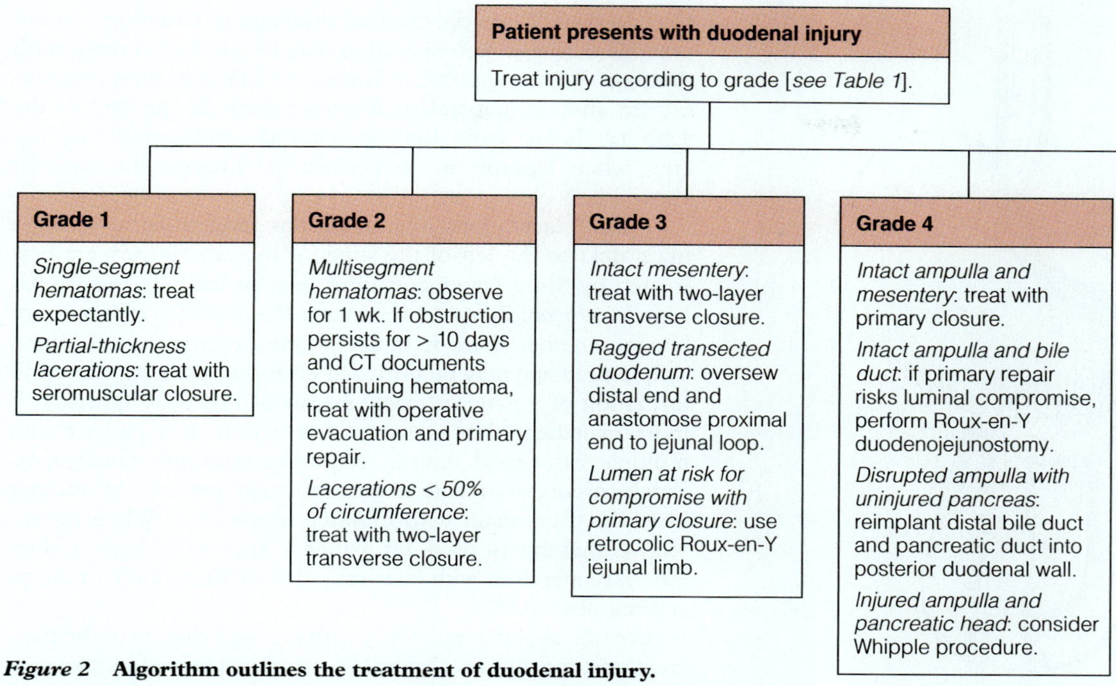

Treatment algorithm for duodenal injury

Patient presents with duodenal injury
Treat injury according to grade [see Table 1].

Grade 1
- *Single-segment hematomas*: treat expectantly.
- *Partial-thickness lacerations*: treat with seromuscular closure.

Grade 2
- *Multisegment hematomas*: observe for 1 wk. If obstruction persists for > 10 days and CT documents continuing hematoma, treat with operative evacuation and primary repair.
- *Lacerations < 50% of circumference*: treat with two-layer transverse closure.

Grade 3
- *Intact mesentery*: treat with two-layer transverse closure.
- *Ragged transected duodenum*: oversew distal end and anastomose proximal end to jejunal loop.
- *Lumen at risk for compromise with primary closure*: use retrocolic Roux-en-Y jejunal limb.

Grade 4
- *Intact ampulla and mesentery*: treat with primary closure.
- *Intact ampulla and bile duct*: if primary repair risks luminal compromise, perform Roux-en-Y duodenojejunostomy.
- *Disrupted ampulla with uninjured pancreas*: reimplant distal bile duct and pancreatic duct into posterior duodenal wall.
- *Injured ampulla and pancreatic head*: consider Whipple procedure.

Grade 5
- *Viable duodenum*: treat with pancreaticoduodenectomy or primary closure with duodenal diversion (i.e., duodenal diverticularization or pyloric exclusion).
- *Devascularized duodenum*: treat with Whipple procedure.

Figure 2 Algorithm outlines the treatment of duodenal injury.

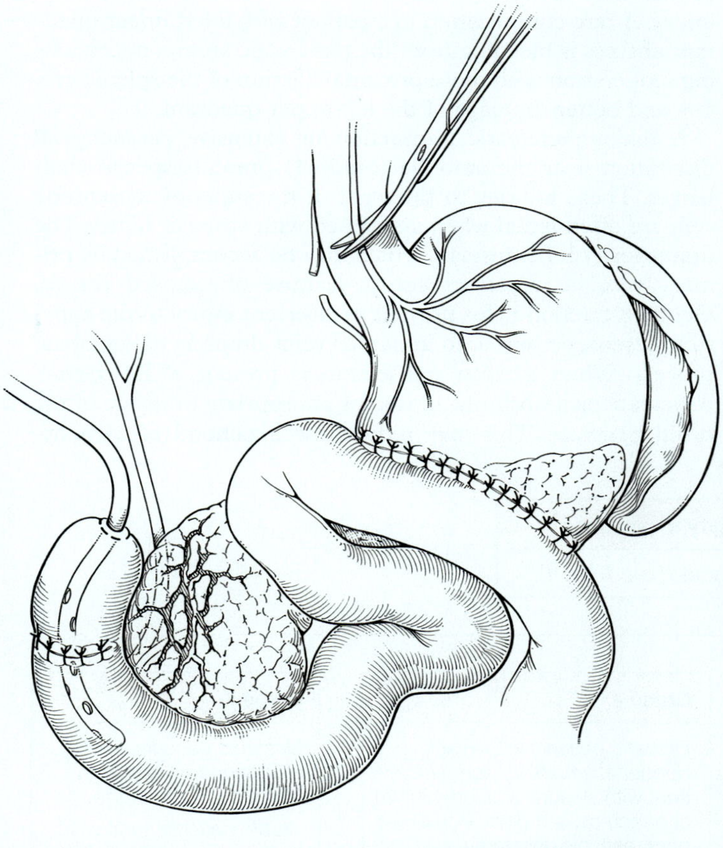

Figure 3 Shown is a grade 4 stellate crack to pancreatic head with a grade 3 (60 percent) transection of the duodenum (D2). After hemostasis is established, it is possible to perform the so-called duodenal diverticularization, consisting of antrectomy with gastrojejunostomy, tube duodenostomy, vagotomy, and peripancreatic drainage. Histamine$_2$ blockade precludes the need for vagotomy.

Injuries to the Pancreas

The treatment of pancreatic injury depends on its grade and extent [see Figure 5 and Table 1].[5] The pancreas is best exposed by dividing the greater omentum just outside the arcades of the gastroepiploic vessels. Assessment of the posterior surface may require mobilization of the inferior border or complete relocation of the spleen and pancreatic tail anteriorly [see Figure 6]. A small hematoma (grade 1) is best treated by unroofing, hemostasis, evacuation, and drainage. Minor bleeding from unnamed vessels is controlled by either electrocoagulation or ligature with fine sutures.

Gentle tension-free tying helps avert iatrogenic injury to the soft pancreatic parenchyma. Careful inspection after hemostasis will confirm the presence of a grade 1 injury, which does not involve a major duct. The site of the unroofed hematoma is left open and drained externally. Closed-suction drainage permits the exit of pancreatic juices. This treatment is recommended for all grade 1 lacerations, whether caused by stabs, gunshots, or blunt trauma. If the fluid drained has a high amylase content, skin will not be digested unless the effluent contains enteric juices that activate pancreatic peptidase.[11]

During a recent five-year period, the surgical services at Detroit Receiving Hospital treated 37 patients with grade 1 pancreatic injury. In all cases, the objectives were hemostasis, minimal debridement (if tiny fragments of loose pancreatic tissue were seen), and external drainage. All of the patients survived. Pancreatitis, defined as an elevated serum level of amylase lasting more than five days, developed in two patients, and a pancreaticocutaneous fistula developed in two patients whose pancreatic drainage lasted more than 14 days. All of the complications resolved with nonoperative supportive care, including parenteral nutrition.

Treatment of larger hematomas or lacerations without duct injury (grade 2 injuries) is similar. Extra care is taken to rule out duct injury and to obtain hemostasis. Once hemostasis has been achieved, the injury is left open and drained. This prac-

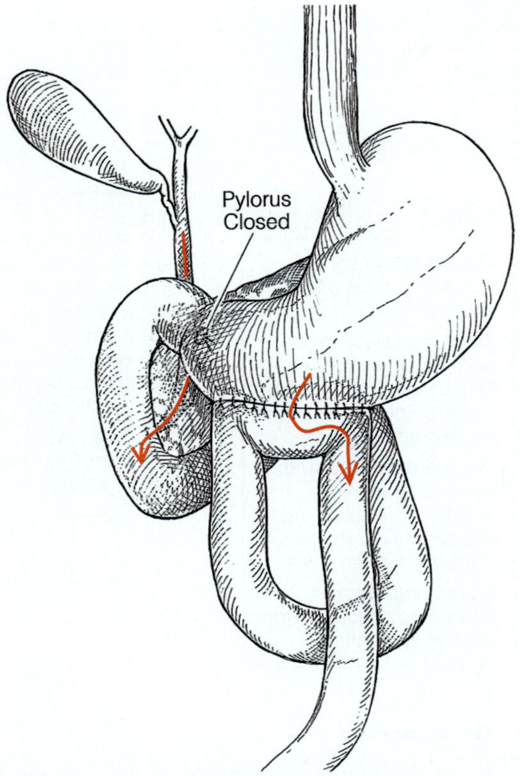

Figure 4 Duodenal exclusion consists of closure of the pylorus from within the stomach, followed by gastrojejunostomy. The procedure eliminates discharge of gastric acid into the duodenum, thus minimizing the stimulation of pancreatic secretion and reducing morbidity if there is breakdown of a repair.

tice helps prevent the development of a pseudocyst, which may occur if tiny ductules leak pancreatic juices within a closed injury.[12,13]

Although the incidence of postoperative pancreatitis (10 percent) or persistent pancreatic drainage (20 percent) seen after grade 2 injury exceeds that seen after grade 1 injury, few patients (three percent) have refractory drainage lasting more than 30 days. When the external drainage system plugs, percutaneous drainage or reoperation may be needed to reestablish drainage. When reoperation is deemed essential for a peripancreatic abscess, dependent drainage through the bed of the 12th rib helps avoid the extensive contamination that occurs when laparotomy is performed through the anterior approach.[13]

Grade 3 lacerations or transections thought to involve the main duct to the left of the superior mesenteric vein are best treated by distal pancreatectomy, with or without splenic salvage [see *Figure 7 and 53 Pancreatic Procedures*].[11,13] If it is not known whether there is injury to the main pancreatic duct, simple drainage may be provided even though it may result in formation of a pancreaticocutaneous fistula. This approach is more expedient than pancreatic resection in a patient with multiple associated injuries requiring multiple transfusions. Total parenteral nutrition permits such patients to recover from the total insult with minimal morbidity.[11] When nonresective therapy is used for patients known to have a duct injury, reoperation with later resection or Roux-en-Y drainage is often needed.[14]

After distal pancreatectomy with primary closure of the pancreatic stump, about 20 percent of patients have drainage lasting longer than two weeks. In most cases, nonoperative supportive therapy leads to resolution. A left upper quadrant abscess may occur, especially in patients with associated colon injury. A rare complication in a patient with a left upper quadrant abscess is bleeding from the pancreatic stump, necessitating reoperation with more proximal ligation of the splenic vessels and better drainage of the left upper quadrant.

A major pancreatic transection or extensive parenchymal disruption near the ampulla (grade 4) presents special challenges. These injuries to the right of the superior mesenteric vein are often lethal when associated with vascular injury. The first priority is hemostasis, which may be accomplished by primary vascular repair or suture ligature of exposed vessels. Gentle retraction helps prevent inadvertent injury to the superior mesenteric vein or to unnamed veins draining the uncinate process. When a clean transection is present, a Roux-en-Y pancreaticojejunostomy allows for appropriate drainage of the distal pancreas. This may reduce the likelihood of carbohy-

Patient presents with injury to pancreas
Treat injury according to grade [see Table 1].

Grade 1 or 2
Treat with unroofing, hemostasis, evacuation, and closed drainage. Control bleeding with either electrocoagulation or suture ligation.
With grade 2 injuries, take extra care to rule out duct injury and obtain hemostasis.

Grade 3
Treat with distal pancreatectomy, with or without splenic salvage. If it is unknown whether duct is injured, simple drainage may be provided instead. When nonresective therapy is given to patients with known ductal injury, reoperation with later resection or Roux-en-Y drainage may be needed.

Grade 4
Diabetic patients with intact duodenal ampullary complex: treat with closure of duodenal rim of pancreas and distal Roux-en-Y pancreaticojejunostomy.
Nondiabetic patients: treat with primary closure of proximal pancreas and distal pancreatectomy.

Grade 5
Unstable patients: treat with duodenal diversion and external drainage.
Stable patients: treat with pancreaticoduodenectomy or Roux-en-Y pancreaticojejunostomy.

Figure 5 Algorithm outlines the treatment of pancreatic injury.

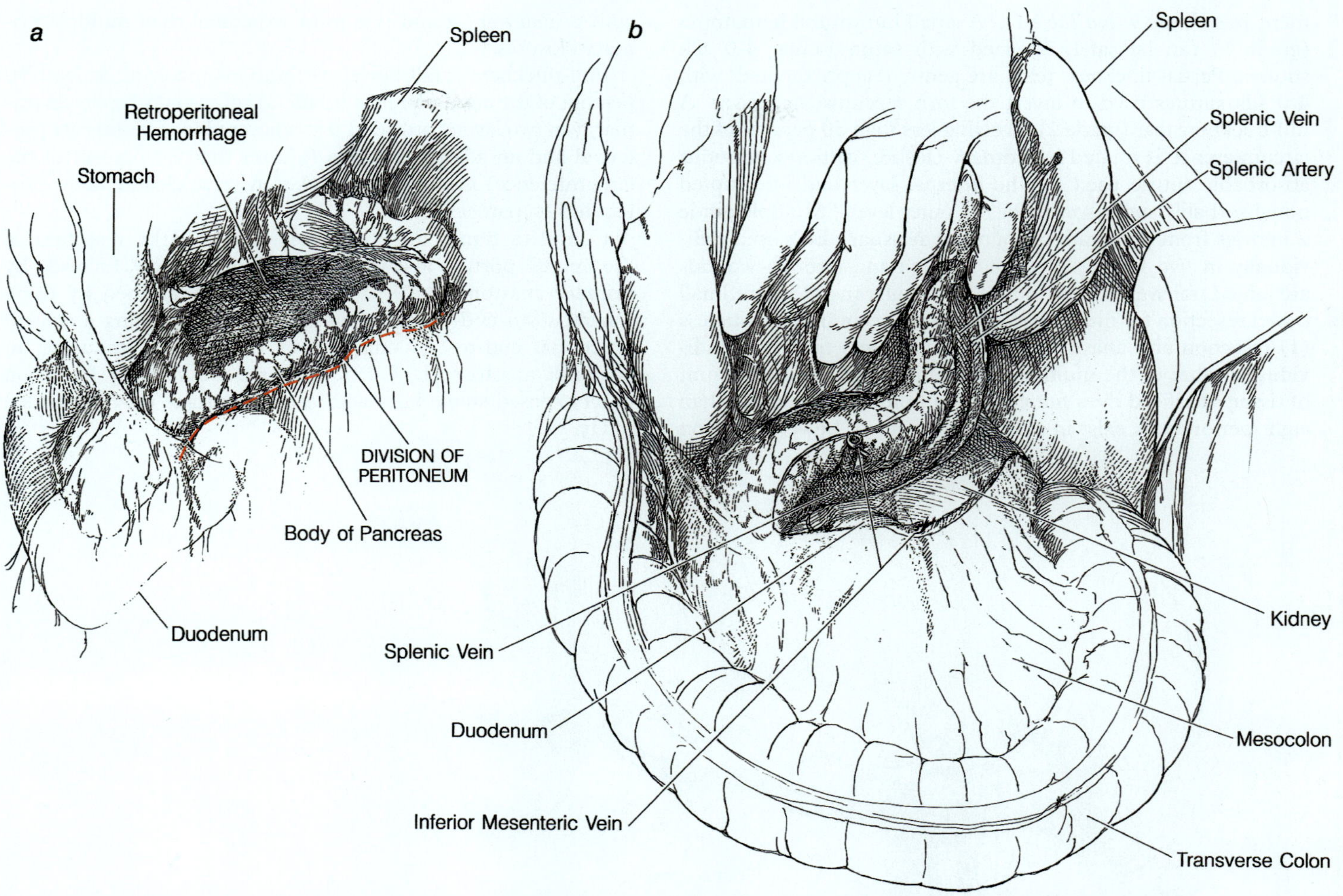

Figure 6 Illustrated is the appearance of a contusion to the body of the pancreas overlying the vertebral column, as seen from the lesser sac (*a*). Such a contusion necessitates mobilization of the pancreas to determine whether a fracture is present and to assess the likelihood of a duct injury. This exposure is best accomplished by dissecting along the inferior border of the gland, dividing the inferior mesenteric vein if necessary, and reflecting the pancreas superiorly (*b*).

drate intolerance in diabetic patients. Simple oversewing of the proximal stump reduces the likelihood that a pancreatic fistula will develop from the transected proximal pancreas [*see Figure 8*]. When the pancreatic head has a stellate laceration that does not extend posteriorly, one should attempt to establish hemostasis and provide for abundant external drainage. Two or more drains are recommended. Although pancreaticoduodenectomy may be used for grade 4 injury, the magnitude of this operation in the midst of pancreatic bleeding argues that it should stay in the hands of the most experienced trauma surgeons.[13,15] Short-term treatment with well-placed drains often permits the patient to recover from the total insult; if a pancreaticocutaneous fistula persists, reoperation can provide definitive intraluminal drainage. When a grade 4 pancreatic injury coexists with a duodenal injury, duodenal diverticularization or duodenal exclusion is recommended.

Grade 5 pancreatic injuries with massive disruption of the pancreatic head (with or without associated duodenal injury) have the highest morbidity and mortality.[13,15] When these injuries result from gunshot or stab wounds, the high incidence of injury to the superior mesenteric vein, the superior mesenteric artery, the inferior vena cava, or the aorta often results in death in the operating room. Once hemostasis has been obtained, the choice of treatment is simple external drainage of the pancreas (for unstable patients) or pancreaticoduodenectomy or Roux-en-Y pancreaticojejunostomy (for stable patients).

Over a five-year period, the surgical services at Detroit Receiving Hospital treated 18 patients with grade 5 pancreatic injury. The treatment regimens varied but included duodenal diverticularization, segmental resection of the duodenum with wide drainage of the pancreatic injury, pyloric exclusion, Roux-en-Y pancreaticojejunostomy, and 95 percent pancreatectomy with external drainage of the remaining pancreas. All patients who survived the hemorrhagic shock survived the procedures, but hospitalization was prolonged. Many of these patients required long-term total parenteral nutrition and additional operations for drainage of abscesses.

Injuries to the Small Bowel

The severity of small bowel injury directs the type of treatment [see Figure 9 and Table 1].[5] A small intramural hematoma (grade 1) can be safely inverted with seromuscular 4-0 silk sutures. Partial-thickness tears are gently reapproximated, with 4-0 silk sutures used to invert the torn seromuscular tissue. A full-thickness tear (grade 2) involving less than 50 percent of the circumference is treated by primary closure, with a continuous absorbable suture used for the internal layer and interrupted nonabsorbable sutures used for the outer layer.[2] Multiple grade 2 injuries from penetrating wounds can usually be closed individually in two layers. Adjacent through-and-through wounds are joined transversely and closed in a similar manner.[16,17] Small bowel resection for multiple injuries is not recommended unless (1) resection and anastomosis would take less time than individual closure of the multiple perforations and (2) the amount of tissue sacrificed does not compromise function. If more than eight perforations exist in a 12 in. segment of bowel, resection with primary anastomosis is more expedient than multiple primary closures.

Full-thickness small bowel perforations involving at least 50 percent of the circumference (grade 3) can usually be closed primarily in two layers, provided that adjacent blood vessels are protected and an adequate lumen (greater than 30 percent of the circumference) is maintained.[18] A transverse closure helps protect lumen patency.

Complete transection (grade 4) is treated by resection of the injured portion and its adjacent blood supply, followed by primary anastomosis.[19,20] This can be accomplished by using a hand-sewn end-to-end technique or by fashioning a stapled functional end-to-end anastomosis (as opposed to using an anatomic anastomosis) [see 55 Intestinal Anastomosis]. Inversion of all exposed staple lines with 4-0 silk sutures provides added safety.

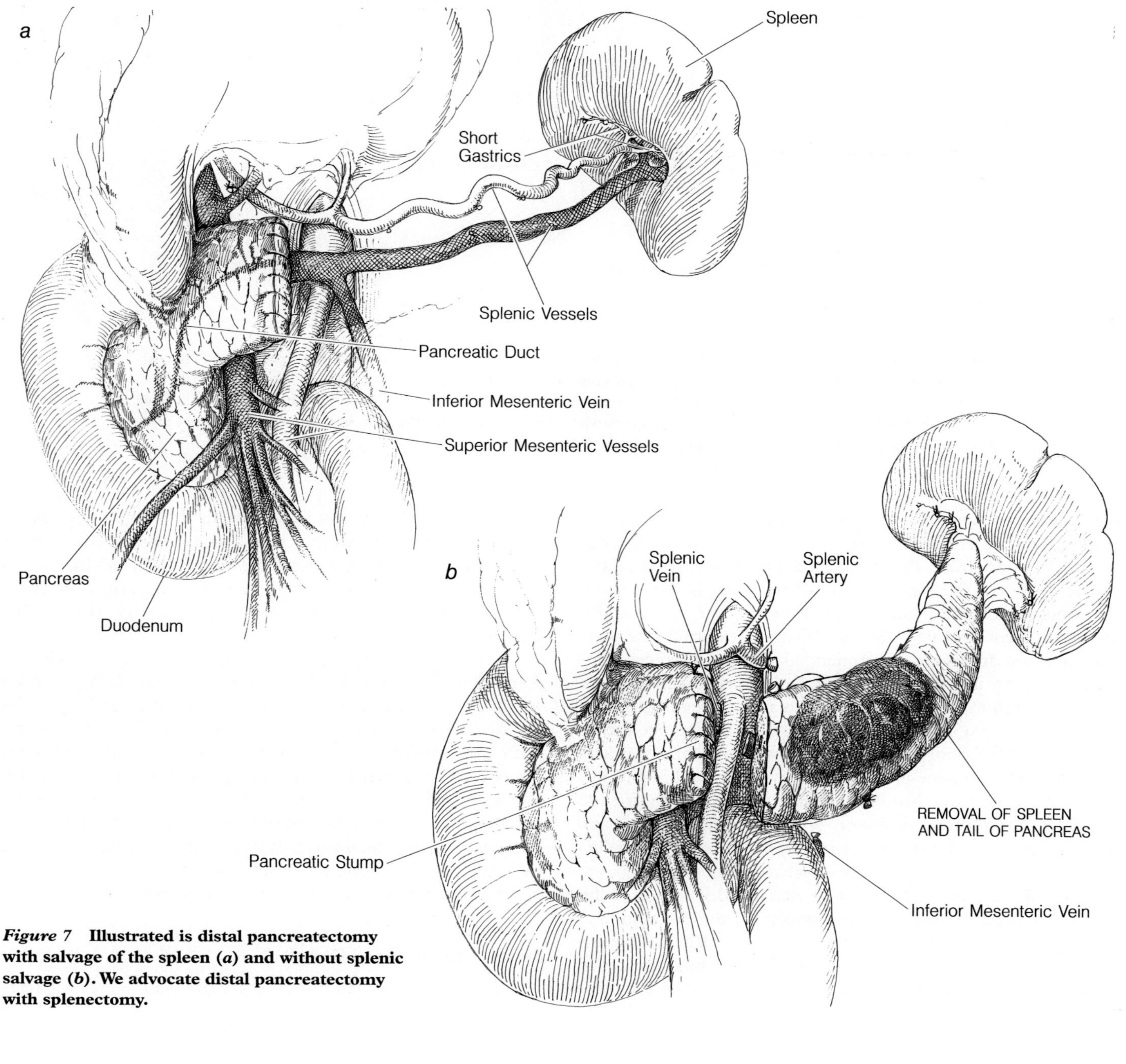

Figure 7 **Illustrated is distal pancreatectomy with salvage of the spleen (*a*) and without splenic salvage (*b*). We advocate distal pancreatectomy with splenectomy.**

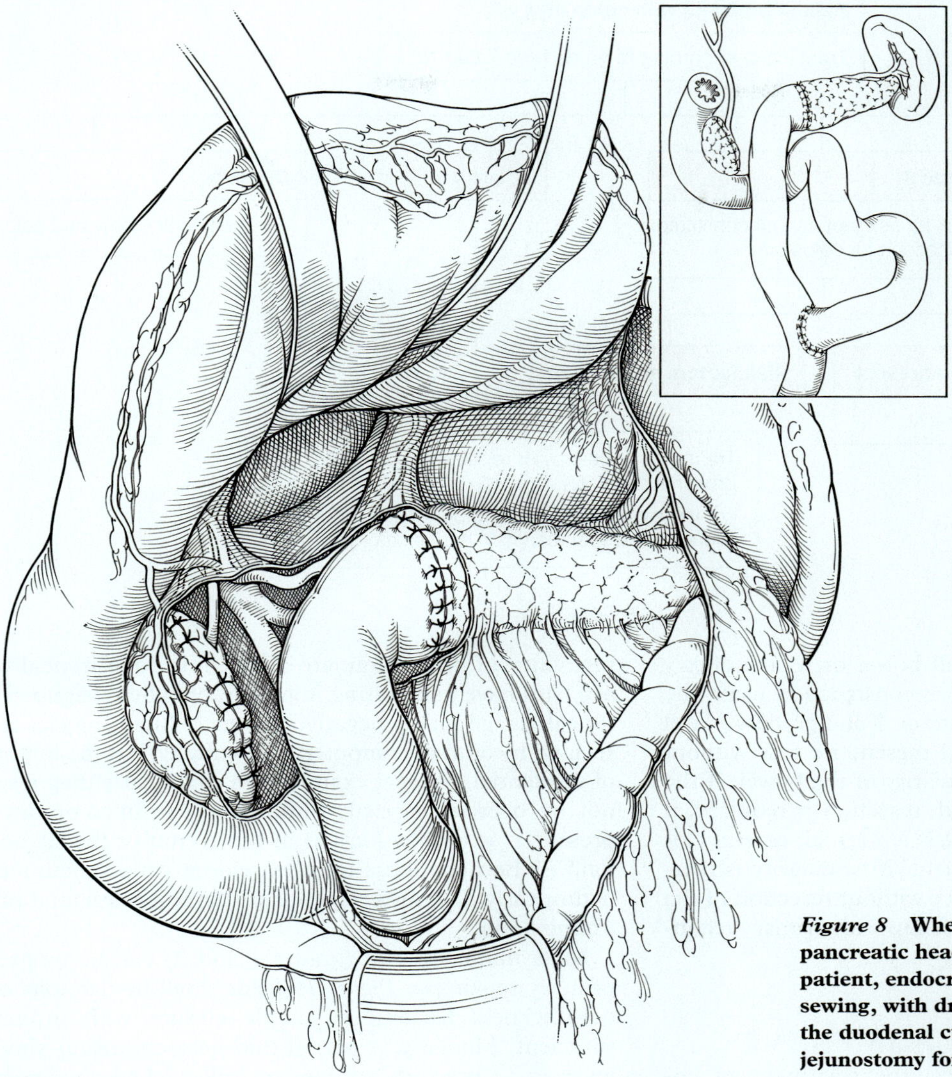

Figure 8 When a grade 4 pancreatic injury to the pancreatic head is sharply demarcated in a diabetic patient, endocrine function can be preserved by oversewing, with drainage of the pancreas along the duodenal curve, and a Roux-en-Y pancreaticojejunostomy for the distal pancreas.

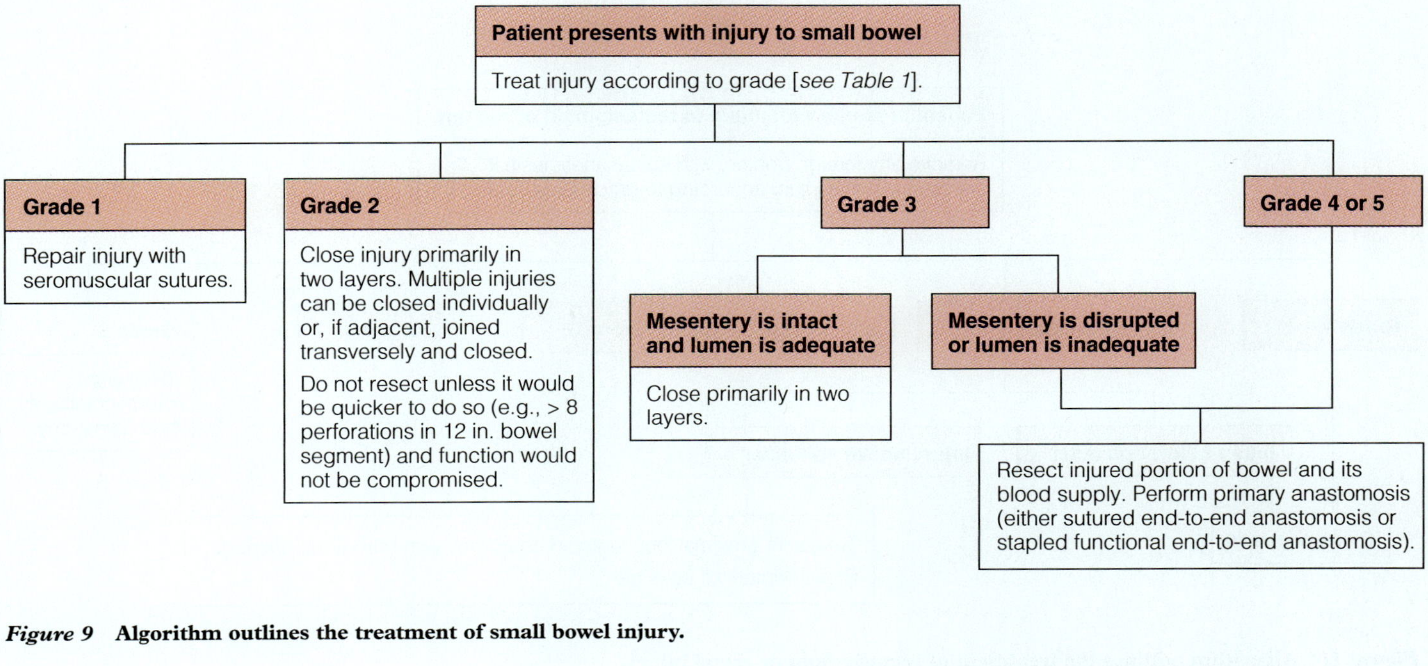

Patient presents with injury to small bowel

Treat injury according to grade [*see Table 1*].

Grade 1
Repair injury with seromuscular sutures.

Grade 2
Close injury primarily in two layers. Multiple injuries can be closed individually or, if adjacent, joined transversely and closed.
Do not resect unless it would be quicker to do so (e.g., > 8 perforations in 12 in. bowel segment) and function would not be compromised.

Grade 3

Mesentery is intact and lumen is adequate
Close primarily in two layers.

Mesentery is disrupted or lumen is inadequate

Grade 4 or 5

Resect injured portion of bowel and its blood supply. Perform primary anastomosis (either sutured end-to-end anastomosis or stapled functional end-to-end anastomosis).

Figure 9 Algorithm outlines the treatment of small bowel injury.

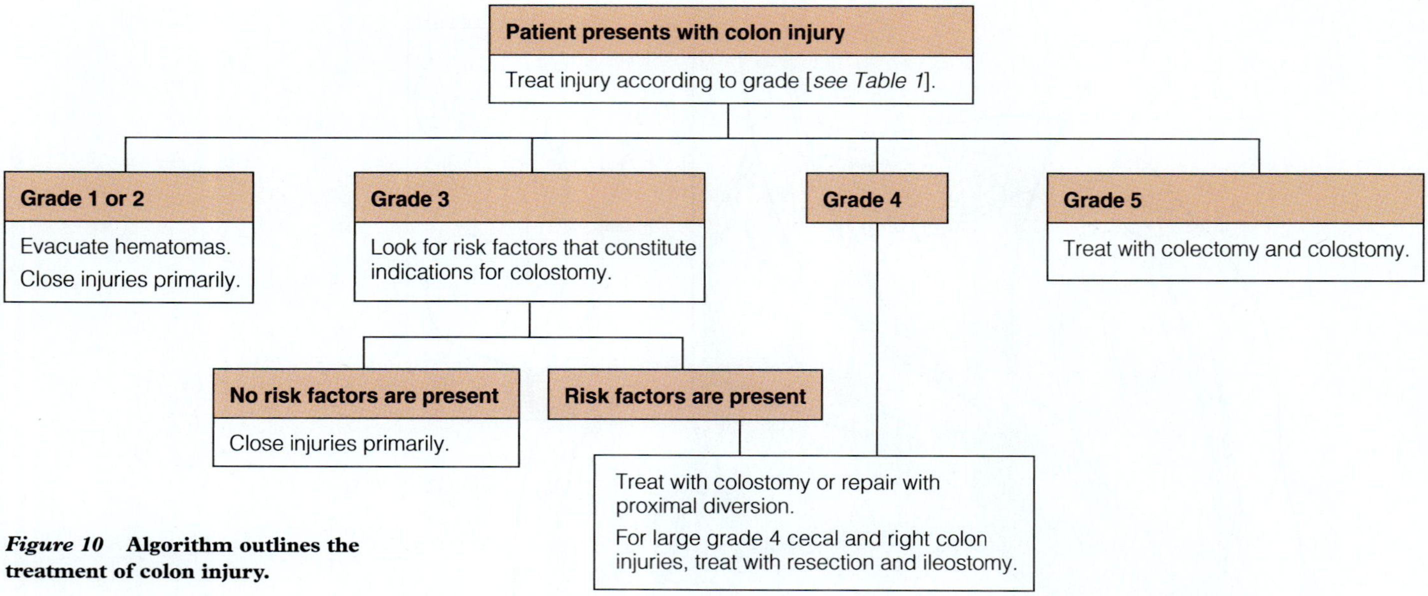

Figure 10 Algorithm outlines the treatment of colon injury.

```
Patient presents with colon injury
Treat injury according to grade [see Table 1].
```
- **Grade 1 or 2**: Evacuate hematomas. Close injuries primarily.
- **Grade 3**: Look for risk factors that constitute indications for colostomy.
  - No risk factors are present: Close injuries primarily.
  - Risk factors are present: Treat with colostomy or repair with proximal diversion. For large grade 4 cecal and right colon injuries, treat with resection and ileostomy.
- **Grade 4**: (see above box)
- **Grade 5**: Treat with colectomy and colostomy.

Extensive destruction of the small bowel or its mesentery (grade 5) necessitates resection and reconstruction using the same techniques recommended for grade 3 and grade 4 bowel injuries.[2,17] Treatment of an isolated mesenteric tear without bowel rupture depends on the vascularity of the bowel. If the bowel is necrotic and devascularized, resection is required; if the bowel remains pink and peristalsis is normal, careful closure of the mesenteric tear is sufficient. If vascularity is marginal, simple closure of the mesentery without resection of the bowel may lead to stenosis; thus, resection with primary reconstruction is recommended.

Injuries to the Colon

As with injuries to other organs, the treatment of colon injury depends on its severity [see Figure 10 and Table 1].[5] Because the ascending, descending, and retrosigmoid segments of the colon are located retroperitoneally, they may still have penetrating injuries even when diagnostic peritoneal lavage yields negative results.[21] Such injuries may be seen with contrast computed tomography, but the importance of sequential physical examination to an early diagnosis cannot be overemphasized. Blunt injury is uncommon; when present, it is usually located in the cecum or the sigmoid colon.[21,22] Because these injuries seldom cause pneumoperitoneum, early diagnosis depends on careful sequential physical examination.

Most minor injuries (grades 1 and 2) can be treated with primary repair [see Figure 10]. For small hematomas or partial-thickness lacerations, simple closure with inversion is sufficient. Similarly, a partial-thickness contusion should be inverted to preclude subsequent full-thickness necrosis with perforation.[21,23] Grade 2 hematomas should be evacuated carefully to prevent full-thickness injury and should be closed

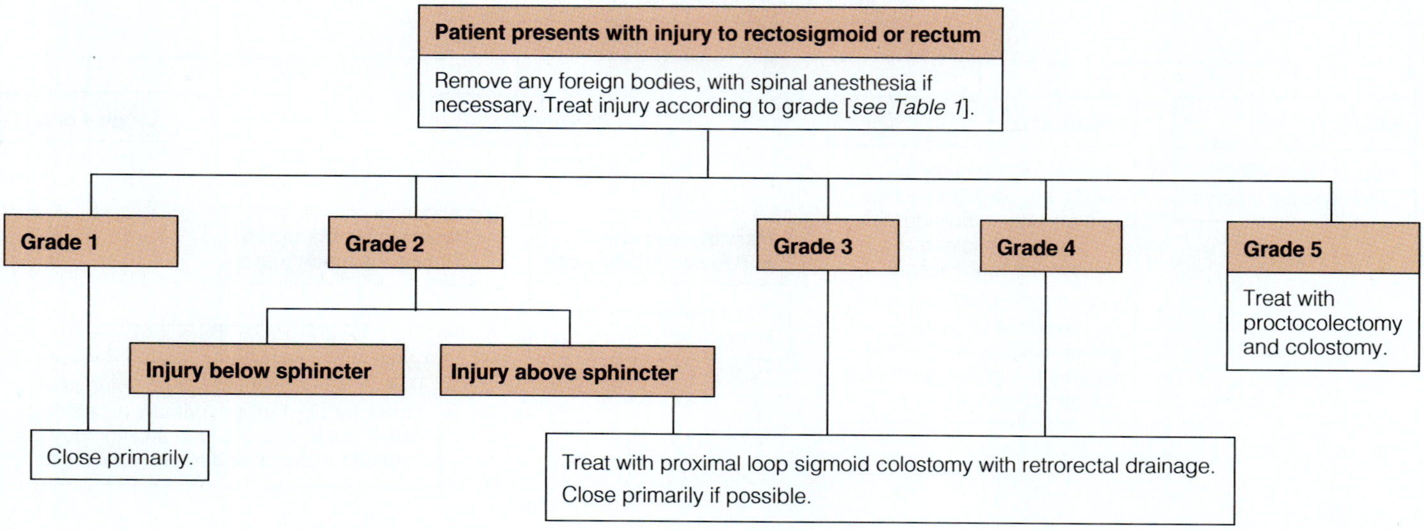

```
Patient presents with injury to rectosigmoid or rectum
Remove any foreign bodies, with spinal anesthesia if necessary. Treat injury according to grade [see Table 1].
```
- **Grade 1**: Close primarily.
- **Grade 2**:
  - Injury below sphincter: Close primarily.
  - Injury above sphincter: Treat with proximal loop sigmoid colostomy with retrorectal drainage. Close primarily if possible.
- **Grade 3**: Treat with proximal loop sigmoid colostomy with retrorectal drainage. Close primarily if possible.
- **Grade 4**: Treat with proximal loop sigmoid colostomy with retrorectal drainage. Close primarily if possible.
- **Grade 5**: Treat with proctocolectomy and colostomy.

Figure 11 Algorithm outlines the treatment of rectosigmoid or rectal injury.

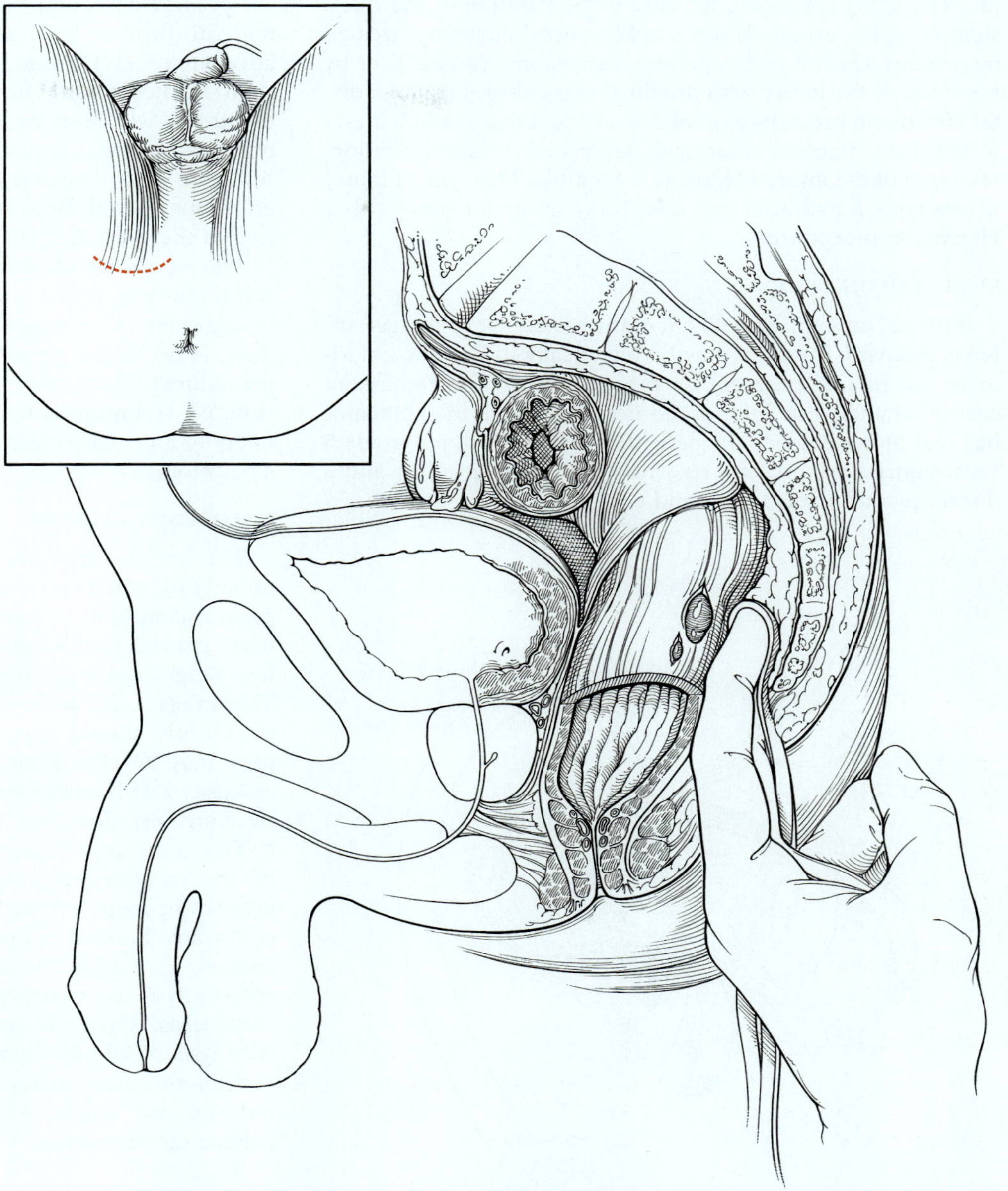

Figure 12 Presacral drainage is provided through a curved incision midway between the anus and the tip of the coccyx. With blunt dissection, two fingers are inserted between the rectum and the hollow of the sacrum. Penrose drains are inserted and sutured to the skin.

primarily. Through-and-through injuries with little or no spill and a minimum of associated injuries can be closed primarily throughout the colon.[23,24]

Because the colon has an increased bacterial level, ranging from 10^6 in the cecum to 10^{13} in the rectum, primary closure of colon injuries is associated with a much greater risk of leakage than primary closure of small bowel perforations. Although many patients are candidates for colostomy, primary closure is preferred for most minor injuries. In a prospective, randomized study of primary closure versus colostomy, Stone and Fabian reported that morbidity was much greater in the colostomy patients.[3] On the basis of these and other studies, primary closure appears to be the preferred technique in patients with the following clinical characteristics: injuries with minimal spill; fewer than three associated injuries; no hypotension; minimal blood loss; a short interval between injury and operation; good colonic vascularity; injury involving no more than 50 percent of the circumference; and an intact abdominal wall.

ROLE OF COLOSTOMY

Colostomy is preferred in patients with one or more of the following clinical characteristics[3,5,21]: a wound involving more than 50 percent of the circumference (grade 3); extensive free peritoneal fecal spill; associated hypotension; a need for multiple transfusions; three or more associated injuries; colonic devascularization (grade 5); a delay of more than six hours between injury and operative intervention; an extensive retroperitoneal hematoma from pelvic fractures; an associated abdominal wall defect; and an associated rectal injury.

Specific methods include exteriorization of the segment of injured colon as a loop colostomy; closure of the injured colon, which is then protected by a proximal colostomy; and resection of the injured colon with a proximal end colostomy and a distal mucous fistula (or the Hartmann closure). Simple exteriorization of the injured colon as a loop colostomy is most effective for serious grade 3 injuries to the right, transverse, left, or sigmoid colon. After the abdomen has been closed, the ostomy is matured primarily to facilitate early fitting with a properly sized appliance. Because exteriorization of the distal sigmoid colon usually is not feasible, such injuries are treated by primary closure with a proximal colostomy (grade 3) or by resection of the injury with proximal end colostomy and a distal Hartmann procedure (grades 4 and 5). For a grade 5 injury to the distal sigmoid colon with associated devascularization, resection of the injured segment is essential. This type of injury necessitates a proximal end colostomy in conjunction with a Hartmann procedure.

RIGHT COLON INJURY

If the cecum or the first 6 cm of the ascending colon has suffered extensive injury, it may be technically difficult to exteriorize the injured segment as a colostomy.[25] The redundant cecum, including its inferior cul-de-sac, may fill the appliance bag and inconvenience the patient. When grade 4 and grade 5 cecal injuries are present, resection with end ileostomy and a distal mucous fistula is safe and effective.

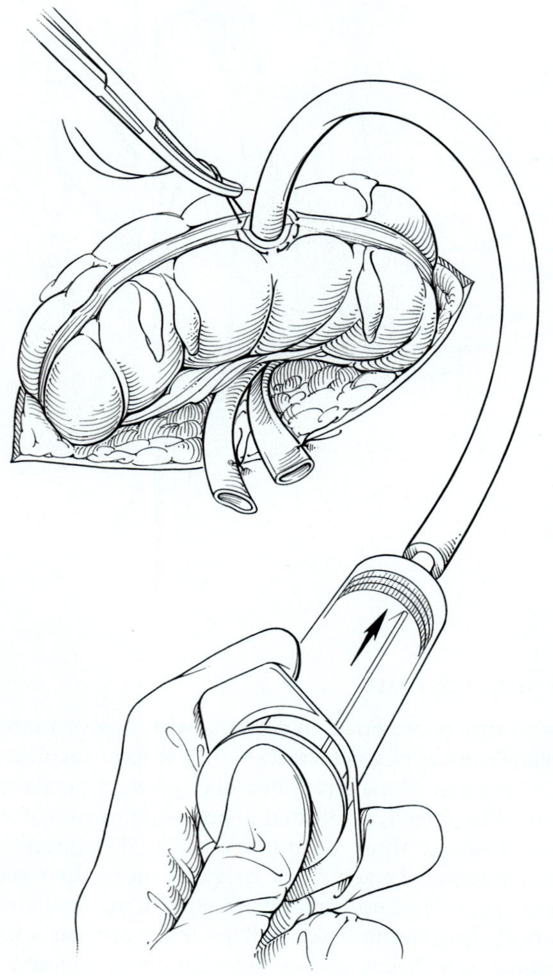

Figure 13 Irrigation of the distal sigmoid colon and rectum reduces soilage of the retrorectal space through unclosed perforations of the rectum as peristalsis returns. At the completion of the operative procedure, a purse-string suture is placed in the sigmoid colostomy and a large Foley catheter passed into the distal limb. The distal limb is irrigated with saline as the anus is held open. The catheter is then removed, and the colostomy is opened and matured.

For large cecal and right colon injuries, right hemicolectomy with primary ileotransverse colon anastomosis has been advocated.[21,24] Despite the excellent results reported with right hemicolectomy and primary anastomosis, we recommend that whenever right colon wounds are so extensive that primary closure cannot be done safely, the best option is resection with ileostomy. Most patients can tolerate a properly constructed Brooke ileostomy with intraoperative fitting of the appliance [see 57 Colorectal Procedures].

The so-called closed-loop exteriorization, in which the colon injury is closed primarily and the injured segment then brought out as a temporary exteriorization for seven to 10 days, is no longer performed. Patients who healed after this procedure probably would have done as well after primary closure. We recommend that whenever there is doubt about the safety of a primary closure, the patient should be treated with a colostomy.

COLOSTOMY CLOSURE

The optimal time for colostomy closure depends on the underlying insult, postoperative morbidity, and the patient's general condition. A patient is ready for a colostomy closure when general health has been restored, appetite has returned, lost weight has been regained, and all wounds have healed. When these criteria are met, mortality associated with colostomy closure should approach zero.[26] Although some colostomies may be closed within days or weeks after injury, those associated with extensive peritonitis and enterocutaneous fistulas are best closed six to 12 months after injury.

The safest way of closing loop colostomies involves resection of the exteriorized loop through an oval-shaped incision around the loop, followed by closure with an end-to-end colocolostomy. Sutures are preferred to the staples in this setting because they allow closure of the ostomy through this pericolostomy incision with less mobilization of the proximal and distal ends. When end colostomies are closed, full laparotomy with lysis of all adhesions is required to provide tension-free end-to-end anastomosis and reapproximation of the mesentery. On the whole, we prefer hand-sewn anastomoses for colonic reconstruction.[26]

Injuries to the Rectosigmoid and Rectum

Rectosigmoid and rectal injuries also vary in severity [see Figure 11 and Table 1].[5,27] The agents of injury include knives, bullets, cars, and rectal obturators such as enema tips, thermometers, and sexual toys. The rectosigmoid colon begins near the sacral promontory and extends to the retrovesical fold, where only the anterior bowel wall is covered with peritoneum. Posterior injuries in this 3 to 5 cm zone are retroperitoneal; below this point, the rectum is completely retroperitoneal.

Small, clean, easily accessible rectosigmoid wounds (types 1 and 2) can be closed primarily if conditions are favorable. Larger wounds require that this segment of bowel be exteriorized or diverted by a proximal colostomy. This can often be accomplished by a proximal sigmoid loop colostomy with primary closure of the rectosigmoid wound.[25,27,28] Massive wounds (grades 4 and 5) in the rectosigmoid junctional zone require excision, with proximal colostomy and a distal Hartmann procedure.

Penetrating rectal injuries can be diagnosed by proctoscopic examination. During laparotomy, the retroperitoneal hematoma associated with rectal injuries often interferes with safe dissection and clear identification of the perforation. Small wounds (grades 1 and 2) can be closed primarily if a proximal colostomy is performed in conjunction with retrorectal drainage. The skin incision for retrorectal drainage is placed between the anus and the coccyx [see Figure 12]. The drain should extend proximal to the perforation. When examination shows that the rectum is filled with stool, the colostomy is opened at the time of operation to facilitate disimpaction and copious distal irrigation with balanced electrolyte solution [see Figure 13]. The anus is kept open only during this irrigation, to facilitate passage of saline and associated stool into an adjacent bucket and to decrease the likelihood that stool will be pushed through the site of injury into retroperitoneal tissues.[26,28] Grade 3 and grade 4 rectal injuries are often more difficult to close primarily; they are usually treated with a proximal colostomy and retrorectal drainage. Massive devascularized grade 5 rectal injuries are rare; they are treated with resection followed by a proximal end colostomy.

Foreign bodies may produce rectal injuries. Although a thermometer is the most common offending agent in pediatric patients, a larger obturator inserted for pleasure is the usual agent in adults. Such obturators include cans, soft drink bottles, light bulbs, vibrators, and other firm objects. When the offending agent is difficult to remove, spinal anesthesia may be helpful. Once the foreign body has been removed, careful endoscopic examination helps rule out intrinsic injury to the upper rectum or rectosigmoid. When transanal extraction is impossible, full laparotomy and gentle pushing of the offending agent from above usually permit safe removal. Repair of full-thickness injuries from these obturators follows the guidelines for other types of penetrating injuries.[26]

Extensive grade 5 rectal injuries associated with close-range shotgun wounds often cause devascularization and intrusion of the bony pelvis. These wounds may require extensive resection of the rectum as well as proximal diversion. Occasionally, these injuries are severe enough to preclude subsequent rectal repair. In rare cases, an industrial accident may result in the same type of extensive injury that is associated with pelvic fractures. For such patients, delayed reconstruction of the rectum may be impossible because of extensive damage to the rectum and the adjacent sacral plexus. Permanent colostomy will be needed in such cases.

References

1. Lucas CE: Splenic trauma: choice of management. Ann Surg 213:98, 1991
2. Wisner DH, Blaisdell FW: Visceral injuries. Arch Surg 127:687, 1992
3. Stone HH, Fabian TC: Management of duodenal wounds. J Trauma 19:334, 1979
4. Kline G, Lucas CE, Ledgerwood AM, et al: Duodenal organ injury severity (OIS) and outcome. Am Surg 60:500, 1994
5. Moore EE, Cogbill TH, Malangoni MA, et al: Organ injury scaling: II. Pancreas, duodenum, small bowel, colon, and rectum. J Trauma 30:1427, 1990
6. Berne CJ, Donovan AJ, White EJ, et al: Duodenal diverticulation for duodenal and pancreatic injury. Am J Surg 127:503, 1974
7. Shorr RM, Greaney GC, Donovan AJ: Injuries of the duodenum. Am J Surg 154:93, 1987
8. Cogbill TH, Moore EE, Feliciano DV, et al: Conservative management of duodenal trauma: a multicenter perspective. J Trauma 30:1469, 1990
9. Degiannis E, Krawczkowski D, Velmahos GC, et al: Pyloric exclusion in severe penetrating injuries of the duodenum. World J Surg 17:751, 1993
10. Vaughan GD 3rd, Frazier OH, Graham DY, et al: The use of pyloric exclusion in the management of severe duodenal injuries. Am J Surg 134:785, 1977
11. Pederzoli P, Bassi C, Falconi M, et al: Conservative treatment of external pancreatic fistulas with parenteral nutrition alone or in combination with continuous intravenous infusion of somatostatin, glucagon, or calcitonin. Surg Gynecol Obstet 163:428, 1986
12. Sugawa C, Lucas CE: The role of endoscopic retrograde cholangiopancreatography in surgery of the pancreas and biliary ducts. Endoscopic Retrograde Cholangiopancreatography. Silvis SE, Rohrmann CA, Ansel HJ, Eds. Igaku-Shoin, New York, 1994, p 3
13. Feliciano DV, Martin TD, Cruse PA, et al: Management of combined pancreatoduodenal injuries. Ann Surg 205:673, 1987
14. Stone A, Sugawa C, Lucas C, et al: The role of endoscopic retrograde pancreatography (ERP) in blunt abdominal trauma. Am Surg 56:715, 1990
15. McKone TK, Bursch LR, Scholten DJ: Pancreaticoduodenectomy for trauma: a life-saving procedure. Am Surg 54:361, 1988
16. Flint LM, Cryer HM, Howard DA, et al: Approaches to the management of shotgun injuries. J Trauma 24:415, 1984
17. Schenk WG 3rd, Lonchyna V, Moylan JA: Perforation of the jejunum from blunt abdominal trauma. J Trauma 23:54, 1983
18. Wisner DH, Chun Y, Blaisdell FW: Blunt intestinal injury: keys to diagnosis and management. Arch Surg 125:1319, 1990
19. Coleman EJ, Dietz PA: Small bowel injuries following blunt abdominal trauma: early recognition and management. NY State J Med 90:446, 1990
20. Sherck J, Shatney C, Sensaki K, et al: The accuracy of computed tomography in the diagnosis of blunt small-bowel perforation. Am J Surg 168:670, 1994
21. Lucas C, Ledgerwood A: Management of the injured colon. Current Surgery 43:190, 1986
22. Ross SE, Cobean RA, Hoyt DB, et al: Blunt colonic injury, a multicenter review. J Trauma 33:379, 1992
23. George SM Jr, Fabian TC, Voeller GR, et al: Primary repair of colon wounds: a prospective trial in nonselected patients. Ann Surg 209:728, 1989
24. Ivatury RR, Licata J, Gunduz Y, et al: Management options in penetrating rectal injuries. Am Surg 57:50, 1991
25. Strada G, Raad L, Belloni G, et al: Large bowel perforations in war surgery: one-stage treatment in a field hospital. Int J Colorectal Dis 8:213, 1993
26. Ledgerwood AM, Lucas CE: Management of colon injuries. Principles and Practice of Trauma Care. Worth MH, Ed. Williams & Wilkins, Baltimore, 1982, p 117
27. Nelken N, Lewis F: The influence of injury severity on complication rates after primary closure or colostomy for penetrating colon trauma. Ann Surg 209:439, 1989
28. Burch JM, Feliciano DV, Mattox KL: Colostomy and drainage for civilian rectal injuries: is that all? Ann Surg 209:600, 1989

Acknowledgments

Figures 1, 2, 5, 9 through 11   Marcia Kammerer.
Figures 3, 8, 12, 13   Susan Brust, C.M.I.
Figures 4, 6, 7   Carol Donner.

30 INJURIES TO THE GREAT VESSELS OF THE ABDOMEN

David V. Feliciano, M.D.

In patients who have injuries to the great vessels of the abdomen, the findings on physical examination generally depend on whether a contained hematoma or active hemorrhage is present. In the case of contained hematomas around the vascular injury in the retroperitoneum, the base of the mesentery, or the hepatoduodenal ligament, the patient often has only modest hypotension in transit or on arrival at the emergency center; the hypotension can be temporarily reversed by the infusion of fluids and may not recur until the hematoma is opened at the time of laparotomy. In the case of active intraperitoneal hemorrhage, the patient typically has significant hypotension and may have a distended abdomen on arrival. Another physical finding that is occasionally noted in association with an injury to the common or external iliac artery is intermittent or complete loss of a pulse in the ipsilateral femoral artery; this finding in a patient with a transpelvic gunshot wound is pathognomonic of an injury to the iliac artery.

Injuries to the great vessels of the abdomen are caused by penetrating wounds in 90% to 95% of cases; accordingly, they are often accompanied by injuries to multiple intra-abdominal organs, including those in the gastrointestinal tract. The general principles governing the sequencing of repairs of injuries to the great vessels and the gastrointestinal tract are outlined elsewhere [see 27 Operative Exposure of Abdominal Injuries and Closure of the Abdomen].

A hematoma [see Figures 1 and 2] or hemorrhage associated with an injury to the abdomen occurs in one of the three zones of the retroperitoneum or in the portal-retrohepatic area of the right upper quadrant [see 27 Operative Exposure of Abdominal Injuries and Closure of the Abdomen]. The magnitude of injury is usually described according to the Abdominal Vascular Organ Injury Scale devised in 1992 by the American Association for the Surgery of Trauma [see Table 1].

Injuries in Zone 1

SUPRAMESOCOLIC

It is helpful to divide midline retroperitoneal hematomas into those that are supramesocolic and those that are inframesocolic. Hematoma or hemorrhage in the midline supramesocolic area of zone 1 is cause to suspect the presence of an injury to the suprarenal aorta, the celiac axis, the proximal superior mesenteric artery, or the proximal renal artery.

When a hematoma is present in the midline supramesocolic area, one usually has time to perform left medial visceral rotation [see Figure 3 and 27 Operative Exposure of Abdominal Injuries and Closure of the Abdomen]. The advantage of this technique is that it allows visu-

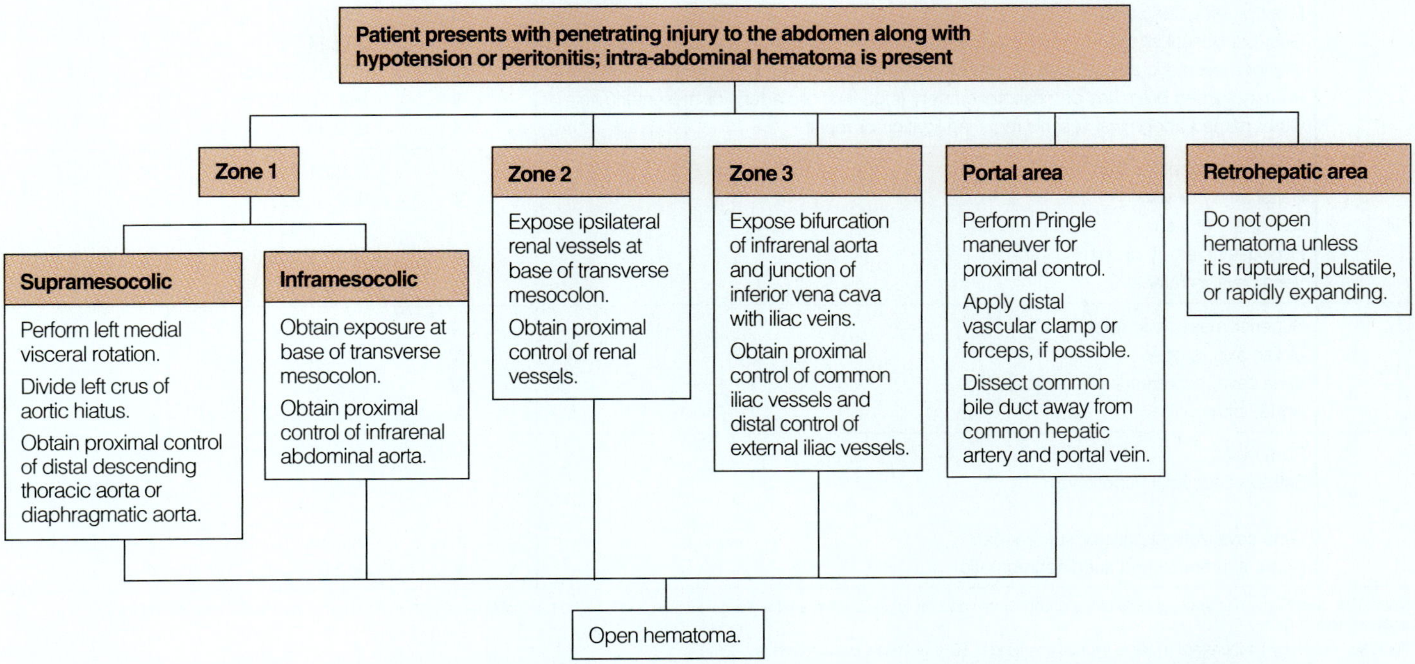

Figure 1 Algorithm illustrates management of intra-abdominal hematoma found at operation after penetrating trauma.

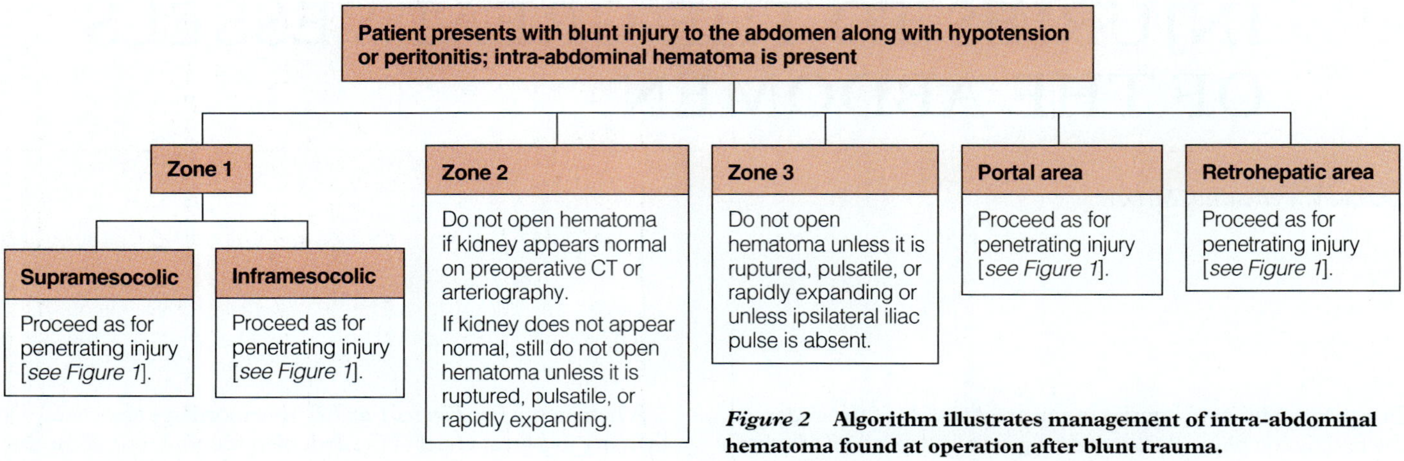

```
Patient presents with blunt injury to the abdomen along with hypotension
or peritonitis; intra-abdominal hematoma is present
```

- **Zone 1**
  - **Supramesocolic**: Proceed as for penetrating injury [see Figure 1].
  - **Inframesocolic**: Proceed as for penetrating injury [see Figure 1].
- **Zone 2**: Do not open hematoma if kidney appears normal on preoperative CT or arteriography. If kidney does not appear normal, still do not open hematoma unless it is ruptured, pulsatile, or rapidly expanding.
- **Zone 3**: Do not open hematoma unless it is ruptured, pulsatile, or rapidly expanding or unless ipsilateral iliac pulse is absent.
- **Portal area**: Proceed as for penetrating injury [see Figure 1].
- **Retrohepatic area**: Proceed as for penetrating injury [see Figure 1].

Figure 2 Algorithm illustrates management of intra-abdominal hematoma found at operation after blunt trauma.

alization of the entire abdominal aorta, from the aortic hiatus of the diaphragm to the common iliac arteries [see Figure 4]. Obvious disadvantages include the 2 to 3 minutes required to complete the maneuver; the risk of damage to the spleen, the left kidney, or the posterior left renal artery as the maneuver is performed; and the anatomic distortion that results when the left kidney and the left renal artery are rotated anteriorly. When the hematoma is near the aortic hiatus of the diaphragm, it may be advisable to leave the left kidney in its fossa, thereby eliminating potential damage to the structure as well as the distortion resulting from rotation. Because of the density of the celiac plexus and the lymphatic vessels surrounding the upper abdominal aorta, this portion of the aorta is difficult to visualize even when left medial visceral rotation has been performed. It is frequently helpful to transect the left crus of the

Table 1 AAST Abdominal Vascular Organ Injury Scale

Grade	Characteristics of Injury	OIS Grade	ICD-9	AIS-90
I	Unnamed superior mesenteric artery or superior mesenteric vein branches	I	902.20/902.39	NS
	Unnamed inferior mesenteric artery or inferior mesenteric vein branches	I	902.27/902.32	NS
	Phrenic artery or vein	I	902.89	NS
	Lumbar artery or vein	I	902.89	NS
	Gonadal artery or vein	I	902.89	NS
	Ovarian artery or vein	I	902.81/902.82	NS
	Other unnamed small arterial or venous structures requiring ligation	I	902.90	NS
II	Right, left, or common hepatic artery	II	902.22	3
	Splenic artery or vein	II	902.23/902.34	3
	Right or left gastric arteries	II	902.21	3
	Gastroduodenal artery	II	902.24	3
	Inferior mesenteric artery, trunk, or inferior mesenteric vein, trunk	II	902.27/902.32	3
	Primary named branches of mesenteric artery (e.g., ileocolic artery) or mesenteric vein	II	902.26/902.31	3
	Other named abdominal vessels requiring ligation or repair	II	902.89	3
III*	Superior mesenteric vein, trunk	III	902.31	3
	Renal artery or vein	III	902.41/902.42	3
	Iliac artery or vein	III	902.53/902.54	3
	Hypogastric artery or vein	III	902.51/902.52	3
	Vena cava, infrarenal	III	902.10	3
IV*†	Superior mesenteric artery, trunk	IV	902.25	3
	Celiac axis, proper	IV	902.24	3
	Vena cava, suprarenal and infrahepatic	IV	902.10	3
	Aorta, infrarenal	IV	902.00	4
V†	Portal vein	V	902.33	3
	Extraparenchymal hepatic vein	V	902.11	3 (hepatic vein) 5 (liver + veins)
	Vena cava, retrohepatic or suprahepatic	V	902.19	5
	Aorta, suprarenal and subdiaphragmatic	V	902.00	4

Note: This classification is applicable to extraparenchymal vascular injuries. If the vessel injury is within 2 cm of the parenchyma of a specific organ, one should refer to the injury scale for that organ.
*Increase grade by I if there are multiple injuries involving > 50% of vessel circumference.
†Reduce grade by I if laceration is < 25% of vessel circumference.
AAST—American Association for the Surgery of Trauma   AIS—Abbreviated Injury Scale   ICD—International Classification of Diseases

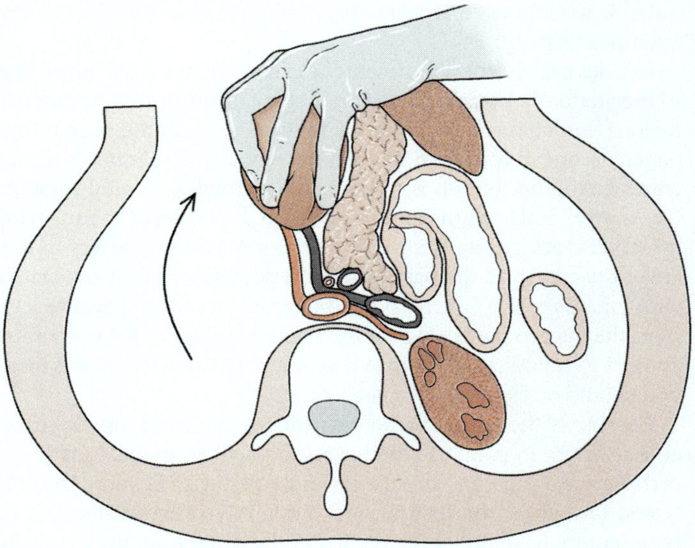

Figure 3 Left medial visceral rotation is performed by means of sharp and blunt dissection with elevation of the left colon, the left kidney, the spleen, the tail of the pancreas, and the gastric fundus.

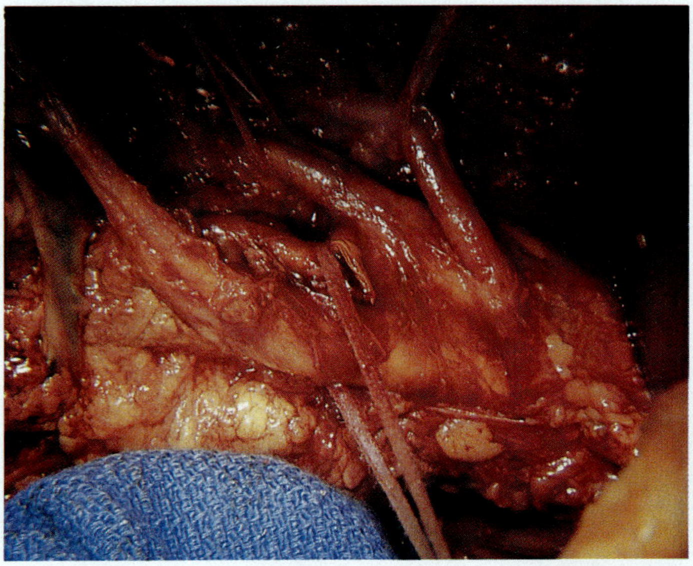

Figure 4 Shown is an autopsy view of the supraceliac aorta and the celiac axis, the proximal superior mesenteric artery, and the medially rotated left renal artery after removal of lymphatic and nerve tissue.

cause of the presence of the anteriorly located celiac axis and superior mesenteric artery. In young trauma patients who are otherwise healthy, ligation and division of the celiac axis allow easier application of the distal aortic clamp and better exposure for subsequent vascular repair.

Small penetrating wounds to the supraceliac abdominal aorta are repaired with a continuous 3-0 or 4-0 polypropylene suture. If two small perforations are adjacent to each other, they can be connected and the defect closed in a transverse fashion. If closure of a perforation would result in significant narrowing of the aorta or if a portion of the aortic wall is missing, patch aortoplasty with polytetrafluoroethylene (PTFE) is indicated. On rare occasions, in patients with extensive injuries to the diaphragmatic or supraceliac aorta, resection of the area of injury and insertion of a vascular conduit are indicated. Even though many of these patients have associated gastric, enteric, or colonic injuries, the most appropriate prosthesis with such a life-threatening injury is a 12 mm or 14 mm Dacron or PTFE graft [*see Figure 6*]. Provided that vigorous intraoperative irrigation is performed after repair of GI tract perforations, that proper graft coverage is ensured, and that perioperative antibiotics are appropriately employed, it is extraordinarily rare for a prosthesis inserted in the healthy aorta of a young trauma patient to become infected.

The aortic prosthesis is sewn in place with a continuous 3-0 or 4-0 polypropylene suture. Both ends of the aorta are flushed before the distal anastomosis is completed, and the distal aortic cross-clamp

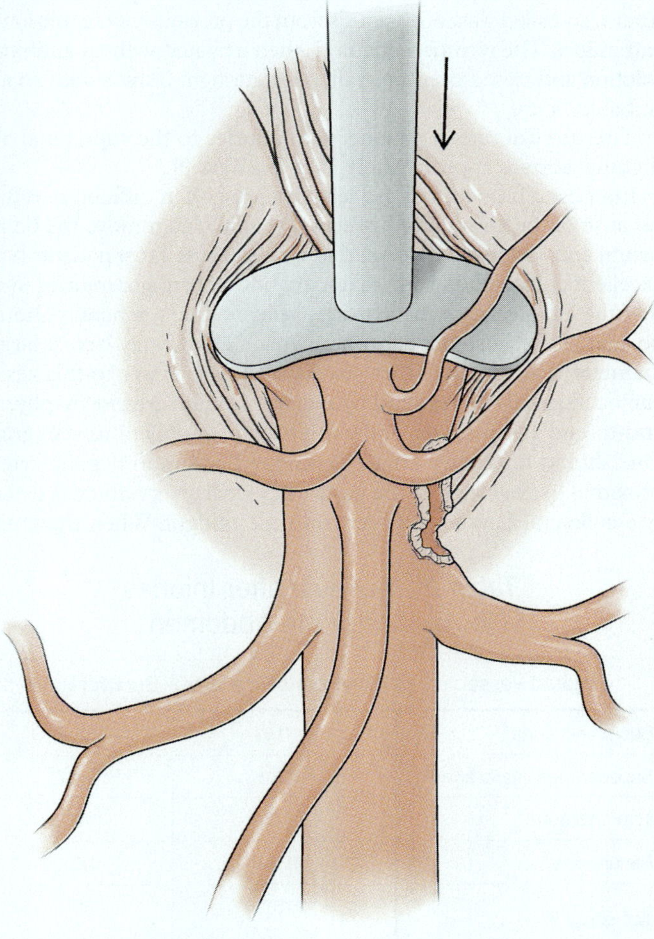

aortic hiatus in the diaphragm at the 2 o'clock position to allow exposure of the distal descending thoracic aorta above the hiatus. Visualization of this portion of the vessel is much easier to achieve than visualization of the diaphragmatic or visceral abdominal aorta below, and an aortic cross-clamp can be applied much more quickly at this level.

Active hemorrhage from the midline supramesocolic area is controlled by packing with laparotomy pads or using an aortic compression device [*see Figure 5*]. An alternative approach is to divide the lesser omentum manually, retract the stomach and esophagus to the left, and manually dissect in the area just below the aortic hiatus to obtain rapid exposure of the supraceliac abdominal aorta. Distal control of the upper abdominal aorta is difficult to obtain be-

Figure 5 An aortic compression device is used to control hemorrhage from the visceral portion of the abdominal aorta.

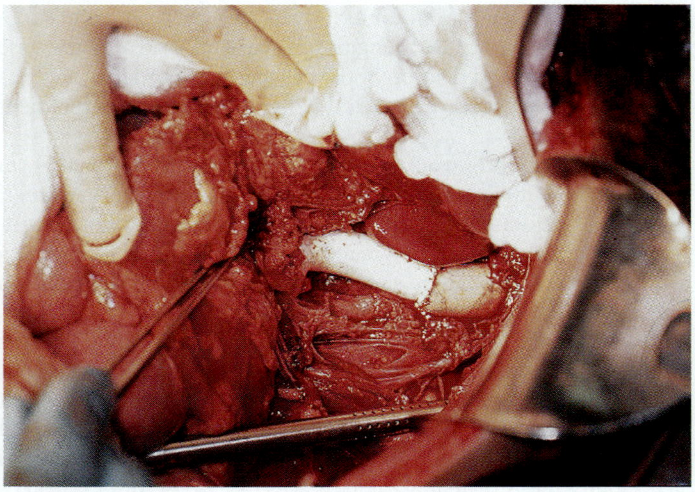

Figure 6 A 22-year-old man with a gunshot wound to the right upper quadrant had injuries to the prepyloric area of the stomach and to the supraceliac abdominal aorta. The aortic injury was managed by means of segmental resection and replacement with a 16 mm polytetrafluoroethylene (PTFE) graft. The patient went home 46 days after injury.

is removed before the final knot is tied to eliminate air from the system. The proximal aortic cross-clamp is removed very slowly as the anesthesiologist rapidly infuses fluids and intravenous bicarbonate to reverse so-called washout acidosis from the previously ischemic lower extremities. The retroperitoneum is then irrigated with an antibiotic solution and closed over the graft in a watertight fashion with an absorbable suture.

The survival rate in patients with injuries to the suprarenal abdominal aorta is approximately 35% [see Table 2].

Injuries to branches of the celiac axis are often difficult to repair because of the amount of dissection required to remove the dense neural and lymphatic tissue in this area. Because most patients have excellent collateral flow in the upper abdomen, major injuries to either the left gastric or the proximal splenic artery generally should be ligated. Because the common hepatic artery may have a larger diameter than either of these two arteries, an injury to this vessel can occasionally be repaired by means of lateral arteriorrhaphy, an end-to-end anastomosis, or the insertion of a saphenous vein graft. One should not worry about ligating the common hepatic artery proximal to the origin of the gastroduodenal artery: there is extensive collateral flow to the liver from the midgut. When the entire celiac axis is injured, it is best to ligate all three vessels and forgo any attempt at repair.

Injuries to the superior mesenteric artery are managed according to the anatomic level of the perforation or thrombosis. On rare occasions, in patients with proximal injuries beneath the neck of the pancreas, one may have to transect the pancreas to obtain proximal control. Another option is to perform left medial visceral rotation (see above) and apply a clamp directly to the origin of the superior mesenteric artery. Injuries to the superior mesenteric artery in this area or just beyond the base of the mesocolon are often associated with injuries to the pancreas. The potential for a postoperative leak from the injured pancreas near the arterial repair has led numerous authors to suggest that any extensive injury to the artery at this location should be ligated [see Figure 7].

Because of the intense vasoconstriction of the distal superior mesenteric artery in patients who have sustained exsanguinating hemorrhage from more proximal injuries treated with ligation, the collateral flow from the foregut and hindgut is often inadequate to maintain the viability of the organs in the distal midgut, especially the cecum and the ascending colon. Therefore, it is safest to place a saphenous vein or PTFE graft on the distal infrarenal aorta, away from the pancreatic injury and any other upper abdominal injuries. Such a graft can be tailored to reach the side or the anterior aspect of the superior mesenteric artery, or it can be attached to the transected distal superior mesenteric artery in an end-to-end fashion without significant tension [see Figure 8]. Soft tissue must be approximated over the aortic suture line of the graft to prevent the development of an aortoenteric fistula in the postoperative period.

In patients with severe shock from exsanguination caused by a

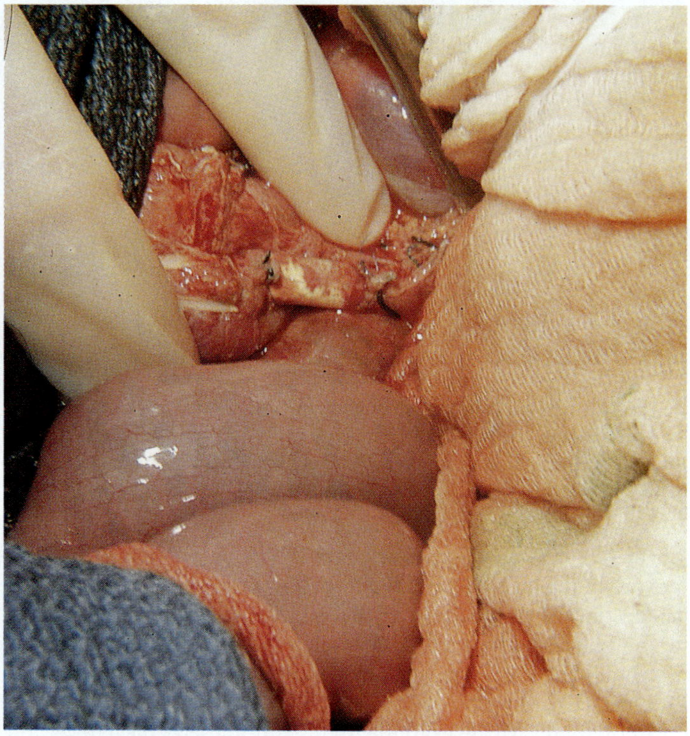

Table 2 Survival after Injuries to Arteries in the Abdomen

Injured Vessel	Survivors/All Patients	Survival Rate (%)
Suprarenal aorta	54/151	35.8
Superior mesenteric artery	67/116	57.7
Infrarenal aorta	39/86	45.3
Renal artery	19/22	86.4
Iliac artery	46/57*	80.7
	145/236†	61.4

*Isolated iliac artery injury.
†Other vascular injury also present.

Figure 7 An 18-year-old man experienced a gunshot wound to the head of the pancreas and the proximal superior mesenteric artery. A Whipple procedure was performed, and a 6 mm PTFE graft was placed in the artery. The artery-graft suture line dehisced secondary to a pancreatic leak on day 30 after injury, and the patient died on day 42.

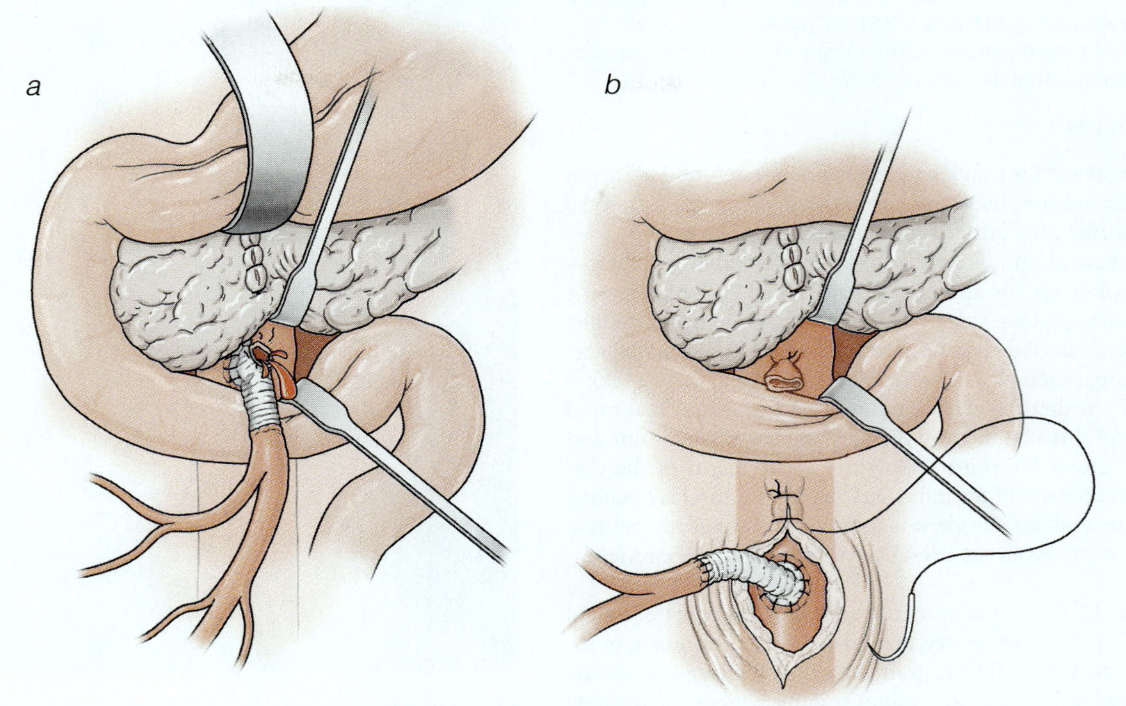

Figure 8 (*a*) When complex grafting procedures to the superior mesenteric artery are necessary, it may be dangerous to place the proximal suture line near an associated pancreatic injury. (*b*) The proximal suture line should be on the lower aorta, away from the upper abdominal injuries, and should be covered with retroperitoneal tissue.

complex injury to the superior mesenteric artery, the injured area should be resected and a temporary intraluminal Argyle, Javid, or Pruitt-Inahara shunt inserted to maintain flow to the midgut during resuscitation in the surgical intensive care unit. When ligation is indicated for more distal injuries to the superior mesenteric artery, segments of the ileum or even the right colon may have to be resected because of ischemia.

The survival rate in patients with penetrating injuries to the superior mesenteric artery is approximately 55% to 60% overall [*see Table 2*] but only 20% to 25% when any form of repair more complex than lateral arteriorrhaphy is necessary.

An injury to the proximal renal artery may also be present under a supramesocolic hematoma or bleeding area. When active hemorrhage is present, control of the supraceliac abdominal aorta in or just below the aortic hiatus must be obtained. When only a hematoma or a known thrombosis of the proximal renal artery is present, proximal vascular control can be obtained by elevating the transverse mesocolon and dissecting the vessel from the lateral aspect of the abdominal aorta. Options for repair of either the proximal or the distal renal artery are described elsewhere [*see* Injuries in Zone 2, *below*].

The superior mesenteric vein is the other great vessel of the abdomen that may be injured in the supramesocolic or retromesocolic area of the midline retroperitoneum. Because of the overlying pancreas, the proximity of the uncinate process, and the close association of this vessel with the superior mesenteric artery, repair of the superior mesenteric vein is quite difficult. As with injuries to the superior mesenteric artery (see above), one may have to transect the neck of the pancreas between noncrushing vascular or intestinal clamps to gain access to a perforation of the superior mesenteric vein. An injury to this vein below the inferior border of the pancreas can be managed by compressing it manually between one's fingers as an assistant places a continuous 5-0 polypropylene suture to complete the repair. When a penetrating injury to the vein has a posterior component, one must ligate multiple collateral vessels entering the vein in this area to achieve proper visualization.

There is now excellent evidence that young trauma patients tolerate ligation of the superior mesenteric vein well when vigorous postoperative fluid resuscitation is performed to reverse the peripheral hypovolemia that results from splanchnic hypervolemia. Typically, ligation is followed almost immediately by swelling of the midgut and discoloration suggestive of impending ischemia. In such cases, closure of the skin with towel clips or sutures only, followed

Table 3 Survival after Injuries to Veins in the Abdomen

Injured Vessel	Survivors/All Patients	Survival Rate (%)
Superior mesenteric vein	75/104	72.1
Inferior vena cava (infrahepatic)	358/497	72.0
Suprarenal	47/79	59.4
Renal	55/84	65.4
Infrarenal	214/275	77.8
Renal vein	38/43	88.4
Iliac vein	123/137*	89.8
	282/404†	69.8
Portal vein	67/134	50

*Isolated iliac artery injury.
†Other vascular injury also present.

by early reoperation, may be necessary to reassure the operating surgeon that the ischemia has not become permanent.

The survival rate in patients with injuries to the superior mesenteric vein is approximately 72% [see Table 3].

INFRAMESOCOLIC

The lower area of the midline retroperitoneum in zone 1 is known as the midline inframesocolic area. Injuries to either the infrarenal abdominal aorta or the inferior vena cava occur in this area.

The infrarenal abdominal aorta is exposed by pulling the transverse mesocolon up toward the patient's head, eviscerating the small bowel to one's own side of the table, and opening the midline retroperitoneum until the left renal vein is exposed. A proximal aortic cross-clamp is then placed immediately inferior to this vessel [see Figure 9]. When there is active hemorrhage from this area, rapid proximal control is obtained by dividing the lesser omentum and applying the cross-clamp just below the aortic hiatus of the diaphragm. Distal control of the infrarenal abdominal aorta is obtained by dividing the midline retroperitoneum down to the aortic bifurcation, taking care to avoid the left-sided origin of the inferior mesenteric artery.

Injuries to the infrarenal aorta are repaired by means of lateral aortorrhaphy, patch aortoplasty, an end-to-end anastomosis, or insertion of a Dacron or PTFE graft. Much as with injuries to the suprarenal abdominal aorta in young trauma patients, it is rarely possible to place a tube graft larger than 12 or 14 mm. Because the retroperitoneal tissue is often thin at this location in young patients, an appropriate option after the aortic repair is to mobilize the gastrocolic omentum, flip it into the lesser sac superiorly, and then bring it down over the infrarenal aortic graft through a hole in the transverse mesocolon. Another option is to mobilize the gastrocolic omentum away from the right side of the colon and then swing the mobilized tissue into the left lateral gutter just below the ligament of Treitz to cover the graft.

The survival rate in patients with injuries to the infrarenal abdominal aorta is approximately 45% [see Table 2].

Injury to the inferior vena cava below the liver should be suspected when the aorta is found to be intact underneath an inframesocolic hematoma, when such a hematoma appears to be more extensive on the right side of the abdomen than on the left, or when there is active hemorrhage coming through the base of the mesentery of the ascending colon or the hepatic flexure. It is certainly possible to visualize the inferior vena cava through the midline retroperitoneal exposure just described (see above); however, most surgeons are more comfortable with visualizing the vessel by mobilizing the right half of the colon and the C loop of the duodenum [see 27 Operative Exposure of Abdominal Injuries and Closure of the Abdomen]. With this right medial visceral rotation maneuver, the right kidney is left in situ unless there is an associated injury to the posterior aspect of the right renal vein, to the suprarenal vena cava, or to the right kidney itself. Right medial visceral rotation, in conjunction with the Kocher maneuver, permits visualization of the entire vena caval system from the confluence of the iliac veins to the suprarenal vena cava below the liver.

For proper exposure of a hole in a large vein such as the inferior vena cava, the loose retroperitoneal fatty tissue must be dissected away from the wall of the vessel. Active hemorrhage coming from the anterior surface of the inferior vena cava is best controlled by applying a Satinsky vascular clamp. If it is difficult to apply this clamp, one should try grasping the area of the perforation with a pair of vascular forceps or two Allis clamps; this step may facilitate safe application of the Satinsky clamp. When the perforation in the

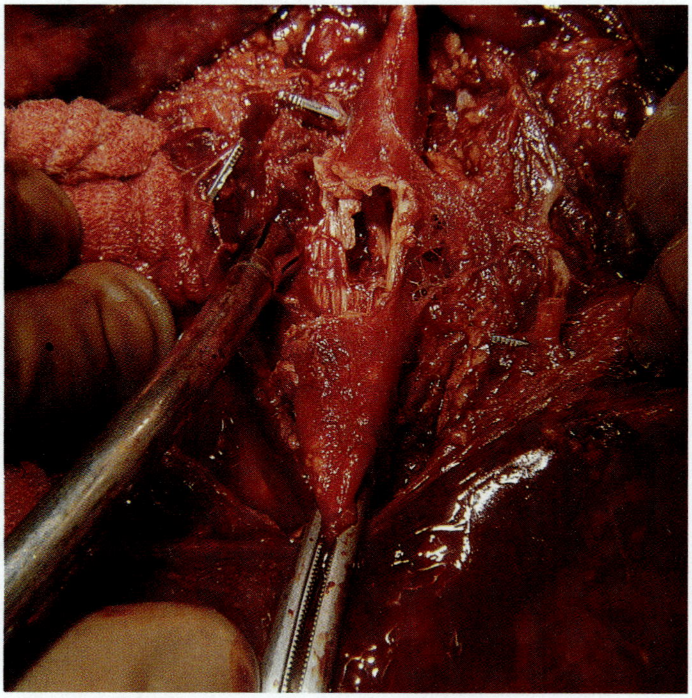

Figure 9 Shown is a gunshot wound to the infrarenal abdominal aorta viewed through standard inframesocolic exposure.

inferior vena cava is more lateral or posterior, it is often helpful to compress the vessel proximally and distally around the perforation, using gauze sponges placed in straight sponge sticks. On occasion, an extensive injury to the inferior vena cava can be controlled only by completely occluding the entire inferior vena cava with large DeBakey aortic cross-clamps. This maneuver interrupts much of the venous return to the right side of the heart and is poorly tolerated by hypotensive patients unless the infrarenal abdominal aorta is cross-clamped simultaneously.

There are two anatomic areas in which vascular control of an injury to the inferior vena cava below the liver is difficult to obtain: (1) the confluence of the common iliac veins and (2) the junction of the renal veins with the inferior vena cava. One interesting approach to an injury to the inferior vena cava at the confluence of the iliac veins is temporary division of the overlying right common iliac artery, coupled with mobilization of the aortic bifurcation to the patient's left. This approach yields a better view of the common iliac veins and the proximal inferior vena cava and makes repair considerably easier than it would be if the aortic bifurcation were left in place. Once the vein is repaired, the right common iliac artery is reconstituted via an end-to-end anastomosis. The usual approach to injuries to the inferior vena cava at its junction with the renal veins involves clamp or sponge-stick compression of the infrarenal and suprarenal vena cava as well as control of both renal veins with Silastic loops to facilitate the direct application of angled vascular clamps. As noted, medial mobilization of the right kidney may permit the application of a partial occlusion clamp across the inferior vena cava at its junction with the right renal vein as an alternative approach to an injury in this area. Another useful technique for controlling hemorrhage from the inferior vena cava at any location is to insert a 5 ml or 30 ml Foley balloon catheter into the caval laceration and then inflate it in the lumen. Once the bleeding is controlled, vascular clamps are positioned around the perforation, and the balloon catheter is removed before repair of the vessel.

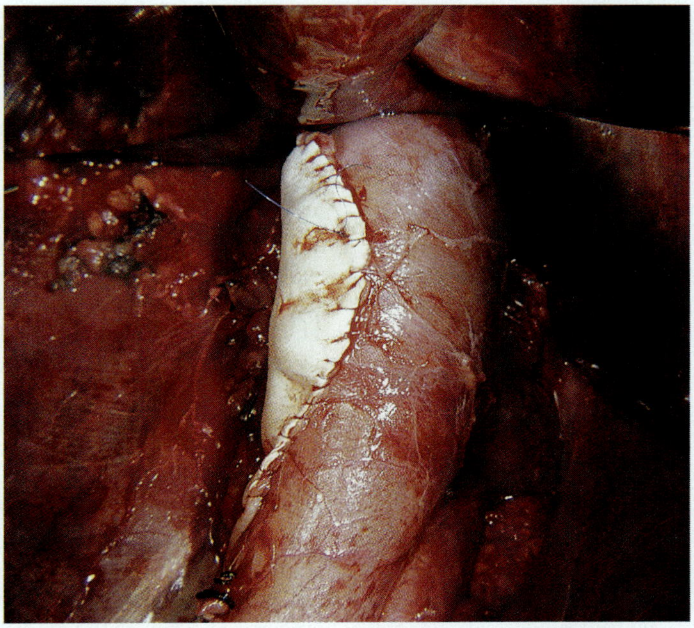

Figure 10 Shown is PTFE patch repair of an injury to the infrarenal inferior vena cava.

Anterior perforations of the inferior vena cava are managed by means of transverse repair with a continuous 4-0 or 5-0 polypropylene suture. Much has been written about visualizing posterior perforations by extending anterior perforations, but in my experience, opportunities to apply this approach have been rare. It is often easier to roll the vena cava to one side to complete a continuous suture repair of a posterior perforation. When both anterior and posterior perforations have been repaired, there is usually a significant degree of narrowing of the inferior vena cava, which may lead to slow postoperative occlusion. If the patient's condition is unstable and a coagulopathy has developed, no further attempt should be made to revise the repair. If the patient is stable, there may be some justification for applying a large PTFE patch to prevent this postoperative occlusion [see Figure 10].

Ligation of the infrarenal inferior vena cava is appropriate for young patients who are exsanguinating and in whom a complex repair of the vessel would be necessary. Such patients require vigorous resuscitation with crystalloid solutions in the postoperative period; in addition, both lower extremities should be wrapped with elastic compression wraps and elevated for 5 to 7 days after operation. Patients who have some residual edema during the later stages of hospitalization despite the elastic compression wraps should be fitted with full-length custom-made support hose. Ligation of the suprarenal inferior vena cava is occasionally necessary when the patient has an extensive injury at this location and appears to be in an irreversible shock state during operation. If the patient's condition improves during a brief period of resuscitation in the SICU, reoperation and reconstruction with an externally supported PTFE graft are necessary to prevent renal failure.

The survival rate in patients with injuries to the inferior vena cava depends on the location of the injury; it ranges from 60% for the suprarenal vena cava to 78% for the infrarenal vena cava.

Injuries in Zone 2

Hematoma or hemorrhage in zone 2 is cause to suspect the presence of injury to the renal artery, the renal vein, or the kidney.

In patients who have sustained blunt abdominal trauma but in whom preoperative intravenous pyelography, renal arteriography, or CT of the kidneys yields normal findings, there is no justification for opening a perirenal hematoma if one is found at a subsequent operation [see Figure 11].

In highly selected stable patients with penetrating wounds to the flank, there are some data to justify performing preoperative computed tomography. On occasion, documentation of an isolated minor renal injury in the absence of peritoneal findings on physical examination makes it possible to manage such patients nonoperatively. In all other patients with penetrating wounds, when a perirenal hematoma is found during initial exploration, the hematoma should be unroofed and the wound tract explored. If the hematoma is not rapidly expanding and there is no active hemorrhage from the perirenal area, one may control the ipsilateral renal artery with a Silastic loop in the midline of the retroperitoneum at the base of the mesocolon [see Figure 12]. Control of the left renal vein can be obtained at the same location; however, control of the proximal right renal vein requires mobilization of the C loop of the duodenum and dissection of the vena cava at its junction with this vessel.

If there is active hemorrhage from the kidney through Gerota's fascia or from the retroperitoneum overlying the renal vessels, no central renal vascular control is necessary. In such a situation, the retroperitoneum lateral to the injured kidney should be opened, and the kidney should be manually elevated directly into the abdominal incision. A large vascular clamp should then be applied directly to the hilar vessels of the elevated kidney to control any further bleeding.

Occasionally, a small perforation of the renal artery can be repaired by lateral arteriorrhaphy or resection with an end-to-end anastomosis. Interposition grafting and replacement of the renal artery with either the hepatic artery (on the right) or the splenic artery (on the left) have been used on rare occasions, but such approaches ordinarily are not indicated unless the injured kidney is the only one the patient has. In patients who have sustained multiple intra-abdominal injuries from penetrating wounds or have undergone a long period of ischemia while other injuries were being repaired, nephrectomy is the appropriate choice for a major renovascular injury, provided that intraoperative palpation has confirmed the presence of a normal contralateral kidney.

The role of renal revascularization in patients who have intimal

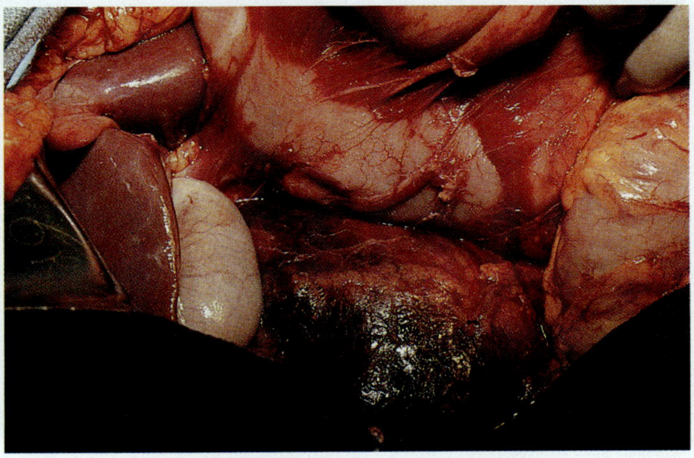

Figure 11 A right perirenal hematoma was not opened at operation, because preoperative abdominal CT documented a reasonably intact kidney.

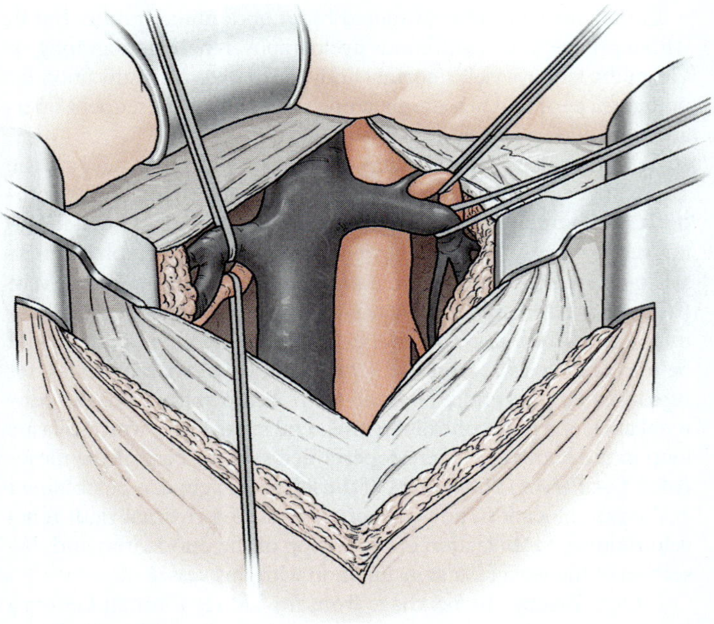

444 — III TRAUMA AND THERMAL INJURY

Figure 12 Midline looping of respective renal vessels is performed before entry into any perirenal hematoma.

tears in the renal arteries as a result of deceleration-type trauma remains controversial. If a circumferential intimal tear is noted on preoperative arteriography but flow to the kidney is preserved, the decision whether to repair the artery depends on whether laparotomy is necessary for other injuries and whether the opportunity for anticoagulation is available. If there are no other significant injuries and flow to the kidney is preserved despite the presence of an intimal tear, anticoagulation and a repeat isotope renogram within the first several days may be justified. If occlusion of the proximal renal artery from blunt deceleration-type trauma is documented, the critical factor for renal salvage is the time from occlusion to revascularization. Renal artery occlusion from deceleration-type trauma that is detected within 12 hours of injury is best treated with immediate operation, resection of the area of intimal damage, and an end-to-end anastomosis performed by an experienced vascular trauma team [*see Figures 13 and 14*]. Given proper exposure and medial mobilization of the kidney, this operation is not technically difficult in a young trauma patient whose renal artery is otherwise normal. The value of renal perfusion during the short period of clamping or decapsulation of the previously ischemic kidney is unclear: few cases of repair of a thrombosis have been reported in the literature. Many patients will experience a prolonged period of renal dysfunction on the side of the arterial repair; they should be followed with isotope renograms in the postoperative period.

The survival rate in patients with injuries to the renal arteries is approximately 86% [*see Table 2*].

Many patients with penetrating wounds to the renal veins are quite stable as a result of the retroperitoneal tamponade described earlier (see above). Once vascular control is obtained with the direct application of clamps, lateral venorrhaphy is the preferred technique of repair. Nephrectomy should be performed if ligation of the right renal vein is necessary to control hemorrhage, whereas the medial left renal vein may be ligated as long as the left adrenal and gonadal veins are intact. It should be noted, however, that in some series, more postoperative renal complications were noted when this maneuver was used on the left side.

The survival rate in patients with injuries to the renal veins is approximately 88% [*see Table 3*].

Injuries in Zone 3

Hematoma or hemorrhage in either lateral pelvic area is suggestive of injury to the iliac artery or the iliac vein.

When lateral pelvic hematoma or hemorrhage is noted after penetrating trauma, compression with a laparotomy pad or the fingers

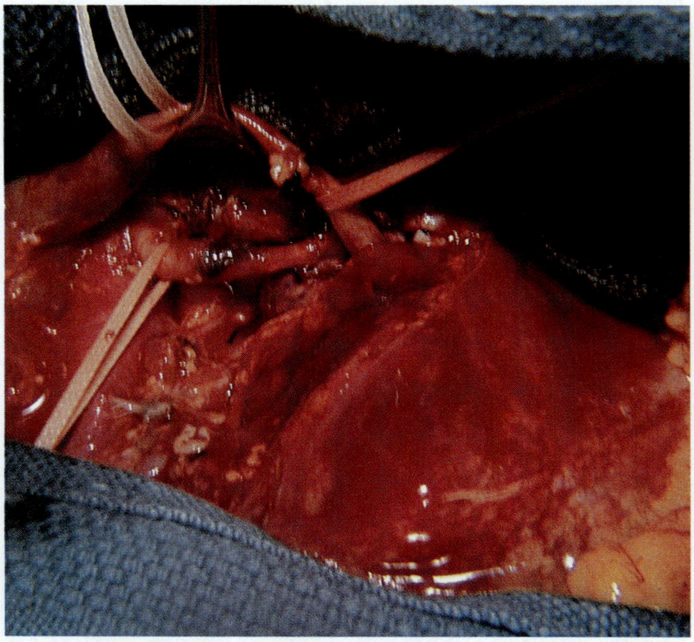

Figure 13 With the left renal vein elevated, a hematoma ring may be noted overlying a blunt intimal tear in an occluded left renal artery.

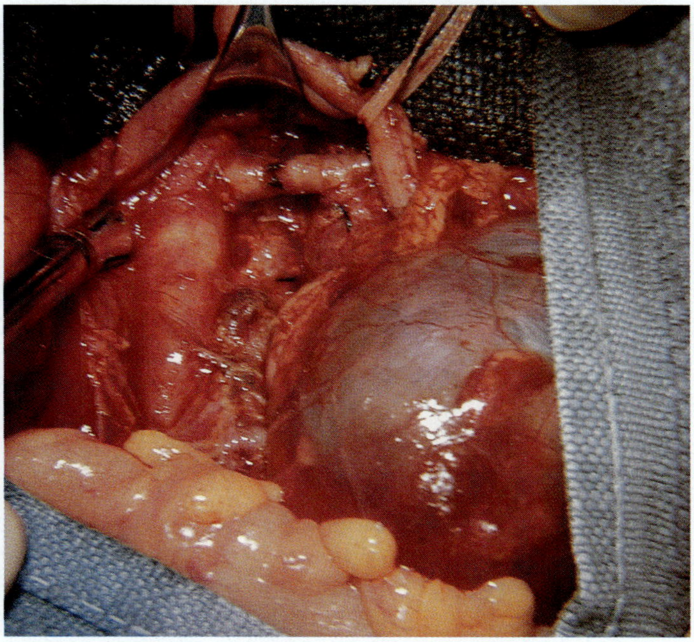

Figure 14 In the same patient as in Figure 13, the intimal tear in the left renal artery was resected, an end-to-end anastomosis was performed, and blood flow to the left kidney was restored.

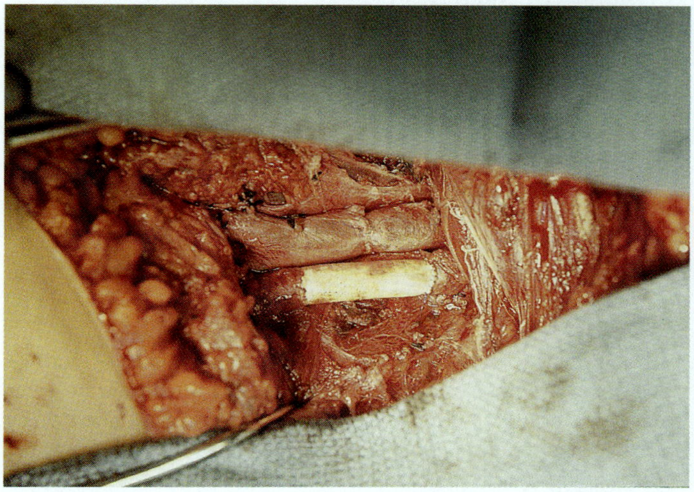

Figure 15 A 24-year-old man experienced a gunshot wound to the left external iliac artery and vein. The arterial injury was repaired with segmental resection and insertion of an 8 mm PTFE graft; the venous injury was repaired with segmental resection and an end-to-end anastomosis.

should be maintained as proximal and distal vascular control is obtained. The proximal common iliac arteries are exposed by eviscerating the small bowel to the right and dividing the midline retroperitoneum over the aortic bifurcation. In young trauma patients, the common iliac artery usually is not adherent to the common iliac vein, and Silastic loops can be passed rapidly around these vessels to provide proximal vascular control. Distal vascular control is most easily obtained where the external iliac artery and vein come out of the pelvis proximal to the inguinal ligament. Even with proximal and distal control of the common or the external iliac artery and vein, there is often continued back-bleeding from the internal iliac artery. Such bleeding is controlled by elevating the Silastic loops on the proximal and distal iliac artery and then either clamping or looping the internal iliac artery, which is the only major branch vessel that descends into the pelvis.

For transpelvic bilateral iliac vascular injuries resulting from a penetrating wound, a technique of total pelvic vascular isolation has been described. Proximally, the abdominal aorta and the inferior vena cava are cross-clamped just above their bifurcations, and distally, both the external iliac artery and the external iliac vein are cross-clamped, with one clamp on each side of the distal pelvis. Back-bleeding from the internal iliac vessels is minimal with this approach.

Ligation of either the common or the external iliac artery in a hypotensive trauma patient leads to a 40% to 50% amputation rate in the postoperative period; consequently, injuries to these vessels should be repaired if at all possible. The standard options for repair—lateral arteriorrhaphy, completion of a partial transection with an end-to-end anastomosis, and resection of the injured area with insertion of a conduit—are feasible in most situations [*see Figure 15*]. On rare occasions, it may be preferable either to mobilize the ipsilateral internal iliac artery to serve as a replacement for the external iliac artery or to transpose one iliac artery to the side of the contralateral iliac artery.

One unique problem associated with repair of the common or the external iliac artery is the choice of technique when significant enteric or fecal contamination is present in the pelvis. In such cases, there is a substantial risk of postoperative pelvic cellulitis, a pelvic abscess, or both, which may lead to blowout of any type of repair.

When extensive contamination is present, it is appropriate to divide the common or external iliac artery above the level of injury, close the injury with a double row of continuous 4-0 or 5-0 polypropylene sutures, and bury the stump underneath uninjured retroperitoneum. If a stable patient has obvious ischemia of the ipsilateral lower extremity at the completion of this proximal ligation, one may perform an extra-anatomic femorofemoral crossover graft to restore arterial flow to the extremity. If the patient is unstable, one should take several minutes to perform an ipsilateral four-compartment below-knee fasciotomy; this step will counteract the ischemic edema that inevitably leads to a compartment syndrome and compromises the early survival of the leg. After adequate resuscitation in the SICU, the patient should be returned to the OR for the femorofemoral graft within 4 to 6 hours.

Injuries to the internal iliac arteries are usually ligated even if they occur bilaterally, because young trauma patients typically have extensive collateral flow through the pelvis.

The survival rate in patients with isolated injuries to the iliac artery exceeds 80% when tamponade is present [*see Table 2*]. If the injury is large and free bleeding has occurred preoperatively, however, the survival rate is only 45%.

Hemorrhage from injuries to the iliac veins can usually be controlled by means of compression with either sponge sticks or the fingers. As noted, division of the right common iliac artery may be necessary for proper visualization of an injury to the right common iliac vein. Similarly, ligation and division of the internal iliac artery on the side of the pelvis yield improved exposure of an injury to an ipsilateral internal iliac vein.

Injuries to the common or the external iliac vein are best treated by means of lateral venorrhaphy with continuous 4-0 or 5-0 polypropylene sutures. Significant narrowing often results, and a number of reports have demonstrated occlusion on postoperative venography. For patients with narrowing or occlusion, as well as for those in whom ligation was necessary to control exsanguinating hemorrhage, the use of elastic compression wraps and elevation for the first 5 to 7 days after operation is mandatory.

The survival rate in patients with injuries to the iliac veins ranges from 70% to 90%, depending on whether associated vascular injuries are present [*see Table 3*].

Injuries in the Porta Hepatis or Retrohepatic Area

PORTA HEPATIS

Hematoma or hemorrhage in the area of the portal triad in the right upper quadrant is cause to suspect the presence of injury to the portal vein or the hepatic artery or of vascular injury combined with an injury to the common bile duct.

If a hematoma is present, the proximal hepatoduodenal ligament should be occluded with a vascular clamp (the Pringle maneuver [*see 28 Injuries to the Liver, Biliary Tract, Spleen, and Diaphragm*]) before the hematoma is entered. If the hematoma is centrally located in the porta, one may also be able to apply an angled vascular clamp to the distal end of the portal structures at their entrance into the liver.

If hemorrhage is occurring, compression of the bleeding vessels with the fingers should suffice until the vascular clamp is in place. Once proximal and distal vascular control is obtained, the three structures in the hepatoduodenal ligament must be dissected out very carefully because of the danger of blindly placing sutures in proximity to the common bile duct [*see Figure 16*].

Injuries to the hepatic artery in this location are occasionally

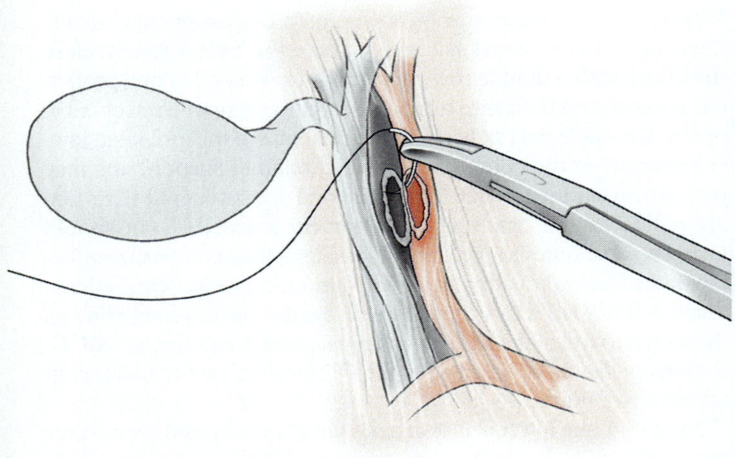

Figure 16 Failure to properly dissect out the structures in the porta hepatis after a penetrating wound led to the creation of an iatrogenic hepatic artery–portal vein fistula, which was corrected after the arrival of the attending surgeon.

amenable to lateral repair, though ligation without reconstruction is ordinarily well tolerated because of the extensive collateral arterial flow to the liver. If an associated hepatic injury calls for extensive suturing or debridement, ligation of the common hepatic artery will certainly lead to increased postoperative necrosis of the hepatic repair. Moreover, ligation of the common hepatic artery, the right or left hepatic artery supplying the injured lobe, and the portal vein branch to that lobe will lead to necrosis of the lobe and will necessitate hepatectomy. Finally, ligation of the right hepatic artery to control hemorrhage should be followed by cholecystectomy.

Because of the large size of the portal vein and its posterior position in the hepatoduodenal ligament, injuries to this vessel are particularly lethal. Once the Pringle maneuver has been performed, mobilization of the common bile duct to the left and of the cystic duct superiorly, coupled with an extensive Kocher maneuver, allows excellent visualization of any injury to this vein above the superior border of the pancreas. When the perforation extends underneath the neck of the pancreas, it may be necessary to have an assistant compress the superior mesenteric vein below the pancreas and then to divide the pancreas between noncrushing intestinal clamps to obtain exposure of the junction of the superior mesenteric vein and the splenic vein.

The preferred technique for repairing an injury to the portal vein is lateral venorrhaphy with continuous 4-0 or 5-0 polypropylene sutures. Complex repairs that have been successful on rare occasions include end-to-end anastomosis, interposition grafting with externally supported PTFE, transposition of the splenic vein, and a venovenous shunt from the superior mesenteric vein to the distal portal vein or the inferior vena cava. Such vigorous attempts at restoration of blood flow are not justified in patients who are in severe hypovolemic shock, for whom ligation of the portal vein is more appropriate. In addition, if a portosystemic shunt is performed in such a patient, hepatic encephalopathy will result because hepatofugal flow will be present in the rerouted or bypassed portal vein. As with ligation of the superior mesenteric vein, it is necessary to infuse tremendous amounts of crystalloids to reverse the transient peripheral hypovolemia that occurs secondary to the splanchnic hypervolemia resulting from ligation of the portal vein.

Since the early 1980s, the survival rate in patients with injuries to the portal vein has been approximately 50% [*see Table 3*].

RETROHEPATIC AREA

Retrohepatic hematoma or hemorrhage is cause to suspect the presence of injury to the retrohepatic vena cava, a hepatic vein, or a renal blood vessel. In addition, hemorrhage in this area may signal injury to the overlying liver [*see 28 Injuries to the Liver, Biliary Tract, Spleen, and Diaphragm*].

If there is a hematoma that is not expanding or ruptured and clearly has no association with the right perirenal area, a tamponaded injury to the retrohepatic vena cava or a hepatic vein is present. Perihepatic packing around the right lobe of the liver for 24 to 48 hours has been shown to prevent further expansion and should be considered.

If hemorrhage is occurring that does not appear to be coming from the overlying liver, the right lobe of the liver should be compressed posteriorly to tamponade the caval perforation. The Pringle maneuver is then applied, and the surgical and nursing team, the anesthesiologist, and the blood blank are notified. Once the proper instruments and banked blood are in the OR, the overlying injured hepatic lobe is mobilized by dividing the triangular and anterior coronary ligaments and then lifted out of the subdiaphragmatic area. On occasion, an obvious perforation of the retrohepatic or suprahepatic vena cava or an obvious area where a hepatic vein was avulsed from the vena cava may be grasped with a forceps or a long Allis clamp; a Satinsky clamp may then be applied. Because of the copious bleeding that occurs as the liver is lifted and the hole in the vena cava sought, the anesthesiologist should start blood transfusions as the lobe is being mobilized.

If the hemorrhage is not controlled after one or two attempts, another technique must be tried. The most common choice is the insertion of a 36 French chest tube or a 9 mm endotracheal tube as an atriocaval shunt [*see 27 Operative Exposure of Abdominal Injuries and Closure of the Abdomen and 28 Injuries to the Liver, Biliary Tract, Spleen, and Diaphragm*]. The shunt can reduce bleeding by 40% to 60%, but vigorous hemorrhage persists until full control of the perforation is obtained with clamps or sutures. An alternative approach is to isolate the liver and the vena cava by cross-clamping of the supraceliac aorta, the porta hepatis, the suprarenal inferior vena cava, and the intrapericardial inferior vena cava. Because profoundly hypovolemic patients usually cannot tolerate cross-clamping of the inferior vena cava, this approach is rarely used.

The retrohepatic vena cava is repaired with continuous 4-0 or 5-0 polypropylene sutures. When the atriocaval shunt is removed from the heart after the vessel has been repaired, the right atrial appendage is ligated with a 2-0 silk tie.

The survival rate in patients undergoing atriocaval shunting and repair of the retrohepatic vena cava who are not in cardiac arrest has ranged from 33% to 50% in recent series.

Damage Control Laparotomy

Patients with injuries to the great vessels of the abdomen are ideal candidates for damage control laparotomy: they are uniformly hypothermic, acidotic, and coagulopathic on completion of the vascular repair, and a prolonged operation would lead to their demise. In such patients, packing of minor or moderate injuries to solid organs, packing of the retroperitoneum, stapling and rapid resection of multiple injuries to the GI tract, consideration of diffuse intra-abdominal packing, and towel-clip closure of the skin are all appropriate. If a towel-clip closure cannot be completed because of distention of the midgut (such as may be seen in association with profound shock or after ligation of the superior mesenteric or portal vein), a temporary silo made from a urologic irrigation bag can be used. The silo can be sewn to the skin edges with a continuous 2-0 polypropylene or nylon suture.

The patient is then rapidly moved to the SICU for further resuscitation. Priorities in the SICU include rapid restoration of normal body temperature, reversal of shock, infusion of intravenous bicarbonate to correct a persistent pH lower than 7.2, and administration of fresh frozen plasma, platelets, and cryoprecipitate when indicated. It is usually possible to return the patient to the OR for removal of clot and packs, reconstruction of the GI tract, irrigation, and reapplication of a towel-clip or silo closure within 48 to 72 hours.

When massive distention of the midgut persists after 7 days of intensive care, the safest approach is to convert the patient to an open abdomen (i.e., without closure of the midline incision) and cover the midgut with a double-thickness layer of absorbable mesh. With proper nutritional support and occasional use of Dakin's solution to minimize bacterial contamination of the absorbable mesh, most patients are ready for the application of a split-thickness skin graft to the eviscerated midgut within 3 to 4 weeks of the original operation for an injury to a great vessel.

Complications

Besides those already mentioned, major complications associated with repair of injuries to the great vessels in the abdomen include thrombosis, dehiscence of the suture line, and infection. Because of the risk of occlusion of repairs in small vasoconstricted vessels (e.g., the superior mesenteric artery), it may be worthwhile to perform a second-look operation within 12 to 24 hours if the patient's metabolic state suggests that ischemia of the midgut is present. Early correction of an arterial thrombosis in the superior mesenteric artery may permit salvage of the midgut.

As noted [see Injuries in Zone 1, *above*], dehiscence of an end-to-end anastomosis or a vascular conduit inserted in the proximal superior mesenteric artery when there is an injury to the adjacent pancreas may be prevented by inserting a distal aorta–superior mesenteric artery bypass graft. To prevent adjacent loops of small bowel from adhering to the vascular suture lines, both lines should be covered with soft tissue (retroperitoneal tissue for the aortic suture line and mesenteric tissue for the superior mesenteric arterial suture line). Also as noted [see Injuries in Zone 3, *above*], when an extensive injury to either the common or the external iliac artery occurs in the presence of significant enteric or fecal contamination in the pelvis, ligation and extra-anatomic bypass may be necessary.

On occasion, vascular-enteric fistulas occur after repair of the anterior aorta or the insertion of grafts in either the abdominal aorta or the superior mesenteric artery. In my experience, such fistulas all occur at suture lines; hence, once again, proper coverage of suture lines with soft tissue should eliminate this complication.

Recommended Reading

Bongard FS, Wilson SE, Perry MO Jr: Vascular Injuries in Surgical Practice. Appleton & Lange, Stamford, Connecticut, 1991

Feliciano DV: Abdominal vessels. The Textbook of Penetrating Trauma. Ivatury RR, Cayten CG, Eds. Williams & Wilkins, Baltimore, 1996

Feliciano DV: Truncal vascular trauma. Vascular Surgery: Theory and Practice. Callow AD, Ernst CB, Eds. Appleton & Lange, Stamford, Connecticut, 1995

Feliciano DV, Burch JM, Graham JM: Abdominal vascular injury. Trauma, 3rd ed. Feliciano DV, Moore EE, Mattox KL, Eds. Appleton & Lange, Stamford, Connecticut, 1996

Feliciano DV, Mattox KL: Thoracic and abdominal vascular trauma. Vascular Surgery: Principles and Practice. Veith FV, Hobson RW II, Williams RA, et al, Eds. McGraw-Hill, New York, 1994

Wilson RF, Dulchavsky S: Abdominal vascular trauma. Management of Trauma: Pitfalls and Practice. Wilson RF, Walt AJ, Eds. Williams & Wilkins, Baltimore, 1996

Acknowledgments

Figures 1 and 2   Marcia Kammerer.

Figures 3, 5, 8, 12, and 16   Tom Moore.

Figures 4 and 9   From "Abdominal Vascular Injury," by D. V. Feliciano, J. M. Burch, and J. M. Graham, in *Trauma*, 3rd ed., edited by D. V. Feliciano, E. E. Moore, and K. L. Mattox. Appleton & Lange, Stamford, Connecticut, 1996. Reproduced by permission.

Table 1   Adapted from "Organ Injury Scaling III: Chest Wall, Abdominal Vascular, Ureter, Bladder, and Urethra," by E. E. Moore, T. H. Cogbill, G. J. Jurkovich, et al, in *Journal of Trauma* 33:337, 1992.

Tables 2 and 3   Data from "Abdominal Vascular Injury," by D. V. Feliciano, J. M. Burch, and J. M. Graham, in *Trauma*, 3rd ed., edited by D. V. Feliciano, E. E. Moore, and K. L. Mattox. Appleton & Lange, Stamford, Connecticut, 1996.

31 INJURIES TO THE UROGENITAL TRACT

Hunter Wessells, M.D., and Jack W. McAninch, M.D.

Hematuria is the hallmark of injury to the urogenital system. Location of the injury and identification of its cause help determine which urologic organs are most likely to have been injured by a particular traumatic event. In penetrating trauma to the abdomen, hematuria signals the need to evaluate the kidneys, ureters, and bladder. Urethral and genital injuries are suspected only with wounds to the pelvis, perineum, and buttocks. When hematuria occurs in association with blunt injuries and pelvic fracture, the entire genitourinary system should be evaluated.

This chapter includes a separate algorithm for each of the major urogenital organs. Injury to both the upper and the lower urinary tract is rare, but a high index of suspicion must be maintained for detection of such an injury. Injury to the female reproductive organs requires special expertise in evaluation and management, particularly if the patient is pregnant or the victim of a sexual assault.

Injuries to the Kidneys

INITIAL EVALUATION

The most reliable sign of injury to the kidney is hematuria, whether microscopic or gross. However, the degree of hematuria is not correlated with the severity of injury, and patients with serious injuries may have no blood in their urine.[1] The same staging system is used to classify both blunt and penetrating injuries [see Figure 1], and the only significant difference in their management is in the initial evaluation [see Figure 2]. For patients with blunt trauma, we recommend the following criteria for radiographic evaluation of injuries to the kidney[2]: adults with microscopic hematuria and systolic blood pressure of at least 90 mm Hg do not require imaging unless serious associated injuries suggest a deceleration injury; all pediatric trauma patients, patients with gross hematuria, and patients with microscopic hematuria and shock require radiographic evaluation; intravenous urography is recommended in hemodynamically stable patients with blunt renal trauma; and in patients requiring computed tomography for the evaluation of other injuries, intravenous pyelography (IVP) is unnecessary.

All penetrating injuries of the kidney require exploration unless a complete radiographic evaluation demonstrates that an injury can be managed nonoperatively. Computed tomography, which is ideal for study of penetrating injuries, should be the first radiographic method used in hemodynamically stable patients.[3] Intravenous urography is adequate for the evaluation of penetrating trauma only if it includes tomography and does not demonstrate poor visualization, an irregular contour, or extravasation, which should prompt further studies or exploration.[4] When CT is not available, angiography is adequate for staging of renal injuries.

All grade 1 and 2 renal injuries, regardless of the mechanism of injury, can be managed without operation. The absolute indications for renal exploration include pulsatile and expanding hematomas and hemodynamic instability resulting from renal injury.[5] In stable patients with adequate staging, grade 3 and nonvascular grade 4 injuries (including devitalized fragments and urinary extravasation) can be observed. In patients requiring laparotomy for associated injuries, we perform renal exploration and reconstruction to reduce the likelihood of delayed complications.[6,7] Shattered kidneys (grade 5) and vascular injuries (grades 4 and 5) require immediate renal exploration. An exception is thrombosis of the renal artery or its branches, which may be treated expectantly if revascularization is not performed expediently in a patient with no associated injuries.

A significant number of patients with a penetrating injury and a minority of those with blunt trauma require immediate laparotomy before they can be evaluated radiographically.[8] Hematuria is the key clinical sign, alerting the surgeon to the possibility of renal injury in inadequately staged patients. In cases of penetrating injury, the presence of a retroperitoneal hematoma should prompt further evaluation. We obtain a single-shot IVP 10 minutes after bolus injection of 150 ml of iodinated contrast material, ensuring the presence of a functioning contralateral unit before exploration. If the injured kidney is imaged adequately and found to be normal, exploration may be omitted. In patients with blunt injuries and gross hematuria or with microscopic hematuria in the presence of shock, intraoperative imaging is required, even in the absence of a retroperitoneal hematoma. If the kidney is not adequately imaged, the possibility of renal artery thrombosis should be considered.

OPERATIVE MANAGEMENT

A midline transabdominal incision permits exploration of the kidneys and abdomen. After areas of bleeding have been packed with laparotomy sponges, the first step is isolation of the renal vasculature before opening Gerota's fascia. This technique, which has reduced our nephrectomy rate, allows rapid control of bleeding from serious injuries.[9] In all renal explorations, regardless of the degree of injury, we begin with isolation of the renal vessels, which is best performed by opening the posterior peritoneum overlying the aorta, preventing premature entry of the retroperitoneal hematoma. Even in the presence of large hematomas, the inferior mesenteric vein serves as a landmark for location of the aorta. Working cephalad along the aorta, the surgeon encounters the left renal vein first and subsequently both renal arteries. The best way to find

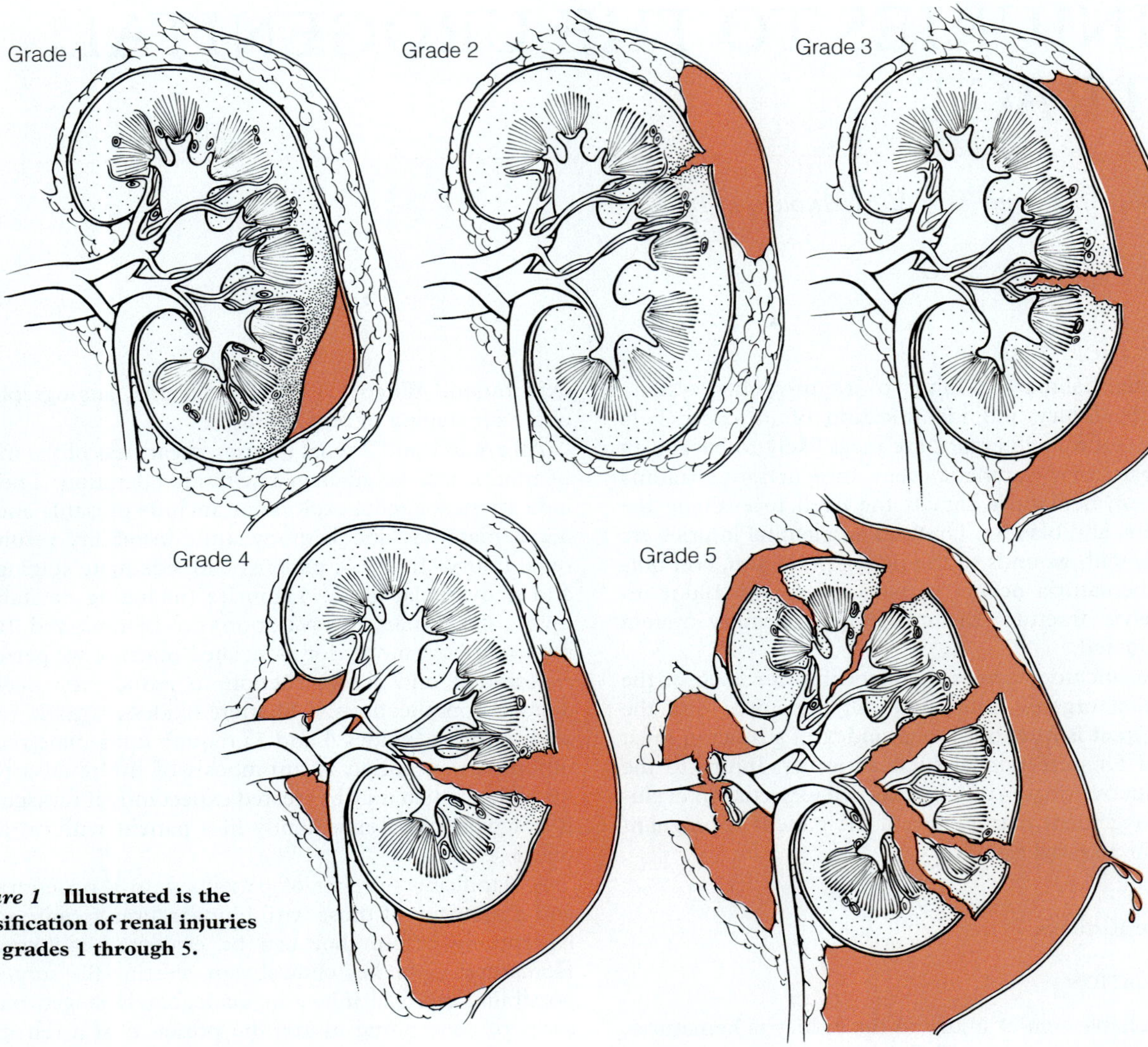

Figure 1 Illustrated is the classification of renal injuries into grades 1 through 5.

the right renal artery is to dissect between the aorta and the vena cava; dissection lateral to the vena cava may lead to inadvertent isolation of a segmental branch of the renal artery. Isolation of the right renal vein may be easier after reflection of the right colon and duodenum. We place vessel loops around the artery and vein, allowing rapid access to the vessels if significant bleeding occurs. The renal vessels can also be approached laterally if the duodenum or left colon has been mobilized.

Gerota's fascia is opened only after vascular isolation. If release of the tamponade effect causes bleeding, we use Rumel tourniquets or vascular clamps to occlude the renal artery and renal vein. Clamping of the renal artery alone usually controls bleeding. If it does not, the surgeon should suspect a venous injury and occlude the vein. It is not routine to cool the surface of the kidney after clamping of the renal artery, because patients with trauma are often hypothermic and coagulopathic. Clamp time should be limited to less than 30 minutes, if possible.

Total exposure of the kidney, by means of sharp and blunt dissection, is necessary to rule out injury to the parenchyma, renal pedicle, and collecting system. The renal capsule can easily be pulled off the parenchyma if dissection is not meticulous. Once the kidney has been delivered into the field, the extent of injury can be assessed and reconstruction can be planned. Renal reconstruction includes debridement of all devitalized tissue, hemostasis, closure of the collecting system, defect coverage, and drainage [see Figure 3]. With these techniques, renal salvage should be possible in close to 90 percent of kidney explorations.[5] Nephrectomy should be reserved for destroyed kidneys that cannot be reconstructed or for serious renal injury associated with other life-threatening injuries, such as vascular or hepatic trauma.

Debridement of devitalized tissue permits reconstruction with healthy tissue and prevents delayed bleeding and urinary extravasation. If the renal capsule is present at the margins of the wound, it should be peeled back and preserved for subsequent closure. A scalpel is used to remove the devitalized renal parenchyma until bleeding occurs at the margin. Polar injuries can be debrided by guillotine amputation of the parenchyma.

Manual compression usually controls bleeding during the ligation of small vessels. Ligation of individual vessels with absorbable monofilament, such as 4-0 chromic, achieves hemostasis. Temporary release of renal artery occlusion for the assessment of hemostasis is not recommended. Ligation of venous bleeding points generally controls adjacent arterial sources.

Once hemostasis is satisfactory, the collecting system should be scrutinized for evidence of injury. If the extent is unclear, 2 to 3 ml of methylene blue can be injected directly into the renal pelvis, while the ureter is occluded, to identify any openings in the collecting system. Open calyxes or infundibula can be closed with running 4-0 absorbable suture. For injuries to the renal pelvis, interrupted closure is more reliable.

The renal capsule can often be used to cover exposed renal parenchyma. The defect in the parenchyma is filled with folded absorbable gelatin sponges or other hemostatic agents, and with interrupted sutures through the capsule but not the parenchyma, the capsule is closed over the bolsters. If the capsule is not available, options include an omental or perinephric fat flap tacked down over the defect, a patch of Dexon or peritoneum, or an entire sac of Dexon wrapped around the kidney, keeping the parenchymal edges well apposed.[5,10]

At the end of the procedure, the kidney should be returned to its location within Gerota's fascia. Drainage of the renal region is recommended, and either a closed-suction or a Penrose drain is acceptable. If there are significant injuries to the collecting system, a Penrose drain is preferable because it does not exert negative pressure on the repair site. Internalized drains and double J stents generally are not necessary for renal injuries. However, major injuries to the renal pelvis or the ureteropelvic junction (UPJ) should be drained with an internalized stent as well as a retroperitoneal drain.

POSTOPERATIVE CARE

Management of patients after operative or nonoperative intervention for renal trauma depends to a large extent on asso-

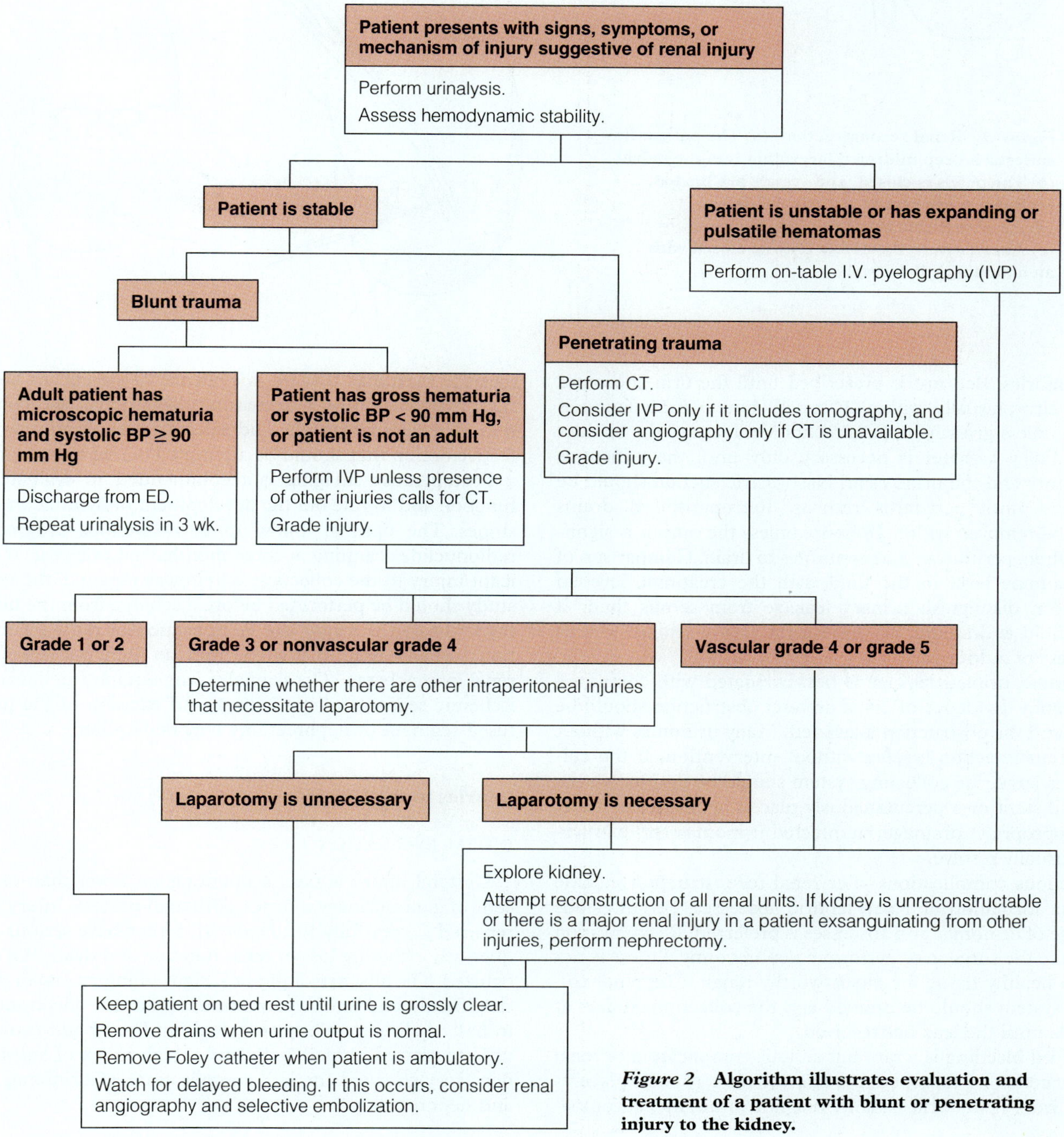

Figure 2 Algorithm illustrates evaluation and treatment of a patient with blunt or penetrating injury to the kidney.

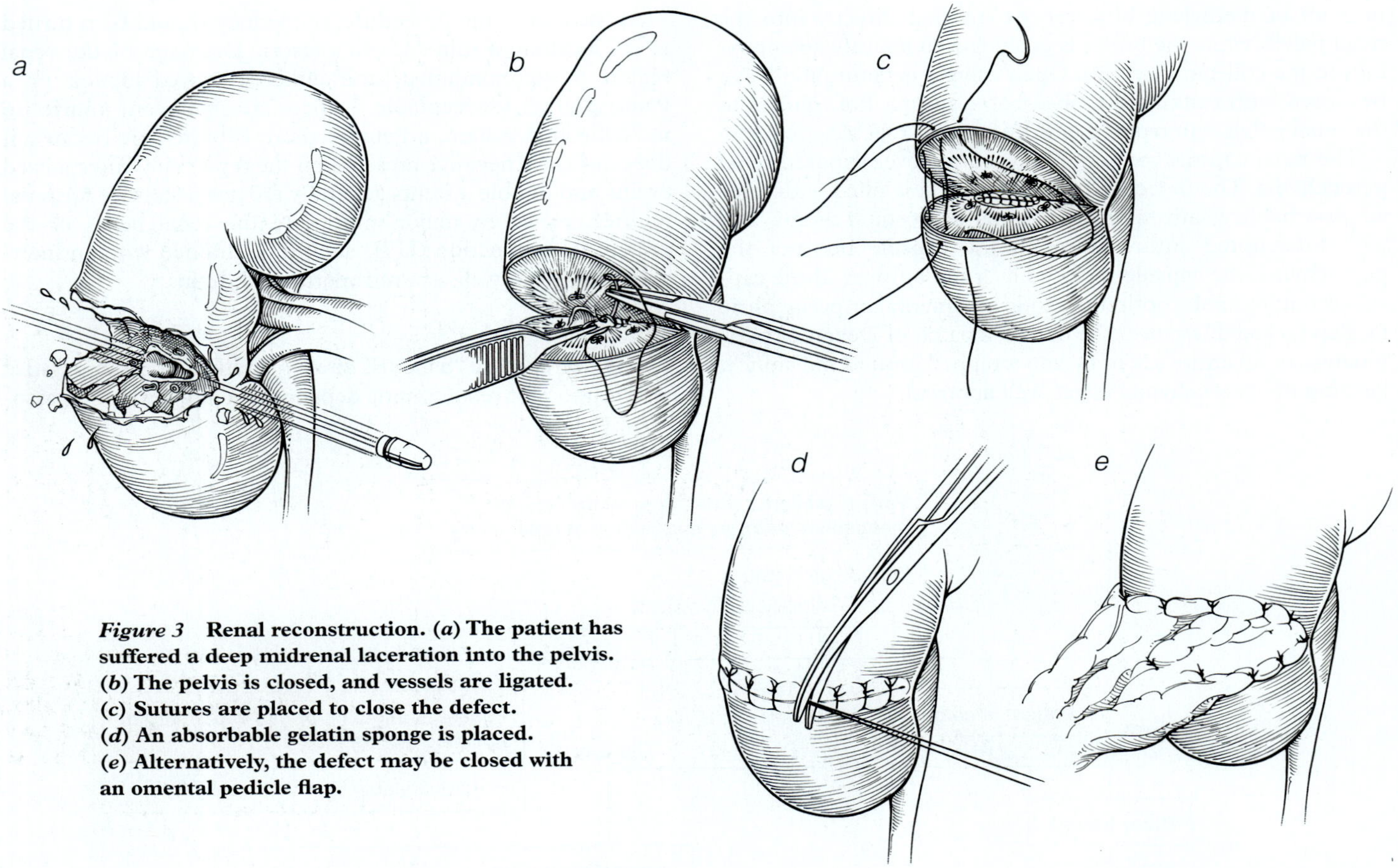

Figure 3 Renal reconstruction. (*a*) The patient has suffered a deep midrenal laceration into the pelvis. (*b*) The pelvis is closed, and vessels are ligated. (*c*) Sutures are placed to close the defect. (*d*) An absorbable gelatin sponge is placed. (*e*) Alternatively, the defect may be closed with an omental pedicle flap.

ciated injuries. Bed rest is prescribed until the urine becomes grossly clear, usually within 24 to 48 hours. Ambulation is allowed unless gross hematuria recurs. Drainage of the bladder with a Foley catheter is necessary only until the patient is ambulatory and the urine clear. Nasogastric suction should be continued until peristalsis returns. Retroperitoneal drains should be removed within 48 hours unless the output is significant. Often, peritoneal fluid continues to drain. Comparison of the creatinine level in the fluid with the creatinine level in serum can distinguish urinary leakage from serous fluid. If serous fluid is draining, we remove the retroperitoneal drains regardless of output.

Persistent urinary leakage is best evaluated with computed tomography. Evidence of distal ureteral obstruction should be sought and the obstruction alleviated. Many urinomas without concurrent infection resolve without intervention. If the collection is large, the collecting system should be drained with a double J stent or a percutaneously placed nephrostomy tube. With appropriate drainage, uninfected urinomas and extravasation usually resolve.

Infectious complications after renal reconstruction include urinoma formation and perinephric abscesses. Percutaneous drainage of urinomas and abscesses is preferred. Reexploration may force the surgeon to perform a nephrectomy if there is not enough healthy tissue for a trustworthy repair. The renal collecting system should be drained and the collection studied at intervals until the leak has resolved.

Delayed bleeding is a rare but serious complication of renal reconstruction or nonoperative management of major lacerations. Gross hematuria usually, but not invariably, accompanies the bleeding. If there is evidence of significant bleeding (i.e., hypotension or a decreasing hematocrit), the combination of renal angiography and selective embolization is an effective option that should be attempted before reexploration.[11]

Postoperative imaging is recommended to evaluate renal function and to rule out the development of hydronephrosis or stones. The optimal follow-up is intravenous urography or radionuclide scanning at three months and one year. If significant injury to the collecting system was repaired, the imaging study should be performed before discharge from the hospital. Hypertension is a rare late complication of renal reconstruction, usually renin-mediated from an ischemic segment of renal parenchyma. Occasionally, angiography delineates the ischemic segment of the kidney, and excision of the nonperfused segment or nephrectomy may be required.

Injuries to the Ureters

INITIAL EVALUATION

Ureteral injury is rare, accounting for fewer than one percent of genitourinary injuries. Although ureteral injury can be repaired successfully [*see Figure 4*], it may have serious consequences, including loss of renal function and death,[12] if unrecognized. The absence of physical signs of injury makes diagnosis difficult, and a delayed presentation is not uncommon. Up to half of all ureteral injuries resulting from blunt trauma are not recognized immediately, and a high index of suspicion is necessary to avoid the late complications of urinoma, sepsis, and nephrectomy.[13]

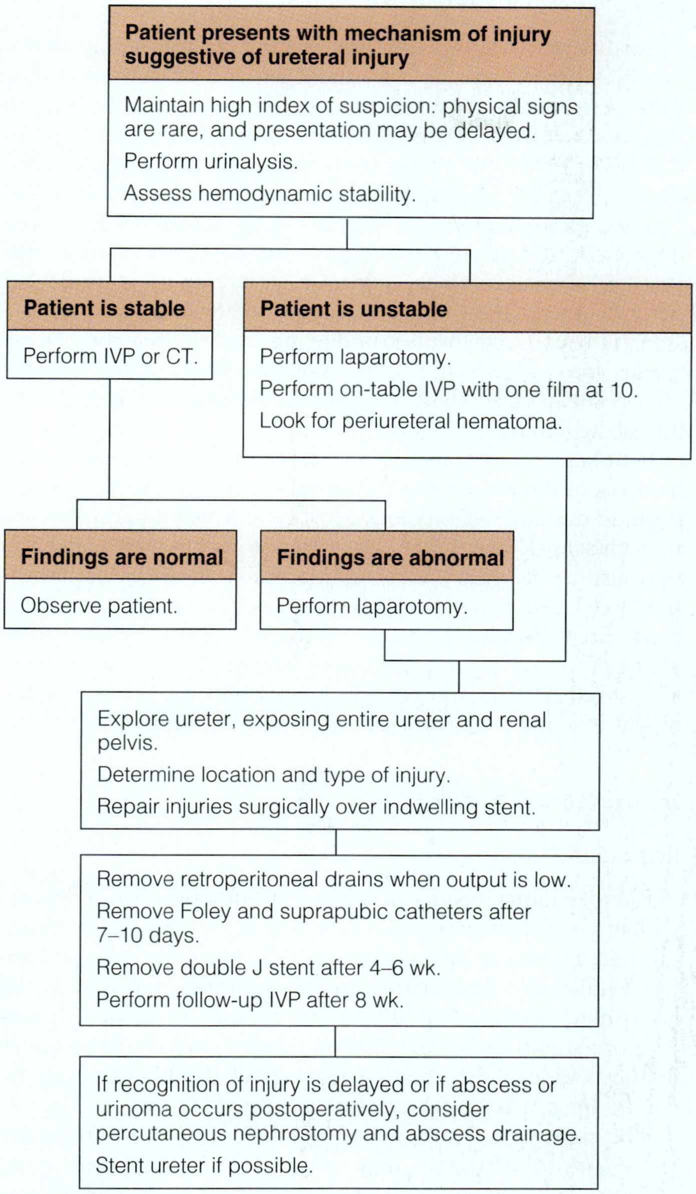

```
┌─────────────────────────────────────────┐
│ Patient presents with mechanism of injury │
│ suggestive of ureteral injury            │
├─────────────────────────────────────────┤
│ Maintain high index of suspicion: physical signs │
│ are rare, and presentation may be delayed. │
│ Perform urinalysis.                      │
│ Assess hemodynamic stability.            │
└─────────────────────────────────────────┘
```

┌──────────────────┐   ┌──────────────────────────────┐
│ Patient is stable│   │ Patient is unstable   │
├──────────────────┤   ├──────────────────────────────┤
│ Perform IVP or CT.│   │ Perform laparotomy.   │
└──────────────────┘   │ Perform on-table IVP with one film at 10. │
                        │ Look for periureteral hematoma. │
                        └──────────────────────────────┘

┌──────────────────┐   ┌──────────────────────────────┐
│ Findings are normal│ │ Findings are abnormal   │
├──────────────────┤   ├──────────────────────────────┤
│ Observe patient. │   │ Perform laparotomy.   │
└──────────────────┘   └──────────────────────────────┘

┌──┐
│ Explore ureter, exposing entire ureter and renal pelvis. │
│ Determine location and type of injury.   │
│ Repair injuries surgically over indwelling stent.   │
└──┘

┌──┐
│ Remove retroperitoneal drains when output is low.   │
│ Remove Foley and suprapubic catheters after 7–10 days. │
│ Remove double J stent after 4–6 wk.   │
│ Perform follow-up IVP after 8 wk.   │
└──┘

┌──┐
│ If recognition of injury is delayed or if abscess or │
│ urinoma occurs postoperatively, consider   │
│ percutaneous nephrostomy and abscess drainage.   │
│ Stent ureter if possible.   │
└──┘

Figure 4 Algorithm illustrates evaluation and treatment of a patient with ureteral injury.

A penetrating wound is the predominant cause of ureteral injury, gunshot wounds being the most common cause and stab wounds the second most common. Deceleration injuries may result in UPJ disruption, especially in children. The pediatric ureter is prone to injury because hyperextensibility of the spine can result in avulsion of the ureter at the UPJ.[14] The patient's history and the physical examination provide little information about ureteral injuries. Signs and symptoms related to associated injuries predominate. In three recent series, gross or microscopic hematuria was present in only 30 to 70 percent of ureteral injuries, making vigilance necessary for diagnosis.[12,13,15]

Intravenous urography or computed tomography should be performed whenever ureteral injury is suspected. Intravenous urography is of variable usefulness in the detection of ureteral injuries, but extravasation of the contrast agent is diagnostic.

Computed tomography does not reveal all renal pelvic and ureteral injuries, and hemodynamic instability may preclude its use in patients with penetrating abdominal trauma.[16]

Ureteral injury may not be suspected until the time of laparotomy, when a hematoma is found near the kidney or ureter. If on-table IVP is not diagnostic, direct inspection of the ureter for injury, contusion, and peristalsis is mandatory. Injection of indigo carmine directly into the collecting system may identify extravasation. All injuries to the ureter should be repaired surgically, unless a delay in diagnosis results in an abscess or a urinoma. For either abscess or urinoma, drainage by percutaneous nephrostomy and ureteral stenting may allow the inflamed ureter to heal, whereas an operative approach may result in nephrectomy.

OPERATIVE MANAGEMENT

Once ureteral injury has been recognized, reconstruction should proceed. Depending on the type of injury and its location, the reconstructive techniques may include debridement of devitalized tissue, a spatulated tension-free anastomosis, watertight mucosal approximation, ureteral stenting, coverage of the repair with vascularized tissue, and appropriate drainage.[12] Stab wounds generally require less tissue debridement than gunshot wounds, and partial transections may be closed primarily.

Disruption or transection of the UPJ is repaired by debridement and primary anastomosis of the renal pelvis and ureter. Penetrating low-velocity injuries require minimal or no debridement. Mobilization of the ureter should be limited to avoid compromising the blood supply. Interrupted 5-0 or 6-0 Vicryl sutures are preferred, and a double J ureteral stent or a nephrostomy tube must be inserted before closure of the anastomosis.

Injuries to the abdominal ureter between the UPJ and the pelvic brim are repaired by ureteroureterostomy [*see Figure 5*]. After debridement, the ends are spatulated on opposite sides, and an interrupted approximation is completed over a double J stent. In cases of overlying colonic, duodenal, or pancreatic injury, the anastomosis may be covered with omentum. Large defects in the abdominal ureter may require transureteroureterostomy, in which the injured ureter is passed behind the mesocolon to the contralateral side. Anastomosis of the injured ureter to a 1 to 2 cm opening in the medial normal ureter can be achieved without tension. With transureteroureterostomy, a stent (usually a 5 French pediatric feeding tube) should cross the anastomosis and be brought out through the normal lower ureter or bladder.

Ureteral injuries below the pelvic brim should be debrided and reimplanted into the bladder. The distal stump is ligated, and after the anterior bladder wall is opened, the proximal end of the ureter is brought through a new hiatus on the back wall of the bladder. The ureter is then spatulated and approximated to the bladder mucosa with interrupted chromic sutures. One 3-0 anchoring stitch should bring the distal apex of the ureter to the muscle and mucosa; the rest of the sutures are 4-0 only, approximating mucosa. A nonrefluxing reimplantation is acceptable in adults. Large defects can be bridged by performing a vesico-psoas hitch, in which the bladder dome is mobilized to bridge the ureteral defect and sewn to the central tendon of the psoas muscle. Three interrupted sutures that enter the detrusor muscle but not the bladder lumen should anchor the dome above the iliac vessels. The dome is mobilized by dividing the obliterated umbilical arteries bilaterally and, if necessary, dividing the contralateral superior vesical artery. Significant bladder or vascular damage may make transureteroureterostomy a more attractive option to avoid further dissection in the injured area. A ureteral stent should be used in all ureteral reimplantations. The bladder is closed in two layers with running 2-0 Vicryl suture, and a drain is placed in the Retzius space.

A retroperitoneal drain is essential in all ureteral reconstructions. A large-bore Foley catheter is sufficient for bladder drainage unless there is coexistent bladder injury or prolonged catheterization is expected. In either of these cases, a suprapubic catheter allows better drainage of clots and, in males, has fewer long-term complications.[17]

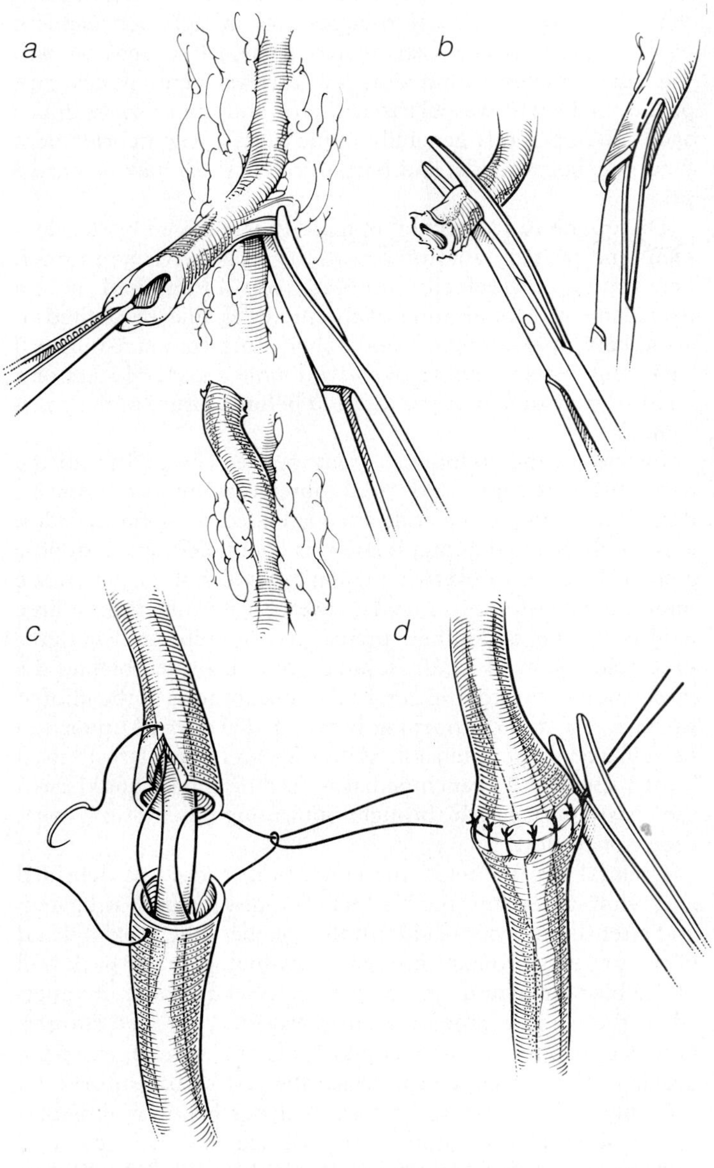

POSTOPERATIVE CARE

Postoperative care of ureteral trauma relates mainly to the manipulation of drains and management of complications. Retroperitoneal drains may have significant output for several days but are removed once the output is minimal. With severe injuries or persistent output from drains, CT or IVP before discharge from the hospital may help rule out the possibility of extravasation. Bladder catheterization is necessary for seven days after ureteral reimplantation. In combined bladder and ureteral reconstructions, contrast cystography is indicated before catheter removal. Cystoscopic removal of the double J stent is usually performed under local anesthesia four to six weeks after operation. Intravenous urography three months after removal of the stent rules out the possibility of asymptomatic obstruction.

Fistula formation, usually the result of distal obstruction or necrosis of the ureter, should be managed by antegrade or retrograde drainage of the collecting system using percutaneous or endoscopic techniques. Drainage of periureteral collection may also be necessary. If recognition of an injury or complication is delayed, reconstruction should not be undertaken for at least three months, to allow resolution of the inflammatory phase of wound healing. Because hydronephrosis may develop as a result of stricture, retroperitoneal fibrosis, or a urinoma, repeat imaging is appropriate one year after injury.

Injuries to the Bladder

INITIAL EVALUATION

Bladder injury occurs in fewer than one percent of trauma patients.[18] Bladder rupture is most often caused by blunt injuries, including injuries resulting from motor vehicle accidents, falls, and direct blows to the abdomen, and is associated with pelvic fracture in 89 percent of cases. Overall, nine percent of patients with a pelvic fracture have an associated injury to the bladder.[19] Penetrating wounds of the bladder may be caused by gunshot, stabs, or pelvic surgery.

The signs and symptoms of bladder injury are nonspecific [see Figure 6]. Patients may complain of suprapubic pain, dysuria, or an inability to void.[20] Physical examination may reveal tenderness in the suprapubic region, ileus, or an acute abdomen. Bladder rupture is associated with gross hematuria in 95 percent of cases; three percent of patients had no hematuria in a series studied by Cass.[21] Laboratory studies are usually inconclusive unless significant reabsorption of urine causes elevated serum creatinine levels.

Bladder rupture is most accurately diagnosed with contrast cystography. Insufficient instillation of the contrast agent, however, yields false negative results. Standard CT is inadequate for the diagnosis of bladder rupture, because the bladder is not sufficiently distended in most patients.

A retrograde cystogram is obtained after an initial scout film by instilling 300 to 400 ml of 25 to 30 percent iodinated contrast through a urethral catheter. An anteroposterior view should be taken with the bladder full and after evacuation. In cases of intraperitoneal bladder injury, extravasation of contrast outlines the bowel loops and may track along the lateral gutters [see Figure 7a]. Extraperitoneal injuries demonstrate flame-shaped extravasation in the pelvis, which may track down into the obturator region, the scrotum, or the thigh [see

Figure 5 Ureteroureterostomy. (*a*) The injured ureter is dissected free. (*b*) The ends are spatulated. (*c*) The ends are approximated over a double J stent. (*d*) The anastomosis is completed with interrupted sutures.

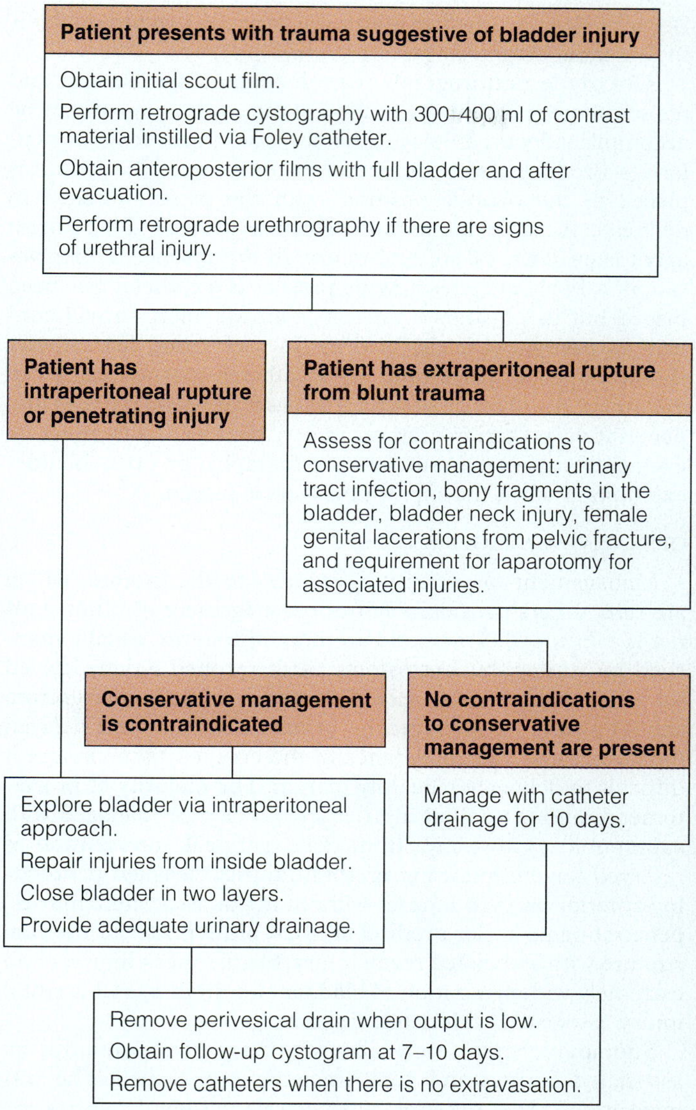

31 INJURIES TO THE UROGENITAL TRACT — 455

hematoma. If the bladder injury is associated with a pelvic fracture in a male patient, the possibility of a urethral injury is 10 to 29 percent and must be excluded.[21] A successfully placed Foley catheter rules out a complete urethral disruption.

All penetrating injuries and all intraperitoneal ruptures of the bladder are managed by bladder exploration and repair. Bladder exploration is always performed via an intraperitoneal approach. In addition to repair of the bladder, exploration makes it possible to rule out associated injuries, ensure the integrity of the ureters by direct visualization, and, in the case of pelvic fracture, avoid entering the pelvic hematoma. Intraperitoneal injuries generally cause a stellate rupture of the dome of the bladder. By enlarging this opening, one can inspect the interior of the bladder to exclude concomitant extraperitoneal injuries, which occur in eight percent of cases.[20]

Figure 6 Algorithm illustrates evaluation and treatment of a patient with bladder injury.

Figure 7b]. Blunt injuries can cause extraperitoneal, intraperitoneal, or combined rupture. The amount of extravasation has no correlation with the degree of injury and should not influence management.[17]

OPERATIVE MANAGEMENT

Extraperitoneal bladder injuries caused by blunt trauma can be managed with catheter drainage for 10 days, unless contraindications exist.[17] After 10 days, cystography should be used to document healing and allow removal of the catheter. If extravasation persists, cystography should be repeated weekly until healing occurs. Contraindications to nonoperative management include urinary infection; the presence of bony fragments in the bladder; bladder neck injury, which may compromise continence; and female genital lacerations associated with pelvic fracture.

If the patient requires laparotomy for associated injuries and is not critically ill, repair of extraperitoneal bladder injuries is recommended to decrease the possibility of infecting the pelvic

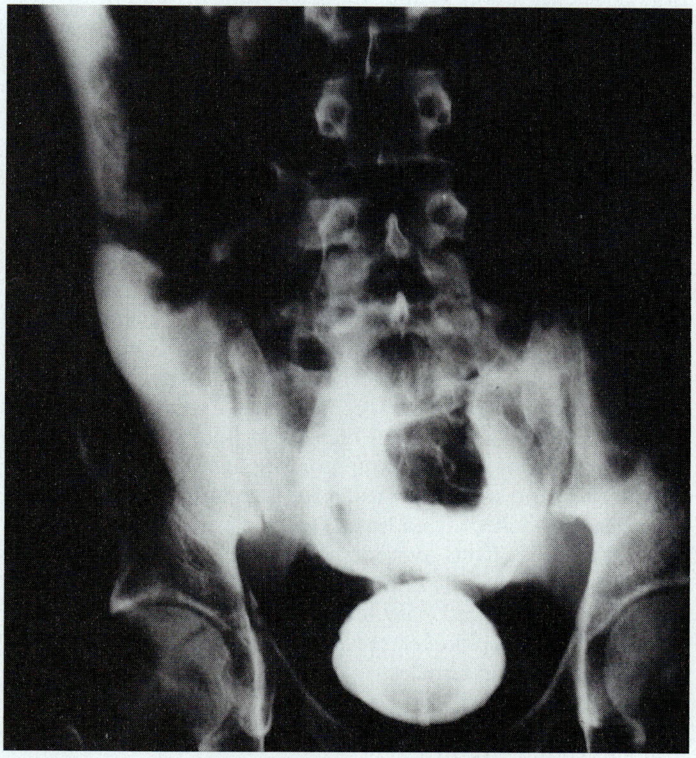

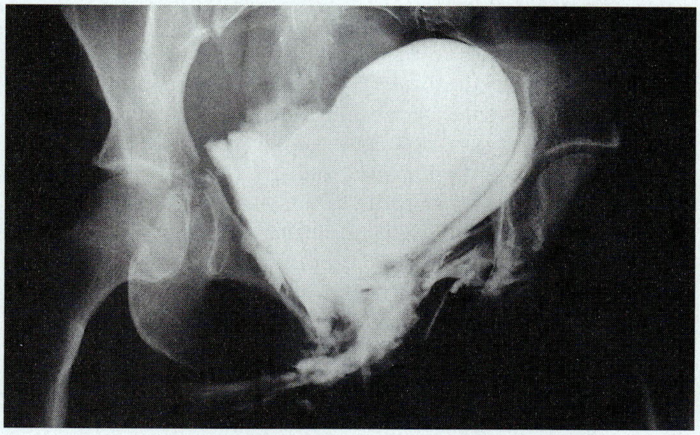

Figure 7 X-rays show intraperitoneal (*a*) and extraperitoneal (*b*) bladder rupture.

Penetrating injuries and extraperitoneal ruptures are approached by opening the bladder with cautery, vertically at the dome or along the anterior surface, and identifying the sites of rupture intravesically. These lacerations are then debrided (rarely necessary) and closed with interrupted 3-0 chromic or Vicryl sutures, which approximate detrusor muscle and mucosa in one layer and provide hemostasis. In patients with gunshot wounds, entrance and exit sites must be identified. The cystotomy is then closed with two layers of running 2-0 or 3-0 Vicryl sutures, the first layer consisting of mucosa and detrusor muscle and the second consisting of detrusor and serosa.

Adequate urinary drainage is essential to successful healing of the repaired bladder. Large-bore (22 French or larger) Foley catheter drainage is adequate if bladder injuries are not extensive and hemostasis is excellent. Gunshot wounds, extensive blunt injuries, and coagulopathy warrant additional drainage with a suprapubic tube, allowing irrigation of clots and proper decompression of the bladder. If suprapubic cystostomy is chosen, a 24 French Malecot catheter placed through a separate site into the bladder is preferred. In addition, a closed-suction or a Penrose drain near the bladder closure, but not overlying the suture line, is recommended. Like the suprapubic tube, the drain should exit through a separate site in the skin.

POSTOPERATIVE CARE

In the majority of patients with a bladder repair, seven days of catheter drainage is sufficient to allow healing. Cystography may be indicated in cases of severe bladder injury or persistent output from drains. The perivesical drain can be removed after the output has decreased to an acceptable rate. Because bladder repair is reliable, complications of bladder injury are related to a delay in diagnosis rather than to postoperative morbidity. Azotemia, ascites, and sepsis may result from an intraperitoneal injury that was overlooked. Because an infected pelvic hematoma can have disastrous effects, nonoperative management of extraperitoneal rupture must be undertaken with caution. Bladder neck injury, if unrecognized, may lead to scarring and incompetence of the proximal sphincter mechanism, with resultant incontinence, especially in females.

Injuries to the Urethra

INITIAL EVALUATION

Almost all injuries to the male urethra are caused by blunt trauma. Posterior urethral (prostatic and membranous urethral) injuries in males occur in five percent of pelvic fractures, which is the most common cause of posterior urethral injury.[22] Anterior urethral (penile and bulbar urethral) injuries are commonly caused by straddle injury but may be the result of penile fracture or penetrating injuries to the genitalia. Penetrating injury to the posterior urethra often leaves the urethral continuity intact. The female urethra is rarely injured, but when it is, it is invariably associated with bladder injury and pelvic fracture.

Blood at the urethral meatus, the classic sign of injury to the male urethra, indicates that urethrography should be performed immediately. Attempts at catheter placement, which may convert incomplete injuries to complete disruptions,[22] are to be condemned in any case of suspected urethral injury. Because signs of urethral injury are variable, urethrography is the essential diagnostic test.

Retrograde urethrography can document the location and nature of urethral injury. Injection of the contrast agent may be accomplished with a Foley catheter placed in the fossa navicularis, a Brodney clamp, or a catheter tip syringe. The patient is placed in the oblique position, with the penis stretched to delineate the anterior urethra. Extravasation of the contrast agent is evidence of urethral injury. In the absence of extravasation, a Foley catheter may be passed. If a catheter has been placed but its position is unclear, contrast injection will confirm its placement in the bladder. In such cases, the catheter should be left in place until a pericatheter contrast study can document the absence of injury. In cases of pelvic fracture and penetrating posterior urethral injury, bladder injury must be excluded via suprapubic tube cystography or open bladder exploration when the suprapubic tube is placed.

OPERATIVE MANAGEMENT

Management of penetrating injuries to the urethra, which are rare, differs considerably from management of blunt trauma [see Figure 8]. Traumatic urethral injuries are usually managed by suprapubic cystostomy, with reconstruction delayed for three to six months. Straddle injuries to the bulbar urethra should always be managed by urinary diversion and delayed repair, because the appearance of the crushed tissue makes it difficult to delineate a healthy margin. The majority of prostatomembranous urethral injuries should also be managed with suprapubic cystostomy. Immediate surgical intervention is reserved for the following urethral injuries: selected penetrating anterior urethral injuries without major associated injuries; penetrating posterior urethral injuries; blunt posterior urethral rupture with associated rectal injury, bladder neck injury, or an extremely wide separation of bladder and urethra; and urethral injury associated with penile fracture.[23]

Suprapubic cystostomy allows urinary diversion until all associated injuries and bony fractures have healed. The vast majority of blunt anterior and posterior urethral injuries are managed with this approach. If laparotomy is not indicated for other injuries, the suprapubic tube may be placed percutaneously under fluoroscopic guidance. A cystogram can then be performed via the suprapubic tube to rule out associated bladder injury. A patient with urethral injury should not be allowed to void (voiding causes urinary extravasation). If open placement of the suprapubic tube is elected, the bladder can be inspected to rule out simultaneous injury, and a cystogram is not necessary.

Suprapubic cystostomy is performed through a lower abdominal incision and an intraperitoneal approach. This approach avoids the pelvic hematoma and allows an anterior vertical incision of the bladder. We lead the suprapubic tube (24 French Malecot or Foley catheter) out the superior aspect of the bladder closure and the inferior aspect of the skin wound in the midline, facilitating subsequent tube changes and reconstructive procedures. The bladder is closed in two layers [see Injuries to the Bladder, Operative Management, above]. In three to six months, a repeat cystogram and a retrograde urethrogram will delineate the residual stricture or rupture defect, which will require repair.

Suprapubic cystostomy should be used for management of penetrating injuries to the anterior urethra if they were caused

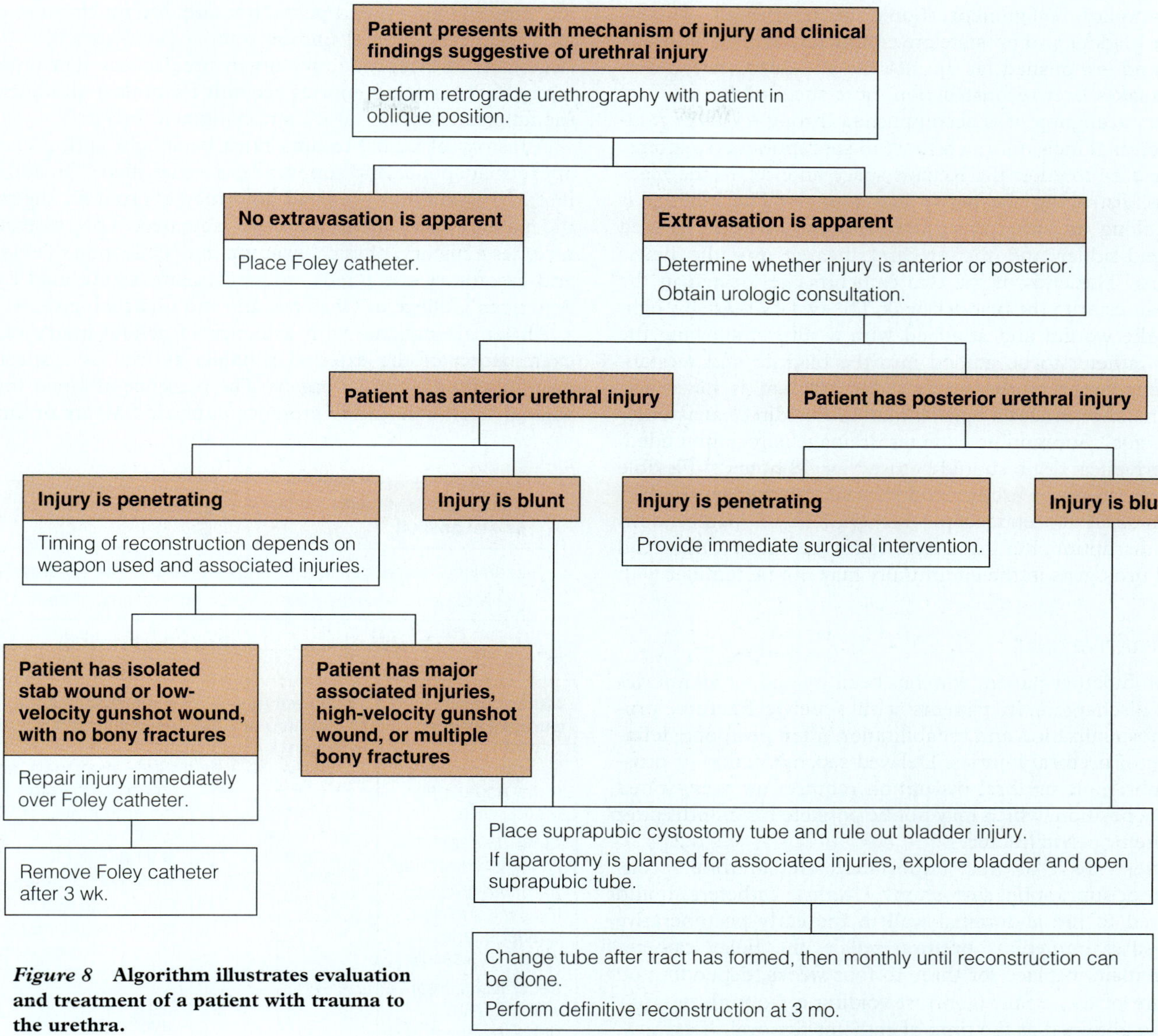

```
                    ┌─────────────────────────────────────────┐
                    │ Patient presents with mechanism of injury│
                    │ and clinical findings suggestive of      │
                    │ urethral injury                          │
                    ├─────────────────────────────────────────┤
                    │ Perform retrograde urethrography with    │
                    │ patient in oblique position.             │
                    └─────────────────────────────────────────┘
```

Figure 8 Algorithm illustrates evaluation and treatment of a patient with trauma to the urethra.

by high-velocity weapons, leading to extensive tissue loss; if they are associated with serious injuries; or if bony fractures prevent use of the lithotomy position. For stab wounds or isolated low-velocity gunshot wounds, the favored approach is primary repair, which is associated with a lower stricture rate.[24]

Penile urethral injuries are approached by making a circumferential distal penile incision and degloving the penis to expose the urethra. Bulbar injuries are approached through a midline perineal incision. In each case, mobilization of the proximal and distal urethra with debridement of devitalized tissue should allow a spatulated end-to-end anastomosis. We use interrupted 6-0 monofilament absorbable suture over a 16 French Foley catheter. Additional drains are usually not necessary, and the wounds can be closed primarily because of the excellent blood supply of the perineum.

Penetrating injuries to the posterior urethra are rare. The prostate acts as a scaffold, preventing total disruption of the prostatic urethra. If contrast agent used during urethrography reaches the bladder, one can assume an incomplete injury. Endoscopic realignment and placement of a Foley catheter may be sufficient treatment of injury to the posterior urethra.

A cystoscope or fluoroscopic guidance is used to place a wire into the bladder, beyond the injury, and a Foley catheter is then advanced over the wire. Positioning is confirmed by contrast instillation. After a month of catheter drainage, a voiding cystourethrogram will document healing.

In cases of prostatomembranous urethral disruption caused by blunt injury, immediate surgical intervention is required in only rare and specific instances. In cases of vascular, rectal, and bladder neck injuries or wide separation of the bladder from the urethra, some authors recommend immediate primary surgical realignment of the urethra.[23] If pelvic exploration is performed for major vascular or orthopedic repair, the urethra can be realigned, and a secondary procedure may not be required.[19] Because of the risk of infection to the pelvic hematoma, simultaneous rectal injury should prompt evacuation of the pelvic hematoma, irrigation, placement of drains, and primary realignment of the urethra. Bladder neck injuries, which may compromise the continence mechanism of the proximal sphincter, require reconstruction in patients with posterior urethral rupture (whose external sphincter has been compromised by the injury). At the time of bladder neck repair, primary realignment should be performed. Finally, when the bladder and prostate are completely avulsed from the urethra and are pushed far up into the abdomen, early intervention makes later reconstruction more successful.

Primary realignment is accomplished through a lower midline abdominal incision. In contrast to suprapubic cystostomy, it is necessary to enter the Retzius space anterior to the bladder, thus disturbing the pelvic hematoma.[25] The bladder is opened along its anterior surface, and catheters are passed from the bladder and the urethral meatus into the pelvic hematoma. The ends of the two catheters are located in the midline anterior to the bladder neck. The two ends are brought up into the wound and attached with a suture, allowing the urethral catheter to be guided into the bladder and reestablishing alignment of the urethra. No traction is necessary, because neither mucosal approximation nor direct anastomosis is the goal. Suprapubic catheter drainage is recommended, and a perivesical drain should be used for 48 hours.[25] Flexible cystoscopy (from the urethra and via a suprapubic approach)[26] has been used for endoscopic realignment of membranous urethral disruption, but these techniques are not in widespread use, and urologists in the community may not be familiar with them.

POSTOPERATIVE CARE

The ambulatory patient who has been treated for all injuries may be discharged. In patients with a pelvic fracture, prolonged hospitalization and rehabilitation often postpone definitive care of urethral injuries. Delayed reconstruction of prostatomembranous urethral disruption requires an exaggerated lithotomy position, which may not be possible for months after long-bone or pelvic fractures.

Catheter care is of great importance after urethral reconstruction or suprapubic cystostomy. Urethral catheters should be secured to the abdominal wall in the early postoperative period. After immediate urethral repair, the Foley catheter should remain in place for three to four weeks, depending on the nature of the repair. Contrast voiding cystourethrography should be obtained at the time of catheter removal. If extravasation is present, the catheter should be replaced for one week and the study repeated. When a suprapubic catheter has been used in addition to a Foley catheter, radiographic studies can be performed via the suprapubic tube.

Patients managed initially with a suprapubic tube alone should have the tube changed after a tract has formed, usually in four weeks, and then monthly until reconstruction can be performed. Stricture formation or complete obliteration of the urethra may be the final result after initial management. Subsequent radiographic studies can indicate whether secondary endoscopic or open procedures are needed. Voiding dysfunction may occur after pelvic fracture and sacral nerve root injury.

Injuries to the Vagina, Uterus, and Ovaries

INITIAL EVALUATION

Injuries to the female genitalia must be regarded as especially morbid because of their association with sexual assault as well as the potential complications of infection and bleeding. Perineal and vaginal injuries, usually the result of blunt trauma, straddle injury, and pelvic fracture, are much more common than cervical and uterine trauma [see Figure 9].[27,28] Enlargement of a reproductive organ predisposes that organ to injury.[29] Penetrating injuries account for almost all injuries to the fallopian tubes, ovaries, and nongravid uterus.[30]

A history of sexual trauma must be sought and, if elicited, appropriate police and support services notified.[27] In addition, if sexual assault has occurred, informed consent for the rest of the patient assessment must be obtained. This assessment includes a history, physical examination, collection of evidence and laboratory specimens, and treatment, as outlined by the American College of Obstetricians and Gynecologists.[31]

All female patients with evidence of genital injury require examination of the external genitalia as well as a speculum examination of internal organs. The presence of blood implies vaginal laceration. In the presence of pelvic fracture or impale-

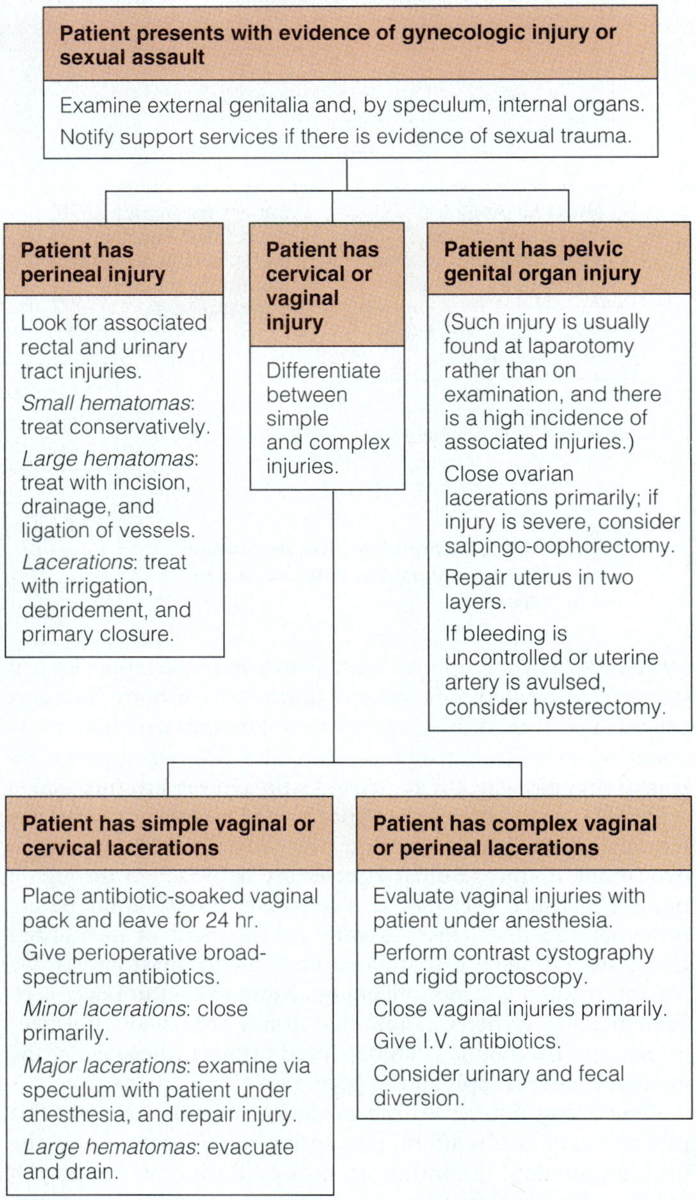

Patient presents with evidence of gynecologic injury or sexual assault

Examine external genitalia and, by speculum, internal organs. Notify support services if there is evidence of sexual trauma.

Patient has perineal injury

Look for associated rectal and urinary tract injuries.
Small hematomas: treat conservatively.
Large hematomas: treat with incision, drainage, and ligation of vessels.
Lacerations: treat with irrigation, debridement, and primary closure.

Patient has cervical or vaginal injury

Differentiate between simple and complex injuries.

Patient has pelvic genital organ injury

(Such injury is usually found at laparotomy rather than on examination, and there is a high incidence of associated injuries.)
Close ovarian lacerations primarily; if injury is severe, consider salpingo-oophorectomy.
Repair uterus in two layers.
If bleeding is uncontrolled or uterine artery is avulsed, consider hysterectomy.

Patient has simple vaginal or cervical lacerations

Place antibiotic-soaked vaginal pack and leave for 24 hr.
Give perioperative broad-spectrum antibiotics.
Minor lacerations: close primarily.
Major lacerations: examine via speculum with patient under anesthesia, and repair injury.
Large hematomas: evacuate and drain.

Patient has complex vaginal or perineal lacerations

Evaluate vaginal injuries with patient under anesthesia.
Perform contrast cystography and rigid proctoscopy.
Close vaginal injuries primarily.
Give I.V. antibiotics.
Consider urinary and fecal diversion.

Figure 9 Algorithm illustrates evaluation and treatment of a female patient with trauma to reproductive organs.

ment injury, vaginal laceration warrants complete evaluation (using cystourethrography, proctoscopy, and laparotomy, as indicated) to rule out associated urinary tract and gastrointestinal injuries. Failure to identify vaginal injury associated with pelvic fracture may lead to abscess formation, sepsis, and death.

OPERATIVE MANAGEMENT

Perineal lacerations in the absence of associated urinary tract and rectal injury can be managed in the emergency department. Only large hematomas must be incised and drained, with ligation of vessels. Lacerations of the vulva may be closed primarily after irrigation and debridement. Interrupted absorbable sutures allow any accumulated fluid to drain and eliminate the need for suture removal. Drains are used if there is a large cavity; if hemostasis is suboptimal, the wound may be left open and packed.[27]

Vaginal and cervical lacerations, the result of either blunt or penetrating injury, may bleed extensively if pudendal vessels are injured.[27] If bleeding is not severe, examination and repair under local anesthesia is possible in the ED. If large lacerations are associated with bleeding and hematoma, speculum examination under anesthesia permits more complete assessment and repair of injuries. Vaginal lacerations should be closed with a running or interrupted absorbable suture that includes mucosal and muscular layers. Antibiotic-soaked vaginal packing should be left in place for 24 hours. Perioperative administration of broad-spectrum antibiotics is sufficient, unless injuries are more complex.

Complex vaginal and perineal lacerations associated with pelvic fracture require much more aggressive management to avoid the morbidity and mortality of open fractures.[27] Evaluation of vaginal injuries under anesthesia, contrast cystography, and rigid proctoscopy are mandatory. The vaginal laceration should be closed with absorbable sutures. Even in the absence of injury to the bladder or rectum, diversion of the urinary and fecal streams should be considered to facilitate care of the wounds.[32] Extraperitoneal bladder rupture associated with vaginal lacerations requires operative repair to prevent infection of pelvic hematoma or the formation of a vesicovaginal fistula. Antibiotic therapy is more prolonged, as appropriate for open fractures.[27] Urologic, gynecologic, and orthopedic consultations are necessary for care of associated injuries.

Injury to the pelvic genital organs is rare in a nongravid patient. Penetrating trauma is the most common cause, and the majority of patients have associated injuries requiring laparotomy.[29] Blunt injury of the nongravid uterus and pelvic organs occurs in the face of preexisting abnormalities; diagnostic peritoneal lavage demonstrates hemoperitoneum in these instances.[30] The uterus, most commonly injured, is repaired with figure-eight sutures or a two-layer closure using Vicryl or chromic sutures.[29] Avulsion of the uterine artery or extensive blast destruction of the uterus may necessitate hysterectomy.[27] When hysterectomy is necessary for trauma, the vaginal cuff may be left open to allow drainage of the operative bed.[33] Lacerations to the ovary or fallopian tube may be managed by primary closure or salpingo-oophorectomy if contralateral structures are normal.

POSTOPERATIVE CARE

Postoperative care should be dictated by the management of associated injuries. After hysterectomy or repair of vaginal lacerations, a vaginal pack should remain in place for 24 hours. Hemorrhage caused by uterine injury has been treated with oxytocin, which increases uterine tone and controls bleeding.[29] Complex lacerations of the perineum may require bowel rest or colostomy to prevent soilage. Fertility after injury to the female reproductive organs is not well documented, but patients must be counseled about the possible adverse consequences of uterine and adnexal trauma.

Injuries to the Gravid Uterus

INITIAL EVALUATION

As a result of the increasing incidence of motor vehicle accidents, six to seven percent of pregnancies are complicated by trauma.[34] Trauma is a leading cause of maternal death, but it more frequently causes death of the fetus.[35-37] Although penetrating injuries are not common, those that do occur are likely to cause uterine and fetal injury because of the size of the uterus.[38] Because of physiologic changes during pregnancy, few signs of injury may be present at initial evaluation, but fetal compromise can easily occur. Conversely, life-threatening hemorrhagic shock may occur with uterine rupture.[33] Maternal survival must remain the first priority, both in initial resuscitation and in the operating room; fetal viability and needs can be managed once the mother's condition has been stabilized.

All pregnant patients suffering traumatic injury require evaluation [see Figure 10]. Ejection from an automobile, presentation in shock, or pelvic fracture increases the likelihood of uterine injury. Estimation of the gestational age is essential for accurate examination of the gravid uterus. Physical signs outlined in the algorithm generally are not useful in determining the status of the fetus. A sterile speculum examination is necessary to evaluate dilation of the cervix and to test for the presence of amniotic fluid.[38] Resuscitation begins by placing the patient in the left lateral decubitus position to minimize obstruction of venous return by the gravid uterus. Once initial evaluation of the mother has been performed, evaluation with external fetal monitoring and real-time ultrasonography provides information on fetal distress, placental abruption, and the general state of the fetus. Most authors agree that real-time ultrasonography gives the most information about the condition of the fetus.[34,39] Kleihauer-Betke testing for fetomaternal hemorrhage has not been predictive of obstetric complications, whereas the maternal Injury Severity Score is correlated with the likelihood of fetal survival.[34,39,40]

Blunt injury and stab wounds to the gravid uterus in a hemodynamically stable female patient should be evaluated by standard methods, with the fetus being shielded as much as possible during radiographic studies but all available modalities being used, including limited computed tomography if indicated.[38] In the absence of significant injuries, the patient and fetus should be observed and evaluated with external fetal monitoring for at least four to six hours. In two studies, all complications developed within this time frame.[34,41] Ruptured amniotic membranes, premature labor, or placental abruption should be managed by the obstetric service.

OPERATIVE MANAGEMENT

Pregnant females who suffer trauma require laparotomy in

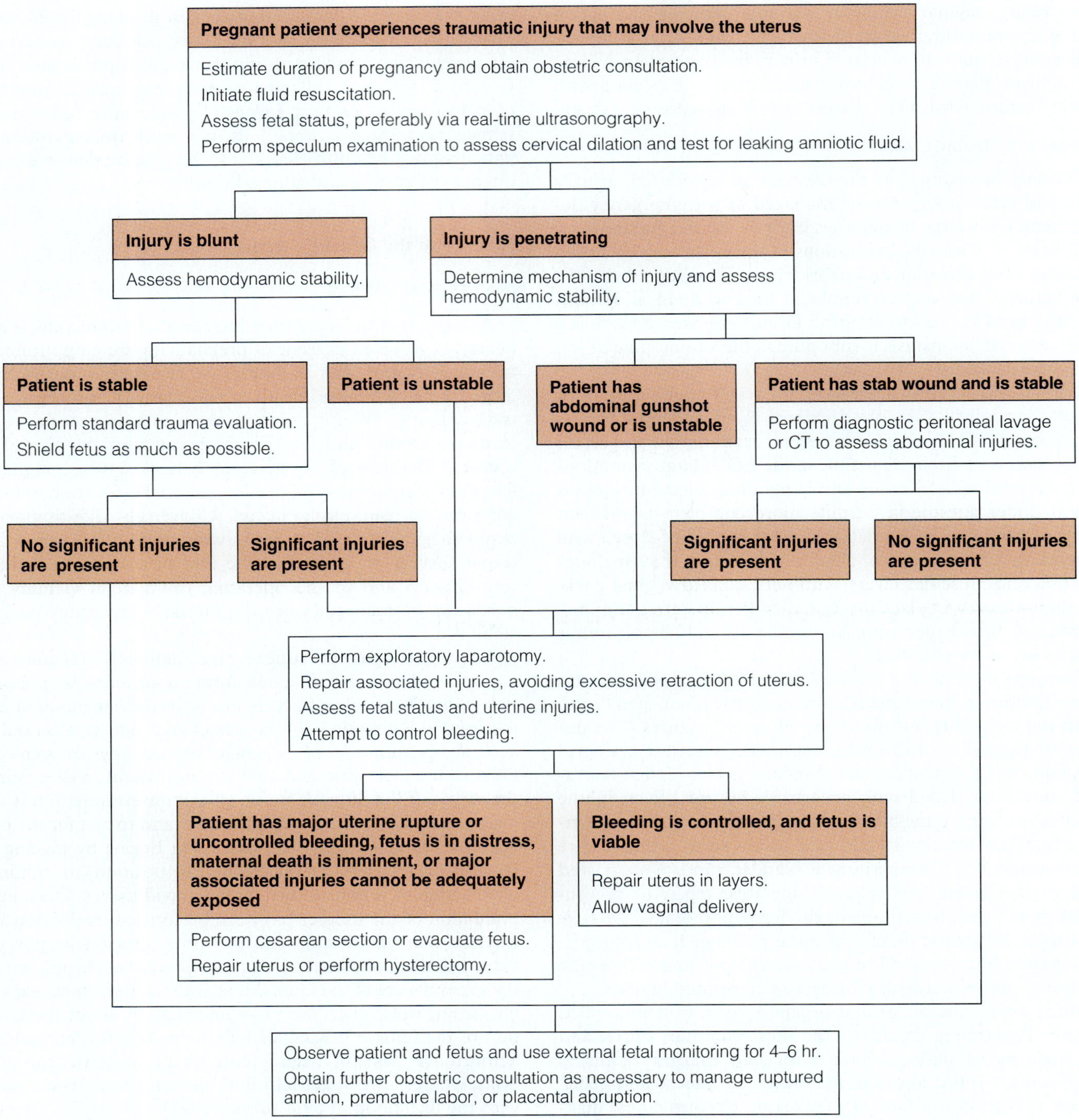

```
┌─────────────────────────────────────────────────────────────────┐
│ Pregnant patient experiences traumatic injury that may involve the uterus │
│ Estimate duration of pregnancy and obtain obstetric consultation. │
│ Initiate fluid resuscitation.                                    │
│ Assess fetal status, preferably via real-time ultrasonography.   │
│ Perform speculum examination to assess cervical dilation and test for leaking amniotic fluid. │
└─────────────────────────────────────────────────────────────────┘
```

Figure 10 Algorithm illustrates evaluation and treatment of a pregnant female with blunt or penetrating injury to the uterus.

the following instances: after a gunshot wound to the abdomen; after a defined associated injury requiring surgery; after a blunt injury or stab wound causes hemodynamic instability; if fetal parts are palpable; and in cases of fetal distress.[38] A midline incision is always selected, and the obstetric consultant should be on hand. Repair of associated injuries can usually be performed by moving the uterus out of the way, permitting subsequent vaginal delivery. Major vascular or rectal injuries may require a cesarean section to provide adequate exposure. Fetal distress or imminent maternal death necessitates an immediate cesarean section. A nonviable fetus, which must be evacuated, is best managed by induced labor at a later date; uterine salvage may be more likely, possibly maintaining reproductive function.[42]

Uterine injuries during pregnancy cause extensive bleeding, but multilayered closure with absorbable sutures should achieve hemostasis. Serious bleeding may be controlled by ligating the hypogastric arteries.[42] In the absence of fetal distress, the abdomen may be closed to allow spontaneous vaginal delivery, even in the perioperative period.[38] If the uterus cannot be sal-

element in the evaluation of scrotal trauma [see Figure 11]. When a straddle injury or penetrating mechanism suggests the possibility of urethral injuries, retrograde urethrography is indicated.

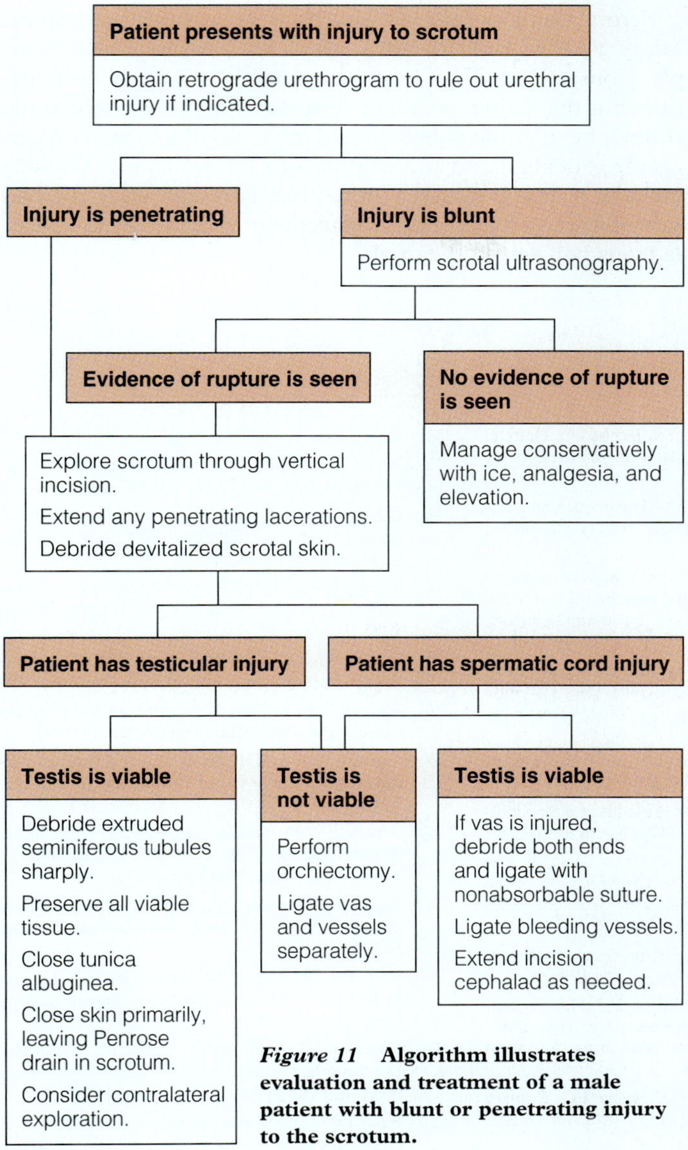

Penetrating scrotal injuries commonly involve not only the testis but also the corpora cavernosa, urethra, and spermatic cord. Because of the excellent blood supply of the scrotal skin, most penetrating injuries may be debrided and closed. Exceptions to this general rule include human and animal bites, which are treated with antibiotics and local wound care (or debridement in cases of severe soft tissue infection).[43]

Rupture of the testicle is often immediately painful, with rapid onset of swelling. Falls, straddle injuries, and direct blows are common mechanisms of injury.[44] However, seemingly minor degrees of trauma may be associated with delayed onset of pain, swelling, and ecchymosis; in this scenario, testicular torsion must be included in the differential diagnosis. Physical signs of rupture include scrotal swelling, tenderness, and ecchymosis. Injury to the scrotal wall or tunica vaginalis may cause significant swelling without rupture of the tunica albuginea of the testis; pelvic hematoma caused by fracture may extend down, resulting in massive scrotal swelling. For these reasons, blunt injury to the scrotum should be evaluated by ultrasonography unless findings of the physical examination are normal.

The ultrasonographic characteristics of testicular rupture include loss of normal homogeneity of the testicular parenchyma, loss of continuity of the tunica albuginea, and intraparenchymal hematoma.[45] A discrete break in the tunica is relatively rare. In cases of pelvic fracture with massive scrotal edema, ultrasonography can document the integrity of the testis and allow conservative management of the swelling. If rupture is not documented, conservative treatment with ice packs, analgesics, and elevation allows resolution of swelling.

OPERATIVE MANAGEMENT

Exploration of the scrotum through a vertical incision allows inspection of the scrotal contents and, when spermatic cord injury is discovered, extension of the incision into the groin. The goal is preservation of testicular parenchyma for endocrine and cosmetic purposes; normal sperm production and transport are not expected after repair of rupture. Clots and extruded seminiferous tubules are debrided with scissors to allow closure of the tunica albuginea over the edematous parenchyma. Running absorbable suture (3-0 Vicryl) is preferred to avoid palpable knots. When spermatic cord injury is detected, the first priority is determination of the viability of the testis. If this is in doubt, a small incision into the tunica albuginea should cause some bleeding; if the testis is cyanotic and does not bleed when cut, orchiectomy should be performed. If only the vas deferens or spermatic vessels are injured, the testis may remain viable. Ligation of the spermatic vessels is performed in the standard fashion; if vasal ligation is necessary, nonabsorbable suture with long tails is preferable, aiding in later identification for reconstruction if infertility ensues.

Because scrotal skin is well vascularized, it can be closed primarily in almost all instances. Exceptions arise if there is a prolonged delay between injury and definitive care or if grossly contaminated wounds are associated with rectal injuries. Hemostasis should be meticulous because the scrotum will

Figure 11 Algorithm illustrates evaluation and treatment of a male patient with blunt or penetrating injury to the scrotum.

vaged because of bleeding or extensive uterine destruction, a cesarean section and hysterectomy are indicated.

POSTOPERATIVE CARE

External fetal monitoring should be offered when the estimated gestational age is greater than 20 weeks and there is no indication for cesarean section. Monitoring should continue for at least six hours after blunt trauma and according to the obstetric recommendations for fetal monitoring after a penetrating injury or laparotomy. $Rh_o(D)$ immune globulin (RhoGAM) should be administered within 72 hours to all Rh-negative mothers, regardless of Kleihauer-Betke test results.[34,35]

Injuries to the Scrotum

INITIAL EVALUATION

Scrotal trauma may result in testicular injury or genital skin loss. Because blunt injuries to the testicle may be difficult to recognize, high-resolution ultrasonography has become a key

expand massively if bleeding occurs; to avoid such complications, we recommend interrupted suture closure of the tunica dartos and skin in two layers, with a Penrose drain brought out through a separate dependent stab wound. Fluffed gauze should be used for dressing, and a scrotal supporter should be used to keep the scrotum elevated. The Penrose drain is removed on the first postoperative day. There are no major restrictions to activity after scrotal surgery, and patients can be discharged once they have recovered from associated injuries.

Scrotal skin loss caused by burns or electrical or mechanical injury usually spares the testis, which has a separate blood supply. Conservative debridement is possible if there is no infection, but the demarcation between viable and nonviable tissue should be identified before extensive debridement.[46] Management depends on the amount of skin remaining. Options include primary closure, immediate coverage with meshed split-thickness skin grafts, or placement of the testes in subcutaneous pouches in the thigh.

References

1. Bright TC, White K, Peters PC: Significance of hematuria after trauma. J Urol 120:455, 1978
2. Mee SL, McAninch JW, Robinson AL, et al: Radiographic assessment of renal trauma: a 10-year prospective study of patient selection. J Urol 141:1095, 1989
3. Bretan PN, McAninch JW, Federle MP, et al: Computerized tomographic staging of renal trauma: 85 consecutive cases. J Urol 136:561, 1986
4. Pollack HM: Renal trauma: imaging and intervention. Problems in Urology 8:199, 1994
5. McAninch JW, Carroll PR, Klosterman PW, et al: Renal reconstruction after injury. J Urol 145:932, 1991
6. Cheng DL, Lazan D, Stone N: Conservative management of type III renal trauma. J Trauma 36:491, 1994
7. Husmann DA, Gilling PJ, Perry MO, et al: Major renal lacerations with a devitalized fragment following blunt abdominal trauma: comparison between nonoperative (expectant) versus surgical management. J Urol 150:1774, 1993
8. Sagalowsky AI, McConnel JD, Peters PC: Renal trauma requiring surgery: an analysis of 185 cases. J Trauma 23:128, 1983
9. McAninch JW, Carroll PC: Renal trauma: kidney preservation through improved vascular control, a refined technique. J Trauma 22:285, 1982
10. Corriere JN Jr, McAndrew JD, Benson GS: Intraoperative decision-making in renal trauma. J Trauma 31:1390, 1991
11. Uflacker R, Paolini RM, Lima S: Management of traumatic hematuria by selective renal artery embolization. J Urol 132:662, 1984
12. Presti JC, Carroll PR, McAninch JW: Ureteral and renal pelvic injuries from external trauma: diagnosis and management. J Trauma 29:370, 1989
13. Boone TB, Gilling PJ, Husmann DA: Ureteropelvic junction disruption following blunt abdominal trauma. J Urol 150:33, 1993
14. Corriere JN Jr: Ureteral injuries. Adult and Pediatric Urology. Gillenwater JY, Grayhack JT, Howards SS, et al, Eds. Mosby–Year Book, St. Louis, 1991, p 491
15. Brandes SB, Chelsky MJ, Buckman RF, et al: Ureteral injuries from penetrating trauma. J Trauma 36:766, 1994
16. Campbell EW, Filderman PS, Jacobs SC: Ureteral injury due to blunt and penetrating trauma. Urology 40:216, 1992
17. Corriere JN Jr, Sandler CM: Management of extraperitoneal bladder rupture. Urol Clin North Am 16:275, 1989
18. Fried FA, Rutledge R: A statewide population-based analysis of the frequency and outcome of genitourinary injury in a series of 215,220 trauma patients. J Urol 153:314A, 1995
19. Corriere JN Jr: Trauma to the lower urinary tract. Adult and Pediatric Urology. Gillenwater JY, Grayhack JT, Howards SS, et al, Eds. Mosby–Year Book, St. Louis, 1991, p 499
20. Peters PC: Intraperitoneal rupture of the bladder. Urol Clin North Am 16:279, 1989
21. Cass AS: Diagnostic studies in bladder rupture: indications and techniques. Urol Clin North Am 16:267, 1989
22. Sandler CM, Corriere JN Jr: Urethrography in the diagnosis of acute urethral injuries. Urol Clin North Am 16:283, 1989
23. Webster GD: Perineal repair of membranous urethral stricture. Urol Clin North Am 16:303, 1989
24. Husmann DA, Boone TB, Wilson WT: Management of low velocity gunshot wounds to the anterior urethra: the role of primary repair versus urinary diversion alone. J Urol 150:70, 1993
25. Devine CJ Jr, Jordan GH, Devine PC: Primary urethral realignment. Urol Clin North Am 16:291, 1989
26. Guille F, Cipolla B, Leveque S, et al: Early endoscopic realignment of complete traumatic rupture of the posterior urethra. Br J Urol 68:178, 1991
27. Knudson MM, Crombleholme WR: Female genital trauma and sexual assault. Abdominal Trauma. Blaisdell FW, Trunkey DD, Eds. Thieme Medical Publishers, New York, 1993, p 311
28. Mandell J, Cromie WJ, Caldamone AA: Sports-related genitourinary injuries in children. Clin Sports Med 1:483, 1982
29. Quast DC, Jordan GL: Traumatic wounds of the female reproductive organs. J Trauma 4:839, 1964
30. Maull KI, Rozycki GS, Pedigo RE: Injury to the female reproductive system. Trauma, 1st ed. Mattox KL, Moore EE, Feliciano DV, Eds. Appleton-Lange, San Mateo, California, 1988
31. Sexual assault. ACOG Technical Bulletin. 101:1, 1987
32. Niemi TA, Norton LW: Vaginal injuries in patients with pelvic fracture. J Trauma 25:547, 1985
33. Shires GT: Trauma. Principles of Surgery, 4th ed. Schwartz SI, Shires GT, Spencer FC, et al, Eds. McGraw-Hill, New York, 1984, p 199
34. Towery R, English TP, Wisner D: Evaluation of pregnant women after blunt injury. J Trauma 35:731, 1993
35. Pearlman MD, Tintinalli JE, Lorenz RP: Blunt trauma during pregnancy. N Engl J Med 323:1609, 1990
36. Fildes J, Reed L, Jones N, et al: Trauma: the leading cause of maternal death. J Trauma 32:643, 1992
37. Esposito TJ, Gens DR, Smith LG, et al: Trauma during pregnancy: a review of 79 cases. Arch Surg 126:1073, 1991
38. Knudson MM: Trauma in pregnancy. Abdominal Trauma. Blaisdell FW, Trunkey DD, Eds. Thieme Medical Publishers, New York, 1993, p 324
39. Drost TF, Rosemurgy AS, Sherman HF, et al: Major trauma in pregnant women: maternal/fetal outcome. J Trauma 30:574, 1990
40. Kissinger DP, Rozycki GS, Morris JA, et al: Trauma in pregnancy: predicting pregnancy outcome. Arch Surg 126:1079, 1991
41. Pearlman MD, Tintinalli JE, Lorenz RP: A prospective controlled study of outcome after trauma during pregnancy. Am J Obstet Gynecol 162:1502, 1990
42. Baker DP: Trauma in the pregnant patient. Surg Clin North Am 62:275, 1982
43. Wolf JS, Gomez R, McAninch JW: Human bites to the penis. J Urol 147:1265, 1992
44. Gomez R: Genital injuries. Problems in Urology 8:279, 1994
45. Fournier GR, Laing FC, McAninch JW: Scrotal ultrasonography and the management of testicular trauma. Urol Clin North Am 16:377, 1989
46. McAninch JW: Management of genital skin loss. Urol Clin North Am 16:387, 1989

Acknowledgments

Figures 1, 3, and 5   Susan Brust, C.M.I. Adapted from originals by P. Stempen.

Figures 2, 4, 6, and 8 through 11   Marcia Kammerer.

32 INJURIES TO THE EXTREMITIES

John T. Owings, M.D., *James P. Kennedy*, M.D., and *F. William Blaisdell*, M.D.

Assessment and Management of Extremity Injuries

Trauma to the extremities falls into two basic categories, penetrating and blunt. After penetrating trauma, the primary problem is vascular or neurologic injury. After blunt traumatic injury, the most common problem is fractures and the soft tissue injuries that accompany them. Nonetheless, high-velocity missile injuries can cause complex bone and soft tissue injuries, and blunt trauma can also cause neurologic and vascular injuries.

Unless active bleeding is present, injuries to the extremities are less urgent than injuries to the trunk, the head, or the neck: most extremity injuries are not immediately life-threatening and thus can be treated more deliberately. If massive hemorrhage occurs, particularly from a proximal extremity, it can usually be controlled by the application of direct pressure over the bleeding area or, if the conformation of the wound permits, by the introduction of a gloved finger for direct control of the bleeding. In either case, the patient should be directly transferred to the operating room.

Initial Assessment, Temporizing of Fracture-Dislocations, and Secondary Evaluation

Assessment of an injured extremity starts with a history, which can be obtained in parallel with the examination. Failure to elicit the patient's bleeding history at the scene from those transporting the patient may result in failure to recognize the presence of a major vascular injury. The mechanism of injury should also be ascertained.

The initial examination should first be directed toward the circulation. Blood pressure and temperature in both the injured limb and its contralateral counterpart should be determined. Distal pulses should be sought; if they are present and bounding, major vascular injury is unlikely. Injured extremities should be compared with their uninjured counterparts because pulse assessment may be difficult in the face of shock resulting from systemic or torso injuries. If the pulses in one extremity differ significantly from those in the other, vascular injury may be present.

If pulses are absent and a joint dislocation or fracture-dislocation is present, then gentle reduction of the dislocation should be carried out without delay. Frequently, a pulseless extremity with a dislocation regains pulses once the fracture or dislocation is reduced. If pulses return after reduction of the dislocation, assessment may continue on to the next priority. If pulses do not return, vascular injury is assumed, and treatment of such injury becomes the immediate priority.

The circulatory examination should be followed first by a quick neurologic examination aimed at assessing motor function in the hands and feet and ascertaining the presence or absence of sensation and later by a proximal examination of sensory and motor function. Gross deformity is pathognomonic of fracture or dislocation, and appropriate x-rays should be obtained that include portions of the joint above and below the area of suspected injury. Before x-rays are obtained, any gross deformities should be gently reduced to yield a more anatomic alignment of the extremity and splinted to relieve any possible compromise of neural or vascular structures. Finally, soft tissue defects should be noted. If considerable oozing is present, particularly in critical areas such as the hand, proximal application of a tourniquet for a few minutes may facilitate examination, permit definitive control of the bleeding point, and help determine whether significant nerve, muscle, or tendon injury has occurred.

Once the patient's condition has fully stabilized and other injuries have been evaluated, a secondary evaluation of the extremities is appropriate after blunt trauma. The shock, pain, and discomfort associated with more severe truncal injuries may mask the presence of significant extremity injuries. Passive motion of the extremity that results in localized discomfort or crepitation is a signal that x-rays are needed. In the absence of fracture or dislocation, specialized films (e.g., motion or stress studies) may be required if major ligamentous disruption is suspected. Any open wound in the extremity that is associated with a fracture is by definition an open fracture and usually must be explored surgically, ideally within six hours of wounding to ensure the removal of any contamination that may have resulted when the bone penetrated the skin.[1] Traumatic penetration of a joint (traumatic arthrotomy) similarly must be expeditiously addressed with prompt irrigation of the joint.

Temporary splinting is in order when definitive treatment of extensive soft tissue injuries, major strains or sprains, or fractures will be delayed. Splints applied in the emergency department must immobilize the injured extremity and prevent movement of the joint above and below the injured area: for example, with a tibial fracture, the leg should be splinted from the toes up to the proximal thigh. Temporary stabilization makes the patient more comfortable and facilitates transfer to the radiology department, the operating room, or elsewhere. Immobilization of long bone fractures also helps prevent further soft tissue damage and decrease wound complications. Because most plaster splints obscure radiographic detail, they are best applied after x-rays have been taken. Cardboard splints can be used to stabilize grossly unstable fractures.

Splints vary in width and thickness according to what is appropriate for the extremity. Generally, 15 layers of plaster are applied for arm splints to prevent breakage at the elbow. This thickness is also appropriate for short leg splints; however, 20 to 25 layers may be required for long leg splints. Before being

Assessment and Management of Extremity Injuries

Patient presents with injury to extremity

Management of life-threatening injuries takes priority.
Elicit history (including bleeding history), and ascertain mechanism of injury.
Compare BP, distal pulses, and T° in injured limb and uninjured counterpart.
Check for paralysis or discomfort on motion.
Apply splints or dressing if treatment of fractures or soft tissue injuries must be delayed.

Fracture-dislocation is present, and extremity is pulseless

Reduce fracture-dislocation.
If pulses return, treat as orthopedic injury. If not, assume vascular injury.

No fracture-dislocation is present, and pulses are relatively normal

Major vascular injury is unlikely.

Signs of vascular injury are present

Pulseless extremity from blunt trauma: perform on-table arteriogram.
Pulseless extremity from penetrating trauma: explore or, if location of injury is uncertain, perform on-table arteriogram.
Extremity with pulses but at high risk for vascular injury: perform duplex Doppler evaluation or arteriogram electively.
Repair injuries identified, ideally via primary repair if ≤ 2 cm is resected. If more must be resected, use autogenous vein or a prosthetic graft.

No signs of vascular injury are present

Neurologic injury is present

Penetrating trauma: treat with early debridement and repair unless wound is heavily contaminated or was caused by a gunshot, in which case repair should be delayed.
Blunt trauma: delay repair to allow for possible return of function; these injuries are often contusions rather than lacerations.

No neurologic injuries are present

Orthopedic injuries are present

Open fractures: debride within 6–8 hr of injury, irrigate with saline, and stabilize. Begin antibiotics in ER [*see Figure 3*].
Closed fractures: stabilize.

No orthopedic injuries are present

applied, the splint should be well padded, especially at its edges and at bony prominences, to prevent abrasions, pressure sores, and burns from the exothermic reactions that occur as fiberglass or plaster hardens. Once it has been applied, the splint should be wrapped in such a way as to prevent constriction and held in place with bias-cut stockinette or a similar material.

The ankle should be placed in as close to a neutral position as possible to prevent an equinus deformity. A neutral position can be achieved with a posterior splint bent at 90° or with sugar tong splints applied to the leg medially and laterally. For long leg splints, the knee should be gently flexed. Upper extremity splints should be applied with the limb in the resting position, the wrist extended 20°, and the phalangeal joints gently flexed. An easy way to remember this position is to imagine the hand holding a glass in a drinking position.

The Robert Jones dressing is a very useful all-purpose compressive dressing that immobilizes the injured extremity, helps control swelling, and prevents circulatory compromise. First, a single layer of cast padding is applied to the skin to prevent irritation. Next, one or two layers of thick cotton batting are applied circumferentially or longitudinally and held in place with a roll of cotton bandage. Finally, a splint is applied and kept in place with an elastic bandage or stockinette.

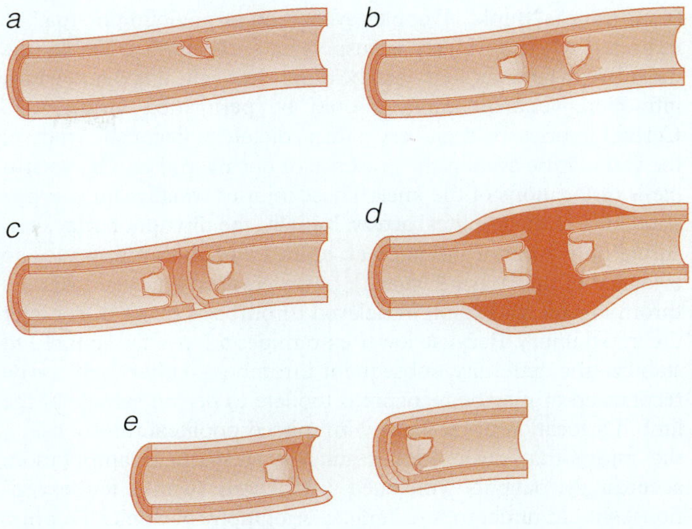

Injuries to Blood Vessels

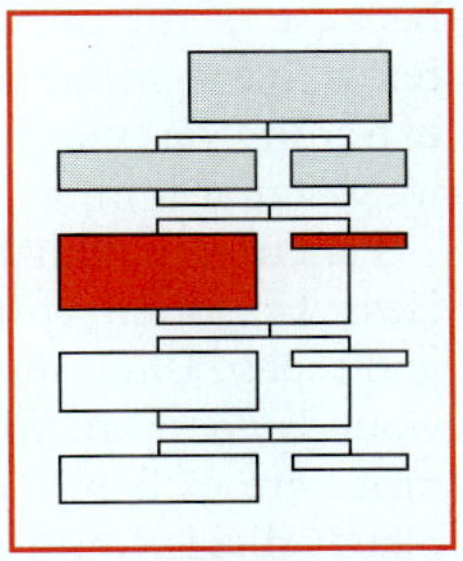

ARTERIES

Arterial injuries in an upper extremity are generally a less demanding problem than corresponding injuries in a lower extremity. The main reasons are, first, that upper extremity vessels have much better collateral flow and, second, that even ischemic upper extremities tend to remain viable except when extensive soft tissue damage is present. Moreover, because arteries and veins are smaller in the upper extremities, life-threatening hemorrhages are less common; exceptions are injuries to the subclavian or axillary arteries, which can cause unexpected exsanguination into the chest or present as intrathoracic bleeding.

Blunt and penetrating trauma usually produce different types of injuries. Injuries from blunt trauma usually result in thrombosis of a vessel. Such injuries are primarily stretch injuries rather than transections [see Figure 1]; as the vessel stretches, the tunica intima and the tunica media are disrupted first, leaving the highly thrombogenic tunica externa to maintain temporary vessel continuity. Penetrating injuries that completely divide the vessel may be manifested by thrombosis rather than hemorrhage. If the vessel is only partially divided, however, it contracts and thus will continue to bleed. Accordingly, partial transections are far more dangerous than complete ones.

Bleeding from injured extremity vessels may be ongoing or, if the patient becomes hypotensive, may stop temporarily, only to resume when resuscitation has been initiated. The urgency with which one approaches this type of hemorrhage is governed by whether there is any ongoing limb-threatening ischemia. If limb-threatening ischemia is present, especially in conjunction with anesthesia and paralysis, the extremity is likely to be nonviable: unless vascular repair can be accomplished within six hours, normal function is unlikely to return. Moreover, attempts at late repair may be associated with reperfusion injury, the consequences of which also can be life-threatening. If, however, the

Figure 1 Shown is an avulsion injury, in which the artery is stretched, resulting either in partial (*a*) or complete (*b*) intimal disruption or in complete intimal or medial disruption (*c*), with or without pseudoaneurysm formation (*d*) and complete separation of all layers of the vessel wall (*e*).

limb is viable (as indicated by normal or modestly delayed capillary refill, normal sensation, and normal muscle function), then management of other injuries may justifiably assume priority.

Penetrating Trauma

Penetrating vascular injuries generally declare themselves readily. As a rule, the location of a presumed vascular injury can be relatively easily determined by simply noting the path of the penetrating object. If there is evidence of thrombosis or ongoing bleeding, a prompt trip to the operating room and an incision placed so as to ensure proximal and distal control are appropriate. If the location of the penetrating injury is obscure or multiple injuries may exist, angiographic or ultrasonographic evaluation may be appropriate. If the extremity is nonviable, arteriography in the operating room is usually preferable to waiting for specific examination in the radiology department. Extremity arteriography in the OR can be performed by injection into the axillary artery (for upper extremity injuries) or the common femoral artery (for lower extremity injuries). Exposure of the x-ray plate immediately after injection of 15 to 20 ml of full-strength contrast material usually results in visualization of the injured area. If it does not, additional films should be obtained; these may be timed according to the progress of the contrast material as estimated from the initial x-ray.

There is considerable controversy regarding whether exploration or angiography is needed when a penetrating injury passes in proximity to a major blood vessel. If the limb appears viable, a duplex Doppler examination may be the best choice: it will identify significant injuries while causing minimal morbidity.[2]

Blunt Trauma

Blunt arterial injuries are more difficult to evaluate than penetrating arterial injuries. With blunt trauma, an artery may be completely disrupted, yet pulses may still be present if sufficient collateral blood flow remains. The injured extremity should be compared with its uninjured counterpart; if there are no major differences, it is unlikely that an arterial injury is present. Because the location of an arterial injury is more difficult to discern in cases of blunt trauma, duplex Doppler evaluation or angiography may be indicated when an injury is suspected. If the limb is viable, the definitive diagnostic study can be done electively. If it is not viable, intraoperative angiography should be performed in the OR. Certain injuries, by their very nature, dictate a diagnostic study of the vasculature even in the presence of normal pulses. One example is dislocations of the knee. These injuries usually cause severe stretching of the popliteal artery. Initially, the disruption may constitute only a minor intimal tear, and examination may reveal no evidence of injury [see Figure 2]; however, these internal tears are thrombogenic and result in delayed thrombosis many hours after the initial injury. Because lower extremities are usually splinted to stabilize the extremity, subsequent thrombosis either may not be recognized or may be recognized too late to permit salvage of the limb. Dislocation of the knee with missed popliteal thrombosis is the injury that most often results in subsequent amputation; accordingly, patients with knee dislocations (with a few exceptions) should undergo screening arteriography or duplex Doppler evaluation before any definitive orthopedic treatment of the limb.[3]

VEINS

In the absence of an associated arterial injury, most venous injuries probably go unrecognized. On the whole, the venous system has excellent collateral circulation, and major secondary hemorrhage is rare. Silent venous thrombosis may be responsible for valve damage or may set the stage for subsequent occlusive thrombosis resulting in limb swelling or thromboembolic problems. In the absence of other indications for exploration of the limb, asymptomatic venous injuries need not be repaired; however, adjusted-dose heparin should be used whenever venous injury is suspected or documented, unless contraindications exist. If there is an associated arterial injury that calls for exposure and operative treatment, the venous injury should be treated simultaneously if the repair is simple. Alternatively, clean ligation may be done; this gives rise to fewer complications than simply ignoring the injury or performing an ill-advised repair of a complex injury. With certain venous injuries, particularly those about the popliteal space or those associated with extensive soft tissue injury, the venous collateral circulation may be inadequate, in which case repair is indicated.

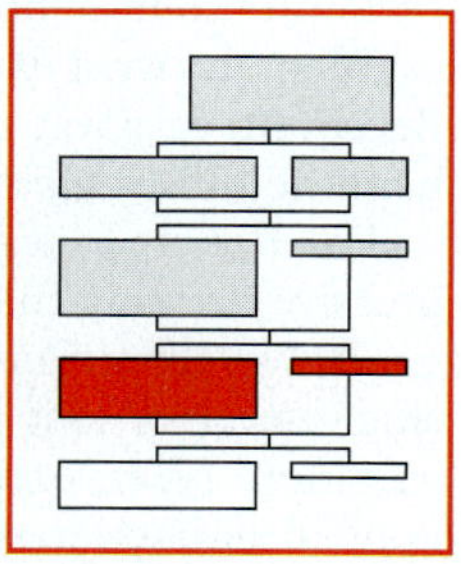

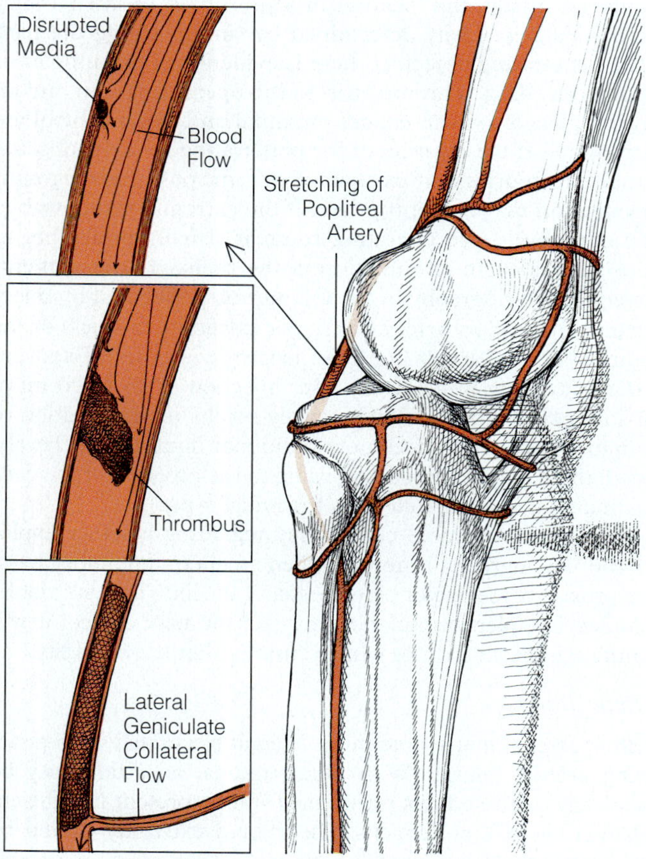

Injuries to Nerves

Nerve injury has always been the most challenging aspect of managing trauma to the extremities. It is the principal factor that accounts for limb loss and permanent disability.[4] Some nerve injuries, such as brachial plexus injuries and nerve root injuries, preclude repair.

Because the upper extremities have less muscle and bone mass and more neurologic structures than the lower extremities do, upper extremity injuries are twice as likely to result in nerve damage as lower extremity injuries are. Furthermore, because of the proximity of the upper extremity nerves to arteries, nerve injuries are more common in patients with upper extremity vascular injuries than in patients with lower extremity vascular injuries.

Penetrating injuries from cuts or stab wounds that result in a clean laceration of a nerve are amenable to early intervention and repair. Blunt injuries and penetrating injuries from gunshot wounds are more difficult to assess and manage. When such injuries are explored, one often finds that the nerve is not completely divided, and it is difficult to identify functional injuries—as opposed to anatomic injuries—through visual inspection. Functional loss does not preclude complete recovery without intervention. If exploration reveals complete division of a nerve, it is difficult to determine how much nerve resection may be required to ensure anastomosis of healthy tissue.

CLASSIFICATION

The most practical guide to classification of nerve injuries is that of Sunderland, which comprises five degrees of nerve injury [see Table 1].

First-degree nerve injury results from either concussion or compression of the nerve; electrical conductivity distal to the lesion is preserved. Surgical repair is not necessary. Recovery is spontaneous and rapid, occurring within days or weeks. Because it does not depend on regeneration of any neural element, recovery is usually complete.

Second-degree nerve injury occurs when the anatomic continuity of the nerve and the Schwann sheath is preserved but the axons are interrupted and must recover by means of axonal regeneration. It is characterized by complete motor, sensory, and autonomic paralysis and progressive muscle atrophy. Surgical repair is not necessary. Recovery from secondary injuries is typically complete unless the injury is so proximal that motor end-plate and sensory receptors atrophy before the axon can grow back. The usual rate of axonal regeneration is approximately 1 mm/day or 1 in/month.

Third-degree nerve injuries involve disruption of endoneural sheaths as well as axons. Thus, when the axons regenerate,

Figure 2 Knee dislocation is a common mechanism of popliteal artery injury.

Table 1 Sunderland's Classification of Injuries to Nerves[13]

Degree of Injury	Anatomic Disruption
First	Conduction loss only, without anatomic disruption
Second	Axonal disruption, without loss of the neurilemmal sheath
Third	Loss of axons and nerve sheaths
Fourth	Fascicular disruption
Fifth	Nerve transection

they may enter the nerve sheaths of other axons, resulting in aberrant regeneration. The loss of the sheath leads to increased intraneural fibrosis, which makes it more difficult for the regenerating axons to penetrate the site of injury. The time needed for functional improvement depends on the distance between the injury site and the end organ.

Fourth-degree injuries involve disruption of nerve fasciculi and cause a greater degree of intraneural scarring. To regain function, axons must grow through the scar and reenter the endoneural sheaths. When fourth-degree injuries are minimal, partial resection with meticulous anastomosis of the fasciculi improves outcome.

Fifth-degree nerve injuries involve transection of the entire peripheral nerve. Invariably, there is considerable epineural and perineural hemorrhage and subsequent scarring. Recovery of neural function is impossible without surgical intervention. Fifth-degree injuries may be limited to a very short section of nerve (as with sharp transection) or may affect a very long segment (as with gunshot injury); they may also be associated with stretch injury or compartment syndrome.

How quickly and successfully the nerves regenerate depends on several factors. One such factor is age: the younger the patient, the faster and more complete the recovery. Another is the type of nerve involved: a pure motor or sensory nerve recovers better than a nerve containing both motor and sensory fibers. Thus, the radial and musculocutaneous nerves, which are primarily motor nerves, recover better than the mixed medial nerves, and the tibial division of the sciatic nerve fares better than the peroneal division. A third factor is the level of nerve injury and the duration of denervation. If regenerating axons take more than 12 months to reach denervated muscle, a significant degree of muscle atrophy will have occurred, and the muscle may remain dysfunctional despite some degree of reinnervation. Even when this is the case, it may still be possible to restore some sensation. For example, repair of a divided ulnar nerve near the axilla or the peroneal nerve above midthigh is unlikely to improve motor function; however, median nerve repair near the axilla or tibial nerve at about midthigh may allow the return of at least some protective sensation.

TREATMENT

Whenever an extremity is injured, careful assessment of motor and sensory function is essential. If other life-threatening cranial or truncal injuries are present, evaluation and treatment of nerve injuries may be deferred until these more urgent problems are dealt with. Before any orthopedic manipulation or treatment of vascular injury, an examination must be conducted to assess the integrity of the nerves.

For lacerating nerve injuries, surgical exploration is often indicated. Generally, if the wound is clean or minimally contaminated, the feasibility of nerve repair can be considered after the more immediate problems (e.g., vascular injuries) are corrected. If the nerve ends appear to have been sharply divided and there is minimal hemorrhage or contusion, immediate repair is appropriate; identification and approximation of nerve fasciculi are more easily accomplished before extraneural scarring obscures nerve anatomy. If, however, the penetrating object is relatively blunt (e.g., a missile), if the injury is dirty, if there is significant soft tissue damage, if associated fractures are present, or if the vascular repair is particularly tenuous, nerve repair should be delayed. In such circumstances, one should clean and debride the wound, identify the nerve ends if they are divided, and fix them in proximity so that they do not retract; the need for subsequent mobilization at the time of repair will thereby be reduced. After the wound has healed, reexploration is indicated for definitive repair about three to four weeks after the injury.

A progressing neurologic deficit is another indication for urgent surgical exploration. Such a deficit may result from a false aneurysm associated with vascular injury or from compartment syndrome attributable to hemorrhage and swelling in a fascial compartment. Emergency nerve decompression for a worsening neurologic deficit involves opening any skin, fascia, or muscle constricting the nerve. The decompressed nerve should be covered with some soft tissue, although delayed skin closure may be necessary if the fascia cannot be closed. In cases of compartment syndrome, fascial closure should not be attempted.

In all instances of blunt trauma, delayed repair (usually two to three months after the injury) is recommended. With neurapraxic lesions, this allows time for recovery, and with axonotmesis lesions, it allows time for possible axonal regrowth through the area of injury. When exploration is delayed, nerve action potential should be recorded intraoperatively to determine whether axonal regeneration has crossed the lesion in continuity. Intraoperative recording of nerve action potentials is much superior to waiting for electromyographic evidence of motor recovery, which requires an average waiting period of six months. If no action potentials are recorded crossing the injury, the nerve is resected proximal and distal to the injury until a normal fascicular pattern is obtained. If possible, the nerve is then primarily reapproximated, the epineurium is sutured, or cable nerve grafts are employed.

Open Fractures and Dislocations

The prognosis after an open fracture is very different from that after a closed fracture; treatment of open fractures is much more complex than treatment of simple fractures or traumatic wounds. The existence of an open fracture means that a great deal of energy has been delivered to the bone to produce soft tissue disruption. Accordingly, it can be inferred that there has been considerable stripping of muscle, periosteum, and ligament from the bone, resulting in relative devascularization, and that varying degrees of contusion, crushing, and devascularization of the associated soft tissues have occurred. All of these events greatly influence the rate of healing, the incidence of nonunion, and the risk of infection.

The basic principles of management for open fractures are aggressive debridement, open wound treatment, soft tissue and bone stabilization, and systemic administration of antibiotics. These principles have reduced the formerly high mortality associated with open fractures to very acceptable levels.

A simple classification for open fractures exists that is well accepted [see Table 2]. High-velocity gunshot wounds and open fractures must be approached somewhat differently from closed fractures because of the force imparted to the soft tissues. A fracture that looks like a grade 1 injury because of a small skin wound may behave as a grade 3 injury because of soft tissue injury. Any open fracture associated with bone loss is treated as a grade 3 injury, as is any grade 1 or grade 2 soft tissue wound that is associated with severe tissue contusion and periosteal stripping. In addition, any fracture associated with gross contamination (e.g., a farmyard injury with vegetable matter or soil within the wound) is treated as a grade 3 injury because of the risk of clostridial infection and clostridial myonecrosis.

EVALUATION

The injured extremity should undergo orthopedic examination, with particular attention paid to evaluation of neural and vascular status. Compartment syndrome [see Compartment Syndrome, below] should be ruled out in patients at risk; as many as 10 percent of open tibial fractures are associated with this syndrome as a result of severe soft tissue injury.

The patient's medical condition before the injury, the time elapsed since the injury, the mechanism of injury, and the presence or absence of associated injuries should be noted. If foreign material that is easily removable can be seen, it should be removed promptly, and a quick saline dump (i.e., pouring 1 to 2 L of saline into the wound to help wash out gross contamination and prevent tissue desiccation) is indicated. If the limb is malaligned, gentle gross reduction should be done to relieve any vascular compromise. A sterile dressing moistened with saline or povidone-iodine should then be applied to the wound, and a few minutes should be spent on securing the wound. Ideally, once the wound is assessed and the dressing applied, the dressing should not be removed until the patient is in the operating room and preparation for operation is initiated. Once a secure dressing has been applied, a temporary splint should be applied to the limb so that the patient can be transported for x-rays if necessary. Cardboard splints are convenient, inexpensive, and disposable and do not interfere with x-rays.

TREATMENT

When a severe open extremity fracture is accompanied by vascular or neurologic injury, the limb may not be salvageable; such an injury may be essentially a traumatic amputation in which the parts remain connected by a bridge of skin. Although some severely injured limbs can be salvaged, those with both neurologic and vascular injury have a high complication rate and a late amputation rate of 78 percent. Often, the best treatment in such cases is immediate amputation.

Every open fracture calls for emergent surgical treatment [see Figure 3]. Ideally, treatment should begin within six hours of injury: the incidence of infection is directly related to delay in initiating treatment. The factors most helpful in reducing infection (the most severe preventable complication) are antibiotic therapy, timely and aggressive surgical debridement, fracture stabilization, and proper treatment of wounds. Tetanus prophylaxis should be given as needed. Cultures should be obtained in the course of debridement because the results may influence subsequent antibiotic therapy. Patients with grade 1 or grade 2 injuries should receive cefazolin in a dosage of 1 g every four hours while in the operating room and 1 g every eight hours afterward. Patients with

Table 2 Gradation of Open Fractures[12]

Grade	Wound Size	Extent of Soft Tissue Damage
1	< 1 cm	No or minimal tissue damage
2	> 1 cm	Moderate tissue damage
3	Any size	Major tissue damage; soft tissue loss; bone loss; gross contamination
3a		Bone can be covered
3b		Bone cannot be covered
3c		Vascular injury

grade 3 fractures or grossly contaminated grade 1 or 2 fractures should receive penicillin and gentamicin as well.

WOUND CARE

For all open fractures, irrigation and debridement in the sterile, controlled environment of the OR are required [see Figure 3]. Even apparently minor injuries, such as minimal grade 1 injuries, benefit from thorough examination. The traumatic wound should be extended in such a way as to be compatible with any fracture fixation that may be necessary, and all devitalized or contused soft tissue should be aggressively debrided back to normal, clean, bleeding tissue. It may be a good idea to have a tourniquet in place, but it should be inflated only long enough to control acute hemorrhage; prolonged inflation leads to further tissue ischemia and eliminates muscle contractility, the best indication of muscle viability. If uncontrollable bleeding is encountered, the tourniquet may be inflated for a few minutes until the bleeding point is located and secured. The fracture ends should be delivered into the wound to facilitate inspection and allow adequate irrigation. Any devitalized, stripped, loose bone fragments that are not crucial to reduction or stabilization should be removed, devascularized bone should be debrided, and bleeding fragments should be carefully handled so as to maintain their attachments to the bone and preserve their vascularity.

A pulsatile lavage system should then be used to irrigate the wound and the bone ends with 8 to 10 L of nornal saline. At this point, tissue specimens should be obtained and sent for culture. Irrigation is completed by adding another 2 L of fluid containing 100,000 units of bacitracin. Any surgically created wound extensions may then be closed; however, the traumatic wound itself should be left widely open. If the wound is small, a portion of the surgical extension should be left open to allow adequate drainage and to prevent the traumatic wound from sealing off prematurely. Every attempt should be made to cover bone, joint surfaces, implants, and sensitive structures (e.g., tendons, nerves, and blood vessels) with available local soft tissue, but this must be done without tension.

After the initial debridement, the antibiotic regimen is continued for 24 to 48 hours. At this point, if the postdebridement cultures are positive, the regimen is changed to include agents that are appropriate for the infecting organism. If the cultures are negative, the antibiotic regimen may be stopped if the wound appears clean. Any patient who has a grade 3 fracture or a grade 1 or 2 fracture with a positive culture should be returned to the OR every 48 hours for repeat irrigation and debridement until the wound appears healthy and clean. Each time the patient is returned to the OR, new tissue cultures are taken and antibiotics restarted. If the bacterial counts on quantitative culture are higher than 10,000/g tissue, wound infection is probable; lower counts tend to reflect colonization

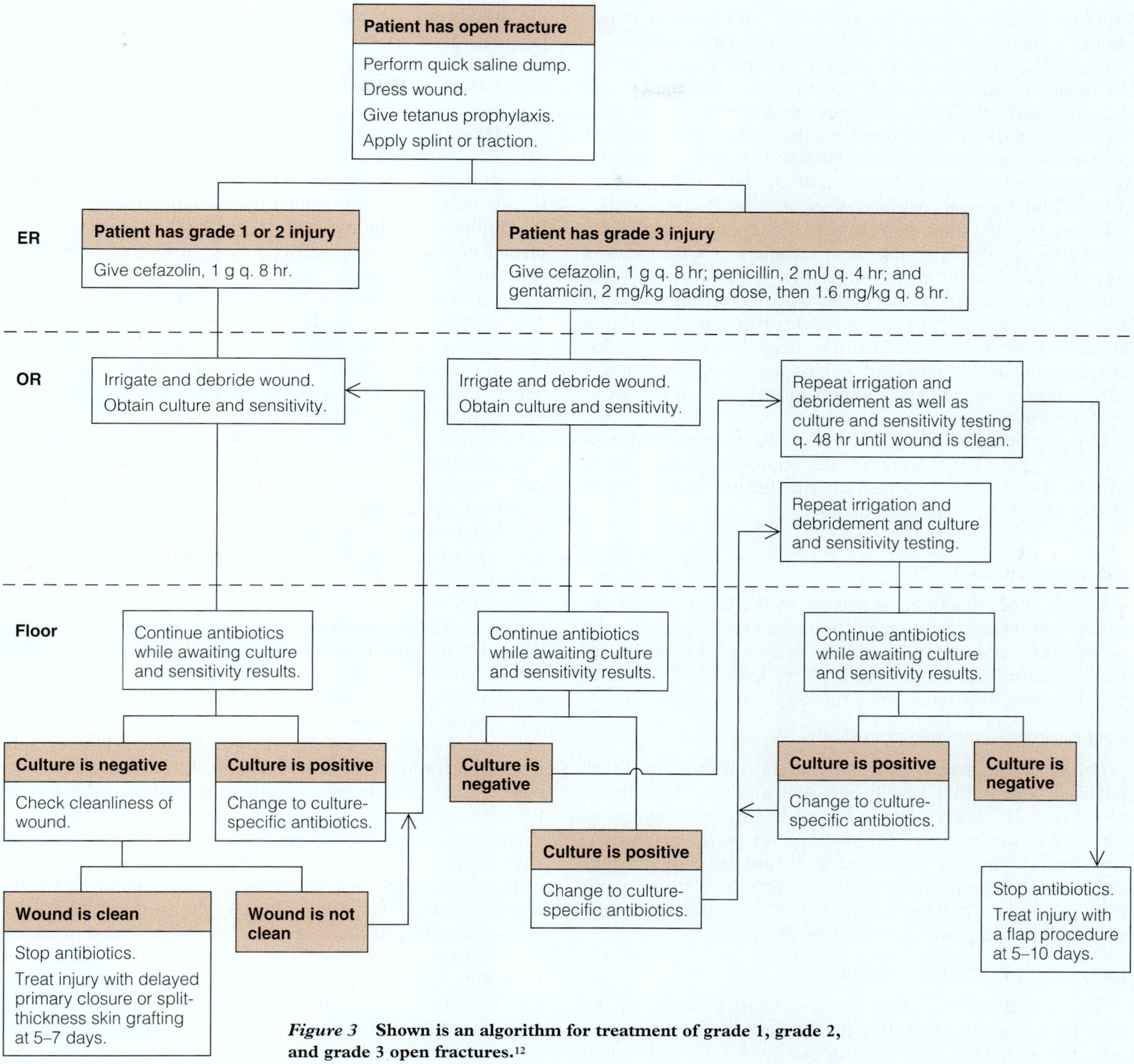

```
                          ┌─────────────────────────────┐
                          │  Patient has open fracture  │
                          │  Perform quick saline dump. │
                          │  Dress wound.               │
                          │  Give tetanus prophylaxis.  │
                          │  Apply splint or traction.  │
                          └─────────────────────────────┘
```

ER

Patient has grade 1 or 2 injury	Patient has grade 3 injury
Give cefazolin, 1 g q. 8 hr.	Give cefazolin, 1 g q. 8 hr; penicillin, 2 mU q. 4 hr; and gentamicin, 2 mg/kg loading dose, then 1.6 mg/kg q. 8 hr.

OR

Irrigate and debride wound. Obtain culture and sensitivity.	Irrigate and debride wound. Obtain culture and sensitivity.	Repeat irrigation and debridement as well as culture and sensitivity testing q. 48 hr until wound is clean.
		Repeat irrigation and debridement and culture and sensitivity testing.

Floor

Continue antibiotics while awaiting culture and sensitivity results.	Continue antibiotics while awaiting culture and sensitivity results.	Continue antibiotics while awaiting culture and sensitivity results.

Culture is negative	Culture is positive	Culture is negative	Culture is positive	Culture is positive	Culture is negative
Check cleanliness of wound.	Change to culture-specific antibiotics.		Change to culture-specific antibiotics.	Change to culture-specific antibiotics.	Stop antibiotics. Treat injury with a flap procedure at 5–10 days.

Wound is clean	Wound is not clean
Stop antibiotics. Treat injury with delayed primary closure or split-thickness skin grafting at 5–7 days.	

Figure 3 Shown is an algorithm for treatment of grade 1, grade 2, and grade 3 open fractures.[12]

rather than infection. In the case of a grade 1 or 2 injury in which the initial culture is negative, the wound may be allowed to close by granulation and secondary intention, or the patient may be returned to the OR in five to seven days for delayed primary closure. For larger wounds, split-thickness skin grafts are often required. For grade 3 wounds, some type of flap is often required for soft tissue coverage. The flap procedure should be done early, five to 10 days after the injury, provided that tissue cultures are negative at this time.

The same protocol used for open fractures is also followed for open dislocations; in addition, the articular surfaces must be kept moist. Cartilage that has been damaged by the force of impact may not be able to tolerate any further insult. Once the dislocation has been reduced with the patient under anesthesia, the joint should be thoroughly irrigated and debrided as required. The capsule of the reduced joint is closed over a suction drain, and the remaining traumatic wound is left open. In patients who have large grade 3 injuries associated with soft tissue loss, coverage for the articular surface may not be available, and immediate reconstruction with local or distal flaps may have to be done to keep articular cartilage viable. In these instances, only the joint cartilage should be covered; the remaining portion of the wound must be left open.

FRACTURE STABILIZATION

Operative fixation of open fractures is an extremely complex issue. Many options are open to the orthopedist, and these options change yearly. For open intra-articular fractures, internal fixation is indicated for better healing of cartilage. This is accomplished via anatomic reduction and lag screw fixation, which allowed early performance of range-of-motion exercises to minimize permanent loss of range of motion. In addition, any open fractures that are associated with massively traumatized limbs, that occur in patients with multiple injuries to multiple systems, or that are associated with vascular injury should be managed with internal fixation if at all possible.

Generally, it is desirable to stabilize the open fracture during the initial operative procedure. Restoring the anatomy through reduction and stabilization improves circulation; promotes healing of bone and soft tissue; reduces inflammation, bleeding, and dead space; and increases revascularization of devitalized tissue. It also results in earlier mobilization of multiply injured trauma patients and improves their overall status.

Isolated grade 1 open fractures that are treated promptly can usually be handled with the same techniques as their closed counterparts, with the exception of open tibial fractures. Grade 2 injuries that occur in ideal circumstances in certain favorable areas (e.g., metaphyseal bone in the forearm and the foot, the humerus, and the femur) can also be treated with the same internal fixation techniques used for closed fractures. Early internal fixation is the optimal method of stabilization for intra-articular fractures.

In other situations, such as those involving open tibial fractures and grade 3 fractures, the safer approach is conservative treatment with either modified internal fixation techniques or immobilization with external fixators.

Closed Fractures

Of the closed fractures, it is those of the lower extremities with which the trauma surgeon should be most concerned: the prognosis for closed upper extremity fractures is excellent, and these fractures are much less likely to have life-threatening complications than fractures of the lower extremities.

UPPER EXTREMITY FRACTURES

On the whole, fractures of the scapula and the clavicle are relatively benign: they usually heal well, and they typically respond to both conservative and open treatment. Fractures of the neck of the humerus, the shaft, or the condyles (particularly the last) may be associated with vascular complications and may call for immediate fixation. Fractures of the forearm, the wrist, and the hand generally respond to conservative measures and have little or no impact on outcome.

LOWER EXTREMITY FRACTURES

The closed fractures that are of greatest concern for the trauma surgeon and that have the greatest potential effect on outcome are fractures of the femur that involve the acetabulum (with or without hip dislocation), standard hip fractures, and fractures of the shaft of the femur. Other, somewhat less worrisome closed fractures of the lower extremities are fractures that involve the tibial plateau in the knee, fractures that involve the tibia or the fibula, and pilon fractures. Fractures and dislocations of the ankle and the foot, though having the potential to affect long-term morbidity when the ankle joint is involved, generally are not of concern in the immediate overall management of the trauma victim.

Acetabular Fracture and Hip Dislocation

Fractures of the acetabulum and hip dislocations have a common mechanism: they are usually the result of auto accidents in which a blow is directed down the axis of the femur with the hip and the knee flexed. The telltale sign of soft tissue injury to the knee in an auto accident victim suggests the possibility of hip injury as well. The converse is also true, in that as many as 25 percent of auto accident victims with posterior hip dislocation also have significant knee injuries. Dislocated hips constitute a pressing orthopedic emergency. Treatment consists of immediate reduction with the patient under general anesthesia to release neurologic compression, restore joint congruency, and reduce any compromise of the femoral head vasculature that may result in aseptic necrosis. This is one situation in which the orthopedist always takes priority over the general surgeon except in the case of impending cardiac arrest. It takes only a few minutes after the induction of anesthesia for the dislocation to be reduced, at which point the case can be turned back over to the general surgeon for definitive treatment of life-threatening emergencies.

Acetabular fractures are of two types. The first type is a fracture associated with hip dislocation; there may be associated cartilage compression with ensuing damage to the joint. The second type results from direct application of force against the pelvis; essentially, it is a pelvic fracture that happens to be intra-articular. The goals of treatment are to obtain anatomic reduction of the articular surfaces and a concentric stable hip joint, to remove intra-articular loose bodies, and to achieve early motion so as to optimize cartilaginous healing. In assessing an acetabular fracture, the most important step is the neurovascular examination, which determines whether any nerve injury has occurred. It is not uncommon to find the nerve entrapped within the sharp edges of a fracture or draped over a displaced fracture under great tension. If a nerve palsy is observed, rapid reduction and stabilization of the fracture are indicated to improve the chances of neurologic recovery. Unless there is an associated hip dislocation, no deformity is noted on examination, but the patient usually complains of deep-seated hip or groin pain. A routine pelvic film usually documents the presence of a fracture; oblique views and computed tomographic scanning permit further localization of the fragments (if necessary) and help determine whether the joint is congruent and the fracture stable.

Although some acetabular fractures (in particular, small chip fractures that have no significant articular component) can be treated with benign neglect, open fixation is usually required if the fracture is displaced or involves the weight-bearing dome of the acetabulum. Fixation may also be necessary for fractures that do not involve the weight-bearing dome if stability is required to prevent recurrent dislocation of the hip. Usually, if an acetabular fracture in a multiply injured patient is displaced severely enough to require internal fixation, intra-articular debris and other indications for open treatment are present. In most situations involving multiple injuries, the best time to fix acetabular injuries is at presentation: at no subsequent point in the early postinjury period will the patient's condition be more favorable and operative fixation easier. If the patient's condition is too unstable to allow immediate fixation, the injury should be treated operatively within five to seven days, before fibrosis and healing begin; once healing has started, mobilization and reduction of the fragments are more difficult. With unstable, displaced fractures, a tibial or femoral traction pin should be inserted if the patient cannot be operated on at presentation or must be stabilized medically before being transferred to a facility that is equipped for operative management of such injuries. In many instances, good reduction can be obtained by using 20 to 30 lb of skeletal traction.

As soon as the patient's level of discomfort has decreased sufficiently, gentle range-of-motion exercise should be started to help mold the cartilage and facilitate its healing. If the

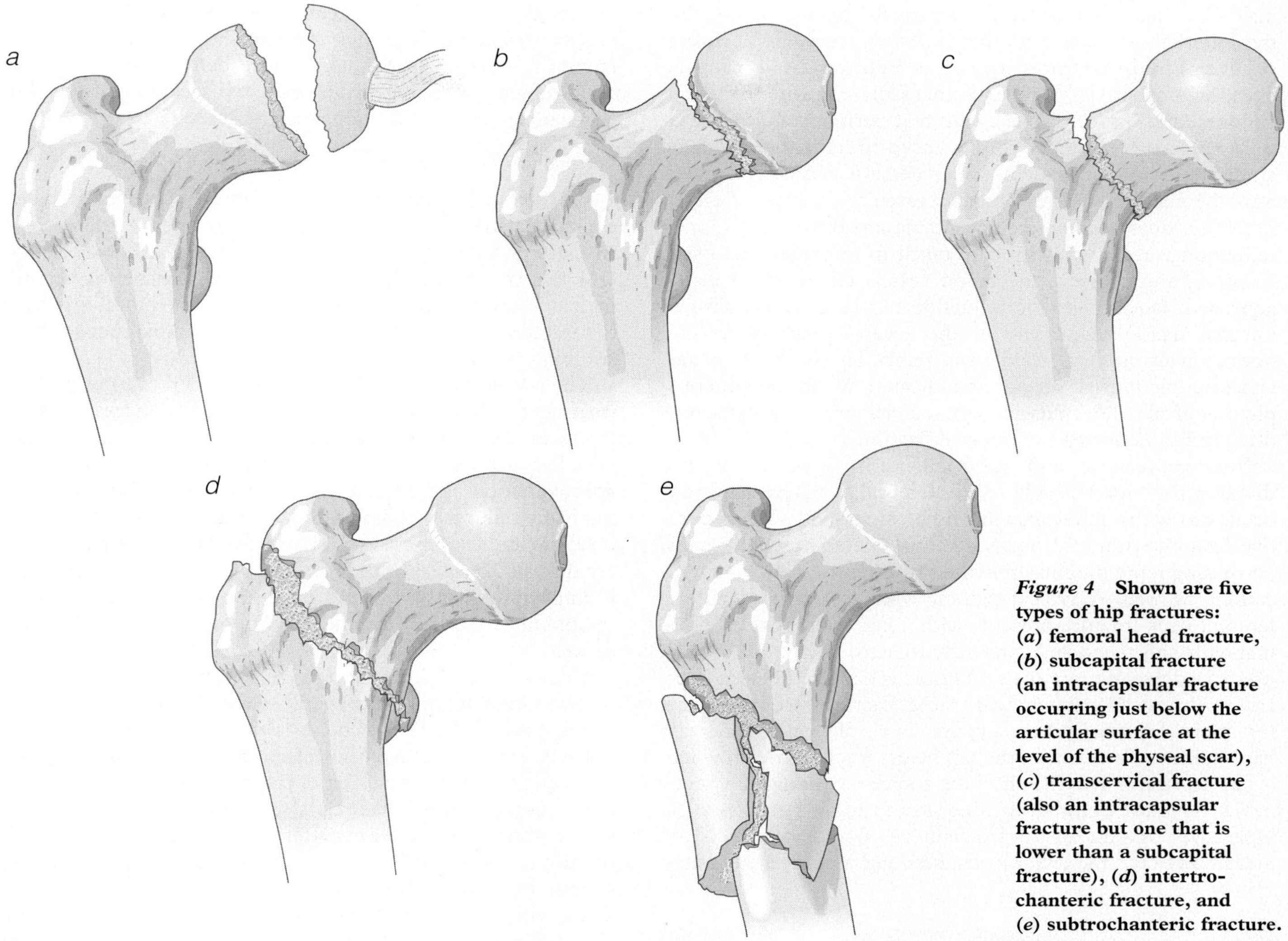

Figure 4 Shown are five types of hip fractures: (*a*) femoral head fracture, (*b*) subcapital fracture (an intracapsular fracture occurring just below the articular surface at the level of the physeal scar), (*c*) transcervical fracture (also an intracapsular fracture but one that is lower than a subcapital fracture), (*d*) intertrochanteric fracture, and (*e*) subtrochanteric fracture.

patient cannot cooperate with these efforts because of other injuries, continuous passive motion exercise can be started by using a mechanical device with an electric motor.

Hip Fracture

Fracture of the hip is one of the most common conditions seen by orthopedists. A substantial force is required to fracture a hip in a young, healthy accident victim, whereas a minor trauma or fall may be sufficient to do so in an elderly osteoporotic female. Hip fractures may be classified according to their anatomic site: (1) femoral head fractures, (2) intracapsular fractures (including subcapital and transcervical femoral neck fractures), (3) intertrochanteric fractures, and (4) subtrochanteric fractures [*see Figure 4*]. Treatment differs slightly from one type to the next; the primary influence on the choice of treatment is whether the all-important blood supply to the femoral head is preserved or disrupted. With intracapsular fractures, there is a significant risk of disrupting the tenuous blood supply to the joint involved. Such disruption leads to nonunion or avascular necrosis, which can be compounded in the hip by collapse of the femoral head.

Fractures of the femoral head are the most devastating of hip injuries and must be handled as surgical emergencies.[5] Once a femoral head fracture is recognized, it must be treated operatively within 24 hours of the injury to achieve optimal results. Closed treatment of such injuries yields uniformly poor results. Although operative treatment is usually necessary to provide the best chance of recovery, the initial trauma often is so great as to preclude good results; at best, good results can be obtained in only 50 percent of cases.[5]

Impaction fractures of the femoral head, however, may be treated in closed fashion with early range-of-motion exercise, particularly if they do not involve a major weight-bearing surface. Internal fixation of these injuries is technically very difficult. Small fracture fragments in the non–weight-bearing inferior portion of the head are probably best excised; large fragments or those involving a significant portion of the weight-bearing dome are best treated with operative fixation. At present, no one form of treatment yields consistently good results. In some patients, particularly physiologically older patients with significant fractures, it may be best to insert a hip prosthesis primarily.

Intracapsular femoral neck fractures carry a high risk of nonunion and avascular necrosis and should be treated on an emergency basis with operative fixation within 12 hours of injury. Even with early optimal surgical treatment, the incidence of avascular necrosis is 20 percent; if near-anatomic reduction is not obtained, the incidence approaches 50 percent.[6] The deformity associated with these fractures is not as great as that associated with extracapsular or intertrochanteric fractures. A typical patient with an intracapsular fracture presents with a shortened, externally rotated, and abducted lower extremity. Traction reduces the pain and, more importantly, may allow increased blood flow across the neck by decreasing the external rotation and thus relieving vascular occlusion resulting from compression of a tight, twisted capsule. Treatment consists of early anatomic reduction with fixation to eliminate the risk of displacement and permit rapid mobilization. Closed reduction of displaced fractures should be attempted with the patient under general anesthesia, and it must be gentle to prevent further vascular damage. If closed reduction does not achieve acceptable anatomic results, open reduction is required, with care taken to minimize soft tissue stripping and preserve the blood vessels encountered in the approach. Once anatomic reduction has been accomplished, internal fixation with any of the several types of fixation devices available (e.g., sliding hip screw devices, blade plates, and multiple pins or screws) is indicated. When the patient is physiologically older than 70 years, a primary hip prosthesis is often indicated instead of internal fixation.

Intertrochanteric and subtrochanteric fractures do not threaten the blood supply to the femoral head, because they occur below the extracapsular ring of vessels. As a rule, operative fixation within 24 hours of injury yields optimal results, permitting rapid mobilization and preventing systemic complications as well. A typical patient with an intertrochanteric femoral neck fracture presents with a limb that appears to be markedly shortened and externally rotated. Traction should be used if a delay of more than 12 hours is expected before operation. Almost all patients with these fractures are candidates for internal fixation; the exception is an elderly patient who had significant arthritis of the hip before the fracture, in whom a hip prosthesis may be the best choice. A sliding hip screw device is most commonly used for fixation [see Figure 5]. Operative fixation of subtrochanteric fractures, which are located between the lesser trochanter and a point 5 cm distally, can be more difficult because high bending forces in the region (resulting from the angular shape of the proximal femur) often lead to implant failure before union. Possible management approaches include cross-locking, intramedullary nailing, and the use of plates and screws.

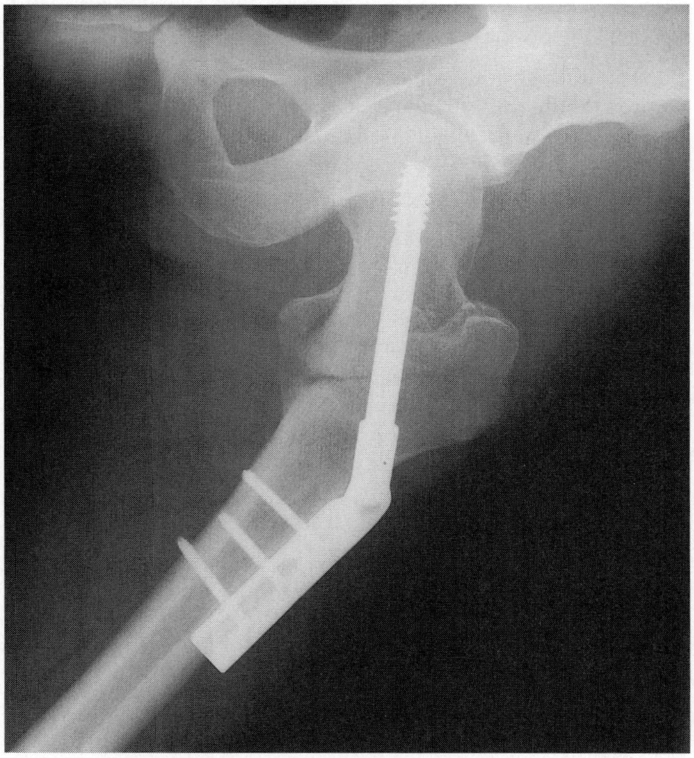

Femoral Shaft Fracture

Fractures of the femoral shaft, like intertrochanteric femoral neck fractures, are associated with significant blood loss. Because of the shape of the thigh, more than 1 L may be lost into this space with little or no external indication. Accordingly, the trauma surgeon must anticipate the blood loss from the fractured femur when formulating the initial management strategy.

The advent of intramedullary nailing has revolutionized the treatment of femoral shaft fractures. With stable femoral shaft fractures that undergo nailing, full weight bearing without crutches is possible within a few days of the operation. Reapproximation of the fracture fragments with nailing also dramatically reduces bleeding into the thigh. Femoral shaft fractures are often associated with injuries to knee ligaments, which are difficult to assess in the presence of the femoral fracture. It is important that, when the patient is under anesthesia for treatment of the fracture, the stability of the knee be assessed as well.

Neurovascular injuries are relatively uncommon with femoral shaft fractures; however, when the fracture is in the distal third of the femur, there is the possibility of injury to either the superficial femoral artery or the popliteal artery as a consequence of the tethering of these vessels against the shaft at the level of the adductor canal [see Figure 6]. The most popular method of immobilizing a femoral fracture for transport is the use of a Hare or Thomas splint. These convenient devices consist of a frame buttressed against the ischial tuberosity, along with a nonwound endstrap about the foot for traction. They effectively immobilize the extremity and lessen patient discomfort, and they need not be removed for x-rays to be taken. These splints do, however, exert some pressure on the foot; therefore, the patient should be placed in skeletal traction to maintain the benefits if immediate operation is not feasible. The skeletal traction pin should be placed in the tibia so that the femur is not contaminated by the pin wound. Its placement in the tibia should be distal to the anterior tubercle so that the entire thigh, including the knee joint, can be prepared for operation without the pin site being included.

Very few tenets in orthopedics are held with such absolute conviction as the tenet that femoral fractures are best treated with intramedullary nailing. Nailing lowers the incidence of respiratory distress syndrome, blood loss, and tissue trauma and reduces the patient's need for narcotics. In a multiply injured patient with a fractured femur, nailing should be done immediately to help control hemorrhage to the fracture site and help stabilize the patient hemodynamically. In one study,[7] multiply injured patients with an injury severity score of 18 or higher who underwent nailing more than 48 hours after the injury had a four times greater incidence of pulmonary complications than a similar group of patients who underwent nailing within 24 hours of injury; in addition, they had a longer average stay in the ICU (7.6 days as opposed to 2.8 days). In a patient who does not have multiple injuries, the timing is not crucial, but nailing is easier to perform if it is done within the first six to 12 hours because after this period, hemorrhage and swelling make reduction more difficult. Although virtually all open femoral fractures

Figure 5 **Hip x-ray shows an intertrochanteric fracture stabilized with a sliding hip screw device.**

are best treated with intramedullary nailing, a plate or an external fixator may be indicated as well in isolated instances.

Femoral fractures were once associated with significant morbidity and mortality but now are among the musculoskeletal injuries with the most predictable results after treatment. Most complications are secondary to technical problems at the time of nailing and therefore can be prevented by paying attention to the technical details.

Fracture and Dislocation of the Knee and the Patella

Knee injuries are common in multiply injured patients, partly because of the vulnerability of this joint to dashboard injuries in auto accidents and to direct trauma in motorcycle accidents.

Intra-articular knee fracture Fractures about the knee that affect the tibial or femoral condyles are as much an injury to the articular surface of the knee joint as they are a fracture of the periarticular bone. Consequently, even if successful bony union has been achieved, the issues of joint alignment, stability, stiffness, and posttraumatic arthritis must still be taken into account to ensure that the clinical result is not compromised. Knee fractures are characterized by local pain, swelling, and crepitation. A hemarthrosis forms when an intra-articular fracture is present. Such a fracture may be suspected when marrow fat globules are present in the hemarthrosis. With any injury about the knee, ligamentous stressing should not be performed until after x-rays confirm that no fracture is present. If the x-rays show a femoral supracondylar or tibial plateau fracture, x-rays of the entire length of the fractured bone should be obtained to rule out the presence of other fractures.

Unstable intra-articular knee fractures should be treated by means of anatomic reduction, rigid fixation, and early motion. Aspiration of a tense hemarthrosis is sometimes required to decompress the joint and relieve pain. The best results are achieved by means of immediate stabilization through rigid internal fixation; however, if treatment must be delayed for a few days after the injury, acceptable results usually can still be achieved. If delayed fixation is to be done, the extremity should be splinted or placed in balanced traction. Femoral condylar fractures, even when they initially are not displaced, should be treated with rigid fixation to minimize the risk of subsequent displacement from muscle forces or knee motion. Rigid fixation allows early motion to facilitate cartilage healing. Unstable or displaced tibial plateau fractures likewise should be treated with rigid fixation and early motion. Tibial plateau compression fractures are the result of an axial load and are displaced by definition. For active individuals, anatomic reduction and fixation allow early motion and yield the best long-term results. Often, bone grafting is required to maintain elevation of the articular surface.

After rigid stabilization of these fractures, the ligamentous structures about the knee should be evaluated via examination or stress films as warranted: as many as 25 percent of plateau fractures are associated with ligamentous injuries.[8] Late knee instability may compromise treatment of tibial plateau fractures and is a major cause of unacceptable results.

Patellar fracture The most common injury to the patella in trauma patients is a stellate comminuted fracture resulting from a direct blow; the second most common is an avulsion fracture that is a rupture of the extensor mechanism. A patient with a fractured patella exhibits soft tissue swelling about the knee as well as hemarthrosis, which may be tense.

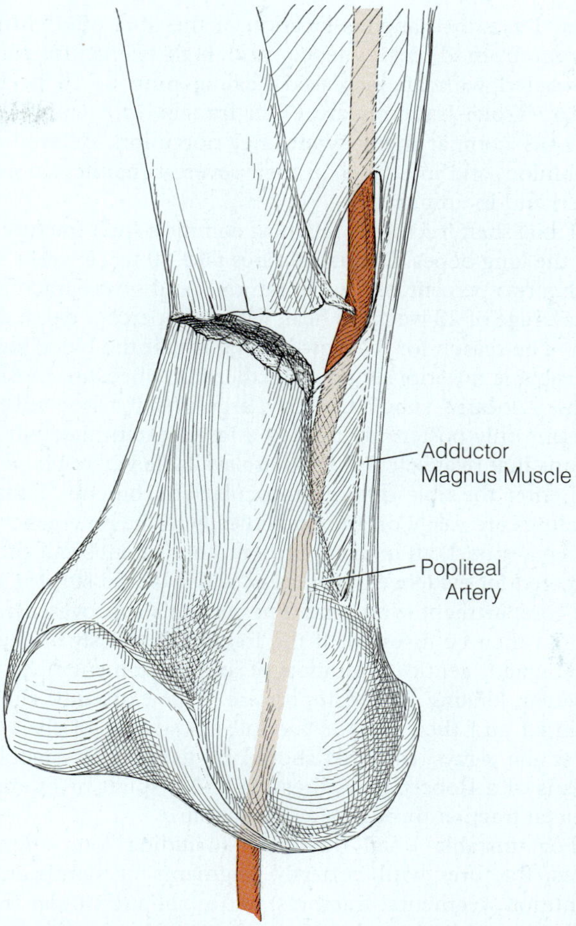

Figure 6 Vascular injuries resulting from blunt trauma to an extremity are usually associated with fracture. Illustrated here is the mechanism of arterial injury in femoral fracture.

Patellar fractures are commonly associated with laceration over the patella; when this is the case, a traumatic arthrotomy must be ruled out. Other injuries, such as cruciate ligament failure and femoral fracture, may be present as well. The most important task in the examination is to make sure that the extensor mechanism is intact. Stellate fractures usually are not associated with extensor ruptures, and the extensor retinaculum keeps many of these fractures from displacing. Avulsion fractures, on the other hand, are associated with tears of the extensor tendon; the patient cannot extend the knee without a lag or perform a straight leg raise against gravity. It may be necessary to infiltrate the joint with local anesthesia so that the patient can attempt the maneuver.

For tensile avulsion fractures, exploration and repair of the fracture are appropriate. Nondisplaced fractures may be treated with a knee immobilizer or a cylindrical cast. Stellate direct blow fractures may be treated initially with simpler immobilization and later with protected motion until the fracture is healed. If the fragments for the joint surface are offset by more than 1 mm, anatomic reduction of the joint surface is necessary to prevent posttraumatic arthritis. Severely comminuted patellar fractures may be irreparable; in such instances, a partial or total patellectomy may be required.

Tibial Fracture, Fibular Fracture, and Pilon Fracture

Tibial fracture Fractures of the tibia are among the most difficult fractures that orthopedic surgeons are called on to treat. The subcutaneous location of the tibia offers little protection from direct violence, and high-energy fractures are associated with an increased healing time in 50 percent of cases.[9] Tibial fractures are often fraught with complications, such as compartment syndrome, nonunion, delayed union, malunion, and infection. In their severest manifestations, they often end in amputation.

Tibial shaft fracture is the most common shaft fracture affecting the long bones. Minor fractures take 10 to 16 weeks to heal, with a two percent delayed union rate, and severe fractures take an average of 23 weeks to heal, with a 60 percent delayed union rate. The reason for the slow healing is that the blood supply to the tibia is notoriously poor; furthermore, because most of the bone is located subcutaneously, a good soft tissue envelope is present only posteriorly and, to a lesser extent, laterally, which means that relatively few areas are available where blood vessels can enter the tibia through muscular attachments. Tibial shaft fractures are easily diagnosed clinically in the emergency room. Whenever such an injury is present, the patient's calf should be palpated for evidence of firmness, which would suggest a possible compartment syndrome. The patient's neurovascular status should then be assessed. If the fracture is grossly angulated or malaligned, gentle restoration of axial alignment helps relieve vascular kinking and compromise. The extremity should be splinted and then x-rayed for full assessment of the fracture. After the x-rays, the tibia should be temporarily stabilized by means of a Robert Jones dressing and a splint or by means of skeletal traction through a calcaneal pin.

For unstable tibial fractures—including long spiral fractures, fractures with butterfly fragments or significant comminution, segmental fractures, and tibial and fibular fractures occurring at the same level—operative fixation is the treatment of choice. For isolated stable tibial fractures in which the fracture line is transverse and there is at least 50 percent bony apposition, long leg casts with weight bearing may be highly successful. If the patient is comatose or has head injuries, operative fixation should be considered, particularly if the patient is agitated or uncooperative.

The standard treatment for tibial shaft fractures—closed, reamed, intramedullary nailing—has a high success rate and a low complication rate. Although the closed technique helps preserve the extraosseous blood supply, the reaming and nailing lead to loss of the intraosseous vasculature that supplies the inner two thirds of the bone. For rotational or axially unstable fractures, interlocking screws may be required. In those unusual circumstances in which the fracture pattern does not permit insertion of an intramedullary rod, a plate or screws may be used; unfortunately, this form of management is associated with a high rate of nonunion. For open fractures with complex wounds, the standard treatment has been external fixation, which permits stabilization of the fracture, allows access to large open wounds, and facilitates nursing care. Currently, however, nonreamed nailing appears be superior to external fixation in this situation: with proper early treatment and aggressive irrigation and debridement, the infection rates are no higher, the complication rate is lower, and the functional end results are better.

Fibular fracture Generally, fibular shaft fractures may be ignored; they heal readily, sometimes so readily that they interfere with the union of associated tibial fractures. Isolated midshaft fibular fractures that do not involve the ankle joint may be treated symptomatically, often without a cast. In some instances, plating the fibular fracture stabilizes an unstable tibial shaft fracture; however, rendering the fibula stable may diminish the cyclic compression that occurs with weight bearing at the site of the tibial fracture and may delay healing. For this reason, in most cases of combined tibial and fibular fracture, the fibula is not stabilized.

Fractures at the distal end of the fibula can be a serious problem if the ankle joint is disrupted. In these circumstances, anatomic reduction (usually with internal fixation) is required to prevent chronic pain or late arthritis from altered joint mechanics. The most common problem associated with proximal fibular head injuries is a peroneal nerve palsy, which usually resolves. If the nerve has been lacerated, however, regeneration may take quite a long time.

Pilon fracture Pilon fracture results from forceful axial compression across the ankle joint, which drives the talus up into the tibial plafond, resulting in a severe intra-articular fracture. It is commonly seen in falls from a height and is usually accompanied by a fracture of the distal fibular diaphysis. Some pilon fractures are so comminuted and severe that reconstruction is technically impossible and primary ankle fusion may be necessary. With severe open fractures, amputation may be required.

Pilon fractures are associated with massive swelling resulting from soft tissue edema and bleeding. Fracture blisters are common. Reconstruction must be done within a few hours of injury; the earlier, the better. If it cannot be done in this period, it must be delayed for five to seven days or longer, until the swelling has decreased. Even with immediate fixation, the swelling can be so great that by the end of the operation, the skin cannot be closed and must be either left open or closed with a skin graft.

The goals of treatment are restoration of ankle joint integrity, congruency and stability, achievement of bony union, and functional painless motion. These are best achieved by means of open reduction and internal fixation, but only if the fracture is amenable to reconstruction. For certain complex fractures, closed treatment may be the only choice.

At best, good surgical technique results in a 50 to 75 percent return to full function. Accordingly, meticulous attention to detail is essential in performing the procedure. The fibula is usually fixed first through a lateral incision, and the tibia is then fixed via an anterior or medial approach. Dissection should be minimized to prevent further soft tissue injury. Any debris present in the joint should be removed. Plates and screws are necessary for stabilization of the fracture. Bone grafting is often required to fill bony defects and voids. If the tibial fracture is not amenable to reconstruction, the fibula may be plated to help bring the tibia out to length, maintain alignment, and afford some stability. If the fracture cannot be immediately fixed, calcaneal pin traction should be used to bring the limb out to length and permit elevation of the leg to decrease swelling. If posttraumatic arthritic pain is severe, delayed ankle fusion may be required.

Compartment Syndrome

Compartment syndrome is defined as high-pressure swelling within a fascial compartment. The forearm and the lower leg are the classic locations for compartment syndrome—any physician who treats trauma patients will encounter compartment syndromes at these sites—but the syndrome may also occur in the hand or the foot or, less commonly, in the shoulder, the upper arm, the buttock, or the thigh. The reason why compartment syndrome is more common in the forearm and the lower leg than in the less classic sites is that the compartments in these anatomic areas have tighter, better-defined fascial boundaries. Many physicians still believe, incorrectly, that compartment syndrome cannot develop in conjunction with an open fracture because the open nature of the injury provides decompression. This is a dangerous assumption: extensive soft tissue injury is in fact a very common accompaniment to an open fracture, and as many as 10 percent of open tibial fractures, for example, are associated with compartment syndrome. Alertness to symptoms and physical findings in patients with open fractures is the key to recognizing compartment syndrome.

Compartment syndrome can have any of several causes. The most common cause is hemorrhage and edema in the damaged soft tissue that accompanies a fracture. A dressing or a cast that is too tight can cause external pressure, as can the eschar from a circumferential burn. Massive soft tissue swelling and edema can occur secondary to various toxins found in venomous snakes, spiders, and scorpions. Unintentional infusion of intravenous fluid outside the vascular space can also cause compartment syndrome. A rarer situation is an iatrogenic compartment syndrome induced by the military antishock trousers; several cases have been reported after ill-advised, prolonged occlusion of the extremity with this garment. Disruption of the venous drainage of a limb may also result in edema and high compartment pressures, as may venous thrombosis.

The classic concept of the etiology of compartment syndrome is that as pressure increases within the compartment, it ultimately reaches that of the venous capillary. At this point, complete venous obstruction occurs, which, if arterial flow should continue, would result in continued escalation of compartment pressure. Inevitably, extensive venous obstruction gives rise to reflex spasm of the accompanying arteries, at which point tissues begin to become ischemic. Muscle can tolerate complete ischemia for three or four hours; after this period, it dies, and limb function is permanently compromised. In advanced ischemia, the microvasculature loses its integrity, with the result that severely ischemic and dead muscle swells and compartment pressure increases. Theoretically, in these circumstances, opening the skin envelope and exposing the dead muscle through fasciotomy would render the tissue vulnerable to infection. With late fasciotomy, when muscle is already necrotic, limb loss occurs primarily as a consequence of loss of skin covering; this consideration should be weighed when fasciotomy is being considered. This issue represents the only significant controversy regarding fasciotomy, which is the treatment of choice for compartment syndrome in all other contexts.

DIAGNOSIS

The key to diagnosis of compartment syndrome is continuous assessment of any extremity injury where there is a chance that the syndrome might develop—for example, fractures of the tibia or the forearm, fractures of the thigh or the upper arm (less likely), and, for that matter, all comminuted fractures associated with severe soft tissue injury. The diagnosis of compartment syndrome is a clinical one: although compartment pressures may be measured, there is no agreement on what constitutes the critical pressure. In fact, it has been shown that there is no specific compartment pressure at which the compartment syndrome occurs. The problem appears to be related more to the difference between the mean arterial pressure and the compartment pressure. As this pressure difference decreases, perfusion of the soft tissues decreases as well, and compartment syndrome occurs. The syndrome is frequently seen when the difference between the mean arterial pressure and the pressure in the involved compartment is less than 40 mm Hg.[10]

The hallmark of the compartment syndrome is the presence of the four Ps: *p*ressure, *p*ain, *p*aresthesia, and intact *p*ulses. On palpation, the compartment will be tense or even boardlike, and this tenseness is usually the critical factor in deciding whether to treat the problem surgically. Pain that is out of proportion to what would be expected for the patient's level of injury and pain that is aggravated by passive stretching of the muscles are also manifestations of compartment syndrome. Muscles are more sensitive to anoxia than nerves are; thus, muscle pain and paralysis occur before paresthesia and anesthesia are noted.

When a patient at risk begins to complain of undue pain, the first step is to remove all circumferential bandages and then split them down to skin to relieve any pressure. If a plaster cast is present, it should be split, spread, or removed; if necessary, maintenance of reduction should be sacrificed. If the clinical picture does not improve after these measures are taken, then a decompressive fasciotomy is indicated.

OPERATIVE TREATMENT

Acute compartment syndrome is treated with wide decompression fasciotomy. To decompress the forearm, two incisions are made, one volar and one dorsal [*see Figure 7*]. A longitudinal dorsal incision provides access to the extensor compartment and the mobile wad. The fascia overlying these compartments must be widely opened. A curvilinear volar incision allows approach to the flexor compartment from a point proximal to the antecubital fossa to the midpalm. Here, too, it is imperative that fascia be widely opened. In severe cases, the deep intramuscular fascia

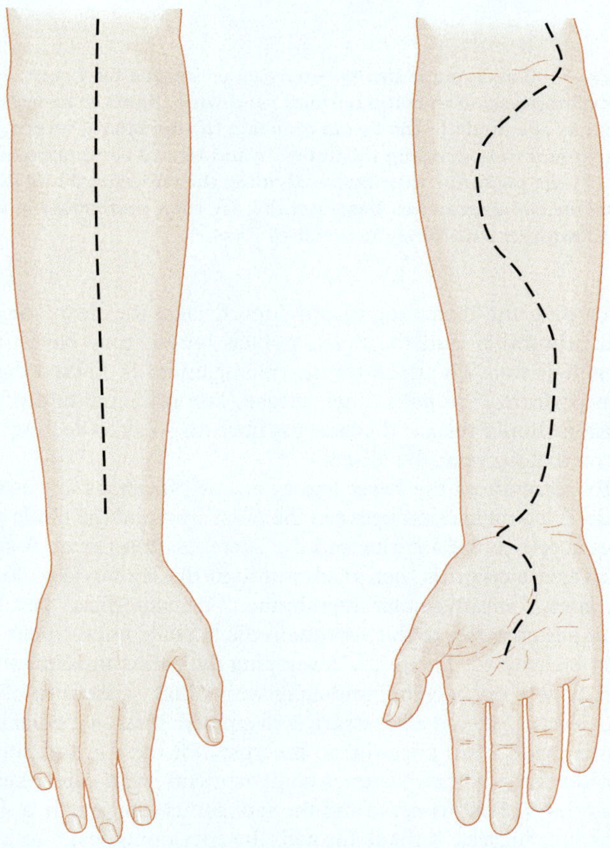

Figure 7 Shown are incisions for forearm decompression in compartment syndrome.

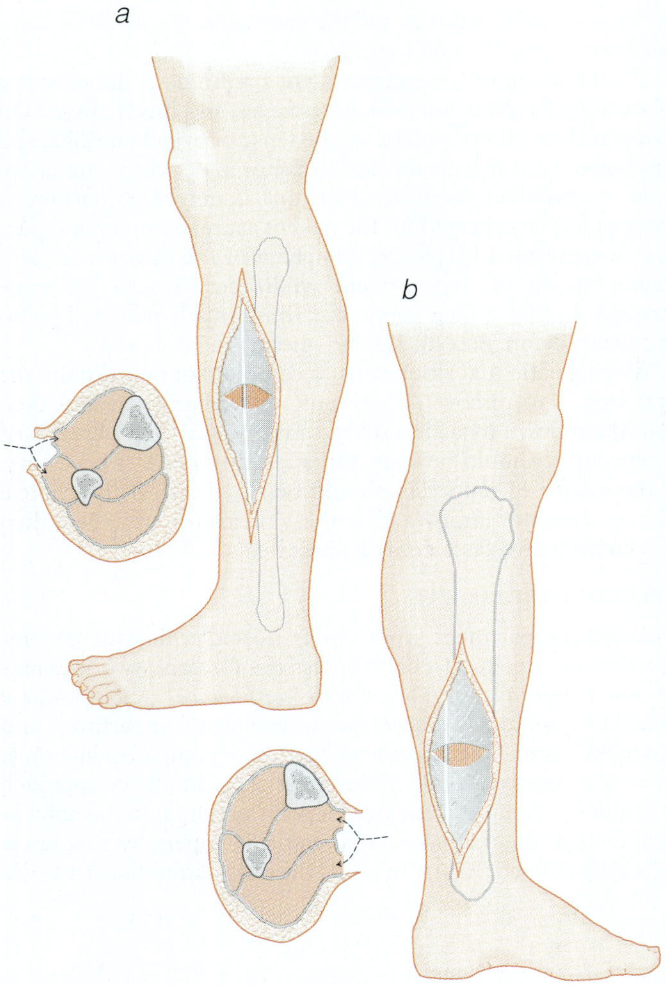

Figure 8 Illustrated is the two-incision technique for lower leg decompression in compartment syndrome. Short transverse incisions are made in the fascia to locate (*a*) the lateral intermuscular membrane dividing the anterior and lateral compartments and (*b*) the posterior membrane dividing the superficial and deep posterior compartments. Fasciotomies are then performed in all four compartments along the dashed lines.

enveloping the flexor digitorum superficialis, the flexor digitorum profundus, and the flexor pollicis longus may have to be opened as well. The thick transcarpal ligament is divided distally to perform a carpal tunnel release. The proximal end of the incision should release the lacertus fibrosus so as to decompress the medial nerve at the elbow.

To decompress the lower leg, again, two incisions are usually made. A lateral incision between the tibial crest and the fibula provides access to the anterior and the lateral compartment. A short transverse incision is then made through the leg fascia to locate the lateral intramuscular membrane. The superficial peroneal nerve lies posterior to this septum in the lateral compartment and must be avoided. The fascia enveloping the two compartments is then widely opened longitudinally with blunt scissors until the muscles are soft and all pressure is dissipated. Next, a medial incision is made 2 cm posterior to the posterior crest of the tibia to provide access to the posterior compartments, with care taken to avoid the saphenous nerve and the saphenous vein. Again, a short transverse incision is made through the enveloping fascia to identify the septum between the deep compartment and the superficial compartment [*see Figure 8*].

After fasciotomy, both fascia and skin are left widely open. The skin defects may be closed with skin grafts, provided that this is done without tension or pressure. Alternatively, the patient may be returned to the OR after the swelling resolves for delayed closure of the skin (again, with fascia left open) or split-thickness skin grafting, as indicated.

Injuries to Soft Tissue

The main types of soft tissue injuries encountered in patients who have experienced trauma to an extremity are abrasions, contusions, lacerations (including avulsion injuries), hemarthrosis, and sprains and strains. All such injuries should be examined with the goal of determining their nature and severity and ruling out underlying injuries to tendons, arteries, or nerves. Local or systemic analgesia or anesthesia may be required for appropriate examination of injuries. The entire area around the wound should then be prepared with an antiseptic solution and thoroughly inspected, palpated, and, if necessary, probed to ascertain the probable depth and direction of the wound. The position the extremity was in when wounded should be kept in mind; it may be critical for identifying injuries to underlying structures.

When examination reveals that a break in the skin has occurred, tetanus prophylaxis should be given in accordance with the patient's immunization history. For minor, clean lacerations that are not associated with other injuries, prompt debridement and irrigation are indicated. Simple wounds and lacerations that are seen and managed within six to eight hours can usually be closed.

Abrasions are generally minor injuries. Typically, there is some ground-in foreign material, which may give rise to subsequent infection and complicate other injuries. Sometimes, abrasions may be treated in the emergency department by anesthetizing the injured area and cleaning it with an antiseptic solution and a soft brush to remove any grit and dirt. For abrasions that are more than 10 cm in diameter and are overtly dirty, however, anesthesia and treatment in the operating room may be required. Once the abraded area is clean, an occlusive, nonadherent dressing should be applied to ease the pain of dressing changes and promote healing.

Contusion is the result of disruption of and hemorrhage into subcutaneous tissue or muscle as a consequence of blunt trauma. Large contusions that contain expanding hematomas may have to be treated with operative debridement and hemostasis; smaller contusions are usually treated with supportive dressings, with or without counterpressure.

Lacerations range in severity from simple full-thickness skin injuries to complex undermining lacerations and flap avulsions. As noted, simple lacerations can generally be treated in the ED with irrigation, debridement, and closure. Contaminated wounds more than six to eight hours old call for a more conservative approach: once the wound is clean, it should be left open for three to four days and then closed by secondary intention. The deeper lacerations seen in avulsion injuries usually call for operative exploration, irrigation, and debridement to ensure removal of devitalized tissue and to minimize the risk of retaining foreign material. In some instances, the wound may have to be extended to permit proper inspection of its depth and to ensure adequate cleaning. Copious irrigation with a pulsatile lavage system dilutes the bacterial load and flushes foreign material from the wound. Because muscle takes sutures poorly, no attempt should be made to close muscles unless major tendinous avulsions have occurred. Once the wound has been cleaned and debrided, closure of the overlying fascia results in close approximation of the muscle ends, particularly if closure is accompanied by suction drainage. In the case of avulsion injuries, the likelihood that the flap will slough is high, particularly if the intact portion of the flap is distally based (that is, if the flap derives its blood supply distally). This problem can be dealt with by removing and defatting the skin, converting it to a full-thickness skin graft, and reapplying it to the injured area (provided that the wound is sufficiently clean).

Any laceration in the vicinity of a joint raises the possibility of traumatic arthrotomy. A long knife blade, a shard of glass, or a jagged piece of metal can travel some distance under the skin and can penetrate a joint. Probing the wound often confirms joint penetration, but it does not necessarily rule it out. Air seen in the joint on x-rays confirms penetration. For other wounds in proximity to synovial joints, an arthrogram should be performed. Saline or dilute methylene blue may be injected into the joint; oozing from the wound confirms arthrotomy. Once arthrotomy is confirmed, irrigation of the wound and the joint should be performed on a timely basis in the OR.

An acute joint effusion that occurs within six to eight hours of injury is usually the result of bleeding. The presence of hemarthrosis can be confirmed by joint aspiration, which is also the treatment of choice. After reoperation, hemarthrosis should be treated with bulky, compressive dressings, ice, elevation, and rest until it resolves.

Sprained ligaments and strained muscles of the extremities rarely necessitate urgent surgical treatment. The diagnosis may not even be apparent until the patient has recovered sufficiently from other injuries to note local discomfort when attempting to bear weight on the extremity. Severe sprains and strains in which gross instability of the joint is apparent may be associated with joint dislocation. As a rule, these more extensive injuries need not undergo urgent surgical repair; repair is usually best done later, on an elective basis. Dislocations associated with vascular injury (most commonly, knee dislocations) may necessitate emergent revascularization procedures. In these situations, joint stabilization or reconstruction may be required to protect the vascular repair.

The Mangled Extremity

One of the more difficult decisions for a trauma surgeon is whether to amputate an extremity with multiple severe injuries. A number of scoring systems have been devised to facilitate this decision; however, most are cumbersome and hence too impractical to be used in the very patients most likely to need them—namely, unstable, multiply injured trauma patients. Although the ultimate usefulness of an extremity is related to the presence of intact neurologic function, the decision on when to amputate versus when to attempt complex repair of the mangled extremity is more appropriately based on the patient's overall condition and the vascular supply to the extremity.

In severely injured patients, dead or devitalized tissue can help precipitate the onset of disseminated intravascular coagulation. It is not uncommon for patients with mangled extremities to manifest the systemic inflammatory response syndrome until the extremity is removed, at which point they recover promptly. For this reason, if a mangled extremity is not an acute threat to the patient during the initial resuscitation, it may be best treated with irrigation and debridement (as described with respect to open fractures) and some form of stabilization. If, however, the extremity has no palpable pulses or does not appear viable, then the decision whether to amputate should be based on the functional prognosis of the extremity, which in turn is based on the presence or absence of nerve injury and the orthopedist's judgment of whether long-term bony stabilization is likely to be achievable.

If the decision is made to attempt salvage of the limb, regular rechecking of both the extremity and the patient's overall condition is essential. If the patient's condition deteriorates significantly or the previous prognostic estimate changes for the worse, amputation should be promptly performed within the first 24 hours.[11]

References

1. Allgöwer M, Border JR: Management of open fractures in the multiple trauma patient. World J Surg 7:88, 1983
2. Knudson MM, Lewis FR, Atkinson K, et al: The role of duplex ultrasound arterial imaging in patients with penetrating extremity trauma. Arch Surg 128:1033, 1993
3. Wagner WH, Calkins ER, Weaver FA, et al: Blunt popliteal artery trauma: one hundred consecutive injuries. J Vasc Surg 7:736, 1988
4. Visser PA, Hermreck AS, Pierce GE, et al: Prognosis of nerve injuries incurred during acute trauma to peripheral arteries. Am J Surg 140:596, 1980
5. Epstein HC, Wiss DA, Cozen L: Posterior fracture dislocation of the hip with fractures of the femoral head. Clin Orthop 201:9, 1985
6. Swiontkowski MF, Winquist RA, Hansen ST Jr: Fractures of the femoral neck in patients between the ages of twelve and forty-nine years. J Bone Joint Surg [Am] 66:837, 1984
7. Bone LB, Johnson KD, Weigelt J, et al: Early versus delayed stabilization of femoral fractures: a prospective randomized study. J Bone Joint Surg [Am] 71:336, 1989
8. Delamarter RB, Hohl M, Hopp E Jr: Ligament injuries associated with tibial plateau fractures. Clin Orthop 250:226, 1990
9. Hoaglund FT, States JD: Factors influencing the rate of healing in tibial shaft fractures. Surg Gynecol Obstet 124:71, 1967
10. Heppenstall RB, Sapega AA, Izanty T, et al: Compartment syndrome: a quantitative study of high-energy phosphorus compounds using ^{31}P-magnetic resonance spectroscopy. J Trauma 29:1113, 1989
11. Roessler MS, Wisner DH, Holcroft JW: The mangled extremity: when to amputate? Arch Surg 126:1243, 1991
12. Chapman MW: Operative Orthopaedics. JB Lippincott, Philadelphia, 1988
13. Sunderland S: Nerves and Nerve Injuries. Churchill Livingstone, Edinburgh, 1978, p 127

Acknowledgments

Figures 1, 4, 7, and 8   Tom Moore.
Figures 2 and 6   Carol Donner.
Figure 3   Marcia Kammerer.

33 BURN CARE IN THE EARLY POSTRESUSCITATION PERIOD

Robert H. Demling, M.D.

Approach to the Burn Patient during the Second to Fifth Days after the Burn

Beginning about 36 hours after injury, major physiologic and biochemical changes occur that differ from earlier alterations [*see 3 Burn Care in the Immediate Resuscitation Period*]. The interval after resuscitation and before the onset of inflammation is generally the most stable period for burn patients. One exception is the patient with a severe inhalation injury, symptoms of which usually become most severe several days after the injury.

Maintenance of Pulmonary Function

ENDOTRACHEAL INTUBATION

Intubation is required for the three Ps:

1. Maintenance of a *patent* airway.
2. *Pulmonary* toilet.
3. *Positive pressure* ventilation.

If edema threatens to compromise airway patency by distortion and compression, intubation is mandatory and should be continued until the upper airway edema begins to resolve, usually between postburn days 2 and 4; elevating the patient's head 30° to 40° allows faster resolution of edema. Oral and facial edema from the burn begins to resolve at this time as well. In the presence of a full-thickness neck burn, tissue edema—including mucosal edema—resolves much more slowly. Positive end-expiratory pressure during this period will help prevent small airway collapse. The injured mucosa is very prone to superinfection because mucosal irritation and increased mucus production persist for several days, whereas clearance is decreased because of the damaged ciliary action of the mucosa. Aggressive mouth care to prevent mucosal infection (particularly with anaerobes) is necessary because aspiration of infected saliva leads to airway infection.

The decision when to extubate is a difficult one because no test of airway patency is foolproof. Laryngoscopy is helpful in that it can determine whether cord edema is present; however, edema of the false cords or the oropharynx, as well as external compression from a neck burn, can impair airway patency even if minimal cord edema is present. As a rule, therefore, extubation should not be performed unless reintubation is technically feasible. If the patient clearly has a severe inhalation injury or a large burn that will necessitate airway protection or ventilatory assistance, a tracheostomy through an unburned or an excised and grafted area of the neck should be done at an early stage (e.g., the first excision and grafting procedure). Percutaneous tracheostomy through unburned skin is an effective approach.

VENTILATION

In the patient without an inhalation injury, lung function during this period is usually surprisingly good if blood volume is not excessively increased. Although massive soft tissue edema is present, lung water measurements are consistently normal or only minimally elevated in both animal and human studies. However, in the presence of inelastic burned tissue and subeschar edema, chest wall compliance may remain significantly decreased. Because the work of breathing is increased, the decreased compliance may result in a diffuse microatelectasis if it is not recognized and aggressively treated.

When initial energy stores are depleted, mechanical ventilatory support may be needed to assist with the increased work load that results from the impaired chest wall function. Although parenchymal pulmonary function may be adequate, it is also important to consider work load and caloric demand before removing ventilatory support. Maintaining the patient in a semierect position improves diaphragmatic function. Oxygen administration to maintain adequate blood oxygen content and tissue oxygen tension is frequently required, for several days at least, after any large burn. Arterial oxygen saturation should be maintained at 90% or greater, preferably with a fraction of inspired oxygen (F_IO_2) of 0.5 or less. In addition, the sequential surgical excisions and wound closure initiated around postburn day 2 or 3 frequently make ventilatory assistance necessary for longer periods because general anesthesia is used every 2 to 3 days and narcotic usage is increased to control postoperative pain, particularly in donor sites. Fluid overload should be carefully avoided to minimize lung dysfunction.

MANAGEMENT OF PULMONARY INJURY

The clearance of soot, mucopurulent exudate, and sloughed mucosa is a major problem during this period, particularly if mucociliary action is impaired by smoke damage. An aggressive surgical approach to the burn wound cannot be undertaken, however, in the absence of good lung function. Airway collapse

Approach to the Burn Patient during the Second to Fifth Days after the Burn

Maintain adequate ventilation

Maintain O$_2$ sat. > 90%, preferably F$_I$O$_2$ < 0.5.
Avoid iatrogenic complications:
- Fluid overload
- Drug-induced hypoventilation

Patient intubated

Maintain ET tube until face, neck, and upper airway edema are adequately resolved.

Assess by laryngoscopy.

Patient not intubated

Continue assessment of airway adequacy for
- Edema
- Secretion clearance
- State of consciousness

No inhalation injury or large chest burn

Extubate when
- Airway edema is resolved
- Patient is alert
- There is no further need for positive airway pressure

Observe closely for pending pulmonary problems:
- Atelectasis
- Fatigue
- Pneumonia

Inhalation injury or large chest burn

Provide positive pressure ventilation as needed.

Remember: Process may worsen during the next 24–48 hr.

Maintain aggressive pulmonary toilet:
- Frequent suctioning
- Position changes
- Bronchodilators

Control infection:
- No prophylactic antibiotics
- Frequent sputum smears and cultures
- Systemic antibiotics with signs of bacterial tracheobronchitis

No inhalation injury or large chest burn

Maintain adequate perfusion

Replace continuing plasma, red blood cell, and evaporative losses.

Maintain
- BP > 90 mm Hg systolic
- Urine output 0.5–1.0 ml/kg/hr
- T° > 37° C

Monitor input and output.

Burns > 20% TBS

Continue I.V. fluid supplementation.

Change fluid to hypotonic salt plus dextrose.

Continue adequate hemodynamic monitoring (BP, pulse, acid-base, urine).

Closely monitor electrolytes, renal function.

Burns < 20% TBS

Can use oral route if patient is extubated, is alert, and has adequate GI function.

Use hemodynamic monitoring as necessary. (The elderly and patients with inhalation injury are at increased risk.)

Patient hemodynamically stable

Watch for ICF to ECF shifts.

Begin nutrition:
- Calories and protein
- Enteral route with peripheral vein supplementation preferred to central line

Patient hemodynamically unstable

Assess for hypervolemia and congestive failure vs. hypovolemia.

Use additional monitoring (e.g., PA catheters) if situation deteriorates.

Hypervolemia or congestive heart failure

Diurese carefully.

Administer inotropes; low-dose dopamine is first choice.

Occasionally, vasodilators are needed; sodium nitroprusside is first choice.

Hypovolemia

Replace blood volume with albumin solution or red blood cells, or both.

Replace evaporative and urine losses with dextrose and hypotonic salt solution.

Consider initiation of nutritional support as soon as feasible

---

Continue wound management

Control infection

Continue chlorhexidine wash.

Avoid body immersion techniques.

Debride loose eschar.

Use topical antibiotics for deep burns.

Do not give prophylactic systemic antibiotics.

Reassess extent or depth of injury

Look for wound conversion.

Maintain perfusion

Continue elevation of burned extremities.

Consider extending escharotomy if perfusion is impaired.

Avoid excessive heat loss

Maintain warm environment.

Use closed dressings.

Provide adequate pain control

Give premedication, followed by small doses of I.V. narcotics.

Use closed dressings; change twice daily in most areas

Treat infection

Biopsy wound to diagnose infection.

Use systemic antibiotics.

Consider changing topical antibiotic (e.g., to mafenide).

Remove eschar more aggressively.

Close the wound

If burn is not infected, begin wound excision and grafting as soon as patient is hemodynamically stable. Use tangential excision for moderate burns of varying depth; use excision to fascia for large full-thickness burns.

and atelectasis will result in an increasing shunt and an increasing risk of bronchopneumonia. Bronchodilators, in particular those delivered by aerosol, are very helpful, along with chest physical therapy and frequent repositioning of the patient. Mechanical ventilatory assistance may be necessary in severe cases.

The clinical magnitude of a chemical injury to the smaller airways becomes much more evident during this period. At the very least, mucosal irritation will persist for several days, causing bronchorrhea, increased coughing, and mucus production. Impairment of the ciliary function of the airway lining leads to a high risk of infection, manifested first (in the next 3 to 4 days) by bacterial tracheobronchitis and subsequently by bronchopneumonia. Bacterial colonization is inevitable. When the injury is severe, the damaged mucosa typically becomes necrotic 3 to 4 days after injury and begins to slough. Increased viscous secretions can lead to distal airway obstruction and atelectasis and can place the patient at high risk for rapidly developing bronchopneumonia.

If the chemical burn to the lung occurs in combination with a body burn, the morbidity and mortality of both processes are substantially higher than they would be otherwise.

Diagnosis

In the first several days after injury, soot continues to be present in the airway secretions. Diffuse rhonchi are usually present once inflammation develops. Wheezing often persists as a result of continued bronchospasm and (more frequently) bronchial edema. Continued coughing, as well as the residual airway edema and bronchospasm, increases the work of breathing, which can lead to fatigue and hypoventilation. Secretions then become tenacious and more difficult to clear. In the most severe airway injuries, rales compatible with edema are noted, especially when concomitant volume overload is present. Bacterial tracheobronchitis is common and is followed by bronchopneumonia in a substantial number of patients; the primary pathogen is usually *Staphylococcus aureus*. The symptom complex includes the following: (1) sputum changing from loose to mucopurulent, (2) evidence of necrotic tissue in sputum, (3) increased work of breathing, (4) altered gas exchange, and (5) infiltrates on radiographs (a late finding). The initial presentation is not necessarily an accurate guide to the magnitude of injury: lung function may be deceptively good on day 2, only to deteriorate rapidly on day 3 or 4.

In general, chest radiographs obtained during this period do not reveal the full severity of the lung damage, because the injury usually is initially confined to the airways. Clinical evidence of continued respiratory compromise—dyspnea, tachypnea, diffuse wheezing, and rhonchi—precedes any radiographic changes. The first radiographic indication of lung damage is usually diffuse atelectasis, pulmonary edema, or bronchopneumonia. Parenchymal changes are late findings.

Treatment

Endotracheal intubation may be necessary if clearance of secretions is inadequate. Ventilatory assistance may also be necessary if the patient is fatigued and if gas exchange is deteriorating. Bronchodilators, particularly those delivered by aerosol [see 3 Burn Care in the Immediate Resuscitation Period], are also helpful, as are frequent changes in position to facilitate postural drainage. Continuously rotating beds are ideal for patients with inhalation injury and large body burns, who often find it difficult to move from side to side because of pain and stiffness from tissue edema; the constant postural drainage helps to remove airway plugs.

Infection surveillance is crucial during this early period so that bacterial bronchitis can be detected before pneumonia develops.

Sputum smears should be obtained, and the character of the sputum should be monitored. Systemic antibiotics are not given prophylactically but are administered when a bacterial process becomes evident; it is important not to wait for obvious radiographic evidence of bronchopneumonia, because the process, once well established, is difficult to reverse. Broad-spectrum antibiotics can be used until susceptibility test results become available and a more specific antibiotic regimen can be instituted.

Maintenance of Hemodynamic Stability

RESTORATION OF BLOOD VOLUME

Although cardiac output may be restored toward normal by fluid resuscitation during the first 24 hours after a burn, blood volume frequently decreases, particularly in the large burn, because of the substantial loss of fluid from the plasma to the interstitial space; edema is maximal at 24 to 36 hours after a burn. Restoration of blood volume is more feasible during the early postresuscitation period. Adequate perfusion pressure must be maintained (i.e., systolic blood pressure greater than 90 mm Hg and urine output 0.5 to 1.0 ml/kg/hr). In the presence of hypovolemia and severe hypoproteinemia (0.5% of normal), plasma protein levels should be restored toward normal to decrease crystalloid needs and to improve gastrointestinal function. Improved gastrointestinal function will be of considerable importance for nutritional support. Protein solutions should be given to replace volume loss [see 3 Burn Care in the Immediate Resuscitation Period]; such solutions should not be administered to patients who are normovolemic or hypervolemic, because volume overload and its complications may result, especially during the fluid mobilization period.

Red blood cells are injured during the burning process and again as a result of the mediator release from burned tissue. Red cell lipid peroxidation is characteristically seen after a burn. The increased fragility leads to a decreased half-life. Red cell hematopoiesis is also markedly impaired. The combination of these processes leads to anemia, beginning during the early postresuscitation period. Red cells should be provided if necessary to maintain a hematocrit of at least 30%, given the increasing oxygen demands in burn patients during this period and the chronic nature of the impaired production.

MAINTENANCE OF FLUID AND ELECTROLYTE BALANCE

A measurable increase in protein permeability in burned tissue vessels persists for days to weeks. The rate of fluid and protein loss into the burned interstitium lessens considerably after the first two postburn days; however, protein loss from the surface of a partial-thickness burn can still be substantial.

After postburn day 2, evaporation from the surface of deep burns becomes a major source of water loss that persists until the wound is closed. Losses are comparable to those expected from an open pan of water with the same surface area. It is possible to calculate a reasonable estimate of water loss from the surface of deep burns [see Table 1].

During the early postresuscitation period, however, intravascular fluid is gained from the resorption of edema fluid. Therefore, continued replacement of free water lost from evaporation and of protein lost into burned tissue and from the burned surface must be balanced against these intravascular fluid gains.

Table 1 Calculation of Evaporative Water Loss and Required Fluid

The patient is a 70 kg male whose burns cover 50% of TBS. His body surface area is 1.7 m².
The patient's output during the previous 24 hours:
    Urine: 2,000 ml
    Nasogastric tube: pulled
Evaporative water loss (ml/hr) = (25 + % TBS burned) × TBS
In this patient: (25 + 50) × 1.7 = 125 ml/hr
    125 ml/hr × 24 hr/day = 3,000 ml/day
Fluid required = evaporative loss + other losses
In this patient: 3,000 ml evaporative loss/day
    + 2,000 ml urine/day
    Fluid required = 5,000 ml/day
Give as 5% dextrose in 0.2% normal saline at ~ 200 ml/hr.

The rate of edema absorption depends on the burn depth and subsequent lymphatic damage. It is rapid in superficial burns, beginning at about day 2 or 3 when lymphatics are intact, but much slower after full-thickness injury.

Sodium requirements are usually minimal because of initial sodium loading and because water loss from evaporation is extensive. Therefore, the preferred crystalloid after the resuscitation period is hypotonic salt plus dextrose. Glucose administration is necessary at this point, however, because glycogen stores are totally depleted. Once glucose is administered and tissue utilization improves, large amounts of potassium must be given as well. Potassium administration will be particularly important once nutritional support is initiated because wound healing and new cell formation will increase potassium utilization. Enteral nutrition should begin as soon as the gastric ileus resolves. Nutrition can be supplemented with central or peripheral vein alimentation until the enteral route becomes totally functional [see 34 Burn Care after the First Postburn Week].

Restoration of blood flow to the burned tissue after resuscitation will result in the resorption of a large load of osmotically active particles made up of solutes from disrupted cells and fragments of denatured proteins. The increased osmotic load is very evident in second-degree burn blisters, which increase dramatically in size and pressure over a period of days. The increased solute load frequently results in an obligate solute diuresis that is manifested by increased output of high–specific gravity urine. It is important that such an increase in urinary output not be mistaken for hypervolemia; therefore, fluids should not be decreased or diuretics initiated. In the diuretic response to hypervolemia, the urine specific gravity is, of course, characteristically low.

TRANSITION FROM HYPOMETABOLISM TO HYPERMETABOLISM

As the hypermetabolic state evolves (beginning at about day 3 or 4), the response of the cardiovascular system changes. Cardiac output begins to increase and exceeds normal values as a hyperdynamic state develops. Mild to modest tachycardia is usually present, partly because of persistently elevated catecholamine levels, which may be even further potentiated by hypothermia, hypoxia, or pain. The tachycardia, however, is usually much less than that seen during the first 24 hours after the burn [see 3 Burn Care in the Immediate Resuscitation Period]. The early increased systemic vascular resistance (SVR) begins to be replaced by SVR that is lower than normal.

It is important to recognize this transition during the postresuscitation period. The hyperdynamic state is characterized by (1) a 50% to 100% increase in oxygen consumption, (2) a 1° to 2° F rise in body temperature, (3) increased gluconeogenesis, (4) increased secretion of anti-insulin hormones (decreased glucose tolerance), and (5) increased catabolism (increased ureagenesis). The increase in oxygen consumption usually peaks 5 to 10 days after the burn. Body temperature tends to increase further as pyrogen is released from the burn wound. The characteristic rise in body temperature makes it more difficult to diagnose the presence of infection.

The increasing oxygen consumption necessitates increasing oxygen delivery by ensuring adequate blood volume, hematocrit, and oxygen saturation (i.e., lung function and cardiac output must be maintained). Lactic acidosis indicates inadequate oxygen delivery, even if P_{aO_2} or oxygen saturation is normal. Oxygen demands are twice normal (100 to 140 ml/min/m² when 50% or more of the total body surface (TBS) has been burned).

Control of Burn Infection

The burn wound is a major site of infection for three reasons: (1) loss of the skin barrier, (2) the presence of dead tissue, and (3) systemic immunosuppression. The stratum corneum is a relatively impermeable barrier to bacterial invasion through the skin. Loss of this barrier as a result of burn injury permits bacteria to populate the underlying tissues. Most of these early colonizing bacteria are endogenous, deriving from heat-injured skin (especially hair follicles, sweat glands, and sebaceous glands), the nares and the oropharynx, the perineum, or stool [see Tables 2 through 4]. The bacteria migrate to the wound by way of wet dressings, immersion in water, hand contact, and, to a lesser extent, aerosolization. The reduced blood flow to the surface of the burn impairs local immune defenses (white blood cells need oxygen to kill bacteria); it also decreases the ability of phagocytes and opsonins to reach the wound. In addition, the wound itself releases a number of immunosuppressive substances that impair both cell-mediated and humoral immunity.

DAILY BURN CARE AND INFECTION CONTROL METHODS

In general, significant bacterial colonization of the burn wound does not occur for several days after injury unless the wound initially is heavily contaminated or inadequately cleaned and treated. The eschar remains intact. Surgical excision of the deep burn is most appropriate during this period because the wound is not yet infected or revascularized [see Wound Closure, *below*].

Wound conversion is common during this period as injured tissue becomes nonviable. Frequent reassessment of the wound is

Table 2 Organisms Most Commonly Recovered from Burn Wounds in First Week

Organism	% of Patients
Staphylococcus aureus	85
β-Hemolytic streptococcus	5
Pseudomonas aeruginosa	25
Escherichia coli	40
Enterococcus	55
Candida albicans	40

Table 3 Findings Distinguishing Colonization of Burn Wound from Invasive Infection

Findings	Colonization	Invasive Infection
Systemic changes	Variable body temperature	Increased body temperature
	WBC count increased, with mild left shift	WBC count either high or low, with pronounced left shift
	Wound may appear either purulent or benign	Wound may appear purulent, or wound surface may appear dry and pale
Bacterial characteristics	Surface bacterial content ranging from trace to large	Surface bacterial content variable
	Usually < 10^5 bacteria/g tissue on biopsy	Usually > 10^5 bacteria/g tissue on biopsy
	No invasion of normal tissue	Invasion of normal tissue

necessary. In addition, continued edema can still lead to excessive increases in tissue pressure, necessitating additional escharotomies. During this period, burned extremities should remain elevated and active and passive range-of-motion exercises should begin.

Evidence of tissue necrolysis remains absent until neutrophils, bacteria, or both proliferate in the eschar, leading to liberation of proteases and breakdown of tissue. Topical antibiotic therapy rehydrates and softens the eschar more rapidly, thereby allowing inflammatory cells to migrate into the subeschar space. Increased bacterial proliferation is then possible if the amount of topical antibiotic is not sufficient.

The epidemiology of burn wound infection seems to indicate that—in the first week, at least—the primary bacteria present are cutaneous organisms and, to a lesser extent, pulmonary and enteric organisms. This predominance of endogenous bacteria is reflected in the early colonization of the wound by gram-positive bacteria, primarily *S. aureus*, followed in several days by the beginning of gram-negative colonization.

Exogenous bacteria are certainly present in any standard critical care unit; these ordinarily resistant organisms become significant pathogens after the normal flora has been altered by the use of systemic antibiotics. The principal mode of cross-contamination with more resistant strains appears to be direct contact; air is a less significant vehicle. Compulsive hand washing between patient contacts is crucial to minimize this problem. Changes of cap, gown, and mask are also very helpful. Sophisticated isolation techniques (e.g., isolators) are not routinely necessary.

Wound Care

In wounds not amenable to early surgical closure or closure with temporary skin substitutes, daily removal of devitalized tissue, wound exudate, and inactive topical agents is important. A number of approaches are used; the primary objective is to maximize wound cleaning while minimizing patient stress. Hydrotherapy is one approach. Adequate pain control [*see* Stress Control, Analgesia and Sedation, *below*] and adequate safeguards against hypothermia are necessary. It has also become clear that immersion in a hydrotherapy tank can result in significant cross-contamination from perineum to wound or from one burned area to another. Therefore, it is recommended that the patient's head be up on a slanted board or that showers be used so that water runs off the wounds, maximizing mechanical debridement and minimizing stagnation. Another approach, which is very effective, is bedside wound care: each portion of the body is cleaned and rewrapped independently, both to minimize pain and to minimize bacterial cross-contamination. When early excision has been performed, bedside wound care is particularly useful to avoid contamination of clean, grafted wounds and donor sites. In addition, vascular catheters can be protected. A warm environment during burn care, preferably 30° to 35° C (86° to 95° F), is necessary to prevent excessive heat loss when the wound is open. Pyrogen release as a result of wound manipulation can be anticipated. Use of antipyretics before wound care is initiated can significantly attenuate this response.

Topical Antibiotics

Topical antibiotics that are sufficiently water soluble to penetrate the burn eschar will temporarily control bacterial growth in the wound [*see* 3 Burn Care in the Immediate Resuscitation Period]. Superficial burns do not require topical antibiotics unless they are heavily contaminated—for example, with ground-in dirt. If the burn is extremely deep (i.e., extending into fat or muscle) or clearly infected, mafenide (Sulfamylon) will be more effective in controlling bacterial growth.

Systemic Antibiotics

Systemic antibiotics are used to treat established infection and are not for prophylaxis. Prophylactic antibiotics for small burns

Table 4 Characteristics of Invasive Burn Wound Infection with Specific Etiologic Organisms

Variable	Infecting Organism		
	S. aureus	*P. aeruginosa*	*C. albicans*
Wound appearance	Loss of wound granulation	Surface necrosis; patchy black	Minimal exudate
Clinical course	Slow onset (days)	Rapid onset (hours)	Slow onset (days)
CNS symptoms	Disorientation	Modest changes	Often no change
Temperature	Marked increase	High or low	Modest changes
WBC count	Marked increase	High or low	Modest changes
Blood pressure	Modest decrease	Often severe decrease	Minimal change
Mortality	5%	20% to 30%	30% to 50%

treated on an outpatient basis have also not been shown to be effective in preventing infection. There are only two exceptions. Low-dose penicillin is indicated during the first 24 to 48 hours if the patient is at particular risk for β-hemolytic streptococcus infection; however, this complication is quite uncommon. Systemic antibiotics are also indicated in the 24 to 48 hours before and after burn wound excision to protect against the effects of a transient bacteremia. The agent is selected on the basis of data from the wound culture. The administration of a dose before surgical wound manipulation, followed by continued doses for 24 hours afterward, is common practice.

Systemic antibiotics play no role in treating wound colonization, simply because the agents are incapable of penetrating the nonviable eschar from beneath in sufficient concentration to control bacterial growth. However, if sufficient bacteria ($\geq 10^5$/g eschar) are present in the wound to cause an invasion of underlying viable tissue by breakdown of tissue defense mechanisms, systemic antibiotics are indicated. Values lower than 10^5/g indicate wound colonization that does not require systemic treatment [see Table 3]. Diagnosis of infection is difficult to make by wound inspection alone. Full-thickness biopsies of the burn wound with determination of quantitative bacteriology are used to detect infection. However, there is considerable variability in results with this method, particularly if only a superficial biopsy is obtained. Inclusion of viable subeschar tissue is necessary to limit the inaccuracies [see Sidebar Technique for Wound Biopsy]. Histologic inspection of the biopsy is a more accurate method for determining tissue invasion.

Wound Closure

Surgical approaches to the management of large surface burns vary. At one extreme is immediate, complete wound excision to fascia and closure with a combination of autografts and skin substitutes within the first week after the burn. Another method is to initiate sequential excision and graftings, beginning about 2 to 4 days after the burn and continuing every 4 to 5 days until wound closure. The latter appears to be the safer and more common approach.

EARLY EXCISION AND GRAFTING

Risk Assessment

Before the decision is made to proceed with wound excision and grafting, two key judgments must be made:

1. Are the patient's cardiopulmonary status and the operative risk such that the potential benefits of the procedure outweigh the risks?
2. What morbidity may be expected if the wound is not rapidly closed? (This judgment takes into consideration the depth of the wound, the extent of loss of function, and the potential effects of wound inflammation on the host [see Table 5].)

General Principles

Four general principles apply to all methods of burn wound excision and grafting.

> **Technique for Wound Biopsy**
>
> The wound should first be washed to remove any superficial exudate. With the use of either a scalpel or a punch biopsy tool, a core of eschar approximately 1 cm in diameter should be taken, which includes obviously viable tissue of the deep margin. The piece should be of uniform diameter to avoid an excessive amount of superficial tissue relative to deep tissue. The biopsy specimen then must be wrapped in a moist sponge and immediately transported to the microbiology or pathology laboratory for processing.

First, the patient must be hemodynamically stable before excision can be considered. Some degree of pulmonary dysfunction may be expected, but it should not be so severe that the patient cannot be safely moved to the operating room and back.

Second, the potential for significant blood loss must be recognized, and adequate amounts of red cells, plasma, and platelets, if indicated, must be available before treatment is begun. The potential for infection must also be recognized: at this stage, the burn is considered a clean-contaminated wound. Preoperative planning should also include perioperative administration of systemic antibiotics. Given that the initial organisms of concern are gram positive, the drug of choice is usually one of the first-generation cephalosporins.

Third, hypothermia must be avoided. Severe hypothermia is a major hazard in burn patients—particularly if coagulation is crucial, as it is when excision is being done. The operating room temperature should be maintained between 75° and 85° F.

Fourth, the stress induced by anesthesia and the operation must be kept at or below a level that the patient can safely tolerate. Because patients with major burns are potentially highly unstable, the time spent in the operating room should be carefully controlled. A reasonable operating time limit, including anesthesia, is 2 hours—less for elderly or compromised patients. It is better to perform several operations of moderate length at intervals of 1 or 2 days than to perform a single lengthy procedure. Blood loss should be carefully controlled to prevent the development of a coagulopathy: no more than 60% of estimated total blood volume should be lost in the course of any one operation. It is usually possible to stay within this limit, given good timing and careful attention to hemostasis (see below). For large excisions, two operating teams, working simultaneously,

Table 5 — Factors Affecting Burn Wound Morbidity

Infants and the elderly tolerate burn inflammation and infection poorly.

Burns in infants and the elderly are usually deep.

Pulmonary dysfunction from smoke inhalation will be accentuated by burn-induced hypermetabolism, inflammation, and infection.

Burns tend to get deeper over the first several days as a result of necrosis of ischemic areas.

Burns caused by direct contact with flames, hot grease, chemicals, or electricity are invariably deeper than first appearances would suggest.

Burns on the lower back, the scalp, the palms, and the soles usually have sufficient remaining dermis to allow primary healing in 3 to 5 wk.

Small burns—even if they are deep dermal 2° or 3° burns—are not life threatening; therefore, the timing of operation can be much more flexible, depending on the risks to the patient.

Large 3° burns are life threatening until closed.

are required: one is responsible for obtaining the skin grafts and maintaining hemostasis from the donor site, and the other is responsible for excising the wound, maintaining hemostasis, and closing the wound. Any blood lost should be replaced with blood products rather than with crystalloid.

Other issues that must be considered in planning burn wound excision include timing of operation and recovery. Appropriate timing of excision in relation to the changes occurring in the wound itself is crucial for minimizing associated risks. There is a marked increase in blood flow to the burn wound, beginning several days after injury and peaking between days 5 and 14. This increase, which parallels the development of wound inflammation, occurs in the viable tissue beneath the eschar. Excision performed after day 5 or 6 should therefore be expected to cause significantly more blood loss than earlier excision. Any clotting abnormalities present at this stage can thus cause major problems. In addition, the wound undergoes colonization by bacteria during the first week, and manipulation of the wound after this period carries an increased risk of bacteremia.

Types of Surgical Excision

There are two types of surgical procedures for removing eschar: tangential excision and excision to fascia. Each type has advantages and disadvantages [see Table 6]. There are also several types of grafts and dressing techniques [see Grafting, below].

Tangential (sequential) excision In tangential excision, the wound is excised in thin layers with a blade held at a very acute angle to the skin surface [see Figure 1]. The objective is to remove only nonviable tissue while sparing as much viable tissue as possible. This is particularly true with patients who have deep dermal burns, in whom every effort should be made to preserve viable dermis. The dermis is responsible for the elasticity of skin, and it provides an excellent base for grafts. Fat is a less suitable base for skin grafts because of its lesser vascularity and because of the difficulty of determining viable fat on inspection.

Excision is performed with a handheld dermatome to which guards of variable thickness (0.008 to 0.020 in) may be attached. Either a Goulian knife [see Figure 1] or a Watson knife is used, depending on the area being excised: the Watson knife, being larger, is used on large, flat surfaces, whereas the Goulian knife is used on curvilinear regions (e.g., bony prominences, fingers, toes, the neck, and, occasionally, the face). Excision over bony surfaces can be facilitated by injecting saline beneath the eschar to flatten the wound and push it away from the bone. For the actual cutting, a back-and-forth motion is used, with very little forward force applied. The depth of the excision is controlled by choosing a guard of the appropriate thickness and by maintaining the blade at the proper angle to the surface. A sharp blade is needed for this procedure, and frequent blade changes are required.

The end point of excision is brisk punctate bleeding and a completely viable wound base [see Figure 2]. Viable dermis is white and shiny; however, one or two large bleeding vessels can make the entire wound look red, which means that careful inspection and considerable experience are needed to assess the adequacy of the wound bed. Nonviable dermis is also white, but punctate bleeding is absent. Nonviable fat is more difficult to recognize because fat often appears to be in better condition than it really is. Healthy fat is light yellow and shiny; any fat that is dark yellow-brown should be removed. It is easy either to underexcise, leaving a poor base for the graft, or to overexcise, thereby removing potentially viable dermis. There is a significant risk of major blood loss, and the procedure must be approached with this risk in mind. Measures must therefore be taken to prepare for the possibility of massive bleeding, and the timing of the procedure must be carefully considered with a view to minimizing this risk [see General Principles, above].

Excision to fascia Excision of the burn wound to fascia is appropriate for patients who have very large full-thickness burns or small deep burns that extend well into fat or underlying tissue. This approach is used when the burn is large but only a limited amount of skin is available for grafting. There are three reasons why excision to fascia is suitable for these settings. First, the end point of excision to fascia is well defined, and graft take is always excellent; therefore, less experience is required to define an adequately excised wound surface. Second, wide-mesh grafts can be used because the fascia appears to be less vulnerable to desiccation than fat or dermis is when covered with a skin substitute. Third, when the procedure is performed early, large amounts of most body areas (except for the face and the perineum) can be excised with only modest blood loss. In the case of the small deep wounds, excision to the depth of the fascia or deeper is required because of the extent of the injury itself.

Excision to fascia involves a combination of sharp dissection, constant tension, and electrocauterization; instruments such as those used for tangential excision are not required. The vessels encountered at the fascial plane are less plentiful and larger than those encountered closer to the skin surface and are much easier to control with the electrocautery and ligatures. If the procedure is performed in the first several days after the burn, when the edema fluid separates fascia from overlying subcutaneous tissue, it is actually very easy. Most of the bleeding derives from the wound edge; often, such bleeding can be controlled and exposure of fat on the wound edge minimized if the skin edge is sutured to the fascia. This form of marsupialization may also decrease the total size of the wound as the edges are pulled

Table 6 Advantages and Disadvantages of Tangential Excision and Excision to Fascia

	Advantages	Disadvantages
Tangential excision	Can be performed rapidly Optimal functional and cosmetic results	Substantial blood loss End point of excision difficult to define Greater risk of underexcision or overexcision Greater need for donor skin for coverage
Excision to fascia	Can be performed rapidly, with relatively little loss of blood End point of excision well defined Tourniquets can be used Wide-mesh grafts can be used Excised areas easily covered with skin substitute	Risk of nerve injury Risk of exacerbating distal edema Risk of exposing joints or tendons Potential cosmetic defect

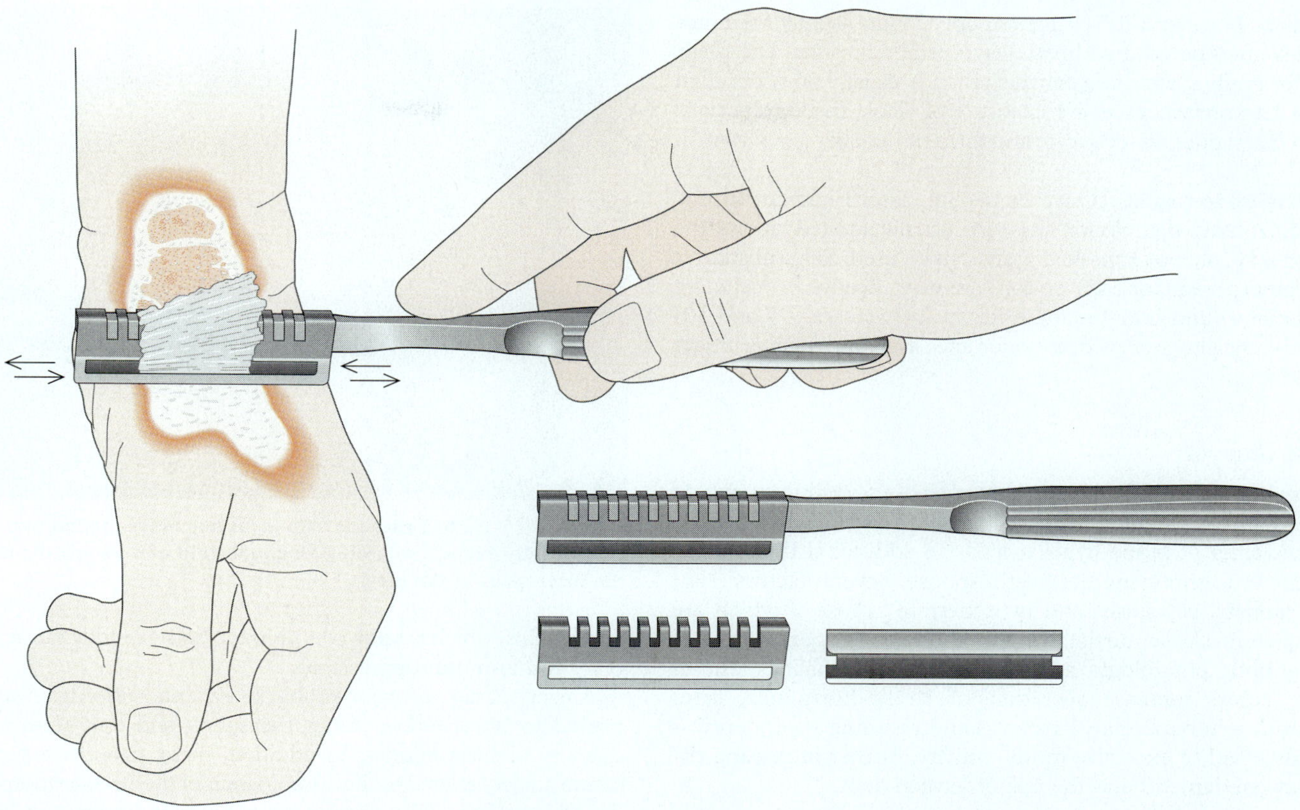

Figure 1 In tangential excision, nonviable tissue is removed in thin layers with a handheld dermatome. Shown at lower right are the components of a Goulian dermatome.

toward the middle. As much as 18% of TBS can be excised with only a 10% to 20% blood loss. Total excision per operation should be limited to 18% to 20% of TBS. Tourniquets may be used when an extremity is being excised to fascia (especially if excision is delayed for several days) because the end point is an anatomic one rather than punctate bleeding (as in tangential excision).

There are a number of disadvantages to this approach that must be carefully weighed against the advantages. The major disadvantage is potential impairment of long-term function of the excised and grafted areas, especially extremities. Removal of superficial veins and lymphatics may result in distal edema; however, in many burn patients, these vessels have already been destroyed by heat. Furthermore, removal of cutaneous nerves leads to impaired sensation in addition to the reduced sensation characteristic of any skin graft in comparison with normal skin, and there is a significant risk of injury to other superficial nerves that have motor function.

The second main disadvantage of fascial excision is cosmetic. A rim of tissue remains at the border between excised and nonexcised tissue and produces a balloonlike effect, especially on the extremities; tapering of the excision at its end points helps minimize this problem. Because fat normally does not regenerate between fascia and skin grafts, the cosmetic defect is persistent, particularly in obese patients. Frequently, fascial excision is combined with tangential excision to maximize the benefits of early wound closure and minimize the complications.

In patients with massive burns, these two disadvantages are outweighed by the excellent graft take and the reliability of the excision end point.

Grafting

Tangential excision Once the wound is excised, the wound bed must be closed. Usually, skin grafts are applied immediately. Meshed skin grafts allow the escape of blood and plasma that would lift a sheet graft off the wound bed. The width of the mesh (e.g., 1.5 to 1 or 3 to 1) depends on the availability of donor skin. Sheet grafts (i.e., nonmeshed grafts) are preferred for the face and

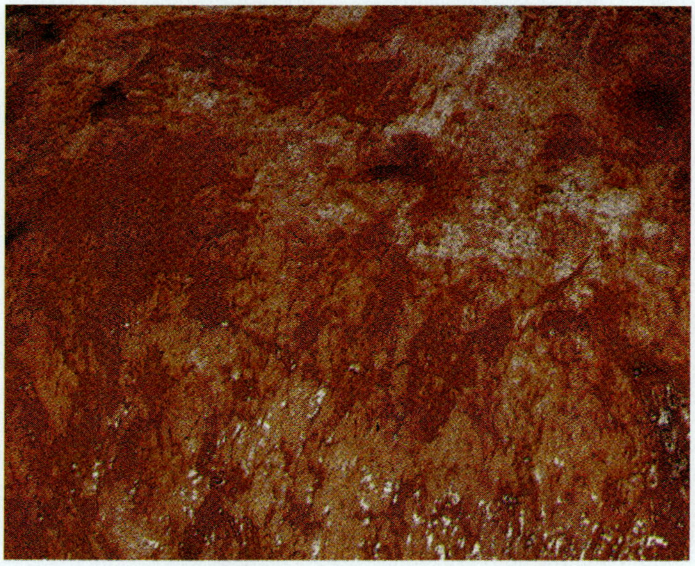

Figure 2 After appropriate tangential excision, brisk punctate bleeding is observed over a completely viable wound base; this is the end point for the procedure.

the hands; however, a 1.5 to 1 mesh opened just slightly for drainage can often be used with excellent cosmetic results. The mesh used for grafting after tangential excision is usually no wider than 1.5 to 1 to prevent excessive exposure of viable tissue (especially fat) so that it does not desiccate and form new eschar [see Figure 3].

Excision to fascia Once excised, the fascial surface must be covered. Given that donor sites are usually limited unless the wound is small, 3 to 1 meshed grafts can be used. Skin substitutes (Biobrane, pigskin, or cadaver skin) are very effective in occluding the fascial wound until the mesh fills in (between days 7 and 10) or until rehealing makes new donor sites available (between days 10 and 14).

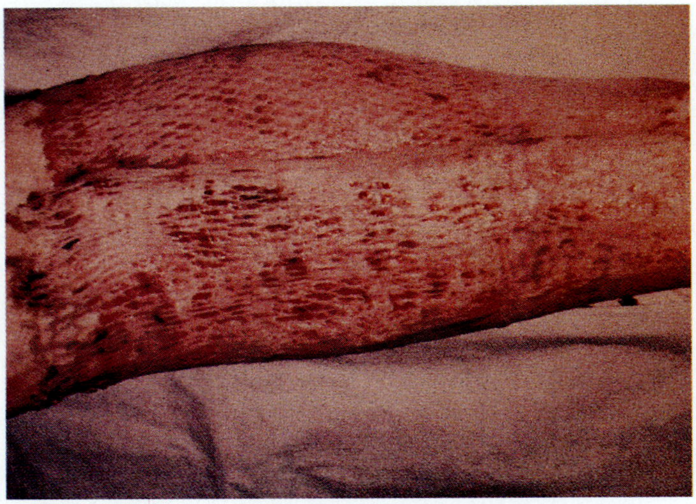

Stress Control

The burn itself initiates the stress response to injury, which includes the development of a marked hypermetabolic state. Hypovolemia or tissue hypoxia leads to additional tissue damage, thereby amplifying the host response. Several factors (e.g., pain, anxiety, psychosis, and hypothermia), most of which are largely controllable, further amplify the stress response, exacerbating both physiologic and metabolic abnormalities. All of these factors increase secretion of stress hormones, catecholamines in particular. Psychosis and resulting sleep deprivation also lead to excessive motor activity, further increasing tissue oxygen demand and the risk of oxygen debt.

HEAT LOSS

The loss of the skin barrier increases the rate of heat loss [see 3 Burn Care in the Immediate Resuscitation Period]. Decreased body temperature is a potent stimulus for catecholamine release. In addition, a core body temperature that falls below what the hypothalamus regards as normal constitutes a strong stimulus for increased heat production (primarily via increased muscle activity).

Heat loss can be controlled by maintaining a warm (30° to 35° C [86° to 95° F]) external environment (e.g., by using radiant overhead heaters), by using occlusive dressings to prevent further convection losses, by minimizing exposure to a wet environment, and by providing adequate oxygen and nutrients. If muscle paralysis proves necessary, the ambient temperature should be further increased, and efforts should be made to achieve additional reduction of heat loss from the wound surface.

HYPERTHERMIA

Severe hyperthermia accentuates the stress response. For every 1° increase in body temperature, oxygen consumption rises by about 5% to 10%. Evaporative water loss increases as well, particularly in patients with large burn wounds. Fluid administration should be stepped up to replace lost water. Nonsteroidal anti-inflammatory drugs may be given; these agents have proved to be very effective in countering hyperthermia in burn patients.

ANALGESIA AND SEDATION

Burn patients experience continuous pain simply from the presence of an open wound. The pain is stimulated by movement and is intensified during dressing changes, debridement, physical therapy, and other burn care–related procedures. Pain increases the stress response and the release of catecholamines, thereby amplifying the hypermetabolic state. The pain-induced increase in sympathetic nervous system activity results in decreased blood flow to skin and soft tissue, which can impair wound healing. Excessive pain also leads to increased release of endogenous endorphins, which is known to produce both hemodynamic instability and immunosuppression.

Anxiety is also a major problem. Patients suffer from anxiety related to uncertainties about the short- and long-term consequences of their injuries. In addition, many patients experience severe anxiety related to the combination of the stress response and the effects of the ICU environment. There is evidence indicating that the stress response, like pain, leads to increased endorphin release, and it has been well documented that several elements of the ICU environment (e.g., noise, sensory deprivation, and lack of day-to-night cycles) have a major impact on the stress response. Frequent disturbances of sleep patterns may lead to disorientation, greater anxiety, and, eventually, a syndrome loosely described as ICU psychosis. Characteristically, patients with ICU psychosis exhibit a marked increase in muscle activity, which further amplifies the stress response and the hypermetabolic state.

Attempts to control pain and anxiety [see Table 7] are required, as well as increased support during the described maneuvers. Relaxation techniques and hypnosis have advantages over narcotics, which suppress gastrointestinal motility and cause other significant side effects.

For severe burns, I.V. narcotics administered by continuous low-dose infusions or on demand can be quite useful. In addition, sedatives such as diazepam and haloperidol are useful for treating anxiety or psychological aberrations. The addition of sedatives to pain medication or hypnosis, biofeedback, or relaxation techniques is also very useful. For chronic burn pain, give narcotics orally, intramuscularly, or intravenously (either intermittently or via low-dose continuous infusion). In addition, administer sedatives to decrease anxiety.

Figure 3 A 1.5 to 1 meshed skin graft has been applied to a tangentially excised wound. Blood and fluid can escape through the interstices of the mesh.

Table 7 Measures for Controlling Pain and Anxiety in Burn Patients

Patient-controlled analgesia
Continuous regional or intravenous infusion
Early use of benzodiazepines for anxiety and of neuroleptics for ICU psychosis
Avoidance of ICU sensory overload

NUTRITIONAL SUPPORT

Hypermetabolism and nutritional support are discussed in more detail elsewhere [see 34 Burn Care after the First Postburn Week and 97 Nutritional Support]. There is, however, one aspect of nutritional management that should be mentioned here—namely, early enteral feeding. Several clinical studies have indicated that initiating enteral feeding soon after the injury (i.e., in the first 48 hours) appears to reduce the degree of subsequent injury-induced hypermetabolism, possibly by preventing early bacterial migration through the gut wall (so-called gut leak). Although the data are not conclusive, it is certainly possible at this point to state that early enteral nutrition is advantageous and that feedings should be started as soon as possible, preferably in the first 48 hours.

GASTRIC pH

Gastrointestinal bleeding from burn stress (i.e., Curling ulcer) was once a major cause of morbidity, but aggressive nutritional support and wound control have decreased this problem. In burn patients as well as in critical care patients in general, maintenance of a gastric pH above 3 has been found to diminish the risk of significant ulceration and bleeding. Scheduled administration of antacids, H_2 receptor blockers, or both can be used to control pH. Continuous tube feeding—or frequent meals, in the absence of a nasogastric tube—is also very effective at decreasing ulceration and maintaining gastric pH at nonulcerogenic levels.

Physical Therapy and Splinting

It is important to maintain as much joint and muscle function as possible during the period of wound closure. If muscle function is not maintained, contraction of the wound by infiltration with myofibroblasts produces permanent impairment of joint motion or a disability requiring extensive reconstructive surgery. Joints must be maintained in the position of function during rest and moved through the limitations of extension, flexion, abduction, and adduction several times a day. Splints are fitted beginning 48 to 72 hours after the burn and refitted as edema resolves.

Recommended Reading

Alexander J: Mechanism of immunologic suppression in burn injury. J Trauma 30:70, 1990

Demling R: Effect of early burn excision and grafting on pulmonary function. J Trauma 24:830, 1984

Desai M, Herdon D, et al: Early burn wound excision significantly reduces blood loss. Ann Surg 211:756, 1990

Dimick P, Heimbach D, Mansen J, et al: Anesthesia assisted procedures in a burn intensive care unit procedure room: benefits and complications. J Burn Care Rehabil 14:446, 1993

Dobke MK, Simoni J, Ninnemann JL, et al: Endotoxemia after burn injury: effect of early excision on circulating endotoxin levels. J Burn Care Rehabil 10:107, 1989

Engrav L, Heimbach D, Reas J, et al: Early excision and grafting vs nonoperative treatment of burns of indeterminate depth. J Trauma 23:1001, 1983

Fuller F, Parrish M, Nance F: A review of dosimetry of silver sulfadiazine cream in burn wound treatment. J Burn Care Rehabil 15:213, 1994

Housinzer T, Lang D, Warden G: A prospective study of blood loss with excisional therapy in pediatric burn patients. J Trauma 34:262, 1993

Hunt J: Is tracheostomy warranted in the burn patient? Indications and complications. J Burn Care Rehabil 7:492, 1986

Lanke K, Liljedahl S: Evaporative water loss from burns, grafts, and donor sites. Scand J Plastic Reconstr Surg 5:17, 1971

Matsumura N, Sugumata A: Aggressive wound closure for elderly patients with burns. J Burn Care Rehabil 15:18, 1994

McDonald W, Deitch E: Immediate enteral feeding in burn patients is safe and effective. Ann Surg 213:177, 1991

Monafo W, Bessey P: Benefits and limitations of burn wound excision. World J Surg 16:37, 1992

Shankowsky H, Callioux L: North American survey of hydrotherapy in modern burn care. J Burn Care Rehabil 15:193, 1994

Acknowledgment

Figure 1   Tom Moore.

34 BURN CARE AFTER THE FIRST POSTBURN WEEK

Robert H. Demling, M.D.

Management of the Burn Patient from 7 Days after the Burn until Complete Wound Closure

Beginning at about postburn day 7, dramatic physiologic and biochemical changes occur, related primarily to the onset of burn wound inflammation. Local and systemic infections also become major factors. The patient with a large burn who was stable during the preceding period frequently becomes unstable again, but the pathophysiologic alterations are much different from those seen during the first postburn week.

Maintenance of Adequate Lung Function

As during the early postresuscitation period, maintenance of pulmonary function is of major importance. There are two reasons for this: first, oxygen demands and carbon dioxide production are increased, and second, infection risks persist from the immunosuppressed state and from any superimposed smoke damage.

MAINTENANCE OF ADEQUATE ARTERIAL OXYGEN SATURATION

Because oxygen demands nearly double during this period in the patient with a major burn, an arterial oxygen saturation of 95% or greater is preferred, especially if it can be maintained with the fraction of inspired oxygen (F_IO_2) below 0.5, to minimize oxygen toxicity. The shunt fraction therefore must be minimized by maintaining both adequate lung volume and adequate blood volume. Atelectasis from hypoventilation or from secretion-induced obstruction of the small airways must be kept to a minimum.

MAINTENANCE OF ADEQUATE TISSUE OXYGENATION

In burn patients, blood volume, cardiac output, and hemoglobin count must be maintained at levels that optimize oxygen delivery to provide for the increased requirements. Oxygen consumption ($\dot{V}O_2$) increases from the normal value of 125 ml/min/m^2 to values approaching 300 ml/min/m^2 in burns exceeding 50% of total body surface (TBS). Pulse rate and cardiac output increase, paralleling the increase in $\dot{V}O_2$. Systemic hypertension is relatively common, as is heart failure, in patients with preexisting cardiac disease, especially the elderly. An obligate urine output of 1 to 2 ml/kg/hr is necessary to remove the increased solute load caused by the hypermetabolic state. Inadequate oxygen delivery is reflected in persistent lactic acidosis or in evidence of early organ failure (in particular, liver dysfunction).

MAINTENANCE OF ADEQUATE MINUTE VENTILATION

The increased carbon dioxide production characteristic of the postburn hypermetabolic state requires a large increase in minute ventilation ($\dot{V}_E$), sometimes twofold or threefold. The increase in $\dot{V}_E$ will depend on how large a portion of the $\dot{V}_E$ is increased dead space ventilation. If excision or grafting is to be performed, the anesthesiologist must be aware that increased ventilation is required to prevent severe hypercapnia.

MECHANICAL VENTILATORY SUPPORT

Frequently, the increased work of breathing necessitates some ventilatory assistance, particularly in the presence of a chest wall burn. Decreased chest wall compliance (in both open and grafted wounds) markedly increases the work necessary to clear the excess carbon dioxide produced. Because oxygen demands are high during this period, mechanical ventilation must be used carefully to allow adequate gas exchange without impeding oxygen delivery. Intermittent mandatory ventilation or, better yet, spontaneous ventilation is preferred to diminish wasted ventilation, provided that adequate energy is available to support the increased work of breathing. In addition, some use of positive end-expiratory pressure (PEEP) may be required to minimize atelectasis. The optimal situation, of course, is adequate spontaneous ventilation, as long as the necessary pulmonary function can be maintained. Any factor that increases carbon dioxide production (e.g., pain, excessive work, or excessive intake of carbohydrate calories) must be controlled.

PULMONARY TOILET

Pneumonia is a major problem during this period, and aggressive maintenance of pulmonary toilet is essential. Among patients in whom the airway mucosal barrier has been injured or actually denuded, pneumonia is particularly frequent and in fact is the major cause of death. The pneumonic process is accentuated by the immunodeficiency state that exists in the presence of the inflamed or infected burn wound.

Careful monitoring of sputum quantity and quality aids in detection of early infection and remains important in preventing the development of a life-threatening pneumonia. In addition, aggressive chest physiotherapy, ambulation, and cough and deep-breathing exercises must be continued until wound closure.

Management of the Burn Patient from 7 Days after the Burn until Complete Wound Closure

Maintain adequate lung function

Avoid hypercapnia and hypoventilation

Maintain adequate alveolar ventilation (CO_2 production is ↑).
Maintain O_2 saturation ≥ 95%.
Ensure adequate nutrition.
Avoid excess CO_2 production.
- Control stress.
- Keep respiratory quotient ≤ 1.

Control lung infection

Maintain pulmonary toilet.
Maintain adequate cough.
Minimize risks of nosocomial infection.

Minimize risks for infection and ARDS

Control potential foci of infection (i.e., lines, wounds, lungs).
Avoid pulmonary edema.
Watch for ↑ volume requirements, ↑ glucose intolerance, and ↑ tachycardia.

Sputum clearance is impaired

Optimize nutrition.
Consider ventilatory support until mechanics improve.

Evidence of lung infection is present

Initiate empirical therapy for nosocomial pneumonia; modify when culture results are available.

If evidence of infection is observed:
- Monitor filling pressure.
- Optimize $\dot{V}O_2$ while avoiding increase in PAWP to > 15 mm Hg.
- Increase ventilatory support.

Maintain adequate nutritional support

Determine total calories required:
- For burn 20%–40% TBS, 30–35 cal/kg/day.
- For burn ≥ 50% TBS, 35–45 cal/kg/day.

Determine protein requirements:
- Establish calorie-to-nitrogen ratio between 100:1 and 150:1.

Replace lost vitamins and trace elements (e.g., vitamin A, vitamin C, and zinc).

Establish appropriate nutrient mix

Of nonprotein calories, give 70% as carbohydrate.
Of final diet, give 55%–60% as carbohydrate, 20%–25% as fat, 20% as protein.

Select appropriate route

Enteral route is preferred, supplemented by parenteral route as needed.
Consider peripheral vein alimentation with increased water needs.

Maintain hemodynamic stability

Replace lost fluids and electrolytes

Estimate evaporative losses (monitor body weight, urine specific gravity, serum osmolarity, and clinical signs of hydration status).
Replenish evaporative losses: ml/hr = (25 + %TBS burn) × m².
Replace lost RBCs and protein.
Monitor electrolyte levels (particularly with nutritional support).

Maintain tissue perfusion

O_2 consumption is 1.5–2 times normal.
Maintain cardiac output at 1.5–2 times normal.
Maintain hematocrit ≥ 30.
Avoid lactic acidosis.

Control stress response

Control the three components of the stress response: (1) systemic inflammation (afferent arc), (2) release of stress hormones (efferent arc), and (3) CNS stimuli such as pain and anxiety (CNS modulation).
Avoid hypothermia:
- Maintain ambient T° ≥ 85° F.
- Minimize heat loss from wound exposure or wet dressings.

Sufficient pain control is essential.
Ensure sufficient sedation to allow for adequate rest.

Burn wound care

Gently debride wound daily.
Graft on clean granulation tissue, if wound is heavily colonized.
Excision should be done cautiously during this period because of increased risks of infection and blood loss.

Control wound infection

Control wound surface bacteria with topical antibiotics.
Treat wound infection with systemic antibiotics.
Monitor plasma levels of antibiotics.

Initiate rehabilitation

Begin and continue joint motion early.
Maintain aggressive muscle-strengthening efforts.
Mobilization should be early and continued.
Apply pressure garments (25 mm Hg) to healed wound.
Use skin moisturizers liberally.

TRACHEOSTOMY

Burn patients are at high risk for lung dysfunction, much of which can be prevented if direct access to excessive secretions can be obtained, the risk of aspirating infected oral secretions can be decreased, and patients can be intermittently rested with partial mechanical support so that the cough reflex can be maintained. A good way of achieving these objectives—given that the time course for correction of a large burn wound or a severe smoke inhalation injury is weeks rather than days—is to perform a tracheostomy. The timing of tracheostomy remains somewhat controversial; however, a tracheostomy through unburned or grafted skin should be considered appropriate if the patient is expected to require an artificial airway for several weeks. Improved pulmonary toilet, enhanced patient comfort, and the elimination of the need for frequent reintubation are all assets. If the high-risk period is short, the burn relatively small, and the patient relatively young, then weaning and extubation are appropriate.

MANAGEMENT OF PULMONARY DYSFUNCTION

Pulmonary problems remain a major cause of morbidity and mortality after the first postburn week. In fact, pulmonary failure and pulmonary infection exceed burn wound infection as causes of death in burn patients. Three major processes occur during this period: (1) nosocomial pneumonia, (2) hypermetabolism-induced respiratory fatigue (power failure), and (3) acute respiratory distress syndrome (ARDS), including low-pressure pulmonary edema. These three processes are closely interrelated. Burn patients are highly vulnerable to infection, particularly after inhalation injury. The hypermetabolic state produces a marked elevation in oxygen requirements and carbon dioxide production; the increased demands placed on the lung as a result may exceed pulmonary functional capacity. ARDS is a severe complication of the septic response; it is very difficult to reverse in burn patients.

Nosocomial Pneumonia

The term nosocomial pneumonia refers to a pneumonia that develops in the hospital in a patient who showed no evidence of lung infection on admission (i.e., to a hospital-acquired pneumonia). Although wound infection, another form of hospital-acquired infection, is more common than nosocomial infection, the latter carries a much higher mortality. Burn patients who have both inhalation injury and a major body burn are at highest risk for nosocomial pneumonia, with the incidence in this population exceeding 50%. This high incidence is attributable to the presence of virulent organisms in the hospital environment and to the immunosuppressed state of burn patients. Once pneumonia is established in a burn patient, it is very difficult to eradicate; consequently, prevention is of primary importance. Preventive measures fall into four main categories: (1) improving systemic host defenses, (2) improving local pulmonary defenses, (3) minimizing oropharyngeal colonization, and (4) minimizing tracheobronchial aspiration [see 103 Early Postoperative Pneumonia].

Hypermetabolism-Induced Respiratory Fatigue (Power Failure)

Several processes may impair oxygenation during this period. The severe catabolism initiated by the inflammatory response can lead not only to extremity weakness but also to chest wall muscle weakness. Chronic pain and anxiety can lead to sleep deprivation and fatigue. Heart failure can lead to lung edema, and growing fatigue can lead to hypoventilation-induced atelectasis. As a rule, however, the major problem during this period is not hypoxemia but hypercapnia. Removal of carbon dioxide is directly dependent on alveolar minute ventilation: if carbon dioxide production doubles, alveolar ventilation must also double to maintain normal arterial oxygen tension (P_aO_2). Increased ventilation means increased work of breathing, especially if compliance is decreased or dead space is increased. Large tidal volumes are necessary to maintain adequate alveolar ventilation because small tidal volumes ventilate little more than dead space. Larger tidal volumes call for greater inspiratory force, and the increased work of breathing must be sustained 24 hours a day. Fatigue may then result in impaired clearance of secretions, which can lead to nosocomial pneumonia (see above) as well as hypercapnia.

Serial measurements of tidal volume, vital capacity, and inspiratory force allow one to detect early deterioration of pulmonary function. Measurement of carbon dioxide production allows one to determine whether production exceeds the value predicted on the basis of the burn size alone. Oxygen consumption can also be measured directly by means of either spirometry or the Fick method, and the respiratory quotient can then be calculated directly [see 92 Use of the Mechanical Ventilator].

Acute Respiratory Distress Syndrome

ARDS is the name given to the clinical manifestations of a number of indirect lung injury states that are characterized by dyspnea, severe hypoxemia, and decreased lung compliance accompanied by radiographic evidence of diffuse bilateral pulmonary infiltrates. Alveolar consolidation with fluid, protein, and inflammatory cells in the presence of normal pulmonary arterial wedge pressure (PAWP) (i.e., low-pressure pulmonary edema) is also a characteristic finding. Altered permeability results in rapid movement of fluid from plasma to the interstitial space without any increase in PAWP.

ARDS caused by burn inflammation and infection carries an extremely high mortality. The major reason why this is so is that the condition will not resolve until the initiating process is removed. Unfortunately, at this point in the postburn period, burn wounds—especially large ones—cannot be readily excised and closed, because of the increased vascularity of the wound, the presence of colonization or infection, and the further debilitation of the patient. Consequently, efforts must be made to prevent ARDS through early removal of as much of the burn wound (which is a potential source of a systemic inflammatory response) as is feasible [see 91 Pulmonary Dysfunction].

Maintenance of Hemodynamic Stability

MAINTENANCE OF ADEQUATE HYDRATION

Evaporative loss is greatest from granulation tissue (with its increased blood supply) and least from a third-degree burn (with its thick eschar). Unhealed donor sites must also be considered in the estimation of evaporative loss. In addition, the increased body temperature characteristic of this period increases evaporative loss. Grafted skin restores much of the barrier, but losses may still be greater than evaporation across normal skin until the graft matures. Estimation of these losses depends on close monitoring of body weight, urine specific gravity, serum osmolarity, and clinical signs of hydration status [see 33 Burn Care in the Early Postresuscitation Period]. Serum sodium is a helpful indicator of the state of hydration. If the value is elevated, more water should be given.

RESTORATION AND MAINTENANCE OF PERFUSION

The Hyperdynamic State

A hyperdynamic state evolves in the postresuscitation period as part of the response to burn injury, peaking about the end of the first postburn week. The degree of hyperdynamism appears to correlate with the degree of initial tissue injury as well as with the degree of initial damage to organs (especially the lungs). The hyperdynamic state is the result of systemic inflammation and the altered hormonal environment: the tissue injury and the secondary inflammatory response it evokes result in increased oxygen demands. Generally, patients remain hemodynamically stable in the postresuscitation period unless volume replenishment is inadequate; however, varying degrees of instability may occur. Physiologic responses range from normal to grossly abnormal or, more specifically, from simple hyperdynamism to the systemic inflammatory response syndrome (SIRS) to septic shock to, finally, the multiple organ dysfunction syndrome (MODS).

It is clear that burn patients who can spontaneously generate a hyperdynamic state in response to injury are capable of supplying enough oxygen to keep up with the increased metabolic demands reflected in increased oxygen consumption. It is also clear that mortality is lower in these patients than in patients who have an oxygen debt. It remains unclear, however, whether patients who cannot spontaneously generate a hyperdynamic response should be artificially maintained in a hyperdynamic state with volume expansion and inotropes, which patients should be so maintained, and what degree of artificial hyperdynamism would be appropriate.

Unfortunately, because of certain direct cellular metabolic changes, lactate concentration is a less sensitive indicator of impaired perfusion in this period than it was in the initial postburn period. Increased quantities of pyruvate are present as a result of the increased glucose utilization. Increased lactate may simply reflect decreased pyruvate utilization. A more reliable indicator of excessive lactate is the lactate-pyruvate ratio. An increase in this ratio would indicate excessive lactate and impaired perfusion. Mixed (or central) venous oxygen saturation may be a less useful monitoring parameter because of inflammation-induced maldistribution of blood flow, which lowers the extraction ratio. Logically, it would appear that maintaining high values for certain physiologic variables might help prevent MODS [see Table 1]; however, this approach has not yet been unequivocally shown to decrease the incidence of MODS during the early stress response.

When bacteria or their by-products are present, a further amplification of the hyperdynamic state occurs, accompanied by increased inflammation; clinical infection may or may not be present. This symptom complex has traditionally been referred to as sepsis but currently is often referred to as SIRS [see Table 2]. The hyperdynamic state persists, but a degree of hemodynamic instability is now present, necessitating both increased fluid infusion and the administration of inotropes to maintain adequate oxygen delivery and perfusion pressure. Cardiac output remains 1.5 to 2.0 times normal, but vascular pressures decrease gradually as a result of a marked downregulation of both alpha and beta agonists by inflammatory mediators, which leads to hypotension and impaired cardiac function.

A modest lactic acidosis may also be present. If the impairment of blood flow is not corrected, the decreased perfusion leads to damage to vital organs. Neurologic changes (usually increased lethargy or confusion attributable to by-products of the metabolic changes) are also evident. As the hemodynamic changes progress, the hyperdynamic state can actually develop into a hypodynamic state.

Methods for Restoring and Maintaining Perfusion

If the patient is incapable of spontaneously increasing oxygen delivery to meet the increased oxygen demands, one may attempt to improve perfusion using the following approaches.

Volume expansion Volume expansion is the initial treatment of choice for restoring perfusion in the hypermetabolic burn patient. This primarily involves raising filling pressure to increase cardiac output as well as to reopen underperfused microcirculatory beds. The specific role of colloids in restoring volume remains unclear; however, it seems reasonable to use them to supplement crystalloids. Albumin has a number of important properties in addition to its ability to maintain plasma colloid oncotic pressure, including antioxidant activity and the ability to bind free fatty acids, oxidants, and endotoxin.

Administration of inotropes Because renal and splanchnic perfusion are often decreased even when overall perfusion appears to be adequate, low-dose dopamine (1 to 3 μg/kg/min) is appropriate for maintaining urine output. Medium-dose dopamine (≥ 4 μg/kg/min) is appropriate for raising the cardiac index when PAWP is normal (14 to 16 mm Hg), and dobutamine

---

Table 1 **Physiologic Values to Be Maintained during the Stress Response to Major Burn Injury**

Cardiac index > 4 L/min/m^2
PAWP 12–16 mm Hg (may have to be as high as 18 mm Hg)
Oxygen delivery 1.5 times normal
Oxygen consumption approximately 1.5 times normal
Normal anion gap (8–12 mEq/L)

Table 2 **Unstable Hyperdynamism: Systemic Inflammatory Response Syndrome**

Clinical and laboratory findings
  Increased temperature, chills
  Warm, dry skin
  Tachycardia, tachypnea
  Blood pressure: usually decreased
  Mental changes
  Urine changes: variable

Laboratory findings
  White blood cell count: increased
  Metabolic acidosis
  Lactate concentration: 1.5–2.0 mmol/L

Physiologic changes
  Increased O_2 consumption, CO_2 production
  Arterial-venous oxygen difference: normal to low
  PAWP: normal to low
  Cardiac output: increased
  Systemic vascular resistance: decreased
  Local microvascular damage

(usually 5 to 10 μg/kg/min), a nearly pure beta agonist, is used when PAWP is elevated (> 16 mm Hg).

Blood transfusion The ideal hemoglobin concentration for restoring perfusion in the hypermetabolic burn patient remains undefined. It is certain that in previously healthy young patients whose condition is stable, 8 g/dl is adequate. In severely burned patients who have MODS to any degree, on the other hand, a value of 10 g/dl is probably a more appropriate goal, especially in view of the impaired ability of critically ill patients to make new red blood cells.

Patients with Established MODS

In patients with established MODS, it is difficult to improve metabolic function simply by increasing oxygen delivery; inotropes are also often ineffective in these individuals. To date, it has not been documented that maintaining a hyperdynamic state by itself has any beneficial effect on survival once secondary MODS is established; it appears that the stress response–induced metabolic abnormalities must also be minimized for outcome to be improved.

CONTROL OF THE SYSTEMIC STRESS RESPONSE

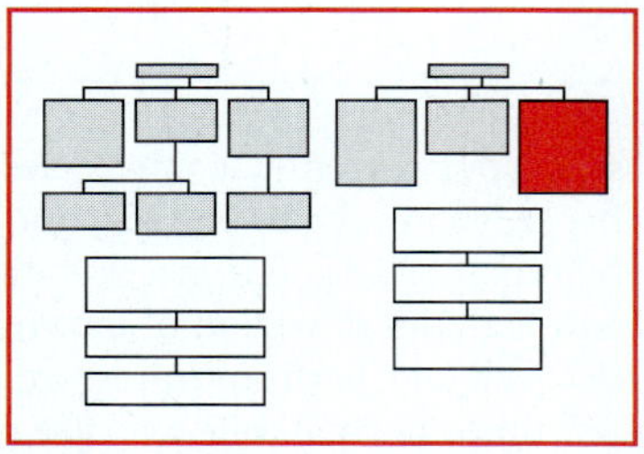

The initial burn insult provokes a reaction on the part of the host. This reaction may be considered a protective mechanism; however, it can in fact produce more injury than the initial insult itself. The components of the stress response are (1) an afferent arc, that is, the inflammatory response; (2) an efferent arc, that is, the release of so-called stress hormones; and (3) a CNS modulation that accentuates the efferent arc, that is, the generation of stimuli such as pain, anxiety, and stress-induced psychosis. The patient's natural response to injury is inflammation, both local and systemic. Although the physiologic manifestations of the stress response are most evident several days after the injury, cellular biochemical changes caused by activation of this response can be seen very early after injury [see Figure 1].

The Afferent Arc: The Inflammatory Response

It has long been known that local inflammation occurs in burn-injured tissue within minutes to hours after injury; it has now also been documented that generalized inflammation also occurs. It is becoming increasingly clear that any severe local tissue trauma can give rise to a massive systemic inflammatory response. Large amounts of cytokines are released soon after major trauma, and inflammatory cells can be found sequestered in the microcirculation in virtually all organs immediately after severe trauma or burn injury. This generalized response appears to be attributable to the systemic activation of a number of inflammatory cascades, including intravascular complement activation. Animal and human studies have found evidence of early tissue oxidant changes, as reflected in elevated levels of circulating lipid peroxides and increased tissue lipid peroxidation.

The inflammatory cell sequestration and adherence to endothelial cells observed initially do not necessarily lead to injury if the inflammatory cells are only primed and not activated. Neutrophils often undergo systemic activation if ischemic or devitalized tissue is not removed or if there is a second insult. Although inflammation begins immediately after injury, physiologic evidence of the systemic response usually is not apparent for several days. The continued presence of devitalized tissue primes the host for a subsequent insult. In addition, the response to any subsequent insult (e.g., endotoxin, vascular catheter bacteremia, or pancreatitis) is amplified, leading to far more tissue damage and hemodynamic instability than would have been expected to result from the same insult in the absence of previous injury or infection.

The observation of this exaggerated response to even modest infection or ischemia on the part of the injured patient has given rise to the so-called two-hit theory of MODS [see Figure 2]. The

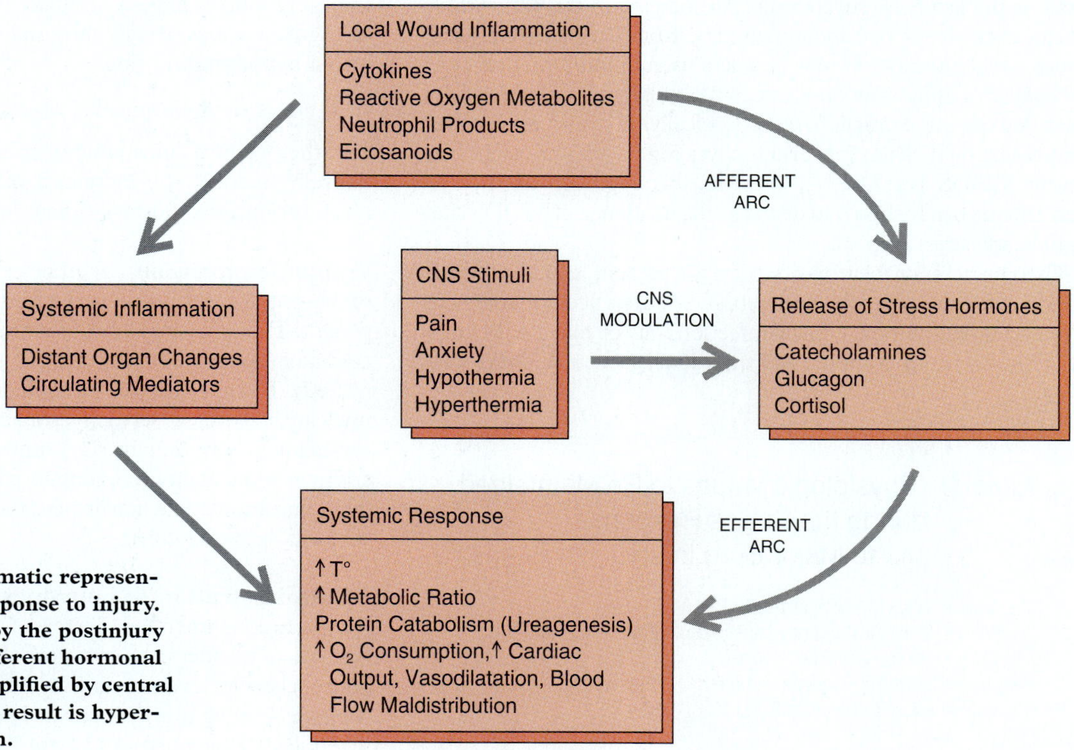

Figure 1 Shown is a schematic representation of the host stress response to injury. The afferent arc initiated by the postinjury inflammation evokes an efferent hormonal response, which can be amplified by central nervous system stress. The result is hypermetabolism and catabolism.

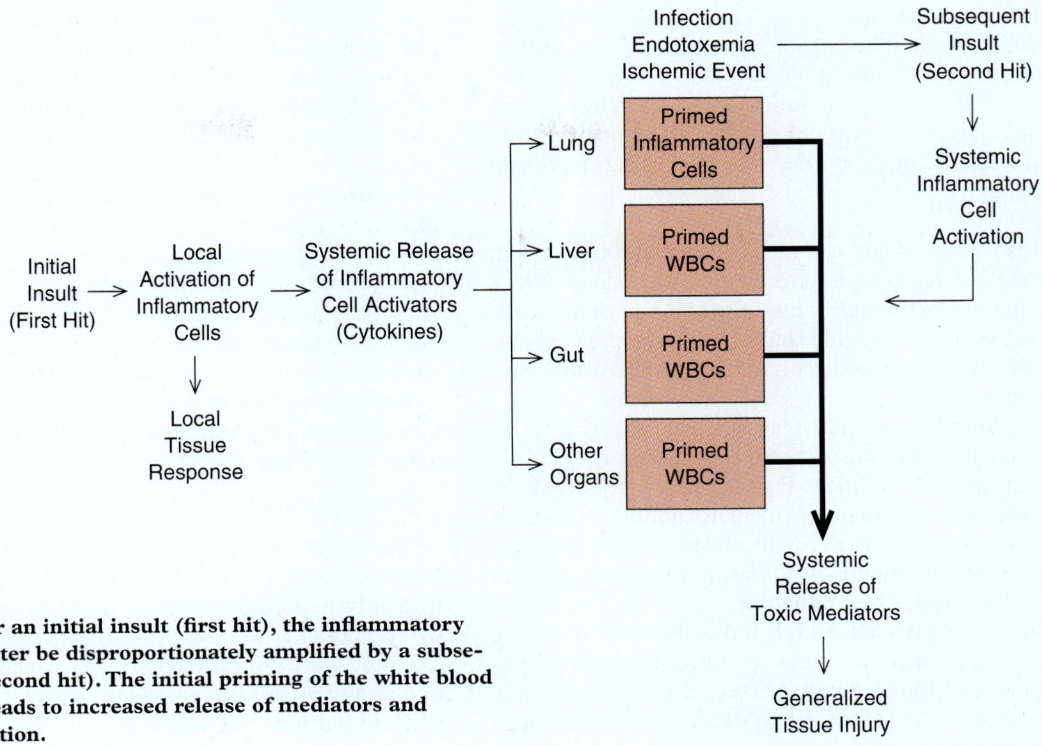

Figure 2 After an initial insult (first hit), the inflammatory response can later be disproportionately amplified by a subsequent insult (second hit). The initial priming of the white blood cells (WBCs) leads to increased release of mediators and systemic activation.

initial burn or smoke inhalation injury—the first hit—induces the inflammatory cells to turn on their metabolic machinery; this process usually is not clinically apparent. A subsequent insult—the second hit—causes the mediator factories to synthesize and release larger quantities of toxic compounds than the degree of the second insult would normally call for; these mediators then produce hemodynamic instability and tissue injury. The most prominent mediators of the stress response are the cytokines. These agents activate the inflammatory process and trigger the release of counterregulatory hormones and other potent vasoactive and cytotoxic mediators.

Cytokines are involved in a number of major responses to injury and infection, including hemodynamic changes, tissue inflammation, wound healing, immune defenses, hypermetabolism, and catabolism. Sustained increases in the activity of some of these agents—tumor necrosis factor (TNF) in particular—are thought to be responsible for the organ dysfunction associated with a persistent, progressive inflammatory response. The major cytokines that play a role in the inflammatory response to injury and infection are TNF, interleukin-1 (IL-1), IL-2, IL-6, and interferon gamma.

Endotoxin Endotoxin is a well-known initiator of inflammation and inflammation-induced disease. It activates the release of a number of mediators, including eicosanoids, oxidants, and cytokines (especially TNF). It also leads to generalized immunosuppression, although the mechanism by which it does so remains undefined.

Endotoxemia is considered to play a major role in the postinjury stress response, even when no obvious source of infection is present. In the absence of clinical infection, endotoxin may be absorbed into the circulation from a colonized wound surface or from a leaky GI tract.

Reactive oxygen metabolites Oxygen radicals are unstable metabolites of oxygen that have an unpaired electron in their outer shell and consequently are potent oxidizing agents; two examples are the superoxide anion (O_2^-) and the hydroxyl anion (OH·). There are other toxic oxygen metabolites that, though not true free radicals, are nonetheless potent oxidants; one example is hydrogen peroxide (H_2O_2). Oxidants are now considered to be involved in several aspects of the response to burn injury and inflammation [see Table 3]. Studies have shown that the systemic inflammatory response seen after severe burns is attributable to systemic activation of complement by OH·. Toxic oxygen metabolites also cause lipid peroxidation in the lungs, liver, kidneys, and other tissues in the early postburn period. Elevated circulating levels of lipid peroxides have been documented in patients who are injured or infected. This early postinjury lipid peroxidation may not result in immediate organ dysfunction, but it may help amplify the response to a second insult by causing the release of more inflammatory cytokines. Tissues injured by oxidants and proteases are much more vulnerable to further injury by a subsequent insult. The degree of oxidant damage is closely correlated with the adequacy of antioxidant defenses. After the process of inflammation and infection is under way, oxygen metabolites are again involved in tissue injury; during this phase, the primary oxidant source is activated white blood cells, with endotoxin playing a major role in the release of these substances.

Table 3 Effects of Reactive Oxygen Metabolites

Alteration of vascular permeability
Lipid peroxidation, altering function
Initiation and perpetuation of local and systemic inflammation
Disruption of interstitial matrix
Impairment of macrophage phagocytosis
Alteration of cellular DNA
Initiation of arachidonic acid metabolism
Red blood cell hemolysis

At present, a number of antioxidants normally present in tissues (e.g., vitamin C, vitamin E, catalase, superoxide dismutase, and glutathione or its substrate, glutamine) are available for clinical use. Other oxidants (e.g., xanthine oxidase inhibitors, iron chelators, and 21-aminosteroids, a new class of agents with iron chelating and antioxidant properties) are also being developed for use in humans.

Eicosanoids Arachidonic acid metabolites play a role in both the early and the late response to burn injury. Arachidonic acid is released from the cell membrane in response to injury or infection. It is metabolized via two enzymatic pathways: (1) the cyclooxygenase pathway, which yields prostaglandins and thromboxanes, and (2) the lipoxygenase pathway, which yields leukotrienes.

After a burn, both the vasodilator prostaglandin I_2 (PGI_2), or prostacyclin, and the vasoconstrictor thromboxane A_2 (TXA_2) are released in great quantities. Prostacyclin increases local blood flow, thereby accentuating mediator-induced vascular leakage. The local increase in TXA_2 increases platelet aggregation and neutrophil margination in the wound microcirculation, thereby also potentiating tissue ischemia.

CNS production of prostaglandin E is thought to be the cause of the fever associated with the stress response. The characteristic maldistribution of blood flow observed in marked systemic inflammation appears to be related to excessive production of TXA_2 or PGI_2 in various vascular beds.

The Efferent Arc: Release of Stress Hormones

Certain characteristic hormonal alterations take place during the stress response to burn injury. There is an early increase in circulating catecholamine levels, and this increase produces the peripheral vasoconstriction, anxiety, and tachycardia observed in the early postburn period. Catecholamine levels appear to correlate directly with the degree of injury. The sympathetic adrenal response—namely, increased $alpha_1$- and $beta_1$-receptor activity—appears to correlate with the degree of subsequent hypermetabolism and increased oxygen demands. Beta-receptor activity predominates in the hyperdynamic state. The increased sympathetic activity generally persists throughout the period of critical illness.

Cortisol and glucagon levels are also increased during critical illness. Both of these agents are considered anti-insulin hormones because they promote gluconeogenesis and glycogenolysis. Cortisol also promotes catabolism.

Insulin not only increases glycogen production and is essential for glucose utilization at the cell level but also is a potent anabolic hormone that facilitates the incorporation of amino acids into protein. Insulin administration improves both glucose utilization and protein synthesis.

Human growth hormone is the most potent anabolic hormone. It induces marked increases in protein synthesis and gluconeogenesis; in addition, unlike insulin, it causes lipolysis and increased utilization of ketone bodies for fuel, sparing skeletal muscle and decreasing the catabolic response to stress. Growth hormone levels typically are lower than normal in the catabolic phase of severe injury.

Metabolic alterations Significant alterations in normal metabolic activity are observed in patients with SIRS [see Table 4]. In addition to increases in circulating levels of inflammatory mediators (particularly macrophage-derived products), there are large, sustained increases in levels of anti-insulin hormones and catabolic hormones (e.g., catecholamines, cortisol, and glucagon). Although insulin levels are increased as well, insulin activity appears to be outweighed by the anti-insulin activity of the catabolic hormones. In hypermetabolic patients, calorie requirements are 50% to 100% higher than normal. Because of the altered metabolism, the compensatory mechanisms normally triggered by starvation are absent, and nutrient utilization is substantially affected.

Acute-phase protein production Hepatic protein synthesis is reprioritized. Production of acute-phase proteins is increased, and production of albumin synthetase is decreased. Acute-phase proteins, which have immunoprotective properties, are released from the liver in response to burn injury, severe smoke inhalation injury, or systemic infection; the specific stimulus appears to be the elevated levels of cytokines (IL-6 and IL-1).

Each acute-phase protein has a characteristic function and duration of action. The downregulation of albumin production results in a hypoalbuminemic state that persists throughout the stress response.

CNS Modulation

The CNS significantly affects the efferent response to a burn. Increased CNS stimulation deriving from pain, anxiety, hypothermia, or hyperthermia amplifies the release of catecholamines, thereby accentuating the hypermetabolic state. Occasionally, patients manifest a stress-induced psychosis, which leads to sleep deprivation and excessive motor activity, thereby further increasing oxygen and nutrient consumption.

Methods for Controlling the Stress Response

Removing the inflammatory focus It is critical to remove deep burned tissue as soon as possible. The objective is to remove a potential inflammatory focus before the host stress response takes hold. Once the hyperdynamic state is clinically present, inflammation is already well established. According to current protocols for preventing secondary MODS, devitalized tissue should be removed even if the patient still appears to be stable.

Modulating release of stress hormones It is essential to minimize the likelihood of further stimuli that will amplify the release of stress hormones, especially catecholamines. Infection must of course be controlled, and further ischemic insults must be avoided (see below). Hypothermia usually is readily controlled. To prevent excessive heat loss during care of the burn wounds, the ambient temperature must be maintained at 30° to 35° C (86° to 95° F). Mild hyperthermia generally is not a major problem, but if body temperature exceeds 103° F, deleterious side effects can result.

Pain control helps prevent excessive release of catecholamines in patients at risk for organ dysfunction. Optimum pain control usually cannot be achieved during initial resuscitation, while patients are still hypovolemic; it is possible only when hemodynamic

---

Table 4 **Major Metabolic Abnormalities with Response to Injury**

Sustained increase in body temperature

Marked increase in glucose demand and therefore strong stimulation of liver gluconeogenesis

Rapid skeletal muscle breakdown caused by demand for amino acid substrate for use as a direct energy source, for gluconeogenesis, and for hepatic acute-phase protein production

Stimulation of the liver to produce large quantities of acute-phase proteins

Absence of ketosis, indicating that fat is not the major calorie source

Unresponsiveness of the rate of gluconeogenesis and catabolism to substrate

stability is restored. Patients require larger and more frequent doses of pain medication after the first postburn week because during this period, they experience increasing tolerance to analgesic agents as a result of long-term use and the increasing pain of the debriding wound [see 3 Burn Care in the Immediate Resuscitation Period and 33 Burn Care in the Early Postresuscitation Period]. Self-administration has been found to be quite useful because the patient's perception of the pain is more accurate than that of the care providers. During the postresuscitation period, high-risk patients should receive continuous epidural analgesia or continuous low-dose narcotic infusion to minimize stress.

Anxiety control is crucial. Close attention must be paid to supporting the neuropsychological status of the patient, especially in the presence of organ dysfunction and SIRS. Adequate sleep periods and the avoidance of sensory overload are essential, especially in the ICU. Administration of benzodiazepines, either intermittently or by continuous infusion, can effectively attenuate anxiety-induced stress. The ICU psychosis syndrome [see 33 Burn Care in the Early Postresuscitation Period] usually must be treated by means of a neuroleptic agent, such as chlorpromazine or haloperidol.

Counteracting or augmenting stress hormone activity
Excessive production of catecholamines occurs in patients with major burns in the later postresuscitation period. This response increases metabolic demands and is responsible for cardiomyopathy, characterized by focal myofiber necrosis. Rapid pulse rate and hypertension are commonly observed. In moderate doses, beta antagonists can reduce the amount of work the heart must perform and actually decrease metabolic demands, especially in patients with head injuries. Oxygen delivery must not be decreased to the point where it fails to meet oxygen demands.

Recent studies suggest that exogenous administration of human growth hormone may be highly beneficial in patients with massive burns. Human growth hormone, 1 to 2 mg/day, has been shown to improve nitrogen balance in normal elderly men. Levels of endogenous human growth hormone are lower than normal in burn patients. When given to such patients in dosages of 5 to 10 mg/day, human growth hormone markedly improved nitrogen retention and increased the rate of wound healing. Exogenous human growth hormone causes more endogenous fat to be used for fuel and reduces protein catabolism. Its use is associated with some complications, namely, a modest (5% to 10%) increase in oxygen consumption, modest hyperglycemia, and positive salt and water retention, especially during the first several days. Efforts are being made to determine how, when, and to which burn patients human growth hormone should be given.

Preventing a second insult As noted (see above), the addition of a second insult to an already primed system evokes an amplified host stress response. To prevent such an occurrence, extreme vigilance and aggressive institution of preventive measures are required in patients who are at high risk for secondary MODS.

Decreasing leakage from the gut Efforts should be made to minimize bacterial translocation and leakage of endotoxin across the impaired gut barrier. A lack of enteral nutrients rapidly leads to mucosal atrophy, especially during the stress response; early enteral nutrition is considered effective in maintaining the mucosal barrier. Several clinical trials have demonstrated that early enteral nutrition—as compared with early parenteral nutrition or delayed enteral nutrition—decreases secondary MODS in burn patients. Placement of a postpyloric feeding tube is becoming an increasingly common practice.

Table 5 Substances with Antioxidant Effects That May Be Given in Nutritional Solutions

Oxidant scavengers
 Vitamin C: 1–2 g/day
 Vitamin E: 400 mg/day
 β-Carotene: 25,000 IU/day
Antioxidant substrate
 Glutamine: 20–30 g/day (required for glutathione synthesis)
Required cofactors
 Selenium: 40 mg/day (cofactor glutathione peroxidase-reductase)
 Zinc: 20 mg/day parenterally (cofactor superoxide dismutase); alternatively, zinc sulfate, 220 mg t.i.d., p.o.

Administering glutamine The amino acid glutamine is the major fuel for the rapidly dividing enterocytes. Injury is often followed by glutamine deficiency as a result of both increased endogenous utilization and decreased exogenous intake. Glutamine is typically absent from central hyperalimentation solutions and standard tube feedings; however, glutamine-enriched enteral and parenteral solutions are now available. The current recommended daily dose of glutamine for adults is 20 to 30 g or 0.5 g/kg.

Using exogenous inhibitors of inflammation Nonsteroidal anti-inflammatory drugs (NSAIDs), particularly ibuprofen, have been shown to attenuate the response to inflammation and endotoxin in humans. Ibuprofen inhibits cyclooxygenase activity, thereby decreasing eicosanoid production. In addition, NSAIDs have antioxidant, anticytokine, and neutrophil-stabilizing properties. Although it is clear that these agents have significant beneficial potential, it has not been determined whether and to what extent they can actually attenuate the stress response and prevent MODS. The use of NSAIDs during the stress response has not led to an increased incidence of renal complications.

Given the deleterious effects of oxidants, the use of agents that prevent or minimize oxidant activity in some fashion is likely to be beneficial [see Table 5]. A host of antioxidants and agents that prevent oxidant release or remove oxidants already released (e.g., vitamin C, vitamin E, and β-carotene) are being used clinically. Optimizing cellular defenses against oxidant activity, particularly by nutritional means, has received considerable attention as a method of preventing inflammation. Marked deficiencies in endogenous antioxidants, resulting from both increased turnover and decreased substrate intake, are known to exacerbate the cellular injury caused by the ongoing inflammatory response. Glutamine, besides being fuel for enterocytes (see above), is also an essential substrate for the endogenous antioxidant glutathione. During critical illness and oxidant stress, tissue glutathione levels decrease.

Nutrition

Adequate nutrition must be provided to meet increased tissue demands by postburn day 7 because early delivery of necessary calories and proteins becomes essential for rapid wound closure and to minimize complications from pulmonary dysfunction and infection. Nutritional support should have begun between postburn days 2 and 5. Increased metabolic activity usually peaks between postburn days 7 and 10, and by then, demands should be completely met.

First, energy requirements must be estimated; second, plans for nutrient delivery must be individually tailored according to each patient's requirement for carbohydrate, protein, and fat.

ENERGY REQUIREMENTS

The goal of nutritional support is to provide the necessary calories to meet energy needs. These needs depend on energy expenditure, measurements of which are based on three components: basal metabolic rate (BMR), muscle activity, and stress-induced energy needs.

Basal metabolic rate describes the energy required to maintain cell integrity at the resting state and at thermoneutrality, which for the burn patient is 28° to 30° C ambient (80° to 88° F). Under these environmental conditions, heat loss is minimized and the need to produce additional metabolic heat to maintain body temperature is absent or greatly attenuated. In normal individuals, environmental temperature below thermoneutrality markedly increases sympathetic activity and caloric requirements. The BMR for humans of various ages has been determined and is widely available in chart form. Body size is the principal factor influencing metabolic rate. Other variables include the age and, to a lesser extent, the sex of the patient.

Muscle activity level is a measure of the average amount of energy used by muscles for daily activity. For patients in an ICU, muscle activity is usually quite limited, and the energy cost is usually considered to be no more than 25% above the BMR. The stress of daily exercise, sitting in a chair, and walking all contribute to the additional energy cost. Energy expenditure in bedridden patients can be markedly increased by excessive muscle activity (e.g., in patients who fight the ventilator, who must work excessively hard to breathe, or who are in a combative, disoriented state). Sedation or, if necessary, muscle paralysis will decrease this component of energy expenditure to almost zero. Prolonged muscle paralysis is not desirable, because muscle tone is necessary to maintain strength and positive nitrogen balance; the latter is particularly important for the muscles of respiration.

The third component on which energy requirements are based is stress-induced energy need. A so-called stress factor defines the hypermetabolism that is induced by the burn. The stress factor is a multiple of the basal metabolic rate (normalized to 1.0); its value takes into consideration the size of the burn injury and the average metabolic response that is seen with this size injury [see Table 6].

Oxygen consumption, carbon dioxide production, or both can be measured directly and the metabolic rate calculated. Direct measurement of calorie requirements with an indirect calorimeter (which essentially involves converting oxygen consumption to calorie expenditure) appears to be more accurate than using a formula to estimate calorie requirements; however, formulas can be very useful as guidelines [see Figure 3].

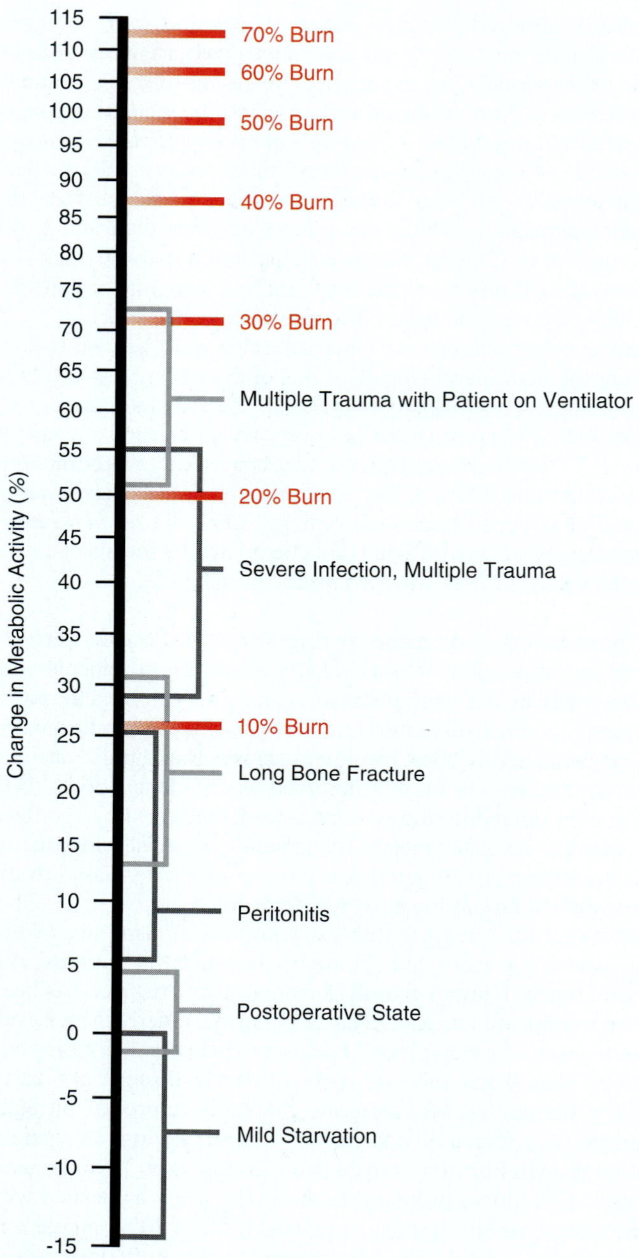

Figure 3 Depicted is the relation between selected injuries and various degrees of change in metabolic activity resulting from these injuries. Major burns cause the largest increases in metabolic rate.

Table 6 Stress Factors

Burn Size (% TBS)	Stress Factor
10	1.25
20	1.50
30	1.70
40	1.85
50	2.00
60–100	2.10

NUTRIENT REQUIREMENTS (CARBOHYDRATE, FAT, AND PROTEIN)

Approximately 70% of estimated nonprotein calorie requirements must be given as glucose to spare nitrogen effectively. If lipid infusions are given, triglyceride levels must be monitored to avoid hypertriglyceridemia. In most burn patients, lipid clearance is not impaired and may in fact be increased. Increasing the proportion of omega-3 fatty acids and decreasing the proportion of omega-6 fatty acids in the infusion may be helpful. Lipids, because of their immunosuppressive effects, should make up no more than 25% of total calories.

When carbohydrates are administered, a large portion is oxidized to carbon dioxide and excreted via the lungs. As the quantity of glucose administered increases, carbon dioxide production rises and the respiratory quotient shifts from 0.7 (reflecting fat oxidation) toward 1.0 (reflecting carbohydrate oxidation). Excess carbohydrate—that is, more than can be primarily oxidized—is converted to fat. When this conversion occurs, the respiratory quotient exceeds 1.0, and the result may be an increased ventilatory load for the patient.

Protein requirements are also calculated in a number of ways. An estimate of 1.5 to 2.0 g of protein per kilogram of body weight can be used for all major burns. A more specific quantitative estimate can be based on a calorie-nitrogen ratio. (The nitrogen content of protein is determined by dividing the amount of protein by 6.25.) A 150:1 ratio is usually used to calculate protein requirements, but some investigators are now proposing that a 100:1 ratio is preferable. Thus, the final diet provides approximately 20% protein, 55% to 60% carbohydrate, and 20% to 25% fat.

VITAMIN AND TRACE-ELEMENT REQUIREMENTS

The burn patient loses a number of vitamins in increased quantities. Vitamins A and C are of particular concern because they are essential for healing. Vitamin A must usually be replaced in a daily dose of 10,000 to 15,000 units and vitamin C in a daily dose of 1 to 2 g. Zinc, a trace element required for healing, is also lost in increased amounts. Replacement is usually 220 mg of zinc sulfate, given orally three times a day. Administering microminerals in the form of a high-potency vitamin-mineral pill or elixir is necessary to provide trace elements.

ADMINISTRATION OF NUTRITION

Nutritional support is best managed during this period by the enteral route, usually with a combination of balanced tube feeding and voluntary intake. Parenteral supplementation through a peripheral vein may be necessary in the patient with a very large burn (i.e., a burn exceeding 50% of TBS). Central venous feedings are occasionally required if the GI tract is not functioning adequately, as sometimes occurs in patients receiving ventilatory assistance or in patients with SIRS.

For patients with large burns (in whom obligate fluid requirements are high), most of the required calories and protein can be infused through a peripheral vein. Enteral feeding via a nasogastric or postpyloric tube can usually be initiated within 2 to 3 days after a burn. As emphasized elsewhere [see 33 Burn Care in the Early Postresuscitation Period], the sooner enteral nutrition can be instituted the better [see 97 Nutritional Support]. Ideally, it should begin on postburn day 1 or 2, with a small feeding tube placed through the duodenum.

Burn Wound Care

DIAGNOSIS AND TREATMENT OF BURN WOUND INFECTION

The primary indication for systemic antibiotics in the treatment of the burn wound is (1) evidence of increased bacterial content (i.e., > 10^5 organism/g tissue or histologic evidence of invasion) or (2) cellulitis or other evidence that the wound is increasing in depth or invading adjacent, noninfected tissue. In addition, systemic antibiotics are indicated in the perioperative period (24 to 48 hours) preceding and following debridement and skin grafting [see 33 Burn Care in the Early Postresuscitation Period]. The initial topical agent is usually silver sulfadiazine. Mafenide, povidone-iodine, gentamicin, and bacitracin are commonly used topical agents when the wound becomes infected or when bacterial overgrowth retards wound healing.

CHANGES IN THE BURN WOUND

By the second postburn week, the burn wound has changed considerably from its state during the first several days. Superficial burns are healing rapidly by this point. Deep second-degree burns are beginning to debride and are becoming much more uncomfortable and prone to infection. Full-thickness burns are now colonized and revascularized, and the eschar is beginning to separate. Deep burns, being now inflamed, hyperemic, and colonized (or infected) with bacteria, must be managed much more gently than in earlier phases. Any vigorous wound manipulation can lead to bacteremia and endotoxemia. Antibiotic-resistant organisms also become more common.

During the first 6 days after the burn, wound inflammation begins and the various components of healing are initiated [see 33 Burn Care in the Early Postresuscitation Period]. In superficial burns, epidermal regeneration is relatively rapid if the wound environment is optimized; this is achieved by providing sufficient amounts of oxygen, nutrients, and wound-healing factors (e.g., vitamin A and vitamin C), by keeping the wound surface from drying out, and by taking steps to prevent infection. The injured dermal elements are usually covered by new epithelium within 2 weeks. The hyperplasia of dermal fibroblasts then begins to resolve, and healing is complete with only modest amounts of collagen deposited. The wound usually becomes relatively pliable with time, and wound contraction is minimal. Superficial second-degree burns typically result in little or no long-term scarring.

The histology of the wound, however, changes dramatically if it has not been closed by 2 weeks after the burn, as would be the case with nongrafted deep dermal or full-thickness burns. Fibroblasts and macrophages become the predominant cells. Large numbers of myofibroblasts—modified fibroblasts that have some of the contractile properties of smooth muscle—also enter the wound. Microfilament bundles can be seen in their cytoplasm, lined parallel to each other and to the direction of contraction. Cells are linked together via extracellular extensions that allow transmission of the contractile forces. This results in a synchronized contractile process similar to that in smooth muscle. More than 75% of the cells in granulating wounds are myofibroblasts; in hypertrophic scars, the number of myofibroblasts present correlates with the rate of wound contraction. Besides leading to contraction, myofibroblasts continue to deposit large quantities of collagen and glycosaminoglycans.

Closure of the wound by reepithelialization or grafting does not eliminate the stimulus for ongoing scar formation. Angiogenesis continues, as does production of mucopolysaccharides and collagen. A marked increase in the proteoglycan content of chondroitin sulfate A can be seen as well. Chondroitin sulfate A, which is usually found in firm tissues such as cartilage, produces a harder, less pliable wound. As myofibroblasts contract, thereby shortening the scar, the deposition of the mucopolysaccharides and ground substances results in the fusion of the collagen fibers in the contracted site. The process of wound contraction leads to joint contractures.

Collagenase is also released by inflammatory cells. Synthesis of new collagen and lysis of old collagen are ongoing processes: any exaggeration of lysis or retardation of synthesis results in the dissolution of the new tissue.

CHANGES IN WOUND CARE

A marked pyrogen release resulting from manipulation of the wound causes a rise in body temperature, which accentuates the stress response and increases oxygen requirements. Use of antipyretics just before burn care begins attenuates the subsequent pyrogen response; the best agent for this purpose appears to be ibuprofen. Quantitative biopsies of the eschar are useful for diagnosing invasive infection and determining whether systemic antibiotics should be added or the topical antibiotic should be changed. Any pockets of suspected purulence below the eschar should be unroofed. Loose eschar should be removed from the wound to lower the bacterial content and to reduce surface exudation and inflammation, which can injure the new tissue being formed. Sharp dissection should not be continued into viable tissue beneath the eschar; if it is continued, substantial blood loss and bacteremia may result. Hypertrophic granulation tissue continues to be formed until the wound is surgically closed. Wound contraction reduces the surface area of the wound somewhat, but at the cost of mobility and function.

SURGICAL MANAGEMENT

As during the early postresuscitation period, surgical management of the burn wound is complicated by both anesthesia-related and wound-related problems.

Anesthesia

After the first postburn week, patients are highly hypermetabolic, and maintenance of anesthesia can be quite complex. The following are the essential components of anesthesia management in burn patients:

1. Airway maintenance and intubation.
2. Provision for increased ventilatory needs.
3. Choice of anesthetic agent.
4. Monitoring.
5. Maintenance of temperature and hemodynamic stability.

It is well known that the skeletal muscle neuromuscular receptors begin to be more sensitive to depolarizing muscle relaxants about 4 or 5 days after a burn injury and that this change results in the release of large amounts of K^+ and potentially fatal hyperkalemia during muscle fasciculations. Depolarizing agents are therefore contraindicated; a nondepolarizing agent is used when paralysis is indicated.

Adequate cardiopulmonary monitoring is extremely important in patients with major burns, who are potentially highly unstable. The relative lack of sites for invasive monitoring—and even for noninvasive monitoring—in these patients calls for considerable ingenuity on the part of the anesthesiologist. Some of the access problems can be avoided by using needle electrocardiographic electrodes, pulse oximetry, and end-tidal carbon dioxide concentrations (obtained from air expired from the ventilator). Advance knowledge of the patient's ventilatory and hemodynamic status and maintenance of preoperative values are essential.

Accurate assessment of blood loss depends on frequent communication between the surgeon and the anesthesiologist. Any blood lost should be replaced with blood products; crystalloid should be given to replace evaporative losses, not blood losses. Blood and blood products should be present in the room before management of a major case begins. The operating room must be warm (at least 80° F), and heating blankets, warm fluids, and similar adjuvants should be available. The operating time should be limited to two hours in patients who have large burns, especially if any significant cardiopulmonary instability is present.

Surgical Procedures

Surgical procedures done in burn patients during the inflammation period should be performed according to the same guidelines that are applicable in the first postburn week [see 33 Burn Care in the Early Postresuscitation Period]: the duration of the operation must be limited, blood loss must be minimized, and the grafted area must be carefully immobilized. The patient must be hemodynamically stable before the operation. Perioperative antibiotics are indicated. The choice of an agent is governed by the results of the preoperative wound culture: if no specific organism predominates, a first-generation cephalosporin is usually preferred because it provides reasonable coverage of Staphylococcus aureus and the more common gram-negative bacteria. S. aureus is the most common organism affecting the skin graft and the donor site.

The wound is colonized with bacteria during this period; thus, the potential for producing significant bacteremia also increases. Certainly, endotoxemia develops and inflammatory mediators are released; SIRS results postoperatively. Perioperative antibiotics help combat the bacteremia but do not block the absorption of endotoxins and pyrogens already present in the wound. If the wound infection cannot be controlled by nonoperative management, limited sequential excision can be lifesaving. The primary caution is to avoid large or long procedures that might have been easily tolerated in the first week but that are not as well tolerated during this period.

Wound Remodeling and Scar Formation

HYPERTROPHIC SCARRING

Pressure is the standard means of controlling hypertrophic scarring and accelerating the maturation process. When dressings are still required, pressure is provided by Ace wraps. Form-fitted pressure garments are used later. The pressure is expected to exceed surface vessel capillary pressure and should reach 25 mm Hg or higher. Pressure immediately reduces hyperemia and wound edema, which in turn prevents blister formation. Over a period of several weeks, a decrease in the chondroitin sulfate content becomes evident, as does a decline in mast cells and myofibroblasts. One theory is that by impeding blood flow to scars, pressure decreases fibroblast and inflammatory cell numbers by means of surface ischemia and thereby decreases overall excess collagen synthesis. In addition, because the water content is decreased, ground substance production is also decreased. The pressure must be continuous to be effective (i.e., about 23 hours every day for up to a year). Therapy with pressure garments is continued until the scar demonstrates complete maturation. Muscle activity and joint motion have been found to be significantly improved when this approach is employed.

It is during this period that permanent skin substitutes are used. There are two types that are commonly used clinically: (1) cultured autologous keratinocytes and (2) bilayer skin with generic dermis covered with the patient's own dermis.

Cultured keratinocytes are used as follows. In the first several days after the burn, the decision is made that cultured keratinocytes will be required to help cover a large burn surface. Full-thickness skin biopsies are then taken for cell preparation, the wound is excised and covered (preferably with cadaver skin), the cells are grown in tissue media for 3 weeks, the skin substitute is removed, the cultured cells are applied, and the area is immobilized. Graft take ranges from 20% to 80%; the best results are obtained with flat surfaces that can be immobilized.

Bilayer skin consists of a dermis, which is absorbed and replaced by the host, and an artificial epidermis in the form of a Silastic sheet, which is eventually replaced by the patient's own epidermis. Bilayer skin, despite its greater potential for providing a dermis and its superior flexibility, is at present less commonly used than cultured keratinocytes, primarily because it is still undergoing developmental changes.

There are a number of experimental skin substitutes in various stages of development. It is likely that before long, skin substitutes will be available that can replace both layers in a predictable fashion.

SKIN LUBRICATION

Because the burn patient's sebaceous glands have been impaired or destroyed, natural skin lubrication is absent; drying, pain, and markedly impaired pliability result. Skin moisturizers will be necessary for months to years to maintain optimal skin function.

Recommended Reading

Alexander W: The role of infections in the burn patient. The Art and Science of Burn Care. Boswick J, Ed. Aspen Publishers, Rockville, Maryland, 1982, p 103

Beeker W: Fungal burn wound infection, a 10 year experience. Arch Surg 126:44, 1991

Bingham H, Gallagher T, Powell R: Early bronchoscopy as a predictor of ventilatory support for burned patients. J Trauma 27:1286, 1987

Bone R, Balk R, Cerra F, et al: Definitions for sepsis and organ failure and guidelines for the use of innovative therapies in sepsis. Chest 101:1644, 1992

Boukoms A: Pain relief in the intensive care unit. J Intens Care Med 3:32, 1988

DeBandt S, Chollet M, Lowry S, et al: Cytokine response to burn injury: relationship with protein metabolism. J Trauma 36:624, 1994

DeBiasse M, Wilmore D: What is optimum nutritional support? New Horizons. Zalaga G, Ed. Society for Critical Care Medicine, Fullerton, California, 1994, p 122

Deitch E: Intestinal permeability is increased in burn patients shortly after injury. Surgery 167:411, 1990

Demling R: Effect of early burn excision and grafting on pulmonary function. J Trauma 24:830, 1984

Demling R: Fluid replacement in burned patients. Surg Clin North Am 67:15, 1987

Demling R, Orgill D: Current concepts and approaches to wound healing. Crit Care Med 16:899, 1988

Demling R, Pomposelli J: Burn wound infection. Surgical Infections: Diagnosis and Treatment. Meakins JL, Ed. Scientific American, Inc, New York, 1994, p 369

Dobke M, Deitch E, Baxter C: Oxidant activity of polymorphonuclear leukocytes after thermal injury. Arch Surg 124:856, 1989

Dong Y, Abdullah K, Yan T, et al: Effect of thermal injury and sepsis on neutrophil function. J Trauma 34:417, 1993

Fong Y, Moldawer L, Shires T, et al: The biologic characteristics of cytokines and their implications in surgical injury. Surg Gynecol Obstet 170:363, 1990

Gatzen C, Scheltinga M, Kimbrough T, et al: Growth hormone attenuates the abnormal distribution of body water in critically ill surgical patients. Surgery 112:181, 1992

Goodwin C, Wilmore D: Surgery and burns. Clinical Nutrition. Paige D, Ed. CV Mosby Co, St Louis, 1988, p 372

Gore D, Honeycutt D, Jahoor F, et al: Effect of exogenous growth hormone on whole body and isolated limb protein kinetics in burned patients. Arch Surg 126:38, 1990

Gottleich M, Warden G: Vitamin supplementation in the patient with burns. J Burn Care Rehabil 11:375, 1990

Hirsch C, Kaemerek R, Stanek K: Work of breathing during CPAP and PSV imposed by the new generation mechanical ventilators. Respir Care 36:815, 1991

Jahoor F, Shangraw RE, Miyoshi H, et al: Role of insulin and glucose oxidation in mediating the protein catabolism of burns and sepsis. Am J Physiol 257:E323, 1989

Jeevandra M, Ramias L, Shamos R, et al: Decreased growth hormone levels in the catabolic phase of severe injury. Surgery 111:495, 1992

Law E, Blecher K, Still J: Enterococcal infections as a cause of mortality and morbidity in patients with burns. J Burn Care Rehabil 15:236, 1994

Machin L, Bendich A: Free radical tissue damage: protective role of antioxidant nutrients. FASEB J 1:441, 1990

Moore E, Jones T: Benefits of immediate jejunostomy feeding after major abdominal trauma: a prospective randomized study. J Trauma 26:874, 1986

Moore F, Haenel J, Moore E, et al: Incommensurate oxygen consumption in response to maximal oxygen availability products post injury multiple organ failure. J Trauma 33:58, 1992

Munster A: Cultured epidermal autograft in the management of burn patients. J Burn Care Rehabil 13:121, 1992

Paxton J, Williamson J: Nutrient substrate: making choices in the 1990s. J Burn Care Rehabil 12:198, 1991

Pinsky M, Matuschak G: A unifying hypothesis of multiple system organ failure: failure of host defense homeostasis. J Crit Care 5:108, 1990

Pruitt B: Infection and the burn patient. Br J Surg 77:1081, 1990

Rodriguez J, Miller C, Till G, et al: Correlation of the local and systemic cytokine response with clinical outcome following thermal injury. J Trauma 34:684, 1993

Servent R, Hansbrough J: Cytotoxicity to human leukocytes by topical antimicrobial agents used for burn care. J Burn Care Rehabil 14:132, 1993

Taddonio T, Thomson P: A survey of wound monitoring and topical antimicrobial therapy practices in the treatment of burn injury. J Burn Care Rehabil 11:423, 1990

Tobin M: Respiratory monitoring. JAMA 264:244, 1990

Wallace B, Caldwell F, Cone J: Ibuprofen lowers body temperature and metabolic rate of humans with burn injury. J Trauma 32:159, 1992

Ward P, Warren J, Johnson K: Oxygen radical inflammation and tissue injury. Free Rad Biol Med 5:403, 1988

Waymack JP, Herndon DN: Nutritional support of the burned patient. World J Surg 16:80, 1992

Wilmore D: Metabolic changes after thermal injury. The Art and Science of Burn Care. Boswick J, Ed. Aspen Publishers, Rockville, Maryland, 1987, p 137

Winchurch R, Thupari J, Munster A: Endotoxemia in burn patients, levels of circulating endotoxins are related to burn size. Surgery 102:808, 1987

Woolf P: Hormonal responses to trauma. Crit Care Med 20:216, 1992

Xia Z, Coolbaugh M, He F, et al: The effects of burn injury on the acute phase response. J Trauma 32:245, 1992

Youn Y, Demling R: The role of mediators in the response to thermal injury. World J Surg 16:30, 1992

Acknowledgments

Figures 1 through 3   Talar Agasyan.

Table 1   Adapted from *Metabolic Management of the Critically Ill*, by D. W. Wilmore. Plenum Publishing Corporation, New York, 1977, p 22.

35 MISCELLANEOUS THERMAL INJURIES

Robert H. Demling, M.D.

Management of Miscellaneous Thermal Injuries

Electrical Injury

Electrical burn injuries account for fewer than 5% of admissions to major burn centers. Compared with skin burns, however, these injuries are much more complex and are associated with higher morbidity and mortality. The mortality is reported to be between 3% and 15%, with about 1,000 deaths a year in the United States attributed to electrical current. More than 90% of injuries occur in males, most of whom are between 20 and 34 years of age. Electrical injuries can be grouped into three categories: high voltage, involving contact with more than 1,000 volts; low voltage, caused by contact with less than 1,000 volts; and those caused by lightning.

HIGH-VOLTAGE INJURY

Diagnosis

The heat generated by arcing (jumping) of a high-voltage current from a high-tension wire toward a human being reaches several thousand degrees and produces a flash skin burn comparable to that caused by any explosion of a volatile substance. The intense heat frequently causes clothes to catch fire, resulting in deep burns of the skin. In the presence of a large skin burn, health care providers may overlook severe injury from an electrical burn. The subsequent soft tissue edema and pain can easily be misinterpreted as the result of thermal injury rather than concomitant damage from the passage of current. Careful history-taking and physical examination are critical to avoiding this error. This type of thermal burn is managed in essentially the same way as any other burn would be [see Figure 1], except that a higher urine output will be necessary if myoglobinuria is present [see Fluid Management, *below*].

Physical evidence of an entrance site [see Figure 2] and of an exit site [see Figures 3 and 4] is pathognomonic of the passage of a significant amount of electrical current through the body. Because the depth of injury and the degree of tissue damage cannot be determined by superficial assessment, victims of electrical injuries must be hospitalized for observation. A history of the event is critical in estimating the extent of injury.

Muscle necrosis Electrical burns more closely resemble crush injuries than thermal burns. Damage below the skin, where the current passes, is usually far greater than the appearance of the overlying skin would indicate [see Table 1]. The immediate damage is caused by heat destruction of cells, which is usually patchy in distribution along the course of the current. Other effects are devascularization, caused by injured blood vessels; tissue infection; and compartment syndrome, with pressure necrosis especially prominent in nerve tissue and muscle enveloped by nonyielding fascia.

Early necrosis does not follow the anatomic division of muscles but is uneven, reflecting the passage of current through the body. In the first few hours after injury, it is difficult to distinguish between normal muscle and muscle that is irreparably damaged but not immediately coagulated. Progressive necrosis is usually evident over the next 4 to 5 days. It is common to find dead muscle in the presence of excellent local blood supply, indicating that the muscle damage is not totally vascular in origin and that the temperature required to kill muscle cells is less than that required to coagulate blood vessels.

Damage to muscle tissues is evident within minutes to hours of injury, when the still perfused muscles begin to swell. The finite boundaries of the fascial envelope cause a rapid increase in tissue pressure; when the microvascular hydrostatic pressure exceeds 25 mm Hg, there is additional ischemia and compression nerve injury in local tissues. Tissue pressure exceeding 30 mm Hg is clearly abnormal and must be decreased to avoid further damage. Edema increases over the next 24 to 48 hours.

Because of current-induced damage to vessels, vascular thrombosis can occur immediately and over the following 3 to 4 days. The progressive devascularization causes additional loss of muscle tissue. The combination of endothelial cell damage and weakening of vessel walls can lead to local thrombosis and tissue hemorrhage. These processes, the uneven nature of the necrosis, and, in particular, the damage to muscles and nerves closest to bone seriously impair function, resulting in a high rate of amputation (30% to 40%). Muscle atrophy and replacement of injured muscle by fibrous tissue cause subsequent dysfunction.

Monitoring

Cardiopulmonary monitoring and supportive care are clearly necessary, given the high incidence of cardiac arrhythmias and pulmonary dysfunction in patients with electrical injuries [see Table 2]. Urinalysis is essential to verify that renal perfusion is adequate and to screen for myoglobinuria, which calls for special management. Measurement of blood gases and the acid-base balance are important for assessment of lung function and peripheral perfusion. Acidosis must be corrected to prevent excess myoglobin in the renal tubules.

Monitoring of peripheral perfusion and palpation of muscle compartments are important for assessment of compartment syndromes caused by muscle edema. Compartment pressure can be monitored by one of the available systems. Indications for fas-

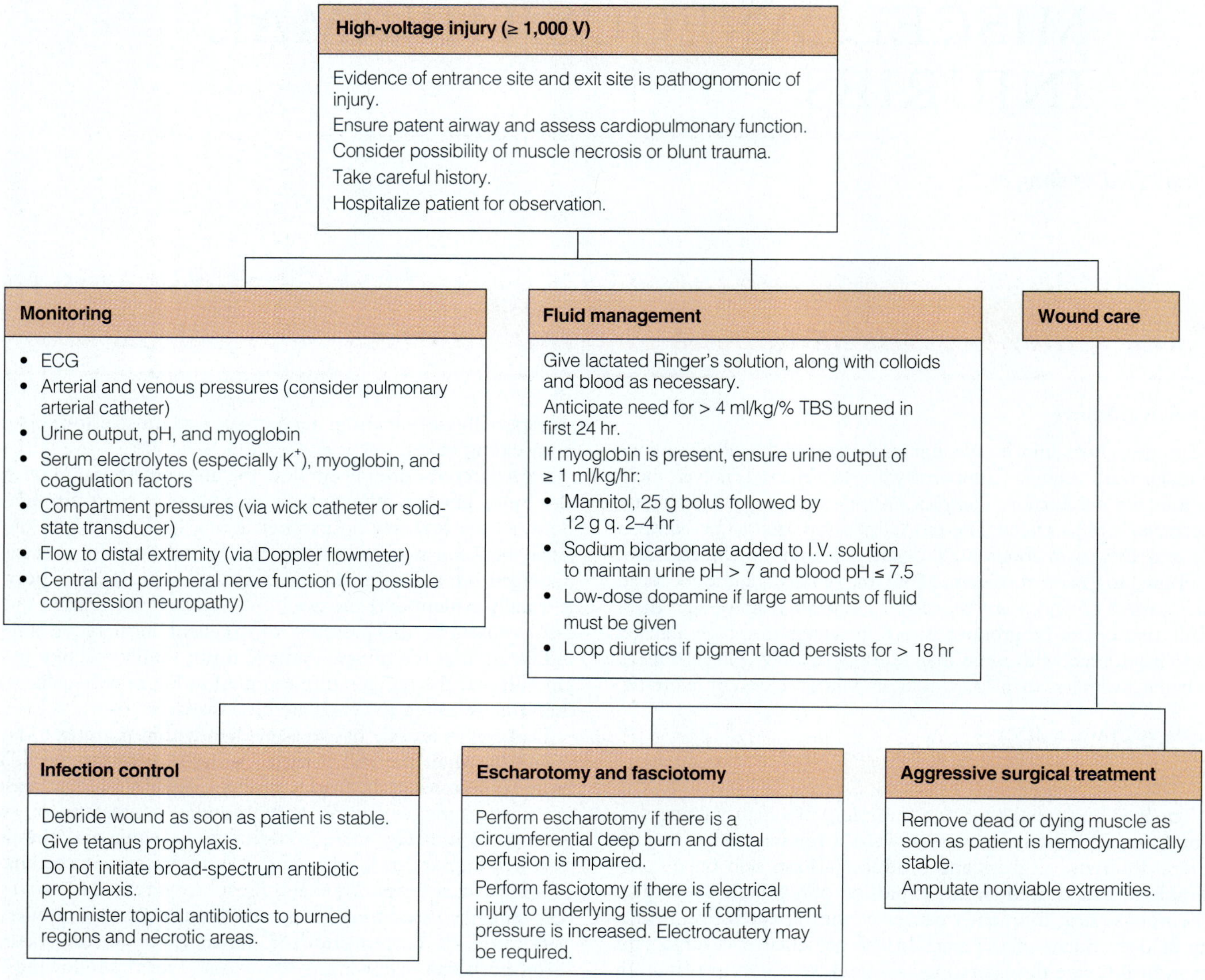

Figure 1 — Algorithm for treatment of high-voltage electrical injury

High-voltage injury (≥ 1,000 V)
- Evidence of entrance site and exit site is pathognomonic of injury.
- Ensure patent airway and assess cardiopulmonary function.
- Consider possibility of muscle necrosis or blunt trauma.
- Take careful history.
- Hospitalize patient for observation.

Monitoring
- ECG
- Arterial and venous pressures (consider pulmonary arterial catheter)
- Urine output, pH, and myoglobin
- Serum electrolytes (especially K^+), myoglobin, and coagulation factors
- Compartment pressures (via wick catheter or solid-state transducer)
- Flow to distal extremity (via Doppler flowmeter)
- Central and peripheral nerve function (for possible compression neuropathy)

Fluid management
- Give lactated Ringer's solution, along with colloids and blood as necessary.
- Anticipate need for > 4 ml/kg/% TBS burned in first 24 hr.
- If myoglobin is present, ensure urine output of ≥ 1 ml/kg/hr:
  - Mannitol, 25 g bolus followed by 12 g q. 2–4 hr
  - Sodium bicarbonate added to I.V. solution to maintain urine pH > 7 and blood pH ≤ 7.5
  - Low-dose dopamine if large amounts of fluid must be given
  - Loop diuretics if pigment load persists for > 18 hr

Wound care

Infection control
- Debride wound as soon as patient is stable.
- Give tetanus prophylaxis.
- Do not initiate broad-spectrum antibiotic prophylaxis.
- Administer topical antibiotics to burned regions and necrotic areas.

Escharotomy and fasciotomy
- Perform escharotomy if there is a circumferential deep burn and distal perfusion is impaired.
- Perform fasciotomy if there is electrical injury to underlying tissue or if compartment pressure is increased. Electrocautery may be required.

Aggressive surgical treatment
- Remove dead or dying muscle as soon as patient is hemodynamically stable.
- Amputate nonviable extremities.

Figure 1 Shown is an algorithm for treatment of high-voltage electrical injury.

---

ciotomy and escharotomy are tissue pressure greater than 40 mm Hg and tissue pressure within 30 mm Hg of diastolic pressure.

The signs of increased compartment pressure include decreased peripheral pulse rate, evidence of nerve compression, paresthesias, decreased sensation or increased pain, and increased muscle turgor. Excessive tissue turgor is the most useful sign of underlying muscle damage and the need for fasciotomy. Motor nerve dysfunction is more difficult to assess because it may be impossible to distinguish nerve damage from muscle damage.

Fluid Management

The principles of fluid management that apply to thermal burns also apply to electrical burns. The primary resuscitation fluid is lactated Ringer's solution (or hypertonic lactated saline), but the unpredictable nature of the tissue damage precludes the use of a standard formula. In general, for a given percentage of total body surface burned, the fluid requirements in patients with electrical burns are 1.5 to 2 times the requirements in patients with skin burns alone, reflecting additional soft tissue injury associated with electrical burns.

The rate of fluid administration is the amount necessary to maintain adequate systemic perfusion. The presence of myoglobin in the urine, other evidence of early renal impairment, or high levels of creatine kinase in plasma indicate the need for adjustments in fluid administration. If the urine is red or reddish black (evidence of massive myoglobin release from muscle), a urine flow of

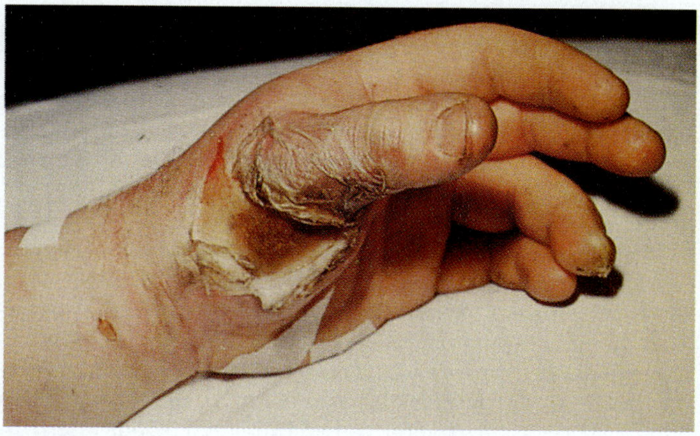

Figure 2 Typical entrance site of high voltage shows desiccation of tissue.

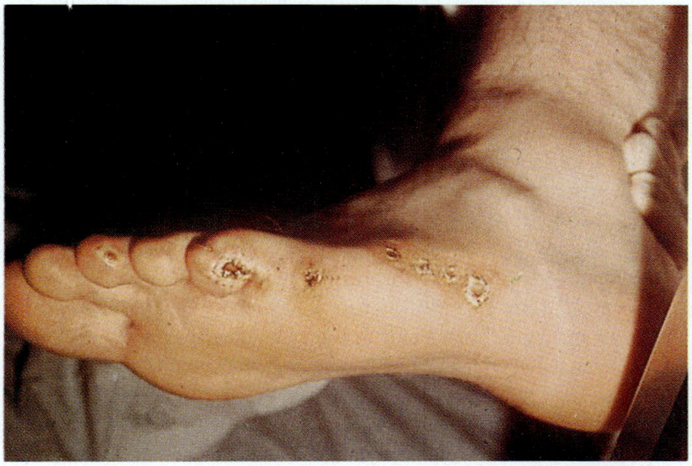

Figure 3 Current often exits the body from the foot, through small, round, punctate areas.

at least 1 ml/kg/hr is needed until the pigment load decreases.

The appropriate treatment regimen is as follows:

1. Mannitol (25 g bolus, followed by 12.5 g every 2 to 4 hours) in addition to fluids until the pigment clears from the urine.
2. Sodium bicarbonate, added to the intravenous solution, to maintain urine pH above 7 without raising blood pH above 7.5.
3. Low-dose dopamine, if excessive amounts of fluid are required to increase renal blood flow and subsequent urine output.
4. Loop diuretics, added to fluid infusion, if the pigment load persists longer than 8 hours.

Infection Control

Infection in areas of tissue necrosis and ischemia begins several days after injury, particularly if a skin burn potentiates cross-contamination from wound to wound. Infection is generally controlled by early wound debridement. Tetanus prophylaxis is required because of the risks of deep tissue necrosis in a relatively anaerobic environment. Prophylactic use of broad-spectrum antibiotics is not indicated, but perioperative antibiotic therapy is, as in the management of thermal burns.

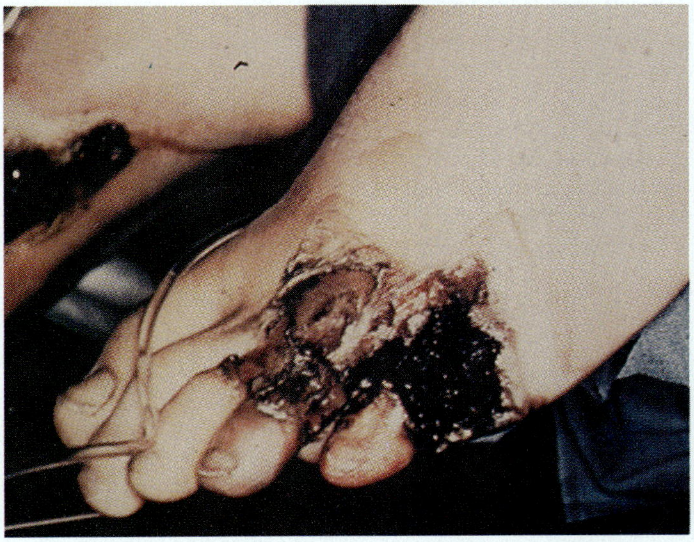

Figure 4 Severe damage was caused at this ground point, where current left the body.

Table 1 Common Complications of Electrical Burns

Ventricular fibrillation and other rhythm abnormalities	Muscle necrosis
Respiratory arrest	Fractures
Seizures	Hemolysis
Coma	Renal failure
Mental changes	Hemorrhage
Hypertension	Limb loss
Retinal detachment	Anemia
Cataract (delayed)	Paresis, complete paralysis, and other neurologic disorders (delayed)

Escharotomy and Fasciotomy

In general, an escharotomy is necessary if there is a circumferential deep burn and any evidence of impaired distal perfusion. Fasciotomy is indicated if there is concomitant electrical injury to underlying tissue and increasing compartment pressure, evident in increased myoglobin levels, rigid muscle compartments, or nerve or vessel compression.

Wound Management

In general, if there are large amounts of necrotic muscle in burns caused by high-voltage contact, treatment must be aggressive, with surgical debridement. These measures minimize subsequent organ dysfunction, infection, and eventual mortality and maximize the salvage of marginal tissue, which is highly susceptible to infection. If gross myoglobinuria is present for several hours, if exit sites are large, if there is mummification of a large entrance wound, or if muscle feels woody, hard, and nonfunctional, a large amount of dead muscle is a virtual certainty.

Early excision of dead muscle is performed as soon as the patient is hemodynamically stable, preferably 1 to 2 days after the injury. The risks of renal failure increase the longer that large amounts of dead and dying muscle remain in the wounds. Muscle of indeterminate viability should be spared, but guillotine amputation should be used on obviously nonsalvageable limbs—a measure that can be lifesaving. After surgery, the wounds should be covered with biologic dressings or moist, dilute antibiotic solutions.

The goal of subsequent surgical procedures is to conserve viable tissue while removing neighboring dead tissue. The uneven nature of injuries makes this approach difficult and time consuming. Small scattered areas of injured muscle will be reabsorbed and replaced by fibrous tissue. A high fever and tachycardia, however, may be physiologic evidence that infected dead tissue remains. The tissue along the bone is often the site of greatest muscle necrosis.

One approach that has shown excellent potential for minimizing long-term disability is early aggressive debridement, followed immediately by reconstruction with rotation flaps and free flaps, if needed, to cover remaining viable tissue, nerves, vessels, and bone.

Managing Entrance and Exit Sites

Entrance and exit sites of electrical current are thermal burns (that is, they are the result of heat generation), but they are more complex than standard skin burns. Heat generated at the skin surface depends on the local resistance to flow. A dry hand in contact with high voltage may generate heat in excess of 1,000° C, leading to mummification at the entrance site. The result is a well-defined charred wound at the site of contact. The skin surface is depressed,

Table 2 Monitoring Patients with Electrical Burns

Evaluation of Systemic Changes	Evaluation of Local Changes
Vital signs Urine output, pH, and myoglobin Serial hematocrits Serum electrolytes (especially K$^+$), myoglobin, and clotting factors	Frequent Doppler ultrasound measurement of blood flow in injured extremity Frequent assessment for nerve compression Frequent palpation of muscle compartments
Consider Arterial line Central line Pulmonary arterial catheter (to monitor perfusion in injured CNS, myocardium, and kidneys) Electrocardiography (to monitor arrhythmias)	*Consider* Measurement of compartment pressures

demonstrating the effect of high temperature on the water content of the tissue. Some entrance wounds may resemble deep flame burns, but in such a case, the injury extends well below the dermis.

If there is moderate exposure to current, the appearance at the exit site is similar to small skin ulcerations, with depressed centers and elevated edges. With passage of a large current, multiple exit sites may be seen along the route of the current, suggesting the effects of an explosion. Pieces of cutaneous tissue may be blown out by the immense energy of the exiting current.

In accordance with the principles used for thermal burns, devitalized tissue below the skin at the entrance and exit sites should be debrided. After 3 to 5 days, residual necrotic tissue should be debrided, and the wounds should be closed with skin grafts or flaps. Tissue defects may necessitate soft tissue coverage by a soft tissue flap. Coverage of large wounds with skin grafts may have to be postponed until the patient's condition is more stable.

Other Effects of High-Voltage Injury

Cardiovascular injury Immediate cardiac arrest is the most common cause of death resulting from electrical injury. The current alters rhythm, leading to fibrillation, or depresses respiration, leading to hypoxia. The immediate mortality associated with passage of a high-voltage current from one hand to the other is 60%. The cardiac arrhythmia is often reversible, however, and cardiac resuscitation should be initiated at the scene of the accident. The most common electrocardiographic changes, other than fibrillation, are sinus tachycardia and nonspecific ST-T wave changes.

Major vessel thrombosis occurs, as does delayed rupture of large vessels, with massive hemorrhage; rupture of these vessels in the absence of surrounding tissue damage indicates low resistance to flow within the vessels. Although rare, aneurysms can occur weeks to months after injury; good follow-up measures should be instituted in the light of this possibility.

Renal injury Renal failure is reported in at least 10% of victims of high-voltage electrical burns. Myoglobin and hemoglobin from damaged muscle and red blood cells can precipitate in the renal tubules, producing acute tubular necrosis. The combination of myoglobin, which is colorless in circulating plasma, and hemoglobin produces pink to red urine. Myoglobin precipitation is accentuated by acid urine and decreased by alkaline urine. Muscle necrosis, which can result in distant organ dysfunction, may affect the kidneys; the low-flow state caused by hypovolemia will aggravate the tissue injury. Another cause of renal vascular damage is direct attack by high-voltage current.

Pulmonary injury The pulmonary abnormalities are the result of CNS-induced hypoventilation and chest wall dysfunction. Impaired respiratory center activity and severe CNS damage lead to hypoventilation, often the cause of immediate death.

Neurologic injury Both immediate and delayed neurologic abnormalities are common. Acute CNS dysfunction—with coma, seizures, motor deficits, and, to a lesser extent, sensory deficits—has been well described. Many of these abnormalities are permanent. Delayed injuries include both peripheral neuropathies and cord damage with paralysis. The mechanisms believed to be responsible for the delayed injuries are delayed vascular thrombosis, leading to ischemia, and progressive demyelination following passage of electrical current through the body.

Orthopedic injury Contact with high-tension current causes severe muscle spasm, which can produce long bone fractures and dislocation at major joints. The next most common orthopedic injury in patients who have been in contact with high-tension sources is heat necrosis of local periosteum, with subsequent production of nonviable bone and sequestration formation. Less common is devascularization of bone, caused by the vascular injury affecting other tissues.

Ocular and otic injury Again, both immediate and delayed injuries are noted. Early changes include conjunctival and corneal burns as well as ruptured eardrums. Late changes, occurring up to 1 year after the injury, include cataract formation, tinnitus, and decreased hearing.

LOW-VOLTAGE INJURY

The most common result of low-voltage injury is a cardiac arrhythmia, especially ventricular fibrillation. This cardiac abnormality can be life threatening because only a small proportion of the population has been trained in cardiopulmonary resuscitation. A less common effect of low-voltage injury is suffocation caused by tetany of chest wall muscles. This effect is less common because it takes several minutes to occur, and assistance is often available to move the patient away from the source of injury. Central nervous system abnormalities, if any, are usually the result of hypoxia caused by cardiopulmonary arrest. Because of the possibility of myocardial injury, it is good practice to hospitalize patients for 24 hours and to observe them with cardiac monitors. Fractures may occur as a result of tetany and muscle spasm from alternating current (AC). Treatment is based on the standard approach to the most common injuries, cardiopulmonary arrest and tetany-induced fractures [*see Figure 5*].

Oral Burns

Low-voltage electricity is the leading cause of electrical injury in children, especially those 1 to 2 years of age [*see Figure 6*]. Sucking an extension cord is responsible for more than half of the injuries, and biting an electrical cord accounts for about 30%. The most common mechanism is the production of an electrical arc by the bared wires, conducted by the child's saliva. Intense local heat is generated, destroying tissues in the mouth. The burn may involve the lip, tongue, or oral mucosa and underlying bone, but the most frequent site is the lip, particularly the commissure area between the upper and lower lips [*see Table 3*]. The burn is typically grayish

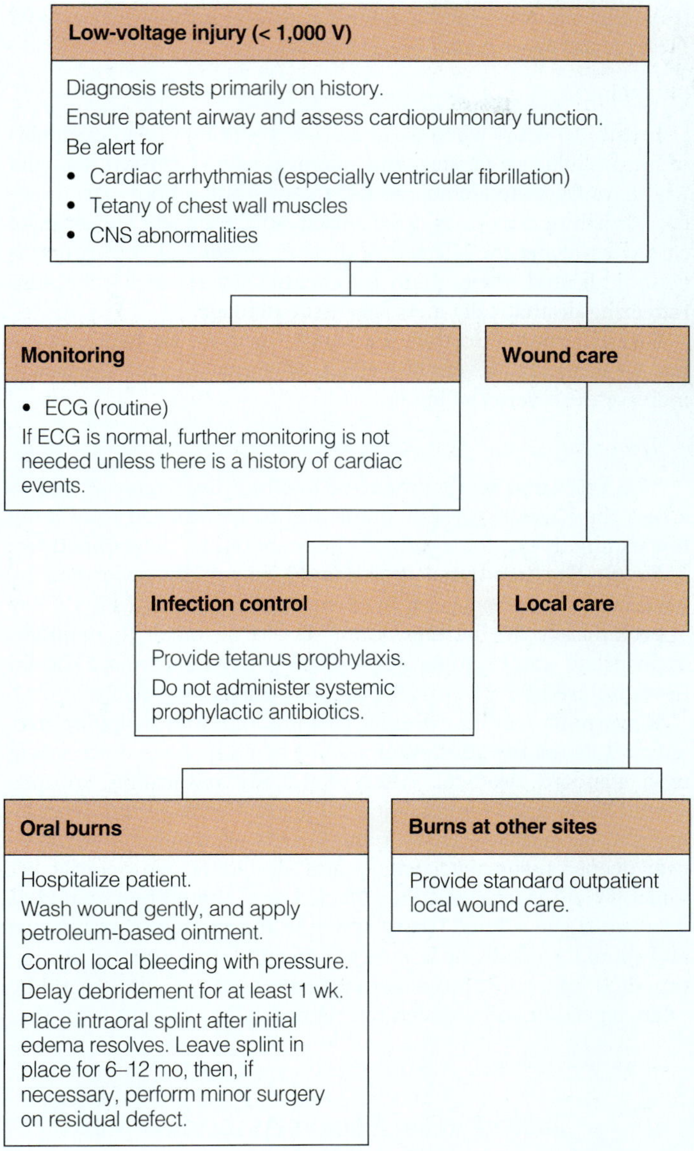

Low-voltage injury (< 1,000 V)

Diagnosis rests primarily on history.
Ensure patent airway and assess cardiopulmonary function.
Be alert for
- Cardiac arrhythmias (especially ventricular fibrillation)
- Tetany of chest wall muscles
- CNS abnormalities

Monitoring
- ECG (routine)
If ECG is normal, further monitoring is not needed unless there is a history of cardiac events.

Wound care

Infection control
Provide tetanus prophylaxis.
Do not administer systemic prophylactic antibiotics.

Local care

Oral burns
Hospitalize patient.
Wash wound gently, and apply petroleum-based ointment.
Control local bleeding with pressure.
Delay debridement for at least 1 wk.
Place intraoral splint after initial edema resolves. Leave splint in place for 6–12 mo, then, if necessary, perform minor surgery on residual defect.

Burns at other sites
Provide standard outpatient local wound care.

Figure 5 Shown is an algorithm for treatment of low-voltage electrical injury.

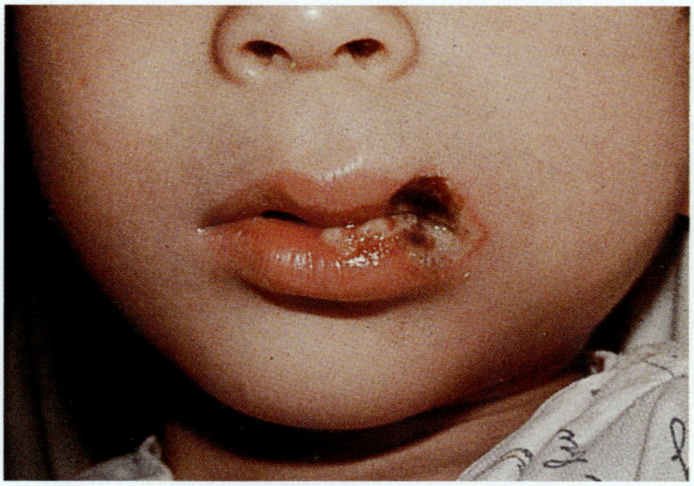

Figure 6 Typical oral burn, caused by biting an electrical cord, shows tissue necrosis at the corner of the mouth.

white and indented at the center because of tissue necrosis. Severe swelling develops as venous thrombosis impedes blood return.

The edema of the lips may be intense, impairing control of saliva. The orbicularis oris muscle is often involved, further impairing control. Edema subsides over the next 5 to 10 days, and local necrotic tissue begins to slough. Bleeding from the labial artery, which occurs in 20% of patients during the period of slough (7 to 21 days), should be anticipated. Granulation tissue then develops, followed by collagen deposition and wound remodeling. Local adhesions and microstomia may develop over a period of 3 to 5 months. Injury to the underlying bone results in dental abnormalities over time.

Hospitalization is recommended to treat the local burn and examine the patient for related injuries. Tetanus prophylaxis is necessary, but systemic antibiotics do not appear to be beneficial. Local wound care consists of gentle washing followed three to four times daily by application of a petroleum-based antibiotic ointment. Feeding by tube, syringe, or a straw is helpful to avoid additional local pressure. Occasionally, vessel ligation is required.

Because the extent of injury cannot be determined for several days, surgical debridement is delayed for at least a week. The present treatment of choice is the placement of a prosthetic intraoral splint after the initial edema resolves, generally 5 to 10 days after the injury. Use of a splint reduces the scarring effect of adhesion formation, thus decreasing the need for cosmetic surgery.

LIGHTNING

Properties and Effects

Lightning is the result of an atmospheric electrical discharge occurring between a positive charge in an upper cloud level and a negative charge at a lower cloud level. A lightning flash occurs when the potential difference between the layers exceeds the insulating properties of air. Air crossed by the lightning is rapidly heated and expands to develop a shock wave, which decays to a sound wave perceived as thunder. The power of a lightning bolt is estimated at 10,000 to 20,000 amperes of current with more than 20 million volts of electromotive force. The four mechanisms of injury are direct strike, flash discharge, ground current, and shock wave.

A direct strike results when a person who is outdoors acts as the grounding site. Mortality is high, with head entry being common. A flash discharge, more common than a direct strike, occurs when the lightning changes direction to hit another object. Injury is still severe, but not as great as in a direct strike.

Ground currents can develop from a strike on the ground. A person standing may generate a sufficient potential difference between legs and ground for current to develop. Overall mortality from lightning injury is about 30%, and approximately two thirds of survivors experience permanent sequelae of the accident.

Table 3 Classification of Electrical Burn of the Lip

Severity	Description
Minor	Injury to less than one third of upper or lower lip, sparing commissure
Moderate	Injury to more than one third of lip, sparing commissure, or injury to commissure alone
Severe	Loss of skin and muscle of more than one third of lip, including commissure

In the phenomenon of flashover, lightning travels along the outside of the conductor—namely, the victim. The current vaporizes skin moisture and destroys clothing but spares the body tissues. The shock wave produced by the heating and expansion of air produces tissue damage comparable to the effects of any large explosion. This form of tissue trauma is often overlooked.

Diagnosis

If the victim is unconscious, if no one witnessed the lightning injury, and if there is no evidence of fire or flames, diagnosis is difficult. Treatment, however, must be based on recognition that the patient was struck by lightning. Understanding of the magnitude of energy involved in the injury minimizes the risk that serious tissue damage, both immediate and delayed, will be overlooked. The general principles of treatment are the same as those for high-voltage electrical burns.

Specific Problems

Cardiovascular injury The direct current of lightning produces myocardial depolarization and arrest. Treatment is supportive.

Central nervous system injury Damage to the CNS is caused by electrical current or by mechanical trauma. At least three fourths of patients with a lightning injury have at least a transient loss of consciousness. More than two thirds experience temporary paralysis of the upper or lower extremities, which resolves over hours to days. Permanent sequelae are common, especially those resulting from anoxia following cardiorespiratory arrest. Treatment is supportive.

Skin injury Injuries to the skin vary from the burns seen after contact with a high-voltage current to a superficial skin abnormality sometimes referred to as feathering or lightning prints. The latter process is characterized by linear fernlike erythematous skin markings that do not blanch. The markings, probably caused by the flashover phenomenon as static electricity is transmitted along the superficial vasculature, fade in several days. Recognition of this skin change in a comatose person can help make the diagnosis of a lightning injury. Treatment of localized deep burns is the same as that of other electrical burns.

Musculoskeletal injury A typical high-tension injury with muscle necrosis is accompanied by compartment syndrome, myoglobinuria, and renal failure. Treatment is the same as that outlined for high-voltage injury.

Ocular and otic injury Lightning may also injure the eyes or the ears. Cataracts are the most common intraocular injury caused by lightning. One type of cataract is traumatic, resulting from the initial concussion; the onset of the second type, which is caused by the current itself, is delayed for several months. Lid lesions from a burn and conjunctivitis are also common. Treatment depends on the injuries produced.

More than 50% of persons struck by lightning have ear injuries, caused by both the concussion (ruptured tympanic membrane) and the current (direct nerve damage). Treatment depends on the specific injuries produced.

Cold Injury

There are three common types of cold injury: tissue-freezing injury (e.g., frostbite), nonfreezing injury (e.g., trench foot and chilblain, or pernio), and hypothermia. Hypothermia is commonly a major complicating factor of cold injury to tissues and is usually the most life-threatening aspect of the injury [*see 98 Fever, Hyperpyrexia, and Hypothermia*].

FROSTBITE

Frostbite occurs when tissue freezes, resulting in the formation of intracellular ice crystals and microvascular occlusion. Patients who have frostbite are able to use the frostbitten body part; however, frostbitten tissue is desensitized, so the patient should take care when using the affected body part. In general, rewarming is contraindicated when there is potential for refreezing because refreezing dramatically increases tissue damage.

Risk factors for frostbite are similar to those for hypothermia [*see Table 4*]. However, the effect of windchill can drastically increase the severity of injury.

Treatment

The first steps in treatment of frostbite [*see Figure 7*] are to assess the patient's overall status and to commence total body rewarming. Next, the depth of injury should be determined [*see Table 5*]. The frostbitten area should be rapidly rewarmed by placing the affected part in a warm-water bath (42° C) for approximately 30 minutes. Care should be taken to maintain appropriate water temperature. A direct dry-heat source should never be used for rewarming, because burns may occur.

Rewarming can be extremely painful, often necessitating narcotics. Tetanus toxoid booster should be administered according to a standard protocol. After total body rewarming, wounds should be assessed for possible cleaning and conservative debridement. Clear blisters may be removed. Hemorrhagic blisters indicate deeper tissue involvement and should be temporarily left intact if fluid is infected. The affected area should be elevated to decrease tissue edema. Use of systemic antibiotics is controversial and should generally be limited to patients with suspected or documented infections. Surgical management of frostbite should be of an expectant and conservative nature, quite different from that

---

Table 4 **Risk Factors Associated with Frostbite Injury**

Flow-related
  Peripheral vascular disease
  Cardiac disease

CNS and mental status
  Dementia; history of psychiatric illness
  Injury to brain or spinal cord

Medications
  Same as with hypothermia—ergot alkaloids, theophylline derivatives (e.g., aminophylline and caffeine), and Fiorinal
  Vasoconstrictors

Age
  Elderly
  Very young

Race
  African Americans at greater risk than whites

Other
  Ethanol ingestion
  Previous cold exposure
  Tobacco use
  Malnutrition

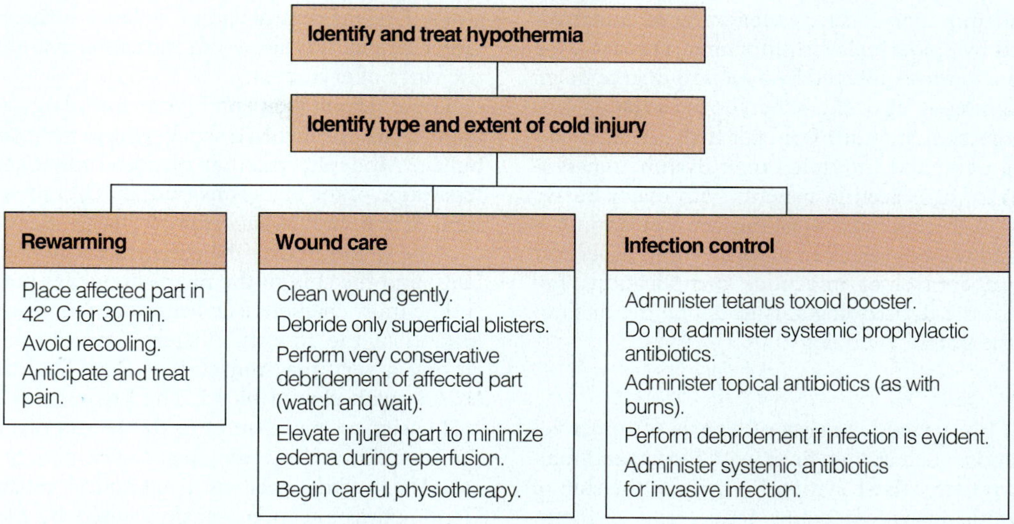

```
┌─────────────────────────────────┐
│ Identify and treat hypothermia  │
└────────────────┬────────────────┘
                 │
┌────────────────┴────────────────┐
│ Identify type and extent of cold injury │
└────────────────┬────────────────┘
```

Rewarming
- Place affected part in 42° C for 30 min.
- Avoid recooling.
- Anticipate and treat pain.

Wound care
- Clean wound gently.
- Debride only superficial blisters.
- Perform very conservative debridement of affected part (watch and wait).
- Elevate injured part to minimize edema during reperfusion.
- Begin careful physiotherapy.

Infection control
- Administer tetanus toxoid booster.
- Do not administer systemic prophylactic antibiotics.
- Administer topical antibiotics (as with burns).
- Perform debridement if infection is evident.
- Administer systemic antibiotics for invasive infection.

Figure 7 Shown is an algorithm for treatment of cold injury.

of a heat burn. Escharotomy is obviously warranted if vascular compromise occurs. Early debridement or amputation may be necessary if the affected tissue is causing an uncontrollable septic response or disseminated intravascular coagulation. Otherwise, surgical intervention consists of conservative debridement and reconstruction, beginning several weeks after injury. This period allows for adequate tissue demarcation and minimizes any viable tissue loss from an aggressive early debridement.

Concomitant fractures or dislocations should be treated when the patient arrives at the emergency room. As with any trauma patient, open fractures warrant immediate intraoperative management.

Adjuvant Therapy

Many forms of adjuvant therapy have been explored. Thromboxane synthetase inhibitors and ibuprofen, a cyclooxygenase inhibitor, appear to be effective in reducing the postwarming inflammatory response by blocking the formation of prostanoids and leukotrienes. Arterial dilators such as reserpine, tolazoline, and nifedipine have also been used but have not been clearly proved to be effective. Antiplatelet and thrombolytic agents such as dextran, heparin, urokinase, and streptokinase have also shown some clinical efficacy. Use of calmodulin antagonists has shown good results.

Attempts at chemical and surgical sympathectomy and, more recently, electrostimulation of the spinal cord have yielded mixed results. Although sympathectomy may offer benefits in decreasing postfrostbite sequelae, it has not been demonstrated to improve tissue salvage.

Long-Term Complications

Sequelae of frostbite vary in severity. Hyperhidrosis, Raynaud's disease, peripheral neuropathy, hypersensitivity to cold, bony deformity, and atrophy of the nails, hair, and muscle are common problems.

IMMERSION FOOT AND TRENCH FOOT

Immersion foot occurs when a foot exposed to nonfreezing temperatures of 10° C or lower loses heat because it is wet and experiences poor vascular flow because it is constricted and immobile. Symptoms include numbness, tingling, pain, and itching. Skin is initially swollen and red and gradually takes on a gray-blue discoloration. The entire foot may appear black, but deep tissue destruction may not be present. After a few days, a hyperemic state sets in. Between 2 and 6 weeks later, these symptoms gradually subside, but the extremity may still be sensitive to cold. Superficial gangrene may be present.

Management is similar to that of second-degree frostbite. Elevation of the foot and careful wound management are essential. Physical therapy is used to maintain range of motion.

CHILBLAIN (PERNIO)

Chilblain occurs when the skin is exposed to cold for extended periods but the core of the body remains warm. For example, mountain climbers, whose skin is exposed to cold but whose body core is kept warm by exertion, are at risk for chilblain. Exposure to dry air that is just above freezing results in superficial ulceration of the skin similar to that seen in second-degree frostbite. As with frostbite, treatment consists of rewarming and very conservative tissue management.

OPHTHALMIC INJURY

Corneal injury caused by freezing of the eye as a result of exposure to high windchill and reflected ultraviolet radiation at high altitudes can cause keratitis with opacification and corneal pitting. Eyewear that screens out ultraviolet radiation and protects the eyes from wind is recommended to prevent corneal injury. Treatment consists of aggressive ophthalmologic intervention with cycloplegia, mydriasis, and antibiotics.

Toxic Epidermal Necrolysis

Toxic epidermal necrolysis (TEN) is not a thermal injury per se but the name given to a group of dermatologic disorders

Table 5   Classification of Frostbite

Degree of Injury	Features
First degree	Hyperemia and edema, without skin necrosis
Second degree	Vesicle formation along with hyperemia, edema, and partial-thickness skin necrosis
Third degree	Full-thickness skin necrosis
Fourth degree	Full-thickness skin necrosis, including necrosis of underlying muscle and bone, with subsequent gangrene

characterized by inflammation-induced separation of epidermis and dermis followed by epidermal skin sloughing. The denuded areas are comparable to those affected by a second-degree burn. Oral mucosal sloughing is also characteristic of TEN. Complications such as infection, malnutrition, negative nitrogen balance, severe wound pain, and multiple organ dysfunction syndrome are identical to those seen in patients with major burns. Mortality is very high if these complications are not optimally managed. Patients should be treated in a burn center, especially for wound care and control of infectious complications [see Figure 8]. The role of the dermatologist is to define the diagnosis and determine the potential etiology.

CLINICAL MANIFESTATIONS

A prodrome of TEN usually consists of signals of upper respiratory tract infection, such as high fever, sore throat, and malaise. Then, 1 to 2 days after these symptoms appear, the skin of the face and extremities usually becomes tender and erythematous. Lesions appear either as large surfaces of red skin or as target lesions that are 2 cm in diameter and consist of concentric rings of erythema.

These lesions soon combine to form large affected areas. In 24 to 96 hours, the involved skin begins to form small blisters or large bullae. Moderate traction of the erythematous skin results in separation of the epidermis from the dermis, a positive Nikolsky's sign. When the bullae rupture, large denuded areas of skin become apparent over the patient's entire body. Fingernails, toenails, and the skin of the palms and soles may also slough.

The most characteristic feature of this disease is severe inflammation of the mouth. Blisters develop on the oral mucosa, leaving a very raw, red surface. The lips may be swollen and crusted with clotted blood. The lesions may be confined to the oral cavity or may extend to the larynx or even to the trachea, the bronchi, and the esophagus. The patient is often unable to eat. The eyelids swell as conjunctival inflammation develops. Conjunctival infection, usually caused by *Staphylococcus aureus*,

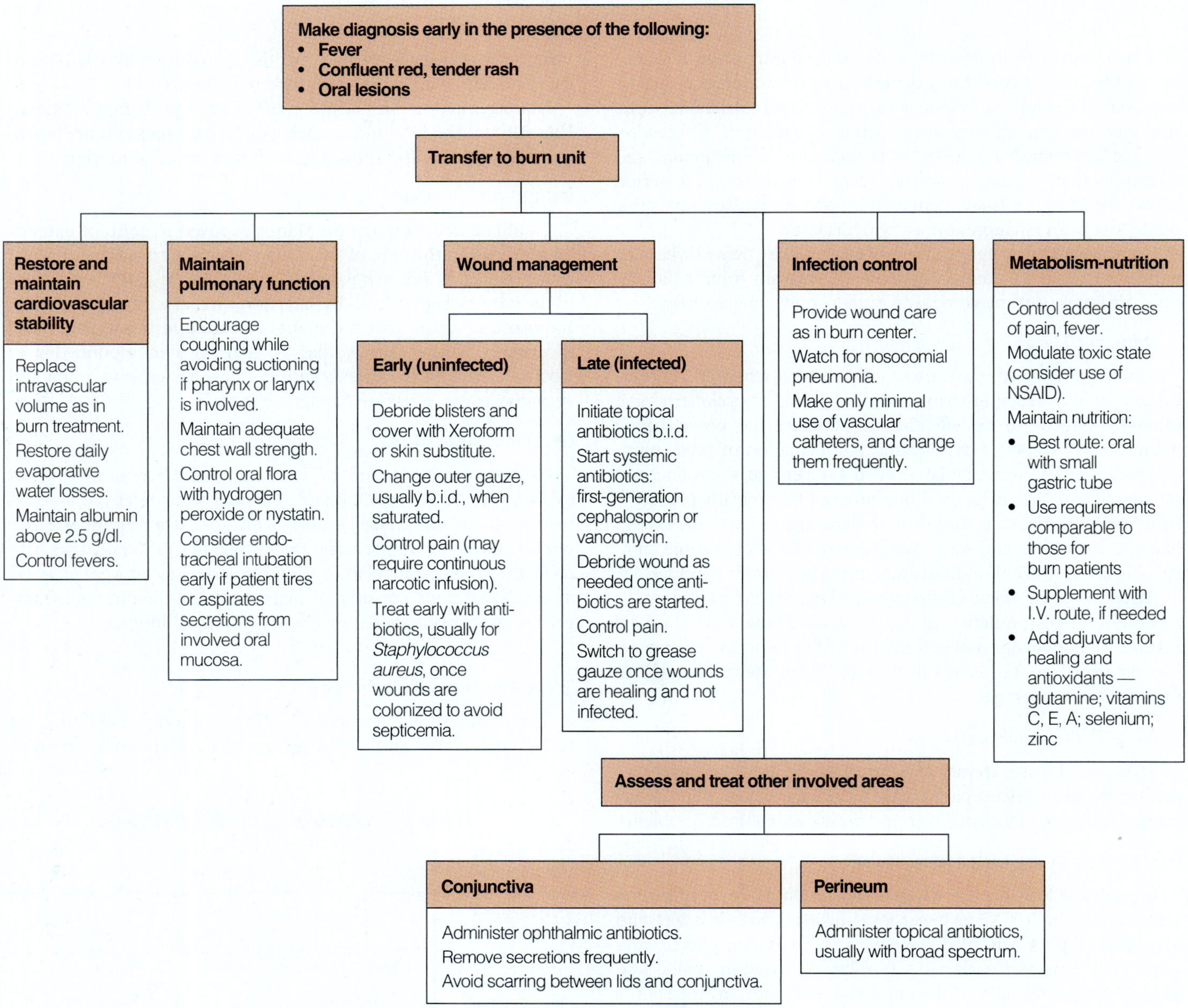

Figure 8 Shown is an algorithm for treatment of toxic epidermal necrolysis (TEN).

may lead to scarring and permanent blindness. The nasal and urethral mucosa may also become inflamed, and erosions can develop on the genital and perianal skin.

Systemic signs of the disease include high fever and leukocytosis. In severe cases, gastrointestinal bleeding is common. Renal failure can also occur as a result of hypovolemia, the septic response, or membranous glomerulonephritis. In up to 50% of cases, there are abnormalities in liver enzymes, including modest increases in aspartate aminotransferase (AST) and alanine aminotransferase (ALT). Bilirubin also shows a modest increase. The mechanism of these increases, which appear to be a part of the toxic component of TEN, is unknown.

TREATMENT

There are three main components to treatment of TEN that should be initiated after the skin sloughing has occurred. The first step is restoration and maintenance of cardiopulmonary stability. The second step is aggressive wound management, similar to that of a massive second-degree burn, in which the emphasis is on optimizing healing and controlling infection. The third step is optimizing nutrition and modulating the hypermetabolic response caused by the toxic elements of the underlying disease process and by the lesion itself. Treatment also includes the use of nutritional supplements to attenuate the inflammation-induced disease.

Restoration of Cardiopulmonary Stability

Lung function is often impaired early as a result of aspirated secretions from involved oral mucosa. Reduced clearance of secretions because of oral pain and overall weakness also impairs lung function. Pain control, rest periods, and aggressive pulmonary toilet to assist the patient's cough are the first line of defense. Suctioning can lead to significant bleeding and should be used either sparingly or only after the patient has an endotracheal tube in place. The patient should be intubated if lung function is progressively impaired by a disease process that is expected to last at least 10 to 14 days. Partial ventilatory assistance is often required if the patient is intubated, because chest wall pain, systemic toxicity, and weakness can severely impair spontaneous ventilatory efforts.

Cardiovascular function is initially impaired as a result of hypervolemia caused by fluid loss into the wounds, increased skin losses, and decreased oral intake. As in the treatment of a burn, intravascular volume replacement and evaporative water replacement are required. Controlling the febrile response will also help decrease fluid losses, vasodilatation, and the resulting hyperadrenergic response. Careful use of nonsteroidal anti-inflammatory drugs is often needed to keep the patient's temperature below 102° F (38.9° C). The use of an ibuprofen or acetaminophen elixir along with antacids is usually successful in lowering temperature.

Wound Management and Infection Control

Early in the course of TEN, the wounds evolve into a skin slough at the epidermal-dermal junction. In severe cases, the basal lamina of the dermis is destroyed. If the patient is seen before the wounds progress to superinfection, the blisters can be removed and the surface covered with an antibiotic grease gauze (e.g., Xeroform), a skin substitute, and then a soft outer gauze dressing to soak up secretions. The advantage of this approach is that the wound becomes occluded, which decreases pain, fluid loss, and risk of superinfection and improves healing rate. The outer gauze should be changed as needed to remove the plasma leak (usually twice a day). Leaving the inner dressing in place optimizes the wound environment for healing and minimizes pain. Cultures of the wound surface and exudate should be performed frequently to monitor for superinfection. If an infection is detected early in the course of TEN (i.e., days 1 to 5), the pathogen is almost always *S. aureus*.

If the wounds are already infected when the patient is first seen, gentle debridement followed by administration of topical antibiotics (e.g., silver sulfadiazine) is required, especially if there is an exudate or eschar on the skin surface. Use of immersion hydrotherapy or showers for these painful superficial wounds may not be feasible, because they may be too painful and because there is a risk that the infection will be spread to clean wounds [see Table 6]. Adequate pain control is essential. Morphine, given as a continuous I.V. infusion or as oral long-acting tablets (e.g., MS Contin), is a good choice.

The role of corticosteroids in the treatment of TEN remains unclear. If started before the skin sloughing occurs, when the disease process is just beginning, corticosteroids can attenuate the process, resulting in less sloughing. However, once vesicles have formed and the separation has occurred, corticosteroids no longer effectively attenuate skin sloughing; in fact, they retard the rate of healing. Aggressive oral care is critical because of the high risk of local mouth infection and consequent wound and lung infection. Early and continued assessment and aggressive management of corneal involvement are required. Administration of ophthalmic antibiotic ointments and gentle breaking of adhesions between conjunctiva and eyelids with a small glass rod are the standard treatment.

Optimizing Nutrition

Nutrition is a major component of care. Total nutrition often cannot be delivered orally because of oral lesions. Delivery of nutrition by a small gastric feeding tube is preferred, if the tube can be accurately placed. If esophagitis is severe, tube placement may be difficult. A nutritional regimen comparable to that prescribed for a person with a large burn is indicated. This regimen includes 30 to 35 calories/kg body weight and a protein content of 1.5 to 2 g/kg body weight. Supplements can be beneficial: additional glutamine (30 g/day) can help heal the gut and skin epithelium and restore cell glutathione levels. In addition, increased daily doses of vitamin C (2 to 4 g), vitamin E (400 units), zinc sulfate (440 mg), selenium (50 mg), and vitamin A (25,000 units) will assist in the wound-healing process and augment tissue antioxidant levels. If adequate nutrition cannot be provided enterally, parenteral supplementation is needed.

Table 6 Wound Management in Toxic Epidermal Necrolysis

Stage and Type of Wound	Treatment
Early, uninfected	Debride blisters Cover wound with Xeroform gauze or skin substitute Cover wound with soft outer gauze dressing; change b.i.d. until drainage decreased Administer antibiotic for *Staphylococcus aureus*, if identified
Late, infected	Debride after initiating systemic antibiotic treatment if infection is invasive Apply topical antibiotics b.i.d.

Discussion

Terminology of Electrical Burns

Familiarity with the appropriate terminology is necessary for an understanding of injuries caused by electrical current [see Table 7].

VOLTAGE AND AMPERAGE

Electrical injuries are classified as low voltage (less than 1,000 volts) and high voltage (usually greater than 1,000 volts). Injuries associated with low voltage are most likely to occur in the home, electrocutions in bathtubs and by electric hair dryers being the most common causes of death associated with low voltage. Injuries caused by high voltage typically occur outdoors, near power sources and lines. Electrical current can arc (jump) 1 in. from a power source or line for every 10,000 volts being carried, so that a person does not have to touch the source to sustain injury.

The severity of injury to tissues depends on the amperage, that is, the amount of current passing through the tissues. Because of the variability of resistance and exposure time, it is impossible to quantify precisely the amperage at the time of an accident, but the amperage can be inferred from the voltage of the source. A low-voltage source is capable of producing serious cardiopulmonary complications and death if a current passing across the chest is strong enough to initiate ventricular fibrillation.

A high-voltage source is usually required to produce tissue necrosis along the path of the current [see Table 8]. The damage is caused by both heat production and direct current. Initial resistance to the flow of current—namely, skin or clothing—is overcome by the heat generated by high voltage. Tissue necrosis occurs with continued contact. Over a short period of time, a dry hand may have sufficient resistance to avoid the passage of current from a low-voltage source. However, contact with several thousand degrees of heat from a high-tension source causes immediate local coagulation and disruption of the electrical barrier. Because water is an excellent conductor, the current can pass more readily through tissues with a high water content. Tissue damage at the contact site can be seen with low voltage as well, again because of local heat generation. A good example is the oral burn seen in children who have bitten an electrical cord.

Besides heat injury, there is tissue damage from the current itself. The mechanism of tissue damage is not completely understood, but there is clearly injury to the nerves, blood vessels, and muscle from the current itself, damaging the cells. When endothelial cells are injured, there is no protection against local clotting and microvascular thrombosis, resulting in tissue devascularization.

RESISTANCE

The resistance of tissues to the passage of current depends in large part on water content, water being a good conductor. In decreasing order, tissue resistance is highest in bone and lower in fat, tendons, skin, muscles, vessels, and nerves. Skin resistance also depends on its moisture content, a moist hand having 10 to 100 times less resistance to the passage of current than a dry hand. With high voltage, however, the current readily passes through all tissues indiscriminately. Heat produced as the current passes is proportional to tissue resistance (heat = $amp^2 \times R$). High voltage can generate local heat of sufficient degree (more than 1,000° C) to cause bone destruction and total coagulation necrosis of surrounding tissues. Heat produced as the current enters and exits the body also leads to coagulation necrosis of the skin and underlying tissues.

PATHWAY OF CURRENT

The pathway of current can be unpredictable, but current generally passes from a point of entry through the body to a grounded site, that is, a site that has lower resistance to flow than does air, which is a poor conductor. Extremely high voltage sources usually exit in multiple areas in an explosive fashion. When current passes from hand to hand or hand to thorax, there is a higher risk of cardiac fibrillation than when current follows a hand-to-foot path. If current passes through the head, it is likely to cause an initial respiratory arrest and subsequent severe neurologic impairment.

Table 7 **Terminology of Electrical Burns**

Voltage (electrical or energy potential) is electromotive force generated by the power source.
Amperage (intensity) is the amount of current flowing per unit of time.
Resistance to flow is measured in ohms.

$$\text{Resistance} = \frac{\text{Voltage}}{\text{Amperage}} \qquad \text{Amperage} = \frac{\text{Voltage}}{\text{Resistance}}$$

Household current = 110 to 220 volts
Residential power lines = 5,000 to 10,000 volts
High-tension wire = Up to 100,000 volts

Heat: Electrical current produces heat when it meets a resistance to flow. This process is defined by Joule's law, with the heat production defined in terms of joules (J): $J = I^2RT$, where I = amperage, R = resistance, and T = contact time

Electrical current produces tissue damage in two ways:
  1. Local generation of heat during passage of current
  2. Direct tissue damage by current

The degree of tissue injury depends on the following:
  Voltage of the source
  Amperage of current passing through the tissues
  Resistance of tissues traversed by current
  Duration of contact
  Pathway of current
  Type of current: alternating (AC) or direct (DC)

Table 8 **Effect of Current on Severity of Injury**

Type of Current	Effect
High-tension source: ≥ 5,000 mA	Destruction of tissue by heat and coagulation Cardiopulmonary failure

Household source:
  60 mA
  30 mA
  5 mA
	
	Cardiac fibrillation
	Respiratory muscle tetany; suffocation
	Pain

mA—milliamperes

TYPE AND DURATION OF CURRENT

Most household current is alternating. Low-voltage AC is more dangerous than direct current (DC) of the same voltage because it produces muscle tetany. The tetany is caused by rapid depolarization and repolarization, impeding attempts at escape from the source of electricity. Injuries caused by high-voltage AC are also more severe than those caused by high-voltage DC, although both have devastating effects. The severity of injury is directly proportional to the duration of current flow, but even brief exposure to high amperage produces massive tissue damage.

Recommended Reading

ELECTRICAL INJURY

Bhatt D, Lee R: Rhabdomyolysis due to pulsed electrical fields. Plast Reconstr Surg 86:1, 1990

Bingham H: Electrical burns. Clin Plast Surg 13:75, 1986

Daniel R, Ballard P, Heroux P, et al: High voltage electrical injury: acute pathophysiology. J Hand Surg 13:44, 1988

Grossman R, Tempereau C: Auditory and neuropsychiatric behavior patterns after electrical injury. J Burn Care Rehabil 14:169, 1993

Grube B, Heimbach P: Acute and delayed neurological sequelae of electrical injury. Electrical Trauma. Lee R, Ed. Cambridge University Press, New York, 1992, p 133

Hiestant D, Colice G: Lightning-strike injury. J Intens Care Med 3:303, 1988

Hunt J, Mason A, Masterson T, et al: The pathophysiology of acute electrical injuries. J Trauma 16:335, 1976

Hunt J, Sato R, Baxter C: Acute electric burns. Arch Surg 115:434, 1980

Lee R, Gaylor D: Role of cell membrane rupture in the pathogenesis of electrical trauma. J Surg Res 44:709, 1988

Lee R, Kolodney M: Electrical injury mechanisms: dynamics of the thermal response. Plast Reconstr Surg 80:663, 1987

Luce E: Electrical injuries. Reconstructive Plastic Surgery. McCarthy, Ed. WB Saunders Co, Philadelphia, 1990, p 110

COLD INJURY

Arregui R, Morandeira JR, Martinez G, et al: Epidural neurostimulation in the treatment of frostbite. PACE Pacing Clin Electrophysiol 12:713, 1989

Beitner R, Chen-Zion M, Sofer-Bassukevitz Y, et al: Treatment of frostbite with the calmodulin antagonists thioridazine and trifluoperazine. Gen Pharmacol 20:641, 1989

Bourne M, Prepcorn M, et al: Analysis of microvascular changes in frostbite injury. J Surg Res 40:26, 1986

Britt LD, Dascombe WH, Rodriguez A: New horizons in management of hypothermia and frostbite injury. Surg Clin North Am 71:345, 1991

Galloway H, Suh JS, Parker S, et al: Radiologic case study: late sequelae of frostbite. Orthopedics 14:191, 1991

Gregory JS, Flancbaum L, Townsend MC, et al: Incidence and timing of hypothermia in trauma patients undergoing operations. J Trauma 31:795, 1991

Heggers J, McCauley R, Robson M: Cold-induced injury: frostbite. Total Burn Care. Herndon D, Ed. WB Saunders Co, Philadelphia, 1996, p 39

Vogel JE, Dellon AL: Frostbite injuries of the hand. Clin Plast Surg 16:565, 1989

TOXIC EPIDERMAL NECROLYSIS

Dajani AS: The scalded-skin syndrome: relation of phage-group II staphylococci. J Infect Dis 125:548, 1972

Keleman J, Cioffi W, McManus W, et al: Burn center care for patients with toxic epidermal necrolysis. J Am Coll Surg 180:273, 1995

Murphy J, Purdue G, Hunt J: Toxic epidermal necrolysis. J Burn Care Rehabil 18:417, 1997

Acknowledgment

Figures 1, 5, 7, and 8   Marcia Kammerer

IV PREOPERATIVE PREPARATION

36 ELEMENTS OF COST-EFFECTIVE NONEMERGENCY SURGICAL CARE

Robert S. Rhodes, M.D., and Charles L. Rice, M.D.

The cost and quality of health care concern all industrialized nations, and the responses to these concerns often reflect each nation's particular culture and philosophy. Health care costs in the United States have risen inexorably since 1960 [see Table 1].[1] A variety of attempts have been made to control this rise in costs, including price controls (during the Nixon administration) and the introduction of the prospective payment system (during the Reagan administration). Because none of the remedies attempted thus far has been successful, the United States has chosen to address these problems through a number of mechanisms loosely referred to as managed care. In addition to reducing fees paid to providers, managed care focuses on the decision-making aspects of health care: about 75% of the costs of health care result from physician recommendations. As a result, managed care has affected both surgeons' income[2] and their autonomy.

The increased role of managed care in medical decision making has raised concerns that managed care is more about managing cost than about managing care. These concerns are fueled by reports of refusal of care, premature discharges, and termination of care. Growing patient dissatisfaction with such management has produced a backlash.[3]

The issues raised by health care professionals and patients have caused attention to be focused on the cost-effectiveness of medical care. In general terms, cost-effectiveness is defined as cost divided by net benefits. The numerator (cost) is expressed in dollars, and the denominator (net benefits) is expressed as beneficial outcomes minus adverse outcomes. Although the primary goal of cost-effectiveness is to maximize benefits in relation to available resources, cost-effectiveness is also a reflection of health care quality.

In this chapter, we outline the basic principles of cost-effectiveness and address some of the complexities involved. (We do not, however, intend this chapter as a cookbook; modern surgical practice is too dynamic and too diverse for such an approach.) We begin by reviewing the strengths and weaknesses of methods used to assess quality and the relation of quality to cost. We then focus on specific skills and attributes that contribute to cost-effective care. Throughout, we emphasize use of electronic reference sources for access to up-to-date information. An appreciation of the principles, strategies, and tactics of cost-effective surgical care should help surgeons to better serve their patients and their profession as well as help reestablish surgeons' authority in surgical care.

Relation between Quality and Cost

To grasp what cost-effective care is, one must, first, possess an adequate definition of quality and, second, understand the relation between quality and cost. These tasks are more problematic than might at first appear. Traditionally, quality was understood in terms of appropriateness. In the light of this understanding, the relation between cost (expenditure) and quality was viewed exclusively as positive: increased health care expenditure was associated

Table 1 U.S. Health Care Expenditures: Selected Years, 1960–1997[1]

Year	Expenditure for Health Services and Supplies ($ billion)	Total Health Care Expenditure ($ billion)	U.S. Population (million)	Expenditure per Capita ($)	GDP ($ billion)	Expenditure as Percentage of GDP (%)
1960	25.2	26.9	190	141	527	5.1
1970	67.9	73.2	215	341	1,036	7.1
1980	235.6	247.3	235	1,052	2,784	8.9
1990	674.8	699.4	260	2,690	5,744	12.2
1994	917.2	947.7	271	3,500	6,947	13.6
1995	963.1	993.7	273	3,637	7,270	13.7
1996	1,010.6	1,042.5	276	3,781	7,662	13.6
1997	1,057.5	1,092.4	278	3,925	8,111	13.5

GDP—gross domestic product

Table 2 Percentage of GDP Spent on Health Care in Selected Countries: 1960, 1990, and 1997[4]

Year	Expenditure as Percentage of GDP (%)						
	Canada	France	Germany	Japan	United Kingdom	United States	OECD Median for 29 Countries
1960	5.5	4.2	4.8	3.0	3.9	5.2	3.8
1990	9.2	8.9	8.7	6.0	6.0	12.6	7.2
1997	9.0	9.6	10.4	7.3	6.7	13.5	7.5

GDP—gross domestic product OECD—Organisation for Economic Co-operation and Development

with increased quality and vice versa. However, appropriateness is difficult to define, and even when it is defined, it is difficult to measure. Without accurate definitions or measurements, the relation between cost and quality becomes somewhat theoretical. Thus, with the traditional view of quality, the strongly held positions of providers, purchasers, and patients regarding health care quality (and their subsequent actions) were actually governed more by perceptions than by data.

Several factors eroded this traditional view. One was the realization that even though the United States spends a larger fraction of its gross domestic product (GDP) on health care than does any other industrialized country [see Table 2], United States citizens are less healthy—often by wide margins—than citizens of comparable countries [see Table 3].[4] Although health status can be significantly influenced by factors outside the health care system (e.g., standard of living, nutrition, sanitation, and safety), the disparity between health care cost and health status in the United States suggested that extravagant health care expenditure did not automatically improve health status.

A second factor, which became apparent before the introduction of managed care, was the growing amount of information on problems with quality in the health care system. For instance, there were data suggesting that one fourth of hospital deaths might be preventable,[5] that one third of hospital procedures might be exposing patients to unnecessary risk, that one third of drugs might not be indicated, and that one third of abnormal laboratory test results might not be followed up by physicians.[6] Reviews of medical records also revealed alarming error rates,[7,8] with as many as half of the adverse events associated with errors in surgical care.

A third factor challenging the traditional relation between quality and cost was the increasing recognition that appropriateness was an insufficient criterion of quality. Without question, some studies of appropriateness had identified valid quality concerns. For instance, researchers at the Rand Corporation, after assessing the appropriateness of carotid endarterectomy, coronary angiography, and upper GI endoscopy, concluded that 32%, 17%, and 17% of these procedures, respectively, were undertaken inappropriately.[9] In another example, an analysis of seven health plans revealed that one in six hysterectomies was inappropriate.[10] Nevertheless, the continued difficulty of measuring appropriateness[11] undermined its value as a standard.[12] For instance, retrospective assessments often judged appropriateness on the basis of outcome alone, without considering processes of care.[13] In addition, appropriateness tended to be judged differently when decisions were made for groups rather than individuals.[14]

A telling blow to the traditional view of the quality-cost relation was the growing awareness of the great disparity in the frequency of surgical procedures within small areas.[15-17] (In addition to these frequency variations, there are also cost variations for seemingly similar services.) The frequency variations proved to be procedure specific. For instance, procedures with highly specific indications (e.g., repair of hip fracture, inguinal herniorrhaphy, and appendectomy) generally exhibited relatively little frequency variation, but carotid endarterectomy, hysterectomy, and coronary angiography exhibited a great deal of variation.[18] The variation also appeared to be related to provider capacity (i.e., number of hospital beds/1,000 persons): one study of the effect of provider capacity on variation noted a close relation between the intensity of local diagnostic testing and invasive cardiac procedures.[19]

Table 3 Health Status and Outcomes in Selected Countries: 1996

	Canada	France	Germany	Japan	United Kingdom	United States	OECD Median for 29 Countries
Percentage of population 65 yr of age or older (%)	12.0	15.4	15.6	14.6	15.6	12.7	14.4
Life expectancy at birth (years)							
Female	81.5	82.0	79.9	83.6	79.3	79.4	80.3
Male	75.4	74.1	73.6	77.0	74.4	72.7	74.0
Infant mortality (per 1,000 live births)	6.0	4.9	5.0	3.8	6.1	7.8	5.8
Potential years of life lost, 1995 (per 100,000 life years)							
Female	3,284	3,092	3,337	2,399	3,616	4,591	3,256
Male	5,451	6,861	6,505	4,443	5,690	8,401	6,281

OECD—Organisation for Economic Co-operation and Development

Several physician factors, such as physician style, a community's so-called practice signature, and physician uncertainty, also appear to be related to variations in the frequency of surgical procedures[20]; this finding lends support to the idea that many medical decisions are based on opinion rather than on evidence.[21] One study even concluded that only about 15% of common medical practices had a documented foundation in any sort of medical research.[22] This conclusion does not necessarily mean that only 15% of care is effective, but it does raise concerns about the lack of hard evidence for most care. In contrast, a subsequent study at a British hospital revealed that 95% of in-hospital surgical patients received treatment based on satisfactory evidence.[23] The different conclusions of these two studies, however, can be accounted for in a number of ways.

Variations in the use of medical services do not correlate with differences in incidence of disease or appropriateness of use.[24] Economic incentives for physicians also appear to have relatively little influence. Thus, there is considerable variation in utilization rates among Veterans Health Administration medical facilities[25] and within countries without fee-for-service reimbursement.

Whether the high utilization rates observed are too high or the low utilization rates are too low is still the subject of debate. The possibility that low frequency of use may reflect restricted access to care is a particular concern, given the association between variation and the ratio of hospital beds to population.[26] Currently, however, the tendency is to believe that the high rates are too high. Moreover, despite the usage variations noted from area to area, providers in each area claim, and often document, equivalent patient health status. This finding led one author to conclude that "marked variability in surgical practices and presumably in surgical judgment and philosophy must be considered to reflect absent or inadequate data by which to evaluate surgical treatment...."[27] The net effect of these developments was to fuel skepticism about the validity of the traditional relation between quality and cost.

The abandonment of the traditional concept of quality as appropriateness was facilitated by the emergence of a new concept of quality,[28] which has three major components: structure (faculties, equipment, and services), process (content of care), and outcomes. This new concept uses many of the industrial quality-control techniques pioneered by W. Edwards Deming and seeks to overcome the shortcomings of the appropriateness criterion. Deming's goal was to minimize quality variations by examining production systems—which, in the case of medicine, are the systems of care. Accordingly, total quality management and continuous quality improvement are increasingly being applied to health care.

This new concept of quality and its relation to cost can be illustrated diagrammatically [see Figure 1].[29] The traditional notion of a positive relation between quality and cost still exists in zones 1 and 2, but the slope of the curve flattens in zone 3 and actually becomes negative in zone 4, where further cost increases are associated with decreased quality. The basis of this effect is that as health care volume increases, the cost-benefit curve flattens but the cost-harm curve does not (i.e., side effects are just as common in patients with mild disease as in those with severe disease).[28] The implication is that reducing use of health care resources in zones 3 and 4 may not detract from quality but actually improve it.

This new concept of quality has intellectual appeal, but like the traditional concept, it remains somewhat theoretical. Because quality itself remains difficult to define, the new construct still oversimplifies the issues. To be more relevant, any definition of the relation of quality to cost should also consider overuse, underuse, and misuse.[30] Despite the shortcomings in definition and measurement, the new three-part concept of quality is widely accepted and has become the template for many profound changes in the United States health care system.

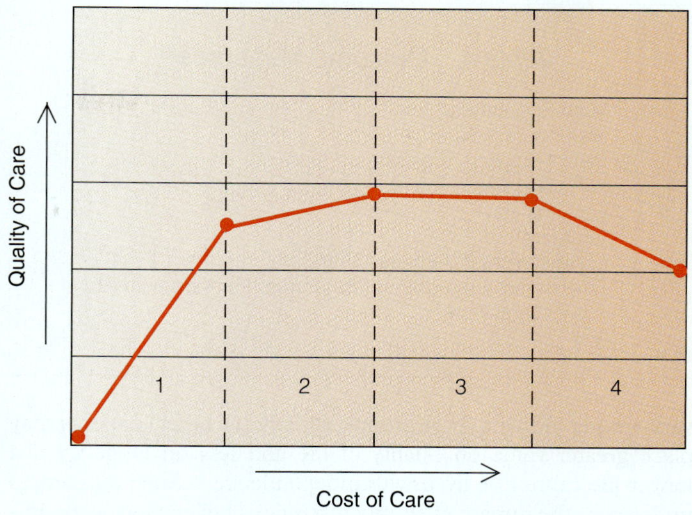

Figure 1 Illustrated is the new concept of quality and cost.[29]

The traditional concept of quality as appropriateness persists today and is at least partly responsible for the fears many patients and health care professionals have about the impact of managed care on quality. The lack of clear data on quality has led to a buyer's market, in which health care purchasers use the apparent similarity in quality, despite variations in frequency and cost, as a rationale for contracting for less expensive care. Purchasers assume that even in an atmosphere of decreasing income and increasing constraints, providers will not knowingly or willingly sacrifice quality. Indeed, they believe that competition may spark a drive to exceed patients' expectations. The medical profession, whose authority was once strong enough to forestall system change, now bears the burden of proof. Practitioners and other providers have become primary targets of those calling for assessment and accountability in health care.

Assessment of Outcome

Of the three components of the new concept of quality, outcome assessment has received the most attention.[30] The list of traditional outcome measures [see Table 4][31] is now being superseded by one that is increasingly diverse. Length of stay, costs, and patient satisfaction are increasingly important. The current focus on treatment outcomes also emphasizes long-term health status. Thus, in addition to the immediate morbidity and mortality of a given procedure, there is interest in long-term functional status.

A preferred measure of these long-term outcomes is the health care quality of life or quality-adjusted life years (QALYs),[32,33] a summary measure of the length of time one experiences a given health status. Of the several systems that quantify this health status,[34] some include objective measures (e.g., functional status), whereas others use subjective estimates of well-being. The latter often involve patients' estimates of the meaningfulness of a given functional status. For instance, patient A may not be able to walk as far as patient B, but one cannot conclude that patient A therefore has a poorer quality of life unless that functional status is placed in a context that is meaningful to patient A.[35]

Although health status is thought to be more easily quantified than appropriateness, its measurement still involves considerable subjectivity. For instance, a given individual's estimate of the future value of an outcome measure may vary with time or according to the specific circumstances at assessment. QALYs may also

Table 4 Outcome Measures[31]

Morbidity/mortality
Recurrence rates
Patient-reported measures of symptoms
Functional status
Length of stay
Charges/costs
Quality-adjusted life years (QALYs)
Emotional consequences of the disease and the treatment
Patient satisfaction

vary among individuals or groups. Elderly (or other) patients may place greater value on quality of life and less on longevity if a longer life cannot be lived with independence.[36] Such differences underscore the impact of ethnicity, religious beliefs, socioeconomic status, and attitudes about health care. Because outcomes have experiential, physiologic, and resource dimensions, patients, providers, and health care purchasers may have entirely different views about which measure is best for judging the outcome of a given intervention. Further complexities may result if there is a discrepancy among measures (e.g., an outcome that is deemed successful by a provider but does not satisfy the patient).

Outcome measures must also take into account health status and severity of illness before treatment,[37] and the necessary adjustments can be difficult. Measuring outcomes may also pose other problems.[38,39] For instance, if outcome measures are valid indices for improving quality of care, the implication is that they must also be intimately related to the processes of care.[30]

Despite concerns that managed care focuses more on cost than on care, managed care organizations are taking significant steps toward assuring quality. At present, the leading organization in this area is the National Committee for Quality Assurance (NCQA) (http://www.ncqa.org). Self-described as a "nonprofit watchdog organization," the NCQA is dominated by the managed care industry it is supposed to evaluate and by large employers. Its two most significant activities are (1) accrediting health care plans and (2) developing and refining the Healthplan Employer Data and Information Set (HEDIS). HEDIS measures focus primarily on utilization and management, but with each revision, more attention is given to the quality of clinical care. Most of the HEDIS measures involve screening, preventive measures (e.g., mammography or smoking cessation), or both.

The Foundation for Accountability (FACCT) (http://www.facct.org) is an independent organization that is establishing standards of care. The National Forum for Health Care Quality Measurement and Reporting (http://www.qualityforum.org) is another important organization. Several recent reports summarize the broader scope of organizational efforts to improve quality in health care.[40-42] Although such efforts will undoubtedly produce some improvements in care, surgeons should recognize that the greatest impact on surgical care is likely to emanate from individual efforts at the grassroots level.

Skills Required for Evidence-Based Decision Making

The most cost-effective care (i.e., the highest-quality care at the lowest cost) will be delivered through evidence-based medical practice. However, such practice requires skills that often are not emphasized during undergraduate and graduate medical education, such as statistical analysis, critical literature analysis, and technology assessment. Acquiring these skills, together with the computer literacy essential for their application, creates the infrastructure for quality improvement.

STATISTICAL ANALYSIS

Statistical analysis is essential for understanding variations in outcomes, interpreting the medical literature, and evaluating one's own performance. Before the Medicare Prospective Payment System and diagnosis-related groups (DRGs) were implemented, hospital Medicare reimbursement was based on cost. Variations in the use of hospital resources were primarily of academic interest and had relatively few fiscal implications. Under prospective payment, however, hospital reimbursement changed to a system based on national averages rather than actual costs. As a result, the Healthcare Financing Administration transferred the concern over the fiscal implications of these cost variations to the hospitals, and private payers now follow Medicare's lead.

The distribution of variation in medical outcomes tends to have a characteristic shape. Instead of having normal distributions, many outcomes, such as cost and length of hospital stay, tend to have skewed distributions, with the tail toward higher costs or longer stay [see Figure 2]. Thus, the mean (or average) value is likely to be greater than the median (or middle) value. However, the overall cluster around the mean or median and the width of the curve vary according to the specific procedure and provider. The longer the tail, the less characteristic of a particular outcome the mean value is. Because the distribution is skewed, the mean is often calculated as the mean of the logarithm of the individual values. This logarithmic average, also known as the geometric mean, is the basis of the length-of-stay calculations of the DRGs.

Currently, the variation in many medical costs and other outcomes is relatively large, often exceeding 200% to 300%. Some of this variation is an expected part of many biologic processes, and some can be accounted for by differences in severity. Consequently, it would probably be difficult to achieve the industry-standard low variation sought by Deming. Still, there is considerable room for improvement [see Assessment of Performance, below].

Health care purchasers are well aware of cost variations among providers and use low-cost providers as benchmarks toward which other providers are expected to strive. These benchmarks, which occupy the extreme left portion of the curve, are considered to

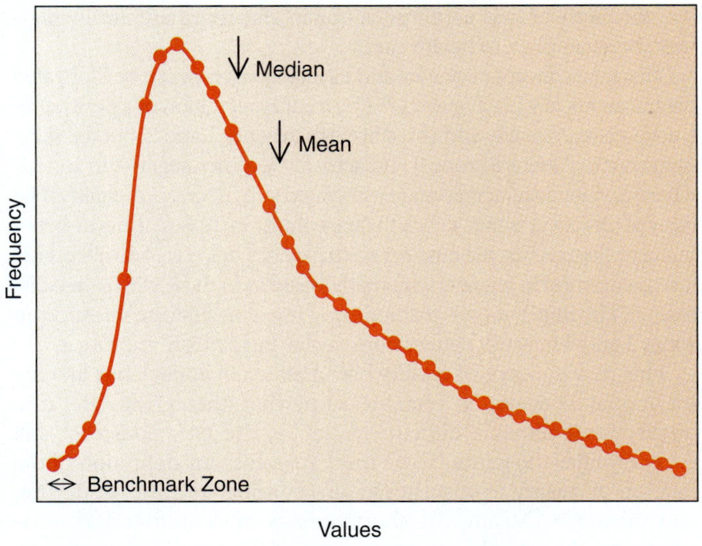

Figure 2 Shown is the skewed distribution curve associated with health care outcomes such as cost or length of stay.

represent best practice and are believed likely to contain lessons for management of similar patients. Such benchmarks, however, often reflect an ideal (i.e., exceptional) patient population rather than a normal one[43]; consequently, applying them to more complicated patients who need more care may increase the risk of adverse outcomes in this setting. Still, understanding the meaning and significance of variation in outcome measures is essential to assessing one's own practice.

Another vital application of statistical analysis to cost-effectiveness is in laboratory and radiologic testing. Such testing accounts for some of the largest increases in health care costs and much of the cost variation. Traditionally, the value of a test was often determined on the basis of its sensitivity (i.e., ability to positively identify patients with a disease) or specificity (i.e., ability to identify patients without a disease).[44] Today, however, these characteristics, by themselves, should no longer be considered sufficient justification for a particular test. The test's value or utility—characteristics that take disease prevalence into account—must also be considered.

For instance, if a test with a 98% sensitivity and a 98% specificity is applied to a group of patients with a disease prevalence of 50% (i.e., a group in which half the patients have the disease being tested for), 245 of every 500 patients tested ($500 \times 0.98 \times 0.5$) will have true positive results and five ($500 \times 0.02 \times 0.5$) will have false positive results. If, however, this same test is applied to 500 members of a population with a disease prevalence of 10%, 49 patients ($500 \times 0.98 \times 0.1$) will have true positive results and nine ($500 \times 0.02 \times 0.9$) will have false positive results. Thus, for a given sensitivity, the ratio of true positives to false positives increases with increasing prevalence of disease in a given patient population, and the opposite holds true as well. Given that most tests are neither as sensitive nor as specific as the one used in this example, the incidence of false positives in the real world is likely to be that much greater. This relation between disease prevalence and the incidence of false positives helps explain why a test with relatively little value as a screening test for a given disease in general practice can be valuable for specialists who see many more patients with that disease.

Increases in diagnostic testing tend to parallel increases in clinically relevant downstream procedures.[45] For instance, there is a known association between the intensity of local diagnostic testing and the frequency of invasive cardiac procedures.[19] Any increase in the number of patients who undergo cardiac catheterization as a result of false positive screening test results increases the number of patients with negative findings who may have complications of catheterization; preoperative evaluation of cardiac function in patients undergoing peripheral vascular surgery provides a specific example. Moreover, the difference in shape between cost-benefit and cost-harm curves demonstrates that besides raising costs, exposing patients to the risks of unnecessary tests may reduce the net benefits of outcomes. The problem of false positives affects both the numerator and the denominator of cost-effectiveness.

Another example of the application of test utility to clinical decision making is found in the functional assessment of incidental adrenal masses.[46] Analysis shows that in the absence of concrete signs and symptoms, measuring specific hormone levels may be of little value. Close inspection of many other routine preoperative tests reveals that they, too, may have little value.[47,48] More selective ordering of tests may be particularly important in capitated systems to minimize the so-called nonfee costs of tests that contribute little or nothing to diagnosis, treatment, or outcome.

Another application of statistical analysis is in clinical decision analysis, in which the effect or impact of each option involved in a medical decision is quantified to yield the probability statistics for that decision. Through the use of a decision tree, the components of decision making (i.e., the underlying assumptions) become explicit, which then enables one to appreciate or discount the role of factors perhaps not previously considered.[49] Thus, clinical decision analysis is valuable for reducing uncertainty and for estimating cost-effectiveness.[50-52] Although some clinicians may be intimidated by the mathematics involved and others may be bothered by what may seem a cookbook approach to health care, it is clear that sensitivity analyses can yield estimates of the importance of specific facets of care that might be difficult to obtain otherwise. Several reviews of surgery-related decision analyses have been published.[53]

CRITICAL LITERATURE ANALYSIS

Surgeons also need to be better at critical literature analysis, which involves both finding evidence on which to base decisions and being able to judge the quality of that evidence. Access to the Internet is essential because of the high number of useful Web sites and the speed of information retrieval. Three Web sites offer a good sampling of the level of information available. MEDLINE and other databases of the National Library of Medicine (http://www.ncbi.nlm.nih.gov/entrez/query.fcgi?db=PubMed), access to which is free, are particularly useful resources. Another site is the Cochrane Collaboration (http://www.update-software.com/ccweb/cochrane/cdsr.htm), an international network of clinicians and epidemiologists who systematically review the best available evidence on medical care.[54] The Cochrane Collaboration includes sources not always accessible through MEDLINE, but a subscription is required. A third useful resource is the British National Health Services Centre for Evidence-Based Medicine (http://cebm.jr2.ox.ac.uk).

Assessing the evidence is as important as finding it. The randomized, controlled trial is often considered the gold standard for evaluating health care, and the number of such trials is growing rapidly.[30] Many such trials pertain to surgery and are accessible through MEDLINE or the Cochrane Collaboration. Yet these trials also have several shortcomings. One is that the methods for reporting them have not been standardized.[55] Another is that stringent inclusion criteria may limit the applicability of the results to certain defined subgroups. Even when it appears that the findings do apply to a particular patient, it may be difficult to reproduce them in a setting that differs from the carefully controlled conditions under which the original trial was conducted. Thus, a test or treatment that is efficacious under the ideal circumstances of a trial may not be effective under less than ideal circumstances.

Carotid endarterectomy provides an excellent example of the crucial distinction between efficacy and effectiveness. Randomized, controlled trials have shown this procedure to be efficacious when performed by surgeons with low perioperative mortality and stroke rates.[56,57] Yet the effectiveness of the procedure depends on continued performance with a similarly low incidence of complications: as the incidence of stroke and other complications increases, carotid endarterectomy may become less effective or entirely ineffective.[58-60] This example illustrates the strong ethical reasons for being familiar with one's results. If patients are to give truly informed consent, they should have access to information about the outcomes their surgeon has achieved in similar patients.

The extent to which results can be generalized is a concern that applies to all studies, not just to randomized, controlled trials. In a study of the value of computed tomography in the diagnosis of appendicitis, the clinical likelihood of appendicitis in 100 patients was estimated by the referring surgeon and assigned to one of four categories: (1) definitely appendicitis (80% to 100%), (2) probably appendicitis (60% to 79%), (3) equivocally appendicitis (40% to 59%), and (4) possibly appendicitis (20% to 39%).[61] These estimates were then compared with the estimated probability of appendicitis determined via CT; the pathology (or lack thereof) was confirmed by operation or recovery. The CT interpretations had a sensitivity of 98%, a specificity of 98%, a positive predictive value of 98%, a negative predictive value of 98%, and an accuracy of 98% for either diagnosing or ruling out appendicitis. The actual incidences of appendicitis in each of the categories were 78%, 56%, 33%, and 44%, respectively. The difference between the true incidence and the initial clinical estimates indicates that surgeons' estimates of outcomes can differ from the actual data. A second point worth emphasizing in this study concerns the extent of cost savings. The authors calculated a savings of $447 per patient; however, costs (and any savings) are likely to vary in conjunction with a number of factors, including surgeons' estimates of the clinical likelihood of appendicitis, the availability of less expensive alternatives to in-hospital observation, and the use of the ED for triage. In this study, 53% of the patients had appendicitis; in other studies, as few as 30% of patients with an admitting diagnosis of appendicitis eventually underwent appendectomy.[62] Thus, the applicability of study results is likely to vary from institution to institution.

Another aspect of literature analysis concerns the distinction between relative and absolute risk reduction. This issue often arises in reports addressing the effectiveness of cancer therapies. A treatment that reduces recurrence from 5% to 4% and one that reduces it from 50% to 40% can both be said to achieve a 20% relative reduction in risk. Clearly, reporting effectiveness in terms of relative improvement may be misleading if the baseline outcome is ignored.[63] Patients' interest in adjuvant therapy (and their willingness to tolerate side effects) may be affected more by absolute reductions in risk than by relative reductions.

Another pitfall in assessing outcomes arises with tests that allow diagnosis at an earlier stage of disease. Earlier diagnosis does not necessarily mean longer survival: it simply means that a patient with presymptomatic disease identified by screening is aware of the condition for a longer time. The equation of earlier awareness with extended survival is referred to as lead-time bias. In general, advances in diagnostic imaging increase the likelihood of such bias and overestimate disease prevalence.[64]

Additional information on critical analysis of the medical literature can be found in a number of excellent references.[21,65-73]

Finally, critical literature analysis is essential for keeping pace with patients' growing access to medical information. There are now more than 15,000 health-related Web sites [see Table 5],[74] and it is estimated that in 1999, well over 20 million adults found health information online. Because some of this information may be inaccurate, misleading, or unconventional,[75] surgeons must be aware of what their patients may know—or, even more to the point, may believe they know.

TECHNOLOGY ASSESSMENT

Explosive technological growth has increased the need for technology assessment. Inarguably, many technological advances have greatly improved surgical care. Moreover, there is a prevailing societal attitude equating the latest with the best, which places considerable pressure on surgeons and hospitals to acquire the newest equipment and techniques, even when these have not been fully tested. Nevertheless, not every new technology proves successful. For example, laser endarterectomy and the use of gastric freezing machines to control upper GI bleeding represented sizable investments in technology but turned out to be of little value.

Surgeons must recognize how factors affecting decisions about technology acquisition contribute to excess capacity within the health care system. The pressure to acquire technology is often strongest in communities with the greatest competition among health care providers. Out of a compulsion to be first, providers often rush to acquire new technology before its value is proved, with other providers, fearing to be left behind, often following right behind. The result can be double jeopardy: if the new technology is unsuccessful, it has added to cost without increasing benefit; if it is successful, more of it will probably be put in place than the community needs. Competition among health care providers can help restrain the growth in health care costs; however, when driven by the so-called technological imperative, it can also contribute to inflationary increases in these costs.

The American College of Surgeons has developed a series of questions to be answered before a new surgical technology is applied to patient care [see Table 6].[76] Although these questions seem both reasonable and straightforward, the answers may be difficult to find, slow in coming, or contradictory. For example, laparoscopic cholecystectomy became rapidly diffused throughout the surgical community before the answers to these questions were known. Fortunately, in this case, the answers appear to be favorable.

An interesting paradox of new technology is that lower cost per procedure may, as a result of increases in volume, actually increase aggregate costs. Such is the case with laparoscopic cholecystectomy.[77] It also exemplifies how patients and purchasers of health care might reach differing opinions as to the "value" of new technology.

Preventive Approaches and Process Measures

COORDINATION OF CARE AND DISEASE MANAGEMENT

Coordination of care is having a growing impact on the quality of medical care. By preventing duplication of tests and unnecessary delays, coordination of care both improves patient satisfaction and saves money. In one analysis, the most frequent cause of delay was scheduling of tests (31%), followed by unavailability of postdischarge facilities (18%), physician decision making (13%), discharge planning (12%), and scheduling of surgery (12%).[78] Given the current patchwork nature of the health care system, however, preventing delays can be difficult and time-consuming. Increased consolidation of health care purchasers may alleviate some of the delays.

The growing number of patients with a given health problem in a single system is also leading to the use of what is known as disease management. This practice, which represents a step beyond coordination of care, involves an explicit, systematic population-based approach that identifies patients at risk, intervenes with specific programs of care, and measures clinical and other outcomes.[79] Disease management is a distinctly preventive approach.

CRITICAL PATHWAYS

Although outcome assessment is the aspect of the new concept of quality that has received the most attention, the importance of structure and process must not be minimized. Some would even argue that measures of process (i.e., what is done to a patient) are more sensitive indicators of quality of care than measures of outcome (i.e., what happens to a patient) because poor outcomes do not occur every time an incorrect decision is made.[39] The concept of process measurement is embodied in critical pathways, an increasingly common method of standardizing treatments of high-volume diagnoses. The purpose of critical pathways is to minimize variation by displaying optimal goals for both patients and providers. Such pathways have been developed by a number of groups and organizations and are available commercially, through surgical societies,[80] and in focused publications.[81] The Agency for

Table 5 Selected Internet Health Care Sites[74]

Site Name	Web Address (URL)	Topics and Formats
Adam.com	www.adam.com	Men's, women's, and children's health, as well as diet and nutrition, first aid, and mental health
AMA Health Insight	www.ama-assn.org/consumer.htm	Easily understood information for consumers, plus the capability to search for physicians, hospitals, and medical subjects
AmericasDoctor.com	www.americasdoctor.com	News, bulletin boards, and shopping, plus the ability to chat one-on-one with a health professional
allHealth.com (formerly BetterHealth)	www.allhealth.com	Magazine-type health coverage
Centers for Disease Control and Prevention	www.cdc.gov	Statistics, news, consumer fact sheets, and other resources on diseases
drkoop.com	www.drkoop.com	Health news and resources for patients
Drug Infonet	www.druginfonet.com	A broad range of pharmaceutical information
Hardin Meta Directory	www.lib.uiowa.edu/hardin/md/index.html	Medical links grouped by category
HealthAnswers.com	www.healthanswers.com	Summaries of health news, a drug database, and "health centers" on specific top
HealthCentral.com	www.healthcentral.com	General interest health site
Healthfinder	www.healthfinder.gov	Government directory of authoritative health information
HealthAtoZ.com	www.healthatoz.com	Family-oriented site with personalization features
InteliHealth	www.intelihealth.com	Joint venture of Aetna and Johns Hopkins, summarizing news and rounding up th latest tools and references
Mayo Clinic Health Oasis	www.mayohealth.org	Timely health information from the Mayo Clinic
Mediconsult.com	www.mediconsult.com	Peer-reviewed educational materials and tailor-made responses from top special
Med Help International	www.medhelp.org	Resources for patients and families
MedicineNet.com	www.medicinenet.com	Health news and resources
Medscape	www.medscape.com	Customized home pages on medical topics for physicians
National Institutes of Health	www.nih.gov/health	Umbrella site for the government's health research institutes, including the Nation Library of Medicine
ThriveOnline	www.thriveonline.com	Magazine-style approach on women's health issues
WebMD	www.webmd.com	Medical news, personalized health information, and support communities; now includes OnHealth

Healthcare Research and Quality (AHRQ) has also established practice guidelines, which are available online (http://www.ahrq.gov or http://www.guideline.gov) or through evidence-based practice centers. The guideline.gov site is part of the National Guideline Clearinghouse, a comprehensive repository for clinical practice guidelines and related materials.

Their current popularity notwithstanding, critical pathways do have limitations. Perhaps the most significant of these is that they focus on quality and efficiency of care *after* the decision has been made to admit the patient or perform a procedure. Another limitation is that standardization per se is not tantamount to quality improvement. A third is that not all guidelines adhere to established methodological standards.[82-85] Summaries of the process of pathway development, implementation, and troubleshooting are readily available elsewhere.[86,87]

Assessment of Performance

Given the impact physician decision making has on health care costs, those who pay these costs will naturally seek to assess physician performance. Surgical interventions are particularly ripe for scrutiny because the costs are easily identified, surgical illnesses generally are of relatively short duration, and outcomes are readily quantified. In contrast, the starting and end points of nonsurgical interventions are often difficult to define.

Calls for assessing surgeon performance are typically met with varying degrees of disinterest or, in some cases, defensiveness. Such was the case roughly 100 years ago in Boston, when E. A. Codman crusaded for hospitals and surgeons to publicize their results.[88] It is human nature for each surgeon to believe that he or she is among the best, but the data clearly show considerable variation in outcomes from one surgeon to another.[89] Health care purchasers and hospitals, equipped with modern information systems, are well aware of this variation; large health care purchasers, in particular, use claims data to create provider performance profiles characterizing hospital and physician costs and outcomes.

The issue is not whether such assessments will be made but who will use them and for what purposes. It seems paradoxical that the data used by purchasers to create these profiles often are not readily available to the surgeons who generate them. Even if surgeons are not aware of their practice profiles, they should be aware that these profiles are likely to have personal economic consequences. One survey of managed care organizations found that in the initial physician selection process, 39% of the organizations were moderately or largely influenced by the physician's previous patterns of costs or utilization, and nearly 70% profiled their member physicians.[90] As health care purchasers merge and expand, their profile data will become increasingly centralized; the use of these profiles as economic credentials is then likely to become more widespread. At least one HMO recently noted that practices with high scores on service and quality indicators attracted significantly more new enrollees than practices with lower scores.[91] By preemptively becoming familiar with their outcome data and with how these data are interpreted and used, surgeons will be better positioned to initiate self-assessment and to respond appropriately to external review.

At present, the main limitation of practice profiles is that they cannot fully account for disease severity factors that affect outcome. The data used to make adjustments for disease severity are usually derived either from claims or administrative data or from medical record review.[92] Medical record review is capable of identifying many more severity factors, but it is much more cumbersome and costly, and it still leaves much of the cost variation unaccounted for.[93] Health care purchasers usually make severity adjustments from claims or administrative data instead; accordingly, the validity of this severity adjustment is particularly distrusted. Moreover, in many claims/administrative databases, the frequency of miscoding may be 10% or higher.

Another limitation of practice profiles is that many of the factors known to affect variations in cost and length of stay are not under surgeons' direct control.[94,95] Patient-related variation may result from age, gender, and cultural, ethnic, and socioeconomic factors extrinsic to the medical care system.[96] Selection bias may also affect reports of outcomes.[97] High rates of inadequate functional health literacy are known to have an adverse effect on compliance (and hence outcomes).[98]

Despite these shortcomings, attempts have been made, and continue to be made, to use currently available methods of severity adjustment to compare providers. These attempts have been associated with considerable controversy. In an early effort, HCFA calculated mortality data for individual hospitals using a risk-adjustment model based on DRGs. After many years, HCFA acknowledged the flaws in the associated mortality model and stopped releasing these data. Subsequently, both HCFA (using Medicare data) and some states publicly disclosed provider-specific data on outcomes of cardiac surgery. Their intent was to educate the public regarding the choice of health care providers. Although these educational efforts used more criteria than were available through DRGs alone,[99,100] the profiles remained highly controversial because they still did not adequately account for all the differences in case severity. Because current severity adjustment may not reflect differences attributable to patient selection, surgeons operating on truly high-risk patients will, all other factors being equal, have poorer outcomes than surgeons operating on truly low-risk patients. However, all other factors may not be equal. If the latter group of surgeons operated on the former group's patients, the outcomes might even be worse, and if the former group operated on the latter group's patients, the outcomes might even be better. Such patient selection among practices is a well-recognized phenomenon.[101]

In addition to these concerns, public release of such data may have unintended consequences. It has been suggested that publicizing provider profiles creates incentives to avoid treating high-risk patients so as to lower risk-adjusted mortality.[102,103] Although consumer guides containing these data appeared to improve quality of care, they also appeared to have limited credibility among cardiovascular specialists.[103] Surveys also indicated that the data were of limited value to the target audience (i.e., patients undergoing cardiac surgery).

Nevertheless, provider report cards are increasingly being made available to the general public. One Web site (http://www.healthgrades.com) contains hospital specialty data on cardiac, orthopedic, neurologic, pulmonary, and vascular surgery. Data on transplantation outcomes are available from the United Network for Organ Sharing (http://www.unos.org). Information on obstetrics and oncology will soon be available at a site that will draw information from the HCFA MEDPAR database.

Two self-assessment projects now under way are worth a brief mention here. One study, under the auspices of the American College of Surgeons,[89,104] compares surgeon outcomes for laparoscopic cholecystectomy, radical prostatectomy, total hip replacement, and lumbar laminectomy by using disease response, patient satisfaction, resource utilization, and severity of illness as the outcome measures. The other study is from the Northern New England Cardiovascular Disease Study Group, which has developed a multi-institutional regional model for the continuous improvement of surgical care.[105] The group possesses certain important characteristics: there is no ambiguity of purpose, the data are not owned by any member or subgroup of members, members have an established safe place to work, a forum is set up for discussion, and regular feedback is provided. Using a systems approach, this group effected a 24% reduction in hospital mortality for cardiac surgery and reduced variation in outcomes among group members. The decrease in mortality was significantly greater than that reported by HCFA and by state report cards on similar procedures. Despite concerns that release of such findings would produce unfavorable publicity, no such reaction occurred. It is noteworthy that the process did not level personal criticism at anyone or attempt to identify the proverbial bad apple. Three important conclusions can be drawn from this study: (1) physician-initiated interventions seem more effective than external review in improving quality, (2) a systems approach to quality improvement is better than the bad-apple approach, and (3) it is possible to conduct quality improvement among practice groups that might otherwise be viewed as competitors.

Table 6 **American College of Surgeons Criteria for Use of New Technology**

Has the new technology been considered adequately tested for safety and efficacy?
Is the new technology at least as safe and effective as existing, proven techniques?
Is the individual proposing to perform the new procedure fully qualified to do so?
Is the new technology cost-effective?

Although self-assessment of quality and cost-effectiveness may seem somewhat daunting, the most difficult step may be the willingness to initiate the process. One must accept from the outset that self-assessment is an ongoing process: as with peeling an onion, the initial step will almost inevitably lead to a more involved procedure. Simple data charts may reveal changes or patterns in a surgeon's outcomes or resource consumption that might not otherwise be obvious.[106] Sometimes, merely standardizing a process is enough to improve outcomes significantly. With time, strategies for optimal practice emerge.[107,108]

A number of studies have reported that increased surgeon or hospital volume is associated with favorable outcomes.[109-114] Such findings led the National Cancer Policy Board of the Institute of Medicine and the National Research Council to conclude that patients requiring complicated cancer operations or chemotherapy should be treated at facilities that perform a large number of these procedures. There also appears to be an inverse relation between hospital volume and cost[115,116]; thus, high-volume institutions may have advantages in both the numerator and the denominator of cost-effectiveness. Similar arguments have been made with regard to the issue of surgical subspecialty training.[117]

One must remember, however, that the data in these studies represent probabilities, not absolute relationships.[118] Thus, one cannot conclude that low volume is always associated with poorer outcomes and high volume with better outcomes. Because some measures can be convincingly assessed only in large patient populations, outcome comparisons can be highly problematic when one is dealing with unusual or infrequent cases. Moreover, the relative importance of hospital volume and surgeon volume may vary with specific procedures: complex, team-dependent procedures (e.g., coronary artery bypass grafting) may be more dependent on hospital volume, whereas less complicated procedures may be more dependent on surgeon volume. A large study of eight common surgical procedures used medical record data rather than claims data but was still unable to establish any correlation between institutional operative volume and postoperative mortality.[119] It therefore remains unclear whether practice makes perfect or perfect makes practice.

The empirical relation between surgical volume and outcome delineated in these studies has prompted discussion of regionalization of care,[120] which has proved effective in trauma care. Given the potential for adverse or unintended consequences, however, some believe that it is too soon to use these data as final determinants of quality.[121]

Economics of Surgical Care

To increase cost-effectiveness, surgeons must understand the basis of costs as well as the essential distinction between costs and charges. Charges reflect the price structure but are a poor reflection of actual cost; therefore, there are often substantial variations among institutions regarding the relation between charges and costs. Even when costs alone are considered, there is often considerable variation with apparently similar services. Such cost variation arises because there are substantial differences in cost attribution, even for a relatively standardized accounting system such as that required by HCFA.

The complexity of calculating costs is expressed in the statement "cost is a noun that never really stands alone."[122] Costs are often categorized according to a decision maker's specific needs. Four general categories of health-related costs are commonly used [see Table 7]. From a surgeon's perspective, perhaps the two most important of these are the traceability of costs and the behavior of cost in relation to output or activity.

Cost traceability is classified as direct or indirect. Examples of direct costs are salaries, supplies, rents, and utilities; examples of indirect costs are depreciation and employee benefits. However, not all costs classified as indirect may actually be indirect. In some situations, they could be defined as direct costs, and the specific classification may depend on the given cost objective.

Cost behavior is a particularly important classification method. Variable costs, such as supplies, change in a constant proportional manner with changes in output; fixed costs do not change in response to changes in volume. Semivariable costs (e.g., utilities) include elements of both fixed and variable costs: there is a fixed basic cost per unit of time but also a direct, proportional relation between volume and cost. Semifixed, or step, costs may change with changes in output; however, the changes are not proportional but occur in discrete steps. An example of a semifixed cost is the number of full-time equivalents (FTEs) required for a particular output. If one FTE can produce 2,000 widgets, every 2,000-unit change in widget output will be associated with a change in labor cost: for every 2,000-unit increment in output, one more FTE is needed (with a concomitant increase in costs), and for every 2,000-unit decrement, one fewer FTE is needed (with a concomitant decrease in costs). Unless the step threshold is attained, costs do not change. Thus, a semifixed cost might be considered either a variable cost or a fixed cost, depending on the size of the steps relative to the range of output. Articles that re-

Table 7 Categories and Types of Hospital Costs

Category	Type	Example or Definition
Traceability to the object being costed	Direct Indirect	Salaries, supplies, rents, and utilities Depreciation and employee benefits
Behavior of cost in relation to output or activity	Variable Fixed Semivariable Semifixed	Supply Depreciation Utilities Number of full-time equivalents per step in output
Management responsibility for control	—	Often limited to direct, variable costs
Future versus historical	Avoidable costs Sunk costs Incremental costs Opportunity costs	Costs affected by a decision under consideration Costs not affected by a decision under consideration Changes in total costs resulting from alternative courses of action Value forgone by using a resource in a particular way instead of in its next best alternative way

port cost analyses of clinical interventions may not include this information, thereby further complicating comparisons. A standardized protocol may help resolve this problem.[123]

One can use cost traceability in conjunction with cost behavior by creating a matrix of the two. For example, variable costs can be direct or indirect, and direct costs can be variable, semivariable, semifixed, or fixed. The subcategory to which a given cost is assigned, however, often depends on whose point of view is assumed—the purchaser, the provider, or the patient.[124,125]

Given the nature of costs, the claim that physicians' decisions affect roughly 75% of health care costs is deceiving. A large proportion of health care expenditure is indeed related to the decision to provide care. In most cases, however, the prime consideration is not whether to provide care but which options for care should be selected. Thus, the only potential savings lie in the relatively small differences between these options. Moreover, physicians can affect costs directly only to the extent that they can influence variable costs, which typically constitute no more than 15% to 35% of hospital costs.[125,126]

Even if physicians alone have less power to affect costs than is commonly believed, it is nonetheless true that there is still substantial variation in costs and considerable room for reduction. For instance, data collected in 1996[127] indicated that whereas best practice in regard to expense per 100 minutes of OR time was $511, the national median was $938—a 46% variance.

Improvement of OR efficiency is a universal goal, and specific methods of addressing this issue have been developed.[128-130] Slow turnover times, a common complaint, are variously attributed to nurses, anesthesiologists, and surgeons themselves. Large inventories to satisfy the preferences of individual surgeons also contribute to higher costs. The emergence of laparoscopy has added new dimensions to this challenge.[131] The issues include reusable versus disposable equipment, the different costs of specific types of equipment used to accomplish the same task, and just-in-time inventory. Major pieces of equipment are often duplicated to allow simultaneous performance of similar cases even if this means that they lie unused much of the time. More efficient use of such equipment reduces costs, but such efficiency requires cooperation and coordination among surgical staff members—something that, to date, has not been widespread.

Many institutions find it difficult to identify and then rectify OR inefficiency. To improve efficiency, the surgical team must think of the OR less as a workshop and more as a factory. Surgeons often have a hard time relinquishing the concept of the surgeon as "captain of the ship" and embracing in its stead the idea that all members of the surgical team have interdependent quality and financial goals. However, even if a surgeon becomes substantially more cost-effective, this change alone may not have much effect if the individual surgeon's cost-effectiveness is offset by high hospital or facility costs.

Although ambulatory surgery is frequently touted as a cost-saving measure, the actual cost savings achieved are likely to depend on existing OR capacity and specific payer issues.[132] Team efforts to reduce the costs of trauma care have been demonstrated to be effective.[133,134] Efforts to reduce ICU costs have also shown considerable potential; a specific example is the use of protocols to guide ventilator weaning.[135,136]

Determination of Cost-Effectiveness

In simple terms, cost-effectiveness reflects the cost of a health care intervention in relation to outcome. It is distinct both from cost-benefit analysis, which assesses return on investment (with both the numerator and the denominator expressed in dollars), and from efficiency, which measures outputs divided by inputs (i.e., productivity). Determining the cost-effectiveness of health care is not simple, because analyses of cost-effectiveness may vary widely with respect to the costs and health effects they consider and consequently may produce very different cost-effectiveness ratios for the same intervention. An investigator's perspective often affects attribution of cost, and the effects of comorbid conditions on cost and outcome are also difficult to sort out.

A 1996 consensus statement on these issues recommended standards for improving study comparability and quality.[33,137,138] The consensus panel advocated that calculations be based on the perspective of society as a whole rather than on that of patients, providers, or purchasers. It concluded that "costs incurred by patients or others, such as outpatient medication or home care after hospital discharge, may be irrelevant from [the purchaser] perspective. They may also disregard some outcomes. For example, it may matter little to the HMO or government program how soon patients return to work after an illness, although it may matter a great deal to individuals, their employers, or the government agency responsible for disability payments." Most surgeons probably agree with this approach.

Cost-effective analysis, by definition, compares two approaches to a given problem. In some cases, the comparison is between two interventions, whereas in others, an intervention is compared with no treatment. The numerator of the cost-effectiveness ratio is the difference in cost, and the denominator is the difference in outcome. A particularly powerful form of cost-effectiveness analysis combines clinical decision analysis with sensitivity analysis. Such models estimate cost-effectiveness and identify the criteria that affect care decisions. They have, for example, been applied to management of penetrating colon trauma[139] and to use of carotid endarterectomy in asymptomatic patients.[140]

Like any ratio, the cost-effectiveness ratio may be affected by changes in either the numerator (costs) or the denominator (quality). In addition, it must be remembered that QALYs (often used in the denominator) comprise two distinct aspects: quality of life and the duration of that quality. Thus, an intervention can achieve cost-effectiveness either through relatively low cost or through a relatively high impact on quality, with the quality impact reflected in quality per se, duration, or both. The relative influence of the numerator and the denominator has been studied with respect to a number of surgical procedures [see Table 8]. The interval from the intervention to the point of measurement also affects the estimate of cost-effectiveness.[141,142] Patients are likely to take a long-term perspective on value, whereas providers and purchasers may focus on the short term (e.g., the term of a health care contract).

Cost-effectiveness analysis may be well suited to examination of concerns that delays in surgical referrals may adversely affect outcomes (e.g., with appendicitis).[143] One report noted that for each 10% increase in the accuracy with which appendicitis was diagnosed, there was a 14% increase in the perforation rate.[144] In this case, the cost (i.e., increased morbidity from perforation) may be the price paid for the benefit derived (i.e., greater diagnostic accuracy). Any upfront savings may be lost in the long run because of more advanced or complicated illness.

Data are available on the relative cost-effectiveness of some common medical interventions [see Table 9].[145] According to these data, the median medical intervention cost is $19,000 per year of life. Currently, many place the cost-effectiveness threshold at roughly $50,000 per year of life saved, but this figure is only a framework for decisions. Such thresholds remain both arbitrary and relative and are not necessarily indicative of an intervention's

Table 8 Cost-Effectiveness Studies of Selected Surgical Procedures

Procedure	$/QALY	Δ QALY	Comment
Carotid endarterectomy in asymptomatic patients[139]	8,000	+0.25	The initial cost of endarterectomy is offset by the high cost of care after a major stroke; the relative cost of surgical treatment increases substantially with increasing age, increasing perioperative stroke rate, and decreasing stroke rate during medical management
Routine radiation therapy after conservative surgery for early breast cancer[167]	28,000	+0.35	The ratio is heavily influenced by the cost of radiation therapy and the quality-of-life benefit that results from a decreased risk of local recurrence
Total hip arthroplasty for osteoarthritis of the hip: 60-year-old woman[168]	117,000 in cost savings	+6.9	The cost savings result from the high cost of custodial care associated with dependency
Total hip arthroplasty for osteoarthritis of the hip: 85-year-old man[168]	4,600	+2	—
Endoscopic versus open carpal tunnel release[169]	195	+0.235	Cost-effectiveness is very sensitive to a major complication such as median nerve injury
Lumbar diskectomy[170]	29,200	+0.43	Cost-effectiveness results from the moderate costs of lumbar diskectomy and its substantial effect on quality of life

QALY—quality-adjusted life year

societal value. The prioritized list of benefits of the Oregon state health plan are not based on a stratified list of $/QALYs but on broad input from stakeholders. This plan initially provoked strong criticism, but after several years of operation, it appears to be functioning well.[146] It is noteworthy that a physician-legislator spearheaded this plan.

Challenges for Academic Health Centers

Academic medical centers are not immune to the current changes in health care[147]: they, too, face special challenges. Traditionally, hospital charges were 15% to 30% higher at these centers than at community hospitals, partly because they provided certain highly specialized services and partly because they subsidized a great deal of teaching, research, and social outreach—activities that were implicitly, if not explicitly, considered valuable by society. Currently, as academic medical centers compete in the open market, they carry the burden of having to subsidize education and research from clinical incomes that are becoming increasingly restricted. Moreover, because of their involvement in teaching and research, these institutions have more specialists than are needed for clinical care alone.[148] Estimates of the network size needed to sustain current faculty levels and income are often physically, if not politically, impractical. Not surprisingly, despite their higher costs, teaching hospitals have demonstrated better outcomes (e.g., with hip fracture),[149] even for rather low-technology interventions.[150]

Information about the potential impact of the changing health care environment on academia and future academic practice is now emerging.[151] A study of medical schools in the United States demonstrated an inverse relation between growth in National Institutes of Health awards and managed care penetration during the past decade.[152] Two other studies indicated that increased competitiveness of health care markets seemed to hinder the capacity of academic health centers to conduct clinical research and foster the careers of young faculty members.[153,154] Graduate medical education, another integral part of academic medical centers' overall mission, is also facing change. Support for such education has traditionally been financed solely through HCFA, but this support is being reduced and may be eliminated entirely.

The implication of these changes is that academic medical centers may lose the capacity for producing the evidence on which cost-effective practice must be based—an event that could be tantamount to eating the proverbial seed corn.[155] Managed care organizations have been reluctant to address this issue, and they have yet to find common ground with academic medical centers.[156] One suggestion for reversing this worrisome trend is to change from a cost-based research mission to a value-based one.[157]

Ethical and Legal Issues

With managed care, health professionals increasingly face conflicts between the ethic of undivided loyalty to patients and the pressure to use clinical methods and judgment for social purposes and on behalf of third parties. Although resolving these tensions is certain to be difficult,[158] the medical profession is no stranger to such conflicts. The vast majority of physicians have avoided the temptations inherent in fee-for-service care, and at least as many appear to be avoiding incentives to undertreat. Physicians must also balance their responsibilities to individual patients with their responsibilities to society as a whole. Although some believe that evidence-based practices derived from large populations may not be readily applicable to individual patients, the rationale for this belief is not clear.

The high costs of the terminal stages of life, particularly among patients who languish in critical care units, are also being scrutinized. In this arena, tremendous expenditures are often incurred to secure even the slightest chance of survival. To avoid the dilemma inherent in a physician's making life-ending decisions, increasing emphasis is being placed on patient self-determination; still, active efforts to follow the choices of patients or their families in this situation have not led to reduced costs or improved outcomes.[159] Some studies suggest that the actual savings may be small.[160]

Professional liability under managed care is an important but complex topic.[161] There is no evidence that increasing use of clinical pathways has increased surgeon liability. There is also little question that competition among surgeons will increase and that health care purchasers are likely to use such competition to help negotiate lower fees. Any collective actions surgeons take against this tactic may render them vulnerable to antitrust action.

Table 9 Cost-Effectiveness of Common Surgical Interventions[144]

Intervention	Cost-effectiveness ($/QALY)
Mammography and breast exam (versus exam alone) annually for women 40–49 yr of age	95,000
Mammography and breast exam (versus exam alone) annually for women 40–64 yr of age	17,000
Postsurgical chemotherapy for premenopausal women with breast cancer	18,000
Bone marrow transplant and high (versus standard) chemotherapy for breast cancer	130,000
Cervical cancer screening every 3 yr for women older than 65 yr	≤ 0*
Cervical cancer screening annually (versus every 3 yr) for women older than 65 yr	49,000
Cervical cancer screening annually for women beginning at age 20	82,000
One stool guaiac colon cancer screening for persons older than 40 yr	660
Colonoscopy for colorectal cancer screening for persons older than 40 yr	90,000
Left main coronary artery bypass graft surgery (versus medical management)	2,300
Coronary artery bypass surgery for octogenarians[171]	10,424
Exercise stress test for asymptomatic men 60 yr of age	40
Compression stockings to prevent venous thromboembolism	≤ 0*
Preoperative chest x-ray to detect abnormalities in children	360,000

*Saves more resources than it consumes.
QALY—quality-adjusted life year

The Future

Although American health care is being reshaped, what the final shape will be is by no means clear, in part because there is no agreement on the best strategies for dealing with the current problems. Marketplace competition is attractive because these forces are familiar and have been effective in other aspects of our economy by redistributing income, providing consumer choice, ensuring producer autonomy, increasing economic efficiency, and generating equity. However, market forces fail to address other important economic and cultural aspects of health care[162]; for example, they are difficult to reconcile with the view of health care as a right, with the often strong inverse relation between illness and the ability to pay for health care, with the great pressure for risk selection among purchasers and providers, and with the asymmetry of knowledge between provider and consumer. As a result, market forces are unlikely to be the sole long-term solution to the current problems in health care.

For the medically indigent, managed care has exacerbated the problems of access to health care, and every indication is that these problems will worsen in the near future. Physicians involved with managed care plans and those who practice in areas with high managed care penetration tend to provide less charity care.[163] Teaching hospitals provide a disproportionate share of care to the medically indigent and consequently have become the safety nets of our health care system. There is great concern that managed care will jeopardize the fragile social contracts under which the faculty at academic medical centers contribute unreimbursed and underreimbursed time.[164]

The high cost of health care is undoubtedly a multifactorial problem, with some factors being inherent in the current system and others resulting from the medicalization of social problems. A quick fix is unlikely. A more prudent policy for improving overall health status might be to redirect health care expenditures toward alleviating the social problems contributing to poor health. The problems of health care for the indigent and the uninsured are integrally related to the dysfunctional aspects of the entire system.

Physicians undoubtedly have a role in the ongoing discussion and debate on the future of the health care system in the United States. The magnitude of their input in this debate may depend on their ability to address the larger issues of quality. Specifically, they must address variation in outcomes and variation in intervention rates. Medical decision making must increasingly be based on evidence. If wide variations persist, especially for procedures with clearly proven indications (e.g., carotid endarterectomy), health care purchasers may choose to reimburse only for proven indications and for surgeons with suitably low morbidity and mortality. Such was the case with pneumoreductive surgery for end-stage chronic pulmonary obstructive disease. This procedure became increasingly popular, but there were no hard data to support its long-term efficacy. HCFA then announced that it would pay for the procedure only if it was performed as part of a clinical trial to prove its efficacy; other payors quickly followed suit.[165]

It is curious that at present, quality is not the foremost concern among health care purchasers: competition over price seems to be a much more urgent issue than competition over quality.[166] It seems logical, however, that at some point concerns about how much is being paid will give way to questions about why something is being paid. If surgeons cannot practice within proven indications, they may have little chance of regaining lost autonomy.

Physicians must embrace the vision that it is possible to have a cost-effective health care system with an acceptable balance of choice, quality, and access. Managed care has disrupted many aspects of the health care system, but this may be but a phase on the path toward a better one. To ensure choice quality and access, surgeons must participate in the process of reform of the health care system. Although it appears that physicians are losing more and more autonomy, they are the only parties with the knowledge and skills needed to address the challenges of identifying cost-effective care. The path toward resolution of these issues is likely to produce some dilemmas (i.e., true conflicts in established ethical principles) and some hard choices (i.e., conflicts between these ethical principles and self-interest). Yet if physicians wish to retain (or even recover) their status, they must maintain the profession's highest priorities: quality of care and patient advocacy.

References

1. Iglehart JK: The American health care system: expenditures. N Engl J Med 340:70, 1999
2. Simon CJ, Born PH: Physician earnings in the managed care environment. Health Aff (Millwood) 15:124, 1996
3. Bodenheimer T: The HMO backlash—righteous or reactionary? N Engl J Med 335:1601, 1996
4. Anderson GF, Poullier J-P: Health spending, access, and outcomes: trends in industrialized countries. Health Aff (Millwood) 18:178, 1999
5. Dubois RW, Brook RH: Preventable deaths: who, how often, and why? Ann Intern Med 109:582, 1988
6. Brook RH, Kamberg CJ, Mayer-Oakes A, et al: Appropriateness of health care for the elderly: an analysis of the literature. Health Policy 14:225, 1990
7. Leape LL, Brennan TA, Laird N, et al: The nature of adverse events in hospitalized patients: results of the Harvard Medical Practice Study II. N Engl J Med 324:377, 1991
8. Gawande AA, Thomas EJ, Zinner MJ, et al: The incidence and nature of surgical adverse events in Colorado and Utah in 1992. Surgery 126:66, 1999
9. Chassin MR, Kosecoff J, Park RE, et al: Does inappropriate use explain geographic variations in the use of health services? A study of three procedures. JAMA 253:2533, 1987
10. Bernstein SJ, McGlynn EA, Siu AL, et al: The appropriateness of hysterectomy: a comparison of care in seven health plans. JAMA 269:2398, 1993
11. Phelps CE: The methodologic foundations of studies of the appropriateness of medical care. N Engl J Med 329:1241, 1993
12. Kassirer JP: The quality of care and the quality of measuring it. N Engl J Med 329:1263, 1993
13. Caplan RA, Posner KL, Cheney FW: Effect of outcome on physician judgments of appropriateness of care. JAMA 265:1957, 1991
14. Redelmeir DA, Tversky A: Discrepancy between medical decisions for individual patients and for groups. N Engl J Med 322:1162, 1990
15. Wennberg J, Gittelsohn A: Variations in medical care among small areas. Sci Am 246(4):120, 1982
16. Chaissin MR, Brook RH, Park RE, et al: Variations in the use of medical and surgical services by the Medicare population. N Engl J Med 314:285, 1986
17. The Dartmouth Atlas of Health Care. American Hospital Publishing, Chicago, 1998
18. Birkmeyer JD, Sharp SM, Finlayson SR, et al: Variation profiles of common surgical procedures. Surgery 124:917, 1998
19. Wennberg DE, Kellett MA, Dickens JD, et al: The association between local diagnostic intensity and invasive cardiac procedures. JAMA 275:1161, 1996
20. Eddy DM: Variations in physician practice: the role of uncertainty. Health Aff (Millwood) 3:74, 1984
21. Muir Gray JA: Evidence-Based Health Care: How to Make Health Policy and Management Decisions. Churchill Livingstone, New York, 1997
22. Williamson JW, Goldschmidt PG, Jillson IA: Medical practice information demonstration project: final report. Office of the Asst Secretary of Health, US Department of Health, Education, and Welfare, contract #282-77-0068GS. Policy Research Inc, Baltimore, 1979
23. Howes N, Chagla L, Thorpe M, et al: Surgical practice is evidence based. Br J Surg 84:1220, 1997
24. Leape LL, Park RE, Solomon DH, et al: Does inappropriate use explain small-area variations in the use of health care services? JAMA 263:669, 1990
25. Ashton CM, Petersen NJ, Souchek J, et al: Geographic variations in utilization rates in Veterans Affairs hospitals and clinics. N Engl J Med 340:32, 1999
26. Health Services Research Group: Small area variations: what are they and what do they mean? Can Med Assoc J 146:467, 1992
27. Bunker JP: Surgical manpower: a comparison of operations and surgeons in the United States and in England and Wales. N Engl J Med 282:135, 1970
28. Donabedian A: The Definition of Quality and Approaches to Its Assessment. Explorations in Quality Assessment and Monitoring, vol 1. Health Administration Press, Ann Arbor, Michigan, 1980
29. Stoline AM, Weiner JP: The New Medical Marketplace: A Physician's Guide to the Health Care System in the 1990s. Baltimore, Johns Hopkins University Press, 1993, p 138
30. Chassin MR, Galvin RW: The urgent need to improve health care quality: Institute of Medicine National Roundtable on health care quality. JAMA 280:1000, 1998
31. Reemtsma K, Morgan M: Outcomes assessment: a primer. Bull Am Coll Surg 82:34, 1997
32. Testa MA, Simonson DC: Assessment of quality of life outcomes. N Engl J Med 334:835, 1996
33. Russell LB, Gold MR, Siegel JE, et al: The role of cost-effectiveness analysis in medicine. JAMA 276:1172, 1996
34. Velanovitch V: Using quality of life instruments to assess surgical outcomes. Surgery 126:1, 1999
35. Leplege A, Hunt S: The problem of quality of life in medicine. JAMA 278:47, 1997
36. Eiseman B: Surgical decision making and elderly patients. Bull Am Coll Surg 81:8, 1996
37. Kreder HJ, Wright JG, McLeod R: Outcomes studies in surgical research. Surgery 121:223, 1996
38. Garvin DA: Afterword: Reflections on the future. Curing Health Care: New Strategies for Quality Improvement: A Report on the National Demonstration Project on Quality Improvement in Health Care. Berwick DM, Godfrey AB, Roessner J, Eds. Jossey-Bass Publishers, San Francisco, 1990, p 159
39. Brook RH, Kamberg CJ, McGlynn EA: Health system reform and quality. JAMA 276:476, 1996
40. Bodenheimer T: The American health care system: the movement for improved quality in health care. N Engl J Med 340:488, 1999
41. Epstein AE: Rolling down the runway: the challenges ahead for quality report cards. JAMA 279:1691, 1998
42. Campion FX, Rosenblatt MS: Quality assurance and medical outcomes in the era of cost containment. Surg Clin North Am 76:139, 1996
43. Rutledge R: An analysis of 25 Milliman & Robertson guidelines for surgery: data-driven versus consensus-driven clinical practice guidelines. Ann Surg 228:579, 1998
44. Rigelman RK: Studying a Study and Testing a Test: How to Read the Medical Literature. Little, Brown & Co, Boston, 1981
45. Verrilli D, Welch GH: The impact of diagnostic testing on therapeutic interventions. JAMA 275:1189, 1996
46. Ross NS, Aron DC: Hormonal evaluation of the patient with the incidentally discovered adrenal mass. N Engl J Med 323:1401, 1990
47. Velanovich V: Preoperative laboratory test evaluation. J Am Coll Surg 183:79, 1996
48. Marcello PW, Roberts PL: "Routine" preoperative studies: which studies in which patients? Surg Clin North Am 76:11, 1996
49. Richardson WS, Wilson MC, Guyatt GH, et al: Users' guides to the medical literature: XV. How to use an article about disease probability for differential diagnosis. JAMA 281:1214, 1999
50. Sox HC, Blatt MA, Higgins MC, et al: Medical Decision Making. Butterworth-Heinemann, Boston, 1988
51. Birkmeyer JD, Welch HG: A reader's guide to surgical decision analysis. J Am Coll Surg 184:589, 1997
52. Millilli JJ, Philiponis VS, Nusbaum M: Predicting surgical outcome using Bayesian analysis. J Surg Res 77:45, 1998
53. Birkmeyer JD, Birkmeyer NO: Decision analysis in surgery. Surgery 120:7, 1996
54. Taubes G: Looking for evidence in medicine. Science 272:22, 1996
55. Meinert CL: Beyond CONSORT: need for improved reporting standards for clinical trials. JAMA 279:1487, 1998
56. North American Symptomatic Carotid Trial Collaborators: Beneficial effect of carotid endarterectomy in symptomatic patients with high-grade carotid stenosis. N Engl J Med 325:445, 1991
57. Executive Committee for the Asymptomatic Carotid Atherosclerosis Study: Endarterectomy for asymptomatic carotid artery stenosis. JAMA 273:1421, 1995
58. Tu JV, Hannan EL, Anderson GM, et al: The fall and rise of carotid endarterectomy in the United States and Canada. N Engl J Med 339:1441, 1998
59. Wennberg DE, Lucas FL, Birkmeyer JD, et al: Variation in carotid endarterectomy in the Medicare population: trial hospitals, volumes, and patient characteristics. JAMA 279:1278, 1998
60. Chassin MR: Appropriate use of carotid endarterectomy. N Engl J Med 339:1468, 1998
61. Rao PM, Rhea JT, Novelline RA, et al: Effect of computed tomography of the appendix on treatment of patients and use of hospital resources. N Engl J Med 338:141, 1998
62. Gill BD, Jenkins JR: Cost-effective evaluation and management of the acute abdomen. Surg Clin North Am 76:71, 1996
63. Wright JC, Weinstein MC: Gains in life expectancy from medical interventions—standardizing data on outcomes. N Engl J Med 339:380, 1998
64. Black WC, Welch HG: Advances in diagnostic imaging and overestimations of disease prevalence and the benefits of therapy. N Engl J Med 328:1237, 1993
65. Naylor CD, Guyatt GH: Users' guides to the medical literature: X. How to use an article reporting variations in the outcomes of health services. JAMA 275:554, 1996
66. Naylor CD, Guyatt GH: Users' guides to the medical literature: XI. How to use an article about clinical utilization review. JAMA 275:1435, 1996
67. Guyatt GH, Naylor CD, Juniper E, et al: Users' guides to the medical literature: XII. How to use articles about health related quality of life. JAMA 277:1232, 1997
68. Drummond MF, Richardson WS, O'Brien BJ, et al: Users' guides to the medical literature: XIII. How to use an article on economic analysis of clinical practice. A. Are the results of the study valid? JAMA 277:1552, 1997
69. O'Brien BJ, Heyland D, Richardson WS, et al: Users' guides to the medical literature: XIII. How to use an article on economic analysis of clinical practice. B. What are the results and will they help me in caring for my patients? JAMA 277:1802, 1997
70. Dans AL, Dans LF, Guyatt GH, et al: Users' guides to the medical literature: XIV. How to decide on the applicability of clinical trials to your patients. JAMA 279:545, 1998
71. Richardson WS, Detsky AS: Users' guides to the medical literature: VII. How to use a clinical decision analysis. A. Are the results of the study valid? JAMA 273:1292, 1995
72. Barratt AA, Irwig L, Glasziou P, et al: Users' guides to the medical literature: XVII. How to use guidelines and recommendations about screening. JAMA 281:2029, 1999

73. Randolph AG, Haynes RB, Wyatt JC, et al: Users' guides to the medical literature: XVIII. How to use an article evaluating the clinical impact of a computer-based clinical decision support system. JAMA 282:67, 1999
74. Davis R, Miller L: Millions scour the Web to find medical information. USA Today, July 14, 1999
75. Soot LC, Moneta GL, Edwards JM: Vascular surgery and the Internet. J Vasc Surg 30:84, 1999
76. Statement on issues to be considered before new surgical technology is applied to the care of patients. Bull Am Coll Surg 80:46, 1995
77. Legorreta AP, Silber JH, Constantino GN, et al: Increased cholecystectomy rate after the introduction of laparoscopic cholecystectomy. JAMA 270:1429, 1993
78. Selker HP, Beshansky JR, Paulker SG, et al: The epidemiology of delays in teaching hospitals. Med Care 27:112, 1989
79. Epstein RS, Sherwood LM: From outcomes research to disease management: a guide to the perplexed. Ann Intern Med 124:832, 1996
80. Gadacz TR, Adkins RB, O'Leary JP: General surgical clinical pathways: an introduction. Am Surg 63:107, 1997
81. Cost Effectiveness in Surgery. Rossi RL, Cady B, Eds. Surg Clin North Am 76:1, 1996
82. Hayward RSA, Wilson MC, Tunis SR, et al: Users' guides to the medical literature. VIII. How to use clinical practice guidelines. A. Are the recommendations valid? JAMA 274:570, 1995
83. Wilson MC, Hayward RSA, Tunis SR, et al: Users' guides to the medical literature. VIII. How to use clinical practice guidelines. B. What are the recommendations and will they help you in caring for your patients? JAMA 274:1630, 1995
84. Shaneyfelt TM, Mayo-Smith MF, Rothwangl J: Are guidelines following guidelines? The methodological quality of clinical practice guidelines in the peer-reviewed medical literature. JAMA 281:1900, 1999
85. Cook D, Giacomini M: The trials and tribulations of clinical practice guidelines. JAMA 281:1950, 1999
86. Pearson SD, Goulart-Fisher D, Lee TH: Critical pathways as a strategy for improving care: problems and potential. Ann Intern Med 123:941, 1995
87. Hoyt DB: Clinical practice guidelines. Am J Surg 173:32, 1997
88. Passaro E, Organ CH: Ernest A. Codman: the improper Bostonian. Bull Am Coll Surg 84:16, 1999
89. Tunner WS, Christy JP, Whipple TL: System for outcomes-based report card. Bull Am Coll Surg 82:18, 1997
90. Gold MR, Hurley R, Lake T, et al: A national survey of the arrangements managed-care plans make with physicians. N Engl J Med 333:1678, 1995
91. Larkin H: Doctors starting to feel report cards' impact. AMA News 42:1, 1999
92. Risk Adjustment for Measuring Health Care Outcomes. Iezzoni LI, Ed. Health Administration Press, Ann Arbor, Michigan, 1994
93. Horn SD, Sharkey PD, Buckle JM, et al: The relationship between severity of illness and hospital length of stay and mortality. Med Care 29:305, 1991
94. Rhodes RS, Sharkey PD, Horn SD: Effect of patient factors on hospital costs for major bowel surgery: implications for managed health care. Surgery 117:443, 1995
95. Kalman PG, Johnston KW: Sociological factors are major determinants of prolonged hospital stay following abdominal aneurysm repair. Surgery 119:690, 1996
96. Salem-Schatz S, Moore G, Rucker M, et al: The case for case-mix adjustment in practice profiling: when good apples look bad. JAMA 272:871, 1994
97. Melton JL: Selection bias in the referral of patients and the natural history of surgical conditions. Mayo Clin Proc 60:880, 1985
98. Williams MV, Parker RM, Baker DW, et al: Inadequate functional health literacy among patients at two public hospitals. JAMA 274:1677, 1995
99. Hannan EL, Kilburn H, Racz M, et al: Improving the outcomes of coronary artery bypass surgery in New York State. JAMA 271:761, 1994
100. Green J, Winfield N: Report cards on cardiac surgeons: assessing New York State's approach. N Engl J Med 332:1229, 1995
101. Rhodes RS, Krasniak CJ, Jones PK: Factors affecting length of stay for femoropopliteal bypass: implications of the DRGs. N Engl J Med 314:153, 1986
102. Chaissin MR, Hannan EL, DeBunno BA: Benefits and hazards of reporting medical outcomes publicly. N Engl J Med 334:394, 1996
103. Schneider EC, Epstein AM: Influence of cardiac surgery performance report cards on referral practices and access to care. N Engl J Med 335:251, 1996
104. Turner WS: Committee on Socioeconomic Issues. Bull Am Coll Surg 83:40, 1998
105. O'Connor GT, Plume SK, Olmstead EM, et al: A regional intervention to improve the hospital mortality associated with coronary artery bypass graft surgery. JAMA 275:841, 1996
106. Hansen FC: What does your future hold: capitation or decapitation? Bull Am Coll Surg 81:12, 1996
107. Ruffin M: Developing and using a data repository for quality improvement: the genesis of IRIS. Jt Com J Qual Improv 21:512, 1995
108. Clare M, Sargent D, Moxley R, et al: Reducing health care delivery costs using clinical paths: a case study on improving hospital profitability. J Health Care Finance 21:48, 1995
109. Sosa JA, Bowman HM, Tielsch JM, et al: The importance of surgeon experience for clinical and economic outcomes from thyroidectomy. Ann Surg 228:320, 1998
110. Sosa JA, Bowman HM, Gordon TA, et al: Importance of hospital volume in the overall management of pancreatic cancer. Ann Surg 228:429, 1998
111. Birkmeyer JD, Finlayson SRG, Tosteson ANA, et al: Effect of hospital volume on in-hospital mortality with pancreaticoduodenectomy. Surgery 125:250, 1999
112. Begg CB, Cramer LD, Hoskins WJ, et al: Impact of hospital volume on operative mortality for major cancer surgery. JAMA 280:1747, 1998
113. Pearce WH, Parker MA, Feinglass J, et al: The importance of surgeon volume and training in outcomes for vascular surgical procedures. J Vasc Surg 29:768, 1999
114. Harmon JW, Tang DG, Gordon TA, et al: Hospital volume can serve as a surrogate for surgeon volume for achieving excellent outcomes in colorectal resection. Ann Surg 230:404, 1999
115. Trends in the concentration of six surgical procedures under PPS and their implications for patient mortality and medicare cost. Technical report #E-87-08. Project Hope, Chevy Chase, Maryland, 1988
116. Gordon TA, Burleyson GP, Tielsch JM, et al: The effect of regionalization on cost and outcome for one general high-risk surgical procedure. Ann Surg 221:43, 1995
117. Porter GA, Soskolne CL, Yakimets WW, et al: Surgeon-related factors and outcome in rectal cancer. Ann Surg 277:157, 1998
118. Houghton A: Variance in outcome of surgical procedures. Br J Surg 81:653, 1994
119. Khuri SF, Henderson WG, Hur K, et al: The relationship of surgical volume to outcome in eight common operations: results from the VA National Quality Improvement Program. Ann Surg 230:414, 1999
120. Luft HS, Bunker JP, Enthoven AC: Should operations be regionalized? the empiric relation between surgical volume and mortality. N Engl J Med 301:1364, 1979
121. Hannan EL: The relation between volume and outcome in health care. N Engl J Med 340:1677, 1999
122. Cleverly WO: Essentials of Healthcare Finance, 2nd ed. Aspen Publishers Inc, Rockville, Maryland, 1986, p 191
123. Balas EA, Kretschmer RAC, Gnann W, et al: Interpreting cost analyses of clinical interventions. JAMA 279:54, 1998
124. Rhodes RS: How much does it cost? how much can be saved? Surgery 125:102, 1999
125. Roberts RR, Frutos PW, Ciavarella GG, et al: Distribution of variable vs fixed costs of hospital care. JAMA 281:644, 1999
126. Taheri PA, Butz DA, Griffes LC, et al: Physician impact on the total cost of care. Ann Surg (in press)
127. The Rising Tide. Emergence of a New Competition Standard in Health Care. Advisory Board Co, Washington, DC, 1996
128. Kanich DG, Byrd JR: How to increase efficiency in the operating room. Surg Clin North Am 76:161, 1996
129. Clockwork Surgery. Re-engineering the Hospital, Vol I. The Advisory Board Company, Washington, DC, 1992
130. The Surgery Capacity Ceiling. Re-engineering the Hospital, Vol II. The Advisory Board Company, Washington, DC, 1992
131. Newman RM, Traverso LW: Cost-effective minimally invasive surgery: what procedures make sense? World J Surg 23:415, 1999
132. Rhodes RS: Ambulatory surgery and the societal cost of surgery. Surgery 116:938, 1994
133. Taheri PA, Wahl WL, Butz DA, et al: Trauma service cost: the real story. Ann Surg 227:720, 1998
134. Taheri PA, Butz DA, Watts CM, et al: Trauma services: a profit center? J Am Coll Surg 188:349, 1999
135. Horst HM, Mouro D, Hall-Jenssens RA, et al: Decrease in ventilation time with a standardized weaning process. Arch Surg 13:483, 1998
136. Thomsen GE, Pope D, East TD, et al: Clinical performance of a rule-based decision support system for mechanical ventilation of ARDS patients. Proc Annu Symp Comput Appl Med Care 1993, p 339
137. Weinstein MC, Siegel JE, Gold MR, et al: Recommendations of the Panel on Cost-Effectiveness in Health and Medicine. JAMA 276:1253, 1996
138. Siegel JE, Weinstein MC, Russell LB, et al: Recommendations for reporting cost-effectiveness analyses. JAMA 276:1339, 1996
139. Brasel KJ, Borgstrom DC, Weigelt JA: Management of penetrating colon trauma: a cost-utility analysis. Surg 125:471, 1999
140. Cronenwett JL, Birkmeyer JD, Nackman GB, et al: Cost-effectiveness of carotid endarterectomy in asymptomatic patients. J Vasc Surg 25:298, 1997
141. Schermerhorn ML, Birkmeyer J, Gould DA, et al: The impact of operative mortality on cost-effectiveness in the UK small aneurysm trial. J Vasc Surg 31:217, 2000
142. Heudebert GR, Marks R, Wilcox CM, et al: Choice of long-term strategy for the management of patients with severe esophagitis: A cost-utility analysis. Gastroenterology 112:1078, 1997
143. Cacioppo JC, Dietrich NA, Kaplan G, et al: The consequences of current restraints on surgical treatment of appendicitis. Am J Surg 157:276, 1989
144. Wen SW, Naylor CD: Diagnostic accuracy and short-term surgical outcomes in cases of suspected acute appendicitis. CMAJ 153:888, 1995
145. Tengs TO, Adams ME, Pliskin JS, et al: Five-hundred life-saving interventions and their cost-effectiveness. Risk Anal 15:369, 1995
146. Bodenheimer T: The Oregon health plan—lessons for the nation. N Engl J Med 337:651, 720, 1997
147. Iglehart J: Support for academic medical centers: revisiting the 1997 Balanced Budget Act. N Engl J Med 341:299, 1999

148. Billi JE, Wise CG, Bills EA, et al: Potential effects of managed care on specialty practice at a university medical center. N Engl J Med 333:979, 1995
149. Taylor DH, Whelan DJ, Sloan FA: The effects of admission to a teaching hospital on the cost and quality of care for Medicare beneficiaries. N Engl J Med 340:293, 1999
150. Kassirer JP: Hospitals, heal yourselves. N Engl J Med 340:309, 1999
151. Simon SR, Pan RJD, Sullivan AM, et al: Views of managed care: a survey of students, residents, faculty, and deans at medical schools in the United States. N Engl J Med 340:928, 1999
152. Moy E, Mazzaschi AJ, Levin RJ, et al: Relationship between National Institutes of Health research awards to US medical schools and managed care market penetration. JAMA 278:217, 1997
153. Campbell EG, Weissman JS, Blumenthal D: Relationship between market competition and the activities and attitudes of medical school faculty. JAMA 278:222, 1997
154. Weissman JS, Saglam D, Campbell EG, et al: Market forces and unsponsored research in academic health centers. JAMA 281:1093, 1999
155. Thompson JC: Seed corn: impact of managed care on medical education and research. Ann Surg 223:453, 1996
156. LaRosa JC, Whelton P, Litwin MS: Academic medicine and managed care: seeking common ground. Acad Med 74:488, 1999
157. Krauss K, Smith J: Rejecting conventional wisdom: how academic medical centers can regain their leadership positions. Acad Med 72:571, 1997
158. Bloche MG: Clinical loyalties and the social purposes of medicine. JAMA 281:268, 1999
159. The SUPPORT Principal Investigators: A controlled trial to improve care for seriously ill hospitalized patients. JAMA 274:1591, 1995
160. Emanuel EJ, Emanuel LL: The economics of dying—the illusion of cost saving at the end of life. N Engl J Med 330:540, 1994
161. Manuel B: Physician liability under managed care. J Am Coll Surg 183:537, 1996
162. Ginsberg E: A cautionary note on market reforms in health care. JAMA 274:1633, 1995
163. Cunningham PJ, Grossman JM, St Peter RF, et al: Managed care and physicians' provision of charity care. JAMA 281:1087, 1999
164. Shea S, Nickerson KG, Tenebaum J, et al: Compensation to a department and its faculty members for teaching of medical students and house staff. N Engl J Med 334:162, 1996
165. Bodily KC: Surgeons and technology. Am J Surg 177:351, 1999
166. Kassirer JP, Angell M: Quality and the medical marketplace—following elephants. N Engl J Med 335:883, 1996
167. Hayman JA, Hillner BE, Harris JR, et al: Cost-effectiveness of routine radiation therapy following conservative surgery for early-stage breast cancer. J Clin Oncol 16:1022, 1998
168. Chang RW, Pellisier JM, Hazen GB: A cost-effectiveness analysis of total hip arthroplasty for osteoarthritis of the hip. JAMA 275:858, 1996
169. Chung KC, Walters MR, Greenfield ML, et al: Endoscopic versus open carpal tunnel release: a cost-effectiveness analysis. Plast Reconstr Surg 102:1089, 1998
170. Malter AD, Larson EB, Urban N, et al: Cost-effectiveness of lumbar discectomy for the treatment of herniated intervertebral disc. Spine 21:1048, 1996
171. Sollano JA, Rose EA, Williams DL, et al: Cost-effectiveness of coronary artery bypass surgery in octogenarians. Ann Surg 228:297, 1998

37 NONEMERGENCY SURGERY: INITIAL EVALUATION, PREOPERATIVE PLANNING, PERIOPERATIVE ISSUES, AND POSTOPERATIVE CARE

Nicolas V. Christou, M.D., and Richard B. Reiling, M.D.

Elements of Preoperative Planning

The objective of preoperative planning for nonemergency surgery is to ensure that the operation is performed with minimal risk and maximum benefit to the patient and, given the current economic climate, in a cost-effective manner. This objective informs all stages of preoperative planning, from the initial visit through clinical and laboratory evaluation to selection of procedure and site.

The purpose of the initial visit is twofold: first, to determine whether there is any known or unsuspected coexisting disease that is sufficiently threatening to delay, modify, or preclude operation; and second, to apprise patient and family of the risks and benefits of the proposed surgical therapy. Postponement of operation is not justified unless the benefits of treating a coexisting disease outweigh the perceived detriments of delay.

A careful history should be taken and a thorough physical examination performed to evaluate the presenting complaint, to screen for related problems, and to assess operative risk. In the first 48 hours after operation (the perioperative risk period), patients are at risk for complications related to anesthesia and to the surgical procedure itself (e.g., myocardial infarction, stroke, respiratory failure, metabolic derangements, and technical problems such as perioperative hemorrhage). From 48 hours to 30 days after operation (the postoperative risk period), a different set of complications (e.g., pulmonary embolism, surgical site infection, peritoneal infection, the systemic inflammatory response syndrome [SIRS], and the multiple organ dysfunction syndrome [MODS]) may become apparent. When evaluating the risk associated with a particular surgical procedure, one must consider the patient's ability to withstand the potential complications of both risk periods [*see* Discussion, *below*]. The available means of evaluating risk during the first period are more standardized than those of evaluating risk during the longer, second period. Patient factors that affect overall risk (encompassing both risk periods) include the nature and duration of the illness necessitating operation, the presence or absence of other underlying illnesses (e.g., pulmonary, cardiovascular, hepatic, and renal), age, nutritional status, and immune competence. Surgical risk factors include the type of anesthesia selected, the operation to be performed, the urgency of the situation, the experience of the surgical team, and the hospital resources available, including special monitoring and critical nursing care. Unfortunately, objective data on the impact of many of these factors are lacking, and as a result, assessment of risk is still largely intuitive and is based on data acquired from the history and the physical examination.

One should select laboratory tests not only to evaluate the primary surgical condition but also to look for risk factors or, if the patient has cancer, to determine the likelihood and degree of metastasis. One should then use this information to determine the direction of subsequent study and the appropriate depth of study before operation. Consultation may follow laboratory testing, depending on the patient's condition and one's own expertise. Long-range preparation for operation includes stabilization of cardiac, pulmonary, vascular, endocrine, and metabolic conditions. Current medications may have to be stopped or supplemented perioperatively.

The trend toward shortened hospital stays has made the timing of admission a matter of concern for patient and surgeon. Many procedures are now done on an ambulatory basis or even in a free-standing ambulatory facility; in other cases, the patient is admitted on the day of operation even though an in-hospital postoperative stay is anticipated. These arrangements, while liberating hospital beds, have forced changes in the surgical approach to preoperative workup and preparation. One no longer has the luxury of becoming acquainted with the patient over a period of several days before the operation. Laboratory tests and x-rays are done on an outpatient basis and must be reviewed before the patient is admitted to determine whether further investigation or correction is necessary. Bowel preparation is started at home. Efforts are made to identify those selected patients who must be admitted at least one day before operation, particularly those who will require invasive preoperative monitoring in the ICU.

Patients referred for surgical management may be seen in one's office, in the emergency department, or in a hospital room. Wherever the first visit takes place, it is important to create an environment in which one can initiate a trusting relationship with the patient in addition to achieving the twofold purpose mentioned earlier.

History and Physical Examination

The history and the physical examination are the most effective means of identifying risk factors associated with coexisting disease. Diagnostically, the history is three times more productive than the physical examination and 11 times more effective than routine laboratory tests. Combined with the physical examination, the history is diagnostic in 75 to 90 percent of patients.[1] Information about the patient's current disease or any other disease processes present helps to guide subsequent testing during the initial visit. The referring physician may have carried out tests that are pertinent to the patient's current illness, and the results of these tests can be extremely useful in planning the operation. Copies of all laboratory test results and radiologic images should be requested. For example, a patient with cholelithiasis may have undergone preoperative ultrasonography, or a patient referred for hepatic resection may have undergone preoperative angiography. The original angiograms, CT scans, barium enema films, and other images should be personally reviewed with a radiologist. A good philosophy to adopt is, if one has not personally seen the test result, one should assume that the test has not been done. In cases of equivocal diagnosis, slides of pathology specimens obtained by the referring physician must be reviewed.

Certain findings in the physical examination are particularly important signals of unsuspected coexisting disease: abnormal blood pressure; abnormal peripheral pulses; systolic heart murmurs; adenopathy; abnormal findings on pelvic, rectal, or breast examination or on lung auscultation; and eye, ear, nose, or throat disorders. Particular attention should be paid to the cardiovascular system, the respiratory system, nutritional status, the endocrine system, the hematologic system, existing infection, current medications, and the social history.

CARDIOVASCULAR SYSTEM

Significant cardiovascular risk factors include angina pectoris, dyspnea and evidence of right-sided or left-sided heart failure, arrhythmias other than sinus arrhythmia, more than five ventricular ectopic beats a minute, aortic stenosis with left ventricular hypertrophy, mitral regurgitation, and previous myocardial infarction.

The risk of intraoperative or postoperative myocardial infarction is much higher in patients who recently had an infarction. In large retrospective reviews, 37 percent of patients experienced reinfarction when they were operated on within three months of an infarction. The incidence of reinfarction decreased to 16 percent when the operation was performed between three and six months after infarction and to 4.5 percent when the operation was performed more than six months afterward.[2] The presence of a murmur is an indication for full evaluation of cardiac function and, in certain cases, for antibiotic prophylaxis.

Likewise, the presence of a carotid thrill or bruit may be an indication for further testing to assess the need for a carotid endarterectomy before elective surgery. Hypertension is frequently associated with increased peripheral resistance, cardiac hypertrophy, increased ventricular stroke work, and impaired renal blood flow. The sudden onset of hypertension or a persistent increase in blood pressure in a patient whose BP has been well controlled by antihypertensive medications may warrant postponement of elective surgery. Selective screening of high-risk patients for primary hyperaldosteronism, pheochromocytoma, renal vascular disease, and Cushing's syndrome should be undertaken.[3-5] Patients with essential hypertension should not undergo elective surgery until their BP is adequately controlled by pharmacological means.

RESPIRATORY SYSTEM

Testing of pulmonary function may be indicated on the basis of physical findings (e.g., cough, wheezing, dyspnea on exertion, rales, or rhonchi) or a history of cigarette smoking. In addition to pulmonary symptoms, a history of cardiac insufficiency, obesity, or poor oral hygiene may be an indication for further study of pulmonary function. Forced inspiratory volume can be directly measured with a handheld spirometer. Limited pulmonary reserve may be revealed by asking the patient to climb one or two flights of stairs.

NUTRITIONAL STATUS

In 1936, Studley demonstrated that weight loss was a basic indicator of operative risk.[6] Loss of more than 12 percent of body weight during the previous six months is frequently associated with postoperative complications, including delayed wound healing, decreased immunologic competence, and inability to meet the demand for respiratory effort. Peripheral edema and signs of specific vitamin deficiency are suggestive of severe malnutrition. Obese patients frequently require operation for conditions such as biliary disease, osteoarthritis, and hernia. Preoperative weight loss is encouraged, but the results are usually disappointing. Morbidly obese patients present specific challenges in preoperative management; they are at particular risk for cardiovascular and respiratory complications, wound infection, and thromboembolism.

ENDOCRINE SYSTEM

Endocrine-related risk factors include hyperthyroidism, hypothyroidism, diabetes mellitus, pheochromocytoma, adrenal insufficiency, and steroid therapy within the previous six months. Certain endocrine conditions should be corrected, or at least stabilized, while the patient awaits admission. Graves' disease, for example, calls for a specific preoperative protocol, including administration of thyroid hormone blockers, iodine, and beta blockers. Hypothyroidism is treated with synthetic thyroid hormone. Patients with pheochromocytoma should not undergo operation until adrenergic blockade is adequate.

HEMATOLOGIC SYSTEM

Clotting abnormalities are best detected by questioning the patient about familial or personal episodes of unusual bleeding.[7] Corroborative findings on physical examination may include petechiae, purpura, or splenomegaly. Risk factors for postoperative phlebothrombosis and, secondarily, pulmonary embolism include hypercoagulability (from antithrombin III deficiency, oral contraceptives, or malignancy), stasis (from obstructed venous outflow, congestive heart failure, or immobility), and vascular endothelial injury (from operation or trauma).

EXISTING INFECTION

Existing infection—in particular, urinary tract infection and pneumonia—must be identified before operation. This is an especially relevant consideration in patients who are to receive a prosthetic implant, such as an artificial heart valve or an aortic graft. Bacteremia resulting from manipulation of an infected urinary tract can predispose to graft infection, which would be catastrophic for the patient. Any infection identified preoperatively in these patients should be treated before elective surgery.

CURRENT MEDICATIONS AND SOCIAL HISTORY

The patient's current medications should be listed and any allergies noted. A careful social history should be obtained to uncover risk factors associated with smoking, alcohol ingestion, and drug abuse. Patients with a significant history of smoking may require further evaluation of cardiac, vascular, and respiratory function. Chronic alcohol ingestion is often associated with CNS and hepatic dysfunction as well as malnutrition. Chronic I.V. drug abuse may be associated with venous thrombosis, hepatitis, acquired immunodeficiency syndrome (AIDS), malnutrition, subacute bacterial endocarditis, and psychiatric disturbance.

Preoperative Tests

The role of routine screening tests has come under review, and fewer tests are now being ordered for otherwise healthy patients undergoing elective procedures.[8] The patient's benefit remains the paramount concern; however, in this cost-conscious era, society exerts pressure on physicians not to order laboratory tests without taking cost and cost-effectiveness into account. Thus, surgeons must know not only the charges for tests but also their performance characteristics, their sensitivity and specificity, their proper sequencing, their risks, and, most of all, their clinical relevance. A test's predictive value depends on its sensitivity (its ability to detect a disease) and its specificity (the probability that the patient has the disease if the test is positive).

The value of routine screening tests both for managing known primary disease and for detecting unsuspected disease has been thoroughly studied[9,10]: the consensus is that routine preoperative laboratory testing is neither useful nor cost-effective. Appropriate selection of preoperative laboratory tests is based on age, gender, the presence or absence of concomitant medical diseases, and the type of operation to be performed. Routine screening tests are diagnostically helpful in only five percent of patients, and they aid in management only nine percent of the time. Sixty percent of patients who undergo routine screening tests show no evidence of recognizable disease.[11] In only 0.22 percent of these patients do the screening tests provide information that influences management.[12]

COMPLETE BLOOD COUNT

A complete blood count (CBC) usually includes determination of the hemoglobin level or the hematocrit, a white blood cell (WBC) count, and a differential count. The CBC is unexpectedly abnormal in three percent of routine hospital admissions.[13,14] Measurement of the hemoglobin concentration is justified in females of any age (the incidence of abnormalities is six to 13 percent) but probably not in males. The WBC count is abnormal in fewer than 0.5 percent of asymptomatic patients whose primary disease is not associated with leukocytosis. Among patients whose total leukocyte count is normal, the differential count contributes to patient care in only 2.8 percent. Healthy pediatric patients five years of age or older who are scheduled for minor surgery do not require routine hemoglobin determinations.[15]

SERUM ELECTROLYTES, BLOOD UREA NITROGEN, AND BLOOD GLUCOSE

The incidence of serum abnormalities on routine admission tests is low. One study found that in only 0.2 percent of hospitalized patients did such tests reveal abnormalities that had not been previously suspected on the basis of the history and the physical examination,[12] and 80 percent of the abnormalities detected were of no clinical significance. Serum electrolyte levels should be routinely determined before operation in patients who are taking diuretics or digitalis, those who have renal disease, those who have heart disease, and those who are vomiting or suffer from disorders in which abnormal electrolyte loss is expected. The frequency of diabetes and the benefits of early detection justify the inclusion of a fasting blood glucose level as a routine test on hospital admission. The overall incidence of diabetes in the general population is about one percent, and about five percent of persons older than 40 years have hyperglycemia. Unexpected abnormalities in blood glucose occur in about 0.4 percent of hospitalized patients.

URINALYSIS

The purpose of a screening urinalysis is to detect unsuspected diabetes, renal disease, or urinary tract infection. The dipstick is a convenient first-line screening study for glucose, blood, or bacteria in the urine. With this method, the incidence of false positive results for hematuria is 13 to 16 percent.[16]

CHEST X-RAY

Of the 52 million chest x-rays obtained annually in the United States, 60 percent are done on a routine basis. Abnormal findings on routine x-rays are rare. The yield is almost negligible in patients younger than 30 years; the incidence of abnormalities begins to reach and exceed 20 percent in patients older than 40 years, but most abnormalities are caused by cardiomegaly. Nineteen percent of abnormalities are related to chronic respiratory disease; most of these are known before the chest x-ray.[17] A lateral view usually does not yield information that significantly affects the diagnosis unless the patient is older than 44 years.[18] Abnormalities detected on a screening chest film seldom alter management. A preoperative chest x-ray does, however, provide a baseline for comparison that may be useful if postoperative complications arise.[19] Accordingly, the indications for posteroanterior and lateral chest x-rays in asymptomatic patients include (1) known pulmonary or cardiac disease, (2) anticipated thoracotomy, (3) age greater than 40 years, (4) high risk for postoperative pulmonary complications, and (5) a positive tuberculin test or high risk for unsuspected tuberculosis or pulmonary infection.

ELECTROCARDIOGRAPHY

Electrocardiography is justified in men older than 40 years and in women older than 55 years.[20] Abnormalities that may affect treatment include ST segment changes suggestive of ischemia, short PR intervals, prolonged QT intervals, and tall, peaked T waves. Atrial fibrillation or flutter, second- or third-degree atrioventricular block, premature ventricular or atrial contractions, left or right ventricular hypertrophy, evidence of a myocardial infarction, a previous abnormal electrocardiogram, and aberrant ventricular conduction may also be indications for treatment alterations.[8,21]

CLOTTING PROFILE

Whether a preoperative clotting profile is appropriate depends in part on the danger of unexpected bleeding: for example, subcutaneous oozing is less threatening than intracranial bleeding. In the absence of clinical evidence of a bleeding tendency, there is only a 0.008 percent probability that a clotting disorder will be present during operation.[22] One study found that although abnormalities in coagulation are common in patients undergoing operations for gynecologic malignancy, preoperative testing for occult coagulopathy provides little clinically useful information.[23] Risk factors in clinical screening include bleeding or clotting problems during a previous operation, a family history of bleeding, and the use of medications that interfere with clotting (e.g., anticoagulants, birth control pills, or nonsteroidal anti-inflammatory drugs). A clotting profile usually includes the prothrombin time, the partial thromboplastin time, and a platelet count. The value of the activated partial thromboplastin time has been challenged. Some abnormality can be expected in 14 percent of preoperative clotting profiles, but 84 percent of these abnormalities are insignificant. A retrospective review of preoperative clotting profiles showed that in 61 to 92 percent of patients, the tests were apparently indicated, but the incidence of abnormalities never exceeded 0.2 percent.[24] Indications for a routine preoperative clotting profile include (1) a history of a bleeding tendency or evidence of abnormal bleeding on physical examination, (2) very young age, because a history of bleeding is necessarily of limited extent in children, and (3) scheduled peripheral vascular or cardiac surgery.

TYPE AND CROSSMATCH

If one anticipates significant blood loss during the procedure, preoperative typing or crossmatching of blood is indicated. Any blood loss amounting to more than 1,000 to 1,500 ml (or 20 ml/kg) should be replaced. A transfusion index, which measures how often transfusions are needed in a given operation, should determine the need for preoperative crossmatching. The risk of acquiring hepatitis or AIDS has prompted critical review of the need for intraoperative transfusions. Formerly, the critical hemoglobin level indicating a need for preoperative transfusion (the so-called transfusion trigger) was considered to be 10 g/dl. More recently, however, a National Institutes of Health consensus panel suggested that a transfusion threshold of 7 g/dl might be permissible.[25,26]

STOOL EXAMINATION FOR BLOOD

The benefit of fecal occult blood testing in patients hospitalized for an elective surgical procedure who have no GI symptoms is uncertain. Preoperative evaluation provides an opportunity to look for blood in the stool as a marker of colorectal cancer. However, even when performed on three specimens and only in patients older than 50 years, the examination has a low yield.[27] The incidence of negative stool examination results among cancer patients is 10 to 30 percent.[28] False positive fecal occult blood test results lead to expenditures for negative GI workups, increased procedural costs, and a diminished success rate for the elective procedure (as a result of delay in performing it). Most studies conclude that routine screening for fecal occult blood is not beneficial in patients hospitalized for any major surgical procedure.[29]

Consultation

With the immense volume of medical information now available, it is difficult for even the most conscientious surgeon to keep abreast of all medical issues relevant to perioperative patient management. The decision to seek consultation should be based on the seriousness of the coexisting disease, the severity of the operation, and the surgeon's expertise in selecting and interpreting second-line tests and planning management accordingly. The common practice of obtaining consultation only to protect against possible litigation or to split fees and gain referrals should be roundly condemned. One prospective, randomized study found that a program of outpatient internal medicine preoperative evaluation significantly decreased preoperative length of stay, had a similar but less pronounced effect on total length of stay, and reduced unnecessary admissions for elective surgery.[30] A small number of high-risk patients may require preoperative and postoperative ICU monitoring. One study found that a structured preoperative consultation with ICU physicians correctly identified patients who needed monitoring and ICU care but did not overutilize scarce and expensive ICU beds.[31]

Selection of Inpatient or Outpatient Procedure

There is little doubt that most operations can be performed in an ambulatory setting. Only those surgical procedures that necessitate extensive postoperative care (e.g., I.V. fluids and medications, intensive monitoring, and prolonged bed rest) are exclusively reserved for inpatients. There is no need for definitive lists that classify operative procedures as either appropriate or unsuitable for the outpatient setting, although it is true that Medicare and other payors may have priorities that must be accepted if reimbursement is to follow. In fact, the American College of Surgeons opposes such lists because "categorizing certain procedures unequivocally as 'ambulatory' does not take into account patient suitability, or give proper weight to surgical judgment."[32] In general, any procedure that does not involve major intervention in the chest or abdominal cavity is suitable for the outpatient setting. Even this rule is not an absolute one: for example, open cholecystectomy would probably be considered a major intervention, but laparoscopic cholecystectomy might not be. The major contraindication to outpatient surgery is the anticipation that postoperative complications—especially hemorrhage or metabolic or cardiopulmonary instability but also severe pain, nausea, or persistent vomiting—would ensue. Pain and nausea, at least, can be reduced through proper management of medications both during and after the surgical procedure.

Certain general temporal guidelines should be kept in mind. An outpatient operative procedure usually should not last longer than two hours, especially if performed with the patient under general anesthesia, and the postoperative recovery period should be no longer than four hours, especially if dismissal from the unit would occur late in the day and it would be difficult to assess the patient at home.

Anesthesia-related issues are relevant as well. A matrix whose purpose was to categorize surgical procedures in relation to anesthetic risk was devised at the Johns Hopkins University Medical School. Although this matrix, which blended the American Society of Anesthesiologists (ASA) physical status classification [see Table 1] with a surgical category system devised at Johns Hopkins [see Table 2],[33] was designed to assist anesthesiologists in performing preoperative evaluations, with a little imagination such a scheme can also be used to evaluate the risk the procedure poses to an individual patient. We have modified this matrix to include those classes and categories of procedures that should not be performed in the ambulatory setting [see Table 3]. Patients in ASA class III or IV must be carefully evaluated. The stability of concurrent disease (e.g., coronary artery disease, insulin-dependent diabetes mellitus, or morbid obesity) must be determined, especially in ASA classes III and IV and surgical categories 3 and 4. Operative mortality and morbidity, not unexpectedly, increase as ASA class increases.[34-36] Many studies support the finding that careful monitoring and improvement of the patient's physical status before operation reduce mortality and morbidity. Therefore, a patient whose physical status is poor before operation should be accepted for outpatient treatment only when one is sure that any concomitant disease is well controlled and that there will be adequate postoperative monitoring and treatment in the patient's home.

Several surgical centers have been gathering outcome data for surgical procedures done in outpatient facilities. For the most part, these data reflect the experience of major teaching facilities and thus of hospital-based units rather than free-standing units or office-based units. Satisfactory data from office-based units are still lacking. A study from Worcester, Massachusetts, compared data from a hospital-based unit with data from a free-standing facility [see Table 4].[37] The findings indicated that patient selection influenced the rate of admission, in that the

Table 1 American Society of Anesthesiologists' Physical Status Classification

Classification	Description	Examples
Class I	Normal, healthy patient	An inguinal hernia in a fit patient or a fibroid uterus in a healthy woman
Class II	Patient with mild systemic disease—a mild to moderate systemic disorder related to the condition to be treated or to some other, unrelated process	Moderate obesity, extremes of age, diet-controlled diabetes, mild hypertension, chronic obstructive pulmonary disease
Class III	Patient with severe systemic disease that limits activity but is not incapacitating	Morbid obesity, severely limiting heart disease, angina pectoris, healed myocardial infarction, insulin-dependent diabetes, moderate to severe pulmonary insufficiency
Class IV	Patient with incapacitating systemic disease that is life threatening	Organic heart disease with signs of cardiac insufficiency; unstable angina; refractory arrhythmia; advanced pulmonary, renal, hepatic, or endocrine disease
Class V	Moribund patient not expected to survive 24 hr without an operation	Ruptured aortic aneurysm with profound shock, massive pulmonary embolus, major cerebral trauma with increasing intracranial pressure
Emergency (E)	Emergency surgery—the suffix "E" is added to denote the poorer status of any patient in one of these five categories who is operated on in an emergency	

rate of admission was significantly higher in the hospital-based unit than in the free-standing unit.

There is a growing body of information supporting the safety of ambulatory surgery. In 1993, for example, researchers from the Mayo Clinic reported on mortality and morbidity in more than 38,000 patients who underwent more than 45,000 surgical procedures in an ambulatory setting.[38] Thirty-three patients either died or experienced major morbidity, and one third of these complications occurred 48 hours or longer after operation. These data were compared with data from the rural community around the Mayo Clinic and matched favorably with predictions of spontaneous occurrences of serious disease (e.g., stroke).

Still, each case must be considered individually. It is unreasonable to assume that all patients should undergo an outpatient procedure for a specific condition (e.g., inguinal hernia) when some of them can be expected to experience postoperative complications. Many hospitals have established procedures for providing overnight accommodations at a lesser charge than a regular admission. Thus, for example, many patients are kept in the facility for 23 hours after a laparoscopic cholecystectomy. Office-based surgical units do not have this flexibility, and it is for this reason that most surgeons now perform major ambulatory surgical procedures in hospital-based units. Office-based surgical units should clearly define emergency procedures for handling patients who have not fully recovered from the procedure and are not ready to return home. Such procedures should involve either a means of transport and admission to an overnight facility or the option of keeping the postanesthesia recovery facility open.

One must advise patients and their families when it is not reasonable to follow the approved procedures of their financial agent. Outside agencies, such as insurance agencies and third-party administrators, must not be permitted to dictate the direction of care, although it is reasonable that they be given an explanation when one does not follow their approved procedures. Such agencies should continually reevaluate their policies of reimbursement to ensure that those policies take realistic account of disease processes and that they satisfy the patients' individual needs as well. They should accept a reasonable concern on the part of the surgeon as justification for hospitalization and should accept the concept that variations of care do exist. Medicare, for example, usually accepts the comorbid diagnosis of cardiac rhythm irregularities as a reason for hospitalization.

Selection of Patients for Inpatient and Outpatient Procedures

Just as inpatient and outpatient procedures must be carefully selected with an eye to difficulty and severity of illness, so too should patients be carefully selected. The following six questions should be asked:

1. Is the facility adequately equipped and appropriate for the intended procedure, and are quality standards maintained?
2. Can the procedure routinely be performed safely without hospital admission?
3. Is the patient at risk for major complications if the operation is performed in the facility?
4. Do concomitant conditions in the patient present unnecessary risks in the intended setting?
5. Will the patient require any special instructions or emotional counseling before the operation?
6. Do the patient and the family accept the concept of outpatient surgery?

Surgeons and anesthesiologists are rapidly gaining experience in managing increasingly more difficult procedures on an outpatient basis. Many procedures that were considered unsafe in an outpatient setting just a few years ago are now commonly being performed in ambulatory centers, and there is mounting evidence that this shift has not increased patient risk.[38-40]

The surgeon is responsible for detecting undiagnosed and unsuspected acute and chronic conditions before operation. The anesthesiologist is also responsible for uncovering potential preoperative problems. In addition, the surgical unit plays a role in determining what types of patients can be treated. Hospital-affiliated units are better able to accept patients who have more serious concomitant illnesses than facilities physically separated from the acute care hospital. Surgeons also tend to select certain patients for in-hospital day surgical units over free-standing day surgical units, as reflected in the higher rate of admission for hospital-based units [see Table 4].[37]

One important caveat is in order when a patient is initially considered for outpatient surgery. If any patient or any responsible relative of the patient does not accept or is extremely critical of nonadmission surgical care and cannot be easily convinced of its advantages, inpatient treatment is indicated, regardless of the policy of the third-party payor. Efforts to coerce the patient or the family to accept outpatient surgery not only engender bad will between physician and patient but also tend to give rise to more postoperative problems (either real or factitious). Third-party payors must accept that some patients will refuse nonadmission surgery. It is the responsibility of third-party payors and their customers (i.e., corporations or employers) to provide adequate information to those covered (i.e., employees and families) about the advantages of outpatient surgery. Such education should be provided well before surgical intervention is sought or needed.

Many studies support the finding that careful monitoring and improvement of the patient's physical status before operation reduce mortality and morbidity. Therefore, one should accept a patient with poor preoperative physical status for outpatient treatment only when one is sure that concomitant disease is well controlled and that there will be adequate postoperative monitoring and treatment in the patient's home.

SPECIFIC PATIENT RISK FACTORS

In evaluating the risk factors for any surgical intervention, the following variables should be considered: (1) the patient's age,

---

Table 2 Surgical Categories

Category 1
Generally noninvasive procedures with minimal blood loss and with minimal risk to the patient independent of anesthesia
  Anticipated blood loss less than 250 ml
  Limited procedure involving skin, subcutaneous, eye, or superficial lymphoid tissue
    Breast biopsy
    Superficial lymph node biopsy
    Removal of minor skin lesions
    Myringotomy tubes
    Circumcision
    Carpal tunnel repair
    Repair of digits without repair to bone
    Retinal surgery
    Cataract extraction
  Entry into body without surgical incision
    Cystoscopy
    Hysteroscopy
    Fiberoptic bronchoscopy
  Excludes the following:
    Open exposure of internal body organs, repair of vascular or neurologic structures, or placement of prosthetic devices
    Entry into abdomen, thorax, neck, cranium, or extremities other than wrist, hand, or digits
    Placement of prosthetic devices
    Postoperative monitored care setting (ICU, ACU)

Category 2
Procedures limited in their invasive nature, usually with minimal to mild blood loss and only mild associated risk to the patient independent of anesthesia
  Anticipated blood loss less than 500 ml
  Limited entry into abdomen, thorax, neck, or extremities for diagnostic or minor therapy without removal or major alteration of major organs
    Diagnostic laparoscopy
    Fallopian tubal ligation
    Laparoscopic lysis of adhesions
    Percutaneous lung biopsy, not including mediastinal structures
    Arthroscopy
    Tonsillectomy
    Adenoidectomy
    Rhinoplasty
    Dilatation and curettage
    Inguinal hernia repair
    Umbilical hernia repair
    Extensive superficial procedure
    Cosmetic surgery to the face or extremities
  Excludes the following:
    Open exposure of internal body organs or repair of vascular or neurologic structures
    Placement of prosthetic devices
    Postoperative monitored care setting (ICU, ACU), with no open exposure of abdomen, thorax, neck, cranium, or extremities other than wrist, hand, or digits

Category 3
More invasive procedures and those involving moderate blood loss with moderate risk to the patient independent of anesthesia
  Anticipated blood loss 500–1,500 ml
  Open exposure of the abdomen
    Hysterectomy
    Myomectomy
    Cholecystectomy
    Resection or reconstructive surgery of the digestive tract
  Reconstructive work on hip, shoulder, knees
    Hip replacement
    Laminectomy
  Excludes the following:
    Open thoracic or intracranial procedure
    Major vascular repair (e.g., aortofemoral bypass)
    Major orthopedic reconstruction (e.g., spinal fusion)
    Planned postoperative monitored care setting (ICU, ACU)

Category 4
Procedures posing significant risk to the patient independent of anesthesia or in one or more of the following categories:
  Procedure for which postoperative intensive care is planned
  Procedure with anticipated blood loss greater than 1,500 ml
  Cardiothoracic procedure
    Cardiac surgery
    Pneumonectomy or lobectomy
  Intracranial procedure
  Major procedure on the oropharynx
    Resection of tumors of the head and neck
    Radical neck dissection
  Major vascular, skeletal, or neurologic repair
    Aortic aneurysm repair
    Major vessel bypass procedure
    Kyphosis repair
    Scoliosis repair
    Procedure on the spinal cord

Table 3 Guidelines for Selection of Outpatient versus Inpatient Surgery

ASA Class	Surgical Category			
	1	2	3	4
I	Outpatient procedure with local anesthesia	Outpatient procedure with general or regional anesthesia	Inpatient procedure	Inpatient procedure
II	Outpatient procedure with local anesthesia*	Outpatient procedure with local, regional, or general anesthesia*	Inpatient procedure	Inpatient procedure
III	Inpatient procedure (unless operation can be done with local anesthesia)*	Inpatient procedure	Inpatient procedure	Inpatient procedure
IV	Inpatient procedure (unless operation can be done with local anesthesia)*	Inpatient procedure	Inpatient procedure	Inpatient procedure

*Patient must be watched carefully.
ASA—American Society of Anesthesiologists.

(2) the proposed anesthetic approach (type and duration), (3) the extent of the surgical procedure (including the surgical site), (4) the patient's overall physiologic status, (5) the presence or absence of concomitant diseases, (6) baseline medications, and (7) the patient's general mental status. The aim should be to return the patient to the preoperative functional level with respect to respiration, cardiovascular stability, and mental status. No deviations should be acceptable. These are the standards used by peer review organizations (PROs) in retroactive evaluation of surgical interventions in Medicare recipients.

Several studies aimed at determining reasons for admission after ambulatory surgical procedures indicate that the major reasons for admission are to an extent related to the patient's preoperative cardiovascular and respiratory status, but the major reason for admission is still uncontrollable nausea and vomiting.[40] Moreover, most complications are related to intraoperative performance and not to the setting of the surgical procedure (outpatient or inpatient). Admission to the hospital after ambulatory surgery because of urinary retention, for example, is related to the use of general anesthesia, the age of the patient, and the use of more than 1,200 ml of I.V. fluids before, during, and after the operation.[41]

When undergoing relatively short procedures, ASA class III (or even class IV) patients are appropriate candidates for ambulatory surgery if their systemic diseases are medically stable.

Age

Extremes of age by themselves automatically increase the ASA classification from I to II. Even though age is not correlated with hospital admission after ambulatory surgery, elderly patients often have concomitant conditions that may have gone unrecognized but should be brought to light before the operation. This is the obvious justification for the higher ASA classification—that is, to make the surgical team aware of the potential increased risk. In addition, the family or social support networks available to elderly patients are often of questionable value and may even pose their own risks after the operation.

Young children—especially neonates—present separate problems that must be independently evaluated by the surgeon and the anesthesiologist.

Preoperative Drug Therapy

Two questions must be answered about a patient taking medication for preexisting disease: First, should the drug or drugs be discontinued or the dosage altered before operation? Second, do the medications necessitate special laboratory evaluations before operation (e.g., a prothrombin time for patients taking anticoagulants)?

Whereas dosages of some medications, such as adrenocorticosteroids, may have to be temporarily increased, certain oral agents may have to be replaced during the immediate perioperative period with agents that can be delivered intravenously. In particular, oral antiarrhythmic drugs (e.g., quinidine sulfate, procainamide, and disopyramide) should be discontinued eight hours before the operation.[42] It is important to note that abrupt withdrawal of clonidine, which is used to treat chronic essential hypertension, is particularly dangerous because it is often associated with an increase in the plasma catecholamine level. Therefore, clonidine should be continued throughout the perioperative period. Patients taking aspirin should be instructed to stop at least one week before elective operation because aspirin's antiplatelet effect lingers for the life of the affected platelets. Patients receiving warfarin require uninterrupted anticoagulation; hence, the drug should only be stopped in the immediate preoperative period, and anticoagulation should not be reversed. Fresh frozen plasma may be required intraoperatively if excessive bleeding occurs. If warfarin is to be discontinued for a longer period, I.V. heparin can be given.

In a study of nearly 18,000 ambulatory surgical patients in a major surgical center, almost 2,000 patients had preexisting systemic disease, and more than 900 of them were taking specific drugs for their disease.[43] Nearly half of these patients were taking at least one antihypertensive medication; a significant number were taking one or more heart medications, including cardiac

Table 4 Admission Rates in Hospital-Based Integrated Surgical Units versus Hospital-Based Free-Standing Surgical Units

Type of Surgical Unit	Cases (N)	Admission Rate
Hospital-based integrated	6,456	4%
Hospital-based free-standing	2,000	0.25%

Data from reference 37.

glycosides, beta blockers, diuretics, antiarrhythmics, vasodilators, and anticoagulants. Other drugs that were being used included insulin and antiasthma medications. However, none of the complications recorded were related to preoperative drug use.

In any case, patients should bring all of their medications—both prescribed and self-administered—on the day of operation.

Hypertension

In general, hypertension should be under control before operation. Monoamine oxidase (MAO) inhibitors should be discontinued, if possible, two weeks before operation because they have unpredictable cardiac effects and may lead to hypertension in patients receiving meperidine or vasopressors. All antihypertensive agents should be continued until the day before operation; beta blockers can be taken on the day of operation.

Heart Disease and Congestive Heart Failure

Patients with serious heart disease or congestive heart failure fall into ASA class III or higher and thus should not be considered for outpatient surgery unless the procedure is a minor one necessitating only local or regional anesthesia. Patients with less serious heart disease should take any cardiac glycosides, beta blockers, or antiarrhythmics that have been prescribed with a small amount of water when they awake on the day of operation.

Bronchopulmonary Disease

Patients with bronchopulmonary disease must be evaluated individually. The degree of impairment is determined by means of a careful history and appropriate testing; a chest x-ray should always be obtained. The history should also reveal factors that initiate attacks of asthma or bronchospasm as well as identify the medications being taken. Many patients with bronchopulmonary disease need steroids and antibiotics preoperatively [*see 71 Pulmonary Insufficiency*].

Diabetes Mellitus

Patients whose diabetes is controlled by oral hypoglycemics or less than 25 units of insulin daily can be adequately managed by withholding the medication on the day of operation. In general, patients with more severe insulin-dependent diabetes mellitus should not undergo outpatient procedures. Those who do are best managed by the administration of a fraction of the insulin dose on the day of operation along with an intravenous dextrose solution (usually a five percent concentration), beginning shortly after the patient's arrival at the surgical facility. The status of these patients is monitored by measuring either the blood glucose level or the urine glucose level, both of which can be easily and rapidly determined at the bedside.

Obesity

In general, moderate to severely obese patients should not undergo outpatient surgery. The hazards and risks of surgery in the obese are often unrecognized. Morbid obesity exerts stress on the cardiopulmonary system, and morbidly obese patients easily become, or already are, hypoxemic. In addition, such patients usually have concomitant preexisting conditions such as diabetes, hypertension, liver disease, or cardiac failure. Moderate obesity increases the ASA classification from I to II; morbid obesity increases it to III. Careful consideration is essential before a morbidly obese patient is released from skilled observation after major anesthesia. Obese children often are not recognized as being at risk. There is some controversy over whether the ability to swallow water in a recovering obese pediatric patient is an acceptable condition for discharge. Tragedies have occurred after minor procedures after a seemingly recovered obese patient was discharged.

Adrenocortical Steroid Therapy

Patients taking adrenocortical steroids for six to 12 months before operation should usually receive supplemental steroids in the preoperative period [*see 73 Adrenal Insufficiency*]. Short-term steroid overdosage has virtually no complications, but inadequate adrenocortical support may have serious repercussions.

Alcohol and Drug Abuse

Alcohol and drug abusers (a category that may also include self-medicated patients and those who are taking a large number of physician-directed medications) are also poor candidates for outpatient surgery. Chronic alcoholism is associated with a number of serious metabolic disorders, and chronic drug abusers often have many medical problems that are related to the habit (e.g., endocarditis, superficial infections, hepatitis, and thrombophlebitis).

Psychotropic Drug Therapy

Except for MAO inhibitors, most psychotropic drugs do not interact with anesthetics.

Psychiatric Illness

Mentally unstable patients are a potential problem even in the best circumstances. A competent adult must be available to provide care after operation. One benefit of outpatient surgery for mentally unstable patients, as for very young and very old patients, is that it allows them to return quickly to a familiar environment, which is desirable when safety can be assured. If safety cannot be assured, admission is indicated.

Selection of Appropriate Site for Procedure

There are four main types of facilities that are used in the performance of outpatient surgical procedures:

1. Office-based surgical units. These include individual surgeons' offices as well as larger group practice units.
2. Free-standing day surgical units. These are often used by managed health care systems and independent contractors.
3. In-hospital day surgical units. These are often associated with inpatient units.
4. In-hospital inpatient units.

At present, the majority of surgical procedures are being performed in a hospital facility. The primary influences on the choice of setting are the type of procedure to be performed and the condition of the patient.

There is still disagreement about whether regulations (i.e., legally imposed standards and guidelines) applying specifically to office-based surgical units are advisable or necessary. It is clear that many individually operated units are delivering cost-efficient, safe, and effective care. The imposition of costly regulations and accreditation processes on such units may be fiscally prohibitive. It is also clear, however, that many such units may well be delivering substandard care. Several institutions are currently involved in devising guidelines, standards, and even regulations. It appears inevitable that society will demand some certification of quality assurance (QA) in the near future. Already, some payors, such as Medicare, are hesitant to reimburse care delivered in nonaccredited facilities.

Hospital-based ambulatory care units that are extensions of inpatient facilities obviously have many advantages for the surgeon and the patient, but they are often less efficient and convenient than other ambulatory facilities. On the other hand, it is easier to assess the safety and quality of hospital-based units, in that the QA function of the hospital must extend to such units. The Joint Commission for Accreditation of Healthcare Organizations (JCAHO) is now well established in the voluntary accreditation process for ambulatory health care facilities as well as for inpatient facilities. Even though accreditation is still voluntary, it is clear that a mandate for some sort of QA for ambulatory facilities already exists. In some cases, reimbursement is limited to surgeons practicing in accredited facilities.

The Office of the Inspector General (OIG) reported on the appropriateness of the surgical setting, the medical necessity of the surgery, and the quality of care performed in physicians' offices.[44] The data were obtained from the 1989 Part B Medicare Annual Data. The results are disturbing: reasonable quality of care was not documented in 20 percent of the medical records, an indication for surgery was not documented in 13 percent, the physician's office was not an appropriate setting for a small number of operations, and procedure codes did not match the operations performed in 16 percent of sample cases. As a result, the OIG has recommended that PROs extend their review to procedures performed in physicians' offices—a recommendation that, although not easily implemented, should impel surgeons to give greater consideration to assurance of quality in their office-based practices.

In 1996, the ACS Board of Governors' Committee on Ambulatory Surgical Care published the second edition of a manual on guidelines for office-based surgery.[45] This manual was designed to provide guidelines, not standards in the manner of the JCAHO. The ACS is not involved in accrediting facilities or setting standards; however, it will continue to monitor and revise the guidelines so that all surgical facilities will be able to demonstrate quality and outcome without incurring prohibitive costs.

Communication with Patient and Family

PREOPERATIVE CONFERENCE

It is essential to discuss the proposed surgical procedure with the patient and the patient's family.[46] The indications for the operation, the essential features of the procedure, its intraoperative and postoperative risks, and any expected changes in normal activities after recovery must be outlined.[47] Questions from the patient or family members should be welcomed rather than discouraged because a thorough understanding of the operation will allay anxiety and stress and make one's explanation of the postoperative course more comprehensible.[48]

It is particularly important that the patient and family have some understanding of the pain and discomfort that the patient may experience.[49] The site of the incision should be indicated to the patient; when appropriate, the patient should be told that significant incisional pain may be likely but that such pain is normal and is rarely associated with a wound-related complication. The patient should also be assured that appropriate analgesia will be provided to reduce, but not eliminate, pain. If an abdominal or thoracic incision is to be made, the patient must be instructed about the necessity for postoperative deep-breathing exercises to prevent atelectasis.[50] The patient must be assured that the medical and nursing staff realize that such manipulations are associated with brief periods of incisional pain. He or she should also be told that coughing and early ambulation will not delay wound healing.

Both family and patient should be told whenever the use of invasive monitoring equipment, I.V. lines, drains, nasogastric tubes, chest tubes, or urinary catheters is likely. If the patient is to be held in the recovery room or the ICU after operation, this environment should be described to him or her, and the family should be notified of the change in location. If postoperative ventilatory support is anticipated, the patient must be told that speaking will be impossible while the endotracheal tube remains in place and that the unsettling sensation of paralysis may be experienced if drugs are required to facilitate toleration of and cooperation with the ventilator. If a pain management team using modern techniques of postoperative analgesia is available, the patient must be told why and how epidural analgesia is to be used and informed about the role and proper use of patient-controlled analgesia (PCA) techniques.[51,52] Finally, the anticipated use of blood products and the potential risk of infection must be discussed, and the opportunity to bank autologous blood for use during the operation must be offered.

Much of this information can be given at the preadmission clinic, where the patient can meet with all the care givers, including the anesthetist, the pain management team, and the nursing staff responsible for postoperative care.[53,54]

Once the operative procedure has been discussed, the follow-up procedures after discharge should be clearly described. Areas of particular concern to the patient[55] include (1) level of activity (e.g., bed rest, walking, climbing stairs, and lifting; driving can usually be resumed after 24 hours); (2) proper methods of bathing (especially how to wash the incision); (3) wound dressing (e.g., when to remove or replace dressings); (4) clothing; (5) use of drugs (e.g., analgesics, laxatives, and sedatives); (6) resumption of medications for existing conditions; and (7) diet.

In addition, one should be prepared to answer questions about when to return to activities such as physical exercise, sexual relations, and work. A full written summary of routine postoperative care and emergency procedures and the names of available physicians should be presented to the patient. This summary will save one the inconvenience of multiple phone calls from the patient as well as lower the risk of bad public relations engendered by patient dissatisfaction. One should be absolutely certain that the patient knows how to obtain emergency care after discharge. The written summary should be reviewed again with the patient at the time of discharge.

OBTAINING INFORMED CONSENT

The concept of informed consent has been legally established in the United States and in most other countries as well.[56,57] It has not been precisely defined but is generally understood to include at least informing the patient of potential complications related to the operation that either are relatively common or, if uncommon, are especially grave [see Sidebar Informed Consent]. Again, questions from the patient and the family should be encouraged, and every attempt should be made to answer these questions accurately. When possible, informed consent should

> ### Informed Consent
>
> Informed consent is an important aspect of surgery, yet the question of precisely what patients want to know before their operation has received relatively little examination. In one study,[137] 50 patients were questioned within three months of an ear, nose, or throat operation. Most of the patients were happy to allow their physicians to determine their treatment, but they wanted information about their condition, the proposed therapy, and any important side effects that might arise. Fifty percent admitted worrying about some aspect of their recent operation. More than two thirds thought that signing a consent form primarily signified agreement to undergo treatment and that it was a legal document; 54 percent thought that there was an important medicolegal aspect to the document. More than half thought that an information sheet would be reassuring; one third thought that it would provoke anxiety; and eight percent thought that it would frighten them away from undergoing the operation. Patients who were most worried about aspects of their operation had a higher mean anxiety score, as did those who thought an information sheet would be either frightening or anxiety-provoking; however, a higher anxiety score was not associated with a desire to know less about the proposed treatment.
>
> Another study[138] assessed the ability of patients to understand and recall information given before written consent to transurethral resection of the prostate was obtained. Some aspects of postoperative management and some complications were less well remembered than others. In particular, 18 percent of the patients could not remember being informed about the possibility of retrograde ejaculation, despite the surgeon's efforts to emphasize this risk. Forty-one percent of patients were not especially concerned about complications, provided that their condition was made better; 54 percent trusted their physician to do the right thing and did not think detailed explanation was important; and 62 percent felt that the main purpose of consent forms was to protect the physician's rights. Most patients still believed that consent forms were necessary.
>
> Other reports indicate that provision of detailed information about the potential complications of general anesthesia does improve patients' knowledge but does not increase their anxiety level.[139,140] Elderly patients and patients with a below-average IQ, impaired cognitive function, or an external locus of control have poor information recall. Consequently, written information may be more useful for these patients if given before admission to hospital.[141]
>
> On the other hand, one study suggests that even a reasonable and prudent surgeon who makes a diligent effort at patient education with the assistance of a professional educator cannot necessarily expect accurate recall or comprehension on the part of the patient or the family members. If this is so, the idea that the doctrine of informed consent typically is fulfilled in the surgical setting may very well be a myth.[142]
>
> The common law has long recognized the right of competent adults to autonomy and self-determination. This right is generally held to include the right to refuse medical and surgical treatment, even when refusal could be severely detrimental to the individual's life and health. Anyone who works with patients in a health care profession may at some time be faced with a patient who will not consent to treatment that, in the best clinical opinion of the physicians responsible for the patient's care, is appropriate, necessary, and in the patient's best interests. There are no clear guidelines determining whether one should treat or not treat in such situations. If the patient remains competent, there will be other opportunities to take the matter up again with him or her as circumstances change; however, if the patient becomes incompetent, a real clinical dilemma arises.

be obtained after such discussions in the presence of an appropriate professional witness. The encounter must be summarized on the hospital chart and should document, at the minimum, (1) explanation of the reasons for the procedure, (2) description of the expected benefit, (3) some indication that the patient understands the risks, and (4) specific plans for monitoring and for preoperative and intraoperative therapy to reduce the risks. Finally, there should be a statement indicating that in the surgeon's judgment, the patient and the family members understood and accepted the operative recommendation.

Performance of the Operation

PREMEDICATION

Premedication is an important adjunct to local and regional general anesthesia[58] [see Table 5]: it can facilitate performance of the procedure by alleviating fear and anxiety and supplementing analgesia. On the other hand, premedication, especially with narcotics, can delay recovery: in fact, patients may actually take longer to recover from premedication and local anesthesia than from general anesthesia. Still, no patient should be denied premedication out of fear that it might delay discharge. Some studies have shown that premedication with agents other than long-acting narcotics does not prolong recovery time[59] [see Table 6]. Narcotic premedications are the usual cause of postoperative nausea and vomiting and one of the major reasons for admission of outpatients to the hospital.

The four major categories of agents used for premedication are (1) anticholinergic drugs, (2) narcotics, (3) sedatives, and (4) antacids and histamine antagonists.

Anticholinergic Drugs

Anticholinergic agents are not routinely indicated for outpatient premedication, because newer anesthetics are less irritating than those previously used and because use of anticholinergic agents may increase the incidence of cardiac irregularities.

Narcotics

Because the primary effect of narcotics is the relief of pain, these agents are time-honored premedications for inpatient procedures; however, their significant side effects limit their usefulness for outpatient procedures. Fentanyl is appropriate for outpatient surgery because of its short duration of action and its limited side effects; it should be given within 30 minutes of the actual induction of

Table 5 Premedications

Class	Drug	Recommended Dose and Route of Administration
Sedative	Diazepam	4–10 mg (0.05–0.15 mg/kg) I.V. or 5–10 mg p.o.
	Droperidol*	2.5–10.0 mg (1–4 ml) I.V. or I.M.
Narcotics	Fentanyl*	1–2 µg/kg I.V. or I.M.
	Sufentanil	0.1–0.25 µg/kg
	Alfentanil	7.5–15.0 µg/kg
	Meperidine†	50–100 mg I.M.

*The combination of droperidol and fentanyl is available as Innovar; each milliliter contains 2.5 mg of droperidol and 50 µg of fentanyl.
†The use of long-acting narcotics such as meperidine and morphine is usually not recommended for outpatient surgery.

Table 6 Premedication and Recovery Time[59]

Type	Number of Patients	Recovery Time* (min)
No premedication	1,015	179 ± 113
Diazepam	98	168 ± 104
Pentobarbital	25	231 ± 88
Narcotics (meperidine, morphine)	388	208 ± 101
Hydroxyzine	92	192 ± 120

*Values are ± SD.

anesthesia. Long-acting narcotics, especially meperidine and morphine, are usually not indicated in the outpatient setting.

As outpatient surgical procedures become more lengthy and complex, larger doses of short-acting narcotics such as fentanyl are being used. As the doses increase, however, the advantages of short-acting drugs over long-acting drugs become less pronounced. Newer short-acting narcotics are now available, but they have side effects of their own.

Sedatives

Most barbiturates are long-acting agents and thus are not indicated for outpatient procedures. Very short acting barbiturates, such as thiopental, are occasionally used during anesthesia. Nonbarbiturate tranquilizers are being used more frequently because they act without causing much sleepiness and because they may reduce the amount of anesthetic required. The phenothiazines and droperidol are powerful antiemetics,[60] and the benzodiazepines (e.g., diazepam) are useful for inducing amnesia and stopping convulsions.

Antacids and Histamine Antagonists

Antacids and histamine antagonists are sometimes used in an effort to diminish the risk of gastric aspiration and the consequent deleterious effects of acidic gastric contents on the respiratory tract, but they have not been proved to be beneficial in this respect. It is important to remember that most of the commonly used antacid preparations are composed of particulate matter, and thus, aspiration of the antacid can itself be a serious problem. Patients who are assumed to be at high risk for aspiration (e.g., diabetic, obese, or pregnant patients) can be premedicated with a nonparticulate antacid, such as sodium citrate. A 50 ml dose of sodium citrate one hour before operation raises the pH to a safe level, at the expense of a slightly increased gastric residual volume.[61]

ANESTHESIA

It is beyond the scope of this chapter to address general anesthesia in depth. We merely note that one should be prepared to meet all of the contingencies that can accompany general anesthesia, especially when anesthesia is delivered by someone other than an anesthesiologist. The patient's cardiac activity, blood pressure, temperature, respiration, and neuromuscular activity should be properly monitored.

Local Anesthetics for Local and Regional Anesthesia

As outpatient surgery has become more popular, there has been an increase in the use of local anesthetics for local and regional control of pain [see 41 Perioperative Effects of Anesthesia and 104 Postoperative Pain]. Local anesthetics are usually administered by the surgeon. It is crucial that the patient accept and be psychologically suited to this type of anesthesia: obviously, local or regional anesthesia can be very disturbing and disruptive when administered inadequately or when given to an emotionally unstable patient. During the preoperative conference [see Preoperative Conference, above], one should make a point of describing how the anesthetic will be administered and what sensations will ensue.

Local anesthetics can be classified into three groups according to their potency and duration of action: (1) low potency and short duration (e.g., procaine and chloroprocaine), (2) moderate potency and intermediate duration (e.g., lidocaine, mepivacaine, and prilocaine), and (3) high potency and long duration (e.g., tetracaine, bupivacaine, and etidocaine) [see Table 7].

Most local anesthetics are administered by infiltration into the extravascular space or, in the case of epidural administration, by injection into cerebrospinal fluid. In some areas, especially the hands, intravascular (intravenous regional) infiltration has been used with considerable success; however, inadvertent intravascular administration of epidural doses of the high-potency agents can lead to life-threatening complications [see Toxicity and Allergy, below]. Although such complications have not been reported in association with inadvertent intravascular administration during infiltration for local anesthesia, it is nevertheless advisable to check carefully to be sure that the injecting needle is not located in an intravascular site. Intravascular injection can usually be prevented by constantly aspirating during infiltration and by infiltrating only when the needle is withdrawn.

Mixing local anesthetics is an effective means of obtaining the advantages of more than one drug at once. At the Lichtenstein Hernia Institute in Los Angeles,[62] patients undergoing repair of

Table 7 Local Anesthetics for Infiltration

Drug		Plain Solutions		Epinephrine-Containing Solutions	
		Maximum Adult Dose (mg)	Duration (min)	Maximum Adult Dose (mg)	Duration (min)
Short-acting	Procaine 1%–2%	800	15–30	1,000	30–90
Intermediate-acting	Lidocaine 0.5%–2.0%	300	30–60	500	120–360
	Mepivacaine 1%–2%	300	45–90	500	120–360
Long-acting	Bupivacaine* 0.25%–5.0%	175	180+	225	240+

*Not recommended for children younger than 12 years.

inguinal hernias receive a 50-50 mixture of one percent lidocaine and 0.5 percent bupivacaine with epinephrine in a 1:200,000 dilution. The maximum therapeutic dose of lidocaine is 300 mg alone and 500 mg with epinephrine; the maximum therapeutic dose of bupivacaine is 175 mg alone and 225 mg with epinephrine. The addition of 1 mEq/10 ml of sodium bicarbonate to the solution shortens the onset time[63] as well as reducing the discomfort by raising the pH. This combination of drugs has several advantages: (1) lidocaine has a rapid onset, whereas bupivacaine prolongs the duration of the effect; (2) the negative chronotropic and inotropic action of lidocaine may well counteract the cardiac excitability of bupivacaine, and (3) use of multiple drugs makes it less likely that the maximum therapeutic dose of any single agent will be exceeded.

Regional anesthesia, also known as peripheral nerve blockade, is generally administered by an anesthesiologist but can be adequately administered by a knowledgeable surgeon.

The use of epinephrine with local anesthetics prolongs the duration of the anesthetic effect without delaying its onset; however, epinephrine should not be used with anesthetics at sites where the vascular supply distal to the site of infusion is marginal (e.g., fingers, toes, the nose, and the external ears). In addition, adrenergic drugs should not be used in unstable cardiac patients unless absolutely necessary. Administration of long-acting local anesthetics (e.g., bupivacaine, 0.25 percent, injected in the skin edges at the end of the procedure) seems to limit postoperative pain and thus to encourage early activity and ambulation. Often, this technique not only postpones pain but reduces it as well. Bupivacaine is not, however, recommended for patients younger than 12 years.

Adjunctive Use of Local Anesthetics to Prolong Anesthetic Effect

It is clear that even when regional or general anesthetics, or both, are employed, adjunctive use of local anesthetics at the end of the procedure prolongs the anesthetic effect. In addition, once the patient realizes that ambulation is possible without discomfort, he or she is more likely to leave the hospital sooner and less likely to need additional postoperative analgesia. Several centers are currently experimenting with administering local anesthetics before operation; the hypothesis—still unproven—is that preoperative administration may result in decreased use of postoperative analgesics and a prolonged anesthetic effect in comparison with administration at the end of the procedure.

Injection of joint capsules with long-acting anesthetics and narcotics (e.g., morphine sulfate) relieves a great deal of postoperative pain.

Bathing of wounds with bupivacaine is a safe and effective method of decreasing postoperative pain.[64] The addition of epinephrine can extend the prolongation of analgesia to 12 hours after operation.

Nonsteroidal Anti-inflammatory Drugs

Some centers use nonsteroidal anti-inflammatory drugs (NSAIDs) to reduce inflammation and thus pain [see 104 Postoperative Pain]. In addition, it has been shown that NSAIDs significantly reduce the need for opioid analgesics after abdominal procedures. Administration of ketorolac over a short period (i.e., five days or less), first at the time of operation (60 mg I.M. in the OR; lower doses for patients weighing less than 50 kg, those older than 65 years, and those with impaired renal function) and then every six hours thereafter (10 to 15 mg p.o.), has improved recovery after many operations, especially perianal and inguinal procedures. Other NSAIDs can be given in transdermal patches (which are not recommended for children) or transnasally.

Toxicity and Allergy

Whenever local anesthetics are used, and especially when they are administered regionally for major nerve blockade, the possibility of systemic toxicity should be considered. Such toxicity often results from inadvertent intravascular injection of these agents, leading to a sudden increase in systemic concentration.[59] The rate of injection is inversely related to the patient's tolerance of the drug: the higher the injection rate, the lower the tolerance. In general, arterial infusion is less likely to cause a toxic reaction than venous infusion because of the delay in circulation through the distal capillary network. Other factors that can lead to toxic reactions are a diminished drug detoxification rate, systemic acidosis, and individual sensitivities, which are highly variable.

In the CNS, toxic reactions range from drowsiness to frank convulsions. One study found that the incidence of mild toxic reactions to local and regional anesthetics was 0.38 percent, and the incidence of convulsions was 0.12 percent.[65] In the cardiovascular system, toxicity is initially manifested by elevated blood pressure; eventually, depression of systemic resistance and myocardial contractility leads to cardiovascular collapse. The myocardial depression associated with intravascular injection of bupivacaine (0.75 percent) for epidural anesthesia has been reported to be strongly resistant to treatment in pregnant women.[66] Systemic toxicity is also manifested by alterations in the metabolic system, such as derangement of acid-base balance. (Respiratory or metabolic acidosis leads to an increased sensitivity to local anesthetics.) All such reactions are best managed by prevention. Constant vigilance is necessary to ensure that inadvertent intravascular injection does not occur at the time of infiltration. Any serious reactions (e.g., convulsions and cardiovascular collapse) that arise despite precautions are treated with standard measures.

Many patients claim to be allergic to anesthetics (which they usually refer to "generically" as Novocain), but true allergic reactions are rare.[67] A careful history of allergic drug reactions should be taken, including reactions to concomitant medications such as epinephrine. It is important to explain to the patient the nature of any reaction that occurs so that if the reaction was not in fact an allergic one, the patient will understand this point and thus will not give a history of allergy to anesthetics in the future.

Allergic reactions are mediated by the release of histamine. Previous exposure to the offending local anesthetic can lead to the production of IgE antibodies, which initiate anaphylaxis on subsequent exposure; however, anesthetics can also initiate complement-mediated release of histamine without previous exposure. Histamine release leads to characteristic symptoms: skin erythema, followed by erythema in various regions of the body and edema of the upper airway. Abdominal cramps and cardiac instability may also be present.

If an allergic reaction occurs, administration of the drug should be stopped immediately. Epinephrine, 5 µg/kg (0.3 to 0.5 ml of a 1:1,000 dilution), should immediately be given either locally or, if the reaction is severe, systemically.[68] Diphenhydramine, 0.5 to 1.0 mg/kg, should also be given systemically. If bronchospasm occurs, aminophylline, 3 to 5 mg/kg I.V., should be administered. Steroids have been used in this setting, but there is little evidence that such therapy is helpful [see Table 8].

One common cause of allergic reactions is sensitivity to paraben derivatives, which are preservatives used in local anesthetics.

Table 8 Treatment of Allergic Reactions to Local Anesthetics

Agent	Route of Administration	Recommended Dose
Epinephrine	Locally or systemically	5 µg/kg (0.3–0.5 ml of 1:1,000 dilution)
Diphenhydramine	Systemically	0.5–1.0 mg/kg
Aminophylline	I.V.	3–5 mg/kg
Corticosteroids	I.V.	1 g

Paraben preservatives resemble para-aminobenzoic acid (PABA), a metabolic breakdown product of ester-type anesthetics (e.g., procaine, benzocaine, and tetracaine). PABA is a member of a class of compounds that are highly allergenic. Patients sensitive to sunscreens containing PABA often show cross-sensitivity to ester-type local anesthetics.

Patients who are allergic to a local anesthetic usually can be safely given a preservative-free anesthetic of unrelated structure. An intradermal skin test, in which 0.1 ml of the anesthetic drug is injected intradermally into the volar aspect of the forearm, may be tried. A negative reaction indicates that the drug probably can be used safely; nevertheless, resources for handling major cardiopulmonary irregularities should be available when anesthetics are used in previously sensitized patients.[68]

Control of Nausea and Vomiting

Many predisposing factors play a role in causing postoperative nausea and vomiting. Not all of these factors can be managed. Nevertheless, it behooves the surgeon and the anesthesiologist to identify patients at risk so as to minimize the incidence of this debilitating syndrome, which is responsible for a large number of hospital admissions after outpatient surgical procedures.

Some of the more common causes of nausea are often overlooked. Pain is in itself capable of causing nausea and vomiting. Accordingly, adequate control of pain must be obtained, and the patient must not be deprived of analgesics under the false assumption that the medications are the only cause of the nausea. Changes in body activity, especially assumption of the upright position by a patient with possible hypotension, can also cause nausea, as is experienced before a vasovagal attack. In some patients who are prone to motion sickness, the sensation of motion is aggravated by the surgical procedure, the anesthetics, and pain. A preoperative history of frequent attacks of motion sickness is often a signal that the patient is prone to nausea and vomiting.

The use of narcotics in premedication, as well as in induction and maintenance of anesthesia, is definitely a cause of increased postoperative nausea and vomiting; however, some of the newer opioid analgesics (e.g., fentanyl, sufentanil, and alfentanil), when given judiciously as premedications [see Table 5], appear to reduce anxiety, decrease anesthetic requirements, and relieve pain in the early postoperative period.[69] One should have a thorough understanding of the proper use of these medications before using them in the ambulatory setting.

Benzquinamide, trimethobenzamide, promethazine, and prochlorperazine have all been used in an effort to control postoperative nausea and vomiting but with only limited success.[70] Droperidol, a long-acting medication that is also used for sedation, has certainly helped to reduce the problem after general anesthesia. It is more effective and reliable in reducing the length of stay in the recovery room while providing reasonable control of the symptoms.[71] The usual dose is 0.625 to 1.25 mg, and the maximum dose is 2.5 mg. Droperidol is a tranquilizer and tends to increase drowsiness; consequently, it should not be used near the time of discharge. Metoclopramide, an agent with central antidopaminergic effects that is similar to droperidol but acts specifically on the upper GI tract, is also used. Metoclopramide is a useful premedication because it also encourages gastric emptying and prevents aspiration; however, it is a short-acting agent and may have to be given again after a long procedure. The usual dose for the average adult patient is 10 to 20 mg. Some centers have tried combining droperidol, 0.625 to 1.25 mg, and metoclopramide, 10 mg, in resistant patients with satisfactory results.[72,73]

Given that a history of motion sickness is a good predictor of increased risk for nausea and vomiting, it is not surprising that dimenhydrinate (familiar to most patients under the name Dramamine) is effective in many cases—in some cases, significantly more effective than droperidol.[74]

Perioperative Monitoring

Perioperative monitoring is a well-established function of anesthesiologists. The presence of a qualified anesthesiologist allows the surgeon to concentrate more closely on the procedure itself and to be reasonably sure that the cardiorespiratory system is being adequately supported by a competent member of the surgical team. The increasing use of sedation and anesthesia to enhance patient comfort during ambulatory surgical procedures places additional responsibility on the surgical team, especially when a qualified anesthesiologist is not present.

Many organizations have attempted to define what is necessary for adequate monitoring when anesthetics and sedatives are delivered in the absence of an anesthesiologist. This issue is a particular concern in relation to gastrointestinal endoscopy because of the critical need to monitor cardiorespiratory parameters during procedures in which sedatives, especially midazolam, are utilized. In a collaborative study with the United States Food and Drug Administration, the American Society of Gastrointestinal Endoscopy demonstrated that reports of serious cardiorespiratory complications are uncommon and that midazolam does not seem to place patients at higher risk for complications than diazepam but that concomitant use of narcotics and the need for emergent procedures do increase the risk of serious cardiorespiratory events.[75]

Similar studies have not been done in ambulatory surgical facilities; however, there are an increasing number of recommendations for the use of pulse oximetry and ECG monitoring during procedures in which sedatives and narcotics are used.[76,77] The British Society of Gastroenterology, for example, has formulated 14 recommendations for standards of sedation and patient monitoring. The Risk Management Committee of the Department of Anesthesia of the Harvard Medical School has also made specific recommendations to anesthesiologists at Harvard-affiliated hospitals who participate in institutional-level committees charged with setting guidelines for such services when they are provided by nonanesthesiologists.[78] These guidelines are presented as educational tools rather than inflexible standards: they offer appropriate objectives for each ambulatory surgical unit to consider and can in fact be easily custom-tailored to specific institutions. Seven variables are addressed:

1. The use of sedatives during diagnostic and therapeutic procedures.
2. Monitoring during sedation.
3. Drug dosage and administration.
4. Sufficient trained personnel availability.
5. Equipment availability.
6. Documentation of the fitness and response of the patient as well as the readiness for release from the ambulatory unit.
7. Use of data that permit audit, review, and revision of the individual unit's guidelines.

The Harvard guidelines clearly define two levels of sedation, conscious and deep. Conscious sedation produces a minimally depressed level of consciousness that "retains the patient's ability to maintain a patent airway independently and continuously and to respond appropriately to physical stimulation and verbal commands." Deep sedation produces a "controlled state of depressed consciousness or unconsciousness from which the patient is not easily aroused and is unable to respond purposefully to physical stimulation or verbal command. This may be accompanied by a partial or complete loss of protective reflexes and an inability to maintain a patent airway independently." Because sedation is not a simple on-off state, one cannot always predict how an individual patient will respond.

The Joint Commission on Accreditation of Healthcare Organizations currently recommends that organizations develop specific protocols that address at least the following five issues:

1. There are sufficient personnel present to perform the procedure and monitor the patient.
2. The equipment is appropriate for care and resuscitation.
3. The monitoring is appropriate to ensure adequate cardiorespiratory function and oxygenation.
4. All aspects of care are documented.
5. Outcomes are monitored.

Each ambulatory surgical unit should, therefore, develop guidelines that are specifically tailored to the types of diagnostic and therapeutic procedures it performs. The types of sedation and anesthesia to be used should be defined first, and then the available guidelines should be customized as appropriate. In a prudently run unit, one would not attempt deep sedation or even the deeper levels of conscious sedation without additional trained personnel, ECG monitoring, and pulse oximetry.

Immediate Postoperative Care

Postanesthesia recovery rooms (PARs) in outpatient facilities are in most cases similar to, if not the same as, those in inpatient surgical units. The standards applying to inpatient facilities also apply to outpatient facilities. The environment, the personnel, and the equipment must be carefully selected and evaluated. As a rule, the PAR is supervised by an anesthesiologist. Satisfactory patient recovery requires the cooperation of the surgeon, the anesthesiologist, the PAR nurse, and the patient.

There are two phases of postoperative outpatient recovery. The first phase is emergence from the effects of the anesthesia and stabilization; this phase is the same for inpatient and outpatient surgery. The second phase is readaptation to the environment after total recovery from the anesthetic. Ideally, the two phases of recovery should take place in separate areas of the unit, although this is not always practical or possible.

A uniform method for assessing a patient's postoperative condition should be used during the critical emergence phase of recovery; several scoring systems have been devised in efforts to standardize reporting.[79-81] Whatever system is used must be simple and comprehensive so as not to distract nurses from patient care but at the same time must provide sufficient information to permit adequate assessment of the patient's postoperative condition. There are five main variables that should be assessed: (1) respiration, (2) circulation, (3) consciousness, (4) skin color, and (5) level of voluntary activity.

Observation during the second phase is crucial for determining whether the patient should be discharged. This phase may be considered complete when coordination returns and the subjective feeling of light-headedness or dizziness disappears. There are a number of methods, mostly involving the testing of psychomotor skills and cognition, that are used to ascertain whether the patient has completed this phase of recovery.

Medications must be used judiciously in the PAR because recovery may be delayed if major narcotics, sedatives, or antiemetics are administered. Supplementation of general anesthesia with fentanyl has successfully reduced postoperative pain for as long as 25 hours.[82] One large surgical clinic found that during the initial recovery phase, I.V. fentanyl, 12.5 µg (0.25 ml) every five minutes to a maximum dose of 50 µg (1.0 ml), was effective for most patients.[83] It should be remembered, however, that the larger the dose of fentanyl, the smaller its advantages over long-acting narcotics [see Performance of the Operation, above].

Discharge

The patient should be discharged only after being observed and evaluated by the discharging physician, who is usually the anesthesiologist. The reasons why it is the anesthesiologist, rather than the surgeon, who generally makes the decision to discharge the patient are (1) that the surgical criteria for discharge are usually met when the operation is completed and (2) that delayed recovery from anesthesia is the most common cause of a prolonged recovery period. Nevertheless, either the surgeon or a representative should always be available until the patient is stable and has been discharged. Neither the anesthesiologist nor the other nonsurgical personnel should be expected to manage postoperative surgical problems, especially bleeding. In addition, a surgical presence is important because the surgeon is almost always the physician responsible for admitting the patient to an inpatient facility if delayed recovery warrants such action.

The ultimate standard for discharge is whether it is medically (as opposed to financially or administratively) advisable to do so. The specific criteria that must be met before the patient is discharged include some of the same criteria governing recovery from any type of anesthesia—in particular, a return to the preprocedure functional level with no deviations accepted with respect to (1) stability of vital signs, including recumbent and orthostatic measurements; (2) stability of respiratory function; (3) full responsiveness and orientation; (4) ability to move voluntarily; and (5) control of nausea, vomiting, and pain. A system has been developed at the University of Toronto—the so-called Post-Anesthesia Discharge Scoring System—that is worthy of consideration.[84]

In addition to returning to the preprocedure functional level, the patient must be verbal and must confirm his or her understanding of the follow-up procedures and the steps to be taken in case of emergency. Verbal explanations should be supplemented with written instructions, and the patient should be given the names of physicians to contact if problems arise. The patient should be discharged only when all of the criteria are met and only when he or she is accompanied by a responsible adult. The patient should not drive home alone.

HANDLING OF POSTDISCHARGE PROBLEMS

Major complications [see Table 9] usually do not arise until after the patient has been discharged. The most common reasons why patients delay seeking help in the postoperative period are (1) that they did not know what to look for, (2) that they did not know the significance of what they found, and (3) that they did not know what to do or whom to contact.[85] Follow-up phone calls or visits are useful for detecting postoperative problems; they also help relieve the anxiety of the patient and the family members. At the very least, such contact reduces the number of panicked or inquiring calls from the patient or the family. It is important, however, that the concerns expressed by the patient and any worrisome signs or symptoms detected by the caller be properly recorded and relayed to a responsible physician, who should then act on them.

Both patient and family will inevitably be concerned about specific aspects of recovery after discharge, such as diet, urinary and bowel function, and wound care. Such concerns are typically addressed before the operation [see Preoperative Conference, above], but it is often a good idea to repeat what was discussed and provide written instructions to allay these concerns further.

Even when given adequate counseling, certain anxious patients require admission for their own peace of mind or that of their families or physicians. It is always safer to admit a patient to the hospital when the potential for a serious problem exists. This point of view must be accepted by the patient and the third-party payor before the procedure is undertaken.

Postoperative Pain Control

Postoperative pain is a significant problem that probably is still underestimated: it contributes to patient discomfort, prolongs recovery time, and contributes to increased use of limited health care resources [see *104 Postoperative Pain*]. It is estimated that standard practices fail to relieve postoperative pain in nearly 50 percent of surgical patients.

A fundamental issue is how to assess the degree of pain present after operation. In the immediate postoperative state, physiologic measurements (e.g., blood pressure, pulse, and respiratory rate) give clues to the patient's experience of pain; however, after recovery from anesthesia, the primary measure of the pain experienced is the patient's own description of the site, type, and level of pain. Accordingly, recognition and assessment of pain demand a certain level of communication between the patient on one hand and the physician and other health care workers (especially nurses) on the other. Without such communication, pain goes unrecognized and thus unrelieved. The considerable difficulty of recognizing pain in comatose or paralyzed patients underscores this point with particular force. In some patients, especially the very young and the very old, innovative techniques are required to achieve the necessary communication.

In ambulatory settings, the mainstay of pain control is pharmacological management. The surgeon's tasks are (1) to select the medication and decide on the route of administration, (2) to determine the initial and maintenance doses, and (3) to assess the

Table 9 Major Complications at a Major Surgical Outpatient Center

Complication	Number of Patients
Hemorrhage	138
Wound infection	24
Other infections	26
Persistent vomiting	11
Phlebitis	8
Laryngospasm (severe)	5
Psychosomatic reactions	4
Drug allergy (urticaria)	3
Perforation of uterus	2
Syncopal episodes	2

Note: data are extrapolated from more than 32,000 patients.

likelihood of side effects and complications. Mild to moderate pain should initially be treated with NSAIDs unless a contraindication is present. Even when they are not effective in themselves, NSAIDs have an opioid-sparing effect. At present, only ketorolac is approved by the FDA for parenteral use. For more severe pain, the use of opioid analgesics is the time-proven approach: these agents almost always provide adequate relief of postoperative pain. If the pain is not relieved by increasing doses of opioid analgesics or if it suddenly intensifies, one should search for a change in the patient's condition that might be the source of the pain (e.g., dehiscence, bleeding, or necrosis). Opioid tolerance or physiologic dependence may occur, but such problems rarely arise in the short administration periods associated with most elective surgical procedures.

The action of opioid analgesics is related to their affinities for opioid receptors in the peripheral and central nervous systems. On the basis of these affinities, these agents are classified as full agonists, as partial agonists, or as mixed agonist-antagonists (which simultaneously activate one type of receptor and block another type). The agonists include morphine, hydromorphone, codeine, oxycodone, and fentanyl; these agents have an affinity for the so-called mu receptor. The mixed agonist-antagonists include pentazocine, butorphanol tartrate, and nalbuphine hydrochloride; these drugs block the mu receptor and activate the so-called kappa receptor.

In many cases, the most commonly used opioids, meperidine and morphine, are given in insufficient doses administered too far apart.[86] In particular, meperidine is rarely effective for longer than two and a half to three hours, and a 75 mg dose is equivalent to only about 5 to 7 mg of morphine. If additional pain relief is needed, it may be advisable initially to decrease the dosing interval of meperidine. This may not be a major issue with ambulatory procedures, however, given that parenteral opioids of any sort are not commonly used in this setting.

PCA is a safe and effective means of providing pain relief. With proper preoperative preparation and postdischarge management, this technique is a useful method of controlling moderate to severe pain after outpatient procedures. Many hospitals provide such services after discharge.

Prolongation of the anesthetic effect with long-acting local anesthetics is discussed in more detail elsewhere [see Anesthesia, above]. The use of epidural injections is not yet a widely accepted practice in the ambulatory setting.

Discussion

Preoperative Assessment to Determine Operative Risk

PERIOPERATIVE RISK PERIOD: THE FIRST 48 HOURS

In the first 48 hours after surgery, the patient is at risk for complications related to anesthesia as well as complications related to the surgical procedure itself. Mortality in the first 48 hours after operation (which are understood to include induction of anesthesia, the intraoperative period, and the immediate postoperative period) has been estimated at approximately 0.3 percent.[87,88] About 10 percent of deaths occur during induction of anesthesia, 35 percent occur intraoperatively, and 55 percent occur during the subsequent 48 hours.[89] Failure to maintain adequate ventilation, aspiration of gastric contents, sudden cardiac difficulty (e.g., arrhythmia), drug-induced myocardial depression, and progressive hypotension (usually from hemorrhage) each account for, on average, 10 to 15 percent of the total 48-hour mortality. Hypoxia has been estimated to play some role in half of all anesthesia-related deaths.[90] The extent to which duration of anesthesia is a risk factor is a more complicated issue.

A 1994 study found that complications caused mainly by the anesthetic procedure occurred in 0.6 percent of patients and that deaths attributable to anesthesia occurred in 0.04 percent.[91] Seriously ill patients (ASA class III or higher) were more likely to be affected by errors and to have a serious negative outcome (e.g., acute myocardial infarction, irreversible cerebral damage, or death) than were more healthy patients (ASA class I or II). One third of the complications attributable to anesthesia were judged to be preventable. The occurrence of cardiopulmonary complications was associated with age greater than 70 years, preoperative clinical signs of ischemic heart disease or recent myocardial infarction, a history of chronic heart failure or chronic obstructive pulmonary disease, and previous major abdominal procedures.

Hypotension before induction of anesthesia is associated with a high incidence of cardiopulmonary morbidity and mortality. The relative incidence of postoperative pulmonary complications in comparable groups of patients is determined primarily by the type of operation performed, with major abdominal procedures being associated with the highest incidence. Regional anesthesia may be less likely to give rise to such complications than general anesthesia, especially in elderly patients with chronic obstructive pulmonary disease who are admitted for major orthopedic procedures. Furthermore, with respect to preventing postoperative complications such as residual neuromuscular blockade, the choice of muscle relaxant is more of a determinant than was manual evaluation of the response to train-to-four nerve stimulation. It is noteworthy that the surgeon's "gut feeling" on completing the operation is still a reasonably good prognostic tool.[92]

Cardiac Risk

The high mortality (60 to 70 percent) associated with postoperative myocardial infarction and the significant threat of heart failure make preoperative cardiac assessment particularly important now that it is possible to improve cardiac function by various surgical and pharmacological methods.[93] Evaluation starts with a careful history and physical examination to identify cardiac risk factors. First-line routine tests include a chest x-ray and ECG. Most surgeons consult a cardiologist before ordering second-line tests. Echocardiography is the second-line test that best documents aortic or mitral valve disease. Aortic stenosis is a particularly ominous finding because of its potential to cause myocardial ischemia during intraoperative hypotension. Third-line studies for ascertaining the threat of valvular disease involve cardiac catheterization, which necessitates two or three days of hospitalization.

The two competing second-line tests for coronary artery disease are the exercise tolerance test and thallium-201 scanning.[94] The exercise tolerance test is being supplanted by more sophisticated imaging techniques but continues to be useful. A positive result from an exercise tolerance test correlates with the presence of coronary artery disease in more than 98 percent of patients with typical angina, in 88 percent of patients with atypical angina, and in 44 percent of patients with noncardiac chest pain.[95] The test has an overall sensitivity of 65 percent and a specificity of 85 percent for coronary artery disease. In men with atypical chest pain, the probability of coronary artery disease is 67 percent but is increased to 88 percent if the exercise test result is positive. If the anginal history is typical, a thallium-201 exercise test is preferable to the standard exercise test.[96] The thallium-201 scan permits visualization of regional myocardial flow, leaving scar tissue unperfused. Its sensitivity for coronary artery disease is 80 percent, and its specificity is 90 percent; thus, it is more efficient than the exercise tolerance test.[97] In particular, the high specificity of the thallium-201 scan makes it preferable to the exercise tolerance test in women with atypical angina, in whom the probability of coronary atherosclerosis is low. Limitations include the high cost and the need for familiarity with the test. Administering dipyridamole along with the thallium-201 scan may increase diagnostic accuracy.

Gated blood-pool scanning is a competitive alternative to thallium-201 scanning.[98] Multiple frames can be rapidly triggered by the QRS complex to yield serial images of technetium-99m–tagged erythrocytes, by means of which distribution of blood flow over the myocardium can be measured. Unlike the thallium-201 scan, the gated blood-pool scan permits visualization of heart wall motion and the ventricular ejection fraction. When performed within two to four days after the onset of chest pain, it has a sensitivity of 89 percent and a specificity of 86 percent for transmural infarction. For visualization of abnormal heart wall motion, its sensitivity is 76 percent and its specificity 95 percent.[99,100] The combination of cardiac catheterization and coronary angiography is the third-line test for coronary artery disease. This combination measures coronary narrowing, for which it has a sensitivity of 88 percent when compared with findings on autopsy.[101,102]

Cardiac disease itself is a better predictor of cardiac death than the ASA scale.[34,103] In both retrospective and prospective studies, patients with recent myocardial infarctions are at greatest risk for postoperative cardiac death. In one large series, the risk of myocardial infarction increased from 0.13 percent in patients without prior infarction to four percent in patients with prior infarction more than six months before operation.[2] In patients who had had an infarction three to six months before, the reinfarction rate rose to 16 percent, and in patients who had had an infarction in the preceding three months, the reinfarction rate was 38 percent.

A 1977 study that used multivariate analysis to detect factors placing surgical patients at risk for cardiac death also found recent myocardial infarction to be an important risk factor.[34] Equally important was the presence of an S_3 gallop or jugular venous distention preoperatively, implying uncompensated congestive heart failure. Preoperative arrhythmia, premature atrial and ventricular contractions, and a heart rhythm other than sinus were also significantly correlated with cardiac death. Age greater than 70 years, certain operations (emergency procedures as well as thoracic, intraperitoneal, or aortic procedures), and significant aortic stenosis all increased the risk of postoperative cardiac death, but to a lesser degree than previous myocardial infarction or congestive heart failure. Using these risk factors, the investigators were able to identify the 1.8 percent of the study group who would sustain 53 percent of the cardiac deaths. When there is a history of myocardial infarction or significant angina, coronary arteriography (followed by coronary bypass surgery when indicated) may well lessen the risk of subsequent major elective surgery.[104]

A 1980 study reported on a system of preoperative staging, based on invasive monitoring, that was developed to reduce operative mortality in elderly patients.[93] The investigators studied 148 consecutive patients who had been cleared for surgery through standard assessment methods. In only 13.5 percent of these patients were measured hemodynamic, respiratory, and oxygen transport function normal. Mild physiologic aberrations that did not necessitate delaying the operation (stage 1) or more severe abnormalities that were indicative of high operative risk (stages 2 and 3) were found in 63.5 percent of the patients. Advanced and incorrigible functional defects (stage 4) were found in the remaining 23 percent, who therefore were considered to be at unacceptably high risk for complications from major procedures done with general anesthesia. All of the stage 4 patients who underwent the planned operations despite the warning died. Comparison of this staging system with the preoperative noninvasive assessment the anesthetists performed using the ASA physical status classification showed a good correlation. For example, all ASA class IV patients had a higher mean pulmonary arterial wedge pressure (PAWP) and high pulmonary vascular resistance, and more than 20 percent died. This noninvasive approach was not as good at predicting mortality as the invasive monitoring technique, in that all of the patients placed in stage 4 by the invasive approach died.

In a later study by the same group,[105] 100 consecutive high-risk elective surgical patients entered a preoperative ICU for a prospective analysis of physiologic assessment, resource utilization, diagnosis-related group (DRG) classification, and outcome. Swan-Ganz catheters were inserted one or two days before operation, and the data obtained were used to compute physiologic profiles and to stage the patients according to previously published criteria. Zero percent of the patients fell into stage 1; 55 percent into stage 2; 41 percent into stage 3; and four percent into stage 4 (which accounted for three of the four total deaths). In 53 percent of the patients, the physiologic profile provided data necessary for preoperative fine tuning: in 37 percent, it identified indications for volume expansion; in 23 percent, for inotropic therapy; and in 17 percent, for pulmonary therapy. Significant differences between stage 2 and stage 3 patients were found with respect to PAWP, right ventricular stroke work, pulmonary vascular resistance, and pulmonary shunt fraction. The patients who died all had advanced liver disease. Invasive preoperative assessment of elderly patients discloses a high incidence of serious physiologic abnormalities, as a result of which operations must be delayed in some cases and canceled in others.

A 1994 study reported a progressive increase in cardiac risk as the overall mean age of the population increases.[106] Parsonnet risk estimates and postoperative lengths of stay were studied for two cohorts of cardiac surgical patients. The first cohort consisted of 287 patients operated on during 1984; the second consisted of all 1,167 patients operated on in the calendar years 1989 to 1991. Mean risk for the patients nearly doubled in this interval, and the risk distribution changed significantly from one skewed toward low-risk patients to a nearly uniform distribution through all risk categories. A high correlation ($r = 0.98$) was identified between the postoperative length of stay and the mean risk estimates for the second patient cohort.

Pulmonary Assessment

The purpose of preoperative pulmonary assessment is to predict which patients are at increased risk for pulmonary complications, in which circumstances such complications may occur, and whether the risk is high enough to be a contraindication to the planned procedure. Prediction, prevention, and treatment of pulmonary complications of surgery have been extensively studied.[107-110] The sequence of hypoventilation, atelectasis, and pneumonia is well known and is estimated to occur in 20 to 40 percent of all postoperative patients. The most useful pulmonary function tests are (1) arterial blood gas values (CO_2 retention correlates best with the need for postoperative ventilatory support), (2) maximum breathing capacity (a capacity less than 50 percent of predicted is associated with a 50 percent postoperative mortality), and (3) maximum midexpiratory flow rate (this measurement correlates with the ability to generate a cough, which is important for preventing postoperative pneumonias).[111]

Risk factors for postoperative pulmonary complications include obesity, age greater than 70 years, a history of smoking, prolonged hospitalization, an anticipated lengthy thoracic or upper abdominal operation, and an ASA score of class I or higher. Chronic obstructive pulmonary disease is the most common concern before operation. It is often present while giving rise to few physical findings and only minimal changes on x-rays. Second-line tests for pulmonary assessment include spirometry with measurement of forced vital capacity (FVC) and forced expiratory volume in one second (FEV_1); from these two measurements, the FEV_1/FVC ratio is calculated. It is often necessary to add a measurement after bronchodilatation.

Patients about to undergo resective surgery of the lung require careful preoperative assessment.[112] Testing modalities used in the preoperative evaluation include spirometry, full pulmonary function tests, measurement of arterial blood gas values, radionuclide lung scanning, exercise testing, invasive measurement of pulmonary arterial pressure, and a variety of studies involving lobar occlusion or lateral position testing. Studies evaluating the utility of these procedures have been reviewed elsewhere.[113] Central to risk assessment for lung resection is the fact that surgery offers the only chance of long-term survival and cure for patients with non–small cell carcinoma of the lung. The challenge, therefore, is to offer surgical treatment to as many patients as possible while minimizing the risk of death from postoperative respiratory failure.

Preexisting respiratory disease may be assessed by means of arterial blood gas analysis, exercise testing, and global and regional lung function testing. Criteria based on these tests have been proposed to aid patient selection before lung resection; however, these criteria do not take into account the beneficial influence of modern anesthesia and postoperative care on outcome. The elimina-

Table 10 Hospital Mortality from All Causes in 4,292 Surgical Patients, Stratified by Admission Skin Test Response

Admission Skin Test Response	N	Outcome	
		Alive (%)	Dead (%)
Reactive	2,509	2,432 (96.9)	77 (3.1)
Relatively anergic	666	593 (89.0)	73 (11.0)
Anergic	1,117	837 (74.9)	280 (25.1)*
Total	4,292	3,862 (88.9)	430 (11.1)

*$\chi^2 = 415.6$; $P < 0.0000001$.

and 17.5 percent mortality). The reduction in mortality for anergic patients over the 20-year study period was attributable primarily to the lower mortality for elective anergic patients (23 percent, 25.1 percent, and 6.3 percent mortality) in comparison with anergic patients in the surgical ICU (34.4 percent, 35.2 percent, and 28.3 percent mortality). Log-linear modeling confirmed this interaction. The logistic regression equation mentioned earlier, generated with data obtained between 1974 and 1981, accurately predicted mortality up to 1989 but overestimated mortality for the period between 1989 and 1994. For example, 18 deaths were predicted to occur in the 249 patients studied in the comorbid analysis carried out between June 1, 1992, and March 31, 1993, but only four deaths actually occurred. Not enough deaths have occurred in elective surgical patients in the hospital database since 1990 to permit the creation of a new logistic model.

CONCLUSION

The primary objective of preoperative evaluation is to detect and manage disease that affects the anticipated operation. The list of possible coexisting diseases is long. For each, the method of evaluation includes the history and the physical examination (with an emphasis on risk factors), followed by first-line, second-line, and third-line laboratory studies if the index of suspicion is high enough to warrant delaying the operation for further study or treatment. Each decision in the evaluation process calls for analysis of existing data in the light of known laboratory test performance, costs, and risks, as well as the clinical relevance of further study to the patient. Preoperative evaluation is an expensive process that is much easier to initiate than to stop. Its proper use requires both knowledge and judgment.

Table 11 Hospital Mortality from All Causes in 2,259 Surgical Patients Who Maintained Admission Skin Test Response in Weekly Sequential Tests

Response to Weekly Sequential Skin Tests	N	Outcome	
		Alive (%)	Dead (%)
Always reactive	1,496	1,475 (98.6)	21 (1.4)
Always anergic	763	490 (44.4)	273 (55.6)*
Total	2,259	1,965 (80.0)	294 (20.0)

*$\chi^2 = 527.4$; $P < 0.00000001$.

Growth of Outpatient Surgery

The recent evolution of health care in response primarily to socioeconomic factors has been spectacular, and the process is by no means complete. The most striking result to date is the emergence of ambulatory surgery as the predominant mode for the delivery of surgical health care. Just a few years ago, it was estimated that more than 40 percent of all operative procedures would be performed in the outpatient setting. By 1995, however, 50 percent of operative procedures were already being performed on an outpatient basis. It is estimated that this number will have approached 60 percent by the end of the 20th century, and even this estimate may be low.

Although the explosive growth of ambulatory surgery was initiated by economic factors, it has had some positive effects on patient care, for the following reasons.

1. Development of new technology. New techniques, such as laparoscopic surgery, minimize the need for hospitalization and decrease the pain and suffering that patients must endure. It is not yet clear, however, that such developments will inevitably lead to a reduction in total health care costs. One study reported that the cholecystectomy rate increased from 1.35 per 1,000 enrollees in an HMO in 1988 to 2.15 per 1,000 in 1990 and that the total cost for cholecystectomies rose by 11.4 percent despite a unit cost savings of 25.1 percent.[135] The authors suggested that these results might be attributable to changing indications for gallbladder operations. It is noteworthy that no increase in the performance of either hernioplasty or appendectomy was recorded.

2. Cost savings achieved by Medicare and other payors. In 1987, Medicare approved over 200 procedures as suitable for ambulatory surgical centers. Currently, more than 900 procedures are so designated, with more procedures being approved every year. Ophthalmologic and gynecologic procedures predominate in ambulatory surgical centers. The endorsement of cost-efficient delivery systems by employers and the reduction of employee benefits by insurers are encouraging employees (as both consumers and patients) to be more cost conscious. When patients are involved in the actual cost of medical care, they tend to accept more efficient modes of delivery. This is even more likely to be the case when they are at risk for the cost of care.

3. Physician concern. The emergence of the concept of managed care has exerted a strong influence on physician involvement in ambulatory surgery. Whether surgeons accept the concept or not, ambulatory surgery is here to stay, and if surgeons desire to participate in the future of health care delivery, they will have to conform to some extent.

4. Patient awareness of quality assurance. Today's patients (or consumers) are more medically knowledgeable than ever before and more concerned with actively seeking out institutions that deliver high-quality and cost-efficient care. Consumers are highly sensitive to the issue of quality, but their definitions of this attribute are not always based on the same criteria that surgeons use.

Economic benefits aside, the major consideration in the movement of surgical activities out of the hospital and into a more convenient and economical environment is how best to ensure that patients continue to receive safe, high-quality care. This consideration must in all circumstances be the primary issue underlying the planning of elective surgery. More and more, third-party payors expect surgical care to be provided to their clients (patients, to us) in a cost-effective environment. On the whole, this is not a bad thing. If, however, they also expect that surgical care can be provided just as cost-effectively to diabetic patients, morbidly obese patients, and patients with serious cardiac or respiratory disease, there is a real danger that patients' welfare could be compromised. Accordingly, it is crucial that all third parties who are not directly involved in the care of the patient permit the surgeon and the anesthesiologist to exercise sound medical judgment in regard to what type of care is needed and where such care can best be delivered. Surgeons must not delegate their responsibility for safeguarding their patients' well-being.

The Health Care Financing Administration, under a cooperative agreement with 3M Health Information Systems, is currently developing a prospective payment system for hospital outpatient services. The result is a patient classification system for outpatient procedures, therapies, and services that consists of approximately 50 so-called ambulatory patient groups (APGs). These APGs are based on groupings of the familiar CPT codes. As of mid-1997, the system had not been finalized.

The American College of Surgeons has issued several statements on ambulatory surgery, the most recent of which appeared in 1983.[136] At that time, the ACS approved "the concept that certain procedures may be performed in an ambulatory surgical facility" but emphasized that "a prime concern about ambulatory surgery is assurance of quality." The report further stated that "a discussion between patient and surgeon about performance of the procedure on an ambulatory basis should result in a mutually agreeable decision."

Outpatient surgery would seem to have an obvious advantage over inpatient surgery with respect to cost savings, especially if the main focus of the comparison is the high charges for one or more days of inpatient care. Such a comparison may be misleading insofar as it suggests that the entire cost of inpatient care can be saved when the procedure is done on an outpatient basis. The hospital inpatient charge reflects the costs of a number of functions associated with early convalescence in the hospital, including nursing, diet, and housekeeping; some of these costs are also associated with immediate postoperative care in the outpatient recovery area and consequently will be reflected in the outpatient facility's bill as well. The comparison may also be misleading insofar as it ignores the implicit costs of outpatient surgery. In some cases, medical personnel perform functions that do not appear on the bill, such as follow-up care, care by phone, and home visits to evaluate recovery, as well as dressing changes and other services similar to those provided by family members or friends. The costs associated with buying or renting durable medical equipment (e.g., beds and commodes), preparing meals, and various other activities must also be taken into account.

Despite the absence of definitive data that convincingly demonstrate significant cost savings from ambulatory surgery (aside from statistics from third-party agencies that seem to show a significant benefit in terms of total agency expenditure), it seems reasonable to assume that reducing inpatient hospitalization is indeed valuable for cost containment. It is to be hoped that the new Medicare regulations mandating evaluation of quality of care in ambulatory surgical centers by professional review organizations will provide definitive statistics for evaluation of actual cost savings. Cost data must be analyzed thoroughly if we are to assess the true contribution of outpatient surgery to cost containment.

Table 12 Hospital Mortality in 4,292 Surgical Patients in a Single Hospital over a 20-Year Period, Stratified by Admission Skin Test Response and Location in Hospital

Admission Skin Test Response	Period	N	Outcome	
			Alive (%)	Dead (%)
All Patients				
Reactive	1973–1979	1,106	1,064 (96.2)	42 (3.8)
	1980–1989	679	658 (96.9)	21 (3.1)
	1990–1994	724	710 (98.1)	14 (1.9)
Relatively anergic	1973–1979	230	194 (84.3)	36 (15.7)
	1980–1989	160	146 (91.2)	14 (8.8)
	1990–1994	276	253 (91.7)	23 (8.3)
Anergic	1973–1979	392	273 (69.6)	119 (30.4)
	1980–1989	307	219 (71.3)	88 (28.7)
	1990–1994	418	345 (82.3)	73 (17.5)
Ward Patients*				
Reactive	1973–1979	896	877 (97.8)	19 (2.1)
	1980–1989	629	611 (97.1)	18 (2.9)
	1990–1994	615	606 (98.5)	9 (1.5)
Relatively anergic	1973–1979	114	106 (93.0)	8 (7.0)
	1980–1989	117	111 (94.9)	6 (5.1)
	1990–1994	163	159 (97.5)	4 (2.5)
Anergic	1973–1979	142	109 (76.8)	33 (23.2)
	1980–1989	199	149 (74.9)	50 (25.1)
	1990–1994	206	193 (93.7)	13 (6.3)
SICU/Trauma Patients†				
Reactive	1973–1979	210	187 (89.0)	23 (11.0)
	1980–1989	50	47 (94.0)	3 (6.0)
	1990–1994	109	104 (95.4)	5 (4.6)
Relatively anergic	1973–1979	116	88 (75.9)	28 (24.1)
	1980–1989	43	35 (81.4)	8 (18.6)
	1990–1994	113	94 (83.2)	19 (16.8)
Anergic	1973–1979	250	164 (65.6)	86 (34.4)
	1980–1989	108	70 (64.8)	38 (35.2)
	1990–1994	212	152 (71.7)	60 (28.3)

*$\chi^2 = 27.4$; $P < 0.000001$.
†$\chi^2 = 3.46$; $P < 0.17$.

References

1. Hampson JR, Harrison MAG, Mitchell JAR, et al: Relative contributions of history-taking, physical examination, and laboratory investigation to diagnosis and management of medical outpatients. Br Med J 2:486, 1975
2. Tarhan S, Moffit EA, Taylor WF, et al: Myocardial infarction after general anesthesia. JAMA 220:1451, 1972
3. Gomez-Sanchez CE, Gomez-Sanchez EP, Yamakita N: Endocrine causes of hypertension. Semin Nephrol 15:106, 1995
4. Ross NS: Epidemiology of Cushing's syndrome and subclinical disease. Endocrinol Metab Clin North Am 23:539, 1994
5. Bickler SW, McMahon TJ, Campbell JR, et al: Preoperative diagnostic evaluation of children with Cushing's syndrome. J Pediatr Surg 29:671, 1994
6. Studley HO: Percentage of weight loss: basic indicator of surgical risk in patients with chronic peptic ulcer. JAMA 106:458, 1936
7. Messmore HL Jr, Godwin J: Medical assessment of bleeding in the surgical patient. Med Clin North Am 78:625, 1994
8. Barnard NA, Williams RW, Spencer EM: Preoperative patient assessment: a review of the literature and recommendations. Ann R Coll Surg Engl 76:293, 1994
9. Macpherson DS: Preoperative laboratory testing: should any tests be "routine" before surgery? Med Clin North Am 77:289, 1993
10. Velanovich V: Preoperative laboratory screening based

on age, gender, and concomitant medical diseases. Surgery 115:56, 1994
11. Krieg AF, Gambino R, Galen RS: Why are clinical laboratory tests performed? When are they valid? JAMA 233:76, 1975
12. Kaplan EB, Shiner LB, Beckman AJ, et al: The usefulness of preoperative laboratory screening. JAMA 253:3576, 1985
13. Carmalt MHB, Freeman P, Stephens AJH, et al: Value of routine multiple blood tests in patients attending the general practitioner. Br Med J 1:620, 1970
14. Macario A, Roizen MF, Thisted RA, et al: Reassessment of preoperative laboratory testing has changed the test-ordering patterns of physicians. Surg Gynecol Obstet 175:539, 1992
15. Roy WL, Lerman J, McIntyre BG: Is preoperative haemoglobin testing justified in children undergoing minor elective surgery? Can J Anaesth 38:700, 1991
16. Mariani AJ, Luangphinith S, Loo S, et al: Dipstick chemical urinalysis: an accurate cost effective screening. J Urol 132:64, 1984
17. Hubbell FA, Greenfield S, Tyler JL, et al: The impact of routine admission chest x-ray films on patient care. N Engl J Med 312:209, 1985
18. Sagel SS, Evens RG, Forrest JV, et al: Efficacy of routine screening and lateral chest x-rays in a hospital-based population. N Engl J Med 291:1001, 1974
19. The Royal College of Radiologists: National study: preoperative chest radiology. Lancet 2:83, 1979
20. Tresch DD: Diagnostic and prognostic value of ambulatory electrographic monitoring in older patients. J Am Geriatr Soc 43:66, 1995
21. Ostrander LD Jr, Brandt RL, Kjelsberg MO, et al: Electrocardiographic finding among the adult population of a total natural community, Tecumseh, Michigan. Circulation 31:888, 1965
22. Suchman AC, Mashlin AI: How well does the activated partial thromboplastin time predict postoperative hemorrhage? JAMA 256:750, 1986
23. Myers ER, Clarke-Pearson DL, Olt GJ, et al: Preoperative coagulation testing on a gynecologic oncology service. Obstet Gynecol 83:438, 1994
24. Rapaport SI: Preoperative hemostatic evaluation: which tests if any? Blood 61:229, 1983
25. Perioperative Red Cell Transfusion: National Institutes of Health Consensus Development Conference Statement, Vol. 7, No. 4, June 27–29, 1988. US Dept of Health and Human Services, Bethesda, Maryland
26. Stehling L, Simon TL: The red blood cell transfusion trigger: physiology and clinical studies. Arch Pathol Lab Med 118:429, 1994
27. Elliot MS, Levenstein JH, Wright JP: Faecal occult blood testing in the detection of colorectal cancer. Br J Surg 71:785, 1984
28. Greegor DH: Diagnosis of large-bowel cancer in the asymptomatic patient. JAMA 201:943, 1967
29. Sonnenberg A, Townsend WF: Preoperative testing for fecal occult blood: a questionable practice. Am J Gastroenterol 87:1410, 1992
30. Macpherson DS, Lofgren RP: Outpatient internal medicine preoperative evaluation: a randomized clinical trial. Med Care 32:498, 1994
31. Varon AJ, Hudson-Civetta JA, Civetta JM, et al: Preoperative intensive care unit consultations: accurate and effective. Crit Care Med 21:234, 1993
32. Ambulatory surgery. ACS Reports. American College of Surgeons, Chicago, August 1983
33. Pasternak LR: Admission patient. Wellcome Trends in Anesthesiology 9(5):3, 1991
34. Goldman L, Caldera DL, Nussbaum SR, et al: Multifactorial index of cardiac risk in noncardiac surgical procedures. N Engl J Med 297:845, 1977
35. Lewin I, Lerner AG, Green SH, et al: Physical class and physiologic status in the prediction of operative mortality in the aged sick. Ann Surg 174:217, 1971
36. Schneider AJL: Assessment of risk factors and surgical outcome. Surg Clin North Am 63:1113, 1983
37. Maini BS: Personal communication
38. Warner MA, Shields SE, Chute CG: Major morbidity and mortality within 1 month of ambulatory surgery and anesthesia. JAMA 270:1437, 1993
39. Laffaye HA: The impact of an ambulatory surgical service in a community hospital. Arch Surg 124:601, 1989
40. Gold BS, Kitz DS, Lecky JH, et al: Unanticipated admission to the hospital following ambulatory surgery. JAMA 262:3008, 1989
41. Petros JG, Rimm EB, Robillard RJ, et al: Factors influencing postoperative urinary retention in patients undergoing elective inguinal herniorrhaphy. Am J Surg 161:431, 1991
42. Pennock JL: Perioperative management of drug therapy. Surg Clin North Am 65:1049, 1983
43. Natof HE: Ambulatory surgery: pre-existing medical problems. Illinois Medical Journal 166:101, 1984
44. Physician Office Surgery (abstr). Project No. 5079. Office of Evaluation and Inspection, Washington, DC, 1993
45. Board of Governors' Committee on Ambulatory Surgical Care: Guidelines for Optimal Office-Based Surgery, 2nd ed. American College of Surgeons, Chicago, 1996
46. Redmond MC: The importance of good communication in effective patient-family teaching. Journal of Postanesthesia Nursing 8:109, 1993
47. Leske JS: Anxiety of elective surgical patients' family members: relationship between anxiety levels, family characteristics. AORN J 57:1091, 1993
48. Laing R, Lam M, Owen H, et al: Perceived risks of postoperative analgesia. Aust NZ J Surg 63:760, 1993
49. Justins DM: Postoperative pain: a continuing challenge. Ann R Coll Surg Engl 74:78, 1992
50. Waisel DB, Truog RD: The benefits of the explanation of the risks of anesthesia in the day surgery patient. J Clin Anesth 7:200, 1995
51. Nowakowski PA: Implementation of an epidural pain management program. J Neurosci Nurs 25:313, 1993
52. Shafer AL, Donnelly AJ: Management of postoperative pain by continuous epidural infusion of analgesics. Clinical Pharmacy 10:745, 1991
53. Rost C: Preparing for surgery: a pre-admission testing and teaching unit. Nursing Management 22:66, 1991
54. Schwartz-Barcott D, Fortin JD, Kim HS: Client-nurse interaction: testing for its impact in preoperative instruction. Int J Nurs Stud 31:23, 1994
55. Davis JE: Surgical considerations. Major Ambulatory Surgery. Davis JE, Ed. Williams & Wilkins Co, Baltimore, 1986, p 105
56. Sangermano C: The Patient Self-Determination Act. Seminars in Perioperative Nursing 1:232, 1992
57. Johnston D, Thomas P: Consent for surgical treatment. Br J Hosp Med 53:211, 1995
58. Philip BK, Covino BG: Local and regional anesthesia. Anesthesia for Ambulatory Surgery, 2nd ed. Wetchler BV, Ed. JB Lippincott Co, Philadelphia, 1991, p 318
59. Meridy HW: Criteria for selection of ambulatory surgical patients and guidelines for anesthetic management: a retrospective study of 1,553 cases. Anesth Analg 61:921, 1982
60. Abramowitz MD, Oh TH, Epstein BS, et al: The antiemetic effect of droperidol following outpatient strabismus surgery in children. Anesthesiology 59:279, 1983
61. Schmidt JF, Schierup L, Banning AM: The effect of sodium citrate on the pH and the amount of gastric contents before general anaesthesia. Acta Anaesthesiol Scand 28:263, 1984
62. Amid PK, Shulman AG, Lichtenstein IL: Local anesthesia for inguinal hernia repair: step-by-step procedure. Ann Surg 220:735, 1994
63. Arthur GR, Covino BG: What's new in local anesthetics? Anesthesiol Clin North Am 6:357, 1988
64. Bays RA, Barry L, Vasilenko P: The use of bupivacaine in elective inguinal herniorrhaphy as a fast and safe technique for relief of postoperative pain. Surg Gynecol Obstet 173:433, 1991
65. Moore DC: Administer oxygen first in the treatment of local anesthetic-induced convulsions (letter). Anesthesiology 53:346, 1980
66. Covino BG: Pharmacology of local anaesthetic agents. General Anaesthesia, 5th ed. Nunn JF, Utting JE, Brown BR Jr, Eds. Butterworths, London, 1989, p 1036
67. Stoelting RK: Allergic reactions during anesthesia. Anesth Analg 62:341, 1983
68. Aldrete JA, Johnson DA: Evaluation of intracutaneous testing for investigation of allergy to local anesthetic agents. Anesth Analg 49:173, 1970
69. Parnass SM: Controlling postoperative nausea and vomiting. Ambulatory Surgery 1:61 1993
70. Cohen SE, Woods WA, Wyner J: Antiemetic efficacy of droperidol and metoclopramide. Anesthesiology 60:67, 1984
71. Wetchler BV, Collins IS, Jacob L: Antiemetic effects of droperidol on the ambulatory surgical patient. Anesthesiol Rev 9:23, 1982
72. Lacroix G, Lessard MR, Trepanier CA: Treatment of postoperative nausea and vomiting: comparison of propofol, droperidol and metoclopramide. Can J Anaesth 43:115, 1996
73. Steinbrook RA, Freiberger D, Gosnell JL, et al: Prophylactic antiemetics for laparoscopic cholecystectomy: ondansetron versus droperidol plus metoclopramide. Anesth Analg 83:1081, 1996
74. Bidwai AV, Meuleman T, Thatte WB: Prevention of postoperative nausea with dimenhydrinate (Dramamine) and droperidol (Inapsine) (abstract). Anesth Analg 68:S25, 1989
75. Arrowsmith JB, Gerstman BB, Fleischer DE, et al: Results from the American Society for Gastrointestinal Endoscopy/U.S. Food and Drug Administration collaborative study on complication rates and drug use during gastrointestinal endoscopy. Gastrointest Endosc 37:421, 1991
76. Singer R, Thomas PE: Pulse oximeter in the ambulatory aesthetic surgical facility. Plast Reconstr Surg 82:111, 1988
77. Bell GD, McCloy RF, Charlton JE, et al: Recommendations for standards of sedation and patient monitoring during gastrointestinal endoscopy. Gut 32:823, 1991
78. Holzman RS, Cullen DJ, Eichhorn JH, et al: Guidelines for sedation by nonanesthesiologists during diagnostic and therapeutic procedures. J Clin Anesth 6:265, 1994
79. Aldrete JA, Kroulik D: A postanesthetic recovery score. Anesth Analg 49:924, 1970
80. Carignan G, Keéri-Szàntò M, Lavellée J-P: Postanesthetic scoring system. Anesthesiology 25:396, 1964
81. Steward DJ: A simplified scoring system for the postoperative recovery room. Can Anaesth Soc J 22:111, 1975
82. Epstein BS, Levy M-L, Thein MH, et al: Evaluation of fentanyl as an adjunct to thiopental-nitrous oxide–oxygen anesthesia for short surgical procedures. Anesthesiol Rev 2:24, 1975
83. Wetchler BV: Problem solving in the post-anesthesia care unit. Anesthesia for Ambulatory Surgery, 2nd ed. Wetchler BV, Ed. JB Lippincott Co, Philadelphia, 1991, p 375

84. Chung F: Are discharge criteria changing? J Clin Anesth 5(suppl 1):64S, 1993
85. Griffith JL, McLaughlin SH: Legal implications. Anesthesia for Ambulatory Surgery, 2nd ed. Wetchler BV, Ed. JB Lippincott Co, Philadelphia, 1991, p 29
86. Marks RM, Sachar EJ: Undertreatment of medical patients with narcotic analgesics. Ann Intern Med 78:173, 1973
87. Marx GF, Mateo CV, Orkin LR: Computer analysis of postanesthetic deaths. Anaesthesiology 39:54, 1973
88. Vacanti CJ, Van Houten RJ, Hill RC: A statistical analysis of the relationship of physiologic status to postoperative mortality in 68,383 cases. Anesth Analg 49:564, 1970
89. Goldstein A Jr, Keats AS: The risk of anesthesia. Anesthesiology 33:130, 1970
90. Rehdar K, Sessler AD, Marsh HM: General anesthesia and the lung. Am Rev Respir Dis 112:541, 1975
91. Pedersen T: Complications and death following anaesthesia. A prospective study with special reference to the influence of patient-, anaesthesia-, and surgery-related risk factors. Dan Med Bull 41:319, 1994
92. Hartley MN, Sagar PM: The surgeon's "gut feeling" as a predictor of postoperative outcome. Ann R Coll Surg Engl 76(6 Suppl):277, 1994
93. Del Guercio LR, Cohn JD: Monitoring operative risk in the elderly. JAMA 4:1350, 1980
94. Younis L, Stratmann H, Takase B, et al: Preoperative clinical assessment and dipyridamole thallium-201 scintigraphy for prediction and prevention of cardiac events in patients having major noncardiovascular surgery and known or suspected coronary artery disease. Am J Cardiol 74:311, 1994
95. Diamond GA, Forester JS: Analysis of probability as an aid in the clinical diagnosis of coronary artery disease. N Engl J Med 300:1350, 1979
96. Weiner DA, Ryan TJ, McCabe CH, et al: Exercise stress testing: correlations among history of angina, ST-segment response and prevalence of coronary-artery disease in the coronary-artery surgery study (CASS). N Engl J Med 301:230, 1979
97. Mahmarian JJ, Mahmarian AC, Marks GF, et al: Role of adenosine thallium-201 tomography for defining long-term risk in patients after acute myocardial infarction. J Am Coll Cardiol 25:1333, 1995
98. Sanford CF, Corbett J, Nicod P, et al: Value of radionuclide ventriculography in the immediate characterization of patients with acute myocardial infarction. Am J Cardiol 49:637, 1982
99. Gibson RS, Watson DD, Taylor GJ, et al: Prospective assessment of regional myocardial perfusion before and after coronary revascularization surgery by quantitative thallium-201 scintigraphy. J Am Coll Cardiol 1:804, 1983
100. Borer JS, Kent KM, Bacharach SL, et al: Sensitivity, specificity, and predictive accuracy of radionuclide cineangiography during exercise in patients with coronary artery disease: comparison with exercise electrocardiography. Circulation 60:572, 1979
101. Levin DC, Fallon JT: Significance of the angiographic morphology of localized coronary stenosis: histologic correlations. Circulation 66:316, 1982
102. Hansing CE: The risk and cost of coronary angiography: I. Cost of coronary angiography in Washington State. JAMA 242:755, 1979
103. Goldman L, Caldera DL, Southwick FS, et al: Cardiac risk factors in non-cardiac surgery. Medicine (Baltimore) 57:357, 1978
104. Scher KS, Tice DA: Operative risk in patients with previous coronary artery bypass. Arch Surg 111:807, 1976
105. Del Guercio LR, Savino JA, Morgan JC: Physiologic assessment of surgical diagnosis-related groups. Ann Surg 202:519, 1985
106. Williams TE Jr, Fanning WJ, Link L, et al: Can we afford to do cardiac operations in 1996? A risk-reward curve for cardiac surgery. Ann Thorac Surg 58:815, 1994
107. Wait J: Southwestern Internal Medicine Conference: preoperative pulmonary evaluation. Am J Med Sci 310:118, 1995
108. Marshall MC, Olsen GN: The physiologic evaluation of the lung resection candidate. Clin Chest Med 14:305, 1993
109. Amesbury SR, Humphrey HJ: Preoperative evaluation of pulmonary function. Hosp Pract (Off Ed) 30:51, 1992
110. Davies JM: Preoperative respiratory evaluation and management of patients for upper abdominal surgery. Yale J Biol Med 64:329, 1991
111. Tisi GM: Preoperative evaluation of pulmonary function. Am Rev Respir Dis 119:293, 1979
112. Thomas SD, Berry PD, Russell GN: Is this patient fit for thoracotomy and resection of lung tissue? Postgrad Med J 71:331, 1995
113. Reilly JJ Jr, Mentzer SJ, Sugarbaker DJ: Preoperative assessment of patients undergoing pulmonary resection. Chest 103:342S, 1993
114. Hirsch CH: When your patient needs surgery: weighing risks versus benefits. Geriatrics 50:26, 1995
115. Surgery in the Aged. Greenfield LJ, Ed. WB Saunders Co, Philadelphia, 1975, p 139
116. Scott DL: Anaesthetic experiences in 1,300 major geriatric operations. Br J Anaesth 33:354, 1961
117. Cole WH: Medical differences between the young and the aged. J Am Geriatr Soc 18:589, 1970
118. Burnett W, McCaffrey J: Surgical procedures in the elderly. Surg Gynecol Obstet 134:221, 1972
119. Weiss AK: The physiology of aging. Surgery in the Aged. Greenfield LJ, Ed. WB Saunders Co, Philadelphia, 1975, p 1
120. The National Halothane Study: A Study of the Possible Association between Halothane and Postoperative Hepatic Necrosis. Bunker JP, Forrest WH, Mosteller F, et al, Eds. National Institute of Health, National Institute of General Medical Sciences, Bethesda, Maryland, 1969
121. Khuri SF, Daley J, Henderson W, et al: The National Veterans Administration Surgical Risk Study: risk adjustment for the comparative assessment of the quality of surgical care. J Am Coll Surg 180:519, 1995
122. Detsky AS, Baker JP, Mendelson RA, et al: Evaluating the accuracy of nutritional assessment techniques applied to hospitalized patients: methodology and comparisons. JPEN 8:153, 1984
123. MacLean LD, Meakins JL, Taguchi K, et al: Host resistance in sepsis and trauma. Ann Surg 182:207, 1975
124. Meakins JL, Pietsch JB, Bubenick O, et al: Delayed hypersensitivity: indicator of acquired failure of host defenses in sepsis and trauma. Ann Surg 186:241, 1977
125. Zinsser H: Studies on the tuberculin reaction and on specific hypersensitivity in bacterial infection. J Exp Med 34:495, 1921
126. Christou NV: Host defense mechanisms in surgical patients: a correlative study of the delayed hypersensitivity skin test response, granulocyte function and sepsis in 2202 patients. Can J Surg 28:39, 1985
127. Christou NV: Predicting septic related mortality of the individual surgical patient based on admission host-defense measurements. Can J Surg 29:424, 1986
128. Adami GF, Terrizzi A, Vita M, et al: The assessment of skin tests in surgery. Surgery in Italy 10:297, 1980
129. Tasseau F, Gaucher L, Nicolas F: Cell mediated immunity studied by skin tests in patients receiving intensive care: prognostic value of repeated tests. Semaine des Hôpitaux 58:781, 1982
130. Brown R, Bankcewicz J, Hamid J, et al: Failure of delayed hypersensitivity skin testing to predict postoperative sepsis and mortality. Br Med J 284:851, 1982
131. Christou NV: Predicting septic related mortality of the individual surgical patient based on admission host-defense measurements. Can J Surg 29:424, 1986
132. Nohr CW, Christou NV, Rode H, et al: In vivo and in vitro humoral immunity in surgical patients. Ann Surg 200:373, 1984
133. Christou NV, Tellado-Rodriguez J, Giannas B, et al: Estimating mortality risk in preoperative patients using immunologic, nutritional and acute phase response variables. Ann Surg 210:69, 1989
134. Christou NV, Meakins JL, Gordon J, et al: The delayed hypersensitivity response and host resistance in surgical patients: 20 years later. Ann Surg 222:534, 1995
135. Legorreta AP, Silber JA, Costantino GN, et al: Increased cholecystectomy rate after the introduction of laparoscopic cholecystectomy. JAMA 270:1429, 1993
136. Ambulatory surgery. ACS Reports. American College of Surgeons, Chicago, August 1983
137. Dawes PJ, Davison P: Informed consent: what do patients want to know? J R Soc Med 87:149, 1994
138. Saw KC, Wood AM, Murphy K, et al: Informed consent: an evaluation of patients' understanding and opinion (with respect to the operation of transurethral resection of prostate). J R Soc Med 87:143, 1994
139. Inglis S, Farnill D: The effects of providing preoperative statistical anaesthetic-risk information. Anaesth Intensive Care 21:799, 1993
140. Dawes PJ, O'Keefe L, Adcock S: Informed consent: the assessment of two structured interview approaches compared to the current approach. J Laryngol Otol 106:420, 1992
141. Lavelle-Jones C, Byrne DJ, Rice P, et al: Factors affecting quality of informed consent. BMJ 306:885, 1993
142. Herz DA, Looman JE, Lewis SK: Informed consent: is it a myth? Neurosurgery 30:453, 1992

38 EVALUATION OF CARDIAC RISK

David A. Fullerton, M.D., Alden H. Harken, M.D., and Keith A. Horvath, M.D.

Preoperative Cardiac Assessment

Assessment of cardiac risk and determination of the level of risk that is acceptable are crucial components of preoperative evaluation. A patient and a physician might be willing to accept substantive operative risks to relieve incapacitating pain or claudication. Conversely, the indication for operation of a pulmonary nodule or an asymptomatic carotid bruit is prolongation of the patient's life. Ultimately, the natural history of the patient's disease must be evaluated and measured against the risk of surgical morbidity and mortality.

Actuarial data on risk-benefit assessment have been developed with persuasive precision by insurance companies for large populations of patients. However, risk analysis in an individual patient is much less a precise science than an art. In 1996, in an effort to clarify some of the issues surrounding assessment of cardiac risk in general surgical patients and vascular surgical patients, the American College of Cardiology and the American Heart Association collaborated with the aim of developing guidelines for perioperative cardiovascular evaluation for noncardiac surgery.[1] In what follows, we outline a stepwise approach that takes these guidelines into account.

Absolute Necessity of Operation versus Indications for Cardiovascular Evaluation

To a patient, an operation is rarely pleasant and almost never risk-free. Accordingly, surgical therapy is proposed only when the anticipated benefits to the patient outweigh the physiologic, psychological, social, and economic risks. Many, if not most, surgeons find it easier to summarize the anticipated benefits of surgery than to rigorously assess the various risks that may militate against operation. Our purpose in this chapter is to examine the tools currently available for analysis of cardiac risk in surgical patients.

An issue that must be addressed early on is the question of whether preoperative cardiac evaluation is indicated at all. Certainly, there are some conditions, such as a perforated viscus or an infected gangrenous foot, that simply obligate surgical intervention even in the face of considerable cardiac risk. When faced with such a condition, one should simply assume that cardiovascular disease is present and then proceed with the operation using invasive monitoring. In the absence of any such absolute indications for operation, however, one should not make this assumption and should address the issue of cardiac risk, beginning with a history and a physical examination.

History and Physical Examination

The most direct method of determining whether a patient has heart disease is by direct questioning. In the absence of a positive history, men are considered at risk for coronary artery disease at age 35 and older, whereas women are considered at risk beginning at age 40.[2,3] Younger men and women who have no history of cardiovascular problems may proceed to operation, on the presumption that there is no unusual cardiac risk. Although the Multiple Risk Factor Intervention Trial was not designed to examine single risk factors, regression analysis revealed that both elevated plasma cholesterol levels and a history of cigarette smoking were significant predictors of coronary disease. These findings may be used to increase the sensitivity of preoperative historical screening.

VALVULAR HEART DISEASE

During preoperative assessment, it is important for the surgeon to ascertain whether valvular heart disease is present and, if it is, to gauge its severity. The surgeon should be concerned primarily with diseases of the aortic valve. In an asymptomatic patient, aortic stenosis is the only valvular lesion that must be excluded. Significant valvular disease should be suspected if there is a history of dyspnea, congestive heart failure, angina, or syncope.

The foundation for diagnosis of significant valvular disease is the physical examination. Electrocardiography will demonstrate evidence of left ventricular hypertrophy. Chest x-ray may or may not show evidence of congestive heart failure or calcification of the aortic valve, and left ventricular hypertrophy or dilatation may be visible. If the history and physical examination suggest significant aortic stenosis, its severity should be quantified by echocardiography and, if necessary, cardiac catheterization.

CONGESTIVE HEART FAILURE

The preoperative history and physical examination must assess the possibility of congestive heart failure. In the three most frequently referenced indices of cardiac risk,[2,4,5] the dominant predictors of perioperative cardiac complications are all accessible via the history and the physical examination: (1) myocardial infarction within six months, (2) cardiac rhythm other than sinus, (3) age greater than 70 years, and (4) evidence of congestive failure (S_3 gallop or jugular venous distention). There is also the stair test, which has resurfaced as the Duke activity status index.[6] Thus, using inexpensive means, one can accurately identify both high-risk and low-risk patients. For these patients, subsequent steps are rel-

Preoperative Cardiac Assessment

Patient scheduled for noncardiac operation may be at risk for cardiac-related complications
Determine whether a condition is present that makes operation absolutely necessary regardless of cardiac risk.

- **Operation is absolutely necessary**
  Proceed with operation with invasive monitoring.

- **Operation is not absolutely necessary**
  Initiate preoperative cardiac evaluation based on patient's age and on presence or absence of a positive history.

  - **Patient is male < 35 yr or female < 40 yr with no history of cardiac disease**
    Proceed with operation without invasive monitoring.

  - **Patient is male > 35 yr or female > 40 yr with no cardiac symptoms**
    Obtain resting ECG.

    - **Resting ECG is negative**
      Proceed with operation with invasive monitoring.

    - **Resting ECG is positive**
      Obtain 12-lead exercise ECG.

  - **Patient has history of heart disease or typical angina**
    Obtain 12-lead exercise ECG.

    - **Exercise ECG is negative**
      Proceed with operation with invasive monitoring.

    - **Exercise ECG is unobtainable, or result is equivocal**
      Obtain exercise thallium scan.

      - **Exercise thallium scan is negative**
        Proceed with operation with invasive monitoring.

      - **Exercise thallium scan is positive**
        Perform cardiac catheterization with coronary angiography.

    - **Exercise ECG is positive for**
      - Angina, or
      - Depression of ST segment > 2 mm, or
      - Ventricular ectopy, or
      - Exercise-induced hypotension

      Perform cardiac catheterization with coronary angiography.

  - **Patient has history of valvular heart disease, dyspnea, fatigue, angina, or syncope**
    Obtain chest x-ray and ECG.

    - **Cardiomegaly or lung markings are evident**
      Obtain echo Doppler ultrasonogram.

      - **Valvular or left ventricular disease is present**
        Perform cardiac catheterization with coronary angiography.

      - **No significant valvular or left ventricular disease is present**
        Proceed with operation with invasive monitoring.

    - **Heart and lungs are normal**
      Proceed with operation with invasive monitoring.

- **Cardiac disease is more significant than original surgical problem**
  Perform cardiac operation.

- **Cardiac disease is less significant than original surgical problem**
  Proceed with operation with invasive monitoring.

atively clear-cut: if cardiac risk is low, one may proceed directly to elective surgery, whereas if it is high, one reevaluates the need for the surgical procedure and then, if the need still exists, proceeds directly to coronary angiography. For intermediate-risk patients, however, subsequent steps are less clear-cut, and various tests may be indicated.

DYSRHYTHMIAS

In the preoperative period, the patient should be asked if he or she has experienced symptoms of dysrhythmia, such as palpitations or syncope. In the physical examination, attention should be directed to the patient's heart rate and rhythm for evidence of irregularity. In addition to these steps, the preoperative electrocardiogram and rhythm strip should be studied for evidence of dysrhythmia.

If the history and physical examination suggest the presence of a dysrhythmia that either was not diagnosed by the electrocardiogram or is severe enough to necessitate further evaluation, the patient should be evaluated by means of continuous ambulatory electrocardiographic monitoring over a 12-hour to 24-hour period.

Dysrhythmias must be well controlled preoperatively. The ventricular response in the patient with atrial fibrillation should be controlled with digoxin. There is no uniformity of opinion regarding the treatment of premature ventricular contraction, but in an otherwise healthy individual, such contractions do not call for preoperative therapy. However, significant dysrhythmias that probably should be treated include the following [see 1 Initial Emergency Management of Noninjured Patients]:

1. Multifocal premature ventricular contractions or nonsustained ventricular tachycardia. These rhythm problems bespeak a diffusely hyperexcitable ventricle. The five most common causes of hyperexcitability are regional ischemia, hypokalemia, hypercalcemia, exogenous (or endogenous) catecholamines, and drug toxicity (typically related to digitalis). Each of these problems is readily diagnosed and treated.
2. Supraventricular tachycardias. These dysrhythmias are runs of narrow–QRS complex rhythms with a ventricular response greater than 100 beats/min. A narrow-complex tachycardia indicates a supraventricular origin. When the tachycardia is generated from a supranodal site, the surgeon may block the node in the short term with adenosine or over the long term with digitalis.

ANGINA PECTORIS

The diagnosis of angina pectoris can usually be made on the basis of the patient's history. The surgeon must be especially alert to the possible presence of variant (Prinzmetal's) angina or the more worrisome unstable angina. Variant angina is characterized by anginal pain at rest, frequently in the early hours of the morning. The patient may, however, experience exertional angina as well. Unstable angina is defined as (1) crescendo angina superimposed on relatively stable angina, (2) angina with minimal exertion and at rest, or (3) angina of new onset (change in a stable anginal pattern during the past six weeks) that is elicited by minimal exertion.[1,2] The significance of unstable angina is that it may be the harbinger of myocardial infarction; the surgeon must therefore be certain of the absence of unstable angina before proceeding with an operation.

Diagnostic Testing

Noninvasive cardiac testing should be reserved for patients who are at moderate risk.[7] Testing of low-risk patients loses its predictive value because of the high incidence of false negative and false positive indicators.

RESTING ELECTROCARDIOGRAM

Most organs do not exhibit dysfunction until stressed. However, for practical and economic purposes, physicians continue to screen patients with a resting ECG. A previous myocardial infarction is accepted as evidence of coronary artery disease. A previous infarction is indicated by the presence of a Q wave 0.04 sec or wider in any of the 12 ECG leads.[1,2] However, the absence of pathological Q waves does not necessarily denote a healthy heart.[8] Although perioperative risk increases with left ventricular hypertrophy or a nonsinus rhythm (which is easily detected by palpating a pulse) and three to four percent of adults exhibit a previously undiagnosed myocardial infarction, the resting ECG is not a powerful predictor of cardiac complications.

The ability to extract information from a communicative patient is extremely important. The patient's willingness or ability to communicate is perhaps the weakest link in the entire algorithm. If a patient denies exertional angina, fatigue, shortness of breath, or syncope and if the resting ECG reveals no evidence of coronary artery disease, the surgeon may proceed with elective surgery. If there is any doubt as to the presence of coronary artery disease, an exercise ECG should be obtained.

AMBULATORY ELECTROCARDIOGRAM

Studies examining the ambulatory ECG indicate that more than 75 percent of patients with diagnosed coronary artery disease exhibit silent (asymptomatic) ischemia.[8] Ambulatory monitoring has determined that silent ischemia occurs in almost all (70 to 100 percent) patients with chronic stable angina. However, in patients without diagnosed coronary artery disease, the ambulatory ECG has both low sensitivity and low specificity for the detection of ischemic heart disease.[8]

If the surgeon uncovers angina that had not been previously diagnosed or a history of chest pain of uncertain etiology, it is appropriate to perform 12-lead exercise testing to confirm the diagnosis and to help evaluate the severity of the disease.

EXERCISE ELECTROCARDIOGRAM

An operative procedure is a stressful hemodynamic insult. If a patient has a history of coronary artery disease, myocardial infarction, typical exercise- or emotion-induced angina, or a positive resting ECG, then it is appropriate to proceed to exercise electrocardiography. Patients with a positive exercise ECG have a significantly higher risk of ischemic heart disease than patients with a negative exercise ECG.[9] One study evaluated thousands of healthy individuals and patients, using data collected by the Seattle Heart Watch.[10,11] These investigations carefully related exercise level to (1) heart rate, (2) heart rate multiplied by systolic blood pressure (rate × pressure product), and (3) calculated total-body oxygen uptake. Four indications of ischemic heart disease were observed:

1. Depression of ST segment (≥ 2 mm).
2. Exercise-induced hypotension (≥ 10 mm Hg fall in systolic blood pressure).

3. Complex ventricular ectopy (≥ 3 consecutive premature ventricular depolarizations).
4. Symptomatic chest pain.

This test is quite specific.[12] In one series,[13] 37 percent of vascular surgical patients with a positive test result experienced a perioperative myocardial infarction, compared with only 1.5 percent of patients with a negative test result. Unfortunately, many vascular surgical patients are unable even to get on the treadmill, and in 40 percent of cases, exercise tolerance testing is nondiagnostic.

RADIOISOTOPE IMAGING

Radioisotope imaging can be valuable in diagnosing coronary artery disease. Currently, thallium-201 is the isotope most frequently used for cardiac imaging. Thallium is concentrated in perfused and viable myocardial cells by the membrane-bound Na^+, K^+-ATPase pumps. Thallium is almost completely extracted from coronary arterial blood by healthy myocardial cells in a single pass. Thus, thallium uptake reflects zones of perfused and viable heart. Decreased or absent thallium uptake indicates myocardial hypoperfusion. A thallium defect (absence of thallium uptake during exercise that fills in at rest) depicts myocardial ischemia.

An exercise thallium scan is accomplished by having the patient perform a standard Bruce protocol exercise test. During exercise, a 2 mCi dose of thallium-201 is administered intravenously for a period of several minutes. Eight-minute thallium cardiac images are obtained during exercise. Three hours later, delayed images are obtained to assess redistribution (filling in) or reperfusion. Again, absence of thallium uptake during exercise delineates regions of nonperfused myocardium. At the three-hour resting scan, regions that fill in are interpreted as having been ischemic during exercise. Zones that do not fill in during the three-hour resting scan are presumed to be dead, nonviable scar tissue.[14]

Many surgical patients who have vascular disease or orthopedic problems cannot exercise hard enough to meet the demands of an exercise study. In addition, patients with conduction defects (e.g., aberrant ventricular conduction, bundle branch block, or accessory atrioventricular bypass tracts [Wolff-Parkinson-White syndrome]) have ECGs that do not permit the analysis of ischemia with or without exercise. For patients who cannot exercise, the adenosine- or dipyridamole-thallium scan has been developed.[15] Adenosine is a potent natural coronary vasodilator. Dipyridamole, also a potent coronary vasodilator, is injected intravenously in a dosage of 0.5 mg/kg over a period of four minutes. After maximal pharmacological coronary vasodilation, thallium-201 is injected, and immediate and three-hour delayed images are obtained. With initial vasodilation by dipyridamole, the entire myocardium should fill in, thereby leaving no opportunity for assessment of redistribution and reperfusion on three-hour resting scan. Thallium images, however, always provide comparisons of uptake in one region with that in an adjacent region. Dipyridamole leads to hyperperfusion of normal zones and therefore to relative hypoperfusion of regions fed by diseased vessels. The three-hour resting image should exhibit redistribution of thallium into these areas of potentially ischemic but viable tissue.

CARDIAC CATHETERIZATION AND CORONARY ANGIOGRAPHY

After initial assessment, if the exercise thallium scan is positive, the 12-lead exercise ECG is positive, or valvular and left ventricular disease appears to be present, then invasive cardiac evaluation is indicated. Not all patients undergoing cardiac catheterization will require cardiac operative intervention. The purpose of the evaluation is to balance the medically controlled cardiac disease against the primary surgical problem. If after cardiac catheterization an operable cardiac problem is identified and this problem is greater than the original or primary surgical problem, then the patient should proceed to cardiac surgical repair. After cardiac operation, the patient's primary surgical problem should be reevaluated. If after cardiac catheterization the patient's identified cardiac disease is less significant or less urgent than the primary surgical problem, the operation for the latter problem should be performed with invasive monitoring.[16]

The High-Risk Patient

Once the preoperative cardiac assessment of a patient at high cardiac risk has been completed and the decision has been made to proceed with operation, the inherent risk of the procedure may be minimized with invasive hemodynamic monitoring and aggressive pharmacological management.

INVASIVE MONITORING

When general anesthesia is planned for a patient with presumed or documented cardiopulmonary dysfunction, techniques should be employed for continuous hemodynamic monitoring:

1. An arterial catheter serves as a means of monitoring systemic pressure and assessing arterial oxygenation (blood gases). Acid-base status may be effectively monitored simply by assessing mixed venous blood gas values.
2. A Foley catheter permits continuous assessment of peripheral organ perfusion. With progressive hemodynamic compromise, peripheral vasoconstriction redistributes the limited blood flow preferentially to the coronary and carotid circulations. Measurement of extremity temperature and urine output may permit estimation of the adequacy of cardiac output.
3. Central venous catheterization permits recognition of right-sided heart filling pressure. In the young trauma victim, this pressure is a valuable assay of total volume status. In the elderly patient with depressed cardiovascular function, the left—not the right—side of the heart is characteristically limiting. Florid pulmonary edema is possible even in the presence of a normal central venous pressure.
4. A pulmonary arterial catheter permits measurement of left ventricular filling pressure, cardiac output, and mixed venous blood gases. A patient normally compensates for decreased systemic oxygen delivery by increasing tissue oxygen extraction. Mixed venous acid-base status relates to arterial acid-base status with clinically relevant precision.[17] To obtain values for arterial carbon dioxide tension (Pco_2) from values for mixed venous Pco_2, one subtracts 5 mm Hg. To obtain arterial pH values from mixed venous pH values, one adds 0.05. The pulmonary arterial catheter has been subjected to a certain amount of high-profile criticism.[18] Although no robust link between surgical outcome and data obtained via the pulmonary arterial catheter has been established,[19] it still appears to be easier to manage high-risk patients with the help of invasive monitoring.
5. ECG monitoring using a single lead can assess heart rate, atrioventricular synchrony, and ventricular ectopy. Continuous 12-lead monitoring is impractical for this purpose. To optimize the search for ST segment abnormalities, the simultane-

Table 1 Cardiac-Related Risk Factors in General and Vascular Surgery

	Risk Factor	Type of Study	Findings	Comments
History	Age	Retrospective: 1,001 patients > 40 yr who underwent general anesthesia[2]	10-fold increase in perioperative cardiac death in patients > 70 yr	
	Peripheral vascular disease	Retrospective: 1,000 patients who underwent cardiac catheterization before vascular surgery[28]	Abdominal aortic aneurysm: 31% with coronary artery disease Cerebrovascular disease: 26% Atherosclerosis obliterans: 21%	Overall, 14% of vascular patients were found to have significant asymptomatic coronary artery disease
	Congestive heart failure (CHF)	Retrospective: 1,001 patients > 40 yr who underwent general anesthesia[33]	35% of patients with preoperative S_3 gallop had perioperative pulmonary edema	Only 6% of patients with a history of CHF but no signs preoperatively had perioperative pulmonary edema
	Cardiac arrhythmia	Retrospective: 566 patients who underwent major vascular procedures[34]	33% of patients with preoperative arrhythmia had cardiac complications, compared with 9% of patients with sinus rhythm	No distinction was made between atrial and ventricular arrhythmias; most prevalent were atrial fibrillation and > 5 PVCs/min
	Recent myocardial infarction (MI)	Retrospective: 587 patients with prior MI who underwent general anesthesia[31]	MI in prior 3 mo: perioperative MI in 27% MI occurred 3–6 mo ago: perioperative MI in 11% MI occurred > 6 mo ago: perioperative MI in 5%	75% of perioperative MIs were silent 69% of perioperative MIs were fatal
Screening Test Results	Positive preoperative ECG	Prospective: 200 patients > 40 yr undergoing abdominal, thoracic, and vascular procedures[35]	Patients with abnormal preoperative ECG were 3.2 times more likely to suffer fatal postoperative MI	In patients with little clinical suggestion of coronary artery disease, ECG is more sensitive than ETT
	Positive exercise tolerance test (ETT)	Retrospective: 808 patients who underwent major vascular procedures[36]	Exercise-induced myocardial ischemia developed in 27% of vascular patients who had no other symptoms of coronary artery disease	ETT may reveal significant coronary artery disease in asymptomatic patients in higher-risk populations (i.e., geriatric and vascular patients)
		Retrospective: 100 patients[37] Prospective: 55 geriatric patients (mean age, 72 yr)[37]	Inability to perform supine bicycle exercise test was the only independent predictor of cardiac complication	
	Reduced ejection fraction (EF)	Prospective, nonrandomized: 100 patients undergoing lower extremity revascularization[38]	EF 56%: no perioperative MI (N = 50) EF 36%–55%: 19% perioperative MI (N = 42) EF 26%–35%: 75% perioperative MI (N = 8)	32% of patients were > 70 yr Reduced EF correlated with perioperative MI, but age, angina, and previous MI did not
	Positive stress or adenosine-dipyridamole-thallium scan	Prospective: 55 patients > 60 yr with high likelihood of coronary artery disease[15]	Cardiac death: 5 patients Angina: 5 patients Myocardial infarction: 1 patient Dysrhythmia: 4 patients	Patients with a positive test result had a higher risk of a perioperative cardiac event ($P < 0.0001$)
Index	Cardiac Risk Index System (CRIS) score	Retrospective: 1,001 patients > 40 yr who underwent general anesthesia[30]	[See Table 2]	[See Table 2]

PVC—premature ventricular contraction

ous and continuous assessment of anterior (V1), lateral (V5), and inferior (II or aVF) leads is recommended.
6. Transesophageal echocardiographic monitoring may permit continuous assessment of ventricular function and regional wall motion abnormalities or ischemia.[20,21]

ADJUSTMENT OF MEDICATIONS

As a rule, all medications should be administered until the time of operation. Moreover, if beta blockers, nitrates, or calcium channel blockers are required for control of heart rate and blood pressure before operation, these medications should be continued throughout the preoperative period. Intravenous propranolol (0.25 to 0.50 mg) or continuous nitroglycerin infusion should be used liberally in the perioperative period to control blood pressure and heart rate. A reluctance to initiate vasoactive medications, such as nitroglycerin or dobutamine, immediately before or during operation has been noted. This hesitancy is not warranted, because once infusion of these medications has begun, it is easy to change the dose. It is important to assume aggressive hemodynamic control continuously before, during, and after operation.

Policies for utilization of hospital beds now place extraordinary pressures on the surgeon to prepare and manage cardiovascular abnormalities outside the hospital. When a patient presents on the morning of an operative procedure with inadequately controlled hypertension (i.e., with a diastolic pressure > 120 mm Hg), it is wise to postpone the operation. Conversely, one study has demonstrated that in the moderately controlled hypertensive patient with a diastolic blood pressure below 120 mm Hg, elective surgery may proceed without increased risk.[22] Indeed, subjective assessment of surgical risk (expressed as a score) with appropriate therapeutic intervention by an experienced anesthesiologist[23] may constitute optimal evaluation, and use of Goldman's cardiac risk index may not enhance evaluation significantly.[2,22]

It is essential to maintain hormonal supplementation during

the operation. One half of the usual daily dose of regular insulin may be given before operation and may be augmented intravenously during the procedure. Thyroid hormone is provided in routine doses. Patients on long-term adrenal corticosteroid therapy should receive supplemental doses the evening before and immediately before operation as well as intraoperatively.

The only exception to the rule that patients' preoperative drug regimens should not be changed during operation applies to patients receiving antidepressants. Administration of these agents should be routinely discontinued before operation. Monoamine oxidase (MAO) inhibitors alter intrinsic catecholamine uptake, with a resultant profound influence on myocardial excitability.[24] Therefore, MAO inhibitors should be discontinued, if possible, two weeks before elective surgery. Similarly, tricyclic antidepressants may have a chronotropic and arrhythmogenic influence in association with halothane and pancuronium.[25] Some safe antidepressant alternatives are available.[25]

PACEMAKERS

The pacemaker-dependent patient presents an important but easily solvable problem. Virtually all surgeons employ electrocautery devices. All currently implanted pacemakers are essentially of the demand type, which are likely to sense the electrocautery signal (which is much like the signal emitted by a microwave oven) and turn off when they sense it. As soon as electrocautery is discontinued, however, the demand pacemaker will resume its normal pacing function. Thus, the electrocautery causes a problem only when it must be in use for protracted, continuous periods. To prevent this intermittent problem, a sterile magnet may be placed over the pacer battery to convert the pacemaker to a fixed-rate mode, or the pacemaker may be reprogrammed to the fixed-rate mode. While the pacemaker is in this fixed-rate mode, it will emit impulses and pace the heart regardless of extraneous electrocautery (or ventricular) activity. Spontaneous ventricular activity with a superimposed paced impulse (R on T phenomenon) is possible but unlikely. Continuous electrocardiographic monitoring is essential while the pacemaker is in the fixed-rate mode. Identification and management of pacemaker malfunctions are discussed elsewhere [see *1 Initial Emergency Management of Noninjured Patients*].

Discussion

Of the 27 million patients who undergo surgical procedures annually in the United States, probably about one third have coexisting coronary artery disease—seemingly a good argument for preoperative evaluation of cardiac risk. For preoperative assessment of anything to be worthwhile, however, a problem must be common, the tools to identify it must be available, and, ultimately, a constructive response must be possible. As of this writing, each of these conditions has been met. It has been argued that a little testing begets more testing at rapidly escalating cost and that surgeons should therefore simply treat all patients as if they had coronary artery disease. Our view, however, is that preoperative cardiovascular assessment can be highly useful if pursued in a practical, cost-effective manner.

The importance of cardiac-related mortality in surgical patients is underscored by the findings of various studies [see *Table 1*]. A multifactorial cardiac risk index system (CRIS) has been developed for cardiac risk assessment in patients undergoing noncardiac operation [see *Table 2*]. The CRIS reflects the high risk of perioperative cardiac complications in patients with evidence of congestive heart failure or recent myocardial infarction. According to the CRIS, any elective operation is contraindicated in patients 70 years of age or older with a third heart sound and evidence of a recent myocardial infarction.[2]

The Framingham Study demonstrated that only five percent of patients who presented with intermittent claudication underwent amputation for gangrene within five years.[26] In contrast, 23 percent experienced symptoms of coronary artery disease within five years, and of this latter group, 13 percent suffered cerebrovascular accidents and 20 percent died. One third of patients who undergo operation for lower extremity vascular disease die of heart disease or stroke within five years. To subject some high-risk patients to noncardiac operation to prolong life may be misdirected.

In the past, some centers performed routine preoperative coronary angiography followed by selective myocardial revascularization in high-risk patients to reduce the risk of cardiovascular complications.[27] A retrospective study of 60 patients who underwent myocardial revascularization and who subsequently underwent 77 operative procedures found that no intraoperative or perioperative mortality occurred in relation to the general operation.[27] Similarly, at the Cleveland Clinic, all patients who presented with abdominal aortic aneurysms or peripheral vascular disease were advised to undergo routine coronary angiography.[28] Forty-one of 68

Table 2 Cardiac Risk Index System (CRIS)[39,40]

	Factors	Points
History	Age > 70 yr	5
	Myocardial infarction in prior 6 mo	10
	Aortic stenosis	3
Physical examination	S_3 gallop, jugular venous distention, or congestive heart failure	11
ECG	Any rhythm other than sinus	7
	> 5 PVCs/min	7
General information	P_aO_2 < 60 mm Hg	3
	P_aCO_2 > 50 mm Hg	3
	K⁺ < 3 mEq/L	3
	BUN > 50 mg/dl	3
	Creatinine > 3 mg/dl	3
	Bedridden	3
Operation	Emergency	4
	Intrathoracic	3
	Intra-abdominal	3
	Aortic	3

Risk of cardiac complications by CRIS class:
    Class I (0–5 points): 1%   Class II (6–12 points): 5%
    Class III (13–25 points): 11%   Class IV (≥ 26 points): 22%

BUN—blood urea nitrogen P_aCO_2—arterial carbon dioxide tension P_aO_2—arterial oxygen tension   PVC—premature ventricular contraction

Table 3 Relation between Use of Aggressive Monitoring with Pharmacological Support and Incidence of Hemodynamic Aberration and Myocardial Reinfarction[33,41]

Monitoring Technique or Drug Employed	No. of Patients	
	Group I (N = 364)	Group II (N = 733)
Direct arterial pressure	137	651
Swan-Ganz catheter	8	607
Vasodilators	24	584
Inotropic agents	94	231
Vasopressors	114	21*
Beta blockers	40	612
Antiarrhythmic agents	18	210

Hemodynamic Aberration	No. of Patients (No. of Reinfarctions)	
	Group I (N = 364)	Group II (N = 733)
Hypotension	38 (4)	12 (9)†
Hypertension	56 (8)	9 (0)
Tachycardia	18 (3)	16 (2)
Tachycardia and hypertension	88 (13)	8 (3)

*Use of vasopressors in group II compared with use in group I, $P < 0.005$.
†$P < 0.05$ compared with other hemodynamic aberrations.

patients with abdominal aortic aneurysms and 26 of 71 patients with aortoiliac occlusive disease had clinical evidence of ischemic heart disease before angiography. Six patients from both groups underwent elective aortic reconstruction after myocardial revascularization; one of these six patients died. Although this strategy has been associated with a reduction in postoperative mortality, routine coronary angiography is impractical and expensive and does involve a certain degree of risk. Indeed, several groups[23,29] have concluded that neither noninvasive nor invasive tests add much to an end-of-the-bed evaluation performed by a seasoned clinical surgeon. When coronary artery bypass grafting and coronary angioplasty are indicated, it is exclusively on the basis of the patient's cardiac symptoms and coronary anatomy, not as measures for enhancing the safety of a planned noncardiac surgical procedure.[29]

The most complete studies of perioperative cardiac mortality have been conducted at the Mayo Clinic. During the late 1960s, the records of more than 32,000 patients who underwent general anesthesia for noncardiac operations were examined.[30] Patients with a history of myocardial infarction who suffered a perioperative myocardial reinfarction exhibited a 54 percent mortality, with 80 percent of the deaths occurring within 48 hours of operation. A decade later, when this study was reevaluated and updated to include new patient records, the incidence of myocardial reinfarction was slightly lower, but the mortality in patients with perioperative reinfarction was 69 percent.[31] The guiding principle of medical therapy for cardiac ischemia is aggressive reduction of myocardial oxygen demand. During unrecognized intraoperative myocardial ischemia, the unsuspecting surgeon violates this principle and stresses the heart, with poor results. Two questions then arise. First, can surgeons identify intraoperative myocardial ischemia and hemodynamic instability? Second, if they can identify these conditions, can they influence perioperative cardiac mortality by means of invasive monitoring and aggressive pharmacological control of hemodynamic status?

Virtually all patients with significant coronary artery disease experience both angina and silent myocardial ischemia during daily life. Insufficient coronary blood flow is to be expected in many of these patients during the stress of operation. It is essential that the surgeon watch for this induced myocardial ischemia during operation and take action to minimize its effects.

Predictably, any hypotension that occurs during anesthesia and operation may result in inadequate blood flow across coronary arterial obstructive lesions. Cardiac pressure work, as opposed to flow work, expends much energy and oxygen. Thus, the combination of tachycardia and hypertension, such as occurs with stress, is dangerous.

The importance of invasive monitoring and pharmacological control in patients undergoing general anesthesia is underscored by the results of a classic comparison of two groups of surgical patients who received different degrees of operative support. In the mid-1970s, 364 patients undergoing general anesthesia (group I) were evaluated retrospectively.[32] This control group was managed without aggressive monitoring or aggressive pharmacological support. From 1977 to 1982, 733 patients (group II) were managed prospectively with frequent invasive monitoring, and aggressive use was made of vasodilators, inotropic agents, vasopressors, beta blockers, and antiarrhythmic agents. The two groups were compared with respect to the incidence of intraoperative hemodynamic aberration and myocardial reinfarction [see Table 3].

All preoperative medications were continued before and during operation. ECG monitors and radial arterial, pulmonary arterial, and urinary catheters were used for all patients considered at risk for cardiac disease. Monitoring was minimized if the procedure was expected to last less than 30 minutes. Monitoring was particularly aggressive for any patient who had had a myocardial infarction during the prior 18 months. Baseline hemodynamic measurements were obtained, and nitroglycerin, dopamine, and phenylephrine infusions were immediately available to maintain systolic pressure, pulmonary arterial pressures, heart rate, cardiac output, and systemic vascular resistance within 20 percent of the preinduction values during the entire procedure. Arterial blood gases, potassium, and blood glucose were corrected frequently; the hematocrit was kept above 30 percent; and urine output was maintained with volume and diuretics. Ventricular ectopy was suppressed with lidocaine and procainamide. Patients were not extubated at the completion of the procedure unless they were awake and alert and had adequate measured tidal volume and vital capacity.

Comparison of the two groups revealed that there was a substantially lower incidence of hemodynamic aberrations in group II, and even though this group had twice as many patients, one half as many reinfarctions were reported (14 in group II versus 28 in group I).

Operation remains a predictable hemodynamic insult. Surgeons can identify patients at increased cardiac risk with clinically useful precision. If these patients are carefully observed for myocardial ischemia and treated aggressively by maintaining blood pressure and heart rate within tight bounds, surgeons can minimize perioperative cardiac morbidity and mortality.

References

1. American College of Cardiology/American Heart Association Task Force Report: Guidelines for perioperative cardiovascular evaluation for non-cardiac surgery. Circulation 93:1278, 1996
2. Mangano DT, Goldman L: Pre-operative assessment of patients with known or suspected coronary disease. N Engl J Med 333:1750, 1995
3. Multiple Risk Factor Intervention Trial Research Group: Coronary heart disease death, nonfatal acute myocardial infarction and other clinical outcomes in the Multiple Risk Factor Intervention Trial. Am J Cardiol 58:1, 1986
4. Detsky AS, Abrams HB, McLaughlin JR, et al: Predicting cardiac complications in patients undergoing non-cardiac surgery. J Gen Intern Med 1:209, 1986
5. Larsen SF, Olesen KH, Jacobsen E, et al: Prediction of cardiac risk in non-cardiac surgery. Eur Heart J 8:179, 1987
6. Nelson CL, Herndon JE, Mark DB, et al: Relation of clinical and angiographic factors to functional capacity as measured by the Duke Activity Status Index. Am J Cardiol 68:973, 1991
7. Fleisher LA, Eagle KA: Screening for cardiac disease in patients having non-cardiac surgery. Ann Intern Med 124:767, 1996
8. Kawanishi DT, Rahimtoola SH: Silent myocardial ischemia. Curr Probl Cardiol 12:509, 1987
9. Bartels C, Bechtel JF, Hossmann V, et al: Cardiac risk stratification for high risk vascular surgery. Circulation 95:2473, 1997
10. Bruce RA: Exercise testing for evaluation of ventricular function. N Engl J Med 296:671, 1977
11. Bruce RA, Hornstein TR: Exercise stress testing in evaluation of patients with ischemic heart disease. Prog Cardiovasc Dis 11:371, 1969
12. Paul SD, Eagle KA: A stepwise strategy for coronary risk assessment for non-cardiac surgery. Med Clin North Am 79:1241, 1995
13. Cutler BS, Wheeler HB, Paraskos JA, et al: Applicability and interpretation of exercise stress testing in patients with peripheral vascular disease. Am J Surg 141:501, 1981
14. Refsnyder T, Bandyk DF, Lanza D, et al: Use of stress thallium imaging to stratify cardiac risk in patients undergoing vascular surgery. J Surg Res 52:147, 1992
15. Mumtaz H, Bomanji JB, Guptka NK, et al: Myocardial perfusion scintigraphy in patients undergoing major non-vascular abdominal surgery. Ann R Coll Surg (Engl) 78:420, 1996
16. Mason JJ, Owens DK, Harris RA, et al: The role of coronary angiography and coronary revascularization before non-cardiac vascular surgery. JAMA 273:1919, 1995
17. Steinberg JJ, Harken AH: Central venous catheter in the assay of acid-base status. Surg Gynecol Obstet 152:221, 1981
18. Dalen JE, Bone RC: Is it time to pull the pulmonary artery catheter? JAMA 276:916, 1996
19. Tuman KJ, Roizen MF: Outcome assessment and pulmonary artery catheterization: why does the debate continue? Anesth Analg 84:1, 1997
20. Practice guidelines for perioperative transesophageal echocardiography. Anesthesiology 84:986, 1996
21. London MJ: Ventricular function and myocardial ischemia: is transesophageal echocardiography a good monitor? Controversies in Intraoperative Echocardiography. Kaplan JA, Ed. WB Saunders Co, Philadelphia, 1997, p 61
22. Goldman L, Caldera DL: Risks of general anesthesia and elective operation in the hypertensive patient. Anesthesiology 50:285, 1979
23. Prause G, Offner A, Ratzenhofer-Komenda B, et al: Comparison of two pre-operative indices to predict perioperative mortality in non-cardiac thoracic surgery. Eur J Cardiothorac Surg 11:670, 1997
24. Wells PH, Kaplan JA: Optimal management of patients with ischemic heart disease for non-cardiac surgery by complementary anesthesiologist and cardiologist interaction. Am Heart J 102:1029, 1981
25. Edwards RP, Miller RD: Cardiac responses to imipramine and pancuronium during anesthesia with halothane or enflurane. Anesthesiology 50:421, 1979
26. Peabody CN, Kannel WB, McNamara PM: Intermittent claudication: surgical significance. Arch Surg 109:693, 1974
27. McCollum CH, Garcia-Rinaldi R, Graham JM, et al: Myocardial revascularization prior to subsequent major surgery in patients with coronary artery disease. Surgery 81:302, 1977
28. Hertzer NR, Beven EG, Young JR: Coronary artery disease in peripheral vascular patients: a classification of 1000 coronary angiograms and results of surgical management. Ann Surg 199:223, 1984
29. Krupski WC, Bensard DD: Pre-operative cardiac risk management. Surg Clin North Am 75:647, 1995
30. Tarham S, Moffitt EA, Taylor WF, et al: Myocardial infarction after general anesthesia. JAMA 220:1451, 1972
31. Steen PA, Tinker JH, Tarhan S: Myocardial reinfarction after anesthesia and surgery. JAMA 239:2566, 1978
32. Rao TLK, Jacobs KH, El-Etr AA: Reinfarction following anesthesia in patients with myocardial infarction. Anesthesiology 59:499, 1983
33. Goldman L: Assessment of perioperative cardiac risk. N Engl J Med 330:707, 1994
34. Cooperman M, Pflug B, Martin EW Jr, et al: Cardiovascular risk factors in patients with peripheral vascular disease. Surgery 84:505, 1978
35. Carliner NH, Fisher ML, Plotnick GD, et al: Routine preoperative exercise testing in patients undergoing major noncardiac surgery. Am J Cardiol 56:51, 1985
36. Arous EJ, Baum PL, Cutler BS: The ischemic exercise test in patients with peripheral vascular disease: implications for management. Arch Surg 119:780, 1984
37. Gerson MC, Hurst JM, Hertzberg VS, et al: Cardiac prognosis in noncardiac geriatric surgery. Ann Intern Med 103:832, 1985
38. Pasternack PF, Imparato AM, Riles TS, et al: The value of radionuclide angiogram in the prediction of perioperative myocardial infarction in patients undergoing lower extremity revascularization procedures. Circulation 72:1113, 1985
39. Goldman L, Caldera DL, Nussbaum SR: Multifactorial index of cardiac risk in noncardiac procedures. N Engl J Med 297:845, 1977
40. Mangano DT, Goldman L: Preoperative assessment of patients with known or suspected coronary disease. N Engl J Med 333:1750, 1995
41. Shah K, Leomann B, Rao T, et al: Reduction in mortality from cardiac causes in Goldman class IV patients. J Cardiothorac Anesth 2:789, 1988

39 PREVENTION OF POSTOPERATIVE INFECTION

Jonathan L. Meakins, M.D., D.Sc., Byron J. Masterson, M.D., and Ronald Lee Nichols, M.D., M.S.

Epidemiology of Surgical Site Infection

Historically, the control of wound infection depended on antiseptic and aseptic techniques directed at coping with the infecting organism. In the 19th century and the early part of the 20th century, wound infections had devastating consequences and a measurable mortality. Even in the 1960s, before the correct use of antibiotics and the advent of modern preoperative and postoperative care, as much as one quarter of a surgical ward might have been occupied by patients with wound complications. As a result, wound management, in itself, became an important component of ward care and of medical education. It is fortunate that many factors have intervened so that the so-called wound rounds have become a practice of the past. The epidemiology of wound infection has changed as surgeons have learned to control bacteria and the inoculum as well as to focus increasingly on the patient (the host) for measures that will continue to provide improved results.

The following three factors are the determinants of any infectious process:

1. The infecting organism (in surgical patients, usually bacteria).
2. The environment in which the infection takes place (the local response).
3. The host defense mechanisms, which deal systemically with the infectious process.[1]

Wounds are particularly appropriate for analysis of infection with respect to these three determinants. Because many components of the bacterial contribution to wound infection now are clearly understood and measures to control bacteria have been implemented, the host factors become more apparent. In addition, interactions between the three determinants play a critical role, and with limited exceptions (e.g., massive contamination), few infections will be the result of only one factor [see Figure 1].

Definition of Surgical Site Infection

Wound infections have traditionally been thought of as infections in a surgical wound occurring between the skin and the deep soft tissues—a view that fails to consider the operative site as a whole. As prevention of these wound infections has become more effective, it has become apparent that definitions of operation-related infection must take the entire operative field into account; obvious examples include sternal and mediastinal infections, vascular graft infections, and infections associated with implants (if occurring within 1 year of the procedure and apparently related to it). Accordingly, the Centers for Disease Control and Prevention currently prefers to use the term surgical site infection (SSI). SSIs can be classified into three categories: superficial incisional SSIs (involving only skin and subcutaneous tissue), deep incisional SSIs (involving deep soft tissue), and organ/space SSIs (involving anatomic areas other than the incision itself that are opened or manipulated in the course of the procedure)[2,3] [see Figure 2].

Standardization in reporting will permit more effective surveillance and improve results as well as offer a painless way of achieving quality assurance. The natural tendency to deny that a surgical site has become infected contributes to the difficulty of defining SSI in a way that is both accurate and acceptable to surgeons. The surgical view of SSI recalls one judge's (probably apocryphal) remark about pornography: "It is hard to define, but I know it when I see it." SSIs are usually easy to identify.

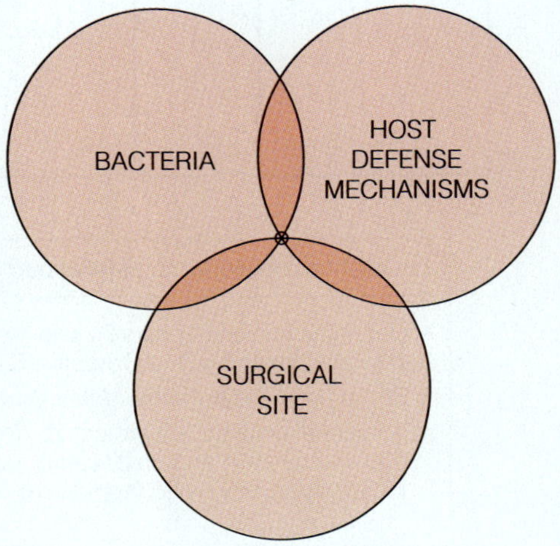

Figure 1 In a homeostatic, normal state, the determinants of any infectious process—bacteria, the surgical site, and host defense mechanisms (represented by three circles)—intersect at a point indicating zero probability of sepsis.

Epidemiology of Surgical Site Infection

```
┌─────────────────────────────────────────────────────┐
│ Wound infection is caused by exogenous or endogenous│
│ bacteria; infection is influenced not only by the   │
│ source of the infecting inoculum but also by the    │
│ bacterial characteristics.                          │
└─────────────────────────────────────────────────────┘
                         │
┌─────────────────────────────────────────────────────┐
│ Ensure that prophylactic antibiotics, if indicated, │
│ are present in tissue in adequate concentrations at │
│ beginning of operation.                             │
└─────────────────────────────────────────────────────┘
```

Endogenous factors or sources of bacteria

- **Remote sites of infection**: Postpone elective operation if possible. Treat remote infection appropriately.
- **Skin**
- **Bowel**

Bacterial characteristics of importance (virulence and antibiotic resistance)

- **Nature and site of operation**: Is the operation
  - Clean
  - Contaminated
  - Clean-contaminated
  - Dirty or infected
- **Size of inoculum required to produce infection**: Varies in different clinical situations.

Exogenous factors or sources of bacteria

- **Operating team–related**
  - Comportment
  - Use of impermeable drapes and gowns
  - Surgical scrub [see Sidebar The Surgical Scrub].
- **Operating room–related**
  - Traffic control
  - Cleaning
  - Air

Surveillance and quality assurance

Preventive measures to control bacteria

- Decontamination of patient's skin [see Sidebar Preoperative Decontamination of the Operative Site]
- Bowel preparation [see Sidebar Bowel Preparation]
- Additional antibiotics if indicated, depending on likelihood of contamination and on bacterial inoculum and properties [see Sidebar Antibiotic Prophylaxis of Infection]

BACTERIA

HOST DEFENSE MECHANISMS

SURGICAL SITE

Factors contributing to dysfunction of host defense mechanisms can be related to surgical disease, to events surrounding the operation, and to the patient's underlying disease.

Surgeon-related

Factors influenced by the surgeon include
- Preoperative decisions
- Timing of operation
- Surgical technique
- Transfusion
- Blood loss
- Duration and extent of operation

Patient-related

Patient-related factors include
- Presence of ≥ 3 concomitant diagnoses
- Presence of underlying disease
- Presence of diabetes
- Age
- Drug use
- Preoperative nutritional status

Surveillance and quality assurance

Local factors influence the susceptibility of the wound environment by affecting the size of the inoculum required to produce infection.

Operating team–related

Factors influenced by the surgeon and operating team include
- Duration of operation
- Maintenance of hemostasis and perfusion
- Avoidance of seroma, hematoma, necrotic tissue, wound drains
- Tissue handling
- Cautery use

Patient-related

- Age
- P_aO_2
- Abdominal procedure
- Tissue perfusion
- Presence of foreign body
- Barrier function

Surveillance and quality assurance

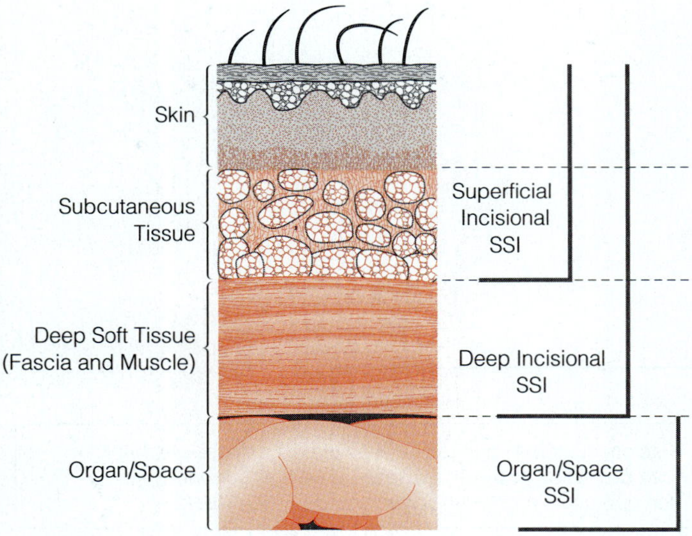

Figure 2 Surgical site infections are classified into three categories, depending on which anatomic areas are affected.[3]

Bacteria

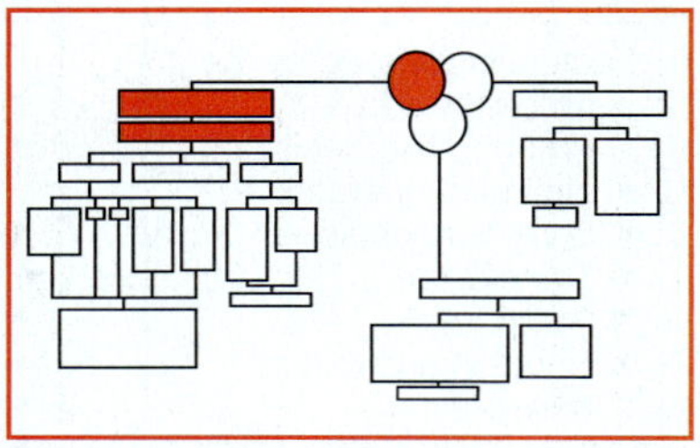

Clearly, without an infecting agent no infection will result. Accordingly, most of what is known about bacteria is put to use in major efforts directed at reducing their numbers by means of asepsis and antisepsis. The principal concept is based on the size of the bacterial inoculum.

Wounds are traditionally classified according to whether the wound inoculum of bacteria is likely to be large enough to overwhelm local and systemic host defense mechanisms and produce an infection [*see Table 1*]. One study showed that the most important factor in the development of a wound infection was the number of bacteria present in the wound at the end of an operative procedure.[4] Another study quantitated this relation and provided insight into how local environmental factors might be integrated into an understanding of the problem [*see Figure 3*].[5] In the years before prophylactic antibiotics as well as during the early phases of their use, there was a very clear relation between the classification of the operation (which is related to the probability of a significant inoculum) and the rate of wound infection.[6,7] This relation has persisted but is now less dominant than it once was; therefore, other factors have come to play a significant role.[8,9]

CONTROL OF SOURCES OF BACTERIA

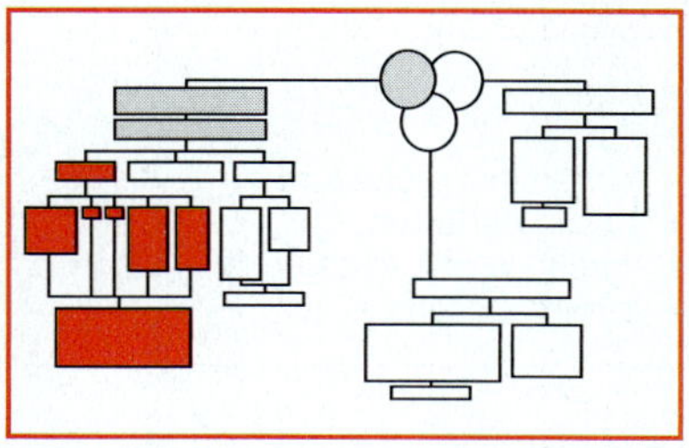

Endogenous bacteria are a more important cause of SSI than exogenous bacteria are. In clean-contaminated, contaminated, and dirty-infected operations, the source and the amount of bacteria are functions of the patient's disease and the specific organs being operated on.

Operations classified as infected are those in which infected tissue and pus are removed or drained, providing a guaranteed inoculum to the surgical site. The inoculum may be as high as 10^{10} bacteria/ml, some of which may already be producing an infection. In addition, some bacteria could be in the growth phase rather than the dormant or the lag phase and thus could be more pathogenic. The heavily contaminated wound is best managed by delayed primary closure. This type of management ensures that the wound is not closed over a bacterial inoculum that is almost certain to cause a wound infection, with attendant early and late consequences.

Patients should not have elective surgery in the presence of remote infection, which is associated with an increased incidence of wound infection.[6] In patients with urinary tract infections, wounds frequently become infected with the same organism. Remote infections should be treated appropriately, and the operation should proceed only under the best conditions possible. If operation cannot be appropriately delayed, the use of prophylactic and therapeutic antibiotics should be considered [*see Sidebar Antibiotic Prophylaxis of Infection and Tables 2, 3, and 4*].

Preoperative techniques of reducing patient flora, especially endogenous bacteria, are of great concern. Bowel preparation, antimicrobial showers or baths, and preoperative skin decontamination have been proposed frequently. These techniques, particularly preoperative skin decontamination [*see Sidebar Preoperative Decontamination of the Operative Site*], may have specific roles in selected patients during epidemics or in units with high infection rates. As a routine for all patients, however, these techniques are unnecessary, time-consuming, and costly in institutions or units where infection rates are low.

The preoperative shave is a technique in need of reassessment. It is now clear that shaving the evening before an operation is associated with an increased wound infection rate. This increase is secondary to the trauma of the shave and the inevitable small areas of inflammation and infection. If hair removal is required,[10,11] clipping is preferable and should be done in the operating room or the preparation room just before the operative procedure. Shaving, if ever performed, should not be done the night before operation.

Bowel preparation [*see Sidebar Bowel Preparation and Tables 5, 6, and 7*] has a clear role in colon and rectal surgery. The suggestion has been made that selective gut decontamination (SGD) may be useful in major elective procedures involving the upper gastrointestinal tract and perhaps in other settings. At present, SGD for prevention of infection cannot be recommended in either the preoperative or the postoperative period.

When infection develops after clean operations, particularly those in which foreign bodies were implanted, endogenous infecting organisms are involved but the skin is the primary source of the infecting bacteria. The air in the operating room and other OR sources occasionally become significant in clean cases; the degree of endogenous contamination can be surpassed by that of exogenous contamination. Thus, both the operating team—surgeon, assistants, nurses, and anesthetists—and OR air have been reported as significant sources of bacteria. In fact, personnel are the most important source of exogenous bacteria.[12-14] In a study by the National Academy of Sciences–National Research Council, ultraviolet light (UVL) was efficacious only in the limited situations of clean and ultraclean cases.[6] There were minimal numbers of endogenous bacteria, and UVL controlled one of the exogenous sources.

Clean air systems have very strong advocates, but they also have equally vociferous critics [*see 40 Preparing the Operating Room*]. It is possible to obtain excellent results in clean cases with implants without using these systems. However, clean

Table 1 National Research Council Classification of Operative Wounds[21]

Clean (class I)	Nontraumatic No inflammation encountered No break in technique Respiratory, alimentary, or genitourinary tract not entered
Clean-contaminated (class II)	Gastrointestinal or respiratory tract entered without significant spillage Appendectomy Oropharynx entered Vagina entered Genitourinary tract entered in absence of infected urine Biliary tract entered in absence of infected bile Minor break in technique
Contaminated (class III)	Major break in technique Gross spillage from gastrointestinal tract Traumatic wound, fresh Entrance of genitourinary or biliary tracts in presence of infected urine or bile
Dirty and infected (class IV)	Acute bacterial inflammation encountered, without pus Transection of "clean" tissue for the purpose of surgical access to a collection of pus Traumatic wound with retained devitalized tissue, foreign bodies, fecal contamination, or delayed treatment, or all of these; or from dirty source

air systems are here to stay. Nevertheless, the presence of a clean air system does not mean that basic principles of asepsis and antisepsis should be abandoned, because endogenous bacteria must still be controlled.

The use of impermeable drapes and gowns has received considerable attention. If bacteria can penetrate gown and drapes, they can gain access to the wound. The use of impermeable drapes may therefore be of clinical importance.[15,16] When wet, drapes of 140-thread-count cotton are permeable to bacteria. It is clear that some operations are wetter than others, but generally, much can be done to make drapes and gowns impermeable to bacteria. For example, drapes of 270-thread-count cotton that have been waterproofed are impermeable, but they can be washed only 75 times. Economics plays a role in the choice of drape fabric because entirely disposable drapes are expensive. Local institutional factors may be significant in the role of a specific type of drape in the prevention of SSI [see 40 Preparing the Operating Room].

PROBABILITY OF CONTAMINATION

The probability of contamination is largely defined by the nature of the operation [see Table 1]. However, other factors contribute to the probability of contamination; the most obvious is the expected duration of the operative procedure, which, whenever examined, has been significant in the wound infection rate.[4,7,8] The longer the procedure lasts, the more bacteria accumulate in a wound; the sources of bacteria include the patient, the operating team (gowns, gloves with holes, wet drapes), the OR, and the equipment. In addition, the patient undergoing a longer operation is likely to be older, to have other diseases, and to have cancer of—or to be undergoing operation on—a structure with possible contamination. A longer duration, even of a clean operation, represents increased time at risk for contamination. These points, in addition to pharmacologic considerations, suggest that the surgeon should be alert to the need for a second dose of prophylactic antibiotics [see Sidebar Antibiotic Prophylaxis of Infection].

Abdominal operation is another risk factor.[8] Significant disease and age play a role in outcome; however, because the major concentrations of endogenous bacteria are located in the abdomen, abdominal operations are more likely to involve bacterial contamination.

In recent years, postoperative contamination of the wound has been considered unlikely. However, one report of SSI in sternal incisions cleaned and redressed 4 hours postoperatively clearly shows that wounds can be contaminated and become infected in the postoperative period.[17] Accordingly, use of a dry dressing for 24 hours seems prudent.

BACTERIAL PROPERTIES

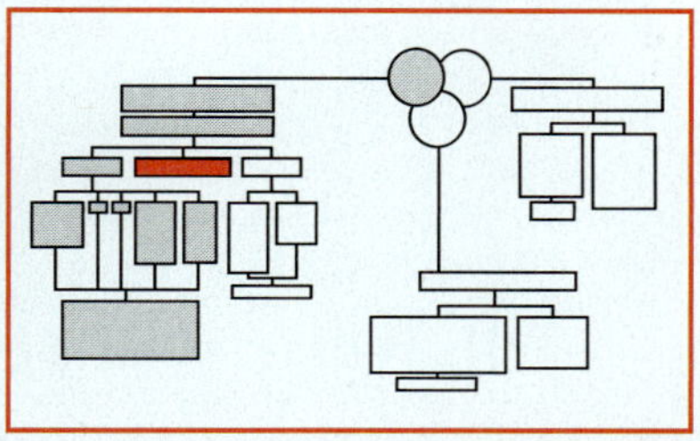

Not only is the size of the bacterial inoculum important; the bacterial properties of virulence and pathogenicity are also significant. The most obvious pathogenic bacteria in surgical patients are gram-positive cocci (e.g., *Staphylococcus aureus* and streptococci). With modern hygienic practice, *S. aureus* should be found mostly in clean cases, with a wound infection incidence of 1% to 2%. Surveillance can be very useful in identifying either wards or surgeons with increased rates. Operative procedures in infected areas

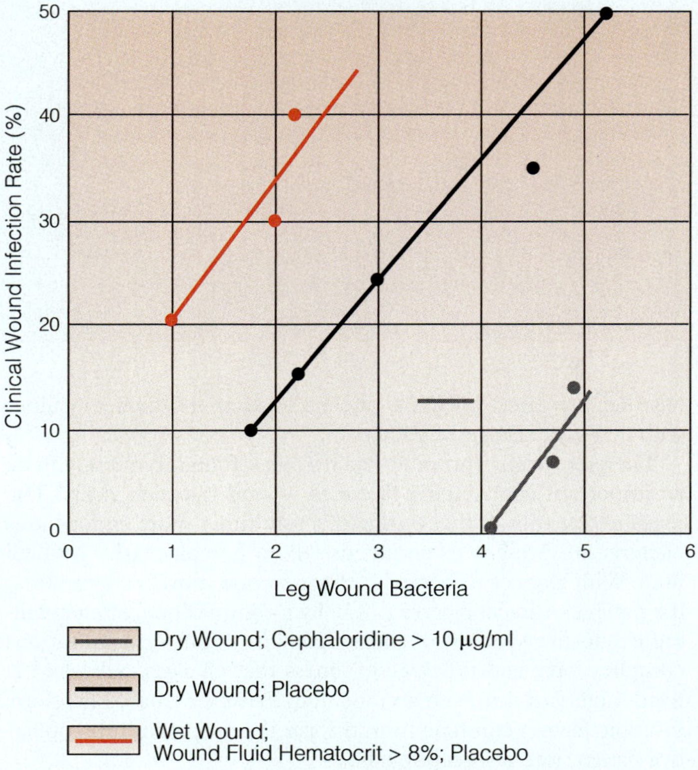

Figure 3 The wound infection rate is shown here as a function of bacterial inoculum in three different situations: a dry wound with an adequate concentration of antibiotic (cephaloridine > 10 μg/ml), a dry wound with no antibiotic (placebo), and a wet wound with no antibiotic (placebo, wound fluid hematocrit > 8%).[5]

Antibiotic Prophylaxis of Infection

Selection

Spectrum. The antibiotic chosen should be active against the most likely pathogens. Single-agent therapy is almost always effective, except in colorectal operations, small-bowel procedures with stasis, emergency abdominal operations in the presence of a polymicrobial flora, and penetrating trauma; in such cases, a combination of antibiotics is usually used because anaerobic coverage is required.

Pharmacokinetics. The half-life of the antibiotic selected must be long enough to maintain adequate tissue levels throughout the operation.

Administration

Dosage, route, and timing. A single preoperative dose that is of the same strength as a full therapeutic dose is adequate in most instances. The single dose should be given I.V. immediately before skin incision. Administration by the anesthetist is most effective and efficient.

Duration. A second dose is warranted if the duration of the operation exceeds either 3 hours or twice the half-life of the antibiotic. No additional benefit has been demonstrated in continuing prophylaxis beyond the day of the operation, and mounting data suggest that the preoperative dose is sufficient. When massive hemorrhage has occurred (i.e., blood loss equal to or greater than blood volume), a second dose is warranted. Even in emergency or trauma cases, prolonged courses of antibiotics are not justified unless they are therapeutic.[50,51,55,56,107]

Indications

CLEAN CASES

Prophylactic antibiotics are not indicated in clean operations if the patient has no host risk factors or if the operation does not involve placement of prosthetic materials. Open heart operation and operations involving the aorta or the vessels in the groin require prophylaxis.

Patients in whom host factors suggest the need for prophylaxis include those who have more than three concomitant diagnoses, those whose operations are expected to last longer than 2 hours, and those whose operations are abdominal.[8] A patient who meets any two of these criteria is highly likely to benefit from prophylaxis. When host factors suggest that the probability of a surgical site infection is significant, administration of cefazolin at induction of anesthesia is appropriate prophylaxis. Vancomycin should be substituted in patients who are allergic to cephalosporins or who are susceptible to major immediate hypersensitivity reactions to penicillin.

When certain prostheses (e.g., heart valves, vascular grafts, and orthopedic hardware) are used, prophylaxis is justified when viewed in the light of the cost of a surgical site infection to the patient's health. Prophylaxis with either cefazolin or vancomycin is appropriate for cardiac, vascular, or orthopedic patients who receive prostheses.

Catheters for dialysis or nutrition, pacemakers, and shunts of various sorts are prone to infection mostly for technical reasons, and prophylaxis is not usually required. Meta-analysis indicates, however, that antimicrobial prophylaxis reduces the infection rate in CSF shunts by 50%.[108] Beneficial results may also be achievable for other permanently implanted shunts (e.g., peritoneovenous) and devices (e.g., long-term venous access catheters and pacemakers); however, the studies needed to confirm this possibility will never be done, because the infection rates are low and the sample sizes would have to be prohibitively large. The placement of such foreign bodies is a clean operation, and the use of antibiotics should be based on local experience.

CLEAN-CONTAMINATED CASES

Abdominal procedures. In biliary tract procedures (open or laparoscopic), prophylaxis is required only for patients at high risk: those whose common bile duct is likely to be explored (because of jaundice, bile duct obstruction, stones in the common bile duct, or a reoperative biliary procedure); those with acute cholecystitis; and those older than 70 years. A single dose of cefazolin is adequate. In hepatobiliary and pancreatic procedures, antibiotic prophylaxis is always warranted because these operations are clean-contaminated, because they are long, because they are abdominal, or for all of these reasons. Prophylaxis is also warranted for therapeutic endoscopic retrograde cholangiopancreatography.[7,9] In gastroduodenal procedures, patients whose gastric acidity is normal or high and in whom bleeding, cancer, gastric ulcer, and obstruction are absent are at low risk for infection and require no prophylaxis; all other patients are at high risk and require prophylaxis. Patients undergoing operation for morbid obesity should receive double the usual prophylactic dose[109]; cefazolin is an effective agent.

Operations on the head and neck (including the esophagus). Patients whose operations are of significance (i.e., involve entry into the oral cavity, the pharynx, or the esophagus) require prophylaxis.

Gynecologic procedures. Patients whose operation is either high-risk cesarean section, abortion, or vaginal or abdominal hysterectomy will benefit from cefazolin. Aqueous penicillin G or doxycycline may be preferable for first-trimester abortions in patients with a history of pelvic inflammatory disease. In patients with cephalosporin allergy, doxycycline is effective for those having hysterectomies and metronidazole for those having cesarean sections. Women delivering by cesarean section should be given the antibiotic immediately after cord clamping.

Urologic procedures. In principle, antibiotics are not required in patients with sterile urine. Patients with positive cultures should be treated. If an operative procedure is performed, a single dose of the appropriate antibiotic will suffice.

---

have an increased infection rate because of the high inoculum with actively pathogenic bacteria.

The preoperative hospital stay has been found frequently to be an important contributing factor to wound infection rates.[7] The usual explanation is that during this stay either more endogenous bacteria are present or commensal flora is replaced by hospital flora. With respect to bacterial changes, one must recognize that the patient's clinical picture is usually a complex one, often entailing exhaustive workup of more than one organ system, various complications, and a degree of illness that changes radically the host's ability to deal with an inoculum, however small. Therefore, multiple factors combine to transform the hospitalized preoperative patient into a susceptible host.

Bacteria with multiple antibiotic resistance can be associated with significant SSI problems. In particular, staphylococci, with their natural virulence, present an important hazard if inappropriate prophylaxis is used. Many surgeons feel it is inappropriate or unnecessary to obtain good culture and sensitivity data on SSIs and instead simply drain infected wounds, believing that they will heal. However, there have been a number of reports of SSIs caused by unusual organisms[14,17,18]; these findings underscore the usefulness of culturing pus or fluid when an infection is being drained. SSIs caused by antibiotic-resistant organisms or unusual pathogens call for specific prophylaxis, perhaps other infection control efforts, and, if the problem persists, a search for a possible carrier or a common source.[12-14,17,18]

SURGEONS AND BACTERIA

The surgeon's perioperative rituals are designed to reduce or eliminate bacteria from the operative field. Many old habits are obsolete [*see Sidebar* The Surgical Scrub *and* 40 Preparing the

Antibiotic Prophylaxis of Infection (continued)

CONTAMINATED CASES

Abdominal procedures. In colorectal procedures, bowel preparation using antibiotics active against both aerobes and anaerobes, along with a parenteral cephalosporin, is recommended. In appendectomy, SSI prophylaxis requires an agent or combination of agents active against both aerobes and anaerobes; a single dose of cefoxitin, 2 g I.V., or, in patients who are allergic to β-lactam antibiotics, metronidazole, 500 mg I.V., is effective. A combination of an aminoglycoside and clindamycin is effective if the appendix is perforated; a therapeutic course of 3 to 5 days is appropriate but does not seem warranted unless the patient is particularly ill. A laparotomy without a precise diagnosis is usually an emergency procedure and demands preoperative prophylaxis. If the preoperative diagnosis is a ruptured viscus (e.g., the colon or the small bowel), both an agent active against aerobes and an agent active against anaerobes are required. Depending on operative findings, prophylaxis may be sufficient or may have to be supplemented with postoperative antibiotic therapy.

Trauma. The proper duration of antibiotic prophylaxis for trauma patients is a confusing issue—24 hours or less of prophylaxis is probably adequate, and more than 48 hours is certainly unwarranted. When laparotomy is performed for nonpenetrating injuries, prophylaxis should be administered. Coverage of both aerobes and anaerobes is mandatory. The duration of prophylaxis should be less than 24 hours. In cases of penetrating abdominal injury, prophylaxis with either cefoxitin or a combination of agents active against anaerobic and aerobic organisms is required. The duration of prophylaxis should be less than 24 hours, and in many cases, perioperative doses will be adequate. For open fractures, management should proceed as if a therapeutic course were required. For grade 1 or 2 injuries, a first-generation cephalosporin will suffice, whereas for grade 3 injuries, combination therapy is warranted; duration may vary. For operative repair of fractures, a single dose of cefazolin may be given preoperatively, with a second dose added if the procedure is long. Patients with major soft tissue injury with a danger of spreading infection will benefit from cefazolin, 1 g I.V. every 8 hours for 1 to 3 days.

DIRTY OR INFECTED CASES

Infected cases require therapeutic courses of antibiotics; prophylaxis is not appropriate in this context. In dirty cases, particularly those resulting from trauma, contamination and tissue destruction are usually so extensive that the wounds must be left open for delayed primary or secondary closure. Appropriate timing of wound closure is judged at the time of debridement. Antibiotics should be administered as part of resuscitation. Administration of antibiotics for 24 hours is probably adequate if infection is absent at the outset. However, a therapeutic course of antibiotics is warranted if infection is present from the outset or if more than 6 hours elapsed before treatment of the wounds was initiated.

Prophylaxis of Endocarditis

Studies of the incidence of endocarditis associated with dental procedures, endoscopy, or operations that may result in transient bacteremia are lacking. Nevertheless, the consensus is that patients with specific cardiac and vascular conditions are at risk for endocarditis or vascular prosthetic infection when undergoing certain procedures; these patients should receive prophylactic antibiotics.[110-114] A variety of organisms are dangerous, but viridans streptococci are most common after dental or oral procedures, and enterococci are most common if the portal of entry is the GU or GI tract. Oral amoxicillin now replaces penicillin V or ampicillin because of superior absorption and better serum levels. In penicillin-allergic patients, clindamycin is recommended; alternatives include cephalexin, cefadroxil, azithromycin, and clarithromycin. When there is a risk of exposure to bowel flora or enterococci, oral amoxicillin may be given; if an I.V. regimen is indicated, ampicillin may be given, with gentamicin added if the patient is at high risk for endocarditis. In patients allergic to penicillin, vancomycin is appropriate, with gentamicin added in high-risk patients. These parenteral regimens should be reserved for high-risk patients undergoing procedures with a significant probability of bacteremia.[114]

In patients receiving penicillin-based prophylaxis because of a history of rheumatic fever, erythromycin rather than amoxicillin should be used to protect against endocarditis.[110] There is no consensus concerning prophylaxis for orthopedic prostheses and acquired infection after transient bacteremia. In major procedures, where the risk of bacteremia is significant, the above recommendations are pertinent.

Operating Room]. Nonetheless, it is clear that surgeons can influence SSI rates.[9] The refusal to use delayed primary closure or secondary closure is an example. Careful attention to the concepts of asepsis and antisepsis in the preparation and conduct of the operation is important. Although no single step in the ritual of preparing a patient for the operative procedure is indispensable, it is likely that certain critical standards of behavior must be maintained to achieve good results.

The measurement and publication of data about individuals or hospitals with high SSI rates have been associated with a diminution of those rates[7,9,19] [*see Table 8*]. It is uncertain by what process the diffusion of these data relates to the observed improvements. Although surveillance has unpleasant connotations, it provides objective data that individual surgeons are often too busy to acquire but that can contribute to improved patient care.

Environment: Local Factors

Local factors influence the development of an SSI because they affect the size of the bacterial inoculum that is required to produce an infection: in a susceptible wound, a smaller inoculum produces infection [*see Figure 2*].

THE SURGEON'S INFLUENCE

Most of the local factors that make a surgical site favorable to bacteria are under the control of the surgeon. Although Halsted usually receives, deservedly so, the credit for having established the importance of technical excellence in the OR in preventing infection, individual surgeons in the distant past achieved remarkable results by careful attention to cleanliness and technique.[20] The Halstedian principles dealt with hemostasis, sharp dissection, fine sutures, anatomic dissection, and the gentle handling of tissues. Mass ligatures, large sutures, necrotic tissue, and the creation of hematomas or seromas must be avoided, and foreign materials must be judiciously used because these techniques and materials change the size of the inoculum required to initiate an infectious process. Logarithmically fewer bacteria are required to produce infection in the presence of a foreign body (e.g., suture, graft, metal, or pacemaker) or necrotic tissue (e.g., that caused by gross hemostasis or injudicious use of electrocautery).

The differences in inoculum required to produce wound infections can be seen in a model in which the two variables are wound hematocrit and the presence of antibiotic [*see*

Table 2 Parenteral Antibiotics Recommended for Prophylaxis of Surgical Site Infection

	Antibiotic	Dose	Route of Administration
For coverage against aerobic gram-positive and gram-negative organisms	Cefazolin	1 g	I.V. or I.M. (I.V. preferred)
If patient is allergic to cephalosporins or if methicillin-resistant organisms are present	Vancomycin	1 g	I.V.
Combination regimens for coverage against gram-negative aerobes and anaerobes	Clindamycin *or* Metronidazole *plus* Tobramycin (or equivalent aminoglycoside)	600 mg / 500 mg / 1.5 mg/kg	I.V. / I.V. / I.V. or I.M. (I.V. preferred for first dose)
For single-agent coverage against gram-negative aerobes and anaerobes	Cefoxitin	1–2 g	I.V.
	Cefotetan	1–2 g	I.V.

Figure 3]. Ten bacteria in the absence of an antibiotic and in the presence of wound fluid with a hematocrit of more than 8% yield a wound infection rate of 20%. In a technically good wound with no antibiotic, however, 1,000 bacteria produce a wound infection rate of 20%.[5]

Drains

The use of drains varies widely and is very subjective. All surgeons are certain that they understand when to use a drain. However, certain points are worth noting. It is now recognized that a simple Penrose drain can function not only as a drainage route but also as an access route for pathogens to the patient.[21] It is important that the operative site not be drained through the wound. The use of a closed suction drain further reduces the potential for contamination and infection.

Duration of Operation

In most studies,[4,7,8] contamination certainly increases with time (see above). Wound edges can dry out, become macerated, or in other ways be made more susceptible to infection (i.e., requiring fewer bacteria for development of infection). Speed and poor technique are not suitable approaches; expeditious operation is appropriate.

Electrocautery

The use of electrocautery devices has been clearly associated with an increase in superficial SSI. However, when the unit is properly used to provide pinpoint coagulation (for which the bleeding vessels are best held by fine forceps) or to divide tissues under tension, there is minimal tissue destruction, no charring, and no change in the wound infection rate.[21]

PATIENT FACTORS

Local Blood Flow

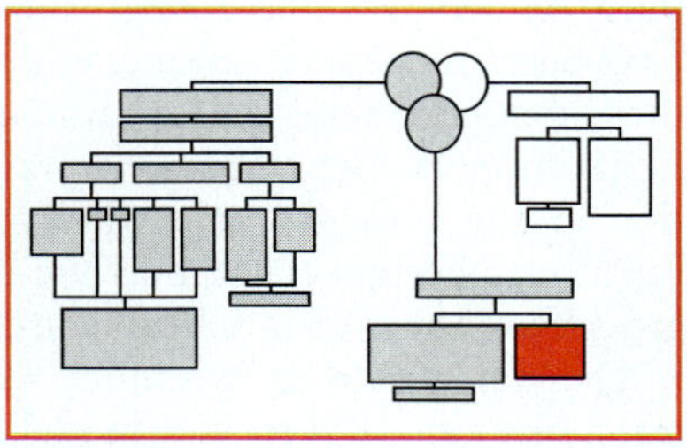

Local perfusion can greatly influence the development of infection, as is seen most easily in the tendency of the patient with peripheral vascular disease to acquire infection of an extremity. As a local problem, inadequate perfusion reduces the number of bacteria required for infection, in part because inadequate perfusion leads to decreased tissue levels of oxygen. Shock, by reducing local perfusion, also greatly enhances susceptibility to infection. Fewer organisms are required to produce infection during or immediately after shock [see Figure 4]. To counter these effects, the arterial oxygen tension (P_aO_2) must be translated into an adequate subcutaneous oxygen level (determined by measuring transcutaneous oxygen tension); this, together with adequate perfusion, will provide local protection by increasing the number of bacteria required to produce infection.

Barrier Function

Inadequate perfusion may also affect the function of other organs, and the resulting dysfunction will, in turn, influence the patient's susceptibility to infection. For example, ischemia-reperfusion injury to the intestinal tract is a frequent consequence of hypovolemic shock and septicemia. Inadequate perfusion of the GI tract may also occur during states of fluid and electrolyte imbalance or when cardiac output is marginal. Experimental studies have associated altered blood flow with breakdown of bowel barrier function—that is, inability of the intestinal tract to prevent bacteria, their toxins, or both from moving from the gut lumen into tissue at a rate too fast to permit clearance by the usual protective mechanisms. A variety of experimental approaches aimed at enhancing bowel barrier function have been studied; at present, however, the most clinically applicable method of bowel protection is initiation of enteral feeding (even if the quantity of nutrients provided does not satisfy all the nutrient requirements) and administration of the amino acid glutamine. Glutamine is a specific fuel for enterocytes and colonocytes and has been found to aid recovery of damaged intestinal mucosa and enhance barrier function when administered either enterally or parenterally.

Advanced Age

Aging is associated with structural and functional changes that render the skin and subcutaneous tissues more susceptible to infection. These changes are immutable; however, they must be evaluated in advance and addressed by excellent surgical technique and, on occasion, prophylactic antibiotics [see Sidebar Antibiotic Prophylaxis of Infection].

Table 3 Conditions and Procedures That Require Antibiotic Prophylaxis against Endocarditis[110,111]

CONDITIONS

Cardiac
  Prosthetic cardiac valves (including biosynthetic valves)
  Most congenital cardiac malformations
  Surgically constructed systemic-pulmonary shunts
  Rheumatic and other acquired valvular dysfunction
  Idiopathic hypertrophic subaortic stenosis
  History of bacterial endocarditis
  Mitral valve prolapse causing mitral insufficiency
  Surgically repaired intracardiac lesions with residual hemodynamic abnormality or < 6 mo after operation

Vascular
  Synthetic vascular grafts

PROCEDURES

Dental or oropharyngeal
  Procedures that may induce bleeding
  Procedures that involve incision of the mucosa

Respiratory
  Rigid bronchoscopy

Incision and drainage or debridement of sites of infection

Urologic
  Cystoscopy with urethral dilatation
  Urinary tract procedures
  Catheterization in the presence of infected urine

Gynecologic
  Vaginal hysterectomy
  Vaginal delivery in the presence of infection

Gastrointestinal
  Procedures that involve incision or resection of mucosa
  Endoscopy that involves manipulation (e.g., biopsy, dilatation, or sclerotherapy) or ERCP

Host Defense Mechanisms

The systemic response is designed to control and eradicate infection. Many factors can inhibit systemic host defense mechanisms; some are related to the surgical disease, others to the patient's underlying disease or diseases and the events surrounding the operation.

SURGEON-RELATED FACTORS

There are a limited number of ways in which the surgeon can improve a patient's systemic responses to surgery [*see 88 Immunomodulation*]. Nevertheless, when appropriate, attempts should be made to modify the host. The surgeon and the operation are both capable of reducing immunologic efficacy; hence, the operative procedure should be carried out in as judicious a manner as possible. Minimal blood loss, avoidance of shock, and maintenance of blood volume, tissue perfusion, and tissue oxygenation all will minimize trauma and will reduce the secondary, unintended immunologic effects of major procedures.

When abnormalities in host defenses are secondary to surgical disease, the timing of the operation is crucial to outcome. With acute and subacute inflammatory processes, early operation helps restore normal immune function. Deferral of definitive therapy frequently compounds problems.

PATIENT FACTORS

Surgeons have always known that the patient is a significant variable in the outcome of operation. Various clinical states are associated with altered resistance to infection. In all patients,

Table 4 Antibiotics for Prevention of Endocarditis[60,110]

Manipulative Procedure	Prophylactic Regimen*	
	Usual	In Patients with Penicillin Allergy
Dental procedures likely to cause gingival bleeding; operations or instrumentation of the upper respiratory tract	*Oral* Amoxicillin, 2.0 g 1 hr before procedure *Parenteral* Ampicillin, 2.0 g I.M. or I.V. 30 min before procedure	*Oral* Clindamycin, 600 mg 1 hr before procedure or Cephalexin or cefadroxil,[†] 2.0 g 1 hr before procedure or Azithromycin or clarithromycin, 500 mg 1 hr before procedure *Parenteral* Clindamycin, 600 mg I.V. within 30 min before procedure or Cefazolin, 1.0 g I.M. or I.V. within 30 min before procedure
Gastrointestinal or genitourinary operation; abscess drainage	*Oral* Amoxicillin, 2.0 g 1 hr before procedure *Parenteral* Ampicillin, 2.0 g I.M. or I.V. within 30 min before procedure; if risk of endocarditis is considered high, add gentamicin, 1.5 mg/kg (to maximum of 120 mg) I.M. or I.V. 30 min before procedure[‡]	Vancomycin, 1.0 g I.V. infused slowly over 1 hr, beginning 1 hr before procedure; if risk of endocarditis is considered high, add gentamicin, 1.5 mg/kg (to maximum of 120 mg) I.M. or I.V. 30 min before procedure[‡]

*Pediatric dosages are as follows: oral amoxicillin, 50 mg/kg; oral or parenteral clindamycin, 20 mg/kg; oral cephalexin or cefadroxil, 50 mg/kg; oral azithromycin or clarithromycin, 15 mg/kg; parenteral ampicillin, 50 mg/kg; parenteral cefazolin, 25 mg/kg; parenteral gentamicin, 2 mg/kg; parenteral vancomycin, 20 mg/kg. *Total pediatric dose should not exceed total adult dose.*
[†]Patients with a history of immediate-type sensitivity to penicillin should not receive these agents.
[‡]High-risk patients should also receive ampicillin, 1.0 g I.M. or I.V., or amoxicillin, 1.0 g p.o., 6 hr after procedure.

Bowel Preparation (continued)

Emergency Colon Operation

Among the clinical conditions that most often necessitate emergency colon operation are acute bleeding, perforated diverticulum or perforated carcinoma, ischemic intestinal disease, obstructing lesions, and trauma involving the colon. Under emergency conditions, the operation must be performed without any bowel preparation because oral antibiotic prophylaxis and mechanical cleansing are either impossible or potentially harmful.

INTRAOPERATIVE LAVAGE

Several techniques for performing intraoperative lavage have been described. In one, 8 to 10 L of saline is introduced into the colon during a period of 20 to 30 minutes through a balloon catheter in the distal ileum; the balloon is inflated to occlude the ileocecal valve. This technique results in uniform cleansing of the unprepared colon; a team approach is necessary to prevent spillage or other mishaps. This method of lavage allowed primary resections and anastomoses in 10 patients who otherwise would have undergone staged procedures (Nichols RL, unpublished data).

PARENTERAL ANTIBIOTICS

Prevention of infectious complications after emergency colon operation depends on proper operative technique, sound judgment, and appropriate choice and administration of parenteral antibiotics.[151] As in elective operation, the antibiotics chosen should be active against both aerobic and anaerobic colonic microflora.[22] They should be given I.V. in appropriate doses, starting shortly before the operation and continuing postoperatively for 1 to 7 days. The duration of administration is governed by the operative findings and by whether the antibiotic regimen is intended to be prophylactic (in which case the antibiotics are given for 1 day) or therapeutic, to manage the intra-abdominal infection for which operation is required (in which case antibiotics are given for 2 days or longer). Many single agents and combinations appear to be equally efficacious and are currently recommended. The choice of an agent or a combination of agents, therefore, depends on local hospital prices, toxicity profiles, and the surgeon's familiarity with the agents. Arguably, potent therapeutic agents such as imipenem have no place in antibiotic prophylaxis before elective colon resection.[152]

TOPICAL ANTIBIOTICS OR ANTISEPTICS

Some surgeons advocate direct application to the wound or irrigation of the wound with either antibiotics or povidone-iodine during colon resection. Solutions containing povidone-iodine should almost never be placed in the peritoneal cavity, because they are likely to be absorbed and subsequently to cause toxic effects.

---

by an interest in self-care, by socioeconomic conditions, or by underlying diseases) or by the surgeon. Of late, considerable attention has been focused on the beneficial effects of daily multivitamin supplements on infectious morbidity in individuals older than 65 years. In addition, there is some evidence that ingestion of certain antioxidants (e.g., beta-carotene, vitamin C, and vitamin E) and trace metals (e.g., selenium and zinc) can enhance host responses to inflammation or infection. A large body of clinical data (particularly in patients with active rheumatoid arthritis) indicates that reducing the quantity of fat in the diet and substituting omega-3 fatty acids (found in high concentrations in fish oil) for omega-6 fatty acids reduces the clinical signs and symptoms of inflammation. Animal studies suggest that similar beneficial effects are observed in the presence of infection; human studies using this approach have yet to be performed. Dietary supplementation with arginine, glutamine, or both also appears to increase resistance to infectious challenge.

Pharmacologic therapy can affect host response as well. Nonsteroidal anti-inflammatory drugs that attenuate the production of certain eicosanoids can greatly alter the adverse effects of infection by modifying fever and cardiovascular effects. Operative procedures involving inhalational anesthetics result in an immediate rise in plasma cortisol concentrations. The steroid response and the associated immunomodulation can be modified by using high epidural anesthesia as the method of choice; pituitary adrenal activation will be greatly attenuated. Some drugs that inhibit steroid elaboration (e.g., etomidate) have also been shown to be capable of modifying perioperative immune responses.

INTEGRATION OF DETERMINANTS

As operative infection rates slowly fall, despite increasingly complex operations in patients at greater risk, it is certain that surgeons are approaching the control of infection with a broader view than simply that of asepsis and antisepsis. It is apparent that this new, broader view must take into account many variables, some of which have no relation to bacteria, but all of which play a role in SSI [see Table 9].

To estimate risk, one must integrate the various determinants of infection in such a way that they can be applied to patient care. Much of this exercise is vague. In reality, the day-to-day practice of surgery includes a risk assessment that is essentially a form of logistic regression, and although not recognized as such, each surgeon's assessment of the probability of whether an SSI will occur takes into account the determining variables:

$$\text{Probability of SSI} = x + a\,(\text{bacteria}) + b\,(\text{environment: local factors}) + c\,(\text{host defense mechanisms: systemic factors})$$

Discussion

Antibiotic Prophylaxis of Surgical Site Infection

It is difficult to understand why antibiotics have not always prevented SSI successfully. Certainly, surgeons were quick to appreciate the possibilities of antibiotics; nevertheless, the efficacy of antibiotic prophylaxis was not proved until the late 1960s.[5] Studies before then had major design flaws, principally the administration of the antibiotic some time after the start of the operation—often in the recovery room. The failure of studies to demonstrate efficacy and the occasional finding that prophylactic antibiotics worsened rather than improved outcome led in the late 1950s to profound skepticism about prophylactic antibiotic use in any operation.

The principal reason for the apparent inefficacy was inadequate understanding of the biology of SSIs. Fruitful study of antibiotics and how they should be used began after physiologic groundwork established the importance of local blood flow, maintenance of local immune defenses, adjuvants, and local and systemic perfusion.[24]

Table 6 Oral and Parenteral Antibiotic Regimens in Patients Receiving Mechanical Cleansing: Prospective Studies, 1983 to 1994

Year	Patients (N)	Neomycin and Erythromycin Base Given to All Patients	Antibiotic	Route	Infection Rate (%)
1983[90]	119	No	Neomycin-erythromycin plus cefazolin Cefoxitin	Oral Parenteral Parenteral	3 12*
1983[148]	241	Yes	No additional antibiotics Cefoxitin	 Parenteral	18 7†
1983[139]	100	No	Cefoxitin Metronidazole-gentamicin	Parenteral Parenteral	12 12*
1983[85]	1,082	Yes	Placebo Cephalothin	Parenteral Parenteral	8 6*
1984[150]	57	Yes	Cefonicid Cefoxitin	Parenteral Parenteral	6 10*
1984[157]	93	No	Neomycin-erythromycin Metronidazole-gentamicin	Oral Parenteral	9 27†
1985[84]	267	No	Tinidazole-doxycycline Tinidazole	Parenteral Parenteral	3 10†
1986[158]	86	No	Moxalactam Metronidazole-gentamicin	Parenteral Parenteral	12 13*
1986[159]	60	No	Neomycin-erythromycin Metronidazole-ceftriaxone	Oral Parenteral	41 10†
1987[160]	100	Yes	Cefazolin Cefoxitin Cefotaxime	Parenteral Parenteral Parenteral	3* 3* 14
1988[82]	239	Variable	Cefotetan Cefoxitin	Parenteral Parenteral	12 8*
1988[161]	119	No	Neomycin-metronidazole plus metronidazole Metronidazole	Oral Parenteral Parenteral	14 28†
1988[162]	102	No	Neomycin-erythromycin plus cefazolin Metronidazole	Oral Parenteral Parenteral	11 32†
1988[91]	310	No	Neomycin-erythromycin plus cefoxitin Cefoxitin	Oral Parenteral Parenteral	5 18†
1989[83]	403	No	Cefoxitin Cefotetan	Parenteral Parenteral	11 9*
1989[163]	54	No	Neomycin-erythromycin Metronidazole-ceftriaxone	Oral Parenteral	4* 7
1990[164]	146	No	Neomycin-erythromycin Cefoxitin Neomycin-erythromycin plus cefoxitin	Oral Parenteral Oral Parenteral	11 12 8
1990[165]	197	Yes	Neomycin-erythromycin Neomycin-erythromycin plus cefoxitin	Oral Oral Parenteral	15 5†
1990[166]	943	No	Cefotaxime-metronidazole Cefuroxime-metronidazole	Parenteral Parenteral	7 7
1992[167]	221	No	Amoxicillin-clavulanate Cefotetan	Parenteral Parenteral	11 13
1993[168]	164	No	Amoxicillin-clavulanate Cefotaxime-metronidazole	Parenteral Parenteral	11 9
1994[169]	128	No	Ampicillin-sulbactam Gentamicin-metronidazole	Parenteral Parenteral	10 11
1994[170]	327	No	Piperacillin plus ciprofloxacin Piperacillin	Parenteral Oral Parenteral	11 23†

*Not significant. †Significant at $P < 0.05$.

Table 7 Parenteral Antibiotics Commonly Used for Broad-Spectrum Coverage of Colonic Microflora

COMBINATION THERAPY OR PROPHYLAXIS

Aerobic Coverage
(to be combined with a drug having anaerobic activity)

Amikacin	Ciprofloxacin
Aztreonam	Gentamicin
Ceftriaxone	Tobramycin

Anaerobic Coverage
(to be combined with a drug having aerobic activity)

Chloramphenicol	Metronidazole
Clindamycin	

SINGLE-DRUG THERAPY OR PROPHYLAXIS

Aerobic-Anaerobic Coverage

Ampicillin-sulbactam	Imipenem-cilastatin*
Cefotetan	Piperacillin-tazobactam
Cefoxitin	Ticarcillin-clavulanate
Ceftizoxime	

*This agent should be used *only* for therapeutic purposes; it should not be used for prophylaxis.

The key antibiotic study, which was conducted in guinea pigs, unequivocally proved the following about antibiotics:

1. They are most effective when given before inoculation of bacteria.
2. They are ineffective if given 3 hours after inoculation.
3. They are of intermediate effectiveness when given in between these times [see Figure 5].[25]

Although efficacy with a complicated regimen was demonstrated in 1964,[26] the correct approach was not defined until 1969.[5] Established by these studies[5,25] are the philosophical and practical bases of the principles of antibiotic prophylaxis of SSI in all surgical arenas: that prophylactic antibiotics must be given preoperatively within 2 hours of the incision, in full dosage, parenterally, and for a very limited period. These principles remain essentially unchanged despite minor modifications from innumerable subsequent studies.[27-30] Prophylaxis for colorectal operations is discussed elsewhere [see Bowel Preparation for Colonic Surgery, below].

PRINCIPLES OF PATIENT SELECTION

Patients must be selected for prophylaxis on the basis of either their risk for SSI or the cost to their health if an SSI develops (e.g., after implantation of a cardiac valve or another prosthesis). The most important criterion is the degree of bacterial contamination expected to occur during the operation. The traditional classification of such contamination was defined in 1964 by the historic National Academy of Sciences–National Research Council study.[6] The important features of the classification are its simplicity, ease of understanding, ease of coding, and reliability. Classification is dependent on only one variable—the bacterial inoculum—and the effects of this variable are now controllable by antimicrobial prophylaxis. Advances in operative technique, general care, antibiotic use, anesthesia, and surveillance have reduced SSI rates in all categories that were established by this classification [see Table 10].[7-9,26]

In 1960, after years of negative studies, it was said, "Nearly all surgeons now agree that the routine use of prophylaxis in clean operations is unnecessary and undesirable."[31] Since then, much has changed: there are now many clean operations for which no competent surgeon would omit the use of prophylactic antibiotics, particularly as procedures become increasingly complex and prosthetic materials are used in patients who are older, sicker, or immunocompromised.

A separate risk assessment that integrates host and bacterial variables (i.e., whether the operation is dirty or contaminat-

The Surgical Scrub

The purpose of cleansing the surgeon's hands is to reduce the numbers of resident flora and transient contaminants, thereby decreasing the risk of transmitting infection. Although the proper duration of the hand scrub is still subject to debate, evidence suggests that a 120-second scrub is sufficient, provided that a brush is used to remove the bacteria residing in the skin folds around the nails.[69] The nail folds, the nails, and the fingertips should receive the most attention because most bacteria are located around the nail folds and most glove punctures occur at the fingertips. Friction is required to remove resident microorganisms, which are attached by adhesion or adsorption, whereas transient bacteria are easily removed by simple hand washing.

Solutions containing either chlorhexidine gluconate or one of the iodophors are the most effective surgical scrub preparations and have the fewest problems with stability, contamination, and toxicity.[65,153] According to one review article, chlorhexidine gluconate (4%) in a sudsing base is the preferred agent because of its initial effectiveness, its residual activity, and its limited toxicity.[154] Another study showed that chlorhexidine gluconate achieves significant, immediate reduction of microorganisms and has persistent and residual efficacy.[155,156] In a comparative study of chlorhexidine gluconate, povidone-iodine, parachlorometaxylenol (PCMX or chloroxylenol), and alcohol, only chlorhexidine gluconate achieved significant antimicrobial efficacy in all parameters.

Alcohols applied to the skin are among the safest known antiseptics, and they produce the greatest and most rapid reduction in bacterial counts on clean skin.[66] A vigorous 1-minute scrub with enough alcohol to wet the hands completely has been shown to be the most effective method for hand antisepsis. A 1-minute immersion or scrub with alcohol is as effective as 4 to 7 minutes of skin preparation with other antiseptics, and washing with alcohol for 3 minutes is as effective as scrubbing for 20 minutes.[66] The main disadvantages of the alcohols are (1) their drying effects on the skin and (2) their volatility and flammability, which necessitate extreme caution when electrosurgery or laser procedures are performed. Although the alcohols are less commonly used in the United States, consistent, immediate, and effective reduction of skin flora makes them useful agents for preoperative skin cleansing.

All variables considered, chlorhexidine gluconate followed by an iodophor appears to be the best option.

Table 8 Effect of Surveillance and Feedback on Wound Infection Rates in Two Hospitals[19]

		Period 1	Period 2*
Hospital A	Number of wounds	1,500	1,447
	Wound infection rate	8.4%	3.7%
Hospital B	Number of wounds	1,746	1,939
	Wound infection rate	5.7%	3.7%

*Periods 1 and 2 were separated by an interval during which feedback on wound infection rates was analyzed.

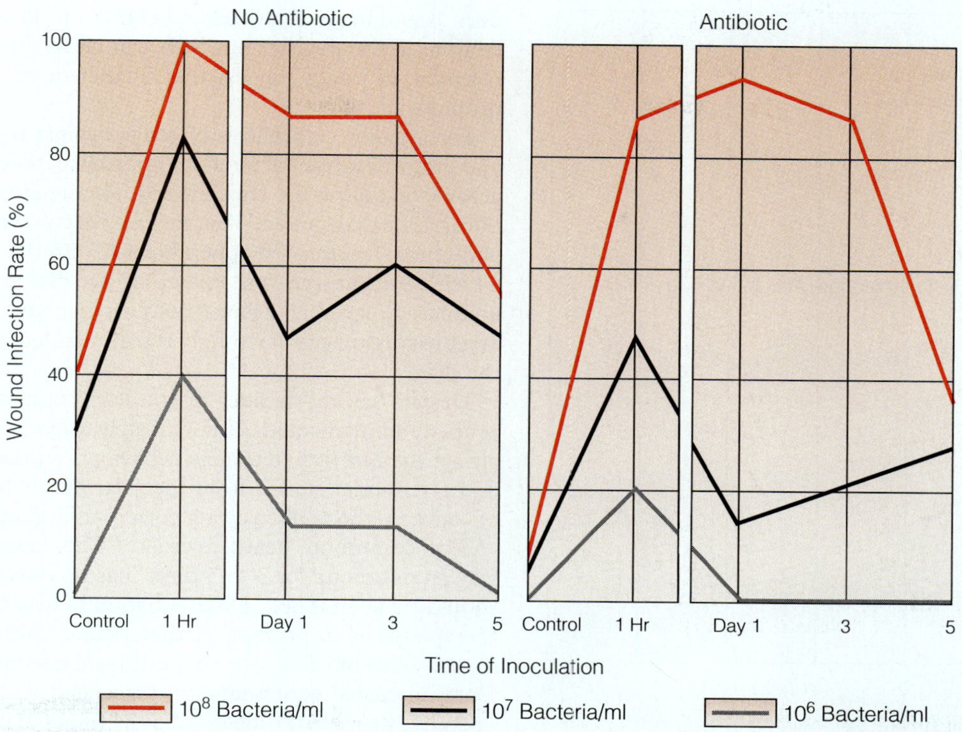

Figure 4 Animals exposed to hemorrhagic shock followed by resuscitation show an early decreased resistance to wound infection. There is also a persistent influence of shock on the development of wound infection at different times of inoculation after shock. The importance of inoculum size (10^6/ml to 10^8/ml) and the effect of antibiotic on infection rates are evident at all times of inoculation.[102]

ed, is longer than 2 hours, or is an abdominal procedure and whether the patient has three or more concomitant diagnoses) segregates more effectively those patients who are prone to an increased incidence of SSI [*see* Integration of Determinants of Infection, *below*]. This approach enables the surgeon to identify those patients who are likely to require preventive measures, particularly in clean cases, in which antibiotics would normally not be used.[8]

It has been implied that antibiotic prophylaxis for two types of clean surgery—hernia repair and breast surgery—represents the standard of practice.[32] However, in the study from which these conclusions were drawn, SSI and urinary tract infection rates were higher than many would have predicted, sample sizes were not large, and potential hazards of widespread antibiotic use were not addressed; neither was the evolution to minimal excisions for breast surgery addressed. Without significantly more supportive data, prophylaxis for clean cases cannot be recommended unless specific risk factors are present.[8,33,34]

Data suggest that prophylactic use of antibiotics may contribute to secondary *Clostridium difficile* disease; caution should be exercised when widening the indications for prophylaxis is under consideration.[35] If local results are poor, surgical practice should be reassessed before antibiotics are prescribed.

ANTIBIOTIC SELECTION AND ADMINISTRATION

When antibiotics are given more than 2 hours before operation, the risk of infection is increased.[30,36] I.V. administration in the OR or the preanesthetic room guarantees appropriate

Table 9 Determinants of Infection and Factors That Influence Wound Infection Rates

Variable	Determinant of Infection		
	Bacteria	Wound Environment (Local Factors)	Host Defense Mechanisms (Systemic Factors)
Bacterial numbers in wound[4]	A		
Potential contamination[4,7,8]	A		
Preoperative shave[7]	A		
Presence of 3 or more diagnoses[8]			C
Age[4,7]		B	C
Duration of operation[4,7,8]	A	B	C
Abdominal operation[8]	A	B	C

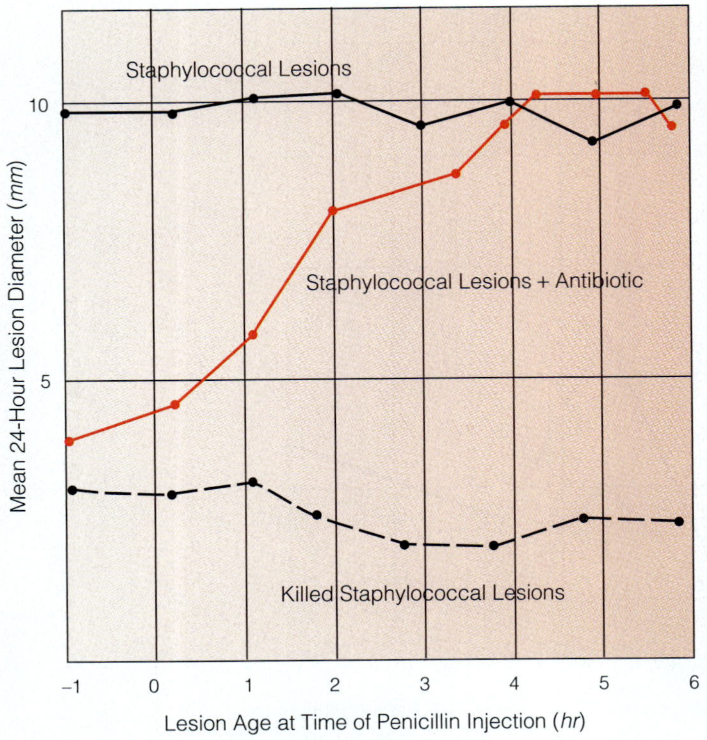

Figure 5 In a pioneer study of antibiotic prophylaxis,[25] the diameter of lesions induced by staphylococcal inoculation 24 hours earlier was observed to be critically affected by the timing of penicillin administration with respect to bacterial inoculation.

levels at the time of incision. The organisms likely to be present dictate the choice of antibiotic for prophylaxis. The cephalosporins are ideally suited to prophylaxis: their features include a broad spectrum of activity, an excellent ratio of therapeutic to toxic dosages, a low rate of allergic responses, ease of administration, and attractive cost advantages. Mild allergic reactions to penicillin are not contraindications for the use of a cephalosporin.[37]

Physicians like new drugs and often tend to prescribe newer, more expensive antibiotics for simple tasks. First-generation cephalosporins (e.g., cefazolin) are ideal agents for prophylaxis. Third-generation cephalosporins are not: they cost more, are not more effective, and promote emergence of resistant strains.[38-40]

The most important first-generation cephalosporin for surgical patients continues to be cefazolin. Administered I.V. in the OR at the time of skin incision, it provides adequate tissue levels throughout most of the operation. A second dose administered in the OR after 3 hours will be beneficial if the procedure lasts longer than that.[36,41] Data on all operative site infections are imprecise, but SSIs can clearly be reduced by this regimen. No data suggest that further doses are required for prophylaxis.

Fortunately, cefazolin is effective against both gram-positive and gram-negative bacteria of importance, unless significant anaerobic organisms are encountered. The significance of anaerobic flora has been disputed,[42] but for elective colorectal operation,[43,44] abdominal trauma,[45,46] appendicitis,[47] or other circumstances in which penicillin-resistant anaerobic bacteria are likely to be encountered, coverage against both aerobic and anaerobic gram-negative organisms is strongly recommended and supported by the data.

Despite several decades of studies, prophylaxis is not always properly implemented. Unfortunately, didactic education is not always the best way to change behavior. Preprinted order forms[48] and a reminder sticker from the pharmacy[49] have proved to be effective methods of ensuring correct utilization.

The commonly heard decision "This case was tough, let's give an antibiotic for 3 to 5 days" has no data to support it and should be abandoned. Differentiation between prophylaxis and therapeusis is important. A therapeutic course for perforated diverticulitis or other types of peritoneal infection is appropriate. Data on casual contamination associated with trauma or with operative procedures suggest that 24 hours of prophylaxis or less is quite adequate.[50-54] Mounting evidence suggests that a single preoperative dose is good care and that additional doses are not required.[55,56]

Trauma Patients

The efficacy of antibiotic administration on arrival in the emergency department as an integral part of resuscitation has been clearly demonstrated.[45] The most common regimens have been (1) a combination of an aminoglycoside and clindamycin and (2) cefoxitin alone. These two regimens or variations thereof have been compared in a number of studies.[22,46,57-59] They appear to be equally effective, and either regimen can be recommended with confidence. For prophylaxis, there appears to be a trend toward using a single drug: cefoxitin[37] or cefotetan.[60] If therapy is required because of either a delay in surgery, terrible injury, or prolonged shock, the combination of an agent that is effective against anaerobes with an aminoglycoside seems to be favored. Because aminoglycosides are nephrotoxic, they must be used with care in the presence of shock.

In all the trauma studies just cited, antibiotic prophylaxis lasted for 48 hours or longer. Subsequent studies, however, indicated that prophylaxis lasting less than 24 hours is appropriate.[52-54,61] Single-dose prophylaxis is appropriate for patients with closed fractures.[62]

Table 10 Historical Rates of Wound Infection

Wound Classification	Infection Rate (%)				
	1960–1962[26] (15,613 patients)	1967–1977[7] (62,937 patients)	1975–1976[8] (59,353 patients)	1977–1981[9] (20,193 patients)	1982–1986[106] (20,703 patients)
Clean	5.1	1.5	2.9	1.8	1.3
Clean-contaminated	10.8	7.7	3.9	2.9	2.5
Contaminated	16.3	15.2	8.5	9.9	7.1
Dirty-infected	28.0	40.0	12.6	—	—
Overall	7.4	4.7	4.1	2.8	2.2

COMPLICATIONS

Complications of antibiotic prophylaxis are few. Although data linking prophylaxis to the development of resistant organisms are meager, resistant microbes have developed in every other situation in which antibiotics have been utilized, and it is reasonable to expect that prophylaxis in any ecosystem will have the same result,[63] particularly if selection of patients is poor, if prophylaxis lasts too long, or if too many late-generation agents are used.

A rare but important complication of antibiotic use is pseudomembranous enterocolitis, which is induced most commonly by clindamycin, the cephalosporins, and ampicillin[35] [see 81 Nosocomial Infection]. The common denominator among different cases of pseudomembranous enterocolitis is hard to identify. Diarrhea and fever can develop after administration of single doses of prophylactic antibiotics. The condition is rare, but difficulties occur because of failure to make a rapid diagnosis.

CURRENT ISSUES

The most significant questions concerning prophylaxis of SSIs already have been answered. Important issues that remain are the proper duration of prophylaxis in complicated cases, trauma, and the presence of foreign bodies. No change in the criteria for antibiotic prophylaxis is required in laparoscopic procedures; the risk of infection may actually be lower in such cases.[64] Cost factors are important and may justify the endless succession of studies that compare new drugs in competition for appropriate clinical niches.

Further advances in patient selection may take place but will require analysis of data from large numbers of patients and a distinction between approaches to infection of the wound, which is only a part of the operative field, and approaches to infections directly related to the operative site. These developments will define more clearly the prophylaxis requirements of patients whose operations are clean but whose risk of wound or operative site infection is increased.

Skin Preparation

As the first line of defense against infection, the skin is remarkable in its complexity and efficiency. Surgeons must respect this organ and carefully manage preparation of both their own skin and their patients' skin. None of the topical antibacterial agents now in use are totally harmless; their destructive effect on the skin's natural defense mechanisms must be recognized and taken into account.

Although the importance of skin preparation cannot be denied, in healthy tissue, a wound contaminated with many microorganisms is amazingly resistant to infection. Admittedly, skin preparation has a relatively minor influence on wound infection as compared with surgical technique and host factors; nonetheless, it consumes OR time and the time of health care personnel, both of which are expensive. Therefore, choosing the most effective agent and method for skin preparation is an important economic decision as well as a surgical decision.

CLEANSING THE SURGEON'S HANDS

Scrubbing

Method The dry microenvironment of the hands is inhabited by coagulase-negative staphylococci and coryneform bacteria. Rubber gloves convert this dry microenvironment to wet skin, causing preferential proliferation of gram-negative resident bacteria.

The question of how long surgeons should scrub their hands has not been definitively answered. There is strong evidence to suggest that the traditional 10-minute scrub should be abandoned. Indeed, almost all the usual application times are probably excessive, given that both alcohol and chlorhexidine gluconate are effective in 60 seconds or less.[65,66] One study evaluated the efficiency of surgical hand disinfection after reduced application times of antimicrobial solutions, including 60% propyl alcohol and preparations containing chlorhexidine gluconate.[67] On the basis of the results of this study, the investigators recommended that surgical hand preparation time be reduced to 3 minutes. Despite such evidence, the hallowed practice of long preoperative scrubs is not easily changed. The Guideline for Handwashing and Hospital Environmental Control, 1985, from the Centers for Disease Control, recommended that before each operation surgeons scrub their hands and arms up to the elbows with an antimicrobial surgical scrub preparation and that the first scrubbing of the day last at least 5 minutes.[68] The recommended length of scrubbing between operations is 2 to 5 minutes. A 98.2% reduction in bacterial counts after a 120-second scrub has been reported,[69] and a 5-minute scrub has been confirmed to be as effective as a 10-minute scrub.[70] In England, a 2- to 3-minute application of antiseptic without using a scrubbing brush is recommended.[71] Shorter hand preparation times are further supported by the rarity of infections resulting from the destruction of bacteria by such applications.[71] The weight of the evidence suggests that a preoperative scrub of at least 120 seconds that includes brushing of the nail and fingertip areas adequately disinfects the hands. It must be remembered, however, that successful preparation of the surgeon's hands is impossible when dermatitis is present.

Agent The ideal surgical scrub preparation should be effective and persistent in reducing the numbers of a broad spectrum of microorganisms without irritating intact skin. Although the question of what level of reduction in microorganisms is sufficient to prevent transmission of infection has never been resolved, at least five commonly used agents or classes of agents have a significant antimicrobial effect: the alcohols, the iodophors, chlorhexidine gluconate [see Table 11], hexachlorophene, and benzalkonium. However, hexachlorophene and benzalkonium need not be considered: they have such problems with stability, contamination, and toxicity that they should not be used. Other agents, such as parachlorometaxylenol and triclosan, have also been used, but these agents as well have various properties that make them less attractive.[66,72]

The most commonly used iodophor is povidone-iodine. A formulation containing 7.5% is widely used as a surgical hand scrub; 10% solutions in applicators and various 2% solutions are also available. Use of iodophors sometimes elicits skin reactions, and as yet little is known about their chronic toxicity. A 5-minute scrub with a povidone-iodine preparation results in absorption of more than four times the normal daily intake of iodine through the skin.[73]

Chlorhexidine gluconate is offered in several formulations, of which the most commonly used is 4% chlorhexidine gluconate in a detergent base. Chlorhexidine gluconate is more persistent than the iodophors and slightly less irritating, but both types of agent are acceptable in this regard.[66] An alcohol-based hand rinse containing 0.5% chlorhexidine gluconate is also used; the rapid effect of alcohol and the persistence of chlorhexidine gluconate would seem to be a particularly desirable combination.

Table 11 Characteristics of Three Topical Antimicrobial Agents Effective against Both Gram-Positive and Gram-Negative Bacteria[66]

Agent	Mode of Action	Antifungal Activity	Comments
Chlorhexidine	Cell wall disruption	Fair	Poor activity against tuberculosis-causing organisms; can cause ototoxicity and eye irritation
Iodine/iodophors	Oxidation and substitution by free iodine	Good	Broad antibacterial spectrum; minimal skin residual activity; possible absorption toxicity and skin irritation
Alcohols	Denaturation of protein	Good	Rapid action but little residual activity; flammable

Studies have shown chlorhexidine gluconate to be a more effective surgical scrub than povidone-iodine. In one trial, chlorhexidine gluconate (4%) detergent caused a greater initial reduction of both resident and transient flora than either povidone-iodine (7.5%) surgical scrub or hexachlorophene (3%) emulsion.[74] Repetitive use of each agent produced a further reduction in resident flora. However, chlorhexidine gluconate was the most effective agent and the only one to reduce transient flora further.

In another comparative study, a solution of 4% chlorhexidine digluconate (British Pharmacopoeia) in a detergent base containing 25% poloxamer 237 and 3.7% dimethyl lauryl amine oxide caused a significantly greater initial reduction in skin flora than a povidone-iodine detergent or 0.75% chlorhexidine detergent.[75] Data from this study on the cumulative effect of multiple applications of antiseptic generally favor chlorhexidine gluconate over povidone-iodine as well.

On hands gloved for 3 hours, chlorhexidine gluconate (4%) detergent reduced microorganisms more persistently than povidone-iodine (10%) detergent.[71] Significant regrowth of bacteria on gloved hands disinfected with povidone-iodine has been documented.[74]

When gloves are used in the operating field, it is important to remember that pathologic changes are produced by surgical glove dusting powders. Several investigators have studied both the anatomic and the cellular changes induced by surgical glove powders and the effects of the powders on adhesion formation.[76,77] The protection of the surgeon's skin—particularly during an operation being performed on a woman of reproductive age—should be accomplished with powder-free gloves.

Skin changes resulting from latex sensitivity have become an increasingly important finding, especially among health care workers. In a study by the Association of Operating Room Nurses, 369 (21%) of 1,738 nurses reported reactions to latex.[78] The most commonly reported localized reaction is contact dermatitis, but more severe systemic reactions have also been documented. At present, there is no safe and effective method of diagnosing latex sensitivity in both health care workers and patients at risk for potentially severe reactions.

On the evidence of almost all the considerable literature on the use of topical agents for preparation of the surgeon's hands and the patient's skin, chlorhexidine gluconate is the most effective agent [see Table 11]. Povidone-iodine is a relatively poor second. Although 70% isopropyl alcohol is effective and inexpensive, it is not heavily marketed: besides being inflammable, it irritates skin with repetitive use.

Washing

The purpose of washing the hands after surgery is to remove microorganisms that are resident, that flourished in the warm, wet environment created by wearing gloves, or that reached the hands by entering through puncture holes in the gloves. On the ward, even minimal contact with colonized patients has been demonstrated to transfer microorganisms.[79] As many as 1,000 organisms were transferred by simply touching the patient's hand, taking a pulse, or lifting the patient. The organisms survived for 20 to 150 minutes, making their transfer to the next patient clearly possible. Viruses have been shown to survive for 20 to 30 minutes on the hands.[80]

A return to the ancient practice of washing hands between each patient contact is warranted. Nosocomial spread of numerous organisms, including *C. difficile*, antibiotic-resistant bacteria, and viruses (e.g., HIV and hepatitis B virus), is a constant threat. As an example, two million or more North Americans are seropositive for HIV, and most of them are unaware of their seroconversion. This likely is the case as well for most other relevant viruses.

Hand washing on the ward is complicated by the fact that overwashing may actually increase bacterial counts. Dry, damaged skin harbors many more bacteria than healthy skin and is almost impossible to render even close to bacteria free. Although little is known about the physiologic changes in skin that result from frequent washings, the bacterial flora is certainly modified by alterations in the lipid or water content of the skin.

Bowel Preparation for Colon Surgery

The results of the numerous studies of antibiotic bowel preparation that have been done [see Table 6] suggest that many different approaches may be equally effective in reducing infection after elective colonic resection. Certain features, however, appear to be common to most of the studies:

1. Oral antibiotic regimens with both aerobic and anaerobic activity (e.g., neomycin–erythromycin base and neomycin-metronidazole) were employed.
2. The oral agents were given in limited doses the day before operation.
3. Addition of systemic antibiotic agents without broad-spectrum coverage to the oral antibiotics generally did not improve the results.
4. Use of broad-spectrum parenteral antibiotic agents alone was associated with a lower infection rate than use of systemic agents with only limited coverage.
5. Addition of a broad-spectrum parenteral antibiotic to the oral antibiotics may further reduce the postoperative infection rate.
6. Parenteral or oral antibiotics should be administered only for short amounts of time during the perioperative period. A single parenteral dose given just before operation may be sufficient.[81-84]

A 5-year cooperative Veterans Administration study of more than 1,000 patients undergoing elective colon operations compared two groups of patients receiving oral neomycin–erythromycin base: one group received only the oral preparation, whereas the other also received parenteral perioperative cephalothin.[85] The infection rates were not significantly different in the two groups and in fact were below 9% in both; however, there was a trend toward lower infection rates in patients receiving both oral and parenteral antibiotics. The authors concluded that if appropriate mechanical cleansing and oral neomycin–erythromycin base therapy are employed, no benefit can be gained from adding parenteral antibiotic prophylaxis. Similar single-hospital studies concluded that the addition of systemic cefazolin to the oral neomycin–erythromycin base preparation did significantly reduce postoperative infections,[86,87] whereas others found no extra benefit from the addition of older systemic antibiotics.[88,89]

Various studies have demonstrated that the duration of colorectal operations affects both the risk of infection and the choice of the optimal preoperative antibiotic preparation. In one study, in operations lasting less than 4 hours, combinations of oral and parenteral antibiotics were not superior to parenteral antibiotics alone; however, in operations lasting longer than 4 hours, combination regimens achieved significantly better results than parenteral agents alone.[90] In another study, combination regimens were found to be superior in operations lasting less than 3 hours and 35 minutes but in which rectal resection was required.[91]

The mechanical cleansing technique employed is a matter of preference. Traditional bowel preparation, if carried out for unnecessarily long periods (3 to 5 days), is associated with less patient compliance and a higher incidence of fatigue and other related symptoms than are other cleansing techniques. Whole gut irrigation as recommended in the past—that is, using large amounts of fluid (10 to 15 L)—should be discouraged. Some authors recommend the use of mannitol in varying concentrations in lavage solutions.[92] Others emphasize that clinical dehydration may develop when 15% mannitol is used or that electrocautery may lead to colonic explosions when mannitol is used without oral antibiotics.[93] Lavage with polyethylene glycol–electrolyte solution appears to be the preferred cleansing method before elective colorectal surgery.[93,94] A study comparing the efficacy of 2-day routine mechanical cleansing with that of lavage performed once on the day before operation demonstrated no difference between the two approaches: 1-day lavage was both safe and economical, and the authors preferred it to 2-day mechanical cleansing.[95] Subsequent studies reported no differences in the adequacy of colon cleansing whether bowel preparation was performed in the inpatient setting or the outpatient setting.[96,97]

Integration of Determinants of Infection

The significant advances in the control of wound infection during the past several decades are linked to a better understanding of the biology of wound infection, and this link has permitted the advance to the concept of SSI.[2] In all tissues at any time, there will be a critical inoculum of bacteria that would cause an infectious process [see Figure 3]. The standard definition of infection in urine and sputum has been 10^5 organisms/ml. In a clean dry wound, 10^5 bacteria produce a wound infection rate of 50% [see Figure 3].[5] Effective use of antibiotics reduces the infection rate to 10% with the same number of bacteria and thereby permits the wound to tolerate a much larger number of bacteria.

All of the clinical activities described are intended either to reduce the inoculum or to permit the host to manage the number of bacteria that would otherwise be pathologic. One study in guinea pigs has shown how manipulation of local blood flow, shock, the local immune response, and foreign material can enhance the development of infection.[98] This study and two others[25,98,99] define an early decisive period of host antimicrobial activity that lasts for 3 to 6 hours after contamination. Bacteria that remain after this period are the infecting inoculum. Processes that interfere with this early response (e.g., shock, altered perfusion, adjuvants, foreign material) or support it (e.g., antibiotics or total care) have a major influence on outcome.

One investigation demonstrated that silk sutures decrease the number of bacteria required for infection.[100] Other investigators used a suture as the key adjuvant in studies of host manipulation,[101] whereas a separate study demonstrated persistent susceptibility to wound infection days after shock.[102] The common variable is the number of bacteria. This relation may be termed the inoculum effect, and it has great relevance in all aspects of infection control. Applying knowledge of this effect in practical terms involves the following three steps:

1. Keeping the bacterial contamination as low as possible via asepsis and antisepsis, preoperative preparation of patient and surgeon, and antibiotic prophylaxis.
2. Maintaining local factors in such a way that they can prevent the lodgment of bacteria and thereby provide a locally unreceptive environment.
3. Maintaining systemic responses at such a level that they can control the bacteria that become established.

These three steps are related to the determinants of infection and their applicability to daily practice. Year-by-year reductions in wound infection rates, when closely followed, indicate that it is possible for surgeons to continue improving results by attention to quality of clinical care and surgical technique, despite increasingly complex operations.[6,9,19-21] In particular, the measures involved in the first step (control of bacteria) have been progressively refined and are now well established.

The integration of determinants has significant effects [see Figures 3 and 4]. When wound closure was effected with a wound hematocrit of 8% or more, the inoculum required to produce a wound infection rate of 40% was 100 bacteria [see Figure 3]. Ten bacteria produced a wound infection rate of 20%. The shift in the number of organisms required to produce clinical infection is significant. It is obvious that this inoculum effect can be changed dramatically by good surgical technique and further altered by use of prophylactic antibiotics. If the inoculum is always slightly smaller than the number of organisms required to produce infection in any given setting, results are excellent. There is clearly a relation between the number of bacteria and the local environment. The local effect can also be seen secondary to systemic physiologic change, specifically shock. One study showed the low local perfusion in shock to be important in the development of an infection.[98,99]

One investigation has shown that shock can alter infection rates immediately after its occurrence [see Figure 4].[102] Furthermore, if the inoculum is large enough, antibiotics will not control bacteria. In addition, there is a late augmentation of infection lasting up to 3 days after restoration of blood volume. These early and late effects indicate that systemic determinants come into play after local effects are resolved. These observations call for further study, but obviously, it is the combined abnormalities that alter outcome.

Table 12 Comparison of Wound Classification Systems[8]

Traditional Wound Classification System	Simplified Risk Index					All from Traditional Classification
	Low Risk	Medium Risk	High Risk			
	0	1	2	3	4	
Clean	1.1	3.9	8.4	15.8		2.9
Clean-contaminated	0.6	2.8	8.4	17.7		3.9
Contaminated		4.5	8.3	11.0	23.9	8.5
Dirty-infected		6.7	10.9	18.8	27.4	12.6
All from SENIC index	1.0	3.6	8.9	17.2	27.0	4.1

SENIC—Study of the Efficacy of Nosocomial Infection Control

Systemic host responses are important for the control of infection. The patient has been clearly implicated as one of the four critical variables in the development of wound infection.[8] In addition, the bacterial inoculum, the location of the procedure and its duration, and the coexistence of three or more diagnoses were found to give a more accurate prediction of the risk of wound infection. The spread of risk is defined better with the SENIC index (1% to 27%) than it is with the traditional classification (2.9% to 12.6%) [see Table 12]. The importance of the number of bacteria is lessened if the other factors are considered in addition to inoculum. The inoculum effect has to be considered with respect to both the number of organisms and the local and systemic host factors that are in play. Certain variables were found to be significantly related to the risk of wound infection in three important prospective studies [see Table 12].[4,7,8] It is apparent that the problem of SSI cannot be examined only with respect to the management of bacteria. Host factors have become much more significant now that the bacterial inoculum can be maintained at low levels by means of asepsis, antisepsis, technique, and prophylactic antibiotics.[103]

Important host variables include the maintenance of normal homeostasis (physiology) and immune response [see 88 Immunomodulation]. Maintenance of normal homeostasis in patients at risk is one of the great advances of surgical critical care.[103] The clearest improvements in this regard have come in maintenance of blood volume, oxygenation, and oxygen delivery.

One group demonstrated the importance of oxygen delivery, tissue perfusion, and P_aO_2 in the development of wound infection.[104] Oxygen can have as powerful a negative influence on the development of SSI as antibiotics can.[105] The influence is very similar to that seen in other investigations. Whereas a P_aO_2 equivalent to a true fractional concentration of oxygen in inspired gas (F_IO_2) of 45% is not feasible, maintenance, when appropriate, of an increased F_IO_2 in the postoperative period may prove an elementary and effective tool in managing the inoculum effect.

Modern surgical practice has reduced the rate of wound infection significantly. Consequently, it is more useful to think in terms of SSI, which is not limited to the incision but may occur anywhere in the operative field; this concept provides a global objective for control of infections associated with a surgical procedure. Surveillance is of great importance for quality assurance; it is discussed in more detail elsewhere [see 108 Infection Control in Surgical Practice]. Reports of recognized pathogens (e.g., *S. epidermidis* and group A streptococci) as well as unusual organisms (e.g., *Rhodococcus* [*Gordona*] *bronchialis*, *Mycoplasma hominis*, and *Legionella dumoffii*) in SSIs highlight the importance of infection control and epidemiology for quality assurance in surgical departments.[12-14,17,18] (Although these reports use the term wound infection, they are really addressing what we now call SSI.) The importance of surgeon-specific and service-specific SSI reports should be clear[7,9,106] [see Table 8] and their value in quality assurance evident.

References

1. Meakins JL: Host defence mechanisms: evaluation and roles of acquired defects and immunotherapy. Can J Surg 18:259, 1975
2. Consensus paper on the surveillance of surgical wound infections. The Society for Hospital Epidemiology of America; The Association for Practitioners in Infection Control; The Centers for Disease Control; The Surgical Infection Society. Infect Control Hosp Epidemiol 13:599, 1992
3. Horan TC, Gaynes RP, Martone WJ, et al: CDC definitions of nosocomial surgical site infections, 1992: a modification of CDC definitions of surgical wound infections. Infect Control Hosp Epidemiol 13:606, 1992
4. Davidson AIG, Clark C, Smith G: Postoperative wound infection: a computer analysis. Br J Surg 58:333, 1971
5. Polk HC Jr, Lopez-Mayor JF: Postoperative wound infection: a prospective study of determinant factors and prevention. Surgery 66:97, 1969
6. Report of an Ad Hoc Committee of the Committee on Trauma, Division of Medical Sciences, National Academy of Sciences–National Research Council: Postoperative wound infections: the influence of ultraviolet irradiation of the operating room and of various other factors. Ann Surg 160(suppl):1, 1964
7. Cruse PJE, Foord R: The epidemiology of wound infection: a 10-year prospective study of 62,939 wounds. Surg Clin North Am 60:27, 1980
8. Haley RW, Culver DH, Morgan WM, et al: Identifying patients at high risk of surgical wound infection: a simple multivariate index of patient susceptibility and wound contamination. Am J Epidemiol 121:206, 1985
9. Olson M, O'Connor M, Schwartz ML: Surgical wound infections: a 5-year prospective study of 20,193 wounds at the Minneapolis VA Medical Center. Ann Surg 199:253, 1984
10. Alexander JW, Fischer JE, Boyajian M, et al: The influence of hair-removal methods on wound infections. Arch Surg 118:347, 1983
11. Olson MM, MacCallum J, McQuarrie DG: Preoperative hair removal with clippers does not increase infection rate in clean surgical wounds. Surg Gynecol Obstet 162:181, 1986
12. Boyce JM, Potter-Bynoe G, Opal SM, et al: A common-source outbreak of Staphylococcus epidermidis infections among patients undergoing cardiac surgery. J Infect Dis 161:493, 1990
13. Mastro TD, Farley TA, Elliott JA, et al: An outbreak of surgical-wound infections due to group A

streptococcus carried on the scalp. N Engl J Med 323:968, 1990

14. Richet HM, Craven PC, Brown JM, et al: A cluster of *Rhodococcus (Gordona) bronchialis* sternal-wound infections after coronary-artery bypass surgery. N Engl J Med 324:104, 1991
15. Moylan JA, Kennedy BV: The importance of gown and drape barriers in the prevention of wound infection. Surg Gynecol Obstet 151:465, 1980
16. Garibaldi RA, Maglio S, Lerer T, et al: Comparison of nonwoven and woven gown and drape fabric to prevent intraoperative wound contamination and postoperative infection. Am J Surg 152:505, 1986
17. Lowry PW, Blankenship RJ, Gridley W, et al: A cluster of legionella sternal-wound infections due to postoperative topical exposure to contaminated tap water. N Engl J Med 324:109, 1991
18. Wilson ME, Dietze C: Mycoplasma hominis surgical wound infection: a case report and discussion. Surgery 103:257, 1988
19. Cruse PJE: Surgical wound sepsis. Can Med Assoc J 102:251, 1970
20. Wangensteen OH, Wangensteen SD: The Rise of Surgery: Emergence from Empiric Craft to Scientific Discipline. University of Minnesota Press, Minneapolis, 1978
21. Cruse PJE: Wound infections: epidemiology and clinical characteristics. Surgical Infectious Disease, 2nd ed. Howard RJ, Simmons RL, Eds. Appleton and Lange, Norwalk, Connecticut, 1988
22. Nichols RL, Smith JW, Klein DB, et al: Risk of infection after penetrating abdominal trauma. N Engl J Med 311:1065, 1984
23. Jensen LS, Andersen A, Fristup SC, et al: Comparison of one dose versus three doses of prophylactic antibiotics, and the influence of blood transfusion, on infectious complications in acute and elective colorectal surgery. Br J Surg 77:513, 1990
24. Miles AA, Miles EM, Burke J: The value and duration of defense reactions of the skin to the primary lodgment of bacteria. Br J Exp Pathol 38:79, 1957
25. Burke JF: The effective period of preventive antibiotic action in experimental incisions and dermal lesions. Surgery 50:161, 1961
26. Bernard HR, Cole WR: The prophylaxis of surgical infection: the effect of prophylactic antimicrobial drugs on incidence of infection following potentially contaminated wounds. Surgery 56:151, 1964
27. Chodak GW, Plaut ME: Use of systemic antibiotics for prophylaxis in surgery: a critical review. Arch Surg 112:326, 1977
28. Di Piro JT, Bivens BA, Record KE, et al: The prophylactic use of antimicrobials in surgery. Curr Probl Surg 20:72, 1983
29. Conte JE Jr, Polk HC Jr: Antibiotic Prophylaxis in Surgery: A Comprehensive Review. JB Lippincott Co, Philadelphia, 1984
30. Classen DC, Evans RS, Pestotnik SC, et al: The timing of prophylactic administration of antibiotics and the risk of surgical-wound infection. N Engl J Med 326: 282, 1992
31. Finland M: Antibacterial agents: uses and abuses in treatment and prophylaxis. RI Med J 43:499, 1960
32. Platt R, Zaleznik DF, Hopkins CC, et al: Perioperative antibiotic prophylaxis for herniorrhaphy and breast surgery. N Engl J Med 322:153, 1990
33. Taylor EW, Byrne DJ, Leaper DJ, et al: Antibiotic prophylaxis and open groin hernia repair. World J Surg 21:811, 1997
34. Platt R, Zucker JR, Zaleznik DF, et al: Prophylaxis against wound infection following hernia or breast surgery. J Infect Dis 166:556, 1992
35. Yee J, Dixon CM, McLean APH, et al: Clostridium difficile disease in a department of surgery: the significance of prophylactic antibiotics. Arch Surg 126:241, 1991
36. Galandiuk S, Polk HC Jr, Jagelman DG, et al: Reemphasis of priorities in surgical antibiotic prophylaxis. Surg Gynecol Obstet 169:219, 1989
37. Kaiser AB: Antibiotic prophylaxis in surgery. N Engl J Med 315:1129, 1986
38. Meijer WS, Schmitz PI, Jeekel J: Meta-analysis of randomized, controlled clinical trials of antibiotic prophylaxis in biliary tract surgery. Br J Surg 77:283, 1990
39. Rotman N, Hay J-M, Lacaine F, et al: Prophylactic antibiotherapy in abdominal surgery: first- vs third-generation cephalosporins. Arch Surg 124:323, 1989
40. Choice of cephalosporins. Med Lett Drugs Ther 32:109, 1990
41. Shapiro M, Muñoz A, Tager IB, et al: Risk factors for infection at the operative site after abdominal or vaginal hysterectomy. N Engl J Med 307:1661, 1982
42. Polk HC Jr: Contributions of alimentary tract surgery to modern infection control. Am J Surg 153:2, 1987
43. Clarke JS, Condon RE, Bartlett JG, et al: Preoperative oral antibiotics reduce septic complications of colon operations: results of prospective, randomized, double-blind clinical study. Ann Surg 186:251, 1977
44. Washington JA III, Dearing WH, Judd ES, et al: Effect of preoperative antibiotic regimen on development of infection after intestinal surgery. Ann Surg 180:567, 1974
45. Fullen WD, Hunt J, Altemeier WA: Prophylactic antibiotics in penetrating wounds of the abdomen. J Trauma 12:282, 1972
46. Gentry LO, Feliciano DV, Lea AS, et al: Perioperative antibiotic therapy for penetrating injuries of the abdomen. Ann Surg 200:561, 1984
47. Heseltine PNR, Yellin AE, Appleman MD, et al: Perforated and gangrenous appendicitis: an analysis of antibiotic failures. J Infect Dis 148:322, 1983
48. Girotti MJ, Fodoruk S, Irvine-Meek J, et al: Antibiotic handbook and pre-printed perioperative order forms for surgical prophylaxis: do they work? Can J Surg 33:385, 1990
49. Larsen RA, Evans RS, Burke JP, et al: Improved perioperative antibiotic use and reduced surgical wound infections through use of computer decision analysis. Infect Control Hosp Epidemiol 10:316, 1989
50. Stone HN, Haney BB, Kolb LD, et al: Prophylactic and preventive antibiotic therapy: timing duration and economics. Ann Surg 189:691, 1978
51. Rowlands BJ, Clark RG, Richards DG: Single-dose intraoperative antibiotic prophylaxis in emergency abdominal surgery. Arch Surg 117:195, 1982
52. Fabian TC, Croce MA, Payne LW, et al: Duration of antibiotic therapy for penetrating abdominal trauma: a prospective trial. Surgery 112:788, 1992
53. Sarmiento JM, Aristizabal G, Rubiano J, et al: Prophylactic antibiotics in abdominal trauma. J Trauma 37:803, 1994
54. Weigelt JA: Role of anaerobic bacteria in antibiotic prophylaxis for trauma. Infect Dis Clin Pract 5(suppl 3):S92, 1996
55. Strachan CJL, Black J, Powis SJA, et al: Prophylactic use of cephazolin against wound sepsis after cholecystectomy. Br Med J 1:1254, 1977
56. Di Piro JT, Cheung RPF, Bowden TA Jr, et al: Single dose systemic antibiotic prophylaxis of surgical wound infections. Am J Surg 152:552, 1986
57. Hofstetter SR, Pachter HL, Bailey AA, et al: A prospective comparison of two regimens of prophylactic antibiotics in abdominal trauma: cefoxitin versus triple drug. J Trauma 24:307, 1984
58. Heseltine PNR, Berne TV, Yellin AE, et al: The efficacy of cefoxitin vs clindamycin/gentamicin in surgically treated stab wounds of the bowel. J Trauma 26:241, 1986
59. Jones RC, Thal ER, Johnson NA, et al: Evaluation of antibiotic therapy following penetrating abdominal trauma. Ann Surg 201:576, 1985
60. Antimicrobial prophylaxis in surgery. Med Lett Drugs Ther 41:75, 1999
61. Dellinger EP: Antibiotic prophylaxis in trauma: penetrating abdominal injuries and open fractures. Rev Infect Dis 13:5847, 1991
62. Boxma H, Broekhuisen T, Patka P, et al: Randomized controlled trial of single-dose antibiotic prophylaxis in surgical treatment of closed fractures: the Dutch Trauma Trial. Lancet 347:1133, 1996
63. Archer GL, Armstrong BC: Alteration of staphylococcal flora in cardiac surgery patients receiving prophylaxis. J Infect Dis 147:642, 1983
64. Illig KA, Schmidt E, Cavanaugh J, et al: Are prophylactic antibiotics required for elective laparoscopic cholecystectomy? J Am Coll Surg 184:353, 1997
65. Casewell MW, Law MM, Desai N: A laboratory model for testing agents for hygienic hand disinfection: handwashing and chlorhexidine for the removal of *Klebsiella*. J Hosp Infect 12:163, 1988
66. Larson E: Guideline for use of topical antimicrobial agents. Am J Infect Control 16:253, 1988
67. Hingst V, Juditzki I, Heeg P, et al: Evaluation of the efficacy of surgical hand disinfection following a reduced application time of 3 instead of 5 min. J Hosp Infect 20:79, 1992
68. Garner JS, Favero MS: CDC guidelines for the prevention and control of nosocomial infections: guideline for handwashing and hospital environmental control, 1985. Am J Infect Control 14:110, 1986
69. Lowbury EJL, Lilly HA, Bull JP: Methods for disinfection of hands and operation sites. Br Med J 2:531, 1964
70. Dineen P: An evaluation of the duration of the surgical scrub. Surg Gynecol Obstet 129:1181, 1969
71. Ayliffe GAJ: Surgical scrub and skin disinfection. Infect Control Hosp Epidemiol 5:23, 1984
72. Sebben JE: Sterile technique and the prevention of wound infection in office surgery: part II. J Dermatol Surg Oncol 15:38, 1989
73. Knolle P, Glöbel B, Glöbel H, et al: Release of iodide from povidone-iodine (PVP-I) in PVP-I preparations: a review of iodide tolerances and a comparative clinical pharmacological study. Proceedings of the International Symposium on Povidone. Digenis GA, Ansell J, Eds. University of Kentucky College of Pharmacy, Lexington, 1983, p 342
74. Peterson AF, Rosenberg A, Alatary SD: Comparative evaluation of surgical scrub preparations. Surg Gynecol Obstet 146:63, 1978
75. Lowbury EJL, Lilly HA: Use of 4% chlorhexidine detergent solution (Hibiscrub) and other methods of skin disinfection. Br Med J 1:510, 1973
76. Ellis H: Pathological changes produced by surgical dusting powders. Ann R Coll Surg Engl 76:5, 1994
77. Tang X-M, Chegini N, Rossi MJ, et al: The effect of surgical glove powder on proliferation of human skin fibroblast and monocyte/macrophage. J Gynecol Surg 10:139, 1994
78. Zaza S, Reeder JM, Luenda EC, et al: Latex sensitivity among perioperative nurses. AORN J 60:806, 1994
79. Casewell M, Phillips I: Hands as route of transmission for Klebsiella species. Br Med J 2:1315, 1977
80. Schürmann W, Eggers HJ: Antiviral activity of an alcoholic hand disinfectant: comparison of the in vitro suspension test with in vivo experiments on hands, and on individual fingertips. Antiviral Res 3:25, 1983
81. Gorbach SL, Condon RE, Conte JE Jr, et al: General guidelines for the evaluation of new anti-infective drugs for prophylaxis of surgical infections. Clin Infect Dis 15(suppl 1):S313, 1992
82. Jagelman DG, Fabian TC, Nichols RL, et al: Single

dose cefotetan versus multiple dose cefoxitin as prophylaxis in colorectal surgery. Am J Surg 155 (suppl 5A):71, 1988

83. Periti P, Mazzei T, Tonelli F, et al: Single dose cefotetan versus multiple dose cefoxitin—antimicrobial prophylaxis in colorectal surgery. Dis Colon Rectum 32:121, 1989
84. Norwegian Study Group for Colorectal Surgery: Should antimicrobial prophylaxis in colorectal surgery include agents effective against both anaerobic and aerobic microorganisms? A double-blind, multicenter study. Surgery 97:402, 1985
85. Condon RE, Bartlett JG, Greenlee H, et al: Efficacy of oral and systemic antibiotic prophylaxis in colorectal operations. Arch Surg 118:496, 1983
86. Stone HH, Hooper CA, Kolb LD, et al: Antibiotic prophylaxis in gastric, biliary and colonic surgery. Ann Surg 184:443, 1976
87. Portnoy J, Kagan E, Gordon PH, et al: Prophylactic antibiotics in elective colorectal surgery. Dis Colon Rectum 26:310, 1983
88. Barber MS, Hirschberg BC, Rice CL, et al: Parenteral antibiotics in elective colon surgery? A prospective, controlled clinical study. Surgery 86:23, 1979
89. Eisenberg HW: The use of new antibiotics in colorectal surgery. Am J Proctol Gastroenterol Colon Rectal Surg 6:9, 1981
90. Kaiser AB, Herrington JL, Jacobs JK, et al: Cefoxitin versus erythromycin, neomycin and cefazolin in colorectal operations: importance of the duration of the surgical procedure. Ann Surg 198:525, 1983
91. Coppa GF, Eng K: Factors involved in antibiotic selection in elective colon and rectal surgery. Surgery 104:853, 1988
92. Jagelman DG, Fazio VW, Lavery IC, et al: A prospective, randomized, double-blind study of 10% mannitol mechanical bowel preparation combined with oral neomycin and short-term, perioperative, intravenous Flagyl as prophylaxis in elective colorectal resections. Surgery 98:861, 1985
93. Beck DE, Harford FJ, DiPalma JA, et al: Bowel cleansing with polyethylene glycol electrolyte lavage solution. South Med J 78:1414, 1985
94. Fleites RA, Marshall JB, Eckhauser ML, et al: The efficacy of polyethylene glycol-electrolyte lavage solution versus traditional mechanical bowel preparation for elective colonic surgery: a randomized prospective, blinded clinical trial. Surgery 98:708, 1985
95. Wolff BG, Beart RW Jr, Dozois RR, et al: A new bowel preparation for elective colon and rectal surgery. Arch Surg 123:895, 1988
96. Frazee RC, Roberts J, Symmonds R, et al: Prospective, randomized trial of inpatient vs. outpatient bowel preparation for elective colorectal surgery. Dis Colon Rectum 35:223, 1992
97. Handelsman JC, Zeiler S, Coleman J, et al: Experience with ambulatory preoperative bowel preparation at The Johns Hopkins Hospital. Arch Surg 128:441, 1993
98. Miles AA, Miles EM, Burke J: The value and duration of defence reactions of the skin to the primary lodgement of bacteria. Br J Exp Pathol 38:79, 1957
99. Miles AA: The inflammatory response in relation to local infections. Surg Clin North Am 60:93, 1980
100. Alexander JW, Alexander WA: Penicillin prophylaxis of experimental staphylococcal wound infections. Surg Gynecol Obstet 120:243, 1965
101. Polk HC Jr: The enhancement of host defenses against infection: search for the holy grail. Surgery 99:1, 1986
102. Livingston DH, Malangoni MA: An experimental study of susceptibility to infection after hemorrhagic shock. Surg Gynecol Obstet 168:138, 1989
103. Meakins JL: Surgeons, surgery and immunomodulation. Arch Surg 126:494, 1991
104. Knighton D, Halliday B, Hunt TK: Oxygen as an antibiotic: a comparison of the effects of inspired oxygen concentration and antibiotic administration on in vivo bacterial clearance. Arch Surg 121:191, 1986
105. Rabkin J, Heurt TK: Infection and oxygen. Problem Wounds: The Role of Oxygen. Davis JC, Heurt TK (Eds). Elsevier, New York, 1987, p 1
106. Olson MM, Lee JT Jr: Continuous, 10-year wound infection surveillance: results, advantages, and unanswered questions. Arch Surg 125:794, 1990
107. Oreskovich MR, Dellinger EP, Lennard ES, et al: Duration of preventive antibiotic administration for penetrating abdominal trauma. Arch Surg 117:200, 1982
108. Langely JM, Le Blanc JC, Drake J, et al: Efficacy of antimicrobial prophylaxis in placement of cerebrospinal fluid shunts: meta-analysis. Clin Infect Dis 17:98, 1993
109. Forse RA, Karam B, MacLean LD, et al: Antibiotic prophylaxis for surgery in morbidly obese patients. Surgery 106:750, 1989
110. Dajani AS, Taubert KA, Wilson W, et al: Prevention of bacterial endocarditis: recommendations by the American Heart Association. JAMA 277:1794, 1997
111. Durack DT: Prevention of infective endocarditis. N Engl J Med 332:38, 1995
112. Prevention of bacterial endocarditis. Med Lett Drugs Ther 32:112, 1990
113. Kaye D: Prophylaxis for infective endocarditis: an update. Ann Intern Med 104:419, 1986
114. Petersen EA: Prevention of bacterial endocarditis. Arch Intern Med 150:2447, 1990
115. Hayek LJ, Emerson JM, Gardner AMN: A placebo-controlled trial of the effect of two preoperative baths or showers with chlorhexidine detergent on postoperative wound infection rates. J Hosp Infect 10:165, 1987
116. Garner JS: CDC guidelines for the prevention and control of nosocomial infections: guideline for prevention of surgical wound infections, 1985. Am J Infect Control 14:71, 1986
117. Hamilton HW, Hamilton KR, Lone FJ: Preoperative hair removal. Can J Surg 20:269, 1977
118. McDonald WS, Nichter LS: Debridement of bacterial and particulate-contaminated wounds. Ann Plast Surg 33:142, 1994
119. Brown TR, Ehrlich CE, Stehman FB, et al: A clinical evaluation of chlorhexidine gluconate spray as compared with iodophor scrub for preoperative skin preparation. Surg Gynecol Obstet 158:363, 1984
120. Ritter MA, French MLV, Eitzen HE, et al: The antimicrobial effectiveness of operative-site preparative agents: a microbiological and clinical study. J Bone Joint Surg [Am] 62A:826, 1980
121. Amstey MS, Jones AP: Preparation of the vagina for surgery: a comparison of povidone-iodine and saline solution. JAMA 245:839, 1981
122. Nichols RL, Condon RE: Preoperative preparation of the colon. Surg Gynecol Obstet 132:323, 1971
123. Bartlett SP, Burton RC: Effects of prophylactic antibiotics on wound infection after elective colon and rectal surgery 1960–1980. Am J Surg 145:300, 1983
124. Nichols RL, Gorbach SL, Condon RE: Alteration of intestinal microflora following preoperative mechanical preparation of the colon. Dis Colon Rectum 14:123, 1971
125. Bowden TA Jr, DiPiro JT, Michael KA: Polyethylene glycol electrolyte lavage solution (PEG-ELS): a rapid, safe mechanical bowel preparation for colorectal surgery. Am Surg 53:34, 1987
126. Burke P, Mealy K, Gillen P, et al: Requirement for bowel preparation in colorectal surgery. Br J Surg 81:907, 1994
127. Santos JCM Jr, Batista J, Sirimarco MT, et al: Prospective randomized trial of mechanical bowel preparation in patients undergoing elective colorectal surgery. Br J Surg 81:1673, 1994
128. Solla JA, Rothenberger DA: Preoperative bowel preparation: a survey of colon and rectal surgeons. Dis Colon Rectum 33:154, 1990
129. Nichols RL: Antibiotic prophylaxis in surgery. Curr Opin Infect Dis 7:647, 1994
130. Nichols RL: Update on preparation of the colon for resection. Current Surg 41:75, 1984
131. Nichols RL, Condon RE, Gorbach SL, et al: Efficacy of preoperative antimicrobial preparation of the bowel. Ann Surg 176:227, 1972
132. Goldring J, McNaught W, Scott A, et al: Prophylactic oral antimicrobial agents in elective colon surgery: a controlled trial. Lancet 2:7943, 1975
133. Matheson DM, Arabi Y, Baxter-Smith D, et al: Randomised multicentre trial of oral bowel preparation and antimicrobials for elective colorectal operations. Br J Surg 65:597, 1978
134. Nichols RL, Condon RE, DiSanto AR: Preoperative bowel preparation: erythromycin base serum and fecal levels following oral administration. Arch Surg 112:493, 1977
135. DiPiro JT, Patrias JM, Townsend RJ, et al: Oral neomycin sulfate and erythromycin base before colon surgery: a comparison of serum and tissue concentrations. Pharmacotherapy 5:91, 1985
136. Panichi G, Pantosti A, Giunchi G, et al: Cephalothin, cefoxitin or metronidazole in elective colon surgery? A single blind randomized trial. Dis Colon Rectum 25:783, 1982
137. Slama TG, Carey LC, Fass RJ: Comparative efficacy of prophylactic cephalothin and cefamandole for elective colon surgery: results of a prospective, randomized, double-blind study. Am J Surg 137:593, 1979
138. Hoffmann CEJ, McDonald PJ, Watts JM: Use of perioperative cefoxitin to prevent infection after colonic and rectal surgery. Ann Surg 193:353, 1981
139. McDonald PJ, Karran SJ: A comparison of intravenous cefoxitin and a combination of gentamicin and metronidazole as prophylaxis in colorectal surgery. Dis Colon Rectum 26:661, 1983
140. Eykyn SJ, Jackson BT, Lockhart-Mummery HE, et al: Prophylactic perioperative intravenous metronidazole in elective colorectal surgery. Lancet 2:761, 1979
141. Feathers RS, Lewis AAM, Sagor GR, et al: Prophylactic systemic antibiotics in colorectal surgery. Lancet 2:4, 1977
142. Nygaard K, Hognestad J: Infection prophylaxis with doxycycline in colorectal surgery: a preliminary report. Scand J Gastroenterol 15(suppl):37, 1980
143. Ivarsson L, Darle N, Kewenter JG, et al: Short-term systemic prophylaxis with cefoxitin and doxycycline in colorectal surgery—a prospective, randomized study. Am J Surg 144:257, 1982
144. Kager L, Ljungdahl I, Malmborg AS, et al: Antibiotic prophylaxis with cefoxitin in colorectal surgery—effect on the colon microflora and septic complications—a clinical model for prediction of the benefit and risks in using a new antibiotic in prophylaxis. Ann Surg 193:277, 1981
145. Song J, Glenny AM: Antimicrobial prophylaxis in colorectal surgery: a systematic review of randomized controlled trials. Br J Surg 85:1232, 1998
146. Peck JJ, Fuchs PC, Gustafson ME: Antimicrobial prophylaxis in elective colon surgery—experience of 1,035 operations in a community hospital. Am J Surg 147:633, 1984
147. Condon RE, Bartlett JG, Nichols RL, et al: Preoperative prophylactic cephalothin fails to control septic complications of colorectal operations: results of controlled clinical trial. Veterans Administration cooperative study. Am J Surg 137:68, 1979
148. Coppa GF, Eng K, Gouge TH, et al: Parenteral and

148. oral antibiotics in elective colon and rectal surgery: a prospective and randomized trial. Am J Surg 145:62, 1983
149. Maki DG, Aughey DR: Comparative study of cefazolin, cefoxitin and ceftizoxime for surgical prophylaxis in colo-rectal surgery. J Antimicrob Chemother 10(suppl C):281, 1982
150. Fabian TC, Mangiante EC, Boldreghini SJ: Prophylactic antibiotics for elective colorectal surgery or operation for obstruction of the small bowel: a comparison of cefonicid and cefoxitin. Rev Infect Dis 6(suppl 4):S896, 1984
151. Nichols RL: Surgical wound infection. Am J Med 91(suppl 3B):54S, 1991
152. Karran SJ, Sutton G, Gartell P, et al: Imipenem prophylaxis in elective colorectal surgery. Br J Surg 80:1196, 1993
153. Aly R, Maibach HI: Comparative antibacterial efficacy of a 2-minute surgical scrub with chlorhexidine gluconate, povidone-iodine, and chloroxylenol sponge-brushes. Am J Infect Control 16:173, 1988
154. Kaul AF, Jewett JF: Agents and techniques for disinfection of the skin. Surg Gynecol Obstet 152:677, 1981
155. Paulson DS: Comparative evaluation of five surgical hand scrub preparations. AORN J 60:246, 1994
156. Proposed recommended practices for surgical hand scrubs. AORN Recommended Practices Committee. AORN J 60:270, 1994
157. Figueras-Felip J, Basilio-Bonet E, Lara-Eisman F, et al: Oral is superior to systemic antibiotic prophylaxis in operations upon the colon and rectum. Surg Gynecol Obstet 158:359, 1984
158. McCulloch PG, Blamey SL, Finlay IG, et al: A prospective comparison of gentamicin and metronidazole and moxalactam in the prevention of septic complications associated with elective operations of the colon and rectum. Surg Gynecol Obstet 162:521, 1986
159. Weaver M, Burdon DW, Youngs DJ, et al: Oral neomycin and erythromycin compared with single-dose systemic metronidazole and ceftriaxone prophylaxis in elective colorectal surgery. Am J Surg 151:437, 1986
160. Jones RN, Wojeski W, Bakke J, et al: Antibiotic prophylaxis of 1,036 patients undergoing elective surgical procedures. Am J Surg 153:341, 1987
161. Playforth MJ, Smith GMR, Evans M, et al: Antimicrobial bowel preparation—oral, parenteral or both? Dis Colon Rectum 31:90, 1988
162. Khubchandani IT, Karamchandani MC, Sheets JA, et al: Metronidazole vs. erythromycin, neomycin and cefazolin in prophylaxis for colon surgery. Dis Colon Rectum 32:17, 1989
163. Kling PA, Dahlgren S: Oral prophylaxis with neomycin and erythromycin in colorectal surgery—more proof for efficacy than failure. Arch Surg 124:705, 1989
164. Stellato TA, Danziger LH, Gordon N, et al: Antibiotics in elective colon surgery: a randomized trial of oral, systemic, and oral/systemic antibiotics for prophylaxis. Am Surg 56:251, 1990
165. Schoetz DJ Jr, Roberts PL, Murray JJ, et al: Addition of parenteral cefoxitin to regimen of oral antibiotics for elective colorectal operations: a randomized prospective study. Ann Surg 212:209, 1990
166. Rowe-Jones DC, Peel ALG, Kingston RD, et al: Single dose cefotaxime plus metronidazole versus three dose cefuroxime plus metronidazole as prophylaxis against wound infection in colorectal surgery: multicentre prospective randomised study. BMJ 300:18, 1990
167. Arnaud JP, Bellissant E, Boissel P, et al: Single-dose amoxycillin–clavulanic acid vs. cefotetan for prophylaxis in elective colorectal surgery: a multicentre, prospective, randomized study. J Hosp Infect 22(suppl A):23, 1992
168. Kwok SPY, Lau WY, Leung KL, et al: Amoxycillin and clavulanic acid versus cefotaxime and metronidazole as antibiotic prophylaxis in elective colorectal resectional surgery. Chemotherapy 39:135, 1993
169. AhChong K, Yip AWC, Lee FCW, et al: Comparison of prophylactic ampicillin/sulbactam with gentamicin and metronidazole in elective colorectal surgery: a randomized clinical study. J Hosp Infect 27:149, 1994
170. Taylor EW, Lindsay G, West of Scotland Surgical Infection Study Group: Selective decontamination of the colon before elective colorectal surgery. World J Surg 18:926, 1994

Acknowledgment

Figures 3 and 4   Albert Miller.

40 PREPARING THE OPERATING ROOM

Ramon Berguer, M.D., Denise Joffe, M.D., Rene Lafreniere, M.D., C.M., James T. Lee, M.D., Ph.D., Joseph LoCicero III, M.D., Edward J. Quebbeman, M.D., Ph.D., H. David Reines, M.D., Cynthia Spry, R.N., M.S.N., and Karen Stanley Williams, M.D.

The operating room should provide an environment that is safe for the patient and efficient for the personnel who work there. These seemingly simple requirements are achieved only by giving attention to many details, including the physical features of the room, the equipment brought into the room, and the procedures followed by surgeons, nurses, anesthesiologists, and other support personnel. These considerations, in turn, must be evaluated for cost-effectiveness, potential for litigation, and, of course, tradition and personal preference.

Physical Aspects of the Operating Room

DESIGN AND CONSTRUCTION

The exact specifications for new construction and major remodeling of ORs are usually dependent on state and local regulations, which commonly incorporate standards published by the U.S. Department of Health and Human Services.[1] In addition to the primary construction standards document published by this agency, a large number of codes and recommendations generated by specialty associations and regulatory agencies also require consideration.[2]

The minimum size recommended for an OR is generally 20 by 20 ft; however, 24 by 24 ft may be needed for specialized cardiac, orthopedic, or neurosurgical procedures that require additional equipment. Generally, an OR should provide enough space for the following: gowning of the operating team, draping of the patient, movement of other personnel without contaminating sterile areas, and accommodation of large pieces of equipment, if necessary. Smaller rooms may be adequate for such procedures as cystoscopy and eye surgery. To ensure optimal scheduling efficiency, all operating rooms should ideally be large and equipped to accommodate any operative procedure; however, construction and maintenance costs would then increase.

Ceiling height should be at least 10 ft to allow for ceiling mounting of operating lights, microscopes, and other equipment. An additional 1 to 2 ft of ceiling height may be needed if x-ray equipment is to be permanently mounted. Conductive flooring is no longer necessary, but the floor should be seamless, hard, and easily cleaned.

A preoperative staging area should be included to allow preparation of the patient and to reduce the amount of time spent in the OR.[3] The staging area, the operating rooms, and the recovery rooms should be in close proximity to the intensive care unit. Unfortunately, as they are typically designed, the patient holding and transfer areas, personnel locker rooms, and, especially, equipment and supply storage areas are often much too small.

TRAFFIC FLOW

Today, floor plans for basic operating suites incorporate the concept of separating clean traffic from dirty traffic; typically, a peripheral corridor with access to a central sterile supply area is constructed around each OR. Consequently, sterile supplies arrive and are stored separately from contaminated materials. Although this concept is theoretically sound, it has not been shown to lower wound infection rates.[2,4] In one study, for example, investigators measured environmental contamination before and after changing from an old operating suite with a single corridor, which received so-called street traffic, to a new operating suite characterized by strictly controlled surgical traffic.[5] Environmental contamination was decreased in the new suite, but the investigators found that the improvement was "substantially less than anticipated." More important, the wound infection rate was unchanged. Furthermore, the considerable traffic back and forth between ORs (the lowest bacterial reservoir in the hospital) and the ICU (the highest bacterial reservoir) has not been shown to increase the risk of septic complications.

The absence of measurable benefit following separation of surgical traffic from the rest of the hospital traffic may be related to several factors:

1. The primary source of perioperative infection is the patient. The secondary source is the OR team. Neither of these sources is influenced by OR traffic-control schemes.

2. It is very difficult to control environmental contamination of horizontal surfaces such as floors. In one study, multiple cultures were obtained from the floors of an operating suite that had separated traffic patterns. The highest degree of contamination was found in the staff changing rooms, and the lowest was found in the public corridor outside the changing rooms.[6] Bacterial counts in the theoretically clean corridor and the dirty corridor were not different. The OR floors had low bacterial counts, obviously caused by frequent washing with detergent, but counts increased rapidly after the first case of the day.

3. The OR staff may not adhere to the traffic-control scheme. In one study, for example, personnel took the shortest route when walking from one point to another.[2]

4. The rate of redispersal of bacteria from the OR floor into the air caused by personnel moving about is either very low or nil, as reported in two studies.[7,8] These investigations also demonstrated that appropriate ventilation rapidly clears bacteria from the air (see below). If these findings are valid, the degree of floor contamination should not contribute to increased infection rates. However, movement of the personnel within the OR (including movement toward or away from the operative field and into or out of the OR) during a procedure does correlate with deposition of colony-forming units of bacteria on settle plates.[9] Movement may be reduced by determining equipment needs in advance, designing proper storage areas in the OR, and instituting policies limiting unnecessary visitation and observation.

AIR HANDLING

The concentrations of airborne particulate matter and bacteria in most ORs are equivalent to concentrations found in specialized clean rooms used in high-tech industries.[10] These low concentrations are achieved by changing room air 20 to 25 times each hour and passing the inflow air through a high-efficiency particulate air (HEPA) filter, which removes 99.97% of particles larger than 0.3 mm in diameter. Thus, the filter efficiently removes bacteria and fungi but not viruses. Bacteria present in OR air exist in association with particles (e.g., skin flakes, floor dust, lint) and dried droplets (e.g., saliva, nasal secretions). With optimal air-handling practices, particle counts can be kept as low as 1 to 5/cu ft, but most ORs have particle counts of 15 to 20/cu ft. The length of time that particles remain suspended in air varies with their size: large particles (100 μm) will fall 10 ft in 10 seconds; however, 10 μm particles, the size of particles that typically carry bacteria,[11] may remain suspended for 17 minutes, and tiny particles (< 3 μm) may remain suspended indefinitely.

Although the OR and its incoming air may be very clean, the numbers of particles and viable bacteria increase substantially once people enter the room because of shedding of skin scales, lint, and other particles.[10,12-15] These particles are then dispersed by the air turbulence caused by people moving about and by heat sources such as lights. Consequently, some investigators recommend increasing the number of air changes per hour to remove even more bacteria and restricting the number of people in the OR and their movements.[12]

Attempts to reduce infection risk further have led to the development of ultraclean air and laminar airflow technologies. However, these approaches are valid only in operations classified as clean, because in other types of operations, the major sources of infection are within the patient and the operative site. The orthopedic literature frequently reports reduced infection rates, particularly for total hip and knee replacement procedures, in ORs equipped with laminar airflow. In one study, for example, the wound infection rate for total hip or knee replacement procedures performed in a conventional operating room was 2.3%.[16] The rate decreased to 0.7% with use of ultraclean air and to 0.6% with use of prophylactic antibiotics. Another institution, however, achieved an infection rate of 1.9% for total hip replacement without using laminar airflow or even HEPA filtration technology.[17]

Although such findings indicate that improvements in the OR environment can reduce wound infection risk, several alternatives to laminar airflow technology exist, including changing operating garments frequently, limiting access to the OR, decreasing talking, updating old ventilation systems, using better skin preparation, and improving surgical technique.[18]

Bacterial viability in the harsh environment of air is limited to a few types of organisms; these include staphylococci, streptococci, bacterial spores, mycobacteria, and various viruses, yeasts, and fungi. Some of these organisms, especially *Aspergillus* and *Legionella*, have caused human infection after growing in hospital ventilation systems. Staphylococci and streptococci, which are frequent causes of postoperative infection, may be transmitted via OR air but are more likely to be spread either by direct contact with the operating team or from an endogenous source within the patient.

Although viable organisms are certainly present in the air of an occupied OR and bacteria are regularly recovered from surgical wounds,[19] organisms recovered from air are often not those that cause wound infection. Many studies that demonstrated reduced infection rates with improvement in air quality failed to show that the organisms eliminated were the causative agents of the previous infections.[20,21] One study analyzed the epidemiology of wound infection before and after the construction of a modern surgical suite that incorporated 20 air changes per hour and controlled traffic flow in the ORs.[5] The investigators found that the most common source of infection was the patient, followed by the surgical personnel. Only infrequently was the OR air implicated as a possible source of infection. They suggested that major changes in air quality would not significantly alter wound infection rates.

Current recommendations for handling OR air are that the air inflow be diffused over the 10 by 10 ft area of ceiling directly over the operating table and that the exhaust sites be located peripherally at the baseboard level. This pattern of airflow may decrease turbulence at the operating table and prevent entrainment of air from the periphery. The pressure in the operating room should be positive (0.125 to 0.25 cm H_2O) relative to the outside corridor to prevent particles and bacteria from entering the room.[4,22]

TEMPERATURE AND HUMIDITY

The ambient temperature of the OR often represents a compromise between the needs of the patient and those of the staff; the temperature desired by staff is itself a compromise between the needs of personnel who are dressed in surgical gowns and those who are not. In Europe and North America, OR temperatures vary from 18° to 26° C (64.4° to 78.8° F). A higher temperature is necessary during operations on infants and burn patients because conservation of body heat is critical in these patients. Generally, surgeons who are actively working and fully gowned prefer a temperature of 18° C (64.4° F), but anesthesiologists prefer 21.5° C (70.7° F).[23]

Humidity in the OR is generally maintained at between 50% and 60%; humidity greater than 60% may cause condensation on cool surfaces, whereas humidity less than 50% may not suppress static electricity.

LIGHTING

Well-balanced illumination in the OR provides the surgeon with a clear view of the operative field, prevents eye strain, and provides appropriate light levels for nurses and anesthesiologists. Much of our factual knowledge of OR illumination has been gained through the efforts of Dr. William Beck and the Illuminating Engineering Society.[24,25] Both the task (operating) light and the general room lights should be flexible, adjustable, and controllable. The ratio of brightness from the center of the operative site to the periphery of the operative site to the periphery of the OR should be 5:3:1. A general illumination brightness of up to 200 footcandles (ft-c) is desirable in new constructions. The lighting sources should not produce glare or undesirable reflection.

The amount of light required during an operation varies with the surgeon and the operative site. In one study, general surgeons operating on the common bile duct found 300 ft-c sufficient; because the reflectance of this tissue area is 15%, the required incident light level would be 2,000 ft-c. Surgeons performing coronary bypass operations required a level of 3,500 ft-c.[25] Surgeons have also expressed preferences for the color of light emitted. Many prefer a light equivalent to 5,000° K, but individual preferences range from 3,500° to 6,500° K. Whether changes in the color of light can improve discrimination of different tissues is unknown.

Other aspects of OR lighting known to vary with surgeon, specialty, and procedure include depth of focus, directionality of the light fixture, ability to decrease shadowing, size of the operative field, and ability to change position or focus of the light in a sterile manner. Light sources that contain multiple elements will continue to emit some light if one element burns out, which is a desirable feature. Ready availability of replacement elements is also desirable.

Another facet of OR lighting is heat production. Heat may be produced by infrared light emitted either directly by the light source or via energy transformation of the illuminated object. The maximum incident light energy value recommended at the wound level is 25,000 µW/cm^2.[24] If several light sources are used to illuminate a wound or if fiberoptic sources are utilized, this value may be exceeded. However, most of the infrared light emitted by OR lights can be eliminated by filters or by heat-diverting dichroic reflectors.

Equipment

Modern surgery uses an ever-increasing number of devices in the OR [see Table 1] to support and protect the patient and to assist the work of the surgical team. All OR equipment should be evaluated with respect to three basic concerns: maintenance of patient safety, maximization of surgical team efficiency, and prevention of occupational injuries.

BASIC CONCERNS

Patient Safety

Patient safety, the first order of business in the OR,[26] begins with proper handling of patients and their tissues, which is particularly important where patients are in direct contact with medical devices. It is imperative that physicians, nurses, and technicians protect patients from injuries caused by excessive pressure, heat, abrasion, electrical shock, chemicals, or trauma during their time in the OR. Equipment must be properly used and maintained because equipment malfunction, especially in life-support or monitoring systems, can cause serious harm.

Surgical Team Efficiency

Despite increased financial constraints, the United States health care system expects high-quality surgical care and access to advanced technology.[27] This goal can be achieved only by increasing the efficiency of surgical operations. Thus, proper storage, maintenance, arrangement, and use of OR equipment are paramount considerations. Both small and large devices used during each operation should be spatially arranged to allow unimpeded flow of persons, supplies, and additional equipment before, during, and after operation. Each member of the surgical team should be able to perform his or her function with minimal delay and the least amount of physical and mental effort. Manufacturers should be encouraged to provide standardized devices for the OR environment, and future OR designs should take into account "human factor" issues so that the myriad devices needed for modern surgery can be most efficiently integrated.

Occupational Injuries

Work-related musculoskeletal injuries are a major cause of decreased productivity and increased litigation costs in the United States.[28] In the OR, occupational injuries can be caused by excessive lifting, improper posture, collision with devices, electrical or thermal injury, puncture by sharp instruments, or exposure to bodily tissues and fluids. Temporary musculoskeletal injuries resulting from poor posture (particularly static posture) or excessive straining are less commonly acknowledged by members of the surgical team but occur relatively frequently during some operations.

To reduce injuries from awkward posture and excessive straining, OR devices should be positioned in an ergonomically desirable manner, so that unnecessary bending, reaching, lifting, and twisting are minimized. Visual displays and monitors should be placed where the surgical team can view them comfortably. Devices that require adjustment during operations should be readily accessible. Placement of cables and tubes across the OR workspace should be avoided if possible. The patient and the operating table should be positioned so as to facilitate the surgeons' work while maintaining patient safety. Lifting injuries can be prevented by using proper transfer technique and obtaining adequate assistance when moving patients in the OR. Thermal, electrical, and mechanical injury can occur if surgical devices and instruments are used improperly or if there are faulty equipment connections, inadequate physical protection, or a cluttered work environment.

OR DEVICES

Life-Support, Anesthetic Delivery, and Monitoring Devices

Life-support, anesthetic delivery, and physiologic monitoring devices are the most important equipment in the OR. These devices are typically integrated into a large, semimobile platform controlled by the anesthesiologist.[29] Power, gas, and data connections for this equipment are often provided via ceiling-mounted columns and should be routed to avoid tangles and hazards. Connections to the patient include the respiratory circuit, I.V. catheters, and monitoring devices such as ECG electrodes and pulse oximetry. More advanced monitoring may require additional bulky equipment for transesophageal echocardiography, electroencephalography, or measurement of somatosensory evoked potentials.

Traditionally, a sterile drape connected to two I.V. poles at the head of the bed (a so-called ether screen) has been used to separate the anesthesiologist's territory from the surgeon's. This arrangement is not necessary and can limit access to the area around the patient, especially when devices such as endoscopic imaging systems and alternative surgical power sources are used. A flexible approach to the arrangement of the anesthetic and surgical teams is most efficient, provided that asepsis and patient safety can be maintained.

Table 1 — Devices Used in the Operating Room

For support of the patient	Anesthesia delivery devices
	Ventilator
	Physiologic monitoring devices
	Warming devices
	I.V. fluid warmers and infusers
For support of the surgeon	Sources of mechanical, electrical, and thermal power, including power tools and electrocautery, laser, and ultrasound instruments
	Mechanical retractors
	Lights mounted in various locations
	Suction devices and smoke evacuators
	Electromechanical and computerized assistive devices, such as robotic assistants
	Visualization equipment, including microscopes; endoscopic video cameras; and display devices such as video monitors, projection equipment, and head-mounted displays
	Data, sound, and video storage and transmission equipment
	Diagnostic imaging devices (e.g., for fluoroscopy, ultrasound, MRI, and CT)
For support of the OR team	Surgical instruments, usually packaged in case carts before each operation but occasionally stored in nearby fixed or mobile modules
	Tables for display of primary and secondary surgical instruments
	Containers for disposal of single-use equipment, gowns, drapes, etc.
	Workspace for charting and record keeping
	Communication equipment

Heating and Insulating Devices

Maintenance of the patient's normal body temperature during anesthesia and operation is important because it decreases complications[30] (although mild hypothermia may have a protective effect in certain situations where cardiac or central nervous system ischemia is unavoidable). All patients undergoing general anesthesia should be considered at risk for hypothermia due to radiation, conduction, convection, and evaporation heat loss.[23] Preventing hypothermia is especially important for infants, the elderly, and burn patients, all of whom have limitations of thermoregulation.

The safest and most effective manner of protecting the patient from hypothermia is to use forced-air warmers with specialized blankets placed over the upper or lower body; alternatively, one may place a warming water mattress under the patient or drape the patient with an aluminized blanket. Second-line therapy for maintaining normothermia is to warm all I.V. fluids. Irrigation fluids used in surgery should always be warmed at or slightly above body temperature before use. Radiant heating devices placed above the operative field may be especially useful during operations on infants. Use of a warmer on the inhalation side of the anesthetic gas circuit can also help maintain the patient's body temperature during an operation.

Electrosurgical Devices

The electrosurgical device is a 500 W radio-frequency generator that is used to cut and coagulate tissue. Although it is both common and necessary in the modern OR, it is also a constant hazard and therefore requires close attention.[31] When in use, the electrosurgical unit generates an electrical arc that has been associated with explosions. This risk has been lessened because explosive anesthetic agents are no longer used; however, explosion of hydrogen and methane gases in the large bowel is still a real—if rare—threat, especially when an operation is performed on an unprepared bowel.[32] Because the unit and its arc generate a broad band of radio frequencies, electrosurgical units interfere with monitoring devices, most notably the electrocardiographic monitor. Interference with cardiac pacemaker activity also has been reported.[33]

The most frequently reported hazard of the electrosurgical unit is a skin burn. Such burns are not often fatal, but they are painful, occasionally require skin grafts, and provide a potential for litigation. The burn site can be at the dispersive electrode, ECG monitoring leads, esophageal or rectal temperature probes, or areas of body contact with grounded objects. The dispersive electrode should be firmly adhered to a broad area of dry, hairless skin, preferably over a large muscle mass.[32]

Lasers

Lasers generate energy that is potentially detrimental. Lasers have caused injuries to both patients and staff, including skin burns, retinal injuries, injuries from endotracheal tube fires, pneumothorax, and damage to the colon and arteries.[34] Some design changes in the OR are necessary to accommodate lasers. The OR should not have windows, and a sign should be posted that indicates that a laser is in use. The walls and ceiling in the room should be nonreflective. Equipment used in the operative field should be nonreflective and nonflammable. The concentration of O_2 and N_2O in the inhaled gases should be reduced to decrease the possibility of fire. In addition, personnel should wear goggles of an appropriate type to protect the eyes from laser damage. A smoke evacuator should be attached to the laser to improve visualization, reduce objectionable odor, and decrease the potential for papillomavirus infection from the laser smoke plume.[35]

Radiologic Devices

Safety requirements during x-ray use must be understood by the surgical team.[36] Unnecessary exposure to radiation should be avoided. Personnel who participate regularly in procedures involving fluoroscopy should wear a badge dosimeter to measure total exposure. If required to remain in the room during exposures, they should stay at the maximal distance from the machine because radiation exposure decreases in proportion to the square of the distance from the source. If these precautions cannot be followed, it is necessary to use lead shielding in the form of lead aprons, thyroid shields, movable leaded barriers for the OR team members to stand behind, or all three. Whenever possible, devices for holding cassettes should be employed, or shielded gloves should be used in the x-ray field.

Portable fluoroscopy units are best employed when the use of x-ray equipment is infrequent. Portable units are awkward to maneuver in a crowded OR and require additional draping to prevent contamination of the surgical field. Fixed x-ray units are more versatile and produce better output; however, they require specialized fluoroscopy OR tables and occupy a significant part of the OR ceiling space. Rooms with built-in x-ray equipment should have lead-lined walls and doors and a separate shielded control booth.

Ultrasonic Devices

Instruments that allow hemostatic division of tissues via high-frequency vibration have become commonplace. So-called ultrasonic scalpels are particularly useful for rapid hemostatic division of vascular pedicles.[37] Ultrasonic dissectors with attached suction are more commonly used for the precise division of vascular solid organs such as the liver.[38] The main advantage of these devices is that no electrical current passes through the tissues. Instead, the instrument tip vibrates ultrasonically to denature proteins, with the result that tissue is divided hemostatically with no risk of burn or electrical shock to OR personnel or the patient. Another advantage is that these devices generate less lateral thermal damage to surrounding tissues than conventional electrocautery devices. Ultrasonic devices require a power generator and are usually pedal operated. The handpieces and connective tubing can be awkward and often require special assembly and cleaning by the surgical scrub nurse.

Powered Devices

The most common powered device in the OR is the surgical table. Central to every operation, this device must be properly positioned and adjusted to ensure the safety of the patient and the efficient work of the surgical team. Manually adjustable tables are simple, but those with electrical controls are easier to manage. OR table attachments, such as the arm boards and leg stirrups used to position patients, must be properly maintained and secured to prevent injuries to patients or staff. During transfer to and from the OR table, care must be taken to ensure that the patient is not injured and that life-support, monitoring, and I.V. systems are not disconnected. Proper transfer technique, personnel assistance, and the use of devices such as rollers will help prevent musculoskeletal injuries to the OR staff during this maneuver.

Other powered surgical instruments common in the OR include those used to obtain skin grafts, open the sternum, and perform orthopedic procedures. Powered saws and drills can cause substantial aerosolization of body fluids, thereby creating a potential infectious hazard for OR personnel.[39,40]

Viewing and Imaging Devices

OR microscopes are required for microsurgical procedures. Floor-mounted units are the most flexible, whereas built-in microscopes are best employed in rooms dedicated to this type of procedure.[41] Microscopes are bulky and heavy devices that can cause obstructions and collision hazards in the OR.

The development of video-assisted surgery in most of the body cavities has had a major impact on modern OR equipment.[42] Laparoscopy, thoracoscopy, arthroscopy, and other minimally invasive video-assisted procedures require a halogen light source and a video camera connected to the endoscope to provide a magnified color image of the operating field. This image is typically displayed for the surgical team on a conventional CRT monitor. Gas or fluid usually must be injected into the cavity being explored via specialized insufflators or pumps. This collection of devices should be arranged (not necessarily together) on wheeled carts or ceiling-mounted booms to facilitate their use and their sterile connection to the surgical field. In all cases, cables and connections should be placed so that OR traffic can flow freely and the surgical team's movements can be relatively unrestricted. All controls and displays must be properly positioned at or below the user's line of sight to allow comfortable and unobstructed viewing.

Today's less invasive operations require more accurate intraoperative assessment of the relevant surgical anatomy through the use of x-ray, computed tomography, magnetic resonance imaging, and ultrasonography. Intraoperative fluoroscopy and ultrasonography are most commonly used for this purpose. Intraoperative ultrasonography requires a high-quality portable ultrasound unit and specialized probes. Depending on the procedure and the training of the surgeon, the presence of a radiologist and an ultrasound technician may be required. The ultrasound unit must be positioned near the patient, and the surgical team must be able to view the image comfortably. In some cases, the image may be displayed on OR monitors by means of a video mixing device. Intraoperative CT and MRI are used less commonly, mostly in neurosurgical cases. Dedicated open radiologic units are usually installed either in the OR proper or immediately adjacent to the OR to permit intraoperative imaging of the selected body area. As image-guided procedures become more commonplace, OR designers will have to accommodate such devices within the OR workspace in a user-friendly manner.

Additional Devices

The use of sequential compression stockings (SCDs), with or without additional medical anticoagulation, has become the standard of care for the prevention of venous thromboembolism in the majority of operations for which direct access to the lower extremities is not required.[43] This is particularly true in operations lasting more than 4 hours with the patient in the lithotomy position. SCDs come in knee-high and thigh-high lengths and must be connected to a powered pump that inflates and deflates the stockings at a prescribed rate. This pump must often be placed near the patient on the floor or on a nearby cart. The pressure tubing from the stockings to the pump must be routed out of the way of the surgical team to prevent hazards and entanglements, particularly during operations requiring perineal access.

Suction devices are ubiquitous in the OR, assisting the surgeon in the evacuation of blood and other fluids from the operative field. A typical suction apparatus consists of a set of canisters on a wheeled base that receive suction from a wall- or ceiling-mounted source. The surgeon's aspirating cannula is sterilely connected to these canisters. Suction tubing is a common tripping hazard in the OR, and the suction canisters fill rapidly enough to require repeated changing.

Portable OR lights or headlights are often used when the lighting provided by standard ceiling-mounted lights is insufficient or when hard-to-see body cavities prove difficult to illuminate. Headlights are usually preferred because the beam is aimed in the direction the surgeon is looking; however, these devices can be uncomfortable to wear for prolonged periods. The fiberoptic light cord from the headset tethers the surgeon to the light source, which can exacerbate crowding near the surgical team.

Case Carts and Instrument Tables

In the case cart system, prepackaged instruments and linen for each scheduled operation are put together in one or more packs on a single cart and delivered from the central sterile supply to the OR area well before the start of the operation. Advocates of this system claim that it increases efficient use of personnel and thereby reduces costs.[44] However, there are no available data that compare the case cart system with the older, traditional method of packing and sterilizing specific instruments for each operation. Less frequently used instruments are kept in nearby fixed or mobile storage modules for ready access when required.

Traditionally, ORs contain a primary instrument table on which all the instruments specified for the operation are laid out, along with a smaller, secondary stand that can be moved to bring the most needed instruments close to the operating field. The primary table is rectangular or curved, is sterilely covered, and is placed close to the scrub nurse or technician. The secondary stand should be movable and adjustable in height (like, for instance, a Mayo stand). Other tables and stands, also sterilely draped, may be used to provide instruments to a second operating team or to support specific instruments and devices (e.g., drills). The most efficient placement of the instrument tables has been a subject of debate over the years, and each team must choose what works best for them. The goal, regardless of the specific placement, is to provide the surgical team with easy and rapid access to primary and secondary instruments and supplies.

The use of disposable instrumentation and drapes has added to the amount of waste generated by modern surgical procedures. Biohazardous waste must be properly disposed of in labeled red disposal bags. Small wheeled containers (so-called kickbuckets) can be useful for collecting small items near the operating field. Small racks or stands with handy impermeable bags for immediate disposal facilitate counting of used surgical sponges and gauze.

Surgical team members usually must complete some administrative tasks in the OR. Often, paper-based charting is used by the circulating nurse to document the details of the procedure and by the physicians to make perioperative notations. The OR should contain a designated area for such paperwork. A small folding desktop in the corner of the OR will suffice; however, physician dictating and charting rooms are sometimes provided adjacent to the surgical suite.

Communication Equipment

Every operation requires communication with the outside. Telephones should be placed in every OR where the circulating nurse can reach them easily without disturbing the surgical team. Most ORs have a computer terminal or a networked personal computer for routine charting options; this should be placed in a proper compact workstation located inside the OR. Information is being transferred in and out of the modern OR in an increasing variety of forms, including live video images and patient physiologic data. Modern OR design must incorporate facilities for safe and efficient communication of data between the surgical team and the outside.

Housekeeping Procedures

FLOORS AND WALLS

Despite detailed recommendations for cleaning the operating room [*see Table 2*],[45] the procedures that are optimal to provide a clean environment for the patient and are still cost-effective have not been critically analyzed.

Only a few studies have attempted to correlate surface contamination of the OR with wound infection risk. In one study, for example, ORs were randomly assigned to either a control group or an experi-

Table 2 OR Cleaning Schedules

Areas requiring daily cleaning	Surgical lights and tracks Fixed ceiling-mounted equipment Furniture and mobile equipment, including wheels OR and hall floors Cabinet and push-plate handles Ventilation grills All horizontal surfaces Substerile areas Scrub and utility areas Scrub sinks
Areas requiring routinely scheduled cleaning	Ventilation ducts and filters Recessed tracks Cabinets and shelves Walls and ceilings Sterilizers, warming cabinets, refrigerators, and ice machines

mental group.[46] The control rooms were cleaned with a germicidal agent and wet-vacuumed before the first case of the day and between cases; in the experimental rooms, cleaning consisted only of wiping up grossly visible contamination after clean and clean-contaminated cases. Both rooms had complete floor cleanup after contaminated or septic cases. The investigators found that bacterial colony counts obtained directly from the floors were lower in the control rooms but that counts obtained from other horizontal surfaces did not differ between the two OR groups. In addition, wound infection rates were the same in the control rooms and the experimental rooms and were comparable with rates reported in other series. Another study found that floor disinfectants decreased bacterial concentration on the floor for only 2 hours; colony counts then returned to pretreatment levels as personnel walked on the floor.[47] These investigators recommended discontinuing routine floor disinfection.

Even when an OR floor is contaminated, the rate of redispersal of bacteria into the air is low, and the clearance rate is high. It is unlikely, therefore, that bacteria from the floor contribute to wound infection. Consequently, routine disinfection of the OR floor between clean or clean-contaminated cases appears unnecessary.

According to the guidelines issued by the Centers for Disease Control and Prevention (CDC) for prevention of surgical site infection, when visible soiling of surfaces or equipment occurs during an operation, an Environmental Protection Agency (EPA)–approved hospital disinfectant should be used to decontaminate the affected areas before the next operation.[48] This statement is in keeping with the Occupational Safety and Health Administration (OSHA) requirement that all equipment and environmental surfaces be cleaned and decontaminated after contact with blood or other potentially infectious materials. Disinfection after a contaminated or dirty case and after the last case of the day is probably a reasonable practice, although it is not supported by directly pertinent data. Wet-vacuuming of the floor with an EPA-approved hospital disinfectant should be performed routinely after the last operation of the day or night.

MACHINES FROM "OUTSIDE"

Recording equipment, monitors, and other devices not routinely used in the operating suite occasionally may be brought in to meet a special need. Such "outside" equipment is often viewed as contaminated, and elaborate rituals of washing or wiping with alcohol or other antibacterial agents are sometimes enforced. However, there are no data to support these practices. It seems reasonable to wipe away visible dust and dirt, but elaborate cleaning of visiting outside equipment that will not come into direct contact with the sterile operative field appears to be unnecessary.

DIRTY CASES

Operations are classified or stratified into four groups in relation to the epidemiology of surgical wound infections.[49] Clean operations are those elective cases in which the GI tract or the respiratory tract is not entered and there are no major breaks in technique. The infection rate in this group should be less than 3%. Clean-contaminated operations are those elective cases in which the respiratory or the GI tract is entered or during which a break in aseptic technique has occurred. The infection rate in such cases should be less than 10%. Contaminated operations are those cases in which a fresh traumatic wound is present or gross spillage of GI contents occurs. Dirty operations include those in which bacterial inflammation occurs or in which pus is present. The infection rate may be as high as 40% in a contaminated or dirty operation.

Fear that bacteria from dirty or heavily contaminated cases could be transmitted to subsequent cases has resulted in the development of numerous and costly rituals of OR cleanup. However, there are no prospective studies and no large body of relevant data to support the usefulness of such rituals. In fact, one study[6] found no significant difference in environmental bacterial counts after clean cases and after dirty ones. Numerous authorities have recommended that there be only one standard of cleaning the OR after either clean or dirty cases.[6,45,50] This recommendation is reasonable because any patient may be a source of contamination caused by unrecognized bacterial or viral infection; more important, the other major source of OR contamination is the OR personnel.

Rituals applied to dirty cases include placing a germicide-soaked mat outside the OR door, allowing the OR to stand idle for an arbitrary period after cleanup of a dirty procedure, and using two circulating nurses, one inside and one outside the room. None of these practices has a sound theoretical or factual basis.

Traditionally, dirty cases have been scheduled after all the clean cases of the day. However, this restriction reduces the efficiency with which operations can be scheduled and may unnecessarily delay emergency cases. There are no data to support special cleaning procedures or closing of an operating room after a contaminated or dirty operation has been performed.[51] Tacky mats placed outside the entrance to an operating room or suite have not been shown to reduce the number of organisms on shoes or stretcher wheels, nor do they reduce the risk of surgical site infection.[52]

Protecting the Patient

POSITIONING

Patient positioning is the responsibility of the entire OR staff. The final position must allow adequate surgical exposure without compromising patient safety.

In many cases, one can use the preanesthesia visit to determine whether the patient will be able to tolerate a position by having him or her assume the anticipated posture and verifying that it is not painful. Occasionally, it may be necessary to modify the desired position. The organ systems most affected by changes in position are the cardiopulmonary system, the musculoskeletal system, and the peripheral nervous system.

Effects on Organ Systems

The cardiovascular system is especially vulnerable to changes in position. For any given position, the effect of gravity on the heart and vascular system created by tilting the bed can cause significant hemodynamic changes.[53] The reverse Trendelenburg position causes pooling of blood in the extremities, leading to a decrease in preload. Compressive leg stockings can help reduce venous pooling when the legs are below the level of the heart. The Trendelenburg position causes an increase in venous pressure that not only can affect the heart but also can cause venous pooling and engorgement in the head, resulting in altered cerebral blood flow and swelling of soft tissue.[54]

The vena cava and, less commonly, the aorta are prone to compression, which can cause dramatic changes in preload and perfusion. Inappropriate positioning of bolsters in the prone position can cause caval and abdominal compression,[53] affecting preload as well as giving rise to increased abdominal venous pressure, which is then transmitted to veins in the spinal canal. This increase in spinal pressure can result in excessive bleeding during operations on the spine.

Excessive pressure on the abdomen caused by surgical factors (e.g., retractors) can also compress the vena cava. Uterine compression in the obstetric patient is one of the most common causes of caval compression.[55] Aortic compression can also develop in these patients[56]; hence, it is vital to ensure left uterine displacement so as not to compromise fetal and maternal perfusion.

The pulmonary system is also vulnerable to position changes. Such changes can alter the ventilation-perfusion ratio and exert significant effects on oxygenation. The most dramatic changes occur in lateral positions, in which the height of the chest wall is highest and the effect of gravity on pulmonary blood flow is greatest. The dependent portions of the lung are most affected by the abdominal contents elevating the diaphragm; decreased pulmonary compliance results. Dead space also increases substantially in the lateral position and can affect measurement of the end-tidal CO_2–arterial CO_2 gradient.[57]

The musculoskeletal and peripheral nervous systems are especially vulnerable to injury because they are prone to compression and stretching. This category of injuries generates a multitude of medicolegal complaints against anesthesiologists.[58] The following are the nerves that are most vulnerable.

1. The peroneal nerve, which may be compressed between the head of the fibula and the support bars of stirrups (in the lithotomy position) or the OR table (in the lateral decubitus position).

2. The femoral nerve, which may be compressed by the inguinal ligament when the hip is in flexed position.

3. The saphenous nerve, which may be injured by pressure over the medial femoral condyle.

4. The obturator nerve, which may be stretched when the hip is in flexion.

5. The brachial plexus, which may be stretched when the arm is above the shoulder plane, stretched by exaggerated rotation of the head away from an extended arm, compressed by axillary structures (in the lateral decubitus position), or compressed by shoulder braces.

6. The ulnar nerve, which may be compressed between the medial humeral epicondyle and the olecranon.

7. The radial nerve, which may be compressed by the humerus.

Regardless of the final position, all pressure points must be protected with padding. For long procedures, extra padding between the patient and the bed provides additional protection against decubitus injury. However, the mechanisms of some injuries are not clear. For example, many cases of ulnar injury (one of the most common causes of litigation) have been demonstrated to have causes unrelated to padding and position of the arm.[59] Men at the extremes of body habitus who require prolonged hospitalization are most likely to be affected despite appropriate supination of the hand and padding of the elbow.

Position may affect other organ systems as well. It is important to ensure that the breasts and genitals are not compressed or pulled. In addition, a soft head support should be used to prevent pressure alopecia.[60] The eyes and ears should be carefully examined. The eyes should be closed, and pressure on the globe should be eliminated. This is especially important in the prone position. Cases of blindness related to pressure on the globe have been reported.[61] Any compression injuries, regardless of the cause, may be exacerbated by hypoperfusion and hypothermia.

Concerns Related to Specific Positions

A number of specific concerns exist regarding specific positions (other than supine), and certain recommendations may be made.

Prone position Cardiac effects can be minimized by avoiding increases in intra-abdominal pressure and vena caval compression. Pulmonary effects can be minimized by ensuring that the abdomen is not compressed, thereby preventing decreases in lung compliance and lung volume. Musculoskeletal effects can be minimized by ensuring that when the patient's arms are up, the axilla is not tense or stretched; if the patient's arms are at his or her side, they should be supinated.

Lateral position Cardiac effects can be minimized by keeping the body flat (so that there is no hydrostatic pressure difference); lateral flexion of the legs can compress the cava. Pulmonary effects can be minimized by addressing any abnormalities in oxygenation and arterial CO_2–end-tidal CO_2 gradient (see above). Musculoskeletal effects can be minimized by ensuring that the cervical spine is aligned with the thoracolumbar spine (to prevent injury and jugular venous compression). Peripheral nervous system effects can be minimized by using an axillary roll to relieve compression of the thorax on the brachial plexus. Adequate padding should be placed on decubitus parts and between the legs.

Sitting position Cardiac effects of note in this position include marked decreases in preload and increases in peripheral and pulmonary vascular resistance and in heart rate (which may be attenuated, depending on the anesthetic). In addition, the risk of air emboli is greatest with the patient in the sitting position.[62] Musculoskeletal effects can be minimized by ensuring that the chin is not forced into the suprasternal notch, which can decrease spinal cord perfusion and venous drainage; cases of tetraplegia and massive swelling of the face and pharynx have resulted.[63,64]

Many other patient positions are commonly used. Most, however, are hybrids of the positions just listed, and their effects on organ systems are a combination of the changes characteristic of the positions from which they derive. It is incumbent on the OR team to ensure that positioning is appropriate: improper positioning can compromise patient care and contribute to multisystem organ dysfunction.

Protecting the Surgeon and Staff

ENVIRONMENTAL HAZARDS

Anesthetic Gases

Anesthetic gases are the most common environmental pollutants in the OR. A study evaluating the distribution of leaked gases in ORs found that anesthesiologists were exposed to the highest levels, although lower levels of gases were detected at the periphery of the room where circulating nurses worked. No OR was completely free of leaks, though exposure could be significantly decreased with proper scavenging.[65]

The major risks of chronic exposure to anesthetic gases are not well known, because many studies of the effects of long-term exposure have yielded inconclusive results. Inhaled agents, such as the halogenated hydrocarbons (e.g., halothane, isoflurane, and enflurane) and nitrous oxide, may be associated with an increased risk of spontaneous abortion among female physicians, nurses, and technicians. Presumably, newer inhaled agents that have not been studied (e.g., desflurane and sevoflurane) have similar effects. Other problems that have been attributed to chronic exposure include an increased incidence of congenital anomalies, liver and kidney disease, and decreased behavioral performance[66-71]; however, the studies supporting the occurrence of these complications are seriously flawed because of their retrospective design, and they induced bias in many participants.[66-71]

Despite the weak scientific evidence for any danger associated with chronic exposure to inhaled anesthetic agents, it is prudent to minimize chronic exposure. The time-weighted exposure limits suggested by the National Institute of Occupational Safety and Health are less than 25 ppm for nitrous oxide, less than 2 ppm for halogenated agents alone, and 0.5 ppm for halogenated agents in combination with nitrous oxide.[72] Scavenging systems can decrease levels by about 90%. If anesthetic vapors are detected by smell, then the levels are at least 33 ppm.[73]

Anesthetic gases may escape into the OR from either anesthetic equipment or the patient. The largest volume of anesthetic gases escapes from the exhalation side of the rebreathing anesthesia circuit via the pop-off valve. Scavenging equipment connects the exhalation side of the rebreathing circuit to a vacuum line, thereby preventing venting of gases into the air. This is a crucial measure used to reduce levels of gases. Although leaks may occur in the anesthetic machine, gas is more likely to come from incomplete isolation of the patient's airway (e.g., from an incompletely sealed ventilation mask, from leaks around endotracheal tubes, or from the patient's mouth after extubation). Meticulous attention to preventing unnecessary leaks from the patient helps decrease the vapor concentration even further.

In many institutions, scavenging is available only in the OR and not in other areas that use anesthetic vapors (i.e., the radiology department). This limited availability should be taken into account in the choice of an anesthetic technique in such areas. Ideally, I.V. anesthesia should be used whenever possible in these situations. Periodically, gas concentrations should be measured in all areas where anesthesia is provided to ensure proper functioning of the anesthesia and scavenging equipment.

Ethylene Oxide

Ethylene oxide (EO), a powerful alkylating agent, is commonly used to sterilize heat- and moisture-sensitive items. EO is a highly penetrating gas with toxic residuals that must be driven from devices that are sterilized. In humans, EO residuals can cause anaphylactic sensitization, contact burns of the skin or the mucous membranes, hemolysis and edema, and other adverse reactions in the respiratory and GI tracts. EO is a known carcinogen.[74]

OSHA has set the permissible exposure limit (PEL) for EO at 1 part EO to 1 million parts of air (1 ppm) as an 8-hour time-weighted average. Sterilization with EO must be followed by lengthy aeration times of 8 to 12 hours or longer in a mechanical aerator to remove toxic residuals. Personnel who operate EO sterilizers must be informed of the associated hazards, and employers are required to provide administrative and engineering controls to protect workers. Annual safety-education programs, badges for monitoring personal exposure, and alarm systems that activate in the event of an EO leak are three such controls.

Originally, EO gas was combined with a chlorofluorocarbon stabilizing agent in a preparation containing 12% EO and 88% chlorofluorocarbons (referred to as 12/88 EO). The chlorofluorocarbons were phased out in December 1995 under the provisions of the Clean Air Act. (Under that legislation, they were classified as a class 1 substance because of scientific evidence linking them to destruction of the earth's ozone layer.) Some states began to require the use of EO abatement technology to reduce the amount of EO being released into ambient air by 90% to 99.9%.

The EO sterilizer is typically located outside the OR, and OR personnel may not be responsible for operating it. It is important, however, that OR personnel be knowledgeable about EO hazards and aeration times and not request or accept less than complete aeration cycles. No matter how pressing the desire to abort the aeration cycle to retrieve an item, it should not be gratified. The composition of the item to be sterilized and the parameters of the aerator determine the length of required aeration. Mechanical aerators generally have standard aeration cycles with an option to extend the cycle as desired. The aeration times supplied by the manufacturer of the item must be strictly adhered to. Although standard aeration times range from 8 to 12 hours, some items require 24 hours or longer.

If a mechanical aerator is not available, aeration with ambient air will extend aeration times to as much as a week or longer. With items not intended for sterilization that are not made of suitable materials, such as children's toys or instruments created in a home workshop, it may be impossible to reach safe levels of residuals.

Because of the hazards associated with EO and the lengthy cycle times, several new sterilization technologies, including liquid peracetic acid and hydrogen peroxide gas plasma, have been introduced. Both technologies offer cycle times of less than 1 hour, and neither requires aeration of sterilized instruments or devices. Liquid peracetic sterilization is a point-of-use process, and the sterilizer is usually installed adjacent to the OR. At the completion of the cycle, items are wet and should be used immediately. Hydrogen peroxide gas plasma, on the other hand, is a dry process. Sterilized items are wrapped and may be either used immediately or stored for future use. The principal by-products of the process are vaporized water and oxygen; because there are no toxic residuals, no aeration is required. The sterilizer may be located in the central processing department; however, many institutions have placed units within the OR. Because of the short cycle time and the lack of toxic residuals, an increasing number of heat- and moisture-sensitive items are now processed by this means.

INFECTIOUS HAZARDS

Awareness of the emergence of new infectious diseases, the increasing prevalence of antibiotic-resistant strains of bacteria, and the ubiquitous presence of infectious viruses with the potential to cause severe and fatal diseases have encouraged health care workers to practice standard and transmission-based precautions on a routine basis to protect both their patients and themselves.

The most common virus, causing the most work-related deaths in health care workers in the United States (200/year), is the hepatitis B virus (HBV), but the one causing the most concern is HIV. Although the risk of acquiring HIV after an accidental parenteral exposure to blood from a known HIV-infected patient is estimated to be 0.3%,[75] the severe and fatal nature of the resulting disease makes HIV transmission a paramount concern.

Currently, there is concern about the incidence of hepatitis C virus. This pathogen is transmitted by percutaneous inoculation from needle sticks, cuts, and open wounds or breaks in the skin and through contact with infectious fluids and materials. Potentially infectious material includes blood, serum, and any other human bodily fluids, tissues, or organs to which the health care worker may be exposed in the practice setting.

In 1991, OSHA formulated its blood-borne pathogens standard, which mandates the use of universal precautions (to reduce the risk of transmission of blood-borne pathogens) and body substance isolation (to reduce the risk of pathogen transmission from moist body substances). The use of universal precautions requires engineering and work-practice controls, provision of personal protective equipment, an exposure-control plan, exposure documentation, methods of compliance, availability of HBV vaccine, postexposure evaluation, labels and warning signs where appropriate, and employee training.

OR practices associated with universal precautions include but are not limited to the following:

1. Precautions to prevent injuries caused by scalpels and other sharp instruments. A hands-free technique is used to create a neutral zone in which sharps are placed instead of being handed directly to scrubbed personnel. Oral confirmation is provided whenever a scalpel or sharp is passed. A needle holder is used to remove scalpel blades from knife handles.

2. Precautions to prevent exposure. Personnel with open lesions do not scrub. Inexperienced health care workers should not scrub when the patient is known to be HIV positive. Pregnant personnel should not participate in operations on patients with AIDS because of the increased risk of exposure to other infectious agents often carried by AIDS patients, particularly cytomegalovirus and *Toxoplasma gondii*, which may have detrimental effects on the developing fetus. Scrubbed personnel wear gowns that are appropriate for the procedure (e.g., gowns with suitable barrier properties when a large amount of potentially infectious material is anticipated). They also wear two pairs of gloves when the procedure is likely to be lengthy and when loss of glove integrity is a significant possibility. Gloves are regularly checked for integrity during a surgical procedure. Scrubbed personnel wear protective eyewear with a splash shield or goggles with side shields. Attire that becomes contaminated is removed as soon as possible and is placed in an appropriate waste container. Specimens are placed in leakproof containers.

All sites of blood spillage and gross soilage from the operative procedure should be cleaned as soon as possible. Spills should be cleaned with a lint-free cloth saturated with a 1:10 solution of household hypochlorite bleach or with a hospital grade EPA disinfectant or detergent-disinfectant.

Transmission-based precautions should be used in addition to standard precautions for patients who are known or believed to be infected with epidemiologically important and highly transmissible pathogens.[76]

Personnel should wear masks when in the presence of patients known to have an infection caused by an airborne pathogen, such as rubella, varicella, or tuberculosis. Such patients should also wear a mask during transport to prevent generation of airborne particles. Elective procedures on patients with active tuberculosis should be delayed until the patient is no longer infectious. If a procedure cannot be delayed, it should be performed in an operating suite with an anteroom, and only necessary personnel should be allowed to enter the room during the operation. If possible, the operation should take place when there are no other patients in the OR or when traffic is minimal.

Table 3 Criteria for Defining a Surgical Site Infection (SSI)[85]

Superficial incisional SSI

Infection occurs within 30 days after the operation, *and* infection involves only skin or subcutaneous tissue of the incisions, *and* at least *one* of the following:

1. Purulent drainage, with or without laboratory confirmation, from the superficial incision
2. Organisms isolated from an aseptically obtained culture of fluid or tissue from the superficial incision
3. At least one of the following signs or symptoms of infection: pain or tenderness, localized swelling, redness, or heat; *and* superficial incision is deliberately opened by surgeon, *unless* incision is culture negative
4. Diagnosis of superficial incisional SSI by the surgeon or attending physician

Do *not* report the following conditions as SSI:

1. Stitch abscess (minimal inflammation and discharge confined to the points of suture penetration)
2. Infection of an episiotomy or newborn circumcision site
3. Infected burn wound
4. Incisional SSI that extends into the fascial and muscle layers (see deep incisional SSI)

Note: Specific criteria are used for identifying infected episiotomy and circumcision sites and burn wounds

Deep incisional SSI

Infection occurs within 30 days after the operation if no implant* is left in place or within 1 yr if implant is in place and the infection appears to be related to the operation, *and* infection involves deep soft tissues (e.g., fascial and muscle layers) on the incision, *and* at least *one* of the following:

1. Purulent drainage from the deep incision but not from the organ/space component of the surgical site
2. A deep incision spontaneously dehisces or is deliberately opened by a surgeon when the patient has at least one of the following signs or symptoms: fever (> 38° C [100.4° F]), localized pain, or tenderness, unless site is culture negative
3. An abscess or other evidence of infection involving the deep incision is found on direct examination, during reoperation, or by histopathologic or radiologic examination
4. Diagnosis of a deep incisional SSI by a surgeon or attending physician

Notes:

1. Report infection that involves both superficial and deep incision sites as deep incisional SSI
2. Report an organ/space SSI that drains through the incision as a deep incisional SSI

Organ/space SSI

Infection occurs within 30 days after the operation if no implant* is left in place or within 1 yr if implant is in place and the infection appears to be related to the operation, *and* infection involves any part of the anatomy (e.g., organs or spaces), other than the incision, which was opened or manipulated during an operation, *and* at least *one* of the following:

1. Purulent drainage from a drain that is placed through a stab wound† into the organ/space
2. Organisms isolated from an aseptically obtained culture of fluid or tissue in the organ/space
3. An abscess or other evidence of infection involving the organ/space that is found on direct examination, during reoperation, or by histopathologic or radiologic examination
4. Diagnosis of an organ/space SSI by a surgeon or attending physician

*National Nosocomial Infection Surveillance definition: a nonhuman-derived implantable foreign body (e.g., prosthetic heart valve, nonhuman vascular graft, mechanical heart, or hip prosthesis) that is permanently placed in a patient during surgery.

†If the area around a stab wound becomes infected, it is not an SSI. It is considered a skin or soft tissue infection, depending on its depth.

HAZARDS DURING PREGNANCY

Pregnant women working in the OR may place the fetus at risk for several work-related complications. Exposure to anesthetic agents has been implicated in an increased risk of spontaneous abortions and congenital anomalies. Exposure to radiation and infectious agents has also been associated with fetal abnormalities.

The evidence that low levels of anesthetic agents give rise to an increased risk of abortions and congenital anomalies is very weak. The published studies are flawed by their retrospective nature, their reporting bias, and their inadequate control of confounding variables such as work-related stress, noise, sleep deprivation, and numerous lifestyle differences among participants.[66-70] In addition, the high incidence of spontaneous abortions in the general population makes differences hard to demonstrate. Furthermore, even if there is a risk to the fetus associated with chronic exposure to anesthetic agents, newer anesthesia machines and improved scavenging systems may make old data hard to extrapolate to today's ORs. Nevertheless, it is prudent for all personnel to minimize exposure to inhaled gases.

As with anesthetic vapor–induced hazards of pregnancy, it is often hard to show a strong causal relationship between radiation exposure in health care workers and adverse effects because the incidence of spontaneous congenital defects, spontaneous mutations, and spontaneous abortions is so high in the general population.[77] The most sensitive gestational period for teratogenesis is between 8 and 17 weeks.[78] Rare consequences of prenatal radiation exposure include a slight increase in the incidence of childhood leukemia, genetic mutations, and spontaneous abortions.[79-82] In addition, there seems to be a definite increase in the incidence of microcephaly and mental retardation.[78,80] Some of these complications may also occur with radiation exposure before conception.[81]

The level of radiation exposure above which the risk of complications increases significantly is unknown, but it has been suggested that exposure not exceed 0.5 cGy for the 9-month gestation period.[82] No single diagnostic study exceeds this maximum. The use of fluoroscopy exposes personnel to the greatest amount of radiation.[82]

Radiation exposure can be avoided or reduced in several ways: the pregnant woman can (1) be assigned to cases in which radiation will not be used or will at least be minimized, (2) leave the room while the x-ray is being taken, (3) use lead aprons and screens (levels of radiation exposure beneath leaded aprons are comparable to environmental exposure),[82] or (4) stay as far from the source as possible (a distance of at least 3 ft is recommended).[83] If radiation film badges are routinely used, the actual risk for an individual will be known and appropriate precautions can be taken to lower exposure.

The dangers of exposure to infectious agents during pregnancy are more concrete.[83,84] Several viral infections, if acquired during pregnancy, can have devastating consequences on fetal development and even result in fetal death. Some may induce chronic illness in the child. These viruses include rubella, cytomegalovirus, varicella-zoster virus (VZV), HBV, and HIV.

The risk of infection can be decreased by ensuring that employee immunization status is up to date. It is recommended that employees be immunized against VZV (if they are not already immune) and HBV, in addition to the standard childhood vaccines.[83,84] Viral infections are common in immunocompromised patients, and caring for these patients may represent an increased risk for pregnant personnel who are not appropriately immunized. It is generally believed, however, that the use of universal precautions will prevent almost all transmission. The viruses are transmitted by close personal contact or contact with secretions, excretions, or blood. Avoidance of these known modes of transmission should provide adequate protection. Some advocate that pregnant women who have never been infected with VZV or who have not been immunized should not care for high-risk patients because of the highly contagious nature of the virus.[83,84] The OR environment is a safe workplace for pregnant women if appropriate safety precautions are adhered to.

Table 4 Site-Specific Classifications of Organ/Space Surgical Site Infection[85]

- Arterial or venous infection
- Breast abscess or mastitis
- Disk space
- Ear, mastoid
- Endocarditis
- Endometritis
- Eye, other than conjunctivitis
- Gastrointestinal tract
- Intra-abdominal, not specified elsewhere
- Intracranial, brain abscess or dura
- Joint or bursa
- Mediastinitis
- Meningitis or ventriculitis
- Myocarditis or pericarditis
- Oral cavity (mouth, tongue, or gums)
- Osteomyelitis
- Other infections of the lower respiratory tract (e.g., abscess or empyema)
- Other male or female reproductive tract
- Sinusitis
- Spinal abscess without meningitis
- Upper respiratory tract
- Vaginal cuff

Asepsis

Infections related to surgical procedures (traditionally referred to as surgical wound infections) have been redefined by the CDC as surgical site infections (SSIs). The current definition classifies such infections as either incisional SSIs or organ/space SSIs [*see Table 3*]. Incisional infections are further classified as superficial incisional SSIs or deep incisional SSIs,[85] and organ/space SSIs are classified by site [*see Table 4*]. The classification of surgical wounds as clean, clean-contaminated, contaminated, or dirty helps determine benchmarks for the development of SSIs.[85] SSIs that occur in clean operations are often caused by bacteria introduced by OR personnel or derived from a source in the patient. This is particularly true of operations in which prosthetic devices or materials are implanted.

Numerous aseptic OR procedures and rituals have been developed to protect patients from environmental sources of infection. These procedures came under scrutiny in the 1990s. A task force, the Hospital Infection Control Practices Advisory Committee (HICPAC), was formed in 1991 under the auspices of the CDC and published its findings in 1999[85]; this document supplants earlier guidelines.[86,87] Part II of the 1999 guidelines comprises a set of recommendations for the prevention of SSIs. Each recommendation has been categorized by HICPAC. Category I recommendations include the subcategories IA (strongly recommended and supported by well-designed studies) and IB (strongly recommended for implementation and supported by some studies). Category II recommendations are suggested for implementation and supported by suggestive clinical epidemiologic studies or a theoretical rationale. The final category, labeled as "no recommendation" or "unresolved issue," includes practices for which there is insufficient evidence or no consensus regarding efficacy. There are, however, certain practices required by federal regulation in these areas (see below). The CDC's position is that all category I recommendations should be accepted by health care facilities. In what follows, we place primary emphasis on this category of recommendation.

SKIN PREPARATION

Because the patient is the most common source of bacteria leading to SSIs, attempts should be made to reduce bacterial counts on the patient's skin. Preventive antiseptic showers or baths decrease skin microbial counts; chlorhexidine gluconate is more effective than povidone-iodine and is most effective when repeat applications are used.[87,88] Although showers have not been shown to reduce the incidence of SSIs, a category IB recommendation is that patients be required to shower or bathe with an antiseptic agent the night before the operative day or just before the operation. This recommendation does not address minimally invasive procedures or procedures restricted to the face or the extremities.

Preoperative shaving with a razor is associated with an SSI rate as high as 5.6% versus 0.6% for those not shaved.[89] Depilatory creams or electric clippers lower preoperative SSI rates significantly,[89-91] but it has not been determined which of these methods is safest. Depilatories occasionally cause cuts, skin irritation, or allergic reactions. The CDC IA recommendation is that hair not be removed preoperatively unless it interferes with the operation. If hair removal is indicated, it should be done with electric clippers immediately before the operation.

An antiseptic should be used for skin preparation.[87] Alcohol is effective, fast acting, and inexpensive, although flammable; it is also drying. Although povidone-iodine is widely used, chlorhexidine gluconate achieves greater reduction in skin microflora and has greater residual activity.[92-94] Great care must be taken when these products are used around mucous membranes and the eyes. The incisional area should be free of gross contamination,[95] and the antiseptic should be applied in concentric circles, beginning in the area of the proposed incision (category II recommendation). There is minimal evidence to support the view that antiseptic-impregnated adhesive drapes or scrubbing all wounds affects the incidence of SSIs.

HAND WASHING

The surgical scrub is traditionally performed before sterile gowns and gloves are donned. At present, it remains unclear what the ideal scrubbing agent is and how long it must be applied. Numerous agents are available. Although alcohol is effective, its irritating effect on skin and its flammability limit its use in the United States. Povidone-iodine and chlorhexidine gluconate are currently the agents of choice among surgical teams.[96] No differences in SSI rates have been associated with particular agents, but chlorhexidine gluconate is known to have greater residual microbial activity than other agents.[17]

Scrubbing for at least 2 minutes has been found to be as effective as the traditional 10-minute scrub.[96] The CDC therefore recommends that surgeons scrub for 2 to 5 minutes (category IB recommendation) with an antiseptic solution up to the elbows. Nails should be kept short and clean before the first scrub of the day.

SURGICAL ATTIRE AND DRAPES

Surgical attire includes scrub suits, hair and shoe covers, gloves, gowns, and masks. Perhaps surprisingly, given conventional wisdom and the experimental data showing that live organisms are shed from the hair, skin, and mucous membranes of OR personnel, there are few controlled studies relating the use of surgical attire to the incidence of SSIs.[97,98] It would seem intuitively obvious that a sterile gown can keep body bacteria from falling into a wound, but small amounts of bacteria still escape from exposed areas. In addition, it would seem obviously prudent to use barriers to minimize patients' exposure to bacteria from OR personnel, but even the use of impermeable plastic gowns and helmets with their own air supply has not been shown to lower the incidence of SSIs significantly.

A two-piece cotton scrub suit composed of pants and a shirt is the standard attire for OR personnel. The use and laundering of scrub suits has not been carefully studied, but the Association of Operating Room Nurses (AORN) recommends that scrubs be changed between operations only when visibly soiled, contaminated, or penetrated by blood or possibly infected matter[99] (category IB recommendation). This practice also meets OSHA regulations. How to launder surgical scrubs and whether a coat is needed to cover scrubs when the person is not in the OR are unresolved issues.

The material used in gowns and drapes must be impermeable to liquids and viruses, comfortable, and cost-effective. Thick plastic fits the bill but is intolerably hot and causes increased sweating. More practical fabrics, both disposable and reusable, are now available. The most common disposable materials are spun-lace cloth (a wood pulp–polyester blend manufactured by the hydroentanglement process) in a spun-bond/melt-blown/spun-bond (SMS) laminate of 100% polypropylene. Formerly, the most commonly reusable fabrics were worn woven cotton or a 50%/50% cotton-polyester blend treated with a water-repellent chemical. However, these fabrics are being replaced by very high thread count polyester fabrics and fabrics made of expanded polytetrafluoroethylene (PTFE).

Gowns vary in their ability to prevent blood strike-through. These variations have been measured in the laboratory and in the OR[100,101] and are determined by the kind of material used and the manufacture and design of the gown. No single type of gown can be recommended as the best for all circumstances. In addition to impermeability, comfort, and cost, the conditions to which the gown will be subjected must also be taken into account. If, for instance, no blood comes in contact with the outside of the gown, then any gown is safe because no blood can strike through; however, if large amounts of blood come in contact with the gown, strike-through is almost inevitable (occurring in 93% of cases), and most gowns will eventually fail. The amount of blood on the outside of the gown is one of the most important factors; however, physical stresses on the fabric (such as abrasion, pressure, or stretching) and increasing the duration of exposure through blood will also degrade gown performance and allow blood strike-through.

Additional barriers used to separate sterile and nonsterile areas during the operative procedure include adhesive plastic barrier sheets and plastic ring drapes. Adhesive incise drapes have been evaluated in several studies; whether or not they are impregnated with iodine, they have not proved superior to standard skin preparation and draping procedures in controlling SSI. However, if the adhesive plastic drape becomes separated from the skin during the operation, the infection rate increases.[17,102] Plastic ring drapes are inserted into the wound to cover the wound edges during a procedure. As with the adhesive plastic drape, use of plastic ring drapes has not been shown to decrease SSI rates.[103]

The final CDC recommendation is to use surgical gowns and drapes that resist liquid penetration and remain effective barriers when wet (category IB recommendation).

The rubber sterile drapes worn by all scrubbed members of the surgical team serve two purposes: (1) they protect patients against transmission of microorganisms from the hands of the team, and (2) they protect the team from the patient's contaminated blood and fluids. If a glove is punctured or torn, it should be changed as promptly as is safe. One study found a 13% incidence of punctured gloves at the end of a procedure but could not correlate this with increases in bacterial counts.[104]

The use of double gloving, the length of the procedure, and the type of procedure affect the penetration rate.[104,105] OSHA recommends that all members of the scrubbed surgical team put on sterile gloves after donning a sterile gown (category IB recommendation).

Surgical masks are traditionally worn to prevent potential bacterial contamination of the operative field. Even this belief has come into question.[106] In a series of studies in which no masks were worn for 6 months, the SSI rate compared favorably with the rates reported in the preceding 4 years, when masks were required.[107] Other studies have demonstrated no patient benefit from masks. Masks, can, however, protect the wearer from inadvertent exposure to bodily fluids and blood. OSHA regulations therefore require masks to be used in combination with protective eyewear (e.g., goggles or glasses with shields) whenever spray, splatter, droplets, or potentially infected fluids may be generated and facial contamination can be reasonably anticipated.[108] In addition, a respirator certified with a protection factor of N95 or higher is required for staff members working directly with patients who have suspected or proven infectious tuberculosis. The recommendation is to wear a mask that fully covers the nose and mouth when entering an OR with sterile instruments exposed and to wear this mask throughout the operation (category IB recommendation, OSHA).

Surgical caps or hoods that fully cover head or facial hair can reduce contamination from the hair and scalp. They are required by OSHA and should be worn on entry into a sterile OR (category IB recommendation).

Although shoe covers have never been shown to decrease SSI rates or bacterial counts in the OR floor,[109] they may protect members of the surgical team from exposure to blood and fluids. OSHA regulations require that shoe covers or boots be worn when gross contamination can reasonably be anticipated (e.g., during orthopedic procedures or in cases of penetrating trauma)[110] (category IB recommendation).

The CDC and AORN recommendations, taken together, represent the best current approaches to codifying the traditions and data available for the OR. Unfortunately, in many cases, the data are insufficient either to support the efficacy of a given OR procedure or to permit a rational choice among alternatives. Acquisition of randomized data is inherently difficult and, for many issues, is unlikely to be forthcoming. The most rational approach to the OR environment combines CDC recommendations and OSHA regulations into a logical, cost-effective, and safe approach to the problems of OR asepsis.

SSI Surveillance

SSI prevention attracts the attention of hospital quality-improvement programs because SSIs, though rarely lethal, result in the expenditure of extra health care dollars.[110] SSI prevention is largely the responsibility of surgeons and other members of surgical teams. With careful use of information obtained by SSI surveillance activity, it may be possible to demonstrate that a practice should more closely address specific SSI prevention techniques. Up-to-date standards for SSI prevention are available from the CDC in a comprehensive, detailed clinical-practice guideline.[85,111]

SSI surveillance entails detection and analysis of SSIs within 30 days of an operation; an infection control nurse is usually in charge of this activity. It is essential to report SSI rates and certain facts regarding each patient with an SSI to surgeons.[112] Such case facts must include whether antibiotic prophylaxis was used correctly, the details of skin wound management, and various characteristics of the patient that may be considered risk factors for SSI development. It is also prudent to gather ancillary information, such as laboratory culture results.

Although it is impossible to establish in scientifically rigorous clinical experiments that performance of SSI surveillance favorably influences SSI risk in practice, there is suggestive evidence to support the notion.[85,110] It is recommended that SSI surveillance information be reported regularly to surgical teams, but there is no evidence that a particular reporting interval for SSI case facts and rates is optimal. Many hospitals with surveillance programs make such reports monthly or quarterly.

Finally, it is not necessary that every kind of operation performed be subjected to SSI surveillance. The CDC recommends focusing SSI surveillance on particular segments of a hospital's surgical caseload, as determined by procedure volume or intrinsic SSI risk.[85]

References

1. Requirements of construction and equipment for hospitals and medical facilities. Health and Human Services Publication (HRS-M-HF-84-1), Rockville, Maryland, 1984
2. Symposium on operating room hazard control. Laufman H, Ed. Arch Surg 107:552, 1973
3. Klebanoff G: Operating-room design: an introduction. Bull Am Coll Surg 64(11):6, 1979
4. Laufman H: The control of operating room infection: discipline, defense mechanisms, drugs, design, and devices. Bull NY Acad Med 54:465, 1978
5. Drake CT, Goldman E, Nichols RL, et al: Environmental air and airborne infections. Ann Surg 185:219, 1977
6. Hambraeus A, Bengtsson S, Laurell G: Bacterial contamination in a modern operating suite: II. Effect of a zoning system on contamination of floors and other surfaces. J Hyg [Camb] 80:57, 1978
7. Hambraeus A, Bengtsson S, Laurell G: Bacterial contamination in a modern operating suite: III. Importance of floor contamination as a source of airborne bacteria. J Hyg [Camb] 80:169, 1978
8. Ritter MA, Sieber JM, Carlson SR: Street shoes vs surgical footwear in the operating room. Infect Surg 3:81, 1984
9. Quraishi ZA, Blais FX, Sottile WS, et al: Movement of personnel and wound contamination. AORN J 38:146, 1983
10. Belkin NL: Clean room technology and aseptic practices in the surgical suite. J Environ Sciences 27:30, 1984
11. Noble WC, Lidwell OM, Kingston D: The size distribution of airborne particles carrying microorganisms. J Hyg 61:385, 1963
12. Sukuki A, Yoshimichi N, Matsuura M, et al: Airborne contamination in an operating suite: report of a five-year survey. J Hyg 93:567, 1984
13. Anderson PA, Hambraeus A, Zettersten U, et al: A comparison between tracer gas and tracer particle techniques in evaluating the efficiency of ventilation in operating theatres. J Hyg 91:509, 1983
14. Fitzgerald RH Jr: Microbiologic environment of the conventional operating room. Arch Surg 114:772, 1979
15. Walter CW, Kundsin RB: The airborne component of wound contamination and infection. Arch Surg 107:588, 1973
16. Lidwell OM, Lowbury EJL, Whyte W, et al: Infection and sepsis after operations for total hip or knee-joint replacement: influence of ultraclean air, prophylactic antibiotics and other factors. J Hyg 93:505, 1984
17. Cruse PJ, Foord R: The epidemiology of wound infection: a 10-year prospective study of 62,939 wounds. Surg Clin North Am 60:27, 1980
18. McQuarrie DG, Glover JL: Laminar airflow systems: a 1991 update. Am Coll Surg Bull 76:18, 1991
19. Howe CW: Bacterial flora of clean wounds and its relation to subsequent sepsis. Am J Surg 107:696, 1964
20. Maki DG, Alvarado CJ, Hassemer CA, et al: Relation of the inanimate hospital environment to endemic nosocomial infection. N Engl J Med 307:1562, 1982
21. Howe CW, Marston AT: Qualitative and quantitative bacteriologic studies on hospital air as related to postoperative wound sepsis. J Lab Clin Med 61:808, 1963
22. Beck WC, Frank F: The open door in the operating room. Am J Surg 125:592, 1973
23. Chinyanga HM: Temperature regulation and anesthesia. Pharmacol Ther 26:147, 1984
24. Beck WC: Choosing surgical illumination. Am J Surg 140:327, 1980
25. Beck WC: Operating room illumination: the current state of the art. Bull Am Coll Surg 66(5):10, 1981

26. Kern KA: The National Patient Safety Foundation: what it offers surgeons. Bull Am Coll Surg 83:24, 1998
27. Fuchs VR: Economics, values, and health care reform. Am Econ Rev 86:1, 1996
28. National Academy of Science/National Institute of Medicine/National Research Council: Work-related musculoskeletal disorders: a review of the evidence. National Academy Press, Washington, DC, 1998
29. Weinger MB, Englund CE: Ergonomic and human factors affecting anesthetic vigilance and monitoring performance in the operating room environment. Anesthesiol 73:995, 1990
30. Schmied H, Kurz A, Sessler DI, et al: Mild hypothermia increases blood loss and transfusion requirements during total hip arthroplasty. Lancet 347:289, 1996
31. AORN Recommended Practices Subcommittee: Recommended practices: electrosurgery. AORN J 41:633, 1985
32. Pearce J: Current electrosurgical practice: hazards. J Med Eng Technol 9:107, 1985
33. Bochenko WJ: A review of electrosurgical units in the operating room. J Clin Eng 2:313, 1977
34. Lobraico RV: Laser safety in health care facilities. An overview. Bull Am Coll Surg 76:16, 1991
35. Gloster HM Jr, Roenigk RK: Risk of acquiring human papillomavirus from the plume produced by the carbon dioxide laser in the treatment of warts. J Am Acad Dermatol 32:436, 1995
36. AORN Recommended Practices Subcommittee: Recommended practices: radiation safety in the operating room (including lasers). AORN J 42:920, 1985
37. Cuschieri A, Shimi S, Banting S, et al: Endoscopic ultrasonic dissection for thoracoscopic and laparoscopic surgery. Surg Endosc 7:197, 1993
38. Hurst BS, Awoniyi CA, Stephens JK, et al: Application of the cavitron ultrasonic surgical aspirator (CUSA) for gynecological laparoscopic surgery using the rabbit as an animal model. Fertil Steril 58:444, 1992
39. Wisniewski PM, Warhol MJ, Rando RF, et al: Studies on the transmission of viral disease via the CO_2 laser plume and ejecta. J Reprod Med 35:1117, 1990
40. Jewett DL, Heinsohn P, Bennett C, et al: Blood-containing aerosols generated by surgical techniques: a possible infectious hazard. Am Ind Hyg Assoc J 53:228, 1992
41. Patkin M: Ergonomics and the operating microscope. Adv Ophthalmol 37:53, 1978
42. Alarcon A, Berguer R: A comparison of operating room crowding between open and laparoscopic operations. Surg Endosc 10:916, 1996
43. Walenga JM, Fareed J: Current status on new anticoagulant and antithrombotic drugs and devices. Curr Opin Pulm Med 3:291, 1997
44. Pitts W: Is a case cart system justified? Hosp Mater Manage Q 8:71, 1986
45. Peers JG: Cleanup techniques in the operating room. Arch Surg 107:596, 1973
46. Weber DO, Gooch JJ, Wood WR, et al: Influence of operating room surface contamination on surgical wounds: a prospective study. Arch Surg 111:484, 1976
47. Daschner F: Patient-oriented hospital hygiene. Infection 38(suppl):243, 1980
48. Mangram AJ, Horan TC, Pearson ML, et al: The Hospital Infection Control Practices Advisory Committee. Guideline for prevention of surgical site infection, 1999. Am J Infect Control 27:98, 1999
49. Report of an Ad-Hoc Committee of the Committee on Trauma, Division of Medical Sciences, National Academy of Sciences-National Research Council: Postoperative wound infections: the influence of ultraviolet irradiation of the operating room and of various other factors. Ann Surg 160(suppl):1, 1964
50. McWilliams RM: There should be only one way to clean up between all surgical procedures. J Hosp Infect Contr 3:64, 1976
51. Nichols RL: The operating room. Hospital Infections, 3rd ed. Bennett JV, Brachman PS, Eds. Little, Brown & Co, Boston, 1992, p 461
52. Ayliffe GA: Role of the environment of the operating suite in surgical wound infection. Rev Infect Dis 13(suppl 10):S800, 1991
53. Martin JT: Patient positioning. Clinical Anesthesia, 2nd ed. Barash PG, Cullen BF, Stoelting RK, Eds. JB Lippincott Co, Philadelphia, 1992
54. Shapiro HM: Intracranial hypertension. Anesthesiol 43:445, 1975
55. Kerr MG, Scott DB, Samuel E: Studies of the inferior vena cava in late pregnancy. Br Med J 1:532, 1964
56. Bieniarz J, Yoshida T, Romero-Salinas G, et al: Aortocaval compression by the uterus in late human pregnancy. IV. Circulatory homeostasis by preferential perfusion of the placenta. Am J Obstet Gynecol 103:19, 1968
57. Wahba RW, Tessler MJ: Misleading end-tidal CO_2 tensions. Can J Anaesth 43:862, 1996
58. Cheney FW, Domino KB, Caplan RA, et al: Nerve injury associated with anesthesia: a closed claims analysis. Anesthesiol 90:1062, 1999
59. Warner MA, Warner ME, Martin J: Ulnar neuropathy. Anesthesiol 81:1332, 1994
60. Abel RR, Lewis GM: Postoperative alopecia. Arch Dermatol 81:72, 1960
61. Alexandrakis G, Lam BL: Bilateral posterior ischemic optic neuropathy after spinal surgery. Am J Ophthalmol 127:354, 1999
62. Venous air emboli in sitting and supine patients undergoing vestibular schwannoma resection. Neurosurgery 42:1282, 1998
63. Dominguez J, Rivas JJ, Lobato RD, et al: Irreversible tetraplegia after tracheal resection. Ann Thorac Surg 62:278, 1996
64. Tattersall MP: Massive swelling of the face and tongue: a complication of posterior cranial fossa surgery in the sitting position. Anaesthesia 39:1015, 1984
65. Brown DG, Wetterstroem N, Finch J: Anesthetic gas exposure: protecting the OR environment. AORN J 41:590, 1985
66. Buring JE, Hennekens CH, Mayrent SL, et al: Health experiences of operating room personnel. Anesthesiol 62:325, 1985
67. Spence AA, Cohen EN, Brown BW Jr, et al: Occupational hazards for operating room-based physicians: analysis of data from the United States and the United Kingdom. JAMA 238:955, 1977
68. Spence AA: Environmental pollution by inhalation anaesthetics. Br J Anaesth 59:96, 1987
69. Tannenbaum TN, Goldberg RJ: Exposure to anesthetic gases and reproductive outcome: a review of the epidemiologic literature. J Occup Med 27:659, 1985
70. Vessey MP: Epidemiological studies of the occupational hazards of anaesthesia—a review. Anaesthesia 33:430, 1978
71. Bruce DL, Bach MJ: Effects of trace anaesthetic gases on behavioral performance of volunteers. Br J Anaesth 48:871, 1976
72. National Institute for Occupational Safety and Health: Criteria for a recommended standard: occupational exposure to waste anesthetic gases and vapors. US Department of Health, Education and Welfare (NIOSH) Publication No. 77-140, Washington, DC, 1977
73. Flemming DC, Johnstone RE: Recognition thresholds for diethyl ether and halothane. Anesthesiol 46:68, 1977
74. Working Committee of the International Agency for Research: Cancer, Feb. 1994. Health Indus Manufac Assoc Bull, Washington, DC, 1994
75. Tokars JI, Marcus R, Culver DH, et al: Surveillance of HIV infection and zidovudine among healthcare workers after occupational exposure to HIV infected blood. Ann Intern Med 118:913, 1993
76. Association of Operating Room Nurses: Recommended practices for standard and transmission-based precautions in the perioperative practice setting. AORN J 69:404, 1999
77. Sever LE, Gilbert ES, Hessol NA, et al: A case-control study of congenital malformations and occupational exposure to low-level ionizing radiation. Am J Epidemiol 127:226, 1988
78. Dunn K, Yoshimaru H, Otake M, et al: Prenatal exposure to ionizing radiation and subsequent development of seizures. Am J Epidemiol 131:114, 1990
79. Draper GJ, Little MP, Sorahan T, et al: Cancer in the offspring of radiation workers: a record linkage study. BMJ 8:1181, 1997
80. Swartz HM, Reichling BA: Hazards of radiation exposure for pregnant women. JAMA 239:1907, 1978
81. Goldberg MS, Mayo NE, Levy AR: Adverse reproductive outcomes among women exposed to low levels of ionizing radiation from diagnostic radiography for adolescent idiopathic scoliosis. Epidemiology 9:271, 1998
82. Krueger KJ, Hoffman BJ: Radiation exposure during gastroenterologic fluoroscopy: risk assessment for pregnant workers. Am J Gastroenterol 87:429, 1992
83. Arnold WP: Environmental safety including chemical dependency. Anesthesia, 3rd ed. Miller RD, Ed. Churchill Livingstone, New York, 1990, p 2409
84. Berry AJ, Katz JD: Hazards of working in the operating room. Clinical Anesthesia, 2nd ed. Barash PG, Ed. JB Lippincott Co, Philadelphia, 1992, p 98
85. Mangram AJ, Horan TC, Pearson ML, et al: The Hospital Infection Control Practices Advisory Committee: guideline for prevention of surgical site infection, 1999. Infect Cont Hosp Epidemiol 20:247, 1999
86. Simmons BP: Guidelines for the prevention of surgical wound infections. Infect Control 3:188, 1982
87. Garibaldi PA: Prevention of intraoperative wound contamination with chlorhexidine shower and scrub. J Hosp Infect 11(suppl B):5, 1988
88. Kaiser AB, Kernodle DJ, Barg NL, et al: Influence of preoperative showers on staphylococcal stain colonization: a comparative trial of antiseptic skin cleansers. Ann Thorac Surg 45:38, 1998
89. Seropian R, Reynolds BM: Wound infections after pre-operative depilatory versus razor preparation. Am J Surg 121:251, 1971
90. Alexander JW, Fischer JE, Boyajian M, et al: The influence of hair removal methods on wound infections. Arch Surg 118:347, 1983
91. Masterson TM, Rodeheaver GT, Morgan RF, et al: Bacteriologic evaluation of electric clippers for surgical hair removal. Am J Surg 148:301, 1984
92. Lowbury EJ, Lilly HA: Use of 4% chlorhexidine detergent solution and other methods of stain disinfection. Br Med J 1:510, 1973
93. Peterson AF, Rosenberg A, Alatary SD: Comparative evaluation of surgical scrub preparations. Surg Gynecol Obstet 146:63, 1978
94. Association of Operating Room Nurses: Recommended practices for skin preparation of patients. AORN J 645:813, 1996
95. Hardin WD, Nichols RL: Handwashing and patient skin preparations. Critical Issues in Operating Room Management. Malangoni MA, Ed. Lippincott-Raven, Philadelphia, 1997, p 133
96. Aly R, Maiboch HI: Comparative antibacterial efficacy of a 2 minute surgical scrub with chorhexidine gluconate, povidone-iodine, and chloroxylenol spongebrushes. Am J Infect Control 16:173, 1998
97. Coop G, Mailhot CB, Zalarm, et al: Cover gowns and the control of operating room contamination. Nurs Rev 35:263, 1986
98. Dineen P: The role of impervious drapes and gowns preventing surgical infection. Clin Orthop 96:210, 1973
99. Best practices for the prevention of surgical site infection. Education Design. Association of Operating Room Nurses, Chicago, 1998

100. Smith JW, Nichols RL: Barrier efficiency of surgical gowns: are we really protected from our patients' pathogens? Arch Surg 126:756, 1991
101. Quebbeman EJ, Telford GL, Hubbard S, et al: In-use evaluation of surgical gowns. Surg Gynecol Obstet 174:369, 1992
102. Lewis DA, Leaper DJ, Speller DCF: Prevention of bacterial colonization of wounds at operation: comparison of iodine-impregnated ('Ioban') drapes with conventional methods. J Hosp Infect 5:431, 1984
103. Nystrom PO, Broome A, Hojer H, et al: A controlled trial of a plastic wound ring drape to prevent contamination and infection in colorectal surgery. Dis Colon Rectum 27:451, 1984
104. McCue SF, Berg EW, Sanders EA: Efficacy of double-gloving as a barrier to microbial contamination during total joint anthroplasty. J Bone Joint Surg 63:811, 1981
105. Dodds RD, Guy PJ, Peacock AM, et al: Surgical glove perforation. Br J Surg 75:966, 1988
106. Tunevall TG, Jorbeck H: Influence of wearing masks on the density of airborne bacteria in the vicinity of the surgical wound. Eur J Surg 158:263, 1992
107. Tunevall TG: Postoperative wound infections and surgical face masks: a controlled study. World J Surg 15:383, 1991
108. US Department of Labor, Occupational Safety and Health Administration: Occupational exposure to bloodborne pathogens: final rule (29 CFR Part 1910.1030). Fed Register 56:64004, 1991
109. Humphreys H, Marshall RJ, Ricketts VE, et al: Theatre over-shoes do not reduce operating theatre floor bacterial counts. J Hosp Infect 17:117, 1991
110. Lee J: Surgical wound infections: surveillance for quality improvement. Surgical Infections. Fry DE, Ed. Little, Brown & Co, Boston, 1995, p 145
111. Horan TC, Gaynes RP, Martone WH, et al: CDC definitions of nosocomial surgical site infections, 1992: a modification of CDC definitions of surgical wound infections. Infect Contr Hosp Epidemiol 13:606, 1992
112. Lee JT, Olson MM: Wound infection surveillance for 85,260 consecutive operations. J Surg Outcomes 2:27, 1999

41 PERIOPERATIVE EFFECTS OF ANESTHESIA

William C. Tullock, M.D., *Charles D. Boucek*, M.D., *Wilbert A. Cusano*, D.O., *and W. David Watkins*, M.D., Ph.D.

The goal of anesthesia is to permit the necessary manipulations of surgery while maintaining the patient's comfort and safety. Modern anesthetics, both local and general, have greatly expanded the scope of possible surgical procedures and increased patients' willingness to undergo surgery. Anesthetics not only alleviate pain and anxiety but also modify homeostatic reflexes. Appropriate anesthetic care maintains artificial physiologic homeostasis despite the stresses of the surgical procedure and the drugs given. Drugs used during the course of anesthesia produce complex physiologic effects that may be further complicated by interactions with the patient's pathophysiology.[1,2] Drug-drug interactions may produce effects unlike those predicted from the known effects of the individual drugs.[3,4] Appropriate management of the physiologic effects, side effects, and interactions of anesthetic agents depends on continuous monitoring, evaluation of the patient's condition, and a comprehensive knowledge of the pharmacology involved.

Every use of anesthetic agents is an exercise in pharmacokinetics (i.e., the disposition of an administered quantity of drug) and pharmacodynamics (i.e., the effects of the drug) [*see 107 Pharmacokinetics in Surgical Practice*]. Although laboratory studies may establish a patient's likely response to a given medication, all studies are predictive only of the average effect on a population. Individual response can be expected to vary along a normal distribution curve. Every anesthetic regimen must be tailored to the individual patient's responses. Appropriate medications and manipulations are applied to counter pain, blood loss, fluid shifts, and temperature alterations. The complexity of the necessary management frequently necessitates the involvement of dedicated anesthetizing personnel, who permit the operating surgeon to concentrate on the surgical procedure itself.

Preoperative Assessment

The preoperative anesthetic assessment includes a review of the patient's history and a physical examination, with special attention given to the airway and the circulatory and respiratory systems. Anesthesia may be provided for patients who are even desperately ill, as long as the increased risks of both surgery and anesthesia in patients with reduced physical status are recognized.[5] Medical consultation for assistance in preoperative and postoperative care may be appropriate for patients with complex medical illnesses, but to speak of medical clearance for surgery is misleading. Few conditions are absolute contraindications to the use of anesthesia, provided that the operation is indicated and that the patient consents. It is essential, however, that needless risk be avoided. Delay or cancellation of an operation on the day of surgery is awkward for all involved, but it may be the best decision when factors such as acute upper respiratory infection or failure to ensure that a patient has not eaten before the operation would needlessly increase the risk associated with anesthesia for an otherwise healthy patient. Through continuing efforts to improve patient management, anesthetic care has evolved to the point where death or serious morbidity attributable solely to anesthesia is rare (approximately one death in 10,000 courses of anesthesia), despite the use of anesthesia in an ever-broadening spectrum of patients.

During the preoperative period, an overall plan for anesthesia is made, including the decision whether to use general anesthesia, regional anesthesia, or local anesthesia, with or without sedation. Plans for dealing with rare but significant potential complications are needed as well. All equipment needed for resuscitation, including that needed for general anesthesia, is always prepared before the procedure is begun. For maximal safety, anesthetic agents are titrated to effect rather than administered by an arbitrary dosing schedule. To achieve the desired result, monitoring and adequate time to establish the effects of incremental doses are required. At the conclusion of the procedure, plans must be made for a gradual step-down in the level of care continuing into the postoperative period.

Premedication

Most patients may safely undergo anesthesia without any premedication. The purpose of premedication is to decrease anxiety, promote hemodynamic stability, reduce oral and gastric secretions, and provide analgesia.[6] After the patient has been medically evaluated, drugs that accomplish these tasks may be useful adjuncts to the anesthetic plan. The choice of premedication warrants careful consideration because the effects of the drugs may extend beyond the completion of the procedure and delay discharge. Heavy sedation is generally undesirable. Patients should be able to answer simple questions and be able to identify themselves.

ANXIETY

Most patients are anxious before undergoing anesthesia and operation. Methods to reduce patient anxiety include preoperative education, relaxation training, and administration of anxiolytic medications—most commonly, benzodiazepines. Anxiolytic medications should be given only after informed consent for anesthesia and operation has been obtained. Respiratory depression, hypoxia, and hypotension may result from an overdose of these medications. These drugs may also cause psychomotor impairment, which may extend into the postoperative period and delay discharge. No epidemiological study has addressed the relation between the lingering effects of anxiolytic agents and the occurrence of accidents, although the chronic use of benzodiazepines is a proven risk factor for falls among elderly patients.[7,8]

HEMODYNAMIC STABILITY

Preoperative administration of clonidine, an α_2-adrenergic agonist, has been shown to reduce intraoperative lability of blood pressure and heart rate.[9] In one study,[10] elderly patients given clonidine, 5 µg/kg orally, 90 to 120 minutes before operation exhibited a reduced cardiovascular response to laryngoscopy with endotracheal intubation. Clonidine reduces the release of catecholamines by acting centrally as well as reduces anesthetic requirements for both potent inhalation anesthetics and narcotics. Clonidine also produces sedation and dry mouth, which may be useful in premedication.

ORAL AND GASTRIC SECRETIONS

Anticholinergic agents, such as atropine and scopolamine, may reduce oral secretions but often cause unpleasant dry mouth. The routine use of anticholinergic drugs preoperatively was necessitated by the use of the anesthetic agent diethyl ether, which irritates the airway and produces copious secretions. Contemporary inhalation anesthetics do not produce irritation severe enough to warrant the routine use of anticholinergic drugs in adults. Anticholinergics may be useful when airway management is expected to be difficult or when an oral surgical procedure is to be performed. H_2-receptor blockers have been used to increase gastric pH and perhaps reduce the volume of residual gastric contents[11] to minimize the risk of aspiration of regurgitated gastric contents. Although the use of H_2-receptor blockers is widespread and costly, their efficacy has been studied only indirectly (by measuring gastric acidity and volume),[12] and the benefit of reducing the morbidity associated with gastric aspiration remains unsubstantiated. As is the case with many rare adverse effects, such as gastric aspiration, studies to prove the efficacy of drug influence would require large patient populations and substantial resources.

ANALGESIA

Patients with painful conditions that are likely to be exacerbated by transport to the operating room may benefit from premedication with narcotics. How effective narcotics actually are in relieving anxiety is controversial. Narcotics may cause nausea, decrease gastric emptying time, and increase gastric volume. In large doses, they may cause decreased respiratory drive with CO_2 retention and hypoxia. Patients with intracranial masses or other conditions in which intracranial pressure may be increased should not receive narcotic premedication, because increased carbon dioxide tension (P_{CO_2}) may raise intracranial pressure.

General Anesthesia

General anesthesia is a drug-induced state of insensibility to painful stimuli characterized by amnesia, analgesia, loss of consciousness, muscle relaxation, and suppression of reflexes.[13] A single inhalation anesthetic, such as halothane, enflurane, or isoflurane, can exert all of these characteristic effects.[14] Alternatively, general anesthesia can be produced by combinations of intravenous drugs that separately provide analgesia, amnesia, and muscle relaxation.

The course of general anesthesia may be characterized by the procedural phase (i.e., induction, maintenance, or emergence) as well as by the stage or depth of anesthesia at any point in time. The first phase, induction, is the transition from the awake state to an unconscious state in which respiratory reflexes and response to noxious stimulation are under the anesthesiologist's control. In the second phase, maintenance, a stable plane of anesthesia permits surgery to be performed. In the third phase, emergence, the patient regains consciousness, reflexes, and homeostatic control.

The effects of anesthetic drugs on the central nervous system occur in a graded fashion as the concentration of the anesthetic in the brain increases. The initial alert state is followed by sedation (stage 1), delirium with increased reflexes (stage 2), and, finally, a stable plane of anesthesia (stage 3). Overdose can lead to cardiovascular collapse (stage 4). The cerebral metabolic rate decreases as the level of consciousness decreases.

INDUCTION

Intravenous drugs are usually preferred for the induction of general anesthesia in adults because they act quickly and are generally well accepted by patients. The duration of stage 2 may be shortened or eliminated by the use of intravenous agents that reduce the coughing, breath-holding, and laryngospasm sometimes observed during this stage. Induction of anesthesia with inhalation anesthetics is frequently preferred in infants and children because of the psychological stress and trauma that may be encountered in the course of establishing intravenous access in an awake, alert pediatric patient.

The combinations and doses of drugs chosen for induction [see Table 1] should be individualized in accordance with the physiologic state and the expected hemodynamic response of each patient. Rapid induction is associated with equally rapid alterations of cardiovascular and respiratory physiology. Decreases in cardiac output and peripheral vascular tone, with a consequent fall in blood pressure, are anticipated cardiovascular effects of the induction of anesthesia. The respiratory effects of anesthesia can be managed through controlled ventilation, either via a face mask or with endotracheal intubation.

Although some surgical procedures may be performed with anesthesia administered by mask, endotracheal intubation may be indicated in patients undergoing procedures involving positions other than supine or lithotomy; most intracranial, intrathoracic, and major intra-abdominal procedures; or any procedure involving major blood loss or a full stomach. Endotracheal intubation causes significant physiologic stress. The resulting catecholamine release may cause hypertension and tachycardia. Myocardial ischemia may also occur as a result of the stress of intubation, especially in patients with left ventricular hypertrophy, a history of hypertension, diabetes, or previous coronary artery disease.[15] Intraoperative ischemia has significant predictive value for perioperative myocardial infarction and death.[16] Multiple-drug regimens, including the use of narcotics, beta blockers, local anesthetics, and vasodilators, have been used to attenuate the physiologic stress of intubation. Drugs that inhibit neuromuscular transmission (muscle relaxants) facilitate intubation and provide skeletal and abdominal muscle relaxation for the surgical procedure [see Table 2] but by themselves are not anesthetics.

Common Problems during Induction

Intubation difficulties Difficulty with intubation may be anticipated in patients who have a limited range of motion of the cervical spine or the temporomandibular joint, a marked overbite, or macroglossia. In adults with an intradental aperture smaller than 4 cm and thyroid cartilage that is less than 5 cm from the chin, endotracheal intubation may be difficult because alignment of the oropharyngeal and pharyngotracheal axes is needed to visualize the vocal cords. Oral intubation may still be difficult in patients without identifiable risk factors. Various techniques, including fiberoptic intubation, retrograde intubation over a guide wire,[17] blind nasal intubation, transtracheal ventilation,[18] and tracheostomy, may be used to facilitate intubation in difficult cases.

Because dental injuries may result from attempts at endotracheal intubation, the teeth should be carefully examined before operation. Patients at special risk include those for whom intubation is expected to be difficult and those with loose or large-capped teeth. Teeth dislodged during intubation must be recovered because aspiration of teeth or tooth fragments could result in obstructive pneumonia.

Table 1 Induction Drugs for General Anesthesia

Agent	Usual Induction Dose	Comments
Thiopental	4–6 mg/kg	Most commonly used induction agent; myocardial depressant and cerebral protective properties noteworthy
Etomidate	0.3 mg/kg	Little reduction in blood pressure; adrenal supression may occur, especially with infusion
Propofol	2 mg/kg	Significant vasodilatation; rapid awakening to alert state; less associated nausea than with other agents; administered in nonbacteriostatic lipid emulsion
Midazolam	0.3 mg/kg	Slower onset and more prolonged sedation, compared with thiopental; frequently used for sedation in lower dosage; may be a vein irritant
Fentanyl Alfentanil Sufentanil	50 µg/kg 150 µg/kg 12 µg/kg	May cause less myocardial depression than nonnarcotic induction agents; prolonged respiratory depression may necessitate postoperative ventilation when full induction dose given; amnesia not reliable unless supplemented with other agents
Ketamine	1–5 mg/kg	Dissociative agent; may cause hallucinations and flashbacks; little decrease in blood pressure, because agent causes release of endogenous catecholamines; myocardial depressant

Laryngospasm Laryngospasm is the spastic reflex closure of the larynx. It may be precipitated by blood, mucus, or foreign bodies contacting the larynx during the early stages of anesthesia, when airway responsiveness is enhanced. This situation may occur either at the induction of anesthesia or after extubation and may lead to hypoxia and death. Laryngospasm is treated with sustained positive airway pressure, which increases the depth of anesthesia, and with neuromuscular-blocking drugs. A technique that frequently helps overcome this obstruction is to subluxate the mandible forward by applying pressure behind the angles of the jaw, thereby widening the pharynx and opening the entrance to the larynx.[19]

Bronchospasm Wheezing, a high-pitched whistling sound during breathing, is commonly observed after the induction of anesthesia. It may be caused by airway obstruction from nonpulmonary disorders or by exacerbations of intrinsic pulmonary disorders, such as asthma. Mechanical causes include endobronchial intubation, an endotracheal tube positioned against the carina, or mechanical obstruction (e.g., mucous plugging, kinking of the tube, or overinflation of the cuff). Any foreign body placed in the trachea may cause reflex bronchospasm. Ventilating with cool, dry air may exacerbate preexisting asthma, much as exercise may. Several anesthetic drugs (e.g., tubocurarine, atracurium, and morphine) increase systemic levels of histamine in a dose-related fashion; histamine increases bronchomotor tone and increases airway resistance to flow.

Wheezing caused by increased bronchomotor tone may be treated with one of the potent inhalation anesthetics, such as isoflurane; these drugs are direct-acting bronchial smooth muscle relaxants. Halothane is also used for bronchodilatation but may sensitize the myocardium to dysrhythmias induced by catecholamines.[20] Concurrent use of a beta-adrenergic agonist, such as inhaled albuterol, or a methylxanthine, such as intravenous aminophylline,[21] should be considered because the inhalation anesthetic will be discontinued at the end of the operation, and wheezing may recur. Administration of parenteral corticosteroids to reduce inflammation should be considered at an early stage because such agents may require some time to be effective.

Aspiration Patients may aspirate gastric contents when anesthesia is induced. Special precautions should be taken to protect the airway if patients may have recently eaten or may have retained secretions (e.g., patients with bowel obstruction, diabetic gastroparesis, or a history of gastric reflux). In these circumstances, rapid-sequence induction of anesthesia may be considered if patients have a normal airway. Patients should hyperventilate on 100 percent oxygen,[22] and indirect compression of the esophagus by manual pressure over the thyroid cartilage (Sellick maneuver)[23] should be initiated, followed by rapid intravenous induction of anesthesia and muscle paralysis to expedite prompt endotracheal intubation. Duplicate equipment, including suction, laryngoscope, endotracheal tubes, and running intravenous infusions, should be available to ensure the safety of this procedure because delays are dangerous once it is started. The risks associated with this procedure involve committing the patient to neuromuscular paralysis without confirmation of airway status and rapidly administering a preestablished dose of an anesthetic with unpredictable influence

Table 2 Neuromuscular-Blocking Drugs

Agent	ED_{95}* (mg/kg)	Onset (min)	Clinical Duration† (min)	Comments
Succinylcholine	0.30	0.7	7	Depolarizing agent; may increase serum potassium 0.5 mEq/L (greater increases in patients with burns, muscle atrophy, and denervation injuries); may increase intracranial pressure
Pancuronium	0.07	3–5	60–90	Vagolytic properties may result in tachycardia and hypertension
Vecuronium	0.06	3–5	20–35	Minimal hemodynamic effects
Pipecuronium	0.07	3–5	50–80	Minimal hemodynamic effects
Atracurium besylate	0.20	3–5	20–35	Histamine release may lead to flushing and hypotension; unique metabolism leads to spontaneous elimination of this drug independently of the renal and hepatic systems
Mivacurium	0.08	3–4	12–20	Shortest duration of nondepolarizing muscle relaxants; histamine release; hypotension
Tubocurarine	0.50	3–5	60–90	Histamine release; hypotension

*ED_{95} is the average dose that causes a 95 percent reduction in muscle strength.
†Clinical duration is defined as the amount of time from clinically effective surgical paralysis to the return of muscle strength to 25 percent of baseline.

on the cardiovascular system. When endotracheal intubation is expected to be difficult, it should be performed while the patient is conscious.

Hypotension A reduction of systemic blood pressure occurs predictably during the induction of general anesthesia. This hypotension may be attributable to vasodilatation or to the bolus effect of a rapid intravenous injection of anesthetic agents on highly vascularized tissues, such as the heart and the brain. In most healthy patients, a 30 percent transient decrease in blood pressure is well tolerated. In patients with known cardiac and cerebrovascular disease, a proportionally smaller decrease in blood pressure is permissible during induction of anesthesia. Several factors may contribute to prolonged or severe hypotension, and these factors should be considered in every patient with cardiac or cerebrovascular disease.

Auscultation of the chest and abdomen can be useful in assessing the patient for tension pneumothorax, endobronchial intubation, and esophageal intubation, which may lead to hypotension. Reduced intravascular volume is common in surgical patients because of the practice of restricting oral fluids during the hours before the operation and other factors, such as bowel preparation, bleeding, and gastric drainage. Because many anesthetics decrease peripheral vascular tone and impair the normal compensatory mechanisms, significant hypovolemia manifests itself as hypotension. Treatment with a rapid intravenous infusion of crystalloid solutions before and during induction of anesthesia may help restore venous return. Adrenergic insufficiency may lead to hypotension resulting from altered vascular response to catecholamines and hypovolemia resulting from salt wasting. This condition is usually caused by exogenously administered corticosteroids. Preoperative administration of replacement therapy may reduce anesthesia-related hypotension.

Because all inhalation anesthetics are myocardial depressants, the dose of an anesthetic should be decreased or discontinued when hypotension occurs. Exogenous vasopressors may be used to restore vascular tone and myocardial contractility. Ephedrine, an adrenergic agonist that acts both directly and indirectly (triggering the release of endogenous catecholamines), is commonly administered intravenously in incremental doses as a temporizing measure while rapid fluid infusion proceeds. In more severe or protracted hypotension, epinephrine and norepinephrine infusions may be warranted. Continuous electrocardiographic monitoring helps diagnose dysrhythmia-related hypotension, which is an unusual but significant cause of perianesthetic hypotension.

Hypertension Increased blood pressure is commonly seen with endotracheal intubation because of catecholamine release. Significant hypertension during anesthesia occurs most commonly in patients with primary or essential hypertension. A mild transient blood pressure elevation is usually not of great concern, because most general anesthetics will reliably lower blood pressure if given in sufficient amounts. However, a hypertensive crisis may occur in the perioperative setting, especially if the patient has preeclampsia, undiagnosed pheochromocytoma, acute clonidine withdrawal, unrecognized use of monoamine oxidase inhibitors,[24,25] or surreptitious cocaine ingestion [see Recovery Issues, Hypertension, below].

MAINTENANCE

The maintenance phase of anesthesia follows the initiation, or induction, phase. Goals during maintenance include provision of optimal operating conditions for the surgeon and amnesia, analgesia, and physiologic stability for the patient. Drugs may be administered intermittently by intravenous injection or continuously by infusion or inhalation to approach steady-state conditions. Commonly, the patient receives nitrous oxide and oxygen supplemented with either a low concentration of a more potent inhalation anesthetic or a narcotic with a neuromuscular blocker. Inhalation anesthetics [see Table 3] as a group are cardiac and respiratory depressants and are associated with decreased blood pressure, lowered cardiac output, and reduced respiratory drive.

A prospective, randomized study of 17,000 patients, designed to identify the occurrence of major perioperative complications (outcome differences) with enflurane, halothane, isoflurane, and fentanyl, was performed. Major adverse outcomes (death, myocardial infarction, and stroke) were so infrequent that no conclusions about relative rates of these events could be drawn.[26] This study did, however, identify differences in other outcomes. Ventricular arrhythmias were more common with halothane, tachycardia was more common with isoflurane, and hypertension and bronchospasm were more common with fentanyl and nitrous oxide. Despite these differences, for most healthy patients, the choice of drug is probably less significant than the care taken in the administration of the drug.

Dysrhythmias

Dysrhythmias are common during anesthesia, partly because of the stresses associated with and the drugs administered during operation and anesthesia. Patients receiving anesthetics undergo continuous electrocardiographic monitoring, which often detects preexisting clinically insignificant dysrhythmias. Not all dysrhythmias detected by ECG during anesthesia require treatment.[27] In the perioperative setting, these dysrhythmias have several potential causes. Appropriate treatment depends on proper diagnosis.[28] Suboptimal lead placement and the potential for artifact resulting from the use of electrocautery units and patient movement may limit the diagnostic value of the intraoperative ECG. Even under optimal circumstances, diagnosis by ECG alone may be uncertain.[29] Tachydysrhythmias are a common response to pain. If adequate analgesia has been achieved, a search for other causes of dysrhythmias should include an assessment of the adequacy of ventilation,[30] mechanical irritation of the heart,[31] metabolic status, and electrolyte status. Whether treatment of dysrhythmias is indicated is partly determined by the associated effects of anesthesia on cardiovascular function. Cardioversion may serve as a rapid treatment but is rarely needed unless cardiovascular collapse is impending. Intravenous lidocaine is administered frequently during anesthesia not only for its antiarrhythmic properties but also to reduce tracheal irritation and to supplement general anesthesia. Other antiarrhythmic agents are used less frequently and for more specific indications.

Significant perioperative bradycardias may be related to beta blockade, vagotonia, and hypoxia. High spinal anesthesia is associated with sympathetic blockade and unopposed vagal stimulation and may necessitate the administration of adrenergic agonists or vagolytic drugs. Potent inhalation anesthetics commonly lead to a benign dose-dependent nodal rhythm with retrograde P waves. Lower doses of the inhalation anesthetic will allow this rhythm to revert to normal sinus rhythm. Only the hypotension associated with nodal rhythm warrants treatment. The presence of heart block should be noted[32-34]; however, bifascicular block usually does not progress to complete heart block during the perioperative period,[35] unless the patient recently had a myocardial infarction.

Positioning

Positioning of the anesthetized patient is the shared responsibility of the surgeon and the anesthesiologist. To prevent tissue injury, bony prominences should be padded and extreme joint positions must be avoided. The patient's position should be carefully assessed to prevent neurovascular compression, stretch injury of nerve roots,[36] and pressure on the breasts, testicles, eyes, and cervical vessels.[37] When the patient's position is being changed, special attention must be paid to prevent falls or the flailing of the arms, the neck, or the legs. Local pressure on the skin may lead to erythema, blistering, sloughing, and late alopecia, especially during lengthy procedures.[38] It may be difficult to avoid compression injury to the skin surface supporting the patient's weight when position changes are contraindicated, as in extended craniotomies.

Surgical positioning may aggravate the physiologic effects of anesthesia. Reduced vascular and muscle tone may lead to pooling of blood and subsequent hypotension and dependent edema. In addition, pneumocephalus may occur after posterior fossa or cervical cord operations if the patient had been in the sitting position during the operation.[39] Intraoperative positioning may also affect postoperative pulmonary complications.[40] Aspiration of retained gastric contents is more common when patients are placed in the prone, the lateral, or Trendelenburg's position and will preferentially involve the most dependent lung segments. Reduction of functional residual capacity (FRC), the volume of gas in the lungs at end expiration during tidal breathing, occurs during general anesthesia. This reservoir of gas permits oxygenation of blood flowing through the pulmonary circuit during the expiratory phase of respiration. When patients are awake and in the erect position, normal intercostal muscle tone helps maintain chest expansion, gravity pulls the abdominal contents away from the diaphragm, and FRC is maximal. When patients are placed in the supine or Trendelenburg's position, the weight of the abdominal contents tends to elevate the diaphragm, further reducing FRC. For patients in the prone position, special care must be taken so that the weight is supported on the thorax and the pelvis rather than on the abdomen; otherwise, each breath will be opposed by the patient's weight. It is important to anticipate how to return the patient to the supine position rapidly should intraoperative resuscitation be necessary.

Table 3 Inhalation Anesthetic Drugs

Agent	MAC*	Comments
Halothane	0.75%	A bronchodilator associated with hepatic dysfunction (rare); sensitizes the myocardium to catecholamines
Enflurane	1.68%	Causes the greatest amount of myocardial depression; renal dysfunction attributable to fluoride ions may occur with prolonged use at a high concentration
Isoflurane	1.05%	Undergoes little metabolism; peripheral vasodilation reduces myocardial depression by unloading the heart and increasing cardiac output
Nitrous oxide	110%	Most rapidly acting inhalation agent; causes little, if any, respiratory depression; low potency requires supplementation with other drugs

*MAC is the minimum alveolar concentration at which 50 percent of patients do not move when the surgical incision is made.

Recall of Intraoperative Events

The incidence of recall of events during general anesthesia is reported to be between 0.2 and 4.0 percent. When the amount of anesthetic administered was limited because of perceived unacceptable risk, as in major trauma, the reported incidence was as high as 43 percent. Measures to diminish the incidence of recall of events during anesthesia and the effects of anesthetic agents on learning and consciousness have been reviewed.[41] Currently, the absence of recall is the only objective criterion for determining unconsciousness. Autonomic responses to surgical stimulation and patient movement are used to judge the clinical depth of anesthesia but are poorly predictive of impending consciousness and recall. Explicit recall may be detected by posing questions such as the following: What is the last thing you remember about the time before the operation? What is the first thing you remember after waking up? Do you remember anything in between? Responses that confirm intraoperative recall should prompt a candid explanation of the possible causes. Consultation with a psychiatrist or psychologist may be warranted if the patient exhibits signs or symptoms of psychic trauma.

Hypothermia

Mild hypothermia (33° to 36° C; 91.4° to 96.8° F) is common during anesthesia and operation because anesthetics reduce metabolic heat production, decrease the temperature at which the activation of thermoregulatory mechanisms occurs, and limit the response of vasoconstriction and nonshivering thermogenesis.[42] Anesthetized patients thus are functional poikilotherms. After induction of anesthesia and vasodilatation, the cool peripheral compartment blood mixes with the central blood and causes its temperature to fall by 0.5° to 1.5° C. Additional cooling often continues, depending on the operating room temperature, the amount of body surface exposed, and the measures taken to actively warm the patient.

Mild hypothermia can cause decreased metabolism and renal excretion of drugs and consequent slow awakening of patients after the operation. Mild hypothermia can also cause a reversible coagulopathy. In addition, shivering in the recovery period[43] increases metabolic stress and exacerbates postoperative pain. Hypothermia can, however, be beneficial during operation: a decrease of 2° to 3° C from normal body temperature may protect against cerebral ischemia.

Heat loss from the skin can be minimized during the operation by using reflective coverings when 60 percent of the body is covered. Active warming with forced-air convective blankets is the most effective method of preventing heat loss from the skin. Circulating water blankets are also effective if placed over the patient. Heat- and moisture-exchanging filters (artificial noses) are useful to slow heat losses from the respiratory system and are about half as effective as heated humidifiers, which actively warm and humidify the inspired gas. Fluid warmers effectively reduce heat loss from large amounts of cold intravenous fluids.

EMERGENCE

At the end of an operation, patients are usually rapidly returned to consciousness. Control of homeostasis is progressively transferred from the anesthesiologist to the awakening patient. Timing is critical because premature emergence from anesthesia can be emotionally stressful and the cardiovascular consequences can be dangerous. Thus, anesthesia should be maintained until the completion of the operation, and analgesia should be continued through the recovery period. The timing and manner in which patients awaken from anesthesia can vary greatly. As concentrations of the anesthetics in the brain lessen, patients pass through a period of altered sensory input, which may cause delirium. Awakening may be delayed because of the effects of anesthetics, hypercapnia, hypothermia, and variable individual responses. Because inhalation anesthetics are eliminated through the lungs, patients require adequate minute ventilation and time for redistribution of these agents from the tissues. Continuous measurement of end-expiratory concentrations of inhalation anesthetics may aid in predicting patients' return to consciousness. The effects of intravenous anesthetics correlate with plasma concentrations, which are largely determined by the process of metabolism and redistribution.

Although specific antagonists for the opiates and, more recently, the benzodiazepine receptors are available, they are infrequently used. The antagonism of narcotics, which may hasten the return of spontaneous ventilation, may also cause the sudden onset of severe pain, leading to hypertension, tachycardia, and stress. Additionally, the duration of effect of benzodiazepines and narcotic antagonists may not match the duration of effect of the agonists. Thus, during the postoperative recovery period, the patient may return unpredictably to a level of consciousness or respiratory depression attained during the operation.

Return of neuromuscular function should precede the regaining of consciousness; otherwise, the patient may experience awareness with paralysis, which can be terrifying. The effect of a nondepolarizing muscle relaxant may be antagonized by administration of a cholinesterase inhibitor as long as the degree of neuromuscular blockade is not profound. To counter the muscarinic side effects of cholinesterase inhibition (bradycardia, salivation, and increased bronchial secretions), an anticholinergic agent should be given simultaneously. A peripheral nerve stimulator should always be used to determine whether neuromuscular function has returned toward normal. Recovery of neuromuscular function is confirmed if the patient can lift his or her head for five seconds.

When the patient emerges from anesthesia, mild hypoventilation will increase arterial carbon dioxide concentrations to a point where respiration is stimulated. Return of spontaneous ventilation normally precedes the patient's return to consciousness. The adequacy of spontaneous respiration is assessed by measuring respiratory rate and tidal volume (minute volume) as well as breathing pattern.

Swallowing reflexes are stimulated by the endotracheal tube or the oral airway but may also be warning signs of impending emesis. The timing of extubation is important to the safety and conduct of anesthesia. Endotracheal extubation should be done either when the patient is deeply anesthetized (stage 3) or, alternatively, when the patient can follow simple commands and protective airway reflexes have returned. Extubation during stage 2 is hazardous because airway reflexes may be hyperactive, and coughing, breath-holding, vomiting, and laryngospasm may occur. The primary purpose of the postanesthesia care unit is to allow patients to further recover from the effects of anesthesia under careful supervision before they are transferred to other locations in the hospital or discharged. The Aldrete postanesthetic recovery room score may be useful for documenting progress toward discharge [see Table 4]. If the patient is to be discharged from the hospital, he or she should have regained orientation and should be able to void urine and assume an upright posture without orthostatic hypotension. A plan for pain control should be established. Finally, patients should be discharged from the hospital on the day of the operation only if the home environment meets the following criteria:

1. The patient must have reliable transportation. A taxi may be acceptable, but mass transit generally is not acceptable, because return to the hospital is difficult if acute complications occur en route.
2. A competent adult care giver should accompany the patient and remain with him or her for 24 hours.
3. Communication by telephone to the medical care system should be possible.
4. Reasonable standards of fitness for habitation should be met (i.e., clean running water, heat, and appropriate sanitation should be available).
5. Access to a pharmacy is usually indicated so that prescribed medications can be obtained.

Local and Regional Anesthesia

For many surgical procedures, local anesthetics can be used to provide regional anesthesia as an alternative or adjunct to general anesthesia. The advantages of local and regional anesthesia are maintenance of consciousness through the operation, minimal recovery from central nervous system depressants, minimal cardiopulmonary effects, no endotracheal intubation, persistent vasodilatation of the operative site, and, possibly, improved postoperative analgesia.

LOCAL ANESTHESIA WITH SEDATION

For many procedures, local anesthetics [see Table 5] may be administered at the site of incision. Conscious sedation may alleviate the patient's fear and anxiety and limit the unpleasantness of prolonged immobility on the operating table. In conscious sedation, intravenous drugs are used to provide a minimally depressed level of consciousness. Patients retain their ability to maintain an airway independently and continuously and to respond appropriately to physical stimulation and verbal commands. Patients should undergo the same preoperative evaluation and preparation for local anesthesia with conscious sedation as for general anesthesia. In fact, conscious sedation may have to be switched to general anesthesia at any time. The presence of anesthesiology personnel in this setting provides the added safety and patient comfort afforded by close monitoring. The primary analgesia for the surgical procedure is provided by the local anesthetic. Attempts to treat surgical pain with excessive doses of sedatives not only are ineffective but also result in the complications that arise from obtundation and respiratory depression. Discharge of a patient after conscious sedation should follow the same guidelines as for general anesthesia.

REGIONAL ANESTHESIA

Local anesthetics may also be administered at sites remote from the surgical incision to produce regional anesthesia. Such blocks involving large body areas may lead to profound physiologic changes [see Table 6]. Consent and preparation guidelines for regional anesthesia should thus be no less stringent than those for general anesthesia. In fact, general anesthesia may be necessary if there is insufficient duration of analgesia or if complications arise from the surgical procedure or the anesthetic technique. The combination of a major regional anesthetic and general anesthesia has become increasingly popular to achieve some of the advantages of both[44]; however, this approach usually requires increased preparation time.

Successful regional anesthesia usually depends significantly on the degree of communication between the surgeon, the patient, and the anesthesiologist. The once-common belief that regional anesthesia is invariably safer than general anesthesia is disputable. Unless continuous regional techniques are used, regional blocks may be inadequate for surgical procedures that may last longer than the duration of action of the local anesthetic. For a patient to receive regional anesthesia, he or she should be psychologically suitable to remain awake or sedated during the operation and cooperative during the anesthetic procedure. The surgeon must be comfortable with confining the operative procedure to the region anesthetized. Even in the hands of the most skilled, experienced anesthesiologist, every regional technique is subject to some degree of failure to provide the intended anesthesia.

Subarachnoid (Spinal) Block

Spinal anesthetics are administered by introducing a small quantity of concentrated local anesthetic into the cerebrospinal fluid in the subarachnoid space, where it anesthetizes the nerves of the cauda equina and the lower spinal cord. The site of needle insertion is usually below the second lumbar interspace in adults to avoid needle injury to the spinal cord. By varying the concentration and the dose of the anesthetic and the patient's position

Table 4 Postanesthetic Recovery Room Score*

Characteristic	Score	Criterion
Activity	2	Moves all four extremities
	1	Moves two extremities
	0	Unable to move any extremities
Respiration	2	Able to breathe deeply and cough freely
	1	Dyspnea; limited respiratory effort
	0	No spontaneous respiratory effort
Circulation	2	SBP within 20% of preoperative pressure; no ECG change
	1	SBP changed by 20%–50% from preoperative pressure; minor ECG changes
	0	SBP more than 50% changed; major ECG changes
Consciousness	2	Full awareness; answering questions
	1	Aroused by hearing name called
	0	No response to auditory stimuli
Color	2	Pink
	1	Pale, dusky, or blotchy
	0	Cyanotic nails, lips, or skin

SBP—systolic blood pressure
*The points scored in each section are added for a maximal possible score of 10.

Table 5 Comparative Pharmacology of Local Anesthetics

Classification	Potency	Onset of Action	Duration of Effect after Infiltration (min)	Maximum Single Dose for Infiltration in Adults* (mg)	Toxic Plasma Concentration (µg/ml)	pK$_a$	Nonionized % pH 7.2	Nonionized % pH 7.4
Esters								
Procaine	1†	Slow	45–60	500	—	8.9	2	3
Chloroprocaine	4	Rapid	30–45	600		8.7	3	5
Tetracaine	16	Slow	60–180	100 (Topical)		8.5	5	7
Amides								
Lidocaine	1‡	Rapid	60–120	300	5	7.9	17	25
Mepivacaine	1	Slow	90–180	300	5	7.6	28	39
Bupivacaine	4	Slow	240–480	175	About 1.5	8.1	11	15
Etidocaine	4	Slow	240–480	300	About 2	7.7	24	33
Prilocaine	1	Slow	60–120	400	5	7.9	17	24

*Increased if solution contains epinephrine.
†Standard of comparison for esters.
‡Standard of comparison for amides.

after injection, some control of the dermatomal distribution of the anesthesia can be achieved.[45] The duration of the spinal block depends on the drug and the dose and may be prolonged by the addition of a vasoconstrictor, such as epinephrine or phenylephrine. Sensory blockade usually proceeds with a caudal-to-rostral dermatomal progression, with sympathetic blockade one to two dermatomes higher. Systemic vascular hypotension may occur unless volume loading with intravenous fluids precedes the block. The use of a subarachnoid catheter to administer small increments of local anesthetic may attenuate the cardiovascular effects and permit repeated drug administration during and after operation. However, the large dural puncture required for insertion of the catheter may cause postspinal headache. Fine-gauge spinal catheters (25 gauge or smaller) were manufactured but were subsequently withdrawn from the market because of their association with cauda equina syndrome.

Epidural Block

An alternative approach to spinal blockade is epidural anesthesia, in which a needle is advanced through the subcutaneous

Table 6 Physiologic Effects of Major Forms of Regional Anesthesia

Effects	Subarachnoid Block	Epidural Block	Plexus Block
Cardiovascular	Rapid onset of vasodilatation; reflex tachycardia; bradycardia may occur if cardiac accelerator fibers are blocked	Slower onset of vasodilatation than with spinal block; systemic absorption of local anesthetic may cause myocardial toxicity	Systemic absorption may cause myocardial toxicity
Respiratory	Loss of chest wall sensation may cause psuedodyspnea; vasodilatation may lead to hypoperfusion of respiratory centers; total spinal block may lead to phrenic paralysis (rare); loss of intercostal muscle tone reduces functional residual capacity	Loss of chest wall sensation may lead to pseudodyspnea; lower incidence of condition than with spinal block	Thoracic interpleural block may reduce diaphragmatic strength; interscalene block may result in transient phrenic nerve paralysis
Renal	Volume loading is necessary to avoid hypotension; urinary retention may occur because of block of normal micturition reflex	Volume loading is necessary to avoid hypotension; urinary retention may require catheterization, especially if narcotics are given	—
Gastrointestinal	Nausea/emesis associated with hypotension and unopposed vagal stimulation may occur	Nausea/emesis is less common than with spinal block	—
Hematologic	Decreased hematocrit and plasma viscosity may occur	Reduced incidence of thrombotic complications relative to general anesthesia (thrombosis of coronary artery, deep vein, or vascular graft)	—

tissue until the epidural space is entered. Local anesthetic solution may be injected either directly or through a catheter inserted through the needle. The use of an epidural catheter permits incremental injection of local anesthetic that is titrated to the desired level of blockade. The catheter may be helpful postoperatively to permit the use of local anesthetics and neuraxial narcotics for analgesia. Because the needle does not penetrate the dura, epidural injection, unlike spinal anesthesia, may be performed above the L2 level with only a small risk of spinal cord injury. Compared with spinal anesthesia, epidural anesthesia has a slower onset of sensory block and a higher incidence of incomplete sensory block. The effective dose of local anesthetic and narcotic is substantially larger with epidural anesthesia, and systemic absorption may approach the toxic threshold.

Plexus Block

Local anesthetics are used for cervical, brachial, and lumbar plexus blocks. The blocks are performed by introduction of the drug into the area immediately surrounding the neural plexus. Many clinicians rely on paresthesias elicited by needle placement as a guide to proper location. Consequently, some patient discomfort during the performance of these blocks is to be expected, and patient cooperation is important to the success of the block. Because sympathetic blockade is usually limited to the innervated region, this form of anesthesia is rarely associated with significant systemic hypotension. However, systemic absorption of local anesthetics administered in recommended doses and the resultant toxic effects, including seizures and cardiovascular collapse, may occur whenever local anesthetics are introduced intravascularly.

COMMON PROBLEMS WITH REGIONAL ANESTHESIA

Inadequate Anesthesia

Inadequate anesthesia after epidural injection may be improved by repeated doses of local anesthetic through the catheter, although areas of intact sensation may persist despite administration of maximal doses. Supplementation with systemic analgesics, including narcotics and subanesthetic concentrations of nitrous oxide, may be sufficient for short procedures, but general anesthesia may ultimately be necessary. Spotty analgesia is less frequent with spinal anesthesia. The extent of spinal block may be increased by placing the patient in Trendelenburg's position shortly after injection. Once a spinal anesthetic has set, it is difficult to modify the extent of blockade. With plexus blocks, areas of intact sensation are not uncommon. Supplementation of the block with a block of a more peripheral nerve or with local anesthetic infiltrated at the site of incision may be useful.

Hypotension

Hypotension after either epidural or spinal anesthesia is commonly caused by relative hypovolemia in conjunction with sensory and motor blockade.[46] Normally, arteries and veins are under moderate vasoconstrictive influence. Local anesthetics block conduction via the efferent fibers of the peripheral sympathetic nervous system located between T1 and L2. This blockade causes hypotension by decreasing both peripheral vascular resistance and venous return. Because sympathetic blockade extends above sensory blockade, sensory block to the fourth thoracic dermatome causes a nearly total blockade of the sympathetic nervous system, including the cardiac accelerator fibers. Mediation of heart rate variability by atrial or arterial baroreceptors may remain partially intact,[47] but bradycardia is common. Treatment with volume loading and a sympathomimetic, such as phenylephrine or ephedrine, is indicated. If hypotension and bradycardia persist after treatment with ephedrine and atropine, epinephrine should be considered. A review of 14 cases of sudden cardiac arrest in healthy patients who had undergone spinal anesthesia recommended that bradycardia and hypotension associated with verbal unresponsiveness be aggressively managed with epinephrine.[48]

Post–Dural Puncture Headache

Post–dural puncture headache (spinal headache) occurs in as many as 11 percent[49] of patients who have had a spinal puncture. The incidence is higher in young healthy patients and increases with the size of the needle used. Post–dural puncture headaches are characterized by position sensitivity, which increases when patients are in an erect posture and abates when patients are supine. These headaches are usually occipital to frontal and may be associated with nausea and altered auditory sensation. Spinal headaches are believed to be caused by alterations of relative cerebrospinal fluid pressure resulting from leakage of cerebrospinal fluid through the dural puncture site. They are treated by providing vigorous hydration, administering analgesics, reassuring the patient, and allowing time for the headache to resolve. Rapid relief is provided by epidural blood patching,[50] in which the patient's own blood is withdrawn from the arm and injected into the epidural space over the site of the dural puncture.[51]

Outpatient Anesthetic Considerations

Outpatient surgery was first used for relatively minor, peripheral procedures that did not last long and involved only minor blood loss and fluid shifts. The degree of complexity of outpatient surgery and anesthesia is continually progressing [see 37 Nonemergency Surgery]. Procedures that have a major impact on nutrition (e.g., bowel surgery), call for close postoperative monitoring, or warrant intensive invasive monitoring and support usually make postoperative hospitalization necessary and cannot be performed on an outpatient basis. The contingency of inpatient admission should always be recognized because even minor complications of operation or anesthesia (e.g., persistent nausea, vomiting, and pain) may be unmanageable in some home settings.

Anesthetic techniques for outpatient surgery can be selected that minimize postoperative nausea and prolonged sedation, both of which may prevent the patient from returning home. However, in such cases, the advantages and disadvantages of these techniques should be weighed carefully in the course of selecting the appropriate anesthetic. Some surgical procedures may be performed with the patient under local anesthesia and intravenous sedation. Intravenous regional anesthetics may be convenient and reliable, but caution must be exercised to prevent the local anesthetic from entering the systemic circulation abruptly. Spinal and epidural anesthetics both carry the risk of headache secondary to dural puncture. General anesthetics are commonly used, but drugs that are slowly cleared from the body should be used sparingly. The recent development of drugs with shorter residual time in the body (e.g., alfentanil, sufentanil, midazolam, propofol, desflurane, and mivacurium) and of new antiemetics (e.g., ondansetron) may significantly reduce the time required for discharge from the outpatient surgical clinic. Before discharge, the patient should have regained orientation, should have stable vital signs, and should have a clear understanding of follow-up procedures.

Recovery Issues

The postanesthesia care unit (PACU) is a special care unit where patients emerge from a surgical and anesthetic state. Its primary purpose is to complete the recovery from the influences of anesthesia. The level and intensity of care are gradually reduced during the recovery period as the patient's level of consciousness and physiologic processes return to baseline levels. Problems commonly encountered in the PACU include nausea and vomiting, pain, hypertension, and respiratory insufficiency.

NAUSEA AND VOMITING

Nausea and vomiting are common after anesthesia and operation, affecting 20 to 30 percent of patients. Viewed by many health care professionals as a minor complication, vomiting is one of the top patient concerns about anesthesia and surgery. It is a common cause of delayed discharge and overnight hospital stay. Hemodynamic alterations, intracranial pressure fluctuations, aspiration, pain, and disruptions of the surgical incisions or repair are other potentially harmful results of vomiting.

The etiology of nausea in the perioperative period is multifactorial.[52] The type and duration of surgery are important risk factors for nausea. Laparoscopic, intra-abdominal, middle-ear, dental, and strabismus surgery are associated with a high incidence of nausea, regardless of the type of anesthetic agents used. Various anesthetics may cause nausea by different mechanisms. For example, narcotics can act directly on the chemoreceptor trigger zone in the brain stem. Volatile anesthetics and nitrous oxide may produce nausea by increasing catecholamine levels. Nitrous oxide may also change middle-ear pressures and stimulate the vestibular system. Propofol, a relatively new intravenous anesthetic, is associated with a lower incidence of nausea than other anesthetics and may have a specific antiemetic effect. Gastric distention caused by positive-pressure ventilation via a face mask may predispose a patient to vomiting. Sudden motion and position changes may cause nausea by vestibular mechanisms or postural hypotension.

Drugs used to treat anesthesia-related nausea block one or more of the four neurotransmitter systems that mediate receptors of the chemoreceptor trigger zone and vagal pathways [see Table 7]. Ondansetron, a novel serotonin antagonist, may be beneficial for prophylaxis and treatment of nausea because it has fewer side effects than metoclopramide and droperidol.[53] Ondansetron is quite expensive, but it may have significant advantages in selected patients whose nausea is intractable.

PAIN

Pain should be recognized and aggressively managed in the perioperative period [see 104 Postoperative Pain]. Surgeons should not overlook conditions for which pain may be a warning sign. Recognizing that clinical surveys continue to show that pain is undertreated, the U.S. Department of Health and Human Services has published a valuable clinical practice guideline, *Acute Pain Management: Operative or Medical Procedures and Trauma*. This document provides a useful review of pharmacological and nonpharmacological pain management.[54]

Because of altered sensorium, postoperative pain may be manifested as restlessness, agitation, hypertension, or tachycardia. In addition to causing patient discomfort, pain causes other detrimental physiologic responses. Tachycardia and hypertension may result in an imbalance between myocardial oxygen supply and demand, which may lead to ischemia. Tachypnea and shallow breathing can result in atelectasis and hypoxemia.

Potent narcotics that act on the mu opioid receptor are commonly given intraoperatively as a component of general anesthesia or as an adjunct to regional anesthesia. Potent narcotics with a relatively short duration of action (e.g., fentanyl, alfentanil, and sufentanil) are often used, yet their effects usually persist into the PACU. The responsibility for titrating the narcotic dosage to alleviate pain is often turned over to the patient after he or she has regained normal sensorium. Patient-controlled analgesia is the name given to on-demand I.V. self-administration of potent narcotics with the aid of a microprocessor-controlled infusion device. The administration of mixed

Table 7 Antiemetic Drugs

Drug	Receptor Site	Dose	Notes
Prochlorperazine	Dopamine	2.5–10 mg I.V.	Sedative, extrapyramidal effects, alpha-adrenergic blocker
Droperidol	Dopamine, histamine	0.01–0.02 mg/kg I.V.	Restlessness, anxiety, sedative, extrapyramidal effects, alpha-adrenergic blocker
Promethazine	Dopamine, muscarinic cholinergic, histamine	12.5–25 mg I.M.	Sedative, extrapyramidal effects
Scopolamine	Dopamine, muscarinic cholinergic, histamine	1.5 mg patch	Sedative, dry mouth, amnesia, hallucinations
Metoclopramide	Dopamine, histamine, serotonin	10 mg I.V.	Extrapyramidal effects (greater in children than in adults)
Ondansetron	Serotonin	0.15 mg/kg I.V.	High cost

agonist-antagonist opioids (e.g., pentazocine, butorphanol, nalbuphine, and buprenorphine) may not produce satisfactory analgesia because of their antagonism of the mu-receptor drugs.

All narcotics cause a dose-dependent depression of the respiratory center in the brain stem. Because narcotics blunt the ventilatory response to carbon dioxide,[55] they cause a characteristically slow and deep respiratory pattern. Should respiratory depression occur, a narcotic antagonist may be given. As little as 0.04 mg of naloxone, a pure narcotic antagonist, has been shown to reverse respiratory depression without reversing the analgesic effects of narcotics. Naloxone should be given cautiously, however, because it can cause hypertension, tachycardia, pulmonary edema, and dysrhythmias. The mechanism of these effects is unclear but may be related to catecholamine discharge.

Narcotics generally cause a reduction in heart rate and have little influence on myocardial contractility, except for meperidine, which may produce tachycardia and reduce myocardial contractility. Narcotics alone usually do not cause hypotension; however, in the presence of hypovolemia or when combined with benzodiazepines, narcotics may produce a significant reduction in blood pressure. This hypotension may result from bradycardia as well as from vasodilatation secondary to decreased sympathetic tone or histamine release. Histamine release is commonly associated with morphine administration, although meperidine has been reported to be more potent in this regard.[56] Histamine release associated with morphine administration is dose related and usually is not a clinically significant problem if morphine is administered intravenously at a rate slower than 5 mg/min.

Narcotics are increasingly being administered via the epidural and intrathecal routes; administration is often initiated intraoperatively. Patients undergoing upper abdominal or thoracic surgery exhibit less pain and better pulmonary function with epidural narcotics than with intravenous morphine.[57] Epidural and intrathecal narcotics seem to be particularly beneficial in patients undergoing prostate and other pelvic surgery. Delayed respiratory depression is a potential side effect that can occur up to six to eight hours after a single dose of epidural morphine. However, this side effect can be detected and treated with proper monitoring of the respiratory rate and the level of sedation. Other side effects of narcotics administered neuraxially and systemically include pruritus, nausea, vomiting, and urinary retention. Urinary retention is a result of increased smooth muscle tone of the detrusor muscle of the bladder and the urethral sphincter.

The nonsteroidal anti-inflammatory drugs (NSAIDs) are another category of analgesics used in the PACU. In particular, ketorolac has gained popularity in treating postoperative pain because it provides satisfactory analgesia without inducing respiratory depression and the other common side effects of narcotics. All NSAIDs are capable of impairing platelet function and thus should be used with caution in patients at risk for prolonged or occult bleeding.

HYPERTENSION

Treatment of hypertension should be directed at the underlying cause. Hypertension in the PACU is commonly caused by untreated pain. Because of the residual effects of anesthetic drugs, patients may be incapable of clearly verbalizing the pain from a surgical site or the discomfort of bladder distention. In addition, anesthesia-related hypoxia and hypercapnia may cause hypertension because of an increase in sympathetic discharge. Drugs that are administered in the perioperative period, such as epinephrine, ketamine, anticholinergics, and cocaine, may also contribute to hypertension. Omission of a patient's normal therapeutic regimen of antihypertensive drugs on the morning of surgery or a patient's withdrawal from alcohol or illicit drugs should be considered. Poorly controlled or uncontrolled essential hypertension may be unmasked in the perioperative period.

RESPIRATORY INSUFFICIENCY

For respiratory insufficiency in the PACU, rapid recognition, thorough evaluation, and appropriate treatment are crucial. Upper airway obstruction is a common cause of respiratory difficulty and may be caused by the tongue and other soft tissue, laryngospasm, foreign bodies, local edema, or paralysis of the recurrent laryngeal nerve. Subglottic edema, which manifests itself as croup or, in severe cases, stridor, may result from the trauma of endotracheal intubation. Wheezing may be a manifestation of pulmonary edema, exacerbated intrinsic asthma, anaphylaxis, or the presence of a foreign body.

Many drugs used to produce anesthesia—narcotics, benzodiazepines, barbiturates, and inhalation anesthetics—can produce a dose-related respiratory depression. The normal ventilatory response to increasing blood levels of carbon dioxide or hypoxia is blunted. Reversal drugs, such as naloxone, flumazenil, and physostigmine, should be administered only by health care professionals who understand the full array of influences the drugs may exert on the postoperative patient.

Incomplete reversal of neuromuscular-blocking drugs may be reflected in decreased vital capacity and inspiratory force. Subjectively, the patient may complain of feeling weak and being unable to inspire deeply. Bedside spirometric measurements may be useful. A sensitive clinical test for evaluating the return of normal neuromuscular function is to ask the patient to sustain a head lift for five seconds. This action has been demonstrated to correlate with an inspiratory pressure of at least -50 cm H_2O, an adequate tidal volume, and appropriate protective airway reflexes.[58] Prolongation of neuromuscular blockade or incomplete antagonism of the neuromuscular blockade may have many causes: overdose of neuromuscular-blocking drugs, hypothermia, hypokalemia, hypermagnesemia, respiratory acidosis, aminoglycoside antibiotics, and phase II blockade after succinylcholine administration.

Malignant Hyperthermia

Malignant hyperthermia is a life-threatening hypermetabolic state that is genetically determined. Although its exact incidence is difficult to determine, it has been estimated to occur in about one in every 14,000 anesthetized children and about one in every 50,000 anesthetized adults. Classically, it is thought of as being triggered by anesthetic agents, most notably succinylcholine and halothane. However, it can also be precipitated by other conditions, such as stress (both psychological and physical) and exercise. Malignant hyperthermia may have a delayed onset and may be first recognized in the PACU. Patients may undergo many courses of anesthesia safely before a malignant hyperthermia crisis occurs.

The risk of malignant hyperthermia is increased in patients with a family history of this condition, Duchenne's muscular dystrophy, central core disease of muscle, King-Denborough syndrome, myotonia congenita, osteogenesis imperfecta, neuroleptic malignant syndrome, or sudden infant death syndrome.

> **Suggested Therapy for Malignant Hyperthermia Emergency: Recommendations of the Malignant Hyperthermia Association of the United States (MHAUS)**
>
> **Acute-Phase Treatment**
>
> 1. Immediately discontinue all volatile inhalation anesthetics and succinylcholine. Hyperventilate with 100 percent oxygen at high gas flows (i.e., at least 10 L/min). The circle system and CO_2 absorbent need not be changed.
> 2. Rapidly administer an initial bolus of dantrolene sodium, 2 to 3 mg/kg, followed by incremental doses up to a total of 10 mg/kg. Continue to administer dantrolene until signs of malignant hyperthermia (e.g., tachycardia, rigidity, increased end-tidal CO_2, and temperature elevation) are controlled. Occasionally, a total dose greater than 10 mg/kg may be needed.
> 3. Administer bicarbonate to correct metabolic acidosis as guided by blood gas analysis. In the absence of blood gas analysis, bicarbonate should be given in a dose of 1 to 2 mEq/kg.
> 4. Simultaneously with the above (point 3), actively cool the hyperthermic patient. Use intravenous iced saline (not lactated Ringer's solution), 15 ml/kg every 15 minutes, three times.
>   a. Lavage the stomach, bladder, rectum, and open cavities with iced saline as appropriate.
>   b. Surface-cool with ice and a hypothermia blanket.
>   c. Monitor closely because overvigorous treatment may lead to hypothermia.
> 5. Dysrhythmias usually respond to treatment of acidosis and hyperkalemia. If they persist or are life threatening, standard antiarrhythmic agents may be used, with the exception of calcium channel blockers, which may cause hyperkalemia and cardiovascular collapse. The safety of lidocaine during malignant hyperthermia has been suggested but not proved. We recommend that it be used cautiously.
> 6. Determine and monitor end-tidal CO_2; arterial, central, or femoral venous blood gases; serum potassium and calcium levels; clotting; and urine output.
> 7. Hyperkalemia is common in the acute phase of malignant hyperthermia and should be treated with hyperventilation, intravenous glucose and insulin (10 units of regular insulin in 50 ml of 50 percent glucose titrated to the potassium level), and bicarbonate. Life-threatening hyperkalemia may also be treated with calcium administration (e.g., calcium chloride, 2 to 5 mg/kg).
> 8. Ensure a urine output greater than 2 ml/kg/hr. Consider central venous or pulmonary arterial monitoring because of the fluid shifts and hemodynamic instability that may occur.
> 9. Boys younger than about nine years who experience sudden cardiac arrest after succinylcholine administration in the absence of hypoxemia should be treated for acute hyperkalemia first. In this situation, calcium chloride administration along with other means should be instituted to reduce the serum potassium level. These patients should be presumed to have subclinical muscular dystrophy.
>
> **Post–Acute-Phase Treatment**
>
> 1. Observe the patient in an ICU setting for at least 24 hours because recrudescence of malignant hyperthermia may occur, particularly after a fulminant case resistant to treatment.
> 2. Administer dantrolene, 1 mg/kg I.V. every six hours, for 24 to 48 hours after the episode. After that, oral dantrolene, 1 mg/kg every six hours, may be used for 24 hours as necessary.
> 3. Monitor the following values until they return to normal (e.g., every six hours): arterial blood gases; creatine kinase, potassium, calcium, and urine and serum myoglobin; clotting; and core body temperature. Central temperature (e.g., rectal and esophageal) should be continuously monitored until stable.
> 4. Counsel the patient and family about malignant hyperthermia and further precautions. Refer the patient to MHAUS. Fill out an adverse metabolic reaction to anesthesia (AMRA) report, available through the North American Malignant Hyperthermia Registry (717-531-6936).
>
> **Caution**
> This protocol may not apply to every patient and must of necessity be altered according to specific patient needs.

Additionally, patients undergoing operations for strabismus or ptosis are at higher risk for malignant hyperthermia.

The biochemical basis for malignant hyperthermia is abnormal calcium metabolism in skeletal muscle. During normal muscle contraction, calcium is released from the sarcoplasmic reticulum into the cell cytoplasm, where it binds to troponin, permitting actin and myosin to interact to produce a contraction. During normal relaxation, calcium reuptake occurs via the sarcoplasmic reticulum. Malignant hyperthermia is characterized as an abnormally high local intracellular calcium concentration, caused by either increased release or decreased reuptake of calcium. The many intracellular calcium-mediated processes proceed without regulation, leading to a consumptive, hypermetabolic state [see 98 Fever, Hyperpyrexia, and Hypothermia].

Early clinical manifestations of malignant hyperthermia may be tachycardia and tachypnea. Other signs include a rise in arterial carbon dioxide tension (P_aCO_2) and end-tidal CO_2, hypertension, dysrhythmias, metabolic acidosis, hyperkalemia, mottled skin, cyanosis, muscle rigidity, and myoglobinuria. The rise in body temperature is usually rapid but may not be alarming until relatively late. Typically, these changes occur shortly after the induction of anesthesia, when one would normally expect a decrease in metabolic rate. Laboratory findings that would support the diagnosis of malignant hyperthermia include elevations in serum creatine kinase and lactate levels, arterial blood gas values indicative of acidosis, and an increase in P_aCO_2 in patients who would otherwise appear to be ventilated adequately.

Prompt diagnosis and appropriate treatment [see Sidebar] can reduce the mortality of malignant hyperthermia from 30 percent to approximately 10 percent. When malignant hyperthermia is suspected, the focus of the surgical team should shift from the operation to the treatment of malignant hyperthermia. All triggering agents should be discontinued immediately, and the patient should be hyperventilated with 100 percent oxygen. The surgical procedure should be canceled or terminated. Specific pharmacological intervention should begin immediately.

Administration of dantrolene is the mainstay of treatment of malignant hyperthermia. Dantrolene reduces intracellular concentrations of calcium by decreasing calcium release from the sarcoplasmic reticulum. The initial dose is 2.5 mg/kg administered intravenously. The maximum dose is debatable: up to 10 mg/kg has been administered successfully, but many believe that higher doses may be needed for reliable prevention of delayed malignant hyperthermia. Doses should be repeated every four hours and continued over the next 12 to 48 hours while the patient is closely monitored in an intensive care setting.

In addition to dantrolene therapy, other important steps should be taken to treat malignant hyperthermia. Acidosis and hyperkalemia should be treated with sodium bicarbonate (1 to 2 mEq/kg I.V.) and combined glucose and insulin, respectively. Active cooling measures, including iced saline solutions for gastric lavage or external ice packs, may be instituted. If dysrhythmias occur, they can be treated in the usual fashion, with one exception: calcium channel blocking agents should not be used in combination with dantrolene, because they may interfere with its actions.

Although no single laboratory test can be considered specific in the diagnosis of an acute malignant hyperthermia episode, several indices of a hypermetabolic state may be useful: serial arterial blood gas values, electrolyte concentrations, lactate levels, and creatine kinase levels. However, peak creatine kinase levels may not be reached until hours after the initial episode. Close monitoring of temperature, end-tidal CO_2, and urine output is important to check the status and treatment of malignant hyperthermia. Cardiovascular instability, coagulopathy, cerebral edema, pulmonary edema, continued metabolic disturbances, rhabdomyolysis, and renal failure may result during the malignant hyperthermia episode and should be considered continually during the course of patient care.

Patients who have had an episode of malignant hyperthermia in the past or have a positive family history for the condition may undergo anesthesia safely, given proper forethought. Advance consultation with an anesthesiologist will allow evaluation of the risk, appropriate consideration of regional techniques, and the selection of drugs not associated with malignant hyperthermia. Full preparations for the perioperative management of malignant hyperthermia, including consideration of prophylactic treatment with dantrolene, can be made.

The Malignant Hyperthermia Association of the United States provides 24-hour phone consultations with physicians for emergencies (209-634-4917).

References

1. Wood M: Plasma drug binding: implications for anesthesiologists. Anesth Analg 65:786, 1986
2. Marty J, Nimier M, Rocchiccioli C, et al: β-Adrenergic receptor function is acutely altered in surgical patients. Anesth Analg 71:1, 1990
3. Cullen DJ, Eger EI II, Stevens WC, et al: Clinical signs of anesthesia. Anesthesiology 36:21, 1972
4. Fennelly M, Galletly DC, Purdie GI: Is caffeine withdrawal the mechanism of postoperative headache? Anesth Analg 72:449, 1991
5. Cullen DJ, Nemeskal AR, Cooper JB, et al: Effect of pulse oximetry, age, and ASA physical status on the frequency of patients admitted unexpectedly to a postoperative intensive care unit and the severity of their anesthesia-related complications. Anesth Analg 74:181, 1992
6. White PF: Pharmacologic and clinical aspects of preoperative medication. Anesth Analg 65:963, 1986
7. Tinetti ME, Speechley M, Ginter SF: Risk factors for falls among elderly persons living in the community. N Engl J Med 319:1701, 1988
8. Ray WA, Griffin MR, Schaffner W, et al: Psychotropic drug use and the risk of hip fracture. N Engl J Med 316:363, 1987
9. Ghignone M, Calvillo O, Quintin L: Anesthesia and hypertension: the effect of clonidine on perioperative hemodynamics and isoflurane requirements. Anesthesiology 67:3, 1987
10. Ghignone M, Noe C, Calvillo O, et al: Anesthesia for ophthalmic surgery in the elderly: the effects of clonidine on intraocular pressure, perioperative hemodynamics, and anesthetic requirement. Anesthesiology 68:707, 1988
11. Manchikanti L, Colliver JA, Marrero TC, et al: Ranitidine and metoclopramide for prophylaxis of aspiration pneumonitis in elective surgery. Anesth Analg 63:903, 1984
12. Manchikanti L, Colliver JA, Marrero TC, et al: Assessment of age-related acid aspiration risk factors in pediatric, adult, and geriatric patients. Anesth Analg 64:11, 1985
13. Prys-Roberts C: Anaesthesia: A practical or impractical construct? (editorial). Br J Anaesth 59:1341, 1987
14. Ueda I, Kamaya H: Molecular mechanisms of anesthesia (review). Anesth Analg 63:929, 1984
15. Hollenberg M, Mangano DT, Browner WS, et al: Predictors of postoperative myocardial ischemia in patients undergoing noncardiac surgery. JAMA 268:205, 1992
16. Raby KE, Barry J, Creager MA, et al: Detection and significance of intraoperative and postoperative myocardial ischemia in peripheral vascular surgery. JAMA 268:222, 1992
17. Audenaert SM, Montgomery CL, Stone B, et al: Retrograde-assisted fiberoptic tracheal intubation in children with difficult airways. Anesth Analg 73:660, 1991
18. Boucek CD, Gunnerson HB, Tullock WC: Percutaneous transtracheal high-frequency jet ventilation as an aid to fiberoptic intubation. Anesthesiology 67:247, 1987
19. Fink BR: Laryngeal complications of general anesthesia. Complications in Anesthesiology. Orkin FK, Cooperman LH, Eds. JB Lippincott, Inc, Philadelphia, 1983
20. Stirt JA, Berger JM, Sullivan SF: Lack of arrhythmogenicity of isoflurane following administration of aminophylline in dogs. Anesth Analg 62:568, 1983
21. Wrenn K, Slovis CM, Murphy F, et al: Aminophylline therapy for acute bronchospastic disease in the emergency room. Ann Intern Med 115:241, 1991
22. Valentine SJ, Marjot R, Monk CR: Preoxygenation in the elderly: a comparison of the four-maximal-breath and three-minute techniques. Anesth Analg 71:516, 1990
23. Georgescu A, Miller JN, Lecklitner ML: The Sellick maneuver causing complete airway obstruction. Anesth Analg 74:457, 1992
24. Michaels I, Serrins M, Shier NQ, et al: Anesthesia for cardiac surgery in patients receiving monoamine oxidase inhibitors. Anesth Analg 63:1041, 1984
25. El-Ganzouri AR, Ivankovich AD, Braverman B, et al: Monoamine oxidase inhibitors: should they be discontinued preoperatively? Anesth Analg 64:592, 1985
26. Forrest JB, Cahalan MK, Rehder K, et al: Multicenter study of general anesthesia: II. Results. Anesthesiology 72:262, 1990
27. Katz RL, Bigger JT Jr: Cardiac arrhythmias during anesthesia and operation. Anesthesiology 33:193, 1970
28. Stewart RB, Bardy GH, Greene HL: Wide complex tachycardia: misdiagnosis and outcome after emergent therapy. Ann Intern Med 104:766, 1986
29. Akhtar M, Shenasa M, Jazayeri M, et al: Wide QRS complex tachycardia: reappraisal of a common clinical problem (clinical review). Ann Intern Med 1:905, 1988
30. Rolf N, Coté CJ: Persistent cardiac arrhythmias in pediatric patients: effects of age, expired carbon dioxide values, depth of anesthesia, and airway management. Anesth Analg 73:720, 1991
31. Voukydis PC, Cohen SI: Catheter-induced arrhythmias. Am Heart J 88:588, 1974
32. Schneider JF, Thomas HE, Kreger BE, et al: Newly acquired right bundle-branch block: The Framingham Study. Ann Intern Med 92:37, 1980
33. Schneider JF, Thomas HE, Kreger BE, et al: Newly acquired left bundle-branch block: The Framingham Study. Ann Intern Med 90:303, 1979
34. McAnulty JH, Rahimtoola SH, Murphy ES, et al: A prospective study of sudden death in "high-risk" bundle-branch block. N Engl J Med 299:209, 1978
35. Bellocci F, Santarelli P, DiGennaro M, et al: The risk of cardiac complications in surgical patients with bifascicular block: a clinical and electrophysiologic study in 98 patients. Chest 77:343, 1980
36. Roy RC, Stafford MA, Charlton JE: Nerve injury and musculoskeletal complaints after cardiac surgery: influence of internal mammary artery dissection and left arm position. Anesth Analg 67:277, 1988
37. Gautier PE, Baele PL, Guerit JM, et al: Changes in somatosensory evoked responses during carotid endarterectomy related to head position. Anesth Analg 73:649, 1991

38. Reuler JB, Cooney TG: The pressure sore: pathophysiology and principles of management. Ann Intern Med 94:661, 1981
39. Toung TJK, McPherson RW, Ahn H, et al: Pneumocephalus: effects of patient position on the incidence and location of aerocele after posterior fossa and upper cervical cord surgery. Anesth Analg 65:65, 1986
40. Lumb AB, Nunn JF: Respiratory function and ribcage contribution to ventilation in body positions commonly used during anesthesia. Anesth Analg 73:422, 1991
41. Ghoneim MM, Block RI: Learning and consciousness during general anesthesia. Anesthesiology 76:279, 1992
42. Sessler DI, Rubinstein EH, Moayeri A: Physiologic responses to mild perianesthetic hypothermia in humans. Anesthesiology 75:594, 1991
43. Macintyre PE, Pavlin EG, Dwersteg JF: Effect of meperidine on oxygen consumption, carbon dioxide production, and respiratory gas exchange in postanesthesia shivering. Anesth Analg 66:751, 1987
44. Saada M, Catoire P, Bonnet F, et al: Effect of thoracic epidural anesthesia combined with general anesthesia on segmental wall motion assessed by transesophageal echocardiography. Anesth Analg 75:329, 1992
45. Atchison SR, Wedel DJ, Wilson PR: Effect of injection rate on level and duration of hypobaric spinal anesthesia. Anesth Analg 69:496, 1989
46. Buckey JC, Peshock RM, Blomqvist CG: Deep venous contribution to hydrostatic blood volume change in the human leg. Am J Cardiol 62:449, 1988
47. Anzai Y, Nishikawa T: Heart rate responses to body tilt during spinal anesthesia. Anesth Analg 73:385, 1991
48. Caplan RA, Ward RJ, Posner K, et al: Unexpected cardiac arrest during spinal anesthesia: a closed claims analysis of predisposing factors. Anesthesiology 68:5, 1988
49. Lybecker H, Møller JT, May O, et al: Incidence and prediction of postdural puncture headache: a prospective study of 1021 spinal anesthesias. Anesth Analg 70:389, 1990
50. DiGiovanni AJ, Dunbar BS: Epidural injections of autologous blood for postlumbar-puncture headache. Anesth Analg 49:268, 1970
51. Casement BA, Danielson DR: The epidural blood patch: are more than two ever necessary? Anesth Analg 63:1033, 1984
52. Watcha MF, White PF: Postoperative nausea and vomiting: its etiology, treatment, and prevention (review). Anesthesiology 77:162, 1992
53. Leeser J, Lip H: Prevention of postoperative nausea and vomiting using ondansetron, a new, selective, 5-HT$_3$ receptor antagonist. Anesth Analg 72:751, 1991
54. Acute Pain Management Guideline Panel. Acute Pain Management: Operative or Medical Procedures and Trauma. Clinical Practice Guideline. AHCPR Pub. No. 92-0032. Agency for Health Care Policy and Research, Public Health Service, U.S. Department of Health and Human Services, Rockville, Maryland, February 1992
55. Weil JV, McCullough RE, Kline JS, et al: Diminished ventilatory response to hypoxia and hypercapnia after morphine in normal man. N Engl J Med 292:1103, 1975
56. Flacke JW, Flacke WE, Bloor BC, et al: Histamine release by four narcotics: a double-blind study in humans. Anesth Analg 66:723, 1987
57. Bromage PR, Camporesi E, Chestnut D: Epidural narcotics for postoperative analgesia. Anesth Analg 59:473, 1980
58. Pavlin EG, Holle RH, Schoene RB: Recovery of airway protection compared with ventilation in humans after paralysis with curare. Anesthesiology 70:381, 1989

V   OPERATIVE MANAGEMENT

42 THYROID AND PARATHYROID PROCEDURES

Gregg H. Jossart, M.D., and Orlo H. Clark, M.D.

Thyroidectomy

OPERATIVE PLANNING

If the patient has had any hoarseness or has undergone a neck operation before, indirect or direct (ideally, fiberoptic) laryngoscopy is essential to determine whether the vocal cords are functioning normally. All patients scheduled for thyroidectomy should be euthyroid at the time of operation; in all other respects, they should be prepared as they would be for any procedure calling for general anesthesia.

Optimum exposure of the thyroid is obtained by placing a sandbag between the scapula and a foam ring under the occiput; in this way, the neck is extended, and the thyroid can assume a more anterior position. The head must be well supported to prevent postoperative posterior neck pain. The patient is placed in a 20° reverse Trendelenburg position. The skin is prepared with 1% iodine or chlorhexidine.

OPERATIVE TECHNIQUE

General Troubleshooting

Thyroid and parathyroid operations should be performed in a blood-free field so that vital structures can be identified. Operating telescopes (magnification: ×2.5 or ×3.5) are also recommended because they make it easier to identify the normal parathyroid glands and the recurrent laryngeal nerve. If bleeding occurs, pressure should be applied. The vessel should be clamped only if (1) it can be precisely identified or (2) the recurrent laryngeal nerve has been identified and is not in close proximity to the vessel.

As a rule, dissection should always be done first on the side where the suspected tumor is; if there is a problem with the dissection on this side, a less than total thyroidectomy can be performed on the contralateral side to prevent complications. There is, however, one exception to this rule: if the tumor is very extensive, the surgeon will sometimes find it easier to do the dissection on the "easy" side first to facilitate orientation with respect to the trachea and the esophagus.

Step 1: Incision and Mobilization of Skin Layers

A Kocher transverse incision paralleling the normal skin lines of the neck is made 1 cm caudad to the cricoid cartilage [see Figure 1]. As a rule, the incision should be about 4 to 6 cm long and should extend from the anterior border of one sternocleidomastoid muscle to the anterior border of the other and through the platysma. Five straight Kelly clamps are placed on the dermis to facilitate dissection, which proceeds first cephalad in a subplatysmal plane anterior to the anterior jugular veins and posterior to the platysma to the level of the thyroid cartilage notch and then caudad to the suprasternal notch. Skin towels and a self-retaining retractor are then applied.

Troubleshooting Placing the incision 1 cm below the cricoid locates it precisely over the isthmus of the thyroid gland. The course of the incision should conform to the normal skin lines or creases. The length of the incision should be modified as necessary for good exposure. Patients with short, thick necks, low-lying thyroid glands, or large thyroid tumors require longer incisions than those with long, thin necks and small tumors. Patients whose necks do not extend also require longer incisions for adequate exposure. A sterile marking pen should be used to mark the midline of the neck, the level at which the incision should be made (i.e., 1 cm below the cricoid), and the lateral margins of the incision (which should be at equal distances from the midline so that the incision will be symmetrical). A scalpel should never be used to mark the neck: doing so will leave an unsightly scar in some patients. To mark the incision site itself, a 2-0 silk tie should be pressed against the neck [see Figure 1].

The upper flap is dissected first by placing five straight Kelly clamps on the dermis and retracting anteriorly and superiorly. Lateral traction with a vein retractor or an Army-Navy retractor

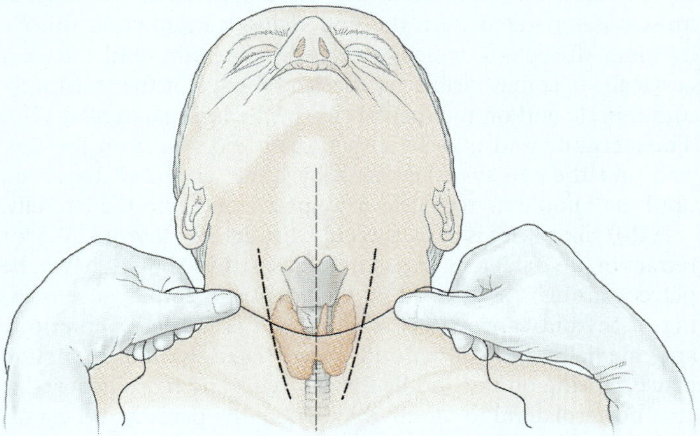

Figure 1 The initial incision in a thyroidectomy is made 1 cm below the cricoid cartilage and follows normal skin lines. A sterile marking pen is used to mark the midline of the neck, the level of the incision, and the lateral borders of the incision. A 2-0 silk tie is pressed against the neck to mark the incision site itself.[2]

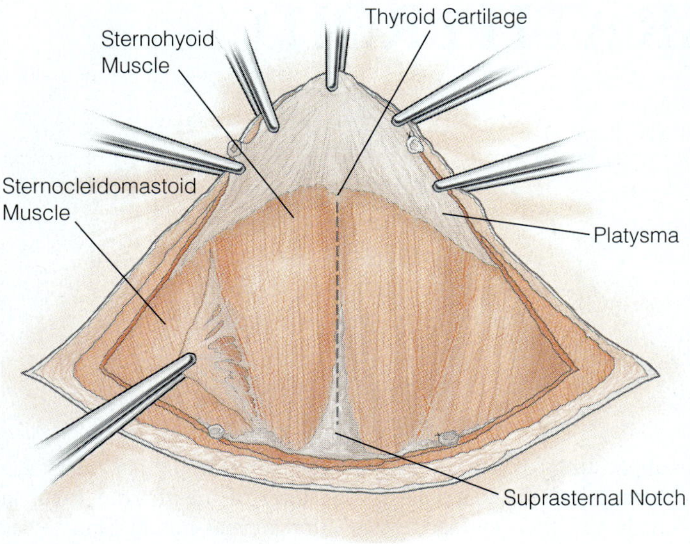

Figure 2 To expose the thyroid, a midline incision is made through the superficial layer of deep cervical fascia between the strap muscles. The incision is begun at the suprasternal notch and extended to the thyroid cartilage.[3]

helps identify the semilunar plane for dissection. This blood-free plane is deep to the platysma and superficial to the anterior jugular veins. Cephalad dissection can be done quickly with the electrocautery or a scalpel, and lateral dissection can be done bluntly. The same principles are applied to dissection of the lower flap. In thin patients, the surgeon must be careful not to dissect through the skin from within, especially at the level of the thyroid cartilage.

Step 2: Midline Dissection and Mobilization of Strap Muscles

The thyroid gland is exposed via a midline incision through the superficial layer of deep cervical fascia between the strap muscles. Because the strap muscles are farthest apart just above the suprasternal notch, the incision is begun at the notch and extended to the thyroid cartilage [*see Figure 2*].

On the side where the thyroid nodule or the suspected parathyroid adenoma is located, the more superficial sternohyoid muscle is separated from the underlying sternothyroid muscle by blunt dissection, which is extended laterally until the ansa cervicalis becomes visible on the lateral edge of the sternothyroid muscle and on the medial side of the internal jugular vein. The sternothyroid muscle is then dissected free from the thyroid and the prethyroidal fascia by blunt or sharp dissection until the middle thyroid vein or veins are encountered laterally.

A 2-0 silk suture is placed deeply through the thyroid lobe for retraction to facilitate exposure. This stitch should never be placed through the thyroid nodule: doing so could cause seeding of thyroid cancer cells. The thyroid is retracted anteriorly and medially and the carotid sheath laterally; this retraction places tension on the middle thyroid veins and helps expose the area posterolateral to the thyroid, where the parathyroid glands and the recurrent laryngeal nerves are situated. The middle thyroid veins are divided to give better exposure behind the upper lobe of the thyroid [*see Figure 3*].

Troubleshooting As a rule, it is not necessary to divide the strap muscles; however, if they are adherent to the underlying thyroid tumor, the portion of the muscle that is adhering to the tumor should be sacrificed and allowed to remain attached to the thyroid. Separation of the sternohyoid muscle from the sternothyroid muscle provides better exposure of the operative field. The middle thyroid veins should be cleaned of adjacent tissues to prevent any injury to the recurrent laryngeal nerve when these veins are ligated and divided. It is always safest to mobilize tissues parallel to the recurrent laryngeal nerve.

Step 3: Division of Isthmus

When a thyroid lobectomy is to be performed, the isthmus of the thyroid gland is usually divided with Dandy or Colodny clamps at an early point in dissection to facilitate the subsequent mobilization of the thyroid gland. The thyroid tissue that is to remain is oversewn with a 2-0 silk ligature. To minimize the chance of invasion into the trachea or to avoid a visible mass in patients with compensatory thyroid hypertrophy, thyroid tissues should not be left anterior to the trachea.

Troubleshooting With larger glands, we divide the isthmus first. This step facilitates the lateral dissection by making the gland more mobile.

Step 4: Mobilization of Thyroid Gland and Identification of Upper Parathyroid Glands

Once the isthmus has been divided, dissection is continued superiorly, laterally, and posteriorly with a small sponge on a peanut clamp. The superior thyroid artery and veins are identified by retracting the thyroid inferiorly and medially. The tissues lateral to the upper lobe of the thyroid and medial to the carotid sheath can be mobilized caudally to the cricothyroid muscle; the recurrent laryngeal nerve enters the cricothyroid muscle at the level of the cricoid cartilage, first passing through Berry's ligament [*see Figure 4*]. The superior pole vessels are individually identified, skeletonized, double- or triple-clamped, ligated, and divided low on the thyroid gland [*see Figure 5*]. To prevent injury to the external laryngeal nerve, the vessels are divided and ligated on the thyroid surface, the thyroid is retracted laterally and caudally, and dissection is carried out on the medial edge of the thyroid gland and lateral to the cricothyroid muscle. The tis-

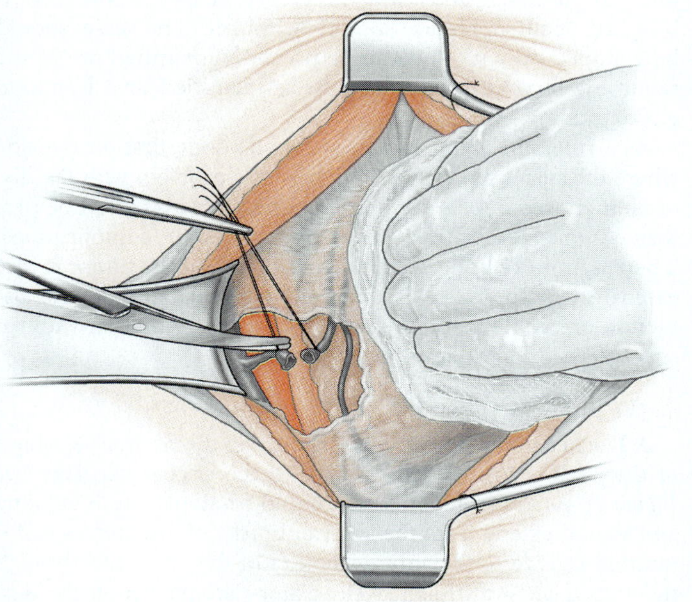

Figure 3 The middle thyroid veins are divided to give better exposure behind the upper lobe of the thyroid.[2]

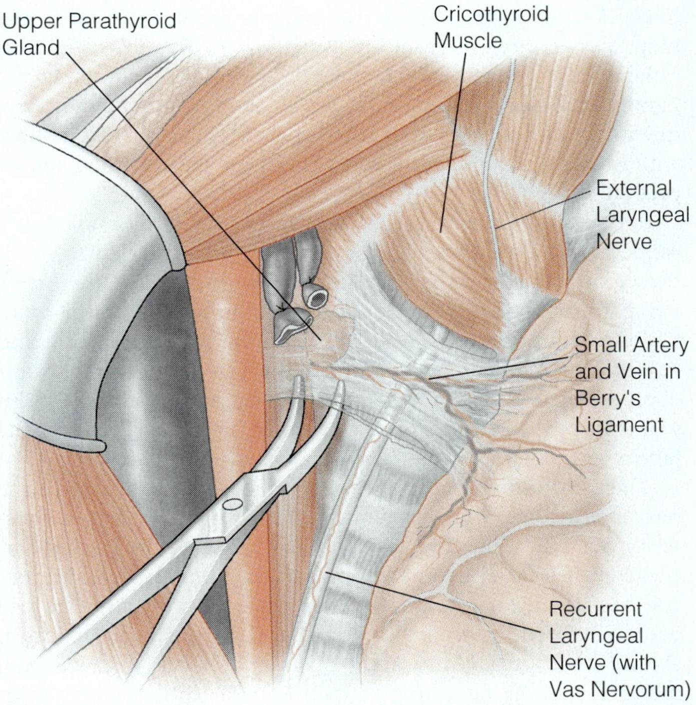

Figure 4 The recurrent laryngeal nerve enters the cricothyroid muscle at the level of the cricoid cartilage, first passing through Berry's ligament.[2]

sues posterior and lateral to the superior pole that have not already been mobilized can now be easily swept by blunt dissection away from the thyroid gland medially and anteriorly and away from the carotid sheath laterally. The upper parathyroid gland is often identified at this time at the level of the cricoid cartilage.

Troubleshooting It is essential to keep from injuring the external laryngeal nerve. This nerve is the motor branch of the superior laryngeal nerve and is responsible for tensing the vocal cords; it is also known as the high note nerve or the Amelita Galli-Curci nerve. In about 80% of patients, the external laryngeal nerve runs on the surface of the cricothyroid muscle; in about 10%, it runs with the superior pole vessels; and in the remaining 10%, it runs within the cricothyroid muscle. Given that this nerve is usually about the size of a single strand of a spider web, one should generally try to avoid it rather than to identify it. Injury to the external laryngeal nerve occurs in as many as 10% of patients undergoing thyroidectomy. The best ways of preventing such injury are (1) to provide gentle traction on the thyroid gland in a caudal and lateral direction and (2) to ligate the superior pole vessels directly on the capsule of the upper pole individually and low on the thyroid gland rather than to cross-clamp the entire superior pole pedicle.

The internal laryngeal nerve is the sensory branch of the superior laryngeal nerve; it provides sensory innervation to the posterior pharynx. Injury to this nerve can result in aspiration. Because the internal laryngeal nerve typically is cephalad to the area of dissection during thyroidectomy and runs cephalad to the lateral portion of the thyroid cartilage, it usually is at risk only when the surgeon dissects cephalad to the thyroid cartilage. Such dissection is necessary only when laryngeal mobilization is performed to relieve tension on the tracheal anastomosis after tracheal resection.

Step 5: Identification of Recurrent Laryngeal Nerves and Lower Parathyroid Glands

When the thyroid lobe is further mobilized, the lower parathyroid gland is usually seen; this gland is almost always located anterior to the recurrent laryngeal nerve and is usually located inferior to where the inferior thyroid artery crosses the recurrent laryngeal nerve [see Figure 6]. The carotid sheath is retracted laterally, and the thyroid gland is retracted anteriorly and medially. This retraction puts tension on the inferior thyroid artery and consequently on the recurrent laryngeal nerve, thereby facilitating the identification of the nerve. The recurrent laryngeal nerve is situated more medially on the left (running in the tracheoesophageal groove) and more obliquely on the right. Dissection should proceed cephalad along the lateral edge of the thyroid. Fatty and lymphatic tissues immediately adjacent to the thyroid gland are swept from it with a peanut clamp, and small vessels are ligated. No tissue should be transected until one is sure that it is not the recurrent laryngeal nerve.

Troubleshooting The upper parathyroid glands are usually situated on each side of the thyroid gland at the level where the recurrent laryngeal nerve enters the cricothyroid muscle [see Figure 6]. Because the recurrent laryngeal nerve enters the cricothyroid muscle at the level of the cricoid cartilage, the area cephalad to the cricoid cartilage is relatively safe.

The right and left recurrent laryngeal nerves must be preserved during every thyroid operation. Although both nerves enter at the posterior medial position of the larynx in the cricothyroid muscle, their courses vary considerably. The right recurrent laryngeal nerve takes a more oblique course than the left recurrent laryngeal nerve and may pass either anterior or posterior to the inferior thyroid artery. In about 0.5% of persons, the right recurrent laryngeal nerve is in fact nonrecurrent and may enter the thyroid from a superior or lateral direction.[1] On rare occasions, both a recurrent and a nonrecurrent laryn-

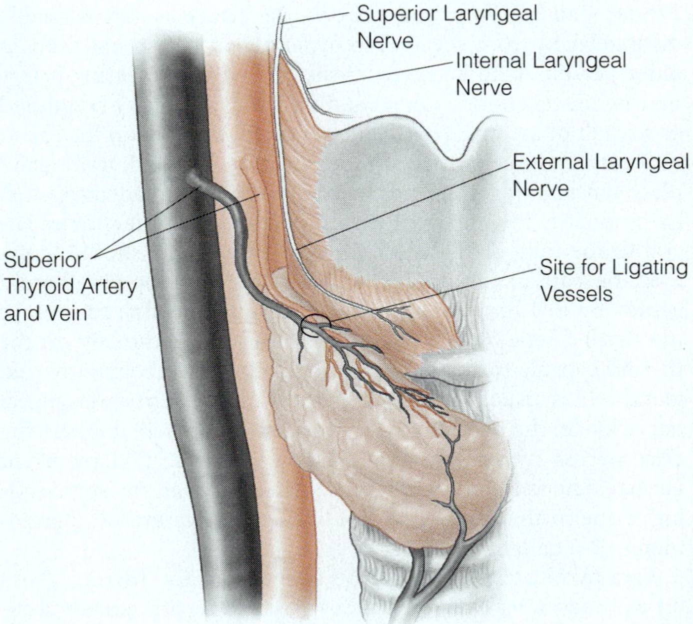

Figure 5 The superior pole vessels should be individually identified and ligated low on the thyroid gland to minimize the chances of injury to the external laryngeal nerve.[2]

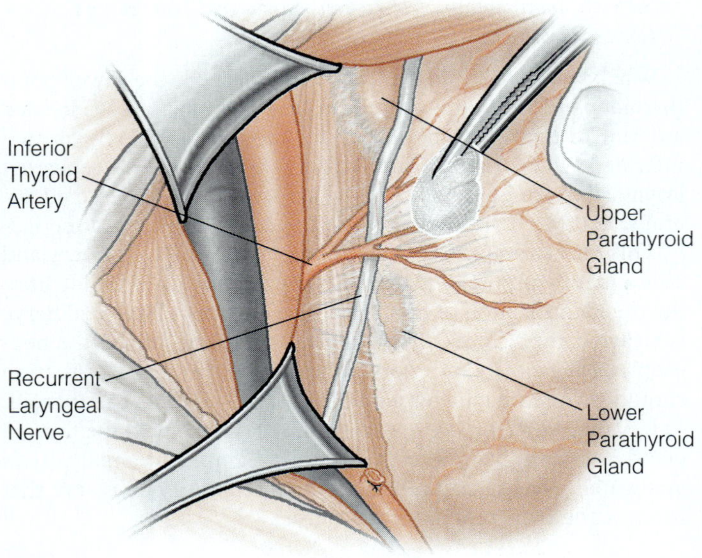

Figure 6 The upper parathyroid glands are usually situated on either side of the thyroid at the level where the recurrent laryngeal nerve enters the cricothyroid muscle. The lower parathyroid glands are usually anterior to the recurrent laryngeal nerve and inferior to where the inferior thyroid artery crosses this nerve.[2]

geal nerve may be present on the right. The left recurrent laryngeal nerve almost always runs in the tracheoesophageal groove because of its deeper origin within the thorax as it loops around the ductus arteriosus. Either recurrent laryngeal nerve may branch before entering the larynx; the left nerve is more likely to do this. Such branching is important to recognize because all of the motor fibers of the recurrent laryngeal nerve are usually in the most medial branch.

In identifying the recurrent laryngeal nerves, it is helpful to remember that they are supplied by a small vascular plexus and that a tiny vessel runs parallel to and directly on each nerve [see Figures 4 and 6]. In young persons, the artery usually is readily distinguished from the recurrent laryngeal nerve; however, in older persons with arteriosclerosis, the white-appearing artery may be mistaken for a nerve, and thus the nerve may be injured as a result of the misidentification. Lateral traction on the carotid sheath and medial and anterior traction on the thyroid gland place tension on the inferior thyroid artery; this maneuver often helps identify the recurrent laryngeal nerve where it courses lateral to the midportion of the thyroid gland. One should, however, be careful not to devascularize the inferior parathyroid glands by dividing the lateral vascular attachments: to remove the thyroid lobe, it is best to divide the vessels directly on the thyroid capsule to preserve the blood supply to the parathyroid glands. It is usually safest to identify the recurrent laryngeal nerve low in the neck and then to follow it to where it enters the cricothyroid muscle through Berry's ligament. The recurrent laryngeal nerves can usually be palpated through the surrounding tissue in the neck; they feel like a taut ligature of approximately 2-0 gauge.

Parathyroid glands should be swept from the thyroid gland on as broad a vascular pedicle as possible to prevent devascularization. When it is unclear whether a parathyroid gland can be saved on its own vascular pedicle, one should biopsy the gland to confirm that it is parathyroid and then autotransplant it in multiple 1 × 1 mm pieces into separate pockets in the ster-

nocleidomastoid muscle. At times, it is preferable to clip the blood vessels running from the thyroid to the parathyroid glands rather than to clamp and tie them. Clipping not only marks the parathyroid gland (which is useful if another operation subsequently becomes necessary) but also enables the gland to remain with minimal manipulation and with its remaining blood supply preserved.

In patients who have extensive thyroid tumors or who require reoperation, extensive scarring is often present. For some of these patients, it is preferable to identify the recurrent laryngeal nerve from a medial approach by dividing the isthmus with Colodny clamps and ligating and dividing the superior thyroid vessels. By carefully dissecting the thyroid away from the trachea, one can identify the recurrent laryngeal nerve at the point where its position is most consistent (i.e., at its entrance into the larynx immediately posterior to the cricothyroid muscle).

The most difficult part of dissection in a thyroidectomy is the part that involves Berry's ligament, which is situated at the posterior portion of the thyroid gland just caudal to the cricoid cartilage [see Figure 4]. A small branch of the inferior thyroid artery traverses the ligament, as do one or more veins from the thyroid gland. If bleeding occurs during this part of the dissection, it should be controlled by applying pressure with a gauze pad. Nothing should be clamped in this area until the recurrent laryngeal nerve is identified. In some patients (about 15%), the peduncle of Zuckerkandl, a small protuberance of thyroid tissue on the right, tends to obscure the recurrent laryngeal nerve at the level of Berry's ligament.

Step 6: Mobilization of Pyramidal Lobe

The pyramidal lobe is found in about 80% of patients. It extends in a cephalad direction, often through the notch in the thyroid cartilage to the hyoid bone. One or more lymph nodes are frequently found just cephalad to the isthmus of the thyroid gland over the cricothyroid membrane (so-called Delphian nodes) [see Figure 7]. The pyramidal lobe is mobilized by retracting it caudally and by dissecting immediately adjacent to it in a cephalad direction. Small vessels are coagulated or ligated.

Step 7: Thyroid Resection

Once the parathyroid glands have been carefully swept or dissected from the thyroid gland and the recurrent nerve has been identified, the thyroid lobe can be quickly resected. For total thyroidectomy, the same operation is done again on the other side.

Troubleshooting The thyroid lobe or gland should be carefully examined after removal. If a parathyroid gland is identified, a biopsy of it should be performed to confirm that it is parathyroid and then autotransplanted. In a thyroid procedure, every parathyroid gland should be treated as if it is the last one, and at least one parathyroid gland should be definitely identified. As a rule, biopsies should not be performed on normal parathyroid glands during a thyroid procedure.

Step 8: Closure

The sternothyroid muscles are approximated with 4-0 absorbable sutures, and a small opening is left in the midline at the suprasternal notch to make any bleeding that occurs more evident and to allow the blood to exit. The sternohyoid muscles are reapproximated in a similar fashion, as is the platysma. The skin is then closed with butterfly clips, which are hemostatic and inexpensive and permit precise alignment of the skin edges. (In children, the skin is closed with a subcuticular stitch and Steri-

Strips instead.) A sterile pressure dressing is applied.

Special Concerns

Invasion of the trachea or the esophagus On rare occasions, thyroid or parathyroid cancers may invade the trachea or the esophagus. As much as 5 cm of the trachea can be resected safely, without impairment of the patient's voice. If the invasion is not extensive and is confined to the anterior portion of the trachea, a small section of the trachea that contains the tumor should be excised, and a tracheostomy may be placed at the site of resection. If the invasion is more extensive or occurs in the lateral or posterior portion of the trachea, a segment of the trachea measuring several centimeters long is resected, and the remaining segments are reanastomosed. To prevent tension on the anastomosis, the trachea should be mobilized before resection, the recurrent laryngeal nerves should be preserved and mobilized from the trachea, and the mylohyoid fascia and muscles should be divided above the thyroid cartilage to drop the cartilage. Pains must be taken not to injure the internal laryngeal nerves during this dissection, given that these nerves course from lateral to medial just above the lateral aspects of the thyroid cartilage. After resection, the trachea is reapproximated with 3-0 Maxon sutures. One or two Penrose drains should be left near the resection site to allow air to exit. The drains are removed after several days, when there is no more evidence of air leakage.

If the esophagus is invaded by tumor, the muscular wall of the esophagus can be resected along with the tumor, with the inner esophageal layer left in place.

Neck dissection for nodal metastases Lymph nodes in the central neck (medial to the carotid sheath) are frequently involved in patients with papillary, medullary, and Hürthle cell cancer. These nodes should be removed without injury to the parathyroid glands or the recurrent laryngeal nerves. In most patients, it is relatively easy to remove all tissue between the carotid sheath and the trachea. In some patients with extensive lymphadenopathy, it is necessary to remove the parathyroids, perform biopsies on them to confirm that they are in fact parathyroid, and autotransplant them into the sternocleidomastoid muscle.

When lymph nodes are palpable in the lateral neck, a modified neck dissection is performed through a lateral extension of the Kocher collar incision to the anterior margin of the trapezius muscle (a MacFee incision). The jugular vein, the spinal accessory nerve, the phrenic nerve, the vagus nerve, the cervical sympathetic nerves, and the sternocleidomastoid muscle are preserved unless they are directly adherent to or invaded by tumor.

In patients with medullary thyroid cancer, a meticulous and thorough central neck dissection is necessary. When a primary medullary tumor is larger than 1 cm or the central neck nodes are obviously involved, these patients will also benefit from a lateral modified radical neck dissection (with the structures just mentioned preserved). During the dissection, all fibrofatty lymph node tissues should be removed from the level of the clavicle to the level of the hyoid bone. The deep dissection plane is developed anterior to the scalenus anticus muscle, the brachial plexus, and the scalenus medius muscle. The phrenic nerve runs obliquely on the scalenus anticus muscle. The cervical sensory nerves can usually be preserved unless there is extensive tumor involvement.

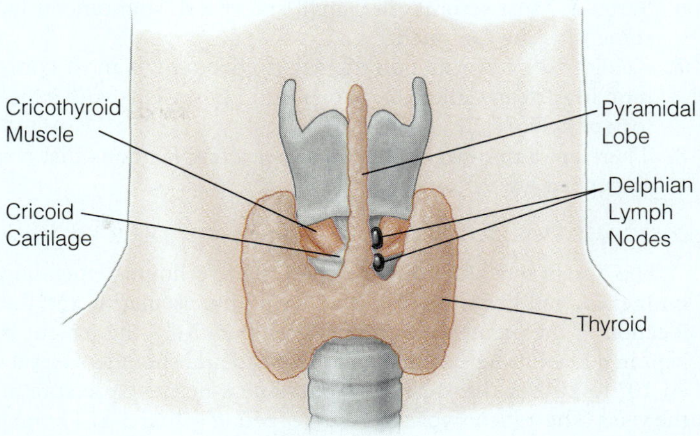

Figure 7 Delphian lymph nodes may be found just cephalad to the isthmus over the cricothyroid membrane.

Median sternotomy A median sternotomy is rarely necessary for removal of the thyroid gland because the blood supply to the thyroid gland, the thymus, and the lower parathyroid glands derives primarily from the inferior thyroid arteries in the neck. Metastatic lymph nodes frequently extend inferiorly in the tracheoesophageal groove into the superior mediastinum; these nodes can almost always be removed through a cervical incision without any need for a sternotomy. On rare occasions, metastatic nodes spread to the aortic pulmonary window and can be identified preoperatively on CT or MRI. If a median sternotomy proves necessary, the sternum should be divided to the level of the third intercostal space and then laterally on one side at the space between the third rib and the fourth. Median sternotomy provides excellent exposure of the upper anterior mediastinum and the lower neck.

COMPLICATIONS

The following are the most significant complications of thyroidectomy.

1. Injury to the recurrent laryngeal nerve. Bilateral injury to the recurrent laryngeal nerve may result in vocal cord paresis and stridor and may have to be treated with a tracheostomy.
2. Hypoparathyroidism. This complication may arise as the result of removal of, injury to, or devascularization of the parathyroid glands. As noted [see Operative Technique, *above*], we recommend leaving parathyroid glands on their own vascular pedicle; however, if one is concerned about possible devascularization of a parathyroid, biopsy should be performed on the gland to confirm its identity and then autotransplanted in 1 × 1 mm pieces into separate pockets in the sternocleidomastoid muscle.
3. Bleeding. Postoperative bleeding can be life threatening in that it can compromise the airway. Any postoperative respiratory distress can be thought of as attributable to a neck hematoma until proved otherwise. Most bleeding occurs within four hours of operation, and virtually all occurs within 24 hours.
4. Injury to the external laryngeal nerve [see Operative Technique, *above*].
5. Infection. This complication is quite rare after thyroidectomy. Any patient with acute pharyngitis should not undergo this procedure.

6. Seroma. Most seromas are small and resorb spontaneously; some must be aspirated.
7. Keloid. Keloid formation after thyroidectomy is most common in African-American patients and in patients with a history of keloids.
8. There are a number of miscellaneous complications that are somewhat less common.

OUTCOME EVALUATION

The duration of a thyroid operation is 1 to 3 hours, depending on the size and invasiveness of the tumor, its vascularity, and the location of the parathyroid glands. Postoperatively, the patient is kept in a low Fowler position with the head and shoulders elevated 10° to 20° for 6 to 12 hours to maintain negative pressure in the veins. The patient typically resumes eating within 3 to 4 hours, and an antiemetic is ordered as needed (many patients experience postoperative nausea and emesis).

The serum calcium level is measured approximately 5 to 8 hours after operation in patients who have undergone bilateral procedures; no tests are required in those who have undergone unilateral procedures. On the first morning after the thyroidectomy, the serum calcium and serum phosphate levels are measured. If the patient is still hospitalized on postoperative day 2, these tests are repeated on the second morning as well. Oral calcium supplements are given if the serum calcium is below 7.5 mg/dl or if the patient experiences perioral numbness or tingling. A low serum phosphate level (< 2.5 mg/dl) usually is a sign of so-called bone hunger and suggests that there is little reason to be concerned about permanent hypoparathyroidism, whereas a high level (> 4.5 mg/dl) should prompt concern about permanent hypoparathyroidism.

The surgical clips are removed on postoperative day 1, and Steri-Strips are applied to prevent tension on the healing wound. Patients usually are discharged on the first day, are given a prescription for thyroid hormone (L-thyroxine, 0.1 to 0.2 mg/day orally) if the procedure was more extensive than a thyroid lobectomy, and are told to take calcium tablets for any tingling or muscle cramps. Patients with papillary, follicular, or Hürthle cell cancer should receive enough L-thyroxine to keep their serum levels of thyroid-stimulating hormone (TSH) below 0.1 mIU/ml. The Steri-Strips are removed on day 10, the pathology is reviewed, and further management is discussed in the light of the pathologic findings. In patients with thyroid cancer, values for serum calcium, TSH, and thyroglobulin are obtained; in patients with coexisting hyperparathyroidism, values for serum calcium, phosphorus, and parathyroid hormone (PTH) are obtained.

Most patients can return to work or full activity in 1 to 2 weeks. Patients with benign lesions who have undergone hemithyroidectomy may or may not require thyroid hormone; those with multinodular goiter, thyroiditis, or occult papillary cancer typically do, whereas those with follicular adenoma typically do not. Patients who have undergone total or near-total thyroidectomy will require thyroid hormone. Patients with papillary or follicular cancer who have undergone total or near-total thyroidectomy appear to benefit from radioactive iodine scanning and therapy. (It is necessary to discontinue L-thyroxine for 6 to 8 weeks and L-triiodothyronine for 2 weeks before scanning.) Those considered to be at low risk (age < 45 years, tumor confined to the thyroid and not invasive, and tumor diameter < 4 cm) may receive radioactive iodine on an outpatient basis in a dose of approximately 30 mCi. Those who are considered to be at high risk should receive approximately 100 to 150 mCi. Long-term (20-year) mortality is about 4% in low-risk patients and about 40% in high-risk patients. Serum thyroglobulin levels should be determined before and after discontinuance of thyroid hormone; such levels are very sensitive indicators of persistent thyroid disease after total thyroidectomy.

Parathyroidectomy

OPERATIVE PLANNING

The preparation for parathyroidectomy is the same as that for thyroidectomy. Patients who have profound hypercalcemia (serum calcium ≥ 12.5 mg/dl) or mild to moderate renal failure should be vigorously hydrated and given furosemide before operation. On rare occasions, such patients require additional treatment—for example, administration of diphosphonates, mithramycin, or calcitonin. Any electrolyte abnormalities (e.g., hypokalemia) should be corrected.

We recommend bilateral exploration for most patients undergoing initial operations for primary or secondary hyperparathyroidism. For some patients with sporadic primary hyperparathyroidism in whom one abnormal gland has been identified by sestamibi scanning, a focused operation using intraoperative PTH assay is an acceptable alternative approach. Preoperative localization studies (e.g., ultrasonography, MRI, sestamibi scanning, and CT scanning) are generally unnecessary: they provide useful information in about 75% of patients, but they are not considered cost-effective, because an experienced surgeon can treat hyperparathyroidism successfully 95% to 98% of the time. Such studies are, however, essential when reoperation for persistent or recurrent hyperparathyroidism is indicated and when a focused approach with intraoperative PTH assay is to be used. We do not believe that using the gamma probe is any better than preoperative sestamibi scanning. All patients requiring reoperation should undergo direct or indirect laryngoscopy before operation for evaluation of vocal cord function.

OPERATIVE TECHNIQUE

Steps 1 through 4

Steps 1, 2, 3, and 4 of a parathyroidectomy are virtually identical to steps 1, 2, 4, and 5 of a thyroidectomy (see above), and essentially the same troubleshooting considerations apply.

Troubleshooting About 85% of people have four parathyroid glands, and in about 85% of these persons, the parathyroids are situated on the posterior lateral capsule of the thyroid. Normal parathyroid glands measure about 3 × 3 × 4 mm and are light brown in color. The upper parathyroid glands are more posterior (i.e., dorsal) and more constant in position (at the level of the cricoid cartilage) than the lower parathyroid glands, which typically are more anteriorly placed (on the posterior-lateral surface of the thyroid gland). Both the upper and the lower parathyroid glands are supplied by small branches of the inferior and superior thyroid arteries in most patients. About 15% of parathyroid glands are situated within the thymus gland, and about 1% are intrathyroidal. Other abnormal sites for the parathyroid glands are (1) the carotid sheath, (2) the anterior and posterior mediastinum, and (3) anterior to the carotid bulb or along the pharynx (undescended parathyroids).

The upper parathyroid glands are usually lateral to the recurrent laryngeal nerve at the level of Berry's ligament; their position makes them generally easier to preserve during thyroidectomy and easier to find during both parathyroid and thyroid surgery. When the upper parathyroids are not found at this site, they often can be found in the tracheoesophageal groove or in the posterior mediastinum along the esophagus. The lower parathyroid glands are almost always situated anterior to the recurrent laryngeal nerves and caudal to where the recurrent laryngeal nerve crosses the inferior thyroid artery; they may be surrounded by lymph nodes. When the lower parathyroids are not found at this site, they usually can be found in the anterior mediastinum (typically in the thymus or the thymic fat).

Step 5: Parathyroid Resection

Abnormal parathyroid glands are removed. In about 80% of patients with primary hyperparathyroidism, one parathyroid gland is abnormal; in about 15%, all glands are abnormal (diffuse hyperplasia); and in about 5%, two or three glands are abnormal and one or two normal. Parathyroid cancer occurs in about 1% of patients with primary hyperparathyroidism. About 50% of patients with parathyroid cancer have a palpable tumor, and most exhibit profound hypercalcemia (serum calcium ≥ 14.0 mg/dl).

Troubleshooting In some patients, parathyroid tumors and hyperplastic parathyroid glands are difficult to find. If this is the case, the first step is to explore the sites where parathyroids are usually located, near the posterolateral surface of the thyroid gland. (About 80% of parathyroid glands are situated within 1 cm of the point where the inferior thyroid artery crosses the recurrent laryngeal nerve.) When a lower gland is missing from the usual location, it is likely to be found in the thymus; this possibility can be confirmed by mobilizing the thymus from the anterior-superior mediastinum. In all, about 15% of parathyroid glands are found within the thymus. If an upper parathyroid gland cannot be located, one should look not only far behind the thyroid gland superiorly but also in a paraesophageal position down into the posterior mediastinum. A thyroid lobectomy or thyroidotomy should be done on the side where fewer than two parathyroid glands have been located and no abnormal parathyroid tissue has been identified. The carotid sheath and the area posterior to the carotid, as well as the retroesophageal area, should also be explored. In rare cases, there may be an undescended parathyroid tumor anterior to the carotid bulb.

Although we do not recommend routine biopsy of more than one normal-appearing parathyroid gland, we do recommend biopsy (not removal) and marking of all normal parathyroid glands that have been identified when no abnormal parathyroid tissue can be found. When four normal parathyroid glands are found in the neck, the fifth (abnormal) parathyroid gland is usually in the mediastinum. The surgeon's responsibility is to make sure during parathyroidectomy that the elusive parathyroid adenoma is not in or removable through the cervical incision used for the initial operation and to minimize complications. The risk of permanent hypoparathyroidism or injury to the recurrent nerve should be less than 2%.

Step 6: Closure

Closure is essentially the same for parathyroidectomy as for thyroidectomy.

COMPLICATIONS

The complications of parathyroidectomy are similar to those of thyroidectomy but occur less often. Patients with a very high serum alkaline phosphatase level and osteitis fibrosa cystica are prone to profound hypocalcemia after parathyroidectomy. In such patients, both serum calcium and serum phosphorus levels are low. In contrast, patients with hypoparathyroidism exhibit low serum calcium levels but high serum phosphorus levels.

OUTCOME EVALUATION

Outcome considerations are essentially the same as for thyroidectomy. The patient should have a normal voice and be normocalcemic. The overall complication rate should be less than 2%.

References

1. Henry JF, Audiffret J, Denizot A, et al: The nonrecurrent inferior laryngeal nerve: review of 33 cases, including two on the left side. Surgery 104:977, 1988
2. Clark OH: Endocrine Surgery of the Thyroid and Parathyroid Glands. CV Mosby, St Louis, 1985
3. Cady B, Rossi R: Surgery of thyroid gland. Surgery of the Thyroid and Parathyroid Glands. Cady B, Rossi R, Eds. WB Saunders Co, Philadelphia, 1991

Acknowledgment

Figures 1 through 7   Tom Moore.

Recommended Reading

Chen H, Sokol LJ, Udelsman R: Outpatient minimally invasive parathyroidectomy: a combination of sestamibi-spect localization, cervical block anesthesia, and intraoperative parathyroid hormone assay. Surgery 126:1016, 1999

Clark OH: Total thyroidectomy and lymph node dissection for cancer of the thyroid. Mastery of Surgery, 2nd ed. Nyhus LM, Baker RJ, Eds. Little, Brown and Co, Boston, 1992, p 204

Clark OH: Total thyroid lobectomy. Atlas of Surgical Oncology. Daly JM, Cady B, Low DW, Eds. CV Mosby Co, St. Louis, 1993, p 41

Gordon LL, Snyder WH, Wians JR, et al: The validity of quick intraoperative hormone assay: an evaluation of seventy-two patients based on gross morphology criteria. Surgery 126:1030, 1999

Irvin GL, Molinari AS, Figuero C, et al: Improved success rate in reoperative parathyroidectomy with intraoperative PTH assay. Ann Surg 229:874, 1999

Tezelman S, Shen W, Shaver JK, et al: Double parathyroid adenomas: clinical and biochemical characteristics before and after parathyroidectomy. Ann Surg 218:300, 1993

43 BREAST PROCEDURES

Barbara L. Smith, M.D., Ph.D., and Wiley W. Souba, M.D., Sc.D.

Since the 1970s, surgical procedures for cancer of the breast have become progressively less extensive while maintaining excellent control of local recurrence. Updates of multiple prospective, randomized trials continue to demonstrate that survival after lumpectomy, axillary dissection, and radiation therapy does not differ significantly from survival after mastectomy.[1-3] Local recurrence rates after lumpectomy and radiation therapy remain in the 10 percent range. At present, there are almost no remaining indications for the Halsted radical mastectomy.

The issue of the precise extent of surgical intervention necessary for evaluation and treatment of breast lesions continues to be reexamined. With the increased availability of screening mammography, a higher proportion of cancers are being detected at a nonpalpable stage (as in situ carcinomas or small invasive lesions), for which long-term survival rates range from 90 to 95 percent or higher. The efficacy of wide local excision without radiation in the treatment of in situ lesions is being investigated, and the need for axillary dissection in the treatment of small invasive cancers and cancers in elderly patients is being reconsidered. Improvements in imaging technology—including more refined mammographic techniques, improved breast ultrasonography, and the development of magnetic resonance imaging (MRI) of the breast—are yielding enhanced diagnostic sensitivity and specificity. Stereotactic and ultrasound-guided core-needle biopsy of nonpalpable breast lesions has proved to be a less invasive and less costly alternative to open surgical biopsy that is appropriate for many patients. Fine-needle aspiration (FNA) biopsy is increasingly replacing open surgical biopsy in the diagnosis of palpable breast malignancies and is proving useful in the diagnosis of many palpable benign lesions as well.

In what follows, we describe our approach to selected common surgical procedures currently employed in the diagnosis and treatment of breast lesions, taking into account various technical and nontechnical issues raised by the growth of new technologies and the evolution of our understanding of the biology of breast diseases.

Breast Biopsy

OPTIONS FOR PALPABLE MASSES

Tissue diagnosis of a palpable breast mass may be obtained by means of FNA biopsy, core-needle biopsy, or open incisional or excisional biopsy. Needle biopsy techniques are less invasive and less costly than open biopsy but are significantly more likely to yield false negative results. The choice of a biopsy technique must be based on the clinical and radiographic features of the lesion.

Fine-Needle Aspiration Biopsy

FNA biopsy is best performed by an experienced operator. It is an appropriate first step in diagnosing most discrete palpable breast masses encountered in clinical practice. The procedure is less useful in evaluating areas of vague thickening or nodularity: such lesions often contain normal tissue mingled with malignant tissue, and the small samples obtained with FNA biopsy may not include any of the malignant cells. FNA biopsy also is not particularly useful for small masses: the mass must be large enough to permit the biopsy needle to be moved back and forth within the lesion without passing out into surrounding normal tissue and contaminating the specimen with excessive amounts of normal cells. FNA biopsy of lesions less than 1 cm in diameter is associated with an unacceptably high rate of sampling error. FNA biopsy is usually the diagnostic procedure of choice for T3 and T4 primary lesions and for chest wall and axillary recurrences for which systemic therapy or irradiation is indicated as the first treatment modality.

Discrete masses discovered on physical examination may be either cystic or solid. Unless previous ultrasonographic examination has shown the mass to be solid, the needle used should be large enough to permit aspiration of potentially viscous fluid if the lesion proves to be cystic (i.e., 20 or 21 gauge). If the mass is known to be solid, a smaller needle (22 to 25 gauge) is sufficient for obtaining diagnostic tissue and will cause the patient less discomfort. For sufficient suction to be generated, a syringe with a capacity no smaller than 10 ml should be used. A variety of syringe holders are available that facilitate application of suction with a single hand.

Technique The skin of the breast is prepared with alcohol or iodine, and the lesion to be biopsied is held steady between the thumb and the index finger of the nondominant hand. A local anesthetic is usually not necessary; if it is used, it should be injected so as to create only a small skin wheal, so that there will be minimal distortion of the approach to the lesion. To facilitate visualization of the collected sample, 1 to 2 ml of air is introduced into the biopsy syringe before the needle enters the skin. The tip of the needle is advanced into the lesion before any suction is applied to minimize collection of tissue outside the lesion. Once the tip is in place, strong suction is applied, and the needle is moved back and forth within the lesion repeatedly along a 5 to 10 mm long track to loosen and collect cells. (This oscillation of the needle along the same track is the most effective way of obtaining a cellular, diagnostic specimen.) The back-

and-forth movement of the needle within the lesion is continued until tissue becomes visible in the hub of the needle. Suction is released while the needle is still within the lesion (again, to prevent collection of contaminating tissue from outside the lesion).

The needle is then withdrawn from the lesion, and its contents are expelled onto prepared glass slides, spread into a thin smear, and fixed according to the preferences of the cytology laboratory. Additional passes through the lesion may be made to ensure that a sufficiently cellular sample has been obtained, and the syringe may be rinsed so that a cell block can be prepared for further analysis. An adhesive bandage is applied to the biopsy site. If the lesion proves to be cystic, all fluid should be aspirated; this should cause the mass to disappear. The fluid need not be sent for analysis unless it is bloody or a palpable mass remains after as much fluid as possible has been aspirated.

The patient is reexamined four to eight weeks after successful aspiration. If the same cyst has recurred, it should be aspirated again and the fluid sent for cytologic analysis.

Interpretation of results Analysis by an experienced cytologist is critical for accurate interpretation of FNA biopsy results. Many cytology laboratories are able to perform immunohistochemical analysis for hormone receptors on FNA specimens if an appropriate fixative has been used. In most cytology labs, the false positive rate for a diagnosis of malignancy in an FNA biopsy of a breast mass is only one to two percent. Thus, a diagnosis of malignancy that is based on cytologic analysis of an FNA specimen may generally be believed, and definitive surgery may be planned without further biopsy. It should be remembered, however, that FNA does not distinguish between invasive and in situ breast cancer; intraoperative frozen section should be performed if necessary to determine the need for axillary dissection.

The false negative rate for identifying breast malignancy, however, is high: FNA fails to diagnose as many as 40 percent of cancers. Any cellular atypia on FNA biopsy is an indication for open biopsy. A diagnosis of normal or fibrocystic breast tissue should also be viewed with suspicion; subsequent open biopsy is usually indicated if the physical examination or a mammogram of the biopsied lesion gives rise to even a minor degree of concern about malignancy. If the cytologic analysis is diagnostic of a specific benign lesion (e.g., a fibroadenoma or a lactating adenoma), it may generally be relied on if it is in keeping with the clinical features of the lesion, and no further workup is necessary. It has been suggested that no further workup is required when the so-called triple negative criteria (a physical examination suggestive of a benign lesion, a normal mammogram, and negative results from FNA biopsy) are present, particularly in younger women.

Core-Needle (Cutting-Needle) Biopsy

As its name suggests, a core-needle biopsy removes a narrow cylinder of tissue from the biopsied lesion. The tissue undergoes standard pathological rather than cytologic analysis; consequently, this technique is preferable if a skilled cytologist is not available for interpretation of FNA biopsy specimens. Nonetheless, FNA biopsy has supplanted core-needle biopsy in the investigation of most palpable lesions. It should be noted that the false negative rate associated with core-needle biopsy for palpable lesions performed without ultrasonographic or stereotactic guidance is as high as or higher than that of FNA biopsy.[4] The technical difficulty of accurately placing and firing the core needle in small mobile lesions or in lesions surrounded by dense fibrocystic tissue makes FNA biopsy preferable in these settings. Core-needle biopsy is, however, ideal for sampling large lesions or chest wall recurrences in which the larger samples permit more detailed pathological analysis and easy determination of hormone receptor levels.

Technique If the mass is palpable, the surgeon can perform the core-needle biopsy in the office. A large needle (usually 14 gauge) is placed either by hand or with a biopsy gun device. A small skin wheal of local anesthetic is usually required, and a nick is made in the skin with a No. 11 blade to permit easy entry of the biopsy needle into breast tissue and into the lesion. As with FNA biopsy (see above), the lesion is held steady in the nondominant hand while the biopsy needle is advanced into the lesion and a core sample obtained.

Interpretation of results Atypia on core-needle biopsy is an indication for open biopsy of the sampled lesion. In addition, any core-needle biopsy (especially one done without stereotactic or ultrasonographic guidance) that yields benign or fibrocystic tissue should be viewed with some suspicion because of the risk of technical or sampling error. Open biopsy should be considered if there is any discordance between a benign core-needle biopsy result and the clinical or mammographic features of the lesion.

Open Biopsy

The vast majority of open breast biopsies are now performed with local anesthesia or local anesthesia with intravenous sedation. General anesthesia is reserved for situations in which multiple lesions must be excised and the amount of local anesthetic required would exceed the maximum safe dose.

Technique Open biopsy incisions should generally be curvilinear and should be placed directly over the lesion to minimize tunneling through breast tissue [*see Figure 1*]. Because the possibility of malignancy must always be taken into account, all open biopsy incisions should also be oriented so that they will be included within any subsequent mastectomy incision. Accordingly, if an open biopsy is to be done at an extremely lateral or medial site, it may be best approached via a radial incision placed over the lesion rather than via a more vertical curvilinear incision.

The incision should be long enough to provide adequate exposure and to ensure that the mass can be excised as a single tissue fragment with a small margin of grossly normal tissue. Specimen margins should be inked by the pathologist. Meticulous hemostasis should be achieved before closure. Deep breast tissue should be approximated only if such approximation does not result in significant deformity of breast contour. A cosmetic subcuticular closure is preferred.

OPTIONS FOR NONPALPABLE MASSES

The increasingly widespread use of screening mammography has led to the identification of more and more nonpalpable breast masses for which tissue diagnosis is required. In most series,[5-7] 15 to 30 percent of such lesions prove to be malignant.

Nonpalpable masses may be approached via core-needle biopsy or open biopsy with wire localization.

Image-Guided Core-Needle Biopsy

Needle biopsy techniques are increasingly being used to diagnose nonpalpable breast lesions. The indications for and limitations of these techniques are still being determined, but certain standards are emerging. In general, FNA biopsy of nonpalpable lesions is inadvisable because of its high false negative rate. Little is lost by attempting an FNA biopsy of a palpable lesion in the office setting, but performing a stereotactic or ultrasound-guided FNA biopsy of a nonpalpable mass carries a significant cost in terms of time, patient discomfort, and expense. The diagnostic accuracy currently achievable with FNA biopsy in this setting does not justify this cost. Consequently, image-guided core-needle biopsy is the preferred approach for needle biopsy of nonpalpable lesions.

In choosing core-needle biopsy, both patient and physician must be comfortable with the fact that the lesion will only be sampled rather than excised, must recognize that the possibility of a sampling error that will cause the examiner to miss the lesion is higher with core-needle biopsy than with open biopsy, and must realize that equivocal findings will necessitate follow-up with open biopsy. The trade-off for these limitations is that core-needle biopsy generally costs less than open biopsy, takes less time, and leaves only a tiny scar.

Stereotactic versus ultrasound-guided biopsy Whenever feasible, core-needle biopsy is performed with ultrasonographic guidance, which permits real-time documentation of needle position within the lesion. Stereotactic mammography-guided core-needle biopsy is performed if the lesion is not visualized ultrasonographically. Stereotactic biopsy is appropriate for lesions that are favorably located within the breast (i.e., that can be stably positioned in the biopsy window of the machine). Lesions very close to the chest wall or the areola may not be accessible to stereotactic biopsy and are best approached via open biopsy with needle localization (see below).

Clustered microcalcifications may be approached by stereotactic core-needle biopsy if the cluster is large enough for calcifications to remain for subsequent wide excision if a malignancy is found. Specimen radiography is done to ensure that calcifications are included in the tissue cores. In planning subsequent treatment after stereotactic core-needle biopsy shows only carcinoma in situ, it should be remembered that the lesion was only sampled and that the biopsy results alone do not rule out an invasive tumor.

Interpretation of results Series comparing the results of stereotactic core-needle biopsy with those of needle-localized open biopsy of the same lesions have shown that core-needle biopsy misses one to 10 percent of lesions.[8-10] There is clearly a learning curve with stereotactic core-needle biopsy: false negative rates are significantly higher among less experienced operators. Core-needle biopsy results must therefore be interpreted with care. Because false positive results are rare, a diagnosis of malignancy may be believed and acted on without further biopsy. As with palpable lesions, however, any finding of atypia is an indication for wire-localized open biopsy. A finding of benign or fibrocystic tissue should also be viewed with some suspicion and interpreted in relation to the lesion sampled. One must decide

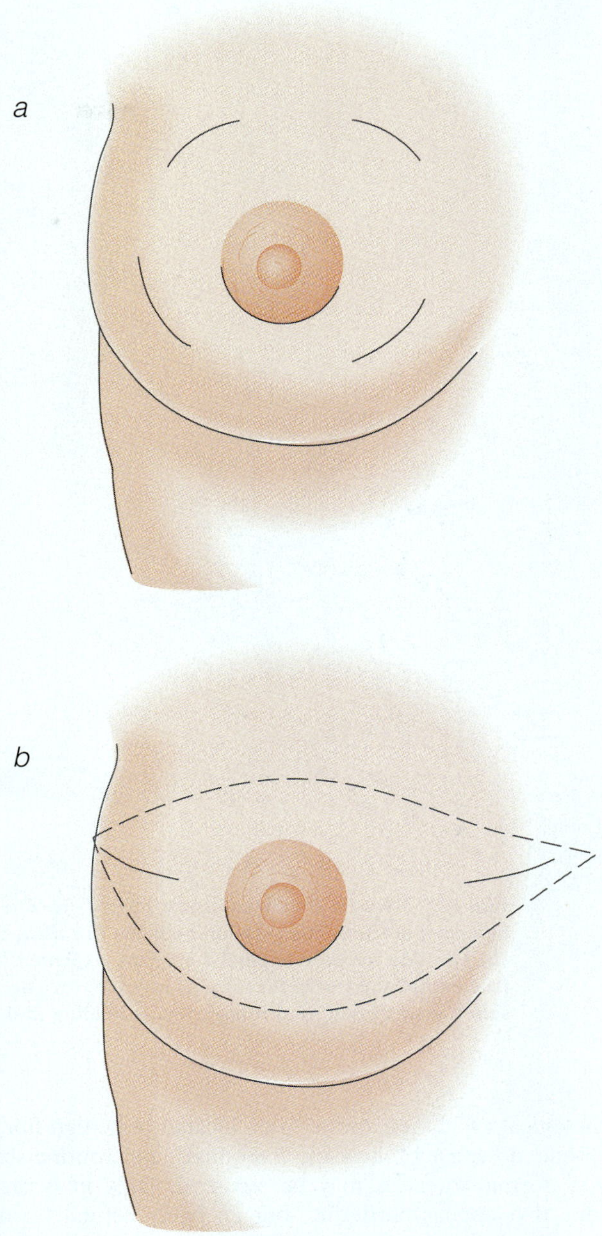

Figure 1 Open breast biopsy. (*a*) In most cases, a curvilinear incision is preferred. If the mass is close to the areola, a periareolar incision may be used. (*b*) Extremely lateral or medial incisions may be radial. In any case, incisions should be placed directly over the lesion and should be oriented so that they will be included within a subsequent mastectomy incision if margins prove positive and mastectomy is indicated.

whether the pathological findings adequately account for the lesion visualized. If any concern remains, open biopsy is indicated.

Follow-up Whether short-interval mammographic follow-up is necessary after core-needle biopsy depends on the pathological findings and the mammographic appearance of the lesion. With a well-circumscribed lesion that pathological evaluation shows to be a fibroadenoma or with calcifications that

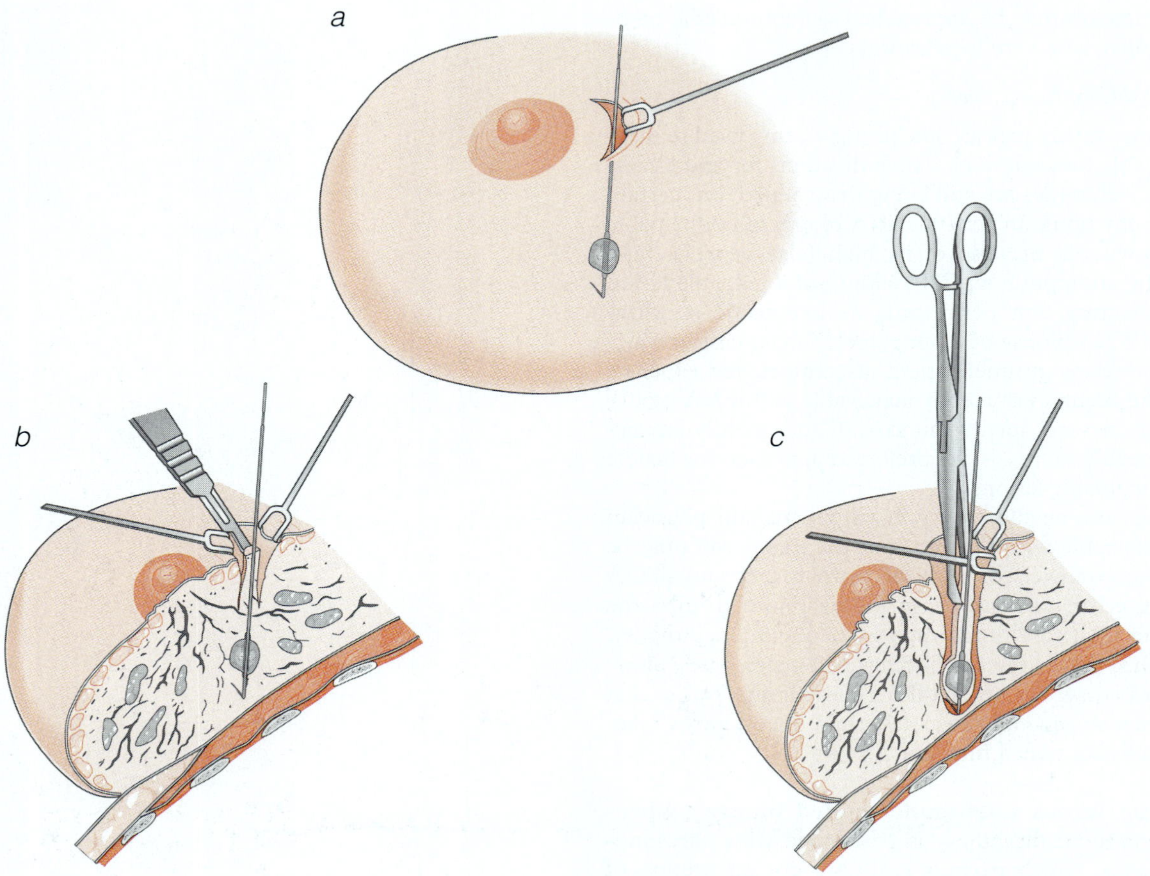

Figure 2 Needle-localized breast biopsy. (*a*) The mammographic abnormality is localized immediately before operation. The relation between the wire, the skin entry site, and the lesion is noted by the surgeon. (*b*) The skin incision is placed over the expected location of the mammographic abnormality. The dissection is accomplished with the wire as a guide. (*c*) The tissue around the wire is removed en bloc with the wire and sent for specimen mammography. Tunneling and piecemeal removal are to be avoided.[11]

pathological evaluation shows to be located in benign fibrocystic tissue, no special follow-up is required, and routine screening at normal intervals may be resumed. Only in occasional lesions that appear borderline but probably benign on mammography and are associated with benign pathological findings are six-month repeat mammograms required to ensure that the lesions remain stable. In general, if the pathological findings are equivocal or discordant with the appearance of the lesion, immediate open excision is preferable to a six-month repeat mammogram. To ensure appropriate follow-up, there should be close communication among the physician ordering the core-needle biopsy, the physician performing the biopsy, and the pathologist analyzing the specimen.

Open Biopsy with Needle (Wire) Localization

As is the case for open biopsy of palpable lesions, the vast majority of needle-localized breast biopsies are now performed with local anesthesia or local anesthesia with intravenous sedation. General anesthesia is reserved for excision of multiple lesions or other special circumstances.

Technique The lesion to be excised is localized by inserting a thin needle and a fine wire under mammographic or ultrasonographic guidance immediately before operation. To facilitate incision placement, images should be sent to the operating room with the wire entry site indicated on them. With superficial lesions, the wire entry site is usually close to the lesion and thus may be included in the incision. With some deeper lesions, the wire entry site is on the shortest path to the lesion and so may still be included in the incision. The incision is placed as directly as possible over the mass to minimize tunneling through breast tissue. Once the incision is made, a core of tissue is excised around and along the wire in such a way as to include the lesion [*see Figure 2*]. (This process is easier and involves less excision of tissue if the localizing wire has a thickened segment several centimeters in length that is placed adjacent to or within the lesion. One then follows the wire itself into breast tissue until the thick segment is reached and only then extends the excision away from the wire to include the lesion in a fairly small tissue fragment.)

With many lesions, the wire entry site is in a fairly peripheral location relative to the position of the lesion, which means that including the wire entry site in the incision would result in excessive tunneling within breast tissue. In such cases, the incision is placed over the expected position of the lesion [*see Figure 3*], the dissection is extended into breast tissue to identify the

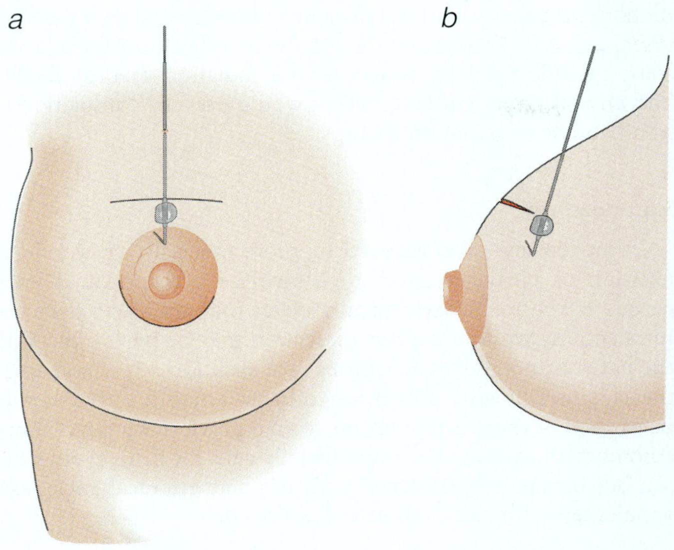

Figure 3 Needle-localized breast biopsy. (*a*) It is sometimes necessary to insert the localizing wire from a peripheral site to localize a deep or central lesion. The incision should be placed directly over the expected location of the lesion, not over the wire entry site. (*b*) Once the skin incision is made, the dissection is extended into breast tissue to identify the wire a short distance from the lesion. The free end of the wire is pulled into the wound, and the biopsy is performed as in Figure 2.

wire a few centimeters away from the lesion itself, and the free end of the wire is pulled up into the incision. A generous core of tissue is then excised around the wire. (Again, this process is easier if the thick segment of the localizing wire is placed adjacent to or within the lesion.)

Radiography should immediately be performed on all wire-localized biopsy specimens to confirm that the lesion has been excised. The patient should remain on the operating table with the sterile field preserved until such confirmation has been received. If the mass was missed and the surgeon has some idea of the likely location of the missed lesion, another tissue sample may be excised immediately. If, however, the surgeon suspects that the wire was dislodged before or during the procedure, the incision should be closed. After the patient has healed sufficiently to be able to tolerate repeat mammography, another mammogram is obtained, and repeat localization and biopsy are performed.

Terminal Duct Excision

Terminal duct excision is the procedure of choice in the surgical treatment of nipple discharge. Local anesthesia with or without sedation (as for breast biopsy) is generally sufficient for this procedure. The goal is to excise the duct from which the discharge arises along with as little additional tissue as possible. To this end, the surgeon should carefully note the precise position of the discharging duct at the time of the initial examination. Ductograms generally are not helpful in directing the surgical procedure and need not be performed.

OPERATIVE TECHNIQUE

The patient is instructed not to attempt to express her discharge for several days before operation. The breast skin is prepared, and drapes are placed. The surgeon then attempts to express the discharge so that the offending duct can be precisely identified. If discharge is obtained, the mark for the incision should be made at the areolar border in the same quadrant, extending for about one third of the areola's circumference [see Figure 4a]. A local anesthetic is then administered, the edge of the nipple is grasped with a forceps, and a fine lacrimal duct probe (000 to 0000) is gently inserted into the discharging duct. An incision is then made as marked at the areolar border, the nipple skin flap is raised, and the duct containing the wire is excised with a margin of surrounding tissue from just below the nipple dermis into the deeper breast tissue [see Figure 4b, c].

If it is not possible to pass the lacrimal duct probe into the discharging duct, the skin incision is made and the nipple skin flap raised as described. The surgeon then bluntly dissects among the subareolar ducts to identify the dark, secretion-filled abnormal duct. If the duct is identified, it is excised along its length from the nipple dermis to a depth of 4 to 5 cm within breast tissue. An option at this point is to incise the duct and insert a lacrimal duct probe to facilitate identification of its course. If no single secretion-filled duct is identified, the entire subareolar duct complex must be excised from immediately beneath the nipple dermis to a depth of 4 to 5 cm within breast tissue [see Figure 5].

In all variants of this procedure, the electrocautery should not be used in the superficial portions of the dissection: it could cause devascularization of the nipple-areola complex and result in an electrocautery artifact that could interfere with patholog-

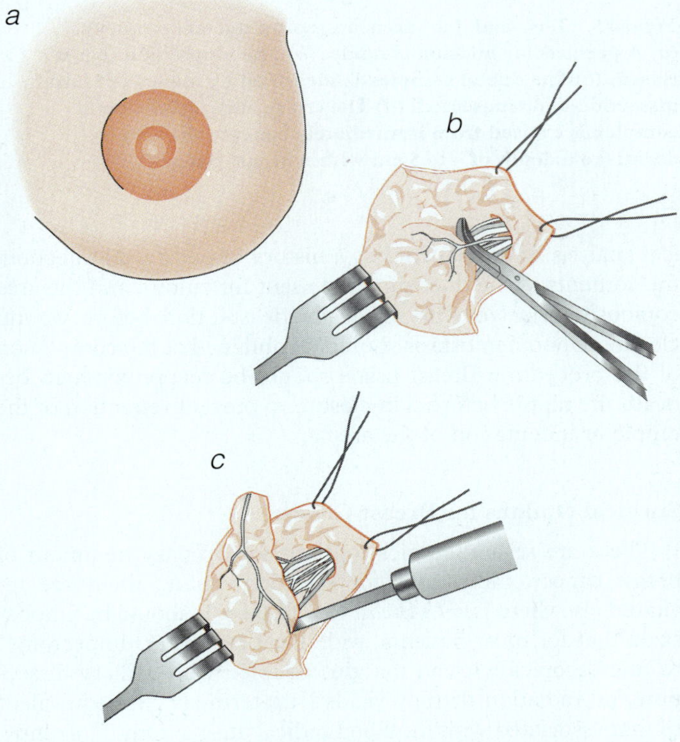

Figure 4 Terminal duct excision (single duct). (*a*) A periareolar incision is made. (*b*) The involved duct is identified by means of blunt dissection. (*c*) The duct is removed along with a core of breast tissue.[12]

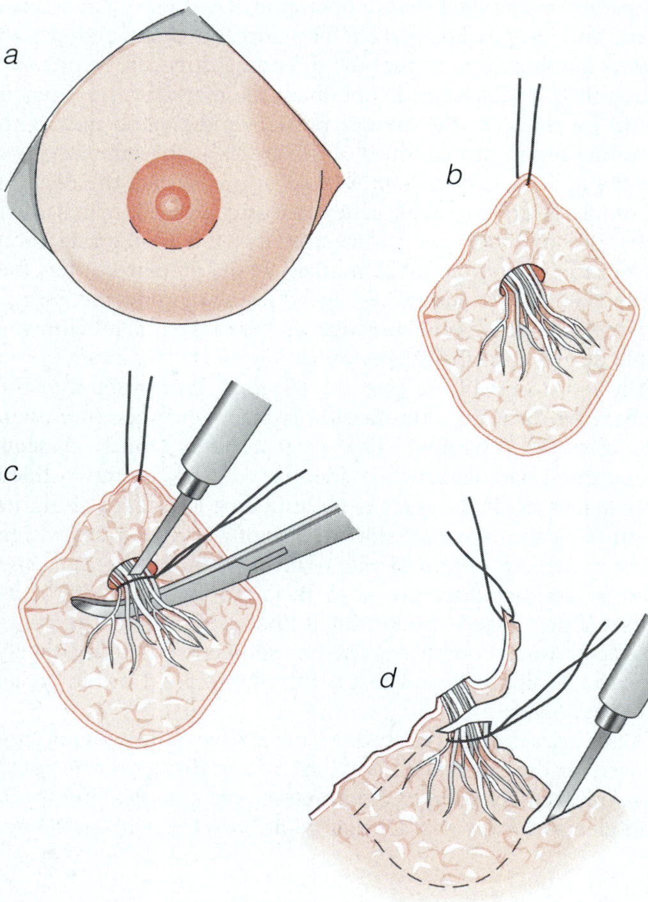

Figure 5 Terminal duct excision (entire ductal complex). (*a*) A periareolar incision is made. (*b*) The nipple skin flap is raised. (*c*) The ductal complex is identified by means of blunt dissection and transected. (*d*) The entire subareolar ductal complex is excised from immediately beneath the nipple dermis to a depth of 4 to 5 cm within breast tissue.[12]

ical analysis. If the patient has a history of periductal infection, the contents of the duct should be sent for culture and the area copiously irrigated with an antibiotic solution before wound closure. Good hemostasis should be obtained at the completion of the procedure. Breast tissue should be reapproximated beneath the nipple before skin closure to prevent retraction of the nipple or indentation of the areola.

Surgical Options for Breast Cancer

There are several surgical options for primary treatment of breast cancer; indications for selecting among them are reviewed elsewhere [*see* 13 Breast Complaints]. It should be emphasized that for most patients, wide local excision (lumpectomy) to microscopically clean margins coupled with axillary dissection and radiation therapy yields long-term survival equivalent to that associated with modified radical mastectomy. Currently, indications for mastectomy include patient preference, inability on the part of the surgeon to achieve clean margins without unacceptable deformation of the remaining breast tissue, the presence of multiple primary tumors, previous chest wall irradiation, pregnancy, and the presence of severe collagen vascular disease (e.g., scleroderma). Nonmedical indications for mastectomy include the lack of access to a radiation therapy facility and any other patient factors that would prevent completion of a full course of radiation therapy.

Lumpectomy

Lumpectomy—also referred to, more precisely, as wide local excision or partial mastectomy—involves excision of all cancerous tissue to microscopically clean margins. Reexcision or lumpectomy without axillary dissection may be performed with the patient under local anesthesia, but sedation or general anesthesia is usually advisable if a significant amount of tissue is to be excised or there is tenderness from a previous biopsy. Lumpectomy with axillary dissection usually calls for general anesthesia, but it may be performed with thoracic epidural anesthesia supplemented by local anesthesia as needed.

OPERATIVE TECHNIQUE

Like open breast biopsy incisions [*see* Breast Biopsy, *above*], lumpectomy incisions should generally be curvilinear, should be placed directly over the lesion, and should also be oriented so as to be included within a subsequent mastectomy incision if margins prove positive [*see Figure 1*]. Extremely lateral or medial incisions may be better approached via a radial incision placed over the lesion. Because accurate assessment of margins is of central importance in a lumpectomy, it is critical that the incision be long enough to allow removal of the specimen in one piece rather than several.

Along with the mass itself, it is generally necessary to remove a 1 to 1.5 cm margin of normal-appearing tissue beyond the edge of the palpable tumor or, if excisional biopsy has already been performed, around the biopsy cavity. In the case of nonpalpable lesions diagnosed via needle biopsy, the position of the lesion must be determined by means of wire localization, and 2 to 3 cm of tissue should be excised around the wire to obtain an adequate margin. The specimen should be oriented by the surgeon and the margins inked by the pathologist; this orientation is useful if reexcision is required to achieve clean margins. Reexcision of any close margins may be performed during the same surgical procedure if the specimen margins are assessed immediately by the pathologist.

In the closure of the incision, hemostasis should be meticulous: a hematoma may delay administration of radiation therapy or chemotherapy. Deep breast tissue should be approximated only if such closure does not result in significant deformity of breast contour. A cosmetic subcuticular closure is preferred.

Axillary Dissection

Axillary dissection for breast cancer includes resection of level I and level II lymph nodes and the fibrofatty tissue within which these nodes lie [*see Figure 6*]. The superior border of the dissection is formed by the axillary vein laterally and the upper extent of level II nodes medially; the lateral border of the dissection is formed by the latissimus dorsi muscle from the tail of the breast to the crossing point of the axillary vein; the medial border is formed by the pectoral muscles and the anterior serratus muscle; and the inferior border is formed by the tail of the breast. Level II nodes are easily removed by retracting the greater and smaller pectoral muscles medially; it is not necessary to divide or remove the smaller pectoral muscle. In general, level III nodes are not removed unless palpable disease is present.

Axillary dissection, either alone or in conjunction with lumpectomy or mastectomy, usually calls for general anesthesia, but it may also be performed with thoracic epidural anesthesia supplemented by local anesthesia as needed. To facilitate identification and preservation of motor nerves that pass through the axilla, the anesthesiologist should refrain from using neuromuscular blocking agents. In the absence of neuromuscular blockade, any clamping of a motor nerve or too-close approach to a motor nerve with the electrocautery will be signaled by a visible muscle twitch.

STRUCTURES TO BE PRESERVED

There are a number of vascular structures and nerves passing through the axilla that must be preserved during axillary dissection [see Figure 7]. These structures include the axillary vein and artery; the brachial plexus; the long thoracic nerve, which innervates the anterior serratus muscle; the thoracodorsal nerve, artery, and vein, which supply the latissimus dorsi muscle; and the medial pectoral nerve, which innervates the lateral portion of the greater pectoral muscle.

The axillary artery and the brachial plexus should not be exposed during axillary dissection. If they are, the dissection has been carried too far superiorly, and proper orientation at a more inferior position should be established. In some patients, there may be sensory branches of the brachial plexus superficial (and, rarely, inferior) to the axillary vein laterally near the latissimus dorsi muscle; injury to these nerves results in numbness extending to the wrist. To prevent this complication, the axillary vein should initially be identified medially, under the greater pectoral muscle. Medial to the thoracodorsal nerve and adherent to the chest wall is the long thoracic nerve of Bell. The medial pectoral nerve runs from superior to the axillary vein to the undersurface of the greater pectoral muscle, passing through the axillary fat pad and across the level II nodes; it has an accompanying vein whose blue color may be used to identify the nerve. If a submuscular implant reconstruction [see Breast Reconstruction after Mastectomy, below] is planned, preservation of the medial pectoral nerve is especially important to prevent atrophy of the muscle.

The intercostobrachial nerve provides sensation to the posterior portion of the upper arm. Sacrificing this nerve generally leads to numbness over the triceps region. In many women, the intercostobrachial nerve measures 2 mm in diameter and takes a fairly cephalad course near the axillary vein; when this is the case, preservation of the nerve will not interfere with node dissection. Sometimes, however, the nerve is tiny, has multiple branches, and is intermingled with nodal tissue that should be removed; when this is the case, one should not expend a great deal of time on attempting to preserve the nerve. If the intercostobrachial nerve is sacrificed, it should be transected with a knife or scissors rather than with the electrocautery, and the ends should be buried to reduce the likelihood of postoperative causalgia.

OPERATIVE TECHNIQUE

The incision for axillary dissection should be a transverse one made in the lower third of the hair-bearing skin of the axilla. For

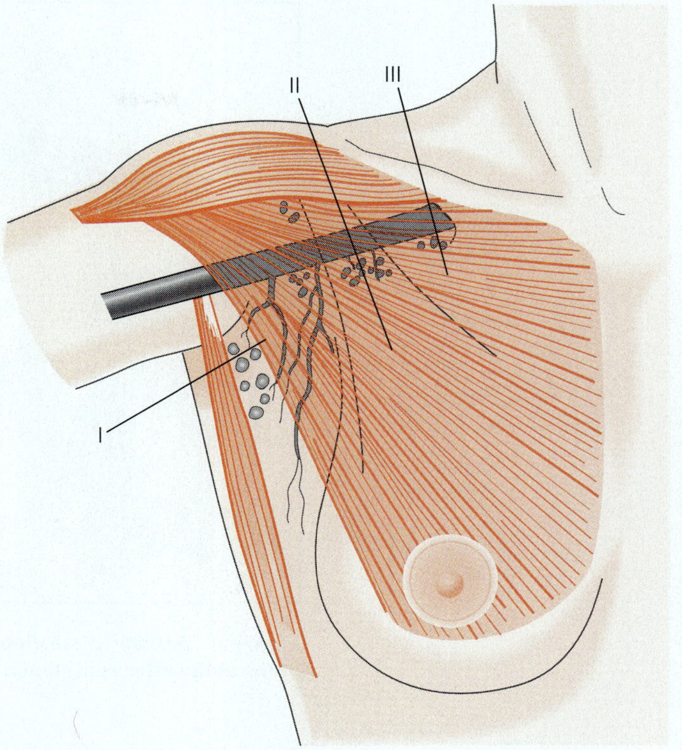

Figure 6 Axillary dissection. Shown are axillary lymph node levels in relation to the axillary vein and the muscles of the axilla (I = low axilla, II = midaxilla, III = apex of axilla).[13]

cosmetic reasons, it should not extend anteriorly onto the greater pectoral muscle; however, it may be extended posteriorly onto the latissimus dorsi muscle as necessary for exposure. Skin flaps are raised to the level of the axillary vein and to a point below the lowest extension of hair-bearing skin, either as an initial maneuver or after the initial identification of key structures.

The key to axillary dissection is obtaining and maintaining proper orientation with respect to the axillary vein, the thoracodorsal bundle, and the long thoracic nerve. After the incision has been made, the dissection is extended down into the true axillary fat pad through the overlying fascial layer. The fat of the axillary fat pad may be distinguished from subcutaneous fat on the basis of its smoother, lipomalike texture. There may be aberrant muscle slips from the latissimus dorsi muscle or the greater pectoral muscle; in addition, there may be an extremely dense fascial encasement around the axillary fat pad. It is important to divide these layers early in the dissection. The borders of the greater pectoral and latissimus dorsi muscles are then exposed, which clears the medial and lateral borders of the dissection.

The axillary vein and the thoracodorsal bundle are identified next. As discussed (see above), the initial identification of the axillary vein should be made medially, under the greater pectoral muscle, to prevent injury to low-lying branches of the brachial plexus. Sometimes, the axillary vein takes the form of several small branches rather than a single large vessel. If this is the case, all of the small branches should be preserved.

The thoracodorsal bundle may be identified either distally at its junction with the latissimus dorsi muscle or at its junction

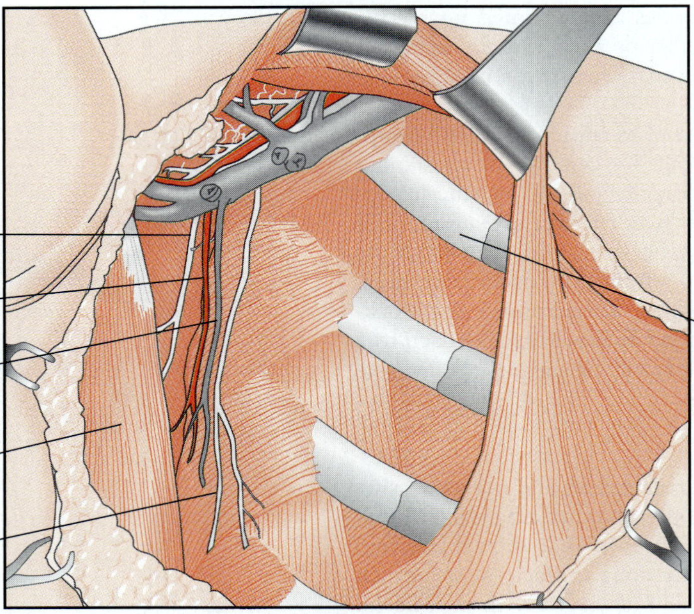

Figure 7 Axillary dissection. Shown is a view of the structures of the axilla after completion of axillary dissection.[14]

with the axillary vein. The junction with the latissimus dorsi muscle is within the axillary fat pad at a point two thirds of the way down the hair-bearing skin of the axilla, or approximately 4 cm below the inferior border of the axillary vein. Occasionally, the thoracodorsal bundle is bifurcated, with separate superior and inferior branches entering the latissimus dorsi muscle; this is particularly likely if the entry point appears very high. If the bundle is bifurcated, both branches should be preserved. The thoracodorsal bundle may be identified at its junction with the latissimus dorsi muscle by spreading within axillary fat parallel to the border of the muscle and looking for the blue of the thoracodorsal vein. The identification is also facilitated by lateral retraction of the latissimus dorsi muscle. The long thoracic nerve lies just medial to the thoracodorsal bundle on the chest wall at this point and at approximately the same anterior-posterior position. It may be identified by spreading tissue just medial to the thoracodorsal bundle and then running the index finger perpendicular to the course of the long thoracic nerve on the chest wall to identify the cordlike nerve as it moves under the finger. Once the nerve is identified, axillary tissue may be swept anteriorly away from the nerve by blunt dissection along the anterior serratus muscle; there are no significant vessels in this area.

The junction of the thoracodorsal bundle with the axillary vein is 1.5 to 2.0 cm medial to the point at which the axillary vein crosses the latissimus dorsi muscle. The thoracodorsal vein enters the posterior surface of the axillary vein, and the nerve and the artery pass posterior to the axillary vein. There are generally one or two scapular veins that branch off the axillary vein medial to the junction with the thoracodorsal vein. These are divided during the dissection and should not be confused with the thoracodorsal bundle.

The axillary vein and the thoracodorsal bundle having been identified, the greater pectoral muscle is retracted medially at the level of the axillary vein, and the latissimus dorsi muscle is retracted laterally to place tension on the thoracodorsal bundle. Once this exposure is achieved, the axillary fat and the nodes are cleared away superficial and medial to the thoracodorsal bundle to the level of the axillary vein. Superiorly, dissection proceeds medially along the axillary vein to the point where the fat containing level II nodes crosses the axillary vein. To improve exposure, the fascia overlying the level II extension of the axillary fat pad should be incised to release tension and expose the lipomalike level II fat. As noted [see Structures to Be Preserved, *above*], the medial pectoral nerve passes onto the underside of the greater pectoral muscle in this area and should be preserved. One or more small venous branches may pass inferiorly from the medial pectoral bundle; particular attention should be paid to preserving the nerve when ligating these venous branches.

The next step in the dissection is to reflect the axillary fat pad inferiorly by dividing the medial attachments of the axillary fat pad along the anterior serratus muscle. Care must be taken to preserve the long thoracic nerve. Because there are no significant vessels or structures in the tissue anterior to the long thoracic nerve, this tissue may be divided sharply, with small perforating vessels either tied or cauterized. Finally, the axillary fat is freed from the tail of the breast with the electrocautery or a knife.

There is no need to orient the axillary specimen for the pathologist, because treatment is not affected by the anatomic level of node involvement. A closed suction drain is placed through a separate stab wound. (Some practitioners prefer not to place a drain and simply aspirate postoperative seromas as necessary.) A long-acting local anesthetic may be instilled into the axilla—a particularly helpful practice if the dissection was done as an outpatient procedure.

Mastectomy

The goal of a mastectomy is to remove all breast tissue,

including the nipple and the areola, while leaving well-perfused, viable skin flaps for primary closure or reconstruction. This is the case whether the mastectomy is performed for treatment of breast cancer or for prophylaxis in high-risk patients. Proper skin incisions and good exposure throughout the procedure are the key components of a well-performed mastectomy. The borders of dissection extend superiorly to the clavicle, medially to the sternum, inferiorly to where breast tissue ends (on the costal margin, below the inframammary fold), and laterally to the border of the latissimus dorsi muscle. The fascia of the greater pectoral muscle forms the deep margin of the dissection and should be removed with the specimen.

Mastectomy usually calls for general anesthesia, but it may be performed with thoracic epidural anesthesia supplemented by local anesthesia as needed. When a simple mastectomy is to be performed in a frail patient for whom general anesthesia poses unacceptable risks (particularly if the patient is elderly and has a narrow-based, pendulous breast), local anesthesia with sedation is appropriate.

OPERATIVE TECHNIQUE

Skin-sparing mastectomy performed in conjunction with immediate reconstruction is discussed elsewhere [see Breast Reconstruction after Mastectomy, below]. In a modified radical or simple mastectomy without reconstruction, the goal is to leave a smooth chest wall that permits comfortable wearing of a bra and a prosthesis. It is important to remove a sufficient amount of skin to ensure that no dog-ears or lateral skin folds are left on the anterior chest wall. This undesirable result can be prevented by extending the incision far enough medially and laterally to remove all skin that contributes to the forward projection of the breast skin envelope.

The incision may be either transverse across the chest wall or angled upward toward the axilla as necessary to include the nipple-areola complex and any incisions from previous biopsies, and care should be taken to make the upper and lower skin flaps of similar length so that there is no redundant skin on either flap [see Figure 8]. The boundaries of the incision can be determined in the following five steps: (1) the lateral and medial end points of the incision are marked, (2) the breast is pulled firmly downward, (3) the upper incision is defined by drawing a straight line from one end point to the other across the upper surface of the breast, (4) the breast is pulled firmly upward, and (5) the lower incision is defined by drawing a straight line from one end point to the other across the lower surface of the breast. The outlined incision is then checked to ensure that it can be closed without either undue tension or redundant skin. (The closure should be fairly snug intraoperatively, when the patient's arm is positioned perpendicular to the torso for exposure, because a significant amount of slack is created when the arm is returned to a more normal position at the patient's side.) The medial and lateral end points of the incision may be adjusted upward or downward to include any previous biopsy incisions in the specimen.

Flaps

In most patients, there is a fairly well-defined avascular plane between subcutaneous fat and breast tissue. This plane is identified by pulling the edges of the incision upward with skin hooks and beginning a flap that is 8 to 10 mm thick and extends approximately 1 cm from the skin edge. After this initial release of the skin edge, the desired plane is developed by applying firm tension to pull breast tissue downward and away from the skin at a 45° angle. The fine fibrous attachments between breast tissue and subcutaneous fat (Cooper's ligaments) are then divided with the electrocautery or a blade, and crossing vessels are coagulated or ligated as they appear. To protect both arterial supply to and venous drainage from the skin flap, one must refrain from excessive ligation or cauterization of vessels on the flap.

Completed mastectomy flaps are perfused through the network of fine subdermal vessels that remains after dissection. The viability of the flaps is determined by their length, the quality of the vessels they contain, the damage sustained by the vessels during the dissection, and the tension imposed by the final closure. For most women, flap viability is not an issue. It is, however, a serious consideration for diabetics and other patients with diffuse small vessel disease. In such patients, flaps should be carefully planned so that they are no longer than necessary and there is no excess tension, and extra care should be taken to preserve flap vessels. Patients should be warned that even with these additional efforts, there may be some necrosis along the edges of the incision. Such necrosis is best treated with gradual debridement of the dark eschar that forms as epithelialization proceeds from viable tissue.

Borders of Dissection

Flaps are raised superiorly to the clavicle, medially to the sternum, inferiorly to where breast tissue ends on the costal margin

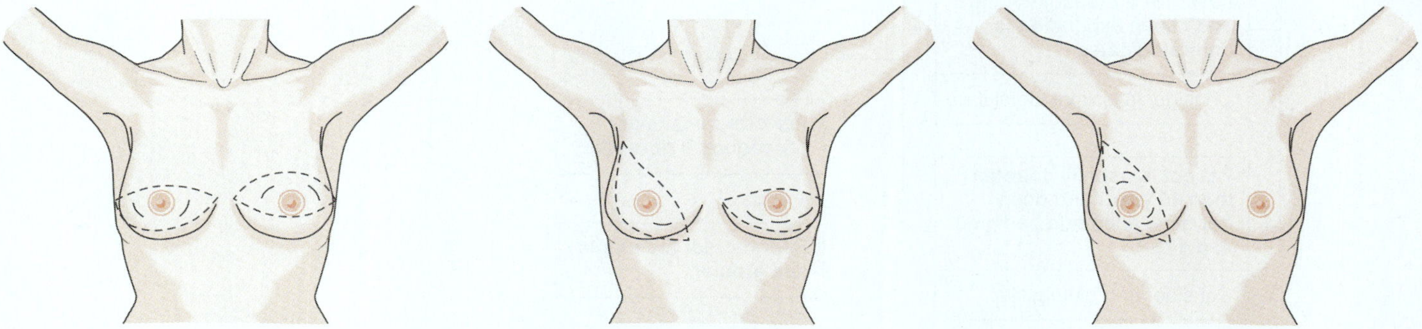

Figure 8 Mastectomy. Shown are common incisions used for mastectomy. Any previous biopsy incisions should have been done in such a way as to be included within the boundaries of the mastectomy incision.[11]

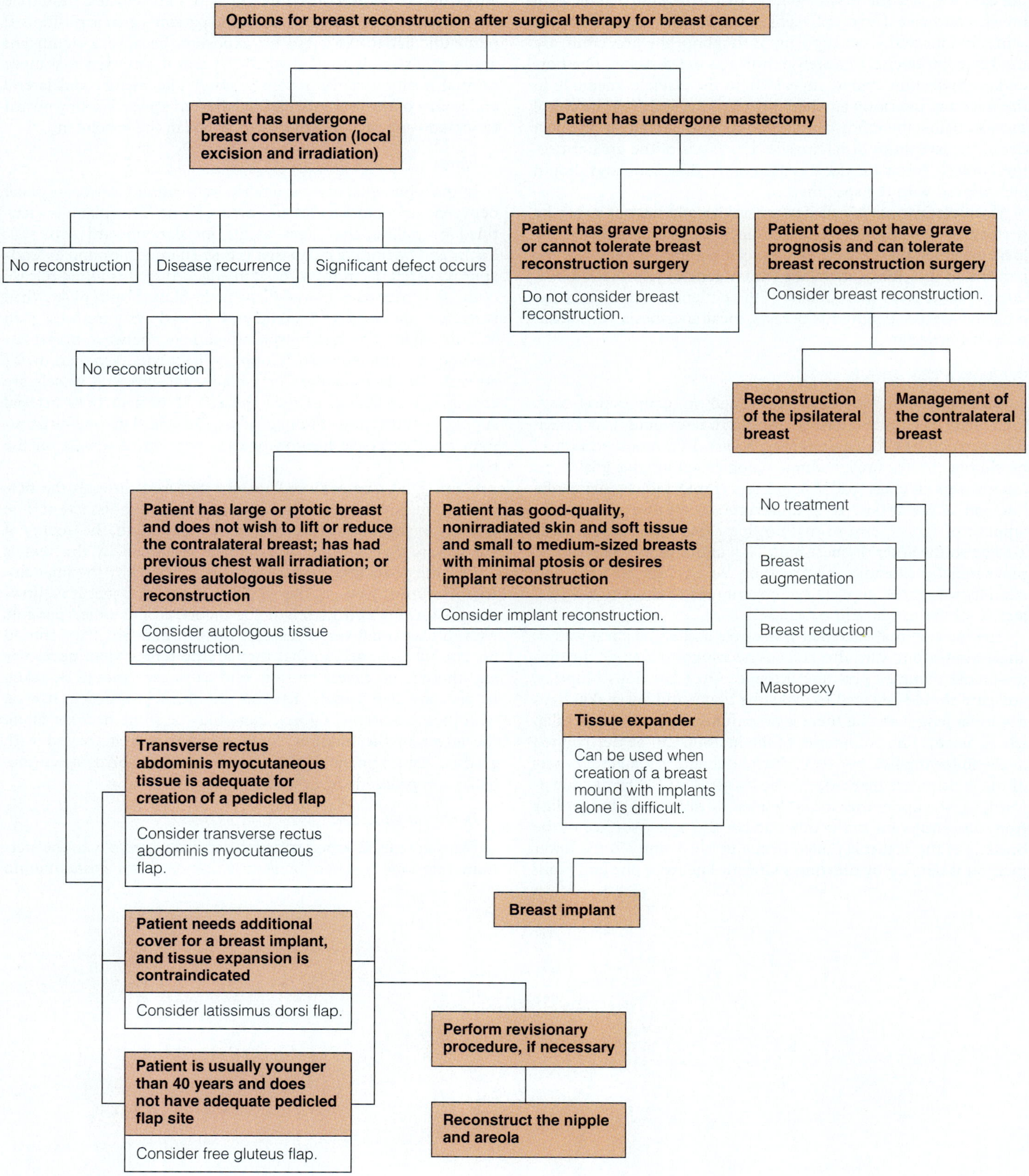

Figure 9 Breast reconstruction after mastectomy. Shown is an algorithm outlining the major steps in breast reconstruction.

(generally below the inframammary fold), and laterally to the border of the latissimus dorsi muscle. The plane between breast tissue and subcutaneous fat is followed down to the greater pectoral muscle and through the pectoral fascia both superiorly and medially. Inferiorly, the fascia of the abdominal muscles is not divided. The greater pectoral muscle, the abdominal muscles, and the anterior serratus muscle form the deep border of the dissection. The pectoral fascia is removed with the breast specimen and may be separated from the muscle with either the electrocautery or a blade.

To maintain the skin tension needed for the development of skin flaps, an assistant holds the flaps taut manually with skin hooks, dull-toothed rakes padded with damp sponges, or Deaver retractors. Care must be taken to obtain adequate tension and exposure so that as much breast tissue as possible can be removed without undue damage to the skin flaps.

Simple versus Modified Radical Mastectomy

Simple mastectomy is performed (1) to treat ductal carcinoma in situ (DCIS), (2) as a prophylactic measure, (3) as a follow-up to lumpectomy and axillary dissection if lumpectomy margins are positive for malignancy, (4) to treat local recurrence of breast cancer after lumpectomy, node dissection, and irradiation, and (5) in elderly patients in whom coexisting medical conditions or other factors constitute contraindications to axillary dissection. Simple mastectomy is also indicated for treatment of sarcomas of the breast: lymphatic spread to axillary nodes is not part of the natural history of this disease.

Modified radical mastectomy is performed to treat invasive breast cancer when (1) there are contraindications to breast preservation or (2) the patient or the physician prefers mastectomy.

Simple mastectomy As described earlier (see above), a skin incision is made, and thin flaps are raised to allow removal of all breast tissue. Laterally, the dissection is extended to the border of the latissimus dorsi muscle, and breast tissue is removed anterior to the long thoracic nerve. The dissection proceeds around the lateral edge of the greater pectoral muscle but stops before entering the axillary fat pad. If one wishes to sample the low axillary nodes (as, for example, in a patient with extensive DCIS of comedo histology), one may remove the lower portion of the axillary fat pad between clamps. (In so doing, one must avoid the long thoracic nerve and the thoracodorsal nerve and keep the dissection low enough to ensure that the intercostobrachial sensory nerve is not damaged.) The breast is then taken off the underlying muscles, and the pectoral fascia is included with the specimen.

A single closed suction drain is placed through a separate stab wound laterally to extend under the lower flap and a short distance upward along the sternal border of the dissection. The skin is closed and a dressing applied according to the surgeon's preference. Early arm mobilization is encouraged.

Modified radical mastectomy The incision is placed and flaps are raised as for simple mastectomy. At the lateral edge of the dissection, the border of the latissimus dorsi muscle is exposed, as is the lateral border of the pectoralis muscle. Some surgeons prefer to proceed with axillary dissection first, leaving the breast attached to the chest wall, whereas others prefer to remove the breast from the chest wall first and then use it to

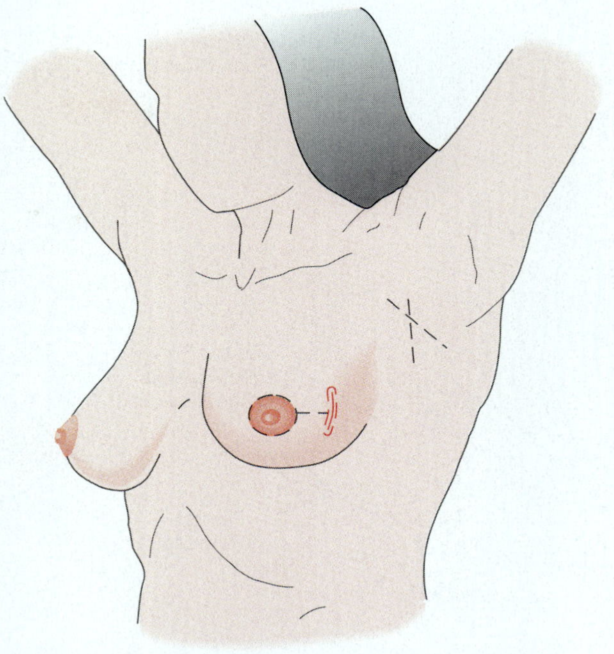

Figure 10 Breast reconstruction after mastectomy. Shown is the recommended placement of incisions for skin-sparing mastectomy. T-shaped incisions extending from the areola to remove previous biopsy incisions may be used if necessary. A separate axillary incision may be necessary when axillary dissection is being done.

provide tension for the axillary dissection. In either case, mechanical or manual retraction of the latissimus dorsi muscle and the greater pectoral muscle generally provides excellent exposure for axillary dissection. The landmarks of the axillary dissection are identified as described earlier [see Axillary Dissection, *above*]. The thoracodorsal bundle can often be seen running along the latissimus dorsi muscle as the muscle is retracted laterally.

Once the axillary dissection has been completed and the breast has been removed from the chest wall, the incision is irrigated and two closed suction drains placed, one in the axilla and another under the lower flap to the midline. The skin is closed and a dressing applied according to the surgeon's preference. Early arm mobilization is encouraged.

Breast Reconstruction after Mastectomy

It is well recognized that immediate breast reconstruction after mastectomy is safe, does not significantly delay subsequent administration of chemotherapy or radiation therapy, and does not prevent detection of recurrent disease. Either implants or autologous tissue may be used in reconstruction. In most cases, the option of breast reconstruction is presented to the mastectomy patient by her breast surgeon during preoperative discussion of mastectomy or, in the case of delayed reconstruction, during follow-up after an earlier mastectomy. The patient, the plastic surgeon, and the oncologic or general surgeon will decide among the several reconstruction options available—implants with tissue expansion, the transverse rectus abdominis myocutaneous (TRAM) flap, the latissimus dorsi myocutaneous flap, and various free flaps—on the basis of patient pref-

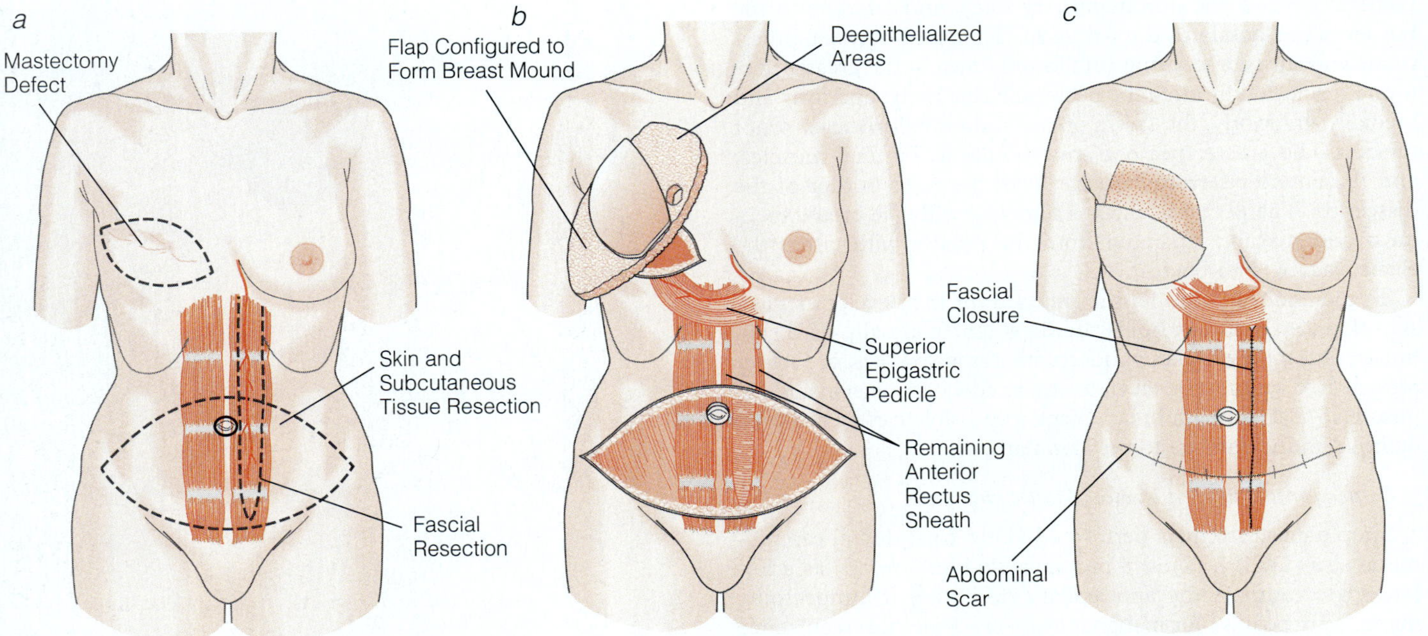

Figure 11 Breast reconstruction after mastectomy. Shown is autologous tissue reconstruction with a transverse rectus abdominis myocutaneous (TRAM) flap. The infraumbilical flap is designed (*a*). The TRAM flap is tunneled subcutaneously into the chest wall cavity. Blood supply to the flap is maintained from the superior epigastric vessels of the rectus abdominis muscle. Subcutaneous fat and deepithelialized skin are positioned under the mastectomy flaps as needed to reconstruct the breast mound (*b*). The fascia of the anterior rectus sheath is approximated to achieve a tight closure of the abdominal wall defect and to prevent hernia formation. The umbilicus is sutured into its new position (*c*).

erence and lifestyle, the availability of suitable autologous tissue, and the demands imposed by any additional cancer therapies required [*see Figure 9*]. Familiarity with the strengths and drawbacks of these reconstruction options facilitates this decision.

OPERATIVE TECHNIQUE

Placement of the incision for mastectomy with immediate reconstruction is determined in discussion with the plastic surgeon. The goal is to preserve as much viable skin as possible for the reconstruction without compromising complete resection of breast and axillary tissue. The nipple and the areola must be included in the resected skin, as must the biopsy incision through which the malignancy was diagnosed [*see Figure 10*]. (One option for removing biopsy incisions while leaving the maximal amount of unaffected skin is to place T-shaped incisions that extend outward from the areola.) FNA and core-needle biopsy incisions are generally not included in the excised skin segment; however, one may, if one wishes, excise a small amount of skin around a core-needle biopsy site. A linear incision should be made as far laterally as necessary to provide adequate exposure for axillary dissection and complete excision of breast tissue. A separate axillary incision may also be used when axillary dissection is being performed [*see Figure 10*]. The extent of dissection should never be compromised in any way for cosmetic reasons.

Reconstruction Options

Implants Perhaps the simplest method of reconstruction is to place a saline-filled implant beneath the greater pectoral muscle and the anterior serratus muscle to recreate a breast mound. Even after a skin-sparing mastectomy, the greater pectoral muscle is usually so tight that unless the patient is small-breasted, expansion of this muscle and the skin is necessary before an implant that matches the opposite breast can be inserted. Serial expansions are performed on an outpatient basis: saline is injected into the expander every 10 to 14 days until an appropriate size has been attained. A second operative procedure is then required to exchange the expander for a permanent implant. A nipple and an areola are constructed at a later date.

The major advantage of implant reconstruction is that there is no need to harvest autologous tissue, and thus the patient is spared the discomfort, scarring, and loss of muscle function that would occur at the donor site. Accordingly, implant reconstructions are commonly performed in patients who require bilateral mastectomies and reconstructions. The initial operative time is significantly shorter for implant reconstruction than for autologous tissue reconstruction, and there is no need for autologous blood donation or transfusion. Hospital stay and recuperation time are also significantly shorter. The main drawbacks are the prolonged time and the multiple office visits required to achieve a symmetric reconstruction if tissue expansion is required and the necessity of a second surgical procedure to place the permanent implant. In addition, the final cosmetic result often is not as good as what can be achieved with autologous tissue reconstruction, and it may deteriorate over time as a consequence of capsule formation or implant migration. The implant-reconstructed breast is significantly firmer than the contralateral breast. The life expectancy of currently available saline implants has not been established, but it may be less than a decade, which means that many patients who have received or are receiving implants may need replacements at some point. Patients who have previously undergone irradiation of the breast or the chest wall may have tissue that cannot be adequately expanded and thus is unsuitable for implant reconstruction. If the final pathological evaluation of the mastectomy specimen indicates that radiation therapy is needed for local control, one may consider irradiating the chest wall before expansion with an expander in place; however, this is not an ideal solution.

Autologous tissue A second approach to reconstruction is to transfer vascularized muscle, skin, and fat from a donor site to the mastectomy defect. The most commonly used myocutaneous flaps are the TRAM flap [see Figure 11] and the latissimus dorsi flap [see Figure 12]. Use of the free TRAM flap is advocated by certain centers; other free-flap options, including the free gluteus flap, are used in special circumstances, when other donor sites are unsuitable.

The major advantage of autologous tissue reconstruction is that it generally yields a superior cosmetic result. Often, the size and shape of the opposite breast can be matched immediately, with no need for subsequent office or operative procedures. The reconstructed breast has a soft texture that is very similar to that of the contralateral breast. In addition, the cosmetic result is stable over time. The main drawbacks are the magnitude of the surgical procedure required for the reconstruction (involving both a prolonged operative time and longer inpatient hospitalization), the need for autologous blood donation or transfusion, and the pain, scarring, and loss of muscle function that arise at the donor site. Smokers and patients with significant vascular disease may not be ideal candidates for autologous tissue reconstruction. Partial necrosis of the transferred flap may create firm areas; on rare occasions, complete necrosis and consequent loss of the flap can occur.

A number of factors are considered in choosing between the TRAM flap and the latissimus dorsi flap. In a TRAM flap reconstruction, the contralateral rectus abdominis muscle is transferred along with overlying skin and fat to create a breast mound. This procedure yields a flatter abdominal contour but calls for a long transverse abdominal incision and necessitates repositioning of the umbilicus. A major advantage of the TRAM flap is that it can provide enough tissue to match all but the largest contralateral breasts. Some patients, however (e.g., those who have undergone an abdominal procedure that compromises the TRAM flap's vascular supply), are not ideal candidates for TRAM flap reconstruction. Postoperative discomfort is greater with TRAM flap reconstruction than with other flap reconstructions because of the extent of the abdominal portion of the procedure. In young, healthy, and motivated patients who require bilateral reconstructions, it is often possible to perform two TRAM flap procedures in the same operation.

In a latissimus dorsi myocutaneous flap reconstruction, the ipsilateral latissimus dorsi muscle is transferred along with overlying skin and fat to create a breast mound. Either a horizontal or a vertical donor site incision may be made on the back. The

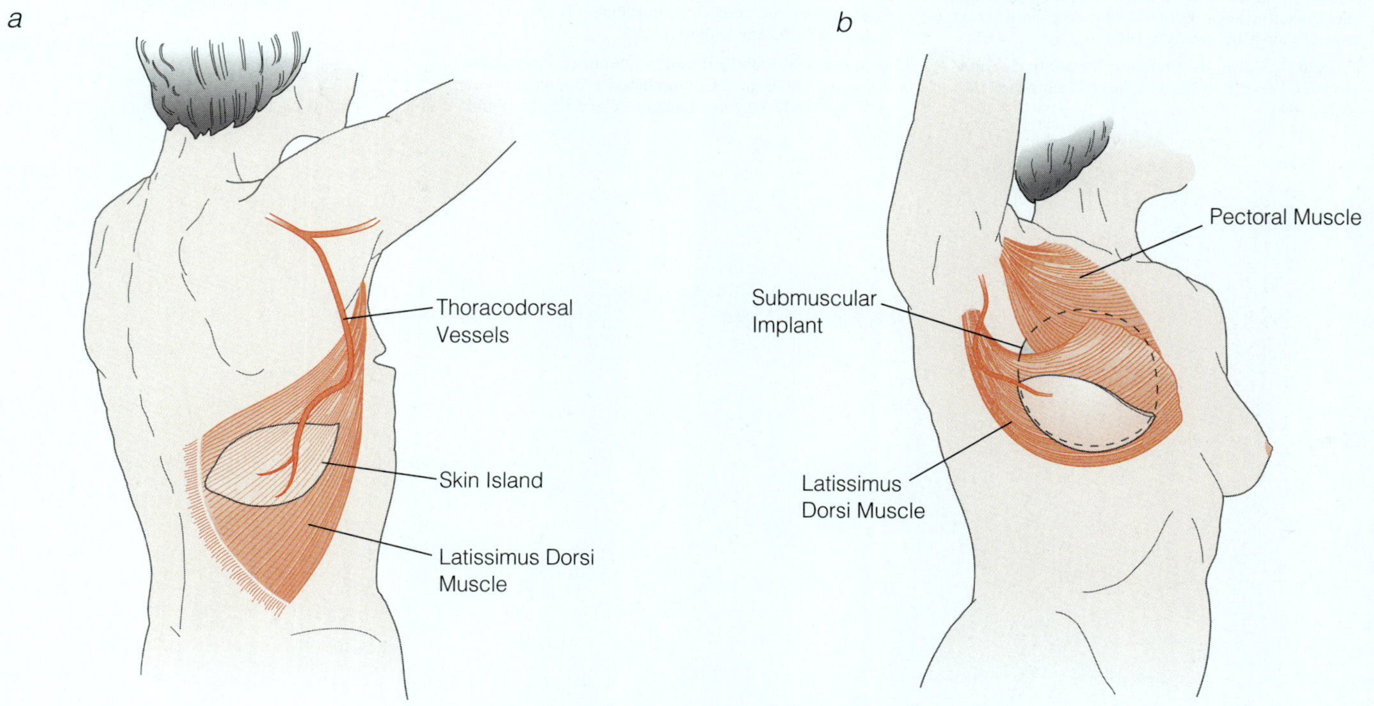

Figure 12 Breast reconstruction after mastectomy. Shown is autologous tissue reconstruction with a latissimus dorsi myocutaneous flap in conjunction with a submuscular implant. (An implant is often required to provide the reconstructed breast with adequate volume and projection.) The myocutaneous flap is elevated; it is important to maintain the blood supply to the flap from the thoracodorsal vessels (*a*). The flap is tunneled subcutaneously to the mastectomy defect (*b*). The latissimus dorsi muscle is sutured to the greater pectoral muscle and the skin of the inframammary fold, so that the implant is completely covered by muscle.

operative technique for the latissimus dorsi flap reconstruction is complex, requiring two intraoperative changes in patient position (from supine to lateral decubitus and from lateral decubitus back to supine for mastectomy, muscle harvest, and final inset of the flap). Patients who have undergone irradiation of the breast, chest wall, or axilla (including irradiation of the thoracodorsal vessels) may not be eligible for this procedure.

A major advantage of the latissimus dorsi flap is that its donor site is associated with less postoperative discomfort than the abdominal donor site of the TRAM flap. In addition, transfer of the latissimus dorsi muscle results in substantially less functional impairment than transfer of the rectus abdominis muscle. A drawback of the latissimus dorsi flap is that in many women, the latissimus dorsi muscle is not bulky enough to provide symmetry with the contralateral breast. In such cases, an implant must be added to the flap to match the size and shape of the opposite breast, which means that the drawback of the implant's limited life span is added to the drawbacks already associated with autologous tissue reconstruction.

Free-flap reconstruction options are utilized primarily when other autologous and implant reconstruction options are not available, do not provide sufficient tissue volume, or have failed. They are more complex procedures, requiring microvascular anastomoses and carrying a higher risk of total flap loss. The two most commonly employed free-flap options are the free TRAM flap and the free gluteus flap.

References

1. Fisher B, Redmond C, Poisson R, et al: Eight-year results of a randomized trial comparing total mastectomy and lumpectomy without irradiation in the treatment of breast cancer. N Engl J Med 320:822, 1989
2. Veronesi U, Luini A, Del Vecchio M, et al: Radiotherapy after breast-preserving surgery in women with localized cancer of the breast. N Engl J Med 328:1587, 1993
3. Sarrazin D, Le M, Rouesse J, et al: Conservative treatment versus mastectomy in breast cancer tumours with mascroscopic diameter of 20 millimetres or less. Cancer 53:1209, 1984
4. Shabot MM, Goldberg IM, Schick P, et al: Aspiration cytology is superior to "Tru-cut" needle biopsy in establishing the diagnosis of clinically suspicious breast masses. Ann Surg 196:122, 1982
5. Gisvold JJ, Martin JK: Prebiopsy localization of nonpalpable breast lesions. AJR Am J Roentgenol 143:477, 1984
6. Meyer JE, Kopans DB, Stomper PC, et al: Occult breast abnormalities: percutaneous preoperative needle localization. Radiology 150:355, 1984
7. Rosenberg AL, Schwartz GF, Feig SA, et al: Clinically occult breast lesions: localization and significance. Radiology 162:167, 1987
8. Dowlatshahi KD, Yaremko ML, Kluskens LF, et al: Nonpalpable breast lesions: findings of stereotaxic needle-core biopsy and fine-needle aspiration cytology. Radiology 181:745, 1991
9. Parker SH, Lovin JD, Jobe WE, et al: Stereotactic breast biopsy with a biopsy gun. Radiology 176:741, 1990
10. Parker SH, Lovin JD, Jobe WE, et al: Nonpalpable breast lesions: stereotactic automated large-core biopsies. Radiology 180:403, 1991
11. Souba WW, Bland KI: Indications and techniques for biopsy. The Breast: Comprehensive Management of Benign and Malignant Diseases. Bland KI, Copeland EM III, Eds. WB Saunders Co, Philadelphia, 1991, p 527
12. Morrow M: Management of common breast disorders. Breast Diseases, 2nd ed. Harris JR, Hellman S, Henderson IC, et al. JB Lippincott, Philadelphia, 1987, p 347
13. Kinne DW: Primary treatment of breast cancer. Breast Diseases, 2nd ed. Harris JR, Hellman S, Henderson IC, et al. JB Lippincott, Philadelphia, 1987, p 347
14. Kinne DW, DeCrosse JJ: Modified radical mastectomy for carcinoma of the breast. Am Surg 48:543, 1982

Acknowledgments

Figures 1, 2, 4 through 8, and 10   Kerry G. Nicholson.

Figure 9   Marcia Kammerer.

Figures 11 and 12   Tom Moore.

44 LYMPHATIC MAPPING AND SENTINEL LYMPH NODE BIOPSY

Douglas Reintgen, M.D., *Fadi Haddad,* M.D., *Solange Pendas,* M.D., *Ni Ni Ku,* M.D., *Claudia Berman,* M.D., *Frank Glass,* M.D., *Jane Messina,* M.D., *and Charles Cox,* M.D.

There is an epidemic of melanoma in the United States: in 1997, 42,000 cases of invasive melanoma and 40,000 cases of melanoma in situ were diagnosed.[1] Moreover, melanoma affects young persons who are in the most productive years of their lives; accordingly, it constitutes a major public health problem. Since the early 1990s, the care of patients with melanoma has changed dramatically with the development of new lymphatic mapping techniques that reduce the cost and morbidity of nodal staging, the emergence of more sensitive assays for occult melanoma metastases, and the identification of interferon alfa-2b as an effective adjuvant therapy for melanoma patients who are at high risk for recurrence. Accurate staging of melanoma patients has become increasingly important in the light of a recent report[2] demonstrating improved survival in patients with T4 (tumor thickness > 4.0 mm) or stage III (nodal metastases) melanoma who were treated with adjuvant interferon alfa-2b.

Breast cancer is one of the most common of the malignancies that surgeons encounter in their practices: approximately 186,000 new cases are diagnosed each year in the United States, and the incidence is likely to increase in the next 10 years because the maturation of the baby-boomer population will result in a larger population at risk. It was one of the first tumors for which adjuvant therapy (i.e., treatment of patients who show no evidence of disease but who are at substantial risk for recurrence and death from the disease) was found to be effective. Most authorities believe that axillary nodal staging is an important part of primary breast cancer therapy in that it facilitates identification of patients who are candidates for more aggressive chemotherapy and enhances regional control of disease—though this view is somewhat controversial, given that most women with invasive breast cancers will receive either adjuvant chemotherapy or hormonal therapy. Complete axillary node dissection, however, is associated with significant morbidity, and physical problems resulting from the dissection are the complaints women voice most frequently after undergoing breast cancer surgery, once they have dealt with the psychological impact of having an incision on their breast or perhaps even losing the breast.

The development of intraoperative lymphatic mapping and selective lymphadenectomy has made it possible to map the lymphatic flow from a primary tumor and to identify its so-called sentinel lymph node (SLN) in the regional basin. Integration of this technique, in association with detailed pathologic examination of the SLN, into the surgical treatment of melanoma and breast cancer offers the potential for more conservative operations that not only result in lower morbidity but also permit more accurate staging. In what follows, we describe the technical aspects of this new approach, as well as certain related issues.

Lymphatic Mapping and SLN Biopsy for Melanoma

RATIONALE

Many factors are known to predict the risk for metastatic disease in melanoma patients. In evaluating treatments for melanoma, it is crucial to take into account prognostic factors that can accurately categorize patients into different risk groups for metastasis. If this is not done, it is difficult or impossible to determine whether differences between treatment regimens (or the absence thereof) are due to the treatments themselves or merely reflect imbalances of prognostic factors.

The presence or absence of lymph node metastases is the single most powerful predictor of recurrence and survival in melanoma patients: the 5-year survival rate is approximately 40% lower in patients who have lymph node metastases than in those who do not. A great deal of time, effort, and money has been expended on identifying prognostic factors based on primary tumor variables (e.g., Breslow's level, ulceration, primary site, and sex); however, multiple regression analyses performed on many collected populations in the literature indicate that once melanoma metastasizes to the regional nodes, such prognostic factors contribute relatively little to the prognostic model compared with the patient's lymph node status. This finding suggests that many melanoma patients might benefit from a nodal staging procedure.

Nodal Staging

Elective lymph node dissection Elective lymph node dissection (ELND) has been the mainstay of the surgeon's armamentarium for nodal staging of melanoma patients. ELND removes clinically negative nodes, as opposed to therapeutic dissection, which removes nodes with gross tumor involvement. Opinions are divided as to whether ELND actually extends survival or whether it is solely a staging procedure. Two prospective, randomized trials failed to demonstrate improved survival in melanoma patients treated with ELND in comparison with patients who underwent wide local excision (WLE) alone as primary surgical therapy.[3,4] Retrospective studies using large databases, however, suggested that there were subpopulations of melanoma patients who did benefit from ELND.[5,6]

The controversy may have been laid to rest by the results of the Intergroup Melanoma Trial, which is the first randomized study to prove enhanced survival after surgical treatment of clinically occult metastatic melanoma. Only patients with intermediate-thickness melanoma (tumor thickness, 1.0 to 4.0 mm) were eligible. In addition, the Intergroup Melanoma Trial was the first prospective study to require preoperative lymphoscintigraphy in all patients to identify and remove all basins at risk for metastasis. Without preoperative lymphoscintigraphy to provide a map for the surgeon, ELND may be misdirected in more than 50% of head and neck dissections and trunk dissections[7]; moreover, so-called in transit nodes (defined as nodes outside the classic anatomic basin between the primary site and the regional nodes), which are equally at risk for metastasis, may be missed in 5% of patients.[8]

In the Intergroup Melanoma Trial, overall survival was not significantly longer in patients who underwent WLE and ELND than in those who underwent WLE of the primary site coupled with observation of the regional basins. There were, however, two well-defined subsets of the ELND group that exhibited a significant increase in overall survival: patients with melanomas 1.1 to 2.0 mm thick and patients younger than 60 years.[9] Stratification by tumor thickness was part of the original design of the trial, but the age-related benefit only became apparent with retrospective subgroup analysis.

Given these results[9] and those of the study that was the impetus for FDA approval of interferon alfa-2b as adjuvant therapy,[2] one can make a strong argument that when the risk of nodal metastasis reaches a certain defined level, a nodal staging procedure should be done. At our institution (H. Lee Moffitt Cancer Center [MCC], Tampa, Florida), that level is considered to have been reached when tumor thickness is 1.0 mm or greater. The nodal staging procedure we recommend and perform is lymphatic mapping and SLN biopsy.

Intraoperative lymphatic mapping and selective lymphadenectomy Intraoperative lymphatic mapping and selective lymphadenectomy were developed as a method of assessing regional lymph node status more accurately than ELND could while reducing both morbidity and expense. This technique relies on two concepts: first, that different regions of the skin have specific patterns of lymphatic drainage to the regional lymphatic basin; and second, that for a given skin region, there is a specific lymph node (i.e., a sentinel lymph node) in the basin to which the cutaneous lymphatic vessels drain first. These concepts were borne out by initial animal studies using

---

Choice of Radiocolloid and Vital Blue Dye for Lymphatic Mapping

Choice of Radiocolloid

Little work has been done to determine which radiocolloid is best suited to either preoperative or intraoperative mapping. The ideal radiocolloid for intraoperative SLN mapping would have small particles (< 100 nm) that are uniformly dispersed, would be highly stable, and would have a short half-life that would not complicate the handling of the excised specimen. Technetium (^{99m}Tc)-labeled compounds, being gamma emitters, satisfy most of these requirements. In a direct comparison between filtered (0.1 μm) ^{99m}Tc-labeled sulfur colloid (^{99m}Tc-SC) and ^{99m}Tc-labeled antimony trisulfide colloid (^{99m}Tc-ATC), which has a particle size of 3 to 30 nm, filtered ^{99m}Tc-SC was transported more quickly to the nodal basin and emitted less radiation to the liver, the spleen, and the whole body.[71] Unfiltered ^{99m}Tc-SC contains relatively large particles (100 to 1,000 nm), and some investigators have found it to migrate more slowly from the injection site; however, other investigators have found it to be slow to flow through the first SLN to higher secondary nodes, which is actually an advantage.

In comparisons between ^{99m}Tc-labeled human serum albumin (^{99m}Tc-HSA), ^{99m}Tc-labeled stannous phyate, and ^{99m}Tc-ATC with respect to lymphoscintigram quality, the last of these provided the best images for preoperative lymphoscintigraphy.[72] In an animal study comparing ^{99m}Tc-HSA and filtered ^{99m}Tc-SC, ^{99m}Tc-SC was actually concentrated in the sentinel lymph node over a period of 1 to 2 hours, whereas ^{99m}Tc-HSA passed rapidly through the SLN.[29] As a result, ^{99m}Tc-SC yielded higher activity ratios at intraoperative mapping, improved the success rate of localization, made the technique easier, and thus was a superior reagent for this application.[28,29]

The Sydney Melanoma Unit (SMU)[73] prefers to use ^{99m}Tc-ATC because it seems to have smaller, more uniform particles that rapidly migrate into the lymphatic channels but still are appropriately trapped and retained by the SLN. At SMU, use of this compound allows injection of the radiocolloid and imaging to be performed the day before operation. These investigators find that hot spots in the regional basin are maintained even if 24 hours have elapsed from the time of the injection. The radioactivity in the basin over the hot spot (i.e., the SLN) is decreased because four half-lives of the technetium have been expended and because some of the radiocolloid has passed through, but the ex vivo activity ratio (i.e., SLN:neighboring non-SLN) is not substantially affected. In the United States, ^{99m}Tc-ATC has been removed from the market and is unavailable for clinical use.

Others investigators have obtained very good intraoperative mapping results with unfiltered ^{99m}Tc-SC; however, they have not obtained good planar images for lymphoscintigraphy and have been unable to identify cutaneous lymphatic flow to any basin in 10% of the patients.[18]

At MCC, we use filtered (0.2 μm) ^{99m}Tc-SC. This particle size gives good images on lymphoscintigraphy and is trapped and concentrated in the SLN over a significant period, so that the hot spot over the SLN actually becomes hotter compared with surrounding tissue for 2 to 6 hours after injection, making the SLN easier to find. It also has an advantage over unfiltered ^{99m}Tc-SC in that it results in less shine-through of radioactivity from the primary site.

Choice of Vital Blue Dye

Several vital blue dyes have been investigated with an eye to their potential applicability to cutaneous lymphatic mapping. Among these are methylene blue (American Regent Lab, Shirley, New York), isosulfan blue, 1% in aqueous solution (Lymphazurin; United States Surgical Corporation, Norwalk, Connecticut), patent blue-V (Laboratoire Guerbert, France), Cyalume (American Cyanamid Company, Bound Brook, New Jersey), and fluorescein dye. All substances tested were known to be nontoxic in vivo and were injected intradermally as provided by the supplier. In a feline study,[10] patent blue-V and isosulfan blue were the most accurate in identifying the regional lymphatic drainage pattern. These dyes entered the lymphatics rapidly, with minimal diffusion into the surrounding tissue. Their bright-blue color was readily visible and allowed easy identification of the exposed lymphatics.

Isosulfan blue has worked extremely well for intraoperative SLN mapping. In some patients with thin skin, the afferent lymphatics can be seen through the skin after the injection of isosulfan blue. In addition, when the dye enters the SLN, it stains part of the node a pale blue, thus clearly distinguishing the SLN from the surrounding non-SLNs. The other dyes have largely been abandoned as unsatisfactory because they diffuse too rapidly into surrounding tissue and are not retained by the lymphatic channels in sufficient concentrations to stain the SLN. The fluorescent dyes fluorescein and Cyalume are readily visualized, but a dark room is necessary for optimal visualization; moreover, because of their diffusion into surrounding tissue, the background fluorescence is unacceptably high. Methylene blue is relatively poorly retained by the lymphatic vessels and thus stains the SLN too lightly.

Use of vital blue dyes has not given rise to any significant complications. Although allergic reactions have been reported on rare occasions in the literature, they have not occurred in large study populations.[14,15] Blue dye can be retained at the primary site for more than a year. The color gradually fades with time; however, patients can be left with a permanent tattoo if the injected dye is not removed with wide local excision (WLE) of the primary site or, in the case of breast cancer, with lumpectomy. Fortunately, in the head and neck area, where a permanent tattoo would be unacceptable, the richness of the cutaneous lymphatics allows rapid clearance of the blue dye from the skin and the subcutaneous tissues. A small amount of residual dye may be left behind after WLE, but this typically disappears rapidly and poses no real problem. All patients report the presence of dye in the urine during the first 24 hours. In some cases, the dye can interfere with transcutaneous oxygen monitoring during anesthesia.

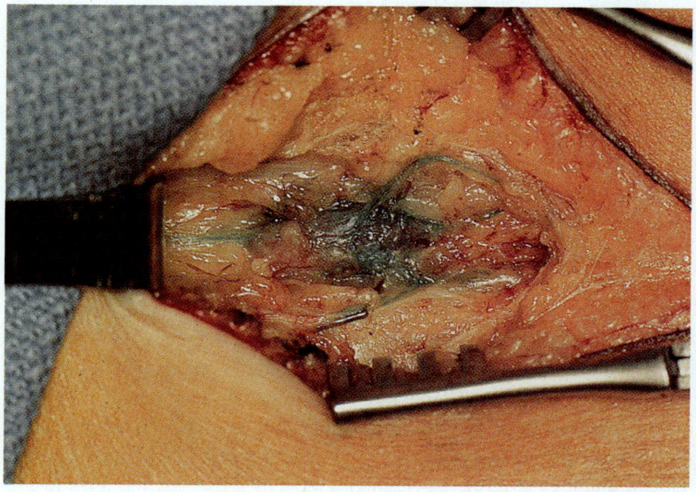

Figure 1 Lymphatic mapping and SLN biopsy for melanoma. Primary sites for both melanoma and breast cancer may have four to six afferent lymphatics emerging from the tumor location, but as the lymphatics travel to the regional basin, they converge into one or two SLNs. Shown are four afferent lymphatics converging into one SLN.

either vital blue dye[10] or radiocolloid[11] (which has been shown to map the same lymphatic pathways and label the same nodes as vital blue dye) [see *Sidebar* Choice of Radiocolloid and Vital Blue Dye for Lymphatic Mapping].

Intraoperative lymphatic mapping and selective lymphadenectomy was initially proposed by Morton and associates,[12,13] who used a vital blue dye method. These investigators showed that the SLN is the first node in the lymphatic basin into which the primary melanoma consistently drains (though not necessarily the closest to the primary). They also hypothesized that the status of the SLN, if it was negative for metastases, would reflect the status of higher nodes (i.e., nodes farther down the lymphatic drainage pathway). Subsequent work on intraoperative mapping and selective lymphadenectomy confirmed that the SLN is the first site of metastatic disease and demonstrated that if the SLN is histologically negative, then the remainder of the lymph nodes in the basin are histologically negative as well.[14,15] These findings suggest that melanoma patients can be accurately staged with procedures that are less extensive than complete dissection.

SLNs can be mapped from different primary site locations, and more than one node in the same basin can be an SLN, depending on the primary site. Fine dermal lymphatic vessels coalesce to form several major lymphatic trunks that eventually drain to the regional lymphatic basin. Because cutaneous lymphatic vessels converge rather than diverge [see *Figure 1*], one can perform intraoperative mapping from various skin sites and still harvest only one or two SLNs from the basin. The small number of specimens facilitates detailed pathologic examination: the pathologist can readily perform serial sections of the nodes and use immunohistochemical methods to look for micrometastatic disease. More intensive pathologic examination of one or two SLNs appears to identify patients with micrometastatic lymph node metastases more accurately than routine examination of all the regional lymph nodes.

Unusual or ambiguous drainage patterns. Lymphoscintigraphy has been used in live patients to map patterns of lymphatic drainage from various primary skin sites. Early assessments of lymphatic flow patterns, such as those of the 19th century anatomist Sappey,[16] were based on anatomic dissections of cadavers and do not accurately reflect lymphatic flow patterns in living humans. The watershed areas of the body are much larger than originally described by Sappey, and there is no clinically predictable lymphatic flow from a melanoma until it is located 10 cm off the midline or 10 cm off Sappey's line (a line running between the umbilicus and L2) [see *Figure 2*]. In addition, the entire head and neck region is a watershed area. Cutaneous lymphatic flow frequently cannot be predicted on the basis of anatomic site, and areas of ambiguous or multidirectional flow are significantly more extensive than classical descriptions predicted.[17]

A number of unusual drainage patterns and pathways have been noted in Australia[17]: 26% of melanomas on the back drained to an in transit node near the scapula in the intermuscular space [see *Figure 3*], 20% of melanomas near the umbilicus drained to an internal mammary node, some posterior scalp melanomas drained to lymph nodes at the base of the neck, and at least one forearm melanoma drained directly to a lymph node in the ipsilateral neck. Krag and coworkers[18,19] have also noted some unusual lymphatic drainage patterns: one melanoma on the right upper back drained directly to a node in the right midclavicular space, almost at the apex of the right lung; another melanoma on the lower back drained to an SLN along the neurovascular bundle under the 12th rib; and two lower extremity melanomas drained to SLNs in the popliteal fossa. At MCC, one primary back melanoma drained directly via different afferent lymphatics to SLNs in both the inguinal and the iliac basin. Finally, some lower extremity lesions may bypass the superficial groin and drain directly into the iliac chain.

PATIENT SELECTION

Selective lymphadenectomy and SLN biopsy are currently being evaluated in a randomized trial sponsored by the National Cancer Institute, the goal of which is to determine whether this surgical strategy by itself extends the survival of the melanoma patient [see Discussion, National Protocols, *below*]. Even if this trial demonstrates no inherent

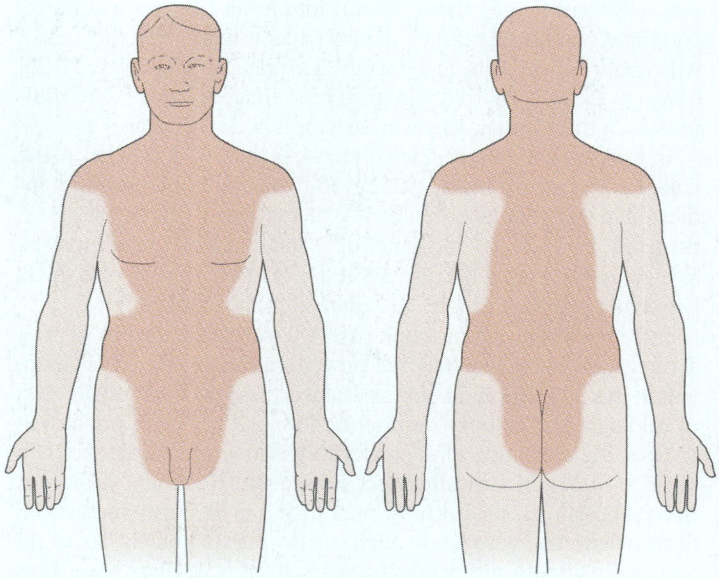

Figure 2 Lymphatic mapping and SLN biopsy for melanoma. The watershed areas of the body where multidirectional cutaneous lymphatic flow is found are much more extensive than classical descriptions predicted. One does not find unidirectional cutaneous lymphatic flow until lesions are 10 cm off the midline or 10 cm off Sappey's line, which runs between the umbilicus and L2. The entire head and neck area is also unpredictable.

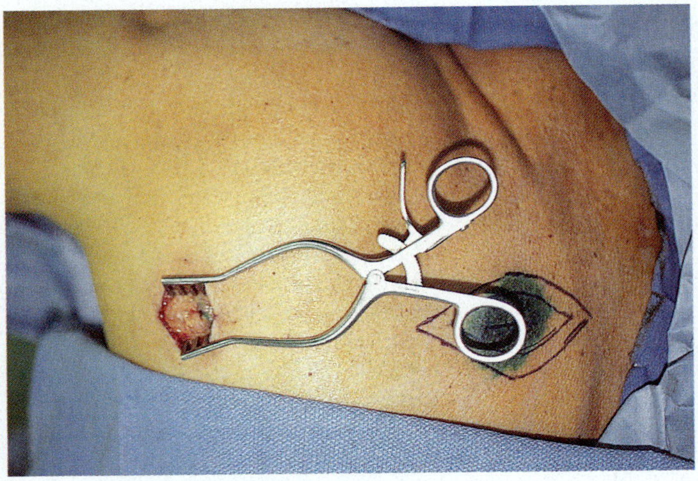

Figure 3 Lymphatic mapping and SLN biopsy for melanoma. Shown is an intermediate-thickness melanoma of the left back in a 40-year-old male. Preoperative lymphoscintigraphy identified flow from the primary site into the left axilla and separate flow into an in transit node located at the tip of the left scapula. Vital blue dye was injected into the dermis around the primary site, and a small incision was made over the tattoo marking the location of the in transit node, which could then be visualized and harvested.

survival benefit, there are additional considerations that support use of the procedure in certain populations. Data from the interferon alfa-2b trial cited earlier[2] suggest that all patients whose melanoma is more than 1.0 mm thick should undergo a nodal staging procedure so that adjuvant therapy can be administered in a selective fashion. If T4N0 patients are removed from the analysis of this trial and only patients with lymph node metastases are considered, disease-free survival (DFS) increases by 82% ($P = 0.0006$) with adjuvant therapy; overall survival increases by 24% as well ($P = 0.006$). Given such a substantial difference in both DFS and overall survival, one would naturally want to offer these patients interferon alfa-2b therapy. Accordingly, one would need to identify patients with nodal metastases who might benefit from such therapy. Lymphatic mapping and SLN biopsy is the least morbid and most cost-effective way of determining which melanoma patients have lymph node metastases.[20]

In female patients with melanomas less than 0.76 mm thick, the risk of nodal metastasis is less than 1%; thus, SLN biopsy is not indicated in this population. In male patients whose primary site is on the trunk, however, the incidence of occult nodal metastases may be as high as 9%, even if the primary lesion is less than 0.76 mm thick; lymphatic mapping may be considered in this population.

In patients whose tumor is 0.76 to 1.0 mm thick, the risk of nodal metastasis is less than 6%; the procedure can be offered as an option in this population. In our experience, these patients usually elect to undergo SLN biopsy despite the low risk of occult nodal metastasis: the morbidity of the procedure is low, and the finding of a positive SLN can radically affect subsequent treatment decisions. Several prognostic factors have been shown to identify patients with thin melanomas who are at higher risk (approximately 10%) for metastatic disease and death at 5 years: tumors at Clark level III or greater, ulcerated primaries, regressed lesions, male gender, and axial melanomas.[21] Patients with these prognostic factors should be treated as if they had thicker lesions, and their SLNs should be harvested even if the primary lesions are less than 0.76 mm thick.

In patients with thick (> 4.0 mm) melanomas, the rate of occult systemic metastasis is 70%, and that of occult nodal metastasis is 60% to 70%. Consequently, in the past, procedures involving the regional nodes (i.e., ELND) were not recommended, because there was no survival benefit. Now that effective adjuvant therapy is available, however, lymphatic mapping and SLN biopsy should be offered to these patients as a staging procedure. Survival is decreased in patients with thick melanomas and documented nodal microscopic disease compared with patients with thick melanomas and no sign of nodal spread[22]; accordingly, some medical oncologists observe T4 patients unless nodal metastasis is documented.

A crucial question to be answered is, what is the standard of surgical care for melanoma patients with tumors thicker than 1.0 mm? Given that five reports in the literature have shown how the histology of the SLN is indicative of the histology of the rest of the nodes in the basin, one can conclude that if the surgeon has adequate support from nuclear medicine and pathology services, there is no need to perform ELND. If such support is unavailable, if intraoperative mapping cannot be done (as, perhaps, when WLE of the primary melanoma has already been performed), or if the results of mapping are equivocal, then the ELND guidelines from the Intergroup Melanoma Surgical Trial[9] should be followed. If this approach is taken, ELND should be guided by preoperative lymphoscintigraphy for identification and dissection of all basins at risk for metastasis.

Finally, previous extensive primary site surgery constitutes a general technical contraindication to lymphatic mapping. Patients who have undergone rotational flap closure or Z-plasty reconstruction are considered ineligible for this procedure.

TECHNIQUE

The technique of intraoperative mapping varies considerably from center to center. We will describe the nuances of the technique as it is performed at MCC, detailing the steps that are important for successful mapping. It cannot be emphasized enough that successful intraoperative SLN mapping requires close collaboration between the surgeon, the nuclear radiologist, and the pathologist, with each member of the team playing a critical role.

An initial caveat regarding the timing of the procedure in relation to WLE is in order. Data from MCC indicate that when lymphatic mapping is done after WLE, the dissection tends to be more extensive than it need have been. More SLNs are removed and more regional basins dissected than when lymphatic mapping is done before WLE; moreover, the rate at which so-called skip metastases are detected appears to be increased. With lymphatic mapping and SLN biopsy becoming the standard of care in the United States for nodal staging to identify melanoma patients who are candidates for adjuvant therapy and a possible survival benefit, it is essential that patient care not be compromised by extensive primary site surgery before lymphatic mapping.

Step 1: Preoperative Lymphoscintigraphy

Patients come to the nuclear medicine suite early on the day of operation and undergo preoperative lymphoscintigraphy with the injection of 450 µCi in 1 ml of filtered technetium-99–labeled sulfur colloid (^{99m}Tc-SC) [see Sidebar Choice of Radiocolloid and Vital Blue Dye for Lymphatic Mapping] per direction of drainage around the primary site. Dynamic scans are performed 5 to 10 minutes after injection of the radiocolloid, and the location of the SLN in the basin is marked with an intradermal tattoo. All regional lymphatic basins at risk for metastatic spread, along with in transit nodes and SLNs, are identified and marked for harvesting.

Comment Preoperative lymphoscintigraphy serves as a road map for planning the surgical procedure and is used for four distinct reasons:

1. To identify all nodal basins at risk for metastatic disease.[7] This is especially important with melanomas of the trunk or the head and neck, whose lymphatic drainage patterns cannot be reliably predicted by clinical judgment or classic anatomic guidelines.[23]

2. To identify any in transit nodes that can be tattooed by the nuclear radiologist for later harvesting [see Figure 4]. An example is afforded by the case of a forearm lesion with an afferent lymphatic vessel flowing to an epitrochlear in transit node and a separate afferent vessel flowing from that node to the axillary basin [see Figure 4a]. The SLNs in both locations were harvested, and only the epitrochlear SLN was histologically positive. In this case, mapping with the blue dye alone would have yielded histologically negative axillary SLNs and understaged the patient. In addition, the tumor containing an epitrochlear in transit node would have been left in place and thus might later have seeded the axillary nodes or distant metastatic sites.

3. To identify the location of the SLN in relation to the rest of the nodes in the basin.[24-26] Because the location of the SLN may vary within a basin, it is important to mark the position of the SLN in reference to other nodes so that harvesting may be done with local anesthesia through a minimal incision. Preoperative lymphoscintigraphy can accomplish this task quite well, especially in the groin and the head and neck area, where the lymph nodes are more superficial. The axilla is the most difficult area to map: here, the best preoperative lymphoscintigraphy can do is to determine whether the node is located anteriorly, posteriorly, superiorly, or inferiorly in the basin. Use of hand-held gamma probes during SLN mapping has reduced the need to mark SLN locations during preoperative lymphoscintigraphy; however, intradermal tattooing to mark the location of the SLN can confirm the site and thereby make the surgical procedure more efficient.

4. To estimate the number of SLNs in the regional basin that will have to be harvested.

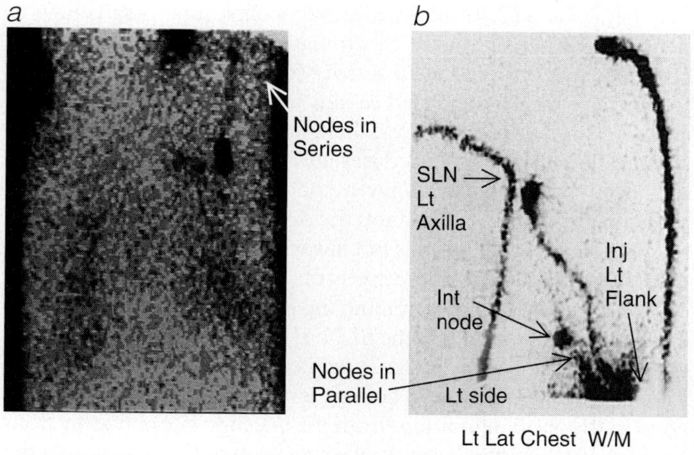

The timing of the injection of the mapping reagent has an impact on the success of the procedure. Whereas vital blue dyes typically travel to the regional basin within a matter of minutes, most radiocolloids are concentrated in the SLN over a period of hours. Activity ratios (see below) for ^{99m}Tc-SC are highest 2 to 6 hours after injection, which is helpful to the surgeon in three respects. First, the higher ratios make the SLN easier to locate. Second, the radiocolloid can be injected by the nuclear radiologist hours before the actual operation, and the surgeon does not need a special license for radioactivity handling. Third, cases are easier to schedule because there is a 2- to 6-hour window during which the intraoperative mapping can be easily accomplished.

Step 2: Intraoperative Lymphatic Mapping and Identification of SLN

The patient is taken to the OR 2 to 6 hours later, and 1 ml of 1% isosulfan blue dye (Lymphazurin) [see Sidebar Choice of Radiocolloid and Vital Blue Dye for Lymphatic Mapping] is injected around the primary site. The primary site and the regional basin are prepared and draped, and 10 minutes is allowed for the vital blue dye to travel to the SLN. Attention is then directed initially to the regional basin. The radioactive hot spot in the regional basin is identified with the hand-held gamma probe, and the in vivo activity ratio (see below) is noted. If shine-through from the residual radioactivity at the primary site is a problem, WLE of the primary may be performed first. An incision is made over the hot spot, and small flaps are created in all directions to allow identification of the blue-stained afferent lymphatic vessels. Surgical dissection is aided by visualization of the stained afferent lymphatic vessel down to the blue-stained node and by the use of the hand-held gamma probe to direct dissection down to the SLN. If, as is sometimes the case, one becomes confused as to what is proximal and what is distal on the afferent lymphatic vessel, the probe can be used to identify the direction of dissection.

Figure 4 Lymphatic mapping and SLN biopsy for melanoma. In transit nodal areas are identified in 5% of melanoma patients; this is the reason why preoperative lymphoscintigraphy is performed for primary sites on either the upper or the lower extremity. In a patient with a melanoma on the left hand (*a*), the injection site and the left hand are raised above the head, and cutaneous lymphatic flow can be seen into an epitrochlear node. This in transit node then emits a lymphatic vessel flowing to the left axilla. By definition, the SLN is the first node in the chain that receives primary lymphatic flow. The epitrochlear node and any axillary nodes are nodes in series. Hence, the epitrochlear node is the SLN and thus is the only node that must be harvested. In a patient with a primary melanoma on the left flank (*b*), there are two separate afferent lymphatics, one leading to an SLN in the left axilla and the other leading to an in transit node on the left flank. These are nodes in parallel in that they both receive primary lymphatic flow from the skin site. Hence, the two nodes are equally at risk for metastatic disease, and both are considered SLNs and must be harvested.

Comment Radiocolloid and vital blue dye mapping techniques are complementary, and there is no reason why the two approaches should not be used simultaneously to improve the chances of locating the SLN successfully. Either may be crucial in a given instance, depending on the location of the primary in relation to the regional basin. If the primary site is close to, overlying, or in a direct line to the basin, so that the gamma probe is likely to encounter shine-through, use of vital blue dye may be the only technique that permits successful mapping. Only 1% to 5% of the injected radiocolloid dose is delivered to the regional basin; thus, even if the radioactivity from the primary site is reduced by performing WLE first, enough radioactivity may remain at that site to increase the background level in the basin to the point where mapping with the radiocolloid alone is impossible. On the other hand, when one is mapping a fatty axilla or the head and neck region, it may be impossible to follow a wisp of blue-stained afferent lymphatic vessel to the SLN. Large flaps are especially to be avoided in the head and neck area because of the surrounding vital structures; in this setting, the ability of the gamma probe to locate the hot spot through the skin before the incision is made is a tremendous advantage.

A key issue with intraoperative radiocolloid mapping is how to define an SLN in terms of accumulated radioactivity. To do this, clinicians must use so-called activity (or localization) ratios. Measurement of the absolute level of radioactivity in a node is not sufficient, because in each harvest, there are a number of crucial variables: different radiocolloid doses are injected at the primary site, the injection is sometimes uneven, the time interval between injection and harvest is not constant, the distance between the primary site and the regional basin is not always the same, and varying degrees of shine-through may be present. The effects of these variables can be eliminated by determining the in vivo activity ratio (i.e., the ratio of the radioactivity in the SLN to the background radioactivity). In vivo radioactivity is measured in counts/10 sec with the SLN fully exposed. Background activity is estimated by counting four areas in the basin equidistant from the injection site and away from the SLN. Also helpful is the ex vivo activity ratio (i.e., the ratio of the radioactivity in an excised SLN to that in an excised neighboring non-SLN), which has the virtue of eliminating all shine-through. At MCC, we define an SLN as a node with an activity ratio of 3:1 or higher in vivo or 10:1 or higher ex vivo. In our experience, 98% of SLNs exhibit these ratios.

Occasionally, pass-through of the blue dye or the radiocolloid occurs but rarely, if ever, to the point where it results in mistaken identification of a higher node as an SLN. That is, one typically does not see non-SLNs that are stained blue or that have activity ratios of 3:1 in vivo or 10:1 ex vivo. When the radiocolloid does pass through the SLN, it is distributed to multiple higher nodes, thereby helping to raise the background radiation level; however, it is not concentrated to any large extent in any one higher node.

Step 3: Removal of SLN

Once the SLN is identified, the entire node is removed by means of sharp dissection or the electrocautery. Afferent and efferent lymphatic vessels proceeding from the SLN, some of which are stained blue, are controlled with hemostatic clips because the electrocautery will not seal these vessels. This measure decreases the risk of postoperative wound seroma. If the opportunity presents itself without the risk of increased morbidity, a neighboring non-SLN may be removed to provide an internal control, and the ex vivo activity ratio may be calculated.

The radioactivity level in the excised SLN is checked with the hand-held gamma probe to confirm that the node has been correctly identified as the SLN. The residual radioactivity in the basin is then checked with the probe to verify that all SLNs have been removed. If radioactivity has not fallen to the background level, the probe should be used to direct additional dissection.

Comment The directed dissection achievable with the help of radio-guided mapping allows the surgeon to perform axillary and head and neck harvests without having to identify the motor nerves running through the basin. A series of 30 head and neck melanoma patients with SLN drainage to the parotid gland[27] showed that the SLNs could be harvested with directed dissection without formal identification of fascial motor nerves. The technique recommended by the authors—which may be adaptable to other basins where dissection passes close to a motor nerve—involved eliminating paralyzing agents with anesthesia, incising the parotid fascia, then, with blunt dissection under gamma-probe guidance, shelling out the SLN in the parotid gland. The success rate of SLN identification in the parotid gland was higher than 90%, and there were no instances of fascial nerve dysfunction. Likewise, in more than 300 axillary SLN mappings at MCC, there has been no evidence of prolonged postoperative thoracic or thoracodorsal dysfunction. Dissections in the posterior cervical triangle are performed similarly when in close proximity to the spinal accessory nerve.

A secondary benefit of radiocolloid mapping is its ability to provide immediate verification that all SLNs have been removed from the lymphatic basin: if all of the radiolabeled SLNs have in fact been excised, the radioactivity in the basin must return to its background level. When only vital blue dye is used for mapping, it often proves necessary to perform further dissection (and create more flaps) to locate additional blue-stained lymphatics and verify that all SLNs have been excised.

In addition, as noted [see Step 1: Preoperative Lymphoscintigraphy, above], the radiocolloid has a much longer retention time than the dye and tends to be concentrated in the SLN. When harvest occurs 2 to 6 hours after injection of the radiocolloid, activity ratios are double what they are when mapping is done immediately after injection.[28,29] In our experience, if one waits until the next day to perform the harvest, one may still be able to identify a hot spot in the basin; however, the radioactivity counts are much lower, and thus, we do not consider this approach ideal.

Step 4: Pathologic Examination of SLN

Once the SLN has been harvested, it is submitted for detailed pathologic examination. The examination may include serial sectioning, immunohistochemical staining with S-100 and HMB-45 monoclonal antibodies, and perhaps reverse transcriptase–polymerase chain reaction (RT-PCR) analysis.

COMPLICATIONS

Complications of lymphatic mapping are rare. All SLN harvests are performed without any postoperative drainage, and this contributes to the low morbidity of the procedure. A seroma develops in about 10% of patients, but it is easily handled with percutaneous aspiration. Surgical site infections are rare, and wound healing is better than with ELND because large flaps are not needed for the dissection.

REPORTED RESULTS

In the initial report by Morton and associates,[12] in which mapping was done with vital blue dye alone, SLNs were successfully identified in 194 of 237 lymphatic basins, and 40 (21%) of the 194 specimens contained metastatic melanoma detected either by routine histologic examination with hematoxylin-eosin staining (12%) or by immunohistochemical staining exclusively (9%). Metastases were present in 47 (18%) of 259 SLNs, whereas non-SLNs were the exclusive site of metastasis in only two of 3,079 nodes from 194 dissections, for a false negative rate of 1% (with nodes rather than patients as the unit of analysis).

Given that lymphatic mapping can be evaluated only in patients with metastatic disease—because these are the only patients in whom a skip metastasis (i.e., a metastasis in which the SLN is histologically negative but nodes farther down the drainage pathway are histologically positive) could be documented—the investigators' findings in these patients are of considerable interest. Of 40 patients with histologically positive nodes, SLN mapping identified 38, for a 5% false negative rate. In 72% of basins, a particular primary site drained to a single SLN; in 20%, to two SLNs; and in 8%, to three or more SLNs. Surgeons successfully identified SLNs in 72% to 96% of attempts, depending on where the surgeons were on the learning curve. Overall, groin mappings were the most successful (89% of attempts); axillary mapping was generally successful as well (78% of attempts). The investigators concluded that a learning curve of 60 cases would be necessary, which meant that the procedure would have to be restricted to major medical centers that treat large numbers of melanoma patients. This caveat notwithstanding, the new technique clearly was capable of accurately identifying patients with occult lymph node metastases who might benefit from radical lymphadenectomy.[12,13]

Surgical trials at several other institutions[8,14,15,18,19] confirmed two essential points. First, nodal metastasis from cutaneous primary sites follows an orderly, nonrandom, progressive pattern. Second, SLNs in the lymphatic basins can be individually identified, and their status reflects the presence or absence of melanoma metastases in the remaining nodes in the basins. In an initial study of 42 patients with intermediate-thickness melanomas,[14] SLN harvesting was followed by complete node dissection to confirm the low incidence of skip metastases in this population. None of the patients in this study had skip metastases: eight had a positive SLN, with the SLN as the only site of disease in seven of the eight, and 34 had a histologically negative SLN, with the rest of the nodes in the basin also histologically negative. Analysis of the results proved that the SLN was the first and favored site of metastatic disease. Preoperative lymphoscintigraphy was performed in this trial to define all basins at risk for metastatic disease, and intraoperative mapping was performed with isosulfan blue dye. The rate of technical failure was 10%.

A trial at the University of Vermont employed radiocolloid for intraoperative mapping after it was determined that in some cases, use of the vital blue dye was difficult if not impossible.[30] The investigators studied 100 patients with melanoma arising at a wide variety of primary sites. All of the patients underwent lymphoscintigraphy 1 to 24 hours before intraoperative mapping and SLN excision. A hand-held gamma probe was used to facilitate accurate identification and removal of the SLNs. Incisions were made directly over the hot spot to minimize dissection; further dissection, if needed, was guided by the probe. The SLNs were successfully located in 98% of the patients, a markedly better result than was obtained in previous reports.

Subsequently, this same melanoma consortium published updated findings.[18] Between February 1993 and October 1994, 121 patients with invasive melanomas and clinically negative nodes were enrolled in a study comparing two different approaches to intraoperative mapping. In one group (64% of patients), mapping involved only injection of a radiocolloid (unfiltered ^{99m}Tc-SC, ^{99m}Tc–human serum albumin [^{99m}Tc-HSA], or Microlite [Dupont, Billerica, Massachusetts]) around the primary site and use of a hand-held gamma probe; the SLN was successfully identified in 97.6% of the patients in this group. In the other group (36% of patients), both vital blue dye and radiocolloid were used. All of the blue-stained SLNs also yielded radioactive hot spots, and in four patients the blue dye was not identified in any of the lymph nodes, which meant that mapping would have been unsuccessful if blue-staining had been the only mapping technique applied. Preoperative lymphoscintigraphy was used in 93% of the patients, with a technical failure rate of 10%. The radiolabeled SLNs could not be successfully imaged in these 12 patients preoperatively, but with the help of the hand-held gamma probe, the SLNs could be identified intraoperatively. This result suggests that a hand-held gamma probe is more sensitive at identifying SLNs than a scintillation camera. The reason may be that the probe accumulates data for scanning the basin in seconds, compared with the 2 to 6 minutes needed for the camera to produce images. This difference probably also explains why multiple nodes are sometimes imaged on preoperative lymphoscintigraphy when 1 to 2 hours have elapsed between radiocolloid injection and imaging. Intraoperative mapping, on the other hand, readily identifies the SLN and does not find multiple nodes to be hot, even when it is done 2 to 4 hours after the lymphoscintigram—provided that ^{99m}Tc-SC is used as the mapping agent.[28] Micrometastatic disease was present in 15 (12.4%) of the 121 patients studied, and the SLN was the only metastatic site in 10 (8.3%). After a minimum follow-up of 220 days, one regional nodal recurrence was observed in an SLN-negative patient.

The addition of intraoperative radiolymphoscintigraphy to vital blue dye lymphatic mapping made SLN localization easier and more widely applicable.[18,28,31] The initial study from MCC making use of this combined approach included 106 consecutive patients with cutaneous melanoma thicker than 0.75 mm at all primary site locations.[28] A total of 200 SLNs and 142 neighboring non-SLNs were harvested from 129 basins; 70% of the SLNs demonstrated blue staining, and 84% were identified as radioactive hot spots. When the two intraoperative mapping techniques were used in conjunction, the SLN could be identified in 96% of the nodal basins sampled. Routine histology identified SLN micrometastases in 15% of patients, and two patients had micrometastatic disease in nodes that were hot but not blue-stained. These data suggest that radiocolloid localization identifies more SLNs, some of which are clinically important in that they contain micrometastatic disease.[28]

Another study used a combination of vital blue dye and radiocolloid (^{99m}Tc-HSA) mapping in a series of 30 patients with melanoma from all primary sites.[31] The SLN stained blue and was the most radioactive site in 27 patients (90%). In five of 13 patients undergoing groin dissection, radiolymphoscintigraphy identified two SLNs in the drainage basin. In each case, the presence of the second inguinal SLN was suggested by the high residual radioactivity after removal of the first node, not by the blue dye; radioactivity decreased to background levels after excision of the second node. The investigators concluded that radiolymphoscintigraphy can be used not only to confirm blue-dye identification of an initial SLN but also to detect additional SLNs that are not easily identified with the dye technique alone.

In a subsequent MCC trial that used isosulfan blue dye and ^{99m}Tc-SC as mapping agents,[25] only patients with a positive SLN underwent complete node dissection. After 3 years of follow-up, two recurrences in regional basins were observed in patients whose previous SLN biopsy was negative. Serial sectioning and immunohistochemical staining of the SLN block found no abnormal cells; however, both patients' SLNs were RT-PCR–positive for messenger RNA (mRNA) for the tyrosinase gene,[32] which suggests the presence of micrometastatic disease that was missed by more conventional tests.

In another study, the Sydney Melanoma Unit reported an 87% success rate in identifying SLNs.[33] There was a pronounced learning curve, in that the success rate for the last 100 patients was 97%. Cutaneous lymphoscintigraphy was performed in 800 melanoma patients and was used to guide subsequent SLN harvesting; 23% of patients were found to have micrometastatic disease. Initially, the SLNs underwent frozen sectioning for occult metastases, but the 9% false negative rate led the investigators to switch to permanent sections, an approach that allowed the pathologist 2 to 5 days to perform a detailed examination. Patients found to have a positive SLN were returned to the OR for complete node dissection. When preoperative lymphoscintigraphy was followed by intraoperative mapping using vital blue-dye staining in conjunction with radiocolloid (^{99m}Tc-ATS) injection and a hand-held gamma probe, a 1.9% false negative rate was reported.

Finally, valuable findings are anticipated from the NCI-sponsored prospective trial now under way [see Discussion, National Protocols, below]. As of fall 1998, survival data from this trial had not been made available.

Patterns of Failure after Negative SLN Biopsy

Several of the earlier studies found that SLN mapping had a false negative rate—defined as a negative SLN with positive higher nodes—of less than 4%, as determined by concomitant formal lymph node dissection[12-15]; however, they did not clearly establish the long-term risk of failure within the mapped nodal basin after a negative SLN alone. This issue was addressed by a joint study from MCC and the M. D. Anderson Cancer Center (Houston, Texas).[34] In this study, patients with cutaneous melanoma whose tumor was at least 1.0 mm thick or was categorized as Clark level IV or higher were eligible for mapping and SLN biopsy. All patients underwent preoperative lymphoscintigraphy, and only those with a histologically positive SLN underwent complete lymphadenectomy. A total of 618 patients underwent mapping with successful identification of at least one SLN; of these, 518 had histologically negative SLNs. After a minimum follow-up of 3 months and a median follow-up of 18 months, 32 (6%) of the 518 patients had recurrent disease; nine (1.7%) of the 518 had their first recurrence in a basin where the SLN was negative at the previous mapping. Patients with a histologically negative SLN had significantly better DFS ($P < 0.001$) and distant disease–free survival ($P < 0.001$) than those with a histologically positive SLN. When SLNs from the nine patients whose SLNs were determined to be free of metastatic disease on initial review were retrospectively reexamined by serial sectioning or immunohistochemistry, occult nodal metastases were present in seven (77%) of the nine. These data established the durable long-term accuracy of lymphatic mapping and SLN biopsy.

Optimal nodal staging requires not only accurate identification of the SLN but also careful examination of the SLN with special pathologic techniques. It is likely that many false negative SLN biopsies do not actually reflect true skip metastases but are the result of micrometastases missed on routine pathologic examination. In the study cited, it is clear, given the subsequent recurrences, that the missed micrometastases represented clinically relevant disease. The recurrences could have been prevented if the SLNs had undergone detailed histologic examination initially, the micrometastases had been found, and complete node dissection had been performed.

Other explanations of false positive SLN biopsies have been proposed. One is that after a negative SLN biopsy, some regional basins are seeded with metastatic cells from in transit metastases or local recurrences. In transit metastasis occurs in 2% to 3% of patients and could be a source of skip metastases.[8]

Clinical Implications

The information generated by all this experience is being used to change the standards for surgical management of melanoma so that only patients with evidence of nodal metastatic disease are subjected to the morbidity and expense of complete node dissection.[3-6] Initial studies showed the usefulness of lymphatic mapping with either vital blue dye or radiocolloid in obtaining such evidence; however, it is now clear that the success rate of SLN identification increases markedly when the two mapping approaches are combined as described [see Technique, above]. A combined mapping approach identifies SLNs both more accurately and more completely: it removes more SLNs and results in a lower incidence of positive nodes on subsequent complete lymph node dissection (CLND).

In 94% of melanoma patients, the SLN is the only site of metastasis. At MCC, we have seen no patients with melanomas less than 2.8 mm thick in whom nodes other than SLNs harbored metastases. It has been hypothesized that a melanoma must reach a certain thickness before it sheds enough cells to involve higher nodes beyond the SLN, and this hypothesis is supported by data from the M. D. Anderson Cancer Center showing no positive higher nodes after a positive SLN biopsy in patients with melanomas less than 2.5 mm thick. It appears that metastatic cells are concentrated in SLNs in much the same way that vital blue dyes and radiocolloids are. Thus, for many melanoma patients (in particular, those whose tumors have not reached the critical thickness just specified), to locate the SLN is essentially to define the limit of metastatic spread. Accordingly, lymphatic mapping, by identifying SLNs (and thus defining the extent of disease) with a high degree of accuracy, can be extremely useful in helping clinicians make more informed therapeutic decisions—for example, regarding eligibility for adjuvant therapy or the possibility of forgoing CLND.

The findings of the studies cited demonstrate that intraoperative lymphatic mapping and SLN biopsy yields accurate pathologic staging, does not lower care standards, decreases morbidity (e.g., lymphedema is absent, and early return to work or normal activity is facilitated), makes possible rational yet less aggressive surgical and adjuvant medical approaches, and reduces costs.[20]

Lymphatic Mapping and SLN Biopsy for Breast Cancer

RATIONALE

For breast cancer, as for most solid tumors, the most powerful prognostic factor is the status of the regional nodes: the presence of regional metastases decreases 5-year survival by approximately 28% to 40%.[35,36] As for melanoma, many prognostic factors for breast cancer have been defined on the basis of primary tumor characteristics, yet regression analyses indicate that such factors add very little to the prognostic model once lymph node status is considered. Hence, the rationale for nodal staging is essentially the same as with melanoma.

Nodal Staging

Currently, surgical management of breast cancer is more conservative than it once was: breast conservation is now considered an acceptable alternative to modified radical mastectomy in as many as two thirds of patients. Management of the axilla in breast cancer patients remains controversial. It is generally accepted that axillary dissection is not indicated for patients with ductal carcinoma in situ (DCIS), because of the low likelihood of axillary node involvement.[37-39] The main point at issue is whether axillary dissection is indicated for patients with small invasive primary lesions. Some authors recommend that patients with T1a lesions be spared a dissection[40]; however, even when an invasive cancer is smaller than 1 cm, a significant percentage (14% to 37%) of patients have axillary nodal metastases.[41,42]

Breast tumors were once thought to have a random nodal metastatic pattern. Accordingly, investigators initially performed sampling procedures of anatomically defined first-station nodal basins in an effort to achieve accurate pathologic staging. These procedures were based on arbitrary assignment of node clusters in the axillary region to various levels (I, II, or III) rather than on intraoperative mapping of the SLN. Unfortunately, this approach led to a high (15%) prevalence of skip metastases (defined in this context as metastases to level II and III axillary nodes without involvement of level I nodes).[43] As a result, investigators abandoned sampling as a nodal staging technique for patients with breast cancer. Subsequent work demonstrated, however, that when lymphatic mapping is performed in patients with upper outer quadrant tumors, about 10% to 15% of them show direct drainage to level II axillary nodes, and skip metastases are not found. In previous studies, these patients would have been classified as having skip metastases; given the available data, it is likely that the earlier investigators simply were using insufficiently accurate staging techniques that were unable to map the SLNs or the levels of the axilla accurately.

More accurate staging involves more than just stage shifting[44]: it can improve survival in the breast cancer population by identifying patients who will gain a survival advantage associated with either the surgical procedure itself (complete axillary dissection)[45] or the accompanying adjuvant therapy.[36] In addition, it keeps a percentage of the population from being exposed to the complications of the more extensive surgical procedure or to the toxicities of the adjuvant therapy. In particular, the ability to limit full axillary lymph node dissection (ALND) to women with documented nodal metastases would be a major advance in the surgical treatment of breast cancer. Now that modern techniques have made breast conservation a viable option for so many women, the main physical complaints patients voice after operation have to do with the side effects of axillary dissection (i.e., lymphedema of the arm and paresthesia). If node-negative patients could be protected from having to experience these side effects, that would be every bit as significant a therapeutic advance as the realization that breast cancer could be treated effectively with lumpectomy and radiation therapy.

PATIENT SELECTION

Any woman with invasive breast cancer is a potential candidate for lymphatic mapping and SLN biopsy. In patients with DCIS, the incidence of nodal metastasis on SLN biopsy with a more detailed examination of the node is 8.4%; in patients with invasive tumors more than 5 cm in diameter, the incidence is 75%. Clinicians must decide for themselves whether these patients should undergo nodal staging; however, at MCC, we routinely offer them the procedure because if nodal metastases are found, the subsequent treatment recommendations will be different.

Contraindications to the procedure are multifocal disease, inflammatory cancer, and extensive previous surgery or radiation therapy (e.g., breast reconstruction with implants above the pectoral muscle).

TECHNIQUE

Step 1: Preoperative Lymphoscintigraphy

Lymphoscintigraphy is performed in much the same way for breast cancer as for melanoma, except that the radiocolloid is injected into the breast parenchyma around the primary tumor. The radioactivity dose is the same as for melanoma (450 μCi), but larger volumes (6 ml) are administered because the breast lymphatics are not as rich as the cutaneous lymphatics. For this reason, the first images are not available until 30 to 40 minutes after injection [*see Figure 5*].

The injection must be diffuse enough around the tumor to allow the radiocolloid to be taken up by the breast lymphatics. If the tumor was detected mammographically, localization wires are placed under either mammographic or ultrasonographic guidance, and the radiocolloid is injected around the wire and the tumor. Injection must not be performed through the localization needle, because the needle will act as a wick, allowing the radiocolloid to flow back out and possibly contaminate the skin. The localization wire is left in place to guide subsequent injection of vital blue dye. If the tumor is palpable, injection is straightforward and is done tightly around the circumference of the tumor. If an excisional biopsy was performed, injection is done under ultrasonographic guidance so that the radiocolloid is placed in the breast parenchyma around the biopsy cavity. If the radiocolloid is placed in the tumor or the biopsy cavity, it will not migrate.

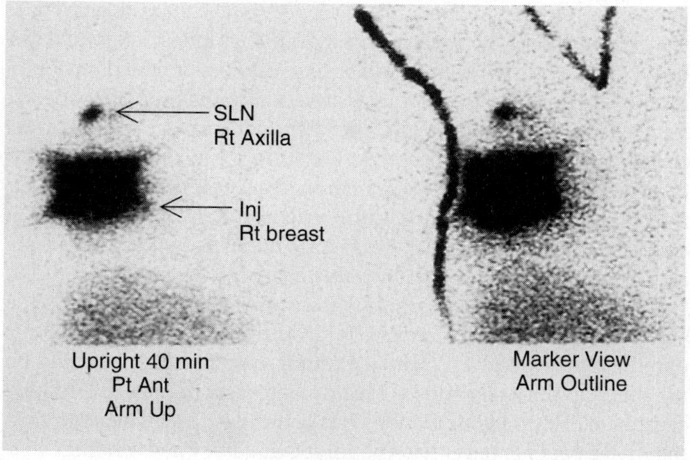

Figure 5 **Lymphatic mapping and SLN biopsy for breast cancer. Whereas flow of the radiocolloid to the SLN takes 5 to 10 minutes for melanoma mapping, it takes 30 to 40 minutes for breast cancer mapping. In addition, the primary site is usually closer to the regional basin in breast cancer than it is in melanoma, and shine-through from the primary site may be a problem. Invariably, the lumpectomy or mastectomy is performed first, followed by axillary SLN harvesting.**

Comment The timing of radiocolloid injection is not highly critical as long as enough time (2 to 6 hours) is allowed between injection and SLN harvesting for the mapping agent to migrate into the SLN. As the radiocolloid migrates, it is concentrated in the SLN. In most cases, this concentration results in an identifiable radioactive hot spot. When this happens, SLN harvesting becomes easier. Axillary hot spots have been identified up to 24 hours after radiocolloid injection, but as with melanoma, waiting until the next day to complete the mapping is not ideal. The advantages of having a wide window of opportunity for SLN harvesting have already been described [*see Lymphatic Mapping and SLN Biopsy for Melanoma, Technique, above*].

It has been suggested that the injection should be done in the skin of the breast above the tumor. The basis for this suggestion is the hypothesis that superficial skin lymphatics merge with deeper breast parenchyma lymphatics. If this is true, it would make breast lymphatic mapping easier, because skin lymphatics are more numerous and cutaneous flow to the regional basin is more rapid. Nevertheless, we are not convinced that skin and deep breast lymphatics really do converge into a single SLN. When lymphoscintigraphy is performed for breast skin melanoma, drainage to both the ipsilateral and the contralateral axilla can be demonstrated in about 20% of cases; however, we have not encountered one case of drainage to the internal mammary nodes from breast cutaneous locations (unpublished data). In contrast, when lymphoscintigraphy is done for breast cancer and the radiocolloid is injected into the breast parenchyma, the mapping agent never crosses the midline. These lymphatic vessels may drain in two directions—to the internal mammary node and to the ipsilateral axilla—but they never drain to the contralateral axilla, as occurs with breast skin melanoma. In addition, there have been cases in which a woman with a melanoma on the skin of the breast underwent WLE and SLN biopsy of an axillary SLN, only to be diagnosed later with a breast cancer in the same breast (unpublished data). Lymphoscintigraphy performed around the breast tumor demonstrated drainage to an axillary SLN that was not removed in conjunction with the earlier mapping for melanoma.

One may question the need to image the patient after radiocolloid injection, given that the standard of care is to stage the patient according to the status of the axillary nodes alone. Lymphoscintigraphy can be used to identify women whose primary tumors drain bidirectionally to the axilla and to the internal mammary nodes. For such patients, it may be appropriate to include the internal mammary nodes in their radiation ports after lumpectomy. The most important potential use of lymphoscintigraphy in breast cancer, however, may be to identify a subgroup of women whose tumors do not drain at all to the axilla and who thus are not at risk for axillary metastases. MCC has a series of 25 patients who fall into this category (unpublished data). Preoperative lymphoscintigraphy showed no axillary drainage. In the OR, vital blue dye and radiocolloid were injected into the breast parenchyma around the primary tumor, but no hot spot could be identified in the axilla and no blue dye appeared. The standard procedure (axillary node dissection) was performed, and it became clear that these patients never had metastatic disease. These findings suggest that axillary dissection may not be indicated if no axillary drainage of the radiocolloid can be detected either preoperatively in the nuclear medicine suite or intraoperatively in the OR and if no hot spots can be identified in the axilla with the sensitive gamma probes. A national trial is now under way that is aimed at evaluating this potential use of lymphoscintigraphy in breast cancer.

Step 2: Intraoperative Lymphatic Mapping and Identification of SLN

Intraoperative lymphatic mapping and SLN identification follow much the same course in breast cancer patients as in melanoma patients. Patients come to the OR 2 to 6 hours after the injection of the radiocolloid in the nuclear medicine suite. If the tumor is palpable, 5 ml of 1% isosulfan blue dye is injected around the circumference of the primary tumor 10 to 15 minutes before the surgical procedure. If the tumor is nonpalpable, the dye is injected around the localization wire left in place after preoperative lymphoscintigraphy. After injection of the vital blue dye, the breast is massaged for 5 minutes to facilitate migration of the mapping agents.

Before a skin incision is made, a hand-held gamma probe is used to identify the most radioactive area in the axilla. If there is sufficient distance between the primary site and the regional basin, isobar levels of radioactivity [*see Figure 6*] are drawn emanating from the primary site, and hot spots of radioactivity are marked along each of the isobars. If possible, the afferent lymphatic is mapped and followed to a hot spot in the axilla that corresponds to the location of the SLN [*see Figure 7*]. A small (2 to 4 cm) axillary incision is made over the hot spot, dissection is directed through the axillary fat with the probe, and the SLN is identified [*see Figure 8*]. Ideally, the SLN should be both hot and blue. If the hot spot corresponds to a cluster of nodes, the blue staining will help distinguish the SLN from the non-SLNs. The in vivo activity ratio is determined to confirm that the node fulfills the criteria of an SLN. Careful dissection is performed to identify the blue-stained afferent lymphatics, which can then be followed to the pale blue–stained SLN or SLNs [*see Figure 8*].

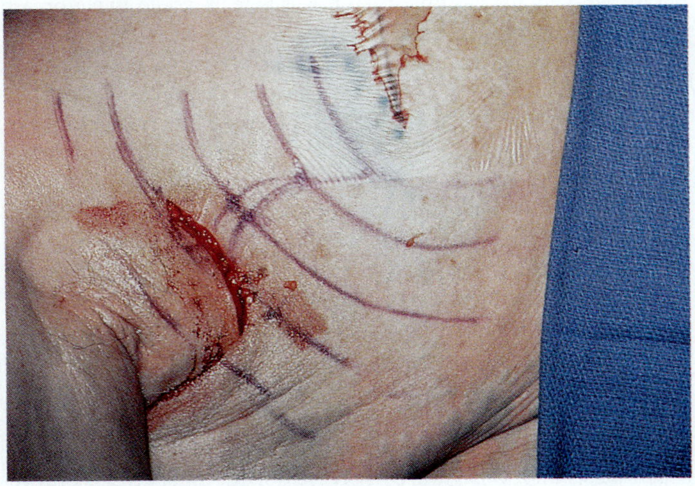

Figure 6 Lymphatic mapping and SLN biopsy for breast cancer. Isobars of radioactivity are drawn equidistant from the primary site (upper right), and hot spots are identified along each of the isobars. These hot spots represent the location of the afferent lymphatic leading to the SLN in the axilla.

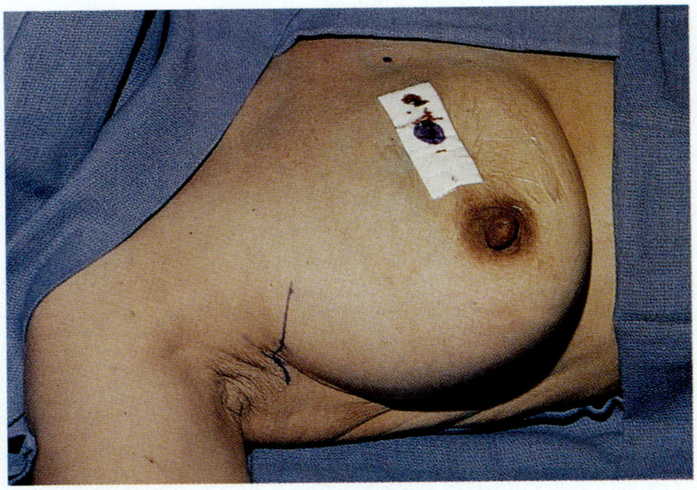

Figure 7 Lymphatic mapping and SLN biopsy for breast cancer. The hand-held gamma probe is used to trace the afferent lymphatic through the skin to a hot spot in the regional basin, under which the SLN is located.

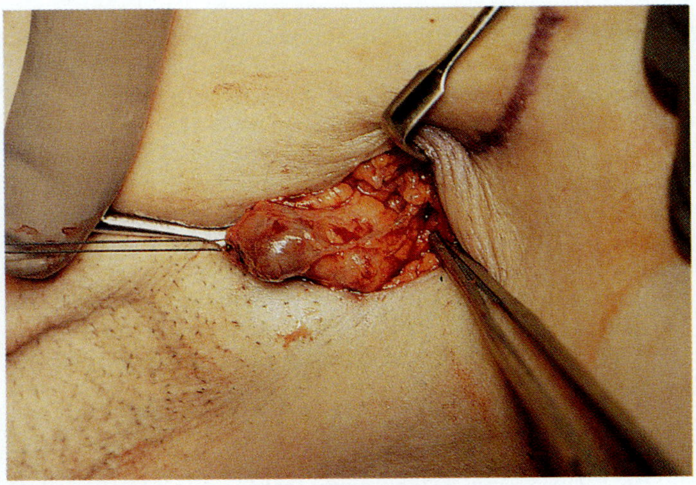

Figure 8 Lymphatic mapping and SLN biopsy for breast cancer. In the same patient as in Figure 7, a small incision is made in the axilla, and with the gamma probe directing the dissection, a blue-stained afferent lymphatic is seen leading into a blue-stained node. This node is hot as well as blue; it is the SLN and is the first site of metastatic disease.

Comment As with melanoma, mapping becomes simpler, more accurate, more complete, and more widely applicable when the vital blue dye method and the radiocolloid method are combined.[46,47] Either method may play a more important role in a given instance, depending on the circumstances. A unique feature of breast lymphatic mapping that makes it more technically demanding than melanoma mapping is that breast cancer primary sites are closer to their regional basins than most melanoma primaries are to theirs. As a result, there may be so much shine-through of radioactivity from the primary site that imaging of the axilla becomes impossible. This may also be the case intraoperatively, when one is trying to identify the axillary SLN, even if lumpectomy is performed first. In such circumstances, vital blue dye mapping takes on a more important role in finding the axillary SLN. On the other hand, radiocolloid mapping takes on a more important role when the blue dye is slow to travel to the regional basin.

In only about 75% of breast mappings can an axillary SLN be imaged with the scintillation camera; however, surgeons may still be able to locate the SLN in the remaining 25% by using the handheld gamma probe (which is more sensitive than the camera) intraoperatively to find the axillary hot spot and direct dissection toward the SLN.

Activity (localization) ratios are used to eliminate uncontrolled variables that might affect identification of an SLN [*see* Lymphatic Mapping and SLN Biopsy for Melanoma, Technique, *above*]. The higher the activity ratio, the easier mapping will be and the more likely it is that SLN harvesting will be successful. A major reason for waiting 2 to 6 hours to allow the radiocolloid to migrate and become concentrated in the SLN before intraoperative mapping is that activity ratios are highest at this point.

A node is considered to be the SLN if it meets one of three criteria:

1. The node is blue.
2. The node has a blue-stained afferent lymphatic leading to it. Occasionally, a node is full of tumor and has a dilated blue-stained lymphatic vessel leading to it, but it does not take up the dye or the radiocolloid readily. This scenario is easily realized intraoperatively because the node is hard. Despite the lack of uptake of the mapping reagent, such nodes must be considered SLNs.
3. The node has an in vivo activity ratio of 3:1 or an ex vivo activity ratio of 10:1.

Step 3: Removal of SLN

Once the SLN is identified, it is removed. A neighboring non-SLN may also be removed so that the ex vivo activity ratio may be calculated. The blue-stained afferent lymphatics that have been visualized are clipped or tied off. The central bed is then reexamined for radioactivity. If radioactivity is 150% of the background level or higher, dissection is continued in search of additional SLNs. The mean number of axillary SLNs removed in breast lymphatic mapping is 2.0/patient.

Step 4: Pathologic Examination of SLN

Once SLNs are dissected away from surrounding tissue, they are bivalved intraoperatively and examined for any gross evidence of metastatic disease. All of the excised nodal tissue is submitted for pathologic evaluation. Tissue contents are classified into three categories: SLNs, adjacent non-SLNs, and axillary contents. SLNs 5 mm or less in maximum diameter are bivalved, and those greater than 5 mm in diameter are serially sectioned at 2 to 3 mm intervals to maximize surface area for touch-print cytology and intraoperative immunohistochemistry (IHC). (To prevent loss of tissue in the cryostat, we do not perform frozen sections of the SLNs.) Imprints are made with a single gentle touch on each cut surface of the SLN. The slides

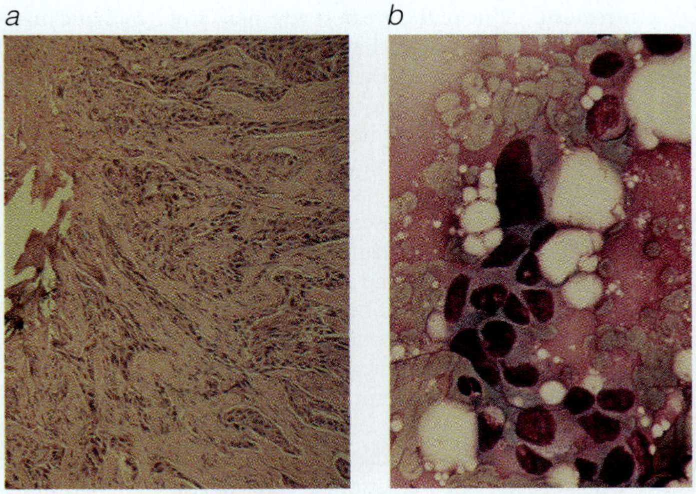

Figure 9 Lymphatic mapping and SLN biopsy for breast cancer. In touch-print cytology, slides are touched to tissue from a "hot" specimen, and cells on the section or the margin are exfoliated onto the slide for cytologic preparation. Shown are (*a*) permanent histology of an infiltrating ductal carcinoma extending down to an inked margin and (*b*) a touch preparation demonstrating bizarre malignant cells from the sampling of the margin. The advantages of this technique are that the entire margin can be sampled and that tissue is not lost in the cryostat.

are air-dried and stained with Diff-Quick stain, then sent for intraoperative interpretation. Approximately 5 to 8 minutes from the specimen's entry into the pathology laboratory, the intraoperative diagnosis (negative, indeterminate, or positive) is rendered. At MCC, we use an intraoperative IHC cytokeratin stain on the cytologic touch imprints as an adjunct to the Diff-Quick stain; this approach may enhance detection of micrometastases, especially with infiltrating lobular carcinoma or well-differentiated (low-grade) ductal carcinoma. If the diagnosis is positive, one can convert to CLND intraoperatively. Primary diagnoses are made and lumpectomy margins examined with the same touch-print cytology technique[48] [*see Figure 9*].

Each SLN is placed in a separate formalin container by the nuclear medicine department staff and quarantined in a dedicated refrigerator with the lumpectomy or mastectomy specimen for 48 hours (six half-lives of technetium-99) to allow decay of the radioisotope. After this period, the SLNs are catalogued, and one or two blocks of tissue per SLN are submitted for permanent histology. Each block is sectioned at one to three levels per slide, depending on the size of the tissue in each block. In addition, any SLNs that appear free of metastasis both grossly and on hematoxylin-eosin staining are stained with IHC using the avidin-biotin complex technique with diaminobenzidine chromogen.

Table 1 Upstaging of Breast Cancer with Lymphatic Mapping and Cytokeratin Staining

Category	IIC with Cytokeratin Stain	Permanent Histology	Permanent Histology with Cytokeratin Stain
True positive	15	40	68
True negative	254	313	313
False negative	35	28	—
False positive	1	0	—

IIC—intraoperative imprint cytology

Comment One of the greatest advantages of lymphatic mapping is that the surgeon gives the pathologist only one or two SLNs, which allows more detailed examination with such procedures as serial sectioning, immunohistochemical staining, and perhaps RT-PCR analysis.[49,50] Incorporating a more detailed examination into routine practice enables clinicians to detect lesser degrees of disease and upstage a number of breast cancer patients. It was once believed that micrometastatic disease in a single lymph node was clinically unimportant in breast cancer patients because such patients were thought to have the same survival as node-negative patients. More recently, this belief has been challenged by studies demonstrating poorer survival in patients who are upstaged with serial sectioning,[51] immunohistochemical staining,[52-54] or RT-PCR analysis.[49,50] In fact, since 1996, immunohistochemical staining and new molecular biology assays for occult metastases have consistently been reported to upstage patients with melanoma,[32] breast cancer,[55] colon cancer,[56] neuroblastoma,[57] prostate cancer,[58] and stomach cancer,[59] and in most cases, this upstaging has proved clinically relevant.

In addition, detailed pathologic examination with these more sensitive techniques may allow a more rational approach to adjuvant chemotherapy. For instance, candidates for such therapy could routinely undergo SLN harvesting, followed by detailed examination of the SLN with immunohistologic staining or RT-PCR, to provide more accurate staging. Adjuvant therapy could then be restricted to patients with solid evidence of metastases, and patients with no evidence of SLN micrometastases could be spared the morbidity and expense of additional therapy. A randomized trial is being proposed to determine whether this approach is viable.

In a series of 255 breast cancer patients who underwent SLN harvesting with detailed pathologic examination at MCC, intraoperative imprint cytology (IIC) with both Diff-Quick and cytokeratin staining was compared with the gold standard, permanent histology with both hematoxylin-eosin and IHC staining[60] [see Table 1]. IIC identified only 50% of the patients with metastatic disease. Another way of stating this result, however, is to say that IIC enabled intraoperative conversion to CLND in 50% of patients with axillary metastatic disease, thereby sparing a substantial number of patients a second trip to the OR. Cytokeratin staining of permanent sections was responsible for the detection of disease in 36.2% of patients with metastases; this disease would have been missed by routine examination of one or two nodal sections and hematoxylin-eosin staining. Detailed examination of SLNs reveals nodal metastases (i.e., upstages) in 9.4% of histologically negative patients[60] [see Figure 10].

In another series from MCC, cytokeratin IHC staining was performed on 196 SLNs from 95 patients with comedo DCIS.[61] Eight of the 95 (8.4%) had positive SLNs. Routine histology identified the metastatic disease in only 2 (25%) of the 8 patients, whereas cytokeratin IHC staining identified metastases in 6 (75%). CLND was performed in seven of the eight patients, and the SLN was the only site of disease in all of them. Previous studies have reported that when CLND is performed in DCIS patients, fewer than 1% turn out to have metastatic disease in the regional basin; accordingly, many clinics have eliminated CLND from primary surgical treatment of these patients. Review of these studies, however, shows that the pathologic examination of the nodes in the CLND specimen was superficial. Lymphatic mapping and SLN biopsy permits a more detailed examination of the one or two nodes most likely to contain disease and, consequently, yields a higher rate of identification of metastases: 2% (2/95) with H&E staining and 6.2% (6/95) with IHC staining in this study.

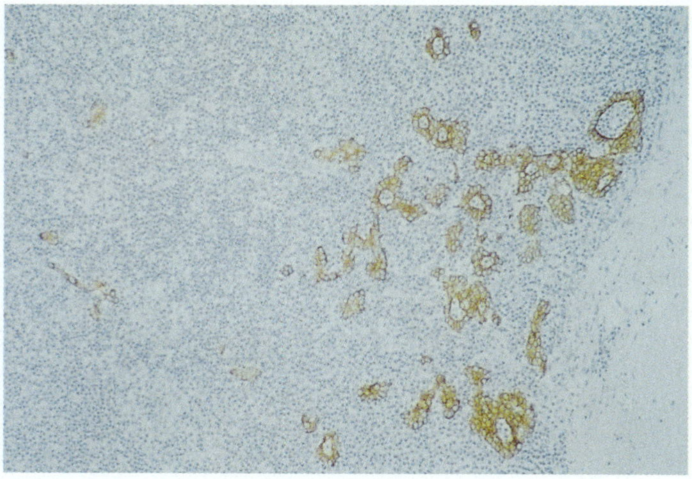

Figure 10 Lymphatic mapping and SLN biopsy for breast cancer. Cytokeratin immunohistochemical staining finds metastatic cells in 9.4% of breast cancer patients whose SLNs are histologically negative on routine examination.

COMPLICATIONS

The complications of the procedure are similar to those of melanoma mapping. Surgical site infections occur in fewer than 1% of cases; a seroma develops in about 10%. In our experience, no patients have complained of paresthesia or lymphedema after lymphatic mapping for breast cancer, in contrast to what is usually noted after CLND.

REPORTED RESULTS

The initial experience with lymphatic mapping and SLN biopsy for breast cancer was gained between April 1994 and December 1995. All patients who presented to the Comprehensive Breast Cancer Program at MCC with suspected breast cancer were evaluated for enrollment into the study.[45] Enrollment criteria included invasive breast cancer documented by fine-needle aspiration (FNA) or core-needle biopsy [see 43 Breast Procedures] rather than excisional biopsy (which meant that the breast lymphatic vessels were unlikely to have been disrupted) and a clinically negative axilla on physical examination. Exclusion criteria included previous incisional or excisional biopsy of the breast cancer [see 43 Breast Procedures], a tumor that could not be adequately localized by palpation or stereotaxis, and pregnancy. A total of 62 women were enrolled in the study; their mean age was 60 years (range, 32 to 81 years). Axillary mapping was successful in 57. Of these 57 patients, 51 (89%) had a histologic diagnosis of invasive ductal carcinoma, four (7%) had invasive lobular carcinoma, one (2%) had invasive medullary carcinoma, and one (2%) had invasive tubular carcinoma. The mean tumor size was 2.2 cm (range, 0.4 to 8.0 cm). Stage I disease was noted in 66% of patients, stage II in 23%, and stage III in 11%.

All 62 patients were scheduled to undergo either lumpectomy and axillary node dissection (63%) or modified radical mastectomy (37%), depending on the clinical presentation and patient preference. Intraoperative lymphatic mapping with isosulfan blue dye and filtered ^{99m}Tc-SC was performed, followed by complete axillary node dissection [see 43 Breast Procedures]. In this way, the skip metastasis rate (and hence the false negative rate) could be calculated. If there was too much shine-through from the primary site, the lumpectomy or mastectomy was performed before the axillary dissection. The SLNs were identified and sent to the pathology laboratory as separate specimens.

An average of 15.5 non-SLNs per patient and 2.2 SLNs per patient were obtained from the 57 women in whom lymphatic mapping was successful. Eighteen (32%) of the 57 had metastatic disease to the axilla; the number of nodes involved ranged from one to seven. In all 18, the SLNs were positive; thus, there were no skip metastases (i.e., no false negatives). In 12 of the 18, the SLN was the only metastatic site. The metastatic distribution was significantly in favor of SLN involvement ($P \leq 0.001$): 55% of the SLNs were positive for metastatic disease, compared with only 5% of the non-SLNs. The ex vivo activity ratio averaged 39.2. Addition of the radiocolloid technique to the vital blue dye technique improved the success rate of mapping from 73% to 92% and increased the average number of SLNs harvested per patient from 1.2 to 2.2. In none of the patients was metastatic disease documented in a hot SLN that was not also stained blue. In 12% of patients (mostly women with upper outer quadrant tumors), lymphatic drainage skipped level I nodes and proceeded directly to level II nodes; no direct drainage to level III nodes was observed.

In 1997, this experience was updated with a report of 466 women with breast cancer who underwent lymphatic mapping and SLN biopsy at MCC after any type of initial diagnostic procedure, including excisional biopsy.[62] Mapping was successful in 440 of the 466. An average of 1.92 SLNs per patient were harvested. One hundred five (23.8%) of the patients had metastases in the SLN; one patient, who had undergone an excisional biopsy, had a skip metastasis, for a false negative rate of less than 1%. Lymphatic mapping was performed in 87 patients with comedo DCIS, and four patients (4.6%) were found to have positive SLNs. As tumor size increased, the number of patients with a positive SLN also increased [see Table 2].

As of fall 1998, this series includes more than 700 patients. The success rate for identifying axillary SLNs remains high (about 95%), and the SLN is positive in 25.3% of patients. No additional skip metastases have been identified. For the last 550 patients, however, the false negative rate is being determined on the basis of nodal recurrence in long-term follow-up after a negative SLN; the reason is that these patients are not undergoing CLND when the SLN is negative.

If mapping fails in vivo, CLND is performed and an attempt is made to identify an axillary hot spot ex vivo. Occasionally, the SLN can be located when the axillary contents are removed and mapped on the back table to eliminate any shine-through. Although this approach exposes the patient to the morbidity of a CLND, it has an important advantage—namely, that if the SLN can be identified, it can be submitted separately to the pathology laboratory for detailed examination and more accurate staging.

At MCC, when excisional biopsy is done before lymphatic mapping, an average of 2.2 SLNs are removed per patient. In 26% of these cases, three or more SLNs are harvested, and this is the population in which the only skip metastasis has occurred. When lymphatic mapping is done with the tumor intact, an average of 1.8 SLNs are removed per patient. In only 16% of these cases are three or more SLNs excised. Excisional biopsy, whether for palpable tumors or for mammographically detected lesions with needle localization, may well become a thing of the past. In the future, when physical examination or mammography suggests the presence of breast cancer, the diagnosis is likely to be made with minimally invasive techniques, such as FNA, core-needle biopsy, and the use of Advanced Breast Biopsy Instrumentation (ABBI; United States Surgical Corporation, Norwalk, Connecticut). Once the diagnosis is made, lymphatic mapping can be done to minimize unnecessary dissection.

Table 2 Tumor Size and Frequency of Positive SLNs

Tumor Size	No. of Patients with Positive SLNs
Tis (ductal carcinoma in situ [DCIS])	4/87 (4.6%)
T1a, T1b < 1.0 cm	18/112 (16.1%)
T1c 1–2 cm	43/131 (32.8%)
T2 2–5 cm	31/76 (40.8%)
T3 > 5 cm	9/12 (75.0%)

Clinical Implications

It has been suggested that axillary dissection should no longer be performed in women with breast cancer[47,63,64]; however, given the importance of regional node status, it makes sense to continue to perform an axillary staging procedure. The problem is that axillary nodal dissection is associated with significant complications that can lengthen hospital stay, increase cost, and cause the patient considerable discomfort.[65-67] There now are numerous reports in the literature[45,68,69] suggesting that lymphatic mapping techniques can be used in breast cancer patients to reduce this morbidity. Initial reports from the John Wayne Cancer Center in Santa Monica, California,[68] (using blue dye only) and the University of Vermont[69] (using radiocolloid only) documented success rates of 65% and 71%, respectively, for SLN identification; combining the two mapping techniques, as is done at MCC, increases the success rate of SLN localization and makes the technique easier and more widely applicable. Those patients who are SLN negative (approximately 75% of all patients) can be spared having to undergo CLND.

As of fall 1998, breast cancer centers across the world had studied more than 1,000 women with breast cancer who had undergone lymphatic mapping and SLN harvesting. The mapping techniques vary slightly from center to center; however, most have attained similarly high success rates, which argues strongly for the viability of the procedure. Sensitivity and diagnostic accuracy rates for SLN identification have consistently been higher than 95%, and the false negative rate has ranged from 0% to 10%. This combined experience suggests that lymphatic mapping has the potential for changing the standards for surgical management of breast cancer in the same way that it has already changed the standards for surgical management of melanoma in the United States.

Discussion

Training and Credentialing

Credentialing criteria for new operative procedures have traditionally been under the jurisdiction of local hospital credentialing committees. When new technology becomes available, adequate training is essential, both to ensure that surgeons can perform the new procedure with confidence and to minimize any medicolegal problems. The American College of Surgeons has a committee (the Committee on Emerging Surgical Technology and Education) that monitors this activity. With some new techniques (e.g., laparoscopic cholecystectomy and image-guided breast biopsy), hospitals have required surgeons to attend formal training courses and to have their first cases proctored by surgeons experienced in the new technique before they are allowed to perform the procedure on their own.

National organizations continue to struggle with the problem of educating and credentialing surgeons to perform new procedures. This problem takes on increasing urgency as medicolegal issues proliferate, as other specialists begin to move into areas once generally considered to be the domain of surgeons (e.g., radiologists doing breast biopsies), and as new technical developments promise to revolutionize surgical care. In an effort to address this problem as it bears on lymphatic mapping, a training network has been established (813-972-8482), with the endorsement of several national organizations, that provides an efficient instructional forum on this new lymphatic mapping technology. The network provides six sites in the United States where teams comprising surgeons, nuclear medicine physicians, and pathologists can meet with local moderators, witness live surgery, interact with surgeons during the procedure, and ask questions of an expert panel. The network also provides mechanisms for gaining hands-on experience with animal laboratories, offers mentoring of initial cases as registrants go back to their institutions, maintains national registries on the World Wide Web so that different experiences with the technique can be compared, and, finally, facilitates the participation of other university and community physicians in national protocols [see National Protocols, below]. Such participation provides a certain degree of protection against medicolegal risk as new technology and procedures are introduced.

The varied experience reported to date provides some idea of the learning curves associated with lymphatic mapping. For melanoma, the learning curve for mapping with vital blue dye alone is about 60 cases, which is more than many surgeons see in their entire career.[12,13] In contrast, gamma probe–guided resection of radiolabeled lymph nodes is readily mastered: even with minimal experience, the success rate of SLN localization approaches 98%.

For breast cancer, it has been suggested that the learning curve for lymphatic mapping is about 30 cases. In all of these first 30 patients, SLN harvesting should be followed by CLND; perhaps 10 of the 30 will have metastatic disease. The success rate for finding the axillary SLN should be 90% or higher, with no more than one skip metastasis identified, before one can consider dropping CLND in SLN-negative patients. More than one surgeon can train on the same case, and the final decision as to when an institution is ready to drop full dissection after a negative SLN should be made in conjunction with the medical and radiation oncologists at the institution as well as with the credentialing committee. More recently, clinicians at MCC have examined the learning curves of five surgeons who performed more than 700 lymphatic mappings to find axillary SLNs in patients with breast cancer.[70] Learning curves were generated for each surgeon by plotting the failure rate against the number of cases. The failure rate was high (20% to 30%) in the first 20 patients but fell rapidly thereafter. The results of the study indicate that 23 cases and 53 cases are required to achieve success rates of 90% and 95%, respectively.

National Protocols

Perhaps the most important national multicenter study addressing lymphatic mapping for melanoma is the Multicenter Selective Lymphadenectomy Trial (Donald Morton, principal investigator), which was initiated under the sponsorship of the NCI (Grant No. PO1 CA29605-12). This trial focuses on the effect of lymphatic mapping and SLN biopsy on survival. Melanoma patients with intermediate or thick tumors (≥ 1.0 mm) are randomly selected to receive either WLE plus observation of the nodal basins or WLE plus SLN harvesting. The study differs from previous studies of ELND in that only some of the patients (i.e., those with a positive SLN) undergo CLND. If this study demonstrates a survival benefit, then there will be two good reasons to perform SLN: (1) to remove the node at highest risk for metastatic disease and (2) to identify patients who are candidates for adjuvant therapy.

The other national trial examining the role of this new procedure in treating melanoma is the industry-sponsored Sunbelt Melanoma Trial, in which 60 institutions across the country, equally divided between university centers and community hospitals, are participating. In this study, melanoma patients whose tumors are at least 1.0 mm thick are undergoing lymphatic mapping and SLN harvesting. SLNs are examined with routine histology, serial sectioning, and immunohistochemical staining. If an SLN is negative on the initial screen, an RT-PCR assay based on a panel of four melanoma-specific markers (at least two of which must be positive for a positive result) is performed. Patients whose SLNs are negative on histology and RT-PCR assay are observed; patients whose SLNs are histologically negative but positive on RT-PCR assay are randomly selected to undergo either observation, CLND, or CLND plus adjuvant interferon alfa-2b. It is conceivable that patients in the second category might have a very small volume of tumor that is confined to the SLN and thus might be cured with SLN harvesting alone, thereby avoiding the side effects attendant on CLND or adjuvant interferon therapy. Another arm of this trial is designed to focus on the role of adjuvant interferon alfa-2b in patients with microscopic nodal disease. In the cooperative group study that found interferon alfa-2b to be effective adjuvant therapy,[2] 85% of the patient population had gross nodal disease. It remains to be determined whether patients with minimal disease in the regional basin (i.e., those with only one positive microscopic SLN) benefit from this adjuvant therapy. As of May 1998, the study had enrolled 300 of the 1,200 patients required.

A trial that is still in the discussion stage would involve the random selection of SLN-positive melanoma patients to undergo either observation of the remaining nodes in the basin plus adjuvant therapy or CLND plus adjuvant therapy. The data suggest that the SLN is the only site of disease in 80% to 94% of cases; thus, the focus of this study would be on defining the role of CLND in patients with microscopic stage III disease documented by SLN biopsy.

Among the national multicenter protocols currently examining the role of SLN biopsy in the management of breast cancer is a trial funded by the Department of Defense (Douglas Reintgen, principal investigator), in which 40 institutions, equally divided between university centers and community or regional hospitals, are participating. The two initial goals of the study are (1) to determine how widely applicable lymphatic mapping is and (2) to assess its accuracy in women who have already undergone excisional biopsy. In addition, SLNs undergo detailed examination that includes more sections, IHC staining, and an RT-PCR assay based on a keratin probe for occult metastases.

In fall 1998, the American College of Surgeons Oncology Group initiated a trial (Armando Giuliano, principal investigator) in which women with invasive breast cancer undergo lymphatic mapping and SLN biopsy. If the SLN is negative, patients are observed and a blinded cytokeratin analysis performed. If the SLN is positive, patients undergo either CLND or observation of the regional basin. It is assumed that all of these women will receive appropriate radiation therapy and postoperative adjuvant therapy. The aims of this trial are (1) to define the role of CLND in women with invasive breast cancer and (2) to begin to assess the clinical relevance of upstaging with IHC.

An interesting industry-sponsored trial of lymphatic mapping and SLN biopsy is scheduled to begin shortly. SLN-positive patients will undergo CLND for determination of the total number of positive nodes; those with fewer than four such nodes will be eligible for the randomization. In one protocol (Douglas Reintgen and Susan Minton, principal investigators), premenopausal women with estrogen receptor–positive tumors will receive four cycles of cyclophosphamide and doxorubicin chemotherapy, then will be randomly selected to receive either tamoxifen or toremifene hormone therapy. In the other protocol (Michael Edwards, principal investigator), postmenopausal women will be randomly selected to receive one or the other hormone therapy. SLN-negative patients will undergo blinded cytokeratin analysis followed by uniform administration of adjuvant therapy. The goals of the two protocols will be (1) to evaluate the role of the new antiestrogen as adjuvant therapy for breast cancer and (2) to study the clinical significance of upstaging with cytokeratin staining. Uniform provision of adjuvant chemotherapy after the procedure will facilitate this analysis and distinguish this trial from the ACS trial.

Finally, a group from the University of Vermont (David Krag, principal investigator) will perform lymphatic mapping and SLN biopsy in women with invasive breast cancer who are undergoing breast conservation. Patients will be randomly selected to undergo either SLN biopsy or CLND. Radiation therapy to the breast and the axilla will be provided to SLN-positive patients with the aim of evaluating the role of such therapy in controlling axillary disease.

Radiation Exposure Guidelines and Policies

The amount of radioactivity injected in the course of lymphatic mapping is minimal: about 450 µCi, on average. By comparison, the amount of radioactivity injected in the course of a typical bone scan is 20 µCi—44 times the lymphatic mapping dose. For the first 100 mappings done at MCC, surgeons and pathologists wore radiation detection badges and rings throughout the procedure, and nuclear medicine technicians swiped the relevant areas in the OR and the pathology laboratory after each case. No significant radiation exposure could be documented. Currently, MCC nuclear medicine technicians routinely come into the OR to calibrate and run the gamma probes, and once the specimen has been removed and processed by the surgeon, they handle the specimen and monitor the radioactivity in each one as it is transported from the OR into the pathology laboratory. A separate room is designated for intraoperative handling of specimens; this is particularly important with breast cancer specimens, for which diagnosis, lumpectomy margin, and SLN status may all be determined intraoperatively. In addition, fresh tissue specimens are removed and snap-frozen for RT-PCR assays and estrogen and progesterone receptor assays. As noted [see Lymphatic Mapping and SLN Biopsy for Breast Cancer, Technique, *above*], specimens are then placed in formalin for 48 hours, stored in a dedicated refrigerator, and later removed for routine processing.

Our experience in handling specimens at MCC notwithstanding, as investigators begin to create lymphatic mapping programs at their own institutions, state regulatory policies must be consulted and procedures put into place to meet each individual state's requirements. Clinicians may have to reinvent the wheel, in a sense, to convince their hospitals and their colleagues that lymphatic mapping and SLN biopsy can be performed safely and results in no significant radiation exposure or health risk.

Cost Considerations

A cost analysis was performed at MCC in an effort to ascertain the impact of lymphatic mapping on both cost and quality of care for patients with malignant melanoma.[20] A series of 98 consecutive patients registered at the Cutaneous Oncology Clinic from July 1993 to August 1994 were entered into the study and separated into four treatment groups, depending on their primary surgical therapy. Group 1 patients (29%) had thin melanomas (< 1.0 mm thick) and underwent 1.0 cm WLE under local anesthesia as outpatients in the clinic. Group 2 patients (13%) underwent WLE and nodal staging by ELND. Group 3 patients (47%) underwent WLE and nodal staging by lymphatic mapping and SLN biopsy under general anesthesia in the OR. As surgeons became comfortable with lymphatic mapping, it became evident that the procedure could be performed with straight local anesthesia, particularly for groin dissections. Group 4 patients (11%) underwent WLE and lymphatic mapping under local anesthesia. CLND was performed in SLN-positive group 3 and group 4 patients, and the costs of the additional surgery were entered into the analysis. The WLEs of the primary sites were closed primarily in all patients. Patients were discharged immediately after the procedure.

Significant cost savings were achieved in group 4 patients compared with group 3 patients ($t = 5.56$; $P = 0.001$); however, no significant cost savings were achieved in group 3 patients compared with group 2 patients ($t = 0.847$; $P = 0.40$). Morbidity was significantly lower in groups 3 and 4, with an earlier projected return to work or normal activity. The study findings suggest that, given an incidence of approximately 42,000 new cases of invasive melanoma in the United States each year, use of lymphatic mapping by itself could save the health care system $116 million annually. This study illustrates that clinicians can maintain quality of care, reduce complications, and lower costs by incorporating this new technique into the care of melanoma patients. These benefits can be achieved without compromising the essential nodal staging data that are the criteria for entry into adjuvant therapy programs—a crucial point, in that adjuvant therapy is offered only to patients whom it has been proved to benefit.

For breast cancer, lymphatic mapping may yield more dramatic cost savings. It is conceivable that the combination of a number of emerging technologies and techniques (e.g., ABBI for image-guided total excision of the tumor, touch-print cytology for making the diagnosis and examining lumpectomy margins, and lymphatic mapping and SLN harvesting for nodal staging) could lead to a scenario where women with mammographic abnormalities can come to the clinic, have their breast lesion diagnosed, and receive at least surgical treatment within a 3- to 4-hour period. With such "one-stop shopping," the patient need not be admitted to a hospital, enter a formal OR, be subjected to general anesthesia, or undergo axillary drainage after CLND.

References

1. Parker SL, Tong T, Bolden S, et al: Cancer statistics 1996. CA 46:5, 1996
2. Kirkwood JM, Strawderman MH, Ernstoff MS, et al: Adjuvant therapy of high-risk resected cutaneous melanoma: the Eastern Cooperative Oncology Group Trial EST 1684. J Clin Oncol 14:7, 1996
3. Veronesi U, Adamus J, Bandiera DC, et al: Inefficacy of immediate node dissection in stage I melanoma of the limbs. N Engl J Med 297:627, 1977
4. Sim FH, Taylor WF, Pritchard DJ, et al: Lymphadenectomy in the management of stage I malignant melanoma: a prospective randomized study. Mayo Clin Proc 61:697, 1986
5. Balch CM, Soong S-J, Milton GW, et al: A comparison of prognostic factors and surgical results in 1,786 patients with localized (stage I) melanoma treated in Alabama, USA, and New South Wales, Australia. Ann Surg 196:677, 1982
6. Reintgen DS, Cox EB, McCarthy KS, et al: Efficacy of elective lymph node dissection in patients with intermediate thickness primary melanoma. Ann Surg 198:379, 1983
7. Norman J, Cruse CW, Wells K, et al: A redefinition of skin lymphatic drainage by lymphoscintigraphy for malignant melanoma. Am J Surg 162:432, 1991
8. Reintgen DS, Albertini J, Berman C, et al: Accurate nodal staging of malignant melanoma. Cancer Control: Journal of the Moffitt Cancer Center 2:405, 1995
9. Balch CM, Soong S, Ross MI, et al: Long-term results of a multi-institutional randomized trial comparing prognostic factors and surgical results for intermediate-thickness melanomas (1.0 to 4.0 mm). Intergroup Melanoma Surgical Trial. Ann Surg Oncol 7:87, 2000

10. Wong JH, Cagle LA, Morton D: Lymphatic drainage of skin to a sentinel lymph node in a feline model. Ann Surg 214:637, 1991
11. Alex JC, Krag DN: Gamma-probe-guided localization of lymph nodes. Surg Oncol 2:137, 1993
12. Morton DL, Wen DR, Wong JH, et al: Technical details of intraoperative lymphatic mapping for early stage melanoma. Arch Surg 127:392, 1992
13. Morton DL, Wen DR, Cochran AJ: Management of early-stage melanoma by intraoperative lymphatic mapping and selective lymphadenectomy or "watch and wait." Surg Oncol Clin North Am 1:247, 1992
14. Reintgen DS, Cruse CW, Berman C, et al: An orderly progression of melanoma nodal metastases. Ann Surg 220:759, 1994
15. Ross M, Reintgen DS, Balch C: Selective lymphadenectomy: emerging role of lymphatic mapping and sentinel node biopsy in the management of early stage melanoma. Semin Surg Oncol 9:219, 1993
16. Sappey MPC: Injection, préparation et conservation des vaisseaux lymphatiques. Thèse pour le doctorat en médecine, No. 241. Paris, Rignoux Imprimeur de la Faculté de Médecine, 1843
17. Uren RF, Hoffman-Giles RB, Shaw HM, et al: Lymphoscintigraphy in high-risk melanoma of the trunk: predicting draining node groups, defining lymphatic channels and locating the sentinel node. J Nucl Med 34:1435, 1993
18. Krag DN, Meijer SJ, Weaver DL, et al: Minimal-access surgery for staging of melanoma. Arch Surg 130:654, 1995
19. Krag D, Meijer S, Weaver D, et al: Minimal access surgery for staging regional nodes in malignant melanoma (abstr). Presented at the 48th Cancer Symposium, Society of Surgical Oncology, Boston, 1995
20. Reintgen DS, Einstein A: The role of research in cost containment. Cancer Control: Journal of the Moffitt Cancer Center 2:429, 1995
21. Slingluff C, Vollmer R, Reintgen D, et al: Lethal thin malignant melanoma. Ann Surg 208:150, 1988
22. Heaton KM, Sussman JJ, Gershenwald JE, et al: Surgical margins and prognostic factors in patients with thick (> 4 mm) primary melanoma. Ann Surg Oncol 5:322, 1998
23. Meyer CM, Lecklitner ML, Logie JR, et al: Technetium-99m sulfur-colloid cutaneous lymphoscintigraphy in the management of truncal melanoma. Radiology 131:205, 1979
24. Godellas CV, Berman C, Lyman G, et al: The identification and mapping of melanoma regional nodal metastases: minimally invasive surgery for the diagnosis of nodal metastases. Am Surg 61:97, 1995
25. Norman J, Wells K, Kearney R, et al: Identification of lymphatic basins in patients with cutaneous melanoma. Semin Surg Oncol 9:224, 1993
26. McCarthy WH, Thompson JF, Uren RF: Minimal access surgery for staging of malignant melanoma (invited commentary). Arch Surg 130:659, 1995
27. Wells K, Reintgen DS, Cruse CW, et al: Parotid gland sentinel lymphadenectomy in malignant melanoma (abstr). Presented at the International Congress on Melanoma, Sydney, Australia, 1997
28. Albertini J, Cruse CW, Rapaport D, et al: Intraoperative radiolymphoscintigraphy improves sentinel lymph node identification in melanoma patients. Ann Surg 223:217, 1996
29. Nathanson SD, Anaya P, Eck L: Sentinel lymph node uptake of two different radionuclides (abstr). Presented at the 49th Cancer Symposium, Society of Surgical Oncology, Atlanta, Georgia, 1996
30. Alex JC, Weaver DL, Fairbank JT, et al: Gamma-probe-guided lymph node localization in malignant melanoma. Surg Oncol 2:303, 1993
31. Essner R, Foshag L, Morton D: Intraoperative radiolymphoscintigraphy: a useful adjunct to intraoperative lymphatic mapping and selective lymphadenectomy in patients with clinical stage 1 melanoma (abstr). Presented at the 47th Cancer Symposium, Society of Surgical Oncology, Houston, Texas, 1994
32. Wang X, Heller R, VanVoorhis N, et al: Detection of submicroscopic metastases with polymerase chain reaction in patients with malignant melanoma. Ann Surg 220:768, 1994
33. Thompson JF, McCarthy WH, Robinson E, et al: Sentinel lymph node biopsy in 102 patients with clinical stage 1 melanoma undergoing elective lymph node dissection (abstr). Presented at the 47th Cancer Symposium, Society of Surgical Oncology, Houston, Texas, 1994
34. Gershenwald J, Thompson W, Mansfield P, et al: Patterns of failure in melanoma patients after successful lymphatic mapping and negative sentinel node biopsy (abstr). Presented at the 49th Cancer Symposium, Society of Surgical Oncology, Atlanta, Georgia, 1996
35. Haagensen CD: Treatment of curable carcinoma of the breast. Int J Radiat Oncol Biol Phys 2:975, 1977
36. Bonadonna G: Conceptual and practical advances in the management of breast cancer: Karnofsky Memorial Lecture. J Clin Oncol 7:1380, 1989
37. Balch CM, Singletary ES, Bland KI: Clinical decision-making in early breast cancer. Ann Surg 217:207, 1993
38. Frazier TG, Copeland EM, Gallaher HS, et al: Prognosis and treatment in minimal breast cancer. Am J Surg 133:697, 1977
39. Silverstein MJ, Rosser RJ, Gierson ED, et al: Axillary lymph node dissection for intraductal carcinoma: is it indicated? Cancer 59:1819, 1987
40. Silverstein MJ, Gierson ED, Waisman JR, et al: Axillary lymph node dissection for T1a breast carcinoma: is it indicated? Cancer 73:664, 1994
41. Baker LH: Breast Cancer Detection Demonstration Project: five-year summary report. CA 32:194, 1982
42. Dewar JA, Sarazin D, Benhamou E, et al: Management of the axilla in conservatively treated breast cancer: 592 patients treated at Institut Gustave-Roussy. Int J Radiat Oncol Biol Phys 13:475, 1987
43. Veronesi U, Rilke F, Luini A, et al: Distribution of axillary nodal metastases by level. Cancer 59:682, 1987
44. Feinstein AR, Sosin DM, Wells CK: The Will Rogers phenomenon: stage migration and new diagnostic techniques as a source of misleading statistics for survival in cancer. N Engl J Med 312:1604, 1985
45. Albertini J, Lyman G, Cantor A, et al: Lymphatic mapping and sentinel node biopsy in the breast cancer patient. JAMA 276:1818, 1996
46. Nathanson SD, Nelson L, Karvelis KC: Rates of flow of technetium 99m-labeled human serum albumin from peripheral injection sites to sentinel nodes. Ann Surg Oncol 3:329, 1996
47. Cady B: The need to reexamine axillary lymph node dissection in invasive breast cancer. Cancer 73:505, 1994
48. Cox C, Nicosia S, Ku NN, et al: Touch preparation cytology of breast lumpectomy margins. Arch Surg 126:490, 1991
49. Noguchi S, Aihara T, Motomura K, et al: Detection of breast cancer micrometastases in axillary lymph nodes by means of reverse transcriptase-polymerase chain reaction. Am J Pathol 148:649, 1996
50. Schoenfeld A, Lugmani Y, Smith D, et al: Detection of breast cancer micrometastases in axillary lymph nodes by using polymerase chain reaction. Cancer Res 54:2986, 1994
51. International Ludwig Breast Cancer Study: Prognostic importance of occult axillary lymph node micrometastases from breast cancers. Lancet 335:1565, 1990
52. Trojani M, de Mascarel I, Bonichon F, et al: Micrometastases to axillary lymph nodes from carcinoma of the breast: detection by immunohistochemistry and prognostic significance. Br J Cancer 55:303, 1987
53. Springall SJ, Rytina ERC, Millis RR: Incidence and significance of micrometastases in axillary lymph nodes detected by immunohistochemical techniques. J Pathol 160:174, 1990
54. Hainsworth PJ, Tjandra JJ, Stillwell RG, et al: Detection and significance of occult metastases in node negative breast cancer. Br J Surg 80:459, 1993
55. Fields K, Moscinski L, Trudeu W, et al: The use of polymerase chain reaction (PCR) for amplification of cytokeratin 19 (K19) to detect bone marrow micrometastases in breast cancer (abstr). Presented at the annual meeting of the American Society of Clinical Oncology, 1994
56. Greeson JK, Isenhart CE, Rice R, et al: Identification of occult micrometastases in pericolic lymph nodes of Duke's B colorectal cancer patients using monoclonal antibodies against cytokeratin and CC49: correlation with long-term survival. Cancer 73:563, 1994
57. Moss TJ, Reynolds CP, Sather HN, et al: Prognostic value of immunocytologic detection of bone marrow metastases in neuroblastoma. N Engl J Med 324:219, 1991
58. Moreno JG, Crose CM, Fisher R, et al: Detection of hematogenous micrometastases in patients with prostate cancer. Cancer Res 52:6110, 1992
59. Maehara Y, Oshiro T, Endo K, et al: Clinical significance of occult micrometastases in lymph nodes from patients with early gastric cancer who died of recurrence. Surgery 119:397, 1996
60. Ku NN: Pathological examination of the sentinel lymph nodes in breast cancer. Handbook on Lymphatic Mapping. Whitman E, Reintgen DS, Eds. R. G. Landes Publishers, Georgetown, Texas (in press)
61. Pendas S, Dauway E, Giuliano R, et al: Upstaging DCIS breast cancer patients using cytokeratin staining of the sentinel lymph nodes (abstr). Presented at the annual meeting of the American Society of Clinical Oncology, 1998
62. Cox C, Pendas S, Cox J, et al: Guidelines for sentinel node biopsy and lymphatic mapping of patients with breast cancer. Ann Surg 227:645, 1998
63. Morrow M: Role of axillary dissection in breast cancer management. Ann Surg Oncol 3:233, 1996
64. Baxter N, McCready D, Chapman JA, et al: Clinical behavior of untreated axillary nodes after local treatment for primary cancer. Ann Surg Oncol 3:235, 1996
65. Lin PP, Allison DC, Wainstock J, et al: Impact of axillary node dissection on the therapy of breast cancer patients. J Clin Oncol 11:1536, 1993
66. Ivens D, Hoe AL, Podd TJ, et al: Assessment of morbidity from complete axillary dissection. Br J Cancer 66:136, 1992
67. Recht A, Houlihan MJ: Axillary lymph nodes and breast cancer: a review. Cancer 76:1491, 1995
68. Giuliano AE, Kirgan DM, Guenther MD, et al: Lymphatic mapping and sentinel lymphadenectomy for breast cancer. Ann Surg 220:391, 1994
69. Krag DN, Weaver DL, Alex JC, et al: Surgical resection and radio localization of the sentinel lymph node in breast cancer using a gamma probe. Surg Oncol 2:335, 1993
70. Cox C, Bass S, Boulware D, et al: Implementation of new surgical technology: outcome measures for lymphatic mapping of breast carcinoma. Ann Surg Oncol 6:553, 1999
71. Tanabe KK: Lymphatic mapping and epitrochlear lymph node dissection for melanoma. Surgery 121:102, 1997
72. Hung JC, Wiseman GA, Wahner HW, et al: Filtered technetium-99m-sulfur colloid evaluated for lymphoscintigraphy. J Nucl Med 36:1895, 1995
73. Uren RF, Nowman RB, Thompson JF, et al: Lymphoscintigraphy in melanoma patients (abstr). Presented at the Sixth World Congress on Cancers of the Skin, Buenos Aires, Argentina, 1995

Acknowledgment

Figure 2   Tom Moore.

45 ULTRASONOGRAPHY: SURGICAL APPLICATIONS

Grace S. Rozycki, M.D.

Although the scientific principles underlying ultrasonography first began to be elucidated in the 19th century [*see Sidebar* Ultrasonography in Surgery: Historical Perspectives], it was not until the second half of the 20th century that this technology could be effectively applied to medicine. In particular, surgeons in the United States have now embraced ultrasonography as a key diagnostic tool in many areas of clinical practice. Because ultrasonography is noninvasive, portable, rapid, and easily repeatable, it is especially well suited to surgical practice. In addition, computer-enhanced high-resolution imaging and multifrequency specialized transducers have made ultrasonography increasingly user friendly, enhancing its applicability to a variety of surgical settings.

Physics and Instrumentation

Before the application of ultrasound devices to patient evaluation is addressed, it is worthwhile to briefly review certain basic physical principles and terminology associated with ultrasonography [*see Tables 1 through 3*].[1-5] Nowhere in diagnostic imaging is the understanding of wave physics more important than in ultrasound diagnostic imaging, because ultrasonography is highly operator dependent. To perform an ultrasound examination correctly, a surgeon must be able to interpret echo patterns, determine artifacts, and adjust the machine appropriately so as to obtain the best images.

In diagnostic ultrasonography, the transducer or probe interconverts electrical and acoustic energy [*see Figure 1*].[6] To accomplish

---

Ultrasonography in Surgery: Historical Perspectives

Ultrasonography has become an important diagnostic modality. Although its potential for medical diagnostic imaging was first recognized in the 1930s and 1940s, when attempts were made to use ultrasound to diagnose brain tumors, it was not until the 1970s that the early pioneering work on ultrasound truly came to fruition. With technological advances, ultrasound machines evolved from large, cumbersome devices that produced suboptimal images to portable, user-friendly, sophisticated instruments that produced detailed and useful images. This evolution required years of research and the marriage of physics with physiology, medicine, engineering, and government.

Milestones in Sound Research

One line of sound research that had a direct bearing on the development of ultrasonography was the invention of SONAR (*SO*und *N*avigation *A*nd *R*anging). The way was paved for this invention by 19th-century inquiries into the measurement of the speed of sound in water. The earliest precursors of SONAR date back to 1838, when Bonnycastle attempted to map the ocean floor by echo-sounding, an operation necessary for the placement of telegraph lines and the safe navigation of large ships. Later, the Swiss physicist Jean-Daniel Colladon[97] determined the speed of sound in water to help confirm his data about the compressibility of liquids. Colladon's experiment, considered the birth of modern underwater acoustics, consisted of striking an underwater bell in Lake Geneva and simultaneously igniting gunpowder. Colladon observed the flash from the gunpowder from 10 miles away, and he also heard the sound of the bell with an underwater trumpet. By measuring the time interval between these two events, he calculated the speed of the sound in Lake Geneva to be 1,435 m/sec, a value that differs from current calculations by only 3 m/sec.[98]

Later, in 1877, John William Strutt published *The Theory of Sound*, which became the foundation for the science of ultrasound. His contributions were deemed so significant that he was appointed to Great Britain's Board of Invention and Research, the body that supervised the development of SONAR during World War I.[99] After the sinking of the *Titanic* and of German U-boats, increased effort was applied to the development of SONAR in the hope that it would help detect underwater objects. It was not until April 1914, however, that iceberg detection was accomplished with the help of Reginald Aubry Fessenden's electromagnetic moving-coil arrangement.[98] Although this technology was well accepted, it was primarily used for underwater signaling and navigation of World War I submarines. In 1915, Constantin Chilowsky, in conjunction with the eminent French physicist Paul Langevin, developed a working hydrophone.[100] This pioneering work considerably enhanced scientists' knowledge of how ultrasound waves were generated and received—an important part of the pulse-echo principle of SONAR. Research and development focusing on underwater acoustics and transducers thrived during this period, and important discoveries were made that advanced the progress of ultrasound technology.

By 1928, with the help of Langevin's contributions, the French ocean liner *Ile de France* had a fully operational device for monitoring the ocean floor and an underwater transmitter for intership communication.[101] The Canadian scientist Donald Sproule led the research efforts that developed the first echo-sounder with a range display for the Canadian navy. Sproule unexpectedly discovered that the echo-sounder not only could display the depth of ocean bedrock but also was capable of detecting schools of fish.[102] This discovery proved to be key for later medical uses of ultrasound.

Another important milestone in sound research was the discovery of piezoelectricity. In 1880, Pierre and Jacques Curie observed that when pressure was applied to crystals of quartz or Rochelle salt, an electric charge was generated that was directly proportional to the force applied to the crystals. The Curies called this phenomenon piezoelectricity, from the Greek word *piezein*, meaning "to press."[97] In addition, they demonstrated the reverse piezoelectric effect that occurred when a rapidly changing electric potential was applied to the crystal and caused it to vibrate. The ultrasound transducers currently in use contain piezoelectric crystals that expand and contract to interconvert electric and mechanical energy; this action is the essence of the ultrasound transducer.

In the post–World War II era, the industrial work of Tom Brown and Ian Donald played a vital role in the development of the first handheld contact ultrasound machine. Donald and colleagues also investigated many of the earliest clinical applications of ultrasound.

Pioneers of Medical Ultrasound

Karl Theodor Dussik, a psychiatrist and neurologist, along with his brother Friederich, a physicist, began studying the clinical uses of ultrasonography in the late 1930s. In 1937, the Dussik brothers used a 1.5

(continued)

this interconversion, the transducer contains the following essential components:

1. An active element. Electrical energy is applied to the piezoelectric crystals within the transducer, and an ultrasound pulse is thereby generated via the piezoelectric effect. The pulse distorts the crystals, and an electrical signal is produced. This signal causes an ultrasound image to form on the screen via the reverse piezoelectric effect.
2. Damping or backing material. An epoxy resin absorbs the vibrations and reduces the number of cycles in a pulse, thereby improving the resolution of the ultrasound image.
3. A matching layer. This substance reduces the reflection that occurs at the transducer-tissue interface. The great difference in density (i.e., the impedance mismatch) between the soft tissue and the transducer results in reflection of the ultrasound waves. The matching material decreases this reflection and facilitates the transit of the ultrasound waves through the body and into the target organ.

Transducers are classified according to (1) the arrangement of the active elements (array) contained within the transducer and (2) the frequency of the ultrasound wave produced. Transducer arrays contain closely packed piezoelectric elements, each with its own electrical connection to the ultrasound instrument.[7] These elements can be excited individually or in groups to produce the ultrasound beam. There are four main transducer arrays: (1) the rectangular linear array, which yields a rectangular image, (2) the curved array, which yields a trapezoidal image, (3) the phased array, a small transducer in which the sound pulses are generated by activating all of the elements in the array, and (4) the annular array, in which the elements are arranged in a circular fashion. The advantage of transducer arrays is that the ultrasound beam can be electronically steered without any moving mechanical parts (except for the annular array) and focused.[7,8] In the clinical setting, this arrangement allows the operator to adjust the focal zone so that he or she can accurately image a large organ (e.g., the liver) while still being able to obtain fine details of a lesion.

The frequency of the transducer is determined by the thickness of the piezoelectric elements within the transducer: the thinner the piezoelectric elements, the higher the frequency.[7,8] Although diagnostic ultrasonography makes use of transducer frequencies ranging from 1 MHz to 20 MHz, the most commonly used frequencies for medical diagnostic imaging are those between 2.5 and 10 MHz [see Table 4]. Ultrasound beams of different frequencies have different characteristics: higher frequencies penetrate tissue poorly but yield excellent resolution, whereas lower frequencies penetrate well but at the cost of compromised resolution. Accordingly, transducers are generally chosen on the basis of the depth of the structure to be imaged.[9] For example, a 7.5 MHz transducer is a suitable choice for imaging a superficial organ such as the thyroid, but a 3.5 MHz transducer would be preferable for imaging a deep structure such as the abdominal aorta.

Ultrasound machines vary in complexity, but each has the following essential components:

Ultrasonography in Surgery: Historical Perspectives *(continued)*

MHz transmitter to record variations in the amplitude of the energy detected in scanning the human brain.[102] Their experiments were deemed to be faulty, however, and research funding for medical uses of ultrasound in the United States was greatly curtailed for the next decade.[102-104]

G. D. Ludwig and F. W. Struthers, working at the Naval Medical Research Institute in Bethesda, Maryland, were among the first investigators to study the use of the pulse-echo technique in biologic tissue; unfortunately, because Ludwig was employed by the military, many of his findings were considered to be restricted information and consequently were not published in medical journals. These studies investigated the transmission velocity of ultrasound waves in slabs of beef and human extremities and determined that the mean propagation speed of ultrasound in soft tissue was 1,540 m/sec. This important achievement had far-reaching consequences that affect how ultrasound software is constructed to this day.

In 1950, the English-trained surgeon John Julian Wild published his preliminary findings on ultrasound-determined bowel wall thickness and the properties of a specimen of gastric cancer.[105] Wild, Donald Neal, and, subsequently, J. M. Reid noted that malignant tissue seemed to be more echogenic than benign tissue.[105,106] Intellectual and financial support for Wild's research was minimal because of his unconventional research methods and his personality differences with his scientific contemporaries. Wild wanted to find immediate clinical applications for ultrasound technology rather than design experiments based on theories. His various difficulties notwithstanding, Wild managed to develop a scanning device that was used to screen patients for breast cancer; he also developed transrectal and transvaginal transducers. With this instrument, he was able to image a brain tumor in a pathology specimen and to localize a brain tumor in a patient after a craniotomy.

Another pioneer from the 1940s, Douglass Howry, played an important role in the development of ultrasound and ultrasonic devices. Working with W. Roderic Bliss, an electrical engineer, Howry began building the first B-mode scanner in 1949. Unlike Wild, Howry was as interested in the behavior of ultrasound waves in tissue as he was in the construction of a functional ultrasound machine. In the early 1960s, W. Wright and E. Meyers joined Howry's research team. The result of this team effort was the production of a direct contact scanner. In 1961, Meyers and Wright incorporated to form Physionics Engineering, and within a year, they produced the prototype for the first handheld contact scanner in the United States.[107] This scanner had an articulated arm with positioning mechanisms at each joint to integrate information obtained from the transducer.

Ian Donald and another gynecologist, John McVicar, along with Tom Brown, an engineer from Kelvin & Hughes Scientific Instrument Company, developed the first contact compound scanner. Donald's contributions were well accepted in the field of medicine: they essentially solidified the concept that ultrasound would have a major role in medical diagnostic imaging.

In 1955, Bernard Jaffe discovered the piezoelectric properties of polarized solid solutions of lead zirconate titanate. This important finding eventually led to smaller and better ultrasound transducers. Inge Edler of Sweden and Carl Hellmuth Hertz were the principal pioneers in the field of echocardiography.

Christian Doppler and the Doppler Effect

Special mention should be made of the Austrian mathematician and physicist Christian Johann Doppler. In 1841, Doppler gave a speech entitled "On the Colored Light of the Double Stars and Certain Other Stars of the Heavens" to an audience consisting of five people and a transcriber.[108] Doppler's treatise proposed that the observed color of a star was caused by a spectral shift of white light that occurred because of the relative motion of the star to the earth. To provide a basis for his theory, Doppler used analogies based on the transmission of light and sound. Although his theory on light was in error, Doppler's theory on the frequency changes in sound waves was correct. The Doppler effect, as the sonic phenomenon he described came to be known, is defined as "the observed changes in frequency of transmitted waves when relative motion exists between the source of the wave and an observer."[108] This theory has been applied to many aspects of science, including astronomy and medicine.

The first application of the Doppler effect in medicine involved the measurement of differences in the transit time between two transducers of ultrasonic waves traveling "upstream" and "downstream" through flowing blood. Since then, research into the clinical use of the Doppler principle has been carried out simultaneously at numerous centers throughout the global scientific community.

Table 1 Ultrasound Physics Terminology Relevant to Ultrasonographic Imaging[4-6]

Term	Definition	Significance
Ultrasound	High-frequency (> 20 KHz) mechanical radiant energy transmitted through a medium	
Frequency	Number of cycles/sec (10^6 cycles/sec = 1 MHz) Diagnostic ultrasound: 1–20 MHz	Increasing frequency improves resolution
Wavelength	Distance traveled by wave per cycle: as frequency becomes higher, wavelength becomes smaller	Wavelength is related to spatial resolution of object: shorter wavelengths yield better resolution but poorer penetration
Amplitude	Strength or height of wave	
Attenuation	Decrease in amplitude and intensity of wave as it travels through a medium; attenuation is affected by absorption, scattering, and reflection	Amplitude and intensity are reduced (attenuated) as waves travel through tissue; time-gain compensation circuit compensates for this attenuation
Absorption	Conversion of sound energy into heat	
Scattering	Redirection of wave as it strikes a rough or small boundary	
Reflection	Return of wave toward transducer	
Propagation speed	Speed with which wave travels through soft tissue (1,540 m/sec)	Propagation speed (determined by density and stiffness of medium) is greater in solids than in liquids and greater in liquids than in gases

1. A monitor (for displaying the ultrasound image).
2. A keyboard (for labeling the image and making adjustments to produce a quality image).
3. A transducer (for interconverting electrical and acoustic energy).
4. An image recorder (for producing copies of the ultrasound images).

Finally, there are three scanning modes, A, B, and M; these modes evolved over several years.[10] A mode (amplitude modulation), the most basic form of diagnostic ultrasonography, yields a one-dimensional image that displays the amplitude or strength of the wave along the vertical axis and the time along the horizontal axis. Therefore, the greater the signal returning to the transducer, the higher the "spike." B mode (brightness modulation), the mode most commonly used today, relates the brightness of the image to the amplitude of the ultrasound wave. Thus, denser structures appear brighter (i.e., whiter, more echogenic) on the image because they reflect the ultrasound waves better. M mode relates the amplitude of the ultrasound wave to the imaging of moving structures, such as cardiac muscle. Before real-time imaging became available, M-mode scanning formed the basis for echocardiography.[10,11]

Clinical Applications of Ultrasonography in Surgical Practice

As an extension of the physical examination, ultrasonography is a valuable adjunct to surgical practice in the office, the emergency department, the operating room, and the surgical intensive care unit. Once surgeons have learned the essential principles of ultrasonography, they can readily build on this experience and extend the use of this technology to various specific aspects of surgery. In what follows, I list and briefly describe several clinical areas in which surgeon-performed ultrasonography has proved to be an effective diagnostic and interventional tool.

BREAST

Ultrasound-directed biopsy of breast lesions is now a common office procedure for general surgeons. The increase in the number of screening mammograms performed since the late 1970s has led to the detection of more nonpalpable breast lesions. The traditional choice for further evaluation of such masses has been open surgical excision, but the yield of malignancies with this approach has been only about 20%.[12-14] Advances in ultrasound technology, including automated biopsy needles and high-resolution transducers,[15] have prompted a surge of interest in fine-needle and core biopsy tissue sampling as an alternative to open biopsy. Such procedures are appealing because they are minimally invasive, are about as accurate as open biopsy,[16] and can be performed by the surgeon in the office setting.

Current indications for breast ultrasonography include (1) evaluation of a nonpalpable, new, or growing mass detected on mammog-

Table 2 Essential Principles of Ultrasound

Principle	Explanation
Piezoelectric effect	Piezoelectric crystals expand and contract to interconvert electrical and mechanical energy
Pulse-echo principle	When ultrasound wave contacts tissue, some of signal is reflected while some is transmitted into tissue; these waves are then reflected to crystals within transducer, generating electrical impulse comparable to strength of returning wave
Acoustic impedance	Acoustic impedance = density of tissue × speed of sound in tissue Strength of returning echo depends on difference in density between two structures imaged: structures of different acoustic impedance (e.g., bile and gallstone) are relatively easy to distinguish from one another, whereas those of similar acoustic impedance (e.g., spleen and kidney) are more difficult to distinguish

Table 3 Terminology Used in Assessment of Ultrasonograms[3,109]

Term	Definition
Echogenicity	Degree to which tissue echoes ultrasonic waves (generally reflected in ultrasound image as degree of brightness)
Anechoic	Showing no internal echoes, appearing dark or black
Isoechoic	Having appearance similar to that of surrounding tissue
Hypoechoic	Less echoic or darker than surrounding tissue
Hyperechoic	More echoic or whiter than surrounding tissue
Resolution	Ability to distinguish between two different structures; spatial resolution improves as frequency increases
Lateral	Resolution transverse to ultrasound wave; relates to width of structure
Axial	Resolution parallel to ultrasound wave; relates to depth of structure

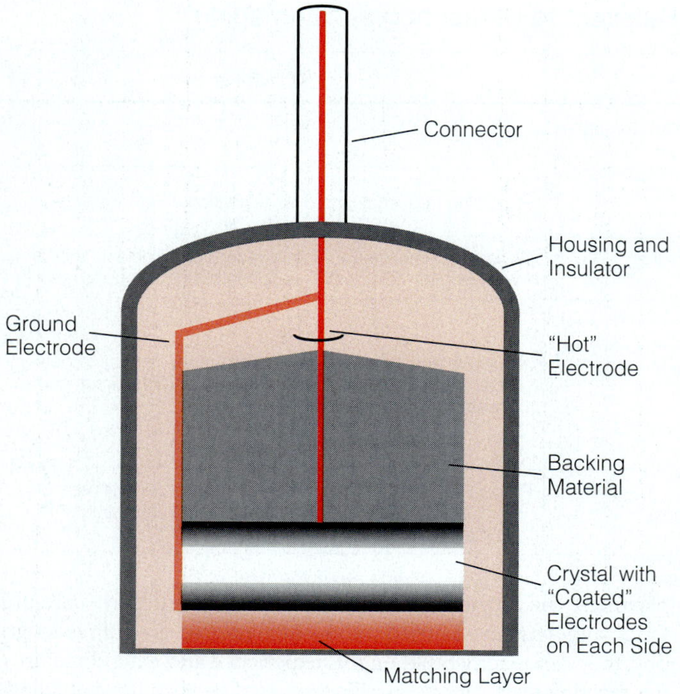

Figure 1 Shown are the basic components of an ultrasound transducer.

Table 4 Clinical Applications of Selected Transducer Frequencies

Frequency	Applications
2.5–3.5 MHz	Renal Aortic General abdominal
5.0 MHz	Transvaginal Pediatric abdominal Testicular
7.5 MHz	Vascular Foreign body in soft tissue Thyroid

raphy, (2) evaluation of duct size in the presence of nipple discharge, (3) assessment of a dense breast or a vaguely palpable mass, (4) differentiation between a solid palpable mass and a cystic one, and (5) guidance of percutaneous drainage of an abscess.[17-21]

GASTROINTESTINAL TRACT

Endoscopic and endorectal ultrasonography have added a new dimension to the preoperative assessment and treatment of many GI lesions. Endoscopic ultrasonography (EUS) involves the visualization of the GI tract via a high-frequency (12 to 20 MHz) ultrasound transducer placed through an endoscope. With the transducer near the target organ, images of the gut wall and the surrounding parenchymal organs can be obtained that are detailed enough to define the depth of tumor penetration with precision and to detect the presence of involved lymph nodes as small as 2 mm. When done preoperatively, EUS is 80% to 90% accurate at predicting the stage of the tumor; if an endoscopically directed biopsy attachment is used, the diagnostic potential is even higher.[22]

Indications for EUS include (1) preoperative staging of GI malignancies, (2) preoperative localization of pancreatic endocrine tumors, particularly insulinomas, (3) evaluation of submucosal lesions of the GI tract, and (4) guidance of imaging during interventional procedures (e.g., tissue sampling and drainage of a pancreatic pseudocyst).[23-25]

Endorectal ultrasonography is used in the evaluation of patients with benign and malignant rectal conditions.[26-34] It is commonly performed with an axial 7.0 or 10.0 MHz rotating transducer that produces a 360° horizontal cross-sectional view of the rectal wall. This special transducer is 24 cm long and is covered with a water-filled latex balloon. After the transducer is advanced above the rectal lesion, the balloon that surrounds the transducer is filled with degassed water to create an acoustic window for ultrasound imaging. The transducer is gradually withdrawn while the examiner views the layers of the rectal wall [see Figure 2] by means of real-time imaging.[35,36] These layers are important landmarks in ultrasonographic staging, just as they are in postoperative pathologic staging. For example, if the middle white line (i.e., the submucosa) is intact, a be-

nign lesion may be removed via a submucosal resection. A classification of preoperative tumor staging called uTNM has been proposed that is analogous to the TNM classification for tumor staging.[37] This classification is based on ultrasonographic determination of the infiltrative tumor depth (the prefix *u* stands for ultrasonography).

The sensitivity of ultrasonography in determining the depth of tumor invasion is about 85% to 90%; however, it can sometimes overestimate the extent of invasion in the presence of tissue inflammation and edema.[28] Further research is needed to assess the accuracy of ultrasonography in detecting recurrent cancer after surgery.[38] Errors in staging are likely to occur with tumors that invade the lamina muscularis mucosae or are associated with inflammation of the lamina propria mucosae.[39] In addition, lesions characterized by ultramicroscopic invasion of the submucosa may be misstaged because the technology currently available cannot provide the fine resolution necessary to assess such invasion.[28,40]

Endoanal ultrasonography is an important part of the evaluation of anal incontinence because it is capable of detecting defects in the internal and external sphincters.[41-45] It is done in much the same way as endorectal ultrasonography, except that the 10 MHz transducer is covered with a sonolucent hard plastic cone instead of a water-filled balloon. Although endoanal ultrasonography does not measure sphincter function, ultrasound-detected sphincter disruption correlates well with pressure measurements[46,47] and operative findings.[45,48] Additional indications for endoanal ultrasonography include evaluation of patients with an exophytic distal rectal tumor (e.g., a villous adenoma) and assessment of patients who have a perianal abscess, fistula in ano, a presacral cyst, or a rectal ulcer.

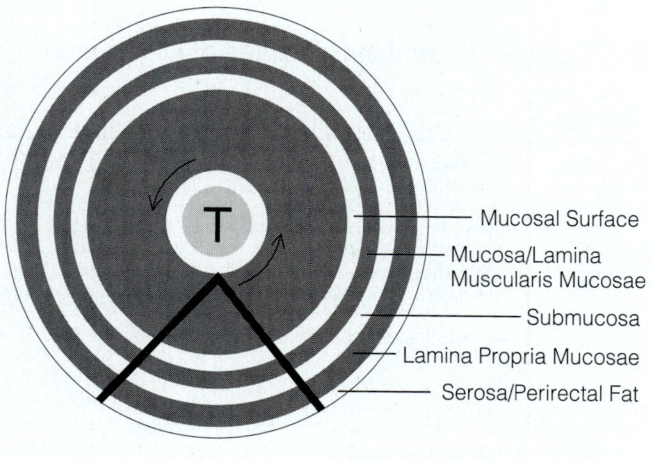

Figure 2 Depicted is the five-layer model of rectal wall anatomy as delineated by endorectal ultrasonography.[110]

ACUTE CONDITIONS

Traumatic

The FAST (Focused Assessment for the Sonographic examination of the Trauma patient) is a rapid diagnostic test developed for the evaluation of patients with potential truncal injuries. Historically, its development is rooted in several fundamental studies that demonstrated the high sensitivity of ultrasonography in detecting small degrees of ascites,[49] splenic injury,[50] and hemoperitoneum in the hepatorenal space and the pelvis.[51] The FAST determines the presence or absence of blood in the pericardial sac and three dependent abdominal regions, including Morison's pouch, the splenorenal recess, and the pelvis.

Nontraumatic

In the acute nontraumatic setting, surgeons are currently using ultrasonography for the following purposes:

1. Assessment for multiple loculations and drainage of a soft tissue abscess.[52,53]
2. Early diagnosis of wound dehiscence through visualization of the fascial defect [see Figure 3].
3. Detection of a foreign body in soft tissue.[54-56]
4. Evaluation of a patient with abdominal pain (e.g., from gallstones).[52,53,57,58]
5. Confirmation of the reduction of an incarcerated hernia through identification of the fascial defect and observation of the reduction occurring with real-time imaging [see Figure 4].[59]
6. Identification of an abdominal aortic aneurysm in a patient who presents with back pain and hypotension. Intramural calcification and intraluminal thrombus are common findings [see Figure 5]. If the aortic aneurysm ruptures into the peritoneal cavity, the FAST can detect the presence of hemoperitoneum.

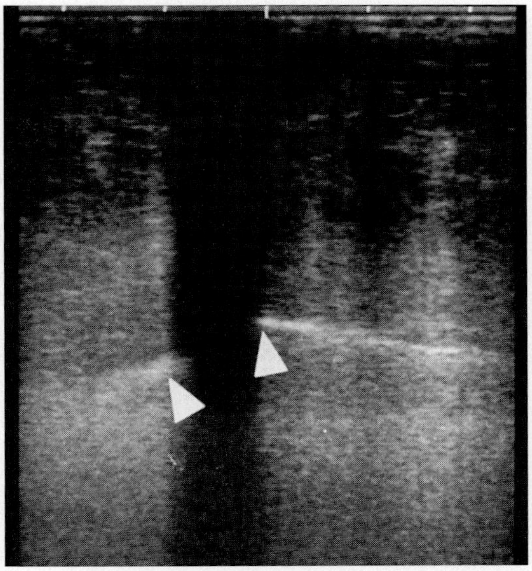

LAPAROSCOPY AND INTRAOPERATIVE USE

Examination with intraoperative or laparoscopic ultrasonography is an integral part of many hepatic, biliary, and pancreatic surgical procedures. With this tool, surgeons can detect previously undiagnosed lesions or bile duct stones,[60] avoid unnecessary dissection of vessels or ducts, clarify tumor margins, and perform biopsy and cryoablation procedures.[61] Compared with preoperative imaging modalities, intraoperative ultrasonography is much more sensitive in detecting malignant or benign lesions.[62] The precision with which intraoperative ultrasonography can delineate small lesions (5 mm) and define their relationship to other structures facilitates resection, reduces operative time, and frequently alters the surgeon's operative strategy.[62-65]

Intraoperative ultrasonography makes use of both contact scanning and so-called standoff scanning for imaging.[66] In contact scanning, the transducer is directly applied to the organ so that the deepest part of the organ is accurately depicted. This technique is most often used for imaging large organs (e.g., the liver). In standoff scanning, the transducer is placed about 1 to 2 cm away from the structure in a pool of sterile saline solution that permits the transmission of ultrasound waves. This technique is often used to image blood vessels, bile ducts, or the spinal cord; it allows good visualization of the structure without compression by the transducer. The size, shape, and type of ultrasound transducer used for intraoperative scanning depend on the anatomic structure to be examined. For example, a pencillike 7.5 MHz transducer is used for scanning the common bile duct, whereas a side-viewing T-shaped 5 MHz transducer is preferable for imaging a cirrhotic liver. Intraoperative ultrasound examinations are conducted systematically to ensure that no subtle pathology is missed and that the examination is reproducible. For example, the liver is imaged sequentially according to a system based on Couinaud's anatomic segments.[67]

Figure 3 Ultrasound image shows midline abdominal wound dehiscence. Transducer orientation is sagittal with respect to long axis of wound. Interruption in horizontal white line (arrows) represents separation of fascia.

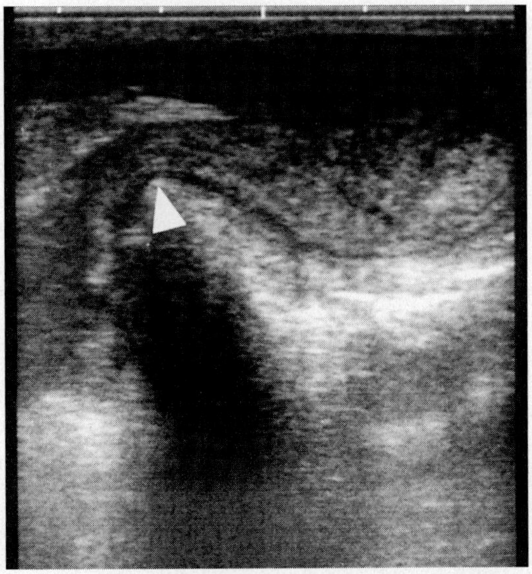

Figure 4 Sagittal ultrasound image shows ventral hernia with fascial defect (arrow).

Similar principles apply to laparoscopic ultrasonography, except that the transducers are made to adapt to the laparoscopic equipment.[68,69] Indications for this modality include detection of common bile duct stones, staging of pancreatic cancer to prevent unnecessary celiotomy, and resection or cryoablation of hepatic metastases.[69]

VASCULAR SYSTEM

Color flow duplex imaging and endoluminal ultrasonography have significantly expanded the diagnostic and therapeutic aspects of vascular imaging. Vascular diagnostic imaging is commonly used for diagnosing arterial disease or deep vein thrombosis (DVT); however, it is also helpful for diagnosing other disorders, such as Raynaud's disease and thoracic outlet syndrome. In the office setting, surgeons use ultrasonography to screen for abdominal aortic aneurysm or to follow patients with a diagnosed aneurysm, because it is capable of detecting change in aortic diameter as small as a few millimeters.[70] In patients who have

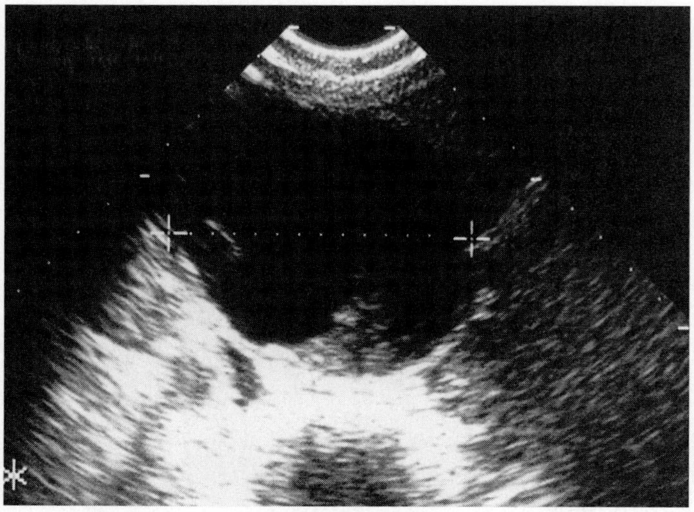

Figure 5 Transverse ultrasound image shows abdominal aortic aneurysm with intraluminal thrombus.

undergone repair of an abdominal aortic aneurysm, color flow duplex imaging is highly specific for the diagnosis of anastomotic false aneurysms. In one study, this modality was compared with B-mode ultrasonography, CT, digital subtraction arteriography, and magnetic resonance imaging and emerged as the diagnostic test of choice when the accuracy, cost, safety, and availability of each method were assessed.[71]

Color flow duplex scanning is also used to examine the patency and size of the portal vein and the hepatic artery in patients who have undergone liver transplantation, to assess the resectability of pancreatic tumors, to diagnose superior mesenteric artery occlusion, and to diagnose a pseudoaneurysm or an arteriovenous fistula after percutaneous arterial catheterization.[72,73] In the acute setting, several investigators have found color flow duplex imaging to be a reliable, time-saving, noninvasive alternative to arteriography for the detection of arterial injury.[74-78]

Duplex imaging of the lower extremity is used to assess the patency of the deep venous system and is capable of detecting DVT reliably.[79] The addition of color flow imaging facilitates the examination by making the artery and its associated vein easier to identify. By performing serial duplex venous ultrasound imaging to detect DVT, one group of investigators was able to identify a subgroup of injured patients who were at highest risk for pulmonary embolism; they suggested that these patients be given DVT prophylaxis and undergo close surveillance with duplex imaging.[79]

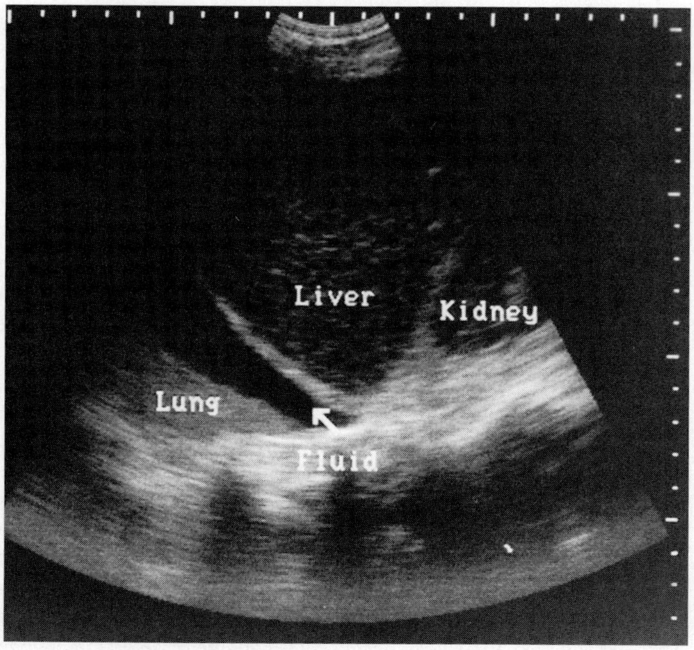

Intraoperative duplex imaging can be used to detect technical errors in vascular anastomoses as well as abnormalities in flow.[80] Arteriography assesses the patency of an anastomosis and measures distal arterial runoff, but it is invasive. Intraoperative duplex imaging, on the other hand, permits rapid visualization of the anatomic and hemodynamic aspects of a vascular reconstruction, and it is noninvasive, easily repeatable, and less time-consuming than arteriography.

SURGICAL INTENSIVE CARE UNIT

Indications for surgeon-performed ultrasonography in the SICU include localization of a central vein or an artery for hemodynamic monitoring[81] and detection of a pleural effusion [*see Figure 6*]. Not only are fewer lateral decubitus x-rays ordered when ultrasonography is done in the SICU, but the safety of thoracentesis is also enhanced when it is performed under ultrasound guidance.[82,83]

General Considerations for Diagnostic Ultrasound Examinations

INSTRUMENTATION

Before an ultrasound examination is performed, the following three steps should be observed:

1. The correct ultrasound machine and transducer should be chosen for the specific type of examination to be done. For example, if a vascular study is to be performed, the machine should have Doppler capability and, ideally, color flow capability as well.
2. The transducer should be chosen according to the structure or organ to be imaged. It must provide both sufficient depth of penetration to image the entire organ and sufficient resolution to allow the examiner to distinguish the details of lesions.
3. Although many machines have preset controls for power and gain, a standard image should be obtained to confirm that the settings are correct for the specific examination being done. For example, the FAST begins with an image of the heart so that blood can be identified and the gain controls adjusted (if necessary) to permit accurate detection of hemoperitoneum.

PATIENT POSITIONING

The patient should be positioned so that all of the images required for a particular examination can be readily obtained. The surgeon should take time to review the scanning planes [*see Figure 7*] and understand the orientation of the patient on the monitor screen in relation to the transducer. It is also important to follow conventional scanning protocols so that when the images are reviewed, a lesion can be accurately located and the scan can be reproduced even by another ultrasonographer. An example of such a protocol is the radial-scanning technique recommended for examination of the breast [*see Technique for Selected Surgical Applications of Ultrasonography, Breast Examination, below*].

DOCUMENTATION

The machine's annotation keys are used to record the patient's name and identification number, the area of interest, and the scanning plane. Most machines have function keys that automate the recording of these data. Furthermore, the internal clock automatically labels each image with the date and time (accurate to 0.01 second).

Figure 6 Sagittal ultrasound image demonstrates pleural effusion.

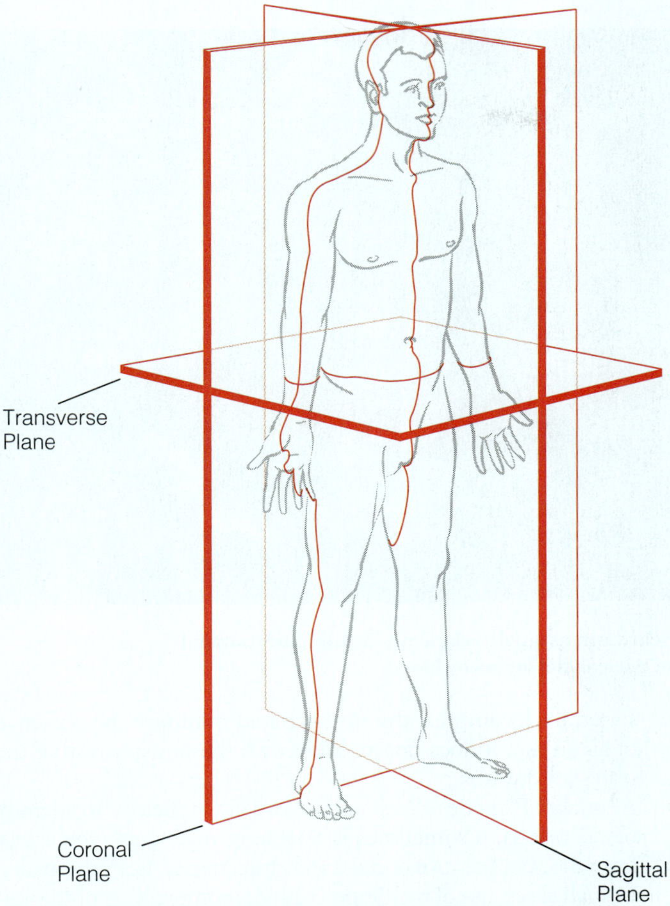

Figure 7 Depicted are scanning planes used in ultrasonography.

TECHNICAL TIPS

The following generic technical tips should prove useful in a wide range of ultrasonographic applications:

1. The ultrasound machine should be inspected according to the guidelines of the institution's department of biomedical engineering to ensure that it is functioning properly.
2. The patient's orientation on the monitor or screen relative to the position of the transducer should be checked by applying gel to the transducer's footprint (i.e., the part of the transducer that is in contact with the patient's skin) and then rubbing the footprint with a finger near the indicator line of the transducer. Motion on the left side of the screen indicates that the transducer is properly oriented.
3. Liberal amounts of gel should be applied to the area being examined. The gel acts as an acoustic coupler, helping to transmit the ultrasound waves and reduce their reflection. If not enough gel has been applied, the waves will not be transmitted properly, and a dark area will appear on the ultrasound image.
4. The transducer should be manipulated with small movements (not wide sweeps), and gentle pressure should be applied initially. This second point is especially important in imaging the breast or the thyroid: the tissues are superficial, and too much pressure can easily compress them and distort the ultrasound image.
5. The gain and time-gain compensation settings should be rechecked for each new examination. For example, after completing a breast examination, the sonographer should not begin an examination of the carotid vessels without confirming that these settings are correct.

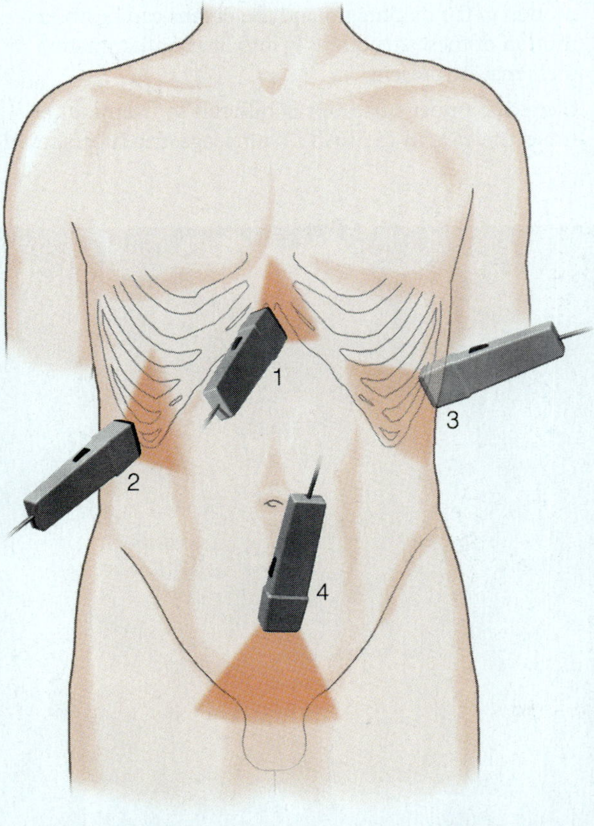

Any hard copies of the ultrasound images that may be required should be printed, saved, and reviewed. Ideally, the ultrasound images should be videotaped, because the dynamic real-time image provides more information than still images, thereby increasing the confidence level associated with each observation.

CONTINUOUS PERFORMANCE IMPROVEMENT

As part of the performance improvement process, ultrasound images should be routinely reviewed, with special attention paid to false positive or false negative examinations. The goal of this process is to help identify any correctable factors associated with such examinations and thereby minimize or prevent their recurrence. Some studies have noted the presence of a pronounced learning curve, as a result of which the sensitivity and specificity initially achieved by new surgeon-ultrasonographers have been relatively low[57,84-86]; however, there is evidence that surgeons' performance may be improved with the help of an ultrasound training course that focuses on those pitfalls of imaging that were found to be problems in the clinical setting. For example, in one study, surgeons learned both to perform examinations correctly and to interpret positive results accurately in patients with minimal as well as pronounced ascites; as a result, they were better able to distinguish relatively subtle differences within the spectrum of positive FAST results.[86] Other suggestions for improving performance are (1) to perform the ultrasound examination initially on normal tissue (as in evaluation of a breast mass) and (2) to perform the examinations on patients with known disease (e.g., a palpable breast mass, ascites, gallstones, or benign pericardial effusion). The rationale for the latter suggestion is that it should help the surgeon learn more rapidly how to recognize lesions with varying degrees of pathology.

Figure 8 FAST. Shown are four transducer positions used in FAST: (1) pericardial area, (2) right upper quadrant, (3) left upper quadrant, and (4) pelvis.[84]

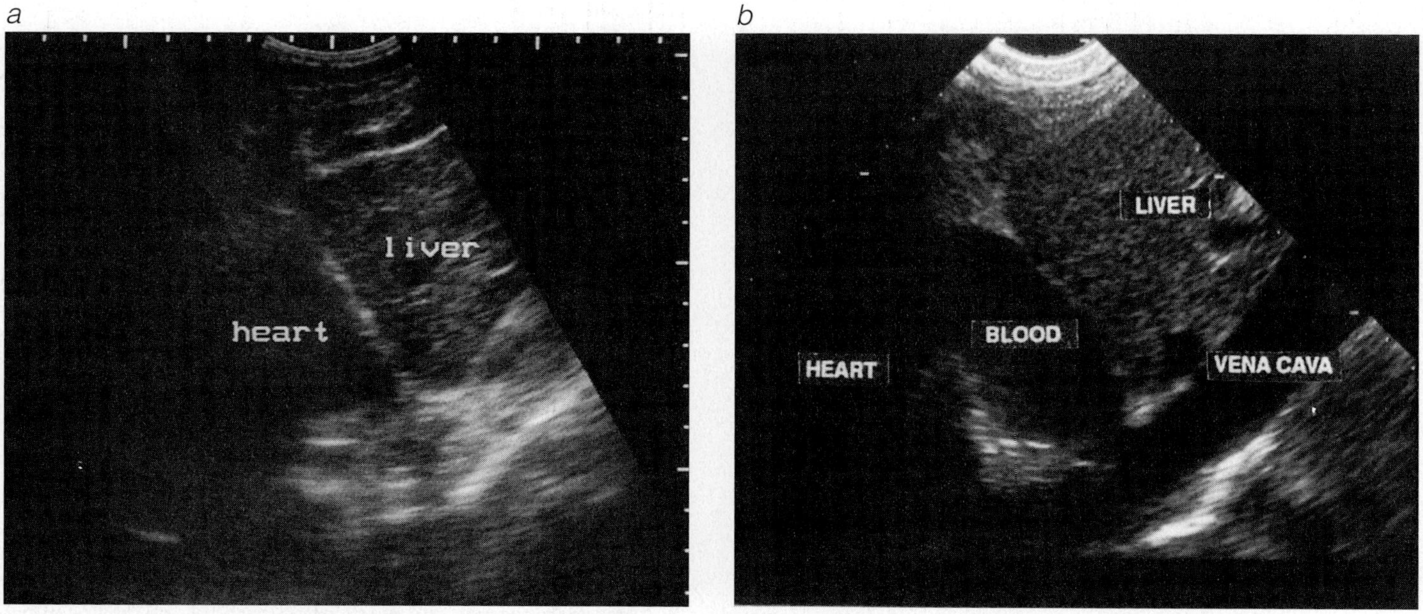

Figure 9 FAST. (*a*) Sagittal ultrasound image of heart shows pericardium as single echogenic (white) line; normal findings. (*b*) Sagittal ultrasound image of heart shows separation of pericardial layers by blood.

6. Normal tissue should be examined ultrasonographically before the sonographer turns to the area of interest. For example, if the goal is to assess an abscess or DVT in one extremity, the first step should be to inspect the other extremity to see what the corresponding normal tissue looks like. This helps to sensitize the examiner to subtle pathologic changes in the abnormal tissue.
7. The patient should be asked to take a deep breath so that the motion of the diaphragm and the organs can be observed. If the motion of these structures is impaired, inflammation or an abscess may be present.
8. If the left upper quadrant is difficult to examine (as is sometimes the case in the FAST), a nasogastric tube should be inserted to decompress the stomach and minimize the presence of air so that it does not interfere with the transmission of the ultrasound waves.
9. Although B-mode ultrasound is usually sufficient to identify blood vessels, it sometimes is unable to distinguish the artery from the vein because of pulsations transmitted from the artery. In such cases, use of the Doppler mode, compression of the vessel (veins compress very easily), or having the patient perform the Valsalva maneuver can help differentiate arterial from venous anatomy. In addition, the vena cava is more readily identified as the patient completes inspiration.
10. A full bladder is needed for pelvic ultrasound examinations: it acts as an acoustic window, facilitating visualization of the pelvic

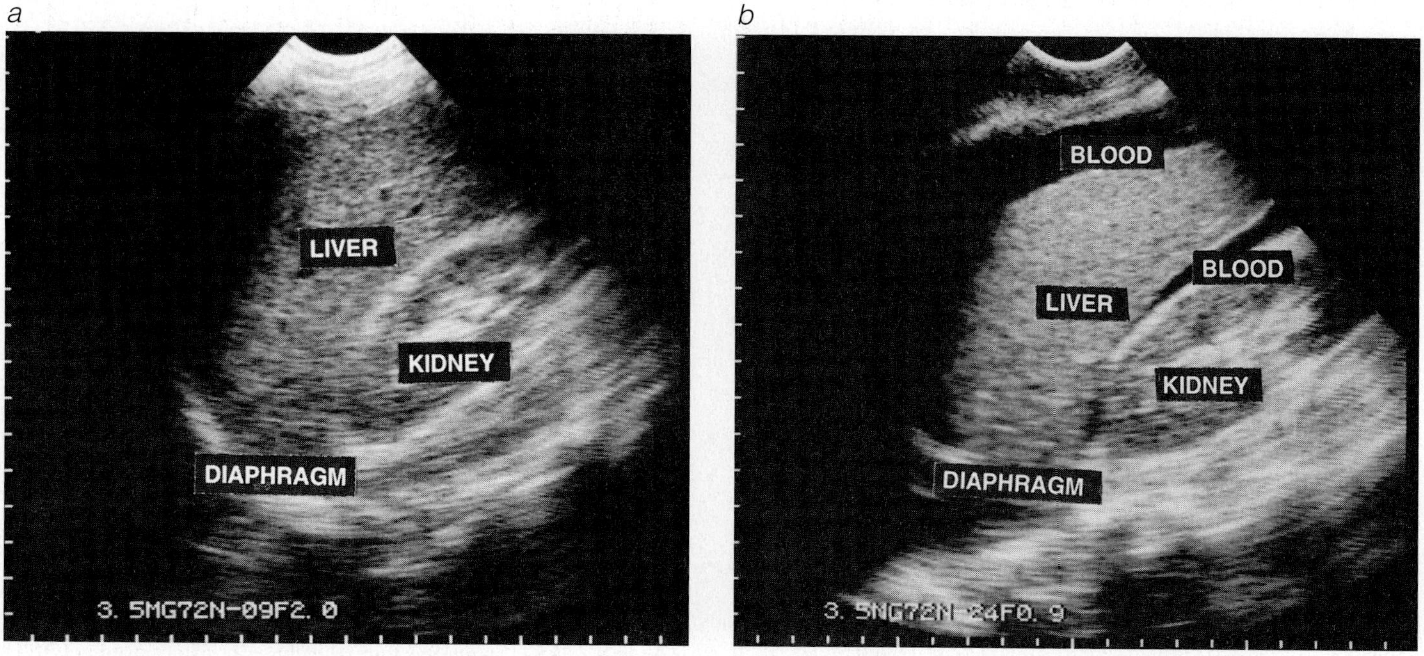

Figure 10 FAST. (*a*) Sagittal ultrasound image of liver, kidney, and diaphragm yields normal findings. (*b*) Sagittal ultrasound image of right upper quadrant shows blood between liver and kidney and between liver and diaphragm.

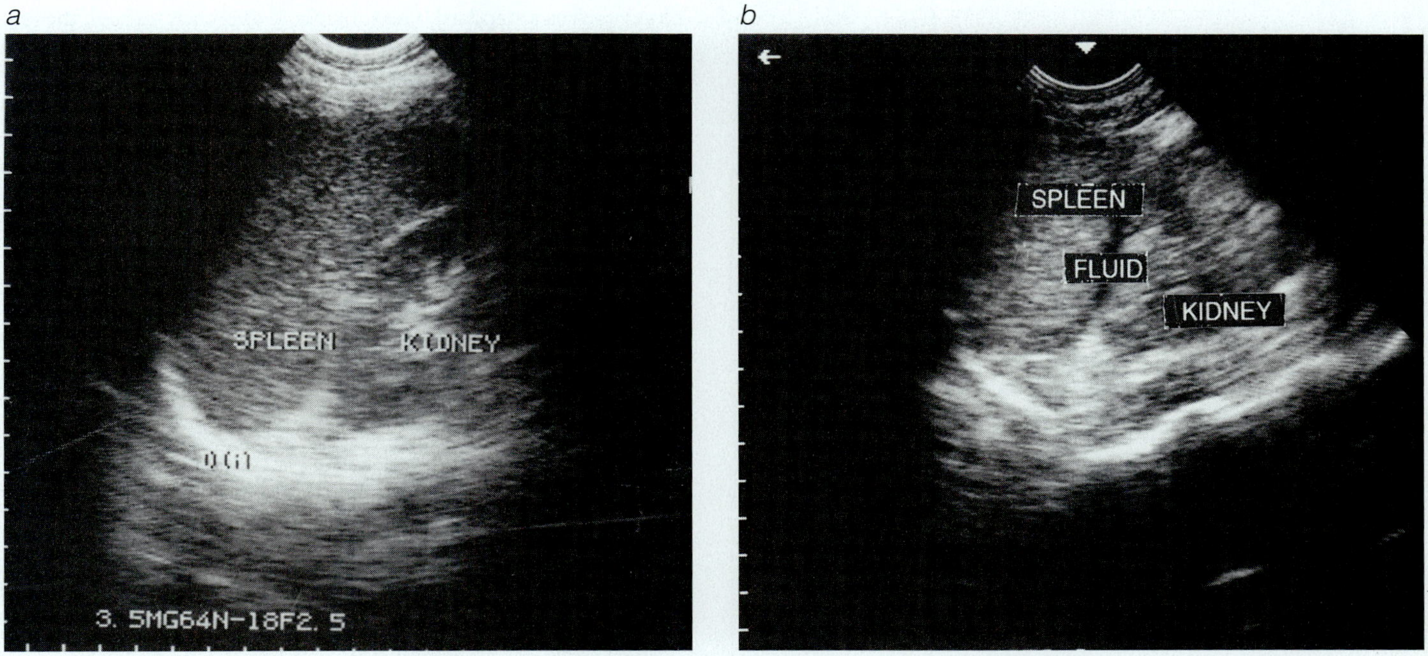

Figure 11 FAST. (*a*) Sagittal ultrasound image of spleen and kidney yields normal findings. (*b*) Sagittal ultrasound image of left upper quadrant shows blood between spleen and kidney.

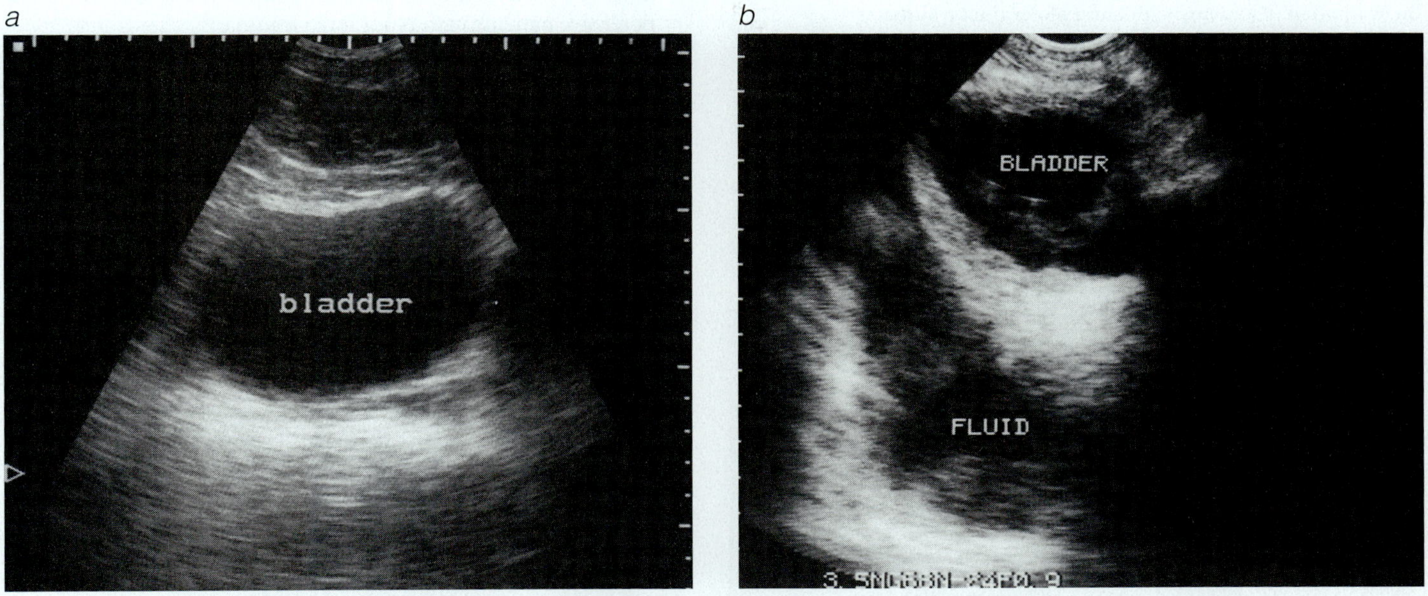

Figure 12 FAST. (*a*) Coronal ultrasound image of pelvis shows full bladder; normal findings. (*b*) Coronal ultrasound image of pelvis shows full bladder surrounded by blood.

structures. It should not, however, be so full that it is overdistended. If the bladder is not full enough, the urinary catheter can be clamped to allow it to fill; if it is too full, the catheter can be unclamped to allow it to drain. In this way, hematomas in the pelvis can be more easily detected.

Technique for Selected Surgical Applications of Ultrasonography

FOCUSED ASSESSMENT FOR THE SONOGRAPHIC EXAMINATION OF THE TRAUMA PATIENT

The FAST is performed during the Advanced Trauma Life Support secondary survey while the patient is in the supine position

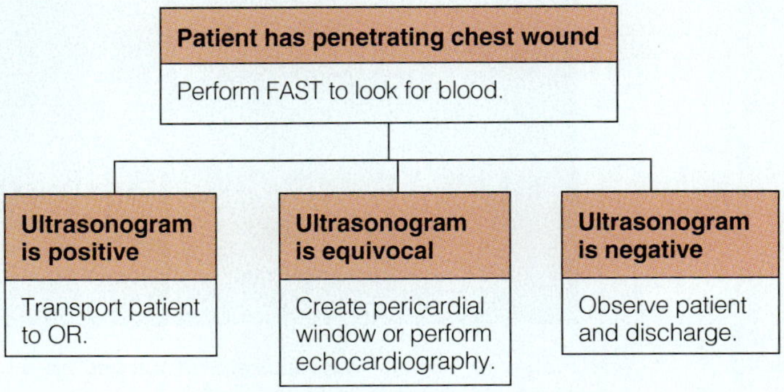

Figure 13 FAST. Shown is an algorithm for use of ultrasonography in evaluation of patients with penetrating precordial wounds.[111]

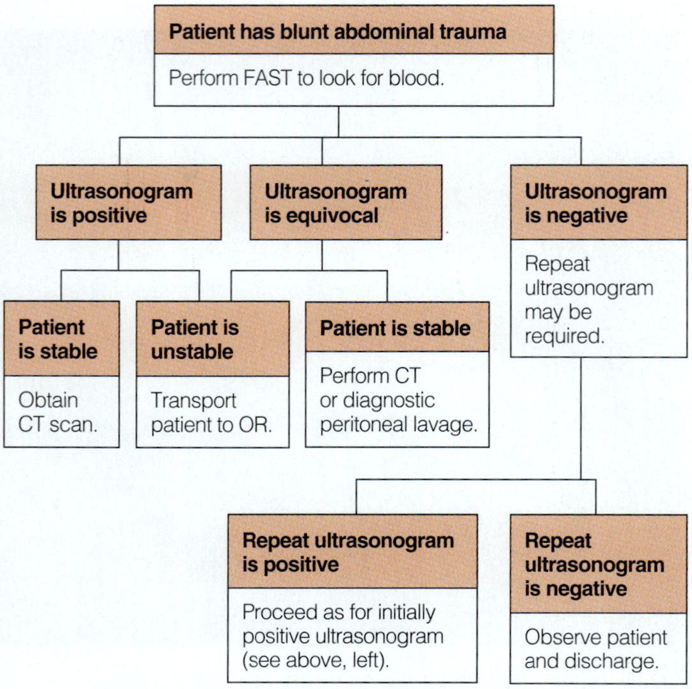

Figure 14 FAST. Shown is an algorithm for use of ultrasonography in evaluation of patients with blunt abdominal trauma.[111]

[see *2 Trauma Resuscitation*]. With the thoracoabdominal area exposed, warmed hypoallergenic, water-soluble ultrasound transmission gel is applied to the abdomen in four specific areas. A focused, limited examination for the detection of blood in these four regions is conducted in sequence as follows: (1) the pericardial area, (2) the right upper abdominal quadrant, (3) the left upper abdominal quadrant, and (4) the pouch of Douglas [see *Figure 8*].

The transducer is oriented for sagittal sections and placed in the subxiphoid region. The heart is then identified, with the density of blood used as a standard. The subxiphoid approach through the longitudinal axis is taken to enable the examiner to identify the heart and to look for blood in the pericardial region [see *Figure 9*].

The transducer is then placed in the right midaxillary line region between the 11th and 12th ribs to enable the examiner to identify the liver, the kidney, and the diaphragm and to look for blood in Morison's pouch [see *Figure 10*].

Next, the transducer is positioned on the left posterior axillary line between the 10th and 11th ribs to enable the examiner to visualize the spleen and the kidney and to look for blood in the space between these organs and posterior to the spleen [see *Figure 11*].

The transducer is then oriented for transverse sections and placed in the midline approximately 4 cm superior to the symphysis pubis to determine whether there is blood around the full bladder [see *Figure 12*].

An analysis of 1,540 injured patients undergoing FAST examinations performed by surgeon-ultrasonographers reached the following conclusions[86]:

1. Ultrasonography should be the initial diagnostic adjunct for the evaluation of patients with precordial wounds and blunt truncal injuries because it is rapid and accurate and augments the surgeon's diagnostic capabilities.

2. Surgeon-performed FAST is most accurate when used for the evaluation of patients with precordial or transthoracic wounds and a possible hemopericardium and for the evaluation of hypotensive patients with blunt torso trauma.

3. Because of the high sensitivity and specificity of ultrasonography when it is used for the evaluation of patients with precordial or transthoracic wounds and hypotensive patients with blunt torso trauma, immediate operative intervention is justified in these patients when the ultrasound examination is positive [see *Figures 13 and 14*].

Although the FAST accurately detects the presence or absence of hemoperitoneum in patients with blunt trauma, it does not readily identify intraparenchymal or retroperitoneal injuries. Therefore, a computed tomographic scan of the abdomen may be needed

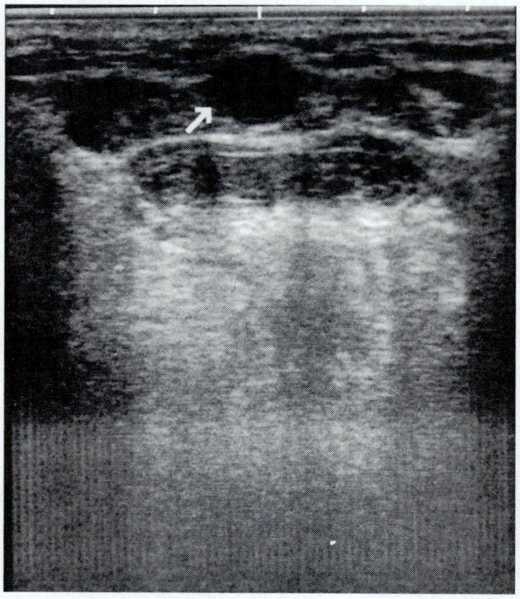

Figure 15 Breast examination. Ultrasound image shows simple cyst (arrow) of breast characterized by sharp, smooth margins and homogeneous, anechoic interior.

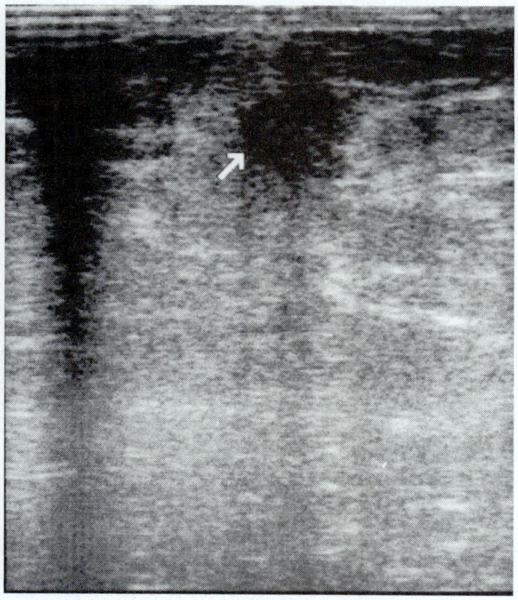

Figure 16 Breast examination. Ultrasound image shows malignant breast lesion (arrow) with indistinct, jagged margins, few internal echoes, and slight posterior shadowing.

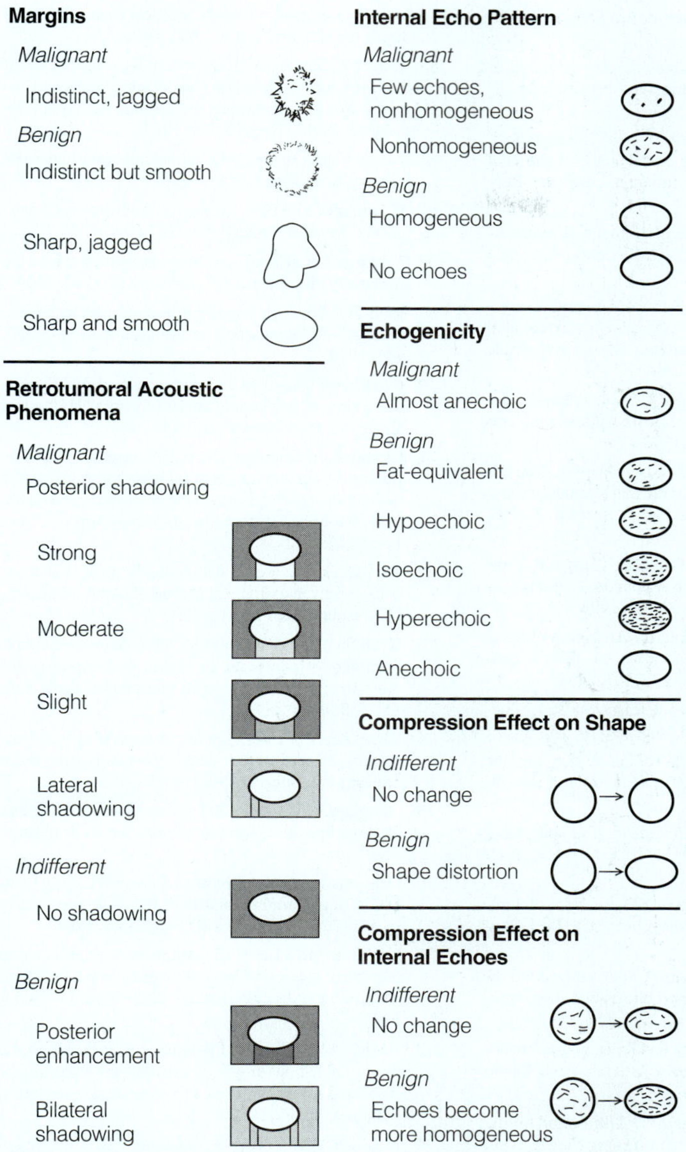

Margins

Malignant
- Indistinct, jagged

Benign
- Indistinct but smooth
- Sharp, jagged
- Sharp and smooth

Retrotumoral Acoustic Phenomena

Malignant
Posterior shadowing
- Strong
- Moderate
- Slight
- Lateral shadowing

Indifferent
- No shadowing

Benign
- Posterior enhancement
- Bilateral shadowing

Internal Echo Pattern

Malignant
- Few echoes, nonhomogeneous
- Nonhomogeneous

Benign
- Homogeneous
- No echoes

Echogenicity

Malignant
- Almost anechoic

Benign
- Fat-equivalent
- Hypoechoic
- Isoechoic
- Hyperechoic
- Anechoic

Compression Effect on Shape

Indifferent
- No change

Benign
- Shape distortion

Compression Effect on Internal Echoes

Indifferent
- No change

Benign
- Echoes become more homogeneous

Figure 17 Breast examination. Shown is a schematic representation of analytic criteria for the interpretation of breast sonograms.[91]

to complement the FAST and reduce the incidence of missed injuries.[84,86-89] There is some evidence that false negative results are more common in patients with pelvic ring fractures, which suggests that CT of the abdomen is routinely indicated in such patients.[90]

The increase in surgeon-performed ultrasound examinations has led to decreased performance of diagnostic peritoneal lavage and CT scanning in the trauma setting. It has become apparent that the FAST can replace central venous pressure monitoring in the diagnosis of hemopericardium and can replace diagnostic peritoneal lavage in the detection of hemoperitoneum in many injured patients. Although CT scanning remains a valuable diagnostic test, the indications for its use in the evaluation of injured patients are now narrower than they once were.

BREAST EXAMINATION

The surgeon must be thoroughly familiar with the ultrasonographic anatomy of normal breast tissue to be able to recognize a mass, discern its ultrasonographic characteristics, and determine whether it is likely to be benign [*see Figure 15*] or malignant [*see Figure 16*].[91,92] Analytic criteria for the interpretation of focal lesions detected on breast ultrasound examinations have been well described and depicted elsewhere [*see Figure 17*].[91]

As noted, breast examination should be done according to a specific scanning protocol. The recommended approach is the radial-scanning technique reported by Teboul.[93] A 7.5 MHz linear-array transducer is used, and the patient is placed in the supine position with the ipsilateral arm behind the head. The transducer is placed at the 6 o'clock position; the breast tissue is scanned, and the transducer is then advanced toward the periphery beyond the breast tissue. Next, the 5 o'clock region is evaluated in the same manner. Each sector (or "hour") of the breast is then scanned in a sequential counterclockwise fashion until the process is completed. Some experts recommend that the nipple be used as a visual pivot point during scanning, remaining in the upper left corner of the monitor throughout the ultrasound examination.[94]

To image the nipple-areola complex, the transducer is placed next to the nipple and angled toward the retroareolar area. Several transverse scans are performed to assess the uniformity of the ligamentous structures and to detect any small tumor that may be present between these structures. Finally, the axilla is scanned with transverse and longitudinal sweeps of the transducer to inspect for lymph nodes.[94]

An important principle in the performance of breast ultrasonography is that the examination must be performed in a consistent and methodical manner so that findings can be accurately described and reproduced. If this principle is followed, a trained examiner can probably identify 80% to 90% of mammographically detected nonpalpable breast masses.[95] One important drawback to remember, however, is that ultrasonography generally will not reveal lesions less than 5 mm in diameter or lesions with an isoechoic appearance.[96]

References

1. Maggio M, Sanders RC: Basic physics. Clinical Sonography: A Practical Guide. Sanders RC, Ed. Little, Brown and Co, Boston, 1991, p 4
2. Hedrick WR, Hykes L, Starchman DE: Ultrasound Physics and Instrumentation. Mosby, St. Louis, 1995, chap 1, p 23
3. Miner NS: Basic principles. Clinical Sonography: A Practical Guide. Sanders RC, Ed. Little, Brown and Co, Boston, 1991, p 33
4. Kremkau F: Diagnostic Ultrasound: Principles, Instrumentation and Exercises. WB Saunders Co, Philadelphia, 1984, chap 2, p 6
5. Hedrick WR, Hykes L, Starchman DE: Ultrasound Physics and Instrumentation. Mosby, St. Louis, 1995, chap 1, p 8
6. Dubinsky T, Horii S, Odwin CS: Ultrasonic physics and instrumentation. Appleton & Lange's Review for the Ultrasonography Examination. Odwin CS, Dubinsky T, Fleischer AC, Eds. Appleton & Lange, Norwalk, Connecticut, 1993, p 8
7. Zagzebski JA: Physics of diagnostic ultrasound. Essentials of Ultrasound Physics. Zagzebski JA, Ed. Mosby, St. Louis, 1996, p 20
8. Hedrick WR, Hykes L, Starchman DE: Ultrasound Physics and Instrumentation. Mosby, St. Louis, 1995, chap 4, p 96
9. Hedrick WR, Hykes L, Starchman DE: Ultrasound Physics and Instrumentation. Mosby, St. Louis, 1995, chap 2, p 55
10. Sanders RC, Miner NS: Introduction. Clinical Sonography: A Practical Guide. Sanders RC, Ed. Little, Brown and Co, Boston, 1991, p 10
11. Kremkau F: Doppler ultrasound: principles and instruments. Ultrasound: Principles, Instrumentation and Exercises. WB Saunders Co, Philadelphia, 1995, chap 7, p 123
12. Sailors DM, Crabtree JD, Land RL, et al: Needle localization for nonpalpable breast lesions. Am Surg 60:186, 1984
13. Wilhelm NC, DeParedes ES, Pope T: The changing mammogram: a primary indication for needle localization biopsy. Arch Surg 121:1311, 1986
14. Miller RS, Adelman RW, Espinosa MH: The early detection of non-palpable breast carcinoma with needle localization: experience with 500 patients in a community hospital. Am Surg 58:193, 1992
15. Schlecht L, Hadijuana J, Hosten N, et al: Ultrasonography of the female breast: comparison 7.5 MHz versus 13 MHz. Akt Radiol 6:69, 1996
16. Saarela AO, Kiviniemi HO, Rissanen TJ, et al: Nonpalpable breast lesions: pathologic correlation of ultra-

16. sonographically guided fine-needle aspiration biopsy. J Ultrasound Med 15:549, 1996
17. Jackson VP: The role of ultrasound in breast imaging. Radiology 177:305, 1990
18. Muttarak M: Abscess in the non-lactating breast: radiodiagnostic aspects. Australas Radiol 40:223, 1996
19. Dempsey PJ: Breast sonography: historical perspective, clinical application, and image interpretation. Ultrasound Q 6:69, 1988
20. Guyer PB, Dewbury KC: Ultrasound of the breast in the symptomatic and x-ray dense breast. Clin Radiol 36:69, 1985
21. Jackson VP, Hendrick RE, Feit SA, et al: Imaging of the radiographically dense breast. Radiology 188:297, 1993
22. Vilmann P, Jacobsen GK, Henriksen FW, et al: Endoscopic ultrasonography with guided fine needle aspiration biopsy in pancreatic disease. Gastrointest Endosc 38:172, 1992
23. Rosch T, Lightdale CJ, Botet JF: Localization of pancreatic endocrine tumors by endoscopic ultrasonography. N Engl J Med 326:1721, 1992
24. Scheiman JM: Endosonography: is it sound for the masses? J Clin Gastroenterol 19:2, 1994
25. Wiersema MJ, Kochman ML, Cramer HM, et al: Real-time endoscopic ultrasound-guided fine-needle aspiration of a mediastinal lymph node. Gastrointest Endosc 39:429, 1993
26. de Lange EE: Staging rectal carcinoma with endorectal imaging: how much detail do we really need? Radiology 190:633, 1994
27. Waizer A, Powsner E, Russo I: Prospective comparative study of magnetic resonance imaging versus transrectal ultrasound for preoperative staging and follow-up of rectal cancer: preliminary report. Dis Colon Rectum 34:1068, 1991
28. Herzog U, von Flue M, Tondelli P, et al: How accurate is endorectal ultrasound in the preoperative staging of rectal cancer? Dis Colon Rectum 36:127, 1993
29. Glaser F, Friedl P, Schlag P, et al: Influence of endorectal ultrasound on surgical treatment of rectal cancer. Eur J Oncol 16:304, 1990
30. Solomon MJ, McLeod RS, Cohen EK: Reliability and validity studies of endoluminal ultrasonography for anorectal disorders. Dis Colon Rectum 37:546, 1994
31. Kusunoki M, Yanagi H, Gondoh N, et al: Use of transrectal ultrasonography to select type of surgery for villous tumors in the lower two thirds of the rectum. Arch Surg 131:714, 1996
32. Beynon J: An evaluation of the role of rectal endosonography in rectal cancer. Ann R Coll Surg Engl 71:131, 1989
33. Milsom JW, Lavery I, Stolfi V, et al: The expanding utility of endoluminal ultrasonography in the management of rectal cancer. Surgery 112:832, 1992
34. Anderson B, Hann L, Enker W, et al: Transrectal ultrasonography and operative selection for early carcinoma of the rectum. J Am Coll Surg 179:513, 1994
35. Saclarides TJ: Endorectal ultrasonography for malignant disease. Ultrasound for the Surgeon. Staren ED, Arregui ME, Eds. Lippincott-Raven, Philadelphia, 1997, p 75
36. Beynon J, Foy DM, Temple LN, et al: The endosonic appearances of normal colon and rectum. Dis Colon Rectum 29:810, 1986
37. Hildebrandt U, Feifel G: Preoperative staging of rectal cancer by intrarectal ultrasound. Dis Colon Rectum 28:42, 1985
38. Romano G, Escercizio L, Santangelo M, et al: Impact of computed tomography vs. intrarectal ultrasound on the diagnosis, resectability, and prognosis of locally recurrent rectal cancer. Dis Colon Rectum 36:261, 1993
39. Hulsmans F, Tio TL, Fockens P, et al: Assessment of tumor infiltration depth in rectal cancer with transrectal sonography: caution is necessary. Radiology 190:715, 1994
40. Sentovitch SM, Blatchford GJ, Falk PM, et al: Transrectal ultrasound of rectal tumors. Am J Surg 166:638, 1993
41. Burnett S, Bartram C: Endosonographic variations in the normal internal anal sphincter. Int J Colorect Dis 6:2, 1991
42. Gantke B, Schafer A, Enck P, et al: Sonographic, manometric and myographic evaluation of the anal sphincter's morphology and function. Dis Colon Rectum 36:1037, 1993
43. Law PJ, Kamm MA, Bartram CI: Anal endosonography in the investigation of faecal incontinence. Br J Surg 78:312, 1991
44. Burnett S, Speakman CT, Kamm MA, et al: Confirmation of endosonographic detection of external anal sphincter defects by simultaneous electromyographic mapping. Br J Surg 78:448, 1991
45. Deen KI, Kumar D, Williams JG: Anal sphincter defects: correlation between endoanal ultrasound and surgery. Ann Surg 218:201, 1993
46. Felt-Bersma RJ, Cuesta MA, Koorevaar M: Anal endosonography: relationship with anal manometry and neurophysiologic tests. Dis Colon Rectum 37:468, 1992
47. Falk PM, Blatchford GJ, Cali RL: Transanal ultrasound and manometry in the evaluation of fecal incontinence. Dis Colon Rectum 37:468, 1994
48. Sultan AH, Kamm MA, Talbot IC: Anal endosonography for identifying external sphincter defects confirmed histologically. Br J Surg 81:463, 1994
49. Goldberg BB, Goodman GA, Clearfield HR: Evaluation of ascites by ultrasound. Radiology 96:15, 1970
50. Asher WM, Parvin S, Virgillo RW, et al: Echographic evaluation of splenic injury after blunt trauma. Radiology 118:411, 1976
51. Chambers JA, Pilbrow WJ: Ultrasound in abdominal trauma: an alternative to peritoneal lavage. Arch Emerg Med 5:26, 1988
52. Parys BT, Barr H, Chantarasak ND, et al: Use of ultrasound scan as a bedside diagnostic aid. Br J Surg 74:611, 1987
53. Peiper HJ, Schmid A, Steffens H, et al: Ultrasound diagnosis in acute abdomen and blunt abdominal trauma. Chirurg 58:189, 1987
54. Blyme PJH, Lind T, Schantz K: Ultrasonographic detection of foreign bodies in soft tissue. Arch Ortho Trauma Surg 110:24, 1990
55. Schlager D, Sanders A, Wiggins D: Ultrasound for the detection of foreign bodies. Ann Emerg Med 20:189, 1991
56. Manthey DE, Storrow AB, Milbourn JM, et al: Ultrasound versus radiography in the detection of soft-tissue foreign bodies. Ann Emerg Med 28:7, 1996
57. Williams RJ, Windsor AC, Rosin RD, et al: Ultrasound scanning of the acute abdomen by surgeons in training. Ann R Coll Surg Engl 76:228, 1994
58. Imhof M, Raunest J, Rauen U, et al: Acute acalculous cholecystitis in severely traumatized patients: a prospective sonographic study. Surg Endosc 6:68, 1992
59. Yokoyama T, Munakata Y, Ogiwara M, et al: Preoperative diagnosis of strangulated obturator hernia using ultrasonography. Am J Surg 174:76, 1997
60. Barteau JA, Castro D, Arregui ME, et al: A comparison of intraoperative ultrasound versus cholangiography in the evaluation of the common bile duct during laparoscopic cholecystectomy. Surg Endosc 9:490, 1995
61. Ravikumar TS, Kane R, Cady B: Hepatic cryosurgery with intraoperative ultrasound monitoring for metastatic colon carcinoma. Arch Surg 102:403, 1987
62. Rafaelsen SR, Kronborg O, Larsen C, et al: Intraoperative ultrasonography in detection of hepatic metastases from colorectal cancer. Dis Colon Rectum 38:355, 1995
63. Machi J, Isomoto H, Kurohiji T, et al: Detection of unrecognized liver metastases from colorectal cancers by routine use of operative ultrasonography. Dis Colon Rectum 29:405, 1986
64. Castaing D, Emond J, Kunstlinger F, et al: Utility of operative ultrasound in the surgical management of liver tumors. Ann Surg 204:600, 1986
65. Kern KA, Shawker TH, Doppman JL, et al: The use of high-resolution ultrasound to locate parathyroid tumors during reoperations for primary hyperparathyroidism. World J Surg 11:579, 1987
66. Machi J, Sigel B: Operative ultrasonography in general surgery. Am J Surg 172:15, 1996
67. Couinaud C: Le Foie, Etudes Anatomiques et Chirurgicales. Masson et Cie, Paris, 1957
68. Schirmer B: Laparoscopic ultrasonography: enhancing minimally invasive surgery. Ann Surg 220:709, 1994
69. John TG: Superior staging of liver tumors with laparoscopy and laparoscopic ultrasound. Ann Surg 220:711, 1994
70. Cook TA, Galland RB: A prospective study to define the optimum rescreening interval for small abdominal aneurysm. Cardiovasc Surg 4:441, 1996
71. Bastounis E, Georgopoulos S, Maltezos C, et al: The validity of current vascular imaging methods in the evaluation of aortic anastomotic aneurysms developing after abdominal aortic aneurysm repair. Ann Vasc Surg 10:537, 1996
72. Turetschek K, Nasel C, Wunderbaldinger P, et al: Power Doppler versus imaging in renal allograft evaluation. J Ultrasound Med 15:517, 1996
73. Wren SM, Ralls PW, Stain SC, et al: Assessment of resectability of pancreatic head and periampullary tumors by color flow Doppler sonography. Arch Surg 131:812, 1996
74. Klyachkin ML, Rohmiller M, Charash WE, et al: Penetrating injuries of the neck: selective management evolving. Am Surg 63:189, 1997
75. Ginzburg E, Montalvo B, LeBlang S, et al: The use of duplex ultrasonography in penetrating neck trauma. Arch Surg 131:691, 1996
76. Demetriades D, Theodorou D, Cornwell E, et al: Evaluation of penetrating injuries of the neck: prospective study of 223 patients. World J Surg 21:41, 1997
77. Knudson MM, Lewis FR, Atkinson K, et al: The role of duplex ultrasound arterial imaging in patients with penetrating extremity trauma. Arch Surg 128:1033, 1993
78. Bergstein JM, Blair JF, Edwards J, et al: Pitfalls in the use of color-flow duplex ultrasound for screening of suspected arterial injuries in penetrating extremities. J Trauma 33:395, 1992
79. Knudson MM, Collins JA, Goodman SB, et al: Thromboembolism following multiple trauma. J Trauma 32:2, 1992
80. Bandyk DF, Mills JL, Gahtan V, et al: Intraoperative duplex scanning of arterial reconstructions: fate of repaired and unrepaired defects. J Vasc Surg 20:426, 1994
81. Gualtieri E, Deppe SA, Sipperly ME, et al: Subclavian venous catheterization: greater success rate for less experienced operators using ultrasound guidance. Crit Care Med 23:692, 1995
82. Sisley AC, Rozycki GS, Ballard RB, et al: Rapid detection of traumatic effusion using surgeon-performed ultrasound. J Trauma 44:291, 1998
83. Kohan JM, Poe RH, Israel RH: Value of chest ultrasonography versus decubitus roentgenography for thoracentesis. Am Rev Respir Dis 133:1124, 1986
84. Rozycki GS, Ochsner MG, Jaffin JH, et al: Prospective evaluation of surgeons' use of ultrasound in the evaluation of trauma patients. J Trauma 34:516, 1993
85. Tso P, Rodriguez A, Cooper C, et al: Sonography in blunt abdominal trauma: a preliminary progress report. J Trauma 33:39, 1992
86. Rozycki GS, Ballard RB, Feliciano DV, et al: Surgeon-performed ultrasound for the assessment of truncal injuries: lessons learned from 1,540 patients. Ann Surg 228:557, 1998
87. Rozycki GS, Ochsner MG, Schmidt JA, et al: A prospective study of surgeon-performed ultrasound as the primary adjuvant modality for injured patient assessment. J Trauma 39:492, 1995

88. Boulanger BR, Brenneman FD, McLellan BA, et al: A prospective study of emergent abdominal sonography after blunt trauma. J Trauma 39:325, 1995
89. Chiu WC, Cushing BM, Rodriguez A, et al: Abdominal injuries without hemoperitoneum: a potential limitation of focused abdominal sonography for trauma (FAST). J Trauma 42:617, 1997
90. Ballard RB, Rozycki GS, Newman PG, et al: An algorithm to reduce the incidence of false-negative FAST examination in patients at high risk for occult injury. J Am Coll Surg 189:145, 1999
91. Leucht W: Analytic criteria for the interpretation of focal sonographic lesions. Teaching Atlas of Breast Ultrasound. Leucht D, Madjar H, Eds. Thieme, New York, 1996, p 23
92. Staren ED: Physics and principles of breast ultrasound. Am Surg 62:103, 1996
93. Teboul M: A new concept in breast investigation: echo-histological acino-ductal 13-analysis or analytic echography. Biomed Pharmacother 42:289, 1988
94. Khattar S, Staren ED: Diagnostic breast ultrasound. Ultrasound for the Surgeon. Staren ED, Arregui ME, Eds. Philadelphia, Lippincott-Raven, 1997, p 85
95. Staren ED: Surgical office-based ultrasound of the breast. Am Surg 61:619, 1995
96. Staren ED, Fine R: Breast ultrasound for surgeons. Am Surg 62:108, 1996
97. Hendee WR: Cross sectional medical imaging: a history. RadioGraphics 9:1155, 1989
98. White DN: Neurosonology pioneers. Ultrasound Med Biol 14:541, 1988
99. Hackmann W: Seek and Strike. Crown, United Kingdom, 1984, p xxiv
100. Hackmann W: Seek and Strike. Crown, United Kingdom, 1984, p 1
101. Hackmann W: Seek and Strike. Crown, United Kingdom, 1984, p 11
102. Hackmann W: Seek and Strike. Crown, United Kingdom, 1984, p 73
103. Meire HB: Basic Ultrasound. John Wiley & Sons, New York, 1995, p 1
104. Wells PNT: Developments in medical ultrasonics. World Med Electron 4:272, 1966
105. Wild JJ: The use of ultrasonic pulses for the measurement of biologic tissues and the detection of tissue density changes. Surgery 27:183, 1950
106. Wild JJ, Reid JM: Diagnostic use of ultrasound. British Journal of Physical Medicine 248, 1956
107. Goldberg BB, Gramiak R, Freimanis AK: Early history of diagnostic ultrasound: the role of American radiologists. AJR Am J Roentgenol 160:189, 1993
108. Maulik D: Doppler Ultrasound in Obstetrics and Gynecology. Springer, New York, 1997
109. Sanders RC, Topper IW: Equipment care and quality control. Clinical Sonography: A Practical Guide. Sanders RC, Ed. Little, Brown and Co, Boston, 1991, p 475
110. Wong WK: Endorectal ultrasonography for benign disease. Ultrasound for the Surgeon. Staren ED, Arregui ME, Eds. Lippincott-Raven, Philadelphia, 1997, p 66
111. Rozycki GS, Shackford SR: Ultrasound: what every trauma surgeon should know. J Trauma 40:1, 1996

Acknowledgments

Figures 1 and 7   Dimitry Schidlovsky.
Figures 2, 13, 14, and 17   Marcia Kammerer.
Figure 8   Tom Moore.

46 THORACOSCOPY

Valerie W. Rusch, M.D.

The technique of thoracoscopy was first described in 1910 by Jacobeus, a Swedish physician who used a cystoscope to examine the pleural space.[1] Although thoracoscopy was initially performed for diagnostic purposes, it later evolved into a therapeutic procedure. During the 1930s and 1940s, it was used to lyse intrapleural adhesions after collapse therapy for tuberculosis. During the 1950s, when effective antituberculous chemotherapy became available, thoracoscopy fell into disuse in the United States[2]; however, it remained popular in Europe, where it was employed in diagnosing and treating problems such as pleural effusion, empyema, traumatic hemothorax, persistent air leakage after pulmonary resection, and spontaneous pneumothorax.[3-5] During the 1970s and 1980s, a few North American surgeons revived the practice of thoracoscopy, both to manage pleural disease and to perform small peripheral lung biopsies in patients with diffuse pneumonitis.

In the first stages of its revival, thoracoscopy was often performed with open endoscopes that were originally designed for other procedures (e.g., mediastinoscopes).[6,7] As optics and lighting systems improved, smaller-caliber endoscopes were created specifically for thoracoscopic applications[8]; however, these instruments were limited in that only one person could visualize the operative field at a given time. In 1991, the application of video technology to thoracoscopy revolutionized the procedure because it allowed several persons to see the operative field simultaneously and to operate together as they would during an open procedure. In addition, the development of endoscopic instruments, particularly endoscopic staplers, enabled surgeons to perform major operations using minimally invasive techniques. The impact of this new technology was so profound that within a 2-year period, traditional thoracoscopic techniques were abandoned in favor of video-assisted thoracic surgery (VATS).[9,10] In what follows, therefore, I focus on current VATS procedures rather than on traditional thoracoscopic techniques. There are numerous accepted diagnostic and therapeutic indications for VATS [see Table 1]. Accordingly, there are numerous operations that can be done by VATS; I describe the most important of these, with the exception of esophageal myotomy and Nissen fundoplication, which are covered elsewhere [see 48 Esophageal Procedures: Minimally Invasive Approaches].

Preoperative Planning

PATIENT PREPARATION AND INTRAOPERATIVE CARE

Patient preparation and positioning are much the same for most VATS procedures. As a rule, the lateral decubitus position offers the best exposure, and it permits easy conversion to a thoracotomy if necessary. There are occasional exceptions to this rule, however, and in such cases, the choice of position is dictated by the procedure planned. For instance, if a cervical mediastinoscopy or a Chamberlain procedure is being performed for lung cancer staging and the pleura must be examined to rule out the presence of metastases, the patient can be left in the supine position and the videothoracoscope introduced through the parasternal incision or a separate inferior incision.[11]

Port placement, the use of so-called access incisions (utility thoracotomies), and instrumentation vary from one procedure to the next. In approximately 20% of patients undergoing VATS, intraoperative conversion to a standard thoracotomy will be necessary for any of several reasons, including extensive pleural adhesions and pulmonary lesions that either cannot be located thoracoscopically or require a

Table 1 Indications and Contraindications for VATS Procedures

Diagnostic indications
  Undiagnosed pleural effusion
  Indeterminate pulmonary nodule
  Undiagnosed interstitial lung disease
  Pulmonary infection in the immunosuppressed patient
  To define cell type in known thoracic malignancy
  To define extent of a primary thoracic tumor
  Nodal staging of a primary thoracic tumor
  Diagnosis of intrathoracic pathology to stage a primary extrathoracic tumor
  Evaluation of intrapleural infection

Therapeutic indications
  Lung
    Spontaneous pneumothorax
    Bullous disease
    Lung volume reduction
    Persistent parenchymal air leak
    Benign pulmonary nodule
    Resection of pulmonary metastases (in highly selected cases)
    Resection of a primary lung tumor (in highly selected cases)
  Mediastinum
    Drainage of pericardial effusion
    Excision of bronchogenic or pericardial cyst
    Resection of selected primary mediastinal tumors
    Esophageal myotomy
    Facilitation of transhiatal esophagectomy
    ? Resection of primary esophageal tumors
    ? Thymic resection
    Ligation of thoracic duct
  Pleura
    Drainage of a multiloculated effusion
    Drainage of an early empyema
    Pleurodesis

Contraindications
  Extensive intrapleural adhesions
  Inability to sustain single-lung ventilation
  Extensive involvement of hilar structures
  Preoperatve induction chemotherapy or chemoradiotherapy
  Severe coagulopathy

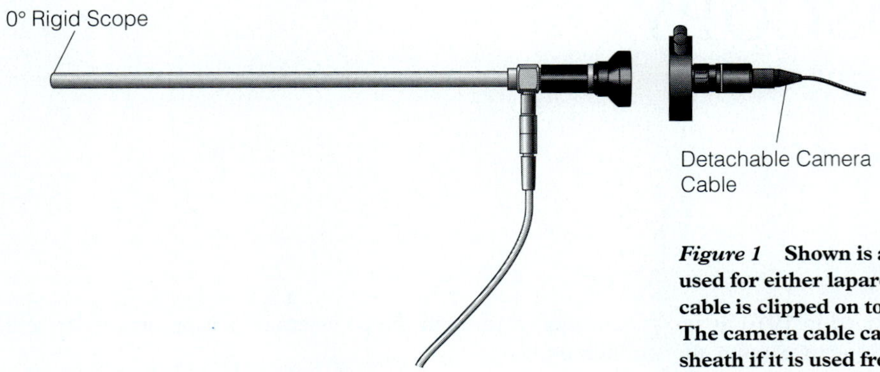

Figure 1 Shown is a forward-viewing (0°) rigid scope that can be used for either laparoscopy or thoracoscopy. A detachable camera cable is clipped on to the eyepiece of the scope for video endoscopy. The camera cable can be sterilized or enclosed within a plastic sheath if it is used frequently.

more extensive resection than can be accomplished endosurgically. With experience, one can learn to predict the likelihood of such conversion in a given case. It is important to discuss this possibility with the patient before operation and to obtain informed consent to conversion. Any patient who is likely to require conversion to a thoracotomy or who may be undergoing lobectomy or pneumonectomy should receive the cardiopulmonary evaluation that is usual for such procedures before VATS is performed.

VATS procedures are performed with the patient under general anesthesia. Very limited operations (e.g., pleural biopsies) can be done with a single-lumen endotracheal tube in place, but most procedures should be performed with single-lung ventilation using a double-lumen endotracheal tube or a bronchial blocker. The degree of intraoperative monitoring needed depends on the extent of the planned procedure and on the patient's general medical condition. Standard monitoring techniques, including pulse oximetry, are always used, but arterial lines are placed selectively. A central venous catheter or a Swan-Ganz catheter is inserted only when the patient's baseline cardiac status demands precise hemodynamic monitoring. A Foley catheter is inserted at the beginning of all VATS procedures to monitor urine output because it is not always possible to predict how long the operation will take or whether conversion to thoracotomy will prove necessary.

INSTRUMENTATION

Instrumentation for VATS comprises (1) video equipment, (2) staplers, (3) thoracic instruments (e.g., lung clamps and retractors) modified for endoscopic use, and (4) various methods of electrocautery, including lasers. Because immediate conversion to thoracotomy is occasionally necessary, a basic set of thoracotomy instruments should be an integral part of a VATS instrument tray.[12]

Video Equipment

Several companies manufacture excellent video systems for thoracoscopy. Minor variations in lighting and optics aside, the basic components of all these systems are similar: a large-screen (21 in.) video monitor, a xenon light source, a video recorder, and a printer for still photography, all mounted together on a cart. A second video monitor, also mounted on a cart, is connected by cable to the main monitor and is placed across from it at the head of the operating table. By using two monitors placed in this manner, both the surgeon and the first assistant can look directly at a video display without having to turn away from the surgical field. Alternatively, a single monitor can be placed at the head of the operating table. The only additional item of equipment necessary for laparoscopy is an insufflator. To maximize cost-efficiency, therefore, hospitals acquiring video monitors and endoscopes should coordinate the choice of this expensive equipment among the specialties using it, including thoracic surgery, general surgery, gynecology, and urology. Hospitals performing many endoscopic procedures may find it advisable to dedicate one or more rooms to video endoscopic surgery and to mount video equipment on the ceilings or walls.

Endoscopes

Most procedures are performed with a forward-viewing (0°) rigid scope; 30°-angled scopes are useful for visualizing the sulci and the superior and posterior mediastinum. The scope is attached to the light source by a light cable and is coupled to the video monitor system by a camera cable [see Figure 1]. Although camera cables can be sterilized, it is best to cover the camera head and cable with a clear plastic bag so that the camera cable can remain in the operating room at all times. Newer videoscopes are now available in which the camera chip is located at the tip of the scope rather than in the connecting camera cable; these will eventually replace the older endoscopes because they provide a sharper image.

Flexible thoracoscopes are also available; these look like a short, heavy version of a flexible bronchoscope but have a more rigid distal end. Some surgeons feel that flexible thoracoscopes enhance their ability to visualize the entire pleural space, but these devices are very expensive and thus continue to be premium purchases for most hospitals.

Trocars for Accessing the Pleural Space

Originally, thoracoscopy made use of trocar cannulas designed for laparoscopy to access the pleural space. These devices are too long and have sharp ends that can injure the lung. Because patients undergoing thoracoscopy are under general anesthesia and have a double-lumen endotracheal tube in place, the cannulas need not maintain an airtight seal, as they do in laparoscopy. Accordingly, modified trocar cannulas called thoracoports, which are shorter than laparoscopy cannulas and have a corkscrew configuration on the outside that stabilizes them within the chest wall, are now routinely used. The trocar is simply a blunt-tipped obturator that facilitates passage of the cannula through the chest wall [see Figure 2a]. Thoracoports are available in several sizes (5, 10.5, 12.0, and 15 mm diameter) to accommodate various instruments.

Staplers

Staplers that cut between two simultaneously applied triple rows of staples (gastrointestinal anastomosis [GIA] staplers) have been developed for endoscopic surgery. They are available in lengths of 30 and 60 mm and in staple depths of 2.5, 3.5, and 4.8 mm [see Figure 2b]. Like their counterparts designed for open procedures, they are disposable multicartridge instruments. The endoscopic GIA stapler with 2.5 mm staples is designed for division of pulmonary vessels. Some surgeons are reluctant to use it on hilar vessels because if the stapler fails mechanically (e.g., cuts without applying both staple lines prop-

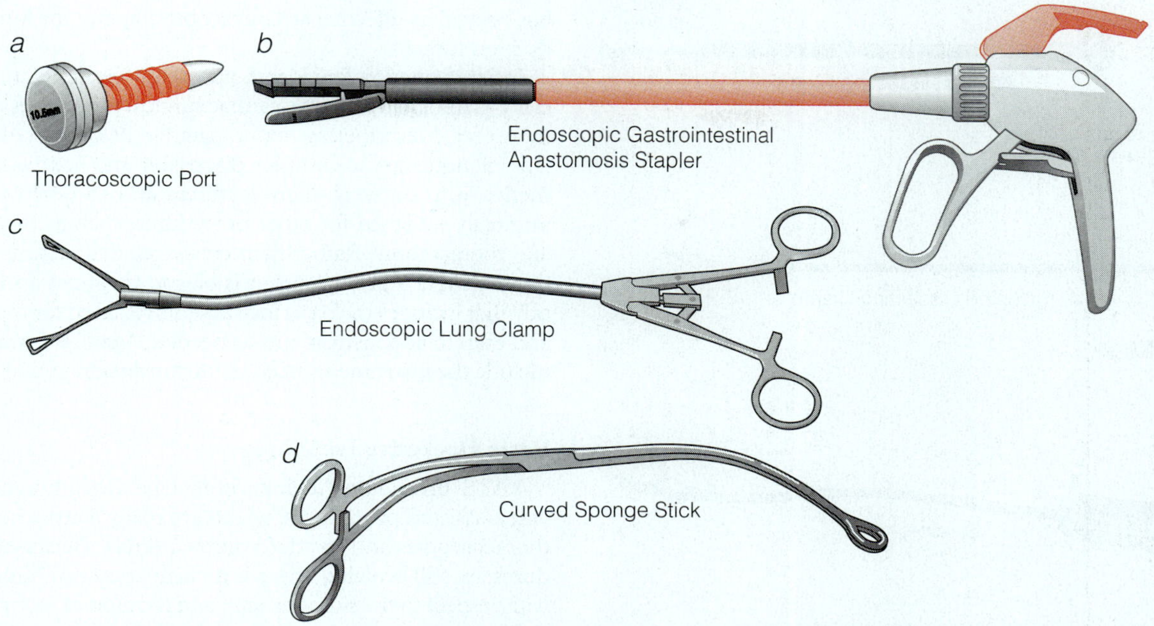

Figure 2 Shown are instruments commonly used during VATS. Modified trocar cannulas, called thoracoports (*a*), facilitate access to the pleural space. They are shorter than the cannulas used in laparoscopy and have a corkscrew configuration on the outside that maintains their position on the chest wall. The trocar is a blunt-tipped plastic obturator that facilitates passage of the cannula through the chest wall. A thin plastic diaphragm stabilizes the position of the instruments or can be removed to facilitate access to the pleural space. Endoscopic GIA staplers that make incisions between two triple rows of staples (*b*) can be inserted through these ports. Like staplers designed for open procedures, endoscopic GIA staplers are disposable multifire instruments that hold three replacements of the staple cartridge. Another instrument that can be inserted through these ports is the nondisposable endoscopic lung clamp (*c*), which is available in various shapes with serrations at the end or along the full length of the clamp. Finally, the port allows insertion of curved sponge sticks (*d*), which have been modified for endoscopic use as lung clamps or lymph node holders.

erly), life-threatening hemorrhage can ensue. Endoscopic staplers that do not cut (TA staplers) are also available. Endoscopic GIA staplers have revolutionized surgeons' ability to perform minimally invasive pulmonary resections. These devices are highly reliable, and because they apply triple rows of staples instead of double rows, they provide excellent hemostasis and closure of air leaks.

Standard stapling instruments are also used during some VATS procedures. They are unnecessary for most pulmonary wedge resections but may be helpful for more complex procedures, such as lobectomies. Standard GIA and roticulator TA staplers are the most practical devices for VATS because they can be inserted and positioned through an access incision.

Instruments

Various types of Pennington and Duval clamps are available [*see Figure 2c*]. Sponge sticks modified by the introduction of various curves and a line of DeBakey-type teeth on the end can also be used as lung clamps or lymph node holders [*see Figure 2d*].

Several retractors have been developed for endoscopic surgery. One such device is a modified Finochietto retractor with long, narrow blades, which is particularly helpful for retracting the chest wall soft tissues in an access incision. Others include vein retractors, the tips of which can be withdrawn into the straight instrument shaft, and the fan retractor, which can be opened and closed like a fan by turning a knob on the end of the retractor. Of these, the fan retractor is the most useful general retractor for thoracoscopic procedures [*see Figure 3*]. Vein retractors are best suited to gentle retraction of hilar or mediastinal structures (e.g., vessels, bronchi, the esophagus, or lymph nodes).

Although biopsy forceps have been specifically created for laparoscopy and thoracoscopy, those used for mediastinoscopy are, in fact, well suited to thoracoscopy. Because laparoscopy instruments were developed before thoracoscopic instruments, many types of grasping forceps are available; however, most are too traumatizing for thoracic surgery. DeBakey forceps, modified for endoscopic use, are the gentlest type available. Various curved and

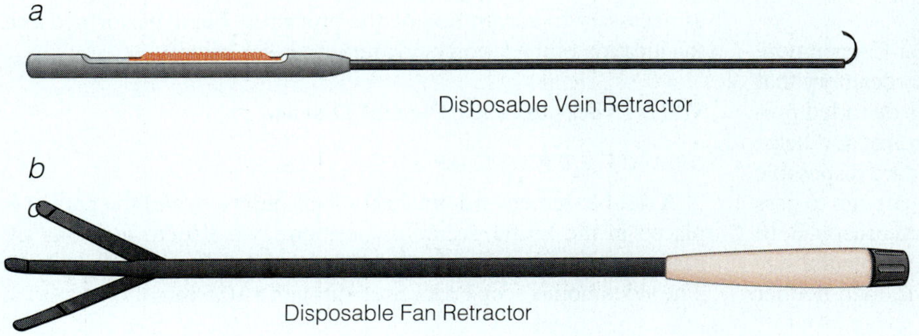

Figure 3 Shown are retractors used for VATS. Vein retractors are best suited for the gentle retraction of hilar or mediastinal structures, such as the vessels, bronchi, esophagus, and lymph nodes. The tip of the disposable vein retractor (*a*) can be extended from or withdrawn into the shaft to allow insertion of the retractor through a 12 mm port. The most useful retractor for general purposes is the fan retractor (*b*). A knob on the end of the handle opens and closes the fan, so that the retractor can be inserted through a port and opened for retraction in the pleural space.

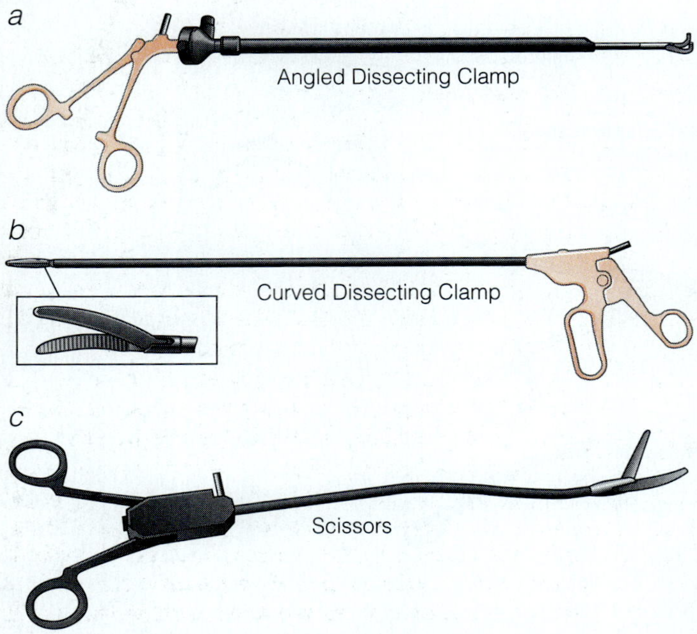

Figure 4 Various right-angle (*a*) and curved (*b*) dissecting clamps are available. On the angled model shown (*a*), the knob close to the handle rotates the shaft of the clamp 360°. Finally, many types of endoscopic scissors (*c*) are available. Some scissors incorporate an attachment for electrocautery so that the surgeon can cut and cauterize simultaneously.

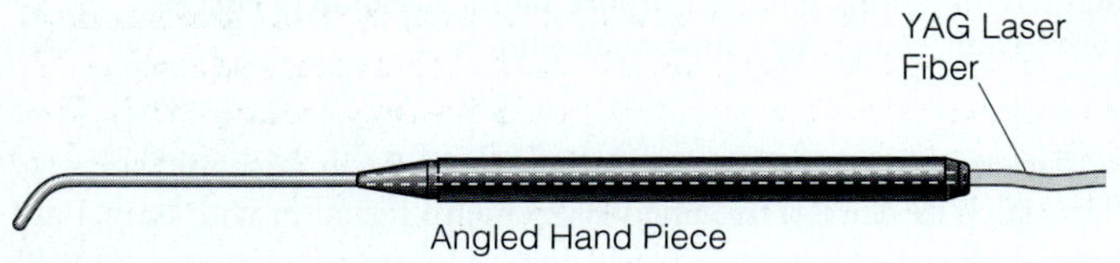

Figure 5 Shown is an angled handpiece through which an yttrium-aluminum-garnet (YAG) laser can be placed during VATS. The handpiece is narrow enough to be used during thoracoscopy as well as during open procedures.

right-angle dissecting clamps, needle holders, and scissors are available. Most scissors have an electrocautery attachment that permits simultaneous cutting and cauterizing [*see Figure 4*]. In addition, standard thoracotomy instruments can be inserted through a minithoracotomy incision and used just as they would be in an open procedure.

The neodymium:yttrium-aluminum-garnet (Nd:YAG) laser is sometimes applied to VATS resection of pulmonary lesions. This is done by inserting the YAG laser fiber through angled or straight handpieces [*see Figure 5*]. Laser-assisted pulmonary resection is helpful in removing lesions on the flat surface of the lung, where a stapler cannot be easily applied.[13]

The argon beam electrocoagulator (ABC) (Birtcher Corporation, Englewood, Colorado) is a noncontact form of electrocautery that provides superb hemostasis on raw surfaces, such as denuded pulmonary parenchyma or the chest wall after pleurectomy, and helps seal air leaks from the surface of the lung.[14] The standard disposable ABC handpiece used for open procedures is narrow enough to pass through a thoracoport and thus may be used for thoracoscopy. Both the YAG laser and the ABC can be used to cauterize the pleural surface for pleurodesis and to ablate bullous disease, though neither

has proved as effective as endoscopic stapling for lung volume reduction surgery.

Instrumentation for videothoracoscopy continues to evolve, especially as minimally invasive cardiac surgical procedures become commonplace. Nevertheless, to put together the best set of instruments, it is still necessary to combine disposable and nondisposable instruments from different manufacturers and to borrow instruments originally designed for other procedures, such as mediastinoscopy and thoracotomy. Rather than create separate instrument trays for different VATS procedures, it is best to maintain a single standard tray that includes the basic instruments required for most operations and then to add instruments as needed. Again, this tray should also include the instruments needed for conversion to thoracotomy.

Basic Operative Technique

VATS procedures include both true videothoracoscopies and video-assisted procedures, which are really a cross between videothoracoscopies and standard thoracotomies. Because VATS procedures are still evolving, there is no firm consensus among surgeons with respect to the number, size, and location of incisions.

The basic videothoracoscopy techniques have been well described.[15] The primary strategy is to place the instruments and the thoracoscope so that all are oriented in the same direction, facing the target disease within a 180° arc [*see Figure 6*]; this positioning prevents mirror imaging. The incisions should also be placed widely distant from each other so that the instruments do not crowd each other. For most procedures [*see Figure 6a*], the videothoracoscope is inserted through a thoracoport placed in the midaxillary line at the seventh or eighth intercostal space. Instruments are introduced through two thoracoports, one placed at approximately the fifth intercostal space in the anterior axillary line and the other placed at the fifth space, parallel to and about 2 to 3 cm away from the posterior border of the scapula. If the procedure is converted to a thoracotomy, the two upper incisions can be incorporated into the thoracotomy incision, and the lower incision can be used as a chest tube site. When a patient is being operated upon for an apical lesion (e.g., bullae causing a spontaneous pneumothorax) [*see Figure 6b*], the camera port can be placed in the fifth or sixth intercostal space, and the instrument ports are also moved higher: one in the axilla and the other higher on the posterior chest wall at approximately the third intercostal space. Depending on the location of the lesion being removed, a fourth port incision may be helpful to permit the introduction of additional instruments.

When the lung has to be palpated so that a small or deep-seated lesion can be located or when complex video-assisted procedures are being performed, a small (about 5 cm) intercostal incision is added to the three port incisions. This utility thoracotomy (access incision) is usually placed in the midaxillary line or in the auscultatory triangle. An infant Finochietto retractor or a Weitlaner retractor is used to retract the soft tissues without actually spreading the ribs [*see Figure 7*].

These basic concepts regarding incision placement are modified as necessary to accommodate the procedure being performed and the location of the lesion being removed (see below).

VATS Procedures for Pleural Disease

OPERATIVE TECHNIQUE

A double-lumen endotracheal tube is inserted, and the patient is placed in the lateral decubitus position. Two 1.5 cm incisions are made, one for the videothoracoscope and one for the instruments. The videothoracoscope is inserted through a 10.5 mm thoracoport at

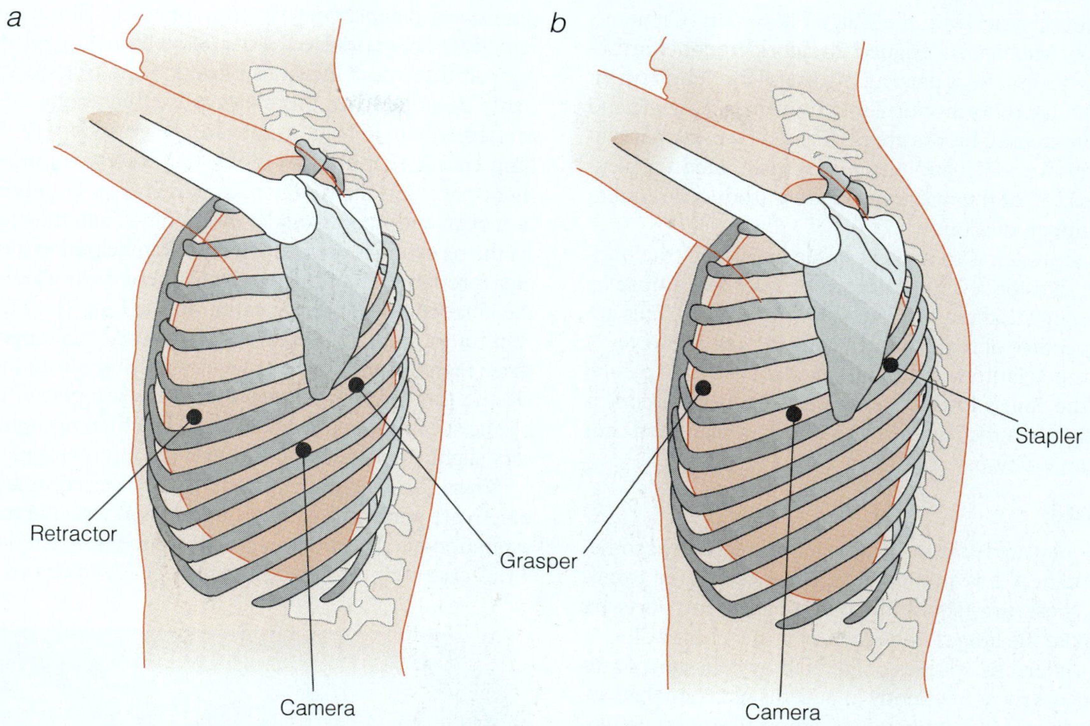

Figure 6 Basic operative technique. Shown is the typical positioning of instruments and the video camera for patients undergoing VATS for a lesion in the superior segment of the left lower lobe of the lung. Instruments are introduced through two port incisions made anteriorly at approximately the fifth intercostal space in the anterior axillary line and posteriorly parallel to and 2 to 3 cm away from the border of the scapula (*a*). For patients undergoing thoracoscopy for apical bullous disease in the left upper lobe of the lung, the camera port can be placed at the fifth or sixth intercostal space, and one instrument port can be inserted in the axilla and the other port inserted higher on the posterior chest wall at approximately the third intercostal space (*b*).

the seventh or eighth intercostal space in the midaxillary line; the instruments are inserted through a port placed a couple of interspaces higher in the anterior axillary line. If talc poudrage is performed, both incisions are reused for placement of chest tubes, with a right-angle tube inserted on the diaphragm through the lower incision and a straight tube inserted up to the apex of the pleural space through the upper incision. The addition of a diaphragmatic chest tube helps prevent loculated basilar fluid collections after a talc pleurodesis. If a thoracotomy is subsequently performed, the upper port site is incorporated into the anterior aspect of the incision, and the lower site can be reused as a chest tube site. Proper placement of port incisions is especially important in patients suspected of having malignant mesothelioma because of the propensity of this tumor to implant in incisions and needle tracks.[8,16,17]

Once the videothoracoscope has been inserted, pleural biopsies are obtained under direct vision by introducing biopsy forceps through a port placed in the upper incision. The mediastinoscopy biopsy forceps is well suited to this task. Pleural fluid is evacuated with a Yankauer or a pool-tip suction device. Fibrinous debris can be removed

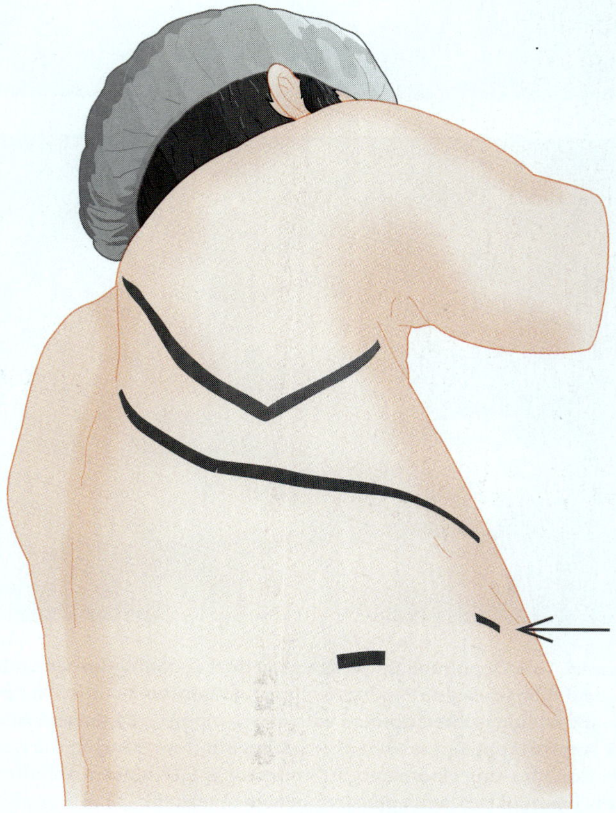

Figure 7 Basic operative technique. Shown are the incisions used for common VATS procedures. The thoracoscope is inserted through the bottom incision. Anterior and posterior incisions are used for the introduction of instruments. Only one additional low anterior incision (arrow) is needed for thoracoscopic pleural procedures. A so-called utility thoracotomy (dotted line) can be added at the fifth intercostal space, if necessary. The tip of the scapula is outlined. These incisions can be incorporated into a standard thoracotomy incision if the VATS procedure is converted to an open procedure.

by irrigating the pleural space with the Water-Pik system (Orthotec, Stryker, Kalamazoo, Michigan) designed for debridement of orthopedic wounds. This technique is particularly useful for debridement and drainage of loculated fibrinopurulent empyemas.[18] At the end of the procedure, intercostal blocks are performed by using a mediastinoscopy aspiration needle, and talc can be insufflated for pleurodesis, if indicated. All of the instruments are introduced sequentially through the upper incision.[19]

An alternative approach is to make a single incision in the midaxillary line at the sixth or seventh intercostal space and to use an operating thoracoscope that incorporates a biopsy forceps. This approach has the advantage of requiring only one incision; however, it does not allow as much latitude in draining or debriding the pleural space. Moreover, the biopsy forceps in an operating thoracoscope is of a smaller caliber than a mediastinoscopy biopsy forceps and thus cannot obtain as large a biopsy specimen.

TROUBLESHOOTING

In patients with loculated effusions, thoracoport placement sometimes must be modified. The preoperative chest computed tomographic scan and chest x-ray should help ensure that the ports are placed in areas where the lung is not adherent to the chest wall.

In some cases, the pleural space is obliterated by adhesions or tumor. This event occurs most frequently in patients who have had severe inflammatory disease (e.g., pneumonia, empyema, or tuberculosis) or extensive pleural malignancy (e.g., locally advanced malignant mesothelioma). Under these circumstances, the anterior thoracoport incision can be extended to a length of 5 to 6 cm, the underlying rib section can be resected, and the parietal pleura can be biopsied directly; a full thoracotomy is not required. If thoracotomy is subsequently warranted for therapeutic reasons (e.g., for pleurectomy, decortication, or extrapleural pneumonectomy for mesothelioma), this small incision can be incorporated into the thoracotomy incision.

VATS Pulmonary Wedge Resection

VATS pulmonary wedge resection has become a standard approach to diagnosing small indeterminate pulmonary nodules, especially those not technically amenable to transthoracic needle biopsy.[20] It is also an accepted method of diagnosing pulmonary infiltrates of uncertain origin, particularly in immunocompromised patients in whom transbronchial biopsy is either unsafe or inappropriate.[21] The role of VATS wedge resection is less well defined in the management of primary lung cancers. It is an appropriate compromise operation for primary lung cancers in patients whose cardiac or pulmonary functional status rules out lobectomy. However, it remains a highly controversial approach to the treatment of pulmonary metastases[22] because improved survival in patients with pulmonary metastases is directly linked to the ability to remove all gross tumor, and VATS does not allow the careful bimanual palpation that is critical to detecting pulmonary metastases too small or too deep to be visible endoscopically.[23-25] Accordingly, most centers reserve VATS for diagnosis rather than treatment of pulmonary metastases.

OPERATIVE TECHNIQUE

Once general anesthesia has been induced and a double-lumen endotracheal tube inserted, the patient is placed in the full lateral decubitus position. It is important to stop ventilation to the lung being operated on as soon as the patient is rotated into the lateral decubitus position so that the lung will be thoroughly collapsed by the time the videothoracoscope is inserted into the pleural space. Small subpleural pulmonary nodules are most easily identified in a fully atelectic lung because they protrude from the surrounding collapsed pulmonary parenchyma, which is softer.[15,16] Most pulmonary wedge resections are performed as true videothoracoscopic procedures using just three port incisions placed in the triangulated manner already described [see Basic Operative Technique, above]. The pulmonary nodules to be removed are grasped with an endoscopic lung clamp (Pennington or Duval) inserted through one instrument port, and the wedge resection is done with repeated application of an endoscopic stapler inserted through the opposite port.[20,26] As the resection is performed, it is often helpful to introduce the stapler through each of the two instrument ports alternately to obtain the correct angle for application to the lung [see Figure 8]. To prevent tumor implantation in the chest wall, small specimens (usually those resected with three or fewer stapler applications) are removed via the thoracoport. Larger specimens are placed in a disposable plastic specimen retrieval bag, which is then brought out through a very slightly enlarged anterior thoracoport incision.

When the wedge resections have been completed, intercostal blocks are performed under direct vision with the mediastinoscopy aspiration needle, and a single chest tube is inserted through the inferior port after the videothoracoscope is withdrawn. The videotho-

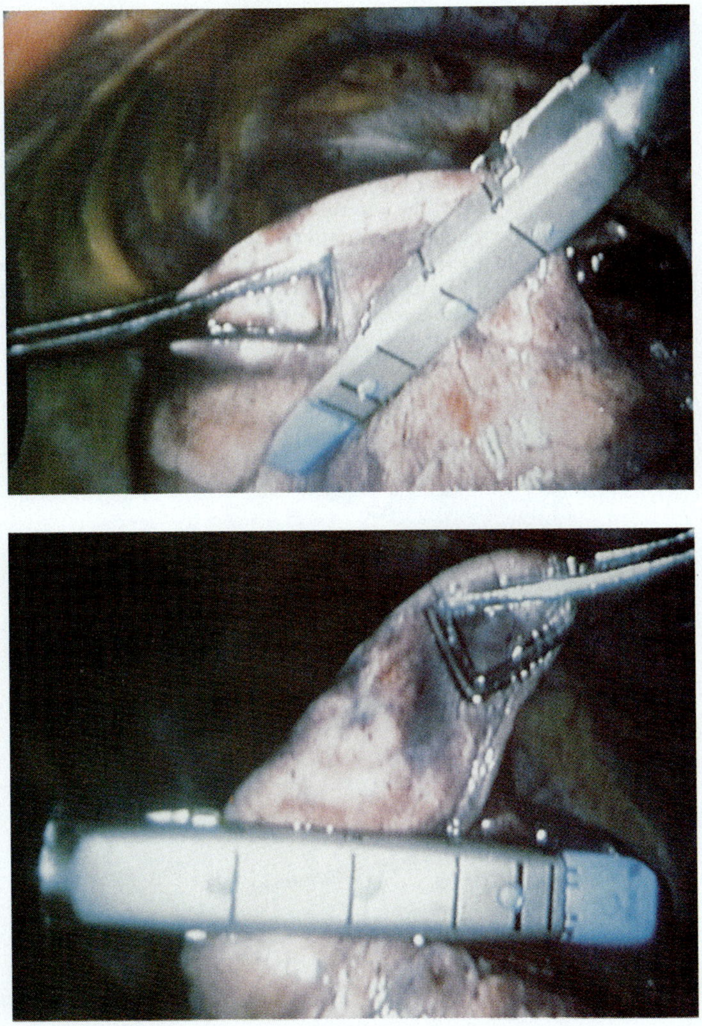

Figure 8 VATS pulmonary wedge resection. A double-lumen endotracheal tube is used to render the lung partially atelectic. The pulmonary nodule is lifted upward with a lung clamp, and the endoscopic GIA stapler is applied to the lung underneath (top). During the wedge resection, the lung clamp and the endoscopic GIA stapler are alternately inserted through opposite ports to obtain the correct angle for performance of the wedge resection (bottom).

racoscope can be placed through the anterior incision to check the position of the chest tube and confirm the reinflation of the lung after the double-lumen endotracheal tube is unclamped. The remaining incisions are then closed with sutures.

TROUBLESHOOTING

Four techniques can be used to locate pulmonary nodules that are either too deep or too small to be easily visible on simple inspection of the lung. All of these should be used in conjunction with a high-quality preoperative CT chest scan to identify the segment of lung in which the nodule is located. First, an endoscopic lung clamp can be gently run across the surface of the lung as an extension of digital palpation.[16,27] With some patience and experience, one can achieve considerable success with this technique. Second, ultrasonographic examination of the collapsed lung can locate deep pulmonary nodules; however, experience with this approach has been very limited.[28] Third, CT-guided needle localization can be used preoperatively if a nodule is likely to be difficult to locate. Localization is accomplished by injecting methylene blue or by inserting a barbed mammography localization needle, which is then cut off at the skin exit site and later retrieved thoracoscopically.[29] Needle localization techniques are effective, but they are also costly and time-consuming and hence are not used by most surgeons. Finally, if careful endoscopic examination of the lung does not reveal the location of a nodule, an access incision is added to the videothoracoscopy.[20,30] Each lobe of the lung is sequentially rotated up to this non–rib-spreading utility thoracotomy for direct digital palpation. This technique almost always allows identification of a nodule when other techniques fail. As the endoscopist gains experience with these techniques, conversion to thoracotomy solely for the purpose of locating a pulmonary nodule is rarely necessary.[31]

Pulmonary nodules located on the broad surface of the lung may not be amenable to wedge resection with an endoscopic stapler. Such nodules can be removed by using the electrocautery, just as in an open thoracotomy. An extension is placed on the handle of the electrocautery, which is then introduced into the pleural space through either a port or an access incision. Another approach is to resect the pulmonary nodule with a laser in either contact or noncontact mode. The potassium-titanyl-phosphate (KTP)/YAG laser is particularly suited to this task because it is capable of both cutting and coagulation. To minimize bleeding and air leakage, raw pulmonary surfaces can be cauterized with either the Nd:YAG laser or the ABC.[13] Numerous types of absorbable sealant patches or materials are also available to control air leaks from raw pulmonary parenchyma.

Occasionally, after a wedge resection, it is necessary to suture together the pleural edges over an area of raw pulmonary parenchyma. The suturing can be done directly through a non–rib-spreading minithoracotomy incision or through port sites. In the latter case, the ports are removed, and a 3-0 Prolene suture is passed through the anterior port site with a standard needle holder. A second needle holder is introduced through the posterior port site and used in place of a forceps to pick up and reposition the needle as it is passed through the lung. The surgeon and the first assistant work together to oversew the lung, in contrast with the normal practice for an open procedure, in which the surgeon uses a needle holder and a forceps to place the sutures.

VATS Procedures for Spontaneous Pneumothorax and Bullous Disease

OPERATIVE TECHNIQUE

VATS is now frequently performed for the management of recurrent spontaneous pneumothorax and for bullous disease.[32,33] The approach is similar to that used for a wedge resection. Three or four port sites are used. The videothoracoscope is inserted at the fifth intercostal space in the midaxillary line. Two other port sites are added at the fourth intercostal space in the anterior and posterior axillary lines.

In patients with spontaneous pneumothorax, the responsible bulla (which is usually apical in location) is identified, and wedge resection is done with an endoscopic stapler.[34,35] Bullae can be excised by applying the stapler across the base of the area of bullous disease. They can also be ablated with the ABC or the Nd:YAG laser, then suture-plicated if necessary; however, this approach may not be as successful over the long term.[36,37]

TROUBLESHOOTING

The placement of port incisions should be determined by the location of the bullae. Because bullous disease is generally apical, port

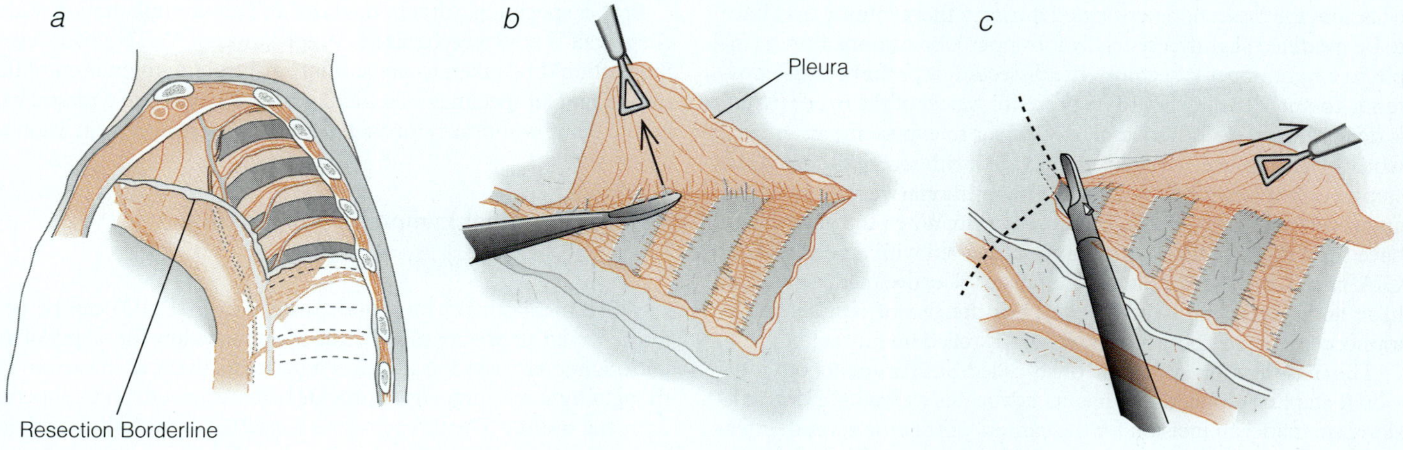

Figure 9 VATS procedures for spontaneous pneumothorax and bullous disease. Limited apical pleurectomy is a useful alternative to chemical pleurodesis in young patients with spontaneous pneumothorax because these patients may need to undergo thoracotomy later in life. Shown is an outline of the pleural resection (*a*) performed in this procedure. The pleura is grasped at the inferior border with forceps and lifted in the avascular layer in a cranial or ventral direction (*b*). A T-shaped incision is made in the pleura at the level of the subclavian artery or the truncus brachiocephalicus. The dissection of the pleural flap thus created is extended in either the ventral or the parasternal direction and in either the apical or the mediastinal direction (*c*).

sites are correspondingly higher than for the average wedge resection (i.e., at the fourth and sixth intercostal spaces rather than at the fifth or sixth and eighth). The precise placement should, however, be determined by pinpointing the disease site or sites on the preoperative chest x-ray and CT scans.

The main problem after resection for bullous disease is prolonged leakage of air from the staple line. This problem can be minimized by applying commercially available sleeves made of bovine pericardium or Gore-Tex (W. L. Gore, Boulder, Colorado) over the arms of the stapler to reinforce the staple line and by performing some form of pleurodesis. Mechanical pleurodesis is done with a small gauze sponge passed through a port site. Some surgeons scarify the pleura by cauterizing it with the ABC or the Nd:YAG laser, but this is not as successful as mechanical pleurodesis. Chemical pleurodesis by talc poudrage is an appropriate option for older patients with emphysema and bullous disease but is unwise in young patients with spontaneous pneumothorax, who might require a thoracotomy later in life.[38] Another option in younger patients is a limited apical pleurectomy [see Figure 9]. Special angulated instruments and blunt dissectors have been designed for this procedure; however, a parietal pleurectomy is also easily performed with combinations of standard blunt and sharp instruments.[39]

VATS Lobectomy and Pneumonectomy

OPERATIVE TECHNIQUE

Although VATS lobectomy is much less frequently performed than VATS pulmonary wedge resection, standard techniques have been developed for it.[40] VATS pneumonectomy, on the other hand, is less well accepted. Both operations are done as video-assisted procedures using a utility thoracotomy, which facilitates the insertion of standard thoracotomy instruments, the extraction of the resected specimen from the pleural space, and the performance of the technically complex aspects of the procedure, including dissection of the hilar vessels and the mediastinal lymph nodes.

Two approaches to lobectomy have been developed. One involves sequential anatomic ligation of the hilar structures, much as in a standard lobectomy,[41,42] and the other involves mass ligation of the pulmonary vessels and the bronchus. Both approaches require at least two port incisions in addition to the utility thoracotomy. The sequential anatomic ligation approach has been well described.[41] On occasion, the dissection performed during a thoracotomy may have to be modified slightly, especially for upper lobe tumors. For example, in a right upper lobectomy, the dissection is performed in a posterior-to-anterior direction. The posterior aspect of the major fissure is divided with an endoscopic GIA stapler to expose the bronchus, which is then isolated, ligated, and divided with an endoscopic GIA stapler or a roticulator TA stapler. The pulmonary artery is ligated and divided, followed by the pulmonary vein. When the hilar vessels have been divided, the minor fissure is divided with an endoscopic GIA stapler, and the specimen is removed. Selective mediastinal and hilar nodal sampling is performed, but the use of cervical mediastinoscopy before thoracotomy is heavily relied on for staging.

The mass ligation approach, or so-called SIS (simultaneous individual stapling) lobectomy, has its advocates as well.[43] Four incisions are made: an incision for the camera port at the seventh intercostal space, a 2 cm incision at the sixth intercostal space in the midaxillary line for the insertion of staplers, and two 3 cm incisions at the fourth intercostal space in the anterior and posterior axillary lines for the insertion of additional instruments. In the initial report of this technique, the bronchus and the pulmonary vessels were ligated separately, but the vessels were stapled en masse.[44] Subsequently, the technique was refined so that the bronchus and the vessels were stapled simultaneously by applying the stapler twice, the first time loosely to obtain closure of the bronchus and the second time more tightly to obtain hemostatic closure of the vessels. Although the early results were satisfactory,[45] concern about the long-term risks of bronchovascular or arteriovenous fistula formation resulting from mass ligation of the hilar structures has prevented universal acceptance of this approach.

A similar approach has been used for VATS pneumonectomy. The thoracoscope is inserted at the seventh intercostal space in the midaxillary line, and a utility thoracotomy is performed at the fourth intercostal space in the same line. Two port sites are then created at the sixth intercostal space in the anterior and posterior axillary lines. The hilar vessels are sequentially isolated, ligated, and divided with endoscopic or standard staplers. The inferior pulmonary vein is done first, followed by the superior pulmonary vein and the pulmonary artery. The bronchus is stapled and divided last.[46,47]

TROUBLESHOOTING

The endoscopic GIA stapler should never be used to divide the hilar vessels: if it fails to fire staples properly, the vessels retract into the pericardium, causing exsanguinating hemorrhage. The hilar vessels can be ligated proximally with a TA stapler, then ligated and divided distally with an endoscopic GIA stapler; alternatively, they can be divided with the scissors after two TA staple rows have been applied. Another option is to doubly ligate or suture-ligate the vessels via the utility thoracotomy, just as is traditionally done during an open procedure.

Most of the reported VATS lobectomies have been performed in patients with stage I lung cancer. If the tumor is invading the chest wall or the mediastinum or if the resection is being performed after induction chemotherapy or chemoradiotherapy, VATS is inappropriate because it does not provide adequate exposure for complex resections, particularly when significant perihilar fibrosis is present. Since a randomized trial comparing VATS lobectomy to lobectomy performed through a standard muscle-sparing thoracotomy incision failed to show any significant difference between the two with respect to hospital stay or perioperative morbidity, enthusiasm for VATS lobectomy has diminished.[48-50] It is never wise to compromise the quality of a cancer resection for the perceived benefit of a shorter hospital stay or less pain.

Proper specimen extraction is critical. Tumor implantation in the chest wall is now a recognized complication of VATS procedures. Steps should be taken to prevent intrapleural fragmentation of the tumor, and all specimens should be carefully placed in a plastic bag before being withdrawn through the utility thoracotomy incision or a port site.[51,52]

VATS Mediastinal Lymph Node Dissection

OPERATIVE TECHNIQUE

VATS mediastinal lymph node dissection (MLND) can be performed as an alternative to a Chamberlain procedure for biopsy of the aortopulmonary window nodes or anterior mediastinal masses and is thought by some surgeons to provide better exposure and a superior cosmetic result.[53] The thoracoscope is inserted at the fifth or sixth intercostal space in the posterior axillary line. Instruments for retracting the lung inferiorly are introduced via a port at the seventh intercostal space in the midaxillary line. Instruments for dissecting the nodes are introduced through ports placed at the fourth intercostal space in the anterior axillary line and in the auscultatory triangle. The lymph nodes are dissected free with graspers, scissors, the electrocautery, and en-

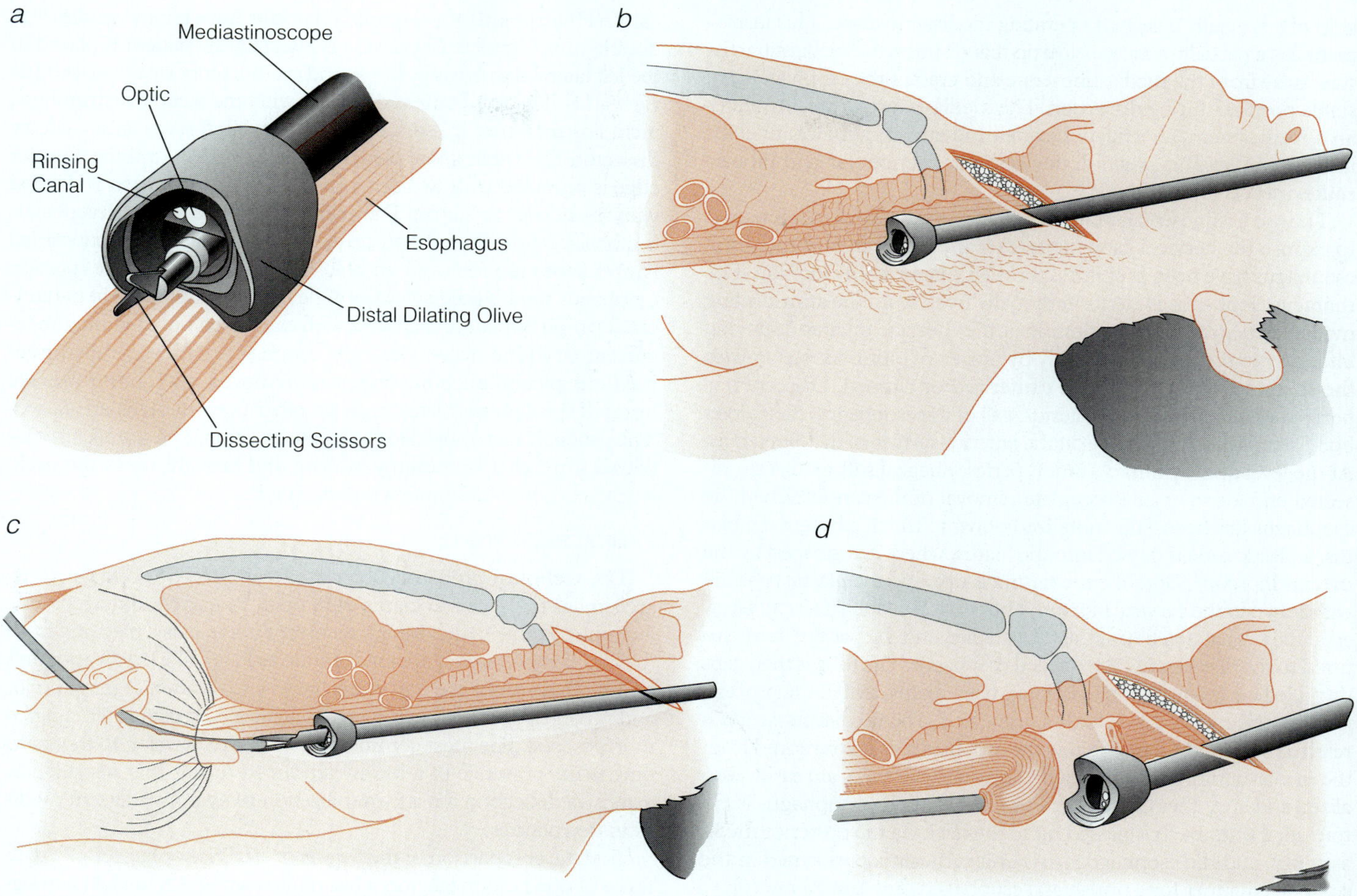

Figure 10 VATS esophagectomy. In the transhiatal approach, a specially designed operating mediastinoscope with an olive-shaped tip (*a*) is used. This tip mechanically distracts the mediastinal tissues away from the mediastinoscope and keeps the esophagus in a stable position during dissection. The scope is shown cradling the esophagus with the dissecting scissors inserted. During periesophageal dissection, the distal dilating olive of the mediastinoscope is placed behind the esophagus (*b*). The olive creates and maintains space by careful probing of the periesophageal areolar tissue. When the esophagus has been fully mobilized down to the diaphragmatic hiatus, a plastic tube is passed into the hiatus, where it is grasped by the mediastinoscope. Both the mediastinoscope and the plastic tube are pulled up from the hiatus (*c*). After esophageal resection with an endoscopic GIA stapler, the esophagus is folded over by using endoscopic control (*d*). Structures still attached to the esophagus are placed in traction, coagulated, and divided.

doscopic hemostatic clips. Curved sponge sticks are ideal lymph node graspers. A similar approach can be used to biopsy other mediastinal nodes, including the paratracheal and periesophageal nodes. This method has become an accepted approach to the surgical staging of esophageal cancer.[54,55] It is harder to do a complete en bloc subcarinal lymph node dissection, though nodal sampling of this region by VATS is certainly feasible, especially when an access incision is used.

TROUBLESHOOTING

Care should be taken not to injure the phrenic nerve as it courses along the superior vena cava on the right and across the anterior aspect of the aortopulmonary window on the left. The vagus nerve should be visualized, and the origin of the recurrent laryngeal nerve should be avoided during dissection. The recurrent laryngeal nerve is most easily injured on the left side, where it passes around the ligamentum arteriosum before traveling under the aortic arch; however, it can also be injured on the right side if MLND is carried too high superiorly along the origin of the innominate artery.

VATS MLND is unwise after induction chemotherapy or chemoradiotherapy because the lymph nodes are often densely adherent to surrounding structures. This is especially true on the right side, where the superior mediastinal lymph nodes become adherent to the superior vena cava and the azygous vein. A thoracotomy, with extensive exposure and sharp dissection, is usually required for a safe and complete MLND.

All lymphatic branches should be ligated during node biopsy or dissection to prevent leakage of chyle. Often, there are large lymphatic branches in the distal right paratracheal area. The thoracic duct can be injured if periesophageal or posterior mediastinal lymph nodes are being removed.

VATS Esophagectomy

OPERATIVE TECHNIQUE

To date, surgeons' experience with thoracoscopic esophageal resection has been limited. VATS esophagectomy can take either a transhiatal or a transthoracic approach.

The technique for VATS transhiatal esophagectomy[56] is a modification of the open technique advocated by Orringer[57] and allows the esophagectomy to be performed entirely under direct vision with the help of a specially designed operating mediastinoscope. This instrument has a partially concave olive tip that distracts the mediastinal tissues away from the mediastinoscope and cradles the esophagus in a stable position during dissection. The mediastinoscope incorporates an optical system, an irrigation canal, and an operating channel for insertion of scissors, suction devices, and monopolar and bipolar cautery forceps.

The mediastinoscope is introduced through the neck incision used to expose the cervical esophagus after the stomach and the distal esophagus have been mobilized through a laparotomy incision. The thoracic esophagus is circumferentially freed from the surrounding mediastinal structures, beginning at the thoracic inlet and moving inferiorly to the hiatus, primarily by means of blunt dissection with the suction device. Vessels are cauterized or clipped. Dissection is performed first along the posterior wall of the esophagus, then along both lateral walls, and finally on the anterior surface of the esophagus. At the level of the primary tumor, periesophageal soft tissues are resected en bloc to ensure complete removal of the cancer. When the esophagus has been fully mobilized down to the diaphragmatic hiatus, a plastic tube is passed into the hiatus, where it is grasped by the mediastinoscope. Both the mediastinoscope and the plastic tube are withdrawn to the cervical incision. The cervical esophagus is transected at the sternal notch with the GIA stapler, and the plastic tube is sutured to the distal end of the divided esophagus. The tube is then gently pulled back down to the diaphragmatic hiatus, and in the process, the thoracic esophagus is folded onto itself. The mediastinoscope is reintroduced and used to follow the esophagus as it is removed from the mediastinum. Any undivided vessels or lymphatics are easily visualized and are either ligated or cauterized. After the esophagus is extracted, the stomach is passed up to the neck via the posterior mediastinum, and the esophagogastric anastomosis is performed in the standard manner for a transhiatal esophagectomy [see Figure 10].

The transthoracic thoracoscopic technique for esophagectomy has been described by several authors.[58-60] One group has refined a clinical VATS technique that is based on results from animal studies.[61] A double-lumen endotracheal tube is inserted, the patient is placed in the left lateral decubitus position, and six thoracoports are placed [see Figure 11]. The soft tissue is dissected with endoscopic instruments, including a 10 mm scissors, a 5 mm grasping forceps, and a cherry dissector. The mediastinal pleura is opened widely, and the anterior edge is retracted with two stay sutures. The azygous vein is divided with an endoscopic stapler. The inferior half of the thoracic esophagus is mobilized away from the aorta and the pericardium. The subcarinal lymph nodes are removed en bloc. The upper third of the thoracic esophagus is mobilized away from the trachea, and the right paratracheal lymph nodes are removed, with care taken not to injure the recurrent laryngeal nerve. Once the esophagus has been fully mobilized, the pleural traction sutures are removed, two chest tubes are inserted through port sites, and the other port incisions are closed. The patient is then moved to the supine position. The stomach is mobilized through a laparotomy incision and brought up to the neck, where a cervical anastomosis is performed.

TROUBLESHOOTING

The technical problems associated with VATS esophagectomy are similar to those associated with open thoracic esophagectomy, including thoracic duct injury, recurrent nerve palsy, bleeding from the intercostal vessels, and anastomotic leakage. The best way of preventing these problems is to obtain good visualization of the superior and posterior mediastinum, which is achieved by using a 30° angled thoracoscope. The most common reason for conversion to thoracotomy is the presence of a locally advanced tumor that necessitates extensive dissection for safe mobilization away from adjacent mediastinal structures.

To date, comparison of the results of VATS esophagectomy with those of open esophagectomy has not shown VATS to yield any significant decrease in major complications, especially postoperative respiratory insufficiency and cardiac arrhythmias. These findings may be attributable in part to the number of port sites required to accomplish a complicated resection and to the necessity of combining VATS with an upper midline laparotomy for mobilization of the stomach.[62,63] As a result, most centers have reverted to standard open transhiatal or transthoracic approaches to esophagectomy.

VATS Pericardial Window

OPERATIVE TECHNIQUE

Some surgeons create a pericardial window by means of VATS as an alternative to taking the subxiphoid approach or the left anterior thoracotomy approach.[64] A double-lumen endotracheal tube is inserted with the patient under general anesthesia, and the patient is rotated into the right lateral decubitus position. Three access sites are used, with the thoracoscope inserted at the seventh intercostal space in the posterior axillary line and instruments introduced through two ports, one at the tip of the scapula and the other at the sixth intercostal space in the anterior axillary line [see Figure 12a]. The pericardium is retracted with a grasper forceps, and the scissors are used to resect 8 to 10 cm² areas of pericardium both anterior and posterior to the phrenic nerve. If indicated, talc pleurodesis can be performed to control an associated pleural effusion. One or two chest tubes are then inserted through the port site incisions.

TROUBLESHOOTING

When a pericardial effusion causes cardiac tamponade, a subxiphoid approach is preferable to VATS for creating a pericardial window because it is safer to perform in a hemodynamically unstable pa-

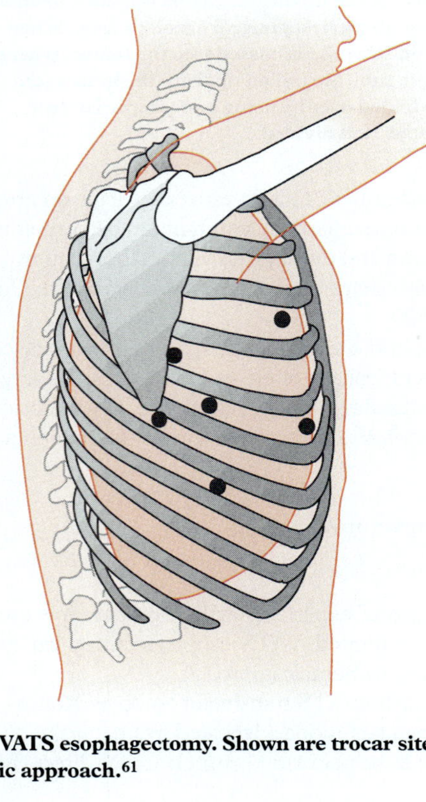

Figure 11 **VATS esophagectomy. Shown are trocar sites for the transthoracic approach.**[61]

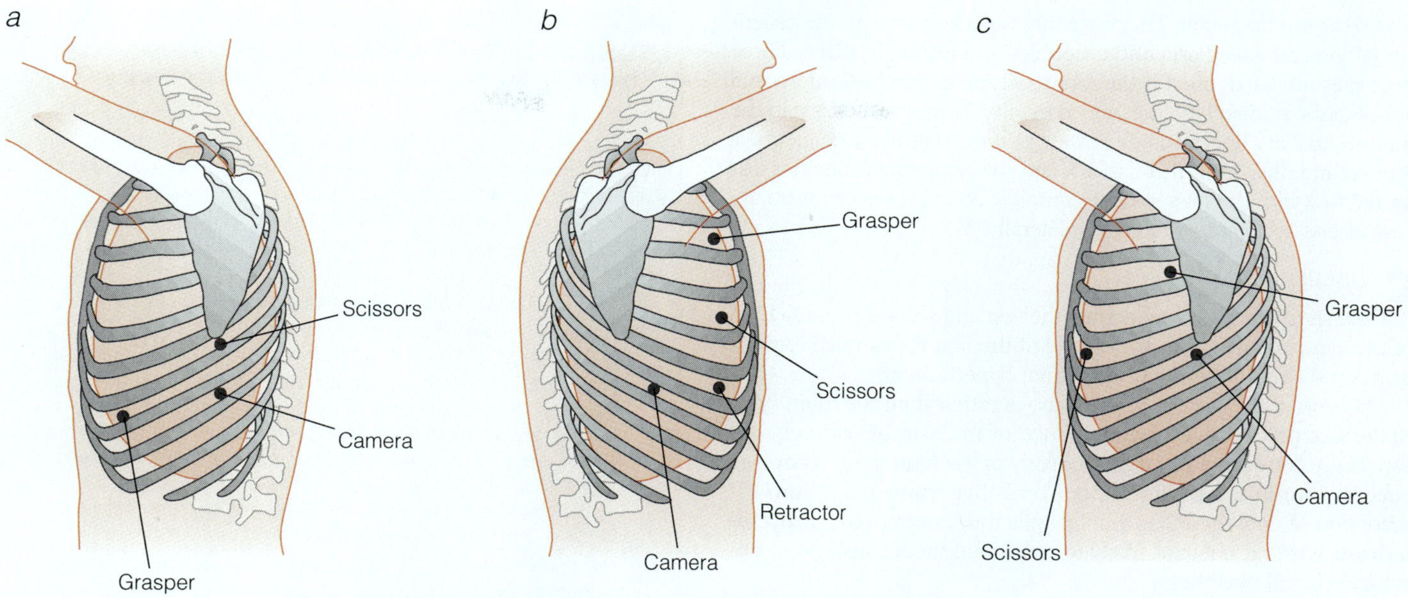

Figure 12 (*a*) VATS pericardial window. Three access sites are used. The thoracoscope is inserted in the posterior axillary line at the seventh intercostal space, the endoscopic scissors are inserted through one port at the tip of the scapula, and the grasper forceps is inserted through another port in the anterior axillary line at the sixth intercostal space. (*b, c*) VATS procedures for mediastinal masses. For posterior masses, the port sites are placed anteriorly (*b*), and the thoracoscope is inserted at the fifth intercostal space in the midaxillary line. A lung retractor is inserted at the sixth intercostal space in the anterior axillary line, and dissecting instruments are inserted at the second and fourth intercostal spaces in the anterior axillary line. For anterior mediastinal masses and thymectomy, the port sites are placed in more posterior locations (*c*). The thoracoscope is introduced at the fifth intercostal space in the midaxillary or the posterior axillary line, and instruments are inserted through one port at the second intercostal space in the midaxillary line and another at the fifth or sixth intercostal space in the anterior axillary line.

tient. A VATS pericardial window is also inadvisable in patients with constrictive physiology or with intrapericardial adhesions discovered at the time of operation. Conversion to an open procedure that includes formal pericardiectomy is advisable under these circumstances.

VATS Procedures for Mediastinal Masses

OPERATIVE TECHNIQUE

VATS has been used to resect masses in all of the mediastinal compartments. VATS resection is an ideal approach to posterior neurogenic tumors that do not extend into the neural canal.[65,66] With the patient in the lateral decubitus position, the operating table is rotated anteriorly, so that the lung falls away from the paravertebral region. The port sites are placed anteriorly: the thoracoscope is inserted at the fifth intercostal space in the midaxillary line, a lung retractor is inserted at the sixth intercostal space in the anterior axillary line, and dissecting instruments are inserted at the second and fourth intercostal spaces in the anterior axillary line [*see Figure 12b*]. The mass is manipulated with a grasper to expose the posteriorly located pedicle, which is then dissected, ligated, and divided with the scissors, clip appliers, and the electrocautery.[67,68]

For removal of anterior mediastinal masses, the port sites are placed in more posterior locations. The thoracoscope is introduced at the fifth intercostal space in the midaxillary or the posterior axillary line, and instruments are inserted through two ports, one at the second intercostal space in the midaxillary line and the other at the fifth or sixth intercostal space in the anterior axillary line [*see Figure 12c*]. The mass is retracted with a grasper and dissected free with a combination of sharp and blunt dissection, clip appliers, and the electrocautery.[69,70]

A similar technique is used to resect medial mediastinal masses, most of which are pericardial or bronchogenic cysts.[71,72] The access sites should be chosen according to the location of the mass on the preoperative CT scan. Generally, however, the triangulated site placement used for pulmonary wedge resections provides more suitable exposure than the site placement used for anterior or posterior mediastinal masses.

TROUBLESHOOTING

The placement of the thoracoports and the positioning of the operative team for the resection of posterior mediastinal tumors or for thoracic diskectomy differ significantly from those for most other VATS procedures. In place of the standard arrangement of trocars in an inverted triangle, the viewing port is placed in the posterior axillary line and the operating ports in the anterior axillary line. The thoracic surgeon and the neurosurgeon both stand on the anterior side of the patient, each viewing a monitor on the opposite side. In addition, a 30° scope is essential for visualizing the intervertebral disk space.[66,68]

Removal of dumbbell neurogenic tumors can be accomplished thoracoscopically if immediately preceded by posterior surgical removal of the spinal component of the tumor by means of laminectomy and intervertebral foraminotomy. Preoperative MRI scanning is crucial for defining the extent of the tumor within the spinal canal.[67] Resection of posterior mediastinal tumors is sometimes associated with significant bleeding from intercostal or spinal arteries; should such bleeding occur, there should be no hesitation in converting to a thoracotomy.

VATS Sympathectomy

OPERATIVE TECHNIQUE

Thoracic sympathectomy is known to be the most effective treatment for upper limb hyperhidrosis, and VATS is now an accepted approach to this operation. The procedure is performed with the patient under general anesthesia and a double-lumen tube in place. Three port sites are used: one for the thoracoscope at the third intercostal space in the midaxillary line, one at the third intercostal space in the anterior axillary line, and one at the tip of the scapula. The pleura is incised and divided from T2 to T5, and the sympathetic chain is dissected free with the scissors. For complete control of upper limb hyperhidrosis, VATS must be done bilaterally.[73,74]

TROUBLESHOOTING

Care should be taken to identify the first and second ribs. Division of the sympathetic trunk at the level of the first rib causes Horner's syndrome and does not reduce palmar hyperhidrosis.

Division of the rami communicantes rather than the main sympathetic trunk reduces the incidence of undesirable side effects, especially compensatory hyperhidrosis of the trunk, but its overall success rate in controlling upper limb hyperhidrosis is lower.[73] Abolition of only the T2 and T3 ganglia may control palmar hyperhidrosis without being as likely to result in unacceptable compensatory truncal sweating.

Postoperative neuralgia is common after VATS sympathectomy. Some authors advocate a 2-day postoperative course of dexamethasone to lower the incidence of this problem.[74]

Miscellaneous VATS Procedures

Several other procedures have been performed by VATS, including ligation of the thoracic duct,[75] examination and repair of the diaphragm after trauma,[76,77] and resection of the adrenal gland.[78] For adrenal resection, three incisions are placed at the ninth or tenth intercostal space, extending from the anterior axillary line to the posterior axillary line. A fan retractor is inserted through a radial incision in the diaphragm and used to retract the perirenal fat. The adrenal gland is dissected free and removed, and the associated vessels are clipped or cauterized.[78]

Cost Considerations

It is hard to estimate the cost-effectiveness of VATS procedures because the instrumentation, the types of procedures performed, and surgical expertise with these operations are all still evolving. Initially, VATS procedures proved expensive, for several reasons (e.g., the cost of purchasing video and endoscopic equipment, the cost of disposable instrumentation, and the need for long operating times as surgeons and nursing staff members gained experience performing these procedures). Soon after VATS was introduced, a study from the Mayo Clinic compared the cost of performing VATS pulmonary wedge resection with that of the same operation done by thoracotomy.[79] The VATS approach was associated with substantially shorter hospital stays but also with increased operating room costs; hence, the use of VATS did not result in any significant overall savings. More recently, however, as some VATS procedures (e.g., pulmonary wedge resection) have become standard operations and more reusable instrumentation has become available, the cost of VATS has undoubtedly decreased. Whether other, more complex procedures (e.g., thoracoscopic esophagectomy) are cost-effective remains to be determined.

Training and Certification in VATS

Thoracoscopy is most frequently performed by thoracic surgeons.[2] In some centers, however, particularly in Europe, pulmonologists became highly experienced in the application of traditional thoracoscopic techniques to the diagnosis of pleural disease. The experience of Boutin epitomizes the involvement of physicians who do not have specific surgical training.[4,8] The development of small-caliber endoscopes that could be used with local anesthesia outside the OR made it easy for nonsurgeons to perform thoracoscopy.

After the 1950s, thoracoscopy was largely forgotten by surgeons and pulmonologists in the United States until the advent of VATS. The dramatic initial popularity of this technique generated considerable debate over whether nonsurgeons should perform VATS in the same way that they performed other invasive endoscopic procedures.[80-82] During this same period, laparoscopic cholecystectomy came to be widely practiced, often by persons who lacked adequate training, and reports of serious complications emerged.

Within this context, the Society of Thoracic Surgeons (STS) and the American Association for Thoracic Surgery (AATS) formed a joint committee to establish standards and guidelines for training and certification in VATS [see Sidebar Statement of the AATS/STS Joint Committee on Thoracoscopy and Video Assisted Thoracic Surgery]. During 1992, this committee organized several courses in VATS that included both didactic sessions and hands-on laboratory experience and that were open to both practicing thoracic surgeons and thoracic surgical residents. As a result, many surgeons were trained in a short time, and VATS was quickly incorporated into thoracic surgical practice and residency training.

Statement of the AATS/STS Joint Committee on Thoracoscopy and Video Assisted Thoracic Surgery[83]

The Councils of the American Association for Thoracic Surgery and The Society of Thoracic Surgeons have formed a Joint Committee on Thoracoscopy and Video Assisted Thoracic Surgery. The purpose of this Committee is to facilitate the education of thoracic surgeons in this new technology and to provide guidelines for appropriate training in and performance of thoracoscopy and video assisted, minimally invasive thoracic surgery.

The following guidelines are recommended by the Joint Committee:

1. In order to ensure optimal quality patient care, thoracoscopy and video assisted thoracic surgery (TVATS) should be performed only by thoracic surgeons who are qualified, through documented training and experience, to perform open thoracic surgical procedures and manage their potential complications. The surgeon must have the judgment, training, and capability to proceed immediately to a standard open thoracic procedure if necessary.

    The preoperative and postoperative care of patients treated by TVATS should be the responsibility of the operating surgeon.

2. It is recommended that TVATS techniques be learned through appropriate instruction:

    a. As part of a formal approved thoracic surgical residency or fellowship program which includes structured and documented experience in these procedures.

    b. For the practicing thoracic surgeon, completion of a course that follows the guidelines approved by the Joint Committee, with hands-on laboratory experience, plus observation of these techniques performed by thoracic surgeons experienced in such procedures.

3. The granting of privileges to perform TVATS remains the responsibility of the credentialing body of individual hospitals.

For the AATS/STS Joint Committee on Thoracoscopy and Video Assisted Thoracic Surgery: Martin F. McKneally, M.D., and Ralph J. Lewis, M.D., co-chairmen; Richard P. Anderson, M.D., Richard G. Fosburg, M.D., William A. Gay, Jr., M.D., Robert H. Jones, M.D., and Mark B. Orringer, M.D.

The important considerations with respect to the training and practice of VATS have been well articulated.[82,83] VATS is not a minor procedure: it is minimally invasive, complex intrathoracic surgery that should be performed only by persons who are familiar with intrathoracic anatomy and pathology and are fully competent to manage complications and make intraoperative decisions in such a way as to ensure safe outcomes for thoracic surgical patients. The complications encountered during thoracoscopic operations are potentially immediately life-threatening, whereas those encountered during other endoscopic procedures usually are not. For that reason, VATS procedures should not be performed by anyone—surgeon or nonsurgeon—who lacks the training and experience to perform immediate thoracotomy and repair intrathoracic injuries.

VATS is now an integral part of the practice of thoracic surgery.[84] The direct involvement of the major thoracic societies in the dispersion of this technology has discouraged the casual and unsafe application of VATS and has promoted an ongoing critical appraisal of VATS procedures.

References

1. Jacobeus HC: The practical importance of thoracoscopy in surgery of the chest. Surg Gynecol Obstet 34:289, 1922
2. Bloomberg AE: Thoracoscopy in perspective. Surg Gynecol Obstet 147:433, 1978
3. Weissberg D, Kaufman M: Diagnostic and therapeutic pleuroscopy: experience with 127 patients. Chest 78:732, 1980
4. Boutin C, Viallat JR, Cargnino P, et al: Thoracoscopy in malignant pleural effusions. Am Rev Respir Dis 124:588, 1981
5. Wihlm JM, Roeslin N, Morand G, et al: Résultats comparés de la ponction, de la biopsie à l'aiguille, de la pleuroscopie et de la thoracotomie dans le diagnostic des pleurésies chroniques. Poumon Coeur 37:57, 1981
6. Rodgers BM, Ryckman FC, Moazam F, et al: Thoracoscopy for intrathoracic tumors. Ann Thorac Surg 31:414, 1981
7. Rusch VW, Mountain C: Thoracoscopy under regional anesthesia for the diagnosis and management of pleural disease. Am J Surg 154:274, 1987
8. Boutin C, Viallat JR, Aelony Y: Practical Thoracoscopy. Berlin, Springer-Verlag, 1991
9. Hazelrigg SR, Nunchuck SK, LoCicero III J: Video Assisted Thoracic Surgery Study Group data. Ann Thorac Surg 56:1039, 1993
10. Krasna MJ, Deshmukh S, McLaughlin JS: Complications of thoracoscopy. Ann Thorac Surg 61:1066, 1996
11. Deslauriers J, Beaulieu M, Dufour C, et al: Mediastinopleuroscopy: a new approach to the diagnosis of intrathoracic diseases. Ann Thorac Surg 22:265, 1976
12. Rusch VW: Instrumentation for video-assisted thoracic surgery. Chest Surg Clin North Am 3:215, 1993
13. Landreneau RJ, Herlan DB, Johnson JA, et al: Thoracoscopic neodymium:yttrium-aluminum garnet laser-assisted pulmonary resection. Ann Thorac Surg 52:1176, 1991
14. Rusch VW, Schmidt R, Shoji Y, et al: Use of the argon beam electrocoagulator for performing pulmonary wedge resections. Ann Thorac Surg 49:287, 1990
15. Landreneau RJ, Mack MJ, Hazelrigg SR, et al: Video-assisted thoracic surgery: basic technical concepts and intercostal approach strategies. Ann Thorac Surg 54:800, 1992
16. Rusch VW, Bains MS, Burt ME, et al: Contribution of videothoracoscopy to the management of the cancer patient. Ann Surg Oncol 1:94, 1994
17. Ohri SK, Oswal SK, Townsend ER, et al: Early and late outcome after diagnostic thoracoscopy and talc pleurodesis. Ann Thorac Surg 53:1038, 1992
18. Angellillo Mackinlay TA, Lyons GA, Chimondeguy DJ, et al: VATS debridement versus thoracotomy in the treatment of loculated postpneumonia empyema. Ann Thorac Surg 61:1626, 1996
19. Hartman DL, Gaither JM, Kesler KA, et al: Comparison of insufflated talc under thoracoscopic guidance with standard tetracycline and bleomycin pleurodesis for control of malignant pleural effusions. J Thorac Cardiovasc Surg 105:743, 1993
20. Landreneau RJ, Hazelrigg SR, Ferson PF, et al: Thoracoscopic resection of 85 pulmonary lesions. Ann Thorac Surg 54:415, 1992
21. Ferson PF, Landreneau RJ, Dowling RD, et al: Comparison of open versus thoracoscopic lung biopsy for diffuse infiltrative pulmonary disease. J Thorac Cardiovasc Surg 106:194, 1993
22. Dowling RD, Keenan RJ, Ferson PF, et al: Video-assisted thoracoscopic resection of pulmonary metastases. Ann Thorac Surg 56:772, 1993
23. McCormack PM, Ginsberg KB, Bains MS, et al: Accuracy of lung imaging in metastases with implications for the role of thoracoscopy. Ann Thorac Surg 56:863, 1993
24. Dowling RD, Ferson PF, Landreneau RJ: Thoracoscopic resection of pulmonary metastases. Chest 102:1450, 1992
25. McCormack PM, Bains MS, Begg CB, et al: Role of video-assisted thoracic surgery in the treatment of pulmonary metastases: results of a prospective trial. Ann Thorac Surg 62:213, 1996
26. Miller DL, Allen MS, Trastek VF, et al: Videothoracoscopic wedge excision of the lung. Ann Thorac Surg 54:410, 1992
27. Normori H, Horio H: Endofinger for tactile localization of pulmonary nodules during thoracoscopic resection. Thorac Cardiovasc Surg 44:50, 1996
28. Shennib H, Bret P: Intraoperative transthoracic ultrasonographic localization of occult lung lesions. Ann Thorac Surg 55:767, 1993
29. Plunkett MB, Peterson MS, Landreneau RJ, et al: Peripheral pulmonary nodules: preoperative percutaneous needle localization with CT guidance. Radiology 185:274, 1992
30. Lewis RJ, Caccavale RJ, Sisler GE, et al: One hundred consecutive patients undergoing video-assisted thoracic operations. Ann Thorac Surg 54:421, 1992
31. Demmy TL, Nielson D, Curtis JJ: Improved method for deep thoracoscopic lung nodule excision. Missouri Med 93:86, 1996
32. Mouroux J, Elkaïm D, Padovani B, et al: Video-assisted thoracoscopic treatment of spontaneous pneumothorax: technique and results of one hundred cases. J Thorac Cardiovasc Surg 112:385, 1996
33. Schramel FMNH, Sutedja TG, Braber JCE, et al: Cost-effectiveness of video-assisted thoracoscopic surgery *versus* conservative treatment for first time or recurrent spontaneous pneumothorax. Eur Respir J 9:1821, 1996
34. Hazelrigg SR, Landreneau RJ, Mack M, et al: Thoracoscopic stapled resection for spontaneous pneumothorax. J Thorac Cardiovasc Surg 105:389, 1993
35. Cole FH Jr, Cole FH, Khandekar A, et al: Video-assisted thoracic surgery: primary therapy for spontaneous pneumothorax? Ann Thorac Surg 60:931, 1995
36. Wakabayashi A: Expanded applications of diagnostic and therapeutic thoracoscopy. J Thorac Cardiovasc Surg 102:721, 1991
37. Wakabayashi A: Thoracoscopic laser pneumoplasty in the treatment of diffuse bullous emphysema. Ann Thorac Surg 60:936, 1995
38. Colt HG, Russack V, Chiu Y, et al: A comparison of thoracoscopic talc insufflation, slurry, and mechanical abrasion pleurodesis. Chest 111:442, 1997
39. Inderbitzi RGC, Furrer M, Striffeler H, et al: Thoracoscopic pleurectomy for treatment of complicated spontaneous pneumothorax. J Thorac Cardiovasc Surg 105:84, 1993
40. Yim APC, Ko K-M, Ma C-C, et al: Thoracoscopic lobectomy for benign diseases. Chest 109:554, 1996
41. Kirby TJ, Mack MJ, Landreneau RJ, et al: Initial experience with video-assisted thoracoscopic lobectomy. Ann Thorac Surg 56:1248, 1993
42. Kohno T, Murakami T, Wakabayashi A: Anatomic lobectomy of the lung by means of thoracoscopy: an experimental study. J Thorac Cardiovasc Surg 105:729, 1993
43. Lewis RJ: Simultaneously stapled lobectomy: a safe technique for video-assisted thoracic surgery. J Thorac Cardiovasc Surg 109:619, 1995
44. Lewis RJ, Sisler GE, Caccavale RJ: Imaged thoracic lobectomy: should it be done? Ann Thorac Surg 54:80, 1992
45. Lewis RJ: Personal communication, 1993
46. Roviaro GC, Rebuffat C, Varoli F, et al: Videoendoscopic thoracic surgery. Int Surg 78:4, 1993
47. Roviaro GC, Varoli F, Rebuffat C, et al: Videothoracoscopic staging and treatment of lung cancer. Ann Thorac Surg 59:971, 1995
48. Landreneau RJ, Hazelrigg SR, Mack MJ, et al: Postoperative pain-related morbidity: video-assisted thoracic surgery versus thoracotomy. Ann Thorac Surg 56:1285, 1993
49. Kirby TJ, Mack MJ, Landreneau RJ, et al: Lobectomy—video-assisted thoracic surgery versus muscle-sparing thoracotomy: a randomized trial. J Thorac Cardiovasc Surg 109:997, 1995
50. Landreneau RJ, Mack MJ, Hazelrigg SR, et al: Prevalence of chronic pain after pulmonary resection by thoracotomy or video-assisted thoracic surgery. J Thorac Cardiovasc Surg 107:1079, 1994
51. Downey RJ, McCormack P, LoCicero III J, et al: Dissemination of malignant tumors after video-assisted thoracic surgery: a report of twenty-one cases. J Thorac Cardiovasc Surg 111:954, 1996
52. Johnstone PAS, Rohde DC, Swartz SE, et al: Port site recurrences after laparoscopic and thoracoscopic procedures in malignancy. J Clin Oncol 14:1950, 1996

53. Landreneau RJ, Hazelrigg SR, Mack MJ, et al: Thoracoscopic mediastinal lymph node sampling: useful for mediastinal lymph node stations inaccessible by cervical mediastinoscopy. J Thorac Cardiovasc Surg 106:554, 1993
54. Krasna MJ: Minimally invasive staging for esophageal cancer. Chest 112(suppl):191S, 1997
55. Krasna MJ, Flowers JL, Attar S, et al: Combined thoracoscopic/laparoscopic staging of esophageal cancer. J Thorac Cardiovasc Surg 111:800, 1996
56. Buess G, Becker HD, Lenz G: Perivisceral endoscopic oesophagectomy. Operative Manual of Endoscopic Surgery. Cuschieri A, Ed. Berlin, Springer-Verlag, 1992, p 149
57. Orringer MB: Transhiatal esophagectomy without thoracotomy for carcinoma of the thoracic esophagus. Ann Surg 200:282, 1984
58. Law S, Fok M, Chu KM, et al: Thoracoscopic esophagectomy for esophageal cancer. Surgery 122:8, 1997
59. Collard J-M, Lengele B, Otte J-B, et al: En bloc and standard esophagectomies by thoracoscopy. Ann Thorac Surg 56:675, 1993
60. Gossot D, Fourquier P, Celerier M: Thoracoscopic oesophagectomy. Ann Chir Gyn Fenniae 83:162, 1994
61. Akaishi T, Kaneda I, Higuchi N, et al: Thoracoscopic en bloc total esophagectomy with radical mediastinal lymphadenectomy. J Thorac Cardiovasc Surg 112:1533, 1996
62. Collard J-M: En bloc and standard esophagectomies by thoracoscopy: update. Ann Thorac Surg 61:769, 1996
63. Peracchia A, Rosati R, Fumagalli U, et al: Thoracoscopic esophagectomy: are there benefits? Semin Surg Oncol 13:259, 1997
64. Mack MJ, Landreneau RJ, Hazelrigg SR, et al: Video thoracoscopic management of benign and malignant pericardial effusions. Chest 103(suppl):390S, 1993
65. Riquet M, Mouroux J, Pons F, et al: Videothoracoscopic excision of thoracic neurogenic tumors. Ann Thorac Surg 60:943, 1995
66. Bousamra M II, Haasler GB, Patterson GA, et al: A comparative study of thoracoscopic vs open removal of benign neurogenic mediastinal tumors. Chest 109:1461, 1996
67. Vallières E, Findlay JM, Fraser RE: Combined microneurosurgical and thoracoscopic removal of neurogenic dumbbell tumors. Ann Thorac Surg 59:469, 1995
68. Mack MJ, Regan JJ, McAfee PC, et al: Video-assisted thoracic surgery for the anterior approach to the thoracic spine. Ann Thorac Surg 59:1100, 1995
69. Yim APC, Kay RLC, Ho JKS: Video-assisted thoracoscopic thymectomy for myasthenia gravis. Chest 108:1440, 1995
70. Knight R, Ratzer ER, Fenoglio ME, et al: Thoracoscopic excision of mediastinal parathyroid adenomas: a report of two cases and review of the literature. J Am Coll Surg 185:481, 1997
71. Hazelrigg SR, Landreneau RJ, Mack MJ, et al: Thoracoscopic resection of mediastinal cysts. Ann Thorac Surg 56:659, 1993
72. Lewis RJ, Caccavale RJ, Sisler GE: Imaged thoracoscopic surgery: a new thoracic technique for resection of mediastinal cysts. Ann Thorac Surg 53:318, 1992
73. Gossot D, Toledo L, Fritsch S, et al: Thoracoscopic sympathectomy for upper limb hyperhidrosis: looking for the right operation. Ann Thorac Surg 64:975, 1997
74. Wong C-W: Transthoracic video endoscopic electrocautery of sympathetic ganglia for hyperhidrosis palmaris: special reference to localization of the first and second ribs. Surg Neurol 47:224, 1997
75. Shirai T, Amano J, Takabe K: Thoracoscopic diagnosis and treatment of chylothorax after pneumonectomy. Ann Thorac Surg 52:306, 1991
76. Lang-Lazdunski L, Mouroux J, Pons F, et al: Role of videothoracoscopy in chest trauma. Ann Thorac Surg 63:327, 1997
77. Spann JC, Nwariaku FE, Wait M: Evaluation of video-assisted thoracoscopic surgery in the diagnosis of diaphragmatic injuries. Am J Surg 170:628, 1995
78. Mack MJ, Aronoff RJ, Acuff TE, et al: Thoracoscopic transdiaphragmatic approach for adrenal biopsy. Ann Thorac Surg 55:772, 1993
79. Allen MS, Deschamps C, Lee RE, et al: Video-assisted thoracoscopic stapled wedge excision for indeterminate pulmonary nodules. J Thorac Cardiovasc Surg 106:1048, 1993
80. Mathur P, Martin WJ Jr: Clinical utility of thoracoscopy. Chest 102:2, 1992
81. Forum: Who should perform thoracoscopy? Chest 102:1553, 1992
82. Thoracoscopy forum, continuing dialogue. Chest 102:1915, 1992
83. McKneally MF, Lewis RJ, Anderson RP, et al: Statement of the AATS/STS Joint Committee on Thoracoscopy and Video Assisted Thoracic Surgery. J Thorac Cardiovasc Surg 104:1, 1992
84. Mack MJ, Scruggs GR, Kelly KM, et al: Video-assisted thoracic surgery: has technology found its place? Ann Thorac Surg 64:211, 1997

Acknowledgment

Figures 1 through 6, 9, 10, and 12   Tom Moore.

47 GASTROINTESTINAL ENDOSCOPY

Jeffrey L. Ponsky, M.D.

Since the beginning of the 1970s, flexible endoscopy of the gastrointestinal tract has been the dominant modality for the diagnosis of gastrointestinal disease. Over the same period, developments in technology and methodology have made possible the use of endoscopy to treat a host of conditions that once were considered to be manageable only by means of open surgical procedures. The integration of flexible endoscopic techniques into the armamentarium of the GI surgeon permits a more multidimensional approach to the treatment of digestive disease. The modern GI surgeon should be conversant in and adept at many of these procedures.

Diagnostic Esophagogastroduodenoscopy

Diagnostic upper GI endoscopy is indicated when a patient has abnormal findings on traditional GI x-ray series, dysphagia, odynophagia, epigastric pain that does not respond to medical therapy, persistent heartburn, or upper GI bleeding; it is also indicated for surveillance of groups at high risk for malignancy and for sampling of GI tissue or fluid. One prepares for the examination by ensuring the patient's hemodynamic stability, having the patient fast for 6 to 8 hours beforehand, and performing conscious sedation, which generally involves applying a topical anesthetic to the posterior pharynx and administering a narcotic and a benzodiazepine intravenously. Monitoring of arterial blood pressure and oxygen saturation throughout the procedure is now standard practice.

TECHNIQUE

With the patient in the left lateral decubitus position, a topical anesthetic is applied to the posterior pharynx and an intravenous sedative administered. The forward-viewing panendoscope—a small-caliber instrument that is long enough to permit examination of the foregut from the mouth to the third portion of the duodenum—is employed.

The endoscope may be introduced either blindly, via finger-guided palpation of the pharynx, or under direct vision. The latter approach is preferable. In this approach, the instrument is advanced slowly until the epiglottis and vocal cords are visualized [*see Figure 1*]; it is then angled posteriorly to the esophageal introitus and gently advanced as the patient is asked to swallow. Insufflation of air is begun to distend the esophagus, which appears as a long, round tube. Frequent peristaltic waves are seen; these are normal. Mucosal surfaces must be closely inspected for signs of ulceration, stricture, tumor, or Barrett's (columnar) epithelium, which manifests itself as orange patches in otherwise pale salmon-pink esophageal (squamous) mucosa. When abnormalities are noted, biopsy, brushing for cytologic evaluation, or both should be performed. Staining of the esophagus with methylene blue may be useful in the search for Barrett's mucosa: the blue dye is avidly absorbed by the intestinal absorptive cells of the columnar epithelium. Darkly stained areas may be biopsied for confirmation.

As the endoscope is advanced, insufflation is continued, and the curve of the lumen is followed to the left as the esophagus traverses the diaphragm to enter the stomach. There is a pinched area where the diaphragm compresses the esophagus; the pinching is exaggerated when the patient is asked to sniff. If gastric folds are seen above this pinched area, a hiatal hernia is present. When the stomach is entered, the tip of the endoscope is elevated so as to center it within the gastric lumen. It should be noted that with the patient lying in the left lateral decubitus position, the stomach is also on its side, with the greater curvature at 6 o'clock, the lesser curvature at 12 o'clock, the posterior wall at 3 o'clock, and the anterior wall at 9 o'clock. Air should be insufflated to distend the stomach fully and permit careful inspection of the mucosal surfaces.

As the instrument is advanced toward the gastric antrum, its tip should be slightly elevated because the stomach has a J shape and the prepyloric region curves upward. The pylorus is normally round and may be seen to open and close with gastric peristalsis. With the tip of the endoscope positioned at the proximal gastric antrum, just under the incisura angularis, a retroflex view of the cardia and the fundus is obtained by elevating the tip of the scope and rotating the shaft to the left. This maneuver provides visual and therapeutic access to the proximal stomach.

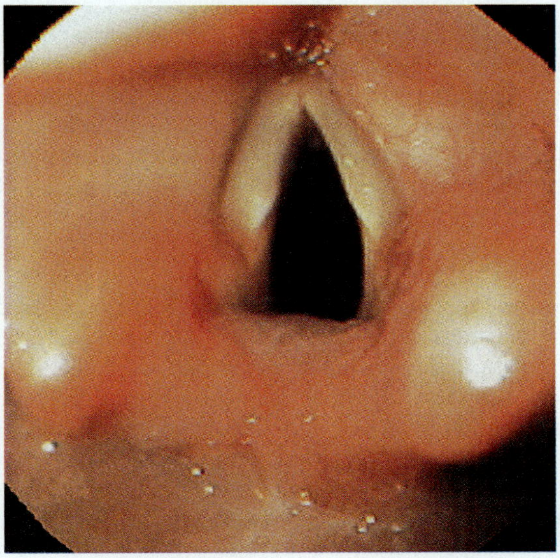

Figure 1 Diagnostic esophagogastroduodenoscopy. As the endoscope is introduced under direct vision, the vocal cords are clearly noted. The esophageal opening is posterior to the cords.

After the stomach has been viewed, the instrument is advanced under direct vision through the pylorus and into the duodenal bulb. Insufflation of air should continue as the scope is pressed against the pylorus to facilitate passage of the instrument. The scope tends to pop into the duodenal bulb rather than slide smoothly; it should be pulled back slightly to allow one to observe the mucosal surfaces of the bulb before moving ahead. Unlike the rest of the small bowel, the duodenal bulb has no semicircular folds. The tip of the scope must be rotated slightly to permit examination of the walls of the bulb. It is advisable to pull the instrument back into the stomach while observing the walls of the bulb and the pyloric channel for lesions; several such withdrawals may be required for full assessment of this area.

Once the duodenal bulb has been examined, the endoscope is advanced just past the bulb to the point where the first duodenal folds are observed. Here, the duodenum turns sharply to the rear and downward as it becomes retroperitoneal. Advancement of the scope into the second portion of the duodenum is one of the few endoscopic maneuvers that cannot be accomplished under direct vision. Because of the sharp angle of the turn, one will experience a moment of so-called red out as the tip of the endoscope touches the mucosa during the turn. To ensure that the turn is accomplished safely, the instrument is advanced as far through the bulb as is possible under direct vision. The control handle of the scope is then rotated approximately 90° to the right as the tip of the scope is turned to the right and angled first upward, then downward. As the second portion of the duodenum appears, the scope is rotated back to its neutral position. When done correctly, the turn is actually quite easy. It should never be forced: if the instrument does not proceed easily into the descending duodenum, the scope should be pulled back and the attempt repeated. Pushing against resistance may result in perforation.

Entering the descending duodenum causes the scope to form a large loop in the stomach. Therefore, once the second portion of the duodenum is successfully entered, the shaft of the instrument is pulled back. Paradoxically, as this movement straightens the gastric loop, it also advances the tip of the instrument deeper into the duodenum. Further advancement of the instrument under direct vision often permits entry into the third or even the fourth portion of the duodenum. Once the distal limit of intubation is reached, the scope is withdrawn and the luminal surfaces carefully examined. Rotating the scope with small right-left movements of the controls and side-to-side movements of the control handle itself will help demonstrate the more subtle details of duodenal anatomy. Often, the upper GI tract is inspected more completely while the instrument is being withdrawn than while it is being advanced.

Mucosal abnormalities should be biopsied; liberal use of brush cytology in combination with biopsy enhances the yield.

COMPLICATIONS

Esophagogastroduodenoscopy is an extremely safe procedure. Perhaps the most common problems associated with the technique arise from the preparatory sedation and analgesia. Respiratory depression and aspiration may occur during the procedure. Careful attention must be paid to the patient's state of consciousness and airway during the endoscopic procedure, appropriate drugs must be available to reverse sedative effects, and a suction apparatus must be ready for use at all times. Blind advancement of the endoscope by force may lead to perforation of the esophagus; this problem may be avoided by taking care never to advance the instrument against resistance.

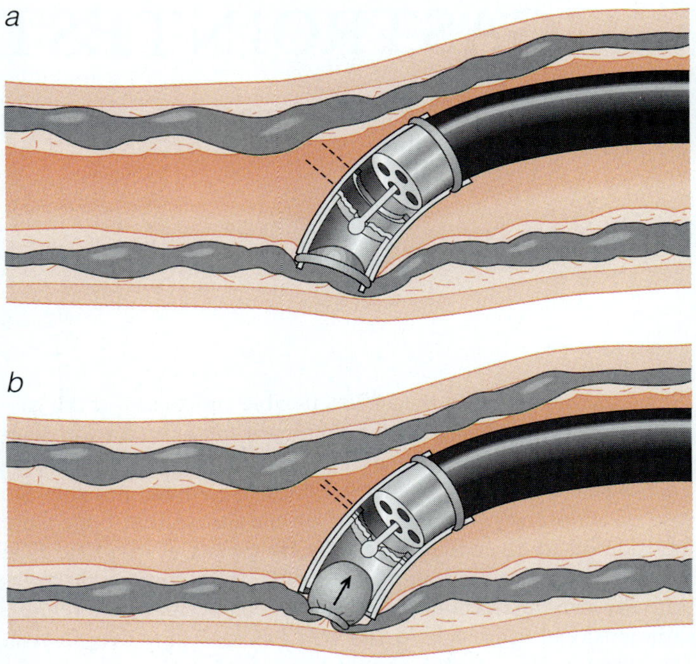

Figure 2 Therapeutic esophagogastroduodenoscopy: control of variceal hemorrhage. (*a*) A plastic tip on the endoscope is used to create a chamber. (*b*) An esophageal varix is suctioned into the chamber, and a rubber band is released around it.

Therapeutic Esophagogastroduodenoscopy

CONTROL OF VARICEAL HEMORRHAGE

In patients with massive upper GI hemorrhage, the first priorities are to establish a secure airway and to ensure hemodynamic stability. These priorities must be addressed before endoscopy is attempted. If the bleeding is thought to be coming from esophageal varices, it is frequently useful to perform endotracheal intubation for control of the airway before the endoscopic intervention.

Technique

A rapid but complete diagnostic upper GI endoscopic procedure is performed to determine whether varices are present and to identify the exact site of hemorrhage. Endoscopic therapy for variceal disease is then delivered by means of either sclerotherapy or rubber band ligation.

Sclerotherapy is commenced in the distal esophagus at the site of active or suspected bleeding: 2 to 3 ml of a sclerosant solution (e.g., sodium tetradecyl sulfate) is injected directly into the lumen of the varix. Additional varices can be treated in the same fashion. After the bleeding has stopped, further therapy is usually delivered at weekly intervals until total variceal obliteration is achieved.

Rubber band ligation of varices has become extremely popular in recent years and has been shown to possess some clear advantages over sclerotherapy [*see Figure 2*]. Originally, multiple passages of the endoscope were required to allow for reloading of the bands; however, newer ligating devices permit ligation of as many as 10 varices with a single passage of the endoscope. As with sclerotherapy, the site of active or suspected bleeding is attacked first; it is most often near the esophagogastric junction. The offending varix is centered in the field of view, and suction is applied to pull it into the ligator cup, which sits on the end of the endoscope. When the varix is deep within the cup, the trigger string on the li-

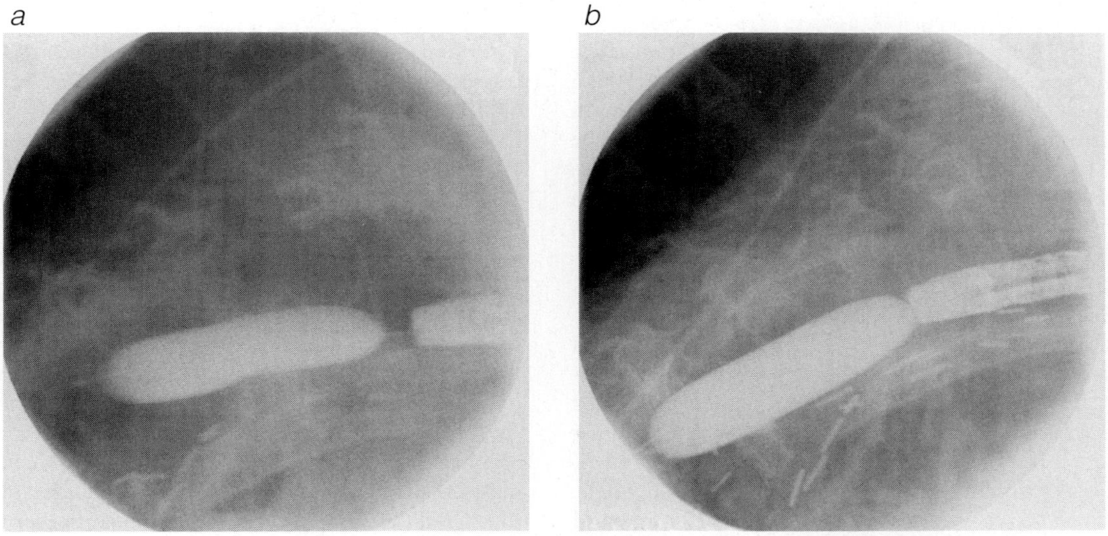

Figure 3 **Therapeutic esophagogastroduodenoscopy: dilation of esophageal strictures. (*a*) A hydrostatic dilating balloon filled with a contrast agent is inflated within the stricture under fluoroscopic guidance. Initially, a "waist" appears at the stricture site. (*b*) Inflation of the balloon is continued until the waist is ablated, which indicates complete dilation of the stricture.**

gator is pulled, and a rubber band is released around the varix. Suction is then released, and the ligated varix is visualized. Additional ligations may be performed at the initial session; follow-up sessions are usually held at weekly intervals until total variceal obliteration is achieved.

Complications

Because aspiration of blood and gastric contents may occur during endoscopic control of variceal hemorrhage, endotracheal intubation must be considered when bleeding is massive. In many cases, general anesthesia will permit adequate airway control and a quiet operating field. Violent patient motion when the injection needle is in a varix may result in perforation of the esophagus. This is a rare complication, however; tearing of the varix, with resultant hemorrhage, is more frequent. Injection of excessive amounts of sclerosant may lead to significant ulceration and necrosis of esophageal tissue. Fever, severe infection, pleural effusion, and subsequent esophageal stricture occasionally occur after sclerotherapy. Ulceration and necrosis of tissue, with subsequent stricture, occur after rubber band ligation as well, but severe infection is less common in this setting.

CONTROL OF NONVARICEAL HEMORRHAGE

Bleeding from peptic ulcer disease, gastritis, or vascular malformations is a common indication for esophagogastroduodenoscopy. Once the patient has been adequately resuscitated, endoscopy should be performed and the entire esophagus, stomach, and duodenum should be examined thoroughly. Before the procedure is begun, the stomach should be vigorously irrigated through a large-bore tube so that as much clotted blood as possible can be evacuated. If a pool of blood is noted in the stomach, the position of the patient should be changed so as to move the pool and permit complete examination of the stomach.

The therapeutic modalities available for control of nonvariceal bleeding include (1) the injection of hypertonic saline, epinephrine (in a 1:10,000 solution), or 98% alcohol, (2) bipolar electrocoagulation, (3) the use of heater probes, (4) argon beam coagulation, (5) the application of acrylic glue, (6) the application of hemostatic clips, and (7) the use of the neodynium:yttrium-aluminum-garnet (Nd:YAG) laser.

Technique

The most popular therapeutic modalities are injection therapy, bipolar coagulation, and the use of the heater probe. Injection therapy is performed around the bleeding lesion to create edema and vasospasm in the area. The bipolar coagulator or the heater probe is applied directly to the bleeding lesion in an attempt to coapt the bleeding vessel as heat is delivered. Frequently, injection therapy is employed in conjunction with coagulation; this combination is very effective.

If there is a clot covering the ulcer base, it must be removed with suction or a snare before coagulation is attempted. If a rapidly bleeding lesion is present, the best approach often is injection therapy in adjacent areas to slow or stop the bleeding, followed by coagulation by direct coaptation. Vascular lesions are often multiple or diffuse, as in so-called watermelon stomach. Such lesions are most effectively treated by means of modalities that can be applied in a spraying fashion, such as the Nd:YAG laser or the argon beam coagulator.

Complications

Nonvariceal hemorrhage is successfully controlled by endoscopic means in more than 90% of cases. At times, however, attempts at endoscopic control may exacerbate the bleeding. Several therapeutic modalities should always be available: one may succeed when another fails. Excessive injection therapy or persistent attempts at coagulation may lead to tissue necrosis and subsequent perforation. Although the argon beam coagulator can injure tissue only to a depth of several millimeters, excessive application may result in massive distention of the bowel if care is not taken to aspirate the constantly infused argon gas frequently. The Nd:YAG laser has the potential to cause full-thickness injury to the gastric wall.

DILATION OF ESOPHAGEAL STRICTURES

When patients complain of dysphagia or odynophagia, prompt endoscopic investigation is warranted. Strictures may be secondary to reflux disease, secondary to caustic burns, or of neoplastic origin.

Technique

Endoscopy is performed in the usual fashion. It is imperative that the endoscope be advanced only under direct vision. When a stricture is encountered, its location, morphology, and length should be determined. Biopsy and cytology specimens should be gathered from the circumference of the stricture. When a stricture is present at the esophagogastric junction and the scope can easily be passed by the stricture, it is helpful to view the area from below with the tip of the scope retroflexed.

Stricture dilation can be accomplished in several different ways and with several different kinds of dilators. One commonly employed method is to use the endoscope to guide the passage of a soft-tipped guide wire through the stricture; the scope is then removed, leaving the wire in place. Subsequently, dilators are passed over the guide wire, usually under fluoroscopic control. Another method for endoscopic dilation of strictures is the use of through-the-scope (TTS) hydrostatic dilating balloons. A balloon of the appropriate inflated diameter (usually no larger than 18 mm or 54 French) is selected, passed through the biopsy channel of the endoscope, and advanced under direct vision until its middle portion passes through the stricture. At the stricture site, the balloon is compressed, giving the appearance of a waist. The balloon is then inflated until the waist is fully expanded [see Figure 3]. Full expansion is verified by fluoroscopic surveillance and the use of contrast to inflate the balloon. This second method is extremely useful for initial dilation of tight strictures in preparation for the use of other, nonendoscopic dilators or the placement of an esophageal stent.

Complications

Dilation of esophageal strictures may result in bleeding (usually minor) or perforation of the esophagus. When a patient experiences severe pain after dilation, a chest x-ray is imperative. The finding of mediastinal or subcutaneous air should prompt the immediate performance of a contrast study with a water-soluble agent to determine whether a perforation is present. Some small perforations can be managed with intravenous antibiotics and observation, but most require surgical therapy. The incidence of perforation can be minimized by avoiding excessive or forceful dilation.

STENTING OF ESOPHAGEAL TUMORS

Under optimal circumstances, esophageal tumors should be treated by means of extirpative surgery. When surgical cure or palliation seems to offer little, placement of an esophageal prosthesis by endoscopic means is a reasonable approach.

Technique

Modern esophageal prostheses are placed under fluoroscopic guidance, frequently after endoscopic balloon dilation of the tumor. During the endoscopic examination, it is useful to inject a small amount of water-soluble contrast material into the muscular wall of the esophagus just above and below the tumor; this enables one to measure the length of the tumor and select the correct stent. Once the tumor has been dilated and marked endoscopically, the scope is removed, and the expandable stent is passed into the esophagus and positioned between the endoscopic injection markings seen on fluoroscopy. The stent is then deployed and allowed to expand [see Figure 4]. The endoscope may then be reintroduced to ensure that the prosthesis is patent and is correctly placed.

Complications

Incorrect positioning of the prosthesis is a frequent problem. Attention to the details of endoscopic marking is very important. Also crucial is correct selection of a stent: stents shorten from both ends as they are deployed, and this must be taken into account in selecting the correct stent length. On occasion, the stent may migrate as a result of tumor-related necrosis or incorrect placement. If it migrates into the stomach, it can usually be captured in a snare and retrieved.

RETRIEVAL OF FOREIGN BODIES

Many ingested foreign bodies pass through the GI tract uneventfully, but a good number must be removed by endoscopic means—in particular, foreign bodies in the esophagus, sharp objects that are likely to perforate the bowel, and objects that do not progress from the stomach.

If the ingested object is of an unfamiliar type, it is an extremely good idea to practice with a similar object outside the patient before attempting endoscopic retrieval. This preparatory step

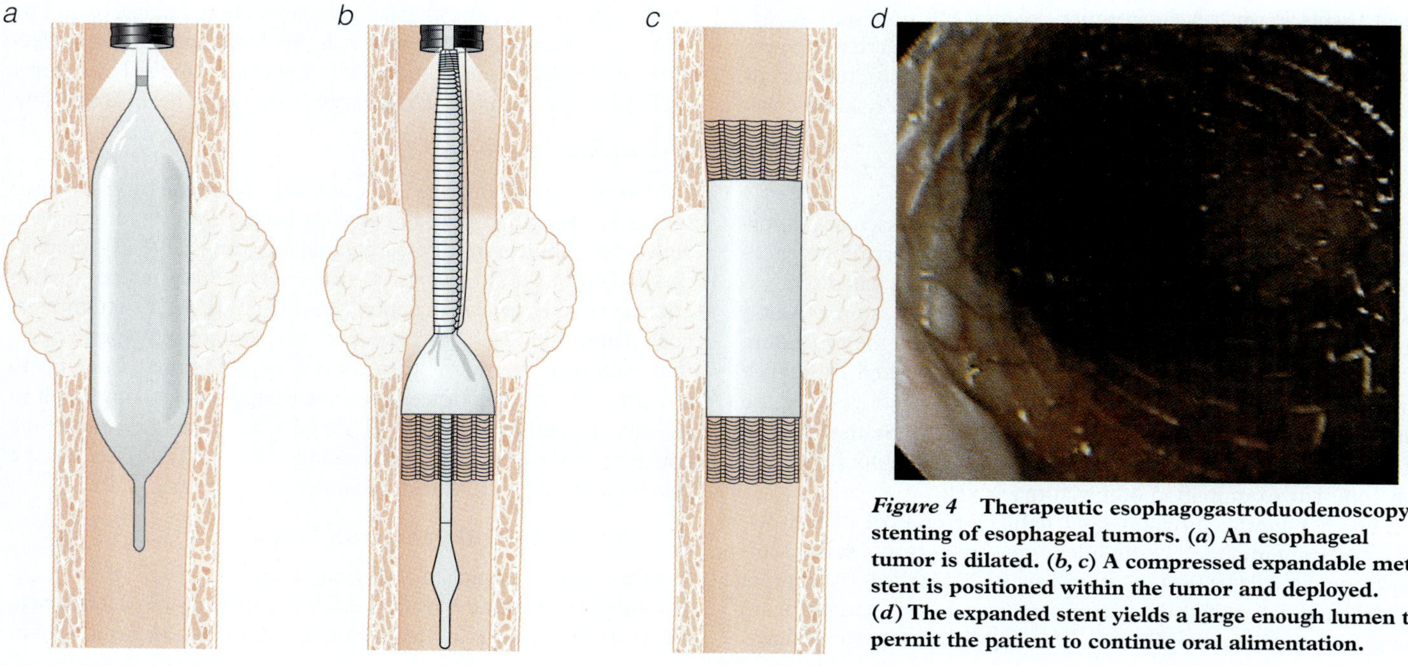

Figure 4 Therapeutic esophagogastroduodenoscopy: stenting of esophageal tumors. (*a*) An esophageal tumor is dilated. (*b, c*) A compressed expandable metal stent is positioned within the tumor and deployed. (*d*) The expanded stent yields a large enough lumen to permit the patient to continue oral alimentation.

allows one to select the most appropriate accessory and technique for removing the object.

Technique

Objects with sharp edges should be removed with the sharp end trailing to prevent perforation. In some cases, this means that the object must be pushed into the stomach and turned around before being removed. If multiple foreign bodies are present or if it is highly likely that the foreign body will injure the esophagus if removed in the standard manner, an overtube should be placed over the scope before insertion. The overtube enables one to pass the instrument several times and retrieve any sharp objects without injuring the esophagus; it also helps ensure that the object is not aspirated into the airway. If the patient is a child, general anesthesia may be advisable.

Perhaps the best method of removing foreign bodies is to surround them with a simple polypectomy snare and secure them in the endoscope's grasp. Meat boluses that form in the esophagus or proximal to a gastric banding may be extremely difficult to dislodge; the use of a variceal ligator cap to produce a suction chamber can be helpful in such situations.

Complications

Endoscopic removal of foreign bodies is extremely safe and effective. Care must be taken to ensure that the esophagus is not injured during removal of the object. If the object is deeply embedded or refractory to removal, a surgical approach is preferred.

PERCUTANEOUS ENDOSCOPIC GASTROSTOMY

Since 1980, endoscopically guided placement of a tube gastrostomy has been widely employed to provide access to the GI tract for feeding or decompression. Indications for percutaneous endoscopic gastrostomy (PEG) include various disease processes that interfere with swallowing, such as severe neurologic impairment, oropharyngeal tumors, and facial trauma. PEG has also been employed to establish a route for recycling bile in patients with malignant biliary obstruction, to provide supplemental feeding in selected patients with inflammatory bowel disease, and to accomplish gastric decompression in patients with conditions such as carcinomatosis, radiation enteritis, and diabetic gastropathy.

Technique

The patient fasts for 8 hours beforehand, and a single prophylactic dose of an antibiotic is administered just before the procedure is begun. The patient is placed in the supine position, a topical anesthetic is applied to the posterior pharynx, and intravenous sedation is begun. A forward-viewing endoscope is passed into the esophagus and advanced into the stomach. The abdomen is prepared in a sterile fashion and draped. The stomach and the duodenum are then inspected.

The room lights are dimmed, and the light of the endoscope is used to transilluminate the abdominal wall so as to indicate a point where the gastric wall and the abdominal wall are in close proximity. Finger pressure is applied to various areas of the abdomen until a spot is identified at which such pressure produces clear indentation of the gastric wall. An endoscopic snare is deployed through the biopsy channel of the endoscope to cover this spot, and a local anesthetic is infiltrated into the overlying skin [*see Figure 5*]. A 1 cm skin incision is made at the chosen spot, and a needle is passed through the incision and into the gastric lumen. The endoscopic snare is tightened around the needle, and a wire

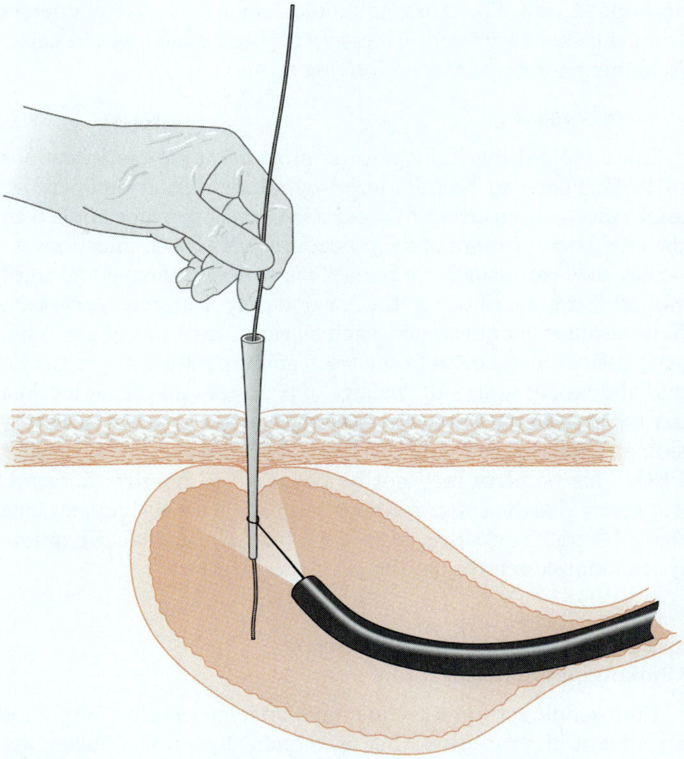

Figure 5 Therapeutic esophagogastroduodenoscopy: percutaneous endoscopic gastrostomy. The first steps in the procedure involve selecting a proper site in the stomach and using a snare to surround a needle that has been passed through the abdominal and gastric walls.

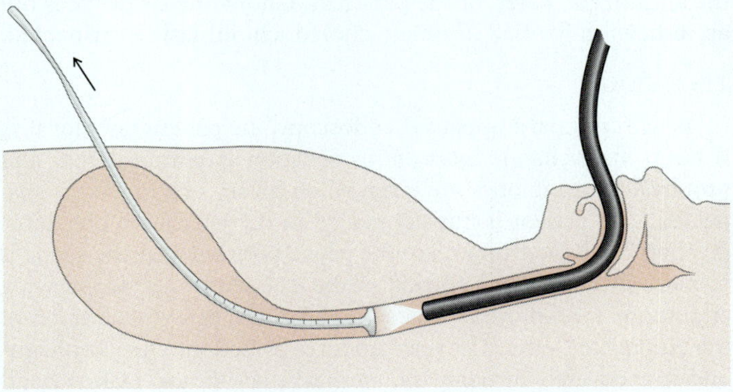

Figure 6 Therapeutic esophagogastroduodenoscopy: percutaneous endoscopic gastrostomy. After the suture is retrieved from the stomach, it is affixed to the gastrostomy tube and used to pull the tube back into the stomach and out the abdominal wall. The gastroscope is reinserted to follow the process and ensure that the final position of the tube is correct.

is passed through the needle and into the gastric lumen. The snare is moved so as to surround the wire, which is then pulled out of the patient's mouth. The gastrostomy tube is fastened to the wire and pulled in a retrograde manner down the esophagus and into the stomach. The gastroscope is subsequently reinserted to ensure that the head of the catheter is correctly positioned against the gastric mucosa [*see Figure 6*].

An outer crossbar is put in place to prevent inward migration of the tube and to hold the stomach in approximation to the abdominal wall. The crossbar should remain several millimeters from the skin to prevent excessive tension, which would cause ischemic necrosis of the underlying tissue.

Complications

Local wound infections are the most common complications of PEG. They can be minimized by administering preoperative antibiotics and ensuring that excessive tension is not applied to the crossbar at the end of the procedure. When such infections do occur, they can usually be treated via simple drainage and local wound care; sacrifice of the gastrostomy is rarely necessary. Several other complications, such as early extrusion of the tube, progressive enlargement of the tract, and separation of the gastric and abdominal walls with leakage of feedings into the abdominal cavity, are also most often attributable to excessive crossbar tension and subsequent ischemia. Gastrocolic fistula can occur after PEG. This problem may not be obvious for months afterward, but severe diarrhea after feedings is grounds for suspicion. Once the PEG tract is mature, gastrocolic fistulas usually close quickly after simple removal of the gastrostomy tube.

Diagnostic Endoscopic Retrograde Cholangiopancreatography

Endoscopic retrograde cholangiopancreatography (ERCP) is an advanced procedure that is technically more challenging than standard upper GI endoscopy; however, it can be mastered by most endoscopists who are willing to dedicate sufficient time to learning the method. ERCP yields a radiologic image of the pancreatic and biliary trees, and in many cases, it provides access for therapy. Indications for ERCP include suspected benign or malignant maladies of the common bile duct (CBD), the ampulla of Vater, or the pancreas. Cholelithiasis per se is not an indication for ERCP unless choledocholithiasis is suspected.

TECHNIQUE

As with standard upper GI endoscopy, the patient fasts for 6 to 8 hours beforehand. Intravenous sedation is administered, and prophylactic antibiotics are given when biliary obstruction is suspected. The patient is initially placed in the left lateral decubitus position but is later rotated to the prone position after the scope is in place in the second portion of the duodenum. A side-viewing endoscope is employed because it allows the best visualization of the ampulla of Vater. The instrument is passed into the esophagus and maneuvered through the stomach, across the pylorus, and into the duodenum. Manipulation of a side-viewing instrument is a bit awkward for the novice but is easily learned.

Once the endoscope is in the second portion of the duodenum, it is pulled back so that the gastric loop is straightened and the tip of the scope occupies a better position with regard to the papilla. This so-called short scope position is generally best for work in the CBD [see Figure 7]. The papilla of Vater (also known as the major duodenal papilla) appears as a small longitudinal nubbin crossing the horizontal semicircular folds of the duodenum, generally in the 12 to 1 o'clock position. At its tip, a small, soft, reticulated area may be noted; this is the papillary orifice. Often, a small mucosal protuberance is seen just proximal and to the right of the papilla of Vater; this is the minor duodenal papilla.

A small plastic cannula is passed through the channel of the endoscope and introduced into the ampullary orifice, and contrast material is injected under fluoroscopic control to provide visualization of the CBD and the pancreatic duct. The two may share a single orifice within the ampulla or may have separate orifices. The CBD exits the papilla in a cephalad direction, tangential to the duodenal wall. The bulge of the ampulla within the duodenum represents the intramural segment of the duct. The orifice of the CBD is typically found at the 11 o'clock position in the ampulla. The pancreatic duct leaves the papilla in a perpendicular fashion. Its orifice is usually in the 1 o'clock area of the papilla [see Figure 8].

COMPLICATIONS

When contrast material is being injected into the pancreatic ductal system, care must be taken to avoid overfilling, which can lead to acinarization, or rupture of the small ductules, with extravasation of contrast material into the pancreatic parenchyma; pancreatitis is a frequent consequence of acinarization. Cholangitis may result when contrast is injected proximal to an obstruction of the biliary tree. When obstruction is demonstrated, drainage of the system by means of stone extraction, stenting, or nasobiliary intubation is important to prevent cholangitis.

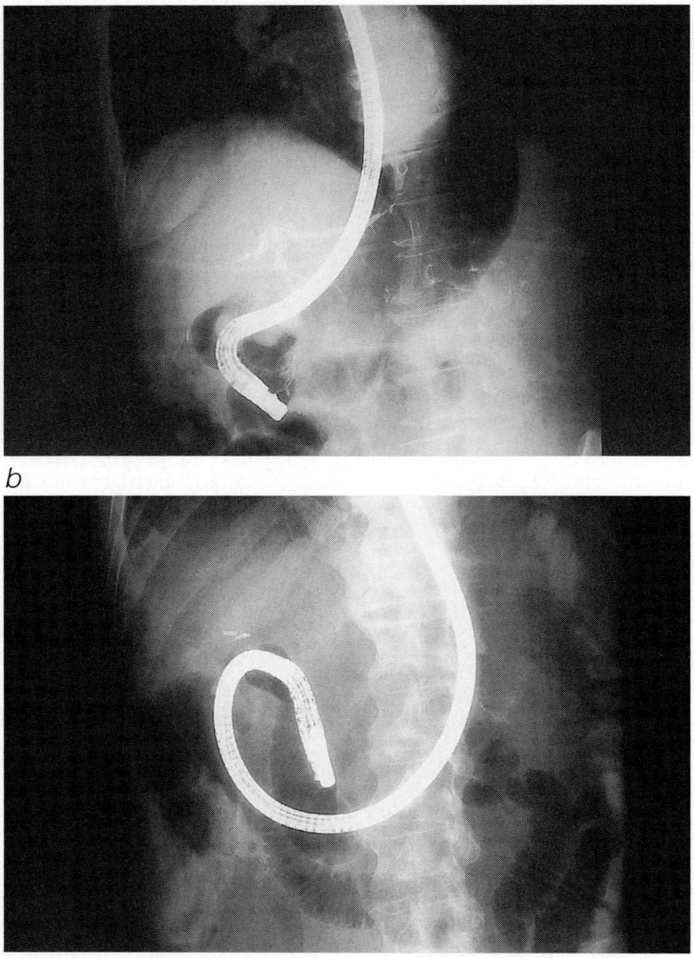

Figure 7 Diagnostic endoscopic retrograde cholangiopancreatography. (*a*) The so-called short scope position, along the lesser curve of the stomach, is usually the most effective in biliary interventions. (*b*) The so-called long scope position may be necessary at times.

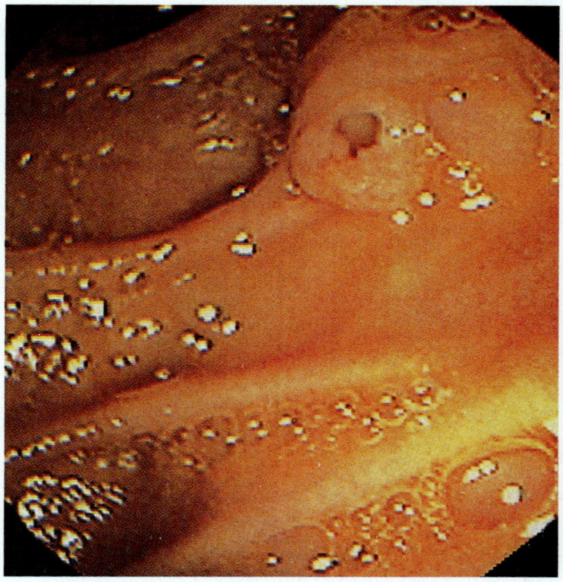

Figure 8 Diagnostic endoscopic retrograde cholangiopancreatography. The so-called long scope position, along the greater curve of the stomach, may be useful in some pancreatic interventions; shown is the pancreatic duct orifice.

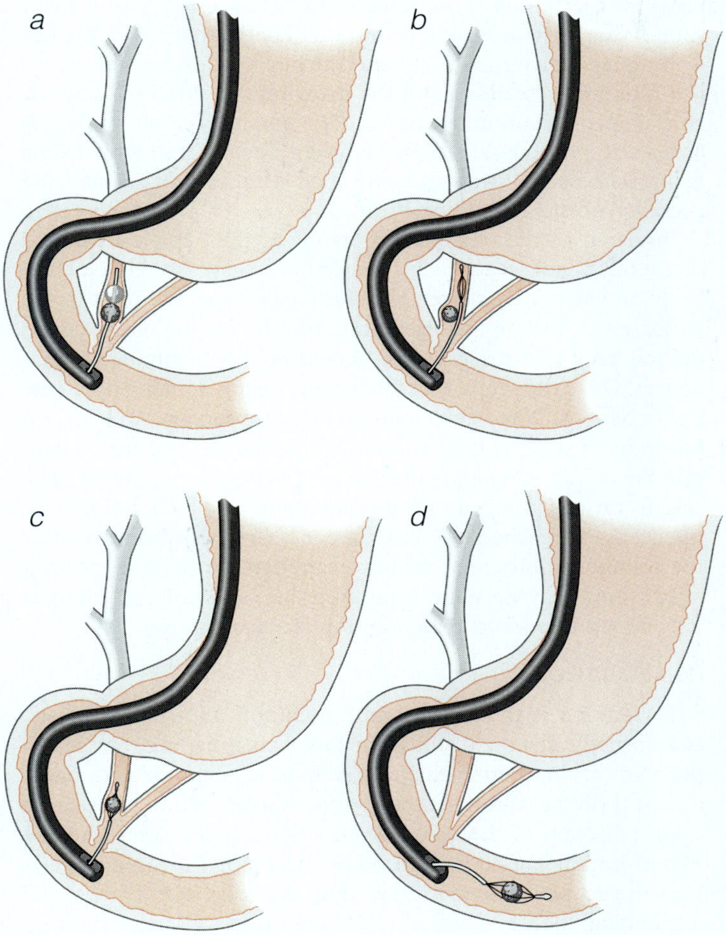

Figure 9 Therapeutic endoscopic retrograde cholangiopancreatography. After endoscopic sphincterotomy, CBD stones may be retrieved with balloons (*a*) or baskets (*b, c, d*).

Therapeutic Endoscopic Retrograde Cholangiopancreatography

Therapeutic interventions that may be accomplished at the time of ERCP include sphincterotomy for ductal access or ampullary stenosis, removal of CBD stones, dilation of benign and malignant biliary strictures, and insertion of stents to maintain ductal patency. Pancreatic duct interventions include removal of stones, bridging of ductal disruptions, and drainage of pseudocysts.

TECHNIQUE

All therapeutic applications of ERCP must begin with selective cannulation of the duct being treated. Frequently, a guide wire is then introduced deep into the duct to provide a means of obtaining access to the duct on an ongoing basis and to ensure correct positioning for intraductal manipulations. After electrosurgical division of the papilla, biliary stones are retrieved with balloon or baskets [*see Figure 9*]. Often, large stones can be captured within the duct in mechanical lithotripsy baskets and crushed before removal.

Strictures should be brushed for cytologic evaluation once they have been traversed by a wire. They may then be dilated with hydrostatic balloons under fluoroscopic guidance and stented [*see Figure 10*]. Plastic stents are used for most benign and many malignant strictures; however, self-expanding metal stents are now being used more frequently for malignant strictures because they remain patent longer [*see Figure 11*].

COMPLICATIONS

Perforation can occur during endoscopic sphincterotomy as a result of extension or tearing of the papilla beyond the junction of the CBD with the duodenal wall. Retroperitoneal or free intraperitoneal air may be seen. In many cases, intravenous antibiotics, hydration, and avoidance of oral intake are sufficient to manage such complications. If the patient's condition deteriorates, surgical exploration is indicated.

Bleeding may also occur with sphincterotomy. It is usually controllable with injection of epinephrine solution (1:10,000), electrocoagulation, or balloon tamponade. Arteriographic embolization of the gastroduodenal artery may be helpful in some cases. As with diagnostic ERCP, pancreatitis may occur, which usually responds to conservative measures.

Diagnostic Colonoscopy

Colonoscopy has become one of the most frequently performed endoscopic examinations. It has revolutionized the diagnosis and treatment of colonic disease and offers the promise of reducing the occurrence of colon cancer. Indications for colonoscopy include iron deficiency anemia, frank or occult rectal bleeding, a history of colonic cancer in the patient or in first-degree family members, a history or suspicion of colonic polyps, inflammatory bowel disease, and a persistent change in bowel habits. Preparation involves purging the bowel mechanically by placing the patient on a clear liquid diet for several days, then giving cathartics and enemas; alternatively, one may use osmotic lavage, in which 1 gal of lavage fluid is administered orally over a period of 4 hours. It is often helpful to administer 10 mg of metoclopramide to enhance gastric motility as preparation begins.

TECHNIQUE

Sedation is accomplished as for upper GI endoscopy, and the patient fasts for 6 to 8 hours before the procedure. With the

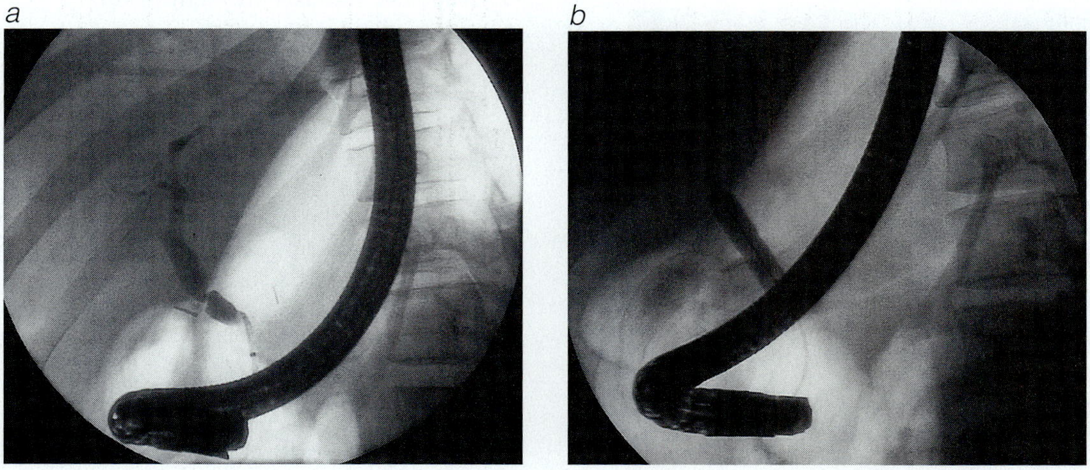

Figure 10 Therapeutic endoscopic retrograde cholangiopancreatography. CBD strictures (*a*), whether benign or malignant, may be dilated effectively with hydrostatic balloons under fluoroscopic guidance (*b*).

patient in the left lateral decubitus position, a rectal examination is performed. This step helps relax the anal sphincter in preparation for insertion of the scope and ensures that low-lying rectal lesions are not overlooked.

The colonoscope is introduced into the rectal vault, and insufflation of air is commenced. The instrument is advanced only when the lumen is clearly apparent. At times, only a portion of the lumen may be visible, but this is usually enough to guide advancement of the scope. Frequently, when the lumen itself is not visible, light reflected onto the colonic folds can guide one to the lumen, with the concavity of the fold indicating the direction of the lumen. In contrast with upper GI endoscopy, in which torsion on the shaft of the endoscope is rarely necessary, such torsion is the rule in colonoscopy. The shaft of the instrument is rotated with the right hand to facilitate straightening and intubation of the colon. By applying torsion to the shaft frequently and pulling back the scope as necessary, one can pleat the colon on the instrument as it is advanced. Pulling back is one of the most useful techniques for advancing the colonoscope through the colon.

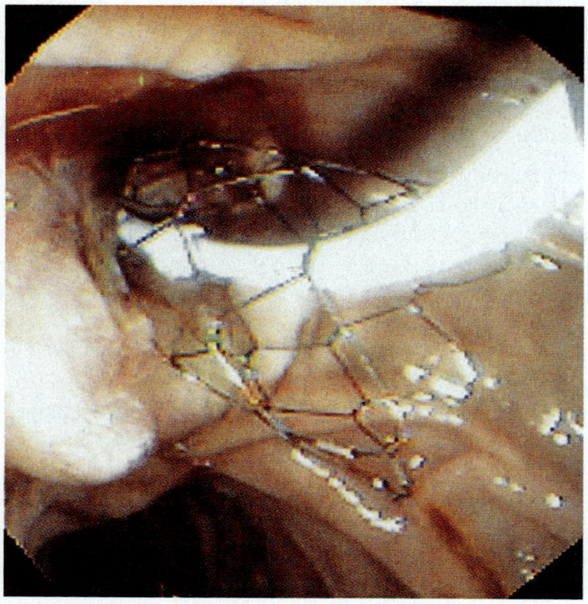

The anatomic landmarks of the colon are characteristic. The sigmoid colon, because of its frequent turns, yields elliptical views of the lumen. The descending colon appears as a long, round tunnel with little haustration. The transverse colon has well-defined triangular folds, and the hepatic flexure may exhibit a blue hue resulting from the proximity of the liver. The cecum is recognized on the basis of the appearance of the ileocecal valve on the lateral wall, the convergence of the colonic taenia to form the cecal strap (the so-called Mercedes sign), and the presence of the appendiceal orifice.

Insertion of the colonoscope as far as the hepatic flexure is rarely difficult. Occasionally, the sigmoid colon presents a challenge, in which case placement of the patient on the back or the abdomen to change the orientation may be helpful. Once again, pulling back and straightening the scope is a highly useful maneuver. Once the scope is in the hepatic flexure looking down the right colon, pulling back, counterclockwise torsion, and the application of suction may all assist in advancing the instrument into the cecum. Changing the patient's position or applying pressure to various points in the abdomen may also be helpful. Once the cecum is reached, the instrument is slowly withdrawn while the colonic parietes are carefully examined. Biopsy and cytologic brushing may be done as appropriate, and colonic contents may be aspirated into a suction trap for examination.

COMPLICATIONS

Perforation is the most common complication of diagnostic colonoscopy. It may result from direct tip pressure, bowing of the shaft of the scope while a large loop is being formed, blowout of a diverticulum secondary to air insufflation, or tearing of an adhesion of the colon to an adjacent structure. The risk of perforation can be minimized by observing the lumen directly as the scope is advanced, avoiding excessive insufflation, and minimizing loop formation. Close attention to patient discomfort is important. If the patient feels poorly after the procedure, an upright chest x-ray, an upright abdominal x-ray, or a lateral decubitus abdominal x-ray should be obtained to determine whether there is any free air, which would indicate a per-

Figure 11 Therapeutic endoscopic retrograde cholangiopancreatography. Self-expanding metal stents may provide effective long-term palliation of malignant biliary obstruction.

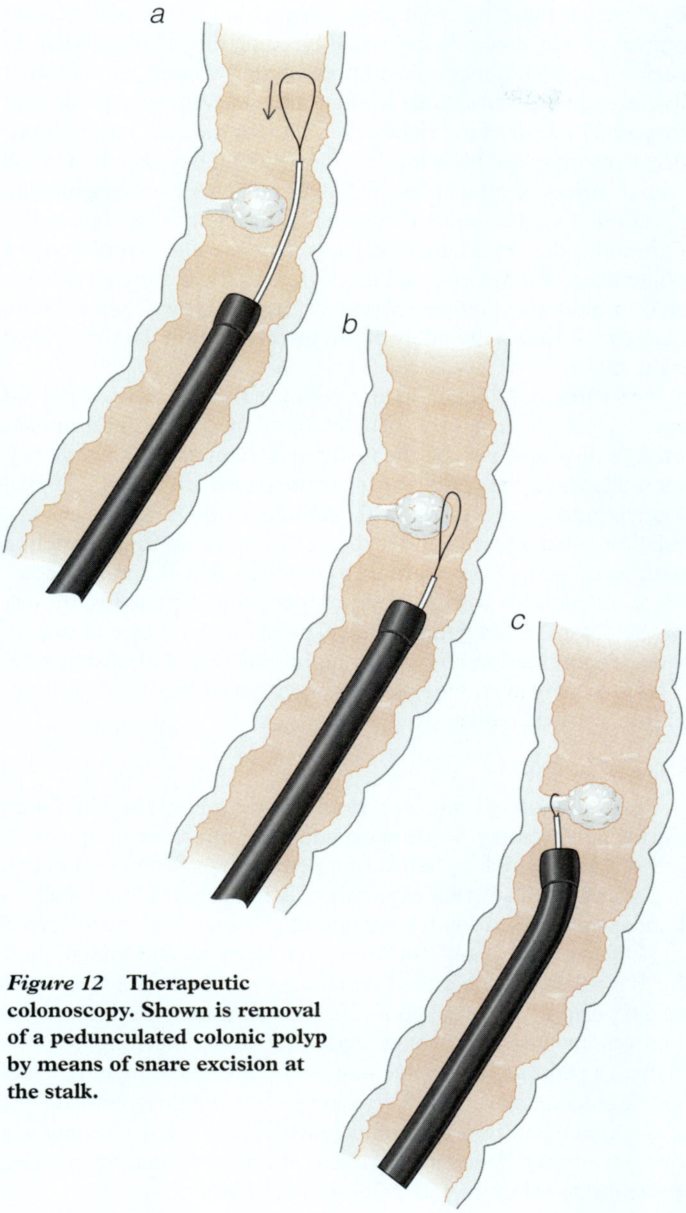

Figure 12 Therapeutic colonoscopy. Shown is removal of a pedunculated colonic polyp by means of snare excision at the stalk.

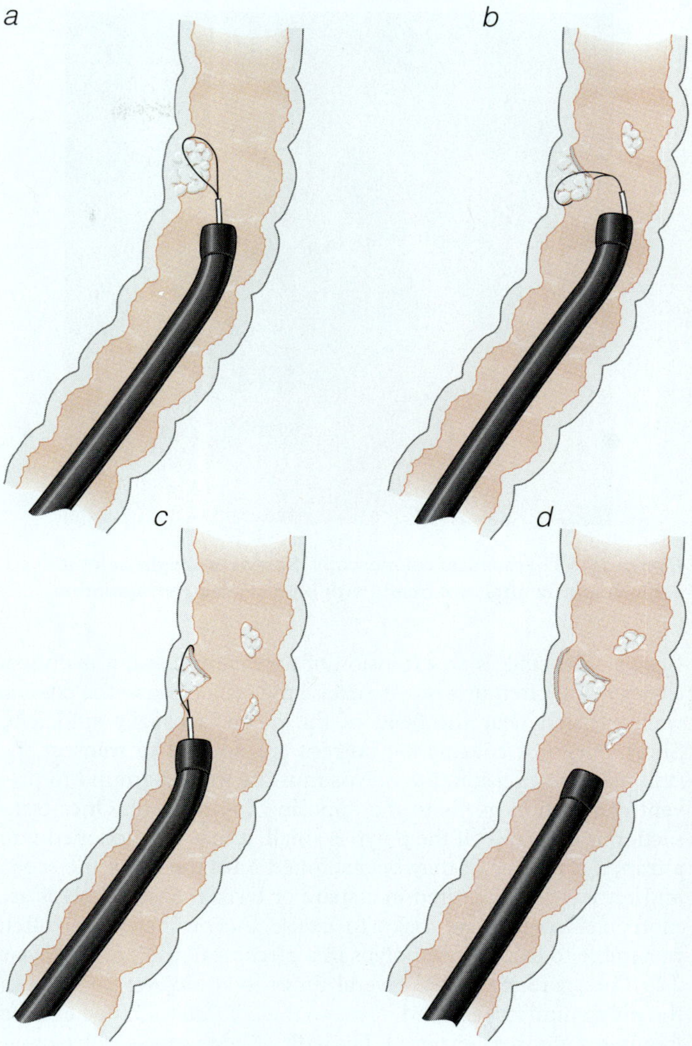

Figure 13 Therapeutic colonoscopy. Illustrated is piecemeal excision of a sessile colonic polyp.

foration. Such situations have been successfully managed by nonoperative means in some cases, but in most cases, prompt operative intervention with primary repair of the perforation is the best approach.

Therapeutic Colonoscopy

By far the most common use of therapeutic colonoscopy is for the excision of polyps. Other applications include control of bleeding, dilation of strictures, and placement of enteral stents.

TECHNIQUE

The development of colonoscopic polypectomy—electrosurgical excision of the polyp with a wire snare—has rendered operative colotomy unnecessary in the management of colonic polyps. Pedunculated polyps are approached by placing the snare over the polyp's head and tightening the loop around the stalk near the junction of the head and the stalk [see Figure 12].

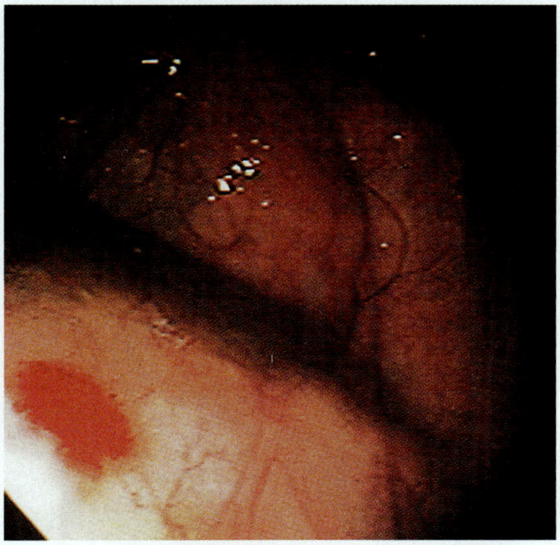

Figure 14 Therapeutic colonoscopy. Shown is an angiodysplasia of the right colon, a frequent cause of lower GI hemorrhage.

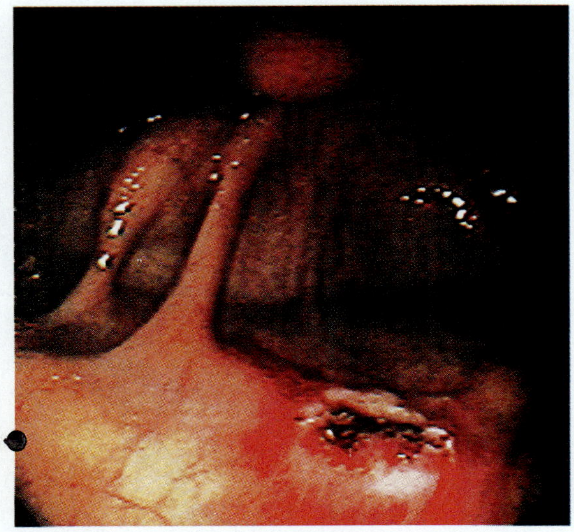

Figure 15 Therapeutic colonoscopy. Shown is a right colonic angiodysplasia after treatment with bipolar electrocoagulation.

Because the stalk is an extension of normal mucosa, it is unnecessary—and often unwise—to excise the stalk close to the colonic wall; excision near the head of the polyp is usually sufficient. Short bursts of coagulating current are applied to transect the stalk. During excision, the polyps must be moved around to prevent conduction burns to the opposing colonic wall. Once transection is complete, if the polyp is small, it may be suctioned into a trap; if it is large, it may be suctioned onto the tip of the scope and retrieved or captured in a snare or basket. Sessile polyps are more challenging and risky to excise. Accordingly, it is often preferable to excise such polyps in a piecemeal fashion [see Figure 13]. The snare is applied several times to successive portions of the polyp until it is excised down to the colonic wall. The excised fragments are then retrieved. Difficult or large sessile polyps may be elevated before excision by injecting epinephrine solution or saline submucosally into the polyp or the surrounding tissue. This maneuver makes transmural injury less likely.

Although the use of colonoscopy to define the site of colonic bleeding is commonplace, its use to treat such bleeding is not. Diverticular bleeding often stops when colonoscopy is done, and only in rare instances is the actual bleeding diverticulum seen. In such cases, injection of epinephrine solution around the mouth of the offending diverticulum is often effective. Angiodysplasias are frequently found in the right colon, though they are rarely identified while they are bleeding [see Figure 14]. They may be treated with a variety of modalities, including bipolar electrocoagulation, injection of a sclerosant solution, and laser therapy [see Figure 15]. Currently, the argon plasma coagulator is often employed for obliteration of these lesions. This device has the advantage of being able to obliterate angiodysplasias with minimal wall penetration, thereby increasing the safety of this intervention in the thin-walled right colon.

Strictures may occur in the colon, as in the rest of the GI tract. Colonic strictures usually develop at an anastomosis, though they may also be the result of ischemia. Hydrostatic balloon dilation is very effective in treating such strictures. The balloon is introduced through the lumen of the endoscope, and dilation is carried out under direct vision, often in conjunction with fluoroscopic observation to confirm that dilation is complete. In patients with fully or almost fully obstructing tumors of the colon, self-expanding metal stents may be placed to provide decompression and at least temporary relief of obstruction. This step may avert emergency surgery or, if the tumor is inoperable, provide palliation.

COMPLICATIONS

Perforation may occur as a result of transmural thermal injury during polypectomy. Some perforations are immediately apparent, but others may not be noticed for several days. When perforation is documented, surgical exploration is indicated. Occasionally, a patient may present with fever and abdominal tenderness several days after polypectomy but show no free air on abdominal films. Such a patient may have a thermal injury to the bowel wall or so-called postpolypectomy syndrome and can usually be treated with intravenous fluids, antibiotics, and observation. Bleeding from the stalk of a pedunculated polyp may occur after excision; it may present immediately or may be delayed until the coagulum on the stalk separates 3 to 5 days after polypectomy. Such bleeding is a rare occurrence. When it does occur, it can be treated by injecting epinephrine solution (1:10,000) into the stalk.

Recommended Reading

Cotton PB, Williams CB: Practical Gastrointestinal Endoscopy, 3rd ed. Blackwell Scientific, Oxford, 1990

Ponsky JL: Atlas of Surgical Endoscopy. Mosby–Year Book, St. Louis, 1992

Schrock T: Colon and rectum: diagnostic techniques. Shackelford's Surgery of the Alimentary Tract. Vol 4: Colon and Anorectum, 3rd ed. Condon R, Ed. Philadelphia, WB Saunders Co, 1991, p 22

Schuman BM, Sugawa C: Diagnostic endoscopy of upper gastrointestinal bleeding. Gastrointestinal bleeding. Sugawa C, Schuman BM, Lucas CE, Eds. Igaku Shoin, New York, 1992, p 222

Venu RP, Geenen JE: Overview of endoscopic sphincterotomy for common bile duct stone. Endoscopic Approach to Biliary Stones. Kozarek RA, Ed. Gastrointest Endosc Clin North Am 1:3, 1991

Acknowledgment

Figures 2, 4a, 4b, 4c, 5, 6, 9, 12, and 13   Tom Moore.

48 ESOPHAGEAL PROCEDURES: MINIMALLY INVASIVE APPROACHES

Marco G. Patti, M.D., *and Carlos A. Pellegrini*, M.D.

The advent and development of minimally invasive techniques has revolutionized the treatment of many diseases, including those that affect the esophagus. During the 1970s and the 1980s, operations for esophageal disorders were often withheld or delayed in favor of less effective forms of treatment in an effort to prevent the postoperative discomfort, the long hospital stay, and the recovery time associated with open surgical procedures. For instance, pneumatic dilatation became the first line of treatment for achalasia, and long-term medical therapy became the preferred approach to gastroesophageal reflux disease, even though studies had shown that surgical management was clearly superior for both diseases.[1,2] Today, however, it is known that the thoracoscopic and laparoscopic procedures currently performed to treat these conditions yield results comparable to those achieved with open procedures while leading to minimal postoperative discomfort, a shorter hospital stay, and a faster return to work.[3-6] Consequently, surgery should be the first line of treatment for achalasia, and it should be considered at an earlier stage in the management of patients with gastroesophageal reflux disease.

In essence, the technical steps in minimally invasive operations on the esophagus are the same as those in the corresponding open procedures. The execution, however, is different: the video-endoscopic operating systems currently in use impose significant perceptual and motor limitations, such as loss of stereopsis, reduced tactile feedback, and decreased range of motion for the instruments. Because of these limitations, most surgeons find laparoscopic and thoracoscopic surgery more challenging than open surgery, and they tend to encounter complications more frequently. Some complications, such as trocar injuries, are unique to the minimally invasive approach; others occur with both open and minimally invasive approaches but tend to be more common with laparoscopy and thoracoscopy.[7]

In what follows, we do not address the standard open esophageal procedures, which are, on the whole, well known and familiar. Instead, we focus on minimally invasive techniques for the treatment of abnormal gastroesophageal reflux and motility disorders of the esophagus.

Laparoscopic Nissen Fundoplication

PREOPERATIVE EVALUATION

All patients being considered for laparoscopic fundoplication to treat gastroesophageal reflux disease should undergo a thorough workup so that the surgeon can tailor the operation to the pathophysiology of each patient's disease.

An upper gastrointestinal series is useful for diagnosing and characterizing an existing hiatal hernia. The size of the hiatal hernia helps predict how difficult it will be to reduce the esophagogastric junction below the diaphragm. In addition, large hiatal hernias are associated with more severe disturbances of esophageal peristalsis and esophageal acid clearance.[8] Esophagograms are also useful for determining the location, shape, and size of a stricture and detecting a short esophagus.

Endoscopy helps establish the degree of esophagitis (if present), the presence or absence of Barrett's esophagus, and the presence or absence of gastric or duodenal pathology.

Esophageal manometry not only provides valuable information about the competence of the lower esophageal sphincter (LES) but also is of key importance for assessing the function of the esophageal body and identifying abnormalities that might influence the choice of procedure.[9,10] If, for example, manometry shows esophageal peristalsis to be normal, a 360° wrap should be performed; this is the most effective way of restoring the competence of the cardia. If, however, the amplitude of peristalsis is less than 40 mm Hg or there are abnormalities in the morphology and propagation of the peristaltic waves, a partial wrap should be performed to prevent postoperative dysphagia and gas bloat syndrome.[9,10]

Because symptoms, radiographic tests, and endoscopy have a sensitivity of only 60 to 70 percent in the diagnosis of gastroesophageal reflux disease, 24-hour pH monitoring should be done before surgical treatment is considered.[11,12] This test quantifies the amount of reflux, determines the correlation between episodes of reflux and symptoms, and provides useful information on the ability of the esophagus to clear gastric refluxate.[13,14] In addition, ambulatory pH monitoring provides baseline data that may prove extremely useful after operation in patients whose symptoms do not respond to the procedure.

OPERATIVE PLANNING

The patient is placed under general anesthesia and intubated with a single-lumen endotracheal tube. Abdominal wall relaxation is ensured by the administration of a nondepolarizing muscle relaxant, the action of which is rapidly reversed at the end of the operation. Adequate muscle relaxation is essential because increased abdominal wall compliance allows increased pneumoperitoneum, which yields better exposure. An orogastric tube is inserted at the beginning of the operation to keep the stomach decompressed; it is removed at the end of the procedure.

The patient is placed in a steep reverse Trendelenburg's position, with the legs extended on stirrups. The surgeon stands between the patient's legs. To keep the patient from sliding as a result of the steep position used during the operation, a bean bag is inflated under the patient [*see Figure 1*], and the knees are flexed only 20° to 30°. A Foley catheter is inserted at the begin-

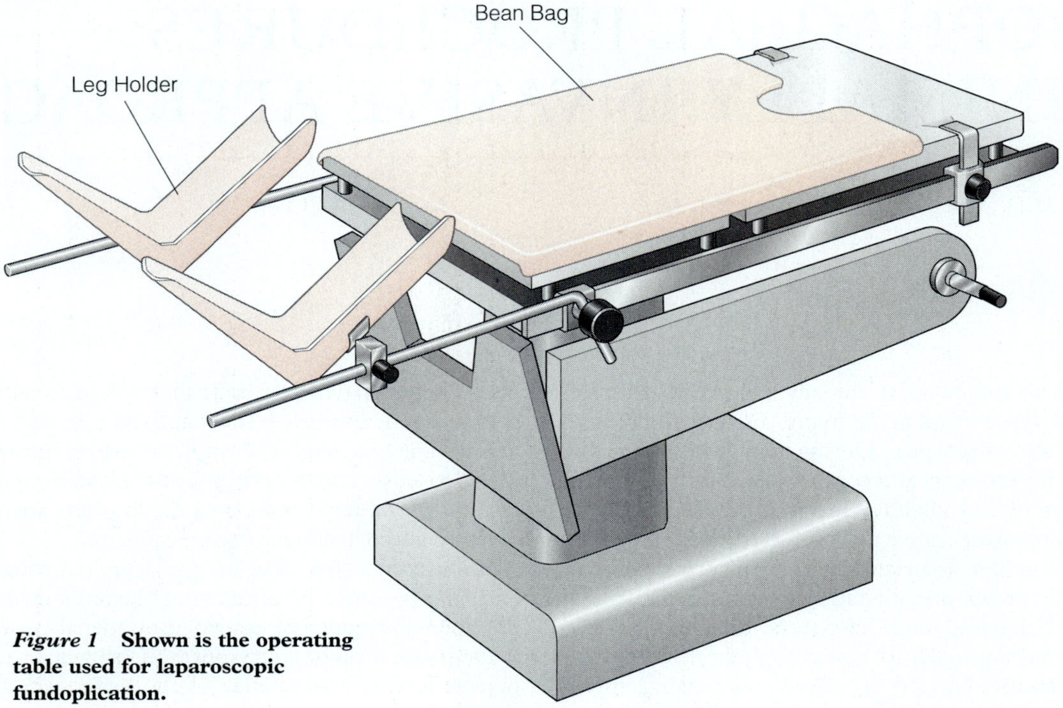

Figure 1 Shown is the operating table used for laparoscopic fundoplication.

ning of the procedure and usually is removed in the postoperative period. Because increased abdominal pressure from pneumoperitoneum and the steep reverse Trendelenburg's position decrease venous return, pneumatic compression stockings are always used as prophylaxis against deep vein thrombosis.

The equipment required for a laparoscopic Nissen fundoplication includes five 10 mm trocars, a 30° laparoscope, a hook cautery, and various other instruments [*see Table 1*]. In addition, we use a three-chip camera system that is separate from the laparoscope.

OPERATIVE TECHNIQUE

In patients with good esophageal motility, we advocate performing a 360° wrap of the gastric fundus around the lower esophagus as described by Nissen, but we always take down the short gastric vessels to achieve what is called a floppy fundoplication. This type of wrap is very effective in controlling gastroesophageal reflux.[1] The operation can be divided into nine key steps as follows.

Step 1: Insertion of the Trocars

Five 10 mm trocars are used for the operation [*see Figure 2*]. Port A is placed about 20 to 25 cm below the xiphoid process, at a point that, in adults of medium body size, is usually 3 to 5 cm above the umbilicus; it can also be placed slightly (2 to 3 cm) to the left of the midline to be in line with the hiatus. This port is used for insertion of the scope. Port B is placed at the same level as port A, but in the left midclavicular line. It is used for insertion of the Babcock clamp; insertion of a grasper to hold the Penrose drain once it is in place surrounding the esophagus; or insertion of the clip applier, the ultrasonic coagulating shears (LaparoSonic Coagulating Shears [LCS], Ultracision Inc., Smithfield, Rhode Island), or both to take down the short gastric vessels. Port C is placed at the same level as the previous two ports but in the right midclavicular line. It is used for insertion of the fan retractor, the purpose of which is to lift the lateral segment of the left lobe of the liver and expose the esophagogastric junction. We do not divide the left triangular ligament. The fan retractor can be held in place by a self-retaining system fixed to the operating table. Ports D and E are placed as high as possible under the costal margin and about 5 to 6 cm to the right and the left of the midline, so that they are about 15 cm from the esophageal hiatus; in addition, they should be placed in such a way that their axes form an angle of 60° to 120°. These ports are used for insertion of the graspers, the electrocautery, and the suturing instruments.

Troubleshooting A common mistake is to place the ports too low in the abdomen, thereby making the operation more

---

Table 1 Instrumentation for Laparoscopic Nissen Fundoplication

Five 10 mm trocars
30° scope
Graspers
Babcock clamp
L-shaped hook cautery with suction-irrigation capacity
Scissors
Laparoscopic clip applier
LaparoSonic Coagulating Shears (LCS®) (Ultracision Inc., Smithfield, RI)
Fan retractor
Needle holder
Penrose drain
2-0 silk sutures
56 French esophageal bougie

difficult. If port C is too low, the fan retractor will not retract the lateral segment of the left lobe of the liver well, and the esophagogastric junction will not be exposed. If port B is too low, the Babcock clamp will not reach the esophagogastric junction, and when the LCS or the clip applier is placed through the same port, it will not reach the upper short gastric vessels. If ports D and E are too low, the dissection at the beginning of the case and the suturing at the end are problematic.

Other mistakes of positioning must be avoided as well. It is important not to place port C too medially, because the fan retractor may clash with the left-hand instrument; the gallbladder fossa is a good landmark for positioning this port. Port A must be placed with extreme caution in the supraumbilical area: its insertion site is just above the aorta, before its bifurcation. Accordingly, we recommend initially inflating the abdomen to a pressure of 20 mm Hg just for placement of port A; increasing the distance between the abdominal wall and the aorta will reduce the risk of aortic injury. We also recommend directing the port toward the coccyx. A Hasson cannula can be used in this location, particularly if the patient has already had one or more midline incisions. In addition, cutting under direct vision to place the trocar can now be accomplished by means of the Visiport (United States Surgical Corporation, Norwalk, Connecticut), which one of us (C.A.P.) always uses for the first insertion site. Maintaining the proper angle (60° to 120°) between the axes of the two suturing instruments inserted through ports D and E is also important: if the angle is smaller, the instruments will cover part of the operating field, whereas if it is larger, depth perception may be impaired. Finally, if a trocar is not in the ideal position, it is better to insert another one than to operate through an inconveniently placed port.

If the surgeon spears the epigastric vessels with a trocar, bleeding will occur, in which case there are two options. The first option is to pull the port out, insert a 24 French Foley catheter with a 30 ml balloon through the site, inflate the balloon, and apply traction with a clamp. The advantage of this maneuver is that the vessel need not be sutured; the disadvantage is that the surgeon must then choose another insertion site. At the end of the case, the balloon is deflated. If some bleeding is still present, it must be controlled with sutures placed from outside under direct vision. The second option is to use a long needle with a suture (e.g., the Endoclose, United States Surgical Corporation, Norwalk, Connecticut), with which one can rapidly place two U-shaped stitches, one above the clamp and one below. The suture is tied outside over a sponge and left in place for two or three days.

Step 2: Division of the Gastrohepatic Ligament; Identification of the Right Crus of the Diaphragm and the Posterior Vagus Nerve

Once the ports are in place, the gastrohepatic ligament is divided. Dissection begins above the caudate lobe of the liver, where this ligament usually is very thin, and continues toward the diaphragm until the right crus is identified. The crus is then separated from the right side of the esophagus by blunt dissection, and the posterior vagus nerve is identified. The right crus is dissected inferiorly toward the junction with the left crus.

Troubleshooting An accessory left hepatic artery originating from the left gastric artery is frequently encountered in the gastrohepatic ligament. On the rare occasions when the pres-

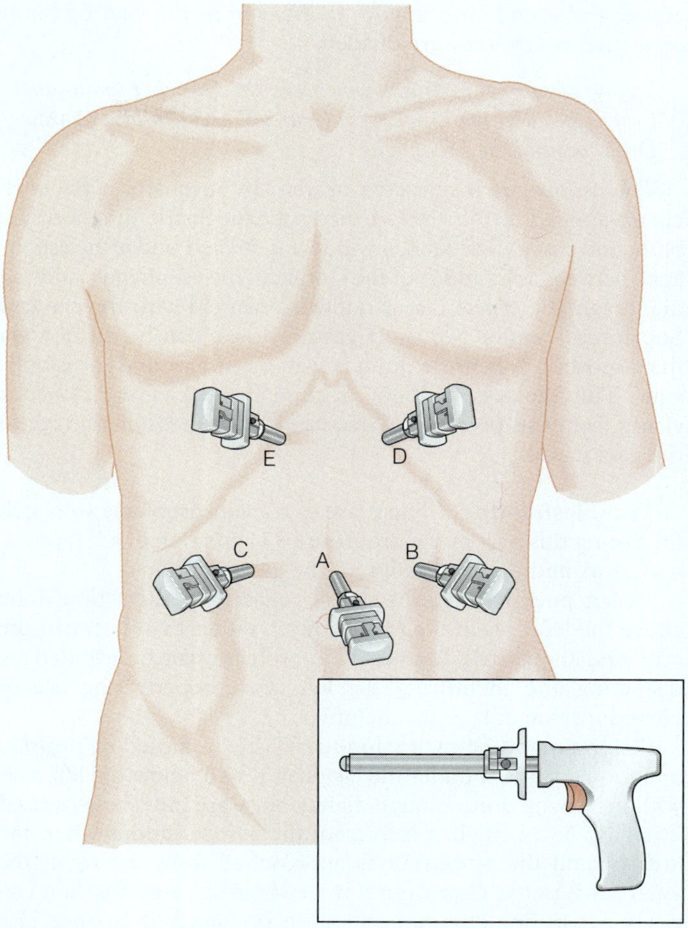

Figure 2 Illustrated is the recommended placement of the trocars for laparoscopic Nissen fundoplication.

ence of this vessel creates problems of exposure, we divide it; to date, its division has not caused problems. When dissecting the right crus from the esophagus, we try to use the electrocautery with particular caution. Because the monopolar current tends to spread laterally, the posterior vagus nerve can sustain damage simply from being in proximity to the device, even when there is no direct contact. The risk of neurapraxia can be reduced by using the cut mode rather than the coagulation mode when the electrocautery is close to the nerve. The cut mode has problems of its own, however, and is not recommended in most laparoscopic procedures. A better alternative is to use bipolar scissors.

Step 3: Division of the Peritoneum and the Phrenoesophageal Membrane above the Esophagus; Identification of the Left Crus of the Diaphragm and the Anterior Vagus Nerve

The peritoneum and the phrenoesophageal membrane above the esophagus are divided with the electrocautery, and the anterior vagus nerve is identified. The left crus of the diaphragm is dissected downward toward the junction with the right crus.

Troubleshooting During this part of the dissection, pains should be taken not to damage the anterior vagus nerve or the esophageal wall. To this end, the nerve should be left attached to the esophageal wall, and the peritoneum and the phrenoesophageal membrane should be lifted from the wall by blunt dissection before they are divided.

Step 4: Creation of a Window between the Gastric Fundus, the Esophagus, and the Esophageal Crura; Placement of a Penrose Drain around the Esophagus

The esophagus is retracted upward by means of a Babcock clamp applied at the level of the esophagogastric junction. Via blunt and sharp dissection, a window is created under the esophagus between the fundus of the stomach, the esophagus, and the diaphragmatic crura. The window is enlarged with the cautery. Sometimes, one or two short gastric vessels can be divided via this exposure. A Penrose drain is then passed around the esophagus. This drain is used for traction instead of the Babcock clamp from this point on to decrease the chances of damage to the gastric wall.

Troubleshooting There are two main problems to watch for during this part of the procedure: (1) creation of a left pneumothorax and (2) perforation of the gastric fundus.

A left pneumothorax is usually caused by dissection done above the left crus in the mediastinum rather than between the crus and the gastric fundus. This problem can be avoided by dissecting and identifying the left crus properly; the use of curved instruments is also helpful.

Perforation of the gastric fundus is usually caused by pushing a blunt instrument under the esophagus and below the left crus without having done enough dissection. Care must be exercised in taking down small vessels from the gastric fundus when the area behind the esophagus is approached from the right: the anatomy is not as clear from this viewpoint, and perforation can easily occur. Sometimes, perforation is caused by the use of a monopolar electrocautery for dissection. An electrocautery burn can go unrecognized during dissection and manifest itself in the form of a leak during the first 48 hours after operation.

Step 5: Division of the Short Gastric Vessels

The clip applier or the LCS is introduced through port B. A grasper is introduced by the surgeon through port D, and an assistant applies traction on the greater curvature of the stomach through port E. Dissection begins at the level of the middle portion of the gastric body and continues upward until the most proximal short gastric vessel is divided and the Penrose drain is reached.

Troubleshooting Again, there are two main problems to watch for during this part of the procedure: (1) bleeding, either from the gastric vessels or from the spleen, and (2) damage to the gastric wall.

Bleeding from the gastric vessels is usually caused by excessive traction or by division of a vessel when the clips are not completely occluding the vessel on both sides. Vessels up to 5 mm in diameter can be taken down with the LCS; this process requires about half of the amount of time needed when only clips are used. The lower blade has a sharp, oscillating inferior edge that must always be kept in view to prevent damage to other structures (e.g., the pancreas, the splenic artery and vein, and the spleen).

Damage to the gastric wall can be caused by a burn from the electrocautery used to dissect between vessels or by traction applied via the graspers or the Babcock clamp.

Step 6: Closure of the Crura

The diaphragmatic crura are closed with interrupted 2-0 silk sutures on a curved needle; the sutures are tied intracorporeally. Exposure during this phase is provided by retracting the esophagus upward and toward the patient's left with the Penrose drain. The lens of the 30° laparoscope is angled slightly to the left by moving the light cable of the scope to the patient's right. The first stitch should be placed just above the junction of the two crura. Additional stitches are placed 1 cm apart, and a space of about 1 cm is left between the uppermost stitch and the esophagus.

Troubleshooting Pains must be taken not to spear the posterior wall of the esophagus with either the tip or the back of the needle. The use of the Endostitch (United States Surgical Corporation, Norwalk, Connecticut) eliminates this hazard and expedites this step. We do not place the bougie inside the esophagus during this part of the procedure; to do so would limit the space available for suturing.

Step 7: Insertion of a Bougie into the Esophagus and through the Esophagogastric Junction

The esophageal stethoscope and the orogastric tube are removed, and a 56 French bougie is inserted by the anesthesiologist. The bougie is passed through the esophagogastric junction under the view provided by the laparoscope. The crura must be snug around the esophagus but not too tight: a closed grasper should be able to slide easily between the esophagus and the crura.

Troubleshooting The most worrisome complication during this step is perforation of the esophagus. This can be prevented by lubricating the bougie and instructing the anesthesiologist to advance the bougie slowly and to stop if any resistance is encountered. In addition, it is essential to remove any instruments from the esophagogastric junction and to open the Penrose drain; these measures prevent the creation of an angle between the stomach and the esophagus, which can increase the likelihood of perforation. The position of the bougie can be confirmed by pressing with a grasper over the esophagus, which will feel full when the bougie is in place.

Step 8: Wrapping of the Gastric Fundus around the Lower Esophagus

The gastric fundus is gently pulled under the esophagus with the graspers. The left and right sides of the fundus are wrapped above the fat pad (which lies above the esophagogastric junction) and held together in place with a Babcock clamp introduced through port B. (The Penrose drain should be removed at this point because it is in the way.) Usually, three 2-0 silk sutures are used to secure the two ends of the wrap to each other. The first stitch does not include the esophagus and is used for traction; the second and the third include a bite of the esophageal muscle. Two coronal stitches are then placed between the top of the wrap and the esophagus, one on the right and one on the left. Finally, two additional sutures are placed between the right side of the wrap and the closed crura. It is important to pass the bougie into the stomach after the first stitch is placed to gauge the size of the wrap. If the wrap seems at all tight, the stitch is removed and repositioned more laterally.

After learning of instances in which the vena cava was injured while the surgeon was looking for the right crus at the beginning of the operation, one of us (C.A.P.) began using a different method—the so-called left crus approach. In this approach, the operation begins with identification of the left crus of the diaphragm and division of the peritoneum and the phrenoesophageal membrane overlying it. The next step is division of the short gastric vessels, starting 8 to 10 cm below the insertion of the phrenogastric ligament and continuing upward to join the area of the previous dissection. When the fundus has been thoroughly mobilized, the peritoneum is divided from the left to the right crus, and the right crus is dissected downward to expose the junction of the right and left crura. With this technique, the vena cava is never at risk. In addition, the branches of the anterior vagus nerve and the left gastric artery are less exposed to danger.

Troubleshooting To determine whether the wrap is going to be floppy, the surgeon must deliver the fundus of the stomach under the esophagus, making sure that the origins of the short gastric vessels that have been transected are seen. Essentially, the posterior wall of the fundus is being used for the wrap. If the wrap remains to the right of the esophagus without retracting back to the left, then it is floppy, and suturing can proceed. If not, the surgeon must make sure that the upper short gastric vessels have been transected. If tension is still present after these maneuvers, it is probably best to perform a partial wrap [see Partial Fundoplication (Guarner Fundoplication), *below*].

Damage to the gastric wall may occur during the delivery of the fundus. Atraumatic graspers must be used, and the gastric fundus must be pulled gently and passed from one grasper to the other. Sometimes, it is helpful to push the gastric fundus under the esophagus from the left. The wrap should measure no more than 2 to 2.5 cm in length and, as noted, should be done with no more than three sutures. The first stitch is usually the lowest one; it must be placed just above the fat pad where the esophagogastric junction is thought to be.

If the anesthesiologist observes that the peak airway pressure has increased (because of a pneumothorax) or that neck emphysema is present (because of pneumomediastinum), the pneumoperitoneum should be reduced from 15 mm Hg to 7 to 8 mm Hg until the end of the procedure. Pneumomediastinum tends to resolve without intervention within a few hours of the end of the procedure. Small pneumothoraces (usually on the left side) tend to reabsorb spontaneously, and thus, the insertion of a chest tube is unnecessary. Larger pneumothoraces (> 20 percent) call for the insertion of a small chest tube (18 to 20 French).

Step 9: Final Inspection and Removal of the Instruments and Ports from the Abdomen

After hemostasis is obtained, the instruments and the ports are removed from the abdomen under direct vision.

Troubleshooting If any areas of oozing were observed during the procedure, they should be irrigated and dried with sponges rolled into a cigarettelike shape before the ports are removed. In addition, if some grounds for concern remain, the oozing areas should be examined after the pneumoperitoneum is decreased to an intra-abdominal pressure of 7 to 8 mm Hg to abolish the tamponading effect exerted by the high intra-abdominal pressure.

All the ports should be removed from the abdomen under direct vision so that any bleeding from the abdominal wall can be readily detected. Such bleeding is easily controlled, either from inside or from outside.

POSTOPERATIVE COMPLICATIONS

A feared complication of laparoscopic Nissen fundoplication is esophageal or gastric perforation. As noted, this complication is caused by traction applied with the Babcock clamp or a grasper to the esophagus or the stomach (particularly when the stomach is pulled under the esophagus) or by inadvertent electrocautery burns during any part of the dissection. A leak will manifest itself during the first 48 hours. Peritoneal signs will be noted if the spillage is limited to the abdomen; shortness of breath and a pleural effusion will be noted if spillage also occurs in the chest. The site of the leak should always be confirmed by a contrast study with barium or a water-soluble contrast agent. Perforation is best handled by means of laparotomy and direct repair. If a perforation is detected intraoperatively, it may be closed laparoscopically.

About 50 percent of patients experience mild dysphagia postoperatively. This problem usually resolves after four to six weeks, during which period patients receive pain medications in an elixir form and are advised to avoid eating meat and bread. If, however, dysphagia persists beyond this period, one or more of the following causes is responsible.

1. Choice of the wrong procedure. In patients who have abnormal esophageal peristalsis (amplitude of peristalsis in the distal esophagus less than 40 mm Hg; abnormal morphology or abnormal propagation of the peristaltic waves), a partial wrap should be performed. A 360° wrap will control reflux, but it will also cause postoperative dysphagia and gas bloat syndrome.
2. A wrap that is too tight or too long. The wrap should be performed without tension over a 56 French bougie. The total length of the wrap should not exceed 2.5 cm.
3. Lateral torsion with corkscrew effect. If the wrap rotates toward the right (either because of tension from intact short gastric vessels or because the fundus is small), a corkscrew effect is created.
4. A wrap made with the body of the stomach rather than the fundus. The relaxation of the lower esophageal sphincter and the gastric fundus is controlled by vasointestinal polypeptide and nitric oxide[15,16]; after fundoplication, the two structures relax simultaneously with swallowing. If part of the body of the stomach rather than the fundus is used for the wrap, it will not relax as the LES does on arrival of the food bolus.

If the wrap slips into the chest, the patient becomes unable to eat and prone to vomiting. A chest radiograph shows a gastric bubble above the diaphragm, and the diagnosis is confirmed by means of a barium swallow. This problem can be prevented by using coronal sutures and by ensuring that the crura are closed securely.

Paraesophageal hernia may occur if the crura have not been closed or if the closure is too loose. In our view, closure of the crura not only is essential for preventing paraesophageal hernia but also is important from a physiologic point of view. Multiple studies have shown that the real sphincteric mechanism is formed by the LES in conjunction with the esophageal crura: the crura work as a kind of extrinsic sphincter, protecting specifically against stress reflux.[17,18] Sometimes, it is possible to reduce the stomach and close the crura laparoscopically. More often, however, because the crural opening is very tight and the gastric wall is edematous, laparoscopic repair is impossible and laparotomy is preferable.

OUTCOME EVALUATION

Outcome evaluation of laparoscopic Nissen fundoplication is discussed elsewhere (see below) in conjunction with outcome evaluation of laparoscopic partial fundoplication.

Partial Fundoplication (Guarner Fundoplication)

PREOPERATIVE EVALUATION AND OPERATIVE PLANNING

Preoperative evaluation and operative planning are essentially the same for partial (or Guarner) fundoplication as for Nissen fundoplication.

OPERATIVE TECHNIQUE

The first seven steps in a Guarner fundoplication are identical to the first seven in a Nissen fundoplication. The wrap, however, differs in that it extends around only 240° to 280° of the esophageal circumference. Once the gastric fundus is delivered under the esophagus, the two sides are not approximated over the esophagus. Instead, 80° to 120° of the anterior esophagus is left uncovered, and each of the two sides of the wrap (right and left) is separately affixed to the esophagus with three 2-0 silk sutures, with each stitch including the muscle layer of the esophageal wall. The remaining stitches (i.e., the coronal stitches and those between the right side of the wrap and the closed crura) are identical to those placed in a Nissen fundoplication.

In patients with poor esophageal body function, a partial wrap is the procedure of choice. In our experience and the experiences of others,[10] this procedure controls gastroesophageal reflux and prevents postoperative dysphagia and gas bloat syndrome.

OUTCOME EVALUATION

When we analyzed the results of our first 70 laparoscopic fundoplications for gastroesophageal reflux disease (including both Nissen and Guarner procedures), we found that the average operating room time was about 190 ± 45 minutes. As we gained more experience and began using the LCS to take down the short gastric vessels, the average operating time decreased: it is now some 45 to 60 minutes shorter. We start patients on a soft mechanical diet on the morning of postoperative day 1 and usually discharge them after 23 to 48 hours. The recovery time for the operation is about seven to 10 days.

At 18 months' follow-up, preoperative symptoms have resolved completely in about 90 percent of patients and have become significantly less severe in the remainder.

Left Thoracoscopic Myotomy

It has been demonstrated that minimally invasive surgical procedures for primary esophageal motility disorders (achalasia, diffuse esophageal spasm, and nutcracker esophagus) yield results that are comparable to those of open procedures but are associated with less postoperative pain and perhaps with a shorter recovery time.[4,5,19,20] In addition, we have shown that thoracoscopic esophageal myotomy is more effective than medical therapy in the treatment of these disorders.[6]

A left thoracoscopic myotomy is the procedure of choice for patients with achalasia and for patients with diffuse esophageal spasm or nutcracker esophagus involving the lower half of the esophagus.

PREOPERATIVE EVALUATION

All patients who are being considered as candidates for a left thoracoscopic myotomy should undergo a thorough and careful evaluation to establish the diagnosis and characterize the disease.[6]

An upper gastrointestinal series is a useful diagnostic test. A characteristic so-called bird beak is usually seen in patients with achalasia. A dilated, sigmoid esophagus may be present in patients with long-standing achalasia. This is a very important finding: myotomy often fails to relieve dysphagia in these patients, and an esophagectomy should therefore be done instead. A corkscrew esophagus in often seen in patients with diffuse esophageal spasm.

Endoscopy is valuable for ruling out the presence of a tumor of the esophagogastric junction, which can mimic the radiographic and manometric manifestations of achalasia. In addition, it is important for ruling out esophagitis because abnormal gastroesophageal reflux can mimic the manometric manifestations of diffuse esophageal spasm or nutcracker esophagus. If the presence of abnormal reflux is confirmed by prolonged pH monitoring, medical or surgical therapy must be directed against reflux.

Esophageal manometry is one of the most useful tests for establishing the definitive diagnosis of a primary esophageal motility disorder. In addition, it is of key importance in ascertaining how much of the esophagus is affected, which in turn determines the surgical approach (i.e., left myotomy versus right myotomy). For example, in patients who have achalasia or diffuse esophageal spasm that is limited to the lower half of the esophagus, we perform a left thoracoscopic myotomy. In patients with nutcracker esophagus involving the entire length of the esophagus, we prefer a long thoracoscopic myotomy performed through the right chest and extending from the diaphragm to the thoracic inlet.

Ambulatory pH monitoring should always be done in patients who have undergone pneumatic dilatation. In our experience, abnormal gastroesophageal reflux develops in about 30 percent of these patients.[21] In patients with achalasia who still complain of dysphagia after pneumatic dilatation and in whom abnormal gastroesophageal reflux has developed, we prefer a laparoscopic approach, which allows a partial fundoplication (i.e., a Dor fundoplication, which is a 180° anterior fundoplication) to be added to the esophageal myotomy.

OPERATIVE PLANNING

The patient is placed under general anesthesia and intubated with a double-lumen endotracheal tube so that the left lung can be deflated during the procedure.

The patient is placed in the right lateral decubitus position over an inflated bean bag, as for a left thoracotomy.

The instrumentation for this procedure is similar to that for a laparoscopic Nissen or Guarner fundoplication. Instead of conventional trocars, we use four or five thoracoports with blunt obturators because insufflation of the thoracic cavity is not required. The myotomy can be performed with either a monopolar hook cautery, bipolar scissors, or an ultrasonically

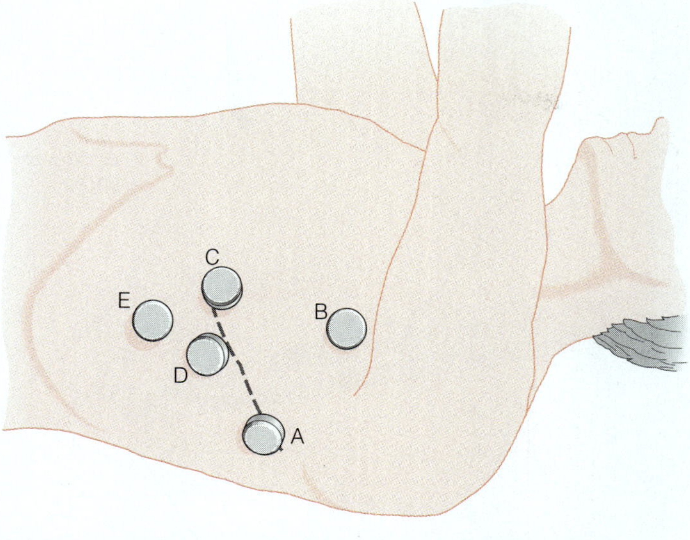

Figure 3 Illustrated is the recommended placement of the thoracoports for a left thoracoscopic esophageal myotomy.

activated scalpel (e.g., the Harmonic Scalpel, Ultracision Inc., Smithfield, Rhode Island). A 30° scope and a 45° scope are essential instruments for the performance of thoracoscopic procedures. In addition, an endoscope is used for intraoperative endoscopy.

OPERATIVE TECHNIQUE

Step 1: Insertion of the Ports

Five ports are usually placed [see Figure 3]. Port A is inserted in the sixth intercostal space about 1.5 to 2 in. behind the posterior axillary line. This port is used for the 30° scope. Port B is placed in the third intercostal space about 0.5 to 1.0 in. anterior to the posterior axillary line. This port is used for the lung retractor. Port C is placed in the sixth intercostal space in the anterior axillary line. It is used for insertion of a grasper. Port D is placed in the seventh intercostal space in the midaxillary line. It is used for insertion of the instrument used for the myotomy. Port E is placed in the eighth intercostal space between the anterior axillary line and the midaxillary line. This port is optional: it is needed in about 30 percent of cases to allow the surgeon to obtain further exposure of the esophagogastric junction by retracting the diaphragm.

Troubleshooting A common mistake is to insert port A too anteriorly. This port must be placed well beyond the posterior axillary line to provide the best angle for the 30° scope. Often, the other ports are placed one or two intercostal spaces too high. This mistake hampers the performance of the most delicate portion of the operation, the myotomy of the distal portion of the esophagus and the stomach.

Sometimes, bleeding occurs from the chest wall as a result of the insertion of the ports. The dripping blood will obscure the operating field, and consequently, it is essential to stop the bleeding before the intrathoracic portion of the procedure is begun. Bleeding can be stopped either by using the cautery from the inside or by applying a stitch from the outside if an intercostal vessel has been damaged.

Step 2: Retraction of the Left Lung and Division of the Inferior Pulmonary Ligament

Once the ports are in place, the deflated left lung is retracted cephalad with a fan retractor introduced through port B. This maneuver places tension on the inferior pulmonary ligament, which is then divided. After the ligament is divided, the fan retractor can be held in place by a self-retaining system fixed to the operating table.

Troubleshooting Before the inferior pulmonary ligament is divided, the inferior pulmonary vein must be identified to prevent a life-threatening injury to this vessel. If oxygen saturation decreases, particularly in patients with lung disease, the retractor should be removed and the lung inflated intermittently.

Step 3: Division of the Mediastinal Pleura and Dissection of the Periesophageal Tissues

The mediastinal pleura is divided, and the tissues overlying the esophageal wall are dissected until the wall of the esophagus is visible. This maneuver varies in difficulty depending on the width of the space between the aorta and the pericardium (which sometimes is very small) and on the size and shape of the esophagus. Large (sigmoid) esophagi tend to curve to the right, which makes identification of the wall difficult. If the esophagus is not immediately apparent, it can be easily identified in the groove between the heart and the aorta by means of transillumination provided by an endoscope [see Figure 4].

Troubleshooting The endoscope placed inside the esophagus at the beginning of the procedure plays an important role. In the early stages of the procedure, it allows identification of the esophagus by transillumination. When the light intensity of the 30° scope is turned down, the esophagus appears as a bright structure. In addition, tilting the tip of the endoscope brings the esophagus into view as it is lifted from the groove between the aorta and the heart.

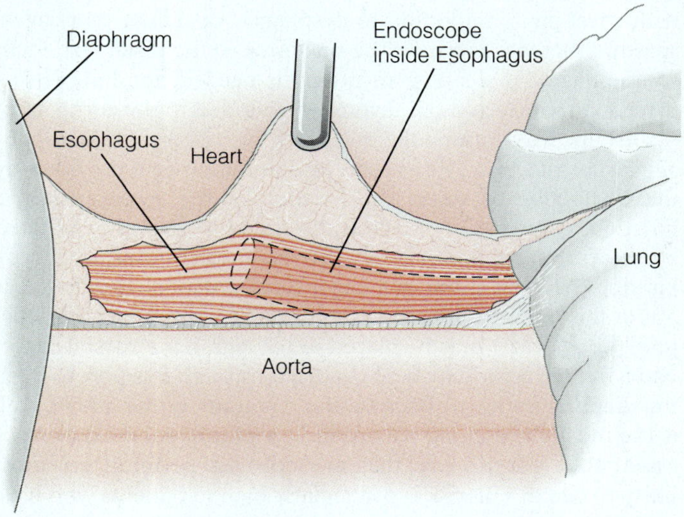

Figure 4 In a left thoracoscopic esophageal myotomy, the esophagus may be identified by means of transillumination from the endoscope.

Step 4: Starting the Myotomy and Reaching the Submucosal Plane

It is helpful to mark the surface of the esophagus along the line through which the myotomy will be carried out. The myotomy is started halfway between the diaphragm and the inferior pulmonary vein. The proper submucosal plane should be reached at a single point before the myotomy is extended; in this way, the likelihood of subsequent mucosal perforation can be reduced.

Troubleshooting The myotomy should not be started close to the esophagogastric junction, because at this level, the layers often are poorly defined, particularly if multiple dilatations or injections of botulin toxin have been performed. It is easier to start 4 to 5 cm above the esophagogastric junction, where the esophageal wall is usually normal. As a rule, we do not open the longitudinal layer first and then the circular layer; we find it easier and safer to try to reach the submucosal plane at one point and then move upward and downward from there. In the course of the myotomy, there is always some bleeding from the cut muscle fibers, particularly if the esophagus is dilated and the wall is very thick. After the source of the bleeding is identified by irrigation, the electrocautery must be used with caution. The most troublesome bleeding comes from the submucosal veins (which are usually large) encountered at the esophagogastric junction. In most instances, gentle compression is preferable to electrocautery. A sponge introduced through one of the ports facilitates the application of direct pressure.

Step 5: Upward and Downward Extension of the Myotomy

Once the mucosa has been exposed, the myotomy can safely be extended proximally and distally [*see Figure 5*]. We usually extend the myotomy for about 5 mm onto the gastric wall, without adding an antireflux procedure.[22] The typical length of the myotomy should be about 6 cm for patients with achalasia.

Troubleshooting Proximally, we extend the myotomy all the way to the inferior pulmonary vein only in cases of vigorous achalasia (high-amplitude simultaneous contractions associated with chest pain in addition to dysphagia) or diffuse esophageal spasm; otherwise, we limit the myotomy to the distal 5 to 6 cm of esophagus. If a longer myotomy is needed, the lung is displaced anteriorly and the myotomy extended to the aortic arch.

Distally, we continue the myotomy for 5 mm past the esophagogastric junction. We use the endoluminal view provided by the endoscope to assess the location of the esophagogastric junction. Often, the stomach is distended by the air insufflated by the endoscope and pushes the diaphragm upward, thereby limiting the view of the esophagogastric junction. If sucking air out of the stomach does not resolve this problem, an additional port (i.e., port E) may be placed in the eighth intercostal space, and a fan retractor may be introduced through this port to push the diaphragm down. Because the myotomy of the gastric wall is the most challenging part of the operation, good exposure is essential. It is at this level that an esophageal perforation is most likely to occur. The risk is particularly high in patients who have undergone pneumatic dilatation or injection of botulin toxin, both of which may lead to the replacement of muscle layers by scar tissue and the consequent loss of the regular planes. Perforations recognized in the operating room can be repaired by thoracoscopic intracorporeal suturing or, if this fails, by thoracotomy and open repair. The gastric fundus can be used to buttress the repair. If it is unclear whether a perforation has occurred, the esophagus should be covered with water, and air should be insufflated through the endoscope; bubbling will be observed over the site of the perforation.

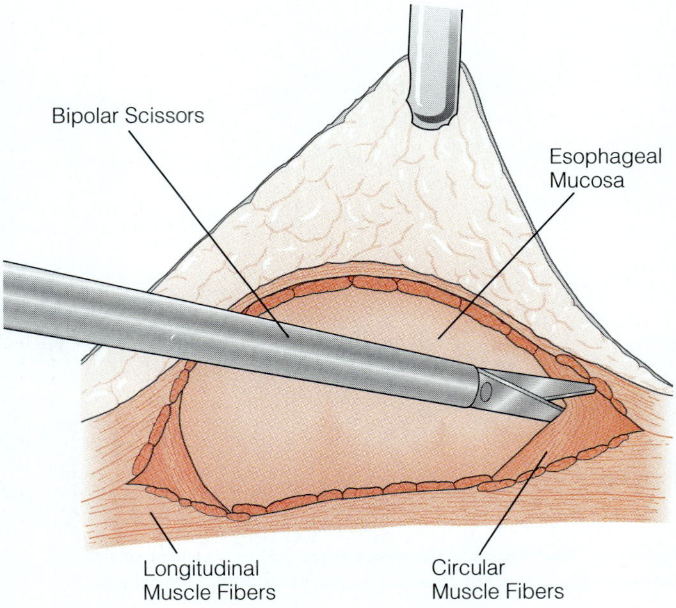

Figure 5 **Shown are the distal and proximal extensions of a left thoracoscopic esophageal myotomy.**

Step 6: Chest Tube Insertion

A 24 French angled chest tube is inserted under direct vision through port D or port E. The ports are removed under direct vision, and the thoracic wall is inspected for bleeding.

POSTOPERATIVE COMPLICATIONS

A common postoperative complication is delayed esophageal leakage, which is most often the result of an electrocautery burn to the esophageal mucosa. The characteristic signals are chest pain, fever, and a pleural effusion on the chest x-ray. The diagnosis is confirmed by an esophagogram. Treatment options depend on the time of diagnosis and on the size and location of the leak. Early, small leaks can be repaired directly. If the site of the leak is high in the chest, a thoracotomy provides the best approach for the repair; if the site is at the level of the esophagogastric junction, a laparotomy provides the best approach, and the stomach can be used to reinforce the repair. If the damage to the esophagus is too extensive to permit repair, a transhiatal esophagectomy is indicated.

Residual dysphagia occurs if the myotomy is not extended far enough onto the gastric wall. To prevent this problem, the distal extent of the myotomy should be assessed by the endoscopist, who will confirm that the myotomy includes 5 mm of the gastric wall. Patients with residual dysphagia must be evaluated by means of esophageal manometry, which will document the extent of and the pressure in the residual high-pressure zone. The myotomy can be easily extended by a laparoscopic approach, and a Dor fundoplication can be added.

Table 2 Results of Thoracoscopic Myotomy in 30 Patients with Achalasia

Results	Patients (% of Total)
Excellent (no dysphagia)	21 (70)
Good (dysphagia < once/wk)	5 (17)
Fair (dysphagia > once/wk)	3 (10)
Poor (persistent dysphagia)	1 (3)

Abnormal gastroesophageal reflux occurs if the myotomy is extended too far onto the gastric wall. Some patients present with heartburn; others are asymptomatic. It is essential to evaluate patients postoperatively with manometry and prolonged pH monitoring. Mild reflux can be treated with acid-reducing medications, particularly in elderly patients. In younger patients, abnormal reflux should be corrected by means of a laparoscopic partial fundoplication (e.g., Dor fundoplication).

OUTCOME EVALUATION

We start patients on a liquid diet the morning of postoperative day 1; on postoperative day 2, we start them on a soft mechanical diet, which is continued for the rest of the first week. We do not routinely obtain an esophagogram before starting feedings. The chest tube is removed after 24 hours if the lung is fully expanded and there is no air leak. Patients are discharged after 48 to 72 hours and are able to resume regular activities in seven to 10 days.

The results obtained with thoracoscopic esophageal myotomy are generally comparable to those obtained with open surgical procedures. Of the first 30 patients with achalasia whom we treated in this fashion, 26 (87 percent) experienced good or excellent results [see Table 2].

Right Thoracoscopic Myotomy

A long myotomy from the diaphragm to the thoracic inlet, performed via a right thoracoscopic approach, is the preferred procedure for patients who have nutcracker esophagus or diffuse esophageal spasm involving the entire length of the esophagus but have normal LES function. On the whole, this procedure is technically simpler than a left thoracoscopic myotomy: because there is no need to go through the esophagogastric junction, perforation, postoperative dysphagia, and abnormal gastroesophageal reflux are largely prevented.

PREOPERATIVE EVALUATION

Preoperative evaluation of patients being considered for right thoracoscopic myotomy is essentially the same as that of patients being considered for left thoracoscopic myotomy.

OPERATIVE PLANNING

Operative planning is similar to that for a left thoracoscopic myotomy. The double-lumen tube is used to deflate the right lung rather than the left.

The patient is placed in the left lateral decubitus position over an inflated bean bag, as for a right thoracotomy.

The instrumentation is identical except for the endovascular 30 mm stapler used to transect the azygos vein. It is essential to have a thoracotomy tray ready in case an emergent thoracotomy is necessary to control bleeding.

OPERATIVE TECHNIQUE

Step 1: Insertion of the Ports

Only port B is inserted where it would be for a left thoracoscopic myotomy. All the other ports are inserted one intercostal space higher because the myotomy need not be extended all the way to the stomach but must be extended to the thoracic inlet. Usually, only four ports are used; however, an additional port can be placed in the fourth intercostal space in the anterior axillary line to facilitate the proximal extension of the myotomy.

Step 2: Dissection of the Periesophageal Tissues and Division of the Azygos Vein

The periesophageal tissues above and below the azygos vein are dissected away from the esophagus. A tunnel is created between the azygos vein and the esophagus with a dissector, a right angle clamp, or both. The azygos vein is then transected with an endovascular 30 mm stapler. (Alternatively, the azygos vein can be spared and simply lifted off the esophagus with umbilical tape.)

Troubleshooting Dissection of the azygos vein is the most critical part of this procedure. We have found that it is easier to transect the azygos vein than to keep the vein lifted away from the esophagus and perform the myotomy under it.

Steps 3, 4, and 5

Steps 3, 4, and 5 of a right thoracoscopic myotomy are virtually identical to steps 4, 5, and 6 of a left thoracoscopic myotomy, with a few minor exceptions. Once the submucosal plane is reached, the myotomy is extended distally to the diaphragm and proximally to the thoracic inlet. The endoscope plays a less critical role in this procedure than in a left thoracoscopic myotomy because the esophagus is easily identified and because the myotomy is not extended through the esophagogastric junction. Instead, we place a 52 to 56 French bougie inside the esophagus. This facilitates the division of the circular fibers and separates the edges of the myotomy nicely.

POSTOPERATIVE COMPLICATIONS

A delayed esophageal leak is the most common postoperative complication. It should be handled as described earlier [see Left Thoracoscopic Myotomy, Postoperative Complications, *above*].

OUTCOME EVALUATION

The postoperative course of patients who have undergone this procedure is usually identical to that of patients operated on for achalasia. Complete relief of chest pain is obtained in about 75 to 80 percent of patients,[6] results comparable to those obtained with open surgical procedures.[23]

References

1. DeMeester TR, Bonavina L, Albertucci M: Nissen fundoplication for gastroesophageal reflux disease. Ann Surg 204:9, 1986
2. Csendes A, Braghetto I, Henriquez A, et al: Late results of a prospective randomised study comparing forceful dilatation and oesophagomyotomy in patients with achalasia. Gut 30:299, 1989
3. Hinder RA, Filipi CJ, Wetscher G, et al: Laparoscopic Nissen fundoplication is an effective treatment for gastroesophageal reflux disease. Ann Surg 220:472, 1994
4. Pellegrini CA, Wetter LA, Patti M, et al: Thoracoscopic esophagomyotomy: initial experience with a new approach for the treatment of achalasia. Ann Surg 216:291, 1992
5. Pellegrini CA, Leichter R, Patti M, et al: Thoracoscopic esophageal myotomy in the treatment of achalasia. Ann Thorac Surg 56:680, 1993
6. Patti MG, Pellegrini CA, Arcerito M, et al: Comparison of medical and minimally invasive surgical therapy for primary esophageal motility disorders. Arch Surg 130:609, 1995
7. The Southern Surgeon Club: A prospective analysis of 1518 laparoscopic cholecystectomies. N Engl J Med 324:1073, 1991
8. DeMeester TR, Lafontaine E, Joelsson BE, et al: Relationship of a hiatal hernia to the function of the body of the esophagus and the gastroesophageal junction. J Thorac Cardiovasc Surg 82:547, 1981
9. Richter JE: Surgery for reflux disease: reflections of a gastroenterologist. N Engl J Med 326:825, 1992
10. Waring JP, Hunter JG, Oddsdottir M, et al: The preoperative evaluation of patients considered for laparoscopic antireflux surgery. Am J Gastroenterol 90:35, 1995
11. Costantini M, Crookes PF, Bremner RM, et al: Value of physiologic assessment of foregut symptoms in a surgical practice. Surgery 114:780, 1993
12. Fuchs KH, DeMeester TR, Albertucci M: Specificity and sensitivity of objective diagnosis of gastroesophageal reflux disease. Surgery 102:575, 1987
13. Kahrilas PJ, Dodds WJ, Hogan WJ: Effect of peristaltic dysfunction on esophageal volume clearance. Gastroenterology 94:73, 1988
14. Patti MG, Debas HT, Pellegrini CA: Clinical and functional characterization of high gastroesophageal reflux. Am J Surg 165:163, 1993
15. Guelrud M, Rossiter A, Souney PF, et al: The effect of vasoactive intestinal polypeptide on the lower esophageal sphincter in achalasia. Gastroenterology 103:377, 1992
16. Tottrup A, Svane D, Forman A: Nitric oxide mediating NANC inhibition in opossum lower esophageal sphincter. Am J Physiol 260:385, 1991
17. Mittal RK, Rochester DF, McCallum RW: Electrical and mechanical activity in the human lower esophageal sphincter during diaphragmatic contraction. J Clin Invest 81:1182, 1988
18. Mittal RK, Rochester DF, McCallum RW: Sphincteric action of the diaphragm during a relaxed lower esophageal sphincter in humans. Am J Physiol 256:139, 1989
19. Shimi S, Nathanson LK, Cuschieri A: Laparoscopic cardiomyotomy for achalasia. J R Coll Surg Edinb 36:152, 1991
20. Shimi S, Nathanson LK, Cuschieri A: Thoracoscopic long oesophageal myotomy for nutcracker oesophagus: initial experience of a new surgical approach. Br J Surg 79:533, 1992
21. Sauer L, Pellegrini CA, Way LW: The treatment of achalasia: a current perspective. Arch Surg 124:929, 1989
22. Ellis FH Jr, Gibb SP, Crozier RE: Esophagomyotomy for achalasia of the esophagus. Ann Surg 192:157, 1980
23. Henderson RD, Ryder D, Marryatt G: Extended esophageal myotomy and short total fundoplication hernia repair in diffuse esophageal spasm: five-year review in 34 patients. Ann Thorac Surg 43:25, 1987

Acknowledgment

Figures 1 through 5 Tom Moore.

49 GASTRIC PROCEDURES

John L. Sawyers, M.D.

In most patients who will undergo gastric procedures, a definitive diagnosis will already have been made by means of esophagogastroduodenoscopy, upper GI tract x-rays, or both. Major gastric procedures are done with the patient under general anesthesia and lying supine on the operating room table.

Initial Incision

The abdomen is opened through an upper midline incision from the left of the xiphoid to the umbilicus. It is not necessary to excise the xiphoid process. Adjacent to the cephalad end of the xiphoid is a small artery that may cause troublesome bleeding; such bleeding can be readily controlled with electrocoagulation. The incision in the linea alba is made with the cutting current of the electrocautery. If further exposure is needed, the incision may be extended around the umbilicus on either side. The wound edges are protected by the application of moist laparotomy pads or a plastic wound protector. A Balfour retractor is then inserted. An upper hand retractor lifts the costal margins to facilitate exposure of the upper abdomen. Some surgeons prefer to use a Buckwalter retractor.

Vagotomy

Since the 1940s, when Dragstedt reintroduced vagotomy as surgical therapy for duodenal ulcer,[1] parasympathetic denervation of the parietal cell mass in the stomach has been the basis for the operative treatment of this disease. Three types of vagotomy—truncal vagotomy, selective vagotomy, and highly selective vagotomy (also known as proximal gastric vagotomy or parietal cell vagotomy)—have been described, all of which result in reduced acid secretion. Of these, selective gastric vagotomy, which denervates the entire stomach but none of the other intra-abdominal organs, is the one that has been least frequently used.

TRUNCAL VAGOTOMY

After entering the abdomen, the surgeon may divide the left triangular ligament of the liver to permit retraction of the left lobe of the liver to the patient's right side. This is not always necessary; often, the left lobe is retracted cephalad. The Weinberg retractor (Joe's hoe) is useful for elevating the left lateral hepatic segment.

The stomach is retracted downward, and the peritoneum overlying the abdominal esophagus is incised transversely. A previously placed nasogastric tube facilitates identification of the esophagus. The esophagus is mobilized circumferentially by a combination of blunt and sharp dissection and encircled with a Penrose drain [*see Figure 1a*]. The drain is passed behind the esophagus either by using a gooseneck clamp or by inserting two fingers posterior to the esophagus and pulling the drain through this opening.

The anterior vagal trunk usually lies on the anterior wall of the esophagus. It can be identified by palpation with a finger as the stomach is retracted caudally with the Penrose drain; it feels like a guitar string. The anterior trunk is mobilized from the esophagus up into the lower mediastinum. Any branches that pass downward toward the esophagogastric junction are divided. A 2 in. segment of the anterior trunk is resected [*see Figure 1b*], and the severed ends are secured with ligating clips or fine (3-0) silk ties.

The posterior vagal trunk is usually larger than the anterior vagal trunk. Its location is variable. Sometimes, it lies directly behind the esophagus and thus is held by the Penrose drain; more often, however, it lies medially and may be found adjacent to the abdominal aorta or in the areolar tissue just medial to the right crus of the diaphragm. Applying traction caudad to the stomach or the Penrose drain will put tension on the posterior vagal trunk, thereby making it easier to identify. As with the anterior trunk, a 2 in. segment is resected [*see Figure 1c*], and the severed ends are secured with ligating clips or silk ties; clips are quicker and easier to use.

Any additional vagal fibers that may arise cephalad to the severed vagal trunks are located and divided. A careful search around the circumference of the esophagus is done to ensure that the vagotomy is complete [*see Figure 1d*].

The esophagus is retracted to the patient's left with the Penrose drain, and the diaphragmatic crura are approximated posterior to the esophagus with one or more heavy (0) silk sutures in such a way that the hiatus is tightened around the esophagus with the indwelling nasogastric tube to a snugness of one finger's breadth.

Because truncal vagotomy denervates the entire stomach (including the gastric antral pyloric pump mechanism), emptying of liquids and solid food is decreased. Gastric stasis may occur; consequently, a drainage procedure (pyloroplasty or gastrojejunostomy) or distal gastric resection (antrectomy) is required.

Transthoracic (Supradiaphragmatic) Vagotomy

Transthoracic truncal vagotomy is usually reserved for cases in which reoperation is necessary because an incomplete previous vagotomy resulted in a recurrent ulcer. The patient is placed on his or her right side, and a left posterior lateral thoracotomy is done in the seventh interspace. The inferior lobe of the left lung is retracted, and the inferior pulmonary ligament is exposed and then divided with the electrocautery. The left lung is either deflated (with a double-lumen endotracheal tube) or retracted upward,

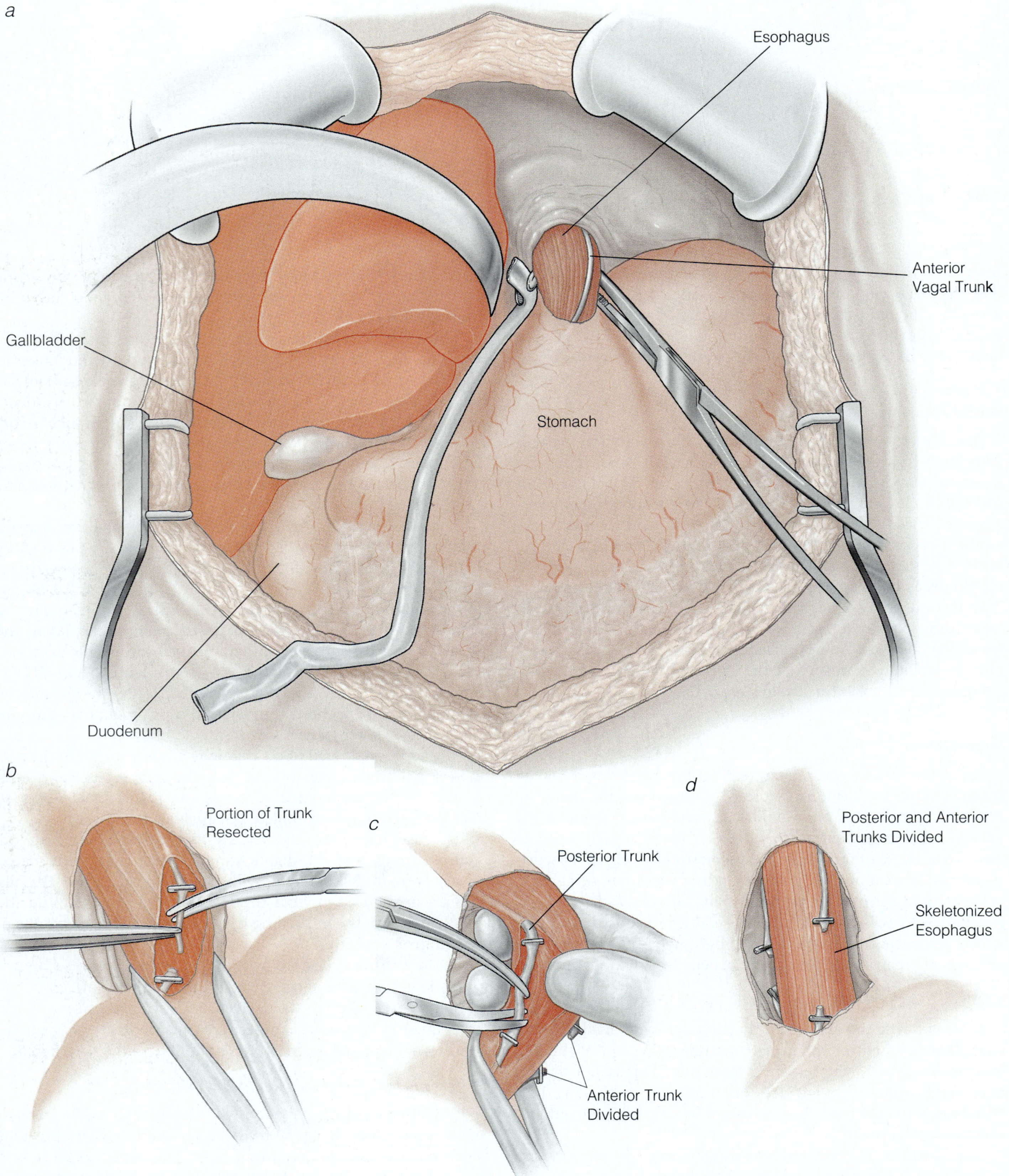

Figure 1 Truncal vagotomy. (*a*) The esophagus is mobilized by blunt and sharp dissection and encircled with a Penrose drain. (*b*) The anterior vagal trunk is identified and mobilized, and a 2 in. segment of the trunk is resected. (*c*) The posterior vagal trunk is identified and mobilized, and a 2 in. segment of this trunk is resected. (*d*) Any additional small vagal fibers are divided, and a careful search is made around the esophagus to confirm that the vagotomy is complete.[23]

and the pleura over the distal esophagus is incised longitudinally. The esophagus is identified by palpating the nasogastric tube previously inserted into the stomach. It is mobilized by blunt dissection until a finger can be passed beneath it. The vagus nerves can then be seen and palpated on each side of the esophageal wall. Because of the patient's rotated position on the table, the left vagus is found on the upper surface of the esophagus, and the right vagus is found beneath the esophagus.

Next, the vagi are freed from the esophagus. At this level, the vagi usually form a single trunk; however, each may consist of two or more fibers. Hence, to be certain of dividing all the fibers, it is advisable to clean all of the adventitia away from the esophagus around its circumference for a length of 5 cm. The vagi are isolated and divided between silk ligatures or ligating clips just above the diaphragm [see Figure 2]. Removal of a segment of nerve is permissible but not necessary. The pleura is then closed over the esophagus.

With the increased use of endoscopic surgical procedures, instruments have been developed that allow transthoracic vagotomy to be performed through a thoracoscope. If no adhesions from a previous thoracotomy are present, the thoracoscopic approach is an easy method of dividing the thoracic vagal nerves. After thoracoscopic vagal nerve resection, the patient may go home the same day or the next day and is spared the discomfort of a thoracotomy incision. This is now my method of choice for transthoracic vagotomy.

HIGHLY SELECTIVE (PROXIMAL GASTRIC) VAGOTOMY

After the anterior and posterior vagal trunks enter the abdomen, the anterior trunk gives off the hepatic vagal branch (or branches) and continues as the anterior gastric nerve of Latarjet, which courses medial to the lesser curvature of the stomach in the anterior leaf of the lesser (or gastrohepatic) omentum. The posterior vagal nerve gives off the celiac branch and continues as the posterior gastric nerve of Latarjet, which parallels the course of the anterior gastric nerve but lies in the posterior leaf of the lesser omentum. These two gastric nerves terminate in fanlike branches that together make up what is called the crow's foot. The crow's foot is located approximately 7 cm proximal to the pylorus along the lesser curvature of the stomach [see Figure 3a]. It is an important anatomic landmark because it coincides with the antral–parietal cell junction.

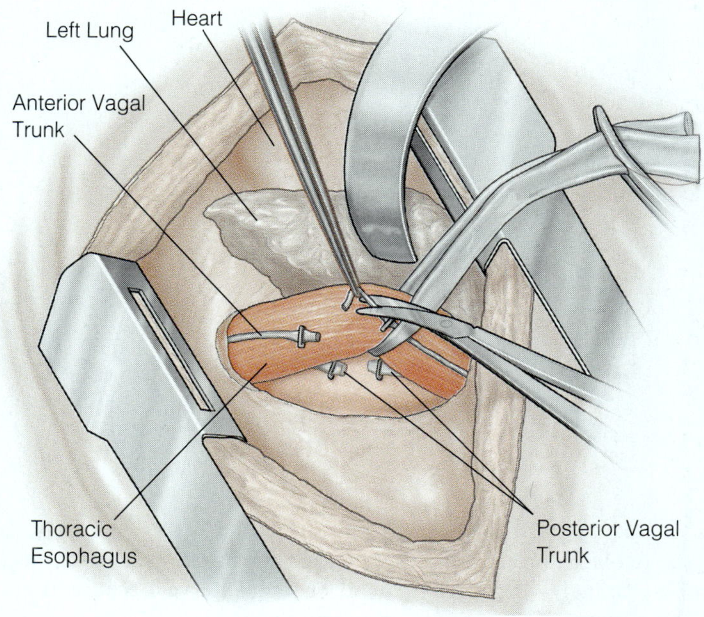

Adequate exposure of the upper abdominal cavity is essential to the performance of a proximal gastric vagotomy. Such exposure may be obtained through an upper midline abdominal incision, as noted [see Initial Incision, above]. An upper hand retractor with two blades is used to lift up the costal margins. The operating table is tilted to place the patient in a head-up (reverse Trendelenburg) position.

The lateral segment of the left lobe of the liver is retracted upward. Some surgeons prefer to incise the left triangular ligament and to retract the lateral segment medially during the dissection of the vagi. The left lobe is returned to its normal location before the abdomen is closed.

The anterior vagal trunk is identified and encircled with a vessel loop; any ancillary anterior nerve trunks should also be identified at this time. The esophagus is then dissected from its bed. An empty sponge forceps is placed parallel to the esophagus and the diaphragmatic crura and used to free the lateral esophagus attachments. The posterior wall of the esophagus is freed by gentle finger dissection, and a narrow Penrose drain is passed around the esophagus. The posterior vagal trunk is then identified; it is usually anterior to the aorta rather than directly behind the esophagus. A second vessel loop is passed around this trunk. Both vagal trunks are kept intact and retracted to the right of the esophagus, which is returned to its normal position with the encircling Penrose drain still in place.

The stomach is then retracted to the patient's left and caudally by applying Babcock clamps to the greater curvature over a previously placed nasogastric tube. The anterior nerve of Latarjet, descending in the lesser omentum to reach the gastric antrum, is visualized. A finger is inserted through the avascular area in the lesser omentum to place tension on the omentum. With the surgeon drawing the lesser omentum to the patient's right and the assistant pulling the greater gastric curvature to the left, the detachment of the anterior leaf of the lesser omentum from the lesser gastric curvature is begun just cephalad to the crow's foot.

The lesser omentum consists of three layers. Each layer contains vessels and nerves that must be divided. First, the anterior layer between the anterior gastric nerve of Latarjet and the lesser gastric curvature is divided from the crow's foot distally up to the esophagogastric junction [see Figure 3a]; second, the middle layer is divided; and third, the posterior layer is divided between the posterior gastric nerve of Latarjet and the lesser gastric curvature [see Figure 3b]. These steps are best done by dividing each individual neurovascular bundle between two hemostats (e.g., Crile clamps) and tying each neurovascular pedicle with fine silk. The temptation to hurry this part of the dissection by incorporating large amounts of tissue in the clamps must be resisted. Hemostatic clips and diathermy coagulation should not be used:

Figure 2 Transthoracic (supradiaphragmatic) vagotomy. Through a left posterior lateral thoracotomy, the vagus nerves are identified, freed from the esophagus, isolated, and divided just above the diaphragm; the pleura is then closed over the esophagus. The procedure may also be performed through a thoracoscope; this is in fact my current method of choice.

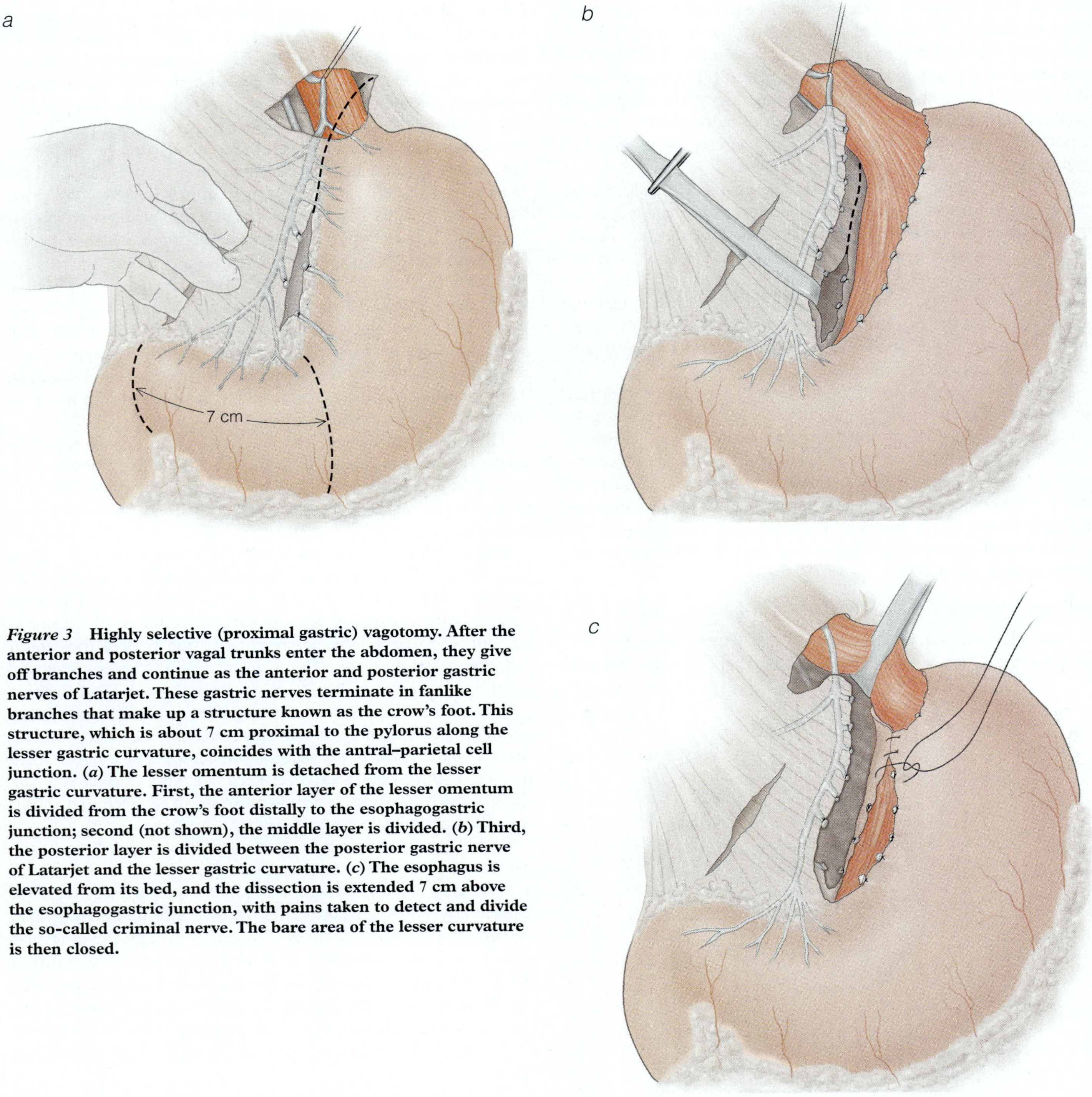

Figure 3 Highly selective (proximal gastric) vagotomy. After the anterior and posterior vagal trunks enter the abdomen, they give off branches and continue as the anterior and posterior gastric nerves of Latarjet. These gastric nerves terminate in fanlike branches that make up a structure known as the crow's foot. This structure, which is about 7 cm proximal to the pylorus along the lesser gastric curvature, coincides with the antral–parietal cell junction. (*a*) The lesser omentum is detached from the lesser gastric curvature. First, the anterior layer of the lesser omentum is divided from the crow's foot distally to the esophagogastric junction; second (not shown), the middle layer is divided. (*b*) Third, the posterior layer is divided between the posterior gastric nerve of Latarjet and the lesser gastric curvature. (*c*) The esophagus is elevated from its bed, and the dissection is extended 7 cm above the esophagogastric junction, with pains taken to detect and divide the so-called criminal nerve. The bare area of the lesser curvature is then closed.

they may result in bleeding, which leads to hematomas in the lesser omentum that obscure visualization of the gastric nerves.

After the lesser gastric curvature is freed from the anterior and posterior gastric nerves of Latarjet up to the esophagogastric junction, the esophagus is elevated from its bed by traction on the Penrose drain. The dissection is extended 7 cm above the esophagogastric junction to sever any vagal fibers supplying the gastric fundus [*see Figure 3c*]. There is usually a constant vagal branch arising from the posterior vagal trunk that courses along the left lateral wall of the esophagus to enter the gastric fundus. This branch—aptly termed the criminal nerve because it so often escapes untouched[2]—must be divided.

Finally, the bare area of the lesser gastric curvature is closed by plicating the anterior and posterior leaves of the lesser omentum with interrupted silk sutures from the esophagogastric junction down to the crow's foot [*see Figure 3c*]. This maneuver is thought to reduce the risk of both lesser curvature necrosis (see below) and vagal sprouting.

I generally do not test the completeness of the vagotomy either by performing pH metering with an intragastric electrode or by observing the color changes on the Congo red test. These tests are tedious, lengthen the operation, and are of questionable value. Intraoperative testing appears to offer no significant advantages.[3]

Rosati and coworkers have recommended resecting about 3 cm of the right gastroepiploic neurovascular bundle along the greater gastric curvature opposite the crow's foot or the upper limit of the pyloric antrum.[4] A vagal branch coming off the pyloric nerve may extend proximally up to the parietal cell mass on the greater curvature. I do not routinely divide the neurovascular bundle at this site.

Complications

Proximal gastric vagotomy has the lowest reported mortality of any operation used to treat duodenal ulcer disease. In one series of 5,000 patients, mortality was 0.26 percent.[5] In 500 patients operated on at Vanderbilt University, mortality was only 0.2 percent; the sole postoperative death was the result of a pulmonary embolus.

An early postoperative complication uniquely associated with proximal gastric vagotomy is lesser curvature necrosis, which occurs during the first week after operation. It may be caused by ligation or electrocoagulation performed too close to the lesser gastric curvature. The area of necrosis is located on the lesser gastric curvature between the antral–parietal cell border and the esophagogastric junction. The incidence of this complication is low, typically less than one percent; it may be further reduced by reperitonealizing the lesser curvature. Early recognition of lesser curvature necrosis can be confirmed by meglumine diatrizoate contrast studies of the stomach. Although reoperation to close the site of perforation is usually successful, there are two reported instances in which gastric resection was necessary in a patient with extensive lesser curvature necrosis.[6]

Dysphagia has been reported as an early complication of proximal gastric vagotomy in 10 to 30 percent of patients.[7] The cause is thought to be the intensive lower esophageal dissection necessary to ensure complete vagal denervation of the parietal cell mass. Postvagotomy dysphagia usually subsides spontaneously in two to three months; in rare instances, esophageal dilation with a Hurst or Maloney bougie may be necessary.

Tears of the splenic capsule occur in about four percent of operations but can usually be controlled with hemostatic agents.

In rare cases, perforation of the esophagus may occur as the surgeon attempts to free the esophagus from the posterior mediastinum by passing the Penrose drain behind the esophagus. If this happens, immediate repair of the perforation with interrupted silk sutures should prevent any esophageal leak. The repair may then be reinforced with fundoplication overlying it.

Because the emptying of solid foods remains normal, the incidence of postgastrectomy sequelae (e.g., dumping, diarrhea, and reflux gastritis) after proximal gastric vagotomy is less than that after gastric operations that destroy the integrity of the pyloric sphincter. No dietary restrictions are required after the operation. Dumping generally is not a problem, nor is postvagotomy diarrhea or alkaline reflux gastritis.

Concern has been expressed about the recurrence rate after highly selective vagotomy. Studies have been published that cover more than 15 years of follow-up. In these studies, ulcer recurrence rates have ranged from two to 23 percent[8]; however, when highly selective vagotomy is done by a surgeon who has extensive experience with the procedure, recurrence rates generally range from five to 10 percent.[9] Proximal gastric vagotomy should not be used to treat pyloric or prepyloric ulcers, because patients with these conditions tend to have higher recurrence rates than those with duodenal ulcers. Recurrent ulcers after proximal gastric vagotomy are likely to respond to medical treatment with H_2-receptor antagonists. If a recurrent ulcer makes reoperation necessary, antrectomy with truncal vagotomy is the procedure of choice.

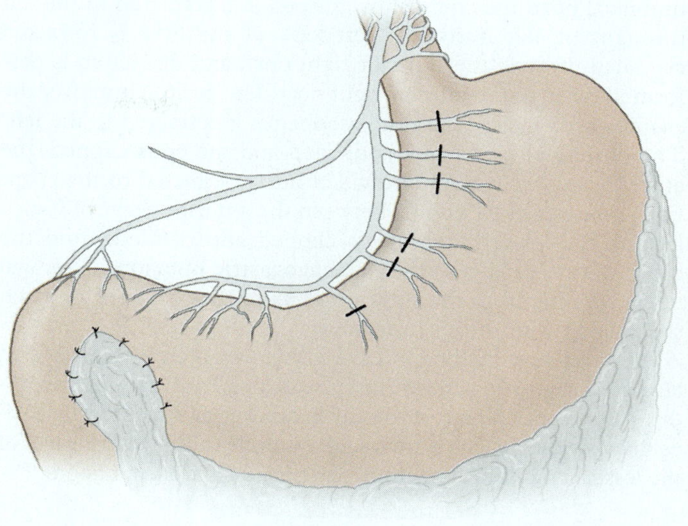

Figure 4 **Patch closure with highly selective vagotomy for perforated duodenal ulcer. An omental patch is placed over the perforation and secured with interrupted 3-0 silk sutures. The peritoneal cavity is thoroughly irrigated, and highly selective vagotomy is performed.**[8]

Patch Closure with Highly Selective Vagotomy for Perforated Duodenal Ulcer

Highly selective vagotomy may be added to patch closure for perforated duodenal ulcer.[10] Highly selective vagotomy prevents undesirable postgastrectomy complications and controls the ulcer diathesis. Omentum is placed over the perforation as a patch and secured with interrupted 3-0 silk sutures [see Figure 4]; closure of the hole with sutures is unnecessary and may narrow the duodenal lumen. After the patch is secured, highly selective vagotomy is performed as described earlier (see above).

LAPAROSCOPIC VAGOTOMY

Techniques have been developed to perform proximal gastric vagotomy through a laparoscope by means of an approach similar to that described earlier [see Highly Selective (Proximal Gastric) Vagotomy, *above*]. Some laparoscopic surgeons prefer to do a posterior truncal vagotomy combined with highly selective vagotomy of the anterior vagal trunk or an anterior seromyotomy.

Laparoscopic highly selective vagotomy is usually done with the patient under general anesthesia and in the reverse Trendelenburg position. Some surgeons prefer the lithotomy position, with the surgeon between the patient's legs. Five trocars are inserted. A 30° telescope is placed through the supraumbilical port; the stomach is grasped and retracted to the left through the left ports; the left lobe of the liver is retracted cephalad through the superior right port; and dissection is performed through the inferior right port. The peritoneum over the esophagus is incised, and the esophagus is retracted to the left. The posterior vagal trunk is divided and the ends clipped; the anterior vagal trunk is not divided but is retracted to the right. Each neurovascular bundle between the anterior nerve of Latarjet and the lesser curvature is clipped and divided, from the crow's foot cephalad to the esophagogastric junction. The vagal fibers running from the anterior trunk to the proximal stomach are divided with the electrocautery.

An alternative method of laparoscopic vagotomy is to perform an anterior gastric seromyotomy with posterior truncal vagotomy.[11] Performing a seromyotomy is quicker and technically easier than dividing each neurovascular bundle in the anterior leaf of the lesser omentum. The immediate results have been good.

Distal Subtotal Gastric Resection (Antrectomy) for Benign Disease

Distal subtotal gastric resection for benign duodenal ulcer usually consists of antral resection in conjunction with truncal vagotomy. The initial abdominal incision is made as previously described [see Initial Incision, above]. After truncal vagotomy is performed, the distal 40 percent of the stomach is excised. Because the antrum extends further cephalad on the lesser curvature, the lesser curvature is divided at a point closer to the esophagogastric junction than to the pylorus, whereas the greater curvature is divided halfway between the pylorus and the fundus [see Figure 5].

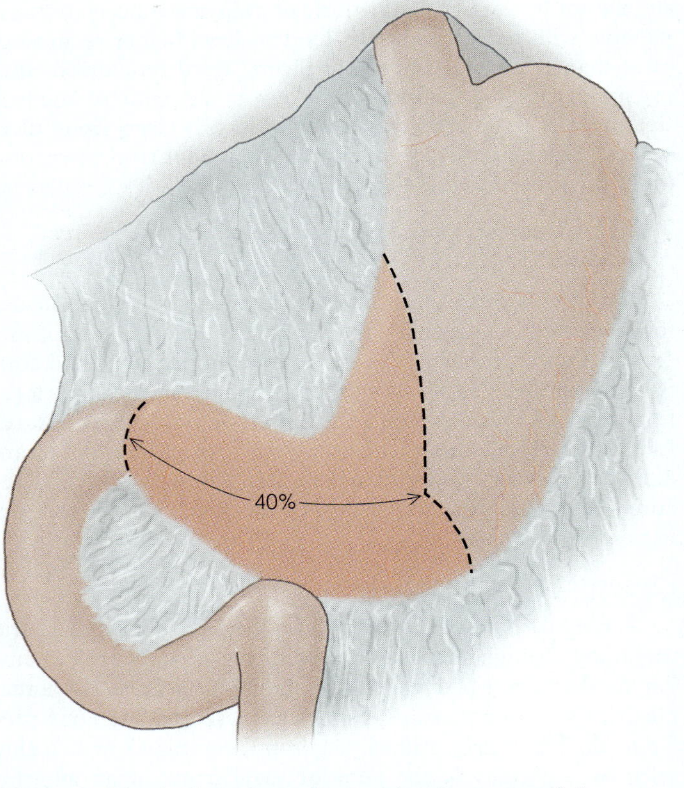

Babcock forceps are placed on the greater gastric curvature, and the organ is lifted up and forward. The arcade of vessels along the middle portion of the greater curvature is divided and ligated with silk. The lesser peritoneal cavity, thus widely opened, is explored, and all fibrous attachments between the posterior gastric wall and the pancreatic pseudocapsule are divided. At this point, an excellent view of the pancreas is obtained, and the organ is carefully inspected for possible adenoma or other pathological findings. The greater curvature is mobilized from the pylorus to a point midway to the fundus. The dissection is extended several centimeters above the incisura angularis on the lesser curvature, and the vessels along the lesser curvature are likewise secured. The descending branch of the left gastric artery is divided and transfixed with silk.

With traction applied to the greater curvature by means of the Babcock forceps, the mobilized stomach is fanned out, and a point along the greater curvature that is approximately midway between the pylorus and the fundus is selected for division; this point is usually just to the right of the first of the vasa brevia. A second point along the lesser curvature that is just proximal to the midway point between the pylorus and the esophagogastric junction is similarly selected for division; this point is usually 3 to 4 cm above the crow's foot.

The stomach is divided between two straight Kocher or Allen clamps placed at right angles to the long axis of the stomach at the selected division point along the greater curvature. The proximal clamp defines the size of the gastroenteric stoma that is to be constructed. A gastrointestinal anastomosis (GIA) stapling device may also be used for this purpose, but I prefer to use the clamps. Next, a TA-60 gastric stapler is placed obliquely along the lesser curvature up to the point previously selected for division. A maneuver that aids in clearing the lesser curvature is to use the left index finger and thumb to place traction medially on the gastrohepatic ligament and to insert a curved hemostat adjacent to the gastric wall, thereby opening a space through which the assistant can place two Kelly clamps across the gastrohepatic ligament in preparation for its division. This piece of tissue, which contains the descending branch of the left gastric artery, is a rather large one and thus is ligated with 2-0 silk. This maneuver quickly clears the lesser curvature and facilitates placement of the linear gastric stapler or GIA stapler. The stomach is then transected at the selected point. The staple line may be inverted with interrupted 3-0 silk sutures.

The resulting gastric remnant assumes a tubular shape. The distal transected stomach is then reflected to the right. At this point, the entire pancreas can again be fully visualized and examined. If traction is applied to the distal transected stomach, the stomach can serve as a handle, and dissection of the pylorus and the duodenal bulb is thereby greatly facilitated. In my experience, this method is much easier and more efficacious than other methods in which the duodenum is mobilized before the stomach is divided. The division is extended distally onto the duodenum far enough to ensure that all antral tissue is removed.

Figure 5 Distal subtotal gastric resection (antrectomy) for benign disease. This procedure usually consists of antral resection combined with truncal vagotomy. After truncal vagotomy, the distal 40 percent of the stomach is excised. The division point on the lesser curvature is more proximal than that on the greater curvature because the antrum extends further cephalad on the lesser curvature.[24]

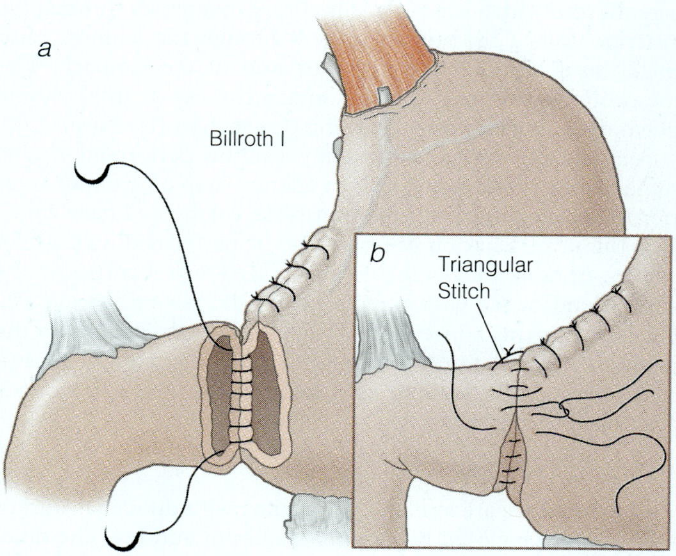

Figure 6 Billroth I gastroduodenostomy. (*a*) The opposing posterior gastric and duodenal walls are approximated with a continuous fine chromic catgut suture that commences in the midline with two separate needles. The suture is continued anteriorly, the opposing anterior walls are inverted with an over-and-over suture (or, alternatively, a Connell inverting suture), and the suture ends are tied in the midline. (*b*) An outer layer of interrupted 4-0 silk sutures is placed, and the angle of sorrow—the potential weak spot—is closed with a triangular stitch.[25]

BILLROTH I RECONSTRUCTION

For establishing gastrointestinal continuity, a Billroth I gastroduodenostomy is the preferred procedure; I have used it in 90 percent of my patients. Gastroduodenostomy offers certain physiologic advantages over gastrojejunostomy: many nutritional studies have indicated that maintaining the duodenum in alimentary continuity causes less loss of fecal fat and nitrogen, enhances iron absorption, and reduces the incidence of reflux gastritis.

A duodenal lumen of normal width, without constriction at or distal to the ulcer, is essential to the performance of an end-to-end gastroduodenostomy. If a satisfactory lumen is not already present, it must be produced surgically; a Horsley longitudinal incision of the anterior duodenal wall is one way of accomplishing this.

The ulcer need not be removed if there is no evidence of cicatricial stenosis at or distal to the site of ulceration in the duodenum. In fact, it is better to leave a difficult penetrating ulcer in situ than to be too aggressive in attempting to remove it: unwarranted aggressive attempts to remove the ulcer may increase mortality and morbidity related to anastomotic leaks, infection, or pancreatitis. When a large penetrating ulcer of the posterior wall is encountered and scarring extends around the entire circumference of the duodenum—particularly if the patient is obese—I often elect to close the duodenal stump with a long anterior wall cuff of duodenum. This long cuff is buttressed to the bed of the ulcer with two inverting layers of catgut sutures, and the pseudocapsule of the pancreas is approximated to the duodenal serosa with interrupted silk sutures. A retrocolic Hofmeister reconstruction using a short afferent loop is then done.

As a rule, the duodenum need not be kocherized except in unusual circumstances: routine use of the Kocher maneuver is neither necessary nor preferred. After the distal stomach is mobilized beyond the pylorus, the gastric pouch is placed in direct apposition to the posterior duodenum. The two structures to be anastomosed must be approximated without the slightest amount of tension. With the distal stomach still attached to the freed duodenum, a row of interrupted seromuscular silk sutures is placed between the posterior gastric wall and the posterior duodenal wall distal to the ulcer site. The so-called rule of nine (according to which the two end sutures are placed first, followed by the middle suture) may be helpful in spacing the sutures. These sutures are rendered taut, and the first assistant approximates the gastric pouch to the posterior duodenal wall by applying gentle traction to the structures. The surgeon then ties the sutures and removes the specimen with the electric cutting current.

A continuous 3-0 chromic catgut suture is placed with two needles through the entire thickness of the posterior gastric and duodenal walls; this placement also serves to approximate the opposing mucosal surfaces [*see Figure 6a*]. The interrupted seromuscular silk sutures placed earlier are held elevated by an assistant as the continuous suture is being placed posteriorly; this maneuver allows improved visualization of the opposing gastric and duodenal mucosae. The continuous catgut suture is started in the middle of the posterior wall, and the posterior row is locked to prevent purse-stringing of the lumen. As the continuous suture is advanced, the interrupted silk sutures are cut close to the knots. The continuous suture is then continued anteriorly, and the opposing gastric and duodenal walls are inverted with an over-and-over suture (or, as some surgeons prefer, a Connell inverting suture). An outer layer of interrupted 4-0 silk completes the anastomosis, and the ends of the suture are tied in the midline. It is essential to close the potential weak spot of the anastomosis—the so-called angle of sorrow—by placing a triangular silk suture at the lesser curve of the anastomosis in such a way as to include both the anterior gastric wall and the posterior gastric wall as well as the lesser curve of the duodenum [*see Figure 6b*]. If there is any appreciable discrepancy between the opposing structures to be anastomosed, the antimesenteric border of the duodenum may be divided for 1 to 2 cm before the anterior row of sutures is completed (Horsley's maneuver). The resulting gastroduodenal stoma is usually just wide enough to admit the surgeon's thumb; it should not be larger.

The nasogastric tube is then irrigated by a member of the OR staff before the abdomen is closed to ensure that all blood clots have been removed from the gastric pouch. I prefer to remove the nasogastric tube after the first 24 hours, provided that the operation has progressed smoothly. At present, I extubate approximately 75 percent of my patients early. If the operation was done on an emergency basis, particularly for an acute ulcer perforation in which there was extensive peritoneal soiling, the tube should be left in place for approximately 72 hours or until the patient expels flatus. In addition, when massive bleeding occurs to the point where the GI tract is filled with blood, adynamic ileus may be anticipated postoperatively, and a few days of nasogastric suction is appropriate.

During the first 72 hours after operation, the patient is given nothing but parenteral fluids. Small amounts of tap water are allowed on postoperative day 4, and a liquid diet usually is begun on day 5. A postgastrectomy diet is begun on day 6 or 7. The patient can get out of bed and walk on postoperative day 1.

BILLROTH II RECONSTRUCTION

A Billroth II gastrojejunostomy may be indicated when technical reasons rule out a Billroth I gastroduodenostomy. The usual indication for a Billroth II procedure is a high gastric resection involving two thirds to three fourths of the stomach.

After the distal end of the stomach is mobilized, the duodenum is divided with a GIA stapler. The duodenal stump may be oversewn with interrupted 3-0 silk sutures. The lesser curve of the gastric reservoir is closed with a stapler (TA-60 or GIA) and oversewn with interrupted 3-0 silk sutures.

A short-loop retrocolic gastrojejunostomy is done by identifying the ligament of Treitz, bringing the proximal jejunum through an avascular space in the transverse mesocolon, and performing a two-layer anastomosis to the clamped greater gastric curvature. The posterior row consists of interrupted 3-0 silk Lembert sutures. The inner layer is sutured with a continuous double-ended 3-0 chromic catgut suture that is begun in the middle of the posterior row, extended around to close the anterior layer with an over-and-over stitch, and locked. If preferred, a Connell inverting suture may be used on the anterior surface. The anastomosis is reinforced with an anterior row of interrupted 3-0 silk sutures. The lesser curvature–jejunum junction is reinforced with a triangular silk suture that passes through the anterior wall of the stomach, then through the jejunum, and finally back through the posterior wall of the stomach. The mesocolon is sutured to the stomach to keep it from sliding down the jejunal limb and causing obstruction [see Figure 7a].

An antecolic gastrojejunostomy can be performed in the same manner by bringing a short afferent loop of jejunum anterior to the omentum and the transverse colon [see Figure 7b].

A Billroth II anastomosis may also be performed with a GIA stapler. An antecolic jejunal loop is placed 2 to 3 cm above the stapled end of the gastric reservoir on the posterior wall. The GIA instrument is inserted through 1 cm stab wounds in the jejunum and the stomach. Firing the stapler creates an anastomosis between the jejunum and the stomach. The stab wounds are closed with silk sutures.

The Difficult Duodenal Stump

Two methods are available for dealing with duodenal stumps that cannot be closed with either staples or sutures. The time-honored method is to insert a 16 French red rubber duodenostomy catheter through the open end of the duodenum. The duodenum is inverted around the catheter with two purse-string sutures and reinforced with omentum. If the duodenal stump has been sutured but there is concern about the closure, a 16 French catheter is inserted through the lateral margin of the

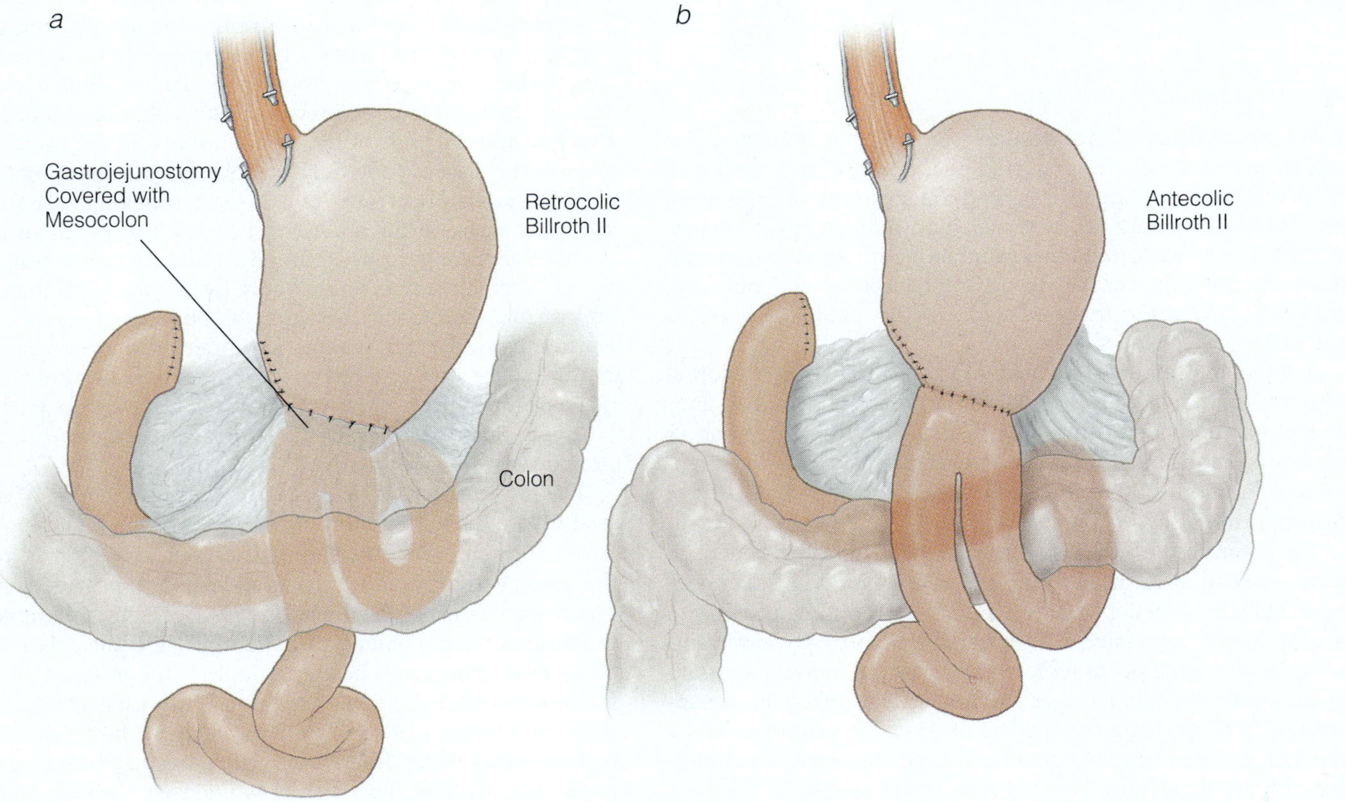

Figure 7 Billroth II gastrojejunostomy. (*a*) A retrocolic Billroth II procedure is done by bringing the proximal jejunum through an avascular space in the transverse mesocolon and anastomosing the jejunum to the greater gastric curvature. The anastomosis is reinforced with an anterior row of interrupted 3-0 silk sutures. As in the Billroth I procedure, the potential weak spot of the anastomosis is closed with a triangular stitch. The mesocolon is then sutured to the gastric wall. (*b*) The antecolic version of the procedure is similar, except that the jejunal loop is brought up anterior to the omentum and the transverse colon.

duodenum by using two inverting sutures, much as in a Stamm gastrostomy [see Stamm Gastrostomy, below]. A closed wound suction (Jackson-Pratt) drain is placed alongside the duodenal stump and brought out through a stab wound.

The other major method of dealing with difficult duodenal stumps is to perform a Roux-en-Y reconstruction.[12] This reconstruction is particularly useful when giant duodenal ulcers, large perforations, or dense inflammatory adhesions involving the duodenal area are present. The isolated Roux limb may be used either as a serosal patch to cover the duodenal defect or as an open end-to-side anastomosis [see Figures 8a and 8b]. Roux-en-Y reconstruction reroutes fluid and gastric contents from the afferent limb, thus reducing intraluminal afferent limb pressure and reducing the tension being applied to the closed duodenal stump. The afferent limb is kept short to prevent obstruction, and anastomotic traps are carefully closed.

Fashioning a Roux-en-Y jejunal limb The ligament of Treitz is identified. The jejunum is divided close to this ligament, but pains must be taken to preserve an arterial arcade to each side of the jejunum. Usually, the jejunum is divided between the first and the second arcade with a GIA stapler. The stapler should be perpendicular to the jejunum rather than at an angle to avoid compromising the vascularity of the ends. It is possible to obtain a longer Roux limb by dividing the mesentery, but again, one arcade must be preserved on each side of the divided jejunum. A Roux limb should be at least 45 cm (18 in.) long to prevent reflux of bile and other alkaline secretions; however, it should not be longer than 60 cm, to prevent delayed transit through the limb (Roux syndrome). Lengths between 45 and 60 cm have been used with considerable success.

Anastomosis of the stomach or the esophagus to the Roux limb is best done to the side of the jejunum, not to the end of the divided jejunum; either stapling or hand suturing in two layers is acceptable. The afferent limb is then stapled with a GIA stapler or sutured in two layers to the Roux limb at least 45 cm from the proximal anastomosis.

A Roux jejunal limb may be a useful method for restoring gastrointestinal continuity after resection of a high-lying gastric ulcer or tumor near the esophagogastric junction on the lesser curvature in cases in which closure of the lesser curvature might compromise the lumen of the esophagus. A Roux-en-Y jejunal limb may be brought up antecolically and anastomosed to the entire open end of the gastric pouch and distal esophagus. This maneuver is called a Csendes gastrojejunostomy.

Total Gastrectomy for Cancer

Total gastrectomy is generally performed through an upper midline incision,[13] although some surgeons prefer a bilateral subcostal incision. Exposure is obtained as outlined earlier [see Initial Incision, above]. The suspensory ligament of the lateral

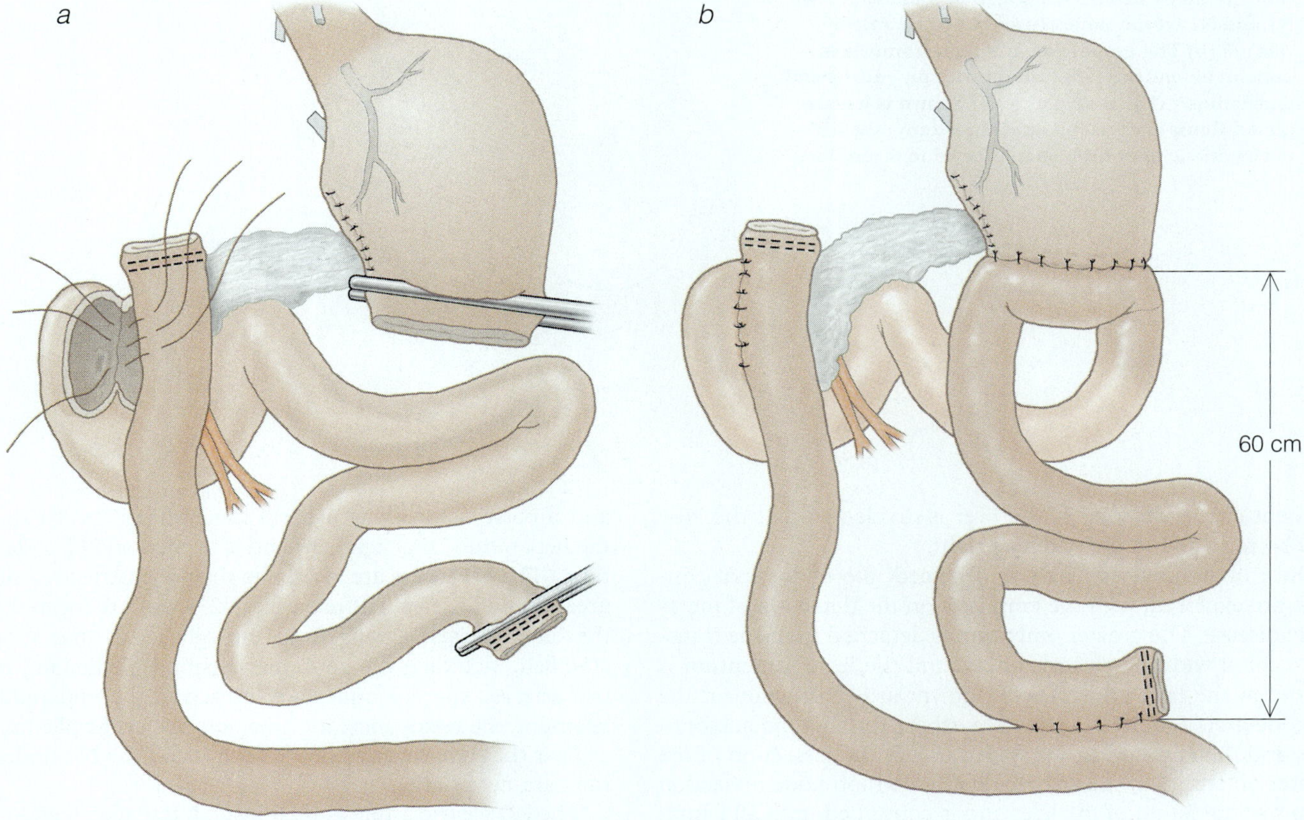

Figure 8 Closure of a difficult duodenal stump with a jejunal limb. (*a*) An isolated Roux jejunal limb may be used either as a serosal patch to cover the duodenal defects or as an end-to-side anastomosis. (*b*) Truncal vagotomy–antrectomy is completed with a Billroth II anastomosis in the Roux duodenojejunostomy. The afferent limb is stapled or sutured to create a Roux limb at least 45 cm long.[12]

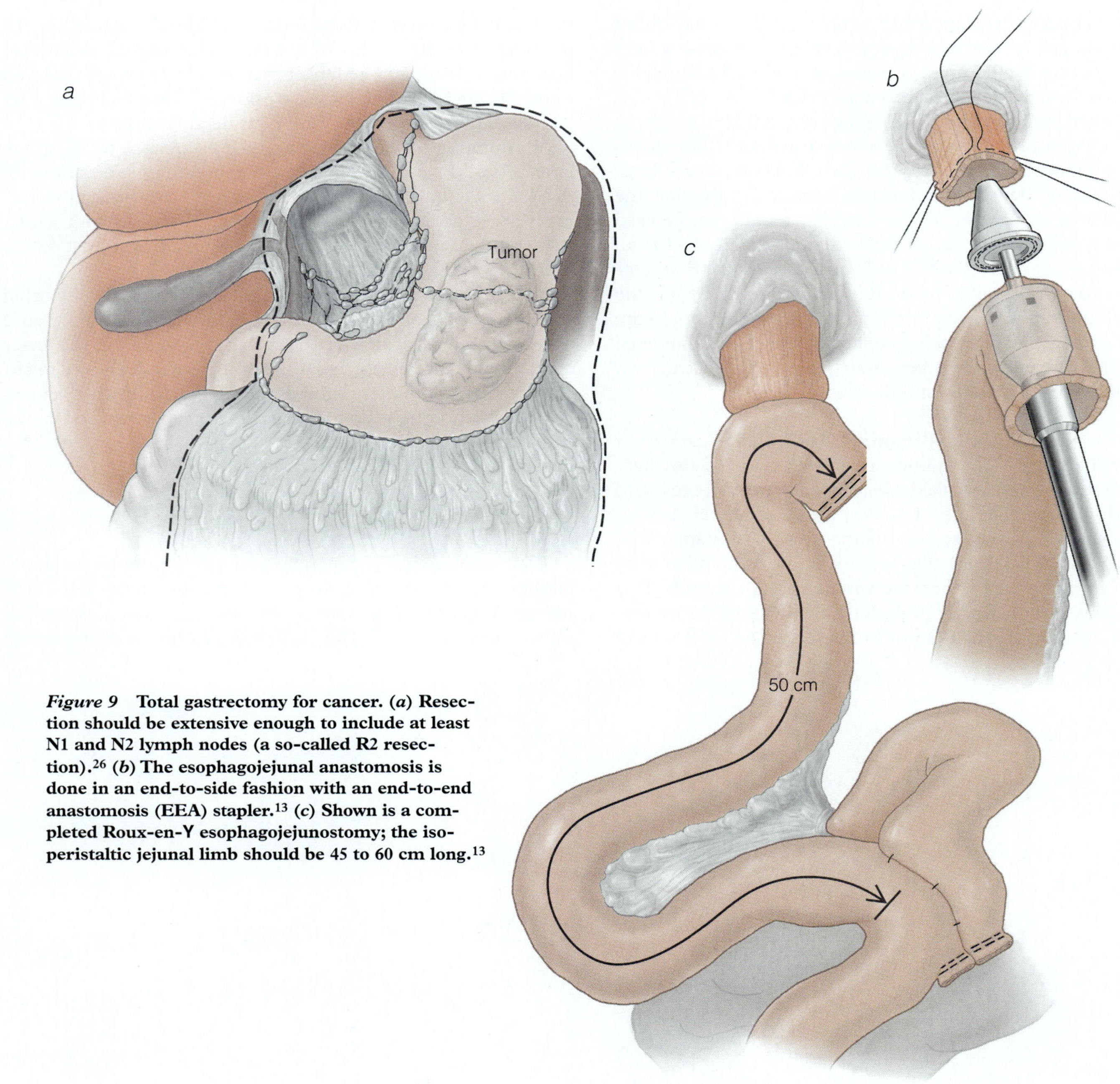

Figure 9 Total gastrectomy for cancer. (*a*) Resection should be extensive enough to include at least N1 and N2 lymph nodes (a so-called R2 resection).[26] (*b*) The esophagojejunal anastomosis is done in an end-to-side fashion with an end-to-end anastomosis (EEA) stapler.[13] (*c*) Shown is a completed Roux-en-Y esophagojejunostomy; the isoperistaltic jejunal limb should be 45 to 60 cm long.[13]

segment of the left lobe of the liver is divided so that the lobe may be retracted to the patient's right.

Once abdominal exposure is obtained, the abdominal contents are explored, with the emphasis on the detection of metastatic disease. The greater omentum is detached from the transverse colon with the electrocautery, and the lesser omentum is incised at the liver and reflected downward. Dissection of the peritoneum is continued upward to expose the abdominal esophagus and then around to the spleen to join the dissection of the greater omentum at the splenic flexure. Lymph node dissection begins at the hilum of the liver and is continued until all lymph nodes, lymphatic vessels, and fatty areolar tissue are stripped from the common bile duct, the portal vein, and the hepatic artery. Further dissection exposes the common hepatic artery and the celiac axis. The preaortic area is cleared of all lymph nodes and areolar tissue. This process skeletonizes the structures in the hepatoduodenal ligament and is termed an N2 node dissection. (The N1 nodes are located in the perigastric area along the greater and lesser curvatures; the N2 nodes are located around the blood vessels arising from the celiac axis that supply the stomach, including the common hepatic, splenic, and left gastric arteries; the N3 nodes are located in the hepatoduodenal ligament, the retropancreatic area, and the celiac plexus, as well as near the superior mesenteric artery; and the N4 nodes are in the para-aortic area.)

The left gastric artery is then ligated, transfixed, and divided. The duodenum is transected 3 cm distal to the pylorus with a GIA stapler and oversewn with interrupted 3-0 silk sutures. The stomach is retracted upward to the left; the resulting excellent exposure of the pancreas permits dissection from the anterior capsule of the pancreas and clearance of the lymph nodes along the splenic artery. The splenic vessels are divided near the caudal end of the pancreas, and the spleen is freed from its ligaments. The abdominal esophagus is then divided about 6 cm above the esophagogastric junction, and the gastrectomy specimen is sent to the surgical pathology laboratory for frozen section examination of the resected margins. This resection includes N1 and N2 nodes and is known as an R2 gastric resection in Japan [see Figure 9a]. (An R0 resection is gastrectomy with incomplete removal of N1 nodes; an R1 resection includes omentectomy along with removal of all N1 nodes; an R3 resection includes removal of all N1, N2, and N3 nodes; and an R4 resection includes removal of all four node groups.)

Alimentary reconstruction takes the form of a Roux-en-Y esophagojejunostomy. The isoperistaltic jejunal limb should be 45 to 60 cm long to prevent alkaline reflux into the esophagus. End-to-end anastomosis should be avoided because the incidence of leakage is unacceptably high, about 16 percent. With end-to-side anastomosis, the incidence of leakage rate is only about two percent, thanks to the superior blood supply.[14] To make an end-to-side esophagojejunal anastomosis, an end-to-end anastomosis (EEA) stapler is inserted through the end of the jejunal segment. The anvil of the stapler is placed in the open end of the esophagus and held in place with a purse-string suture [see Figure 9b]. After the anastomosis is done, the excess portion of the jejunal limb is stapled with a linear stapling device and excised. The proximal jejunum is then anastomosed to the isoperistaltic jejunal limb in an end-to-side fashion with sutures or a GIA stapler [see Figure 9c].

The esophageal connection to the jejunum may be accomplished by creating a jejunal pouch.[15-17] A 1989 review of a century's worth of literature on the pathophysiological and nutritional effects of various types of gastric replacement pouches after total gastrectomy concluded that Roux-en-Y esophagojejunostomy was adequate for reconstructing the alimentary tract and that complicated pouches are not needed.[18] The author did, however, advocate further study of the use of distal jejunojejuneal pouches at Roux-en-Y sites.

Fat and protein malabsorption caused by failure of adequate food intake is often seen after total gastrectomy. This condition abates with time. Initially, patients with end-to-side Roux-en-Y esophagojejunostomies must eat a number of small meals in the course of the day, but after a few months, they can usually resume eating three regular meals a day. With a Roux-en-Y esophagojejunostomy, the transit of food through the small intestine is slower than normal. The proximal jejunum limb does not act as a reservoir, but because it empties rapidly during eating, patients are able to eat a normal-sized meal. The only nutrient that must be replaced on a continuing basis after total gastrectomy is vitamin B_{12}, which is given to prevent megaloblastic anemia.

Subtotal Gastrectomy for Cancer

Cancers in the gastric antrum or the distal third of the stomach are becoming less frequent but still account for about one third of all gastric adenocarcinomas.[19] Because these tumors tend to cause obstruction, they are generally diagnosed earlier than proximal gastric carcinomas (which, in contrast, are increasing in frequency).

Radical distal subtotal gastrectomy that includes regional lymph node removal is the operation of choice for distal gastric carcinoma [see Figure 10]. Resection of 75 to 80 percent of the stomach, including the lesser curvature, leaves enough of a gastric reservoir to minimize postgastrectomy sequelae. My preference is to perform this procedure through an upper abdominal incision [see Initial Incision, above]. The duodenum is divided 3 cm distal to the pylorus with a GIA stapler. The duodenal stump may be oversewn. The stomach is divided at least 6 cm proximal to gross tumor. Frozen-section histologic examination is performed to evaluate the surgical margins before alimentary reconstruction. The greater and lesser omenta are removed. The lymph nodes in the pyloric area, along the common hepatic artery, and in the celiac axis are excised with the stomach. The left gastric artery is divided at its origin. The spleen and the tail of the pancreas are not removed. Gastrointestinal continuity is established via the Schoemaker modification of the Billroth II anastomosis; some surgeons, however, prefer to perform a Billroth I anastomosis or a Roux-en-Y gastrojejunostomy in this setting.

Stamm Gastrostomy

Gastrostomy may be indicated either for gastric decompression or for gastric tube feeding. At present, most tube gastrostomies are performed percutaneously with the aid of an endoscope; however, if stricture or tumor prevents passage of an endoscope into the stomach or previous abdominal operations make percutaneous tube placement hazardous, then an open abdominal procedure may be done to insert a gastrostomy tube with the Stamm technique.

A 7 to 8 cm upper midline abdominal incision is made, and the stomach is grasped with two Babcock clamps. Two concentric

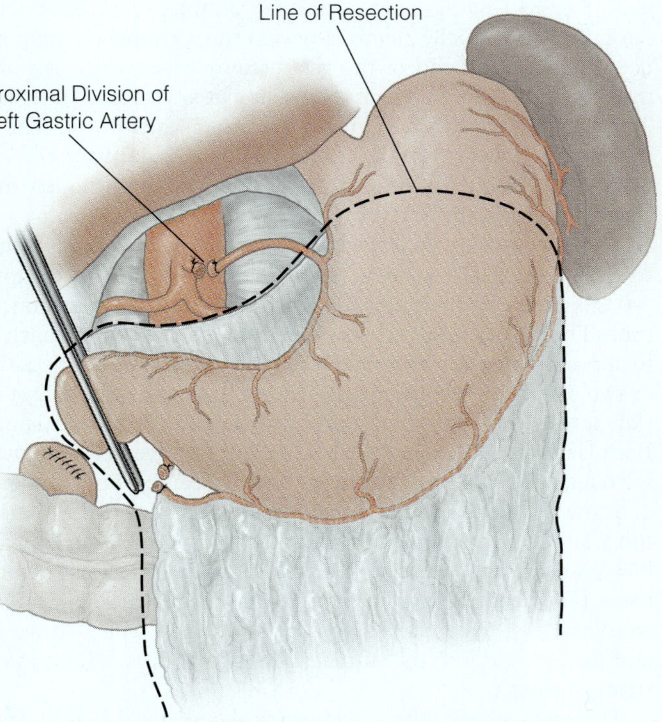

Figure 10 Radical distal subtotal gastrectomy for cancer. From 75 to 80 percent of the stomach is resected, including the lesser gastric curvature, and regional lymph nodes are removed.[26]

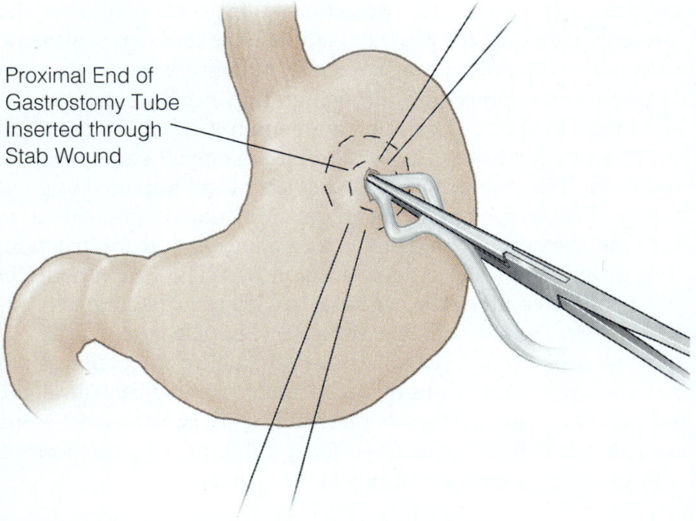

Figure 11 Stamm gastrostomy. Two concentric purse-string sutures are placed on the anterior gastric wall, about 2.5 cm apart. A Malecot or mushroom catheter is inserted into the stomach through an opening made in the center of the inner suture. A stab wound in the left upper abdominal quadrant serves as the exit site for the tube.[27]

purse-string sutures of 2-0 silk are placed on the anterior gastric wall, about 2.5 cm apart. An opening into the stomach is made with the electrocautery in the center of the inner purse-string suture. A Malecot or mushroom catheter (about 24 French) is inserted into the gastric opening [*see Figure 11*]. The inner purse-string suture is tied, then the outer purse-string suture. A stab wound is made with the electrocautery in the left upper abdominal quadrant. A Kelly clamp is passed through this opening and used to grasp the end of the gastrostomy tube, which is pulled through the abdominal wall. The skin exit site should be at least 2 cm from the costal margin and not too far laterally, so that the stomach is not distorted; a useful guideline is to place the stab wound at a point about one third of the way from the left midclavicular line at the costal margin to the umbilicus.

The anterior gastric wall around the gastric opening is affixed to the abdominal wall near the exit site with four interrupted 2-0 silk sutures, one suture to each quadrant surrounding the tube. The gastrostomy tube is then used to pull the stomach up to approximate the abdominal wall, and the sutures are tied. One or two 3-0 nylon sutures are placed in the skin, tied loosely at the skin level, wrapped spirally around the tube, and tied snugly. Because these sutures may be left in place for several weeks, nylon is preferred to silk, which is more likely to cause skin irritation.

Some surgeons like to suture omentum around the gastrostomy site to protect against leaks, but I find this practice troublesome and unnecessary. In addition, some surgeons prefer to use a Foley catheter for the gastrostomy tube. A Foley catheter would be first inserted through the abdominal wall stab wound and then placed into the stomach through the concentric purse-string sutures.

The gastrostomy tube is connected to straight drainage. If the tube is to be used for nutritional purposes, feedings are initiated when normal gastric emptying resumes, which is usually within 24 hours.

Pyloroplasty

Pyloroplasty is performed after truncal vagotomy for duodenal ulcer disease or after esophagectomy. It is appropriate only if the anterior surface of the pylorus is minimally involved and the duodenum is mobile enough to make the operation technically feasible.

WEINBERG PYLOROPLASTY

Heineke in 1886 and Mikulicz[20] in 1888 independently described a pyloroplasty in which a longitudinal incision was made through the pylorus, extending from the distal antrum to the proximal duodenum, and the incision was closed transversely in two layers, which resulted in ablation of the continuity of the pyloric sphincter and an increase in the diameter of the outlet of the pylorus. Weinberg[21] modified the closure so that it consisted of only one layer of nonabsorbable sutures; this resulted in a larger opening through the pyloric channel.

My approach to this procedure is as follows. The pylorus is identified, and the duodenum is mobilized by Kocher's maneuver. If the location of the pylorus is difficult to determine, a small incision should be made in the area of the pylorus; once entrance into the stomach or the duodenum is achieved, the pyloric ring can usually be located by palpation from the inside. Two traction sutures are placed about 1 cm apart on the anterior surface of the pylorus. A longitudinal incision is made between the two traction sutures, extending 2.5 to 3.5 cm proximally onto the antrum and a similar distance distally onto the duodenum. Any bleeding that occurs is controlled with electrocoagulation. To ensure adequate closure and a good outlet, the longitudinal incision must be made very carefully. Some surgeons extend the incision slightly further on the gastric side than on the duodenal side; this practice may yield better alignment when the incision is closed transversely. The total length of the incision should be at least 5 cm to ensure that the outlet is adequate after transverse closure. Generally, however, the incision should not be longer than 7 cm, or the surgeon may find it difficult to close the incision transversely without applying excessive tension.

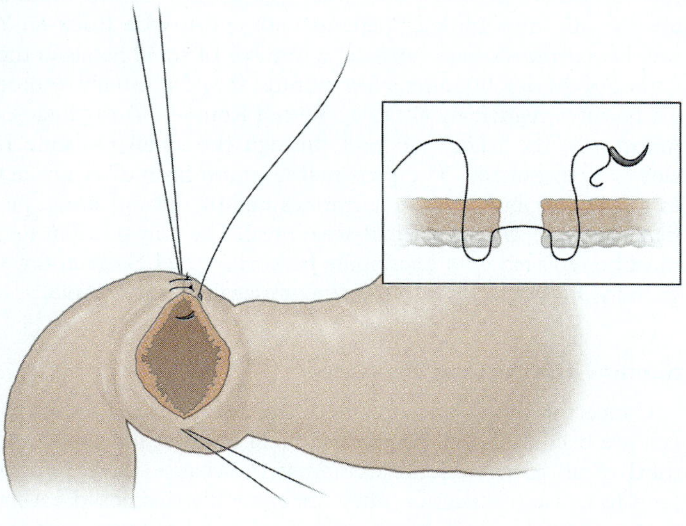

Figure 12 Closure of a Weinberg pyloroplasty. A pyloroplasty may be closed with the Gambee stitch, as shown. Once all of the sutures have been placed, they are tied.[28]

I prefer to close a pyloroplasty with the Gambee stitch[22] [see Figure 12]. The suture is started from the serosa of the stomach and passed through all layers, including the mucosa. It is then passed back through the mucosa to the junction of the submucosa and the muscularis on the gastric wall. Mucosal approximation between the stomach and the duodenum is obtained by next passing the suture on the duodenal side from the junction of the submucosa and the muscularis through the mucosa, then back through all layers of the duodenal wall from the mucosa to the serosa. Once all of the sutures have been placed, they are tied; this helps invert the mucosa and improves the approximation of the serosal surfaces. A simple full-thickness stitch that incorporates more of the serosal surface than of the mucosal surface is also an effective technique for closing a pyloroplasty.

References

1. Dragstedt KR, Owens FM Jr: Supra-diaphragmatic section of the vagus nerves in treatment of duodenal ulcer. Proc Soc Exp Biol Med 53:152, 1943
2. Grassi G, Orecchia C: A comparison of intraoperative tests of completeness of vagal section. Surgery 75:155, 1974
3. Amdrup E, Anderson D, Jenson HE: Parietal cell (highly selective or proximal gastric) vagotomy for peptic ulcer disease. World J Surg 1:19, 1977
4. Rosati I, Serantoni C, Cianni PA: Extended selective proximal vagotomy: observations on a variant in technique. Chir Gastroenterol 10:33, 1976
5. Johnston D: Operative mortality and post-operative morbidity of highly selective vagotomy. Br Med J 5:545, 1975
6. Kennedy T, Magill P, Johnston GW, et al: Proximal gastric vagotomy, fundoplication and lesser curve necrosis. Br Med J 1:1455, 1979
7. Guelrud M, Zambrand-Ricones V, Simon C, et al: Dysphagia and lower esophageal sphincter abnormalities after proximal gastric vagotomy. Am J Surg 149:232, 1985
8. Sawyers JL, Goligher JC: Proximal gastric vagotomy. Surgery of the Stomach, Duodenum and Small Intestine, 2nd ed. Scott HW Jr, Sawyers JL, Eds. Blackwell Scientific Publications, Boston, 1992, p 510
9. Jordan PH, Thornby J: Should it be parietal cell vagotomy or selective vagotomy-antrectomy for treatment of duodenal ulcer: a progress report. Ann Surg 205:572, 1987
10. Sawyers JL, Herrington JL Jr: Perforated duodenal ulcer managed by proximal gastric vagotomy and suture plication. Ann Surg 185:656, 1977
11. Taylor TV, Gunn AR, MacLeod DAD, et al: Anterior lesser curve seromyotomy and posterior truncal vagotomy in the treatment of chronic duodenal ulcer. Lancet 2:846, 1982
12. Herrington JL Jr, Bluett MK: The surgical management of recurrent ulceration. Contemporary Surgery 28(2):15, 1986
13. Sawyers JL: Gastric carcinoma. Curr Probl Surg, Feb 1995, p 153
14. Inberg MV, Linna MI, Scheinin TM, et al: Anastomotic leakage after excision of esophageal and high gastric carcinoma. Am J Surg 122:540, 1971
15. Hunt CJ: Construction of food pouch from segment of jejunum as substitute for stomach in total gastrectomy. Arch Surg 64:601, 1952
16. Lawrence W: Reservoir construction after total gastrectomy: an instructive case. Ann Surg 155:191, 1962
17. Paulino F, Roselli A: Carcinoma of the stomach: with special reference to total gastrectomy. Curr Probl Surg, Dec 1973, p 1
18. Nadrowski L: Is a gastric replacement reservoir essential with total gastrectomy? Pathophysiologic update. Current Surgery 46:276, 1989
19. Cady B, Rossi R, Silverman ML, et al: Gastric adenocarcinoma: a disease in transition. Arch Surg 124:303, 1989
20. Mikulicz J, 1886: Cited in Mikulicz J: Zur operativen Behandlung des stenosier enden Magengeschwures. Arch Klin Chir 37:79, 1888
21. Weinberg JA, Stempien SJ, Movius JJ, et al: Vagotomy and pyloroplasty in treatment of duodenal ulcer. Am J Surg 92:202, 1956
22. Gambee LP: A single layer open intestinal anastomosis applicable to the small as well as the large intestine. West J Surg 59:1, 1951
23. Cameron JA: Atlas of Surgery, Vol 2. Mosby–Year Book, St. Louis, 1994
24. Scott HW Jr, Sawyers JL, Gobbel WG Jr, et al: Definitive surgical treatment in duodenal ulcer disease. Curr Probl Surg, Oct 1968, p 11
25. Herrington JL Jr: Vagotomy and antrectomy. Surgery of the Stomach, Duodenum and Small Intestine, 2nd ed. Scott HW Jr, Sawyers, JL, Eds. Blackwell Scientific Publications, Boston, 1992, p 533
26. Scott HW Jr, Longmire WP, Gray GF: Carcinoma of the stomach. Surgery of the Stomach, Duodenum and Small Intestine, 2nd ed. Scott HW Jr, Sawyers, JL, Eds. Blackwell Scientific Publications, Boston, 1993, p 333
27. Sabiston DC Jr: Atlas of General Surgery. WB Saunders Co, Philadelphia, 1994, p 231
28. Sawyers JL: Selective vagotomy and pyloroplasty. Mastery of Surgery. Nyhas LM, Baker RS, Eds. Little, Brown, Boston, 1984, p 525

Reviews

Atlas of General Surgery. Sabiston DC Jr, Ed. WB Saunders Co, Philadelphia, 1994

Atlas of Surgery, Volume 2. Cameron JL, Ed. Mosby–Year Book, St Louis, 1994

Acknowledgment

Figures 1 through 12   Tom Moore.

50 GASTRIC PROCEDURES FOR MORBID OBESITY

Eric J. DeMaria, M.D., and Harvey J. Sugerman, M.D.

It is clear that severe obesity is associated with a significant increase in morbidity[1] and a decreased life expectancy.[2] Morbid obesity has been shown to have a significant genetic basis.[3,4] To date, attempts to manage morbid obesity with medical weight reduction programs have met with an unacceptably high incidence of recidivism.[5] The approach that has had the greatest and longest-lasting success in achieving weight loss is bariatric surgery.

Choice between Gastric Bypass and Gastric Restriction

The gastric operations performed for morbid obesity include gastric bypass (GBP) procedures and gastric restrictive procedures (i.e., gastroplasty). Randomized, prospective trials have conclusively shown that GBP is as effective for weight control as jejunoileal (JI) bypass and results in significantly fewer complications.[6,7] JI bypass is associated with a substantial incidence of both early complications (e.g., acute cirrhosis, electrolyte imbalance, and fulminant diarrhea)[8] and late complications (e.g., cirrhosis, interstitial nephritis, arthritis, enteritis, nephrocalcinosis, and recurrent oxalate renal stones).[9] If evidence of cirrhosis, renal failure secondary to interstitial nephritis, or other complications mandates reversal of a JI bypass, the patient, if not extremely ill, should be converted to a GBP; otherwise, all the lost weight is sure to be regained, and the obesity-related comorbidity will return. Admittedly, however, many patients have done well after JI bypass and do not need to have the operation reversed.

Several randomized, prospective trials have found that horizontal gastroplasty yields poorer results than GBP.[10-12] Failure of horizontal gastroplasty has generally been attributed to technical causes, such as enlargement of the proximal pouch or the stoma or disruption of the staple line. Vertical banded gastroplasty (VBG) was developed by Mason in the hope that it would solve these technical problems and yield weight loss comparable to that seen after GBP without incurring the significant risk of iron, calcium, and vitamin B_{12} deficiencies associated with GBP. Although VBG appears to be an excellent procedure from a technical point of view,[13] one randomized, prospective trial found it to be significantly less effective than standard GBP.[14] In this trial, patients addicted to sweets lost much more weight after GBP than after VBG because they experienced symptoms of dumping syndrome when ingesting sweets. The failure rate was high after VBG because these patients experienced no difficulties when eating candy or drinking nondietetic sodas.

Two subsequent randomized, prospective trials confirmed the superiority of GBP.[15,16] Furthermore, weight loss after GBP appears to continue for as long as 10 years after operation: in the average patient, weight loss amounts to about two thirds of excess weight at 1 to 3 years after operation, three fifths at 5 years, and more than half in years 5 through 10.[17,18] It has been suggested that standard, or proximal, GBP will fail in 10% to 15% of patients because these patients will frequently nibble on high-fat snacks (e.g., corn chips, potato chips, and buttered popcorn). Such patients may have to be converted to a combined restrictive and malabsorptive procedure, such as partial biliopancreatic bypass (BPB).[19]

The original BPB involves hemigastrectomy and anastomosis of the distal 250 cm of intestine to the stomach; the bypassed small intestine is reanastomosed to the ileum 50 cm from the ileocecal valve. However, BPB has been associated with a high incidence of deficiencies of fat-soluble vitamins, hypocalcemia-induced osteoporosis, and protein-calorie malnutrition.[20] These nutritional deficiencies may be more common in the United States, where fat intake is high, than in many other countries. In Italy, for example, starch intake (as in pasta) probably outstrips fat intake; still, a number of Italian patients have had to be readmitted for parenteral nutrition and extension of the common absorptive intestinal tract because of refractory malnutrition. In some patients, it might be possible to convert a failed proximal GBP into a modified BPB with a 150 cm absorptive ileal limb; however, these patients also must be monitored carefully for deficiencies of fat-soluble vitamins, osteoporosis, and malnutrition.

Superobese patients, defined as those whose weight is 225% of ideal body weight or greater or whose body mass index (BMI) is 50 kg/m^2 or higher, will lose, on average, only about half of their excess weight, rather than two thirds, after standard GBP. In these patients, a 150 cm proximal Roux-en-Y procedure (so-called long-limb GBP [*see* Proximal Gastric Bypass, Operative Technique, *below*]) has been found to increase weight loss to two thirds of excess weight without causing an increase in nutritional complications.[21]

Preparation for Operation

Many surgeons, fearing increased perioperative morbidity and mortality, hesitate to operate on morbidly obese patients. It is true that such patients are at greater risk for complications and adverse results. Nevertheless, severely obese patients can undergo major abdominal surgery for weight loss with a remarkably low complication rate and a low mortality. These results, however, can only be achieved if a comprehensive program for preoperative and postoperative surgical care is rigorously planned and followed. The key elements of preparation for operation in the morbidly obese patient are discussed in greater detail elsewhere [*see* 69 *Obesity*].

Vertical Banded Gastroplasty

OPERATIVE TECHNIQUE

The first step in VBG is to make a circular stapled opening in the stomach 5 cm from the esophagogastric junction. A 90 mm bariatric stapler with four parallel rows of staples is then applied once between this opening and the angle of His. (At this point, ac-

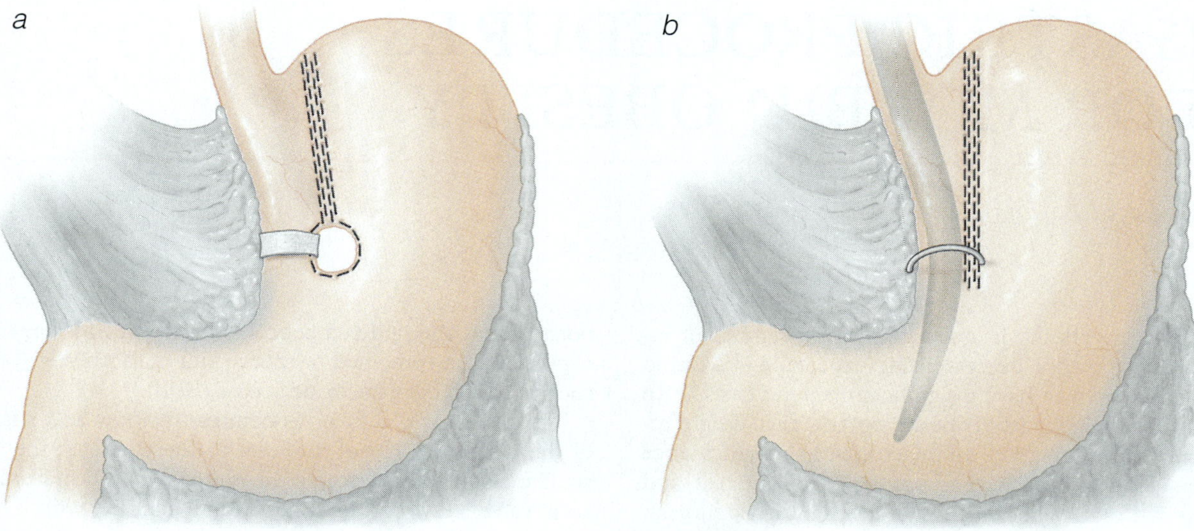

Figure 1 Vertical banded gastroplasty. Depicted are (*a*) standard VBG and (*b*) Silastic ring gastroplasty, a variant of VBG in which the stoma is reinforced with a Silastic tube.

cording to Mason, the originator of the procedure, the volume of the pouch should be measured by means of an Ewald tube placed by the anesthetist; ideally, pouch volume should be 15 ml.) Next, a strip of polypropylene mesh is wrapped around the gastrogastric outlet on the lesser curvature and sutured to itself—but not to the stomach—in such a way as to create an outlet with a circumference of 5 cm for the small upper gastric pouch [*see Figure 1a*]. Some surgeons have used a stomal outlet 4.5 cm in circumference, but this smaller outlet has not led to better weight loss; in fact, many patients with the 4.5 cm outlet exhibit maladaptive eating behavior, drinking high-calorie liquids because meat tends to get caught in the small stoma.

Silastic ring gastroplasty [*see Figure 1b*] is a variant of VBG that uses a vertical staple line and a stoma reinforced with Silastic tubing.

COMPLICATIONS

Complications of VBG include erosion of the polypropylene mesh used to restrict the gastroplasty stoma into the gastric lumen, enlargement of the pouch, stomal stenosis, reflux esophagitis, and mild vitamin deficiencies.[22] To date, mesh erosion has been infrequently observed after VBG. Pouch enlargement is fairly common with horizontal gastroplasty but is much less likely to occur with VBG, in which the vertical staple line is placed in the thicker, more muscular part of the stomach. In addition, stomal diameter remains fixed with the mesh band. If mesh erosion, pouch enlargement, stomal stenosis, disabling GI reflux, or recurrent vomiting occurs, it is probably best to convert the patient to GBP. In particular, patients with a Silastic ring VBG may exhibit intractable vomiting of solid foods with no evidence of mechanical obstruction. In our experience, conversion of these patients to GBP yields good results and eliminates the vomiting problem. Finally, vitamin deficiencies may be prevented by having VBG patients take a multivitamin daily for life.

Laparoscopic Adjustable Gastric Banding

Gastric banding is another form of gastroplasty, in which a polypropylene or Silastic band is placed around the stomach just below the esophagogastric junction. In several series, gastric banding has had markedly variable results with respect to achievement of weight loss. Furthermore, it has been associated with slipping or kinking of the banded stoma, obstruction at the band, and intractable vomiting.

In the past few years, laparoscopic approaches to gastric banding have been developed and brought into use at a number of centers around the world. Laparoscopic adjustable gastric banding is potentially a significant advance over open gastric banding procedures, primarily because of the adjustability of the band. Open gastric banding procedures have used a variety of materials to constrict the gastric lumen and carry a recognized risk of postoperative nausea and vomiting that do not respond to any treatment short of reoperation. The adjustable gastric band (BioEnterics, Carpinteria, California) used in the laparoscopic procedure [*see Figure 2*] is a silicone device with an inflatable reservoir that can be inflated or deflated postoperatively through a subcutaneous port placed deep in the abdominal wall for percutaneous access. Saline is injected into or withdrawn from the reservoir through the port to adjust gastric luminal diameter, as measured by barium contrast evaluations. Thus, if intractable vomiting develops, saline can easily be removed from the band to alleviate the problem; similarly, if the patient fails to lose weight after operation, additional saline may be injected into the band to narrow the gastric lumen further.

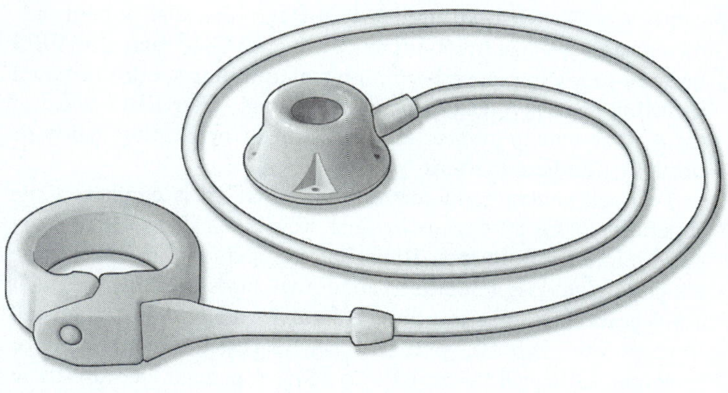

Figure 2 Laparoscopic adjustable gastric banding. Shown is the adjustable gastric banding device used in the procedure.

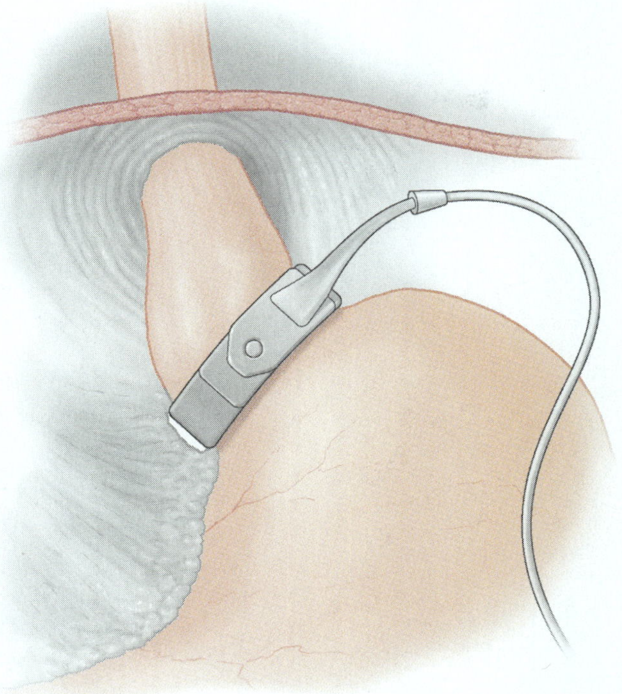

Figure 3 Laparoscopic adjustable gastric banding. Once in the correct position on the proximal stomach, the adjustable band is locked into place.

At present, use of the laparoscopically placed adjustable gastric band is not approved by the Food and Drug Administration (FDA). The FDA has, however, authorized a prospective trial involving 300 patients at seven centers in the United States. Enrollment in this initial trial is now complete; after a mandatory 3-year follow-up period, currently under way, the FDA plans to consider approval of this implantable device. No outcome data have been reported yet.

OPERATIVE TECHNIQUE

Laparoscopic adjustable gastric banding is performed by using a six-port technique. Initial abdominal access is obtained via a supraumbilical trocar, and the remaining five ports are placed sequentially along the right and left costal margins. The liver is retracted via the right lateral port, and the proximal stomach is visualized via a laparoscope inserted through the subxiphoid port. A 20 ml balloon catheter is placed perorally into the proximal stomach to define an appropriately small pouch size. Dissection is then begun at the equator of the balloon with a hook electrocautery placed immediately alongside the gastric wall. The retrogastric tunnel should be above the posterior peritoneal reflection so that the free space of the lesser sac posterior to the stomach is not entered. Additional dissection is carried out laterally at the angle of His to open the peritoneum and start clearing a plane behind the proximal stomach. Once the plane is completely cleared from the lesser curve to the angle of His, a specially designed implement is inserted behind the stomach and used to grasp the tubing of the banding device and pull it around the stomach. The banding device is then locked into place at a spot overlying a pressure-sensitive location on the specially designed balloon catheter; this step allows one to confirm that the band is properly closed in the correct position and that the lumen is sufficiently tightened [*see Figure 3*]. The band tubing is then brought through the left midclavicular trocar port, which is placed via the left midclavicular line subcostal trocar incision and fixed to the abdominal wall fascia with sutures. The tubing is connected to the reservoir, which is filled with saline.

TROUBLESHOOTING

It is essential to place the band properly during the initial procedure. Early results suggest that the proximal pouch must be very small to optimize weight loss. In addition, proper placement minimizes—though it does not eliminate—the risk of band slippage and the complications thereof.

It remains controversial whether posterior fixation of the band is necessary to prevent band slippage. Anterior fixation is routinely performed, with interrupted sutures of nonabsorbable

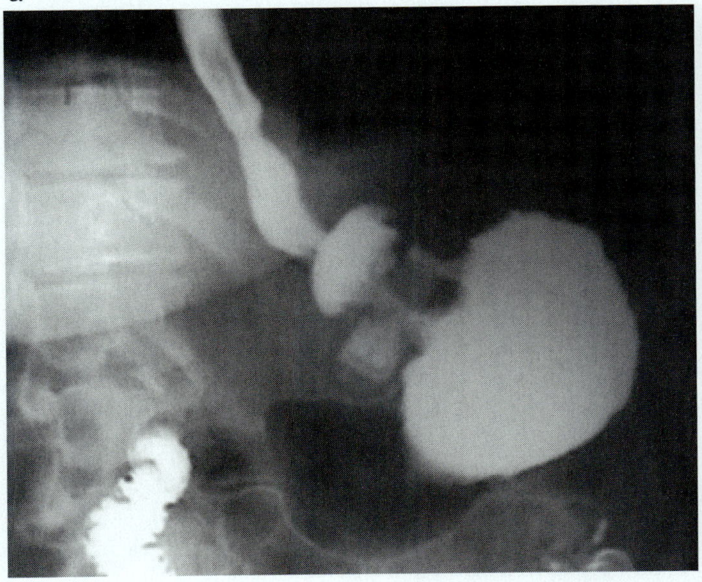

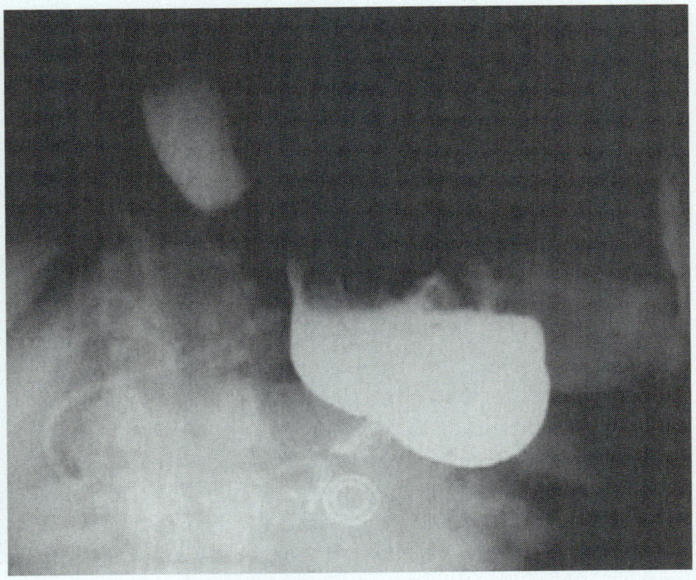

Figure 4 Laparoscopic adjustable gastric banding. Contrast studies illustrate (*a*) a normally positioned laparoscopic adjustable gastric band and (*b*) a slipped band.

material placed between the distal and the proximal stomach to allow tissue to be apposed over the band and held in place. Several techniques have been suggested for posterior fixation of the band, but they are more difficult than anterior fixation techniques. If, as recommended (see above), the band is tunneled above the peritoneal reflection posteriorly, posterior fixation may not be necessary.

Although laparoscopic adjustable gastric banding appears easier than many of the procedures done to treat obesity, there is a definite learning curve. A number of surgical misadventures have been reported, including gastric perforation, splenic injury, and malposition of the band.

COMPLICATIONS

Band slippage (usually posterior rather than anterior) may occur even after proper placement, resulting in intolerance of oral intake and vomiting. Such complaints are an indication for an upper GI series, which usually reveals dilatation of the proximal pouch and rotation of the band [see Figure 4]. Initial treatment consists of evacuating all saline from the band. Frequently, however, the proximal pouch does not return to its normal size, and symptoms recur or fail to resolve. Laparoscopic or open revision of the banding procedure is then required; if the patient also has not lost a sufficient amount of weight, conversion to GBP may be recommended. It is noteworthy that band erosion into the stomach, a not infrequent complication of the use of mesh in VBG or in the Angelchik prosthesis for gastroesophageal reflux treatment, has not been frequently reported to date. Longer follow-up will be necessary to evaluate the true extent of this risk.

As after any form of gastroplasty, the patient may fail to lose weight or may regain lost weight. Inappropriate eating behaviors (e.g., intake of high-calorie sweets) are the most likely cause. If obesity-related comorbid conditions persist, conversion to proximal GBP is appropriate.

OUTCOME EVALUATION

How successful laparoscopic adjustable gastric banding is at achieving weight loss over the long term remains unclear. The adjustability and reversibility of the operation, as well as the decreased disability that results, make it attractive to both patients and physicians. The procedure appears to avoid some of the major postoperative complications associated with open gastric bypass procedures (e.g., incisional hernia, marginal ulcer, and stomal stenosis. Band slippage remains a major postoperative concern, however, though the incidence of slippage does appear to decrease as one's experience with the procedure increases. More significant, there appears to be a high frequency of failed weight loss—as high as 15% to 20% of all patients undergoing the procedure and possibly even higher. European and Australian data confirm that there is a significant failure rate but also suggest that the remaining patients achieve a degree of weight loss approaching that seen with proximal GBP. Whether these reports will withstand the scrutiny of long-term follow-up remains to be seen.

Laparoscopic adjustable gastric banding may come to play an important role in the management of some morbidly obese patients in the United States. If it receives the authorization of the FDA, it may quickly become a frequently performed surgical procedure. On the basis of our participation in the clinical trial, we believe that at present, it is premature to authorize general use of this implantable banding device. It is undeniable, however, that in the United States, the prevalence of severe obesity is increasing at an alarming rate. This worrisome increase, coupled with the disappointingly poor results of medical therapy, the observation that more than 30,000 of these banding devices have already been implanted in patients worldwide, and the potential political consequences of failure to allow use of a potentially helpful device, may spur the FDA to approve laparoscopic adjustable gastric banding prematurely.

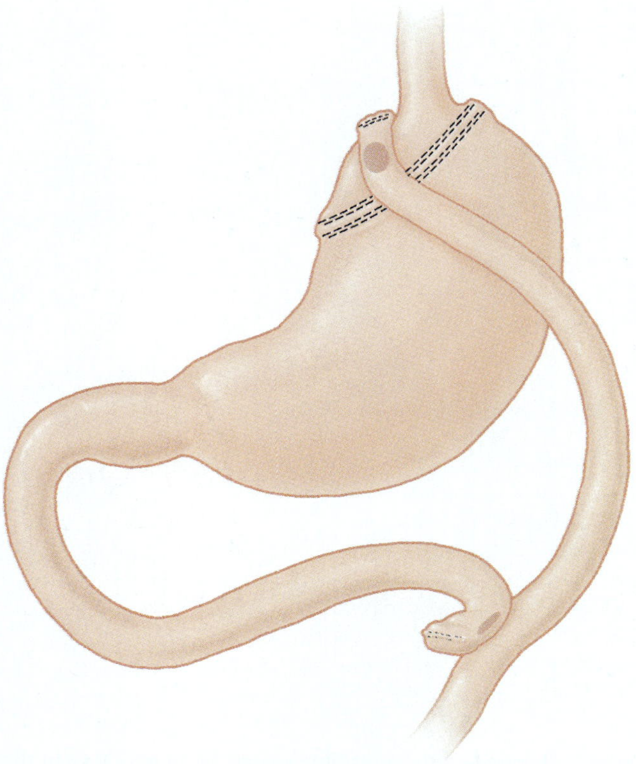

Figure 5 **Proximal gastric bypass. Depicted is the completed procedure.**

Proximal Gastric Bypass

Proximal GBP results in greater weight loss than the gastric restrictive procedures (see above) and carries a lower incidence of weight regain; consequently we consider it the superior procedure. Our focus since the beginning of the 1990s has been on developing techniques for minimizing complications after proximal GBP. In our view, any surgeon currently performing this procedure ought to be able to achieve a gastrojejunal anastomotic leakage rate lower than 5%; many groups, in fact, report rates lower than 3%. In addition, we believe that other postoperative complications (e.g., acute dilatation of the excluded portion of the stomach) are usually preventable if strict attention is paid to mastering the technical aspects of the operation.

Compared with the version of GBP we perform at our institution, the original GBP created a much larger proximal gastric pouch and a much wider anastomotic opening, and it was often associated with inadequate weight loss. In our version of GBP, three superimposed 55 or 90 mm staple lines are placed across the proximal stomach in such a way as to create a gastric pouch no larger than 30 ml with a 45 cm Roux limb and a stoma no larger than 1 cm [see Figure 5].

OPERATIVE TECHNIQUE

Step 1: Initial Incision and Abdominal Exploration

Once the patient is anesthetized, the abdomen receives a thorough, careful cleansing with Betadine and is draped in a sterile fashion. An upper midline incision is made and extended through the fascia alongside the xiphoid process to facilitate cephalad exposure. We routinely carry the incision down to the supraumbilical area. The deep layer of subcutaneous fat can often be separated bluntly with aggressive lateral traction applied by the surgeon and the assistant, and the midline usually can then be identified for fascial incision. We use the electrocautery to enter the abdominal cavity and often encounter a thick layer of subfascial preperitoneal fat before entry into the peritoneal cavity. Abdominal exploration is undertaken in every patient, including examination of the liver for possible signs of liver disease. Other incidental findings may become apparent as well.

Troubleshooting On a number of occasions, we have discovered unexpected significant liver disease at the time of operation. If the patient has cirrhosis without portal hypertension, one should perhaps proceed with bypass if the patient's comorbid conditions make it mandatory; liver transplantation carries increased risk in morbidly obese patients. The gallbladder should be palpated for gallstones, which, if found, we consider an indication for cholecystectomy at the time of the bypass procedure. If there are no visual or palpable gallbladder abnormalities, we use intraoperative ultrasonography to examine the gallbladder and perform cholecystectomy if small stones, sludge, or polyps are identified.

It is not unusual to discover previously unrecognized conditions during GBP, primarily because symptoms may not be obvious in morbidly obese patients and because their large size tends to make radiologic imaging difficult or even impossible. For example, intraoperative discovery of pelvic cysts and tumors is not uncommon in obese female patients. Such lesions may be excised during GBP; on occasion, if they appear benign and their location prevents safe excision, they may be managed with careful follow-up.

Step 2: Mobilization of the Esophagus

The bypass procedure itself is begun by mobilizing the distal esophagus and encircling it with a soft rubber drain 0.5 in. in diameter. The gastrohepatic omentum is bluntly entered at a point overlying the caudate lobe, with care taken to look for and avoid injury to an aberrant left hepatic artery. The phrenoesophageal ligament overlying the anterior and lateral distal esophagus is sharply incised to facilitate subsequent blunt mobilization of the distal esophagus. To prevent esophageal injury, the nasogastric tube is carefully palpated within the lumen of the esophagus during mobilization, and blunt dissection proceeds widely around this important landmark. Laterally, dissection must be at the level of the esophagus or higher.

Troubleshooting If dissection is too low laterally, it may result in blunt injury to the short gastric vessels, bleeding, and the need for urgent splenectomy, which is no easy task in a morbidly obese patient. In addition, it may lead to creation of an inappropriately large pouch by keeping the surgeon from recognizing that some of the stomach is above the level at which the encircling rubber drain is placed.

Step 3: Division of the Mesentery and Dissection around the Stomach

Once the esophagus is mobilized, the assistant's left hand is placed through the gastrohepatic omental opening behind the stomach wall on the lesser curvature. The space between the first and second branches of the left gastric artery is then identified as a landmark for location of the gastric staple line, both to ensure that the pouch created is no larger than 30 ml and to prevent

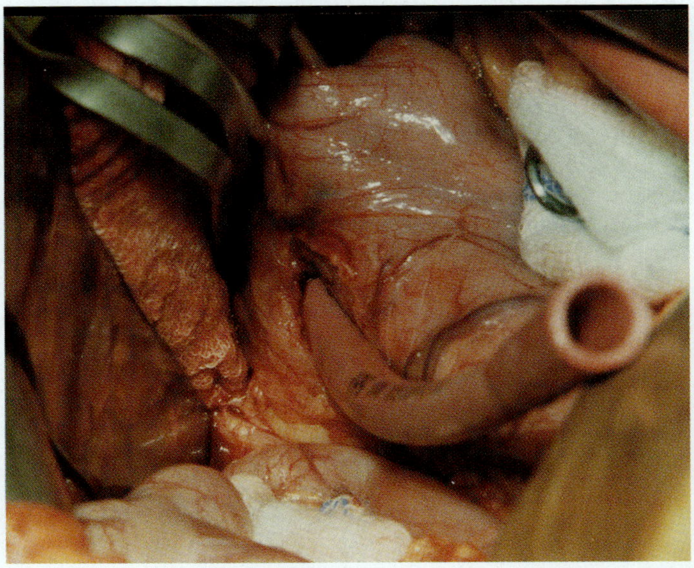

Figure 6 Proximal gastric bypass. After dissection of the avascular tissue on the posterior gastric wall, a red rubber catheter is passed through the resulting space to encircle the stomach.

injury to the left gastric artery, which usually runs cephalad to this location. With the surgeon's posterior finger pressing anteriorly to place tension on the tissue, a fine-tip right-angle clamp and the electrocautery pencil are used to divide the mesentery carefully at this level immediately alongside the stomach wall so as to create a mesenteric opening that will admit a large right-angle clamp. The avascular tissue on the posterior wall of the stomach is then bluntly dissected between the opening in the gastrohepatic omentum and the lateral angle of His, which is identified by the encircling rubber drain. The blunt tip of a large 28 French red rubber tube is placed behind the stomach in a medial-to-lateral direction along this dissected path to encircle the stomach [*see Figure 6*]. The open end of the red rubber tube is subsequently brought through the previously created mesenteric opening with a large right-angle clamp. The stomach is now ready for stapling, and the red rubber tube serves as a guide for introduction of the stapler. At this point, all intraluminal tubes and devices (e.g., the nasogastric tube and the esophageal stethoscope) are removed from the esophagus by the anesthetist.

Troubleshooting When a tube is inadvertently stapled within the stomach, excising it from the staple line can become a technical nightmare. To remove the stapled tube, it is usually necessary to transect the stomach, thereby creating the potential for significant injury to the gastric tissue and possibly compromising the eventual anastomosis.

Step 4: Creation and Mobilization of the Roux Limb and Jejunojejunostomy

The ligament of Treitz is identified, and the jejunum is measured to a point 45 cm beyond the ligament, where the jejunum is divided with a stapler. An 8 to 12 cm segment of jejunum is resected at this point to create a larger mesenteric defect, which we believe facilitates mobilization of the limb to the proximal stomach. Mesenteric dissection is carried posteriorly in fat with the sequential application of clamps until further dissection appears either unnecessary for mobilization or unwise (i.e., likely to cause mesenteric vascular injury).

A side-to-side jejunojejunostomy is then created with a 60 mm linear stapler either 45 cm beyond the initial point of jejunal division, for standard proximal GBP, or 150 cm downstream, for the long-limb modification of the procedure used in superobese patients [see Choice between Gastric Bypass and Gastric Restriction, above]. It is important not to narrow the efferent lumen at the jejunojejunostomy site, particularly with the long-limb modification, in which the lumen at the distal end of the Roux limb may be quite small. The enterotomies made to allow placement of the stapler can usually be closed with a 55 mm stapler loaded with 3.5 mm staples; however, if stapling would cause undue narrowing of the lumen, the closures should be handsewn instead.

Troubleshooting We generally proceed to mobilization of the Roux limb before committing to stapling the stomach so that we can determine whether the limb can be extended to reach the proximal stomach without tension being placed on it. In those rare cases in which the mesentery is too foreshortened to permit the limb to reach the proximal stomach, we advocate changing the procedure to VBG rather than creating a gastrojejunal anastomosis under tension and incurring the increased risk of leakage.

Step 5: Gastric Stapling and Gastrojejunostomy

The Roux limb is brought through the mesentery of the transverse colon with blunt dissection and then brought up to the proximal stomach. The 55 or 90 mm stapler, loaded with 4.8 mm staples, is guided behind the stomach by inserting its open-mouthed end into the lumen of the previously positioned red rubber tube. Once it is determined that the staple line will reach completely across the stomach and that the stomach is not folded on itself, the stomach is stapled three times in such a way that the three staple lines are superimposed [see Figure 7].

A 1 cm anastomosis is created between the proximal stomach pouch and the Roux limb, with an outer layer composed of interrupted 3-0 silk sutures and an inner layer composed of a continuous absorbable 2-0 polyglycolic acid (Dexon) suture. When the posterior aspect of the anastomosis is complete, a 30 French dilator is placed with the patient under anesthesia and is guided through the anastomosis by the surgeon to ensure that the stoma has the appropriate diameter [see Figure 8]. The anterior aspect of the anastomosis is then completed.

Troubleshooting A significant concern for many bariatric surgeons has been a high incidence of staple line disruption causing failed weight loss or weight regain; in one series, the incidence of such disruption was 35%. To minimize this risk, some surgeons advocate transecting the stomach. This is done by inserting two parallel TA-90 staplers and cutting between them with a scalpel after the staplers are fired. Other surgeons, however, prefer to oversew the staple line. By using the technique of three superimposed staple lines, we have decreased the incidence of staple line disruption to less than 2%; consequently, we believe that gastric transection is unnecessary on a routine basis (though occasionally useful in selected cases) and may increase the risk of the procedure. Another advantage of gastric transection besides reduction of staple line disruption is that it allows the Roux limb to be brought up to the gastric pouch via a retrocolic and retrogastric tract, which is significantly shorter and places less tension on the limb. This approach is particularly helpful in severely obese patients with a fatty and foreshortened mesentery, in whom it is difficult to free the Roux limb sufficiently to reach the proximal stomach without tension. The possibility that gastric transection may prove helpful in a specific patient is another reason why it is advisable to delay stapling the stomach until the Roux limb is mobilized.

Step 6: Assessment of the Anastomosis

When the entire anastomosis is complete, the dilator is removed and the tip of an 18 French nasogastric tube is advanced by the anesthetist and carefully guided through the anastomosis by the surgeon. The Roux limb is occluded with the assistant's left hand or with an atraumatic intestinal clamp, and the anesthetist injects a series of 10 ml aliquots of methylene blue dye through the nasogastric tube to determine whether the anastomosis is leaking. A total of 30 to 60 ml of methylene blue must usually be injected; lesser amounts will not stress the suture line enough to constitute an adequate test.

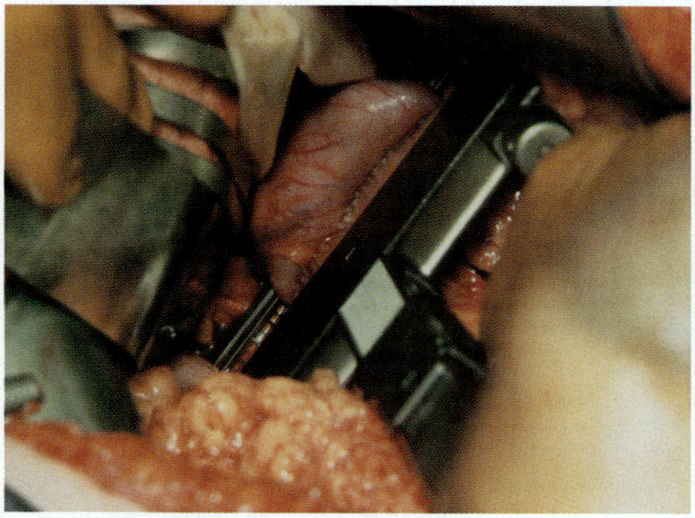

Figure 7 Proximal gastric bypass. The stomach is stapled to create the small proximal pouch. The stapler is fired three times to create three superimposed staple lines, thereby decreasing the risk of staple line disruption.

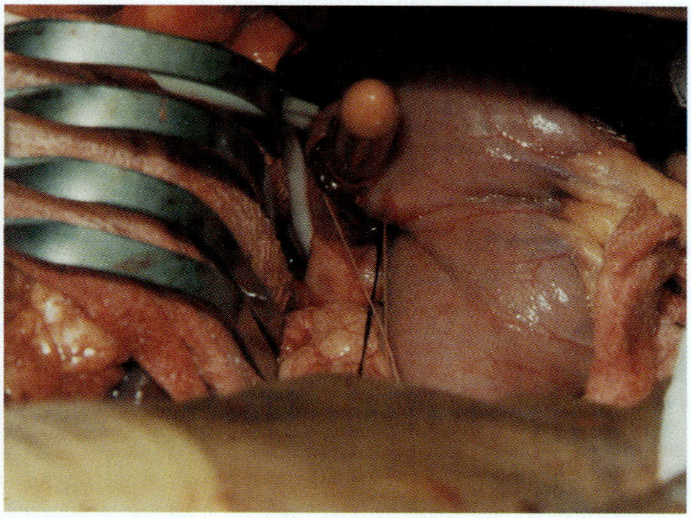

Figure 8 Proximal gastric bypass. When the posterior aspect of the gastrojejunal anastomosis has been completed, a 30 French dilator is placed through the stoma to confirm that the opening is correctly sized.

Troubleshooting When an intraoperative leak is identified, we oversew the area of leakage with silk sutures until injection of additional methylene blue dye via the nasogastric tube yields no further leakage. The most difficult area to repair is the posterior suture line, which is quite close to the gastric staple line. Posterior leaks are usually repaired by reinforcing the posterior suture line with additional sutures between the excluded stomach and the jejunal limb; often, we oversew the entire posterior suture line. In addition, a viable pedicle of omentum may be mobilized and placed around the anastomosis for additional reinforcement. Closed suction drains may also be placed in this area, both to detect possible postoperative leakage and to control a postoperative fistula.

Finally, a gastrostomy tube is placed in the excluded portion of the stomach. This measure provides postoperative decompression, which should prevent the development of undue tension on the Roux limb as a result of gastric distention, and establishes a route for enteral feeding if a fistula develops. Fortunately, such fistulas are rare. When they do occur, they often heal if (1) they are well drained, (2) there is no distal obstruction or local abscess, and (3) the patient is receiving nutritional support with no oral intake. A gastrostomy tube should also be placed in the distal gastric pouch when extensive adhesions from a previous procedure or a difficult gastric reoperation prevents postoperative dilatation of the pouch.

Step 7: Closure

When the absence of leakage is confirmed or when any leaks identified have been controlled, the tip of the nasogastric tube can be positioned further down in the Roux limb and left to continuous suction overnight. All mesenteric defects—at the jejunojejunostomy, at the mesocolon, and behind the Roux limb—are then closed to prevent a Petersen hernia. The abdominal fascia is reapproximated with a continuous No. 2 nonabsorbable suture, subcutaneous tissues are irrigated with a crystalloid solution containing 1% neomycin, and the skin is closed with skin staples. No subcutaneous sutures or drains are used in routine cases.

COMPLICATIONS

Proximal GBP is associated with a significant incidence of stomal stenosis and with marginal ulcer.[23] The former responds to endoscopic stomal dilatation, and the latter usually responds to H_2 receptor blocker or proton pump inhibitor therapy.

Iron, vitamin B_{12}, and folic acid deficiencies may occur but can usually be corrected with oral supplements[22]; accordingly, GBP patients, like VBG patients, should be advised to take a multivitamin daily for life. Compared with VBG, GBP results in significantly lower serum hemoglobin and iron concentrations. This is primarily a problem in menstruating women. All menstruating women who have undergone GBP should be treated prophylactically with supplemental oral ferrous sulfate, 325 mg/day. As many as six iron tablets a day may be required if menstrual bleeding is heavy. On occasion, intramuscular iron injections or, rarely, hysterectomy may be necessary. The risk of vitamin B_{12} deficiency is higher after GBP than after VBG, but this condition can be prevented with supplemental oral vitamin B_{12}, 500 mg/day. A few patients may require (or prefer) monthly B_{12} injections, which they can learn to administer themselves.

Concerns have been expressed that GBP can lead to other divalent cation deficiencies. We have not encountered zinc deficiencies 5 to 9 years after GBP. We have, however, observed calcium deficiencies leading to osteoporosis, which may take many years to become manifest and may not be biochemically evident because of normal serum calcium levels. We therefore recommend that all our GBP patients take oral calcium supplements. Magnesium deficiencies should be treated with $MgSO_4$ supplementation.

Nutritional deficiencies do not appear to be a greater problem with long-limb GBP than with standard proximal GBP. We do monitor patients for possible malabsorption of the fat-soluble vitamins A, D, and E after long-limb GBP.

BPB may be associated with all of the complications seen after GBP. In addition, patients who undergo BPB may experience diarrhea, severe protein malnutrition (manifested as hypoalbuminemia), and deficiencies of vitamins A (manifested as severe night blindness), D (manifested as severe osteoporosis), and E.[20] Hypoalbuminemia may respond to oral pancreatic enzymes but often must be treated with total parenteral nutrition. In some patients, it may prove necessary to lengthen the absorptive intestinal tract from 50 cm to 200 cm.

OUTCOME EVALUATION

In our series of 672 open proximal GBP procedures,[17] we reported a 1.2% incidence of anastomotic leak with peritonitis, a 4.4% incidence of severe wound infection (defined as infection serious enough to delay hospital discharge), an 11.4% incidence of minor wound infections and seromas (which were easily treated at home), a less than 1% incidence of gastric staple line disruption with the use of three superimposed applications of a 90 mm linear stapler, a 15% incidence of stomal stenosis, a 13% incidence of marginal ulcer, a 16.9% incidence of incisional hernia, and a 10% incidence of cholecystitis necessitating cholecystectomy. Gallstones developed in 32% of the GBP patients who had a normal intraoperative gallbladder ultrasonogram within 6 months of surgery, and sludge was observed in another 10%. In a multicenter randomized prospective trial,[24] we and others were able to reduce the incidence of gallstones within 6 months of GBP from 32% to 2% by giving patients ursodeoxycholic acid, 300 mg twice daily. Gallstone formation is very rare beyond 6 months. The operative mortality in our series was less than 1%. Patients with respiratory insufficiency of obesity had a 2.2% operative mortality, whereas those without pulmonary dysfunction had a 0.4% mortality.

Neither the data from our randomized, prospective trial nor the data from selective studies support the contention that VBG is safer than GBP. Although GBP includes one more anastomosis than VBG, complications such as leaks and peritonitis occur with both operations. A common criticism of GBP is that it is difficult to evaluate the distal gastric pouch and duodenum after the operation. Such evaluation, however, can be done in 75% of patients by means of retrograde passage of an endoscope into the duodenum and the stomach and in others by means of percutaneous distal distention gastrography (DeMaria EJ, Sugerman HJ, unpublished data, 2000). To our knowledge, bleeding from either the distal gastric pouch or a duodenal ulcer has occurred in only one of our more than 1,200 GBP patients. In one patient, a perforation of the proximal gastric pouch developed after administration of high-dose nonsteroidal anti-inflammatory medication. Gastric mucosal metaplasia of the bypassed portion of the stomach was noted in 5% of patients after retrograde endoscopy, a finding that has raised concerns regarding the risk of carcinoma arising at that location. However, tens of thousands of these procedures have been performed since 1967, and only one case of cancer in the bypassed stomach has been reported to date. We have also had one such case but have not published it.

Laparoscopic Gastric Bypass

Laparoscopic gastric bypass is a relatively new alternative to standard open GBP. One would anticipate that laparoscopic GBP would yield much the same weight loss results as open

GBP but with less pain, reduced disability, and a shorter hospitalization period. In addition, one would anticipate a decrease in major wound infections as well as fewer incisional hernias. On the face of it, it seems likely that the laparoscopic procedure, though more expensive, would be cost-effective, but proving it is so will probably require an analysis of long-term follow-up that documents decreased subsequent hospitalizations for wound infections, hernia repairs, and complications of intra-abdominal adhesions (e.g., bowel obstruction), given that early results cannot demonstrate a dramatic reduction in the length of hospitalization after the procedure. If the additional benefit of reduced disability-related absence from work is realized, this would help reduce overall costs as well.

TOTAL INTRACORPOREAL LAPAROSCOPIC GASTRIC BYPASS

Laparoscopic GBP poses significant technical challenges, even for surgeons with advanced laparoscopic skills. Most of the variations seen at different institutions are related to creation of the gastrojejunal anastomosis, with most groups favoring the use of a circular rather than a linear stapler. The anvil of the circular stapler may be placed within the proximal gastric pouch either by means of flexible upper GI endoscopy, through an approach similar to the snare-and-wire technique used for placement of a percutaneous endoscopic gastrostomy (PEG) tube, or by means of a gastrotomy of the pouch for intra-abdominal anvil placement followed by staple closure of the gastrotomy. Peroral placement of the stapler's anvil can be problematic: even the small 21 French anvil is hard to pass through the proximal esophagus in some patients. Nevertheless, we will describe this approach in some detail because it seems to be favored by most surgeons at present and it is easier to perform.

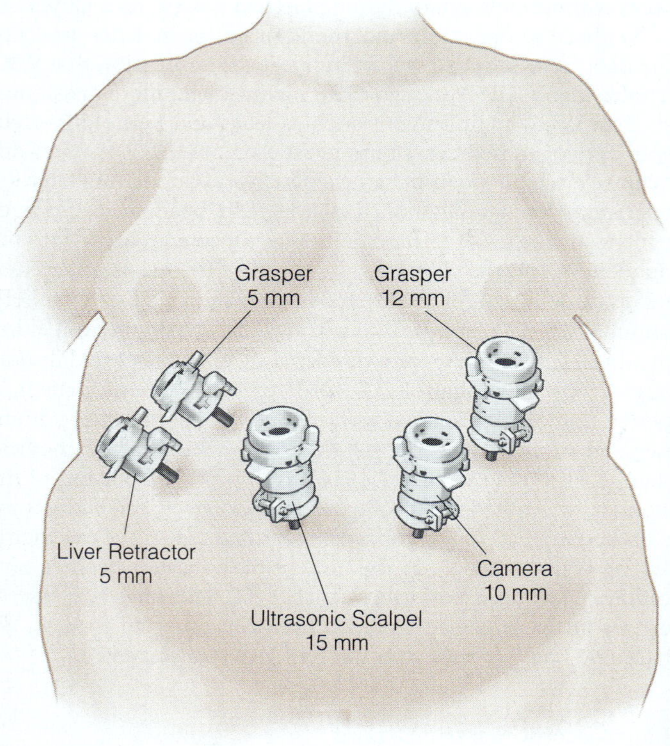

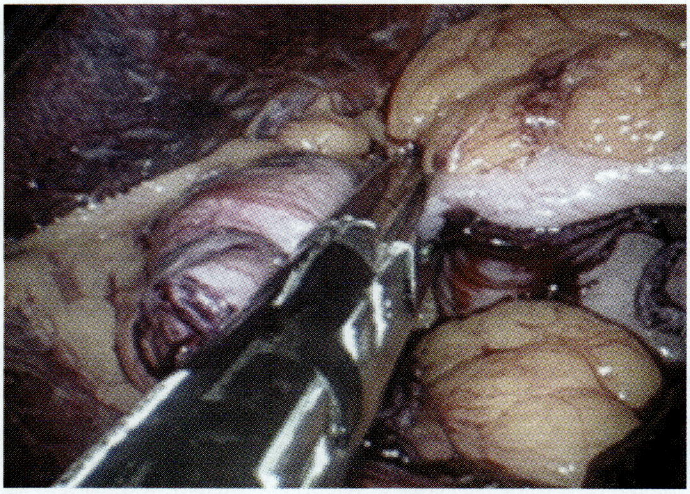

Figure 10 Laparoscopic gastric bypass: total intracorporeal approach. Much as in open GBP, a linear endoscopic GIA stapler is fired three times to transect the stomach and create the gastric pouch.

Operative Technique

Step 1: initial access and trocar placement Initial access to the abdomen is obtained through a left subcostal incision with either a Veress needle or a commercially available device that allows direct vision through the scope while a 12 mm trocar is inserted. Gas is then insufflated into the abdomen to a pressure of 15 mm Hg; on occasion, a pressure of 18 mm Hg may be necessary. Additional trocars are placed in specific locations [see Figure 9]. To retract the liver, we employ a metal Nathanson liver retraction device anchored to the bed, which is inserted after a 5 mm sharp trocar is used to enter the abdominal cavity and peritoneum and removed. If the left lateral segment of the liver is very large (as in patients with steatosis), additional liver retraction may be necessary.

The falciform ligament is then dissected from the anterior abdominal wall with an ultrasonic scalpel. This dissection allows the trocar incision to be placed quite high in the epigastrium, which facilitates proximal gastric exposure. A 12 mm port placed in the right paramedian position near the costal margin serves as the surgeon's primary operative port; two lateral subcostal 5 mm ports allow both surgeon and assistant to employ two-handed techniques for the entire procedure.

Step 2: dissection around the stomach and creation of the gastric pouch Dissection is performed along the lesser curvature of the stomach between the neurovascular bundle and the gastric wall; the ultrasonic scalpel is the best instrument for this purpose. Dissection posterior to the stomach is performed in the avascular free plane of the lesser sac. Additional dissection along the lesser curvature is not recommended, because it may increase the devascularization of the pouch. Further dissection is done with the ultrasonic scalpel at the angle of His to create a connection with the posterior gastric space. A linear endoscopic gastrointestinal anastomosis (GIA) stapler loaded with 3.5 mm staples in 60 mm cartridges is then used to transect the stomach and create the proximal gastric pouch; three firings are usually necessary [see Figure 10].

Step 3 (circular stapling): placement of the stapler in the gastric pouch As noted (see above), surgeons use several different techniques to complete the gastrojejunal anastomosis.

Figure 9 Laparoscopic gastric bypass: total intracorporeal approach. Shown are the trocar incision sites for laparoscopic GBP.

Initially, we employed the technique reported in Wittgrove's original description of the procedure,[25] which involved passing the anvil of a circular stapler down the patient's esophagus in a manner resembling placement of a PEG tube. With this approach, the next step in the procedure is to have an assistant perform flexible upper GI endoscopy of the gastric pouch. The pouch wall is transilluminated by the endoscope light, and a site is chosen for the gastrojejunostomy. The endoscopist then places an endoscopic snare, which can be seen pressing against the tissue of the pouch wall. A small opening is made in the pouch with the electrocautery scissors so that the snare can be pushed through the gastric wall at this location. The snare is then used to grasp a wire placed through a needle across the abdominal wall in the left abdomen, and snare and wire are withdrawn through the mouth along with the scope.

The anvil of the stapler is attached to the end of the wire that was drawn through the mouth, and the surgeon pulls on the other end of the wire to deliver the anvil through the mouth, down the esophagus, and into the gastric pouch, where it can be visualized. The electrocautery attached to the scissors is used to enlarge the opening in the gastric wall slightly, and the stem of the stapler is then brought through the gastrotomy. To prevent anastomotic leakage after stapling, the gastrotomy should be no larger than the diameter of the stem; if it is too large, it can be closed around the stem by placing one or two simple sutures.

Troubleshooting. Difficulty in passing the anvil perorally may arise at the level where the trachea separates from the esophagus in the deep pharynx. This difficulty can usually be overcome either by having the endoscopist perform a jaw-thrust maneuver or by placing a large laryngoscope blade deep in the pharynx to make the anvil visible in the proximal esophagus and then nudging the anvil forward with either the tip of the blade or a McGill forceps. Deflating the endotracheal tube balloon may also help. Occasionally, we use the large esophageal dilator to place pressure on the tip of the anvil. Given the potential for esophageal injury if the anvil will not advance, it is important not to apply excessive force. We have seen a case in which the anvil became lodged in the proximal esophagus beyond the laryngoscopic view and the long suture holding it broke; retrograde passage of an esophageal dilator was required to dislodge the anvil. Other surgeons who use wire to draw the anvil down the esophagus have identified nontransmural esophageal injuries on postoperative contrast studies or have seen subcutaneous emphysema in the neck after operation.

Step 3 (linear stapling) Currently, we prefer a technique in which a linear stapler, rather than a circular one, is used to create the gastrojejunal anastomosis. In this approach, therefore, we proceed directly from creation of the gastric pouch to creation of the Roux limb for subsequent anastomosis to the pouch.

Step 4: creation and mobilization of the Roux limb and jejunojejunostomy In most reports of laparoscopic GBP, regardless of how the gastrojejunostomy is done, the approach to creating the Roux limb is essentially the same. The patient is placed in a supine position, and graspers are used to bring the omentum upward into the upper abdomen so that the transverse colon and the underlying mesocolon are exposed. Graspers are then placed on the transverse mesocolon and used to elevate it anteriorly so that the ligament of Treitz is exposed. The position of the ligament of Treitz is confirmed by careful manipulation and verification that the bowel is attached to the retroperitoneum at this location; this may be a more difficult task in patients who have previously undergone abdominal procedures.

With the help of a measuring instrument inserted into the abdomen, the small bowel is measured to a point 30 to 40 cm from the ligament of Treitz, where it is transected with the endoscopic GIA stapler, loaded with 2.5 mm staples. A 0.5 in. Penrose rubber drain is sutured to the cut end of the Roux limb so that it is not confused with the other cut end of the bowel. The Roux limb is then measured to a length of 45 to 60 cm. (As in open GBP, the Roux limb may have to be significantly longer—up to 150 cm—if the long-limb modification is being performed.) The afferent side of the previously transected small bowel is then attached with a simple absorbable suture to the proposed jejunojejunostomy site on the Roux limb. Intracorporeal suturing is facilitated by using an automatic suturing device. Positioning is important: the afferent limb should be kept to the patient's left, with the Roux limb more medial.

A small enterotomy is then made in preparation for passage of the linear stapler, loaded with 2.5 mm staples in a 60 mm cartridge, into the bowel. Two sutures are placed, one anterior to the enterotomy and the other posterior, to help manipulate the bowel onto the stapler. The stapler is then fired, creating a 60 mm side-to-side anastomosis. A third suture is placed at the midpoint of the enterotomy, and all three sutures are grasped to facilitate closure of the enterotomy with another application of the linear stapler. Once completed, the anastomosis is inspected both for integrity and for possible narrowing. At this point, anterior traction is applied to the three sutures to facilitate placement of interrupted or continuous sutures to close the mesenteric defect.

Next, a retrocolic, retrogastric tunnel (which we consider clearly superior to an antecolic approach) is created so that the Roux limb can be advanced to the proximal stomach for anastomosis. The ligament of Treitz is once again identified by lifting the transverse mesocolon anteriorly, and a spot 1 to 2 cm anterior and to the left of the ligament is chosen as the starting point for dissection with the ultrasonic scalpel. The middle colic artery should be visualized medial to this point of entry into the mesocolon. The goal of the dissection is to identify the posterior wall of the stomach, which may be difficult in patients who are extremely obese, have a fatty, foreshortened mesocolon, or have previously undergone abdominal surgery. Once the stomach is visible, it is grasped and elevated through the mesocolic window, and the end of the Penrose drain is grasped and brought through the mesocolic defect into the lesser sac. When the Penrose is in place in the lesser sac, the omentum is pulled down from the epigastrium to allow visualization of the drain, now posterior to the divided distal stomach. The Penrose drain is grasped, and the patient is placed back into a steep reverse Trendelenburg position. Traction is applied to the Penrose drain to deliver the cut end of the Roux limb up into the lesser sac for anastomosis.

Troubleshooting. Some surgeons place the Roux limb in the antecolic position and divide the fatty omentum with the ultrasonic scalpel to decrease the tension on the limb. This technique appears to be inferior to the retrocolic approach, in that it does not decrease the tension on the limb and the anastomosis sufficiently and it necessitates more aggressive transection of the small bowel mesentery to achieve adequate mobilization. For these very reasons, many bariatric surgeons do not favor the antecolic approach during open GBP; thus, to use this approach during laparoscopic GBP violates a basic principle of modern surgery, according to which the application of minimally invasive techniques to an operation must not compromise the quality of the procedure. There are also some surgeons who prefer to create a loop gastrojejunostomy, thus avoiding the technical challenges of creating a Roux limb laparoscopically. This approach was abandoned years ago in open GBP because of postoperative bile reflux and an increased severity of complications resulting from high output of digestive juices when a leak occurs at the gastrojejunal anastomosis; it should be abandoned in laparoscopic GBP as well. We firmly believe that the practice of using such suboptimal methods for the purpose of performing this complex operation more expeditiously is poorly conceived and is to be condemned.

Step 5 (circular stapling): gastrojejunostomy In the circular stapling technique, the stapled end of the Roux limb is open to permit introduction of the stapler. The 12 mm trocar site in the left upper quadrant is dilated so that the circular stapler can be inserted through the abdominal wall without the need for a trocar; lubrication is helpful for this step. The stapler then cannulates the Roux limb. This step is facilitated by holding the open mouth of the limb in three locations, with one of the three holds involving traction on the Penrose drain previously sutured to the bowel. The stapler is advanced 3 to 4 cm down the limb, and the spike on the stapler is brought through the antimesenteric portion of the bowel by unscrewing the stapler under direct vision. Once the stapler has been opened completely, it is laparoscopically joined to the anvil and the gastric pouch, then closed and fired.

Once fired, the stapler is removed from the abdominal wall, and a balloon trocar device is used to close the dilated abdominal wall opening. A single firing of the endoscopic GIA stapler, loaded with 2.5 mm staples, is often all that is required to reclose the cut end of the small bowel. Interrupted or continuous absorbable sutures are then placed around the stapled anastomosis for added security.

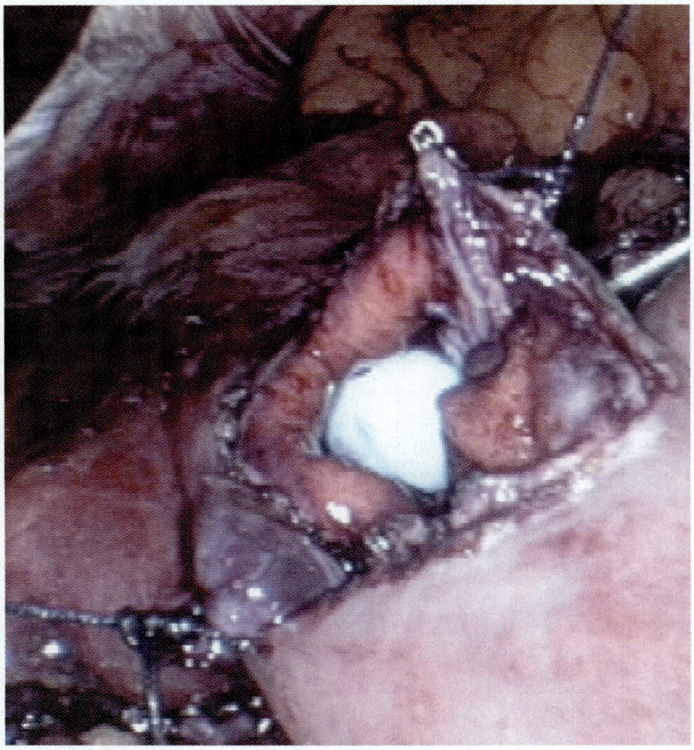

Figure 11 **Laparoscopic gastric bypass: total intracorporeal approach. A 30 French dilator is placed into the proximal gastric pouch before closure of the gastrojejunal anastomosis with the endoscopic GIA stapler.**

Step 5 (linear stapling): gastrojejunostomy For the linear stapling technique that we currently prefer, it is not necessary to dilate a trocar site, which appears to increase postoperative pain. Two holding sutures are placed to secure the antimesenteric Roux limb to the posterior gastric pouch toward the lesser curvature. Between the two sutures, an enterotomy and a gastrotomy are performed that are large enough to admit the jaws of the endoscopic GIA stapler, which is loaded with 3.5 mm staples in a 30 mm cartridge for a side-to-side anastomosis [*see Figure 11*]. Applying traction to the sutures facilitates placement of the stapler into the lumen of the bowel and the stomach by means of the same techniques employed in creation of the jejunojejunostomy. A 30 French dilator is then passed into the pouch by the anesthetist and guided through the anastomosis by the surgeon under direct vision to maintain the appropriate stomal diameter (10 to 12 mm) during closure of the open end. Placement of a third suture between the first two holding sutures allows anterior traction and facilitates amputation of the tissue to close the openings. The stapler, loaded with 3.5 mm staples in a 60 mm cartridge, should be placed so as to amputate a significant amount of tissue during this closure; the esophageal dilator preserves the stomal diameter.

We have found that using the linear GIA stapler simplifies the procedure, decreases operative time, and eliminates the concerns about injury to the body of the esophagus that arise with passage of the circular stapler.

Step 6: assessment of the anastomosis In every case, regardless of which stapling technique is employed, flexible upper GI endoscopy is performed to assess the anastomosis. The Roux limb is occluded with an intestinal clamp to prevent excessive bowel and distal gastric dilatation. The patient is placed in the supine position, and the area around the anastomosis is irrigated with saline; the presence of air bubbles, easily detectable in the irrigant, indicates that the anastomosis is leaking. In most cases, we are able to distend the pouch and the Roux limb tightly, and we reinforce even tiny air leaks with additional sutures. The anastomosis and the staple lines are visualized, and the endoscope is navigated through the anastomosis into the Roux limb whenever possible. After adequate visualization and testing, the gas is suctioned from the intestine, the Roux limb is unclamped, and the endoscope is removed.

Step 7: closure Finally, a 10 mm closed suction drainage tube is placed adjacent to the anastomosis to permit monitoring for postoperative leaks. This drain is removed after the patient begins oral intake if an upper GI series reveals no postoperative leakage [*see Figure 12*]. The liver retractor is removed under direct vision to ensure that no bleeding occurs. Trocar sites 10 mm in diameter or larger are closed by using a needle suture passer to place 0 absorbable sutures under direct endoscopic visualization. Skin wounds are closed with skin staples or absorbable subcutaneous sutures.

HAND-ASSISTED LAPAROSCOPIC GASTRIC BYPASS

Because total intracorporeal laparoscopic GBP is such a challenging technical adventure, we initially developed a technique for a hand-assisted version of the procedure based on work done by others.[26] We viewed this technique as a bridge to the total intracorporeal approach, in that it enabled us to learn the technical aspects of a difficult, highly advanced laparoscopic procedure while enjoying the security provided by the presence of an intra-abdominal hand for palpation and manipulation during the procedure. This added security is the major advantage of the hand-

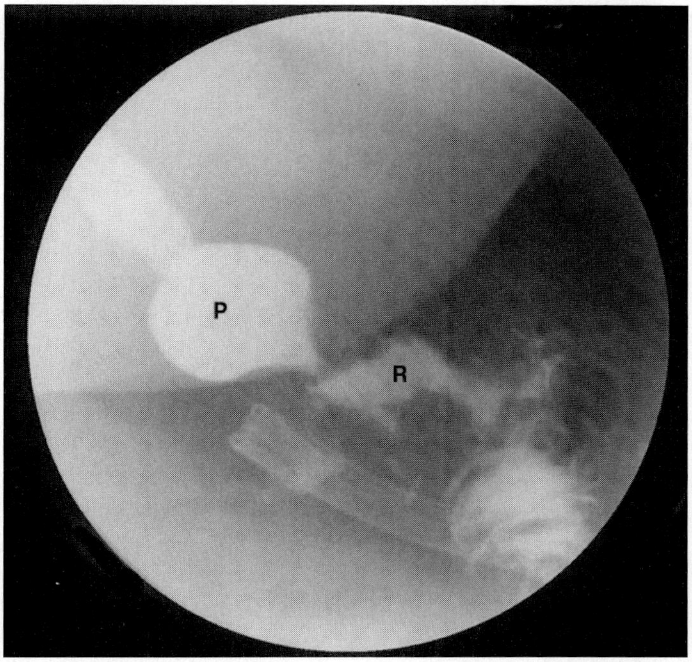

Figure 12 Laparoscopic gastric bypass: total intracorporeal approach. Flexible upper GI endoscopy is performed to assess the completed anastomosis.

assisted approach. The major disadvantage is the potential for complications at the incision used for manual access. The complications seen at this site are reminiscent of those seen after open GBP, including major wound infection, dehiscence, and hernia formation. In our series of hand-assisted laparoscopic GBP procedures, we have seen one major wound infection in the hand incision and one instance of postoperative fascial dehiscence.

Operative Technique

Step 1: initial access and placement of the hand-assisted device A left subcostal incision is made, a Veress needle is inserted, and gas is insufflated into the abdomen to a pressure of 15 mm Hg. A periumbilical location for a midline incision is then identified. This incision will allow insertion of the hand at a later point in the procedure; thus, its length in centimeters should roughly correspond to the surgeon's glove size. To provide the assisting hand with access to the abdomen, we use a device called the Pneumo Sleeve (Dexterity Surgical, Inc., Roswell, Georgia). This device includes a ring system at one end. Once pneumoperitoneum is obtained, the ring is glued to the skin of the abdominal wall in such a way that the proposed line of incision is in the middle of the ring.

Step 2: creation and mobilization of the Roux limb, jejunojejunostomy, and creation of the gastric pouch With the ring of the Pneumo Sleeve secured to the skin, the small midline incision is opened and extended directly through the midline fascia. The pneumoperitoneum is released as this incision is opened, and the ligament of Treitz is identified by palpation. Retractors are placed into the incision, and the Roux limb is constructed with an open surgical technique. The small bowel is mobilized into the wound to the extent possible and is transected 20 to 30 cm from the ligament of Treitz. A side-to-side stapled jejunojejunostomy is then constructed with an open technique. In our experience, using an endoscopic GIA stapler rather than a traditional surgical stapler for this step is both technically superior and more cost-efficient.

Once the anastomosis is created and the enterotomy is closed, the mesenteric defect is sutured in the usual fashion with an open technique. A Penrose drain is sutured to the cut end of the Roux limb. The surgeon, standing on the patient's left side, attaches the Pneumo Sleeve to the nondominant hand and places this into the abdominal cavity. Pneumoperitoneum is reestablished. The ligament of Treitz can then be manually identified, and a blunt mesocolic dissection into the retrogastric space can be performed. This manipulation can be visualized through a laparoscope with the placement of additional trocars, including two in the right subcostal area (as in total intracorporeal laparoscopic GBP); we usually place the laparoscope through a left subcostal trocar site. The Penrose drain is then grasped with the surgeon's fingers and advanced through the mesocolic tunnel into the retrogastric space. The hand is then brought anterior to the stomach, and the patient is placed in a steep reverse Trendelenburg position.

The Nathanson liver retractor is inserted through a subxiphoid puncture as described earlier [*see* Total Intracorporeal Laparoscopic Gastric Bypass, *above*] and positioned to allow visualization of the esophagogastric junction and proximal stomach. The gastrohepatic ligament is bluntly opened, and the surgeon's hand is extended behind the stomach into the lesser sac to retrieve the Penrose drain. The hand is then used to facilitate the mesenteric dissection on the lesser curvature of the stomach 2 to 3 cm from the esophagogastric junction. An endoscopic GIA stapler loaded with 3.5 mm staples in 60 mm cartridges is fired three times to create the gastric pouch (as in total intracorporeal laparoscopic GBP).

Step 3: gastrojejunostomy Again, the gastrojejunal anastomosis can be created with either a circular stapler or a linear stapler [*see* Total Intracorporeal Laparoscopic Gastric Bypass, *above*]. The Roux limb is manipulated into view with the surgeon's hand. In the circular stapling technique, the stapler is placed into the Roux limb with the help of the intra-abdominal hand so that it can be opened, penetrating the antimesenteric portion of the bowel, and joined to the anvil in the gastric pouch. The hand also facilitates removal of the circular stapler, which is occasionally difficult.

Step 4: assessment of the anastomosis The open end of the Roux limb is then stapled closed, and flexible upper GI endoscopy is performed as in total intracorporeal laparoscopic GBP, with the hand (rather than an intestinal clamp) occluding the limb to allow insufflation and testing of the anastomosis. Additional absorbable sutures can be placed around the anastomosis for added security; we use an automatic suturing device such as the Endostitch (United States Surgical, Norwalk, Connecticut) for this purpose. If the sutures are left long, the surgeon can actually tie knots intra-abdominally, using the sleeved hand in a one-handed technique.

Step 5: closure Except for the hand incision, closure is accomplished in the same way as for total laparoscopic GBP. Although the hand incision is small, it may be difficult to close in severely obese patients who have a thick layer of subcutaneous fat. We use a continuous fascial closure with a heavy No. 1 or 2 nonabsorbable suture.

POSTOPERATIVE CARE

The basic principles of care after bariatric surgery [*see* Postoperative Management, *below*] generally apply to laparoscopic cases as well, but with some differences. Unlike patients who have undergone open GBP, those who have undergone laparoscopic GBP do not have a nasogastric tube left in place. In addition, a contrast study of both the pouch and the anastomosis is ordered on postoperative day 1. A water-soluble contrast agent is initially used for this study, followed by barium if no leak or abnormality is identified. The patient may then begin to drink small amounts of liquids and may advance to a pureed diet with no sugar or concentrated sweets as soon as he or she can tolerate it. Discharge usually takes place 2 or 3 days after operation.

COMPLICATIONS

The complications observed to date after laparoscopic GBP include the usual problems that occur in some patients after open GBP, including marginal ulcer and stenosis at the gastrojejunal anastomosis necessitating dilatation. We have seen one gastrogastric fistula leading to a treatment-resistant marginal ulcer. The major advantage of laparoscopic GBP over open GBP is likely to be reduced wound complications (e.g., major wound infection and incisional hernia). We have seen several relatively minor trocar site infections but none carrying the long wound care disability characteristic of a major wound infection after open GBP. In our experience to date, weight loss with laparoscopic GBP is identical to that with open GBP.

Postoperative Management

For optimal results after bariatric surgery, postoperative management must be as well planned as preoperative preparation. The basic principles of postoperative care, including intubation, ambulation, feeding, and monitoring for complications (e.g., anastomotic leakage, abdominal catastrophe, acute gastric distention, and internal hernia), are discussed more fully elsewhere [see 69 Obesity].

FAILED WEIGHT LOSS AND WEIGHT REGAIN

A postoperative problem that deserves special mention is the risk of failed weight loss or weight regain. This is one of the greatest problems associated with bariatric surgery and may arise after any gastric procedure for morbid obesity. Approximately 20% of VBG patients have difficulty with solid foods and come to exhibit a maladaptive eating behavior involving frequent ingestion of high-calorie liquid carbohydrates; in about 10% of VBG patients, the procedure fails for this reason. We have converted 53 VBG patients to GBP.[27] After VBG, the average loss of excess weight was 31 ± 5%; 2 years after conversion to GBP, it was 67 ± 2%, a value virtually identical to that in our primary GBP group. Thirteen patients became sweets eaters and had lost only 15 ± 5% of their excess weight more than 1 year after VBG, though there were no radiographically demonstrated problems with the procedure; 1 year after conversion to GBP, they had lost an average of 78 ± 11% of their excess weight.

Inadequate weight loss is also seen in GBP patients. In some, stomal dilatation eventually develops after the procedure; however, no correlation between stomal size and weight loss has been demonstrated for GBP patients, and reoperation to make the pouch or the stoma smaller has not yielded any benefit when the initial procedure has failed. In our experience, failure of GBP is generally due either to the loss or absence of dumping syndrome symptoms in a small percentage of patients, leading to resumption of high-calorie sweets ingestion, or, more often, to frequent ingestion of high-fat junk foods (e.g., potato or corn chips, microwave popcorn, or peanut butter crackers) that crumble easily and empty quickly from the pouch, thereby keeping the patient from feeling full. Repeated dietary counseling over a period of years is required to educate patients to eat low-calorie, high-fiber foods (e.g., raw carrots, broccoli, cauliflower, apples, and oranges) that will stay in the small gastric pouch longer and provide a sensation of early satiety.

Our philosophy is to make clear to patients, well in advance of the operation, that bariatric surgery is designed to help them help themselves. Obesity is easily beaten by surgical treatment, but to maintain the victory, patients must continue to make good food choices and exercise appropriately for the rest of their lives. In our experience, patients who begin to eat more than 1,100 kcal/day will begin to gain weight; even if weight gain is only 0.5 lb/month, this amounts to 6 lb/year, or 60 lb in 10 years. We strongly believe, therefore, that bariatric surgical patients need lifelong nutritional counseling to optimize the results of surgical management of morbid obesity.

References

1. Van Itallie TB: Obesity: adverse effects on health and longevity. Am J Clin Nutr 32:2723, 1979
2. Drenick EJ, Bale GS, Seltzer F, et al: Excessive mortality and causes of death in morbidly obese men. JAMA 243:443, 1980
3. Stunkard AJ, Foch TT, Hrubec Z: A twin study of human obesity. JAMA 256:51, 1986
4. Stunkard AJ, Sorensen TIA, Hanis C, et al: An adoption study of human obesity. N Engl J Med 314:193, 1986
5. Johnson D, Drenick EJ: Therapeutic fasting in morbid obesity: long-term follow-up. Arch Intern Med 137:1381, 1977
6. Griffen WO, Young VL, Stevenson CC: A prospective comparison of gastric and jejunoileal bypass procedures for morbid obesity. Ann Surg 186:500, 1977
7. Buckwalter JA: A prospective comparison of the jejunoileal and gastric bypass operations for morbid obesity. World J Surg 1:757, 1977
8. Halverson JD, Wise L, Wazna MF, et al: Jejunoileal bypass for morbid obesity: a critical appraisal. Am J Med 64:461, 1978
9. Hocking MP, Duerson MC, O'Leary PJ, et al: Jejunoileal bypass for morbid obesity: late follow-up in 100 cases. N Engl J Med 308:995, 1983
10. Pories WJ, Flicinger EG, Meelheim D, et al: The effectiveness of gastric bypass over gastric partition in morbid obesity: consequences of distal gastric and duodenal exclusion. Ann Surg 196:389, 1982
11. Lechner GW, Elliott DW: Comparison of weight loss after gastric exclusion and partitioning. Arch Surg 118:685, 1983
12. Linner JH: Comparative effectiveness of gastric bypass and gastroplasty: a clinical study. Arch Surg 117:695, 1982
13. Mason EE: Vertical banded gastroplasty for obesity. Arch Surg 117:701, 1982
14. Sugerman HJ, Starkey JV, Birkenhauer R: A randomized prospective trial of gastric bypass versus vertical banded gastroplasty for morbid obesity and their effects on sweets versus non-sweets eaters. Ann Surg 205:613, 1987
15. Hall JC, Watts JM, O'Brien PE, et al: Gastric surgery for morbid obesity: the Adelaide Study. Ann Surg 211:419, 1990
16. MacLean LD, Rhode BM, Sampalis J, et al: Results of the surgical treatment of obesity. Am J Surg 165:155, 1993
17. Sugerman HJ, Kellum JM, Engle KM, et al: Gastric bypass for treating severe obesity. Am J Clin Nutr 55(suppl 2):560S, 1992
18. Pories WJ, MacDonald KG Jr, Morgan EJ, et al: Surgical treatment of obesity and its effect on diabetes: 10-year follow-up. Am J Clin Nutr 55(suppl 2):582S, 1992
19. Scopinaro N, Bachi V: Evoluzione del bypass biliopancreatico parziale per l'obesita. Minerva Chir 39:1299, 1984
20. Liszka TG, Sugerman HJ, Kellum JM, et al: Risk/benefit considerations of distal gastric bypass. Int J

Obes 12(suppl A):604, 1988

21. Brolin RE, Kenler HA, Gorman JH, et al: Long-limb gastric bypass in the superobese: a prospective randomized study. Ann Surg 215:387, 1992
22. MacLean LD, Rhode BM, Shizgal HM: Nutrition following gastric operations for morbid obesity. Ann Surg 198:347, 1983
23. Sanyal AJ, Sugerman HJ, Kellum JM, et al: Stomal complications of gastric bypass: incidence and outcome of therapy. Am J Gastroenterol 87:1165, 1992
24. Sugerman HJ, Brewer WH, Shiffman ML, et al. A multi-center, placebo-controlled, randomized, double-blind, prospective trial of prophylactic ursodiol for the prevention of gallstone formation following gastric bypass-induced rapid weight loss. Am J Surg 169:91, 1995
25. Wittgrove AC, Clark GW, Schubert KR: Laparoscopic gastric bypass: Roux-en-Y technique and results in 75 patients with 3-30 month follow-up. Obes Surg 6:500, 1996
26. Naihoth T, Gagner M: Laparoscopically assisted gastric bypass surgery using Dexterity Pneumo Sleeve. Surg Endosc 11:830, 1997
27. Sugerman HJ, Kellum JM, DeMaria EJ, et al: Conversion of failed or complicated vertical banded gastroplasty to gastric bypass in morbid obesity. Am J Surg 171:263, 1996

Acknowledgment

Figures 1, 2, 3, 5, and 9   Tom Moore.

51 BILIARY TRACT PROCEDURES

Bernard Langer, M.D., and Bryce R. Taylor, M.D.

Over the past few decades, remarkable advances in imaging technology have been made that allow more accurate diagnosis of biliary tract diseases and better planning of surgical procedures and other interventions aimed at managing these conditions. Operative techniques have also improved as a result of a better understanding of biliary and hepatic anatomy and physiology. In what follows, we describe common operations performed to treat diseases of the biliary tract, emphasizing details of operative planning and intraoperative technique and suggesting specific strategies for preventing common problems. It should be remembered that complex biliary tract procedures are best done in specialized units where surgeons, anesthetists, intensivists, and nursing staff all are accustomed to handling the special problems and requirements of these patients undergoing such procedures.

General Considerations

PREOPERATIVE PREPARATION

Imaging Studies

It is essential to define the pathological anatomy accurately before embarking on any operation on the biliary tract. Extensive familiarity with the numerous variations of ductal and vascular anatomy in this region is crucial. High-quality ultrasonography and computed tomography are noninvasive and usually provide excellent information regarding mass lesions, the presence or absence of ductal dilatation, the extent and level of duct obstruction, and the extent of vessel involvement. Cholangiography—either percutaneous transhepatic cholangiography (PTC) or endoscopic retrograde cholangiopancreatography (ERCP)—can supply more detailed information about ductal anatomy and is used when CT and ultrasonography yield insufficient information. Angiography should not be used routinely to create a road map of the blood supply: it is appropriate only when vessel involvement is suspected on the basis of other imaging studies and confirmation is required to determine resectability. Magnetic resonance imaging and MRI cholangiography, which are noninvasive, may also provide valuable information.

Management of Biliary Obstruction

Although jaundice by itself does not increase operative risk, biliary obstruction has secondary effects that may increase operative mortality and the incidence of complications. There is little evidence to support the practice of routine preoperative biliary drainage in all jaundiced patients, but there are some elective situations in which preoperative drainage is required.

Infection Patients with clinical cholangitis, whether spontaneous or induced by duct intubation (via PTC or ERCP), should be treated with biliary drainage and appropriate antibiotics until they are infection free; the recommended duration of treatment is at least three weeks. In addition, perioperative antibiotic prophylaxis with cefazolin or another agent with a comparable spectrum of activity should be employed routinely before any intervention or operation involving the biliary tract. For certain patients with biliary tract infection (e.g., associated with choledocholithiasis), urgent surgical decompression may be necessary, especially if antibiotics and endoscopic or transhepatic drainage are not immediately effective.

Renal dysfunction The combination of a high bilirubin level and hypovolemia is a significant risk factor for acute renal failure, which can occur in the presence of a number of additional factors, such as acute infection, hypotension, and the infusion of contrast material. Patients with biliary obstruction should therefore be well hydrated before undergoing angiographic or operative procedures. In patients with acute renal dysfunction secondary to biliary obstruction, decompression of the bile duct until renal function returns to normal is advisable before any major elective procedure for malignant disease.

Impaired immunologic function or malnutrition Patients with long-standing biliary obstruction have impaired immune function and may become malnourished. Decompression of the bile duct until immune function and nutritional status are restored to normal is indicated before any major elective procedure is undertaken; this may take as long as four to six weeks.

Coagulation dysfunction Prolonged bile duct obstruction may lead to significant deficits in clotting factors. These deficits should be corrected with fresh frozen plasma and vitamin K before an operative procedure is begun. Even if there is no measurable coagulation dysfunction, vitamin K should be given to all patients with obstructive jaundice at least 24 hours before operation to replenish their depleted vitamin K stores.

POSITIONING

The patient is placed in the supine position on an operating table that can be rotated and elevated. An x-ray cassette and machine should be available during major resections. Slight elevation of the right portion of the chest with an intravenous bag facilitates exposure of the liver and the biliary structures. A choledochoscope and equipment for intraoperative ultrasonography should also be available. Access to a pathology department that can perform cytologic or frozen section examination of tissue is essential in operations intended as treatment of malignant disease.

EXPOSURE OF SUBHEPATIC FIELD

A right subcostal incision provides excellent exposure for most open procedures on the gallbladder and biliary tract. For more extensive resections or reconstructions, the right subcostal incision can be extended laterally below the costal margin and across the midline to the left as a chevron incision. In patients with very narrow costal margins, a vertical midline incision may be more suitable for limited operations on the gallbladder and biliary tract, and a combination of a chevron incision and a midline vertical extension to the xiphoid may be required for more extensive operations. In any case, the incision must be long enough to allow sufficient visualization for safe performance of the procedure.

Adequate exposure and lighting are essential. The best retractors are those that can be fixed to the table while remaining flexible in terms of placement and angles of retraction. Modern high-intensity lights with focusing capabilities and headlamps are especially useful when the surgeon wears magnifying glasses.

Good access to the hepatoduodenal ligament and the structures in the porta hepatis is critical. In patients who have never undergone an abdominal procedure, identification of these structures is straightforward. In patients who have undergone previous operations or have a local inflammatory process, however, there may be considerable obliteration of planes. If this is the case, the following techniques may be useful in defining the anatomy.

1. *Using the falciform ligament as a landmark.* In reoperative surgery, the key to opening up the upper abdomen is the falciform ligament. This structure should be found immediately after the opening of the abdominal wall and retracted superiorly. The omentum, the colon, and the stomach are then dissected inferiorly, and a plane that leads to the hepatoduodenal ligament and the porta hepatis is thereby opened.
2. *Taking the right posterolateral approach.* When the colon and the duodenum are adherent to the undersurface of the right lobe of the liver, separation may be difficult. In most patients, an open space remains that can be approached by sliding the left hand posteriorly to the right of these adhesions and into the (usually open) subhepatic space in front of the kidney and behind the adhesions. Anterior retraction allows identification of the adherent structures by palpation and permits dissection of the adhesions in a lateral-to-medial direction. The undersurface of the liver is thus cleared, and the hepatoduodenal ligament can be approached.
3. *Taking the lesser sac approach.* Ordinarily, the foramen of Winslow is open, and the left index finger can be passed through it from the right subhepatic space. When the foramen of Winslow is obliterated, however, one should approach it from the left, dividing the lesser omentum and passing an index finger from the lesser sac behind the hepatoduodenal ligament to reopen the foramen of Winslow by blunt dissection.
4. *Using the round ligament to find the true porta hepatis.* Patients who have already undergone one or more operations on the bile duct often have adhesions between the hepatoduodenal ligament and segment IV of the liver. If one dissects this area via the anterior approach, one may think that the actual porta hepatis has been reached but notice that the hepatoduodenal ligament looks unusually short. In most cases, one can find the true porta more easily by tracing the round ligament to the point where it joins the left portal pedicle (including the ascending branch of the left portal vein) and then following that to the right along the true porta. The adhesions between the hepatoduodenal ligament and segment IV can then be more easily divided from the left than from the front.
5. *Using aids to dissection.* Usually, structures in the hepatoduodenal ligament can be identified by palpation and inspection. In cases in which such identification is not easily accomplished, an intraoperative Doppler flow detector may be useful in identifying the hepatic artery and the portal vein, intraoperative ultrasonography may be helpful in identifying the bile duct as well as vessels, and needle aspiration may also be used before the duct is incised if there is any doubt about its location. Either blunt or sharp dissection is effective in this area. Our preference is to use a long right-angle clamp (Mixter) to obtain exposure in a layer-by-layer fashion; we then electrocoagulate or ligate and divide the exposed tissue.

TECHNICAL ISSUES IN BILIARY ANASTOMOSIS

As a rule, biliary anastomoses, whether of duct to bowel or of duct to duct, heal very well provided that the principles of preservation of adequate blood supply, avoidance of tension, and accurate placement of sutures are followed. In preparing the bile duct for anastomosis, it is essential to define adequate margins while avoiding excessive dissection that might compromise the blood supply to the duct. In repairs that follow acute injuries, it is important to resect crushed or devascularized tissue; however, in late repairs, it is not necessary to resect all scar tissue as long as an adequate opening can be made in the proximal obstructed duct through normal healthy tissue and as long as mucosa, rather than granulation tissue, is present at the duct margin. The length of the corresponding opening in the jejunal loop should be smaller than the bile duct opening, because the bowel opening tends to enlarge during the procedure.

Mucosa-to-mucosa apposition is essential for good healing and the prevention of late stricture. Sutures should be of a monofilament synthetic material (preferably absorbable) and should be as fine as is practical (e.g., 5-0 for a normal duct and 4-0 for a thickened duct). Because the bile duct wall has only one layer, biliary anastomoses should all be single layer. Sutures should pass through all layers of the bowel, taking sizable bites of the seromuscular layer and much smaller bites of the mucosa, and should take moderate-sized (1 to 3 mm, depending on duct diameter) bites in the bile duct. Interrupted sutures are used when access is difficult or the duct is small; running sutures, when it is easy and the duct is larger. Sutures should be securely placed but should not be so tight as to injure the tissues. Magnification with loupes is particularly useful in anastomosing small ducts. Stents are not routinely required for biliary anastomoses, and drainage of the operative field is seldom necessary.

There are several principles of suture placement that can be applied to most biliary anastomoses, whether end to side or side to side. When the bile duct opening has a vertical configuration (as in side-to-side choledochoduodenostomy or choledochojejunostomy), stay sutures are placed inferiorly and superiorly in the duct and at corresponding points in the intestine. Traction is placed on these sutures to line up the adjacent walls. The right side of the anastomosis is done first; the bowel is then rotated

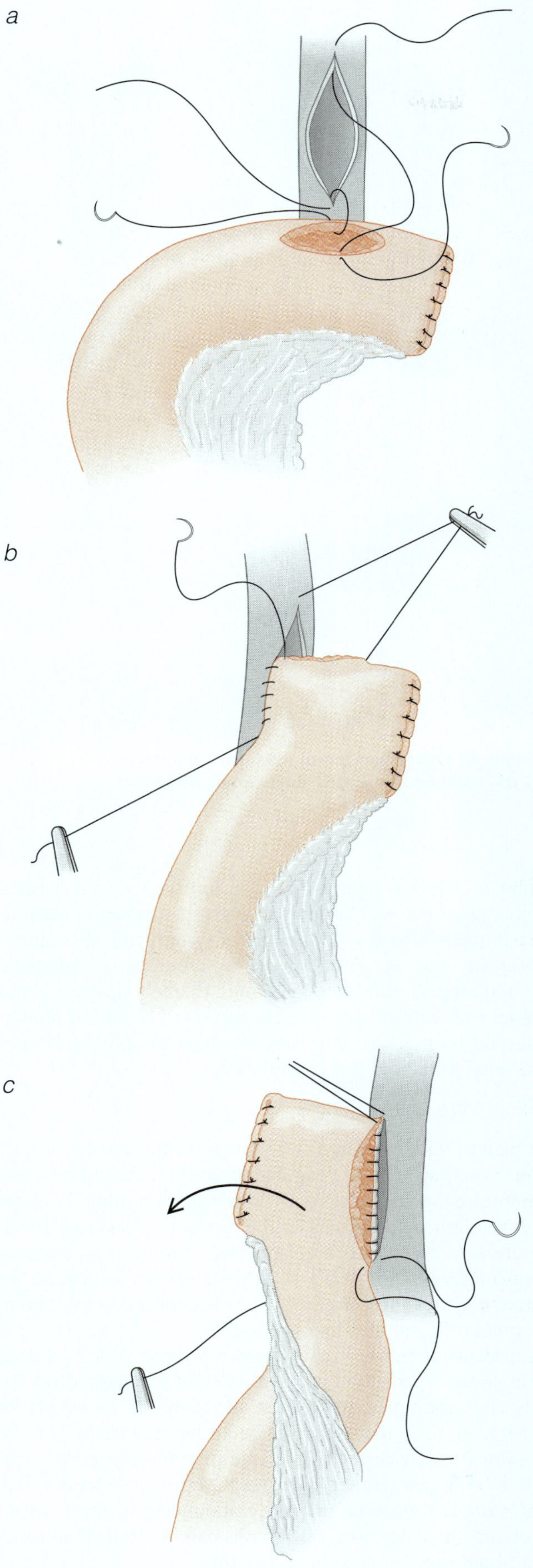

Figure 1 Technical issues in biliary anastomosis. Shown is a side-to-side choledochojejunostomy using a vertical incision in the bile duct. The same technique can be used for choledochoduodenostomy or end-to-side choledochojejunostomy. (*a*) Inferior and superior corner sutures are placed. (*b*) The right side of the anastomosis is sewn. (*c*) The bowel is rotated 180° so that the left side is exposed. The left side of the anastomosis is then sewn.

180°, and the other side is completed [*see Figure 1*]. It is often easier to sew about two thirds of the right wall and two thirds of the left wall, leaving the anterior third of the circumference (the easiest part) to be closed last. This technique can also be used for end-to-side choledochojejunostomy and allows all the knots to be tied outside the lumen. When the bile duct opening lies transversely, as in bifurcation reconstruction, lateral stay sutures are placed first, and the posterior wall stitches are placed from inside the lumen. If interrupted sutures are used, they are all placed individually before any of them are tied, with the untied tails carefully arranged in order. When the posterior wall sutures have been tied, the anterior wall can then be sutured with either running or interrupted sutures [*see Figure 2*].

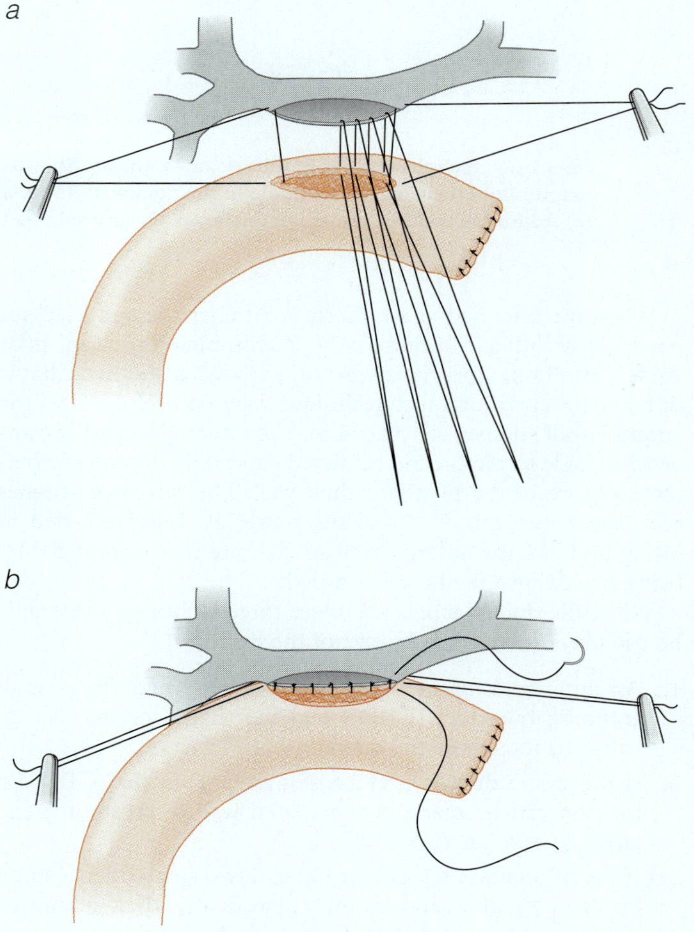

Figure 2 Technical issues in biliary anastomosis. Shown is an end-to-side choledochojejunostomy using a transverse opening in the bile duct. This technique can be used at any level. (*a*) Corner sutures and posterior wall sutures are all placed before being tied. (*b*) The posterior wall is completed, and the anterior wall is sewn.

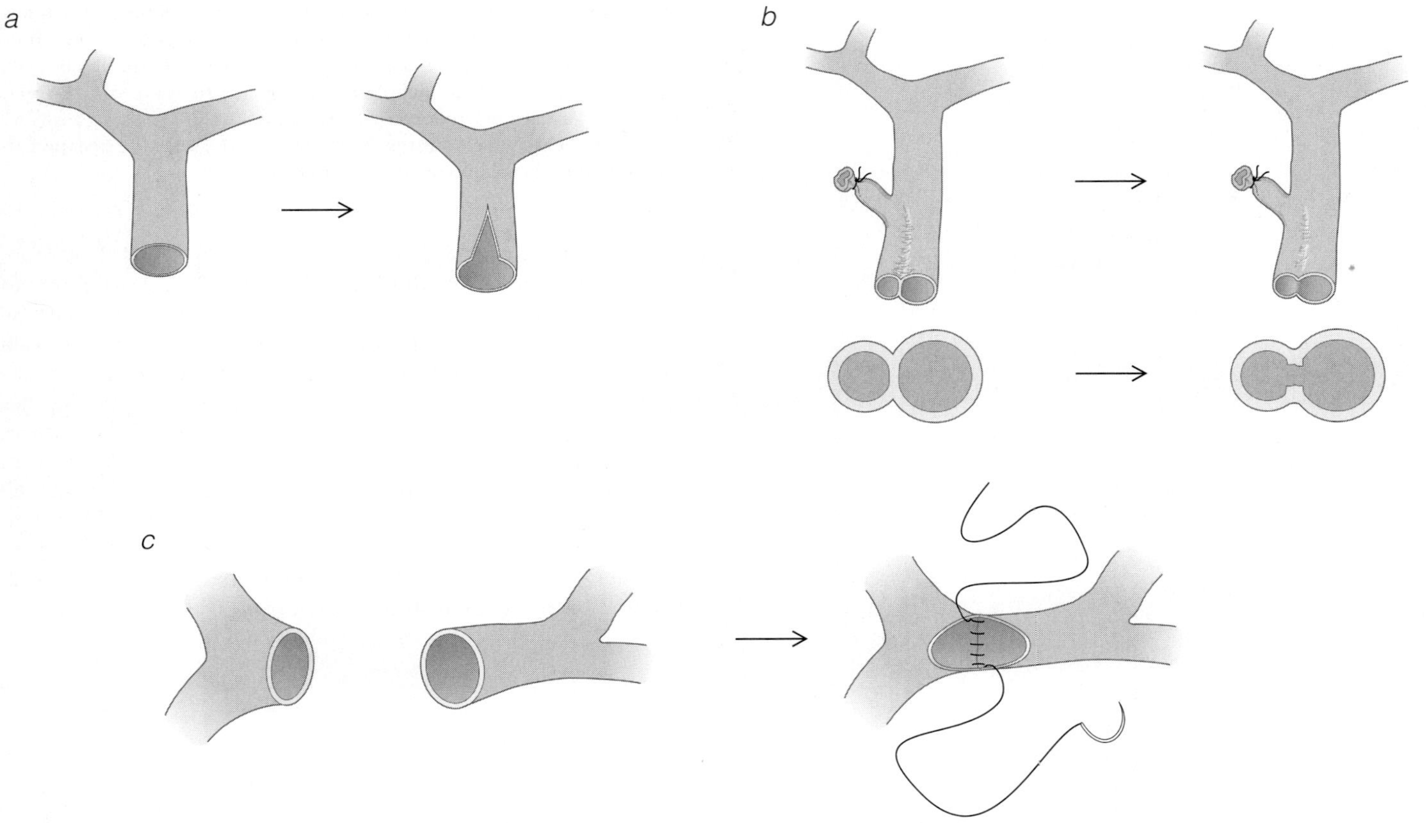

Figure 3 Technical issues in biliary anastomosis. Shown are three methods of enlarging a small duct. (*a*) An anterior longitudinal incision can be made in the duct wall. (*b*) A wall shared by the CBD and the cystic duct can be divided. (*c*) Adjoining walls of two small ducts can be sutured together.

When the intended anastomosis is intrahepatic and access is particularly difficult because of some combination of an unfavorable position, a previous scar, or, perhaps, a stiff liver that is difficult to retract, another technique may be useful. All of the anterior wall stitches are placed into the duct, grouped together on a single retractor, and retracted superiorly to promote better exposure of the posterior duct wall. The posterior stitches are placed into the duct and the bowel as described, tied in order, and cut; the anterior wall stitches are then completed by being placed into the bowel and tied.

When the duct is small, there are three techniques that may be useful for increasing the size of the lumen.

1. An anterior longitudinal incision can be made in a small common bile duct (CBD), and the sharp corners can be trimmed to enlarge the opening [*see Figure 3a*].
2. If the cystic duct is present alongside a divided CBD, an incision can be made in the shared wall to create a single larger lumen [*see Figure 3b*].
3. If the bifurcation has been resected, two small ducts can be brought together and sutures placed into their adjoining walls to form a single larger lumen [*see Figure 3c*].

CONSTRUCTION OF ROUX LOOP

When the jejunum is used for long-term biliary drainage, a self-emptying Roux loop is used to prevent reflux of small bowel content into the biliary system. In the creation of the loop, it is important to select a segment of jejunum with a well-defined vascular arcade that will be long enough to support a tension-free anastomosis. If access to the biliary system will be required in the future (e.g., in an operation for recurrent intrahepatic stones), the loop should be long enough to allow fixation to the abdominal wall with nonabsorbable sutures. The site of attachment should be marked with metallic clips to facilitate future percutaneous puncture and cannulation.

POSTOPERATIVE CARE

In a patient with impaired liver function, the results of liver function tests, particularly coagulation studies, should be carefully monitored postoperatively. Transient worsening of these results is not unusual, especially if the procedure was long. Moderately elevated results from coagulation studies (e.g., international normalized ratio [INR] < 2.0) are not an indication for treatment with fresh frozen plasma or concentrated coagulation factors unless clinical bleeding is evident.

Postoperative infections may occur as a result of biliary tract contamination, especially if a bile duct stent was placed preoperatively. Antibiotic prophylaxis with broad-spectrum agents for periods longer than usual for perioperative treatment may be appropriate in such cases. If postoperative fever occurs, especially if it is accompanied by unusual pain and tenderness, imaging studies should be promptly obtained and fluid collections sought. In most cases, bile or pus can be drained satisfactorily through percutaneously placed tubes.

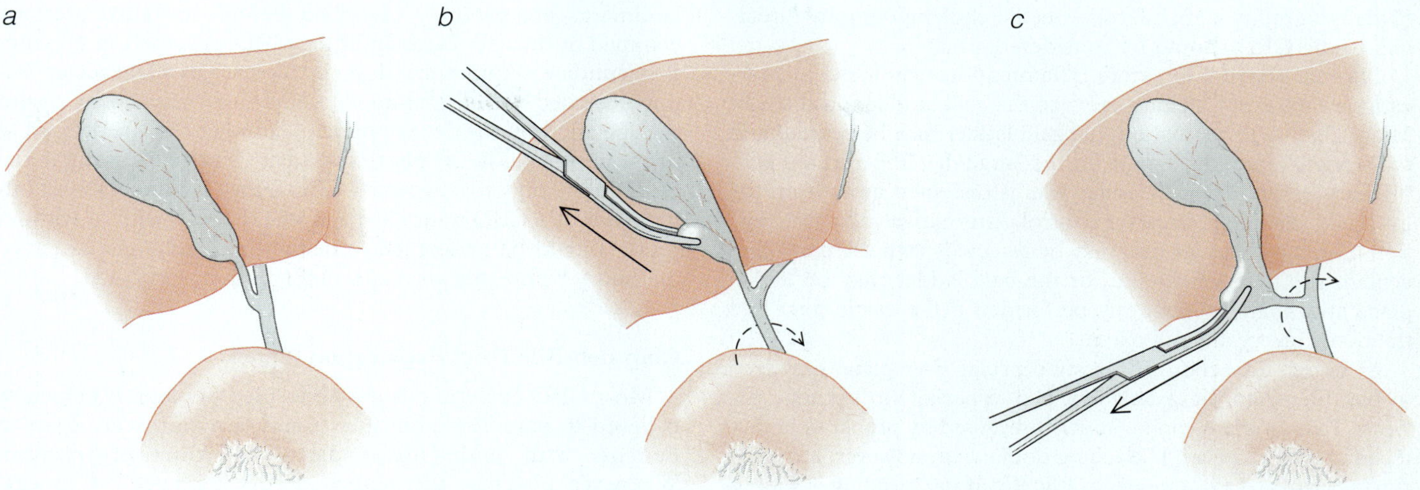

Figure 4 Open cholecystectomy. (*a*) Shown are the resting positions of the cystic duct and the CBD (with Calot's triangle closed). (*b*) Improper upward retraction of Hartmann's pouch lines up the CBD and the cystic duct so that one can easily encircle the CBD or clamp the cystic duct and the CBD. (*c*) Correct downward and rightward retraction opens Calot's triangle; dissection proceeds lateral to the CBD.

Open Cholecystectomy

Most of the cholecystectomies done for gallstone disease are performed laparoscopically [*see 52 Laparoscopic Cholecystectomy*]. The decision between the laparoscopic approach and the open approach is based largely on operator experience and the technology available. The open method is more likely to be used in pregnant patients and patients with portal hypertension, acute cholecystitis, or multiple adhesions. It is also used when the presence of a tumor is suspected, when a cholecystostomy has already been done, and when there is a recognized cholecystenteric fistula. Surgeons should not be reluctant to choose the open approach whenever they feel, for any reason, that it is safer in a given situation than the laparoscopic approach.

OPERATIVE TECHNIQUE

Step 1: Identification of Anatomic Structures

The important anatomic structures must be identified and the common anatomic variations kept in mind. The cystic duct and the cystic artery are identified by retracting the duodenum to the left and retracting Hartmann's pouch downward and to the right [*see Figure 4*]. The cystic node is the landmark for the position of the cystic artery. The window in Calot's triangle can then be opened between the cystic artery and the liver bed, and the fatty and areolar tissue can be cleared away from the cystic duct and the cystic artery via sharp and blunt dissection. Verification of the identity of the cystic duct is more safely accomplished by dissecting proximally to the duct's junction with the gallbladder neck than by dissecting distally to its junction with the CBD.

Step 2: Cholangiography

Cystic duct cholangiography is ordered routinely by some surgeons and selectively by others. It is mandatory if there is any question about local anatomy or if CBD exploration is contemplated (e.g., for possible choledocholithiasis). Visualization of the CBD on cholangiography is facilitated by elevating the patient's left side on an I.V. fluid bag to prevent superimposition of the bile duct image on the lumbar spine.

Step 3: Excision of Gallbladder

The gallbladder can be removed in either a prograde or a retrograde fashion. The dissection must stay close to the gallbladder wall to minimize the risk of injury to the right hepatic artery (which may be coursing close to Hartmann's pouch) and prevent entry into the subcapsular plane of the liver (which results in bleeding, especially in cirrhotic patients). The cystic artery and the cystic duct must be cleared around their entire circumference before being divided. Once divided, they can be either ligated or occluded with a carefully applied clip. Postoperative drainage is not routinely used.

TROUBLESHOOTING

In the face of chronic inflammation, the planes may be obscured, rendering dissection difficult. The cystic duct may be shortened and the relationship to the common duct poorly defined. In this situation, manual palpation of the cystic duct may allow identification of the relevant structures, especially after one has rolled the tissues between finger and thumb to squeeze out the liquefied fat and edema fluid [*see Figure 5*]. This technique is especially useful in the presence of acute cholecystitis. When chronic fibrosis is present and the structures cannot be readily identified either visually or with palpation, it may be better to open the gallbladder, remove the stones, and then identify the cystic duct by using a sound in the gallbladder. In the face of extensive scarring or inflammation of the gallbladder neck, removal of the gallstones accompanied by cholecystostomy may be safer than continued dissection without landmarks.

On occasion, it may not be possible to cannulate the cystic duct. In this situation, the cystic duct can be dissected distally, with care taken to ensure that there are no cystic duct stones, and the incision in the duct can be enlarged and dilated gently with sounds. If cannulation is not possible and cholangiography is mandatory, needle cholangiography directly into the CBD should be considered.

Chronic scarring or severe inflammation may make identification of the correct plane between the gallbladder and the liver impossible. In this situation, the gallbladder may be opened and the stones removed. Then, with the surgeon's finger in the gallbladder lumen, the gallbladder wall is dissected away from the liver, with the finger used for control. Alternatively, the free portion of the gallbladder wall may be resected, with the part adjacent to the liver left in situ, or the gallbladder may be left in place and a cholecystostomy performed if the cystic duct and the cystic artery are still patent.

As noted, dissection in the subcapsular liver plane may lead to bleeding from the gallbladder bed, especially in cirrhotic patients. This problem can be largely prevented by proper operative technique (see above). If bleeding does occur, however, it usually can be managed without great difficulty. If the bleeding is venous and comes from the liver parenchyma, local pressure should be applied, along with Surgicel or Avitene packing. Surface cauterization is appropriate for smaller vessels, and sutures may be required in cirrhotic patients. If the bleeding is arterial, one should not use the electrocautery or clamps indiscriminately until the source of the bleeding has been accurately identified. A Pringle maneuver should be performed, initially with the fingers and then with a noncrushing clamp, to identify the exact source of the arterial bleeding. The bleeding is then controlled with a hemostat, a small clip, or fine sutures, as appropriate.

COMPLICATIONS

Postoperative infection and bleeding are uncommon complications unless problems were encountered in the course of the operation. Injury to the biliary tract is also an uncommon complication; it can almost always be prevented if the anatomic landmarks are carefully identified before any structures are clamped or divided. Ligation of the CBD will result in obstructive jaundice within a few days. In the case of a transected but not occluded CBD, abdominal symptoms may be mild and nonspecific, and the development of jaundice may be delayed as bile accumulates in the peritoneal cavity. The most useful initial test in a patient with suspected CBD injury is a radiolabeled biliary scan. If a CBD injury is diagnosed, ERCP (with or without PTC) should be performed to define the nature and extent of the injury before any corrective intervention is initiated.

Common Bile Duct Exploration (Open)

Most CBD explorations are performed in patients known or believed to have common duct stones; a minority are done in patients with undiagnosed distal bile duct obstruction. Whenever possible, the nature of the pathological process should be confirmed via cholangiography before exploration is begun.

OPERATIVE TECHNIQUE

Step 1: Identification of Anatomic Structures and Evaluation of CBD

All of the important anatomic structures, including the CBD, the hepatic artery, and the duodenum, must be clearly seen. In a patient undergoing CBD exploration for the first time, the duct usually is easily identified by its slightly greenish-blue color, which is visible through the peritoneum, especially if the patient is thin. In a reoperative situation, exposure of the CBD may be somewhat more involved [see General Considerations, Exposure of Subhepatic Field, above]. A limited Kocher maneuver allows the surgeon, standing on the patient's left and using

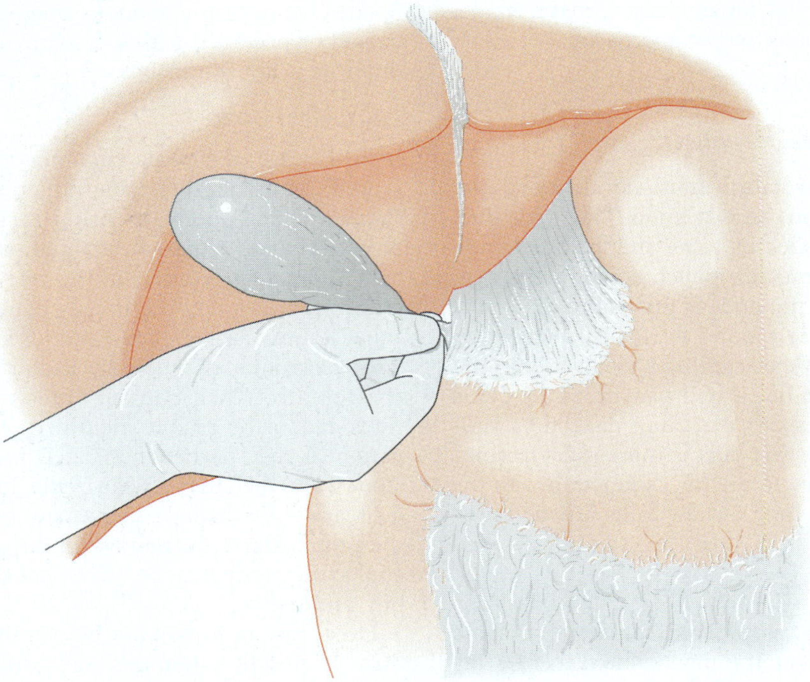

Figure 5 Open cholecystectomy. Shown is the right finger–thumb technique for identifying the cystic duct and the cystic artery.

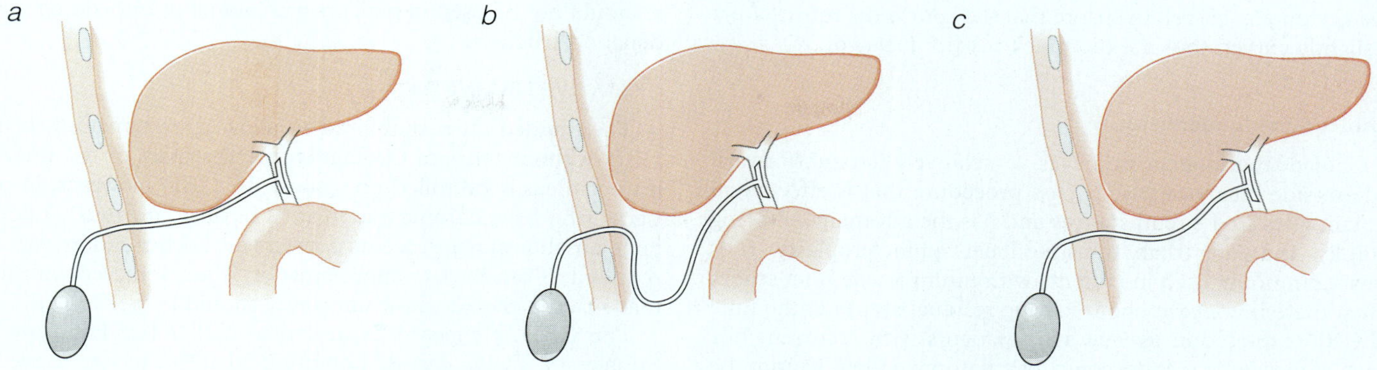

Figure 6 CBD exploration (open). Proper placement of a T tube is shown. The route the tube takes should be neither straight (*a*) nor very curved (*b*) but only slightly curved (*c*).

the left hand, to palpate the distal CBD between the fingers behind the pancreatic head and the thumb in front of it. Preoperative evaluation of the duct is desirable; if it is not possible, preexploration cholangiography is advisable, especially in the case of stone disease.

Step 2: Entry into CBD

The CBD is opened by making a vertical incision on its anterior surface to avoid the main arterial blood supply, which runs vertically at the 3 o'clock and 9 o'clock positions. The incision may be facilitated by placing two stay sutures in the duct wall. The opening is then enlarged with scissors to accommodate the largest palpable stone and any exploring instruments required. If the duct is small, care must be taken to avoid the back wall.

Step 3: Extraction of Stones

Many stones can be removed with gentle manual manipulation of the duct. This is done first, and the duct is then irrigated proximally and distally through a 12 or 14 French catheter to wash out mobile stones before any instruments are inserted. Stone forceps, baskets, and balloon catheters are used to retrieve stones identified via palpation, cholangiography, or choledochoscopy. The patency of the ampulla is confirmed by gentle passage of a 3 French sound or a filiform catheter through the ampulla and into the duodenum. Dilation of the ampulla with sounds is potentially dangerous and is never indicated.

Step 4: Choledochoscopy

Choledochoscopy facilitates stone extraction with a Fogarty balloon catheter or a Dormia basket and is the most reliable method of verifying complete removal. A flexible fiberoptic choledochoscope yields a good view of the intrahepatic ducts and the distal CBD; in most patients, a rigid right-angle choledochoscope or nephroscope also provides adequate visualization.

Step 5: Closure and Postoperative Care

The incision in the CBD is usually closed over a T tube so that immediate cholangiography can be done to confirm that the duct is clear. If there is concern that some stones might have been left behind, a 14 French T tube should be left in place to allow extraction of stones through the tube tract at a later date. The T tube should take a slightly curved route from the CBD to the abdominal wall—that is, curved enough to prevent dislodgment from the duct by abdominal wall movement but not so curved as to make subsequent percutaneous stone removal difficult [see Figure 6].

The T tube is left to free drainage until gastrointestinal function has resumed. The follow-up cholangiogram is obtained on postoperative day 4 or 5, and if there is free passage of contrast material into the duodenum with gravity flow only, the tube can be clamped. The T tube may be removed after 14 days (four weeks if the patient is receiving steroids or immunosuppressive agents), provided that the follow-up cholangiogram is normal. If retained stones are discovered on follow-up cholangiography, the T tube should be left in place for a total of four weeks, and the stones should then be removed through the T tube tract or, if this approach fails, via ERCP.

Drainage of the subhepatic space is not routinely required; however, a drain may be left in place if the CBD closure is insecure or if there is concern about persistent distal CBD obstruction.

TROUBLESHOOTING

Impacted stones, either at the ampulla or in the intrahepatic ducts, may resist the usual removal techniques (i.e., manipulation, baskets, and balloon catheters). Distal stones should be removed via transduodenal sphincterotomy at the time of the open operation; proximal stones may be left behind for later retrieval via the T tube tract under direct fluoroscopic control, sometimes with additional help via the transhepatic route.

Instrument injuries can result from excessively vigorous or persistent efforts to retrieve or dislodge impacted stones. For example, a Fogarty balloon catheter can rupture an intrahepatic duct if overinflated, and it can strip duct mucosa if traction is applied when it is overinflated. A Dormia basket can perforate a duct wall if forced past an impacted stone. A CBD sound can make a false passage into the duodenum, the pancreas, or the retroperitoneum if it is forced past an impacted stone or through a tight ampulla of Vater. The primary solution to these problems is simple prevention. All instrument manipulations in the CBD must be done gently. The maxim "If it doesn't go easily, you're in the wrong place" is appropriate here.

The T tube may migrate out of the CBD if there is not enough slack in the tube between the anchoring stitches in the CBD and the abdominal wall as a result of patient movement or abdominal distention. Accordingly, it is important, as noted [see Operative Technique, *above*], to ensure that the course the tube follows is slightly curved (but not too much so) [*see Figure 6*].

Choledochoduodenostomy

Choledochoduodenostomy is a relatively straightforward side-to-side biliary-enteric bypass procedure that is effective in certain restricted circumstances and has the advantage of being simpler and safer than transduodenal sphincteroplasty. It is most commonly used in patients with multiple bile duct stones when there is concern about leaving residual stones at the time of CBD exploration as well as in patients with recurrent bile duct stones when endoscopic papillotomy either cannot be done or has been unsuccessful. It is also used in patients with benign distal biliary obstruction (e.g., from chronic pancreatitis) and occasionally in patients with malignant distal CBD obstruction whose life expectancy is short. Choledochoduodenostomy works best if the CBD is at least 1 cm in diameter; it should not be used in patients with actual or impending duodenal obstruction.

OPERATIVE TECHNIQUE

The duodenum is mobilized to allow approximation to the CBD without tension. Ordinarily, the first part of the duodenum can easily be rolled up against the CBD; however, in patients who have chronic pancreatitis or have previously undergone an abdominal procedure, extensive kocherization may be required. If satisfactory approximation is not achieved with this maneuver, a choledochojejunostomy should be performed.

The CBD is exposed as described earlier [*see* Exposure of Subhepatic Field, *above*]. Longitudinal incisions are made in both the duodenum and the duct [*see Figure 1*], and the anastomosis is carried out as described previously [*see* Technical Issues in Biliary Anastomosis, *above*].

COMPLICATIONS

Late closure or stricture of the anastomosis may occur if the CBD is small or malignant disease is present. Alternative methods of biliary decompression should be considered in these situations.

Cholangitis related to the presence of food in the CBD distal to the anastomosis (so-called sump syndrome) is an uncommon occurrence. The larger the anastomosis, the smaller the likelihood that this complication will occur.

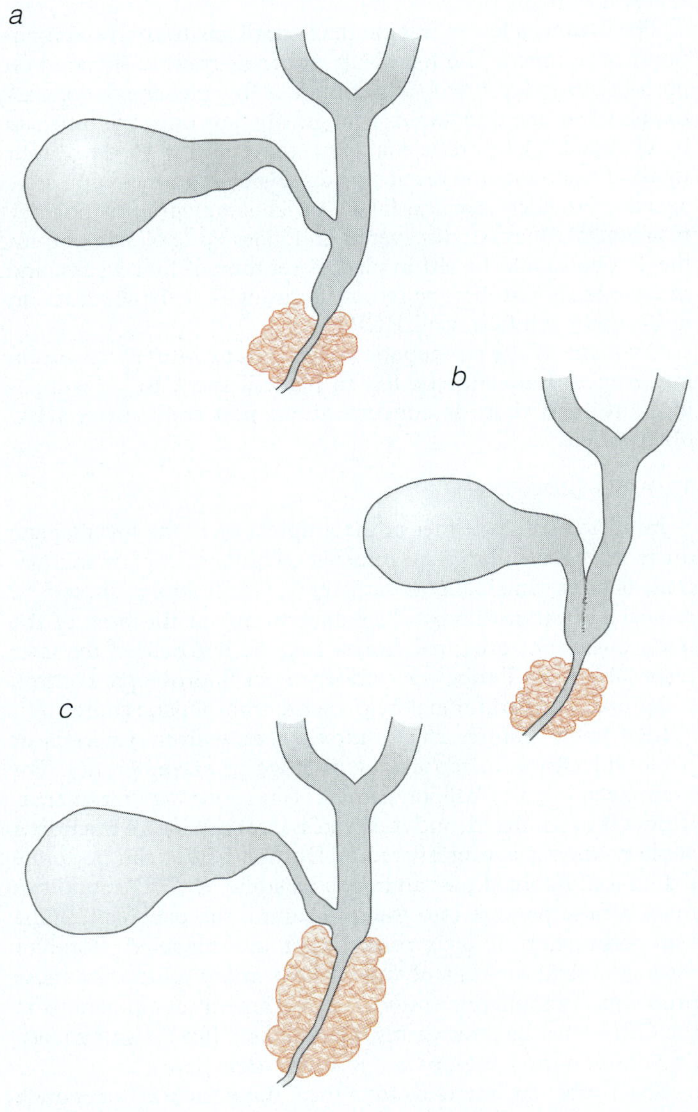

Cholecystojejunostomy

Cholecystojejunostomy may be performed to treat malignant biliary obstruction in selected patients who are found to be unresectable at operation and whose life expectancy is expected to be short. Occasionally, it is indicated for patients in whom endoscopic or percutaneous stenting has been unsuccessful. This operation is not the preferred procedure for long-term decompression.

Laparoscopic cholecystojejunostomies have been performed; however, this procedure is still evolving and should be attempted only by surgeons with a high level of expertise.

OPERATIVE TECHNIQUE

Step 1: Verification of Feasibility of Procedure

The cystic duct must be patent. Its junction with the CBD must be at least 1 cm above the tumor obstruction [*see Figure 7*]. The suitability of the anatomy for cholecystojejunostomy may have been verified by cholangiography preoperatively; if not, intraoperative cholangiography via the gallbladder or the CBD is mandatory. If one still cannot be certain that the operation is feasible, the CBD should be opened and a choledochoenterostomy performed. The finding of a bile-filled gallbladder is not sufficient evidence that the patient is a suitable candidate for a cholecystojejunostomy. The gallbladder should be normal: there should be no evidence of cholecystitis or stones. Normal status is verified by inspection, palpation, and, if necessary, needle cholecystography. Finally, for the anastomosis to be feasible, one should be able to approximate the jejunum to the gallbladder easily.

Step 2: Preparation for Anastomosis

A site near the fundus is selected for the anastomosis, and an appropriate segment of proximal jejunum is anchored to the

Figure 7 Cholecystojejunostomy. Cholangiography is essential for determining whether the anatomy is suitable (*a*) or unsuitable (*b,c*) for the procedure.

gallbladder with two fine stay sutures in anticipation of a transverse incision in the gallbladder and a longitudinal incision in the antimesenteric border of the bowel.

Step 3: Anastomosis

A 2 cm opening is made in the gallbladder and the adjacent segment of the jejunum, and a single-layer anastomosis is constructed with a continuous monofilament absorbable suture.

Step 4: Optional Additional Procedures

A Roux loop, rather than a simple jejunal loop, may be used in the construction of the choledochojejunostomy, and a gastrojejunostomy [see 49 Gastric Procedures] may be added in patients with pancreatic head cancer in whom duodenal obstruction is either present or anticipated in the near future.

COMPLICATIONS

Bile leakage may occur if there is excessive tension on the anastomosis. In addition, jaundice may persist if there is unrecognized cystic duct obstruction resulting from inflammation or an unnoticed stone in the cystic duct or the gallbladder. Recurrent jaundice is usually the result of extension from an obstructing tumor that has involved the cystic duct–common bile duct junction.

Choledochojejunostomy

Choledochojejunostomy, one of the most commonly performed biliary tract procedures, is done to provide biliary drainage after CBD resection, repair of ductal injury, or relief of benign or malignant stricture. To reduce the likelihood of reflux of intestinal contents into the biliary tract, a Roux-en-Y jejunal loop is usually used for the anastomosis [see General Considerations, Construction of Roux Loop, above]. If long-term access to the biliary tract is required (e.g., in patients with recurrent intrahepatic strictures or stones), the Roux limb may be anchored to the abdominal wall rather than left free in the abdominal cavity.

When the operation is performed after CBD resection, an end-to-side choledochojejunostomy using the proximal transected duct is made. When the operation is performed for bile duct obstruction resulting from tumor or stricture and no resection has been performed, a side-to-side anastomosis is constructed.

OPERATIVE TECHNIQUE

Step 1: Preparation for Anastomosis

Preparation for an end-to-side anastomosis includes resection of any crushed or devitalized tissue. The CBD should be trimmed back to healthy, viable, bleeding duct wall. If the lumen of the duct is small, a short incision on the anterior wall will effectively increase its circumference to facilitate the anastomosis [see Figure 3a]. If the CBD has been transected at the level of the cystic duct, the lumina of the CBD and the cystic duct may be combined by incising and oversewing their common wall [see Figure 3b].

If a side-to-side anastomosis is being performed for stricture or tumor, the proximal duct is almost always dilated and has thicker walls, and thus a vertical incision is made on the anterior surface. When the procedure is being done for malignant disease, the incision should be made as high as possible above the malignancy to delay the eventual obstruction of the anastomosis by tumor growth.

Step 2: Anastomosis

When the duct is large, a secure, tension-free anastomosis can be constructed by means of the techniques previously illustrated [see Figures 1 and 2]. When the duct is small, extra efforts must be made to place sutures carefully to prevent narrowing of the lumen.

TROUBLESHOOTING

It is essential to preserve the blood supply to the CBD. Adequate debridement of injured ducts is mandatory even if this means extending the resection of the duct to the bifurcation. Incisions should not be made in the medial or lateral portions of the CBD, where the major longitudinal blood supply is found. Finally, extensive mobilization of the duct from the surrounding tissues should be avoided so as to preserve the ductal blood supply.

Meticulous surgical technique is critical for ensuring good healing and preventing stricture. The finest suture material that will do the job should be employed, and magnifying devices should be used to facilitate the accurate placement of sutures. In very small ducts, the temporary placement of a small T tube at the anastomosis will allow most of the circumference to be completed without the risk of either picking up the opposite wall or placing sutures incorrectly. The T tube is then removed and the anastomosis completed. Routine use of postoperative stents is unnecessary but may be helpful in those rare cases in which mucosal apposition cannot be accomplished.

COMPLICATIONS

The main complications of choledochojejunostomy are bile leakage, late stricture, and recurrent jaundice as a result of tumor extension [see Cholecystojejunostomy and Choledochoduodenostomy, above].

Transduodenal Sphincteroplasty

Transduodenal sphincteroplasty is often indicated when an impacted stone at the ampulla of Vater cannot be removed via choledochotomy. It is also sometimes useful for clarifying the nature of an obstructive process at the ampulla, definitively treating ampullary stenosis, and gaining access to the main pancreatic duct if ERCP has been unsuccessful. Pancreatic sphincteroplasty may be added in selected cases.

OPERATIVE TECHNIQUE

Step 1: Exposure of Ampulla

Mobilization of the duodenum and the pancreatic head is necessary for obtaining exposure of the lateral portion of the second part of the duodenum. The ampulla is located by palpation, which may be facilitated by passage of a sound down the CBD, out the ampulla, and into the duodenum. A longitudinal incision is made on the lateral surface of the duodenum; it should be at least 3 cm long to ensure good exposure. The duodenal edges are retracted gently. Crushing forceps should not be used; they may cause hematomas.

Step 2: Cannulation

If the bile duct has been opened, cannulation of the CBD is done from above. A metal sound may be used; alternatively, a filiform catheter with a flexible follower may be inserted, and the ampulla can then be gently cannulated and elevated into the

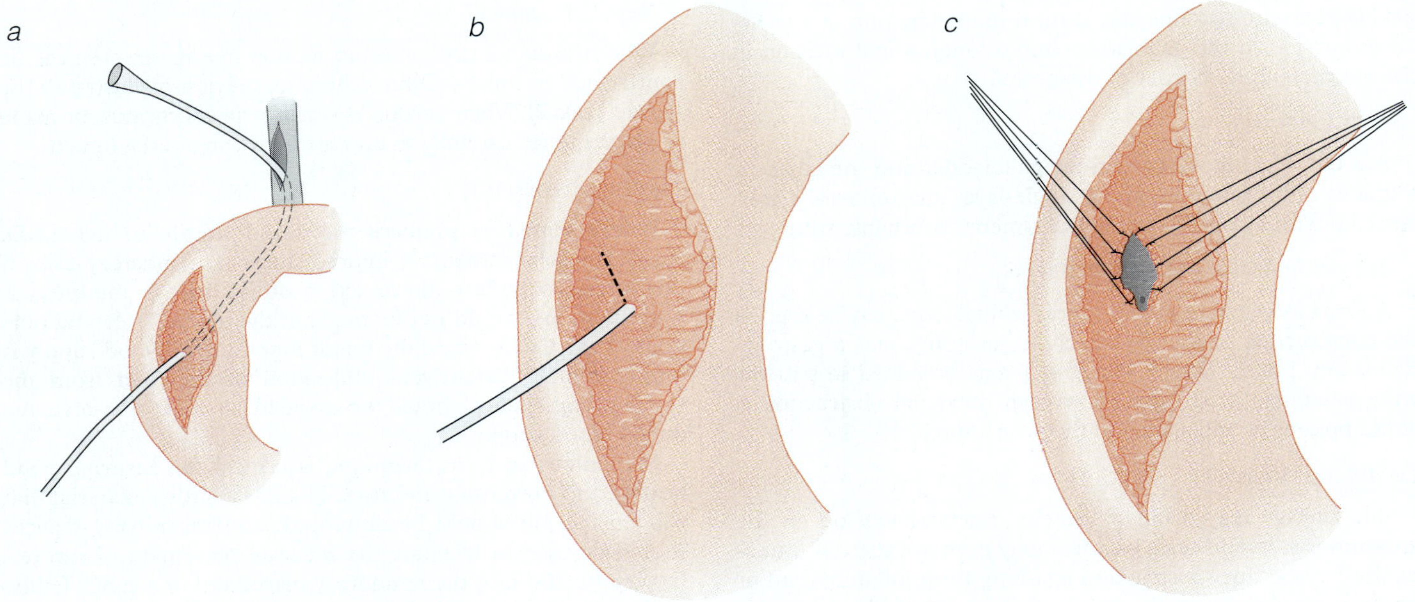

Figure 8 Transduodenal sphincteroplasty. (*a*) A longitudinal incision is made in the duodenum, and a filiform catheter and a follower are used to find and elevate the ampulla. (*b*) An incision is made at the 11 o'clock position with scissors or a scalpel. (*c*) Interrupted sutures are placed through the bile duct wall and the duodenal wall. Lateral traction is applied.

field [*see Figure 8*]. This step facilitates accurate placement of an incision in the ampulla. If the duct has not been opened, cannulation is accomplished from below with a sound. Use of a grooved director may simplify the sphincterotomy.

Step 3: Sphincteroplasty

To prevent injury to the pancreatic duct, the incision in the ampulla is placed at the 11 o'clock position with either scissors or a scalpel rather than the electrocautery. A so-called cut-and-sew approach, using interrupted 5-0 monofilament absorbable sutures placed 2 mm apart, is followed. The incision is started at the papillary orifice and extended above the ampullary sphincter. The sutures should include both the bile duct and the duodenal wall. Once the sutures have been placed, lateral traction is applied to provide exposure of the bile duct lumen and to make each subsequent step in the cut-and-sew procedure easier. The pancreatic duct opening (usually found at the 4 o'clock position) must be identified and protected from being incorporated in the sutures.

Step 4: Exploration of CBD

Exploration of the bile duct should be completed from below with sounds and choledochoscopy to ensure that all stones are removed. If the presence of a tumor is suspected, biopsies of any suspicious areas should be performed.

Step 5: Closure and Postoperative Care

The duodenum is then closed in the direction in which the incision was made. This can be done in either one or two layers, provided that care is taken to prevent inversion and preserve the luminal diameter. Routine drainage is not necessary unless there is concern about the duodenotomy closure or the choledochotomy closure. If a T tube has been left in place, a cholangiogram should be obtained before it is removed.

TROUBLESHOOTING

There may be an impacted stone at the distal end of the CBD that prevents cannulation from either above or below. Such a stone can usually be felt through the duodenal wall, in which case a vertical incision can be made in the medial duodenal wall directly onto the stone. Once the stone has been extracted, the incision can be extended down through the ampulla with a sound used as a guide.

Occasionally (e.g., in some patients with chronic pancreatitis), a long stricture of the CBD may extend above the ampulla. In such cases, the sphincteroplasty may have to be extended proximally to the point where it communicates with the retroperitoneal space. This will not be a problem as long as the duodenum-to-CBD repair is carefully executed. If the obstruction cannot be managed with an extended sphincteroplasty, a different decompressive procedure, such as choledochojejunostomy or choledochoduodenostomy, must be chosen.

Postoperative pancreatitis may develop if there was excessive manipulation of the ampulla, if the electrocautery was used at the ampulla, or if the pancreatic duct orifice is occluded by one of the sphincteroplasty sutures.

Choledochal Cyst Resection

Choledochal cysts are generally categorized according to the Todani classification [*see Figure 9*]. More than 80 percent are type I cysts that involve the CBD in its accessible portion. The following discussion addresses the resection of type I cysts and those type IV cysts that include the proximal right or left hepatic ducts.

Most choledochal cysts are related to an abnormal junction of the pancreatic duct and the distal CBD. Preoperative cholangiography to clarify the anatomy is important for preventing injury to the pancreatic duct, especially when an intrapancreatic

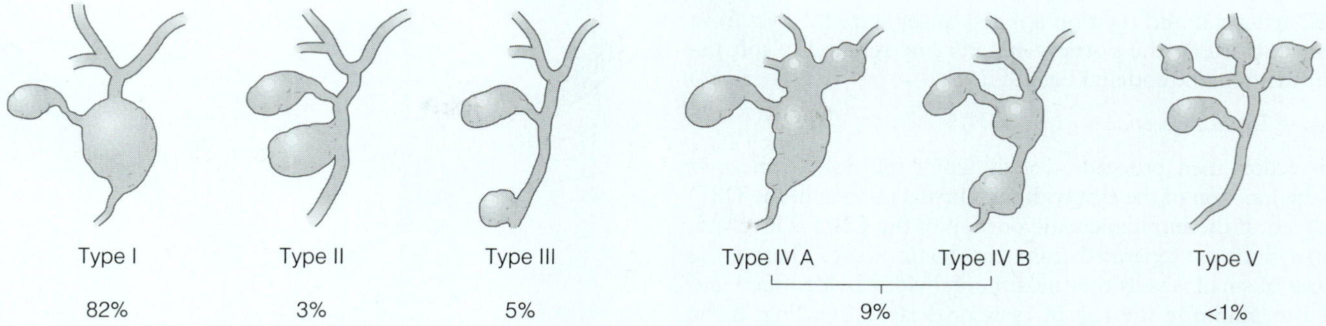

Figure 9 Choledochal cyst resection. Illustrated is the Todani classification of choledochal cysts.

Type I — 82%
Type II — 3%
Type III — 5%
Type IV A / Type IV B — 9%
Type V — <1%

resection may be required. Occasionally, intraoperative cholangiography is required to clarify abnormal anatomy.

Patients may be symptomatic as a result of stones within the cyst, infection, or malignancy, any of which is an indication for operation. Because of the high incidence of such conditions and the extremely high mortality associated with carcinoma in this setting, prophylactic cyst resection seems justified even in asymptomatic patients.

The objectives of treatment are (1) to remove the cyst completely, along with the gallbladder and any stones that remain in the bile ducts proximal to the cyst, and (2) to achieve free biliary drainage. Resection of a choledochal cyst may be made more difficult by several factors, such as previous operations, recurrent bouts of infection and inflammation in the cyst, and portal hypertension, which may develop as a result of long-standing cholangitis or portal vein thrombosis.

OPERATIVE TECHNIQUE

Resection of a choledochal cyst may be difficult and bloody, especially if inflammation is present. In addition, dissection of a choledochal cyst in its intrapancreatic portion may be hazardous because of the vascularity of this region and the difficulty of identifying anatomic structures.

Step 1: Clarification of Anatomy

The proximal and distal extent of the cyst and the presence or absence of stones or tumor may be determined preoperatively, as noted, but in many cases, intraoperative verification of the findings is necessary. Intraoperative cholangiography can be carried out by inserting a catheter through the gallbladder, by directly needling the cyst, or both. If cholangiography does not yield an accurate definition of the anatomy of the cyst, the cyst may then be opened and digital exploration and choledochoscopy used to clarify the anatomy.

Step 2: Initial Dissection

If the gallbladder is still in place, it is dissected free of the liver and left attached to the cyst via the cystic duct, then retracted to the right. If the patient has already undergone a cystoenteric anastomosis, this should be taken down at the beginning of the procedure, and the opening in the bowel should be carefully closed.

Step 3: Mobilization of Cyst

As noted, the vascularity of the region and the presence of inflammation may render dissection difficult. Rather than cleaning off the hepatic artery and the portal vein and dissecting them off the cyst, the surgeon should find a plane immediately adjacent to the wall of the cyst and remain close to it [*see Figure 10*]. This approach differs significantly from the corresponding approach in resection of a bile duct malignancy [*see Bile Duct Resection for Tumor, Operative Technique, below*]. If necessary, the cyst may be opened and the dissection continued with a finger inside the cyst to yield a more accurate definition of its boundaries. The cyst should be cleared circumferentially in the middle third of the CBD so that a tape can be

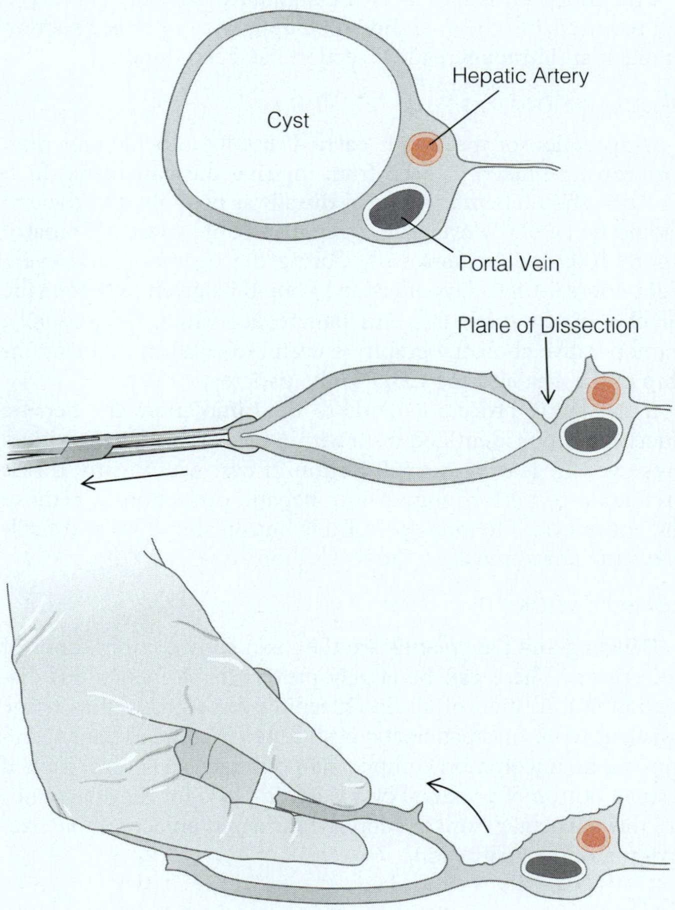

Figure 10 Choledochal cyst resection. Illustrated is the proper plane of dissection in removal of a choledochal cyst. If necessary, dissection can be done with a finger inside the cyst.

passed around it and traction applied to separate the cyst from the hepatic artery, the portal vein, and any remaining soft tissue in the hepatoduodenal ligament.

Step 4: Distal Dissection

Dissection then proceeds distally along the wall of the cyst until the junction of the cyst with the normal portion of the CBD is reached. If the intrapancreatic portion of the CBD is involved, the cyst must be separated from pancreatic tissue. There are a number of small vessels that must be individually identified and ligated to minimize the risk of early or delayed bleeding. If the cyst is close to the pancreatic duct junction, considerable care must be exercised not to injure the pancreatic duct.

Step 5: Proximal Dissection

If the proximal common hepatic duct is normal, it is transected above the cyst. If the cystic dilatation includes the bifurcation, a small button of proximal cyst is usually left attached to the intrahepatic ducts [*see Figure 11*].

Step 6: Reconstruction

Reconstruction is accomplished via an end-to-side anastomosis to a Roux jejunal loop to minimize the likelihood of reflux of enteric contents into the biliary tract.

Step 7: Closure

The abdomen is closed in the standard fashion. Stenting is not required, but the area should be drained with closed suction drains if an intrapancreatic resection has been done.

TROUBLESHOOTING

If dissection of the cyst is carried distally into the pancreas, care must be taken to keep from injuring the pancreatic duct. The cyst should be transected as distally as possible, and the end should be carefully oversewn with absorbable sutures. Somatostatin, 100 µg subcutaneously during the operation and every eight hours for five days afterward, should be given to reduce the likelihood of pancreatitis and pancreatic fistula. Occasionally, intraoperative cholangiography is useful to confirm the relationship of the cyst and the CBD to the pancreatic duct.

If the cystic process extends to the bifurcation, the hepatic ducts should be identified from within the cyst and their orifices preserved by leaving a small button of cyst wall in situ; this is preferable to performing an intrahepatic dissection to remove the entire cyst. The presence of this button simplifies and facilitates the anastomosis to the Roux loop.

COMPLICATIONS

Bleeding and pancreatitis are the main early complications of cystectomy. These can be largely prevented by meticulous dissection and ligation of all fine bleeding vessels as well as tissue adjacent to an intrapancreatic cyst. Late stricture of the anastomosis is an uncommon complication but may occur, especially if a small button of proximal cyst is left in place for the anastomosis; this particular complication is considered an acceptable hazard in a difficult situation.

OUTCOME

The immediate expected outcome is the relief of pain, jaundice, and cholangitis and the return of liver function to normal. The long-term expected outcome is the absence of any recurrence of symptoms of stone disease, cholangitis, or malignancy. Because of the rarity of this condition, no good data on the recurrence rate of problems are available.

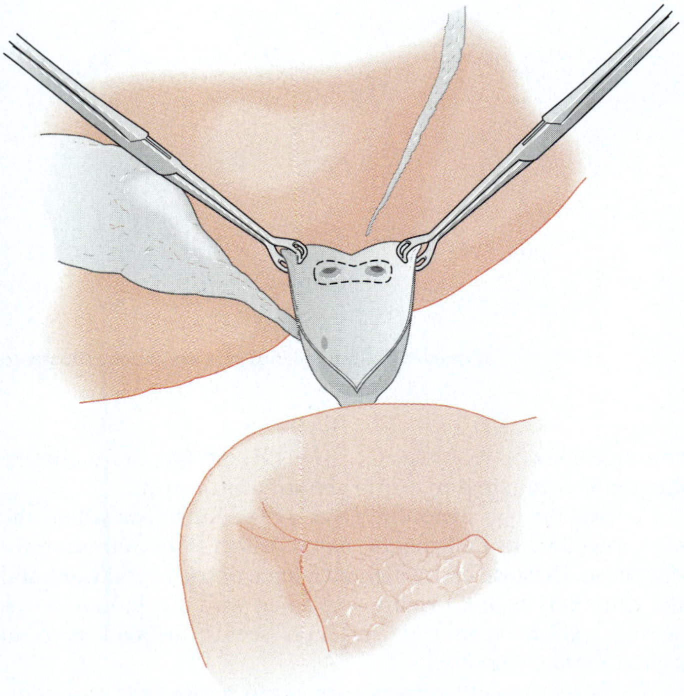

Figure 11 Choledochal cyst resection. If a cyst extends proximally past the bifurcation (e.g., a type IVa cyst), it may be necessary to open the cyst widely to identify the hepatic duct orifices. A small button of cyst wall is left attached to the hepatic ducts.

Bile Duct Resection for Tumor

The most common bile duct tumor is adenocarcinoma. Because this tumor responds poorly to irradiation and chemotherapy, surgical resection offers the best opportunity for cure. The appropriate operative approach depends on the location and extent of the tumor [*see Figure 12*]. Tumors in the distal third of the CBD (the pancreatic portion) are treated by means of the Whipple procedure [*see 53 Pancreatic Procedures*]. Those in the middle third or the proximal third are treated by means of bile duct resection, with or without liver resection (see below).

There are certain basic principles underlying bile duct resection for tumor that must be followed. First, the proximal extent of the tumor must be identified so that the correct procedure can be planned. Preoperative PTC is usually required, often bilaterally. Some authors advocate bilateral percutaneous drainage to facilitate intraoperative dissection. We do not routinely use preoperative drainage tubes, because of the risk of cholangitis.

Second, given that bile duct tumors spread by local extension to lymphatics, along perineural spaces, and directly into the liver, wide local excision beyond the visible edges of the tumor is required in the performance of curative resections. In proximal tumors, this often involves resection of the adjacent portion of the liver. The principles of en bloc resection beyond tumor margins must be closely adhered to: dissection into or even close to the tumor must be avoided.

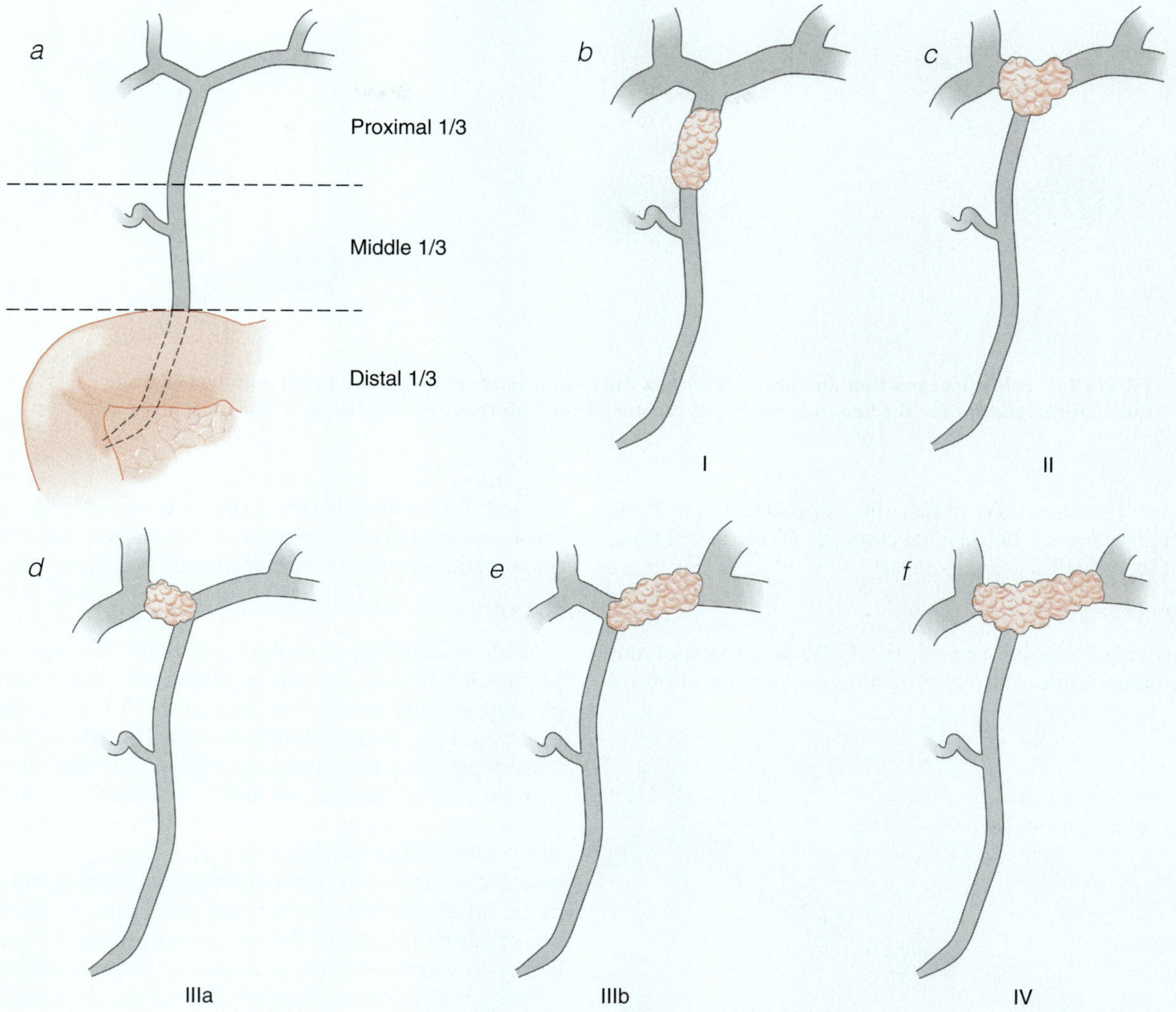

Figure 12 Bile duct resection for tumor. The appropriate operation depends on the location and extent of the tumor. (*a*) Broadly, tumors may be localized to the proximal third, the middle third, or the distal third of the biliary tract. (*b through f*) Proximal tumors may be further categorized according to the Bismuth classification.

Third, intraoperative biopsy of the tumor should not be done, because of the difficulty of making a firm pathological diagnosis on the basis of frozen section examination and because of the risk of tumor dissemination.

Finally, given that liver resection is required in some cases, one must be careful to preserve enough healthy liver tissue to allow regeneration of the remnant. If there has been long-standing obstruction, biliary drainage on the side to be preserved is important for recovery of function in that portion of the liver. Some authors advocate preoperative portal vein embolization on the contralateral side to stimulate hepatic regeneration in the segments to be preserved, especially if the future remnant is marginal in size.

OPERATIVE TECHNIQUE

Step 1: Assessment of Resectability

Before any dissection of the tumor or the CBD is done, a careful search for peritoneal metastases is undertaken. Spread within the liver is evaluated via palpation and intraoperative ultrasonography. Lymph nodes are assessed in the immediate and secondary drainage areas. Biopsies of any suspicious areas outside the planned resection margins are carried out. If tumor is found, stenting or a bypass procedure is indicated.

During dissection, determination of resectability is often difficult, especially with respect to assessment of tumor extension into the liver and the degree of vessel involvement. Therefore, any firm commitment to resection (e.g., dividing the blood supply) should be deferred until resectability is confirmed.

The gallbladder is mobilized from the liver bed by entering the usual plane superficial to the liver capsule without dissecting or dividing the cystic artery and the cystic duct. Exposure is improved by mobilizing the gallbladder and, if necessary, emptying the gallbladder of bile. The gallbladder can also be used as a retractor on the bile duct.

Dissection is then begun from below. The common hepatic artery and the portal vein are identified just above the neck of the pancreas and circumferentially cleared of all tissue. Dissection then proceeds proximally, with the hepatic artery retracted to the left and the portal vein to the right. Adjacent areolar tissue, nerve trunks, and lymph nodes are left in place around the CBD and

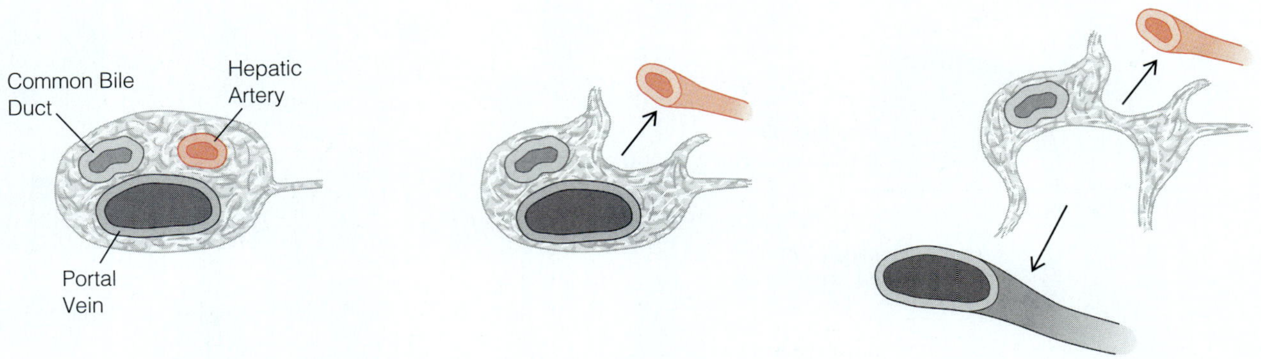

Figure 13 Bile duct resection for tumor. Shown is the proper plane of dissection in the removal of a bile duct cancer. Except for the hepatic artery and the portal vein, all tissue stays with the CBD to be resected.

the tumor [*see Figure 13*]. As noted, this approach differs from that used in resection of choledochal cysts [*see* Choledochal Cyst Resection, Operative Technique, *above*].

Step 2: Division of CBD

Once resectability is confirmed, the CBD is divided at the level of the pancreas. A clamp is placed on the upper end of the divided duct, which is then used as a retractor to facilitate the most proximal dissection of the CBD and the tumor away from the hepatic artery and the portal vein [*see Figure 14*].

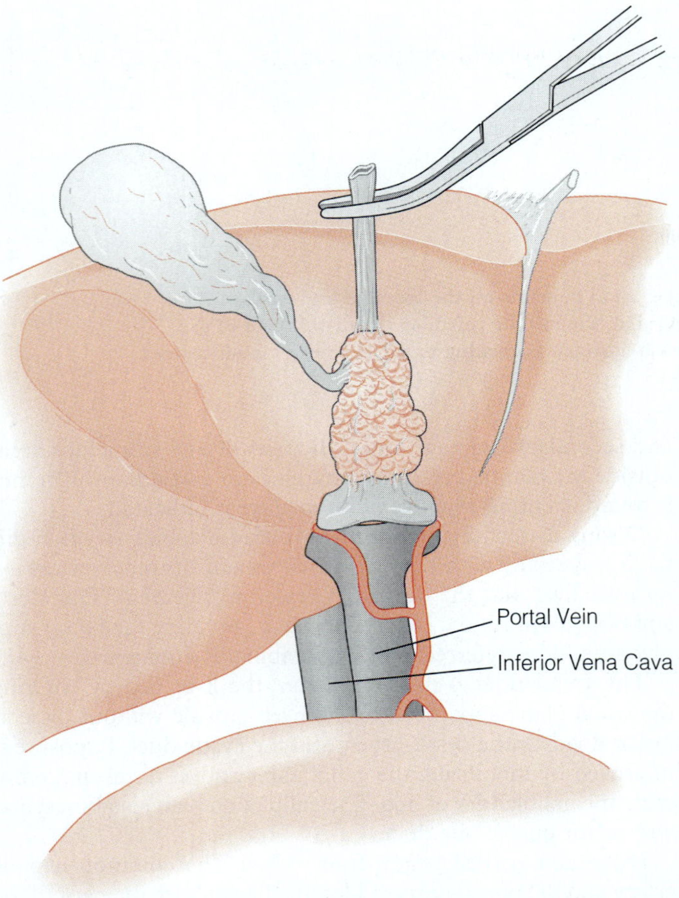

Step 3: Proximal Dissection

With middle-third tumors or Bismuth type I proximal tumors, it is usually possible to palpate the proximal tumor margin and identify uninvolved right and left hepatic ducts. If this is not the case, the possibility of a type II or III tumor should be considered, and complete excision of the bifurcation, with or without part of the liver, should be planned.

The hepatic artery is dissected by retracting the vessel anteriorly and to the left, dividing and ligating the cystic artery where it originates from the right hepatic artery, and clearing all tissue off the right and left branches at least 1 cm proximal to the proximal margin of the tumor. Involvement of the right or left hepatic artery by tumor is almost always a sign of extensive spread on the corresponding side and an indication for resection of that half of the liver.

The portal vein is dissected by retracting the bile duct and the tumor anteriorly and the hepatic artery to the left. All tissue is then cleanly dissected away from the portal vein to expose the bifurcation and the region proximal to it [*see Figure 14*]. At this point, the duct may be found to be tethered down to the caudate lobe by several small branches. If these branches are clearly proximal to the tumor, they are divided and carefully ligated, and the caudate lobe is preserved. If there is tumor in this area, the caudate lobe is resected along with the bifurcation tumor.

The level at which the proximal bile ducts are transected depends on the proximal extent of the tumor. For all middle-third tumors that are at least 1 cm beyond the bifurcation, proximal resection should be at or above the level of the bifurcation [*see Figure 15*]. For type I or type II proximal tumors, proximal resection should include all of the bifurcation along with portions of the right and left bile ducts out to the first major branch [*see Figure 16*].

With type III or IV proximal tumors, the proximal extent of the tumor cannot be determined in both right and left ducts unless the main pedicles are dissected out of the liver. Because these tumors tend to infiltrate locally, such dissection is not advisable. A decision on whether liver resection is indicated should be made at an early stage so that the chances of a cure are not compromised. Intraoperative ultrasonography may help

Figure 14 Bile duct resection for tumor. When resectability is confirmed, the CBD is transected at the duodenum. The proximal portion of the divided duct is retracted anteriorly, and the CBD is cleaned off the portal vein up to a point above the bifurcation.

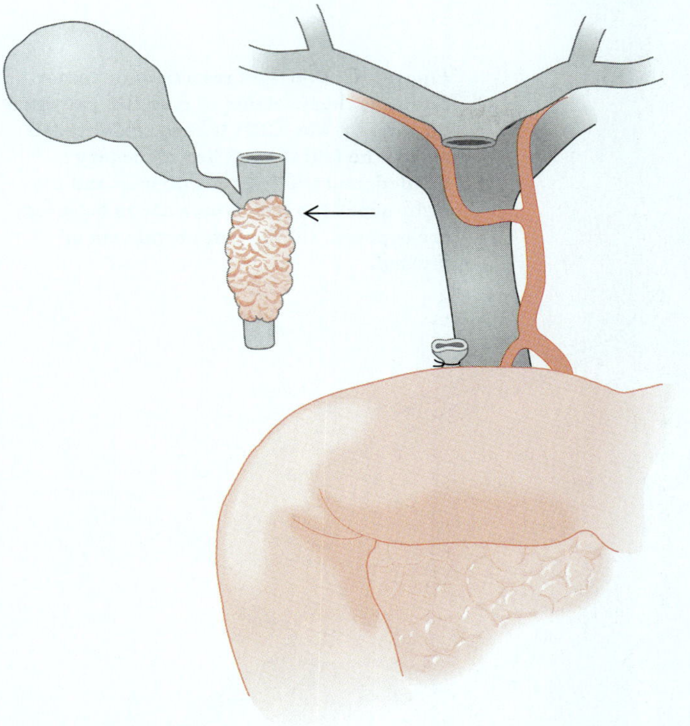

verify the extent of tumor at this point in the operation. Any major liver resection for type III or IV bile duct cancer should include the caudate lobe [see Figure 17].

Once the decision to resect part of the liver has been made, the operation consists of dissecting the hepatic artery and the portal vein branch to the part of the liver to be saved away from the tumor area. The hepatic artery and the portal vein branch to the side to be resected are then divided; this allows the tumor to be retracted further and provides better exposure of the duct to the side to be preserved [see Figures 18 and 19]. In selected cases, resection of an involved portal vein bifurcation may be carried out at this point [see Figure 20]; an end-to-end anastomosis is then fashioned.

The point at which the hepatic parenchyma will be divided is marked, and the parenchymal transection is performed. Division of the hepatic duct (or ducts) to the part of the liver being preserved is done as far from the tumor as possible.

Step 4: Reconstruction

After resection of the bifurcation or intrahepatic bile ducts, an intrahepatic cholangiojejunostomy is performed [see Intrahepatic Cholangiojejunostomy, below]. The duct tissue is usually healthy enough and the duct lumen large enough to

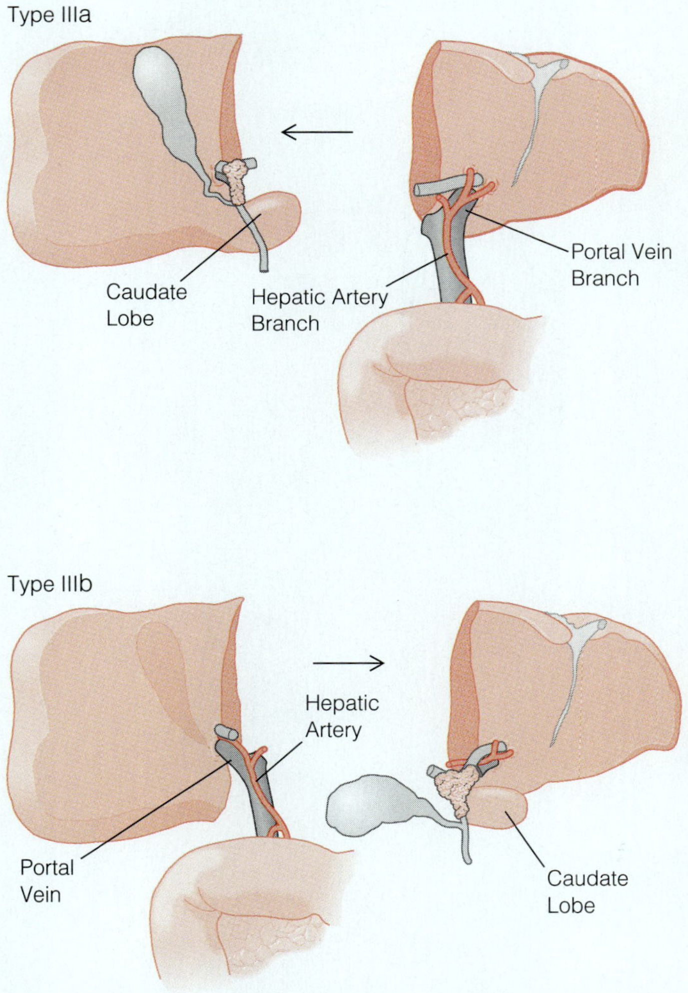

Figure 15 Bile duct resection for tumor. Illustrated is the level of resection for middle-third tumors. The CBD is resected from the pancreas to the bifurcation. Reconstruction is accomplished via Roux-en-Y choledochojejunostomy.

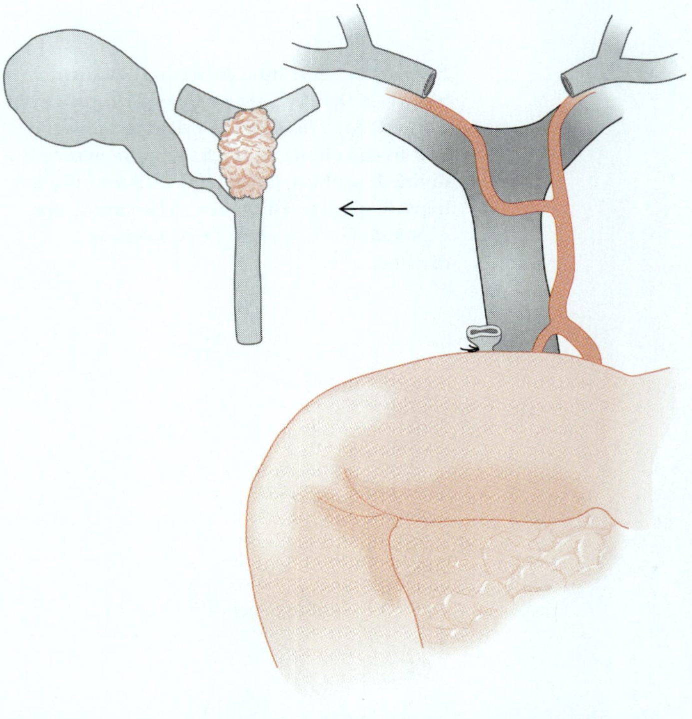

Figure 16 Bile duct resection for tumor. Illustrated is the level of resection for type I proximal tumors. The CBD is resected from the pancreas to a point above the bifurcation. Reconstruction is accomplished via Roux-en-Y hepaticojejunostomy (involving either one or two separate anastomoses).

Figure 17 Bile duct resection for tumor. Illustrated is the extent of liver resection for type III tumors.

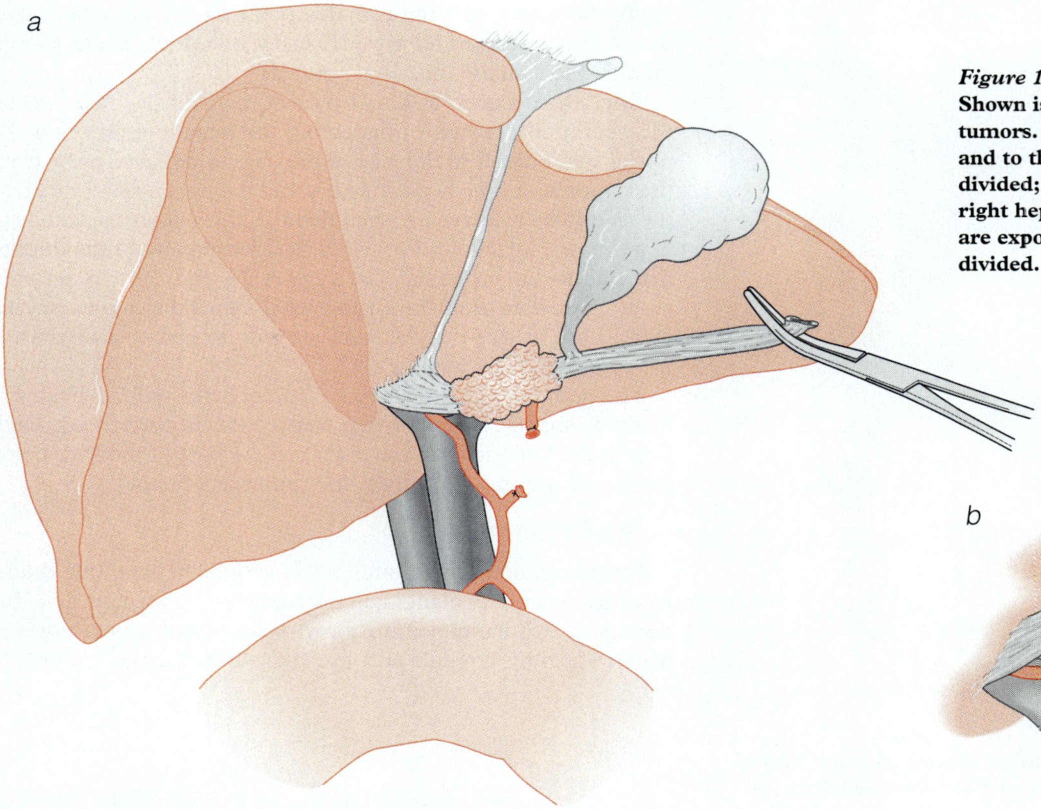

750 — V OPERATIVE MANAGEMENT

Figure 18 Bile duct resection for tumor. Shown is the resection of type IIIb proximal tumors. (*a*) The CBD is retracted upward and to the left; the left hepatic artery is divided; and the right portal vein and the right hepatic artery, which are to be saved, are exposed. (*b*) The left portal vein is divided.

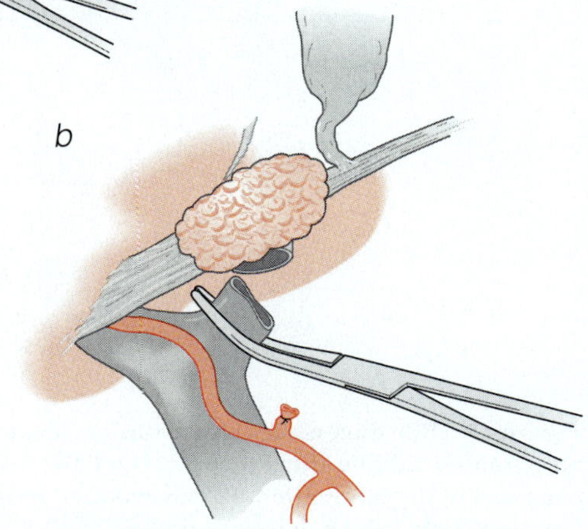

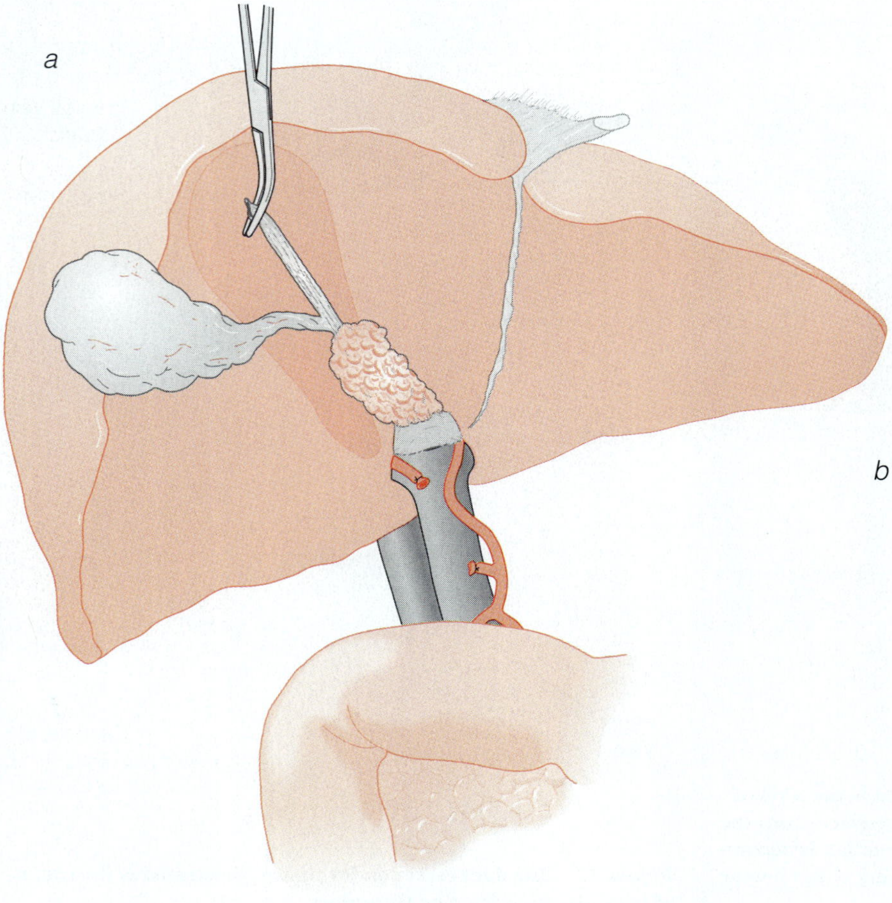

Figure 19 Bile duct resection for tumor. Shown is the resection of type IIIa proximal tumors. (*a*) The CBD is retracted upward and to the right; the right hepatic artery is divided; and the left portal vein and the left hepatic artery, which are to be saved, are exposed. (*b*) The right portal vein is divided.

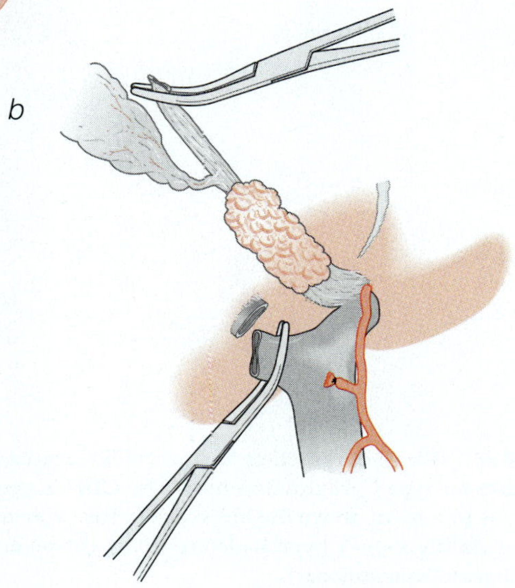

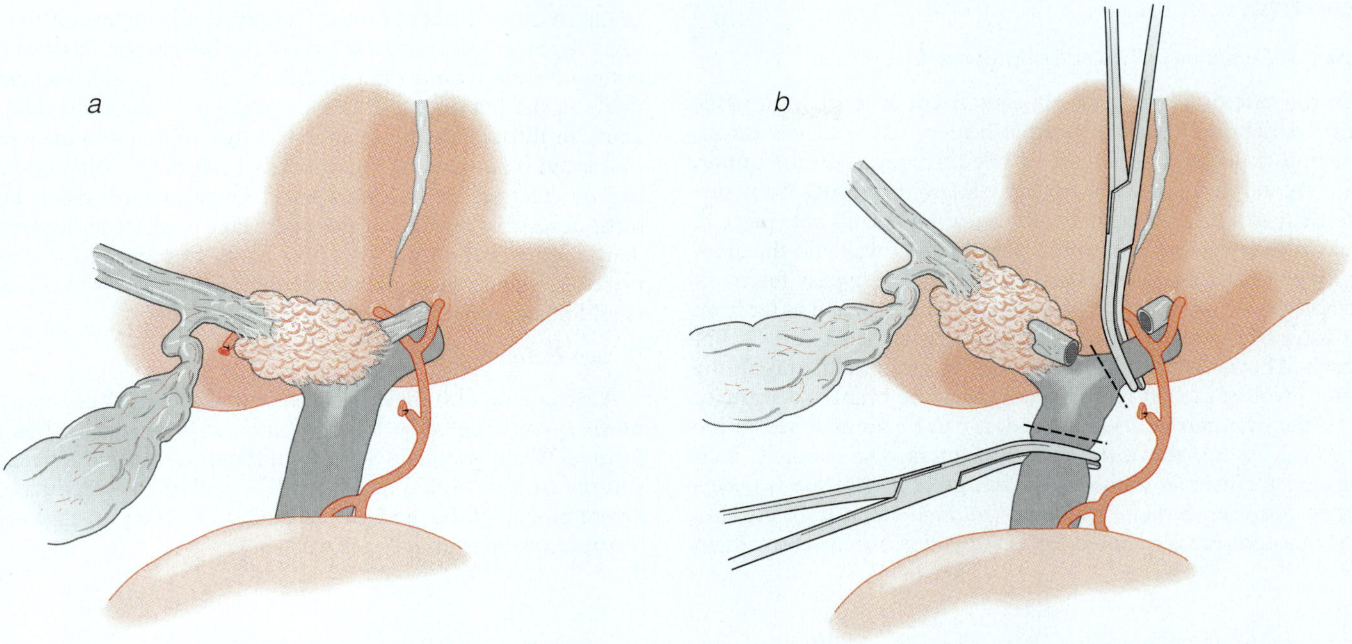

Figure 20 Bile duct resection for tumor. (*a*) Occasionally, a type III or IV proximal tumor will involve the portal vein bifurcation. (*b*) Shown is the resection of an involved portal vein bifurcation. Reconstruction is accomplished in an end-to-end fashion.

allow mucosa-to-mucosa repair without stenting. Some authors place transhepatic tubes through these anastomoses to facilitate postoperative treatment with internal radiation sources; however, there is no evidence that this practice reduces local recurrence or prolongs survival.

Step 5: Closure and Postoperative Care

The abdomen is closed in the standard fashion, and closed suction drains are placed. Liver function is monitored, particularly when a major liver resection has been done. Mild abnormalities in coagulation test results are common, and soluble coagulation factors are given only if there is evidence of bleeding.

COMPLICATIONS

Bile leakage, bleeding, and infection are the most important complications of bile duct resection for tumor. Parahepatic collections are treated with percutaneous drainage, and significant early bleeding is usually best managed by reexploration.

Intrahepatic Cholangiojejunostomy

Intrahepatic cholangiojejunostomy is commonly performed after resection of the bifurcation for a more proximal tumor; it is also performed to manage injury or stricture at the level of the bifurcation and to bypass an unresectable bifurcation tumor.

Because the ducts are smaller, have thinner walls, and are more adherent to the areolar tissue of the pedicles than either the portal vein branches or the hepatic artery branches, dissection of the ducts must be more meticulous. Magnification is an important aid, particularly in dealing with undilated ducts. Good exposure is essential; if necessary, the liver may be split to allow adequate visualization, access, and lighting. Anatomic mucosal suturing can be achieved in most situations. In rare instances, excessive inflammation, scarring, or tumor makes such suturing impossible, in which case periductal sutures are used and a stent is placed. As described [*see* General Considerations, Technical Issues in Biliary Anastomosis, *above*], separate ducts that are close together can be first sutured together at their adjacent walls to create a single larger proximal duct lumen so that a safer anastomosis can be created [*see* Figure 3*c*].

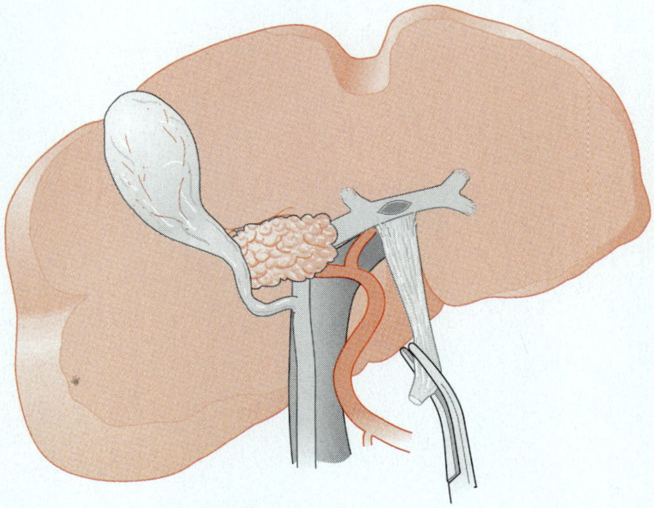

Figure 21 Intrahepatic cholangiojejunostomy. If a tumor involves the left main hepatic duct, the branch of the duct that supplies segment III of the liver may be used instead for anastomosis to the jejunum. This branch may be approached in the umbilical fissure, above the round ligament. Incision into the liver or wedge excision may be necessary to ensure adequate exposure.

OPERATIVE TECHNIQUE

Step 1: Definition of Tissues for Anastomosis

In the case of injury, crushed, cauterized, or devitalized tissue must be debrided back to normal healthy tissue before reconstruction is begun. In the case of bile duct resection for tumor, there should be no attempt to clear a length of duct from surrounding areolar or liver tissue; the suturing should take place in situ, with the stitches passed through the duct wall and the areolar tissue of the portal pedicles. In the case of bypass for unresectable cancer, the duct being used should be opened as far from the tumor as possible. The left main hepatic duct can be approached between the bifurcation and the umbilical fissure. If the tumor involves the left main hepatic duct, the branch to segment III of the liver can be used instead; it can be approached in the umbilical fissure, above the round ligament. Occasionally, incision into the liver or excision of a wedge of liver tissue is necessary to provide adequate exposure [*see Figure 21*]. If an intrahepatic anastomosis is required for a bifurcation stricture, resection of the stricture is not necessary; however, it is important to identify a normal duct above the level of the bifurcation. If there is no communication from right to left, a horizontal incision can be made in the left duct and carried across into the right duct just above or through the bifurcation stricture so that a single anastomosis can be made that incorporates both ducts. Duct openings can be enlarged by making a small longitudinal incision in the most accessible portion of the duct. This is easier to accomplish in the left hepatic duct (because of its extrahepatic transverse position) than in the right hepatic duct (which tends to run lateral and posteriorly directly in the liver substance).

Step 2: Anastomosis

A Roux loop of sufficient length to make a tension-free anastomosis is constructed. A biliary-enteric anastomosis is then performed. When adequate access is difficult to obtain, interrupted sutures are first placed in the anterior wall of the bile duct to allow retraction of that wall and facilitate accurate placement of interrupted sutures in the back wall.

Recommended Reading

Bismuth H, Nakache R, Diamond T: Management strategies in resection for hilar cholangiocarcinoma. Ann Surg 215:31, 1992

Bornman PC, Terblanche J: Subtotal cholecystectomy: for the difficult gallbladder in portal hypertension and cholecystitis. Surgery 98:1, 1985

Braasch JW, Rossi RL: Reconstruction of the biliary tract. Surg Clin North Am 65:273, 1985

Fry DE: Surgical techniques in the management of distal biliary tract obstruction. American Surgeon 49:138, 1983

Gallinger S, Gluckman D, Langer B: Proximal bile duct cancer. Advances in Surgery, vol 23. Cameron JL, Ed. Year Book Medical Publishers, St. Louis, 1990, p 89

Lillemoe KD, Pitt HA, Cameron JL: Current management of benign bile duct strictures. Advances in Surgery, vol 25. Cameron JL, Ed. Year Book Medical Publishers, St. Louis, 1992, p 119

Russell E, Hutson DG, Guerra JJ Jr: Dilatation of biliary strictures through a stomatized jejunal limb. Acta Radiologica: Diagnosis 26:283, 1985

Smadja C, Blumgart LH: The biliary tract and the anatomy of biliary exposure. Surgery of the Liver and Biliary Tract. Blumgart LH, Ed. Churchill Livingstone, New York, 1988, p 11

Stain SC, Guthrie CR, Yellin AE, et al: Choledochal cyst in the adult. Ann Surg 222:128, 1995

Strom PR, Stone HH: A technique for transduodenal sphincteroplasty. Surgery 92:546, 1982

Acknowledgment

Figures 1 through 21   Tom Moore.

52 LAPAROSCOPIC CHOLECYSTECTOMY

Gerald M. Fried, M.D., and Liane S. Feldman, M.D.

Cholecystectomy is the treatment of choice for symptomatic gallstones because it removes the organ that contributes to both the formation of gallstones and the complications ensuing from them. The morbidity associated with cholecystectomy is attributable to injury to the abdominal wall in the process of gaining access to the gallbladder (i.e., the incision in the abdominal wall and its closure) or to inadvertent injury to surrounding structures during dissection of the gallbladder. Efforts to diminish the morbidity resulting from laparotomy have led to the development of laparoscopic cholecystectomy, made possible by improvements in optics and video technology.

Philippe Mouret performed the first laparoscopic cholecystectomy in France in 1987; by 1992, 90% of cholecystectomies in the United States were performed laparoscopically. Compared with open cholecystectomy, the laparoscopic approach has dramatically reduced hospital stay, postoperative pain, and convalescent time. However, rapid adoption of laparoscopic cholecystectomy as the so-called gold standard for treatment of symptomatic gallstone disease was associated with complications, including an increased incidence of major bile duct injuries.

Since 1993, there have been several new developments in laparoscopic cholecystectomy. Improved optics and equipment, combined with improved laparoscopic skills, have reduced the list of absolute contraindications to laparoscopic cholecystectomy. Many surgeons now begin with a laparoscopic approach for virtually all patients, including pregnant patients and those with acute cholecystitis, intra-abdominal adhesions, or cirrhosis. Laparoscopy is converted to open cholecystectomy only if necessary. Because many surgeons have become more comfortable with laparoscopic approaches to the removal of stones from the common bile duct (CBD), the pendulum is swinging away from endoscopic retrograde cholangiopancreatography (ERCP) and endoscopic sphincterotomy (ES) in some institutions. Magnetic resonance cholangiopancreatography (MRCP) and laparoscopic ultrasonography, where available, have reduced reliance on intraoperative cholangiography. Miniaturization of instruments to 2 mm in diameter may decrease the morbidity associated with incisions. The pressure to reduce hospital stays has also led to the adoption of outpatient cholecystectomy in many centers.

The primary goal of laparoscopic cholecystectomy is removal of the gallbladder with minimal risk of injury to the bile ducts and surrounding structures. Our approach is designed to maximize the safety of both routine and complicated laparoscopic cholecystectomies. In this chapter, we describe our approach and discuss current indications and techniques for imaging and exploring the CBD.

Preoperative Evaluation

To plan the surgical procedure, assess the likelihood of conversion to open cholecystectomy, and determine which patients are at high risk for CBD stones, the surgeon must obtain certain data preoperatively. Useful information can be obtained from the patient's history, from imaging studies, and from laboratory tests.

PREOPERATIVE DATA

History and Physical Examination

A good medical history provides information about associated medical problems that might affect the patient's tolerance of pneumoperitoneum. Patients with cardiorespiratory disease may have difficulty with the effects of CO_2 pneumoperitoneum on cardiac output, lung inflation pressure, acid-base balance, and the ability of the lungs to eliminate CO_2. Most bleeding disorders can also be identified by a good medical history. A disease-specific history is important in identifying patients in whom previous episodes of acute cholecystitis may make laparoscopic cholecystectomy more difficult, as well as those at increased risk for choledocholithiasis (e.g., those who have had jaundice, pancreatitis, or cholangitis).

Physical examination identifies patients whose body habitus is likely to make laparoscopic cholecystectomy difficult, such as the morbidly obese and small, muscular patients. Abdominal examination also reveals any scars, stomas, or hernias that are likely to necessitate the use of special techniques for trocar insertion.

Imaging Studies

Ultrasonography is highly operator dependent, but in capable hands, it can provide useful information. It is the best test for diagnosis of cholelithiasis, and it can usually determine the size and number of stones. Large stones indicate that a larger incision in the skin and the fascia will be necessary to retrieve the gallbladder. Multiple small stones suggest that the patient is more likely to require operative cholangiography (if a policy of selective cholangiography is practiced) [*see* Operative Technique, Step 5: Intraoperative Cholangiography, *below*]. The presence of a shrunken, thickened gallbladder on ultrasound examination is a significant predictor of conversion to open cholecystectomy. The presence of a dilated CBD or CBD stones preoperatively is predictive of choledocholithiasis. Other intra-abdominal pathologic conditions, either related to or separate from the hepatic-biliary-pancreatic system, may be identified before operation and may direct laparoscopic evaluation and biopsy.

Preoperative imaging studies of the CBD may allow the surgeon to identify patients with CBD stones before surgery and then to attempt stone clearance by means of ES (preoperatively or postoperatively) or planned operative clearance of the CBD by laparoscopic or open techniques. These techniques also provide an anatomic map of the extrahepatic biliary tree, identifying unusual anatomy preoperatively and helping the surgeon plan a safe operation. Such imaging may involve ERCP [*see 47 Gastrointestinal Endoscopy*] and MRCP [*see* Figure 1]. ERCP may be performed

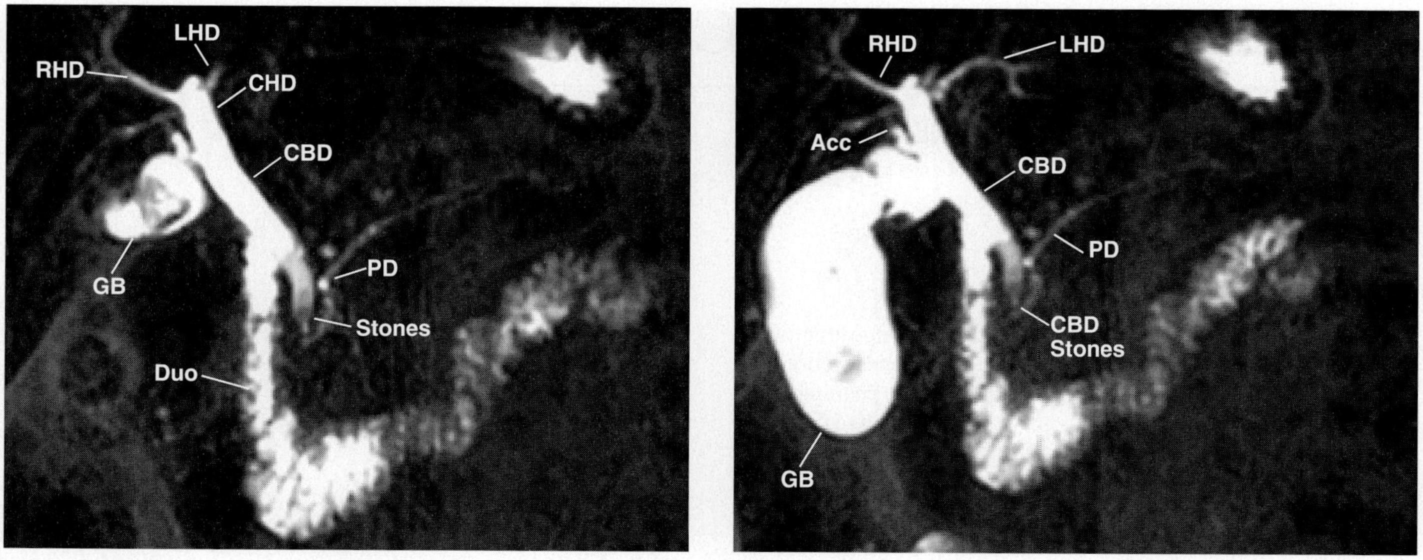

Figure 1 Laparoscopic cholecystectomy. Preoperative MRCP alerts the surgeon to abnormal anatomy and the presence of stones in the distal CBD. (Acc—accessory duct entering common hepatic duct near neck of gallbladder; CHD—common hepatic duct; Duo—duodenum; GB—gallbladder, containing stones; LHD—left hepatic duct; PD—pancreatic duct; RHD—right hepatic duct)

simultaneously with a therapeutic procedure (i.e., endoscopic sphincterotomy) if stones are identified in the CBD. MRCP has an advantage over ERCP in that it is noninvasive and does not make use of injected iodinated contrast solutions. Most surgeons would probably recommend that preoperative cholangiography be performed selectively in patients with clinical or biochemical features associated with a high risk of choledocholithiasis. The specific modality used in such a case varies with the technology and expertise available locally.

Laboratory Tests

Preoperative blood tests are important for evaluation of liver function and for detection of unsuspected abnormalities of renal function, electrolyte balance, or coagulation. Abnormal liver function test results may reflect choledocholithiasis or primary hepatic dysfunction.

SELECTION OF PATIENTS

Patients Eligible for Outpatient Cholecystectomy

Patients in good general health who have a reasonable amount of support from family or friends are eligible for outpatient cholecystectomy, especially if they are at low risk for conversion to laparotomy [*see* Special Problems, Conversion to Laparotomy, *below*]. These patients can generally be discharged home from the recovery room 6 to 12 hours after surgery, provided that the operation went smoothly, their vital signs are stable, they are able to void, they can manage at least a liquid diet without vomiting, and their pain can be controlled with oral analgesics.

Technically Challenging Patients

Before performing laparoscopic cholecystectomy, the surgeon can predict which patients are likely to be technically challenging. These include patients who have a particularly unsuitable body habitus, those who are at high risk for multiple and dense peritoneal adhesions, and those who are likely to have distorted anatomy in the region of the gallbladder.

Morbidly obese patients present specific difficulties [*see* Special Considerations in Obese Patients, *below*]. Small, muscular patients have a noncompliant abdominal wall, resulting in a small working space in the abdomen and necessitating high inflation pressures to obtain reasonable exposure.

Patients with a history of multiple abdominal operations, especially in the upper abdomen, and those who have a history of peritonitis are likely to pose difficulties because of peritoneal adhesions. These adhesions make access to the abdomen more risky and exposure of the gallbladder more difficult.

Patients who have undergone gastroduodenal surgery, those who have any history of acute cholecystitis, those who have a long history of recurrent gallbladder attacks, and those who have recently had severe pancreatitis are particularly difficult candidates for laparoscopic cholecystectomy. These patients have dense adhesions in the region of the gallbladder, the anatomy is distorted, the cystic duct may be foreshortened, and the CBD may be very closely and densely adherent to the gallbladder. These patients are a challenge to the most experienced laparoscopic surgeon. When such problems are encountered, conversion to open cholecystectomy should be considered early in the operation.

Predictors of Choledocholithiasis

Common bile duct stones may be discovered preoperatively, intraoperatively, or postoperatively. The surgeon's goal is to clear the ducts but to use the smallest number of procedures with the lowest risk of morbidity. Thus, before elective laparoscopic cholecystectomy, it is desirable to group patients at low, medium, and high risk for choledocholithiasis according to clinical parameters [*see* Preoperative Data, *above*]. Subsequent investigational and interventional strategy depends on the expertise locally available, as there have been no randomized trials demonstrating an advantage of one approach over another [*see Figure 2*].

In our institution, where MRCP is available and reliable and where ERCP achieves greater than 90% stone clearance, we recommend the following approach: preoperative ERCP and sphincterotomy (if required) for high-risk patients (those who have clinical jaundice or cholangitis, hyperbilirubinemia, a dilated CBD, or visible choledocholithiasis on ultrasonography) and MRCP or intraoperative fluoroscopic cholangiography for moderate-risk patients (those who have mildly elevated serum bilirubin levels, ele-

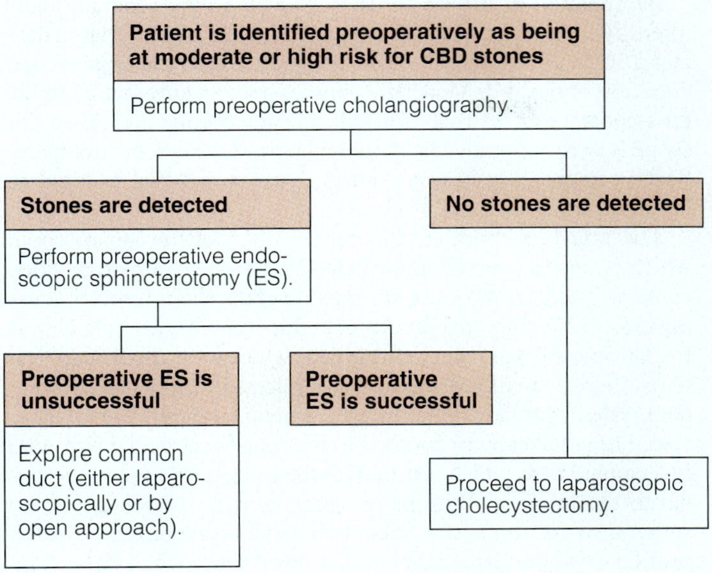

Figure 2 Laparoscopic cholecystectomy. Shown is an algorithm outlining the use of preoperative cholangiography in patients at moderate or high risk for CBD stones.

vated alkaline phosphatase concentrations, pancreatitis, or multiple small gallstones). Patients at low risk for CBD stones do not routinely undergo cholangiography.

Contraindications

There are few absolute contraindications to laparoscopic cholecystectomy. Certainly, no patient who poses an unacceptable risk for open cholecystectomy should be considered for laparoscopic cholecystectomy, because there is always the possibility that conversion will become necessary. Of the relative contraindications, surgical inexperience is the most important.

Neither ascites nor hernia is a contraindication to laparoscopic cholecystectomy. Ascites can be drained and the gallbladder visualized. Large hernias may present a problem, however, because with insufflation, the gas preferentially fills the hernia. Patients with large inguinal hernias may require an external support to minimize this problem and the discomfort related to pneumoscrotum. Patients with umbilical hernias can have their hernias repaired while they are undergoing laparoscopic cholecystectomy. For such patients, the initial trocar should be placed by open insertion according to the Hasson technique [*see* Operative Technique, Step 1: Placement of Trocars and Accessory Ports, *below*], with pains taken to avoid injury to the contents of the hernia. The sutures required to close the hernia defect can be placed before insertion of the initial trocar. A similar technique can be applied to patients with incisional hernias, although for large incisional hernias, laparoscopic cholecystectomy may have no advantages over open cholecystectomy if a large incision and dissection of adhesions are required. Patients with stomas may also undergo laparoscopic cholecystectomy, provided that the appropriate steps are taken to prevent injury to the bowel during placement of trocars and division of adhesions.

Patients with cirrhosis or portal hypertension are at high risk for morbidity and mortality with open cholecystectomy. If absolutely necessary, laparoscopic cholecystectomy may be attempted by an experienced surgeon. The risk of bleeding can be minimized by rigorous preoperative preparation, meticulous dissection with the help of magnification available through the laparoscope, and use of the electrocautery.

Patients with bleeding diatheses, such as hemophilia, von Willebrand's disease, and thrombocytopenia, may undergo laparoscopic cholecystectomy. They require appropriate preoperative and postoperative care and monitoring, and a hematologist should be consulted.

Questions have been raised about whether laparoscopic cholecystectomy should be performed in pregnant patients; it has been argued that the increased intra-abdominal pressure may pose a risk to the fetus. Because of the enlarged uterus, open insertion of the initial trocar is mandatory, and the positioning of other trocars may have to be modified according to the position of the uterus. Despite these potential problems, safe performance of laparoscopic cholecystectomy and other laparoscopic procedures in pregnant patients has been described in the surgical and gynecologic literature.

Operative Planning

PROPHYLACTIC ANTIBIOTICS

Some surgeons recommend routine preoperative administration of antibiotics to all patients undergoing laparoscopic cholecystectomy. The rationale for this recommendation is that inadvertent entry into the gallbladder is not uncommon and can lead to spillage of bile or stones into the peritoneal cavity. Other surgeons, however, recommend using the same guidelines for antibiotic prophylaxis in patients undergoing laparoscopic cholecystectomy as in those undergoing open cholecystectomy. Although resolution of this controversy awaits proper prospective trials, we recommend selective use of antibiotic prophylaxis for patients at highest risk for bacteria in the bile, including those with acute cholecystitis, CBD stones, previous instrumentation of the biliary tree, and age greater than 70 years.

PROPHYLAXIS OF DEEP VEIN THROMBOSIS

During laparoscopic surgery in the upper abdomen, exposure is enhanced by positioning the patient in the reverse Trendelenburg's position. This position, coupled with the positive intra-abdominal pressure generated by CO_2 pneumoperitoneum and the vasodilatation induced by general anesthesia, leads to venous pooling in the lower extremities. This consequence may be minimized by using antiembolic stockings or by wrapping the legs with elastic bandages. Subcutaneous heparin may be used for patients considered to be at increased risk for deep vein thrombosis (DVT) [*see* 70 Thromboembolic Problems]. There has not yet been convincing evidence, however, that the incidence of DVT increases with laparoscopy compared with open surgery.

PATIENT POSITIONING

The patient should be positioned so as to optimize exposure of the gallbladder and to give the surgeon, the camera operator, and the assistant easy access to the patient and a clear view of the video monitor or monitors. There should be a direct line from the surgeon to the laparoscope to the gallbladder. This can be accomplished with the patient in the supine position and the surgeon on the patient's left (North American positioning) [*see Figure 3a*] or with the patient in low stirrups and the surgeon on the patient's left or between the patient's legs (European positioning) [*see Figure 3b*].

With North American positioning, in which the patient is supine, the camera operator usually stands on the patient's left to the left of the surgeon, while the assistant stands on the patient's right. The video monitor is positioned on the patient's right above the level of the costal margin. If a second monitor is available, it should be positioned on the patient's left to the right of the surgeon, where the assistant can have an unobstructed and comfortable view.

Exposure can be improved by tilting the patient in the reverse Trendelenburg's position and by rotating the table with the patient's right side up. Gravity pulls the duodenum, the colon, and the omentum away from the gallbladder, thereby increasing the working space available in the upper abdomen.

The operating room table should allow easy access for a fluoroscopic C-arm, to facilitate intraoperative cholangiography. The table cover should be radiolucent.

EQUIPMENT

The equipment required for laparoscopic cholecystectomy [see Table 1] includes the following: an optical system, an electronic insufflator, trocars (cannulas), surgical instruments, and hemostatic devices.

Optical System

The optical system consists of a laparoscope, a high-intensity light source, a miniature (3/4 in.) video camera and camera box, and a high-resolution video monitor. A videotape recording system is optional but desirable. A video printing system and digital-image capturing system are also valuable for documentation of operative findings.

The laparoscope can provide either a straight, end-on (0°) view or an angled (30° or 45°) view. Scopes that provide an end-on view are easier to learn to use, but angled scopes are more versatile. Scopes with a 30° viewing angle cause less disorientation than those with a 45° angle and are ideal for laparoscopic cholecystectomy. Excellent 30° angle scopes are currently available in 10 mm, 5 mm, and 3.5 mm sizes.

Illumination in the abdomen is provided by a separate high-intensity light source (usually xenon or metal halide) that generates 150 to 300 watts. The light is conducted to the laparoscope via a fiberoptic cord. Most light sources have an automatic brightness-control system that will reduce light output the closer the scope is to the operative field, thereby diminishing reflective glare. Some cameras also have a control that can be used to regulate light output.

The image is conducted to the eyepiece of the laparoscope, which in turn is coupled to the video camera. The miniature video camera systems now in use are capable of excellent resolution using either one chip or three. In one-chip systems, a single chip is responsible for red, blue, and green, whereas in three-chip systems, there is a chip for each of the colors. In most cases, three-chip systems provide better images, albeit at a significantly higher cost. The small camera coupled to the scope is attached by a wire to a camera box, which synthesizes the images and sends the signal to the monitor. Buttons on some camera models allow the surgeon to control accessories such as video recorders or video printers or to perform camera functions such as white-balancing, activation of filters, digital enhancement, or controlling gain.

The monitor is a 13 to 19 in. high-resolution medical-grade video monitor. The quality of the monitor is usually rated in terms of the number of lines that can be resolved per inch. The best monitors currently available have a resolution of approximately 600 lines/in.

The resolution and quality of the final image depend on (1) the brightness of the light source; (2) the integrity of the fiberoptic cord used to convey the light; (3) clean and secure connections between the light source and the scope; (4) the quality of the laparoscope (glass-rod lens systems are preferred), the camera, and the monitor; and (5) correct wiring of the components. The distal end of the scope must be kept clean and free of condensation; bile, blood, or fat will reduce brightness and distort the image.

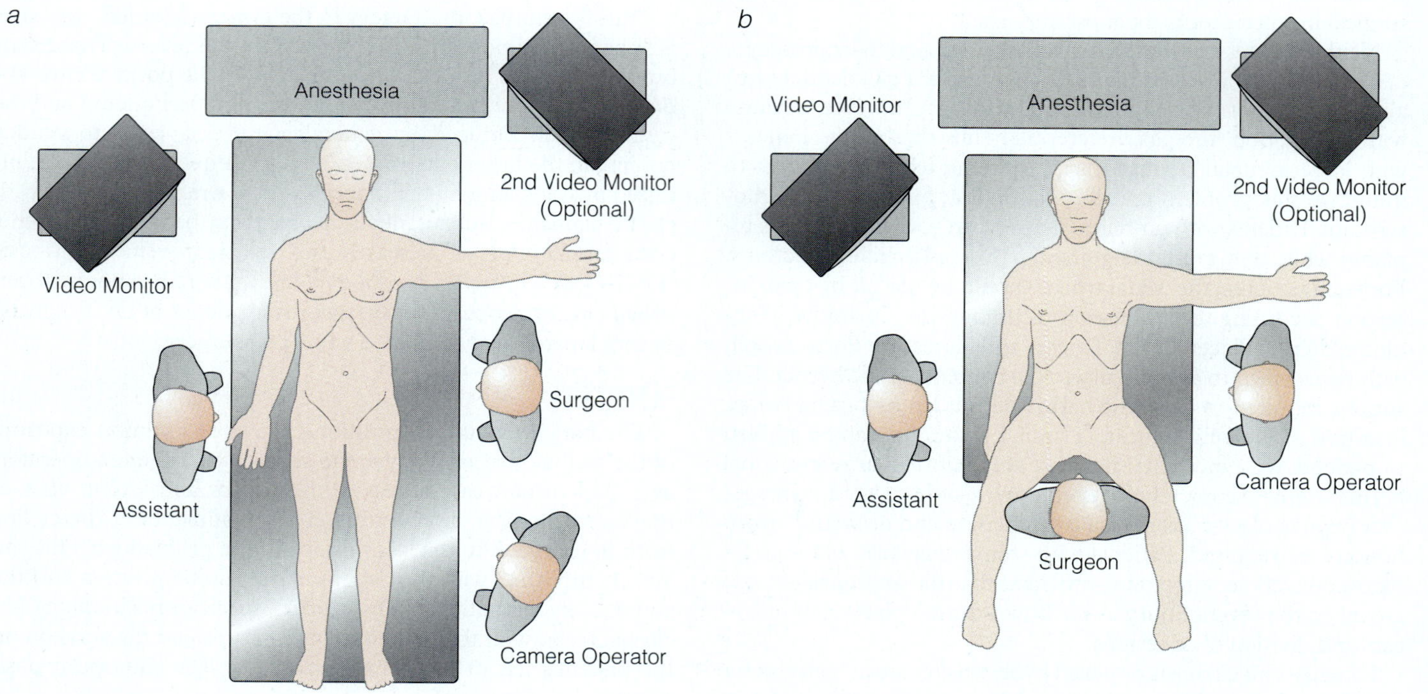

Figure 3 Laparoscopic cholecystectomy. A patient undergoing laparoscopic cholecystectomy should be positioned so as to allow easy access to the gallbladder and a clear view of the monitors. Shown are the positions of the surgeon, the camera operator, and the assistant in the OR according to (*a*) North American positioning and (*b*) European positioning.

Table 1 Equipment for Laparoscopic Cholecystectomy

Instrument/Device	Number	Size	Comments

Laparoscopic cart
  High-intensity halogen light source (150–300 watts)
  High-flow electronic insufflator (minimum flow rate of 6 L/min)
  Laparoscopic camera box
  Videocassette recorder (optional)
  Digital still image capture system (optional)			

Laparoscope	1	5–10 mm	Available in 0° and angled views; we prefer to use a 30° 5 mm diameter laparoscope
Atraumatic grasping forceps	2–4	2–10 mm	Selection of graspers should allow surgeon choice appropriate to thickness and consistency of gallbladder wall; insulation is unnecessary
Large-tooth grasping forceps	1	10 mm	Used to extract gallbladder at end of procedure
Curved dissector	1	2–5 mm	Should have a rotatable shaft; insulation is required
Scissors	2–3	2–5 mm	One curved and one straight scissors with rotating shaft and insulation; additional microscissors may be helpful for incising cystic duct
Clip appliers	1–2	5–10 mm	Either disposable multiple clip applier or 2 manually loaded reusable single clip appliers for small and medium-to-large clips
Dissecting electrocautery hook or spatula	1	5 mm	Available in various shapes according to surgeon's preference; instrument should have channel for suction and irrigation controlled by trumpet valve(s); insulation required
High-frequency electrical cord	1		Cord should be designed with appropriate connectors for electrosurgical unit and instruments being used
Suction-irrigation probe	1	5–10 mm	Probe should have trumpet valve controls for suction and irrigation; may be used with pump for hydrodissection
10-to-5 mm reducers	2		Allows use of 5 mm instruments in 10 mm trocar without loss of pneumoperitoneum; these are often unnecessary with newer disposable trocars and may be built into some reusable trocars
5-to-3 mm reducer	1		Allows use of 2–3 mm instruments and ligating loops in 5 mm trocars
Ligating loops			
Endoscopic needle holders	1–2	5 mm	
Cholangiogram clamp with catheter	1	5 mm	Allows passage of catheter and clamping of catheter in cystic duct
Veress needle	1		Used if initial trocar is inserted by percutaneous technique
Allis or Babcock forceps	1–2	5 mm	Allows atraumatic grasping of bowel or gallbladder
Long spinal needle	1	14-gauge	Useful for aspirating gallbladder percutaneously in cases of acute cholecystitis or hydrops

The camera will last longer if it is not sterilized. During the operation, it can be placed in a sterile, disposable plastic bag.

Insufflator

To provide the exposure required for the procedure, it is necessary to create a working space within the abdomen by insufflating gas under positive pressure. CO_2 is preferred because of its high solubility in water and because it does not support combustion when the electrocautery is used for hemostasis. The CO_2 should be insufflated with an electronic pump capable of a flow rate of at least 6 L/min; most current systems have a maximum flow rate of 10 L/min or higher. The insufflator is connected to one of the trocars by means of a flexible tube and a stopcock.

When intra-abdominal pressure drops below a preset value (usually about 15 mm Hg), gas flow begins at the preset rate. The insufflator should provide digital readouts of the actual gas flow rate, the actual intra-abdominal pressure, and the total amount of CO_2 used during the procedure. It should also have a control for adjusting maximum flow rate and a control for setting the pressure above which gas flow is automatically shut off. An audible alarm should sound when the measured pressure exceeds a certain preset value.

When multiple trocars are used, as they are in laparoscopic cholecystectomy, there is a certain unavoidable loss of gas around and through the trocars. The insufflator rapidly replaces this gas. Because the rate of gas flow is influenced by the diameter of the port through which the gas is infused, insufflators capable of flow rates higher than 6 L/min are rarely used to their full potential. Insufflators that can provide heated gas minimize heat loss and fogging.

Trocars

Access to the abdominal cavity is gained via trocars inserted percutaneously. To minimize loss of pneumoperitoneum, these trocars are equipped with valves and gaskets. They are available in a variety of sizes; selection depends on the external diameter of the instruments to be placed through them.

For cholecystectomy, most surgeons prefer to use a 10/12 mm trocar at the umbilicus because a large opening is required for extraction of the gallbladder. The other trocars can be between 2 and 12 mm, depending on the size of the laparoscope, grasping forceps, and clip applicators being used. The conventional technique uses 10/12 mm trocars at the umbilicus and for the epigastric operating port and 5 mm trocars for the graspers. If a 5 mm laparoscope is used, the epigastric port size can be reduced to 5 mm; a clip applicator with a 10 mm diameter can be placed through the umbilical port after the laparoscope is moved to the epigastric port. If a 5 mm clip applicator is available, it can be used through the epigastric port and viewed through the 5 mm scope at the umbilicus. If instruments 5 mm in diameter are inserted through a 10 mm trocar, a reducer is required to minimize leakage of gas.

Currently, 2 mm instrumentation is becoming increasingly popular. The grasping instruments, scissors, and dissectors currently available work well. The 2 mm laparoscopes, available in the 0° configuration, do not have the same image quality as larger scopes. Other limitations of the 2 mm trocars include the impossibility of passing clip applicators, suction devices, and instruments with curved tips (such as hooks and curved dissectors) through them. With the combination of a 10 mm umbilical trocar, 5 mm epigastric operating port, and 2 mm ports for grasping forceps, there is no significant loss of optical quality or flexibility in the selection of operating instruments, trocar size is minimized, and the cosmetic result is excellent.

Surgical Instruments

The choice of surgical instruments from the large array now available is clearly a personal one. Many instruments are available in both disposable and reusable forms. Reusable instruments tend to be sturdier and better designed, but their design may rapidly become obsolete, and like reusable trocars, they must be checked periodically. Disposables are more current in design, are consistently sharp, and are excellent to have as backups in case nondisposables break down. Instruments are also available in both insulated versions (to allow use of the electrocautery) or noninsulated versions (to reduce maintenance costs).

A minimal set of instruments for laparoscopic cholecystectomy would include graspers, dissectors, clip applicators, scissors, a dissecting electrocautery hook or spatula (or both), probes, reducers, ligating loops, a Veress needle, needle holders, and a cholangiography catheter system [see Table 1]; other instruments may be considered as options.

For clip applicators, curved scissors, and curved dissectors, a rotatable shaft can afford the surgeon more comfortable and convenient working angles. The shaft should be easily locked once it is at the appropriate angle so that it will not rotate when the instrument is in use.

Suction and irrigation probes are available with either trumpet valves or stopcock attachments. Reusable instruments must be checked periodically to ensure that the valves do not stick or leak. Irrigation can be provided under pressure by means of a commercial pump system, a system that uses high-pressure gas, or a pressure bag like those used for infusion of blood products. If a pressure bag is used, it should be pressurized to approximately 300 mm Hg, and either normal saline or lactated Ringer's solution can be used as an irrigant.

Hemostatic Devices

Hemostasis can be achieved with monopolar or bipolar electrocautery. Electrocautery units are widely available, safe, inexpensive, and familiar to all surgeons, and they provide excellent hemostasis. A monopolar electrocautery can be connected to most available instruments; however, bipolar electrocauterization will likely prove to be safer, and laparoscopic instruments designed to be used with a bipolar electrocautery are being developed. With a monopolar electrocautery, depth of burn is less predictable, current can be conducted through noninsulated instruments and trocars, and any area of the instrument that is stripped of insulation may conduct current and result in a burn. Caution is essential when the electrocautery is used near hemostatic clips; delayed sloughing may occur.

Electrocauterization should be avoided near the CBD because delayed bile duct injuries and leaks may occur as a result of sloughing from a burned area and devascularization of the duct. Electrocauterization should also be used carefully near the bowel and when intra-abdominal adhesions are being taken down. In addition to attaching the electrocautery to dissecting forceps and scissors, the surgeon can use various cautery probes, classified according to whether the tip has the shape of a hook or a spatula. Either L-shaped or J-shaped hooks may be used, according to the surgeon's preference. The use of hand-activated cautery probes and the presence of a channel that allows suction and irrigation through the cautery probes are especially convenient.

Operative Technique

STEP 1: PLACEMENT OF TROCARS AND ACCESSORY PORTS

Placement of Initial Trocar

The initial step in laparoscopic cholecystectomy is the creation of pneumoperitoneum and the insertion of an initial trocar through which the laparoscope can be passed. This is a critical step in the procedure because complications resulting from improper placement may cause serious morbidity and death. The surgeon may use either a percutaneous technique or an open technique. We prefer the open technique, which eliminates the risks inherent in the blind puncture.

Percutaneous technique As the first step in percutaneous insertion, a small curvilinear incision is made in the area of the umbilicus and extended downward through the subcutaneous fat. A Veress needle is then inserted through the fascia and the peritoneum into the abdominal cavity [see Figure 4a]. This is best accomplished by elevating the abdominal wall and slightly angling the needle toward the pelvis, with the patient in Trendelenburg's position. The tip of the needle should be directed toward the hollow of the sacrum. Entry of the Veress needle into the peritoneal cavity can usually be confirmed by a popping sensation as the resistance of the peritoneum is overcome. A 10 ml syringe should then be attached to the needle and aspiration attempted. If the aspirate contains any blood or bowel contents, the needle is clearly in an inappropriate position.

If the aspirate is clear, the next step is to confirm proper positioning by means of the saline drop test [see Figure 4b]. The surgeon then attaches the electronic insufflator to the Veress needle and begins inflating the abdomen at a rate of approximately 1 L/min. The intra-abdominal pressure should be very low when insufflation is started, usually about 2 to 5 mm Hg; high pressure suggests improper needle placement. As the abdomen is distended with carbon dioxide, the surgeon should percuss the abdomen to ensure even distribution of the gas. When a pressure of approximately 15 mm Hg is reached (which requires about 5 L of gas in an average-sized patient), the Veress needle is withdrawn, and a sharp 10/12 mm trocar is percutaneously inserted through the

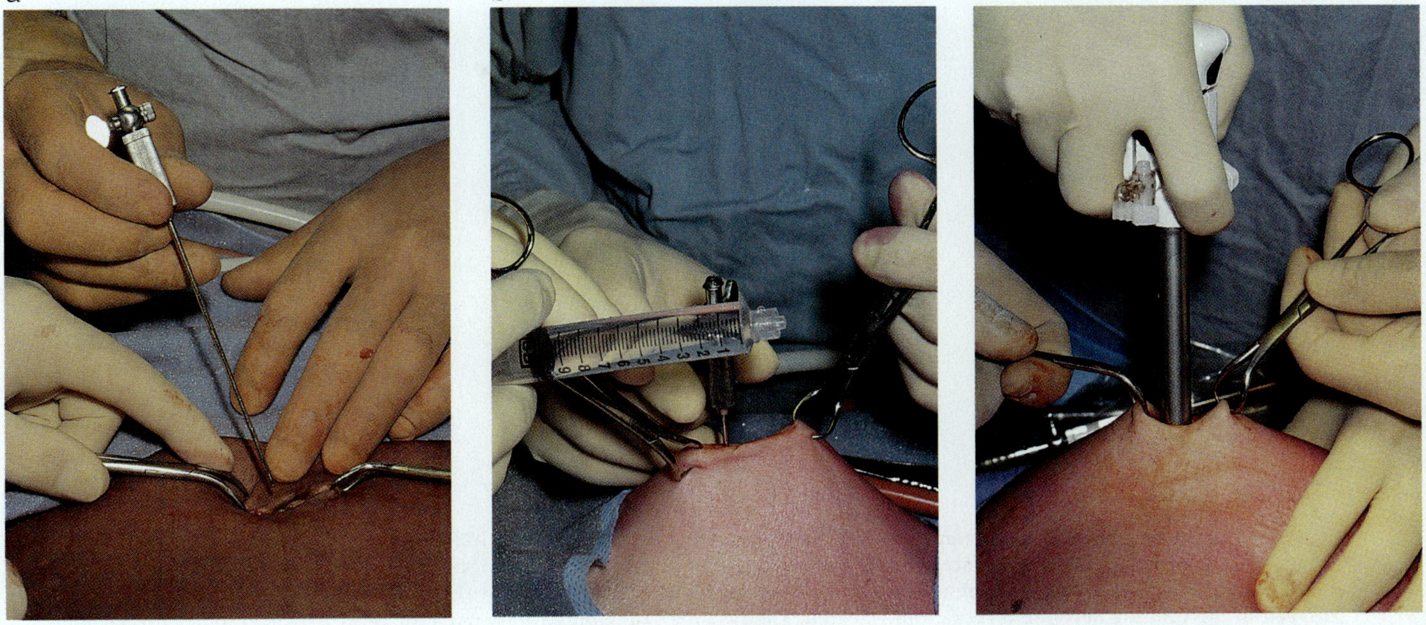

Figure 4 Laparoscopic cholecystectomy. Illustrated is percutaneous placement of the initial trocar. (*a*) A Veress needle is used for percutaneous entry into the peritoneal cavity. It is angled toward the sacral hollow (where the distance from the anterior to the posterior abdominal wall is greatest) and toward an area below the bifurcation of the aorta. This space can be enlarged by tilting the patient in Trendelenburg's position, allowing the free intestinal loops to fall cephalad. (*b*) With the stopcock on the Veress needle in the closed position, a drop of saline is placed into the hub of the needle. The stopcock is then opened and the abdominal wall elevated. Lifting the abdominal wall creates negative pressure in the peritoneal cavity. Thus, if the tip of the needle is properly positioned within the cavity, the drop of saline should be drawn into the abdomen. (*c*) The abdominal wall is elevated, and a sharp 10/11 mm trocar is inserted into the peritoneal cavity along the same path as the Veress needle. Disposable trocars with a retracting plastic sheath provide further protection against perforation of viscera or vessels.

same incision into the abdominal cavity, following the same route as the needle. Because this procedure is done in a blind fashion, it may be advisable to enhance its safety by using disposable trocars with a spring-loaded protective plastic mechanism [*see Figure 4c*]. Once the initial trocar is inserted, proper positioning is confirmed by placing the laparoscope. Insufflation of CO_2 through the trocar resumes, maintaining pneumoperitoneum.

Open insertion technique The advantage of the open technique is that the trocar is inserted into the peritoneal cavity under direct vision; no Veress needle is required. Although it is certainly possible to injure the bowel inadvertently when placing the trocar, the injury almost always can be identified immediately and usually can be repaired easily through the same incision. Injury to the blood vessels or the bladder should virtually never occur with the open technique.

The umbilical skin is elevated with a sharp towel clip, and a 1 cm incision is made just inferior to the umbilicus [*see Figure 5a*]. Dissection is carried down through the subcutaneous tissue. The skin flap is raised, and a raphe can be seen connecting its undersurface to the midline fascia of the abdominal wall. The raphe is followed down to the fascia, which is then elevated between vertically placed forceps and incised [*see Figure 5b*]. The peritoneum is grasped next and pulled up into the wound, where it is incised. Entry into the abdominal cavity is easily confirmed by inserting a finger or a blunt instrument into the peritoneum [*see Figure 5c*]. Stay sutures are then placed on either side of the fascial incision, and a blunt olive-tipped 10/12 mm trocar, designed to occlude the fascial defect around it, is placed into the abdomen under direct vision. These sutures are then used to fasten the trocar to the wound and to prevent any leakage of gas. Because proper positioning of the trocar is obvious and needs no further confirmation, pneumoperitoneum can be created rapidly. The additional time expended on the dissection needed for insertion of the trocar is more than outweighed by the increased speed with which pneumoperitoneum is created. The stay sutures can also be used at the end of the procedure to close the fascial defect.

Scars

Patients who have previously undergone abdominal surgery are at risk for adhesions, both to the undersurface of the abdominal wall and intra-abdominally. Adhesions to the undersurface of the abdominal wall make access to the abdominal cavity potentially hazardous, particularly when the percutaneous method is used for placement of the initial trocar. Scars from previous operations may affect insertion of the initial trocar, depending on its orientation and location. If a patient has a scar in the lower abdomen (e.g., from a Pfannenstiel's incision or an incision in the right lower quadrant for an appendectomy), the position of the initial trocar need not be changed. If the scar is in the upper abdomen, the initial trocar may be inserted below the umbilicus in the midline. If there is a long midline scar that is impossible to avoid, careful dissection of the peritoneum through a somewhat longer vertical incision than usual affords safe access to the peritoneum in most cases.

An alternative is to insert the initial trocar high in the epigastrium or in the right anterior axillary line, where bowel adhesions are less likely to be present. The laparoscope is inserted through this trocar and used to examine the undersurface of the old scar for a clear site near the umbilicus where a 10 mm trocar can be

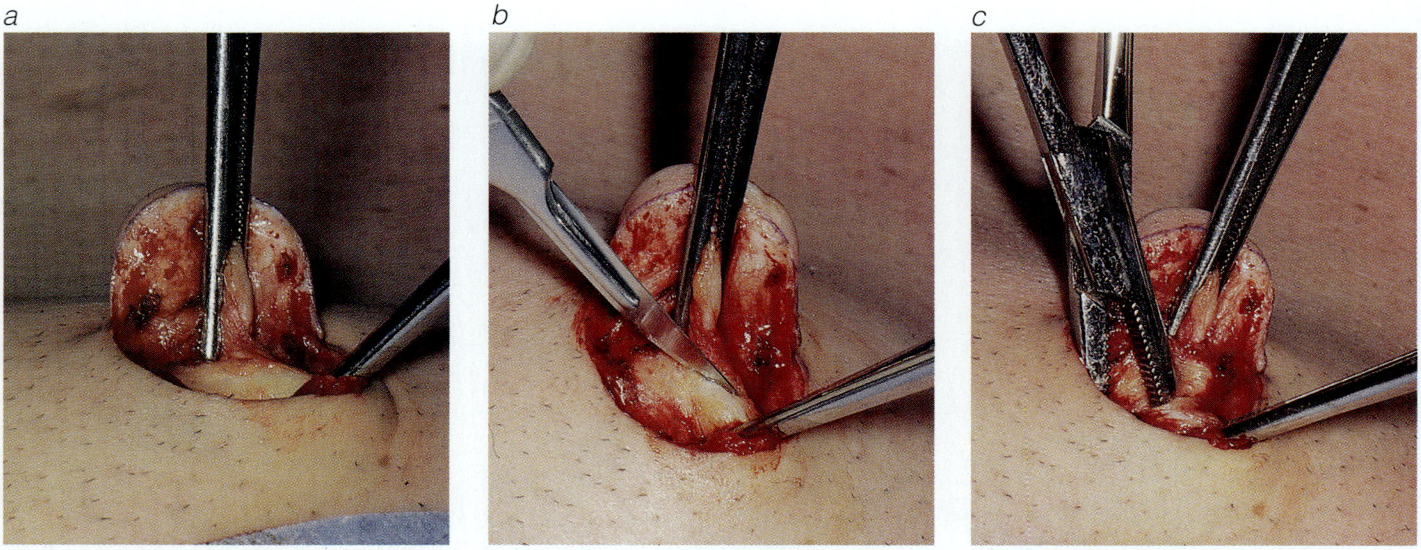

Figure 5 Laparoscopic cholecystectomy. With the open insertion technique, the initial trocar is placed under direct vision. (*a*) The umbilical skin is elevated with a sharp towel clip. A curvilinear incision is made in the inferior umbilical fold. The skin flap is elevated, and the raphe leading from the dermis to the fascia is thereby exposed. (*b*) The fascia is grasped in the midline between forceps and elevated. The fascia and the underlying peritoneum are incised under direct vision. (*c*) A blunt instrument is placed into the peritoneum to ensure that the undersurface of the peritoneum is free of adhesions. The opening can be enlarged sufficiently to allow placement of a blunt 10/11 mm trocar.

placed. Previous laparoscopy, which rarely creates significant intra-abdominal adhesions, rarely necessitates modification of trocar insertion.

Some surgeons still prefer to use the percutaneous insertion method even in patients who have had multiple abdominal operations. In these cases, the Veress needle should be inserted well away from any old scars. After pneumoperitoneum has been obtained, a trocar can be placed at the site. If a 5 mm laparoscope is available, a 5 mm port can be used. The anterior abdominal wall should then be inspected so that appropriate sites for the other trocars can be selected.

The surgeon should also consider the reason for the previous surgery. For example, a patient who underwent an appendectomy for perforating appendicitis may have had diffuse peritonitis and may have adhesions well away from the old scar.

Placement of Accessory Ports

In most cases, four ports are necessary. The first port is used for insertion of the laparoscope; the remaining ports are used for insertion of grasping forceps, dissectors, and clip applicators. The precise position of the accessory ports depends on the surgeon's preference, the patient's body habitus, and the presence or absence of previous scars or intra-abdominal adhesions. To have a rigid approach to port placement is inappropriate: placement of the trocars determines exposure to the site of operation, and improper placement will haunt the surgeon throughout the case. In some cases, a fifth trocar is required to elevate a floppy liver or to depress or retract the omentum or a bulky hepatic flexure of the colon. In trocar placement, as in patient positioning, European practice tends to differ from North American practice [*see Figure 6*].

Most surgeons elect to place one of the grasping forceps on the fundus of the gallbladder through an accessory port that is placed approximately in the anterior axillary line below the level of the gallbladder. Because the level of the gallbladder varies from patient to patient, the placement of this accessory port should not be decided on until the gallbladder is visualized. If the gallbladder is low lying and the trocar is placed too high, it is difficult for the surgeon to achieve the appropriate angle of retraction. As a rule, positioning the trocar in the anterior axillary line approximately halfway between the costal margin and the anterosuperior iliac spine provides the appropriate exposure. A 2 or 5 mm port usually suffices at this site because its only function is to allow retraction of the gallbladder. In some cases of acute cholecystitis, however, placement of a 10 mm port might be preferable, so that a 10 mm Babcock instrument can be inserted and used to grasp the gallbladder without tearing it.

A second accessory port (also 2 or 5 mm) allows the surgeon to grasp the gallbladder in the area of Hartmann's pouch for retraction. This port is usually positioned just beneath the costal margin. Some surgeons prefer it to be approximately at the midclavicular line; others prefer it to be higher and more medial, just to the right of the falciform ligament and as high as possible.

The main operating port should be 5 or 10 mm in diameter so that clip applicators can be readily placed through it and the laparoscope can be moved to this position at the end of the procedure. The positioning of this port is determined by the surgeon's preference and, in particular, by the body habitus of the patient. To obtain the best visualization of the instrument passed through the operative port, the instrument should be at an angle of about 90° to the angle of view of the laparoscope; this is usually best achieved by placing the trocar at about the same horizontal level as the gallbladder, or slightly higher. Some surgeons prefer to place the operative port in the midline, to the right of the falciform ligament; others prefer to place it to the left of the falciform, passing the trocar underneath and elevating the ligament with the trocar.

Surgeons should be encouraged to use both hands when performing laparoscopic cholecystectomy. One hand should control the grasping forceps holding Hartmann's pouch, so that the gallbladder can be moved to provide the surgeon with the best possible exposure. The other hand should control the dissecting instruments placed through the operative port.

Special considerations in obese patients Obese patients pose specific problems that affect port placement. The problems

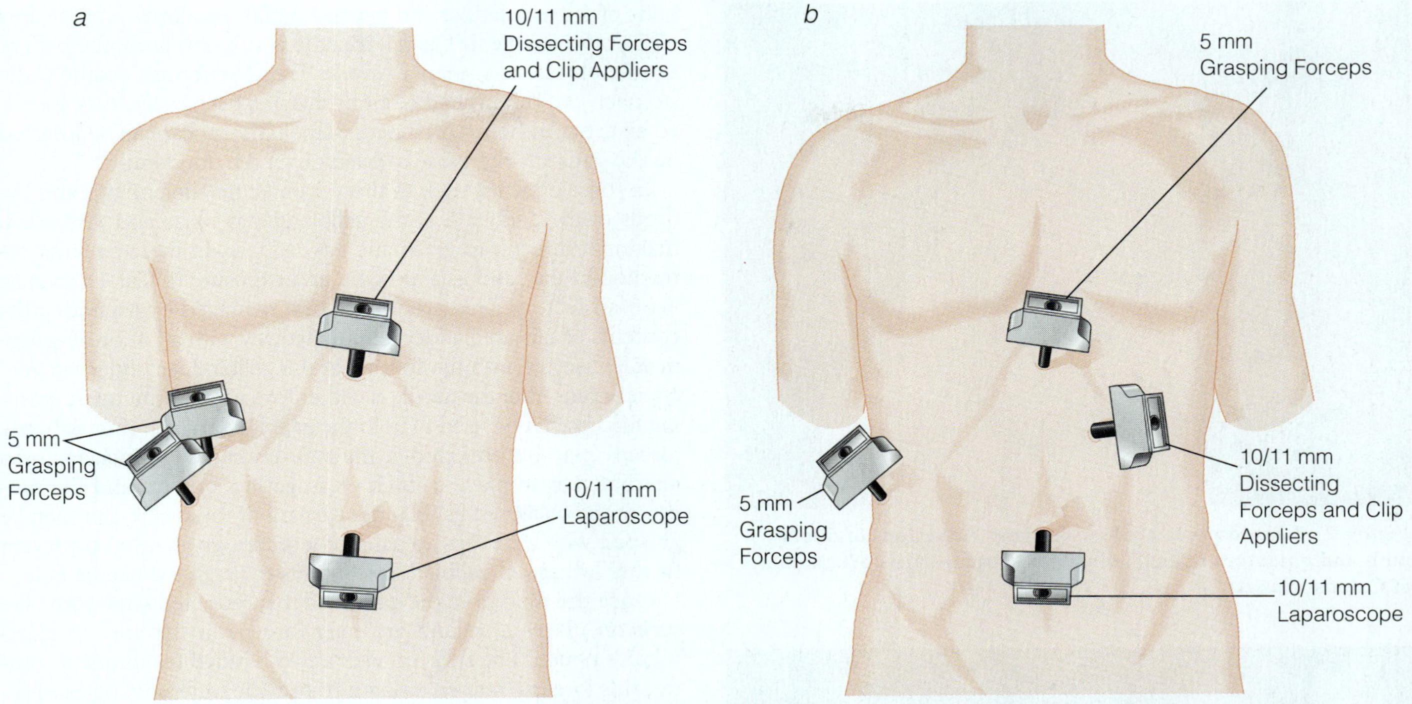

Figure 6 Laparoscopic cholecystectomy. Illustrated are the differences between typical North American practice (*a*) and typical European practice (*b*) with respect to the placement of the trocars and the instruments inserted through each port.

may be related to the thick abdominal wall, the large amount of intra-abdominal fat, or both. A thick abdominal wall makes it more difficult to rotate the trocar around the normal fulcrum point in the abdominal wall. Consequently, it is essential to place the trocar at the angle most likely to be used during the procedure. When a trocar is tunneled through the abdominal wall, more of the cannula is within the abdominal wall than if the trocar had been placed perpendicularly; this results in inflexibility of the trocars. If the trocars are not easily rotated, the instruments placed through them will be difficult to manipulate smoothly. Thus, in the patient with a very thick pannus, a standard-length trocar may be too short. Displacement of trocars can lead to insufflation into the abdominal wall and consequently to subcutaneous emphysema, which further thickens the abdominal wall and hinders exposure.

To prevent such problems, special extra-length trocars designed for morbidly obese patients have been developed and are commercially available. It may also be necessary to place the trocars closer to the area of the gallbladder to ensure that the operating instruments can reach the gallbladder. For example, the initial port may have to be placed above the umbilicus.

In the obese patient, the bulky falciform ligament and the large omentum may adversely affect exposure. A 30° laparoscope may help the surgeon see over the omentum and the high-lying hepatic flexure of the colon. In some cases, it is useful to place a fifth port so that the surgeon can retract the hepatic flexure downward. When the fat forms a layer enveloping intra-abdominal organs, other problems arise—in particular, the difficulty of identifying the anatomic landmarks through the fat. When the electrocautery is used, the heat melts the fat and causes it to sizzle and spray onto the lens of the laparoscope, resulting in a blurry image. To prevent this, the camera operator should pull the scope slightly away from the operative field while the electrocautery is being used, then advance the scope during dissection.

Given that obese patients are more difficult candidates for open cholecystectomy and have a higher complication rate with laparotomy, the advantages of laparoscopic cholecystectomy in these individuals justify the effort needed to overcome the technical problems.

STEP 2: EXPOSING THE GALLBLADDER AND CALOT'S TRIANGLE

Dissection of Adhesions

Adhesions must be dissected to afford the surgeon an unimpeded view of the gallbladder through the laparoscope. Not all intra-abdominal adhesions must be taken down, just enough of them to allow entry of accessory trocars under direct vision and thus permit access to the gallbladder. This process is facilitated by pneumoperitoneum, which provides traction on adhesions to the abdominal wall, and by the magnification provided by the optical system, which allows identification of the avascular plane of attachment.

The most difficult problem is positioning of the dissecting instruments so that they can reach the undersurface of the anterior abdominal wall. A rigid trocar inserted through the anterior abdominal wall cannot be rotated enough to allow scissors passed through this port to cut adhesions to the anterior abdominal wall. In such cases, one or two trocars should be placed laterally, near the anterior axillary or midaxillary line. Instruments passed through these ports can easily be angled parallel to the anterior abdominal wall, and the adhesions can then be dissected without difficulty.

Bowel adhesions should be taken down with endoscopic scissors at their insertion to the abdominal wall, where they are least vascular. Electrocauterization, generally unnecessary, should be avoided because of the risk of thermal injury to the bowel. Interloop adhesions, which rarely interfere with exposure of the gallbladder, need not be dissected. Frequently, adhesions to the gallbladder occur as a reaction to inflammatory attacks [*see Figure 7*]. They are usually relatively avascular. Dissection of these adhesions should begin at the fundus of the gallbladder and should then proceed down toward the neck of the gallbladder. The best way to take them down is to grasp the gallbladder with one grasping forceps at the site where the adhesions attach, gradually placing traction on the adhesions with the

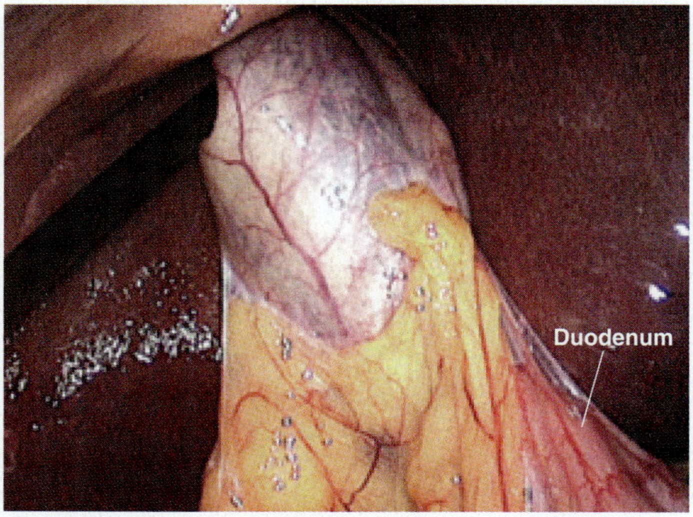

Figure 7 Laparoscopic cholecystectomy. Adhesions of duodenum and omentum to gallbladder wall obscure view of structures of Calot's triangle.

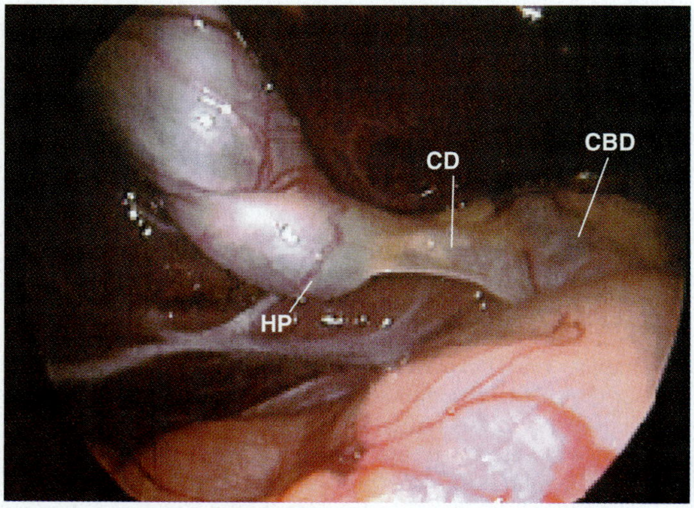

Figure 8 Laparoscopic cholecystectomy. Initial view of gallbladder and related structures is facilitated by appropriate tilting of the operating table. Hartmann's pouch (HP), the cystic duct (CD), and the common bile duct (CBD) can be readily identified before any dissection.

body of the gallbladder and permits initial visualization of the area of Calot's triangle. If Calot's triangle is still obscured, the patient can be placed in a steeper reverse Trendelenburg's position, the stomach can be emptied of air by use of a nasogastric tube inserted by the anesthetist, or, if necessary, a fifth trocar can be inserted on the patient's right side to push down the duodenum.

In some patients, such as those with acute cholecystitis and hydrops of the gallbladder, the gallbladder is tense and distended, making it difficult to grasp and easy to tear. In these patients, retraction of the fundus is difficult, and exposure of Calot's triangle is unsatisfactory. This problem is best managed by aspirating the contents of the gallbladder percutaneously with a 14- or 16-gauge needle inserted into the fundus of the gallbladder under laparoscopic vision. After the needle is withdrawn, a large atraumatic grasping forceps can be used to hold the gallbladder; a 10 mm Babcock forceps may be preferred if the wall is markedly thickened. An alternative is to place a stitch or a ligating loop around the fundus of the collapsed gallbladder; the tail of the suture can then be grasped with a forceps to achieve a secure grip and also prevent further leakage of gallbladder contents through the needle hole.

Once the fundus of the gallbladder is retracted superiorly, the surgeon places a second grasping forceps in the area of Hartmann's pouch. The surgeon uses a two-handed technique to control this forceps, maneuvering it to provide different angles of access to Calot's triangle. Initially, lateral and inferior traction are placed on Hartmann's pouch, opening up the angle between the cystic duct and the common ducts [see Figure 9], avoiding their alignment [see Figure 10].

A large stone impacted in the gallbladder neck may impede the surgeon's ability to place the second forceps on Hartmann's pouch. This problem can usually be managed by dislodging the stone early in the operation, as follows: the gallbladder should be grasped as low as possible with one grasping forceps; a widely opening dissecting instrument, such as a right-angle dissector, a Babcock forceps, or a curved dissector, is used to dislodge the stone and milk it up toward the fundus; with the same forceps or another large grasper, the stone is held up and away from the neck of the gallbladder, and appropriate retraction is provided.

If the stone cannot be disimpacted, an instrument can be used to elevate the infundibulum of the gallbladder superiorly, allowing

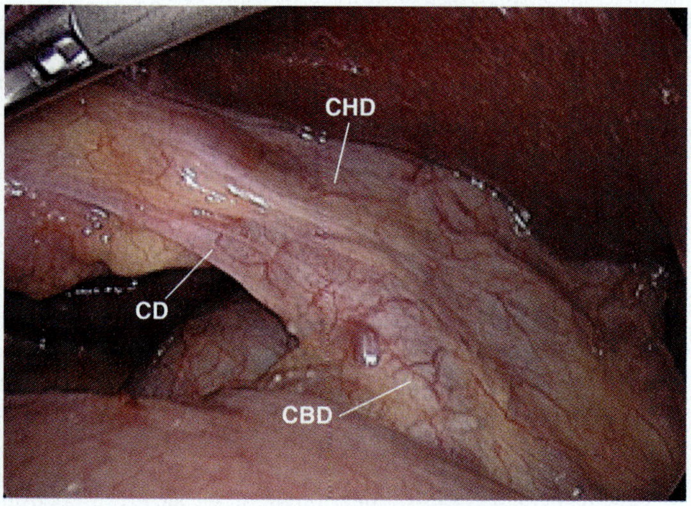

other hand. Usually, the adhesions will peel down in an avascular plane. Dissection should continue until all adhesions to the inferolateral aspect of the gallbladder have been taken down. It is not necessary to divide adhesions between the superior surface of the liver and the undersurface of the diaphragm unless they impede superior retraction of the liver.

Exposing Calot's Triangle

Obtaining adequate exposure of Calot's triangle is an integral step in a cholecystectomy. First, the patient is placed in reverse Trendelenburg's position, with the table rotated toward the left side. The next maneuver is elevation of the fundus of the gallbladder and right liver toward the patient's right shoulder. One grasping forceps, inserted through the most lateral port and held by an assistant, is placed on the fundus of the gallbladder [see Figure 8], and the gallbladder is retracted superiorly and laterally above the right lobe of the liver. This maneuver straightens out folds in the

Figure 9 Laparoscopic cholecystectomy. The area of Hartmann's pouch is retracted laterally. The cystic duct (CD) is seen at an angle to the common hepatic duct (CHD) and the common bile duct (CBD).

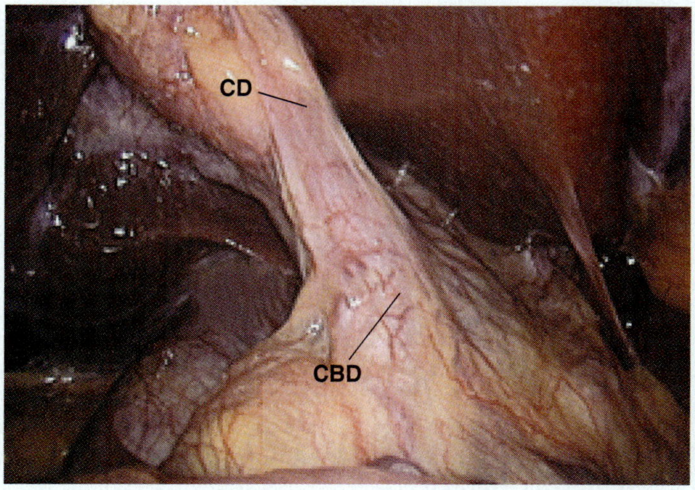

Figure 10 Laparoscopic cholecystectomy. In this case, the gallbladder is retracted cephalad. The cystic duct (CD) can be seen running in the same direction as the common bile duct (CBD). The CBD may be misinterpreted as being the cystic duct and consequently is at risk for injury.

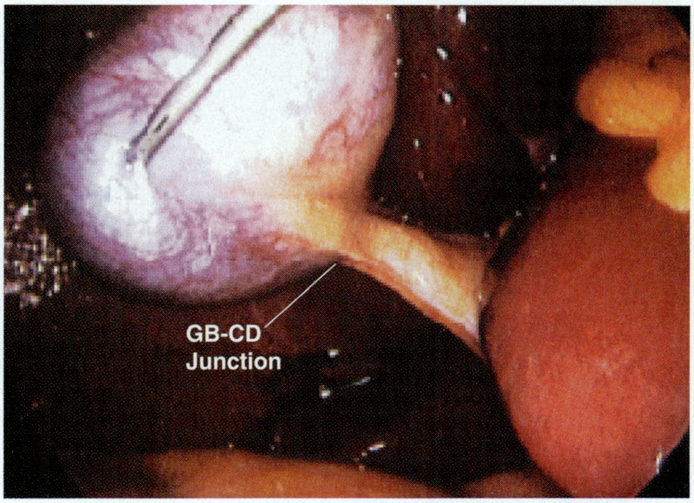

Figure 11 Laparoscopic cholecystectomy. The gallbladder–cystic duct (GB-CD) junction can be identified as lateral traction is applied to the area of Hartmann's pouch.

a curved dissector, the surgeon gently teases away peritoneum attaching the neck of gallbladder to the liver posterolaterally to visualize the funneling of the neck of the gallbladder into the cystic duct [*see Figure 13*]. Only the posterior layer of peritoneum is dissected; care must be taken not to dissect deeply in this area because of the risk of injury to the cystic artery [*see Figure 14*].

Once the funneling of the gallbladder into the cystic duct has been identified, the area of Hartmann's pouch should be again pulled laterally and inferiorly so that the anterior peritoneum can be dissected, while the 30° scope is angled to view the area. The two-handed technique facilitates the surgeon's movement between the posterior and anterior aspects of Calot's triangle, providing complete visualization. Dissection should always take place at the gallbladder–cystic duct junction, staying close to the gallbladder to avoid inadvertent injury to the CBD. A curved dissecting forceps is used to strip the fibroareolar tissue just superior to the cystic duct. The superior border of the cystic duct can then be identified and the cystic duct gently and gradually dissected [*see Figure 15*].

When traction is placed in the manner described above, the cystic artery tends to run parallel to the cystic duct and somewhat cephalad to it. The artery can often be identified by noting its close relation to a lymph node in this area. Complete dissection of the area between the cystic duct and artery develops a window through which the liver should be seen. The cystic duct is then encircled with a curved dissecting instrument or an L-shaped hook. Downward traction should be applied to the cystic duct to open this window and ensure that there is no ductal structure running through this space in Calot's triangle to join the cystic duct (i.e., the right hepatic duct).

Dissection of Calot's triangle should be completed before the cystic duct is clipped or divided. This is best accomplished by dissecting the neck of the gallbladder from the liver bed. Unequivocal identification of the gallbladder–cystic duct junction is imperative. The cystic duct should be dissected only for a length that will permit secure placement of two clips; it is not necessary, and indeed may be hazardous, to attempt to identify the cystic duct–common duct junction.

The cystic artery is exposed next [*see Figure 16*]. A small vein can usually be identified in the space between the cystic duct and the cystic artery; this vein can usually be pulled up anteriorly and

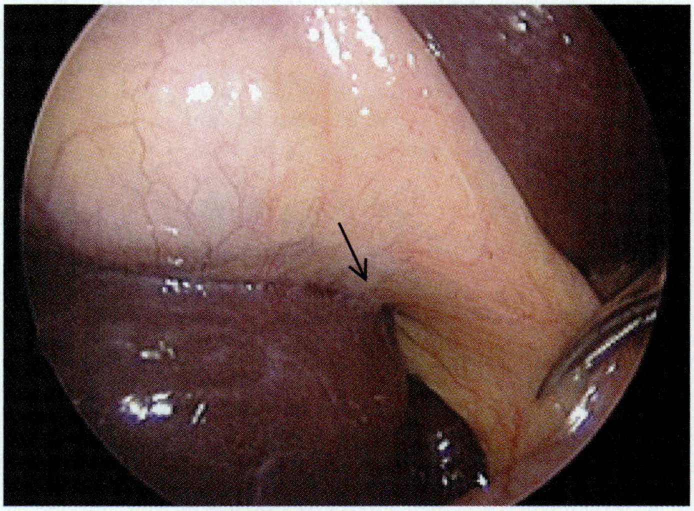

exposure of the cystic structures. Alternatively, one can attempt to crush the stone, but small pieces of the stone may fall into the cystic duct. A third option is to place a stitch in Hartmann's pouch and grasp the end of the stitch to provide exposure.

STEP 3: STRIPPING THE PERITONEUM

The key to avoiding injury to the major ducts during laparoscopic cholecystectomy is accurate identification of the junction between the gallbladder and the cystic duct [*see Figure 11*]. Unless the gallbladder–cystic duct junction is immediately obvious upon examination of Calot's triangle anteriorly, our approach is to begin the dissection of Calot's triangle posteriorly [*see Figure 12*]. From this approach, the insertion of the gallbladder neck into the cystic duct is usually more clearly identified, especially with the aid of a 30° laparoscope. The exposure is obtained by retracting Hartmann's pouch superomedially and is facilitated by looking from below with a 30° scope.

Dissection should always start high on the gallbladder and hug the gallbladder closely until the anatomy is identified clearly. Using

Figure 12 Laparoscopic cholecystectomy. A view from below with a 30° laparoscope demonstrates the point for beginning dissection (arrow), where the gallbladder funnels down to its junction with the cystic duct.

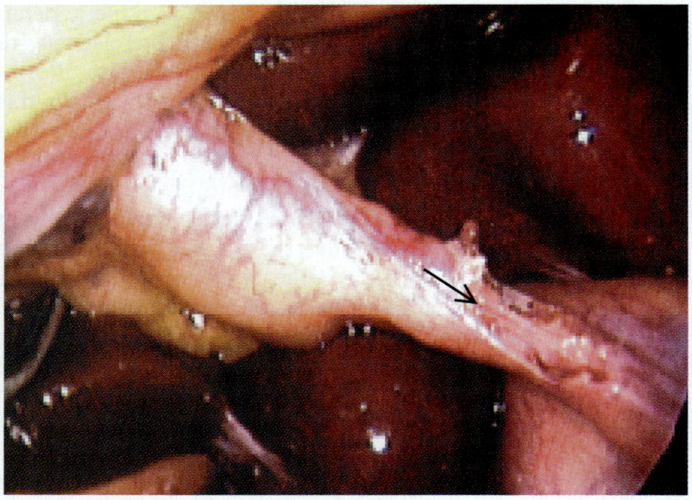

Figure 13 Laparoscopic cholecystectomy. The peritoneum is dissected from the gallbladder–cystic duct junction (arrow), as seen from below through a 30° angled laparoscope.

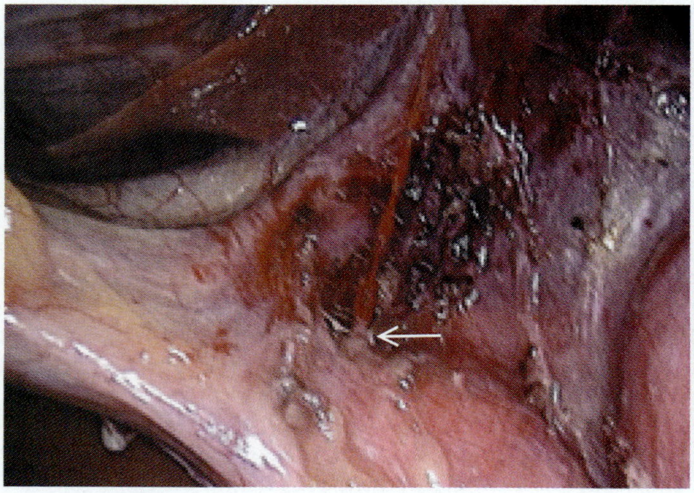

Figure 14 Laparoscopic cholecystectomy. Arterial bleeding can be seen (arrow) from a branch of the cystic artery injured during dissection from the posterior approach.

artery safely if bleeding occurs. Electrocauterization should be avoided near the cystic duct and all clips. Electrical current will be conducted through clips and may result in delayed sloughing of the duct or a clip. Delayed injuries to the CBD may be caused by a direct burn to the duct or by sparking from noninsulated instruments or clips during dissection.

Control of a Short or Wide Cystic Duct

Edema and acute inflammation may lead to thickening and foreshortening of the cystic duct, with subsequent difficulties in dissection and ligature. If the duct is edematous, clips may cut through it; if the duct is too wide, the clip may not occlude it completely. A modified clipping technique can be employed, with placement of an initial clip to occlude as much of the duct as possible. The portion of the duct that is occluded by this clip is then incised. A second clip is placed flush with the first one in such a way as to occlude the rest of the duct. Because this technique is not always possible, the surgeon should be familiar with techniques for

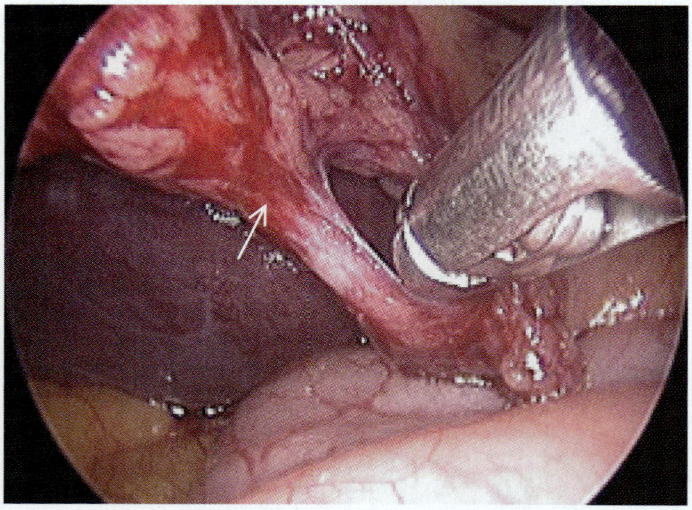

Figure 15 Laparoscopic cholecystectomy. The superior border of the cystic duct has been dissected. The funneling of the gallbladder into the cystic duct is clearly seen (arrow).

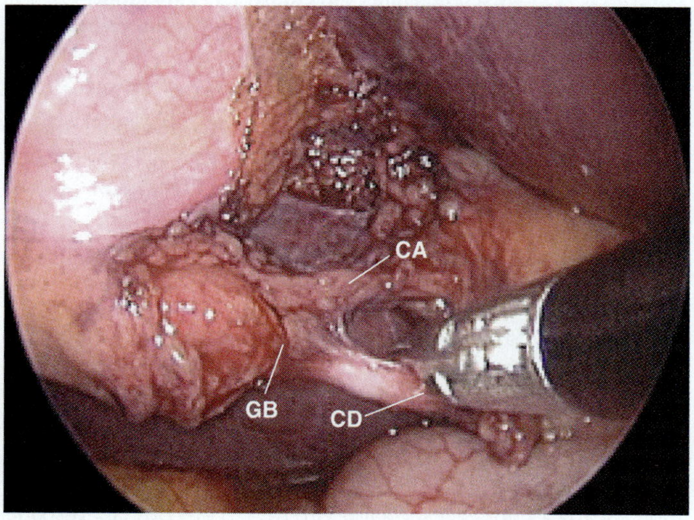

cauterized. Because dissection is done near the gallbladder, it is not unusual to encounter more than one branch of the cystic artery. Each of these branches should be dissected free of the fibroareolar tissue. Care should also be taken to ensure that the right hepatic artery is not inadvertently injured as a result of being mistaken for the cystic artery.

STEP 4: CONTROL AND DIVISION OF THE CYSTIC DUCT AND CYSTIC ARTERY

At this point, the cystic duct is clipped on the gallbladder side, and a cholangiogram is obtained if desired [*see* Step 5: Intraoperative Cholangiography, *below*]. If a cholangiogram is not desired, three or four clips should be placed on the cystic duct and the cystic duct divided between them. Two or three hemostatic clips are placed on the cystic artery, and it is divided. It is prudent to incise the artery partially before transecting it completely to ensure that the clips are secure and that there is no pulsatile bleeding. Once the artery is completely divided, the proximal end will retract medially and it will become more difficult to expose and control the

Figure 16 Laparoscopic cholecystectomy. Dissection of the triangle of Calot further exposes the cystic duct (CD) and the cystic artery (CA) near their entry into the gallbladder (GB) in preparation for clipping and division.

ligating the duct with either intracorporeal or extracorporeal ties. It is extremely helpful to know how to tie extracorporeal ties so that the cystic duct can be ligated in continuity before it is divided. In some cases, the duct can be divided, held with a forceps, and controlled with a ligating loop. If there is concern about secure closure of the cystic duct, a closed suction drain may be placed. If inflammation, as in cholecystitis, has caused the duct to be shorter than usual, dissection must be kept close to the gallbladder to avoid inadvertent injury to the CBD. A short cystic duct is often associated with acute cholecystitis. Patient blunt dissection with the suction-irrigation device may be the safest technique.

Stones in the Cystic Duct

Stones in the cystic duct may be visualized or felt during laparoscopic cholecystectomy. Every effort should be made to milk them into the gallbladder before applying clips. Placing a clip across a stone may push a fragment of the stone into the CBD and will increase the risk that the clip will become displaced, leading to a bile leak. If the stone cannot be milked into the gallbladder, a small incision can be made in the cystic duct (as is done for cholangiography), and the stone can usually be expressed and retrieved.

STEP 5: INTRAOPERATIVE CHOLANGIOGRAPHY

Whether intraoperative cholangiography should be performed routinely is still controversial. Advocates believe that this technique enhances understanding of the biliary anatomy, thus reducing the risk of injury to bile ducts. As yet, however, there are no objective data to confirm this impression. Cholangiography is not a substitute for meticulous dissection, and injuries to the CBD can occur before cystic duct dissection reaches the point at which cholangiography can be performed. Catheter-induced injuries and perforations of the biliary tree have been reported, and cholangiograms have been misinterpreted. On the other hand, one of the main advantages of cholangiography is that injuries can be recognized during the operation and promptly repaired. Another advantage of routine cholangiography is that it helps develop the skills required for more complex biliary tract procedures, such as transcystic common bile duct exploration.

The two methods of laparoscopic cholangiography differ in their technique for introducing the cholangiogram catheter into the cystic duct. In both approaches, a clip should be placed at the junction of the gallbladder and the cystic duct and a small incision made in the anterior wall of the cystic duct. In the first technique, a specially designed 5 mm cholangiogram clamp (the Olsen clamp) with a 5 French catheter is inserted via a subcostal trocar. For easy guidance of the catheter into the incision in the cystic duct, the catheter should be parallel, rather than perpendicular, to the cystic duct. This angle is facilitated by placing the subcostal port directly below the costal margin, near the anterior axillary line. A fifth trocar may occasionally be needed if exposure is lost when one of the grasping forceps is removed to allow passage of the cholangiogram clamp. The clamp and catheter are then brought to the cystic duct under direct vision, and the catheter is steered into the duct [*see Figure 17*]. The clamp is then closed, holding the catheter in position and sealing the duct to avoid extravasation of dye.

In the second method, the cholangiogram catheter is introduced percutaneously through a 12- to 14-gauge catheter, inserted subcostally as described above. The surgeon then grasps the cholangiogram catheter and directs it into the cystic duct. A hemostatic clip is applied to secure the catheter in place. If passage of the catheter into the cystic duct is prevented by Heister's valve, a guide wire can be passed initially.

If the cystic duct is tiny and it is anticipated that cannulation will be difficult or impossible, the gallbladder can be punctured,

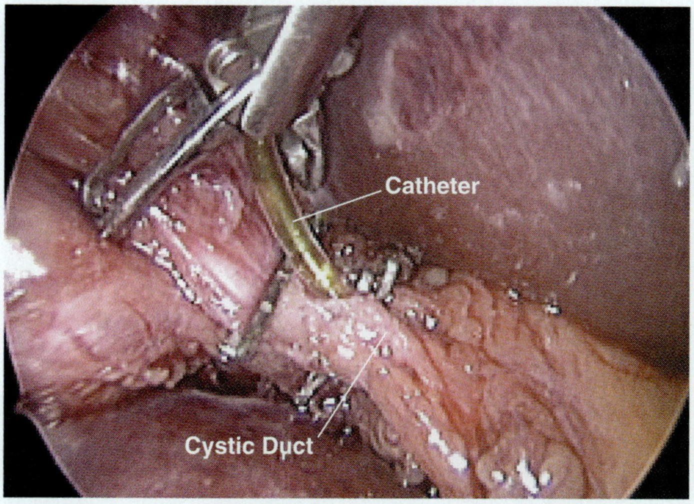

Figure 17 Laparoscopic cholecystectomy. The cystic duct has been clipped, a small incision has been made for placement of the cholangiogram catheter, and the catheter has been advanced through the specialized cholangiogram clamp into the cystic duct.

the bile aspirated, and the contrast material injected through the gallbladder until the biliary tree is filled.

The cannulas and operating instruments should be positioned so as not to obstruct the view of the biliary tree. If the cannulas cannot be positioned outside the x-ray window, radiolucent cannulas should be used, or the cannulas should be removed and replaced after the cholangiogram. A cholangiogram that does not visualize the biliary tree from the liver to the duodenum is inadequate.

Fluoroscopy with hard-copy film is the ideal way of obtaining cholangiograms [*see Figure 18*]. After the C-arm is positioned, with the surgeon protected behind a lead screen, full-strength (60%) contrast is slowly injected under fluoroscopic control. Complete visualization of the biliary tree, including the right and left hepatic ductal systems as well as the distal duct, is mandatory. Once the cholangiogram is obtained, the catheter is removed, and the cystic duct is double-clipped and transected.

Laparoscopic Ultrasonography

A new technology for intraoperative study of the biliary tree is laparoscopic ultrasonography. Recent studies have confirmed that it is as accurate as fluoroscopic cholangiography for intraoperative detection of stones in the CBD. Furthermore, laparoscopic ultrasonography is more rapid and less invasive than fluoroscopic cholangiography, does not require cystic duct cannulation, and does not use radiation. With a 7.5 MHz linear-array 10 mm transducer, ultrasound examination of the biliary tree is done via the epigastric port, placing the transducer directly on the porta hepatis structures. The number, size, and location of stones, as well as the diameter of the CBD, can be reliably determined.

STEP 6: DISSECTION OF THE GALLBLADDER FROM THE LIVER BED

The next step is to dissect the gallbladder from the liver bed. The gallbladder is grasped near the cystic duct insertion and pulled down toward the right anterosuperior iliac spine, placing the areolar tissue between the gallbladder and liver anteriorly on the stretch. The areolar tissue is cauterized with an L-shaped hook dissector, and the dissection is carried upward as far as possible for as long as there is sufficient exposure. When exposure begins to diminish, the cystic duct end of the gallbladder should be pulled up toward or

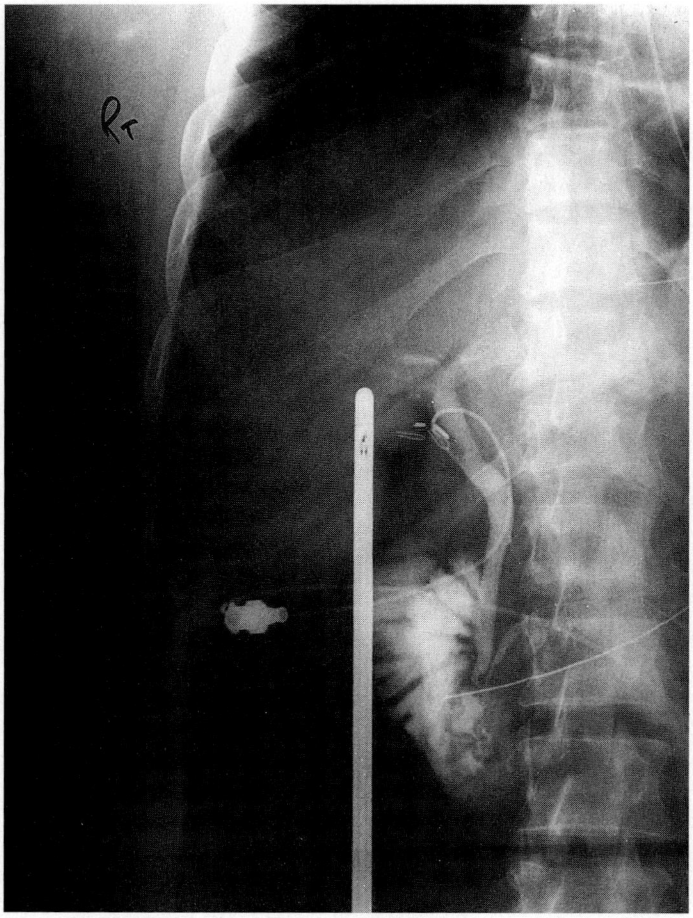

Figure 18 **Laparoscopic cholecystectomy. Shown is a normal intraoperative cholangiogram.**

over the left lobe of the liver to expose the posteroinferior attachments of the gallbladder. It is sometimes helpful to apply downward and lateral traction on the forceps grasping the fundus. Bleeding during this stage generally indicates that the surgeon has entered the wrong plane and dissection has entered the liver. Bleeding can usually be readily controlled with the electrocautery.

Dissection continues until the gallbladder is attached only by a small piece of peritoneum at the fundus. Before the last attachment to the gallbladder is completely divided, the vital clips should be reinspected to ensure that they have not slipped off, and the operative field should be checked for hemostasis. The final attachment to the gallbladder is then divided. The gallbladder should be placed over the right lobe of the liver and laterally so that it can be found again to be retrieved. The grasping forceps on the gallbladder should not be removed.

Perforation of the Gallbladder

The gallbladder may be accidentally breached at some point in the operation, with the result that bile and stones are spilled into the peritoneal cavity. Efforts should be made to suction the spilled bile, which accumulates in the suprahepatic space, the right subhepatic space, and the lower abdomen because of the patient's position. Each of these areas should be irrigated and the effluent aspirated until it is clear.

Stones should be located and removed whenever possible. An effective way of removing small stones is to irrigate the subhepatic space copiously. Cholesterol stones usually float on the irrigation fluid and can then be suctioned through a 10 mm suction probe or through a 32 French chest tube passed through the 10 mm operating port. Unfortunately, small stones may be lost in the omentum or between bowel loops. In such cases, it is probably appropriate to leave the stones within the peritoneum rather than perform a laparotomy to attempt to retrieve them. However, there have been reports of serious morbidity, including intra-abdominal abscess, fistula, empyema, and bowel obstruction, resulting from lost stones.

If the gallbladder is perforated and it seems likely that multiple stones will be spilled, the surgeon should introduce a sterile bag into the peritoneal cavity, placing it close to the perforation. Spilled stones can then be transferred immediately into the bag. After the gallbladder is removed from the liver bed, it too is placed in the bag, affording some protection to the wound when it is removed from the abdominal cavity.

STEP 7: EXTRACTION OF THE GALLBLADDER

The laparoscope is moved to the epigastric port, and a large-tooth grasping forceps is inserted through the umbilical port to grasp the gallbladder at the area of the cystic duct. Under direct vision, the gallbladder is then retrieved and pulled out as far as possible through the umbilical port. It is sometimes necessary to stretch the fascial opening with a Kelly clamp or to aspirate bile from the gallbladder. It is far preferable to enlarge the incision than to have stones or bile spill into the abdominal cavity from a ripped gallbladder. All of the other ports are then removed from the abdominal wall under direct vision to ensure that there is no bleeding. All residual CO_2 should be removed to prevent postoperative shoulder pain. The fascial opening at the umbilicus should be sutured closed to prevent subsequent herniation, and all skin incisions should be closed.

Need for Drainage

The decision to place a drain after laparoscopic cholecystectomy should be governed by the same principles applied to patients undergoing open cholecystectomy. There are two main indications for drainage: (1) the cystic duct was not closed securely, and (2) the CBD was explored by either a direct or a transcystic approach.

Placement of a drain is easily accomplished. A closed suction-type drain can be inserted intra-abdominally through the 10 mm operative port. A grasping forceps placed through the right lateral port is used to pull one end of the drain out through the abdominal wall. The other end of the drain is then positioned according to the surgeon's preference, usually in the subhepatic space.

Complications

INTRAOPERATIVE COMPLICATIONS

Veress Needle Injury

A syringe must always be attached to the Veress needle, and fluid must be aspirated before insufflation is initiated: failure to do so may lead to insufflation into a vessel and consequently to massive gas embolism. If the aspirate from the syringe attached to the Veress needle contains copious amounts of blood, immediate laparotomy is indicated. Major vascular injury may have occurred. Because the problem at this point is a needle injury, it can usually be repaired easily and without serious sequelae.

Puncture of the bowel by a Veress needle is usually signaled by aspiration of bowel contents through the needle. If this occurs, the needle should be withdrawn and the approximate course and direction of the puncture remembered. The initial trocar should then be inserted by means of the open technique, under direct vision, to ensure that the undersurface of the abdominal wall is free of adherent bowel. Once pneumoperitoneum is created, careful examination of the abdomen through the laparoscope is imperative. In most cases, either further leakage of bowel contents, staining of the serosal surface with bowel contents, or an ecchymosis on the serosal surface of the bowel helps the surgeon locate the site of the bowel injury. If ecchymosis is present without spillage of bowel contents, the bowel loop should be marked with a suture and reinspected at the end of the procedure. If ongoing leakage of bowel contents is noted, the injured loop of bowel can be grasped with an atraumatic forceps and gently withdrawn through an enlarged umbilical incision. The small hole can then be easily sutured, the bowel returned to the peritoneal cavity, and the laparoscopic cholecystectomy completed.

Improper placement of the Veress needle into the omentum, the retroperitoneum, or the preperitoneal space may also occur. In each of these cases, high inflation pressures, uneven distribution of the gas on percussion, or marked subcutaneous emphysema may be a helpful clue. If incorrect placement of the insufflation needle is not recognized, it will not be possible to create a safe intraperitoneal space; subsequent blind insertion of the trocar may then result in injury to an intraperitoneal structure.

Trocar Injury

Trocar injury to blood vessels or bowel is much more dangerous than Veress needle injury to the same structures. Major vascular injuries virtually never occur when trocars are placed under direct vision; however, they remain a potentially lethal—though rare—complication of percutaneous trocar insertion. If active bleeding follows removal of the trocar from the cannula, prompt laparotomy is mandatory; if bleeding passes unnoticed and insufflation begins, massive air embolism will result. At the time of laparotomy, both the anterior and the posterior wall of the vessel must be examined after proximal and distal control of the vessel have been obtained.

Bowel injuries can result from either percutaneous or open insertion of the initial trocar. With open insertion, the bowel injury should be immediately obvious and can be repaired after pulling the injured bowel through an enlarged umbilical incision. Laparoscopic cholecystectomy can then proceed. Bowel injuries caused by percutaneous insertion of the trocar may occur even in the absence of adhesions to the abdominal wall. They can be managed in the same way. The one caveat is that it is possible to spear the bowel in a through-and-through fashion so that when the laparoscope is inserted through the trocar, the view is normal and the injury is not recognized. This type of injury can be diagnosed only if the laparoscope is repositioned to the operative port at some time during the procedure, and the undersurface of the umbilical site is carefully examined. This step is mandatory during the course of the operation, preferably early.

Bleeding

Abdominal wall Bleeding from the abdominal wall can usually be prevented by careful placement of the trocars. The abdominal wall should be transilluminated before percutaneous trocar insertion and the larger vessels avoided. If a vessel is speared, the cannula usually tamponades the bleeding reasonably effectively during the procedure.

Once the procedure is completed, each trocar is removed under direct vision. If bleeding follows the removal of a trocar, the puncture hole is occluded with digital pressure to maintain pneumoperitoneum; a figure-eight stitch is then placed under direct vision. The stitch can be removed the next day, before the patient is discharged. Alternatively, the surgeon may place a Foley catheter through the trocar site with a stylet, inflate the balloon, and place traction on the catheter for 4 to 6 hours.

Omental or mesenteric adhesions Omental adhesions to the gallbladder can generally be bluntly teased from their attachments to the gallbladder, keeping the plane of dissection close to the gallbladder, where they are less vascular. Adhesions to the liver should be taken down with cautery to avoid capsular tears. Persistent bleeding from omental adhesions is unusual but can be managed with electrocauterization (taking care to avoid damage to the duodenum or colon) or the application of hemostatic clips or a pretied ligating loop.

Cystic artery branch Arterial bleeding encountered during dissection in Calot's triangle is usually due to loss of control of the cystic artery or one of its branches. Biliary surgeons must be aware of the many anatomic variations in the vasculature of the gallbladder and the liver. Because the main cystic artery frequently branches, it is common to find more than one artery if dissection is maintained close to the gallbladder. If what seems to be the main cystic artery is small, a posterior cystic artery may be present and may need to be clipped during the dissection.

Prevention of arterial bleeding begins with careful and complete dissection of the artery before clipping and by inspection of the clips to ensure that they are placed completely across the artery without incorporating additional tissue, such as a posterior cystic artery or right hepatic artery. When arterial bleeding is encountered, it is essential to maintain adequate exposure and to avoid blind application of hemostatic clips or cauterization. The laparoscope should be withdrawn slightly so that the lens is not spattered with blood. The surgeon should then pass an atraumatic grasping forceps through a port other than the operating port and attempt to grasp the bleeding vessel. It may be necessary to insert an additional trocar for simultaneous suction-irrigation. Once proximal control is obtained, the operative field should be suctioned and irrigated to improve exposure. Hemostatic clips are then applied under direct vision. Conversion to open cholecystectomy is indicated whenever bleeding cannot be promptly controlled laparoscopically.

Liver bed Bleeding from the liver bed may be encountered when the wrong plane is developed during dissection of the gallbladder. Patients who have portal hypertension or a coagulopathy are at particularly high risk for this complication. Control of bleeding requires good exposure, accomplished via lateral and superior retraction of the gallbladder; hence, all bleeding should be controlled before the gallbladder is detached from the liver bed. Most liver bed bleeding can be controlled with the electrocautery, and it should be controlled as it is encountered to allow exposure of the specific bleeding site. Either a hook-shaped or a spatula-shaped coagulation electrode is effective. Finally, if oozing continues, oxidized cellulose can be placed as a pack through the operative port and pressure applied on the raw surface of the liver.

POSTOPERATIVE COMPLICATIONS

If a patient (1) complains of a great deal of abdominal pain requiring administration of systemic narcotics, (2) has a high or prolonged fever, or (3) develops an ileus and is unable to eat for more than 24 hours, an intra-abdominal complication may have occurred. Blood should be drawn so that the white cell count, the hemoglobin concentration, liver function, and the serum amylase levels can be assessed. Abdominal ultrasonography may help diagnose dilated intrahepatic ducts and subhepatic fluid collections [see Figure 19].

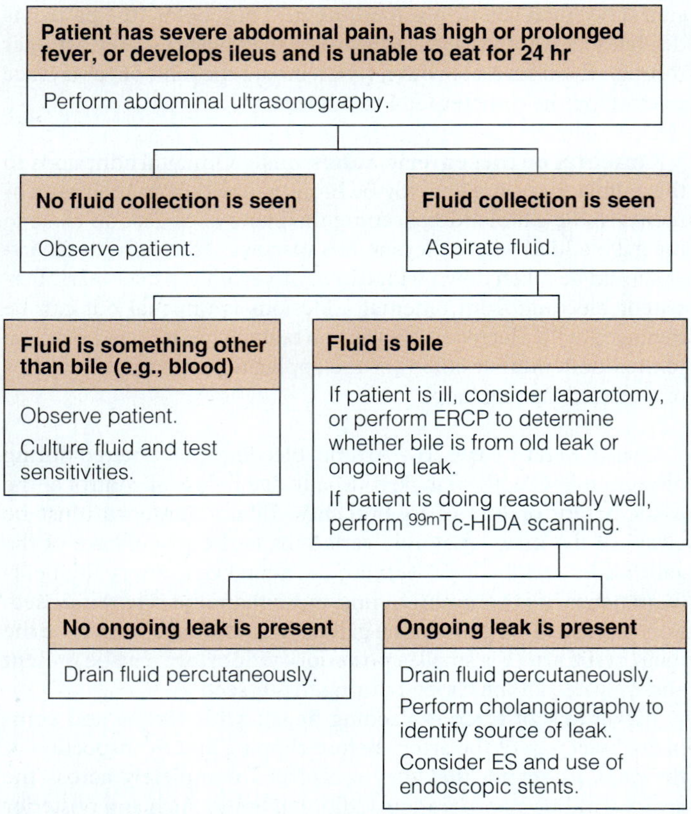

Fluid Collection or Bile Leak

When a fluid collection is seen, it should be aspirated percutaneously under ultrasound guidance. If the fluid is blood and the patient is hemodynamically stable and requires no transfusion, observation of the patient and culture of the fluid are usually sufficient. If the fluid is bile and the patient is ill, immediate laparotomy should be considered; alternatively, if the appropriate facilities are available, MRCP or ERCP may be performed to identify the site of bile leakage, determine whether obstruction is also present, and assess the integrity of the extrahepatic biliary tree. If the bile ducts are in continuity and the bile is coming from the cystic duct stump or a small lateral tear in the bile duct, endoscopic sphincterotomy, with or without stenting, usually controls the leak. Percutaneous placement of a drain under ultrasound guidance allows control of the bile leakage and measurement of the quantity of fluid present.

Fever

Postoperative fever is a common complication of laparoscopic cholecystectomy. As noted, it may be indicative of a postoperative complication such as a bile collection or bile leakage. Other common reasons for postoperative fever (e.g., atelectasis) should also be considered.

Abnormal Liver Function

When postoperative blood tests indicate significantly abnormal liver function, possible causes include injury to the biliary tree and retained CBD stones [see Figure 20]. Cholangiography is required, even if it was performed intraoperatively. If MRCP or ERCP yields normal results, observation is sufficient; the abnormalities may be attributable to a passed stone or drug-related cholestasis. If stones are present, ES can usually solve the problem. If ERCP demonstrates extravasation of bile, it is important to establish whether the common duct is in continuity. If the duct is interrupted, early reoperation, ideally at a specialized center, is the best option. If the duct is in continuity, endoscopic and radiologic techniques may successfully resolve the problem without substantial morbidity. Percutaneous drainage is instituted to control the fistula, and sphincterotomy or stenting is useful to overcome any resistance at the sphincter of Oddi. Any retained stones causing distal obstruction should also be removed.

Special Problems

CONVERSION TO LAPAROTOMY

Conversion from laparoscopy to laparotomy may be required in any case of laparoscopic cholecystectomy, in accordance with the judgment of the surgeon. Conversion is usually necessitated by an inability to identify important anatomic structures in the region of the gallbladder. Distorted anatomy may be the result of previous surgery, inflammation, or anatomic variants. Conversion may also be required because of an intraoperative complication, such as bleeding, injury to the bowel, or bile leakage. Clearly, the appropriate surgical judgment is to convert before a complication occurs.

Several authors have looked at ways to predict the probability of conversion on the basis of preoperative information. It is clearly useful to stratify patients on the basis of their likelihood of conversion. This information is useful in selecting patients for laparoscopic cholecystectomy in an outpatient versus hospital setting, in determining the resources required in the operating room, and in assisting patients in planning their work and family needs around the time of surgery.

Factors found to be predictive of an increased probability of conversion include the following: acute cholecystitis, either at the time

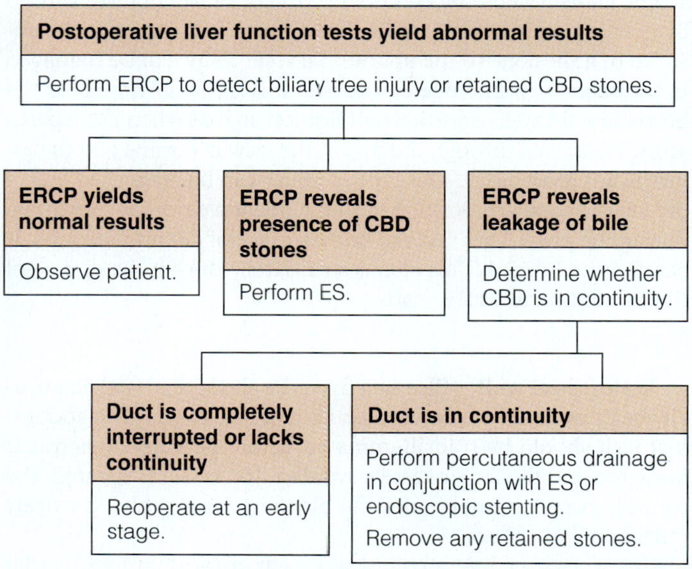

Figure 19 Laparoscopic cholecystectomy. Shown is an algorithm outlining a screening approach that is often useful when the patient shows signs (e.g., pain, fever, or ileus) that are suggestive of a postoperative intra-abdominal complication, such as fluid collection or bile leakage.

Figure 20 Laparoscopic cholecystectomy. Shown is an algorithm outlining an approach to abnormal liver function test results after laparoscopic cholecystectomy.

of surgery or at any point in the past; age greater than 65 years; male sex; and thickening of the gallbladder wall to more than 3 mm as measured by ultrasonography. Other factors more variably associated with an increased likelihood of conversion are obesity, previous upper abdominal surgery (especially gastroduodenal), multiple gallbladder attacks over a long period of time, and severe pancreatitis. Factors not associated with an increased likelihood of conversion are jaundice, previous endoscopic sphincterotomy, previous lower abdominal surgery, stomas, mild pancreatitis, and diabetes.

On the basis of our data, a 45-year-old woman with no history of acute cholecystitis and no thickening of the gallbladder wall has a probability of conversion lower than 1%; such a patient is a good candidate for laparoscopic cholecystectomy in an outpatient setting. Conversely, a 70-year-old man with acute cholecystitis and ultrasound evidence of gallbladder wall thickening would have a risk of conversion estimated at 30%; this patient would be better managed in a traditional hospital environment.

ACUTE CHOLECYSTITIS

The safety and efficacy of laparoscopic cholecystectomy for the treatment of acute cholecystitis have been demonstrated in several series. Acute cholecystitis presents several technical problems that must be addressed if laparoscopic cholecystectomy is to be performed safely. It should also be recognized that the probability of conversion to laparotomy is greatly increased in these circumstances. There appears to be no advantage to delaying surgery in these patients, even if the patient improves rapidly with nonoperative management. Many patients return within a short time with recurrent attacks, and delaying surgery does not reduce the probability of conversion.

Technical difficulties associated with cholecystectomy for acute cholecystitis include dense adhesions, the increased vascularity of tissues, difficulty in grasping the gallbladder, an impacted stone in the gallbladder neck or cystic duct, shortening and thickening of the cystic duct, and close approximation of the common duct to the gallbladder wall.

When performing laparoscopic cholecystectomy in patients with acute cholecystitis, the surgeon should not hesitate to insert additional ports, such as for a suction-irrigation apparatus. Because the tense, distended gallbladder is difficult to grasp reliably, it should be aspirated through the fundus early in the procedure, as described above. If the graspers fail to grasp the wall or cause it to tear, exposure of Calot's triangle can be achieved by propping up or levering the neck of the gallbladder and right liver with a blunt instrument. This maneuver is also useful when an impacted stone in the neck of the gallbladder precludes grasping of the gallbladder in the area of Hartmann's pouch. Dense adhesions that may be present between the gallbladder and the omentum, duodenum, or colon should be dissected bluntly, as with a suction tip. Because the tissues are friable and vascular, oozing may be encountered, but cautery should not be applied before the vital structures in Calot's triangle are identified. Instead, one should move to another area of dissection, allowing most of the oozing to coagulate on its own. Liberal use of suction and irrigation will keep the operative field free of blood.

When identifying anatomic structures, it is important to keep dissection close to the gallbladder wall, working down from the gallbladder toward Calot's triangle. Dissection of the lower part of the gallbladder from the liver bed early in the operation may aid in identification of the gallbladder neck–cystic duct junction (analogous to an open, retrograde dissection). The surgeon should be aware that edema and acute inflammation may cause foreshortening of the cystic duct. If the anatomy cannot be identified, preliminary cholangiography through the emptied gallbladder may indicate the position of the cystic duct and the CBD.

Often, the obstructing stone responsible for the acute attack is in the neck of the gallbladder; thus, the cystic duct will be normal and easily secured with clips. If the stone is in the cystic duct, it must be removed before the duct is clipped or ligated. A thickened, edematous cystic duct is better controlled by ligation, using an extracorporeal tie or a ligating loop, than by clipping. If closure of the cystic duct is tenuous, closed suction drainage is advisable. Obviously, conversion to open cholecystectomy is indicated if the anatomy remains obscure. Conversion should also be considered if no progress is made after a predesignated period of time—for example, 15 minutes—because at this point, it is unlikely that the surgeon will make any headway.

COMMON BILE DUCT STONES

Identification of Patients at Risk

About 10% of all patients undergoing cholecystectomy for gallstones will also have choledocholithiasis. To select from the various diagnostic and therapeutic options available for management of choledocholithiasis, it is helpful to know preoperatively whether the patient is at high, moderate, or low risk for stones. Patients with obvious clinical jaundice or cholangitis, a dilated CBD, or stones visualized in the CBD on preoperative ultrasonography are likely to have choledocholithiasis (risk > 50%). Patients who have a history of jaundice or pancreatitis, elevated preoperative levels of alkaline phosphatase or bilirubin, or ultrasound evidence of multiple small gallstones are somewhat less likely to have choledocholithiasis (risk, 10% to 50%). Patients with large gallstones, no history of jaundice or pancreatitis, and normal liver function are unlikely to have choledocholithiasis (risk < 5%).

Diagnostic and Therapeutic Options

One argument for routine intraoperative cholangiography is that it is a good way of identifying unsuspected CBD stones. However, more selective approaches to diagnosing choledocholithiasis make use of preoperative cholangiography, either via MRCP or, more invasively, ERCP [see 47 Gastrointestinal Endoscopy]. Preoperative identification of choledocholithiasis allows the surgeon to attempt preoperative clearance of the CBD by means of ES or intraoperative clearance during laparoscopy, depending on the expertise of the surgeon. Preoperative cholangiography is suggested when the patient's history and the results of laboratory and diagnostic tests suggest that there is a moderate or high risk of common duct stones. It is our practice that patients at high risk for CBD stones undergo ERCP and ES if warranted. For patients at moderate risk, an MRCP is done first, followed by therapeutic ERCP if the MRCP suggests common duct stones; intraoperative cholangiography can also be used to identify choledocholithiasis.

When stones are detected during the operation, the options include laparoscopic transcystic duct exploration, laparoscopic choledochotomy and CBD exploration, open common bile duct exploration, and postoperative ERCP/ES. If a single small (2 mm) stone is visualized, it can probably be flushed into the duodenum by flushing the CBD via the cholangiogram catheter and administering 1 to 2 mg of intravenous glucagon to relax the sphincter of Oddi. Even if a stone of this size does not pass intraoperatively, it will usually pass on its own postoperatively.

Laparoscopic Transcystic Exploration of the Bile Duct

Accessing the biliary tree The first step is to review the cholangiogram. The size of the cystic duct, the site of insertion of the cystic duct into the CBD, and the size and location of the CBD stones all contribute to the success or failure of transcystic exploration of the CBD. For example, transcystic exploration is extremely challenging in a patient who has a long, spiraling cystic duct with a medial insertion. The size of the stones to be removed dictates the approach to the CBD: stones smaller than 4 mm can usually be retrieved in fluoroscopically directed baskets and generally do not necessitate cystic duct dilatation; larger stones (4 to 8 mm) are retrieved under direct vision with the choledochoscope.

The first step is insertion of a hydrophilic guide wire through the cholangiogram catheter into the CBD, under fluoroscopic guidance. The cholangiogram catheter is then removed. If the largest stone is larger than the cystic duct, dilatation of the duct is necessary, not only for passage of the stone but also to allow passage of the choledochoscope, which may be 3 to 5 mm in diameter.

Dilation is accomplished with either a balloon-dilator or sequential plastic dilators. Because plastic dilators may cause the cystic duct to split, balloon dilation is recommended. A balloon 3 to 5 cm in length is passed over the guide wire and positioned with its distal end just inside the CBD and its proximal end just outside the incision in the cystic duct. The balloon is then inflated to the pressure recommended by the manufacturer and observed closely for evidence of shearing of the cystic duct. The cystic duct should not be dilated to more than 8 mm in diameter. Larger stones in the CBD can be fragmented with electrohydraulic or mechanical lithotripsy, if available, or they may be removed via choledochotomy.

Once dilation is completed, the guide wire may be removed or left in place to guide passage of a choledochoscope or baskets. When the choledochoscope is used, a second incision in the cystic duct, close to the CBD, will avoid Heister's valve and allow removal of the guide wire. If baskets are used, a 6 French plastic introducer sheath may be inserted through the trocar used for cholangiography into the cystic duct. This sheath is especially useful if multiple stones must be removed.

Fluoroscopic wire basket transcystic bile duct exploration Stones smaller than 2 to 4 mm that do not pass with irrigation through the cholangiocatheter after injection of intravenous glucagon can usually be retrieved using a 4 French or 5 French helical stone basket passed into the CBD over a guide wire, under fluoroscopic guidance. The baskets can be passed alongside the cholangiocatheter or inserted via a plastic sheath replacing the cholangiocatheter. The basket is opened in the ampulla of Vater, pulled back into the CBD, and rotated clockwise until the stone is entrapped. The stone and basket are then removed together. A Fogarty catheter should not be used, because the stones are likely to be pulled up into the hepatic ducts, where they are much more difficult to remove.

Endoscopic transcystic bile duct exploration When stones are 4 to 8 mm in diameter, the helical stone basket wires are generally too close together to permit retrieval. Hence, choledochoscopic basketing is utilized. A 7 to 10 French choledochoscope with a working channel is either passed over the guide wire or inserted directly into the cystic duct. Because the usual grasping forceps may damage the choledochoscope, forceps with rubber-covered jaws should be used. A separate camera should be inserted onto the choledochoscope, and the image it produces can be displayed on the monitor by means of an audiovisual mixer (picture within a picture) or displayed on a separate monitor.

Once the choledochoscope enters the cystic duct, warm saline irrigation is begun under low pressure to distend the common duct and provide a working space. The choledochoscope usually enters the CBD rather than the common hepatic duct. When a stone is seen, a 2.4 French straight four-wire basket is inserted through the operating port. The stones closest to the cystic duct are removed first, by advancing the closed basket beyond each stone, opening the basket, and pulling the basket back, trapping the stone. The basket is then closed and pulled up against the choledochoscope so that they can be withdrawn as a unit. Multiple passes may be required until the duct is clear. A completion cholangiogram is done to ensure that the duct is clear and to rule out proximal stones. The dilated, traumatized cystic duct is ligated with a ligating loop rather than a hemostatic clip. If drainage is required, a red rubber catheter can be inserted into the CBD via the cystic duct.

Because of the angle created by the cephalad and superior retraction of the gallbladder, it may be difficult to pass the choledochoscope into the proximal ducts. If a common hepatic duct stone is seen on the cholangiogram, the patient is placed in steep reverse Trendelenburg's position. In this position, any nonimpacted stones may fall into the distal duct for retrieval. If stones remain entrapped, the surgeon may attempt to pass the choledochoscope proximally, but a long or spiral cystic duct renders this almost impossible. If the anatomy is more conducive, a fifth port can be introduced between the umbilicus and right costal margin; it may be possible to retract the cystic duct inferiorly, allowing the endoscope to pass proximally.

Laparoscopic Common Bile Duct Exploration

Stones larger than 1 cm in diameter, as well as most stones in the common hepatic ducts, will not be retrievable with the techniques described above. Ductal clearance can be achieved via choledochotomy if the duct is dilated and the surgeon has exceptional laparoscopic skills, including experience with intracorporeal knot tying. The anterior wall of the CBD is bluntly dissected for a distance of 1 to 2 cm. When small vessels are encountered, it may be preferable to apply pressure and wait for hemostasis rather than attempt to apply cautery in this area. Two stay sutures are placed in the common duct. An additional 5 mm trocar is placed in the right lower quadrant for insertion of an additional needle driver. The 4-0 sutures are lubricated with mineral oil to avoid sawing of the tissue. A small choledochotomy (a few millimeters longer than the circumference of the largest stone) is made using curved microscissors while the stay sutures are elevated. A flexible or rigid choledochoscope is then inserted and warm saline irrigation instituted. Additionally, baskets or Fogarty catheters can be used to withdraw the calculi. Subsequently, a 12 or 14 French latex T-tube is fashioned with short limbs, placed entirely intraperitoneally to avoid escape of CO_2, and positioned in the CBD. The choledochotomy is then closed with interrupted stitches of 4-0 braided absorbable sutures. The first suture is placed right next to the T-tube, securing it distally, and the second at the most proximal end of the choledochotomy; lifting these sutures helps in placement of additional sutures. Intracorporeal knots are preferred to avoid sawing of the delicate tissues. The end of the T-tube is then pulled out through a trocar, and cholangiography is performed after completion of the procedure.

53 PANCREATIC PROCEDURES

John L. Cameron, M.D.

Pylorus-Preserving Pancreaticoduodenectomy (Whipple Procedure)

The peritoneal cavity is entered through an upper midline incision, and the abdomen is thoroughly explored. The head of the pancreas (containing a walnut-sized mass) and the duodenum are extensively mobilized out of the retroperitoneum via the Kocher maneuver. (This extensive kocherization allows one to palpate the superior mesenteric artery to confirm that the tumor has not extended from the uncinate process to involve the vessel. It is distinctly unusual for the tumor to extend directly posteriorly into the aorta or the inferior vena cava.) If there is no evidence of local or regional spread to serosal surfaces or the liver, the gallbladder is mobilized out of the liver bed. The common hepatic duct is identified by palpating for the previously placed percutaneous transhepatic catheter and is then divided [*see Figure 1*]. A complete rim of the duct is sent for frozen section examination. The percutaneously placed catheter is extracted from the distal biliary segment and retracted cephalad.

Once the common hepatic duct has been divided, the anterior surface of the portal vein is easily and quickly identified. If one finds the appropriate plane directly on the anterior surface of the portal vein, one can easily pass the index finger of the left hand on top of it posterior to the first portion of the duodenum and the neck of the pancreas; usually, there are no veins joining the anterior surface of the portal vein, and the maneuver can be carried out with no resistance. (If this maneuver is difficult, the gastroduodenal artery should be identified where it comes off the common hepatic artery, cleaned, triply clamped, divided, and triply ligated with 2-0 silk. When this is done, part of the tunnel through which the index finger is slipped is unroofed, and separation of the portal vein from the posterior aspect of the first portion of the duodenum and the neck of the pancreas typically is much easier.)

The third portion of the duodenum is then further kocherized until the superior mesenteric vein is identified [*see Figure 2*]. The superior mesenteric vein is cleaned along its anterior

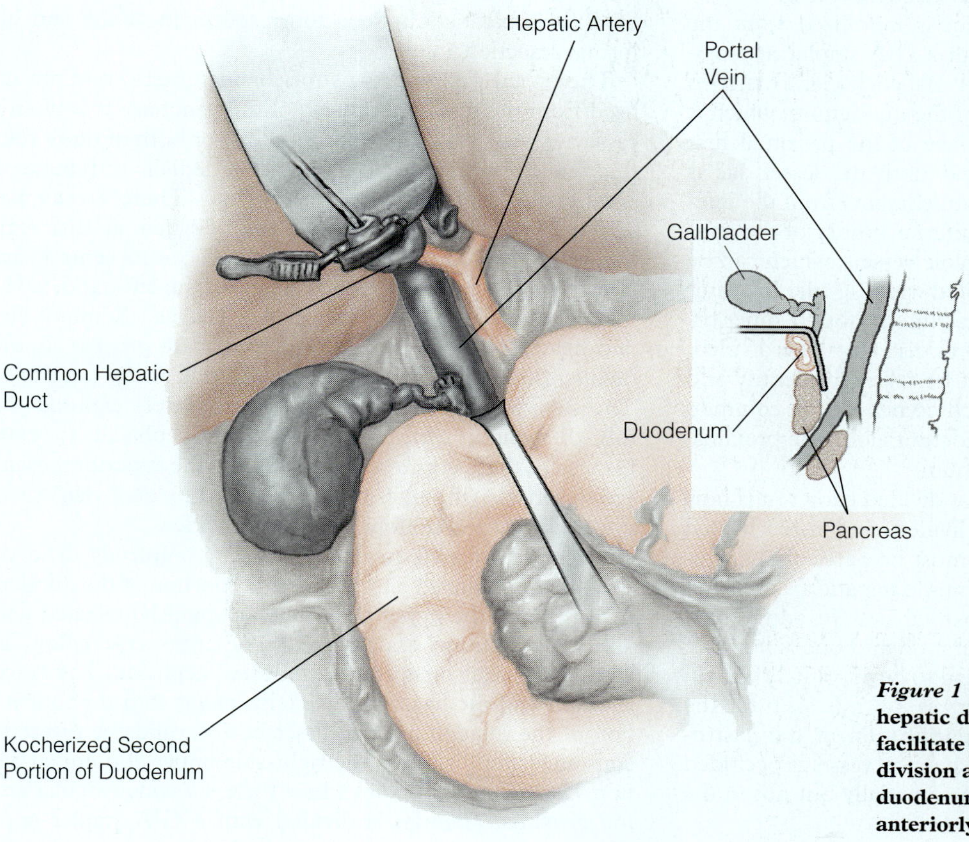

Figure 1 Whipple procedure. The common hepatic duct is divided at an early stage to facilitate identification of the portal vein. This division also untethers the first portion of the duodenum and allows it to be retracted anteriorly.[2]

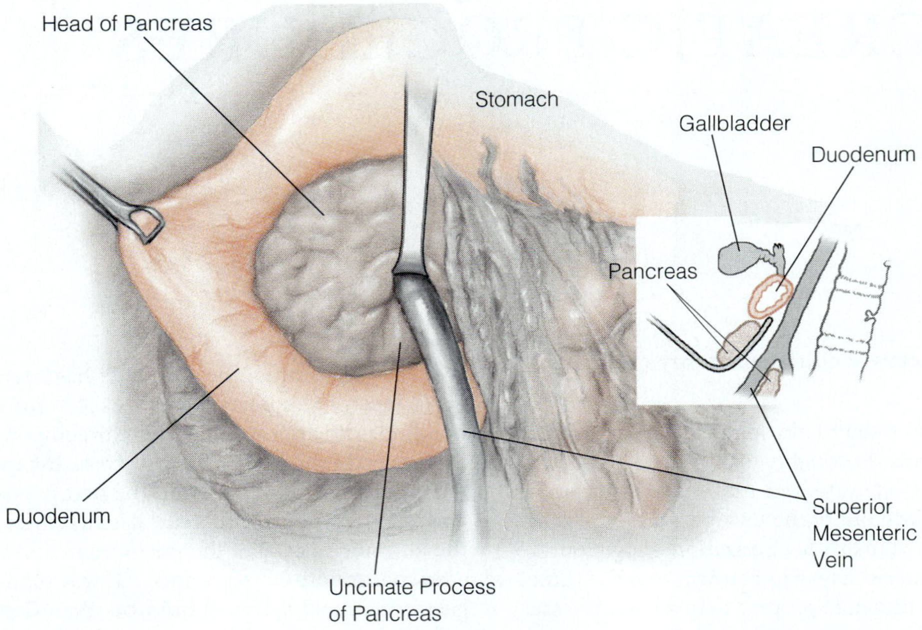

Figure 2 Whipple procedure. Kocherization of the duodenum is continued along the third portion until the superior mesenteric vein is reached. This vein can then be easily cleaned up to its connection with the portal vein.[2]

surface under the neck of the pancreas up to its connection with the portal vein. (Identification of the superior mesenteric vein is far easier by this anterior approach than by the traditional route through the lesser sac and is associated with virtually no blood loss.) At this point one can be virtually certain about the resectability of the lesion; if it is resectable, further steps are taken that commit one to a pancreaticoduodenectomy.

The first portion of the duodenum is mobilized from the neck of the pancreas and divided with a GIA stapler approximately 2 cm distal to the pylorus. A Babcock clamp is then placed on the proximal first portion of the duodenum, which is reflected medially. The posterior surface of the proximal first portion of the duodenum is dissected until the lesser sac is entered. At this point, the soft tissue attachments from the inferior border of the duodenum to the inferior border of the pancreas are divided; the right gastroepiploic vessels, which can be sizable, are clamped, divided, and ligated with 2-0 silk. In a similar fashion, the soft tissue areolar attachments found superiorly are divided with the electrocautery or else clamped, divided, and ligated with 3-0 silk. (Care must be taken to identify and preserve the right gastric artery, which comes off the common hepatic artery and actually joins the foregut along the proximal part of the first portion of the duodenum.)

If the gastroduodenal artery was not divided earlier, it is now identified, cleaned, triply clamped, divided, and triply ligated with 2-0 silk. (During this step, one must be particularly careful to ensure that the lumen of the common hepatic artery is not encroached upon by one of the proximal ties. In addition, if angiography was not done before operation and one is not sure that the anatomy is classic, it is essential to be absolutely certain that an anomalous right hepatic artery is not mistaken for the gastroduodenal artery. Definitive identification of the gastroduodenal artery is relatively simple: when the vessel is occluded with a vessel loop, the pulse disappears caudally but not in the cephalad direction.)

The neck of the pancreas is divided with the electrocautery. A rush of pancreatic juice is the signal that the enlarged pancreatic duct has been divided. A 1 mm thick complete cross section of the pancreas is taken at this time and sent for frozen section examination. (Margins should be sent for frozen section as they become available so that one is not delayed in proceeding with the reconstruction while the pathologist takes the margin off the pancreaticoduodenectomy specimen at the end of the formal resection.)

The portal vein and the superior mesenteric vein are mobilized from the uncinate process of the pancreas. It is often necessary to wrap vessel loops around one or both of these veins so that one can retract them far enough medially to remove them completely from the uncinate process. (There are amazingly few veins that must be ligated and divided in this region.) Dissection should proceed until the superior mesenteric artery, clearly palpable with the index finger of the left hand, is visualized. The uncinate process is divided between Reinhoff clamps and ligated with 2-0 silk ties. The uncinate process should be divided flush with the superior mesenteric artery [*see Figure 3*]. The superior mesenteric artery is completely exposed during this dissection, which proceeds from cephalad to caudad. Generally, there is one large vein joining the superior mesenteric vein inferiorly (the inferior pancreaticoduodenal vein) that one must dissect free, doubly ligate, and divide.

After the uncinate process has been completely divided, the specimen is attached only by the third portion of the duodenum. At this point, the upper abdomen is copiously irrigated with an antibiotic solution and packed. The transverse colon, along with the greater omentum, is reflected cephalad. The proximal jejunum and the ligament of Treitz, along with the fourth portion of the duodenum, are dissected free, and the dissection is continued until it meets the right-side upper abdominal dissection. At a convenient point where there is a wide vascular arcade, the proximal jejunum is divided with a GIA stapler approxi-

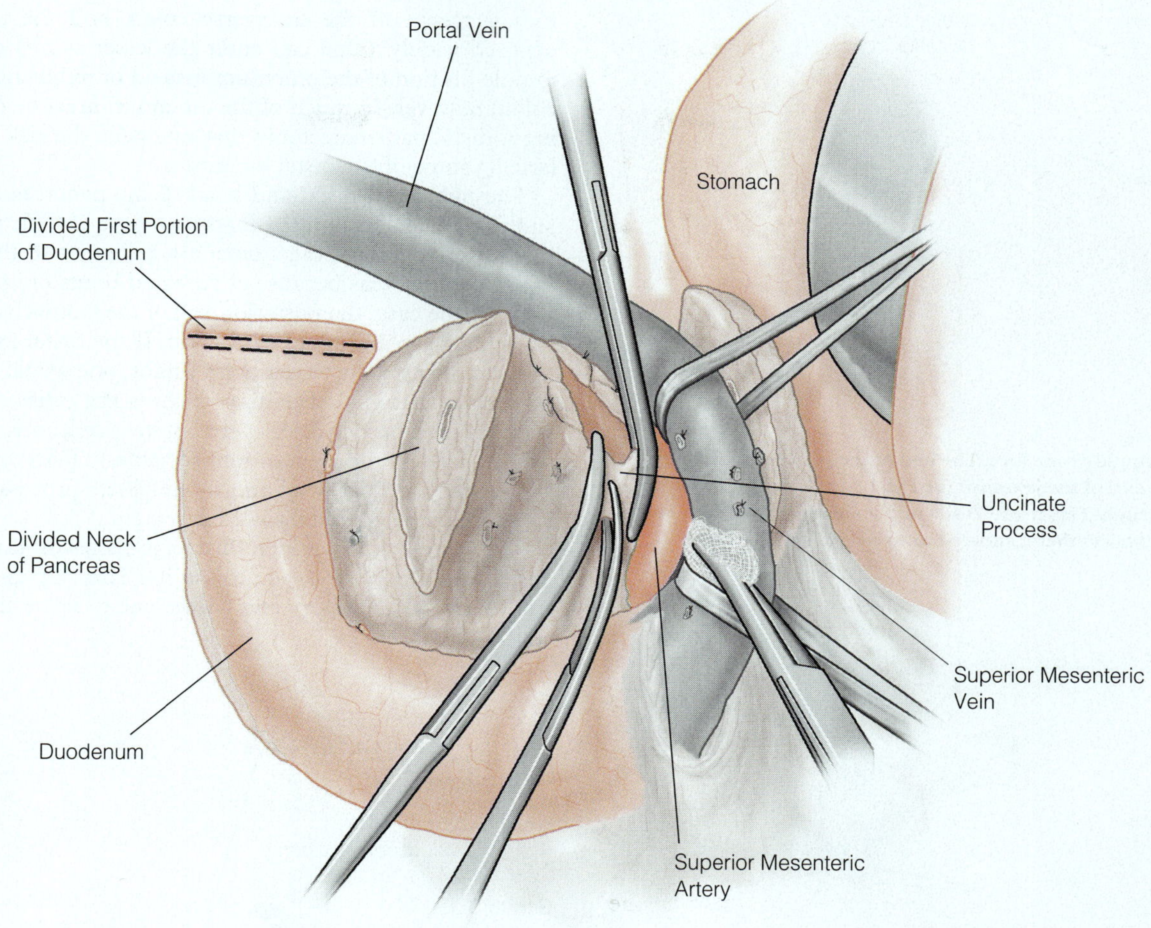

Figure 3 Whipple procedure. The uncinate process is divided flush with the superior mesenteric artery.[3]

mately 4 to 5 in. from the ligament of Treitz. The proximal jejunum is then grasped with a Babcock clamp and retracted cephalad. The mesentery to the proximal jejunum is divided between Reinhoff clamps and ligated with 2-0 silk. When the mesentery is completely divided, the specimen is free and can be removed from the operative field.

The proximal jejunum is then brought up through a rent in the transverse mesocolon. An end-to-end pancreaticojejunostomy is performed in which the end of the pancreas is invaginated into the end of the jejunum for approximately 1 to 1.5 in. This anastomosis is performed with an outer interrupted layer of 3-0 silk and an inner continuous layer of 3-0 absorbable synthetic suture material [*see Figure 4*]. (The inner layer incorporates the dilated pancreatic duct with several throws, both posteriorly and anteriorly.)

Approximately 3 in. distal to the pancreaticojejunostomy, an end-to-side hepaticojejunostomy (common hepatic duct to jejunum) is performed with a single interrupted layer of 4-0 absorbable synthetic suture material [*see Figure 5*]. Once the posterior layer has been placed and secured, an enterotomy is performed with the electrocautery. The anastomosis is decompressed with the previously placed biliary catheter. (Preoperative placement of a transhepatic biliary catheter percutaneously to provide decompression of the biliary tree permits one to be more flexible in planning the pancreaticoduodenectomy. In par-

ticular, it allows more time for preoperative preparation of patients who have been in a septic state or nutritionally depleted. Moreover, it obviates T tube placement at the time of operation. Furthermore, if the patient has recently undergone surgical exploration for obstructive jaundice at another institution—as approximately 40 percent of the patients at my institution have—the presence of a previously inserted biliary catheter allows one to proceed with the identification and division of the common hepatic duct without delay.)

Approximately 6 in. distal to the biliary-enteric anastomosis, an end-to-side duodenojejunostomy is performed with an inner continuous layer of 3-0 absorbable synthetic suture material and an outer interrupted layer of 3-0 silk [*see Figure 6*].

The abdomen is copiously irrigated with an antibiotic solution. The jejunal loop is tacked to the rent in the transverse mesocolon with interrupted 4-0 silk sutures. The defect in the retroperitoneum previously occupied by the third portion of the duodenum is closed with a continuous 4-0 silk suture. A closed suction Silastic drain is placed posterior to the hepaticojejunostomy and brought out through a stab wound in the right upper quadrant. The pancreaticojejunostomy is drained with two closed suction Silastic drains, one placed posteriorly and one placed anteriorly directly upon the anastomosis; the two drains are brought out through separate stab wounds in the left upper quadrant. The abdomen is closed with multiple interrupted No. 1

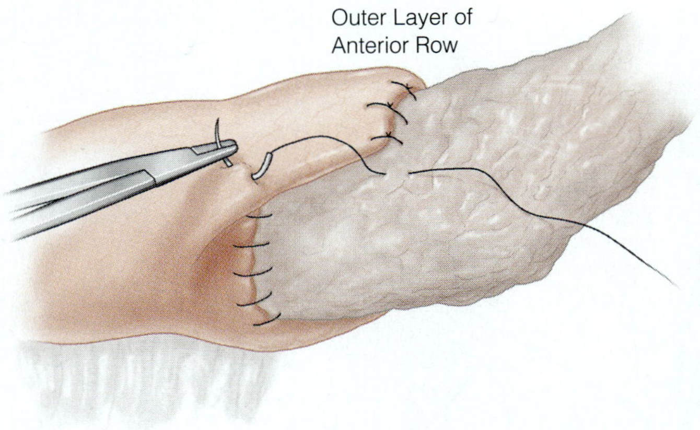

Figure 4 Whipple procedure. The end of the pancreas is invaginated into the end of the jejunum for 1 to 1.5 in. This is done with an outer interrupted layer of 3-0 silk and an inner continuous layer of 3-0 absorbable synthetic suture material.[3]

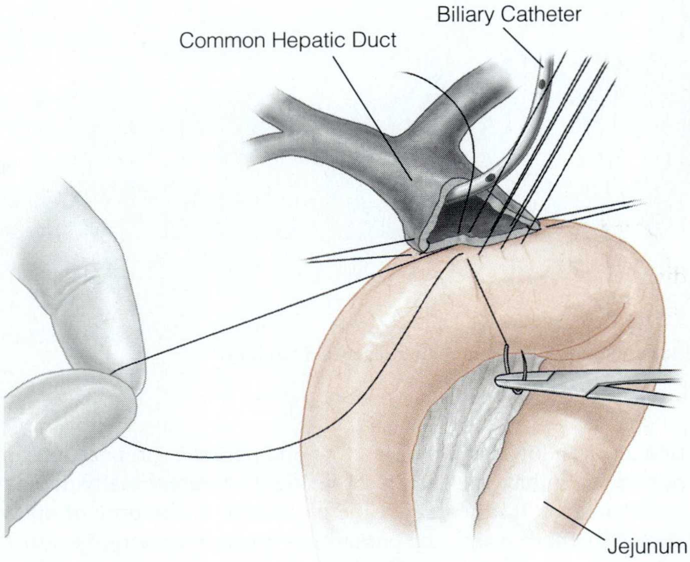

Figure 5 Whipple procedure. The common hepatic duct is anastomosed to the jejunum in an end-to-side fashion with a single layer of 4-0 interrupted absorbable synthetic sutures.[3]

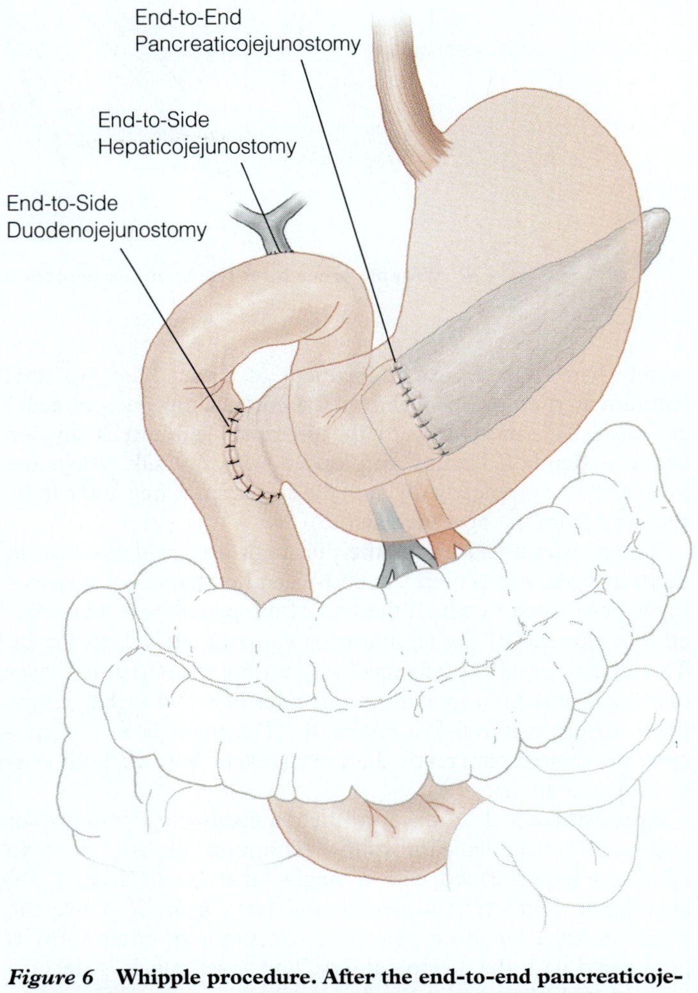

Figure 6 Whipple procedure. After the end-to-end pancreaticojejunostomy and the end-to-side hepaticojejunostomy, the duodenum is anastomosed to the jejunum in an end-to-side fashion with an inner continuous layer of 3-0 absorbable suture material and an outer interrupted layer of 3-0 silk.[3]

tum is taken off the transverse colon, and the lesser sac is exposed widely. (One can enter the lesser sac by dividing the middle portion of the omentum instead of removing it from the colon; however, so much of the omentum must be divided during a distal pancreatectomy that one runs the risk of devascularizing some of the distal omentum.)

The tail, body, neck, and head of the pancreas are exposed and examined. (In some patients who have chronic pancreatitis, the posterior wall of the stomach is adherent to the body and tail of the pancreas because of repeated bouts of inflammation. If this is the case, the posterior wall of the stomach is mobilized via both sharp and blunt dissection. If the distal pancreatectomy were being done to remove a tumor, one would also have to be certain that vital structures such as the celiac axis and the superior mesenteric vessels were not involved; such involvement would render the lesion unresectable.) The duodenum is kocherized, and the head and the uncinate process of the pancreas are palpated and visualized.

The splenic artery is identified as it comes off the celiac axis, and a vessel loop is placed around it. (This step gives one control of the splenic artery and allows one to ligate it early in the

monofilament sutures placed through and through all muscle and fascial layers. The subcutaneous tissues are irrigated with an antibiotic solution and closed with a continuous 3-0 absorbable synthetic suture. The subcuticular layer is closed with a continuous 4-0 absorbable synthetic suture. Steri-Strips are applied.

At the termination of the procedure, the biliary catheter is connected to bile bag drainage for three or four days and then internalized with a stopcock. It is removed at the patient's first follow-up clinic visit, approximately one month after operation.

Distal Pancreatectomy for Chronic Pancreatitis

The peritoneal cavity is entered through an upper midline incision, and the abdomen is thoroughly explored. The omen-

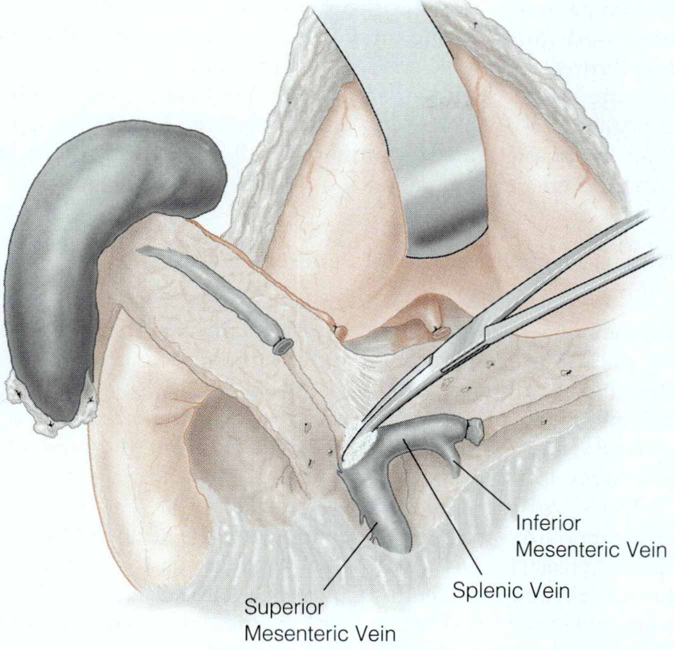

Figure 7 Distal pancreatectomy. The splenic vein is divided just distal to its junction with the inferior mesenteric vein and then dissected away from the posterior surface of the pancreas from this point up to where it joins the superior mesenteric vein to form the portal vein.[3]

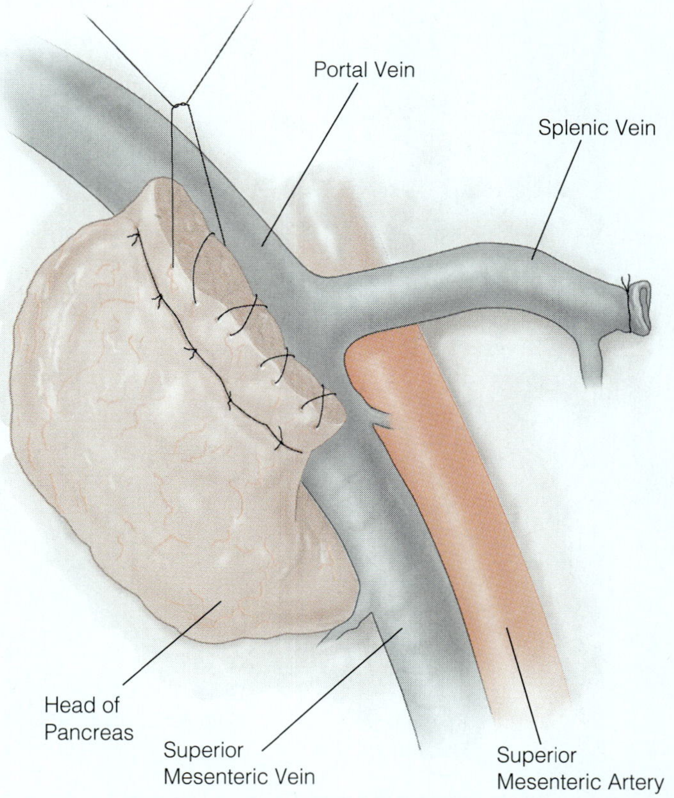

Figure 8 Distal pancreatectomy. A row of overlapping horizontal mattress sutures is placed in the neck of the pancreas just proximal to where it is to be divided, the neck is divided with the electrocautery, and a row of figure-eight sutures of 3-0 absorbable synthetic suture material is placed over the end of the pancreas.[3]

procedure if bleeding should occur. Occasionally, patients with chronic pancreatitis have a thrombosed splenic vein and left-side portal hypertension. If this is the case, there are usually multiple collateral vessels leading from the spleen to the stomach via the vasa brevia and involving the omentum. In such circumstances, it is usually preferable to triply ligate and divide the splenic artery early in the procedure.)

The spleen is mobilized out of the retroperitoneum. (This task is made easier if a splenic pack has been placed beneath the left flank of the patient to elevate the left retroperitoneum before preparation and draping. The spleen is retracted toward the midline with the left hand; it should be compressed medially toward the spine rather than retracted anteriorly. As one opens up the retroperitoneum with the electrocautery, the assistant, standing to the left of the patient, grasps the retroperitoneal serosa. Once the serosa has been entered, the retroperitoneum usually consists of loose areolar tissue that is easily mobilized. One must be careful not to dissect too deep and injure the kidney or its vessels.)

The tail of the pancreas is mobilized out of the retroperitoneum via both sharp and blunt dissection. The omental attachments anterior to the hilum of the spleen are divided between Kelly clamps and ligated with 2-0 silk. (The line of division is easily determined if the omentum has previously been completely taken off the transverse colon. As the division extends up toward and then along the greater curvature of the stomach, the vasa brevia are encountered and are doubly clamped, divided, and ligated.) The splenic flexure of the colon is carefully dissected away from the inferior pole of the spleen, and the peritoneal attachments that make up the lienocolic ligament are divided.

The tail and body of the pancreas are further mobilized out of the retroperitoneum by retracting the spleen and the tail of the pancreas medially. (In the course of this mobilization, one must be careful not to injure the left adrenal gland, which often occupies a fairly superficial position in the retroperitoneum, anterior and medial to the superior pole of the left kidney.) The splenic vein is easily identified in the middle portion of the posterior aspect of the pancreas. The inferior mesenteric vein, which joins the splenic vein at the middle of the body of the pancreas, is identified in the retroperitoneum just lateral to the ligament of Treitz. (Although the inferior mesenteric vein can be divided and ligated with impunity, one should try to preserve it.)

Further mobilization of the pancreas to the midline exposes the point where the splenic artery comes off the celiac axis. (Whereas the splenic vein invariably resides in a groove in the middle portion of the posterior surface of the gland, the splenic artery usually runs along the superior aspect of the gland and is easily identified by palpation where it arises from the celiac axis.) The splenic artery is triply clamped, divided, and triply ligated with 2-0 silk near its point of origin. (If the artery is particularly large, it may be suture ligated also.)

The junction of the inferior mesenteric vein and the splenic vein is identified, and the splenic vein is mobilized just distal to this junction. (Because the splenic vein resides in a groove or trough on the posterior aspect of the pancreas, one must be careful when mobilizing the splenic vein out of the pancreatic parenchyma. There are many small venous branches that can be injured if the mobilization is not done fastidiously enough.) The splenic vein is triply clamped, divided, and triply ligated with 3-0 silk just distal to its junction with the inferior mesenteric vein. The splenic vein is then mobilized from the posterior surface of the pancreas from this point onward to its junction with the superior mesenteric vein and the portal vein [see Figure 7].

The portal vein and the superior mesenteric vein are carefully dissected away from the undersurface of the neck of the pancreas. (At the neck, the pancreas is often very thinned out and narrow before expanding into the substantially thicker head and uncinate process.) A row of overlapping horizontal mattress sutures of 3-0 absorbable synthetic material is placed in the neck of the pancreas just proximal to the point where it is to be divided. (Using large needles that have been straightened makes this task simple even if the head-neck junction through which the needles are passed is thickened.) The neck of the pancreas is then divided with the electrocautery. A row of figure-eight sutures of 3-0 absorbable synthetic suture material is placed over the end of the pancreas [see Figure 8]. If the pancreatic duct can be identified, it should be separately oversewn with a figure-eight or mattress suture (again, of 3-0 absorbable synthetic suture material).

The abdomen is copiously irrigated with an antibiotic solution. The pancreatic remnant is drained with a closed suction Silastic drain brought out through a stab wound in the left upper quadrant. There is no need to drain the splenic bed. The abdominal wall is closed with a single layer of interrupted No. 1 nonabsorbable synthetic monofilament sutures placed through and through all muscle and fascial layers. The subcutaneous tissues are irrigated with an antibiotic solution and closed with a continuous 3-0 absorbable synthetic suture. The subcuticular layer is closed with a continuous 4-0 absorbable synthetic suture. Steri-Strips are applied.

Ninety-Five Percent Distal Pancreatectomy

In a 95 percent distal pancreatectomy for chronic pancreatitis, the initial part of the procedure is identical to the initial part of the distal pancreatectomy for chronic pancreatitis just described (see above), up to the point where the spleen and the tail and body of the pancreas have been mobilized and the splenic artery and the splenic vein divided. From this point, one continues as follows.

The superior mesenteric vein and the portal vein are extensively mobilized from the undersurface of the neck and head of the pancreas [see Figure 9a]. Vessel loops are passed around the portal vein and the superior mesenteric vein, and the vessels are retracted to the left. The two veins are then dissected away from the uncinate process of the pancreas, which passes posterior to

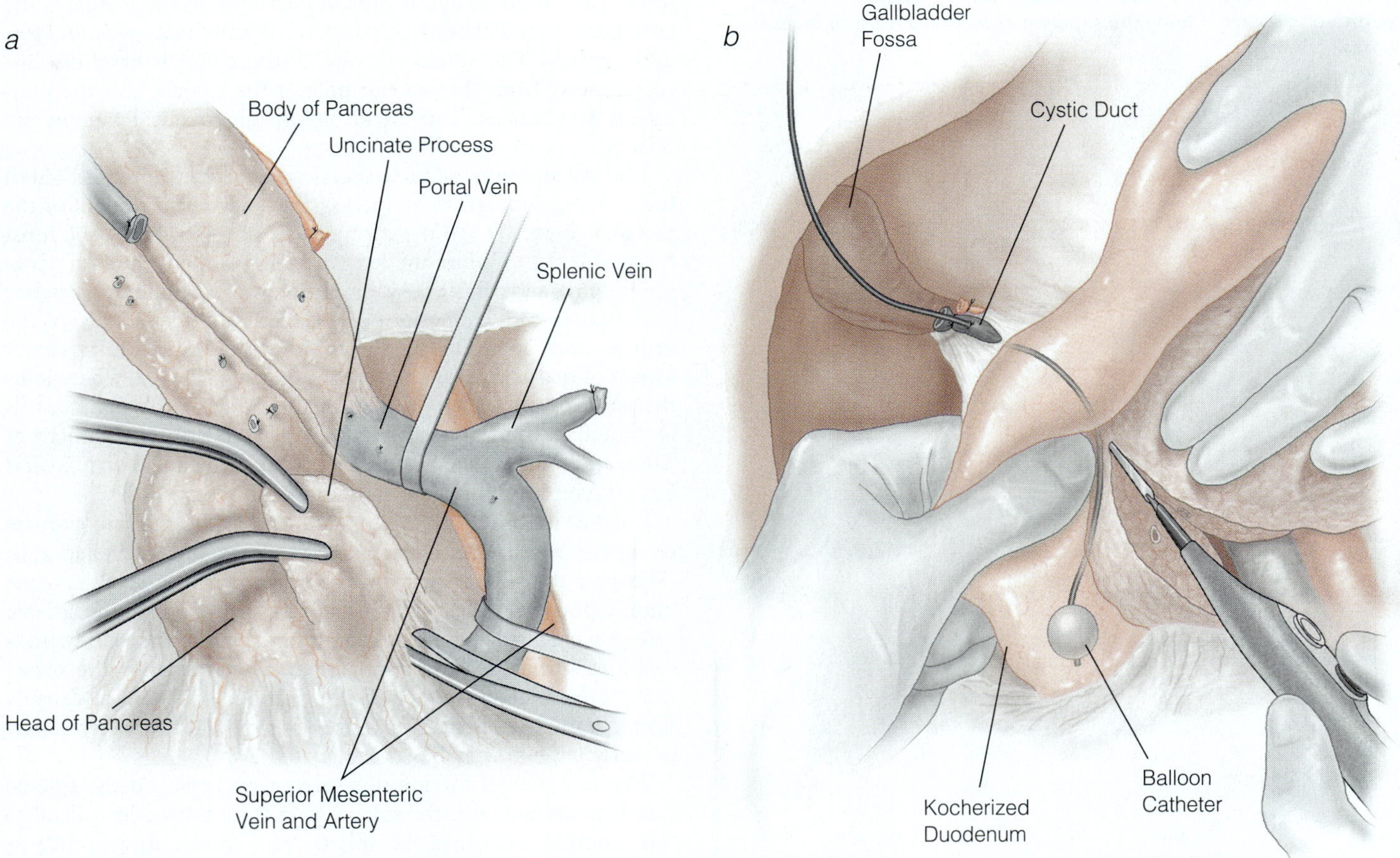

Figure 9 Ninety-five percent distal pancreatectomy. (*a*) The superior mesenteric vein and the portal vein are dissected away from the undersurface of the neck and head of the pancreas. Next (not shown), the two vessels are encircled with vessel loops, retracted to the left, and dissected away from the uncinate process. (*b*) The gallbladder is mobilized, a balloon catheter is passed through the cystic duct and into the duodenum, and the balloon is inflated to keep the catheter in place. The course of the common duct can be identified by palpating the catheter. This step helps prevent injury to the common duct when the pancreas is divided.[3]

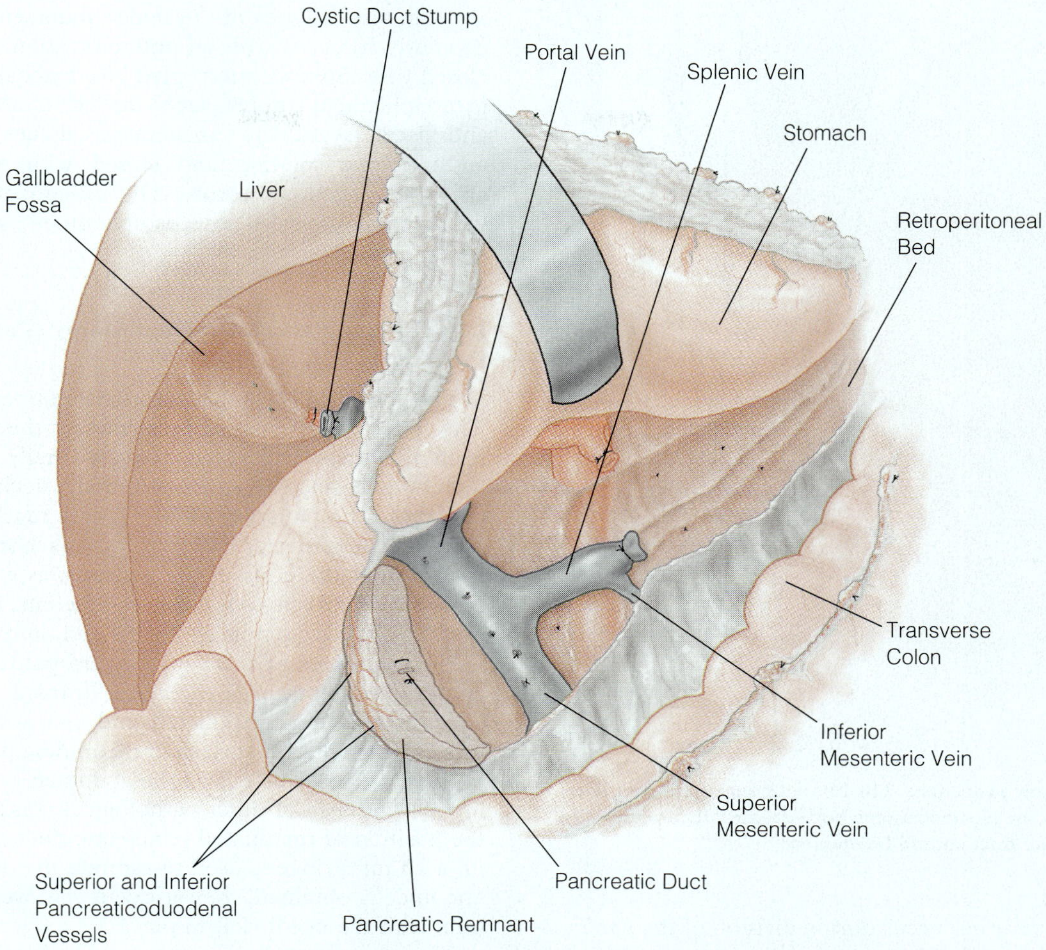

Figure 10 Ninety-five percent distal pancreatectomy. The pancreas is divided in the C loop of the duodenum, a small remnant of pancreatic tissue is left, and the specimen is removed from the operative field.[3]

the superior mesenteric vein. The gallbladder is mobilized, and a biliary Fogarty catheter is passed through an opening in the cystic duct, down through the common duct and the ampulla of Vater, and into the duodenum. The balloon is inflated to keep the catheter in place [see Figure 9b]. (Placement of the catheter makes it easier to palpate the course of the common duct through the posterior aspect of the head of the pancreas, thereby helping to prevent injury to this structure when the head of the pancreas is divided. If the gallbladder has already been removed in a previous operation, a transhepatic biliary catheter should be placed percutaneously before operation.)

The anterior superior pancreaticoduodenal artery and the anterior inferior pancreaticoduodenal artery are identified in the duodenal pancreatic groove. (In performing a 95 percent pancreatectomy, it is essential to preserve these vessels so as to prevent ischemia to the duodenum.) The portal vein and the superior mesenteric vein are further mobilized from the uncinate process and retracted medially until the superior mesenteric artery can be palpated. (It is best to identify the superior mesenteric artery where it comes off the aorta. This is easily accomplished if the duodenum and the head of the pancreas have been extensively mobilized well to the left of the aorta.)

The uncinate process is divided by cleaning the superior mesenteric artery and dividing the areolar attachments between the tip of the uncinate process and the artery. (This is most easily done from the left side of the operating table by the surgeon, who can keep the left hand both anterior and posterior to the uncinate process while cleaning the superior mesenteric artery with a clamp in the right hand.) The uncinate process, which terminates flush with the superior mesenteric artery, is then completely cleaned and separated from the artery along its entire length. Because there are many small vessels that pass from the artery into the uncinate process, all tissues should be clamped with Reinhoff clamps and ligated with 2-0 silk.

The pancreas is then divided in the C loop of the duodenum and removed from the operative field [see Figure 10]. (This step varies in difficulty depending on the extent to which the head of the pancreas is involved by the chronic inflammatory process. If the head is extremely thick and the Fogarty catheter in the bile duct is difficult to palpate, a larger, wider segment of pancreas must be left in the duodenal C loop; if the head is smaller and less diseased, most of the pancreatic tissue can be excised, preferably with the electrocautery. Often, the safest approach is to leave perhaps a 2 cm rim of pancreas in the C loop initially and then to remove the specimen from the operative field. This 2 cm rim can then be gradually reduced by shaving off a series of 1 to 2 mm segments—with the caution that the course of the common bile duct must be carefully identified to prevent injury.

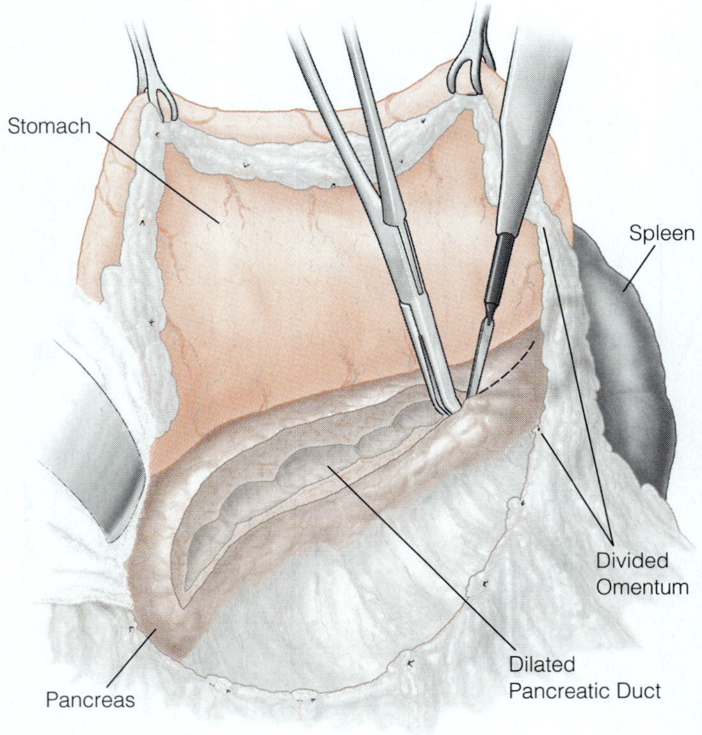

Figure 11 Puestow procedure. The dilated pancreatic duct is filleted open with the electrocautery both proximally and distally. At least 6 cm of the duct should be opened.[3]

If a bile duct injury does occur during division of the pancreatic head, a T tube should be inserted in the common bile duct and a cholangiogram performed. If the injury is small and tangential, it may be reparable with simple sutures; if it is substantial, a hepaticojejunostomy may be necessary. An intermediate repair would be to anastomose a Roux-en-Y jejunal loop around the area of injury in the duodenal C loop.)

The biliary Fogarty catheter is removed from the cystic duct, which is then clamped. The cystic duct is ligated with 3-0 silk. The pancreatic duct is oversewn with 3-0 absorbable synthetic suture material.

The rim of pancreas in the duodenal C loop is drained with closed suction Silastic drains, which are brought out through separate stab wounds in the upper abdomen. The abdomen is copiously irrigated with an antibiotic solution. The wound is closed with multiple interrupted No. 1 nonabsorbable synthetic monofilament sutures placed through and through all muscle and fascial layers. The subcutaneous tissues are irrigated with an antibiotic solution and closed with a continuous 3-0 absorbable synthetic suture. The subcuticular layer is closed with a continuous 4-0 absorbable synthetic suture. Steri-Strips are applied.

Longitudinal Pancreaticojejunostomy (Puestow Procedure)

The abdomen is entered through an upper midline incision. The lesser sac is entered by removing the greater omentum from the transverse colon along virtually its entire length, thereby exposing the entire tail, body, neck, and head of the pancreas. The pancreas often appears markedly fibrotic and scarred. The posterior wall of the stomach may be adherent to a portion of the body of the pancreas as a result of multiple episodes of inflammation; if it is adherent, it is easily dissected free. The duodenum is kocherized, and the head and the uncinate process of the pancreas are palpated from both an anterior and a posterior direction. In many cases, the pancreatic duct is markedly dilated and can actually be palpated through the anterior surface in the middle portion of the body of the pancreas. The rest of the abdomen is explored to check for the presence of other pathological conditions. To confirm the position of the dilated pancreatic duct, a 20-gauge needle on a 10 ml syringe is used to aspirate the duct. Once pancreatic juice is obtained, the syringe is removed from the needle hub, with the needle left in place.

The pancreatic duct is entered by dividing the pancreatic parenchyma with the electrocautery on either side of the needle. A large right-angle clamp is then inserted, and the duct is filleted open with the electrocautery both proximally and distally [*see Figure 11*]. Small pancreatic ductal concretions are carefully removed. (Experience has demonstrated that at least 6 cm of the duct must be opened to yield a good chance of long-term success. Ideally, if the duct is dilated all the way out to the tail, it can be filleted open virtually to the tip of the pancreas. In the proximal direction, the duct can easily be opened as far as the neck of the pancreas. Beyond this point, however, the duct passes posteriorly and inferiorly into the head of the pancreas;

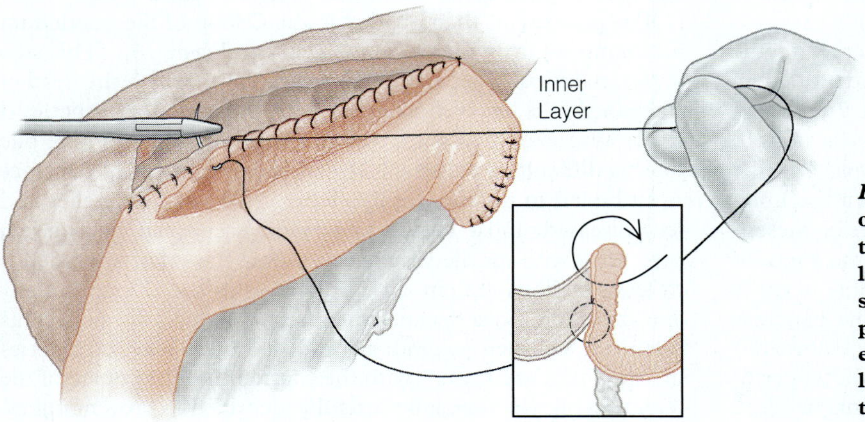

Figure 12 Puestow procedure. When the diameter of the dilated pancreatic duct is 1 cm or wider, a side-to-side pancreaticojejunostomy should be done in two layers. Once an outer layer of interrupted 3-0 silk sutures is placed between the jejunal loop and the pancreatotomy, an enterotomy is made along the entire length of the jejunal suture line, and an inner layer consisting of a continuous 3-0 absorbable synthetic suture is placed.[3]

because the head can be very thick, opening up the duct any further can be difficult.)

A Bakes dilator is passed proximally through the open pancreatic duct, down through the pancreatic duct in the unopened head, through the ampulla of Vater, and into the duodenum. (If a Bakes dilator cannot be passed into the duodenum, the duodenum should be opened and a sphincteroplasty performed, so that by working both from within the duodenum and from within the open pancreatic duct, the patency of the entire pancreatic duct can be ensured.)

A Roux-en-Y jejunal loop approximately 60 cm long is constructed. The most proximal loop of jejunum in which there is a good vascular arcade is selected. A 2 cm segment of this loop is cleaned and divided with a GIA stapler. The small bowel mesentery is divided between clamps down through the arcade vessel and is ligated with 3-0 silk. The end of the distal jejunum is oversewn with a layer of 3-0 silk Lembert sutures. A 60 cm length is then measured. Alimentary tract continuity is reestablished by means of an end-to-side jejunojejunostomy, in which the most proximal portion of the divided jejunum is anastomosed to the side of the Roux-en-Y jejunal loop 60 cm distally with an inner continuous layer of 3-0 absorbable synthetic suture material and an outer interrupted layer of 3-0 silk. The defect in the small bowel mesentery is closed with a continuous 4-0 silk suture.

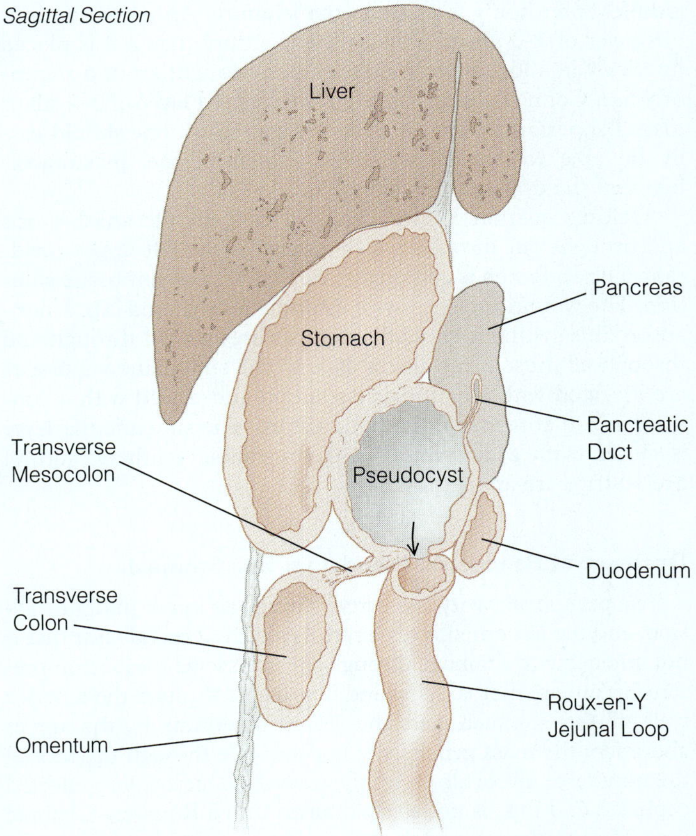

Figure 13 Drainage of pancreatic pseudocyst into Roux-en-Y jejunal loop. The transverse mesocolon is usually the most inferior and dependent part of a pancreatic pseudocyst; thus, drainage through the transverse mesocolon into a Roux loop is usually the ideal approach.[3]

The Roux-en-Y jejunal loop is brought up into the lesser sac in a retrocolic position through a small rent in the transverse mesocolon. A side-to-side pancreaticojejunostomy is performed in two layers. Before the Roux loop is opened, an outer interrupted layer of 3-0 silk is placed between the jejunal loop and the pancreatotomy, passing through the capsule of the pancreas and out through the opened pancreatic parenchyma along the inferior border of the pancreas. When this layer is complete, an enterotomy approximately 2 mm from the jejunal suture line is made along the entire length of this line. Starting at the distal pancreatic tail, an inner continuous layer of 3-0 absorbable synthetic suture material is placed in an over-and-over locking fashion through the entire wall of the jejunum and the entire divided surface of the pancreas and into the duct [*see Figure 12*]. The inner layer of the superior suture line is placed in an over-and-over fashion without locking, again with a continuous 3-0 absorbable synthetic suture. The outer layer of the superior suture line consists of interrupted 3-0 silk sutures placed in a Lembert fashion. (When the pancreatic duct is dilated to a diameter of 1 cm or greater, a two-layer anastomosis is possible and is in fact preferred. However, when the diameter of the duct is between 5 mm and 1 cm, a two-layer anastomosis is generally difficult, and a one-layer anastomosis is preferred. A single layer of interrupted 3-0 silk sutures is placed so that the knots are tied on the outside. This is easily accomplished with the superior suture line. With the inferior suture line, which is placed first, the suture passes from outside inward on the pancreas and then from inside outward on the jejunum. In a single-layer side-to-side pancreaticojejunostomy, the jejunotomy must be performed before any sutures are placed.) The Roux-en-Y jejunal loop is then tacked to the rent in the transverse mesocolon with interrupted 4-0 silk sutures.

The longitudinal pancreaticojejunostomy anastomosis is drained with closed suction Silastic drains that are placed on either side of the anastomosis and brought out through separate stab wounds in the left upper quadrant. The abdomen is copiously irrigated with an antibiotic solution. The midline incision is closed with a single interrupted layer of No. 1 nonabsorbable synthetic monofilament sutures passed through and through all muscle and fascial layers. The subcutaneous tissues are irrigated with an antibiotic solution and closed with a continuous 3-0 absorbable synthetic suture. The subcuticular layer is closed with a continuous 4-0 absorbable synthetic suture. Steri-Strips are applied.

Drainage of Pancreatic Pseudocyst into a Roux-en-Y Jejunal Loop

The peritoneal cavity is entered through a midline incision, and the abdomen is explored. Typically, a substantial mass that is cystic and easily ballotable is palpable posterior to the stomach. The duodenum and the head of the pancreas are kocherized so that the head may be palpated both anteriorly and posteriorly. The physical characteristics of chronic pancreatitis are usually present. The body and the tail of the pancreas are palpated as well; the pancreas is usually fibrotic, firm, and somewhat enlarged. The rest of the abdomen is explored to check for the presence of other pathological conditions. (At this point, the size and configuration of the cyst are compared with the size and configuration on the preoperative CT scan. If the CT scan shows a unilocular solitary cyst and if, at the time of

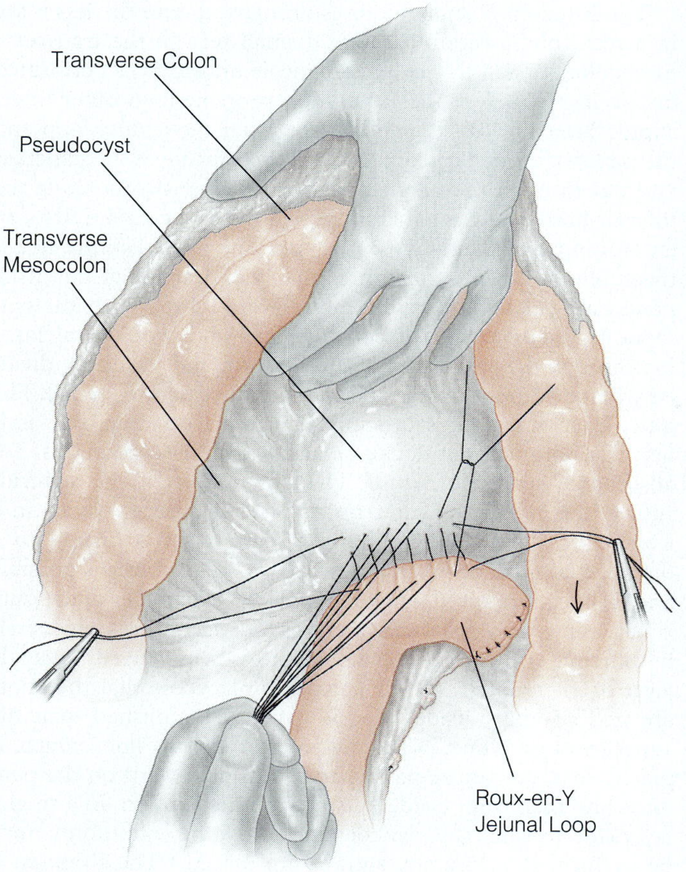

Figure 14 Drainage of pancreatic pseudocyst into Roux-en-Y jejunal loop. The outer posterior layer of the side-to-side cystojejunostomy comprises a series of 3-0 silk sutures placed through and through the jejunal loop and the transverse mesocolon.[3]

laparotomy, there appears to be a mass that coincides exactly with what is seen on the CT scan, there is no need to enter the lesser sac. The lesion can be drained into a Roux-en-Y jejunal loop through the transverse mesocolon, and the lesser sac need not be explored. Most pseudocysts are formed by anterior disruptions of the main pancreatic duct. When pancreatic sections leak out into the lesser sac, the body walls off the leak through its inflammatory response. The transverse mesocolon becomes adherent to the posterior wall of the stomach, which in turn becomes adherent to other adjacent structures in and around the retroperitoneum, and the leak is sealed off. Thus, the transverse mesocolon is usually the inferior and most dependent portion of the pseudocyst, and this site is the ideal location for drainage [see Figure 13].)

The transverse colon is retracted cephalad, and the cyst is easily visualized and palpated through the transverse mesocolon. The location of the cyst is confirmed by aspirating pancreatic juice through the transverse mesocolon with a 10 ml syringe and a 20-gauge needle. (One must be careful to identify and avoid the middle colic vessels.) A 60 cm long Roux-en-Y jejunal loop is constructed. The proximal jejunum is divided with a GIA stapler at the first convenient arcade. The small bowel mesentery is divided down through the arcade. The distal end of the jejunum is inverted with an interrupted layer of 3-0 silk Lembert sutures.

Alimentary tract continuity is reestablished by means of an end-to-side jejunojejunostomy, in which the proximal jejunum is anastomosed to the side of the Roux-en-Y jejunal loop 60 cm from the inverted end. This anastomosis is performed with an inner continuous layer of 3-0 absorbable synthetic suture material and an outer interrupted layer of 3-0 silk. The rent in the small bowel mesentery is closed with a continuous 4-0 silk suture.

A side-to-side cystojejunostomy is performed with an outer interrupted layer of 3-0 silk and an inner continuous layer of 3-0 absorbable synthetic suture material. The posterior outer layer of the anastomosis consists of a series of 3-0 silk sutures passed through and through the jejunal loop and through and through the transverse mesocolon (which is the inferior wall of the pseudocyst) [see Figure 14]. The suture line should be approximately 1 to 2 in. long. After the posterior layer has been secured, a cystotomy is performed with the electrocautery. An ellipse of cyst wall is removed and sent for frozen section examination. (No matter how convinced one is that one is dealing with a pseudocyst, a specimen from the cyst wall should always be sent for frozen section examination. Cystic neoplasms can masquerade as pancreatic pseudocysts; a substantial proportion of patients with cystic neoplasms initially undergo exploration and drainage procedures under the assumption that the lesion is inflammatory instead of neoplastic. If no epithelial lining is found on frozen section examination, one can assume that a pancreatic pseudocyst is present and proceed accordingly.) A parallel enterotomy is made in the jejunum. An inner continuous layer of 3-0 absorbable synthetic suture material is placed inferiorly in a locking fashion and then brought around superiorly in a Connell stitch. An outer interrupted layer of 3-0 silk is placed superiorly. With the cyst decompressed, one should easily be able to palpate a sizable lumen in the anastomosis between the cyst and the jejunal loop.

A closed suction Silastic drain is left near the anastomosis and brought out through a stab wound in the left upper quadrant. The abdomen is copiously irrigated with an antibiotic solution. The wound is closed with multiple interrupted No. 1 nonabsorbable synthetic monofilament sutures placed through and through all muscle and fascial layers. The subcutaneous tissues are irrigated with an antibiotic solution and closed with a continuous 3-0 absorbable synthetic suture. The subcuticular layer is closed with a continuous 4-0 absorbable synthetic suture. Steri-Strips are applied.

Drainage of Pancreatic Pseudocyst into Stomach

The peritoneal cavity is entered through an upper midline incision, and the abdomen is explored. Typically, a pseudocyst that is not amenable to drainage through the transverse mesocolon presents as a mass that is cystic and is palpable through the anterior wall of the stomach and the lesser omentum in the upper abdomen; the mass generally is not palpable through the root of the transverse mesocolon with the transverse mesocolon reflected cephalad and thus is not easily drained into a Roux-en-Y jejunal loop. The duodenum and the head of the pancreas are kocherized and the head of the pancreas is palpated. Signs of chronic pancreatitis are invariably present. The body and tail of the pancreas are palpated through the transverse mesocolon and show changes characteristic of chronic inflammation. The rest of the abdomen is explored to check for the presence of other pathological condi-

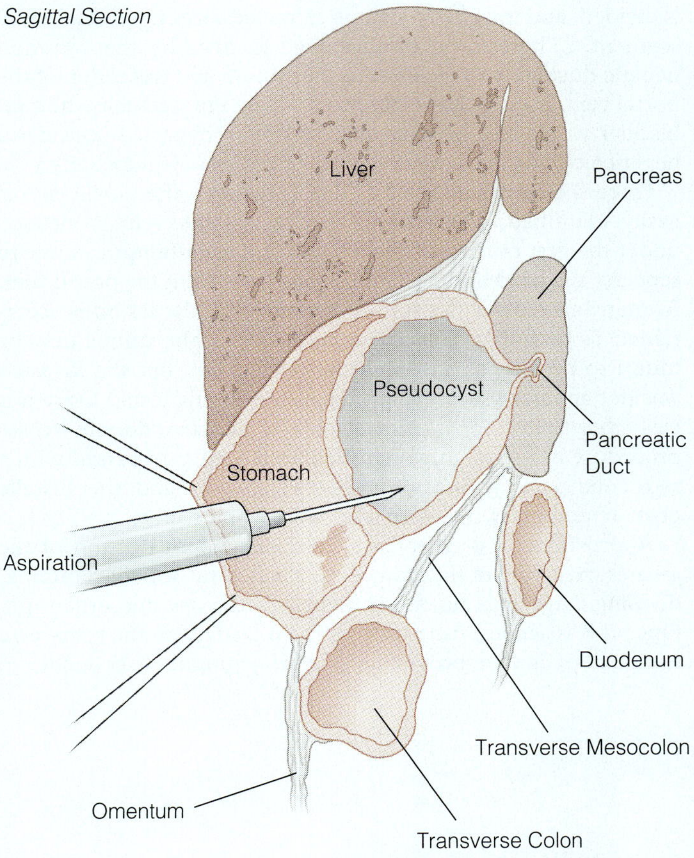

Figure 15 **Drainage of pancreatic pseudocyst into stomach. The location of the pseudocyst is confirmed by aspirating pancreatic juice through the back wall of the stomach.**[3]

tions. (A cyst that is situated high in the abdomen and presents more through the lesser omentum is not accessible to dependent drainage with a Roux-en-Y loop through the transverse mesocolon. Because bringing a Roux-en-Y loop anterior to the stomach to drain the cyst through the lesser omentum is unsatisfactory, such cysts are best drained into the stomach.)

Stay sutures of 3-0 silk are placed in the body of the stomach. A transverse gastrotomy is made with the electrocautery. The cyst wall is easily palpable through the posterior wall of the stomach. The location of the cyst is confirmed by aspirating pancreatic juice through the back wall of the stomach with a 10 ml syringe and a 20-gauge needle [*see Figure 15*]. (The mass palpated at the time of operation is compared with the cyst as it appears on the preoperative CT scan. If the CT scan shows a solitary unilocular cyst that corresponds to the palpable mass identified at the time of laparotomy, one can be certain that the cyst is solitary and can be drained effectively into the stomach.)

A transverse incision is made with the electrocautery through the posterior wall of the stomach, through the cyst wall, and into the pseudocyst. It is often desirable to leave the 20-gauge needle in place and to perform the posterior wall gastrotomy on either side of the needle. An ellipse of cyst wall is sent for frozen section examination. (Again, no matter how obvious it seems that one is dealing with an inflammatory cyst, a portion of the cyst wall should always be sent for frozen section examination to rule out a neoplasm.) A continuous locking suture of 3-0 absorbable synthetic material is placed through and through the posterior wall of the stomach and the anterior wall of the cyst [*see Figure 16*]. (This step may or may not actually be important for achieving long-term patency of the opening between the cyst and the posterior wall of the stomach, but it does ensure good

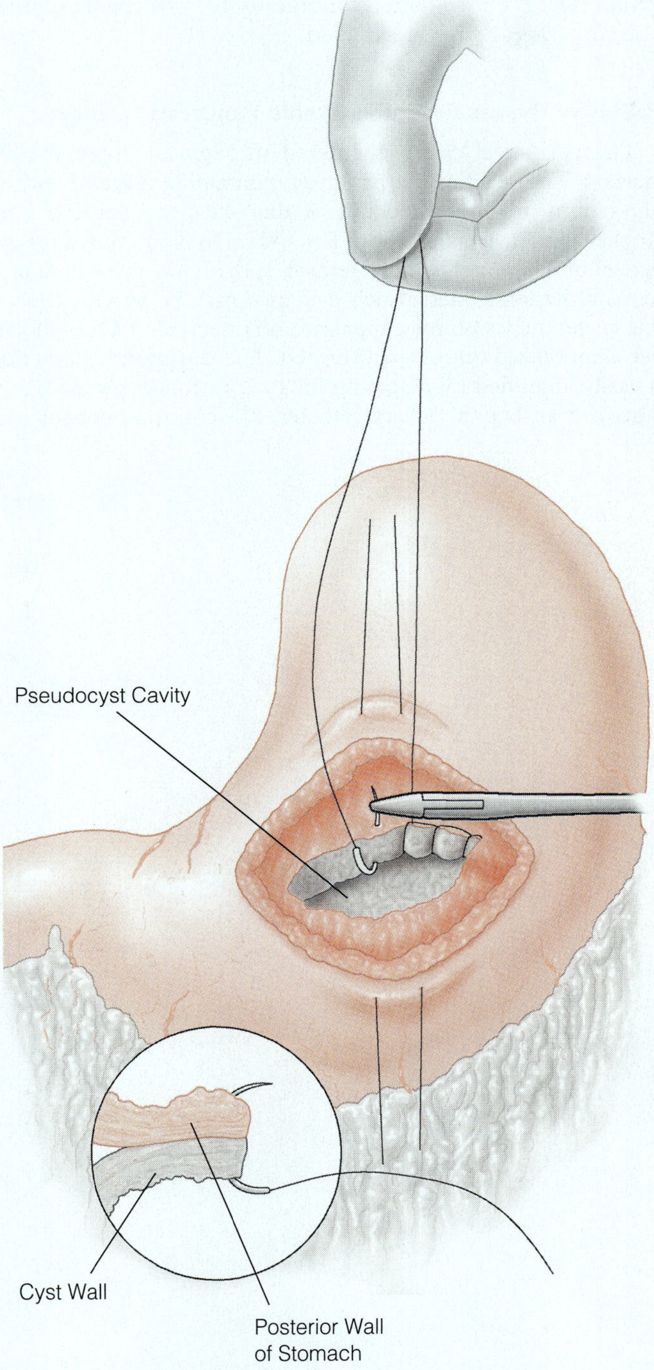

Figure 16 **Drainage of pancreatic pseudocyst into stomach. Once an incision has been made through the posterior wall of the stomach, through the cyst wall, and into the pseudocyst, a continuous locking 3-0 absorbable synthetic suture is placed through and through the posterior wall of the stomach and the cyst wall.**[3]

hemostasis.) The anterior gastrotomy is closed with an inner continuous layer of 3-0 absorbable synthetic suture material in a Connell stitch and an outer interrupted layer of 3-0 silk.

The abdomen is copiously irrigated with an antibiotic solution. The wound is closed with a single layer of interrupted No. 1 nonabsorbable synthetic monofilament sutures. The subcutaneous tissues are irrigated with an antibiotic solution and closed with a continuous 3-0 absorbable synthetic suture. The subcuticular layer is closed with a continuous 4-0 absorbable synthetic suture. Steri-Strips are applied.

Palliative Bypass for Unresectable Pancreatic Cancer

The peritoneal cavity is entered through an upper midline incision. The head of the pancreas (containing a mass) and the duodenum are mobilized out of the retroperitoneum via the Kocher maneuver. The rest of the abdomen is examined for evidence of liver metastases, serosal spread, or involvement of regional lymph nodes. (Such evidence may be absent; thus, at this stage, the lesion may appear to be resectable.) The gallbladder is mobilized out of the liver bed. The common hepatic duct is easily identified by palpating for the previously placed percutaneous transhepatic biliary catheter. The common hepatic duct is divided, and the biliary stent is extracted from the distal biliary segment. (There is no disadvantage to dividing the common hepatic duct early to facilitate identification and dissection of the portal vein. Even if the lesion proves to be unresectable, the gallbladder would not be used for the biliary bypass. I consider a hepaticojejunostomy preferable to a cholecystojejunostomy.)

Once the common hepatic duct is divided, the portal vein is easily identified. The anterior surface of the vein is cleaned under the first portion of the duodenum. An attempt is made to separate the head and neck of the pancreas from the portal vein. In many cases, it is not until this point that the lesion is ascertained to be unresectable. (As an example, the tumor may be found to be directly invading the portal vein, but the invasion was not apparent from the preoperative staging tests.) Once it is clear that the tumor is unresectable, a palliative double bypass procedure is begun, in which the duodenum is bypassed with a retrocolic gastrojejunostomy [see Figure 17] and the distally obstructed biliary tree with a hepaticojejunostomy.

Approximately 4 cm of the most dependent portion of the greater curvature of the stomach is cleaned by doubly clamping, dividing, and ligating attachments of the greater omentum. Once this is accomplished, a small rent is made in the transverse mesocolon, and a proximal loop of jejunum is brought up

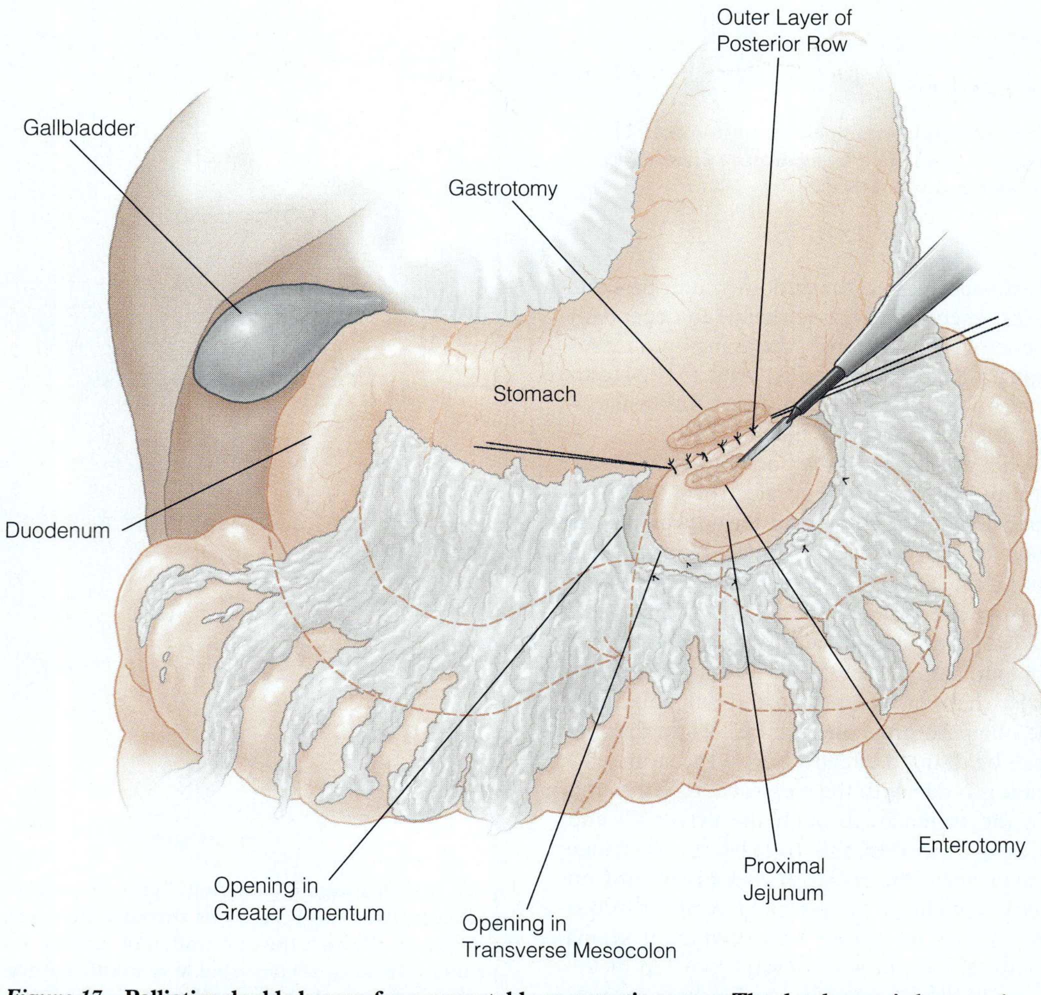

Figure 17 Palliative double bypass for unresectable pancreatic cancer. The duodenum is bypassed with a retrocolic gastrojejunostomy.[3]

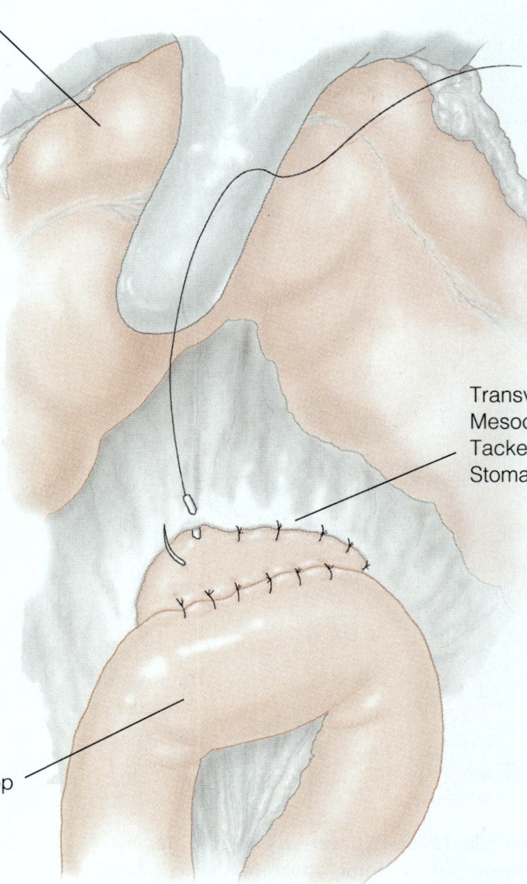

Figure 18 Palliative double bypass for unresectable pancreatic cancer. Once the retrocolic gastrojejunostomy is complete, the anastomosis is tacked to the rent in the transverse mesocolon on the gastric side with interrupted 4-0 silk sutures.[3]

theoretical possibility that if a common channel is present, pancreatic secretions might reflux up the distal biliary tree and out into the peritoneal cavity.)

Approximately 1 ft. distal to the gastrojejunostomy, a loop of jejunum is brought up into the right upper quadrant through a second rent in the transverse mesocolon. An end-to-side hepaticojejunostomy is performed [see Figure 20]. The posterior row is placed first; this is done with one layer of interrupted 4-0 absorbable synthetic sutures. Once the posterior row is complete, a small enterotomy is made, and the percutaneous transhepatic biliary catheter is placed into the jejunum to decompress the biliary anastomosis. The anterior row is then placed; this is done with one layer of interrupted 4-0 absorbable synthetic sutures.

A side-to-side anastomosis is performed between the afferent jejunal loop leading to the biliary anastomosis and the efferent jejunal loop leading from it [see Figure 20]. This short side-to-side anastomosis is placed below the rent in the transverse mesocolon. It is performed with an inner continuous layer of 3-0 absorbable synthetic suture material and an outer interrupted layer of 3-0 silk. The two limbs are tacked to the rent in the transverse mesocolon to prevent herniation.

The lesser omentum is divided, and a chemical splanchnicectomy is performed by injecting 20 ml of 50 percent alcohol into the celiac plexus on either side of the aorta at the level of the celiac axis [see Figure 20]. The level of the celiac axis is

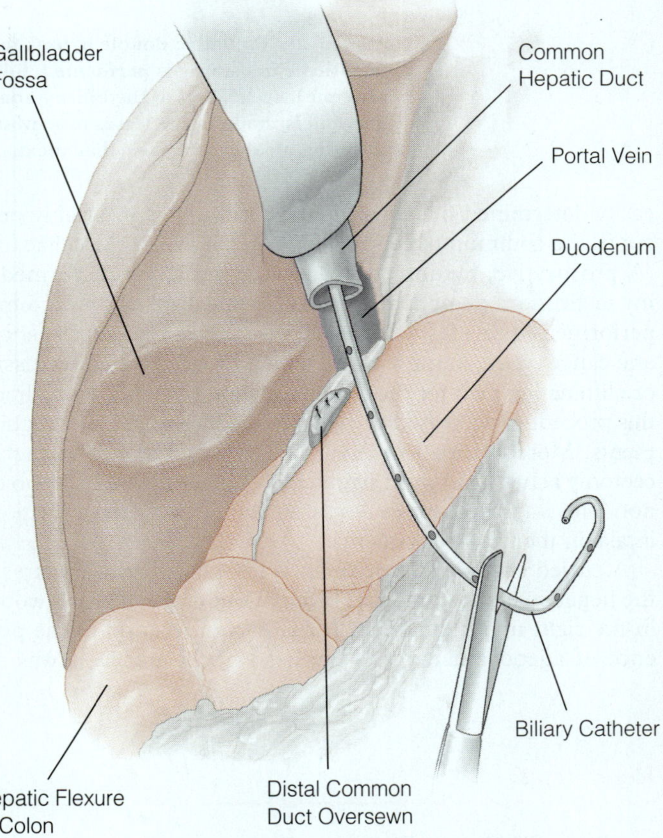

through this rent and anastomosed to the greater curvature of the stomach in a side-to-side fashion. The anastomosis is performed with an outer interrupted layer of 3-0 silk and an inner continuous layer of 3-0 absorbable synthetic suture material. (Ordinarily, palliative duodenal bypasses for pancreatic cancer are performed by carrying out an anterior gastrojejunostomy. Unfortunately, delayed gastric emptying is frequent after an anterior gastrojejunostomy. A posterior gastroenterostomy virtually eliminates this complication. Historically, surgeons have been reluctant to perform posterior gastroenterostomies for pancreatic cancer, fearing that tumor growth would occlude the anastomosis; however, at my institution, we have performed well over 100 posterior gastroenterostomies in this setting and have yet to demonstrate any tumor ingrowth into the anastomosis.) Once the posterior gastroenterostomy is complete, the anastomosis is tacked to the rent in the transverse mesocolon on the gastric side with multiple interrupted 4-0 silk sutures [see Figure 18]. (The purpose of this step is to prevent the afferent and efferent jejunal limbs from herniating up through the rent in the transverse mesocolon and becoming obstructed.)

The gallbladder is removed, and the distal biliary segment is oversewn with interrupted 3-0 silk sutures [see Figure 19]. (The distal biliary segment is routinely oversewn because there is a

Figure 19 Palliative double bypass for unresectable pancreatic cancer. The common duct is divided distally, the gallbladder is removed, and the distal biliary segment is oversewn with interrupted 3-0 silk sutures.[3]

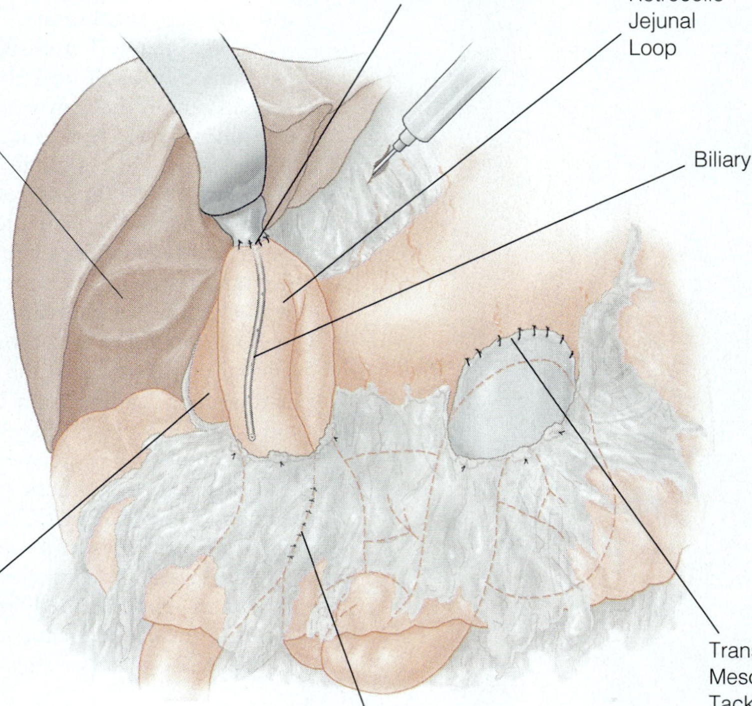

Figure 20 Palliative double bypass for unresectable pancreatic cancer. An end-to-side hepaticojejunostomy is performed, followed by a side-to-side jejunojejunostomy between the afferent loop leading to the biliary anastomosis and the efferent loop leading from it. An opening is made in the lesser omentum, and a chemical splanchnicectomy is performed by injecting alcohol into the celiac plexus.[3]

easily determined by palpating the thrill that is invariably present in the common hepatic artery as it comes off the celiac axis. (A prospective, randomized, double-blind study performed at my institution[1] demonstrated that chemical splanchnicectomies performed in this fashion in patients with unresectable pancreatic cancer were, in most cases, markedly effective in decreasing or eliminating pain for the remaining months of life. In addition, this procedure decreased or eliminated patients' narcotic requirements. Moreover, patients who underwent chemical splanchnicectomy actually survived significantly longer than those who did not. The improved survival was attributed to better nutritional intake in the pain-free patients.)

A closed suction Silastic drain is left posterior to the area of the hepaticojejunostomy and brought out through a stab wound in the right upper quadrant. If tissue confirmation of the presence of adenocarcinoma of the head of the pancreas was not obtained preoperatively, it should be obtained during operation. As a rule, this is most easily accomplished by performing a needle biopsy with a Tru-Cut needle transduodenally. The abdomen is irrigated with an antibiotic solution and then closed with multiple interrupted No.1 nonabsorbable synthetic sutures placed through and through all muscle and fascial layers. The subcutaneous tissues are irrigated with an antibiotic-containing saline solution and closed with a continuous 3-0 absorbable synthetic suture. The subcuticular layer is closed with a continuous 4-0 absorbable synthetic suture. Steri-Strips are applied.

The percutaneous transhepatic biliary stent, which is placed on the day before operation, is left connected to dependent bile bag drainage for four days after operation. After cholangiography demonstrates that the anastomosis is intact, the stent is internalized. It is removed at an outpatient visit, generally about six weeks after operation.

References

1. Lillemoe KD, Cameron JL, Kaufman HS, et al: Chemical splanchnicectomy in patients with unresectable pancreatic cancer: a prospective randomized trial. Ann Surg 217:447, 1993
2. Cameron JL: Rapid exposure of the portal and superior mesenteric veins. Surg Gynecol Obstet 176:395, 1993
3. Cameron, JL: Atlas of Surgery, Vol 2. Mosby–Year Book, St. Louis, 1994

Acknowledgments

Figures 1 and 2 Tom Moore.
Figures 3 through 20 Tom Moore. Original illustrations by Corinne Sandone.

The phrenicocolic ligament courses laterally from the diaphragm to the splenic flexure of the colon; its upper portion is called the phrenicosplenic ligament. The attachment of the lower pole on the internal side is called the splenocolic ligament. Between these two, a horizontal shelf of areolar tissue, known as the sustentaculum lienis, is formed on which the inferior pole of the spleen rests. The sustentaculum lienis is often molded into a sac that opens cephalad and acts as a support for the lower pole. This structure, often overlooked during open procedures, is readily visible through the laparoscope. The phrenicocolic ligament, the splenocolic ligament, and the sustentaculum lienis are usually avascular, except in patients who have portal hypertension or myeloid metaplasia.

A 1937 study found that the tail of the pancreas was in direct contact with the spleen in 30% of cadavers.[16] A subsequent report confirmed this finding and added that in 73% of patients, the distance between the two structures was no more than 1 cm.[17] Care must be exercised to avoid damage with the electrocautery during dissection as well as damage with the linear stapler in the course of en masse ligation of the splenic hilum (a maneuver more easily performed via the lateral approach to laparoscopic splenectomy).

Operative Technique

LATERAL APPROACH

This approach was first described in connection with laparoscopic adrenalectomy and is currently used for most laparoscopic splenectomies.[18] At present, the only indication for the anterior approach to laparoscopic splenectomy is the presence of massive splenomegaly or a megaspleen. Typically, this alternative approach is taken when a spleen reaches or exceeds 23 cm in length or 3 kg in weight.

Step 1: Placement of Trocars

The patient is placed in the right lateral decubitus position, much as he or she would be for a left-side posterolateral thoracotomy. The operating table is flexed and the kidney bolster raised to increase the distance between the lower rib and the iliac crest. Usually, four 12 mm trocars are used around the costal margin so that the camera, the clip applier, and the linear stapler can be interchanged with maximum flexibility [see Figure 4]. The trocars must be far enough apart to permit good working angles. Some advantage may be gained from tilting the patient slightly backward; this step gives the operating team more freedom in moving the instruments placed along the left costal margins, especially during lifting movements, when it is easy for instrument handles to touch the operating table. For the same reason, it is also advisable to place the anterior or abdominal side of the patient closer to the edge of the operating table.

A local anesthetic is infiltrated into the skin at the midpoint of the anterior costal margin, and a 12 mm incision is made. The first trocar is inserted under direct vision, and a symmetrical 15 mm Hg pneumoperitoneum is created. The locations of the remaining trocars are determined by considering the anatomic configuration in relation to the size of the spleen to be excised. In most cases, the fourth posterior trocar cannot be inserted until the splenic flexure of the colon has been mobilized. Accordingly, the procedure is usually started with three trocars in place.

Troubleshooting *Open insertion of first trocar.* After years of using the Veress needle, we now prefer the open method of inserting the first trocar. It is true that use of the Veress needle is for the most part safe; however, the small number of catastrophic complications that occur with blind methods of first trocar insertion are more and more difficult to justify. Admittedly, these complications are infrequent, and thus, it is unlikely that even a large randomized trial would be able to show any significant differences between various methods of first trocar insertion. Nevertheless, even though complications occur with the open method of first trocar insertion as well, they are very uncommon and tend to be limited to trauma to the intestine or the omental blood vessels; they do not have the same serious consequences as the major vessel injury that may arise from blind trocar insertion.

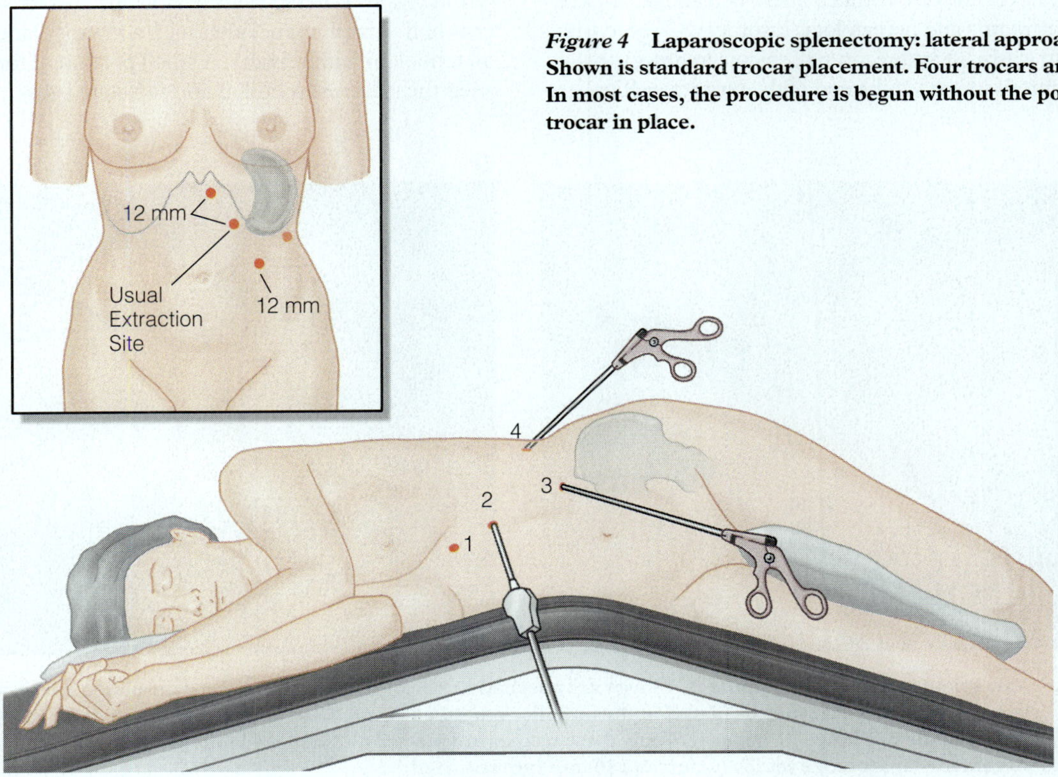

Figure 4 Laparoscopic splenectomy: lateral approach. Shown is standard trocar placement. Four trocars are used. In most cases, the procedure is begun without the posterior trocar in place.

Alternative trocar placement. More experienced surgeons (or those simply wishing to make the procedure easier) may choose to replace one or two 12 mm trocars with 5 mm trocars [see Figure 5a]. The procedure can also be performed with only three trocars. In leaner patients, one of the trocars can be inserted into the umbilicus to gain a cosmetic advantage. The advent of needlescopic techniques has made it possible to replace some of the 5 and 12 mm trocars with 3 mm trocars. The ultimate (i.e., least invasive) technique, usually reserved for lean patients with ITP and normal-size spleens, involves one 12 mm trocar placed in the umbilicus and two 3 mm trocars placed subcostally [see Figure 5b]. This approach requires two different camera-laparoscope setups, so that a 3 mm laparoscope can be interchanged with a 10 mm laparoscope as necessary to permit application of clips or staplers through the umbilical incision once the dissection is completed. The specimen is then retrieved through the umbilicus. Because the use of 3 mm laparoscopes is accompanied by a decrease in available intra-abdominal light and focal width, a meticulously bloodless field and sophisticated surgical judgment are critical for successful performance of needlescopic splenectomy.

Step 2: Search for and Retrieval of Accessory Spleens

The camera is inserted, and the stomach is retracted medially to expose the spleen. Then a fairly standard sequence is followed. A thorough search is then made for accessory spleens. To maximize retrieval, all known locations of accessory spleens should be carefully explored [see Figure 6]. Any accessory spleens found should be removed immediately; they are considerably harder to locate once the spleen is removed.

Troubleshooting It is especially important to retrieve accessory spleens from patients with ITP, in whom the presence of overlooked accessory spleens has been associated with recurrence of the disease. Remedial operation for excision of missed accessory spleens has been reported to bring remission of recurrent disease; such operation can be performed laparoscopically. The overall retrieval rate for accessory spleens should fall between 15% and 30%.

Splenic activity has been demonstrated after open and laparoscopic splenectomy for trauma and hematologic disorders[19,20]; accordingly, it is advisable to wash out and recover all splenic fragments resulting from intraoperative trauma at the end of the procedure. This step is particularly important for patients with ITP, in whom intraoperative trauma to the spleen is thought to contribute to postoperative scan-detectable splenic activity. As of this writing, we have recovered accessory spleens in 33% of ITP cases treated laparoscopically.

Step 3: Control of Vessels at Lower Pole, Demonstration of "Splenic Tent," and Incision of Phrenicocolic Ligament

The splenic flexure is partially mobilized by incising the splenocolic ligament, the lower part of the phrenicocolic ligament, and the sustentaculum lienis. The incision is carried slightly into the left side of the gastrocolic ligament. This step affords access to the gastrosplenic ligament, which can then be readily separated from the splenorenal ligament to create what looks like a tent. This maneuver cannot be accomplished in all cases, but when it can be done, it simplifies the procedure considerably. The walls of this so-called splenic tent are made of the gastrosplenic ligament on the left and the splenorenal ligament on the right, and the floor is made up of the stomach. In fact, this maneuver opens the lesser sac in its lateral portion (a point that is better demonstrated with gentle upward retraction of the splenic tip) [see Figure 7].

The branches of the left gastroepiploic artery are controlled with the electrocautery or with clips, depending on the size of the branches. The avascular portion of the gastrosplenic ligament, situated between the gastroepiploic artery and the short gastric vessels, is then incised sufficiently to expose the hilar structures in the splenorenal ligament. To accomplish this, the lower pole is gently elevated; in this position, the spleen almost retracts itself as it naturally falls toward the left lobe of the liver. At this point, the surgeon can usually assess the geography of the hilum and determine the degree of difficulty of the operation. The fourth trocar, if needed, is then placed posteriorly under direct vision, with care taken to avoid the left kidney. Caution must also be exercised in placing the trocars situated immediately anterior and posterior to the iliac crest. The iliac crest can impede movement and hinder upward mobilization of structures if the trocars are placed over it rather than in front of or behind it [see Figure 8].

Finally, the phrenicocolic ligament is incised all the way to the left crus of the diaphragm, either with a monopolar electrocautery with an L hook or with scissors. A small portion of the ligament is left to keep the spleen suspended and facilitate subsequent bagging. The

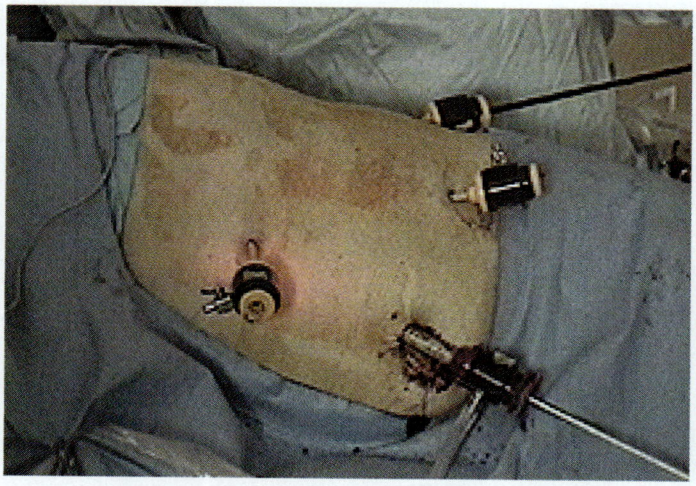

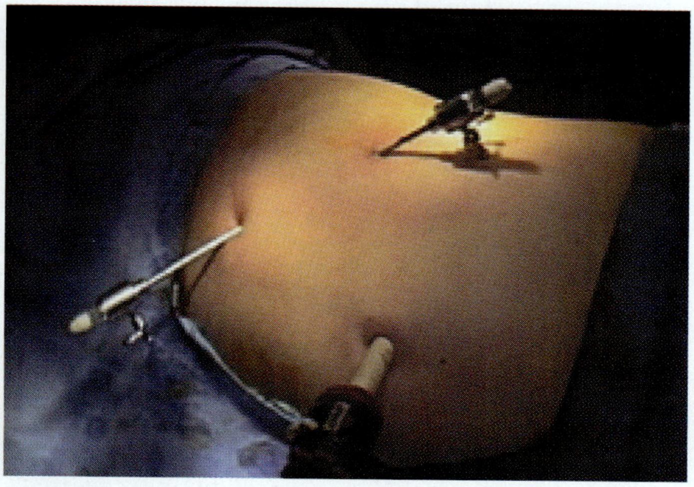

Figure 5 Laparoscopic splenectomy: lateral approach. Shown are alternative trocar placements. (*a*) In some patients (e.g., thin patients with normal-size spleens), a 12 mm trocar may be placed in the umbilicus to gain a cosmetic advantage, and most of the other trocars may be downsized to 5 mm. (*b*) In the needlescopic approach, only three trocars are placed: a 12 mm trocar in the umbilicus and two 3 mm subcostal trocars. Two camera-laparoscope setups (3 mm and 10 mm) are required.

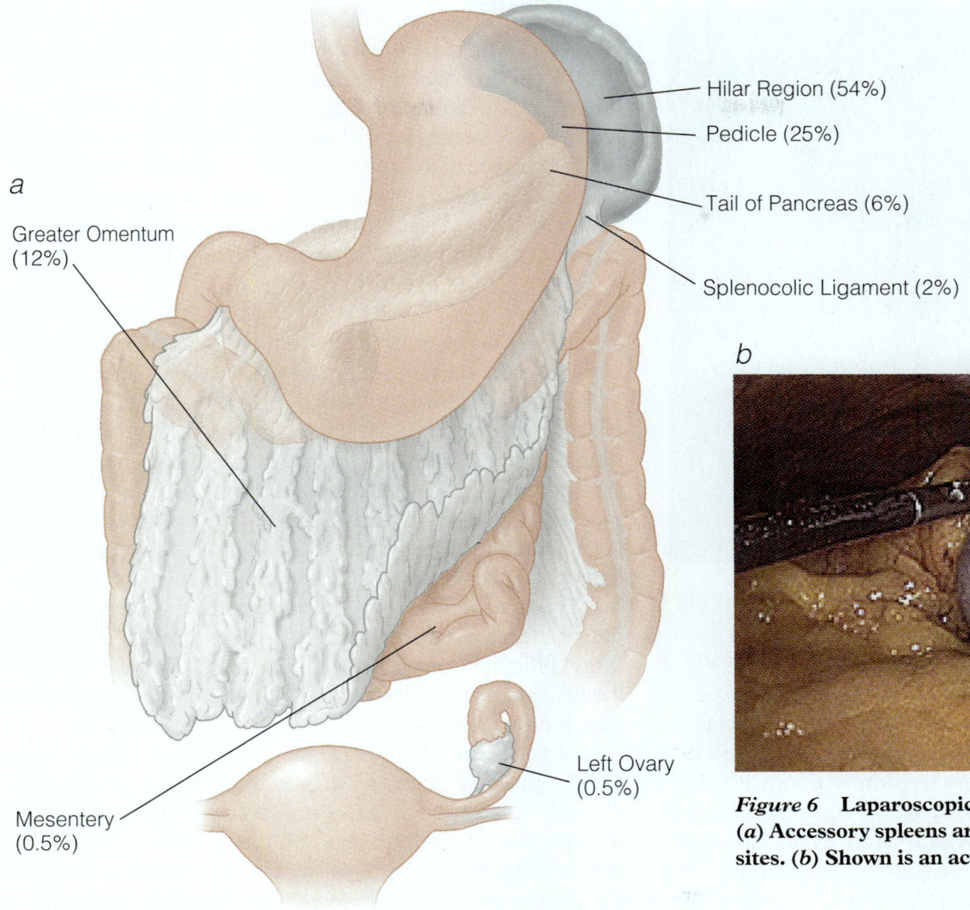

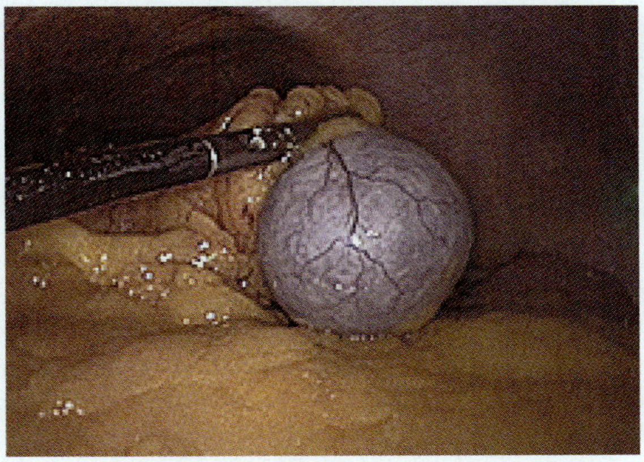

Figure 6 Laparoscopic splenectomy: lateral approach. (*a*) Accessory spleens are known to occur at specific sites. (*b*) Shown is an accessory spleen.

phrenicocolic ligament is avascular except in patients with portal hypertension or myeloproliferative disorders (e.g., myeloid metaplasia). Leaving 1 to 2 cm of ligament all along the spleen side facilitates retraction and handling of the spleen with instruments.

Troubleshooting Remarkably few instruments are needed for laparoscopic splenectomy [*see Figure 9*]: most of the operation is done with three reusable instruments. A dolphin-nose 5 mm atraumatic grasper is used to elevate and hold the spleen. It is also used to separate tissue planes and vessels with blunt dissection because its atraumatic tip is easily insinuated between tissue planes. A gently curved 5 mm fine-tip dissector (Crile or Maryland) and a 10 mm 90° right-angle dissector are the only other tools required for cost-efficient dissection.

When a powered instrument is called for, we use a monopolar electrocautery with an L hook or a gently curved scissors [*see Figure 9*]. An ultrasonic dissector can also be used.

Step 4: Dealing with Splenic Hilum and Tailoring Operative Strategy to Anatomy

It is advisable to base one's operative strategy on the specific splenic anatomy. If a distributed anatomy is present, the splenic branches are usually dissected and clipped. This is not only the least costly approach but also the simplest, in that the vessels are spread over a wider area of the splenic hilum and are easier to dissect and separate [*see Figure 10*].

A magistral anatomy lends itself more to a single use of the linear stapler, provided that the tail of the pancreas is identified and dissected away when required. When possible, a window is created above the hilar pedicle in the splenorenal ligament so that all structures can be included within the markings of the linear stapler under direct vision [*see Figure 11*]. The angles provided by the various trocars make this maneuver much easier via the lateral approach than via the anterior approach. Dissection continues with individual dissection and clipping of the short gastric vessels; occasionally, these vessels can also be taken en masse with the linear stapler. So far, we have not used sutures in this setting, except once to control a short gastric vessel that was too short to be clipped safely. This portion of the operation is performed while the spleen is hanging from the upper portion of the phrenicocolic ligament, which has not yet been entirely cut.

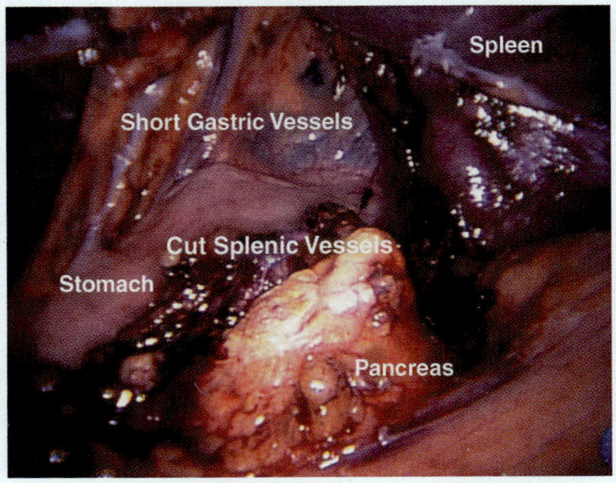

Figure 7 Laparoscopic splenectomy: lateral approach. The so-called splenic tent is formed by the gastrosplenic and splenorenal ligaments laterally and the stomach below.

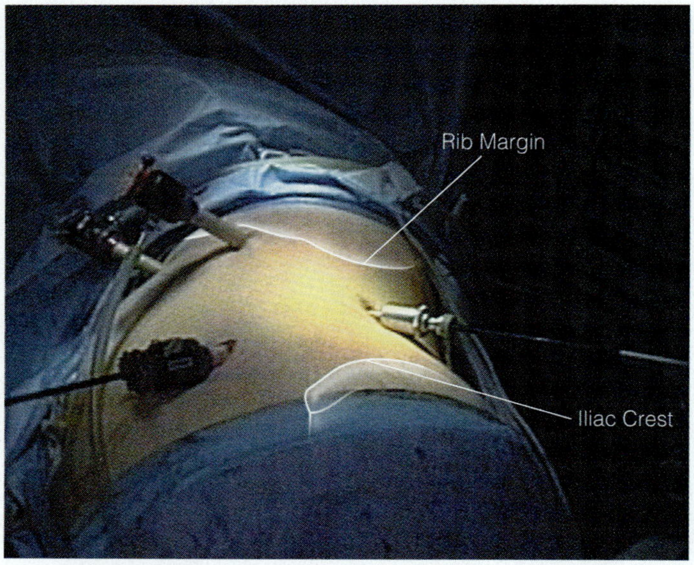

Figure 8 Laparoscopic splenectomy: lateral approach. Shown is the recommended trocar placement around the iliac crest.

Troubleshooting It is at this point in the procedure that experience in designing the operative strategy pays off in reduced operating time. Because of the many variations in size, shape, vascular patterns, and relations to adjacent organs, spleens are almost as individual as fingerprints. Accordingly, an experienced spleen surgeon learns to keep an open mind with regard to operative strategy and must be able to call on a wide range of skills to facilitate the procedure.

The surgeon should start by looking at the internal surface of the spleen. If the splenic vessels cover more than 75% of the internal surface (as is the case in 70% of patients), a distributed anatomy is present, which means that the spleen can be expected to have more vessels spread out over a wider area. The number of splenic branches is also related to the presence of notches on the spleen surface. With a distributed vascular anatomy, the vessels tend to be easier to dissect and isolate and thus can be readily (and cost-effectively) controlled with clips. On the other hand, if the splenic vessels entering the spleen cover only 25% to 35% of the inner surface of the hilum (30% of patients), the pattern is magistral. In such cases, the hilum is more compact and fewer vessels can be expected, especially if the surface of the spleen is smooth and without notches. With a magistral vascular anatomy, the vessels can usually be controlled with a single application of the vascular stapler across the hilum, provided that the tail of the pancreas can be protected.

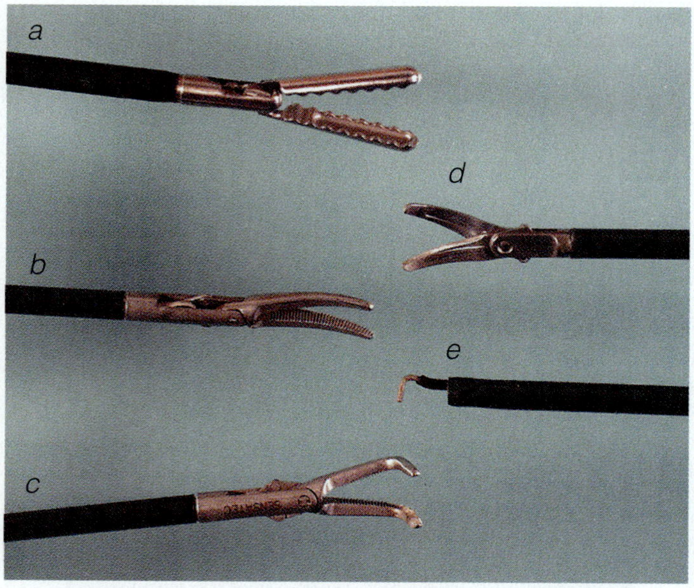

Step 5: Extraction of Spleen

A medium-size or large heavy-duty plastic freezer bag, of the sort commercially available in grocery stores, is used to bag the spleen. This bag is sterilized and folded, then introduced into the abdominal cavity through one of the 12 mm trocars [*see Figure 12*]. The bag is unfolded and the spleen slipped inside to prevent splenosis during the subsequent manipulations. Grasping forceps are used to hold the two rigid edges of the bag and to effect partial closure. Bagging is facilitated by preserving the upper portion of the phrenicocolic ligament. After final section of the phrenicocolic ligament and any diaphragmatic adhesions present, extraction is performed through one of the anterior port sites. Extraction through a posterior site is more difficult because of the thickness of the muscle mass; usually, the incision must be opened, and more muscle must be fulgurated than is desirable.

The subcostal or umbilical incision through which extraction is to take place is extended slightly. A grasping forceps is inserted through the extraction incision to hold the edges of the bag inside the abdomen. Gentle traction on the bag from outside brings the spleen close to the peritoneal surface of the umbilical incision and then out of the wound [*see Figure 13*]. Specimen retrieval bags have been developed that can accommodate a normal-size spleen and thus make bagging much easier, but they are costly.

A biopsy specimen of a size suitable for pathologic identification is obtained by incising the splenic tip. The spleen is then fragmented with finger fracture, and the resulting blood is suctioned. The remaining stromal tissue of the spleen is then extracted through the small incision, hemostasis is again verified, and all trocars are removed. No drains are used. The incisions are closed with absorbable sutures and paper strips. After verification of hemostasis, the trocar sites are closed with absorbable sutures and paper strips.

Troubleshooting The freezer bags can be more easily introduced into the abdomen if they are pulled in rather than pushed in [*see Figure 12*]. This may be accomplished by bringing out a 5 mm toothed grasper through the introduction trocar from another properly angled trocar, grasping the specimen bag, and pulling the bag back down through the trocar.

Slipping the spleen into a freezer bag is also an acquired skill that takes some time to master. It is an important skill that is useful in many other instances where specimen retrieval is needed (e.g., in procedures involving the gallbladder, the appendix, the adrenal glands, or the colon). In addition, it is highly cost-effective, in that these commercially available bags cost only a few cents each. Admittedly, laparoscopic retrieval bags are easier to use, but their substantially higher cost can become a factor in a busy minimally invasive surgery unit. We recently started to use a powerful suction machine (−70 mm Hg) and a custom-made sharp beveled 10 mm cannula to suction splenic tissue from the plastic retrieval bag [*see Figure 14*].

ANTERIOR APPROACH

The anterior approach is seldom used nowadays; however, it remains the preferable approach in some patients with massive spleno-

Figure 9 Laparoscopic splenectomy: lateral approach. Laparoscopic splenectomy can be done with a few basic instruments: (*a*) a 5 mm laparoscopic grasper, (*b*) a 5 mm laparoscopic dissector, (*c*) a 10 mm right-angle dissector, (*d*) a curved laparoscopic scissors, and (*e*) a monopolar electrocautery with an L hook.

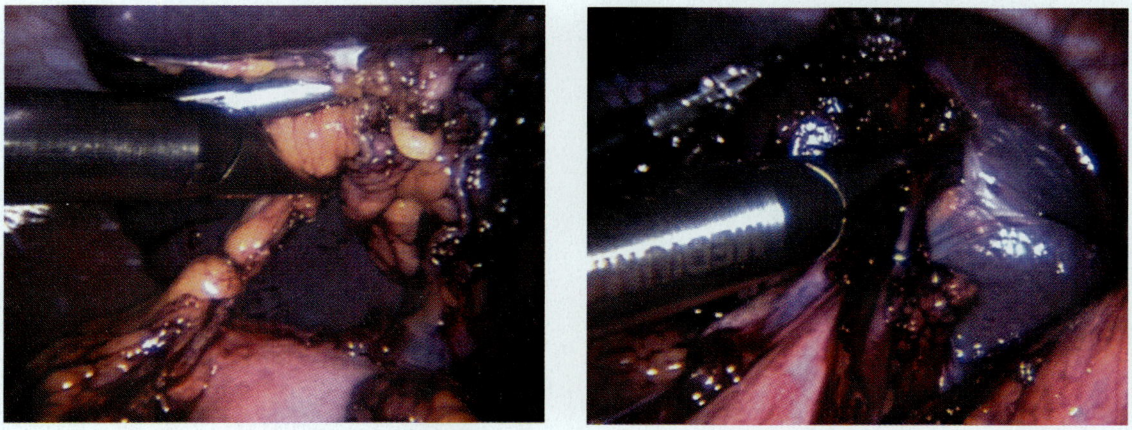

Figure 10 Laparoscopic splenectomy: lateral approach. (*a, b*) Clipping is well suited to controlling short gastric or gastroepiploic vessels. It is also appropriate for distributed-type splenic vasculatures, in which more splenic vessels are spread over a wider area of the hilum.

megaly (21 to 30 cm long) and all patients with megaspleens (> 30 cm or > 3 kg). Very large spleens are extremely heavy and difficult to manipulate with laparoscopic instruments, and it is complicated to lift them so as to gain access to the phrenicocolic ligament posteriorly. The anterior approach can also be considered if another procedure (e.g., cholecystectomy) is being contemplated; alternatively, in this situation, the lateral approach can be used, and the patient can be repositioned for the secondary procedure.

Step 1: Placement of Trocars

Under general anesthesia, the patient is placed in a modified lithotomy position to allow the surgeon to operate between the patient's legs and to allow the assistants to stand on each side of the patient. The procedure is performed through five trocars in the upper abdomen [*see Figure 15*], with the patient in a steep Fowler position with left-side elevation. A 12 mm trocar is introduced through an umbilical incision, and a 10 mm laparoscope (0° or 30°) is connected to a video system. A 12 mm trocar is placed in each upper quadrant, and two 5 mm trocars are inserted close to the rib margin on the left and right sides of the abdomen. Alternatively, trocars can be deployed in a semicircle away from the left upper quadrant. Trocar sites are carefully selected to optimize working angles. The 12 mm ports are used to allow introduction of clip appliers, staplers, or the laparoscope from a variety of angles as needed.

Troubleshooting With increasing experience, we find that we prefer to do as many laparoscopic splenectomies as possible via the lateral approach because it is so much easier, even with spleens that are longer than 20 cm and are readily palpable. The decision is arbitrarily made on the basis of estimated available working space. If the spleen comes too close to the iliac crest or the midline, the anterior approach should be taken instead.

Step 2: Isolation of Lower Pole and Control of Blood Supply

The left hepatic lobe is retracted, and the stomach is retracted medially to expose the spleen. Accessory spleens are searched for, and the phrenicocolic ligament, the splenocolic ligament, and the sustentaculum lienis are incised near the lower pole with an electrocautery and a hook probe or with scissors. Vascular adhesions—frequently found on the medial side of the spleen—are cauterized. The gastrocolic ligament is carefully dissected close to the spleen, and the left gastroepiploic vessels are ligated one by one with metallic clips or, if small, simply cauterized. The upper and lower poles of the spleen are gently lifted with one or both palpators (placed through the 5 mm ports) to expose the splenic hilum and the tail of the pancreas within the splenorenal ligament, thereby facilitating individual dissection and clipping of all the branches of the splenic artery and vein close to the spleen. The short gastric vessels are then identified and ligated with clips or, occasionally, with staples. No sutures are used. Alternatively, the splenic artery itself can be isolated and clipped within the lesser sac before extensive dissection of the lower pole and suspensory ligaments.

When preoperative splenic artery embolization is employed [*see* Preoperative Splenic Artery Embolization, *below*], the dissection plane is situated between the sites of distal embolization of splenic artery branches and the site of proximal embolization of the splenic artery itself. Because of the segmental and terminal distribution of splenic arteries, it is easy to determine the devascularized portions of the spleen: these segments exhibit a characteristic grayish color, whereas the vascularized segments retain a pinkish hue. When the organ is completely isolated, it is left in its natural cavity, and hemostasis is verified.

Troubleshooting If one elects first to clip the splenic artery within the lesser sac, there are a few precautions that must be taken. First, the clipping must be done distal to the pancreatica magna artery to prevent pancreatic injury. Second, one must make sure that the splenic artery proper is clipped, not one of its branches (e.g., the superior terminal branch). This is an easy mistake to commit with the distributed type of splenic vasculature [*see Figure 1*] because the splenic artery itself is short and the branches can take off very early. Third, one must always keep in mind the possibility of an anastomotic branch between the major splenic branches, as described by Testut.[13] Should a major terminal branch be clipped rather than the splenic artery proper, there will be no spleen ischemia if such an anastomosis is present [*see Figure 1*].

Yet another challenge posed by the anterior approach is that if bleeding occurs, the blood tends to pool in the area of the hilum and obscure vision even more, whereas in the lateral approach, the blood tends to flow away from the operative field. One quickly learns that there is a steep price to pay for cutting corners during the dissection. The dissection must be meticulous, especially behind branches of the splenic vein.

Step 3: Extraction of Spleen

Given that the anterior approach is now used only in cases of

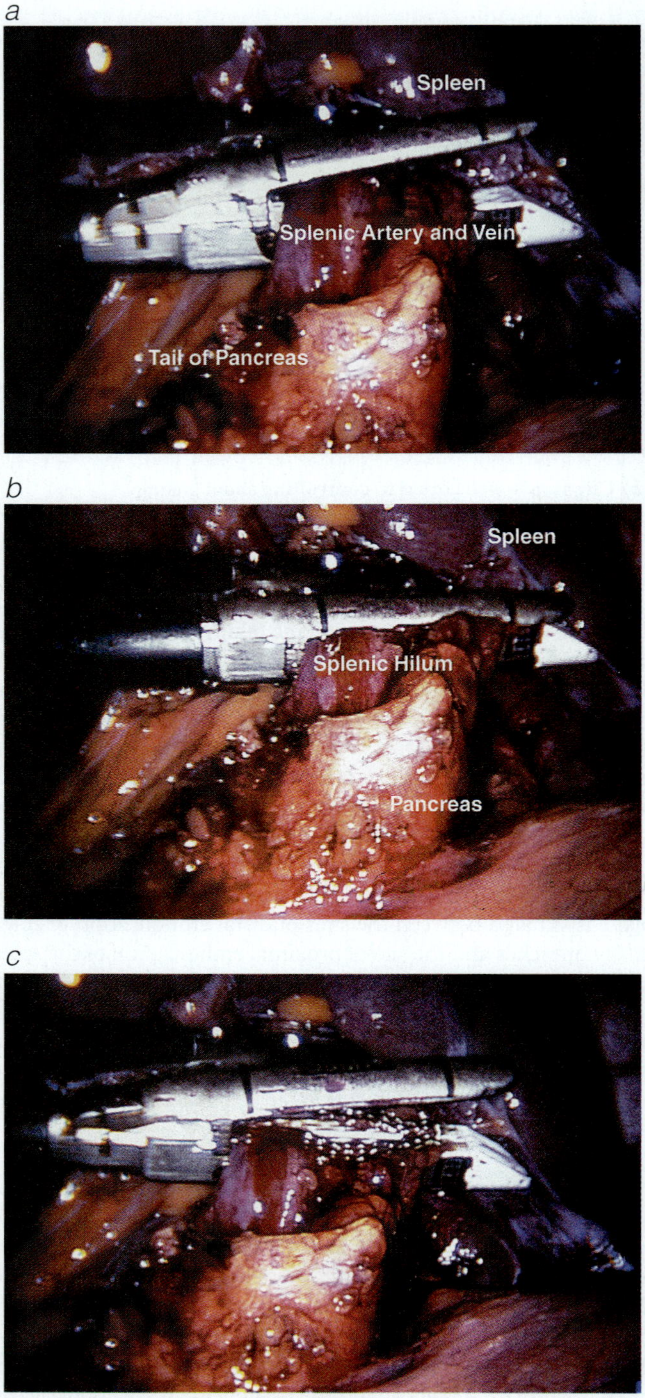

796 — V OPERATIVE MANAGEMENT

Figure 11 **Laparoscopic splenectomy: lateral approach.** (*a through c*) Stapling is particularly well suited to the compact hilum found in the magistral-type distribution of splenic vessels. As shown, all of the vascular structures are within the stapler markers, and the tail of the pancreas is well protected.

massive splenomegaly or megaspleen, bagging can be problematic. The largest commercially available freezer bag we have seen measures 27 by 28 cm, and the largest spleen we have been able to bag in one of them was 24 cm long. Furthermore, an accessory extraction incision is often required; a Pfannenstiel incision gives better cosmetic results, but a left lower quadrant incision can also be used. A plastic sleeve designed to maintain pneumoperitoneum is also a useful adjunct for vessel dissection and extraction in patients with very large spleens.

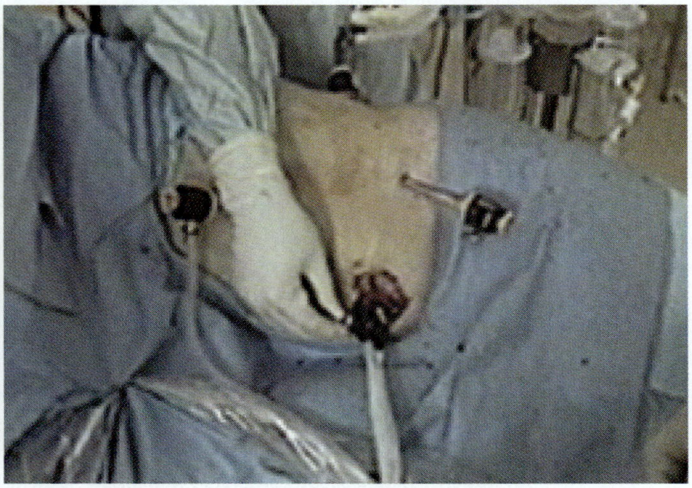

Figure 12 **Laparoscopic splenectomy: lateral approach.** Illustrated is the introduction of a sterile freezer bag for specimen extraction via the pull method. A toothed grasper is passed across the abdomen between two trocars and brought out through the 12 mm umbilical trocar site. This grasper is used to pull the extraction bag back into the abdomen.

If the spleen cannot be bagged, it may be fragmented in the pelvis before extraction, provided that the abdomen is copiously washed and cleaned of any residual spleen fragments before closure to prevent splenosis. Most patients with large spleens have hematologic malignancies; thus, residual splenic activity is not as crucial an issue in these patients as it would be in others.

Troubleshooting Many surgeons advocate the use of pneumatic sleeves as an adjunct to laparoscopic splenectomy. Most such sleeves require at least a 7.5 cm incision for introduction. In our view, use of these sleeves tends to work against the ultimate goal of minimally invasive surgery, which is to produce good surgical outcomes with as little trauma as possible; however, it can be a very helpful aid while one is learning laparoscopic splenectomy as well as in certain special circumstances (e.g., laparoscopic splenectomy for large spleens).

The incision for the pneumatic sleeve may be placed either transversely in the right upper quadrant or vertically in the upper midline. Alternatively, a Pfannenstiel incision may be employed: it has

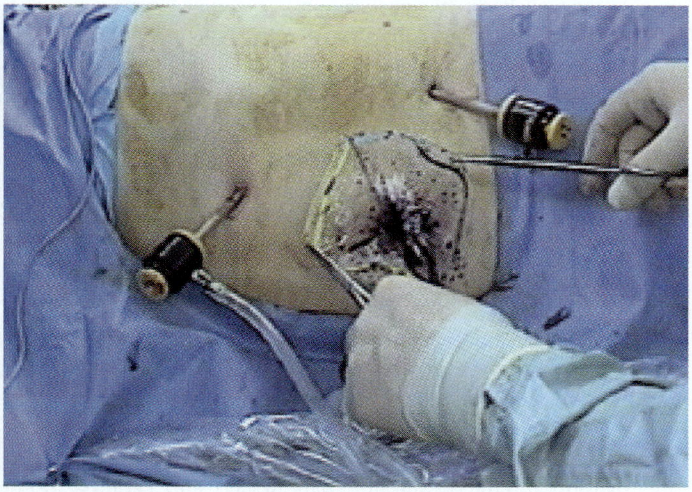

Figure 13 **Laparoscopic splenectomy: lateral approach.** Shown is the position of the specimen bag position before finger fragmentation or pulp suction.

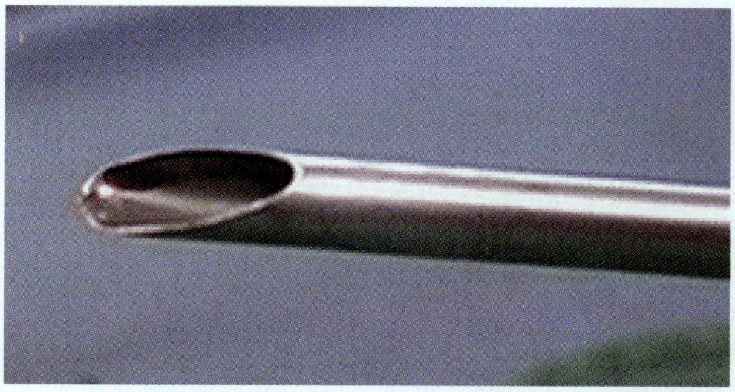

Figure 14 Laparoscopic splenectomy: lateral approach. A beveled 10 mm suction cannula is used for subcapsular volume reduction in patients with megaspleens. This custom-made suction cannula can also be used to aspirate splenic pulp from the plastic retrieval bag during laparoscopic splenectomy in patients with normal-size or moderately enlarged spleens.

cosmetic advantages over upper abdominal incisions and may result in fewer pulmonary complications. Use of the pneumatic sleeve may facilitate hilar dissection by improving retraction (especially in the upper pole) and by guiding placement of linear staples or clips. It may also facilitate retraction of enlarged spleens to improve access to all of the suspensory ligaments.

LAPAROSCOPIC PARTIAL SPLENECTOMY

Concern regarding the risk of OPSS has encouraged the practice of preserving splenic tissue and function whenever possible. For this reason, partial splenectomy has occasionally been indicated for treatment of benign tumors of the spleen and for excision of cystic lesions.[21] Its use has been described in connection with the management of type I Gaucher disease, cholesteryl ester storage disease, chronic myelogenous leukemia, and thalassemia major as well as the staging of Hodgkin disease.[22,23] Partial splenectomy has also been an option in the management of splenic trauma when the patient's condition is stable enough to permit the meticulous dissection required for the operation.[24,25]

Operative Technique

Like standard laparoscopic splenectomy, laparoscopic partial splenectomy is performed with the patient in the right lateral decubitus position. Trocar placement is similar as well. The splenocolic ligament and the lower part of the phrenicocolic ligament are incised to permit mobilization of the lower pole of the spleen. If the lower portion of the spleen is to be excised, branches of the gastroepiploic vessels supplying the lower pole are dissected and clipped close to the parenchyma. An appropriate number of penultimate branches of the inferior polar artery are then taken in such a way as to create a clear line of demarcation between normal spleen and devascularized spleen. This process is continued until the desired number of splenic segments are devascularized. Next, a standard monopolar electrocautery is used to score the splenic capsule circumferentially, with care taken to ensure that a 5 mm rim of devascularized splenic tissue remains in situ; this is the most important technical point for this procedure [*see Figure 16*]. The incision is then carried into the splenic pulp. Atraumatic intestinal graspers are also used to fracture the splenic pulp in a bloodless fashion. The laparoscopic L hook and scissors provide excellent hemostatic control.

Once the spleen has been allowed to demarcate, resection is remarkably bloodless, provided that the 5 mm rim of ischemic tissue is left in place. Complete control of the splenic artery is not required before splenic separation, because division occurs in an ischemic segment of spleen.[9] The feasibility of leaving portions of ischemic spleen in situ has been demonstrated in a large prospective, randomized trial involving partial splenic embolization as primary treatment of hematologic disorders.[26]

If the superior pole is to be removed, the phrenicocolic ligament must be incised almost entirely so that the spleen can be easily mobilized and the proper exposure achieved. The short gastric branch-

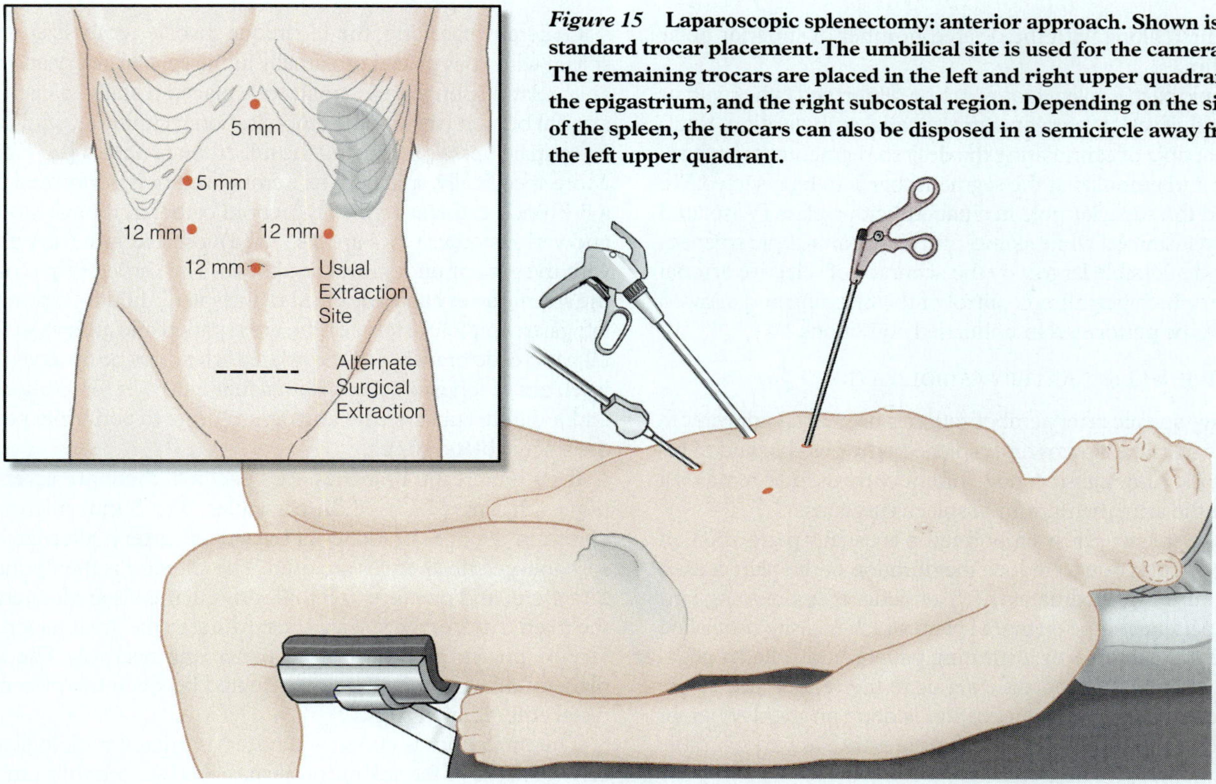

Figure 15 Laparoscopic splenectomy: anterior approach. Shown is standard trocar placement. The umbilical site is used for the camera. The remaining trocars are placed in the left and right upper quadrants, the epigastrium, and the right subcostal region. Depending on the size of the spleen, the trocars can also be disposed in a semicircle away from the left upper quadrant.

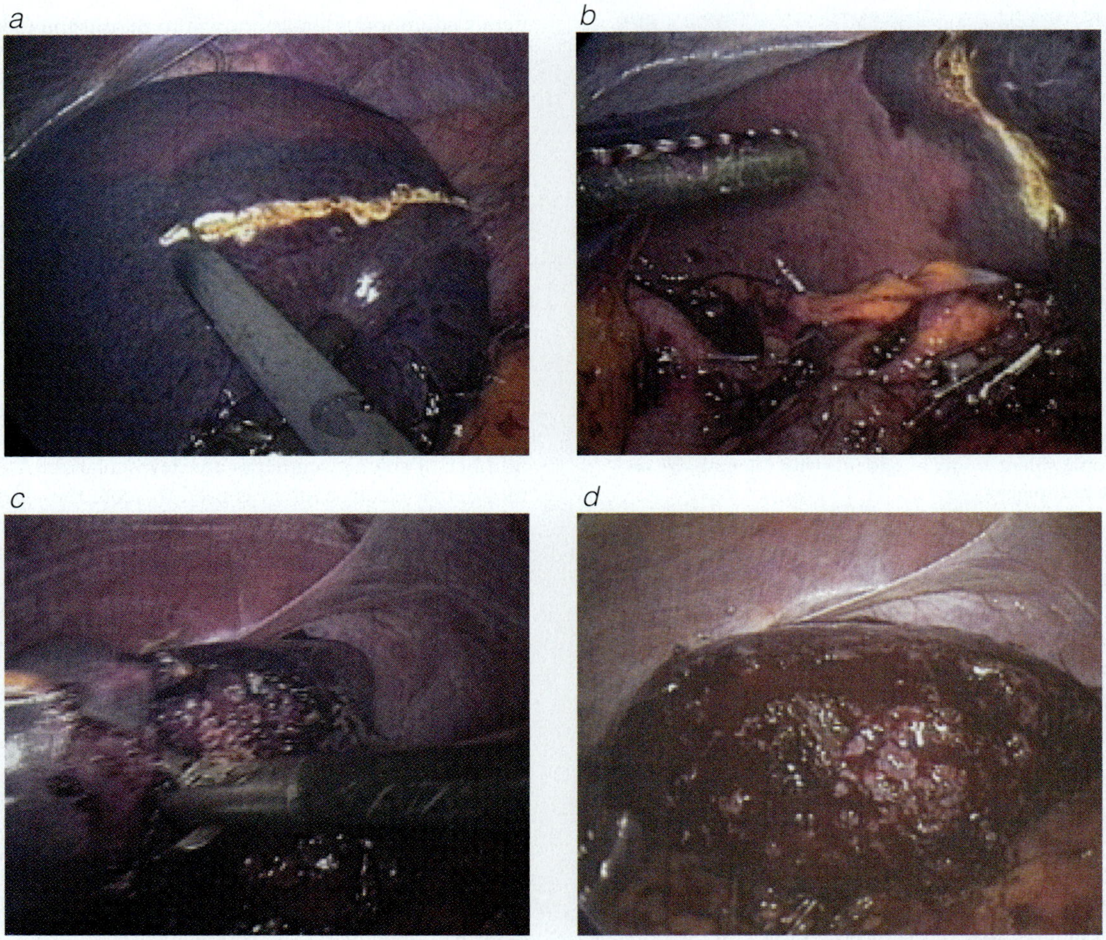

Figure 16 Laparoscopic splenectomy: partial splenectomy. (*a, b*) The splenic capsule is scored with the monopolar cautery, and a 5 mm margin of devitalized tissue is left. (*c*) The splenic pulp is fractured with an atraumatic grasper. The electrocautery with the L hook is also used to control parenchymal bleeding. (*d*) Shown is the cut surface of the spleen after transection. The operative field remains remarkably dry.

es are taken first, along with the desired number of superior polar artery branches.

Laparoscopic partial splenectomy can be performed either with or without the aid of selective preoperative arterial embolization. Radiologists are capable of cannulating the desired segmental splenic arterial branch and embolizing the segment that is to be resected. We have removed the superior pole in a patient with a class IV isolated splenic injury sustained while skiing[8]; partial laparoscopic splenectomy was made possible largely by the accuracy of selective arterial embolization, which permitted control of the bleeding and allowed laparoscopy to be performed in unhurried conditions.[27]

PREOPERATIVE SPLENIC ARTERY EMBOLIZATION

Preoperative splenic artery embolization is used as an adjuvant in a few patients to make laparoscopic splenectomy possible and to reduce blood loss. Although it is now infrequently used, it remains a useful tool in the armamentarium of spleen surgeons.

Preoperative splenic artery embolization is usually performed on the morning of operation to reduce the duration of the pain caused by the procedure. Approximately 45% of patients undergoing embolization experience some degree of pain, which is easily controlled by administering narcotics or instituting patient-controlled analgesia. In some patients, thrombosis extends to the venous side of the splenic blood supply when embolization is done on the day before operation. Whether this occurrence translates into any measurable advantage remains to be determined.

Generally speaking, the technique involves embolization of the spleen with coils placed proximally in the splenic artery and absorbable gelatin sponges and small coils placed distally in each splenic arterial branch (the double embolization technique), with care taken to spare vessels supplying the tail of the pancreas [*see Figure 17*]. More specifically, splenic artery embolization is performed through a 5 French catheter (typically a cobra catheter, though sidewinder and various other types are also used) inserted into the right groin with the patient under local anesthesia. The catheter tip is placed in the splenic artery and advanced to the splenic hilum proximal to the left gastroepiploic artery (or the great pancreatic artery) so that distal pancreatic branches of the splenic artery can be observed. At this level, either iohexol 65% or iothalamate 60% is forcefully injected and a digital substraction angiogram done to verify the pattern of the splenic blood supply.

If no pancreatic branches are opacified, there are several techniques that may be used. In particular, 3 to 5 mm microcoils are placed in the hilar branches of the splenic artery; alternatively, absorbable gelatin sponges are used. The catheter is then pulled back 2 to 4 cm, and one or two 5 to 8 mm microcoils are launched into the main trunk of the splenic artery distal to the great pancreatic artery to prevent pancreatitis or pancreatic necrosis. The surgical plane of dissection is therefore situated between the proximal and distal embolization sites.

The procedure is ended when it is estimated radiologically that 80% or more of the splenic tissue has been successfully embolized.

In most cases, successful embolization is achieved with both proximal and distal emboli; in a minority of cases, it is achieved with proximal emboli alone or with distal emboli alone.[28]

Troubleshooting Preoperative splenic artery embolization is safe, provided that two main principles are adhered to. First, embolization must be done distal to the great pancreatic artery to minimize pancreatic damage. Second, neither microspheres nor absorbable gelatin powder should be used, because particles of this small size may migrate to unintended target organ capillaries and cause tissue necrosis; only coils and absorbable gelatin sponge fragments should be used. If these precautions are taken, embolization is safe and remains a useful tool for difficult cases.

Postoperative Care

Postoperative care for patients who have undergone laparoscopic splenectomy is usually simple. The nasogastric tube inserted after induction of general anesthesia is removed either in the recovery room, once stomach emptying has been verified, or the next morning, depending on the duration and the degree of technical difficulty of the procedure. The urinary catheter is usually removed before the patient leaves the recovery room. The patient is allowed to drink clear fluids on the morning after the operation; when clear fluids are well tolerated, the patient is allowed to proceed to a diet of his or her choice.

If the patient has no history of ulcer or dyspepsia, a 100 mg indomethacin suppository is inserted before induction of anesthesia and again every 12 hours for a total of three to five doses. Postoperative pain medication is given on an individualized basis with a view to ensuring complete patient comfort. Meperidine injections (1 mg/kg) are administered during the first night, followed by oral acetaminophen (1 g every 6 hours). If pain is not well controlled, coanalgesia with an NSAID is added; this combination produces the best results. Because of its side effects (i.e., nausea, vomiting, abdominal fullness, and constipation), codeine is currently avoided if at all possible. When indomethacin is used, prophylactic doses of subcutaneous heparin are avoided on empirical grounds, especially if the platelet count is low or platelet function is abnormal.

Patients receiving I.V. cortisone are given oral steroids on postoperative day 1 after an overlap I.V. injection; thereafter, steroids are gradually tapered. Patients are allowed to shower 48 hours after surgery and are advised to keep the paper strips covering the trocar incisions in place for 7 to 10 days. No drains are used. No limitations are imposed on physical activity, and patients are allowed to tailor their activities to their degree of asthenia or discomfort.

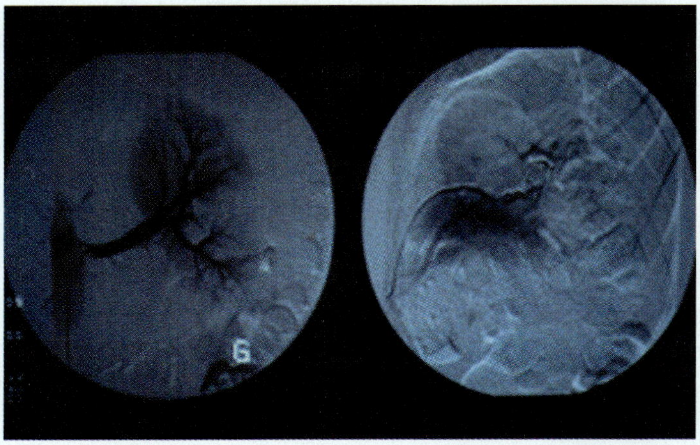

Complications

Postoperative complications directly related to splenectomy include intraoperative and postoperative hemorrhage; left lower lobe atelectasis and pneumonia; left pleural effusion; subphrenic collection; iatrogenic pancreatic, gastric, and colonic injury; and venous thrombosis.[24-31]

Successful laparoscopic splenectomy depends to a large extent on proper preparation. Recognition of anatomic elements and their arrangement is paramount. As with other laparoscopic procedures, the keys are avoiding complications and minimizing technical misadventures. Vascular structures should be cleanly isolated and dissected from surrounding fat; they then can usually be controlled with two clips proximally and distally. Staplers should be used with care and should not be applied blindly. The stapler tip should be clearly seen to be free of tissue before it is closed; otherwise, hemorrhage from partial section of a major splenic branch might occur after the instrument is released. Blind application of the stapler may also result in damage to the tail of the pancreas, which often lies in close proximity to the inner surface of the spleen. If both clips and a linear stapler are used, it is vital to prevent interposition of clips in the staple line, which will cause the stapler to misfire and possibly to jam.

Improper use of the electrocautery during the procedure can cause iatrogenic injury to the stomach, the colon, or the pancreas. In a smoke-filled environment, where controlling vessels is difficult and time consuming, blind fulguration of fat in the hilum can lead to bleeding. Structures close to the lower pole in the gastrocolic ligament can be approached more aggressively, but not those in the hilum. To prevent arcing and spot necrosis, which may result in delayed perforation and sepsis, the instrument should be activated only in proximity to the target organ.

The assistants also play an important role in preventing complications. All instruments, including those handled by assistants, should be moved under direct vision. Especially in the anterior approach, retraction of the liver and stomach and elevation of the spleen require constant concentration if lacerations and subsequent hemorrhage or perforation are to be avoided.

Special Considerations

EXTRACTION OF SPECIMENS

Spleens removed via the anterior approach are extracted through the umbilical trocar site after finger fragmentation in a plastic bag. It is rarely necessary to enlarge the umbilical incision to more than 2 or 3 cm. When the lateral approach is used, extraction is more easily performed through one of the ports situated anteriorly. This extraction site also requires little or no enlargement. On occasion, for a spleen longer than 20 cm, a 7.5 to 10 cm Pfannenstiel incision is made, and the operator's forearm is introduced into the abdomen to deliver the spleen into the pelvis for extraction in large fragments under direct vision. Pneumatic sleeves may also be used to facilitate hand-assisted surgery. The abdomen is copiously irrigated before closure.

Special mention should be made of laparoscopic splenectomy in patients with malignant disease. If lymphoma or Hodgkin disease is suspected, neither preoperative splenic artery embolization nor finger fragmentation in a plastic bag should be performed, for fear of

Figure 17 Laparoscopic splenectomy: splenic artery embolization. Shown are splenic angiograms of a patient with thrombotic thrombocytopenic purpura before (left) and after (right) splenic artery embolization with 3 cm, 5 cm, and 7 cm coils and absorbable gelatin sponge fragments.

making the histologic diagnosis difficult. Extraction of intact spleens through a small left subcostal or median incision has also been employed when preservation of tissue architecture is required. The various techniques of fragmentation and extraction of splenic tissue during laparoscopic splenectomy should be discussed and agreed on with the pathologist ahead of time to ensure that proper pathologic diagnoses are not compromised by either necrotic tissue (in the case of preoperative splenic artery embolization) or altered tissue architecture (in the case of finger fragmentation), especially if malignancy is suspected but not proven. In practice, however, we have found that the diagnosis is made preoperatively in more than 90% of patients with benign and malignant hematologic disease; hence, the issue rarely arises.

MASSIVE SPLENOMEGALY AND MEGASPLEENS

Massive splenomegaly is defined as the presence of a spleen with an interpole length exceeding 20 cm on ultrasonography or a weight exceeding 1,000 g. Laparoscopic removal of spleens of this size is fraught with problems, mostly related to the size of the organ and its components. Large spleens, besides being heavy and hard to manipulate, carry a high risk of serious hemorrhage. Consequently, preoperative splenic artery embolization is sometimes done beforehand because it helps control arterial flow preoperatively. If embolization is performed long enough before operation, it may even be possible to control the venous side of the blood supply through retrograde thrombosis; that blood clots are occasionally expelled from sections of splenic veins during laparoscopic splenectomy attests to the occurrence of this phenomenon. Finding a sensible way to retrieve the specimen also presents an important challenge.

When a spleen longer than 20 cm is to be removed, some modifications must be made to the technique of laparoscopic splenectomy. Once sectioning of the vessels and the suspensory ligaments is complete, a 7.5 to 10 cm Pfannenstiel incision is made at the pubic hairline. Through this incision, hand revision of the operative site under laparoscopic control can be accomplished, and if necessary, any remaining vessels or ligamentous attachments can be sectioned under video control. Adequate pneumoperitoneum can be maintained with the forearm placed through the lower abdominal incision. Whenever possible, the spleen is placed in a plastic bag; however, to date, we have not been able to bag a spleen longer than 24 cm.

That extraction of a very large specimen requires fragmentation of the spleen in the pelvis and extraction through a Pfannenstiel incision raises the possibility of postoperative splenosis. To minimize this problem, after reconstitution of the pneumoperitoneum, the abdomen is copiously irrigated and reviewed for fragments of spleen and accessory spleens, which can be done very thoroughly with laparoscopy.[32]

For a long time, we had no success with laparoscopic splenectomy for spleens longer than 30 cm (i.e., megaspleens): our conversion rate was 100%. Currently, we use preoperative embolization for these spleens. We also take the anterior approach, using five trocars, and are experimenting with a technique for subcapsular volume reduction with a sharp beveled 10 mm suction cannula connected to a powerful –70 mm Hg aspirator. Megaspleens are next to impossible to move with laparoscopic instruments, and the space constraints make our usual laparoscopic approaches futile. We therefore insert the –70 mm Hg aspirating cannula into the spleen and proceed to reduce the splenic volume so that the spleen can be sectioned into more manageable pieces that can be bagged and extracted in the usual fashion. At present, it is too early to tell whether laparoscopic splenectomy will have a place in the management of megaspleens.

Outcome Evaluation

No randomized, prospective trials comparing open splenectomy with laparoscopic splenectomy have yet been conducted. At present, such trials are unlikely to be held, for a variety of reasons. For one thing, randomization is difficult with procedures that are still in evolution. At one end of the spectrum, laparoscopic splenectomy is done for patients with ITP, who usually are relatively healthy and have normal-size spleens. In many of these patients, needlescopic instruments (< 3 mm) can be used in conjunction with a single 12 mm port site in the umbilicus. This approach permits hospital discharge within 24 hours of operation in a significant number of cases. At the other end of the spectrum, laparoscopic splenectomy is done for patients with myeloid metaplasia and spleens longer than 30 cm. In this setting, a laparoscopic approach poses formidable challenges, and the optimal technique and its justification remain to be determined. The window of opportunity for randomized comparative trials may have been lost.

Large case series and nonrandomized comparative trials, however, have consistently reported better outcomes from laparoscopic splenectomy than from open splenectomy.[33-40] For example, in one set of 528 patients [see Table 2],[35-38] the rate of postoperative pneumonia was 1.1% (6/528), and no subphrenic abscesses occurred as postoperative complications. Many surgeons who have completed the learning curve associated with the procedure feel that there is still room for improvement regarding complication rates and length of stay for pa-

Table 2 Clinical Results of Laparoscopic Splenectomy

Authors	N	ITP/Non-ITP	Conversion Rate (%)	OR Time (min)	Morbidity (%)	Mortality (%)	Length of Stay (days)	Accessory Spleen Present (%)
All diagnoses								
Katkhouda et al (1998)[37]	103	67/36	3.9	161	6	0	2.5	16.5
Targarona et al (2000)[35]	122	54/68	7.4	153	18	0	4.0	12
Park et al (2000)[36]	203	129/74	3.0	145	9	0.5	2.7	12.3
Poulin et al (2001)[38]	100	50/50	8.0	180	15	4	3.0	25
ITP								
Trias et al (2000)[39]	48	—	4.2	142	12	N/A	4.0	11
Poulin et al (2001)[38]	51	—	3.9	160	5.9	0	2.0	32
Malignancy								
Schlachta et al (1999)[40]	14	—	21	239	18	9	3.0	—
Trias et al (2000)[39]	28	—	14*	171	28	N/A	5.5	—

*71% required accessory incision because of spleen size.

tients with ITP and other relatively benign conditions necessitating laparoscopic splenectomy. The more serious conditions and the mortality seen in conjunction with the procedure tend to occur in patients with advanced hematologic malignancies or mega-spleens. In such cases, most of the adverse results are related to the disease state rather than to the operation, and it remains to be seen whether laparoscopic splenectomy will have a positive effect on outcome.

One of the great attractions of minimally invasive surgery has been the prospect of significant cost reductions. At this early point in the development of laparoscopic splenectomy, however, we are reluctant to place too much trust in premature cost analyses that do not take into account the "work in progress" nature of minimally invasive surgery. Most surgeons can now perform most cases of laparoscopic splenectomy with simplified trays of reusable instruments. Our basic laparoscopic tray contains a few instruments and two sizes of reusable clip appliers with inexpensive clips. As noted [see Operative Technique, above], clips are used for distributed-type spleens, single-use linear staplers mostly for magistral-type spleens. To reduce costs, ultrasonic dissectors are rarely used. In addition, the use of commercially available freezer bags instead of laparoscopic retrieval bags further reduces the cost of specimen extraction. Finally, even if intraoperative costs are higher with laparoscopic splenectomy, our experience is that the increase is offset by reductions in postoperative stay.

We, like most authorities, believe that as a surgeon gains experience with laparoscopic splenectomy, operating time tends to fall until it approaches that of open splenectomy. We also concur with many authors who have suggested that once laparoscopic splenectomy is mastered, use of blood products tends to decrease substantially.

References

1. Cole F: Is splenectomy harmless? Surg Gynecol Obstet 133:98, 1971
2. Johnston GB: Splenectomy. Ann Surg 48:50, 1908
3. Campos Cristo M: Segmental resections of the spleen: report on the first eight cases operated on. O Hosp (Rio) 62:205, 1962
4. Upadhyaya P, Simpson JS: Splenic trauma in children. Surg Gynecol Obstet 126:781, 1968
5. Delaitre B, Maignien B: Splénectomie par voie laparoscopique, 1 observation. Presse Médicale 20:2263, 1991
6. Carroll BJ, Phillips EH, Semel CJ, et al: Laparoscopic splenectomy. Surg Endosc 6:183, 1992
7. Thibault C, Mamazza J, Létourneau R, et al: Laparoscopic splenectomy: operative technique and preliminary report. Surg Laparosc Endosc 2:248, 1992
8. Poulin EC, Thibault C, DesCôteaux JG, et al: Partial laparoscopic splenectomy for trauma: technique and case report. Surg Laparosc Endosc 5:306, 1995
9. Seshadri PA, Poulin EC, Mamazza J, et al: Technique for laparoscopic partial splenectomy. Surg Laparosc Endosc 10:106, 2000
10. Goerg C, Schwerk WB, Goerg K, et al: Sonographic patterns of the affected spleen in malignant lymphoma. J Clin Ultrasound 18:569, 1990
11. Poulin EC, Thibault C: The anatomical basis for laparoscopic splenectomy. Can J Surg 36:485, 1993
12. Michels NA: The variational anatomy of the spleen and splenic artery. Am J Anat 70:21, 1942
13. Testut L: Traité d'anatomie humaine, 7th ed. Librairie Octave Doin, Paris, 1923, p 942
14. Lipshutz B: A composite study of the coeliac axis artery. Ann Surg 65:159, 1917
15. Henschen C: Die chirurgische Anatomie der Milzgefüsse. Schweiz Med Wochenschr 58:164, 1928
16. Ssoson-Jaroschewitsch A: Zür chirurgischen Anatomie des Milzhilus. Zeitsch f. d. ges. Anat I Abt 84:218, 1937
17. Baronofsky ID, Walton W, Noble JF: Occult injury to the pancreas following splenectomy. Surgery 29:852, 1951
18. Gagner M, Lacroix A, Bolte E, et al: Laparoscopic adrenalectomy: the importance of a flank approach in the lateral decubitus position. Surg Endosc 8:135, 1994
19. Gigot JF, Jamar F, Ferrant A, et al: Inadequate detection of accessory spleens and splenosis with laparoscopic splenectomy: a shortcoming of the laparoscopic approach in hematologic diseases. Surg Endosc 12:101, 1998
20. Nielsen JL, Ellegard J, Marqversen J, et al: Detection of splenosis and ectopic spleens with 99mTc-labeled heat damaged autologous erythrocytes in 90 splenectomized patients. Scand J Haematol 27:51, 1981
21. Pachter HL, Hofstetter SR, Elkowitz A, et al: Traumatic cysts of the spleen: the role of cystectomy and splenic preservation: experience with seven consecutive patients. J Trauma 35:430, 1993
22. Guzetta PC, Ruley EJ, Merrick HFW, et al: Elective subtotal splenectomy: indications and results in 33 patients. Ann Surg 211:34, 1990
23. Hoeckstra HJ, Tamminga RY, Timens W: Partial instead of complete splenectomy in children for the pathological staging of Hodgkin's disease. Ned Tijdschr Geneeskd 137:2491, 1993
24. Sheldon GF, Croom RD, Meyer AA: The spleen. Textbook of Surgery, 14th ed. Sabiston DC, Ed. WB Saunders Co, Philadelphia, 1991, p 1108
25. Jalovec LM, Boe BS, Wyffels PL: The advantages of early operation with splenorrhaphy versus nonoperative management for the blunt splenic trauma patient. Am Surg 59:698, 1993
26. Mozes MF, Spigos DG, Pollak R, et al: Partial splenic embolization, an alternative to splenectomy: results of a prospective randomized study. Surgery 96:694, 1984
27. Poulin E, Thibault C, Mamazza J, et al: Laparoscopic splenectomy: clinical experience and the role of preoperative splenic artery embolization. Surg Laparosc Endosc 3:445, 1993
28. Poulin EC, Mamazza J, Schlachta CM: Splenic artery embolization before laparoscopic splenectomy: an update. Surg Endosc 12:870, 1998
29. Hoeffer RA, Scullin DC, Silver LF, et al: Splenectomy for hematologic disorders: a 20 year experience. J Ky Med Assoc 89:446, 1991
30. Ly B, Albrechtson D: Therapeutic splenectomy in hematologic disorders. Effects and complications in 221 adult patients Acta Med Scand 209:21, 1981
31. Macrae HM, Yakimets WW, Reynolds T: Perioperative complications of splenectomy for hematologic disease. Can J Surg 35:432, 1992
32. Poulin EC, Thibault C: Laparoscopic splenectomy for massive splenomegaly: operative technique and case report. Can J Surg 38:69, 1995
33. Poulin EC, Mamazza J: Laparoscopic splenectomy: lessons from the learning curve. Can J Surg 41:28, 1998
34. Cathode N, Hurwitz MB, Rivera RT, et al: Laparoscopic splenectomy: outcome and efficacy in 103 consecutive patients. Ann Surg 228:568, 1998
35. Targarona EM, Espert JJ, Bombuy E, et al: Complications of laparoscopic splenectomy. Arch Surg 135:1137, 2000
36. Park AE, Birgisson G, Mastrangelo MJ, et al: Laparoscopic splenectomy: outcomes and lessons learned from over 200 cases. Surgery 128:660, 2000
37. Katkhouda N, Hurwitz MB, Rivera RT, et al: Laparoscopic splenectomy: outcome and efficacy in 103 consecutive patients. Ann Surg 228:568, 1998
38. Poulin EC, Schlachta CM, Mamazza J: Unpublished data, February 2001
39. Trias M, Targarona EM, Espert JJ, et al: Impact of hematological diagnosis on early and late outcome after laparoscopic splenectomy: an analysis of 111 cases. Surg Endosc 14:556, 2000
40. Schlachta CM, Poulin EC, Mamazza J: Laparoscopic splenectomy for hematologic malignancies. Surg Endosc 13:865, 1999

Acknowledgment

Figures 1, 3, 4, 6a, and 15   Tom Moore.

55 INTESTINAL ANASTOMOSIS

Zane Cohen, M.D., and Barry Sullivan, M.D.

Intestinal anastomosis is one of the most commonly performed intra-abdominal procedures [see *Sidebar* Intestinal Anastomosis: Historical Perspective]. It is required to reestablish gastrointestinal continuity after surgical resection, traumatic disruption, or bypass procedures. There are several principles that are crucial for obtaining successful results [see Table 1]. Of these, surgical technique is widely regarded as the most important for maintaining anastomotic integrity, given that intersurgeon rates of anastomotic breakdown vary by as much as a factor of 60.[1] Anastomotic leakage greatly increases the morbidity and mortality associated with surgical procedures. It has been shown to double the length of hospital stay and increase the chance of dying threefold to 10-fold.[2] Dehiscence, when it occurs, has been associated with one fifth to one third of all postoperative deaths in patients who underwent intestinal anastomosis.[3] Reported leakage rates range from 1.5 percent[4] to 2.2 percent,[5] depending on the type of anastomosis performed and the clinical scenario (i.e., elective or emergency).

Unfortunately, anastomotic dehiscence can occur even in ideal circumstances. This unwelcome fact has stimulated a great deal of debate regarding the reliability of various methods and approaches. In what follows, we address certain fundamental technical issues in the performance of an intestinal anastomosis and attempt to summarize what is known about how these issues relate to the reliability of various anastomotic techniques. We also describe our own approach to performing certain of these procedures [see Operative Technique for Selected Anastomoses, *below*].

Intestinal Anastomotic Healing

The process of intestinal anastomotic healing mimics that of wound healing elsewhere in the body in that it can be arbitrarily divided into an acute inflammatory (lag) phase, a proliferative phase, and, finally, a remodeling or maturation phase. As Halsted[6] demonstrated, most of the bowel wall's strength is provided by the collagenous connective tissue layer in the submucosa [see Figure 1]. Collagen is thus the single most important molecule for determining intestinal strength, which makes its metabolism of particular interest for understanding anastomotic healing.

Collagen is secreted from fibroblasts in a monomeric form called tropocollagen; this is a large stiff molecule that can be visualized by electron microscopy. Collagen itself can be divided into subtypes on the basis of differences in composition (i.e., different combinations of α_1 and α_2 chains). Type I predominates in mature organisms; type II is found primarily in cartilage; and type III is associated with type I in remodeling tissue and in elastic tissues such as the aorta, the esophagus, and the uterus. Synthesis of collagen is an intracellular process that occurs on polysomes. A critical stage in collagen formation is the hydroxylation of proline to produce hydroxyproline; this process is believed to be important for maintaining the three-dimensional triple-helix conformation of mature collagen, which gives the molecule its structural strength. The amount of collagen found in a tissue is indirectly determined by measuring the amount of hydroxyproline, although no significant statistical correlation between hydroxyproline content and objective measurements of anastomotic strength has ever been demonstrated.[7] Vitamin C deficiency results in impaired hydroxylation of proline and the accumulation of proline-rich, hydroxyproline-poor molecules in intracellular vacuoles.

The degree of fiber and fibril cross-linking relates to the maturity of the collagen and is probably important in determining the overall strength of the scar tissue. Of equal importance is the orientation of the fibers and their weave. The bursting pressure of anastomoses has often been used to gauge the strength of the healing process. This pressure has been found to increase rapidly in the early postoperative period, reaching 60 percent of the strength of the surrounding bowel by three to four days and 100 percent by one week.[8,9]

Collagen synthesis is a dynamic process that is dependent on the balance between synthesis and collagenolysis. Degradation of mature collagen begins in the first 24 hours and predominates for the first four days. By one week, collagen synthesis is the dominant force, particularly proximal to the anastomosis. After five to six weeks, there is no significant increase in the amount of collagen in a healing wound or anastomosis, though turnover and thus synthesis are extensive. The strength of the scar continues to increase for many months after injury. Local infection increases collagenase activity and reduces levels of circulating collagenase inhibitors.[10,11]

Collagen synthetic capacity is relatively uniform throughout the large bowel but less so in the small intestine: synthesis is significantly higher in the proximal and distal small intestine than in the midjejunum. Overall collagen synthetic capacity is somewhat less in the small intestine. Although no significant difference has been found between the strength of ileal anastomoses and that of colonic anastomoses at four days, colonic collagen formation is much greater in the first 48 hours.[12] It is noteworthy that the synthetic response is not restricted to the anastomotic site but appears to be generalized to a significant extent.[13]

Factors Influencing Incidence of Anastomotic Breakdown

ASSOCIATED DISEASES AND SYSTEMIC FACTORS

Resections for Crohn's disease appear to carry a significant risk of anastomotic dehiscence (12 percent in one prospective study[5]) even when macroscopically normal margins are obtained. Strictureplasty has therefore become an attractive alternative to resectional management of Crohn's disease even in the presence of moderately long strictures, diseased tissue, or sites of previous anastomoses.

The glucocorticoid response to injury may attenuate physio-

Intestinal Anastomosis: Historical Perspective

Intestinal anastomosis has a long history. Hippocrates is known to have referred to intestinal suturing as early as 460 B.C., and Celsus is reported to have written about using the glover's stitch to suture colonic perforations and close intestinal fistulas between 30 B.C. and 30 A.D.[73] In the second century, Galen, probably the most influential physician of the time, took a different view, opposing intestinal anastomosis because of the significant risks of stricture and subsequent obstruction. Unfortunately, this view prevailed throughout most of Europe during the Dark Ages. Toward the end of the first millennium, Abulkasim of the Muslim school was experimenting with the so-called ant closure, in which the pincers of ants were allowed to grasp the two intestinal edges to be joined and bring the edges together; the bodies of the ants were then pinched off, and the subsequent spasm of the pincers kept the edges apposed. This closure is considered by many to be the forerunner of the Michel clip, which was developed later in France. Abulkasim also experimented with the glover's stitch for closing enterotomies, using sheep-gut filaments as sutures.

In the 11th century, the School of Salerne was founded by the so-called Four Masters. These physicians reviewed the principles of Hippocrates and Celsus regarding closure of intestinal injuries, maintenance of aseptic technique, and wound closure. They devised a method of closure that made use of a variety of stents to prevent the stricture so feared by Galen. These stents were made of a number of different materials, including elder wood and goose trachea. The Four Masters were also the first to use interrupted sutures as opposed to the glover's stitch. This new practice reduced the incidence of stricture further and, coupled with the use of stents, caused less narrowing of the intestinal lumen. The sutures themselves were not tied; in fact, they were brought out through the skin to be removed once healing had been achieved.

The Four Masters greatly influenced a contemporary group of Benedictine monks, who used dried animal intestine as the stent of choice along with removable sutures. The Four Monks closure, as it became known, was practiced throughout many parts of Europe for nearly a century. In the 12th century, however, Papal ordinances forbade members of the clergy to perform surgical procedures on the grounds that doing so distracted them from ministering to the souls of their flocks. As a result, the somewhat less well educated barbers became the practitioners of surgery. This development was accompanied by a return to Galenic principles, including the use of the running glover's stitch. The high incidence of leakage and obstruction that resulted soon led the barbers to abandon intestinal procedures, except for repair of partial transverse or colonic wounds. Attempts were made to close bowel injuries and to approximate the repaired area to the abdominal wall or to other organs with the goal of imitating natural adhesion formation. In the 1700s, Palfyn and Peyronie brought the closed intestinal injury out into the wound so that if primary healing failed to occur, an enterocutaneous fistula would develop; this was the first description of a rudimentary stoma. Verduc and von de Wyl carried this principle to its logical conclusion and developed the so-called artificial anus for use in cases of complete transection. In 1730, Ramdohr intussuscepted one segment of bowel into another, fixing it in place with a single transfixing suture. The resultant mucosa-to-serosa coaptation healed poorly and exhibited a high leakage rate.

Stoma formation and stenting with removable sutures followed by approximation to the abdominal wound remained the standards of care until as recently as the 19th century, when Larrey first described his attempts at a two-layer anastomosis. These attempts were followed closely by Travers's description in 1812 of an agglutination substance that was necessary to approximate the wounded intestinal edges. Meanwhile, Bell was experimenting with the baseball stitch and a tallow plug stent that was ultimately melted by body heat, and Lembert at the Charité de Paris was describing the use of interrupted inverting sutures to obtain serosa-to-serosa apposition. Lembert used fine-caliber silk sutures that incorporated all layers except the mucosa and were left in situ. An interesting historical note is that another French surgeon, Jobert, had actually described a full-thickness interrupted inverting stitch for intestinal anastomoses two years earlier, but he was not nearly as vocal a proponent of his approach as Lembert was of his. Many other surgeons were experimenting with different methods of closure throughout the 19th century. For example, Henroz described a self-securing system of metallic rings that was the precursor of the modern Murphy's button or Valtrac system, and Wolfer described a secure two-layer interrupted method of anastomosis.

---

logic responses to other mediators whose combined effects could be deleterious to the organism.[14] In animal experiments, wound healing, as measured by bursting pressure of an ileal anastomosis one week after operation, was strongly influenced by the maintenance level of corticosterone.[15] Optimal healing occurred at a plasma corticosterone level that maintained maximal nitrogen balance and corresponded to the mean corticosterone level of normal animals. Both supranormal and subnormal cortisol levels resulted in significantly impaired wound healing, probably through different mechanisms. It is believed that slow protein turnover is responsible for delayed anastomotic healing in adrenalectomized animals,[16] whereas negative nitrogen metabolic balance is responsible for increased protein breakdown and delayed healing in animals with excess glucocorticoid activity.[15] Nonsteroidal anti-inflammatory drugs (NSAIDs) may help increase anastomotic bursting pressure by decreasing perianastomotic inflammation,[17,18] but this effect has not been well studied.

Systemic factors such as diabetes mellitus, anemia, vitamin deficiencies, malnutrition (hypoalbuminemia), exposure to ionizing radiation, and systemic chemotherapy all may influence the rate of anastomotic healing.

PATIENT PREPARATION

Patients must be fit and stable to maximize the chances that the intestinal anastomosis will heal uneventfully. Ideally, patients should be well nourished, should have a minimum of active intercurrent illness, and should receive adequate preoperative antibiotic prophylaxis steroid coverage as required [see 73 Adrenal Insufficiency], and bowel preparation.

At least two studies have suggested that mechanical bowel preparation may not be essential for successful healing.[19,20] In one of these, a series of 72 patients underwent elective colonic anastomosis without any mechanical bowel preparation and a single preoperative dose of intravenous antibiotics.[19] No anastomotic dehiscence was observed, nor were any differences in wound infection rates (8.3 percent) or overall mortality (2.7 per-

---

Table 1 **Principles of Successful Intestinal Anastomosis**

Well-nourished patient with no systemic illness
No fecal contamination, either within the gut or in the surrounding peritoneal cavity
Adequate exposure and access
Well-vascularized tissues
Absence of tension at the anastomosis
Meticulous technique

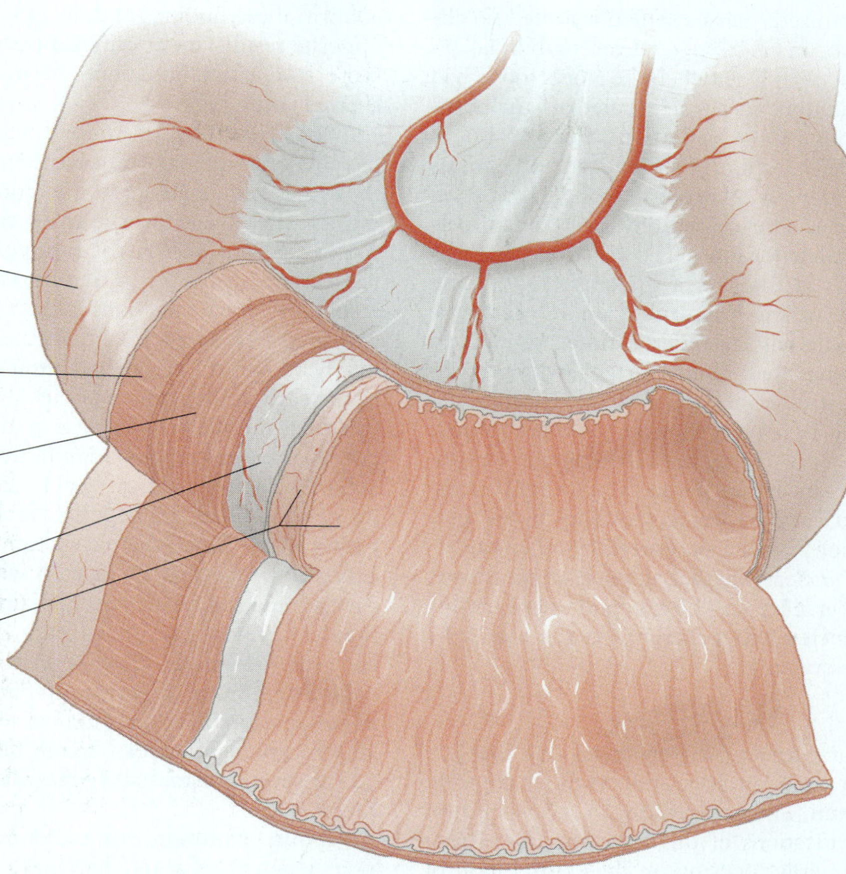

Figure 1 Shown are the tissue layers of the jejunum. Most of the bowel wall's strength is provided by the submucosa.

Labels: Serosa (Visceral Peritoneum); Longitudinal Muscle Layer; Circular Muscle Layer; Submucosa; Mucosa

cent) noted in comparison with published reports of series of patients who underwent full bowel preparation.

On the other hand, a 1989 study reported significantly increased anastomotic bursting pressure and reduced anastomotic dehiscence rates in dogs that underwent mechanical bowel cleansing before low anterior resection.[21] This observation was further supported by a study showing that increasing fecal loading impaired colonic anastomotic healing in rats and by one showing that adding oral erythromycin and kanamycin to bowel preparation led to significantly increased bursting pressure at seven days after operation.[22] In addition, a number of clinical series have been published in which inadequate bowel preparation clearly increased the incidence of anastomotic complications.[23,24]

At our institution, two bottles of Fleet enema are given at 9:00 A.M. and 7:00 P.M. on the day before operation. Patients receive only clear fluids for 24 hours before operation, remain on NPO status after midnight, and then receive tap water enemas on the morning of surgery (for colon and rectal procedures). Neomycin, 500 mg orally, and metronidazole, 500 mg orally, are given at 1:00 P.M., 2:00 P.M., and 10:00 P.M. on the day before operation, and routine I.V. antibiotic prophylaxis is provided on an on-call basis to the OR. Perioperative steroid coverage is important in those patients who may have adrenal suppression as a result of long-term or high-dose steroid therapy. Heparin is administered subcutaneously two hours before operation to all patients scheduled to undergo intestinal anastomosis.

TYPE AND LOCATION OF ANASTOMOSIS

As a rule, for any given technique, the location of the anastomosis seems not to influence the overall leakage rate. The one exception is low anterior anastomoses, which are associated with leakage rates ranging from 4.5 percent to an incredible 70 percent.[21,23]

Animal studies have demonstrated improved transmission of the intestinal migrating myoelectric complex (MMC) across hand-sewn end-to-end anastomoses in comparison with stapled or sewn side-to-side or end-to-side anastomoses or stapled functional end-to-end anastomoses.[25] This may be of importance to patients with diseases affecting small bowel motility.

Hand-Sewn versus Stapled Anastomoses

Stapled anastomoses are said to heal by primary intention, whereas sutured anastomoses are said to heal by secondary intention, though further experimentation is needed to confirm this distinction.[26] Titanium staples are ideal for tissue apposition at anastomotic sites because they provoke only a minimal inflammatory response and provide immediate strength to the cut surfaces during the weakest phase of healing. Initially, tissue eversion at the stapled anastomosis was a major concern, given that everted hand-sewn anastomoses had previously been shown to be inferior to inverted ones; however, the greater support and improved blood supply to the healing tissues associated with stapling tend to counteract the negative effects of eversion. In fact, one study found that bursting strength for canine colonic end-to-end anastomoses was six times greater when the procedure was performed with an end-to-end anastomosis (EEA) stapler than when it was done with hand-sewn interrupted Dacron sutures.[27] Another study demonstrated a significantly reduced radiographic anastomotic leakage rate with staples applied by an EEA stapler as opposed to a double layer of hand-sewn sutures.[28]

Various prospective randomized trials have demonstrated no differences in clinical and subclinical leakage rates, length of hospital stay, or overall morbidity.[29-31] Even when the anastomosis had to heal under adverse conditions (e.g., carcinomatosis, malnutrition, previous chemotherapy or radiation therapy, bowel obstruction, anemia, or leukopenia), no significant differences were apparent between stapled anastomoses and hand-sewn ones. Stapling did, however, shorten the time required to perform the procedure, especially for low pelvic anastomoses.

Cancer recurrence rates at the site of the anastomosis have been reported to be higher or lower depending on the technique used. Certainly, suture materials engender a more pronounced cellular proliferative response than titanium staples do, particularly with full-thickness sutures as opposed to seromuscular ones,[32] and malignant cells have been shown to adhere to suture materials.[33] One clinical report suggested that stapling anastomoses after resection for cancer can reduce anastomotic recurrence by 40 percent and cancer-specific mortality by 50 percent.[34] This finding has not yet been supported by other work.

At present, it remains unclear whether stapling or suturing is safer from an oncologic perspective. The exception is a very low rectal anastomosis, in which a better margin can sometimes be obtained through double-stapling.

Unusual Techniques

In 1892, Murphy[35] introduced a two-part metal stud that was designed to hold wound edges in apposition without suturing until adhesion had occurred. Thereafter, the stud was voided via the rectum. Several modifications of this technique have been described since then, primarily focusing on the composition of the rings or stents. In 1968, Hopcroft[36] described a casein prosthesis that ultimately dissolved under the influence of intestinal proteolytic enzymes. In 1977, Sognen and associates[37] described a mixture of gelatin and barium sulfate that was molded into a tubular stent for use in veterinary surgery. This structure was meant to provide a firm base for suturing and to shorten the time required for anastomosis; the purpose of the barium was to facilitate radiographic localization of the stent in the postoperative period. More recently, dissolvable polyglycolic acid systems have been developed. These so-called biofragmentable anastomotic rings leave a gap of 1.5, 2.0, or 2.5 mm between the bowel ends to prevent ischemia of the anastomotic line.

The use of adhesive agents such as methyl-2-cyanoacrylate to approximate the divided ends of intestinal segments has been studied.[38] There was only a moderate inflammatory response at the wound, which persisted for two to three weeks. Leakage rates were high, however, and many technical problems remained (e.g., how to stabilize the bowel edges while they underwent adhesion).

CONTROVERSIAL AREAS

The question of the importance of inversion (as described by Lembert in the early 1800s) versus eversion of the anastomotic line has been a controversial one. It has been argued that the traditional inverting methods ignore the basic principle of accurately opposing clean-cut tissues. Halsted,[6] in 1887, was the first to clearly demonstrate the importance of the submucosa as the strength layer of intestinal anastomoses. He initially proposed an interrupted extramucosal technique, which has since been assessed in retrospective[1] and prospective[5] reviews and found to have a low leakage rate (1.3 to 6.0 percent) in a wide variety of circumstances. A 1969 study reported greater anastomotic strength, less luminal narrowing, and less edema and inflammation in everted small intestinal anastomoses in dogs.[39] Subsequent laboratory and clinical studies have not been able to confirm these findings and, in fact, have often yielded quite the opposite results: lower bursting pressure,[40] slower healing,[41] and more severe inflammation[42] have all been associated with an everted suture line.

The advisability of routine nasogastric decompression in patients undergoing a procedure involving an intestinal anastomosis has remained somewhat controversial over the years. In retrospective[43] and prospective[44] randomized controlled trials, routine use of a nasogastric tube conferred no significant advantage. There was, in fact, a trend toward an increased incidence of respiratory tract infections in patients who underwent routine gastric decompression.[45] Nonetheless, one study found that nearly 20 percent of patients required insertion of a gastric tube in the early postoperative period.[44] We no longer place nasogastric tubes routinely; however, it is still important to be alert to the potential for gastric dilatation in these patients.

There has been a great deal of controversy regarding the ability of abdominal drainage to "protect" the anastomosis. Even before World War I, the old dictum "when in doubt, drain" was called into question by Yates,[46] who wrote that the peritoneal cavity could not be effectively drained because of adhesions and rapid sealing of the drain tract. Six decades later, one study showed a dramatic increase in the incidence of anastomotic dehiscence (from 15 percent to 55 percent) after the placement of perianastomotic drains in dogs.[47] This increase was associated with a significant increase in mortality. Yet another study reported the severe inflammatory reaction caused by drains at anastomoses.[48]

At our institution, intra-abdominal drains are occasionally used when it appears that there is a specific area (e.g., the pelvis) where there is a higher than usual risk that a fluid collection will develop (e.g., after a very low anterior resection or a coloanal anastomosis without diversion). Rectal tubes are commonly employed after subtotal colectomy for acute colitis and after two-stage pelvic pouch procedures.

Hand-Sewn Sutures: Technical Issues

CHOICE OF SUTURE MATERIAL

Sutures act as foreign bodies in the anastomosis and thus produce an inflammatory reaction.[7] One study that examined the relative efficiency of absorbable and nonabsorbable material concluded that the strength of the anastomosis, expressed as a percentage of normal tissue strength, was essentially the same regardless of the type of suture used. Other studies that examined the amount of inflammation induced at the anastomosis by various types of sutures found that polypropylene (Prolene), catgut, and polyglycolic acid (Dexon) were equivalent in this regard.[49,50] Silk, however, produced a significantly greater cellular reaction at the anastomosis, and the reaction persisted for as long as six weeks.[50] A 1975 study reported on a series of 41 patients who underwent low anterior resection involving a primary side-to-end colorectal anastomosis with 5-0 stainless steel wire.[51] The investigators believed that this material was ideal because of its strength and relative inertness within the tissues and supported their claims with a relatively low clinical leakage rate (7.3 percent).

The ideal suture material—one that causes minimal inflammation and tissue reaction while providing maximum strength during the lag phase of wound healing—has not yet been discovered. Clearly, however, monofilament and coated braided sutures represent an advance over silk and other multifilament materials.

CONTINUOUS SUTURES VERSUS INTERRUPTED SUTURES

Both continuous and interrupted sutures are commonly used in fashioning intestinal anastomoses [see Figure 2]. No randomized trials have addressed the question of whether interrupted sutures have a significant advantage over continuous sutures in a single-layer anastomosis; however, retrospective reviews have not revealed any such advantage.[52-54] Animal studies, on the other hand, have found that perianastomotic tissue oxygen tension was significantly less with continuous sutures than with interrupted sutures.[55] This finding was correlated with an increased anastomotic complication rate and impaired collagen synthesis and healing in a rat model.[56]

SINGLE-LAYER ANASTOMOSES VERSUS DOUBLE-LAYER ANASTOMOSES

Double-layer anastomoses were described in the literature before single-layer ones. They are fairly uniform and consist of an inner layer of continuous or interrupted absorbable sutures and an outer layer of interrupted absorbable or nonabsorbable sutures [see Figure 3]. Traditionally, double-layer anastomoses have been considered more secure; however, for some time, single-layer anastomoses have been performed in difficult locations (e.g., low in the pelvis or high in the chest) or in difficult circumstances (e.g., in a patient who is unstable or has multiple intraabdominal injuries) with good results. Moreover, work from the 1980s suggests that the single-layer technique has significant inherent advantages.[56-59]

Double-layer anastomoses were long believed to be essential for safe healing of the wound; however, subsequent pathological analysis of these anastomoses revealed microscopic areas of necrosis and sloughing of the tissues incorporated in the inner layer as a result of strangulation.[60] Animal studies have confirmed that single-layer anastomoses take less time to create,[61] cause less narrowing of the intestinal lumen,[57-62] foster more rapid vascularization[56] and mucosal healing, and increase the strength of the anastomosis (as measured by the bursting pressure) in the first few postoperative days.[61] Nonetheless, although clinical studies have fairly consistently demonstrated that single-layer anastomoses are associated with improved postoperative return to normal bowel function (as measured by bowel sounds, passage of flatus, and return to oral intake),[42,63] nonrandomized studies of anastomotic leakage rates have not shown any differences between single- and double-layer anastomoses in this regard.[64-66]

Some authors still favor double-layer anastomoses when the tissues are very edematous or friable, are under minimal tension, or lie in highly vascular areas (e.g., the stomach). There are no data to indicate that this practice yields superior results.

Staples: Technical Issues

CHOICE OF STAPLER

Surgical stapling devices were first introduced in 1908 by Hültl. Besides the EEA stapler already mentioned, the types most commonly used are the gastrointestinal anastomosis (GIA) stapler and the transverse anastomosis (TA) stapler. Most stapling devices place two double staggered rows of B-shaped staples and can simultaneously cut between the rows. Staplers may be used to create functional (GIA plus TA) or true anatomic (EEA) end-to-end anastomoses as well as side-to-side anastomoses.

In a functional end-to-end anastomosis, two cut ends of bowel (either open or stapled closed) are placed side by side with their blind ends beside each other. A cutting linear stapler (GIA) is then used to fuse the two bowel walls into a single septum with two double staggered rows of staples and to create a lumen between the two bowel segments by dividing this septum between the rows. A noncutting linear stapler (TA) is then used to close the defect at the apex of the anastomosis. The cut and stapled edges of the bowel should be inspected for adequacy of hemostasis before the apex is closed. Some authors suggest cauterizing these edges to ensure hemostasis.[67] However, given that electrical current may be conducted along the metallic staple line to the rest of the bowel, it is probably easier and safer simply to underpin bleeding vessels with a fine absorbable suture. It is also important to offset the two inverted staple lines before closing the apex.[68]

True anatomic end-to-end stapled anastomoses may be fashioned with a linear stapler by triangulating the two cut ends, then firing the stapler three times in intersecting vectors to achieve complete closure [see Figure 4]. The creation of end-to-end anastomoses has been considerably facilitated by the development of the EEA stapler. This device places two double circular rows of staples from the inside of the intestinal lumen and cuts between them to create a directly apposed, inverted, stapled end-to-end anastomosis.

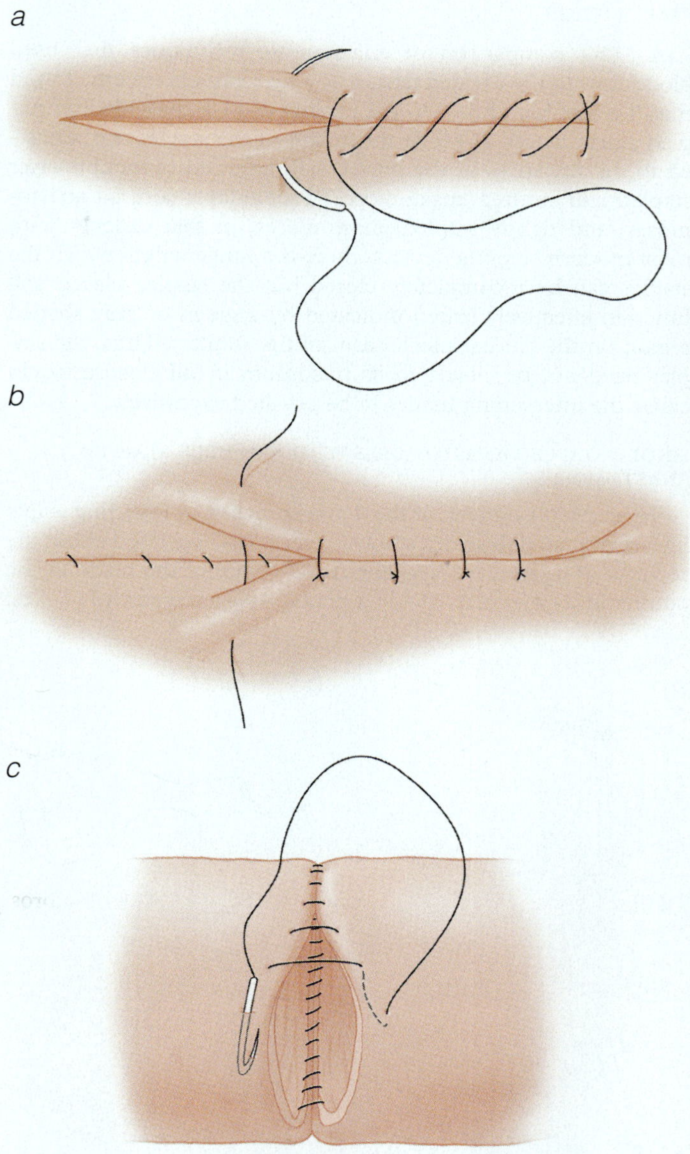

Figure 2 Shown are stitches commonly used in fashioning intestinal anastomoses: (*a*) the continuous over-and-over suture, (*b*) the interrupted Lembert suture, and (*c*) the Connell suture.

STAPLE HEIGHT

A 1987 comparison of anastomotic techniques that used blood flow to the divided tissues as a measure of outcome found that the best blood flow to the healing site was provided by stapled anastomoses in which the height of the staples was adjusted to the thickness of the bowel wall, followed by double-layer stapled and sutured anastomoses, double-layer sutured anastomoses, and tightly stapled anastomoses, in that order.[69] With most modern stapling devices, there is a range within which the stapler can be incompletely closed but the staples placed still function effectively (often indicated by a green or gray shaded region on the closing mechanism of the stapler). Thus, the stapler need not be closed to its maximum if full closure would cause the intervening tissues to be crushed excessively.

SINGLE-STAPLED ANASTOMOSES VERSUS DOUBLE-STAPLED ANASTOMOSES

To accomplish many of these anastomoses, intersecting staple lines are created. Initially, some concern was expressed about the security of these areas and about the ability of the blade in the cutting instruments to divide a double staggered row of staples. Subsequent animal studies, however, demonstrated that even though nearly all (> 90 percent) of the staple lines that were subsequently transected by a second staple line contained bent or cut staples, the integrity of the anastomosis was not compromised in any way, nor was its healing adversely affected.[29,70]

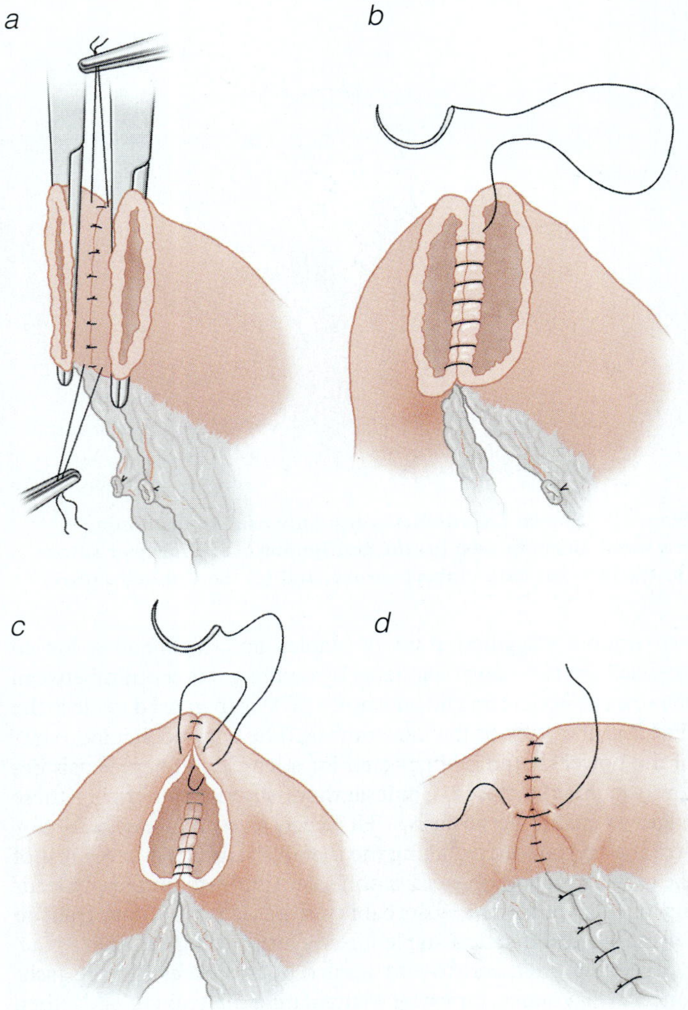

Operative Technique for Selected Anastomoses

In what follows, we describe our approach to several operative procedures involving intestinal anastomosis. These procedures are intended not as an exhaustive list but as a representative selection that illustrates the principles already discussed.

A general note about the cosmetic aspect of these procedures is appropriate here. After any of these operations, a close visual inspection of the entire circumference of the anastomosis should be performed. As a general principle, if the divided ends appear well opposed, then the anastomosis is probably sound.

INCISION AND EXPOSURE

Currently, most laparotomies are performed through a standard midline incision with the patient supine and level. Adequate exposure is obtained by ensuring that the skin incision is long enough and using retractors such as a Buchwalter or a Gibson/Balfour type. In procedures involving the small intestine, only the segment of bowel being worked on should be brought out of the abdomen into the operative field; the remainder should be kept warm and tension free inside the abdominal cavity. In colonic procedures, the small intestine may be packed into the left upper quadrant or the right flank region with a damp pack.

The small intestine is quite mobile, and it is rarely difficult to expose a given loop unless adhesions or other disease processes are tethering the bowel. Adequate mobility of the colon is obtained by incising the peritoneal reflection along the white line of Toldt, preferably with a coagulating electrocautery to maintain a bloodless field, and reflecting the retroperitoneal structures posteriorly. For a tension-free primary colonic anastomosis, the splenic and hepatic flexures often must be mobilized.

For rectal procedures, the patient should be placed in Allen stirrups in the lithotomy position. Care must be taken to position the legs and feet properly and secure them so as to prevent pressure points that could lead to ulcers, thrombosis, or neurapraxia. The legs should not be spread too widely or flexed excessively; however, if an EEA stapler is to be used, sufficient maneuvering room must be left between the stirrups. Placing the patient in a 30° Trendelenburg's position and packing the small bowel superiorly also help keep the operative field in the pelvis clear.

BOWEL RESECTION

The technique of bowel resection will not be reviewed in great detail here; a brief summary should suffice. (Colonic resection is covered extensively elsewhere [see 57 Colorectal Procedures].) Appropriate resection margins must be obtained to provide adequate clearance of the lesion or diseased segment. The most important consideration in this regard is the blood supply to the region in question; this is clearly more of an issue in colonic resections than in small bowel resections, given the ample vascular supply of the small bowel. The segment may be removed by first clearing away all mesenteric and serosal attachments with a coagulating electrocautery, then dividing the bowel proximally and distally with either a cutting linear stapler, a combination of a noncutting linear stapler and a crushing bowel clamp, or two

Figure 3 Double-layer end-to-end anastomosis. (*a*) Interrupted Lembert stitches are used to form the posterior outer layer. (*b*) A full-thickness continuous over-and-over stitch is used to form the posterior inner layer. (*c*) A Connell stitch is used to form the anterior inner layer. (*d*) Interrupted Lembert stitches are used to form the anterior outer layer.

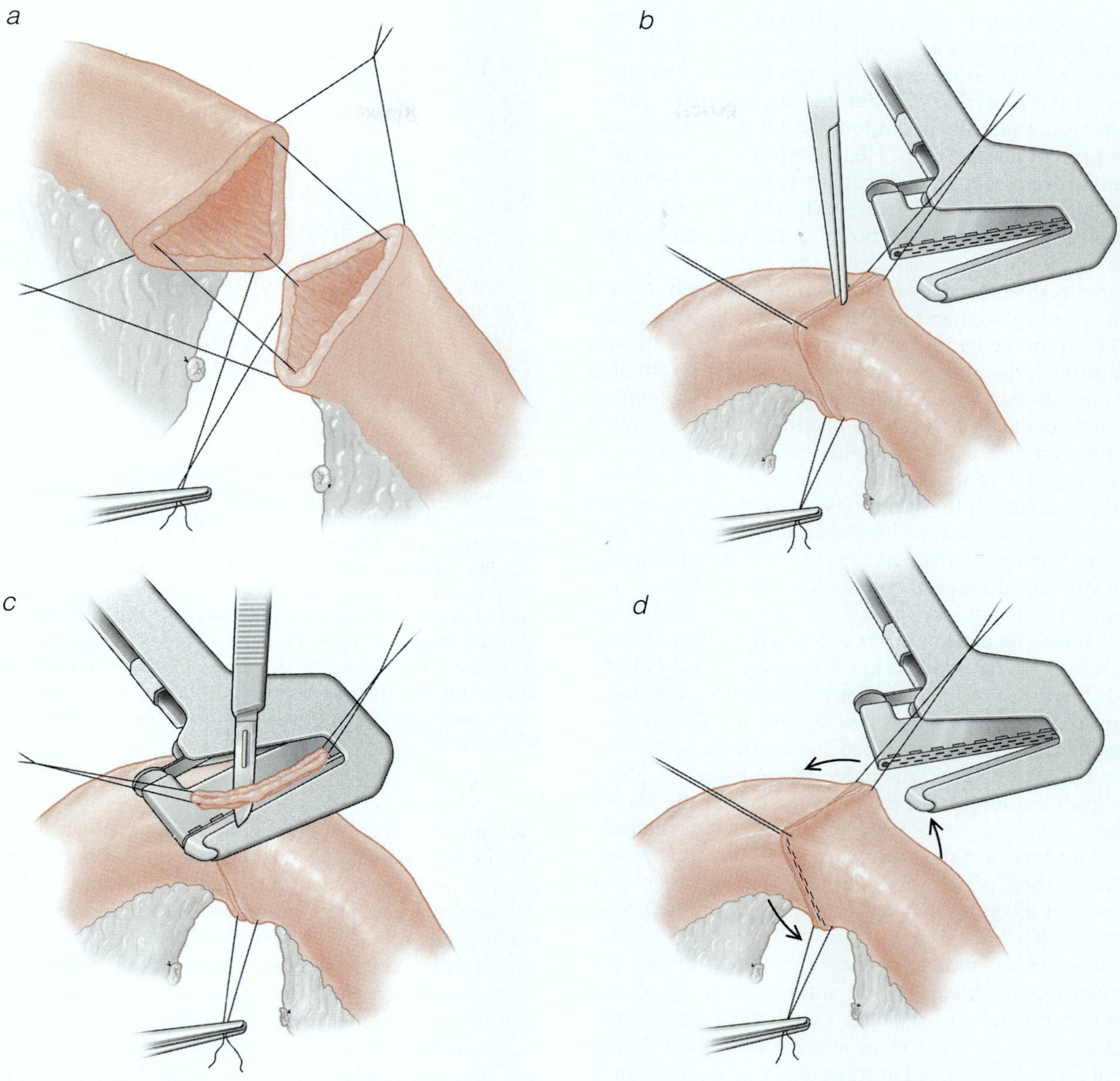

Figure 4 End-to-end anastomosis with linear noncutting stapler. (*a*) The bowel ends are triangulated with three traction sutures. (*b*) A noncutting linear stapler (TA) is placed between two of the sutures. (*c*) The stapler is closed and the excess tissue excised. (*d*) The bowel is rotated, and steps *b* and *c* are repeated twice more to close the remaining two sides of the triangle.

crushing bowel clamps and a knife or scissors. The tissue to be used for the anastomosis must be well vascularized, viable, and free of its fatty attachments. The pinch-burn technique is particularly useful in clearing the mesenteric attachments close to the bowel wall itself; ties often bunch tissues excessively, resulting in angulation or distortion of the free edge of the intestine. In the pelvis, an angulated noncutting linear stapler is often used to obtain as much length as possible distal to the lesion. The proximal rectum is clamped with a crushing bowel clamp, and a long knife is used to transect the rectum.

Special mention should be made of the technique of strictureplasty, which is used for a number of benign small bowel strictures (especially those resulting from Crohn's disease) as a means of avoiding small bowel resection and anastomoses. In this procedure, the bowel is opened longitudinally and closed transversely with a single layer of 2-0 polyglycolic acid sutures in a Connell stitch. Excellent functional results have been achieved with this technique.

SINGLE-LAYER SUTURED EXTRAMUCOSAL SIDE-TO-SIDE ENTEROENTEROSTOMY

A side-to-side small bowel anastomosis [*see Figure 5*] may be performed as a bypass procedure when no resection is done, when there is a discrepancy in the diameter of the two ends to be anastomosed, or when the anatomy is such that the most tension-free position for the anastomosis is with the two bowel segments parallel (as in a Finney strictureplasty). The operative field is exposed and prepared as described (see above). The bowel is milked of its contents, and noncrushing bowel clamps are placed proximal and distal to the site of anastomosis, with care taken not to impinge on the mesentery. The two loops in question must lie comfortably within the abdomen, without tension, and must be exposed in such a manner as to minimize or at least contain spillage of intestinal content if it occurs. The field is walled off with clean sponges or packs, and the loops are laid side by side.

Two stay sutures of 3-0 polyglycolic acid are placed approximately 3 in. apart on the inner aspect of the antimesenteric border. A 2 in. enterotomy is made on each loop with an electrocautery or a blade on the inner aspect of the antimesenteric border. If an electrocautery is used, care must be taken not to injure the mucosa of the posterior wall during this maneuver; placement of a hemostat into the enterotomy to lift the anterior wall will usually prevent this problem. Hemostasis of the cut edges is ensured, and the remaining enteric contents are gently suctioned out. A Betadine-soaked Harris gauze pad may be used at this point to cleanse the lumen of the bowel in the perianastomotic region.

A full-length seromuscular and submucosal stitch of 4-0 polyglycolic acid is placed and tied on the inside approximately 0.25 to 0.5 in. from the far end of the enterotomies. The stitch is not passed through the mucosa: to do so would add no strength to the anastomosis and would hinder epithelialization by rendering the tissue ischemic. A hemostat is placed on the short end of the tied suture, and the assistant applies continuous gentle tension to the long end of the suture. An over-and-over stitch is started in the direction of the surgeon; small bites are taken, and proper inversion of the suture line is ensured with each pass through tissue. When the proximal ends of the enterostomies are reached, this so-called baseball stitch is continued almost completely around to the anterior wall of the anastomosis. A single Connell stitch may be used to invert this anterior layer. Another full-length seromuscular and submucosal suture of 4-0 polyglycolic acid is then inserted and tied at the same location in the posterior wall as the first. If the two sutures are placed close enough together, the short ends need not be tied together and may simply be cut off. The remainder of the posterior wall is sewn away from the surgeon in the same manner as the portion already sewn, and the corners are approximated with the baseball stitch. The anterior wall is then completed with this second suture, either in the Connell stitch or in an over-and-over stitch with the assistant inverting the edges before applying tension to the previous stitch.

When the defect is completely closed, the two sutures are tied across the anastomotic line. The stay sutures are removed, and the anastomosis is carefully inspected. Often, there is no mesenteric defect to close in a side-to-side anastomosis, but if there is one, it should be approximated at this point with continuous or interrupted absorbable sutures, with care taken not to injure the vascular supply to the anastomosis.

DOUBLE-LAYER SUTURED END-TO-SIDE ENTEROCOLOSTOMY

The patient is positioned and control of the operative field obtained as described (see above). The bowel loops are isolated with clean sponges, and noncrushing bowel clamps are used as needed to prevent excessive spillage of intestinal contents. This procedure is often performed when there is a significant discrepancy in luminal diameter between the two segments to be joined, as in ileocolic anastomoses. The distal bowel or colon is divided with a cutting stapler so that a blind end is left. Some surgeons underpin or bury this staple line, although this practice is probably unnecessary. The proximal cut end of the intestine is similarly closed either with staples after division with a cutting linear stapler or with a crushing bowel clamp. This proximal end is brought into apposition with the side of the distal bowel segment at a point no further than 1 to 2 in. from the blind end of the distal segment; this proximity to the cut end is important for prevention of the blind loop syndrome [see Figure 6].

Stay sutures of 3-0 polyglycolic acid are placed between the serosa of the proximal limb about 0.5 to 0.75 in. from the clamp and the serosa of the distal limb. Interrupted seromuscular sutures of 3-0 polyglycolic acid are then placed between these

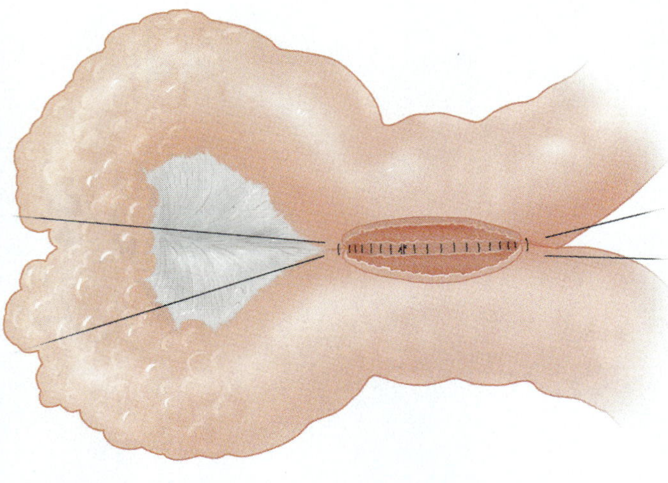

Figure 5 Single-layer sutured extramucosal side-to-side enteroenterostomy. A full-length suture is started in the back wall and run through the seromuscular and submucosal layers in the direction of the surgeon; the corners of the enterotomy are approximated with a baseball stitch, and a single Connell stitch is used to invert the anterior layer. A second suture is started at the same spot on the posterior wall and run in the opposite direction, again through all layers except the mucosa; the corners of the enterotomies are approximated with a baseball stitch, and the suture is continued in either the Connell stitch or the over-and-over stitch to complete the anterior wall of the anastomosis.

stay sutures, spaced about eight to 16 to the inch. These stitches may be tied sequentially or snapped and tied once they are all in place. It is crucial not to apply excessive tension, which could cut the seromuscular layer or render it ischemic. Suction is then readied. The staple line or crushed tissue on the proximal limb is cut off with a coagulating electrocautery or a knife; this maneuver opens the lumen of the proximal limb. All residual intestinal content is gently suctioned.

An enterotomy or colotomy is created on the distal limb opposite the open lumen of the proximal bowel. A full-thickness suture of 3-0 polyglycolic acid is inserted in the posterior wall at a point close to the far end of the enterotomy and run in an over-and-over stitch back toward the surgeon. The corner is rounded with the baseball stitch, and when the anterior wall is reached, the Connell stitch is used. A second full-length 3-0 suture is started at the same point on the posterior wall as the first, and the short ends of the two sutures are tied together and cut. This second suture is then run away from the surgeon to complete the posterior wall, and the anterior wall is completed with the Connell stitch. The two sutures are then tied across the anastomotic line.

A second series of interrupted seromuscular stitches is then placed anteriorly in the same fashion as the seromuscular stitches placed in the posterior wall. It is important not to narrow either lumen excessively by imbricating too much of the bowel wall into this second layer. The lumen of the anastomosis is palpated to confirm patency, and the mesenteric defect is closed if possible with either continuous or interrupted absorbable sutures.

DOUBLE-STAPLED END-TO-END COLOANAL ANASTOMOSIS

Preoperative mechanical and antibiotic bowel preparation is performed, and the patient is optimized medically. The patient is placed in stirrups in the lithotomy position and prepared as described (see above). Laparotomy is performed and colonic and rectal mobilization carried out as described (see above). The patient is then placed in Trendelenburg's position, with the small intestine packed into the upper abdomen and a Gibson retractor placed to provide adequate exposure.

The proximal resection margin is determined and cleared of its mesenteric attachments and its appendices epiploicae with the electrocautery. The operative field is prepared, and the colon is divided between crushing bowel clamps. An angled linear noncutting stapler is fired across the distal resection margin, and another bowel clamp is placed proximal to it. The rectum is divided with a long-handled knife, with care taken to avoid plunging the blade into the pelvic sidewall, which could cause significant neurovascular damage. The specimen is removed and the stapler withdrawn. Adequate pelvic hemostasis is ensured.

Once sufficient mobilization has been achieved, a noncrushing bowel clamp is placed on the colon 10 to 15 cm proximal to the margin, and the crushing clamp is removed. (At this stage, some thought should be given to creating an 8 to 10 cm colonic J pouch, which may improve functional outcome after low anastomoses, especially in the early postoperative period in older patients.) A whip-stitch (or purse-string suture) of 2-0 polypropylene is placed around the colotomy, and the anvil from the appropriately sized curved EEA (C-EEA) stapler is inserted into the open end and secured in place by tying the suture [see Figure 7]. The proximal bowel clamp is removed. A digital rectal examination is performed by the assistant, who may also, if desired, gently wash out the rectal stump with a dilute Betadine solution. The stapler, with its trocar attachment in place, is then inserted into the anus under the careful guidance of the surgeon. The pointed shaft is brought out through or adjacent to the linear staple line, and the sharp point is removed. The peg from the anvil in the proximal colon is snapped into the protruding shaft of the stapler, and the two edges are slowly brought together. The colonic mesentery must not be twisted, and the ends must come together without any tension whatsoever. The stapler is fired, and a distinctive crunching sound is heard. The anvil is then loosened the appropriate amount, and the entire mechanism is withdrawn through the anus. Finally, the proximal and distal rings of tissue are carefully inspected to confirm circumferential closure of the staple line.

The pelvis is then filled with body-temperature saline, and a Toomey syringe is used to insufflate the neorectum with air. The surgeon watches for bubbling in the pelvis as a sign of leakage from the anastomosis. A rectal tube may then be inserted by the assistant or may be placed at the end of the case.

When the anastomosis is very low or there is some concern about healing, a drain may be placed in the pelvis behind the staple line; however, as noted [see Controversial Areas, above], this practice has not been shown to be beneficial and may in fact impair healing. Some surgeons prefer to protect the anastomosis with a temporary covering loop ileostomy, though recent data suggest that this may not be necessary.[71,72]

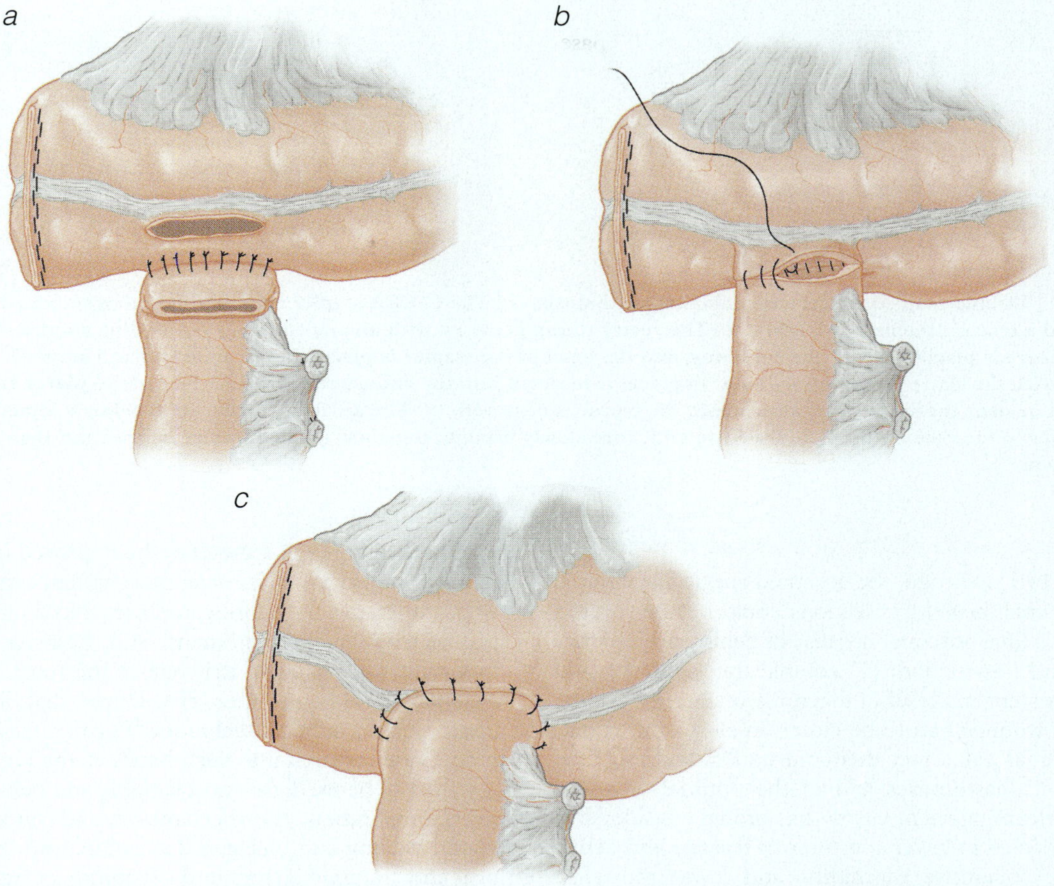

Figure 6 Double-layer sutured end-to-side enterocolostomy. (*a*) The proximal bowel end is stapled, interrupted Lembert stitches are used to form the posterior outer layer, and a colotomy is made. (*b*) Two continuous sutures are used to form the inner layer of the anastomosis; the posterior portion is done with the over-and-over stitch, the anterior with the Connell stitch. (*c*) Interrupted Lembert stitches are used to form the anterior outer layer.

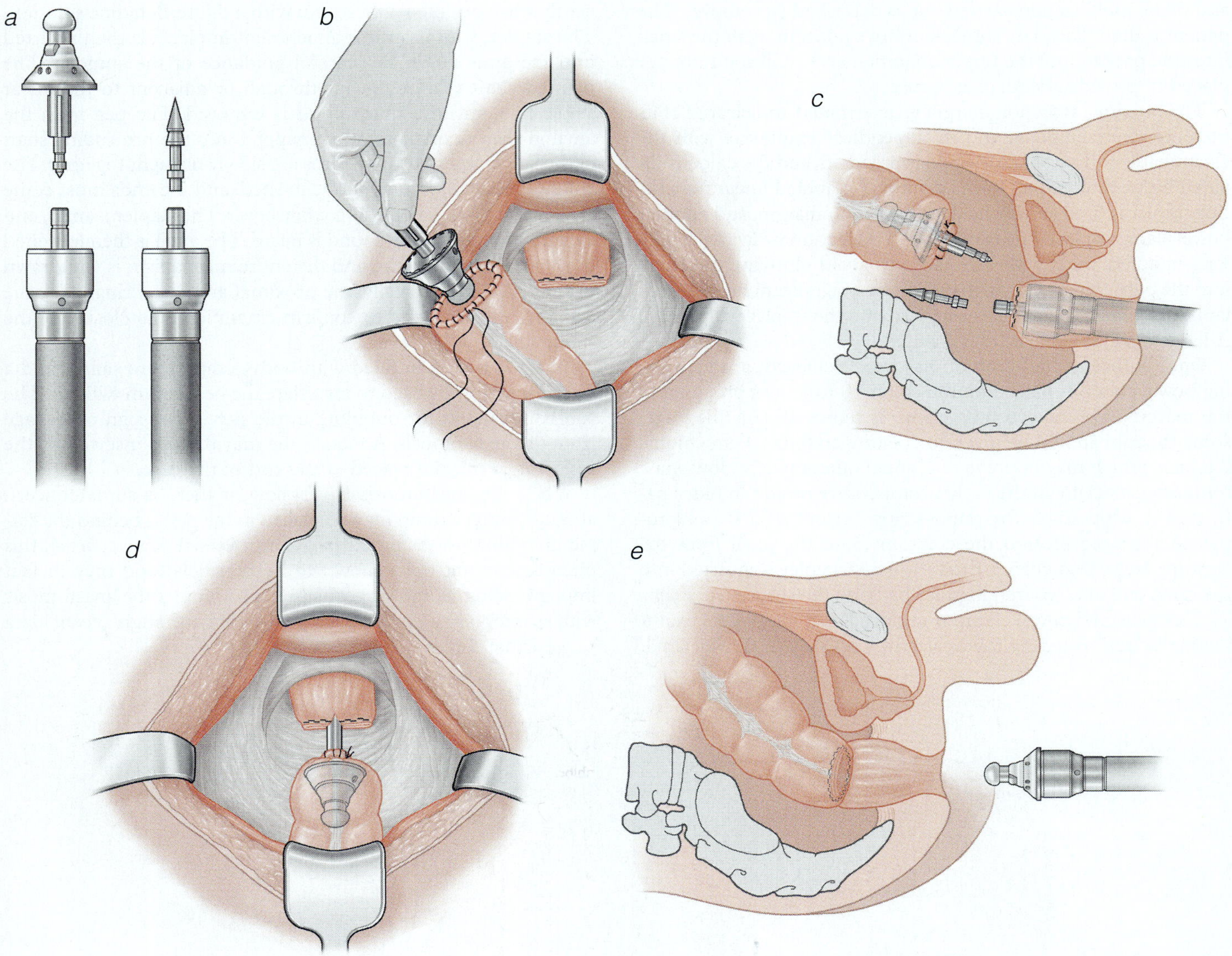

Figure 7 Double-stapled end-to-end coloanal anstomosis. (*a*) The C-EEA stapler comes with both a standard anvil (left) and a trocar attachment (right). (*b*) The rectal stump is closed with an angled linear noncutting stapler. A pursestring suture is placed around the colotomy, and the anvil of the stapler is placed in the open end and secured. (*c*) The stapler, with the sharp trocar attachment in place, is inserted into the anus, and the trocar is made to pierce the rectal stump at or near the staple line, after which the trocar is removed. (*d*) The anvil in the proximal colon is joined with the stapler in the rectal stump, and the two edges are slowly brought together. (*e*) The stapler is fired and then gently withdrawn.

Conclusion

As far back as 190 years ago, the accepted surgical standards dictated that (1) small bowel transections could not be sutured primarily without a fatal outcome because of dehiscence or stricture formation and obstruction; (2) colonic transections could be sutured over a stent made of autogenous or foreign tissues; and (3) intestinal wounds had to be closed in close approximation to the abdominal wall. Since then, our understanding of the healing of surgical anastomoses and of the optimal technical approaches to performing them clearly has grown considerably. This growth is reflected in lower anastomotic leakage and dehiscence rates, lower operative morbidity, and lower mortality.

Some would argue that much of the improved outcome is attributable to improved anesthesia, more potent antibiotics, and better postoperative monitoring and care. No doubt there is a good deal of truth to this argument. Still, however, we believe it is important to emphasize that one of the most significant determinants of outcome after procedures that include intestinal anastomosis is surgical technique. For this reason, it is essential to continue research into such issues as the best suture material or stapler to be used, the most suitable and best-tolerated type of bowel preparation, the mechanisms and variables involved in wound healing and collagen deposition, and the importance of local and systemic factors in determining overall outcome.

References

1. Smith SRG, Connolly JC, Crane PW: The effect of surgical drainage materials on colonic healing. Br J Surg 69:153, 1982
2. Debas HT, Thompson FB: A critical review of colectomy with anastomosis. Surg Gynecol Obstet 135:747, 1973
3. Schrock TR, Deveney CW, Dunphy JE: Factors contributing to leakage of colonic anastomoses. Ann Surg 177:513, 1973
4. Matheson NA, McIntosh CA, Krukowski ZH: Continuing experience with single layer appositional anastomosis in the large bowel. Br J Surg 72(suppl):S104, 1985
5. Carty NJ, Keating J, Campbell J, et al: Prospective audit of an extramucosal technique for intestinal anastomosis. Br J Surg 78:1439, 1991
6. Halsted W: Circular suture of the intestine—an experimental study. Am J Med Sci 94:436, 1887
7. Hastings JC, Van Winkle W, Barker E, et al: Effects of suture materials on healing of wounds of the stomach and colon. Surg Gynecol Obstet 140:701, 1975
8. Wise L, McAlister W, Stein T, et al: Studies on the healing of anastomoses of small and large intestines. Surg Gynecol Obstet 141:190, 1975
9. Hesp F, Hendriks T, Lubbers E-J, et al: Wound healing in the intestinal wall: a comparison between experimental ileal and colonic anastomosis. Dis Colon Rectum 24:99, 1984
10. Hawley PJ, Hunt TK, Dunphy JE: Aetiology of colonic anastomotic leaks. Proc R Soc Med 63:28, 1970
11. Hawley PJ, Faulk WP: A circulating collagenase inhibitor. Br J Surg 57:900, 1970
12. Martens M, Hendriks T: Postoperative changes in collagen synthesis in intestinal anastomoses of the rat: differences between small and large bowel. Gut 32:1482, 1991
13. Martens M, deMan B, Hendriks T, et al: Collagen synthetic capacity throughout the uninjured and anastomosed intestinal wall. Am J Surg 164:354, 1992
14. Munck A, Guyre M, Holbrook N: Physiological functions of glucocorticoids in stress and their relation to pharmacological actions. Endocrinol Rev 5:25, 1984
15. Matsusue S, Walser M: Healing of intestinal anastomoses in adrenalectomized rats given corticosterone. Am J Physiol 263:R164, 1992
16. Quan Z, Walser M: The effect of corticosterone administration at varying levels on leucine oxidation and whole body protein synthesis and breakdown in adrenalectomized rats. Metabolism 40:1263, 1991
17. Letwin E, Williams HTG: Healing of intestinal anastomosis. Can J Surg 10:109, 1967
18. Gadacz T, Menguy RB: Effects of anti-inflammatory drug oxyphenbutazone on the rate of wound healing and the biochemical composition of wound tissue. Surgery Forum 18:58, 1967
19. Irving AD, Scrimgeour D: Mechanical bowel preparation for colonic resection and anastomosis. Br J Surg 74:580, 1987
20. Hughes ESR: Asepsis in large bowel surgery. Ann R Coll Surg Engl 51:347, 1972
21. O'Dwyer PJ, Conway W, McDermott EWM, et al: Effect of mechanical bowel preparation on anastomotic integrity following low anterior resection in dogs. Br J Surg 76:756, 1989
22. Leveen HH, Wapnicks S, Falk D: Effects of prophylactic antibiotics on colonic healing. Am J Surg 131:47, 1976
23. Goligher JC, Graham NG, DeDombal FT: Anastomotic dehiscence after anterior resection of the rectum and sigmoid. Br J Surg 57:109, 1970
24. Irvin T, Goligher J, Johnston D: A randomized prospective clinical trial of single-layer and two layer inverting intestinal anastomoses. Br J Surg 60:457, 1973
25. Hocking M, Carlson R, Courington K, et al: Altered motility and bacterial flora after functional end-to-end anastomosis. Surgery 108:384, 1990
26. O'Donnell AF, O'Connell PR, Royston D, et al: Suture technique affects perianastomotic colonic crypt cell production and tumour formation. Br J Surg 78:671, 1991
27. Greenstein A, Rogers P, Moss G: Doubled fourth-day colorectal anastomotic strength with complete retention of intestinal mature wound collagen and accelerated deposition following full enteral nutrition. Surgery Forum 29:78, 1978
28. Bubrick MP: Effects of technique on anastomotic dehiscence. Dis Colon Rectum 24:232, 1981
29. Brennan SS, Pickford IR, Evans M, et al: Staples or sutures for colonic anastomosis—a controlled clinical trial. Br J Surg 69:722, 1982
30. Lafrenier R, Ketcham AS: A single layer open anastomosis for all intestinal structures. Am J Surg 149:797, 1985
31. Beart RW, Kelly KA: Randomised prospective evaluation of the EEA stapler for colorectal anastomoses. Am J Surg 141:143, 1981
32. Akyol AM, McGregor JR, Galloway DJ, et al: Recurrence of colorectal cancer after sutured and stapled large bowel anastomoses. Br J Surg 78:1297, 1991
33. O'Dwyer P, Ravikumar TS, Steele G: Serum dependent variability in the adherence to tumour cells to surgical sutures. Br J Surg 72:466, 1985
34. Everett WG, Friend PJ, Forty J: Comparison of stapling and hand-suture for left-sided large bowel anastomosis. Br J Surg 73:345, 1986
35. Murphy JB: A contribution to abdominal surgery, ideal approximation of abdominal viscera without suture. North American Practitioner 4:481, 1892
36. Hopcroft SC: An absorbable intestinal prosthesis for rapid intestinal anastomosis. Expl Med Surg 26:9, 1968
37. Sogren E, Birkeland R, Sohlberg S: A gelatine prosthetic aid for intestinal anastomosis. Journal of Small Animal Practice 18:529, 1977
38. Ballantyne GH: The experimental basis of intestinal suturing: effect of surgical technique, inflammation and infection on enteric wound healing. Dis Colon Rectum 27:61, 1984
39. Getzen L: Intestinal anastomoses. Curr Probl Surg, August 1969, p 3
40. Kratzer GL, Onsanit T: Single layer steel wire anastomosis of the intestine. Surg Gynecol Obstet 139:93, 1974
41. Ravitch MM, Steichen FM: Techniques of staple suturing in the gastrointestinal tract. Ann Surg 175:815, 1972
42. Brunius U, Zederfeldt B: Efffects of antiinflammatory treatment on wound healing. Acta Chir Scand 129:462, 1965
43. Burg R, Geigle C, Faso J, et al: Omission of routine gastric decompression. Dis Colon Rectum 21:98, 1978
44. Reasbeck P, Rice M, Herbison G: Nasogastric intubation after intestinal resection. Surg Gynecol Obstet 158:354, 1984
45. Argov S, Goldstein I, Barzilai A: Is routine use of a nasogastric tube justified in upper abdominal surgery? Am J Surg 139:849, 1980
46. Yates JL: An experimental study of the local effects of peritoneal drainage. Surg Gynecol Obstet 1:473, 1905
47. Berliner SD, Burson LC, Lear PE: Use and abuse of intraperitoneal drains in colon surgery. Arch Surg 89:686, 1964
48. Manz CW, LaTendresse C, Sako Y: The detrimental effects of drains on colonic anastomoses. Dis Colon Rectum 13:17, 1970
49. Koruda MJ, Rolandelli RH: Experimental studies on the healing of colonic anastomoses. J Surg Res 48:504, 1990
50. Munday C, McGinn FP: A comparison of polyglycolic acid and catgut sutures in rat colonic anastomoses. Br J Surg 63:870, 1976
51. Khubchandani IT: Low end-to-side rectoenteric anastomosis with single-layer wire. Dis Colon Rectum 18:308, 1975
52. Irvin T, Goligher J: Aetiology of disruption of intestinal anastomoses. Br J Surg 60:461, 1973
53. Olsen GB, Letwin E, Williams HTG: Clinical experience with the use of a single-layer intestinal anastomosis. Can J Surg 56:771, 1969
54. Sarin S, Lightwood RG: Continuous single-layer gastrointestinal anastomosis: a prospective audit. Br J Surg 76:493, 1989
55. Shandall A, Lowndes R, Young HL: Colonic anastomotic healing and oxygen tension. Br J Surg 72:606, 1985
56. Jiborn H, Ahonen J, Zederfeldt B: Healing of experimental colonic anastomoses: the effect of suture technique on collagen metabolism in the colonic wall. Am J Surg 139:406, 1980
57. Khoury GA, Waxman BP: Large bowel anastomosis: I. The healing process and sutured anastomoses: a review. Br J Surg 70:61, 1983
58. Abramowitz H: Everting and inverting anastomoses: an experimental study of comparative safety. Rev Surg 28:142, 1971
59. Polglase AL, Hughes ESR, McDermott FT, et al: A comparison of end-to-end staple and suture colorectal anastomosis in the dog. Surg Gynecol Obstet 152:792, 1981
60. O'Neil P, Healey JEJ, Clark RI, et al: Nonsuture intestinal anastomosis. Am J Surg 104:761, 1962
61. Orr NWM: A single layer intestinal anastomosis. Br J Surg 56:77, 1969
62. Templeton JL, McKelvey STD: Low colorectal anastomoses: an experimental assessment of two sutured and two stapled techniques. Dis Colon Rectum 28:38, 1985
63. Goligher J, Morris C, McAdam W: A controlled trial of inverting versus everting intestinal suture in clinical large-bowel surgery. Br J Surg 57:817, 1970
64. Fielding LP, Stewart Brown S, Blesowsky L, et al: Anastomotic integrity after operations for large bowel cancer: a multicentre study. Br Med J 282:411, 1980
65. Leob MJ: Comparative strength of inverted, everted and endon intestinal anastomoses. Surg Gynecol Obstet 125:301, 1967
66. Undre AR: Enteroplasty: a new concept in the management of benign strictures of the intestine. Int Surg 68:73, 1983
67. Chassin JL, Rifkind KM, Turner JW: Errors and pitfalls in stapled gastrointestinal tract anastomoses. Surg Clin North Am 64:441, 1984
68. Ravitch MM: Intersecting staple lines in intestinal anastomoses. Surgery 97:8, 1985
69. Chung RS: Blood flow in colonic anastomoses: effect of stapling and suturing. Ann Surg 206:335, 1987
70. Julian TB, Ravitch MM: Evaluations of the safety of end-to-end stapling anastomoses across linear stapled closure. Surg Clin North Am 64:567, 1984
71. Gorfine SR, Gelernt IM, Bauer JJ, et al: Restorative proctocolectomy without diverting ileostomy. Dis Colon Rectum 38:188, 1995
72. Grobler SP, Hosie KB, Keighley MR: Randomised trial of loop ileostomy in restorative proctocolectomy. Br J Surg 79:903, 1992
73. Semm N: Enteroraphy: its history, technic and present status. JAMA 21:215, 1893

Acknowledgment

Figures 1 through 7   Tom Moore.

56 APPENDECTOMY

Hung S. Ho, M.D.

The vermiform appendix was first depicted in anatomic drawings in 1492 by Leonardo da Vinci and was first described as an anatomic structure in 1521 by Jacopo Berengari da Carpi, a professor of human anatomy at Bologna. Appendicitis became recognized as a surgical disease when the Harvard University pathologist Reginald Heber Fitz reported his analysis of 257 cases of perforating inflammation of the appendix and 209 cases of typhlitis or perityphlitis at the 1886 meeting of the Association of American Physicians. In this landmark paper, Fitz correctly pointed out that the frequent abscesses in the right iliac fossa were often due to perforation of the vermiform appendix, and he referred to the condition as appendicitis.[1] Among his classic observations of the disease was his emphasis on the "vital importance of early recognition" and its "eventual treatment by laparotomy." It was not until 1894 that Charles McBurney first described the surgical incision that bears his name and the technique of appendectomy that was to become the gold standard for appendectomy throughout the 20th century.[2]

Although appendectomy has traditionally been done—and largely continues to be done—as an open procedure, there has been increasing interest in laparoscopic appendectomy since the beginning of the 1990s. In what follows, I describe both approaches to the operation and briefly discuss factors affecting the choice between them.

Choice between Open and Laparoscopic Appendectomy

There have been 20 formally conducted prospective, randomized trials comparing laparoscopic appendectomy with open appendectomy. Of these, 17 were published as full manuscripts in English [see Table 1], two as full manuscripts in German, and one as an abstract in English. The 17 full reports published in English involved a total of 1,960 patients, of whom 1,035 were randomly selected to undergo laparoscopic appendectomy and 925 to undergo open appendectomy.[3-19] Similar incidences of histologically normal appendix were found in the two groups (14.4% with laparoscopic appendectomy versus 14.5% with open appendectomy). The conversion rate was 9% (range, 0% to 20%). Laparoscopic appendectomy was associated with a lower incidence of postoperative wound infection than open appendectomy was (2.9% versus 7.4%), but it was also associated with a higher incidence of postoperative intra-abdominal abscess (1.9% versus 0.8%). The length of stay was slightly shorter after laparoscopic appendectomy than after open appendectomy (3.0 days versus 3.7 days). In men with suspected acute appendicitis, laparoscopic appendectomy has no major advantage over open appendectomy.[10,11] In women of reproductive age and in equivocal cases, laparoscopy may be valuable as a diagnostic tool, but the practice of not removing a normal-looking appendix during exploration for right lower quadrant pain is controversial. Laparoscopic appendectomy appears to offer the potential benefit of less postoperative adhesion formation, but the evidence is inconclusive in the light of the short follow-up times reported in these trials, and the higher incidence of intra-abdominal abscess formation is cause for concern.

As of early 1999, the gold standard for surgical treatment of acute appendicitis remained open appendectomy as described by McBurney in 1894. Meta-analysis of prospective, randomized trials showed that although laparoscopic appendectomy is at least as safe as the corresponding open procedure, it is more time-consuming and more costly. Moreover, it is questionable whether the benefits of laparoscopic appendectomy in terms of postoperative pain, time to resumption of oral feeding, length of hospital stay, return to normal preoperative activities, and the incidence of surgical site infection outweigh the doubled incidence of postoperative intra-abdominal abscess formation. Further randomized clinical studies focusing on the efficacy of laparoscopic appendectomy as a diagnostic tool and on the incidence of postoperative intra-abdominal abscess and adhesion formation are needed, as are additional cost analyses. At present, the only patients for whom laparoscopic appendectomy appears to offer significant advantages are female patients of childbearing age, obese patients, and patients with an unclear diagnosis [see Figure 1].

Open Appendectomy

With the patient in the supine position, general anesthesia is induced and the abdomen is prepared and draped in a sterile fashion so as to expose the right lower quadrant. The skin incision is made in an oblique direction, crossing a line drawn between the anterior superior iliac spine and the umbilicus at nearly a right angle at a point about 1 in. from the iliac spine. This point, McBurney's point, is approximately one third of the way from the iliac spine to the umbilicus [see Figure 2]. The subcutaneous fat and fascia are incised to expose the external oblique aponeurosis. A slightly shorter incision is made in this structure; first, a scalpel is used, and then the incision is extended with scissors in the direction of the fibers of the muscle and its tendon in such a way that the fibers are separated but not cut. The fibers of the internal oblique and transversalis muscles are separated with a blunt instrument at nearly a right angle to the incision on the external oblique aponeurosis. The parietal peritoneum is lifted up, with care taken not to include the underlying viscera, and is opened in a transverse fashion with a scalpel. This incision is then enlarged transversely with scissors. When greater exposure is required, the lateral edge of the rectus sheath is incised and the rectus abdominis muscle retracted medially without being divided [see Figure 3].

A foul smell or the presence of pus on entry into the peritoneum is an indication of advanced appendicitis. The free peritoneal fluid is collected for bacteriologic analysis. The appendix is located by following the cecal taeniae distally. The inflamed appendix usually feels firm and turgid. The appendix, together with the cecum, is delivered into the surgical incision and held with a Babcock tissue forceps. If this step proves difficult, the appendix can sometimes be swept into the field with the surgeon's right index finger as gentle traction is maintained on the cecum with a small, moist gauze pad held in the left hand [see Figure 4]. Care should be taken at this point not to avulse the friable and

Table 1 Results of 17 Prospective, Randomized Trials Comparing Laparoscopic Appendectomy with Open Appendectomy

Study Authors	Procedure	No. of Patients	Negative Appendix [No. (%)]	Conversion to Open Procedure [No. (%)]	Wound Infection [No. (%)]	Intra-abdominal Abscess [No. (%)]	Length of Stay (days)
Attwood[3]	LA	30	5 (16.7)	2 (6.7)	0	0	2.5
	OA	32	1 (3.1)	NA	1 (3.1)	0	3.8
Tate[4]	LA	70	9 (12.9)	14 (20)	7 (10)	1 (1.4)	3.5
	OA	70	10 (14.3)	NA	10 (14.3)	0	3.5
Kum[5]	LA	65	10 (15.4)	0	0	0	3.2
	OA	72	11 (15.3)	NA	5 (6.9)	0	4.2
Frazee[6]	LA	38	6 (15.8)	2 (5.3)	0	0	2.0
	OA	37	6 (16.2)	NA	0	0	2.8
Ortega[7]	LA	167	30 (18)	11 (6.6)	4 (2.4)	6 (3.6)	2.6
	OA	86	13 (15.1)	NA	11 (12.8)	0	2.8
Martin[8]	LA	88	5 (5.7)	13 (14.8)	3 (3.4)	3 (3.4)	2.2
	OA	81	18 (22.2)	NA	6 (7.4)	3 (3.7)	4.3
Hansen[9]	LA	86	7 (8.1)	7 (8.1)	2 (2.3)	0	3.0
	OA	72	16 (22.2)	NA	8 (11)	0	3.0
Mutter[10]	LA	50	3 (6)	6 (12)	0	2 (4)	4.9
	OA	50	3 (6)	NA	0	0	5.3
Cox[11]	LA	33	4 (12.1)	5 (15.2)	0	0	2.9
	OA	31	4 (12.9)	NA	2 (6.5)	0	3.8
Lejus[12]	LA	32	5 (15.6)	0	0	0	3.0
	OA	31	4 (12.9)	NA	0	0	3.0
Williams[13]	LA	21	5 (23.8)	2 (9.5)	1 (4.8)	0	2.4
	OA	18	3 (16.7)	NA	1 (5.6)	0	2.8
Hart[14]	LA	44	13 (29.5)	4 (9.1)	3 (6.8)	3 (6.8)	3.2
	OA	37	7 (18.9)	NA	3 (8.2)	0	3.0
Reiertsen[15]	LA	56	14 (25)	2 (3.6)	8 (14.3)	2 (3.6)	3.5
	OA	52	10 (19.2)	NA	9 (17.3)	2 (3.8)	3.2
Laine[16]	LA	25	9 (36)	2 (8)	1 (4)	0	2.7
	OA	25	7 (28)	NA	1 (4)	0	2.3
Macarulla[17]	LA	106	11 (10.4)	9 (8.5)	1 (0.9)	1 (0.9)	3.4
	OA	104	8 (7.7)	NA	5 (4.8)	0	4.8
Kazemier[18]	LA	97	8 (8.2)	12 (12.4)	0	0	3.7
	OA	104	11 (10.6)	NA	6 (5.8)	1 (1)	4.4
Minne[19]	LA	27	5 (18.5)	2 (7.4)	0	2 (7.4)	1.1
	OA	23	2 (8.7)	NA	0	1 (4.3)	1.2
Total	**LA**	**1,035**	**149 (14.4)**	**93 (9)**	**30 (2.9)**	**20 (1.9)**	**3.0**
	OA	**925**	**134 (14.5)**	**NA**	**68 (7.4)**	**7 (0.8)**	**3.7**

LA—laparoscopic appendectomy OA—open appendectomy

possibly necrotic appendix. To deliver a retrocecal appendix, it may be necessary to mobilize the ascending colon partially by dividing the peritoneum on its lateral side, starting from the terminal ileum and proceeding toward the hepatic flexure.

The mesoappendix, containing the appendicular artery, is divided between clamps and ligated with 3-0 absorbable sutures [*see Figure 5*]. The appendix is held up with a Babcock tissue forceps, and its base is crushed with a straight mosquito arterial forceps. The mosquito forceps is then opened, moved up the appendix, and closed again. The base of the appendix is doubly ligated with 2-0 absorbable sutures at the point where it was crushed, so that a cuff of about 3 mm is left between the forceps and the tie. The appendix is divided by running a scalpel along the underside of the forceps. The mucosa of the appendiceal stump is fulgurated with the electrocautery. The stump is not routinely invaginated into the cecum. In those rare cases in which the viability of the appendiceal base is in question, a 2-0 absorbable purse-string suture is placed in the cecum, and the stump is invaginated as the suture is tied. The operative field is checked for hemostasis. In cases of perforated appendicitis, the right paracolic gutter and pelvis are thoroughly aspirated to ensure that any collected pus or particulate material is removed.

The peritoneum is then closed with a continuous 3-0 absorbable suture. The fibers of the transversalis muscle and the internal oblique muscle fall together readily, and their closure can be completed with two 3-0 absorbable ligatures. The external oblique aponeurosis

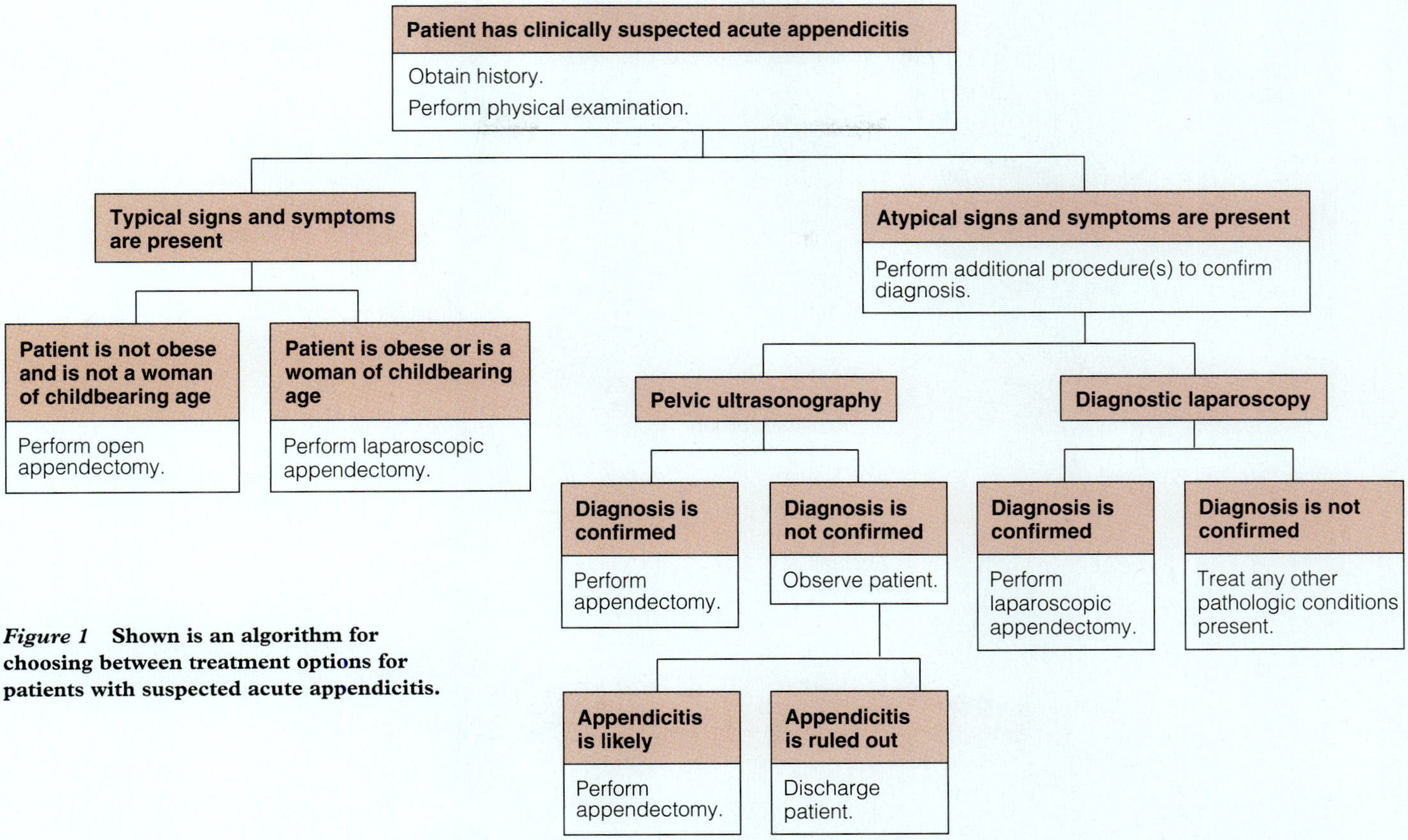

Figure 1 Shown is an algorithm for choosing between treatment options for patients with suspected acute appendicitis.

is closed from end to end with a continuous 2-0 absorbable suture. Scarpa's fascia is approximated with interrupted 3-0 absorbable sutures, and the skin is closed with a continuous subcuticular 4-0 absorbable suture and reinforcing tapes. If the wound has been grossly contaminated, the skin is loosely approximated with Steri-Strips, which can easily be removed postoperatively if surgical site infection or abscess develops. An alternative approach is to leave the skin and the subcutaneous tissue open but dressed with sterile nonadherent material and then to perform delayed primary closure with Steri-Strips on postoperative day 4 or 5.

Laparoscopic Appendectomy

The patient is placed in the supine position, with both arms tucked along the sides, and general anesthesia is induced. Decompression with a temporary nasal or orogastric tube should be routine, as should placement of a Foley catheter and use of lower extremity sequential compression devices. The monitors are placed on the opposite side of the operating table toward the foot, so that both the surgeon and the assistant can view the procedure at all times. The surgeon should stand on the patient's left side, with the assistant (who operates the camera) near the patient's left shoulder [see Figure 6].

The abdomen is prepared and draped in a sterile fashion so as to expose the entire abdomen. A three-port approach is routinely used [see Figure 6]. All skin incisions along the midline are made vertically to allow a more cosmetically acceptable conversion to laparotomy, should this become necessary. The suprapubic port must be large enough to accommodate the laparoscopic stapler (usually 12 mm); the other two ports can be smaller (e.g., 5 or 10 mm). The ports are placed as far away from the operative field as possible to permit the application of a two-handed dissection technique. The use of a 25° or 30° angled scope facilitates operative viewing and dissection. With the patient pharmacologically relaxed and in Trendelenburg's position, a Veress needle is inserted into the peritoneal cavity at the base of the umbilical ligament.

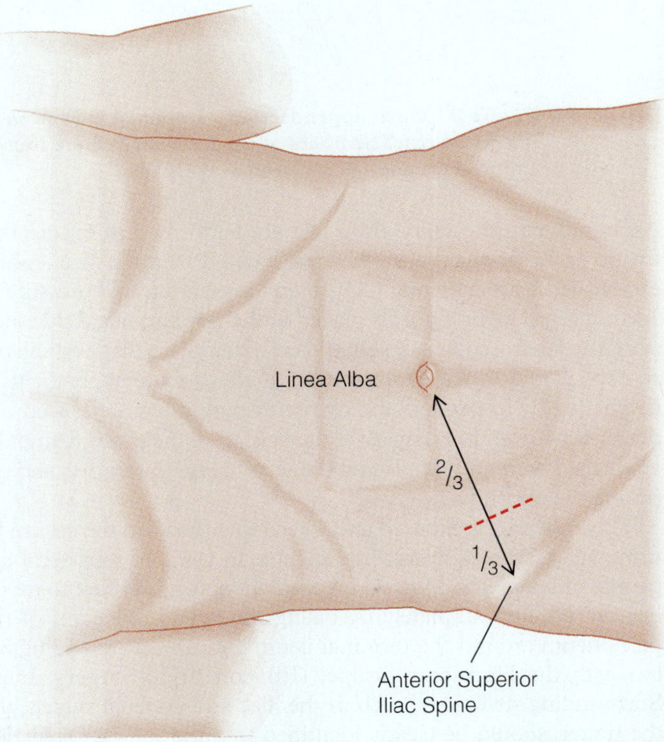

Figure 2 Open appendectomy. Shown are McBurney's point and McBurney's incision.

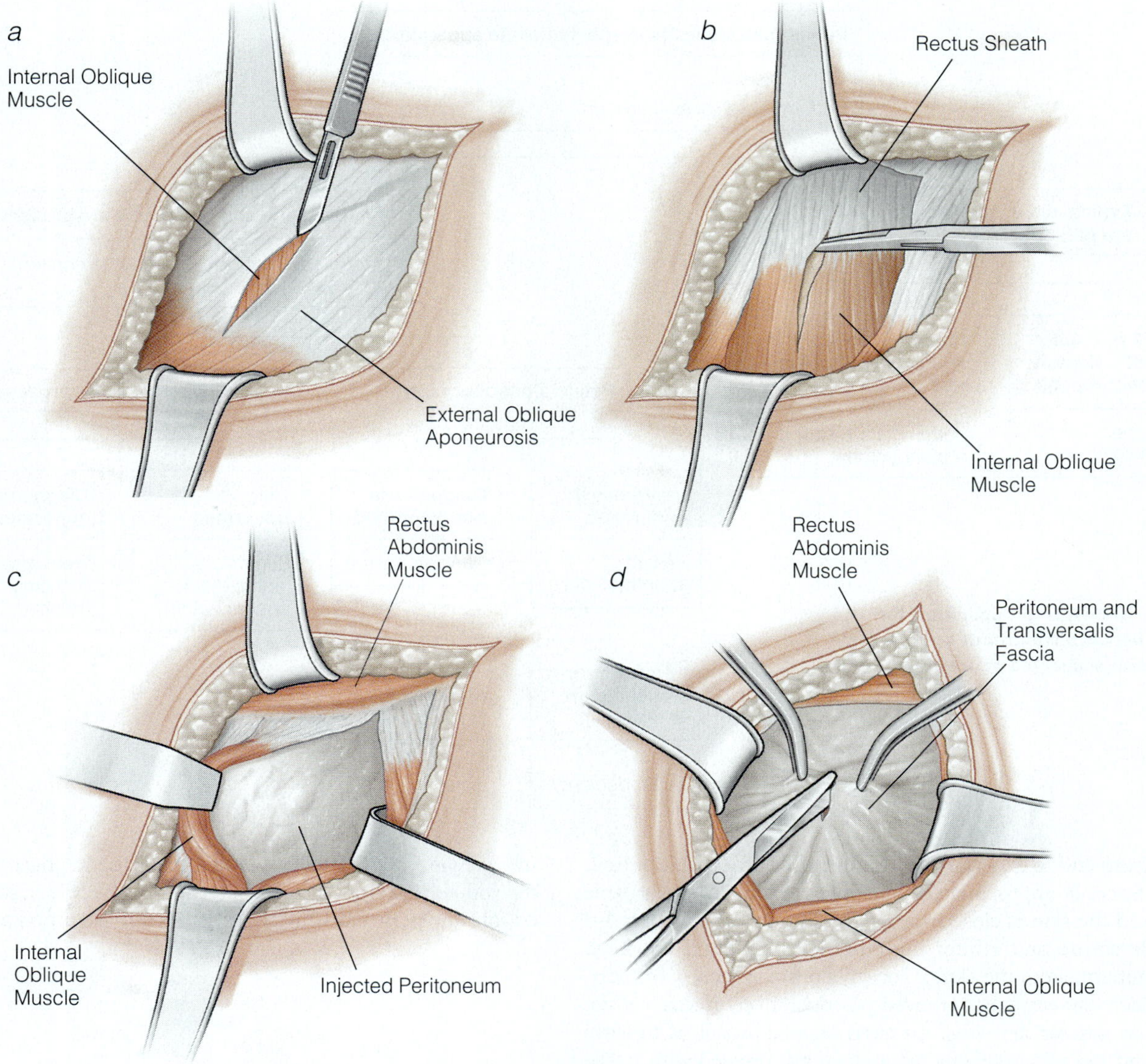

Figure 3 Open appendectomy. Depicted is exposure of the abdominal cavity. The external oblique aponeurosis is opened (*a*). The fibers of the internal oblique muscle are separated bluntly (*b*). The parietal peritoneum is exposed (*c*) and opened transversely (*d*).

Aspiration and the saline-drop test are performed to ensure that the tip of the needle is correctly positioned. Pneumoperitoneum is established by insufflating CO_2 to an intra-abdominal pressure of 14 mm Hg. The first port is placed at the infraumbilical skin incision, the laparoscope is inserted, and a complete diagnostic laparoscopy is performed. Once the diagnosis of acute appendicitis is confirmed by inspection, the two remaining ports are placed under direct vision. In many cases, however, the diagnosis cannot be confirmed without first placing the second and third ports and exposing the appendix.

The appendix is exposed and traced to its base on the cecum by using an atraumatic retracting forceps. In cases of retrocecal appendix or severe appendiceal inflammation, it is best first to mobilize the cecum completely by taking the lateral reflection of the peritoneum around the terminal ileum and up the ascending colon with the Harmonic Scalpel (Ethicon Endo-Surgery, Inc.). Surrounding structures, such as the iliac and gonadal vessels and the ureter, should be clearly identified to avoid injury. Dissection of the appendix can then begin. The tip of the appendix is grasped and retracted anteriorly toward the anterior abdominal wall and slightly toward the pelvis; the mesoappendix is thus exposed in a triangular fashion. A window between the base of the appendix and the blood supply is created with a curved dissecting forceps. The mesoappendix is divided either with hemostatic clips and scissors or with a laparoscopic gastrointestinal anastomosis (GIA) stapler loaded with a vascular cartridge [*see Figure 7*]. If a window on the mesoappendix cannot be safely created because of intense inflammation, antegrade dissection of the blood supply is necessary. The Harmonic Scalpel is a handy (albeit expensive) instrument for this purpose. Endoscopic hemostatic clips usually suffice to control the small branches of the appendicular artery during the course of this dissection.

The base of the appendix is then cleared circumferentially of any adipose or connective tissue and is divided with a laparoscopic GIA stapler loaded with an intestinal cartridge [*see Figure 8*]. To ensure an adequate closure away from the inflamed appendiceal wall, a small portion of the cecum may have to be included within the stapler. To ensure proper placement of the stapler and to prevent injury to the right ureter or the adjacent small bowel, the tips of the stapler must be clearly visualized before the instrument is closed.

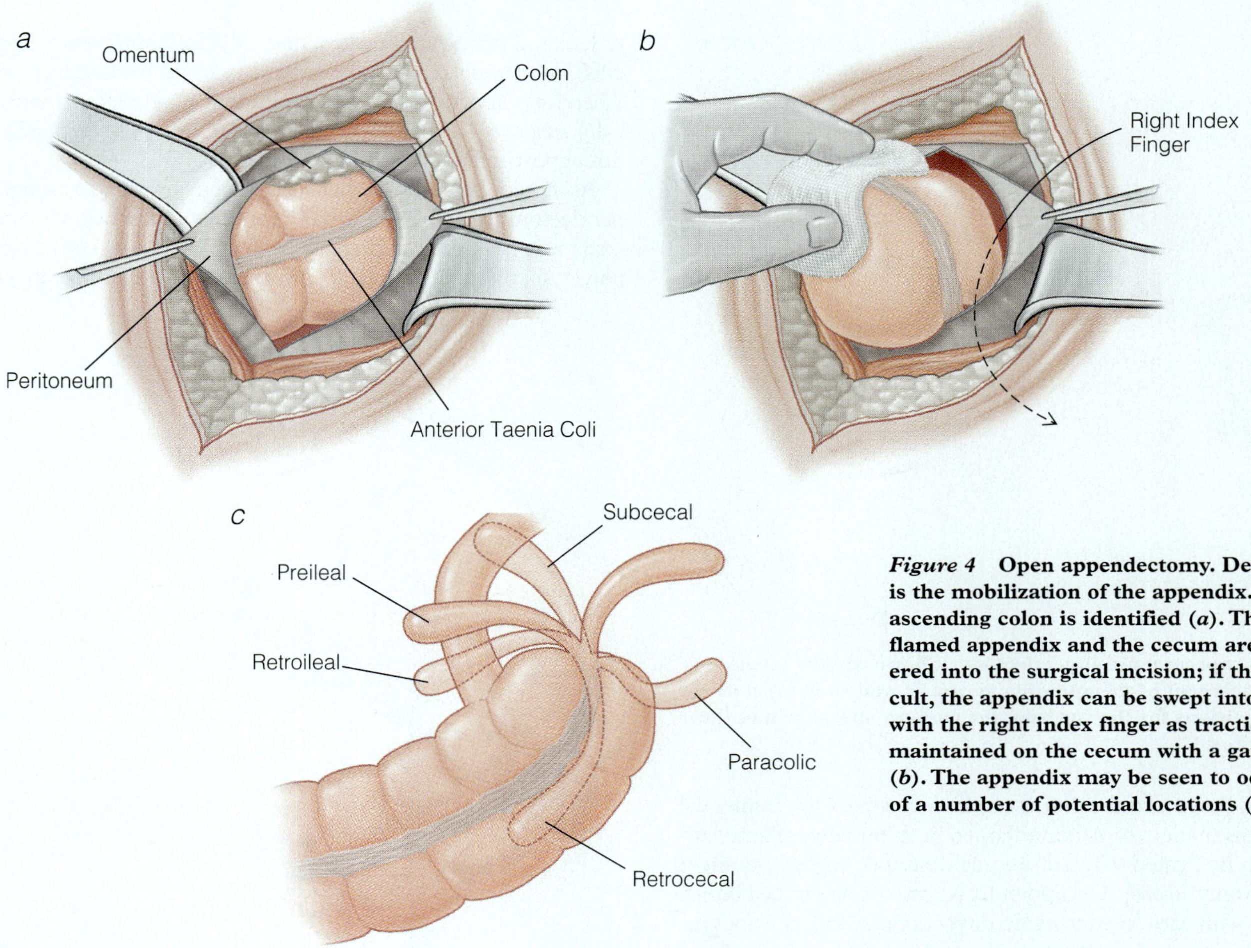

Figure 4 Open appendectomy. Depicted is the mobilization of the appendix. The ascending colon is identified (*a*). The inflamed appendix and the cecum are delivered into the surgical incision; if this is difficult, the appendix can be swept into the field with the right index finger as traction is maintained on the cecum with a gauze pad (*b*). The appendix may be seen to occupy any of a number of potential locations (*c*).

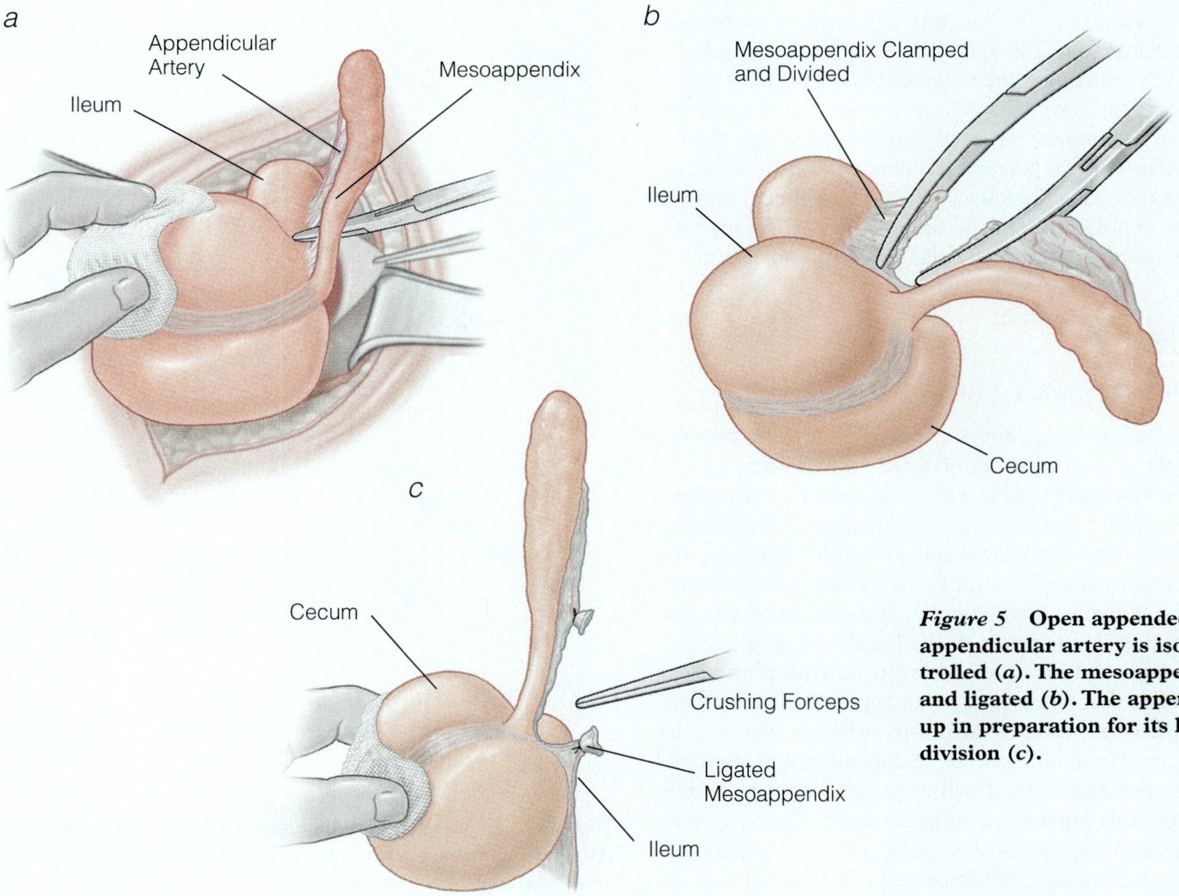

Figure 5 Open appendectomy. The appendicular artery is isolated and controlled (*a*). The mesoappendix is divided and ligated (*b*). The appendix is held up in preparation for its ligation and division (*c*).

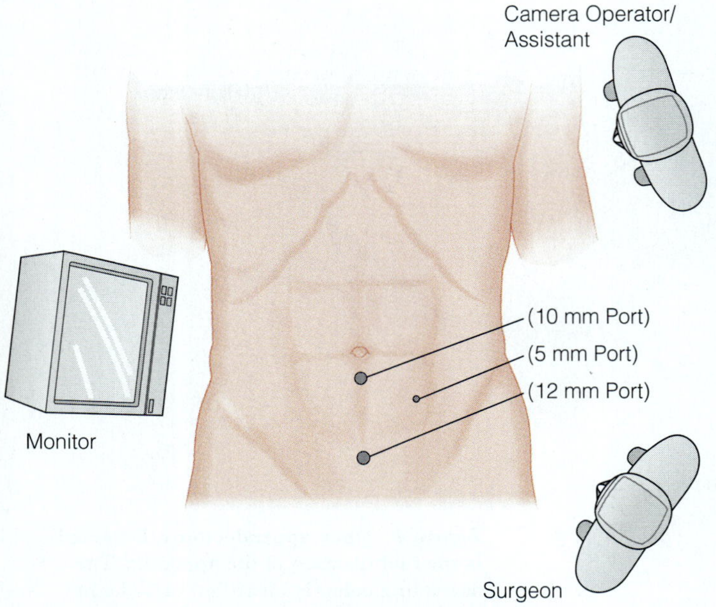

Figure 6 Laparoscopic appendectomy. Shown are the positioning and placement of the operative ports, as well as the recommended positions for the surgeon, the camera operator, and the video monitor.

The angled scope and the roticulator laparoscopic GIA stapler will facilitate this maneuver. A noninflamed or minimally inflamed appendix can be ligated with sutures, as described earlier [*see* Open Appendectomy, *above*]. The appendix is removed from the abdominal cavity, with care taken to avoid direct contact with the abdominal wall. A mildly inflamed appendix can be delivered through one of the larger ports; a severely inflamed appendix is often too big and hence should be delivered in a specimen retrieval bag [*see Figure 9*].

The operative field is irrigated and aspirated dry. Hemostasis is confirmed, and the cecum is inspected to ensure proper closure of the appendiceal stump. The ports are removed under direct vision, the absence of back-bleeding from the port sites is confirmed, and the abdomen is completely decompressed. All fascial defects larger than 5 mm are closed with 0 absorbable sutures. The skin incisions are reapproximated with either staples or a subcuticular 4-0 absorbable suture.

Special Considerations

THE HISTOLOGICALLY NORMAL APPENDIX

The incidence of histologically normal appendix in patients with clinical signs and symptoms of acute appendicitis ranges from 8% to 41%.[20-30] Nonetheless, appendectomy relieves symptoms in the vast majority of these patients. When extensive sectioning is done on histologically normal specimens, it often happens that a focus of inflammation is found in only a few serial sections. This condition is known as focal appendicitis—so called because the polymorphonuclear infiltration is confined to a single focus, while the remaining appendix is devoid of any polymorphonuclear cells.[31] It is not clear that all cases of acute appendicitis arise from this focal inflammation; however, such inflammatory foci may be the earliest recognizable manifestations of appendicitis in some so-called negative appendectomies. Furthermore, a substantial proportion of histologically normal appendices removed from patients with clinical signs and symptoms of acute appendicitis exhibit significantly increased expression of tumor necrosis factor–α and interleukin-2 mRNA (a sensitive marker of inflammation in appendicitis) in germinal centers, the submucosa, and the lamina propria.[32] Therefore, appendectomy is recommended in patients with clinically suspected acute appendicitis even when the appendix does not appear inflamed during exploration.

As noted [*see* Choice between Open and Laparoscopic Appendectomy, *above*], 17 formally conducted prospective, randomized trials published in English between 1992 and 1997 that compared laparoscopic appendectomy with open appendectomy found

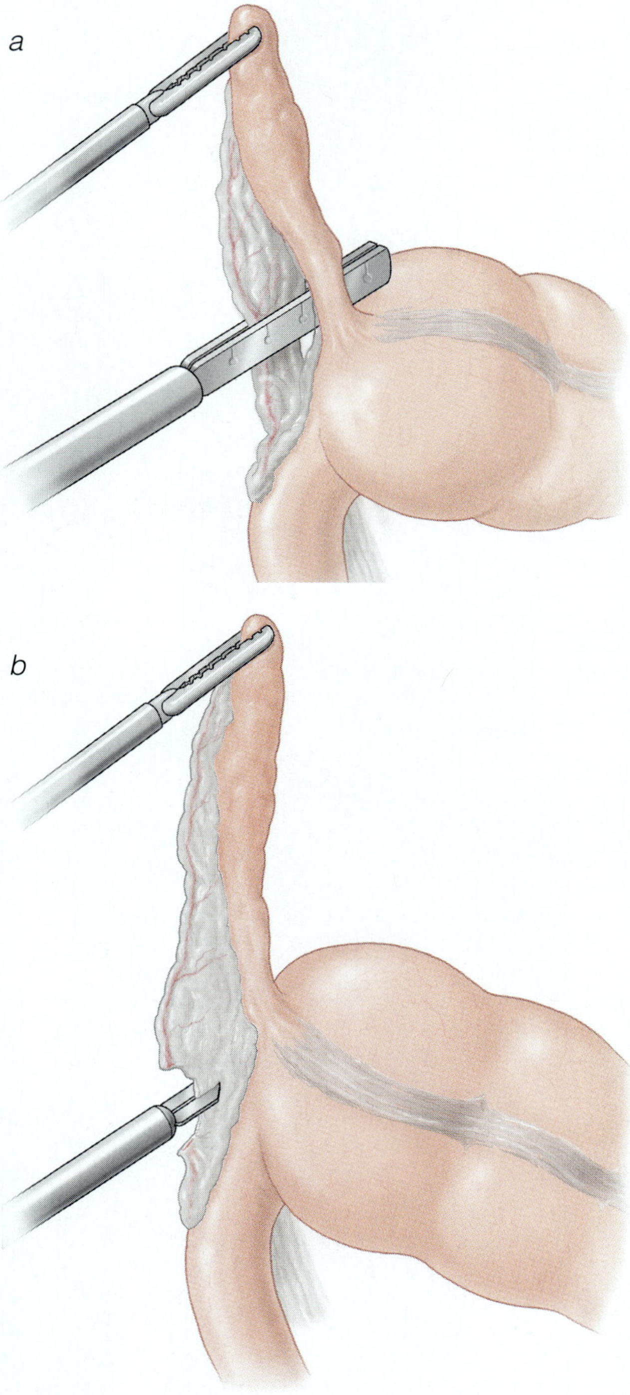

Figure 7 Laparoscopic appendectomy. The mesoappendix is divided either with a laparoscopic GIA stapler (*a*) or with hemostatic clips and scissors (*b*).

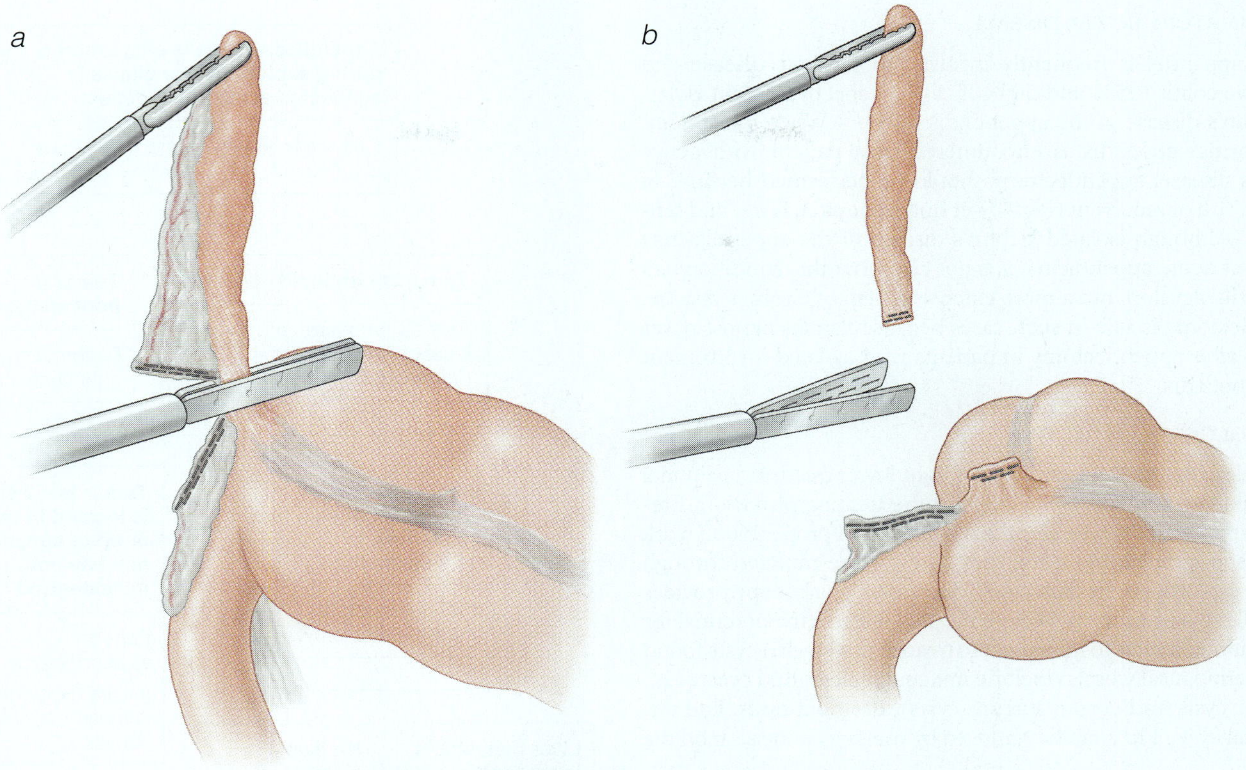

Figure 8 Laparoscopic appendectomy. The mesoappendix having been divided (*a*), the base of the appendix is cleared circumferentially and divided with a GIA stapler (*b*).

no differences with respect to the incidence of histologically normal appendix in patients with clinically suspected acute appendicitis[3-19]: the incidence ranged from 7.7% to 36% (average, 14.4%) with laparoscopic appendectomy and from 3.1% to 28% (average, 14.5%) with open appendectomy [*see Table 1*].

APPENDICEAL NEOPLASM

Neoplastic lesions of the appendix are found in as many as 5% of specimens obtained with routine appendectomy for acute appendicitis.[33-36] Most are benign. Preoperative detection of such conditions is rare, and intraoperative diagnosis is made in fewer than 50% of cases. Appendectomy alone may be curative for appendiceal mucocele, localized pseudomyxoma peritonei, most appendiceal carcinoids, and other benign tumors. Definitive management of an appendiceal mass unexpectedly encountered during exploration for clinically suspected acute appendicitis depends on whether the tumor is carcinoid, its size and location, the presence or absence of metastatic disease, and histologic and immunohistochemical findings [*see Figure 10*].

Benign neoplasms of the appendix include mucosal hyperplasia or metaplasia, leiomyomas, neuromas, lipomas, angiomas, and other rare lesions. Appendiceal adenomas tend to be diffuse and to have a predominant villous character. Mucus-producing cystadenomas predispose to appendiceal mucocele, sometimes accompanied by localized pseudomyxoma peritonei. These lesions are rarely symptomatic and are often encountered incidentally during operation; however, they may also be clinically manifested as acute appendicitis, torsion, intussusception, ureteral obstruction, or another acute condition. If the base of the appendix is free of disease, appendectomy alone is sufficient treatment.

Malignant tumors of the appendix primarily consist of carcinoids and adenocarcinomas; altogether, they account for 0.5% of all gastrointestinal malignancies.[37] The incidence of malignancy in the appendix is 1.35%.[33] Metastasis to the appendix is rare. Carcinoids are substantially more common than adenocarcinomas in the appendix: as many as 80% of all appendiceal masses are carcinoid tumors. Overall, carcinoid tumors are found in 0.5% of all appendiceal specimens, and appendiceal carcinoid tumors account for 18.9% of all carcinoid lesions.[38] These tumors are predominantly of neural cellular origin and have a better prognosis than all other intestinal carcinoid tumors, which typically are of mucosal cellular origin. If the tumor is less than 2 cm in diameter, is located within the body or the tip of the appendix, and has not metastasized, appendectomy is the treatment of choice. If the lesion is at the base of the appendix, is larger than 2 cm in diameter, or has metastasized, right hemicolectomy is indicated. In addition, secondary right hemicolectomy is indicated if the tumor is invasive, if mucin production is noted, or if the tumor is found to be of mucosal cellular origin at final pathologic examination.[39,40] Patients with metastatic appendiceal carcinoid tumors appear to have a far better prognosis than those with other types of metastatic cancers.[39] Therefore, hepatic debulking for symptomatic control is indicated and justified in cases of liver metastasis.

Primary adenocarcinoma of the appendix is rare, and as yet there is no firm consensus regarding prognosis, treatment of choice, and outcome.[41] Currently, the recommended treatment is right hemicolectomy: a 1993 study found that this approach resulted in an overall 5-year survival rate of 68%, compared with 20% when appendectomy alone was performed.[40] The prognosis is determined by the degree of tumor differentiation and by the histologic stage. As many as one third of these patients have a second primary neoplasm, which will be located within the GI tract about half the time.

Finally, nonepithelial appendiceal tumors, though extremely rare, occur as well. Such lesions include malignant and Burkitt's lymphomas, smooth muscle tumors, granular cell tumors, ganglioneuromas, and Kaposi's sarcoma.

INFLAMMATORY BOWEL DISEASE

The appendix is frequently involved in Crohn's disease and ulcerative colitis (25% and 50% of cases, respectively), but isolated Crohn's disease of the appendix is rare.[42-45] When a histologically normal appendix is encountered in a patient with active Crohn's disease, appendectomy should be performed because of the high risk of recurrent right lower quadrant pain, fever, and tenderness. Although isolated Crohn's disease of the appendix may present as acute appendicitis, it is not clear that this condition will necessarily develop into a more extensive form of Crohn's disease. Appendectomy is safe in such cases because fistulas almost never develop after appendectomy in patients with isolated involvement of the appendix.

GYNECOLOGIC CONDITIONS

It is clear that the presentation of right lower quadrant pain in a female patient remains a challenge to the treating physician. Frequently, the causes can be identified by means of proper blood work or ultrasonography, but often they can only be revealed through surgical exploration. In such cases, diagnostic laparoscopy provides an excellent view of the pelvic organs, and it offers the potential for easy continuation on to laparoscopic treatment. Ovarian cysts found in premenopausal women include unilocular clear fluid cysts (e.g., follicular cysts and corpus luteum cysts), dermoid cysts, and endometrial cysts. They can be removed by making an incision on the ovary and separating the cyst from the ovarian cortex. Dermoid cysts should be removed in toto to prevent chemical peritonitis. Endometrial cysts are best evaporated with the laser: complete removal is very difficult and sometimes impossible. Torsion of the fallopian tube or the ovary can be reversed by gentle detorsion of the organ with atraumatic forceps. If there is no evidence of ischemia, no further therapy is indicated. If there is gangrene with no indication of recovery, resection is indicated. If the organ shows partial recovery within 10 minutes after the pedicle is untwisted, a second-look laparoscopy is indicated in 24 hours. Pelvic inflammatory disease should be treated on an individualized basis in accordance with the degree of inflammation, the patient's age and desire to have children, and the microbiologic findings.

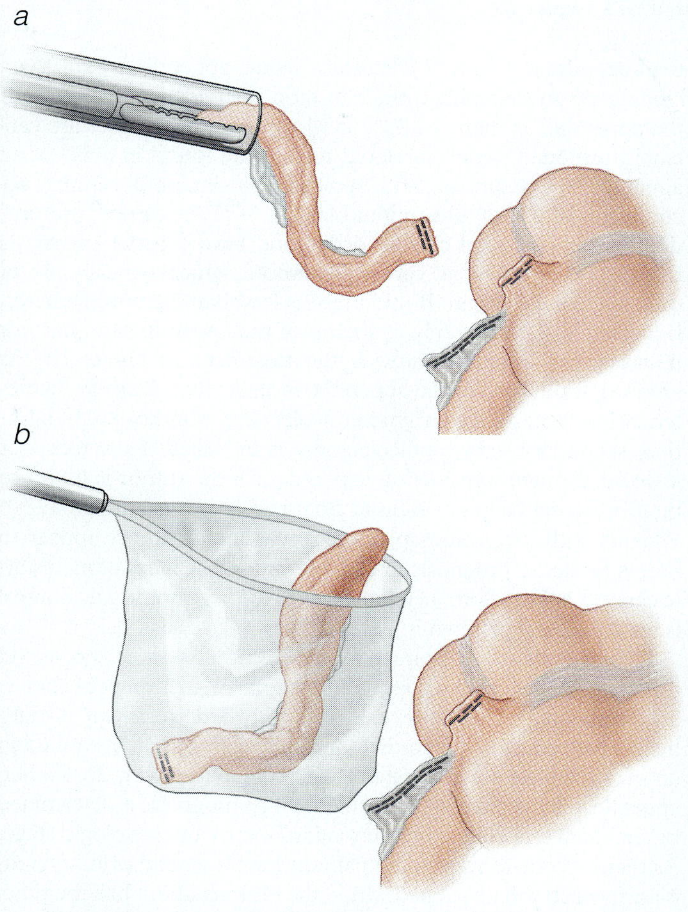

Figure 9 Laparoscopic appendectomy. The specimen is delivered either through one of the larger ports (*a*) or in a specimen retrieval bag (*b*).

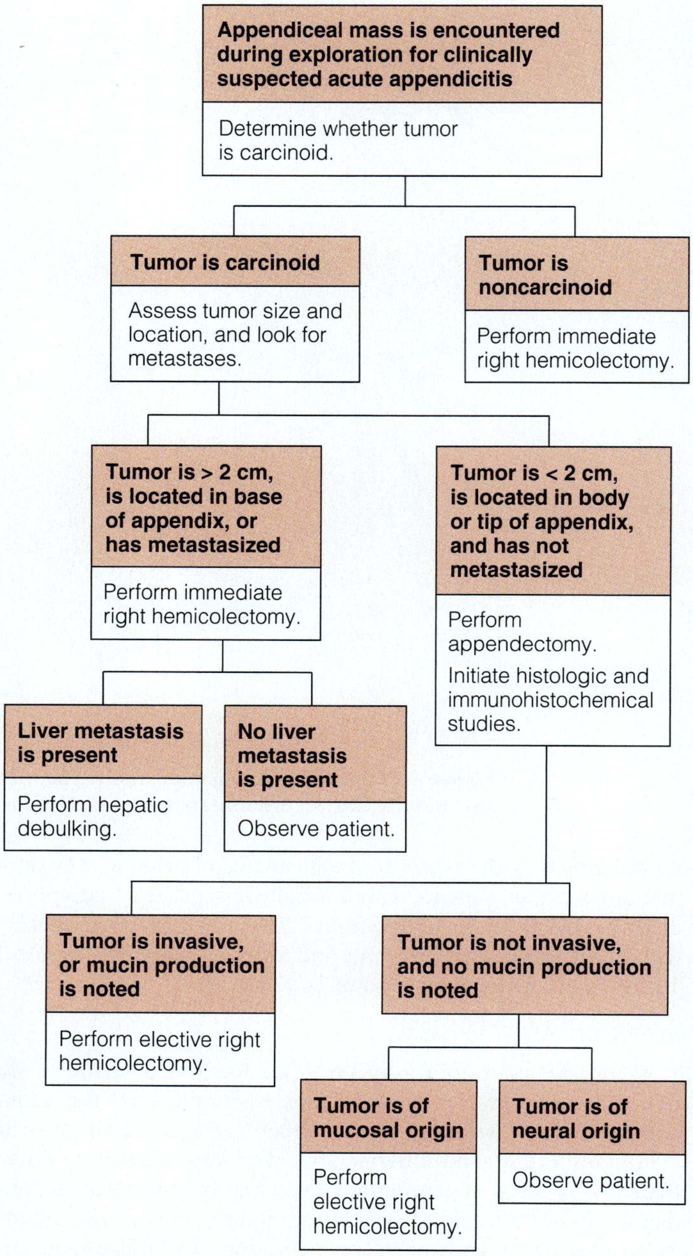

Figure 10 Shown is an algorithm for the management of an appendiceal mass encountered during exploration for clinically suspected acute appendicitis.

References

1. Fitz RH: Perforating inflammation of the vermiform appendix with special reference to its early diagnosis and treatment. Trans Assoc Am Physicians 1:107, 1886
2. McBurney C: The incision made in the abdominal wall in cases of appendicitis, with a description of a new method of operating. Ann Surg 20:38, 1894
3. Attwood SEA, Hill ADK, Murphy PG, et al: A prospective randomized trial of laparoscopic versus open appendectomy. Surgery 112:497, 1992
4. Tate JJT, Dawson JW, Chung SCS, et al: Laparoscopic versus open appendectomy: prospective randomised trial. Lancet 342:633, 1993
5. Kum CK, Ngoi SS, Goh PMY, et al: Randomized controlled trial comparing laparoscopic and open appendicectomy. Br J Surg 80:1599, 1993
6. Frazee RC, Roberts JW, Symmonds RE, et al: A prospective randomized trial comparing open versus laparoscopic appendectomy. Ann Surg 219:725, 1994
7. Ortega AE, Hunter JG, Peters JH, et al: A prospective, randomized comparison of laparoscopic appendectomy with open appendectomy. Am J Surg 169:208, 1995
8. Martin LC, Puente I, Sosa JL, et al: Open versus laparoscopic appendectomy: a prospective randomized comparison. Ann Surg 222:256, 1995
9. Hansen JB, Smithers BM, Schache D, et al: Laparoscopic versus open appendectomy: prospective randomized trial. World J Surg 20:17, 1996
10. Mutter D, Vix M, Bui A, et al: Laparoscopy not recommended for routine appendectomy in men: results of a prospective randomized study. Surgery 120:71, 1996
11. Cox MR, McCall JL, Toouli J, et al: Prospective randomized comparison of open versus laparoscopic appendectomy in men. World J Surg 20:263, 1996
12. Lejus C, Dellie L, Plattner V, et al: Randomized, single-blinded trial of laparoscopic versus open appendectomy in children. Anesthesiology 84:801, 1996
13. Williams MD, Collins JN, Wright TF, et al: Laparoscopic versus open appendectomy. South Med J 89:668, 1996
14. Hart R, Rajgopal C, Plewes A, et al: Laparoscopic versus open appendectomy: a prospective randomized trial of 81 patients. Can J Surg 39:457, 1996
15. Reiertsen O, Larsen S, Trondsen E, et al: Randomized controlled trial with sequential design of laparoscopic versus conventional appendicectomy. Br J Surg 84:842, 1997
16. Laine S, Rantala A, Gullichsen R, et al: Laparoscopic appendectomy—is it worthwhile? a prospective, randomized study in young women. Surg Endosc 11:95, 1997
17. Macarulla E, Vallet J, Abad JM, et al: Laparoscopic versus open appendectomy: a prospective randomized trial. Surg Laparosc Endosc 7:335, 1997
18. Kazemier G, de Zeeuw GR, Lange JF, et al: Laparoscopic versus open appendectomy: a randomized clinical trial. Surg Endosc 11:336, 1997
19. Minne L, Varner D, Burnell A, et al: Laparosopic versus open appendectomy: prospective randomized study of outcomes. Arch Surg 132:708, 1997
20. Boerema WJ, Burnand KG, Fitzpatrick RI: Acute appendicitis. Aust NZ J Surg 51:165, 1981
21. Chang AR: An analysis of the pathology of 3,003 appendices. Aust NZ J Surg 51:169, 1981
22. Knight PJ, Vassy LE: Specific diseases mimicking appendicitis in childhood. Arch Surg 116:744, 1981
23. Pieper R, Kager L, Nasman P: Acute appendicitis: a clinical study of 1,018 cases of emergency appendectomy. Acta Chir Scand 148:51, 1982
24. Arnbjornsson E, Asp NG, Westin SI: Decreasing incidence of acute appendicitis, with special reference to the consumption of dietary fiber. Acta Chir Scand 148:461, 1982
25. Blind PJ, Dahlgren ST: The continuing challenge of the negative appendix. Acta Chir Scand 152:623, 1986
26. Lau WY: Correlation between gross appearence of the appendix and histological examination. Ann R Coll Surg Edinb 70:336, 1988
27. Budd JS, Armstrong CP: The correlation between gross appearance at appendix and histological examination. Ann R Coll Surg Edinb 70:395, 1988
28. Blair PM, Bugis PS, Turner LJ, et al: Review of the pathologic diagnosis of 2,216 appendectomy specimens. Am J Surg 165:618, 1993
29. Dahlstom JE, MacArthur EB: *Enterobius vermicularis:* a possible cause of symptoms resembling appendicitis. Aust NZ J Surg 64:692, 1994
30. Pearl RH, Hale DA, Molloy M, et al: Pediatric appendectomy. J Pediatr Surg 30:173, 1995
31. Truji M, Puri P, Reen DJ: Characterization of the local inflammatory response in appendicitis. J Pediatr Gastroenterol Nutr 16:43, 1993
32. Wang Y, Reen DJ, Puri P: Is a histologically normal appendix following emergency appendicectomy always normal? Lancet 347:1076, 1996
33. Collins DC: 71,000 human appendix specimens: a final report, summarizing 40 years' study. Am J Proctocol 14:265, 1963
34. Chan W, Fu KH: Value of routine histopathological examination of appendices in Hong Kong. J Clin Pathol 40:429, 1987
35. Lenriot JP, Hugier M: Adenocarcinoma of the appendix. Am J Surg 155:470, 1988
36. Gupta SC, Gupta AK, Keswani NK, et al: Pathology of tropical appendicitis. J Clin Pathol 42:1169, 1989
37. Thomas RM, Sobin LH: Gastrointestinal cancer. Cancer 75:154, 1995
38. Modlin IM, Sandor A: An analysis of 8305 cases of carcinoid tumors. Cancer 79:813, 1997
39. Moertel CG, Weiland LH, Nagorney DM, et al: Carcinoid tumor of the appendix: treatment and prognosis. N Engl J Med 317:1699, 1987
40. Gouzi JL, Laigneau P, Delalande JP, et al: Indications for right hemicolectomy in carcinoid tumors of the appendix. Surg Gynecol Obstet 176:543, 1993
41. Nitecki SS, Wolff BG, Schlinkert R, et al: The natural history of surgically treated primary adenocarcinoma of the appendix. Ann Surg 219:51, 1994
42. Yang SS, Gibson P, McCaughey RS, et al: Primary Crohn's disease of the appendix. Ann Surg 189:334, 1979
43. Jahadi MR, Shaw ML: The pathology of the appendix in ulcerative colitis. Dis Colon Rectum 19:345, 1976
44. Ruiz V, Unger SW, Morgan J, et al: Crohn's disease of the appendix. Surgery 107:113, 1990
45. Goldblum JR, Appelman HD: Appendiceal involvement in ulcerative colitis. Mod Pathol 5:607, 1992

Acknowledgments

Figures 1 and 10   Marcia Kammerer.
Figures 2 through 9   Tom Moore.

57 COLORECTAL PROCEDURES

Theodore R. Schrock, M.D.

Total Colectomy with Ileorectal Anastomosis

OPERATIVE PLANNING

Total colectomy involves resection of the entire colon with oversewing of the rectum or construction of an ileorectal anastomosis.[1] Candidates for this operation include certain patients with inflammatory bowel disease, familial adenomatous polyposis, hereditary nonpolyposis colorectal cancer syndromes, chronic constipation, or severe lower gastrointestinal hemorrhage [see 19 *Lower Gastrointestinal Bleeding*].[2-5] The operation is performed in two stages in patients with fulminant colitis, severe inflammation of the rectum, pelvic abscess, or severe associated disease. Some surgeons perform total colectomy with ileorectal anastomosis via a laparoscopic or laparoscopic-assisted approach; however, in what follows, I address only conventional open techniques.

OPERATIVE TECHNIQUE

Step 1: Positioning and Incision

The lithotomy position, with the lower extremities in Lloyd-Davies leg rests or Allen universal stirrups, has the advantage of providing good access to the anus. The rectum can be examined and irrigated with saline before preparation and draping, and intraoperative colonoscopy, stapling maneuvers, and inspection of the anastomosis for integrity can be performed.

The positioning of the surgical team depends on the experience and the anticipated role of the assistants. If the first assistant is able to dissect under the surgeon's guidance, the surgeon should stand on the patient's left side, a position that gives the surgeon control of retraction and exposure of the right colon and the transverse colon. (I assume this arrangement in the description of the procedure.) When working on the left colon, the assistant retracts with one hand and dissects with the other, while the surgeon displays the tissues to be incised laterally. In the teaching environment, positions sometimes shift around the table.[1]

A midline incision is standard, but a transverse incision below the umbilicus is feasible in slender patients and in patients with long-standing inflammatory bowel disease, which often shortens the colon and the mesocolon.

Step 2: Mobilization and Removal of the Colon

The sigmoid colon is occluded with an encircling ligature of heavy material (e.g., umbilical tape) to prevent perineal soilage from distal passage of colonic contents.

Mobilization of the colon usually begins on the right side. The surgeon pinches the peritoneal surfaces together lateral to the cecum to protect the bowel from injury, and the peritoneum is incised very close to the cecal wall. The surgeon inserts the left index finger into the defect, retracting the cecum and the ascending colon medially while the lateral peritoneum is incised [see *Figure 1*]. The white line of Toldt is ignored on the right side, and the peritoneum is incised as close to the colon as possible. (Incising the peritoneum close to the wall of the right colon makes it unlikely that the surgeon will incise Gerota's fascia and dissect into perinephric fat.) The cecum is pulled laterally, and the medial layer of peritoneum of the distal ileal mesentery is incised proximally as far as necessary. The right ureter is identified.

As the hepatic flexure is approached, the duodenum appears, and the mesocolon is detached from it by dividing filmy tissue containing tiny vessels. In patients with benign disease, separation of the mesocolon from the duodenum up to the pancreas is unnecessary, but it does facilitate division of the mesocolon. In patients with cancer, full mobilization is necessary to ensure that vessels are ligated close to their origin. Hepatic flexure attachments contain vessels of varying size, some of which are large enough to necessitate ligation.

At this point, the surgeon must decide whether to preserve the greater omentum or to remove it. If the omentum is to be preserved, it is detached from the transverse colon; if it is to be removed, the gastrocolic ligament is serially divided and ligated. (I prefer to excise the greater omentum with the colonic specimen because the omentum causes obstruction of the small bowel after total colectomy much more frequently than it does after segmental colectomy.)

The lesser sac is entered to the left of the midline. (One should do this before the hepatic flexure is taken down completely and then work down to the right.) In the lesser sac, adhesions of the stomach to the transverse mesocolon are lysed, the gastrocolic ligament is serially divided and ligated outside the gastroepiploic vessels [see *Figure 2*], and the hepatic flexure is approached from the left. The mesocolon is left intact until it is fully separated from the gastrocolic, duodenal, and pancreatic attachments. The ileocolic, right colic (if present), and middle colic vessels are then divided at a level determined by the pathological problem being treated [see *Figure 3*]. (Some surgeons preserve the ileocolic vessels in case a pelvic pouch is possible later; however, because I deliberately divide the ileocolic vessels when constructing an ileoanal pouch, I do not preserve them when fashioning an ileorectal anastomosis.) The ileum is divided at the ileocecal valve with a linear cutting stapler or between intestinal clamps.

Once the dissection has reached the distal transverse colon, the sigmoid colon is mobilized so that the splenic flexure can be approached from the left. The sigmoid colon and the mesocolon are retracted to the right by the assistant, who remains on the patient's right side. Adhesions of the appendices epiploicae, the colon, and the mesocolon to the parietal peritoneum are divided. (This must be done in a bloodless plane. No fat should be

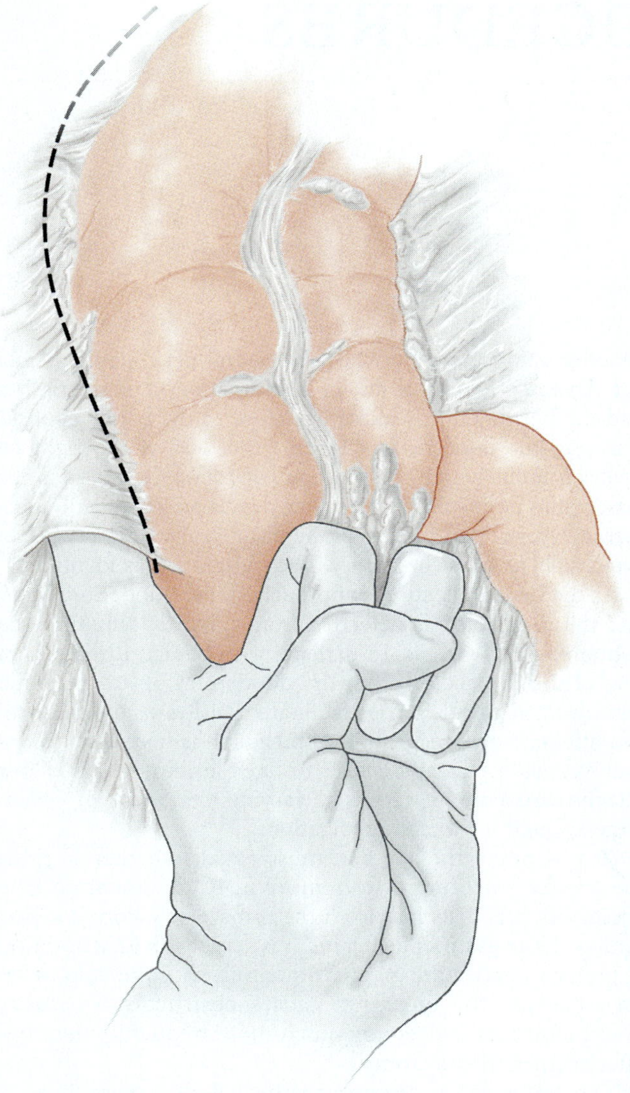

Figure 1 Total colectomy with ileorectal anastomosis. The surgeon inserts the left index finger into the peritoneal defect, retracting the cecum and the ascending colon medially while the lateral peritoneum is incised as close to the colon as possible.[1]

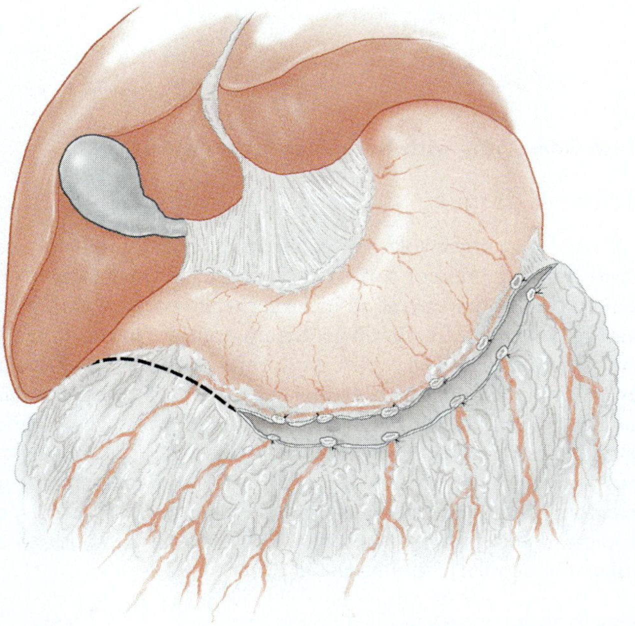

Figure 2 Total colectomy with ileorectal anastomosis. The gastrocolic ligament is serially divided and ligated outside the gastroepiploic vessels, and the hepatic flexure is approached from the left.[1]

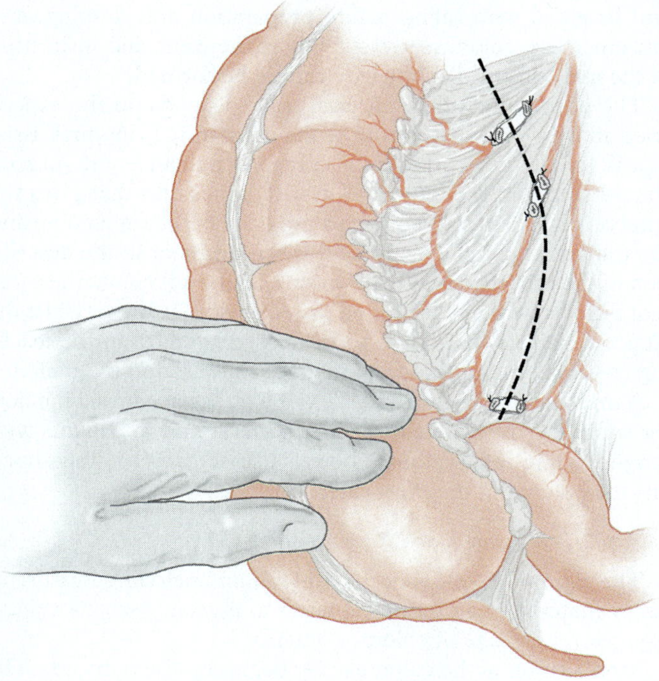

toneal attachments of the descending colon are incised a little at a time. (If the colonic attachments are divided all the way to the splenic flexure first, one can stray too far laterally and even end up within Gerota's fascia. The surgeon can insert one or two fingers into the space behind the peritoneum to display the next cut in mobilizing the sigmoid colon. There is no fat in the proper plane; if one is cutting through fat, one is in the wrong plane.)

The sigmoid colon is then pulled farther to the right, and the mesosigmoid is incised at its base. (The incision should be made on the left side, medial to the left ureter. If the ureter is not seen through the intact posterior parietal peritoneum, it should be visible after this incision is made.) The peritoneal incision is extended longitudinally, parallel to the course of the ureter, and the ureter is swept laterally. (Care should be taken to avoid the sympathetic nerves on the surface of the aorta, about 1 cm posterior to the superior hemorrhoidal vessels; injury to these nerves can cause ejaculatory impairment. In men with benign disease, there is no need to risk such impairment. Accordingly, dissection in the vicinity should be minimized once the ureter is seen and protected.)

The splenic flexure is taken down by approaching it from the left, from below, and from behind. The colon and the mesocolon are separated from Gerota's fascia, and the lateral peri-

Figure 3 Total colectomy with ileorectal anastomosis. The ileocolic, right colic, and middle colic vessels are ligated and divided at a level called for by the pathological problem being treated.[1]

portion for incision [*see Figure 4*]. It is important that the path of dissection remain within a few millimeters of the colon as the flexure is taken down. In this way, one follows the plane of attachment of the omentum, which is relatively avascular.) These maneuvers separate the omentum from the colon. If the omentum is to be removed, the remaining portion of the gastrocolic ligament must be divided and ligated so that a connection can be made with the plane established earlier.

The anterior layer of the peritoneum of the transverse mesocolon must be incised to take the splenic flexure down. Behind this thin layer, of course, lie the mesocolic vessels, which must be ligated. In patients with malignant disease, the inferior mesenteric artery and vein are divided and ligated (usually separately) after the left colic vessels are divided. In men with colitis or another benign disease, it is preferable to divide the left colic vessels and then the sigmoidal branches, leaving the inferior mesenteric vessels intact to obviate dissection in the vicinity of the sympathetic nerves. If the inferior mesenteric vessels must be divided, dissection should be carried out as close to them as possible to minimize the risk of nerve injury. The peritoneum on the right side of the base of the mesosigmoid is incised to facilitate vascular division.

The vessels at the rectosigmoid are divided close to the rectal wall in men with benign disease, and the proximal rectum is prepared for transection by division of the mesorectum. (The rectosigmoid is a 4 cm long transitional zone at the sacral promontory, where the taeniae coli merge into a confluent circular muscle coat and the lumen widens.) The rectum is divided between clamps.

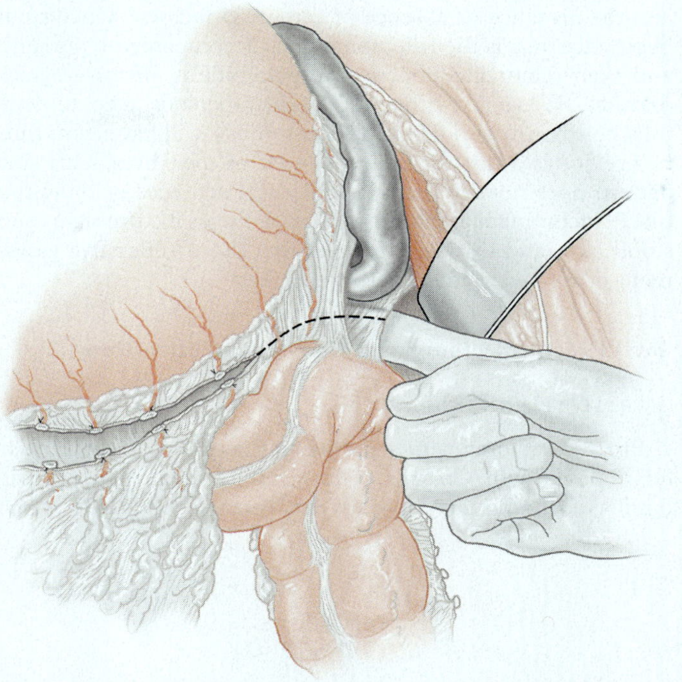

Step 3: Ileorectal Anastomosis

Whether an ileorectal anastomosis should be done by hand suturing or by stapling and whether it should be end-to-end or side-to-end are matters of personal preference. My own predilection is for a side-to-end stapled anastomosis, as described here.

A basic problem in ileorectal anastomosis is that the ileal lumen is substantially smaller than the rectal lumen. When performing an end-to-end anastomosis, one can obviate the luminal discrepancy problem by making an antimesenteric slit in the ileum to enlarge it. Another way of obviating the problem is to construct a side-to-end ileorectal anastomosis, either with sutures or with staples (see below). (One caveat is that side-to-end stapling of a very small ileum to a very large rectum seems to bunch up the ileal wall. Although the anastomosis generally heals well and functions satisfactorily, it may not look quite right to the eye. For this reason, I usually hand suture if the luminal discrepancy is very great.)

In a side-to-end stapled ileorectal anastomosis [*see Figure 5*], the stapled end of the ileum is arranged with the cut edge of the mesentery to the patient's right. A 0 polypropylene purse-string suture is placed on the rectal stump. (A finer suture might break when it is tied.) A divot large enough to accommodate the intraluminal stapler is excised from the antimesenteric wall of the ileum. (I generally prefer to use the largest intraluminal stapler available—31 or 33 mm, depending on the manufacturer—but sometimes the next smaller size seems to fit better.) The anastomosis should be about 1 cm from the stapled stump of the ileum. (It should not be so close that the zone between is devascularized.) A 2-0 polypropylene purse-string suture is placed on the ileal defect. The stapler is inserted through the anus and opened, and the distal purse-string suture is tied. (The stapler should have

Figure 4 Total colectomy with ileorectal anastomosis. The surgeon can insert one or two fingers into the space behind the peritoneum to display the next portion for incision. The avascular plane is within a few millimeters of the colon as the flexure is taken down.[1]

a flat anvil: if the anvil has a protruding knob, it will bump into the opposite wall.) The shaft is separated, and the anvil is secured in the ileum by tying the proximal purse-string suture. The stapler is then reassembled and fired. Two intact rings of tissue ("doughnuts") should be obtained. The anastomosis is checked for integrity by inserting a rigid sigmoidoscope through the anus and insufflating air with the pelvis filled with saline.

Step 4: Completion

The edge of the ileal mesentery is sutured to the retroperitoneal surface to eliminate the potential hernial defect. Drains are not required. A diverting loop ileostomy is rarely necessary with this procedure.

COMPLICATIONS

Ileus can be prolonged after total colectomy [*see 17 Intestinal Obstruction*]. Obstruction of the small bowel after total colectomy can be minimized by excising the omentum and closing the mesenteric defect. Anastomotic leakage after ileorectal anastomosis is more common in patients with inflammatory bowel disease than in patients with other conditions; in any case, the incidence of this complication should be lower than four percent. Large leaks necessitate reoperation, takedown of the anastomosis, closure of the rectal stump, and end ileostomy until conditions are right for reconnection of the bowel. Small leaks may be managed nonoperatively.

OUTCOME

Return of function depends on the indication for the operation, the presence or absence of rectal disease, the patient's age, and the presence or absence of comorbid factors.[6] Once stools begin, diarrhea is the rule, sometimes accompanied by urgency and even minor incontinence. Loperamide is effective against diarrhea. Generally, otherwise healthy persons who undergo total colectomy with ileorectal anastomosis will have from three to five stools a day for the remainder of their lives. This stool pattern does not interfere with physical activities or daily routine.[7] Incontinence should not be a lingering problem once stools slow and thicken, provided that the preoperative assessment of sphincter adequacy was correct.

Total Proctocolectomy with Conventional Ileostomy

OPERATIVE PLANNING

Proctocolectomy with a permanent ileostomy is appropriate for patients with Crohn's colitis and for some patients with familial adenomatous polyposis or ulcerative colitis who are not candidates for restorative proctocolectomy because of obesity, advanced age, or the presence of cancer in the distal rectum.

Preoperative education of the patient regarding the ileostomy is essential. Either an enterostomal therapist or the surgeon should, if possible, select the site for the stoma with the patient supine, standing, and sitting [see 105 Stomal Care]. The ileostomy must pass through the rectus sheath and must be located away from depressions and elevations. The ideal site is nearly always in the right lower quadrant.

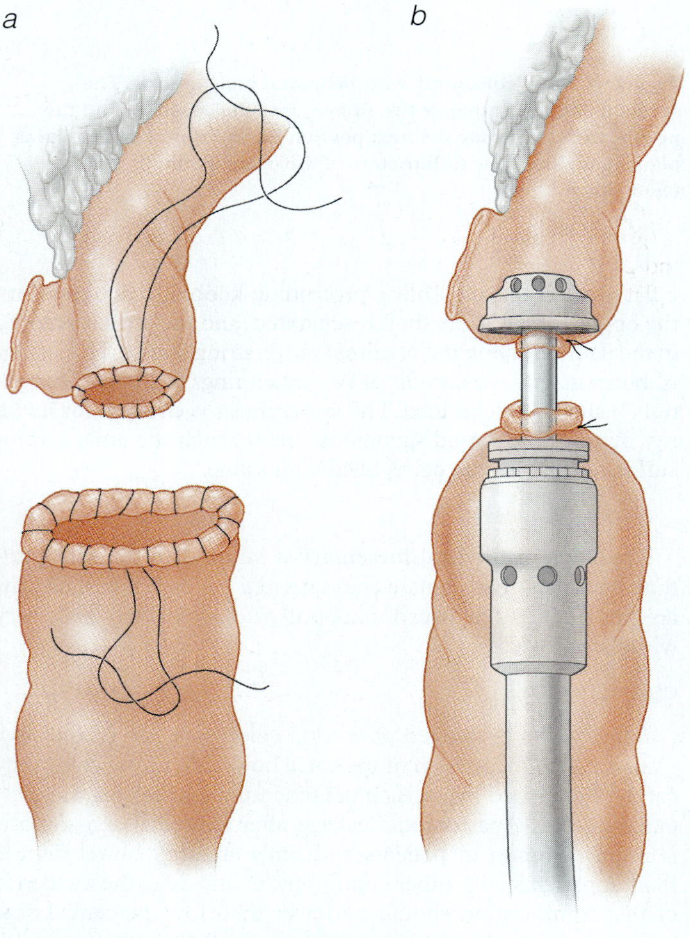

OPERATIVE TECHNIQUE

Step 1: Positioning

If the operation is to be performed by two teams, the lithotomy position obviously is necessary. If the entire operation is to be performed by a single surgeon, the patient can be repositioned after the abdomen is closed. The anus is closed with a heavy purse-string suture.

Step 2: Creation of Ileostomy Aperture

The first step in creating the ileostomy aperture is to excise a circle of skin about 2.5 cm in diameter.[8] (This aperture should be made before incising the abdominal incision so as to maintain normal alignment of the layers of the abdominal wall.) My preferred technique is to grasp the skin with a Kocher clamp and elevate it strongly, then to excise a disk of skin with a heavy curved scissors oriented in the longitudinal direction; stress along Langer's lines converts an elliptical aperture on the vertical axis to a circular opening. Dermis that was crushed but not excised is removed with the electrocautery. (Admittedly, this method looks crude, but it nearly always results in a perfect circle.)

The fat is spread with a clamp, not excised. Dead space is not desirable at an ileostomy site. The anterior rectus sheath is incised longitudinally, the rectus is separated with a clamp, and the posterior rectus sheath is exposed. A moist sponge is stuffed into this space, and the aperture is completed after the main abdominal incision is made. (Care should be taken not to injure the inferior epigastric vessels.)

Step 3: Colectomy and Preparation of Ileal Mesentery

Colectomy is carried out as described earlier [see Total Colectomy with Ileorectal Anastomosis, above]. (It is important to prepare the ileal mesentery in such a way that the bowel projects straight ahead and is not curved by tension on the mesentery. The ileal mesentery is divided in an L fashion so that the blood supply is preserved but the tissue that is to be brought through the abdominal wall is thinned [see Figure 6].)

Step 4: Pelvic Dissection

Dissection proceeds close to the rectal wall until well below the sacral promontory.[9] (In this way, one can usually keep from injuring the sympathetic nerves of the superior hypogastric plexus—that is, the presacral nerves. These nerves lie at the level of the aortic bifurcation and divide into the left and right hypogastric nerves, which extend into the pelvis.[10])

The technique of posterior dissection has changed. In the classical method, the presacral connective tissue was incised for a short distance, the surgeon's hand was inserted, and the mesorectum was separated from the endopelvic fascia by blunt dissection; the separation created a characteristic sucking sound.[11] (This technique crudely tears the soft tissues in what the surgeon can only hope is the proper plane, sometimes

Figure 5 Total colectomy with ileorectal anastomosis. (*a*) In a side-to-end stapled ileorectal anastomosis, a 0 polypropylene purse-string suture is placed on the rectal stump. A divot is excised from the antimesenteric wall of the ileum, and a 2-0 polypropylene purse-string suture is placed on the ileal defect. (*b*) An end-to-end or intraluminal stapler is inserted through the anus and opened, and the distal purse-string suture is tied. The proximal purse-string suture is tied to secure the anvil in the ileum. The stapler is then reassembled and fired.[1]

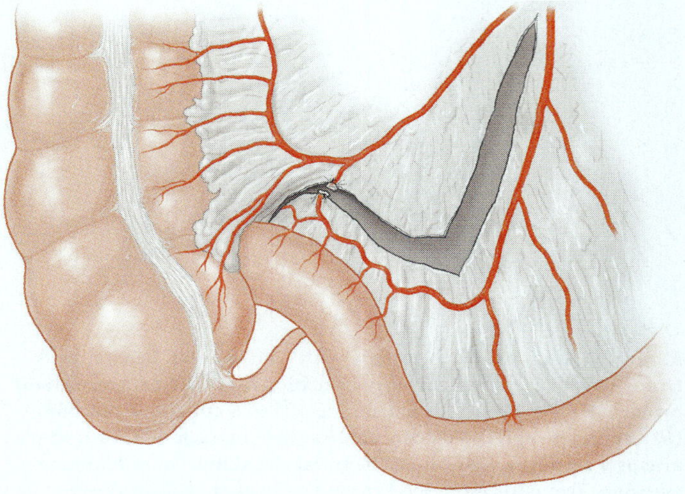

Figure 6 Total proctocolectomy with conventional ileostomy. The ileal mesentery is divided in an L fashion to thin the tissue that will be brought through the abdominal wall. After the ileocolic vessels are divided and ligated, the mesentery is incised toward the bowel about 1 cm away from the vessels to be preserved; this plane is crossed by no important vessels. The mesenteric incision is then extended at a right angle toward the ileocecal area. Transillumination shows the vessels that must be divided so that the edge of the ileum at the cecum can be reached; there are usually two of these.[8]

under direct vision. (This dissection is bloodless or nearly so, and it rarely results in injury to the presacral veins.) Posterior dissection is carried down to the surface of the levator muscles. The pelvic peritoneum is incised bilaterally 1 cm or more medial to the ureters, and the two incisions are connected anteriorly. In men, the rectum is separated from the anterior structures posterior to Denonvilliers' fascia; the seminal vesicles and the prostate are separated from the rectum by blunt dissection or electrocauterization. In women, the rectum is separated from the vagina. If no cancer is present, the lateral dissection should be close to the wall of the rectum. The surgeon's left hand retracts the rectum strongly to the left as the right hand dissects the right side of the pelvis, and the assistant provides the same exposure on the left side. The lateral ligaments are divided completely down to the levators. Either electrocauterization or serial ligation is appropriate.

Step 5: Proctectomy (Perineal Phase)

In patients with benign disease, an intersphincteric proctectomy is performed to minimize the risk of autonomic neurologic sequelae [see Figure 7]. In some patients with extensive fistulas, this method is not advantageous or even possible, and an extrasphincteric proctectomy must be done.

For an intersphincteric proctectomy, an elliptical incision is made around the anus over the intersphincteric groove, an easily palpable landmark just at the anal verge. Pennington clamps on the skin edges facilitate retraction. The incision is deepened with the electrocautery or with scissors to display the white fibers of the internal sphincter muscle running circumferentially. (The plane between the internal and external sphincters is fairly obvious laterally and posteriorly because the external sphincter is skeletal muscle and therefore reddish.[10]) Circumferential dissection continues proximally as the longitudinal muscle fibers are cut. Posteriorly, the external sphincter and the puborectalis sling are retracted until the pelvic space is entered by incision through Waldeyer's fascia. The specimen is delivered posteriorly, and the remaining anterior attachments are severed.

injuring the presacral veins, the pelvic nerves, or both. Consequently, it should be abandoned except in the most difficult situations, such as in obese men in whom there is limited visibility of the posterior pelvis.) In the method I now use, the rectum is pulled forward with a deep pelvic retractor, and the loose areolar tissue between the intact mesorectum and the intact endopelvic fascia is cut with the electrocautery or with scissors

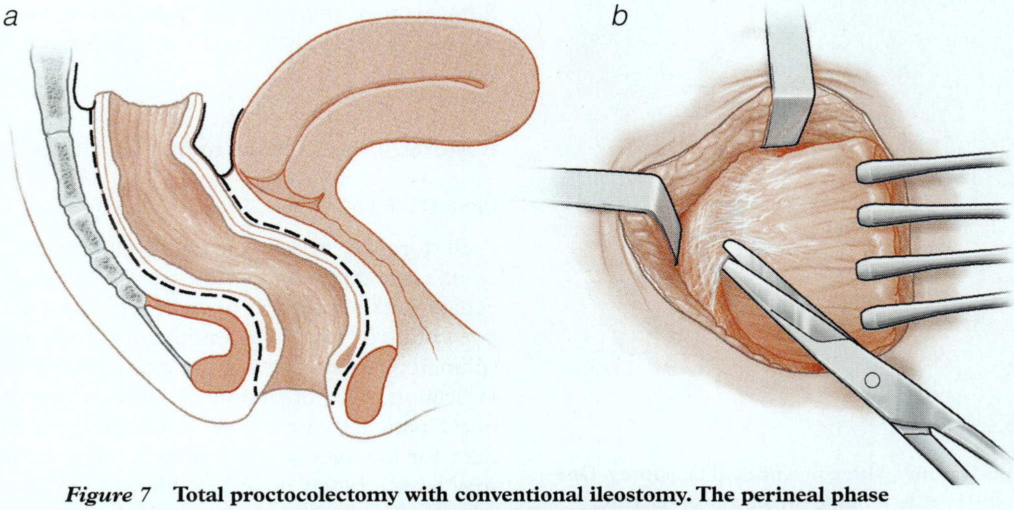

Figure 7 Total proctocolectomy with conventional ileostomy. The perineal phase usually involves the performance of an intersphincteric proctectomy. (*a*) The pelvic dissection is accomplished from the abdomen, and the perineal dissection preserves the external sphincters and the levators. (*b*) The internal and external sphincters are separated circumferentially by dividing the longitudinal muscle fibers of the gut, which lie in this plane. The specimen is delivered posteriorly (not shown), and the remaining anterior attachments are severed.[9]

Step 6: Closure of Perineal Wound

Sump drains are placed into the pelvic space through the buttocks rather than through the perineal wound itself. The levator muscles are approximated with absorbable sutures, and the soft tissues are closed in layers. The skin is closed with a subcuticular suture. (Primary closure should not be attempted in the presence of anorectal abscesses or complex fistulas.) The pelvic peritoneal floor is closed from the abdominal side with absorbable sutures.

Step 7: Fashioning of Ileostomy

The ileal stump is brought through the aperture so that it projects straight ahead about 5 to 6 cm above the skin.[8] The lateral gutter should be closed to prevent herniation of small bowel around the stoma [see Figure 8]. It is unnecessary to suture the bowel to fascia.

A Brooke-type everting ileostomy is fashioned by placing interrupted 4-0 absorbable sutures between the full thickness of the ileal wall and the subcuticular tissue [see Figure 9]. One suture in each quadrant also grasps a seromuscular bite of ileum at the skin level. (This facilitates eversion.) The completed stoma should project about 2.5 cm above the skin level. An appliance is placed immediately.

COMPLICATIONS

Early postoperative complications from ileostomy construction include ischemia, paraileostomy abscess, and intestinal obstruction from herniation of small bowel through the gutter.

Perineal wounds may become infected or fail to heal for other reasons. Persistent perineal sinus is a difficult problem that may occur in as many as 50 percent of patients with Crohn's colitis, especially if complex abscesses and fistulas were present at the time of operation.

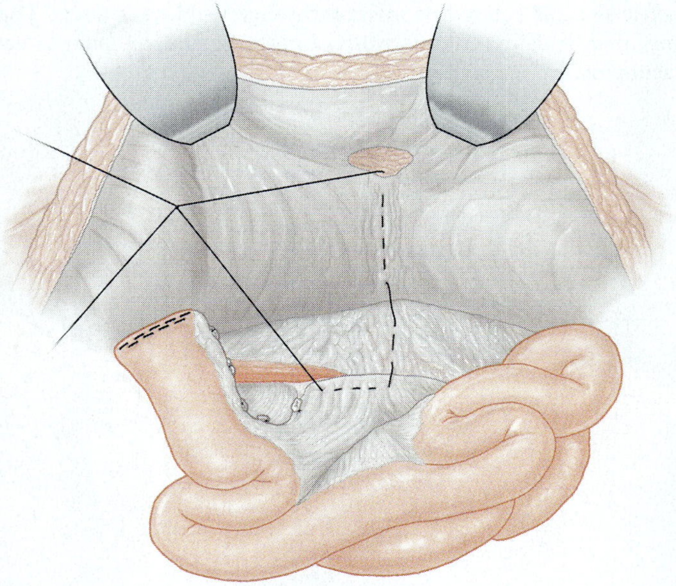

Figure 8 Total proctocolectomy with conventional ileostomy. One method of closing the gutter uses a purse-string suture passing laterally from the ileostomy aperture to the parietal peritoneum, the retroperitoneal tissue (with care taken to avoid the ureter), and the edge of the mesentery to a point about 8 cm from the ileal stump. The suture is tied and then continued cephalad to the duodenum.[8]

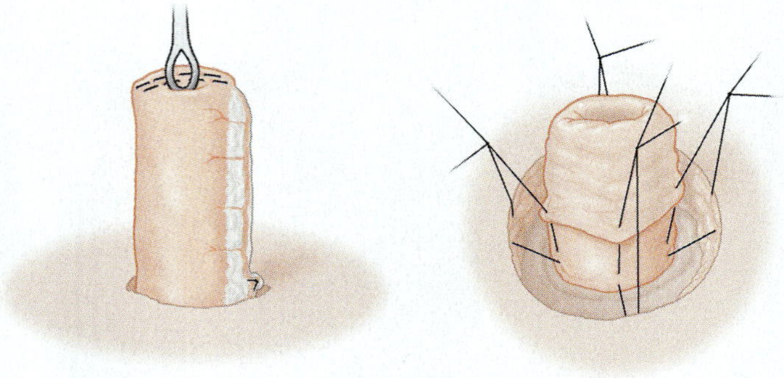

Figure 9 Total proctocolectomy with conventional ileostomy. A Brooke-type everting ileostomy is fashioned. (*a*) The ileum should project straight ahead for a distance of 5 to 6 cm above the skin. (*b*) One interrupted 4-0 absorbable suture in each quadrant also grasps a seromuscular bite of ileum at the skin level to facilitate eversion. Two additional interrupted sutures (not shown) are placed in each quadrant between the full thickness of the ileal wall and the subcuticular tissue.[8]

Postoperative bladder dysfunction is common but is usually transient.

OUTCOME

Operative mortality for proctocolectomy with ileostomy is less than one percent in elective settings; it is higher when the procedure is done on an emergency basis. Long-term sequelae include a variety of ileostomy complications, such as retraction, stenosis, prolapse, and paraileostomy hernia. Approximately 90 percent of patients with a permanent ileostomy are reasonably content, but much depends on the availability of alternatives when the initial operative decision was discussed. Some patients who experience physical or psychological problems with a conventional ileostomy are candidates for conversion to a continent ileostomy (Kock pouch).

As many as 15 percent of men who undergo proctocolectomy for benign disease exhibit some postoperative change in sexual function; only about one percent become totally impotent. Some women experience dyspareunia as a result of pelvic fibrosis; others experience sexual dysfunction as a result of altered body image.

Restorative Proctocolectomy with Ileoanal Pouch

OPERATIVE PLANNING

Restorative proctocolectomy—complete resection of the colon and rectum and anastomosis of an ileal pouch to the anal canal—is the operation of choice for most patients with ulcerative colitis or familial adenomatous polyposis.[3,12,13] Good anal sphincter function is a requisite. Crohn's disease is a contraindication. The operation is difficult but usually possible in obese patients. There is no absolute upper age limit for candidacy for this procedure; however, many elderly, infirm persons may have a better quality of life with an ileostomy. In patients who are acutely ill or malnourished, are receiving huge doses of steroids, or have a significant complication (e.g., perforation), the procedure should be staged.

Whether to perform rectal mucosectomy as part of the procedure is controversial at present. The approach described here involves excising all of the columnar epithelium and restoring continuity with a double-stapling technique that renders mucosectomy unnecessary in most patients.[14] The main advantage of this approach is that it minimizes the risk of minor functional impairment resulting from the direct trauma to the sphincters associated with mucosectomy and from the anal dilatation necessary to obtain exposure for mucosectomy. (Insertion of a self-retaining retractor that can be cranked open to improve exposure is risky. Although such devices yield a good view, they can damage the sphincters, often permanently.) The disadvantage of not performing mucosectomy is that one may leave behind some diseased columnar epithelium, which could remain inflamed in patients with ulcerative colitis or become malignant in patients with colitis or polyposis.[15]

OPERATIVE TECHNIQUE

Step 1: Positioning

The patient is positioned as for total proctocolectomy with ileostomy.

Step 2: Colectomy and Preparation of Ileal Mesentery

Colectomy is carried out as in total proctocolectomy with ileostomy. (Again, it is important to prepare the ileal mesentery in an L fashion as described for proctocolectomy with ileostomy. Some surgeons preserve the ileocolic vessels, but I do not: if these vessels are divided and the mesentery is prepared properly, the pouch will reach the anus in nearly every instance. It is also important to mobilize the base of the mesocolon and the small bowel mesentery in the hepatic flexure area all the way to the pancreas. Attachments to the duodenum are lysed thoroughly. The peritoneum should be incised on the medial side of the small bowel mesentery all the way up as well.) The ileum is divided with a linear cutting stapler flush with the ileocecal valve.

The ability of the proposed pouch to reach the anus is tested by grasping the ileum about 15 cm proximal to the stapled stump and pulling it to the pubis. If it reaches or extends beyond the lower edge of the pubic bone, there will be no problem; if it does not extend to the lower edge of the pubis, it probably will still reach the anus, but there may be some tension. (A diverting ileostomy may be advisable.) If additional length is needed, it can be obtained via relaxing incisions through the peritoneum of the mesentery on both sides. (Some surgeons divide mesenteric vessels to gain length, but I have never found this step necessary.) Construction of the pouch is deferred until the colectomy is completed.

Step 3: Proctectomy

The abdominal and pelvic portions of the operation are carried out as described for total proctocolectomy with ileostomy. The rectum is mobilized to the levator muscles circumferentially, but one does not stop at this point: the bowel is dissected from the enveloping puborectal muscles posteriorly and laterally and from urogenital structures anteriorly. (This portion of the large bowel is actually the anal canal. It is lined by columnar epithelium in the upper 1 cm and by transitional epithelium in the lower 1 cm down to the dentate line, though there is anatomic variation in this regard. The pelvic staple line should be in the anal canal rather than the rectum so that diseased mucosa will not be left behind. The surgeon can judge the adequacy of distal mobilization by inserting a finger into the anus from the perineum with the other hand in the pelvis. It is possible to mobilize all the way to the dentate line in most persons, but the intent is to staple across the anal canal 1.0 to 1.5 cm proximal to the dentate line. The end-to-end stapler removes another 1 cm. An assistant can apply pressure to the perineum with a fist, but this is seldom necessary.)

The anal canal is closed off with a right-angle stapler. (I use a 30 mm stapler. If a 30 mm device is too small to close the anal canal across its entire width, one may be certain that mobilization has not been carried far enough distally. The stapler must be aligned so that the distance above the anal verge is uniform.) A crushing intestinal clamp is applied above the stapler, and the bowel is divided and removed. When the stapler is detached, the stump of the anal canal slips within the puborectal muscle.

Step 4: Construction of Ileal Pouch

A J pouch is constructed by approximating two 15 cm limbs measured proximally from the closed end of the ileum [*see Figure 10*]. (The J pouch and the W pouch are favored over other types that once were more popular.[16] Of the two, I prefer the J pouch because it functions as well as the W pouch and is simpler to construct.[17]) Three or four sutures are placed to align the limbs for side-to-side stapling. A divot is excised from the apex of the J with scissors, and an 80 mm linear cutting stapler is inserted with the anvil in one limb and the cartridge in the other. The stapler is fired and reloaded, and the bowel is bunched up in an accordionlike manner for the second firing. Two applications of the stapler are sufficient to construct a pouch 15 cm long.

A 2-0 polypropylene purse-string suture is placed on the cut edge of the apex of the J pouch, and the anvil of an end-to-end stapler is inserted and secured as the purse-string suture is tied. (I prefer to use the largest stapler available—31 or 33 mm—in the hope that all of the staple line on the anal canal stump will thereby be excised to minimize the possibility of leaving an ischemic corner.)

Step 5: Ileoanal Anastomosis

The end-to-end stapler is inserted into the anus with the spike withdrawn into the cartridge. (It is helpful to insert a sequence of progressively larger stapler sizers into the anus to ensure that the anus can accommodate the stapler and also to show the anal canal stump from the pelvic side. At this point, one must be certain that there is adequate separation from surrounding structures, especially the vagina. I find it essential to insert the stapler into the anus with both hands and then to manipulate it into place with the left hand while palpating the anal canal stump with the right hand in the pelvis. The contamination from this maneuver is a small price to pay for the assurance that the stapler is resting firmly against the stump of the anal canal circumferentially. The entire head of the stapler does not slip into the anal canal above the sphincters, as is normally the case in colorectal anastomoses; instead, the stapler rests within the anal sphincters because the anastomosis is so low. If the stapler is not properly positioned, staples may be fired through empty space rather than through tissue.)

The stapler is opened, and the spike is allowed to penetrate the anal stump adjacent to the staple line. The cut edge of the small bowel mesentery is placed toward the patient's right, and a quick check is done to make sure that the pouch has not been rotated 360°. The stapler is then closed and fired. (Before the stapler is closed, one should be sure that the vagina is adequately cleared away and thus will not be caught in the anastomosis. As the stapler is closed, there is inevitably some rotation of the pouch and its mesentery, but this does not seem to cause any problem.)

Two intact doughnuts should be obtained. The anastomosis is tested by palpation and by direct inspection with a rigid sigmoidoscope inserted into the anus. A noncrushing clamp is placed across the ileum above the pouch, and a pool of saline is placed in the pelvis. Air is insufflated to test for leaks. Leaks can usually be repaired by suturing through the anus (see below). In some patients, a diverting ileostomy may be advisable (see below).

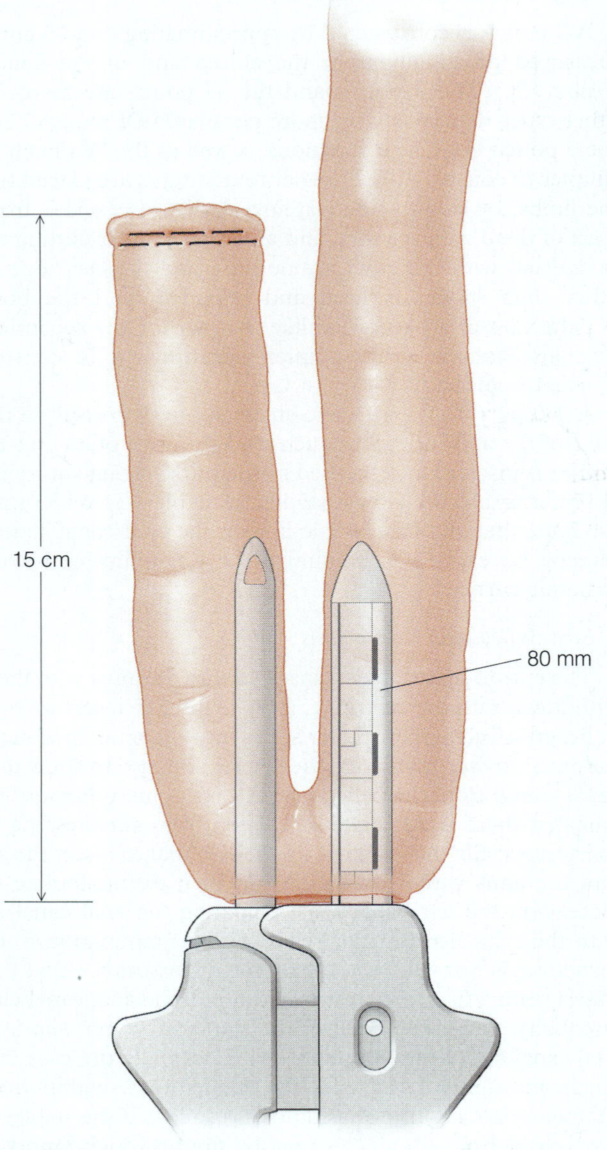

Step 6: Optional Steps

Placement of transanal purse-string suture If, for some reason, one cannot use the stapler or if there has been a mishap in the course of the operation (e.g., entry into the lumen), the procedure can be salvaged by transanal placement of a purse-string suture. (This step can be difficult for surgeons who lack experience with the technique. Exposure is limited, and bleeding can obscure the view. A headlight is essential. Separate instruments should be available for the perineal operator.)

Two Gelpi retractors are placed to evert the anus, and a Hill-Ferguson retractor is inserted to expose the anoderm and the epithelium of the anal canal above the dentate line. The full thickness of the wall of the anal canal is incised with a curved scissors in the posterior midline about 1 cm above the dentate line. This incision should provide entry into the pelvic dissection space if the earlier dissection was extended low enough. The entire circumference of the anal canal is divided, and the purse-string suture is placed through the full thickness of the bowel. (I prefer to start this suture in the posterior midline so that it will be easier to tie with the stapler in place. A curved needle holder is helpful.) The Hill-Ferguson retractor is moved to bring successive portions of the circumference into view. The stapler is inserted and opened, and the shaft is reattached. The distal purse-string suture is tied. The stapler is then closed and fired. (This method is more likely to yield incomplete distal doughnuts.)

Construction of diverting ileostomy If there is concern about anastomotic integrity or the patient's healing capacity, a diverting ileostomy should be constructed. (Diverting loop ileostomy was once routine for all restorative proctocolectomy patients, but I no longer do it in low-risk patients whose anastomosis looks satisfactory and does not leak on testing.[18]) If an ileostomy is constructed, it can be taken down in about two months.

Step 7: Completion

Drains are inserted into the pelvis from the abdominal side. The edge of the small bowel mesentery is sutured to the retroperitoneum down to the pelvic brim; it is usually impossible to complete this closure.

COMPLICATIONS

The main complications of this procedure are abscess, anastomotic leakage, and so-called pouchitis. Most abscesses are related to minor anastomotic leaks that are contained in a small area; they tend to be small and easily drained. Large anastomotic or pelvic abscesses or fistulas are uncommon; they may result in failure of the procedure if corrective steps cannot salvage the pouch. So-called cuff abscesses are a complication of mucosectomy in which infected fluid accumulates in the space between the denuded rectal muscle tube and the ileal pouch.

Anastomotic leaks are usually masked by the presence of a diverting ileostomy. They may be revealed by imaging studies before the ileostomy is taken down, or they may remain undetected until the fecal stream is reestablished. If a diverting ileostomy is not performed, leaks become clinically evident in the first few postoperative days; if leakage is significant, laparotomy with ileostomy is the only recourse. Since I abandoned routine initial ileostomy, I have encountered significant anastomotic leakage in only three percent of 95 patients, and other surgeons have reported similar results.[14]

Pouchitis is a late postoperative complication that presumably is related to bacterial overgrowth in the stagnant pouch contents.

Figure 10 Restorative proctocolectomy with ileoanal pouch. Shown is the construction of a J pouch. Two 15 cm limbs, measured proximally from the closed end of the ileum, are aligned; sutures (not shown) may help hold the alignment for stapling. A divot is excised from the apex of the J with scissors. An 80 mm linear cutting stapler is inserted through the resulting opening with the anvil in one limb and the cartridge in the other. Two applications of the stapler are sufficient to construct a 15 cm pouch.

It is rare in patients with familial adenomatous polyposis and consequently is believed to be related in some way to inflammatory bowel disease.[19] Perhaps 25 percent of patients with an ileoanal pouch experience pouchitis at some point. The typical manifestations are cramps and diarrhea (sometimes bloody); occasionally, there are systemic symptoms (e.g., fever or arthralgia). The pouch appears inflamed on endoscopy, but this finding is deceptive because some asymptomatic pouches appear red and friable also. Treatment with antibiotics (e.g., metronidazole or a cephalosporin) is usually successful. In a few patients, medical management fails and the pouch must be excised.

OUTCOME

The average patient has about five stools a day after restorative proctocolectomy, but stool frequency may range from two to 10 a day without complications. Minor seepage is common in the first weeks after operation, but significant fecal incontinence is uncommon. With the techniques currently in use, infection, pouchitis, incontinence, and other problems lead to failure in about five percent of patients.[20]

Low Anterior Resection with Coloproctostomy

OPERATIVE PLANNING

Anterior resection is the procedure of choice for most cancers in or above the midrectum. The goal is to excise the portion of the rectum that contains the tumor and to remove the entire mesorectum as well as pararectal tissue containing lymphatic vessels and lymph nodes. Good technique is critical for minimizing the likelihood of recurrence in the pelvis.

Tumor Assessment

Resection and anastomosis are anatomically impossible when the distal edge of the cancer is lower than about 5 cm above the anal verge (3 cm above the dentate line). In practice, many midrectal cancers that are large, deeply invasive, or poorly differentiated cannot be dealt with by anterior resection either. If the tumor can be moved at all before dissection is begun, it can usually be excised; however, fixity on digital palpation is not a reliable sign that the tumor is unresectable. Computed tomography, magnetic resonance imaging, and endorectal ultrasonography may be helpful. The patient's body habitus and preferences should be taken into account. Sometimes, the final decision regarding sphincter preservation can be made only during the operation. Occasionally, the potential for anastomosis cannot be assessed until the rectum has been mobilized. Extension into the urogenital structures may be apparent, and it should be possible to determine whether the anterior structures (the uterus or the vagina in particular) must be resected en bloc to effect cure.

Excision of the primary tumor is the most effective way of palliating rectal adenocarcinoma. Prevention or relief of tenesmus is a goal worth pursuing, even in patients with distant metastases. Tenesmus is not relieved by fecal diversion, nor is it reliably eliminated by radiation therapy or other forms of local treatment.

OPERATIVE TECHNIQUE

Step 1: Positioning

The patient should be placed in the lithotomy position in Lloyd-Davies leg rests or Allen universal stirrups. Rectal examination is performed to confirm the preoperative assessment of the tumor, and the rectum is irrigated with saline to eliminate any residual stool.

Step 2: Mobilization of Sigmoid and Mesosigmoid

The distal sigmoid is occluded with an encircling umbilical tape to prevent movement of luminal contents from the proximal colon into the rectum and intraluminal migration of malignant cells from the primary rectal cancer into the portion of colon to be retained.

The sigmoid colon and the mesocolon are dissected away from peritoneal attachments, and the left base of the mesosigmoid is incised medial to the ureter as described for total colectomy with ileoanal anastomosis. The splenic flexure is taken down partially or completely, with the redundancy of the sigmoid and the level of the tumor kept in mind. The peritoneum at the base of the mesosigmoid on the right is incised, and the incision is continued cephalad toward the duodenum for a variable distance, depending on the planned level of vessel ligation. (Care should be taken not to injure the preaortic sympathetic nerves during this step. In addition, it is vital that the colon be mobilized in such a way that the proximal end of the bowel will reach the rectal stump with no tension. There must be no compromise on this point.)

Step 3: Ligation of Vessels

There is some controversy regarding the level at which vessels should be ligated during curative resection of rectal cancer. Some surgeons ligate just below the origin of the left colic artery; others ligate at the origin of the inferior mesenteric artery to remove the few nodes that remain with ligation more distally. The data consistently indicate, however, that the level of ligation does not influence survival rates. Today, most surgeons ligate the inferior mesenteric vessels just distal to the origin of the left colic artery.[21]

The mesocolon is divided radially to the point at which the surgeon plans to transect the colon. The colon may be transected either at this point or after the pelvic dissection has been completed.

Step 4: Pelvic Dissection

Dissection is carried out under direct vision. In men, the anterior plane of dissection is anterior to Denonvilliers' fascia if the cancer is nearby; if the lesion is more proximal, dissection can be posterior to Denonvilliers' fascia. In women, the rectum is separated from the vagina, but if there is an anterior lesion invading the vagina, the posterior vaginal wall must be excised. It may be possible to restore colorectal continuity in this situation; however, adjacent suture lines should be avoided, and abdominoperineal resection (see below) may be safer.

The aim of lateral dissection is to leave the pelvis devoid of lateral soft tissue. (To this end, one should remove all of the node-bearing tissue all the way to the pelvic sidewall but not external to the parietal pelvic fascia. One can ligate the middle hemorrhoidal vessels close to the pelvic sidewall and still achieve complete extirpation of soft tissues if this maneuver is conducted under direct vision.) The lateral ligaments are completely divided down to the levator muscles, with the bilobed so-called lipoma of the mesorectum left intact.

Step 5: Removal of Mesorectum

If the tumor is in the midrectum (especially if it is in the distal portion), one should excise the entire mesorectum rather than dissect through it to reach the rectal wall. (Residual tumor in the mesorectum is an important cause of local recurrence.) At the levator muscles, the rectal lumen is small, no more than 2.5 to 3.0 cm in diameter; above that point, the rectal lumen enlarges substantially.

Step 6: Anastomosis

Colorectal anastomosis The anastomosis may be done either by hand suturing or by stapling. (Because hand suturing a low anastomosis is tedious, I prefer either the double-staple technique or an open stapled approach.)

In a double-stapled coloproctostomy, the lumen above the planned line of transection is occluded with a right-angled crushing bowel clamp. The distal anorectum is irrigated transanally with dilute povidone-iodine to destroy malignant cells. A 30 mm right-angle ligating stapler (or a device of comparable size) is positioned and fired. (If dissection of the mesorectum is incomplete or if all of the pararectal tissue has not been divided, the 30 mm ligating stapler will not close off the entire rectal stump. One can usually tell when this problem is likely to arise, because the tissue grasped by the stapler will feel unusually bulky. The solution is to remove the stapler without firing it and then to dissect more completely.) The rectum is divided sharply between the stapler and the crushing clamp. A purse-string suture is applied to the colonic stump proximally, and an intraluminal or end-to-end stapler is inserted through the anus. (With a large stapler—31 or 33 mm—one can usually excise the entire original rectal staple line. Anastomotic leakage can arise from a tiny devascularized corner if a smaller device is used.)

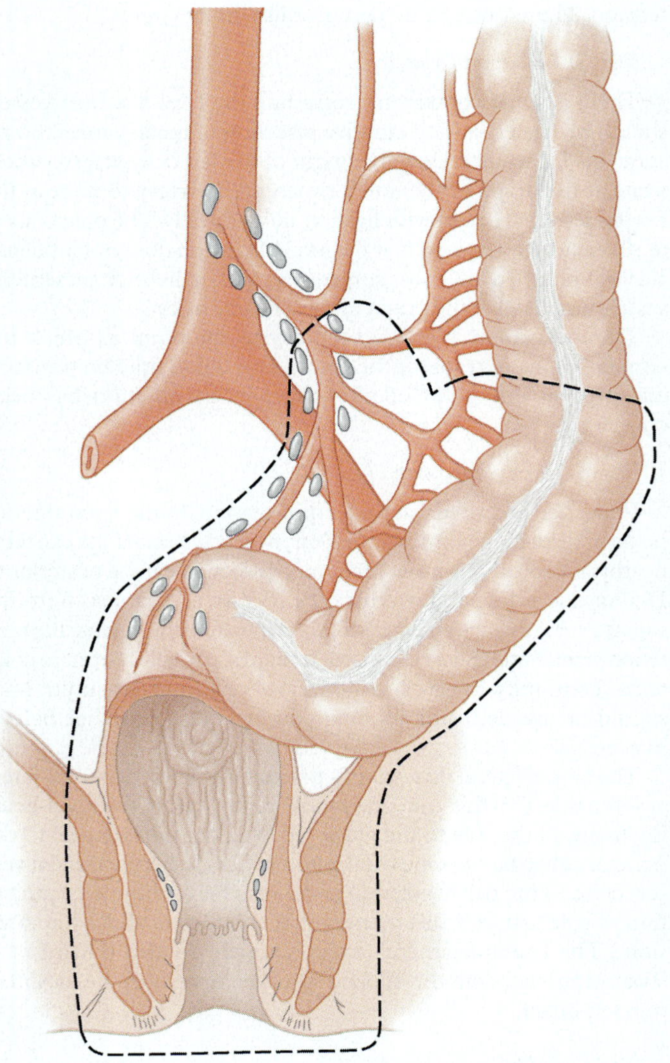

Alternatively, a purse-string suture can be placed distally by hand. (If the rectum is transected deeply in the pelvis, currently available mechanical purse-string appliers do not work well.) The rectum is occluded with a clamp proximal to the proposed site of transection, and the distal portion is irrigated as described for double stapling. The proximal clamp is placed immediately above the planned site of transection so that the bowel can be divided on the distal side flush with the clamp. A beaver blade scalpel with a long handle is used to incise into the rectal lumen in the center, and placement of the purse-string suture is begun with only a portion of the lumen open. (If the rectum is completely divided before the suture is begun, the stump will retract and the mucosa will pout, making the task of suturing unnecessarily difficult.) The rectal transection is completed gradually as the suture is continued.

The anastomosis is tested by digital rectal examination and inspection through a rigid sigmoidoscope as described for ileoanal anastomosis. Drains are placed through a stab wound in the left lower quadrant.

Coloanal anastomosis When a tumor lies in the distal portion of the midrectum but is still high enough for a margin to be obtainable, one may avoid abdominoperineal resection by performing a coloanal anastomosis. (Coloanal anastomosis is contraindicated in patients with impaired sphincters and persons with infirmities that prevent ready access to bathroom facilities.) Usually, the final decision is made during the operation. This procedure can be performed by means of the double-staple technique or by placing a purse-string suture transanally. Dissection within the levator muscles and the stapling procedure itself are performed as described for restorative proctocolectomy.

COMPLICATIONS

The incidence of clinically significant anastomotic leakage is about four percent. This complication is more common after colorectal anastomoses than after colonic anastomoses, in part because the rectum is devoid of serosa. Tension on the anastomosis is an important—and avoidable—precipitating factor. Infected pelvic fluid can erupt into the lumen and create a leak. Devascularization of a corner of the rectal stump in the double-stapling method can also cause anastomotic leakage.

Anastomotic stricture is usually the consequence of a leak, but membranous stenosis can develop in stapled anastomoses. This is rarely a significant problem if large-caliber staplers are used. Digital or sigmoidoscopic stretching of a membranous stenosis usually solves the problem permanently.

OUTCOME

Long-term survival of cancer patients after low anterior resection depends on the tumor stage; it should be no different from survival after abdominoperineal resection if patients are selected properly.

Figure 11 Abdominoperineal resection. The extent of the resection is outlined.[22]

The results of very low colorectal or coloanal anastomoses are sometimes functionally unsatisfactory. Mucous leakage is not uncommon. Bowel habits are unpredictable, and patients may experience irregularity and urgency.

Abdominoperineal Resection

OPERATIVE PLANNING

Abdominoperineal resection (APR) is the standard procedure for cancers of the distal rectum that are too low to permit preservation of the sphincter [see Figure 11].[22] Whether APR is appropriate in a given setting depends on the characteristics of the tumor and the general condition of the patient. The tumor is assessed as described for low anterior resection. Ascites is a strong contraindication to APR because ascitic leak through the perineal wound may be troublesome or even fatal if it leads to peritonitis. Palliative APR is worthwhile in many instances.

A colostomy site is selected, and the educational process is begun preoperatively.

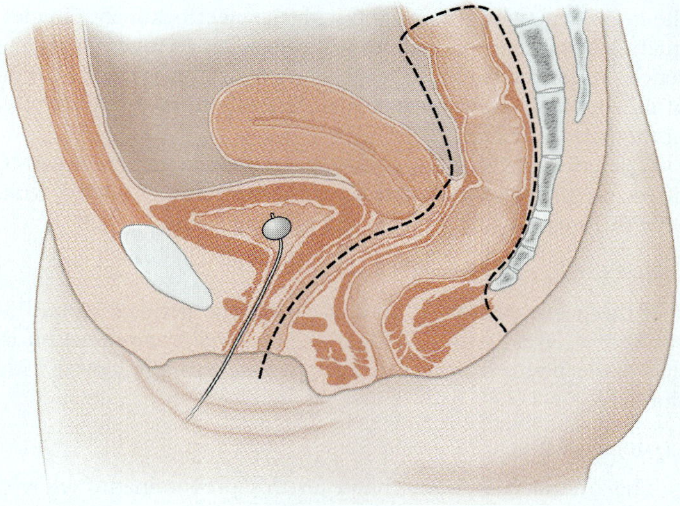

OPERATIVE TECHNIQUE

Step 1: Positioning

How the patient is positioned depends on whether APR is to be done in separate stages by a single team or synchronously by two teams. (The synchronous technique is more efficient, but a second experienced surgeon is needed to perform the perineal dissection.) If the two-stage approach is selected, the patient is supine for the abdominal phase and in the lithotomy position or the left lateral decubitus position for the perineal phase. The lateral decubitus position is more cumbersome because the patient must be turned, but it provides superb exposure of the anterior structures. In a difficult patient with an extensive tumor on the anterior wall, the lateral decubitus position is recommended. If the synchronous approach is selected, the patient is in the lithotomy position. If it is certain that APR will be done, the anus is closed with a purse-string suture of heavy material; two sutures should be placed, one within the other. (If there is no doubt about the need for a colostomy, the colostomy aperture is made before the main abdominal incision, as described for total proctocolectomy with ileostomy.)

Step 2: Pelvic Dissection

It is unnecessary to take down the splenic flexure. In men, the anterior pelvic dissection plane is anterior to Denonvilliers' fascia. In women with anterior rectal cancer, the posterior vaginal wall is included with the specimen [see Figure 12]. Hysterectomy is usually advisable in this situation.

Step 3: Closure of Pelvic Peritoneal Floor

If the operation is done in separate phases, the sigmoid is divided at this point, and the distal stump is covered with a rubber glove secured with an umbilical tape. The specimen is placed in the pelvis, and the pelvic peritoneum is closed. (If the entire specimen does not fit into the pelvic space, the bowel must be divided again, but this must not be done too close to the tumor.) If the synchronous approach is used, the specimen is passed through the posterior aspect of the perineal wound to the perineal operator. (Some surgeons do not close the pelvic peritoneum routinely; in a few patients, it is impossible to close this layer because of previous pelvic surgery or irradiation. With

Figure 12 Abdominoperineal resection. In women with anterior rectal cancer, the posterior vaginal wall is included with the specimen. Hysterectomy (not shown) is often done as well.[22]

the pelvic peritoneal floor open, the small bowel falls into the pelvis, but this occurrence probably does not increase the incidence of intestinal obstruction.[21] If postoperative radiation therapy is likely, the pelvic peritoneal floor should be closed, and if there is insufficient peritoneum for this purpose, either omentum or Dexon mesh can be used to create a floor.[22])

Step 4: Colostomy

A conventional sigmoid colostomy is made by bringing the colon straight through the rectus muscle.[8] Once this is done, a space is left lateral to the colon through which small bowel can herniate and become obstructed; this space should be closed. Alternatively, the colostomy can be placed extraperitoneally.[11] The main advantage of the extraperitoneal approach is the complete obliteration of the lateral space. Unfortunately, hopes that extraperitoneal colostomy would result in fewer paracolostomy hernias have not been realized. (The peritoneum is tightly adherent to the fascia at the lateral border of the rectus. Creation of the extraperitoneal tunnel goes easily up to this point, beyond which the peritoneum can be torn easily and may have to be repaired with sutures. Accordingly, the pelvic peritoneum should not be closed until the colon is brought through the tunnel. On the whole, the advantages of extraperitoneal colostomy do not seem to justify the additional time and effort.)

Although protrusion above the skin level is essential for an ileostomy, it is not necessary with a colostomy.

Step 5: Perineal Dissection (Perineal Phase)

An elliptical incision encompassing the anus is made with a scalpel or the electrocautery. The incision is extended through the ischiorectal fat in such a way that much—but not all—of this tissue is included with the specimen. Large rake retractors are used to expose the levator muscles.

The anococcygeal raphe is incised just anterior to the coccyx. (Amputation of the coccyx is unnecessary in routine cases.) With the anus retracted forward, the white Waldeyer's fascia is exposed and incised transversely. The pelvic dissection space is thus entered. The surgeon can insert one or two fingers to locate the levator muscles for division with the electrocautery. (Inadequate levator excision seldom leads to local or regional recurrence; unless the tumor is deeply invasive at this level, a margin of iliococcygeal muscle can be left laterally to facilitate closure of the perineal wound.)

When the levator muscles have been divided, the specimen is delivered through the posterior part of the perineal wound, with only the anterior attachments left to be severed.

Step 6: Closure of Perineal Wound

If the pelvic peritoneal floor is closed, the perineal wound is sutured in layers with drainage.[23] If bacterial contamination is heavy, the perineal wound is left open or partially closed with drainage.

COMPLICATIONS

The overall complication rate in this predominantly elderly patient population is 35 percent, but most of the complications—such as atelectasis and postoperative urinary retention—are relatively minor.[9,21,22] Operative mortality ranges from zero to 7.3 percent; most contemporary series report mortalities of two to three percent.[22] The majority of deaths are from cardiovascular complications and pulmonary embolism. Surgical complications leading to death are increasingly uncommon in experienced hands.

Intraoperative hemorrhage most commonly arises from injury to the presacral veins. Bulky tumors, previous radiation therapy, a narrow pelvis, and obesity make this complication more likely. If presacral veins are torn, bleeding may stop with pressure. If pressure is ineffective, the bleeding can sometimes be controlled by electrocauterization or ligation with fine sutures; however, if the vessel is torn where it emerges from the bone, these measures may not be effective. (Special metal tacks are manufactured for the purpose of controlling bleeding from these vessels, but I have never found it necessary to use them.) The last resort would be to pack the pelvis and then to return to the operating room later to remove the pack.

Injury to the left ureter must be repaired immediately. The urethra is vulnerable to injury during the anterior perineal dissection; fortunately, such injury is rare. Injury to the urethra should be repaired primarily, and a suprapubic cystostomy tube should be placed.

The rectum can be torn during the posterior pelvic dissection or during the perineal phase. The greatest concern is contamination of the field by malignant cells; bacterial contamination is also problematic but is less worrisome. In the event of entry into the rectal lumen, the field should be irrigated thoroughly with water, a tumoricidal agent (e.g., dilute povidone-iodine), or both.

Colostomy complications include necrosis, retraction, and paracolostomy abscess.

Perineal wound complications occur in about 15 percent of patients who undergo APR for rectal cancer; the most common such complication is persistent perineal sinus.[23] Perineal hernia is uncommon after APR but is more likely to occur if the levator muscles are excised widely.

OUTCOME

Late colostomy complications are mainly limited to paracolostomy hernia. Prolapse is an uncommon complication of a sigmoid colostomy.[8]

Sexual dysfunction in men after APR is usually neurogenic, but advanced age and psychological factors may play a role as well.[24] Total impotence occurs in 15 to 40 percent of men after APR.[21] Sexual dysfunction in women may result from psychological problems related to altered body image. Dyspareunia, presumably arising from pelvic fibrosis, is reported by as many as 50 percent of women after APR.[24]

References

1. Schrock TR: Total colectomy and ileorectal anastomosis. Mastery of Surgery, 3rd ed. Nyhus LM, Baker RJ, Fischer JE, Eds. Little, Brown & Co, Boston (in press)
2. Arnaud J-P, Bergamaschi R: Emergency subtotal/total colectomy with anastomosis for acutely obstructed carcinoma of the left colon. Dis Colon Rectum 37:685, 1994
3. Melville DM, Ritchie JK, Nicholls RJ, et al: Surgery for ulcerative colitis in the era of the pouch: the St Mark's Hospital experience. Gut 35:1076, 1994
4. D'Emilia JC, Rodriguez-Bigas MA, Petrelli NJ: The clinical and genetic manifestations of hereditary nonpolyposis colorectal carcinoma. Am J Surg 169:368, 1995
5. Beckwith PS, Wolff BG, Frazee RC: Ileorectostomy in the older patient. Dis Colon Rectum 35:301, 1992
6. Bender J, Wiencek R, Bouwman D: Morbidity and mortality following total abdominal colectomy for massive lower gastrointestinal bleeding. Am Surg 57:536, 1991
7. Nugent KP, Spigelman AD, Phillips RKS: Life expectancy after colectomy and ileorectal anastomosis for familial adenomatous polyposis. Dis Colon Rectum 36:1059, 1993
8. Schrock TR: Ileostomy and colostomy. Gastrointestinal Surgery. Fromm D, Ed. Churchill Livingstone, New York, 1985, p 669
9. Schrock TR: Inflammatory diseases of the colon and rectum. Gastrointestinal Surgery. Fromm D, Ed. Churchill Livingstone, New York, 1985, p 541
10. Gordon PH, Nivatvongs S: Principles and Practice of Surgery for the Colon, Rectum, and Anus. Quality Medical Publishing, St. Louis, 1992
11. Goligher JC: Surgery of the Anus, Rectum and Colon, 4th ed. Baliere, Tindell and Cassell Ltd, London, 1984
12. Binderow SR, Wexner SD: Current surgical therapy for mucosal ulcerative colitis. Dis Colon Rectum 37:610, 1994
13. McIntyre PB, Pemberton JH, Wolff BG, et al: Comparing functional results one year and ten years after ileal pouch-anal anastomosis for chronic ulcerative colitis. Dis Colon Rectum 37:303, 1994
14. Sugerman HJ, Newsome HH: Stapled ileoanal anastomosis without a temporary ileostomy. Am J Surg 167:58, 1994
15. Lavery IC, Sirimarco MT, Ziv Y, et al: Anal canal inflammation after ileal pouch-anal anastomosis: the need for treatment. Dis Colon Rectum 38:803, 1995
16. Sagar PM, Taylor BA: Pelvic ileal reservoirs: the options. Br J Surg 81:325, 1994
17. Utsunomiya J, Shoji Y: Surgical management of total ulcerative colitis and familial adenomatous polyposis. J Formos Med Assoc 94:213, 1995
18. Gorfine SR, Gelernt IM, Bauer JJ, et al: Restorative proctocolectomy without diverting ileostomy. Dis Colon Rectum 38:188, 1995
19. Ruseler-van Embden JGH, Schouten WR, van Lieshout LMC: Pouchitis: result of microbial imbalance? Gut 35:658, 1994
20. Kohler L, Troidl H: The ileoanal pouch: a risk-benefit analysis. Br J Surg 82:443, 1995
21. Rothenberger DA, Wong WD: Abdominoperineal resection for adenocarcinoma of the low rectum. World J Surg 16:478, 1992
22. Schrock TR: Abdominoperineal resection—technique and complications. Cancer of the Colon, Rectum, and Anus. Cohen AM, Winawer SJ, Eds. McGraw-Hill, New York, 1995, p 595
23. Campos RR, Ayllon JG, Paricio PP, et al: Management of the perineal wound following abdominoperineal resection: prospective study of three methods. Br J Surg 79:29, 1992
24. Cunsolo A, Bragaglia RB, Manara G, et al: Urogenital dysfunction after abdominoperineal resection for carcinoma of the rectum. Dis Colon Rectum 33:918, 1990

Acknowledgment

Figures 1 through 12   Tom Moore.

58 LAPAROSCOPIC COLECTOMY

Babak N. Rad, M.D., and Robert W. Beart, Jr., M.D.

The growing emphasis on minimally invasive approaches in modern surgery has forced surgeons to reevaluate traditional approaches to proven procedures. Laparoscopic cholecystectomy, laparoscopic appendectomy, and laparoscopic inguinal and incisional herniorrhaphy all have proved to be viable alternatives to their open counterparts.[1] Their success has led to the application of laparoscopy to bowel surgery in an effort to reduce the morbidity associated with conventional open colon resections. There is now considerable published evidence indicating that laparoscopic colectomy is both safe and effective and has certain advantages over open techniques—namely, decreased operative morbidity, decreased pain, shorter length of stay, more rapid return to work, and improved cosmesis.[1-3]

Laparoscopic bowel surgery does require that surgeons acquire a new set of skills. Thus, it should not be surprising that the natural human tendency to resist change has, to date, limited its utilization. If, however, encouraging recent study findings are confirmed by trials now under way, it is likely that laparoscopic colectomy will become the treatment of choice in the future.

Indications

Accepted indications for laparoscopic colectomy include most of the benign colonic diseases (e.g., colorectal polyps, rectal prolapse, diverticular disease, inflammatory bowel disease, intestinal stomas for diversion, cecal or sigmoid volvulus, and symptomatic colonic lipomas).[2] The role of laparoscopic bowel resection in the management of malignant colonic disease, however, remains controversial. Specifically, there are questions about the incidence of port-site recurrence and about long-term survival rates that have not yet been answered.[3-6] These questions have provided the impetus for a number of prospective, randomized studies in several countries. Currently, at least seven such trials are under way, most of which are being conducted at multiple centers. Results from these studies should be forthcoming in the next few years.

Operative Planning

No patient should undergo laparoscopic bowel surgery without a defined diagnosis. Colonoscopy, barium enemas, and computed tomography are all potentially useful in determining the diagnosis before operation; the choice of diagnostic modality should be governed by the patient's initial presenting signs and symptoms. The distance from the tumor to the anal verge is readily measured in the course of colonoscopy, but such measurement does not always result in accurate identification of the corresponding segment of diseased bowel intraoperatively. Furthermore, with the exception of the ileocecal valve (which remains a constant and easily identifiable landmark), the general shape and curves of the colon are indistinct. Therefore, it is recommended that India ink tattooing be used to mark lesions located in segments of the bowel outside the area of the ileocecal valve, thereby facilitating intraoperative localization of the tumor.

Patients who have a history of severe cardiopulmonary disease, hepatic disease, coagulopathy, significant respiratory compromise, or a complex colonic disorder (e.g., obstruction, contained perforation, or colovesical fistula) should not be considered for laparoscopic colectomy, nor should patients who are known to have extensive intra-abdominal adhesions. Patients who have tumors larger than 8 to 10 cm in diameter are also unsuitable candidates for laparoscopic colectomy. Larger specimens inevitably require larger incisions for removal; accordingly, patients with large tumors would benefit from having an appropriately sized incision in place from the beginning of the operation.

Before operation, the surgeon must recognize that the laparoscopic colectomy may have to be converted to an open procedure, and he or she must discuss this possibility with the patient. Standard bowel preparation is provided. An epidural catheter is placed to facilitate postoperative pain control, which is an important consideration for the first 2 days after laparoscopic bowel surgery.

Operative Technique

RIGHT HEMICOLECTOMY

Step 1: Positioning of Patient and Operative Team

The patient is initially placed supine on the operating table. Because the position of the patient is changed several times during the operation, some form of restraining device should be employed to minimize the possibility of a fall; we favor the use of a beanbag that is secured to the table. Pneumatic compression stockings are placed on the patient to minimize the risk of deep vein thrombosis. After induction of general anesthesia, a nasogastric tube and a Foley catheter are placed to decompress the bladder and the stomach so that these organs will not be perforated when the trocars are inserted. The abdomen is then prepared and draped in the usual fashion.

The surgeon and the camera operator stand to the left of the patient, the assistant surgeon and the nurse to the right. The monitors are placed on either side of the patient, adjacent to the shoulders. With this configuration, all members of the operative team can easily view the operative field [*see Figure 1*].

Step 2: Placement of Trocars

We use a standardized trocar placement for all colectomies [*see Figure 2*]. A 12 mm Hasson trocar is inserted through the rectus muscle and into the abdominal cavity via a small left upper quadrant incision placed 3 to 4 cm below the costal margin. The trocar is secured with sutures, and the abdomen is insufflated with CO_2 to achieve pneumoperitoneum. We use a pressure of 10 to 12 mm Hg to minimize the risk of pneumatosis, which can involve the entire body (presumably as a result of dissection through the extraperitoneal tissue planes, which are opened during the operation). After a complete survey of the peritoneal cavity, including the liver, three

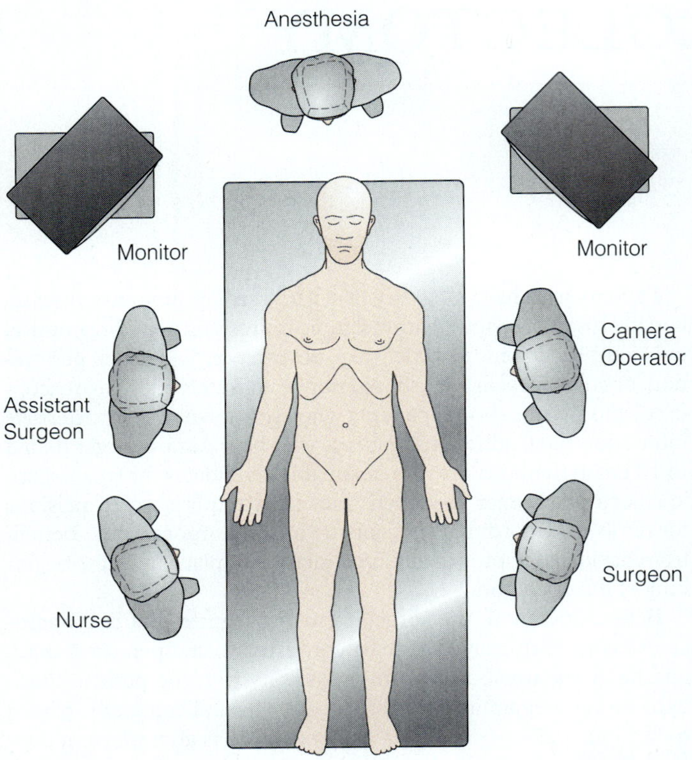

Figure 1 Laparoscopic colectomy: right hemicolectomy. Shown is the recommended positioning of the operating team.

additional ports are inserted under direct vision. A 10/12 mm port is placed at the suprapubic location. (Here and at the first site, we recommend the use of 10/12 mm ports to minimize the risk of postoperative port-site herniation.) Two 5 mm ports are placed at sites where stomas could be placed in a conventional procedure. We tend to use a 0° scope for viewing the pelvis, but many surgeons prefer a 30° angled scope. Attempts should be made to close all 10/12 mm ports at the end of the operation.

Step 3: Mobilization of Ascending Colon

The patient is placed in the Trendelenburg position, maximally rotated to the left. This positioning causes the small bowel to fall away from the right colon and allows visualization of the colonic mesentery. Dissecting scissors are inserted through the suprapubic port, and a grasper is inserted through the 5 mm port in the left lower quadrant. The surgeon, standing on the patient's left, operates these two instruments using a two-handed technique. The assistant uses a grasper to retract the peritoneum, taking care not to grasp the bowel but instead to grasp the mesentery or the peritoneum to place the tissues on traction.

The surgeon begins the dissection by incising the peritoneum along the cecum [*see Figure 3*]. The appendiceal and terminal ileal attachments are easily visualized and similarly divided. The bowel is then bluntly reflected from the retroperitoneum. At this point, the ureter can usually be identified in the retroperitoneum. The bowel is further mobilized medially by means of blunt dissection. The dissection is extended upward to the hepatic flexure, and the transverse colon is mobilized as necessary for the diseased bowel segment to be resected. For complete dissection of the transverse colon, it may be necessary to put the patient in the reverse Trendelenburg position. Additional dissection of the colon can also be done under direct vision during the removal of the specimen. The duodenum can usually be visualized during this mobilization.

Step 4: Dissection

The bowel is returned to its normal position, the mesentery is grasped, and the medial aspect of the colon and the ileocolic vessels are placed on traction. With traction placed on the mesentery, the ileocolic vessels are easily visualized. The key technical point here is that on each side of the mesenteric vessels, there exists a clear avascular space, which can be rapidly and readily dissected back into the previously dissected retroperitoneum to create a window [*see Figure 4*]. Once this window is complete, the vessels are isolated and can be controlled with minimal difficulty. The artery and the vein can usually be identified at their origin, separated, and individually clipped. The right colic vessels are then similarly exposed and clipped.

With the dissection of the bowel complete, attention is turned to mobilization and division of the ileocolic and right colic vessels. Once this is accomplished, the bowel is completely mobile and can be retrieved through the abdominal wall. To facilitate creation of the anastomosis, the attachments of the terminal ileum must be completely divided; if this is not done, the surgeon will find it difficult to bring the bowel through the abdominal wall.

Step 5: Anastomosis and Closure

A 5 cm incision is made at the right lower quadrant port site and extended downward through the muscle. Hemostatic techniques must be used: no bleeding should be allowed to occur through this incision. The bowel can then be grasped and brought through the wound with relative ease. Once the bowel is outside the abdomen, any additional mesenteric dissection and ligation that may be needed can be completed under direct vision. Before creating the anastomosis, the surgeon must ensure that the bowel has not been rotated; this can be accomplished by maintaining the orientation of the bowel as it is brought out through the abdominal wall.

The bowel is then divided and reanastomosed either with staples or with sutures. It is not necessary to close the mesenteric defect. The bowel is returned to the peritoneal cavity, and the abdominal wound is closed in layers. The peritoneal cavity is reinsufflated, laparoscopically inspected for hemostasis, and irrigated. The cannulas are removed under direct vision, and the 10/12 mm port sites are closed. Finally, the skin is closed with a subcuticular absorbable suture and Steri-Strips.

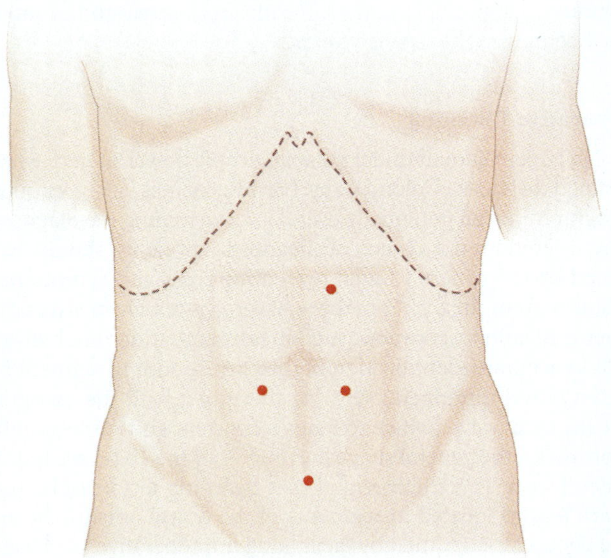

Figure 2 Laparoscopic colectomy: right hemicolectomy. Standard port placement.

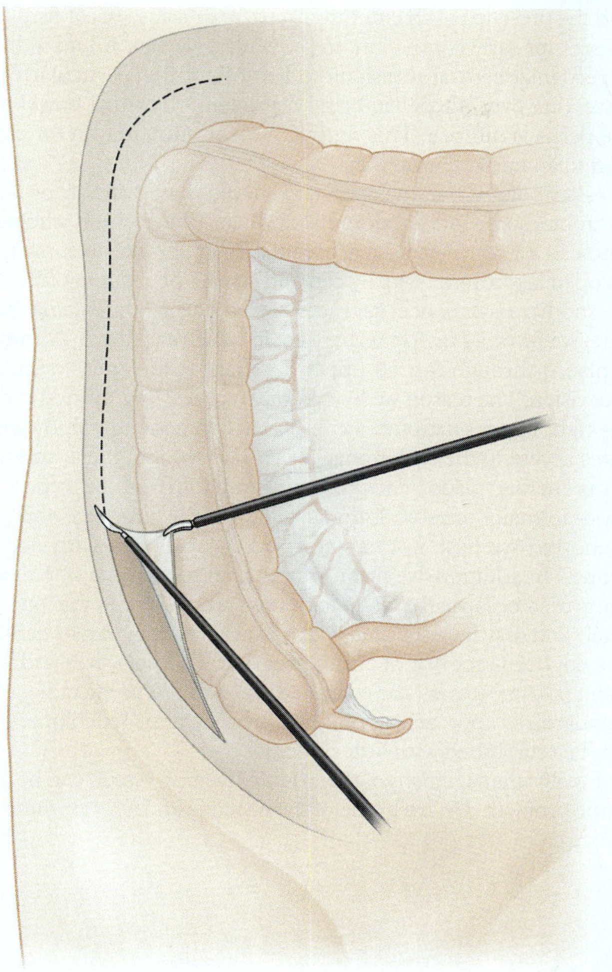

Figure 3 Laparoscopic colectomy: right hemicolectomy. Right colon mobilization.

the peritoneum incised along the white line of Toldt. Once the peritoneum has been incised, the colon can be mobilized by blunt reflection off the retroperitoneum.

As in a right hemicolectomy, the ureter must be identified. As a rule, the gonadal vessels appear first, then the ureter. After the ureter is carefully identified and dissected away from the mesentery, the bowel is again laid laterally. To ensure adequate length, the splenic flexure should be mobilized in much the same way as the hepatic flexure.

Step 4: Dissection

After the bowel is returned to its normal anatomic location, the mesentery is grasped and the inferior mesenteric vessels identified. Using the avascular space around the origin of the vessels, the surgeon creates a window that extends laterally to the previously dissected plane. Once the pedicle is isolated, the fat around the vessels can be stripped, and the artery and the vein can be individually controlled and clipped. We use large clips, placing two on the aortic side of the vessels and one on the distal side. In dividing large arteries, it is best to cut partway through the artery and then remove tension from the vessel to make sure that the clips are correctly applied [*see Figure 6*]; alternatively, the pedicle can be divided with a vascular endoscopic stapler. The choice of approach is a matter of individual preference.

Step 5: Anastomosis and Closure

Once the inferior mesenteric artery is ligated, the left colic artery may be divided, depending on which bowel segment is to be removed. A 5 cm incision is then made at the port site in the left lower quadrant. The bowel is grasped and brought up through the incision. The entire bowel can usually be seen, and any additional mesentery can be divided. The bowel is then divided and reanastomosed by means of standard anastomotic techniques. When the anastomosis is complete, the bowel is returned to the abdominal cavity. The fascia is closed in two layers with continuous absorbable sutures, and the skin is closed with a subcuticular absorbable suture.

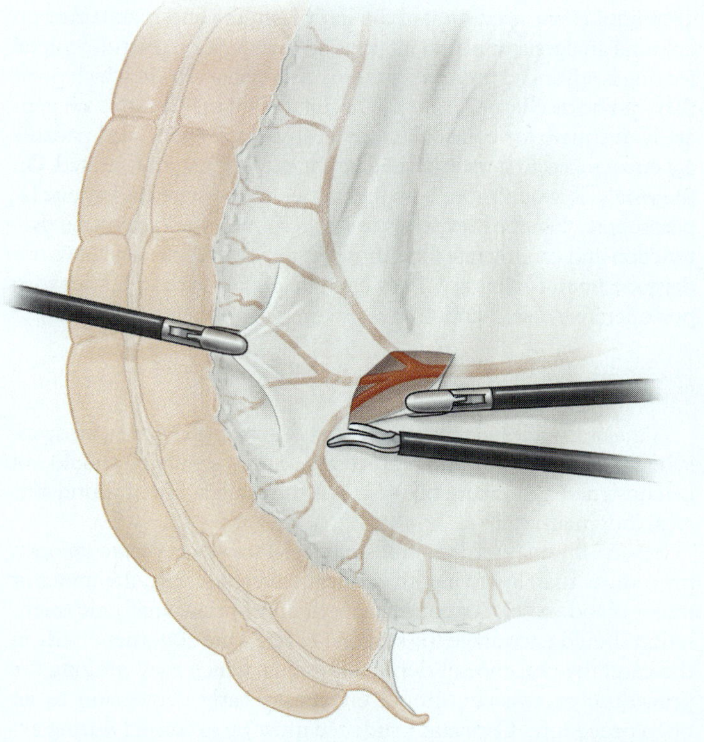

LEFT HEMICOLECTOMY AND SIGMOID RESECTION

Step 1: Positioning of Patient and Operative Team

Initial positioning and preparation of the patient are essentially the same as for a right hemicolectomy (see above). The position of the operative team differs somewhat, in that the surgeon and the nurse stand to the right of the patient, and the camera operator and the assistant stand to the left [*see Figure 5*]. The monitors are placed in the same locations as for a right hemicolectomy.

Step 2: Placement of Trocars

As in a right hemicolectomy, a Hasson trocar is placed in the left upper quadrant via a small incision over the rectus muscle 3 to 4 cm below the costal margin. After pneumoperitoneum is established through this trocar, three additional ports are inserted under direct vision in the same locations used for a right hemicolectomy.

Step 3: Mobilization of Descending Colon

The patient is placed in a steep Trendelenburg position, maximally rotated to the right. For the initial dissection, the laparoscope (either 0° or 30°) is placed in the left upper quadrant port. As the assistant retracts the peritoneal attachments laterally to the left, the surgeon, using the electrified scissors in the suprapubic port and the grasper in the right lower quadrant port, retracts the descending colon cephalad and to the right. The dissection commences along the peritoneal reflection of the sigmoid and descending colon, with

Figure 4 Laparoscopic colectomy: right hemicolectomy. Right colon mesenteric dissection.

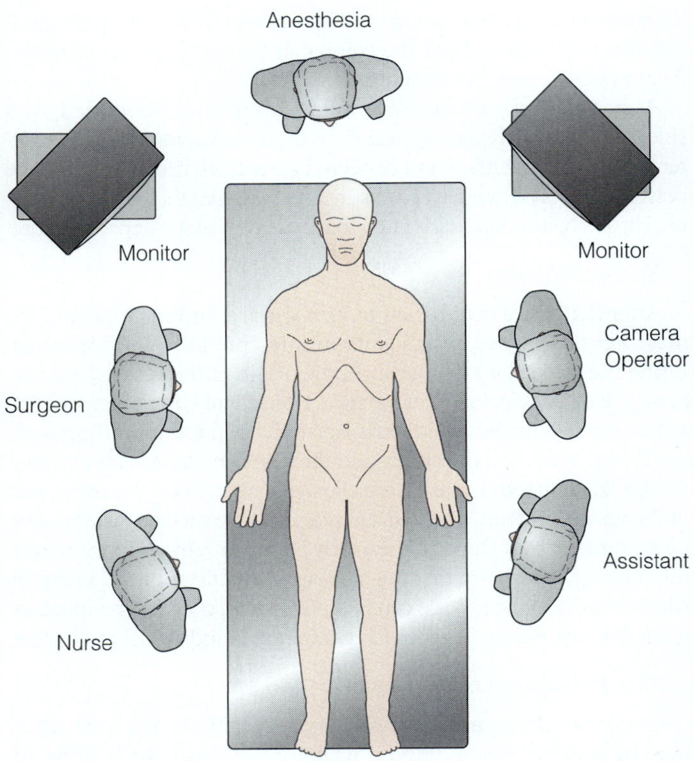

Figure 5 Laparoscopic colectomy: left hemicolectomy and sigmoid resection. Shown is the recommended positioning of the operating team.

and the presence of an enterotomy, structure, abscess, or fistula may all prompt early conversion. In particular, we have found it difficult to recognize serosal abrasions and enterotomies, particularly when dissecting over the pelvic brim. Dissecting the small bowel out of the pelvis is difficult. This finding is a common reason for conversion to an open laparotomy.

A key point is that the operation should not be unduly prolonged by troublesome intra-abdominal findings. The decision whether the case can be completed laparoscopically or should be converted to an open laparotomy usually can and should be made rapidly.

Another issue concerns trocar placement. When placing the trocars, we favor a Hasson technique, in which the initial 12 mm port is placed through the left upper quadrant rectus muscle under direct vision. The reason we have come to prefer this location is that in the right upper quadrant, the falciform ligament frequently complicates access to the abdominal cavity. The second, third, and fourth ports are then placed under direct vision. Initial studies reported injuries to major intra-abdominal vessels in the course of port placement, but we have not encountered this problem with our technique.[7] In addition, we favor minimizing the number of 10/12 mm ports used because the larger incisions can be difficult to repair accurately and may be associated with bowel herniation. Bowel herniation has not been reported at 5 mm port sites. The port sizes and instrument sizes necessary for colonic dissection are predictable; thus, a standardized approach, as outlined [see Operative Technique, above], can be established with little difficulty.

Finally, management of the primary feeding vessels can be an irksome problem. On each side of the ileocolic and inferior mesenteric

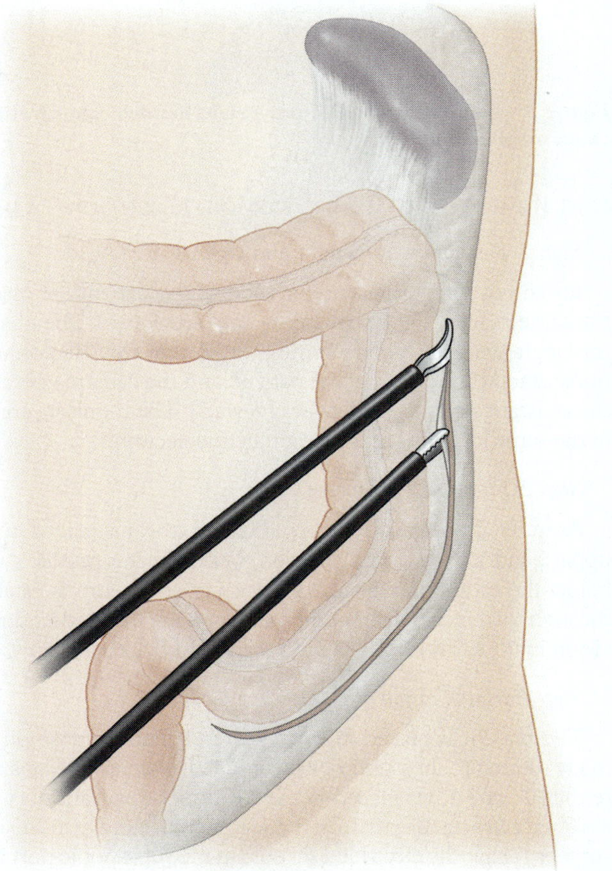

Postoperative Care

Postoperative care of patients who have undergone laparoscopic colectomy should be similar to that of patients who have undergone open colectomy; however, a shorter recovery period is to be expected with the less invasive procedure. As a rule, patients are started on clear liquids in the evening of the day of surgery and maintained on epidural analgesia until oral intake is adequate. Subsequently, enteral feeding is advanced until patients are on a regular diet, at which point they can be discharged from the hospital. Oral medications are generally adequate for controlling any postoperative pain, and patients are encouraged to pursue desired activities to the extent tolerated. On the whole, it is our impression that patients who have undergone laparoscopic colectomy experience less respiratory and immune dysfunction and can tolerate food more rapidly than those who have undergone open colectomy. They can usually be discharged between postoperative days 3 and 4.

Troubleshooting

A major troubleshooting issue is that of conversion of a laparoscopic bowel resection to an open procedure. Such conversion should not be construed as a failure but rather as the application of sound surgical judgment.

Several findings or conditions may lead to conversion to an open procedure. Inability to identify critical structures (e.g., the ureter or major blood vessels) or concern about appropriate anatomic orientation should encourage the surgeon to open the abdomen. Early in the case, the presence of dense adhesions, which may prolong the procedure excessively, should encourage early conversion to an open procedure. Care and prudence must be exercised during extensive adhesiolysis. In addition, lack of adequate exposure, poor hemostasis, disorientation, inadequate resection or reconstruction,

Figure 6 Laparoscopic colectomy: left hemicolectomy and sigmoid resection. Sigmoid mesentery and pelvic dissection.

vessels, there is a large avascular window. We take advantage of this predictable anatomic finding and aggressively dissect and isolate these vessels. Our usual practice is to separate the vein from the artery with a right-angle dissecting clamp and clip them separately. Occasionally, a fibrotic sheath prevents this separation, in which case we use an endovascular stapler to occlude and divide the vessels.

Complications

Complications associated with laparoscopic colectomy include major vessel injuries and enterotomies (both recognized and unrecognized). These can generally be minimized and managed through careful troubleshooting (see above).

A potential complication that has given rise to considerable concern is recurrence at port sites after laparoscopic colectomy for cancer. Anecdotal reports of wound and port-site recurrences after laparoscopic colon cancer resection were widely published in the early 1990s. A growing body of experience suggests that such recurrences are rare: the average incidence appears to be about 1%, which is comparable to the recurrence rates reported after open procedures.[3-6] Nevertheless, the anecdotal reports of port-site recurrence after laparoscopic colon resection led to a resurgence of the theory that tumoricidal agents may prevent such recurrence. Jacobi and associates found that taurolidine combined with heparin decreased tumor cell growth in a rat model.[8] Basha and coworkers showed that 5% pyrrolidone iodine mixed with 0.5% chloramine killed almost all tumor cells in vitro and prevented their growth in vivo.[9] We demonstrated that povidone decreased tumor cell growth in laparoscopic ports in a murine model.[10] If these results can be confirmed by other studies, placement of a tumoricidal agent in the incisions or on the trocars to prevent port-site recurrence may well become the standard of care.

The best way of putting the issue of port-site recurrence to rest is to perform a prospective, randomized study comparing laparoscopic colectomy with open colectomy in patients with colon cancer. In 1995, the National Cancer Institute initiated a multicenter study designed to address this issue and others having to do with safety, staging, and 5-year survival rates. The results of this study should be available in 2003. The general consensus in the United States is that until the results are in hand, laparoscopic colectomies for cancer should be performed at those centers involved in the study.

Outcome Evaluation

To date, laparoscopic approaches have been most successful for right hemicolectomy, sigmoid resection, and stoma formation. Abdominoperineal resection is also easily and safely performed with laparoscopic techniques.

Studies have found that laparoscopic colectomy results in decreased short-term morbidity, decreased abdominal wall trauma, earlier tolerance of food, shortened hospital stays, and reduced pain and narcotic requirements.[11] It has also been reported that surgical blood loss and the need for transfusions are reduced and that postoperative cell-mediated immunity and neutrophil function are improved.[12,13] There appear to be less immunosuppression after laparoscopic colectomy and, therefore, greater resistance to tumor regrowth (theoretically, at least). Because of the overall improvement in function, patients can return to normal activities and work more quickly.

With respect to short-term outcome, laparoscopic colectomy is comparable to open colectomy. No major differences in the number of lymph nodes resected or the length of bowel resected have been found between the two approaches; there is a trend toward greater length of bowel resection in open colectomy, but the difference is not statistically significant.[14,15] No significant cost differences between the two procedures have been documented: the decreased length of stay associated with laparoscopic colectomy is effectively balanced by the increased operating expenses. If, however, the rate of conversion to open colectomy is high (i.e., > 20%), the cost of laparoscopic surgery may be higher than that of open surgery.

At present, there is a great deal of interest in the use of laparoscopy to resect colon cancers and to minimize the short-term morbidity associated with treatment of malignant diseases. There has been sufficient research into and experience with laparoscopic treatment of colorectal cancer to show that it is a feasible modality offering the same advantages as laparoscopic treatment of benign colonic disease. The heart of the current debate surrounding the application of laparoscopy to malignant colonic disease is the question of how a laparoscopic approach might affect long-term patterns of recurrence and survival.[3,5,6]

Concerns regarding the efficacy of laparoscopic colectomy for cancer have centered on the completeness of the bowel and lymph node resections. As noted, multiple studies have shown no differences between laparoscopic colectomy and open colectomy with respect to proximal and distal margins of resection or the adequacy of lymph node dissection. Most of the concerns regarding the incidence and pattern of recurrence after laparoscopic treatment were generated early in surgeons' experience with laparoscopic colectomy, and subsequent studies tended not to find substantial differences. However, further studies that include long-term follow-up to determine the adequacy of resection and the comparability of cure rates are needed to assess any changes in the long-term staging and survival patterns after laparoscopic colectomy.

References

1. Beart RW Jr: Laparoscopic colectomy: status of the art. Dis Colon Rectum 37(suppl):S47, 1994
2. Monson JRT, Hill ADK, Darzi A: Laparoscopic colonic surgery. Br J Surg 82:150, 1995
3. Ramos JM, Gupta S, Anthone GJ, et al: Laparoscopy and colon cancer: is the port site at risk? a preliminary report. Arch Surg 129:897, 1994
4. Paik PS: Abdominal incision tumor implantation following pneumoperitoneum laparoscopic procedure vs. standard open incision in a syngeneic rat model. Dis Colon Rectum 41:419, 1998
5. Wexner SD, Cohen SM: Port site metastases after laparoscopic colorectal surgery for cure of malignancy. Br J Surg 82:295, 1995
6. Lacy AM, Garcia-Valdecasas JC, Pique JM, et al: Short-term outcome analysis of a randomized study comparing laparoscopic vs open colectomy for colon cancer. Surg Endosc 9:1101, 1995
7. Nordestgaard AG, Bodily KC, Osborne RW Jr, et al: Major vascular injuries during laparoscopic procedures. Am J Surg 169:543, 1995
8. Jacobi C, Ordemann J, Bohm B, et al: Inhibition of peritoneal tumor cell growth and implantation in laparoscopic surgery in a rat model. Am J Surg 174:359, 1997
9. Basha G, Penninckx F, Geboes K, et al: Tumoricidal activity of antiseptics with assessment of cell viability in mice with severe combined immunodeficiency. Tumour Biol 18:213, 1997
10. Hoffstetter W, Ortega A, Chiang M, et al: The effects of topical tumoricidals on port site recurrence of colon cancer. J Soc Laparoendosc Surg (in press)
11. Chen HH, Wexner SD, Iroatulam AJN, et al: Laparoscopic colectomy compares favorably with colectomy by laparotomy for reduction of postoperative ileus. Dis Colon Rectum 43:61, 2000
12. Harmon GD, Senganore AJ, Kilbride MJ, et al: Interleukin-6 response to laparoscopic and open colectomy. Dis Colon Rectum 37:754, 1994
13. Kloosterman T, Von Blomberg ME, Borgstein P, et al: Unimpaired immune function after laparoscopic cholecystectomy. Surgery 113:424, 1994
14. Kockerling F: Prospective multicenter study of the

quality of oncologic resections in patients undergoing laparoscopic colorectal surgery for cancer. Dis Colon Rectum 41:963, 1998

15. Hida J, Yasutomi M, Maruyama T, et al: The extent of lymph node dissection for colon carcinoma: the potential impact on laparoscopic surgery. Cancer 80:188, 1997

Recommended Reading

Beart RW Jr: Increased tumor establishment and growth after laparotomy vs laparoscopy in a murine model (invited commentary). Arch Surg 130:653, 1995

Dorrance HR, Oien K, O'Dwyer PJ: Effects of laparoscopy on intraperitoneal tumor growth and distant metastases in an animal model. Surgery 126:35, 1999

Fleshman JW, Wexner SD, Anvari M, et al: Laparoscopic *vs.* open abdominoperineal resection for cancer. Dis Colon Rectum 42:930, 1999

Hewitt PM: Laparoscopic-assisted vs. open surgery for colorectal cancer. Dis Colon Rectum 41:901, 1998

Huguet EL, Earnshaw JJ, Heather BP: Major vascular injury during laparoscopy. Br J Surg 84:1479, 1997

Liberman MA, Phillips EH, Carroll BJ, et al: Laparoscopic colectomy vs traditional colectomy for diverticulitis: outcome and costs. Surg Endosc 10:15, 1996

Schwandner O, Schiedeck THK, Bruch HP: Advanced age—indication or contraindication for laparoscopic colorectal surgery? Dis Colon Rectum 42:356, 1999

Solomon MJ, Egan M, Roberts RA, et al: Incidence of free colorectal cancer cells on the peritoneal surface. Dis Colon Rectum 40:1294, 1997

Wolf JS Jr, Stoller ML: The physiology of laparoscopy: basic principles, complications and other considerations. J Urol 152:294, 1994

Acknowledgment

Figures 1 through 6   Tom Moore.

59 ANAL PROCEDURES

Ira J. Kodner, M.D.

Operative Management of Hemorrhoids

In recent years, the frequency of hemorrhoid surgery has diminished significantly. More patients seem to be achieving adequate symptomatic relief by means of bowel control medications and improved diet (e.g., increased intake of fiber, fruit, vegetables, and grain). It is probable that both for these reasons and because more and better patient information is available, fewer patients today have hemorrhoids that progress to a stage advanced enough to necessitate operative treatment for relief of symptoms.

OPERATIVE PLANNING

It is important to distinguish between internal and external hemorrhoids [see Figure 1]. Internal hemorrhoids are treated to relieve specific symptoms, including prolapse and bleeding, not simply because hemorrhoidal tissue was seen on routine examinations. Prolapsing tissue occasionally results in maceration of the perianal skin that may not be clearly evident at the time of examination, especially if the patient is in the prone position. External hemorrhoids are treated because they thrombose and cause pain. There are no other symptoms of the anorectum that should be attributed to the presence of hemorrhoids [see Table 1]; in particular, difficulties with bowel movements (e.g., straining, the need for digital evacuation of the rectum, and cramping abdominal pain) must not be ascribed to hemorrhoids.

Before embarking on the surgical treatment of hemorrhoids, one must always rule out neoplastic disease, compromise of the immune system, and defective clotting mechanisms. The patient's general health status and ability to tolerate pain and an operative procedure should also be taken into account. The postoperative response to anorectal surgery varies enormously among patients. For example, young men tend to strain to have bowel movements after anorectal procedures, and this tendency can lead to bleeding and disruption of postoperative healing. These patients often benefit from the administration of parenteral pain medication for the first 12 to 24 hours after operation, which usually requires hospitalization. Elderly patients, on the other hand, prefer not to be in the hospital. For these patients, single elastic ligation of individual clusters of internal hemorrhoids is performed in the outpatient office.

The next step is to determine the appropriate procedure for the patient. The options include (1) elastic ligation of internal hemorrhoids, (2) excision of thrombosed external hemorrhoids, (3) complete excisional hemorrhoidectomy, and (4) elastic ligation of internal hemorrhoids combined with excision of external hemorrhoids. One should always consider whether complete sigmoidoscopy, rigid or flexible, will be necessary at the time of the procedure and whether anal sphincterotomy will be indicat-

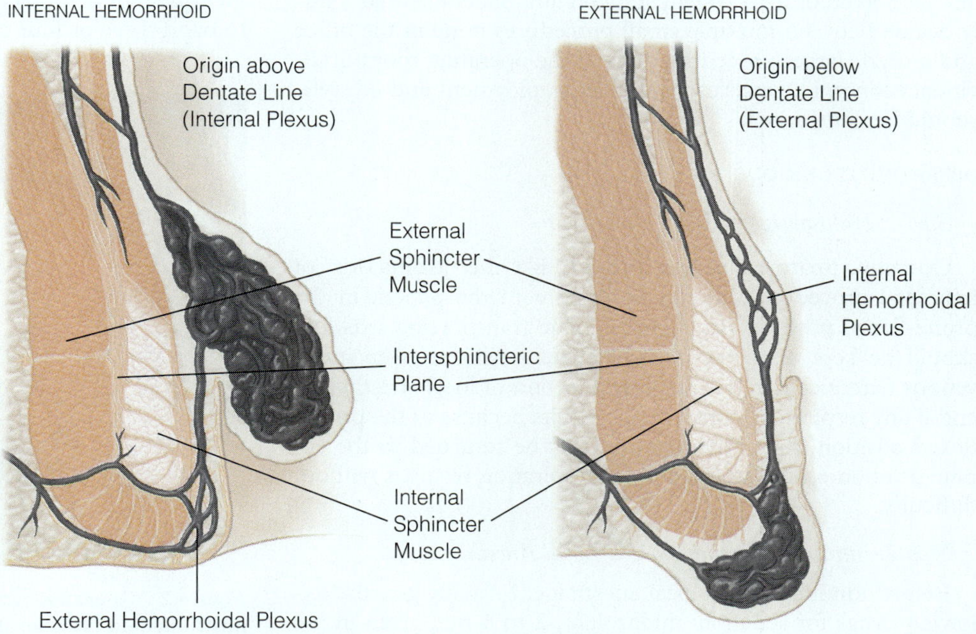

Figure 1 Operative management of hemorrhoids. A key issue is the differentiation of internal hemorrhoids from external hemorrhoids. Internal hemorrhoids (*left*) originate from the internal hemorrhoidal plexus, above the dentate line. External hemorrhoids (*right*) originate from the external hemorrhoidal plexus, below the dentate line.

Table 1 Anal Symptoms Mistakenly Attributed to Hemorrhoids

Symptoms	Cause
Pain and bleeding after bowel movement	Ulcer/fissure disease
Forceful straining to have bowel movement	Pelvic floor abnormality (paradoxical contraction of anal sphincter)
Blood mixed with stool	Neoplasm
Drainage of pus during or after bowel movement	Abscess/fistula, inflammatory bowel disease
Constant moisture	Condyloma acuminatum
Mucous drainage and incontinence	Rectal prolapse
Anal pain with no physical findings	*Caution:* possible psychiatric disorder

ed, especially in young men with a history of straining. This second consideration is important because many patients are treated for hemorrhoids when in fact their primary disease is anal ulcer/fissure disease, the symptoms of which are pain and some bleeding at defecation. These are not symptoms that can be attributed to hemorrhoids. If a patient undergoes hemorrhoid surgery when the primary disease is anal fissure, proper healing will be impeded.

Finally, one should explain the procedure and its attendant risks to the patient in the outpatient office because in most cases, given the restrictions imposed by health care insurers and managed care administrators, one will not see the patient again until the operating room on the day of operation. Specific complications to be discussed preoperatively include urinary retention, bleeding, and infection. In the event that several symptomatic hemorrhoids are present, surgeon and patient should jointly decide between multiple small procedures done in the office and a single larger procedure done in the operating room. Individual economic concerns, as well as employment and lifestyle, should be considered.

OPERATIVE TECHNIQUE

Step 1: Positioning

Operative treatment of hemorrhoids, like the vast majority of anorectal procedures, should be done with the patient in the prone-flexed position [*see Figure 2*]. The transporting stretcher should be kept in the room. The patient will be given intravenous narcotics to allow painless injection of local anesthetics, and if any respiratory compromise results because of the prone-flexed position, the patient can quickly be returned to the supine position on the stretcher until respiration resumes without difficulty.

Step 2: Intravenous Sedation and Local Anesthesia

Before administering a local anesthetic, I usually give the following drugs for sedation: midazolam, 2 to 5 mg, given in the holding area for sedation and amnesia; alfentanil, 0.5 to 1 mg, or fentanyl, 50 to 100 µg, for analgesia to help alleviate the discomfort of the local anesthetic injection; and propofol, 20 to 50 mg, or methohexital, 20 to 50 mg, to achieve patient cooperation with the injection. Sedation is followed by the injection into perianal tissue of 40 ml of bupivacaine (0.5 percent) along with a buffer that is added immediately before injection (0.5 ml of 8.4 percent sodium bicarbonate [1 mEq/ml] added to 50 ml of local anesthetic). If resection is anticipated, epinephrine (1:200,000) is usually included with the local anesthetic. I find that hyaluronidase is not helpful, even for acutely thrombosed, prolapsed hemorrhoids. To achieve adequate local anesthesia, 5 ml of bupivacaine is injected into the subcutaneous tissue in each quadrant of the tissue immediately surrounding the anus [*see Figure 3a*]. Next, 10 ml of local anesthetic is injected deep into the sphincter mechanism on each side of the anal canal [*see Figure 3b*].

Step 3: Anoscopy or Sigmoidoscopy

Either anoscopy or sigmoidoscopy, or both, should be performed at this point if neither procedure was done before the operation.

Step 4: Sphincterotomy

As noted, sphincterotomy should always be considered, especially if a hypertrophic band of the lower third of the internal sphincter muscle persists after the local anesthetic has been injected and an anoscope has been inserted. It is always best to obtain permission to do this beforehand on the operative consent form.

Step 5: Treatment of Hemorrhoids

Elastic ligation of internal hemorrhoids This is a very safe operation because by the nature of the banding procedure [*see Figure 4*], bridges of normal mucosa are maintained between treated clusters of hemorrhoids. Any clusters of tissue with squamous metaplasia and obviously friable internal hemorrhoids can be treated in this manner. I find that these tissue clusters are not always confined to the three classic positions identified for hemorrhoids and that in many cases it is necessary to band three or four clusters. If the bands do not stay on, then

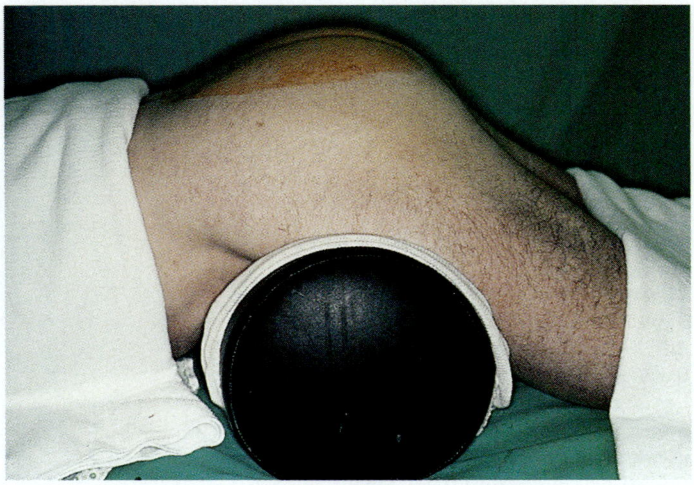

Figure 2 **Operative management of hemorrhoids. The patient is positioned on the operating table in the prone-flexed position, with a soft roll under the hips.**

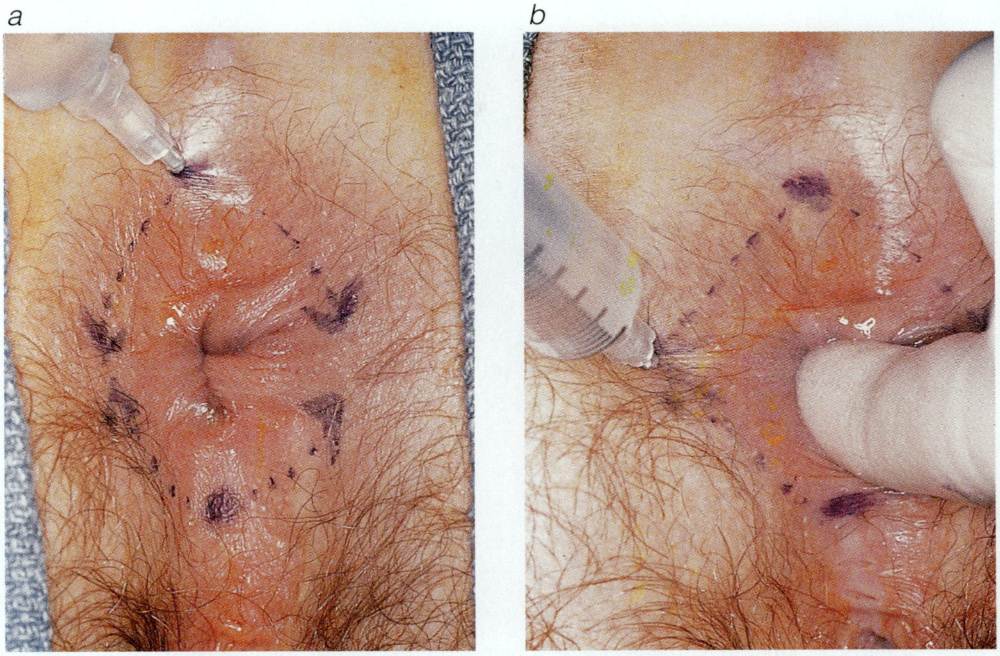

Figure 3 Operative management of hemorrhoids. (*a*) Five milliliters of bupivacaine is injected into subcutaneous tissue. (*b*) Ten milliliters of local anesthetic is injected deep into the sphincter muscle on each side of the anal canal.

the tissue probably need not be treated and no further action need be taken.

I use two rubber bands on each cluster. If one of them breaks, bleeding is unlikely to occur, because the tissue rapidly becomes edematous and necrotic. It is important that the placement of the rubber band be proximal to the mucocutaneous junction; if it is not, the procedure will be too painful, given the extensive innervation of the skin. On the other hand, the band should not be placed so proximally as to incorporate the full thickness of the rectal wall; to do so can be risky for patients in whom difficulties with bowel movements indicate the presence of intussusception or some other pelvic floor abnormality. Occasionally, the friable tissue gives rise to a suspicion of cancer. If this is the case, rubber bands may be placed at the base, and the tip may be excised for biopsy.

Excision of residual external hemorrhoids Residual external hemorrhoids are rarely treated as a primary problem: true symptoms are few, and the main indication for treatment is maintenance of hygiene. In addition, I find that much of the

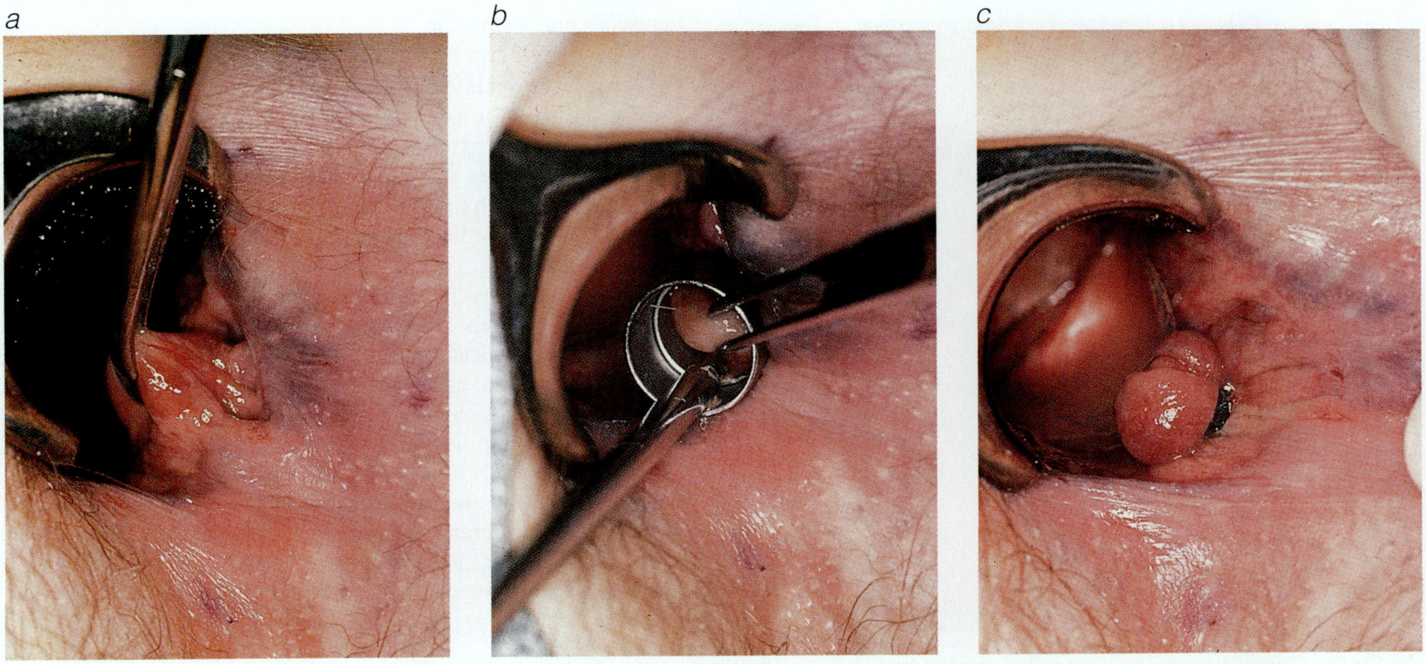

Figure 4 Operative management of hemorrhoids. Shown is the elastic ligation technique for internal hemorrhoids. (*a*) The hemorrhoidal tissue is identified. (*b*) The hemorrhoid is grasped and pulled through the drum. (*c*) The elastic band is applied to the base of the hemorrhoid.

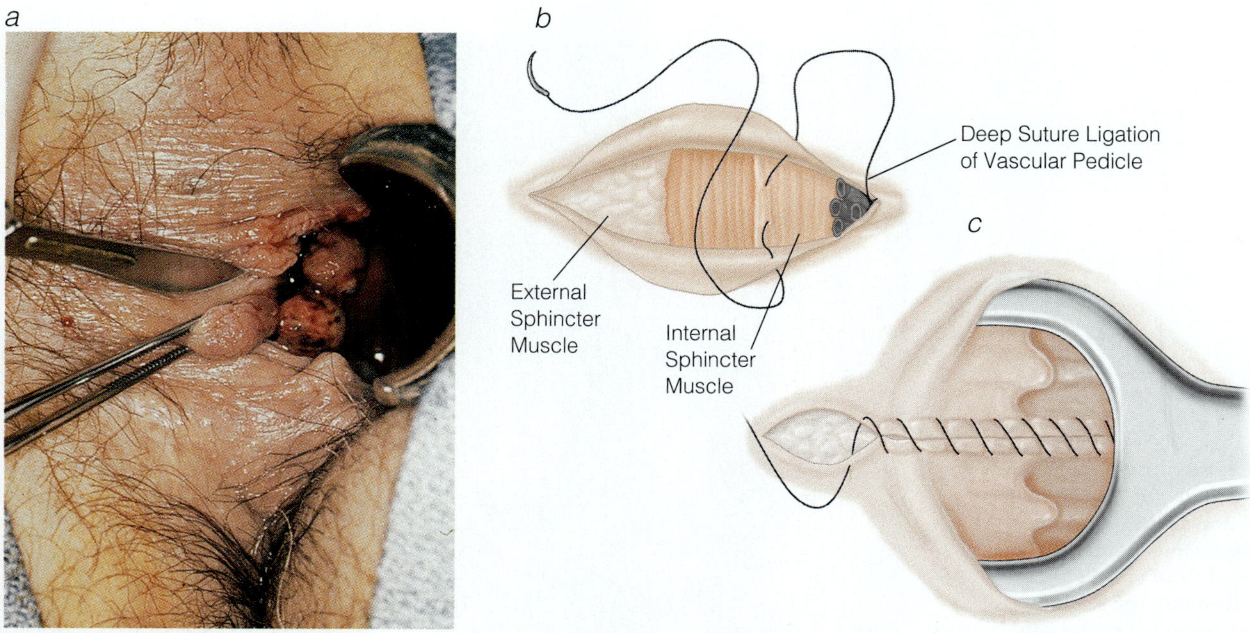

Figure 5 Operative management of hemorrhoids. Shown is an excisional hemorrhoidectomy. (*a*) An elliptical incision is made in the perianal skin. (*b*) A continuous suture is used in a three-point placement in such a way as to incorporate skin edges and muscle. (*c*) The elliptical defect is closed and the dead space obliterated.

external tissue is pulled in when the internal hemorrhoids are ligated. Accordingly, I do the internal ligation first and then excise any residual symptomatic external tissue. An elliptical incision is made in the perianal skin, with care taken to protect the underlying sphincter muscle and avoid the previously placed elastic band [*see Figure 5a*]. Although the perianal skin is very forgiving, it is essential to protect the anoderm; this is achieved through careful placement of the rubber band. The elliptical defect is then closed with a continuous absorbable suture in a three-point placement to obliterate the underlying dead space [*see Figure 5b, c*]. The suture is tied loosely to allow for swelling. There is no need for separate ligation or coagulation of the small bleeding vessels; this problem is obviated by the continuous suture. It is important not to use slowly absorbable suture material, because it may give rise to infection in this highly susceptible tissue. I prefer to use 3-0 chromic catgut on an exaggeratedly curved needle.

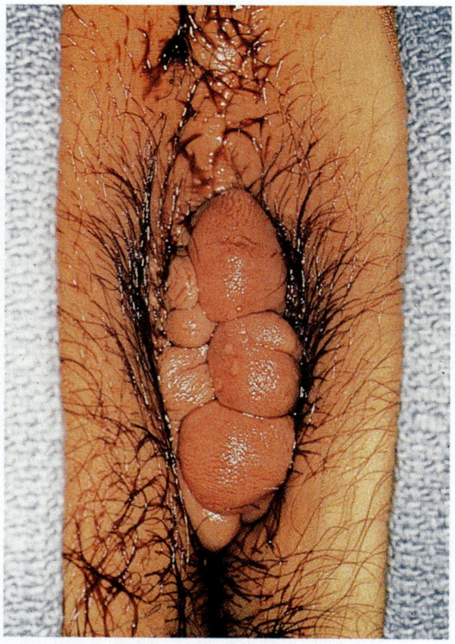

Complete excisional hemorrhoidectomy This procedure is indicated in patients who have large combined internal and external hemorrhoids, patients who are receiving anticoagulants, and patients who have massive edema and thrombosis, as seen in the postpartum rosette of tissue [*see Figure 6*]. I find that even massive edema generally resolves after the local anesthetic is injected and the muscle is allowed to relax. Resolution of edema then permits identification of the specific clusters of hemorrhoids, which can be isolated with a forceps and excised via an elliptical incision. Care must be taken to preserve the underlying muscle, especially in the anterior region in women. I use 3-0 chromic catgut with a deep stitch at the apex and a continuous three-point suture that is extended on the perianal skin [*see Figure 5b*]. It is important to preserve a bridge of anoderm between the areas of excision. I know of no indications for a radical circumferential procedure (the so-called Whitehead procedure); in fact, I see numerous patients who are seeking a remedy for the stenosis and ectropion that frequently occur after this radical operation [*see Figure 7*].

Figure 6 Operative management of hemorrhoids. Massive edema and thrombosis, as seen in the postpartum rosette of tissue, can be reduced after a local anesthetic is injected and the muscle is allowed to relax.

Step 6: Postoperative Care

Immediately after the procedure—in fact, after any anorectal procedure—antibiotic ointment and a gauze pad are applied.

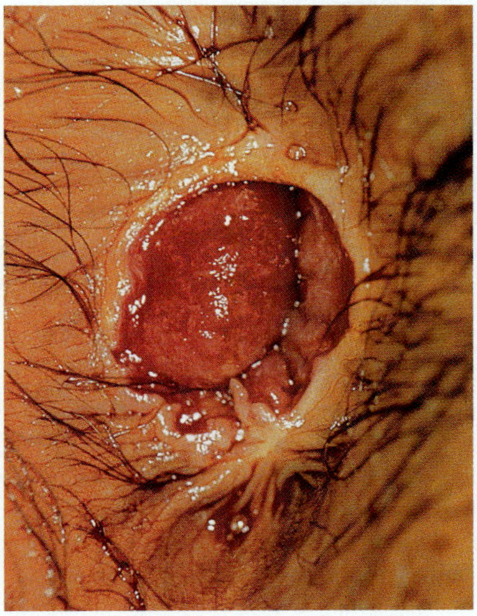

Figure 7 Operative management of hemorrhoids. Stenosis and ectropion often result from radical circumferential (Whitehead) procedures.

Pressure dressings are unnecessary. Only a very small amount of adhesive tape should be used, so as to prevent traction avulsion of the perianal skin, an event for which we surgeons too often avoid responsibility by ascribing it to a "tape allergy" on the part of the patient.

TROUBLESHOOTING

The most fundamental way of preventing problems is to make an accurate diagnosis. Surgical treatment of hemorrhoids in a patient whose main disease process is Crohn's disease, a pelvic floor abnormality, or ulcer/fissure disease inevitably yields inferior results. It is especially important to recognize the anal pain and spasm of ulcer/fissure disease because in patients with this condition, excision of hemorrhoidal tissue without sphincterotomy leads to increased pain and poor wound healing.

I prefer to operate with the patient in the prone-flexed position, using local analgesia supplemented by intravenous medication. I have found over the years that with this approach, patients retain no unpleasant memories from the operating room experience, and good pain control is achieved in the immediate postoperative period.

In the postoperative period, efforts must be made to minimize straining on the part of the patient. To accomplish this, pain must be kept at a low level. I prefer to give only parenteral pain medication, in relatively high doses, on the first night. The patient and the nursing staff must be cautioned that the first sensation of pain, especially after elastic ligation of hemorrhoids, is the urge to defecate. This urge is an indication that pain medication should be given. The patient must not sit on the toilet and strain; to do so is likely to result in extrusion of the recently ligated tissue.

At least 20 percent of patients experience some degree of urinary retention. If this occurs, an indwelling catheter should be placed. In-and-out straight catheterization is contraindicated. No bladder stimulants should be given: such agents encourage straining and increase the risk of complications.

Bulk-forming agents and stool softeners are started in the immediate postoperative period. I encourage patients to take warm soaks, either in a bathtub or in a shower, rather than try to squeeze into the disposable sitz-bath mechanisms provided by the hospitals, which are often too small. I also encourage patients to sit on soft cushions rather than the rubber rings marketed for postoperative care; the rings seem to cause more dependent edema and pain.

COMPLICATIONS

Bleeding

Either immediate or delayed bleeding may occur after hemorrhoid surgery. Bleeding within the first 12 to 24 hours after the operation represents a technical error. The only management is to return the patient to the operating room, with good anesthesia and adequate visualization, so that the bleeding site can be suture ligated. Frequently, spinal or epidural anesthesia is necessary because the patient is too uncomfortable, and the tissue perhaps too edematous, to allow local anesthesia. Bleeding within five to 10 days after the operation usually results from sloughing of the eschar created by suturing or elastic ligation. This delayed bleeding is usually minimal, and the patient is encouraged to rest and to take stool softeners. If the bleeding is significant, examination with adequate anesthesia is indicated to allow cauterization or suture ligation of the bleeding site.

It is important to discourage patients from taking aspirin-containing compounds in the postoperative period, and it is especially important to follow patients taking systemic anticoagulants closely. I prefer to treat these patients with excisional hemorrhoidectomy so that sutures can be placed; in this way, I avoid the risk that the elastic-ligated tissue will slough after five to 10 days.

Infection

Infection is unusual after hemorrhoidectomy because perianal tissue is normally well vascularized and extremely resistant to infection despite constant bombardment by bacteria. When it does occur, it is most likely to be in an immunocompromised patient—that is, one who has a blood dyscrasia, diabetes, or AIDS or has recently undergone chemotherapy. In my view, it is imperative to obtain at least a complete blood count and a chemistry profile before embarking on anorectal procedures; abnormal results militate against elective hemorrhoid surgery.

Any local focus of infection noted in the postoperative period must be drained. I have seen this only when slowly absorbable suture material was used, which is the reason why I have returned to using 3-0 chromic catgut. Postoperative perianal infection can be severe and life-threatening, and it is therefore critically important to be familiar with its symptoms and to treat it intensively. Frequently, such infection is initially manifested by pain that is greater than anticipated, urinary retention, and fever. These symptoms have occasionally been reported after elastic ligation of hemorrhoids. In this event, it is critical that the patient be seen emergently, the elastic bands removed, the patient hospitalized, and parenteral administration of antibiotics begun. In retrospect, I find that all such patients whom I have seen had preoperative symptoms of a pelvic floor abnormality with difficulty in defecation—not clear symptoms of hemorrhoids.

Urinary Retention

Urinary retention is apparently caused by reflex spasm of the pelvic musculature, which may not become evident until the local anesthesia wears off. Often, a patient still under the influence of local anesthesia seems to be doing exceedingly well for the first few hours after operation, only to go into urinary retention later that night. It may be helpful to reduce the fluid load in the perioperative period. When a patient has trouble urinating, an indwelling urinary catheter should be placed and left in place for at least 12 hours. This, in my view, is one of the major reasons for in-hospital observation after treatment of more than one cluster of hemorrhoids. Placement of the indwelling catheter is of particular importance for the patient's well-being, even if it is not looked on with favor by managed care administrators. Urinary retention is a frightening experience for the patient to undergo at home. What is more, if placement of an indwelling catheter is postponed for 12 to 24 hours, recovery may be delayed. Again, it is important to remember that urinary retention may be an early sign of pelvic infection.

Stricture

Stricture, with or without ectropion, results from circumferential excision of hemorrhoids. I mention this point only to discourage the performance of this procedure.

OUTCOME EVALUATION

Because hemorrhoids are treated only when symptoms—bleeding, prolapse, pain, and difficulty with hygiene—are present, success is determined simply by the extent to which the symptoms are alleviated. If other symptoms were present before operation and persist after the procedure, the primary diagnosis should be called into question. Many elderly patients with a single prolapsing hemorrhoid that causes bleeding or maceration of the perianal skin are well served by outpatient ligation; occasionally, there is a second cluster that requires treatment some months later.

The basic point is that any patient treated surgically for hemorrhoids should experience symptomatic relief. With newer surgical techniques and improved methods of postoperative management, there is no reason for the patient to experience the severe pain described by those who have undergone extensive excisional procedures.

Operative Management of Abscess and Fistula

The conditions that cause infectious processes in the anoperineum are cryptoglandular abscess and fistula, Crohn's disease, and hidradenitis suppurativa [*see Sidebar* Disease Processes That Cause Anorectal Abscess and Fistula in Ano]. Accurate

---

Disease Processes That Cause Anorectal Abscess and Fistula in Ano

Cryptoglandular Abscess and Fistula

This condition results from obstruction of the duct of a gland, the body of which resides in the intersphincteric plane. The orifice of the gland is at the base of the crypt. The disease process has both an acute aspect and a chronic aspect.

Abscess is the acute process of the disease. The anatomy is complex because of the tissue planes in the anorectal-perineal area.[2] Surgical drainage, or at least surgical evaluation, is always necessary. Attempts to manage this condition medically can result in progressive tissue destruction and life-threatening infection. It is also essential always to be alert to the possibility of an immunocompromised state. Normally, the anoperineum is quite resistant to microbial invasion; however, in immunocompromised patients, infection can be life-threatening.

Fistula is the chronic process of the disease. Persistent inflammation results in the formation of tracts from the anal duct to the anoperineal skin or to the inside of the rectum. These tracts can take extremely complex courses. For this reason and because of the complicated tissue planes of dissection, surgical treatment must be carefully planned: the status of the sphincter mechanism may be jeopardized if inappropriate surgical techniques are employed to open a fistula tract.

Crohn's Disease

Anal and perineal infection is a major factor in the clinical course of one third of all patients who have Crohn's disease. The main pathological process is full-thickness penetration of Crohn's ulcers, occurring at any location in the anal canal (as opposed to uncomplicated cryptoglandular abscess or fistula, which is usually found posteriorly or anteriorly in the midline). The infection associated with Crohn's disease can be massive but is surprisingly well tolerated by the patient. The infectious process can be progressively destructive to the sphincter and the surrounding tissue. Patients are at lifelong risk for severe diarrhea and loss of rectal distensibility; accordingly, meticulous preservation of the sphincter mechanism is crucial.

The incisional surgical procedures usually employed for infectious foci in the anal canal may be too hazardous, and excisional procedures are never indicated. Given that Crohn's disease tends to persist and recur, long-term drainage may be necessary. Medical management is useful and efficacious, but it should be provided in combination with surgical consultation and drainage of abscesses. Because patients with anal Crohn's disease usually exhibit some degree of intestinal involvement as well, it is important to evaluate the remainder of the GI tract, especially the rectum, before embarking on any surgical treatment of the anus.

Hidradenitis Suppurativa

This condition is caused by blockage and disruption of the apocrine sweat glands in the perianal and perineal tissue. It gives rise to destructive infected sinus tracts in the perineal tissue. Although the destruction can be profound, there is no connection with the intestinal tract (either the rectum or the anus). No specific pathological diagnosis can be made, because all that is left is the destructive fibrotic reaction to the content of the ruptured gland. Hidradenitis suppurativa occurs in persons with seborrheic skin and those who perspire profusely; it often involves the axillary, suprapubic, and inguinal areas as well as the perineum.

Because the lesions are actually sinus tracts in the skin, therapy involves simply incising the tracts; biopsy is appropriate at some point during the course of management.

Sepsis Resulting from Immunocompromised State

Anoperineal infection in an immunocompromised patient is a very serious and possibly life-threatening situation. Because this part of the body is so highly contaminated, failure of immune barriers can be disastrous. This condition is seen in patients who have diabetes, human immunodeficiency virus infection, or other forms of blood dyscrasias and in patients who have undergone chemotherapy. It is diagnosed on the basis of its symptoms: the clinical findings may be obscured by the absence of pus resulting from leukopenia.

Treatment involves aggressive antibiotic therapy, careful examination with the patient under anesthesia, extremely conservative drainage procedures, and biopsy of the tissue (leukemic infiltrates are occasionally found). The potential consequences of failing to recognize and treat this condition are serious enough to warrant evaluation of all patients with perineal infection for the immunocompromised state before any treatment is undertaken or before they are discharged from the surgeon's supervision.

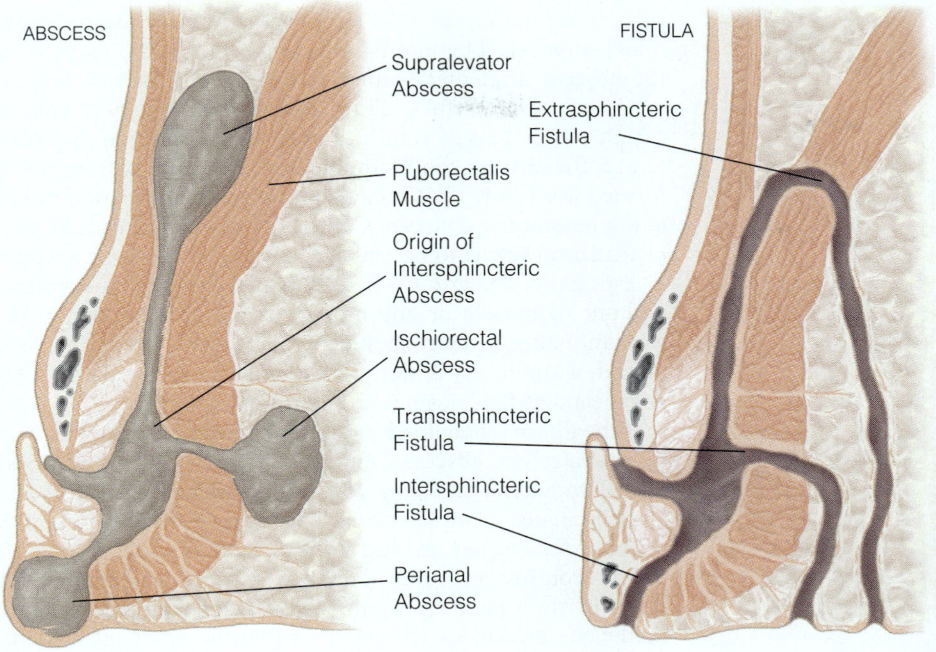

Figure 8 Operative management of abscess and fistula. Abscess and fistula are, respectively, the acute aspect and the chronic aspect of a single disease process. Acute inflammation can lead to different types of abscesses (*left*), depending on the direction in which the inflammation extends. Chronic inflammation leads to communication of the abscess sites with the surface—that is, fistula tracts (*right*).

diagnosis is essential for proper surgical management. Although these conditions may appear similar at times, each one is managed somewhat differently.

OPERATIVE PLANNING

The most important initial step is to determine the activity and severity of the disease process and the immune status of the patient. For example, a large, fluctuant abscess surrounded by erythema, induration, and superficial necrosis of the skin in an insulin-dependent diabetic is a surgical emergency. On the other hand, a chronic abscess or fistula that drains periodically over a matter of months is not nearly as urgent a problem. Multiple fistula tracts to the perineum in a patient with Crohn's disease require that one perform an adequate study of the intestinal tract and the sphincter mechanism before attempting definitive surgical treatment. It is important to determine the etiology of the process whenever possible. Unfortunately, the determination cannot always be made without examination under anesthesia, during which treatment as well as diagnosis could be accomplished, and this complicates the obtaining of informed consent and the choice of anesthesia.

It is also important to gain as accurate a picture as possible of the complexity of the disease process; this facilitates the planning of the procedure, the choice of anesthesia, and the selection of the information given to patient and family before treatment. For example, in the absence of other significant health problems, a small, well-localized, low intersphincteric abscess often can be easily drained with the patient under local anesthesia if an internal opening can be seen preoperatively on anoscopy, although on occasion even this procedure calls for spinal or epidural anesthesia. (It should be remembered that use of the prone-flexed position [*see Figure 2*], which is my preference, makes general anesthesia more difficult.) Multiple infected tracts associated with undrained infectious foci in a case of rectal Crohn's disease necessitate examination with the patient under spinal or epidural anesthesia. The treating surgeon should perform careful anoscopy and sigmoidoscopy and conservative temporary drainage procedures until consultation with a specialist can be arranged. Severe destruction and suspected deep tissue necrosis, especially in immunocompromised patients, may necessitate extensive resection of tissue and perhaps a completely diverting colostomy.

Bowel preparation should include mechanical cleansing and antibiotics but may not be possible when the situation is urgent (as is most often the case). Appropriate antibiotic coverage (i.e., agents effective against gram-negative organisms and anaerobes) is indicated for all but the simplest cases, with special consideration given to patients who require prophylaxis because of cardiac disease or the presence of prosthetic material.[1] Usually, a urinary catheter should be inserted before operation, especially if the infectious process is located in the anterior region in a man, where the urethra is at risk for injury.

OPERATIVE TECHNIQUE

Many technical elements are common to all operations for conditions that cause infectious processes in the perineum. The patient should be in the prone-flexed position, with the buttocks taped apart. Conduction anesthesia (spinal, caudal, or epidural) is usually required. The perineum should be examined carefully with an eye to areas of infection or external drainage sites. Endoscopic examination of the anus, the rectum, and the vagina should be undertaken to search for primary inflammatory bowel disease, internal openings of the fistula, or vaginal openings of the fistula.

Cryptoglandular Abscess and Fistula

The abscess must be located and characterized because drainage will depend on the location of the abscess, the course of the fistula tract, and any related infectious processes [*see Figure 8*]. It is important not to create a fistula through the levator plate of the pelvic floor. This means that an abscess with a low origin must be drained low, with care taken to avoid iatrogenic perforation of the rectum, and an abscess with a high origin (e.g., a high intersphincteric abscess) must be drained high by incising the rectal wall (not a procedure for the occasional rectal surgeon). The internal opening—that is, the crypt where the abscess originated—must be sought; this is best done by anoscopy, very careful probing, and sigmoidoscopy to rule out a high source (e.g., Crohn's disease). If the internal opening is found, the abscess can be drained or a fistulotomy can be performed [see Figure 9]. With a fistulotomy, determination of safety is a paramount concern. Careful consideration must be given to which muscle is to be cut. The anterior location in a woman is especially precarious. If the fistula involves a significant amount of muscle or any muscle in the anterior region in a woman, either a seton should be placed or a drain should be placed without disruption of the muscle in preparation for advancement flap closure of the internal opening.

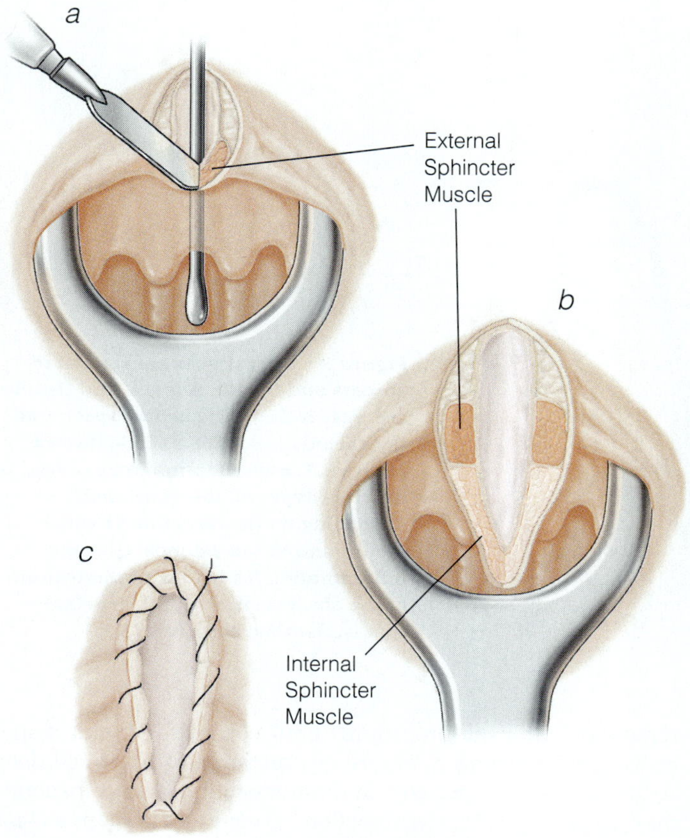

If the internal opening is not found, one should not make one by probing. The abscess should be drained with a mushroom-tipped catheter [see Figure 10]; this is preferable to unroofing and eliminates painful packing. The catheter can be left in place for an extended period, and it permits subsequent injection of dye or contrast material. Once the mushroom catheter is in place in the operating room, the surgeon can inject diluted methylene blue to search again for internal openings, which, if found, allow one to consider fistulotomy. The drain is usually sutured in place. The patient should be seen a few days after the operation to confirm that the abscess is adequately drained. After two weeks, the patient is seen in the office, and Betadine is injected through the drain while the inside of the anal canal is inspected via an anoscope. If an internal opening is seen, then fistulotomy is planned. If no internal opening is seen (as is the case in about 50 percent of patients), the drain should be removed one week later. This allows any irritant effect of the Betadine to resolve and prevents the abscess from recurring.

If the fistula tract is known to have an external opening and fistulotomy is planned, the following approach should be considered. First of all, fistulectomy is never indicated. Fistulotomy is performed rarely and with great caution in the face of Crohn's disease. To perform the fistulotomy, one must first find the internal opening. In this regard, Goodsall's rule is often helpful: external fistula openings anterior to the midanal line are usually connected to internal openings via short, straight tracts, whereas external openings posterior to this line usually follow a curved course to internal openings in the posterior midline. Dilute methylene blue is injected through the external opening, often via a plastic intravenous catheter. Careful probing, perhaps with a lacrimal duct probe, is then carried out. If the internal opening still cannot be found, a drain is placed so that the surgeon can return at another time to search for the internal opening. If the internal opening is found, a probe is passed and an effort is made to determine how much muscle and which muscle must be transected to accomplish the fistulotomy and how much muscle will remain to maintain continence [see Figure 11]. If the surgeon is not sure of the extent of muscle involvement or of how safe a fistulotomy would be, the infectious process should be drained, and either the patient should be referred to a specialist or plans should be made for an advancement flap procedure to close the internal opening. If a fistulotomy is done, a biopsy specimen should be obtained from the infected tract, and the tract should be marsupialized to prevent premature healing of the superficial aspect.

Special problems A cryptoglandular abscess that

Figure 9 Operative management of abscess and fistula. Shown is a fistulotomy in a patient with cryptoglandular abscess/fistula. (*a*) The fistula tract is carefully probed, a decision is made about which muscle and how much muscle to cut, and the tract is incised. (*b*) Once the tract is open, the involved crypt is excised. (*c*) The defect is marsupialized by sewing skin to the tract.

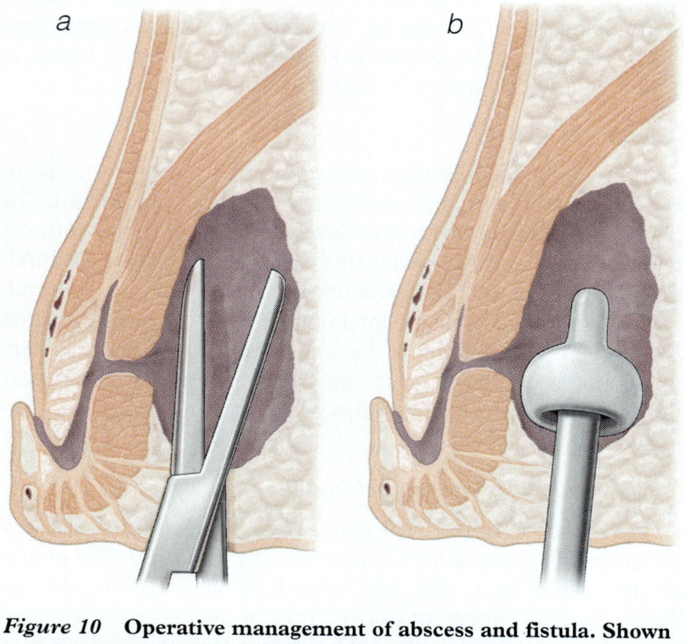

Figure 10 Operative management of abscess and fistula. Shown is drainage of an ischiorectal abscess. Such abscesses may be palpated above the anorectal ring, even though their location is more inferior. (*a*) The abscess is incised. (*b*) A mushroom-tipped catheter is placed.

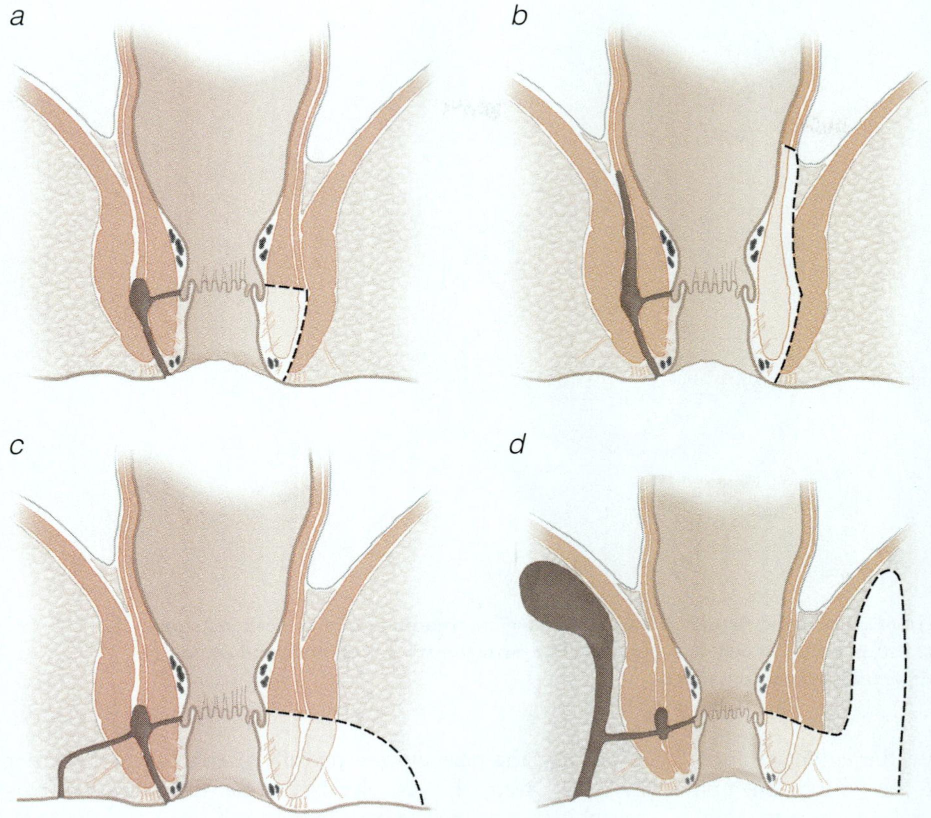

Figure 11 Operative management of abscess and fistula. Shown are examples of the different types of fistulotomies indicated for some of the many types of fistulas: intersphincteric fistula with a simple low tract (*a*), intersphincteric fistula with a high blind tract (*b*), uncomplicated transsphincteric fistula (*c*), and transsphincteric fistula with a high blind tract (*d*). In each image, the left half of the drawing shows the disease process, and the right half illustrates the recommended operation.

extends into the posterior anal and posterior rectal spaces is often missed as a source of infection. Diagnosis of such abscesses typically involves bidigital examination, often with the patient under anesthesia; needle aspiration may be required as well. Fistulotomy in this area often necessitates opening large amounts of tissue, including partial transection of the sphincter muscle; the tract may also have to be marsupialized. If one is unsure of the anatomy or has never done the procedure before, the abscess should be drained as simply as possible and the patient referred to a specialist.

The so-called horseshoe abscess [*see Figure 12*] results from an undiagnosed posterior-space abscess that has dissected laterally and may have been drained several times through the lateral extension into the ischiorectal fossa. This condition is cured by opening the posterior space and placing a long-term lateral drain, after which healing proceeds by secondary intention (the so-called Hanly procedure). The drain should not be removed until there is solid healing in the posterior midline; this may take weeks or even months.

Crohn's Abscess and Fistula

The goals of treatment are to drain and control the focus of infection, to preserve sphincter function, to plan and implement a staged approach to preservation of anorectal function, and to make the correct diagnosis. To these ends, careful identification of the location and course of the abscess and any associated fistulas is essential; this is accomplished via endoscopic dye injection, probing, and vaginoscopy. The safest approach, in my view, is to place mushroom catheters in abscesses and complicated fistula tracts or, in some cases, to use setons to allow drainage of the fistulas (not to cut through the tissue, which is often the intended result of seton placement) [*see Figure 13*]. For optimal resolution of inflammation at the site of the internal opening in anticipation of a possible advancement flap procedure, perirectal mushroom catheters are preferable to setons placed through the internal opening. Superficial fistula tracts may occasionally be managed with fistulotomy if the Crohn's disease is otherwise inactive. Sphincterotomy is never indicated in a patient with Crohn's disease if severe infection is present or the disease is active. When a patient is known or believed to have Crohn's disease, biopsy of the edematous external skin tags that are often present can be a good way of finding granulomatous tissue to confirm the diagnosis.

Hidradenitis Suppurativa

Patients with infected fistula tracts or abscesses secondary to hidradenitis suppurativa must be positioned in such a way as to allow visualization of and access to all tracts. This is crucial because some of the tracts may extend into the scrotum, the labia, the inguinal areas, or the suprapubic area. Conduction anesthesia is important in that it covers broad areas of the perineum; adequate local anesthesia is impossible unless one is dealing with very small, isolated tracts.

The definitive therapeutic surgical procedure is incision (rather than excision) of these often extensive inflammatory tracts [*see Figure 14*]. The surgeon should do as much as possible at one time, with the understanding that it is not unusual to leave a few tracts undrained or to return later to address new areas of dissection. Because the primary disease process does not involve the sphincter, intestinal diversion is rarely indicated. Biopsy is indicated because on rare occasions, these long infected tracts exhibit malignant changes or result from an anal

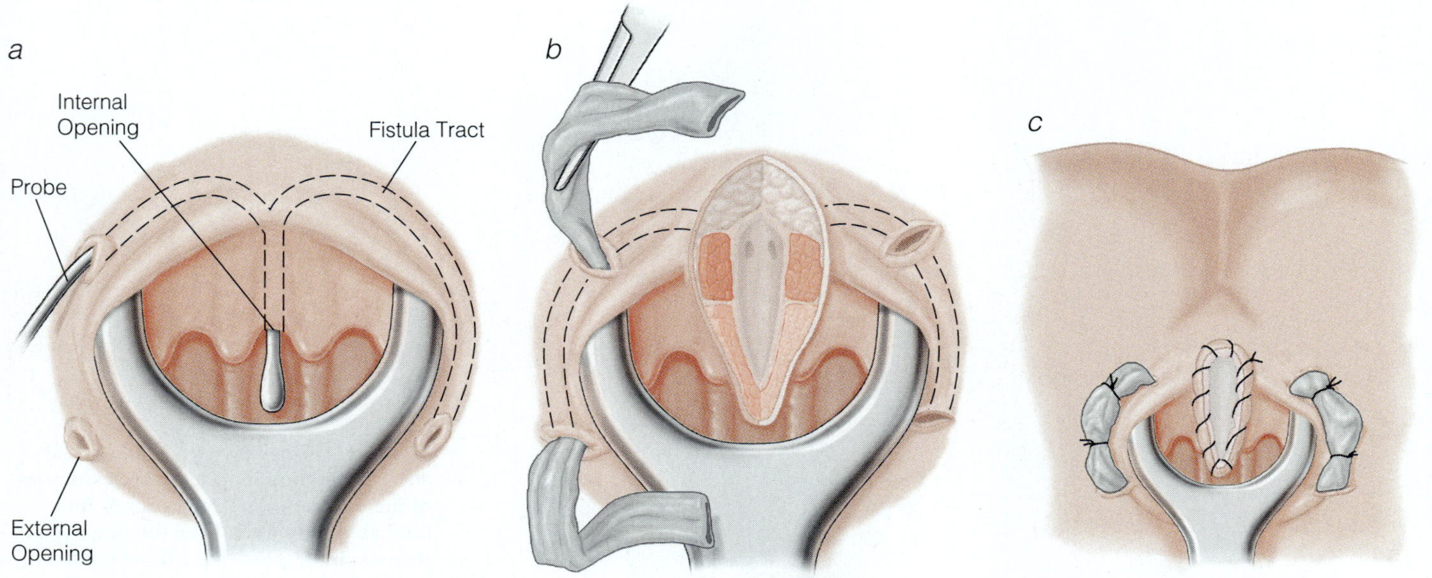

Figure 12 Operative management of abscess and fistula. Shown is the surgical treatment of a horseshoe fistula. (*a*) The main posterior tract of the fistula is identified by probing. (*b*) The posterior tract is opened, and drains are placed laterally. (*c*) The posterior tract is marsupialized.

malignancy. The perineal skin can tolerate the extensive incisions necessary to cure the process. Special precautions must be taken not only to preserve the sphincter itself but also to avoid damaging the neurovascular bundle that enters the anus from the posterolateral aspect. In male patients, efforts must be made to avoid the urethra during incision in the anterior midline; to this end, a Foley catheter should always be placed before the surgical procedure is begun. Because so many incised skin edges remain after treatment of extensive hidradenitis, it is imperative to achieve adequate hemostasis. The disposable suction cautery units currently available can be especially helpful for this purpose. The wounds may be either left open or loosely packed until good granulation tissue forms.

Bathing the perineum, especially after a bowel movement, is helpful. Often, showers are better for this purpose than the portable minuscule sitz baths commonly used. For patients who have undergone extensive procedures, twice-daily trips to a whirlpool bath (often located in the physical therapy department) are helpful. Despite the multiple lengthy incisions, there is usually little pain, and most of the postoperative care can be done at home. Adequate follow-up is necessary to treat residual or new areas of disease before the dissection becomes extensive again. Care must be taken, especially in the operating room, to search for the infected tracts, which may contain little pus and may be apparent only as indurated cords within the perineal skin.

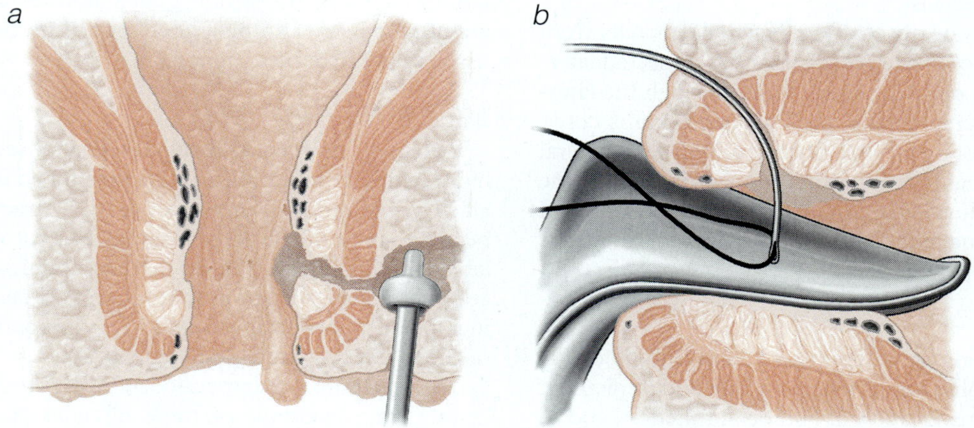

Figure 13 Operative management of abscess and fistula. Shown are alternatives for treating Crohn's abscess or fistula. In Crohn's disease, multiple perianal and perineal fistulas and abscesses may be seen, often in atypical locations. (*a*) Abscesses may be drained by placing a small mushroom-tipped catheter as close to the anus as possible. A Malecot catheter should not be used. (*b*) In some settings, it is appropriate to place a seton between internal and external openings. This seton may then be left in situ for a time for drainage and for prevention of further disease progression.

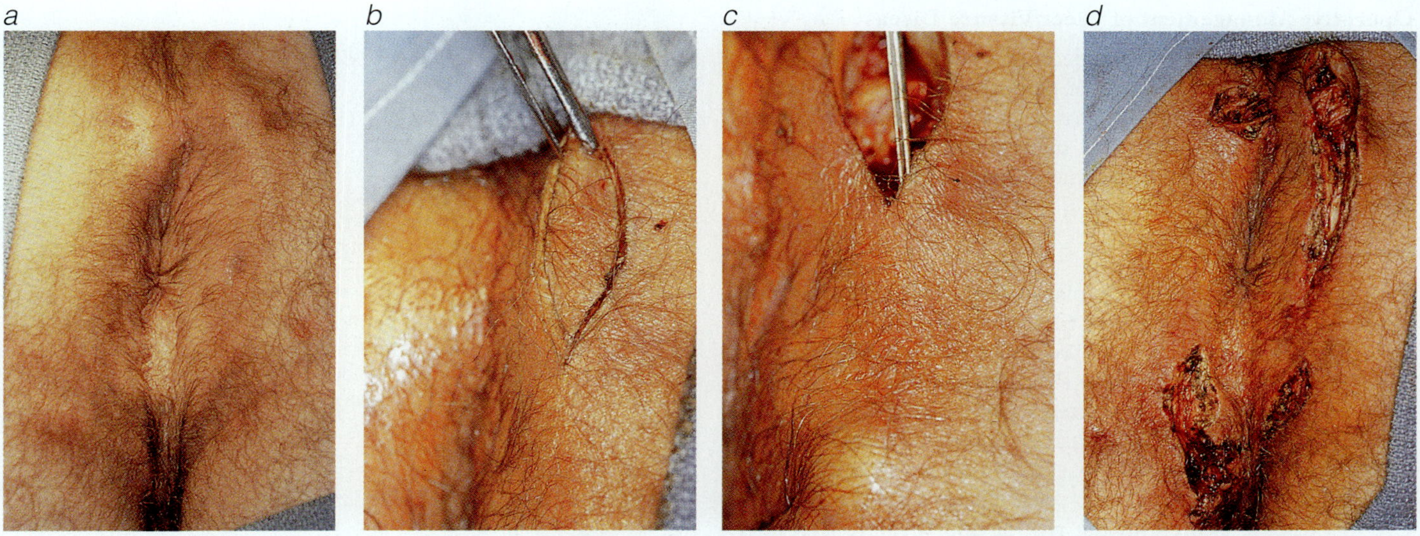

Figure 14 Operative management of abscess and fistula. In this patient, the causative condition is hidradenitis suppurativa. (*a*) Multiple openings of sinus tracts can be seen and extensive indurated tracts palpated. (*b*) Abscesses are unroofed. (*c*) Indurated tracts are probed. (*d*) All tracts are identified and incised.

TROUBLESHOOTING

Most of the important steps for avoiding problems have already been described in the course of addressing preoperative planning and operative technique (see above). The goals in the treatment of all of the processes associated with anorectal abscess and fistula in ano are to preserve sphincter function, to control acute infection, and to eliminate the source of the infection. If it is likely that sphincter function will be compromised at all, a baseline level of sphincter function (including the status of muscles and nerves) must be determined before any surgical procedure is initiated. One should never hesitate to perform an examination with the patient under anesthesia and to inject dilute methylene blue to delineate the extent and location of the infectious process.

Anyone embarking on surgical management of such processes must keep in mind the option of performing an advancement flap procedure to close the internal opening, especially in the anterior region and most particularly in women. If such a procedure is planned, initial drainage should be done external to the rectum with a mushroom catheter rather than through the internal opening with a seton. Simple 3-0 chromic catgut should be used to marsupialize fistula tracts because employing the newer, less quickly absorbable materials may lead to a chronic nidus that gives rise to ongoing infection. Patients should be watched closely in the immediate postoperative period to ensure that all infection is controlled. Not uncommonly, a superficial collection is drained, but a deeper abscess remains that must be sought more aggressively.

One should always take into account the risk of anoperineal infection in immunocompromised patients. Given that the anatomy of the anal tissue planes is complex and can be rendered even more so by multiple surgical procedures, one should not venture beyond one's level of expertise. One should never hesitate to drain an infectious focus with a simple mushroom-tipped catheter and, if appropriate, refer the patient to a colon and rectal surgical specialist who is trained to manage complex anoperineal infectious processes safely and definitively.

COMPLICATIONS

Complications occur if one or more of the goals just mentioned (see above) have not been achieved. Persistent or recurrent infection is seen with some frequency. In patients with cryptoglandular abscess or fistula, infection usually results from failure to locate the internal opening or to discover a deep posterior midline abscess; such failure is often seen in patients with a horseshoe abscess, in whom repeated lateral drainage procedures may have been undertaken without the primary cavity in the posterior anal or posterior rectal space being discovered and dealt with.

In patients with Crohn's disease, infection can persist if a deeper pocket or extension has gone undiscovered or if the disease has recurred, leading to further penetration and infection in the anoperineum or the perirectal tissue. Extensive examination with the patient under anesthesia, including transrectal ultrasonography or CT scanning, may be required to determine the source and extent of the infection. It is always possible that the infection derives from a superlevator abscess secondary to intestinal disease; consequently, a detailed evaluation of the intestinal tract is indicated in patients with Crohn's disease.

In patients with hidradenitis suppurativa, the most common problems are a residual undrained tract and recurrent disease. Again, examination with the patient under anesthesia and repeated drainage are called for. Because this disease process does not originate in the rectum, care must be taken not to enter the rectum or to cut any of the nerves entering the anus from the posterolateral aspect. It has been reported anecdotally that very chronic or persistent fistula tracts may eventually exhibit malignant changes (squamous cell carcinoma); for this reason, such tracts should be biopsied.

OUTCOME EVALUATION

No sophisticated surveillance is necessary: if drainage persists or some degree of incontinence develops, the patient usually will volunteer the information freely. Either of these complaints could be an indication for a detailed examination, including a sophisticated evaluation of sphincter function.

Operative Management of Ulcer/Fissure Disease

Ulcer and fissure are two aspects of a single anorectal disease process with an unclearly defined pathophysiology [see Figure 15]. Accurate diagnosis is crucial [see Sidebar Ulcer/Fissure Disease: Diagnosis and Treatment]. Not uncommonly, patients are treated for hemorrhoids when the true primary condition is ulcer/fissure disease.

OPERATIVE PLANNING

Fundamental concerns in planning the operation—besides confirming the diagnosis—are to verify that there are no other conditions that could threaten complete healing of an incision in the anal tissue and to make sure that there is no significant incontinence before the sphincterotomy.

For example, a history of diarrhea compatible with the presence of inflammatory bowel disease indicates the need for further evaluation to eliminate the possibility of Crohn's disease; if Crohn's disease is present, the risk of poor healing is greater, and it will be necessary to preserve all of the available sphincter function of the anus for a long period. As another example, a woman who has borne children by vaginal delivery and has any degree of incontinence should undergo manometry, ultrasonography, and perhaps electromyography to confirm that the sphincter is not compromised by a mechanical or neurologic deficiency. Yet another example is a patient with irritable bowel syndrome or a pelvic floor abnormality who experiences a multitude of difficulties with bowel movements. It is important to recognize such conditions and to advise the patient of the need for special attention to maintain adequate bowel function in the postoperative period.

It is essential to clearly explain the nature of the operative procedure (i.e., the incision of a portion of the internal sphincter mechanism) to the patient and to warn him or her that minor incontinence of flatus may persist for as long as a few months postoperatively. To be fair, significant incontinence is highly unusual: in fact, most patients experience very rapid relief of their often distressing symptoms. One should also advise the patient that any other anal procedures that may be indicated (e.g., elastic ligation of internal hemorrhoids or excision of symptomatic external hemorrhoids) can and should be accomplished at the time of sphincterotomy, with or without excision of the anal ulcer, and that he or she should take three to five days off from work. The risk of urinary retention, pain, and bleeding must also be discussed. In planning the operative procedure and immediate postoperative care, one must take into account the patient's specific needs, idiosyncrasies, and home environment. Some patients are comfortable undergoing the procedure completely on an outpatient basis, whereas others clearly need to be admitted for short-term observation and

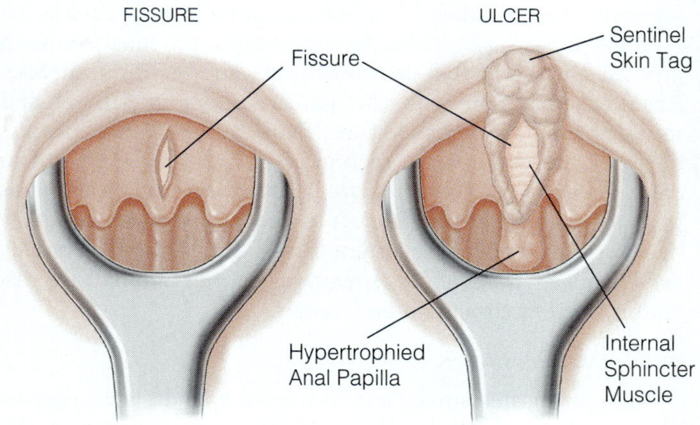

Ulcer/Fissure Disease: Diagnosis and Treatment

This condition is a very common one; however, the pathophysiology remains unclearly defined. Like abscess and fistula, it has an acute phase and a chronic phase.

A fissure (the acute phase) results from a tear in the tissue at the mucocutaneous junction of the anal canal. The cause is usually a hard bowel movement that stretches the anal opening and tears the tissue. In fact, fissures are also seen in patients with persistent diarrhea (especially in patients who have undergone the once popular jejunoileal bypass procedure for morbid obesity). The anal canal has an extremely rich blood supply, and most fissures heal with bowel control (i.e., bulk-forming agents and stool softeners), warm soaks, and mild analgesics. Patients must be assured that although the condition is extremely painful and is associated with some degree of bleeding, it is not a significant health threat.

For reasons that are not clear, perhaps as many as 50 percent of fissures do not heal spontaneously. As the opening persists, the surrounding tissue becomes hypertrophied and the process extends into the underlying internal sphincter muscle as an ulcer (the chronic phase) with a sentinel hemorrhoidal tag and a hypertrophied anal papilla (the triad of findings typical of an anal ulcer). Spasm and hypertrophy of the lower third of the internal sphincter muscle of the anal canal are always associated with this condition. Many believe, as I do, that spasm of this involuntary muscle results in diminishment of the blood supply to the anal canal and subsequent poor healing of the acute tear. It seems that as the process persists, the ulcer burrows deeper. The condition then becomes more painful, and the muscular spasm evolves into actual hypertrophy. At present, optimal therapy is based on the principle of incising the hypertrophied band of muscle, releasing the spasm, and improving the relative ischemia, thus allowing the injury to heal.

Ulcer/fissure disease can usually be diagnosed on the basis of the typical history of sudden onset of anal pain (often with a tearing sensation) and bleeding. Symptoms are usually exacerbated during bowel movements and may go on for weeks to months with intermittent healing and recrudescence of the process as the ischemia prevents solid, definitive healing. Diagnosis is complicated in that digital rectal examination can be extremely painful, and most physicians do not have the equipment and skills to perform an adequate anoscopic examination. If examination is too painful, local anesthesia may be necessary. Diagnosis can be facilitated by passage of a lubricated cotton swab to look for the typical streak of blood from the ulcer.

Medical treatment is often begun before the specific diagnosis can be verified. I usually try two weeks of medical therapy, often including topical antibiotics and anti-inflammatory suppositories or foam preparations. Once the diagnosis is confirmed, it becomes the patient's choice whether or when to undergo surgical treatment. I explain that the reason for the operation is to relieve discomfort, not to cure a life-threatening condition; however, I also point out that once significant spasm and hypertrophy of the sphincter are identified, definitive cure is unlikely unless a sphincterotomy is performed.

Some reports have described adequate healing of ulcer/fissure disease after multiple applications of dilute nitroglycerin paste to the anal canal. The place of this relatively new nonsurgical approach in the management of this disease remains to be defined.

Figure 15 Operative management of ulcer/fissure disease. Anal fissure (*left*) and anal ulcer (*right*) are, respectively, the acute aspect and the chronic aspect of a single disease process.

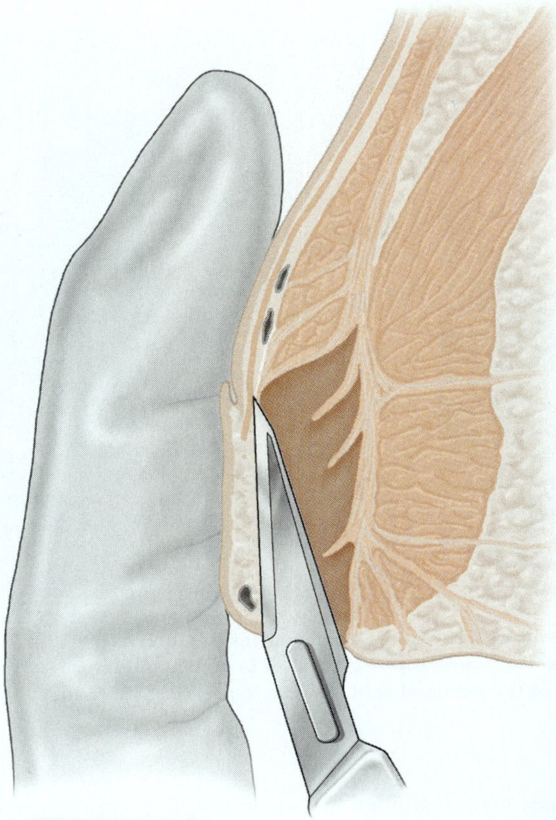

59 ANAL PROCEDURES — 855

band of the lower third of the internal sphincter muscle is clearly identified. If this band is not a distinctly identifiable entity, sphincterotomy should not be performed. The ulcer or fissure itself need not be present, because the disease may be in a relatively inactive state at the time of surgery.

Rigid or flexible sigmoidoscopy should then be performed if it was not done in the immediate preoperative period. The primary purpose of this step is to make sure that no features of Crohn's disease are visible in the rectum. When the endoscopic examination is complete, I usually repeat the preparation of the anal opening.

A 1 cm incision is made in the posterior lateral aspect of the perianal skin, hemostasis is obtained, and a delicate dissection is done with a curved hemostat in the intersphincteric plane. The posterior midline is avoided because healing in this position may result in scar tissue that interferes with perfect continence (the so-called keyhole deformity). The white hypertrophied band of muscle is then elevated into the wound with a curved hemostat. If a rent is made in the anal mucosa, it must be repaired with 3-0 chromic catgut. The band of muscle is then incised with the electrocautery, and pressure is maintained for a few minutes to ensure hemostasis. Digital examination confirms adequate transection of the band. The skin is left open.

Attention is then directed to the ulcer, which may be excised sharply in an elliptical fashion so as to incorporate the entire triad of the ulcer (i.e., the ulcer itself, the sentinel hemorrhoidal tag, and the hypertrophied anal papilla) while avoiding additional transection of the underlying muscle. If I excise the ulcer complex, I usually close the wound with a continuous three-point suture of 3-0 chromic catgut to obliterate any dead space and thus to lower the risk of postoperative infection.

Any additional anal surgery required is then completed, the surgical site is covered with antibiotic ointment, and a very light gauze bandage is applied with a minimum of tape and traction on the perianal skin.

TROUBLESHOOTING

To perform this simple procedure well, one must have a clear understanding of the surgical anatomy of the anal canal and must be able to clearly identify the internal sphincter, the intersphincteric groove, and the external sphincter muscle. The hypertrophied band of muscle must be accurately identified and cleanly transected. No attempt should be made to extend or amplify the procedure by stretching the anal canal and thus bursting the muscle.

Although the procedure and anatomy are simple, the best way of learning the operation is to watch an experienced surgeon perform it. I do not believe this procedure can be learned through reading alone.

COMPLICATIONS

Because the internal sphincter muscle is responsible for resting, involuntary continence, injury to this structure can lead to nocturnal incontinence. Again, special caution is advised with respect to the anterior aspect of the anoperineum in women. On the other hand, incising the posterior midline can also lead to the keyhole deformity, which may cause prolonged anal seepage because of the configuration of the scar tissue; a good analogy is a bent rim on a tubeless tire. It is tempting to close the tiny skin incision at the site of sphincterotomy, but I think it should be left open to reduce the already low risk of infection.

Figure 16 Operative management of ulcer/fissure disease. Shown is the closed approach to posterior lateral internal sphincterotomy. A No. 11 blade is inserted in the intersphincteric groove and moved upward to the level of the dentate line. Medial movement of the blade divides a portion of the internal sphincter muscle. The anoderm and the other anal muscles are not divided.

parenteral administration of pain medication.

When possible, I keep patients on a liquid diet for 24 hours before operation and use small, self-administered enemas to empty the rectum immediately before the procedure. I advise patients to discontinue any aspirin-containing products and any other anticoagulants, if possible, at least 10 days beforehand.

OPERATIVE TECHNIQUE

Operative treatment of ulcer/fissure disease consists of a posterior lateral internal anal sphincterotomy, in which the internal sphincter is divided but the external sphincter, the anoderm, and the longitudinal muscle remain intact. I generally prefer to place the patient in the prone-flexed position with the buttocks taped apart and adequate local anesthesia in place. The operation can then be performed in one of three ways: (1) as a closed procedure involving the use of a No. 11 blade and digital palpation of the muscle [see Figure 16], (2) as an open procedure without direct visualization of the muscle, or (3) as an open procedure with clear identification of the muscle before its transection. The third option is the one I prefer.

An open procedure with visualization of the muscle is done as follows [see Figure 17]. The first step is anoscopy, preferably with a medium Hill-Ferguson instrument. The hypertrophied

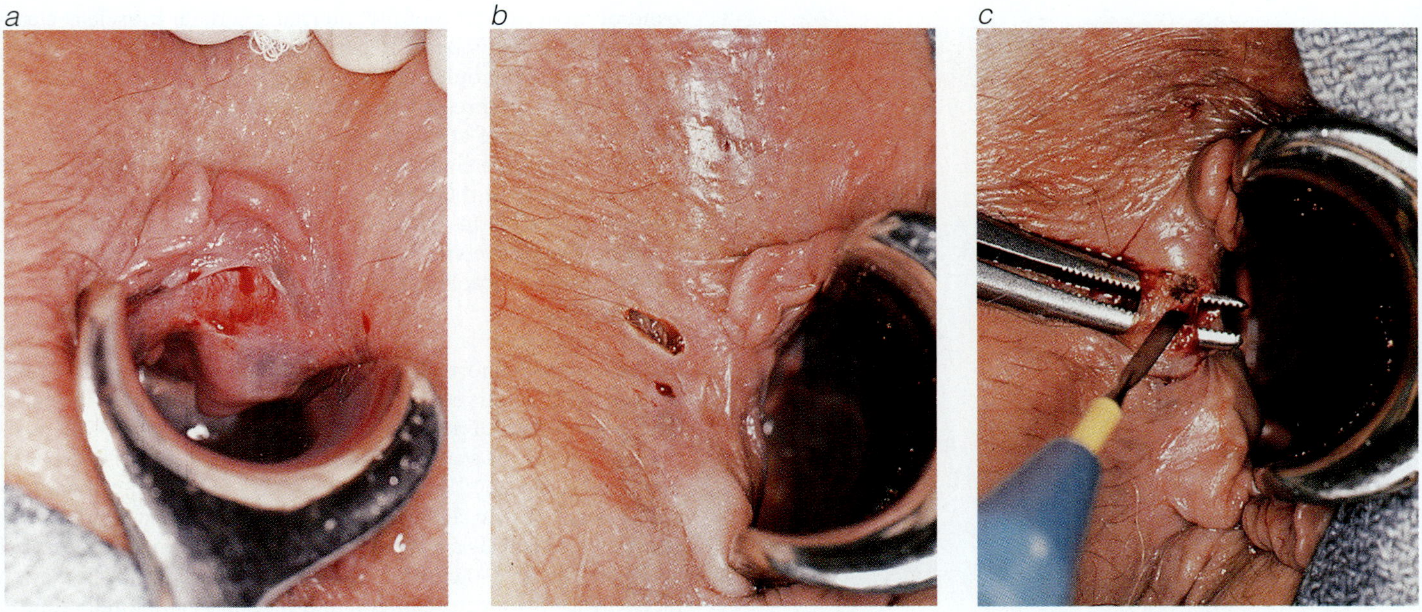

Figure 17 Operative management of ulcer/fissure disease. Shown is the open approach to posterior lateral internal sphincterotomy. (*a*) **The triad of the ulcer complex is visualized. (*b*) Once the hypertrophied band of internal sphincter muscle is identified, a 1 cm incision is made in the posterolateral aspect of the perianal skin. (*c*) The hypertrophied band is elevated into the wound and divided with the electrocautery.**

There should be very little postoperative pain. If the patient does complain of significant pain, especially in the presence of fever or urinary hesitancy, one must assume that infection is present in the anoperineum, a structure that is normally highly resistant to microbial invasion. Urgent evaluation, removal of sutures, antibiotic therapy, bowel rest, placement of a urinary catheter, and very close observation in the hospital are indicated.

The major causes of complications are misevaluation of the disease process (especially overlooking the presence of Crohn's disease) and failure to fully understand the anatomy of the continence mechanism of the anal canal. If too much of the internal sphincter muscle is cut, if this muscle is already compromised, or if the external sphincter muscle is transected by mistake, the patient will be rendered incontinent. On the other hand, if not enough of the internal muscle is transected, the ulcer will not heal and the symptoms will persist.

Overall, the single most common cause of complications that I have observed is the failure even to suspect, much less diagnose, ulcer/fissure disease as the source of a patient's symptoms. I frequently see patients who seem to have failed to heal months after a hemorrhoidectomy. When their symptoms are reviewed and a thorough examination performed, it becomes apparent that the underlying disease process was always ulcer/fissure disease rather than hemorrhoids and that the hemorrhoidectomy only intensified the anal pain and bleeding. These patients are finally cured when an adequate sphincterotomy is performed.

In very rare instances, drainage continues at the site of the sphincterotomy. If drainage persists for weeks, the patient should be examined under appropriate anesthesia, and the focus of infection should be opened. This is essentially equivalent to a very superficial fistulotomy.

OUTCOME EVALUATION

Again, no sophisticated surveillance is necessary: when the patient returns two weeks after the procedure, free of pain and bleeding and able to have bowel movements without difficulty, one may be sure that an acceptable outcome has been achieved. Digital rectal examination should confirm good healing and normal sphincter tone (both while resting and while contracting). For additional confirmation, I have patients continue to take bulk-forming agents and stool softeners and then examine them one month later to verify that healing is complete.

References

1. Practice parameters for antibiotic prophylaxis to prevent infective endocarditis or infected prosthesis during colon and rectal endoscopy. Standards Practice Task Force, American Society of Colon and Rectal Surgeons. Dis Colon Rectum 35:277, 1992
2. Kodner IJ, Fry RD, Fleshman JW, et al: Colon, rectum and anus. Principles of Surgery, 6th ed. Schwartz SI, Ed. McGraw-Hill, New York, 1994

Recommended Reading

Corman ML: Colon and Rectal Surgery, 3rd ed. JB Lippincott Co, Philadelphia, 1993

Fry RD, Kodner IJ: Anorectal disorders. Clin Symp 37:6, 1985

Gordon PH, Nivatvongs S: Principles and Practice of Surgery for the Colon, Rectum and Anus. Quality Medical Publishers, St. Louis, 1992

Keighley MRB, Williams NS: Surgery of the Anus, Rectum and Colon, Vols 1 and 2. WB Saunders, London, 1993

Kodner IJ: Differential diagnosis and management of benign anorectal diseases. Gastrointestinal Diseases Today 5:8, 1996

Kodner IJ, Fry RD, Fleshman JW, et al: Colon, rectum and anus. Principles of Surgery, 6th ed. Schwartz SI, Ed. McGraw-Hill, New York, 1994

Standards Practice Task Force, American Society of Colon and Rectal Surgeons: Practice parameters for treatment of fistula-in-ano. Dis Colon Rectum 39:1361, 1996

Acknowledgment

Figures 1, 5b, 5c, 8 through 13, 15, and 16   Tom Moore.

60 OPEN REPAIR OF HERNIAS OF THE ABDOMINAL WALL

George E. Wantz, M.D.

Hernias of the abdominal wall are a major recurrent surgical problem. New techniques, modifications of established methods, and even the introduction of synthetic prosthetic screens have not perfected the repair of this type of hernia. Another factor affecting the outcome of a hernia, as in all operations, is the skill and experience of the surgeon.

Classification of Hernias of the Groin

Traditionally, hernias of the groin have been described and classified on the basis of the anterior clinical presentation of the hernial sac (i.e., indirect inguinal, direct inguinal, and femoral). From the posterior, however, this classification is irrelevant because only the neck of the hernial sac and the parietal defect can be seen [*see Figure 1*].

Many attempts to classify hernias and to stage the degree of parietal deterioration have been devised.[1-5] Unfortunately, although the intent of such categorization is to promote a common surgical understanding, the classifications are incomplete and lack unanimity. Until accord is reached, hernias should be described on the basis of the volume of the sac and the location, size, and type of the parietal defect (e.g., a large indirect inguinal hernia with a 3 cm parietal defect).

Fruchaud[6] introduced a concept that unified the various hernias of the groin and simplified our understanding of them. Rather than defining hernias by their clinical presentation, he defined them by their origin and emphasized that all hernias of the groin, no matter the type, begin in a single weak area he called the myopectineal orifice (MPO). Until recently, this concept of groin hernias was little appreciated by surgeons in English-speaking countries.[6,7]

The MPO, a bony muscular framework, is bridged and bisected by the inguinal ligament, traversed by the femoral vessels and the spermatic cord, and sealed on its inner surface by the transverse fascia (endopelvic fascia). The integrity of the MPO depends on the strength of the transverse fascia. A hernia occurs when a peritoneal sac protrudes through the MPO; failure of the transverse fascia to retain the peritoneum is the fundamental cause of all hernias of the groin.

The inguinal ligament along with its recurved lacunar-shaped insertion on the pecten, although only loosely attached to the underlying structures, strongly braces the MPO, serves as the dividing line separating inguinal from femoral hernias, and defines the medial border of the orifice of the femoral canal.

A persistent processus vaginalis peritonei predisposes men and women to indirect inguinal herniation. The descent of the testicle through the abdominal wall predisposes men to direct inguinal herniation. This passage weakens the superior portion of the MPO and changes the function of the inferior portion of the internal oblique abdominal muscle from that of a protective muscle that embraces the floor of the inguinal canal to that of a suspensory muscle of the testicle (cremaster muscle) that embraces the spermatic cord. In women, the increased diameter of the true pelvis compared with that in men proportionately widens the femoral canal and probably predisposes them to femoral herniation.

Essentials of Groin Hernioplasty

Restoring the integrity of the MPO prevents peritoneal protrusion and repairs the hernia. This task may be accomplished in two fundamentally different ways: (1) repairing the parietal defect and (2) replacing the deficient transverse fascia with a synthetic prosthesis.

Access to the MPO may be anterior, through a groin incision, or posterior, through an abdominal incision [*see Figure 2*]. Exposure of the bony and musculoaponeurotic borders of the MPO by the anterior approach requires dissection of the inguinal canal, spermatic cord, and sensory nerves of the groin; by the posterior approach, only reflection of the peritoneum is necessary.

Tension on the suture line is the enemy of successful hernia surgery and must be diligently avoided. Suture tension causes tissue necrosis and, hence, parietal defects and recurrences. It also increases postoperative pain. Sutures must never be drawn up so tightly as to indent tissues.

Permanent synthetic prostheses, usually in the form of a mesh, are now widely employed in the management of hernias of the abdominal wall. At first, there was concern that synthetic prostheses would act like foreign bodies and would easily become infected, but they have not proved to be the bugbear surgeons previously thought they might be.

Finally, recurrence rates may not be a proper measure of the success of classic and prosthetic hernioplasties, because too many variables are involved in hernia recurrence. The outcome of hernia repair depends on the quality of the surgery, the integrity of the tissues, and the amount of suture tension, not on the chosen technique.

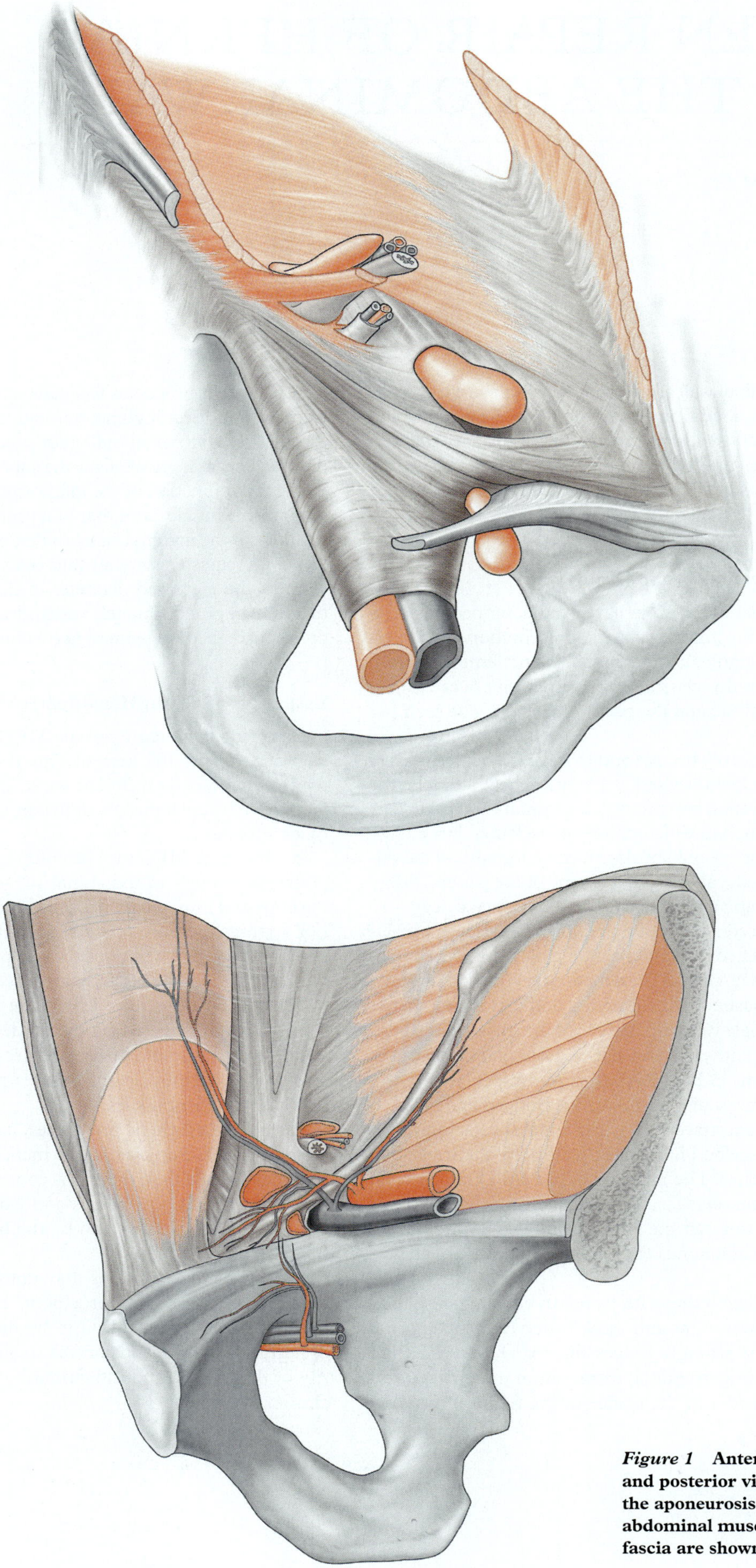

Figure 1 Anterior view (top) and posterior view (bottom) of the aponeurosis of the transverse abdominal muscle and the transverse fascia are shown.[53]

Classic Hernioplasties

The classic hernioplasties remain popular and produce excellent results (overall recurrence rates of one to three percent) when expertly performed in appropriate patients.[8-10] Knowledge of the classic hernioplasties is important because they embody the surgical principles and techniques applicable to prosthetic repair.

Only three classic hernioplasties are still in use: the Marcy repair, also known as the simple ring closure; the Bassini repair, either in its original form or in the form developed at the Shouldice Hospital in Toronto; and the Cooper's ligament repair, also known as the McVay-Lotheissen hernioplasty. The three hernioplasties preserve the shutter mechanism of the deep inguinal ring and the obliquity of the inguinal canal; they differ only in the extent to which the MPO is repaired.

OPERATIVE TECHNIQUE

The classic hernioplasties have three stages, namely, dissection, repair, and closure. All use an anterior groin incision.

Dissection

The object of the dissection is to eliminate the hernial sac and to expose the parietal defect in the innermost aponeuroticofascial layer of the abdominal wall. The dissection is performed in several steps. First, the inguinal canal is opened; the ilioinguinal

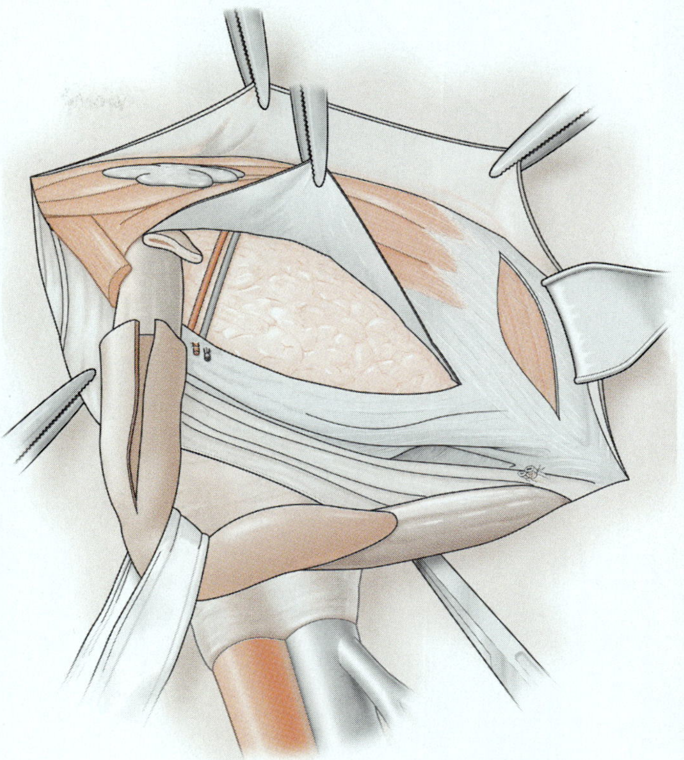

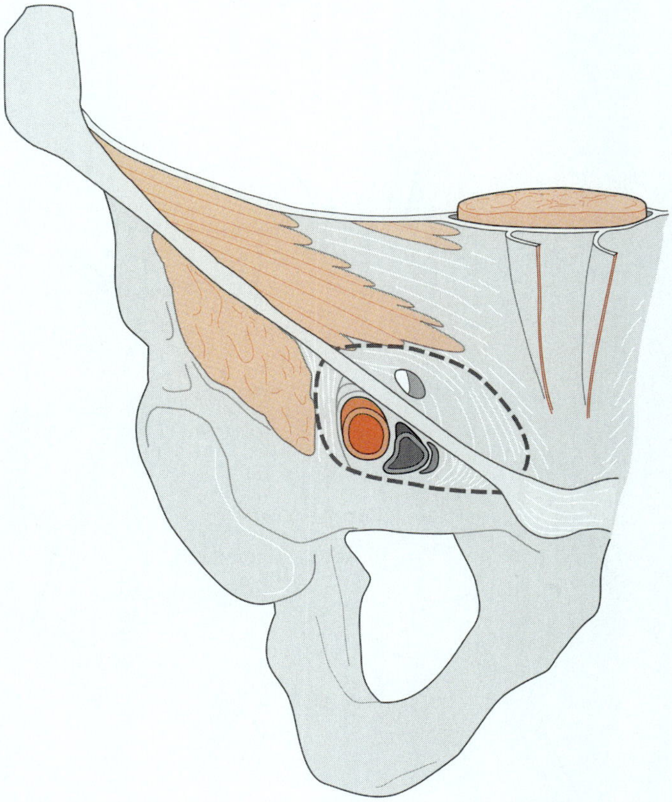

Figure 2 Shown is the anterior view of the myopectineal orifice of Fruchaud. This bony muscular framework is bounded by the iliopsoas muscle, the oblique abdominal muscles, the rectus abdominis muscle, and the pecten of the pubis. It is traversed by the femoral vessels and spermatic cord, bridged by the inguinal ligament, and sealed on the inside by the transverse fascia. Failure of the transverse fascia to retain the peritoneum is the fundamental cause of all hernias of the groin.[53]

Figure 3 Shown is complete anterior dissection of the groin. The spermatic cord has been mobilized and held aside with a Penrose drain. The cremaster muscle and cremaster neurovascular bundle have been divided to enhance the view of the innermost aponeuroticofascial layer of the abdomen. The posterior wall of the inguinal canal has been divided from the deep inguinal ring medially toward the pubic tubercle to a point at which healthy muscle is reached. This division destroys the deep inguinal ring. The transverse aponeurotic arch is an important structure in the repair of hernias and cannot be seen unless the medial flap of the posterior wall is reflected. If a McVay-Lotheissen repair is anticipated, it is also necessary to excise the outlined portion of the iliopubic tract for full exposure of Cooper's ligament and the medial edge of the femoral sheath [see Figure 4e].

The aponeurosis of the external oblique muscle is retracted medially to reveal the aponeurosis of the internal oblique muscle. Relaxing incisions are made by vertically incising the aponeurosis of the internal oblique muscle over the belly of the rectus abdominis muscle.

A simple indirect hernial sac is merely divided near the deep inguinal ring, and the distal portion is allowed to remain in situ undissected from the spermatic cord. The proximal portion is dissected from the cord and adjacent structures, ligated or not, and allowed to retract. The spermatic cord should never be dissected beyond the pubic tubercle for fear of damaging the delicate veins of the pampiniform plexus and causing testicular atrophy. The exception to this would be a sliding indirect inguinal hernia when an abdominal viscus is actually a part of the wall of the indirect hernial sac. Sliding indirect hernial sacs and all direct inguinal hernial sacs are simply inverted. Femoral hernial sacs are usually ligated below the inguinal ligament because they are vascular and often contain a lymph node.

860 — V OPERATIVE MANAGEMENT

a

b

c

d

Figure 4 (*a*) **The Marcy hernioplasty.** The deep inguinal ring is tightened and returned to normal size by one or two permanent synthetic monofilament sutures (often called Marcy sutures) placed medially in the transverse aponeurotic arch and laterally in the iliopubic tract or femoral sheath. (*b*) **The Bassini hernioplasty.** Bassini divided the floor of the inguinal canal as illustrated in Figure 3. Many surgeons omit this step. The three-layer repair consists of approximating with interrupted sutures the internal oblique abdominal muscle, the transverse abdominal muscle, and the transverse fascia to the inguinal ligament and iliopubic tract. (*c*) **The Shouldice-Bassini hernioplasty.** The floor of the inguinal canal is repaired by imbrication of the innermost aponeuroticofascial layer of the abdominal wall. The iliopubic tract is fastened to the undersurface of the transverse aponeurotic arch, and the free edge of the transverse aponeurotic arch is attached to the shelving edge of the inguinal ligament with a single continuous to-and-fro monofilament suture. Suturing begins near the pubic tubercle, continues to the deep inguinal ring, and then returns to the starting point. (*d*) The surgeons at the Shouldice Hospital also place a to-and-fro continuous suture affixing the internal oblique abdominal muscle to the inguinal ligament. Most enthusiasts of the technique consider the second suture to be superfluous and therefore leave it out. Sutures should not grasp the periosteum of the pubic tubercle, because this may cause residual postoperative pain. (*e*) **The McVay-Lotheissen hernioplasty.** This repair consists of attaching the transverse aponeurotic arch to Cooper's ligament, the medial side of the femoral sheath, and the anterior femoral sheath with interrupted sutures. The suture affixing the transverse aponeurotic arch to the medial edge of the femoral sheath is called the transition suture. Relaxing incisions are mandatory.[53]

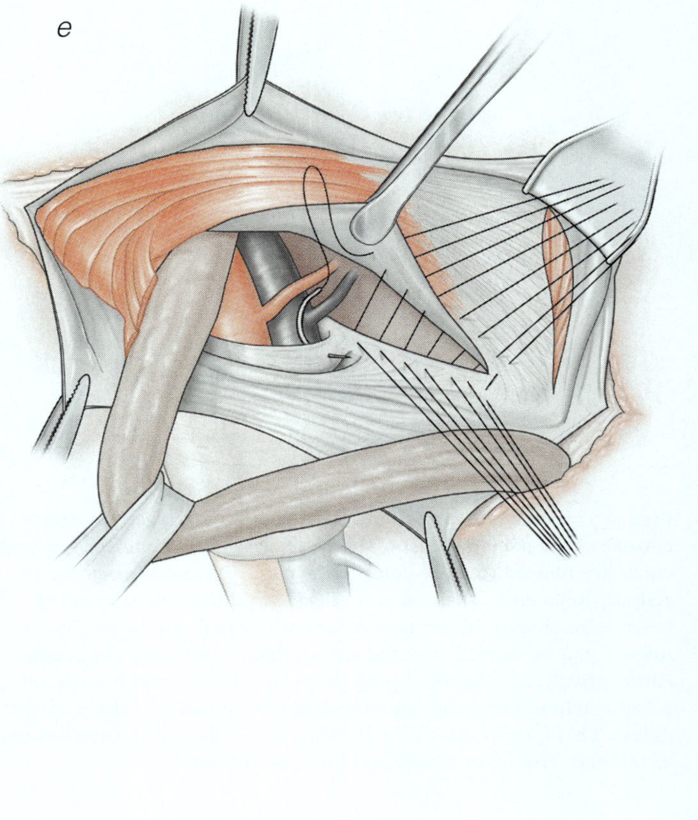

nerve is preserved, if possible; the cremaster muscle and neurovascular bundle are divided to expose the deep inguinal ring; and the spermatic cord is mobilized. Then, the posterior wall of the inguinal canal is divided and excised to the extent that it is weak, and the transverse aponeurosis is assessed. Finally, the peritoneal sac is eliminated, cord lipomata are removed, and a relaxing incision is made [*see Figure 3*].

Division of the cremaster muscle and division of the posterior wall of the inguinal canal are very important steps that many surgeons omit even today, although Bassini routinely performed them and surgeons at the forefront of inguinal hernia repair have repeatedly emphasized their importance.[11] Also important are relaxing incisions, which are required in the Cooper's ligament hernioplasty and are strongly recommended in the Bassini and Shouldice-Bassini hernioplasties. They are not needed in the Marcy repair.

Hernial sacs need not be excised: direct hernial sacs are merely inverted, and indirect hernial sacs are divided near their neck. The proximal sac is dissected from adjacent tissues and may or may not be ligated. The sac is then allowed to retract. The distal sac remains undissected and in situ but should be slit along the avascular border to prevent fluid accumulation. Sliding indirect hernias must be dissected from the spermatic cord and then inverted.

Repair

Common to the repair of all inguinal hernias in men is reconstruction of the deep inguinal ring. The ring cannot be made so tight that it strangles the spermatic cord, because the lateral border of the ring is elastic, muscular, indistinct, undefinable, and nonpalpable. What the surgeon apparently palpates as the deep inguinal ring is actually the inguinal canal, the diameter of which is always reduced when the inguinal ligament is used in the repair. Failure to reconstruct the medial border of the ring adequately is the chief cause of recurrences of indirect hernias. In women, the round ligament should be divided and the deep inguinal ring completely closed.

Marcy hernioplasty The Marcy repair is indicated in men and women with minimally damaged inguinal floors [*see Figure 4a*].[12,13]

Bassini and Shouldice-Bassini hernioplasties The Bassini and Shouldice-Bassini hernioplasties repair the area of the MPO that is superior to the inguinal ligament, that is, the deep inguinal ring and Hesselbach's triangle. Currently, the Shouldice-Bassini hernioplasty is very popular, produces exceptional results, and is used to manage most indirect and direct inguinal hernias in men. (The Marcy repair remains the most popular procedure in women.)

In the Bassini repair, the triple layer that consists of the internal oblique abdominal muscle, the transverse abdominal muscle, and the transverse fascia is approximated to the iliopubic tract and the shelving edge of the inguinal ligament with interrupted permanent sutures [*see Figure 4b*]. This differs markedly from the Bassini operation traditionally performed by North American surgeons, in which the posterior wall is plicated beneath sutures approximating the internal oblique muscle and conjoint tendon to Poupart's ligament. In the Shouldice-Bassini repair, the same myoaponeurotic layers are approximated, not edge to edge with interrupted sutures but by precise layered imbrication with continuous sutures [see Figure 4c and d].[8,14-16]

The Bassini repair and the Shouldice-Bassini repair are considered nonanatomic because the transverse aponeurosis is sutured to the inguinal ligament. This criticism is academic because the repairs work. Those who object to using the inguinal ligament to repair the MPO favor instead edge-to-edge approximation of the transverse aponeurotic arch and the iliopubic tract. The technique is called the iliopubic tract repair to distinguish it from the Bassini and Shouldice-Bassini repairs, which are inguinal ligament repairs.[17,18]

Cooper's ligament hernioplasty The Cooper's ligament hernioplasty (McVay-Lotheissen repair) addresses the three areas that are most vulnerable for herniation in the MPO, namely, the deep inguinal ring, Hesselbach's triangle, and the femoral canal. Therefore, the Cooper's ligament repair is used to manage femoral hernias and large indirect and direct inguinal hernias.[19-22]

The repair is accomplished by suturing the transverse aponeurotic arch to Cooper's ligament medially and to the femoral sheath laterally [see Figure 4e]. To expose Cooper's ligament and the medial border of the femoral sheath, the medial portion of the iliopubic tract must be excised [see Figure 3]. This extra step in the dissection is important because it allows the accurate placement of sutures. Relaxing incisions are mandatory in this repair.[23]

Although many enthusiasts employ this repair routinely, McVay himself used it in only about half of the hernioplasties he performed; in patients with smaller defects, he essentially used the Marcy repair.[9] The popularity of the McVay repair has declined in recent years because the operation is more difficult to perform and is associated with more postoperative pain than other repairs. Nevertheless, it is a neat and anatomic procedure.

Closure

The classic hernioplasties are completed by approximating the aponeurosis of the external oblique abdominal muscle. This process closes the inguinal canal and reassembles the superficial inguinal ring. The suture should include the distal stump of the divided cremaster muscle so that the testicle is pulled up.

SPECIAL CONSIDERATIONS

Bilateral inguinal hernias are usually repaired simultaneously because repairing them separately does not improve recurrence rates. Direct hernias are usually bilateral and inherently have a higher recurrence rate than indirect hernias do. This fact has led to the false conclusion that the simultaneous performance of bilateral hernioplasties is associated with increased suture line tension and, therefore, increased recurrence rates. If a hernial sac other than a small indirect one must be removed from the spermatic cord, simultaneous contralateral inguinal hernia repair should not be performed, because bilateral testicular atrophy may occur [see Dissection, *above*, and Complications of Groin Hernioplasty, *below*]. Obesity per se is not a contraindication for elective inguinal hernioplasty or a cause of recurrence. However, inguinal hernioplasty is more difficult in obese patients, and general or regional anesthesia is usually required.

In women, femoral hernias with small parietal defects are repaired subinguinally through an anterior groin incision by a few simple sutures (Bassini technique) [see Figure 5] or are corked with

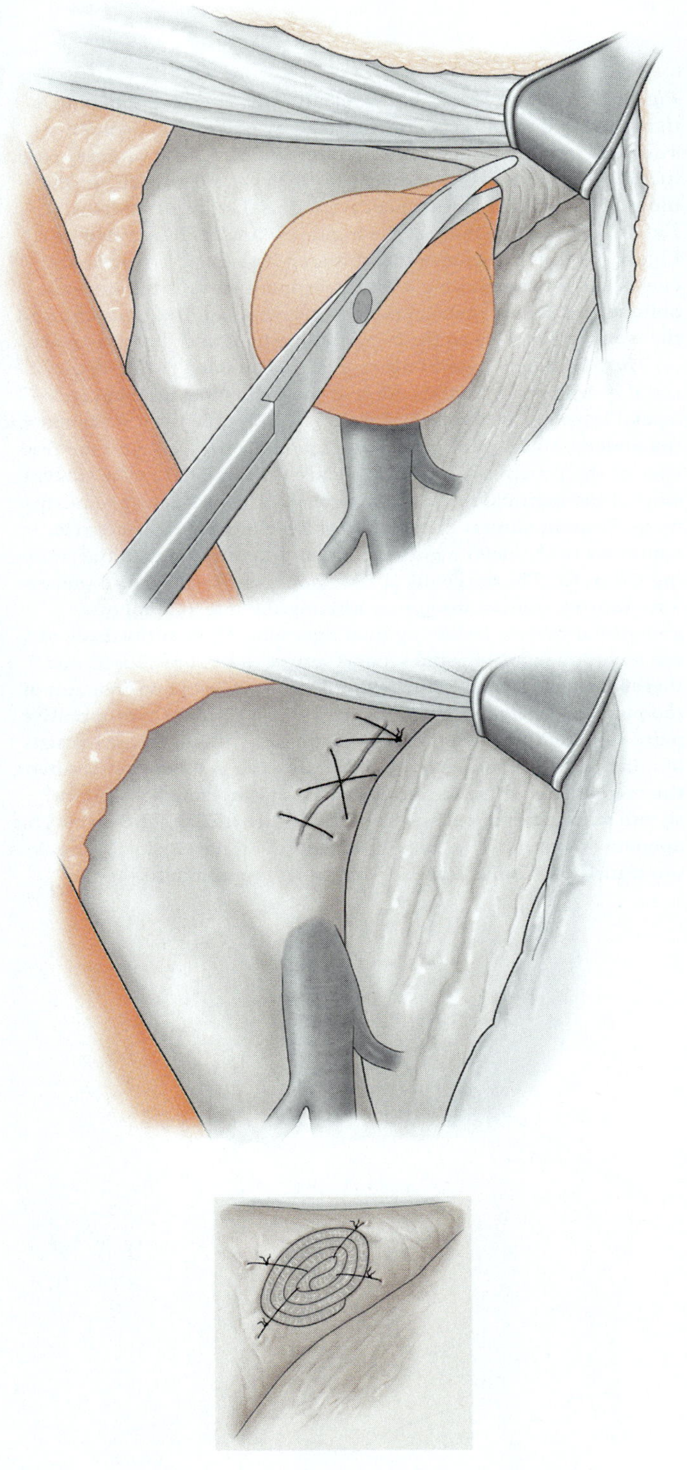

Figure 5 Femoral hernias in women can be managed by simple closure of the parietal defect. The lacunar ligament and the femoral canal are incised (top) to enlarge the canal and make it easier to reduce the hernia. The defect is closed (middle) with a running to-and-fro absorbable suture. A flap of fascia from the pectineal muscle can be turned over the suture line to reinforce the repair. Alternatively, a cylindrical plug (bottom) constructed from a 2.0 to 2.5 cm strip of polypropylene mesh can be sutured in the parietal defect. This type of repair, by itself, is not indicated in men because of the high risk of an associated inguinal hernia.[53]

a cylindrical polypropylene prosthetic plug [see Lichtenstein's Tension-Free Hernioplasty, below]. The Cooper's ligament hernioplasty or a properitoneal prosthetic repair [see Figure 5] should be used to repair large femoral hernias in women and all femoral hernias in men, because the latter are usually associated with inguinal hernias. Strangulated femoral hernias should be corrected with a properitoneal repair because this approach provides direct access to the constricting femoral orifices, easy release of the entrapped bowel by incision of the iliopubic and lacunar ligaments, and ample room for bowel resection.[24,25]

In indirect hernias in infants, children, and some young adults, the MPO is not damaged, and a classic repair is unnecessary; simply eliminating the sac repairs the hernia. The operation known as high ligation of the sac consists of opening the inguinal canal and, without mobilizing the spermatic cord, identifying and tracing the sac proximal to the deep inguinal ring and ligating and dividing it there.

CRITIQUE OF THE CLASSIC REPAIRS

The classic hernioplasties have several disadvantages:

1. Considerable experience and skill are required to obtain a recurrence rate of one to two percent.
2. The classic repairs are inadequate for the repair of recurrent hernias.
3. Some unwanted tension will always be present.
4. The problem of continued tissue deterioration is not addressed.
5. There will always be some patients with very poor tissues and some with connective tissue diseases.

These disadvantages have caused many surgeons to use synthetic soft tissue prostheses.

Prosthetic Hernioplasty

Prosthetic hernioplasties are beginning to replace the classic hernioplasties, and a wide variety of permanent synthetic prostheses are readily available. In prosthetic hernioplasty, biomaterials are used to patch or plug the parietal defects, to reinforce the classic repairs, and to replace the transverse fascia (endoabdominal fascia). Enthusiasm for the prosthetic repairs has been stimulated by reports of good results, aggressive promotion by the manufacturers of the prostheses, and recognition in the surgical community that prosthetic infection is not as large a problem as surgeons once thought it was.

SPECIAL CONSIDERATIONS

Synthetic Prostheses for Abdominal Hernioplasty

The permanent synthetic soft tissue prostheses commonly used in hernia surgery are composed of one of the following materials: polypropylene, the polyester Dacron, and expanded polytetrafluoroethylene (Teflon). These materials have replaced the inconvenient biologic grafts, such as fascia lata, and are generally well tolerated.

Marlex mesh, Prolene mesh, and Trelex Natural mesh are composed of loosely knitted monofilament strands of polypropylene. They are semirigid, slightly elastic, and relatively heavy materials that buckle when bent in two directions at once. They have granular surfaces that grip tissue and prevent prosthesis wandering before incorporation occurs. The three meshes resemble one another and may be used interchangeably.

Surgipro mesh is an open knitted mesh composed of braided strands of polypropylene. Its physical properties resemble those of the knitted monofilament polypropylene meshes, for which it may be substituted.

Mersilene and Lars meshes are open knitted meshes composed of braided strands of Dacron. In contrast to the polypropylene meshes, Dacron meshes are soft, supple, flexible, highly compliant and conforming, elastic in one direction only, and very light. They also have grainy surfaces that grip tissues and prevent the prostheses from wandering when they are not sutured in place.

Gore-Tex is not a mesh but an impervious and pliable material made from Teflon. A patented process expands the material at microscopic intervals so that extremely tiny and complex channels are created that pass completely through the material. Fibroblasts and collagen fibers grasp the material by penetrating these crevices. Gore-Tex is soft, supple, slightly elastic, and smooth.

Absorbable synthetic prostheses are occasionally needed in hernia surgery. The most commonly used materials are Vicryl and Dexon mesh, both of which may be knitted or woven. Vicryl is made from polyglactin 910 acid, Dexon from polyglycolic acid.

Tissue Response

The prostheses made of polypropylene and polyester desirably incite fibroplasia with only minimal inflammation. Therefore, they become quickly integrated into soft tissues. However, the ability to incite fibroplasia can be detrimental if these prostheses are placed intraperitoneally. Troublesome and tightly binding abdominal adhesions may form that are difficult to divide and can cause intestinal obstruction and fistulization.

Binding intra-abdominal adhesions can be prevented by interposing the omentum between an intraperitoneal permanent prosthesis and the abdominal viscera. An absorbable prosthesis made of tightly woven or knitted Vicryl or Dexon may be substituted for the omentum or for peritoneum and posterior rectus abdominis sheath when these structures cannot be approximated. The absorbable prostheses (e.g., those made from Vicryl or Dexon) also cause adhesions. However, they may prevent the viscera from becoming dangerously grafted to the permanent prosthesis because integration of the permanent prosthesis in the mesothelial tissues occurs before the absorbable prosthesis disappears.

Gore-Tex is inert and does not incite fibroplasia or inflammation. Consequently, integration is delayed and may take at least 40 days. This property plus the constant peristaltic intestinal motion usually prevents the formation of adhesions between Gore-Tex and the intestine when the material is placed intraperitoneally.

Infection of a Permanent Prosthesis

All the nonabsorbable synthetic materials can become sequestered, act like a foreign body, and aggravate and prolong infections. Theoretically, mesh made of braided fibers should tolerate infection less well than that made of single strands. Braided yarn contains microscopic interstices 1 to 2 μm in diameter that should conceal bacteria and cellular debris from macrophages, which are 10 mm in diameter, and from tissue fluids that contain antibiotics. In clinical practice, however, this phenomenon happens infrequently. Braided, knitted polyester mesh, such as Mersilene, tolerates infection as well as a nonbraided, solid-fiber, polypropylene mesh, such as Marlex. If either mesh is infected, incorporation rather than rejection usually can be expected, provided that treatment is timely; the wound does not also contain silk, cotton, or coated, heavy-braided Dacron sutures; and the prosthesis is not floating free in the wound but is in firm contact with healthy tissues.

The Dacron yarn in Mersilene and Lars mesh is very fine and pure and is unlike the Dacron sutures, which are heavier and have a reputation for being readily rejected and behaving like foreign bodies. Sutures made from Dacron are typically not pure and are coated with another substance to ensure that they do not drag during their passage through the tissues.

Gore-Tex, although inert, is virtually intolerant of infection because of the delay in integration that occurs when this material is used. When infection occurs in a space that contains Gore-Tex, the material must be removed because the material will not become incorporated in the tissues before bacteria have contaminated the material and occupied microscopic crevices too small for phagocytes to enter.

Management of infection The management of infected wounds that contain a synthetic prosthesis is relatively easy and requires simple application of sound surgical principles. Superficial infection in a wound containing a prosthesis that is positioned deep to the subcutaneous tissues usually can be expected to heal without incident.

Infections involving a prosthesis require vigorous and aggressive treatment. The prosthesis must be exposed without delay; failure to do so leads to chronic sinus formation. Local treatment consists of irrigating away purulent material; lysing cellular, fibrous, and fibrinous debris; and destroying the infectious agent. Interventions such as irrigation with saline or Dakin's solution and application of honey or granulated sugar and topical antimicrobial substances are all useful. Complete incorporation can usually be expected with polypropylene or polyester meshes within three to four weeks of the time when the infection is first recognized. Administration of systemic antibiotics is, of course, also essential.

Delayed infections involving nonabsorbable prostheses may occur months or even years after prosthesis implantation. The cause of delayed infections usually cannot be determined. In delayed infections, reintegration of the prosthesis, regardless of the type, infrequently occurs, and excision of sequestered portions is necessary. Only the sequestered mesh need be removed. Chronically draining sinus tracts involving nonabsorbable prostheses are managed similarly.

Prophylaxis of infection Prophylaxis of infection is essential. Rigid sterile conditions, precise and meticulous surgical technique, and avoidance of seromas and hematomas with the use of closed suction drains are important. When large pieces of mesh are used, broad-spectrum antibiotics should be administered intravenously shortly before the operation begins and should be continued after the operation until the closed suction drains are removed. Topical antibiotics and antimicrobial agents are also commonly used intraoperatively. However, antibiotic prophylaxis is not commonly used in hernia repairs in which small prostheses are used.

Inflammatory granulomas are occasionally encountered during prosthetic hernioplasties for recurrent inguinal and incisional hernias. Gram's staining at the time of operation is not always reliable; consequently, if a granuloma is encountered, a synthetic prosthesis should not be implanted.[26]

Patients with completely integrated soft tissue prostheses are not customarily given preoperative prophylactic antibiotics. They are not at increased risk for infection, as are patients with prostheses that are not integrated into the soft tissues, such as artificial hips and heart valves.

OPERATIVE TECHNIQUE

Anterior Prosthetic Hernioplasty

The anterior groin incision is well known to all surgeons; consequently, it is not surprising that this incision is also the one most commonly used to implant a prosthesis. Usually, the prosthesis is placed on top of the posterior wall of the inguinal canal, although behind it would seem to be the proper site [see Posterior (Properitoneal) Prosthetic Hernioplasty, *below*]. Variations and combinations of the following techniques are common.

Lichtenstein's tension-free hernioplasty Synthetic soft tissue patch prostheses have been used for years to buttress the classic repairs, but they have not significantly improved the results. However, when the prosthesis is implanted without a formal repair, thereby obviating tension, results improve dramatically [see *Figure 6*].[27] Lichtenstein credited this original idea to R. Newman of Rahway, New Jersey, but it was Lichtenstein and his associates who championed the tension-free patch hernioplasty and who first reported very favorable results with this technique in a large number of patients.

Lichtenstein, who recognized the importance of tension, was already promoting a tension-free prosthetic plug repair for femoral hernias and for recurrent direct and indirect inguinal hernias. He advocated the use of this technique in situations in which the parietal defect was fibrous, circumscribed, and not too large [see *Figure 7*].[28] Lichtenstein borrowed the idea of the plug hernioplasty from Cheatle, who in 1921 plugged the parietal defect of a femoral hernia with a coil of saphenous vein.[24]

The semirigid knitted polypropylene meshes are the preferred prostheses for Lichtenstein's tension-free patch hernioplasties because they handle well, are easily tailored to the patient, and become integrated quickly. Some surgeons like the feel and the texture of Gore-Tex and prefer it to polypropylene, even though integration is slow with the former.

Originally, Lichtenstein used a 10×5 cm swatch of mesh in his repairs. However, because of recurrences, Lichtenstein's associates now advise using a larger prosthesis (12×6 to 8 cm) and circumcising the cremaster muscle for a snugger fit at the deep inguinal ring. Some proponents of the tension-free patch hernioplasty are concerned about the possibility of indirect hernia recurrences and place a polypropylene cone or an umbrella plug in the deep inguinal ring to ensure against this possibility [see Gilbert's Sutureless Hernioplasty, *below*].

The plug employed by Lichtenstein for plug hernioplasty is cylindrical and is made from a 2.0 to 2.5 cm tightly wound strip (or strips) of polypropylene mesh. The plug must occlude the aponeurotic defect completely and must be fixed flush to the defect with four or more permanent synthetic sutures. Polyester and Gore-Tex are not suitable materials for the plugs: polyester meshes are too soft, and coiled Gore-Tex plugs will not be completely integrated. Incompletely integrated prostheses have an increased chance of becoming secondarily infected.

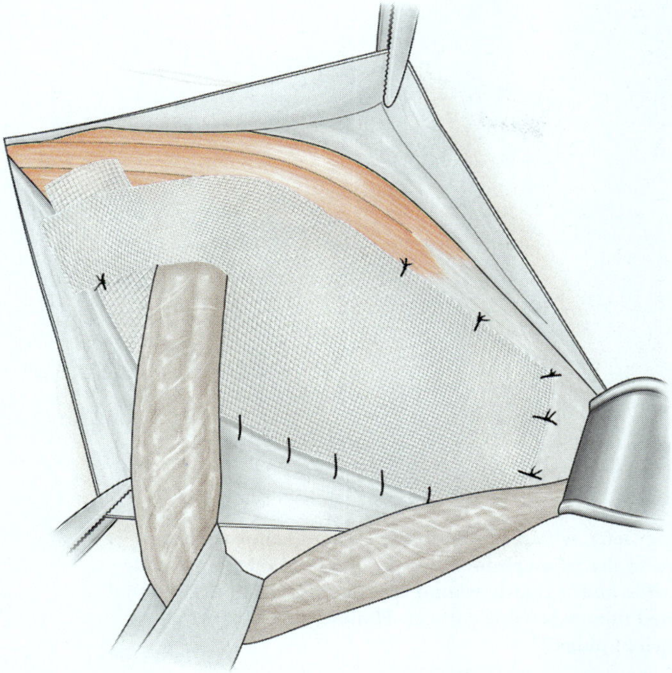

Figure 6 Lichtenstein's tension-free repair for primary hernia. The repair consists of a polypropylene patch laid over the posterior wall of the inguinal canal. The patch is tailored to the patient from a 12 × 8 cm swatch and has a slit to accommodate the spermatic cord. The prosthesis should extend 1.5 to 2.0 cm medial to the pubic tubercle and well lateral to the deep inguinal ring. The patch is sutured to the rectus abdominis sheath and the inguinal ligament. To ensure a snug fit at the deep inguinal ring, Lichtenstein's associates recommend circumcising the cremaster muscle at the level of the ring and crossing the legs of the mesh. The overlapped mesh is fixed with a single suture that grasps the lower edge of both mesh legs and the shelving edge of the inguinal ligament. In lieu of circumcision of the cremaster muscle, a cone plug of polypropylene mesh (like that used by Gilbert) may be placed in the deep inguinal ring [*see Figure 8*]. In a direct hernia, the hernial sac is inverted without tension and secured with a synthetic absorbable suture to ensure a smooth surface on which to place the mesh patch. Once placed, the mesh patch is secured by synthetic absorbable sutures.[53]

Tension-free patch hernioplasties are usually not recommended for recurrent hernias, because remobilization of the spermatic cord greatly increases the chance of testicular atrophy. However, the plug technique does not require remobilization of the spermatic cord, and only a small anterior groin incision directly over the parietal defect is necessary. Local anesthesia is helpful in hernioplasties for recurrent hernias in which plugs have been used, because the hernia can be revealed to the surgeon when the patient coughs. Plug repair for fibrous, small, well-circumscribed indirect and direct defects is very effective. However, recurrent hernias with large or multiple parietal defects are preferably managed by a posterior properitoneal prosthetic repair.

There has been widespread acceptance of the Lichtenstein tension-free patch hernioplasty because postoperative pain is minimal and because the procedure is easy to perform with the patient under local anesthesia. Detractors point out that the technique is not foolproof and that long-term results are not yet known. Furthermore, even the recommended larger patch does not cover all of the MPO, it contains a slit for potential peritoneal protrusion, it is on the external side of the parietal defect, and it frequently does not fit, because the space is too small or is occupied by a traversing sensory nerve.

Gilbert's sutureless hernioplasty Gilbert placed a 6 × 6 cm cone-shaped swatch of polypropylene mesh through the deep inguinal ring of a patient with a minimally dilated ring and a small indirect hernial sac. Quite astonishingly, the patient could not expel the prosthesis or the hernial sac by coughing and straining. Recognizing the therapeutic possibilities of this observation, Gilbert added to the cone in the deep inguinal ring an unsutured flat patch of polypropylene mesh placed on the floor of the inguinal canal and thereby created the so-called sutureless hernioplasty [*see Figure 8*].[29,30] A slit in the lateral edge of the patch is made to accommodate the spermatic cord.

Gilbert surmised that the gathered mesh unfolded in the properitoneal space and blocked the entrance to the deep inguinal ring. He therefore called the prosthesis an umbrella plug. However, the cone-shaped plug need not unfold in the properitoneal space to be effective, because the textured polypropylene mesh adheres to adjacent tissues and obliterates the entrance of the deep inguinal ring even before integration occurs. Cone-shaped occlusive plugs should always be supplemented with an onlay patch because by themselves, the plugs may deform, collapse, and cease to contain the peritoneal sac.

Gilbert minimizes the dissection of the groin in his technique. The cremaster muscle and vessels are not divided, and the lipomata of the cord and the small, indirect hernial sacs are merely returned to the properitoneal space. The sutureless hernioplasty is used chiefly for indirect hernias with only minimal enlargement of the deep inguinal ring. However, indirect hernias with dilated deep inguinal rings may be managed with this technique if the ring is tightened with one or two Marcy sutures. The repair is simple and produces excellent results.

Rutkow and Robbins adapted Gilbert's sutureless technique to the repair of all types of groin hernias.[31,32] For indirect hernias with patulous deep inguinal rings, a large polypropylene mesh cone plug is implanted in the ring and fixed at the perimeter with interrupted absorbable synthetic sutures. Direct inguinal hernias are similarly managed. Direct hernias are incised at the circumference of the neck to expose properitoneal fat before the cone is implanted and sutured to the fringe of the defect. Combined indirect and direct inguinal hernias are treated with two cone plugs. Plugs are also used in the treatment of femoral and recurrent hernias.

The repairs are completed with a flat piece of polypropylene mesh laid over the inguinal floor. The mesh has a slit at the lateral end that is closed with a suture after it accommodates the spermatic cord. In this procedure, as in Gilbert's original procedure, the dissection of the groin is kept to a minimum. The repairs are easily performed with unassisted local anesthesia, and recovery is fast.

These new and clever repairs are finding favor because they are simple to perform and produce minimal postoperative pain. They are criticized because the onlayed patch is not sutured in place, may not cover the MPO sufficiently, and contains a slit. Furthermore, the cones in the direct and indirect spaces can become deformed by the contracture of the enveloping scar tissue; as they lose their shape, they may fail to occlude the parietal defects. This

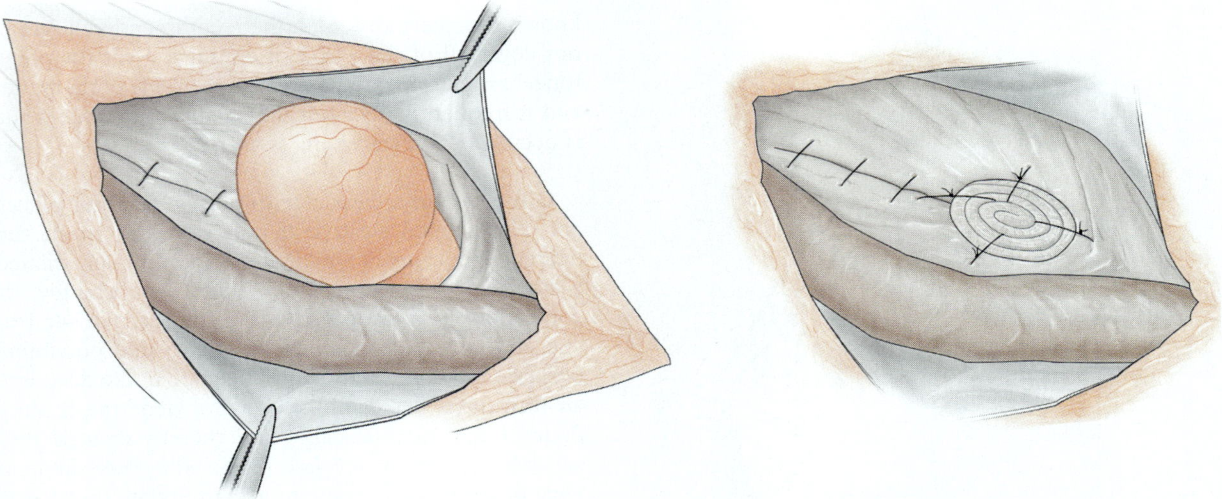

Figure 7 Lichtenstein's recurrent hernia repair. The hernial sac (left), which will be in the subcutaneous tissues under the external oblique aponeurosis, is exposed and returned to the properitoneal space. The plug (right) is made of a strip (or strips) of polypropylene mesh that is 2.0 to 2.5 cm wide and is tightly wound to a diameter that fits snugly in the defect. The plug is fixed in place by four or more interrupted nonabsorbable sutures. Hollow cone-shaped plugs can deform and are not a suitable substitute for the solid cylindrical plugs.[53]

phenomenon has been observed with Lichtenstein's cylindrical plugs that were not tightly rolled and fitted.

Posterior (Properitoneal) Prosthetic Hernioplasty

The properitoneal space is the logical site in which to implant a prosthesis. The prosthesis is held in place by intra-abdominal pressure. It is remote from the relatively avascular subcutaneous tissues and is therefore relatively immune to superficial infection. The myopectineal orifice can be patched or plugged and hernioplasties buttressed with a prosthesis implanted from the posterior approach in the same way as from the anterior approach [*see Figure 9*].[33,34] Although the properitoneal space can be reached through an anterior groin incision, an abdominal incision is preferable because it enables dissection of the inguinal canal to be completely bypassed.

Stoppa's giant prosthetic reinforcement of the visceral sac Stoppa proposed treating hernias of the groin through the use of a large, permanent prosthesis that essentially replaced the transverse fascia.[35-37] The prosthesis adheres to the visceral sac and renders the peritoneum inextensible, so that peritoneum cannot protrude through the MPO or adjacent areas of weakness; repair of the defect in the abdominal wall is then unnecessary. The repair is tension free and sutureless. The operation is technically known by the descriptive phrase "giant prosthetic reinforcement of the visceral sac" (GPRVS), but it is commonly called the Stoppa procedure. Stoppa's innovative and revolutionary properitoneal prosthetic technique was unique: for the first time, hernia repair was focused on retaining the peritoneum rather than on closing the aponeurotic defect.

GPRVS is performed bilaterally or unilaterally. Bilateral GPRVS entails the insertion of a single large prosthesis into the properitoneal space of both groins through a midline or Pfannenstiel's incision [*see Figure 10*].[35,37] The procedure requires general or regional anesthesia and, sometimes, an overnight stay in the hospital. The procedure is ideal for patients with

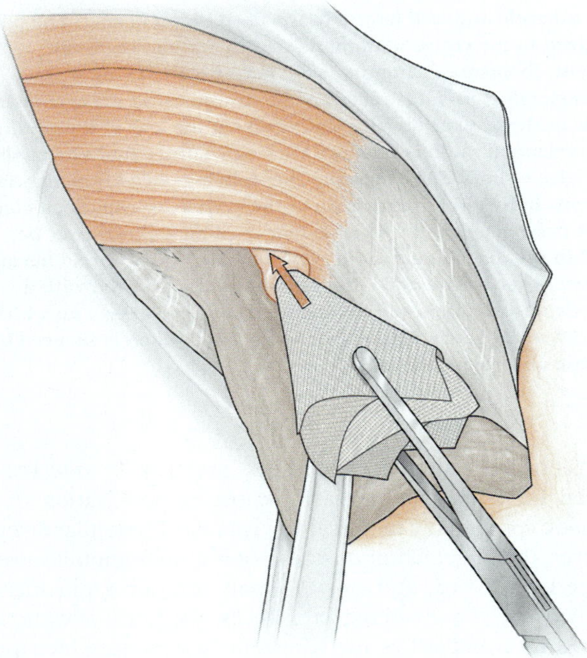

Figure 8 Gilbert's sutureless hernioplasty. A swatch of polypropylene mesh (6 × 6 cm) is folded into a cone-shaped plug and placed through the deep inguinal ring. The gathered mesh unfolds in the properitoneal space and occludes the deep inguinal ring. Cone-shaped plugs do not have to pass through the deep inguinal ring and into the properitoneal space to be an effective barrier, provided they are sutured in place. Another swatch of mesh slit to accommodate the spermatic cord is tailored to cover the floor of the inguinal canal. Some surgeons use a single suture to fix the distal end of the swatch to the rectus abdominis sheath.

bilateral recurrent hernias, bilateral direct primary hernias, hernias associated with connective tissue disorders, and hernias resulting from fractures of the pelvis. It is quick and exceptionally easy to perform, even in obese patients, for whom it may be the preferred hernioplasty when bilateral hernias are present.

Unilateral GPRVS was developed for use in day surgical centers.[38] The preferred entry route is through a transverse lower quadrant abdominal incision, but an anterior groin incision can be used instead [see Figure 11].[39] Because the abdominal incision circumvents the dissection of the inguinal canal, it is the method of choice for recurrent inguinal hernia in men who have undergone classic and prosthetic anterior repairs. Local anesthesia is suitable for most patients undergoing anterior unilateral GPRVS but only for selected patients undergoing the posterior unilateral procedure.

Ordinarily, a large prosthesis in the properitoneal space requires a slit to accommodate the spermatic cord at the deep inguinal ring [see Figure 9]. The slit, which is sutured closed around the elements of the cord, partially holds the prosthesis in place, but it is also a potential site for peritoneal protrusion. However, a slit in the mesh becomes unnecessary if the elements of the spermatic cord—the vas deferens and the testicular vessels—are dissected from the peritoneum, to which they are attached by a lamina of transverse fascia. Then, the elements of the cord can lie against the wall of the pelvis, and the properitoneal prosthesis will cover them, the deep inguinal ring, and the MPO completely. This technique, called parietalization of structures of the spermatic cord, was devised by Stoppa and facilitates properitoneal prosthetic implantation [see Figure 11].[35,37,39]

Mersilene is the prosthesis of choice for GPRVS because it is supple and elastic, it stays in place without sutures, it conforms to the complex curvature of the pelvis, and it induces prompt fibroblastic integration. In GPRVS, the prosthesis is placed with long abdominal clamps. The prosthesis may be attached with sutures to the anterior abdominal wall, but it is otherwise not fixed.

If prostheses made from materials other than Mersilene are used, peripheral fixation is usually necessary. The polypropylene meshes are too stiff to conform by intra-abdominal pressure alone, and Gore-Tex wanders before integration occurs. The use of sutures and staples in the retroperitoneal space is not recommended, because they may inadvertently include a vital structure, such as a nerve or a blood vessel. For these reasons, Mersilene is the only material recommended for use in GPRVS.

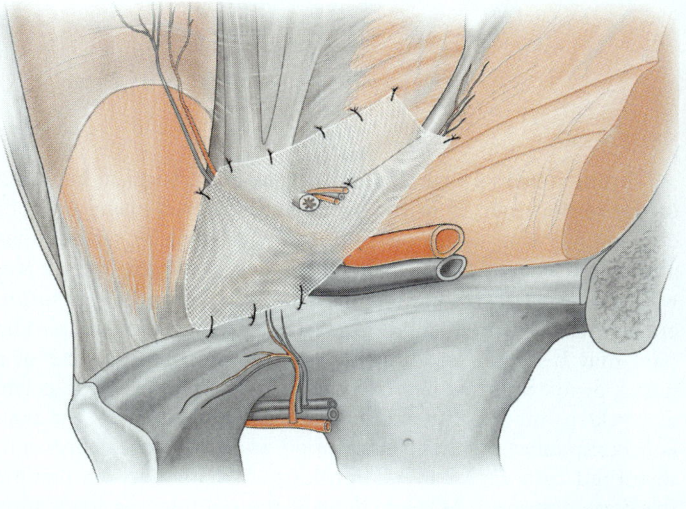

Recurrences after GPRVS occur as a result of technical mishaps—most often an incorrectly sized, shaped, and positioned prosthesis (usually the prosthesis is too small). Another pitfall is an insufficiently cleaved properitoneal space that does not admit the large prosthesis. In these instances, the prosthesis buckles, crimps, and fails to smoothly extend far beyond the MPO when the implantation clamps are withdrawn. Surplus properitoneal fat should be excised because it can pass in and out of a parietal defect and mimic a peritoneal protrusion exactly. Usually, the dissection of the properitoneal space is bloodless, but if it is not or if there is a large retained hernial sac, closed suction drainage is necessary. Hematomas and seromas delay integration, are a good medium for the growth of bacteria, and can also dislodge the unsutured mesh.

Recurrences after GPRVS are usually approached anteriorly and are managed by adding a prosthetic extension to the existing prosthesis. Alternatively, another permanent prosthesis can be implanted transabdominally.

GPRVS is an efficient, anatomic, sutureless, and tension-free repair. It may be the ultimate hernioplasty; when it is correctly performed, all hernias of the groin are cured, even the prevascular femoral hernias. Recovery is very fast and discomfort minimal. GPRVS is the technique I prefer to use for recurrent hernias and for all primary hernias in men when regional or general anesthesia is used.

Complications of Groin Hernioplasty

Testicular atrophy[40-43] and residual neuralgia[44,45] are the important and dreaded complications unique to inguinal hernioplasty. They are more common after anterior hernia repairs than after posterior repairs and are very likely to initiate malpractice suits.

TESTICULAR ATROPHY

Testicular atrophy is a sequela of ischemic orchitis. The clinical manifestations of ischemic orchitis develop insidiously, do not become apparent for two to five days after the hernioplasty, and are frequently misinterpreted at presentation. The testicle and spermatic cord become swollen, hard, tender, painful, and retracted. The process lasts six to 12 weeks and may resolve completely or may end in testicular atrophy. The return of the testicle to normal size and shape does not mean that the process is complete. On occasion, atrophy of the testicle does not become apparent for as long as a year. Gangrene is unusual, and orchiectomy is rarely necessary.

Ischemic orchitis is caused by thrombosis of the spermatic cord, and the testicular pathology is intense venous congestion. The thrombosis is induced by surgical trauma to the cord, especially that associated with the dissection performed to completely remove a large indirect hernial sac. The spermatic cord must always be handled gently, and surgical trauma to the cord must be kept to a minimum. The cord should not be dissected beyond the pubic tubercle, and scrotal pathology should not be dealt with at the time of hernia repair. Trauma to the spermatic

Figure 9 Posterior patch prosthetic hernioplasty. The prosthesis is fixed with synthetic permanent sutures to Cooper's iliopectineal ligament inferiorly and to the abdominal wall superiorly. A slit in the mesh accommodates the spermatic cord.[53]

a

cord, especially to the delicate veins of the pampiniform plexus, is the paramount cause of testicular atrophy after inguinal hernioplasty.[40,41] Dissection of an indirect hernial sac in the scrotum damages the delicate veins of the pampiniform plexus, initiates the thrombosis, and coincidentally disrupts the collateral circulation [*see* Dissection, *above*].

No known successful preventive treatment exists for testicular atrophy. Antibiotics, anti-inflammatory drugs, and massive doses of steroids are often given. Fortunately, the incidence of testicular atrophy can be minimized by reducing surgical trauma to the spermatic cord through such measures as avoiding excision of the distal part of an indirect hernial sac; avoiding dissection beyond the pubic tubercle; and avoiding redissection of an inguinal canal and spermatic cord in patients who are predisposed to the complication by a previous anterior hernioplasty, vasectomy, hydrocelectomy, or other inguinal or scrotal surgery. In these situations, posterior properitoneal prosthetic hernioplasty is the preferred alternative.

NEURALGIA

Chronic residual neuralgia may result from surgical handling of the sensory nerves in the groin during hernioplasty or from constricting scar tissue or adjacent inflammatory granulomas after hernioplasty. The intraoperative trauma to the nerve, whether caused by division, stretching, contusion, or suture entrapment, is usually not appreciated at the time it occurs. The pain may be localized, diffuse, projected along the course of a nerve, or referred to a nearby site. It may develop early or as late as weeks to months after the operation. In most cases, the pain is accompanied by changes in mood and behavior; depression, disturbed interpersonal relationships, and inability to resume work are common. Management of the neuralgia is frustrating and complicated and benefits from a multidisciplinary approach.

A well-known cause of nociceptive (somatic) residual neuralgia is a neuroma. A neuroma results from a proliferation of nerve fibers outside the neurilemma of a partially or completely divided nerve. The pain from a neuroma varies in intensity, may be induced by

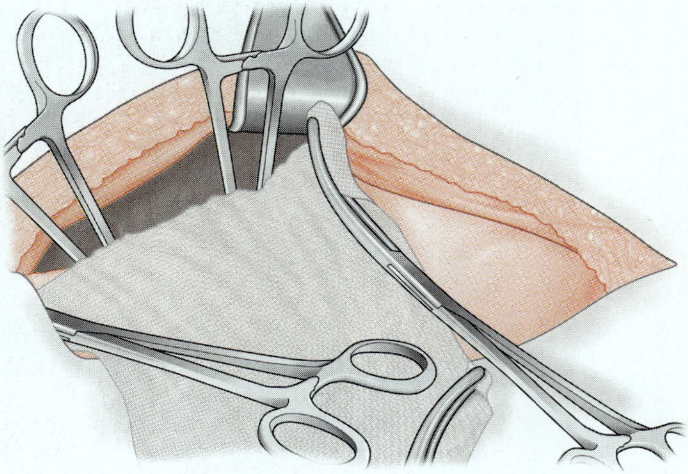

Figure 10 Bilateral giant prosthetic reinforcement of the visceral sac. (*a*) A large prosthesis is implanted via a midline or a Pfannenstiel incision. The mesh envelops the visceral sac of both groins and extends far beyond the borders of the myopectineal orifice (dotted line). The prosthesis is chevron-shaped and arranged so that the stretch is transverse. The width equals the distance between the anterior superior iliac spines minus 2 cm in a normal patient but can be larger in an obese patient. The vertical dimension equals the distance between the umbilicus and the symphysis. The tails of the chevron are exaggerated to ensure a firm grip of the visceral sac.[53] (*b*) Wide cleavage of the properitoneal space is necessary and easy. The pedicle of an indirect hernial sac is encircled, the sac divided, and the visceral sac closed.[53] (*c*) The vas deferens and the testicular vessels are dissected from the parietal peritoneum. When freed, they will lie against the parietal wall of the pelvis (parietalization), and the prosthesis will cover the entire MPO without a slit having to be made for the cord.[53] (*d*) The prosthesis is implanted by long (30 cm) Wiley or Rochester-Pean clamps, so that it smoothly envelops the visceral sac. The large dead space may require drainage. The prosthesis is fixed with a single suture to the umbilical fascia only.[35]

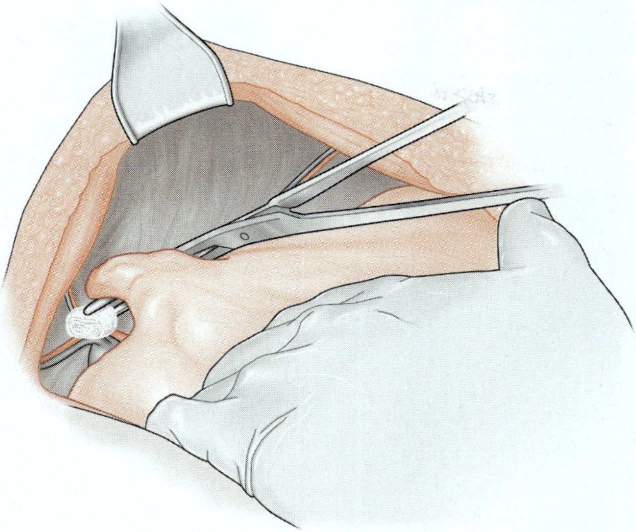

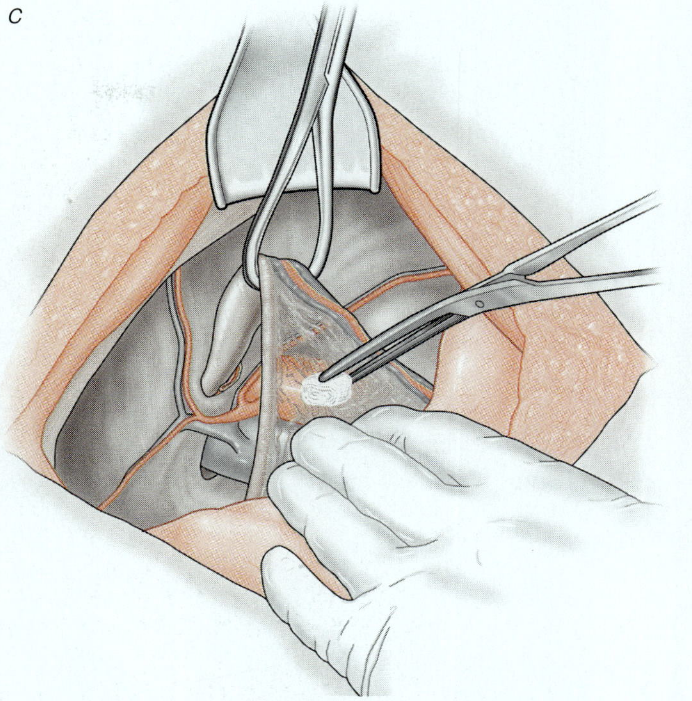

changes in position, and is without spontaneous paroxysmal exacerbations. Hyperesthesia is detectable in the area of the lesion, and tapping the site may produce a severe shooting pain.

Deafferentation (central) chronic pain differs from the pain of a neuroma. It is burning and permanent, with intermittent paroxysmal exacerbations. The area of involvement is anesthetic at first but becomes hyperesthetic. Typically, the onset of deafferentation pain is delayed for about a week after the injury, and tapping the site does not produce exquisite pain.

The management of residual neuralgia is often difficult. Neurolysis of the involved nerve may afford relief, especially if it is instituted early. The involved nerve may be identified by local anesthetic nerve blocks. The iliohypogastric and ilioinguinal nerves can be blocked and divided in the groin. However, a foolproof method of blocking the genitofemoral nerve in the groin does not exist; neuralgia from this nerve is identified by blocking L1 and L2 paravertebrally. Division of the genitofemoral nerve is performed through a flank incision. Other adjunctive therapy includes administration of analgesics, antidepressants, anticonvulsants, and anxiolytic drugs and transcutaneous electrical stimulation. Injections of steroids in the involved area are sometimes helpful.

The prevention of nerve injury is important because the treatment of neuralgic complications is often unsuccessful. Fortunately, such complications are rare. The sensory nerves should be preserved if possible; however, this is not always possible, and some small, not readily visible nerves are invariably divided. Occasionally, major branches of the sensory nerves or the nerve trunks themselves must be divided to accomplish the hernioplasty. Division (usually with ligation) of the genital branch of

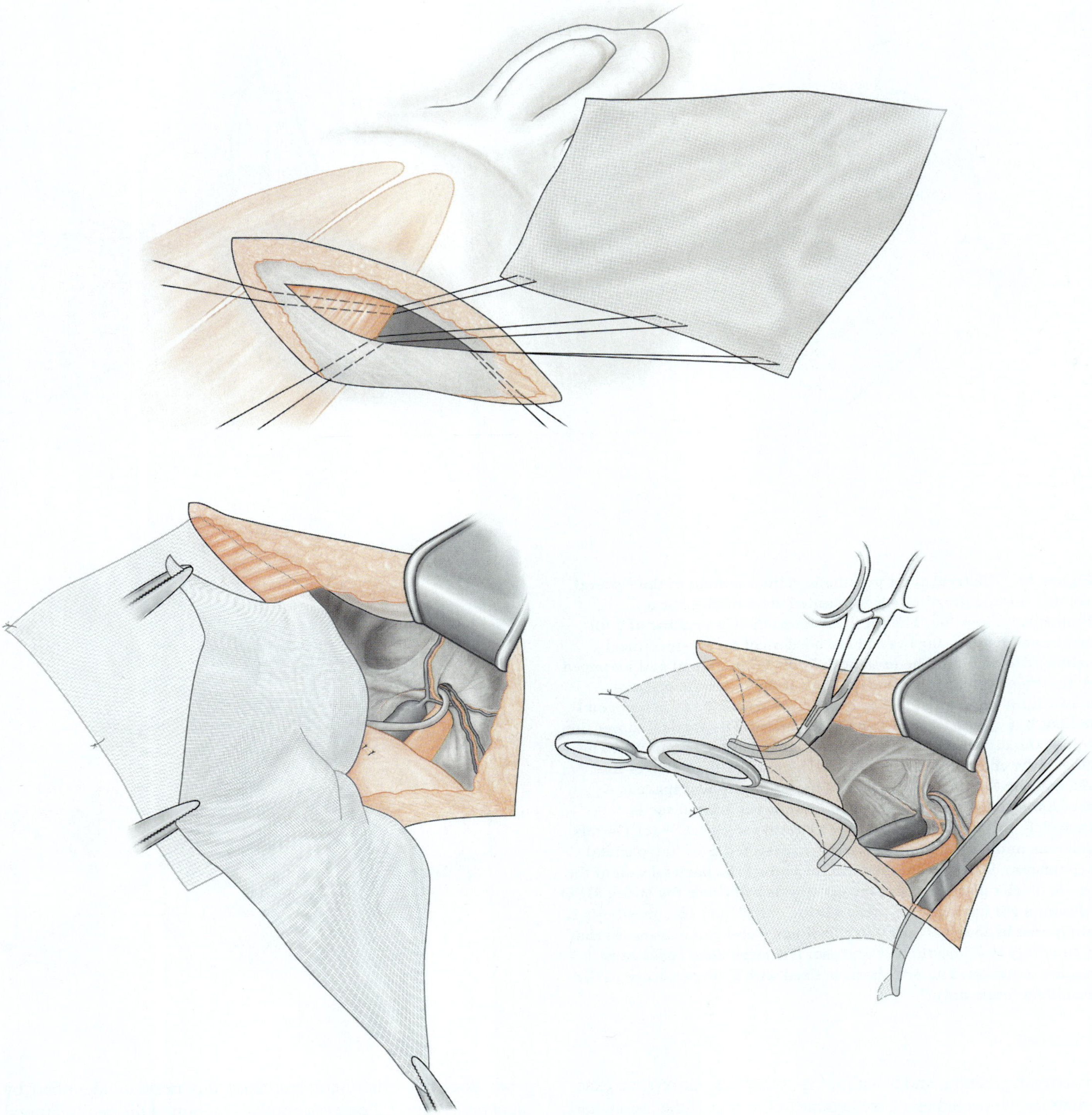

Figure 11 Unilateral giant prosthetic reinforcement of the visceral sac. The prosthesis is shaped somewhat like a diamond and is arranged so that it stretches transversely. It is important that the inferior edge be wider than the superior edge (by 2 to 4 cm) and that the lateral side be longer than the medial side. The long lateral inferior corner ensures a solid prosthetic grip on the lateral visceral sac. The width of the prosthesis at the superior edge equals the distance from the midline to the anterior superior iliac spine minus 1 cm, and the vertical length is approximately 14 cm. The prosthesis is drawn into place (top) under the rectus abdominis muscle and the abdominal wall by three absorbable sutures that affix the prosthesis to the midline, the semilunar line, and the oblique muscles near the anterior superior iliac spine. The abdominal wall is retracted (bottom, left) to expose the properitoneal space. The superior portion of the prosthesis is implanted deep into the muscles of the properitoneal space. Clamps are ready to implant the prosthesis inferiorly. The distal prosthesis is implanted (bottom, right) with long (30 cm) Wiley or Rochester-Pean clamps and positioned so that the prosthesis envelops the peritoneum.

the genitofemoral nerve is routine in most anterior groin hernioplasties. This process virtually never produces genital nerve neuralgia, which suggests that complete division of the nerve may be less likely to cause residual neuralgia than other types of nerve trauma. Most nerves require ligation to control bleeding. Fortuitously, the ligature may also confine neuroma formation to within the neurilemma.

Noninguinal Abdominal Wall Hernias

UMBILICAL AND EPIGASTRIC HERNIAS

Umbilical hernias are common in infants and close spontaneously without special treatment if the diameter of the aponeurotic defect is 1.5 cm or less. However, repair is indicated in infants with hernial defects greater than 2.0 cm in diameter and in all children whose umbilical hernia is still present at three to four years of age.

Umbilical hernias in adults are acquired and require repair. They have no relation to umbilical hernias in children. Strangulation of the colon and omentum is fairly common, and rupture occurs in chronic ascitic cirrhosis, in which case an emergency portal decompression is necessary.

Small umbilical hernias are merely closed with a to-and-fro continuous nonabsorbable suture or a small polypropylene plug. Large umbilical hernias should be managed with a prosthetic repair that resembles the prosthetic repair for incisional hernia. The classic repair for umbilical hernias is the Mayo hernioplasty. In this operation, a vest-over-pants imbrication of the superior and inferior aponeurotic segments is performed. However, the Mayo hernioplasty is infrequently used because the results are not as satisfactory as those achieved with the prosthetic repairs.

Epigastric hernias occur between the decussating fibers of the linea alba above the umbilicus. They are managed in the same way as umbilical hernias.

SPIGELIAN HERNIAS

Spigelian hernias are ventral hernias that occur along the subumbilical portion of Spieghel's semilunar line and through Spieghel's fascia.[46] Spigelian hernias are rare, and unless they are large, these hernias are difficult to diagnose because they are

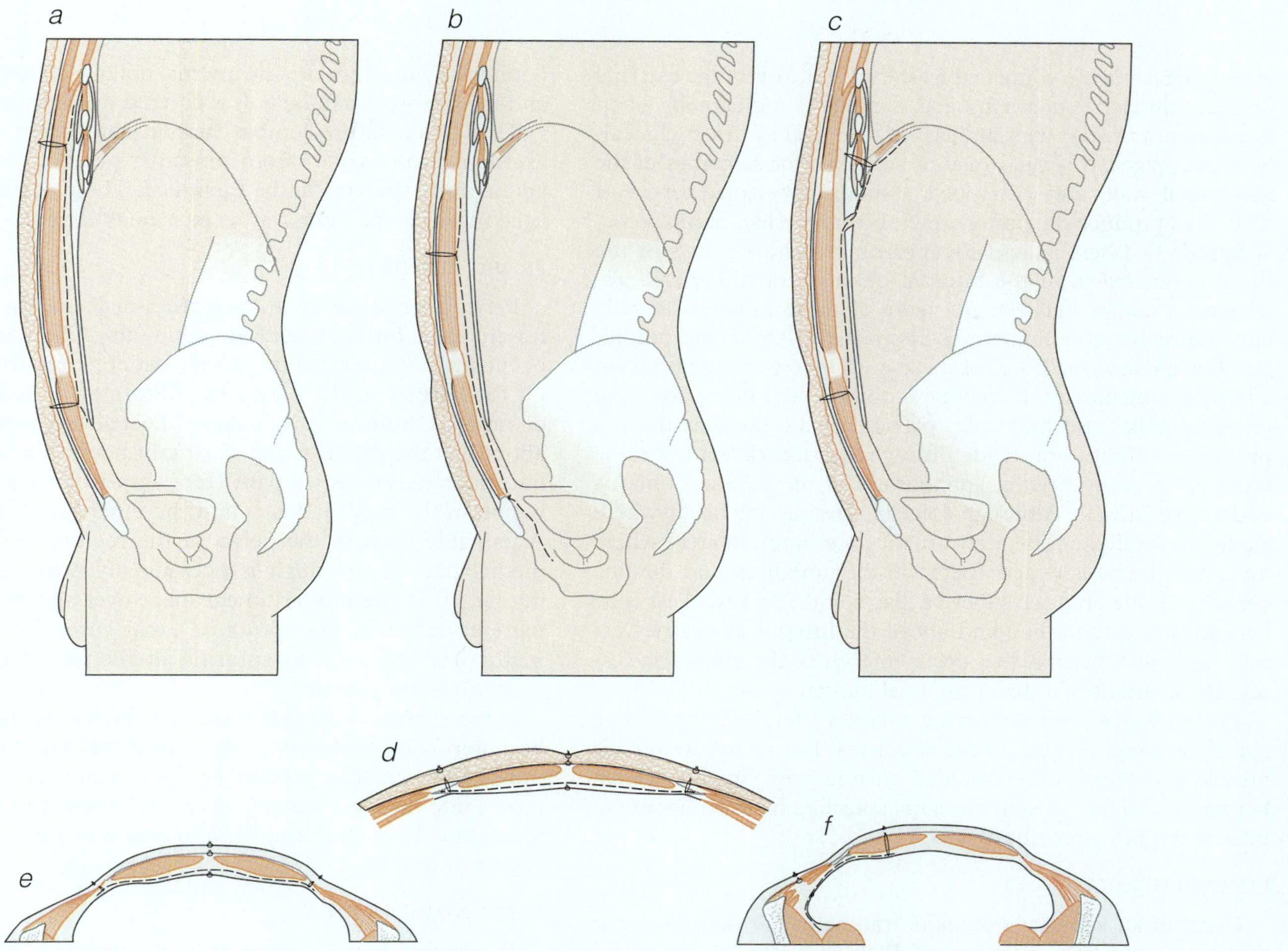

Figure 12 Rives-Stoppa incisional hernia repair. Parasagittal views showing the site of implantation of the prosthesis (broken line) and suture fixation in (*a*) supraumbilical midline incisional hernias, (*b*) subumbilical midline incisional hernias, and (*c*) subcostal incisional hernias. Cross sections of the abdominal wall anatomy show the implantation of the prosthesis (broken line), the lateral extent of the prosthesis, and suture fixation in the (*d*) epigastric region, (*e*) hypogastric region, and (*f*) right lower quadrant (appendectomy).

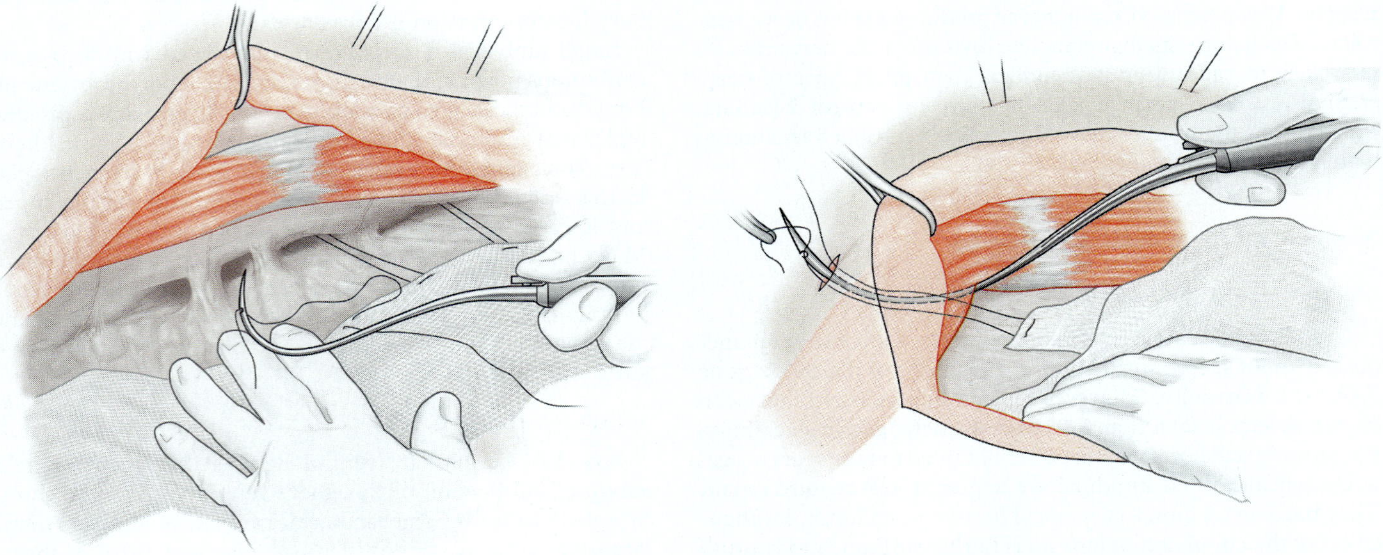

Figure 13 Mesh placement for repair of incisional hernia. The retromuscular space has been dissected (left), exposing the intercostal vessels and nerves. A Reverdin suture needle (right) facilitates the placement of the sutures for prosthetic fixation.

interparietal and are contained by the aponeurosis of the external oblique muscle. Sonography and computed tomography often reveal symptomatic spigelian hernias too small to detect clinically. Large spigelian hernias may be mistaken for sarcomas of the abdominal wall, and entrapped anterior cutaneous nerves of T10–T12 produce discomfort resembling spigelian herniation.

Spieghel's fascia is actually aponeurotic and consists of the fused aponeuroses of the internal oblique and transverse abdominal muscles between the belly of these muscles laterally and the rectus abdominis muscle medially. Above the umbilicus, the aponeurotic fibers of these muscles crisscross and form a fairly strong barrier. Below the umbilicus, the fibers are more or less parallel and may split, permitting the peritoneum and properitoneal fat to protrude through a slitlike defect but to be retained by the overlying aponeurosis of the external oblique abdominal muscle. Although spigelian hernias occur anywhere along the semilunar line, they are most common in areas where Spieghel's fascia is widest (between the umbilicus and the line connecting the anterior superior iliac spines) and weakest (just beneath the arcuate line and above the inferior epigastric vessels). Spigelian hernias that occur inferior to the epigastric vessels are a variant of a direct inguinal hernia.

The neck of a spigelian hernia enlarges laterally by spreading apart the broad muscles of the abdomen. The rectus abdominis muscle and sheath inhibit medial enlargement. Small spigelian hernias are simply closed, but large spigelian hernias that are in muscle require a prosthesis.

LUMBAR HERNIAS

Congenital, spontaneous, and traumatic herniations occur through Grynfeltt's superior and Petit's inferior lumbar triangles. They are very rare and are impossible to repair successfully without a prosthesis or a myoaponeurotic flap. Petit's triangle is upright and is bounded by the latissimus dorsi, the external oblique abdominal muscle, and the iliac crest. It is covered by the superficial fascia only. Grynfeltt's triangle is inverted and is bounded by the 12th rib, the internal oblique abdominal muscle, and the sacrospinal muscle. It is covered by the latissimus dorsi.

The large, diffuse lumbar hernias that occur after kidney excision result in part from muscular paralysis; as a rule, no aponeurotic defects can be identified. These hernias are managed in much the same way as incisional hernias.

PELVIC HERNIAS

Pelvic hernias occur in the obturator fossa, the greater and lesser sciatic foramen, and the perineum. All are very rare and occur mainly in cachectic elderly patients, especially women. Of the hernias in the pelvis, the obturator hernia is the most common. Obturator hernias are almost always strangulated. In about half the patients with obturator hernias, pressure on the obturator nerve causes pain (Howship-Romberg sign) in the region of the hip, the knee, and the inner aspect of the thigh. A palpable mass in the pelvis or the rectum or in the upper medial part of the thigh is occasionally noted. A prosthesis implanted in the properitoneal space over and far beyond the parietal defect in the obturator canal cures the hernia. This method is preferred to suturing of the defect unless septic conditions are present.

Perineal hernias occur through the pelvic diaphragm and may be anterior or posterior to the superficial transverse perineal muscle. The anterior perineal hernia is seen only in women and passes into the labia majora, whereas the posterior perineal hernia enters the ischiorectal fossa in men and passes close to the vagina in women.

PARASTOMAL HERNIAS

Parastomal hernias interfere with colostomy irrigations and the adhesion of stomal appliances. Paracolostomy hernias are more common than paraileostomy hernias, and both are likelier to occur when the stoma emerges through the semilunar line rather than through the rectus abdominis sheath. Parastomal hernias, therefore, are usually lateral to the ostomy.

Moving the stoma to a new location is often the easiest method of management of parastomal hernias. A prosthesis should be used in the repair; otherwise, the operation is likely to fail because the belt muscles lateral to the ostomy lack sufficient aponeurosis. The prosthesis may be implanted extramuscularly on the aponeurotic abdominal wall in the subcutaneous space, retromuscularly or intraperitoneally [see Major Incisional Hernias, below].

Leslie's technique for parastomal hernia repair is easy and effective.[47] In this operation, an incision is made well away from the stoma and the stoma appliance. The skin and subcutaneous tissue are dissected from the abdominal wall and reflected to expose the bowel and the parietal defect. The defect is then closed with sutures. A 12 × 15 cm Mersilene prosthesis is partially slit to accommodate and embrace the bowel. The mesh positioned around the bowel in the subcutaneous tissues is spread out over the repair and the anterior abdominal wall, where it is fixed with staples or sutures. Closed suction drainage is essential until prosthetic integration is assured.

Sugarbaker's parastomal hernioplasty repairs the hernia from within the abdomen without disturbing the stoma.[48] A polypropylene mesh sandwiched between two layers of an absorbable mesh (or, alternatively, a swatch of Gore-Tex) is shaped and sutured to the perimeter of the parietal defect intraperitoneally. The prosthesis creates a flap valve that ensures against recurrence. Success is wholly dependent on the integrity of the sutures unless the prosthesis significantly overlaps the edges of the defect. Sugarbaker's repair should not be used for parastomal hernias involving an ileal conduit, because the method may cause dysfunction by kinking the bowel or ureters.

MAJOR INCISIONAL HERNIAS

Major incisional hernias are serious surgical problems. They have an inordinate tendency to enlarge, are frequently formidable to repair, and are usually accompanied by serious conditions. Patients with incisional hernias are usually obese. In fact, obesity and infection are the two principal causes of this condition. The weight of the panniculus adiposus literally pulls apart the surgical incision, and subsequent wound healing is hampered by infection. Hypertension, cardiac and renal disorders, diabetes, and purulent intertrigo commonly accompany obesity and increase the morbidity associated with the repair.

Pathophysiology

The loss of integrity of the abdominal wall reduces intraabdominal pressure and causes serious pathophysiological disturbances, which Rives appropriately termed eventration disease.[49] The salient abnormality resulting from abdominal weakness is respiratory dysfunction. A large incisional hernia produces paradoxical respiratory abdominal motion similar to that seen in a flail chest. Diaphragmatic function becomes inefficient: the diaphragm no longer contracts against the abdominal viscera but forces them into the hernial sac instead. Appraisal of respiratory function and blood gases is essential.

The detachment of the tendinous insertion of the broad belt muscles of the abdomen aggravates midline incisional hernias. The muscles retract, pull apart the parietal defect, and cause the normally horizontal rectus abdominis muscle to assume a vertical position. Contraction of the rectus abdominis muscle then causes the abdominal viscera to be expelled rather than retained. Ultimately, atrophy, fatty degeneration, and fibrosis of the lateral muscles ensue and make tendinous reinsertion of the belt muscle by the midline approximation of the linea alba difficult. In some midline hernias, actual loss of the abdominal wall may occur as a result of infections, trauma, and repeated laparotomies. However, in most cases, the loss of substance is more apparent than real.

In long-standing large incisional hernias, the viscera are displaced from their normal positions in the abdomen and cannot be restored to them. In such cases, reduction of the viscera at operation can cause death by compression of the inferior vena cava and by respiratory failure caused by forced elevation and immobilization of the diaphragm. The introduction of pneumoperitoneum by Goni Moreno in 1947 made these formerly inoperable hernias reparable.[50]

Reduced intra-abdominal pressure from the hernia also causes edema of the mesentery and stasis in the splanchnic venous system and the inferior vena cava. Distention and atony of the hollow viscera occur and, in conjunction with decreased ability to increase intra-abdominal pressure, produce difficulties with micturition and bowel movements. Back pain is a common complaint and results from lordosis that is caused by retraction of the belt muscles and decreased efficiency of the rectus abdominis muscle.

The skin and subcutaneous tissues overlying large incisional hernias are stretched and damaged, and the skin becomes atrophic, hypoxic, and devoid of subcutaneous fat. Spontaneous ulcerations develop that are typically solitary and occur at the apex of the hernia. These ulcerations are often misdiagnosed as pressure sores. They resist healing, and intensive local and systemic antimicrobial therapy must be administered to prevent infectious complications at the time of hernioplasty.

Obese patients with large incisional hernias are especially at risk for postoperative infectious complications, respiratory dysfunction, and pulmonary emboli.[26] Preoperative and postoperative prophylaxis for these problems is essential.

Progressive pneumoperitoneum is a useful technique to prepare patients for incisional hernioplasty.[51] It overcomes some of the problems associated with eventration disease and enables some patients with massive irreducible incisional hernias to undergo the operation. Pneumoperitoneum stretches the abdominal wall and intra-abdominal adhesions, facilitates the return of the viscera to the abdomen, and improves diaphragmatic function.

The technique of pneumoperitoneum is simple. Air is injected into the peritoneal cavity through a pneumoperitoneum needle that is inserted with the aid of local anesthesia. Insufflation continues until the patient experiences shortness of breath or shoulder pain. At first, the patient may tolerate only small amounts of air; sometimes, as much as 2 to 4 L may be insufflated initially. Thereafter, air is added at one- to three-day intervals as needed. The pneumoperitoneum is maintained for 10 to 20 days. The patient is ready for operation when palpation reveals flabbiness in the flanks. Inability of the patient to tolerate pneumoperitoneum is a contraindication for incisional hernioplasty.

Incisional Hernioplasty

The object of incisional hernioplasty is anatomic reconstruction of the abdominal wall. This process includes closure of the parietal defect, restoration of normal intra-abdominal pressure, and, in midline hernias, tendinous reinsertion of the lateral abdominal muscles.

Most small incisional hernias are managed by simple closure of the aponeurotic defect. However, large incisional hernias with aponeurotic defects greater than 10 cm in diameter have a strong tendency to recur. Repairs performed by edge-to-edge approximation of aponeurosis or by imbrication frequently fail: recurrence rates have been estimated to be as high as 50 percent. Consequently, most incisional hernias and all recurrent incisional hernias call for the insertion of a prosthesis. The Rives-Stoppa procedure is the preferred method for accomplishing the objectives of incisional hernioplasty.[36,49,52] It is applicable to all types of abdominal incisional hernias, including postnephrectomy lumbar hernias.

The Rives-Stoppa incisional hernioplasty consists of implanting a very large Mersilene prosthesis deep to the muscles of the abdominal wall on top of the posterior rectus abdominis sheath or peritoneum [see Figure 12]. The prosthesis extends far beyond the borders of the myoaponeurotic defects and initially is firmly held in place by intra-abdominal pressure (Pascal's principle) and later by fibrous ingrowth. The prosthesis prevents peritoneal eventration in two ways: by rendering the visceral sac indistensible and by solidly uniting and consolidating the abdominal wall. The technique therefore employs the same concept and principles as Stoppa's properitoneal inguinal hernioplasty and likewise is referred to as GPRVS.

The knitted elastic Mersilene prosthesis is arranged so that it expands vertically and is inextensible horizontally. The mesh must extend beyond the lateral borders of the aponeurotic defect by 8 to 10 cm. The distance inferiorly and superiorly is less critical and requires only 4 to 5 cm. Above the umbilicus, the linea alba interferes with the midline placement of the prosthesis, and a slit in the middle of the superior edge of the prosthesis is necessary to allow the prosthesis to protrude upward within the rectus abdominis sheath on either side of the linea alba.

Peripheral fixation by sutures or staples is usually advisable. The preferred technique for fixation is that developed by Rives, in which the mesh is attached to the abdominal wall with traction-fixation sutures every 5 to 6 cm with the aid of the Reverdin suture needle [see Figure 13]. The lateral traction sutures also advantageously stretch the retracted belt muscles, retain the peritoneum, and facilitate midline approximation. Fixation sutures are not needed when the prosthesis extends deep into the space of Retzius or far into the iliac fossa. When the retromuscular space is undissectable, the prosthesis must be implanted intraperitoneally. The intraperitoneal prosthesis must be prevented from touching the viscera either by the omentum or by an absorbable synthetic prosthesis. Likewise, an absorbable prosthesis is used to substitute for the posterior rectus abdominis sheath when the sheath cannot be approximated.

Aponeurotic closure of the parietal defect is important. The midline closure can withstand greater tension because the prosthesis, not the suture line, ultimately unites the abdomen. However, when necessary, tension can be reduced by the use of 1 cm vertical relaxing incisions arranged quincuncially in the rectus abdominis sheath. Each row of overlapping relaxing incisions expands the sheath 1 cm. Long relaxing incisions above the umbilicus are not recommended and should never be made below the umbilicus. Aponeurotic approximation is usually achievable. When it is not, a second absorbable or nonabsorbable prosthesis inlaid in the aponeurotic defect ensures stability of the abdominal wall during the healing process; usually, this inability to achieve approximation occurs in the region of the xiphoid or the symphysis. Dead space created by large prostheses always calls for closed suction drainage to prevent seroma and hematoma formation and to allow quick fibrous incorporation of the prosthesis in the abdominal wall.

References

1. Gilbert AI: An anatomic and functional classification for the diagnosis and treatment of inguinal hernia. Am J Surg 157:331, 1989
2. Nyhus LM, Klein MS, Rogers F: Inguinal hernia. Curr Probl Surg 73:407, 1991
3. Nyhus LM: Clinical update: individualization of hernia repair: a new era. Surgery 114:1, 1993
4. Bendavid R: The TSD classification: a nomenclature for groin hernias. GREPA 15:9, 1993
5. Schumpelick V, Treutner KH, Arlt G: Inguinal hernia repair in adults. Lancet 344:375, 1994
6. Fruchaud H: Le Traitement Chirurgical des Hernies de L'Aine Chez L'Adulte. G Doin, Paris, 1956
7. Fruchaud H: Anatomie Chirurgicale des Hernies de L'Aine. G Doin, Paris, 1956
8. Glassow F: Inguinal hernia repair using local anaesthesia. Ann R Coll Surg Engl 66:382, 1984
9. Halverson K, McVay CB: Inguinal and femoral hernioplasty: a 22-year study of the authors' methods. Arch Surg 101:127, 1970
10. Wantz GE: The Canadian repair: personal observations. World J Surg 13:516, 1989
11. Wantz GE: The operation of Bassini as described by Attilio Catterina. Surg Gynecol Obstet 168:67, 1989
12. Griffith CA: The Marcy repair of indirect inguinal hernia. Surg Clin North Am 51:1309, 1971
13. Griffith CA: The Marcy repair revisited. Surg Clin North Am 64:215, 1984
14. Glassow F: The surgical repair of inguinal and femoral hernias. Can Med Assoc J 108:308, 1973
15. Shearburn EW, Myers RN: Shouldice repair for inguinal hernia. Surgery 66:450, 1969
16. Wantz GE: The Canadian repair of inguinal hernia. Hernia, 3rd ed. Nyhus LM, Condon RE, Eds. JB Lippincott Co, Philadelphia, 1989, p 236
17. Madden JL, Hakim S, Agorogiannis AB: The anatomy and repair of inguinal hernias. Surg Clin North Am 51:1269, 1971
18. Condon RE: The anatomy of the inguinal region and its relation to groin hernia. Hernia, 3rd ed. Nyhus LM, Condon RE, Eds. JB Lippincott Co, Philadelphia, 1989, p 18
19. McVay CB: A fundamental error in current methods of inguinal herniorrhaphy. Surg Gynecol Obstet 74:746, 1942
20. McVay CB: Inguinal hernioplasty: common mistakes and pitfalls. Surg Clin North Am 46:1089, 1966
21. McVay CB: The anatomic basis for inguinal and femoral hernioplasty. Surg Gynecol Obstet 139:931, 1974
22. Rutledge RH: Cooper's ligament repairs: a 25-year experience with a single technique for all groin hernias in adults. Surgery 103:1, 1988
23. McVay CB: The anatomy of the relaxing incision in inguinal hernioplasty. Quarterly Bulletin of the Northwestern University Medical School 36:245, 1962
24. Cheatle GT: An operation for inguinal hernia. BMJ 2:1025, 1921
25. Henry AK: Operation for femoral hernia by a midline, extraperitoneal approach with a preliminary note on the use of this route for reducible inguinal hernia. Lancet 1:531, 1936
26. Houck JP, Rypins EB, Sarfeh IJ, et al: Repair of incisional hernia. Surg Gynecol Obstet 169:397, 1989
27. Lichtenstein IL, Shulman AG, Amid PK, et al: The tension-free hernioplasty. Am J Surg 157:188, 1989
28. Lichtenstein IL, Shore JM: Simplified repair of femoral and recurrent inguinal hernias by a "plug" technic. Am J Surg 128:439, 1974
29. Gilbert AI: Sutureless repair of inguinal hernia. Am J Surg 163:331, 1992
30. Gilbert AI: Inguinal hernia repair: biomaterials and sutureless repair. Perspect Gen Surg 2:113, 1991
31. Rutkow IM, Robbins AW: "Tension-free" inguinal herniorrhaphy: a preliminary report on the "mesh plug" technique. Surgery 114:3, 1993
32. Robbins AW, Rutkow IM: The mesh-plug hernioplasty. Surg Clin North Am 73:501, 1993
33. Read RC: Bilaterality and the prosthetic repair of large recurrent inguinal hernias. Am J Surg 138:788, 1979

34. Nyhus LM, Pollak R, Bombeck TC, et al: The preperitoneal approach and prosthetic buttress repair for recurrent hernia. Ann Surg 208:733, 1988
35. Stoppa RE, Rives JL, Warlaumont CR, et al: The use of Dacron in the repair of hernias of the groin. Surg Clin North Am 64:269, 1984
36. Stoppa RE: The treatment of complicated groin and incisional hernias. World J Surg 13:545, 1989
37. Stoppa RE, Warlaumont CR: The preperitoneal approach and prosthetic repair of groin hernia. Hernia, 3rd ed. Nyhus LM, Condon RE, Eds. JB Lippincott Co, Philadelphia, 1989, p 199
38. Wantz GE: Giant prosthetic reinforcement of the visceral sac. Surg Gynecol Obstet 169:408, 1989
39. Wantz GE: The technique of giant prosthetic reinforcement of the visceral sac performed through an anterior groin incision. Surg Gynecol Obstet 176:497, 1993
40. Fong Y, Wantz GE: Prevention of ischemic orchitis during inguinal hernioplasty with 6454 hernioplasties in male patients. Surg Gynecol Obstet 174:399, 1992
41. Wantz GE: Testicular atrophy and chronic residual neuralgia as risks of inguinal hernioplasty. Surg Clin North Am 73:571, 1993
42. Wantz GE: Testicular atrophy as a risk of inguinal hernioplasty. Surg Gynecol Obstet 154:570, 1982
43. Wantz GE: Ambulatory surgical treatment of groin hernia: prevention and management of complications. Curr Probl Surg 3:311, 1986
44. Chevrel JP, Gatt MT: The treatment of neuralgias following herniorrhaphy: a report of 47 cases. Postgrad Gen Surg 4:142, 1992
45. Starling JR, Harms BA: Diagnosis and treatment of genitofemoral and ilioinguinal neuralgia. World J Surg 13:586, 1989
46. Spangen L: Spigelian hernia. World J Surg 13:573, 1989
47. Leslie D: The parastomal hernia. Surg Clin North Am 64:407, 1984
48. Sugarbaker PH: Prosthetic mesh repair of large hernias at the site of colonic stomas. Surg Gynecol Obstet 150:577, 1980
49. Rives J: Major incisional hernias. Surgery of the Abdominal Wall. Chevrel JP, Ed. Springer-Verlag, New York, 1986, p 116
50. Goni Moreno I: Chronic eventrations and large hernias. Surgery 22:945, 1947
51. Raynor RW, DelGuercio LRM: The place for pneumoperitoneum in the repair of massive hernia. World J Surg 13:581, 1989
52. Wantz GE: Incisional hernioplasty with Mersilene. Surg Gynecol Obstet 172:129, 1991
53. Wantz GE: Atlas of Hernia Surgery. Raven Press, New York, 1991
54. Wantz GE: Abdominal wall surgery. Principles of Surgery, 6th ed. Schwartz SI, Shires GT, Spencer FC, eds. McGraw-Hill, New York, 1994, p 1517

Reviews

Chevrel JP: Surgery of the Abdominal Wall. Springer-Verlag, New York, 1986

Devlin HB: Management of Abdominal Hernias. Butterworth, London, 1988

Lichtenstein IL: Hernia Repair Without Disability, 2nd ed. Ishiyaku Euroamerica, St. Louis, 1986

Nyhus LM, Condon RE: Hernia, 3rd ed. JB Lippincott Co, Philadelphia, 1989

Schumpelick V, Zinner M: Atlas of Hernia Surgery. BC Decker, Philadelphia, 1990

Skandalakis JE, Gray SW, Mansberger AR, et al: Hernia: Surgical Anatomy and Technique. McGraw-Hill, New York, 1989

Wantz GE: Atlas of Hernia Surgery. Raven Press, New York, 1991

Acknowledgment

Figures 1 through 13   Tom Moore.

61 LAPAROSCOPIC HERNIA REPAIR

Liane S. Feldman, M.D., and Marvin J. Wexler, M.D.

The introduction of video-assisted minimal access surgery has dramatically altered patient care over the past decade. Certain laparoscopic procedures, including cholecystectomy and antireflux procedures, have shown obvious benefits (e.g., more rapid and less painful recovery) and have been readily and universally adopted. Others, particularly laparoscopic inguinal hernia repair (first described by Ger in 1990[1]), remain controversial. Laparoscopic inguinal herniorrhaphy has shown a great deal of promise; however, concurrently with its development, open anterior herniorrhaphy has evolved into a tension-free, often sutureless mesh repair that is easily performed with the patient under local anesthesia and that is also associated with rapid recovery and low recurrence rates.[2] Thus, to gain acceptance, laparoscopic inguinal hernia repair must be shown to provide a significant advantage over the tension-free open repair now in use.

The two most common techniques for laparoscopic inguinal hernia repair both involve the insertion of mesh into the preperitoneal space; one makes use of a transabdominal preperitoneal (TAPP) approach, the other a totally extraperitoneal (TEP) approach. Both approaches would appear to offer potential advantages, such as reduced postoperative pain, shortened convalescence, quicker and more accurate assessment and repair of bilateral groin hernias simultaneously, and, in the case of recurrent hernia, avoidance of previously dissected and technically difficult scarred areas. In practice, however, these advantages are not invariably realized: a laparoscopic approach is not always minimally invasive, and various disadvantages accrue from the current requirement for general anesthesia, the need to traverse the abdominal cavity in the TAPP technique, and the increase in operating room time and costs.[3]

Meticulous attention to surgical technique is essential. Because surgeons may be unfamiliar with inguinal anatomy as viewed from inside the abdomen and because the potential for complications necessitating laparotomy is increased with the laparoscopic approach, surgeons must be proficient in laparoscopic techniques and must have a precise knowledge of anatomic relations in the region of the groin as seen from the peritoneal surface.

Since the late 1990s, laparoscopic video techniques have also been increasingly applied to the repair of incisional hernias.[4-8] Laparoscopic repair of large incisional hernias resembles open repair in that mesh is inserted to cover the defect in the abdominal wall fascia. A laparoscopic approach is theoretically attractive because an open approach usually necessitates a large incision as well as extensive and tedious wide dissection to expose the abdominal wall defect, resulting in considerable postoperative pain and a risk of wound complications—problems that a laparoscopic approach to the defect from within might minimize.

It may be many more years before we can determine the true safety and efficacy of laparoscopic herniorrhaphy and establish the correct indications for its use. In the meantime, every repair performed should be subjected to careful classification, documentation, and quality-of-life assessment. Surgeons should not perform laparoscopic herniorrhaphy simply because it is novel or potentially economical: they should perform this procedure only when convinced that it is anatomically and physiologically correct and logical.

In what follows, we discuss laparoscopic repair of both inguinal and incisional hernias. In addition to describing current operative techniques, we address inguinal surgical anatomy, preoperative planning, and complications. Finally, we review selected trials measuring the results of laparoscopic repair against those of open repair and comparing the outcomes of TAPP repair with those of TEP repair.

Laparoscopic Inguinal Hernia Repair

LAPAROSCOPIC INGUINAL ANATOMY

To most surgeons, inguinal anatomy as viewed through the laparoscope appears unfamiliar. The surgical perspective on the pelvic anatomy from the intraperitoneal view has been best described by Skandalakis and coworkers[9] and has been elegantly demonstrated in cadaver dissections by Spaw and colleagues,[10] whose work forms the basis of the descriptions we present in this chapter. Excellent descriptions of the preperitoneal space by Wantz[11] and Condon[12] are also worthy of review.

During laparoscopic herniorrhaphy, a number of structures that are usually visible during open herniorrhaphy (e.g., the inguinal ligament, the pubic tubercle, the lacunar ligament, and the ilioinguinal and iliohypogastric nerves) are not seen initially. Conversely, a number of structures that are visible only after significant dissection in the open approach are easily viewed through the laparoscope [see Figure 1]. Identification of the iliopubic tract, Cooper's ligament, and the transverse abdominal arch is mandatory to ensure proper coverage and securing of prosthetic material margins. The obliterated umbilical artery, a structure not encountered in the anterior approach to open herniorrhaphy, must be divided or retracted medially to afford visualization and dissection of the pubic tubercle, Cooper's ligament, and often the entire Hesselbach's triangle.

Peritoneum Intact

Four important landmarks should be seen at initial laparoscopic inspection of the inguinal region [see Figure 2]: the spermatic vessels, the obliterated umbilical artery (also referred to as the medial umbilical ligament or bladder ligament by various authors), the inferior epigastric vessels (also referred to as the lateral umbilical ligament), and the external iliac vessels.

Spermatic vessels The testicular artery and vein descend from the retroperitoneum, travel directly over and slightly lateral to the external iliac artery, and enter the internal spermatic ring posteriorly. These vessels are covered only by the peritoneum and are usually well visualized as flat structures in the abdominal cavity that assume a cordlike appearance when joined by the vas def-

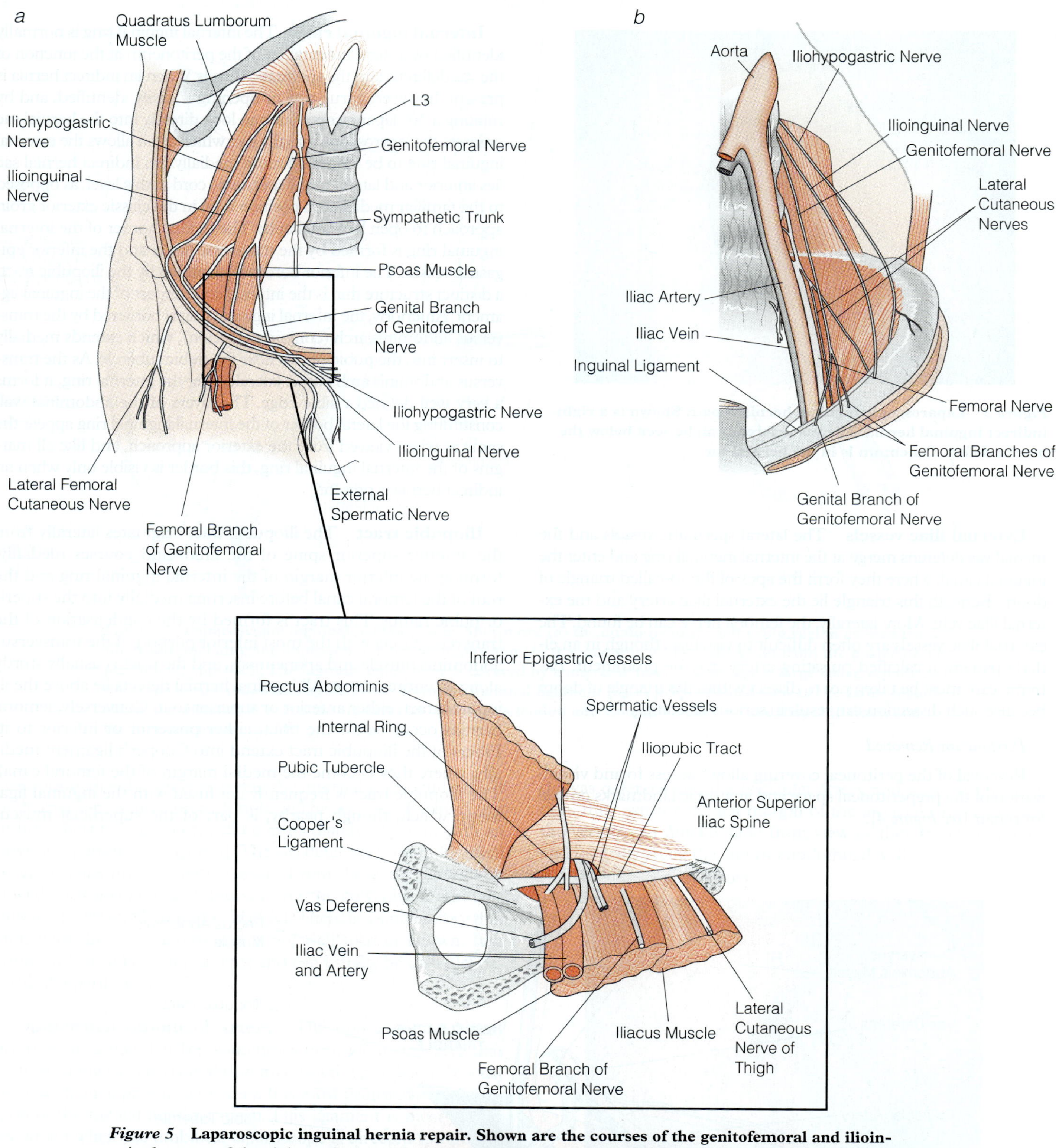

Figure 5 **Laparoscopic inguinal hernia repair.** Shown are the courses of the genitofemoral and ilioinguinal nerves of the right groin (*a*) and of the left groin (*b*). Inset shows the preperitoneal anatomy of the right groin, as seen by the laparoscopic surgeon.

loaponeurotic layer, which is not seen laparoscopically. The iliopubic tract is part of the deep layer.

Cooper's ligament Cooper's ligament is a condensation of the transverse fascia and the periosteum of the superior pubic ramus lateral to the pubic tubercle. It can be seen only from within the abdominal cavity once the peritoneum is opened and deflected inferiorly, but a considerable amount of preperitoneal fat must often be cleaned off the ligament before it can be seen. Initially, it is often easier to palpate the ligament than to see it, but once the ligament has been identified and cleaned, its glistening white fibers are apparent. Care must be taken during dissection to avoid the tiny branches of the obturator vein that often run along the ligament's surface. The iliopubic tract inserts into the superior ramus of the pubis just lateral to Cooper's ligament, blending into it.

Femoral canal The femoral canal is seen only in the presence of a femoral hernia in the most medial aspect of the femoral triangle. The anterior and medial borders are bounded by the iliopubic tract, the posterior border is formed by the pectineal fascia, and the lateral border is formed by the femoral sheath and vein.

Trapezoid of disaster. Another area worthy of careful attention is the so-called trapezoid of disaster, containing the genitofemoral, ilioinguinal, iliohypogastric, and lateral cutaneous nerves of the thigh, which innervate the spermatic cord, testicle, scrotum, and upper and lateral thigh, respectively. A detailed knowledge of their anatomic course and careful avoidance of the nerves are essential [*see Figure 5*].

Genitofemoral nerve. The genitofemoral nerve arises from the first and second lumbar nerves; pierces the psoas muscle and fascia at its medial border opposite L3 or L4; descends under the peritoneum, on the psoas major muscle; and divides into a medial genital and a lateral femoral branch. The femoral branch descends lateral to the external iliac artery and the spermatic cord, passing posteroinferior to the iliopubic tract and into the femoral sheath to supply the skin over the femoral triangle. The genital branch crosses the lower end of the external iliac artery and enters the inguinal canal through the internal inguinal ring with the testicular vessels. This branch supplies the coverings of the spermatic cord down to the skin of the scrotum. The genitofemoral nerve is the most visible of the cutaneous nerves and is sometimes confused with the testicular vessels if the latter are not well appreciated in their more medial position.

Ilioinguinal and iliohypogastric nerves. When dissected from the anterior position, the ilioinguinal and iliohypogastric nerves lie between the external oblique and the internal oblique muscles above the internal inguinal ring and descend the spermatic cord. In the abdomen, the ilioinguinal and iliohypogastric nerves arise from the 12th thoracic and first lumbar nerve roots, are more laterally located, and run subperitoneally, emerging from the lateral psoas border to pierce the transversus abdominis muscle near the iliac crest and then pierce and course between the internal oblique and the external oblique muscles close to the internal inguinal ring. Aberrant branches sometimes descend with the genital nerve. The ilioinguinal nerve supplies a small cutaneous area near the external genitals.

Lateral cutaneous nerve of the thigh. Supplying the front and lateral aspect of the thigh, the lateral cutaneous nerve of the thigh arises from the second and third lumbar nerves and emerges at the lateral border of the psoas. There, it descends deep to the peritoneum on the iliac muscle and only comes to lie in a superficial position 3 cm below the anterosuperior iliac spine.

PREOPERATIVE EVALUATION

History and Physical Examination

Preoperative assessment is necessary to determine whether a patient is a suitable candidate for laparoscopic herniorrhaphy. A careful surgical history, including both previous hernia repairs and other procedures (particularly those involving the lower abdomen), should be elicited. A cardiovascular history should also be obtained and risk factors for general anesthesia determined.

Physical examination should confirm the presence of an inguinal hernia. If the patient reports a history of a bulge but no hernia is felt on physical examination, an occult hernia may be presumed. If doubt exists, herniography is indicated. Ultrasonography may be helpful for distinguishing an incarcerated groin hernia from other causes of inguinal swelling (e.g., lymphadenopathy).

Selection of Patients

Indications With the evolution of the open anterior approach to tension-free prosthetic mesh repair, determining which patients will benefit significantly from laparoscopic herniorrhaphy becomes increasingly important. One may choose either (1) to offer laparoscopic repair to all hernia patients in the belief that it is an inherently superior procedure or (2) to reserve laparoscopic repair for specific indications. We prefer the latter choice, believing that these patients are best served when the surgeon has several approaches at his or her command that can be applied to and, if necessary, modified for individual circumstances.

In our opinion, primary unilateral hernias are best treated with an open anterior tension-free repair, preferably with the patient under local or regional anesthesia; possible exceptions include manual laborers and athletes who desire a rapid return to vigorous physical activity and who may benefit from the absence of a sizable incision. We generally reserve laparoscopic inguinal herniorrhaphy for the following clinical situations:

1. Recurrent hernias after previous anterior repair. In such cases, a laparoscopic approach allows one to avoid the scar tissue and distorted anatomy present in the anterior abdominal wall by performing the repair through unviolated tissue, thereby reducing the risk of damage to the vas deferens or the testicular vessels.
2. Bilateral hernias or a unilateral hernia when the presence of a contralateral hernia is strongly suspected. In such cases, a laparoscopic approach allows one to repair both hernias simultaneously and perhaps more rapidly without having to make additional incisions.
3. Repair of an inguinal hernia concurrent with another laparoscopic procedure, provided that there is no contamination of the peritoneal cavity.

Contraindications We do not treat incarcerated hernias laparoscopically. In patients to whom general anesthesia may pose an increased risk, we prefer open anterior repair using local or regional anesthesia. In infants and young children with indirect hernias, for whom repair of the posterior canal wall is unnecessary, we recommend high ligation of the sac via the anterior approach.

Previous lower abdominal surgery, though not an absolute contraindication, may make laparoscopic dissection difficult. In particular, with respect to TEP repair, previous abdominal wall incisions may make it impossible to safely separate the peritoneum from the abdominal parietes for entry into the extraperitoneal plane. Previous surgery in the retropubic space of Retzius, as in prostatic surgery, is a relative contraindication that is associated with an increased risk of bladder injury[13] and other complications.[14]

OPERATIVE PLANNING

Preparation

General anesthesia administered by inhalation is routinely used. Prophylactic antibiotics are unnecessary. The patient is instructed to void before surgery, which means that preoperative bladder catheterization is unnecessary.

Patient Positioning

The patient is placed in the supine position with both arms tucked against the sides. The anesthesia screen is placed as far toward the

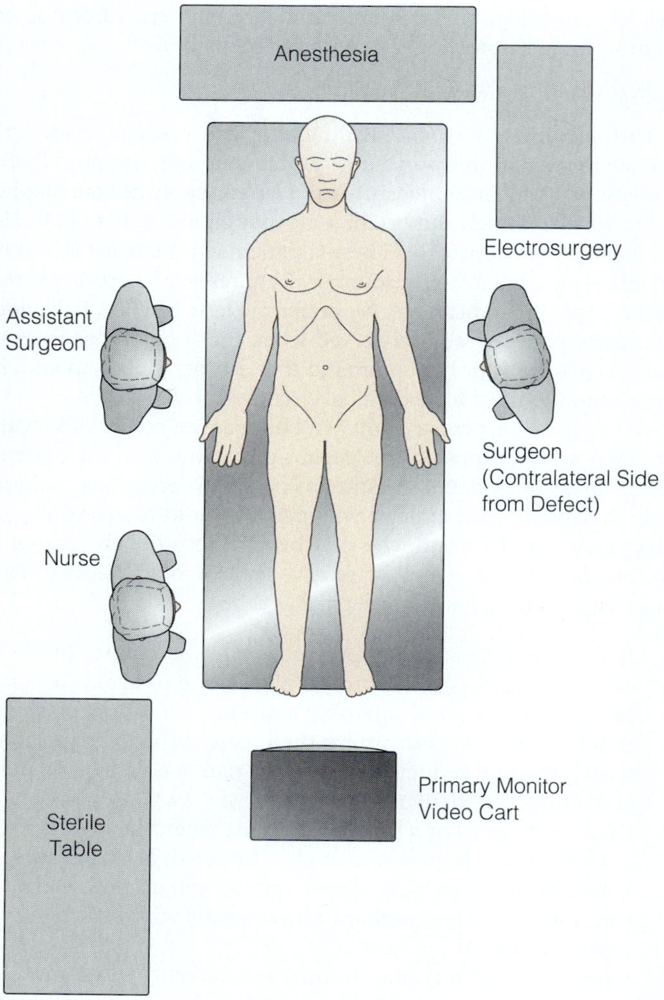

Figure 6 Laparoscopic inguinal hernia repair. Shown is one of several possible OR setups. The surgeon stands on the side contralateral to the defect, with a nurse on the ipsilateral side. The assistant surgeon stands opposite the surgeon. This positioning may vary, depending on the surgeon's preference and handedness, the visibility of the defect, and the type of defect present, as well as on the prominence of the medial umbilical ligament and the need for its retraction.

head of the table as possible to allow the surgeon a wide range of mobility with the laparoscope. The skin must be prepared and draped so as to allow exposure of the entire lower abdomen, the genital region, and the upper thighs because manipulation of the hernial sac and the scrotum is frequently necessary. After the laparoscope has been introduced, the patient is placed in a deep Trendelenburg position so that the viscera will fall away from the inguinal areas. Further bowel manipulation is rarely necessary, except to reduce hernial contents. Rotation of the table to elevate the side of the hernia can provide additional exposure, if necessary. A single video monitor is placed at the foot of the bed, directly facing the patient's head.

The surgeon usually begins the repair while standing on the side contralateral to the defect; the assistant surgeon stands opposite the surgeon, and the nurse stands on the ipsilateral side [see Figure 6]. Once the key anatomic landmarks and the hernial defect are located and defined, the surgeon should be able to move to either side of the patient, and the surgeon or the assistant should be able to move the camera and the instruments to the ports of preference, the choice of which depends on optimum exposure, angle, right- or left-handedness, and the designated role of the assistant surgeon as either camera operator or surgical assistant. A two-handed technique provides a distinct technical advantage and also eliminates the need for an additional surgical assistant.

Equipment

Because inguinal hernias occur in the anterior abdominal wall, visualization through the umbilicus requires angling the laparoscope close to the horizontal plane. The view is paralleled anteriorly by the surface of the lower abdominal wall, which may make visualization with a 0° laparoscope difficult. In addition, an indirect hernia is a three-dimensional tubular defect that can be well visualized in its entirety only with an angled lens. For these reasons, we recommend routine use of an oblique, forward-viewing 30° laparoscope. Excellent 30° laparoscopes are currently available in 10 mm, 5 mm, and 3 mm sizes.

A basic set of instruments for laparoscopic hernia repair should include graspers, dissectors, curved scissors, a suction-irrigation device, a hook cautery, and needle drivers. In addition, we use a multifire stapler to fix the mesh and close the peritoneum (though it is certainly possible to use sutures instead). Either a circular tacker or a linear stapler can be employed; both are available in 10 mm and 5 mm sizes. We prefer the linear stapler.

In a TEP repair, besides the equipment needed for a TAPP repair, a blunt trocar is required for gaining access to the preperitoneal space. An operative laparoscope is needed as well. Alternatively, special preperitoneal distention balloon (PDB) systems [see Operative Technique, Totally Extraperitoneal Repair, below] are also frequently used to develop the preperitoneal space.

OPERATIVE TECHNIQUE

As noted (see above), there are two principal techniques of laparoscopic inguinal hernia repair. The TAPP repair involves insufflating the peritoneal cavity, penetrating the abdomen with trocars, incising the peritoneum overlying the defect, and closing the peritoneum after the repair with a piece of mesh placed in the preperitoneal space. The TEP repair, on the other hand, involves gaining access to the preperitoneal space via trocars placed in a space created between the fascia and the peritoneum, insufflating that space, and placing a piece of mesh between the underside of the anterior abdominal wall and the peritoneum.

We will not describe the intraperitoneal onlay mesh (IPOM) technique, in which polypropylene mesh is fixed directly onto the peritoneum intra-abdominally. This approach has been abandoned by most surgeons out of fear of complications related to adhesions and possible erosion of the mesh into bowel.[3,15]

Transabdominal Preperitoneal Repair

Step 1: placement of trocars Pneumoperitoneum is established through a small vertical infraumbilical incision. Either a closed approach, using a Veress needle, or an open (Hasson) approach, using a 10/12 mm trocar, may be employed. We prefer the open technique, in which the first trocar is inserted into the peritoneal cavity under direct vision. This approach usually prevents injuries to the major blood vessels; although it does not completely prevent bowel injuries, it does facilitate discovery and repair of such injuries.

CO_2 is then insufflated into the abdomen to a pressure of 15 mm Hg. The angled laparoscope is introduced, and both inguinal areas are inspected. Two 10/12 mm accessory ports are then placed at the lateral border of each rectus abdominis muscle at the level of the umbilicus to allow placement of the camera and the instruments [see Figure 7]. The 10/12 mm lateral ports can be

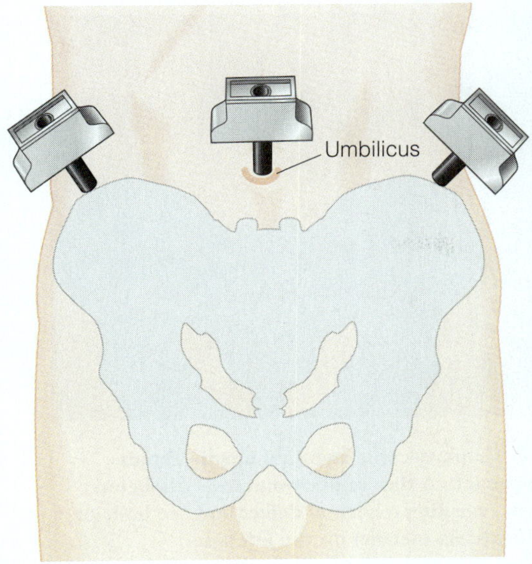

Figure 7 Laparoscopic inguinal hernia repair: TAPP approach. Shown is standard trocar placement for TAPP repair. Usually, three trocar sites are used. The laparoscope is inserted through the umbilical trocar, and two additional trocars are placed in the right and the left midabdomen. To ensure that the first trocar is not placed too close to the surgical field, the first trocar should be placed either in the umbilicus or immediately above it. The two lateral trocars should be placed lateral to the rectus sheath to prevent bleeding and postoperative muscle spasms. At least one trocar must be 10/12 mm to allow insertion of the mesh.

replaced with 5 mm ports if 5 mm instruments and a 5 mm laparoscope are available. To facilitate port placement, the abdominal wall is transilluminated with the laparoscope so as to delineate the border of the rectus abdominis muscle, which can be difficult to define in muscular or obese males. Additional care is taken to keep from puncturing the large subcutaneous veins that are frequently present in this region. Failure to transilluminate the abdominal wall can result in placement of the trocar through the rectus muscle, which can cause troublesome bleeding.

Step 2: identification of anatomic landmarks The four key anatomic landmarks mentioned earlier [*see* Laparoscopic Inguinal Anatomy, Peritoneum Intact, *above*]—the spermatic vessels, the obliterated umbilical artery (medial umbilical ligament), the inferior epigastric vessels (lateral umbilical ligament), and the external iliac vessels—are identified on each side. In the presence of an indirect hernia, the internal inguinal ring is easily identified by the presence of a discrete hole at the junction of the vas deferens and the testicular vessels. Identification of a direct hernia can be more difficult [*see Figure 8*]. A direct hernia sometimes appears as a complete circle or hole and sometimes as a cleft, and at other times it is completely hidden by preperitoneal fat and the bladder and umbilical ligament. Visualization can be particularly difficult in obese patients, who may have considerable lipomatous tissue between the peritoneum and the transversalis fascia, or in patients whose hernia consists of a weakness and bulging of the entire inguinal floor rather than a distinct sac. For adequate definition of this type of hernia and deeper anatomic structures, the peritoneum must be opened, a peritoneal flap developed, and the underlying fatty layer dissected.[16] Direct hernial defects are often situated medial to the ipsilateral umbilical ligament, and retraction or even division of this structure is sometimes necessary. Traction on the ipsilateral testicle can demonstrate the vas deferens when visualization is obscured by overlying fat or pressure from the pneumoperitoneum.

Step 3: creation of peritoneal flap The curved cautery scissors or the hook cautery is used to create a peritoneal flap by making a transverse incision along the peritoneum, beginning just above the upper border of the internal inguinal ring and extending medially above the pubic tubercle and laterally 2 cm beyond the internal inguinal ring [*see Figure 9*]. Extreme care must be taken to avoid the inferior epigastric vessels. Bleeding from the epigastrics can usually be controlled by cauterization, but application of hemostatic clips may be necessary on occasion. Another solution is to pass percutaneously placed sutures above and below the bleeding point while applying pressure to the bleeding vessel so as not to obscure the field of vision.

If the monopolar cautery is used to create the peritoneal flap, the entire uninsulated portion of the instrument must be visible at all times. Unlike laparoscopic cholecystectomy, in which the liver acts as a safe backdrop for scatter and dissection is anterosuperior to the colon, laparoscopic herniorrhaphy may bring bowel loops in contact with instruments, an occurrence that can be particularly dangerous if current is applied to a long-nosed forceps or grasper and a backdrop is lacking. The medial umbilical ligament must be retracted for me-

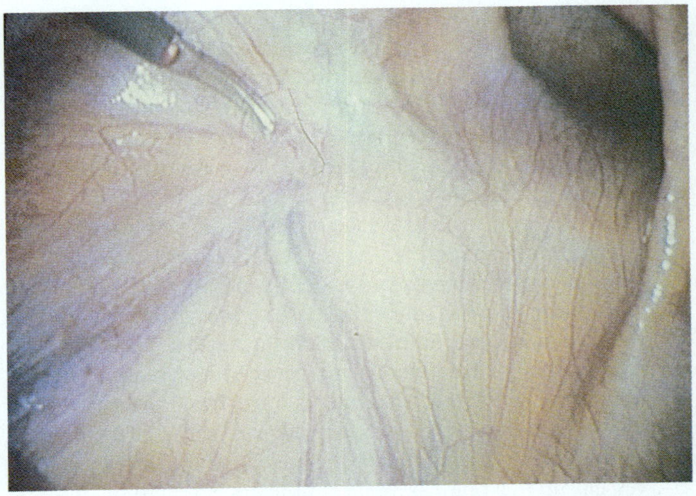

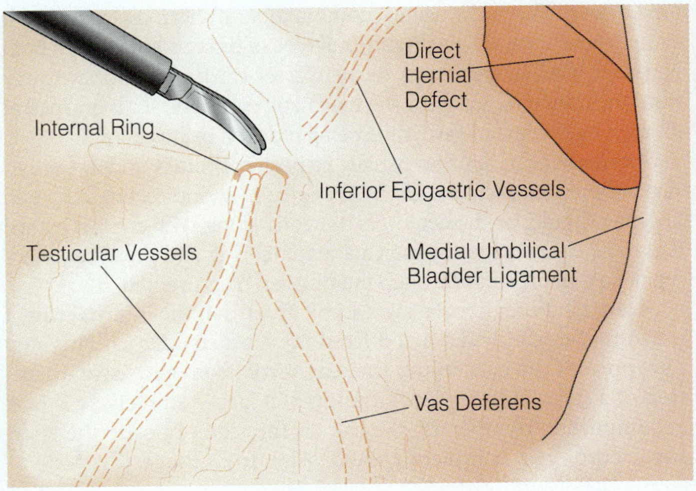

Figure 8 Laparoscopic inguinal hernia repair: TAPP approach. Shown is a left direct inguinal hernia with the peritoneum intact. The dissector indicates the intact internal ring.

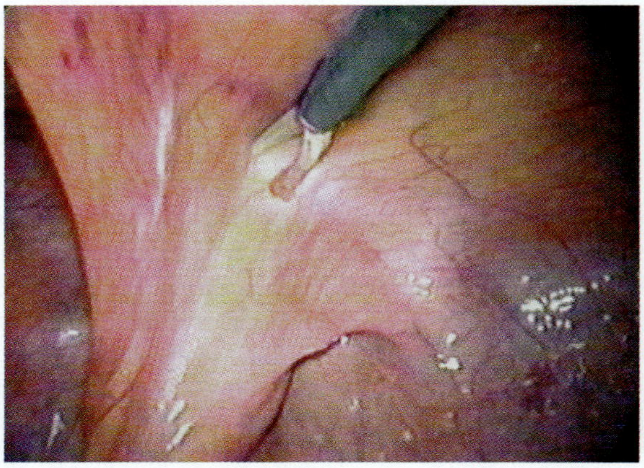

Figure 9 Laparoscopic inguinal hernia repair: TAPP approach. Shown is dissection of a left direct inguinal hernia. The hernial sac is inverted and the peritoneum incised superior to the sac.

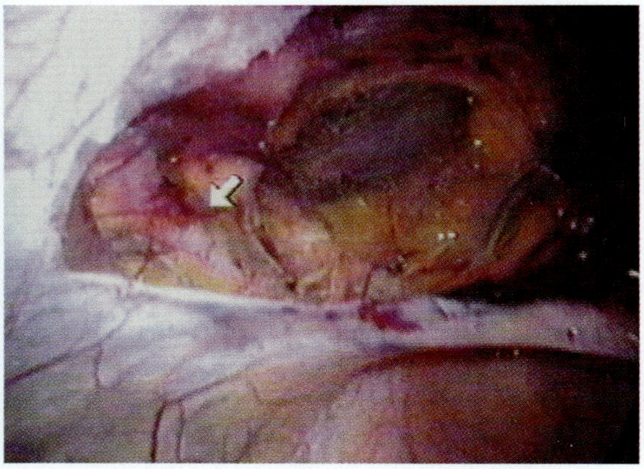

Figure 10 Laparoscopic inguinal hernia repair: TAPP approach. A flap of peritoneum is dissected downward, revealing a hernial defect and the inferior epigastric vessels (arrow) on the left side.

dial dissection and may have to be divided. Division of this structure does not have any negative sequelae; however, one should be aware that the obliterated umbilical artery may still be patent and should use the cautery or clips.

The incised peritoneum is grasped along with the attached preperitoneal fat and the peritoneal sac and is dissected caudad with blunt and sharp dissection to create a lower peritoneal flap [*see Figure 10*]. Dissection must stay close to the abdominal wall. A significant amount of preperitoneal fat may be encountered, and this should remain with the peritoneal flap so that the abdominal wall is cleared. When the correct preperitoneal plane is entered, dissection is almost bloodless and easily carried out. A smaller superior peritoneal flap is then created, exposing the posterior rectus muscle and the transversus abdominis arch. Scissors, if used, should always have cautery capability so that bleeding from the multiple small vessels beneath the peritoneum can be prevented.

Step 4: dissection of hernial sac The hernial sac, if present, is removed from Hesselbach's triangle or the spermatic cord and surrounding muscle through inward traction, countertraction, and blunt dissection with progressive inversion of the sac until the musculofascial boundary of the internal inguinal ring and the key deep anatomic structures are identified. An endoscopic Kitner dissector or a 2 × 2 in. piece of gauze on a grasper facilitates blunt dissection of the preperitoneal space. We prefer using a combination of sharp dissection with cautery scissors and a push-and-pull type of dissection in which both hands are used. In most cases, the hernial sac can be slowly drawn away from the transverse fascia or the spermatic cord. The sac is grasped at its apex and pulled inward, thus being reduced by inversion.

Spermatic cord lipomas usually lie posterolaterally and are extensions of preperitoneal fat. In the presence of an indirect defect, such lipomas should be dissected off the cord along with the peritoneal flap to lie cephalad to the internal inguinal ring and the subsequent repair so that prolapse through the ring can be prevented.

A large indirect hernial sac can be divided at the internal ring if it cannot be readily dissected from the cord structures. This step may prevent the cord injury that can result from extensive dissection of a large indirect sac. Division of a large indirect sac is best accomplished by opening the sac on the side opposite the spermatic cord, then completing the division from the inside.[13]

Step 5: reidentification and exposure of landmarks Once the peritoneal flap has been created, the key anatomic landmarks mentioned earlier [*see* Laparoscopic Inguinal Anatomy, Peritoneum Removed, *above*] must be identified and exposed so that neurovascular structures can be protected from injury and the tissues required for reliable mesh fixation can be located. The pubic tubercle is often more easily felt than seen. Cooper's ligament is initially felt and subsequently seen along the pectineal prominence of the superior pubic ramus as dissection continues laterally and fatty tissue is swept off to expose the glistening white structure. Care must be taken to avoid the numerous small veins that often run on the surface of the ligament as well as to avoid the occasional aberrant obturator artery. The iliopubic tract is initially identified at the inferior margin of the internal inguinal ring, with the spermatic cord above, and is then followed in both a medial and a lateral direction. Minimal dissection is carried out inferior to the iliopubic tract so as not to injure the genitofemoral nerve, the femoral nerve, and the lateral cutaneous nerve of the thigh [*see Figure 11*].

Step 6: placement of mesh A 10 × 6 cm sheet of polypropylene mesh is tapered at its medial end, rolled into a cigarette shape and introduced into the abdomen through the 10/12 mm umbilical trocar. Prolene mesh is preferable to Marlex mesh because it is less dense, conforms more easily to the posterior inguinal wall, and has larger pores, which facilitate visualization and subsequent securing with staples. The inherent elasticity and resiliency of Prolene mesh allow it to unroll easily while maintaining its form. The mesh is used to cover the direct space (Hesselbach's triangle), the indirect space, and the femoral ring areas (i.e., the entire inguinal floor). We do not routinely make a slit in the mesh for the cord, because recurrences through the slits have been noted. An alternative is the double-buttress technique, in which a piece of mesh with a slit and a central opening is placed first and a second, uncut piece is then placed on top of the first for added security and reinforcement.[17]

Although not all surgeons consider fixation of the mesh necessary, it is our practice to staple the mesh to prevent any migration. We use an endoscopic multifire hernia stapler to secure the mesh, beginning at the pubic tubercle and proceeding laterally. The upper margin is tacked first to the rectus muscle and the transversus abdominis fascia and arch, with care taken to stay 1 to 2 cm above the level of the internal inguinal ring and avoid the inferior epigastric vessels, up to a point several centimeters lateral to the internal inguinal ring or the indirect hernial defect. Extending mesh fixation to the anterior iliac spine is neither necessary nor desirable. A

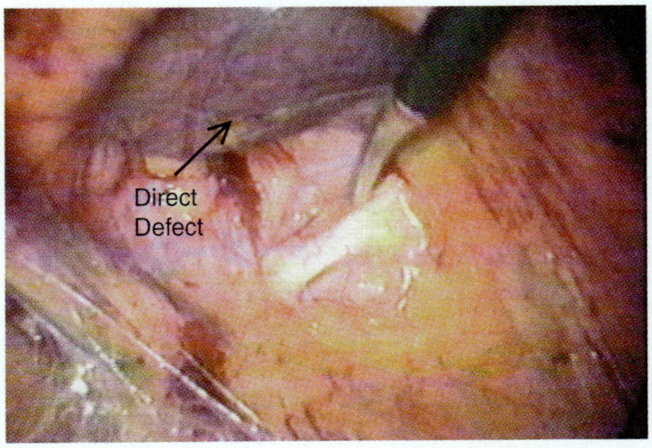

Figure 11 Laparoscopic inguinal hernia repair: TAPP approach. Dissection of the preperitoneal space on the left side allows identification of the anatomic landmarks. The dissector points to the iliopubic tract inferior to the direct hernial defect.

two-handed technique is recommended for staple placement: one hand is on the stapler, and the other is on the abdominal wall, applying external pressure to place the wall against the stapler. The stapler itself is frequently pushed against the tissues and used as a spreader and palpator; however, it must not be forced too deeply into the abdominal wall superolateral to the spermatic cord so as not to entrap the sensory nerves inadvertently. The stapler can be moved from the left port to the right port, depending on which position more readily allows placement of the staples perpendicular to the mesh and the abdominal wall.

Once the superior margin is fixed, any excess mesh can be trimmed with scissors; however, this step is rarely necessary with a 10 × 6 cm swatch. Fixation of the inferior margin is then easily accomplished, beginning at the pubic tubercle and moving laterally along Cooper's ligament. The mesh is lifted frequently to ensure adequate visualization of the spermatic cord. Care is taken to avoid the adjacent external iliac vessels, which lie inferiorly. Lateral to the cord structures, all staples are placed superior to the iliopubic tract to prevent subsequent neuralgias involving the lateral cutaneous nerve of the thigh or the branches of the genitofemoral nerve. If the surgeon can palpate the stapler through the abdominal wall with the nondominant hand, the stapler is above the iliopubic tract. When an indirect hernia is present, staples are placed circumferentially to the entire musculoaponeurotic ring of the hernia, which can usually be visualized through the pores of the polypropylene mesh. The mesh should lie flat at the end of the procedure [see Figure 12].

For bilateral repairs, we prefer to make two peritoneal incisions and use two pieces of mesh rather than the single large piece advocated by some authorities; we find that this approach makes the mesh easier to manipulate.

Step 7: closure of peritoneum The peritoneal flap, including the redundant inverted hernial sac, is placed over the mesh, and the peritoneum is reapproximated with the tacker by precocking and partially closing the stapler, then hooking the peritoneum on one side and drawing it to the other side [see Figure 13]. Reduction of intra-abdominal pressure and external abdominal wall pressure facilitates a tension-free reapproximation. Alternatively, the peritoneum can be sutured over the mesh, but in most surgeons' hands, this closure takes longer.

Step 8: closure of fascia and skin The peritoneal repair is inspected to ensure that there are no major gaps that might result in exposure of the mesh and subsequent formation of adhesions. The trocars are then removed under direct vision, and the pneumoperitoneum is released. The fascia at the 10/12 mm port sites is closed with 2-0 Prolene sutures to prevent incisional hernias. The skin is closed with 4-0 absorbable subcuticular sutures.

Totally Extraperitoneal Repair

The extra-abdominal preperitoneal approach to laparoscopic hernia repair, developed by McKernan,[18] attempts to duplicate the open preperitoneal repair described by Stoppa[19-21] and Wantz.[11,22] In a TEP repair, the trocars are placed preperitoneally in a space created between the fascia and the peritoneum. An operating laparoscope provides access to the preperitoneal space of the groin, where the mesh repair is effected. Ideally, none of the preliminary exploratory trocars penetrates the peritoneum, and the dissection remains in the extra-abdominal plane at all times.

Patient preparation and positioning are much the same as in a TAPP repair. The surgeon stands on the side opposite the hernia.

Step 1: creation of preperitoneal space With the patient in the Trendelenburg position, the fascia is opened through a 1 cm infraumbilical transverse incision placed slightly toward the side of the hernia, which helps one avoid inadvertently opening the peritoneum. An index finger is inserted on the medial aspect of the exposed rectus muscle and slid over the posterior rectus sheath. A

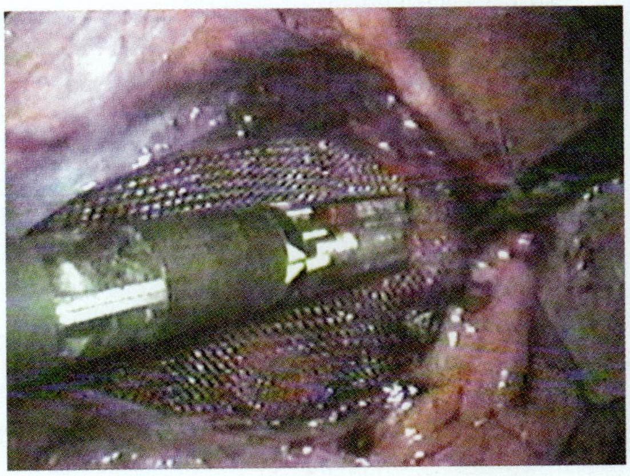

Figure 12 Laparoscopic inguinal hernia repair: TAPP approach. The mesh is stapled in place.

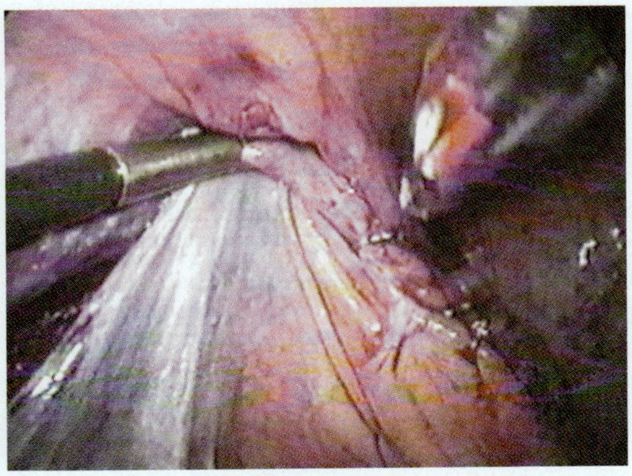

Figure 13 Laparoscopic inguinal hernia repair: TAPP approach. The peritoneum is stapled over the mesh.

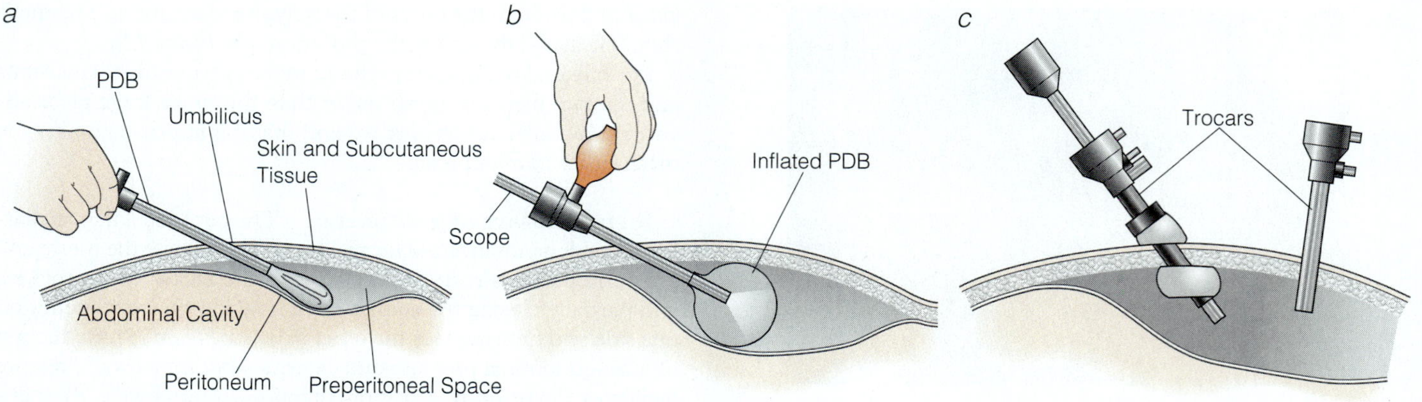

Figure 14 Laparoscopic inguinal hernia repair: TEP approach. Shown is the preperitoneal distention balloon (PDB) system. The PDB is introduced into the preperitoneal space (*a*). As it is tunneled inferiorly toward the pubis, the PDB is inflated under laparoscopic vision (*b*). Once the preperitoneal space is created, the PDB is removed and replaced with a blunt-tip trocar. The preperitoneal space is insufflated under low pressure, additional trocars are placed, and the repair is completed (*c*).

preperitoneal tunnel between the rectus abdominis muscles and the peritoneum is created in the midline with blunt finger dissection. A blunt 10/12 mm trocar is then secured in the preperitoneal space with fascial stay sutures.

An operating laparoscope is inserted through the trocar with a blunt 5 mm probe in the operating channel. Insufflation of the preperitoneal space is begun while the probe depresses the peritoneum and develops the preperitoneal space down to the pubis under direct vision, with the rectus muscles seen anteriorly and the peritoneum posteriorly. Maximum inflation pressure is 8 to 10 mm Hg to prevent disruption of the peritoneum or development of extensive subcutaneous emphysema.

TEP repair can be facilitated by using a preperitoneal distention balloon (PDB) system (Origin Medsystems, Inc., Menlo Park, California). This system consists of a trocar with an inflatable balloon at its tip, which is used to develop the preperitoneal space by atraumatically separating the peritoneum from the abdominal wall. The PDB is inserted into the preperitoneal space below the umbilicus by means of an open Hasson technique and is tunneled inferiorly toward the internal inguinal ring. The preperitoneal working space is developed by gradual inflation of the balloon to a volume of 1 L; the transparency of the balloon permits constant visualization throughout the distention process. Once the working space is created, the PDB is removed and replaced with a blunt sealing trocar. The preperitoneal space is then reinsufflated to a pressure of 8 to 10 mm Hg [see Figure 14].

After the peritoneum is dissected away from the rectus muscle, a midline 5 mm trocar is inserted just above the pubis under direct vision, and a 10/12 mm trocar is placed halfway between the pubis and the umbilicus [see Figure 15], with care taken not to penetrate the peritoneum. The risk of intraperitoneal entry can be minimized by blunt dissection down to the fascia with a hemostat after the skin incision. If the peritoneum is penetrated, the resulting pneumoperitoneum can reduce the already limited working space. One can try to repair the rent with a suture, but if such repair is unsuccessful, the loss of working space may necessitate conversion to a TAPP approach.

Step 2: dissection of hernial sac The operating laparoscope is replaced by a 45° laparoscope, which facilitates exposure and visualization of this region. Wide dissection of the preperitoneal space is then undertaken with blunt graspers in a two-handed technique, with the grasper in the left hand depressing the peritoneum. The pubis, Cooper's ligament, and the inferior epigastric vessels are located. If a direct hernia is present, the sac and the preperitoneal contents are carefully dissected away from the fascial defect, with care taken not to enter the peritoneal cavity. The peritoneum is then further dissected cephalad to expose the internal ring and any indirect hernial sac. A small indirect hernial sac is dissected off the spermatic cord and reduced or amputated with an endoscopic ligating loop after reduction of its contents has been ensured. A large indirect hernial sac is transected and closed, with the distal sac left in place and not ligated.

For hernias that are not readily reduced, McKernan[23] suggests making an incision in the groin above the pubis down to the external oblique aponeurosis and severing the adhesions between the sac and the external ring. If this measure does not work, the sac

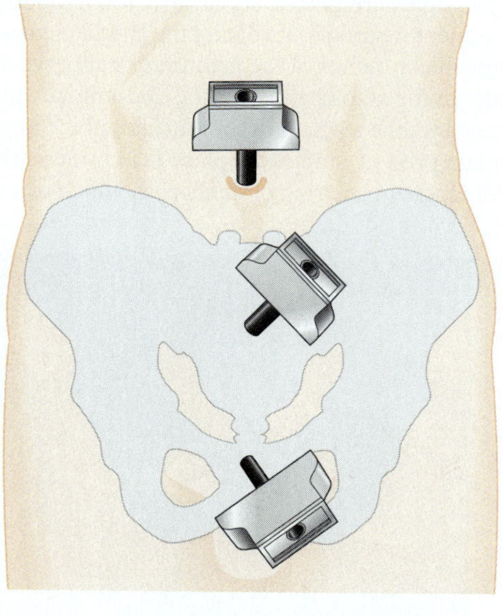

Figure 15 Laparoscopic inguinal hernia repair: TEP approach. Shown is standard trocar placement for TEP repair. As in TAPP repair, three trocar sites are used. One trocar is placed in the umbilicus; the second is placed in the midline, midway between the umbilicus and the pubis; and the third is placed above the pubic arch. The trocars should not penetrate the peritoneum.

can be opened through the incision and the adhesions within the sac lysed. If the hernia still cannot be reduced, the TEP repair is abandoned in favor of an anterior approach.

Step 3: placement of mesh A 10 × 15 cm piece of Prolene mesh is incised vertically, and a 1 cm hole is created centrally for the spermatic cord. The mesh is then folded in half horizontally, with sutures at each corner to maintain the fold, then inserted through the umbilical trocar and drawn behind the cord structures. Once the mesh is well positioned, with the spermatic cord seated in the central hole, the corner sutures are divided, and the mesh is unfolded against the anterior abdominal wall. As in a TAPP repair, the mesh is tacked to key structures, including the pubic tubercle, Cooper's ligament, and the iliopubic tract inferiorly and anteriorly to the posterior aspect of the rectus abdominis muscle. The opening in the mesh is then closed with staples, with great care taken not to compromise cord structures. The mesh must lie flat. No staples are placed inferior to the iliopubic tract lateral to the internal ring. For bilateral hernias, two identical repairs are done, and the two mesh patches are tacked together at the pubis. An additional piece of mesh may be placed cephalad to the pubis for reinforcement.

A major advantage of the TEP approach is avoidance of entry into the peritoneal cavity and thus of the potential risk of adhesions and bowel obstruction. In practice, however, breaches in the peritoneum are common, resulting in decreased operating space and a compromised view of the anatomic structures as pneumoperitoneum ensues. In addition, even when intraperitoneal entry is avoided, the small amount of working space inherent in the nature of the technique can cause the surgeon great difficulty and confusion. For these reasons, considerable experience is required and caution advised before TEP repair is attempted.

Step 4: closure The operative site is inspected for hemostasis. The trocars are removed under direct vision with release of the insufflated CO_2. The fascia at trocar sites larger than 10 mm is closed with 2-0 Prolene sutures, and the skin is closed with subcuticular sutures.

POSTOPERATIVE CARE

Patients are observed in the recovery room until they are able to ambulate unassisted and to void; if they are unable to void at the time of discharge, in-and-out catheterization is performed. Patients are advised to resume their usual activities as they see fit; driving a car is permitted the next day. Outpatient prescriptions for acetaminophen and codeine are given, and follow-up visits in the surgical clinic are scheduled for day 7 after operation. Patients who live alone, who have had an intraoperative complication, who have significant nausea or vomiting, or have unexplained or inordinate pain are admitted overnight.

DISADVANTAGES AND COMPLICATIONS

Disadvantages

Need for general anesthesia The need for pneumoperitoneum and thus for general anesthesia in laparoscopic herniorrhaphy is sometimes considered a major disadvantage. Nausea, dizziness, and headache are more common in the recovery room after TAPP repair than after Lichtenstein repair.[24] It is not necessarily true, however, that local or regional anesthesia is safer than general anesthesia.[25] Anesthesiologic studies critically appraising anesthetic techniques for hernia surgery have shown the choice of general anesthesia over local or regional anesthesia to be safe and, in many cases, advantageous, particularly in patients who are in poor health. Furthermore, TEP repair has been successfully done with patients under epidural[26] and local[27] anesthesia.

Lower cost-effectiveness The costs of laparoscopic repair exceed those of open repair.[24,28-33] For the most part, the differences are accounted for by longer operative time and the use of disposable equipment. Operative time decreases with experience, and disposable trocars and scissors can be replaced with reusable instruments. Suturing the mesh and peritoneum saves the cost of the stapler but requires more operative time.

The higher operative costs of laparoscopic repair notwithstanding, economic impact studies to date have not shown either approach to be clearly more cost-effective. In terms of effectiveness, the laparoscopic approach fares better on most patient-based outcome measures, including pain and convalescence; however, it remains to be seen whether these savings in disability offset the higher operative costs. One randomized study suggested that the total costs of laparoscopic repair were actually lower than those of the Lichtenstein repair when lost workdays were taken into account.[34]

Complications

Most randomized trials comparing laparoscopic repair with open mesh repair have found comparable numbers of total complications in the two groups [see Table 1]. Four studies reported fewer overall complications after laparoscopic repair.[24,32,35,36] In general, although intraoperative complications are more common and potentially more serious in the laparoscopic approach, particularly when a TAPP repair is chosen, postoperative complications tend to be less common.

Complications of access to peritoneal cavity A TAPP hernia repair exposes the patient to several potentially serious risks related to the choice of the transabdominal route. Trocar injuries to the bowel, the bladder, and vascular structures can occur during the creation of the initial pneumoperitoneum or the subsequent insertion of the trocars. Use of an open insertion technique to create the pneumoperitoneum should eliminate major vascular injuries as well as make identification and repair of bowel injuries simpler than they would be with the closed technique. Another complication related to trocar sites is incisional hernia, which can lead to postoperative bowel obstruction.[37]

The use of the transabdominal route also exposes the patient to the risk of adhesions and the potential for late bowel obstruction. Fortunately, evidence from study of herniorrhaphy in pigs[38] and from extensive gynecologic application of laparoscopy in humans over many years suggests that adhesions form significantly less often after laparoscopic procedures than after open procedures.

Complications of dissection Injuries occurring during dissection are often linked to inexperience with laparoscopic inguinal anatomy. If serious enough, they can necessitate laparotomy. Conversion of a laparoscopic procedure to an open one, however, is regarded more seriously in herniorrhaphy patients than in cholecystectomy patients. In laparoscopic cholecystectomy, conversion to laparotomy is acceptable and expected in 4% to 5% of cases, and common bile duct injury is a recognized complication of both open and laparoscopic cholecystectomy. In contrast, some of the complications encountered in laparoscopic herniorrhaphy never occur in classic open anterior herniorrhaphy, and conversion to laparotomy to correct a complication arising during laparoscopic herniorrhaphy is not acceptable. Fortunately, such conversion is rare: in more than 800 laparoscopic herniorrhaphies reported by 19 institutions in a multicenter phase II study, only one bladder injury and one bowel perforation requiring laparotomy for repair were documented.[15]

Table 1 Selected English-Language Randomized Controlled Trials Comparing Laparoscopic with Open Mesh Repairs

Study Authors	Technique Employed	N	OR Time Needed for Unilateral Repairs (min)	Less Early Pain after Laparoscopic Repair?	Complications*	Recovery† (days)	Recurrences (No.)	Cost
Payne et al (1994)	TAPP	48	68	NA	12%	8.9	0	$3,093
	Lichtenstein	52	56		18%	17‡	0	$2,494‡
Wright et al (1996)	TEP	60	58	Yes‡	15	NA	NA	NA
	Lichtenstein	60	45‡		43			
Champault et al (1997)	TEP	51	NA	Yes‡	4%	17	3	NA
	Stoppa	49			30%‡	35‡	1	
Paganini et al (1997)	TAPP	52	67	No	27%	15	2	$1,249
	Lichtenstein	56	48‡		27%	14	0	$306‡
Wellwood et al (1998)	TAPP	200	45	Yes‡	316	5	0	£747
	Lichtenstein	200	45		452‡	8‡	0	£412‡
Zieren et al (1998)	TAPP	80	61	No	19%	3	0	$1,211
	PP	80	36‡		15%	4	0	$124‡
Khoury (1998)	TEP	150	32	Yes‡	13%	8	4	
	PP	142	31		23%‡	15‡	4	
Johansson et al (1999)	TAPP	205	65	Yes‡	66	18	4	5,988 SEK
	Stoppa	204	38		49	24‡	11	350 SEK
MRC (1999)	TAPP/TEP	468	58	NA	30%	10	7	LH £314
	Mixed open§	460	43‡		44%‡	14‡	0‡	more

*Complications are expressed as percentage of patients affected or total number of complications, as reported in the individual studies.
†Definition of recovery varies from study to study.
‡$P < 0.05$.
§Lichtenstein in 94%.
LH—laparoscopic herniorrhaphy   NA—not available   PP—plug-and-patch   TAPP—transabdominal preperitoneal   TEP—totally extraperitoneal

The most common vascular injuries in laparoscopic inguinal herniorrhaphy are those involving the inferior epigastric vessels and the spermatic vessels. The external iliac, circumflex iliac, profunda, and obturator vessels are also at risk. A previous lower abdominal operation is a risk factor.[13] The source of any abnormal bleeding during the procedure must be quickly identified. All vessels in the groin can be ligated except the external iliac vessels, which must be repaired.[13]

Injuries to the urinary tract can also occur. Four bladder injuries requiring repair were documented in a collected series of 762 laparoscopic repairs by different surgical groups.[39] Bladder injuries are most likely to occur when the space of Retzius has been previously dissected (e.g., in a prostatectomy). Renal and ureteral injuries can result from poorly placed trocars. Any urinary tract injuries identified intraoperatively should be repaired immediately. Often, however, these injuries are not apparent until the postoperative period, when they present as lower abdominal pain, renal failure, ascites, dysuria, or hematuria—all of which should be investigated promptly. Although indwelling catheter drainage may constitute sufficient treatment of a missed retroperitoneal bladder injury, intraperitoneal injuries are best treated by direct repair via either laparoscopy or laparotomy.

Complications related to mesh   Complications related to the use of mesh include infection, migration, adhesion formation, and erosion into intraperitoneal organs. Such complications usually become apparent weeks to years after the initial repair, presenting as abscess, fistula, or small bowel obstruction.

Mesh infection is very rare. Phillips and colleagues collected information on 2,559 North American patients and found only one patient who required removal of an infected mesh after an IPOM repair.[40] Estour and Mouret reviewed 7,340 patients from 22 European groups and found only seven patients with reported mesh infections.[41] Mesh infection usually responds to conservative treatment with antibiotics and drainage. On rare occasions, the mesh must be removed; this may be accomplished via an external approach. It is noteworthy that removal of the mesh does not always lead to recurrence of the hernia, a finding that may be attributable to the resulting fibrosis.[42]

Mesh migration may lead to hernia recurrence. In a TAPP repair, appropriate stapling of the mesh should reduce this possibility. In a TEP repair, stapling does not appear to be necessary to prevent migration.[43,44]

The risk that adhesions to the mesh will form is substantially augmented if the mesh is left fully exposed to the bowel, as in the case with the IPOM technique. Even with the TAPP approach, the long-term durability and effectiveness of the sometimes flimsy peritoneal coverage have been questioned. Over the past 25 years, however, extensive intraperitoneal use of polypropylene mesh in abdominal wall reconstruction has rarely led to adhesions causing bowel obstruction. Nonetheless, either small bowel[40] or omentum[33] can be incarcerated at a defect in the peritoneal closure site, and reoperation may be required.

Urinary complications   Injuries to the urinary tract aside [*see* Complications of Dissection, *above*], urinary retention, urinary tract infection, and hematuria are the most common complications. Avoidance of bladder catheterization reduces the incidence of these complications, but urinary retention still occurs in 1.5% to 2.0% of patients. General anesthesia and the administration of large volumes of I.V. fluids may also predispose to retention.

Vas deferens and testicular complications Wantz[45] believes that the most common cause of postoperative testicular swelling, orchitis, and ischemic atrophy is surgical trauma to the testicular veins (i.e., venous congestion and subsequent thrombosis). Because spermatic cord dissection is minimized with the laparoscopic approach, the risk of groin and testicular complications resulting from injury to cord structures and adjacent nerves should be reduced. When the hernial sac is left undisturbed, there is less trauma to the cord, its vessels, and adjacent nerves.

Most testicular complications, such as swelling, pain, and epididymitis, are self-limited. Testicular pain occurs in about 1% of patients after laparoscopic repair,[34] an incidence comparable to that seen after open repair.[46] A similar number of patients experience testicular atrophy,[32] for which there is no specific treatment.

The risk of injury to the vas deferens appears to be much the same in laparoscopic repair as in open repair.[13] If fertility is an issue, the cut ends should be reapproximated if the injury is recognized intraoperatively.

Postoperative groin and thigh pain Unlike patients who undergo open anterior herniorrhaphy, in whom discomfort or numbness is usually localized to the operative area, patients who undergo laparoscopic repair occasionally describe unusual but specific symptoms of deep discomfort that are usually positional and are often of a transient, shooting nature suggestive of nerve irritation. The pain is frequently incited by stooping, twisting, or movements causing extension of the hip and can be shocklike. Although these symptoms can frequently be elicited in the early postoperative period, they are usually transient. If a neuralgia is present in the recovery room, however, prompt reexploration is the best approach.[13]

Persistent pain and burning sensations in the inguinal region, the upper medial thigh, or the spermatic cord and scrotal skin region occur when the genitofemoral nerve or the ilioinguinal nerve is stimulated, entrapped, or unintentionally injured. When these symptoms persist, they may result in severe morbidity.[47] A more worrisome symptom is lateral or central upper medial thigh numbness, which is reported in 1% to 2% of patients and often lasts several months or longer. Whether this numbness is related to staple entrapment, fibrous adhesions, cicatricial neuroma, or mesh irritation is unknown. Numbness and paresthesia of the lateral thigh are less frequent and are related to the involvement of fibers of the lateral cutaneous nerve. These problems can be prevented by paying careful attention to anatomic detail and technique.[48] After performing 50 cadaveric dissections to determine the relation of the nerves to the internal ring, Rosen and coworkers concluded that both the genitofemoral nerve and the lateral cutaneous nerve of the thigh will be protected in all cases if no staples are placed further than 1.5 cm lateral to the edge of the internal ring.[49]

A great deal of attention has rightly been focused on the risk of nerve injury with laparoscopic hernia repair as well as on ways of preventing it. At the same time, it is important to note that pain and numbness, including thigh numbness, can also occur after open repair and may in fact be more common in that setting than was previously realized. In one study, groin pain lasting longer than 1 month was present in 8% of patients after Lichtenstein repair but in no patients after TAPP.[33] A randomized study of 928 patients found that 1 year after operation, the laparoscopic group had a lower rate of persistent groin pain than the open mesh group (30% versus 37%) and a similar incidence of thigh numbness (14% versus 11%).[32]

Miscellaneous complications Early postoperative examination of patients who have undergone laparoscopic hernia repair frequently reveals groin bogginess, a cough impulse, and deep tenderness over the internal inguinal ring, particularly when the hernia was indirect and when the hernial sac was left in situ.[50] True hydroceles are rare. Well-defined, confined masses 1 to 3 cm in diameter are often palpated at the external inguinal ring or near the pubic tubercle. These typically represent hematomas,[50] which are more common when the sac has been dissected in a TAPP repair. Unlike the diffuse hematomas seen with open repair, these hematomas are very well defined and usually asymptomatic; however, they are very slow to disappear. These findings often mimic those of recurrent hernia and call for careful follow-up. Lipomas of the spermatic cord, if left unreduced in patients with indirect hernias, may produce a persistent groin mass and a cough impulse that mimic recurrence, especially to an uninitiated examiner. These lipomas are always asymptomatic.

OUTCOME EVALUATION

Although there is a large body of literature on laparoscopic inguinal hernia repair—including a variety of randomized controlled trials—the benefits of the laparoscopic approach have not yet been clearly defined or widely accepted. One reason may be that the literature can be difficult to summarize and understand. For example, studies have reported conflicting results: several randomized, controlled trials suggested that the laparoscopic technique offered little benefit,[28,29,34,51,52] but many trials reached the opposite conclusion.[24,30-33,35,36,43,53-57] Furthermore, different trials have compared different operations: TAPP repair, TEP repair, or a mixture of the two, on one hand, against open mesh repair, open sutured repair, or a mixture of the two, on the other hand.

Given the low morbidity and relatively short convalescence already associated with the conventional operation, demonstration of any significant improvements that might be associated with the laparoscopic operation would probably require large study samples. Thus, combining existing studies may be illuminating. In a meta-analysis that included studies performed up to March 1997, Chung and Rowland grouped 18 trials according to the operations compared.[58] In group 1, laparoscopic repair (TAPP, in most cases) was compared with open tension-free repair. In group 2, laparoscopic repair was compared with open sutured repair. In group 3, laparoscopic repair was compared with a mixture of open operations ("at the discretion of the surgeon"). In all comparisons, the laparoscopic operation took longer to perform. Compared with sutured repair, laparoscopic operation yielded significantly less postoperative pain and a significantly shorter recovery. Compared with tension-free repair, however, laparoscopic repair showed no significant advantage with respect to pain but resulted in a slightly shorter recovery (though the reduction was of marginal statistical significance). The results of the meta-analysis suggest that the postoperative course of open tension-free repair is different from that of open sutured repair, with the former clearly resulting in less postoperative pain and a shorter recovery. In that open tension-free repair uses mesh, it resembles laparoscopic repair more closely than open sutured repair does and thus is probably a more relevant comparison procedure. Accordingly, we will briefly review the findings of a number of recent studies that compare laparoscopic inguinal herniorrhaphy with open mesh repair.

Laparoscopic Repair versus Open Mesh Repair

At least 12 prospective, randomized trials comparing laparoscopic repair with open tension-free mesh repair were published in English between 1994 and 1999,[24,28-36,46,59] nine of which are summarized elsewhere [see Table 1]. The heterogeneity of the studies' designs (particularly with respect to the different types of repairs done and the different outcome measures assessed) makes direct comparisons difficult. For example, the laparoscopic methods used included TAPP repair alone (eight studies[24,28-31,33,34,59]), TEP repair alone (three studies[35,36,46]), and a combination of TAPP and TEP repair (one study[32]). The open methods used included Lichtenstein repair with local anesthesia (four studies[24,28,33,34]), Lichtenstein repair with general anesthesia (four studies[30,32,46,59]), open Stoppa preperitoneal repair with general anesthesia (two studies[31,35]), plug-and-patch repair with local anesthesia (one study[29]), and plug-and-patch repair with general anesthesia (one study[36]). Most of the studies included bilateral along with unilateral hernias.[24,28,32,33,35,36,46] The considerable differences between these 12 studies notwithstanding, several suggestive patterns do emerge.

Convalescence time The most significant short-term outcome measure after hernia repair is convalescence time, defined as the time required for the patient to return to normal activities. One of the most frequently cited benefits of laparoscopic herniorrhaphy is the patient's rapid return to unrestricted activity, including work. Most of the randomized studies comparing laparoscopic with open mesh repair, including the four largest, report a significantly shorter convalescence time after laparoscopic repair.[24,30-33,35,36] For example, in a study of 400 patients specifically designed to detect differences in convalescence at various defined levels, Wellwood and coworkers found that the self-reported time to return to normal household and social activities was significantly shorter after TAPP repair than after Lichtenstein repair with local anesthesia.[24] In a large multicenter cooperative trial of 928 patients in which TAPP or TEP was compared mainly with tension-free mesh repair, the laparoscopic group returned to normal social activities significantly faster than the open group (10 days versus 14 days).[32]

Convalescence time, particularly time off work, is a complex outcome measure that varies as much with patient expectation, motivation, and disability coverage as it does with surgical morbidity.[33,60] Moreover, measurement of convalescence is subject to bias if the assessor is not blinded to the treatment arm. Finally, the operating surgeon may not assess outcome in the same way as other unbiased observers[61] or the patients themselves would.

Postoperative pain After laparoscopic repair, most patients experience minimal immediate postoperative pain and have little or no need for analgesics after postoperative day 1. In addition, patients are generally able to perform some exercises better after laparoscopic repair than after Lichtenstein repair.[33] That patients experience less postoperative pain after laparoscopic repair than after open mesh repair has been reported in several randomized studies.[24,30,31,35,36,46] A meta-analysis of more than 500 patients in five trials, however, found that postoperative pain, measured on the basis either of analgesic administration or of ratings on a visual analog scale (VAS), was not significantly less after TAPP repair than after open tension-free repair.[58] Zieren and colleagues found no difference in postoperative pain assessed by VAS between 80 patients undergoing TAPP repair and 80 patients undergoing open plug-and-patch repair; however, both groups had significantly lower VAS scores than did 80 patients undergoing Shouldice repair[29]— a finding consistent with almost all of the reports comparing laparoscopic repair with open sutured repair.[43]

Quality of life The studies that have assessed quality of life immediately after hernia repair have tended to favor the laparoscopic approach, albeit marginally. Using the SF-36 (a widely accepted general health–related quality-of-life questionnaire), Wellwood and coworkers found that at 1 month, greater improvements from baseline were apparent in the laparoscopic group in every dimension except general health; however, by 3 months, the differences between the two groups were no longer significant.[24] The MRC group also found no differences in any SF-36 domains at 3 months after operation.[32] Filipi and associates, using the Sickness Impact Profile, found some benefit to the laparoscopic approach.[59]

Bilateral hernias Laparoscopy allows simultaneous exploration of the abdominal cavity and diagnosis and treatment of bilateral groin hernias as well as of coexisting femoral hernias (which are often unrecognized preoperatively), without added risk or disability. Many surgeons avoid performing simultaneous bilateral repair during an open procedure because of the resulting increase in swelling, pain, disability, operative time, and the risk of infection and recurrence. One retrospective study found that simultaneous repair of bilateral hernias via the laparoscopic approach resulted in a shorter convalescence time and a quicker return to work than a modified Shouldice repair.[62] In a prospective, randomized study, Paganini and colleagues found in subgroup analysis that the mean operative time did not differ significantly between bilateral laparoscopic repair and bilateral open mesh repair (85.7 ± 32.2 minutes for TAPP repair versus 75.9 ± 43.3 minutes for open repair).[28] Further prospective, randomized trials designed to compare simultaneous bilateral open tension-free repair with bilateral laparoscopic repair should be undertaken.

Hernia recurrence Open mesh repair has been associated with long-term recurrence rates of 1% or less, even when not performed by hernia specialists.[63,64] If the laparoscopic approach is to be a viable alternative to open repair, it should have comparable results.

In fact, the short-term experience with laparoscopic hernia repair is encouraging. Case series of TAPP and TEP repairs demonstrate recurrence rates ranging from 0% to 2%, with especially low recurrence rates reported after TEP repair.[65] Of the 12 randomized studies of laparoscopic repair versus open mesh repair mentioned earlier (see above), only one found a significant difference in recurrence rates, reporting seven recurrences in 468 laparoscopic patients and no recurrences in 460 open repairs.[32] All seven recurrences occurred in patients who underwent TAPP repair, even though TAPP accounted for only 21% of the laparoscopic repairs.

Most reported recurrences after laparoscopic herniorrhaphy come at an early stage in the surgeon's experience with this procedure and soon after operation.[15] The majority can be attributed to (1) the surgeon's imperfect understanding of the preperitoneal anatomy and the anatomic landmarks for mesh fixation, which leads to inadequate preperitoneal dissection; (2) use of an inadequately sized patch, which fails to provide support for the entire inguinal area, including direct, indirect, and femoral spaces; or (3) staple failure. Secure fascial fixation of the prosthesis is a paramount concern, particularly with TAPP repair; accurate stapling technique, with careful placement of each staple, is vital to prevention of recurrence.

Once a hernia recurs after an initial open repair, laparoscopic repair may be a particularly suitable treatment approach.[66] Normal anatomic and cord structures are not distorted by scar tissue in the preperitoneal space, dissection planes are unmarred, and the risk of causing testicular damage is reduced. The recurrence is usually very well seen and better defined from the peritoneal aspect, and the entire myopectineal inguinal floor can be reinforced and repaired without tension and without the need to use scarred or weakened tissue, which predisposes to further recurrence. Unfortunately, there are few controlled studies that have examined recurrent hernias exclusively. In one randomized study of 79 patients in which TAPP repair of recurrent hernias was compared with open preperitoneal repair, patients experienced less pain and had a shorter convalescence after TAPP repair; however, there were seven recurrences after TAPP repair and only one after open repair.[67]

Transabdominal Preperitoneal Repair versus Totally Extraperitoneal Repair

The TAPP approach is easier to learn and perform than the TEP approach, and even experienced laparoscopic hernia surgeons report more technical difficulties with the latter.[68] Nonetheless, there is a growing body of literature to suggest that TEP repair, by avoiding entry into the peritoneal cavity, provides significant advantages over TAPP repair.[3] In particular, the TEP approach should eliminate trocar site hernias, small bowel injury and obstruction, and intraperitoneal adhesions to the mesh. Kald and colleagues consecutively performed TAPP repairs in 339 patients and TEP repairs in 87 patients, then followed the patients for a mean of 23 and 7 months, respectively.[69] Time off work was shorter after TEP. In the 426 patients studied, 15 major complications were noted, including one death, two bowel obstructions, one severe neuralgia, three trocar site hernias, one epigastric artery hemorrhage, and seven recurrences; all except the epigastric artery hemorrhage occurred in the TAPP group. It is possible, however, that these results can be partly explained by the learning curve, in that the TAPP repairs were all done before the TEP repairs. That six TAPP recurrences occurred in the first 31 cases, whereas only one occurred in the subsequent 395 patients, lends support to this possibility.

In a study comparing 733 TAPP repairs with 382 TEP repairs, 11 major complications occurred in the TAPP group (two recurrences, six trocar hernias, one small bowel obstruction, and two small bowel injuries), whereas only one recurrence and no intraperitoneal complications occurred in the TEP group.[70] Seven TEP procedures were converted to TAPP procedures. Time off work was equal in the two groups but was prolonged in patients receiving compensation. As in the Kald study, the TAPP patients were followed longer than the TEP patients, and the TAPP cases occupied the first part of the learning curve. To avoid this type of selection bias would require a randomized study.

Not all surgeons are convinced that TEP repair is the laparoscopic procedure of choice. Cohen and coworkers compared 108 TAPP repairs with 100 TEP repairs.[68] Although the TEP repairs were done only by surgeons who were already familiar with TAPP repair, many of the surgeons still encountered technical difficulties and problems with landmark identification. Overall, complications did not occur significantly more frequently in either group, but they seemed more severe in the TAPP group: four trocar site hernias, one bladder injury, and six seromas were noted in the TAPP group, compared with one cellulitis and six seromas in the TEP group. The authors concluded that because TAPP repair is easier and does not increase complications significantly, it is an "adequate" procedure. The sample size may have been too small to permit detection of small differences in complication rates.

Laparoscopic Incisional Hernia Repair

Incisional hernias develop in approximately 2% to 11% of patients undergoing laparotomy.[71,72] It has been estimated that 90,000 ventral hernia repairs are carried out in the United States every year.[4] Open incisional hernia repair can be a difficult procedure and may carry a high morbidity. Without prosthetic mesh, repair of large incisional hernias is associated with recurrence rates as high as 50%; in addition, it can be associated with significant complications and a substantial hospital stay.

Laparoscopic repair of incisional hernia was initially described in 1992,[8] and it remains an emerging procedure. Taking a laparoscopic approach allows the surgeon to minimize the abdominal wall incisions, avoid extensive flap dissection and muscle mobilization, and eliminate the need for drains in proximity to the mesh, thereby potentially achieving decreases in pain, recovery time, and duration of hospitalization as well as lower rates of surgical site infections. In addition, the improved visualization of the abdominal wall associated with the laparoscopic view may result in better definition of the defect, the discovery of unrecognized hernia sites, and improved adhesiolysis. If this improved visualization permits more precise and accurate placement and tailoring of the mesh, recurrence rates may also be decreased.

Laparoscopic incisional hernia repair is best suited for repairing large incisional hernias, which may be defined as any incisional hernia in which the smallest diameter is greater than 3 cm. With these large defects, prosthetic material must be used to ensure tension-free repair of the hernia, which reduces the risk of recurrence. Smaller hernias can usually be repaired without mesh, often on an outpatient basis; there is little to be gained by adopting a laparoscopic approach to these defects. Both upper abdominal and lower abdominal incisions are amenable to a laparoscopic approach. The so-called Swiss cheese hernia, which comprises multiple small defects, is particularly well suited to this approach: open repair would necessitate a large incision for access to the multiple fascial defects. Incarcerated hernias can also be approached laparoscopically; however, the suspected presence of compromised bowel is an absolute contraindication. An abdomen that has undergone multiple operations and contains dense adhesions presents a challenge in terms of both access to the abdominal cavity and access to the hernia site. If the surgeon cannot obtain safe access to the peritoneal cavity for insufflation, a laparoscopic approach is contraindicated.

To date, very few comparative trials focusing on laparoscopic incisional herniorrhaphy have been reported. We will therefore concentrate on the technique we currently employ for the repair.

OPERATIVE PLANNING

Preparation

Formal mechanical and antibiotic bowel preparation is administered if it is suspected that there is incarcerated bowel in the hernia. With the patient straining, the edges of the hernia defect are marked on the skin whenever possible. If the defect is in the lower abdomen, a Foley catheter is placed in the bladder. Prophylactic antibiotics are not routinely administered. The procedure is performed with the patient under general anesthesia.

Positioning

The patient is placed in the supine position with the arms extended. If the hernia is in the midline, the surgeon can stand on either side of the patient, with the monitor directly opposite. Initially, the assistant stands on the same side as the surgeon; however, he or she may later have to move to the opposite side to help with dissection and stapling. A second monitor on the opposite side of the table is useful. If the defect is subcostal, the surgeon may prefer to operate from between the patient's legs, with a monitor at the head of the bed.

Equipment

Because laparoscopic incisional hernia repair leaves the mesh exposed to the intraperitoneal cavity, some concern has arisen about the risk of adhesion formation and fistulization if polypropylene mesh is used. A polytetrafluoroethylene (PTFE) prosthesis would have a reduced propensity for adhesion formation and could be more safely placed in an intraperitoneal position, but PTFE is much harder to manipulate laparoscopically than polypropylene and is a less effective scaffold for ingrowth of collagen. We currently use Composix mesh (Bard, Davol Inc., Cranston, Rhode Island), which consists of PTFE on the side facing the peritoneal cavity and two layers of polypropylene mesh on the side facing the abdominal wall. This mesh marries the strength of Marlex with the safety of PTFE.

Additional special equipment used for incisional hernia repair includes 2-0 nonabsorbable sutures, a Keith needle, a 2 mm suture passer, a sterile marking pen, and a stapler (typically, a 12 mm 65° device that uses 4.8 mm staples). Atraumatic bowel instruments are required to reduce incarcerated intestines without injuring them. An ultrasonic scalpel is useful if extensive adhesiolysis is required: it helps expedite the procedure while improving hemostasis.

OPERATIVE TECHNIQUE

In essence, the repair consists of the intraperitoneal placement of a large piece of mesh so that it overlaps the defect in the fascia and the abdominal wall. The defect is not closed. The mesh is anchored with a minimum of four subcutaneously tied transfascial sutures placed at the four corners and is further secured between the sutures with intraperitoneally placed staples.

Step 1: Placement of Trocars

Because of the probability of extensive intra-abdominal adhesions, we begin with open insertion of a blunt 12 mm trocar. This trocar is inserted laterally, at the level of the middle of the hernia, rather than in the midline, even though doing so necessitates dissecting through several layers of muscle.

A 30° scope is then inserted. As in inguinal repair, an angled scope is essential because dissection and repair are done on the undersurface of the anterior abdominal wall, which cannot be adequately visualized with a 0° scope. Laparoscopy is performed and the hernial defect identified. Two additional 5 mm ports are then placed on the same side as the surgeon. These ports are placed superior and inferior to the initial trocar and should be located as far laterally as possible, with care taken to ensure that the downward movement of the instruments is not limited by the iliac crest or the thigh. Lateral placement is necessary to optimize exposure of the abdominal wall.

Once all adhesions to the abdominal wall have been dissected sufficiently (see below), a fourth port can be placed on the opposite side to facilitate adhesiolysis and mesh fixation. As noted, some of the ports can be 5 mm, depending on the caliber of the instruments available. Ultimately, port placement depends on the hernia's location, the patient's body habitus, and the surgeon's preference.

Step 2: Exposure of Hernial Defect

The edges of the hernial defect are exposed by reducing the contents of the hernia into the abdominal cavity. All adhesions from bowel or omentum to the abdominal wall in the vicinity of the defect must be transected. This dissection may be performed with cautery scissors or a hook cautery. An ultrasonic scalpel may be useful for optimizing hemostasis if extensive vascularized adhesions are encountered. It is not necessary to excise or reduce the hernial sac itself [see Figure 16].

Step 3: Tailoring of Mesh

The contours of the hernia defect are marked as accurately as possible on the exterior abdominal wall; the edges may be delineated with a combination of palpation and visualization. A rough pictorial representation of the swatch of mesh that will be required is then drawn on the skin around the hernial defect, with care taken to overlap the edges of the defect by at least 2 cm on all sides [see Figure 17]. This template is measured, and the mesh swatch is cut to its dimensions. The four corners of the swatch and those of its representation on the abdominal wall are numbered clockwise from 1 to 4 for later orientation. A mark is made on the inner side of the mesh so that the surgeon can easily determine which side is to face the peritoneum once the mesh is inserted into the peritoneal cavity. A 2-0 Prolene suture is tied in each corner of the mesh swatch, and both ends are left about 15 cm long. Thicker suture material is not easily passed through the abdominal wall.

The mesh swatch is rolled as tightly as possible around a grasping forceps, then introduced into the peritoneal cavity. Small swatches can be inserted through a 12 mm trocar[4]; for larger pieces, we remove a large trocar, enlarge the incision, and insert the mesh directly into the abdomen. The trocar is then repositioned.

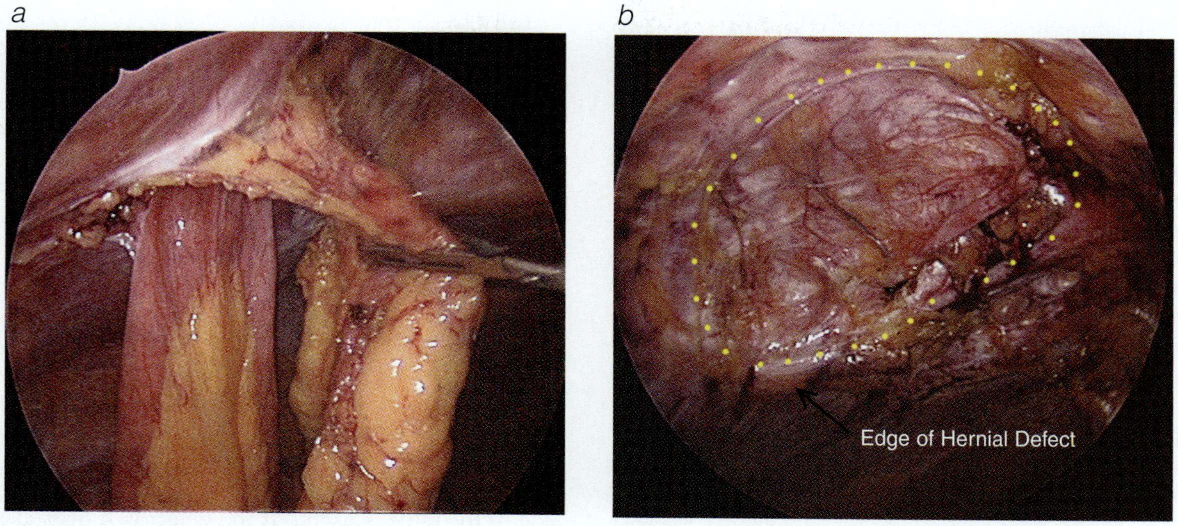

Figure 16 Laparoscopic incisional hernia repair. (*a*) Shown is dissection of incarcerated small bowel and omentum from an incisional hernia. (*b*) After adhesiolysis, the edges of the defect can be seen.

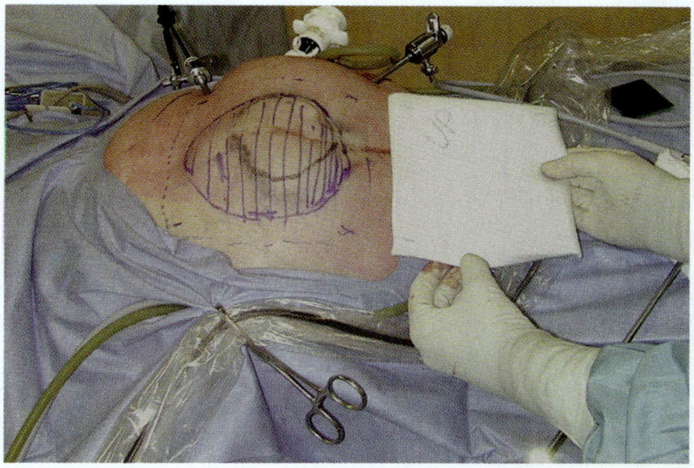

Figure 17 Laparoscopic incisional hernia repair. An outline of the hernial defect is drawn on the abdominal wall, with a 2 cm margin marked around the defect to serve as a template for tailoring the mesh. The four corners of the mesh swatch and of the template are numbered to facilitate orientation of the mesh once it is inside the peritoneal cavity. Patient's head is to the left.

Step 4: Fixation of Mesh

Once the mesh swatch has been introduced into the abdomen, it is unfurled and spread out, with the previously placed corner sutures facing the fascia and oriented so that the four numbered corners are aligned with the numbers marked on the abdominal wall. Small skin incisions are then made in two lateral corners. Through each of these incisions, a suture passer is inserted to grasp one tail of the previously placed 2-0 Prolene suture and pull it out through the abdominal wall, then reintroduced through the incision to pull out the second tail. Each suture is then tied and buried in the subcutaneous tissue so as to anchor the mesh to the fascia and maintain its proper orientation. Once two corners are secured, the mesh is spread out tautly and the other two corners secured in a similar fashion. A stapler is then used to tack the mesh circumferentially at 1 cm intervals [*see Figure 18*].

If multiple defects are present over a large area, we overlap multiple swatches of mesh rather than use a single large swatch, which is cumbersome to manipulate laparoscopically.

Step 5: Closure

The pneumoperitoneum is released. The fascia at any trocar site larger than 10 mm is closed. The skin is then closed with subcuticular sutures.

POSTOPERATIVE CARE

The Foley catheter is removed at the end of the procedure. Patients are admitted to the hospital. Oral intake is begun when bowel sounds are present and there is no abdominal distention; when this state is reached varies according to the extent of adhesiolysis and bowel manipulation required to liberate the contents of the hernial sac. Patients are discharged when a full diet is tolerated. Patients are warned that fluid may accumulate at the hernia site. Any fever or redness should be reported.

OUTCOME EVALUATION

Several series of laparoscopic incisional hernia repairs have been reported. In preparation for a randomized trial, Toy and colleagues described 144 patients at multiple centers who were operated on with a standardized technique and followed prospectively.[4] The mean operating time was about 2 hours. Two enterotomies were made intraoperatively. The most common postoperative complication was wound seroma, which occurred in 23 patients (16%). Surgical site infection occurred in five patients (3%). Two patients required removal of the mesh. One experienced bowel obstruction. Recurrences were observed in eight cases (6%) after a mean follow-up of 222 days. In a study of 122 laparoscopic incisional hernia repairs reported by Franklin and associates, there was one recurrence after a mean follow-up of 30.1 months.[6]

Park and colleagues compared 56 prospective laparoscopic incisional hernia repairs with 49 open incisional hernia repairs assessed through retrospective chart review.[7] The groups were comparable in terms of patient characteristics and hernia size. Although the mean operating time was longer in the laparoscopic group (95.4 minutes versus 78.5 minutes), the postoperative length of stay was significantly shorter after laparoscopic repair than after open repair (3.4 days versus 6.5 days). Overall, there were significantly fewer complications after laparoscopic repair. There were fewer recurrences after laparoscopic repair than after open repair (six versus 17); the mean follow-up time was 24.1 months, but follow-up was significantly longer after open repair, for which the data were collected retrospectively.

Carbajo and colleagues compared 30 laparoscopic incisional hernia repairs with 30 open repairs in a randomized trial.[5] There were no intraoperative complications in the laparoscopic group and two enterotomies in the open group. The mean operating time was significantly shorter in the laparoscopic group (87 minutes versus 111.5 minutes), as was the postoperative length of stay (2.23 days versus 9.06 days). One patient in each group required reoperation for bowel obstruction; in the laparoscopic group, this complication was attributable to incarceration of the bowel between the mesh and the abdominal wall. There were fewer wound complications in the laparoscopic group. After a minimum follow-up of 18 months, no recurrences were noted in the laparoscopic group and two in the open group.

Although the results of other large randomized trials are not available yet, preliminary work suggests that the laparoscopic approach to the repair of large incisional hernias is highly promising. The laparoscopic approach seems to confer the well-known benefits of other video-assisted procedures (e.g., quicker recovery) while comparing favorably to the open operation in terms of complication and recurrence rates.

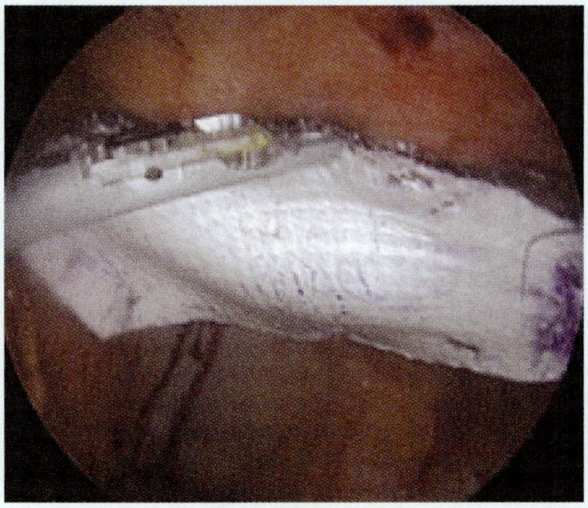

Figure 18 Laparoscopic incisional hernia repair. The mesh is secured to the peritoneum with sutures and staples.

References

1. Ger R, Monroe K, Duvivier R, et al: Management of indirect hernias by laparoscopic closure of the neck of the sac. Am J Surg 159:370, 1990
2. Robbins AW, Rutkow IM: Mesh plug repair and groin hernia surgery. Surg Clin North Am 78:1007, 1998
3. Crawford DL, Phillips EH: Laparoscopic repair and groin hernia surgery. Surg Clin North Am 78:1047, 1998
4. Toy FK, Bailey RW, Carey S, et al: Prospective, multicenter study of laparoscopic ventral hernioplasty: preliminary results. Surg Endosc 12:955, 1998
5. Carbajo MA, Martin del Olmo JC, Blanco JI, et al: Laparoscopic treatment vs open surgery in the solution of major incisional and abdominal wall hernias with mesh. Surg Endosc 13:250, 1999
6. Franklin ME, Dorman JP, Glass JL, et al: Laparoscopic ventral hernia repair. Surg Laparosc Endosc 8:294, 1998
7. Park A, Birch DW, Lovrics P: Laparoscopic and open incisional hernia repair: a comparison study. Surgery 124:816, 1998
8. LeBlanc KA, Booth WV: Laparoscopic repair of incisional abdominal hernias using expanded polytetrafluorethylene: preliminary findings. Surg Laparosc Endosc 3:39, 1992
9. Skandalakis JE, Gray SW, Skandalakis LJ, et al: Surgical anatomy of the inguinal area. World J Surg 13:490, 1989
10. Spaw AT, Ennis BW, Spaw LP: Laparoscopic hernia repair: the anatomic basis. J Laparoendosc Surg 1:269, 1991
11. Wantz GE: Atlas of Hernia Surgery. Raven Press, New York, 1991
12. Condon RE: The anatomy of the inguinal region and its relation to groin hernia. Hernia, 3rd ed. Nyhus LM, Condon RE, Eds. JB Lippincott Co, Philadelphia, 1989, p 18
13. Memon MA, Fitzgibbons RJ: Laparoscopic inguinal hernia repair: transabdominal (TAPP) and totally extraperitoneal (TEP). The SAGES Manual. Scott-Connor CEH, Ed. Springer, New York, 1999
14. Ramshaw BJ, Tucker JG, Conner T, et al: A comparison of the approaches to laparoscopic herniorrhaphy. Surg Endosc 10:29, 1996
15. Fitzgibbons RJ Jr, Camps J, Cornet DA, et al: Laparoscopic inguinal herniorrhaphy: results of a multicenter trial. Ann Surg 221:3, 1995
16. Arregui ME. Transabdominal retroperitoneal inguinal herniorrhaphy. Operative Laparoscopy and Thoracoscopy. MacFayden BV, Ponsky JL, Eds. Lippincott-Raven, Philadelphia, 1996
17. Felix H, Michas C: Double buttress laparoscopic herniorrhaphy. J Laparoendosc Surg 3:1, 1993
18. McKernan JB, Laws HL: Laparoscopic repair of inguinal hernias using a totally extraperitoneal prosthetic approach. Surg Endosc 7:26, 1993
19. Stoppa R, Warlaumont C, Verhaeghe P, et al: Dacron mesh and surgical therapy of inguinal hernia. Chir Patol Sper 34:15, 1986
20. Stoppa R, Warlaumont CR: The preperitoneal approach and prosthetic repair of groin hernias. Hernia, 3rd ed. Nyhus LM, Condon RE, Eds. JB Lippincott Co, Philadelphia, 1989
21. Stoppa R: The treatment of complicated groin and incisional hernias. World J Surg 13:545, 1989
22. Wantz GE: Giant prosthetic reinforcement of the visceral sac. Surg Gynecol Obstet 169:408, 1989
23. McKernan JB: Extraperitoneal inguinal herniorrhaphy. Operative Laparoscopy and Thoracoscopy. MacFayden BV, Ponsky JL, Eds. Lippincott-Raven, Philadelphia, 1996
24. Wellwood J, Sculpher MJ, Stoker D, et al: Randomized clinical trial of laparoscopic versus open mesh repair for inguinal hernia: outcome and cost. BMJ 317:103, 1998
25. Amado WJ: Anesthesia for hernia surgery. Surg Clin North Am 73:427, 1993
26. Ferzli G, Sayad P, Hallak A, et al: Endoscopic extraperitoneal hernia repair: a 5-year experience. Surg Endosc 12:1311, 1998
27. Ferzli G, Sayad P, Vasisht B: The feasibility of laparoscopic extraperitoneal hernia repair under local anesthesia. Surg Endosc 13:588, 1999
28. Paganini AM, Lezoche E, Carle F, et al: A randomized controlled clinical study of laparoscopic vs. open tension-free inguinal hernia repair. Surg Endosc 12:979, 1998
29. Zieren J, Zieren H, Jacobi CA, et al: Prospective randomized study comparing laparoscopic and open tension-free inguinal hernia repair with Shouldice's operation. Am J Surg 175:330, 1998
30. Heikkinen T, Haukipuro K, Leppälä J, et al: Total costs of laparoscopic and Lichtenstein inguinal hernia repairs: a prospective study. Surg Lap Endosc 7:1, 1997
31. Johansson B, Hallerbäck B, Glise H, et al: Laparoscopic mesh *versus* open preperitoneal mesh *versus* conventional technique for inguinal hernia repair. A randomized multicenter trial (SCUR Hernia Repair Study). Ann Surg 230:225, 1999
32. The MRC Laparoscopic Groin Hernia Trial Group: Laparoscopic versus open repair of groin hernia: a randomised comparison. Lancet 354:185, 1999
33. Payne JH, Grininger LM, Isawa MT, et al: Laparoscopic or open inguinal herniorrhaphy? a randomized prospective trial. Arch Surg 129:973, 1994
34. Heikkinen TJ, Haukipuro K, Hulkko A: A cost and outcome comparison between laparoscopic and Lichtenstein hernia operations in a day-case unit: a randomized prospective study. Surg Endosc 12:1199, 1998
35. Champault GG, Rizk N, Catheline J-M, et al: Inguinal hernia repair. Totally preperitoneal laparoscopic approach versus Stoppa operation: randomized trial of 100 cases. Surg Lap Endosc 7:445, 1997
36. Khoury N: A randomized prospective controlled trial of laparoscopic extraperitoneal hernia repair and mesh-plug hernioplasty: a study of 315 cases. J Laparoendosc Surg 8:367, 1998
37. Phillips EH, Arregui ME, Carroll BJ, et al: Incidence of complications following laparoscopic hernioplasty. Surg Endosc 9:16, 1995
38. Salerno GM, Fitzgibbons RJ Jr, Filipi CJ: Laparoscopic inguinal hernia repair. Surgical Laparoscopy. Zucker KA, Ed. Quality Medical Publishing, St Louis, 1991
39. MacFayden BV Jr, Arregui M, Corbitt J, et al: Complications of laparoscopic herniorrhaphy. Surg Endosc 7:155, 1993
40. Phillips EH, Arregui M, Carroll BJ, et al: Incidence of complications following laparoscopic hernioplasty. Surg Endosc 9:16, 1995
41. Estour E, Mouret PH: Cure laparoscopique des hernies de l'aine. J Coelio Chir 16:15, 1995
42. Avtan L, Avci C, Bulut T, et al: Mesh infections after laparoscopic inguinal hernia repair. Surg Laparosc Endosc 7:192, 1997
43. Leim NSL, Van der Graaf Y, van Steensel CJ, et al: Comparison of conventional anterior surgery and laparoscopic surgery for inguinal hernia repair. N Engl J Med 336:1541, 1997
44. Ferzli GS, Frezza EE, Pecorato AM Jr, et al: Prospective randomized study of stapled versus unstapled mesh in a laparoscopic preperitoneal inguinal hernia repair. J Am Coll Surg 188:461, 1999
45. Wantz GE: Ambulatory surgical treatment of groin hernia: prevention and management of complications. Problems in General Surgery 3:311, 1986
46. Wright DM, Kennedy A, Baxter JN, et al: Early outcome after open versus extraperitoneal endoscopic tension-free hernioplasty: a randomized clinical trial. Surgery 119:552, 1996
47. Starling JR, Harms BA: Diagnosis and treatment of genitofemoral and ilioinguinal neuralgia. World J Surg 13:586, 1989
48. Kraus MA: Nerve injury during laparoscopic inguinal hernia repair. Surg Laparosc Endosc 3:342, 1993
49. Rosen A, Halevy A: Anatomical basis for nerve injury during laparoscopic hernia repair. Surg Laparosc Endosc 7:469, 1997
50. Wexler MJ, Meakins JL, Garzon J: Laparoscopic groin hernia repair: preliminary results from a prospective clinical trial. Can J Surg 36:384, 1993
51. Lawrence K, McWhinnie O, Goodwin, et al: Randomized controlled trial of laparoscopic vs. open repair of inguinal hernia: early results. Br J Surg 311:981, 1995
52. Bassell JR, Baxter P, Riddell F, et al: A randomized controlled trial of laparoscopic extraperitoneal hernia repair as a day surgical procedure. Surg Endosc 10:495, 1996
53. Kald A, Anderberg B, Carisson P, et al: Surgical outcome and cost-minimization analyses of laparoscopic and open hernia repair: a randomised prospective trial with one-year follow up. Eur J Surg 163:505, 1997
54. Kozol R, Lange PN, Kosir N, et al: A prospective randomized study of open vs. laparoscopic inguinal hernia repair. Arch Surg 132:292, 1997
55. Stoker DL, Spiegelhalter DJ, Singh R, et al: Laparoscopic versus open inguinal hernia repair: randomised prospective trial. Lancet 343:1243, 1994
56. Schrenk P, Woisetschlager R, Reiger R, et al: Prospective randomized trial comparing postoperative pain and return to physical activity after transabdominal preperitoneal, total preperitoneal, or Shouldice technique for inguinal hernia repair. Br J Surg 83:1563, 1996
57. Vogt DM, Curet MJ, Pitcher DE, et al: Preliminary results of a prospective randomized trial of laparoscopic onlay versus conventional inguinal herniorrhaphy. Am J Surg 169:84, 1995
58. Chung RS, Rowland DY: Meta-analysis of randomized controlled trials of laparoscopic vs conventional inguinal hernia repairs. Surg Endosc 13:689, 1999
59. Filipi CJ, Gaston-Johansson F, McBride PJ, et al: An assessment of pain and return to normal activity: laparoscopic herniorrhaphy vs open tension-free Lichtenstein repair. Surg Endosc 10:983, 1996
60. Barkun JS, Keyser EJ, Wexler MJ, et al: Short-term outcomes in open vs. laparoscopic herniorrhaphy: confounding impact of worker's compensation on convalescence. J Gastrointest Surg 3:575, 1999
61. Barkun JS, Barkun AN, Sampalis JS, et al: Randomized controlled trial of laparoscopic versus mini cholecystomy. Lancet 340:1116, 1992
62. Krähenbühl L, Schäfer M, Schilling M, et al: Simultaneous repair of bilateral groin hernias: open or lap-

63. Lichtenstein IL, Shulman AG, Amid PK: The cause, prevention, and treatment of recurrent groin hernia. Surg Clin North Am 73:529, 1993
64. Robbins AW, Rutkow IM: Mesh plug repair and groin hernia surgery. Surg Clin North Am 78:1007, 1998
65. Lowham AS, Filipi CJ, Fitzgibbons RJ, et al: Mechanisms of hernia recurrence after preperitoneal mesh repair: traditional and laparoscopic. Ann Surg 225:422, 1997
66. Memon MA, Rice D, Donohue JH: Laparoscopic herniorrhaphy. J Am Coll Surg 184:325, 1997
67. Beets GL, Dirksen CD, Go PM, et al: Open or laparoscopic preperitoneal mesh repair for recurrent inguinal hernia? A randomized controlled trial. Surg Endosc 13:323, 1999
68. Cohen RV, Alvarez G, Roll S, et al: Transabdominal or totally extraperitoneal laparoscopic hernia repair? Surg Laparosc Endosc 8:264, 1998
69. Kald A, Anderberg B, Smedh K, et al: Transperitoneal or totally extraperitoneal approach in laparoscopic hernia repair: results of 491 consecutive herniorrhaphies. Surg Laparosc Endosc 7:86, 1997
70. Felix EL, Michas CA, Gonzalez MH Jr: Laparoscopic hernioplasty: TAPP vs TEP. Surg Endosc 9:984, 1995
71. Hesselink VJ, Luijendik RW, de Wilt JHW, et al: An evaluation of risk factors in incisional hernia recurrence. Surg Gynecol Obstet 176:228, 1993
72. Santora TA, Roslyn JJ: Incisional hernia. Surg Clin North Am 73:557, 1993

Acknowledgment

Figures 1, 4 through 7, 8 (right), 14, and 15   Tom Moore.

62 VASCULAR AND PERITONEAL ACCESS

Bernard Montreuil, M.D., Laurie Morrison, M.D., Lawrence Rosenberg, M.D., Ph.D., and Carl Nohr, M.D., Ph.D.

Vascular Access via Arteriovenous Fistulas

The number of patients with end-stage renal disease (ESRD) in the United States increased steadily through the 1990s, reaching 300,000 by the end of 1997.[1] Extracorporeal dialysis of blood was introduced in 1943 by Kolff and associates[2]; however, application of this approach was hindered by the requirement for repeated and routine access to the circulation. The full potential of hemodialysis for patient salvage was realized only after the introduction of the external arteriovenous (AV) shunt by Quinton and colleagues in 1960[3] and of the endogenous AV fistula (AVF) by Brescia and coworkers in 1966.[4] The subsequent introduction of synthetic vascular prostheses has permitted continued access in patients who have exhausted peripheral venous sites[5]; however, the long-term performance of such prostheses remains inferior to that of autogenous fistulas. The creation and maintenance of functioning vascular access, along with the associated complications, constitute the most common cause of morbidity, hospitalization, and cost in patients with end-stage renal disease.

The ideal vascular access route permits a flow rate that is adequate for the dialysis prescription (≥ 300 ml/min), can be used for extended periods, and has a low complication rate. The native AVF remains the gold standard. In 1997, the National Kidney Foundation Dialysis Outcome and Quality Initiative (NKF-DOQI)[6] organized multidisciplinary work groups that evaluated all available data on vascular access and concluded that quality of life and overall outcome could be improved significantly for hemodialysis patients if two primary goals were achieved:

1. Increased placement of native AVFs: a minimum of 50% of new dialysis patients should have primary AVFs.
2. Detection of dysfunctional access before thrombosis of the access route occurs.

OPERATIVE PLANNING

At least 4 to 6 weeks—preferably 3 to 4 months—is required for a native AVF to heal and mature before it can be used. Therefore, access planning should be done early in the course of progressive renal failure. Patients should be referred for surgical treatment when creatinine clearance approaches 25 ml/min, the serum creatinine level reaches 4 mg/dl, or dialysis is likely to be necessary within 1 year. Every effort should be made not to puncture forearm veins, particularly the cephalic veins of the nondominant arm; the dorsal hand veins may be used for venipuncture. Subclavian vein catheterization should also be avoided because of the risk of central vein stenosis, which may preclude the use of any part of the ipsilateral arm for vascular access.

Assessment of Venous System

A history of subclavian vein cannulation or transvenous pacemaker placement is associated with a 10% to 40% rate of central vein stenosis or thrombosis.[7] Previous injuries or operative procedures involving the arm, the neck, or the chest, including previous vascular access, also may give rise to significant venous abnormalities. Physical signs of venous outflow obstruction include extremity edema, differences in arm size, and development of collateral veins. All of these historical and physical findings call for investigation by means of phlebography or color flow duplex scanning.[8] Central vein stenosis greater than 50% is a contraindication to creation of an ipsilateral distal AVF: it is a predictor of venous hypertension and edema in the arm and of poor function in the fistula.

Selection of the ideal vein for access is facilitated by distending the veins with a tourniquet around the upper arm. In particular, the cephalic vein is palpated from the region of the anatomic snuffbox to the area above the elbow. Percussion of the vein is performed to confirm that it is patent and to rule out stenosis from previous venipuncture. The fingertips of one hand are positioned over the vein at the elbow, and the vein is gently tapped distally with the other hand. If the vein is patent and of substantial diameter, a fluid wave is felt over the proximal vein.

Assessment of Arterial System

A history of arterial trauma or catheterization, diabetes mellitus, or peripheral arterial disease may be associated with chronic damage to the arterial system. Physical examination involves palpation of the pulses (including both brachial and axillary pulses) and comparison of blood pressure in the arms. A difference of more than 20 mm Hg between the two sides suggests proximal arterial occlusive disease, which may cause the AVF to fail as a result of inadequate inflow. An Allen test is also performed to confirm that the palmar arch is patent, to determine which artery is the dominant vascular supply to the hand, and to ensure that the ulnar artery can support the hand if the radial artery must be divided. Any abnormality on physical examination should be further investigated by means of arterial studies in the vascular laboratory; in select cases, angiography may be indicated.

Noninvasive Preoperative Assessment

Systematic use of noninvasive evaluation in the vascular laboratory permits objective assessment of arterial and venous conduits. If necessary, venous conduits other than the cephalic and basilic veins may be identified,[9] and both arterial and venous segments may be mapped with skin marks to facilitate the operative procedure. The aims are to increase the use of autogenous fistulas and to raise the early and late patency rates by decreasing the use of suboptimal veins and arteries.

Complete noninvasive assessment includes segmental pressure measurements of the upper extremity, arterial waveform recording, and arterial and venous duplex studies. A tourniquet should be placed on the arm, and tapping and stroking maneuvers should be used to distend the vein maximally. Established criteria [see Table 1] are then applied to determine whether venous outflow and arterial inflow are likely to be satisfactory.

Choice of Type of AVF

Multiple varieties of AV fistulas have been used in hemodialysis patients. According to the NKF-DOQI report,[6] the order of preference for AV fistulas in patients requiring long-term hemodialysis is as follows:

1. Wrist (radiocephalic) primary AV fistula.
2. Elbow (brachiocephalic) primary AV fistula.

If neither of these can be constructed, access may be achieved via either of the following:

3. AV graft of synthetic material.
4. Transposed brachiobasilic AV fistula.

All of these fistulas should be established in the nondominant arm, if possible.

The distal radiocephalic AVF remains the gold standard in terms of ease of creation and long-term results. Its advantages considerably outweigh its disadvantages—namely, a higher primary failure rate (10% to 15%) and a long maturation time (1 to 4 months). Radiocephalic AVFs may be constructed either in the anatomic snuff-box or just above the wrist crease. Although the radial artery is smaller in the snuff-box than it is at the classical Brescia-Cimino fistula site, the long-term results at the two sites are comparable if only arteries of adequate diameter are used.[10]

An alternative method of creating an AVF in the forearm that was not mentioned in the NKF-DOQI report is vein transposition.[11] Preoperative duplex ultrasonography often identifies veins that, except for their deep subcutaneous location, are suitable for AVF formation. In addition, the basilic vein in the forearm is often spared and is frequently suitable for AVF formation; however, use of this vein in situ for needle cannulation and hemodialysis may necessitate placing the forearm in an uncomfortable position. In the great majority of cases, such veins can be successfully transposed to a superficial tunnel in the midportion of the volar aspect of the forearm, and the resulting fistula theoretically has the same advantages as a radiocephalic fistula in terms of long-term patency and complication rates. This aggressive approach to autogenous forearm fistula formation also has the advantage of preserving more proximal vessels for future access placement.

If duplex ultrasonography does not identify an adequate forearm vein conduit, a brachiocephalic primary AVF is the next choice. It is easy to create and has the advantage of providing higher blood flow than the wrist fistula. The cephalic vein in the upper arm, because of its position and superficial location, is easy to cannulate and easily covered (a potential cosmetic benefit). The elbow AVF has a theoretical advantage in diabetic patients, in whom medial calcification of the distal radial artery commonly prevents the gradual arterial dilatation required for full maturation of a radiocephalic fistula. In fact, some authors[12] consider an upper-arm autogenous AVF (either a brachiocephalic or a transposed basilic vein fistula) the preferred approach in this particular subgroup of patients. Disadvantages of brachiocephalic fistulas include higher frequencies of arm swelling and steal syndrome than are seen with forearm fistulas.

If the cephalic vein in the upper arm is unsuitable, the remaining options include a prosthetic graft and transposed basilic vein. An AVF using transposed basilic vein has all the attributes of an autogenous fistula and consequently is preferred to a graft despite being more difficult to create. Its protected, deep subfascial position and large caliber make it a high-quality conduit for hemodialysis access. Its advantages over a prosthetic graft include the avoidance of the distal venous anastomosis (which causes the majority of stenoses in synthetic graft fistulas) and higher primary and secondary patency rates.[13,14] Flow rates are high in basilic vein fistulas because of the large size of the vein, and the infection rate is relatively low. Furthermore, thrombosis of a brachiobasilic fistula does not compromise the integrity of the axillary vein and thus does not preclude subsequent use of a prosthetic conduit at the same site.

If no veins in either upper extremity are suitable for a native AVF, then the use of prosthetic material should be considered. Two options are available. First, if a segment of vein at least 15 cm long is available but is too far from the artery to be used in the creation of a fully native fistula, a jump graft can be constructed between the artery and the vein, and the arterialized vein can be used as the needle conduit for dialysis. Second, the graft itself can be used as the needle conduit for dialysis. The data currently available suggest that extruded polytetrafluoroethylene (ePTFE) is preferable to other biologic and synthetic materials: ePTFE grafts are less likely to disintegrate with infection, they are more widely available, they remain patent longer, and they are easily handled by surgeons. Grafts may be placed in straight, looped, or curved configurations on either the forearm or the upper arm.

OPERATIVE TECHNIQUE

Autogenous AVFs

Radiocephalic fistula The arm is placed on an arm board in 90° of abduction. A tourniquet is applied to the upper arm to distend the cephalic vein, and the vein's course is marked on the skin. The tourniquet is then released.

Local anesthesia using 0.5% or 1% lidocaine without epinephrine is usually adequate for construction of an autogenous AVF at the wrist or the antecubital fossa. General anesthesia may depress cardiac output and thus may, by reducing fistula flow, exert a negative impact on the success of the fistula. Conversely, brachial or supraclavicular regional anesthesia may cause peripheral vasodilatation and thus increase arterial blood flow.

Table 1 **Noninvasive Criteria for Selection of Upper-Extremity Arteries and Veins for Dialysis Access Procedures[9]**

Venous examination
- Venous luminal diameter ≥ 2.5 mm for autogenous AVFs, ≥ 4.0 mm for bridge AV grafts
- Absence of segmental stenoses or occluded segments
- Continuity with the deep venous system in the upper arm
- Absence of ipsilateral central vein stenosis or occlusion

Arterial examination
- Arterial luminal diameter ≥ 2.0 mm
- Absence of pressure differential ≥ 20 mm Hg between arms
- Patent palmar arch

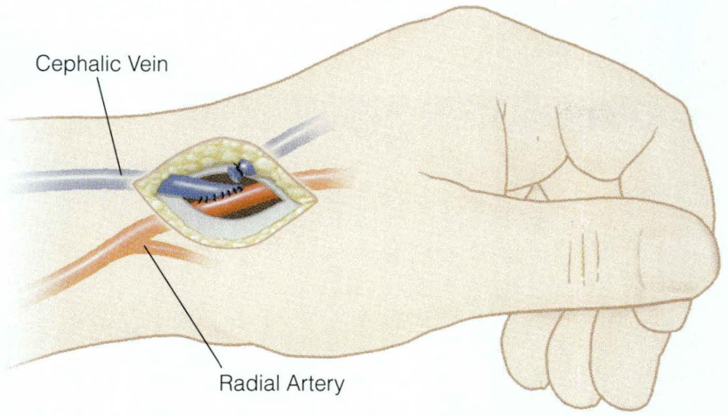

Figure 1 Vascular access via AVFs: radiocephalic fistula. Shown is the anatomic snuff-box fistula, with the end of the cephalic vein anastomosed to the side of the radial artery.

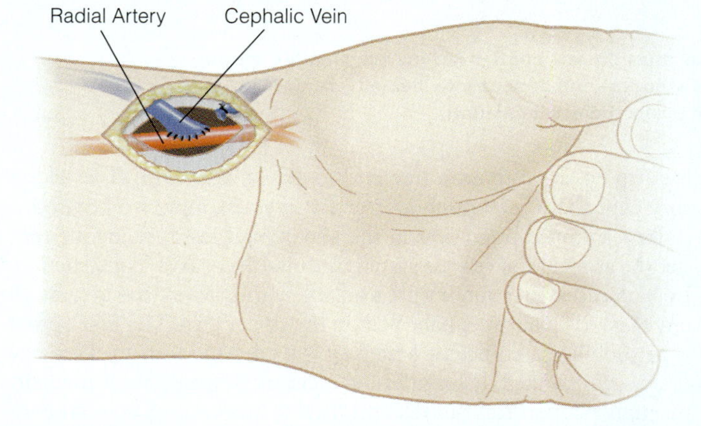

Figure 2 Vascular access via AVFs: radiocephalic fistula. Shown is the Brescia-Cimino fistula. An incision is made midway between the radial artery and the cephalic vein, and the end of the vein is anastomosed to the side of the artery.

A longitudinal incision is placed either in the anatomic snuff-box, between the tendons of the extensor pollicis longus and the extensor pollicis brevis [*see Figure 1*], or midway between the cephalic vein and the radial artery, proximal to the wrist skinfold [*see Figure 2*]. In the anatomic snuff-box, the cephalic vein overlies the radial artery, so that minimal mobilization is required to approximate the two vessels. Slightly more mobilization is required to approximate the cephalic vein to the radial artery above the wrist without kinking or twisting. A comparable length of radial artery, found under the deep fascia, is also isolated. Care is taken to preserve the superficial branch of the radial nerve, which lies lateral to the radial artery and is separated from it by the brachioradialis muscle.

Four types of anastomoses can be constructed: side to side, end of vein to side of artery, end to end, and end of artery to side of vein. The side-to-side anastomosis [*see Figure 3a*] yields the highest flow through the fistula but may be associated with venous congestion of the hand. Over time, arterial pressure may render the valves of the distal vein incompetent, resulting in retrograde flow toward the hand and venous hypertension. The end of artery–side of vein anastomosis [*see Figure 3b*] also presents a risk of venous hypertension. This configuration reduces the risk of distal steal by preventing retrograde flow into the fistula, but at the price of lower flow through the fistula. Of the four options, the end of artery–end of vein variation [*see Figure 3c*] produces the least distal arterial steal and venous hypertension but yields the lowest flow.

The preferred configuration of the anastomosis is end of vein to side of artery [*see Figure 3d*]. Dividing the vein reduces the risk of venous congestion in the hand; moreover, by allowing retrograde flow from the distal radial artery and the ulnar artery into the vein, which contributes approximately 30% of the total flow of the fistula, this approach yields maximal blood flow through the fistula. There is a risk of steal syndrome with such fistulas, but this problem is easily corrected by ligating the radial artery distal to the fistula, thereby converting the anastomosis to an end-to-end configuration.

Vascular control is obtained with small vessel loops or Heifets clamps. Heparinization is not needed unless the artery is an end artery. A 1 cm arteriotomy is performed, and the vein is ligated and divided distally and tailored to match the arteriotomy. Coronary dilators are then inserted gently to verify patency and to ensure that the vessel lumina are large enough: the artery should easily admit a 2 mm dilator; the vein, a 3 mm dilator. The vessels are then anastomosed in the desired configuration with a fine continuous monofilament suture (6-0 or 7-0 polypropylene) placed by means of standard techniques. The vessels can be probed with the coronary dilators before the anastomosis is completed, to confirm that the vein is not twisted or to overcome any arterial spasm. Once vascular control is released, a thrill should be easily felt over the fistula and for a moderate distance along the venous conduit. The skin is closed with an absorbable suture.

Vein transposition in the forearm The artery and the vein selected for the primary AVF are identified and mapped preoperatively by means of duplex ultrasonography. Positioning and anesthetic considerations are essentially the same as for a radiocephalic fistula.

A longitudinal incision is made directly over the mapped vein, beginning at its distal end and extending toward the antecubital fossa for a distance of at least 15 cm [*see Figure 4a*]. The vein is gently skeletonized and mobilized by ligating and dividing all side branches. The targeted artery (either the radial or the ulnar) is identified and dissected through a separate incision. A superficial subcutaneous tunnel is made between the two incisions with a blunt tunneling instrument, and the vein is passed through the tunnel [*see Figure 4b*]. The vein should be marked along its length with a marking pen before tunneling; this step provides a usual visual check that allows the surgeon to confirm that the vein is not twisted as it passes through the tunnel. A 1 cm anastomosis is then carried out in the same fashion as for a radiocephalic fistula (see above).

Brachiocephalic fistula After adequate local anesthesia, a transverse incision is made 1.5 cm distal to the antecubital crease[15] to expose the superficial antecubital venous system [*see Figure 5a*]. If the median cubital vein is patent, sufficiently wide, and in continuity with the cephalic vein, it is dissected so that the perforating branch of the antecubital venous system (vena mediana cubiti profunda) can be located. The bicipital aponeurosis is divided, and the perforating branch is followed down to the deep system. In the process, the brachial artery is also exposed, as are the origins of the radial and ulnar arteries.

Once the patient is fully heparinized, the confluence of the brachial vein and the perforating vein is identified, and part of the brachial vein is excised so as to form a venous patch. The perforating vein is gently dilated, so that any valves are rendered incompetent, and the proximal median cubital vein is ligated to prevent diversion of blood flow into the basilic vein. The perforating vein is then anastomosed to the brachial artery in an end-to-side fashion [*see Figure 5b*].[16] To prevent subsequent steal syndrome, the arteriotomy should be no larger than 5 to 6 mm.

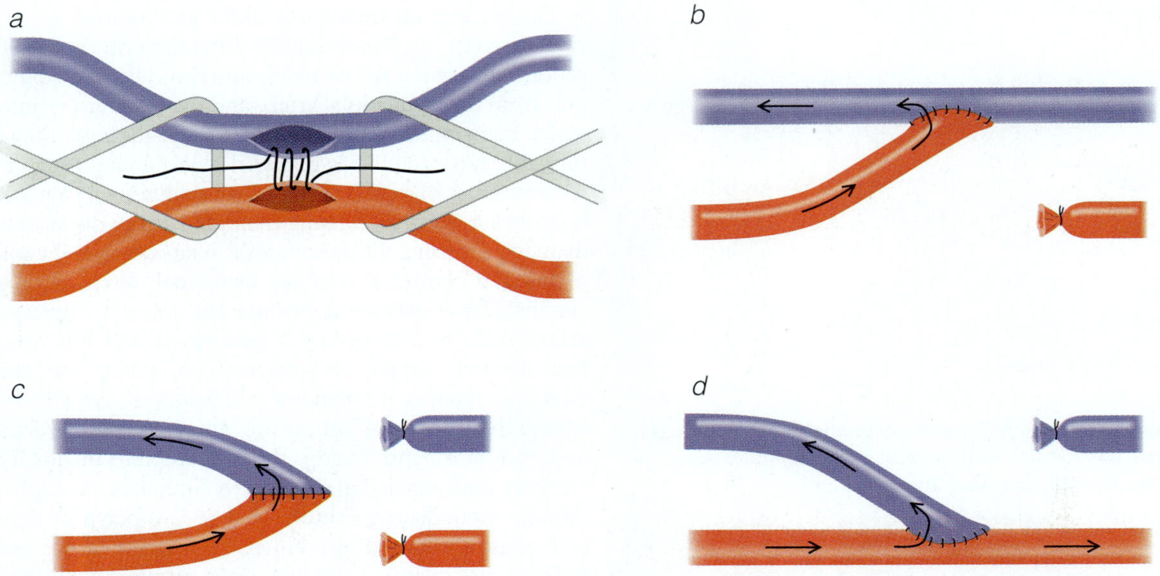

Figure 3 Vascular access via AVFs: radiocephalic fistula. Four anastomotic configurations are possible for an autologenous radiocephalic fistula: (*a*) side of artery to side of vein, (*b*) end of artery to side of vein, (*c*) end of artery to end of vein, and (*d*) end of vein to side of artery (the preferred configuration).

Other techniques may be used if the perforating vein is very large or very small. If the perforating vein is 5 mm or more in diameter, it may be anastomosed directly to the artery without a patch. If the vein is less than 2.5 mm in diameter, it should not be used; instead, the median cubital vein should be ligated and divided and the cephalic end of the vein anastomosed directly to the brachial artery in an end-to-side fashion [see Figure 5c]. If the median cubital vein is too small, the incision is extended laterally and proximally to allow mobilization of the cephalic vein. The length of this incision depends on the extent to which the cephalic vein must be mobilized to ensure a tension-free end-to-side anastomosis. The accessory cephalic vein, though located far laterally, may also be used.

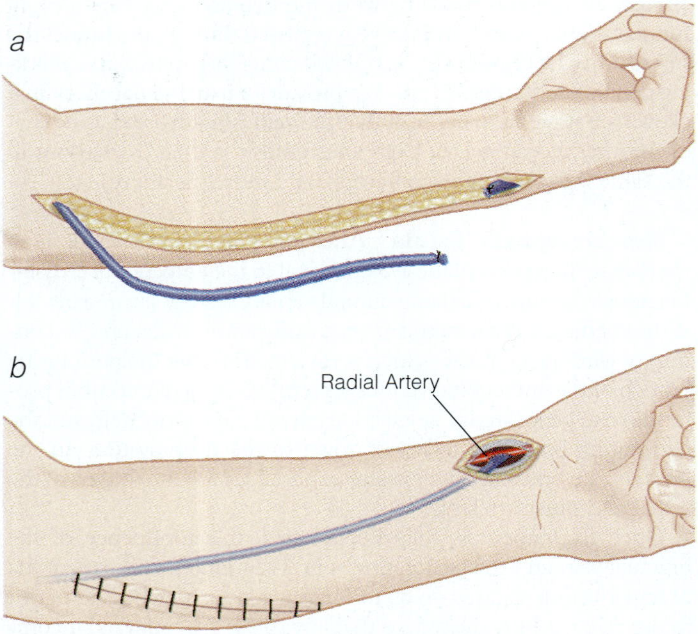

Repeated venipunctures in the antecubital fossa frequently render the antecubital venous system unsuitable for AVF construction. In such cases, two options are available if the patient has at least 15 cm of good-quality cephalic vein in the upper arm. The first option is to mobilize a sufficient length of the cephalic vein in the distal upper arm through a longitudinal incision, to transpose it medially through a superficial tunnel, and then to anastomose it in an end-to-side fashion to the brachial artery, which has been exposed above the elbow through a separate incision. The second, which avoids extensive dissection of the cephalic vein, is to place two short longitudinal incisions over the brachial artery and the cephalic vein a few centimeters above the elbow crease, to tunnel a short segment of 6 mm ePTFE graft between the two incisions, and to anastomose the ePTFE graft to both the brachial artery and the cephalic vein in an end-to-side fashion [see Figure 6].[17] The cephalic vein is used as the needle conduit for this type of bridge AV graft.

Brachiobasilic fistula The technique for constructing a brachiobasilic fistula was described first by Dagher and associates in 1976[18] and then by Logerfo and colleagues in 1978.[19] Local anesthesia can be used, but an axillary block eases the procedure considerably.

An oblique incision overlying the median basilic vein is made in the antecubital fossa, and the vein is mobilized. The brachial artery is exposed as usual by dividing the bicipital aponeurosis. The incision is extended along the medial aspect of the upper arm (the so-called hockey-stick incision), and the basilic vein is mobilized from beneath the fascia, with care taken to preserve the medial cutaneous nerve of the forearm [see Figure 7a]. The basilic vein usually pierces the brachial fascia just below the middle of the upper arm, then parallels the course of the brachial artery and vein while remaining superficial to them. At the axillary level, the basilic vein joins the brachial vein to form the axillary vein; this junction constitutes the proximal limit of the dissection.

The distal end of the conduit vein may consist of either the basilic vein or a section of the median cubital vein, which is already exposed. All venous tributaries are ligated and divided. Once this is done, the vein is divided distally, and its anterior surface is

Figure 4 Vascular access via AVFs: vein transposition in the forearm. (*a*) The selected vein, identified by duplex ultrasonography, is completely mobilized. (*b*) The vein is transposed through a superficial tunnel in the midportion of the volar aspect of the forearm and anastomosed to the radial artery in an end-to-side fashion.

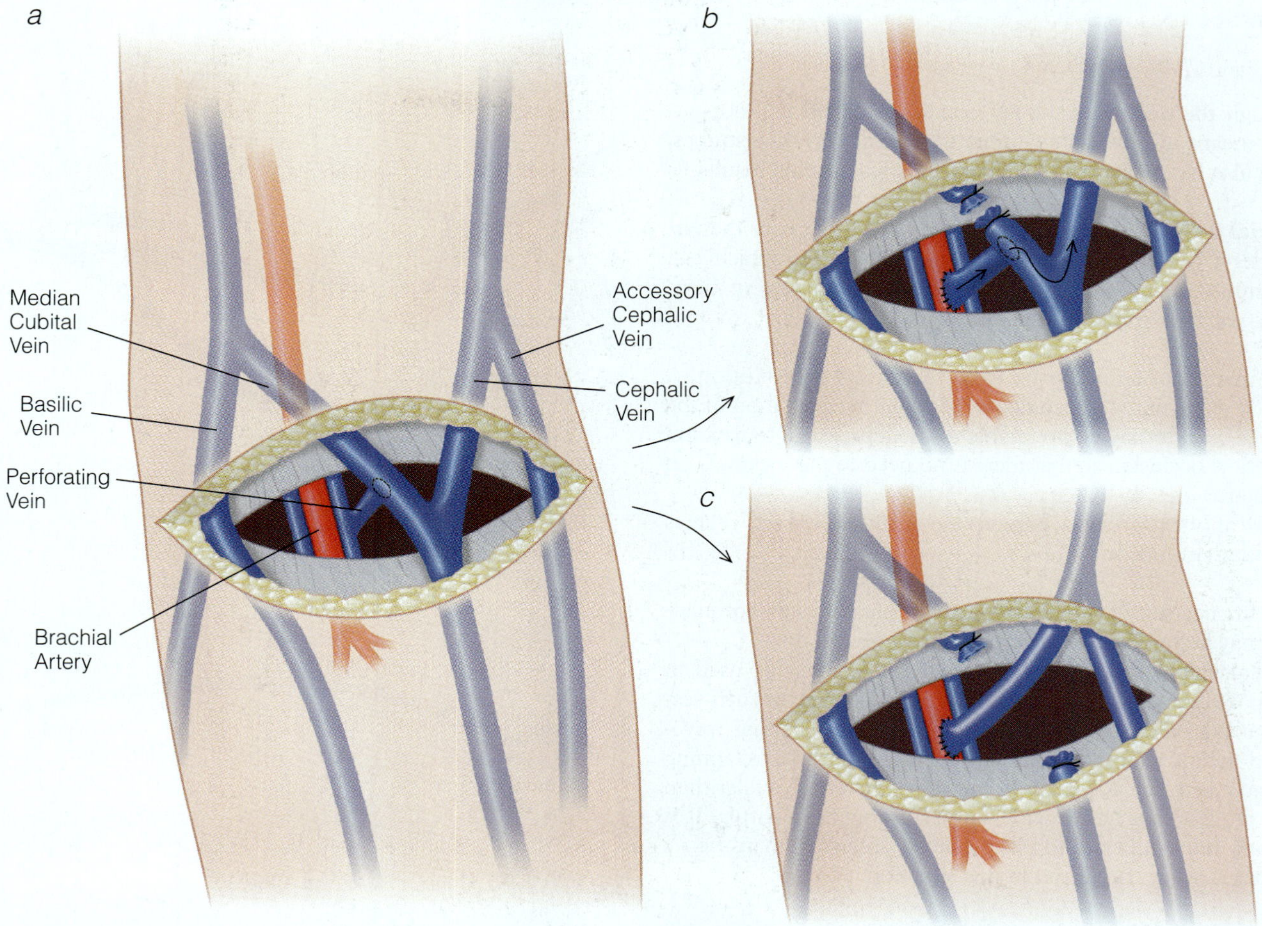

Figure 5 Vascular access via AVFs: brachiocephalic fistula. (*a*) A transverse incision exposes the antecubital venous system (including the perforating branch) and the brachial artery under the bicipital aponeurosis. (*b*) An end-to-side anastomosis is made between the perforating vein and the brachial artery. (*c*) If the perforating vein is too small, the cephalic vein is mobilized and anastomosed to the brachial artery in an end-to-side fashion.

marked to help the surgeon avoid axial rotation during transposition. The vein is then passed through a subcutaneous tunnel on the anterior surface of the arm and anastomosed in an end-to-side fashion to the brachial artery in the antecubital fossa with 6-0 or 7-0 polypropylene [*see Figure 7b*]. This transposition places the vein in a more superficial location and positions it anterolaterally on the arm, thereby facilitating cannulation during hemodialysis sessions. Closure involves approximating the fascia and the subcutaneous tissue in two separate layers.

A modification of the procedure just described is the so-called elevated basilic vein arteriovenous fistula.[20] In this variant, the vein is left in situ rather than transposed anterolaterally, but it is elevated by closing the deep fascia and the subcutaneous tissue beneath the vein. The brachial artery anastomosis is created, and the overlying skin is reapproximated with clips or interrupted sutures. Although the vein remains in its medial location, its new superficial position facilitates cannulation for dialysis.

Bridge AV Grafts

Bridge AV graft procedures involve placing an interposition graft between an artery and a vein and using that graft as the needle conduit for dialysis. In the forearm, the most common configurations are loop grafts between the brachial artery and an antecubital vein (including the brachial veins)[21] and straight bridge AV grafts from the radial artery to an antecubital vein. Most studies report superior patency rates with a loop configuration.[22] Adequate results may be obtained with a straight graft in the forearm if the radial artery is at least 2.5 to 3.0 mm in diameter.

Secondary options for bridge AV graft construction include a variety of unusual configurations, including reverse grafts between the axillary artery and the brachial or the antecubital vein and axilloaxillary grafts, which may be looped in the upper arm or may cross the sternum. It is also possible to construct a looped graft between the proximal superficial femoral artery and the proximal saphenous vein or a straight, reversed graft between the distal superficial femoral or popliteal artery and the proximal saphenous or femoral vein [*see Figure 8*]. Such lower-limb AV grafts are associated with an increased risk of potentially life- or limb-threatening infection and thus are used only as a last resort.

Either local anesthesia or axillary block is usually appropriate for upper-extremity bridge AV grafts. A single dose of a cephalosporin should be given before the procedure. Separate longitudinal incisions are placed to expose the artery and the vein—except when the procedure involves the brachial artery and the antecubital venous system, which are better exposed through a single transverse incision. A 6 mm or a tapered 4 to 7 mm ePTFE graft is then passed through a superficial tunnel between the two incisions. Both anastomoses are constructed in an end-to-side fashion, beginning with the venous side. Systemic heparinization is used if an end artery is occluded for the arterial anastomosis.

TROUBLESHOOTING

Autogenous AVFs

Although the quality of the AV conduit is assessed preoperatively by means of physical examination and noninvasive studies, it should also be confirmed intraoperatively for optimal results.

Arterial inflow Normally, a strong pulse is felt over the targeted artery; however, dissection may cause spasm, which can render intra-operative assessment difficult. The following three measures will help minimize this problem:

1. Elimination of epinephrine from the anesthetic solution.
2. Gentle dissection and avoidance of direct manipulation of the arterial wall. It may be preferable to use a proximal tourniquet for inflow occlusion so that there is no need to place clamps on small arteries.
3. Local application of a papaverine solution, which relaxes vascular smooth muscle.

If spasm occurs, gentle probing of the artery with coronary dilators may help relieve the spasm and restore full flow.

Stiff, calcified arteries can sometimes be successfully used in the creation of fistulas, but it is difficult to assess flow in such vessels. Quantitative and qualitative analyses of the arterial waveform and the intraluminal diameter by means of duplex scanning can help confirm the adequacy of the vessel. Arteries smaller than 1.5 mm are less likely to provide sufficient flow for a fistula. It is particularly important not to place clamps on calcified arteries; a tourniquet is always preferred in this situation.

Venous outflow A venous diameter of at least 2.5 to 3.0 mm is required for successful maturation of an autogenous fistula. The diameter of the target vein should be known preoperatively from the duplex examination and should be confirmed intraop-

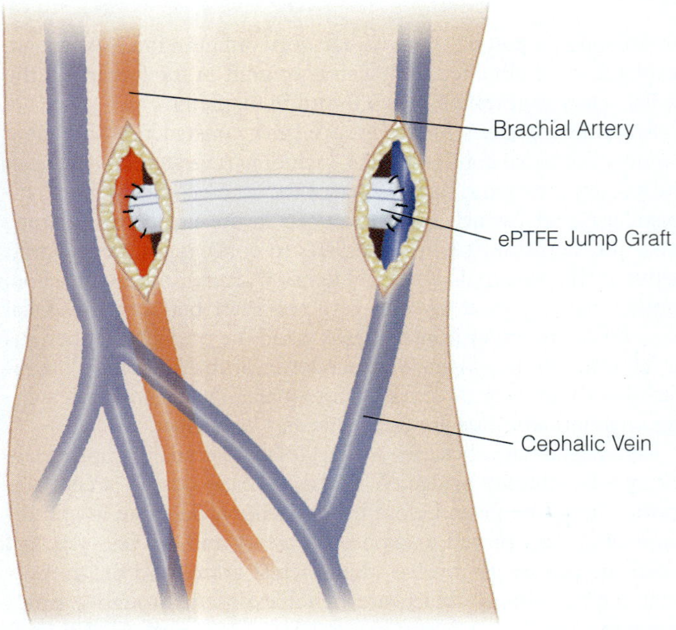

Figure 6 Vascular access via AVFs: brachiocephalic fistula. If the antecubital venous system is unsuitable for AVF construction, one option is to place an ePTFE interposition graft between the brachial artery and the cephalic vein.

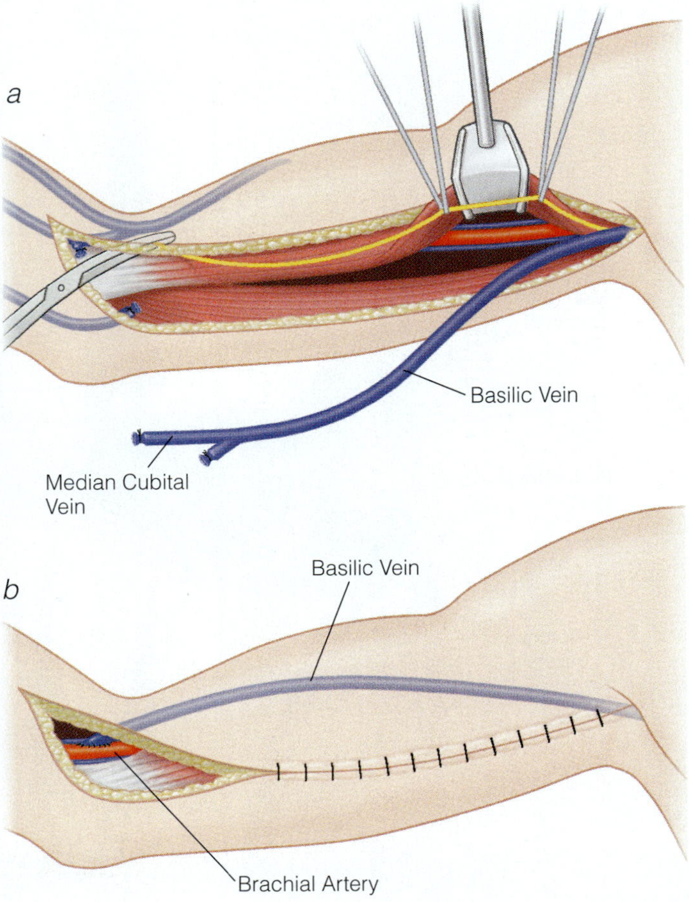

Figure 7 Vascular access via AVFs: brachiobasilic fistula. (*a*) The basilic vein is completely mobilized from underneath the fascia in continuity with a section of the median cubital vein in the antecubital fossa. (*b*) The vein is transposed in a subcutaneous tunnel on the anterior surface of the arm and anastomosed to the brachial artery in an end-to-side fashion.

eratively by calibration with coronary dilators. No attempt should be made to dilate the vein, however, because endothelial injury may result.

Webs, thickened valve leaflets, and areas of sclerosis from previous phlebitis or punctures are common in upper-extremity veins and may be the cause of poor venous outflow and fistula failure. Passage of the coronary dilator helps to localize such obstructive lesions, which should be corrected when found. The patency of the proximal vein can be demonstrated by free flow of injected heparinized saline or by successful passage of a Fogarty catheter. The evoked thrill is also a useful maneuver: intermittent, pulsatile injection of saline into the vein, mimicking arterial flow, should produce a palpable thrill over the proximal vein.[23] The absence of an evoked thrill suggests the presence of stenosis or areas of thickened, nondistensible vein wall proximally. Intraoperative phlebography is indicated in any doubtful situation.

AV anastomosis Both the artery and the vein should be mobilized sufficiently to ensure that the anastomosis is tension-free once completed. As noted (see above), marking the most superficial aspect of the vein with a sterile pen before mobilization helps ensure that the vein is not rotated when it is approximated to the artery. The ideal anastomosis is constructed by transecting the vein just distal to a bifurcation and using the branch vessel as

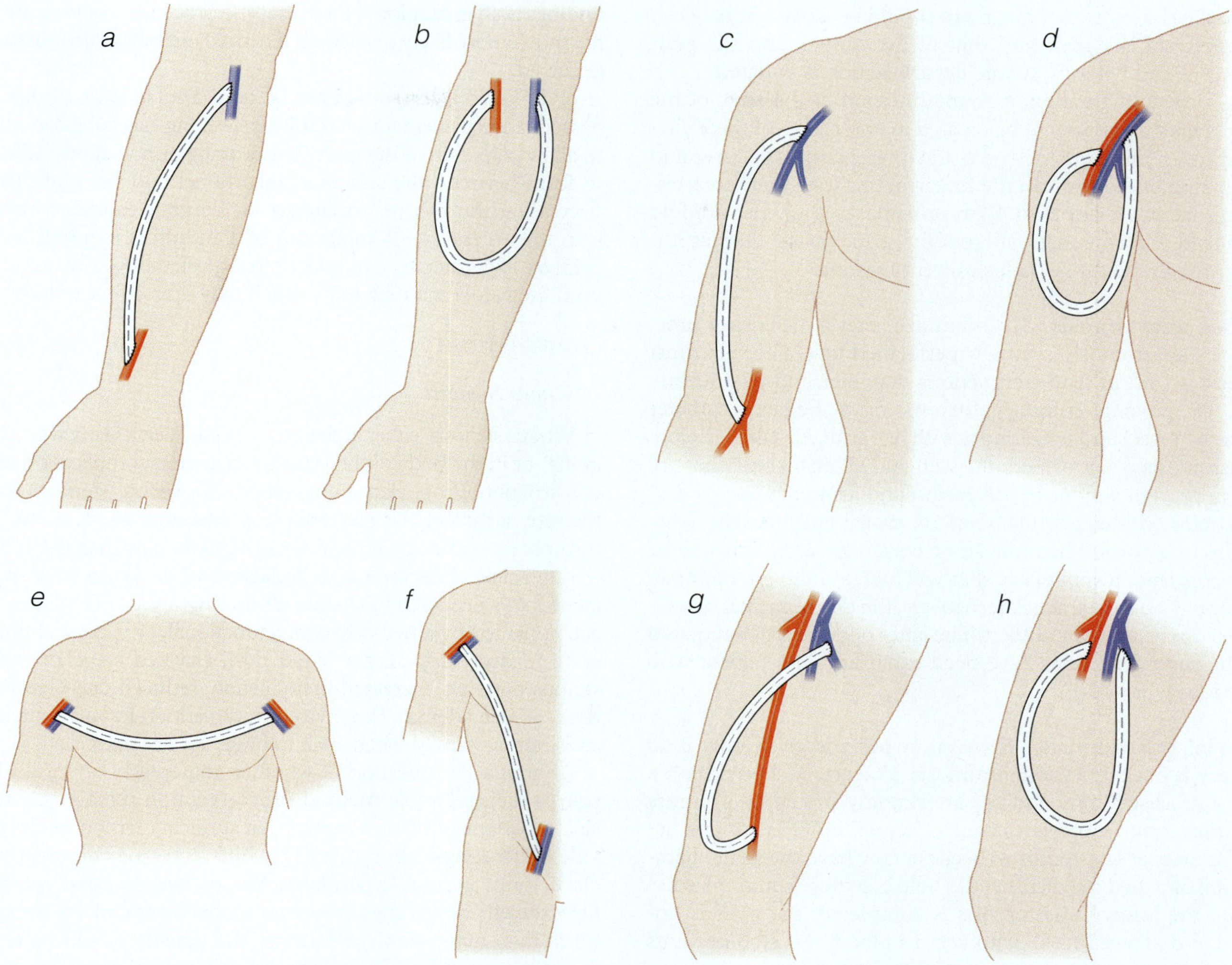

Figure 8 Vascular access via AVFs: bridge AV grafts. Options for bridge graft construction include (*a*) straight forearm AV graft, (*b*) loop forearm AV graft, (*c*) brachioaxillary AV graft, (*d*) loop axilloaxillary AV graft, (*e*) axillary artery–contralateral axillary vein AV graft, (*f*) axillary artery–iliac vein AV graft, (*g*) distal superficial femoral or popliteal artery–saphenous vein AV graft, and (*h*) proximal superficial femoral artery–saphenous vein loop AV graft.

a patch. Such a spatulated venous conduit facilitates the anastomosis and minimizes the risk of anastomotic stenosis.

For a distal AVF, the anastomosis should be about 10 mm long to ensure that a gradual increase in flow through the fistula can occur. An anastomosis that is too small may impair the normal dilation of the artery and the vein. For AVFs in the antecubital space and the upper arm, in contrast, the arteriotomy should be limited to 5 to 6 mm to prevent excessive shunting.

The anastomosis can be performed with standard vascular techniques. However, construction of the anastomosis with a single continuous suture may have a purse-string effect; accordingly, the use of two separate running sutures may be preferable for small vessels. Interrupted stitches are preferable for very small vessels. Loupes and microvascular instruments are helpful in this setting.

When the anastomosis is completed, vascular control should be released from the proximal vein and the distal artery first; the resultant back-bleeding will confirm the patency of the palmar arch and reveal any major anastomotic defects. Gentle compression is usually sufficient to obtain hemostasis. Any additional sutures deemed necessary should be placed with great caution because of the risk that they may narrow the anastomosis.

The presence of a pulse rather than a thrill in the arterialized vein indicates inadequate outflow, whereas the absence of either a thrill or a pulse indicates poor inflow. The draining vein should be examined for kinking, twisting, or compression by a fibrous band. If the vein appears to be satisfactory, the anastomosis and the distal vein are inspected and probed with dilators through a venous side branch or a transverse phlebotomy. If no abnormality is identified, the fistula is examined with I.V. contrast studies and fluoroscopy. Focal lesions may be corrected by placement of a vein patch or a short interposition graft or by resection and primary reanastomosis. Alternatively, a short segment of the vein may be excised and the anastomosis repositioned more proximally.

AV Grafts

Skin incisions Incisions should be placed so that neither the graft nor the anastomoses lie directly beneath them. Proper placement reduces the risk of skin erosion, minimizes the risk that the graft will become infected if a surgical site infection occurs, and maximizes the length of conduit available for needle insertion. The subcutaneous tissue and skin should be closed in separate layers to minimize the risk of graft infection in the event of skin dehiscence.

Tunneling The tunnel should be made atraumatically with a Kelly-Wick bidirectional tunneler. It should be superficial to the muscle fascia but no more than 5 mm beneath the skin surface. To decrease the risk of hematoma, there should be a close fit between the diameter of the graft and that of the tunnel, and the graft should be placed before systemic heparinization is initiated.

For a loop configuration, a counterincision at the apex of the tunnel permits the tunnel to be created in two passes of the Kelly-Wick tunneler. This approach gives the tunnel a smooth curve and limits kinking of the graft. In the forearm, this transverse counter-incision is usually made 3 to 4 cm proximal to the wrist skinfold [*see Figure 9*]. Careful observation of the stripe on the graft as it is passed through the tunnel helps prevent twisting.

Venous anastomosis To minimize arterial occlusion time, the venous anastomosis is usually performed first. The vein must be at least 4 mm in diameter; venous diameter and patency are verified by passing coronary dilators or a Fogarty catheter through the vessel and irrigating it with heparinized saline. Before the anastomosis is performed, the vein and all distal branches are ligated to prevent venous hypertension and arm edema.

If no veins of adequate diameter are available, either two adjacent veins or a portion of a transverse communicating vein can be used to construct a venoplasty that will increase the net diameter of the venous outflow tract. Alternatively, the deep brachial or axillary veins can be used for outflow. The latter option is often required when the superficial veins have been exhausted in a patient who has previously had AVFs.

Arterial anastomosis Systemic heparin is given only if an end artery is occluded for anastomosis. The artery should have a lumen of at least 3 mm, and the arteriotomy should be no more than 6 mm long to prevent distal ischemia. ePTFE sutures are useful for arterial anastomoses: because they have the same diameter as the attached needles, needle-hole bleeding is minimized.

Before the arterial anastomosis is completed, the graft is unclamped and allowed to fill with venous blood; this step prevents air embolism when arterial control is released. When the anastomosis is complete, a thrill should be palpable over the venous outflow tract rather than directly over the graft.

Graft type The choice between a tapered 4 to 7 mm ePTFE graft and a 6 mm straight graft is a matter of personal preference. The tapered graft was introduced to reduce the incidence of steal syndrome by increasing the resistance to flow through the prosthesis; however, it has not been shown to provide consistent protection from ischemic complications. Both types of graft are also available in either a standard or a thin-wall configuration; the only randomized study published to date reported superior results with the standard configuration.[24] Stretch ePTFE appears to yield better results than the older, nonstretch grafts.[25]

FOLLOW-UP

Upon discharge, the patient is instructed to elevate the arm so as to reduce edema. Regular hand and arm exercise, though not of proven benefit, is nonetheless recommended until the fistula matures.

Physical examination of the fistula, including inspection and palpation for pulse and thrill, should be done on a weekly basis. The patient should also be advised to seek prompt medical attention if the quality of the thrill changes. Normally, a thrill is palpable throughout the cardiac cycle, though it is more intense during systole. Disappearance of the diastolic component of the thrill is generally a consequence of outflow obstruction. Such obstruction (usually from venous or anastomotic stenosis) may also cause intensification of the thrill or bruit. In addition, diminished flow or outflow stenosis may cause the thrill to be converted to a pulse. Any of these abnormal findings is an indication for a diagnostic procedure: salvage attempts are much more likely to succeed if carried out before thrombosis has occurred.

ePTFE AV grafts should not be used until at least 14 days have passed since placement or until the swelling has subsided enough to allow palpation of the graft. This waiting period allows adhesions to form between the subcutaneous tunnel and the graft, thereby decreasing the risk of hematoma in the graft tunnel, which may ruin the access site. A minimum of 1 month is required before a primary AVF may be cannulated. It is preferable, however, to wait until the fistula matures fully, which may take 3 to 4 months.

COMPLICATIONS

Venous Stenosis

Venous stenosis, either at the anastomosis (particularly with ePTFE grafts) or in the body of the vein, is a common complication of AVF construction. Prophylactic intervention for venous stenoses reduces the rate of thrombosis and graft loss, and stenoses detected before thrombosis occurs are more responsive to therapy than those detected afterward. Intervention is indicated when stenosis of 50% or greater (documented by duplex ultrasonography or fistulography) is accompanied by a hemodynamic, functional, or clinical abnormality (e.g., decreased access blood flow, elevated static or dynamic venous pressure, increased recirculation, reduced delivered dialysis dose, or arm edema). Prophylactic intervention for anatomic stenosis is not warranted when such findings are absent.[26]

Although the question of whether angioplasty or surgical revision is the preferable method of intervention remains controversial, experience to date suggests that surgical revision tends to provide better long-term results. This difference may derive from the elasticity of intimal hyperplastic lesions, whose rapid recoil may limit the efficacy of angioplasty. As a rule, if angioplasty is required more than twice within 3 months, the patient should be referred for surgical revision. Treatment options include patch angioplasty for localized or anastomotic stenoses, bypass for longer stenoses, relocation of the venous anastomosis to a new vein, and resection of the stenotic segment with interposition grafting.

Central venous stenosis Stenotic or occlusive lesions of the central veins develop in as many as 40% of patients who have previously undergone subclavian hemodialysis catheter placement for temporary vascular access.[7] When a vascular access graft or fistula is placed distal to these lesions, they may become symptomatic,

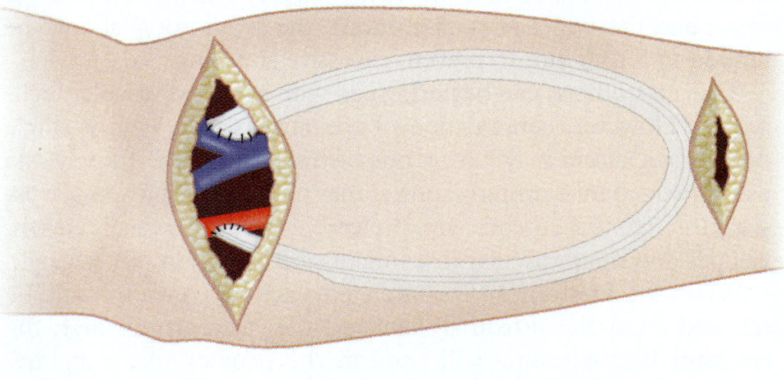

Figure 9 Vascular access via AVFs: bridge AV grafts. With a loop forearm graft, tunneling of the graft is facilitated by making an incision 1.5 cm distal to the elbow crease to expose the brachial artery and the antecubital venous system, followed by a counterincision at the apex of the tunnel 3 to 4 cm proximal to the wrist skinfold.

resulting in venous hypertension, arm edema, low access flow, or thrombosis. Percutaneous intervention with transluminal angioplasty is the preferred treatment; the tendency for central venous stenosis to recur soon after treatment[27] may be circumvented by the addition of a stent. Stents are particularly helpful for treating rigid or kinked stenoses, for sealing dissections or circumscribed perforations, and for reestablishing the patency of chronically occluded veins. Surgical repair of central venous obstruction is a major undertaking and is reserved for those occasional cases in which percutaneous procedures have failed in a patient with no alternative access site.

Arterial Stenosis

Arterial stenosis is relatively uncommon. It should be corrected if it is associated with diminished access flow and elevated arterial prepump pressure. Arterial stenosis may be suspected even before dialysis is initiated if a patent vein does not enlarge significantly within several weeks of fistula creation. Angiography provides a definitive diagnosis. Stenosis of the distal artery, the anastomosis, or the distal vein is best treated with reanastomosis proximal to the stenotic area. More proximal stenosis may have to be treated with conventional arterial reconstruction.

Early Thrombosis

Early thrombosis is defined as thrombosis occurring within 3 months of access construction. It is usually the result of technical factors or of inadequate assessment of the arterial or venous conduit. The following are the most common causes of early thrombosis:

1. Inadequate arterial inflow caused by proximal arterial disease.
2. Narrowing of the anastomosis during construction.
3. Kinking or twisting of the vein proximal to the anastomosis or in a subcutaneous tunnel.
4. Undetected occlusion of venous outflow.
5. Compression of the fistula by a hematoma resulting from either inadequate hemostasis during the procedure or early puncture of the fistula with subsequent extravasation of blood.

If early thrombosis is thought to be caused by technical complications and not by the use of marginal vessels, reexploration is worthwhile. Reexploration usually involves takedown of the anastomosis, thrombectomy of the conduit, reevaluation of both arterial inflow and venous outflow, corrective measures as needed, and reanastomosis. Both autogenous AVFs and AV grafts may be profitably reexplored. With an autogenous AVF, reexploration should be done within 24 hours of thrombosis to minimize ischemic endothelial injury.

Late Thrombosis

Autogenous AVFs Little information is available on success rates for treatment of thrombosis in autogenous AVFs; however, it seems that neither percutaneous nor surgical techniques offer good results. Thrombosis of an autogenous AVF most commonly results from an aneurysm of the fistula, hyperplastic stenosis at the anastomosis or in the vein just distal to the anastomosis, fibrosis at an area of repeated needle punctures, or kidney transplantation.

The surgical approach should include exposure of the vein just distal to a clinically apparent or suspected venous stenosis. The vein is opened longitudinally and the thrombus evacuated. Adequacy of venous outflow is assessed with a Fogarty catheter or coronary dilators. If a segment less than 4 mm in diameter is encountered, the problem is corrected with patch angioplasty, vein bypass, or resection and primary anastomosis. (The last of these three approaches is often easy to perform because the tortuosity of the vein allows easy mobilization and length extension.) Central vein stenosis is corrected with intraoperative balloon angioplasty.

When the venous side of the AVF is in satisfactory condition, the thrombus is removed from the arterial limb. Any suspected anastomotic or proximal arterial stenosis should be corrected [see AV Grafts, *below*]. If the thrombosis resulted from a fistula aneurysm containing adherent thrombus, the aneurysm should be repaired to prevent its recurrence.

AV grafts About 85% of AV graft thromboses are caused by stenosis of the venous anastomosis or of the draining vein (as a result of intimal hyperplasia), and most instances of graft loss are attributable to such stenosis. Treatment of a thrombosed graft has only a 10% chance of success if the underlying venous stenosis is not addressed. Although arterial stenoses are less common causes of late thrombosis, they should be sought out and corrected as well. Before treatment is initiated, information about recent graft performance should be obtained. Signs of venous or outflow stenosis include increasing venous resistance and prolonged bleeding from puncture sites. Inadequate flow rates and increased negative pressures during dialysis are associated with stenosis of the arterial inflow. Hypotension or excessive graft compression can explain spontaneous thrombosis in a previously well-functioning graft.

Graft thrombosis may be corrected either with surgical thrombectomy or with pharmacomechanical or mechanical thrombolysis. On the whole, technical success and long-term patency rates are similar for the two approaches, though there is some evidence for a trend toward longer primary patency with surgical management.[28] The choice between these two approaches continues to be controversial, and the decision should generally be based on local expertise. To date, neither surgical treatment nor endovascular management has produced unassisted patency rates higher than 50% at 6 months. If graft thrombosis occurs repeatedly in a given patient, plans for a new access site should be considered.

If surgical treatment is chosen, it should be carried out in an operating suite with the capacity for intraoperative fluoroscopy. Unless preoperative findings indicate that an arterial lesion is present, the incision is made at the venous anastomosis, and an adequate length of graft and outflow vein is mobilized. A transverse graftotomy is made within 1 or 2 mm of the suture line, any clot found on the venous side is removed with suction and a forceps, and the anastomosis is inspected. The anastomosis is calibrated but not dilated: if a 5 mm dilator passes easily through the venous anastomosis, then thrombectomy alone is often sufficient treatment. A 4 French Fogarty catheter is passed proximally into the right atrium and pulled back slowly with the balloon inflated to check for proximal venous stenosis and to evacuate clot. Any abnormality encountered is an indication for operative phlebography. The presence of a venous abnormality does not rule out the possibility of a coexisting arterial defect; both should be corrected if found.

After the venous anastomosis is examined, a 4 French Fogarty catheter is used to evacuate any clot in the graft itself. Thrombectomy at the arterial anastomosis is delayed until any structural problems in the body of the graft are corrected; this delay permits the structural corrections to be carried out in a bloodless field. Narrowing in the body of the graft is usually caused by fibrous material adherent to the wall, which can be removed with the aid of a curette, an endarterectomy instrument, or suction. Once the body of the graft is clear, any thrombus present at the arterial anastomosis is removed. Free passage of the Fogarty balloon catheter suggests that there is no arterial anastomotic stenosis. The arterial anastomosis may be examined under direct vision if necessary to

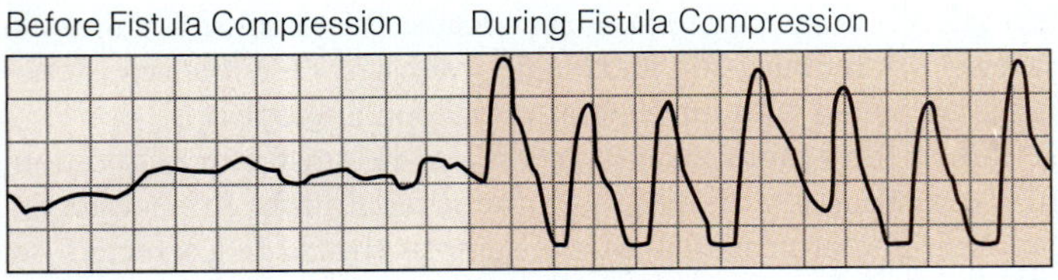

Figure 10 Vascular access via AVFs. Shown are digital photoplethysmographic waveforms on an arm with steal syndrome before and during fistula compression.

ensure complete removal of the compacted thrombus at the arterial end of the graft.

The graft is filled with heparinized saline before the arterial or the venous anastomosis is repaired. When the arterial side of the graft is involved, a new arterial anastomosis usually suffices to solve the problem. A new arterial site proximal to the old one is selected, and either the graft is moved to the new site or a new free segment is added.

More commonly, the defect is at the venous anastomosis. In this case, the graftotomy is extended longitudinally through the anastomosis. If the stenosis is short, smooth, and hyperplastic, a small patch angioplasty is adequate for repair. If the stenosis is long or if the vein is sclerotic, revision to a new venous outflow site is preferred. The graft can be reanastomosed to another nearby vein, or the stenosis can be bypassed by anastomosing an ePTFE graft of appropriate size to a more proximal segment of the original vein. Joints may be crossed if necessary, in which case an externally supported prosthesis is used.

Steal Syndrome

The incidence of symptomatic steal syndrome has been reported to be approximately 2% for autogenous AVFs and as high as 4% for AV grafts. Ischemic complications result from preferential diversion of arterial flow into the low-pressure venous outflow of the fistula. When collateral arterial flow is inadequate or when proximal or distal occlusive arterial disease is present, distal ischemia occurs. In some cases, the flow into the venous side of the fistula is sufficient to induce reversal of the flow in a portion of the artery distal to the fistula, a phenomenon referred to as steal. Unfortunately, there is no reliable method of predicting the development of symptomatic steal after the construction of an autogenous AVF or AV graft.

The ischemia is usually mild and is characterized by coldness, numbness, and pain during dialysis. In most cases, the problem resolves without treatment within a few weeks. If the patient experiences constant pain, severe numbness, a nonhealing ischemic fissure, digital cyanosis or gangrene, or finger contracture, the ischemia should be corrected. The differential diagnosis of vascular steal syndrome includes the neuropathies of uremia and diabetes as well as secondary hyperparathyroidism. Carpal tunnel syndrome—an uncommon but distinct condition occurring in hemodialysis patients—presents with symptoms similar to those of vascular steal but can be differentiated from steal on the basis of the characteristic electromyographic findings.

A classic indicator of clinically significant steal is that digital pulse waves are absent or markedly diminished on digital photoplethysmography (PPG) or pulse volume recordings (PVR) but rise to normal amplitude and contour when the fistula is compressed [see Figure 10]. Digital pressures lower than 50 mm Hg and a digital-brachial index lower than 0.47 are also indicative of clinically significant distal ischemia.[29] A significant difference in segmental or digital pressure between the two arms with the fistula compressed may be indicative of superimposed arterial disease proximal or distal to the fistula, in which case arteriography is indicated before surgical correction. Identification of reversed flow distal to the fistula on duplex studies is not, in itself, sufficient reason to conclude that clinically significant steal is present: steal is a common phenomenon and is a physiologic consequence of the rheology of the fistula in 73% of autogenous AVFs and 92% of AV grafts.[30]

The goal of treatment is to reduce steal to a level where there is both adequate residual flow volume for dialysis and adequate perfusion to the hand to eliminate ischemic symptoms. Treatment options include the following:

1. Elimination of the fistula. This is the simplest form of treatment and invariably corrects ischemia; however, it raises the vexing problem of reestablishing access in another extremity.
2. Reducing the flow but maintaining patency. Usually, this option involves narrowing a portion of the access to reduce flow. One technique for accomplishing this narrowing is to excise an elliptical portion of the graft or vein just distal to the anastomosis and reapproximate the edges or to plicate the graft or outflow vein with mattress or continuous sutures[31] [see Figure 11a through c]. Another technique is to band the fistula or graft with a crossed ePTFE band.[32] The tails of the band are secured with hemostatic clips, and once the appropriate degree of narrowing has been achieved, the clips are held in place with a figure-eight suture of 5-0 polypropylene [see Figure 11d]. Both techniques should narrow the outflow over a fairly long distance ($\geq$ 1 cm). A third technique involves interposing a small-diameter (4 mm) ePTFE graft between the artery and the vein or graft[33] [see Figure 11e]; however, this technique does not allow progressive calibration of the narrowing to achieve the desired hemodynamic result.
3. Ligation of the source of steal, with distal revascularization when necessary. When steal occurs in a patient who has a radiocephalic fistula at the wrist with flow reversal in the radial artery distal to the fistula (documented by duplex scans) and whose ulnar artery and palmar arch are patent and competent to perfuse the hand, it is easily treated by ligating the radial artery distal to the fistula.[34] The effect of this treatment is easily demonstrated by compressing the radial artery distal to the fistula, which should relieve the ischemia. With a more proximal fistula, in which ligation of a terminal artery would inevitably result in severe distal ischemia, the distal artery is ligated and an arterial bypass established from a point 5 cm proximal to the fistula to a point just distal to the ligation [see Figure 12]. This so-called distal revascularization–interval ligation (DRIL) procedure, originally reported by Schanzer and coworkers,[35] is an elegant way of both preserving adequate flow through the fistula and reversing the ischemia. The pathway of steal is eliminated, and antegrade flow into the extremity is restored through the bypass. This technique is particularly helpful when concomitant arterial stenosis proximal or distal to the fistula contributes to the distal ischemic process, because the bypass can be positioned so as to bypass the arterial stenosis as well.

With any of these techniques, intraoperative assessment is required to ensure adequate residual flow volume in the fistula (assessed by intraoperative duplex scanning) and adequate distal perfusion (assessed by evaluation of digital PPG or PVR waveforms). The goal is to achieve a digital pressure of at least 60 mm Hg, a digital-brachial index of 0.6 or greater, and a residual flow of at least 300 ml/min in the fistula (a level of flow that is adequate both for hemodialysis and for maintenance of patency).[36]

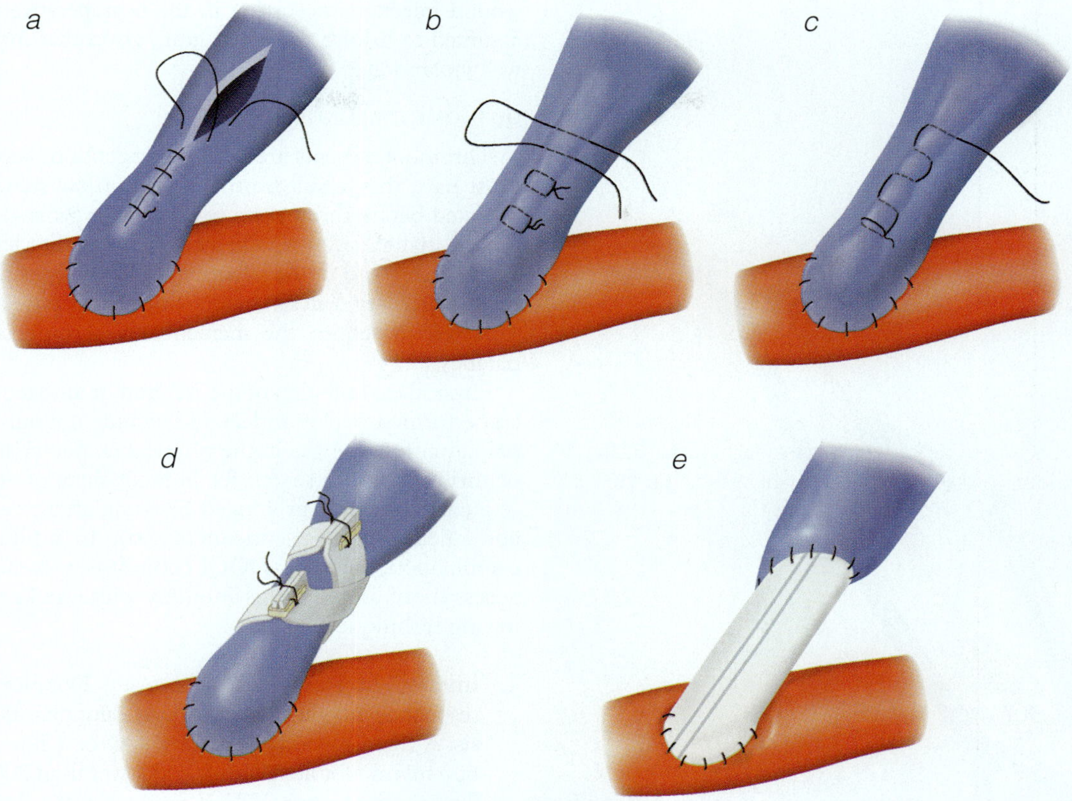

Figure 11 Vascular access via AVFs. One option for treating steal is to decrease blood flow in the access conduit. Methods that may be used include (*a*) excision of a portion of the vein or graft, (*b*) plication with mattress sutures, (*c*) plication with continuous sutures, (*d*) placement of a crossed ePTFE band with application of hemostatic clips, and (*e*) interposition of a 4 mm ePTFE graft.

Inadequate Maturation of the Vein

Failure of a fistula to mature may result from either inadequate inflow or venous abnormality. Physical examination combined with Doppler ultrasonography or fistulography should identify the underlying cause. If stenosis is not identified in a nonmaturing radiocephalic fistula, venous side branches may be draining critical flow from the primary vessel; ligation of these branches sometimes leads to successful maturation. Median cubital vein ligation may be attempted, as may temporary banding of the main venous channel in the antecubital fossa. Banding is accomplished by narrowing the vein with a 3-0 Vicryl tie over a 4 mm probe. The Vicryl resorbs in 3 to 4 weeks, during which period it is hoped that the increased resistance to flow will cause dilatation of the vein.[37] If none of these measures succeed, another access site should be sought.

True Aneurysm (Autogenous AVFs)

Aneurysmal dilatation of the vein develops in 5% to 8% of autogenous AVFs as a result of high pressure applied to a vein wall weakened by repeated punctures. Usually, the course of such aneurysms is benign and does not preclude use of the fistula; however, large aneurysms containing mural thrombus have been reported to cause late thrombosis and embolization. On rare occasions, progressive enlargement can compromise circulation to the skin above the aneurysmal vein, leading to incomplete hemostasis when the needle is withdrawn and ultimately to graft rupture. Skin compromise and progressive enlargement are therefore indications for surgical correction. Surgical revision is also recommended if the aneurysm involves the arterial anastomosis or is associated with stenosis of the venous outflow.

Options for revision include total excision of the aneurysm with primary reanastomosis, exclusion of the aneurysm with vein bypass grafting, and partial excision in which part of the vein wall is kept as the arterial conduit. The last option frequently results in early recurrence as the vein wall continues to weaken and dilate with time.

Pseudoaneurysm (AV Grafts)

Pseudoaneurysms occur in prosthetic AV grafts and are usually small and asymptomatic. They can be prevented by allowing sufficient time after graft placement to ensure firm fibrous encapsulation of the graft and by avoiding repeated needle insertion at the same site. On occasion, however, pseudoaneurysms are precipitated by underlying venous stenosis, which should be documented and corrected whenever present. Urgent surgical repair is indicated if the pseudoaneurysm is expanding rapidly or is causing ischemia of the overlying skin. Elective repair is indicated if the diameter of the false aneurysm is more than twice that of the graft.

Infection

Infection is the second most common cause of loss of AV access, occurring in 0% to 3% of autogenous AVFs and 6% to 25% of AV grafts. Infection may be acquired during surgery or cannulation of the conduit and is most often caused by *Staphylococcus aureus*.

Autogenous AVFs Infection of an autogenous AVF should be treated aggressively with 6 weeks of antibiotic therapy, much as subacute bacterial endocarditis would be. Local measures, such as

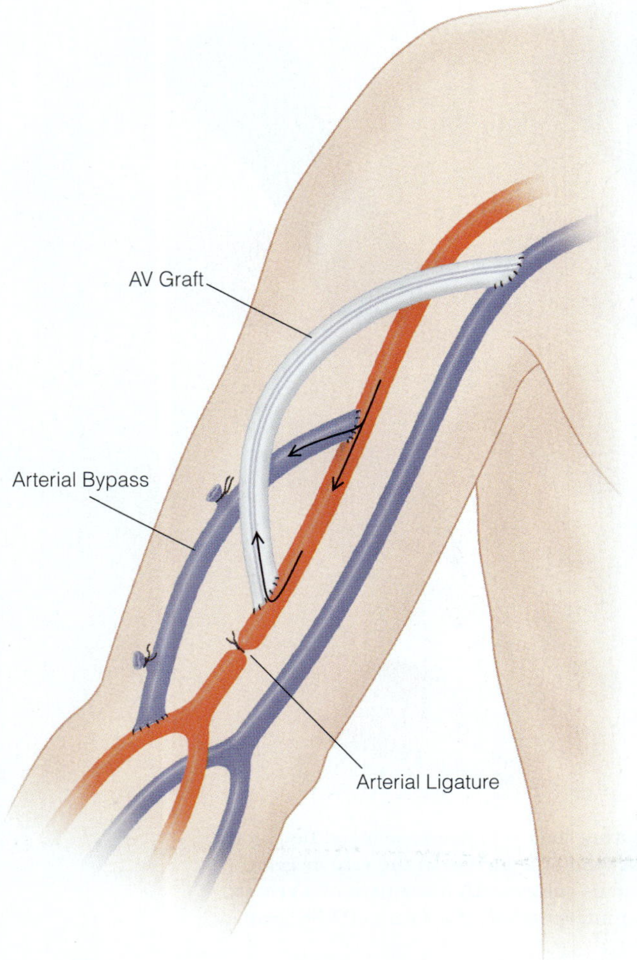

Figure 12 Vascular access via AVFs. Another option for treating steal is to ligate the source. Shown is the so-called DRIL procedure, which involves arterial ligation distal to the takeoff of the AV graft or the autogenous AVF and arterial bypass from a point 5 cm proximal to the fistula to a point just distal to the ligation.

drainage of a perifistular abscess, may be necessary. In rare instances, infection-induced anastomotic pseudoaneurysm or septic emboli necessitate takedown of the fistula.

AV grafts Generally, both antibiotic therapy and surgical treatment are necessary for cure. An antibiotic regimen that covers gram-negative organisms, staphylococci, and streptococci should be given until culture results are available. In most cases, complete excision of the prosthetic graft is required,[38] along with vein patch reconstruction of the artery. If the anastomosis is not grossly involved, a small cuff of ePTFE may be left on the arterial side and used to close the arterial defect; this does not seem to alter the prognosis.

In selected cases of well-localized infection, it is possible to resect only the infected portion of the graft and to restore the continuity of the fistula by placing a new conduit in a clean subcutaneous tunnel away from the infected area. A useful approach to managing an infected forearm loop graft is to resect the graft and reconstruct the fistula with an immediate anastomosis between the artery and the arterialized vein remaining after graft excision. Superficial surgical wound infections occurring in the postoperative period can sometimes be treated successfully with aggressive local debridement in combination with systemic administration of antibiotics. Deeper wound infections occurring in the postoperative period must be assumed to involve the entire graft, given that the graft is not yet well incorporated.

OUTCOME EVALUATION

Thrombotic events are the leading cause of access loss. For the most part, they result from venous outflow stenosis that can be detected before thrombosis occurs. An organized monitoring approach that includes regular assessment of the clinical parameters of the access and of the adequacy of the dialysis should be implemented in every dialysis center.[6] Such a proactive approach can be expected to reduce the incidence of thrombosis and increase patency.

Physical examination of the AV graft or autogenous AVF should be performed weekly and should include not only inspection and palpation for changes in the physical characteristics of the pulse or thrill but also a search for indirect signs of graft dysfunction (e.g., arm swelling, prolonged bleeding after needle withdrawal, and aneurysm or pseudoaneurysm). In addition to physical examination, the NKF-DOQI committee recommended routine access monitoring at least monthly with one or more of the following techniques:

1. Intra-access flow assessment using Doppler flow, magnetic resonance imaging, or ultrasound dilution online during dialysis. A trend toward decreasing flow or a flow rate lower than 600 ml/min for an AV graft and lower than 200 to 300 ml/min for an autogenous AVF is predictive of a high likelihood of access stenosis and eventual thrombosis.
2. Static or dynamic venous pressure measurement. Progressively increasing pressures or pressures that exceed the threshold value determined by each center's own protocol are predictive of significant venous outlet stenosis.
3. Urea and nonurea recirculation measurement. Recirculation is defined as the percentage of flow that is recirculated from the venous line into the dialyser inflow by retrograde blood flow through the fistula. A recirculation value exceeding 10% to 20% is significant and usually indicates low arterial blood flow or venous stenosis.
4. Delivered dialysis dose. A decrease is associated with venous outflow stenosis.
5. Arterial prepump pressure. An elevated negative pressure is a sign of inflow insufficiency.

Vascular Access via Percutaneous Catheters

Percutaneous venous catheterization is a useful method of gaining immediate access to the circulation; however, it is associated with significant risks, and the use-life of this type of access is shorter than that of AVFs. Percutaneous catheterization should be reserved for patients with acute renal failure who have an immediate need for dialysis and for patients with chronic renal failure in whom a permanent vascular or peritoneal access route either cannot be established or has not yet matured.

OPERATIVE PLANNING

Patient Assessment

A history is taken, a physical examination is performed, laboratory data are reviewed, and radiologic studies are ordered as for AVFs [*see* Vascular Access via Arteriovenous Fistulas, *above*]. Any finding that might affect the integrity of the central venous system should be noted.

A history or physical signs of previous central venous catheterization, a history of major injury or operation in the area where the catheter is to be inserted, a body mass index greater than 30 or less than 20, and an increasing number of insertion attempts are all known risk factors for perioperative complications from the insertion of venous access devices.[1] If there is any question about the patency of the central venous system, duplex scanning[39] or phlebography is indicated.

On physical examination, the surgeon should note the patient's body type, assess the flexibility of the patient's neck and shoulders, and evaluate the patient's ability to tolerate Trendelenburg's position without dyspnea or discomfort. Chest x-rays are reviewed to verify the patient's pleuropulmonary status and to identify any bony deformities.

The only laboratory study absolutely necessary is a complete blood count (including the platelet count and the differential count); prothrombin and partial thromboplastin times are required if the patient is receiving anticoagulant therapy. The effects of warfarin or heparin should be reversed before the procedure; patients with platelet counts lower than 50,000/mm³ should undergo platelet transfusion immediately before and during catheter placement.[40]

Choice of Type of Catheter

The catheters best suited for hemodialysis are high-flow, large-diameter (12 French or larger) devices with external ports. Silicone catheters are more flexible, are less likely to give rise to injury or thrombosis, and remain patent longer than polyethylene, polyvinyl chloride, and polytetrafluoroethylene catheters. Silicone catheters are available in both noncuffed (temporary) and cuffed (semipermanent) double-lumen configurations through which flow rates of 250 ml/min or higher can be achieved [see Figure 13]. The venous and arterial orifices are separated by 1 to 2 cm; recirculation is thereby limited to 5%.

Noncuffed (temporary) catheters Noncuffed catheters can be percutaneously inserted into the internal jugular, subclavian, or femoral vein without the need for fluoroscopic guidance. They are suitable for immediate use and provide acceptable flow rates (250 ml/min). Their main disadvantages are their high rates of infection, thrombosis, and venous stenosis and their short use-life (2 to 3 weeks). For these reasons, noncuffed catheters should be reserved for patients in whom access is expected to be needed for less than 3 weeks, and they should be inserted no earlier than required.

Cuffed (semipermanent) catheters Cuffed catheters are placed in a subcutaneous tunnel under fluoroscopic guidance. They are free of some of the shortcomings of noncuffed catheters; in particular, they are associated with lower infection rates and permit higher flow rates. Cuffed catheters are preferred when temporary access is required for longer than 3 weeks, particularly for patients in whom a primary AV fistula is maturing but who require immediate hemodialysis. Semipermanent catheters have been used for as long as 4 years, but long-term follow-up data on large numbers of patients is lacking.[41] Most patients readily accept this approach to dialysis: cuffed catheters allow so-called no-needle dialysis with high flow rates, they eliminate the problem of vascular steal, and they have no effect on cardiac function. In addition, patients appreciate that the access site is hidden from view, does not limit physical activity, and does not require particular care between treatments.

Choice of Insertion Site

The subclavian veins have given way to the right internal jugular (IJ) vein as the preferred site of primary central access. This site

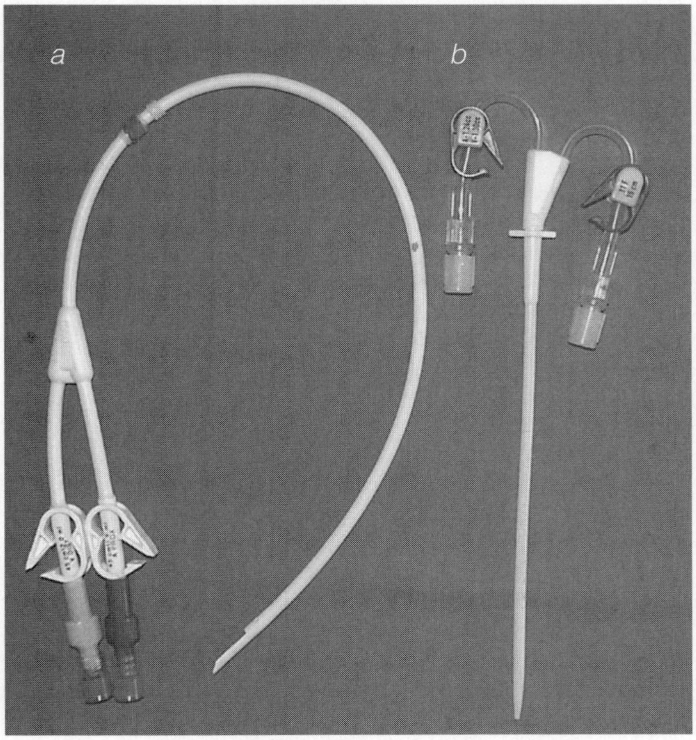

Figure 13 Vascular access via percutaneous catheters. Catheters used for hemodialysis include (*a*) cuffed double-lumen (semipermanent) catheters, introduced by means of the peelaway sheath technique, and (*b*) noncuffed double-lumen (temporary) catheters, introduced by means of the Seldinger technique.

has four main advantages: (1) it offers a consistent, predictable anatomic location with palpable landmarks, (2) it provides a short, straight course to the superior vena cava, (3) success rates are high, and (4) the risk of complications is diminished in comparison with other catheter insertion sites.[42] Of particular importance is that the risk of subclavian vein stenosis is decreased; this complication is a major concern for dialysis patients, who may require subsequent construction of an AVF in the ipsilateral arm. The right IJ vein is preferable to the left IJ vein as an access site because the latter calls for longer catheters, which increase the risk of kinking and diminish flow rates. The left IJ approach is also associated with a high rate of stenosis or thrombosis of the left brachiocephalic vein and may hinder subsequent use of the left arm for an AVF. Placement of the catheter in a subclavian vein either via the percutaneous approach or via cutdown on the cephalic vein should be reserved for cases in which neither jugular vein can be used.[6]

The right IJ vein can be catheterized percutaneously, or it can be surgically exposed and catheterized via direct needle puncture or phlebotomy (venous cutdown). The cutdown approach on the internal jugular vein or the external jugular vein allows greater control over the vessel than the percutaneous approach does and is preferred in patients who have a bleeding diathesis, patients whose body habitus or venous anatomy limits percutaneous access, and patients in whom a percutaneous attempt at placement has failed.

A less commonly used approach is femoral vein catheterization. It is technically easy and has few immediate complications, but it necessitates hospitalization (because the patient cannot ambulate) and is associated with high infection rates that limit use of the catheter to 5 days. Alternatively, access to the inferior vena cava can be gained by cannulating the greater saphenous, inferior epigastric, right gonadal, and lumbar veins. It is also possible to cannulate the azygos vein and the right atrium directly via thoracotomy.

OPERATIVE TECHNIQUE

Right Internal Jugular Vein Approach

Step 1: patient preparation Noncuffed catheters may be inserted at the bedside; cuffed catheters should be inserted in a standard OR with facilities for fluoroscopy.

The anatomy is surveyed before preparation and draping. Important anatomic landmarks include the sternal notch, the clavicle, and the sternocleidomastoid (SCM) muscle. The carotid artery should be palpated lateral to the trachea, under the medial (sternal) head of the SCM. The IJ vein lies lateral and slightly anterior to the carotid artery, between the sternal head and the clavicular head of the SCM muscle.

The patient is placed supine in Trendelenburg's position so that the neck veins are distended and the risk of air embolism is minimized. The head is extended and turned slightly to the left to expose the right side of the neck and keep the chin from interfering with the procedure. The neck should not be overextended or overrotated, however, because either of these actions flattens out the vein, making it more difficult to cannulate, and may increase the risk of arterial puncture by causing the internal jugular vein to overlie the carotid artery.

Step 2: cannulation of right IJ vein The jugular vein is located with a 22-gauge finder needle. This needle is left in place and used to guide the subsequent placement of an 18-gauge needle, through which the guide wire is passed. Use of the smaller needle minimizes the consequences of arterial or pleural puncture occurring during blind attempts at venous puncture.

After local anesthesia is administered, the fingers of the left hand are gently positioned on the carotid pulse to provide an anatomic landmark. The right hand locates the IJ vein by applying negative pressure to the 22-gauge finder needle mounted on a 5 ml syringe [*see Figure 14*]. The needle is inserted at the apex of the triangle formed by the two heads of the SCM muscle and directed toward the ipsilateral nipple at an angle of 30° from the plane of the skin. Alternatively, the needle may be inserted under the medial border of the SCM muscle and directed toward the thoracic inlet while the carotid artery is dislocated medially, or it may be inserted under the lateral border of the SCM muscle and directed toward the contralateral nipple.

Once the vein is located, the syringe is disconnected from the finder needle, which is left in place. The vein is then repunctured with an 18-gauge needle oriented parallel to the finder needle. When venous backflow is obtained, the 18-gauge needle is reoriented at a more acute angle to the skin and is advanced 2 to 3 mm. The syringe is disconnected and the needle hub occluded to prevent air embolism. A 0.035-in. guide wire with either a J tip or a flexible straight tip is then inserted through the needle, and the needle is withdrawn over the wire.

Troubleshooting. Because of the predictable anatomic location of the right IJ vein, the first attempt at cannulation is successful in the majority of cases. If the first attempt fails, the finder needle should be withdrawn and its tip reoriented slightly laterally; however, the needle should not be entirely withdrawn from the skin puncture site. An orderly, systematic search performed in this manner often identifies the vein while posing little risk of carotid artery injury as long as the carotid artery remains palpable medially. To avoid lacerating deep structures, the needle orientation should be changed only when the needle is inserted very superficially. If the vein cannot be located after several passes of the needle, the finder needle is withdrawn completely and the anatomy reassessed. Alternative puncture sites can be attempted. In difficult cases, cannulation may be carried out under ultrasound guidance, or a cutdown can be performed on the external or IJ vein through a small transverse incision.

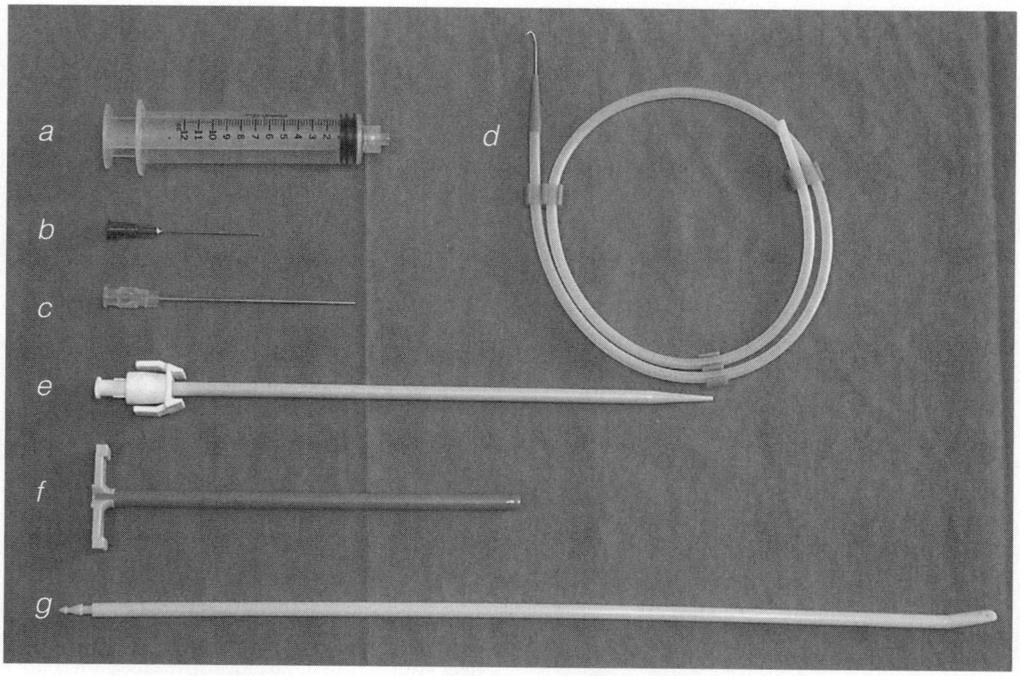

Figure 14 Vascular access via percutaneous catheters. The equipment used in percutaneous catheter insertion includes (*a*) a 5 ml syringe, (*b*) a 22-gauge finder needle, (*c*) an 18-gauge needle, (*d*) a guide wire, (*e*) a dilator, (*f*) a peelaway sheath, and (*g*) a plastic subcutaneous tunneler.

When the 18-gauge needle is advanced, the lumen of the jugular vein is often compressed, with the result being that the needle may transfix both front and back walls almost simultaneously. The needle tip should be advanced only slightly beyond the expected depth, then slowly withdrawn, with gentle aspiration maintained on the syringe. Entry into the vein is confirmed by the sudden and easy return of venous blood.

Pulsatile back-bleeding of bright-red blood from the needle usually indicates arterial puncture. If any doubt exists, the aspirated blood can be compared with a simultaneously obtained arterial sample, or the 18-gauge needle can be connected to a pressure transducer. Whenever there is any possibility of arterial puncture, it is preferable to withdraw the needle rather than take the risk of creating a large hole in the artery with a dilator.

The guide wire should be inserted with caution because any forceful movement can result in perforation of the vein wall. The risk is minimized by using a soft-tipped or J-tipped wire. The wire should advance easily into the vein without resistance; if it does not, the guide wire and the needle should be withdrawn together to ensure that the tip of the guide wire is not sheared off and does not embolize.

Step 3 (Seldinger technique): insertion of noncuffed catheter A small nick is made at the point where the guide wire enters the skin [see Figure 15]. The dilator is passed over the wire only far enough to enter the vein; it is then removed, and the catheter is inserted over the wire. The catheter tip should be placed in the superior vena cava, above the right atrial junction. This position is typically 15 to 18 cm from the puncture site if the catheter is placed in the right IJ vein; an additional 3 to 5 cm is required for the left IJ approach. The guide wire is then retrieved, venous blood is aspirated from both ports, and each lumen is flushed with heparinized saline. The catheter is anchored to the skin.

Troubleshooting. Dilators are relatively inflexible, and their stiffness increases with size. Consequently, they can easily perforate the vein wall if inserted deeper than the point of entry into the vein. Catheters may also cause perforation, though less commonly. The risk of catheter-related perforation is increased with the left IJ approach and the subclavian approach because catheters inserted from the left side must traverse the innominate vein and enter the superior vena cava at an acute angle, and this course increases the possibility that the tip of the catheter will perforate the right lateral wall of the superior vena cava. No resistance should be felt when the catheter is inserted. In addition, the guide wire should move freely within the catheter during insertion; such free movement suggests that the catheter is not compressing the wire against the wall of the vein.

Manual control of the guide wire must be maintained at all times; without such control, pushing a catheter or dilator over the wire can cause the wire to be completely advanced into the vein.

Inadvertent placement of a dilator or catheter into the carotid artery makes a large hole in the vessel wall, thereby creating the potential for substantial bleeding when the device is removed. In such cases, the catheter should be left in the artery, and a vascular surgeon should be consulted.

Step 3 (peelaway sheath technique): insertion of cuffed catheter A small transverse incision is made at the point where the guide wire enters the skin. Once adequate local anesthesia is achieved, a subcutaneous tunnel is created between the guide-wire entry point and a site on the chest wall at least 10 cm away [see Figure 16]. The position of the catheter is estimated by laying the catheter out along its intended tract; the course forms an inverted U, with the apex at the entry point of the guide wire and the tip of the catheter 5 cm caudad to the angle of Louis (at the second or third intercostal space). The position of the Dacron cuff is noted, and a stab wound is made in such a way that the cuff will be positioned in the subcutaneous tunnel, 2 cm from the wound. This placement simplifies removal of the catheter, prevents the cuff from eroding through the skin, and reduces the incidence of inadvertent catheter dislodgment. The exit wound should be at least 3 to 4 cm from the nipple-areola complex to allow space for the dressing.

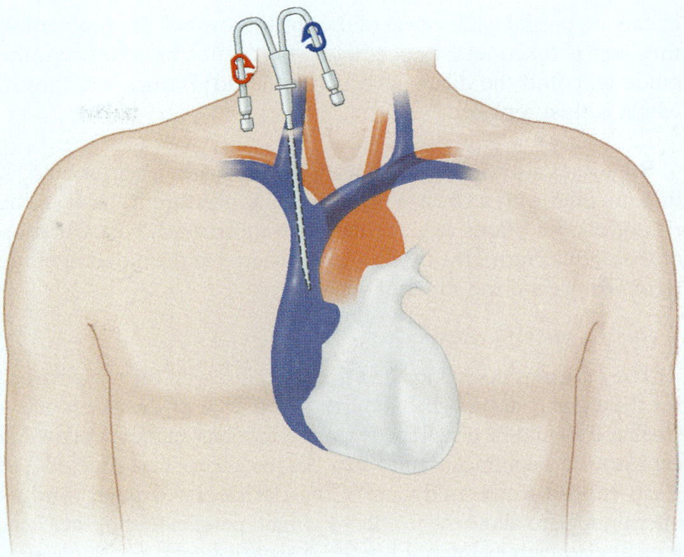

Figure 15 Vascular access via percutaneous catheters: Seldinger technique. Shown is a noncuffed (temporary) catheter inserted in the right IJ vein.

A plastic subcutaneous tunneler is attached to the catheter and used to pull the catheter through the tunnel so that the tip emerges adjacent to the guide wire. The venous dilator is then inserted over the wire to effect entry into the vein. Once entry is effected, the dilator is removed and inserted into the peelaway sheath, and sheath and dilator are introduced together into the vein over the guide wire. The guide wire and the dilator are removed, and the open end of the peelaway sheath is occluded with the fingers to prevent air embolism and bleeding. The flushed catheter is then inserted into the peelaway sheath and its position confirmed via fluoroscopy. When the catheter is well positioned, the peelaway sheath is cracked, peeled apart, and removed. Both lumina are tested for easy aspiration of blood and irrigated with heparinized saline. The two incisions are closed with absorbable sutures, and an adequate dressing is applied.

Troubleshooting. Because the procedure is performed under fluoroscopic guidance, fluoroscopy should be used to confirm that the position of the guide wire is satisfactory before the catheter is inserted. If the guide wire is not satisfactorily positioned, a 14-gauge plastic I.V. catheter is placed over the wire into the vein, and the wire is removed and repositioned through the catheter.

The peelaway sheath must be inserted to its full length, which means that the dilator must be inserted to its full length as well. Bending the dilator and the sheath into a gentle curve that matches the curve of the vein minimizes the risk of venous wall perforation, particularly if the left IJ approach or the subclavian vein approach is used.

If resistance is encountered when the catheter is inserted through the sheath, the usual cause is a kink in the sheath. In most instances, partial withdrawal of the sheath resolves the problem. If this step is taken and the catheter still cannot be advanced, the guide wire and the dilator can be reinserted through the sheath, which is then replaced.

Step 4: evaluation The location of the catheter tip should be documented with a chest x-ray after the procedure. To reduce the risk of complications (e.g., central vein thrombosis or perforation of the right atrium), the tip should be located at the junction of the right atrium and the superior vena cava.[43]

Subclavian Vein Approach

The patient is positioned and prepared in much the same way as for the right IJ approach. The arms should be at the sides, and a small roll should be placed between the shoulder blades to allow full exposure of the infraclavicular area. An insertion site is selected 2 to 3 cm caudad to the midpoint of the clavicle, far enough from its inferior edge to allow the needle to remain parallel to the clavicle as it passes beneath its inferior border. A slightly lateral position is preferred to prevent kinking of the peelaway sheath or compression of the soft silicone catheter between the clavicle and the first rib.

Local anesthesia should include the clavicular periosteum. The 18-gauge needle should be advanced into the space between the clavicle and the first rib in the direction of a finger placed in the suprasternal notch. The needle is oriented as horizontally as possible, and the bevel of the needle is oriented downward to decrease the risk that the guide wire will pass upward into the ipsilateral IJ vein.

Careful technique helps prevent pneumothorax and puncture of the subclavian vein. For example, "walking" the tip of the needle down the clavicle, so that it passes as closely underneath the clavicle as possible, reduces the risk of deep puncture and thus of pneumothorax. The rate of complications is directly related to the number of puncture attempts made; consequently, if the subclavian vein is not punctured on the second or third attempt, one should resist the temptation to make additional needle thrusts.

Once the vein is cannulated, the catheter may be inserted by means of either the Seldinger technique or the peelaway sheath technique as previously described [see Right Internal Jugular Vein Approach, *above*].

A chest x-ray will confirm the positioning of the tip of the catheter and the presence or absence of kinking. It will also rule out so-called pinch-off, which is a narrowing or notching of the catheter as it passes through the tight space between the clavicle and the first rib that may result in transection and embolization of the catheter tip.

Femoral Vein Approach

Femoral venipuncture is performed below the inguinal ligament just medial to the palpated femoral arterial pulse. The catheter is inserted by means of the Seldinger technique. The catheter should be at least 19 cm long to reach the inferior vena cava, thereby minimizing recirculation.

COMPLICATIONS

Early Complications

In more than 5% of catheter insertions, the catheter is improperly positioned. Such malpositioning may cause central venous perforation, venous thrombosis, or device malfunction. The most common positioning error is entry of a subclavian catheter into the ipsilateral IJ vein; less commonly, the catheter tip may inadvertently be placed in an axillary, internal mammary, azygos, or hepatic vein. Placement of the tip within the more cephalad portion of the superior vena cava at an obtuse angle to the venous wall or directly in the heart increases the risk of perforation. Catheter malpositioning is diagnosed by means of fluoroscopy or chest x-ray; management involves immediate repositioning of the catheter with the help of guide wires and fluoroscopy.

Guide-wire embolism can be prevented by being careful not to withdraw the wire through the 18-gauge needle, which can shear off the tip of the wire. Catheter embolism, though rare, may occur when a subclavian venous catheter is inserted too medially and as a consequence is compressed between the costoclavicular ligament, the clavicle, and the first rib. Such compression may lead to biomaterial fatigue, fracture of the catheter, or embolization. Embolized portions of a guide wire or catheter should be removed by means of interventional radiologic techniques to prevent thrombotic complications.

Air embolism occurs when air is inadvertently aspirated into the patient's venous system while the catheter is being inserted, removed, or used. It is easily prevented by using a fingertip to cover all potential communication sites between the venous lumen and the outside air, including the needle hub before guide-wire insertion, the open end of the peelaway sheath just before catheter insertion, and the disconnected external ports of catheters. Patients whose pulmonary status is compromised or who have aspirated large volumes of air may experience respiratory distress. Cardiovascular collapse, caused by obstruction of right ventricular outflow by gas bubbles, can also result. Auscultation may reveal a characteristic millwheel precordial murmur. The patient should be placed in the left lateral decubitus position with the foot of the table elevated so as to trap the air pocket away from the right ventricular outflow tract, and immediate ventilatory support for hypoxemia should be instituted.

Internal hemorrhage may occur at any site, usually as a result of perforation of a central venous or arterial structure during needle puncture or insertion of a guide wire, a dilator, or a catheter. Mediastinal hemorrhage, manifested by mediastinal widening on chest x-ray, occurs in fewer than 1% of all insertions.[44] It is usually self-limited in that the bleeding generally tamponades before hemodynamic compromise occurs.

If both a vascular structure and the parietal pleura are lacerated, hemothorax may result. The chest x-ray will suggest the diagnosis. Treatment includes placement of a thoracostomy tube and early consultation with a thoracic surgeon. Fortunately, the bleeding ceases spontaneously in most cases.

Pericardial tamponade, the most lethal complication of central venous catheterization, may arise as a consequence of perforation into the pericardial space, either through the wall of the vein or

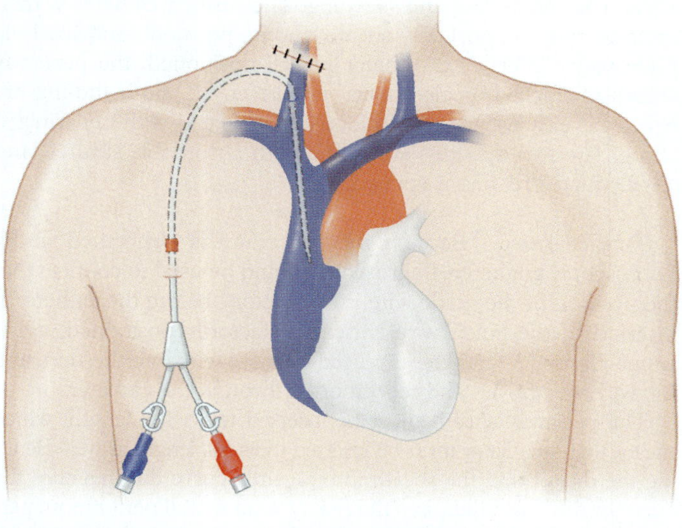

Figure 16 Vascular access via percutaneous catheters: peelaway sheath technique. Shown is a cuffed (semipermanent) catheter inserted in the right IJ vein and placed in a subcutaneous tunnel.

through the heart. It can occur immediately, or it can appear hours to days later as a result of delayed perforation by the catheter tip. Proper positioning of the catheter tip is the key to preventing pericardial tamponade. Treatment involves pericardiocentesis, creation of a pericardial window, or median sternotomy, depending on the patient's clinical status.

Cardiac arrhythmias are frequent during catheter insertion: atrial and ventricular arrhythmias occur in as many as 41% and 11% of patients, respectively.[45] These arrhythmias are usually benign; fewer than 1% call for cardioversion.

Pneumothorax occurs in 1% to 4% of attempts at percutaneous catheter placement. The incidence varies according to the experience of the operator and the site selected; in particular, it is higher with the subclavian approach. The presence of pneumothorax may be suggested by air in the syringe during attempts at vein cannulation and may be confirmed by chest x-ray. If the pneumothorax is asymptomatic, with less than 25% lung collapse, it can be treated conservatively; if it is large, symptomatic, or increasing in size, placement of a thoracostomy tube is indicated. Tension pneumothorax is an unusual but important complication that calls for immediate chest tube decompression.

Inadvertent puncture of a lymphatic duct may occur during left subclavian vein or left IJ vein catheterization in patients with hepatic portal hypertension or superior vena caval obstruction. The diagnosis is usually made when clear or milky fluid is aspirated in the syringe during vein cannulation; however, if the duct is punctured at the junction with the vein, the appearance of blood mixed in with the lymphatic fluid may mask the complication. Once lymphatic duct puncture is recognized, the procedure should be abandoned, and pressure should be applied to the site until lymphorrhagia abates. If the complication is recognized late on the basis of spontaneous leakage of lymph around the catheter, either the catheter can be removed or the leak can be stopped with a purse-string suture around the catheter. If persistent fluid drainage, subcutaneous edema, mediastinal enlargement, or chylothorax is noted, the leak is ongoing, and the catheter should be removed.

Late Complications

Central venous thrombosis Catheter-associated central venous thrombosis is more common than was once believed. It is often asymptomatic because of the rich venous collateral circulation in the area. Central venous thrombosis has been estimated to occur in 13% to 35% of catheter insertions[46] and to carry less than a 10% risk of pulmonary embolism and a 19% risk of postphlebitic syndrome. The incidence of catheter-associated thrombosis is correlated with the following factors:

1. Placement site. The incidence of thrombosis or stenosis is as high as 38% with subclavian vein catheters but less than 10% with IJ vein catheters.
2. Site of catheter entry. Surgical cutdown causes less endothelial injury than percutaneous puncture and dilation of the vein and may therefore be less likely to cause thrombosis.
3. Catheter tip position. Catheters placed high in the superior vena cava, near the brachiocephalic vein, are more likely to cause thrombosis.
4. Catheter size. Larger, stiffer catheters are more likely to traumatize the endothelium and to obstruct flow.
5. Catheter material. Silicone is less thrombogenic than other materials.
6. Duration of catheter placement. The incidence of thrombosis increases with the duration of catheter placement.
7. Underlying hypercoagulable state.
8. Associated catheter infection.

The diagnosis is easily made by means of duplex scanning or phlebography. Treatment involves removal of the catheter and administration of anticoagulant therapy. Asymptomatic patients who have no alternative sites for venous access should undergo anticoagulation without removal of the catheter. Thrombolytic therapy through the catheter, though never evaluated in a prospective randomized study, may be useful if the thrombosis is new or symptomatic, is progressing in the face of standard therapy, or is associated with catheter occlusion in a patient with no alternate site of venous access.

Catheter malfunction Catheter malfunction is the most common noninfectious complication of central venous catheterization. Malfunction is defined as either (1) failure to achieve a blood flow rate of at least 300 ml/min on two consecutive occasions or (2) failure to achieve a blood flow rate of 200 ml/min on a single occasion. In addition, partial or complete so-called withdrawal occlusion, in which solutions can be infused but blood cannot be withdrawn, may occur, as may complete occlusion.

Early catheter malfunction is usually caused by improper positioning of the catheter tip proximal to the distal superior vena cava, positioning of the tip against the venous wall, or subcutaneous kinking of the catheter. The precise cause can be determined via chest x-ray and contrast study. Malpositioning of the catheter tip can be corrected by using a tip deflector wire inserted through the lumen of the catheter, by snaring the catheter via the femoral approach and repositioning it, or by replacing the catheter.

Late catheter malfunction is usually caused by intraluminal thrombi; less commonly, it may be caused by extraluminal thrombi (e.g., fibrin tails or sheaths enveloping the distal portion of the catheter) or central venous thrombosis. Most late catheter dysfunction can be successfully managed with thrombolytic therapy. Thrombolysis with urokinase should be attempted first because of its high success rate (up to 90%) and its ease of administration.[47] Multiple protocols have been described. Typically, 5,000 units of urokinase, in a volume sufficient to fill the catheter lumen (usually 1.2 ml), is injected in each port and left in place for 20 to 30 minutes. The urokinase is then withdrawn, and another attempt is made to flush the line. The procedure can be repeated if necessary; the dose and the incubation time may be increased if desired because the urokinase is unlikely to reach the circulation. If catheter function fails to improve, imaging of the catheter with infused contrast material will allow identification and correction of other problems. Residual thrombus in the catheter lumen can be treated by means of intracatheter urokinase infusion (20,000 U/lumen/hr for 6 hours), catheter embolectomy, or catheter exchange over a guide wire. Fibrin sheaths around the catheter can be treated by means of urokinase infusion, fibrin sheath stripping with a snare,[48] or catheter exchange.

Catheter infection Infection is the most common complication of venous catheterization for vascular access, occurring in as many as 30% to 40% of patients. It is also one of the leading causes of catheter removal and morbidity in dialysis patients. Gram-positive bacteria, principally *S. aureus* and *S. epidermidis*, are the most commonly isolated organisms, though gram-negative bacteria and fungi may also be involved.

The clinical spectrum of catheter infection includes exit-site infection, tunnel infection, systemic line sepsis, and suppurative thrombophlebitis.

Exit-site infection. The characteristic signals are localized erythema, induration, tenderness, and exudate at the catheter exit site. Systemic symptoms are absent, and blood cultures are negative.

Treatment involves local wound care and application of topical antibiotics. The catheter need not be removed.

Tunnel infection. If the inflammatory process extends along the entire course of the subcutaneous tunnel, a more extensive cellulitic process, with or without purulent discharge, results. Initially, tunnel infection can be treated with parenteral antibiotics and local measures; however, it usually does not respond to this regimen, and removal of the catheter is often required. If a new catheter is called for, it should use a different tunnel and exit site.

Systemic line sepsis. This condition is manifested by systemic symptoms and signs of bacteremia in a patient who has a central venous catheter in place but exhibits no local evidence of catheter or tunnel infection and has no other identifiable source of infection. It is defined on the basis of the following two criteria: (1) in comparison with peripheral blood, a 10-fold increase in colony-forming units (CFU)/ml blood drawn from the catheter, or (2) in the absence of a positive peripheral blood culture, more than 1,000 CFU from blood drawn through the device. Empirical I.V. antibiotic treatment (including coverage for penicillin-resistant staphylococci) should be administered through the catheter. This measure will eliminate the clinical sepsis syndrome in 70% of patients. Once the antibiotics are discontinued, however, there is a 40% risk of reinfection; for this reason, catheter exchange over a guide wire, using the same tunnel and exit site, is recommended once bactericidal levels have been obtained[49] and the sepsis syndrome has resolved. I.V. antibiotics should be continued for 3 weeks thereafter. If the patient is unstable or still symptomatic after 24 to 36 hours of antibiotic therapy, removal of the catheter is mandatory. The catheter should also be removed if fungemia is suspected or confirmed.

Suppurative thrombophlebitis. When arm edema occurs in addition to systemic sepsis, suppurative thrombophlebitis of a great vein should be suspected. The diagnosis may be confirmed by means of duplex scanning or contrast phlebography. Treatment involves catheter removal, systemic I.V. antibiotic therapy, and heparin anticoagulation and is successful in more than 50% of patients. Vein excision is associated with significant morbidity and consequently is not indicated. Patients who do not respond to treatment can be treated with vena caval filter placement and central vein thrombectomy.

OUTCOME EVALUATION

To improve dialysis outcomes and to maintain or improve quality of care for dialysis patients, percutaneous catheterization should be performed only in selected cases. Given that percutaneous catheterization is associated with higher complication rates, morbidity, and mortality than AV fistulization, the goal should be to use percutaneous catheters in fewer than 10% of hemodialysis patients requiring long-term vascular access. In those cases in which central catheter placement is the best available option, the use of a consistent technique by skilled operators should, according to the NFK-DOQI, reduce the risk of serious complications necessitating intervention to 2% or lower.

Peritoneal Access

OPERATIVE PLANNING

Patient Assessment

For short-term peritoneal access, little formal patient assessment is required. The insertion site should be away from any areas of soft tissue infection and as far from any abdominal scars as is practical.

For long-term peritoneal access, more thorough patient assessment is required. Peritoneal dialysis is absolutely contraindicated in patients who have lost more than 50% of their peritoneal surface area. This degree of loss occurs in some patients who have previously undergone extensive intra-abdominal surgery or have had peritonitis or inflammatory bowel disease. Nonetheless, many patients who have undergone operation have a peritoneal cavity that either is usable for dialysis as is or could be made usable by lysis of adhesions. Patients who have previously undergone intra-abdominal vascular procedures are not candidates for peritoneal dialysis unless the graft is not accessible to the dialysate, so that episodes of peritonitis will not result in graft infection. In addition, adhesions are to be expected in such patients, and preparations to deal with them should be made when catheter insertion is being planned. If active local or distant bacterial infection is present, a permanent catheter should not be inserted until the infection has completely resolved. Advanced age is not a contraindication to peritoneal dialysis, but if the procedure is to be performed in an ambulatory setting, the patient must have sufficient motivation, dexterity, and mental capacity. A prolapsed rectum or uterus is considered a contraindication. Relative contraindications include very large polycystic kidneys, cutaneous stomas, and abdominal hernias. In patients with umbilical or groin hernias, herniorrhaphy may be done either before or at the time of catheter insertion. After herniorrhaphy, it is probably best not to use the catheter for several weeks; a small volume of heparin should be infused every other day while the site of the repair heals.

Choice of Type of Catheter

The catheters used for short-term access to the peritoneal cavity, as in diagnostic peritoneal lavage or short-term peritoneal dialysis, are constructed of rigid plastic and have no Dacron cuff. They may be inserted either percutaneously or under direct vision through small cutdown incisions; the preferred location is the midline.

To obtain long-term access to the peritoneal cavity for chemotherapeutic purposes, the surgeon may elect to place a subcutaneous reservoir to which a catheter is attached in such a way that the unattached end enters the peritoneal cavity. (The same devices are also sometimes used to obtain long-term nondialysis venous access.) The reservoir is accessed with special Huber-point needles; between uses, it is filled with heparinized saline. Alternatively, the surgeon may insert a Dacron-cuffed Silastic catheter [*see* Operative Technique, Step 1: Insertion of Catheter, *below*].

For long-term peritoneal dialysis, transcutaneous catheters made of silicone and equipped with one or two Dacron cuffs are used. These devices are available in a variety of configurations: the intra-abdominal portion may be straight or curved or may have plastic disks attached to it, and the subcutaneous portion may be straight or bent [*see Figure 17*]. The preferred configuration is a pigtail catheter with a preformed bend in the subcutaneous portion.

OPERATIVE TECHNIQUE

General Principles

Long-term peritoneal dialysis catheters may be inserted by means of percutaneous, laparoscopic, or cutdown techniques. Certain general principles apply to all these approaches. The double-cuffed catheter should be placed so that the catheter tip is in the pelvis, the inner cuff is in the rectus abdominis muscle (or adjacent to the linea alba), and the outer cuff is in the subcutaneous tissues. The exit site chosen should permit the patient to see the site to provide local care and should cause minimal interference with clothing. The catheter should exit the skin pointing in a caudal direction;

use of special curved or bent catheter configurations facilitates this. Nearly all patients need only local anesthesia; however, patients who have undergone abdominal operation should be prepared for general anesthesia in case extensive lysis of adhesions is required for satisfactory catheter placement.

What follows is a description of the most commonly used approach to insertion of a long-term peritoneal dialysis catheter, namely, use of a cutdown technique with the patient under local anesthesia [see Figure 18].

Step 1: Insertion of Catheter

Catheter insertion and exit sites are chosen so as to avoid old scars, belt lines, and possible future transplantation incisions. Full sterile precautions are taken. A local anesthetic is infiltrated at the catheter insertion site, and an incision is made down to the anterior rectus sheath. This incision is opened longitudinally, the rectus abdominis muscle is split, and the posterior rectus sheath is exposed. A purse-string suture of 2-0 absorbable material is placed in the posterior rectus sheath, and a small incision is made in the peritoneum.

The catheter is inserted into the peritoneal cavity and directed into the pelvis; if a curled catheter is used, it is directed by means of a lubricated straight metal rod. The inner cuff is positioned just outside the posterior rectus sheath, and the purse-string suture is tied. With the ends of the purse-string suture providing traction, the posterior sheath is held up, and a free tie of absorbable material is placed around the tented-up peritoneum and catheter to keep the insertion site watertight. The barrel of a 50 ml syringe full of saline is then attached to the catheter. When the syringe barrel is held above the abdomen, the fluid should flow freely into the abdomen by gravity alone. Conversely, when the syringe barrel is placed in a dependent position, the fluid should flow rapidly and freely out of the peritoneal cavity and back into the barrel. This test confirms that catheter position is satisfactory.

Troubleshooting The possibilities for error during placement are numerous: the catheter may be misdirected into the upper abdomen, it may be placed in a pocket of adhesions and blocked from reaching the greater peritoneal cavity, or it may be kinked in the abdomen, in muscle, or in the subcutaneous fascia. Plain radiographs sometimes facilitate recognition of incorrect placement. Surgical management—involving reexploration of the catheter insertion site, laparoscopy, or simple removal of the catheter and replacement at another site—is usually necessary if catheter malpositioning is not recognized at the time of the initial insertion.

Step 2: Tunneling of Catheter

The catheter is then tunneled to the exit site. It should emerge from the skin pointing in a caudal direction; this is more easily achieved with a catheter that has a preformed bend. The anterior sheath is closed snugly around the catheter, with the inner felt cuff left in the rectus abdominis muscle. The skin is closed with subcuticular sutures. If the catheter is to be used immediately, dialysis tubing is connected and a dressing is applied. If the catheter is not to be used immediately, 50 ml of saline containing 5,000 units of heparin is placed in the peritoneal cavity and the catheter is capped; this procedure is repeated every other day until dialysis begins.

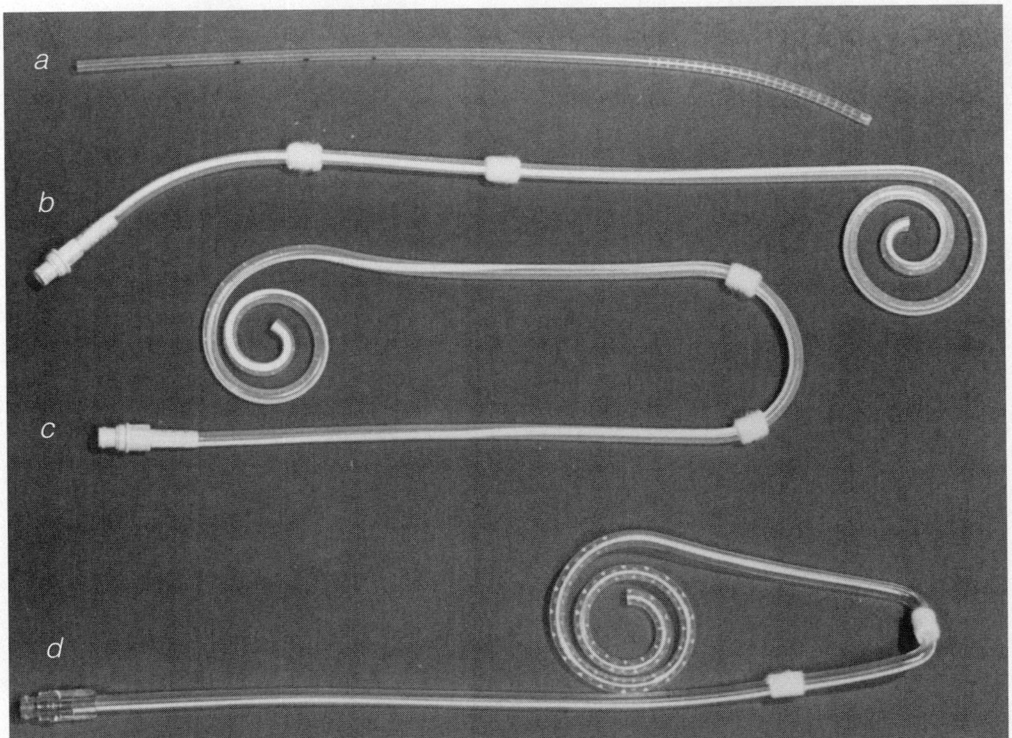

Figure 17 Peritoneal access. Four types of peritoneal access catheters are shown: (*a*) a rigid catheter without a cuff, designed for temporary use, (*b*) a pigtail silicone catheter with a straight subcutaneous portion, (*c*) a pigtail silicone catheter with a curved subcutaneous portion, and (*d*) a pigtail silicone catheter with a preformed bend in the subcutaneous portion, which is currently the preferred configuration.

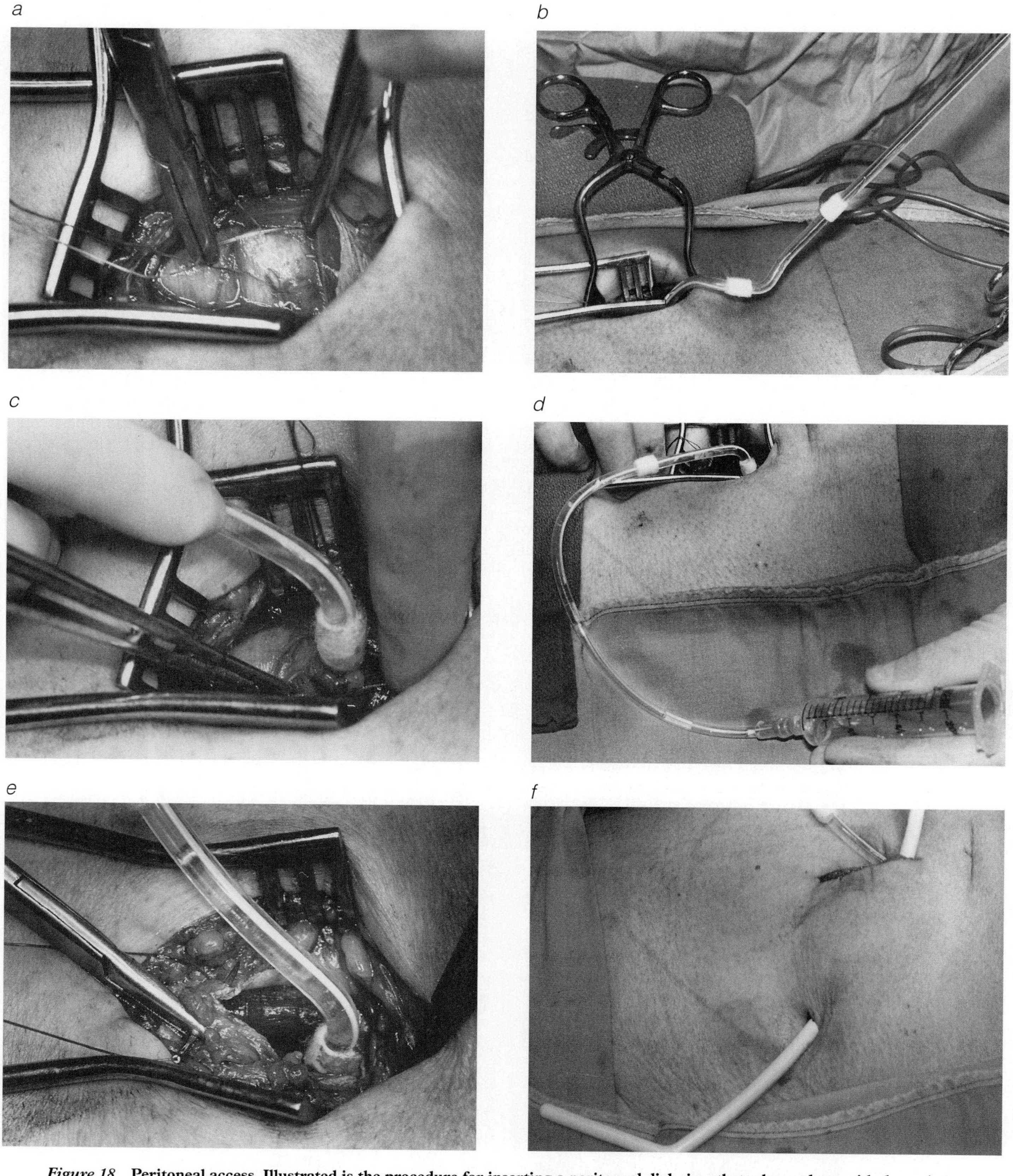

Figure 18 Peritoneal access. Illustrated is the procedure for inserting a peritoneal dialysis catheter by cutdown with the patient under local anesthesia. (*a*) A local anesthetic is infiltrated, the anterior rectus sheath is opened, the rectus abdominis muscle is split, and a purse-string suture is placed in the posterior rectus sheath. (*b*) With the stylet in place, the catheter is inserted in the direction of the pelvis (left). (*c*) With the inner cuff at the level of the rectus abdominis, the purse-string suture is tied and reinforced with an additional circumferential free tie around the peritoneum, if possible. (*d*) A flow test is performed to confirm satisfactory catheter position. (*e*) The anterior rectus sheath is closed over the inner cuff. (*f*) The catheter is tunneled to the exit site so that it emerges pointing inferiorly (left), with the outer cuff in the subcutis.

Step 3: Maintenance of Catheter

Maintenance of the catheter involves use of sterile dressings until the skin sites are healed, after which time a routine of skin cleansing and dressing is maintained. Whenever the catheter is disconnected, sterile precautions are taken to limit the possibility of contamination.

Step 4: Removal of Catheter

A Tenckhoff catheter is removed as follows. First, a local anesthetic is infiltrated into the original insertion site, and the inner Dacron cuff is dissected out of the rectus abdominis muscle (or the linea alba) with the electrocautery. Next, the catheter is divided and the abdominal portion removed. The rectus sheath (or the linea alba) is repaired with sutures, and the incision is closed. The subcutaneous cuff is then dissected out from the outside, and the outer portion of the catheter is removed. Finally, the insertion site is debrided, and the small skin opening is left to heal by second intention.

Troubleshooting Infection of the catheter tunnel or the Dacron cuffs necessitates some modification of this technique. If both the inner Dacron cuff and the outer are infected, salvage is impossible and the entire catheter must be removed. Areas of gross infection are treated with drainage and debridement and left open to heal by second intention. If alternative temporary peritoneal access for dialysis is available, a new catheter is not placed until the skin has healed completely. If no alternative temporary access is available, it may be necessary to insert a new catheter simultaneously at another site that is distant from the original infected location.

If only the outer cuff is infected and no other sites are available for subsequent catheter replacement, salvage may be attempted as follows: the outer cuff is dissected out of the subcutaneous tissue, the Dacron is shaved off, and this portion of the catheter is left outside the skin. This approach may allow resolution of the infection; however, it makes the inner cuff the sole barrier to deep infection and thus should not be used when alternative access is possible.

Special Considerations

Peritoneal access in children The technical considerations for peritoneal access in children are much the same as those for peritoneal access in adults. There are, however, some significant differences. If a Tenckhoff catheter is to be used in a child weighing less than 20 kg (44 lb), it should have only one Dacron cuff, which should be placed in the rectus abdominis muscle. The appropriate length for the catheter must be determined; this is done by measuring the size of the child from the point of insertion to the pelvic basin. Leaks should be prevented by ligating the peritoneum underneath the purse-string suture in the posterior rectus sheath [see Step 1: Insertion of Catheter, *above*]. General anesthesia is usually required. Postoperative dialysis volumes are selected according to patient size.

Alternative technology Laparoscopic techniques have also been developed for placement of peritoneal catheters. These techniques employ the standard 5 to 10 mm diameter trocars commonly used for laparoscopic procedures.[50] The catheter is inserted into the abdomen through a large cannula. One problem with this technique is that it is difficult to confirm that the deep cuff is placed within the musculature until after the cannula is removed. Moreover, despite the excellent visualization of the peritoneal cavity achieved with catheters placed in this manner, there is a high incidence of pericatheter leakage. Alternatively, one may resort to new techniques using specially designed equipment, such as the Y-Tec 2.2 mm–diameter Peritoneoscope, which always positions the deep cuff tightly within the musculature.[51] In fact, randomized, controlled studies have indicated that catheters placed via peritoneoscopy survive approximately twice as long as catheters placed via traditional surgical dissection.[52] Furthermore, such procedures can always be performed at the bedside with local anesthesia or in an outpatient setting.

COMPLICATIONS

The following are the most significant early complications of peritoneal access procedures:

1. Injury to intra-abdominal organs, most commonly the small bowel, the colon, the bladder, and the fallopian tubes. Immediate exploration is necessary.
2. Leakage of peritoneal dialysate soon after catheter placement. This complication is caused by inadequate closure of the peritoneum around the catheter.
3. Incorrect catheter placement, usually manifested by relatively good inflow but poor outflow.
4. Intra-abdominal bleeding, signaled by a bloody dialysate. Although most episodes of intra-abdominal bleeding are minor and self-limited and consequently do not call for transfusion or specific intervention, investigation to determine the underlying cause is warranted.

The following are the most significant late complications of procedures for peritoneal access:

1. Intra-abdominal bleeding. The most common causes of such bleeding are related to menstruation and ovulation.
2. Erosion of the outer cuff of the catheter through the skin. This complication can be treated by dissecting the remaining cuff completely out of the subcutaneous tissues and shaving off the Dacron [see Operative Technique, Step 4: Removal of Catheter, *above*]. Because this approach, as noted, leaves only the inner cuff as a barrier to infection, it is usually advisable to treat outer-cuff erosion by removing the catheter completely and replacing it at another site.
3. Catheter breakage. If more than 2 cm remains outside the skin, special repair kits may be used to splice a new external catheter piece onto the original catheter.
4. Tunnel infections. Such infections are typically associated with contamination and infection of the outer cuff. The most common causative organisms are *Staphylococcus* species and *Pseudomonas* species.[53] Nasal carriage of *Staphylococcus* is a risk factor for tunnel infections, and pretreatment with rifampin may help decrease the risk.[54] Although many tunnel infections can be controlled with several weeks of antibiotic therapy and some can even be cured, most eventually necessitate removal of the catheter, especially if there is concomitant peritonitis.[55]
5. Catheter malfunction. Late catheter malfunction is uncommon. Complete obstruction of both inflow and outflow is generally attributable to fibrin plugs and can be corrected by infusing streptokinase. Good inflow coupled with poor outflow frequently signals wrapping of the catheter by omentum. This problem can be corrected by performing an omentectomy either laparoscopically or in an open fashion via a low midline incision.

OUTCOME EVALUATION

When peritoneal dialysis catheter function is poor shortly after operative placement, possible causes to be suspected include misdirection into the upper abdomen, kinking, previous abdominal adhesions, and omental obstruction of the catheter. Most of these complications present with satisfactory inflow but poor drainage.

Plain radiographs of the abdomen (or contrast studies if the catheter is not radiopaque) may reveal the problem. Sometimes, the complications respond to enemas (which may alter the location of the catheter) and to persistent attempts to achieve satisfactory exchange. Frequently, however, abdominal exploration via a lower midline incision is required, followed by omentectomy, redirection of the catheter, or catheter replacement. If omental wrapping of the catheter is the problem, the entire omentum should be removed to prevent a recurrence. General anesthesia is often necessary, though in some cases, certain of these procedures can be done with the patient under local anesthesia with sedation or under regional anesthesia. Laparoscopy has also been used to diagnose and treat peritoneal dialysis catheter dysfunction; general anesthesia is usually required.

References

1. US Renal Data System: USRDS 1999 Annual Data Report. The National Institute of Health, National Institute of Diabetes and Digestive and Kidney Disease. Am J Kidney Dis 34(suppl 1):540, 1999
2. Kolff WJ, Berk HT, ter Welle M, et al: The artificial kidney: a dialyzer with a great area. 1944. J Am Soc Nephrol. 8:1959, 1997
3. Quinton WE, Dillard DH, Scribner BH: Cannulation of blood vessels for prolonged hemodialysis. Trans Am Soc Artif Intern Organs 6:104, 1960
4. Brescia MJ, Cimino JE, Appell K, et al: Chronic hemodialysis using venipuncture and surgically created arteriovenous fistula. 1966. J Am Soc Nephrol 10:193, 1999
5. Baker LD, Johnson JM, Goldfarb D: Expanded polytetrafluoroethylene (PTFE) subcutaneous arteriovenous conduit: an improved vascular access for chronic hemodialysis. Trans Am Soc Artif Intern Organs 22:382, 1976
6. National Kidney Foundation DOQI: Clinical Practice Guidelines for Hemodialysis Vascular Access. Am J Kidney Dis 30(suppl 3):S150, 1997
7. Schwab SJ, Quarles LD, Middleton JP, et al: Hemodialysis-associated subclavian vein stenosis. Kidney Int 33:1156, 1988
8. Passman MA, Criado E, Farber MA, et al: Efficacy of color duplex imaging for proximal upper extremity venous outflow obstruction in hemodialysis patients. J Vasc Surg 28:869, 1998
9. Silva MB, Hobson RW, Pappas PJ, et al: A strategy for increasing use of autogenous hemodialysis access procedures: impact of preoperative noninvasive evaluation. J Vasc Surg 27:302, 1998
10. Marx AB, Landmann J, Harder FH: Surgery for vascular access. Curr Probl Surg 28(1):15, 1990
11. Silva MB, Hobson RW, Pappas PJ, et al: Vein transposition in the forearm for autogenous hemodialysis access. J Vasc Surg 26:981, 1997
12. Hakaim AG, Nalbandian M, Scott T: Superior maturation and patency of primary brachiocephalic and transposed basilic vein arteriovenous fistulae in patients with diabetes. J Vasc Surg 27:154, 1998
13. Matsuura JH, Rosenthal D, Clark M, et al: Transposed basilic vein versus polytetrafluoroethylene for brachial-axillary arteriovenous fistulas. Am J Surg 176:219, 1998
14. Coburn MC, Carney WI: Comparison of basilic vein and polytetrafluoroethylene for brachial arteriovenous fistula. J Vasc Surg 20:896, 1994
15. Gracz KC, Ing TS, Soung L, et al: Proximal forearm fistula for maintenance hemodialysis. Kidney Int 11:71, 1977
16. Bender MHM, Bruyninckx CMA, Gerlag PGG: The brachiocephalic elbow fistula: a useful alternative angioaccess for permanent hemodialysis. J Vasc Surg 20:808, 1994
17. Polo JR, Vazquez R, Polo J, et al: Brachiocephalic jump graft fistula: an alternative for dialysis use of elbow crease veins. Am J Kidney Dis 33:904, 1999
18. Dagher FJ, Gelber R, Ramos E, et al: The use of basilic vein and brachial artery as an A-V fistula for long term hemodialysis. J Surg Res 20:373, 1976
19. LoGerfo FW, Menzoian JO, Kumaki DJ, et al: Transposed basilic vein-brachial arteriovenous fistula: a reliable secondary-access procedure. Arch Surg 113:1008, 1978
20. Humphries AL, Colborn GL, Wynn JJ: Elevated basilic vein arteriovenous fistula. Am J Surg 177:489, 1999
21. Benedetti E, Del Pino A, Cintron J, et al: A new method of creating an arteriovenous graft access. Am J Surg 171:369, 1996
22. Santaro TD, Cambria RA: PTFE shunts for hemodialysis access: progressive choice of configuration. Semin Vasc Surg 10:166, 1997
23. Lazarides MK, Staramos DN, Tzilalis VD, et al: Evoked thrill: a simple intraoperative maneuver predicts early patency of arteriovenous fistulas. J Vasc Surg 27:750, 1998
24. Lenz BJ, Veldenz HC, Dennis JW, et al: A three-year follow-up on standard versus thin wall ePTFE grafts for hemodialysis. J Vasc Surg 28:464, 1998
25. Tordoir JH, Hofstra L, Bergmans DC, et al: Stretch versus standard expanded PTFE grafts for hemodialysis access. Vascular Access for Hemodialysis IV. Henry ML, Ferguson RM, Eds. WL Gore & Associates and Precept Press, Chicago, 1995, p 277
26. Lumsden AB, MacDonald MJ, Kikeri D, et al: Prophylactic balloon angioplasty fails to prolong the patency of expanded polytetrafluoroethylene arteriovenous grafts: results of a prospective randomized study. J Vasc Surg 26:382, 1997
27. Shoenfeld R, Hermans H, Novick A, et al: Stenting of proximal venous obstruction to maintain hemodialysis access. J Vasc Surg 19:532, 1994
28. Marston WA, Criado E, Jacques PF, et al: Prospective randomized comparison of surgical versus endovascular management of thrombosed dialysis access grafts. J Vasc Surg 26:373, 1997
29. DeMasi RJ, Gregory RT, Sorrell KA, et al: Intraoperative noninvasive evaluation of arteriovenous fistulae and grafts: "the steal study." J Vasc Tech 18:192, 1994
30. Kwun KB, Schanzer H, Finkler N, et al: Hemodynamic evaluation of angioaccess procedures for hemodialysis. Vasc Surg 13:170, 1979
31. Odland MD, Kelly PH, Ney AL, et al: Management of dialysis-associated steal syndrome complicating upper extremity arteriovenous fistulas: Use of intraoperative digital photoplethysmography. Surgery 110:664, 1991
32. Mattson WJ: Recognition and treatment of vascular steal secondary to hemodialysis prostheses. Am J Surg 154:198, 1987
33. West JC, Evans RD, Kelley SE, et al: Arterial insufficiency in hemodialysis access procedures: reconstruction by an interposition polytetrafluoroethylene graft conduit. Am J Surg 153:300, 1987
34. Bussel JA, Abbott JA, Lim RC: A radial steal syndrome with arteriovenous fistula for hemodialysis. Ann Intern Med 75:1657, 1971
35. Schanzer H, Schwartz M, Harrington E, et al: Treatment of ischemia due to "steal" by arteriovenous fistula with distal artery ligation and revascularization. J Vasc Surg 7:770, 1988
36. Shemesh D, Mabjeesh NJ, Abramowitz HB: Management of dialysis access-associated steal syndrome: use of intraoperative duplex ultrasound scanning for optimal flow reduction. J Vasc Surg 30:193, 1999
37. Beathard GA, Settle SM, Shields MW: Salvage of the nonfunctioning arteriovenous fistula. Am J Kidney Dis 33:910, 1999
38. Zibari GB, Rohr MS, Landreneau MD, et al: Complications from permanent hemodialysis vascular access. Surgery 104:681, 1988
39. Haire WD, Lynch TG, Lieberman RP, et al: Duplex scans before subclavian vein catheterization predict unsuccessful catheter placement. Arch Surg 127:229, 1992
40. Whitman ED: Complications associated with the use of central venous access devices. Curr Probl Surg 33:324, 1996
41. Dunea G, Domenico L, Gunnerson P, et al: A survey of permanent double-lumen catheters in hemodialysis patients. ASAIO Trans 37:M276, 1991
42. Chimochowski GE, Worley E, Rutherford WE, et al: Superiority of the internal jugular over the subclavian access for temporary hemodialysis. Nephron 54:154, 1990
43. The Food and Drug Administration Task Force: Precautions necessary with central venous catheters. FDA Drug Bulletin 15:6, 1989
44. Mansfield PF, Hohn DC, Fornage BD, et al: Complications and failures of subclavian-vein catheterization. N Engl J Med 331:1735, 1994
45. Stuart RK, Shikora SA, Akerman P, et al: Incidence of arrhythmia with central venous catheter insertion and exchange. J Parenter Enteral Nutr 14:152, 1990
46. Horattas MC, Wright DJ, Fenton AH, et al: Changing concepts of deep venous thrombosis of the upper extremity: report of a series and review of the literature. Surgery 104:561, 1988

47. Suchoki P, Conlon P, Knelson M, et al: Silastic cuffed catheters for hemodialysis vascular access: thrombolytic and mechanical correction of HD catheter malfunction. Am J Kidney Dis 28:279, 1996
48. Crain MR, Mewissen MW, Ostrowski GJ, et al: Fibrin sleeve stripping for salvage of failing hemodialysis catheters: techniques and initial results. Radiology 198:41, 1996
49. Schaffer D: Catheter-related sepsis complicating long-term, tunnelled central venous dialysis catheters: management by guidewire exchange. Am J Kidney Dis 25:593, 1995
50. Douglas AF, Deardon DA, Barclay CA, et al: Laparoscopic insertion of CAPD catheters. Proceedings of the 3rd International Congress on Access for Dialysis. Maastricht, 1997
51. Ash SR: Bedside peritoneoscopic peritoneal catheter placement of Tenckoff and newer peritoneal catheters. Adv Peritoneal Dialysis 14:1, 1998
52. Gadallah MF, Pervez A, El-Shahawy M, et al: Peritoneoscopic versus surgical placement of Tenckhoff catheters: a prospective study on outcome. J Am Soc Nephrol 7:A0904, 1996
53. Prevention of peritonitis in CAPD (editorial). Lancet 337:22, 1991
54. Piraino B: A review of *Staphylococcus aureus* exit-site and tunnel infections in peritoneal dialysis patients. Am J Kidney Dis 16:89, 1990
55. Holley JL, Bernardini J, Piraino B: Risk factors for tunnel infections in continuous peritoneal dialysis. Am J Kidney Dis 18:344, 19

Acknowledgments

Figures 1 through 9, 11, 12, 15, and 16 Jean Montreuil, B.Ing, M.Sc. Digitized and adapted by Tom Moore.

63 CAROTID ARTERIAL PROCEDURES

Wesley S. Moore, M.D.

The rationale for operating on patients with carotid artery disease is to prevent stroke. It has been estimated that in 50% to 80% of patients who experience an ischemic stroke, the underlying cause is a lesion in the distribution of the carotid artery, usually in the vicinity of the carotid bifurcation. It would follow, then, that appropriate identification and surgical intervention could significantly reduce the incidence of ischemic stroke.

Carotid endarterectomy for both symptomatic and asymptomatic carotid artery stenosis has been extensively evaluated in prospective, randomized trials. Symptomatic patients have been studied in the North American Symptomatic Carotid Endarterectomy Trial (NASCET),[1] the European Carotid Stenosis Trial (ECST),[2] and the symptomatic carotid stenosis trial from the Veterans Affairs (VA) Cooperative Studies Program.[3] The results of all three trials conclusively demonstrate that symptomatic patients with greater than 50% stenosis on arteriography are at substantially lower risk for stroke after carotid endarterectomy than control subjects receiving medical management alone. Asymptomatic patients with hemodynamically significant stenosis also benefit from surgical treatment: the Asymptomatic Carotid Atherosclerosis Study (ACAS)[4] and the asymptomatic carotid stenosis trial from the VA Cooperative Studies Program[5] show that the risk of both transient ischemic attacks (TIAs) and stroke is markedly lower in patients treated with carotid endarterectomy and best medical management than in control subjects treated with best medical management alone.

Surgical reconstruction of the carotid artery yields the greatest benefits when done by surgeons who can keep complication rates to an absolute minimum. The majority of complications associated with carotid arterial procedures are either technical or judgmental; accordingly, in what follows, I emphasize the procedural details that I consider particularly important for deriving the best short- and long-term results from surgical intervention.

Preoperative Evaluation

PATIENT SELECTION

Indications for carotid artery surgery can be divided into two major categories: (1) asymptomatic critical stenosis and (2) symptomatic hemodynamically significant stenosis.[6]

Asymptomatic Critical Stenosis

ACAS and the VA asymptomatic carotid stenosis study both found that in patients with diameter-reducing stenosis of 60% or greater on angiography, carotid endarterectomy resulted in fewer fatal and nonfatal strokes over a 5-year period than nonoperative treatment with best medical management alone. It is important to keep in mind that there are several different ways of measuring stenosis [*see 12 Asymptomatic Carotid Bruit*]. The 60% figure cited by ACAS and the VA study was determined according to the North American method rather than the European method. Moreover, it was determined by means of contrast angiography rather than duplex ultrasonography (DUS) or magnetic resonance imaging. If the decision for carotid endarterectomy is to be based on DUS, some conversion of values is required. A patient who has an 80% to 99% stenosis on DUS can generally be assumed to have a diameter-reducing stenosis of at least 60% on angiography; a stenosis that is less than 80% on DUS may fall short of a 60% diameter-reducing stenosis on angiography.

Symptomatic Hemodynamically Significant Carotid Stenosis

Transient ischemic attacks Both NASCET and ECST found that symptomatic patients with hemodynamically significant stenoses experienced fewer fatal and nonfatal strokes after carotid endarterectomy combined with best medical management than after best medical management alone, provided that the perioperative morbidity and mortality from stroke was 6.0% or less. Thus, patients with monocular or hemispheric TIAs are good candidates for carotid endarterectomy. Global ischemic attacks have also been used as an indication for carotid endarterectomy. This practice has not been evalutated in clinical trials; it is usually justified on the basis of the ACAS data alone.

Prior stroke Patients who have previously experienced a hemispheric stroke but who are not disabled and have made a reasonable recovery are also good candidates for carotid endarterectomy if they have a hemodynamically significant stenosis.

IMAGING

Indications for Carotid Duplex Scanning

Identification of a carotid lesion that can be treated with endarterectomy usually begins with a carotid duplex scan. Indications for carotid duplex scanning fall into three main categories: symptoms, signs, and risk factors. Symptoms include classic TIAs and strokes that give rise to clinical suspicion of carotid bifurcation disease. The primary sign is the presence of a carotid bruit on auscultation. Risk factors include cigarette smoking, hypertension, diabetes mellitus, hypercholesterolemia, peripheral vascular disease, and coronary artery disease. As the number of risk factors present increases, the likelihood of associated carotid bifurcation disease increases exponentially.

Other Considerations in Symptomatic Patients

Patients who present with focal ischemic symptoms are likely to have associated carotid bifurcation disease; however, other pathologic conditions (e.g., emboli of cardiac origin, aortic arch disease, intracranial vascular disease, coagulopathy, and brain tumors) can also be responsible for focal symptoms. Accordingly, a complete workup of a symptomatic patient should include cardiac evaluation as well as intracranial imaging.

Additional Arterial Imaging

The accuracy of carotid duplex scanning is highly dependent on the technician performing it and on the laboratory where it is done. A carefully performed carotid duplex scan is often the most accurate indicator of carotid bifurcation disease; however, a hastily or carelessly performed scan can result in overestimation of the extent of the carotid bifurcation disease. For this reason, additional imaging studies (e.g., MRI, computed tomographic angiography, and, when there is serious doubt, contrast angiography) may be indicated.

Operative Planning

Before operation is scheduled, the general health of the patient must be assessed, with particular attention paid to cardiac and pulmonary status. Given that many patients with carotid artery disease are hypertensive or diabetic, good preoperative control of diabetes mellitus and blood pressure is mandatory. Finally, to reduce the risk of thromboembolic complications, patients should receive antiplatelet drugs (e.g., aspirin) up to and on the day of operation.

ANESTHESIA

Surgery on the cervical portion of the carotid artery may be performed with the patient under either general or cervical block anesthesia. Both techniques have their advocates, their advantages, and their disadvantages.

The advantages of general anesthesia include a quiet operative field, maximal patient comfort, good airway control, and convenient blood gas management. In addition, general anesthesia may lead to improved cerebral blood flow and give better protection against reduced blood flow during carotid clamping. The disadvantages of general anesthesia include blood pressure swings during induction and the inability to monitor the patient's conscious response to carotid clamping. Some reports also suggest that the incidence of cardiac complications is higher during general anesthesia than during cervical block anesthesia.

The main advantage of cervical block anesthesia is the ability to monitor cerebral function during carotid clamping: an awake patient can be engaged in conversation and can be asked to carry out motor activities of the extremities. The disadvantages of cervical block anesthesia include possible patient discomfort, restlessness, and intolerance of the longer operations that are sometimes necessary for technical reasons. Another disadvantage is that on occasion, a patient cannot tolerate carotid clamping and demonstrates an immediate neurologic deficit with clamp application. Such an occurrence heightens the anxiety level of the surgical team, thereby increasing the risk that they will commit technical errors in the rush to place an internal shunt.

Besides considering the inherent advantages and disadvantages of these two anesthetic techniques with respect to the patient, it is important to consider their advantages and disadvantages with respect to individual surgical practice. A given surgeon may well work better and achieve better results with one technique or the other.

Whichever anesthetic approach is used, all patients should have a radial arterial line in place to allow continuous blood pressure monitoring as well as provide access for determining blood gas levels. As a rule, there is no need to place a central venous line or a right heart catheter, except in patients with marginal cardiac function.

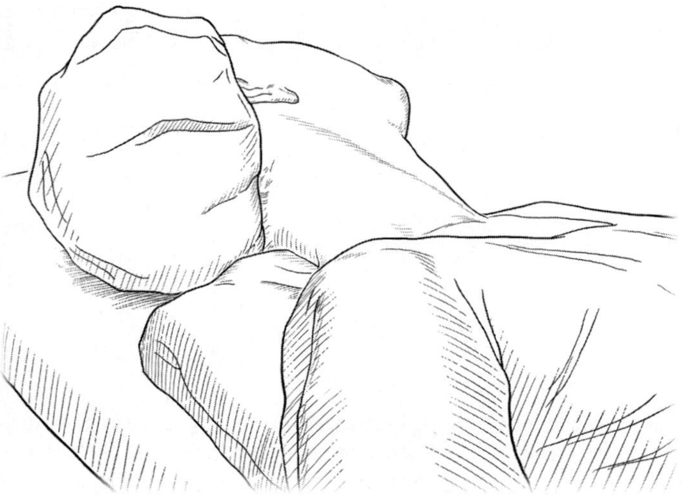

Figure 1 Carotid arterial procedures. Shown is the recommended patient positioning.

PATIENT POSITIONING

Proper positioning of the patient is necessary to provide optimal exposure of the neck from the clavicle up to the mastoid process on the side of the proposed operation [*see Figure 1*]. The patient is placed in the supine position with a folded sheet under the shoulders to induce a mild degree of neck extension. Excessive neck extension should be avoided, however, because it places tension on the artery and actually hinders rather than facilitates exposure. This potential problem can be addressed by placing one or more towels under the head to adjust the neck to the optimal degree of extension. The patient's head is then turned away from the side of the operation to improve cervical exposure further. Finally, the table top may be rotated slightly away from the side of the operation so as to provide a flat surgical field. The head of the table may be elevated slightly if the patient's blood pressure is adequate; this step helps

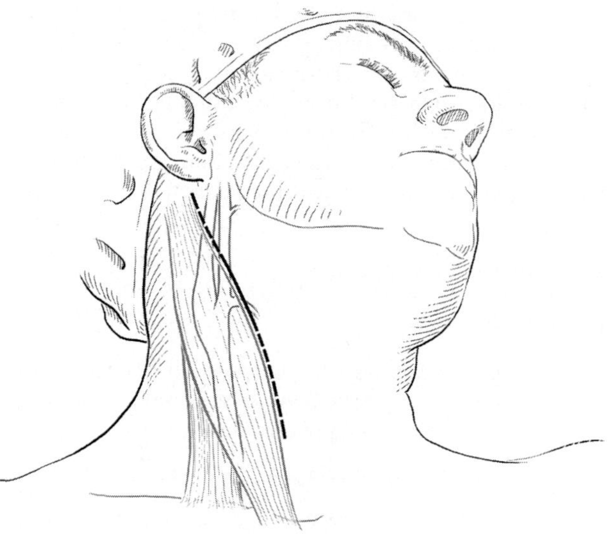

Figure 2 Carotid arterial procedures. The incision most commonly used to expose the cervical carotid artery is a vertical one placed along the anterior margin of the sternocleidomastoid muscle and centered over the presumed location of the carotid bifurcation. It may be extended proximally or distally, depending on where the carotid bifurcation turns out to be.

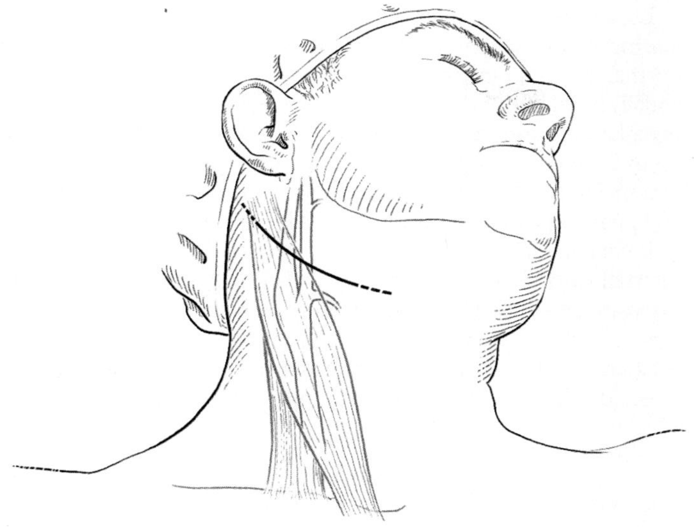

Figure 3 Carotid arterial procedures. An alternative incision to the vertical incision is a transverse incision along a skin crease in the vicinity of the carotid bifurcation.

lower venous pressure and reduce venous bleeding during the operation [*see Figure 1*].

Operative Technique

STEP 1: INITIAL INCISION

Either of two incisions may be used for exposure of the cervical carotid artery. The more common choice is a vertical incision placed along an imaginary line that extends from the sternoclavicular junction to the mastoid process, paralleling the anterior margin of the sternocleidomastoid muscle as well as the course of the carotid artery and the contents of the carotid sheath [*see Figure 2*]. The incision is centered over the presumed location of the carotid bifurcation. The advantage of this incision is that it provides optimal exposure of the cervical carotid artery and can readily be extended either proximally or distally along the aforementioned imaginary line to give additional exposure when needed (e.g., when the carotid bifurcation is unusually high). The disadvantage of this incision is that it runs against Langer's lines; thus, if a keloid occurs, it is likely to be in an unsightly position. In most patients, the incision heals to a fine line, and it usually is not noticeable once healing is complete.

The alternative to the vertical incision is a transverse incision that is placed in a skin crease on the anterior portion of the neck and then curved toward the mastoid process posteriorly [*see Figure 3*]. Skin flaps are raised in a subplatysmal layer, and the incision is deepened along the anterior border of the sternocleidomastoid muscle. The advantage of this alternative incision is that it may be more cosmetically acceptable; however, its inferior portion frequently crosses the neck anteriorly, which may make it more visible than an incision confined to the line of the sternocleidomastoid muscle would be. The disadvantage of this incision is that it requires the raising of skin flaps, which takes additional time and may limit the extent of any proximal exposure that may be required.

STEP 2: EXPOSURE OF CAROTID ARTERY

Once the incision through the platysmal layer has been completed, an avascular areolar plane is developed along the anterior border of the sternocleidomastoid muscle for the full length of the incision so as to expose the carotid sheath. The internal jugular vein is usually the most visible vessel, and the carotid sheath is opened along this vessel's anterior border. The common facial vein, which drains into the internal jugular vein, is a relatively constant landmark. Because the common facial vein is the venous analogue of the external carotid artery, it can generally be used as a guide to the position of the carotid bifurcation [*see Figure 4*]. On occasion, a patient has several accessory facial veins instead of a single common facial vein. The common facial vein or the accessory facial veins are then divided between ligatures so that the jugular vein can be retracted laterally. The common carotid artery and the carotid bifurcation lie immediately beneath the divided facial veins.

At this point, care must be taken to look for the vagus nerve. This nerve is usually located posterior to the common carotid artery, but it is sometimes rotated into a more superficial position. Another important neurologic structure in this area is the ansa cervicalis, which is formed by the junction of fibers from the hypoglossal (12th cranial) nerve and fibers from the first cervical nerve and which continues inferiorly as a single trunk, providing innervation to the strap muscles. This nerve should be spared if possible, but it can be divided without significant sequelae if it interferes with optimal exposure of the carotid bifurcation. One convenient method of separating the nerve from the artery is to divide the fibers running from the first cervical nerve to the ansa cervicalis; when this is done, the nerve is readily mobilized and retracted anteriorly away from the carotid artery.

The perivascular plane of the common carotid artery is then entered, and the common carotid artery is circumferentially mobilized. The common carotid artery is palpated against a right-angle clamp to determine the proximal extent of the atherosclerotic plaque. If possible, the common carotid artery should be mobilized proximal to the plaque until a circumferentially soft portion of that vessel is

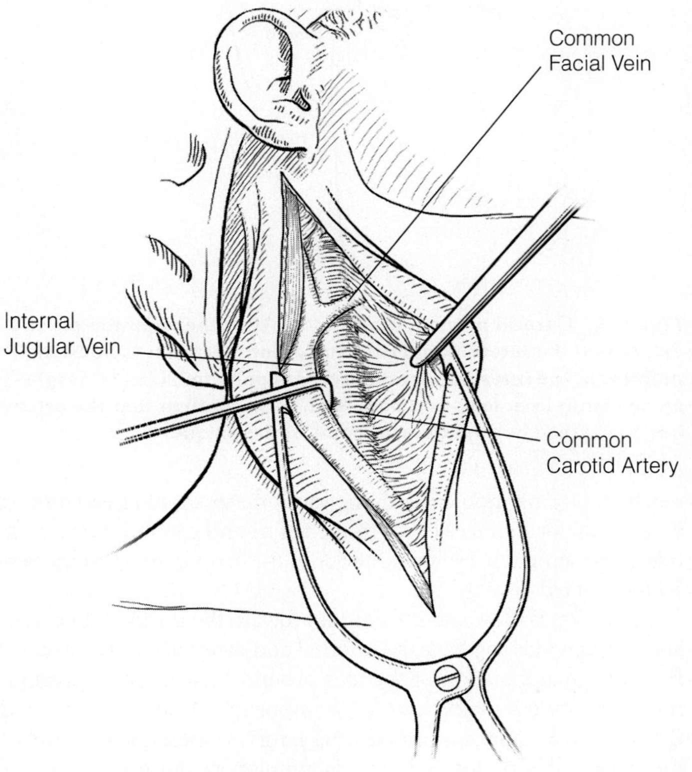

Figure 4 Carotid arterial procedures. After the sternocleidomastoid muscle is mobilized off the carotid sheath, the jugular vein is identified. The perivascular plane along the jugular vein is opened until the common facial vein is exposed.

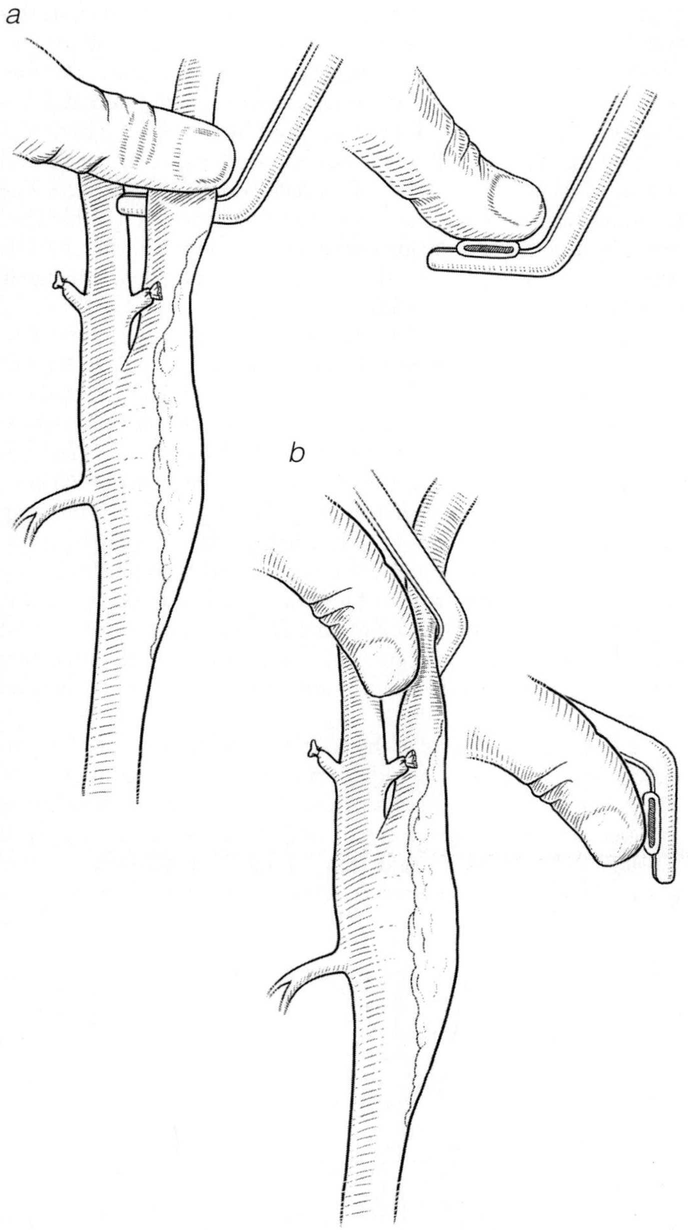

Dissection should then continue distally beyond the bulb of the internal carotid artery to a point where the internal carotid artery is normal. At this point, the relevant portion of the vessel is circumferentially mobilized and palpated against a right-angle clamp in at least two planes to confirm that the atheromatous plaque does not reach up to the level of the proposed clamping [*see Figure 5*]. Once this is accomplished, the external carotid artery is mobilized beyond the end point of plaque extension in a similar manner.

If the patient has a high carotid bifurcation or if the plaque in the internal carotid artery extends further distally than usual, a more extensive exposure of the carotid bifurcation, the internal carotid artery, or both is required. To provide such exposure, the skin incision is extended all the way to the mastoid process. The sternocleidomastoid muscle is fully mobilized up to the mastoid process, with reached. During mobilization, the vagus nerve should be identified in its usual location posterior to the vessel and carefully protected; this nerve sometimes spirals anterior to the carotid artery as the vessel is dissected distally.

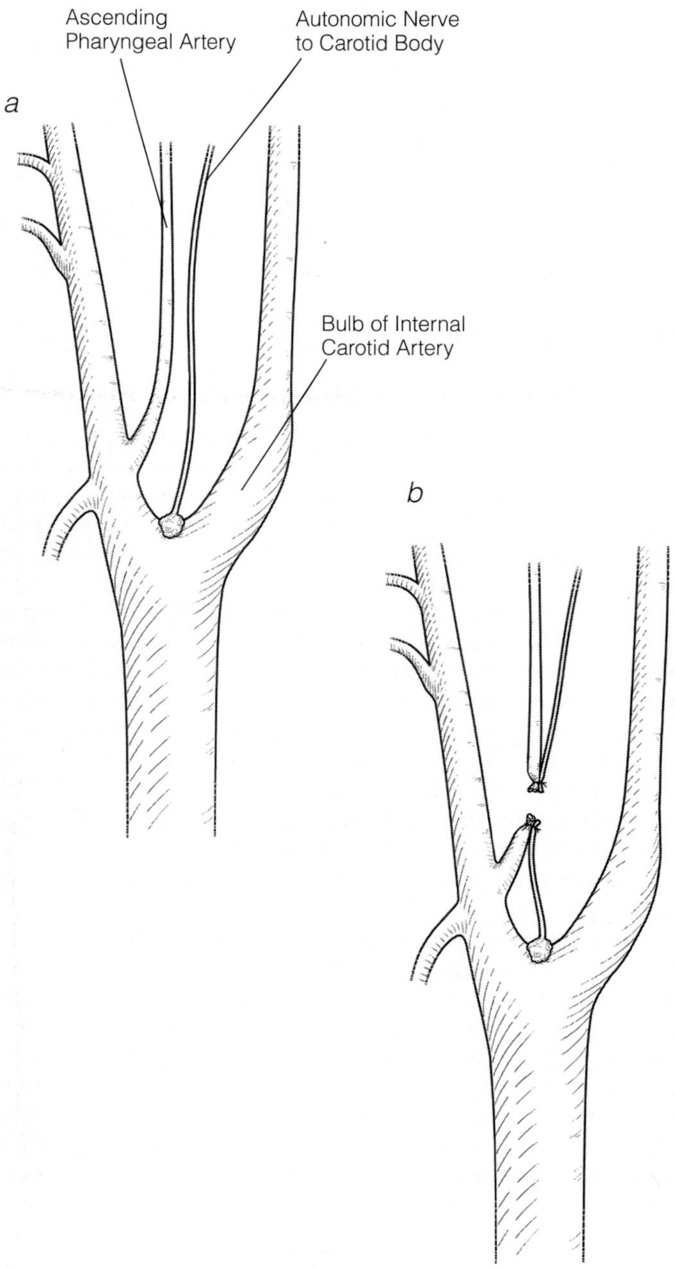

Dissection is then extended distally toward the carotid bifurcation and continued along both the internal and external carotid arteries. Excessive manipulation of the area around the carotid bifurcation must be avoided. In particular, it is important to be careful around the bulb of the internal carotid artery: this is where the majority of the plaque will be located, and manipulation can easily dislodge plaque or thromboembolic material. With exposure of the carotid bifurcation, the hypoglossal nerve may come into view. Care should be taken not to injure this nerve, though it may have to be mobilized to permit sufficient distal exposure of the internal carotid artery.

Figure 5 **Carotid arterial procedures. After the common carotid artery and the internal and external carotid arteries have been mobilized, the internal carotid artery is palpated against a right-angle clamp in at least two planes (*a, b*) to confirm that the artery has been freed beyond the end point of the plaque.**

Figure 6 **Carotid arterial procedures. Once the common, internal, and external carotid arteries are fully mobilized, the structures between the internal and external carotid arteries (*a*) are divided (*b*) to allow the carotid bifurcation to drop down.**

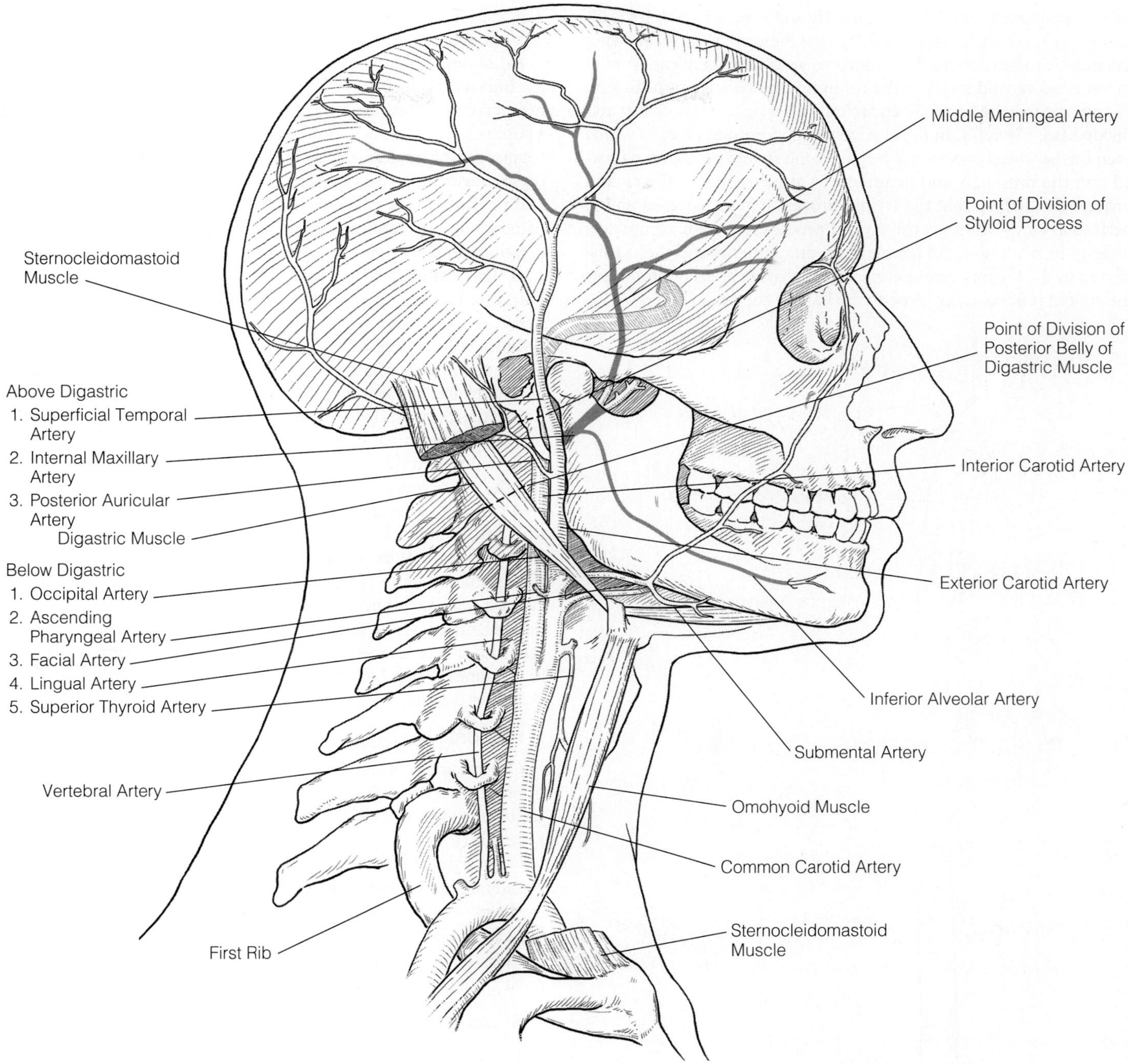

Figure 7 Carotid arterial procedures. Division of the posterior belly of the digastric muscle yields additional exposure of the internal carotid artery. If the internal carotid artery must be mobilized all the way to the base of the skull, further distal exposure is obtained by separating the attachments of the ligaments to the styloid process and dividing the styloid process.

care taken to look for the spinal portion of the accessory (11th cranial) nerve as it enters the sternocleidomastoid muscle on the medial surface. With the sternocleidomastoid muscle fully mobilized and retractors in place, the internal carotid artery can then be further exposed.

The jugular vein is mobilized up toward the base of the skull, with care taken to look for additional accessory facial branches, which must be divided between ligatures so that the jugular vein can be fully mobilized and moved posteriorly. The perivascular plane of the internal carotid artery is carefully defined, and the artery is gently mobilized with a sharp-tipped clamp applied in a spreading motion; in this way, the more distal portion of the internal carotid artery can be mobilized downward. If the vessel is still insufficiently mobile, then the nerve to the carotid body and the ascending pharyngeal artery within the crotch between the internal and external carotid arteries are mobilized and divided between ligatures. These two structures often serve as a de facto suspensory ligament for the carotid bulb; dividing them allows the carotid bifurcation to drop down and permits further downward traction of the internal carotid artery as the vessel is gently mobilized distally [*see Figure 6*].

Once the internal carotid artery is further exposed distally and the hypoglossal nerve is mobilized along its vertical portion and moved anteriorly, the posterior belly of the digastric muscle is encountered.

An areolar plane is developed posteriorly and superiorly along the inferior margin of the posterior belly of the digastric muscle, allowing the muscle to be mobilized anteriorly to yield additional exposure of the internal carotid artery. If the resulting exposure is not sufficient, the muscle may be carefully encircled with a right-angle clamp and divided [see Figure 7]. In those relatively uncommon cases in which even further distal exposure is required, the styloid process is palpated and the muscular and ligamentous attachments to the styloid process divided, so that the styloid process can be exposed with a periosteal elevator. Once the styloid process has been completely freed of its muscular and ligamentous attachments and the cranial nerves in the vicinity have been identified and carefully protected, the styloid process is cut close to the base of the skull [see Figure 7].

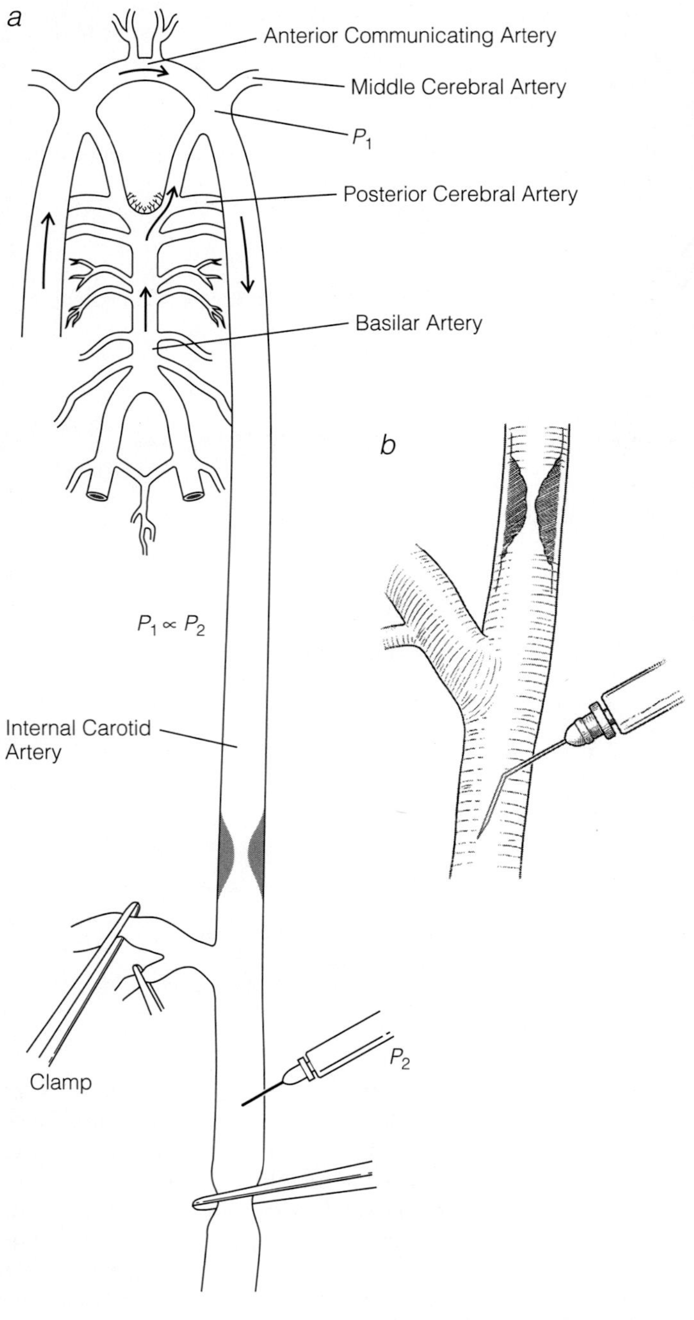

This step yields optimal exposure of the internal carotid artery all the way to the base of the skull.

Additional adjunctive measures for more extensive exposure of the internal carotid artery have been described. These include subluxation or dislocation of the mandible,[7] wiring of the mandible into a subluxed position, and division of the ramus of the mandible with rotation of the mandible away from the base of the skull. In my view, these measures are unnecessary, provided that the sternocleidomastoid muscle and the jugular vein have been adequately mobilized, the plane around the internal carotid artery has been developed, and the carotid bifurcation has been released.

A significant risk associated with extended exposure of the internal carotid artery is possible injury to the vagus nerve, the accessory nerve, or the hypoglossal nerve. Retraction of the vagus nerve may produce either temporary or permanent vocal cord palsy, and extensive retraction of or injury to the hypoglossal nerve causes denervation of the ipsilateral side of the tongue, manifested by tongue deviation to the ipsilateral side on protrusion or difficulty with mastication or swallowing. In addition, posterior exposure of a high carotid bifurcation may result in injury to branches of the glossopharyngeal (ninth cranial) nerve.

A common error in carotid artery mobilization is failure to recognize that the plaque in the internal carotid artery extends beyond the upper limit of the arterial exposure. It is far better to anticipate this problem before clamping and opening the artery than to discover it afterward and be forced to mobilize the vessel after it has been clamped. Once the common carotid and internal carotid arteries have been mobilized sufficiently, they are encircled with umbilical tapes; Rumel tourniquets are used if an internal shunt is required or desired.

STEP 3: CEREBRAL CIRCULATORY SUPPORT

Clamping of the carotid artery necessarily results in interruption of blood flow through the vessel. Patients who have good collateral circulation via the contralateral carotid artery or the vertebral arteries generally (though not always) tolerate the temporary interruption of flow through the clamped artery well.[8] Patients who have inadequate collateral blood flow require cerebral circulatory support, usually in the form of placement of an internal shunt. There are three basic approaches to shunt use: (1) routine use of an internal shunt, (2) selective use of an internal shunt, and (3) routine avoidance of shunting in an attempt to minimize clamp time.

Shunting Options

Routine shunting In approximately 10% of patients undergoing carotid artery surgery, collateral blood flow is inadequate and temporary use of an indwelling shunt is necessary to prevent brain damage; in the remaining 90%, collateral blood flow is adequate and clamping generally well tolerated, and shunting is therefore unnecessary. Clearly, routine use of an internal shunt takes care of the 10% of patients who require shunts. Its disadvantage is that it is an additional procedure that carries its own complications, to which not only the 10% of patients who require shunting but also the 90% who do not are subjected. The potential complications associated with placement of a shunt include intimal injury (including the raising of an intimal flap), atheroma embolization (if atheromatous material is scooped up during shunt placement), and air embolization (if air bubbles are trapped within the shunt and not recognized).

Selective shunting Selective placement of a shunt has an advantage over routine placement in that the procedure and its potential complications are limited to the 10% of patients who actually re-

Figure 8 **Carotid arterial procedures. (*a*) Shown is a graphic representation of the measurement of internal carotid artery back-pressure. (*b*) The needle is bent at a 45° angle before being inserted into the common carotid artery.**

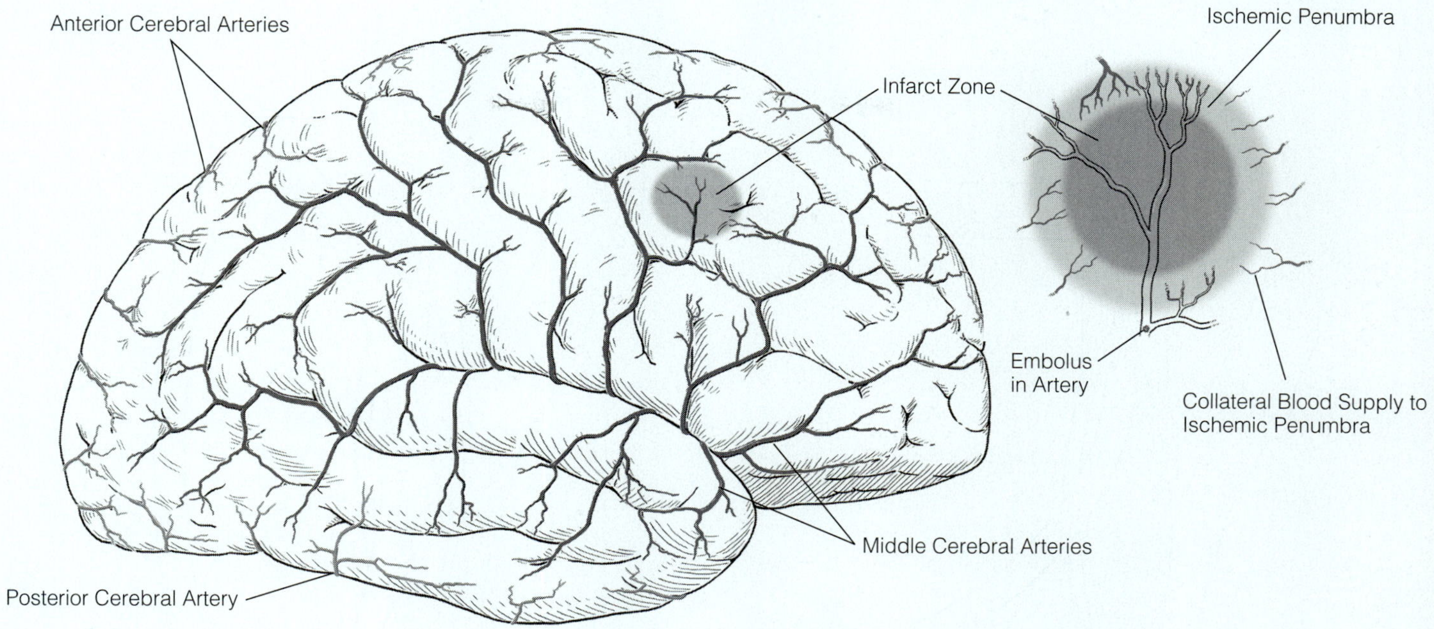

Figure 9 Carotid arterial procedures. When a thromboembolic fragment occludes a cortical arterial branch, a central infarct zone develops, surrounded by an ischemic zone that derives some residual blood supply from collateral vessels. In this zone, known as the ischemic penumbra, the residual blood supply is sufficient to maintain viability.

quire a shunt. Its main disadvantage is that the methods used to identify patients who require shunting may not be entirely reliable.

Selective identification of patients who require shunting can be accomplished in several ways. The most direct—and perhaps safest—method is to employ local or cervical block anesthesia so that the effect of temporary carotid clamping can be assessed in a conscious patient; if clamping leads to a neurologic deficit, then the patient clearly requires an internal shunt. Other methods of identifying patients who require a shunt make use of techniques such as continuous electroencephalographic monitoring, measurement of somatosensory evoked potential, and monitoring of middle cerebral blood flow with transcranial Doppler ultrasonography.

A useful method of determining the adequacy of collateral cerebral blood flow is measurement of back-pressure in the internal carotid artery.[9] Back-pressure has been shown to be a good index of the adequacy of collateral blood flow, and it correlates well with the safety of temporary clamping and thus with the necessity of placing an internal shunt. Back-pressure is measured by placing into the common carotid artery a needle that is connected to pressure tubing and a pressure transducer. The tip of the needle is bent at a 45° angle. Systemic blood pressure is measured, and clamps are placed on the common carotid artery proximal to the needle and on the external carotid artery. The residual pressure in the common carotid artery, which is in continuity with the internal carotid artery, is then allowed to equilibrate; the resulting pressure reading represents internal carotid artery back-pressure [*see Figure 8*]. It has been determined that patients with back-pressures higher than 25 mm Hg can tolerate temporary clamping without incurring brain damage.

Selective shunting is also appropriate for patients who have previously had strokes, regardless of the degree of neurologic recovery. In these patients, a central area of cerebral infarction is surrounded by a zone of relatively ischemic tissue—the so-called ischemic penumbra. The ischemic penumbra is made up of live and potentially functional brain tissue, but its viability is highly dependent on maximization of cerebral perfusion pressure through collateral channels. Accordingly, any interruption of carotid circulation, regardless of the degree of collateral circulation present, may threaten the ischemic penumbra and extend the infarct [*see Figure 9*]. In my opinion, all carotid endarterectomy patients with prior strokes should receive shunts on a routine basis.

Routine avoidance of shunting The advantage of routinely avoiding the use of shunts is that the technical issues and potential complications associated with the additional procedure are avoided entirely. The disadvantage is that unshunted patients with poor collateral blood flow may sustain ischemic brain damage, particularly if the clamp time turns out to be longer than was anticipated.

Technique of Shunt Placement

Internal shunts must be placed with great care if shunt-associated complications are to be avoided. Of the various shunts currently available, I prefer the Javid shunt, which is tapered, has smooth leading edges, and possesses external bulbous circumferential extensions that permit it to be held in place with a circumferential Rumel tourniquet, thereby minimizing the chances of inadvertent dislodgment. Optimal placement of an internal shunt may be achieved by means of the following steps [*see Figure 10*].

After the patient has been adequately heparinized and the artery clamped and opened, the distal portion of the internal shunt is placed into the internal carotid artery. A clamp is placed on the shunt and briefly opened to allow back-bleeding; good back-bleeding confirms that the shunt is lying free in the lumen of the internal carotid artery. The shunt is then secured by tightening a Rumel tourniquet, and the bulbous portion of the shunt is engaged to prevent dislodgment.

Next, the proximal portion of the shunt is placed into the common carotid artery. As this is done, the clamp is removed from the shunt so that backflow from the shunt will dislodge any loose material and air within the common carotid artery. The shunt is then re-

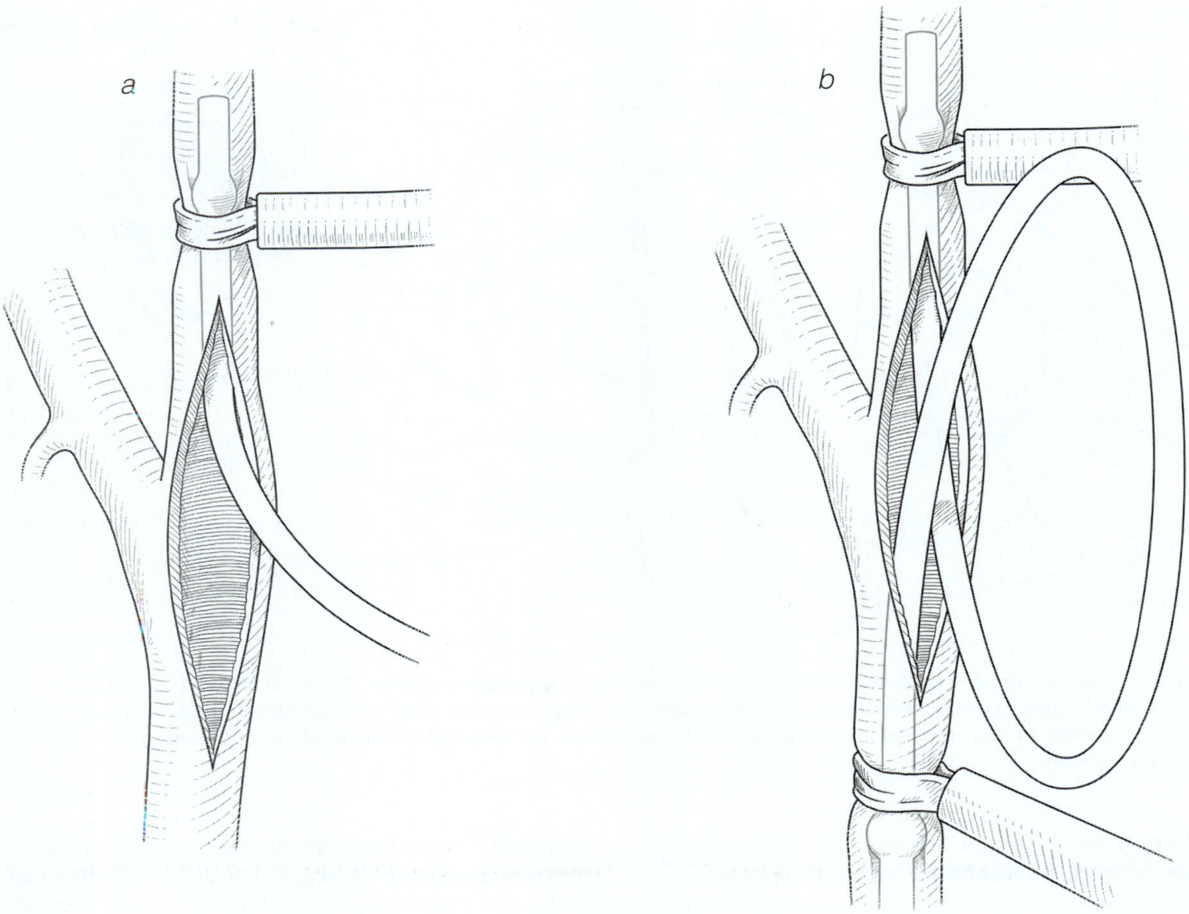

Figure 10 Carotid arterial procedures. Shown is the technique of shunt placement, first distally (*a*) and then proximally (*b*).

clamped, and the clamp is removed from the common carotid artery as the proximal portion of the shunt is passed into that vessel.

When the proximal portion of the shunt is in the proper position in the common carotid artery, it is secured by tightening a Rumel tourniquet on the vessel. The clamp on the shunt is then slowly opened so that the surgeon can observe flow through the translucent device and thus verify that no solid particles or air bubbles are passing through it. Because the shunt is relatively long, the surgeon has a reasonable amount of time in which to observe flow. If any particles or air bubbles are identified, the shunt can be quickly clamped, removed from the common carotid artery, and back-bled, and the procedure can then be repeated.

Once the shunt is secured in place and open, its length and redundancy allow it to be easily manipulated medially and laterally; endarterectomy can then be performed without the encumbrance of an inlying shunt.

STEP 4: RECONSTRUCTION OPTIONS

There are four principal reconstructions involving the common carotid artery and the carotid bifurcation: (1) conventional open carotid endarterectomy with either patch angioplasty or primary closure, (2) eversion endarterectomy, (3) reconstruction for proximal lesions of the common carotid artery, and (4) reconstruction for recurrent stenosis with resection of the carotid bifurcation and grafting.

Open Carotid Endarterectomy

Once the carotid bifurcation has been fully mobilized both proximal and distal to the lesion, systemic anticoagulation with heparin is initiated. I generally give 5,000 units, an amount that is sufficient to produce adequate anticoagulation for the duration of carotid clamping but is not large enough to necessitate heparin reversal on completion of the operation. If internal carotid artery back-pressure is to be used to determine whether the patient requires an internal shunt, then it is measured at this time. If cerebral electrical activity is to be the determinant, then the internal, external, and common carotid arteries are clamped and electrical activity is monitored (e.g., via EEG) with the clamps in place. If electrical changes are noted with clamping, an internal shunt is required.

Arteriotomy The common carotid artery and the carotid bifurcation are rotated so as to be positioned for an arteriotomy that begins on the common carotid artery and extends through the bulb of the internal carotid artery to a point 180° opposite the flow divider [*see Figure 11*]. This incision effectively bivalves the carotid bulb, thus making possible a more accurate primary or patch closure. The arteriotomy continues through the plaque and extends well up into the internal carotid artery, beyond the visible end point of the atherosclerotic plaque.

Plaque removal A dissection plane separating the atherosclerotic intima from the media and the adventitia is then developed with a sharp-bladed dissector. As a rule, it is easiest to begin the endarterectomy at the point where the plaque is bulkiest. At this point, the medial fibers are usually gone, but as the dissection continues both proximally and distally, more normal medial tissue may be seen. It is important to develop the dissection plane between the intima and the media if possible because doing so permits the creation of a feathered end point distally as dissection proceeds into a relatively normal portion of the internal carotid artery [see Figure 12]. If the dissection plane is between the media and the adventitia, a feathered end point is much harder to achieve. Failure to achieve a feathered end point often results in a sharp shelf at the internal carotid artery level, which increases the risk of subsequent intimal dissection when blood flow is restored.

Once the dissection plane is complete on one side of the arteriotomy at the level of the common carotid artery, a right-angle clamp is gently inserted into the plane and advanced through it to the opposite side of the arteriotomy, thereby separating the plaque from the arterial wall around the entire circumference of the vessel. The clamp is then gently spread and brought downward to complete the circumferential dissection of the plaque proximally. The proximal end point of plaque dissection is obtained by cutting the intima with a No. 15 blade.

With the same depth of dissection now existing on both sides of the open common carotid artery, dissection then continues distally up to the carotid bifurcation. At this point, the plaque within the external carotid artery is carefully separated in a circumferential fashion. This is usually done by using a sharp mosquito clamp until all of the plaque has been separated from the vessel wall and dissection has reached normal intima. The freed plaque is gently grasped with the opened mosquito clamp, traction is applied, and the distal end point of plaque dissection in the external carotid artery is obtained.

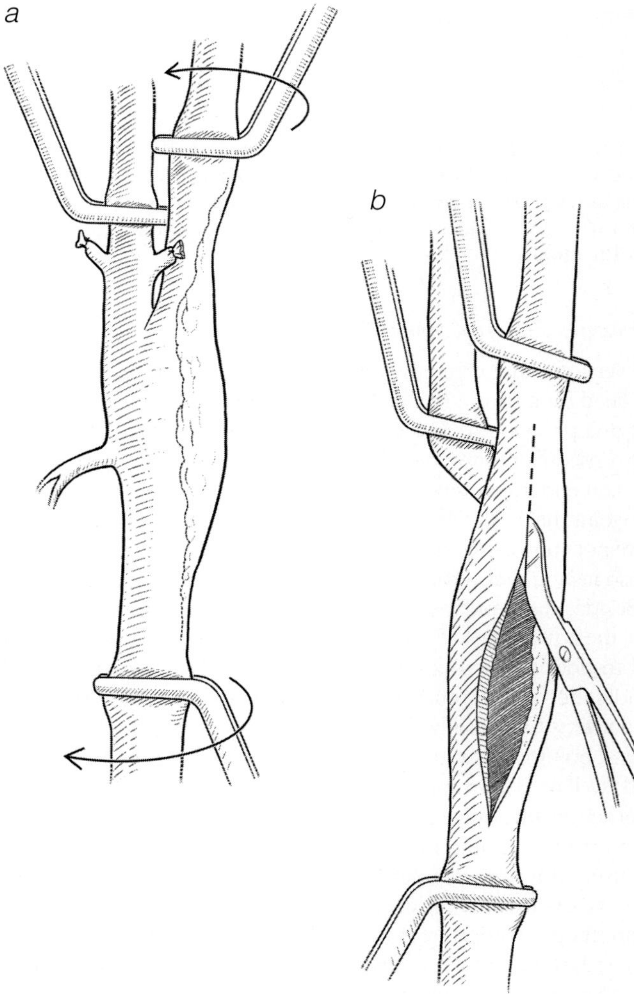

Dissection then continues up the internal carotid artery, with care taken to leave normal intima behind. Often, the plaque becomes a relatively narrow tongue of atheroma on the posterior wall of the internal carotid artery. If the edge of the atheromatous plaque is followed to its end, a tapered, feathered end point can be achieved.

Irrigation and clearing of debris After removal of the specimen, the intimectomized surface is vigorously irrigated with heparinized saline. Any medial debris present is carefully removed. The distal end point is irrigated to determine whether there is a residual flap that might lead to subsequent intimal dissection; if there is a flap, it is carefully removed. If there is a sharp shelf at the distal end point, it is usually an indication that the endarterectomy has not been carried far enough distally. When this is the case, the arteriotomy should be lengthened so that the endarterectomy can be extended to a point where the intima is completely normal. If the patient has a very high carotid bifurcation, very distal plaque, or both and further dissection is impeded by the base of the skull, it may be necessary to secure the distal end point with tacking sutures. Tacking sutures should be used only in exceptional circumstances because their use may lead to healing abnormalities or to the presence of platelet aggregate material that can cause thromboembolic or occlusive complications.

Once the intimectomized surface is completely clear of debris, the lumen of the external carotid artery should be visually inspected to confirm that all overlying dissected intima has been cleared. Any residual dissected intima can be gently teased out with a mosquito clamp. Once the vessel is completely clear, preparation is made for closure of the arteriotomy.

Closure of arteriotomy If the arteriotomy is relatively short and extends only up to the central portion of the bulb of the internal carotid artery, it can usually be closed primarily with a continuous 6-0 polypropylene suture. Placing very small stitches close together in the internal carotid artery should minimize the risk of vessel narrowing.

If the vessel is relatively small or the arteriotomy was extended well up on the internal carotid artery to ensure a complete endarterectomy, the arteriotomy should be closed with a patch angioplasty. Of the several patch options available, the basic choice is between a prosthetic patch and an autogenous patch composed of a segment of saphenous vein obtained from an extremity. The relative merits of autogenous and prosthetic patches have been extensively debated in the literature, but no definitive conclusions have been reached. One of the disadvantages of an autogenous patch is that surgeons tend to use the entire open portion of the saphenous vein, which then dilates further under arterial pressure, leading to an artery of aneurysmal proportions. Another disadvantage is the potential for patch blowout, which, though rare, has been reported in several series. The main disadvantage of a prosthetic patch is the risk of infection, but this is extremely low.

At present, it would appear that a prosthetic patch is at least as acceptable as an autogenous patch, and the prosthetic patch has an additional advantage in that there is no need to remove a normal saphenous vein segment from an extremity. Prosthetic patches can be composed of either fabric or polytetrafluoroethylene (PTFE). Fabric patches now come impregnated with either collagen or gelatin to make them leakproof; PTFE patches do not leak on the surface, but they are prone to leakage at suture needle puncture sites.

Figure 11 Carotid arterial procedures: open endarterectomy. Clamps are applied to the common, internal, and external carotid arteries, and the structures are rotated (*a*) so that an arteriotomy can be made in the common carotid artery 180° opposite the flow divider (*b*).

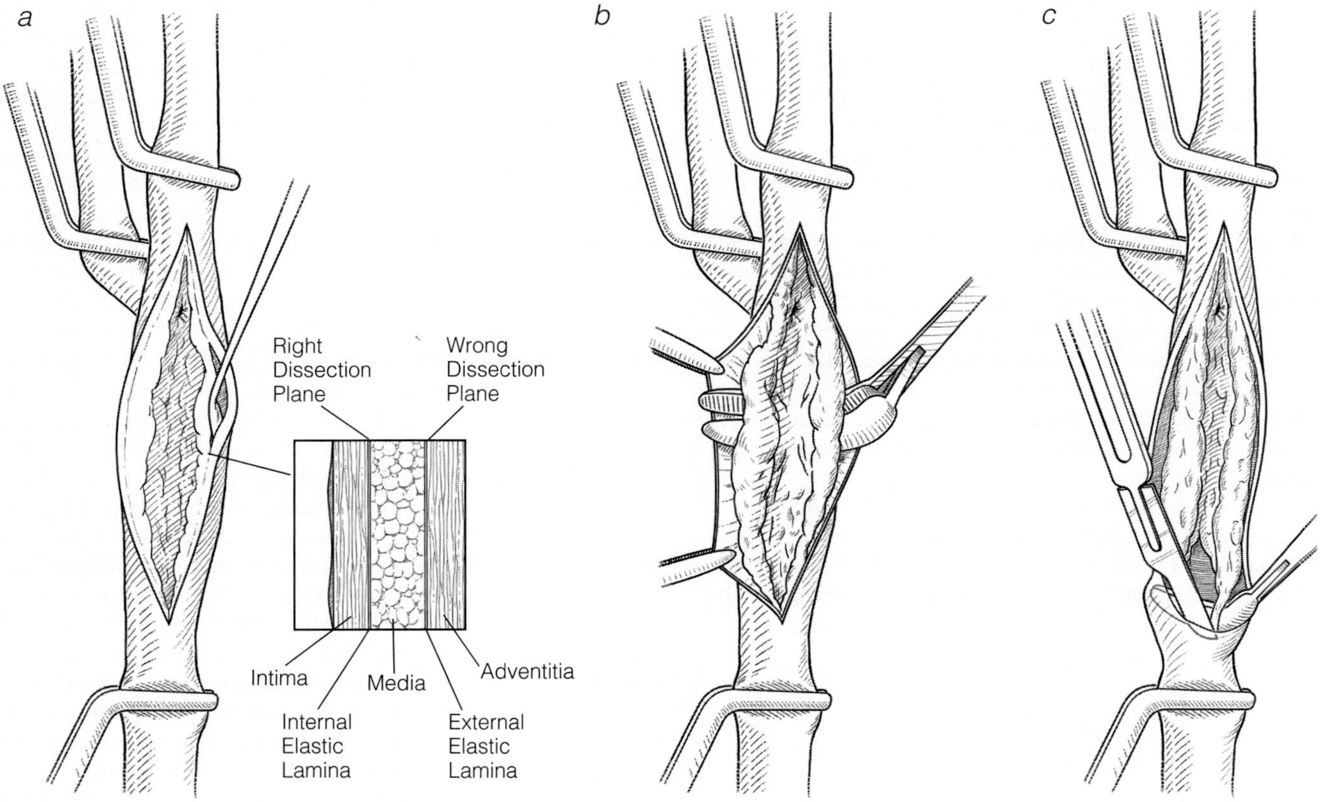

Figure 12 **Carotid arterial procedures: open endarterectomy. (*a*) The endarterectomy plane is started at the point where plaque is thickest and ideally is developed between the diseased intima and the media. Dissection proceeds both proximally and distally along one side of the arteriotomy. (*b*) Once dissection is complete on one side, a right-angle clamp is used to establish the same plane on the opposite side. (*c*) The end point of proximal dissection is established by sharp division of the plague against the clamp.**

Patch size is a crucial consideration: it is important that the patch be neither too wide nor too narrow. If the patch is too narrow, it will not provide the additional material needed to restore the carotid bifurcation to a normal diameter. If the patch is too wide, it will provide too much additional material and create what virtually amounts to a carotid aneurysm; this would represent a significant disadvantage to the patient in terms of flow dynamics and the risk of producing laminated thrombus in the most dilated portion of the carotid bulb. My preference is to use a 6.0 mm wide collagen-impregnated fabric patch for patch angioplasty.

Whichever patch is selected is cut to length, beveled at each end, and sewn in place with a continuous 6-0 polypropylene suture.

Before completion of the closure, the internal carotid artery and the external carotid artery are back-bled, and the common carotid artery is flushed. The arteriotomy is then completely closed. Removing the clamp on the internal carotid artery allows blood flow to fill the carotid bulb and permits one last internal flush. The origin of the internal carotid artery is then occluded with a vascular forceps, and the clamps are removed first from the external carotid artery and then from the common carotid artery to allow resumption of blood flow. After several heartbeats, the forceps on the origin of the internal carotid artery is removed, and blood flow through the internal carotid artery is restored. There may be some leakage of blood along the suture line, which can usually be controlled with the placement of thrombin-soaked absorbable gelatin sponge. If any obvious defect is noted between sutures, an additional stitch should be placed.

Eversion Endarterectomy

Eversion endarterectomy was designed and developed to eliminate the need for a suture line on the internal carotid artery, in the hope that doing so would reduce the incidence of myointimal hyperplasia and consequent restenosis. There is evidence to suggest that the use of eversion endarterectomy has led to some reduction in the incidence of myointimal hyperplasia, but the data are controversial and certainly are not conclusive. Nonetheless, the technique may well have merit, and it should be a part of the vascular surgeon's armamentarium.

Besides the avoidance of a suture line on the internal carotid artery, the advantages of eversion endarterectomy include the simple end-to-side anastomotic closure and the possibility of managing a redundant internal carotid artery by moving it down the common carotid artery. One disadvantage is the potential difficulty of achieving an end point in cases in which the bifurcation is high or plaque extends well up the internal carotid artery toward the base of the skull. Another disadvantage arises with patients who require an internal shunt, in that it is not possible to keep an internal shunt in place for the entire duration of an eversion endarterectomy. Yet another disadvantage is that the distal end point cannot be viewed as clearly as it can in open endarterectomy. A fourth disadvantage is that eversion endarterectomy is poorly suited to cases in which the internal carotid artery is relatively small and contracted and thus better treated with patch angioplasty.

Eversion and plaque dissection After the carotid bifurcation is fully mobilized, the internal, external, and common carotid arteries are clamped. A circumferential incision is placed in an oblique fashion at the junction of the common carotid artery and the bulb of the internal carotid artery to permit division of the bulbous portion of the internal carotid artery from the common carotid [see Figure 13]. The edges of the adventitia of the bulb of the internal carotid artery are grasped, and the outer layers of the vessel wall are gradually everted away from the plaque. Eversion continues cephalad until it reaches the end point of the atherosclerotic lesion, which is marked by presence of a thin, filmy intima that clearly separates from the specimen, leaving normal vessel behind. The plaque in the common carotid artery and the external carotid artery is then [removed] in the traditional manner; the opening in the [common carotid] artery may be extended proximally to facilitate this [end]arterectomy.

[Division] and reanastomosis The internal carotid artery is [restored] to its normal anatomic position, and an anastomosis [between] the end of the divided bulb of the internal carotid artery [and the] common carotid artery is fashioned with a continuous 6-0 [p]ropylene suture. If the internal carotid artery is redundant [see [Spe]cial Considerations, below], the arteriotomy on the common ca[ro]tid artery is extended proximally and the arteriotomy on the medial aspect of the bulb of the internal carotid artery is extended distally so that the carotid bifurcation may be advanced between the internal and common carotid arteries to eliminate the redundancy.

Reconstruction for Proximal Lesions of Common Carotid Artery

Lesions at the origin of the common carotid artery, either at the level of the aortic arch (in the case of the left common carotid artery) or at the innominate bifurcation (in the case of the right common carotid artery), are relatively rare but do occur. Such lesions may arise either in isolation or in combination with carotid bifurcation disease. They can be managed by dividing the common carotid artery and transposing it to the adjacent subclavian artery, provided that there is no occlusive disease in the ipsilateral subclavian artery.

Exposure and mobilization If the lesion at the origin of the common carotid artery is the only one being treated, both the common carotid artery and the subclavian artery should be exposed through a supraclavicular incision that parallels the clavicle. If a carotid bifurcation lesion is present in conjunction with the lesion at the origin of the common carotid artery, the supraclavicular incision is supplemented with a vertical incision along the sternocleidomastoid muscle to permit exposure of the carotid bifurcation. Exposure of the bifurcation has already been addressed (see above); accordingly, I focus here on exposure of the subclavian artery and the proximal common carotid artery.

A supraclavicular incision is placed approximately 1.5 fingerbreadths above the clavicle and centered over the lateral head of the sternocleidomastoid muscle. The lateral head of the sternocleidomastoid muscle is divided, and the scalene triangle is defined. The scalene fat pad is mobilized off the anterior scalene muscle. The phrenic nerve is identified, mobilized off the scalene muscle, and gently retracted. A plane is developed with gentle dissection between the posterior portion of the anterior scalene muscle and the underlying subclavian artery, and the anterior scalene muscle is divided. Division of the muscle exposes the underlying subclavian artery, a sufficient length of which can then be mobilized in the perivascular plane to permit an anastomosis.

The jugular vein is identified at the medial aspect of the incision and mobilized anteriorly and medially to expose the common carotid

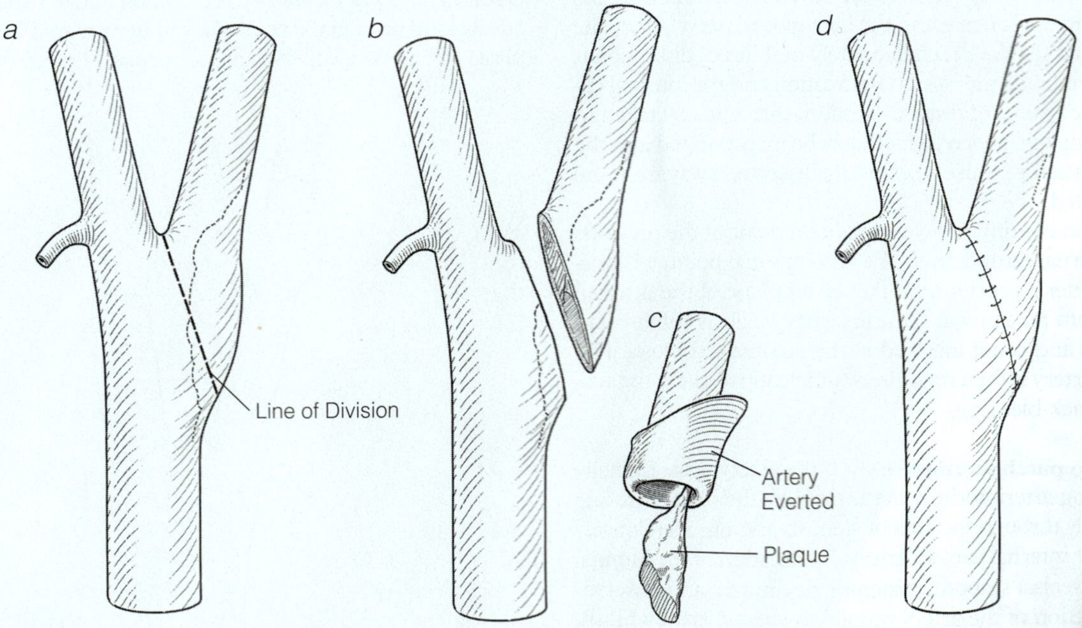

Figure 13 Carotid arterial procedures: eversion endarterectomy. (*a, b*) The internal carotid artery is divided from the common carotid artery in an oblique line. (*c*) The divided internal carotid artery is everted on itself so that it can be separated from the underlying plaque. Eversion proceeds distally until the plaque end point is encountered, and the plaque is removed from the internal carotid artery. Proximal endarterectomy of the common carotid artery and endarterectomy of the external carotid artery are then carried out. (*d*) Once all of the plaque has been removed, the internal carotid artery is reverted and an end-to-side anastomosis is fashioned between the common carotid artery opening and the internal carotid artery.

id artery. The vagus nerve is identified and carefully protected. The common carotid artery is then mobilized both proximally and distally; proximal mobilization should extend as far behind the sternoclavicular junction as the surgeon can comfortably manage.

Transection and anastomosis The common carotid artery is clamped proximally and distally, then divided; the proximal portion of the vessel is oversewn. The transected common carotid artery is brought posterior to the jugular vein in the vicinity of the subclavian artery. The subclavian artery is clamped proximally and distally, a longitudinal arteriotomy is made, and a small ellipse of subclavian arterial tissue is removed. The end of the common carotid artery is then sewn to the side of the subclavian artery with a continuous 6-0 polypropylene suture.

Before completion, the vessels are back-bled and flushed. Once the anastomosis is complete, blood flow is restored, first to the distal subclavian artery and then to the common carotid artery.

Reconstruction for Recurrent Carotid Stenosis

For an initial recurrence of carotid stenosis that primarily results from myointimal hyperplasia, conversion to a patch angioplasty is generally the best treatment. For second or third recurrences or for recurrences that develop in spite of patch angioplasty, resection of the carotid bifurcation with interposition grafting between the common carotid artery and the normal distal internal carotid artery is the best treatment.

Exposure and mobilization Exposure of a carotid bifurcation for treatment of recurrent carotid stenosis can be challenging. The original skin incision is reopened, and dissection is carried down through the scar tissue to the common carotid artery. The common carotid artery is sharply dissected from the surrounding scar tissue, with the dissection plane kept close to the adventitia to minimize the risk of injury to the vagus nerve and the hypoglossal nerve. Once the common carotid artery has been adequately mobilized, dissection is extended to include the carotid bifurcation and the internal carotid artery. In the course of distal dissection, care must be taken to identify the hypoglossal nerve, which may be incorporated into the scar; this structure must be carefully dissected away from the artery.

Dissection continues beyond the end point of the previous endarterectomy of the carotid artery. Beyond this end point, it is usually easy to find a previously undissected plane of the internal carotid artery. Moving upward, the artery typically is soft around the bifurcation but involved in the recurrent stenosis. The internal carotid artery is mobilized sufficiently to allow the surgeon...

Patch angioplasty If the artery was originally closed primarily, an incision is made through the old suture line and extended through the area of stenosis and onto a relatively normal portion of the internal carotid artery. Exploration of the luminal surface typically reveals a glistening neointima, and observation of the transition zone reveals an area where a whitish, fibrous plaque has been incorporated as a result of myointimal hyperplasia. It is difficult to reendarterectomize such a lesion because the lesion is not, in fact, plaque but rather the end result of a cascade of events that will recur if endarterectomy is reinitiated. Accordingly, the neointima should be carefully protected. A patch angioplasty, extending from the common carotid artery to the relatively normal portion of the internal carotid artery, is usually sufficient to treat the lesion.

Resection of carotid bifurcation with interposition grafting If the stenosis is recurring for the second or third time or the artery was originally closed with a patch, the surgeon should proceed with resection and interposition grafting. In most cases, it is necessary to sacrifice the external carotid artery. The internal carotid artery is divided distal to oversew its origin. The internal carotid artery is divided proximal to the hyperplastic lesion, the common carotid artery is divided proximally, and the diseased specimen is removed.

I prefer to use 6.0 mm thin-walled PTFE for the interposition graft. The internal carotid artery distally and the common carotid artery proximally are spatulated by making vertical incisions approximately 6.0 mm in length. The PTFE graft is appropriately sized both proximally and distally, and beveled or spatulated. Carotid arterial anastomoses are performed, first to the internal carotid artery and then to the common carotid artery.

Before completion, the vessels are back-bled and flushed; once the anastomoses are complete, blood flow is reestablished.

Some surgeons may be tempted to use autogenous saphenous vein for the interposition graft. To use such grafts would appear, on the face of it, to be a good idea; in fact, it is a mistake. For reasons not clearly understood, the use of autogenous saphenous vein in the neck has an extremely poor track record, yielding unacceptably high rates of recurrent stenosis and occlusion in comparison with the use of prosthetic grafts.

Special Considerations

Fibromuscular dysplasia of internal carotid artery Fibromuscular dysplasia of the internal carotid artery is a congenital or acquired lesion that has been subdivided into four pathologic varieties, of which the most common is medial fibroplasia. On contrast angiography, medial fibroplasia has a characteristic appearance, resembling a string of beads in the extracranial portion of the internal carotid artery [*see Figure 14*]. A common initial manifestation is a relatively loud bruit in the neck of a young woman. Fibromuscular dysplasia can cause symptoms of monocular or hemispheric TIAs, or it

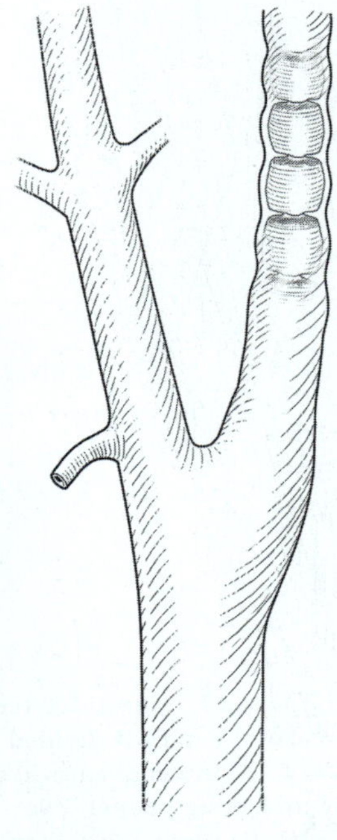

Figure 14 **Carotid arterial procedures: repair of fibromuscular dysplasia. Depicted is the so-called string of beads deformity of the cervical portion of the internal carotid artery, which is characteristic of medial fibroplasia.**

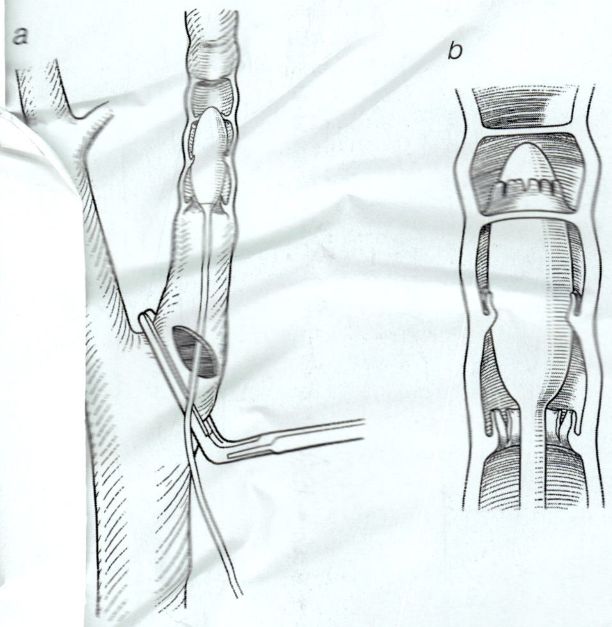

tion, about the same number of patients have associated intracranial aneurysms that should be checked for by means of intracranial imaging studies.

Once the carotid bifurcation has been suitably mobilized and it has been established that no associated atheromatous plaque is present, a small transverse incision is made on the bulb of the internal carotid artery, with flow being maintained between the common and external carotid arteries. Serial intraluminal dilatations are then performed with coronary artery dilators of progressively increasing diameter [see Figure 15]. The first dilator (usually 2.5 mm in diameter) is passed up the carotid artery to the base of the skull under digital control. The dilator is then withdrawn, and the artery is back-bled to flush out any fractured segments. The next larger dilator (3.0 mm in diameter) is passed in a similar fashion. Dilatation is repeated with progressively larger dilators (3.5, 4.0, and possibly 4.5 mm in diameter) to complete the procedure.

The transverse arteriotomy is closed with 6-0 polypropylene suture material and flow is reestablished. A completion angiogram verifies that the dysplastic segment is fully restored.

Coiling or kinking of internal carotid artery Redundancy of the internal carotid artery, often resulting in a 360° coil of the high cervical portion of the internal carotid artery, is usually thought to be developmental in origin [see Figure 16a]. Elongation of the internal carotid artery, which often results in kinking of the vessel, is believed to be related to the degenerative changes that occur with aging and atherosclerosis [see Figure 16b]. Both of these phenomena, in and of themselves, are usually asymptomatic; exceptions occur when an atheromatous plaque develops at the apex of the coil or when kinking of the internal carotid artery is accentuated with changes in head position in a patient who depends on relatively normal blood flow through that vessel. Redundancy of the internal carotid artery often becomes a technical consideration during standard surgical treatment of a carotid bifurcation atheroma. When redundancy occurs, it must be appropriately dealt with to prevent postoperative complications.

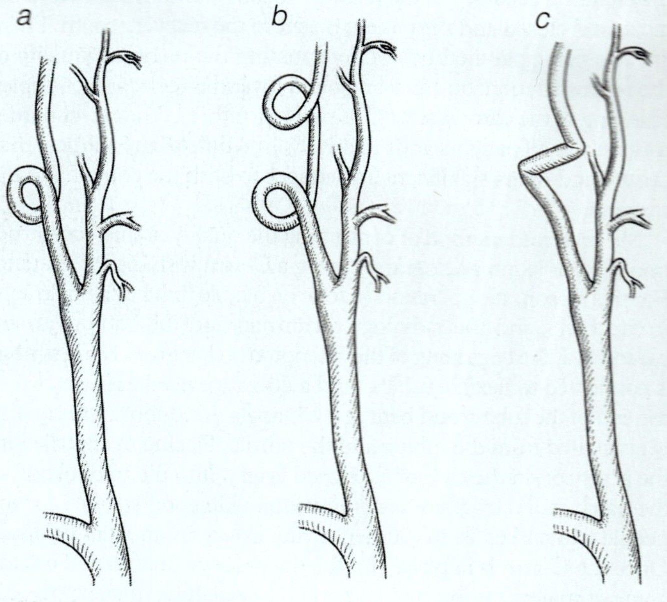

Figure 15 Carotid arterial procedures: repair of fibromuscular dysplasia. (*a*) The proximal portion of the internal carotid bulb is mobilized, a transverse arteriotomy is made, and a coronary dilator is passed into the internal carotid artery and advanced up the artery to the base of the skull. (*b*) The small septa in the internal carotid artery are disrupted by the advancing probe.

go on to cause a stroke, usually as a consequence of a dissection resulting in thrombotic occlusion. If symptoms develop, they can generally be controlled by means of antiplatelet drugs. Currently, the only indication for surgical intervention is the persistence of symptoms despite antiplatelet therapy.

Treatment of fibromuscular dysplasia has evolved in recent years. The first attempts at surgical repair involved a total resection of the internal carotid artery coupled with interposition of a graft (usually composed of saphenous vein). This technique is now largely abandoned because of the extensive surgical dissection required and the substantial risk of cranial nerve injury; its only remaining application is in cases where there is associated aneurysmal dilatation in the dysplastic segment that calls for resection and graft interposition. At present, the two most popular modes of therapy both involve intraluminal dilatation with disruption of the small septa within the artery. One mode achieves intraluminal dilatation via an open approach, and the other achieves the same end via a percutaneous approach that includes balloon angioplasty. Dilatation and fracturing of the intraluminal septa often result in the release of particles of septal tissue, which in turn can lead to cerebral embolization and infarction. Consequently, open methods, which enable the surgeon to flush out the disrupted segments, are usually favored.

In symptomatic patients with fibromuscular dysplasia, the carotid bifurcation may be exposed in the usual manner. If there is significant redundancy of the internal carotid artery, as documented by preoperative imaging, the artery should be mobilized relatively extensively so that it can be straightened by downward traction before intraluminal dilatation is begun. If, on the other hand, the artery is relatively straight, only minimal mobilization is required. It should be kept in mind that approximately 25% of patients with fibromuscular dysplasia have associated atheromatous disease of the carotid bifurcation that must be dealt with at the time of operation. In addi-

Figure 16 Carotid arterial procedures: repair of coiling or kinking of the internal carotid artery. (*a, b*) Redundancy of the internal carotid artery can result in one or more 360° coils in the vessel. (*c*) Degenerative atheromatous changes of the internal carotid artery can cause elongation with associated kinking or buckling.

Anticipated redundancy of the internal carotid artery at the time of carotid bifurcation endarterectomy can usually be managed with a patch angioplasty. Provided that the arteriotomy extends beyond the apex of the kink, the patch should smooth out the curvature of the redundant vessel and eliminate the kink. If it appears that internal carotid artery redundancy is greater than can be corrected by an elongated patch, then detachment of the internal carotid artery followed by eversion endarterectomy and reimplantation is indicated.

If the arteriotomy has already been closed when it becomes apparent that a kink is present, the problem may be dealt with by mobilizing the external carotid artery sufficiently and then resecting a segment of the common carotid artery and pulling down on the carotid bifurcation with a new end-to-end anastomosis to straighten the redundant internal carotid artery [see Figure 17]. Segmental resection of the internal carotid artery itself combined with end-to-end repair has also been described; this approach is less desirable, being more technically demanding and hence more subject to technical error.

Patients with coiling of the internal carotid artery may present a more difficult problem. If the atheromatous plaque involves only the first portion of the internal carotid artery and the vessel beyond that first portion is relatively normal up to the point where coiling begins, the surgeon can simply avoid the problem by leaving the smooth coil in place and not carrying out an extensive distal dissection. If, on the other hand, it appears that there may be plaque in the coil, then the entire coil must be dissected free, and the patient is left with a very redundant internal carotid artery that must be dealt with. Once again, the best method of managing the problem is to resect the redundant segment of the internal carotid artery, with or without eversion endarterectomy, and to reimplant the internal carotid artery onto the distal common carotid artery at the point of transection.

Upon completion of the reconstruction, a completion angiogram should be obtained to verify that the coiling or kinking has been adequately treated.

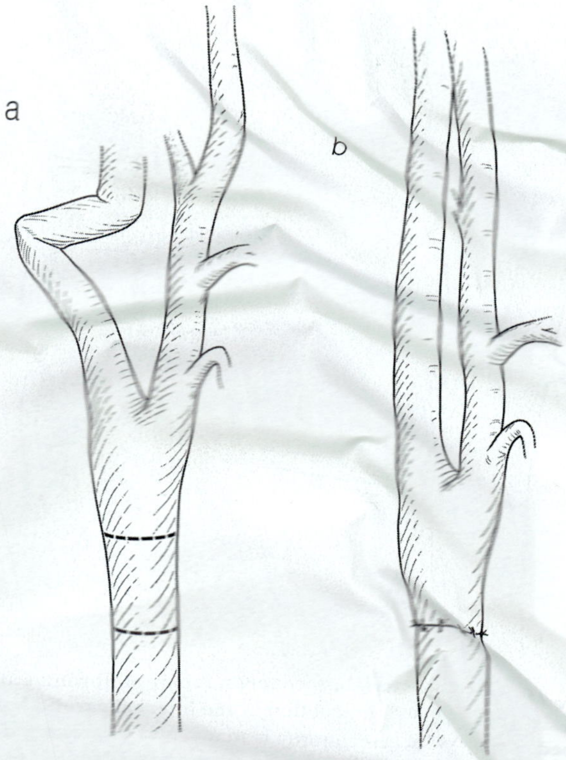

STEP 5: COMPLETION IMAGING

Given that the majority of neurologic complications after carotid artery surgery are attributable to technical error, it is imperative that the technical accuracy of the reconstruction be confirmed before the incision is closed and the patient is sent to the recovery room. There are two principal methods of determining the technical quality of the reconstruction: on-table angiography and direct-contact duplex scanning of the carotid artery. To perform either of these techniques routinely in all patients adds relatively little time to the surgical procedure and offers significant advantages to both the patient and the surgeon.[10,11]

My preferred method of confirming the quality of the reconstruction is completion angiography using a C-arm with digital imaging. For this reason, the operation is done on a table that has angiographic capability, and the radiology technician and the equipment are called for at the beginning of the arteriotomy closure. A 10 ml syringe is connected to flexible tubing, and a 20-gauge needle is attached to the end of the tubing and bent at a 45° angle. Air bubbles are carefully evacuated from the tubing and the needle. Placing the needle into the artery or, in the case of a patched artery, into the midportion of the patch in a retrograde fashion will provide good stability for the needle, which lies in the lumen of the artery in an axial position. Once the C-arm is in place and the fluoroscopy unit turned on, the contrast material is injected by hand. The resulting image of the carotid bifurcation can be continuously replayed until maximal radiographic opacity of the carotid bifurcation and the intracranial circulation has been attained. The image is then carefully inspected for defects at the end points in the internal and external carotid arteries.

Intimal defects in the internal carotid artery are unusual, though

Figure 17 Carotid arterial procedures: repair of coiling or kinking of the internal carotid artery. Kinking or redundancy of the internal carotid artery can be managed by mobilizing the external carotid artery, then resecting a segment of the common carotid artery (*a*). The surgeon can then draw down the carotid bifurcation for a new primary anastomosis (*b*).

not unknown. Defects in the external carotid artery are more common because the endarterectomy is essentially done in a blind or closed manner. Defects in the external carotid artery are matters of concern because they may lead to thrombus formation in the external carotid artery; if the thrombus propagates proximally, it may embolize up the internal carotid artery and cause a stroke.[12] For this reason, if a defect is found in the external carotid artery, it is repaired at the time of the operation. To accomplish the repair, clamps are placed on the external carotid artery proximally at its origin and distally beyond the intimal flap. A transverse arteriotomy is made in the external carotid artery to permit identification and removal of the intimal flap. Once the flap has been carefully removed, the transverse arteriotomy is closed with two or three interrupted 6-0 polypropylene sutures and flow is restored.

Completion angiography also has the advantage of permitting the surgeon to image the intracranial circulation. Now that many operations are being performed on the basis of preoperative carotid duplex scanning, intracranial imaging is typically unavailable beforehand, which means that the status of the intracranial circulation with respect to atherosclerotic lesions in the area of the siphon or the middle cerebral artery or with respect to intracranial aneurysms is usually unknown at the start of the procedure. A completion angiogram gives the surgeon the opportunity to rule out these lesions by looking not only at the area around the reconstruction but also at the intracranial circulation.

An alternative to completion angiography is DUS. DUS can be a highly satisfactory way of examining the area of reconstruction, provided that the operating room has duplex scanning capability and that a technologist is available to operate the equipment. Standard B-mode imaging, in conjunction with Doppler ultrasonography, can accurately identify patent or compromised internal and external carotid arteries.

Once the surgeon has confirmed that a good technical reconstruction has been achieved, preparations can be made for closure.

STEP 6: CLOSURE

The dissected area around the reconstructed carotid artery is carefully irrigated with an antibiotic solution, and the wound is meticulously inspected for hemostasis. Even when good hemostasis has been achieved, it is my practice to place a drain overnight—specifically, a 7.0 mm Jackson-Pratt drain brought out through a small separate stab wound. The platysmal layer is closed with a continuous 3-0 absorbable suture, and the skin is closed with a continuous 4-0 subcuticular absorbable suture. A clear adhesive plastic dressing is applied to the skin, and the patient is sent to the recovery room.

Postoperative Management

The main patient variables to be evaluated in the postoperative period are neurologic status, blood pressure, and wound stability.

On awakening from anesthesia, the patient is carefully observed with a view to determining gross cerebral function on the basis of response to commands and movement of extremities. When the patient is fully awake, vagus nerve and hypoglossal nerve function can be tested.

Blood pressure monitoring is of critical importance after carotid endarterectomy. It is essential first to decide on an acceptable blood pressure range for the patient and then to ensure that this pressure is maintained: neither hypertension nor hypotension is acceptable. Patients with severe carotid bifurcation disease who have undergone carotid endarterectomy temporarily lose autoregulation on the side of the operation; therefore, hypertension can result in reperfusion injury to that side of the brain, ranging all the way from simple headache to fatal intracerebral hemorrhage.

The surgical site should be carefully observed for possible wound expansion resulting from hematoma formation. Even when good hemostasis is achieved and a drain is in place, there is still the possibility of delayed bleeding leading to hematoma and airway compromise. If an expanding hematoma is noted, the safest response is to return the patient to the OR so that the hematoma can be evacuated and a bleeding site sought. The earlier this is done, the better.

If the patient is neurologically intact, blood pressure is well controlled, and there is no evidence of an expanding hematoma, then the remaining postoperative care can be provided in a regular hospital room. It is seldom necessary to observe the patient in the intensive care unit, as was once standard practice.

Follow-up

Periodic follow-up examination is essential. There are two major areas of concern: (1) the possibility of recurrent stenosis on the operated side and (2) the possibility of disease developing or progressing in the contralateral carotid artery. It is my practice to see the patient approximately 3 weeks after carotid endarterectomy. In that visit, the patient is examined for quality of wound healing and the presence or absence of carotid bruit on both the operated side and the contralateral side, and a carotid duplex scan is performed. If at this time there are no grounds for concern about the contralateral side, scanning is done only on the side of the operation. The scan serves to establish the new baseline and confirms that the carotid reconstruction is satisfactory. The new baseline is then used as the basis for assessing patient status during subsequent follow-up.

The next patient visit takes place 6 months after operation, at which time a bilateral carotid duplex scan is performed. If the operated side continues to be normal and there are no major problems on the contralateral side, the patient is seen again at the 1-year anniversary of the procedure. If examinations yield satisfactory results at this time, the patient may thereafter be seen at 1-year intervals, with bilateral carotid duplex scanning done at each visit.

Alternatives to Direct Carotid Reconstruction

Stented balloon angioplasty of the carotid bifurcation and the common carotid artery is currently under investigation as an alternative to direct carotid reconstruction. Several phase I studies have been published. Some report unacceptably high incidences of perioperative stroke, but others report complication rates comparable to those of carotid endarterectomy. It appears that a state of clinical equipoise exists. A prospective, randomized trial comparing carotid endarterectomy with stented balloon angioplasty in symptomatic patients is under way. It is anticipated that the trial will be completed by 2006.

References

1. Beneficial effect of carotid endarterectomy in symptomatic patients with high-grade carotid stenosis. North American Symptomatic Carotid Endarterectomy Trial Collaborators. N Engl J Med 325:445, 1991
2. MRC European Carotid Surgery Trial: interim results for symptomatic patients with severe (70-99%) or with mild (0-29%) carotid stenosis. European Carotid Trialists' Collaborative Group. Lancet 337:1235, 1991
3. Mayberg MR, Wilson SE, Yatsu F, et al: Carotid endarterectomy and prevention of cerebral ischemia in symptomatic carotid stenosis. Veterans Affairs Cooperative Studies Program 309 Trialist Group. JAMA 266:3332, 1991
4. Endarterectomy for asymptomatic carotid artery stenosis. Executive Committee for the Asymptomatic Carotid Atherosclerosis Study. JAMA 273:1421, 1995
5. Hobson RW II, Weiss DG, Fields WS, et al: Efficacy of carotid endarterectomy for asymptomatic carotid stenosis. The Veterans Affairs Asymptomatic Cooperative Study Group. N Engl J Med 328:221, 1993
6. Moore WS, Barnett HJM, Beebe HG, et al: Guidelines for carotid endarterectomy—a multidisciplinary consensus statement from the Ad Hoc Committee, American Heart Association. Circulation 91:566, 1995
7. Fisher DF Jr, Clagett GP, Parker JI, et al: Mandibular subluxation for high carotid exposure. J Vasc Surg 1:727, 1984
8. Moore WS, Yee JM, Hall AD: Collateral cerebral blood pressure—an index of tolerance to temporary carotid occlusion. Arch Surg 106:520, 1973
9. Moore WS, Hall AD: Carotid artery back pressure—a test of cerebral tolerance to temporary carotid occlusion. Arch Surg 99:702, 1969
10. Blaisdell FW, Lim R Jr, Hall AD: Technical results of carotid endarterectomy: arteriographic assessment. Am J Surg 114:239, 1967
11. Schwartz RA, Peterson GJ, Noland KA, et al: Intraoperative duplex scanning after carotid reconstruction: a valuable tool. J Vasc Surg 7:260, 1988
12. Moore WS, Martello JY, Quiñones-Baldrich WJ, et al: Etiologic importance of the intimal flap of the external carotid artery in the development of post-carotid endarterectomy stroke. Stroke 21:1497, 1990

Recommended Reading

Eastcott HHG, Pickering GW, Robb C: Reconstruction of internal carotid artery in a patient with intermittent attacks of hemiplegia. Lancet 2:994, 1954

Matsumoto GH, Cossman D, Callow AD: Hazards and safeguards during carotid endarterectomy: technical considerations. Am J Surg 133:485, 1977

Mock CN, Michael PL, McRae RG, et al: Selection of the approach to the distal internal carotid artery from the second cervical vertebra to the base of the skull. J Vasc Surg 13:846, 1991

Moore WS: Surgery for Cerebrovascular Disease, 2nd ed. WB Saunders Co, Philadelphia, 1996

Sundt TM, Sharbrough FW, Anderson E, et al: Cerebral blood flow measurements and electroencephalogram during carotid endarterectomy. J Neurosurg 41:310, 1974

Acknowledgment

Figures 1 through 17   Tom Moore.

64 REPAIR OF INFRARENAL ABDOMINAL AORTIC ANEURYSMS

Frank R. Arko, M.D., and Christopher K. Zarins, M.D.

An arterial aneurysm is defined as a permanent localized enlargement of an artery to a diameter more than 1.5 times its expected diameter. Aneurysms are classified according to morphology, etiology, and anatomic site. The most common morphology is a fusiform, symmetrical, circumferential enlargement that involves all layers of the arterial wall. A saccular morphology is also seen, in which aneurysmal degeneration affects only part of the arterial circumference.

The most common cause of an arterial aneurysm is atherosclerotic degeneration of the arterial wall. The pathogenesis is a multifactorial process involving genetic predisposition, aging, atherosclerosis, inflammation, and localized activation of proteolytic enzymes. Most aneurysms occur in elderly persons, and the prevalence rises with increasing age. Aneurysms also occur in genetically susceptible individuals with Ehlers-Danlos syndrome or Marfan syndrome. Other causes include tertiary syphilis and localized infection resulting in a mycotic aneurysm.

Aneurysms of the infrarenal aorta are by far the most common arterial aneurysms encountered in clinical practice today: they are three to seven times more common than thoracic aneurysms and affect four times as many men as women.[1] Abdominal aortic aneurysms (AAAs) have a tendency to enlarge and rupture, causing death. In the United States, AAAs result in approximately 15,000 deaths each year and are thus the 13th leading cause of death in the United States.[2,3] The only way to reduce the death rate is to identify and treat aortic aneurysms before they rupture.

Preoperative Evaluation

IDENTIFICATION OF RISK FACTORS

For successful surgical reconstruction of AAAs, any significant comorbidities that would increase the risk of operative repair must be identified and managed at an early stage. Patients undergoing the procedure usually are elderly and often have coexisting cardiac, pulmonary, cerebrovascular, renal, or peripheral vascular disease. The major anesthetic risk factors for elective resection of AAAs are similar to those for other major intra-abdominal operations; in particular, they include inadequate cardiopulmonary and renal function. Patients with unstable angina or angina at rest, a cardiac ejection fraction of less than 25%, a serum creatinine concentration higher than 3 mg/dl, or pulmonary disease (manifested by oxygen tension < 50 mm Hg, elevated carbon dioxide tension, or both on room air) are considered to be at high risk.[4,5]

Myocardial ischemia is the most common cause of perioperative morbidity and mortality after arterial reconstruction of the aorta. Optimization of preoperative medical management, perioperative invasive monitoring, and long-term risk factor modification are all facilitated by an accurate preoperative cardiac evaluation. Such evaluation may include transthoracic echocardiography, exercise stress testing, myocardial scintigraphy, stress echocardiography, and coronary angiography; each test has its own merits and limitations with regard to clinical risk assessment. To reduce the mortality associated with resection of AAAs, it is necessary not only to identify high-risk groups but also to institute appropriate preoperative, intraoperative, and postoperative alterations in patient care. Patients who have severe coronary disease (manifested by unstable angina, ischemic congestive heart failure, or recent myocardial infarction [MI]) benefit from invasive cardiac evaluation and possibly from preliminary coronary intervention.

With intensive perioperative monitoring and support in place, resection of AAAs has been successfully performed even in high-risk patients, with operative mortalities of less than 6%.[6-8]

CONFIRMATION OF DIAGNOSIS AND DETERMINATION OF ANEURYSM SIZE

Physical examination suffices for detection of most large aneurysms. To determine the exact size of the aneurysm as well as to identify smaller aneurysms, however, more objective methods are available and should be used. Determination of the size of the aneurysm is extremely important because size is the most important determinant of the likelihood of rupture and plays a crucial role in subsequent management decisions. Imaging modalities commonly employed to diagnose and measure aneurysms include duplex ultrasonography (DUS), aortography, computed tomography, and magnetic resonance imaging.

The main advantages of DUS are its ready availability in both inpatient and outpatient settings, its low cost, its safety, and its good performance; many studies have documented the ability of DUS to establish the diagnosis and accurately determine the size of AAAs [see Figure 1].[9-11] The primary limitations of DUS are that imaging of the thoracic and suprarenal aorta is poor, that the quality of the images is considerably lower in the presence of obesity or large amounts of intestinal gas, and that it must be performed by a skilled imaging technician.

Aortography yields excellent images of the contours of the aortic lumen, but it is not a reliable method for determining the diameter of an aneurysm or even for establishing its presence, because the mural thrombus within the aneurysm tends to reduce the lumen to near-normal size. Nonetheless, aortography can be helpful in determining the extent of an aneurysm, especially when there is iliac or suprarenal involvement, defining associated arterial lesions involving the renal and visceral arteries, and detecting lower-extremity occlusive disease. There are risks associated with aortography that place some restrictions on its use. Among these risks are the potential renal toxicity resulting from the use of contrast agents. In addition, manipulation of catheters through the laminated mural thrombus increases the risk of distal embolization. Finally, local arterial complications may arise at the arterial puncture site.

CT provides reliable information about the size of the entire aorta, thereby allowing accurate determination of both the size and the extent of the AAA [see Figure 2]. Spiral CT scanning permits identification of the visceral and renal arteries and their relationship to the aneurysm. With the administration of I.V. contrast material, the aor-

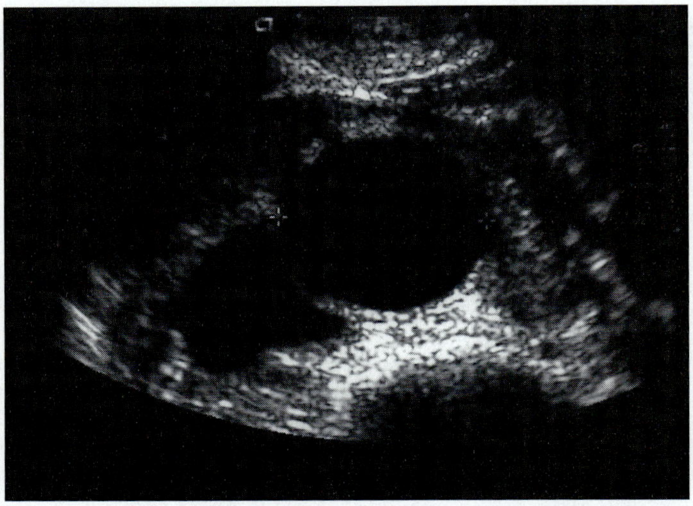

Figure 1 Duplex ultrasonography may be used as a screening test as well as to determine the actual size of the aneurysm.

tic lumen, the amount and location of mural thrombus, and the presence or absence of retroperitoneal hematoma can all be assessed [*see Figure 3*]. Overall, spiral CT scanning is currently the most useful imaging method for evaluation of the abdominal aorta.

MRI is also useful in preoperative evaluation of aortic aneurysms.[12,13] It employs radiofrequency energy and a magnetic field to produce images in longitudinal, transverse, and coronal planes. The advantages of MRI over CT are that no ionizing radiation is administered, multiplane images can be obtained, and no nephrotoxic contrast agents are used.

CLASSIFICATION OF PATIENTS FOR ELECTIVE OR URGENT REPAIR

Patients may usefully be classified into three categories according to how they present for repair: (1) elective patients, (2) symptomatic patients, and (3) patients with ruptured aneurysms.

Elective aneurysm repair is recommended for asymptomatic patients who have aneurysms 5.0 cm in diameter or larger, who have an acceptable level of operative risk, and who have a life expectancy of 1 year or more. Furthermore, elective operation should be considered for patients with aneurysms smaller than 5.0 cm who are not at high operative risk if they are hypertensive or live in a remote area where proper medical care is not readily available. Repair is also appropriate for aneurysms that are between 4.0 and 5.0 cm in diameter and have shown growth of more than 0.5 cm on serial images in less than 6 to 12 months. Peripheral embolization originating from the aneurysm is an indication for repair, regardless of the size of the aneurysm.

Urgent operation is indicated for patients with symptomatic aneurysms, regardless of the size of the aneurysm. Such patients typically present with abdominal or back pain. Sometimes, the back pain radiates to the groin, much as in ureteral colic; this pain may be elicited by palpating the aneurysm. In most cases, DUS, CT, and MRI will reliably detect the presence of periaortic blood; however, the absence of this finding should not delay operation, because actual rupture of the aneurysm can occur at any time.

Emergency operation is indicated for almost all patients with known or suspected rupture of an aneurysm.

Operative Planning

Preoperative planning is essential for a successful outcome after repair of an infrarenal AAA. Like the choice between elective and urgent or emergency repair, operative planning is governed by the presentation of the patient. In patients with ruptured aneurysms, diagnosis is immediately followed by operative repair. In patients with symptomatic aneurysms, the amount of preoperative imaging done is balanced against the risk of impending rupture. In patients presenting for elective repair, it is generally possible to perform extensive imaging to determine whether the repair is best done via an endovascular approach or a standard open approach. Current preoperative imaging methods utilizing CT angiography obviate several common pitfalls. The recent introduction of endovascular techniques for excluding an aneurysm should not alter the patient selection criteria for aneurysm repair. Endovascular grafting does introduce certain morphologic criteria into the process of patient selection, in that stent grafting is appropriate only for patients in whom the infrarenal neck and the iliac arteries are suitable.

Given that the long-term outcome of endovascular grafting is currently unknown, younger patients who are at low operative risk and are expected to survive into the long term are typically better served with open surgical repair. In addition, patients who require additional abdominal or pelvic revascularization procedures, who have small or diseased access vessels, or who have short (< 10 mm) or tortuous infrarenal necks are not candidates for endovascular grafting and should undergo open surgical repair instead.

Preoperative preparation to optimize cardiopulmonary function, administration of preoperative antibiotics, and intraoperative hemodynamic monitoring with appropriate fluid management can significantly reduce the risks associated with AAA repair. Before aortic cross-clamping, appropriate volume loading, combined with vasodilatation, is carried out to help prevent declamping hypotension.

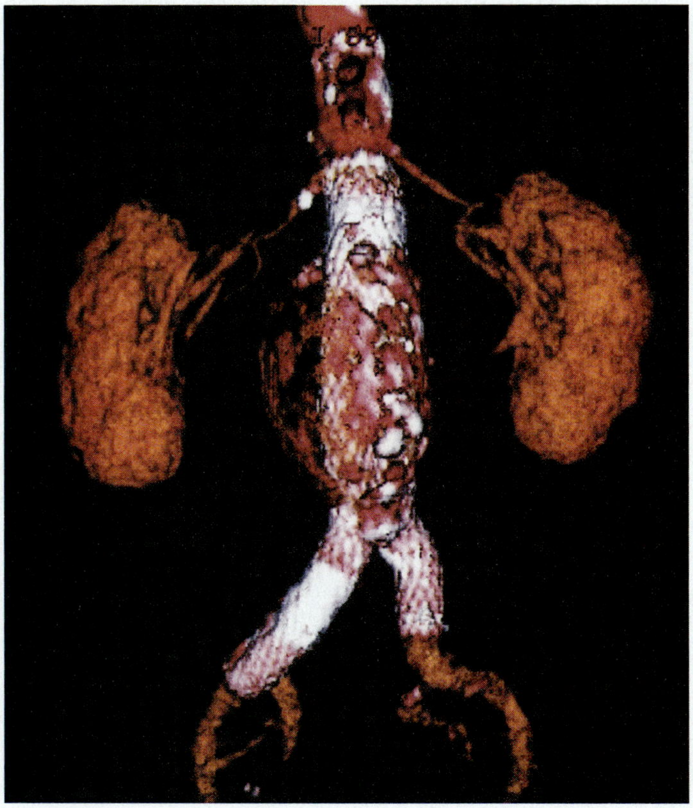

Figure 2 Shown is a CT angiogram providing a three-dimensional reconstruction of an infrarenal AAA after endovascular repair. Of particular interest is the relation of the graft to the renal arteries and the hypogastric arteries distally.

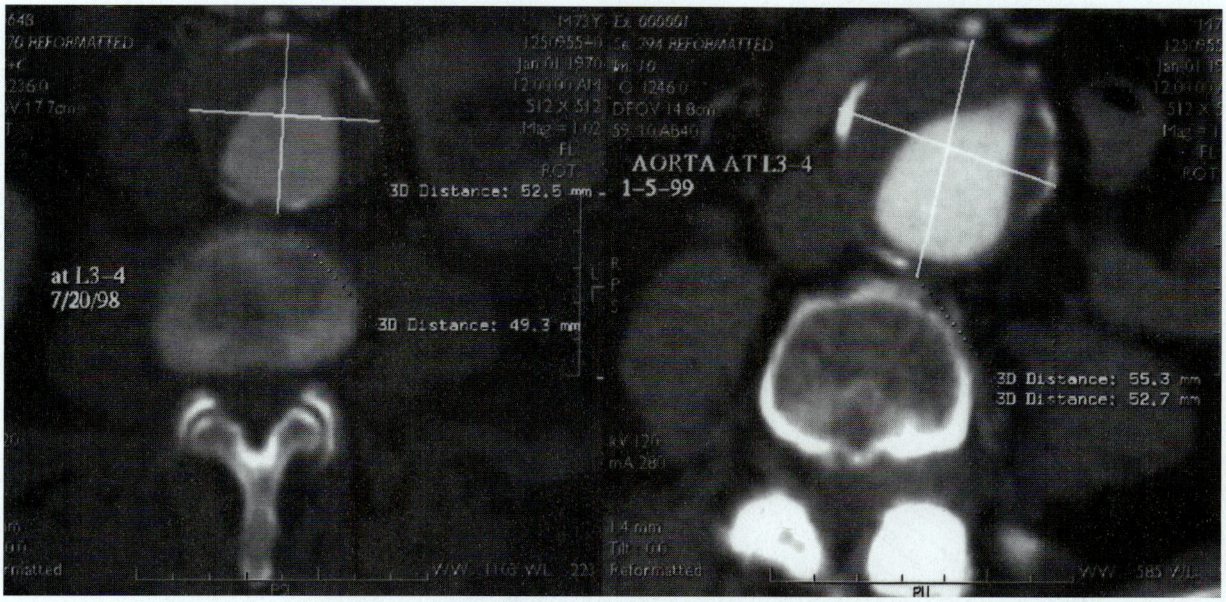

Figure 3 CT scanning assesses the size of the aneurysm, the amount of mural thrombus present, and the relation of other intra-abdominal structures to the aneurysm.

Operative Technique

OPEN REPAIR

Step 1: Initial Incision and Choice of Approach

Open surgical repair of infrarenal AAAs is performed through a transperitoneal or retroperitoneal exposure of the aorta with the patient under general endotracheal anesthesia. The aneurysm may be exposed through either a long midline incision (for the transperitoneal approach) or an oblique flank incision (for the retroperitoneal approach) [see Figure 4a]. An upper abdominal transverse incision may also be used for either retroperitoneal or transperitoneal exposure. The results with the two exposures are equivalent. The transperitoneal approach is preferred when exposure of the right renal artery is required and when access to the distal right iliac system or to intra-abdominal organs is necessary. The retroperitoneal exposure offers advantages when extensive peritoneal adhesions, an intestinal stoma, or severe pulmonary disease is present and when there is a need for suprarenal exposure. Use of the retroperitoneal approach has been associated with a shorter duration of postoperative ileus, a lower incidence of pulmonary complications, and a reduction in length of stay in the ICU.

Step 2 (Transperitoneal Approach): Exposure and Control of Aorta and Iliac Arteries

When the transperitoneal approach is used, the small bowel (including the duodenum) is retracted to the right, and the retroperitoneum overlying the aneurysm is divided to the left of the midline [see Figure 4b]. The duodenum is completely mobilized, and the left renal vein is identified and exposed. The normal infrarenal neck, which is just below the left renal vein, is then exposed and encircled for proximal control. Both common iliac arteries are then mobilized and controlled, with care taken to avoid the underlying iliac veins and ureters that cross over at the iliac bifurcation [see Figure 5]. If the common iliac arteries are aneurysmal, then both the internal and the external iliac arteries are controlled. The inferior mesenteric artery is then dissected out and controlled for possible reimplantation into the graft after the aneurysm has been repaired.

Step 2 (Retroperitoneal Approach): Exposure and Control of Aorta and Iliac Arteries

When the retroperitoneal approach is taken, a transverse left abdominal or flank incision is made, and the peritoneum is reflected anteriorly. The left kidney usually is left in place but may be mobilized anteriorly to expose the posterolateral aorta. Exposure of the right iliac system can be achieved by dividing the inferior mesenteric artery early in the course of dissection. The aorta and the iliac arteries are controlled in essentially the same fashion regardless of the type of incision used.

Step 3: Opening of Aneurysm and Creation of Proximal Anastomosis

Systemic anticoagulation with I.V. heparin is then performed. After sufficient time (3 to 5 minutes) has elapsed to permit adequate circulation, the infrarenal neck and the iliac arteries are clamped. To prevent distal embolization, the distal clamps should be applied before the proximal aortic clamp. The aneurysm is then opened longitudinally, the mural thrombus is removed, and back-bleeding lumbar arteries are oversewn. Depending on its degree of backflow and on the patency of the hypogastric arteries, the inferior mesenteric artery may be either ligated or clamped and left with a rim of aortic wall for subsequent reimplantation [see Troubleshooting, below].

The aortic neck is then partially or completely transected, and an appropriately sized tubular or bifurcated graft is sutured to the aorta with a continuous nonabsorbable monofilament suture [see Figure 6]. When the proximal aortic neck is very short, suprarenal aortic clamping may be required for performance of the proximal anastomosis. If suprarenal clamping is necessary, the security of the proximal anastomosis should be verified, and the clamp should then be moved onto the graft below the renal arteries as soon as possible to minimize renal ischemia. If the aorta is especially weak or friable, the anastomosis may be supported with Teflon-felt pledgets.

Step 4: Creation of Distal Anastomosis

When the aneurysm is confined to the aorta, the distal anastomosis is performed by suturing a straight tube graft to the aortic bi-

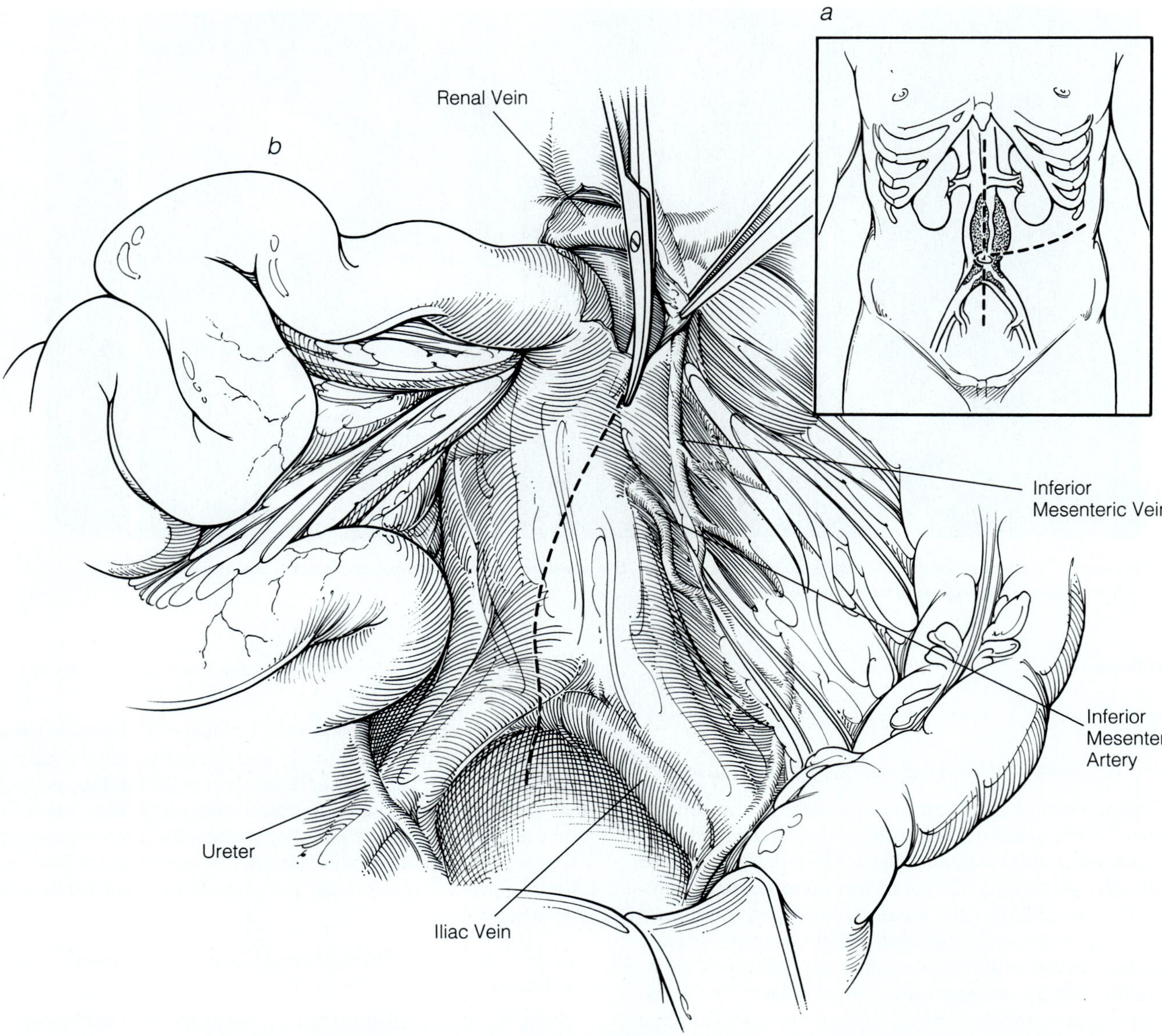

Figure 4 Open repair of infrarenal AAAs. (*a*) For the transabdominal approach to the abdominal aorta, a midline or transverse incision is appropriate. For the retroperitoneal approach, an oblique flank incision may be used. (*b*) The small intestine (including the duodenum) is retracted laterally after the ligament of Treitz is mobilized, and the retroperitoneum is incised in the midline. The left renal vein is the landmark for the infrarenal neck.

furcation [*see Figure 7*]; straight tube graft reconstructions are used about 30% of the time. Distally, the dissection should avoid the fibroareolar tissue overlying the left common iliac artery because this tissue contains branches of the inferior mesenteric artery and the autonomic nerves that control sexual function in men.

When the aneurysm extends into the common iliac arteries, the distal anastomosis is accomplished by suturing a bifurcated graft to the distal common iliac arteries or, in the case of significant occlusive disease, to the common femoral arteries. In these situations, control of the iliac arteries is best achieved by mobilizing the external and internal arteries and clamping them individually [*see Figure 8*]. It is sometimes easier to control iliac artery back-bleeding by using intraluminal balloon catheters and oversewing the common iliac arteries from within the opened aortic or iliac aneurysms. Care must be taken not to injure the accompanying venous structures or the ureters, which cross anterior to the iliac bifurcation. Every effort should be made to ensure perfusion of at least one hypogastric artery to help minimize the risk of postoperative left colon ischemia.

Declamping hypotension may occur after reperfusion of the lower extremities. It is essential to maintain communication with the anesthesiologist so that blood and fluid replacement can be adjusted in anticipation of lower-extremity reperfusion. Even though the graft and vessels are flushed and back-bled before distal flow is reestablished, it is preferable first to establish flow into one of the hypogastric arteries so as to minimize the chances of distal embolization to the legs.

Before the abdomen is closed, adequate perfusion of the lower extremities and the left colon should be ensured via either direct inspection or noninvasive monitoring. The open aneurysm sac is then sutured closed over the aortic graft to separate the graft from the duodenum and the viscera [*see Figure 9*]. This step reduces the risk of aortoenteric fistula.

Troubleshooting

If the inferior mesenteric artery is small and back-bleeding is adequate, it may be ligated [*see Figure 10a*]; however, if the vessel is large or back-bleeding is meager, it should be reimplanted. Reimplantation of the inferior mesenteric artery can be accomplished with relative ease by using the Carrel patch technique. After the graft has been completely sewn to the aorta, a partial occluding clamp is placed on the main body of the graft or on one of the limbs. An opening in the graft is then created, and an end-to-side anastomosis [see Figure 10b]—with an interposition graft added if necessary [see Figure 10c]—is used to reconstruct the inferior mesenteric artery. This anastomosis is created with a continuous monofilament suture.

ENDOVASCULAR REPAIR

Endovascular repair was introduced during the 1990s as a less invasive approach to treating infrarenal AAAs. In this approach, a stent-graft is placed endoluminally via bilateral groin incisions; thus, there is no need for a major abdominal incision and aortic clamping. Early results are promising: blood loss is decreased, hospital stay is shortened, and earlier return to function is achieved. Not all patients are candidates for endovascular repair, however. In September 1999, the United States Food and Drug Administration approved two stent-graft devices for use in surgical management of

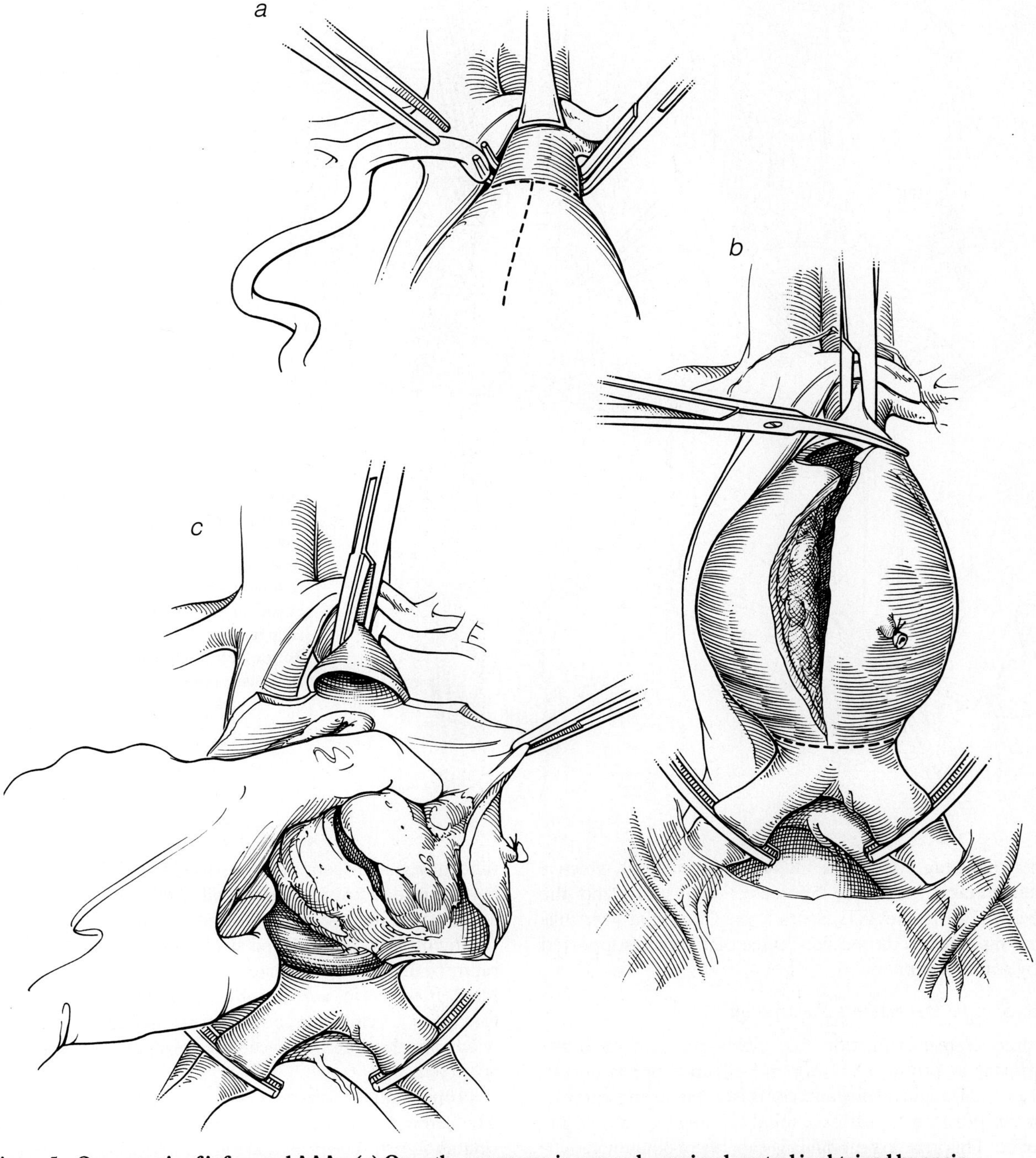

Figure 5 Open repair of infrarenal AAAs. (*a*) Once the aneurysm is exposed, proximal control is obtained by encircling the proximal neck with an umbilical tape or heavy Silastic. The inferior mesenteric artery is identified and then either clamped or ligated for possible reimplantation at the end of the procedure. (*b*) The iliac arteries are dissected free, systemic heparin anticoagulation is instituted, and distal control is obtained, followed by proximal control to prevent distal embolization. The aneurysm sac is then opened longitudinally. (*c*) All mural thrombus is removed, and the proximal and distal necks of the aorta are incised.

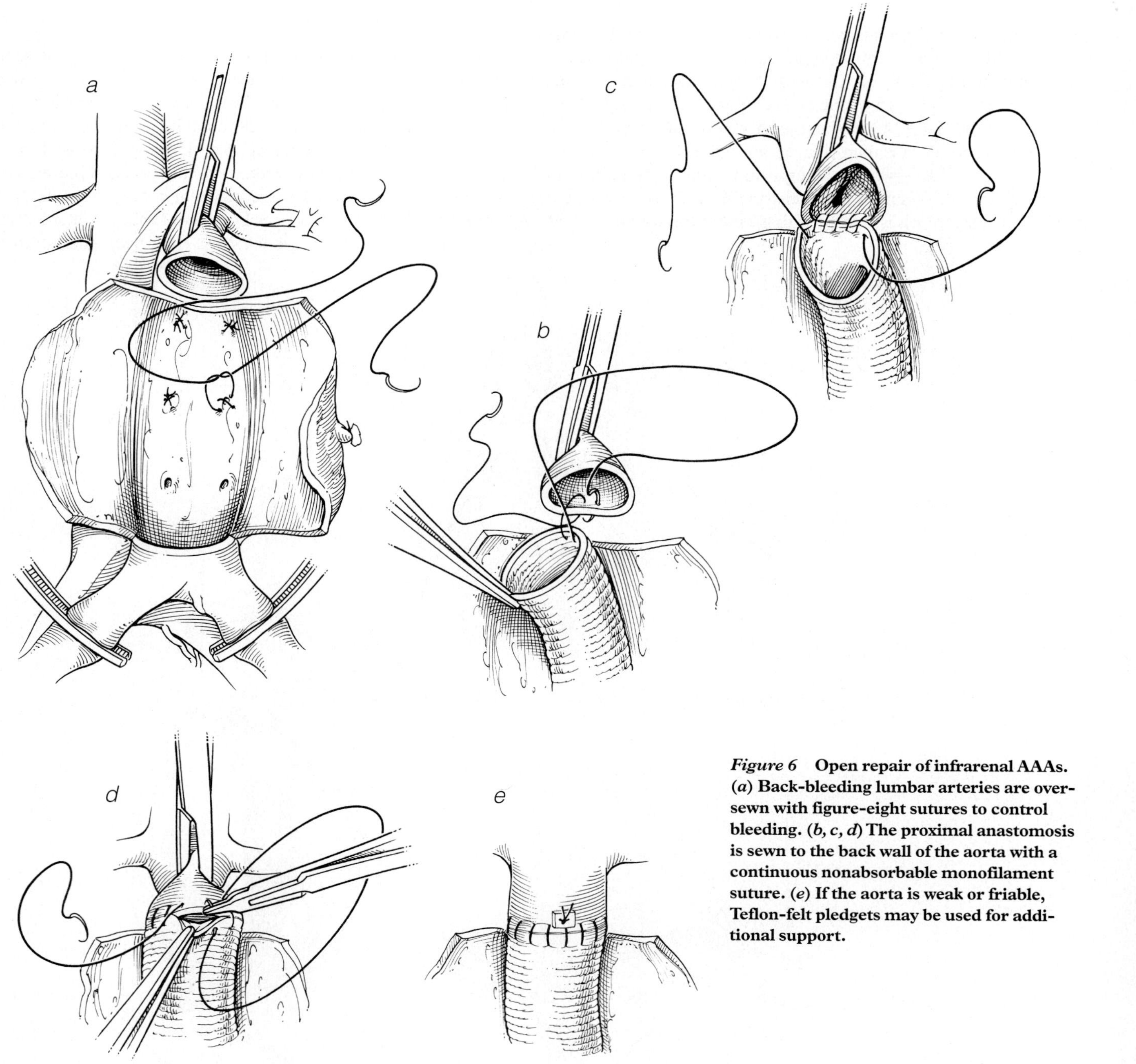

Figure 6 **Open repair of infrarenal AAAs.** (*a*) Back-bleeding lumbar arteries are oversewn with figure-eight sutures to control bleeding. (*b, c, d*) The proximal anastomosis is sewn to the back wall of the aorta with a continuous nonabsorbable monofilament suture. (*e*) If the aorta is weak or friable, Teflon-felt pledgets may be used for additional support.

AAAs: the Ancure device (Guidant, Indianapolis, Indiana), which is a balloon-expandable one-piece bifurcated stent-graft, and the AneuRx device (Medtronic AVE, Santa Rosa, California), which is a self-expanding bifurcated modular device that is fully supported externally by a nitinol stent.

Procedure-Specific Preoperative Preparation

Precise preoperative evaluation that yields accurate measurements will result in proper planning and effective prevention of problems. Both CT angiography and contrast biplane angiography are used for this purpose. Of the two, spiral CT angiography is currently preferred. This imaging modality is capable of obtaining high-quality images of the vascular anatomy and reconfiguring them into detailed three-dimensional images. For optimal evaluation, images should be obtained at 3 mm intervals from the celiac artery to the femoral arteries. Spiral CT angiography accurately defines the proximal and distal characteristics of the AAA as well as detects any significant renal, visceral, or iliac occlusive disease. It is particularly helpful in defining the infrarenal neck between the renal arteries and the proximal portion of the aneurysm.

Angiography is employed as a complement to spiral CT angiography in this setting. An arteriogram is useful in that it helps define renal, mesenteric, and distal arterial anatomy; helps characterize tortuosity, calcification, and stenoses in access arteries; and helps determine the angles between the aorta, the proximal neck, and the aneurysm.

Proper patient selection is mandatory for successful outcome. The common femoral arteries must be large enough to accept a 22 French sheath. The proximal infrarenal aortic neck must be suitable for device implantation—that is, its diameter must be between 16 and 25 mm, and it must be longer than 10 mm. The common iliac artery implantation should be at least 10 mm above the hypogastric artery, and the iliac artery diameter must be between 8 and 15 mm. In patients with iliac artery aneurysms, it is possible to land the end

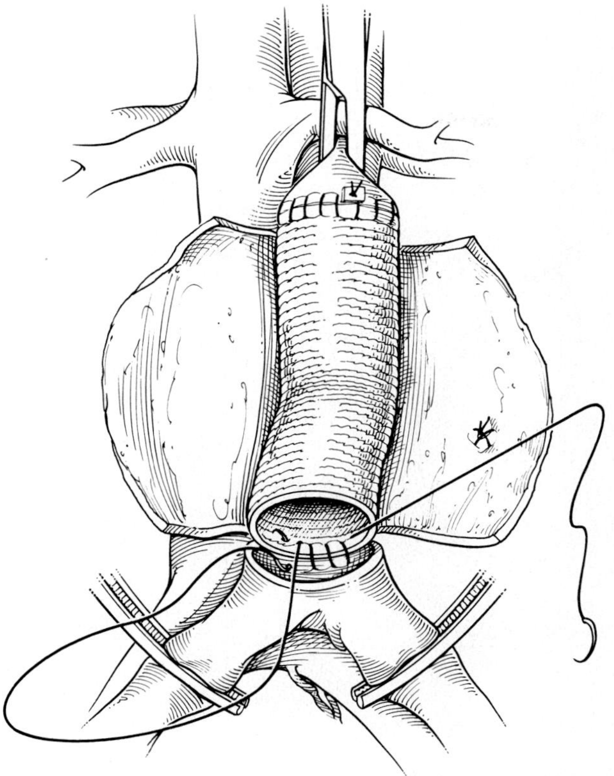

Figure 7 Open repair of infrarenal AAAs. When the aneurysm does not extend into the iliac arteries, a straight tube graft is used. The distal anastomosis is completed with a continuous suture. Before completion of the anastomosis, the graft is flushed by back-bleeding the iliac arteries and flushing the proximal anastomosis.

of the stent in the external iliac artery and thereby exclude one internal iliac artery; however, exclusion of both internal iliac arteries should be avoided so as to prevent ischemic sequelae.

Technique for Device Implantation

The methods and technical principles we briefly describe here derive from the personal experience one of us (C.K.Z.) has accumulated with more than 150 modular implants. The ensuing technical description is not intended to be exhaustive, nor is it meant as a substitute for the instructions provided by the manufacturer.

The patient is placed under epidural or general anesthesia. Bilateral femoral artery cutdowns are performed through transverse groin incisions to allow exposure of the common femoral artery from the inguinal ligament to the femoral bifurcation. Proximal control of the femoral arteries is obtained with umbilical tapes. Systemic anticoagulation with I.V. heparin is instituted to prolong the activated clotting time (ACT) to greater than 250 seconds. The ACT is monitored and maintained at this level throughout the procedure, and additional heparin is given as needed.

The femoral arteries are cannulated with an 18-gauge needle, and 0.035-in. guide wires are placed bilaterally under fluoroscopic guidance; 10 French sheaths are then placed over the two guide wires and advanced into the aneurysm under fluoroscopic guidance. A superstiff 0.035-in. guide wire 260 cm in length is inserted into the thoracic aorta, usually from the right limb. In the contralateral iliac artery, a pigtail catheter is placed just above the level of the renal arteries, and an initial roadmapping aortogram is obtained. The 10 French sheath in the right femoral artery is exchanged for a 22 French sheath, which is placed over the superstiff guide wire and carefully advanced into the proximal infrarenal aorta under fluoroscopic guidance. The main stent-graft module, which is chosen on

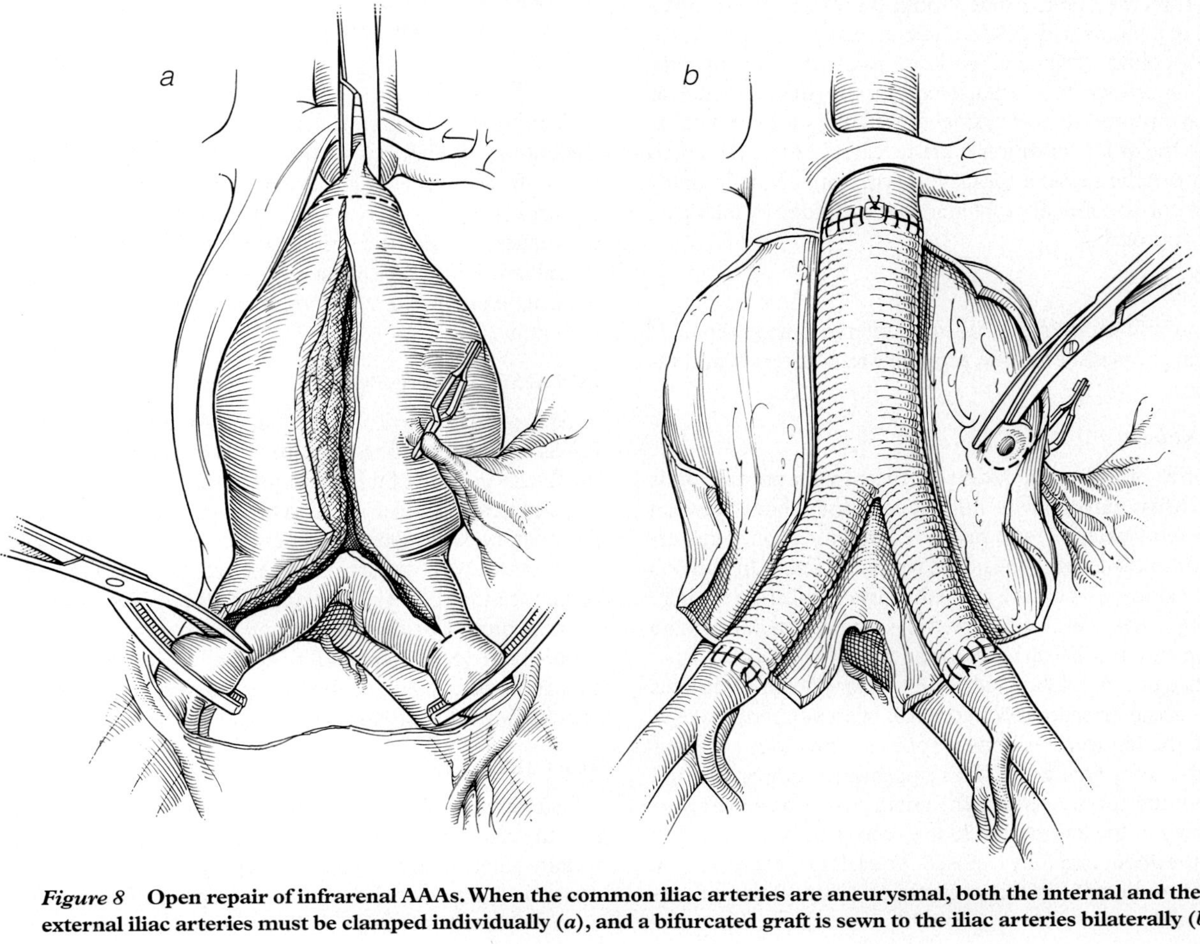

Figure 8 Open repair of infrarenal AAAs. When the common iliac arteries are aneurysmal, both the internal and the external iliac arteries must be clamped individually (*a*), and a bifurcated graft is sewn to the iliac arteries bilaterally (*b*).

the basis of preoperative measurements, is then advanced over the guide wire and through the delivery sheath into the perirenal aorta [see Figure 11a]. A second aortogram is performed to verify the position of the renal arteries. Under fluoroscopic guidance, the stent-graft is then gradually deployed by retracting the outer sheath and allowing the graft to expand, and it is positioned directly below the level of the renal arteries [see Figure 11b].

Once the main bifurcation module has been deployed, the 10 French sheath in the contralateral iliac artery is pulled back, and a 0.035-in. angled hydrophilic wire and a guide catheter are inserted into the contralateral limb of the bifurcation module. The hydrophilic wire is then exchanged for a superstiff guide wire, over which a 16 French sheath is advanced into the contralateral limb under fluoroscopic guidance. The contralateral limb is then advanced through the sheath into the contralateral limb and deployed [see Figure 11c]. A final aortogram is then performed to confirm that a satisfactory technical result has been achieved [see Figure 11d]. Proximal and distal extender cuffs may be placed if necessary. The femoral arteriotomies are repaired, and lower-extremity perfusion is reestablished.

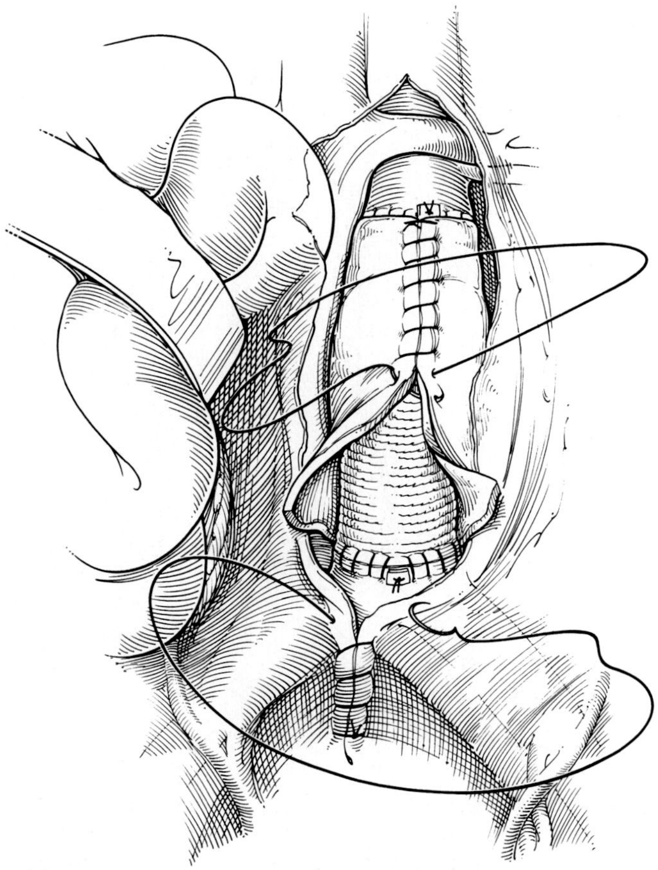

Special Considerations

CONCURRENT DISEASE PROCESSES

At times, a concurrent disease process complicates repair of an AAA. The most common problems encountered are hepatobiliary, pancreatic, gastrointestinal, gynecologic, and genitourinary disorders. Careful evaluation of the situation is necessary to determine whether to treat the two disease entities concurrently. As a rule, the more life-threatening disorder is treated first.

There are three key points that should be remembered in the management of patients with AAAs and concurrent diseases. First, a careful preoperative diagnostic workup usually detects any concomitant disease processes. Second, in emergency situations such as ruptured or symptomatic aneurysms, the aneurysm always takes priority unless the other condition is life-threatening and the aneurysm is clearly not the cause of the critical symptoms. Finally, many concomitant intra-abdominal problems can be avoided by taking an endovascular approach.

ANATOMIC VARIANTS

Several anatomic variants may be encountered during repair of AAAs, including horseshoe kidney, accessory renal arteries, and venous anomalies.

Horseshoe Kidney

The incidence of horseshoe kidney in the general population is less than 3%. Most patients with horseshoe kidneys have between three and five renal arteries.[14] To preserve renal function, renal arteries arising from the aneurysm should be reimplanted. In patients with horseshoe kidneys who have more than five renal arteries, there often are multiple small accessory arteries, some of which originate from the aneurysm, the iliac arteries, or both.

The presence of a horseshoe kidney may complicate—but does not preclude—an anterior approach to repair of an infrarenal AAA.[15] In such cases, the left retroperitoneal approach provides excellent exposure of the infrarenal aorta. This approach requires that the surgeon dissect the space between the aneurysm and the left portion and isthmus of the kidney; the kidney can then be reflected to the right and the aneurysm fully exposed. The left ureter crosses the iliac arteries from the right in this position, and duplication of ureters may be noted.

Figure 9 Open repair of infrarenal AAAs. Once the anastomoses have been completed and adequate flow to the lower extremities and the left colon has been confirmed, the open aneurysm sac is sutured closed over the aortic graft.

Venous Anomalies

A number of different venous anomalies may be observed in the course of AAA repair; however, the overall incidence is quite low. Left renal vein variants, such as retroaortic left renal veins and circumaortic venous rings, are the most commonly seen venous anomalies.[16] Azygous continuation of the inferior vena cava and bilateral inferior vena cava have also been noted. Unnecessary bleeding can be prevented by means of careful dissection and meticulous technique.

INFLAMMATORY ANEURYSM

Approximately 5% of infrarenal AAAs are inflammatory.[17] These AAAs have a dense fibroinflammatory rind that typically adheres to the fourth portion of the duodenum; they may also involve the inferior vena cava, the left renal vein, or the ureters. Patients with inflammatory AAAs typically experience abdominal or flank pain and may present with weight loss. The erythrocyte sedimentation rate is usually elevated as well. Inflammatory aneurysms rarely rupture, because most are symptomatic and consequently are treated before rupture can occur. Repair of inflammatory aneurysms poses technical problems because of the involvement of adjacent structures. A retroperitoneal approach is usually advocated for these aneurysms.

RUPTURED ANEURYSM

Infrarenal AAAs can rupture freely into the peritoneal cavity or into the retroperitoneum. Free rupture into the peritoneal cavity is usually anterior and is typically accompanied by immediate hemodynamic collapse and a very high mortality. Retroperitoneal ruptures are usually posterior and may be contained by the psoas muscle and adjacent periaortic and perivertebral tissue. This type of rupture may occur without significant blood loss initially, and the patient may be hemodynamically stable.

When an aortic aneurysm ruptures, immediate surgical repair is indicated. If the patient is unstable and either an abdominal aortic aneurysm was previously diagnosed or a palpable abdominal mass is present, no further evaluation is necessary and the patient should be taken directly to the OR. If the patient is stable and the diagnosis is questionable, CT scanning may be performed to confirm the presence of an aneurysm and determine its extent, the site of the rupture, and the degree of iliac involvement. Bedside ultrasonography may also be used for quick confirmation of the presence of an AAA.

Surgical repair of ruptured aneurysms is performed via a transperitoneal approach. In cases of contained rupture, supraceliac control should be achieved before infrarenal dissection; once the neck of the aneurysm has been dissected free, the aortic clamp may be moved to the infrarenal level. In cases of free rupture, efforts to obtain vascular control may include compression of the aorta at the hiatus and infrarenal control with a clamp or an intraluminal balloon. Once proximal and distal control have been achieved, the operation is conducted in much the same way as an elective repair.

Outcome Evaluation

The mortality associated with repair of AAAs has been greatly reduced by improvements in preoperative evaluation and perioperative care: leading centers currently report death rates ranging from 0% to 5%.[18] Mortality after repair of inflammatory aneurysms and after emergency repair of symptomatic nonruptured aneurysms continues to be somewhat higher (5% to 10%), primarily as a consequence of less thorough preoperative evaluation. The mortality associated with endovascular repair of AAAs is 1% to 3%—that is, essentially equivalent to that associated with open repair in selected patients.

Overall morbidity after elective aneurysm repair ranges from 10% to 30%. The most common complication is myocardial ischemia, and MI is the most common cause of postoperative death. Mild renal insufficiency is the second most frequent complication, occurring after 6% of elective aneurysm repairs; however, severe renal failure necessitating dialysis is rare in this setting. The third most common complication is pulmonary disease; the incidence of postoperative pneumonia is approximately 5%.

Postoperative bleeding may occur as well. Common sources of such bleeding include the anastomotic suture lines, inadequately recognized venous injuries, and coagulopathies resulting from intraoperative hypothermia or excessive blood loss. Any evidence of ongoing bleeding is an indication for early exploration.

Lower-extremity ischemia may occur as a result of either emboli or thrombosis of the graft and may necessitate reoperation and thrombectomy. So-called trash foot may also develop when diffuse microemboli are carried into the distal circulation.

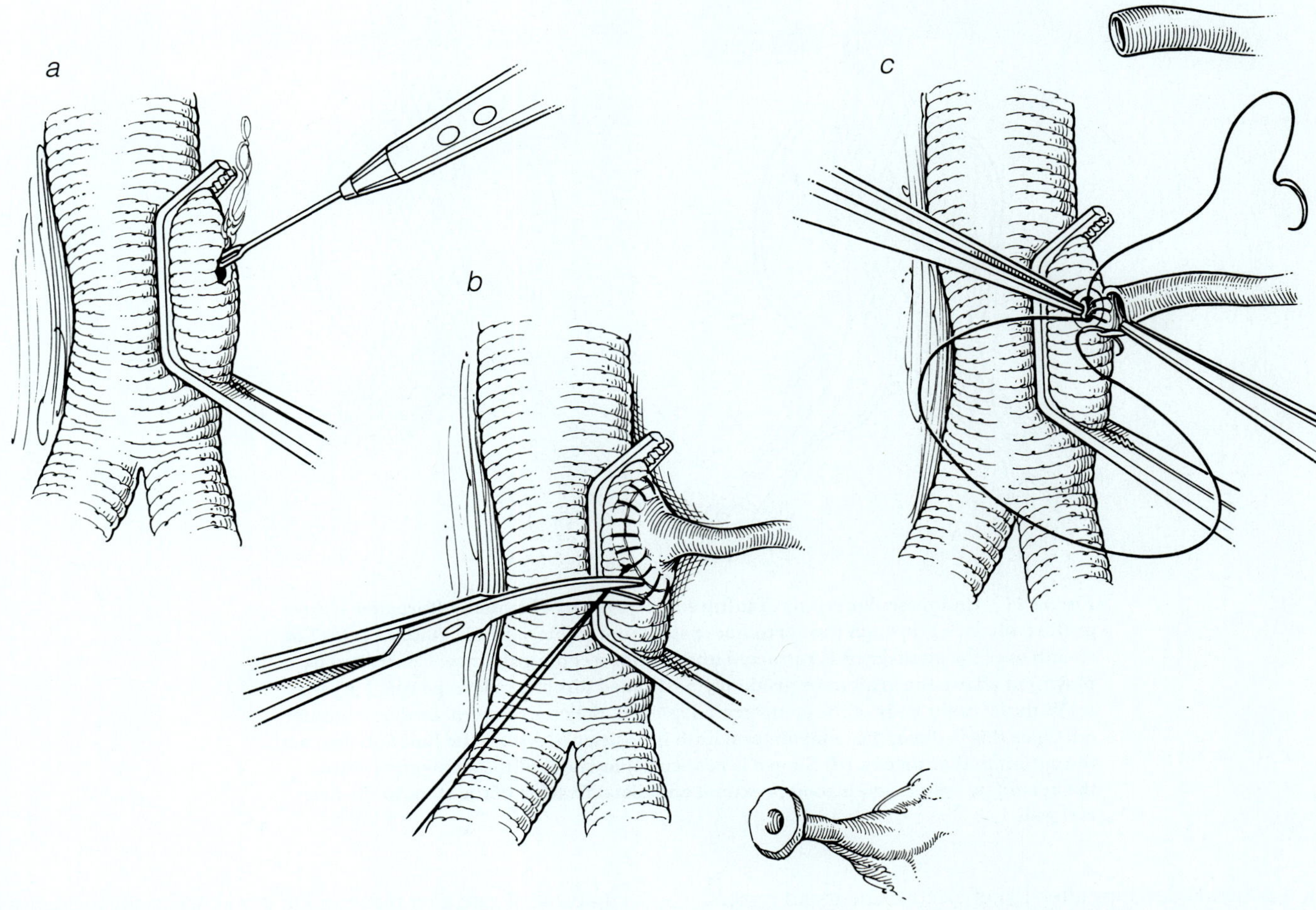

Figure 10 Open repair of infrarenal AAAs. (*a*) A small, adequately back-bleeding inferior mesenteric artery may be ligated. (*b*) A large or meagerly back-bleeding inferior mesenteric artery should be reimplanted. A side-biting clamp is applied to the graft, and an end-to-side anastomosis is created with a fine monofilament suture. (*c*) If the inferior mesenteric artery is not long enough for a direct anastomosis, an interposition graft—either a segment of a vein or a prosthetic graft—may be used for added length.

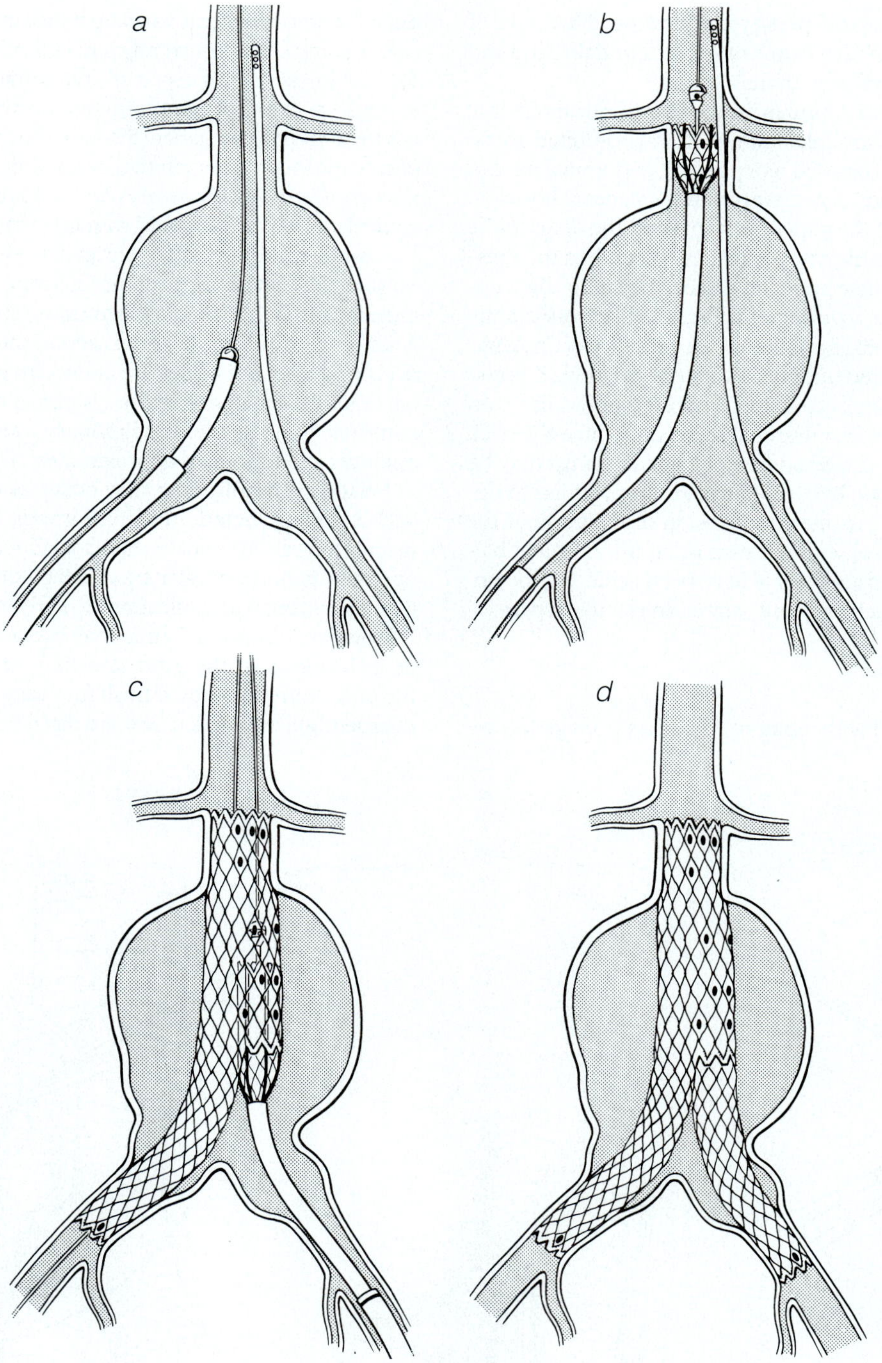

Figure 11 Endovascular repair of infrarenal AAAs. (*a*) The main bifurcated stent-graft is advanced through the aortoiliac system under fluoroscopic guidance. (*b*) The sheath over the stent-graft is retracted under fluoroscopic guidance. Controlled deployment allows the graft to be gradually positioned directly below the renal arteries. (*c*) With the main body of the stent-graft deployed, the contralateral limb is cannulated. Once this is done, the contralateral limb is positioned within the junction gate and the common iliac artery. (*d*) Shown is proper deployment of the stent-graft within the aortoiliac system, with good proximal and distal fixation of the stent to the arterial wall.

Colon ischemia develops after 1% of elective aneurysm repairs. Patients usually present with bloody diarrhea, abdominal pain, a distended abdomen, and leukocytosis. Diagnosis is confirmed by sigmoidoscopy, which reveals mucosal sloughing. In cases of transmural colonic necrosis, colon resection and exteriorization of stomas are warranted.

Paraplegia is rare after repair of infrarenal AAAs: the incidence is only 0.2%. Most instances of paraplegia occur after repair of a ruptured aneurysm or when the pelvis has been devascularized. The majority of patients recover at least some degree of neurologic function.

Late complications—such as pseudoaneurysms at the suture lines, graft or graft limb thrombosis, and graft infection—may occur but are extremely rare. Graft infection may be associated with graft-enteric fistula and is notoriously difficult to diagnose and treat.

Long-term survival in patients who have undergone successful AAA repair is reduced in comparison with that in the general population. The 5-year survival rate after AAA repair is 67% (range, 49% to 84%), compared with 80% to 85% in age-matched control subjects, and the mean duration of survival after AAA repair is 7.4 years. Part of the difference in survival can be attributed to associated coronary disease in patients with aneurysms. Late deaths result primarily from cardiac causes.

References

1. Taylor LM, Porter JM: Basic data related to clinical decision-making in abdominal aortic aneurysms. Ann Vasc Surg 1:502, 1980
2. Bickerstaff LK, Hollier LH, Van Peenen HJ, et al: Abdominal aortic aneurysm: the changing natural history. J Vasc Surg 1:6, 1984
3. Melton L, Bickerstaff L, Hollier LH, et al: Changing incidence of abdominal aortic aneurysms: a population based study. Am J Epidemiol 120:379, 1984
4. Darling RC, Messina CR, Brewster DC, et al: Autopsy study of unoperated aortic aneurysms. Circulation 56(suppl 2):161, 1977
5. Thurmond AS, Semler JH: Abdominal aortic aneurysm. Incidence in a population at risk. J Cardiovasc Surg 27:457, 1986
6. Whittemore AD, Clowes AW, Hechtman HB, et al: Aortic aneurysm repair reduced operative mortality associated with maintenance of optimal cardiac performance. Ann Surg 120:414, 1980
7. Pairolero PC: Repair of abdominal aortic aneurysms in high-risk patients. Surg Clin North Am 69:755, 1989
8. Stokes J, Butcher HR: Abdominal aortic aneurysms: factors influencing operative mortality and criteria of operability. Arch Surg 107:297, 1973
9. Quill DS, Colgan MP, Summer DS: Ultrasonic screening for the detection of abdominal aortic aneurysms. Surg Clin North Am 69:713, 1989
10. Bluth EI: Ultrasound of the abdominal aorta. Arch Intern Med 144:377, 1994
11. Gomes MN, Choyke PL: Preoperative evaluation of abdominal aortic aneurysms: ultrasound or computed tomography? J Cardiovasc Surg 28:159, 1987
12. Amparo EG, Hoddick WK, Hricak H, et al: Comparison of magnetic resonance imaging and ultrasonography in the evaluation of abdominal aortic aneurysms. Radiology 154:451, 1985
13. Lee JKT, Ling D, Heiken JP, et al: Magnetic resonance imaging of abdominal aneurysms. Am J Roentgenol 143:1197, 1984
14. Papin E: Chirurgie du rein. Anomalies du rein. Paris, G. Doin, 1928, p 205
15. Zarins CK, Gewertz BL: Atlas of Vascular Surgery. New York, Churchill Livingstone, 1988, p 56
16. Trigaux JP, Vandroogenbroek S, De Wispelaere JF, et al: Congenital anomalies of the inferior vena cava and left renal vein: evaluation with spiral CT. J Vasc Interv Radiol 9:339, 1998
17. Crawford JL, Stowe CL, Safi HJ, et al: Inflammatory aneurysms of the aorta. J Vasc Surg 2:133, 1985
18. Crawford ES, Saleh SA, Babb JW 3d, et al: Infrarenal abdominal aortic aneurysm: factors influencing survival after operation performed over a 25-year period. Ann Surg 193:699, 1981

Acknowledgment

Figures 4 through 11   Susan Brust, C.M.I.

65 LOWER-EXTREMITY AMPUTATION FOR ISCHEMIA

William C. Pevec, M.D.

Patients with infected, painful, or necrotic lower extremities can be restored to a better functional level by means of a properly selected and performed amputation. This procedure should be considered reconstructive and restorative. In what follows, I address amputations across the toe, the forefoot, the leg, and the thigh. Because Symes' amputations and hip disarticulations are seldom appropriate on ischemic limbs, I omit discussion of these procedures.

General Preoperative Planning

Selecting the appropriate level of amputation is of primary importance for healing and preservation of function. For an ambulatory patient who has either a palpable pulse over the dorsal pedal or posterior tibial arteries or a functioning infrainguinal arterial bypass graft, amputation on the foot (either toe amputation or transmetatarsal amputation) is appropriate. For an ambulatory patient who has a palpable femoral pulse and a patent profunda femoral artery, whose skin is warm at least to the level of the ankle, and who has no skin lesions on the proposed amputation flaps, amputation below the knee is appropriate. For a nonambulatory patient who has ischemic rest pain, ulceration, or gangrene, amputation above the knee is appropriate. Arterial reconstruction is not indicated if the extremity is nonfunctional. Below-the-knee amputation does not offer nonambulatory patients any functional advantage; moreover, it is less likely to heal and often results in a flexion contracture at the knee that leads to pressure ulceration of the stump. Above-the-knee amputation depends on pulsatile flow into the ipsilateral internal iliac artery for successful healing. Above-the-knee amputation is also necessary for a patient whose skin is cool at or above the midcalf or who has skin lesions at or proximal to the midcalf.

Several adjunctive measurements (e.g., transcutaneous oxygen tension and segmental arterial pressure) have been used to select the level of amputation but have not proved particularly helpful. Generally, these adjuncts can reliably determine a level of amputation at which healing is virtually assured, but they cannot reliably determine the level at which an amputation will not heal. Consequently, reliance on such measures to select the level of amputation will result in an unnecessarily high percentage of more proximal amputations.

In most cases, definitive amputation can be accomplished in a single stage. Local cellulitis can usually be controlled beforehand with bed rest and systemic administration of antibiotics. Undrained pus or recalcitrant cellulitis, however, must be treated with debridement and drainage in advance of definitive amputation. This can be accomplished with local soft tissue debridement, single-toe amputation, or guillotine amputation across the ankle.

Careful preoperative medical assessment is essential. Lower-extremity amputation for ischemia is associated with a mortality of 4.5% to 16%,[1-5] owing to the poor overall condition of the patient population. Accordingly, optimization of cardiac and pulmonary function and control of systemic infection are mandatory.

Finally, the timing of elective amputation is crucial. Because the loss of a limb is a difficult and frightening thing for a patient to accept, there is a natural tendency to delay amputation for as long as possible. This tendency is understandable but must be weighed against the potential problems associated with delay, such as poor preoperative pain control, which leads to an increased incidence of postamputation phantom limb pain, and extended preoperative immobility, which leads to physical deconditioning and makes prosthetic limb rehabilitation more difficult. A preoperative consultation with a physiatrist can allay some of the patient's anxiety by addressing the expected postoperative course of rehabilitation and thereby removing some of the fear of the unknown.

Toe Amputation

Amputation of the toe can be done either across a phalanx or across a metatarsal bone; the latter procedure is commonly referred

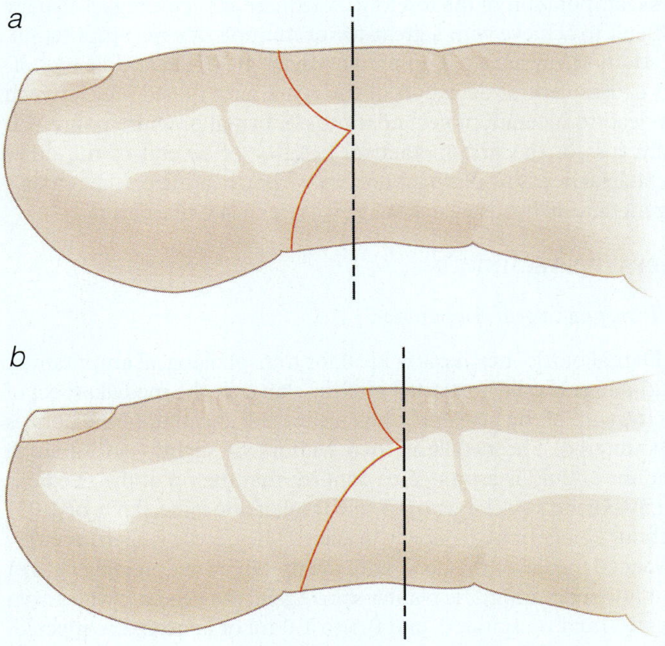

Figure 1 Toe amputation: transphalangeal amputation. Transphalangeal amputation can be performed either with dorsal and plantar flaps of equal length (*a*) or with a plantar flap that is longer than the dorsal flap (*b*). The phalanx is transected at the level of the apex of the skin flaps (dashed line). The bone is transected through the shaft of the phalanx, never across the joint.

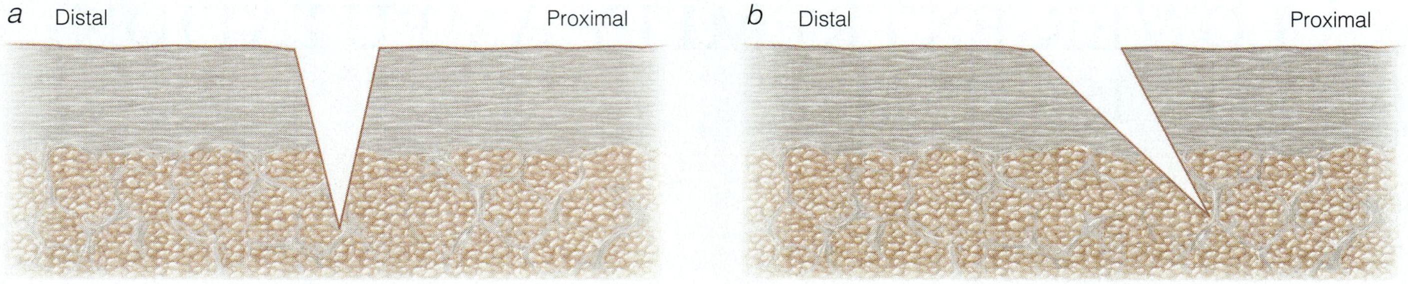

Figure 2 In a lower-extremity amputation, the skin is always incised perpendicular to its surface (*a*). Given the varying contours encountered during extremity amputation, it can be difficult to maintain the perpendicular orientation of the scalpel; however, an incision that undermines the proximal skin flap (*b*) will devascularize the epidermis and lead to necrosis of the suture line.

to as a ray amputation. Many of the perioperative issues are essentially similar for the two approaches; however, indications and operative details differ somewhat and thus will be described separately.

OPERATIVE PLANNING

As noted (see above), for a toe amputation to heal properly, there must be either a palpable pulse over the dorsal pedal or posterior tibial artery or a functioning bypass graft to an infrapopliteal artery. If tissue necrosis or infection is confined to the distal or middle phalanx, transphalangeal amputation is appropriate; if tissue loss or necrosis involves the proximal phalanx, ray amputation is indicated. If tissue necrosis or infection extends over the metatarsophalangeal joint, either transmetatarsal amputation of the entire forefoot or below-the-knee amputation is usually necessary (see below).

Multiple transphalangeal amputations are functionally well tolerated. If, however, ray amputation of the great toe or of more than one smaller toe is called for, it is preferable to perform a transmetatarsal amputation of the forefoot. Adequate skin coverage is usually difficult to achieve with a great-toe or multiple-toe ray amputation. In addition, ray amputation of more than one of the middle toes often causes central deviation of the remaining outside toes, which can lead to ulcerations secondary to abnormal pressure points. Finally, loss of the first metatarsal head or of several of the other metatarsal heads results in abnormal weight-bearing on the remaining metatarsal heads, which may give rise to late ulceration.

OPERATIVE TECHNIQUE

Transphalangeal Amputation

Digital block anesthesia is ideal for transphalangeal amputation. A 25-gauge needle is inserted into the skin over the medial aspect of the dorsum of the proximal phalanx and advanced until the bone is encountered. The needle is then withdrawn slightly, and a small amount of fluid is aspirated to confirm that the tip of the needle is not in a blood vessel. Next, 0.5 to 1.0 ml of lidocaine, 0.5% or 1.0% without epinephrine, is slowly injected. The needle is then carefully advanced medial to the bone until the tip can be felt pressing against (but not puncturing) the plantar skin. Again, the needle is withdrawn slightly, fluid is aspirated, and 0.5 to 1.0 ml of lidocaine is injected. The same technique is repeated on the lateral aspect of the proximal phalanx. In this way, all four digital nerve branches are blocked. If multiple toe amputations are required, an ankle block, epidural anesthesia, spinal anesthesia, or general anesthesia can be used.

An incision is made to create dorsal and plantar skin flaps. Typically, these flaps are equal in length [see Figure 1a]; however, depending on the location of the skin lesion, either the dorsal flap or the plantar flap can be left longer [see Figure 1b]. Care must be taken not to create excessively long flaps, which may lack sufficient perfusion for healing, or to create undermined bevels with the scalpel [see Figure 2], which will lead to epidermolysis of the suture line.

The incision is extended down to the phalanx, and the soft tissues are gently separated from the bone with a small periosteal elevator. All tendons and tendon sheaths are debrided because the poor vascularity of these tissues may compromise the healing of the toe. The phalanx is transected at the level of the apices of the skin incisions [see Figure 1]. Care must be taken not to leave the remaining bone segment too long: this places undue tension on the skin flaps and is a primary cause of poor healing. The best way of transecting the phalanx is to use a pneumatic oscillating saw. Manual bone cutters can splinter the bone, and manual saws can cause extensive damage to the soft tissues. The bone is always transected across the shaft: because of the poor vascularity of the articular cartilage, disarticulation across a joint typically leads to poor healing.

Hemostasis is achieved with absorbable sutures and limited use of the electrocautery. Excessive tissue manipulation and electrocauterization should be avoided. The skin edges are carefully approximated with simple interrupted nonabsorbable monofilament sutures; perfect apposition is necessary to maximize the potential for primary healing. The sutures must not be placed too close to the skin edges, because the heavily keratinized skin of the foot is easily lacerated. The final step is the application of a soft dressing.

Ray Amputation

For ray amputation, spinal, epidural, or general anesthesia can be employed. A so-called tennis racket incision is made—that is, a straight incision along the dorsal surface of the affected metatarsal bone coupled with a circumferential incision around the base of the toe [see Figure 3a]. The goal is to save all available viable skin on the toe; this skin is used to ensure a tension-free closure, and any excess skin can be debrided later, at the time of closure. Again, undermined bevels are avoided. The incision is taken down to the bone, and the soft tissues are separated from the distal metatarsal bone with a periosteal elevator. Dissection must be kept close to the affected metatarsal head to prevent injury to the adjacent metatarsophalangeal joint, which can lead to necrosis of the adjacent toe. The metatarsal bone is transected across the shaft with a pneumatic oscillating saw [see Figure 3b]. The tendons and the tendon sheaths are debrided.

Meticulous hemostasis is achieved with absorbable sutures and limited use of the electrocautery. The skin is approximated with simple interrupted nonabsorbable monofilament sutures. If sufficient viable skin was preserved, a flap of plantar skin is rotated dorsally, and the incision is closed in the shape of a Y [see Figure 4a]. Alternatively, the medial and lateral edges are shifted, one proximally and the other distally, the corners are trimmed, and the incision is

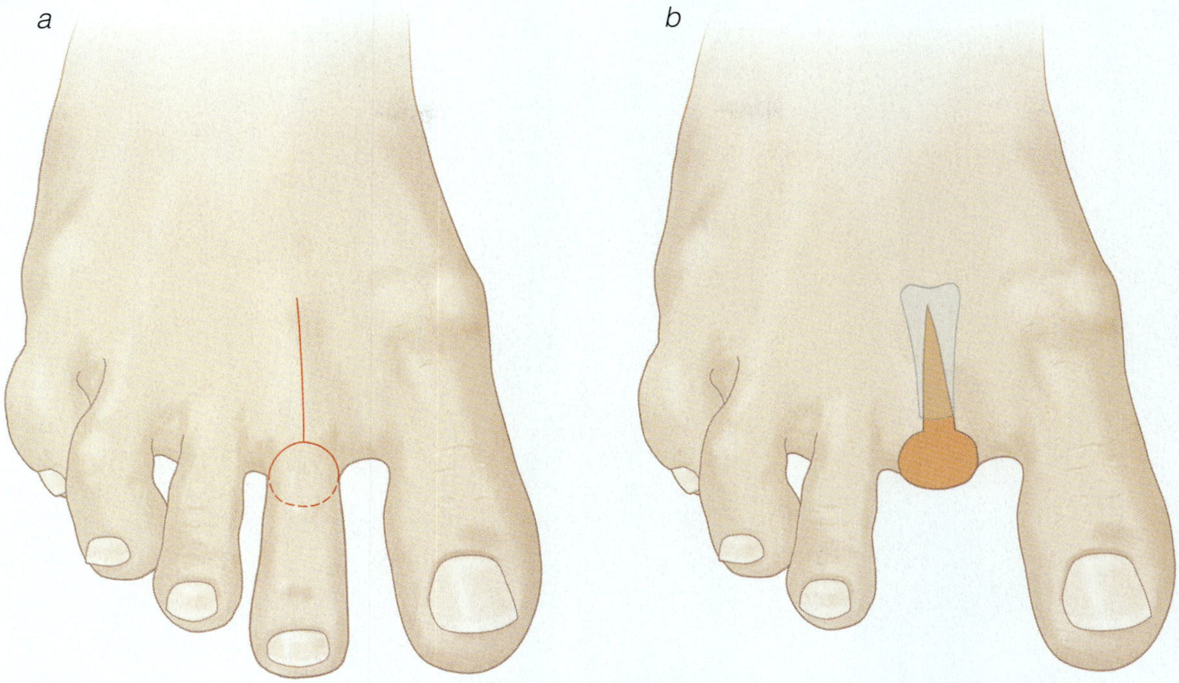

Figure 3 Toe amputation: ray amputation. (*a*) A longitudinal incision is made along the dorsum of the shaft of the metatarsal bone of the affected toe. A circumferential incision is then made around the phalanx. The circumferential incision should be placed as distal on the toe as there is viable skin so that as much skin as possible is retained for closure of the wound. (*b*) The metatarsal bone is transected across its shaft, proximal to the metatarsal head; the joint is never disarticulated.

closed in a linear fashion [*see Figure 4b*]. A soft supportive dressing is applied.

COMPLICATIONS

Complications of toe amputation include bleeding, infection, and failure to heal. Because even a small amount of bleeding under the skin flaps can prevent proper healing, meticulous hemostasis is mandatory. In most cases, infection and failure to heal are attributable to poor patient selection and poor surgical technique; the usual result is a more proximal amputation.

OUTCOME

For optimal healing, there must be an extended period (2 to 3 weeks) during which no weight is borne by the foot that underwent toe amputation. Once healing is complete, the patient should be able to walk normally, with no need for orthotic or assist devices. Beginning ambulation too early can disrupt healing flaps and necessitate more proximal amputation, which lengthens the hospital stay and increases long-term disability. For these reasons, toe amputation in patients with arterial occlusive disease is not an outpatient procedure. Patients are kept on bed rest and instructed in techniques (e.g., use of a wheelchair, a walker, or crutches) that allow them to function without stepping on the foot that was operated on. Hospital discharge is delayed until such techniques are mastered.

Transmetatarsal Amputation

OPERATIVE PLANNING

As noted (see above), transmetatarsal amputation is indicated if there is tissue loss in the forefoot involving the first metatarsal head, two or more of the other metatarsal heads, or the dorsal forefoot. It is contraindicated if there is extensive skin loss on the plantar surface of the foot or on the dorsum proximal to the midshaft of the metatarsal bones. The peroneus longus and peroneus brevis muscles insert on the proximal portions of the fourth and fifth metatarsal bones; if these insertions are sacrificed, inversion of the foot results, eventually leading to chronic skin breakdown from the side of the foot repeatedly striking the ground during ambulation. Transmetatarsal amputation is also contraindicated if there is a preexisting footdrop (peroneal palsy).

OPERATIVE TECHNIQUE

Spinal, epidural, or general anesthesia may be employed. Placement of a tourniquet on the calf is a useful adjunctive measure. This step greatly reduces intraoperative blood loss. More important, the bloodless operative field that results allows more accurate assessment of tissue viability and hence more precise selection of the level of amputation; in a field stained with extravasated blood, it is easy to leave behind nonviable tissue that will doom the amputation. Use of a tourniquet is, however, contraindicated in patients who have a functioning infrapopliteal artery bypass graft.

After sterile preparation and draping, the leg is elevated to help drain the venous blood, and a sterile pneumatic tourniquet is placed around the calf, with care taken to pad the skin under the tourniquet and to position the tourniquet over the calf muscles, where it will not apply pressure over the fibular head (and the common peroneal nerve) or other osseous prominences. The tourniquet is then inflated to a pressure higher than the systolic blood pressure. In patients who do not have diabetes mellitus, a tourniquet inflation pressure of 250 mm Hg is typically employed; in patients who have diabetes mellitus and calcified arteries, a pressure of 350 to 400 mm Hg is preferred.

An incision is made across the dorsum of the foot at the level of the middle of the shafts of the metatarsal bones, extending medially and laterally to the level of the center of the first and fifth metatarsal bones, respectively [*see Figure 5*]. The dorsal incision is curved prox-

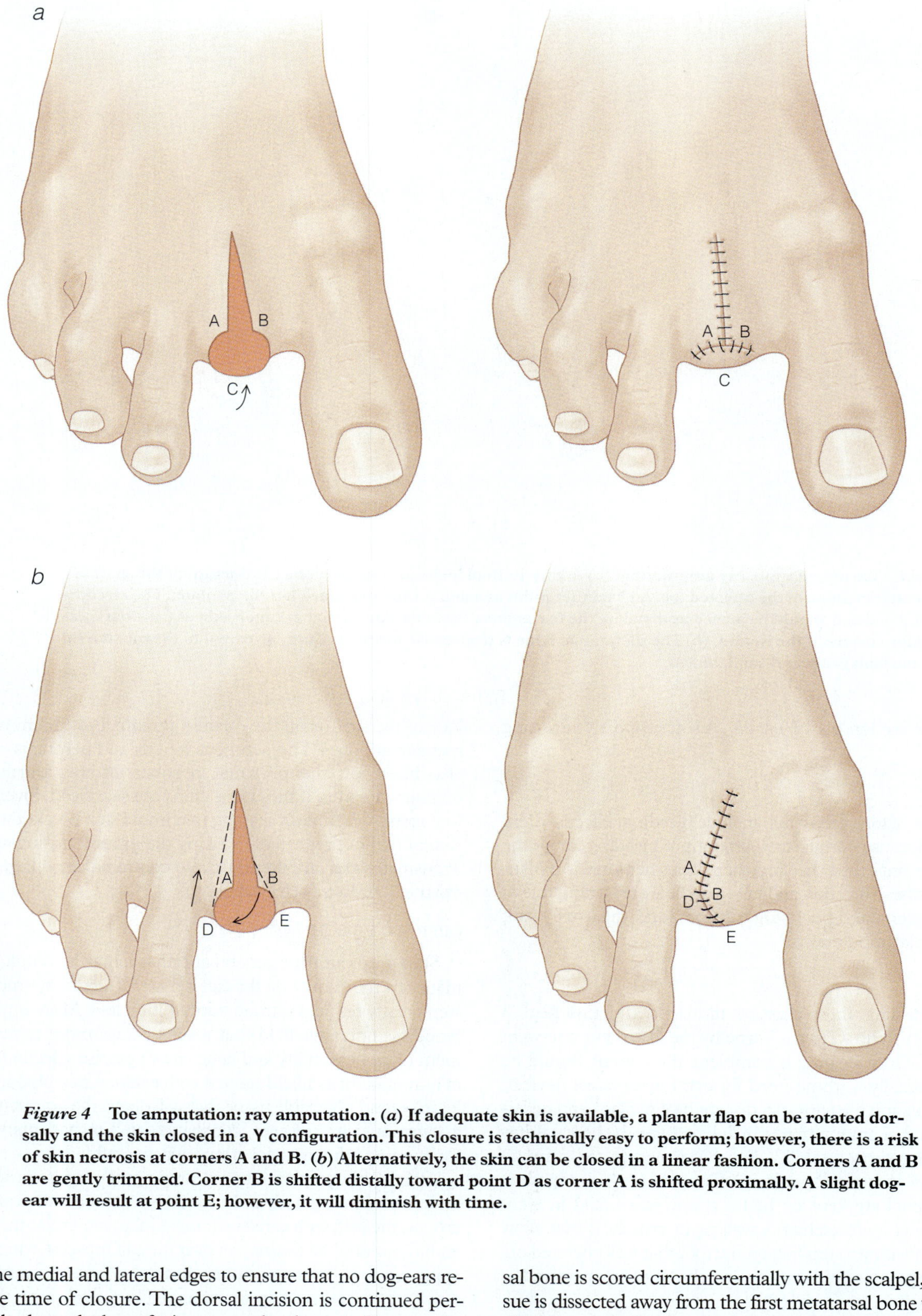

Figure 4 Toe amputation: ray amputation. (*a*) If adequate skin is available, a plantar flap can be rotated dorsally and the skin closed in a Y configuration. This closure is technically easy to perform; however, there is a risk of skin necrosis at corners A and B. (*b*) Alternatively, the skin can be closed in a linear fashion. Corners A and B are gently trimmed. Corner B is shifted distally toward point D as corner A is shifted proximally. A slight dog-ear will result at point E; however, it will diminish with time.

imally at the medial and lateral edges to ensure that no dog-ears remain at the time of closure. The dorsal incision is continued perpendicularly through the soft tissues on the dorsum down to the metatarsal bones. The plantar incision is extended distally to a point just proximal to the toe crease. Care is taken not to bevel the skin incisions.

A plantar flap is created by making an incision with the scalpel adjacent to the metatarsophalangeal joints; the incision is then carried more deeply to the level of the midshafts of the metatarsal bones on their plantar surfaces. The periosteum of the first metatarsal bone is scored circumferentially with the scalpel, and the soft tissue is dissected away from the first metatarsal bone with a periosteal elevator to a point about 1 cm proximal to the dorsal skin incision. The first metatarsal bone is then transected perpendicular to its shaft at the level of the dorsal skin incision with a pneumatic oscillating saw. This process is repeated for each individual metatarsal bone, with care taken to follow the normal contour of the forefoot by cutting the lateral metatarsal bones at a level slightly proximal to the level at which the more medial bones are transected. All visible digital arteries are clamped and tied with absorbable ligatures. If a

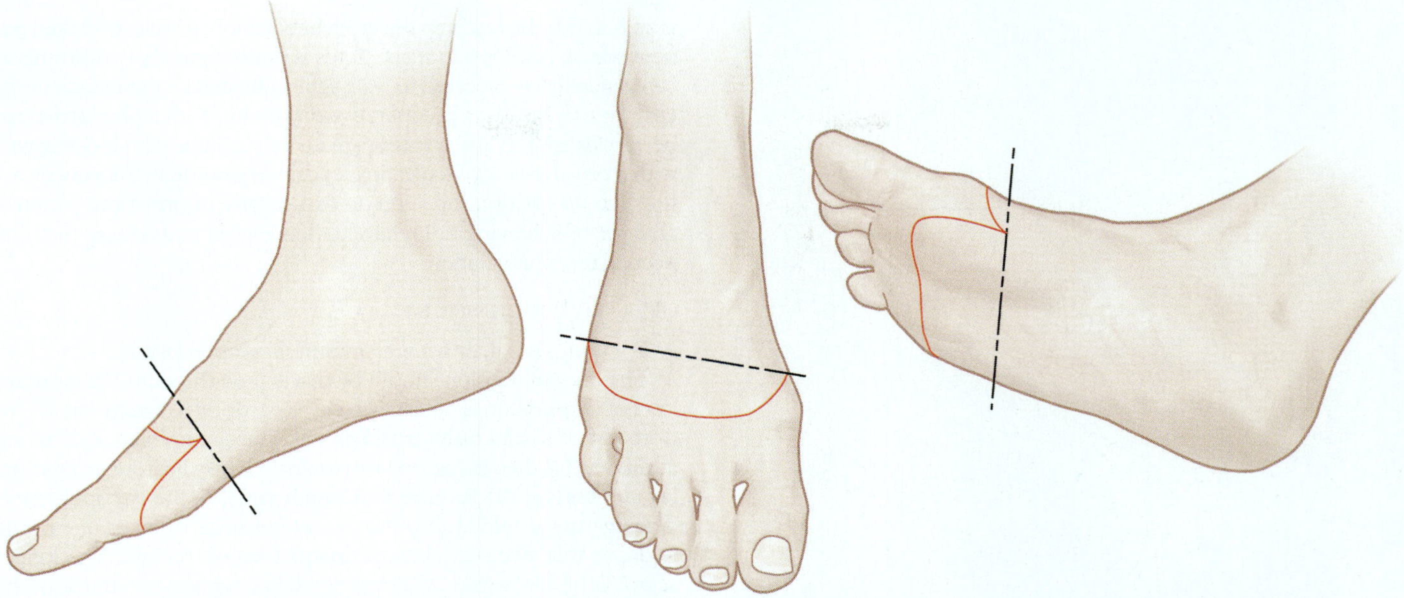

Figure 5 Transmetatarsal amputation. The skin incisions are shown from various angles. The metatarsal shafts are divided in their midportions (dashed line). The metatarsal bone transection is at the level of the apices of the skin incision, and the lateral metatarsal bones are cut slightly more proximally than the medial metatarsal bones, in a pattern reflecting the normal contour of the forefoot.

tourniquet was used, it is deflated at this time. All tendons and tendon sheaths are debrided from the wound.

Meticulous hemostasis is achieved with absorbable sutures and limited use of the electrocautery. Any sharp edges on the metatarsal bones are smoothed with a rongeur or a rasp. The wound is irrigated to flush out devitalized tissue and thrombus. The plantar flap is trimmed as needed. The dermis is approximated with simple interrupted absorbable sutures, and the knots are buried. Because the edge of the plantar flap is generally longer than the edge of the dorsal flap, the sutures must be placed slightly farther apart on the plantar flap than on the dorsal flap if perfect alignment is to be obtained. It is imperative to achieve the correct skin alignment with the dermal suture layer. Once this is accomplished, the skin edges are gently and perfectly apposed with interrupted vertical mattress sutures of nonabsorbable monofilament material. Finally, a soft supportive dressing with good padding of the heel is applied; casts and splints are avoided because of the risk of ulceration of the heel or over the malleoli.

COMPLICATIONS

If a tourniquet is not used, intraoperative blood loss can be substantial; the blood pools in the sponges and drapes, often out of the anesthesiologist's field of view. Consequently, good communication between the surgeon and the anesthesiologist is crucial for preventing ischemic complications secondary to hemorrhage.

Postoperative complications include bleeding, infection, and failure to heal, all of which are likely to result in more proximal amputation. They can best be prevented by means of careful patient selection and meticulous surgical technique.

OUTCOME

For proper healing, postoperative edema must be avoided and the plantar flap protected against shear forces. To prevent swelling, the patient is kept on bed rest with the foot elevated for the first 3 to 5 days. This step is particularly important if the transmetatarsal amputation was performed simultaneously with arterial reconstruction, which carries a high risk of reperfusion edema of the foot. After 3 to 5 days, the patient is instructed in techniques for moving in and out of the wheelchair without stepping on the foot. The foot that was operated on should not bear any weight at all for at least 3 weeks; early weight-bearing may disrupt the healing of the plantar flap and necessitate more proximal amputation.

Once healed, patients should be able to walk independently with standard shoes. There is, however, a risk that they may trip over the unsupported toe of the shoe. In addition, the pushoff normally provided by the toes is lost after transmetatarsal amputation, and this change results in a halting, flat-footed gait. These problems can be obviated by using an orthotic shoe with a steel shank (to keep the toe of the shoe from bending and causing tripping) and a rocker bottom (to provide a smooth heel-to-toe motion).

Guillotine Ankle Amputation

OPERATIVE PLANNING

Guillotine amputation across the ankle is indicated when a patient presents with extensive wet gangrene that precludes salvage of a functional foot (e.g., wet gangrene that destroys the heel, the plantar skin of the forefoot, or the dorsal skin of the proximal foot). In such patients, initial guillotine amputation through the ankle is safer than extensive debridement: the operation is shorter, less blood is lost, the risk of bacteremia is reduced, and better control of infection is possible. Guillotine amputation is also indicated in patients with foot infections who have cellulitis extending into the leg. Transection at the ankle, perpendicular to the muscle compartments, tendon sheaths, and lymphatic vessels, allows effective drainage and usually brings about rapid resolution of the cellulitis of the leg, thus permitting salvage of the knee in many cases in which the knee might otherwise be unsalvageable.

OPERATIVE TECHNIQUE

General anesthesia is preferred; regional anesthesia is relatively contraindicated for critically ill patients who are in a septic state. Anesthesia is required for no more than 15 to 20 minutes.

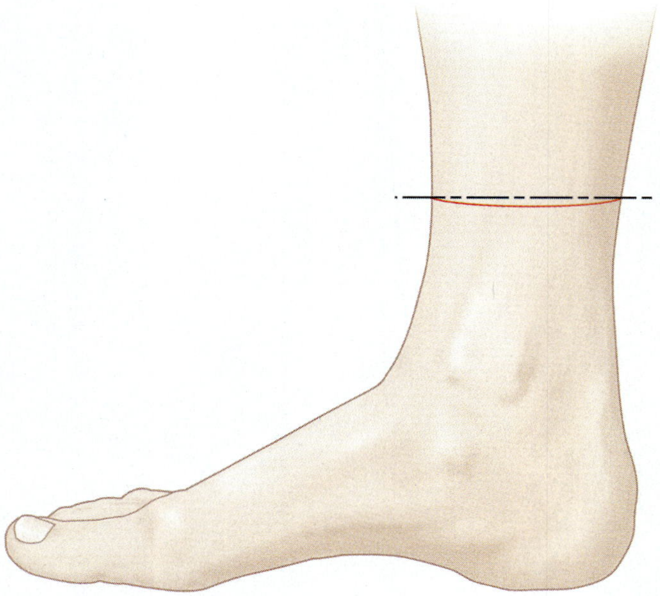

Figure 6 Guillotine ankle amputation. The skin incision is made circumferentially at the narrowest portion of the ankle. The bones are then transected at the same level (dashed line).

A circumferential incision is made at the narrowest part of the ankle (i.e., at the proximal malleoli) regardless of the level of the cellulitis [*see Figure 6*]. This placement takes the line of incision across the tendons, thereby preventing bleeding from transected muscle bellies. The incision is then carried through the skin and soft tissues to the bone. If the arteries are patent, the assistant applies circumferential pressure to the distal calf. The distal tibia and fibula are then divided with a Gigli saw. Hemostasis is achieved with suture ligation and electrocauterization. A moist dressing is applied.

OUTCOME

After the procedure, the patient is kept on bed rest and given systemic antibiotics. Formal below-the-knee amputation can be performed when the cellulitis resolves, usually within 3 to 5 days. Routine dressing changes are unnecessary—first, because they are painful, and second, because the decision to proceed with formal below-the-knee amputation is based on the extent of the cellulitis in the calf, not on the appearance of the transected ankle.

Below-the-Knee Amputation

OPERATIVE PLANNING

Below-the-knee amputation is indicated when the lower extremity is functional but the foot cannot be salvaged by arterial reconstruction or by amputation of one or more of the toes or the forefoot. Healing can be expected if there is a palpable femoral pulse with at least a patent deep femoral artery, provided that the skin is warm and free of lesions at the distal calf. Before formal below-the-knee amputation, infection should be controlled with antibiotic therapy, debridement, and, if indicated, guillotine amputation. It is advisable to obtain consent to possible above-the-knee amputation beforehand in case unexpected muscle necrosis is encountered below the knee.

As with any amputation, the surgeon's preoperative interaction with the patient should be as positive as possible. A constructive perspective to convey is that the amputation, though regrettably necessary, is in fact the first step toward rehabilitation. A well-motivated patient whose cardiopulmonary status is not too greatly compromised can generally be expected to walk again, albeit at an increased energy cost. In this regard, a preoperative discussion with a physiatrist can be very helpful, as can a meeting with an amputee who is doing well with a prosthesis. By inculcating a positive attitude in the patient before the procedure, the surgeon can greatly improve the patient's chances of achieving full rehabilitation as well as decrease the time needed for rehabilitation.

OPERATIVE TECHNIQUE

Epidural, spinal, or general anesthesia is appropriate.

The lines of incision should be marked on the skin. The primary level of amputation is determined by measuring a distance of 10 cm from the tibial tuberosity [*see Figure 7*]. The circumference of the leg at this level is then measured by passing a heavy ligature around the leg and cutting the ligature to a length equal to the circumference. The ligature is folded into thirds and cut once more at one of the folds, so that two segments of unequal length remain. The longer segment of the ligature, which is equal in length to two thirds of the leg's circumference 10 cm below the tibial tuberosity, is used to measure the anterior transverse incision; this incision is centered not on the tibial crest but on the gastrocnemius-soleus muscle complex. The shorter segment, which is one third of the leg's circumference at this level, is used to measure the posterior flap; the line of the posterior incision runs parallel with the gastrocnemius-soleus complex. To prevent dog-ears, the medial and lateral ends of the anterior transverse incision are curved cephalad before meeting the posterior incision, and the distal corners of the posterior incision are curved as well [*see Figure 7*].

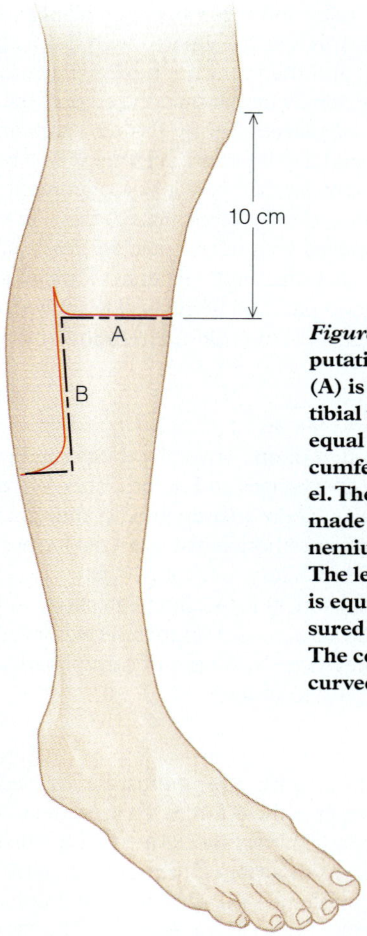

Figure 7 Below-the-knee amputation. The transverse incision (A) is made 10 cm distal to the tibial tuberosity. Its length is equal to two thirds of the circumference of the leg at that level. The posterior incision (B) is made parallel with the gastrocnemius-soleus muscle complex. The length of the posterior flap is equal to one third of the measured circumference of the leg. The corners of the incisions are curved to avoid dog-ears.

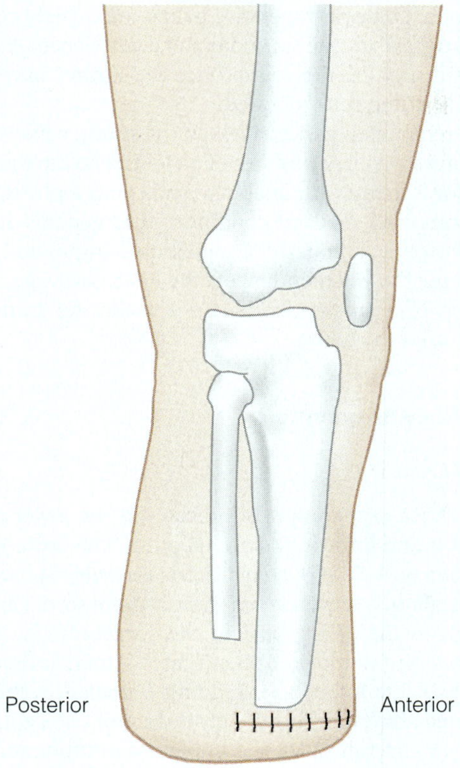

Figure 8 Below-the-knee amputation. In this lateral view of the right leg, the tibia is beveled anteriorly, and the anterior portion is smoothed with a rasp. The fibula is transected at least 1 cm proximal to the level of transection of the tibia.

Blood loss can be reduced by using a sterile pneumatic tourniquet. A gauze roll is passed around the distal thigh. The leg is elevated to drain the venous blood, and the tourniquet is applied over the gauze roll. The tourniquet is inflated to a pressure of 250 mm Hg (350 to 400 mm Hg if the patient has heavily calcified arteries). The assistant elevates the leg, and the incision on the posterior flap is made first, followed by the anterior transverse incision; this sequence helps prevent blood from obscuring the field while the incisions are being made. The incisions are carried fully through the dermis, and the skin edges are allowed to separate and expose the subcutaneous fat. Care is taken to keep the scalpel perpendicular to the skin so as not to bevel the incision, which can lead to necrosis of the epidermal edges [see Figure 2].

The anterior muscles are transected with the scalpel in a direction parallel to the transverse skin incision. The tibia is scored circumferentially, and a periosteal elevator is used to dissect the soft tissues away from the tibia for a distance of approximately 3 to 4 cm. The tibia is then transected just proximal to the transverse skin incision. Dividing the tibia more than 1 cm proximal to the anterior skin incision will cause the thin skin of the anterior leg to be pulled taut over the cut end of the tibia by the weight of the posterior flap, thereby leading to skin ulceration. The tibia is transected perpendicularly, with a cephalad bevel of the anterior 1 cm to keep from creating a sharp point at the tibial crest [see Figure 8]. The tibia can be transected with either a Gigli saw or an oscillating saw; because of the unpleasant sound of the power saw, the Gigli saw is preferred if the patient is under regional anesthesia. Sedation should be augmented in awake patients before division of the tibia. Benzodiazepines provide good sedation and amnesia.

The lateral muscles are divided, and the fibula is scored circumferentially. A periosteal elevator is used to dissect the soft tissues away from the fibula to a point 2 to 3 cm cephalad to the level at which the tibia was transected. The fibula is then transected with a bone cutter at least 1 cm cephalad to the tibial transection level. The distal end of the tibia is lifted with a bone hook, and division of the posterior muscles is completed with an amputation knife. The specimen is then handed off the field.

The anterior tibial, posterior tibial, and peroneal arteries and veins are clamped, and the tourniquet is released. Clamps are placed on all other bleeding vessels. The posterior tibial and sural nerves are placed on gentle traction and clamped proximally. The distal nerves are transected, and the proximal nerves are allowed to retract into the soft tissues so as to prevent painful neuromas at the end of the stump. All clamped structures are then ligated with absorbable ligatures. The nerves are ligated because their nutrient vessels can bleed significantly. The distal anterior tip of the tibia is smoothed with a rasp to decrease the risk of skin ulceration over this osseous prominence. The stump is gently irrigated to remove all thrombus and devitalized tissue and to reveal any bleeding sites that may have been missed. Electrocauterization is rarely necessary.

The deep muscle fascia—not the Achilles tendon—is approximated with simple interrupted absorbable sutures, with care taken to align the posterior flap with the anterior incision. The dermis is approximated as a separate layer with simple interrupted absorbable sutures; if correctly placed, the dermal sutures should take all tension off the skin. The skin edges are then accurately apposed with interrupted vertical mattress sutures composed of monofilament nonabsorbable material. A carefully padded posterior splint or cast is applied to prevent flexion contracture.

COMPLICATIONS

The most common complications after below-the-knee amputation are bleeding, infection, and failure to heal, all of which are likely to result in a more proximal amputation, frequently accompanied by loss of the knee. Prevention of these complications depends on careful patient selection, preoperative control of infection, and meticulous surgical technique.

To walk with a prosthetic leg, the patient must be able to fully extend and lock the knee; thus, flexion contracture at the knee is a major complication. Such contractures are usually attributable either to poor pain control or to noncompliance with knee extension exercises. Good perioperative analgesia is of vital importance because knee flexion is the position of comfort and the patient will be unwilling to extend the knee if doing so proves too painful. To maintain knee extension, the patient should be placed in either a cast or a splint in the early postoperative period. Once postoperative pain has abated, the splint or cast can be removed. At this point, the patient must be taught extension exercises, in which the quadriceps muscles are contracted to maintain the length of the hamstring muscles. If a patient spends all of his or her time in a sitting position with the knee flexed, a flexion contracture will quickly develop. Once this happens, the patient may find it very difficult to regain full knee extension, and without full knee extension, prosthetic limb rehabilitation is impossible.

Phantom sensation is a common complication after below-the-knee amputation but is rarely of any consequence. Phantom pain, on the other hand, can be devastating. Sometimes, phantom pain develops as a consequence of unintentional suggestions made to the patient by medical personnel who fail to distinguish between the two entities. For example, a patient remarks to a medical attendant that he or she can still feel the amputated foot and toes, and the attendant suggests in response that the patient has phantom pain; the patient then focuses on the sensation and exaggerates the severity of

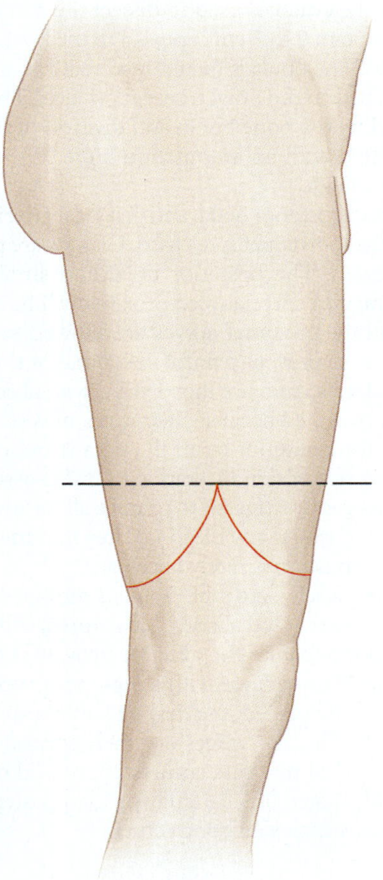

Figure 9 Above-the-knee amputation. Broadly based anterior and posterior flaps are created. The femur is transected along the dashed line, at the apices of the skin flaps. The skin flaps and the level of transection of the femur can be placed more proximally if clinically indicated.

the foot and toe discomfort, setting up a cycle of ever-worsening pain. This scenario is even more likely if the patient has had prolonged ischemic rest pain before the amputation. Phantom pain can be prevented by (1) encouraging early amputation in a patient with a hopelessly ischemic foot (while taking into account the patient's need to come to grips with the prospect of amputation), (2) providing good pain control in the early postoperative period, and (3) assuring the patient that phantom sensation after a below-the-knee amputation is common and that any discomfort in the foot immediately after the operation period will vanish once he or she begins walking again with a prosthetic leg.

Ulceration of the skin over the transected anterior portion of the tibia is another serious complication that may preclude successful prosthetic limb fitting. This complication is also best managed through prevention, which depends on meticulous surgical technique. As noted (see above), the anterior tibial crest must be carefully beveled and smoothed at the level of transection, and the tibia must not be transected more than 1 cm proximal to the anterior skin incision.

OUTCOME

Shortly after the amputation, the patient should be encouraged to start working on strengthening the upper body; upper-body strength is critical for making transfers and for using parallel bars, crutches, or a walker. In patients who have preoperative intractable ischemic rest pain, postoperative administration of epidural analgesia can break the cycle of pain. Once postoperative pain is adequately controlled, patients are taught to transfer in and out of a wheelchair. A compression garment is used on the stump once the sutures have been removed and the stump is fully healed.

Prosthetic rehabilitation begins when the stump achieves a conical shape. Unfortunately, a number of patients who have undergone amputation for ischemia are unable to walk with a prosthetic limb because of comorbid medical conditions and general debility. In many cases, however, even if full ambulation is impossible, patients can maintain relative independence if the knee is salvaged by using a combination of a prosthetic leg and a walker for transfers and movement around the house.

Above-the-Knee Amputation

OPERATIVE PLANNING

Above-the-knee amputation is indicated if the lower extremity is unsalvageable and there is no femoral pulse. The presence of pulsatile flow into a well-developed ipsilateral internal iliac artery usually ensures healing, but even when there is more severe arterial occlusive disease in the pelvis, healing can sometimes be achieved. Above-the-knee amputation is also indicated if there is tissue necrosis or uncontrollable infection extending cephalad to the midleg. Above-the-knee amputation is the procedure of choice in the case of gangrene or ulceration of a completely nonfunctional lower extremity.

OPERATIVE TECHNIQUE

Epidural, spinal, or general anesthesia may be used.

For the best functional results, it is desirable to keep the femur as long as possible. A longer stump improves the prognosis for prosthetic limb rehabilitation and provides better balance for sitting and transfers. Healing potential, however, is lower with a longer stump; therefore, if the pelvic circulation is severely compromised, a shorter stump should be fashioned.

Anterior and posterior flaps of equal length are marked on the skin. The flaps should be wide and long [see Figure 9], and their apices should be centered on the line dividing the anterior and posterior muscle compartments. The posterior incision is made first to minimize the presence of blood in the operative field. The anterior incision is made second and carried through the anterior muscles in a plane parallel to the skin incision. The skin incisions are carried through the dermis, and the skin edges are allowed to separate and expose the subcutaneous fat; as in other amputations, they should be perpendicular to the skin surface so as not to undermine the skin.

If the superficial femoral artery is patent, the artery and vein are isolated and clamped after the sartorius muscle is divided but before the remainder of the anterior muscles are divided. The femur is scored circumferentially. The soft tissues are dissected away from the femur to the level of the apices of the flaps, and the femur is divided with an oscillating saw at this level. If the end of the resected femur extends beyond the apices of the flaps, the wound cannot be closed without tension. The posterior flap is completed with an amputation knife, and the specimen is handed off the field.

All bleeding points are clamped and tied with absorbable sutures. The sciatic nerve is placed on gentle traction, clamped, divided, and ligated, and the transected nerve is allowed to retract into the muscles. The deep fascia is approximated with interrupted absorbable sutures, with adjustments made for any discrepancy in length between the two flaps. The dermis is approximated with interrupted absorbable sutures; the dermal sutures should take all tension off

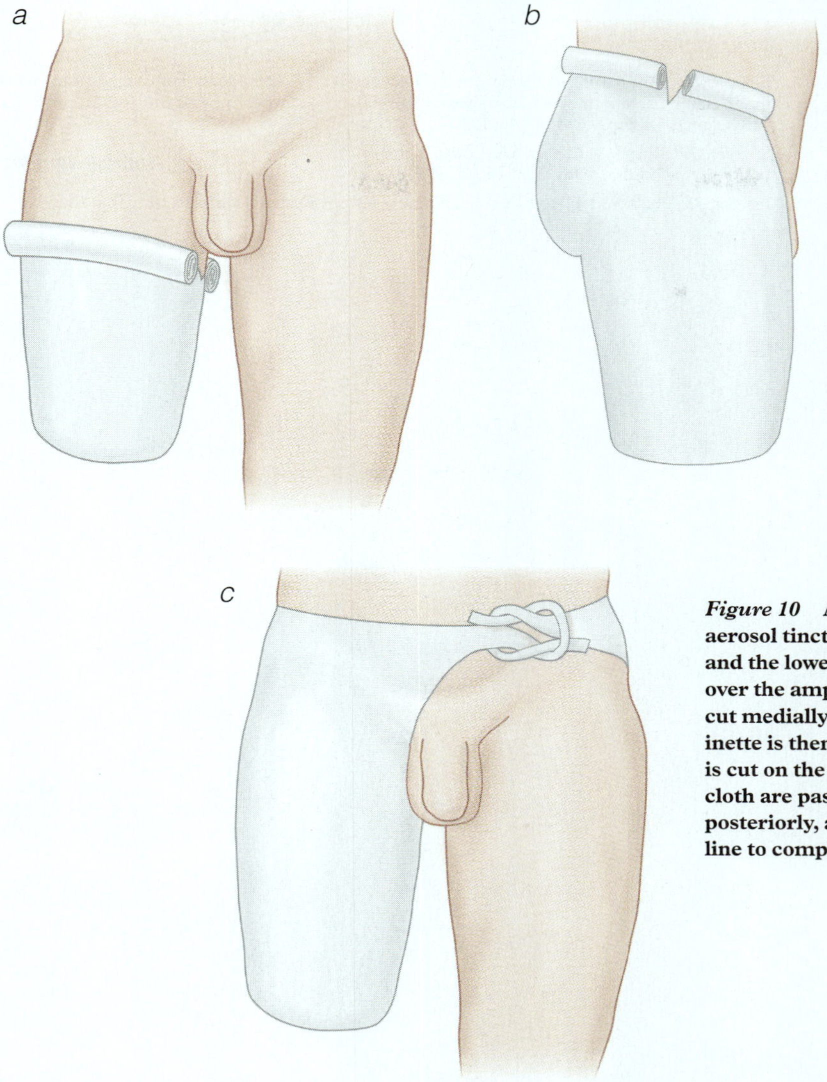

Figure 10 Above-the-knee amputation. (*a*) After an aerosol tincture of benzoin is applied to the thigh, the hip, and the lower abdomen, a 4 in. wide stockinette is rolled over the amputation stump. The cuff of the stockinette is cut medially at the groin. (*b*) The remainder of the stockinette is then rolled laterally up over the hip, and the cuff is cut on the lateral midline. (*c*) The two resulting strips of cloth are passed around the waist, one anteriorly and one posteriorly, and these strips are tied on the anterior midline to complete the dressing.

the skin. The skin edges are then carefully apposed with interrupted vertical mattress sutures.

A nonadherent dressing is placed on the suture line and covered with dry, fluffed gauze bandages. An aerosol tincture of benzoin is sprayed on the thigh, the hip, and the lower abdomen. When the benzoin is dry, a cloth stockinette with a diameter of 4 in. is stretched over the stump [*see Figure 10*]. The cuff of the stockinette is cut medially at the groin, and the stockinette is rolled laterally above the hip, where the cuff is then cut on the midaxillary line. This process yields two strips of cloth, one anterior and one posterior, which are passed around the patient's waist and tied on the anterior midline.

If the patient is a candidate for prosthetic limb rehabilitation, a traction rope is passed through a hole cut in the distal end of the stockinette and tied. The traction rope is hung over the end of the bed and tied to a 5 lb weight; this step helps prevent flexion contracture at the hip.

The stockinette need not be removed for the wound to be inspected. A window is cut in the distal end of the stockinette, and the gauze is removed. Once the incision has been inspected, fresh gauze is applied, and the window in the stockinette is closed with safety pins.

COMPLICATIONS

Postoperative complications include bleeding, infection, and failure to heal, all of which are likely to result in the need for surgical revision of the amputation stump. Control of preoperative infection and meticulous surgical technique and hemostasis are necessary to prevent these complications.

Flexion contracture of the hip is a major complication of above-the-knee amputation. Such contractures preclude successful prosthetic limb rehabilitation. In dealing with this complication, prevention is far more effective than treatment: once a flexion contracture at the hip becomes fixed, it is very difficult to reverse. If a patient is a candidate for prosthetic limb rehabilitation, the traction weight mentioned earlier (see above) can be very helpful. As soon as postoperative pain is controlled, the patient should be taught to spend three periods daily in a prone position to help extend the hip. He or she should then be taught exercises for maintaining range of motion in the hip before prosthetic limb rehabilitation is initiated. Flexion contracture of the hip is less of a problem in nonambulatory patients; however, it can still lead to wound breakdown and chronic skin ulceration.

OUTCOME

Once postoperative pain has abated, patients are mobilized to wheelchair transfers. The prognosis for successful prosthetic limb ambulation in patients undergoing above-the-knee amputation for ischemia is very poor.

References

1. Reichle FA, Rankin KP, Tyson RR, et al: Long-term results of 474 arterial reconstructions for severely ischemic limbs: a fourteen year follow-up. Surgery 85:93, 1979
2. Maini BS, Mannick JA: Effect of arterial reconstruction on limb salvage. Arch Surg 113:1297, 1978
3. Ellitsgaard N, Andersson AP, Fabrin J, et al: Outcome in 282 lower extremity amputations: knee salvage and survival. Acta Orthop Scand 61:140, 1990
4. Stewart CPU, Jain AS, Ogston SA: Lower limb amputee survival. Prosthet Orthot Int 16:11, 1992
5. Inderbitzi R, Buttiker M, Pfluger D, et al: The fate of bilateral lower limb amputees in end-stage vascular disease. Eur Vasc Surg 6:321, 1992

Acknowledgment

Figures 1 through 10   Tom Moore.

66 ORGAN PROCUREMENT

Charles M. Miller, M.D., Felix T. Rapaport, M.D., and Thomas E. Starzl, M.D., Ph.D.

Approach to the Potential Organ Donor

Preliminary Steps

When a patient presents with severe neurologic insult, initial efforts should be directed at saving the injured patient by minimizing cerebral swelling and possible brain herniation [see 23 Injuries to the Central Nervous System]. Often, this is best accomplished by strict fluid restriction and the administration of diuretics and mannitol. However, one of the key advances in clinical organ transplantation has been improved identification and early referral of potential organ donors. Any patient who has suffered severe brain damage should be considered for organ donation. Causes of such damage include external trauma, motor vehicle accidents, falls, assaults, spontaneous intracerebral hemorrhages, drownings, hangings, primary brain tumors, drug overdoses, and sudden infant death syndrome.

A neurologist, a neurosurgeon, or both should be consulted early in the evaluation of a patient with a severe neurologic insult. Such consultation will be important in an eventual diagnosis of brain death, which can be made on clinical criteria alone[1] but is often confirmed by means of electroencephalography,[2] occasionally by means of a cerebral blood flow scan,[3] and sometimes by means of both. Clinical criteria of brain death include deep coma, lack of spontaneous movement, a positive apnea test, and no response to painful stimuli. In addition, cranial nerve reflexes, such as the oculocephalic reflex (tested with the doll's-eyes maneuver) and the oculovestibular reflex (tested with the caloric test), should be absent. Brain-dead patients have fixed, dilated pupils and do not have protective corneal reflexes. Spinal reflexes may still be present because they do not involve the higher centers of the brain or the brain stem.[4,5] If the patient has stable cardiovascular function, the clinical criteria of brain death usually are documented twice within an interval of six to 12 hours before a final declaration of death is made [see 9 Coma, Seizures, Cognitive Impairment, and Brain Death].

As soon as the possibility of donation is established, the local organ procurement agency should be contacted. (The telephone numbers of these agencies are available in most intensive care units.) The procurement coordinator then evaluates the patient's potential for organ donation, assists in the administrative details necessary for declaration of death, and acts as intermediary between the hospital and the donor's family.

When brain death is confirmed, the attending physician or neurologist should make a pronouncement in the patient's chart and complete the death certificate. The physician, procurement coordinator, or both may then formally request consent to donation from the family, making sure that the family members have complete and separate understandings of each of the two distinct issues involved—namely, the diagnosis of brain death and the process of organ procurement.

Donor Evaluation and Management

With the declaration of brain death, efforts must be redirected toward protecting the organs to be transplanted rather than the now dead brain. Usually, primary therapy entails aggressive rehydration. In addition, the procurement coordinator must clearly establish the adequacy of each organ to be used, according to well-recognized sets of standard criteria (see below). A detailed medical history must be obtained that includes the cause of the brain damage as well as the donor's age, height, weight, and blood type. Assessment of acute physiologic status can be made by measuring blood pressure, central venous pressure (CVP), urine output, and arterial blood gases. Serologic analysis must be done for syphilis (Venereal Disease Research Laboratory [VDRL]), hepatitis B surface antigen (HB_sAg), hepatitis B core antibody (HB_cAb), hepatitis C virus (HCV), and cytomegalovirus,[6] as well as for human immunodeficiency virus (HIV)[7] and human T cell lymphotropic virus type I (HTLV-I); otherwise, recipients may be infected with these organisms.

A kidney donor can be between six months and 75 years of age. Levels of serum creatinine and blood urea nitrogen (BUN) should be normal, although elevations may be caused by dehydration or other adverse but reversible acute states. If dehydration is responsible, BUN and creatinine levels should fall after adequate fluid replacement.

Kidneys can be preserved after nephrectomy for up to 72 hours. Thus, there may be time for tissue typing and matching before kidneys are sent to recipients in distant cities. However, the chances that a kidney will function immediately in the recipient diminish greatly with storage for more than 24 hours.

The pancreas may be safely preserved for as long as 20 hours.

With newer preservation solutions, the liver may now be safely preserved for up to 20 hours. Time constraints are more rigid for the thoracic organs, however, and they should be transplanted within six hours after removal from the donor.

There is no consensus on the upper age limit for donors of extrarenal organs. Although an arbitrary limit of 40 to 45 years

Approach to the Potential Organ Donor

Patient has severe neurologic insult

Perform complete neurologic exam. Treat for cerebral edema, if present.

Patient has no signs of cerebral or brain stem function

Consult neurologist or neurosurgeon. Contact local procurement agency.

Neurologist or neurosurgeon confirms and makes formal pronouncement of brain death

Death certificate should be completed.
Request for donation is made by physician, local procurement coordinator, or both.

Consent obtained; patient becomes potential organ donor

Redirect therapy to donor organs. If donor is unstable, resuscitate with appropriate rehydration. Evaluate medical history and physiologic status. Screen for HB_sAg, HB_cAb, HCV, VDRL, HIV, HTLV-I, and CMV.

Evaluate each potential organ

Kidney donors

Kidneys can be preserved after nephrectomy for up to 72 hr. Criteria for donors are flexible:
- Age > 6 mo but < 75 yr.
- Normal or correctable levels of BUN and serum creatinine.

Pancreas donors

Pancreas can be preserved up to 20 hr. Donors can be as young as 10 yr or as old as 45 yr.

Liver donors

Livers can be preserved for up to 18 hr. Donors may be as old as 85 yr. Near-normal or normalizing levels of AST, ALT, and bilirubin should be documented.

Heart and heart-lung donors

Thoracic organs can be preserved for 4 to 6 hr. Donors may be as old as 60 yr. Criteria include the following: no history of cardiac disease; near-normal chest x-ray; no significant abnormality of ECG, echocardiography, or isoenzyme levels; negative Gram's stain and cultures of sputum.

Consult regional and national lists for renal and extrarenal organ placement

Contact the Organ Center of the United Network for Organ Sharing: 1-800-292-9537. Organize and coordinate donor operation.

Move donor to operating room

Include anesthetic team in management of donor. Carry out multiorgan harvesting.

Successful procurement

Store kidneys to await crossmatch. Transport extrarenal organs to transplant centers for back-table preparation and transplantation.

of age had been used to exclude donors, many recent reports have shown that livers have been safely and successfully used from donors as old as 85 years,[8] and hearts can be successfully transplanted from donors as old as 60 years.[9]

If the liver is under consideration for donation, normal or near-normal serum aspartate aminotransferase (AST), serum alanine aminotransferase (ALT), and bilirubin levels must be documented. A history of hepatitis or alcoholism is a warning sign but not necessarily a contraindication to liver transplantation. Very obese donors can be problematic for liver recovery: there is a high likelihood of macrovesicular steatosis that may preclude safe transplantation.

Heart and heart-lung donors must have no history of cardiac disease and should have a normal chest x-ray, electrocardiogram, and physical examination. The arterial oxygen tension (P_aO_2) of heart-lung donors should be 350 mm Hg during ventilation with a fraction of inspired oxygen (F_IO_2) of 1. Sputum cultures and Gram's stains should be negative. In trauma cases, tests of cardiac isoenzymes should also yield negative results.

ABO blood group and organ size are important factors in placing extrarenal organs. Ideally, a liver donor should be slightly smaller than the proposed recipient, but large variations on this generalization may occur, according to the size of the recipient liver that is to be removed. Size is a special concern in pediatric liver transplantation. Because small baby donor organs are scarce, most pediatric centers reduce the size of adult organs by performing right hepatic lobectomies or right hepatic trisegmentectomies and implanting the left lobe itself or the left lateral segment.[10-12] In addition, to maximize the donor potential, partition of the liver into the right lobe and the left lateral segment with subsequent implantation into two separate recipients is becoming more popular. These practices address both the restrictions of size and the scarcity of both pediatric and adult organ donors.

In heart transplantation, the organ of the donor usually should be slightly larger than that of the recipient because cardiomegaly is a common finding in the recipient. The height, weight, and chest circumference of the heart-lung recipient must closely match those of the donor. The donor team is responsible for accumulating the information on which wise recipient selection can be based.

During the evaluation, the donor must be maintained in a stable physiologic state.[13] Basic monitoring should include an arterial line for blood pressure monitoring and blood gas surveillance, a central venous pressure monitor, and an indwelling urinary catheter to measure urine output. Because the basic physiologic situation rarely, if ever, improves in brain-dead patients, the interval between pronouncement of death and procurement surgery should be kept as short as possible. If a donor is unstable, aggressive therapy must be directed at maintaining adequate circulation, ventilation, and diuresis. If the donor is dehydrated from earlier efforts to prevent cerebral edema, rapid repletion is required with crystalloid solutions, colloid solutions, or both.

One relatively simple guide to fluid therapy is to maintain the central venous pressure between 6 and 8 mm Hg if a normal systemic blood pressure can be achieved. However, brain death is sometimes associated with severe neurogenic shock and peripheral vasodilatation. In such cases, the peripheral vascular resistance will not support a normal systemic blood pressure, no matter how well the heart is loaded. In these patients, vasopressors, such as dopamine, should be added to restore normal blood pressure. Norepinephrine bitartrate (Levophed) should be used judiciously and metaraminol bitartrate (Aramine) should be avoided because they produce severe visceral and renal vasoconstriction and may injure the organs to be transplanted.

Respiratory care of the potential donor is the same as that of any ventilator-dependent patient in an intensive care setting. Chest x-rays should be obtained at least once a day. Frequent endotracheal suctioning must be done, good pulmonary toilet must be maintained at all times, and arterial blood gases must be monitored frequently. Oxygen saturation should be maintained at no less than 95 percent by adjusting the F_IO_2 settings on the ventilator [see 92 Use of the Mechanical Ventilator]. Levels of positive end-expiratory pressure (PEEP) greater than 5 cm H_2O are not recommended, because the higher levels increase intrathoracic and right atrial pressures, which in turn may cause hepatic parenchymal congestion and preclude the use of the liver.

A stable brain-dead donor should produce urine at a rate of at least 1 ml/kg/hr. The most common cause of oliguria is hypovolemia. If the CVP is low, further fluid resuscitation is in order. In some instances, however, oliguria may be the result of acute heart failure that is secondary to excessive fluid resuscitation, and osmotic and loop diuretics, such as mannitol and furosemide, will be needed.

When trauma to the brain is severe, pituitary function often fails. The resulting absence of antidiuretic hormone causes diabetes insipidus, and a large volume diuresis ensues, which can lead to severe volume depletion and donor instability. Most cases of diabetes insipidus can be handled simply by replacing the urine output intravenously with half-normal saline. Serum electrolytes must be monitored frequently during such treatment because hypernatremia can easily be produced. If fluid replacement cannot keep up with the diuresis, intravenous vasopressin may be given, but only with great caution, because the resulting vasoconstriction can cause severe end-organ ischemia.

Coordination of Donor and Recipient Activities

After the donor has been identified, studied, and stabilized, the procurement team contacts regional transplant programs about their needs for renal and extrarenal organs and inquires about needs in other parts of the country. A national computer registry of potential recipients of renal and extrarenal organs is maintained by the Organ Center at the United Network for Organ Sharing (UNOS). (The 24-hour UNOS number is 1-800-292-9537.)

Potential recipients of extrarenal organs are categorized according to ABO blood group, weight, acceptable weight range of the donor, distance the recipient team is willing to travel for procurement, length of time the patient has been on the transplant list, and medical urgency status. Sharing of all organs is based on the principle that organs should be allocated first within the local area, then within a specific geographic region, and finally nationally if no suitable recipients can be found locally or within the region. An exception to this rule exists for renal graft allocation. For kidneys, when there is a six-antigen match (i.e., a perfect histocompatibility match between a donor and a recipient on all six HLA-A, HLA-B, and HLA-DR antigens) or when there is at least phenotypic identity between a donor and a prospective recipient, the kidney must be offered to the matched recipient regardless of geographic location.

Within each of these geographic distributions, whether it is local, regional, or national, organs are shared according to computerized point systems, which are based on a variety of parameters that are slightly different for each organ concerned. A potential kidney recipient may accumulate points for time on the waiting list, the degree of histocompatibility match between donor and recipient, and the degree of previous antibody sensitization. There is no allocation of points for medical urgency in kidney recipients. The variables in the point system for liver recipients include blood type compatibility, time on the waiting list, and medical urgency on a scale of 1 to 4, with 4 being the least urgent and 1 being the most urgent. Finally, distribution of thoracic organs is based on principles similar to those governing distribution of livers. However, there are only two categories of medical urgency in heart and heart-lung recipients. A status 1 recipient is a critically ill patient in the intensive care unit receiving either pressor or mechanical heart support. Status 2 includes all other patients who are waiting either at home or in the hospital but outside of an ICU.

Once recipients for extrarenal organs have been identified, the local procurement team must coordinate the arrival of the participating recovery teams, schedule the operating room for donor surgery, and maintain the stability of the donor. With the recent proliferation of experienced extrarenal transplant centers throughout the United States, it is becoming more common for donor operations for extrarenal organs, especially the liver, to be performed by expert local procurement teams.[14] In the past, the recipient institution was required to send a donor team to retrieve the liver. This change has improved the coordination of the retrieval process, reduced the transportation costs associated with long-distance procurements, and helped ease the burden on the recipient team.

With cooperation from all participants, including promptness, the different procurement teams will arrive as the donor is transported to the operating room. Before actual operation, the renal and extrarenal procurement teams should coordinate their techniques and preferences to avoid unseemly conflicts during a multiple-organ harvest.

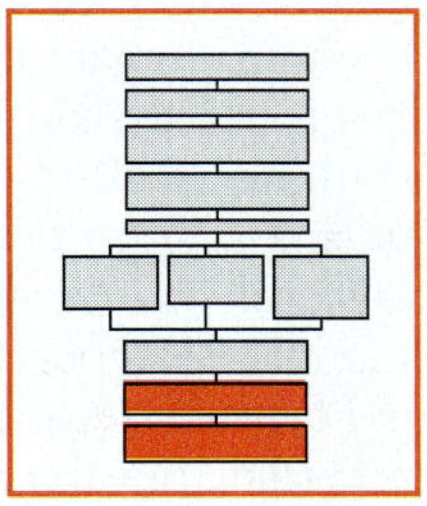

The Donor Operation

When the donor is brought to the operating room, the anesthetic team begins to participate in donor management. If spinal reflexes persist in the donor, a muscle relaxant such as pancuronium bromide should be administered.

The operation for multiple-organ procurement must proceed in such a way that the kidneys, the pancreas, the liver, the heart, the heart and the lung, or various combinations of these or other organs can be removed without any of them being jeopardized. The basic principle of the procedure is to carry out preliminary dissection of the great vessels of the abdomen and chest. The aorta is isolated at preplanned levels to allow crossclamping, so that the organs to be removed can be core-cooled in situ with cold intra-aortic and intraportal infusions (see below).[15] Thus, warm ischemia will be avoided in the donor organs. This technique has been adopted as an international standard. The most refined version of this procedure,[16] commonly known as the rapid-flush technique, can be completed in less than an hour, from beginning to end.

To start, a complete midline incision is made from the suprasternal notch to the pubis [see Figure 1]. If a heart team is on hand for cardiectomy, the pericardium is opened and the heart is inspected. Very minimal dissection is required to prepare the heart for removal. The superior vena cava and the aorta are encircled with tapes to allow eventual occlusion of the inflow and outflow tracts. The heart team can complete its preliminary work in 10 to 15 minutes.

The abdominal team, which consists of hepatic and renal surgeons, then proceeds. The left triangular ligament of the liver is incised, the esophagus is held to the left with a finger, and a longitudinal incision is made in the diaphragmatic crura, between the retrohepatic inferior vena cava and the esophagus [see Figure 2]. The aorta is encircled with a tape at this level.

At this point, the abdominal team's decision on how to proceed is based on the physiologic status of the donor. If the donor

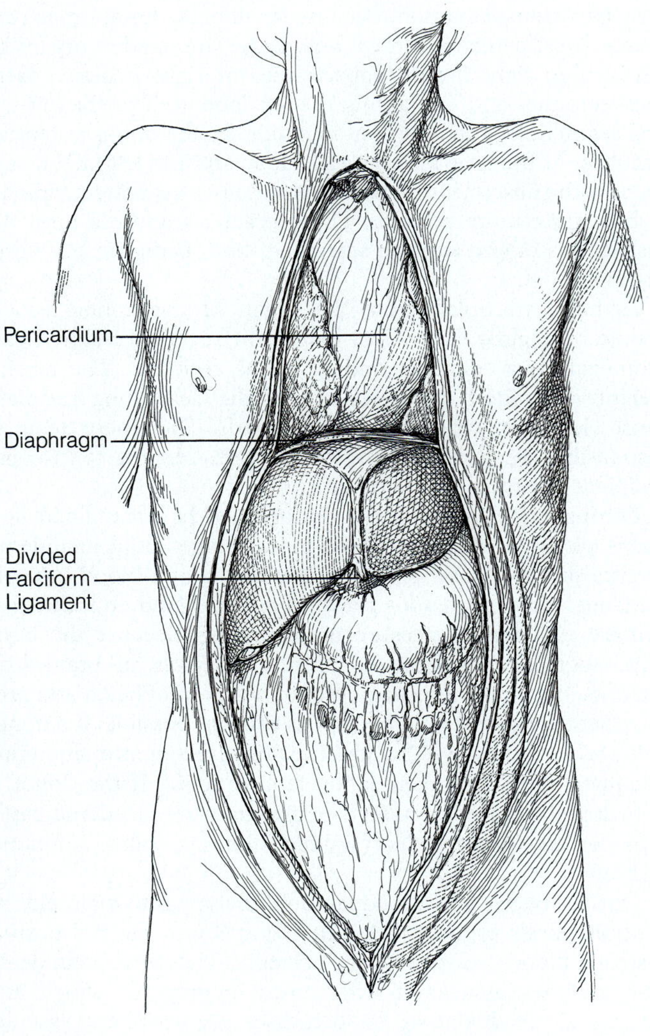

Figure 1 The incision used for multiple-organ procurement is made from the suprasternal notch to the pubis, as illustrated here.

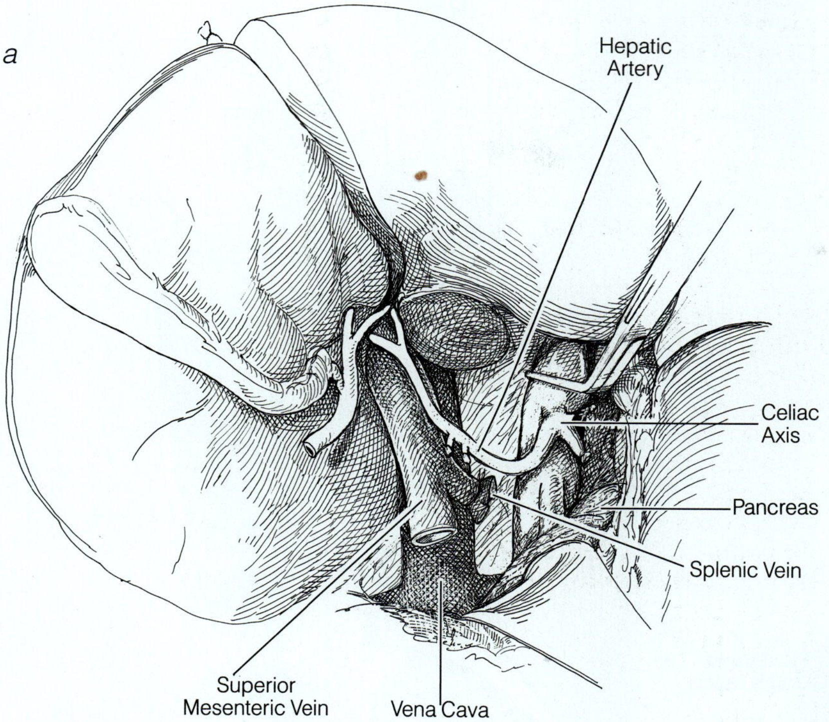

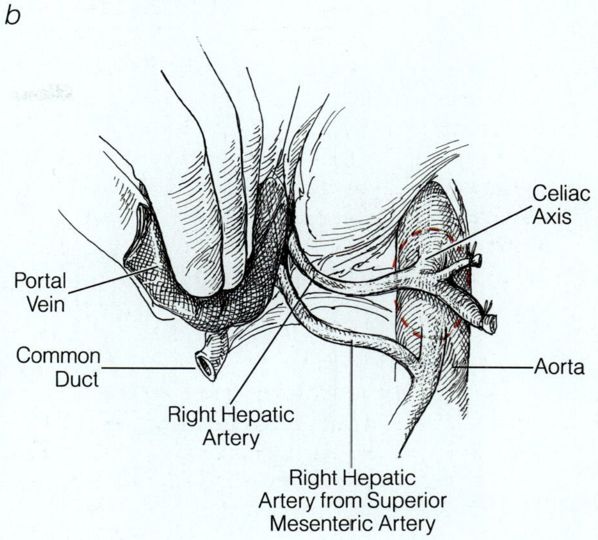

Figure 6 Hilar transection completed (*a*). With the superior mesenteric vein and the splenic vein cut, the portal vein may be folded superiorly with a finger so that an anomalous right hepatic artery may be found posterior to the portal vein (*b*).

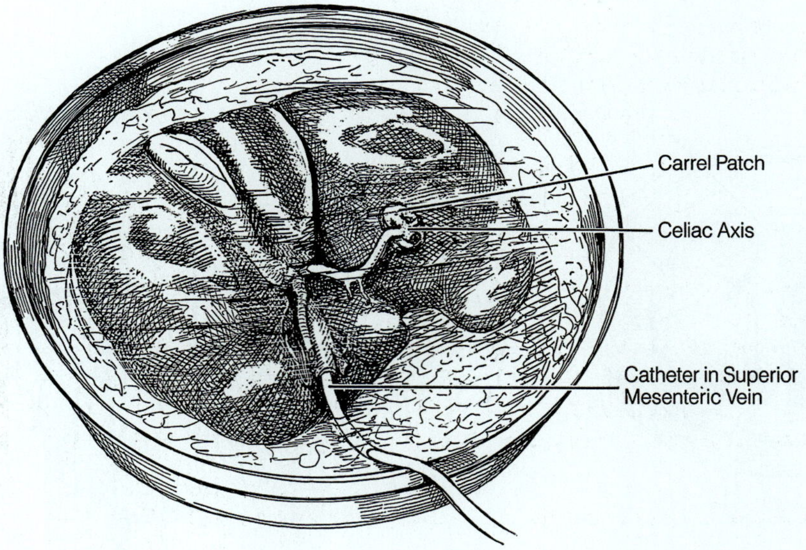

Figure 7 The aortic Carrel patch and the portal cannula used to infuse chilled preservation solution are shown in this illustration of an excised liver in an ice basin.

1.5 L of University of Wisconsin (UW) preservation solution.[17] The organ is subsequently packed in the effluent that remains in the sack and kept refrigerated in a standard ice chest.

The organ is transported to the recipient hospital, where it is cleaned and prepared for transplantation in a formal back-table procedure that takes approximately 30 minutes.

Removal of the cold and bloodless liver requires 15 to 30 minutes, but during most of this time, effective cold perfusion of the kidneys in situ continues through the aortic cannula. With the liver out of the field, the two kidneys can be removed en bloc; this process takes an additional five to 10 minutes. Removal is best accomplished from below upward [*see Figure 8*].

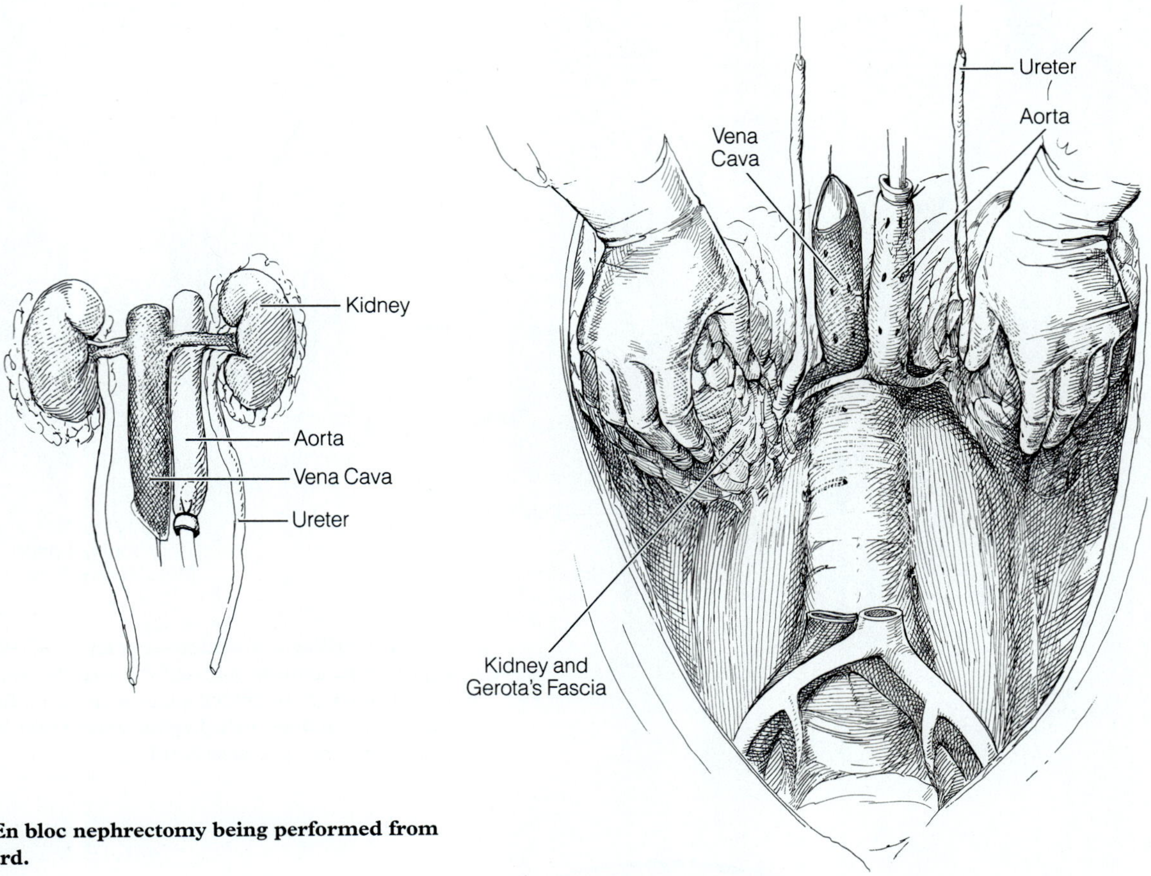

Figure 8 En bloc nephrectomy being performed from below upward.

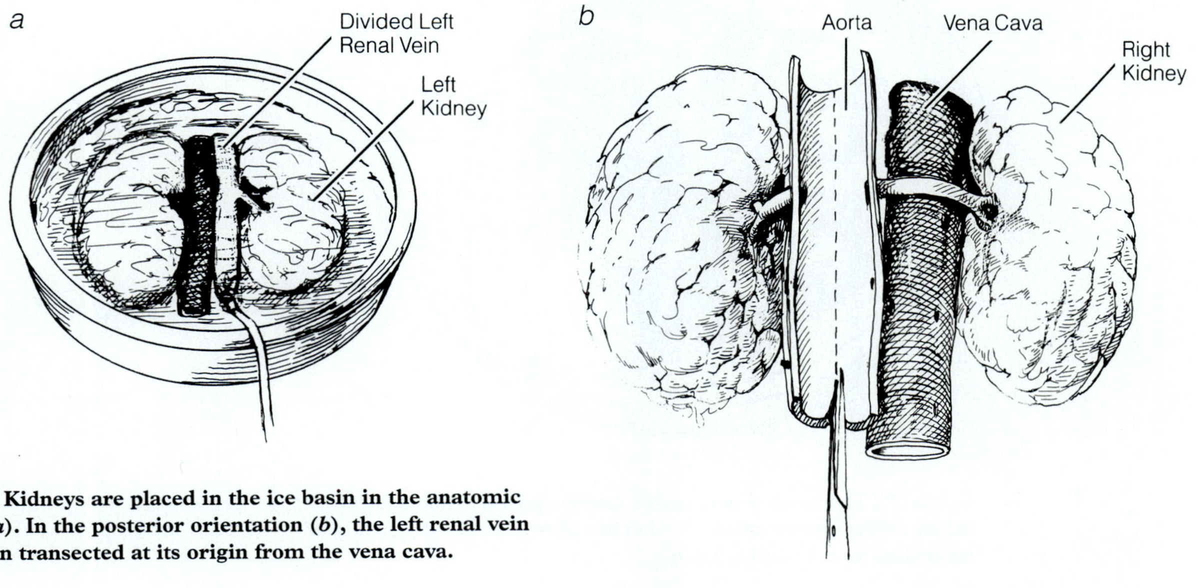

Figure 9 Kidneys are placed in the ice basin in the anatomic position (*a*). In the posterior orientation (*b*), the left renal vein can be seen transected at its origin from the vena cava.

After the kidneys are removed, they are immersed in an ice bath and reperfused with preservation solution either individually or through the aorta. If the kidneys are to be separated, the left renal vein is transected flush at the point where it enters the inferior vena cava [*see Figure 9*]. The kidneys are then turned over so that the posterior wall of the aorta is accessible. Inserting one blade of a scissors into the aortic lumen, the surgeon incises the posterior wall of the aorta at the midline. A perfect guide to the line of aortic incision is the row of lumbar arteries. Then, having an internal view of the renal arterial branches passing laterally, the surgeon incises the anterior wall of the aorta longitudinally from the inside. If continuous perfusion is planned for later preservation of the organs, aortic flaps can be fashioned during separation of the kidneys and used for

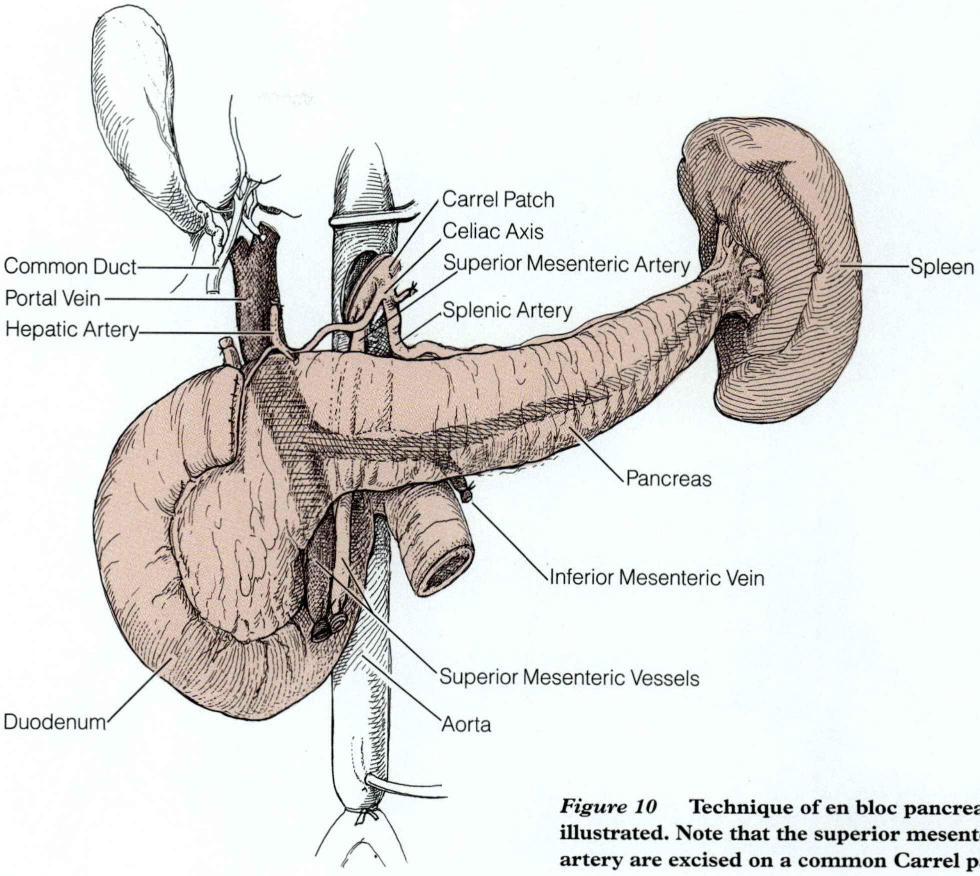

Figure 10 Technique of en bloc pancreaticoduodenectomy is illustrated. Note that the superior mesenteric artery and celiac artery are excised on a common Carrel patch of aorta.

closure so that cannulas need not be placed directly into the renal arteries. Final dissection of the kidneys is performed on a back table at the recipient hospital.

Total or segmental pancreatectomy can be part of the multiple-organ procurement procedure [*see Figure 10*]. The technique differs in details but not in principle from that of the procedures described (see above). The dissection is almost always accomplished before in situ flushing and may require between one and a half and three and a half hours to complete. If the whole pancreas is to be transplanted, a Carrel patch, including the celiac axis and the superior mesenteric artery, can be taken from the abdominal aorta [*see Figure 10*]. This procedure ensures better vascularization of the pancreas graft, and the natural superior-to-inferior pancreaticoduodenal arterial anastomoses are vascularized from both directions.

It was once thought that simultaneous whole organ pancreas and liver recovery could not be done (because both procedures called for retention of the celiac axis and the portal vein), but safe techniques now exist for dividing the vasculature of these organs. The use of free iliac vein and arterial grafts has allowed successful transplantations of liver and pancreas from a single donor.[18] It is now UNOS policy to encourage utilization of both organs from appropriate donors, although many liver teams approach these donors with trepidation because of the lengthy dissection and associated risks of graft nonfunction. For most diabetics, pancreas transplantation is something of a luxury because of the option of insulin administration, whereas for patients who require liver transplantation, no alternative exists. Therefore, if an anomaly in the donor precludes successful procurement of both the liver and the pancreas, the liver team takes priority.

With the improved technique that makes possible the use of the liver and the whole pancreas, the liver retains almost all of the portal vein, and the short portal vein of the pancreatic specimen is lengthened with an iliac vein graft from the donor [*see Figure 11*]. The donor celiac axis, proximal hepatic artery, and superior mesenteric artery stay with the pancreas. The hepatic artery retained with the liver is lengthened with a free iliac artery graft. Obviously, many variations of this technique are possible with the use of free iliac artery and vein grafts.

The arteries and veins of a multiple-organ donor can be put to many other uses. After all the organs have been removed and packaged, segments of the remaining iliac arteries and veins are routinely removed [*see Figure 12*] and placed in a cold tissue culture solution for refrigeration. The thoracic aorta and pulmonary artery may also be harvested under special circumstances. Vascular grafts can be lifesaving in the event of unexpected technical problems in hepatic recipients, approximately 25 percent of whom require portal vein or hepatic arterial homografts. Vascular grafts are also often employed for reconstruction of renal vessels or for other purposes, including potential pancreas vessel reconstruction.

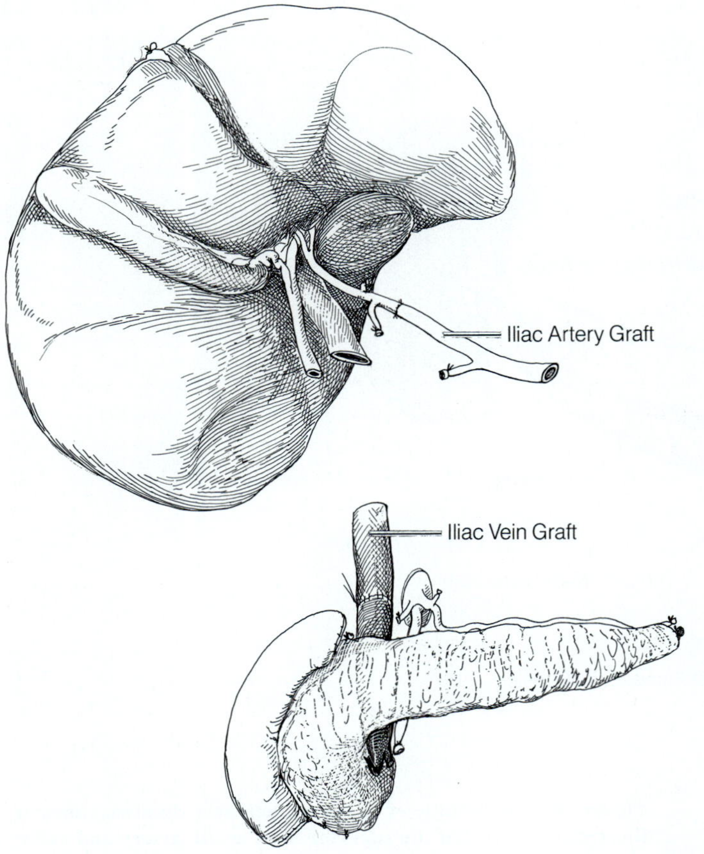

Figure 11 The addition of an iliac artery graft to the hepatic artery and an iliac vein graft to the portal vein of the pancreas graft allows the use of both organs from a single donor.

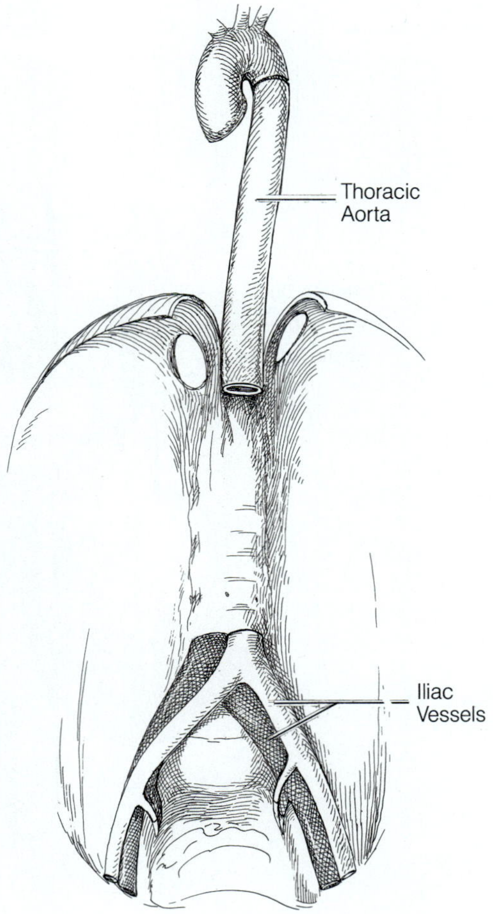

Figure 12 After organs have been removed and packaged, segments of iliac arteries, veins, and thoracic aorta are routinely removed, as illustrated here.

Discussion

Principles and Limitations of Current Methods of Organ Preservation

Despite its importance and despite recent advances, organ preservation remains the least developed component of transplantation technology. Preservation techniques begin with the intraoperative infusion of cold fluids; the paramount objective is to avoid warm ischemia. Cooling of organs by intravascular infusions of chilled lactated Ringer's solution at the time of circulatory arrest was first introduced into the laboratory for experimental liver transplantation more than a quarter of a century ago. The procedure was promptly applied clinically to the preservation of kidneys and other organs. Such cooling lengthens the duration of organ viability and allows subsequent application of more sophisticated preservation measures.

Lactated Ringer's solution is low in potassium and nearly isotonic. In 1969, researchers documented that chilled solutions with an electrolyte composition similar to that in cells, such as Collin's solution, extended the permissible time limit of cold renal ischemia beyond that achievable with isotonic solutions.[19] The same effect was demonstrated in livers.[20] Cardiac surgeons have cooled the heart with various cardioplegic solutions having potassium concentrations of 20 mEq/L or greater.

From 1969 to 1987, these high-potassium preservation solutions were the only means available for inexpensive cold-storage preservation of transplanted organs. In 1987, the University of Wisconsin solution was introduced.[17] This solution immediately extended safe preservation times for the liver and pancreas and provided improved function as well. The allowable cold ischemia time for the liver increased from eight to 18 hours or longer, and pancreas preservation was increased to 20 hours with excellent postoperative function. UW solution is a complex multiconstituent solution, the components of which address a number of theoretical issues in organ preservation. Although the exact function of each constituent in the solution is unknown, it is felt that the parenchymal cells of the liver, pancreas, and kidney are impermeable to the large anion in the solution, lactobionic acid, and that this prevents the cellular swelling that can complicate all forms of hypothermic preservation. UW solution receives its oncotic support from the complex starch hydroxyethyl starch rather than from dextrose or the other complex sugars used in the older solutions. Finally, there are a variety of components, including glutathione, raffinose, and allopurinol, that act as free radical scavengers and help prevent reperfusion injury.[21] UW solution is now internationally accepted as a universal flush and preservation solution, although preference for it over isotonic saline as a flush solution is controversial. Its application to cardiac preservation has been studied extensively in the laboratory, and it has become a popular substitute for potassium-based cardioplegic solutions in cardiac preservation. One of the most profound impacts of UW solution has been felt by liver transplant surgeons, who can temporally separate the complex donor and recipient operations and perform them in an unrushed, meticulous fashion without jeopardizing organ function.

Highly sophisticated and costly techniques for continuous perfusion of these organs exist, but they have been widely used only for kidney grafts. The continuous perfusion technique for kidneys as originally described used an asanguineous and oncotically controlled fluid.[22] The method has proved to be a good one but has not markedly improved the quality of renal preservation in the first 48 hours over that provided by the simpler infusion-and-slush method. In the future, better continuous perfusion techniques may extend preservation time for all organs.

Even with UW solution, it is still essential to appreciate how unpredictable the outcome of a transplantation can be with any of the currently available preservation techniques. The unknown extent to which the donor has suffered organ ischemia caused by the processes of injury and dying contributes to this unpredictability. All experienced transplant surgeons have been dismayed to observe that homografts retrieved from seemingly ideal donors occasionally do not function, whereas organs obtained under seemingly adverse conditions may function perfectly. One study has documented this phenomenon particularly well for liver transplants[23]; no correlation could be found between liver recipient outcome and the use of ideal versus less than ideal donors. What is urgently needed is a simple, discriminating predictive technique for assessing organ viability before the ruthless biologic test of actual transplantation is performed.

Medical, Ethical, and Legal Considerations

THE RETRIEVAL TEAM

Because the stakes are so high in terms of recipient survival, the technical elements of the organ procurement operation must be constantly reassessed. Much attention is now given to the specific training of the donor, or retrieval, surgeon. When kidneys were the only organs transplanted, transplant centers often assigned organ retrieval to local surgeons whose experience was limited to only the occasional case. Frequently, the penalty for this practice was a prolonged period of acute tubular necrosis in the transplanted kidney, with the attendant risks and mortality. The enormously increased sophistication of today's multiple-procurement procedures make this approach undesirable and probably indefensible from the medicolegal standpoint. In addition, it is important to emphasize that surgeons should not delegate to nonphysicians the actual task of excising organs for transplantation from cadaver donors. Today, most transplant centers tend to delegate organ procurement operations to highly trained surgeons with a specific interest and training in transplantation surgery and organ preservation. Only in this way has it been possible for teams from different institutions to retrieve organs from common donors and to work harmoniously and effectively together. This development reflects the maturation of the field of transplantation.

THE ROLES OF GOVERNMENT AND THE PRIVATE SECTOR

Organ harvesting was once an uncommon, hurried, poorly standardized surgical exercise in which kidneys (or, rarely, other organs) were rapidly excised from a donor whose heart had just stopped beating.[1] The establishment of irreversible neurologic injury, or brain death, as actual death[24] has made it possible for surgeons to procure organs from heart-beating cadavers in a well-organized manner. Legislation sanctioning the concept of brain death has been passed in 44 states, and judicial precedent exists in the other six.[25]

Despite these developments, skepticism, fear, and anxiety regarding the concept of brain death persist.[26] Brain death must be clearly and fully explained to the relatives of a potential donor to allay the common fear that lifesaving measures may be prematurely terminated to gain rapid access to organs for transplantation. This is never the case. The physician in charge of the initial care of the donor is responsible for determining and making the pronouncement of brain death, with the collaboration of experts in the neurosciences. He or she in no way participates in the donation and harvesting procedures. Conversely, the transplant surgeons cannot participate in the determination of death.

The Uniform Anatomical Gifts Act (UAGA), passed by Congress in 1973, has been adopted in some form in all 50 states.[27] This act states that organ donation is a voluntary gift made by either the donor or the family. The UAGA does not include the concept of presumed consent, whereby organs may be removed automatically unless the next of kin objects. Presumed consent has been practiced in many European countries with some success, and strong ethical arguments have been advanced in its favor.[28] The concept of presumed consent has not gained a foothold in transplantation in the United States.

Despite passage of brain-death legislation and of the UAGA, there is still an acute shortage of cadaveric renal and extrarenal organs, which has been aggravated by the burgeoning success of transplantation. Several factors contribute to this shortage. Some physicians do not wish to face the failure implicit in the death of their patients, do not want to burden a grieving family further by requesting donation, are aware of certain religious taboos about organ donation, or have an unrealistic fear of legal recriminations.

The Surgeon General of the United States has made several recommendations for solving these problems, including systematic public education and education of physicians, nurses, and paramedical personnel; recruiting support from the religious community; and sharper delineation of the exact conditions to be met for a pronouncement of brain death.[29] Another strategy for increasing organ donation has been to encourage the signing of donor cards and other forms of living wills.[30]

The organ shortage has prompted a new kind of legislative initiative called required request. Required-request laws have been passed in almost half the states. These laws mandate that each hospital systematically approach the families of all patients who die under circumstances that might make solid-organ donation possible. With such laws, physicians and hospital staff are protected from charges of callousness for asking a grieving family for donation, they are relieved of the fear of legal recrimination, and they can work within an organized administrative channel. Unfortunately, these required-request laws have not been consistently honored and therefore have not helped increase the supply of organs. New initiatives aimed at encouraging voluntary reporting of all deaths by the hospital to the local organ procurement organization, so as not to miss any potential donors, have been tried in pilot programs in a few regions, with promising results.

In 1984, Congress enacted legislation authorizing a task force to study issues in organ procurement and distribution and provided for the creation and funding of an Organ Procurement and Transplant Network (OPTN). In 1986, the federal government awarded the OPTN contract to the United Network for Organ Sharing. Under the terms of the contract, UNOS operates a computer-matching system designed to aid in systematic placement of renal and extrarenal organs and to ensure equitable allocation of organs throughout the country. In addition, UNOS is to keep careful data on all harvested organs to analyze and define patterns of organ procurement in the United States so that resources for future development can be better allocated. In the distribution of extrarenal organs, UNOS acts in an advisory capacity to the organ procurement agency managing a specific donor by supplying a prioritized list of acceptable recipients.

In the first version of this chapter, published in early 1989, we speculated about how this system would change, as more surgeons were trained in extrarenal organ procurement, as regional centers proliferated, as involvement of personnel at the new centers increased, and as additional demands for equitable allocation of organs were made on the distribution network. We predicted that as more powerful immunosuppression and preservation techniques were developed and tissue typing and matching became better understood, smaller organ procurement regions in the country would coalesce into larger, more centralized territories to increase the pool of potential local recipients, improve equity, and ultimately improve transplantation outcomes.

Unfortunately, the system has not evolved as far as we hoped it would have by now. The urgency imposed by current organ preservation techniques is made more pressing by continued reliance on complex tissue typing for renal allocation; these factors place a real strain on any kidney distribution and sharing system covering a large region. Although the restrictive limits of preservation and the logistics of allocation are not as burdensome for the extrarenal organs, influential segments of the transplantation community have resisted any movement to larger regional or national sharing, continuing to rely on the standard renal distribution algorithms despite the clear advantages of larger distribution regions (especially with regard to fairness and justice for patients).

For better or for worse, transplantation of all organs has achieved the level of mass clinical application, even though the field of transplantation has yet to gain full recognition as an established science. Consequently, federal and state governments continue to have a strong interest in regulating transplantation medicine. We agree that the government should collaborate with the transplantation community in developing new health policies; however, we believe that overregulation could stifle the progress of transplantation. The emphasis should be on constructive collaboration, not on domination, but this balance has proved difficult to achieve. Political machinations such as the opposition expressed by the transplantation community to realistic proposals for a true national retrieval and sharing system can have extremely negative repercussions for transplantation medicine and can provoke a demand for greater governmental intervention so as to ensure equity and fairness. The result may be efforts on the part of government to regulate the criteria for patient treatment. Political guidelines must not be allowed a role in judging a candidate's suitability for transplantation. Physicians cannot ethically accept any but strict medical criteria in selecting organ recipients.[31,32]

Since the early 1960s, knowledge in the field of transplantation medicine has grown almost exponentially. The tremendous potential of this field continues to depend on broad research aimed at solving a wide variety of problems in the laboratory and at the bedside as well as on resolution of the issues and controversies that transplantation has generated for the public and the medical community.

References

1. A definition of irreversible coma. Report of the Ad Hoc Committee of the Harvard Medical School to examine the definition of brain death. JAMA 205: 337, 1968
2. Silverman D, Saunders MG, Schwab RS, et al: Cerebral death and the electroencephalogram. Report of the Ad Hoc Committee of the American EEG Society on EEG Criteria for Determination of Cerebral Death. JAMA 209:1505, 1968
3. Goodman JM, Heck LL: Confirmation of brain death at bedside by isotope angiography. JAMA 238:966, 1977
4. Ivan LP: Spinal reflexes in cerebral death. Neurology 23:650, 1973
5. Ropper AH: Unusual spontaneous movements in brain-dead patients. Neurology 34:1089, 1984
6. Goldsmith J, Montefusco CM: Nursing care of the potential organ donor. Critical Care Nurse 5:22, 1985
7. Tzakis AG, Cooper MH, Dummer SJ, et al: Transplantation in HIV+ patients. Transplantation 49:354, 1990
8. Emre S, Schwartz ME, Altaca G, et al: Safe use of hepatic allografts from donors older than 70 years. Transplantation 62:62, 1996
9. Teperman L, Podesta L, Mieles L, et al: The successful use of older donors for liver transplantation. JAMA 262:2837, 1989
10. Otte JB, de Ville de Goyet J, Sokal E, et al: Size reduction of the donor liver is a safe way to alleviate the shortage of size-matched organs in pediatric liver transplantation. Ann Surg 211:146, 1990
11. de Hemptinne B, Salizzoni M, Tan KC, et al: The technique of liver size reduction in orthotopic liver transplantation. Transplant Proc 20(suppl 1):508, 1988
12. Broelsch CE, Emond JC, Thistlethwaite JR, et al: Liver transplantation including the concept of reduced size liver transplants in children. Ann Surg 208:410, 1988
13. Montefusco CM, Mollenkopf FP, Kamholz SL, et al: Maintenance protocol for potential organ donors in multiple organ procurement. Hospital Physician 20:9, 1984
14. Miller CM, Teodorescu V, Harrington M, et al: Regional procurement and export of hepatic allografts for transplantation. Mt Sinai J Med 57:93, 1990
15. Starzl TE, Hakala TB, Shaw BW, et al: A flexible procedure for multiple cadaveric organ procurement. Surg Gynecol Obstet 158:223, 1984
16. Starzl TE, Miller C, Broznick B, et al: An improved technique for multiple organ harvesting. Surg Gynecol Obstet 165:343, 1987
17. Kalayoglu M, Sollinger HW, Stratta RJ, et al: Extended preservation of the liver for clinical transplantation. Lancet 1:617, 1988
18. Sollinger HW, Vernon WB, D'Alessandro AM, et al: Combined liver and pancreas procurement with Belzer-UW solution. Surgery 106:685, 1989

19. Collins GM, Bravo-Shugarman M, Terasaki PI: Kidney preservation for transportation. Lancet 2:1219, 1969
20. Benichou J, Halgrimson CG, Weil R III, et al: Canine and human liver preservation for 6–18 hours by cold infusion. Transplantation 24:407, 1977
21. Belzer FO, Southard JH: Principles of solid-organ preservation by cold storage. Transplantation 45:673, 1988
22. Belzer FO, Ashby BS, Dunphy JE: 24-hour and 72-hour preservation of canine kidneys. Lancet 2:536, 1967
23. Makowka L, Gordon RD, Todo S, et al: Analysis of donor criteria for the prediction of outcome in clinical liver transplantation. Trans Proc 19:2378, 1987
24. Guidelines for the Determination of Death: Report of the Medical Consultants on the Diagnosis of Death to the President's Commission for the Study of Ethical Problems in Medicine and Biomedical and Behavioral Research. JAMA 246:2194, 1981
25. Gunby P: Panel ponders organ procurement problem. JAMA 250:455, 1983
26. Lee PP, Kissner P: Organ donation and the uniform anatomical gift act. Surgery 100:867, 1986
27. Sadler AM, Sadler BL, Stason EB, et al: Transplantation—a case for consent. N Engl J Med 280:862, 1969
28. Caplan AL: Sounding board—ethical and policy issues in the procurement of cadaver organs for transplantation. N Engl J Med 311:981, 1984
29. Koop CE: Increasing the supply of solid organs for transplantation. Public Health Rep 98:566, 1983
30. Overcast TD, Evans RW, Bowen LA, et al: Problems in the identification of potential organ donors. JAMA 251:1559, 1984
31. Starzl TE, Hakala T, Tzakis A, et al: A multifactorial system for equitable selection of cadaveric kidney recipients. JAMA 257:3073, 1987
32. Starzl TE, Gordon RD, Tzakis A, et al: Equitable allocation of extrarenal organs: with special reference to the liver. Transplant Proc 20:131, 1988

Acknowledgment

Figures 1 through 12   Carol Donner.

67 PLASTIC SURGICAL RECONSTRUCTION

David A. Hidalgo, M.D., and Joseph J. Disa, M.D.

Approach to Surgical Reconstruction

Acute Reconstruction

EVALUATION AND INITIAL TREATMENT OF THE OPEN WOUND

Problem wounds are characterized by one of the following: large size that precludes direct primary closure, gross infection or uncertain bacteriologic status, or threatened loss of critical structures exposed as a result of insufficient soft tissue coverage. Surgically created wounds, which generally pose less of a problem from a bacteriologic standpoint than traumatic wounds, are best managed by an immediate coverage procedure when direct closure is impossible.

Traumatic wounds are more difficult to evaluate than surgical wounds for several reasons. First, in traumatic wounds, the potential for infection is high because of the environment in which the wound is created, the mechanism of injury, and the time that elapses before operative intervention. Second, the mechanism of injury (e.g., crush, avulsion, or gunshot) may extend the zone of injury beyond what is immediately apparent [see Figure 1]. Serious postoperative infection may develop in these cases if definitive wound coverage is provided in the absence of adequate debridement. Third, the long-term functional prospects for the injured part are a key determinant in selecting the method of acute treatment. However, accurate assessment of the chances for recovery of specific structures within the wound is often difficult immediately after injury.

The initial step in the management of problem wounds is to decide whether the wound is suitable for immediate soft tissue coverage. Wounds that are surgically created during the course of an elective procedure are almost always best treated with primary definitive coverage. Traumatic wounds that present within an hour or two of injury and have a minimal crush component are also best treated with a primary definitive coverage procedure after thorough operative debridement.

Injuries with a significant crush component and exposure of critical structures such as nerves, vessels, tendons, or bone are best treated more aggressively. In these cases, thorough debridement requires considerable surgical experience because the tendency is to debride inadequately. The degree of accuracy to which tissue viability can be assessed varies among different types of tissue. For example, skin can be evaluated by its color, the nature of its capillary refill, the quality of its dermal bleeding, or its bleeding response to pinprick. After intravenous fluorescein injection, skin viability can also be assessed qualitatively, by using a Wood's light, or quantitatively, by using a dermofluorometer. Muscle is the most difficult tissue to evaluate. Color, capillary bleeding, and contractile response to stimulation are not always reliable indicators of muscle viability. In severe injuries, they can be misleading. Inadequate debridement may lead to severe consequences resulting from infection. Therefore, serial debridement at 24-hour intervals is essential to establish accurately the limits of muscle injury. Efforts should be made during debridement to preserve tissues such as major nerves and blood vessels unless they are severely contused. These structures are vital for function and are of small mass compared with other tissues (e.g., skin, fat, and muscle) at risk for necrosis and subsequent infection.

Wound debridement, therefore, should involve careful analysis of the injury from an anatomic point of view; debridement should not consist of indiscriminate excision of blocks of tissue. Between debridement procedures, the wound should be treated with sterile dressings but in an open manner (i.e., without closure by sutures and with wet-to-dry dressings changed three to four times a day). A definitive soft tissue coverage procedure should then be performed as soon after the initial injury as wound conditions permit. When thorough debridement and definitive coverage can be completed within less than a week, the wound will generally heal uneventfully. Inadequate debridement frequently results in the loss of any additional tissue invested to achieve acute soft tissue coverage. The wound becomes grossly infected, and important functional structures within the wound are reexposed.

Infected surgical wounds, neglected wounds, or other complex wounds in which initial wound management fails should be debrided and then treated by open methods. Proper care of these wounds is achieved by a multifaceted approach aimed at converting established gross infection to a much lower level of bacterial contamination, which is then compatible with successful secondary wound closure.

Debridement   Devitalized tissue provides an ideal culture medium for bacteria and isolates them from host defense mechanisms. Surgical debridement must be performed as often as necessary to remove all necrotic tissue.

High-pressure irrigation   A useful adjunct to debridement is high-pressure irrigation, which has been shown experimentally to decrease wound infection rates significantly.[1] The necessary pres-

Acute reconstruction is indicated

Evaluate and treat open wound.
Select coverage procedure to achieve healed wound and avoid infection.
Defer treatment of functional problems for secondary reconstruction.

Wound does not contain exposed bone, cartilage, nerve, or tendon but cannot be closed directly

Apply a skin graft.

Wound is small defect but is in an area where graft contracture is not desirable (e.g., face, hand, or flexion crease)

Apply full-thickness skin graft; donor sites include the ear, upper eyelid, neck, and groin.

Wound has a large surface area or is a small wound in a noncritical area

Apply split-thickness skin graft.

Wound is known to be significantly contaminated

Apply meshed split-thickness skin graft or consider delayed skin graft replacement and open treatment of wound until bacteriologic status is clear.

Secondary reconstruction of chronic defect is indicated

Defect is a small localized scar or a focal scar contracture

Revise with Z-plasty or other local tissue rearrangement procedure.

There is a shortage of skin and subcutaneous tissue only, but skin graft coverage is not desirable

Use tissue expanders (except on hand or foot).

One or more of the following conditions is present:
- Composite defect
- Functional defect of muscle or bone
- Contour deformity
- Unstable soft tissue coverage of vital structure
- Inadequate soft tissue coverage for bone or nerve grafting

Repair with free or local flap.

Approach to Surgical Reconstruction

Bone, cartilage, nerve, or tendon is exposed and cannot be covered by direct wound closure
Perform flap coverage procedure.

Local donor site meets needs and is not involved in the primary process
Use local flap.
- *Small or clean wound:* use local skin flap if possible.
- *Large or contaminated wound:* use regional myocutaneous flap.

Local flap is not possible or would not provide appropriate tissue
Use free flap.
- If wound is clean and thin flap is desired, apply skin or fascial free flap.
- If wound is large or contaminated, apply muscle or myocutaneous free flap.

Muscle flaps require coverage with a meshed split-thickness skin graft.

Head or neck defect
- *Small facial defect with no facial features involved:* use Z-plasty, Limberg flap, or other advancement flap of cheek or forehead.
- *Large defect of neck or lower head:* use regional myocutaneous flap of trapezius, latissimus dorsi, or pectoralis major muscle.

Chest or back defect
In most cases, use regional myocutaneous flap (e.g., pectoralis major, rectus abdominis, latissimus dorsi, or trapezius muscle).

Arm defect
Cover large wounds above the elbow with latissimus dorsi muscle transposed as a pedicled flap.

Hand defect
Free flaps are preferred, but pedicled distant skin flaps from the chest or abdomen are also acceptable. Defects of the digits can be covered with cross-finger flaps or, for tip injuries, with thenar flaps.

Abdominal defect
Use regional flap (e.g., tensor fasciae latae, rectus femoris, or rectus abdominis muscle).

Gluteal or perineal defect
Use regional myocutaneous flap (e.g., gluteus maximus, gracilis, tensor fasciae latae, or biceps femoris).

Thigh, knee, or leg defect
- *Thigh defect:* use regional muscle flap (e.g., tensor fasciae latae, rectus femoris, vastus lateralis, or vastus medialis muscle).
- *Defect of knee or proximal leg:* use gastrocnemius muscle flap.
- *Proximal or midleg defect:* use soleus muscle flap.

Foot defect
- *Plantar:* close defect of weight-bearing heel or midsole with medially based skin rotation flap raised superficial to plantar fascia or with other myocutaneous or fasciocutaneous plantar flap. Cover limited defect of distal plantar surface with toe flap.
- *Posterior heel, Achilles tendon, malleoli:* use either extensor digitorum brevis muscle as pedicled flap or lateral calcaneal artery flap.

Head or neck defect
- *Large defect of scalp or upper face:* cover with latissimus dorsi, scapular, or rectus abdominis free flap.
- *Floor of the mouth:* replace with forearm free flap.
- *Mandible:* reconstruct with various composite free flaps of bone and skin.
- *Oropharynx or cervical esophagus:* use jejunum free flap or forearm flap.

Forearm defect
Cover large forearm wound with free flap of rectus abdominis, scapular, or latissimus dorsi muscle.

Hand defect
- *Exposed tendons on the dorsum:* cover with temporalis fascia free flap.
- *Defect of the web space:* correct with lateral arm free flap.

Knee or leg defect
- *Major wound of the popliteal fossa:* use free flap if the blood supply to the gastrocnemius muscle is compromised.
- *Defect of the lower third of the leg:* use latissimus dorsi, rectus abdominis, scapular, or gracilis free flap.

Foot defect
- *Plantar:* repair very large defect with muscle free flap covered with a skin graft.
- *Dorsum:* use fascial free flap and overlying skin graft, or use thin skin free flap.

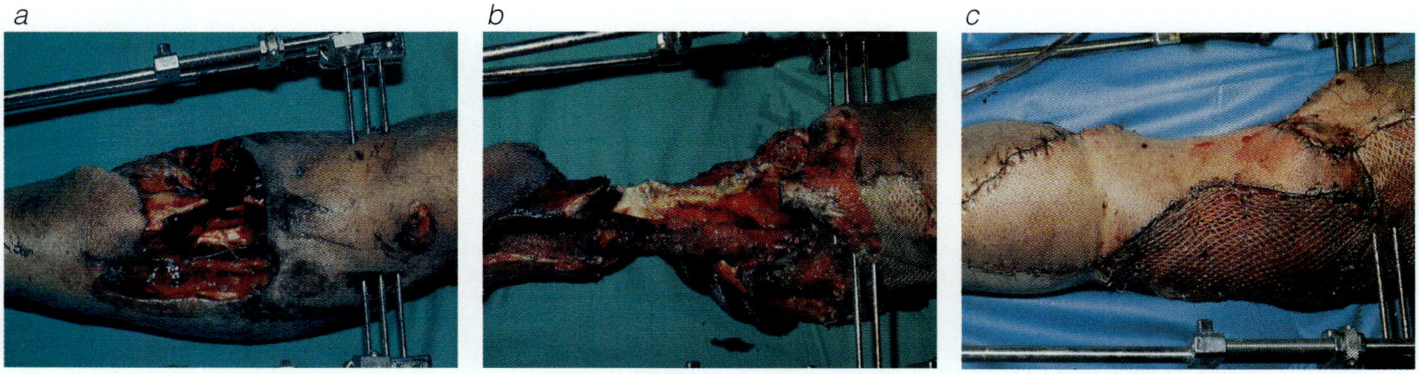

Figure 1 (*a*) A so-called bumper injury of the leg is shown after initial debridement and bony stabilization (two days after injury). After the second debridement (*b*), the true extent of devitalization of bone and soft tissue is apparent (four days after injury). (*c*) A latissimus dorsi free flap has been used to reconstruct the soft tissue defect (five days after injury).

sure of 8 psi can be achieved by forceful irrigation through a 35 ml syringe fitted with a 19-gauge needle. Low-pressure irrigation with a bulb-type syringe, for example, has not proved to be beneficial.

Bacterial counts The degree of bacterial wound contamination can be accurately quantified. The standard technique of quantitative bacteriology requires several days to complete. In addition to a count, it provides identification and antibiotic sensitivities of the organism. Quantitative bacteriology can also be performed using the rapid slide technique, which provides valuable information about the wound within 20 minutes.[2]

The level of bacterial contamination has been shown to be a significant predictor of outcome in wound closure by either skin-graft or flap-coverage techniques. According to the golden-period principle of wound closure, a minimum time interval is necessary for bacteria to proliferate to a certain threshold level. Studies show that contaminated wounds take a mean time of about five hours to reach a level of 10^5 bacteria per gram of tissue. Attempts to close wounds that have counts higher than 10^5/g of tissue will fail 75 to 100 percent of the time, whereas wounds with lower counts are successfully closed more than 90 percent of the time.[3] β-Hemolytic streptococci are an exception in that much lower concentrations of these organisms consistently result in failure of wound closure. When a β-hemolytic streptococcus is the dominant isolate, the wound should generally be treated openly until cultures become negative.

Systemic antibiotics The role of systemic antibiotics in wound management is not clearly defined. Broad-spectrum antibiotics should be given in cases of severe trauma or established, uncontrolled infection. They may also be useful for minor wounds that cannot be closed within three hours of injury.

Topical antibiotics Certain antibiotics provide broad-spectrum activity when applied topically. Neomycin used at a concentration of 10 mg/ml or a combination of bacitracin, 50 U/ml, and polymyxin B, 0.05 mg/ml, will kill most common wound pathogens. These solutions can be used when wet dressings are indicated.

Topical antiseptics A variety of topical antiseptics have been used empirically in wound care. Critical examinations have revealed, however, that these solutions are detrimental to wound healing when used in the concentrations usually recommended. Povidone-iodine (1 percent), hydrogen peroxide (3 percent), acetic acid (0.25 percent), and sodium hypochlorite (0.5 percent) all have been shown to be lethal to fibroblasts as well as bacteria. More dilute concentrations of povidone-iodine (0.001 percent) and sodium hypochlorite (0.005 percent) have been shown to be effective against bacteria while being safe for fibroblasts.[4] A number of these agents also inhibit normal white blood cell function in the wound.

Wet dressings Open wounds are treated with wet dressings, generally consisting of gauze soaked in saline or an acceptable topical antiseptic. Wet-to-wet dressings prevent desiccation of exposed vital structures or freshly placed skin grafts. Wet-to-dry dressings are useful for assisting in daily wound debridement. These dressings are allowed to dry on the wound; when they are removed, adherent fibrinous debris is removed with the dressing. Wet dressings of either type should be changed at least three times a day.

Small wounds can be expected to close by contraction and secondary epithelialization after appropriate open management with the techniques described. Large wounds will improve with aggressive open care but will then stabilize into a chronic state of wound colonization of varying degrees. A soft tissue coverage procedure is then necessary to complete closure in these cases.

SELECTION OF THE COVERAGE PROCEDURE

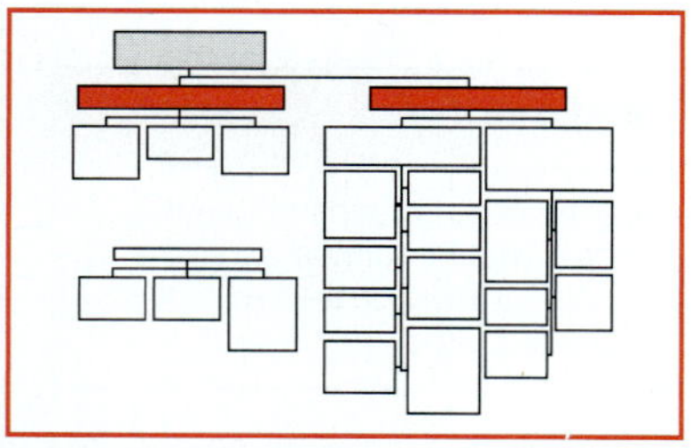

The goals of coverage procedures in the management of acute as well as chronic wounds are to achieve a healed wound and to avoid infection. The treatment of functional problems is generally deferred for secondary reconstruction. The method of coverage depends on whether vital structures, such as vessels, tendons, nerves, and bone, are exposed in the wound. If no vital structures are exposed, skin-graft coverage is indicated. Skin grafts can also be used over tendon if the paratenon is intact, over nerve if the epineurium is intact, and over bone if the periosteum is intact. Skin grafts are the most expendable type of soft tissue available for the coverage of open wounds. They allow the wound to heal completely and set the stage for secondary reconstruction, during which more valuable tissue can be used to achieve other goals at minimal risk.

When vital structures are exposed in the wound, a flap is preferred because it provides more substantial soft tissue coverage of the structure. The choice of flap depends on the location of the wound and on its overall size, depth, and topographic configuration (see below).

Skin Grafts

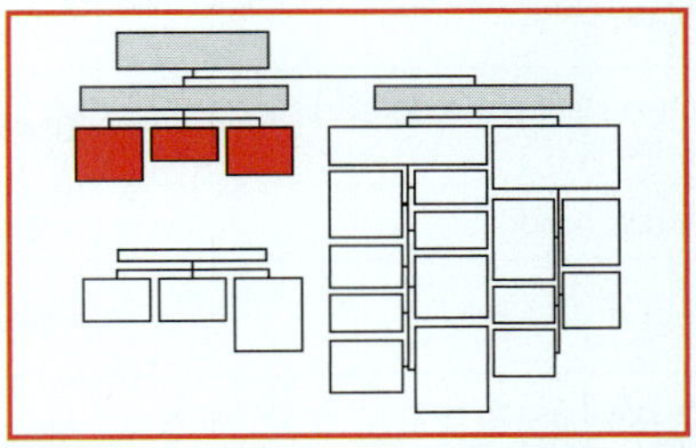

Skin grafts may be either partial thickness (i.e., split thickness) or full thickness. Split-thickness grafts are preferred for wounds with a large surface area. Full-thickness grafts are suitable only for small defects because their donor sites must be closed primarily; the most common donor sites for full-thickness grafts are the ears, upper eyelids, neck, and groin. Full-thickness grafts contract less with time than split-thickness grafts and are therefore particularly suitable for wounds of the hands, extremity flexion creases, nose, eyelids, and other areas of the face.

Successful healing of skin grafts requires immobilization of the recipient site to prevent shearing in the plane between the graft and the wound bed [see Postoperative Care, below]. However, although complete immobilization is desirable, the required dressings may preclude observation of a wound that is known to be significantly contaminated. In such cases, a meshed split-thickness graft is indicated, and the wound should be treated in an open fashion. A meshed graft can be placed directly over the muscle of a flap and secured over its irregular contour with staples [see Figure 2]. Because the graft is meshed, serum can escape between the interstices and there is little risk of separation from the underlying tissue. A meshed graft is also less vulnerable to disruption by shear forces. An additional advantage of a meshed graft is that it permits the wound to be treated with wet dressings if there is still risk for infection. A mesh expansion ratio of 1.5 : 1.0 is generally preferred, except when the surface area of the wound is very large and the availability of donor sites is limited.

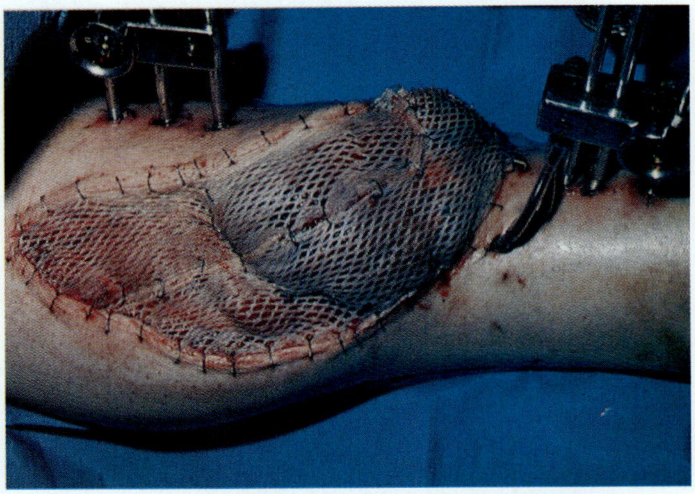

Figure 2 A meshed (1.5 : 1.0 ratio) skin graft has been secured to the irregular contour of a muscle free flap with staples. No additional immobilization of the graft is needed. The interstices of the graft allow free drainage of serous exudate from the muscle.

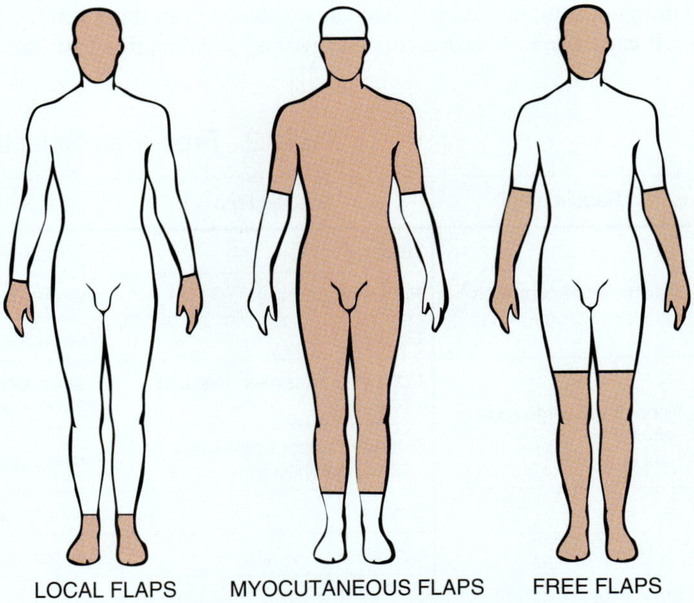

Flap-Coverage Procedures

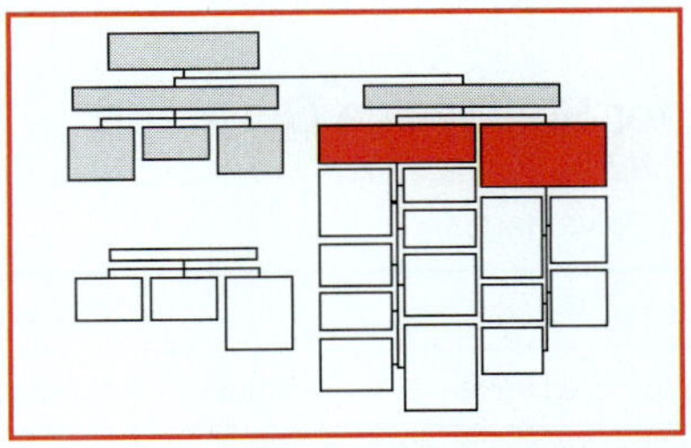

Flaps consist of tissues that have a self-contained vascular system. They permit a more substantial transfer of tissue bulk than do skin grafts and may consist of either skin and subcutaneous tissue, fascia, muscle, bone, or a combination of several of these tissue types. Local flaps consist of tissue that is mostly detached from surrounding tissue but retains enough connection to preserve an adequate blood supply to the entire flap. Local flaps are either transposed, rotated, or advanced into adjacent defects for purposes of reconstruction. Free flaps are totally detached and have their blood supply reconnected at the recipient site by surgically performed microvascular anastomoses between recipient-site blood vessels and the major vessels that supply the flap.

Local Flaps versus Free Flaps

The choice between a local flap and a free flap is determined by the amount and the type of tissue needed, as well as by the availability of flaps in the immediate area of the wound [see Figure 3]. Availability of local flaps, in turn, is determined by the nature of the regional blood supply. The vascular anatomy of a particular area determines the availability of arterialized skin flaps, fasciocutaneous flaps, myocutaneous flaps, and other forms of composite flaps. Local flaps can be grouped regionally by the types of tissue that they provide [see Table 1].

A local flap is generally preferred over a free flap if the two provide similar tissue, primarily because of the additional effort required to move a free flap. A free-flap procedure commonly takes twice as long as a local-flap procedure. The preference for local flaps does not result from fear of performing microvascular anastomoses—experienced surgeons accomplish free tissue transfer with success rates higher than 95 percent.

Figure 3 Regional alternatives in flap selection are illustrated. Defects in the central portion of the body are treated with myocutaneous flaps primarily; defects of the peripheral areas are treated with either local flaps or free flaps. In some areas, several options exist, and the choice is influenced by the size of the defect and the specific tissue requirements.

Table 1 Selection of Local Flaps by Region and Tissue Type

Site	Skin Flaps	Muscle and Myocutaneous Flaps	Fascial and Fasciocutaneous Flaps
Head and neck	Scalp; forehead; nasolabial; cervicofacial; Mustardé; eyelid; lip	Trapezius; latissimus dorsi; pectoralis major	Superficial and deep temporal fascia
Chest and back	Lateral thoracic; deltopectoral	Trapezius; pectoralis major; latissimus dorsi; rectus abdominis (superiorly based)	Scapular
Arm	Medial arm (Tagliacozzi)	Latissimus dorsi; pectoralis major	Lateral arm; forearm
Hand	Cross-finger; thenar; neurovascular island; fingertip advancement	—	Forearm
Abdomen and perineum	Groin	Rectus abdominis (inferiorly based); tensor fasciae latae; rectus femoris; gracilis	Medial thigh
Gluteal area	Sacral; thoracolumbar	Gluteus maximus; gracilis; tensor fasciae latae; biceps femoris	Gluteal thigh
Thigh	—	Tensor fasciae latae; rectus femoris; vastus lateralis; vastus medialis; gracilis; biceps femoris; rectus abdominis	Anterior thigh; anteromedial thigh; posterior thigh
Knee and proximal leg	—	Gastrocnemius	Saphenous artery; posterior calf
Midleg	—	Soleus; tibialis anterior	Anterior leg; lateral leg; posterior leg
Distal leg	—	—	—
Foot	Dorsalis pedis; plantar rotation; lateral calcaneal artery; plantar V-Y	Flexor digitorum brevis; abductor hallucis; abductor digiti minimi; extensor digitorum brevis	—

Free flaps are indicated in areas where local flaps are unavailable, such as in the distal third of the leg, or when an extremely large flap is needed but is unavailable locally. When regional donor sites are affected by the primary process, free tissue transfer allows healthy, well-vascularized tissue to be brought into the compromised area. Moreover, if free tissue is transferred, the size of the wound is not extended, because the donor site is not contiguous but instead is located at a distance from the wound.

If expertise in microvascular surgery is available, free flaps are frequently a first-line choice. Free flaps allow selection of the appropriate type of tissue in the most suitable size and configuration for the specific reconstructive problem. Compared with free flaps, local flaps are inefficient ways of moving tissue because only a small portion of a local flap actually reaches the defect itself. The choice of donor site is greater with free flaps because the limitations imposed by local availability are avoided.

Free flaps used in acute reconstruction can be grouped into three major types [see Table 2]. The soft tissue coverage requirements of

Table 2 Free Flap Selection for Soft Tissue Coverage*

Requirement	Specific Flap	Advantages	Disadvantages
Reliable workhorse flaps	Latissimus dorsi	Ideal pedicle[†]; ease of dissection	Awkward patient positioning
	Rectus abdominis	Ideal pedicle; supine position; ease of dissection	No major disadvantages
	Scapular	Ideal pedicle; skin flap only	Awkward patient positioning
Flaps of very large surface area	Combined latissimus dorsi and scapular	Independent component inset[‡]; primary donor-site closure possible; ideal pedicle	Awkward patient positioning
	Extended tensor fasciae latae and partial quadriceps	Supine position; large skin flap component	Donor-site healing[§]; pedicle configuration[‖]
Small flaps	Gracilis	Small muscle	Small vessels
	Lateral arm	Thin, sensate; convenient for hand trauma	Small vessels; donor-site scar
	Forearm	Thin skin flap; ideal pedicle	Minor hand morbidity; poor donor-site appearance
	Temporalis fascia	Thinnest flap; ideal coverage for exposed tendons[¶]; can transfer hair-bearing scalp	Variable donor-site scar alopecia

*Includes only the more commonly used free flaps for purposes of comparison.
[†]Characterized by large-diameter vessels and long pedicle length.
[‡]Each part can be arranged and sewn into the wound separately.
[§]Donor-site closure requires a skin graft, which may result in delayed healing.
[‖]Pedicle enters middle of undersurface of flap.
[¶]Permits tendon gliding underneath if used on dorsum of the hand or of the foot.

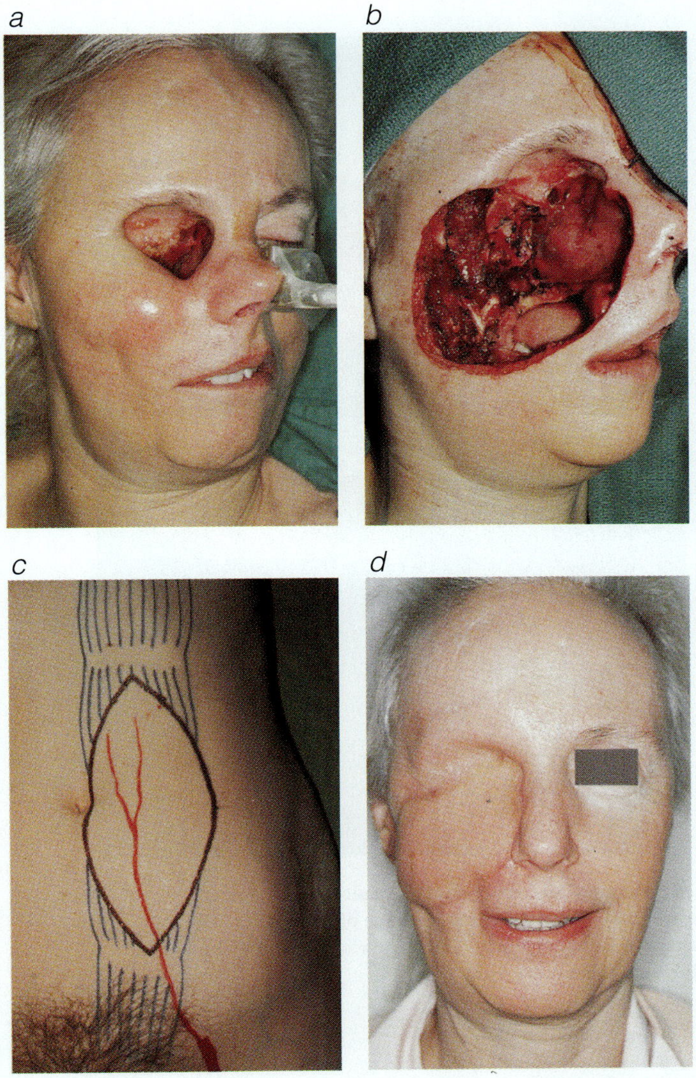

Figure 4 (*a*) A facial tumor has recurred following previous orbital exenteration. (*b*) The defect has been resected. Local flaps and regional myocutaneous flaps are not available for this defect. (*c*) The design for a rectus abdominis myocutaneous free flap is shown. This flap can be designed in other sizes and configurations depending on specific needs. The vascular pedicle is long and of large diameter, and the flap is easily accessible in the supine patient. (*d*) Soft tissue coverage with a reasonable restoration of facial contour has been achieved.

most wounds can be met by so-called workhorse free flaps. These flaps typically have the advantages of large size, ease of dissection, and a vascular pedicle that is long and of large diameter. The disadvantages, such as awkward patient positioning for flap harvest, are minor. Most workhorse flaps consist of muscle with an optional skin component; they are the flaps of choice for contaminated wounds [*see Figure 4*]. A second group of free flaps is useful for acute reconstruction of unusually large wounds. These flaps consist of combined vascular territories supplied by a single vascular pedicle. A third category consists of smaller free flaps that provide tissue that is superior in either amount or type to the local flaps that are otherwise available. An additional advantage of these flaps is that they tend not to be bulky. They are frequently used in areas such as the head, hands, distal third of the leg, and feet [*see Figure 5*].

Regional Alternatives in Flap Selection

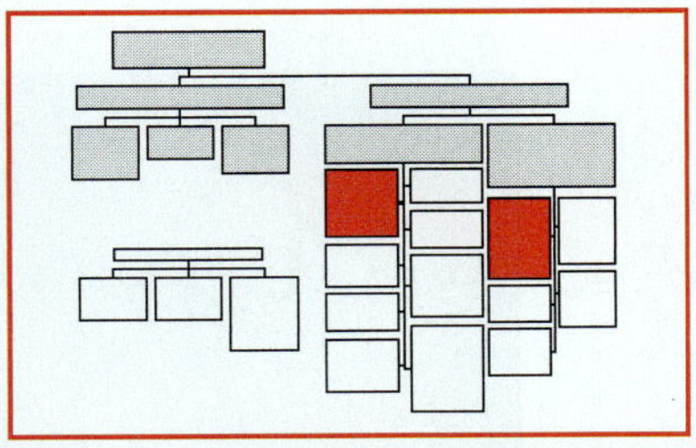

Head, neck Facial defects of small to moderate size are best treated with local skin flaps. A variety of flaps are available for reconstruction of limited defects of the eyelids, cheeks, nose, and mouth.[5-7] Small facial defects that do not directly involve the facial features can often be closed with several types of flaps that rearrange the existing tissue in the area—for example, Z-plasty [*see Secondary Reconstruction, Small Localized Scar, below*] or a Limberg flap. Tissues that are difficult to match, such as those of the eyelids or lips, can often be reconstructed with flaps that borrow tissue from their opposite, intact counterparts; the Abbe lip flap is such a flap [*see Figure 6*].

For coverage of some large defects in the head and neck region, the trapezius, latissimus dorsi, and pectoralis major muscles can be used. Each muscle can be raised with an optional skin island. These flaps are generally too bulky to be used on the face, and their reach is limited when used as pedicled flaps: none of them can cover major portions of the scalp or comfortably reach the upper face.

Latissimus dorsi, scapular, and rectus abdominis free flaps are useful for very large defects of the scalp or upper face. Smaller defects of the scalp are best treated with local scalp flaps.

Other free flaps of a specialized nature are superior for reconstruction of the floor of the mouth and mandible, even though local myocutaneous flaps will reach this area. For example, the forearm free flap based on the radial artery is quite thin and pliable and therefore provides an ideal replacement for the floor of the mouth. Composite free flaps that contain both bone and skin, such as those taken from the scapula, ilium, radius, and fibula, provide tissue of the appropriate type and proper configuration for defects of the lower face in which the mandible must be reconstructed along with the intraoral lining, the external skin, or both.

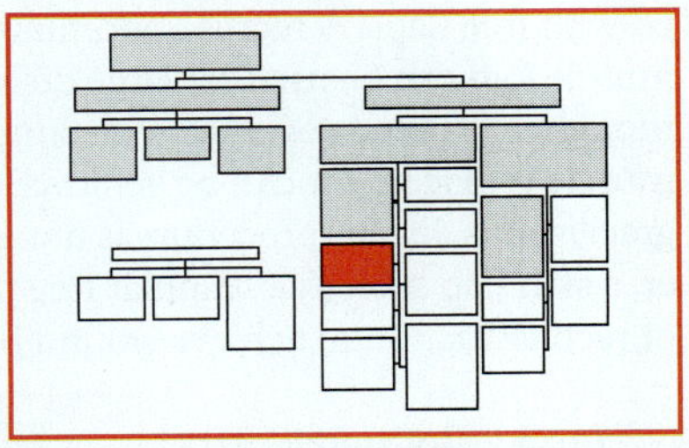

Chest, back Most defects of the chest and back are amenable to treatment with local myocutaneous flaps because of the wide arc of rotation of muscles located in these areas.[8] Midline sternal wounds can be covered with either pectoralis major or rectus abdominis muscle flaps; lateral chest defects with latissimus dorsi or pectoralis major muscle flaps; and midline back defects with latissimus dorsi or trapezius muscle flaps. Both the pectoralis and latissimus muscles can be divided from their primary vascular supply while retaining their intercostal supply and folded over as local flaps to cover midline defects anteriorly and posteriorly, respectively.

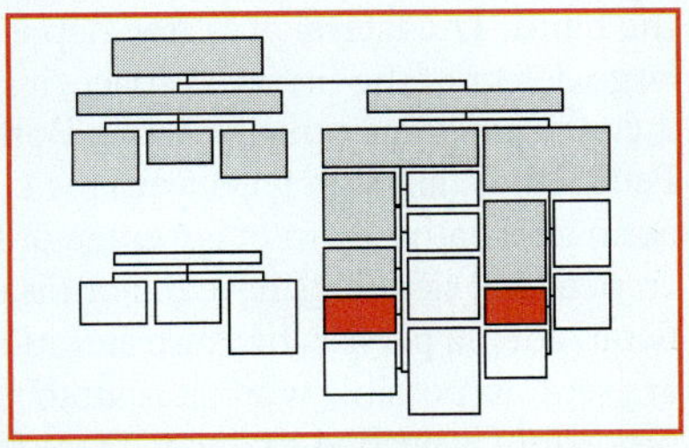

Arm, forearm Large wounds above the elbow can be covered with a latissimus dorsi myocutaneous flap transposed as a pedicled flap, provided that the vascular pedicle of the muscle has not been affected by the injury. Forearm wounds that require flap closure are best treat-

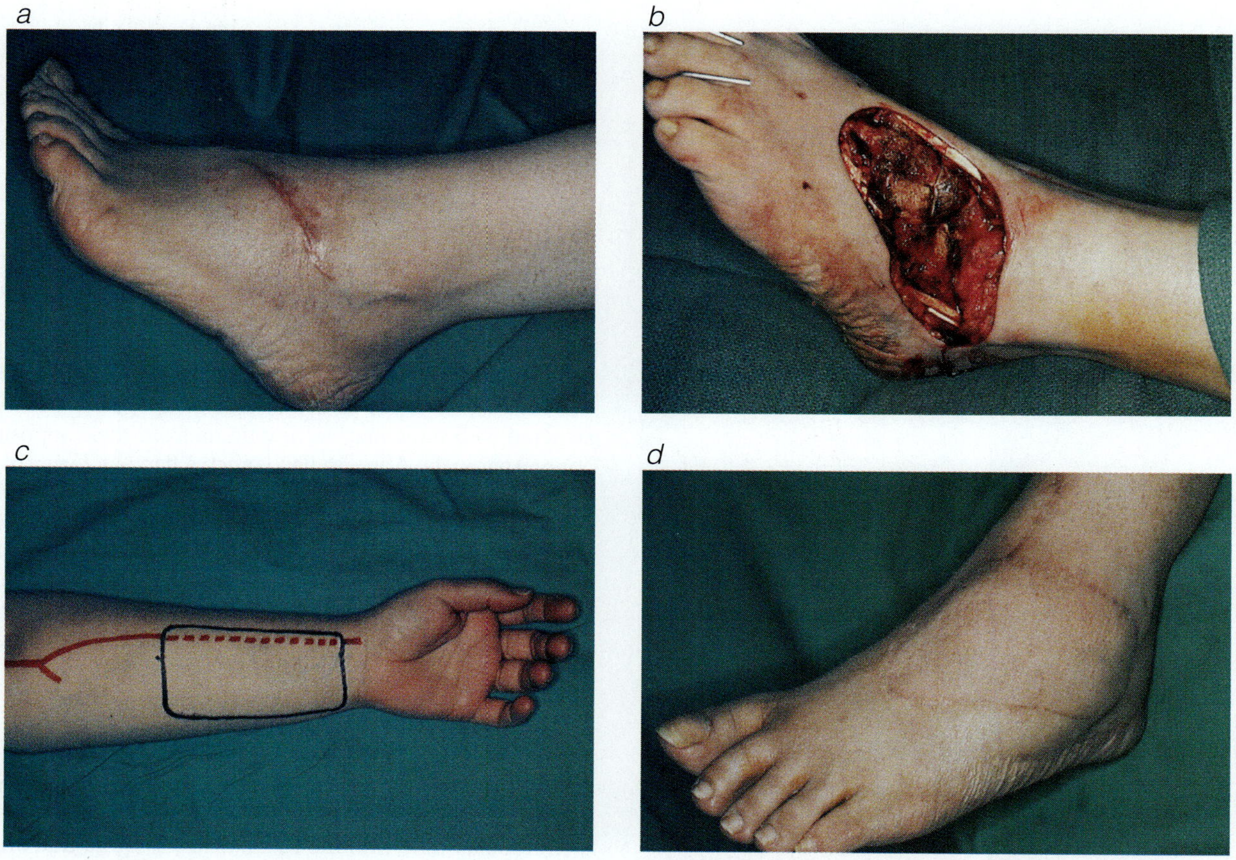

Figure 5 (*a*) A soft tissue sarcoma has recurred in the scar of a previous excision. Reexcision of the defect (*b*) has exposed bone and tendons. No regional flaps are available for satisfactory coverage of this defect. The forearm (*c*) is a source of small, thin free flaps. (*d*) Flap transfer has been completed. The radial artery and venae comitantes have been anastomosed to their dorsalis pedis counterparts.

ed with free flaps. A rectus abdominis, scapular, or latissimus dorsi muscle flap can be used for large defects of the arm or forearm. Although soft tissue coverage with simultaneous functional forearm muscle replacement can be achieved with a single flap such as the gracilis muscle, this procedure is not generally recommended; rather, a skin flap such as a scapular free flap is preferred as a first stage of reconstruction to achieve wound healing.

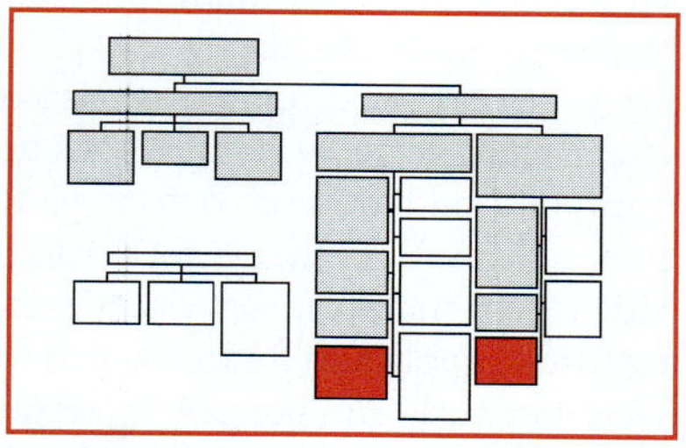

Hand Both free flaps and pedicled skin flaps are useful for soft tissue coverage of hand wounds. The temporalis fascia free flap is particularly thin and is ideal for coverage of exposed tendons on the dorsum of the hand. The lateral arm free flap is ideal for reconstruction of a large defect of the first web space; it has sensory potential because it contains a large sensory nerve. Both of these free flaps are small. Pedicled distant skin flaps from the chest or abdomen are available as an alternative form of coverage of sizable hand defects. However, pedicled skin flaps have major disadvantages: wound care is difficult, edema persists because elevation and movement of the hand are seldom possible while it is attached to the trunk, and a second procedure is needed to divide these flaps.

Digital injuries with exposed tendons can be closed with a variety of cross-finger flaps of skin and subcutaneous tissue raised from either the volar or extensor aspect of an adjacent digit. Because these flaps do not contain a great deal of subcutaneous tissue, they are preferred for coverage of digits proximally, where a thick subcutaneous pad is not essential. The thenar flap is useful for fingertip injuries in which the soft tissue pad of the fingertip is lost and bone is exposed. This flap provides an ideal pulp replacement as well as better sensory recovery than skin grafts. Fingertip injuries can also be closed with several types of V-Y advancement flaps that can be raised from either the volar or lateral surfaces of the end of the finger.

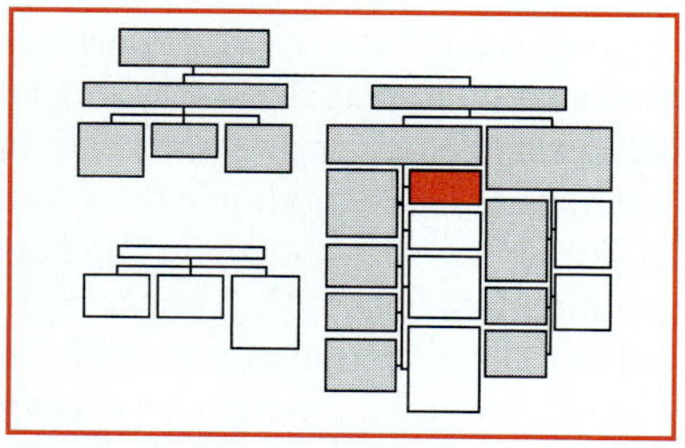

Abdomen Defects of the abdominal wall that require flap closure are best treated with local muscle flaps such as the tensor fasciae latae and rectus femoris from the thigh. The rectus abdominis also can occasionally be transposed to cover an abdominal defect. Each of these flaps is harvested along with skin, although a large tensor fasciae latae flap will probably require skin-graft closure of the donor site. The tensor fasciae latae flap has the advantage of including the thickened deep fascia (iliotibial band) of the thigh, which can provide additional strength for abdominal wall closure.

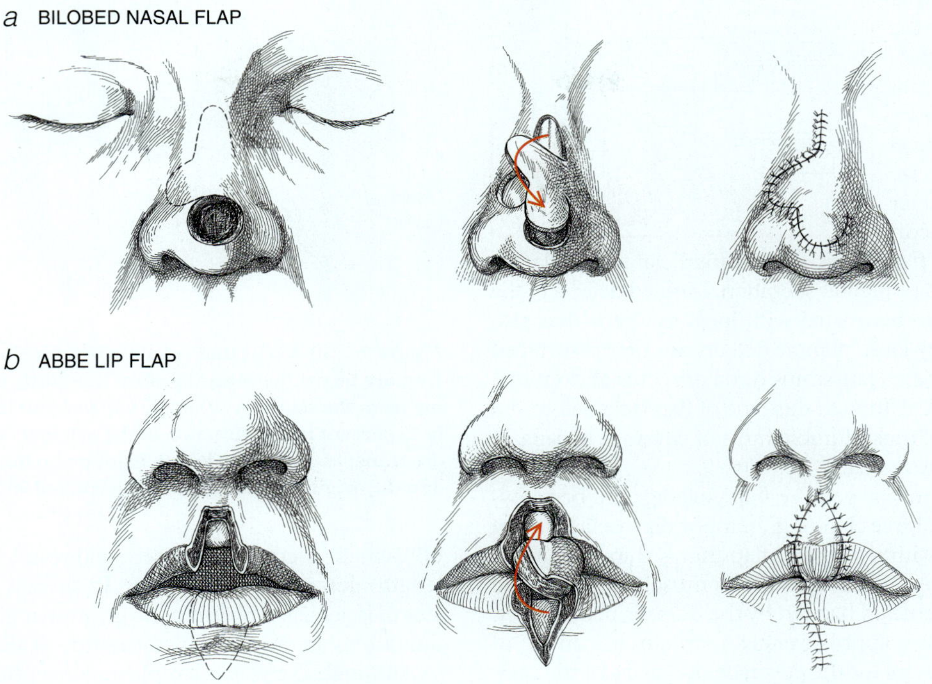

a BILOBED NASAL FLAP

b ABBE LIP FLAP

Figure 6 To close small facial defects, the bilobed nasal flap (*a*) and a variety of local flaps take advantage of skin laxity that exists in certain directions. Specialized tissues such as lip (*b*) and eyelid are frequently reconstructed with the same type of tissue borrowed from the opposite side.

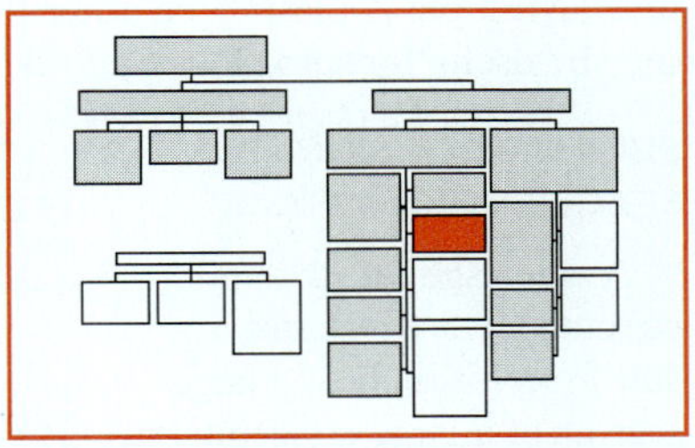

Gluteal area, perineum Local muscle flaps with or without skin are indicated for defects in this area. They are preferable to large, random-pattern advancement skin flaps from the posterior thigh and thoracolumbar rotation skin flaps. The gluteus maximus muscle, for example, can be used as a rotation, V-Y advancement, or turnover flap in the treatment of pressure sores. As a turnover flap, it can be proximally or distally based, or it can be split along its longitudinal axis so that only a portion of it is used. Also useful for covering defects in the gluteal area and the perineum is the myofasciocutaneous gluteal-thigh flap, a combination of a gluteus muscle flap and a fasciocutaneous flap from the posterior thigh that is supplied by an extension of the inferior gluteal artery. Because of its size and location, the gracilis muscle is well suited for coverage of defects of the perineum. The gracilis and biceps femoris muscles are generally secondary choices for the treatment of pressure sores over the ischium. The tensor fasciae latae muscle is frequently used for treating open wounds over the greater trochanter. The entire quadriceps muscle can be used to close defects resulting from hemipelvectomy.

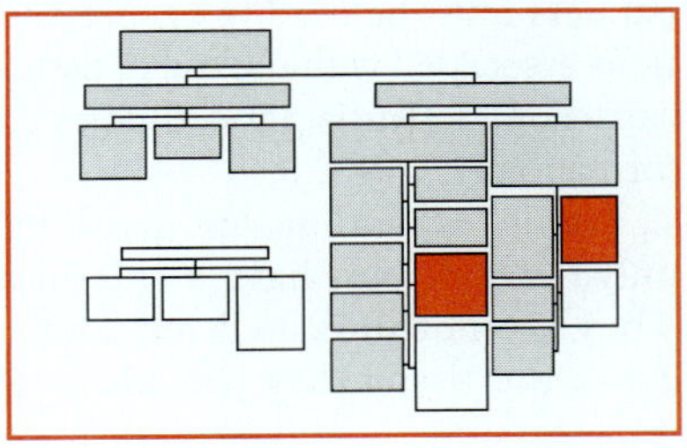

Thigh Flaps are rarely required for soft tissue coverage in the thigh area, because critical vital structures are located deep within the thigh and are rarely exposed by injury or by surgical procedures. A number of regional muscle flaps are available, however, including the tensor fasciae latae, rectus femoris, vastus lateralis, and vastus medialis muscles. The gracilis and posterior thigh muscles are rarely used in this area. An anterior defect with exposure of the femoral vessels can be covered with either an ipsilateral or a contralateral rectus abdominis myocutaneous flap. A number of smaller local skin flaps that are supplied with blood from the deep fascia can be raised over portions of the thigh; except for the posterior thigh flap, however, the clinical usefulness of these flaps remains to be demonstrated.

Knee, proximal leg, midleg The two heads of the gastrocnemius muscle can be used either together or independently to cover defects of the knee and proximal leg. The soleus muscle is useful for coverage of defects of the proximal leg and midleg. Local flaps should not be used for major leg wounds if the extent of the injury suggests involvement of the muscle donor site. Instead, a free flap should be used to bring healthy tissue into the area. Therefore, free flaps are a first choice, for example, for coverage of major wounds of the popliteal fossa, knee, and proximal leg that involve the sural artery blood supply to the gastrocnemius muscle.

Skin flaps fed by the fascial blood supply can also be raised over the leg.[9] A number of fasciocutaneous flaps have been described in this area, but they tend to be smaller than muscle flaps and generally less reliable. These flaps are longitudinally oriented over the course of the anterior tibial artery or the peroneal artery. The maximum length at which such fasciocutaneous flaps are safe and their specific applications have not been well established.

Foot The foot is as complex as the hand and the face in that it is composed of separate regions, each of which has a unique set of alternatives for reconstruction. These regions include the plantar surface; the dorsum; and the posterior (non–weight-bearing) heel, Achilles tendon, and malleoli.

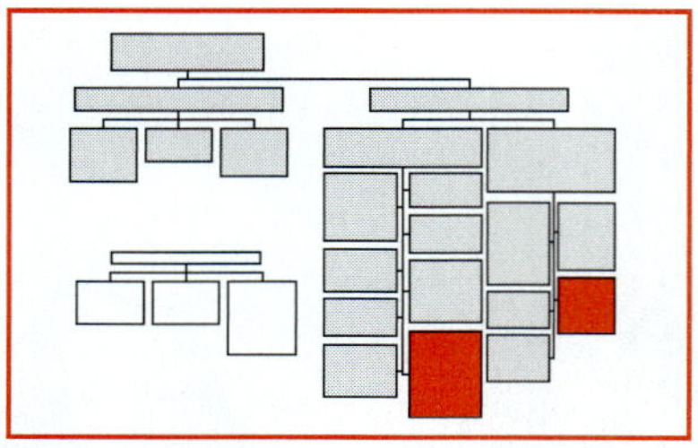

Superficial defects that lie completely within the non–weight-bearing portion of the midsole do not need flap coverage. Defects of the weight-bearing heel and midsole area that are less than 6 cm in diameter can be closed with a medially based skin rotation flap that is raised superficial to the plantar fascia.[10] This flap maintains plantar sensation. Limited defects of the distal plantar surface can be treated with local toe flaps that also maintain sensation. Very large plantar defects are best resurfaced with a muscle free flap (e.g., latissimus dorsi or rectus abdominis) covered with a skin graft. Although this type of flap lacks sensation, it appears to provide the most durable form of coverage because it is able to resist shear forces well.[11]

Defects of the dorsum that require flap coverage are best covered either with a fascial free flap (e.g., temporalis fascia) and an overlying skin graft or with a skin free flap that is thin (e.g., from the forearm). The extensor digitorum brevis muscle can be raised from the dorsum as a pedicled flap fed by the dorsalis pedis artery. This flap, which measures approximately 5 × 6 cm, has an arc of rotation that makes it useful for the coverage of defects of the malleolus or the Achilles tendon area. A narrow transposition skin flap fed by the lateral calcaneal artery is useful for coverage of defects approximately 3 cm in diameter that lie over the Achilles tendon or the non–weight-bearing posterior heel.

Secondary Reconstruction

Selection of the proper method for secondary reconstruction requires analysis of the type and extent of tissue deficiency that is present. Superficial defects may require replacement or supplementation of only skin and subcutaneous tissue, whereas more complex defects may require replacement of several types of tissue. Specialized tissue such as vascularized nerve (i.e., a nerve free flap) or intestine may be necessary to provide a functional reconstruction in some cases (see below).

SMALL LOCALIZED SCAR

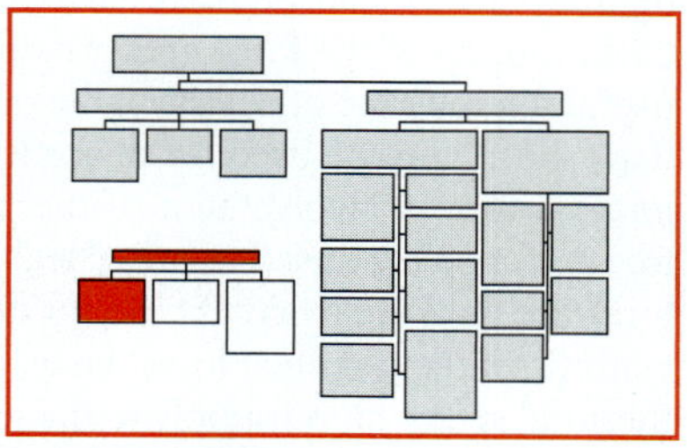

When small localized scars need reconstruction, soft tissue coverage is generally sufficient and poses no threat of breakdown leading to exposure of important structures. Instead, the reconstructive problem is generally functional in nature. An example is a tight scar band across a flexion crease, commonly seen after a burn injury. A local procedure that rearranges the existing tissue can relieve the tension by making more tissue available in one direction, although the amount of tissue in the area is not actually increased.

The Z-plasty is an example of such tissue rearrangement [see Figure 7]. Two triangular flaps are designed to have a common, or central, limb aligned in the direction that needs to be lengthened. Each of the other two limbs is equal in length to the central limb and diverges from it at an equal angle varying from 30° to 90°. After the flaps are transposed, length is gained in the desired direction, and the original Z is rotated 90° and reversed. An angle of

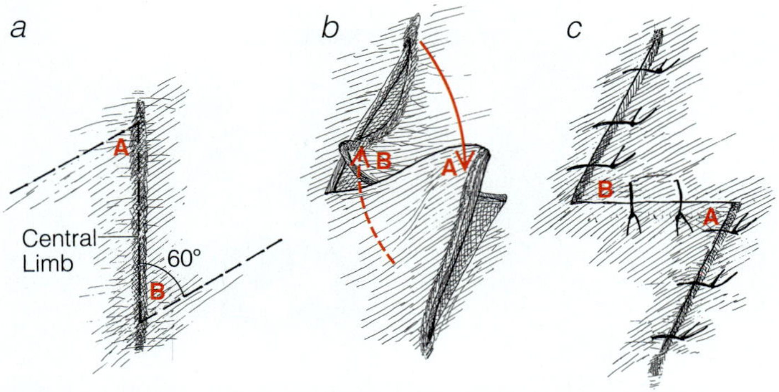

Figure 7 (*a*) A scar that requires lengthening to eliminate a contracture forms the central limb of a Z-plasty design. Incisions diverging from the scar at a 60° angle will yield an increase of approximately 75 percent in the direction of the original central limb. (*b*) The flaps are transposed. (*c*) The length from top to bottom has been increased, and the original Z design has been rotated 90° and reversed.

60°, which is commonly used, will result in a 75 percent gain in length along the central limb. In theory, the maximum gain in length is achieved by using the greatest angle possible, but practical limitations are imposed by the nature of skin elasticity.

Although Z-plasty is simple in conception, experience is necessary for the surgeon to realize the limitations of the technique and appreciate the subtleties of proper design. Important considerations in the use of Z-plasty include the proper length of the central limb and the proper orientation of the limbs so that the new central limb formed after transposition is parallel to the skin tension lines. Multiple Z-plasties or other procedures, such as W-plasty, may be useful for some localized scars.

SHORTAGE OF SKIN AND SUBCUTANEOUS TISSUE

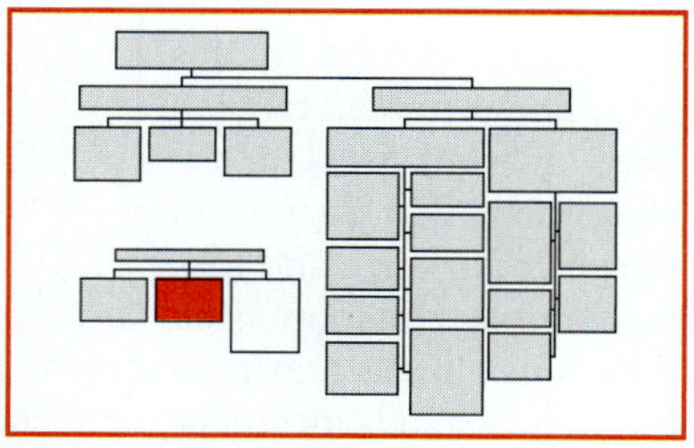

A shortage of skin and subcutaneous tissue may result from excision of a large scar or of a large congenital defect such as a nevus. Mastectomy commonly leaves a shortage of skin that prevents creation of a breast mound. In these cases, extra tissue can be created locally with the use of tissue expanders. These devices are inflatable plastic reservoirs of various shapes and volumes that are implanted under the skin. The skin over the expander is stretched during a period of several weeks as the expander is gradually filled by percutaneously injecting saline into an incorporated or remote fill port. The expander is then removed as a second procedure, and the expanded area of skin is advanced to cover the defect.

A number of important principles govern the use of tissue expanders. The expanders must be placed in such a way as to allow expansion to occur only in normal skin adjacent to the defect and not in the defect itself. A sufficiently large expander or multiple expanders must be used to ensure adequate expansion. Complications associated with the use of tissue expanders include infection, extrusion, deflation, flipped ports (remote type), and hematoma formation.[12]

Tissue expanders are used in secondary reconstruction only; they do not have a role in acute wound management. They are not indicated for contour defects (see below), because the tissue they provide is of only two dimensions and is deficient in bulk. Nor is expanded tissue adequate for coverage of chronically exposed structures such as bone. Tissue expanders do not provide adequate replacement tissue to establish a suitable bed for nerve or bone grafting. Therefore, they are not a substitute for flaps in general.

The scalp is an ideal location for the use of tissue expanders because no equivalent substitute for this type of hair-bearing tissue exists. Expanders work effectively when implanted over the hard calvarium and are useful in cases of burn alopecia and large nevi involving the scalp. Expanders are also useful for breast reconstruction, for carefully selected large lesions of the face, and for certain scars of the limbs. They are generally not indicated for use in the hands or feet. Although some local flap donor sites, such as the forehead, can be expanded before flap transfer, there is a loss of tissue pliability that appears to limit the usefulness of this particular application.

COMPLEX DEFECTS

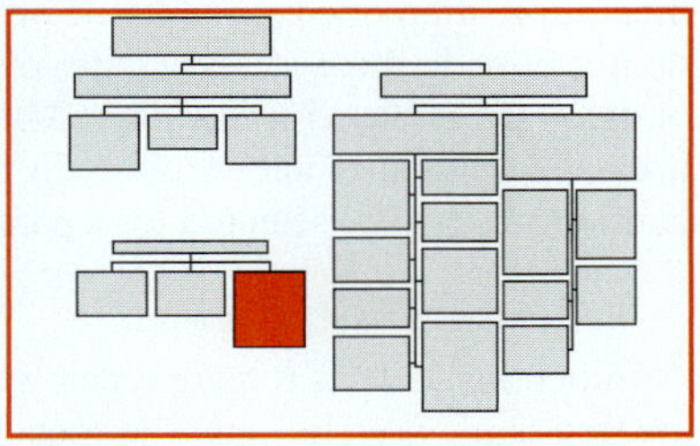

Certain reconstructive problems require substantial amounts of tissue of one or more types or of a very specialized type. Either local or free flaps are used to meet these tissue requirements.

Composite Defect

A composite defect may result from resection of an intraoral carcinoma with loss of the mandible and either the lining of the mouth or external skin. Another example is a crush injury of the leg with loss of soft tissue and a segment of weight-bearing bone. These defects require that a composite flap be brought to the area to

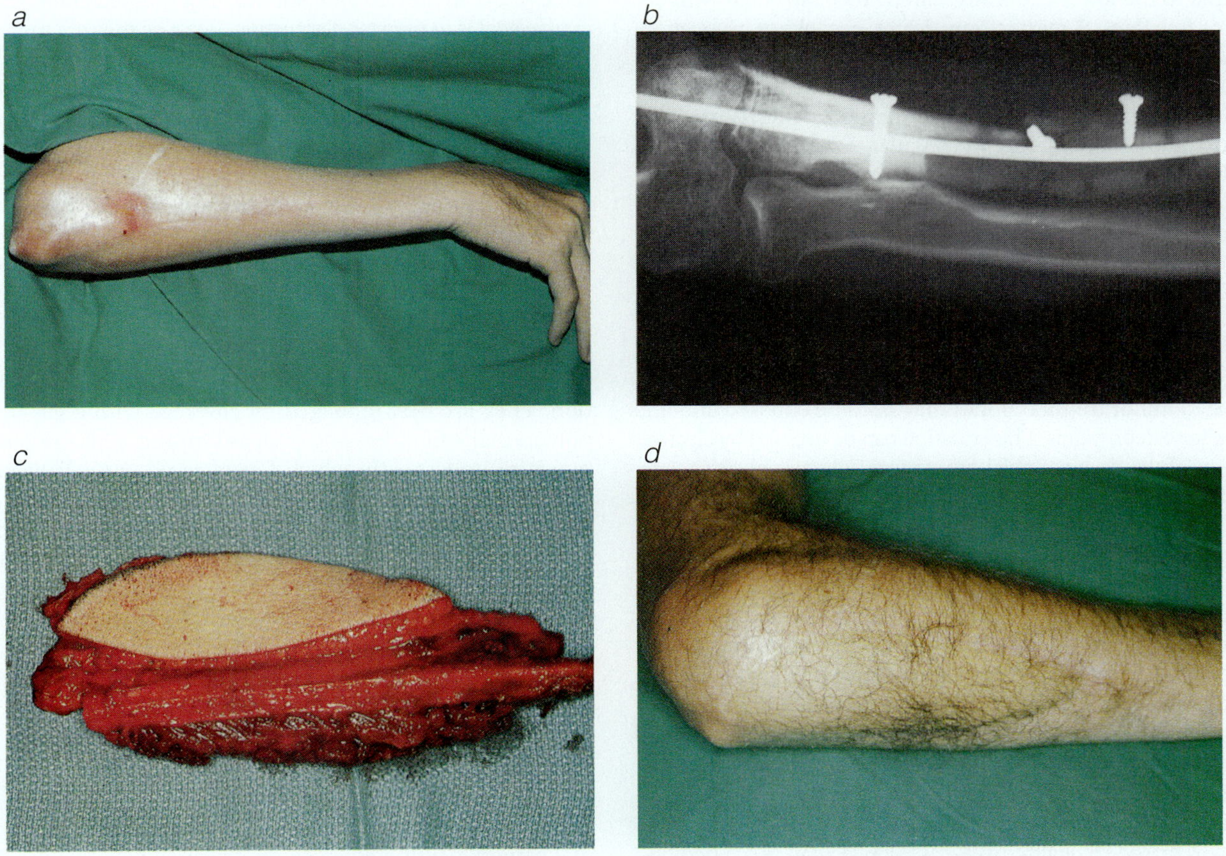

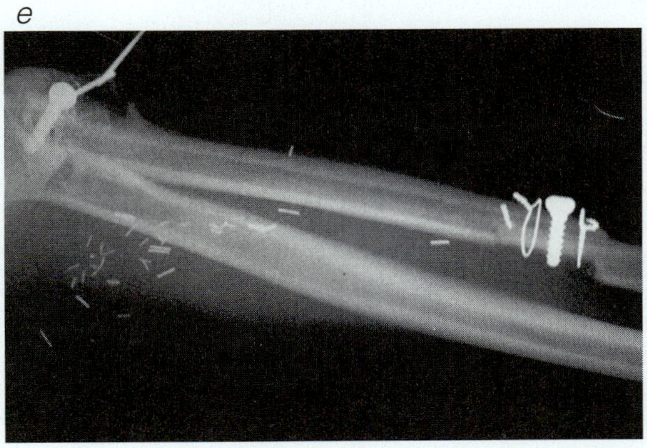

Figure 8 (*a*) A chronic draining sinus of the ulna with poor overlying soft tissue coverage is shown. Simultaneous replacement of both bone and overlying soft tissue with a composite tissue flap is needed. (*b*) A radiograph shows nonunion of the ulna with orthopedic hardware. A fibular free flap (*c*) provides bone and skin in the appropriate amount and configuration for replacement of the affected tissues in a single stage. (*d*) The segment of ulna and overlying skin has been replaced. A radiograph (*e*) shows the vascularized fibula in place.

meet more than one type of tissue deficiency. Local flaps generally do not provide the necessary types of tissue or permit the freedom of design possible with free flaps. The wide variety of free flap donor sites that exists allows tissue in the appropriate quantity and configuration to be selected for a particular defect [see Figure 8].

Functional Defect

Functional defects require repair with specialized flaps. Free flaps are frequently used because the specific tissue requirements usually cannot be satisfied by a local flap. A functional defect may result, for example, in the cervical esophagus from tumor resection or in the forearm from Volkmann's contracture. A segment of small intestine can repair the esophageal defect; transfer of a vascularized and innervated muscle such as the gracilis can replace forearm muscle.[13]

Contour Deformity

Contour defects, such as those that result from mastectomy or from trauma to the lower extremity, can be reconstructed with either local or free flaps. A mastectomy defect, because of its location on the chest, is suitable for reconstruction with one of several myocutaneous flaps from either the back or the abdomen. A free flap from the abdomen or the gluteal area is another alternative. The best reconstructive solution for a particular person is determined by variables such as body habitus and the size and configuration of the contralateral breast.

A contour defect of the lower extremity is best reconstructed with a large myocutaneous free flap that provides tissue of sufficient quantity and flexibility to allow sculpting into the appropriate shape.

Unstable Soft Tissue Coverage

Marginal soft tissue coverage (e.g., skin grafts) may break down after repeated minor trauma. Bones may become exposed and are then at risk for osteomyelitis. This situation can be avoided by elective replacement of the tissue at risk with a more substantial soft tissue covering. As in acute reconstruction, local flaps are the first choice for lesions of the trunk or the proximal extremities, whereas free flaps are often more appropriate for lesions of the distal extremities.

Soft tissue coverage is sometimes inadequate even in a healed wound. For example, certain procedures, such as nerve or bone grafting, require an ideal soft tissue bed to promote adequate graft revascularization. In some cases, it may be necessary first to replace the existing soft tissue coverage as a first-stage procedure before grafting a bone or nerve gap. A skin or muscle flap is most commonly used in these cases. This problem is most common in areas such as the distal extremities, where native soft tissue coverage is not overly abundant and is easily lost from trauma or tumor resection. Free flaps are usually chosen to provide a healthy, well-vascularized soft tissue bed before further functional reconstruction is undertaken.

Postoperative Care

SKIN GRAFTS

The postoperative fate of a skin graft is largely determined by the circumstances of the wound (especially the presence or absence of infection) and the technical execution of the grafting procedure. Successful healing of skin grafts requires immobilization of the recipient site for five to seven days. Immobilization can be accomplished with tie-over bolsters; on extremities, skin grafts can be further immobilized with plaster casts. Proper immobilization is critical for graft survival because it prevents shearing in the plane between the graft and the wound bed. After five to seven days of immobilization, either a gauze dressing such as Xeroform or a lubricating antibiotic ointment should be applied for another five to seven days.

Grafts that are treated by closed methods (i.e., tie-over bolsters) are carefully observed for evidence of infection. Developing erythema or suppuration is an indication for immediate removal of the bolster dressing and inspection of the graft. A graft threatened by infection may be saved by switching to an open method of graft care with wet dressings changed three to four times a day.

Nonmeshed grafts may form a hematoma or seroma that will prevent the graft from taking. Fluid accumulation should be evacuated by puncturing the graft or by rolling cotton-tipped swabs over it until the fluid escapes from under its edges. Survival of the entire graft is possible if fluid is meticulously evacuated within the first few days after graft placement.

Meshed grafts are not subject to the problem of fluid accumulation, nor are they as vulnerable as nonmeshed grafts to the shear forces that can prevent graft survival. For meshed grafts, the postoperative goal is to prevent desiccation, because they are more exposed to the environment. Gauze dressings such as Xeroform should be placed over the graft and changed once a day. After two weeks, the dressings can be discontinued, but the graft should be kept well lubricated with either a skin cream or cocoa butter.

Meshed grafts that are placed over wounds at high risk for infection should be aggressively managed postoperatively with wet dressings changed three or four times a day. The dressing changes will not interfere with graft take and will maximize graft survival in the face of heavy bacterial contamination.

Management of Skin-Graft Donor Sites

The donor sites of split-thickness grafts heal by epithelialization. They are best managed by coverage with a gas-permeable polyurethane film dressing such as Op-Site. This dressing retains moisture underneath, which favors rapid epithelialization. It is also impermeable to bacteria. It is placed on the donor site after removal of the skin graft, and the area is wrapped with an overlying dressing for 48 hours to prevent formation of a seroma or hematoma under the Op-Site. The outer dressing is then removed, and the Op-Site is left in place for as long as two weeks. This plastic dressing is painless and much better tolerated than more traditional forms of dressing such as Xeroform gauze, which is left to dry out and spontaneously separate.[14]

LOCAL FLAPS

The postoperative care of local flaps is not complex. Flap healing is supported by adequate nutrition and maintenance of a normal hemodynamic state, including normal blood volume. Tension must not be placed on the flap. Tension can develop in flaps on the trunk by changes in patient position or in flaps on the limbs by loss of immobilization. The tip of any local flap is generally not only its most valuable portion but also its most vulnerable area. At the tip, the blood supply is the most precarious, and the detrimental effects of tension are magnified. Unfortunately, no pharmacological agents are of proven benefit in preventing progressive necrosis of a flap with failing circulation. Any flap necrosis that might develop should be minimized by preventing infection of the necrotic tissue. Necrotic tissue must therefore be debrided after the extent of tissue loss becomes clear. Portions of the flap that are undergoing demarcation but do not appear to be actively infected can be protected by the application of a topical antibiotic such as silver sulfadiazine cream (Silvadene).

FREE FLAPS

Survival of free flaps, unlike that of local flaps, tends to be an all-or-none phenomenon. Careful postoperative monitoring of flap circulation is essential because flap failure is likely to be the result of a problem at the vascular anastomoses. Flaps are usually monitored for seven days. However, the most critical time for free-flap monitoring is the first six to eight hours because the majority of vascular crises usually occur within this period. Early detection and aggressive investigation of such crises generally allow a flap to be salvaged.

Maintenance of normal blood volume and treatment of hypothermia are important in the early postoperative period to avoid vascular spasm. Spasm causes flaps to appear pale and to exhibit a significant temperature drop.

Free flaps should be monitored on an hourly basis during the early postoperative period. Most free flaps include an exposed skin island, which facilitates evaluation of the flap circulation. The flap is observed for color and for capillary refill. A pale flap generally indicates arterial insufficiency; however, the normal, lighter color of certain donor sites, such as the abdomen, can be misleading. Flaps with venous insufficiency are characteristically blue in color and exhibit rapid capillary refill. Bleeding from the edges of a flap is common in the presence of venous hypertension.

Surface temperature probes are used to monitor free flaps that have a skin island. The advantages of this method are simplicity and reliability. One probe is placed on the flap and another on a nearby area to serve as a control. The flap surface temperature is generally less than the control temperature by 1.0° to 2.5° C. A progressive widening of the temperature difference is ominous and requires critical assessment of the flap circulation. The absolute temperature of the flap probe is also significant: a flap temperature greater than 32° C indicates healthy circulation, whereas a temperature between 30° and 32° C indicates marginal circulation and a temperature less than 30° C usually indicates a vascular problem. In a healthy flap, temperature fluctuations may be caused by a dislodged probe, an exogenous heat source (such as a lamp), cooling of one of the probes from an oxygen mist mask, or cleaning of the flap skin with alcohol (which results in a precipitous drop in skin temperature).

To confirm the presence of an anastomotic problem, flap circulation is assessed directly by a full-thickness puncture of the flap skin with a 19- or 20-gauge needle. If flap circulation is healthy, a drop of bright-red blood should appear at the puncture site within a few seconds, and another drop should appear each time the previous drop is wiped away by an alcohol swab. The failure of blood to appear or the delayed appearance of a clear, serous ooze instead of blood is an indication of arterial insufficiency. Vigorous, dark bleeding confirms a venous problem. Flaps that are pale as a result of vascular spasm are difficult to assess because their bleeding response to needle puncture is poor despite intact anastomoses. Whenever uncertainty exists, however, surgical exploration should be undertaken because the entire flap is in jeopardy.

Free flaps without skin islands are more difficult to monitor accurately. Muscle flaps can be followed in much the same way as skin free flaps by inserting needle temperature probes directly into the muscle belly. A healthy muscle free flap is red in color and typically has a serous ooze between the interstices of the overlying meshed skin graft. A flap with an arterial problem quickly becomes dry and dark in appearance. A muscle flap with a venous problem becomes dark and engorged with blood and exhibits bleeding from its surface and perimeter. A muscle free flap can be punctured with a needle to assess the quality of the bleeding if its circulatory status is unclear.

Fascial free flaps covered with skin grafts are more difficult to assess. They tend to transmit body core temperature readily because they are quite thin; therefore, needle temperature probes are generally unreliable. It is often possible in these cases either to observe the arterial pulsations in the flap directly or to monitor them with a conventional Doppler device.

Some free flaps are completely buried beneath the skin. Others, such as intraoral skin free flaps, are equally difficult to monitor postoperatively. Specialized transplants, such as jejunum, are particularly vulnerable to short periods of anoxia and are not likely to be salvageable by the time a problem is recognized. Alternative methods of monitoring buried free flaps are being developed, although they are not in wide clinical use. One example is the implantable Doppler monitor. This device is placed in direct contact with the artery distal to the anastomosis to obtain a continuous Doppler signal.

PATIENT POSITIONING

Extremities that are recipient sites for skin grafts or flaps should always be maintained above heart level for a minimum of one week postoperatively. Lower extremities with skin grafts or free flaps, particularly below the knee, should remain elevated for a minimum of 10 days to two weeks. Patients should be mobilized in a progressive manner, beginning with brief periods of limb dangling. Premature ambulation of patients with lower-extremity skin grafts can result in loss of the skin graft despite an early appearance of complete graft take. Free flaps exhibit venous engorgement when placed in a dependent position up to several weeks postoperatively. Such engorgement is generally not dangerous, although patients with free flaps below the knee should be gradually mobilized in the same fashion as patients with skin grafts in this location.

Free flaps in the head and neck area require that the patient's head motion be restricted somewhat for the first few days. It is important that electrocardiographic leads and tracheostomy tube ties not compress the external jugular vein if it was used as a recipient vessel for anastomosis. If central lines are required postoperatively, they should be placed on the contralateral side of the neck.

Discussion

Wound Healing

The wound healing process consists of several identifiable phases [see 8 Acute Wound Care]. The first phase is an inflammatory response that includes both vascular and cellular components. The second stage is fibroplasia, during which collagen deposition by fibroblasts increases the tensile strength of the wound. The maturation phase of wound healing begins at about three weeks, when the rate of collagen degradation begins to balance the rate of collagen production. The previously random arrangement of collagen fibers becomes more organized, and the type I to type III collagen ratio returns to normal. The wound gradually progresses from a raised, indurated, red scar to a mature form that is flat, soft, lighter in color, and of increased tensile strength. The maturation phase continues for more than a year.

Contraction of open, so-called granulating wounds is caused by myofibroblasts, modified fibroblasts that have smooth muscle characteristics. The number of myofibroblasts within the wound has been found to be proportional to the rate at which the wound contracts.[15,16] These cells are scattered throughout the wound and pull the edges of the wound toward the center. Skin grafts inhibit wound contraction, apparently by accelerating the life cycle of the myofibroblast.

Skin Grafts

Split-thickness skin grafts include the epidermis and only a portion of the dermis, whereas full-thickness skin grafts include the entire dermis. Skin grafts contract to a degree that is related to their thickness. After their harvest from donor sites, full-thickness grafts will contract to a surface area as small as 40 percent of their original surface area, whereas split-thickness grafts contract only about half as much. This reduction in area, referred to as primary contraction, is a passive phenomenon caused by elastic tissue within the graft. Secondary contraction occurs as a graft heals at the recipient site. Full-thickness grafts undergo minimal secondary contraction, whereas split-thickness grafts contract to a degree that is inversely proportional to their dermal content. In other words, thick split-thickness grafts contract less than thin split-thickness grafts.

Skin grafts gradually regain sensation by reinnervation from the wound bed. Thick grafts and healthy wound beds contribute to greater sensory recovery. However, the degree of sensation after healing is complete does not equal that of normal skin. Graft thickness also affects recovery of certain other functions of normal skin, such as secretion from sweat glands and sebaceous glands, and of hair growth. These processes will be active only in full-thickness and thick split-thickness grafts. Secretion from sweat glands depends on sympathetic reinnervation of the graft and follows the sweat pattern of the recipient site. Sebaceous glands, on the other hand, secrete independently of graft reinnervation by the recipient bed. Thin split-thickness skin grafts tend to be quite dry because they contain inadequate numbers of functioning sebaceous glands, which are more abundant in thicker grafts.

GRAFT REVASCULARIZATION

A phase of serum imbibition lasts for the first two days after placement of a skin graft. During this period, the graft is nourished by passive absorption of nutrients from serum in the recipient bed and not by direct vascular perfusion. The graft gains as much as 40 percent of extra weight because of fluid absorption. Vessels within the graft gradually dilate and fill with static columns of blood. A fibrin network in the wound bed causes graft adherence during this early phase.

The next phase in revascularization is a period of inosculation, during which anastomoses are formed between vessels in the graft and those in the wound bed. It is not clear, however, whether connections are established between existing vessels in the recipient bed and graft or whether new vessels grow into the graft from the recipient bed. Both processes may occur, and both may be important in graft revascularization. In any case, circulation is sluggish during the third and fourth postoperative days but gradually increases during the fifth and sixth postoperative days to become essentially normal by day 7.[17]

Lymphatic drainage from the graft is established at approximately the same rate as the circulation of blood. Lymphatic flow is present by the fifth to sixth postoperative day, and the graft starts losing the extra fluid weight it has gained. The graft begins to resume its normal weight by the ninth postoperative day.

FACTORS AFFECTING GRAFT SURVIVAL

Hematoma formation beneath a skin graft is the most common cause of graft failure. Blood accumulation interferes with graft adherence as well as with both imbibition and inosculation. Early evacuation of blood from beneath a skin graft can result in graft survival. Shear forces that result from inadequate immobilization cause graft failure by preventing or disrupting developing communications between vessels of the graft and the recipient bed. Infection of the recipient bed makes the bed unsuitable for grafting, and such infection is another major cause of graft failure. Proteolytic enzymes produced by microorganisms destroy the fibrin bond between the graft and recipient bed. Bacteria such as β-hemolytic streptococci and *Pseudomonas* are particularly virulent because they produce high levels of plasmin and other proteolytic enzymes. The type of organism present may actually be a more important factor in graft failure than the number of organisms.[18]

HEALING OF DONOR SITES

Donor sites for split-thickness grafts heal by reepithelialization. Epithelial cells from remaining portions of skin appendages, such as hair follicles, sebaceous glands, and sweat glands, migrate across the exposed dermis to establish a new epidermis. Donor sites for thin grafts heal more rapidly and leave less of a scar than those for thick grafts, which take longer to heal and can be associated with significant scarring. The epidermis of a healed donor site is fully differentiated within three to four weeks. The dermis shows little evidence of regeneration, however. An occlusive dressing such as Op-Site promotes more rapid healing of the donor site than coverage with fine mesh gauze.[14]

Flaps

FLAP NOMENCLATURE

Flaps are described by the types of tissue that they contain, their blood supply, and the method by which they are moved from the donor to the recipient site. Flaps commonly consist of skin and subcutaneous tissue alone. However, they may also consist of skin combined with either muscle, fascia, or bone; in these cases, the flaps would be called myocutaneous, fasciocutaneous, or osteocutaneous, respectively. Flaps of skin and subcutaneous tissue that contain a known major artery are described as axial-pattern, or arterialized, skin flaps. If such a flap is raised at the donor site and remains attached only by the vascular pedicle, it is termed an island flap. The same flap is termed a free flap if the vascular pedicle is severed, the flap is transferred to a distant recipient site, and its circulation is restored by microvascular anastomoses. Local flaps may be called either rotation, advancement, or transposition flaps, depending on how they are moved to reach their recipient sites. The combination of several descriptive terms provides a more complete characterization of flaps. For example, a muscle and skin flap that is rotated to cover an adjacent soft tissue defect is termed a myocutaneous rotation flap, and a skin and bone flap used to reconstruct a distant composite defect is termed an osteocutaneous free flap.

FLAP BLOOD SUPPLY

Plastic surgical reconstruction has evolved with the improved understanding of how blood is supplied to various body tissues. The earliest flaps in common use were skin flaps described as having a so-called random-pattern type of circulation [*see Figures 9 and 10*],[19] because they were supplied by the subdermal capillary plexus rather than by a major, named vessel. The precarious nature of the

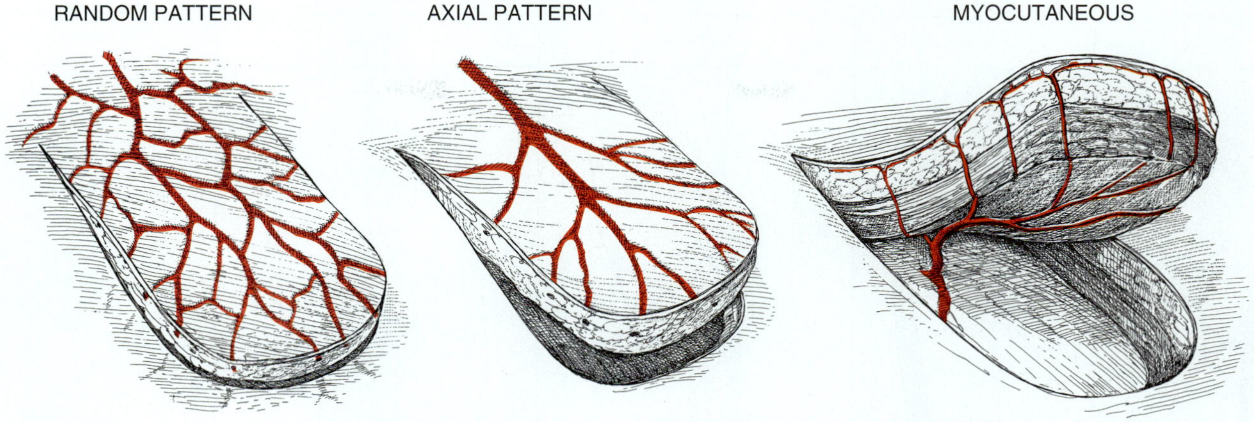

RANDOM PATTERN **AXIAL PATTERN** **MYOCUTANEOUS**

Figure 9 A random-pattern skin flap is supplied by a subdermal plexus of small vessels that do not have an axial orientation. An axial-pattern skin flap is designed parallel to the axis of a known major subcutaneous artery. It can have a greater length:width ratio because its blood supply is more reliable. A myocutaneous flap derives the blood supply of its skin component from vertical perforators from the underlying muscle. The skin can be completely isolated over the muscle as an island.

blood supply of such flaps severely limited flap design and resulted in a preoccupation with maintaining suitable length:width ratios. Greater length:width ratios became possible after the empirical discovery that a more vigorous circulation develops in flaps raised in stages.[20] The reason for this delay phenomenon is accommodation to ischemia, but the precise mechanism is still not well understood.

The next advance in flap technology was the identification of several body sites where a sizable artery coursed directly to a specific cutaneous territory. The groin was the first region where this

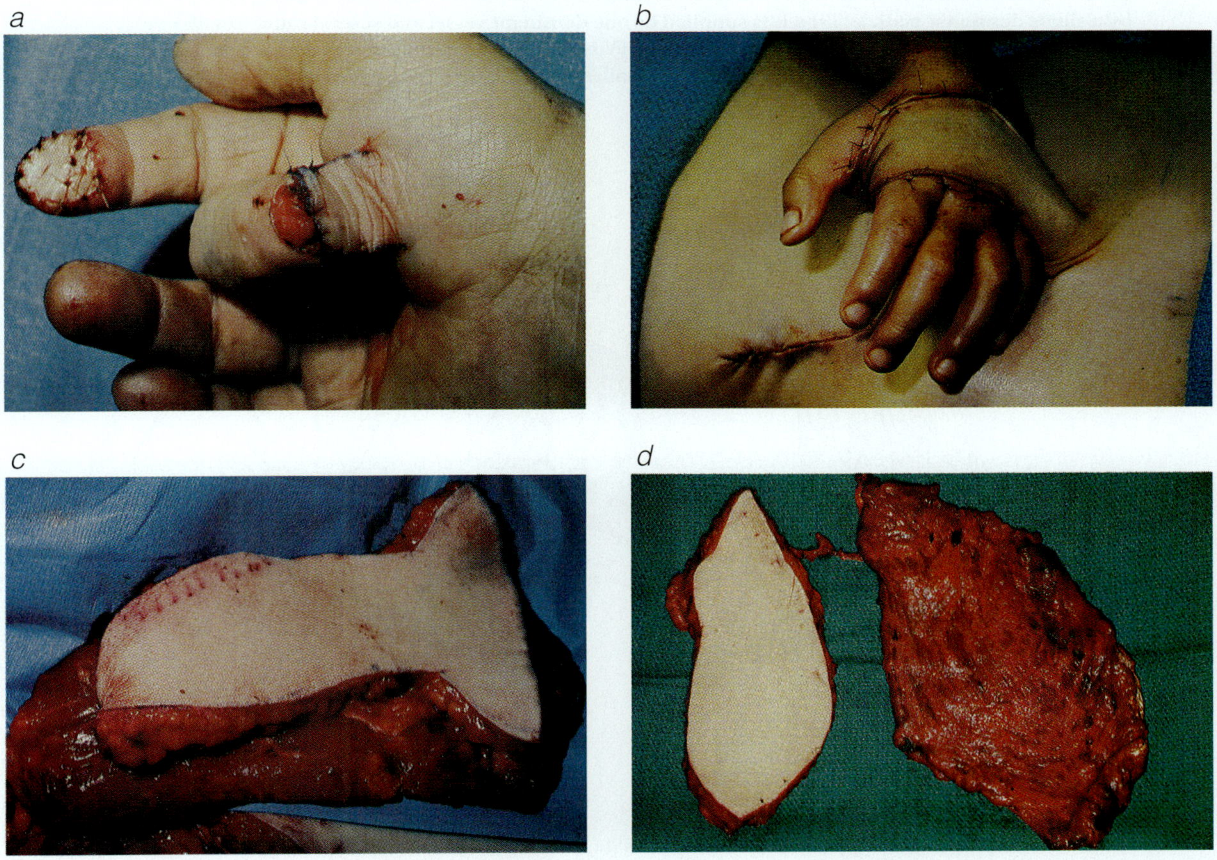

a

b

c

d

Figure 10 The blood supply of random-pattern skin flaps is quite limited, and only small flaps, such as thenar flaps (*a*), are consistently reliable. (*b*) An axial-pattern skin flap is shown. The skin and subcutaneous tissue of a myocutaneous flap (*c*) can exist as a complete island because the blood supply is derived from vertical muscular perforators. (*d*) A large free flap of scapular area skin and the entire latissimus dorsi muscle are shown. The subscapular vessels that connect the two will supply both components of the flap after microvascular anastomoses.

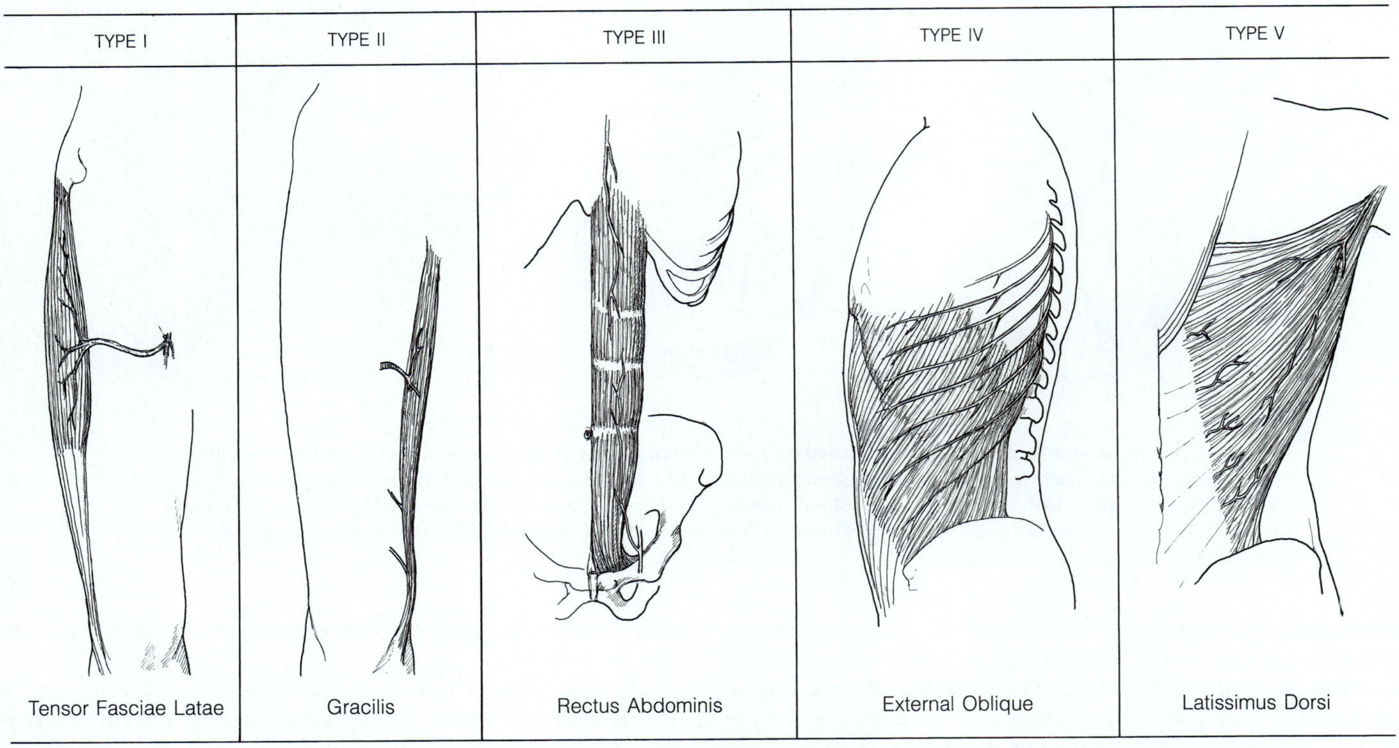

TYPE I	TYPE II	TYPE III	TYPE IV	TYPE V
Tensor Fasciae Latae	Gracilis	Rectus Abdominis	External Oblique	Latissimus Dorsi

Figure 11 Schematized are the five basic patterns of blood supply to muscle. Individual muscles are classified on the basis of the dominance, number, and size of the vessels that supply them. Type I is supplied by a single dominant pedicle. Type II is supplied by one dominant vessel and several much smaller vessels. Type III is supplied by two dominant pedicles. Type IV is supplied by multiple vessels of similar size. Type V is supplied by one dominant pedicle and several smaller segmental vascular pedicles.

arrangement was carefully described, and it remains a useful source of flaps for selected applications. Because longer flaps can be made in areas where the blood supply has an axial pattern [see Figures 9 and 10], the length:width ratio and delay phenomenon became less important issues in flap design.[21] Identification of a specific vessel as the supply for a certain territory of tissue allows so-called islanding of this tissue from the donor site except for the vascular connection, which is preserved. Such island flaps have greater mo-

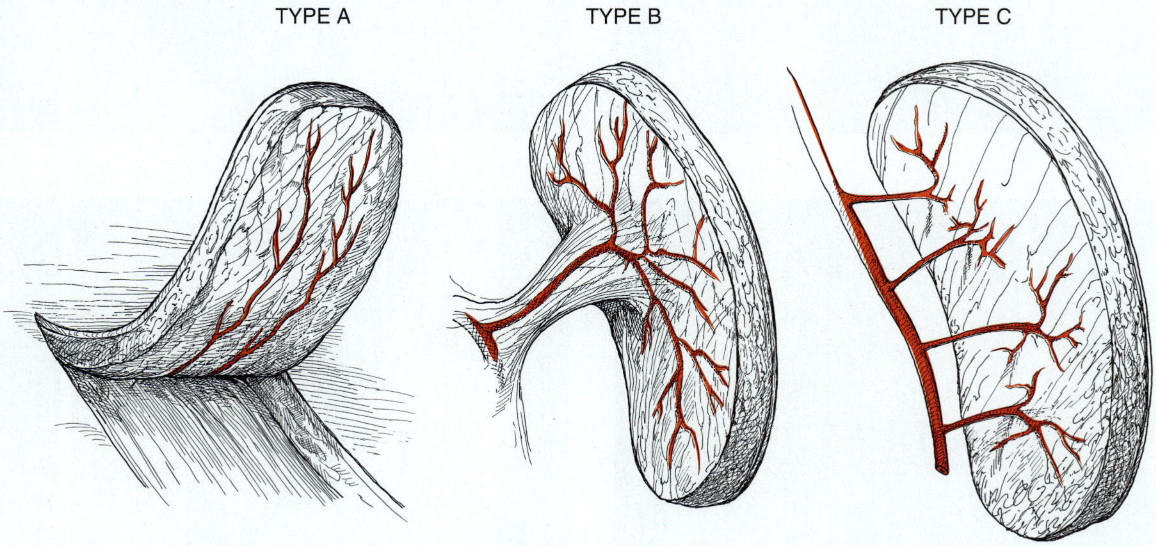

TYPE A   TYPE B   TYPE C

Figure 12 At least three types of fasciocutaneous flaps exist, categorized by blood supply configuration. Type A is supplied by multiple small, longitudinal vessels that course with the deep fascia. These flaps must retain a base of a certain width and cannot be raised as an island (e.g., longitudinally oriented flaps of skin and fascia on the lower leg). Type B is supplied by a single major vessel within the fascia (e.g., scapular flap). Type C is supplied by multiple perforating segments from a major vessel that courses through intermuscular septa (e.g., forearm flaps).

bility than do flaps that have a more significant soft tissue attachment to the donor site.

Another major advance in flap technology was an understanding of the important myocutaneous blood supply, a network of vessels that perforate muscles vertically and supply overlying cutaneous territories. These perforators are not necessarily the exclusive supply to the skin in a specific region, but they are able to support the skin entirely when other sources of blood supply are eliminated [see Figure 9]. This arrangement assumed great clinical significance when it was recognized that a skin flap could be designed as an island that is based on a muscle blood supply [see Figure 10] and that such an island could be safely moved anywhere within the arc of rotation of the particular muscle once the muscle was detached from its origin, its insertion, or both.[22]

The revolution in myocutaneous flaps took place in the 1970s. A systematic study of the blood supply to the muscle itself became important in the clinical application of the myocutaneous flap principle. Investigation of the body musculature showed that there were at least five basic patterns of blood supply to muscle, distinguished by the existence of and balance between primary pedicles and secondary sources of supply [see Figure 11]. Some muscles can be rotated or transposed as myocutaneous flaps on the basis of either their dominant or secondary blood supply (e.g., pectoralis major and latissimus dorsi). Some muscles have two dominant supplies and can be transposed on either one (e.g., rectus abdominis). Other muscles do not reliably support skin territories supplied by minor pedicles (e.g., gracilis).

Other patterns of cutaneous blood supply were later recognized and quickly assumed clinical importance. The discovery that larger skin flaps can be raised if the deep fascia is included led to more careful study of fascial blood supply. Fasciocutaneous flaps with high length:width ratios can be reliably raised on the trunk, arms, and legs. The blood supply of deep fascia appears to consist of both a deep and a superficial fascial plexus. These fascial vessels connect both to perforating vessels from the underlying muscles and to the subcutaneous tissue vessels above them.[23] At least three types of fasciocutaneous flaps have been described that are based on the nature of the fascial blood supply to the skin [see Figure 12].[24]

In some areas, fascia supplies overlying subcutaneous tissue and skin in a more direct fashion. This arrangement of fasciocutaneous blood supply is most evident in the extremities. There, direct branches from major vessels course through intermuscular septae to reach the deep fascia. The overlying skin and subcutaneous tissue are supplied by these so-called septocutaneous perforators. The forearm has become an important donor site clinically because thin septocutaneous flaps that are fed by the radial artery can be raised either as pedicled or free flaps. Other examples of fasciocutaneous flaps include the lateral arm septocutaneous flap, fed by the profunda brachii artery; the scapular flap, fed by the circumflex scapular artery; and the fibular osteofasciocutaneous flap, fed by the peroneal artery.

FLAP RESISTANCE TO INFECTION

Skin flaps, myocutaneous flaps, and fasciocutaneous flaps have been shown experimentally to vary in their resistance to bacterial infection.[25] Random-pattern skin flaps are not as resistant as myocutaneous flaps. The cutaneous portions of myocutaneous and of fasciocutaneous flaps have similar levels of resistance, but the muscle component of myocutaneous flaps is more resistant than the fascial component of fasciocutaneous flaps in situations where the flap lies over a focus of infection within the wound. Muscle therefore appears to be the type of flap most resistant to infection. Such resistance is of clinical significance in cases of exposed bone with chronic osteomyelitis, for example. This condition can be successfully treated by debridement and immediate coverage with a muscle flap.

FREE FLAPS: THE CONCEPT OF NO-REFLOW

Free tissue transfer is unique in that the flap is completely ischemic for a given period. How long ischemia can be tolerated without resultant flap failure (despite technically satisfactory microvascular anastomoses) is an important clinical question. An increasing duration of ischemia has been associated experimentally with obstruction to blood flow in the microcirculation.[26,27] This obstruction results from cellular edema, increased interstitial fluid pressure, and sludging of blood and thrombus formation. This phenomenon is initially reversible but becomes irreversible as the duration of ischemia increases. After 12 hours of ischemia under experimental conditions, obstruction to blood flow has been demonstrated to be complete, preventing successful reperfusion of the flap. How long uninterrupted ischemia can safely continue is not precisely known clinically, and evidence suggests that the ischemic tolerance of specific types of tissue varies. For example, flaps that are primarily bone are more durable than muscle or bowel flaps. Evidence gained by clinical experience has shown that up to four hours of ischemia is safely tolerated by most free flaps.

TISSUE EXPANSION

Histologic changes of expanded skin include thinning of the dermis but not of the epidermis,[28] suggesting a permanent net gain in epidermal tissue only. The mitotic rate in the epidermis has been shown to increase with expansion, but the mechanism for this increase is unclear.[29]

The circulation of expanded skin also changes. An increase in vascularity of expanded tissue is partially explained by the fact that tissue expansion is a form of delay procedure. However, experimental studies suggest that an increased potential for flap survivability is directly attributable to the expansion process and not merely to its delay component.[30-32] The fibrous capsule that forms around the prosthesis during expansion appears to contribute to the increased vascularity of these flaps, and the increased pressure around the expander may stimulate angiogenesis.

References

1. Stevenson TR, Thacker JG, Rodeheaver GT, et al: Cleansing of the traumatic wound by high pressure syringe irrigation. Journal of the American College of Emergency Physicians 5:17, 1976
2. Edlich RF, Rodeheaver GT, Thacker JG: Technical factors in the prevention of wound infection. Surgical Infectious Diseases. Simmons R, Howard R, Eds. Appleton-Century-Crofts, East Norwalk, Connecticut, 1981
3. Robson MC, Heggers JP: Delayed wound closures based on bacterial counts. J Surg Oncol 2:379, 1970
4. Lineaweaver W, Howard R, Soucy D, et al: Topical antimicrobial toxicity. Arch Surg 120:267, 1985
5. Jackson IT: Local Flaps in Head and Neck Reconstruction. CV Mosby, St Louis, 1985
6. Spinelli HM, Forman DL: Current treatment of posttraumatic deformities: residual orbital, adnexal, and soft-tissue abnormalities. Clin Plast Surg 24:519, 1997
7. Luce EA: Reconstruction of the lower lip. Clin Plast Surg 22:109, 1995
8. Mathes SJ, Eshima I: The principle of muscle and musculocutaneous flaps. Plastic Surgery, Vol 1. McCarthy JG, Ed. WB Saunders Co, Philadelphia, 1990, p 379

9. Taylor GI, Giantoutsos MP, Morris SF: The neurovascular territories of the skin and muscles: anatomic study and clinical implications. Plast Reconstr Surg 94:1, 1994
10. Hidalgo DA, Shaw WW: Reconstruction of foot injuries. Clin Plast Surg 13:663, 1986
11. May JW Jr, Halls MJ, Simón SR: Free microvascular muscle flaps with skin graft reconstruction of extensive defects of the foot: a clinical and gait analysis study. Plast Reconstr Surg 75:627, 1985
12. Bennett RG, Hirt M: A history of tissue expansion: concepts, controversies, and complications. J Dermatol Surg Oncol 19:1066, 1993
13. Shaw WW: Microvascular free flaps: the first decade. Clin Plast Surg 10:3, 1983
14. Smith DJ Jr, Thomson PD, Bolton LL: Microbiology and healing of the occluded skin-graft donor site. Plast Reconstr Surg 91:1094, 1993
15. McGrath MH, Hundahl SA: The spatial and temporal quantification of myofibroblasts. Plast Reconstr Surg 69:975, 1982
16. Rudolph R: Inhibition of myofibroblasts by skin grafts. Plast Reconstr Surg 63:473, 1979
17. Vasconez HC: Skin grafts. Mastery of Plastic and Reconstructive Surgery, Vol 1. Cohen M, Ed. Little, Brown & Co, Boston, 1994, p 45
18. Teh BT: Why do skin grafts fail? Plast Reconstr Surg 63:323, 1979
19. Daniel RK, Kerrigan CL: Skin flaps: an anatomical and hemodynamic approach. Clin Plast Surg 6:181, 1979
20. Cederna PS, Chang P, Pittet-Cuenod BM, et al: The effect of the delay phenomenon on the vascularity of rabbit abdominal cutaneous island flaps. Plast Reconstr Surg 99:183, 1997
21. Milton SH: Pedicled skin-flaps: the fallacy of the length:width ratio. Br J Surg 57:502, 1970
22. McCraw JB, Vasconez LO: Musculocutaneous flaps: principles. Clin Plast Surg 7:9, 1980
23. Tolhurst DE, Haeseker B, Zeeman RJ: The development of the fasciocutaneous flap and its clinical applications. Plast Reconstr Surg 71:597, 1983
24. Cormack GC, Lamberty BG: Arterial Anatomy of Skin Flaps. Churchill Livingstone, Edinburgh, 1987
25. Gosain A, Chang N, Mathes S, et al: A study of the relationship between blood flow and bacterial inoculation in musculocutaneous and fasciocutaneous flaps. Plast Reconstr Surg 86:1152, 1990
26. Kerrigan CL, Stotland MA: Ischemia reperfusion injury: a review. Microsurgery 14:165, 1993
27. Kirschner RE, Fyfe BS, Hoffman LA, et al: Ischemia-reperfusion injury in myocutaneous flaps: role of leukocytes and leukotrienes. Plast Reconstr Surg 99:1485, 1997
28. Johnson TM, Lowe L, Brown MD, et al: Histology and physiology of tissue expansion. J Dermatol Surg Oncol 19:1074, 1993
29. Olenius M, Johansson O: Variations in epidermal thickness in expanded human breast skin. Scand J Plast Reconstr Hand Surg 29:15, 1995
30. Babovic S, Angel MF, Im MJ, et al: Effects of tissue expansion on secondary ischemic tolerance in experimental free flaps. Ann Plast Surg 34:593, 1995
31. Matturri L, Azzolini A, Riberti C, et al: Long-term histopathologic evaluation of human expanded skin. Plast Reconstr Surg 90:636, 1992
32. Olenius M, Dalsgaard CJ, Wickman M: Mitotic activity in expanded human skin. Plast Reconstr Surg 91:213, 1993

Acknowledgment

Figures 3, 6, 7, 9, 11, and 12   Carol Donner.

VI SPECIAL PERIOPERATIVE PROBLEMS

68 DIABETES MELLITUS

Maha F. Ansara, M.D., Philip E. Cryer, M.D., and David W. Scharp, M.D.

Perioperative Management of the Diabetic Patient

Patients with diabetes have a 50 percent chance of undergoing surgical procedures during their lifetime.[1] In the past, operation in these patients was associated with a mortality of four to 13 percent,[2,3] usually attributed to cardiovascular complications. This statistic suggests the risks of performing operative procedures in diabetic patients. Any improvement in this situation has probably been offset by the increasing age of patients with diabetes and the larger variety of procedures they undergo.

The perioperative management of diabetic patients is complicated by the metabolic abnormalities of the disease and, if present, the effects of atherosclerotic disease, diabetic nephropathy, and autonomic neuropathy. There is also an increased risk of postoperative wound infection.

Nomenclature

The term insulin-dependent diabetes mellitus (IDDM) is applied to all forms of diabetes in which exogenous insulin is required to prevent diabetic ketoacidosis, regardless of the etiology. IDDM is not, however, synonymous with type I diabetes, which is the term applied to diabetes that results from autoimmune destruction of beta cells, regardless of whether the destruction is sufficient to cause ketoacidosis. The term non–insulin-dependent diabetes mellitus (NIDDM) can be applied to any form of diabetes in which endogenous insulin production is sufficient to prevent diabetic ketoacidosis. NIDDM is not synonymous with type II diabetes; the latter term should be restricted to patients with NIDDM who do not have autoimmune destruction of beta cells (type I diabetes), diabetes secondary to pancreatic disease, or other hyperglycemic conditions. Thus, IDDM is distinguished from NIDDM on the basis of the need for exogenous insulin for survival, whereas type I diabetes is distinguished from type II on the basis of the presence of autoimmune beta cell destruction.

Type I diabetes accounts for approximately three percent of all new cases of diabetes diagnosed each year in the United States. Although type I is much less common in the general population than type II, it is by no means rare among children and young adults. The estimated annual incidence of new cases of type I diabetes in children is one per 7,000, making this disorder three to four times more common than chronic childhood diseases such as cystic fibrosis, peptic ulcer, juvenile rheumatoid arthritis, and leukemia and nearly 10 times more common than nephrotic syndrome, muscular dystrophy, or lymphoma.

After 20 years of age, the yearly incidence of type I diabetes decreases to five per 100,000. The incidence is similar in men and women, lower in African Americans than in whites, and still lower in Latinos, Asian Americans, and Native Americans. Two to five percent of the siblings of persons with type I diabetes will acquire the disorder; among identical twins, one of whom has type I diabetes, concordance rates are only 50 percent.

Criteria for Diagnosis

Possible causes of perioperative hyperglycemia [*see Table 1*] must be carefully evaluated before operation. Diabetes is diagnosed de novo in a significant number of patients admitted for routine procedures. The measurement of blood glucose, glycosylated hemoglobin, or even urine glucose in outpatients could lead to earlier diagnosis, preventing last-minute detection of diabetes. If perioperative hyperglycemia is diagnosed in the hospital, major procedures should be delayed until patients have received proper metabolic and cardiovascular assessment. For patients with mild glycemic disturbances and those undergoing minor procedures, metabolic adjustments can be made quickly.

Fasting plasma glucose levels greater than 140 mg/dl (7.8 mmol/L) or random plasma glucose levels in excess of 200 mg/dl (11.1 mmol/L) are indicative of diabetes. Other signs and symptoms are polyuria, polydipsia, polyphagia, weight loss, and blurred vision. If the fasting plasma glucose levels are below 140 mg/dl (7.8 mmol/L), the diagnosis may be established by the results of an oral glucose tolerance test [*see Table 2*].

Table 1 **Possible Causes of Perioperative Hyperglycemia**

Diabetes mellitus
- Insulin-dependent (IDDM)
- Non–insulin-dependent (NIDDM)

Impaired glucose tolerance (secondary diabetes mellitus)
- Pancreatic disease
- Endocrinopathies (e.g., acromegaly, Cushing's syndrome, pheochromocytoma, glucagonoma, and primary aldosteronism)
- Chemical agents (e.g., estrogen, glucocorticoids, catecholamines, certain antihypertensive agents, thiazides, and psychoactive agents)
- Insulin-receptor abnormalities (e.g., acanthosis nigricans)
- Genetic disorders (e.g., hyperlipidemia, Huntington's disease, and muscular dystrophies)
- Miscellaneous conditions (e.g., malnutrition)

Perioperative Management of the Diabetic Patient

Diabetic patient is scheduled to undergo operation

Perform patient evaluation:

History: Look for recent fluctuations in blood glucose levels; consider timing and dosages of current medications; watch for diabetic complications (e.g., neuropathy, nephropathy, peripheral vascular disorders, cardiac disease).

Physical examination: Assess eyes, skin, neurologic system, and cardiovascular system.

Laboratory tests: Measure levels of plasma glucose (after fasting and 2 hr after eating), HbA_{1c}, electrolytes, ketones, serum creatinine; obtain blood gas values; perform ECG with Valsalva maneuver to rule out cardiac autonomic neuropathy.

Before operation

Monitor metabolic status: If glycemic control is not achieved before admission, schedule admission for 12–16 hr before operation to allow time to optimize control of diabetes. Target values for blood glucose are < 125 mg/dl (fasting) and < 180 mg/dl (postprandial). If emergency operation is required in a patient with a severe metabolic derangement, provide 6–8 hr of intensive treatment. Substitute intermediate-acting insulins for long-acting and, in NIDDM, short-acting sulfonylureas for long-acting. Discontinue metformin. Correct any dehydration.

Assess cardiovascular and renal systems: Watch particularly for cardiac autonomic neuropathy. On ECG, ratio of longest RR interval to shortest during Valsalva maneuver is normally ≥ 1.21; 1.11–1.20 is borderline, and ≤ 1.10 is abnormal. Look for hypoglycemia (in patients taking beta blockers) and thrombosis. Measure BUN, serum creatinine, electrolytes, and urine protein. Consider monitoring central venous pressure or pulmonary arterial wedge pressure.

During operation

Administer insulin, glucose, or both.

Elective major procedures

If patient has type I diabetes, takes insulin for type II, or has type II that is not controlled by drugs or diet, give glucose and short-acting insulin. Target value for blood glucose is between 125 and 200 mg/dl.

Minor procedures

If patient fasted, withhold morning dose of insulin or oral hypoglycemic agent, give short-acting insulin every 2–4 hr, and resume normal dosing after procedure. If patient ate breakfast, give normal morning does, give 4 U of short-acting insulin if blood glucose > 250 mg/dl, and resume normal dosing after procedure.

Emergency procedures

If emergency operation precipitates metabolic decompensation, manage patient conservatively at first, emphasizing correction of any underlying metabolic cause. If problem is metabolic, it should resolve or improve in 3–4 hr; if it is surgical, it will remain the same or worsen over the same period.

Prevent renal dysfunction: Use contrast agents with caution, choosing the least invasive procedure that will provide adequate data; give mannitol and furosemide from 1 hr before to 6 hr after the study; give saline in D5W with potassium.

After operation

Administer insulin and glucose: Infusion should be continued until patient can tolerate oral feeding. If patient is receiving TPN, give insulin only.

Assess cardiovascular and renal systems: If patient is older, has long-standing type I diabetes, or has heart disease, perform serial ECGs. Watch for MI and orthostatic hypotension. Monitor BUN and serum creatinine levels, ensure adequate hydration, and correct any electrolyte abnormalities.

Evaluation of the Diabetic Patient

HISTORY

In the preoperative history, attention should be directed to any recent fluctuation in blood glucose as well as to the type of therapy used to control the patient's diabetes. Inquiries should cover the timing and dosage of medication, especially if the patient is using a long-acting insulin or an oral hypoglycemic. The degree of control of diabetes in the perioperative period, which has an impact on the patient's postoperative recovery, could be affected by certain medications, such as antihypertensive agents. The presence of diabetic complications (e.g., neuropathy, peripheral vascular disorders, nephropathy, and cardiac disease) should be documented because they may have serious effects during and after operation.

The incidence of peripheral neuropathy increases with the age of the patient and the duration of diabetes.[4] Diabetic neuropathies, which mimic many syndromes, should be considered in the differential diagnosis of all patients who are candidates for operation. Patients with cardiac autonomic neuropathy, who are at risk for sudden cardiorespiratory arrest, may have orthostatic hypotension that is not associated with tachycardia, evidence of peripheral neuropathy, and manifestations of other autonomic neuropathies such as nocturnal diarrhea and gustatory sweating.[5]

Diabetic nephropathy alters the clearance of numerous drugs and increases the renal threshold for glucose, making it possible for a patient to produce a urine sample that is negative for glucose even though the plasma glucose level is higher than 300 mg/dl. This condition should be suspected if the patient has overt proteinuria, hypertension, or decreasing insulin requirements. Diabetic nephropathy increases the risk of acute renal failure after the administration of iodinated contrast agents. In some patients, contrast-associated renal failure results in permanent impairment of kidney function, necessitating dialysis.

PHYSICAL EXAMINATION

Specific areas for attention on physical examination are the eyes, the skin, and the neurologic and cardiovascular systems.

Diabetic retinopathy is often asymptomatic in its most treatable stages. Unfortunately, only 45 percent of the diabetic population receives adequate ophthalmic care.[6] Retinopathy rarely occurs in patients who have had type I diabetes for less than five years; after 10 years, however, some degree of retinopathy is present in 60 percent. Proliferative diabetic retinopathy (PDR) is unusual before the disorder has been present for 10 years but is present in 26 percent of type I diabetes patients after 15 years. Diabetic retinopathy is present in approximately 20 percent of patients with type II diabetes at the time of diagnosis; after 15 years, the percentage increases to 60 to 85 percent. PDR is present in three to four percent of the patients who have had type II diabetes for less than four years; after 15 years, five to 20 percent of type II diabetes patients have PDR.[6] Cataracts are four to six times more likely to develop at a young age.

The progressive signs of diabetic retinopathy are the formation of microaneurysms, the development of new vessels elsewhere on the retina (with or without periretinal or vitreous hemorrhage), contraction of the vitreous humor, and retinal detachment. Diabetic macular edema, which occurs at any level of diabetic retinopathy, is best detected by stereoscopic examination of macules with a slit-lamp biomicroscope or a funduscope. Diabetic macular edema may be associated with nonproliferative diabetic retinopathy, which is manifested by formation of retinal microaneurysms, hard exudate, and intraretinal microvascular abnormalities. The nonproliferative form may advance to proliferative diabetic retinopathy, in which new vessels form, with or without preretinal or vitreous hemorrhage. Panretinal photocoagulation has beneficial effects for all eyes threatened by retinopathy.

Diabetic dermopathy is characterized by multiple hyperpigmented macules on the extensor surface of the distal lower extremities. The individual lesions are oval or circular, ranging in size from 0.5 to 2.0 cm, and are sometimes associated with atrophy and scaling. These skin changes, also referred to as shin spots or pigmented pretibial patches, occasionally occur in persons with no evidence of glucose intolerance. Except for its appearance, the dermopathy is generally asymptomatic. No effective treatment has been described.

Table 2 Diagnostic Criteria for Diabetes Mellitus, Gestational Diabetes, and Impaired Glucose Tolerance

Diabetes mellitus

In nonpregnant adults, diagnosis should be restricted to those meeting *one* of the following criteria:
- Random plasma glucose level ≥ 200 mg/dl *plus* classic signs and symptoms of diabetes mellitus.
- Fasting plasma glucose level ≥ 140 mg/dl on at least two occasions
- Fasting plasma glucose level < 140 mg/dl *plus* sustained elevated plasma glucose levels during at least two oral glucose tolerance tests. The 2-hr sample and at least one other from the first 2 hr after a 75 g glucose dose should be ≥ 200 mg/dl. Oral glucose tolerance testing is not necessary if the patient has a fasting plasma glucose level ≥ 140 mg/dl.

In children, diagnosis should be restricted to those meeting *one* of the following criteria:
- Random plasma glucose level ≥ 200 mg/dl *plus* classic signs and symptoms of diabetes mellitus.
- Fasting plasma glucose level ≥ 140 mg/dl on at least two occasions *plus* sustained elevated plasma glucose levels during at least two oral glucose tolerance tests. The 2-hr sample and at least one other from the first 2 hr after a glucose dose (1.75 g/kg of ideal body weight, up to 75 g) should be ≥ 200 mg/dl.

Gestational diabetes

The diagnosis can be made if, on two occasions, oral intake of 100 g of glucose results in plasma glucose values that are (1) ≥ 105 mg/dl while the patient is fasting or (2) ≥ 190 mg/dl at 1 hr, ≥ 165 mg/dl at 2 hr, or ≥ 145 mg/dl at 3 hr postprandially.

Impaired glucose tolerance

In nonpregnant adults, the diagnosis should be restricted to those meeting *all* of the following criteria:
- Fasting plasma glucose level < 140 mg/dl.
- 2-hr oral glucose tolerance test result between 140 and 200 mg/dl.
- Intervening oral glucose tolerance test result ≥ 200 mg/dl.

In children, the diagnosis should be restricted to those who have *both* of the following:
- Fasting plasma glucose concentration < 140 mg/dl.
- 2-hr oral glucose tolerance test result > 140 mg/dl.

Necrobiosis lipoidica diabeticorum (NLD) is characterized by red to red-brown to violet plaques that enlarge, often becoming yellow at the center. The overlying skin is usually shiny and transparent because of epidermal atrophy. In 90 percent of patients, this condition is most likely to occur on the shins, but it can also be found on the scalp, face, arms, and trunk. NLD lesions, especially in the distal lower extremities, may ulcerate. There is no well-established treatment for the condition, but some success has been reported with pentoxifylline (400 mg three times daily), dipyridamole (50 to 75 mg three or four times daily) plus low-dose aspirin (325 mg/day), and intralesional corticosteroids (5 mg/ml of triamcinolone acetonide). With triamcinolone acetonide, there may be breakdown of skin lesions.[7]

Lipodystrophy may appear as atrophic or hypertrophic lesions that are thought to be caused by a local response to insulin administration. Use of a less antigenic form of insulin, deeper insulin injections, and frequent changes of injection sites are recommended. When subcutaneous fat has disappeared, improvement has been reported after the injection of purified insulin into the edge of the lipoatrophy.

In tissues affected by vascular insufficiency, minor trauma may lead to infection. Patients with peripheral sensory neuropathy may not be aware of these minor injuries and may fail to treat them. Infections may undermine extensive amounts of tissue, especially in the feet or at pressure points (bedsores). These infections are caused by both aerobic and anaerobic organisms.

The peripheral polyneuropathy of diabetes is distributed in a stocking-glove pattern. The lancinating pain of diabetic radiculopathy is dramatic and can mimic abdominal pain caused by other disorders. Confirmation of the diagnosis of diabetic neuropathy may depend on electromyography and, in rare cases, nerve biopsy.

LABORATORY TESTS

Plasma levels of glucose should be measured while the patient is fasting and two hours after he or she has eaten; long-term diabetic control can be assessed by measurement of glycosylated hemoglobin (HbA_{1c}) concentrations. The potential for metabolic disturbances can be gauged from measurement of electrolyte and ketone levels and arterial blood gas values. Serum creatinine levels can be used to monitor renal function, and an ECG performed in conjunction with the Valsalva maneuver can rule out cardiac autonomic neuropathy.

Preoperative Management

METABOLIC MONITORING

All diabetic patients who are candidates for elective surgical procedures require careful preoperative assessment, including metabolic monitoring [see Table 3]. Ideally, diabetic patients achieve glycemic control before being admitted to the hospital. It may be more realistic, however, to schedule admission for 12 to 16 hours before the operation to allow time to optimize metabolic control in all insulin-dependent patients and in non–insulin-dependent patients who have inadequate metabolic control. In general, preoperative blood glucose targets should be less than 125 mg/dl (6.9 mmol/L) during fasting and less than 180 mg/dl (10.0 mmol/L) postprandially. If emergency operation is required in patients with severe metabolic derangements (diabetic ketoacidosis or hyperosmolar nonketotic states), six to eight hours of intensive treatment usually improves their general condition. This brief period permits clarification of the diagnosis in patients with acute abdominal pain, which may be the consequence of diabetic ketoacidosis rather than the so-called surgical abdomen.

The current practice in preparing diabetic patients for operation is to stop all use of long-acting insulins (Ultralente preparations), replacing them with intermediate-acting insulins (the neutral protamine Hagedorn [NPH] or Lente preparations). In patients with NIDDM, use of long-acting sulfonylureas such as chlorpropamide and glyburide should be stopped because of the risk of hypoglycemia; a short-acting preparation should be substituted. Use of metformin should be stopped because of the risks of lactic acidosis when renal function is impaired, as it may be during any procedure requiring anesthesia. Chronically hyperglycemic patients are frequently dehydrated, and this condition must be corrected before operation.

CARDIOVASCULAR AND RENAL ASSESSMENT

Coronary artery disease and hypertensive vascular disease are common in diabetic patients. Thorough evaluation of a patient's cardiovascular condition should include careful assessment of the autonomic nervous system because of the known risks of cardiorespiratory arrest in patients with auto-

---

Table 3 **Preoperative Assessment and Preparation of the Diabetic Patient**

Assessment
 Cardiovascular
  History (hypertension, angina, infarction)
  Blood pressure
  Full examination, including peripheral pulse rates
  Electrocardiogram
 Neurologic
  Peripheral neuropathy
  Autonomic examination: RR interval
 Renal
  Proteinuria
  Serum creatinine levels
  Urinalysis
 Metabolic
  Home glucose control
  Glycosylated hemoglobin
  Electrolytes (sodium, potassium)

Preparation
 Patients with insulin-dependent diabetes mellitus (IDDM)
  Stop administration of long-acting insulin
  Substitute b.i.d. intermediate-acting insulin (NPH or Lente) combined with t.i.d. regular insulin before meals
 Patients with non–insulin-dependent diabetes mellitus (NIDDM)
  Stop administration of long-acting sulfonylureas (e.g., chlorpropamide), but substitute a short-acting one if necessary
  Stop administration of metformin
  Reinforce dietary advice

nomic neuropathy. Cardiac autonomic neuropathy can usually be diagnosed preoperatively by means of electrocardiography. One method calculates the ratio of the longest RR interval to the shortest RR interval during the Valsalva maneuver. The normal ratio is 1.21 or higher, a borderline ratio is 1.11 to 1.20, and an abnormal ratio is 1.10 or lower.[8] (Occasionally, however, older nondiabetic patients have a ratio lower than 1.03.) The poor prognosis of patients with cardiac autonomic neuropathy, in whom mortality reaches 50 percent within 2.5 years of diagnosis,[9] may influence the decision to perform an elective procedure in this group.

Well-controlled hypertension does not pose special risks during operation, but hypoglycemia may develop without warning in patients receiving beta blockers, who should be monitored accordingly. Patients with type I diabetes (resulting from autoimmune destruction of beta cells) who use beta blockers are also at greater risk for prolonged episodes of insulin-induced hypoglycemia. All diabetic patients are at increased risk for thrombosis. Unless its use is specifically contraindicated, 5,000 units of heparin should be administered subcutaneously every eight to 12 hours to diabetic patients who are confined to bed, whether before or after operation.

Measurement of blood urea nitrogen, serum creatinine, electrolytes, and urine protein should be performed before operation. Azotemic patients may have problems with fluid management, and monitoring of central venous or pulmonary arterial wedge pressure may be necessary. Hyperkalemia, often seen in patients with mild to moderate kidney failure, can precipitate acute cardiac arrhythmia. This metabolic finding usually results from hyporeninemic hypoaldosteronism. Hypokalemia, if present, may be aggravated by use of insulin and glucose therapy.

Intraoperative Management

METABOLIC EFFECTS OF OPERATION AND ANESTHESIA

Surgical procedures and anesthesia have profound metabolic effects that are exacerbated by insulin deficiency or hyposecretion and by insulin insensitivity. The effects of operation are amplified in patients who are in a catabolic state, as are diabetic patients with poor metabolic control.

During anesthesia and operation, endogenous insulin secretion is suppressed but the plasma levels of counterregulatory hormones (glucagon, epinephrine, cortisol, and growth hormone) increase in nondiabetic as well as diabetic patients. The increased secretion of these hormones in the setting of low insulin levels stimulates hepatic glucose production. In nondiabetic persons, major procedures are frequently associated with blood glucose levels of 150 to 200 mg/dl (8.3 to 11.1 mmol/L). In diabetic persons, the metabolic abnormality varies according to the extent and duration of the surgical procedure and the impairment of insulin secretion.

Two studies in patients with stable IDDM have shown blood glucose levels rising from about 180 mg/dl (10.0 mmol/L) to about 270 mg/dl (15.0 mmol/L) postoperatively, with ketone body levels rising to about twice the levels in nondiabetic control subjects.[10,11] The situation is similar metabolically even in patients with NIDDM who undergo minor procedures that generate relatively little stress—blood glucose levels rising to 180 mg/dl (10.0 mmol/L), with higher than normal levels of ketone bodies and free fatty acids.[12]

Autonomic neuropathy can cause severe hypotension during induction of anesthesia. Diabetic nephropathy complicates fluid management, usually resulting in electrolyte abnormalities. All diabetic patients are at higher risk for postoperative myocardial infarction, which is often asymptomatic. Poor nutrition and impaired phagocytosis make diabetic patients more susceptible to infection and slower to heal.

INSULIN AND GLUCOSE ADMINISTRATION

Elective Major Procedures

In a patient undergoing general anesthesia, regardless of the duration of the operation, infusion of insulin and glucose is recommended if the patient has type I diabetes, takes insulin for type II diabetes, or uses drugs or diet therapy (or both) but has not achieved satisfactory control of type II diabetes. Several methods of insulin administration have been recommended for use during the perioperative period. Most of the protocols include the intravenous administration of short-acting insulin and five to 10 percent glucose.

In some of the protocols, the glucose and insulin are administered in a single infusion. The advantage of this approach is that if the glucose infusion is accidentally disconnected or obstructed, the insulin infusion is as well, so that the risk of hypoglycemia is eliminated. The disadvantage of this method is that it is impossible to change the delivery rate of one agent without changing the delivery rate of the other. The administration of insulin and glucose in separate bags but through the same vein (that is, piggybacked) allows either infusion rate to be changed without affecting the other. The insulin infusion rate is progressively increased, and the glucose infusion rate is progressively decreased, according to the capillary blood glucose levels, measured hourly [see Table 4]. With this protocol, a blood glucose level in the range of 125 to 200 mg/dl (6.9 to 11.1 mmol/L) is easily maintained during the entire perioperative period. Close observation of blood glucose levels and prompt adjustment of insulin and glucose delivery are mandatory to achieve a stable blood glucose level. Electrolyte supplementation is administered via a separate infusion.

In patients who are fluid restricted or those receiving large amounts of other solutions, 10 percent dextrose in water (D10W) can be substituted for the five percent dextrose (D5W) solution. If D10W is not available, it can be made by adding 100 ml of 50 percent dextrose in water (D50W) to 1 L of D5W. D50W can be administered in the central line in patients with severe congestive heart failure or end-stage renal disease, whose fluid intake is severely restricted. For a person weighing 70 kg, this corresponds to a glucose infusion rate of 2 mg/kg/min. Clinical judgment dictates changes in the infusion protocol as necessary, the glucose infusion rate remaining constant while the insulin infusion rate is modified. The blood glucose level must be monitored hourly. Capillary blood glucose levels can be measured with glucose oxidase strips and a reflectance meter in the operating and recovery rooms. With appropriate adjustments of the insulin-glucose infusion algorithm, blood glucose levels will remain between 125 and 200 mg/dl (6.9 and 11.1 mmol/L).

Table 4 Representative Protocol for Insulin-Glucose Infusion during the Perioperative Period

1. Infuse 5% dextrose in water (D5W) I.V. via pump.
2. Make insulin solution with 0.5 U/ml of short-acting insulin (i.e., 250 U of regular insulin in 500 ml of normal saline). Administer in piggyback fashion via infusion pump into D5W infusion.
3. After initiating glucose-insulin infusion, stop all subcutaneous insulin therapy.
4. Measure capillary blood glucose levels every hour.
5. On the basis of hourly blood glucose levels, adjust each infusion according to the following schedule:

Blood Glucose (mg/dl)	Insulin Infusion (ml/hr)	Insulin Infusion (U/hr)	D5W Infusion (ml/hr)
< 70*	1.0	0.5	150
71–100	2.0	1.0	125
101–150	3.0	1.5	100
151–200	4.0	2.0	100
201–250	6.0	3.0	100
251–300	8.0	4.0	75
> 300	12.0	6.0	50

*Give 10 ml D5W I.V. and repeat blood glucose measurement 15 min later.

abdomen, it is crucial to ascertain whether there may be a metabolic cause for the condition. The sensible approach is to manage the patient conservatively at first, with an emphasis on metabolic correction. If the problem is metabolic, it should resolve or improve in three to four hours; a surgical problem will remain the same or worsen in three to four hours.

PREVENTION OF RENAL DYSFUNCTION

Injudicious use of contrast agents can cause permanent impairment of renal function, necessitating dialysis. In patients with preexisting renal disease, certain measures can prevent contrast-associated renal failure. These include selection of the least invasive procedure that will provide adequate diagnostic information. The following recommendations can be used for patients whose serum creatinine is at or above 2 mg/dl (≥ 176.9 mmol/L) at baseline: one hour before the contrast study, begin infusing 20 ml/hr of a solution of 500 ml of 20 percent mannitol with 200 mg of furosemide added; continue this infusion uninterrupted for six hours after completion of the study; and give 0.5 N saline in D5W with 30 mEq/L of potassium to replace the urine output. Although this regimen has not been validated by controlled studies, it appears to be safe. Many clinicians recommend the use of nonionic low-osmolar contrast agents in diabetic patients with renal insufficiency to reduce the risk of significant renal ischemia, but there is no evidence justifying the considerable cost of the newer agents.[13]

Minor Procedures

Diabetic patients who fast before minor operations (for example, endoscopy or procedures performed with the patient under local anesthesia) should omit the morning dose of insulin or oral hypoglycemic agent. Their capillary blood glucose level should be measured every two to four hours. Supplemental subcutaneous short-acting insulin can be administered according to a variable insulin schedule, and the usual insulin or oral agent can be taken after the procedure [see Table 5]. This method of administration, which is associated with unpredictable absorption and variable plasma insulin levels, is restricted to surgical patients undergoing minor procedures and should not be used in patients undergoing major operations.

Emergency Procedures

Diabetic patients may be more likely than nondiabetic patients to undergo emergency operation, which can cause rapid metabolic decompensation with dehydration, hyperglycemia, and ketoacidosis. Uncontrolled diabetes may also be precipitated in patients with no history of diabetes. Management depends, to a large extent, on the patient's metabolic condition. In a patient with a so-called surgical

Table 5 Management of Diabetes in Patients Undergoing Minor Surgical Procedures[20]

If patient fasted

1. Withhold morning dose of insulin or oral agent.
2. Measure capillary blood glucose level before procedure and every 2–4 hr thereafter.
3. Give short-acting insulin every 2–4 hr, as follows:

Blood Glucose (mg/dl)	Short-Acting Insulin (U)
< 150	0
151–200	2
201–250	3
251–300	5
> 300	6

4. After procedure, give usual dose of insulin or oral agent.

If patient ate breakfast

1. Give normal morning dose of insulin or oral agent.
2. Measure blood glucose levels before and after procedure.
3. Give supplemental 4 U of short-acting insulin if blood glucose level exceeds 250 mg/dl.
4. After prodecure, give usual afternoon dose of insulin or oral agent.

Postoperative Management

INSULIN AND GLUCOSE ADMINISTRATION

After a minor procedure, a diabetic patient should receive glucose and insulin by infusion until the metabolic condition is stable and oral feeding can be tolerated. To prevent ketosis, the insulin and glucose infusions should be continued for at least one hour after the administration of subcutaneous short-acting insulin. After a major procedure, the patient should receive glucose and insulin infusions until he or she is able to take solid food without difficulty. The regimen of multiple subcutaneous injections of short-acting insulin before meals and intermediate-acting insulin twice daily is recommended during the first 24 to 48 hours after cessation of the insulin and glucose infusions and before resumption of the patient's usual insulin regimen [see Table 6].

Total parenteral nutrition (TPN), often required during the postoperative period, can cause serious metabolic derangements in diabetic patients. A variable insulin infusion schedule [see Table 4], with hourly determinations of blood glucose, is recommended under these circumstances, but additional glucose is not needed, because it is included in the TPN solution. Initially, the insulin should be given as a continuous infusion separate from the TPN solution. Once a stable dose of insulin is reached (usually within 24 to 48 hours), the total amount of insulin required over 24 hours can be added to the TPN bag. This amount may be high—often more than 100 units daily. At this point, capillary blood glucose levels can be measured every two to four hours.

CARDIOVASCULAR AND RENAL ASSESSMENT

Serial postoperative electrocardiograms are recommended for older diabetic patients, those with long-standing type I diabetes, and those with known heart disease. Postoperative myocardial infarction, which may be silent, has a high mortality. When the patient begins to walk, the possibility of orthostatic hypotension must be considered.

Careful monitoring of blood urea nitrogen and serum creatinine levels facilitates the detection of acute kidney failure, which may occur after procedures involving the administration of iodinated contrast material. If a contrast agent is used, the patient should be well hydrated before and after the procedure. Electrolyte abnormalities, such as elevated or decreased levels of potassium, must be treated aggressively.

INFECTION

Wound infection is common in diabetic patients with poor metabolic control. Impaired granulocyte function, resulting from hyperglycemia, may predispose to bacterial infections. If autonomic neuropathy is present, it may lead to difficulty in postoperative voiding, which increases the risk of urinary tract infection. Poor circulation as a result of macroangiopathy or microangiopathy can also contribute to the likelihood of postoperative infection.

Tight metabolic control during the perioperative period can decrease the risk of postoperative infection. If wound infections occur, they are usually caused by mixed flora, including aerobic and anaerobic organisms such as *Escherichia coli*, Enterobacteriaceae, various streptococci, *Staphylococcus aureus*, and *Bacteroides fragilis*. Several organisms produce gas, resulting in crepitation in patients with the so-called diabetic foot. This must be distinguished from the much less common and more acutely devastating clostridial gas gangrene and necrotizing fasciitis.

Surgical debridement and drainage, if needed, should be performed early. Cultures should be obtained during drainage procedures and, ideally, before antibiotic therapy is started. However, it may be preferable to initiate empirical therapy for the most likely organisms until the results of cultures are available. Swarming of *Proteus* organisms may obscure other pathogens on culture plates. Unless the patient is clearly manifesting a septic response, aminoglycosides should not be used because of their nephrotoxicity and the likelihood that diabetic patients may have underlying kidney disease. If severe infections do not respond to antibiotic therapy, the presence of *Candida* or other fungal species [see 85 Fungal Infection] should be suspected.

Table 6 Postoperative Management When Diabetic Patient Can Take Solid Food

1. Continue intravenous insulin-glucose infusion for 1 hr after subcutaneous administration of insulin dose.
2. Measure capillary blood glucose before meals, at 10:00 P.M., and at 3:00 A.M. If the patient is hypoglycemic at 3:00 A.M., reduce the insulin dose at 10:00 P.M.
3. Administer preprandial short-acting insulin according to the following variable-dosage schedule:

Blood Glucose (mg/dl)	Short-Acting Insulin (U)			
	Breakfast	Lunch	Dinner	10:00 P.M.
< 70	3	2	2	0
71–100	4	3	3	0
101–150	6	4	4	0
151–200	8	6	6	0
201–250	10	8	8	1
251–300	12	10	10	2
> 300	14	12	12	3

4. Administer 10–20 U of intermediate-acting insulin at 10:00 P.M. (in addition to the dose of short-acting insulin scheduled for this time).
5. Provide three meals and three snacks, for a total of 20 to 30 kcal/kg/day.

Discussion

Developments in Diabetic Management

PREVENTION OF INSULIN-DEPENDENT DIABETES MELLITUS

Diabetologists' ultimate goal is to find a means of preventing diabetes. It is now known that IDDM is an autoimmune disorder strongly associated with the class II alleles DR3 and DR4, and it is thought that alleles of the HLA-DQ β chain are primarily responsible for susceptibility (and resistance) to autoimmune destruction of beta cells. This theory has generated a series of studies on immunosuppression induced by cyclosporine, azathioprine, or steroids in patients newly diagnosed with IDDM, with the goal of delaying or preventing the autoimmune destruction of beta cells. Cyclosporine has proved to be relatively effective in delaying insulin dependence and inducing prolonged remission, but diagnosis must be made during the prediabetes phase because more than 90 percent of beta cells have been destroyed by the time IDDM is diagnosed.

There are ethical obstacles to using broad-spectrum immunosuppression in patients at risk for IDDM, because conventional insulin therapy has increased the life expectancy of patients with this disorder. The Barts Windsor study[14] has shown that islet cell antibodies develop many years before the onset of clinical diabetes in the nondiabetic siblings of patients with IDDM. A series of studies from New Zealand,[14] largely uncontrolled and unconfirmed, suggest that nicotinamide induces remission in patients with newly diagnosed IDDM and delays the onset of diabetes in antibody-positive nondiabetic children. Additional studies are needed to substantiate these findings.

The prospect of being able to intervene in the prediabetic state is an exciting one, but it must be remembered that these early studies are limited in scope, focusing on first-degree relatives (even though familial cases of diabetes constitute a minority of all cases) and relying on strategies that are not totally harmless. Immunosuppression and administration of nicotinamide, subcutaneous insulin, oral insulin, and glutamic decarboxylase have been proposed as means of intervention. Even subcutaneous insulin is not totally harmless, and nicotinamide, though a natural substance, was used in these studies in doses higher than the recommended daily allowance. Well-designed multicenter studies are needed for the development of acceptable means of preventing IDDM.

INSULIN PUMPS

Results of the Diabetes Control and Complications Trial[15] (DCCT) may prompt many physicians to advocate intensive insulin therapy. The DCCT clearly demonstrated that intensive therapy delays the development and progression of retinopathy, nephropathy, and neuropathy. Hypoglycemic reactions, however, were more frequent in the group receiving intensive therapy than in the conventional-therapy group.

Insulin pump therapy or continuous subcutaneous insulin infusion (CSII) is a highly adjustable method offering type I diabetes patients an alternative to multiple daily injections. Effective use of intensive insulin therapy requires that the health care provider possess a great deal of knowledge about diabetes and that the patient, the family, and the health care team be highly motivated. Before beginning treatment with an insulin pump, the patient and health care provider should be familiar with the following features of intensive insulin therapy in general and pump therapy in particular:

1. The patients most likely to achieve improved glycemic control with insulin pump therapy are those who monitor their capillary blood glucose concentration at least four times daily.

2. Target levels of blood glucose should be selected with care to reduce the risk of hypoglycemia. Pump therapy per se does not increase the frequency of serious hypoglycemia, but attempts to achieve blood glucose values within the normal range substantially increase the risk of serious hypoglycemia—a danger in patients who are unaware of their hypoglycemic states.

3. Care of the skin at infusion sites must be meticulous. Patients with a history of recurrent staphylococcal skin infections and those who are nasal carriers may be at higher risk.

4. Plugging of infusion sets and leaks in infusion-set connections are common. These problems can be identified with self-monitoring of blood glucose and corrected with adjustment of the infusion system, but ketoacidosis may occur if interruption of insulin delivery is not detected. An insulin syringe and vial should be kept for backup.

5. Insulin pump therapy demands more time, effort, and money than treatment with conventional injections. Many people develop a sense of well-being while using a pump, but those with a history of emotional problems or stress may not be able to cope with the increased demands of intensive insulin therapy.

Initiating Pump Therapy in Type I Diabetes Patients

Before using the pump, the patient should practice loading and programming the unit and changing infusion sets. The best sites are usually far from bony prominences and belt lines. The infusion set is secured with an occlusive dressing or paper tape and is generally changed every two to three days to prevent infection.

Pump therapy is often initiated during a two- to three-day hospital stay. In general, blood glucose targets are 80 to 140 mg/dl (4.4 to 7.8 mmol/L) for the average of values taken before each meal and at bedtime. Target averages for pregnant patients are usually somewhat lower, generally not exceeding 100 mg/dl (5.5 mmol/L). Targets for patients who have been unaware of their hypoglycemia or who have a history of recurrent severe hypoglycemia should be higher, at least at the beginning of infusion pump therapy.

If pump therapy is started outside the hospital, a friend or relative should be available to assist in the event of serious hypoglycemia. The patient should be instructed not to undertake unusual activity for several days, until approximate insulin doses have been established.

The initial programming of insulin dosages is based on the total daily prepump dosages, as follows:

1. The basal rate is initially set at 50 percent of the total prepump dosage. Breakfast, lunch, dinner, and bedtime boluses are initially written as 16, 12, 16, and 6 percent, respectively, of the total prepump insulin dosage. Capillary blood glucose concentrations are checked before each meal and at bedtime, and basal and bolus doses are altered by 10 to 20 percent every one to two days to move toward target values.

2. The basal rate is adjusted to achieve the target fasting blood glucose level, with mealtime boluses adjusted to achieve similar values before the next meal. Peak blood glucose elevations between meals can be blunted by giving the premeal bolus 30 to 45 minutes before eating.

3. A prebreakfast increase in blood glucose may require a preprogrammed basal rate step-up in the early morning, but multiple complex changes in basal rate throughout the day are usually not necessary. In general, the proportion of insulin delivered over 24 hours should begin at approximately 50 percent of the total for the basal and bolus modes, allowing for flexibility in delivering bolus doses. Increases in basal rate and bolus doses are usually required if hyperglycemia occurs during intercurrent illness.

Benefits

Approximately 90 percent of patients changing from two conventional injections daily to insulin pump therapy achieve improved glycemic control. Fifty percent of patients using pumps achieve at least temporary normalization of glycosylated hemoglobin concentration, and 15 percent are able to maintain normal yearly averages of glycosylated hemoglobin for at least three years.[16] Most patients appreciate the greater flexibility of intensive insulin therapy, which matches insulin administration to variations in diet and exercise.

Complications

Insulin therapy is not without complications. In approximately 30 percent of patients, infections develop at infusion sites, usually caused by coagulase-positive *S. aureus*. Cellulitis is often responsive to dicloxacillin (250 mg orally four times daily for one week). Abscesses should be incised and drained promptly. Ketoacidosis is the second most common acute complication of pump therapy, occurring in 15 percent of patients using pumps in one large series. Capillary blood glucose levels should be measured four times daily. If the patient's blood glucose level exceeds 240 mg/dl (13.3 mmol/L), the infusion set should be checked. If the blood glucose level remains elevated after one to two hours, the infusion set should be changed. The infusion set should also be changed if the patient becomes ill unexpectedly and the blood glucose level exceeds 240 mg/dl (13.3 mmol/L).[17] Finally, CSII therapy, like any other intensive insulin regimen, may be associated with an increased incidence of hypoglycemic reactions.

Although insulin pumps more closely approximate the physiologic secretion of insulin than other methods of insulin administration do, they have some of the drawbacks of conventional regimens. The appearance of insulin in the circulation is not regulated by the plasma glucose concentration, and absorption from subcutaneous injection sites is variable and unpredictable. These shortcomings limit the efficacy and safety of pump therapy when attempts are made to approach a normal metabolic state.

PANCREAS AND ISLET TRANSPLANTATION

The DCCT sponsored by the National Institutes of Health established that more intensive insulin therapy reduces the risk of multiorgan microvascular and macrovascular complications.[15] This reduced risk is accompanied, however, by a threefold increase in serious hypoglycemic episodes that necessitate the intervention of another person. In addition, the treatment goal of normal glycosylated hemoglobin levels has not been achieved, which suggests that alternatives to intensive insulin therapy would be beneficial if normoglycemia could be achieved without these risks.

Pancreas transplantation clearly achieves normoglycemia and normal glycosylated hemoglobin levels, with a 75 percent rate of one-year graft function (comparable to the success achieved with kidney or liver transplantation).[18] This approach, unfortunately, necessitates lifelong immunosuppression, with engraftment only in patients with end-stage complications. Thus, although pancreas transplantation provides normoglycemia in patients requiring immunosuppression, it is not an option for most diabetic patients.

Islet transplantation has recently advanced from a technique used in laboratory animals to one that has achieved insulin independence in a few patients.[19] Although islet transplantation offers normoglycemia to a few recipients, its use, like that of pancreas transplantation, is limited to immunosuppressed individuals. This cellular transplant, however, has the potential of being protected from the immune system by means of immunoisolation (e.g., encapsulated islets) or the development of tolerance. Additional study will be required before islet transplantation can be offered to more patients with diabetes.

References

1. Root HF: Preoperative medical care of the diabetic patient. Postgrad Med 40:439, 1966
2. Galloway JA, Shuman CR: Diabetes and surgery: a study of 667 cases. Am J Med 34:177, 1963
3. Alberti KGMM, Marshall SM: Diabetes and surgery. Diabetes Annual/4. Alberti KGMM, Krall LP, Eds. Elsevier Science Publishers, Amsterdam, 1988, p 248
4. Clements RS Jr: Diabetic neuropathy—new concepts of its etiology. Diabetes 28:604, 1979
5. Fraser DM, Campbell IW, Ewing DJ, et al: Peripheral and autonomic nerve function in newly diagnosed diabetes mellitus. Diabetes 26:546, 1977
6. Aiello LM, Cavallerano JD: Ocular complications. Therapy for Diabetes Mellitus and Related Disorders. Lebovitz HE, Ed. American Diabetes Association, Alexandria, Virginia, 1991, p 226
7. Bolognia JL, Braverman IM: Skin and subcutaneous tissues. Therapy for Diabetes Mellitus and Related Disorders. Lebovitz HE, Ed. American Diabetes Association, Alexandria, Virginia, 1991, p 204
8. Page MM, Watkins PJ: Cardiorespiratory arrest and diabetic autonomic neuropathy. Lancet 1:14, 1978

9. Ewing DJ, Campbell IW, Clarke BF: Mortality in diabetic autonomic neuropathy. Lancet 1:601, 1976
10. Alberti KG, Thomas DJ: The management of diabetes during surgery. Br J Anaesth 51:693, 1979
11. Walts LF, Miller J, Davidson MB, et al: Perioperative management of diabetes mellitus. Anesthesiology 55:104, 1981
12. Thompson J, Husband DJ, Thai AC, et al: Metabolic changes in the non–insulin-dependent diabetic undergoing minor surgery: effect of glucose-insulin-potassium infusion. Br J Surg 73:301, 1986
13. Bennett WM: Drug-induced renal dysfunction. Therapy for Diabetes Mellitus and Related Disorders. Lebovitz HE, Ed. American Diabetes Association, Alexandria, Virginia, 1991, p 241
14. Alberti KG: Preventing insulin dependent diabetes mellitus (editorial). BMJ 307:1435, 1993
15. The effect of intensive treatment of diabetes on the development and progression of long-term complications in insulin-dependent diabetes mellitus. Diabetes Control and Complications Trial Research Group. N Engl J Med 329:977, 1993
16. Skyler JS: Insulin treatment. Therapy for Diabetes Mellitus and Related Disorders. Lebovitz HE, Ed. American Diabetes Association, Alexandria, Virginia, 1991, p 127
17. Mecklenburg RS, Benson EA, Benson JW Jr, et al: Acute complications associated with insulin infusion pump therapy: report of experience with 161 patients. JAMA 252:3265, 1984
18. Sutherland DER, Gruessner A, Moudry-Munns K: Analysis of United Network for Organ Sharing (UNOS) United States of America (USA) Pancreas Transplant Registry data according to multiple variables. Clinical Transplants 1992. Terasaki PI, Cecka JM, Eds. UCLA Tissue Typing Laboratory, Los Angeles, 1992, p 45
19. Hering BJ, Browatzki CC, Schultz A, et al: Clinical islet transplantation—registry report, accomplishments in the past and future research needs. Cell Transplantation 2:269, 1993
20. Surgery: practical guidelines for diabetes management. Clinics in Diabetes 5:49, 1987

69 OBESITY

Harvey J. Sugerman, M.D.

Approach to the Morbidly Obese Patient

Many surgeons are afraid to operate on the morbidly obese patient (i.e., a patient whose weight is 100 lb greater than ideal body weight or who has a body mass index [BMI] greater than 35 kg/mg²) because they presuppose a marked increase in perioperative morbidity and mortality. Although the morbidly obese patient is certainly at greater risk, this risk can be markedly reduced by paying careful attention to detail in preoperative and postoperative care. The increased risks encountered in these patients include wound infection, dehiscence, thrombophlebitis, pulmonary embolism, anesthetic calamities, acute postoperative asphyxia in patients with obstructive sleep apnea syndrome (SAS), acute respiratory failure, right ventricular or biventricular cardiac failure, and missed acute catastrophes of the abdomen, such as an anastomotic leak. In a series of about 2,000 gastric procedures for morbid obesity itself, we have observed the following incidence of complications: wound infection that delayed hospital discharge, 5%, as well as minor infections or seromas in an additional 10%; clinically apparent phlebitis, 0.4%; clinically diagnosed fatal pulmonary embolism, 0.15%; and pneumonia, 0.5%. We reported a 0.4% operative mortality. Although many of these patients had severe preoperative morbidity (respiratory insufficiency, pseudotumor cerebri, or insulin-dependent diabetes), the risks of complication approach the risks associated with major abdominal operation in nonobese patients. In what follows, I focus on issues that the surgeon should carefully consider when operating on an extremely overweight patient.

Cardiac Dysfunction

Morbidly obese patients are at significant risk of coronary artery disease as a result of an increased incidence of systemic hypertension, hypercholesterolemia, and diabetes. Because of this increased risk for cardiac dysfunction, preoperative electrocardiography should be performed on all obese patients 20 years of age or older.

Most morbidly obese patients have minimal evidence of cardiac dysfunction as detected by Swan-Ganz catheterization. Markedly elevated pulmonary arterial pressure (PAP) and pulmonary arterial wedge pressure (PAWP) values will frequently be noted in patients with the respiratory insufficiency of obesity, especially those with obesity hypoventilation syndrome (OHS) [see Respiratory Insufficiency, Obesity Hypoventilation Syndrome, *below*].[1] Intubation and ventilation in these patients will often be followed by a vigorous diuresis, and it is not unusual for a patient to lose 50 lb or more of retained fluid. In a few obese patients, acute respiratory insufficiency will be caused by a greatly expanded central blood volume and heart failure. Abnormal blood gas values in these individuals will be corrected by vigorous diuresis alone. As with most other abnormalities related to morbid obesity, weight loss will also correct cardiac dysfunction.

Respiratory Insufficiency

Morbidly obese patients may suffer from obstructive SAS or OHS. The simultaneous presence of SAS and OHS is known as the pickwickian syndrome [see Discussion, Respiratory Insufficiency of Obesity, *below*].[2-4]

SLEEP APNEA SYNDROME

SAS is a potentially fatal complication of morbid obesity. A diagnosis of SAS should be suspected when there is a history of loud snoring, frequent nocturnal awakening with shortness of breath, and daytime somnolence. It is estimated that 2% of middle-aged women and 4% of middle-aged men in the United States workforce have SAS, and the incidence is markedly higher in the severely obese.[5] Patients will often admit to falling asleep while driving and waking up with their car on the road's median strip or bumping its guardrail. It is extremely important that trauma surgeons be aware of the relation between obesity and somnolence should a morbidly obese patient be seen in the emergency room after an automobile accident in which he or she fell asleep at the wheel. Elective patients with suspected sleep apnea syndrome should undergo preoperative polysomnography at a sleep center to confirm the diagnosis. Medications are usually ineffective. Stimulants, such as methylphenidate hydrochloride (Ritalin), should not be used. If a patient has more than 25 apneic episodes per hour of sleep or has cardiac arrhythmias in association with apnea, treatment by nocturnal nasal continuous positive airway pressure (nasal CPAP) should be provided. If the patient does not respond with elimina-

Approach to the Morbidly Obese Patient

Patient is morbidly obese (current weight at least 100 lb > ideal body weight, body mass index ≥ 35 kg/m², or both)

Increased risks include
- Missed abdominal catastrophe
- Respiratory failure
- Cardiac failure
- Anesthetic calamities
- Pulmonary embolism
- Internal hernia
- Acute gastric distention
- Wound infection
- Postoperative asphyxia
- Dehiscence
- Thrombophlebitis

Evaluate cardiopulmonary status preoperatively

Patient reports loud snoring, frequent nocturnal awakening, and daytime somnolence, or trauma victim has fallen asleep at the wheel

Suspect sleep apnea syndrome (SAS).
Confirm SAS by polysomnography in elective patients. Provide nocturnal nasal CPAP if apneic episodes are ≥ 25/hr of sleep or are associated with arrhythmias. If patient does not respond to — or does not tolerate — CPAP, perform tracheostomy with extra-long tube.

Patient has heart failure or extreme shortness of breath

Suspect obesity hypoventilation syndrome (OHS).
OHS is confirmed by $P_aO_2 \leq 55$ mm Hg or $P_aO_2 \geq 47$ mm Hg
- If PAWP ≥ 18 mm Hg, try I.V. furosemide.
- If PAP ≥ 40 mm Hg, consider insertion of Greenfield vena caval filter.
- If Hb ≥ 16 g/dl, phlebotomize to Hb of 15 g/dl.

Give prophylaxis against thromboembolism, induce anesthesia, and intubate

Administer regular or low-molecular-weight heparin 30 min preoperatively and at appropriate intervals thereafter until the patient is ambulatory.
Use intermittent sequential venous compression boots during anesthesia induction and throughout operation.
Two anesthesia personnel are required for induction and intubation of patients with SAS or OHS (one to hold the mask and one to squeeze the ventilation bag).
Insert oral airway after administration of succinylcholine and sodium pentobarbital. Ventilate with 100% O_2 for several minutes before intubation. If intubation is unsuccessful, reinsert oral airway and ventilate with a mask. Patient should be in reverse Trendelenburg's position.

In the recovery room, keep patient in reverse Trendelenburg's position

---

Patient does not have respiratory insufficiency of obesity

Extubate in recovery room when patient is fully alert and ventilatory effort is adequate; return patient to room.

Patient has SAS

In the absence of OHS, wean and extubate the day after operation. If patient was on nasal CPAP before operation, reinstitute on second night after operation. Monitor for prolonged apnea or arrhythmia; if either occurs, awaken patient.

Patient has OHS

Continue mechanical ventilation after operation until pain of breathing resolves. Wean to preoperative arterial blood gas levels; several days may be required.

Encourage early postoperative ambulation

Use intermittent sequential venous compression boots until patient is fully ambulatory.

Maintain high index of suspicion for recognition of abdominal catastrophes

Guarding, tenderness, and rigidity may be absent. Signs of infection (fever, tachypnea, tachycardia) may be absent. Acute respiratory failure may be secondary to peritonitis. Radiographic contrast studies and laparotomy may be indicated even when clinical signs are few.

tion of the apneic episodes or cannot tolerate nasal CPAP, a tracheostomy should be performed. An extra-long tracheostomy tube is usually necessary because of the depth of the trachea in the morbidly obese patient.

OBESITY HYPOVENTILATION SYNDROME

OHS should be suspected in patients who present with heart failure or extreme shortness of breath. Diagnosis is confirmed when the patient's arterial oxygen tension (P_aO_2) is 55 mm Hg or less or the arterial carbon dioxide tension (P_aCO_2) is 47 mm Hg or greater. These patients often have marked elevations in mean PAP, mean PAWP, or both, as well as severe polycythemia. In patients with obesity hypoventilation syndrome, a Swan-Ganz catheter should be inserted as part of the preoperative evaluation. If PAWP is 18 mm Hg or greater, diuresis with intravenous furosemide is indicated. In many of these patients, however, an elevated PAWP is necessary to maintain adequate cardiac output; such patients do not have congestive heart failure, despite a markedly elevated filling pressure [see Discussion, below]. Little can be done for the pulmonary hypertension that is seen in many of these patients; raising the P_aO_2 above 60 mm Hg usually will not lower PAP acutely.

Polycythemia can significantly increase the incidence of phlebothrombosis. If the hemoglobin (Hb) concentration is 16 g/dl or greater, phlebotomy to a concentration of 15 g/dl should be performed to reduce the postoperative risk of venous thrombosis. If PAP is 40 mm Hg or greater, consideration should be given to prophylactic insertion of a Greenfield vena caval filter because of the high risk of a fatal pulmonary embolism in these patients.[6] Placement of this filter can be a challenge because the appropriate landmarks cannot be identified in the operating room with fluoroscopy. It is necessary before operation to tape a quarter to the patient's back over the second lumbar vertebra with the aid of fixed radiographs and then during operation to aim for the quarter with the insertion catheter, using fluoroscopy. Because these patients are usually too heavy for angiography tables, the Greenfield filter usually cannot be inserted percutaneously in the radiology department.

Embolism

The risk of deep vein thrombosis [see 70 Thromboembolic Problems] increases with a prolonged operation or a postoperative period of immobilization, and it increases even further in the morbidly obese patient. Standard or low-molecular-weight heparin should be administered subcutaneously 30 minutes before operation and at appropriate intervals thereafter (depending on the type of heparin used) for at least 2 days or until the patient is ambulatory. Because respiratory function in the morbidly obese patient is greatly enhanced with the reverse Trendelenburg's position, intermittent sequential venous compression boots should be used to counteract the increased venous stasis and the propensity for clotting. It is important that the intermittent venous compression boots be used before induction of anesthesia and throughout the operative procedure. Compression boots are usually part of a standard preoperative protocol in gastric procedures for weight control; their use should not be unintentionally neglected in preparation for other elective or emergency procedures on morbidly obese patients. As noted (see above), prophylactic insertion of a Greenfield vena caval filter should be considered in OHS patients with a high PAP.

Anesthesia in Patients with Respiratory Insufficiency

Morbidly obese patients can be intimidating to the anesthesiologist because they are at significant risk for complications from anesthesia, especially during induction. The risk is particularly great for obese patients with respiratory insufficiency. An obese patient often has a short, fat neck and a heavy chest wall, which make intubation and ventilation a challenge. If endotracheal intubation proves difficult, however, these patients can usually be well ventilated with a mask. Awake intubation can be performed, with or without fiberoptic aids, but is quite unpleasant and unnecessary.

It is extremely important that at least two anesthesia personnel be present during induction and intubation for patients with respiratory insufficiency of obesity. An oral airway is inserted after muscle paralysis with succinylcholine and sodium pentobarbital induction. One person elevates the jaw, hyperextends the neck, and ensures a tight fit of the mask, using both hands. To ensure adequate oxygen delivery, a second person compresses the ventilation reservoir bag, using two hands because of the resistance to air flow from the poorly compliant, heavy chest wall. After ventilation with 100% oxygen for several minutes, intubation is attempted. If difficulties are encountered within 30 seconds, the steps above should be repeated until the patient has been successfully intubated. A volume ventilator is required during operation. Placing the patient in the reverse Trendelenburg's position expands total lung volume and facilitates ventilation[7]; however, the reverse Trendelenburg's position increases lower extremity venous pressure and therefore mandates the use of intermittent sequential venous compression boots [see Embolism, above]. It is helpful to monitor blood gases through a radial arterial line or digital pulse oximeter.

Postoperative Management

After operation, the obese patient should be kept in the reverse Trendelenburg's position and should not be extubated until he or she is fully alert and showing evidence of adequate ventilatory effort [see 92 Use of the Mechanical Ventilator]. In the absence of respiratory insufficiency, most obese patients can be extubated in the OR or the recovery room and returned to a standard hospital room.

Patients with SAS, however, should be managed with overnight mechanical ventilation in the ICU. In the absence of concomitant OHS, they can usually be weaned and extubated the day after operation. Patients who were receiving ventilatory support with nasal CPAP before operation should have this treatment reinstituted the second night after operation; monitoring for prolonged apnea should be continued in the ICU or in a stepdown unit with digital oximetry. If apnea occurs, simply waking the patient should correct the problem. Patients who required tracheostomy can also usually be weaned from the ventilator the morning after operation.

Patients with OHS require prolonged mechanical volume ventilation until the pain of breathing resolves. One cannot expect such patients to manifest normal arterial blood gas levels, and they should be weaned to their preoperative values. This weaning process may require several days. It is important that these patients remain in the reverse Trendelenburg's position to maximize diaphragmatic excursion. Positive end-expiratory pressure (PEEP) ventilation may be detrimental in patients with OHS because it can overdistend alveoli, thereby leading to capillary compression, decreased cardiac output, and increased dead space, all of which can exacerbate retention of carbon dioxide.

Swan-Ganz catheters, inserted preoperatively in patients with severe OHS, are useful in monitoring postoperative intravascular volume and oxygen delivery status. Excessive diuresis or restriction of fluids should be avoided [see Discussion, below].

It is extremely important to encourage early postoperative ambulation for the morbidly obese patient. These patients have surprisingly little pain, and it is not unusual to see them walking in the afternoon or early evening after a major abdominal procedure. If the patients have been advised preoperatively of the merits of early postoperative ambulation and know it is for their own welfare, they are usually willing to cooperate.

Complications of Gastric Surgery for Obesity

Current gastric procedures for obesity include gastric bypass (GBP) and gastroplasty, in which the stomach is stapled so as to create small and large pouches connected via a small stoma. The procedures themselves are described in more detail elsewhere [see 50 Gastric Procedures for Morbid Obesity]; the following are some of the main complications associated with any abdominal operation in a severely obese patient.

ABDOMINAL CATASTROPHE

It may be very difficult to recognize an abdominal catastrophe in patients who are very young, very old, or morbidly obese or who are receiving high doses of steroids. The obese patient, for example, may present in the emergency room with a perforated duodenal ulcer or a ruptured diverticulum, complaining of abdominal pain, and yet on abdominal examination have no evidence of peritoneal irritation (no guarding, tenderness, or rigidity). This situation has been well documented in patients in whom an anastomotic or gastric leak has developed after operation for morbid obesity.[8] Symptoms include shoulder pain, pelvic or scrotal pain, back pain, tenesmus, urinary frequency, and, of great importance, marked anxiety. Signs of infection (e.g., fever, tachypnea, and tachycardia) may be absent. Patients with peritonitis often have clinical symptoms and signs suggesting a massive pulmonary embolus: severe tachypnea, tachycardia, and sudden hypotension. Such acute pulmonary failure is probably secondary to sepsis-induced acute respiratory distress syndrome (ARDS). Thus, peritonitis must be suspected in any morbidly obese patient with acute respiratory failure.

Because a high index of suspicion of peritonitis is required to detect the condition in morbidly obese patients, radiographic contrast studies with water-soluble agents such as diatrizoate meglumine (Gastrografin) may be indicated even when there are few clinical signs. If a perforated viscus is suspected, an exploratory laparotomy may be necessary despite normal findings on radiographic contrast study.

INTERNAL HERNIA

GBP places patients at risk for internal hernia with a closed-loop obstruction, leading to bowel strangulation. There are three potential locations for these internal hernias: the Roux-en-Y anastomosis; the opening in the transverse mesocolon through which the retrocolic Roux limb is brought; and the Petersen hernia, which is located behind the retrocolic Roux limb. The primary symptom of an internal hernia is periumbilical pain, usually in the form of cramping consistent with visceral colic. These internal hernias may be very difficult to diagnose. An upper gastrointestinal radiographic series is often normal, providing a false sense of security. The resulting assumption that no problem exists may be devastating for the patient should bowel infarction occur as a consequence of closed-loop obstruction. One should always carefully inspect the plain abdominal radiograph for the abnormal placement or spreading of the Roux-en-Y anastomotic staples. The safest course of action in patients with recurrent attacks of periumbilical pain is abdominal surgical exploration.

ACUTE GASTRIC DISTENTION

After GBP, massive gaseous distention occasionally develops in the distal bypassed stomach; this can lead to a gastric perforation or disruption of the gastrojejunostomy. The primary symptoms of this complication are hiccups and a bloated feeling. Massive gastric dilatation can lead to severe left shoulder pain and shock. The problem is usually secondary to edema at the Roux-en-Y anastomosis but can also be secondary to a mechanical problem. The diagnosis is made by means of an urgent upright abdominal radiograph, which reveals the markedly dilated and air-filled bypassed stomach. Occasionally, the stomach is filled with fluid, and the diagnosis may be more difficult. In those few cases in which the dilatation is primarily caused by air, the problem can be relieved by percutaneous transabdominal skinny-needle decompression with subsequent passage of gas and gastric and biliopancreatic juices through the Roux-en-Y anastomosis. Should the dilatation recur or the patient be in serious difficulty, an emergency laparotomy with insertion of a gastrostomy tube should be performed and the jejunojejunostomy evaluated. If a patient has extensive adhesions from previous abdominal surgery, a gastrostomy tube should be inserted at the time of GBP to prevent gastric dilatation.

Diabetes Mellitus

Type 2 (non–insulin-dependent) diabetes mellitus, a nonketotic form of diabetes that is usually noted after age 40, is markedly exacerbated by obesity. Patients with this type of diabetes often require large amounts of insulin for blood glucose control because of a significant reduction in insulin receptors. It is not unusual, however, to note a complete absence of the requirement for insulin in the immediate postoperative period in morbidly obese patients. Therefore, insulin should be withheld on the morning of operation. There is often a marked reduction in the requirement for insulin throughout the postoperative period and even at discharge in morbidly obese patients who have undergone GBP, probably because of increased release of gastric inhibitory peptide (GIP) from the proximal small bowel. Therefore, regular subcutaneous insulin should be administered to GBP patients according to a sliding scale after operation until insulin requirements can be determined. Before discharge, the patient should be taking an appropriate dose of neutral protamine Hagedorn (NPH) or Lente insulin but must perform frequent finger-stick blood glucose determinations afterward, given that the need for insulin will decrease progressively with weight loss.

In one study of 23 patients with type 1 (insulin-dependent) diabetes mellitus who underwent gastric bariatric operation, the average requirement for insulin decreased from 74 units/day before operation to 8 units/day after operation.[9] Fourteen of the 23 patients were able to discontinue insulin completely, 11 by the time of discharge from the hospital 1 week after operation. These benefits were maintained during long-term follow-up to 39 months and were a result of a major decrease in insulin resistance that was associated with decreased food intake as well as weight loss.

Wound Care

Morbidly obese patients have been reported to have an increased risk of wound infection and dehiscence. However, the incidence of these complications in this group of patients can be very low. In a randomized, prospective trial comparing a running, continuous absorbable No. 2 polyglycolic acid suture with a No. 28 stainless-steel wire in morbidly obese patients who weighed an average of 320 lb, there was no significant difference in complications, including the incidence of incisional hernia, between the types of closure.[10] However, the running absorbable suture closure required significantly less time. Similar results comparing continuous with interrupted sutures have been noted by others.[11] Subcutaneous sutures should not be used, because the subcutaneous fat becomes reapproximated during skin closure, and subcutaneous sutures have been found to increase the risk of wound infection.[12] Obese patients undergoing clean-contaminated intestinal procedures should be given a parenteral antibiotic immediately before the operation and for only 24 hours after the operation[13]; it is important to note that morbidly obese patients should receive a double dose of prophylactic antibiotics because of the increased volume of distribution. If a gastric or gallbladder operation is planned, only aerobic bacterial coverage is necessary; a colon operation will necessitate anaerobic coverage as well.

It has been our experience that the incidence of incisional hernia is much higher in morbidly obese patients than in thin patients with ulcerative colitis who are taking large doses of corticosteroids and who undergo the same fascial wound closure with running No. 2 polyglycolic acid sutures.[14] This increased risk in morbidly obese patients is probably secondary to the increased intra-abdominal pressures (IAP) present in patients with central, or android, obesity.[15]

Obese diabetic patients are at risk for rapidly spreading panniculitis secondary to mixed aerobic and anaerobic organisms.[16] Subcutaneous gas and extensive necrosis, which usually does not involve the underlying muscle, are often present. It is uncommon to culture clostridia from these wounds. Even after extensive and repeated debridement, mortality remains high [see 21 *Soft Tissue Infection*].

Other Obesity-Related Diseases

GALLSTONES

Approximately one third of morbidly obese patients either have had a cholecystectomy or may have had gallstones noted at the time of another intra-abdominal operative procedure, such as gastric operation for morbid obesity. Preoperative evaluation of the gallbladder may be technically quite difficult in morbidly obese patients because gallstones may be missed with either ultrasonography or oral cholecystography. Intraoperative sonography is probably much more accurate. Should stones be present in a patient undergoing gastric operation for obesity, the gallbladder should be removed. In the past, obese patients with intermittent attacks of biliary colic were told to lose weight before an elective cholecystectomy for fear of significant morbidity and mortality from an elective operation. This attitude is no longer valid, because among the large numbers of obese patients who now undergo major elective abdominal procedures, morbidity is similar to that seen in thin patients if appropriate precautions are taken. Furthermore, obese patients have great difficulty losing large amounts of weight by diet alone and should be allowed to undergo definitive corrective operative procedures before weight reduction.

Rapid weight loss may lead to the development of gallstones in 25% to 40% of patients who undergo GBP. The risk of cholelithiasis in this setting can be reduced to 2% by administering ursodeoxycholic acid, 300 mg orally twice daily.[17]

PSEUDOTUMOR CEREBRI

Pseudotumor cerebri is an unusual complication of morbid obesity that is associated with benign intracranial hypertension, papilledema, blurred vision, headache, and elevated cerebrospinal fluid pressures.[18] It has been our experience that patients with pseudotumor cerebri are not at any additional perioperative risk and that cerebrospinal fluid does not have to be removed before anesthesia and major abdominal operation. Weight reduction will cure pseudotumor cerebri.[19,20]

DEGENERATIVE OSTEOARTHRITIS

Degenerative osteoarthritis of the knees, hips, and back is a common complication of morbid obesity. Weight reduction alone may greatly reduce the pain and immobility that afflict these patients, although the damage may be so extensive that a total joint replacement may be desirable. However, joint replacement in patients who weigh more than 250 lb is associated with an unacceptable incidence of loosening.[21] Weight reduction by means of a gastric bariatric operation may be the most sensible initial approach, to be followed by joint replacement after weight loss if pain and dysfunction persist.

Discussion

Morbidity Associated with Central Fat Deposition

Much has been written about the increased health risks inherent in central, or android, fat deposition as compared with peripheral, or gynoid, fat deposition. It is thought that in the former, the increased metabolic activity of mesenteric fat is associated with increased metabolism of amino acids to sugar, which leads to hyperglycemia and hyperinsulinism. Hyperinsulinism gives rise to increased sodium absorption and hypertension. Furthermore, central obesity has been linked to hypercholesterolemia. Hence, these patients have a significantly higher incidence of diabetes, hypertension, hypercholesterolemia, and gallstones[22]—which explains the higher mortality of the apple distribution of body fat as compared with the pear distribution. In the past, fat distribution was measured on the basis of the waist-to-hip ratio; however, computed tomography scans have shown that abdominal circumference is a more accurate measurement of central fat distribution.[23] We have found that morbidly obese women have significantly increased IAP and that this is associated with stress and urge overflow urinary incontinence.[24] With weight loss comes a significant decrease in bladder pressure and correction of incontinence. We have found IAP, as reflected in bladder pressure, to be closely correlated with sagittal abdominal diameter but not with waist-to-hip ratio (many morbidly obese patients have both central and peripheral obesity). We have also found that the increased IAP associated with central obesity may cause additional comorbid factors, including venous stasis ulcers, OHS, gastroesophageal reflux, and inguinal and incisional hernias.

Respiratory Insufficiency of Obesity

Obese patients are at risk for respiratory difficulties, which may be present before operation or may be exacerbated by an operation. The term pickwickian syndrome (which derives from *The Posthumous Papers of the Pickwick Club*, by Charles Dickens) was resurrected from the late 1800s to describe a morbidly obese man 52 years of age who fell asleep in a poker game while holding a hand containing a full house.[2] He was taken to the hospital by friends who presumed he was ill. The pickwickian syndrome is now known to comprise two pulmonary syndromes associated with morbid obesity: obstructive SAS and OHS.[3]

Patients with SAS suffer from repeated attacks of upper airway obstruction during sleep. The cause is probably related to a large, fat tongue as well as to excessive fat deposition in the uvula, pharynx, and hypopharynx. The normal genioglossus reflex is depressed, but this depression may be secondary to the excessive weight of the tongue. These patients are notorious snorers. As a result of inadequate stage IV and rapid eye movement (REM) sleep, they are markedly somnolent during the day.

Patients with SAS are at great risk for acute upper airway obstruction and respiratory arrest after operation and general anesthesia. A high index of suspicion is necessary before operation. Patients with severe SAS often have ventricular arrhythmias and sinus arrest during their apneic episodes, thereby placing them at even greater risk. A history of heavy snoring, early morning headaches, frequent awakening at night with shortness of breath, severe daytime somnolence (including falling asleep at the wheel), and frequent headaches should prompt further study. The syndrome is confirmed by sleep polysomnography, which is available at sleep centers in most major cities.

In most instances, severe SAS can be treated with nocturnal nasal CPAP. With this technique, air flowing through a nasal mask against a constant airway resistance enters the nasal pharynx and pushes the tongue forward to prevent recurrent obstruction.[25] The pressure can be adjusted for each patient. Unfortunately, many patients cannot tolerate the device, because it is cumbersome and noisy and tends to dry out the upper airway, although dryness can be prevented with an inexpensive room humidifier. If nasal CPAP cannot be tolerated by the patient, or if it is ineffective and the problem is severe (i.e., causing cardiac arrhythmias or severe hypoxia), tracheostomy is indicated. This procedure can be very difficult and dangerous and therefore should not be relegated to the youngest house officer in a surgical residency program. Because of the extremely deep neck in obese patients, a standard tracheostomy tube is usually inadequate, and a special tube with a deep bend should be used.

OHS is a condition associated with morbid obesity in which an individual suffers from hypoxemia and hypercapnia when breathing room air while awake but resting.[26] Spirometry reveals decreases in forced vital capacity, residual lung volume, expiratory reserve volume, functional residual capacity, and maximum minute volume ventilation, usually without obstruction to airflow [see Figure 1]. The most profound decrease is that in expiratory reserve volume; it is probably secondary to increased intra-abdominal pressure and a high-riding diaphragm. Thus, these patients have restrictive rather than obstructive pulmonary disease. The decreased expiratory reserve volume implies that many alveolar units are collapsed at end-expiration, which leads to perfusion of unventilated alveoli, or shunting. Patients with OHS often are heavy smokers or have additional pulmonary problems, such as asthma, sarcoidosis, idiopathic pulmonary fibrosis, or recurrent pulmonary emboli. One study of patients who underwent operation for morbid obesity showed no statistically significant difference in weight between those who had OHS and those who did not.[3]

As a result of chronic and severe hypoxemia, patients with OHS are often markedly polycythemic. The polycythemia further increases their already significant risk for venous thrombosis and pulmonary embolism. Because we have had several patients who later had a subclavian venous thrombosis and one patient who probably had a transient sagittal sinus thrombosis, patients with OHS should probably undergo phlebotomy to a hemoglobin concentration of 15 g/dl before elective operation.

Chronic hypoxemia also leads to pulmonary arterial vasoconstriction and severe pulmonary hypertension[1,27] and eventually to right-sided heart failure or cor pulmonale with neck vein distention, tricuspid valvular insufficiency, right upper quadrant tenderness secondary to acute hepatic engorgement, and massive peripheral edema. Such patients may also have significantly elevated PAWP, which suggests left ventricular dysfunction.[1] All morbidly obese patients should have preoperative determinations of blood gas values. If an abnormality is detected, spirometry can be performed, although it would probably be of little additional diagnostic value. If arterial blood gas measurement reveals severe hypoxemia (i.e., $P_aO_2 \leq 55$ mm Hg), severe hypercapnia ($P_aCO_2 \geq 47$ mm Hg), or both, the patient should undergo Swan-Ganz catheterization. If PAWP is 18 mm Hg or greater, intravenous furosemide should be administered for diuresis before elective operation. However, some patients may require a high ventricular filling pressure. A low cardiac output and hypotension may follow diuresis, necessitating volume reexpansion. If mean PAP is 40 mm Hg or greater, consideration should be given to the prophylactic insertion of a Greenfield inferior vena caval filter [see Thrombophlebitis, Venous Stasis Ulcers, and Pulmonary Embolism in the Morbidly Obese Patient, *below*].

It is highly probable that some of the elevated PAP and PAWP measurements are caused by the increased IAP in the morbidly obese[15,28] [see Figure 2]. This leads to an elevated diaphragm, which in turn increases intrapleural pressure and thereby PAP and PAWP; if the pleural pressure is measured with an esophageal transducer, the transmyocardial pressure can be estimated. For this reason, these patients may require a markedly elevated PAWP to maintain an adequate cardiac output, and excessive diuresis may lead to hypotension. The same reasoning may be applied to a patient with a distended abdomen resulting from peritonitis and pancreatitis in whom what seem to be unusually high cardiac filling pressures are

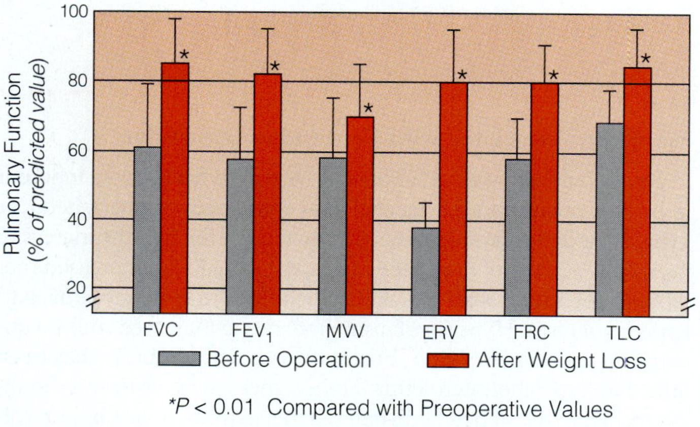

*$P < 0.01$ Compared with Preoperative Values

Figure 1 Impaired pulmonary function in the morbidly obese improved significantly after weight loss induced by gastric operation.[3]

necessary. Therefore, one must rely on relative changes in cardiac output in response to either volume challenge or diuresis to determine the optimal PAWP in morbidly obese patients.

Patients with OHS respond rapidly to supplemental oxygen. However, oxygen administration is occasionally associated with significant CO_2 retention, which necessitates intubation and mechanical ventilation. Because their pulmonary disease is restrictive rather than obstructive, these patients are usually easy to ventilate without high peak airway pressures. Arterial blood gases need not return to normal before extubation; it is only necessary that they return to their preoperative values. These values are achieved, on average, 4 days after major upper abdominal operation, when the patients no longer have abdominal pain.[3]

It is important to emphasize that morbidly obese patients, especially those with respiratory insufficiency, should be placed in the reverse Trendelenburg's position to maximize diaphragmatic excursion and to increase residual lung volume.[7] These patients will often complain of air hunger and respiratory distress when they lie supine. So-called breaking of the bed at the waist may exacerbate the problem by pushing the abdominal contents into the chest, thereby raising the diaphragm and further reducing lung volumes. Placing these patients in the leg-down position may predispose them to venous stasis, phlebitis, and pulmonary embolism, which should be offset with intermittent venous compression boots [see Thrombophlebitis, Venous Stasis Ulcers, and Pulmonary Embolism in the Morbidly Obese Patient, *below*].[29]

Both SAS and OHS can be completely corrected with weight reduction after gastric operation for morbid obesity: the nocturnal apneas resolve, the P_aO_2 rises, and the P_aCO_2 falls to normal as lung volumes improve.[3]

Cardiac Dysfunction in the Morbidly Obese Patient

Cardiac dysfunction in the morbidly obese patient is usually associated with respiratory insufficiency of obesity, especially OHS.[2] Elevated PAP in these patients may be secondary to hypoxemia-induced pulmonary arterial vasoconstriction, to elevated left atrial pressures secondary to left ventricular dysfunction, or to a combination of these; they may also be secondary to the increased pleural pressures arising from an elevated diaphragm secondary to increased IAP.[1,28,29] It is unusual for morbidly obese patients without respiratory insufficiency to experience significant cardiac dysfunction in the absence of severe coronary artery disease. Morbidly obese patients often have systemic hypertension, which can aggravate left ventricular dysfunction; however, mild left ventricular dysfunction can be documented in many morbidly obese patients in the absence of systemic hypertension.[30,31] Circulating blood volume, plasma volume, and cardiac output increase in proportion to body weight.[31] Massively obese patients may occasionally present with acute heart failure: it is reasonable to assume that the enormous metabolic requirements of such patients can present a greater demand for blood flow than the heart can provide. Vigorous diuresis will often correct such acute heart failure. Significant weight loss will correct pulmonary hypertension [see Figure 3] as well as left ventricular dysfunction associated with respiratory insufficiency.[1,32]

Thrombophlebitis, Venous Stasis Ulcers, and Pulmonary Embolism in the Morbidly Obese Patient

Morbidly obese individuals have difficulty walking; tend to be sedentary; have a large amount of abdominal weight resting on their inferior vena cava; and have increased intrapleural pressure, which impedes venous return.[27,28] All of these conditions increase the tendency toward phlebothrombosis. The patient is most at risk when immobilized in the supine position for long periods in the operating room. These patients have also been shown to have low levels of antithrombin III, which may increase their tendency toward venous thrombosis.[33] It has also been suggested that starvation, particularly in the postoperative period, may be associated with high levels of free fatty acids, which may predispose to perioperative thrombotic complications.[34]

Intermittent venous compression boots have been shown in randomized trials to reduce the incidence of deep vein thrombosis.[29] Administration of low-dose subcutaneous heparin must be started immediately before operation. However, because morbidly obese patients show a significant improvement in pulmonary function when placed in the reverse Trendelenburg's position,[7] and because this position further increases venous pressure in the legs and the tendency toward stasis, it is preferable to use this position and intermittent venous compression boots. All patients, but especially the

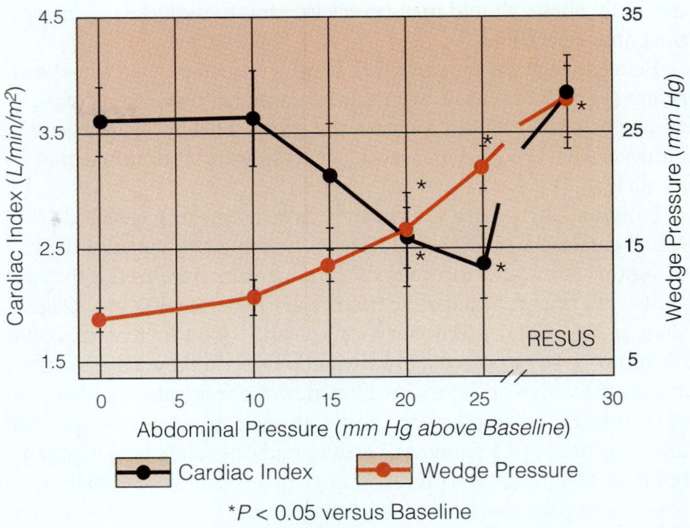

Figure 2 In a porcine model,[28] raising IAP caused cardiac index to fall and PAWP to rise. At an IAP of 25 mm Hg, saline was given to restore intravascular volume; cardiac index returned to baseline levels, but PAWP remained elevated. (IAP—intra-abdominal pressure; PAWP—pulmonary arterial wedge pressure)

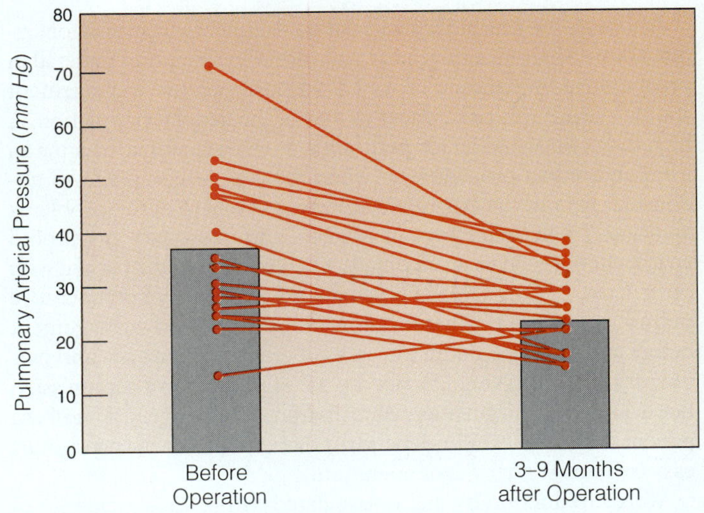

Figure 3 Mean pulmonary arterial pressure was significantly improved in 18 patients 3 to 9 months after gastric surgery–induced weight loss of 42% ± 19% of excess weight.[1]

morbidly obese, should make every attempt to walk during the evening after operation.

Because pulmonary embolism is quite unusual when the appropriate precautions have been taken, acute air hunger, tachypnea, and hypoxemia should suggest the equal likelihood that sepsis-induced ARDS is present secondary to an intra-abdominal anastomotic leak.

Patients with severe OHS often have noticeably elevated PAP, which can lead to right-sided heart failure and can increase the risk of venous stasis and thrombosis. Investigators have noted that patients with primary idiopathic pulmonary hypertension are at significant risk for fatal pulmonary embolism.[5] For this reason, it has been our policy to place a prophylactic Greenfield vena caval filter in patients with respiratory insufficiency of obesity and a mean PAP of 40 mm Hg or greater. With this approach (in which a vena caval filter was used in 15 patients), we have had one fatal pulmonary embolus in 156 patients with respiratory insufficiency of obesity who have undergone gastric bariatric procedures. The fatality was a patient whose mean PAP was initially 40 mm Hg but fell to 35 mm Hg with diuresis and who was not considered to require a filter.

Venous stasis ulcers can be quite difficult to treat in a thin individual; they are almost impossible to cure in a patient with morbid obesity [see Figure 4]. The most important goal in management of these ulcers is weight loss, which almost invariably leads to healing of the ulcer, probably as a result of decreased IAP.

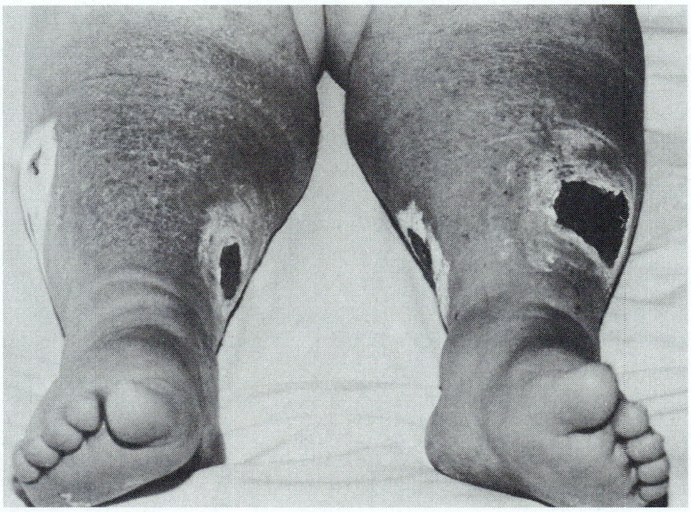

Pseudotumor Cerebri in the Morbidly Obese Patient

Pseudotumor cerebri (also known as idiopathic intracranial hypertension) associated with obesity is almost certainly secondary to increased IAP. The rise in IAP causes a rise in intrathoracic pressure, which in turn raises central venous pressure and PAWP [see Figure 2], thus decreasing venous drainage from the brain.[28] This sequence of events has been reproduced in a porcine model.[35] The elevated intracranial pressure (ICP) can be prevented by means of median sternotomy and pleuropericardiotomy [see Figure 5].[36] In humans studied 3 years after weight-reduction surgery, surgically induced weight loss was associated with a significant decrease in ICP (from 353 ± 35 mm H₂O to 168 ± 12 mm H₂O; $P < 0.001$) and with relief of headache and pulsatile tinnitus.[19,20]

Conclusion

Although the morbidly obese patient is potentially at risk for significant perioperative morbidity and mortality, attention to detail in preoperative preparation as well as in postoperative management should reduce this risk almost to that of the general population. A high index of suspicion for peritonitis must be maintained after an intra-abdominal procedure or when the patient complains of abdominal pain in the emergency room. Awareness of the problems associated with respiratory insufficiency in obese patients should enable the surgeon to avoid pitfalls when managing the patient with obstructive SAS or OHS. These patients may require preoperative pulmonary arterial catheterization for optimal fluid management before and after operation. The risks of venous thrombosis and pulmonary embolism are high, but the use of intermittent compression boots and early ambulation can minimize the dangers. The obese patient with non–insulin-dependent diabetes has been surprisingly easy to manage after major operation.

Weight reduction by diet is associated with a 95% incidence of recidivism. The average morbidly obese patient can be expected to lose two thirds of the excess weight within 1 year after a standard GBP or, if superobese, after a long-limb gastric bypass. Furthermore, recent reports note that this weight loss is long-lasting and averages 60% of excess weight at 5 years and more than 50% of excess weight up to 10 years after operation. This weight loss is associated with the correction of insulin-dependent diabetes, obstructive SAS, OHS, pseudotumor cerebri, hypertension, chronic venous stasis ulcers, stress incontinence, gastroesophageal reflux, and female sex hormone abnormalities, which may be related to dysmenorrhea, infertility, hirsutism, and an increased risk of endometrial carcinoma. Weight loss can markedly improve the patient's self-image and employability. Because techniques for operation for morbid obesity continue to change as understanding of pathophysiology improves, it is important for surgeons to keep abreast of the latest developments.

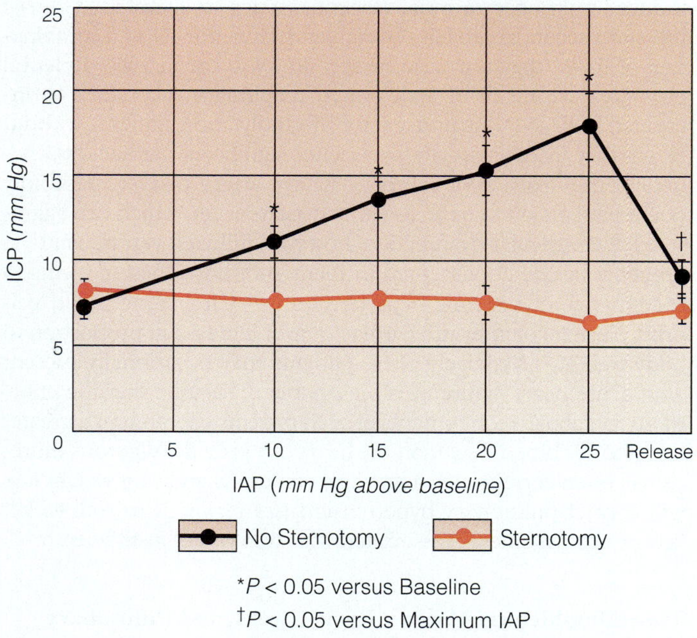

Figure 4 This chronic venous stasis ulcer was present for several years in a morbidly obese patient. Healing promptly followed weight loss induced by a gastric operation.

Figure 5 In a porcine model,[36] IAP was increased to 25 mm Hg in 12 animals, of which three underwent median sternotomy and pleuropericardiotomy (red line) and nine did not (black line). Sternotomy and pleuropericardiotomy prevented the expected increase in ICP. (ICP—intracranial pressure)

References

1. Sugerman HJ, Baron PL, Fairman RP, et al: Hemodynamic dysfunction in obesity hypoventilation syndrome and the effects of treatment with surgically induced weight loss. Ann Surg 207:604, 1988
2. Burwell CS, Robin ED, Whaley RD, et al: Extreme obesity associated with alveolar hypoventilation—a pickwickian syndrome. Am J Med 21:811, 1956
3. Sugerman HJ, Fairman RP, Baron PL, et al: Gastric surgery for respiratory insufficiency of obesity. Chest 89:81, 1986
4. Sugerman HJ, Fairman RP, Sood RK, et al: Long-term effects of gastric surgery for treating respiratory insufficiency of obesity. Am J Clin Nutr 55(2 suppl):597S, 1992
5. Young T, Palta M, Dempsey J, et al: The occurrence of sleep-disordered breathing among middle-aged adults. N Engl J Med 328:1230, 1993
6. Greenfield LJ, Scher LA, Elkins RC: KMA-Greenfield® filter placement for chronic pulmonary hypertension. Ann Surg 189:560, 1979
7. Vaughan RW, Bauer S, Wise L: Effect of position (semirecumbent versus supine) on postoperative oxygenation in markedly obese subjects. Anesth Analg 55:37, 1976
8. Mason EE, Printen KJ, Barron P, et al: Risk reduction in gastric operations for obesity. Ann Surg 190:158, 1979
9. Herbst CA, Hughes TA, Gwynne JT, et al: Gastric bariatric operation in insulin-treated adults. Surgery 95:209, 1984
10. McNeill PM, Sugerman HJ: Continuous absorbable vs interrupted nonabsorbable fascial closure: a prospective, randomized comparison. Arch Surg 121:821, 1986
11. Richards PC, Balch CM, Aldrete JS: Abdominal wound closure: a randomized prospective study of 571 patients comparing continuous vs. interrupted suture techniques. Ann Surg 197:238, 1983
12. De Holl D, Rodeheaver G, Edgerton MT, et al: Potentiation of infection by suture closure of dead space. Am J Surg 127:716, 1974
13. Stone HH, Hooper CA, Kolb LD, et al: Antibiotic prophylaxis in gastric, biliary, and colonic surgery. Ann Surg 184:443, 1976
14. Sugerman HJ, Kellum JM, Reines HD, et al: Incisional hernia: greater risk with morbidly obese than steroid dependent patients; low recurrence rate with prefascial polypropylene mesh repair. Am J Surg 171:80, 1996
15. Sugerman H, Windsor A, Bessos M, et al: Intra-abdominal pressure, sagittal abdominal diameter, and obesity co-morbidity. J Intern Med 241:71, 1997
16. Rouse TM, Malangoni MA, Schulte WJ: Necrotizing fasciitis: a preventable disaster. Surgery 92:765, 1982
17. Sugerman HJ, Brewer WH, Shiffman ML, et al: A multicenter, placebo-controlled, randomized, double-blind, prospective trial of prophylactic ursodiol for the prevention of gallstone formation following gastric-bypass-induced rapid weight loss. Am J Surg 169:91, 1995
18. Corbett JJ, Mehta MP: Cerebrospinal fluid pressure in normal obese subjects and patients with pseudotumor cerebri. Neurology 33:1386, 1983
19. Sugerman HJ, Felton WL, Salvant JB, et al: Effects of surgically induced weight loss on pseudotumor cerebri in morbid obesity. Neurology 45:1655, 1995
20. Sugerman HJ, Felton WL III, Sismanis A, et al: Gastric surgery for pseudotumor cerebri associated with severe obesity. Ann Surg 229:634, 1999
21. Goldin RH, McAdam L, Louie JS, et al: Clinical and radiologic survey of the incidence of osteoarthritis among obese patients. Ann Rheum Dis 35:349, 1976
22. Kissebah AH, Vydelingum N, Murray R, et al: Relation of body fat distribution to metabolic complications of obesity. J Clin Endocrinol Metab 54:254, 1982
23. Kvist H, Chowdhury B, Grangard U, et al: Total and visceral adipose-tissue volumes derived from measurements with computed tomography in adult men and women: predictive equations. Am J Clin Nutr 48:1351, 1988
24. Bump RC, Sugerman HJ, Fantl JA, et al: Obesity and lower urinary tract function in women: effect of surgically induced weight loss. Am J Obstet Gynecol 167:392, 1992
25. Sullivan CE, Issa FG, Berthon-Jones M, et al: Reversal of obstructive sleep apnoea by continuous positive airway pressure applied through the nares. Lancet 1:862, 1981
26. Rochester DR, Enson Y: Current concepts in the pathogenesis of the obesity hypoventilation syndrome: mechanical and circulatory factors. Am J Med 57:402, 1974
27. Alexander JK, Amad KH, Cole VW: Observations on some clinical features of extreme obesity, with particular reference to cardiorespiratory effects. Am J Med 32:512, 1962
28. Ridings PC, Bloomfield GL, Blocher CR, et al: Cardiopulmonary effects of raised intra-abdominal pressure before and after volume expansion. J Trauma 39:1168, 1995
29. Coe NP, Collins RE, Klein LA, et al: Prevention of deep vein thrombosis in urological patients: a controlled, randomized trial of low-dose heparin and external pneumatic compression boots. Surgery 83:230, 1978
30. Kaltman AJ, Goldring RM: Role of circulatory congestion in the cardiorespiratory failure of obesity. Am J Med 60:645, 1976
31. De Divitiis O, Fazio S, Petitto M, et al: Obesity and cardiac function. Circulation 64:477, 1981
32. Alpert MA, Terry BE, Kelly DL: Effect of weight loss on cardiac chamber size, wall thickness and left ventricular function in morbid obesity. Am J Cardiol 55:783, 1985
33. Batist G, Bothe A, Bern M, et al: Low antithrombin III in morbid obesity: return to normal with weight reduction. JPEN 7:447, 1983
34. Printen HJ, Miller EV, Mason EE, et al: Venous thromboembolism in the morbidly obese. Surg Gynecol Obstet 147:63, 1978
35. Bloomfield GL, Ridings PC, Blocher CR, et al: Effects of increased intra-abdominal pressure upon intracranial and cerebral perfusion before and after volume expansion. J Trauma 40:936, 1996
36. Bloomfield GL, Ridings PC, Blocher CR, et al: A proposed relationship between increased intra-abdominal, intrathoracic, and intracranial pressure. Crit Care Med 25:496, 1997

Acknowledgments

Figures 1 and 3 Albert Miller.
Figures 2 and 5 Marcia Kammerer.

70 THROMBOEMBOLIC PROBLEMS

F. William Blaisdell, M.D., and John T. Owings, M.D.

Approach to Venous Thromboembolism

Superficial Thrombophlebitis

CLINICAL MANIFESTATIONS

Superficial thrombophlebitis has several characteristic clinical manifestations [see Figure 1]. Pain is usually present, and slight swelling of the extremity can be seen, with most of the edema occurring over the course of the involved vein. Unless the patient is obese, with a heavy layer of subcutaneous tissue, a palpable, very tender subcutaneous cord is usually found; the presence of this cord is pathognomonic of the disease. There is usually some edema in the adjacent subcutaneous tissue and erythema in the overlying skin. The main conditions to be considered in the differential diagnosis are cellulitis and streptococcal lymphangitis. For both conditions, there should be a proximal source (e.g., an open wound); neither condition will be associated with a palpable cord or with evidence of increased superficial collateral circulation.

If there is overt limb swelling (i.e., one limb is at least several centimeters larger in diameter than the other) in a patient who appears to have superficial phlebitis, associated deep thrombophlebitis should be assumed, and appropriate treatment [see Deep Thrombophlebitis, below] should be initiated.

Superficial thrombophlebitis, which is largely a benign disease, is often overtreated out of fear that infection may be contributing to the phlebitis. It is therefore important to differentiate between sterile superficial thrombophlebitis and septic superficial thrombophlebitis. The two are often confused because they may have many of the same manifestations (e.g., redness and induration).

STERILE THROMBOPHLEBITIS

Sterile thrombophlebitis can be assumed with minimal risk of misdiagnosis if there has been no invasion in or near the superficial vein involved. The condition is best treated not with immobilization of the patient or the extremity but with administration of aspirin (one tablet daily) or dipyridamole (50 mg four times daily).

If the phlebitis persists or continues to extend and there is significant morbidity, interruption of the vein may be appropriate, particularly when a lower extremity saphenous vein is involved. This is especially true when the phlebitis is affecting a previously varicose vein; because these dilated veins can accommodate a large amount of clot, considerable disability can result. The choice of treatment is between interrupting the vein above the area of palpable thrombosis and stripping and removing the vein. The second alternative carries a higher morbidity than simple interruption, but it can be used effectively when there are associated varicosities and the thrombosis is not responding to treatment. Stripping of the channels above and below the phlebitic process as well as the phlebitic area itself will remove the risk of extension of the phlebitis and subsequent recurrence.

SEPTIC THROMBOPHLEBITIS

When the vein has been invaded or when there are systemic manifestations of severe infection (e.g., fever and an elevated white blood cell count), septic thrombophlebitis is likely. In addition, the induration, tenderness, and redness over and along the course of the vein are usually more extensive than with sterile thrombophlebitis.

If the phlebitis is associated with an intravenous catheter, the device should be removed, the tip cultured, and the patient's response observed [see 81 Nosocomial Infection]. If the patient has no overt systemic signs of infection, treatment is similar to that of sterile phlebitis. If the patient has systemic signs, antibiotics should be administered; if a skin organism is the presumed source of infection, antistaphylococcal drugs are appropriate. If the patient is a drug addict or the phlebitis is associated with a contaminated wound, blood samples for culture and a Gram's stain should be obtained by aspirating the vein with a small syringe and needle. Specific antibiotic therapy directed toward the organisms seen on Gram's stain or culture should then be instituted.

If the patient is in a toxic state from presumed septic phlebitis in a subcutaneous vein or is not responding to treatment, it may be appropriate to ligate the vein, to drain it by cutting down on the phlebitic process with the patient under local or general anesthesia and laying the vein open, or to combine ligation with drainage. Moist compresses are then applied, the area is immobilized, and antibiotics are administered. Heparin may occasionally be of value, particularly when the process appears to be extending into the deep venous system (e.g., into the saphenofemoral junction).

Deep Thrombophlebitis

CLINICAL MANIFESTATIONS

Deep thrombophlebitis can involve either obstructive clots, which affect the drainage of venous blood from an extremity, or nonobstructive clots, which are relatively asymptomatic [see Figure 2]. Obstructive clots may also occur in association with nonobstructive clots. The latter are more dangerous because they are not circumferentially attached to the vein wall, do not elicit much vein inflammation, and are prone to embolization—the lethal complication of deep thrombophlebitis.

Deep thrombophlebitis may be divided into three main forms: nonocclusive thrombophlebitis, occlusive thrombophlebitis, and phlegmasia cerulea dolens (massive thrombophlebi-

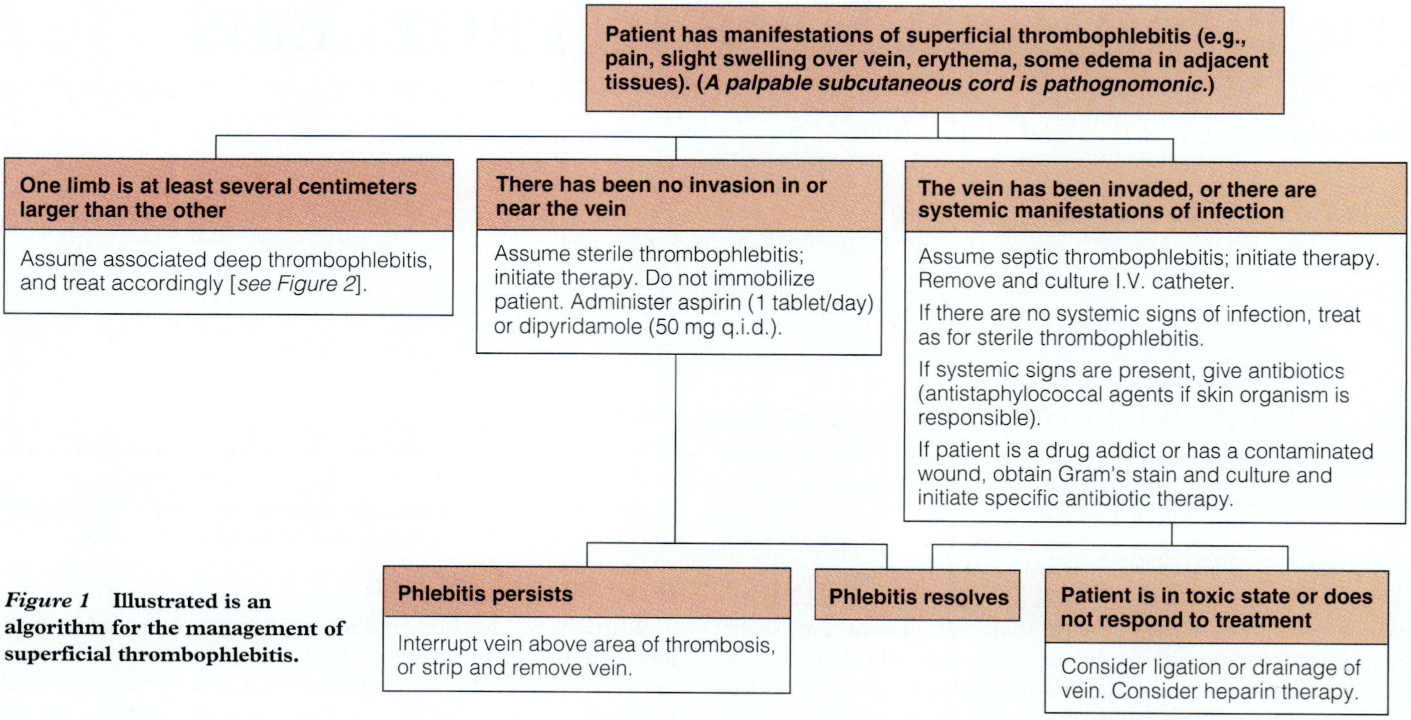

Figure 1 Illustrated is an algorithm for the management of superficial thrombophlebitis.

[Algorithm flowchart:]

- **Patient has manifestations of superficial thrombophlebitis (e.g., pain, slight swelling over vein, erythema, some edema in adjacent tissues). (*A palpable subcutaneous cord is pathognomonic.*)**

  - **One limb is at least several centimeters larger than the other**
    - Assume associated deep thrombophlebitis, and treat accordingly [*see Figure 2*].

  - **There has been no invasion in or near the vein**
    - Assume sterile thrombophlebitis; initiate therapy. Do not immobilize patient. Administer aspirin (1 tablet/day) or dipyridamole (50 mg q.i.d.).

  - **The vein has been invaded, or there are systemic manifestations of infection**
    - Assume septic thrombophlebitis; initiate therapy. Remove and culture I.V. catheter.
    - If there are no systemic signs of infection, treat as for sterile thrombophlebitis.
    - If systemic signs are present, give antibiotics (antistaphylococcal agents if skin organism is responsible).
    - If patient is a drug addict or has a contaminated wound, obtain Gram's stain and culture and initiate specific antibiotic therapy.

  - **Phlebitis persists**
    - Interrupt vein above area of thrombosis, or strip and remove vein.

  - **Phlebitis resolves**

  - **Patient is in toxic state or does not respond to treatment**
    - Consider ligation or drainage of vein. Consider heparin therapy.

tis). Each form gives rise to different clinical problems and therefore is discussed separately.

NONOCCLUSIVE THROMBOPHLEBITIS

Nonocclusive thrombophlebitis, sometimes referred to as phlebothrombosis, is a frequent complication in postoperative surgical patients. Unfortunately, its presence all too often is not suspected until an embolic complication occurs. In many instances, it is the development of pulmonary embolism that precipitates the search for asymptomatic deep vein thrombosis. There may be absolutely no manifestations of clot on clinical examination, or there may be some nonspecific swelling in an extremity; rarely is there sufficient pain or tenderness to suggest the presence of deep thrombophlebitis. Consequently, it is essential to be aware of the major risk factors for this condition [*see Table 1*].

When thrombophlebitis develops or appears likely to develop in an outpatient, every effort should be made to determine the cause because apparent spontaneous onset of this condition is often the manifestation of a congenital clotting tendency that will necessitate lifelong treatment [*see* Approach to Acquired and Congenital Thrombotic Syndromes, *below*]. Conversely, when risk factors for deep thrombophlebitis (e.g., injury, the postoperative state, or systemic infection) are identified in a hospitalized patient, it can be assumed that the etiology is acquired and that the clotting tendency will be reversed when the patient recovers from his or her illness. If there is no contraindication to anticoagulation, moderate- or high-dose heparin therapy can be initiated on an empirical basis. Even if tests reveal no clot at the moment, the patient remains at risk for thrombophlebitis.

Once anticoagulant therapy is begun, the diagnosis, if not already clinically obvious, should be verified. The differential diagnosis includes muscle contusion, plantar muscle rupture, gastrocnemius muscle rupture, ruptured Baker's cyst, popliteal artery aneurysm, arthritis of the knee or the ankle, cellulitis, and myositis. The gold standard for diagnosis of deep thrombophlebitis is phlebography. However, study of the entire lower extremity venous system often involves injection of dye not only at the foot or ankle level but also at the groin level so that the iliac and femoral veins can be adequately visualized. This approach is uncomfortable for the patient and is associated with morbidity; in critically ill ICU patients, it may not be feasible. For these reasons, noninvasive techniques of evaluating the veins are favored.

The most sensitive noninvasive technique is iodine-125 (^{125}I)–labeled fibrinogen scanning. This test is so efficient at detecting small calf vein thrombi that it frequently detects minor disease that is of little or no clinical significance. Calf vein thrombi, by themselves, are almost always clinically insignificant: although they occur in as many as 30 to 40 percent of hospitalized patients, they usually resolve spontaneously. It is thrombi in the major deep veins of the thigh and the pelvis that place the patient at high risk for morbidity and mortality. Clots in these vessels are not diagnosed well by ^{125}I-labeled fibrinogen scanning. In addition, this technique yields false positives in patients who have had bleeding or inflammation. Consequently, this study, despite its sensitivity, is no longer used in most centers.[1-3]

Various modifications of plethysmographic techniques have been used.[4,5] For instance, impedance plethysmography measures alterations in calf circumference by recording changes in electrical impedance. These techniques are strictly noninvasive and are accurate only when there is at least 50 percent obstruction of the lumen of a deep vein. The presence of large collateral vessels may result in a false negative test result as well.

Doppler ultrasonography can be performed quickly and easily. It measures alterations in venous flow velocity during compression and during respiratory excursion. Interpretation of the results, however, requires considerable experience. Because Doppler ultrasonography is a physiologic method that depends on alterations in flow and the presence of obstruction, it has the same drawbacks as plethysmography.[4]

Real-time B-mode (duplex) ultrasonography, originally developed to visualize extracranial cerebrovascular disease, has recently proved valuable in detecting deep thrombophlebitis.[4,6,7] B-mode ultrasonography can actually visualize the thrombus within a vessel. Inability to obliterate the vein with probe compression is additional evidence of thrombus. Often, experienced users can even differentiate between new and old thrombi: the former are compressible, whereas the latter are not.

B-mode ultrasonography is quite sensitive and specific in patients with suspected deep vein thrombosis; the addition of color flow imaging may further enhance its diagnostic qualities. Its sensitivity is similar to that of impedance plethysmography, and it has in fact become the noninvasive procedure of choice for assessment of clot in the neck and the extremity vessels. Unfortunately, it is less specific above the axilla and the inguinal ligament because in these regions it is difficult to compress the vessels. B-mode ultrasonography is particularly valuable for detecting associated conditions that may confuse the diagnosis (e.g., muscle hematomas or a popliteal cyst).[7]

Ultimately, ascending phlebography is the most accurate method of assessment.[8,9] This approach requires cannulation of a vein of the foot; if the iliac veins are not well visualized or the vena cava is suspect, it may be necessary to inject the contrast agent into the femoral vein [see Figure 3]. If a good contrast study fails to demonstrate the presence of clot, venous thrombophlebitis is effectively ruled out.

Once nonocclusive phlebitis is diagnosed, the treatment of choice is medium-dose heparin anticoagulation. After three or four days, depending on the response, heparin can be replaced with an oral anticoagulant, such as warfarin. If anticoagulation is contraindicated because of the presence of fresh wounds or a bleeding disorder, low-molecular-weight dextran may be of some benefit.

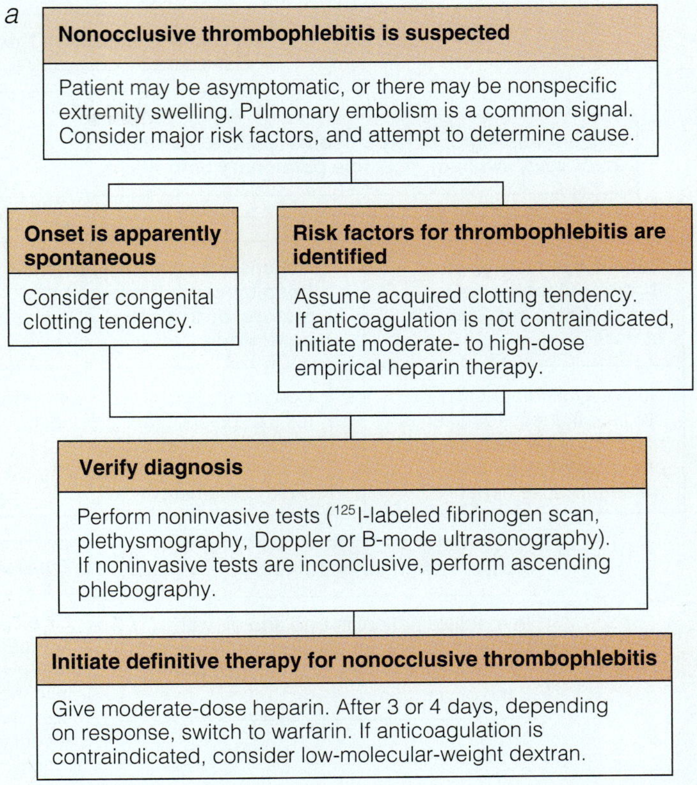

OCCLUSIVE THROMBOPHLEBITIS

Leg Thrombophlebitis

In the lower extremity, deep thrombophlebitis that produces venous obstruction is usually associated with swelling; however, if good collateral circulation or duplicate veins are present, especially in the thigh, only local manifestations of inflammation may be apparent. The typical findings include pain and tenderness over the involved veins as well as swelling in the distal limb (which may be minimal with the patient in the supine position). The differential diagnosis is essentially the same as for nonocclusive thrombophlebitis. Lower leg occlusive thrombophlebitis is characterized by pain, swelling, and tenderness of the limb in the segment below the phlebitic process. In addition, lower extremity thrombophlebitis can be associated with pulmonary embolism: free-floating clot may occur in conjunction with occlusive (inflammatory) clot, although the latter is inevitably firmly adherent to the vein wall.

If the entire leg is swollen, the proximal portion of the clotting process must be in the iliac veins. If both legs are involved, involvement of the cava is likely. If the swelling is limited to the lower leg below the knee, the thrombotic problem is probably in the superficial femoral vein. If the manifestation is simply calf tenderness with only minimal to moderate swelling, then the thrombus is probably limited to the sural vein, the gastrocnemius vein, or both.

If the patient has a history of thrombophlebitis, is hospitalized, and has risk factors for deep thrombophlebitis, it is appropriate to begin treatment with moderate-dose heparin without ordering further diagnostic studies if there is no contraindication to anticoagulation. If the patient is an outpatient, if the patient is hospitalized but has no risk factors for deep thrombophlebitis, or if there appears to be a potential contraindication to anticoagulation, then the diagnosis should be confirmed by means of the same techniques that are recommended for nonocclusive thrombophlebitis. In such patients, the accuracy of noninvasive assessment is excellent because any clot present must be occlusive. Impedance plethysmography, Doppler and B-mode ultrasonography, and phlebography can all be used with confidence. If diagnostic studies yield equivocal results and phlebography is difficult or impossible, treatment should proceed as if the diagnosis had been confirmed.

a

Nonocclusive thrombophlebitis is suspected

Patient may be asymptomatic, or there may be nonspecific extremity swelling. Pulmonary embolism is a common signal. Consider major risk factors, and attempt to determine cause.

Onset is apparently spontaneous

Consider congenital clotting tendency.

Risk factors for thrombophlebitis are identified

Assume acquired clotting tendency. If anticoagulation is not contraindicated, initiate moderate- to high-dose empirical heparin therapy.

Verify diagnosis

Perform noninvasive tests (^{125}I-labeled fibrinogen scan, plethysmography, Doppler or B-mode ultrasonography). If noninvasive tests are inconclusive, perform ascending phlebography.

Initiate definitive therapy for nonocclusive thrombophlebitis

Give moderate-dose heparin. After 3 or 4 days, depending on response, switch to warfarin. If anticoagulation is contraindicated, consider low-molecular-weight dextran.

Figure 2 Illustrated are algorithms for the management of deep thrombophlebitis. The treatment approach depends on whether the thrombophlebitis is nonocclusive (*a*), occlusive (*b*), or massive (*c*). [*Figure continues on p. 1016.*]

Table 1   Risk Factors for the Development of Acute Deep Thrombophlebitis

Hypercoagulability
   Congenital hypercoagulability
   Malignancy
   Oral contraceptives
   Polycythemia
   Thrombocytosis
Venous stasis
   Immobility
   Varicose veins
   Advanced age
   Congestive heart failure
   Obesity
Endothelial injury
   Trauma
   Recent surgery
   Severe infection

b

```
Signs of occlusive thrombophlebitis are present
```

Patient has signs of leg phlebitis (pain, tenderness over vein, swelling, possible pulmonary embolism)

- **Patient has history of thrombophlebitis, is hospitalized, and has risk factors**
  Do not await diagnostic studies. If anticoagulation is not contraindicated, begin empirical treatment with moderate-dose heparin.

- **Patient is outpatient, patient is hospitalized but has no risk factors, or treatment is contraindicated**
  Confirm diagnosis via noninvasive tests or phlebography. If these modalities are inconclusive, proceed as if diagnosis had been confirmed.

- **Initiate definitive treatment**
  Immobilize patient in bed and elevate leg (with or without elastic compression). Give moderate-dose heparin, followed by 6 mo of warfarin.

Patient has signs of arm phlebitis (pain, tenderness over vein, swelling); may be relatively asymptomatic

- **Patient has no systemic signs of infection**
  Assume that patient has sterile thrombophlebitis. If diagnosis is in doubt, utilize noninvasive tests or phlebography.

- **Patient has systemic signs of infection**
  Assume that patient has septic thrombophlebitis.

- **Treat sterile thrombophlebitis**
  Give moderate-dose heparin immediately. Consider lytic therapy. If arm veins are compressed after lytic therapy or spontaneous recovery from thrombosis, consider first-rib resection.

- **Treat septic thrombophlebitis**
  Remove any foreign body, culture tip, and do a Gram's stain of any clot. Give moderate-dose heparin. Give broad-spectrum antibiotics until organism is identified, then initiate specific antibiotic therapy.

  - **Phlebitis resolves**
  - **Phlebitis persists**
    Consider ligation or drainage of vein.

c

- **Signs of phlegmasia cerulea dolens are present**
  Limb is massively swollen, bluish, and mottled distally. Gangrene is noted. Acute fluid losses may lead to hypovolemic shock.

- **Treat phlegmasia cerulea dolens**
  Replace fluids and elevate limb. Give high-dose heparin.

  - **Phlebitis resolves**
  - **Phlebitis persists**
    Consider thrombectomy.

The treatment of choice is immobilization in bed, elevation of the limb (with or without elastic compression), and moderate-dose heparin, usually followed by three to six months of warfarin therapy. If the episode is mild, recovery is usually prompt. If the pain and swelling do not respond promptly to anticoagulation, either the diagnosis is wrong or the anticoagulation is inadequate [see General Principles of Anticoagulation and Lytic Therapy, below]. The combination of lytic therapy and heparin anticoagulation may be superior to heparin anticoagulation alone, leading to better clearance of clot from the valves with improved function and less risk of postphlebitic syndrome.[10]

Arm Thrombophlebitis

For all practical purposes, deep thrombophlebitis of the upper extremity involves only the axillary, the subclavian, or the innominate vein (or a combination thereof). Involvement of the superior vena cava is rare; when it does occur, it is usually in chronic conditions, such as malignancy in the mediastinum and long-term venous catheterization. Arm thrombophlebitis is characterized by pain and swelling in the involved limb with tenderness over the involved vein. In many instances, however, the condition is relatively asymptomatic: because of the excellent collateral circulation in the arm, particularly about the shoulder, the thrombosis must be extensive to produce marked swelling.

Spontaneous onset of axillary or subclavian vein thrombosis can occur in association with thoracic compression syndromes or as a complication of so-called Saturday night palsy (the result of an alcoholic's sleeping with his or her axilla compressed by the arm of a chair); investigation into the etiology [see Table 2], which includes the acquired and congenital clotting disorders [see Approach to Acquired and Congenital Thrombotic Syndromes, below] in the absence of mechanical factors that might explain the condition, is called for. The onset of swelling, tenderness, or fever in a patient with a central venous catheter is an indication for removal of the foreign body. If the patient is not bacteremic or febrile, if there has been a foreign body in the vein, and if the problem developed spontaneously, the presumption is that he or she has a sterile thrombophlebitis.

Subclinical nonocclusive clot is probably of little significance because documented pulmonary embolism from the upper extremity is quite rare. For this reason, the need for diagnosis of thrombophlebitis is less compelling in the upper extremity than in the lower extremity. Most of the noninvasive tests described earlier [see Nonocclusive Thrombophlebitis, above] usually yield positive results when the upper extremity is involved.[8] Moreover, catheterization of the distal veins is easy, and phlebography is relatively uncomplicated. These techniques should be used whenever the diagnosis is in doubt.

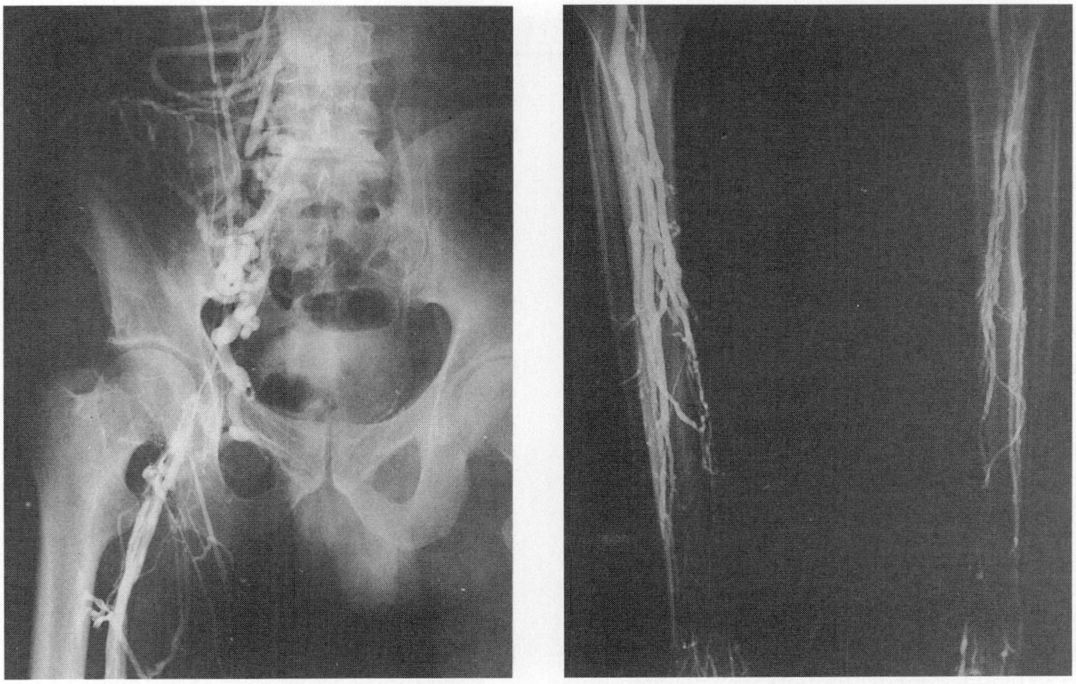

Figure 3 Shown is a phlebogram of the lower extremities. Injection of dye into the dorsal foot veins demonstrated occlusion of the iliac veins with excellent pelvic collateral circulation.

The morbidity of symptomatic upper extremity venous thrombosis can be quite significant. Thus, if the patient presents with massive swelling of the upper limb, moderate-dose heparin anticoagulation should be initiated immediately, and consideration should be given to lytic therapy (i.e., streptokinase, urokinase, or tissue plasminogen activator [t-PA]) [see General Principles of Anticoagulation and Lytic Therapy, below].[10] If phlebography shows compression of arm veins at the thoracic inlet after lytic therapy or spontaneous recovery from the thrombotic process, first-rib resection may be indicated, particularly if positional morbidity is present.

Septic deep thrombophlebitis is more common in the upper extremity than in the lower extremity. This is so primarily because the upper extremity veins are more frequently catheterized, as well as because they are the vessels most often used by drug addicts. If the phlebitis occurs in a critical care setting and there is an intravenous catheter in the vein at the time of clinical manifestations of fever and sepsis, the foreign body should be removed immediately, the tip cultured, and a Gram's stain done on any clot present. Broad-spectrum antibiotics (e.g., gentamicin, 80 mg four times daily, or metronidazole, 500 mg four times daily) should be administered until the organism can be identified and more specific antibiotic therapy instituted. Moderate-dose heparin anticoagulation is the primary treatment unless strictly contraindicated.

Ligation and drainage are not as practical for deep veins as they are for superficial veins, but one or the other, or both, may be indicated on rare occasions if the process does not respond to conventional therapy within three or four days and marked swelling and fever persist. Drainage is done on the most accessible portion of the phlebitic process. For ligation, the proximal end of the obstructive process should be identified via surgery or phlebography and the vein then ligated proximally.

PHLEGMASIA CERULEA DOLENS

Phlegmasia cerulea dolens is most apt to occur in dehydrated, cachectic patients and is usually superimposed on another critical illness, such as peritonitis or terminal malignancy. It can involve either the upper or the lower extremity but more commonly affects the latter. The swelling is severe because of massive thrombosis of all the main channels and their collateral vessels. In the lower extremity, there is usually simultaneous thrombosis of the iliac, the femoral, the common femoral, and the superficial femoral vein. The limb is massively swollen, bluish, and mottled in its most distal portion. Eventually, the limb becomes nonviable as arterial flow stops because of intense arterial vascular spasm associated with massive venous outflow obstruction. The clinical problem is compounded by acute massive fluid loss into the limb that can result in hypovolemic shock.

Treatment involves massive fluid replacement, elevation of the limb, and high-dose heparin anticoagulation. If the patient does not respond, thrombectomy may be considered, provided that the associated disease does not carry a fatal prognosis.[11] The procedure is best done via the transfemoral route with a limited incision so that anticoagulation can be continued postoperatively. If anticoagulation cannot be continued after thrombectomy, the thrombophlebitis will immediately recur.

Table 2 Etiology of Upper Extremity Thrombophlebitis

Congenital hypercoagulability
Thoracic outlet syndrome
Axillary vein compression
Stress injury
Central venous catheters
Mediastinal malignancy
Shoulder trauma

Approach to Pulmonary Embolism

All authorities agree that pulmonary embolism is a grossly underdiagnosed disease. In the United States, pulmonary embolism is believed to be associated with approximately 200,000 deaths a year, and it is probable that most episodes of pulmonary embolism (perhaps as many as 90 percent) are unsuspected because they are clinically insignificant or are misdiagnosed as other conditions.[1-3,12] Clinical manifestations include dyspnea, hemoptysis, pleurisy, heart failure, and cardiovascular collapse; however, each of these symptoms or signs is also associated with a number of other conditions [see Table 3]. The risk factors for pulmonary embolism in postoperative patients are similar to those for thrombophlebitis [see Table 4].

It is worthwhile to distinguish pulmonary embolism from pulmonary infarction. Of the approximately 10 percent of all emboli that are recognized clinically, only 10 percent are associated with pulmonary infarction.[13] Because the collateral circulation of the lung is excellent, obstruction of the larger pulmonary arteries rarely leads to death of lung tissue. When pulmonary infarction does occur, the diagnosis is usually obvious; hemoptysis, pleuritic chest pain, and a wedge-shaped density on chest x-ray are the classic manifestations. In most patients with pulmonary embolism (i.e., those who do not have pulmonary infarction), the chest x-ray is relatively normal.

From the standpoint of clinical diagnosis and treatment, pulmonary embolism is best classified as minor (or suspected) pulmonary embolism, moderate pulmonary embolism, or catastrophic pulmonary embolism [see Figure 4].

Minor Pulmonary Embolism

Minor pulmonary embolism undoubtedly occurs frequently in critically ill medical and surgical patients.[12] Manifestations may include transient tachypnea, with perhaps a slight change in blood gas values, and cardiac irritability, with frequent premature beats or tachyarrhythmias.[14-16] These changes may resolve in a few moments, and the patient may then appear perfectly normal. In these circumstances, it is probable that the embolus either is small or is composed of relatively fresh clot that produces only transient obstruction when it enters the pulmonary vascular tree.

If risk factors for pulmonary embolism are present [see Table 4], the differential diagnosis should be considered[15]; this includes acute respiratory distress syndrome, aspiration, atelectasis, heart failure, pneumonia, and systemic infection. If the diagnosis is not obvious but the risk of pulmonary embolism is substantial and there is no contraindication to anticoagulation, moderate-dose heparin therapy should be instituted while the diagnostic tests are being selected and performed. (Alternatively, one can simply assume the diagnosis of pulmonary embolism and continue therapy for as long as the patient is at risk.)

If pulmonary embolism is unlikely, if the risk from anticoagulation is high, or if there are other serious conditions in the differential diagnosis that are likely and cannot be ruled out, then specific studies should be ordered. These consist of laboratory studies for intravascular coagulation and noninvasive peripheral vascular studies to document the presence or absence of clot in leg veins, ventilation-perfusion lung scanning, or venous or pulmonary angiography.

Most patients with pulmonary embolism will have laboratory evidence of intravascular coagulation; however, the coagulation process may also be activated by severe infection, very recent soft tissue trauma, or devitalization of tissue. The most accurate tests for detection of intravascular clotting are the test for the presence of fibrin degradation products (FDPs) and that for the presence of D-dimer, which is the particle cleaved off cross-linked (clotted) fibrin. The latter test is more specific because the presence of D-dimer signals the fibrinolytic breakdown of cross-linked fibrin, whereas fibrin degradation products can result from fibrinolytic dissolution of fibrinogen as well as fibrin.[16,17] High levels of both FDPs and D-dimer constitute strong indirect evidence of intravascular clotting. Although such a finding does not necessarily establish the diagnosis of pulmonary embolism, it strongly suggests the presence of clot somewhere in the vascular system and the need for anticoagulation, if only to prevent subsequent clotting complications. If both tests yield negative results, the probability of clotting anywhere in the vascular system is low. It must be remembered, however, that with both tests, fibrinolysis must be relatively intact for a positive result to be possible; if fibrinolysis is defective, these tests could, in theory, yield negative results even in the presence of clotting.

Noninvasive assessment (e.g., duplex scanning) aimed at detecting clot in the major leg veins may facilitate diagnosis. When definitive evaluation that includes phlebography is done, as many as 70 percent of patients with pulmonary embolism are found to have clot in the thigh or abdominal veins. This finding

Table 3 Clinical Features of Pulmonary Embolism: Differential Diagnosis

Clinical Feature	Other Conditions Associated with Feature
Dyspnea	Aspiration Atelectasis Pneumonia Pneumothorax Pulmonary edema Systemic infection
Heart failure	Cardiac tamponade Intracardiac injury Myocardial contusion Myocardial infarction
Hemoptysis	Bronchial injury Pulmonary contusion Tracheal erosion Unsuspected neoplasm
Pleurisy	Chest wall injury Pneumonia Pneumothorax Subphrenic inflammation
Cardiovascular collapse	Air embolism Cardiac tamponade Hypovolemia Myocardial infarction Severe hypoxemia Systemic infection Tension pneumothorax

Table 4 Risk Factors for Pulmonary Embolism
Major surgery
Surgical complications
Severe trauma
Lower extremity fractures
Obesity
Immobilization
Old age
Previous thrombotic events
Heart failure

in itself is usually an indication for treatment, even if pulmonary embolism is not present.

The initial enthusiasm for the use of lung scans to diagnose or screen for pulmonary embolism has receded somewhat.[18,19] It was thought that a negative scan rules out pulmonary embolism; however, in one study,[18] patients with negative or near-negative scans (14 percent of the total) still had a four percent incidence of pulmonary embolism when they were evaluated by means of angiography. A high-probability scan, on the other hand, did establish the presence of pulmonary embolism: the diagnosis was verifiable in 86 percent of cases when pulmonary angiography was done concomitantly.[18] Unfortunately, patients with high-probability scans accounted for only 13 percent of the total and only 40 percent of those who later proved to have embolism. In the low- to moderate-probability group, which contained 72 percent of the patients with possible pulmonary embolism, 21 percent of the patients in the group proved to have pulmonary embolism on angiography. Although most of the patients with pulmonary embolism had scans ranging from low to moderate probability, so too did most of the patients in whom pulmonary embolism was initially suspected on clinical grounds but later excluded. Overall, therefore, whereas the sensitivity of scanning is high (96 percent), the specificity is low (10 percent). Even if patients with negative or near-negative scans are excluded, most patients will still require pulmonary angiography to confirm the diagnosis.

Because patients who are critically ill tolerate diagnostic testing poorly, pulmonary angiography is a more appropriate initial study in these patients than lung scanning; at present, it is the gold standard for diagnosis[1,3,20] [see Figure 5]. If the pulmonary angiogram is done immediately after the clinical episode, particularly if the patient is still symptomatic, a negative result rules out pulmonary embolism. However, pulmonary emboli frequently lack integrity and break up quickly. Thus, if the patient improves or recovers before the angiogram is done, the implication is that the clot was minimal, that it has disappeared into the microcirculation, or that it has been disposed of by the natural lytic process. Because angiography is not reliable in diagnosing clot in the subsegmental arteries,[21] a negative angiogram in a patient who is no longer symptomatic does not

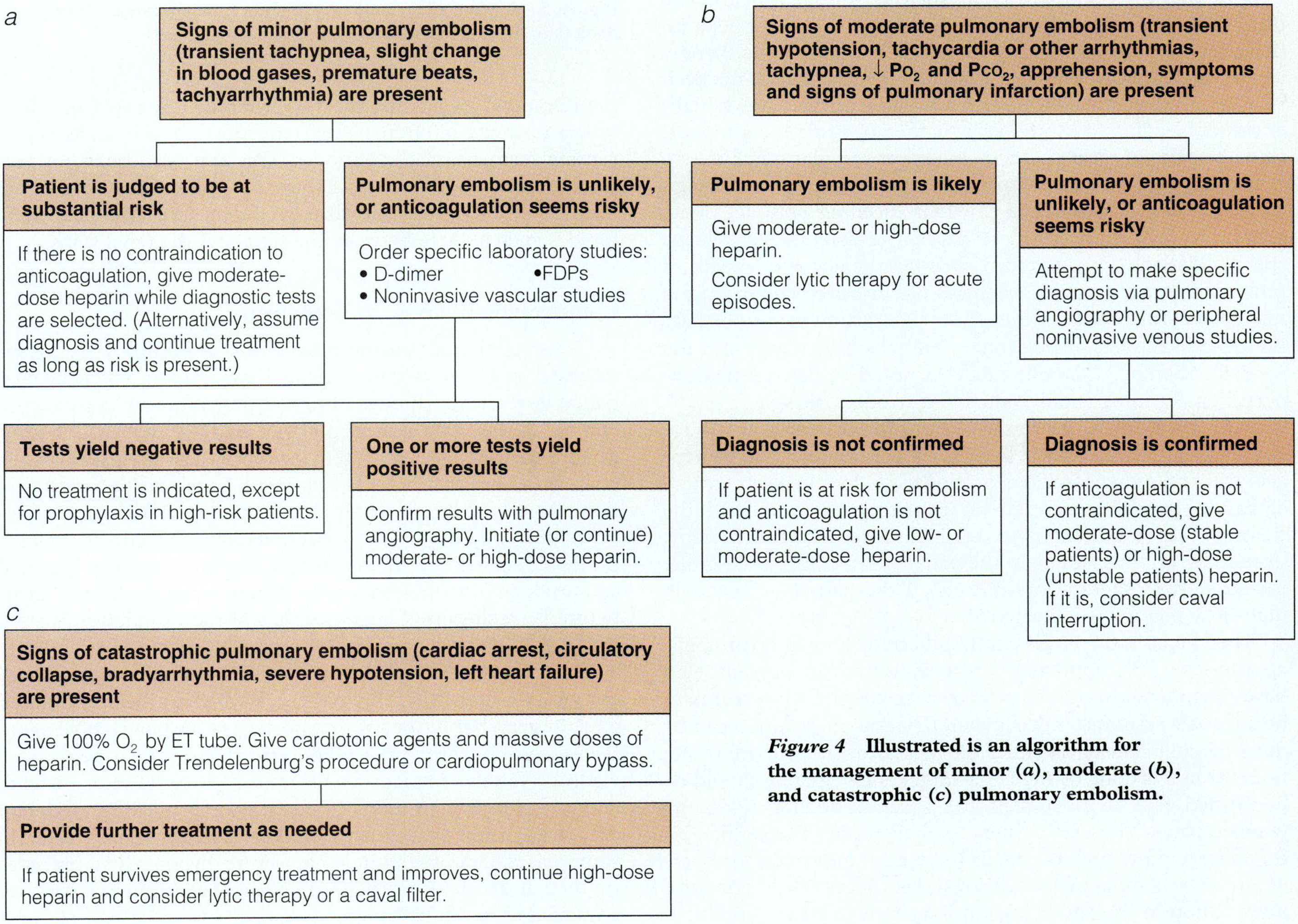

a

Signs of minor pulmonary embolism (transient tachypnea, slight change in blood gases, premature beats, tachyarrhythmia) are present

- **Patient is judged to be at substantial risk**
  If there is no contraindication to anticoagulation, give moderate-dose heparin while diagnostic tests are selected. (Alternatively, assume diagnosis and continue treatment as long as risk is present.)

- **Pulmonary embolism is unlikely, or anticoagulation seems risky**
  Order specific laboratory studies:
  • D-dimer   •FDPs
  • Noninvasive vascular studies

  - **Tests yield negative results**
    No treatment is indicated, except for prophylaxis in high-risk patients.

  - **One or more tests yield positive results**
    Confirm results with pulmonary angiography. Initiate (or continue) moderate- or high-dose heparin.

b

Signs of moderate pulmonary embolism (transient hypotension, tachycardia or other arrhythmias, tachypnea, ↓ Po_2 and Pco_2, apprehension, symptoms and signs of pulmonary infarction) are present

- **Pulmonary embolism is likely**
  Give moderate- or high-dose heparin.
  Consider lytic therapy for acute episodes.

- **Pulmonary embolism is unlikely, or anticoagulation seems risky**
  Attempt to make specific diagnosis via pulmonary angiography or peripheral noninvasive venous studies.

  - **Diagnosis is not confirmed**
    If patient is at risk for embolism and anticoagulation is not contraindicated, give low- or moderate-dose heparin.

  - **Diagnosis is confirmed**
    If anticoagulation is not contraindicated, give moderate-dose (stable patients) or high-dose (unstable patients) heparin. If it is, consider caval interruption.

c

Signs of catastrophic pulmonary embolism (cardiac arrest, circulatory collapse, bradyarrhythmia, severe hypotension, left heart failure) are present

Give 100% O_2 by ET tube. Give cardiotonic agents and massive doses of heparin. Consider Trendelenburg's procedure or cardiopulmonary bypass.

Provide further treatment as needed

If patient survives emergency treatment and improves, continue high-dose heparin and consider lytic therapy or a caval filter.

Figure 4 Illustrated is an algorithm for the management of minor (*a*), moderate (*b*), and catastrophic (*c*) pulmonary embolism.

rule out a pulmonary embolus, although it can establish the degree of patency of the pulmonary vasculature, which affects the prognosis. Alternative studies using magnification or balloon occlusion techniques may eventually be able to diagnose clot in vessels as small as 2 mm in diameter. Conceivably, studies of this type may show that some perfusion defects documented by scanning actually are related to pulmonary embolism.[21,22]

If all diagnostic tests for pulmonary embolism yield negative results, treatment may not be indicated, except for prophylaxis in patients at risk. If the tests are suggestive or indicative of pulmonary embolus, heparin anticoagulation should be continued at a moderate to high dosage, depending on the clinical significance of the embolic episode.

Moderate Pulmonary Embolism

The manifestations of moderate pulmonary embolism include transient hypotension, tachycardia or other cardiac arrhythmias, tachypnea with a significant fall in arterial oxygen tension and carbon dioxide tension, apprehension, and symptoms or signs of pulmonary infarction.[14,16] There may be signs of right heart failure as documented by increased central venous pressure, right ventricular heave, and an accentuated pulmonic second sound. Electrocardiography is rarely helpful in the differential diagnosis. Although acute right axis deviation, new incomplete right bundle branch block, and changes in S_1, Q_3, or T_3 are thought to characterize this disorder, they are found in only a small percentage of patients with proven pulmonary embolism.

If the diagnosis is probable and there are no likely alternative diagnoses, anticoagulant therapy (moderate- to high-dose heparin, depending on the symptoms) should be initiated. Lytic therapy can be used for acute episodes; however, its mortality has not been significantly lower than that of heparin, and it carries a much higher risk of bleeding.[1,3] Moreover, lytic therapy is often contraindicated because of recent surgery, injury, or vascular punctures.

If there is a relative contraindication to anticoagulation (e.g., an acute surgical wound, a previous bleeding episode, or an allergic reaction to heparin) or alternative diagnoses are likely, specific diagnosis is required. This is best achieved by means of pulmonary angiography. Peripheral noninvasive venous studies may be helpful because if they show significant venous obstruction, the likelihood of pulmonary embolism increases and the need for therapy is documented. As noted earlier, ventilation-perfusion scanning is only valuable if strongly positive.

If the diagnosis is not confirmed but the patient is at risk for embolic complications and there is no contraindication to heparin therapy, either low-dose or moderate-dose heparin anticoagulation should be initiated.[23,24] If the diagnosis is verified, the treatment is moderate-dose to high-dose heparin therapy, depending on the stability of the patient. If the patient is stable, moderate-dose therapy is sufficient; if the patient is unstable, high-dose therapy is indicated.[25-28]

When heparin therapy is contraindicated, caval interruption is appropriate. This approach is also indicated for patients who have documented pulmonary embolism despite what seems to be adequate systemic anticoagulation. Caval interruption can be done percutaneously via either the jugular or the femoral route; however, if it is done by the latter route, phlebography should be performed first to document the absence of clot along the planned route. The use of filters, such as those of Greenfield, is the most popular method.[29-31] If there is an indication for operation or a complication develops that necessitates operative intervention in the abdomen, caval ligation or caval clipping at the infrarenal level is the most appropriate therapy. Caval ligation at the juxta-infrarenal level is the most certain means of preventing further embolic episodes. This approach does not produce an area of relative stasis above the clip or ligature; clot has been shown to propagate through filters and embolize when there is such an area between the filter and the renal veins.

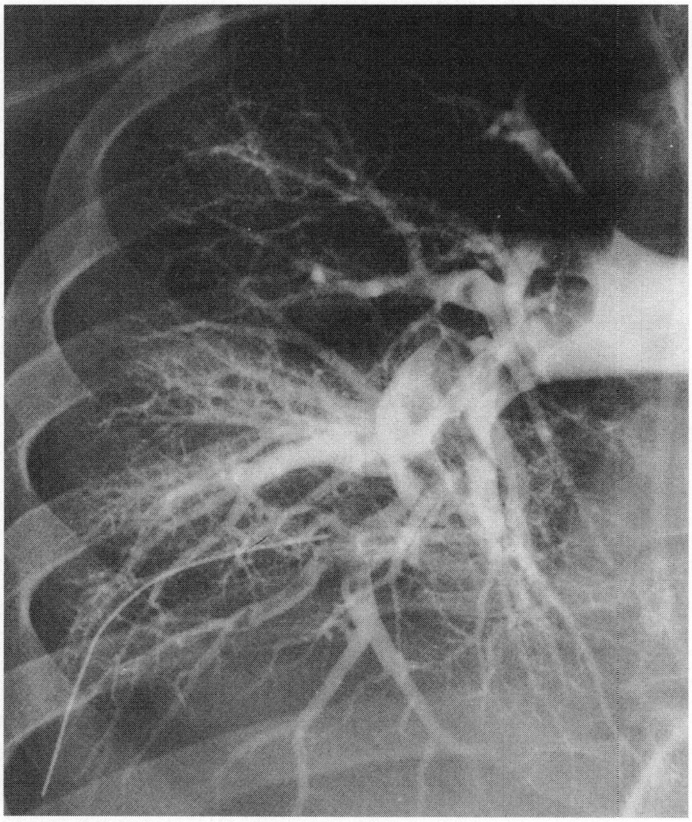

Figure 5 **A pulmonary angiogram shows nonequivocal filling defects in multiple arteries.**

Catastrophic Pulmonary Embolism

Catastrophic pulmonary embolism is most apt to be superimposed on a critical illness or a major operation. The peak incidence is seven to 10 days after the procedure or the onset of clinical illness. The reason for this delay is that a clot must mature in the vascular system before it has integrity when it embolizes, and this process requires a considerable amount of time. As noted earlier, fresh clot breaks up readily and disappears promptly into the microvasculature, and thus it tends to produce transient problems; mature clot is resistant to lysis and can produce acute pulmonary obstruction and acute right heart failure.[14] Occlusion of large portions of the vasculature is associated with hemodynamic catastrophe.

Typically, the clinical onset of catastrophic pulmonary embolism comes when the patient, having just been mobilized after surgery, has his or her first postoperative bowel movement. If in the course of the bowel movement the patient performs a vigorous Valsalva maneuver, the great abdominal veins distend, and any clot present tends to be stripped loose. If a large clot embolizes, immediate collapse and cardiac arrest may result; in some cases, bradyarrhythmia or severe hypotension precedes the actual arrest. Immediate emergency treatment comprises administration of 100 percent oxygen by endotracheal tube, massive doses of heparin, and, if cardiac arrest occurs, cardiopulmonary resuscitation. A Swan-Ganz catheter should be inserted as soon as possible so that the effects of therapy can be monitored. Cardiotonic agents (e.g., dopamine, 2.0 to 5.0 μg/min, or dobutamine, 2.5 to 10.0 μg/kg/min) should be administered to strengthen myocardial function. If sudden arrest occurs in circumstances that permit emergency thoracotomy, Trendelenburg's procedure can be performed; however, this procedure is rarely indicated and even more rarely successful. If the patient survives the initial emergency treatment and improves, high-dose heparin therapy should be continued and lytic therapy considered.[27,29]

Approach to Arterial Embolism

Arterial embolism has been much less common in recent decades, thanks to a decreased incidence of congenital heart disease, improved prevention of rheumatic heart disease, and better initial treatment of acquired heart disease.[32-34] The manifestations of arterial embolism result from sudden occlusion of a major artery, which characteristically is associated with overt clinical catastrophe (because previously patent arteries generally have very little collateral circulation). Sudden catastrophic arterial thrombosis can also occur, as a consequence of sudden elevation of an arteriosclerotic plaque; however, in most instances, the onset of arterial thrombosis is gradual, the danger is less, and the condition is easily distinguished from arterial embolism [see Table 5]. Spontaneous thrombosis of small arteries can be a complication of congenital clotting syndromes and autoimmune states [see Approach to Acquired and Congenital Thrombotic Syndromes, below]. Because arterial thrombosis is almost invariably superimposed on underlying occlusive disease, it will not be discussed further here.

The most common site for an embolic lodgment is the common femoral bifurcation[32-34] [see Figure 6]. Next in incidence is the aortoiliac region, followed by the popliteal artery and the brachial artery. The carotid bifurcation may be involved 20 to 25 percent of the time, but embolic lodgment at this site may be difficult to distinguish from occlusion secondary to carotid atherosclerosis. The superior mesenteric arterial circulation and the renal arterial circulation are involved five to 10 percent of the time, but as with carotid bifurcation involvement, the source of the occlusion may be hard to ascertain. Diagnosis of superior mesenteric arterial embolism is often delayed until the bowel is irreversibly damaged. The true incidence of renal artery involvement is more difficult to determine. Because of the bilaterality of the kidneys and because an isolated embolus typically has little or no impact on renal function, the diagnosis sometimes is not made.

When arterial embolism is likely or probable, two steps should be taken simultaneously: treatment should be begun, and an attempt should be made to determine the source of the embolus. Treatment involves immediate initiation of anticoagulation with heparin in moderate to high dosages (depending on the severity of the symptoms), followed by specific treatment for the site of lodgment. Discussion of specific diagnosis and treatment will be limited to visceral embolism and extremity embolism because these are the types of arterial embolism most often seen by the surgeon in the emergency setting. Carotid artery embolism is rarely managed surgically in the initial stages.

In most cases, arterial emboli have their origin in the heart; less commonly, they derive from the great vessels [see Figure 7]. If the patient is known to have an underlying cardiac disorder, such as atrial fibrillation, myocardial infarction, valvular heart disease, or thrombus formation on an artificial heart valve, then it can be assumed that the heart is the source. If cardiac evaluation, including ultrasonography, yields negative results, the large blood vessels are the probable source. The most common kind of embolic material is thrombus from aortic aneurysms or debris associated with atherosclerosis (usually involving the abdominal aorta). Ultrasonography can be rapidly performed in most environments; if there is evidence of aneurysm, the patient can be evaluated further with CT scanning. Alternatively, aortography may reveal atherosclerotic irregularities that explain the source of the embolic event.

Visceral Embolism

Early diagnosis of visceral arterial occlusion depends on a high degree of suspicion. When abdominal pain develops suddenly in a patient who is in the arteriosclerotic age group, has underlying heart disease, or is known to be at risk for embolism, the diagnosis should be suspected. Typically, in the first few hours, the pain is out of proportion to the clinical findings; on examination, the abdomen seems relatively normal, and only after several hours have passed is some tenderness apparent [see Figure 8]. If the patient is seen acutely and the diagnosis is suspected, immediate operative intervention is indicated. On rare occasions, arteriographic evaluation of the visceral circulation may be indicated if the index of suspicion is low or if nonocclusive causes (e.g., low cardiac output or shock-induced mesenteric venous thrombosis) are likely.

Mesenteric arterial occlusion is usually diagnosed late. After six to eight hours of ischemia, the diagnosis becomes obvious when abdominal tenderness and rebound develop and the patient becomes hemodynamically unstable. Mucus mixed with blood (currant jelly stool) is the characteristic finding on rectal examination if the colon is ischemic; often, however, gross, dark blood is found.

When the diagnosis of mesenteric arterial occlusion is suspected or documented, urgent laparotomy is indicated. If the diagnosis is made at an early stage and the bowel is still viable, mesenteric embolectomy or autogenous vein aortomesenteric bypass is indicated. If the intestine has been deprived of circulation for many hours, it is usually no longer viable; the only possible treatment may be resection of the dead portion of bowel. More often

Table 5 Differentiation of Arterial Embolism and Arterial Thrombosis

	Arterial Embolism	Arterial Thrombosis
History	Preexisting symptoms of vascular disease uncommon Sudden onset usual Symptoms usually severe	Preexisting symptoms of vascular disease common Sudden onset uncommon Symptoms usually moderate
Examination	Opposite limb usually normal Chronic skin changes absent Ischemia profound (no preexisting collateral)	Usually vascular disease in opposite limb Chronic skin changes usual Ischemia moderate (preexisting collateral)

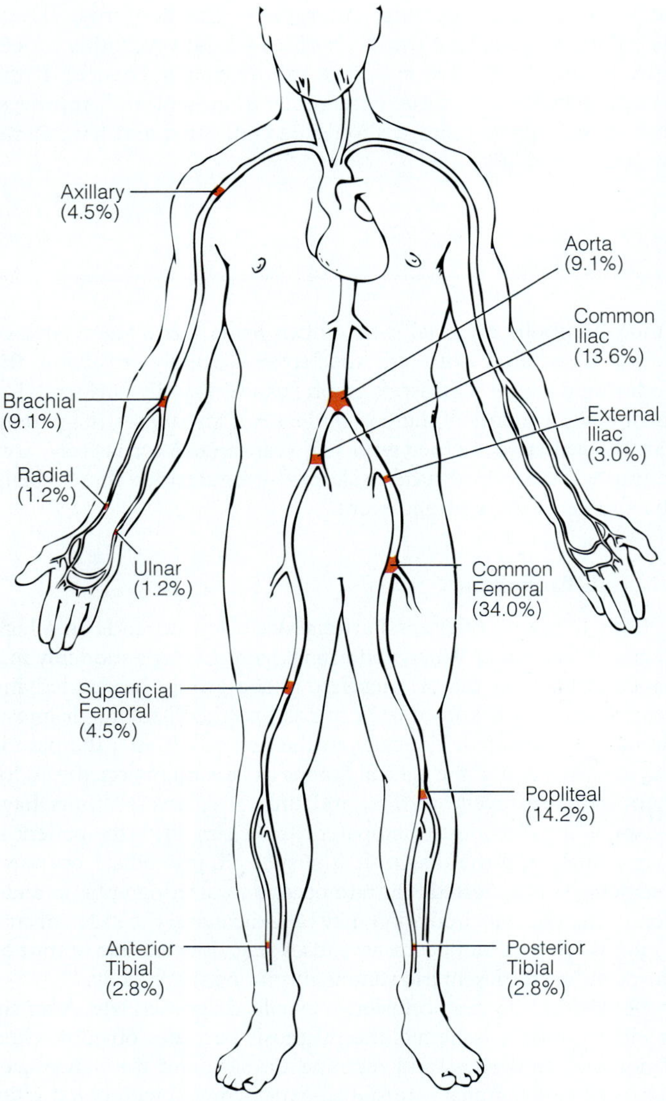

Figure 6 **Arterial embolism occurs with varying frequency in different peripheral arteries. The most common sites of embolic lodgment are shown.**

Axillary (4.5%)
Aorta (9.1%)
Common Iliac (13.6%)
Brachial (9.1%)
External Iliac (3.0%)
Radial (1.2%)
Ulnar (1.2%)
Common Femoral (34.0%)
Superficial Femoral (4.5%)
Popliteal (14.2%)
Anterior Tibial (2.8%)
Posterior Tibial (2.8%)

after surgery and continued for two to three days, provided that no bleeding complication develops. Because long-term prophylactic anticoagulation is indicated, the patient should be transferred to warfarin after this initial period of heparin therapy.

Renal arterial embolism is usually manifested by the onset of flank pain, with or without microscopic hematuria, in a patient at risk for embolism. These findings constitute an indication for further diagnostic evaluation with renal scanning, arteriography, or both. Failure to identify blood flow on the renal scan and the demonstration of arterial occlusion on arteriography are indications for treatment. Once the diagnosis is made, the therapeutic choice is between moderate-dose heparin anticoagulation, direct catheter infusion of a thrombolytic agent, and surgery. If the kidney appears viable, surgical treatment involves exploration combined with restoration of circulation by embolectomy or autogenous vein aortorenal bypass; if the kidney is not viable, exploration is combined with nephrectomy.

Extremity Embolism

Arterial embolism to a limb results in acute limb ischemia, manifested by pain, paralysis, or anesthesia in the involved extremity [see Figure 9]. The presence of anesthesia, paralysis, or both is an indication of nonviability if allowed to persist. If the patient is seen promptly (within six to eight hours), immediate restoration of the circulation by means of thromboembolectomy is indicated, followed by high-dose heparin and then warfarin. If, however, more than six to eight hours has passed, the muscles are firm, and the skin is blue and mottled, then the process is unlikely to be reversible[35-37]; if it is reversible, it carries a high risk of mortality secondary to the reperfusion syndrome. In such cases, the best treatment is high-dose heparin anticoagulation for two to three days. This regimen allows sharp demarcation of the nonviable region from the rest of the limb, which permits successful amputation at the lowest possible level—ideally, no higher than just below the knee.

Pain and coldness coupled with retained sensation and muscle function indicate that the limb is still viable. When these signs and symptoms are first noted (usually in the emergency room), anticoagulation should be initiated with a large bolus of heparin (10,000–20,000 units) as the limb is evaluated. If the limb is viable when anticoagulation is begun, viability will improve as collateral flow is mobilized.[38] It is important not only to treat the initial ischemia but also to minimize the possibility of recurrent embolism. The heparin dosage, which should be high initially, can gradually be titrated downward over a period of two or three days, after which the patient can be transferred to warfarin.[39]

If the patient has minimal disability in the limb after this treatment, he or she should be followed and anticoagulation continued as clinically appropriate. The source of the embolus should be identified and treated if possible. If the patient has moderate or severe disability in the ischemic limb, elective revascularization can be carried out later.

than not, the entire portion of the bowel supplied by the mesenteric artery is nonviable, and the condition is untreatable. If the bowel appears to be marginally viable, resection should be conservative, the mesenteric artery should be repaired if possible, and a second-look operation should be performed within 24 hours to reassess the viability of the remaining portion of the bowel.

In addition, the attempts to determine the source of the embolus that were begun earlier (see above) should be continued, and the underlying condition should be corrected if possible. Low- or moderate-dose heparin anticoagulation should be initiated (if not contraindicated by operation) 24 to 48 hours

General Principles of Anticoagulation and Lytic Therapy

Heparin Anticoagulation

LOW-DOSE HEPARIN

Low-dose heparin therapy is usually initiated with a 3,000 to 5,000 unit bolus given intravenously.[40] Next, 1,000 units/hr is given by continuous intravenous infusion; this method of administration permits more precise control than subcutaneous administration. The activated partial thromboplastin time (PTT) should be elevated to at least five points above the normal value for the laboratory involved and should be maintained at this level for

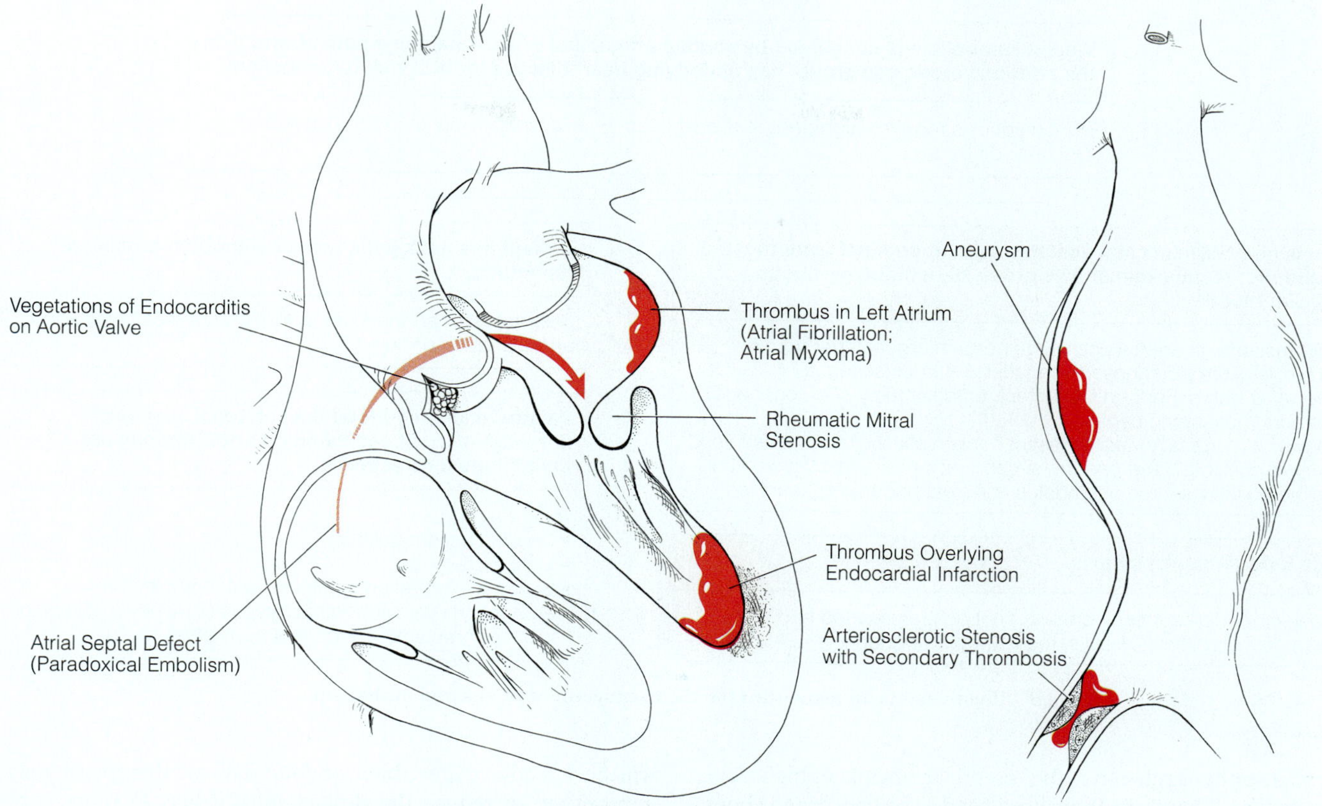

Figure 7 Most arterial emboli originate in the heart; less commonly, emboli arise in the great vessels.

the entire period of risk for clotting. If the initial PTT is more than five points above the laboratory's normal value, the heparin dosage should be gradually titrated downward to maintain the PTT at the appropriate level. If the patient is able to take nourishment and if anticoagulation for a week or longer is appropriate, warfarin therapy can be started in parallel with heparin anticoagulation, and heparin can be discontinued when the prothrombin time (PT) reaches a standard international ratio of about 2.0 to 3.0 [see Oral Anticoagulation, Dosage, below]. When the patient is active and mobile, anticoagulation with heparin or warfarin can be discontinued.

MODERATE-DOSE HEPARIN

Moderate-dose heparin could also be referred to as conventional anticoagulation.[41-43] This regimen may be appropriate for patients with non–life-threatening clotting complications (e.g., pulmonary embolism causing minimal morbidity or deep thrombophlebitis). Before therapy is begun, a clotting battery should be performed, consisting of the PTT, the PT, the platelet count, and levels of fibrinogen, antithrombin III, FDPs, fibrin monomer, and D-dimer. High fibrinogen levels and platelet counts are seen in patients with chronic clotting syndromes,[44] probably representing overcompensation for increased utilization. Elevated levels of fibrin monomer indicate low-grade clotting, and elevated levels of FDPs and D-dimer suggest clotting and activation of fibrinolysis. If these tests all strongly suggest intravascular clotting, high-dose heparin may be more appropriate initially, unless it is contraindicated by imminent or very recent surgery or by the presence of open lesions.

In the average patient, moderate-dose heparin anticoagulation begins with an arbitrary dose, 10,000 units, followed by continuous intravenous administration at a rate sufficient to double the PTT. This rate varies greatly but averages about 2,000 units/hr. When dosages higher than 2,000 units/hr are required, preexisting antithrombin depletion is highly probable.

Tight control of heparin therapy is not as important as monitoring the patient for evidence of bleeding and platelet depletion. Clinical evidence of bleeding does not necessarily contraindicate continuing anticoagulation. Minimal amounts of blood may be lost in the urine or through the GI tract; if the patient has a clear-cut need for anticoagulation, these minor bleeding complications should be accepted. Only when transfusion is indicated to maintain the hematocrit must the risk-benefit ratio of continuing therapy be considered. At that point, if the risks of bleeding seem to outweigh the benefits of anticoagulation, heparin can be discontinued or reduced to the low-dose level. One of the most important aspects of monitoring is watching for falls in hematocrit that indicate significant bleeding. The most common sites for hemorrhagic complications are surgical wounds and the retroperitoneum. The latter is a silent area.

HIGH-DOSE HEPARIN

High-dose heparin therapy consists of the administration of arbitrary large doses of heparin without regard to PTT monitoring. The PTT is used only to ensure that the heparin is having an appropriate effect. The maximum PTT that can be measured by our laboratory is 150 seconds; in high-dose heparin treatment, the PTT should be greater than this value. Given that a fully anticoagulated patient cannot form clot at all, the PTT in this circumstance theoretically should be infinite.

In most patients, high-dose therapy begins with a 20,000 unit I.V. bolus, followed by infusion of 5,000 units/hr I.V. Such high dosages are necessary in most patients with arterial ischemia to produce complete anticoagulation and prevent distal propagation of clot.[38,39,45-47] Clinical evidence of improved collateral circulation in a patient being treated for arterial ischemia or venous thrombosis is a sign that the dosage is adequate. Pulmonary function should improve in patients being treated for pulmonary embolism.

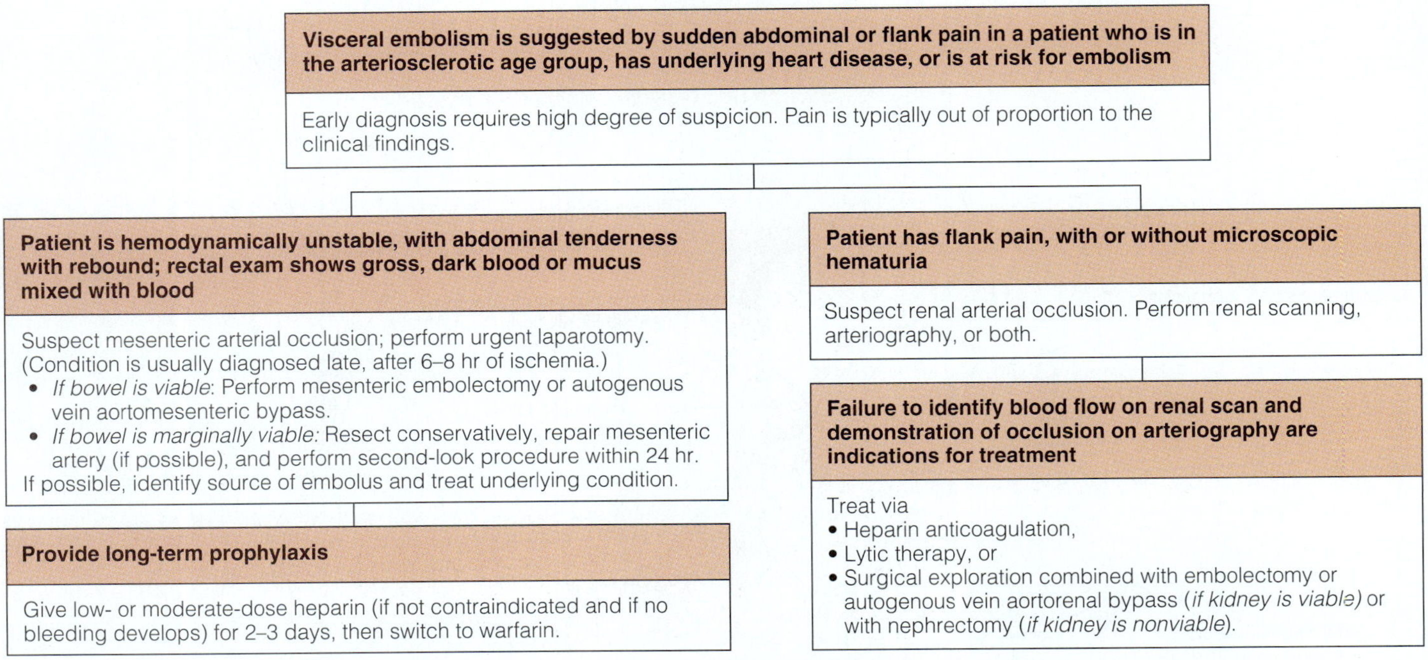

```
┌─────────────────────────────────────────────────────────────────────────┐
│ Visceral embolism is suggested by sudden abdominal or flank pain in a   │
│ patient who is in the arteriosclerotic age group, has underlying heart  │
│ disease, or is at risk for embolism                                     │
├─────────────────────────────────────────────────────────────────────────┤
│ Early diagnosis requires high degree of suspicion. Pain is typically    │
│ out of proportion to the clinical findings.                             │
└─────────────────────────────────────────────────────────────────────────┘
```

Patient is hemodynamically unstable, with abdominal tenderness with rebound; rectal exam shows gross, dark blood or mucus mixed with blood

Suspect mesenteric arterial occlusion; perform urgent laparotomy. (Condition is usually diagnosed late, after 6–8 hr of ischemia.)
- *If bowel is viable*: Perform mesenteric embolectomy or autogenous vein aortomesenteric bypass.
- *If bowel is marginally viable:* Resect conservatively, repair mesenteric artery (if possible), and perform second-look procedure within 24 hr.

If possible, identify source of embolus and treat underlying condition.

Provide long-term prophylaxis

Give low- or moderate-dose heparin (if not contraindicated and if no bleeding develops) for 2–3 days, then switch to warfarin.

Patient has flank pain, with or without microscopic hematuria

Suspect renal arterial occlusion. Perform renal scanning, arteriography, or both.

Failure to identify blood flow on renal scan and demonstration of occlusion on arteriography are indications for treatment

Treat via
- Heparin anticoagulation,
- Lytic therapy, or
- Surgical exploration combined with embolectomy or autogenous vein aortorenal bypass (*if kidney is viable*) or with nephrectomy (*if kidney is nonviable*).

Figure 8 **Illustrated is an algorithm for the management of visceral embolism.**

Complete anticoagulation is the essential principle of high-dose heparin therapy. Therefore, there is no need to be concerned about an upper limit for the dosage: if the patient cannot clot, doubling or even tripling the dosage will not, in theory, increase the risk of bleeding. Moreover, because the incidence of bleeding is very low in the first two or three days of therapy, regardless of the heparin dosage,[46,47] high initial dosages will not be associated with an unacceptable risk of bleeding. After the heparin has been observed to have an effect and the prolonged PTT has been documented, the high dosage should continue for at least 24 hours. The dosage can then be decreased by 500 to 1,000 units/hr in the next 24 hours. If the clinical effect is maintained and the patient continues to improve, the dosage can be decreased once again in the following 24 hours by another 500 to 1,000 units/hr. In theory, if all clotting has stopped, levels of natural antithrombins (which are depleted by clotting) should recover, and lower dosages of heparin will be effective. After three or four days of therapy, it may be appropriate to reduce the dosage still further, to more conventional levels, such as the moderate level described earlier [*see* Moderate-Dose Heparin, *above*].

If the improvement initially noted is lost, the dosage should be increased to its previous level, and the elevated dosage should be maintained for several days before any attempt is made to reduce it again. Careful monitoring of the platelet count and the hematocrit is appropriate. The hematocrit should be monitored at least four times a day, and heparin should be discontinued or the dosage reduced only when the risks posed by bleeding and transfusion exceed the benefits provided by anticoagulation. In a monitored environment, patients very rarely die of hemorrhage; rather, they die of the consequences of the clotting. The primary hemorrhagic risk is intracranial bleeding. Fortunately, this is a quite rare complication of heparin anticoagulation. The risk of

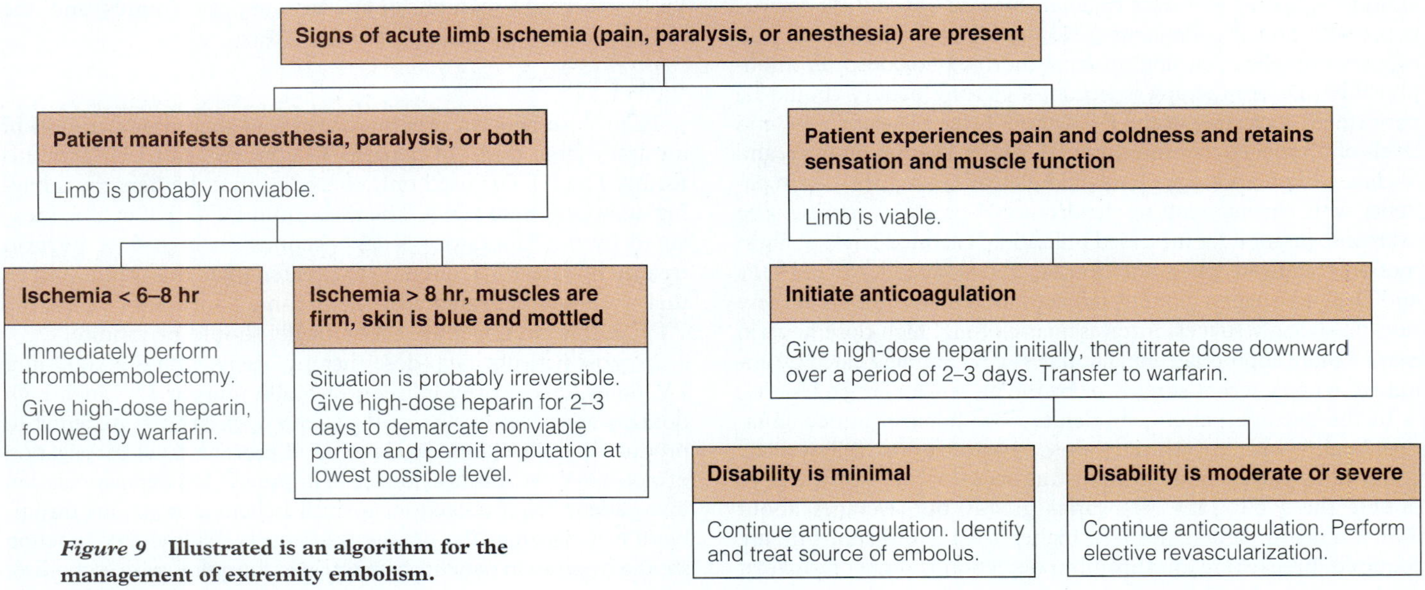

Signs of acute limb ischemia (pain, paralysis, or anesthesia) are present

Patient manifests anesthesia, paralysis, or both

Limb is probably nonviable.

Ischemia < 6–8 hr

Immediately perform thromboembolectomy. Give high-dose heparin, followed by warfarin.

Ischemia > 8 hr, muscles are firm, skin is blue and mottled

Situation is probably irreversible. Give high-dose heparin for 2–3 days to demarcate nonviable portion and permit amputation at lowest possible level.

Patient experiences pain and coldness and retains sensation and muscle function

Limb is viable.

Initiate anticoagulation

Give high-dose heparin initially, then titrate dose downward over a period of 2–3 days. Transfer to warfarin.

Disability is minimal

Continue anticoagulation. Identify and treat source of embolus.

Disability is moderate or severe

Continue anticoagulation. Perform elective revascularization.

Figure 9 Illustrated is an algorithm for the management of extremity embolism.

intracranial bleeding is greatest in elderly patients, particularly women[42]; however, it is small in comparison with the obvious risks posed by the clotting episode. Nevertheless, the existence of the risk makes it appropriate to use high-dose heparin primarily in life-threatening conditions.

COMPLICATIONS

Two forms of acute heparin-induced thrombocytopenia have been reported.[48-51] Mild thrombocytopenia occurs in two to five percent of patients two to 15 days after the initiation of therapy. The platelet count usually remains at about 100,000/mm³, and treatment can be continued without undue risk of bleeding. Severe thrombocytopenia is much less frequent. It usually occurs about seven to 14 days after the initiation of heparin therapy (perhaps depending on the type of heparin being used) and is reversible once the drug is discontinued. This severe form of heparin-induced thrombocytopenia has been associated with thrombotic complications, including arterial thrombosis with platelet fibrin clots, which may cause myocardial infarction or stroke or necessitate amputation of the limb. Thrombocytopenia appears to be less common when porcine rather than bovine heparin is used.

Unlike warfarin, heparin does not cross the placenta and has not been associated with fetal malformations; therefore, it is the drug of choice for thrombotic complications of pregnancy. Heparin can be administered for periods of three to six months by subcutaneous injection in an outpatient setting. Osteoporosis and spontaneous vertebral fractures can occur with long-term administration.[52] Thrombocytopenia excepted, allergic reactions to heparin are rare.

An extremely rare complication of heparin therapy is adrenal hemorrhage, which can result in adrenal insufficiency[42] [*see 73 Adrenal Insufficiency*]. If acute adrenal insufficiency is suspected, anticoagulant therapy should be discontinued, and high-dose steroid therapy, preferably with hydrocortisone, should be initiated. Treatment should not be delayed until laboratory confirmation can be obtained. CT scanning may be useful in diagnosing this condition. Heparin may also suppress aldosterone synthesis, especially with prolonged use.[42]

REVERSAL OF HEPARIN EFFECT

The anticoagulant effect of heparin disappears within hours after the drug is discontinued. If the effect must be reversed quickly, the patient should be given protamine sulfate intravenously. Protamines are low-molecular-weight basic charged proteins that are isolated from fish sperm. They bind tightly to heparin in vitro and neutralize its anticoagulant effect.[42,43] Protamine sulfate also interacts in vivo with platelets, fibrinogen, and other plasma proteins and may have an anticoagulant effect of its own. Therefore, it should be given in the smallest dosages that are still capable of producing the desired result—typically, about 1 mg of protamine sulfate for every 100 units of heparin remaining in the patient. Protamine sulfate should be administered slowly over a period of five to 10 minutes; rapid infusion can cause shortness of breath, flushing, bradycardia, hypotension, or anaphylaxis. On rare occasions, in patients previously sensitized to protamine (e.g., diabetics), massive platelet aggregation can occur, as manifested by catastrophic arterial thrombosis.

Oral Anticoagulation

Warfarin is the prototypical oral anticoagulant; the agents in this class have much the same effects, differing primarily with respect to potency and duration of action.[42,43]

Table 6 **Recommendations for Use of Varying Dosages of Warfarin**

The dosage of warfarin is regulated by monitoring the INR. A less intense therapeutic range (INR = 2.0 to 3.0, corresponding to a PT 1.3 to 1.5 times normal with a WHO-designated thromboplastin) is appropriate for the following applications:

1. The prevention of venous thromboembolism in high-risk patients.
2. The treatment of venous thrombosis and pulmonary embolism after an initial course of heparin.
3. The prevention of systemic embolism (a) in patients with tissue heart valves, (b) in selected patients with atrial fibrillation, (c) in patients with acute anterior wall myocardial infarction, and (d) in patients with valvular heart disease.

A more intense therapeutic range (INR = 3.0 to 4.5, corresponding to a PT 1.5 to 2.0 times normal with a WHO-designated thromboplastin) is appropriate for patients with mechanical prosthetic valves and patients with recurrent systemic embolism.

INR—international normalized ratio PT—prothrombin time WHO—World Health Organization

---

DOSAGE

Historically, the dosage of warfarin has been regulated by monitoring the PT. A PT that is 1.5 to 2.5 times the normal value (11 or 12 seconds) has generally been considered to represent the optimal therapeutic level. However, wide variation in the PT has been reported because of the different thromboplastins used by different laboratories.[53] The World Health Organization (WHO) has recommended converting the PT ratio into an international normalized ratio (INR) so that all laboratory assessments will be comparable. This involves comparing the various thromboplastins with a single standard, a WHO-designated human brain thromboplastin. An INR of 2.0 to 3.0 corresponds to a PT that is 1.3 to 1.5 times normal and represents a moderate dose; an INR of 3.0 to 4.5 corresponds to a PT that is 1.5 to 2.0 times normal and represents a high dose. When bleeding and recurrence rates were measured in patients with high-dose and moderate-dose INRs, the incidence of bleeding was 20 percent in the first group versus five percent in the second, and the therapeutic benefit was equivalent in the two groups.[53] Consequently, the lower ratios are recommended for all but extremely high-risk patients[53] [*see Table 6*].

Initially, the daily dose of warfarin required to increase the INR to between 2.0 and 3.0 is estimated and administered. The INR is then checked every morning. If a sudden overshoot of the target INR range occurs, the warfarin dosage is reduced. If the INR has not reached or surpassed 1.5 after the third warfarin dose, the dosage should be increased. The maintenance dosage averages approximately 5 mg/day but may range from 2.5 to 7.5 mg/day. Warfarin tablets come in three sizes (2.5, 5, and 7.5 mg); however, it is safer to use a single tablet size (e.g., 5 mg) throughout treatment because patients can become confused when tablet size is varied. Thus, if a patient requires 7.5 mg, 5 mg, and 2.5 mg on successive days, he or she can simply take one and a half tablets, one tablet, and half a tablet.

While the maintenance dosage is being determined, the INR should be checked daily. Once the patient stabilizes, the INR can be checked less often: twice weekly for the first few weeks, once weekly for the next several months, and once monthly thereafter if the patient is stable. The patient should be cautioned about drug interactions. If the dosages of other medications are changed, the impact on the INR should be investigated and the warfarin dosage adjusted as appropriate.

DRUG INTERACTIONS

The patient's response to warfarin is affected not only by various bodily factors but also by interactions with numerous drugs [see Table 7]. Interactions are most dangerous when the drugs administered in parallel are taken intermittently.[42,43] Increased metabolic clearance of the drug, secondary to activation of hepatic enzymes, can result from administration of barbiturates, rifampin, or phenytoin; chronic use of alcohol; ingestion of large amounts of vitamin K; and rich foods. Elevated levels of coagulation factors during pregnancy also decrease the effectiveness of the drug.

Decreased metabolism or displacement from protein binding sites caused by phenylbutazone, sulfinpyrazone, metronidazole, disulfiram, allopurinol, cimetidine, amiodarone, or acute intake of ethanol can increase the INR and increase the risk of hemorrhage. Relative deficiency of vitamin K, resulting from inadequate diet or the elimination of the intestinal flora by antimicrobial agents, may have similar effects.

There are some serious interactions that increase the risk of bleeding without altering the INR. These include inhibition of platelet function by drugs such as aspirin and gastritis or gastric ulceration induced by anti-inflammatory drugs.

COMPLICATIONS

Bleeding is the major toxic complication of oral anticoagulation. Whereas tight control of heparin therapy is usually not crucial, tight control of warfarin therapy is definitely necessary to minimize bleeding complications. Bleeding is rare when the INR is kept below 3; when bleeding does occur, it suggests a preexisting lesion. If the bleeding is minor, the warfarin dosage should be adjusted, and if it is major, the drug may have to be discontinued. As with heparin, the risk of intracerebral or subdural hematoma is greater in patients older than 50 years. If the patient shows any sign of hemorrhage, the next dose of anticoagulant should be withheld and the PT measured. For continued or serious bleeding, 5 to 10 mg of vitamin K_1 oxide (phytonadione) I.V. is an effective antidote. Several hours may pass before significant improvement in hemostasis becomes apparent, and 24 hours or longer may be needed for maximal effect. If immediate restoration of hemostatic competence is necessary, levels of vitamin K–dependent coagulation factors can be raised by giving fresh frozen plasma, 10 to 20 ml/kg body weight. Vitamin K_1 oxide should be given simultaneously.

Because administration of warfarin during pregnancy can cause birth defects and abortion, it is contraindicated under these circumstances. Warfarin-induced skin necrosis is a rare complication of oral anticoagulant therapy.[50] First noted in 1943, this syndrome is characterized by the appearance of skin lesions shortly after treatment is initiated. It may be the result of depressed protein C and S levels.

Lytic Therapy

Although heparin is used primarily as an anticoagulant, there is evidence that it may also promote lysis of clot. This phenomenon has been observed in vivo, and a sophisticated group of experiments utilizing cultured mesothelial cells has shown that when heparin is added, these cells are also capable of lysing fibrin.[54] However, lytic therapy is generally understood to refer to administration of streptokinase, urokinase, or tissue plasminogen activator.[42,43,55-58] These agents act by different mechanisms on the endogenous fibrinolytic system to convert plasminogen to plasmin [see 5 Bleeding and Transfusion]. Streptokinase indirectly promotes plasmin formation by combining with plasminogen to form streptokinase-plasminogen complexes that are converted to streptokinase-plasmin complexes. These activator complexes convert residual plasminogen to plasmin.[42,58] Urokinase directly cleaves a peptide bond in the plasminogen molecule to form plasmin. Tissue plasminogen activator binds to fibrin via lysine binding sites at the N-terminal.

The thrombolytic agents are most effective when treatment can be initiated in a matter of hours. Lytic therapy is worth attempting when the clot has been present for less than one week, particularly if it has been present for less than three days. When lytic therapy is begun, heparin therapy usually is temporarily discontinued because of the theoretical possibility of increased bleeding risk; anticoagulation may be resumed immediately upon completion of lytic therapy. If, however, the problem is immediately life threatening (e.g., myocardial infarction or massive pulmonary embolism), anticoagulation should probably be carried out in parallel with lytic therapy to prevent rethrombosis.

INDICATIONS AND CONTRAINDICATIONS

The indications for lytic therapy are being extended.[58] Streptokinase and urokinase are being used for venous thrombotic conditions, such as symptomatic obstruction of major veins in the upper extremities. The morbidity of axillary vein thrombosis can be considerable; clearance of clot may not only help restore patency but also help identify the underlying cause, if it is unknown. In the lower extremities, more thorough clearance of clot should, in theory, help restore valve function and prevent so-called postphlebitic syndrome.[57,59]

Lytic therapy is also of some use in patients with arterial embolism. Although acute arterial ischemia may become irreversible before lytic agents can take effect, the ability of these agents to clear clot from peripheral bypass grafts and arterial venous shunts may not only result in restoration of vascular

Table 7 Factors Influencing Response to Warfarin

Factors Leading to Increased Response	Factors Leading to Decreased Response
Drugs	Drugs
Allopurinol	Barbiturates
Amiodarone	Cholestyramine
Aspirin	Diuretics
Cephalosporins	Ethanol (chronic use)
Cimetidine	Phenytoin
Clofibrate	Rifampin
Disulfiram	Vitamin K
Ethanol (acute intoxication)	Foods
Heparin	Green leafy vegetables
Metronidazole	Bodily factors
Sulfinpyrazone	Hereditary resistance
Trimethoprim-sulfamethoxazole	Hypometabolic states
Bodily factors	Pregnancy
Age	Uremia
Congestive heart failure	
Dietary inadequacy	
Hypermetabolic states	
Intestinal flora loss	
Liver disease	

function but also permit identification of the lesion that precipitated the embolism. Lytic agents may also clear clot sufficiently to permit correction of underlying anatomic defects by means of balloon angioplasty or local surgical procedures.[58]

There are several contraindications that preclude the use of thrombolytic therapy: surgery in the previous 10 days, serious gastrointestinal bleeding in the previous three months, a history of hypertension, an active bleeding or hemorrhagic disorder, a previous cerebrovascular accident, or an active intracranial process. As with heparin, the risk of intracranial bleeding is increased in older patients. Use of t-PA appears to be associated with a higher risk than use of streptokinase or urokinase.

STREPTOKINASE

Streptokinase is a 47 kd protein produced by β-hemolytic streptococci. Because streptokinase is not an endogenous protein, circulating antibodies to it are often already present in plasma; these antibodies result from previous streptococcal infections. When streptokinase is administered via a traditional intravenous infusion, a loading dose must be given to overcome these antibodies. It is essential to ensure that the desired therapeutic effects are achieved. This is done by documenting a rise in the thrombin time (TT), a fall in the fibrinogen level, or an abrupt rise in the D-dimer level. At times, a large loading dose may be necessary to overcome the inactivating antibodies. Once the antibodies are depleted, the half-life of streptokinase is about 80 minutes.

Because streptokinase may deplete circulating plasminogen after a few hours, the optimal therapeutic approach may be to administer it for six hours by continuous infusion every 24 hours for a period of two or three days and then to administer heparin in the intervals between streptokinase infusion.

UROKINASE

Urokinase is a 34 kd globulin that was originally found in human urine and is now isolated from cultured human cells. It has a half-life of 15 minutes and is metabolized by the liver. For catheter clearance, a solution containing 5,000 units/ml should be infused into the obstructed tubing. Like streptokinase, urokinase lacks fibrin specificity and therefore produces a systemic lytic state. Its primary disadvantage is that it costs far more than streptokinase.

TISSUE PLASMINOGEN ACTIVATOR

Tissue plasminogen activator is an enzymatic glycoprotein composed of 527 amino acids that is produced from a human melanoma cell line by means of recombinant DNA technology. The half-life of t-PA is approximately four minutes; it is metabolized by the liver, and approximately 80 percent of the dose is excreted in the urine within 18 hours. It is not antigenic and does not promote antibody formation. Theoretically, t-PA should be somewhat more specific for fibrin clot than urokinase or streptokinase: t-PA invades clot locally, and the t-PA that reaches the systemic circulation is largely deactivated by circulating t-PA inhibitor. In practice, however, the effects of t-PA have not been clinically distinguishable from those of urokinase. Like urokinase, t-PA is extremely expensive.

TECHNIQUE OF ADMINISTRATION

Several methods of administering thrombolytic therapy are currently in use. The traditional method, venous infusion, has been widely used to treat coronary artery thrombosis[60]; however, it has shown only modest effectiveness against peripheral arterial occlusion and is associated with a high rate of hemorrhagic complications.[61] Over time, administration of thrombolytic agents has evolved to become more focused on the site of occlusion, particularly with the development of intra-arterial infusion techniques. A 1974 study reported success with lower total doses of streptokinase administered directly into the occluded artery.[62] The theoretical advantages of this approach were (1) that it decreased the systemic dose of the thrombolytic drug and the concomitant risk of bleeding and (2) that it improved the local effect, as demonstrated by increased 90-minute patency rates. Since that study, intra-arterial infusions have been provided either via a drip proximal to the thrombosis or via a pulse spray directly into the clot through a specialized catheter.

For patients with acute occlusion of a peripheral artery, direct infusion of urokinase into the affected artery in a dosage of 4,000 IU/min for four hours, then in a dosage of 2,000 IU/min for up to 48 hours, has proved as efficacious as immediate surgery.[63] The survival and amputation rates associated with this method of therapy are not significantly different from those associated with a standard primary surgical approach.

Use of thrombolytic agents as the primary therapy has both advantages and disadvantages. One advantage is that it gives the surgeon time to optimize the patient's condition for the stress of an operative procedure. Another is that once the thrombus has been dissolved, it may be easier to identify the underlying atherosclerotic lesion, which would permit better operative planning. The concurrent disadvantages are that there is a one to two percent rate of bleeding at the skin insertion site for the catheter as well as a similar rate of arterial thrombosis at the site where the catheter enters the arterial tree.

Thrombolytic therapy for acute pulmonary embolism has a number of attractive theoretical benefits; however, clinical trials have not shown that such therapy has any significant practical advantages, except in patients who are hemodynamically unstable as a result of an embolus. In these patients, thrombolysis, compared with heparin alone, achieves greater improvements in intermediate end points, such as right ventricular function, but does not increase survival.[64]

MONITORING

Although monitoring of thrombolytic therapy is less standardized than monitoring of anticoagulant therapy, there are several principles that should be followed. First, the effect should be monitored from both a clinical and a laboratory perspective. Clinical monitoring involves following improvements in the angiographic images. Laboratory monitoring has three components. First, D-dimer levels should be measured; a marked increase should be noted, signaling that cross-linked fibrin is undergoing breakdown. Second, adequate stores of the effector protein plasminogen should be documented; without plasminogen, none of the thrombolytic drugs are effective. Third, fibrinogen levels should be followed to prevent exhaustion of native clotting. Most authorities recommend that thrombolytic therapy be discontinued once fibrinogen levels fall below 50 mg/dl. Previously, the TT had been used for monitoring thrombolysis; however, given the current recommendation for concurrent use of heparin,[60] the TT is of little value in this setting.

COMPLICATIONS

The major toxicity of all three thrombolytic agents is hemorrhage. The incidence of bleeding is many times higher after lytic therapy than after anticoagulant therapy and is dependent on both the dosage and the duration of lytic therapy. With careful administration of thrombolytic agents, the incidence of major hemorrhage is less than five percent and the incidence of intracranial hemorrhage is less than one percent.[58] Hemorrhage is the result of two factors: (1) the lysis of physiologic thrombi occurring at sites of vascular injury (e.g., venipuncture sites) and (2) a systemic lytic state caused by the systemic formation of plasmin, which results in fibrinogenolysis and destruction of other coagulation proteins, especially factors V and VIII.

A potential major complication is distal embolism of partially lysed clot. In theory, this possibility should contraindicate use of these agents to treat thrombus in the heart or in the cerebrovascular system.[58] Surprisingly, dislodgment of intracardiac clot as a result of lytic therapy is rare.

There are several adverse reactions that are caused by streptokinase but not by urokinase or t-PA. When streptokinase was first produced, it was associated with a very high incidence of antigenicity and severe pyrogenic reactions. The current purified formulation is relatively free of pyrogens and has a reduced incidence of allergic side effects. It is still antigenic, however, and its use may cause allergic reactions or, in rare instances, anaphylaxis resulting from the presence of preformed streptococcal antibodies. Streptokinase may also induce the formation of additional antibodies that eliminate the possibility of retreatment. In contrast, patients may be re-treated with urokinase as often as necessary with minimal risk of allergic reactions.

Approach to Acquired and Congenital Thrombotic Syndromes

It is well known that certain patients seem to have a tendency to clot spontaneously. Although it has long been postulated that so-called hypercoagulability states exist, such states have been difficult to document except on clinical grounds. Over the past several decades, however, a clearer picture of the nature of these clotting tendencies has emerged.[65] A major impetus for this development was the recognition of the role of antithrombins in exposing clotting. If an antithrombin deficiency exists and clotting goes unchecked, the activation of a clotting cascade could theoretically progress to clotting throughout the entire vascular system. Another important discovery in the understanding of thrombotic syndromes was the recognition of natural lytic substances in the blood that tends to remove the clot after clotting has occurred. Deficiencies of these lytic substances may also exist and may result in a clinical thrombotic tendency. Both types of deficiency can be either acquired or congenital.

Screening

When the etiology of a clotting episode is unclear, the family history should be reviewed for evidence of a congenital disorder. If the history is negative, the patient should be screened for the acquired disorders; if it is positive or if initial screening for acquired disorders yields negative results, the patient should be screened for the congenital disorders [see Figure 10].

ACQUIRED CLOTTING CONDITIONS

Screening for acquired clotting conditions [see Table 8] is based on the history, physical examination, and laboratory assessment. The history should include medications, diseases, and surgical procedures or other injuries.[66-68] Examination may disclose causes of hypercoagulability.[69] Soft tissue injury, for example, whether from surgery, injury, or vascular damage, is a potent activator of the coagulation system. If the injury is severe enough, as in a mangled extremity, it may by itself be capable of causing a severe acquired coagulopathy. The problem is usually obvious, but on occasion, detailed study may be necessary to identify tissue damage or ischemic injury to bowel or extremities. Hypovolemia—especially hypovolemic shock—markedly reduces the clotting time: blood from a patient in profound shock may clot instantaneously in the syringe as it is being drawn. The breakdown of red cells in a hemolytic transfusion reaction can cause clotting. Severe infection, especially from gram-negative organisms, is a potent activator of coagulation.[70]

Laboratory screening may facilitate the diagnosis. A complete blood count may document the presence of polycythemia or leukemia. Thrombocythemia may be a manifestation of a hypercoagulable disorder, and thrombocytopenia after the administration of heparin raises the possibility of intravascular platelet aggregation. A prolonged PTT is suggestive of lupuslike anticoagulant. The presence of increased levels of D-dimers, FDPs, or fibrin monomers in the plasma may document the presence of low-grade intravascular coagulation.

CONGENITAL CLOTTING CONDITIONS

Congenital clotting tendencies can result from deficiencies in thrombosis inhibitors (antithrombin III, protein C, protein S, and possibly heparin cofactor II), dysfibrinogenemias, or dysfibrinolysis (defects in fibrinolysis) [see Table 9]. Most of the congenital clotting defects are transmitted as an autosomal dominant trait. A negative family history, however, does not preclude inherited thrombophilia, because the defects have a low penetrance and fresh mutations may have occurred.

Initial Laboratory Assessment

If the TT and the euglobulin clot lysis time are used in initial laboratory assessment, the following approach, described by Rodgers and Shuman,[71] can be taken.

If the TT is prolonged, dysfibrinogenemia is likely. Further assessment using the reptilase test and specific functional assays for fibrinogen will confirm the diagnosis (see below).

A prolonged euglobulin clot lysis time is suggestive of dysfibrinolysis. This possibility can be verified by applying a tourniquet. If venous blood specimens are taken before and after 10 to 20 minutes of venous occlusion midway between systolic and diastolic pressure, the second specimen should show a shorter lysis time because the application of the tourniquet activates t-PA. If a fibrinolytic defect is evident, the nature of the defect can be determined by means of specific assays for plasminogen, t-PA, and t-PA inhibitor (see below).

If the TT and the euglobulin clot lysis time are normal, specific tests for the antithrombins (antithrombin III, protein C, protein S, and heparin cofactor II) should be carried out (see below).

Specific Causes of Thrombotic Tendency

Dysfibrinogenemia More than 100 qualitative abnormalities of fibrinogen (dysfibrinogenemias) have been reported.[72] Dysfibrinogenemias are inherited in an autosomal dominant manner, with most patients being heterozygous. Most patients with dysfibrinogenemia have either no clinical symptoms or symptoms of a bleeding disorder; a minority (about 11 percent) have clinical features of a recurrent thromboembolic disorder, either venous or arterial.[73,74] Congenital dysfibrinogenemias associated with thrombosis account for about one percent of cases of unexplained venous thrombosis occurring in young individuals. The most commonly observed functional defect in dysfibrinogenemias associated with thrombosis is abnormal fibrin monomer polymerization combined with resistance to fibrinolysis. In recently described cases, decreased binding of plasminogen and increased resistance to lysis by plasmin have been noted.

In addition to the routine prolongation of the TT, patients who have dysfibrinogenemia associated with thromboembolism may also have a prolonged INR. The diagnosis is confirmed if the reptilase time is also longer than normal. When measured with clotting techniques, fibrinogen levels may be slightly or moderately low; however, when measured immunologically, levels may be normal or even increased.

Dysfibrinolysis The plasma fibrinolytic system can be impaired by inherited deficiencies of plasminogen, defective release of t-PA from the vascular endothelium, and high plasma levels of regulatory proteins such as t-PA inhibitors.[74,75] In addition, a deficiency of factor XII (contact factor) may induce failure of fibrinolysis activation.

Inherited plasminogen deficiency is believed to be only rarely responsible for unexplained deep thrombophlebitis in young patients. The defect is transmitted as an autosomal dominant trait. In heterozygous persons with a thrombotic tendency, plasminogen activity is about one half the normal level (normal, 3.9 to 8.4 µmol/ml. As noted earlier, the euglobulin clot lysis time is prolonged. Functional assays should be carried out, and there should be full transformation of plasminogen into plasmin activators. Several commercial methods are now available.

The important role of t-PA inhibitors in the regulation of fibrinolysis is now well defined.[75,76] Two such inhibitors have been purified, t-PA inhibitor I and t-PA inhibitor II. In normal plasma, t-PA inhibitor I is the primary inhibitor for both t-PA and urokinase. Release of t-PA inhibitor I by platelets results in locally increased concentrations where platelets accumulate. The ensuing

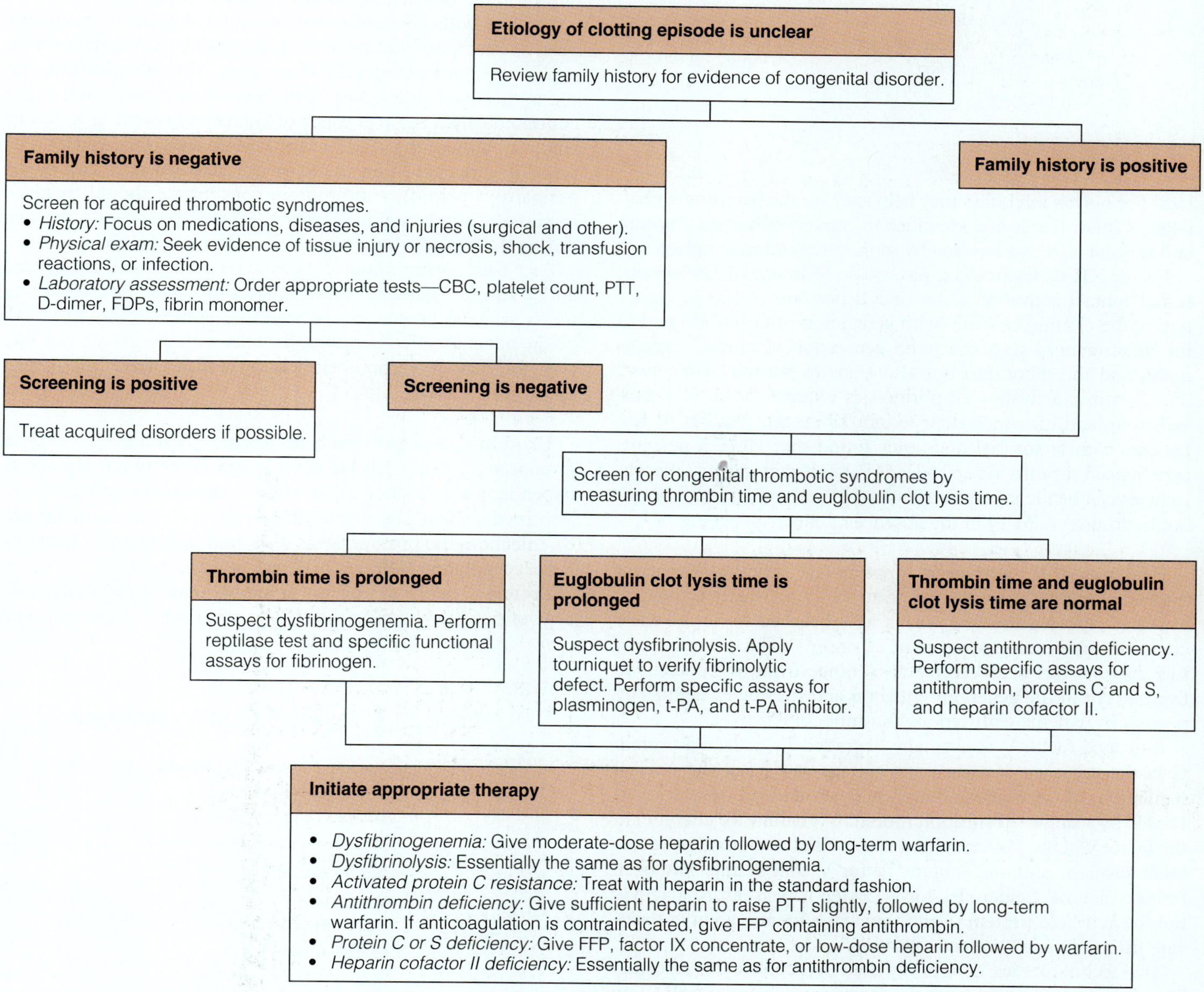

Figure 10 Illustrated is an algorithm for screening for acquired and congenital thrombotic syndromes. The direction screening should take depends on the family history.

Table 8 Etiology of Acquired Hypercoagulability

Tissue and cellular damage
    Shock
    Trauma
    Surgery
    Tissue necrosis
    Transfusion necrosis
Drugs
    Estrogens
    Drug reactions and interactions
    Heparin platelet antibody
    Warfarin
Disease
    Blood dyscrasias
    Cancer
    Diabetes
    Homocystinuria
    Hyperlipidemia
    Presence of lupuslike anticoagulant
    Severe infection
Pregnancy

---

local fibrinolysis inhibition may help stabilize the hemostatic plug. t-PA inhibitor II was first identified in extracts of human placenta and is present in and secreted by monocytes and macrophages.

Factor XII deficiency is a rare cause of impaired fibrinolysis. Initial contact activation of factor XII not only results in activation of the clotting cascade (with generation of thrombin) and of the inflammatory response (with generation of kinins, complement, and thromboxane) but also leads to plasmin generation. This intrinsic activation of fibrinolysis requires factor XII, prekallikrein, and high-molecular-weight kininogen. Studies of 121 patients with factor XII deficiency found that 10 (8.3 percent) experienced thrombotic episodes.[72] Patients with factor XII deficiencies can be identified by a prolonged activated partial thromboplastin time (aPTT) in the absence of clinical bleeding.[65,71]

Resistance to activated protein C The resistance of human clotting factors to inactivation by activated protein C was first reported in 1993 and is now believed to be the most common inherited procoagulant disorder.[77] The prevalence of this disorder has been estimated to range from one percent to five percent in the general population and may be as high as 45 percent in patients with venous thromboembolism.[78]

Activated factor V is normally degraded by activated protein C in the presence of membrane surface as part of the normal regulation of thrombosis. Activated protein C resistance is caused by a single substitution mutation (guanine for adenine) in the factor V gene. This mutation is passed in an autosomal dominant fashion, and the mutant factor V that results has been termed factor V Leiden. Factor V Leiden is resistant to inactivation by activated protein C and thus has a greater ability to activate thrombin and accelerate clotting.

Two techniques are commonly used to diagnose this disorder. The first is a functional assay that compares a standard aPTT to one performed in the presence of exogenous activated protein C. If the latter aPTT does not exhibit significant prolongation, then the patient is probably resistant to activated protein C. The second technique involves analysis of the patient's DNA with a polymerase chain reaction to detect the mutation directly.

Antithrombin deficiency Antithrombin III (now termed simply antithrombin because there is no antithrombin I or II) is a 65 kd protein that decelerates the coagulation system by inactivating activated factors.[79,80] Its principal activity is to inactivate factor Xa and thrombin; it also inactivates activated factors XII, XI, and IX. Antithrombin therefore acts as a scavenger of activated clotting factors. Its activity is enhanced 100-fold by the presence of heparans on the endothelial surface and 1,000-fold by administration of exogenous heparin.

Antithrombin deficiency is one of the more common congenital hypercoagulable states.[79] Its prevalence is approximately 0.01 to 0.05 percent in the general population and two to four percent in patients with venous thrombosis. The trait is passed on as an autosomal dominant trait, with the heterozygous genotype being incompatible with life. Antithrombin-deficient patients are at increased risk for thromboembolism when their antithrombin activity falls below 70 percent of normal.[81]

Patients with congenital antithrombin deficiency frequently present after a stressful event, such as childbirth, surgery, or trauma. These patients usually have deep thrombophlebitis but sometimes have pulmonary embolism. If anticoagulation is not contraindicated, the treatment of choice is heparin at a dosage sufficient to raise the aPTT to the desired level, followed by warfarin. If anticoagulation is contraindicated (as it is during the peripartum period), antithrombin concentrate should be given to raise the antithrombin activity to 80 to 120 percent of normal during the period when anticoagulants cannot be given.

Acquired antithrombin deficiency is now a well-recognized entity. In most patients undergoing severe systemic stress (e.g., major surgical procedures or trauma), antithrombin levels fall below normal.[82] Furthermore, patients with the classic risk factors for venous thromboembolism tend to have the lowest antithrombin levels.

Protein C and protein S deficiency Protein C is a 62 kd glycoprotein with a half-life of six hours. Because it is vitamin K dependent, a deficiency will develop in the absence of vitamin K. Acquired protein C deficiency is seen in liver disease, malignancy, infection, the postoperative state, and disseminated intravascular coagulation (DIC).[11]

Protein C deficiency occurs in approximately four to five percent of patients younger than 40 to 45 years who present with

Table 9 Congenital Clotting Disorders

Deficiencies in thrombosis inhibitors
    Antithrombin III deficiency
    Proteins C and S deficiency
    Activated protein C resistance
Dysfibrinogenemias
Dysfibrinolysis
    Hypoplasminogenemia
    Impaired release of t-PA
    High levels of t-PA inhibitor
    Factor XII deficiency

unexplained venous thrombosis.[83] It is transmitted as an autosomal dominant trait, and the family history is usually positive for a clotting tendency.

Protein C levels range from 70 to 164 percent of normal in patients who do not manifest a clotting tendency; levels below 70 percent of normal are associated with a thrombotic tendency. The most appropriate tests for screening, however, are functional assays, because there are cases of dysfunctional protein C deficiency in which levels of protein C antigen are normal but levels of protein C activity are low, and these would not be detected by the usual immunoassays.

Protein S is a vitamin K–dependent protein that functions as a cofactor for activated protein C by enhancing protein C–induced inactivation of activated factor V. The incidence of protein S deficiency is similar to that of protein C deficiency: about five percent of young patients with unexplained venous thrombosis.[83] Like protein C deficiency, it is transmitted as a dominant trait, and the family history is often positive for a thrombotic tendency.

Treatment

Treatment of a clinical hypercoagulable state involves both prophylaxis [see Discussion, Prophylaxis of Thromboembolism, below] and specific treatment.[84] Prophylaxis in postoperative patients consists primarily of maintaining good hydration, ensuring normal cardiac output, and early mobilization. Administration of low-dose heparin, use of intermittent pneumatic compression, administration of low-molecular-weight dextran, or any combination of these may also be appropriate for a specific patient.

Treatment of thromboembolism associated with dysfibrinogenemia involves moderate-dose heparin anticoagulation followed by long-term warfarin anticoagulation.

Treatment of thromboembolic disorders associated with abnormalities of fibrinolysis is essentially the same as that of dysfibrinogenemia. It is possible that patients with these qualitative plasminogen defects and acute massive thrombotic events might not respond to fibrinolytic treatment with urokinase or streptokinase.

Patients with activated protein C resistance who present with venous thrombosis should be treated with heparin in the standard fashion. They also should receive genetic counseling and refrain from using oral contraceptives.

Treatment of antithrombin deficiency associated with active clotting involves initiating anticoagulation with the appropriate doses of heparin so as to ensure a significant rise in the PTT. Warfarin is the drug of choice for long-term prophylaxis and should be given in a dose sufficient to maintain an INR of 2.0 to 3.0. For patients with a contraindication to anticoagulation, a purified form of antithrombin is available that can be administered directly. Patients with acquired antithrombin deficiency should receive prophylaxis for thromboembolism in the form of heparin in dosages sufficient to raise the aPTT five seconds above the upper limit of the normal laboratory value.

Treatment of the clotting states related to protein C or protein S deficiency involves administering fresh frozen plasma or factor IX concentrate. Low-dose heparin followed by warfarin may be appropriate for long-term treatment.

Discussion

Development of Venous Thrombosis

PATHOPHYSIOLOGY

In 1856, Virchow described a triad of factors that predisposed to venous thrombosis: venous stasis, endothelial damage, and hypercoagulability.[85] Whether all three are required to induce an intravascular thrombotic episode or not, it is certainly true that when all three factors are present, the tendency toward clotting is overwhelming.

Vascular stasis occurs primarily in the great veins of the body, which constitute the blood reservoirs; at any given moment, approximately 70 percent of the total blood supply is contained in the venous system. Muscular activity, with the resultant compression of the great veins, is the pump that promotes return of blood to the heart. When a portion of the body is immobilized, the blood flow slows, and there is a tendency toward stagnation in the veins draining that region. In one experiment, contrast material was administered through the dorsal vein of the foot to patients who had no history of venous disease.[86] The dye tended to be retained in the valve pockets of the thigh and calf veins and in the venous saccules of the calf muscles. Moreover, in supine, completely immobilized patients, the clearance time of the dye was 21 minutes in the thigh and 27 minutes in the lower leg. The retention of dye was substantially reduced by both muscle contractions and elevation of the leg by 15° or more.[87] Patients who suffer from quadriplegia, paraplegia, or hemiplegia have an increased incidence of thrombosis in the paralyzed limbs; in fact, thrombosis is almost universal in this group of patients.[88] Inactivity also results in a relative paralysis of the lytic system, which further encourages propagation of thrombus.[89,90]

Although there is no question that endothelial damage is associated with a thrombotic tendency, it is uncertain whether or how this component of Virchow's triad plays a significant role in the tendency toward venous thrombosis. Certainly, whenever the endothelium of a blood vessel has been directly injured by trauma or by placement of a prosthetic graft or other surgery, blood is exposed to a thrombogenic surface. Exposure of basement membranes to the circulation results in platelet adhesion, platelet release reaction, platelet aggregation, thrombin generation, and clot formation. A 1974 study found no microscopic damage to valve pockets in patients with venous thrombosis.[91] A later study, however, suggested that hypoxic injury to the endothelium plays a role in the formation of deep thrombophlebitis.[92] The endothelium in the venous valve cusp receives little or no oxygen from the adjoining avascular tissue and depends on the oxygen content of the blood. In hypokinetic conditions, oxygen supply to the valve cusp endothelium is reduced. The investigators sampled oxygen tension (Po_2) values in various areas of the valve pocket and in the saphenous vein of humans undergoing operations to remove varicose veins. They found that the Po_2 in the deepest part of the valve pocket was lower than that in the saphenous vein and concluded that venous thrombi were initiated as a result of hypoxic endothelial damage. The investigators postulated that freshly oxygenated leukocytes and platelets adhere more readily to hypoxic endothelium and that the damaged endothelium therefore was the initiating site of thrombus formation. One could also speculate that hypoxic damage to endothelium interferes with the release of plasminogen activator, thereby allowing any clotting process that is initiated to progress.

Hypercoagulability, the third factor in the triad, undoubtedly plays a large role in thrombogenesis. Acquired and congenital disorders that promote the hypercoagulable state are present in surgical patients and surgical disease states, particularly trauma and vascular disease. As noted earlier [see Approach to Acquired and Congenital Thrombotic Syndromes, above], this hypercoagulable state could result from depletion of antithrombins, compromise of the lytic system, or the entrance of procoagulants into the bloodstream from injured tissues. Precipitation of clot would tend to occur in areas of stasis or sites of endothelial damage.

Most spontaneous venous clots occur in the deep venous system of the lower half of the body. In immobilized postoperative patients, the initial site of most thrombus formation appears to be the valve pockets, where flow is stagnant and eddies form. Thrombi grow by the progressive deposition of layers of thrombotic material, forming in the direction of blood flow. Initially, the thrombus is attached at the point of origin on the vessel wall, with the tail floating freely in the lumen. Most clots that form in this manner promptly lyse or fragment and break loose. Small fragments that reach the pulmonary vascular system lyse and disappear. If persistent stasis is present, antithrombin activity is reduced, or lytic activity is impaired, the clot will continue to grow. It may elicit an inflammatory response in the vein wall and become circumferentially adherent (and therefore obstructive), or it may remain primarily free floating, except for a localized attachment.

Alternatively, the clot may take a combined form, with some portions adherent and the propagating tail free floating, depending on how much vein wall inflammation the thrombus induces. Obstructive clot may well propagate backward down the vein, aggravating the obstruction by blocking collateral vessels.

Normally, the hydrostatic pressure on the arterial side of the capillary loop is approximately 30 mm Hg, that on the venous side is approximately 12 mm Hg, and that in the surrounding external tissue is approximately 2 to 3 mm Hg. Venous hypertension caused by obstructive clot raises the hydrostatic pressure in the distal venous capillary bed, thereby increasing the transfer of fluid from the vascular compartment into the interstitium. Eventually, the interstitial extravasation of fluid increases tissue tension and counterbalances Starling forces, preventing further accumulation of fluid.

Leg swelling causes passive muscle engorgement and dilation of muscle fibrils. These, in turn, activate pain receptors located in the muscle spindle and account for the muscle discomfort. Stretching the muscle aggravates the discomfort—hence, the positive Homans' sign (pain in the calf on forced dorsiflexion of the foot).

Stable clot does not release inflammatory mediators, but actively proliferating clot releases serotonin, histamine, thromboxane, and other mediators. These activate vein wall afferent receptors and account for most of the pain and the tenderness in the vein containing the thrombus. Inflammatory mediators pass through the vein wall and, in the superficial veins, are associated with redness and swelling of the overlying skin.[3]

INCIDENCE

It is estimated that 2.5 million people a year suffer from deep thrombophlebitis.[93] The incidence of deep thrombophlebitis in surgical patients varies widely depending on the method of study. In a review of eight series in which venography or autopsy was used to verify the diagnosis, the incidence of deep thrombophlebitis ranged from 18 to 90 percent (average, 42 percent).[94]

Estimates of the incidence of pulmonary embolism also vary widely, but reviews suggest that about 700,000 individuals suffer from this complication each year and that about 200,000 die as a result.[1,2] In the absence of prophylaxis, fatal pulmonary embolism has been reported in four to seven percent of hip surgery patients and in 0.1 to 0.8 percent of general surgery patients.[1,95] In about 40 to 60 percent of patients who die of pulmonary embolism, the diagnosis is not made clinically. Pulmonary embolism may be responsible for as many as five percent of postoperative deaths, and it may occur in as many as 25 percent of patients admitted to the hospital.[96,97] Pulmonary infarction occurs in about 10 percent of patients with clinical evidence of pulmonary embolism.[13]

Development of Arterial Embolism

PATHOPHYSIOLOGY

The sequential changes secondary to sudden vascular occlusion can be clearly followed when the site of embolic lodgment is in a major artery. Sudden obstruction of a vessel leads to immediate accretion of platelets and clot on the embolus and the downstream release of inflammatory mediators, including histamine, serotonin, thromboxane, complement, and kinins. These mediators cause reflex spasm in all the vessels distal to the obstruction, and the skin becomes pale, cold, and ischemic. The spasm is actually protective to an extent, in that it prevents propagating thrombus from filling the lumina of the main vessels distal to the obstruction. Most of the small side branches of these main channels essentially close.[39]

A small, thin string of clot may propagate, but if collateral flow subsequently develops, there is room for nutritive blood flow alongside the thrombotic cord. If collateral flow is not sufficient to meet the minimal nutritional needs of the organ or limb, function will be lost in the critical tissues, particularly those most distal to the obstruction. Ischemia of sensory nerves of the extremities will result in numbness and anesthesia. Muscle will become paralyzed and nonfunctional. If collateral flow is subsequently mobilized in response to stimulation by the low pressures distal to the obstruction, this event may be sufficient to ensure viability; the numbness may improve and muscle function may return even if the limb remains pale and cool.

If collateral flow continues to be inadequate, the tissues distal to the obstruction ultimately die. The initial manifestations of irreversibility are loss of tone in smooth muscle that has been in spasm and microvascular dilation, usually occurring after six to eight hours of ischemia. When an extremity is involved, there will be bluish mottling of the overlying skin, which signals that capillaries have reopened and vascular stasis is present[35] [see Figure 11]. Initially, the bluish mottling is patchy and varies in its location; finally, however, it becomes confluent. At this point, major feeding channels thrombose, and muscle goes into rigor, becoming firm, hard, and patchily necrotic.[36,37] In absolute ischemia associated with thigh tourniquet shock, muscle starts to die at approximately three hours, and extensive areas of necrosis are present by six to eight hours.[37] At this point, attempts to open major channels and extract thrombus will be unsuccessful because clotted branches of the main arterial channels feeding dead or markedly ischemic tissue will not accept flow. Moreover, clot will begin to accumulate in the venules and major veins, further compromising capillary flow. Finally, the limb becomes irreversibly ischemic, as indicated by failure of the bluish areas of the skin to blanch with pressure.

It should be remembered that skin can tolerate prolonged periods of ischemia much better than any of the underlying structures (except perhaps bone and tendon) can: irreversible thrombosis of skin capillaries occurs only after 24 hours of ischemia. Theoretically, therefore, late reestablishment of circulation to an ischemic extremity could be associated with death of muscle and irreversible damage to nerves, but the skin could still be viable. In the final analysis, limbs are lost when the skin is lost, not when muscle is lost. This is a crucial point when fasciotomy is under consideration.

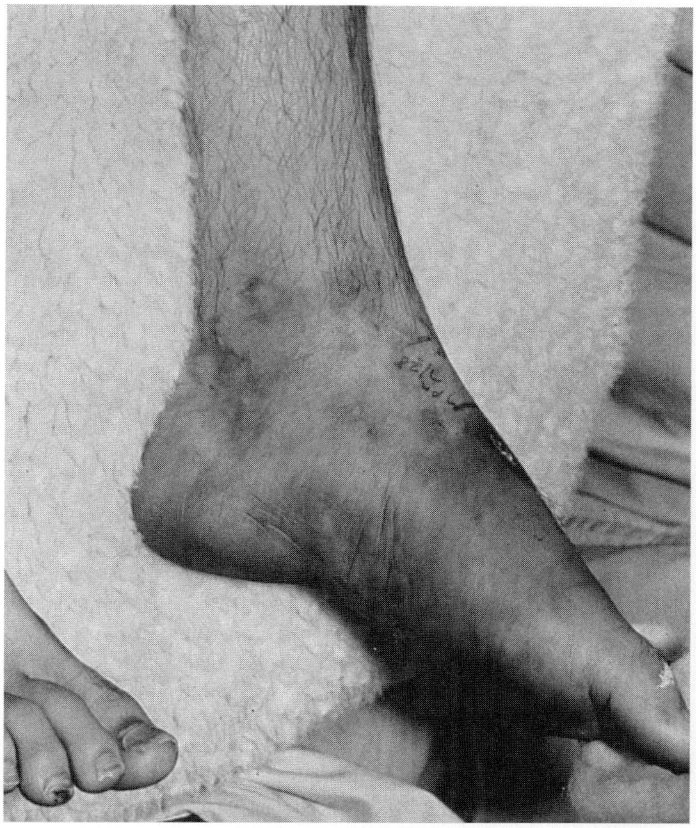

Figure 11 The bluish, mottled appearance of the skin of the left foot and ankle denotes irreversible ischemia.

OUTCOME CONSIDERATIONS

The act of extracting clot and restoring circulation, especially when done on the lower extremity through a femoral incision with the patient under local anesthesia,[98] seems benign; however, the literature clearly documents a high mortality associated with embolic occlusion in an extremity.[99-103] This average mortality has improved very little in recent years.

Almost all studies of extremity embolic occlusions that are associated with low mortalities document the importance of heparin anticoagulation given preoperatively, intraoperatively, and postoperatively.[39,104] If reperfusion can be reestablished before the organ is irreversibly damaged—preferably while it is still completely viable—then systemic morbidity will be acceptable and the end result optimal.

Both the bowel and skeletal muscle remain viable for six to eight hours after interruption of circulation. After six or eight hours of profound ischemia, attempts to revascularize major segments of bowel or extremities in which there is a large mass of ischemic muscle tissue not only meet with little success in reestablishing flow but also carry a high risk of mortality from the reperfusion insult.[105-109] In advanced ischemia involving the entire lower leg below the knee, reperfusion will result in death for most older patients, and in advanced ischemia of the entire leg, reperfusion will be life threatening for even young patients.

There are two main problems associated with reperfusion. The first is the acute metabolic problem produced by reperfusion of a large mass of ischemic tissue. There is an obligatory diffuse vascular dilation in the ischemic limb, and the dilated vascular bed can temporarily sequester large volumes of blood when flow is initially reestablished. Peripheral resistance is lost, and reperfusion flow can be three times normal or even greater, creating a demand for increased cardiac output that a patient with poor cardiac reserve may be incapable of meeting.[107] Large quantities of potassium and lactate are washed out of the distal circulation[106]; serum potassium may reach critically high levels when the mass of tissue reperfused is equivalent to an entire leg. These high levels, coupled with systemic acidosis from lactate release, can compromise myocardial function.

Fresh clot that formed in the venous system during stasis is washed out into the systemic circulation and is eventually filtered out by the lung. This clot, along with inflammatory mediators released from devitalized cells in the ischemic limb, induces diffuse systemic inflammation, increased vascular permeability, and third-spacing (transudation of fluid into the extravascular space). Pulmonary function is impaired, and the hypovolemia caused by the third-spacing may result in systemic organ damage.[105,107,108] Systemic release of myoglobin and other tissue procoagulants leads to systemic hypercoagulability and thus to intravascular coagulation. Intravascular coagulation results in further release of inflammatory mediators and, on rare occasions, disseminated intravascular coagulation with diffuse, uncontrollable hemorrhage. Thrombotic renal cortical necrosis may lead to renal shutdown.

The second problem associated with reperfusion of severely ischemic limbs is fascial compartment swelling. When fasciotomy is carried out on these ischemic limbs, dead muscle is usually found. The question that must then be answered is whether the compartmental swelling resulted from permeability alterations in viable muscle or whether the muscle was irreversibly damaged and capillary permeability increased as a direct result of the vascular occlusion. The answer has important implications for treatment. On one hand, if it is only irreversibly ischemic muscle that swells enough to produce high compartmental pressures, opening the skin and the fascia to relieve pressure would expose dead muscle. In theory, this should increase the risk of loss of limb because exposed nonviable muscle inevitably becomes infected. On the other hand, if viable muscle is being compromised by the swelling, early exposure should prevent muscular death and facilitate salvage of extremities. It is of therapeutic interest that in one study, early administration of heparin to animals with ischemic limbs markedly diminished local vascular permeability and muscle swelling.[110]

There is no question that when compartment syndromes involve primary swelling resulting from high venous pressure, direct hemorrhage, or muscle contusion, fasciotomy is beneficial. If, however, the muscle is already dead or irreversibly ischemic secondary to the proximal arterial occlusion, fasciotomy is not beneficial and might even be harmful. We have found that when fasciotomy is required to relieve high compartmental pressures after proximal arterial occlusion, limb loss is extremely high, and significant mortality may be expected. For this reason, our policy—admittedly a controversial one—is not to do fasciotomy routinely after restoration of extremity blood flow. If revascularization is carried out within six to eight hours, severe muscle swelling is rare. Moreover, attempts to enhance reperfusion of severely ischemic or dead muscle by means of fasciotomy may increase mortality. It is better to risk the loss of a limb than the loss of a patient.

INCIDENCE

The incidence of arterial embolism is much lower than it once was[34]; however, reliable figures are not currently available. In most series, the incidence of cerebral embolism is not well documented, because it is often confused with other causes of stroke—in particular, local atherosclerotic obstruction and intracranial hemorrhage.[34]

Prophylaxis of Thromboembolism

The optimal means of treating a thromboembolic event is to prevent its occurrence. This is particularly true for certain groups known to be at high risk for thromboembolic complications.[111,112] Patients older than 60 years should be considered for prophylaxis if they are about to undergo major surgery or are significantly injured. Immobilized patients are at high risk for thromboembolism because prolonged immobilization results in stasis in lower leg veins. Any patient with a major injury (particularly a pelvic fracture) is at risk for thromboembolism as well, perhaps because the trauma may involve stretch injuries to pelvic and iliac veins, which then become the source of thrombus. Finally, any patient with a history of a spontaneous thrombotic event, either after surgery or de novo, is at high risk for subsequent thromboembolism.

There are a number of techniques that can be used to prevent thromboembolic complications. The most effective of these is early ambulation. It is known and universally accepted that surgical patients immobilized for prolonged periods have a very high incidence of thrombotic events.[2,93-95,111] Elastic stockings have been used for decades as prophylaxis for thromboembolism. Unfortunately, most commercial stockings neither fit adequately nor provide adequate compression; thus, they probably offer little or no benefit.[2] Low-molecular-weight dextran, which lowers blood viscosity and inhibits platelet aggregation, is helpful in certain instances but is not completely protective.[112] In theory, it should prevent arterial clots (which are primarily composed of platelets) more effectively than venous clots (which are primarily composed of fibrin). Dextran may provide a fair degree of prophylaxis. A 2 unit priming dose is given in the first 24 hours, followed by 1 unit/day for three or four days in the postoperative period.

A newer modality that seems to have a significant impact on the incidence of thromboembolic complications is intermittent pneumatic compression. The original rationale for this technique was based on the concept that massage of the lower legs would empty the veins and improve venous efflux. This rationale was faulty in that venous efflux cannot possibly be increased unless arterial influx is increased in parallel, which, of course, is not the case. Moreover, the clots that cause fatalities form in the large veins of the upper thigh and the pelvis, and massage of the calf and the lower thigh would do nothing for these veins. Although intermittent pneumatic compression does not have the effect originally predicted, it probably has a more important one: massage of the leg veins is known to activate t-PA and thus the fibrinolytic system,[113] thereby providing not only local but also systemic benefit. Massage of upper extremities decreases clotting in lower extremity veins, and massage of one leg decreases clotting in the other leg. As a result, intermittent pneumatic compression has proved to be a safe, although somewhat uncomfortable, method of preventing clots in patients who are immobilized for prolonged periods. It has found particular favor in critical care units, where other forms of prophylaxis are inapplicable or contraindicated.[111]

Finally, there is prophylactic anticoagulation. A major British study of thromboembolic prophylaxis in patients undergoing surgical therapy for hip fractures found that subcutaneous administration of 5,000 units of heparin two or three times daily before, during, and after the operation was not associated with a significantly increased incidence of bleeding and substantially lowered the incidence of thromboembolic complications.[95] This low-dose protocol has been criticized as being insufficiently individualized for specific high-risk patients. The mode of action of low-dose heparin is to markedly augment the antithrombotic effect of antithrombin[114]; therefore, if antithrombin levels are reduced, low-dose heparin might not be effective, and moderate-dose heparin might be more appropriate in high-risk settings.

Recently, a new form of heparin has appeared on the market: low-molecular-weight heparin. This form of heparin uses the same pentasaccharide chain to potentiate the effects of antithrombin (thereby achieving anticoagulation) as unfractionated (standard) heparin does. Like unfractionated heparin, it is ineffective if antithrombin levels have been depleted. The main advantage of low-molecular-weight heparin is that it has a more dependable half-life and bioavailability than unfractionated heparin. For this reason, it has been given without any monitoring of the drug's effect or the patient's plasma heparin levels.

Several clinical trials in Europe and in the United States have documented the efficacy of low-molecular-weight heparin. The majority of the trials have been in patients undergoing elective hip[115,116] or knee operations; however, a few have addressed other patient populations, such as trauma patients.[117] In these studies, the rates of deep thrombophlebitis for patients receiving unmonitored low-molecular-weight heparin therapy have, for the most part, been compared with those of patients receiving either placebo[115] or so-called minidose heparin therapy[116,117] (5,000 units of unfractionated heparin given subcutaneously twice or three times daily). Several studies from the 1980s have shown the superiority of so-called adjusted-dose heparin therapy to either placebo or the minidose approach.[118,119] (The adjusted-dose approach is identical to the low-dose approach described earlier [see General Principles of Anticoagulation and Lytic Therapy, Heparin Anticoagulation]; we use the latter term to clarify the relation of this approach to the other two regimens that we recommend, moderate dose and high dose.)

From the available information on low-molecular-weight heparin, it appears that it can be recommended for both elective and emergency trauma patients in place of placebo or minidose heparin. Whether it is superior to adjusted-dose therapy with unfractionated heparin remains uncertain. An unmonitored low-molecular-weight heparin regimen is clearly simpler to manage than an adjusted-dose unfractionated heparin regimen. In settings where compliance with monitoring and dose-adjusting protocols is an issue, unmonitored low-molecular-weight heparin therapy may well be preferable because it may lead to improved compliance.

Warfarin may be used instead of heparin in some patients.[112,120] Warfarin anticoagulation must be started three or four days before the surgical procedure, and the patient must be able to continue taking oral medications in the immediate postoperative period. Consequently, this approach is of limited value for abdominal procedures, although it has proved to be a useful alternative to heparin for orthopedic procedures. The INR should be kept below 3.0 to prevent excessive bleeding. Warfarin is not as easy to regulate tightly as heparin, and it is not as easily turned on and off; that is, several days are needed for the therapeutic effect to be achieved and several more days for the effect to wear off. Recently, it has been shown that use of low-dose warfarin (as little as 1 mg/day) may offer prophylactic benefit.[120]

Rationale for Varying Heparin Dosage

For many years after the introduction of heparin therapy into surgery in 1936,[121-123] the dosages used were arbitrary. In 1955, however, a series of experiments in dogs showed that when a ligature was applied to the jugular vein and sufficient heparin administered to increase the clotting time of blood in a test tube to 2.5 times normal (corresponding to a Lee-White clotting time of 20 to 30 minutes), thrombus formation was prevented distal to the ligature.[124] Because the prolonged periods of observation necessary for the Lee-White clotting time are not practical in modern clinical laboratories, other tests, such as the activated PTT and the activated clotting time, have been introduced; these represent practical modifications to the original Lee-White clotting time. An activated PTT of 1.5 to 2.0 times normal and an activated clotting time of 200 seconds are considered to be therapeutically equivalent to a Lee-White clotting time of 30 minutes.

Heparin therapy is still plagued by several misconceptions. One is that the extent of anticoagulation is necessarily correlated with prolongations of the activated PTT or the activated clotting time.[38,45,125] All the experimental studies on which this misconception is based are concerned with anticoagulation in normal animals or normal humans, who have normal levels of antithrombins.

Another misconception is the idea that pathological bleeding correlates directly with the prolongation of the clotting time and that bleeding complications can be prevented by tight control of anticoagulation. In fact, there is no evidence of any correlation between the bleeding risk and the anticoagulatory effect.[46,47,125] In normal patients, anticoagulation for as long as three or four days is rarely associated with bleeding unless a prior sensitivity to heparin has been induced.

Still another misconception is the idea that a relative degree of anticoagulation can be achieved that effectively counteracts the clotting yet is free of the risk of bleeding. The fallacy of this idea is best illustrated by considering the therapeutic problem presented by the ischemic limb. An ischemic limb is, to an extent, isolated from the circulation. This means that a dose of heparin that is sufficient to produce the desired anticoagulation, according to conventional measures, may be relatively ineffective in the ischemic area, distal to the obstruction. For therapeutic purposes, it is the clotting status in the ischemic area that is crucial; therefore, conventional monitoring, which provides information only about the clotting status in a peripheral vein,[38] must be disregarded. To ensure adequate anticoagulation in the involved limb, arbitrary high doses of heparin are required.[39] Similar principles apply to the treatment of major pulmonary embolism. Downstream from the embolus, the inflammatory products released by the proximal clot will result in both vascular and bronchiolar spasm. These inflammatory mediators also impair collateral circulation and potentiate clotting in the region of vascular stasis. Administration of high doses of heparin is necessary to prevent further propagation of clot distal to where the embolism is lodged.[126]

Determination of the optimal heparin dose is further complicated by the fact that the shock state itself markedly augments the clotting tendency. Two hundred years ago, Hewson observed that when he bled patients, "the blood that emerged last clotted first, the blood that emerged first clotted last."[127] Nearly every clinician who works with shock patients has noted that in some instances, the blood of the patient clots in the syringe before it can be placed in the anticoagulant. Presumably, this is a survival mechanism, in that enhanced spontaneous thrombosis would result in prompter cessation of hemorrhage.

Out of frustration at the apparent unreliability of current tests of clotting status, one of us (F.W.B.) and others measured the survival of radioactive-labeled fibrinogen as a means of documenting the effectiveness of anticoagulation under various experimental and clinical conditions.[38,45,68] In patients on cardiopulmonary bypass or extracorporeal membrane oxygenation, the fibrinogen half-life remained abnormal despite what appeared to be adequate anticoagulation according to the activated PTT. Dosages three times as large as the "adequate" dosage were required to normalize the fibrinogen half-life and to anticoagulate the patient fully. In a canine study, the adequacy of anticoagulation after administration of thrombin and thrombin-heparin was assessed according to both the activated PTT and the half-life of fibrinogen.[55] Once again, the fibrinogen half-life remained grossly abnormal despite what appeared to be adequate anticoagulation according to the activated PTT.

In all the experiments, particularly the clinical ones, it was apparent that when full anticoagulation was obtained in a clinical clotting situation, vascular spasm decreased, as manifested by improvement in collateral flow. When adequate anticoagulation was achieved in an ischemic limb, the level of demarcation inevitably dropped, and the pain decreased.[45-47] In venous thrombotic conditions, the findings were even more dramatic: when adequate anticoagulation was achieved, pain inevitably disappeared, and swelling and signs of inflammation improved within hours.[46,47] An interesting corollary of this finding is that in patients with venous thrombosis, conventional doses of anticoagulant controlled in a conventional fashion were associated in most instances with immediate improvement,[45] whereas in patients with arterial ischemia, this was almost never true—much higher doses of anticoagulant were required than the conventional tests suggested.[38,39]

Therefore, to meet the varying needs of patients with thromboembolic complications, we use three degrees of heparin anticoagulation: low dose, moderate dose, and high dose [see General Principles of Anticoagulation and Lytic Therapy, Heparin Anticoagulation, *above*].

References

1. Hirsh J, Hull RD: Venous Thromboembolism: Natural History, Diagnosis, and Management. CRC Press, Boca Raton, Florida, 1988
2. Bergqvist D: Postoperative Thromboembolism: Frequency, Etiology, Prophylaxis. Springer-Verlag, New York, 1983
3. LeClerk JR: Venous Thromboembolic Disorders. Lea & Febiger, Philadelphia, 1991, pp 54, 176
4. Bergqvist D, Bergentz SE: Diagnosis of deep vein thrombosis. World J Surg 14:679, 1990
5. Hirsh J: Reliability of non-invasive tests for the diagnosis of venous thrombosis (editorial). Thromb Haemost 65:221, 1991
6. Krupski WC, Bass A, Dilley RB, et al: Propagation of deep venous thrombosis identified by duplex ultrasonography. J Vasc Surg 12:467, 1990
7. Lensing AW, Prandoni P, Brandjes D: Detection of deep-vein thrombosis by real-time B-mode ultrasonography. N Engl J Med 320:342, 1989
8. Haire WD, Lynch TG, Lund GB: Limitations of magnetic resonance imaging and ultrasound directed (duplex) scanning in the diagnosis of subclavian vein thrombosis. J Vasc Surg 13:391, 1991
9. Barnes RW, Nix ML, Barnes CL: Perioperative asymptomatic venous thrombosis: role of duplex scanning versus venography. J Vasc Surg 9:25, 1989
10. Hirsh J, Turpie AG: Use of plasminogen activators in venous thrombosis. World J Surg 14:688, 1990
11. Lord RS, Chen FC, DeVine TJ, et al: Surgical treatment of acute deep venous thrombosis. World J Surg 14:694, 1990
12. Smith GT, Dammin GJ, Dexter L: Postmortem arteriographic studies of the human lung in pulmonary embolization. JAMA 188:143, 1964
13. Dalen JE, Haffajee CI, Alpert JS 3rd, et al: Pulmonary embolism, pulmonary hemorrhage and pulmonary infarction. N Engl J Med 296:1431, 1977
14. Moser KM, Hull R, Saltzman HA, et al: Recent advances in diagnosis of pulmonary embolism and deep venous thrombosis. Am Rev Respir Dis 138:1046, 1988
15. Coon WW: Risk factors in pulmonary embolism. Surg Gynecol Obstet 143:385, 1976
16. Boneu B, Bes G, Pelzer H, et al: D-dimers, thrombin antithrombin III complexes and prothrombin fragments 1 + 2 diagnostic value in clinically suspected deep vein thrombosis. Thromb Haemost 65:28, 1991
17. Speiser W, Mallek R, Koppensteiner R: D-dimer and

TAT measurement in patients with deep venous thrombosis: utility in diagnosis and judgment of anticoagulant treatment effectiveness. Thromb Haemost 64:196, 1990
18. PIOPED Investigators: Value of ventilation/perfusion scan in acute pulmonary embolism: results of prospective investigation of pulmonary embolism diagnosis (PIOPED). JAMA 263:2753, 1990
19. Hull RD, Hirsh J, Carter CJ, et al: Diagnostic value of ventilation-perfusion lung scanning in patients with suspected pulmonary embolism. Chest 88:819, 1985
20. Hull RD, Raskob GE, Hirsh J: The diagnosis of clinically suspected pulmonary embolism: practical approaches. Chest 89:4175, 1986
21. Ferris EJ, Holder JC, Lim WN, et al: Angiography of pulmonary emboli: digital studies and balloon-occlusion cineangiography. Am J Roentgenol 142:369, 1984
22. Hull RD, Hirsh J, Carter CJ, et al: Pulmonary angiography, ventilation lung scanning, and venography for clinically suspected pulmonary embolism with abnormal perfusion lung scan. Ann Intern Med 98:891, 1983
23. Atik M, Broghamer WL Jr: The impact of prophylactic measures on fatal pulmonary embolism. Arch Surg 114:366, 1979
24. Collins R, Scrimgeour A, Yusuf S, et al: Reduction in fatal pulmonary embolism and venous thrombosis by perioperative administration of subcutaneous heparin: overview of results of randomized trials in general, orthopedic, and urologic surgery. N Engl J Med 318:1162, 1988
25. Geerts WH: Pulmonary embolism. Conn's Current Therapy 1992. Rakel RE, Ed. WB Saunders Co, Philadelphia, 1992, p 179
26. Moser KM: State of the art: pulmonary embolism. Am Rev Respir Dis 115:829, 1977
27. Thomas DP: Therapeutic role of heparin in acute pulmonary embolism. Curr Ther Res 18:21, 1975
28. Silver D: Pulmonary embolism: prevention, detection and nonoperative management. Surg Clin North Am 54:1089, 1974
29. Rohrer MJ, Scheidler MG, Wheeler HB, et al: Extended indications for placement of an inferior vena cava filter. J Vasc Surg 10:44, 1989
30. Fink JA, Jones BT: The Greenfield filter as the primary means of therapy in venous thromboembolic disease. Surg Gynecol Obstet 172:253, 1991
31. Wells I: Inferior vena cava filters and when to use them. Clin Radiol 40:11, 1989
32. Zimmerman JJ, Fogarty TJ: Acute arterial occlusion. Textbook of Surgery: The Biological Basis of Modern Surgical Practice, 13th ed. Sabiston DC, Ed. WB Saunders Co, Philadelphia, 1986, p 1904
33. Imparato AM, Riles TS: Peripheral arterial disease. Principles of Surgery, 5th ed. Schwartz SI, Shires GT, Spencer FC, Eds. McGraw-Hill Book Co, New York, 1989, p 933
34. Haimovici H: Peripheral arterial embolism: a study of 330 unselected cases of embolism of the extremities. Angiology 1:20, 1950
35. Stallone RJ, Blaisdell FW: Analysis of morbidity and mortality from arterial embolectomy. Surgery 65:207, 1969
36. Dunant JH, Edwards WS: Small vessel occlusion in the extremity after various periods of arterial obstruction: an experimental study. Surgery 73:240, 1973
37. Mullick S: The tourniquet in operations upon the extremities. Surg Gynecol Obstet 146:821, 1978
38. Blaisdell FW, Graziano CJ, Effeney DJ: In vivo assessment of anticoagulation. Surgery 82:827, 1977
39. Blaisdell FW, Steele M, Allen RE: Management of acute lower extremity arterial ischemia due to embolism and thrombosis. Surgery 84:822, 1978
40. Leyvraz PF, Richard J, Bachmann F, et al: Adjusted versus fixed dose heparin in the prevention of deep vein thrombosis after hip replacement. N Engl J Med 309:954, 1983
41. Rooke TW: Deep venous thrombosis of the extremities. Conn's Current Therapy 1992. Rakel RE, Ed. WB Saunders Co, Philadelphia, 1992, p 289
42. Majerus PW, Broze GJ Jr, Miletich JP, et al: Anticoagulant, thrombolytic and antiplatelet drugs. Goodman & Gilman's The Pharmacological Basis of Therapeutics. Goodman AG, Rall TW, Nies AS, et al, Eds. Pergamon Press, New York, 1990, p 1311
43. USP DI, Drug Information for the Health Care Professional, Vol IB. The United States Pharmacopeial Convention, Inc, Rockville, Maryland, 1992, pp 1505, 2357, 2658
44. Owen CA Jr, Bowie EJ, et al: Chronic intravascular coagulation syndromes: a summary. Mayo Clin Proc 49:673, 1974
45. Blaisdell FW, Graziano CJ: Assessment of clotting by the determination of fibrinogen catabolism. Am J Surg 135:436, 1978
46. Conti S, Daschbach M, Blaisdell FW: A comparison of high-dose versus conventional-dose heparin therapy for deep vein thrombosis. Surgery 92:972, 1982
47. Kashtan J, Conti S, Blaisdell FW: Heparin therapy for deep venous thrombosis. Am J Surg 140:836, 1980
48. Silver D, Kapsch DN, Tsoi EK: Heparin induced thrombocytopenia, thrombosis and hemorrhage. Ann Surg 198:301, 1983
49. Becker PS, Miller VT: Heparin-induced thrombocytopenia. Stroke 20:1449, 1989
50. Celoria GM, Steingart RH, Banson B, et al: Coumarin skin necrosis in a patient with heparin-induced thrombocytopenia: a case report. Angiology 39:915, 1988
51. Walker AM, Jick H: Predictors of bleeding during heparin therapy. JAMA 244:1209, 1980
52. Ginsberg JS, Kowalchuk G, Hirsh J, et al: Heparin effect on bone density. Thromb Haemost 64:286, 1990
53. Hirsh J, Poller L, Deykin D, et al: Optimal therapeutic range for oral anticoagulants. Chest 95(2 suppl):5s, 1989
54. Grulich-Henn J, Preissner KT, Müller-Berghaus G: Heparin stimulates fibrinolysis in mesothelial cells by selective induction of tissue plasminogen activator but not plasminogen activator inhibitor-1 synthesis. Thromb Haemost 64:420, 1990
55. Blaisdell FW: Hemostasis and thrombosis. Vascular Surgery: A Comprehensive Review, 2nd ed. Moore WS, Ed. Grune & Stratton, New York, 1986, p 909
56. Meyerovitz MF, Goldhaber SZ, Reagan K, et al: Recombinant tissue-type plasminogen activator versus urokinase in peripheral arterial and graft occlusions: a randomized trial. Radiology 175:75, 1990
57. Turpie AG: Thrombolytic agents in venous thrombosis. J Vasc Surg 12:196, 1990
58. Marder VJ, Sherry S: Thrombolytic therapy: current status. N Engl J Med 318:1585, 1988
59. Goldhaber SZ, Buring JE, Lipnick RJ, et al: Pooled analyses of randomized trials of streptokinase and heparin in phlebographically documented acute deep venous thrombosis. Am J Med 76:393, 1984
60. The effects of tissue plasminogen activator, streptokinase, or both on coronary-artery patency, ventricular function, and survival after acute myocardial infarction. The GUSTO Angiographic Investigators. N Engl J Med 329:1615, 1993
61. Amery A, Deloof W, Vermylen J, et al: Outcome of recent thromboembolic occlusions of limb arteries treated with streptokinase. Br Med J 4:639, 1970
62. Dotter CT, Rosch J, Seaman AJ: Selective clot lysis with low-dose streptokinase. Radiology 111:31, 1974
63. Ouriel K, Veith FJ, Sasahara AA: Thrombolysis or peripheral arterial surgery: phase I results. TOPAS investigators. J Vasc Surg 23:64, 1996
64. Meyer GJ, Sors H, Charbonnier B, et al: Effects of intravenous urokinase versus alteplase on total pulmonary resistance in acute massive pulmonary embolism: a European multicenter double-blind trial. The European Cooperative Study Group for Pulmonary Embolism. J Am Coll Cardiol 19:239, 1992
65. Schafer AI: The hypercoagulable states. Ann Intern Med 102:814, 1985
66. Baehner RL: Alterations in blood coagulation with trauma. Pediatr Clin North Am 22:289, 1975
67. Jansson IG, Hetland O, Rammer LM, et al: Effects of phospholipase C, a tissue thromboplastin inhibitor, on pulmonary microembolism after missile injury of the limb. J Trauma 28:S222, 1988
68. Effeney DJ, McIntyre KS, Blaisdell FW, et al: Fibrinogen kinetics in major human burns. Surg Forum 29:56, 1978
69. Blaisdell FW: Acquired and congenital clotting syndromes. World J Surg 14:664, 1990
70. Hauptman JG, Hassouna HI, Bell TG, et al: Efficacy of antithrombin III in endotoxin induced disseminated intravascular coagulation. Circ Shock 25:111, 1988
71. Rodgers GM, Shuman MA: Congenital thrombotic disorders. Am J Hematol 21:419, 1986
72. Rocha E, Paramo JA, Aranda A, et al: Congenital dysfibrinogenemias: a review. Ric Clin Lab 15:205, 1985
73. Liu Y, Lyons RM, McDonagh J: Plasminogen San Antonio: an abnormal plasminogen with a more cathodic migration, decreased activation and associated thrombosis. Thromb Haemost 59:49, 1988
74. Nilsson IM, Ljungner H, Tengborn L: Two different mechanisms in patients with venous thrombosis and defective fibrinolysis: low concentration of plasminogen activator or increased concentration of plasminogen activator inhibitor. Br Med J 290:1453, 1985
75. Kruithof EK, Gudinchet A, Bachmann F: Plasminogen activator inhibitor 1 and plasminogen activator inhibitor 2 in various disease states. Thromb Haemost 59:7, 1988
76. Juhan-Vague I, Roul C, Alessi MC, et al: Increased plasminogen activator inhibitor activity in non insulin dependent diabetic patients—relationship with plasma insulin. Thromb Haemost 61:370, 1989
77. Dahlbäck B, Carlsson M, Svensson PJ: Familial thrombophilia due to a previously unrecognized mechanism characterized by poor anticoagulant response to activated protein C: prediction of a cofactor to activated protein C. Proc Natl Acad Sci USA 90:1004, 1993
78. Bertina RM, Reitsma PH, Rosendaal FR, et al: Resistance to activated protein C and factor V Leiden as risk factors for venous thrombosis. Thromb Haemost 74:449, 1995
79. Egeberg O: Inherited antithrombin deficiency causing thrombophilia. Thrombosis et Diathesis Haemorrhagica 13:516, 1965
80. High KA: Antithrombin-III, protein-C, and protein-S: naturally occurring anticoagulant proteins. Arch Pathol Lab Med 112:28, 1988
81. Bauer KA, Goodman TL, Kass BL, et al: Elevated factor Xa activity in the blood of asymptomatic patients with congenital antithrombin deficiency. J Clin Invest 76:826, 1985
82. Owings JT, Bagley M, Gosselin R, et al: Effect of critical injury on plasma antithrombin activity: low antithrombin levels are associated with thromboembolic complications. J Trauma 41:396, 1996
83. Gladson CL, Scharrer I, Hach V, et al: The frequency of type I heterozygous protein-S and protein-C deficiency in 141 unrelated young patients with venous thrombosis. Thromb Haemost 59:18, 1988
84. Blaisdell FW: What's new in clotting and anticoagulation. Progress in Vascular Surgery. Najarian JS, Delaney JP, Eds. Year Book Medical Publishers, Chicago, 1988, p 75
85. Virchow R: Gesammelte Abhandlungen zur wissenschaftlichen Medizin. Von Meidingersohn, Frankfurt am Main, Germany, 1856
86. McLachlin AD, McLachlin JA, Jory TA, et al: Venous stasis in the lower extremities. Ann Surg 152:678, 1960
87. McLachlin J, Paterson JC: Some basic observations

on venous thrombosis and pulmonary embolism. Surg Gynecol Obstet 93:1, 1951
88. Cope C, Reyes TM, Skversky NJ: Phlebographic analysis of the incidence of thrombosis in hemiplegia. Radiology 109:581, 1973
89. Dooijewaard G, deBoer A, Turion PN, et al: Physical exercise induces enhancement of urokinase-type plasminogen activator (u-PA) levels in plasma. Thromb Haemost 65:82, 1991
90. Hansen J-B, Wilsgård L, Olsen JO, et al: Formation and persistence of procoagulant and fibrinolytic activities in circulation after strenuous physical exercise. Thromb Haemost 64:385, 1990
91. Sevitt S: The structure and growth of valve-pocket thrombi in femoral veins. J Clin Pathol 27:517, 1974
92. Hamer JD, Malone PC, Silver IA: The P_{O_2} in venous valve pockets: its possible bearing on thrombogenesis. Br J Surg 68:166, 1981
93. Dunmire SM: Pulmonary embolism. Emerg Med Clin North Am 7:339, 1989
94. Shackford SR, Moser KM: Deep venous thrombosis and pulmonary embolism in trauma patients. J Intensive Care Med 3:87, 1988
95. Kakkar VV, Stringer MD: Prophylaxis of venous thromboembolism. World J Surg 14:670, 1990
96. Bell WR, Simon TL: Current status of pulmonary thromboembolic disease: pathophysiology, diagnosis, prevention and treatment. Am Heart J 103:239, 1982
97. Sabiston DC Jr: Pathophysiology, diagnosis and management of pulmonary embolism. Am J Surg 138:384, 1979
98. Fogarty TJ, Cranley JJ, Krause RJ, et al: A method for extraction of arterial emboli and thrombi. Surgery 116:241, 1963
99. Gregg RO, Chamberlain BE, Myers JK, et al: Embolectomy or heparin therapy for arterial emboli. Surgery 93:377, 1983
100. Ricotta JJ, Scudder PA, McAndrew JA, et al: Management of acute ischemia of the upper extremity. Am J Surg 145:661, 1983
101. Jivegård L, Holm J, Bergqvist D: Acute lower limb ischemia: failure of anticoagulant treatment to improve one month results of arterial thromboembolectomy: a prospective randomized multi-center study. Surgery 109:610, 1991
102. Kendrick J, Thompson BW, Read RC, et al: Arterial embolectomy in the leg: results in a referral hospital. Am J Surg 142:739, 1981
103. Balas P, Bonatsos G, Xeromeritis N, et al: Early surgical results on acute arterial occlusion of the extremities. J Cardiovasc Surg 26:262, 1985
104. Dale WA: Differential management of acute peripheral arterial ischemia. J Vasc Surg 1:269, 1984
105. Stallone RJ, Lim RC Jr, Blaisdell FW: Pathogenesis of the pulmonary changes following ischemia of the lower extremities. Ann Thorac Surg 7:539, 1969
106. Haimovici H: Proceedings: myopathic-nephrotic-metabolic syndrome associated with massive acute arterial occlusions. J Cardiovasc Surg 14:589, 1973
107. Kontaxis AN, Skalkas G, Sechas M, et al: Proceedings: effect of acute arterial ischemia of the extremities on cardiac and pulmonary functions. J Cardiovasc Surg 14:605, 1973
108. Anner H, Kaufman RP, Valeri CR, et al: Reperfusion of ischemic lower limbs increases pulmonary microvascular permeability. J Trauma 28:607, 1988
109. Jivegård L, Holm J, Schersten T: Acute limb ischemia due to arterial embolism or thrombosis: influence of limb ischemia versus pre-existing cardiac disease on postoperative mortality rate. J Cardiovasc Surg 29:32, 1988
110. Hobson RW 2nd, Neville R, Watanabe B, et al: Role of heparin in reducing skeletal muscle infarction in ischemia-reperfusion. Microcirc Endothelium Lymphatics 5:259, 1989
111. Blaisdell FW: Preventing postoperative thromboembolism. West J Med 151:188, 1989
112. Reilly DT: Prophylactic methods against thromboembolism. Acta Chir Scand Suppl 550(suppl):115, 1989
113. Skillman JJ, Collins RE, Coe NP, et al: Prevention of deep vein thrombosis in neurosurgical patients: a controlled randomized trial of external pneumatic compression boots. Surgery 83:354, 1978
114. Rosenberg RD: Action and interactions of antithrombin and heparin. N Engl J Med 292:145, 1975
115. Turpie AG, Levine MN, Hirsh J, et al: A randomized controlled trial of a low-molecular-weight heparin (enoxaparin) to prevent deep-vein thrombosis in patients undergoing elective hip surgery. N Engl J Med 315:925, 1986
116. Levine MN, Hirsh J, Gent M, et al: Prevention of deep vein thrombosis after elective hip surgery: a randomized trial comparing low molecular weight heparin with standard unfractionated heparin. Ann Intern Med 114:545, 1991
117. Geerts WH, Jay RM, Code KI, et al: A comparison of low-dose heparin with low-molecular-weight heparin as prophylaxis against venous thromboembolism after major trauma. N Engl J Med 335:701, 1996
118. Leyvraz PF, Richard J, Bachmann F, et al: Adjusted versus fixed-dose subcutaneous heparin in the prevention of deep-vein thrombosis after total hip replacement. N Engl J Med 309:954, 1983
119. Owings JT, Blaisdell FW: Low-dose heparin thromboembolism prophylaxis. Arch Surg 131:1069, 1996
120. MacCallum PK, Thomson JM, Poller L: Effects of fixed minidose warfarin on coagulation and fibrinolysis following major gynaecological surgery. Thromb Haemost 64:511, 1990
121. Crafoord C: Preliminary report on post-operative treatment with heparin as a preventive of thrombosis. Acta Chir Scand 79:407, 1937
122. Murray GDW, Jaques LB, Perrett TS, et al: Heparin and the thrombosis of veins following injury. Surgery 2:163, 1937
123. Murray GDW, Best CH: The use of heparin in thrombosis. Ann Surg 108:163, 1938
124. Wessler S, Morris LE: Studies in intravascular coagulation: IV. The effect of heparin and dicumarol on serum-induced venous thrombosis. Circulation 12:553, 1955
125. Wessler S, Gitel SN: Heparin: new concepts relevant to clinical use. Blood 53:525, 1979
126. Holm HA, Finnanger B, Hartmann A, et al: Heparin treatment of deep venous thrombosis in 280 patients: symptoms related to dosage. Acta Med Scand 215:47, 1984
127. Gulliver G: The Works of William Hewson. Printed for the Sydenham Society, London, 1846, p 5

71 PULMONARY INSUFFICIENCY

Robert H. Bartlett, M.D.

Approach to Pulmonary Insufficiency

Prevention of Postoperative Pulmonary Insufficiency

Pulmonary insufficiency is the most common complication occurring after operative procedures. It ranges in incidence from five to 50 percent and in severity from minor atelectasis to lethal acute respiratory distress syndrome (ARDS). The lungs are extremely vulnerable in the postoperative period because both ventilation (the anatomy and physiology of breathing) and pulmonary circulation (the anatomy and physiology of the pulmonary endothelium and interstitium) are affected by all the events surrounding tissue injury, anesthesia, and tissue dissection.[1] Abnormal ventilation leads to alveolar collapse, decreased functional residual capacity (FRC), and atelectasis. Abnormal capillary homeostasis leads to lung edema. ARDS comprises a combination of atelectasis and edema, with edema predominating. The term ARDS will be used sparingly in this discussion, to describe the occurrence of pulmonary edema caused by increased capillary permeability.

This discussion will describe the care of patients at risk for pulmonary complications, including the clinical presentation, pathogenesis, prevention, recognition, and treatment of pulmonary insufficiency. Atelectasis and lung edema will be considered as separate events, although it is obvious that the two abnormalities can and do occur simultaneously in the postoperative period. Disorders of the pulmonary parenchyma will be emphasized, as opposed to pulmonary insufficiency secondary to such conditions as cardiac disease, thromboembolism, and central nervous system depression, all of which are covered elsewhere. This discussion is limited to mild pulmonary insufficiency; major insufficiency is discussed elsewhere in this text [see 91 Pulmonary Dysfunction].

Preoperative Pulmonary Function Testing

Preoperative assessment of respiratory status is important because identification of high-risk patients can minimize the incidence of pulmonary complications. The history is the most valuable step. Indications for detailed study of pulmonary function include exercise intolerance, dyspnea on exertion, wheezing, cigarette smoking, cough, and sputum production.

Physical examination should include auscultation and percussion of the lung bases during tidal breathing and maximal inspiration to detect hypoventilation in weak or debilitated patients and hyperinflation in patients with chronic airway disease. The presence of wheezing, rales, or rhonchi should trigger further examination. Any signs of cardiac insufficiency, obesity, clubbing, tobacco stains, or poor oral hygiene are all relative indications for more detailed pulmonary function testing. A chest x-ray should be considered part of the routine physical examination for any patients with an abnormality detected from the history or the physical examination, any patient scheduled to undergo a thoracotomy, and any patient at risk for cardiac or pulmonary disease because of age (i.e., persons older than approximately 60 years).

As part of every physical examination, the patient should be instructed to inhale to the maximum, followed by a vigorous forced expiration (a vital capacity maneuver). Observation of the chest and the sound of the forced expiration can enable the surgeon to estimate the volume of inspiration (in normal adults, at least 1 L/50 kg), forced expiration (in normal adults, at least 2 L/50 kg), and expiratory flow (most of the exhaled volume should come out in the first second without wheezing). The forced expiratory volume (or vital capacity) and the maximum voluntary ventilation (MVV, or maximal breathing capacity) can be directly measured with a handheld turbine spirometer.

Strength and endurance can be estimated by stair climbing.[2] A patient who cannot climb two flights of stairs at a steady pace without dyspnea may have respiratory, cardiac, or joint disease or may be too obese, too weak, too sedentary, or too debilitated to manage mild exercise. Whatever the cause, more detailed evaluation is indicated.

Breathing maneuvers to accomplish maximal inflation must be carefully taught to the patient preoperatively [see Postoperative Measures to Prevent Pulmonary Insufficiency, Routine Measures, *below*]. Most patients cannot learn breathing exercises in a painful, narcotized, postoperative state.

Pulmonary function tests (e.g., spirometry) should be performed whenever the history, physical examination, or bedside tests indicate major abnormalities of pulmonary function. The measurements obtained for tidal volume, inspiratory capacity, vital capacity (total and timed intervals), and MVV are compared with tables for normal persons of the same age, sex, and size and the values reported as percentages of the predicted normal. Values of 80 to 120 percent of what was predicted are considered normal. If these tests of lung volume and flow are within the normal range, the risk of pulmonary complications is small—although the tests do not measure endurance. Abnormally high values are not important. Values below 70 percent of predicted indicate one or more of the following: a low expiratory flow rate indicative of small airway or obstructive lung disease, a low vital capacity indicative of loss of lung vol-

Approach to Pulmonary Insufficiency

Assess pulmonary function preoperatively

Review history; perform physical exam. Evaluate for wheezing, rales, and rhonchi; cough and sputum production; cardiac insufficiency; and obesity. Estimate volume of inspiration, forced expiration, and expiratory flow.
Obtain chest x-ray if abnormality is detected, thoracotomy is planned, or patient is at risk for cardiac or pulmonary disease because of age (e.g., > 60 years).
If pulmonary dysfunction is suspected:
- Measure tidal volume, inspiratory capacity, vital capacity, and maximum voluntary ventilation.
- Obtain baseline blood gas measurements.
- In special circumstances: Measure functional residual capacity. Assess for chronic fibrotic disease. Obtain ventilation-perfusion lung scan if pulmonary resection is contemplated.

Correct abnormalities, and prepare patient before operation

Teach breathing maneuvers, and exercise patient's respiratory muscles.
Reduce risk factors (e.g., smoking).
Assess effects of bronchodilators in patients with bronchospasm.
Provide adequate nutrition.
Augment left ventricular function pharmacologically if signs of LV failure exist.

Follow a pulmonary prophylaxis regimen during and after operation

Inflate all alveoli regularly:
- Use breathing exercise with incentive spirometer. Use intermittent positive pressure breathing (IPPB) if necessary.
- Use mechanical ventilation in high-risk patients.
- Use bronchodilators for bronchospasm.

Maintain normal body fluid volume and composition:
- Give blood and fluids as needed, but not excessively.
- If fluid overload is unavoidable, diurese when stable.

Minimize the risk of venous thrombosis and pulmonary embolism.

Postoperative pulmonary insufficiency does not develop

Postoperative pulmonary insufficiency develops (e.g., dyspnea, tachypnea, tachycardia, confusion, cyanosis, abnormal x-ray)

Rule out mechanical limitation of breathing, bronchospasm, pulmonary embolism, congestive heart failure, and hypovolemia.
Evaluate for atelectasis or pulmonary edema.
General support: Give O_2 during preliminary investigations (10–20 L/min by cannula or mask).
(**Caution:** in patients with preexisting pulmonary disease, supplemental O_2 may result in CO_2 narcosis.)

Treat atelectasis

Establish large-volume inflation via deep breathing exercises. If unsuccessful, try IPPB without intubation.
Initiate chest physiotherapy and postural drainage. Administer hydration, nebulized bronchodilators, and mucolytic drugs via airway. Perform bronchoscopy or tracheal suctioning as indicated.
If ventilation is still inadequate: Intubate and initiate mechanical ventilation. Provide nutritional support. Treat coexisting lung edema and lung infection. Maintain fraction of inspired oxygen < 60% and airway pressure < 40 cm H_2O.

Treat increased lung water

Decrease pulmonary hydrostatic pressure by improving left ventricular function pharmacologically. (Monitor changes in cardiac output.)
Reduce total extracellular fluid volume by forced diuresis, dialysis, or hemofiltration.
Increase plasma oncotic pressure by administering colloids during diuresis.
Establish and maintain normal pulmonary microvascular integrity by treating any extrapulmonary site of infection or inflammation.

ume, and localized or generalized muscle weakness. If the expiratory flow is abnormally low, spirometry should be repeated after the administration of aerosolized bronchodilators. Low expiratory flow that improves after bronchodilation indicates bronchospasm, which will require special management during and after operation. An MVV value below 50 percent of predicted correlates most closely with the incidence of postoperative pulmonary complications. The MVV may be abnormally low for many reasons both pulmonary and nonpulmonary.[3]

Arterial blood gas measurements are obtained only if major pulmonary dysfunction is suspected, and they serve primarily as a baseline for postoperative comparison and for decisions regarding postoperative ventilation rather than as a screening test for inadequate pulmonary function. Arterial carbon dioxide tension (P_aCO_2) greater than 45 mm Hg at rest indicates significant alveolar hypoventilation. If the cause is muscular weakness, bronchospasm, or chronic bronchitis, it should be treated before any elective operation. If the arterial oxygen tension (P_aO_2) is less than 70 mm Hg, the patient has one or more of the following: a significant right-to-left shunt, a diffusion block, or ventilation-perfusion mismatch—usually the last. These three causes of hypoxemia can be further identified on the basis of the patient's response to breathing 100 percent oxygen, but this evaluation requires special equipment (a face mask or nasal catheter is not satisfactory), and the effort is generally not worthwhile in preoperative assessment.

More detailed tests of pulmonary function are needed only in special circumstances. The most useful measurement is of functional residual capacity. An FRC greater than 120 percent of predicted indicates air trapping from small airway disease or bronchospasm. These conditions should be treated before any elective operation. An FRC less than 50 percent of predicted indicates loss of lung volume, which may be caused by atelectasis, pneumonia, pleural effusion, or congestive heart failure. Measurement of diffusing capacity by carbon monoxide inhalation is not helpful. When severe fibrotic lung disease is suspected, diffusion can be measured by determination of P_aO_2 while the patient is breathing air and of P_aO_2 while the patient is breathing 100 percent oxygen. Oxygen consumption, CO_2 production, and the respiratory quotient are measurements of systemic metabolism rather than of pulmonary function; therefore, although these measurements may be very helpful in preoperative detection of sepsis or in planning nutritional therapy, they are generally not useful as measurements of pulmonary function. Ventilation-perfusion scan should be added to the regimen of routine preoperative testing in any patient with evidence of compromised pulmonary function in whom pulmonary resection is contemplated.

In summary, history, physical examination, and chest x-ray are sufficient means of preoperative pulmonary assessment in almost all patients. Patients at risk for pulmonary complications, as identified by history or examination, should undergo simple spirometry (pulmonary function testing) to identify abnormalities that can be corrected before elective operations. Arterial blood gases should be measured preoperatively in patients with major respiratory dysfunction to serve as a baseline for postoperative management.

Preoperative Correction of Abnormalities

If the planned operation is totally elective, as much time as is necessary should be spent measuring lung function, correcting the abnormalities and conditions that may predispose to pulmonary complications, and improving physical conditioning, including breathing. This is particularly true in patients with preexisting cardiopulmonary disease. Patients should be advised in the preoperative period to train for a major operation as one would train for an athletic event. The respiratory muscles should be exercised and specific breathing maneuvers learned.

Factors that may decrease the efficiency of ventilation should be corrected, including smoking, gross obesity, and existing bacterial infection, particularly chronic bronchitis. Patients with bronchospasm should become accustomed to bronchodilator treatment preoperatively, and the effect of bronchodilators on pulmonary mechanics should be directly measured, particularly in patients with known bronchospastic disorders, such as asthma.

Preoperative preparation should include adequate nutrition to ensure normal total serum protein concentration and a normal plasma oncotic pressure; inotropic support should be provided if signs of left ventricular failure exist.

The patient with preexisting lung disease requires special consideration. Preparation related to bronchospasm or to chronic bronchitis has been discussed. The patient in whom acute pulmonary insufficiency, increased lung water, or atelectasis is secondary to an acute disorder such as pancreatitis or systemic sepsis will often improve during the operation and with postoperative mechanical ventilation. The condition of the patient with severe chronic obstructive pulmonary disease should be improved as much as possible by means of bronchodilators, therapy for chronic bronchitis, nutritional support, and breathing and coughing training. If the pulmonary disorder is very severe (if P_aO_2 is < 50 mm Hg with the patient breathing room air or if carbon dioxide retention is evident), prolonged postoperative intubation and mechanical ventilation should be anticipated, and the patient should be advised accordingly.

Intraoperative Measures to Prevent Pulmonary Complications

Intraoperatively, several factors may minimize the risk of postoperative pulmonary complications. The operation itself may directly improve pulmonary function (e.g., by repairing an incompetent mitral valve or a large abdominal wall hernia) or may eliminate factors that of themselves are causing pulmonary insufficiency (e.g., empyema, a foreign body, or dead tissue).

Abdominal incisions should be planned to minimize postoperative pain and to maintain the strength of the abdominal wall for forced inspiration. Transverse incisions should be used whenever possible, particularly in patients with chronic heavy sputum production who will need to cough excessively after the operation. Gastrostomy should be considered to avoid prolonged nasogastric intubation. Bone fragments should be manipulated as gently as possible to avoid marrow embolism. Veins under negative pressure (e.g., in the brain) must be managed carefully to avoid air embolism. If the patient has a history of pulmonary embolism or existing deep vein thrombosis in the legs, prophylactic inferior vena cava plication should be considered when abdominal procedures are performed.

The method of anesthesia may be important in preventing pulmonary complications. Local or spinal anesthesia would seem to be preferred to avoid the respiratory depression of general anesthetic agents. However, general anesthesia gives the anesthesiologist control over the airway with the opportunity to provide optimal inflation and ventilation. In general, the patient who is at high risk for pulmonary complications is best managed with general anesthesia. Epidural anesthesia combined with light general anesthesia intraoperatively and continued for the first few days after operation is ideal for high-risk patients.[4]

During long procedures, alveoli will begin to collapse unless regularly inflated.[5] Sustained inflation to 20 ml/kg or an airway pressure of 30 cm H_2O should be done hourly. Overload with crystalloid fluid should be avoided. Generally, blood or plasma losses that exceed 10 percent of the blood volume should be replaced with blood or plasma. Moderate amounts of saline-type solutions are permissible, but caution should be observed. Saltwater overload does not cause pulmonary insufficiency, but if the pulmonary endothelium is injured, the edematous patient is primed for pulmonary edema.

Mechanical ventilation should be continued postoperatively until the adequacy of spontaneous ventilation has been clearly established. The action of paralytic drugs should be reversed completely and a vital capacity at least twice the tidal volume documented before extubation.

Postoperative Measures to Prevent Pulmonary Insufficiency

ROUTINE MEASURES

In the recovery room, the endotracheal tube should be maintained in place as long as necessary. Patients with preexisting pulmonary dysfunction or those at high risk for pulmonary complications may need to remain intubated and be maintained on mechanical ventilation for hours or days after operation. The well-ventilated alveolus is less susceptible to humoral capillary damage than is the atelectatic alveolus.[6] Elderly, debilitated patients and patients with extensive trauma, multiple fractures, pancreatitis, dead tissue, or severe peritonitis are commonly left intubated and are maintained on mechanical ventilation for at least 12 hours postoperatively. When the patient is fully alert and awake, when perfusion and cardiac status are stable, and when the blood and extracellular fluid volumes are demonstrated to be normal, then the patient is ready for spontaneous ventilation and extubation.

Deep breathing exercises, clearing of sputum and mucus, and avoidance of prolonged periods in the supine position must begin in the recovery room. Profound hypoventilation, ventilation-perfusion imbalance, and the resultant hypoxemia are the rule in the patient awakening from anesthesia. For this reason, moderate amounts (5 to 10 L/min) of supplemental oxygen are commonly administered to all patients in the recovery room. This precaution is wise for the first hour or two after anesthesia, but it is actually prophylactic only against hypoxic arrhythmias and may actually be slightly detrimental to lung function by suppressing whatever deep breathing may result from moderate degrees of hypoxemia. Consequently, supplemental oxygen should not be administered for more than a few hours after anesthesia unless oximetry indicates significant hypoxemia.

Airway cleaning, suctioning, expectorant drugs, mist inhalation, and mucolytic agents are all useful in patients with preexisting chronic bronchitis or thick, tenacious tracheobronchial secretions. However, these maneuvers and agents may not be necessary in patients who can adequately inflate their lungs by means of inspiratory maneuvers. A compulsion to force patients to cough dominates much of the thinking on postoperative pulmonary care. Coughing may be necessary in patients with chronic bronchitis. In general, however, coughing maneuvers are painful, and they are unnecessary if the lung remains well ventilated.

Breathing maneuvers and devices designed to encourage those maneuvers are important adjuncts to postoperative care.[7] Because shallow breathing, the lack of spontaneous deep breaths, and alveolar collapse are the steps that lead to postoperative pulmonary complications, respiratory maneuvers must emphasize maximal lung inflation. Breathing out (i.e., with coughing, tracheal stimulation, or so-called blow bottles) does nothing to accomplish alveolar inflation, except perhaps for the preparatory inspiration the patient may take before that maneuver. The greater the emphasis placed on the inhaled volume and the inspiratory pressure, the more effective the maneuver will be.

Deep inspiratory maneuvers can be performed spontaneously[8] or with a device that indicates the volume inhaled and rewards the patient's efforts, such as an incentive spirometer. The regular performance of deep breathing exercises using an incentive spirometer has been shown to decrease the incidence of pulmonary complications after laparotomy from about 30 percent to about 10 percent.[7-9]

Another method of preventing postoperative atelectasis is application of continuous positive airway pressure (CPAP) with a tightly fitting face mask.[10] Initial reports of the benefits of this technique show improved alveolar inflation. The potential complications of mask CPAP—gastric distention, vomiting and aspiration, and patient discomfort—did not occur in the initial series but remain a cause for concern. This technique, perhaps combined with intermittent positive pressure breathing (IPPB)—so-called mask IPPB—may prove useful in the management of patients who are extubated but who cannot or will not breathe deeply.

If the patient cannot do deep breathing inspiratory exercise voluntarily, inflation can be achieved with a mechanical ventilator attached to a mouthpiece (IPPB). To be effective, IPPB must be based on volume rather than pressure and should be done frequently (hourly while the patient is awake). In previous studies, infrequent, pressure-limited IPPB did not prevent atelectasis, and this technique was largely abandoned.[11] Properly administered, however, intermittent positive pressure breathing is a very useful method of preventing and treating atelectasis.

Frequent change of position and early ambulation will minimize fluid collection in the dependent portions of the lung. Adequate nutrition should be maintained postoperatively. If the patient must go without enteral feeding for more than four or five days, parenteral nutrition will be required to maintain the strength of the respiratory muscles. Fluids must be managed carefully to avoid overloading the extracellular space and diluting the serum proteins.

Pulmonary thromboembolism from the deep veins of the leg or pelvis is a constant threat in the postoperative period. Obese patients, immobilized patients, and patients with cancer are at particularly high risk. Several methods have been proposed to prevent deep vein thrombosis [see 70 Thromboembolic Problems], including administration of anticoagulants or drugs that inhibit platelet function, application of pressure to the legs by means of plastic wraps or stockings, and frequent active or passive exercises for the lower leg. Regular muscle exercise and early ambulation are the easiest of these maneuvers, have the fewest complications, and are advised for all postoperative patients.

Postoperative analgesia should be planned to decrease pain without depressing ventilation. Intramuscular narcotics may suppress deep breathing and contribute to atelectasis. In high-risk patients, therefore, intermittent local or regional blocks, intrathecal narcotics, and catheter epidural analgesia are the preferred methods of pain control[12] [see 104 Postoperative Pain].

PREEXISTING LUNG DISEASE

Patients with chronic disease of the airways or of the pulmonary parenchyma have less pulmonary reserve; consequently, acute respiratory failure may develop after they suffer a minimal insult to the lung. The patient with emphysema or asthma presents an interesting problem. Because of the primary disease, the residual volume and functional residual capacity are abnormally expanded. The patient is protected to a small extent against alveolar collapse secondary to shallow breathing. The affected alveoli are difficult to ventilate, however, even with maximal effort. The dead space is abnormally large, so that the minute ventilation must be higher than normal just to achieve normal carbon dioxide excretion. In addition, carbon dioxide excretion and oxygenation may be decreased because of the presence of alveolar destruction, fibrosis, or bulae. Shallow breathing in such a patient will not produce atelectasis, as would occur in the normal lung, but rather carbon dioxide retention and hypoxemia. Supplemental oxygen may reverse the hypoxemia, but carbon dioxide narcosis may result, particularly if the patient is also sedated with narcotics or anesthetics.

Chronic bronchitis narrows the small airways, increasing susceptibility to inadequate inflation and alveolar collapse. Heavy cigarette smoking has the same effect. For these conditions, treating the airways before elective procedures (with antibiotics or the cessation of smoking, respectively) is advisable. Severe restrictive disease from pulmonary fibrosis, pleural thickening or fibrosis, or chest wall deformities predisposes the patient to atelectasis.

Patients with acute respiratory failure may require operation; in fact, the respiratory failure may be secondary to the indication for operation (e.g., abscess, ischemic tissue, or long-bone fracture). Such patients come to operation with a decreased FRC and increased pulmonary water [see Discussion, Pathogenesis of Postoperative Pulmonary Insufficiency, below]. The respiratory failure may improve with operative resolution of the primary condition, but if improvement in pulmonary function does not occur, these patients cannot afford any worsening of alveolar collapse or pulmonary edema. In these patients, further deterioration of pulmonary function must be prevented by means of prolonged postoperative ventilatory support and by fine-tuning of the hydrostatic pressure and colloid osmotic pressure in relation to cardiac output and blood volume.

Clinical Presentation of Postoperative Pulmonary Insufficiency

At any time during the first week after a major operation, a patient may manifest the syndrome of pulmonary insufficiency: dyspnea, tachypnea, tachycardia, fever, confusion, and cyanosis. Although the most likely causes of this syndrome are atelectasis and edema, the first step in evaluating the patient is to rule out mechanical limitation of breathing, acute bronchospasm, pulmonary thromboembolism, congestive heart failure, and hypovolemia [see Table 1]. Mechanical limitation of breathing may be caused by gastric or intestinal distention, ascites, pneumothorax, hydrothorax, or splinting of the chest wall because of pain or rib fractures. Mechanical limitation of breathing is diagnosed by physical examination and chest x-ray and treated by removing the limitation.

Bronchospasm occurs in patients with a history of asthma. The diagnosis is made by finding wheezes on physical examination and hyperinflation on x-ray. Treatment consists of the administration of bronchodilators.

Pulmonary embolism is the first consideration when the onset of pulmonary insufficiency is sudden, but it is the least common cause. Small, lobar pulmonary emboli rarely cause symptoms. The patient who is symptomatic from embolism has had a major embolism or a series of minor emboli occluding more than 50 percent of the pulmonary circulation. It is usually easy to differentiate pulmonary embolism from atelectasis by clinical examination and evaluation of blood gases [see Table 1].

Congestive heart failure in the postoperative period may be an exacerbation of a chronic condition or acute cardiac failure secondary to myocardial infarction. In either case, the diagnosis is made by physical and x-ray examination of the chest. The initial management of acutely ill patients with heart failure includes diuresis, administration of supplemental oxygen, review of records of body weight and fluid balance, and transfer to the intensive care unit for more invasive monitoring. In the patient who is fluid overloaded, pulmonary arterial monitoring may be required to differentiate cardiogenic from capillary-injury pulmonary edema.

Hypovolemia is often first manifested by dyspnea, and postoperative shortness of breath should always raise the question of occult bleeding or third-space sequestration. Clinical examination indicates findings of hypovolemia. The chest x-ray is usually clear, and blood gases demonstrate normal oxygenation and carbon dioxide clearance with metabolic acidosis.

In postoperative pulmonary insufficiency caused by atelectasis or edema, physical examination shows diminished breath sounds over one or both lung bases. Rales and rhonchi may be heard in the middle and lower lung fields. Although tidal volume is normal, vital capacity (judged or actually measured) is decreased. Chest x-ray demonstrates incomplete lung inflation, usually with overt collapse or consolidation apparent in the lower lobes. If the pulmonary abnormality is predominantly the result of lung edema, a diffuse increase in lung density is seen, which, when combined with irregular inflation, is often described as

Table 1 Differential Diagnosis of Postoperative Dyspnea

	Atelectasis/Edema	Pulmonary Embolism	Bronchospasm	Congestive Heart Failure
Lung bases	Not aerated	Clear	Wheezes	Rales
Chest x-ray	Consolidation, general edema	Clear, ↑ Diameter of main pulmonary artery	Hyperinflated	Hydrostatic edema, ↑ Diameter of main pulmonary artery
Central venous pressure	Normal	Elevated	Normal	Elevated
Pulmonary arterial wedge pressure	Normal	Normal or low	Normal or high	High
Arterial P_{O_2} (breathing air) (mm Hg)	40–60	40–80	70–90	40–60
Arterial P_{O_2} (breathing O_2) (mm Hg)	50–100	100–300	200–300	100–300
Arterial P_{CO_2}	Low	Normal or low	High	Normal or high
Lung scan	Regional ischemia	Regional ischemia	± Normal	± Normal
Pulmonary angiogram	Normal	Diagnostic	Normal	Normal

diffuse fluffy infiltrates. This finding can usually be differentiated from radiographic findings of cardiogenic pulmonary edema, which are more apparent in the lower and middle lung fields when the x-ray is taken with the patient sitting or standing. Measurement of arterial blood gases while the patient is breathing air demonstrates hypoxemia, hypocapnia, and respiratory alkalosis.

Supplemental oxygen supplied by nasal catheter or face mask with high-flow oxygen (10 to 20 L/min) supplies approximately 40 percent inspired oxygen (regardless of the settings on the equipment). Supplemental oxygen reverses the hypoxemia caused by ventilation-perfusion mismatch, pulmonary embolism, or cardiogenic pulmonary edema, typically resulting in a P_aO_2 greater than 150 mm Hg. In contrast, supplemental oxygen has a minor effect on hypoxemia caused by atelectasis, with the P_aO_2 typically rising from the 40s to the 80s. Fever and mild leukocytosis often accompany atelectasis, and the differential diagnosis between atelectasis and pneumonia is based primarily on continuing signs of infection without another obvious source, combined with pathogenic organisms on sputum culture. Thickened or copious bronchial secretions may be present in any postoperative patient, particularly if the patient has had endotracheal intubation and general anesthesia during operation. Bronchial secretions are neither the cause nor the result of atelectasis. However, sputum samples should be acquired from every patient with pulmonary complications for Gram's staining and culture.

Treatment of Postoperative Pulmonary Insufficiency Caused by Atelectasis or Edema

GENERAL SUPPORT

Beginning during the preliminary clinical and laboratory examinations, supplemental oxygen should be supplied by nasal cannula or a face mask at 10 to 20 L/min. Special precautions must be taken in patients who have a history of severe pulmonary disease with preoperative hypoxemia and hypercapnia, because supplemental oxygen may correct the hypoxemia but diminish the respiratory drive and result in carbon dioxide narcosis. The patient should be positioned in a way that maximizes diaphragmatic excursion—that is, sitting but not hunched forward; the stomach and abdomen must not be distended.

TREATMENT OF ATELECTASIS

The cornerstone of treatment aimed at alveolar inflation [see Figure 1] is to establish large volume inflation by instituting deep breathing exercises [see Postoperative Measures to Prevent Pulmonary Insufficiency, above]. If adequate volumes cannot be generated by the patient in this manner, then mechanical assistance is necessary, initially with IPPB with a mechanical ventilator, without intubation. Mechanical assistance must be done with direct exhaled-volume measurement and often requires high pressures (30 cm H_2O) with the IPPB device. All of the inflation techniques of mechanical ventilation (positive end-expiratory pressure, sighs, inspiratory hold, CPAP) can be used in patients who have not been intubated [see 92 Use of the Mechanical Ventilator].

When an area of lung is not ventilated, mucus secreted in the bronchi draining from that segment may become thickened and impacted and hinder efforts at reexpansion. This mucus should be cleared by chest physical therapy (percussion) and postural drainage. Hydration and nebulized bronchodilator and mucolytic drugs may be administered via the airway. Coughing will help expel mucus from airways that have been inflated distally but will not dislodge mucus from airways leading to nonventilated areas of the lung. In this situation, mucus must be removed directly by means of bronchoscopy or tracheal suction.

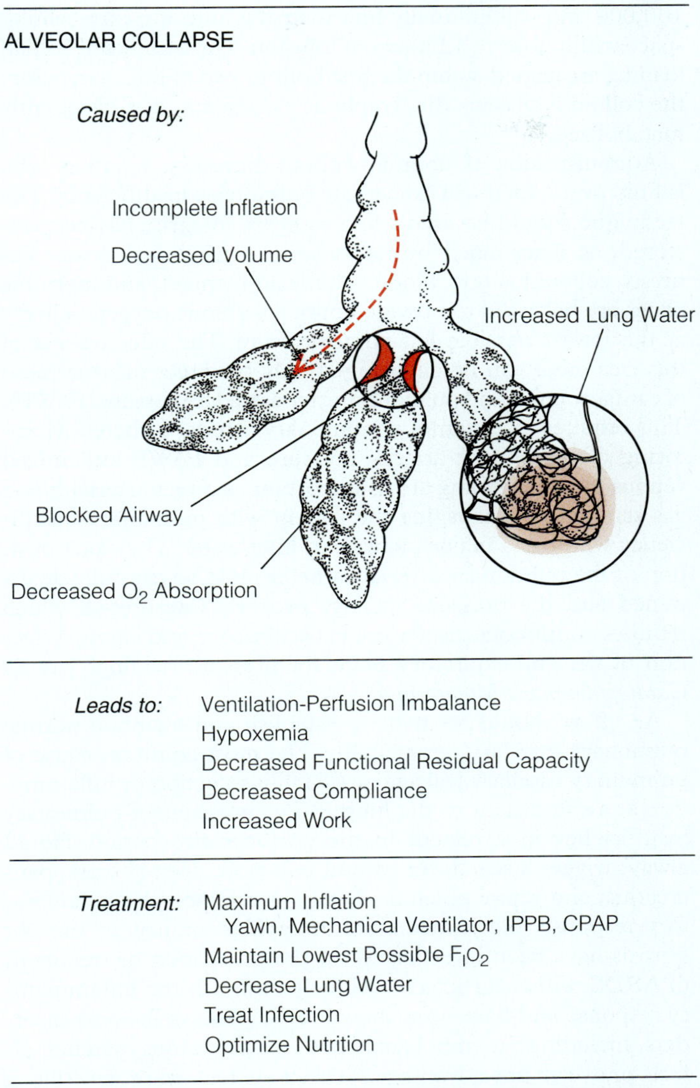

ALVEOLAR COLLAPSE

Caused by:

Incomplete Inflation
Decreased Volume
Increased Lung Water
Blocked Airway
Decreased O_2 Absorption

Leads to: Ventilation-Perfusion Imbalance
Hypoxemia
Decreased Functional Residual Capacity
Decreased Compliance
Increased Work

Treatment: Maximum Inflation
   Yawn, Mechanical Ventilator, IPPB, CPAP
Maintain Lowest Possible F_IO_2
Decrease Lung Water
Treat Infection
Optimize Nutrition

Figure 1 Illustrated are causes and effects of alveolar collapse in postoperative pulmonary insufficiency. (IPPB = intermittent positive pressure breathing; CPAP = continuous positive airway pressure; F_IO_2 = fraction of inspired oxygen.)

Tracheal suctioning should be done only if thick mucus cannot be removed with simple methods.[13] The catheter is passed through the nose, verified as passing through the larynx by a change in voice, and connected to oxygen at 5 L/min. Then, 5 ml of saline is injected, and the oxygen is reconnected for several coughing breaths. Suction is applied for no longer than 10 seconds; then, oxygen is resumed. This process is repeated for one to five minutes until the suction return is clear. Electrocardiographic monitoring should be done during and after suctioning. Atropine is given for bradycardia.

In adults, the value of endotracheal suctioning lies primarily in its stimulation of deep breathing associated with the vigorous coughing it produces. Deep breathing can be easily accomplished by other means, however, without the potential vagal complications associated with tracheal suctioning. Routine tracheal suctioning has no rational place in the care of adult patients postoperatively.

Flexible fiberoptic bronchoscopy[14] is preferable to blind tracheal suctioning in the management of atelectasis. Topical anesthesia is administered, and an endotracheal tube is placed without balloon inflation. Bronchoscopy is performed to examine the airways and clear mucus from the atelectatic area. Use of the endotracheal tube facilitates repeated removal and reinsertion of the bronchoscope, which may be necessary if mucus is too thick to be aspirated through the small suction lumen.

If adequate ventilation cannot be established with the methods described earlier, endotracheal intubation and continuous mechanical ventilation are indicated; specific indications are (1) an inspiratory force during a Müller's maneuver of less than 20 cm H_2O, (2) a vital capacity less than twice the tidal volume, (3) a respiratory rate consistently greater than 30, or (4) severe hypoxemia (P_aO_2 < 50 mm Hg, breathing room air). If any one of these indications cannot be reversed, intubation and mechanical ventilation should be considered [see 92 *Use of the Mechanical Ventilator*].

If supplemental oxygen has been instituted for the general support of the patient, the amount of oxygen should be kept as low as possible to avoid displacing nitrogen from alveoli and causing absorption atelectasis. Nutritional support should be instituted and a positive nitrogen balance achieved to maintain the strength of respiratory muscles and to optimize host defenses. The amount of nutrition should be based on the measured expenditure of energy to avoid overfeeding, particularly with carbohydrates; carbon dioxide produced in response to excess carbohydrates may add to the pulmonary insufficiency.[15]

TREATMENT OF EDEMA

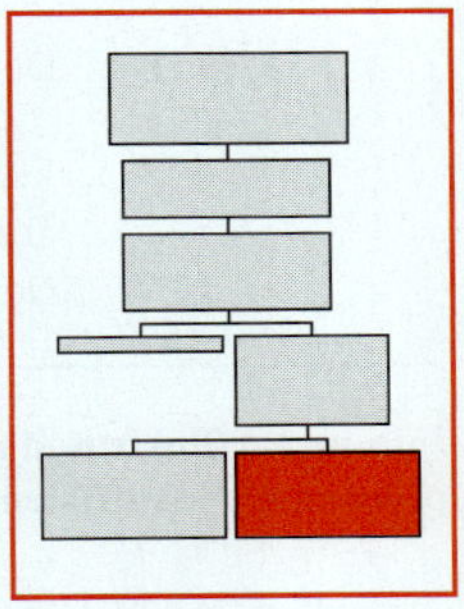

The amount of lung water can be reduced by decreasing the entire extracellular fluid space, decreasing the hydrostatic pressure in the pulmonary capillary bed, and increasing the plasma oncotic pressure without increasing the oncotic pressure in the interstitial fluid of the lung [see *Figure 2*]. Mechanical positive pressure ventilation is not a means of decreasing lung water. In fact, positive end-expiratory pressure actually increases lung water slightly, probably by stretching the pulmonary tissue.[16] Mechanical ventilation improves gas exchange in patients with pulmonary edema by overcoming the ventilation-perfusion mismatch associated with bronchodilator or alveolar thickening, but it does not decrease lung water.

If the patient is in renal failure, total extracellular fluid volume must be reduced by forced diuresis, dialysis, or hemofiltration. Diuresis is induced with a potent diuretic such as furosemide or mannitol. The course of diuresis is followed by daily measurement of body weight and hourly measurement of fluid intake and output. Usually, the patient with postoperative pulmonary insufficiency will be found to be 4 to 5 kg overloaded, primarily with extracellular fluid. Diuresis and negative fluid balance greatly improve the chance of survival in patients with pulmonary edema.[17,18]

Adequate treatment of pulmonary edema must include removal of the excess extravascular fluid (i.e., returning the patient to his or her baseline weight). A major decrease in total extracellular fluid volume will be accompanied by a minor decrease in pulmonary extracellular fluid volume, but even this change may be enough to improve pulmonary function greatly.

INCREASED LUNG WATER

Caused by:

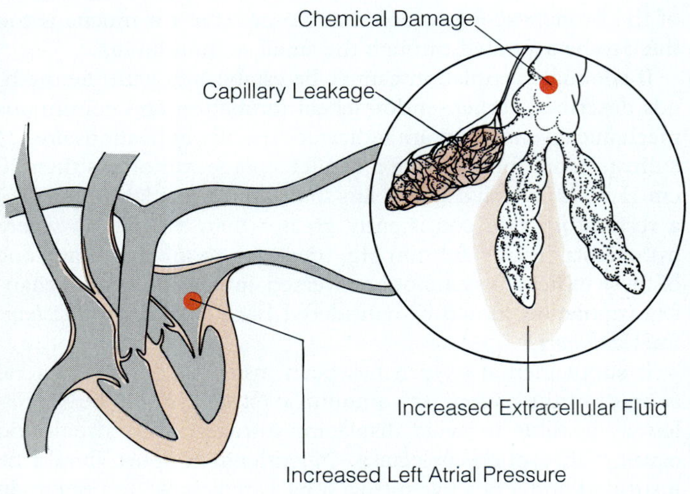

- Chemical Damage
- Capillary Leakage
- Increased Extracellular Fluid
- Increased Left Atrial Pressure

Leads to: Increased Pulmonary Vascular Resistance
Decreased Functional Residual Capacity
Ventilation-Perfusion Imbalance
Infection

Treatment: Decrease Extracellular Fluid
Diuresis, Decrease Intake
Increase Plasma Oncotic Pressure
Treat Capillaries
Decrease Hydrostatic Pressure

Figure 2 Illustrated are effects of lung water in postoperative pulmonary insufficiency.

If the patient becomes hypovolemic because of diuresis, blood volume should be expanded with red blood cells (if the patient is anemic) or colloid solutions; a net loss of sodium and water should be maintained. Diuretic agents will remove water, sodium, and potassium at differing rates, so that all must be monitored carefully and frequently. Usually, water is removed in excess of electrolytes, so that with extreme, forced diuresis a hypernatremic, hyperosmotic state results. Serum sodium concentrations should be monitored closely, and diuresis should be discontinued when the serum sodium level is between 140 and 150 mEq/L.

Diuresis concentrates serum proteins and results in increased plasma oncotic pressure. Diuresis should be combined with colloid loading to further increase plasma oncotic pressure transiently and force the movement of fluid from the extravascular to the intravascular space. The colloids should be administered during the course of diuresis, because most agents used for colloid loading, such as albumin, have a molecular weight between 50,000 and 100,000 and will gradually find their way into the extracellular space within four to 12 hours of infusion. The benefits of colloid loading are gained within the first hour or two of infusion, before the colloid load joins the lymphatic system and is subsequently metabolized.[19]

Administration of albumin without diuresis to a patient who is fluid overloaded will exacerbate pulmonary insufficiency. The technique should be used when capillary integrity has been restored, as determined by response to small initial doses. Diuresis, colloid loading, blood volume adjustment, and inotropic drugs are balanced to provide optimal systemic oxygen delivery at the lowest possible left atrial pressure. The effectiveness of this treatment can be determined only by direct measurement of cardiac output and pulmonary arterial wedge pressure (PAWP). This requires insertion of a pulmonary arterial catheter. Monitoring of pulmonary arterial pressure and PAWP and mixed venous blood sampling are as important as direct arterial blood gas sampling in managing the patient with pulmonary insufficiency who has a major increase in lung water. The exact position of the pulmonary arterial catheter must be carefully determined and the pressure tracings properly interpreted, which requires continuous display on an oscilloscope and careful selection of the end-expiratory point for pressure readings [*see 89 Cardiopulmonary Monitoring*].

An effort should be made to establish and maintain normal pulmonary capillary permeability. The most common cause of pulmonary capillary leakage or ARDS is infection or inflammation at a site distant to the lungs.[20] The presence of pulmonary insufficiency in a patient in the postoperative period should always trigger a search for wound infection, deep abscess, pancreatitis, and septic phlebitis. Drugs that inhibit the inflammatory response, block mediators of capillary injury, or prevent fibrosis have been investigated for the prevention or treatment of ARDS. Glucocorticoids definitely diminish the inflammatory response and have been shown to be effective in some disorders, including fat embolism,[21] but the deleterious systemic effects outweigh any advantage.[22] Drugs such as ibuprofen[23] block production of inflammatory mediators more specifically than do steroids. Drugs that inhibit the action of specific mediators (e.g., antihistamines,[24] superoxide dismutase, and catalase[25]) are under investigation in the treatment of lung edema.

Vigorous treatment of alveolar collapse can lead to lung injury and exacerbate lung edema (see below). Specifically, inspired oxygen concentrations greater than 60 percent and airway pressures greater than 40 cm H_2O should be carefully avoided.[26] With these precautions in mind, efforts at maintaining alveolar expansion are an important component of the treatment of interstitial lung edema. The well-ventilated lung appears to be more resistant to capillary injury than the atelectatic lung.

Bacterial infection often complicates atelectasis and edema, and it may occur as a primary event after operation. The progression from atelectasis to pneumonia can be difficult to identify because pulmonary infiltration and consolidation, fever, leukocytosis, and sputum production occur in both conditions. This differential diagnosis is one of the most difficult in postoperative care; decisions must be based on repeated examination of the patient and the sputum [*see 103 Early Postoperative Pneumonia*].

Discussion

Pathogenesis of Postoperative Pulmonary Insufficiency

VENTILATION AND PULMONARY MECHANICS

After any major operation, changes occur in lung function. These changes occur in all patients but are not detected on routine examination.[27,28] Aside from shallow tidal ventilation and some decreased breath sounds at the lung bases, most patients show no signs of respiratory abnormality. On direct measurement, lung volumes are decreased (particularly residual volume, expiratory reserve volume, functional residual capacity, and vital capacity). Compliance is decreased because of the decrease in FRC. The work of breathing is increased for the same reason: more pressure is required to inhale a given volume into the decreased lung air space. Further evidence that alveoli are not being ventilated is the presence of absolute or relative arterial hypoxemia, which occurs when the patient is breathing room air or 100 percent oxygen and which indicates transpulmonary shunting (i.e., nonventilated alveoli are being perfused).[29]

These changes in lung function are present immediately after operation, then evolve slowly over one to two days, and return to normal in most patients [see Figure 3]. The extent and duration of abnormality are related to the site of operation, the duration of operation and anesthesia, the quality of postoperative care, and preexisting pulmonary status. The extent and duration are greatest for those operations on the thorax and upper abdomen and progressively decrease for operations situated more distally and more superficially on the body structures. These changes may occur after only one to two hours of general anesthesia if careful attention is not paid to maximal lung inflation during anesthesia. Such changes are superimposed on the patient's preexisting lung status. If, for example, operation is required for complications of pancreatitis two weeks after the onset of disease, the patient may already have pleural effusions, increased pulmonary capillary permeability, and existing transpulmonary shunting and will not tolerate further deterioration of lung function. Likewise, the patient with preexisting chronic obstructive pulmonary disease with high airway resistance, maximal work of breathing, and minimal functional lung tissue may retain carbon dioxide postoperatively if the work of breathing is only slightly increased. Advanced age itself is not a cause of lung dysfunction,[30] but elderly patients may have chronic lung disease or cardiac disease and thus be at greater risk for pulmonary failure. More importantly, the elderly patient may be weak, and weak respiratory muscles predispose to alveolar collapse.

Several factors contribute to these changes in pulmonary function, but shallow breathing with incomplete alveolar inflation is the common denominator.[31] If spontaneous deep breaths to maximal lung inflation are eliminated from the pattern of breathing, alveolar collapse begins within one hour and progresses rather rapidly to produce significant transpulmonary shunting.[32] Several studies have shown that patterns of spontaneous deep breaths are abnormal in postoperative patients because of severe pain, anesthetics, or narcotics.[28] Supporting this observation is the fact that the postoperative changes in lung function can be returned toward normal by instituting maximal-inflation deep breathing exercises at regular intervals.[33,34] Excessive tracheobronchial secretions, aspiration of oral or gastric contents, and intraoperative fluid overload can contribute to the postoperative lung abnormalities described earlier.

Within two to four days after operation, it becomes clear whether the pattern of decreased lung volume and shunting is returning to normal or progressing [see Figure 3]. Decreased lung volume is detectable as decreased breath sounds on physical examination, and atelectatic areas may be visible on chest x-ray. Shunt-produced hypoxemia leads to an increased ventilatory rate and the sensation of dyspnea.

Severe hypoxemia may cause cyanosis. Atelectasis causes fever and pooling of mucus in nonventilated areas, leading to an apparent increase in sputum production. Against the background of changes that normally accompany major operations, a more complete picture of pulmonary pathophysiology in the surgical patient can be drawn.

Abnormal ventilation will lead to atelectasis as outlined earlier. The typical postoperative pattern of tidal breathing without spontaneous deep breaths is a good example of this phenomenon. A patient lying on his or her back in bed will preferentially ventilate the superior lobes while the blood will flow preferentially to dependent lobes. This ventilation-perfusion imbalance itself will result in hypoxemia; if it progresses over time, lower lobe alveoli begin to collapse in the pathogenetic pathway. Alveolar collapse will occur in any patient who remains in one position for a prolonged period and in whom the pattern of breathing is that of shallow tidal ventilation. It should be emphasized that normal tidal breaths delivered with a mechanical ventilator will similarly lead to alveolar collapse if regular maximal inflations are not carried out.[4]

EDEMA AND THE PULMONARY INTERSTITIUM

Increased pulmonary hydrostatic pressure, decreased plasma oncotic pressure, and increased capillary permeability may all occur in the surgical patient. All of these states will cause increased pulmonary extravascular water and deterioration of lung function. Edema is the hallmark of ARDS.[35] Edema causes atelectasis in the dependent lung simply by the weight of the fluid.[36,37] This effect can often be reversed by prone positioning of the patient.[38]

Fluid flux is a net function of the hydrostatic pressure that tends to force fluid out of the vascular space, on the one hand, and the oncotic pressure that tends to pull fluid in, on the other hand. High hydrostatic pressure or low plasma oncotic pressure will result in accumulation of fluid in the extravascular space [see Figure 3]. If the pulmonary endothelium is damaged, fluid may leak into the extracellular space at normal hydrostatic or oncotic pressures (the acute respiratory distress syndrome). Pulmonary vascular resistance increases because of periarteriolar cuffing. Ventilation-perfusion imbalance is created by peribronchiolar and alveolar compression. Shunting occurs if the alveoli become completely collapsed or filled with fluid. Finally, boggy atelectatic areas of lung are ideal breeding grounds for bacterial pulmonary infection.

In the normal course of treatment or resuscitation, well-intentioned interventions may result in increased lung water. For example, when blood or plasma is replaced with crystalloid, that fluid must equilibrate into the entire extracellular space, including that in the lung. This effect is compounded by the

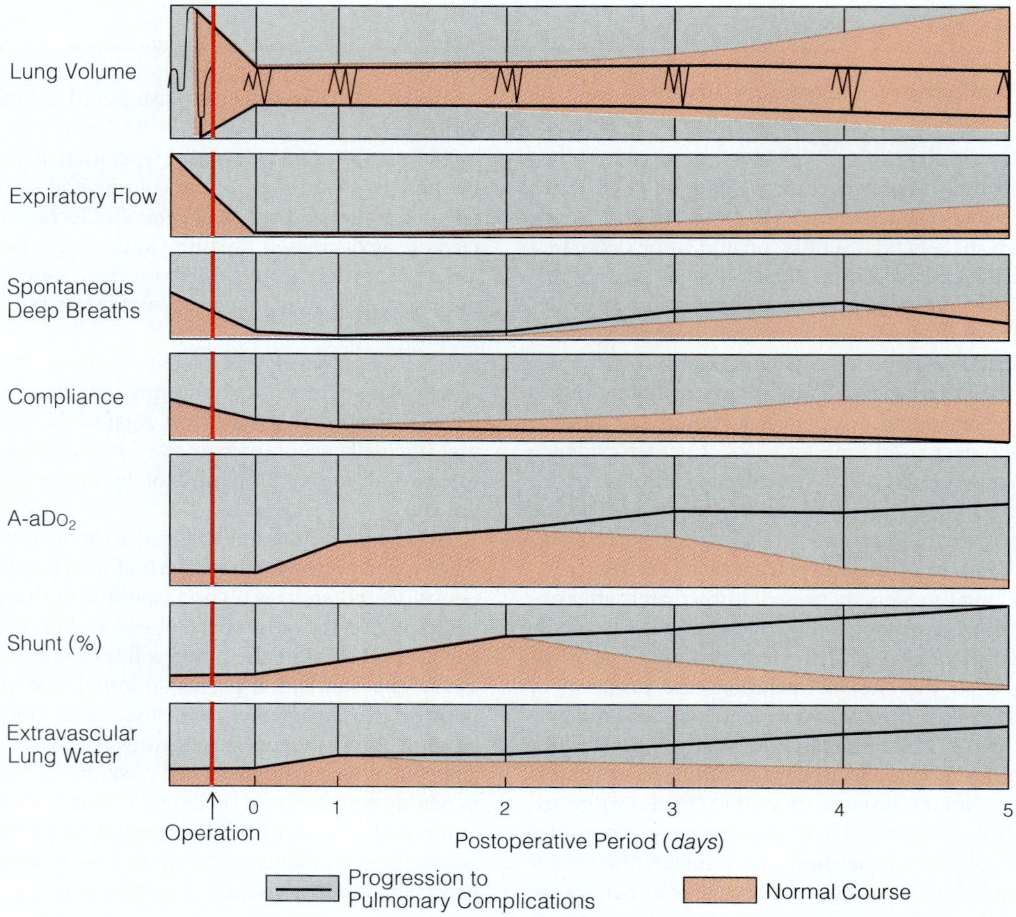

Figure 3 Shaded areas represent normal changes in pulmonary function after an operation. Solid lines represent progression to pulmonary insufficiency. (A-aDo$_2$ = alveolar-arterial difference in oxygen.)

reduced oncotic pressure that results when protein is lost or replaced with non–colloid-containing fluids. When plasma proteins are diluted in this way, lung interstitial proteins are also diluted; thus, the oncotic gradients stay unchanged,[39] whereas the entire extracellular space expands.

The pulmonary capillary endothelium is the first major vascular bed to be exposed to toxic substances arising from peripheral organ metabolism or perfusion of ischemic or infected tissue. The venous effluent from underperfused tissue arrives directly at the lung, where pulmonary capillary damage occurs. Humoral substances (e.g., lysosomal enzymes) and bacterial endotoxin or particulate materials (e.g., microemboli, platelet aggregates, and fat particles) may lodge in the pulmonary capillary bed.

As these materials are cleared, leaky pulmonary capillaries are left behind, with a resulting accumulation of extravascular fluid despite normal hydrostatic pressure. The pulmonary effects of materials released into the venous blood in shock sets in motion a particularly vicious circle. The increased pulmonary vascular resistance and hypoxia that result from the pulmonary capillary damage lead to a decrease in cardiac output and peripheral oxygen delivery, which adds to the shock state and perpetuates the pulmonary lesion.

Left ventricular failure with increased left atrial pressure will result in pulmonary transcapillary transudation, which may be subtle or grossly obvious, as in congestive heart failure with overt pulmonary edema. Left ventricular pressures may waver at the point of high left atrial pressure for short periods—even minutes—resulting in a transient increase in lung water, and then return to a balanced state. This situation may not lead to severe pulmonary edema in itself, but it probably places the lung in a more vulnerable position when minor capillary damage coexists.

The pulmonary interstitium is particularly vulnerable to the events surrounding an operation. Saltwater infusion usually greatly exceeds losses and increases the extracellular space. Bleeding and venous compression may cause hypotension and necessitate blood transfusion. Mediators from sterile tissue injury or bacterial invasion may injure the pulmonary capillary endothelium. Transient myocardial depression may cause hydrostatic pulmonary edema. With all of these factors, it is remarkable that there is no primary change in lung water volume after uncomplicated operations, even operations including cardiopulmonary bypass.[40] Nonetheless, it should be remembered that the patient usually leaves the operating room overloaded with fluid and primed for the development of lung edema.

Summary

The pathogenesis of pulmonary failure in surgical patients can be characterized as a decrease in functional residual capacity and an increase in interstitial fluid. Decreased FRC is caused by inadequate alveolar inflation; prevention and treatment are aimed at maximal inflation. Pulmonary edema is caused by cardiac failure, fluid overload, and increased capillary permeability; it is prevented and treated by maximizing cardiac function and systemic oxygen delivery, avoiding extracellular space overload, and treating conditions that lead to altered pulmonary capillary permeability. Understanding these aspects of pulmonary pathophysiology and using such understanding to guide prevention and treatment should decrease mortality and morbidity from postoperative pulmonary complications.

References

1. Bartlett RH: Pulmonary pathophysiology in surgical patients. Surg Clin North Am 60:1323, 1980
2. Bolton JWR, Weiman DS, Haynes JL, et al: Stair climbing as an indicator of pulmonary function. Chest 92:783, 1987
3. Tisi GM: Preoperative evaluation of pulmonary function: validity, indications, and benefits. Am Rev Respir Dis 119:293, 1979
4. Cuchieri RJ, Morran CG, Howie JC, et al: Postoperative pain and pulmonary complications: comparison of three analgesic regimens. Br J Surg 72:495, 1985
5. Bendixen HH, Bullwinkel B, Hedley-Whyte J: Atelectasis and shunting during spontaneous ventilation in anesthetized patients. Anesthesiology 25:297, 1964
6. Tilson MD, Bunke MC, Smith JW, et al: Quantitative bacteriology and pathology of the lung in experimental Pseudomonas pneumonia treated with positive end-expiratory pressure (PEEP). Surgery 82:133, 1977
7. Bartlett RH, Gazzaniga AB, Geraghty TR: Respiratory maneuvers to prevent postoperative pulmonary complications: a critical review. JAMA 224:1017, 1973
8. Roukema JA, Carol EJ, Prins JG: The prevention of pulmonary complications after upper abdominal surgery in patients with noncompromised pulmonary status. Arch Surg 123:30, 1988
9. Bartlett RH: Incentive spirometry. Current Respiratory Care. Kacmarek RM, Stoller JK, Eds. BC Decker, Philadelphia, 1988, p 38
10. Greenbaum DM, Millen JE, Eross B, et al: Continuous positive airway pressure without tracheal intubation in spontaneously breathing patients. Chest 69:615, 1976
11. Bartlett RH: Respiratory therapy to prevent postoperative pulmonary complications. Respiratory Intensive Care. Pierson DJ, Ed. Daedalus Enterprises, Dallas, 1986, p 369
12. Bromage PR, Camporesi E, Chestnut D: Epidural narcotics for postoperative analgesia. Anesth Analg 59:473, 1980
13. Demers RR: Complications of endotracheal suctioning procedures. Respir Care 27:453, 1982
14. Ratliff JL: Bronchoscopy in respiratory care. Surg Clin North Am 60:1497, 1980
15. Kemper M, Weissman C, Askanazi J, et al: Metabolic and respiratory changes during weaning from mechanical ventilation. Chest 92:979, 1987
16. Parker JC, Hernandez LA, Peevy KJ: Mechanisms of ventilator-induced lung injury. Crit Care Med 21:131, 1993
17. Simmons RS, Berdine GG, Seidenfeld JJ, et al: Fluid balance and the adult respiratory distress syndrome. Am Rev Respir Dis 135:924, 1987
18. Mitchell JP, Schuller D, Calandrino FS, et al: Improved outcome based on fluid management in critically ill patients requiring pulmonary artery catheterization. Am Rev Respir Dis 145:990, 1992
19. Skillman JJ, Parikh BM, Tanenbaum BJ: Pulmonary arteriovenous admixture: improvement with albumin and diuresis. Am J Surg 119:440, 1970
20. Seidenfeld JJ, Pohl DF, Bell RC, et al: Incidence, site, and outcome of infections in patients with the adult respiratory distress syndrome. Am Rev Respir Dis 134:12, 1986
21. Schonfeld SA, Ploysongsang Y, DiLisio R, et al: Fat embolism prophylaxis with corticosteroids: a prospective study in high-risk patients. Ann Intern Med 99:438, 1983
22. Bernard GR, Luce JM, Sprung CL, et al: High-dose corticosteroids in patients with the adult respiratory distress syndrome. N Engl J Med 317:1565, 1987
23. Johnson A, Malik AB: Pulmonary transvascular fluid and protein exchange after thrombin-induced microembolism: differential effects of cyclooxygenase inhibitors. Am Rev Respir Dis 132:70, 1985
24. Leeman M, Boeynaems JM, Degaute JP, et al: Administration of dazoxiben, a selective thromboxane synthetase inhibitor, in the adult respiratory distress syndrome. Chest 87:726, 1985
25. Flick MR, Hoeffel JM, Staub NC: Superoxide dismutase with heparin prevents increased lung vascular permeability during air emboli in sheep. J Appl Physiol 55:1284, 1983
26. Kolobow T, Moretti MP, Fumagalli R, et al: Severe impairment in lung function induced by high peak airway pressure during mechanical ventilation: an experimental study. Am Rev Respir Dis 135:312, 1987
27. Lee AB, Kinney JM, Turino G, et al: Effects of abdominal operations on ventilation and gas exchange. J Natl Med Assoc 61:164, 1969
28. Okinaka AJ: The pattern of breathing after operation. Surg Gynecol Obstet 125:785, 1967
29. Julien M, Lemoyne B, Denis R, et al: Mortality and morbidity related to severe intrapulmonary shunting in multiple trauma patients. J Trauma 27:970, 1987
30. Bartlett RH: The respiratory system in the elderly. Surgical Care of the Elderly. Meakins JL, McClaran JC, Eds. Year Book Medical Publishers, Chicago, 1988, p 121
31. Zikria BA, Spencer JL, Kinney JM, et al: Alterations in ventilatory function and breathing patterns following surgical trauma. Ann Surg 179:1, 1974
32. Caro CG, Butler J, Dubois AB: Some effects of restriction of chest cage expansion on pulmonary function in man: an experimental study. J Clin Invest 39:573, 1960
33. Bartlett RH, Krop P, Hanson EL, et al: Physiology of yawning and its application to postoperative care. Forum on Fundamental Surgical Problems 21:222, 1970
34. Ward RJ, Danziger F, Bonica JJ, et al: An evaluation of postoperative respiratory maneuvers. Surg Gynecol Obstet 123:51, 1966
35. Bernard GR, Artigas A, Brigham KL, et al: The American-European consensus conference on ARDS: definitions, mechanisms, relevant outcomes and clinical trial coordination. Am J Respir Crit Care Med 149:818, 1994
36. Pelosi P, D'Andrea L, Vitale G, et al: Vertical gradient of regional lung inflation in adult respiratory distress syndrome. Am J Respir Crit Care Med 149:8, 1994
37. Gattinoni L, D'Andrea L, Pelosi P, et al: Regional effects and mechanism of positive end-expiratory pressure in early adult respiratory distress syndrome. JAMA 269:2122, 1993
38. Lamm WJE, Graham MM, Albert RK: Mechanism by which the prone position improves oxygenation in acute lung injury. Am J Respir Crit Care Med 150:184, 1994
39. Demling RH, Manohar M, Will JA, et al: The effect of plasma oncotic pressure on the pulmonary microcirculation after hemorrhagic shock. Surgery 86:323, 1979
40. Shires GT III, Peitzman AB, Albert SA, et al: Response of extravascular lung water to intraoperative fluids. Ann Surg 197:515, 1983

Acknowledgments

Figures 1 and 2   Dana Burns-Pizer.
Figure 3   Albert Miller.

72 RENAL DYSFUNCTION

Nicholas L. Tilney, M.D., Julian L. Seifter, M.D., and Robert J. Rizzo, M.D.

Perioperative Management of the Patient with Renal Failure

Renal failure is defined as a general loss of kidney function with (1) alterations in volume regulation and ionic composition of body fluids and (2) inadequate excretion of metabolic wastes. Clinical manifestations vary depending on the extent and rate of functional decline: patients with acutely deteriorating kidneys become symptomatic earlier than those who have adapted to progressive chronic renal failure (CRF).[1] The three stages of renal dysfunction are diminished renal reserve (creatinine clearance > 30 ml/min), renal failure (creatinine clearance 10 to 30 ml/min), and uremia (creatinine clearance < 10 ml/min).[2]

Patients with diminished renal reserve are typically asymptomatic. With the onset and progression of renal failure, the following may occur: hypertension, anemia, carbohydrate intolerance, hyperuricemia, hypertriglyceridemia, acidosis, hyperphosphatemia, hypocalcemia, and hyponatremia. (Hyperkalemia occurs infrequently at this stage unless myonecrosis or hemolysis is present or the patient receives a depolarizing muscle relaxant during operation.) Care must be taken in patients with worsening renal failure to prevent or treat acute surgical stresses—for example, hypotension, infection, or use of nephrotoxic agents—that may further diminish renal function. Finally, as will be described, virtually every major organ system is adversely affected in patients with uremia, who often present with malaise, weakness, nausea, vomiting, weight loss, and edema.[3]

When evaluating a surgical patient with renal compromise or impending or established renal failure, the surgeon should first obtain answers to the following questions:

1. What are the extent and rate of progression of renal failure?
2. Is renal failure acute or chronic? If acute, to what degree is it reversible? What contributing factors are present, if any, and how can they be corrected?
3. What steps must be taken to prevent further renal injury?
4. What steps must be taken to minimize and manage perioperative complications?

Extent and Rate of Progression of Renal Failure

The seriousness of the patient's renal dysfunction may not be apparent from symptoms or physical examination. Acute renal failure (ARF) rarely produces the physical findings of severe chronic uremia, so its extent is best ascertained by laboratory evaluation.

Several methods are used to assess glomerular and tubular function. The glomerular filtration rate (GFR) is the most practical measure of renal function. GFR may be estimated clinically by measuring blood urea nitrogen (BUN), the serum creatinine concentration, or creatinine clearance. BUN depends on several variables, including GFR, the rate of urea production, and the rate of tubular reabsorption of urea. Urea production is increased by extrarenal factors, such as blood in the GI tract, a high-protein diet or intravenous nutrition, and administration of glucocorticoid hormones, which stimulate gluconeogenesis and protein catabolism.[4] Furthermore, tubular reabsorption of urea is increased by low urine output and volume depletion. An elevated BUN should not be equated with a low GFR.

The serum creatinine level is affected by GFR as well as by the rate of production and tubular secretion of creatinine.[5] In contrast to BUN levels, the rate of creatinine production is relatively constant in an individual because it depends primarily on products of muscle breakdown and only minimally on increased protein ingestion. Thus, a muscular male with renal dysfunction may have high serum creatinine values, whereas a small female with severe renal failure may have only minor elevations. Creatinine production also decreases with age (by 1 ml/min every year after 35 years of age[6]) secondary to diminished muscle mass and in proportion to diminished GFR associated with normal aging; therefore, normal creatinine concentrations in elderly individuals do not reflect the same GFR as they would in younger patients. Because the rate of tubular secretion in normal kidneys is also relatively constant, it does not interfere with the inverse correlation between the GFR and serum creatinine concentrations. GFR has been estimated for males by the following formula (for females, the calculated value is decreased by 15 percent[7]):

$$\text{GFR (ml/min)} = \frac{(140 - \text{age}) \times \text{weight (kg)}}{72 \times \text{serum creatinine}}$$

This formula assumes a stable creatinine concentration and thus should not be used in the setting of ARF, where the creatinine concentration is rising. On the other hand, estimation of the GFR by measuring creatinine clearance [see 93 Acute Renal Failure] does not require a stable creatinine concentration or correction for age, but it does require accurate collection of urine. (Normal values for men are from 90 to 130 ml/min; for women, normal values are from 80 to 125 ml/min.)[8] Because creatinine is secreted preferentially by the renal tubules in renal failure, estimates of the GFR based on creatinine clearance can be too high by as much as 20 percent in normal individuals and by 50 percent when the GFR is reduced to 10 percent of normal.[9] In addition, certain conditions increase the serum creatinine con-

Perioperative Management of the Patient with Renal Failure

Clinical or laboratory data suggest renal dysfunction

Determine creatinine clearance.

Diminished renal reserve (creatinine clearance > 30 ml/min)

Patients are typically asymptomatic.

Renal failure (creatinine clearance 10–30 ml/min)

Symptoms include hypertension, anemia, carbohydrate intolerance, hyperuricemia, hypertriglyceridemia, acidosis, hyperphosphatemia, hypocalcemia, and hyponatremia.

End-stage uremia (creatinine clearance < 10 ml/min)

Symptoms include malaise, weakness, nausea, vomiting, weight loss, and edema.

Patient has oliguria, tachycardia, hypotension, high urine osmolality, $FE_{Na} < 1$

Seek prerenal cause of renal failure (e.g., by measuring pulmonary arterial wedge pressure, cardiac output, and systemic vascular resistance). Correct to extent possible.

$FE_{Na} > 3$

Seek and correct postrenal cause of renal failure by bladder catheterization, ultrasonography, retrograde or intravenous pyelography, CT scan, retrograde cystoscopy, or percutaneous measures.

Renal failure persists after prerenal and postrenal factors have been excluded

Seek intrarenal cause of renal failure on the basis of history, physical examination, and laboratory studies, including x-rays or ultrasonography. Distinguish between acute and chronic intrarenal failure.

Prevent further acute renal injury

Maintain adequate urine output (≥ 0.5 ml/kg/hr) and cardiac output; correct volume deficits, and control hypertension. Monitor weight and input/output daily. If oliguria persists, give mannitol or loop diuretic. Maintain alkaline urine, avoid nephrotoxins, hydrate adequately, adjust medication dosages, treat UTI aggressively, and restrict dietary protein.

Preoperative management

If patient is uremic, give broad-spectrum prophylactic antibiotics. Patients on chronic steroid therapy may require higher doses.

Emergency operation: Treat hyperkalemia aggressively by giving 5–10 ml of 10% calcium chloride I.V. over 2 min; other treatments are sodium bicarbonate (44 mEq I.V. over 5 min), glucose (250 ml of 20% dextrose), insulin (10–25 U/ml I.V. over 30 min), and Kayexalate (25–50 g) with sorbitol (100 ml of 20% solution). Remove excess intravascular fluid by plasmapheresis. Give packed RBCs to correct anemia and sodium bicarbonate to correct acidosis.

Elective operation: If patient is unstable or on chronic dialysis, dialyze against low-potassium bath. Otherwise, correct fluid, electrolyte, and metabolic abnormalities conservatively.

Anesthesia

Halothane can be used without complications; pancuronium, tubocurarine, gallamine, and methoxyflurane are contraindicated. Treat hypotension judiciously with colloid infusions. Dialysis patients may not tolerate local anesthesia.

Postoperative management

Monitor fluids, electrolytes, and pH. Pericardial rub and asterixis are ominous signs. Institute prophylactic dialysis early. Use fractional or regional heparinization. Give diet high in carbohydrates and essential amino acids or their α–ketoanalogues; urea may be used as a source of nonessential amino acids. Consider continuous renal replacement therapy. Modify medication dosages.

centration and decrease creatinine clearance without altering GFR.[10] For example, ketones[11] and some cephalosporins[12] produce spuriously elevated values for serum creatinine by interfering with its assay, and cimetidine[13] and trimethoprim-sulfamethoxazole[14] inhibit the tubular secretion of creatinine.

Several isotopic methods, including measurement of iodine-125–iothalamate clearance, are available for precise measurement of GFR.

Classification of Renal Failure and Correction of Reversible Factors

ACUTE RENAL FAILURE

Potentially reversible acute renal failure may be categorized as prerenal, postrenal, or intrarenal in origin [see Table 1].[15]

Prerenal factors decrease renal perfusion; they include volume depletion, cardiac failure, systemic vasodilatation, and renovascular obstructive disease. The patient typically presents with oliguria, tachycardia, and hypotension (except for the patient with renovascular disease, who is typically hypertensive). The urinary sediment is unremarkable, and urine osmolality is high. An isolated urine sample with a sodium concentration of less than 10 mEq/L indicates good tubular function and suggests a prerenal mechanism for the renal dysfunction.

The fractional excretion of sodium (FE_{Na}) provides a good assessment of prerenal states; it is often low (less than one percent) because of sodium and water conservation by the kidneys [see 93 Acute Renal Failure].[16] A spot urine sample rather than a timed collection may be employed to determine FE_{Na}. Measurements of pulmonary arterial wedge pressure, cardiac output, and systemic vascular resistance also assist in the diagnosis of ARF[17] and indicate the direction of subsequent therapy. Correction of prerenal conditions should be aggressive to prevent ischemic renal injury. A special circumstance occurs in the setting of volume depletion or renal arterial stenosis when angiotensin-converting enzyme (ACE) inhibitors or angiotensin II antagonists are used. Reversible oliguria and azotemia develop because of a fall in glomerular pressure that follows dilatation of the efferent arterioles. This development reflects failure of normal autoregulatory function; volume repletion and discontinuance of the drug are required for resolution.

Postrenal factors are typically caused by mechanical complications and are usually secondary to urinary tract obstruction or extravasation. Bladder catheterization will relieve or rule out urethral or bladder outlet obstruction. Ultrasonography is most helpful in documenting upper urinary tract obstruction, which may be relieved acutely by retrograde cystoscopy or percutaneous means. Urinary extravasation, as in a patient with a ruptured bladder, is associated with hematuria and may be assessed by means of intravenous or retrograde pyelography or CT scans. It should be noted that the radiopaque dyes used for contrast studies are not without potential hazards. Intravenous urography contrast agents may cause renal failure in patients with multiple myeloma or diabetes mellitus as well as in those with other renal diseases.

If ARF persists even after prerenal and postrenal factors have been excluded or corrected, the presence of intrarenal disease must be considered [see Table 1]. Differentiation between acute and chronic causes of intrarenal failure may require a thorough clinical evaluation [see Table 2].[3] The causes of acute intrarenal failure may be categorized according to the site of the primary parenchymal abnormality—tubules, glomeruli, vessels, interstitium, papillae, or cortex.[15]

1. The most common cause of ARF in surgical patients is acute tubular necrosis (ATN) from systemic infection, ischemia, or exposure to nephrotoxins[18]; patients with ATN are rarely hypertensive. The urine sediment classically shows pigmented, granular casts; heme pigment may reflect ATN from hemoglobinuria caused by a transfusion reaction or from myoglobinuria caused by a crush injury or muscle ischemia.[19] In rhabdomyolysis, serum creatine phosphokinase levels are elevated.[20] Nonsteroidal anti-inflammatory agents are a common cause of renal failure, particularly in dehydrated patients.
2. Acute glomerulonephritis often follows systemic infection or collagen vascular disease and is associated with hematuria, proteinuria, hypocomplementemia, and hypertension.
3. Vasculitides involving glomeruli present in much the same way as acute glomerulonephritis, but serum complement levels are normal. Other signs of systemic diseases may be present. A test for antineutrophil cytoplasmic antibodies should be performed.
4. The urine sediment in interstitial nephritis from medication allergy or pyelonephritis may contain eosinophils and mononuclear leukocytes.
5. Acute papillary necrosis may be precipitated by analgesic abuse, diabetes, or urinary tract infection or obstruction; sloughed papillae may lodge in the ureter, creating painful obstruction.[21]
6. Acute cortical necrosis is particularly likely to occur in an obstetric patient as a consequence of profound shock and disseminated intravascular coagulation after a complicated labor and delivery.[22]
7. Atheroembolic disease is an important cause of subacute renal failure in patients who have undergone vascular procedures or have received anticoagulants.

Most patients with ARF are oliguric, producing urine volumes of less than 400 ml/day, although nonoliguric (high-output) renal failure is not uncommon and is characteristic of aminoglycoside-related ATN.[23] Complete anuria suggests bilateral renal artery occlusion, obstructive uropathy, cortical necrosis, or rapidly progressive glomerulonephritis. Severe disease or obstruction of a single kidney and inadvertent ureteral ligation during a difficult retroperitoneal surgical dissection should be ruled out as causes of acute anuria.

CHRONIC RENAL FAILURE

Irreversible, progressive CRF has many possible causes, including glomerulonephritis, hypertensive nephrosclerosis, diabetic nephropathy, tubulointerstitial disease, obstructive uropathy, chronic pyelonephritis, polycystic kidney disease, and congenital hypoplasia.[24] Consequently, the differential diagnosis requires a complete clinical evaluation [see Table 2].[3] The history should record symptoms of urinary tract dysfunction, systemic diseases that could affect the kidneys, exposure to nephrotoxins or infectious agents, and family history of renal disease. The physical exam should evaluate blood pressure, the retinas, the cardiovascular system, and the kidneys—including the presence or absence of renal artery bruits. Urine volume is not usually helpful in evaluating CRF. Many patients continue to excrete urine, at least until dialysis is begun. Broad casts that are granular and

Table 1 Classification of Acute Renal Failure

Prerenal
- Volume depletion
  - Dehydration (i.e., from cutaneous or gastrointestinal losses or renal losses in adrenal insufficiency)
  - Hemorrhage (i.e., from trauma, surgery, childbirth, or gastrointestinal lesions)
  - Fluid redistribution (i.e., from trauma, crush injury, burns, pancreatitis, peritonitis, sepsis, or hypoalbuminemia)
- Cardiac failure (i.e., from myocardial or valvular causes, arrhythmia, or tamponade)
- Systemic vasodilatation (i.e., from sepsis, anaphylaxis, neurogenic shock, anesthesia, or antihypertensive medications)
- Renovascular obstructive disease
  - Arterial (e.g., arteriosclerosis, embolism, dissection, fibromuscular dysplasia, vasculitis, or disease related to aortic or any retroperitoneal operation)
  - Venous (e.g., renal vein thrombosis)

Postrenal
- Obstructive uropathy
  - Renal pelvis and ureters (i.e., from calculus, tumor, clot, papillae, infection, trauma, or retroperitoneal fibrosis)
  - Bladder and urethra (i.e., from calculus, bladder or prostatic tumor, clot, trauma, benign prostatic hypertrophy, neuropathic bladder, obstructed bladder catheter, or phimosis)
- Extravasation (i.e., from trauma)

Intrarenal
- Acute tubular necrosis
  - Ischemia
  - Nephrotoxins
    - Endogenous: pigments (myoglobin and hemoglobin), crystals (uric acid, calcium phosphate, and oxalate), or tumors (tumor lysis syndrome and myeloma)
    - Exogenous: antibiotics (aminoglycosides, cephalosporins, sulfonamides, and amphotericin B), anesthetics (methoxyflurane and enflurane), chemotherapeutic and immunosuppressive agents (e.g., cisplatin and cyclosporine), contrast media, organic solvents (heavy metals, poisons, or other chemicals), and dextran
- Glomerulonephritis
  - Postinfectious (e.g., associated with streptococcal, pneumococcal, viral, and shunt infections and abdominal abscesses)
  - Membranoproliferative
  - Rapidly progressive (e.g., associated with lupus erythematosus, Goodpasture's syndrome, polyarteritis nodosa, Wegener's granulomatosis, Schönlein-Henoch purpura)
  - Serum sickness
  - Thrombotic microangiopathy (e.g., hemolytic-uremic syndrome or thrombotic-thrombocytopenic purpura) and other microvascular diseases (e.g., scleroderma, malignant hypertension, radiation, and disseminated intravascular coagulation)
- Vasculitides (e.g., polyarteritis nodosa, hypersensitivity angiitides, scleroderma, hemolytic-uremic syndrome, coagulopathy, radiation, diffuse intravascular coagulation, eclampsia, malignant hypertension, or thrombotic-thrombocytopenic purpura)
- Interstitial nephritis
  - Drugs (e.g., penicillin, cephalosporins, sulfonamides, rifampin, nonsteroidal anti-inflammatory drugs, thiazides, cimetidine, and interferon)
  - Infection
    - Direct invasion (e.g., by *Staphylococcus*, viruses, or fungi)
    - Indirect effects (e.g., of streptococcal or pneumococcal infection, typhoid, or diphtheria)
  - Infiltration (lymphoma, leukemia, or sarcoidosis)
  - Idiopathic
- Papillary necrosis (e.g., associated with analgesics, infection, obstruction, or diabetes)
- Acute cortical necrosis (e.g., profound shock, often associated with complicated pregnancy or septic abortion)
- Atheroembolic syndrome (renal failure with lower extremity ischemia)

waxy are often seen in the urine sediment, reflecting compensatory hypertrophy of surviving nephrons.

Prevention of Further Renal Injury

Prevention of further acute renal injury is a priority in the perioperative care of patients with CRF. Because prerenal and postrenal complications may be superimposed on the already compromised renal function of a previously asymptomatic patient, factors that may precipitate ARF must be eliminated. By reversing these factors, the surgeon may gain time before the patient's kidneys fail completely and dialysis becomes necessary.

In an acute situation, the patient with renal failure needs close monitoring of daily weight and input/output measurements and hourly urine volume measurements, via an indwelling bladder catheter. An output of at least 0.5 ml/kg/hr should be maintained. Renal perfusion should be optimized by correcting volume deficits and maintaining adequate cardiac output. Unless it is controlled, severe hypertension may worsen preexisting renal failure; overzealous use of antihypertensive medication may also be deleterious, particularly in patients with renal vascular disease.[23,25]

Table 2 Findings Suggestive of Chronic Rather Than Acute Renal Failure

History
  Symptoms of uremia
  Hypertension
  Hematuria or proteinuria
  Abnormal blood chemistry values (elevated urea nitrogen or creatinine levels)

Physical examination
  Debility
  Alopecia
  Excoriations and yellow pallor of skin
  Peripheral neuropathy
  Conjunctival calcification
  Band keratopathy
  Gynecomastia, testicular atrophy, or both

Laboratory examination*
  Anemia on presentation (only if there is no history of acute blood loss)
  Low urinary sodium level or high urine osmolarity (either suggests prerenal azotemia)

X-rays or ultrasonography
  Bilateral small kidneys
  Other evidence of long-standing renal dysfunction (e.g., chronic obstruction, pyelonephritis, or polycystic kidney disease)
  Bone changes of secondary hyperparathyroidism (e.g., osteitis fibrosa cystica, osteomalacia, or osteosclerosis)

*Urinary sodium values are informative only if they are low; urine osmolarity is informative only if the value is high. The remainder of the serum chemistry values are not helpful, because they may be altered in both acute and chronic renal failure.

Autoregulation of renal blood flow, which is an important self-protective mechanism in renal hypoperfusion, is mediated by renal prostaglandins and the renin-angiotensin system.[26] Therefore, use of ACE inhibitors, for instance, may lead to further deterioration in renal function.[27] As an alternative, low-dose dopamine—1 to 3 µg/kg/min, as often used primarily in the cardiac surgical setting to prevent or attenuate ATN—augments renal blood flow with minimal influence on cardiac output.[28] Dopamine should be administered with caution, however, because of the potential for arrhythmogenesis. It should be discontinued if the desired effect on urine flow rate is not obtained.

If oliguria persists despite correction of prerenal and postrenal factors, an early trial of mannitol[29] or a loop diuretic[30] may initiate diuresis and convert oliguric to nonoliguric renal failure.[23] In a volume-expanded patient who responds to diuretics, constant infusion of furosemide at a rate of 5 to 10 mg/hr may be attempted. Mannitol increases intravascular volume and stimulates an osmotic diuresis; loop diuretics alter tubular reabsorptive mechanisms and may diminish intravascular volume. Thus, mannitol may be used to increase urine flow when intravascular volume can tolerate the osmotic load, and diuretics are appropriate when intravascular volume is high (or when the patient has been receiving diuretics for an extended period and is dependent on them). Mannitol is especially useful in the setting of rhabdomyolysis. When renal blood flow may be compromised intraoperatively (e.g., during cardiac or aortic operation), prophylactic use of mannitol or furosemide has been suggested for inducing diuresis.[31] However, in individuals whose intravascular volume is already low, diuretics may precipitate additional renal injury by causing further volume decreases.

Several other perioperative precautions may prevent the worsening of compromised renal function.

1. Maintenance of an alkaline urine to diminish free heme pigment, which can be directly toxic to tubular cells (a urine pH > 6 usually discourages dissociation of heme from hemoglobin or myoglobin[32]).
2. Avoidance of nephrotoxins, with levels of potentially nephrotoxic agents (e.g., aminoglycoside antibiotics) carefully maintained in the nontoxic range.
3. Adequate hydration before[33] and during surgical exposure to protect against the nephrotoxicity of contrast agents, aminoglycosides, antineoplastic agents, heme pigment, and hypercalcemia.[34]
4. Smaller doses of medications for elderly patients, whose GFR is lower given the same serum creatinine level.[35]
5. Aggressive treatment of urinary tract infections and other factors that may cause deterioration of kidney function.[34]
6. Dietary protein restriction, which may slow the progression of renal failure by decreasing glomerular hyperfiltration.[36,37]

Perioperative Complications of Renal Failure

Both elective and emergency operations can be performed in patients with renal failure, provided that physiologic homeostasis is reestablished by judicious and aggressive perioperative dialysis.[38,39] Dialysis particularly improves abnormalities of hemostasis that are caused largely by platelet dysfunction[40]; however, anticoagulants and antiplatelet medications that are used to maintain patency of arteriovenous fistulae may also contribute to excessive bleeding [*see* Discussion, Hematologic System, *below*]. In addition, heparin may still be active in patients undergoing operation soon after hemodialysis, and heparin rebound may occur because of the shorter action of protamine in relation to heparin.[41] Abnormal prothrombin times are correctable by means of fresh frozen plasma or vitamin K, although such measures are usually unnecessary; in fact, angioaccess devices commonly thrombose after operation. Attention to intraoperative hemostasis and technique is also important for a successful outcome.

For the uremic patient, whose host defense mechanisms are often altered or depressed,[42] broad-spectrum antibiotics should be administered perioperatively to prevent infection.[43] In patients receiving long-term steroid therapy, coverage with stress steroids may be required [*see* 73 *Adrenal Insufficiency*].

PREOPERATIVE CONSIDERATIONS IN ELECTIVE SURGERY

Preoperative preparation of the stable renal failure patient for elective surgery is routine. For the unstable patient, however, preoperative dialysis should be performed to correct volume overload; requirements depend on the severity of renal failure and the potential extent of the operative procedure.[1] Patients on long-term maintenance dialysis are usually dialyzed the day before and the day after operation, most often against a low-potassium bath in anticipation of the increased intraoperative release of potassium that occurs secondary to muscle relaxant administration,[44] tissue manipulation and breakdown, and blood transfusions.[1] Patients in whom acute renal failure develops require earlier and more aggressive dialysis, particularly if they are hypercatabolic.[3]

Indications for dialysis before elective surgery are less clear in patients with compromised renal function who do not yet require maintenance dialysis.[1] Conservative correction of fluid, electrolyte, and metabolic abnormalities usually suffices unless the condition necessitating operation could possibly increase catabolism and the potential for uremic complications. Asymptomatic patients who have a normal physical examination and reasonable blood chemistries usually do not require preoperative dialysis, but this prophylactic treatment should be employed at the first sign of need.

PREOPERATIVE CONSIDERATIONS IN EMERGENCY SURGERY

If dialysis cannot be performed preoperatively, evidence of hyperkalemia should prompt aggressive treatment by other methods.[1] Aggressive measures are especially necessary in hypercatabolic patients who have suffered trauma or severe burns, because these patients may experience a rapid elevation of serum potassium levels. In these patients, prompt initiation of aggressive dialysis may be lifesaving. In addition, administration of calcium may be necessary. Calcium (5 to 10 ml of 10 percent calcium chloride solution I.V. over a two-minute period) directly antagonizes the cardioplegic effects of hyperkalemia and allows time for instituting less dramatic measures:

1. Sodium bicarbonate (44 mEq I.V. over a five-minute period), glucose (250 ml of 20 percent dextrose), and insulin (10 to 25 U I.V. over a 30-minute period) all drive extracellular potassium into cells.
2. Sodium polystyrene sulfonate (Kayexalate), a potassium-binding ion exchange resin, can be given orally every three to four hours in doses of 25 to 50 g administered with 100 ml of 20 percent sorbitol to decrease constipation. (Given alone, Kayexalate can cause extensive colonic concretions that may be difficult to remove. For this reason, Kayexalate and aluminum-containing phosphate binders should not be given simultaneously.) Alternatively, 50 g of Kayexalate with 50 g of sorbitol in 200 ml of water can be given every one to two hours as a retention enema; however, this treatment should be avoided in the immediate postoperative period because of the potential hazard of colonic necrosis.[45]

Preoperative correction of other renal failure abnormalities can be done more leisurely. Excess intravascular fluid can be removed by plasmapheresis, packed red blood cells can be used to correct anemia and to establish some hematologic reserve, and sodium bicarbonate can be given to correct acidosis as well as to reduce hyperkalemia[1]—provided that volume status will allow the sodium load.

ANESTHETIC CONSIDERATIONS

Some neuromuscular blockers (particularly pancuronium and tubocurarine) can potentiate both acidosis and hyperkalemia, so their use is contraindicated in anesthetic management of the patient with renal failure. Gallamine is also contraindicated because it is excreted by the kidneys and is not dialyzable. Halothane has been used frequently and without complications as a general anesthetic in patients with compromised kidney function. Methoxyflurane is nephrotoxic and is no longer used.[46]

Because extracellular fluid volume may be decreased immediately after dialysis, hypotension that occurs after the induction of general anesthesia should be treated judiciously with colloid infusions.[47] In addition, the hemodialysis access site must be protected; the involved upper arm should never be used for blood pressure measurement or I.V. infusion. Finally, patients on dialysis tend to be very anxious and typically have undergone several operative procedures, so they may require general or regional anesthesia in situations in which local anesthesia is usually used.

POSTOPERATIVE CONSIDERATIONS

All general principles of postoperative care apply to renal failure patients, with some exceptions[1] and additional considerations.

Fluids, electrolytes, and acid-base balance should be monitored closely. Because levels of toxins are increased and their clearance is decreased, uremic manifestations may worsen rapidly. The development of a pericardial rub or asterixis are two clues that uremia may be worsening. Prophylactic dialysis should be instituted early, before complications of advanced uremia develop.[1] It is usually initiated the day after operation because heparinization is thought to be less dangerous than the bleeding disorders that result from a buildup of uremic toxins. To prevent hemorrhage at the operative dissection site (a potential but uncommon complication), fractional or regional heparinization is used during dialysis.

Cardiac failure may occur secondary to ischemic coronary artery disease, a common problem in elderly patients on dialysis.[48] Hypotension may result from abnormal receptor function[49] or from volume depletion, sepsis, tamponade, or myocardial ischemia. Another cause of hypotension is the removal of vasopressive agents after bilateral nephrectomy.[50]

Wound healing, particularly healing of serosal surfaces,[51] may be delayed in renal failure patients. An exteriorized bowel may not seal to the abdominal wall, intestinal anastomoses may leak, and intraperitoneal infection or perforation may occur in the absence of fever or in the presence of a diminished leukocyte response. The common bile duct may be very slow to heal; T tubes should be left in for several weeks. Thus, the surgeon should be slow to remove nasogastric tubes, some wound drains, and skin or retention sutures but aggressive in treating suspected surgical complications.[1]

Protein malnutrition impairs both wound healing and immunity. Nutritional support with a diet high in carbohydrates and essential amino acids (or their alpha ketoanalogues) has been shown to limit protein catabolism without eliciting uremic symptoms.[37] Endogenous urea may be used as a source of nonessential amino acids for protein synthesis.[52] In undernourished patients, protein-containing nutrition should not be withheld to maintain a low BUN. It is better to provide nitrogen via amino acids and then to dialyze if necessary. Techniques for continuous renal replacement therapy are now available. These procedures (e.g., continuous arteriovenous and venovenous hemodialysis) are particularly useful in hypercatabolic patients in the ICU, who require large volumes of replacement fluid and intravenous nutrients.

Drug dosages should be modified in renal failure patients. Consideration should be given to the absence of renal excretion and the possible dialytic removal of medications.[53] Consideration should also be given to the potential systemic toxicity of medications. For example, meperidine should not be given to patients with renal failure because of the possibility of serious neurologic sequelae.

Discussion

Pathophysiological Mechanisms in Renal Failure

The pathophysiological mechanisms in renal failure include the progression of kidney disease and the effects of the uremic syndrome on metabolism and the major body systems. The general pathophysiology of renal failure has been thoroughly reviewed elsewhere [see 93 Acute Renal Failure].

PROGRESSION OF KIDNEY DISEASE

The progression of kidney disease is related to underlying aggravating factors, which may include dehydration, infection, obstruction, poorly controlled hypertension, and intrarenal deposition of crystals.[54] In addition, the processes of adaptation may actually induce further damage. Progressive glomerulosclerosis may develop in the normal nephrons that remain after surgical removal of large amounts of kidney tissue.[55] Both the rate of progression of injury and the magnitude of the glomerular hemodynamic changes in the remaining nephrons correlate directly with the proportion of tissue removed. Moderate dietary protein restriction may blunt adaptive hyperperfusion and hyperfiltration of the kidney remnants, thus limiting further glomerular injury.[56]

Treatment with ACE inhibitors, which decrease arteriolar and glomerular capillary pressures, also limits glomerular injury in patients with diabetic and nondiabetic renal disease.[57]

THE UREMIC SYNDROME

The uremic syndrome is a clinical state resulting from loss of renal function; regulation of body fluid volume and ionic composition, excretion of endogenous and exogenous metabolic wastes, and participation in endocrine metabolic processes are subsequently impaired. The resulting adverse effects hamper a range of intracellular and systemic body processes.

The Effects of Uremia on Major Organ Systems

Although severe uremia can impair the function of most major body systems, the most obvious and profound effects seldom occur today because of prompt and aggressive treatment. These effects must be considered, however, when patients with CRF are evaluated for surgery.

Cardiovascular system Cardiovascular complications are responsible for more than half of the deaths in patients with chronic renal disease,[58] primarily because of the frequency of severe atherosclerosis in this population.[59,60] Cardiac hypertrophy is common, often occurring secondary to hypertension. Deposition of calcium and oxalate crystals may cause decreased myocardial function, leading to congestive heart failure, arrhythmias, and, sometimes, sudden death.[61]

Potential myocardial toxins include phenol,[62] parathyroid hormone, and cobalt.[63] Large arteriovenous fistulas used for dialysis access may also contribute to high-output myocardial failure.[64] Improvement of myocardial function with dialysis has been correlated specifically with increased plasma levels of calcium.[65]

Pericarditis may present as chest pain, fever, pericardial friction rub, or acute cardiovascular collapse; hypotension, jugular venous distention, and pulsus paradoxus may appear during dialysis secondary to hemopericardium and pericardial tamponade. Constrictive pericarditis also may result in circulatory instability.[66] The etiology of uremic pericarditis is unknown, but it may be a response to uremic toxins, fluid overload, or infection.[67]

Pericardial effusion can be diagnosed by ultrasonography, tamponade by equalization of atrial pressures, and constrictive pericarditis by angiography and catheterization.[68] Aggressive dialysis is indicated for uremic patients with pericarditis, and fluid balance must be carefully managed. Acute tamponade or enlarging effusions call for drainage, and constrictive pericarditis may necessitate pericardiectomy.[69]

Pulmonary system Abnormal pulmonary function in renal failure patients is associated with anemia, fluid overload, and the direct effects of toxins on pulmonary tissue.[70] In the uremic lung, increased densities in the perihilar and inner lung zones form a butterfly appearance on x-ray.[71] As pulmonary vascular permeability increases,[72] pulmonary edema may occur with relatively low pulmonary arterial pressures.[73,74]

In uremic pneumonitis, membranes formed within alveoli and fibrin deposited in the interstitium eventually give rise to interstitial fibrosis.[75] Restrictive pulmonary insufficiency may occur secondary to diffuse pulmonary calcification.[76] Fibrinous pleuritis, which may also cause a restrictive defect, responds to dialysis and thoracentesis; only rarely is surgical decortication required.[77]

Gastrointestinal system Severe uremia may alter the entire GI tract from nasopharynx to rectum because urea diffuses into the lumen and is converted to ammonia by bacterial urease. The result may be edema, hemorrhage, ulceration, or necrosis.[78] Constipation is a common problem in dialysis patients, who are also being given phosphate binders; fecal impactions may become massive, and they occasionally cause serious problems. Patients on dialysis also have an increased propensity for the development of adynamic ileus and diverticulosis; perforation of diverticula is very common and is a possibility in any renal failure patient with abdominal discomfort.[79,80] Prompt Gastrografin enema and removal of the involved segment with formation of an end colostomy have been very effective in reducing mortality from this condition[81]; CT scan of the colon has been helpful in diagnosing diverticulitis.[82] Phosphate enemas should be avoided in patients with renal failure because of the risk of severe, acute hyperphosphoremia. The regenerative capacity of the liver is diminished in renal failure,[83] and albumin and protein synthesis is decreased.[84] The incidence of hepatitis C has been reported to be nearly 60 percent in hemodialysis patients, and hepatitis B incidence is increased as well.[85]

Peptic ulcer disease is not uncommon in patients with renal failure. Magnesium-containing antacids may cause severe hypermagnesemia and should therefore be avoided. Cimetidine carries a significant risk of neurotoxicity in renal failure patients. In addition, such patients may experience gastroparesis, particularly if they are diabetic. Amyloidosis, which may develop in long-term dialysis patients, may involve the stomach and lead to GI bleeding.

Endocrine system Metabolism of vitamin D is markedly altered by diminished renal conversion of 25-hydroxyvitamin D_3 to its most active metabolite, 1,25-dihydroxyvitamin D_3.[86] The resulting decrease in intestinal calcium absorption contributes to the development of secondary hyperparathyroidism, as does hyperphosphatemia caused by decreased excretion of phosphate by the kidneys.[87] Renal failure patients require calcium carbonate, both as a source of calcium and as a phosphate binder when given at mealtime. 1,25-dihydroxyvitamin D_3 should be administered to hypocalcemic patients after the serum phosphate level has been normalized. This step will lower the parathyroid hormone level; an appropriate parathyroid hormone level is approximately two to three times the normal one. Severe metabolic acidosis should be corrected by giving bicarbonate to diminish bone loss.

Hematologic system Anemia is common among renal failure patients, many of whom have hematocrits in the range of 20 to 25 percent. Decreased production of red blood cells is almost always a feature of the anemia of renal failure. The rate of red cell production by the marrow is determined by erythropoietin elaboration in the kidneys [see Figure 1]. Whereas individuals with normal kidney function generally employ compensatory mechanisms in the presence of mild hemolysis, those with renal failure cannot compensate for hemolysis, because decreased production of erythropoietin by the diseased kidneys impairs erythropoiesis in the marrow.[88] (In normal kidneys, endothelial cells in the proximal tubules or peritubular capillaries in the cortex and the outer medulla are thought to produce most of the renal erythropoietin.[89] Synthesis is stimulated by renal hypoxia.) In renal disease, the normal physiologic response to anemia—that is, a homeostatic increase in marrow erythropoiesis—cannot occur. Patients with end-stage renal disease have serum erythropoietin levels that are within normal ranges for healthy, nonanemic individuals; in anemic patients with normal renal function, however, serum erythropoietin levels may be markedly increased and therefore are not useful for predicting the response to exogenous erythropoietin.

Blood losses from the GI tract, menstruation, multiple laboratory determinations, or even dialysis itself can also contribute to anemia. It has been estimated that the average dialysis patient loses about 2.5 L of blood a year, and this figure does not include occasional large losses caused by rupture of the dialysis coil, bleeding from access devices, or surgical procedures.[90]

Patients with uremia also have increased bleeding tendencies, even though their prothrombin times, partial thromboplastin times, and platelet counts are usually normal.[91] Heparin anticoagulation during dialysis, combined with abnormal platelet function, may predispose the patient to epistaxis, hemopericardium, intracranial hemorrhage, retroperitoneal bleeding, and other complications.[92-94] Subdural hematoma may mimic dialysis disequilibrium syndrome.

The most important clotting defect in uremia—one that correlates directly with the severity of renal failure—involves platelet dysfunction, which is measured as decreased release of platelet factor 3 and diminished platelet aggregation and adhesiveness and which is believed to be related to the presence of guanidinosuccinic acid, a dialyzable toxin in uremic plasma.[95] Phenolic acid, cyclic adenosine triphosphate (cATP), hypermagnesemia, and elevated prostacyclin levels may be toxic to platelets; peritoneal dialysis markedly inhibits these adverse effects.

On the other hand, the nephrotic syndrome (usually associated with membranous glomerulonephritis in patients who are not yet in end-stage renal failure) has been associated with a hypercoagulable state that may produce renal vein thrombosis; antithrombin III deficiency may become significant when the serum albumin level has fallen to less than 2 mg/dl.[96,97] Anticoagulation may be necessary to prevent thrombosis, but the condition may be resistant to heparin. Hemodialysis may induce a transient thrombocytopenia through contact activation on dialyzer membranes, but antiplatelet agents such as short-acting prostacyclins can block this effect.

Operative blood loss secondary to platelet dysfunction is rare if the patient is well dialyzed.[98] However, the use of heparin during dialysis and the extended use of coumadin or antiplatelet drugs to maintain the patency of dialysis accesses may potentiate intraoperative blood loss. In addition, even if heparinization is regional during the preoperative dialysis, heparin rebound may occur during operation.[99] Therefore, the surgeon must be aware of the type and the degree of preoperative anticoagulation. The effects of heparin can generally be reversed intraoperatively by the intravenous infusion of protamine; the prothrombin times of patients on long-term coumadin regimens can be normalized by the administration of vitamin K. More urgent reversal can be accomplished with fresh frozen plasma. Occasionally, blood loss is excessive even when such coagulation defects have been reversed, particularly with retroperitoneal dissection for procedures on the abdominal aorta or the iliac arteries. The surgeon must also be aware of the increased likelihood of clotting of the arteriovenous fistula postoperatively.

Treatment of anemia in patients with end-stage renal disease should include iron replacement if iron stores are depleted, as determined by measuring transferrin iron saturation (a value of < 20 percent signals depletion). Until the 1990s, blood transfusions were the mainstay of therapy. Since then, however, recombinant erythropoietin has come to play a prominent role. The availability of recombinant human erythropoietin constitutes a tremendous advance in the care of patients with end-stage renal disease. The drug largely eliminates the need for transfusions, thereby not only improving the anemia but also avoiding the acute and chronic hazards of transfusion (viral infection and iron overload).[100,101] Recombinant human erythropoietin also corrects clotting changes.[100,101] Indeed, most patients who are now receiving erythropoietin have normal bleeding times. The drug has other benefits as well, including increased energy level, greater exercise tolerance, and improved overall well-being.

The most effective approach to uremic bleeding is prevention by means of adequate dialysis. Regional heparinization may be

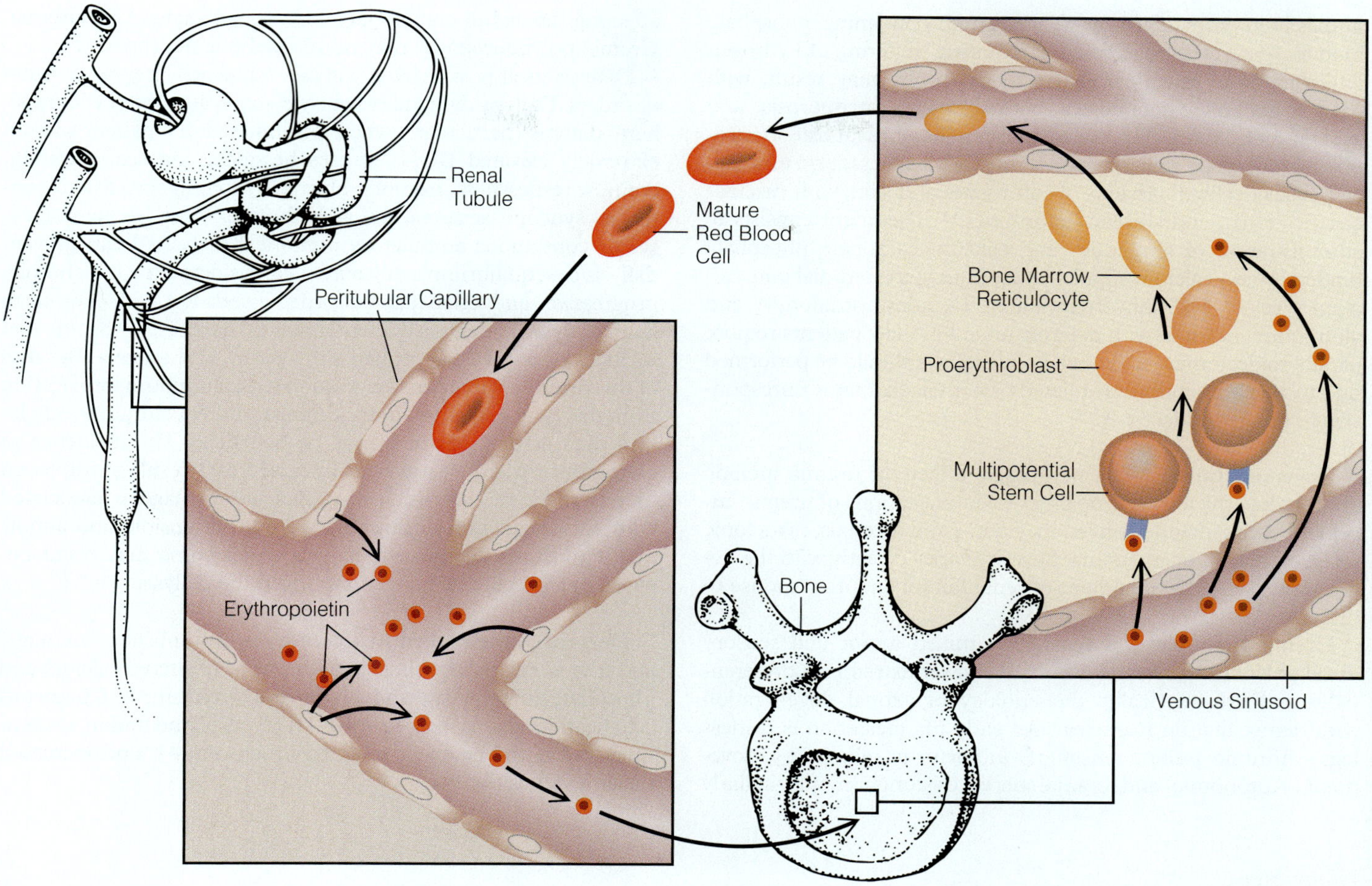

Figure 1 The rate of red cell production in the marrow is determined by erythropoietin elaboration in the kidneys. In normal kidneys, as shown here, endothelial cells in the tubules or peritubular capillaries are thought to produce most of the renal erythropoietin. Synthesis is stimulated by renal hypoxemia. (The hypoxemia would not necessarily be caused by anemia. It could, for example, be the result of dwelling at high altitudes.) In the marrow, the erythropoietin binds to erythroid progenitors, stimulating their differentiation and proliferation. In patients with renal failure, decreased production of erythropoietin by the diseased kidneys impairs erythropoiesis in the marrow. Red cell morphology is unaffected, however.[142]

used with good results; patients come to surgery after dialysis with their clotting ability reasonably intact. Cryoprecipitate, conjugated estrogens, and 1-desamino-8-D-arginine vasopressin (DDAVP) may be administered postoperatively as needed to correct bleeding disorders; conjugated estrogens may take several days to influence bleeding times.[102] In most cases, however, none of these measures are necessary if dialysis is adequate.

Immune system Alteration of leukocyte and immunologic function in renal failure patients is thought to contribute to their increased susceptibility to infection.[43] Neutrophil counts are usually normal but may decrease transiently after hemodialysis because of leukocyte sequestration in pulmonary capillaries, possibly related to complement activation.[103] Chemotaxis of granulocytes and phagocytes is also depressed, both by inhibitors in uremic serum[104] and by an intrinsic cell defect,[105] and it is worsened by hemodialysis (although less so by peritoneal dialysis). Transplantation restores depressed chemotaxis.[105,106]

In some patients, lymphocytopenia with impaired cellular immunity develops.[107] T cell function is depressed by uremic serum but improved by dialysis.[108] B cell–mediated antibody response to some stimuli may also be attenuated,[109] although serum immunoglobulin levels are not always decreased[110] and response to vaccines is usually normal.[111]

Musculoskeletal system Myopathy in renal failure may be secondary to malnutrition,[112] hyperparathyroidism,[113] abnormal vitamin D metabolism,[114] or aluminum accumulation[115]; correction requires 1,25-dihydroxyvitamin D_3 administration,[116] aluminum chelation,[115] or renal transplantation. Uremic bursitis may be a result of generalized serositis.[117] The olecranon bursa of the access arm has an increased predilection for bursitis from prolonged pressure on the bed or chair during hemodialysis.[118] The incidence of tendon ruptures increases in association with hyperparathyroidism,[119] in which crystal deposition[120] and septic arthritis are common.[121] Dialysis amyloidosis is a debilitating condition that includes arthropathy and is attributable to retention of β_2-macroglobulin in tissues.

Bone demineralization may result from altered vitamin D metabolism and secondary hyperparathyroidism,[122,123] aluminum intoxication from dialysate or aluminum-containing phosphate binders,[124] or metabolic acidosis requiring buffering of hydrogen ion with bone salts.[125] Renal osteodystrophy may result, with osteitis fibrosis, osteomalacia, osteosclerosis, osteoporosis, and growth retardation. Physical manifestations of renal osteodystrophy include bone pain, proximal muscle weakness, pruritus, calciphylaxis (ischemic lesions of soft tissues and skin, with vascular calcifications), and skeletal deformities.[123] Treatment consists of administration of aluminum and calcium carbonate phosphate binders[126] and calcium supplements,[127] an increased dialysate calcium level,[128] 1,25-dihydroxyvitamin D_3 administration,[129] and aluminum chelation with deferoxamine.[130] A few patients require parathyroidectomy,[131] although bone biopsies should be performed first to rule out aluminum-related osteomalacia that is unresponsive to parathyroidectomy.[132]

Nervous system The neurologic effects of uremia include encephalopathy and neuropathy.[133] Manifestations of uremic encephalopathy include confusion, tremor and asterixis, myoclonic seizures, delirium, and coma. Severity varies directly with the degree and rate of development of renal failure and its response to dialysis.

Uremic neuropathy is typically a mixed motor and sensory distal polyneuropathy that affects the lower extremities preferentially and symmetrically; the etiology of axonal degeneration with demyelination is unclear. An early manifestation is restless legs syndrome: pulling sensations and pruritus relieved by movement. Autonomic and cranial nerve dysfunction, particularly affecting the eighth cranial nerve, is also associated with uremia. Uremic polyneuropathy may mimic diabetic neuropathy.

Dialysis itself is associated with several central nervous system disorders. Dialysis dysequilibrium syndrome, associated with rapid hemodialysis (particularly when it is initiated in a patient with an extremely elevated BUN), causes headache, nausea, vomiting, cramps, restlessness, tremors, blurred vision, hypertension, confusion, syncope, seizures, and arrhythmias. Short, frequent dialyses or continuous ambulatory peritoneal dialysis[134] can prevent dialysis dysequilibrium syndrome. Dialysis dementia is a chronic, progressive, and often fatal disorder associated with long-term hemodialysis[135]; dialysis dementia may be part of a syndrome that includes osteomalacia, proximal myopathy, and anemia. Because of this disorder's frequent association with aluminum intoxication from dialysate contamination, administration of aluminum chelators such as deferoxamine may be beneficial. The incidence of aluminum toxicity has in fact decreased as a result of improved management of dialysis. Intracranial hemorrhage is associated with anticoagulation during dialysis,[93] hypertension, and abnormal hemostasis. Nonketotic hyperosmolar coma may occur because of high glucose concentrations in the dialysate.[136]

Dermal system Pruritus commonly complicates uremia[137] and may be related to skin gland atrophy or to altered calcium and phosphate metabolism and hyperparathyroidism.[138] Cutaneous calcification also causes pruritus.[139] Hyperpigmentation is common and is the result of retained urochromes[140] and increased melanin deposition.[141]

References

1. Lazarus JM, Morgan AP, Tilney NL: Patients with chronic renal failure: general management and acute surgical illness. Surgical Care of the Patient with Renal Failure. Tilney NL, Lazarus JM, Eds. WB Saunders Co, Philadelphia, 1982, p 1
2. Vincent F: Preoperative and postoperative care: renal disease. Handbook of Surgery. Schrock TR, Ed. Jones Medical Publications, Greenbrae, California, 1985, p 47
3. Bellomo R, Parkin G, Love J, et al: A prospective comparative study of continuous arteriovenous hemodiafiltration and continuous venovenous hemodiafiltration in critically ill patients. Am J Kidney Dis 21:400, 1993
4. Morgan DB, Carver MF, Payne RB: Plasma creatinine and urea:creatinine ratio in patients with raised plasma urea. Br Med J 2:929, 1977
5. Bjornsson TD: Use of serum creatinine concentrations to determine renal function. Clin Pharmacokinet 4:200, 1979
6. Rowe JW: Clinical research on aging: strategies and directions. N Engl J Med 297:1332, 1977
7. Cockcroft DW, Gault MH: Prediction of creatinine clearance from serum creatinine. Nephron 16:31, 1976
8. Wallach J: Interpretation of Diagnostic Tests, 3rd ed. Little, Brown & Co, Boston, 1981, p 96
9. Carrie BJ, Golbetz HV, Michaels AS, et al: Creatinine: an inadequate filtration marker in glomerular diseases. Am J Med 69:177, 1980
10. Brezis M, Rosen S, Epstein RH: Acute renal failure. The Kidney. Brenner BM, Rector FC Jr, Eds. WB Saunders Co, Philadelphia, 1986, p 735
11. Nanji AA, Campbell DJ: Falsely elevated serum creatinine values in diabetic ketoacidosis: clinical implications. Clin Biochem 14:91, 1981
12. Guay DR, Meatherall RC, Macauley PA: Interference of selected second and third generation cephalosporins with creatinine determination. Am J Hosp Pharm 40:435, 1983
13. Larsson R, Bodemar G, Kagedal B, et al: The effects of cimetidine (Tagamet) on renal function in patients with renal failure. Acta Med Scand 208:27, 1980
14. Shouval D, Ligumsky M, Ben-Ishay D: Effects of co-trimoxazole on normal creatinine clearance. Lancet 1:244, 1978
15. Thadhani R, Pascual M, Bonventre JV: Acute renal failure. N Engl J Med 334:1448, 1996
16. Espinel CH: The FE_{Na} test: use in the differential diagnosis of acute renal failure. JAMA 236:579, 1976
17. Shah DM, Browner BD, Dutton RE, et al: Cardiac output and pulmonary wedge pressure: use for evaluation of fluid replacement in trauma patients. Arch Surg 12:1161, 1977
18. Pascual J, Liano F, Ortuno J: The elderly patient with acute renal failure. J Am Soc Nephrol 6:144, 1995
19. Flamenbaum W, Gehr M, Gross M, et al: Acute renal failure associated with myoglobinemia and hemoglobinemia. Acute Renal Failure. Brenner BM, Lazarus JM, Eds. WB Saunders Co, Philadelphia, 1983, p 269
20. Gabow PA, Kaehny WD, Kelleher SP: The spectrum of rhabdomyolysis. Medicine (Baltimore) 61:141, 1982
21. Abuelo JG: Diagnosing vascular causes of renal failure. Ann Intern Med 123:601, 1995
22. Donahue JF: Acute bilateral cortical necrosis. Acute Renal Failure. Brenner BM, Lazarus JM, Eds. WB Saunders Co, Philadelphia, 1983, p 252
23. Lieberthal W, Levinsky NG: Treatment of acute tubular necrosis. Semin Nephrol 10:571, 1990
24. Wineman RJ: Endstage renal disease. Dial Transplant 7:1034, 1978
25. Mattern WD, Sommers SC, Kassirer JP: Oliguric acute renal failure in malignant hypertension. Am J Med 52:187, 1972
26. Henrich WL, Anderson RJ, Berns AS, et al: The role of renal nerves and prostaglandins in control of renal hemodynamics and plasma renin activity during hypotensive hemorrhage in the dog. J Clin Invest 61:744, 1978
27. Bonventre JV: Mechanisms of ischemic acute renal failure. Kidney Int 43:1160, 1993
28. Davis RF, Lappas DG, Kirklin JK, et al: Acute oliguria after cardiopulmonary bypass: renal functional improvement with low-dose dopamine infusion. Crit Care Med 10:852, 1982
29. Bonventre JV, Weinberg JM: Kidney preservation ex vivo for transplantation. Annu Rev Med 43:523, 1992
30. Cantarovich F, Galli C, Benedetti L, et al: High dose frusemide in established acute renal failure. Br Med J 4:449, 1973
31. Barry SR, Cohen A, Knochel JP, et al: Mannitol infusion: II. The prevention of acute functional renal failure during resection of an aneurysm of the abdominal aorta. N Engl J Med 264:967, 1961
32. Braun SR, Weiss FR, Keller AI, et al: Evaluation of the renal toxicity of heme proteins and their derivatives: a role in the genesis of acute tubular necrosis. J Exp Med 131:443, 1970
33. Bush HL, Huse JB, Johnson WC, et al: Prevention of renal insufficiency after abdominal aortic aneurysm resection by optimal volume loading. Arch Surg 116:1517, 1981
34. Better OS, Stein JH: Early management of shock and prophylaxis of acute renal failure in traumatic rhabdomyolysis. N Engl J Med 322:825, 1990

35. Rowe JW, Andres R, Tobin JD, et al: The effect of age on creatinine clearance in men: a cross sectional and longitudinal study. J Gerontol 31:155, 1976
36. Maschio G, Oldrizzi L, Tessitore N, et al: Effects of dietary protein and phosphorus restriction on the progression of early renal failure. Kidney Int 22:371, 1982
37. Abel RM, Beck CH Jr, Abbott WM, et al: Improved survival from acute renal failure after treatment with intravenous essential L-amino acids and glucose: results of a prospective double blind study. N Engl J Med 288:695, 1973
38. Hampers CL, Bailey GL, Hager EB, et al: Major surgery in patients on maintenance hemodialysis. Am J Surg 115:747, 1968
39. Brenowitz JB, Williams CD, Edwards WS: Major surgery in patients with chronic renal failure. Am J Surg 134:765, 1977
40. Rabiner SF: The effect of dialysis on platelet function of patients with renal failure. Ann NY Acad Sci 201:234, 1972
41. Hampers CL, Balufox MD, Merrill JP: Anticoagulation rebound after hemodialysis. N Engl J Med 275:776, 1966
42. Goldblum SE, Reed WP: Host defenses and immunologic alterations associated with chronic hemodialysis. Ann Intern Med 93:597, 1980
43. Burke JF: The use of preventive antibiotics in clinical surgery. Am Surg 39:6, 1973
44. Koide M, Waud BE: Serum potassium concentration after succinylcholine in patients with renal failure. Anesthesiology 36:142, 1972
45. Lillemoe KD, Romolo JL, Hamilton SR, et al: Intestinal necrosis due to sodium polystyrene (Kayexalate) in sorbitol enemas: clinical and experimental support for the hypothesis. Surgery 101:267, 1987
46. Crandell WB, MacDonald A: Nephropathy associated with methoxyflurane anesthesia. JAMA 205:798, 1968
47. Gillies IDS: Anaemia and anaesthesia. Br J Anaesth 46:589, 1974
48. Lazarus JM, Lowrie EG, Hampers CL, et al: Cardiovascular disease in uremic patients on hemodialysis. Kidney Int 7(suppl 2):167, 1975
49. Lazarus JM, Hampers CL, Lowrie EG, et al: Baroreceptor activity in normotensive and hypertensive uremic patients. Circulation 47:1015, 1973
50. Lazarus JM, Hampers CL, Bennett AH, et al: Urgent bilateral nephrectomy for severe hypertension. Ann Intern Med 76:733, 1972
51. Nayman J: Effect of renal failure on wound healing in dogs: response to hemodialysis following uremia induced by uranium nitrate. Ann Surg 164:227, 1966
52. Giordano C: Use of exogenous and endogenous urea for protein metabolism in normal and uremic subjects. J Lab Clin Med 62:231, 1963
53. Bennett WM: Altering drug dosage in patients with diseases of the kidney and liver. Clinical Uses of Drugs in Patients with Kidney and Liver Disease. Anderson RJ, Schrier RW, Eds. WB Saunders Co, Philadelphia, 1981, p 16
54. Harris RC, Meyer TW, Brenner BM: Nephron adaptation to renal injury. The Kidney. Brenner BM, Rector FC Jr, Eds. WB Saunders Co, Philadelphia, 1986, p 1553
55. Shimamura T, Morrison AB: A progressive glomerulosclerosis occurring in partial five-sixths nephrectomized rats. Am J Pathol 79:95, 1975
56. Hostetter TH, Olson JL, Rennke HG, et al: Hyperfiltration in remnant nephrons: a potentially adverse response to renal ablation. Am J Physiol 241:F85, 1981
57. Anderson S, Meyer TW, DeGraphenreid RL, et al: Control of glomerular hypertension preserves glomerular structure and function in rats with renal ablation (abstr). Clin Res 32:564A, 1984
58. Lindner A, Charra B, Sherrard DJ, et al: Accelerated atherosclerosis in prolonged maintenance hemodialysis. N Engl J Med 290:697, 1974
59. Bonomini V, Feletti C, Scolari MP, et al: Atherosclerosis in uremia: a longitudinal study. Am J Clin Nutr 33:1493, 1980
60. Green D, Stone NJ, Krumlovsky FA: Putative atherogenic factors in patients with chronic renal failure. Prog Cardiovasc Dis 26:133, 1983
61. Terman DS, Alfrey AC, Hammond WS, et al: Cardiac calcification in uremia: a clinical, biochemical and pathologic study. Am J Med 50:744, 1971
62. Lee JC, Downing SE: Negative inotropic effects of phenol on isolated cardiac muscle. Am J Pathol 102:367, 1981
63. Pehrsson SK, Lins LE: The role of trace elements in uremic heart failure. Nephron 34:93, 1983
64. Ahearn DJ, Maher JF: Heart failure as a complication of hemodialysis arteriovenous fistula. Ann Intern Med 77:201, 1972
65. Henrich WL, Hunt J, Nixon JV: Increased ionized calcium and left ventricular contractility during hemodialysis. N Engl J Med 310:19, 1984
66. Lindsay J Jr, Crawley IS, Callaway GM Jr: Chronic constrictive pericarditis following uremic hemopericardium. Am Heart J 79:390, 1970
67. Drüeke T, Le Pailleur C, Zingraff J, et al: Uremic cardiomyopathy and pericarditis. Adv Nephrol 9:33, 1980
68. Bailey GL, Hampers CL, Hager EB, et al: Uremic pericarditis: clinical features in management. Circulation 38:582, 1968
69. Collins HA, Killen DA, Gobbel WG Jr, et al: Pericardiectomy for uremic pericardial tamponade. Ann Thorac Surg 9:327, 1970
70. Mujais SL, Sabatini S, Kurtzman NA: Pathophysiology of the uremic syndrome. The Kidney. Brenner BM, Rector FC Jr, Eds. WB Saunders Co, Philadelphia, 1986, p 1587
71. Doniach I: Uremic edema of the lungs. AJR Am J Roentgenol 58:620, 1947
72. Crosbie WA, Snowden S, Parsons V: Changes in the lung capillary permeability in renal failure. Br Med J 4:388, 1972
73. Gibson DG: Haemodynamic factors in the development of acute pulmonary oedema in renal failure. Lancet 2:1217, 1966
74. Craddock PR, Fehr J, Brigham KL, et al: Complement and leukocyte mediated pulmonary dysfunction in hemodialysis. N Engl J Med 296:769, 1977
75. Bleyl U, Sander G, Schindler T: The pathology and biology of uremic pneumonitis. Intensive Care Med 7:193, 1981
76. Firooznia H, Pudlowski R, Golimbu C, et al: Diffuse interstitial calcification of the lungs in chronic renal failure mimicking pulmonary edema. Am J Radiol 129:1103, 1977
77. Gilbert L, Ribot S, Frankel H, et al: Fibrinous uremic pleuritis: a surgical entity. Chest 67:53, 1975
78. Mason EE: Gastrointestinal lesions occurring in uremia. Ann Intern Med 37:96, 1952
79. Bailey GL, Griffiths H, Lock JP, et al: Gastrointestinal abnormalities in uremia (abstr). Am Soc Nephrol 5:5, 1971
80. Adams PL, Rutsky EA, Rostand SG, et al: Lower gastrointestinal tract dysfunction in patients receiving long-term hemodialysis. Arch Intern Med 142:303, 1982
81. Misra MK, Pinkus GS, Birtch AG, et al: Major colonic diseases complicating renal transplantation. Surgery 73:942, 1973
82. Morris J, Stellata TA, Lieberman J, et al: The utility of computed tomography in colonic diverticulitis. Ann Surg 204:128, 1986
83. Chen TS, Leevy CM: Liver regeneration and uraemia. Br J Exp Pathol 54:591, 1977
84. Grossman SB, Yap SH, Shafritz DA: Influence of chronic renal failure on protein synthesis and albumin metabolism in rat liver. J Clin Invest 59:869, 1977
85. Dienstag JL, Stevens CE, Szmuness W: The epidemiology of non-A, non-B hepatitis: emerging patterns. Non-A, Non-B Hepatitis. Gerety RJ, Ed. Academic Press, Orlando, Florida, 1981, p 119
86. Brickman AS, Coburn JW, Massry SG, et al: 1,25-dihydroxy-vitamin D3 in normal man and patients with renal failure. Ann Intern Med 80:161, 1974
87. Arnaud CD: Hyperparathyroidism and renal failure. Kidney Int 4:89, 1973
88. Eschbach JW, Adamson JW: Anemia of end-stage renal disease (ESRD). Kidney Int 28:1, 1985
89. Eschbach JW: The anemia of chronic renal failure: pathophysiology and the effects of recombinant erythropoietin. Kidney Int 35:134, 1989
90. Hocken AG, Marwah PK: Iatrogenic contribution to anaemia of chronic renal failure. Lancet 1:164, 1971
91. Carvalho AC: Bleeding in a uremia: a clinical challenge (editorial). N Engl J Med 308:38, 1983
92. Guild WR, Bray G, Merrill JP: Hemopericardium with cardiac tamponade in chronic uremia. N Engl J Med 257:230, 1957
93. Talalla A, Halbrook H, Barbour BH, et al: Subdural hematoma associated with long-term hemodialysis for chronic renal disease. JAMA 212:1847, 1970
94. Galen MA, Steinberg SM, Lowrie EG, et al: Hemorrhagic pleural effusion in patients undergoing chronic hemodialysis. Ann Intern Med 82:359, 1975
95. Llach F, Arieff AI, Massry SG: Renal vein thrombosis and nephrotic syndrome. Ann Intern Med 83:8, 1975
96. Kauffmann RH, Veltkamp JJ, Van Tilburg NH, et al: Acquired antithrombin III deficiency and thrombosis in the nephrotic syndrome. Am J Med 65:607, 1978
97. Stein IM, Cohen BD, Kornhauser RS: Guanidinosuccinic acid in renal failure, experimental azotemia and inborn errors of the urea cycle. N Engl J Med 280:926, 1969
98. Rabiner SF: The effect of dialysis on platelet function of patients with renal failure. Ann NY Acad Sci 201:234, 1972
99. Hampers CI, Blaufox MD, Merril JP: Anticoagulation rebound after hemodialysis. N Engl J Med 275:776, 1966
100. Eschbach JW: The anemia of chronic renal failure: pathophysiology and the effects of recombinant erythropoietin. Kidney Int 35:134, 1989
101. Lim VS, DeGowin RL, Zavala D, et al: Recombinant human erythropoietin treatment in pre-dialysis patients: a double-blind placebo-controlled trial. Ann Intern Med 110:108, 1989
102. Tolkoff-Rubin NE, Pascual M: Chronic renal failure. Scientific American Medicine, Vol 2. Rubenstein E, Federman DD, Eds. Scientific American, Inc., New York, 1997, Sect 10, Subsect X, p 11
103. Craddock PR, Fehr J, Dalmasso AP, et al: Hemodialysis leukopenia: pulmonary vascular leukostasis resulting from complement activation by dialyzer cellophane membranes. J Clin Invest 59:879, 1977
104. Clark RA, Hamory BH, Ford GH, et al: Chemotaxis in acute renal failure. J Infect Dis 126:460, 1972
105. Salant DJ, Glover AM, Anderson R, et al: Depressed neutrophil chemotaxis in patients with chronic renal failure and after renal transplantation. J Lab Clin Med 88:536, 1976
106. Greene WH, Ray CR, Mauer SM, et al: The effect of hemodialysis on neutrophil chemotactic responsiveness. J Lab Clin Med 88:971, 1976
107. Touraine JL, Touraine F, Revillard JP, et al: T-lymphocytes and serum inhibitors of cell-mediated immunity in renal insufficiency. Nephron 14:195, 1975

108. Holdsworth SR, Fitzgerald MG, Hosking CS, et al: The effect of maintenance dialysis on lymphocyte function: I. Haemodialysis. Clin Exp Immunol 33:95, 1978
109. Boulton-Jones JM, Vick R, Cameron JS, et al: Immune responses in uremia. Clin Nephrol 1:251, 1973
110. Stoloff IL, Stout R, Myerson RM, et al: Production of antibody in patients with uremia. N Engl J Med 259:320, 1958
111. Pabico RC, Douglas RG, Betts RF, et al: Influenza vaccination of patients with glomerular diseases. Ann Intern Med 81:171, 1974
112. Delaporte C, Bergström J, Broyer M: Variation in muscle cell protein of severely uraemic children. Kidney Int 10:239, 1976
113. Mallette LE, Patten BM, Engel WK: Neuromuscular disease in secondary hyperparathyroidism. Ann Intern Med 82:474, 1975
114. Schott GD, Wills MR: Muscle weakness in osteomalacia. Lancet 1:626, 1976
115. Floyd M, Ayyar DR, Barwick DD, et al: Myopathy in chronic renal failure. Q J Med 43:509, 1974
116. Henderson RG, Russell RG, Ledingham JG, et al: Effects of 1,25-dihydroxycholecalciferol on calcium absorption, muscle weakness, and bone disease in chronic renal failure. Lancet 1:379, 1974
117. Handa SP: Uremic bursitis. Ann Intern Med 89:723, 1978
118. Cruz C, Shah SV: Dialysis elbow: olecranon bursitis from long term hemodialysis. JAMA 238:243, 1977
119. Lotem M, Bernheim J, Conforty B: Spontaneous rupture of tendons. N Engl J Med 266:969, 1962
120. Mirahmadi KS, Coburn JW, Bluestone R: Calcific periarthritis and hemodialysis. JAMA 223:548, 1973
121. Matthews M, Shen FH, Lindner A, et al: Septic arthritis in hemodialyzed patients. Nephron 25:87, 1980
122. Mason RS, Lissner D, Wilkinson M, et al: Vitamin D metabolites and their relationship to azotaemic osteodystrophy. Clin Endocrinol (Oxf) 13:375, 1980
123. Coburn JW, Slatopolsky E: Vitamin D, parathyroid hormone and renal osteodystrophy. The Kidney. Brenner BM, Rector FC Jr, Eds. WB Saunders Co, Philadelphia, 1987, p 1657
124. Wills MR, Savory J: Aluminum poisoning: dialysis encephalopathy, osteomalacia, and anaemia. Lancet 2:29, 1983
125. Litzow JR, Lemann J Jr, Lennon EJ: The effect of treatment of acidosis on calcium balance in patients with chronic azotemic renal disease. J Clin Invest 46:280, 1967
126. Slatopolsky E, Weerts C, Lopez S, et al: Calcium carbonate is an effective phosphorus-binder in dialysis patients. Kidney Int 27:173, 1985
127. Meyrier A, Marsac J, Richet G: The influence of a high calcium carbonate intake on bone disease in patients undergoing hemodialysis. Kidney Int 4:146, 1973
128. Regan RJ, Peacock M, Rosen SM, et al: Effect of dialysate calcium concentration on bone disease in patients on hemodialysis. Kidney Int 10:246, 1976
129. Brickman AS, Sherrard DJ, Jowsey J, et al: 1,25-Dihydroxycholecalciferol: effect on skeletal lesions and plasma parathyroid hormone levels in uremic osteodystrophy. Arch Intern Med 134:883, 1974
130. Ackrill P, Ralston AJ, Day JP, et al: Successful removal of aluminum from patients with dialysis encephalopathy (letter). Lancet 2:692, 1980
131. Wilson RE, Hampers CL, Bernstein DS, et al: Subtotal parathyroidectomy in chronic renal failure. Ann Surg 174:640, 1971
132. Hodsman AB, Sherrard DJ, Wong EGC, et al: Vitamin-D-resistant osteomalacia in hemodialysis patients lacking secondary hyperparathyroidism. Ann Intern Med 94:629, 1981
133. Arieff AI: Neurological manifestations of uremia. The Kidney. Brenner BM, Rector FC Jr, Eds. WB Saunders Co, Philadelphia, 1986, p 1731
134. Arieff AI: Dialysis disequilibrium syndrome: current concepts on pathogenesis. Controversies in Nephrology. Schreiner GE, Winchester JF, Eds. Georgetown University Press, Washington, DC, 1982, p 367
135. Flendrig JA, Kruis H, Das HA: Aluminum and dialysis dementia (letter). Lancet 1:1235, 1976
136. Arieff AI, Carroll HJ: Nonketotic hyperosmolar coma with hyperglycemia: clinical features, pathophysiology, renal function, acid-base balance, plasma-cerebrospinal fluid equilibria and the effects of therapy in 37 cases. Medicine (Baltimore) 51:73, 1972
137. Rosen T: Uremic pruritus: a review. Cutis 23:790, 1979
138. Massry SG, Puputzer MM, Coburn JW, et al: Intractable pruritus as a manifestation of secondary hyperparathyroidism in uremia. N Engl J Med 279:697, 1968
139. Androgue HJ, Frazier MR, Zeluff B, et al: Systemic calciphylaxis revisited. Am J Nephrol 1:177, 1981
140. Scoggins RB, Haran WR: Cutaneous manifestations of hyperlipidemia and uremia. Postgrad Med 41:537, 1967
141. Aronin N, Liotta AS, Schickmanter B, et al: Impaired clearance of beta-lipotropin in uremia. J Clin Endocrinol Med 53:797, 1981
142. Hatch FE: Reversing the anemia of renal failure. Hosp Pract 25(25A):25, 1990

Acknowledgment

Figure 1 Dana Burns-Pizer.

73 ADRENAL INSUFFICIENCY

Valerie J. Halpin, M.D., and Jeffrey A. Norton, M.D.

Recognition and Management of Adrenal Insufficiency

Adrenal glucocorticoid or mineralocorticoid insufficiency is a rare clinical problem. It may be the direct result of a primary adrenal lesion (primary adrenal insufficiency), or it may be secondary to an abnormality in the pituitary or the hypothalamus (secondary adrenal insufficiency) (see below). Either primary or secondary adrenal insufficiency may lead to so-called adrenal crisis (acute adrenal insufficiency) perioperatively if the hypothalamus-pituitary-adrenal (HPA) axis is unable to generate an appropriate stress level of cortisol [see Discussion, below]. Adrenal crisis is an uncommon occurrence; however, if adrenal insufficiency is left untreated, the consequences may be severe.[1,2] Accordingly, it is essential that surgeons know how to recognize adrenal insufficiency and how to identify those patients who will benefit from perioperative glucocorticoid coverage.

Recognition and Classification

A fundamental issue is how to determine which patients need perioperative adrenal steroid replacement and which do not. Involved in this issue is the question of whether the insufficiency is primary or secondary [see Sidebar Causes of Primary and Secondary Adrenal Insufficiency]. The initial clues should come from the history and the physical examination. Patients who have been receiving prednisone or another steroid preparation [see Table 1] for extended periods after organ transplantation or as treatment for systemic diseases such as systemic lupus erythematosus or rheumatoid arthritis are at risk for secondary adrenal cortical insufficiency. Their serum cortisol levels are unlikely to increase in response to surgical stress. Patients who are receiving small doses of prednisone every other day or who have received a short course of high-dose corticosteroid therapy in the recent past are at lesser risk for secondary insufficiency. They may be able to generate an appropriate stress cortisol response during some procedures.

On physical examination, persons with secondary insufficiency may be identified by various clinical features of Cushing's syndrome or hypercortisolism (e.g., hypertension, diabetes, weight gain, truncal obesity, hirsutism, muscle weakness, osteoporosis, striae, buffalo hump, and easy bruising).

Persons with primary adrenal insufficiency or Addison's disease may be identified by their thin, hyperpigmented appearance and by various characteristic complaints (e.g., fatigue, weakness, nausea, abdominal pain, diarrhea, postural dizziness, myalgias, and arthralgias).

It is essential to be alert for any signs of possible adrenal crisis. Patients in acute adrenal crisis present with a constellation of symptoms that may include unexplained hypotension, fever, nausea, vomiting, abdominal pain, weakness, or dizziness. These symptoms are not unique to acute adrenal insufficiency and may resemble those of severe infection. In fact, the clinical picture of adrenal crisis may mimic that of septic shock. Acute blood loss, severe dehydration, significant infection, or any of a number of other stressful conditions may precipitate an adrenal crisis. Patients at risk for acute hypocortisolism include those who have active tuberculosis, those who are actively bleeding, and those who are receiving maintenance glucocorticoid therapy after a recent adrenalectomy for correction of hypercortisolism.

Management

ADRENAL CRISIS

If the diagnosis of adrenal crisis is suspected, hydrocortisone should immediately be given intravenously, and steps should be taken to correct precipitating factors.

First, blood is drawn and sent for measurement of serum levels of cortisol, glucose, sodium, potassium, blood urea nitrogen (BUN), and creatinine. A complete blood count is obtained. Treatment then proceeds before the laboratory results come in. A 200 mg bolus of hydrocortisone is rapidly administered intravenously, followed by infusion of glucose and saline to correct dehydration and maintain volume. If the patient has acute adrenal insufficiency, there should be a rapid response to I.V. hydrocortisone: blood pressure should return to normal within one to two hours. If there is no response to the hydrocortisone bolus, adrenal crisis is unlikely. Steroid therapy is discontinued, and a search for another cause of the clinical condition is initiated.

If the patient is improving clinically and the results of the

Recognition and Management of Adrenal Insufficiency

History or physical examination is suggestive of adrenal insufficiency

Clues include a history of steroid use; clinical features of Cushing's syndrome or hypercortisolism (hypertension, diabetes, weight gain, truncal obesity, hirsutism, muscle weakness, osteoporosis, striae, buffalo hump, easy bruising); a thin, pigmented appearance; and various characteristic complaints (fatigue, weakness, nausea, abdominal pain, diarrhea, postural dizziness, myalgia, arthralgia).

Be particularly alert for signs or symptoms of acute adrenal insufficiency (adrenal crisis): unexplained hypotension, fever, nausea, vomiting, abdominal pain, weakness, dizziness.

Attempt to determine whether insufficiency is primary (caused by damage to adrenal) or secondary (caused by inadequate adrenal stimulation) [see Sidebar Causes of Primary and Secondary Adrenal Insufficiency].

Patient exhibits signs or symptoms of adrenal crisis

Treat immediately

Draw blood for measurement of serum cortisol, glucose, Na^+, K^+, BUN, and creatinine. Obtain CBC. *Do not wait for lab results to return.*

Give 200 mg bolus of hydrocortisone I.V., followed by glucose and saline infusion.

Patient does not respond to hydrocortisone

Discontinue steroids.
Search for another cause of clinical condition.

Patient responds to hydrocortisone, and lab results support diagnosis

Continue hydrocortisone, first at 100 mg q. 8 hr for 2 days, then 50 mg q. 8 hr for 2 days, then 25 mg q. 8 hr for 2 days, and finally 15 mg/m²/day.

If patient has primary insufficiency, give fludrocortisone, 0.1–0.2 mg/day, when hydrocortisone dosage < 50 mg/day.

When patient stabilizes, perform ACTH test to confirm diagnosis.

Determine cause of adrenal crisis.

Patient has known or suspected adrenal insufficiency

Patient has primary adrenal insufficiency or secondary insufficiency from long-term steroid therapy

Serum cortisol < 20 μg/dl with < 7 μg/dl increase over baseline

HPA axis function is abnormal. Steroid supplementation is necessary.

Determine amount of steroid coverage needed according to magnitude of surgical procedure

Major procedure

Give hydrocortisone, 100–150 mg I.V., before operation.

Continue hydrocortisone, first at 50 mg I.V. q. 8 hr for 2 days, then 25 mg I.V. q. 8 hr for 3 days.

If there are no complications, resume usual steroid dosage.

Procedure of moderate magnitude

Give hydrocortisone, 50–75 mg I.V., before operation.

Give an additional 50–75 mg over remainder of operative day.

Give 50–75 mg on postoperative day 1.

Resume usual steroid dosage on postoperative day 2.

Minor procedure

Give hydrocortisone, 25 mg I.V., before operation.

Give usual daily dose on operative day.

Resume usual steroid dosage on postoperative day 1.

Patient once took steroids but no longer does or else is taking low doses every other day

Perform ACTH stimulation test.

Serum cortisol > 20 µg/dl with > 7 µg/dl increase over baseline

HPA axis function is normal. No steroid supplementation is necessary.

Patient is undergoing surgical correction of endogenous hypercortisolism

Glucocorticoid replacement is always necessary. Do *not* give steroids preoperatively.

Give hydrocortisone, 100 mg I.V., intraoperatively once tumor or second adrenal is removed.

Initiate replacement therapy, first at 50 mg I.V. q. 8 hr for 2 days, then 25 mg I.V. q. 8 hr for 3 days, and finally 12–15 mg/m^2/day.

Patient underwent unilateral adrenalectomy

Replacement therapy continues until HPA axis function returns.

Perform ACTH stimulation test 6 mo after procedure and every 3–6 mo thereafter to determine when steroids can be discontinued.

Patient underwent bilateral adrenalectomy

Replacement therapy continues on permanent basis.

When hydrocortisone dosage < 50 mg/day, give fludrocortisone, 0.1 mg/day.

Causes of Primary and Secondary Adrenal Insufficiency

Primary Insufficiency

In primary adrenal insufficiency, the adrenal cortex is incapable of producing sufficient amounts of adrenal hormones, usually because of a disease process that destroys the adrenal gland. Secretion of both glucocorticoids and mineralocorticoids is deficient. Although primary adrenal insufficiency is rare, its etiology is varied. In the industrialized world, autoimmune disease is the most common cause. There are two associated autoimmune polyendocrine syndromes, type 1 and type 2. Type 1 includes adrenal insufficiency, hypoparathyroidism, mucocutaneous candidiasis, and, less commonly, hypogonadism, pernicious anemia, chronic active hepatitis, and alopecia. Type 2 is associated with autoimmune thyroid disease, diabetes mellitus, and adrenal insufficiency.

Worldwide, tuberculosis remains the most prominent cause of hypocortisolism. Other granulomatous diseases, such as sarcoidosis and some fungal infections, may exhibit a similar clinical picture. Primary adrenal insufficiency may occur in association with adrenal hemorrhage; it is usually attributable to anticoagulation or severe infection but may also be seen after trauma or severe hypertension. Adrenal metastases from a primary lesion elsewhere are not unusual, but metastases rarely cause inadequate adrenocortical function. The cancers most often associated with adrenal metastases are breast cancer, lung cancer, stomach cancer, colon cancer, melanoma, and lymphoma.

Other possible causes of primary adrenal insufficiency are congenital disorders, the acquired immunodeficiency syndrome (AIDS), and the demyelinating syndromes, including adrenoleukodystrophy and adrenomyeloneuropathy.

Secondary Insufficiency

In secondary adrenal insufficiency, hypocortisolism is caused by inadequate stimulation of the adrenal gland. Mineralocorticoid production is normal because aldosterone secretion is regulated via the renin-angiotensin system, independently of pituitary adrenocorticotropic hormone (ACTH) secretion. The etiology of secondary adrenal insufficiency has three main components: adrenal suppression after the administration of exogenous glucocorticoid or ACTH, adrenal suppression after the surgical correction of endogenous hypercortisolism, and ACTH insufficiency resulting from abnormalities of the hypothalamus or the pituitary gland.

The most common specific cause of secondary adrenal insufficiency is long-term prescription of exogenous glucocorticoids to treat other diseases. Any patient receiving glucocorticoids on a daily basis just before operation is clearly at risk for adrenal insufficiency. Furthermore, any patient who has taken the equivalent of 20 to 30 mg/day of prednisone [see Table 1] for longer than five consecutive days in the previous 12 months is at risk.[18] It is difficult to know in advance which patients will experience hypothalamus-pituitary-adrenal (HPA) axis suppression: neither the glucocorticoid dosage nor the duration of therapy is predictive of the eventual degree of adrenal suppression.[8] Because patients may not think to mention steroid therapy that started and stopped several months ago, the surgeon must make a point of inquiring about steroid use if the patient has a medical problem that is commonly treated with glucocorticoids (e.g., asthma, rheumatoid arthritis, autoimmune diseases, collagen vascular diseases, or immunosuppression in transplant recipients).

Pituitary failure can also lead to secondary adrenal insufficiency, but it is a much less common cause. In patients who have undergone transsphenoidal surgery, decreased production of ACTH may occur and may result in secondary adrenal insufficiency.

---

initial laboratory evaluation support the diagnosis, glucocorticoid replacement is continued. (Laboratory findings consistent with the diagnosis of acute adrenal crisis include a serum cortisol level lower than 20 μg/dl, hyponatremia, hyperkalemia, hypoglycemia, and azotemia. The complete blood count may show anemia, leukopenia, lymphocytosis, and eosinophilia.) After the initial bolus of hydrocortisone, hydrocortisone is given intravenously at a dosage of 100 mg every eight hours for two days. The hydrocortisone dosage is reduced by half every two days, first to 50 mg I.V. every eight hours and then to 25 mg I.V. every eight hours. Finally, a replacement regimen is initiated at a dosage of 15 mg/m²/day. Patients with primary adrenal insufficiency require mineralocorticoid replacement (fludrocortisone, 0.1 to 0.2 mg/day) when the hydrocortisone dosage is less than 50 mg/day.

Once the patient's condition is stable, the diagnosis of adrenal crisis is confirmed by means of an adrenocorticotropic hormone (ACTH) stimulation test [see Table 2]. Finally, the cause of the adrenal crisis is determined.

KNOWN OR SUSPECTED ADRENAL INSUFFICIENCY

Patients known to have primary adrenal insufficiency or chronic secondary adrenal insufficiency caused by long-term glucocorticoid treatment for another disease process must receive glucocorticoid treatment during surgical procedures. On the other hand, patients who had previously been treated with glucocorticoids but are no longer taking them and patients who are currently receiving glucocorticoids in low doses every other day may in fact be able to generate an appropriate stress cortisol response during operation and consequently may not need perioperative

Table 1 Selected Corticosteroid Preparations

Preparation	Equivalent Doses (mg)	Glucocorticoid Activity*	Mineralocorticoid Activity*
Short-acting (8–12 hr)			
Hydrocortisone	20	1	1
Cortisone	25	0.80	0.80
Intermediate-acting (12–36 hr)			
Prednisone	5	4	0.80
Prednisolone	5	4	0.80
Methylprednisolone	4	5	0
Triamcinolone	4	5	0
Long-acting (36–54 hr)			
Betamethasone	0.60	25	0
Dexamethasone	0.75	30	0
Mineralocorticoid			
Fludrocortisone	—	10	125

*Ranked on a scale rating hydrocortisone as 1.

Table 2 — ACTH Stimulation Test

1. Measure baseline serum cortisol level
2. Give 250 μg of ACTH by I.V. bolus or I.M. injection
3. Draw blood, and measure serum cortisol level 30 and 60 min after administration of ACTH
4. Interpret results:
   - If serum cortisol level > 20 μg/dl and an increase > 7 μg/dl is noted after ACTH administration, HPA axis function is normal
   - If serum cortisol level < 20 μg/dl and an increase > 7 μg/dl is noted after ACTH administration, HPA axis function is abnormal

glucocorticoid replacement. If enough time is available before an elective surgical procedure, an ACTH stimulation test can be performed to ascertain whether the stress response is abnormal and thus whether glucocorticoid replacement is called for. If the ACTH stimulation test yields normal results, then HPA axis function is adequate and there is no need for any perioperative steroid coverage.

If, however, the ACTH test yields abnormal results or the patient is known to have chronic adrenal insufficiency, the amount of cortisol coverage required must be assessed. This assessment is made on the basis of the magnitude of the surgical procedure (i.e., major, moderate, or minor). The stress response to surgery ranges from minimal elevation of the cortisol level after minor procedures to a total cortisol production of 200 mg/day after major procedures.[3-5] Perioperative steroid coverage should approximate the expected stress cortisol response but need not exceed it.[6] If the patient's maintenance glucocorticoid dosage equals or exceeds the expected stress cortisol production, he or she may receive the maintenance dosage equivalent of cortisol preoperatively, with no additional supplementation. Preferably, cortisol should be administered intravenously in an easily hydrolyzable form (e.g., hydrocortisone hemisuccinate or hydrocortisone phosphate).

Coverage for major, moderate, and minor procedures is provided as follows. Patients undergoing major surgical procedures (e.g., the Whipple procedure, esophagogastrectomy, coronary artery bypass grafting, and thoracotomy) should receive 100 to 150 mg of hydrocortisone intravenously before operation. Hydrocortisone coverage is continued at a dosage of 50 mg I.V. every eight hours for two days. The dosage is then reduced to 25 mg I.V. every eight hours for an additional three days. After this period, the usual dosage may be resumed, provided that there are no complications. Patients undergoing surgical procedures of moderate magnitude (e.g., cholecystectomy, appendectomy, joint replacement, colectomy, and hysterectomy) should receive hydrocortisone, 50 to 75 mg I.V., before operation and then an additional 50 to 75 mg I.V. over the remainder of the day of the operation. Another 50 to 75 mg I.V. is given on postoperative day 1, and the usual steroid dosage may be resumed on postoperative day 2. Patients undergoing procedures done under local anesthesia (e.g., herniorrhaphy and dental procedures) should receive hydrocortisone, 25 mg I.V. (or the equivalent), preoperatively on the day of the procedure; the usual dosage may be resumed on postoperative day 1.

Adrenal Insufficiency after Surgical Correction of Endogenous Hypercortisolism

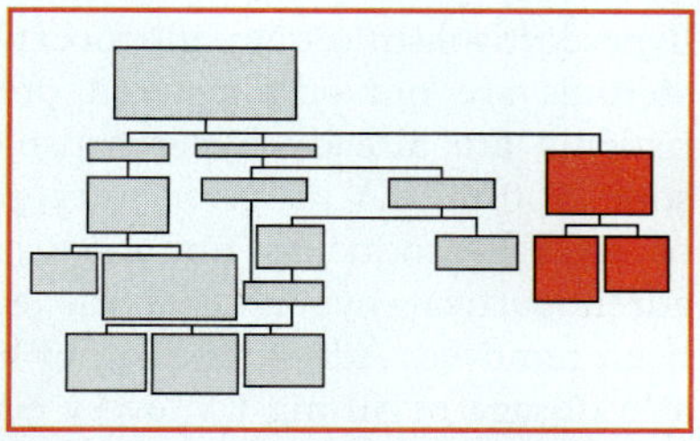

Cushing's syndrome is a hypercortisolemic state that results either from overproduction of cortisol by an adrenocortical adenoma or carcinoma or from overproduction of ACTH by a pituitary tumor or another ACTH-producing tumor. The hypercortisolemia causes suppression of the HPA axis in much the same way that long-term steroid use does, via suppression of the hypothalamus or the pituitary gland [see Figure 1]. Adrenal insufficiency is manifested after surgical removal of the tumor.

All patients undergoing surgical treatment of endogenous

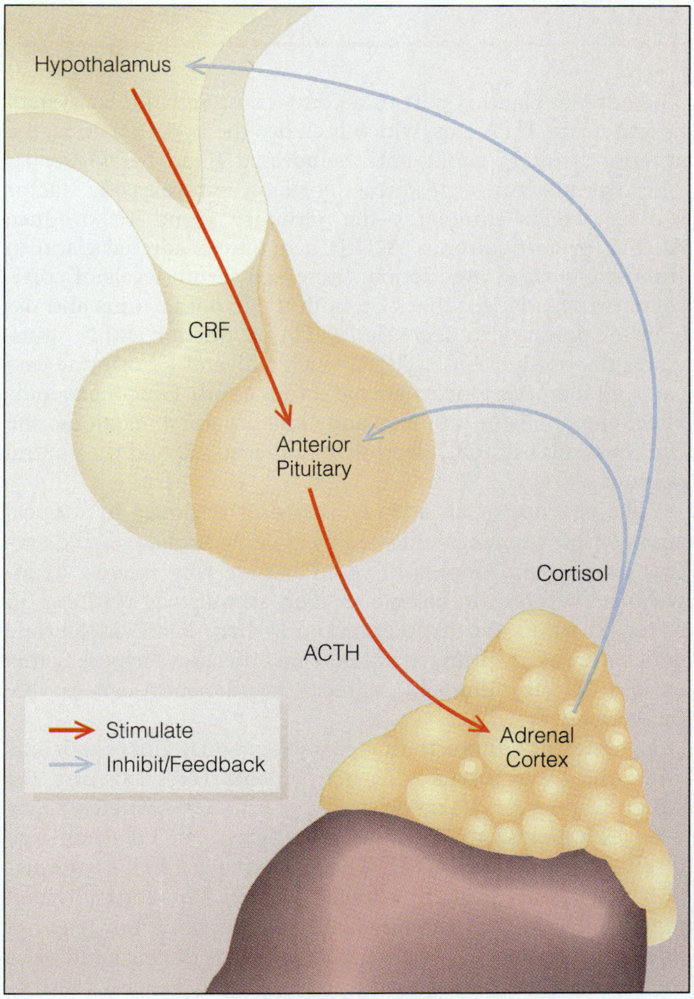

Figure 1 Shown is a schematic representation of the hypothalamus-pituitary-adrenal (HPA) axis. The hypothalamus produces corticotropin-releasing factor (CRF), which stimulates the pituitary to release adrenocorticotropic hormone (ACTH), or corticotropin. ACTH acts on the adrenal, stimulating production of cortisol. When serum levels of cortisol rise, negative feedback prompts the pituitary and the hypothalamus to decrease ACTH production.

hypercortisolism require glucocorticoid replacement. Corticosteroids are not administered preoperatively, because these patients are already hypercortisolemic. Instead, hydrocortisone, 100 mg I.V., is given intraoperatively once the cortisol- or ACTH-producing tumor—or, in patients with primary adrenocortical hyperplasia, the second adrenal gland—has been removed. Administration of hydrocortisone is continued at a dosage of 50 mg I.V. every eight hours for two days and then at a dosage of 25 mg I.V. every eight hours for an additional three days. The final replacement dosage is 12 to 15 mg/m^2/day. This dosage may be adjusted as necessary to prevent symptoms and signs of adrenal insufficiency. All patients should be advised to wear a medical identification bracelet notifying health care workers that adrenal insufficiency may result from any condition that evokes the stress response.

In patients who have undergone unilateral adrenalectomy for hypercortisolemia, replacement therapy continues until the hypothalamus-adrenal-pituitary axis recovers. To assess the status of the hypothalamus-adrenal-pituitary axis, an ACTH stimulation test is performed six months after operation and again every three to six months thereafter until the cortisol response returns to normal (> 20 μg/dl and a > 7 μg/dl increment over baseline levels). Once the response is normal, the daily replacement dosage of steroids can be rapidly tapered and eventually discontinued.[7] In patients who have undergone bilateral adrenalectomy, replacement hydrocortisone therapy continues indefinitely. Mineralocorticoid replacement is also required when the hydrocortisone dosage is less than 50 mg/day; the standard starting regimen is fludrocortisone acetate, 0.1 mg/day orally. Normal serum sodium and potassium levels, normal blood pressure, and the absence of postural hypotension indicate that replacement therapy is efficacious. Again, patients should be advised to wear a medical identification bracelet.

Discussion

The adrenal gland is part of a complex interglandular system known as the HPA axis, which includes the hypothalamus, the anterior pituitary gland, and the adrenal gland [see Figure 1]. The hypothalamus produces corticotropin-releasing factor (CRF), which stimulates the pituitary gland to produce ACTH, or corticotropin. ACTH acts on the adrenal gland to stimulate cortisol production. Increased serum levels of cortisol exert negative feedback on both the hypothalamus and the anterior pituitary to decrease ACTH production. Stress stimulates the production of CRF, which activates a hormone cascade to increase glucocorticoid production. Glucocorticoids affect metabolism, immune and inflammatory reactions, the cardiovascular system, electrolyte homeostasis, and the central nervous system.

The absence of an adequate cortisol response to surgical stress or infection is manifested by hypoglycemia, reduced cardiac output, and decreased vascular tone with relative hypovolemia. Vasopressin release is then stimulated, resulting in water retention and hyponatremia. If there is an aldosterone deficiency, as in primary adrenal insufficiency, hyperkalemia ensues. If left untreated, adrenal insufficiency can be life threatening.

Long-term administration of exogenous glucocorticoids alters the usual interactions between the HPA axis and the stress response. Glucocorticoids given at pharmacological dosages suppress the hypothalamic release of CRF and the pituitary release of ACTH. The inadequate adrenal stimulation that results leads to adrenal atrophy. The adrenal gland may be able to maintain adequate daily function but may not be able to produce sufficient glucocorticoids during conditions that evoke a maximal stress response, such as general anesthesia and major surgical procedures. The HPA axis may recover if the glucocorticoid dosage is reduced to maintenance levels or if glucocorticoids are given in low doses every other day; however, neither low dosages, shortened duration of therapy, nor an every-other-day regimen guarantees recovery of the normal glucocorticoid stress response.[8] HPA axis testing, specifically the ACTH stimulation test [see Table 2], must be done unless stress doses of glucocorticoids are administered.

Endogenous hypercortisolism, or Cushing's syndrome, affects the hypothalamus and pituitary in much the same way as long-term administration of exogenous glucocorticoids. The HPA axis is suppressed immediately after operation and in the postoperative period. In patients receiving maintenance glucocorticoid therapy (hydrocortisone, 12 to 15 mg/m^2/day), the time to recovery of HPA axis function ranges from nine months to two years.[7] Assessment of the HPA axis by means of ACTH testing should begin six months after operation and should be repeated every three to six months thereafter until normal function has been regained. Once adrenal function has returned to normal, as defined by a normal ACTH stimulation test result, maintenance hydrocortisone therapy can be discontinued. Thus, the ACTH stimulation test can be used as a guide to the optimal duration of postoperative glucocorticoid replacement after the resection of a cortisol-secreting tumor.[7]

There is evidence to suggest that some patients receiving exogenous glucocorticoids may not require perioperative stress-dose glucocorticoid coverage.[9-11] This evidence derives from studies in which patients underwent surgery without any glucocorticoid coverage and experienced no untoward effects; however, because the incidence of adrenal insufficiency is so low, the effect of steroid coverage could not be defined with certainty on the basis of the relatively small numbers of patients included in these studies. In one animal study, subphysiologic levels of cortisol replacement had detrimental effects on clinical outcome (including increased mortality) after cholecystectomy in adrenalectomized primates.[2] Given the impossibility of predicting the degree of HPA suppression and the adequacy of the patient's cortisol response to surgical or anesthetic stress, one cannot assume that the patient will be able to generate the necessary physiologic levels of cortisol. Therefore, either HPA axis function must be assessed via an ACTH stimulation test or steroids must be administered perioperatively in amounts approximately equivalent to the expected stress glucocorticoid response.[12]

Some investigators have suggested that elements of the surgical stress response may actually be detrimental to the patient.[13] The production of neuroendocrine hormones (including cortisol) and the local release of cytokines increase metabolism, heart rate, and coagulability and alter immune function. As a consequence, the stress response may increase cardiac and vascular morbidity and foster postoperative immunosuppression and infection. A few studies have examined the results of modifying the biochemical parameters of the stress response.[14-17] It has been clearly demonstrated that the cortisol response is modified—and, in some cases, completely abolished—by epidural anesthesia. Studies comparing stress response and postoperative morbidity in patients undergoing general anesthesia with those in patients undergoing epidural anesthesia suggest that epidural anesthesia has a beneficial effect.[17] At present, the data are insufficient to establish a clear relation between reduction of the stress response and reduction of cardiac and vascular morbidity. More work is necessary to elucidate which components of the stress response are beneficial and which are not. The results of such work may have a significant bearing on the necessity of perioperative cortisol replacement. Until the effects of the surgical stress response can be further defined, perioperative steroid coverage must be continued. Studies have also shown, however, that the glucocorticoid dosage can be significantly reduced when the surgical procedure is one that evokes a relatively minor stress response.[6]

References

1. Kehlet H: Clinical course and hypothalamic-pituitary-adrenocortical function in glucocorticoid-treated surgical patients. FADL's Forlag, Copenhagen, 1976
2. Udelsman R, Ramp J, Gallucci WT, et al: Adaptation during surgical stress—a reevaluation of the role of glucocorticoids. J Clin Invest 44:539, 1986
3. Udelsman R, Norton J, Jelenich SE, et al: Responses of the hypothalamic-pituitary-adrenal and renin-angiotensin axis and the sympathetic system during controlled surgical and anesthetic stress. J Clin Endocrinol Metab 64:986, 1987
4. Peterson RE: The miscible pool and turnover rate of adrenocortical steroids in man. Recent Prog Hormone Res 15:231, 1959
5. Peterson RE, Nokes G, Chen PS, et al: Estrogens and adrenocortical function in man. J Clin Endocrinol Metab 20:495, 1960
6. Salem M, Tainsh RE Jr, Bromberg J, et al: Perioperative glucocorticoid coverage: a reassessment 42 years after emergence of a problem. Ann Surg 219:416, 1994
7. Doherty G, Nieman LK, Cutler GB Jr, et al: Time to recovery of the hypothalamic-pituitary-adrenal axis after curative resection of adrenal tumors in patients with Cushing's syndrome. Surgery 108:1085, 1990
8. Schlaghecke R, Kornely E, Santen RT, et al: The effect of long-term glucocorticoid therapy on pituitary-adrenal responses to exogenous corticotropin-releasing hormone. N Engl J Med 326:226, 1992
9. Bromberg JS, Alfrey EJ, Barker CF, et al: Adrenal suppression and steroid supplementation in renal transplant recipients. Transplantation 51:385, 1991
10. Roberts C, LaFond J, Fitt CT, et al: New patterns of transplant nephrectomy in the cyclosporine era. J Am Coll Surg 178:59, 1994
11. Friedman RJ, Schiff CF, Bromberg JS: Use of supplemental steroids in patients having orthopaedic operations. J Bone Joint Surg 77A:1801, 1995
12. Kehlet H, Binder C: Value of an ACTH test in assessing hypothalamic-pituitary-adrenocortical function in glucocorticoid-treated patients. Br Med J 2:147, 1973
13. Kehlet H: The surgical stress response: should it be prevented? Can J Surg 34:565, 1991
14. Downing R, Davis I, Black J, et al: Effect of intrathecal morphine on the adrenocortical and hyperglycaemic responses to upper abdominal surgery. Br J Anaesth 58:858, 1986
15. Rittmaster R, Cutler GB Jr, Sobel DO, et al: Morphine inhibits the pituitary-adrenal response to ovine corticotropin-releasing hormone in normal subjects. J Clin Endocrinol Metab 60:891, 1985
16. Engquist A, Brandt MR, Fernandes A, et al: The blocking effect of epidural analgesia on the adrenocortical and hyperglycemic responses to surgery. Acta Anaesth Scand 21:330, 1977
17. Liu S, Carpenter RL, Neal JM: Epidural anesthesia and analgesia, their role in postoperative outcome. Anesthesiology 82:1474, 1995
18. Axelrod L: Glucocorticoid therapy. Medicine (Baltimore) 55:39, 1976

Acknowledgment

Figure 1 Seward Hung.

74 NON-AIDS IMMUNOSUPPRESSION

Carl Nohr, M.D., Ph.D.

Approach to Patients with Host Defense Defects

Evaluation of Host Defense Mechanisms in Surgical Patients

Immunosuppression is a biologic state characterized by detrimental alterations in aspects of host anatomy and physiology normally dedicated to defense against infections and malignancy. Because of the invasive nature of surgery and because defects in systemic immunity have been observed in most major illnesses, it is reasonable to state that all, or nearly all, surgical patients are immunosuppressed at some point. The nature and degree of immunosuppression in a particular patient is the sum of several disease-related or iatrogenic changes.

An understanding of normal immune mechanisms is important to the recognition of immunodeficiency. Host defense mechanisms may be broadly categorized as either local or systemic. Local host defenses include epithelial coverings, specialized cells, and secretions. Systemic defense mechanisms include phagocytic cells as well as complement, humoral, and cell-mediated immune mechanisms. There are major interactions at many levels between the various local and systemic immune processes. Comprehensive descriptions of actual immune processes appear elsewhere.[1] The following sections of this chapter are limited to the clinical and laboratory evaluation of host defense defects [see Figure 1].

Immunodeficiency may be primary or acquired secondary to illness or iatrogenic intervention. In most primary immunodeficiency diseases, defects in systemic host defenses can be clinically detected and have a clear relation to the kinds of infection for which the patient is at risk. In the more common acquired immunodeficiencies, however, the relation of host defense defects to the pathogenesis of infections is generally less clearly defined. Nevertheless, tests of immune function can help define underlying defects in local and systemic host defense mechanisms in patients with an acquired increased susceptibility to local and systemic infection with or without the septic response.

LOCAL HOST DEFENSES

The human body is a complex tube covered by skin and lined with mucosa. Various mechanical, cellular, microbiological, and biochemical properties of these coverings account for local host defense mechanisms.[1] When these coverings are broken or disrupted, the defense mechanisms may be compromised. Evaluation of breaks in local host defenses thus begins with determining the location and number of invasive devices or procedures and the duration of their use. Such interventions include endotracheal tubes, tracheostomies, nasogastric tubes, bladder catheters, and central venous catheters. Intracranial pressure monitors, chest tubes, drains, external fixation devices, and implanted prostheses also produce changes in local host defenses.

The presence and condition of burn wounds, fistulas, decubitus ulcers, and open or closed surgical wounds should be noted.

Mechanical aspects of the urinary, respiratory, and gastrointestinal systems should be evaluated. Obstruction or stasis in any of the lumina of these systems will alter the local microflora and change the efficacy of local secretions and ciliated and phagocytic cells, thus predisposing to invasive infection. The condition of the gastrointestinal system is especially important in this regard because the gut may be the major source of bacterial infection resulting in sepsis and organ failure in critically ill surgical patients.[2,3]

Changes in local microflora are important considerations, especially in hospitalized patients. Prolonged hospitalization results in gram-negative colonization.[4] Changes in gastric pH can allow overgrowth of some bacterial species.[5] Prolonged broad-spectrum antibiotic treatment is associated with fungal superinfection. Although changes in the local microflora can be evaluated by culture of body fluids and mucosal surfaces, the status of many other important aspects of local immunity cannot be determined reliably by clinical means at present. Measurement of cellular and immunoglobulin contents of respiratory, urinary, and gastrointestinal secretions is not clinically feasible. Evaluation of local defenses of the peritoneum, which are very important to the control of the septic response to infection, is also not feasible.[6]

SYSTEMIC HOST DEFENSES

For purposes of study, systemic immunity may be classified as either antigen specific or nonspecific. Humoral immunity and cell-mediated immunity provide antigen-specific immunity, whereas phagocytes and complement provide nonspecific immunity. There are many interactions between these arbitrary divisions. At the present time, little therapy is available for most of the deficiencies discussed (see below), with the exception of some primary immunodeficiencies. Immunomodulation is an active area of research, however, and the biologic description of acquired immunodeficiencies will assume increasing importance as corrective methodologies evolve [see 88 *Immunomodulation*].

Approach to Patients with Host Defense Defects

Surgical patient manifests defects in host defense

Assess present state of patient's local and systemic defenses.

Take history, and perform physical examination, radiologic and laboratory studies, and specific tests of immune function.

Significant immunosuppression is present

Treat any correctable immunodeficiency (e.g., by administering immunoglobulin for defects in B cell function or by reducing dosage of immunosuppressive agents in patients receiving such therapy).

Immunity is slightly impaired

Optimize overall medical and surgical care to help restore immune function

Reassess need for invasive devices.

Remove any infected foreign bodies.

Restore blood volume, and optimize tissue perfusion.

Treat any fistulas, decubitus ulcers, or other wounds.

Correct any underlying nutritional deficiency.

Provide surgical intervention as appropriate: e.g., drain abscesses, resect tumors, and excise burns, if present.

Diagnose and treat any local or systemic infections.

Assess need for vaccination.

Use prophylactic antibiotics when indicated.

For patients who are receiving immunosuppressive therapy, institute appropriate prophylaxis to prevent specific complications.

Optimize renal function, using dialysis if necessary.

Correct hyperglycemia in patients with diabetes mellitus.

Institute therapy to optimize cardiac function.

Candidate for transplantation is to be deliberately immunosuppressed

Perform preimmunosuppression workup, including:
- History and physical examination
- Blood work
- Radiologic studies
- Nuclear medicine scans
- Other studies and tests

Workup should address the following:
- Nervous system
- Cardiovascular system
- Respiratory system
- Digestive system
- Genitourinary system
- Musculoskeletal system
- Endocrine system
- Dermal system
- Hematologic system
- Immune system
- Preexisting infection
- Nutritional state
- Psychological, social, and financial assessment

Patient has no invasive infection or malignant disease

Treat any underlying correctable conditions (e.g., local infection around foreign bodies).

Provide appropriate prophylaxis to prevent complications.

Patient has active invasive infection or malignant disease

Do not proceed with immunosuppression.

Proceed with transplantation, and institute immunosuppressive therapy

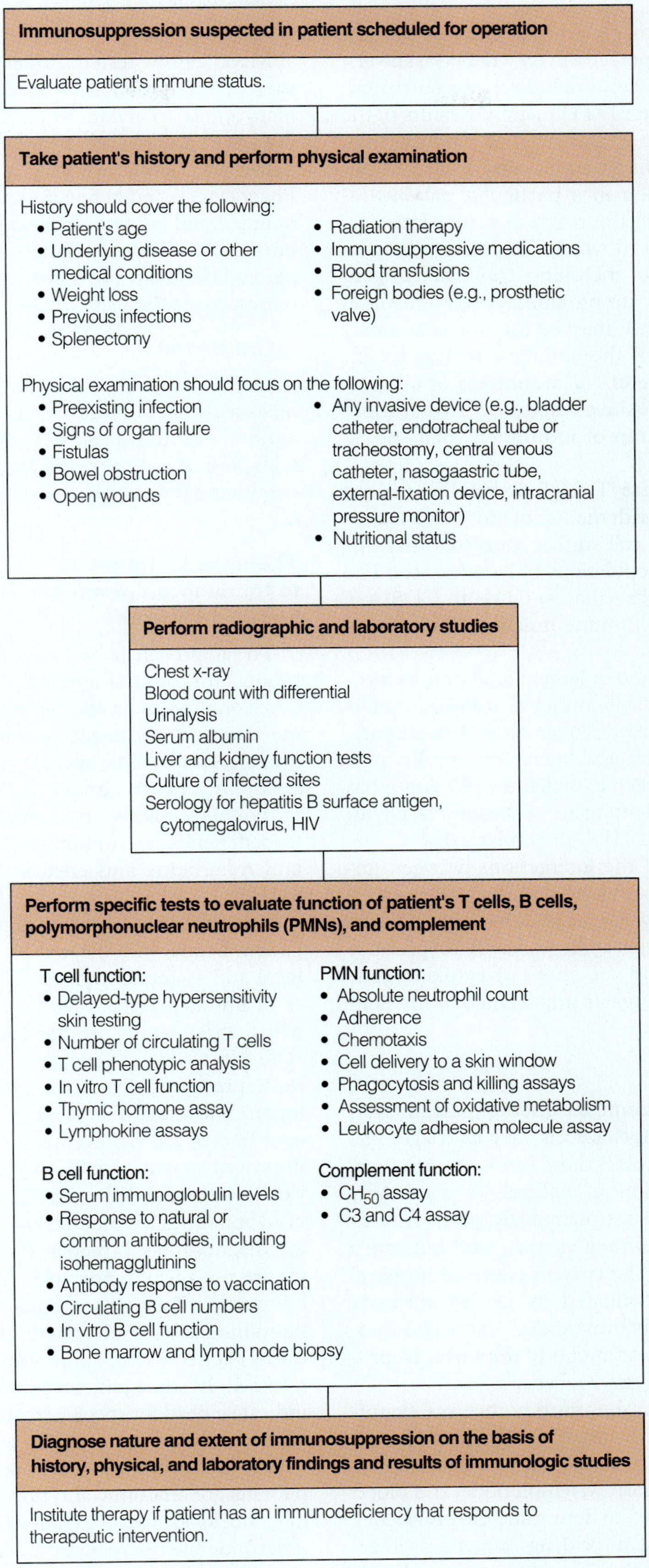

Immunosuppression suspected in patient scheduled for operation

Evaluate patient's immune status.

Take patient's history and perform physical examination

History should cover the following:
- Patient's age
- Underlying disease or other medical conditions
- Weight loss
- Previous infections
- Splenectomy
- Radiation therapy
- Immunosuppressive medications
- Blood transfusions
- Foreign bodies (e.g., prosthetic valve)

Physical examination should focus on the following:
- Preexisting infection
- Signs of organ failure
- Fistulas
- Bowel obstruction
- Open wounds
- Any invasive device (e.g., bladder catheter, endotracheal tube or tracheostomy, central venous catheter, nasogaastric tube, external-fixation device, intracranial pressure monitor)
- Nutritional status

Perform radiographic and laboratory studies

Chest x-ray
Blood count with differential
Urinalysis
Serum albumin
Liver and kidney function tests
Culture of infected sites
Serology for hepatitis B surface antigen, cytomegalovirus, HIV

Perform specific tests to evaluate function of patient's T cells, B cells, polymorphonuclear neutrophils (PMNs), and complement

T cell function:
- Delayed-type hypersensitivity skin testing
- Number of circulating T cells
- T cell phenotypic analysis
- In vitro T cell function
- Thymic hormone assay
- Lymphokine assays

B cell function:
- Serum immunoglobulin levels
- Response to natural or common antibodies, including isohemagglutinins
- Antibody response to vaccination
- Circulating B cell numbers
- In vitro B cell function
- Bone marrow and lymph node biopsy

PMN function:
- Absolute neutrophil count
- Adherence
- Chemotaxis
- Cell delivery to a skin window
- Phagocytosis and killing assays
- Assessment of oxidative metabolism
- Leukocyte adhesion molecule assay

Complement function:
- CH_{50} assay
- C3 and C4 assay

Diagnose nature and extent of immunosuppression on the basis of history, physical, and laboratory findings and results of immunologic studies

Institute therapy if patient has an immunodeficiency that responds to therapeutic intervention.

Figure 1 Illustrated is a diagnostic approach to suspected immunosuppression in a patient scheduled for operation.

Cell-Mediated Immunity

The most useful test of cell-mediated immunity in surgical patients is the delayed-type hypersensitivity (DTH) skin-test reaction.[7] Many disease processes, including malnutrition,[8] cancer,[9] and thermal injury,[10] alter DTH testing. Results of the test provide a global assessment of host defense function that, together with age, sex, and serum albumin, can be used to calculate the probability of infection in a particular patient.[11,12] DTH is assessed by determining the reaction to the intradermal injection of several antigens to which the patient presumably has had previous exposure, including *Candida* antigen, *Trichophyton* antigen, tuberculin, streptokinase-streptodornase, and mumps antigen. The response may be measured at either 24 or 48 hours after injection of the antigens. It may be expressed as the sum of the diameters of induration of all antigens, or it may be defined as a positive response if two or more antigens produce more than 5 mm of induration each [*see 37 Nonemergency Surgery*].

The next echelon of tests evaluates T cell function. Populations of T cells are measured precisely with the use of monoclonal antibodies. These antibodies bind to cell surface receptors that distinguish between functional subpopulations of lymphocytes. The ratio of helper to suppressor T cells—that is, $CD4^+$ to $CD8^+$—is frequently used as a measure of immune function. The normal ratio is 1.8:2.2.

Testing of in vitro T cell function is largely a laboratory process that measures the capacity of mononuclear cells to proliferate, produce lymphokines, or become killer cells after stimulation in culture. Several stimulating agents are used in this process. Such stimulants include antigen to which the cell donor has been previously exposed and T cell mitogens—for example, phytohemagglutinin, concanavalin A, or HLA-dissimilar cells.

With greater understanding of the interactions between immunologically active cells, it is possible to define more precisely the communication signals between cells. Although not yet clinically routine, the study of the ability of cells to produce normal amounts of cytokines and the study of cytokine gene expression will, in time, assume greater importance in the definition of immunosuppression.

Humoral Immunity

As a first measure of humoral immune function, serum levels of IgG, IgM, and IgA are measured. Levels vary with age; IgA and IgM are absent in neonates unless there has been intrauterine infection. Next, determination of natural or commonly occurring antibodies—for example, isohemagglutinins or antibody to diphtheria, tetanus, or common viruses—will indicate a past humoral immune response. The current status of humoral immune function can best be evaluated by testing antibody response to active vaccination. Tetanus toxoid[13] and pneumococcal vaccine[14] may be used to test antibody responses to protein and polysaccharide antigens, respectively.

In-depth investigation of humoral immunity involves examination of cell surface markers and in vitro B cell function. B cells are characterized by the presence of surface immunoglobulin or other cell surface markers. Bone marrow, lymph node, and blood mononuclear cells may be examined to determine the prevalence of B cells. Spontaneous and mitogen- or drug-induced proliferation of B cells in vitro, as well as their maturation into plasma cells that produce immunoglobulin, may be studied by a variety of research laboratory methods.[8]

Neutrophil Function

Most of the functions of polymorphonuclear neutrophils (PMNs) can be tested. Adherence, a first step in ingress toward sites of inflammation, is tested by measuring the attachment of neutrophils to nylon wool. Chemotaxis, the directed motion toward a stimulus, can be quantitated by several techniques. Cell delivery to skin abrasions is a useful test of phagocyte function. Phagocytosis and killing assays measure the ability of host PMNs to ingest and kill test organisms. Oxidative metabolism of PMNs, important to normal function, can be measured with myeloperoxidase assay, nitroblue tetrazolium reduction, or chemoluminescence studies.[8]

Complement

Overall integrity of the complement cascade is determined by measuring the amount of serum needed to lyse 50 percent of antibody-coated sheep red cells; this measurement is called the CH_{50} test. An abnormal CH_{50} is followed by assay of individual complement components, usually C3 and C4.

Therapeutic Approach to Immunocompromised Surgical Patients

The approach to the care of the immunocompromised surgical patient focuses on ways of promoting wound healing and host resistance to infection. At present, there is little specific anti-immunosuppressive treatment for the broad-based acquired immunodeficiencies seen in surgical patients. Management therefore depends on minimizing immunosuppressive procedures and treatments and ensuring that overall care is as good as possible.

The surgical approach to the care of the immunocompromised patient begins with a complete evaluation of the present state of local and systemic immunity. The possibility of reduced dosages of immunosuppressive medications is considered in cases in which these drugs are the cause of the immunocompromised state. (In transplant recipients, the benefits of decreasing immunosuppressive medications must be balanced against the risk of allograft rejection.) The need for invasive devices is reviewed. Foreign bodies are removed if infected. Physiologic conditions are improved by restoring blood volume and optimizing tissue perfusion. Nutritional deficiencies are corrected. Fistulas, decubitus ulcers, and other wounds are treated. Local and systemic infections are diagnosed and treated. Prophylactic or therapeutic antibiotics are used when indicated. Appropriate measures are instituted to stop ongoing hemorrhage so transfusion requirements can be minimized. Abscesses are drained, malignancies treated, and burns excised where appropriate. The need for any vaccination is assessed. In some patients, evaluation of systemic immunity may indicate a need for specific treatment—for example, immunoglobulin infusions.

The first two goals of immunomodulatory therapy in surgical patients are anatomic and physiologic restoration and assurance of good local microcirculation. Host anatomy and physiology determine the microenvironmental milieu in which wound healing and antimicrobial resistance mechanisms operate. Regional blood flow, concentration of protein and hormones in plasma and interstitial fluid, tissue oxygenation, and other systemic physiologic parameters determine not only the microenvironmental conditions in which defense mechanisms operate but also the ability of the body to produce resistance factors and deliver them to inflammatory sites. All treatments, procedures, and agents designed to restore and maintain normal anatomy and physiology are therefore useful in the care of the immunosuppressed patient.

Restoration of nutritional status by oral or intravenous feeding has been shown to be beneficial for several abnormalities of host defense,[8] including skin-test reactivity; lymphocyte transformation, serum immunoglobulin levels, specific antibody responses, and neutrophil chemotaxis may also be restored in this manner. For patients with a functional intestinal tract, enteral feeding is preferred over parenteral nutrition [see 97 Nutritional Support].

Although surgical intervention is generally immunosuppressive, it can help restore immune function by treating disease. For example, the depressed DTH test responses of cancer patients, which are associated with an increased risk of infection and mortality, can be improved by tumor resection.[15,16] Correction of biliary tract disease, bowel obstruction, hypovolemia, and visceral abscesses can also improve responses to DTH tests.[17] Similarly, early burn excision decreases immunosuppression. Care in administering prophylactic antibiotics, handling tissue, and controlling contamination and blood loss will produce the best outcomes.

Two aspects of the host response to bacterial infection—a critical interval termed the decisive period and the so-called inoculum effect—are of special importance to the timing of surgical intervention. After subcutaneous injection of bacteria in guinea pigs, there is a decisive period of only a few hours during which the administration of antibiotics can prevent the development of infection and the septic response.[18] The inoculum effect describes the important observation that a large inoculum (i.e., large numbers of bacteria) is more likely to cause invasive infection than a small inoculum. Incorporating the concepts of a decisive period during the process of infection and an inoculum effect is an important aspect of the philosophy of surgical care. Minimizing the quantity and duration of bacterial contamination through early diagnosis and definitive surgical therapy is important in the care of the immunocompromised patient.

Some preexisting illnesses—for example, renal failure or diabetes mellitus—are also immunosuppressive. Because these abnormalities are regarded as part of an acquired immunodeficiency syndrome caused by illness, optimization of organ system function should also help restore immune function. The restoration of red cell mass, use of dialysis, correction of hyperglycemia, and treatment of heart failure are examples of general care that can improve local and systemic host defense and wound-healing mechanisms.

Vaccination, either active or passive, is an important topic in the care of the immunocompromised patient. Live vaccines, such as those for smallpox, measles, rubella, polio (oral vaccine), mumps, and yellow fever, must not be given to immunosuppressed patients. Vaccination against tetanus, diphtheria, pneumococcus, and meningococcus is permitted, as is subcutaneous vaccination for polio, all with the same indications as in nonimmunosuppressed patients. In immunosuppressed patients, there is one additional indication for vaccination with pneumococcal and meningococcal polysaccharide—namely, patients who have been splenectomized or who are scheduled to undergo splenectomy. In the latter case, the vaccine is preferably administered two weeks before splenectomy.

Passive vaccination against gram-negative organisms may be available soon. Gram-negative bacterial organisms are antigenically complex, but many share a common core glycolipid antigen system. Polyclonal or monoclonal antibodies to this moiety may be useful in the management of bacterial infection in the immunocompromised surgical patient.[17] Vaccination may also be useful in viral infections other than polio. Vaccine against cytomegalovirus (CMV) has undergone clinical trial but is not universally used. Passive vaccination with CMV hyperimmune globulin or prophylactic administration of ganciclovir may be more practical approaches to the prevention of CMV infections in transplant recipients.[19-21] Early treatment with ganciclovir, rather than universal prophylaxis, in patients with positive surveillance cultures for CMV may also be effective in reducing the incidence and severity of symptomatic infection.[22]

The use of drugs and other agents specifically intended to improve host defense mechanisms is at present experimental. In general, such agents act by removing suppressor influences, replenishing supplies of endogenous host defense factors, restoring deficient mechanisms to normal, or hyperstimulating already functioning host defense mechanisms.[17]

Prophylaxis of certain disease processes is a special topic in the care of immunocompromised patients. Several measures are commonly used or are under study for the prevention of complications in such patients [see Table 1].

SPECIAL CONSIDERATIONS

Prevention of infection is preferable to treatment. However, if clinical illness develops, outcome will be determined by the speed with which a specific diagnosis is reached and the correct therapy instituted.

Approach to Suspected Infection

Several factors must be considered in the workup of a possibly infected immunosuppressed patient [see Table 2]. Two aspects of infection in the immunosuppressed patient are especially important. One is the effect of immunosuppression on the presentation of infections and on their natural history and response to treatment. The other is the increased susceptibility of so-called septic patients to infections by opportunistic microorganisms [see Table 3]. When a diagnosis of infection is being considered in febrile allograft recipients, it is important to remember that other causes of fever, such as rejection and malignancy, may also be present.

Signs and symptoms of many infectious processes are altered or absent in immunosuppressed patients. Low-grade fever, confusion, acidosis, tachypnea, unexplained third-space fluid loss, or tachycardia may be the only manifestations of infection and should be worked up and treated vigorously. It is frequently appropriate to treat speculatively with antibiotics early while pursuing aggressive diagnostic procedures. This approach is especially important in neutropenic patients. Failure to respond to therapy indicates the need for more aggressive diagnostic procedures and changes in antibiotic treatment.

All body fluids and tissue specimens must be studied microbiologically and, frequently, histologically for conventional bacteria, viruses, acid-fast bacteria, fungi, and protozoa. DNA hybridization may be useful in the diagnosis of latent infection in cells.

Table 1 Prevention of Complications in Immunosuppressed Patients

Complication	Preventive Measure
Bacteremia	Preimmunosuppressive dental work Prophylaxis for later dental work Low-bacterial-content diet ? Protected environment ? Gut decontamination
Pneumocystis pneumonia	Trimethoprim-sulfamethoxazole
Listeria infection	Trimethoprim-sulfamethoxazole
Nocardia infection	Trimethoprim-sulfamethoxazole
Mycobacterium infection	Isoniazid
Cryptococcus infection	Fluconazole
Urinary tract infections	? Preimmunosuppressive nephrectomy for chronic pyelonephritis (in renal transplant candidates) Trimethoprim-sulfamethoxazole
Hepatitis A	? Postexposure prophylaxis with hyperimmune globulin
Hepatitis B	Vaccination
Cytomegalovirus infection	Avoid seropositive-to-seronegative transplants ? Vaccination ? Hyperimmune globulin ? Prophylactic acyclovir or ganciclovir
Varicella-zoster virus	Hyperimmune globulin
Influenza	Vaccination
Influenza A	? Amantadine prophylaxis
Postsplenectomy infection with septic response	Nonoperative treatment Splenic salvage Pneumococcal polysaccharide vaccine Meningococcal polysaccharide vaccine ? Prophylactic antibiotics
Candidal esophagitis	Nystatin swish and swallow
Peptic ulcer disease	Avoidance of acetylsalicylic acid and anti-inflammatory agents Antacids H_2-receptor antagonists
Acute cholecystitis	Preimmunosuppressive cholecystectomy
Perianal ulceration	Stool softeners Antiseptic lotions
Skin carcinoma	Avoidance of sun exposure Use of sunscreens
Osteopenia	Antiresorptive therapy

Wound infections in transplant recipients are caused by common pathogens such as *Staphylococcus* species and mixed bacterial species. They may present, however, with very few local findings as long as years after operation. Diagnostic aspiration of fluid collections is helpful [*see Table 4*].

Mycobacterial or fungal infection of the skin may cause ulcerated, nodular lesions. Although some fungi produce characteristic skin lesions, biopsy may be necessary to distinguish species of *Candida, Torulopsis, Histoplasma, Cryptococcus, Aspergillus, Blastomyces, Actinomyces,* and *Nocardia*. If such organisms are found, systemic infection should be strongly suspected and probably treated even if unproved. Viral infections of the skin are common. Herpes simplex usually causes characteristic vesicular mucocutaneous lesions, whereas varicella-zoster causes chicken pox or shingles. In the immunocompromised patient, either of these viruses may produce disseminated disease as well. Amebic infections may also present initially as skin infection before progressing to systemic infection. Biopsy is diagnostic.

Headache, seizures, altered mentation, or focal neurologic signs suggest central nervous system infection. Viral encephalitis and viral, bacterial, or fungal meningitis are possible. Computed tomographic scanning, with or without infusion of a contrast agent, can rule out space-occupying lesions such as abscess or lymphoma. Funduscopic examination may show evidence of local or systemic infection. For some viral encephalitides, an electroencephalogram or magnetic resonance imaging is diagnostically useful. The most important test for CNS infection, however, is lumbar puncture. Specimens must be stained with Gram's stain and India ink stain and examined for cell count, protein content, and the presence of cryptococcal and bacterial antigens. Finally, brain biopsy may be necessary. *Cryptococcus, Listeria,* and *Aspergillus* are the most important causes of meningitis.

Infection of the cardiovascular system is suggested by bacteremia, new heart murmurs, worsening of congestive heart failure, mycotic aneurysms, or metastatic infarcts or abscesses. Blood cultures and echocardiography are the mainstays of diagnosis.

Any conventional bacteria or mycobacteria may cause pneumonia in the immunosuppressed patient. The major opportunistic agents are CMV, *Aspergillus, Nocardia, Cryptococcus,* and *Pneumocystis* species. This variety of microorganisms in immunosuppressed patients requires a more aggressive diagnostic approach than in nonimmunosuppressed patients. Patterns of infiltration, consolidation, or cavitation on chest radiographs may suggest specific etiologies but are not diagnostic. Detection of *Aspergillus* on throat and nasopharyngeal cultures may indicate the presence of invasive infection caused by this organism elsewhere. Although chest radiographs, sputum examination and culture, thoracentesis, nuclear scanning, and CT scanning are useful in the diagnosis of pneumonitis and empyema, bronchoscopy is frequently required to provide an accurate and timely diagnosis. Minimal abnormalities on chest radiograph, pulmonary function studies, or blood gas measurement should be taken as indications for bronchoscopy. Bronchoalveolar lavage specimens are examined for *Pneumocystis* species, viral inclusion bodies, and CMV antigen, and they are cultured for bacteria, mycobacteria, viruses, and fungi. Transtracheal aspiration can also be used but may be complicated by bleeding and cervical cellulitis. Transbronchial biopsy, open-lung biopsy, and video thoracoscopic lung biopsy are final steps if the diagnosis has not been made.[23,24]

Table 2 Components of Workup for Infection in Immunocompromised Patients

Patient Subgroup	Components of Workup
All patients	History Review travel, exposure to illness, animal contact Physical examination Blood count and differential count Serum electrolyte levels Liver profile Serum amylase levels Serum cryptococcal antigen Culture of blood, sputum, nasopharyngeal secretions, and urine for aerobes, anaerobes, viruses, and fungi Serum titers of antibodies to herpes simplex virus, cytomegalovirus, and Epstein-Barr virus Chest x-ray ECG Arterial blood gas concentrations
Patients with cutaneous or systemic symptoms or signs	Skin biopsy Fine-needle aspiration Bone marrow aspiration
Patients with neurologic symptoms or signs	Ophthalmoscopic examination CT scan of head MRI scan of head EEG Examination and culture of CSF: cell count, protein content, glucose level, India ink stain, Gram's stain, cryptococcal antigen, bacterial antigens Brain biopsy
Patients with sinus symptoms or signs	Sinus x-rays CT scan of sinuses Sinus aspiration
Patients with cardiac symptoms or signs	Echocardiogram Myocardial biopsy
Patients with pulmonary symptoms or signs	Lung scan CT scan Pulmonary function tests Transtracheal aspiration Bronchoscopy: viral inclusion bodies; cytomegalovirus antigen; culture for bacteria, fungi, and viruses Thoracocentesis: cell count; protein content; glucose level; LDH level; Gram's stain; cytology; culture for bacteria, fungi, and viruses Pleural biopsy Transbronchial lung biopsy Open or thoracoscopic lung biopsy
Patients with abdominal symptoms or signs	Upper and lower endoscopy: biopsy; culture for bacteria, fungi, and viruses Contrast studies of upper and lower GI tract Ultrasonography of abdomen CT scan of abdomen Paracentesis or aspiration
Patients with urinary tract symptoms or signs	Ultrasonography of native and transplanted kidneys Cystoscopy
Patients with bone or joint symptoms or signs	Joint aspiration: cell count; glucose level; Gram's stain; culture for bacteria, fungi, and viruses

Table 3 Common Opportunistic Infectious Agents in Immunosuppressed Patients

Bacteria
  Brucella species
  Legionella species
  Listeria monocytogenes
  Mycobacterium avium–intracellulare
  Nocardia asteroides
  Mycobacterium tuberculosis
  Salmonella species
  Chlamydia species

Fungi
  Aspergillus species
  Candida species
  Cryptococcus neoformans
  Histoplasma capsulatum
  Rhizopus species

Protozoa and parasites
  Cryptosporidium species
  Giardia lamblia
  Isospora belli
  Pneumocystis carinii
  Strongyloides stercoralis
  Toxoplasma gondii
  Trypanosoma species

Viruses
  Cytomegalovirus
  Epstein-Barr virus
  Herpes simplex
  Herpes zoster

Sinusitis may present as fever and headache and can be diagnosed by means of radiographs, CT scanning, and aspiration. There are special problems in the diagnosis of gastrointestinal or abdominal infection in the immunosuppressed patient. Evaluation of the oropharynx and esophagus is performed by physical examination and endoscopy. Inspection of the mucosa and biopsy will usually yield a diagnosis of either candidal or viral (CMV or herpes simplex) esophagitis. Systemic treatment of either viral or fungal esophagitis is frequently necessary.

Inflammatory intra-abdominal conditions may not be revealed by history and physical examination. An absence of free intraperitoneal air is not enough to rule out perforation in immunosuppressed patients with infection. A contrast swallow with a water-soluble agent, followed by barium if initially negative, is a definitive test for upper intestinal perforation. A similar diagnostic approach is used for colon perforation. Ultrasonography or CT scanning is used to rule out fluid collections in the abdomen, which are almost invariably present in patients with acute abdominal diseases. Acalculous cholecystitis can be diagnosed by ultrasonography and treated by percutaneous drainage.[25] Paracentesis or radiologically guided aspiration may be useful in cases in which there is demonstrable intra-abdominal fluid but no clear indication for laparotomy [see Table 4].

Viral infections and hepatotoxic drugs such as azathioprine account for most episodes of hepatitis in immunocompromised patients. Most cases of hepatitis are clinically indolent, but hepatic failure and death from systemic opportunistic infection can occur.[26]

Infections in the genitourinary tract can usually be diagnosed by urinalysis, urine culture, and ultrasonography. In renal transplant recipients, infection can occur in either transplanted or native kidneys. Asymptomatic viral excretion in the urine is common after transplantation. Candiduria is also common, especially in diabetic immunosuppressed patients, but it usually reflects colonization rather than invasive infection [see 85 Fungal Infection].

Bone and joint infections are caused by either normal pathogens, mycobacterial organisms, or fungi. Persistent sampling of effusions with appropriate microbiological workup is needed.[27]

Management of Neutropenia

Neutropenic patients are a special challenge.[28] The most common cause of important neutropenia is chemotherapy. The white blood cell nadir usually occurs from 10 to 20 days after the start of chemotherapy. Infections produce few local signs of a septic response because there are not enough granulocytes to produce classic signs of inflammation or pus. Asymptomatic pneumonia may present with only slight abnormalities on x-ray. Similarly, urinary tract infection may produce bacteremia without significant symptoms. Mucocutaneous viral infections or dental caries can provide a portal of entry for gram-negative bacteria. Fungal superinfections are common and usually develop after broad-spectrum antibiotic treatment. Diagnosis of invasive fungal sepsis is sometimes difficult, and a clinical response to systemic antifungal treatment may be the best evidence that such an infection is present. Invasive fungal infection is often detected at autopsy.

Perirectal pain may occur in neutropenic patients and is usually caused by ulceration, fissure, or abscess. Diagnosis of a rectal abscess is difficult and may require observation of the clinical response to antibiotics and local treatment. Aspiration of the abscess, which usually yields watery fluid, or examination under anesthesia may be useful. Fluctuance is an indication for drainage.

Even without evidence of primary infection, bacteremia is common.[29] Most of the organisms implicated in bacteremia are derived from the patient's endogenous flora, some of which is acquired nosocomially. These findings suggest that bacteremia originates in the gut or from colonized body surfaces. The classic signs and symptoms of bacteremia are frequently absent in the leukopenic patient, who may present with only hyperventilation or an altered mental state. Immediate institution of broad-spectrum antibiotic therapy is indicated.

Leukocyte transfusions may be useful in the management of neutropenic patients.[29] Most neutrophil functions are preserved in storage up to 24 hours. Clinical studies of efficacy, however, have been hampered by problems of cell isolation and patient variability.[17] The use of colony-stimulating factors for reducing the duration and severity of neutropenia is more promising.[30]

To prevent neutropenic bacteremia, it may be useful to decontaminate the intestine by administering oral nonabsorbable antibiotics, such as combinations of oral nystatin, an aminoglycoside, and polymyxin, while the patient follows a diet containing foods of low bacterial content.[31] However, the benefit of this approach has not yet been proved. A total protected environment has been tried in the care of the neutropenic patient. Sterilized air is provided to the patient, who is decontaminated with skin antiseptics and nonabsorbable antibiotics. The room is sterilized with disinfectants. Although this approach reduces the number of infections, they still occur. At present, bone marrow transplant recipients are candidates for a protected

Table 4 Therapy for Opportunistic Infectious Agents in Immunosuppressed Patients

Organism	Recommended Agent
Central nervous system	
Cryptococcus neoformans	Amphotericin B plus flucytosine
Herpes simplex	Acyclovir
Listeria monocytogenes	Ampicillin or trimethoprim-sulfamethoxazole
Mycobacteria	Multiple drug combinations
Nocardia species	Sulfonamide
Toxoplasma gondii	Trisulfapyrimidines or sulfadiazine plus pyrimethamine
Varicella-zoster	Acyclovir
Gastrointestinal tract	
Cytomegalovirus	Ganciclovir
Cryptosporidium species	None available
Giardia lamblia	Quinacrine or metronidazole
Isospora belli	Trimethoprim-sulfamethoxazole
Salmonella species	Ciprofloxacin, ceftriaxone, trimethoprim-sulfamethoxazole, or chloramphenicol
Lungs	
Aspergillus species	Amphotericin B
Candida species	Fluconazole or amphotericin B
Cryptococcus neoformans	Amphotericin B plus flucytosine
Cytomegalovirus	Ganciclovir
Gram-negative bacteria	Aminoglycoside plus cephalosporin or aminoglycosides plus penicillin
Herpes simplex	Acyclovir
Histoplasma capsulatum	Amphotericin B
Legionella species	Erythromycin
Mycobacterium avium–intracellulare	Combined treatment with antituberculous and antimicrobial agents
Mycobacterium tuberculosis	Antituberculous agents
Pneumocystis carinii	Trimethoprim-sulfamethoxazole or pentamidine
Varicella-zoster	Acyclovir or vidarabine
Oropharynx and sinuses	
Aspergillus species	Fluconazole or amphotericin B
Candida species (esophagus)	Fluconazole or amphotericin B
Candida species (mouth)	Nystatin suspension, clotrimazole troches, oral ketoconazole, or oral fluconazole
Cytomegalovirus	Ganciclovir
Herpes simplex	Acyclovir
Rhizopus species	Fluconazole or amphotericin B
Strongyloides species	Thiabendazole
Skin	
Papillomavirus	Podophyllin, fluorouracil, or interferon
Varicella-zoster	Acyclovir

environment; indications for use in the care of other immunosuppressed patients have not yet been established.[31]

In the granulocytopenic patient, systemic infections with both gram-negative and gram-positive organisms occur. The early institution of empirical therapy before definitive identification of the infection site or causative organism will reduce the risk of mortality. Several antibiotic regimens have been shown to be effective. Patients who are neutropenic and febrile for more than one week while receiving antibacterial therapy should be considered to have a fungal infection and should be treated with systemic antifungal antibiotics. If no source of infection is found, treatment may be stopped when the neutrophil count has returned to normal. If a discrete focus is found, local treatment should be given and the antibiotic therapy continued.

Special acute abdominal conditions requiring surgical intervention occur in neutropenic patients. Neutropenic enterocolitis is characterized by fever, abdominal pain, and tenderness occurring during periods of neutropenia.[32] It is probably a bacterial infection of the wall of the large or small bowel. It may cause hemorrhage in the bowel wall, ischemia, and perforation, frequently accompanied by bacteremia. The condition is treated initially with bowel rest and antibiotics, but laparotomy should be done at any sign of clinical deterioration, an acute abdomen, or free air. Early recognition by frequent physical examination, abdominal radiography, and ultrasonography or CT scanning, followed by surgical intervention, will produce a better outcome than protracted nonoperative care. As is true for other causes of gastrointestinal perforation in the immunocompromised patient, resection and exteriorization is preferred to anastomosis unless conditions are optimal in terms of the patient's condition, expected course of neutropenia, timing after perforation, spillage, and degree of peritoneal reaction.[33]

Evaluation of Patients before Immunosuppressive Therapy

An immunosuppressed state is sometimes deliberately created—for example, to prevent allograft rejection in transplant recipients. Such patients undergo a preimmunosuppression workup [*see Table 5*] that has six objectives: full investigation of the primary disease, optimization of physiologic status, treatment of infections, discovery of occult malignancy, minimization of risk of posttransplant complications, and complete psychological, social, and financial evaluation. Details of the first and last objectives are not considered here. For the other objectives, an organ systems approach is used.

The presence of active invasive infection or active malignant disease is a contraindication to transplantation and immunosuppressive therapy. It is not yet known how much time should elapse between treatment of malignancy and the beginning of immunosuppressive therapy. It seems reasonable to wait until recurrence of malignancy is unlikely, prove that the patient is free of tumor, and proceed after advising the patient that immunosuppressive medication may reactivate malignancy.

Transplantation is also inadvisable when the patient's physiologic state predicts operative mortality, when the anatomic setting is inadequate for technical success, and when the patient has severe psychological, social, or financial problems without evident support or solution.

Table 5 Components of Preimmunosuppression Workup

History
  Review of underlying disease
  Surgical history
    Peptic ulcer surgery
    Cholecystectomy
    Nephrectomy
    Splenectomy
    Cardiac surgery
  Medical history
    Cardiac disease
    Pulmonary disease
    Renal disease
    Parenchymal disease
    Urosepsis
    Gastrointestinal disease
    Cholelithiasis
    Peptic ulcer disease
    Infectious diseases
    Malignancies
    Blood transfusions
    Vaccinations
      Hepatitis B
      Pneumococcal polysaccharide
  Review of current medications
Physical examination
  General examination
  Neurologic examination
  Cardiopulmonary examination
  Abdominal examination
  Breast examination
  Genitourinary examination
  Complete skin examination
Blood work
  ABO and HLA type
  Mixed lymphocyte culture
  Cytotoxic antibody determination
  Complete blood count
  Platelet count
  Prothrombin time and partial thromboplastin time
  Bleeding time
  Electrolytes, urea nitrogen, and creatinine
  Serum calcium and phosphate
  Hepatic enzymes and bilirubin
  Serum albumin, transferrin, and total protein
  Serum protein electrophoresis
  Uric acid, cholesterol, and triglycerides
  Arterial blood gases
  Hepatitis B surface antigen, hepatitis B antibody and core antibody
  Cytomegalovirus, herpes simplex virus, herpes zoster virus, and Epstein-Barr virus titers
  Human immunodeficiency virus test
  VDRL
Radiologic studies
  Chest radiography
  Upper gastrointestinal series
  Gallbladder ultrasonography
  Barium enema
  Voiding cystourethrography
  Doppler examination of abdominal vessels
  Skeletal survey
  Coronary angiography
  Sinus radiography
  CT scan of head, chest, or abdomen
Nuclear medicine scans
  Thallium stress test
  Myocardial kinetic scan
  Liver-spleen scan
  Bone densitometry scan
Other studies and tests
  Electrocardiography
  Treadmill test
  Pulmonary function studies
  Noninvasive vascular laboratory studies
  Urinalysis
  Creatinine clearance
  Quantitative protein excretion
  Hormonal studies
  Occult blood screening
  Upper or lower endoscopy
  Cystometry
  DTH skin testing (includes PPD)
  Pap smear and cervical swab for herpes
  Examination of stool for bacteria, ova, and parasites
  Cultures of urine, stool, and throat for viruses and bacterial pathogens
  Dental consultation
  Ophthalmologic consultation
  Neurologic evaluation
  Psychosocioeconomic consultation

NERVOUS SYSTEM

Examination of the central and peripheral nervous systems should be supplemented by diagnostic tests as indicated to investigate degenerative, vascular, malignant, or infectious processes. The brain and spinal cord can be evaluated by CT and MRI scanning. Cerebrospinal fluid examination may be necessary to rule out demyelinating diseases or infections. Electromyography or the study of visually evoked potentials is necessary in some cases. Ophthalmologic examination should be performed to rule out infectious processes in the eye and to determine the state of the fundus and optic nerve before immunosuppressive therapy is begun. Visual field testing may be useful in the diagnosis of demyelinating diseases and other disease states. Autonomic nervous function is assessed with tests of gastric emptying, the presence or absence of orthostatic hypotension, and heart-rate responses to standing, the Valsalva maneuver, and deep inspiration.

CARDIOVASCULAR SYSTEM

History and physical examination of the heart should focus on determining the presence of intrinsic heart or valvular disease and the functional state of the cardiovascular system. If the cardiac history reveals ischemic heart disease or underlying disease with accelerated atherosclerosis, a treadmill or thallium exercise test should be done. Cardiac performance should also be measured with a gated scan. Because extensive cardiac morbidity occurs after transplantation, preoperative coronary angiography should be considered in patients with a positive cardiac history. At present, however, it is unknown whether the indications for coronary artery dilatation or bypass surgery are different for pretransplant patients than for other patients with ischemic heart disease. The peripheral vascular system is also evaluated. Ischemia in upper and lower extremities should be corrected if possible to diminish the risk of infection in the extremities and a septic response. Carotid arteries should be examined and tested according to usual criteria.

RESPIRATORY SYSTEM

The respiratory system must be able to survive operation and must be free from infection and malignancy. Evaluation should include a chest x-ray, pulmonary function tests, and, if indicated, bronchoscopy, CT scanning of the chest, and lung biopsy. Patients with a history of bronchopulmonary disease must be in the best possible condition before operation. Preoperative chest physiotherapy, bronchodilators, and antibiotics are used to ensure fitness [see 71 Pulmonary Insufficiency].

DIGESTIVE SYSTEM

Evaluation of the digestive system begins with dental consultation. Necessary dental work should be performed before immunosuppression. This work frequently involves multiple extractions to minimize the risk of oral infection.

The esophagus may be examined with either contrast radiography or endoscopy. Candidal esophagitis, which is likely to worsen after immunosuppression, should be treated with nystatin, ketoconazole, or, in severe cases, systemic amphotericin B.[34] Disruption of the esophageal mucosal barrier resulting from reflux esophagitis should be decreased with the usual antireflux treatments.

There is no clear solution to the problem of peptic ulcer disease in potential transplant recipients. Available data are from renal transplant studies.[35] The risk of posttransplant ulcer complications is five to 10 percent, but this risk is doubled in patients who have a pretransplant history of peptic ulcer disease.[36] Mortality in those who develop such complications is high.[34] Various protocols have been used for prophylactic gastric surgery. It is not clear, however, that the rate of posttransplant gastroduodenal complications can be decreased by prophylactic surgery.[36] Antacid prophylaxis, however, probably is effective. Although potentially immunostimulatory, cimetidine has also been used effectively for ulcer prevention.[35] Until further data have been accumulated, the following measures are recommended. In asymptomatic patients, routine workup for peptic ulcer disease is optional. Good-risk patients with a definite history of recurrent or complicated ulcer disease should have acid-reducing surgery before immunosuppressive therapy is initiated. Other patients with inactive ulcer disease may be treated with cimetidine before and after transplantation, and all patients should receive antacid prophylaxis.

Prophylactic cholecystectomy has been suggested for patients with asymptomatic gallstones. The justification for this procedure is to eliminate the risk of postoperative cholecystitis and to avoid possible diagnostic confusion in cases in which jaundice or pancreatitis develops after transplantation. In one study, pretransplant cholecystectomy was associated with a lower incidence of morbidity and mortality than surgical treatment for complications of cholelithiasis after transplantation.[37] However, this approach is not universally accepted at present.

Although postoperative pancreatitis is known to occur after transplantation and immunosuppression,[35] there is no predictive or preventive preoperative workup. The functional status of the liver should be evaluated with blood tests and CT scanning if necessary. The presence of infectious or noninfectious hepatitis should be determined by serologic studies, and disease activity should be staged by follow-up blood tests, biopsy, or both.

Infectious or malignant disease of the colon should be ruled out. Screening tests include stool culture, examination for ova and parasites, and tests for occult blood. If test results are positive, barium enema or colonoscopy (or both) is indicated. Digital examination of the rectum is performed to find local pathological lesions, such as fissures, hemorrhoids, or malignant tumors, that may require treatment before the transplantation procedure is undertaken.

GENITOURINARY SYSTEM

Renal function is evaluated by measurement of creatinine clearance, quantitative tests for proteinuria, and renal biopsy if necessary [see 72 Renal Dysfunction]. Upper and lower urinary tract infections must be treated. In the case of renal transplantation, pretransplant bilateral nephrectomy may be necessary to eliminate a potential source of infection. Indications for nephrectomy include pyelonephritis and severe ureterovesical reflux, with dilatation of the renal pelvis. Lesser degrees of ureterovesical reflux, polycystic kidney disease, and hypertension are less frequent indications.[38] Bladder infections in anuric patients may be treated with systemic antibiotics with or without antibiotic irrigation.

In women, a gynecologic examination, including a Papanicolaou test and cervical swab for bacterial and viral pathogens, should be performed before immunosuppressive therapy.

MUSCULOSKELETAL SYSTEM AND ENDOCRINE SYSTEM

Steroids occasionally cause avascular necrosis of the hip.[35] Existing skeletal disorders should be studied before transplantation. A suggestive history or physical signs of thyroid or adrenal hyperfunction or hypofunction should be followed by laboratory testing. Thyroid nodules, which are potentially malignant, should be a special focus of physical examination. In some potential recipients, assessment of calcium metabolism with parathyroid hormone assays, skeletal surveys, and bone scans is indicated.

DERMAL SYSTEM

The entire body surface should be examined for malignancies and present or potential sources of infection. All boils and other skin infections should be treated before transplantation. Diffuse skin diseases such as psoriasis should be as fully treated as possible. Anal condylomata, which may contain squamous cell carcinoma, should be removed.[39] Diabetic patients and those with peripheral vascular disease are especially likely to acquire foot infections and should have their feet evaluated. They should be instructed to wear loose-fitting shoes, trim toenails square, and apply lanolin creams frequently.

HEMATOLOGIC SYSTEM

Complete blood count and peripheral smear should be done; abnormal results may call for a bone marrow examination. If the patient has undergone splenectomy or if an underlying disease has resulted in splenic dysfunction, the patient should receive pneumococcal and meningococcal polysaccharide vaccines.

IMMUNE SYSTEM

Unless there is evidence of primary immunodeficiency, little specific treatment is currently available for abnormal immunity. A comprehensive workup before deliberate immunosuppressive therapy is therefore not useful. If desired, however, the acquired immune abnormalities associated with organ failure could be studied [see Table 1].

INFECTIOUS DISEASES

The patient should be examined and treated for bacterial, fungal, viral, and protozoan diseases. Bacterial infections of the CNS, lungs, blood, urinary system, and skin require conventional surgical and antibiotic treatment.

Mycobacterial Infection

Mycobacterial infections are of special concern. Administration of steroids to a patient with latent tuberculosis may precipitate active infection. Patients are screened by history; physical examination of the neck, chest, and abdomen; chest and bone x-rays; urinalysis and urine culture; and skin testing. Active tuberculosis should be treated with conventional therapy: double or triple chemotherapy for 24 months before transplantation, if possible. Patients with positive tuberculin skin tests but no evidence of active infection are given prophylactic isoniazid after immunosuppressive medication is started.

Fungal Infection

Most fungal infections occur in patients who are already seriously immunosuppressed. Candidal esophagitis and cystitis, however, may occur in patients awaiting transplants who are not severely immunosuppressed, especially diabetic patients and patients receiving antibiotics. Oral nystatin may be effective in mild cases of candidal esophagitis, but severe candidal esophagitis should be treated with ketoconazole or with a short course of systemic amphotericin B. Candidal cystitis requires correction of motor abnormalities of the bladder, if possible [see 85 Fungal Infection].

Viral Infection

The experience of the recipient's immune system with viral infections can be evaluated serologically. Titers of antibody to CMV, herpes simplex virus (HSV), varicella-zoster virus (VZV), Epstein-Barr virus (EBV), hepatitis B surface antigen (HB_sAg), and human immunodeficiency virus (HIV) are determined. CMV titers may influence the subsequent management of immuno suppression or prophylaxis against CMV. Titers to herpes simplex virus and varicella-zoster virus are mostly useful as baseline measurements for later testing. A positive titer for HB_sAg requires complete evaluation of liver function. It has not been established, however, whether patients with negative tests for HB_sAg should be vaccinated against hepatitis B. A positive test for HIV has a controversial impact. Asymptomatic individuals who are positive for HIV have a life expectancy that may justify transplantation with lifesaving organs such as the heart or liver. As in other patients with similar life expectancy, transplantation may not be justifiable when the organ failure can be treated by other means.

Foreign Bodies

Peritonitis in peritoneal dialysis patients should be treated [see 82 Peritonitis and Intra-abdominal Abscesses]; if the infection resolves, transplantation is not contraindicated. If bacterial infections arise around implanted devices, the devices often must be removed before the infection will resolve. In some patients, persistent local infection of hemodialysis shunts, indwelling bladder catheters, and Tenckhoff catheters may be treated by removal of the devices at the time of transplantation and administration of systemic antibiotics.

Local infection around transcutaneous foreign bodies, such as shunts and catheters, can become systemic after immunosuppression or may result in diffuse skin colonization, increasing the risk of wound infection. If possible, all such transcutaneous devices should be removed or local infection controlled before immunosuppression. If only bacterial colonization is present, it is reasonable to remove the device involved at the time of transplantation and to begin antibiotic therapy.

NUTRITIONAL STATE

Malnutrition is frequently present in patients with organ failure and generally worsens the outcome of operation. Despite the lack of clear data, it seems reasonable, when possible, to determine and correct the patient's nutritional state before transplantation. DTH skin testing, anthropometry, measurement of serum proteins, and body composition studies are used to evaluate the patient's nutritional status preoperatively. Treatment may include tube feeding or parenteral nutrition to restore body cell mass before transplantation [see 97 Nutritional Support].

PSYCHOLOGICAL, SOCIAL, AND FINANCIAL ASSESSMENT

Potential organ recipients must be psychologically, socially, and financially capable of undergoing transplantation. Discrete criteria depend on the organ being transplanted, local programs for care and support of transplant patients, and availability of financial assistance.

References

1. Howard RJ, Simmons RL: Surgical Infectious Diseases, 2nd ed. Appleton & Lange, East Norwalk, Connecticut, 1988
2. Border JR, Hassett JM: Multiple systems organ failure: history, pathophysiology, prevention, and support. Trauma, Sepsis, and Shock: The Physiological Basis of Therapy. Clowes GHA Jr, Ed. Marcel Dekker, New York, 1988, p 335
3. Marshall JC, Christou NV, Horn R, et al: The microbiology of multiple organ failure: the proximal gastrointestinal tract as an occult reservoir of pathogens. Arch Surg 123:309, 1988
4. Johanson WG Jr, Pierce AK, Sanford JP, et al: Nosocomial respiratory infections with gram-negative bacilli: the significance of colonization of the respiratory tract. Ann Intern Med 77:701, 1972
5. Giannella RA, Broitman SA, Zamcheck N: Influence of gastric acidity on bacterial and parasitic enteric infections. Ann Intern Med 78:271, 1973
6. Hau T: Local host defense in the peritoneal cavity. Surgery and Immunity 2:1, 1989
7. Christou NV: Host-defence mechanisms in surgical patients: a correlative study of the delayed hypersensitivity skin-test response, granulocyte function and sepsis. Can J Surg 28:39, 1985
8. Meakins JL, Nohr CW: Assessment of immunologic responsiveness. Nutrition and Metabolism in the Surgical Patient. Kirkpatrick JR, Ed. Futura Publishing Co, Mt Kisco, New York, 1983, p 107
9. Kirkpatrick JR, Meakins JL, Wilson RF: Gastrointestinal disease: fistulas and malignancy. Nutrition and Metabolism in the Surgical Patient. Kirkpatrick JR, Ed. Futura Publishing Co, Mt Kisco, New York, 1983, p 385
10. Kirkpatrick JR, Meakins JL: The burn patient. Nutrition and Metabolism in the Surgical Patient. Kirkpatrick JR, Ed. Futura Publishing Co, Mt Kisco, New York, 1983, p 425
11. Christou NV: Predicting septic related mortality of the individual surgical patient based on admission host-defence measurements. Can J Surg 29:424, 1986
12. Tellado-Rodriguez J, Christou NV: Clinical assessment of host defense. Surg Clin North Am 68:41, 1988
13. Nohr CW, Christou NV, Rode H, et al: In vivo and in vitro humoral immunity in surgical patients. Ann Surg 200:373, 1984
14. Nohr CW, Latter DA, Meakins JL, et al: In vivo and in vitro humoral immunity in surgical patients: antibody response to pneumococcal polysaccharide. Surgery 100:229, 1986
15. Eilber FR, Morton DL: Impaired immunologic reactivity and recurrence following cancer surgery. Cancer 25:362, 1970
16. Meakins JL, Christou NV, Shizgal HM, et al: Therapeutic approaches to anergy in surgical patients: surgery and levamisole. Ann Surg 190:286, 1979
17. Nohr CW, Meakins JL: Biological response modifiers. Surgical Infection in Critical Care Medicine. Meakins JL, Ed. Churchill Livingstone, New York, 1985, p 309
18. Miles AA, Miles EM, Burke J: The value and duration of defence reaction of the skin to the primary lodgement of bacteria. Br J Exp Pathol 38:79, 1957
19. Snydman DR, Werner BG, Heinze-Lacey B, et al: Use of cytomegalovirus immune globulin to prevent cytomegalovirus disease in renal-transplant recipients. N Engl J Med 317:1049, 1987
20. Suthanthiran M, Strom TB: Renal transplantation. N Engl J Med 331:365, 1994
21. Snydman DR, Rubin RH, Werner BG: New developments in cytomegalovirus prevention and management. Am J Kidney Dis 21:217, 1993
22. Goodrich JM, Mori M, Gleaves CA, et al: Early treatment with ganciclovir to prevent cytomegalovirus disease after allogeneic bone marrow transplantation. N Engl J Med 325:1601, 1991
23. Rubin RH, Greene R: Etiology and management of the compromised patient with fever and pulmonary infiltrates. Clinical Approach to Infection in the Compromised Host. Rubin RH, Young LS, Eds. Plenum Publishing Corp, New York, 1988, p 131
24. Bensard DD, McIntyre RC Jr, Waring BJ, et al: Comparison of video thoracoscopic lung biopsy to open lung biopsy in the diagnosis of interstitial lung disease. Chest 103:765, 1993
25. Klimbert S, Hawkins I, Vogel SB: Percutaneous cholecystostomy for acute cholecystitis in high-risk patients. Am J Surg 153:125, 1987
26. Dienstag JL: Viral hepatitis in the compromised host. Clinical Approach to Infection in the Compromised Host. Rubin RH, Young LS, Eds. Plenum Publishing Corp, New York, 1988, p 325
27. Peterson PK, Simmons RL: Infections in organ transplant recipients. Principles and Practice of Infectious Diseases, 2nd ed. Mandell GL, Douglas RG, Bennett JE, Eds. John Wiley & Sons, New York, 1985, p 1676
28. Joshi JH, Schimpff SC: Infections in special hosts: infections in the compromised host. Principles and Practice of Infectious Diseases, 2nd ed. Mandell GL, Douglas RG, Bennett JE, Eds. John Wiley & Sons, New York, 1985, p 1644
29. Young LS: Gram-negative sepsis. Principles and Practice of Infectious Diseases, 2nd ed. Mandell GL, Douglas RG, Bennett JE, Eds. John Wiley & Sons, New York, 1985, p 452
30. Rusthoven J: The potential role of recombinant hematopoietic colony-stimulating factors in preventing infections in the immunocompromised host. Can J Infect Dis 2:74, 1991
31. Pizzo PA: Empiric therapy and prevention of infection in the immunocompromised host. Principles and Practice of Infectious Diseases, 2nd ed. Mandell GL, Douglas RG, Bennett JE, Eds. John Wiley & Sons, New York, 1985, p 1680
32. Kemeny MM, Brennan MF: The surgical complications of chemotherapy in the cancer patient. Curr Probl Surg 24:609, 1987
33. Cosimi AB: Surgical aspects of infection in the compromised host. Clinical Approach to Infection in the Compromised Host. Rubin RH, Young LS, Eds. Plenum Publishing Corp, New York, 1988, p 649
34. Frick T, Fryd DS, Goodale RL, et al: Incidence and treatment of candida esophagitis in patients undergoing renal transplantation. Am J Surg 155:311, 1988
35. Vincenti F, Parfrey PS, Briggs W: Skeletal, gastrointestinal, hepatic, and hematologic disorders following kidney transplantation. Renal Transplantation. Garovoy MR, Guttman RD, Eds. Churchill Livingstone, New York, 1986, p 233
36. Bansky G, Huynh Do U, Largiadèr F, et al: Gastroduodenal complications after renal transplantation: the role of prophylactic gastric surgery in hyperacid kidney allograft recipients. Clin Transpl 1:209, 1987
37. Graham SM, Flowers JL, Schweitzer E, et al: The utility of prophylactic laparoscopic cholecystectomy in transplant candidates. Am J Surg 169:44, 1995
38. Briggs JD: The recipient of a renal transplant. Kidney Transplantation. Morris PJ, Ed. Grune & Stratton, London, 1984, p 59
39. Penn I: Cancers of the anogenital region in renal transplant recipients: analysis of 65 cases. Cancer 58:611, 1986
40. Rosen FS, Cooper MD, Wedgewood RJP: The primary immunodeficiencies (pts 1 and 2). Medical Progress 311:235, 300, 1984
41. Delafuente JC: Immunosenescence: clinical and pharmacologic considerations. Med Clin North Am 69:475, 1985
42. Kishimoto S, Tomino S, Mitsuya H, et al: Age-related decline in the in vitro and in vivo syntheses of anti-tetanus toxoid antibody in humans. J Immunol 125:2347, 1980
43. Ceuppens JL, Goodwin JS: Regulation of immunoglobulin production in pokeweed mitogen-stimulated cultures of lymphocytes from young and old adults. J Immunol 128:2429, 1982
44. Tsukayama D, Breitenbucher R, Steinberg S, et al: Polymorphonuclear leukocyte, T-lymphocyte, and natural killer cell activities in elderly nursing home residents. Eur J Clin Microbiol 5:468, 1986
45. Chandra RK, Kutty KM: Immunocompetence in obesity. Acta Paediatr Scand 69:25, 1980
46. Nohr CW, Tchervenkov JI, Meakins JL, et al: Malnutrition and humoral immunity: short-term acute nutritional deprivation. Surgery 98:769, 1985
47. Horita M, Suzuki H, Onodera T, et al: Abnormalities of immunoregulatory T cell subsets in patients with insulin-dependent diabetes mellitus. J Immunol 129:1426, 1982
48. Hill HR, Augustine NH, Rallison ML, et al: Defective monocyte chemotactic responses in diabetes mellitus. J Clin Immunol 3:70, 1983
49. Beam TR, Crigler ED, Goldman JK, et al: Antibody response to polyvalent pneumococcal polysaccharide vaccine in diabetes. JAMA 244:2621, 1980
50. Goldblum SE, Reed WP: Host defenses and immunologic alterations associated with chronic hemodialysis. Ann Intern Med 93:597, 1980
51. Glassock RJ: Nutrition, immunology, and renal disease. Kidney Int 24(suppl 16):S194, 1983
52. Fernandez LA, Laltoo M, Fox RA: A study of T cell populations in alcoholic cirrhosis and chronic alcoholism. Clin Invest Med 5:241, 1982
53. Havens WP Jr, Myerson RM, Klatchko J: Production of tetanus antitoxin by patients with hepatic cirrhosis. N Engl J Med 257:637, 1957
54. Bagby GC Jr: Leukopenia. Cecil Textbook of Medicine. Wyngaarden JB, Smith LH, Eds. WB Saunders Co, Philadelphia, 1988, p 961
55. Orgill D, Demling RH: Current concepts and approaches to wound healing. Crit Care Med 16:899, 1988
56. Meuleman J, Katz P: The immunologic effects, kinetics, and use of glucocorticosteroids. Med Clin North Am 69:805, 1985
57. Cupps TH, Edgar LC, Thomas CA, et al: Multiple mechanisms of B cell immunoregulation in man after administration of in vivo corticosteroids. J Immunol 132:170, 1984
58. Hobbs CH, McClellan RO: Radiation and radioactive materials. Casarett and Doull's Toxicology: The Basic Science of Poisons, 2nd ed. Casarett LJ, Doull J, Eds. Macmillan Publishing Co, New York, 1980, p 497
59. Christou NV, McLean APH, Meakins JL: Host defense in blunt trauma: interrelationships of kinetics of anergy and depressed neutrophil function, nutritional status, and sepsis. J Trauma 20:833, 1980

60. Salo M: Effects of anaesthesia and surgery on the immune response. Trauma, Stress and Immunity in Anesthesia and Surgery. Watkins J, Salo M, Eds. Butterworth Publishers, Stoneham, Massachusetts, 1982, p 211
61. Moudgil GC: Update on anaesthesia and the immune response. Can Anaesth Soc J 33:S54, 1986
62. Wu H-S, Little AG: Perioperative blood transfusions and cancer recurrence. J Clin Oncol 6:1348, 1988
63. Bohnsack JF, Brown EJ: The role of the spleen in resistance to infection. Annu Rev Med 37:49, 1986
64. Hau T: Infections of the liver and spleen. Surgical Infectious Diseases, 2nd ed. Howard RJ, Simmons RL. Appleton & Lange, East Norwalk, Connecticut, 1988, p 659
65. Wilson RE: Surgical Problems in Immuno-Depressed Patients. WB Saunders Co, Philadelphia, 1984
66. Sheil AGR: Cancer after transplantation. World J Surg 10:389, 1986
67. Hanto DW, Najarian JS: Advances in the diagnosis and treatment of EBV-associated lymphoproliferative diseases in immunocompromised hosts. J Surg Oncol 30:215, 1985
68. Kelly GE, Sheil AGR, Taylor R: Nonspecific immunological studies in kidney transplant recipients with and without skin cancer. Transplantation 37:368, 1984
69. Birkeland SA: Immune monitoring of tumor development after renal transplantation. Cancer 55:988, 1985
70. Penn I: Cancer in the immunosuppressed organ recipient. Transplant Proc 23:1771, 1991
71. Hanto DW: Polyclonal and monoclonal posttransplant lymphoproliferative diseases (LPD). Clin Transpl 6:227, 1992
72. Harid IR, Strong RW, Hartley LCJ, et al: Skin cancer in Caucasian renal allograft recipients living in a subtropical climate. Surgery 87:177, 1980
73. Napolitano LM, Chernow B: Guidelines for corticosteroid use in anesthetic and surgical stress. Int Anesthesiol Clin 26:226, 1988
74. Salem M, Tainsh RE Jr, Bromberg J, et al: Perioperative glucocorticoid coverage: a reassessment 42 years after emergence of a problem. Ann Surg 219:416, 1994

75 THE ELDERLY SURGICAL PATIENT

James M. Watters, M.D., and Jacqueline C. McClaran, M.D.

Perioperative Management of the Elderly Patient

Principles of Surgical Care in the Elderly

Management of surgical illness in geriatric patients is different from that in younger patients and typically more complex. Assessment of surgical problems and physiologic status of the elderly must take into account (1) the marked variability of the changes associated with advancing age, both among individuals and among different organ systems in an individual, (2) changes in the incidence, prevalence, and natural history of certain disease processes, and (3) the increased likelihood of multiple medical diagnoses and polypharmacy.[1]

These factors and others may alter the presentation of surgical illness: symptoms may be diminished in intensity, nonspecific, indirect, or atypical and therefore may be inappropriately ignored or attributed simply to advanced age. Patients may postpone seeking medical attention, or physicians may fail to recognize the gravity of an acute surgical condition if pain, fever, and acute-phase responses are blunted [*see* Alterations in Clinical Presentation, *below*]. Furthermore, it may be difficult to obtain the details of the history if the patient is confused or suffers from impaired hearing or memory.

Both the potential benefits and the risks of surgical treatment are more difficult to assess in the elderly. Assumptions about physiologic status and primary treatment goals that are reasonable in younger patients may not be appropriate in older patients. Often, the major concern of elderly patients is whether they will be able to enjoy an independent life after surgery to at least the extent they did before. Consequently, such patients may find a radical procedure that offers potential cure less desirable than a more conservative procedure (or endoscopic, percutaneous, or nonoperative treatment) that relieves pain or other symptoms, largely restores function, and allows a return to normal surroundings. On the other hand, an aggressive early approach may obviate later procedures and prevent associated morbidity. A thorough knowledge of treatment alternatives and their risks, a close familiarity with the natural history of the disease in relation to life expectancy, and a clear understanding of the patient's goals are paramount in surgical decision making in the elderly.

The risks associated with surgical treatment depend on the nature of the proposed procedure and on the patient's physiologic and medical status [*see* Discussion, Assessment of Risks, *below*]. Whereas minor elective procedures done with the patient under local anesthesia can be performed safely regardless of age, emergency thoracotomy and laparotomy are associated with significant mortality in the elderly. Mortality from emergency procedures is markedly higher than mortality from elective procedures. Elective surgery may therefore be indicated when it can be predicted that complications will develop and emergency intervention will be necessary. Cardiovascular and pulmonary complications remain important causes of postoperative mortality in the elderly, much more so than in younger patients.

Advancing age is accompanied by predictable changes in virtually every organ system and by a tendency toward a decline in physiologic reserve and in the ability to maintain homeostasis [*see* Discussion, Patterns of Change in Body Composition, Organ Systems, and Integrated Responses, *below*]. Nevertheless, the geriatric population is a very heterogeneous one. Some elderly persons are wholly independent, have maintained moderate levels of physical activity throughout their lives, have preserved lean body mass and cardiopulmonary function, and have physiologic responses similar to those of younger individuals; in these patients, the risks associated with surgical illness and treatment are relatively low. At the opposite extreme, some elderly persons have multiple illnesses, are capable of only limited activity and independence, and suffer from cardiovascular and pulmonary disease; in these patients, the surgery-associated risks are substantial. Although mortality from surgery, trauma, and systemic infection increases consistently with age, it seems likely that physiologic status is a more fundamental determinant. As one surgeon put it as long ago as 1907, "In deciding for or [against] operation we depend upon the condition of the heart, the arteries, the lungs, and kidneys, rather more than the number of years the patient has lived."[1] Recognition of the heterogeneity of the geriatric population and a careful assessment of physiologic and functional status are essential to surgical care of the elderly.

Eight factors are critical for obtaining the best outcome from surgical treatment of elderly patients. These factors are (1) careful preoperative preparation of the patient and optimization of medical and physiologic status, (2) appropriate anesthesia and physiologic monitoring, (3) recognition of alterations in clinical pharmacology, (4) minimization of the postoperative stresses of hypothermia, hypoxemia, and pain, (5) prevention of alterations in blood pressure and heart rate, (6) avoidance of perturbations of fluid, electrolyte, and acid-base status, (7) careful surgical technique, and (8) optimization of functional level [*see Sidebar* Achievement of Optimal Functional Level]. The importance of these factors will be discussed below.

Achievement of Optimal Functional Level

Optimal functional level is the goal of all diagnostics, therapeutics, and management in the elderly.[215-217] According to a 1988 statement by the American College of Physicians, "maintenance of the patient's functional well-being is a fundamental goal of medical practice. Assessment of the impact of illness on physical, mental, and psychosocial functioning is an essential element of clinical diagnosis, a major determinant of therapeutic choices, a measure of their efficacy, and a guide in the planning of long-term care for the dependent elderly."[218]

Functional level assessment is intrinsic to geriatric care and should be practiced throughout the perioperative period to predict rehabilitation potential, to estimate biologic reserve, to follow progress, to signal complications, to identify appropriate social supports at discharge,[219,220] and to ensure discharge.[221] Functional level assessment is known to improve diagnostic and therapeutic outcomes.[222] Recognition of functional impairment leads to identification of previously undiagnosed conditions that may be treatable preoperatively or managed perioperatively.[223] Another justification for functional assessment is that disease states do not correlate as well with severity of impairment in elderly patients as they do in younger adults even when clinical judgment has provided a reliable estimate of degree of aging and all disease states are known.[224-227]

The recent surgical literature reflects a growing awareness of functional outcomes, both specific outcomes related to pathology and surgery and general ones related to patients' day-to-day activities and self-satisfaction.[228-234]

For optimal assessment of functional level, surgeons need a fast, simple tool that is suitable for all stages of management (preoperative, perioperative, and postoperative), that correlates well with measures of cardiovascular, pulmonary, and renal function, and that identifies patients who will achieve maximum postoperative function and who need community supports at discharge. Unfortunately, no such tool exists; surgeons will probably have to develop one themselves. In the meantime, the traditional Goldman and American Society of Anesthesiologists (ASA) biologic assessments can be complemented with functional assessments borrowed from the medical, psychiatric, and social science literatures.[235]

There are actually hundreds of functional assessment tools, some of which have been validated for use in the geriatric population and some of which were specifically developed for elderly patients. These tools have various goals, ranging from predicting social supports to monitoring deterioration.[219,221,236,237] Most of them address one or more of the following areas: mobility, falls and balance, continence, cognition, emotional and affective status, nutrition, homeostasis, basic activities of daily living (ADL), instrumental ADL, environment, and social supports. The various functional level scales cover items ranging from disability, handicap, and incapacity to independence and from ability to self-development and self-realization.

Of the functional assessment tools available, perhaps the most comprehensive and positive in orientation is the OARS (Older Americans Retirement Survey), which was developed at Duke University for use in community-dwelling seniors.[238] The OARS assesses the following functional dimensions: social resources, economic resources, mental health, physical health, and ADL. It is valid and reliable in elderly populations.

A functional assessment that is practical in surgical settings is offered by the Katz index of basic ADL, which identifies six areas of function, from the most primitive to the most sophisticated, in the following order: feeding, continence, transferring, toileting, dressing, and bathing. The Katz index is reliable, valid, simple, and quick. It yields a comprehensive picture when coupled with a measure of instrumental ADL and a measure of mental status.[239-242] This battery of tests can be carried out reliably many times by several different health professionals at various stages of surgical care.

The instrumental ADL that should be measured as a complement to the Katz index include meal preparation, food shopping, use of telephone, use of public or private transport, occupation, and banking. For example, does the patient drive his or her own car, take the bus unaccompanied, or both? Does the patient still work or have a part-time volunteer job? Does the patient go to the bank and keep his or her own accounts without help? The functional scale that best covers these items is the Lawton and Brody instrumental ADL test.[243]

Finally, cognitive function should be assessed, preferably with the Folstein Mini-Mental State examination [*see 9 Coma, Seizures, Cognitive Impairment, and Brain Death*].

It is worth remembering that assessments of basic and instrumental ADL and cognition do not explain why a particular function is impaired but simply describe how well a patient is functioning at a given time. Any functional impairment is a signal that further assessment to identify correctable pathological conditions is indicated. When areas of compromised function have been identified before an elective procedure, it may be wise to request a period of rehabilitation to maximize functional level before admission. For example, continence training may be provided by a community health nurse; gait and mobility training may be provided by a geriatric physiotherapist. Complementary assessments by the family physician, a psychiatrist, or a geriatrician may help identify ways of achieving maximal function preoperatively.

There are no good data on the impact of surgery on ADL and functional level. In general, however, it is not expected that a preoperative functional impairment will be improved postoperatively unless the surgical intervention was specifically designed to address the impairment. For example, if mobility is compromised by an inguinal hernia, it is reasonable to expect the patient to resume his or her own banking after herniorrhaphy.

The nursing team should be made aware of the patient's functional deficits in the OR, in recovery, and in the ward afterwards. To some degree, they may be able to compensate for disability in the surgical environment and may even prevent additional disability. For example, a patient who is encouraged to wear glasses and a hearing aid in recovery is more cooperative and better oriented and is ready for step-down to the ward. Nurses who compensate for patient deafness by ensuring that he or she sees their lips when they speak and by speaking slowly and clearly can report patient level of consciousness more accurately.[57,244]

ALTERATIONS IN CLINICAL PRESENTATION

The manifestations of surgical illness in the elderly may be considerably different from those in young or middle-aged individuals.[2] Multiple medical disorders are often present, and the symptoms of acute surgical illness may be masked.[3] The central nervous system is particularly sensitive to the effects of drugs and disease, and the presentation of surgical and medical illness may be nonspecific (e.g., lethargy, confusion, or agitation) or indirect (e.g., an unexplained fall).[4,5] Relative inactivity may limit the manifestations of important cardiac, pulmonary, or peripheral vascular disease. The patient, the family, or the surgeon may inappropriately attribute relevant symptoms to the supposedly inevitable changes of advancing age. Memory or hearing impairment may make it difficult to obtain a reliable history. To ensure effective communication, the surgeon may have to make an extra effort when taking the history and reviewing the medical records.

Elderly patients may have a higher pain threshold than younger individuals. Older patients presenting with acute abdominal pain are more likely than younger individuals to require surgical intervention.[6] The localization of abdominal pain in patients with peritonitis may not be as reliable; elderly patients with appendicitis are less likely than younger patients to have pain localized to the right lower quadrant.[7] Abdominal pain is a less frequent presentation of colorectal carcinoma in geriatric patients than in younger patients.[2] These observations suggest that pain is a particularly important symptom in the elderly and that its degree is not necessarily an adequate indication of the gravity of the underlying problem.[8] The perception of pain is complex, however; situational factors and expectations may have a major impact on reactions to injury.

Although febrile responses are generally intact, fever may be less marked in elderly individuals with infectious or inflammatory processes, particularly those older than 80 years. Hypothermia is more common in elderly patients who are seriously ill than in younger patients.[9]

The prevalence and natural history of some pathological processes, as well as their clinical manifestations, may be altered in the geriatric population. For example, elderly patients presenting with appendicitis are more likely to have gangrenous or perforated appendicitis than younger patients are. It is not clear whether this finding reflects a change in the onset of symptoms, a difference in the evolution of the pathological process, or a delay in seeking medical attention. Similarly, elderly patients with symptomatic gallstones are more likely than younger patients to present with perforation, empyema, or gangrene of the gallbladder, acute cholecystitis, or cholangitis and are more likely to require urgent surgery.[10] The natural history and presentation of some carcinomas differ in the geriatric population.[2,5] The importance of malignancy as a cause of surgical illness in the elderly is indicated by its increasing prevalence with age, the high proportion of surgical procedures related to malignancy, and its frequency as a cause of death in surgical patients.[11-13]

Trauma

The management of trauma is typically more complex and challenging in elderly patients than in younger ones.[14] The prevalence of preexisting medical conditions increases with age, and such conditions are associated with longer hospital stays and higher mortality after injury.[15,16] Mechanisms of injury change in relative frequency with age, as do the types of injuries that result from a given physical insult and the outcomes that follow a given injury. In the Major Trauma Outcome Study (MTOS), for example, falls were the predominant mechanism of injury among patients 65 years of age or older, but they were relatively infrequent in younger patients[17] [see Table 1].

Motor vehicle crashes are the most common mechanism of injury in younger patients and remain the second most common in older patients. The circumstances and nature of motor vehicle crashes tend to differ in the elderly. Crashes involving older drivers occur mainly in daytime and close to home and more often result from errors of judgment or perception than from high speed, aggressive driving, loss of vehicle control, or the use of alcohol.[23] Older drivers are more likely to be in crashes involving right-of-way conflicts, improper turning or starting, and failure to recognize or obey traffic signals.[19,20] Older drivers are also more likely to be involved in multivehicle side-impact collisions.[21-23]

The direction of impact influences both the pattern of injuries sustained and mortality.[23] In one study, injuries to the face and the lower extremities were significantly more common in drivers involved in frontal collisions, whereas injuries to the chest, the abdomen, and the pelvis were more frequent in left lateral impacts.[23] Mortality was nearly doubled in left lateral impacts; this increase was independent of both Injury Severity Score and driver age.

The pattern of injuries resulting from a given physical insult also seems to differ to some extent in the elderly: older drivers have a higher incidence of chest injuries, specifically rib and sternal fractures.[22,24] Greater chest wall stiffness and osteoporotic changes may predispose older persons to rib fractures after relatively minor trauma. Rib fractures or even flail chest may sometimes occur in the elderly without the significant underlying pulmonary contusion that would be anticipated in a younger patient.[25,26] Striking age-related increases in fractures of the vertebrae, the hip, and the distal forearm have been documented, and the pivotal role of osteoporosis in such fractures is well recognized.[27] Burn injuries are more common in the elderly, and these injuries tend to be more severe in terms of both surface area and depth; moreover, inhalation injury is more likely.[28] As a consequence, mortality is higher and hospi-

Table 1 Incidence of Specific Mechanisms of Injury and Associated Mortality[17]

	≥ 65 Years		< 65 Years	
	Incidence (%)	Mortality (%)	Incidence (%)	Mortality (%)
Fall	46.0	11.7	11.0	6.0
Motor vehicle accident	28.2	20.7	33.5	9.6
Pedestrian hit by vehicle	10.0	32.6	7.9	13.5
Stab wound	2.6	17.3	11.9	4.7
Gunshot wound	5.5	52.1	13.0	19.5
Motorcycle accident	0.4	11.8	7.7	11.9
Other	7.0	13.8	14.9	5.4
Unknown	0.3	19.0	0.1	9.8

tal stay longer in the elderly.[28] The increased risk for burn injury may be attributable to a diminished sense of smell, impaired hearing or vision, or reduced mobility and reaction time. The tendency to more severe injury may be attributable to age-related changes in skin morphology.[28]

Because elderly persons are, in general, less sensitive to deviations from physiologic norms and less able to maintain homeostasis, they tend to be less able to maintain adequate perfusion of vital organs after injury. Thus, elderly patients are more likely to arrive in the emergency room hypotensive, cold, and in shock after a given injury than younger patients are. Presumably, reduced homeostatic capacity contributes to the overrepresentation of the elderly among immediate and early trauma deaths as well as among late deaths related to infection and multiple organ dysfunction syndrome. In one study, no elderly patient with a Trauma Score (TS) lower than 7 survived long enough to be admitted to a hospital.[29] Resuscitative measures, though identical in principle to those taken in younger patients, must be carried out with an eye to the physiologic limitations of the elderly, particularly the need for volume loading to achieve increases in cardiac output. Preexisting medical conditions must be identified rapidly via history taking, physical examination, and investigative studies as needed, and information about previous medication use should be obtained. Because thermoregulatory mechanisms are less efficient in the elderly, measures should be taken to minimize ongoing heat loss from exposure and administration of cool fluids and to prevent the adverse effects of hypothermia.

Unfortunately, even an apparently good physiologic status in the emergency room (at least as reflected in the TS or the Revised Trauma Score [RTS]) does not guarantee survival for the elderly trauma patient: mortality in elderly patients with high TS or RTS is many times higher than that in younger patients with comparable scores.[17,30,31] MTOS data demonstrate that case-fatality rates are uniformly higher in patients 65 years of age or older than in younger patients for every injury mechanism for which sufficient data were available.[32] Mortality was consistently higher for each range of Injury Severity Scores and for each injury severity–body region combination. Patients 65 years of age or older accounted for 30 percent of the deaths that were unexpected according to Trauma Score Revised Injury Severity Score (TRISS) projections despite representing only eight percent of the MTOS study population. Complications (pulmonary, cardiovascular, and infectious) were also more common in the older patients[17,32]; the difference was most striking among patients with mild to moderate injury. Others have noted the high incidence in the elderly of respiratory complications (including pneumonia) as well as cardiac complications that are relatively uncommon in younger patients.[33,34]

Although elderly patients are less likely to survive their injuries and be discharged than younger patients are, several reports indicate that many older survivors will ultimately return to a satisfactory level of function and independence.[25,33-37] Variations in functional recovery and placement status result from a number of factors besides the specific mechanism and nature of the injury. For example, family and social support systems have been shown to be important for achieving discharge-to-home and optimal functional recovery in patients with isolated hip fracture, and some authors have reached similar conclusions with reference to trauma in the elderly in general.[38,39] Very advanced age, preinjury

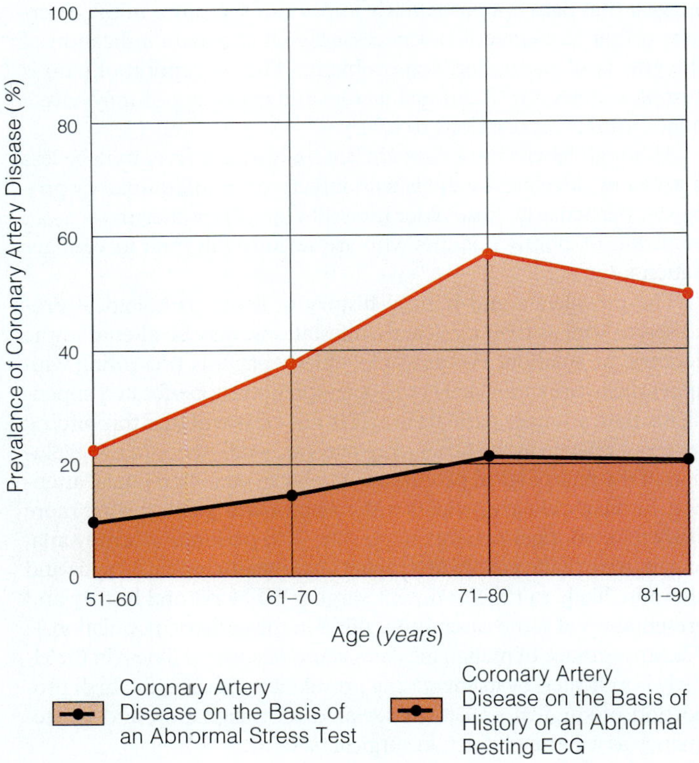

Figure 1 Shown is an estimate of the prevalence of coronary artery disease in men between 51 and 90 years of age.[266]

placement, preinjury functional status, and preexisting medical conditions are also likely to influence postinjury rehabilitation. Injury-causing falls may, in some instances, be a reflection of important underlying problems, such as drop attacks or a poor physical state. The adverse impact of serious head injury on early and delayed mortality has been reported in a number of studies.[31,33,35-37] Admission to an ICU, even if the stay is longer than two weeks and even if mechanical ventilation is necessary, does not preclude a very good functional recovery in the majority of survivors.[25,33-35]

Preoperative Management

ASSESSMENT AND OPTIMIZATION OF PHYSIOLOGIC AND MEDICAL STATUS

The most frequent potentially preventable causes of death are those related to the cardiovascular and pulmonary systems. It is worthwhile to pay particular attention to the preoperative assessment of these systems.

Assessment of the Cardiovascular System

The prevalence of coronary artery disease increases with age: significant coronary artery disease is present at autopsy in more than 50 percent of individuals older than 70 years [see *Figure 1*]. According to the Cardiac Risk Index, major risk factors for postoperative cardiovascular complications include myocardial infarction in the previous six months, uncompensated congestive heart failure, aortic stenosis, nonsinus rhythm or the occurrence of more than five premature ventricular contractions per minute at any time, diabetes, and age greater than 70 years [see 38 Evaluation of Cardiac Risk].[40] Although age greater than 70 years was one of the factors on which the Cardiac Risk Index was based, its weighting in the index is relatively small. Evaluation of the cardiovascular system in the elderly patient includes a history, a physical examination, electrocardiography, and chest x-rays. Myocardial infarction is unaccompanied by recognized symptoms in as many as 10 percent of elderly patients; dyspnea and syncope are relatively prominent manifestations.[41] The incidence of postoperative myocardial infarction is low (0.1 to 0.2 percent) in patients with no evidence of previous heart disease.[42,43] In one study, postoperative cardiac ischemic events, but no cardiac deaths, occurred in 3.1 percent of patients (two of 64) without clinical markers of cardiac disease who underwent major vascular operation; however, age greater than 70 years was identified as one predictor of such events. Age was not a predictor of postoperative myocardial infarction in a study of 12,654 surgical patients or of myocardial reinfarction in another study.[42,44] Claudication, stroke, and transient ischemic attacks with related physical findings are important markers of peripheral vascular disease and its sequelae. Whether patients with chronic stable angina are at increased risk for perioperative complications after noncardiac surgery is a controversial issue, although such appears to be the case in patients with symptomatic peripheral vascular disease.[45] Patients with unstable angina rarely present for elective noncardiac surgery; complete evaluation and treatment of the coronary artery disease should be undertaken if at all possible. The likelihood of perioperative myocardial ischemia and infarction, arrhythmias, and cardiac death is increased when nitrates, beta blockers, and calcium channel blockers are discontinued preoperatively.[45]

Clinical assessment of cardiac status may be unsatisfactory in patients with limitations in physical activity (e.g., patients with claudication or arthritis), in which case further investigation may be appropriate. Dipyridamole-thallium scintigraphy is a sensitive screening test for detecting ischemic heart disease and predicting postoperative cardiovascular complications [see 38 Evaluation of Cardiac Risk].

The high risk associated with surgery in patients with overt congestive heart failure is clear, and all but the most urgent procedures should be postponed.[45] The risk of postoperative cardiac complications appears to be substantially lower when congestive heart failure is well controlled preoperatively than when it is not. Preoperative diuresis should not be so vigorous that it results in dehydration and contributes to hypotension at anesthetic induction.

The unexpected preoperative finding of mild to moderate essential hypertension (diastolic blood pressure ≤ 110 mm Hg) should not delay surgery; however, the possibility of end-organ injury, associated coronary artery disease, and secondary hypertension must be taken into account.[46] Preoperative hypertension may be associated with an increased likelihood of postoperative cardiac complications, although there are conflicting data on this point.[40,42,45,46] Because preoperative control of blood pressure may lessen hemodynamic instability during anesthesia, antihypertensive medications should be continued up to the beginning of the procedure. Significant intraoperative hypotension is strongly linked with postoperative cardiac complications and death [see Intraoperative Management, below].[43,44,47]

Patients who have a systolic murmur suggestive of aortic stenosis should undergo further evaluation whether they have symptoms (e.g., syncope, dyspnea, or angina) or not.

Preexisting arrhythmias, especially frequent premature ventricular contractions or rhythms other than sinus rhythm, are usually believed to reflect underlying cardiac disease and are associated with an increased incidence of postoperative cardiac ischemia and congestive heart failure.[45] Prophylactic antiarrhythmic therapy is not helpful and should be avoided except in patients with a history of sustained ventricular arrhythmia. Patients without underlying coronary disease do not appear to be at increased risk.

Assessment of Pulmonary Function

Elderly patients are at particular risk for postoperative respiratory complications, even those who are in good general health [see Discussion, Patterns of Change in Body Composition, Organ Systems, and Integrated Responses, below]. Consequently, it is vital to recognize limitations in respiratory function and to institute preoperative measures to counteract them. Respiratory assessment should routinely include a history focusing on habitual level of activity, presence of dyspnea or cough, smoking habits, and previous deep venous thrombosis or pulmonary embolus as well as a physical examination and chest x-rays. Dyspnea may reflect ischemic cardiac disease in the elderly. Routine preoperative chest x-rays are more likely to reveal abnormalities in elderly patients than in younger ones; however, the influence of such findings on perioperative management is unclear.[48]

Simple spirometry is the most useful pulmonary function test and should be used as a screening test in patients with suspected obstructive lung disease, patients scheduled for thoracic or upper abdominal surgery, and patients older than 70 years.[49] The effect of bronchodilators on flow rates should be determined if flow rates are low. When the history and the physical examination suggest pulmonary dysfunction and spirometric findings are abnormal, the risk of postoperative pulmonary complications appears to be increased.[50] An arterial blood gas analysis should be obtained in patients with significantly abnormal results on spirometry.[51] Other factors predisposing to pulmonary complications, such as obesity and smoking, must also be taken into account.[49]

Patients of any age with abnormal pulmonary function are at increased risk for postoperative pulmonary complications, and there are many reasons to anticipate such complications in the aged patient; however, there is no well-defined lower limit of function that contraindicates operation.[50] Elevated arterial carbon dioxide tension (P_aCO_2) presumably reflects a marked loss of pulmonary function and limitation of reserve; preoperative P_aCO_2 greater than 45 mm Hg has been associated with an increased incidence of postoperative respiratory complications.[52] In another study, the finding of preoperative P_aCO_2 greater than 50 mm Hg mandated a postoperative period of mechanical ventilation.[51] Hypercapnia may be a less significant contraindication if it is due to a correctable condition, such as infection, bronchospasm, or central alveolar hypoventilation.

In 42 patients (mean age, 71 years) with a forced expiratory volume in one second (FEV_1) of 0.3 to 1.0 L (11 to 59 percent of predicted) who underwent elective operation with general or regional anesthesia, postoperative use of mechanical ventilation was best predicted by preoperative dyspnea at rest and arterial hypoxemia.[53] FEV_1 was considered to have only limited predictive value, perhaps serving best as a screening test. In a study of patients with an FEV_1 of less than 1 L who underwent predominantly abdominal and pelvic procedures, the authors concluded that reduced FEV_1 (FEV_1 < 1 L or 50 percent of predicted), with or without hypoxemia, should not contraindicate operation, although postoperative monitoring in an ICU was advocated.[51]

Smoking should be stopped as far in advance of operation as possible, ideally at least eight weeks beforehand. Patients with poorly controlled wheezing should be identified and treated. Bronchodilators such as inhaled beta-adrenergic agents, oral theophylline, and, occasionally, oral steroids may be required. Gram's staining and culture of sputum, physiotherapy, and administration of broad-spectrum antibiotics may be indicated in individuals who have a productive cough. Elective procedures should be delayed for four to six weeks in patients who have significant upper respiratory infection or pneumonia. Planned postoperative mechanical ventilation should be considered for—and discussed with—patients who have serious pulmonary dysfunction. The nature of the proposed operation and anesthesia must be taken into account. Thoracic and upper abdominal procedures carry the highest risks of postoperative pulmonary complications.

Assessment of Renal Function

The progressive decline in renal function that occurs with advancing age has been well described[54] and appears to be more consistent than changes in other organ systems [see Discussion, Management Considerations throughout the Perioperative Period, *below*]. Because of predictable decreases in skeletal muscle mass—and therefore in creatinine production—the serum creatinine concentration is likely to remain within the laboratory normal range despite the substantial concurrent decreases in the glomerular filtration rate (GFR) that occur. Increased serum creatinine concentrations reflect a marked impairment of renal function. The glomerular filtration rate is best assessed by the determination of creatinine clearance [see Figure 2].

Nonsteroidal anti-inflammatory drugs (NSAIDs) have a number of potentially detrimental effects on the kidneys of older patients.[55] Prostaglandin inhibition may allow unopposed vasoconstriction and marked decreases in renal blood flow and glomerular filtration rate in hypovolemic states, which in turn may result in acute renal failure. In addition, NSAIDs potentiate hyponatremia and hyperkalemia through their effects on the renin-angiotensin-aldosterone system and may cause acute interstitial nephritis.

Consideration of Other Risk Factors

Advanced age is a well-recognized risk factor for the development of postoperative deep venous thrombosis (DVT). Objective surveillance or prophylaxis of DVT, or both, should therefore be considered in elderly surgical patients [see 70 Thromboembolic Problems]. Advanced age is also a risk factor for the development of surgical site infection: patients older than 66 years are six times more likely to have infections of clean wounds than are patients one to 14 years of age.[56]

PSYCHOLOGICAL PREPARATION

Psychological factors are of considerable importance in pre-

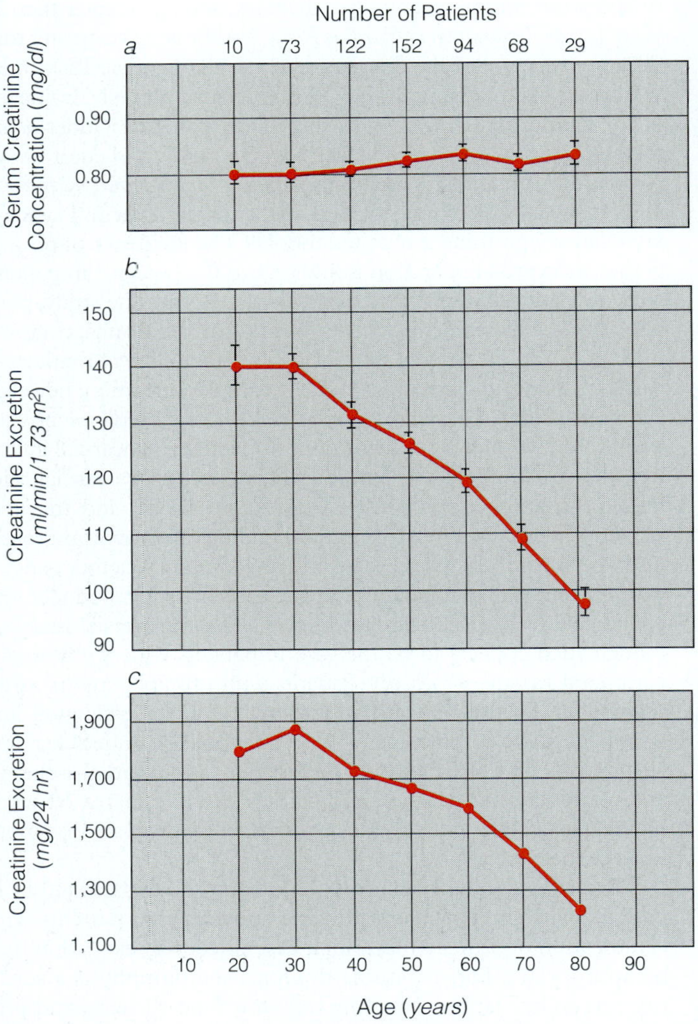

Figure 2 Illustrated are cross-sectional differences in serum creatinine concentration, creatinine clearance, and creatinine excretion.[267]

paring the elderly patient for operation [see *Sidebar* Establishing Rapport with the Elderly Patient]. Preoperative patient education has been shown to enhance patient confidence and to hasten the resumption of activities of daily living (ADL) after operation.[57] Acute mental stress has been associated with myocardial ischemia in patients with coronary artery disease. The ischemia was reflected in wall motion abnormalities observed on radionuclide ventriculography, was frequently silent, and was similar in magnitude to that induced by exercise but occurred at a lower heart rate.[58] Preoperative reassurance and education of the patient have been shown to reduce anxiety and the postoperative need for narcotic analgesics. Preoperative teaching probably also improves patient compliance with and the effectiveness of postoperative chest physiotherapy and other respiratory maneuvers.[51] Postoperative psychological adjustment has been shown to be enhanced by the physician's caring attitudes, as displayed, for example, in preoperative diagnostic interviews with breast cancer patients, who perceived the actual information given in the interviews as the less important component.[59]

> **Establishing Rapport with the Elderly Patient**
>
> The surgeon's personal rapport with the patient remains an important element of healing. The patient tends to interpret every aspect of preoperative, intraoperative, and postoperative care—including physiotherapy, nursing, and the ward routine as well as the surgical skills and knowledge displayed—as part of the surgeon's treatment. Older patients are often more in awe of physicians than are younger patients and thus may attribute almost shamanic powers to the surgeon. Such beliefs may be a valuable therapeutic aid.[219]
>
> The elderly generations comprise more disparate styles, cultures, vocabularies, and individual differences than any other generational group. It is therefore especially important that the surgeon attempt to understand and empathize with each patient's attitudes, beliefs, concerns, and modes of communication, some of which have been retained from an earlier time. The result will be a more confident patient, and confident elderly patients have been shown to experience fewer complications.[225,236] Enhanced feelings of control and autonomy on the part of the patient correlate with a shorter hospital stay. These feelings can be promoted by specific behaviors on the part of the surgeon:
>
> - Never call the patient by his or her first name, even if the patient calls you by yours. Never use "dear," "granny," or any other diminutive or familiar name.
> - Address the patient, not the accompanying family member.
> - When you speak to the patient, keep your expression calm, smile, bring your face close, and do not turn away. Speak slowly and distinctly, but do not raise your voice.
> - Pause from time to time to permit the patient to speak. Do not allow the accompanying family member to fill all the pauses.
> - To interrupt or to bring the patient back to the subject you want to discuss, touch him or her slowly on the hand or arm and repeat the question.
> - Ask the patient if he or she understands what you have said.
> - Ask the patient how he or she feels about what you have said, and address any concerns raised.
>
> It is essential to avoid the appearance of haste or carelessness. If the surgeon is calm and supportive, the patient is likely to be calm and confident. Such nonverbal messages are more important to elderly persons than to younger adults and are perceived as more valuable than the actual information given.[63]
>
> Confused, demented, or depressed elderly patients are not the only ones who benefit from reassuring nonverbal messages. This style of interaction may be used, for instance, with an active 70-year-old CEO who has sandwiched an appointment with the surgeon between a board meeting and a golf game, even if it seems somewhat exaggerated under the circumstances. Later, when the patient feels confused and cold, cannot see, hear, or smile normally, and has just suffered the indignity of a catheter, he or she will remember the respectful healing behaviors, and the surgeon-patient rapport will be enhanced.
>
> Finally, it should be remembered that aged persons are subject to psychological, physical, and financial abuse. The surgeon should ask the patient directly about these potential problems and should, if necessary, request social and psychiatric assessment and legal intervention.

PLANNING CONVALESCENCE

Convalescence should be planned before operation, with full consideration given to both the potential impact of planned surgery on function and the possible duration of functional impairment. During convalescence, the patient has not only medical needs but also personal needs (e.g., clothing to be washed, cooking to be done, and living space to be cleaned). Arrangements must be made to meet these personal needs.

In elderly individuals, the lack of any immediate family contributes not only to very long hospital stays but also to the requirement for nursing home placement at discharge. These trends hold true regardless of surgical procedure, surgical service of admission, diagnosis, age, and gender. The adjusted odds ratio for very long hospital stays is 1.85 in patients with no adult child. The adjusted odds ratios for requirement for nursing home placement at discharge are 2.59 in patients with no spouse, 3.27 in patients with no adult child, and 8.47 in patients with neither.[60]

The caretaker is typically a daughter 50 to 70 years of age or a frail elderly spouse. The caretaker often has a wide range of concerns in addition to the elderly parent or spouse who is the surgical candidate. These might include holding down a job, helping her adult children through graduate school, minding her grandchildren, maintaining the traditional homemaker's role, and planning financially for her own retirement. Accordingly, she should plan to do one or more of the following: (1) hire a full-time housekeeper for her parent, (2) miss some work, or (3) arrange for convalescent care for a few weeks after the operation.

If family members are reluctant to participate in planning convalescence or arranging for live-in help or community support, they should be warned that they may eventually need to take as much as eight weeks off from work to compensate for temporary and minor functional lapses on the part of the patient. For reasons not well understood, the elderly patient may not feel quite like himself or herself postoperatively.

During convalescence, which may go on for weeks after discharge, family members should save their energy for those personal support activities in which they cannot be replaced (e.g., visits and telephone conversations). They should not spend disproportionate amounts of time and effort on activities that another person could be paid to perform, such as washing sheets or delivering provisions. In this way, the family may avoid burnout or family stress, either of which may lead to neglect of the elderly member or to early placement.

The elderly patient should be advised to cultivate healthy habits preoperatively, such as exercising and having regular, balanced meals. Finally, the patient should come to the hospital prepared for an active postoperative period, bringing his or her clothes, jogging suit, shoes, walker or cane, hearing aid, glasses, pictures of loved ones, radio, and calendar.

INFORMED CONSENT AND ASSESSMENT OF COMPETENCE

Inherent in the idea of informed consent is that each patient has both the right to be informed about the therapeutic options available and the right to consent to intervention or nonintervention. Obtaining informed consent is more complicated with elderly patients than with younger ones for several reasons: first, older patients may be psychologically or physically dependent on someone else; second, they may be overly deferential to (or suspicious of) the surgeon; third, they may be demented but nonetheless competent to accept or reject a surgical choice. Occasionally, an elderly patient is capable in all the usual areas of function but acts irrationally when asked to accept or forgo a surgical intervention. When told that complications are rare, an older patient may believe the risk to be higher than a younger person would.[61] Older patients may be less interested in obtaining information about complications than younger patients are[62,63]; however, giving detailed information about anesthesia risk does not appear to raise their anxiety level.[64]

The term competence, as used in this discussion, is defined simply as the capacity to understand the available options and their consequences and the ability to choose freely among these options.[65,66] Competence may refer to either clinical status or legal status. It should be remembered that guidelines allowing a parent or guardian to speak for a child or for a mentally challenged person cannot be generalized to apply to a frail elderly individual whom the surgeon may consider clinically incompetent but who has not yet been determined to be legally incompetent.

To maximize the possibilities for informed consent, the surgeon should arrange to spend some time with the patient, even if the patient seems completely demented. The patient should be asked the following questions:

1. Do you feel comfortable with the idea of surgery?
2. Do you understand what is planned?
3. Do you have any questions for me?

Only after these questions have been answered satisfactorily should the patient be reassured that surgery is in his or her best interests. If the patient is unaccompanied, the surgeon should ask permission to speak with the spouse, a child, or anyone who may be assisting the patient either before or after the surgical procedure. The surgical plan is reviewed with family members and repeated to the patient in the presence of the family. Included in the review should be expectations for the patient's capacity to function in the immediate postoperative period as well as the amount of family support that will be required. Finally, the surgeon should make it very clear to both the patient and the family that although family members can help the patient to understand the available choices, they do not have the right to make the final decision, even if the patient is completely dependent and demented, unless they can prove that they are the patient's legal representatives, appointed by the court specifically for health care, including surgery. Definitions and terminology vary among jurisdictions.

When the patient's competence is uncertain, assessment by a psychogeriatrician may be helpful, as may assessments by a geriatrician, a social worker, and the patient's family physician. Some variation of opinion is to be expected because the issue of competence is not a simple one. For example, a patient may be incompetent to manage money but competent to accept operation. Alternatively, a patient may have a borderline status and experience diurnal fluctuations in cognition. A 1994 study of 2,100 internists, surgeons, and psychiatrists concluded that "the common clinical practice of relying on expert medical opinion may introduce bias and produce inaccurate results that undermine patient autonomy."[67] Surgeons performed almost as well as psychiatrists on theoretical issues of competence but surpassed their psychiatric colleagues in the practical application of competence assessment. Practical solutions and common sense must prevail. The patient's values, both cultural and personal, must be taken into account.

When the patient is deemed incompetent, the next step is to establish legal incompetence. Most provinces, states, and hospitals require two psychiatric opinions to declare incompetence and to place the patient under legal guardianship. The efforts of a social worker are usually vital to this process, which can be accomplished immediately in urgent situations, usually through the director of professional services. The patient comes under the protection of the state, which may delegate the role of legal representative to the private sector in the form of family guardianship or the so-called committee of the person. These private-sector guardians are then overseen by the state.

Hospital personnel and family members should be aware that in most North American jurisdictions, power of attorney does not constitute legal guardianship. Power of attorney concerns management of certain delegated acts, such as writing checks and buying and selling certain properties. In fact, as soon as a person becomes incompetent, whether clinically or legally, power of attorney is invalid, because the person is no longer able to decide how these acts should be delegated.

It is vital to consult with, to educate, to reassure, and to work with the family when surgical decisions must be made about a demented elderly patient. Questions to the family should focus on gathering relevant information, such as what the patient's wishes would probably be if he or she could express them and what the patient's functional and biologic status was before the current surgical problem. The family must understand that such questions constitute a request not for permission but rather for information that will help the surgeon in the management of the demented patient.

If the family is the legal representative for health care and refuses operation but the surgeon feels strongly that surgical intervention is in the patient's best interest, legal review should be requested. This request may place the surgeon in a difficult position. In fact, it may relieve some of the burden of decision making carried by the most responsible family member, who may blame herself or be blamed by her siblings for everything that goes wrong with the aging parent in the remaining years of life, regardless of whether the problem is related to the surgical intervention.

Rarely, it may happen that even when the patient has been declared legally incompetent, the legal representative for health care has signed the consent form, hospital administrators and the psychogeriatric consultant are supportive of the decision to operate, the family is supportive of the patient, and the patient seems to accept surgery, the patient will adamantly refuse to go to the operating room on the morning of the operation. In such cases, although the surgeon has the right to proceed with the operation and would not be faulted for insisting on it, it is probably best to cancel the procedure and reschedule it for the next day. The presence of someone the patient trusts, such as an old friend or a minister, through the perioperative period may allow the frail elderly demented patient to tolerate the procedure and the surgical milieu.

Finally, when surgical intervention is considered neither urgent nor life threatening, the surgeon may be frustrated waiting for the courts to appoint a legal representative for health care. If so, the help of other knowledgeable and action-oriented professionals, such as the family physician, a psychogeriatrician, or a social worker, may be valuable. New, more flexible mechanisms are being explored in various jurisdictions for management of the well-being of the patient who has lost some autonomy. The newer mechanisms include durable power of attorney, health care proxy, living wills, and judicial advisers. The surgeon's consultants should be able to assist in selecting the most appropriate mechanism, depending on the patient's medical status, prognosis, and family support and on local laws.

Intraoperative Management

POSITIONING

Because elderly patients commonly have diminished ranges of joint motion, particular attention must be paid to how they are positioned for surgery. The use of regional or general anesthesia may allow positioning that would be uncomfortable and beyond the usual range of motion were the patient not anesthetized. Postoperative back pain is a well-recognized complication of the use of the lithotomy position in the elderly. The remarkable prevalence of osteoporosis and the high incidence of related fractures in the geriatric population emphasize the fragility of these patients and the importance of gentleness and care in turning and positioning them, particularly when discomfort and protective musculoskeletal reflexes have been suppressed by anesthesia. In addition, the skin of elderly individuals is easily injured by tape, adhesive electrodes, cautery pads, and warming blankets. Careful padding is necessary to prevent localized pressure, which may result in nerve compression and injury to the skin, and to maintain appropriate positioning throughout anesthesia. The head and neck should also be kept in a position that is comfortable and limits hyperextension so that cerebral blood flow is not compromised.

ANESTHESIA

Studies of anesthetic technique as an independent risk factor in the elderly are limited.[68] Most studies of patients with cardiac disease have demonstrated no differences attributable to anesthetic technique.[45] Particular anesthetic techniques are appropriate for specific surgical procedures; the choice of technique will depend on the nature of the procedure, the coexisting diseases (if any), and the personality of the patient. The most important factor may be the experience and specific skills of the attending anesthesiologist.

Ideally, anesthesia permits safe, efficient, and stress-free performance of a surgical procedure and a rapid, uneventful return to normal function. Specific concerns in the elderly patient are (1) avoidance of hemodynamic instability, (2) maintenance of a favorable myocardial oxygen supply-demand ratio, (3) minimization of postoperative impairment of respiratory function, and (4) minimization of postoperative alterations in mental function. The strong relation between intraoperative hypotension and postoperative morbidity and mortality has been well established[42-44,47]: for example, when mean blood pressure decreases by one third or more from preoperative values for 10 minutes or longer, the risk of cardiac death is increased fivefold. Intraoperative tachycardia is also associated with myocardial ischemia.[45] The combination of tachycardia and hypotension may be particularly hazardous in the elderly patient.

General Anesthesia

General anesthesia allows the surgeon to perform prolonged operations with a secure airway and necessary monitoring devices in place and without discomfort to the patient. It may be particularly appropriate in the confused or agitated patient. The decrease in blood pressure that may occur at induction and the increases at intubation, incision, and emergence may be extreme on occasion and on the whole appear to be more marked in older patients than in younger ones.[69]

Advancing age is accompanied by reduced vital capacity, increased physiologic dead space, decreased efficiency of coughing, increased ventilation-perfusion mismatch, decreased ventilatory and cardiovascular responses to hypoxemia and hypercapnia, and decreased arterial oxygen tension (P_aO_2) at rest [see Discussion, Patterns of Change in Body Composition, Organ Systems, and Integrated Responses, *below*]. General anesthesia and abdominal surgery are accompanied by decreases in functional residual capacity (FRC), FEV_1, and vital capacity. In addition, the normal compensatory increase in diaphragmatic excursion in the supine position is impaired during controlled ventilation with paralysis; as a result, there is increased ventilation in the upper portions of the lungs and a more marked ventilation-perfusion mismatch.[69] Thus, the decreases in pulmonary function that follow abdominal operation under general anesthesia exacerbate the changes associated with aging [see Figure 3].[69] As a result, the decrease in resting P_aO_2 that occurs with aging is exaggerated postoperatively.[70]

High doses of various opiates and opioids have been shown to limit increases in circulating stress hormones, energy expenditure, blood glucose, and heart rate during cardiac and abdominal surgery and after burn injury.[71-73] These and other observations indicate the role of the central nervous system in mediating many of the metabolic responses to stress. Inhibition of these responses does not appear to be detrimental when the patient is carefully monitored and given appropriate cardiopulmonary support; such inhibition minimizes increases in myocardial oxygen demand and may allow major surgical procedures to be done more safely in certain patients (e.g., those with severe cardiac disease).

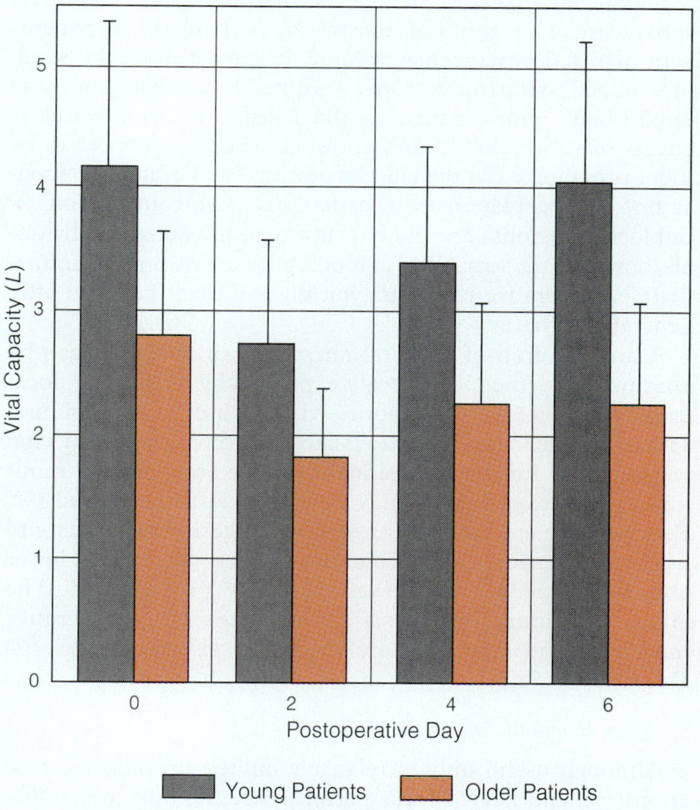

Figure 3 Abdominal operations with general anesthesia induce decreases in vital capacity that can persist in older patients; these decreases exacerbate the respiratory changes associated with aging.[135]

Regional Anesthesia: Subarachnoid and Epidural Anesthesia

Although it requires a greater degree of patient cooperation, regional anesthesia has several potential advantages over general anesthesia. It allows the patient to remain awake and thus gives the surgeon and the anesthesiologist the opportunity to assess alterations in mental state and the onset of chest pain as indicators of physiologic derangement. In addition, the patient's ability to maintain appropriate ventilation, to cough effectively, and to clear respiratory secretions remains unimpaired unless anesthesia is higher than midthoracic dermatome levels.

Postoperative respiratory function may be improved as well. Diaphragmatic function during the first 24 hours after upper abdominal surgery with general anesthesia can be improved by a thoracic epidural block to T4 with bupivacaine. Patients undergoing lower extremity surgery under general anesthesia exhibit more marked decreases in arterial oxygen tension (from the preoperative period to one hour after operation) than those receiving subarachnoid anesthesia[74,75]; however, no difference in mortality has been observed.[74,76] Epidural anesthesia has also been associated with diminished intraoperative blood loss during hip replacement and prostatectomy and with a lower incidence of postoperative deep venous thrombosis after these procedures. There is often less postoperative confusion after epidural anesthesia than after general anesthesia, depending on the doses of narcotics, sedatives, or anticholinergics that are also given.[75,77,78] Depending on the surgical procedure, use of regional anesthesia may allow the prompt resumption of preoperative medication and diet.

Significant hypotension may occur after the induction of subarachnoid or epidural anesthesia, particularly in patients with depleted intravascular volume. It is most often the result of reduced sympathetic tone, peripheral vasodilatation, and diminished venous return to the heart. The cardiovascular effects of subarachnoid and epidural anesthesia appear to be more pronounced in the elderly, presumably because compensatory reflex responses (particularly vasoconstriction in unblocked regions) are less effective than in younger individuals; however, the variability in blood pressure during the immediate postoperative period is typically less than that seen after general anesthesia.

Administration of epidural anesthesia or analgesia can be continued in the postoperative period by delivering local anesthetic agents or narcotics via an indwelling epidural catheter. When this is done, postoperative decreases in vital capacity and functional residual capacity are generally minimized, and oxygenation may be significantly improved.[79,80] Perioperative epidural anesthesia or analgesia also appears to limit stress responses to certain procedures, particularly lower abdominal, pelvic, and lower extremity procedures.[81] The effects of epidural anesthesia and analgesia on postoperative morbidity and mortality are discussed elsewhere [see 104 Postoperative Pain].

Other Regional Anesthesia

Although useful only in relatively limited procedures, local anesthesia and nerve blocks permit earlier ambulation, earlier resumption of a normal diet, and earlier voiding and provoke less postoperative nausea than general anesthesia does. Local anesthetics have a prolonged half-life in the elderly; toxicity may be reflected in myocardial depression and commonly involves the central nervous system, manifesting itself as numbness of the tongue, light-headedness, loss of consciousness, and generalized seizures. Intravenous regional anesthesia in the elderly may be complicated by the rapid influx of local anesthetics into the systemic circulation after release of the tourniquet.

INTRAOPERATIVE MONITORING

The principles of intraoperative physiologic monitoring are the same in elderly patients as in young ones [see 89 Cardiopulmonary Monitoring], but such monitoring is perhaps of even greater importance in the geriatric population because of limitations in cardiovascular and pulmonary function and a diminished ability to maintain fluid, electrolyte, acid-base, and temperature homeostasis. In the awake patient, alterations in mental state may reflect acute abnormalities in electrolyte or glucose status as well as changes in oxygen delivery to the central nervous system. Periodic measurement of blood pressure by cuff and continuous electrocardiographic monitoring are essential. Automated blood pressure measurement and continuous noninvasive monitoring of respiratory rate, peripheral tissue oxygenation (with an oxygen saturation monitor), end-tidal carbon dioxide tension, and body temperature should be considered in all patients. Monitoring urine output with an indwelling urinary catheter is appropriate when a procedure is prolonged and when the need for significant fluid administration is anticipated.

The decision to employ invasive hemodynamic monitoring should be based on the results of the preoperative assessment of the patient's medical and physiologic status in relation to the proposed surgical procedure rather than on age alone. Cannulation of blood vessels may be more complicated and risky in elderly patients than in younger ones.

The relation between intraoperative hemodynamic instability and ischemic cardiac events in high-risk patients is very clear. One aim of invasive monitoring is to prevent or limit such perturbations; apparent reductions in the rate of myocardial reinfarction when an operation is performed less than six months after infarction may be attributable to the use of aggressive perioperative hemodynamic monitoring.[44,82] Some investigators believe that in patients older than 65 years, important abnormalities of cardiac, pulmonary, and oxygen transport physiology occur that are not identified by conventional methods of assessment but can be identified by invasive hemodynamic monitoring.[83,84] The use of invasive monitoring is nearly routine in aortic procedures and in cases in which acute changes in circulating volume and hemodynamics are anticipated, regardless of the patient's age. The incidence of pulmonary artery rupture is very low overall (0.2 percent of catheterizations), but the risk is increased if the patient is older than 60 years, if pulmonary hypertension is present, if the catheter tip occupies a distal position in the pulmonary artery, or if the balloon is overinflated.[85]

MANAGEMENT OF HYPOTHERMIA

A fall in core temperature is common in patients undergoing surgery, whether general or regional anesthesia is used. It depends in part on the nature and length of the procedure and on the ambient temperature. In addition, the extent of the hypothermia increases with advancing age.[86,87] One group of investigators reported that patients older than 60 years were admitted to and discharged from the recovery room with lower core temperatures than younger patients and that hypothermia lasted longer and shivering was more common in older patients.[87] Temperature returned toward normal more slowly in patients who had received regional anesthesia than in those who had been given general anesthesia.

Shivering may be accompanied by a severalfold increase in oxygen consumption,[88-90] which imposes a substantial additional burden on the cardiac and pulmonary systems in the immediate postoperative period.[88,89] If the oxygen transport system is unable to meet the increased oxygen demand, myocardial ischemia may result. Hypothermia should be minimized or prevented in the operating room by controlling room temperature, minimizing exposure of body surfaces, warming intravenous fluids and ventilator gases, and using active warming devices, such as a warming blanket, as needed. The opportunity to restore an appropriate core temperature without excessive metabolic stress and cardiac work is a reason to consider postoperative ventilation and sedation, with or without paralysis.

Postoperative Management

RESPIRATORY CARE

Elderly patients are predisposed to postoperative respiratory complications, respiratory failure, and resultant inadequate oxygen transport for many reasons. Such complications remain an important cause of death in this population. Resting arterial oxygen tension and content decrease progressively with advancing age, and the further decrease associated with operation is most marked in the elderly. In addition, the ventilatory responses to both hypoxia and hypercapnia are blunted in older persons. Postoperative hypothermia is more prominent in the elderly, and oxygen demand is markedly increased by postoperative shivering. Abdominal procedures with general anesthesia induce decreases in vital capacity and FEV_1 that last as long as two weeks after operation[79,91]; similar declines in lung volume accompany aging. The combined result is increased closure of small airways, ventilation-perfusion mismatch, and an increased alveolar-arterial oxygen gradient. Impairment of diaphragm function after upper abdominal procedures results in a shift in ventilation away from dependent portions of the lung.[92-94] Because of stiff chest walls and diminished elastic lung recoil, elderly patients are more reliant on diaphragmatic function than younger patients and are therefore more vulnerable to respiratory compromise.[95] Protective airway reflexes are less sensitive in the elderly, mucociliary transport is less efficient, and coughing is less effective because strength, elastic recoil of the lungs, vital capacity, and maximum expiratory flow rate are all diminished. The use of parenteral narcotics for postoperative analgesia has been associated with striking episodic falls in P_aO_2; the increased sensitivity of the elderly to narcotics may further predispose them to such hypoxemia. The presence of significant coronary artery disease in a substantial number of older persons underscores the importance of maintaining adequate oxygen delivery and avoiding excessive myocardial oxygen demand in the perioperative period.

Effective postoperative analgesia with epidural narcotics or local anesthetics is associated with a partial reversal of the decreases in vital capacity and functional residual capacity and appears to be superior to parenteral narcotic analgesia in this regard.[79] The supine position in elderly patients is accompanied by the closure of small airways in dependent areas of the lung, resulting in ventilation-perfusion mismatch, an increased alveolar-arterial oxygen gradient, and hypoxemia. For this reason, besides providing adequate analgesia, the surgeon should encourage early resumption of physical activity. Changing from the supine to the sitting position increases functional residual capacity and improves gas exchange in patients who have undergone abdominal surgery.[96] Incentive spirometers, breathing exercises, and intermittent positive-pressure breathing are of some benefit in reducing pulmonary complications after upper abdominal surgery and may help shorten the hospital stay.[97,98] These aids are probably most valuable when used on a regular and frequent basis by patients who are at high risk for pulmonary complications. Supplemental oxygen via a mask or nasal prongs should be routinely provided to elderly patients who have undergone abdominal or thoracic procedures for a period of several days or until physical mobility is restored—that is, until functional residual capacity is returning to preoperative values, ventilation and perfusion are better matched, and oxygen delivery is more reliable.

High-dose narcotic anesthesia, with its abrogation of stress responses and its limitation of increases in myocardial work, may necessitate a period of postoperative ventilation. Postoperative mechanical ventilation for up to 24 hours may be useful in elderly patients who have undergone abdominal or thoracic procedures under general anesthesia and who are at high risk for postoperative pulmonary or cardiac complications. Mechanical ventilation may be used prophylactically to ensure the adequacy of respiratory gas exchange during the early postoperative period, when anesthetic effects on cardiopulmonary function are dissipating, body temperature is returning toward normal, and major shifts of fluid between body water compartments are occurring. Despite the potential benefits of prophylactic mechanical ventilation, the impairment of pulmonary defenses associated with endotracheal intubation and ventilation and the potential for development of respiratory infection and ventilator dependence increase with time; early weaning is therefore indicated.

CARDIOVASCULAR MONITORING

Cardiovascular complications are also a major cause of postoperative death in elderly patients. The assessment of cardiac risk should be the basis for the decision whether to initiate cardiovascular monitoring in the perioperative period. It is in the first 48 to 96 hours after operation that the most significant shifts in fluid between body compartments occur, the onset of congestive heart failure is most frequent, and the hemodynamic abnormalities contributing to myocardial ischemia are most readily identified and treated. When invasive hemodynamic monitoring has been initiated in the operating room, consideration should be given to continuing it during this period. In studies of patients of varying ages, myocardial infarction and reinfarction have tended to occur in the early postoperative period, often painlessly. Continuous monitoring of ST segment changes in the postoperative period may prove to be a sensitive method for detecting myocardial ischemia and determining whether intensive therapy is needed. Data and observations from many studies suggest the need for frequent clinical assessment and continuous electrocardiographic monitoring for at least three days and possibly as long as six days postoperatively in elderly patients who are at high risk for postoperative cardiac complications.

PAIN MANAGEMENT

Analgesia plays a critical role in allowing early resumption of physical activity, increasing lung volumes, and improving respiratory gas exchange after operation. In addition, postoperative pain is itself a stimulus to the elaboration of stress hormones and stress responses. Activation of the sympathoadrenal axis and other mediators results in increases in overall metabolic demand and in myocardial work. These increases serve no obvious beneficial purpose in the postoperative patient and may be detrimental in some individuals.

Alternatives in the management of postoperative pain are discussed in detail elsewhere [see 104 Postoperative Pain]. Of particular note in elderly patients is the reported CNS stimulation induced by multiple doses of meperidine, which is attributed to accumulation of the metabolite normeperidine; meperidine should therefore be used with caution in these patients. The volume of distribution of morphine is smaller in the elderly patient, plasma and tissue drug levels are greater for a fixed dose, and the drug disappears more slowly from the cerebrospinal fluid; these differences would account for the more marked respiratory depression and other CNS effects observed in older patients [see Discussion, Management Considerations throughout the Perioperative Period, below]. Plasma morphine concentration and morphine clearance also depend on renal function.[99] Elderly patients reportedly obtain greater relief of pain from constant narcotic doses and show more marked CNS depression at given blood levels of benzodiazepines than younger patients do.[100,101] Parenteral administration of narcotics may be associated with profound arterial oxygen desaturation ($S_aO_2 < 80$ percent), particularly in older patients and particularly during sleep, and in fact, the parenteral narcotics may not provide optimal relief of pain.[80,102]

NSAIDs have been used in combination with narcotics and other analgesics in the management of postoperative pain; side effects include renal vasoconstriction and gastritis.[103] Such agents should be used with caution in elderly surgical patients. Patient-controlled techniques may be appropriate for the elderly patient who understands and is able to self-administer analgesic medication (usually intravenously). In one study of elderly patients undergoing major procedures, patient-controlled analgesia was associated with improved pain relief and a lower incidence of postoperative confusion and pulmonary complications when compared with as-needed intramuscular narcotic administration.[104]

OPTIMIZING FUNCTIONAL LEVEL

The goal of postoperative care is maximum function. Achievement of optimal functional level depends on three principal areas—mobility, continence, and cognition—and on how these areas are integrated with the six basic activities of daily living during hospitalization [see Table 2].

Each patient should have a program designed to enhance independence in performing activities of daily living at every stage of recovery. Occasionally, postoperative ADL function may exceed preoperative ADL function, either because the surgery has direct effects on function or because the patient had been unnecessarily limited (by self, family, or care givers) preoperatively.[105] All stages of step-down care must be individually tailored and modified when medical conditions are present that might inhibit progress.

Mobility

Mobility and appropriate sensory stimulation should be maximized before and after operation. Even healthy elderly patients have lost a good deal of their muscle strength; for example, the average 80-year-old woman in good health is at or near the limits of her quadriceps strength when rising from a low, armless seat.[106] The continued loss of strength that accompanies immobility may have marked functional consequences. Elderly patients are at increased risk for atelectasis and other pulmonary complications after operation, and early mobilization helps minimize the incidence of these complications [see Table 3]. Cardiovascular deconditioning occurs regardless of

Table 2 Hierarchy of Sociobiological Function*[245]

Feeding	Independence is defined as getting food from the plate or its equivalent to the mouth
Continence	Independence is defined as complete self-control of urination and defecation
Transferring	Independence means that the patient can move in and out of bed, chair, or wheelchair without assistance and with or without mechanical supports (e.g., walker or cane)
Toileting	Independence means that the patient decides when to go the toilet (either by the clock in a toilet-training program or by recognizing the biologic urge), can get on and off the toilet unassisted, can clean self, and can arrange clothing appropriately; if the patient is not fully continent, independent toileting includes emptying any bedpan or commode used in care, managing pads, and washing soiled clothing unassisted
Dressing	Independence means that the patient chooses seasonally appropriate clothing and puts things on in proper order, managing fasteners and any prosthesis
Bathing	Independence means getting in and out of the bath as well as deciding to bathe at appropriate intervals

Note: this assessment system does not consider *why* the patient does not do the activity.
*Modified from the Katz index of primary social biologic function.[224,245]

Table 3 Potential Complications of Immobility[272]

Skin	Pressure sores
Musculoskeletal	Muscular deconditioning and atrophy Contractures Bone loss (osteoporosis)
Cardiovascular	Deconditioning Decreased plasma volume Orthostatic hypotension Venous thrombosis, embolism
Pulmonary	Decreased ventilation Atelectasis Aspiration pneumonia
Gastrointestinal	Anorexia Constipation Fecal impaction, incontinence
Genitourinary	Urinary infection Urinary retention Bladder calculi Incontinence
Metabolic	Negative nitrogen balance Impaired glucose tolerance Altered drug phamacokinetics
Psychological	Sensory deprivation Dementia, delirium Depression

age: the decrease in cardiac output on standing may be considerable after a period of prolonged bed rest and may be accompanied by orthostatic hypotension and tachycardia.[107] Maximum oxygen consumption, cardiac output, and stroke volume at maximum exercise are all lower after prolonged immobilization.[108,109] Bed rest for two weeks is also accompanied by a significant decrease in tissue sensitivity to insulin in healthy individuals.[110]

Although bed rest is associated with an increased incidence of DVT (as is advancing age), most patients with DVT have other risk factors, which suggests that immobilization may not be the sole factor responsible. Constipation and fecal impaction are frequent in immobilized patients as a result of alterations in gastrointestinal motility (related to inactivity and medications), lack of privacy, and the use of bedpans. Decubitus ulcers are well-recognized complications of immobility to which the elderly are predisposed because of diminished subcutaneous fat and decreased skin elasticity.

Beginning in the immediate postoperative period, full passive range-of-motion exercises of all joints should be undertaken daily, even after the patient is able to sit up in a chair and walk a short distance in the corridor. These interventions not only conserve the patient's capacity for mobility but also help prevent bedsores. The surgeon may need to insist on the involvement of a physiotherapist during the recovery period.[111]

Once awake, the patient who requires glasses or a hearing aid should wear them at all times. As soon as the patient is able to sit in a chair, he or she should wear shoes, preferably solid, comfortable jogging shoes with Velcro closures. The patient should wear regular clothes, preferably a jogging suit, as soon as possible. (Sometimes, elderly women must be persuaded that such attire is chic. An outfit in an attractive, vibrant color and a matching accessory may be sufficiently convincing if offered as a gift from a family member.) A walker, a cane, or a wheelchair should be kept at the bedside and used as the physiotherapist advises. The patient should be encouraged to walk the full length of the hall each day. Intravenous lines should not prohibit these activities but may necessitate accompaniment. Periods of activity should be systematically alternated with rest periods. The primary nurse is the care giver best equipped to ensure that this routine is maintained.

These rehabilitation and maintenance efforts must be carried out in the surgical ward [*see Sidebar* Creating a Geriatrically Adapted Hospital Milieu]. There is no point to sending a frail elderly person down to the physiotherapy/occupational therapy department: the patient will not learn to integrate the new skills into a daily routine. Older persons must work like athletes in the postoperative period. A training effect can be noted in skeletal muscle and in the cardiovascular and pulmonary systems. Accordingly, elderly patients deserve continual congratulations and encouragement.

Aggressive rehabilitation instituted early will certainly lead to better function at discharge. However, a general surgical ward that properly serves elderly patients will also show a higher incidence of hip fracture and minor injuries. These risks must be accepted by staff, patients, and family.

Persistent difficulty with mobility is not a normal consequence of aging. A definitive diagnosis should be sought and definitive therapy for the problem identified; management of immobility should be undertaken simultaneously.

Continence

Efforts to help the patient achieve and maintain continence should begin preoperatively and should be reestablished postoperatively as soon as possible. Systematic toileting (every two hours) should be initiated by the primary nurse, even before the catheter is removed, to maintain bowel function and toileting habits. Catheters should be removed as soon as possible and should not be relied on for monitoring of input and output. Nurses should respond promptly to patient requests for toileting. If urinary incontinence recurs or persists, the toileting interval should be shortened until continence is achieved and then should be lengthened. If urinary continence cannot be established in 48 hours, residual urine should be measured, urinalysis should be performed, and a urine specimen should be sent for culture. Other metabolic causes of urinary incontinence should be sought and urodynamic studies carried out.

Stool incontinence (with or without diarrhea) should be considered secondary to impaction, until proved otherwise, even if there is no fecalith palpable on digital examination. Bowel care must be the responsibility of the surgeon and primary nurse. A step-down program for encopresis should be started aggressively with enemas, followed by stool softeners and bulk agents, with suppositories as needed, and toileting one hour after each meal as well as in response to urge. A behavioral program should be developed with the patient, who should participate in maintaining the toileting schedule and recording performance. Rewards, even trivial ones such as stick-on stars for clean, dry days and big stars for clean, dry days and nights, can make the program more attractive and enjoyable for the patient and the staff.

It is worth remembering that incontinence is never a normal consequence of aging. In every case, it should be explained by a specific diagnosis, managed, and treated.

Cognition

Cognition should be maximized and maintained throughout the perioperative period. The goals must be individualized at each stage. Continuing ongoing assessment and stimulation is the key. The Folstein Mini-Mental State (MMS) examination is a valid, quick, and reliable assessment tool that identifies organic as well as functional lapses. It is designed for elderly patients and is suitable for repeat assessment [see 9 Coma, Seizures, Cognitive Impairment, and Brain Death].

Confusion that persists in the face of a normal or unchanged MMS score is probably a delirium secondary to pain, pain medications or other medications (e.g., cimetidine), or underlying conditions (e.g., hypercalcemia, hyperglycemia, hyperthyroidism, vitamin B_{12} deficiency—with or without anemia—folate deficiency, neurosyphilis, tuberculosis, cancer, and postoperative infection).

In a dark, soundless, weightless chamber without aural, visual, sensory, or vestibular cues, young, fit adults undergoing training as astronauts are known to have a high incidence of transitory psychosis, presumably caused by the intense isolation and lack of stimulation. The elderly hospitalized patient who is medicated, deprived of glasses or a hearing aid, and restrained in a dim light may exhibit a similar response, provoked by isolation and lack of cueing. The sensory deprivation characteristic of even brief confinement in a typical hospital setting may be accompanied by changes in affect, impaired cognition and intellectual function, and perceptual distortions in the elderly patient.

All staff members who have contact with older patients, including housekeeping personnel and technicians, should be taught to continually provide them with orienting cues, such as the weather, the season, the day of the week, the name of the hospital, and their own name and function. Many of the interventions described in the discussions of mobility, continence, and activities of daily living have the added advantage of increasing the amount of appropriate sensory stimulation provided to the patient and thereby contributing to improved cognition.

Confusion, dementia, and cognitive deficits are not normal consequences of aging. Their presence is an indication for diagnostic and therapeutic intervention.

Activities of Daily Living

Patients should groom and dress themselves entirely as soon as they are out of recovery; this includes putting on aids and prostheses. Self-medications should be introduced gradually, starting as soon as possible after recovery, and should be reviewed twice daily by the nursing staff. Dosette boxes and calendars are useful assists. Unit dose pharmacy management has no place in geriatric care because it systematically teaches dependence.

The independence of the hospitalized elderly patient is continually undermined. To begin with, insisting on patient independence takes extra nursing time: it is quicker and easier to do things for patients than it is to instruct them. In addition, patients themselves often sabotage nurses' efforts to foster independence, arguing that because they are old and sick they should not be expected to do much for themselves. Consequently, nurses who encourage self-care sometimes have patients who feel neglected and who may even become resentful and uncooperative; in some cases, an unhappy family may even complain to the administration.

Families are not naturally helpful in mobilization. Instead, they often insist on doing things for geriatric patients even while scolding them for not doing more for themselves. Families must be taught by nurses and physiotherapists exactly how the elderly persons are to get out of a chair and how far and how often they are to walk.

Persistent stepwise encouragement to regain autonomy is perhaps the most beneficial service nurses can offer elderly surgical patients in the postoperative period. A word from the surgeon to the patient and family may gain the nurse and physiotherapist the patient's willing cooperation. If behavioral problems persist, a behaviorist, a psychiatrist, a geriatrician, or the patient's family physician should be consulted.

Optimizing Functional Level: Summary

The surgeon should not make the mistake of assuming that paying attention to the patient's functional level in basic ADL is the responsibility solely of the rehabilitation unit or the convalescent unit. Orientation, mobility, and ADL all are significantly and systematically compromised in the traditional surgical ward in just a few days. Once function is lost, even long-term rehabilitation cannot ensure that it will be recaptured.

Other patient skills to be demonstrated before discharge should match the environment to which the patient is going. Stair walking and ability to use a stove and a washing machine should be demonstrated in the surgical ward. Occupational and physical therapists should routinely follow geriatric surgical patients and should integrate planning with the nursing staff. Elderly patients are less likely than younger patients to integrate the skills demonstrated during rehabilitation in a traditional occupational/physical therapy work area or gymnasium into the performance of activities of daily living on the ward and, later, at home. Home visits by the occupational and physical therapists are useful components of assessment and rehabilitation.

Creating a Geriatrically Adapted Hospital Milieu

In this day of shortened hospital stays, increased use of day surgery and noninvasive techniques, and greater willingness on the part of older individuals to accept surgical interventions, the daily hospital census is likely to show a higher proportion of elderly patients. With the graying of North American surgical units must come the development of a milieu that is suited to the elderly client. The goals of design should be (1) to minimize the loss of function inherent to bed rest and hospital routine, (2) to encourage initiative, (3) to maximize safety, (4) to shorten length of stay, and (5) to guarantee successful discharge to the appropriate setting. It is a mistake to believe that geriatric interventions can be accomplished after discharge to a rehabilitation or convalescence unit or even after transfer to a special geriatric unit; that is far too late. Geriatric rehabilitation and maintenance of function must be as integral to tertiary care university hospitals as they are to rehabilitation institutes. Architectural design and nursing routine must reflect these goals. Surgical geriatric units are among the high-tech measures of the next millennium for which surgeons must lobby.[65,222,225]

Structural Elements

The structural elements required for a geriatrically adapted surgical environment are manifold. Corridors should be well lit, preferably at the baseboards. All patient areas should be well lit during the daytime. Common areas should be slightly less well lit in the evenings and at night, with baseboard lighting maintained. This technique not only provides day and night cues but also minimizes glare for patients with cataracts, glaucoma, or other conditions that impair dark-light adjustment. Lighting should not cause glare on the floor, and polishing of floors should be prohibited. Floors should be constructed from impact-absorbing tiles or covered with low-pile nonskid washable rugging.[246] No confusing visual patterns should be evident. The floor should be easily distinguishable from the walls by color or shade. Handrails that fit the function of the hand (rather than the architect's concept of beauty) should line the corridors.[247] Chairs should be grouped in twos and threes along the length of the corridor. The chairs should be chosen by the geriatric physiotherapist. In general, they should be approximately 17 in. high, washable, relatively straight, and skidproof and should have arms and padded seats.

Each patient area should be clearly delineated. The patient's own bedroom area should be seen as private territory and treated as such. This rule holds even for very demented patients.[248] Function and orientation are better when each patient has a safe, private place to go. The patient's name should be on the door, and each door frame should be a different color. Ideally, each patient should have a single room with a television monitor and a call bell to the nursing station. It is a myth that the risk of accident in a demented elderly person is diminished by the presence of other elderly people in the room. More often, demented elderly patients present a hazard to each other. Five percent of elderly hospitalized patients who suffer a fall are tripped or knocked down by another patient, who usually is also elderly and cognitively impaired. Each patient should have some familiar objects from home on display, such as pictures of loved ones, a clock, or a radio. Other objects, such as a comforter or a teddy bear, may be present if they make the patient more comfortable.

Each patient room should have a full-length mirror to encourage patients to pay attention to walking and personal appearance. The patient's bedside chair should be more comfortable and attractive than the bed. Each bed should have colorful, highly textured blankets, which are thought to enhance the awareness, orientation, and comfort of elderly patients. (They have a quite different effect on younger adults, who feel calmer and get to sleep more easily in a pale, smooth, cool bed.) The patient's telephone, calendar, walker or cane, glasses, and hearing aid should be visible and reachable from the bed and the chair.[249]

Each unit should have a number of water beds or air mattresses available for use at the discretion of the nursing staff, and a bath bed should be available for the temporarily totally dependent patient. Generally, standard electric hospital beds are suitable for elderly patients. If possible, toward the end of the hospital stay, patients should receive a substitute bed that is low, without rails, and more like their beds at home. Patients should make this bed every day. Bed rails, in general, are no more advisable for elderly patients than for younger ones. Bed rails are a form of restraint and are considered to be a medical order to treat a specific condition. Bed rails that are not indicated cause more falls than they prevent, and the consequences of these falls are more serious than those of slipping out of bed (which is rare in any case).[250]

All bathrooms should have doors wide enough for wheelchair access, should meet standards for wheelchair space, and should be equipped with grab bars. Mirrors should tilt down so that the patient can perform grooming and washing while seated at the sink. Bathroom doors should slide into the wall rather than swing either into the bathroom or into the corridor. All door handles should be at wheelchair height. There should be no bathroom sills or door sills of any kind in a geriatrically adapted surgical unit.

Every general surgical ward should have a dining room. Progression to the point of being able to go to the dining room for meals, even if only in a wheelchair, should be an important part of step-down care. The dining room should be brightly lit, with comfortable chairs and nice tablecloths (bedsheets are perfectly acceptable substitutes). As a rule, each patient should sit at his or her own place for each meal. Patients should be grouped at the tables by cognitive level. A common dining room allows one nurse to help many patients at once and motivates patients to do things for themselves. It is also convenient for the dietitian, allowing him or her to verify intake for several patients at a glance.

An information board that provides information about the day, the date, the weather, and any significant holiday or political event should be posted near the nursing station. An individual patient board should state when and where various procedures (such as physiotherapy or x-rays) are scheduled so that patients who are able to get to the right areas themselves can take the initiative to do so.

There should also be a common room for reading, television, afternoon tea, and other special scheduled activities. A family room should be available for interviews, grieving, and education. Common spaces should contain plants, birds, magazines, and simple games. A donation closet for shoes, functional aids, and clothing is a desirable resource in the geriatric surgical ward, where fluid retention or weight loss may make it impossible for patients to wear their own clothes. A washing machine and a stove or a practice kitchen should be available in the service.

Remarkably, most space and program revisions designed for disabled or elderly persons tend to improve the quality of life for younger, more able patients as well. For example, large doors to public bathrooms, grab bars, and access ramps make for attractive, modern environments that are comfortable for everyone. If the facility to be converted is old and does not lend itself to renovation, much can be done with paint and lighting alone to simplify the routine of the elderly patient.

The last day of hospitalization can take place in a miniapartment just outside the surgical unit's fire doors. Such an arrangement enhances patient self-confidence before discharge and allows step-down care while preserving the continuum of nursing care.

Geriatric Staffing and Special Programs

It is advisable to have additional personnel in the geriatric surgical ward. A geriatrically trained resource nurse who is knowledgeable about geriatric care plans should be an integral part of the surgical unit staff, even in hospitals with attentive consulting geriatric teams.[251] Higher nurse-patient ratios, early occupational and physiotherapy assessments for selected patients, and recreation therapy programs will improve function and safety and shorten length of stay.[252]

Primary nursing—a system in which each patient has one specific nurse assigned for all aspects of care—integrates the on-unit management plans of the surgeon, the occupational therapist and the physiotherapist, social services, the psychiatrist, and consultants; maximizes bedside nursing time; and is the most effective method of delivering nursing care for all patients. Surgical units have resisted primary nursing because specialized surgical nursing functions and the usual surgical length of stay

(continued)

> **Creating a Geriatrically Adapted Hospital Milieu** (continued)
>
> prevent maximum benefit from being achieved. In elderly patients—especially very old, frail patients—however, the benefits (e.g., superior functional level at discharge, lower rate of readmission, and shorter lengths of stay) outweigh the inconvenience. Primary nursing does require good nurse-to-nurse communication, so that the surgeon never hears such uninformative remarks as "I don't know; she's not my patient. Her nurse won't be in until Saturday."
>
> Social supports provided by volunteers, such as pet therapy programs, music therapy programs, and adopt-a-grandparent programs, all help alleviate boredom, stimulate and orient the elderly person, motivate both patient and family, and shorten hospital stay.
>
> All hospital routines should be reliable and regular. Periods of activity (e.g., physical therapy) should alternate with rest periods. Breakfast, lunch, tea, and dinner should be served at the same time every day. Special events should occur consistently on the same days of the week at the same time and should be clearly posted.
>
> In all health care markets, both the average age and the proportion of frail elderly patients are increasing. For optimal care of the growing numbers of elderly patients, maintenance and rehabilitation therapies must be integrated with traditional surgical and medical care to maximize function and quality of life. In hospitals that are not prepared to integrate geriatric maintenance therapies into their usual routines, complication rates will be higher and hospital stays longer for older patients. Such an integrated approach does incorporate the very real risks associated with rehabilitation and step-down care, such as fractures and self-medication errors. On the whole, however, these problems are no more common in geriatrically adapted units than in traditional wards; they merely occur for different reasons.[253,254]

Discussion

Management Considerations throughout the Perioperative Period

CLINICAL PHARMACOLOGY

Use of both prescription and nonprescription drugs is heavy in the geriatric population: in the United States, individuals 65 years of age or older account for 20 to 25 percent of the annual expenditure for drugs, even though they represent only about 11 percent of the population.[112] One Canadian study reported that as many as 77 percent of individuals 65 years of age or older were receiving prescription medication; in another series, 27 percent of the elderly patients studied were receiving an average of eight different prescription drugs.[113,114]

Table 4 Age-Related Changes with Potential Relevance to Pharmacology[273]

Pharmacological Parameter	Age-Related Changes
Absorption	Decreased absorptive surface, splanchnic blood flow, and gastric acidity Altered gastrointestinal motility
Distribution	Decreased total body water, lean body mass, and serum albumin Increased body fat Altered protein binding
Metabolism	Decreased liver blood flow, enzyme activity, and enzyme inducibility
Excretion	Decreased renal blood flow, glomerular filtration rate, and tubular secretory function
Tissue sensitivity	Altered receptor number, receptor affinity, second-messenge function, and cellular and nuclear responses

The incidence of adverse drug reactions increases with age and is two to three times greater in patients 60 years of age or older than in those 30 years of age or younger.[112,115] This may reflect increased use of drugs (particularly drugs with a low therapeutic index, such as digoxin) by older patients, polypharmacy and the resultant interactions, the presence of multiple and more severe diseases in the elderly, and aging-associated alterations in pharmacokinetics and pharmacodynamics [*see Table 4*]. Noncompliance probably is no more frequent in elderly patients than in younger ones, occurring in one third to one half of cases. Most instances of noncompliance may actually be underadherence, which is indeed an appropriate response to adverse drug effects on occasion.[112,116] Compliance may be improved by simplifying dosage schedules, reducing the number of medications, and providing clear written and verbal instructions.[116]

Pharmacological considerations include both pharmacokinetics and pharmacodynamics. The term pharmacokinetics refers to the absorption, distribution, protein binding, metabolism, and excretion of drugs and their metabolites (drug disposition), whereas the term pharmacodynamics refers to the interaction of drugs with receptors and the resulting desired or undesired physiologic responses (drug response). Alterations in both pharmacokinetics and pharmacodynamics are predictable to a degree and must be taken into account whenever a drug is given to an elderly patient.[112,116]

Most clinically relevant drugs given orally are absorbed by passive diffusion across the very extensive surface area of the proximal small bowel. Absorption of these drugs is unimpaired in the elderly, although gastric acid secretion may be decreased and gastric emptying diminished. Changes in body composition, specifically an increase in the proportion of body fat and a decrease in the proportion of lean tissue [*see Patterns of Change in Body Composition, Organ Systems, and Integrated Responses, below*], may influence the distribution of drugs: the volume of distribution of relatively water-soluble drugs tends to decrease, and that of more fat-soluble drugs tends to increase. Altered distribution influences the elimination half-life of drugs, but it does not affect steady-state blood levels with multiple dosing if hepatic and renal drug clearances are unchanged.

Clearance of drugs primarily excreted by the kidneys declines predictably with advancing age and the concomitant decrease in the glomerular filtration rate. Creatinine clearance is a much more reliable marker of the GFR than serum creatinine concentration, which depends on muscle mass as well. Drugs for which the dosage must be adjusted according to the patient's renal function include aminoglycosides, vancomycin, penicillins, cephalosporins, digoxin, cimetidine, and procainamide. Age-related differences in the pharmacokinetics of renally excreted drugs, including the aminoglycosides, are unlikely when the creatinine clearance is greater than 80 ml/min/1.73 m².[112] Drug levels should be monitored, particularly when drugs with a low therapeutic index are used.

Clearance of drugs by the liver depends on the delivery of the drug (i.e., on hepatic blood flow) and on the activity of biotransforming enzymes. Clearance of drugs that are metabolized relatively slowly is dependent on the function of hepatic enzymes; since hepatic mass decreases with age, clearance of such drugs tends to be reduced.[116,117] Hepatic blood flow also decreases with age: it is 40 to 45 percent less in elderly persons than in young adults, which results in diminished flow-dependent clearance.[117] Age-related reductions in the clearance of diazepam, chlordiazepoxide, theophylline, and propranolol have been suggested on the basis of decreased hepatic biotransformation (whether dependent on blood flow or on enzyme function). Such reductions may be more pronounced in males. Plasma levels of drugs cleared in a flow-dependent fashion may be higher when hepatic blood flow is further decreased, as it is in conditions such as congestive heart failure or chronic liver disease.[116]

The effects of age on the actions of drugs at target sites have not been extensively studied. Reductions in the number of beta-adrenergic receptors may contribute to the diminished effectiveness of sympathetic agonists in the elderly.[118] Synthesis of vitamin K–dependent clotting factors may be more strongly inhibited in older patients at a given plasma warfarin concentration.[119] The elderly also exhibit more marked CNS depression at given blood levels of benzodiazepines.[101]

FLUID, ELECTROLYTE, AND ACID-BASE HOMEOSTASIS

Elderly patients are less able to restore and maintain acid-base, fluid, and electrolyte homeostasis during surgical illness. Compensatory mechanisms that can be relied on in younger patients function less rapidly in older ones. Renal handling of salt and water is less efficient, the physiology of aldosterone and vasopressin is altered, and renal and other mechanisms of acid-base regulation are limited. As a result, elderly patients are less able to maintain the integrity of the extracellular space and other fluid compartments when challenged. Careful management, based on an understanding of physiologic mechanisms, is necessary if extreme abnormalities of fluid, electrolyte, and acid-base status are to be avoided.

The minimum requirement for water is increased in older patients as a result of increased insensible losses through thinned skin and impairment of the concentrating ability of the kidneys. Thirst is an important response to fluid deprivation, but it is known to be diminished in the elderly.[120] In one study, thirst after a 24-hour period of water deprivation was less in healthy elderly males (67 to 75 years of age) than in younger subjects (20 to 31 years of age), despite higher circulating vasopressin levels and higher plasma osmolality; urine osmolality was lower in the first group as well.[121] Hypothalamic responsiveness to osmotic signals appears to increase with age, as manifested by increased release of vasopressin from the posterior pituitary.[122] Unlike the response to osmotic signals, however, the vasopressin response to volume-pressure changes is blunted in the elderly.[123] Renin responses to sodium restriction and postural changes are diminished in older patients, and circulating aldosterone levels are decreased as a result of diminished adrenal sensitivity to both renin-angiotensin and local sodium-potassium signals.[124,125]

Renal blood flow decreases progressively with advancing age, and the GFR falls rapidly after the fifth or sixth decade. The ability of older persons to conserve or excrete water or solute is further reduced by the diminished efficiency of tubular processes, which is a result of decreased osmotic stratification in the medulla and decreased responsiveness to vasopressin.[126] One group of investigators found that healthy young subjects demonstrated a marked decrease in urine flow and a moderate increase in urine osmolality in response to 12 hours of water deprivation, whereas healthy elderly subjects were unable to decrease urine flow or urine osmolality.[127] Sodium conservation is similarly impaired: the half-time to the achievement of sodium equilibrium in the face of sodium restriction is significantly longer in healthy individuals older than 60 years than in younger individuals.[128] Thus, inefficient renal conservation of salt and water exacerbates hypovolemic states in the elderly patient, and the onset of oliguria may be delayed.

A fall in the GFR also accounts for the decreased ability of the kidneys in the elderly to excrete an acute load of salt or water, predisposing to extracellular fluid volume expansion.[129] Hyponatremia coupled with water intoxication is a serious disorder in the elderly, presenting as anorexia, weakness, lethargy, confusion, and, if severe, seizures or coma. The elderly are prone to excessive secretion of antidiuretic hormone (ADH), particularly during the stress of surgical illness; this excessive ADH secretion is accompanied by extracellular fluid expansion, hyponatremia, and inappropriately concentrated (i.e., less than maximally dilute) urine despite normal renal function.[129]

Although the pH of body fluids is normally only slightly affected by age, the efficiency of acid-base homeostasis is decreased in the elderly.[126] For example, elderly persons (72 to 93 years of age) take twice as long to eliminate an acid load as younger individuals (17 to 35 years of age) do.[130] Maintenance of normal pH depends on chemical buffer systems in body fluids, alterations in ventilation and elimination of carbon dioxide, and renal excretion of excess acid or base.[131] The slight decreases in extracellular volume and in bicarbonate concentration that occur in the elderly may limit the capacity of rapid chemical buffering systems. Similarly, decreased plasma volume and lean body mass and bone demineralization decrease the availability of slower buffers such as plasma and intracellular proteins and hydroxyapatite.[126] Bicarbonate buffering depends on the rapid elimination of carbon dioxide by the lungs. Neither P_aCO_2 nor minute ventilation changes with age: increased physiologic dead space is compensated for by a decreased metabolic rate and carbon dioxide production. Ventilatory responses to hypercapnia are significantly diminished in healthy elderly persons[132]; however, because ventilation is increased and eucapnia maintained during exercise in the elderly,[133] physiologic pH buffering by respiratory mechanisms probably will not be limited except perhaps in the face of a very large acid load.

Renal regulation of acid-base status is based on the variable reabsorption of bicarbonate, the elimination of hydrogen ions in the form of titratable acid, and the regeneration of extracellular bicarbonate accompanying the deamination of glutamine and the synthesis of ammonia.[126] The capacity of each of these mechanisms is presumably limited by the diminished effective renal mass in the elderly.[134] Although the efficiency of bicarbonate reabsorption is maintained and is adequate for handling an acid load, a decreased GFR results in decreased presentation of bicarbonate to the proximal tubule and delayed elimination of bicarbonate in response to an alkaline load. The major buffer used for the generation of titratable acid is phosphate, which is less available in the distal nephron of the aged kidney, primarily as a result of a decreased GFR. The deamination of glutamine in the distal tubule provides ammonia (NH_3), which combines with secreted hydrogen ions to form ammonium (NH_4^+) and is then excreted with chloride and other tubular anions; this process is accompanied by a net increase in bicarbonate in the extracellular fluid. These processes are less effective in the elderly because the capacity of the aged kidney to deaminate glutamine is decreased and lower plasma aldosterone levels limit the exchange of sodium and hydrogen in the distal segment.

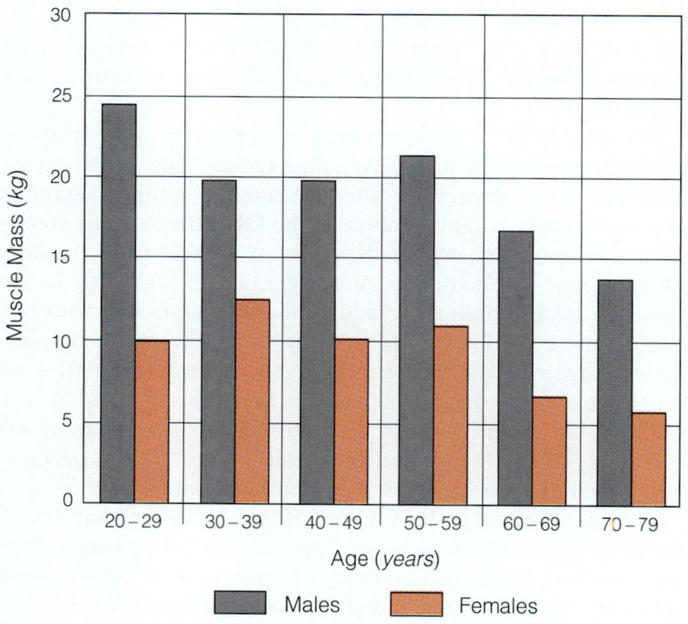

NUTRITIONAL SUPPORT

Fasting, at least for brief periods, is commonplace in hospitalized patients and is associated with a negative net nitrogen balance. Host responses to major operations and acute surgical illnesses are characterized by an accelerated breakdown of skeletal muscle with a net release of amino acids supporting a variety of accelerated metabolic processes. Such losses of muscle protein may be uniquely detrimental in elderly patients. Lean body mass and body cell mass both decrease considerably with normal aging, largely because of declining muscle mass: a loss of 40 percent of muscle mass or more is typical between young adulthood and the age of 80 years and is accompanied by a comparable decrease in strength [see Figure 4]. Thus, during prolonged or severe illness, the rapid erosion of muscle mass may reduce an elderly patient's muscle strength to critical levels and may limit the period during which metabolic demands can be met endogenously. For example, the recovery of strength after major abdominal operation in older patients is substantially impaired compared with that in young patients[135] [see Figure 5]. Early provision of nutritional support should be considered in elderly patients who are not taking in sufficient nutrients in the form of a regular diet.

The typical diets followed by older persons may provide adequate vitamins and trace minerals in the absence of stress, though it is worth remembering that there is a general lack of information about specific requirements in the elderly. Stores may be limited, however, and deficiencies may arise during illness.[136,137] For example, plasma zinc concentration decreases after injury and other stresses, partly as a result of increased urinary losses. Zinc deficiency has been associated with impaired wound healing and depressed immune function. Skeletal muscle holds the largest store of zinc. The decrease in muscle bulk in the elderly, coupled with the inadequate zinc intake and impaired absorption reported in this age group, suggests that zinc supplementation may play an important role in the nutritional support of these patients. Decreased serum levels of a number of vitamins have been observed after burn injury, and increased requirements for several vitamins and minerals that may affect immune function, wound healing, and antioxidant defenses have been demonstrated during acute stress states.[138] Daily supplementation of the diets of healthy elderly subjects with physiologic amounts of various vitamins and trace elements has been shown to enhance immune function and reduce the rate of clinical infection.[139] Early vitamin and trace element supplementation (i.e., within the first 24 to 48 hours) should be considered in all elderly patients, particularly in nonelective settings.

Voluntary food intake is often inadequate in hospitalized elderly patients. Several trials have suggested that nutritional supplementation has a beneficial effect on outcome after hip fracture.[140-142] In one randomized, controlled study of overnight nasogastric feeding, hospital stay and rehabilitation were shortened in the fed group, particularly among the most malnourished patients, in whom an improvement in hospital mortality approached statistical significance.[140] One third of patients randomly assigned to supplementation were fed for five days or less because of intolerance of the nasogastric tube or death. In another study, patients were randomly assigned to either oral nutritional supplementation at 8 P.M. each evening or no supplement.[141] Supplementation was associated with a reduced hospital stay and less frequent unfavorable outcomes. The supplements were well tolerated and did not lead to a decrease in voluntary intake. Thus, voluntary nutrient intake should be carefully assessed and nutritional supplementation considered even when the elderly patient is allowed a full diet,

Figure 4 A substantial portion of the muscle mass present in young adulthood is lost by 70 years of age. Age-related declines in muscle strength have been documented as well.[150]

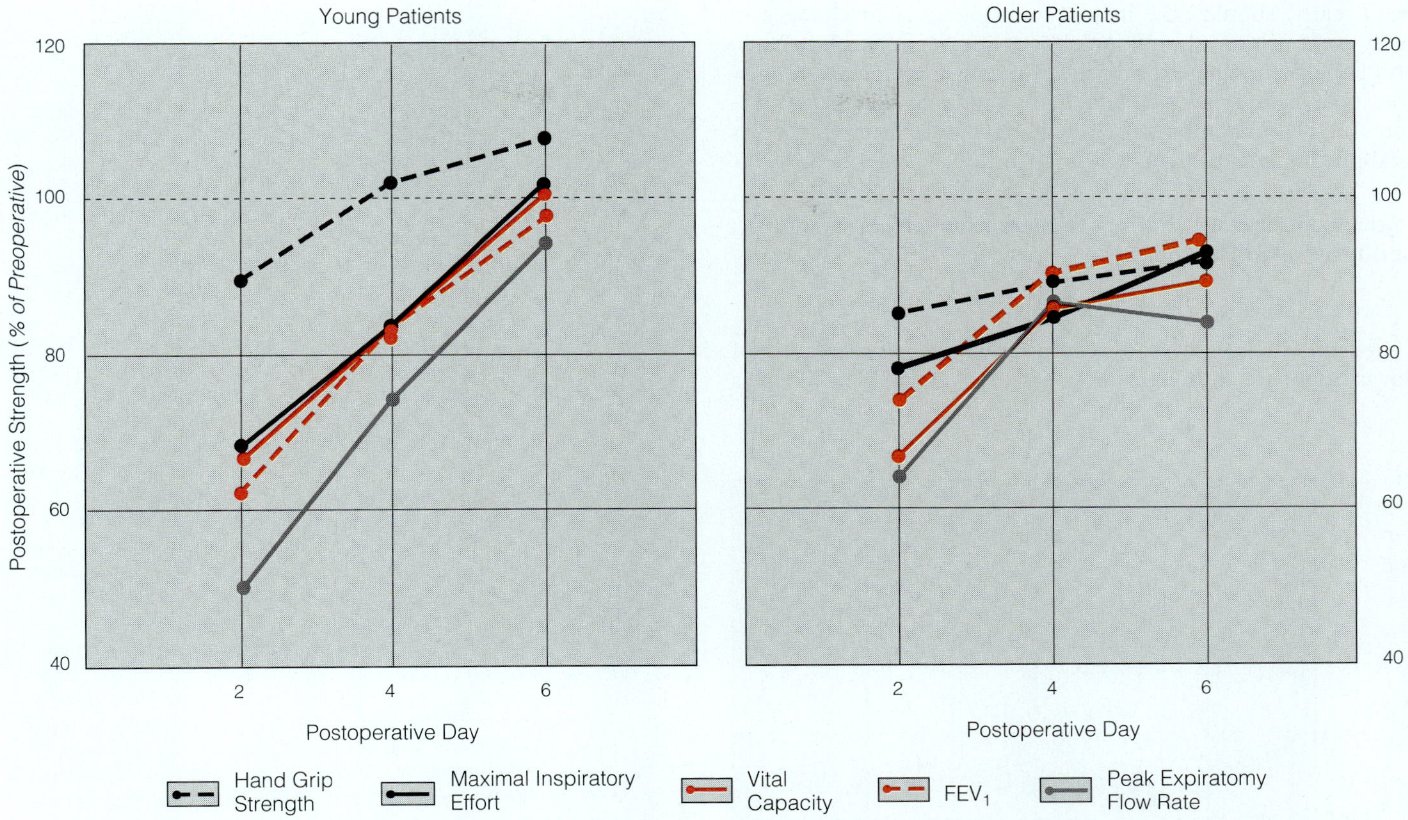

Figure 5 Illustrated is the recovery of postoperative strength (assessed with respect to five variables) in younger and older patients.[135]

particularly if preexisting nutritional deficits are identified.

Enteral feeding should be initiated promptly in any elderly patient whose voluntary intake is not adequate. If the patient's nutritional state is suboptimal or if he or she has an acute surgical illness, at least 50 percent of energy and protein requirements should be provided by the third to the fifth day after admission, and full support should be provided by the seventh day. Parenteral feeding, either peripheral or central, may be used alone or as an adjunct when prescribed nutrients cannot be fully administered by the enteral route. Energy intake and expenditure in healthy individuals tend to decrease in parallel with advancing age as a result of diminished metabolic body size (i.e., body cell mass) and reduced activity[143] [*see Figure 6 and Sidebar* Long-Term Effects of Physical Activity]. The number of calories provided to elderly surgical patients should reflect these changes, although of course the considerable variability among individuals must be taken into account as well. Protein intake should normally be 1 to 2 g/kg/day, depending on the severity of the primary illness and the nature of the associated disease states. Supplementation with arginine has been shown to improve experimental wound healing and immune function in healthy elderly subjects, possibly via growth hormone and insulinlike growth factor–1 (IGF-1) secretagogue activity.[144] Provision of nutritional support via enteral and parenteral routes is discussed in detail elsewhere [*see 97 Nutritional Support*].

The need for nutritional support appears to be greater in elderly patients than in well-nourished younger patients; however, such support may be less efficacious and less well tolerated because of the combined influences of aging and critical illness on intermediary metabolism. Glucose tolerance decreases with normal aging, and enteral or parenteral feeding may result in marked hyperglycemia, particularly when coupled with the insulin resistance that accompanies trauma and critical illness.[145,146] Additionally, insulin responses to glucose loads are markedly diminished in the elderly after injury[145] [*see Figure 7*]. Renal clearance of glucose is normally an important defense against hyperglycemia; however, a reduced glomerular filtration rate and an increased renal threshold for glucose make elderly patients even more prone to hyperglycemia. Uncontrolled hyperglycemia resulting from either an enteral or a parenteral glucose load may give rise to hyperosmolar nonketotic coma, in which serum osmolarity and glucose are markedly elevated in association with a solute diuresis, dehydration, coma, and inappropriately low insulin and ketone levels. This condition is corrected by rehydration and insulin administration. Hyperglycemia may limit the administration of calories provided in the form of glucose even when insulin is used. Fat emulsion may be used as an alternative energy source in parenteral feeding, but plasma triglyceride levels should be monitored because they tend to increase with age and because lipid clearance may be altered.[147] Decreased serum growth hormone and IGF-1 responses to feeding have been reported in older trauma patients.[148,149] Growth hormone is a potent anabolic hormone, many of whose metabolic effects are mediated by IGF-1.

Nutritional support of the elderly trauma patient should

begin early, should take into account age-related changes in body composition, should include appropriate micronutrients, and should anticipate diminished glucose tolerance. Administration of insulin may well be required and may, along with factors such as recombinant growth hormone, offer particular anabolic benefits to the elderly patient.

Patterns of Change in Body Composition, Organ Systems, and Integrated Responses

CHANGES IN BODY COMPOSITION

Specific changes in body composition are characteristic of advancing age, although they are not inevitable. Whereas weight remains more or less stable, fat mass tends to increase and lean body mass tends to decrease.[150] Lean body mass comprises body cell mass—defined as the "component of body composition containing the oxygen-consuming, potassium-rich, glucose-oxidizing, work-performing tissue"[151]—and extracellular mass. Body cell mass decreases an average of 23 percent in men and 25 percent in women from the third to the eighth decade.[150] Besides decreasing in absolute terms, body cell mass declines as a proportion of lean body mass; this decline is largely accounted for by diminished skeletal muscle mass [see Figure 7]. Forty to 45 percent of the muscle mass present in young adulthood is lost by the time a person reaches 70 years of age.[150] At the same time, muscle strength is lost as well.[152,153] Reductions in FEV_1 and maximal midexpiratory flow rate occur with advancing age; these reductions are partially attributable to a decrease in the strength of the respiratory musculature.[154] Together with decreased physical activity, changes in body composition contribute to decreased resting energy expenditure and therefore to decreased requirements for calories.

The changes in body composition and muscle function appear to be at least partially determined by the level of habitual physical activity. For example, body weight and proportion

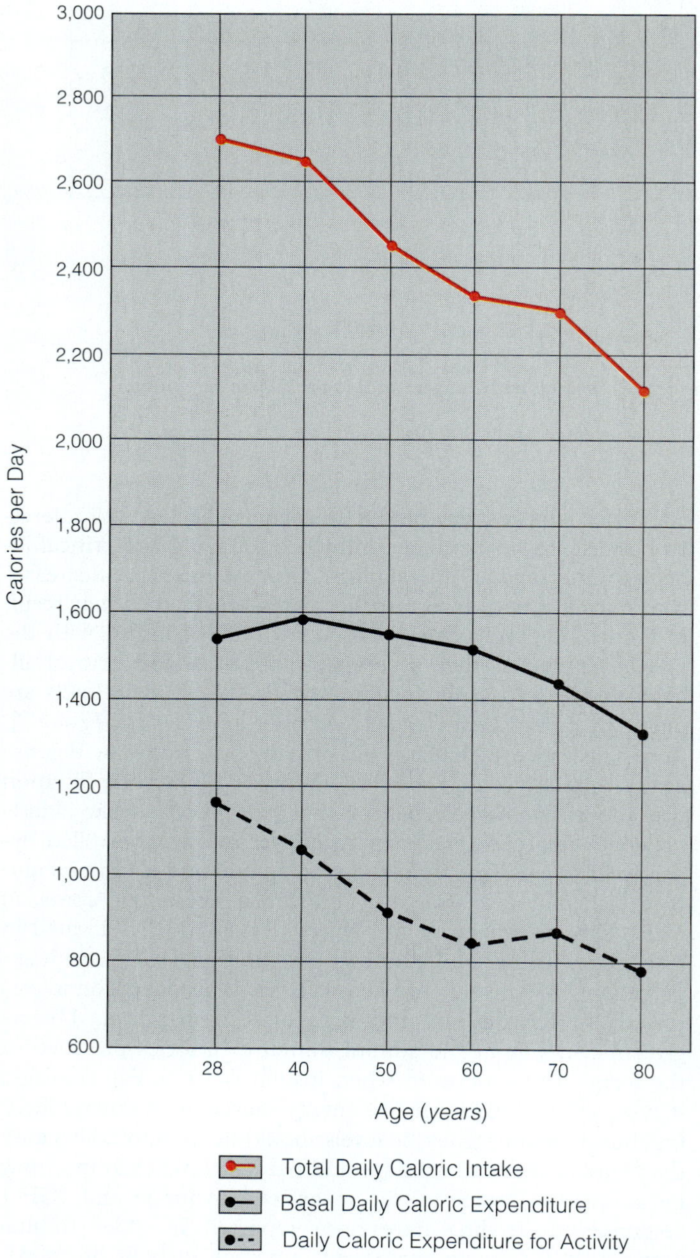

Long-Term Effects of Physical Activity

Many of the physiologic changes considered to be inevitable effects of aging may in fact be attributable to the decline in habitual levels of physical activity typically seen in older persons as well as to dietary, environmental, and psychosocial factors.[147,191] For example, the degree of carbohydrate intolerance observed in the elderly is strongly associated with levels of physical activity and fitness.[255] Moreover, physical training has been shown to increase insulin sensitivity in young males as well as improve glucose tolerance in older individuals.[256,257]

Reduced activity and diminished body cell mass, particularly muscle mass, can account for decreases in resting energy expenditure with age. A sedentary lifestyle appears to limit maximal oxygen consumption as well: longitudinal studies of maximal oxygen consumption during treadmill exercise demonstrate a decline that is two to three times greater in sedentary persons than in those participating in a weekly running program.[174] Older athletes also appear to avoid the decrease in maximum stroke volume and oxygen extraction during exercise that occur in sedentary individuals.[258] With physical conditioning such that 70 to 85 percent of maximal heart rate is achieved for 20 to 40 minutes three times a week for several weeks, heart rate and blood pressure are less for a given workload, and peripheral resistance and myocardial oxygen demand are also less.[259] Rates of coronary artery disease and myocardial infarction are lower among individuals participating in consistent vigorous exercise.[260,261] In college alumni, overall mortality (especially from cardiovascular and respiratory disease) has been demonstrated to be inversely related to energy expenditure on physical activity up to a level of 3,500 kcal/week.[262] The cardiovascular benefits of fitness depend on long-term habitual exercise, but the trainability of older individuals has been well demonstrated.[259,261] In addition, fractures related to osteoporosis appear to be less frequent in more active populations, and habitual moderate exercise may slow the progression of osteoporosis.[263,264]

Thus, long-term moderate physical activity slows the decline of a number of physiologic functions associated with aging, may contribute to increased longevity, may ease the completion of activities of daily living, and may allow longer retention of the ability to live independently.[259,265]

Figure 6 Depicted are the daily intake and expenditure of calories in normal males of various age groups.[268,269]

of fat were constant in a cross-sectional study of lumberjacks 20 to 70 years of age, in contrast to the gradual increase in weight and body fat seen in males with sedentary occupations.[155] Another study found that the body composition of male endurance athletes 50 to 75 years of age was very similar to that of younger athletes, whereas both untrained individuals and visually matched lean older individuals had significantly higher levels of body fat.[156] One group of investigators demonstrated increased muscle strength and a modest but significant decrease in body fat in elderly males who underwent six weeks of training as well as significant increases in minute ventilation during exercise and vital capacity.[157] Another group observed a 10 percent increase in lean tissue, a 17 percent decrease in skin-fold thickness, a four to five percent increase in body potassium, and an apparent halting of age-related decreases in bone calcium during a one-year physical-training program in individuals in their seventh decade.[158] Another investigator, who studied age-related muscle fiber atrophy in males 25 to 65 years of age, found that muscle fiber size and strength increased after twice-weekly exercise for 15 weeks, particularly in the older subjects.[159]

CHANGES IN ORGAN SYSTEMS

Aging is associated with a variety of predictable morphologic, functional, and pathological changes in major organ systems. Such changes have been best described for cardiovascular, respiratory, and renal systems, which are also the systems most relevant to perioperative care.

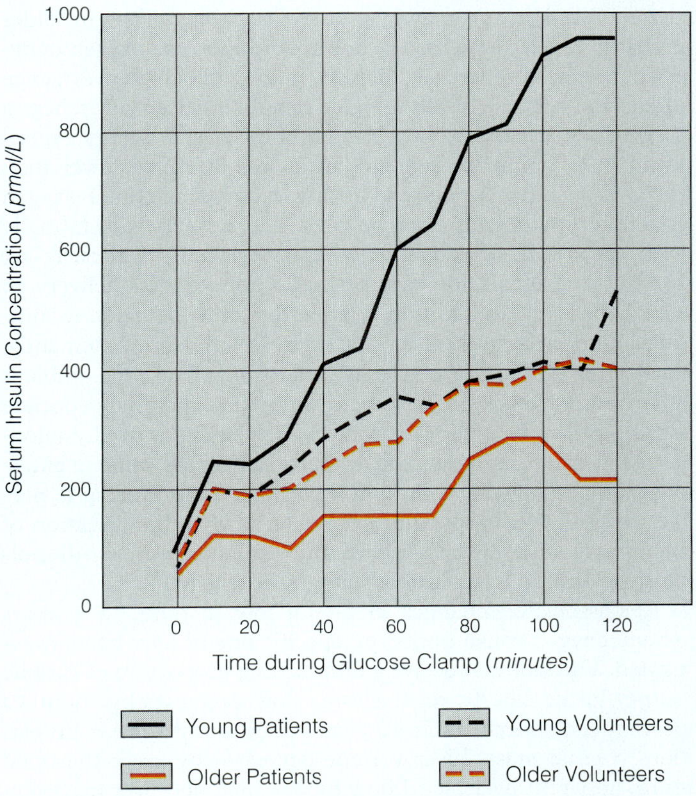

Figure 7 Shown are serum insulin responses to glucose loading (during glucose clamp).[145]

CHANGES IN INTEGRATED RESPONSES

Oxygen Delivery and Consumption

The earliest physiologic responses to tissue injury are directed at restoring and maintaining the perfusion of vital organs. These responses rely on rapid activation of the sympathoadrenal axis by signals from the site of injury and from baroreceptors and chemoreceptors. Blood flow to the skin and skeletal muscle is decreased by peripheral vasoconstriction, and cardiac output is redistributed to vital tissues. With advancing age, however, the efficiency of many of these critical responses is diminished, even in healthy individuals. Baroreflex sensitivity is decreased in the elderly, presumably as a result of reduced arterial distensibility.[160] Vasoconstrictor responses are also reduced, probably because of alterations in autonomic neural pathways.[161] In addition, an age-associated decline in the inotropic and chronotropic effects of beta-adrenergic stimulation has been well described.[162] Thus, diminished arterial compliance, impaired vasoconstriction, altered autonomic function and sensitivity to catecholamines, and decreased baroreflex sensitivity all may limit the maintenance of cardiovascular homeostasis.

Delivery of oxygen to the tissues may be impaired in the elderly at every step of the oxygen transport pathway and may be inadequate when oxygen demands are increased.[126,163] Ventilatory responses to both hypoxia and hypercapnia are diminished. The alveolar-arterial oxygen gradient increases, and P_aO_2 progressively declines. There is substantial variation in most cardiac variables among older individuals, reflecting aging, atherosclerotic and other disease, and various lifestyle factors that interact and influence cardiovascular function in ways that are often difficult to disentangle.[162] Cardiac output declines approximately one percent a year, beginning in the fourth decade, when unselected individuals are studied.[126] Progressive decreases in resting stroke volume and cardiac output with increasing age have been observed in individuals without clinical evidence of cardiovascular disease, both at rest and during exercise[164,165]; in addition, older subjects have had larger arteriovenous oxygen differences and increased arterial lactate concentrations. However, the older individuals in such studies may well have had clinically occult cardiovascular disease or deconditioning resulting from long-standing limitations of physical activity (e.g., from time spent in nursing homes), and the use of invasive measurement techniques may have influenced observations.

More recent studies of nonsedentary individuals who were screened with resting and stress electrocardiography and dipyridamole-thallium scanning have demonstrated that older individuals, assessed noninvasively, maintain resting cardiac output, heart rate, stroke volume, and ejection fraction[162] [see Figure 8]. Stiffening of the aorta and of more peripheral vessels tends to be associated with increased peripheral vascular resistance. A normal modest increase in left ventricular wall thickness with aging is exaggerated in persons with hypertension and coronary artery disease. Myocardial relaxation is typically prolonged, and early diastolic filling is slowed and delayed with advancing age.[162,166] Left ventricular end-diastolic volume at rest tends to be increased, with more rapid filling later in diastole; this tendency is associated with left atrial enlargement and an enhanced contribution to filling from atrial contraction.[167] Resting pulmonary arterial pressure and pulmonary vascular resistance increase moderately.[168]

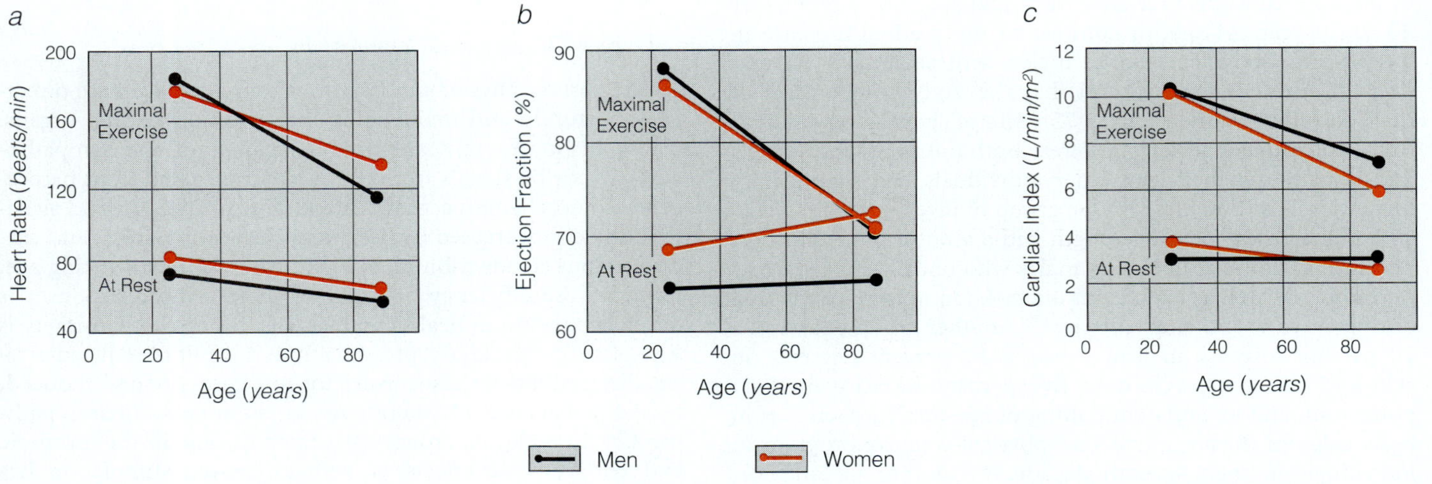

Figure 8 Shown are linear regressions on age of (*a*) heart rate, (*b*) ejection fraction, and (*c*) cardiac index at rest and during maximal cycle ergometry in healthy, sedentary male and female volunteers who had been screened to exclude clinical hypertension and occult coronary artery disease.[270]

Cardiovascular responses to exercise have been studied in detail and provide insight into the responses associated with acute surgical illness. The maximum heart rate achieved during exercise diminishes consistently with age, whereas changes in stroke volume index are variable (reflecting occult coronary artery disease, fitness level, heart size, and body composition) and maximum cardiac index tends to decline.[162] Older persons who are free of cardiovascular disease rely more on increases in stroke volume to achieve increases in their cardiac index during exercise than younger persons do.[169] Thus, end-diastolic volume index tends to increase in older subjects; decreases in end-systolic volume index and increases in ejection fraction are less prominent than in young individuals[162,170] [*see Figure 9*]. In one study of generally healthy subjects who were not extensively screened, the likelihood of ventricular wall motion abnormalities during exercise rose consistently with age.[170] In an older study of subjects with varying levels of habitual activity, the incidence of ECG abnormalities during and after maximal exercise increased with age and was much higher than the incidence at rest.[164]

The response of healthy older individuals to an increase in afterload differs from that of young subjects: significant left ventricular dilatation occurs, and contraction begins from a greater preload than in young subjects, presumably as a reflection of a diminished contractile reserve in the older subjects.[171] The diminution of the inotropic, chronotropic, and arterial vasodilating effects of beta-adrenergic stimulation with advancing age may contribute to many age-related changes in cardiovascular function.[162] Isoproterenol infusion results in lesser increases in heart rate, left ventricular ejection fraction, and cardiac index in older persons than in younger ones.[172] Dobutamine augments cardiac output and stroke volume to a much lesser extent in elderly patients with decompensated congestive heart failure than in younger patients and provides no additional hemodynamic benefit at infusion rates higher than 5 mg/kg/min.[173]

Thus, older patients are predisposed to hemodynamic compromise related to tachyarrhythmias, atrial fibrillation, increased afterload, and coronary artery disease. Increased end-diastolic volume and stroke volume are compensatory mechanisms that maintain cardiac output in the face of other limitations, and appropriate filling volumes must be achieved. Inotropic drugs may be less beneficial in the elderly, and agents that are nonvasoconstricting (e.g., dobutamine) or have nonadrenergic mechanisms of action (e.g., amrinone) may be useful. Agents that reduce afterload (e.g., angiotensin-converting enzyme inhibitors) may also play a greater role in older patients. Elderly patients are less able to increase oxygen delivery in the face of increased demand and, with a high prevalence of coronary artery disease, are at risk for myocardial ischemia if demands are excessive. Although increases in energy expenditure in hospitalized patients are generally much lower than those in healthy individuals during exercise, maximal oxygen consumption during exercise does decline very substantially with age.[174] It is probably not appropriate to arbitrarily set supranormal goals for cardiac index and oxygen delivery in elderly patients. In addition, every effort must be made to minimize unnecessary stresses that increase metabolic demands, such as hypothermia, shivering, exposure to a cool ambient environment, hypovolemia, acidosis, pain, and inappropriate weaning from ventilatory support. The principles of physiologic and invasive hemodynamic monitoring are the same in elderly patients as in the young; however, such monitoring is perhaps even more important in the elderly when the direction of therapy is unclear because of the limitations in cardiopulmonary function and homeostatic mechanisms.

Age-associated changes in blood flow to (and, to a lesser extent, oxygen consumption in) specific organs have been investigated. The kidneys receive a diminishing proportion of cardiac output in the elderly; renal plasma flow decreases by about 10 percent each decade after 40 years of age and decreases in relation to renal mass. Liver volume decreases by more than one third, apparent liver blood flow by one half, and liver perfusion by one fifth from age 24 to age 91.[117] Cerebral blood flow, blood volume, and oxygen consumption decrease approximately 0.50 percent a year in pure gray and white matter regions, whereas

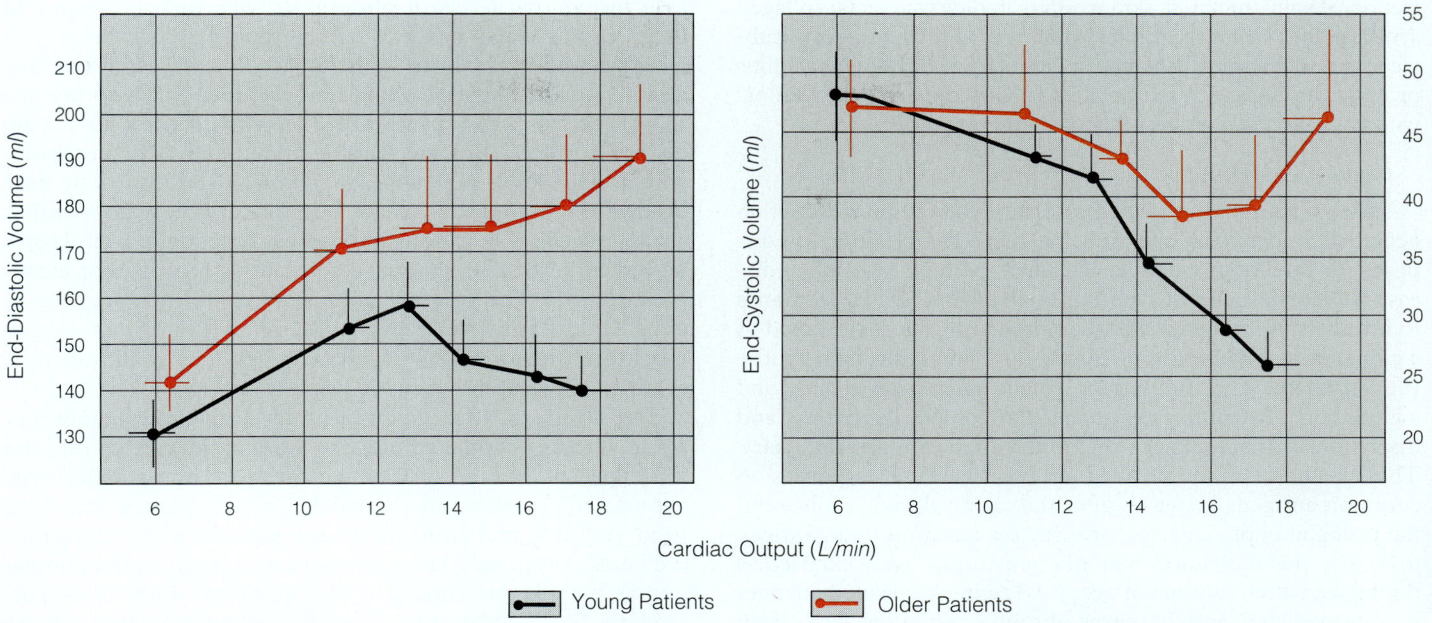

Figure 9 Depicted are relations between end-diastolic volume, end-systolic volume, and cardiac output in young and older patients at rest and during graded upright bicycle exercise.[271]

the oxygen extraction ratio does not change or changes to a minor degree.[175] Skeletal muscle blood flow at rest appears to be unaffected by age, but maximal blood flow after exercise is diminished in older subjects.[176,177] Average skin blood flow decreases by 30 to 40 percent from age 20 to age 70.[178]

Thermoregulation

The endogenous temperature set point is typically elevated after operation or injury and during sepsis, and ambient temperature is often kept inappropriately low in hospital patient care areas. Alterations in vasomotor activity are normally relied on in the range of temperatures between those that elicit shivering and those that cause sweating. When the core temperature is lower than the thermoregulatory set point and heat conservation is inadequate, shivering is initiated to generate heat. Shivering may be accompanied by a severalfold increase in oxygen consumption, which would constitute a substantial metabolic load. When the core temperature falls below 34° C (93.2° F), thermoregulation becomes impaired, metabolic activity slows, and further decreases in temperature are more rapid. The hypothermic myocardium is prone to intractable arrhythmias that may be triggered by minimal stimulation. Conditions associated with secondary hypothermia, such as hypothyroidism and diabetes mellitus, may be more frequent (or more frequently undiagnosed) in the elderly. The management of hypothermia and hyperthermia is discussed in detail elsewhere [see 98 Fever, Hyperpyrexia, and Hypothermia].

The elderly, particularly those older than 80 years, are less sensitive to alterations in environmental temperature and less able to maintain thermal homeostasis.[179] These limitations result in a higher incidence of hypothermia and heatstroke, a lower maximum body temperature during febrile illness, and more marked and prolonged falls in body temperature with surgery.[9,86,87,89,179]

Mechanisms of heat conservation, production, and offloading are less efficient in the elderly. Sensitivity to changes in ambient temperature is less precise, and behavioral responses are delayed. Vasoconstrictor responses to a cold stimulus are depressed in some elderly individuals, and shivering is delayed.[180] Moreover, the capacity for metabolic heat production by shivering is limited by the reduced muscle mass characteristic of the aged. With decreased blood flow in the skin, reduced sweat gland density, and delayed and diminished sweating responses, the elderly are less able to offload heat and reduce body temperature than younger individuals are.[126]

Malnutrition may predispose to hypothermia and accidental injury. In a study of 744 elderly women with fractures of the neck of the femur, most of those who were very thin had a core temperature lower than 35° C (95.0° F) on admission, whereas most of those who were well nourished had a temperature higher than 36° C (96.8° F).[181] The increase in the incidence of fractures in cold weather was greatest among the very thin; the finding that most injuries occurred indoors suggested that impaired thermoregulation in the malnourished individuals resulted in hypothermia, lack of coordination, and subsequent injury. In a study of elderly patients exposed to a range of ambient temperatures after femur fracture, vasoconstrictor responses were generally maintained, but whereas patients who were well nourished could increase metabolic heat production appropriately, those who were undernourished (by anthropometric measurements) could not.[182]

Wound Healing

Advanced age is often cited as a risk factor for impaired wound healing, although not consistently. Any such association is probably attributable to a higher prevalence of specific risk factors in the elderly, such as malnutrition, malignancy, uremia, diabetes mellitus, and atherosclerosis. Studies of healthy, well-nourished volunteers have shown minor delays in the epithelialization of split-thickness skin wounds in older subjects; collagen synthesis in subcutaneous implants was similar in young subjects and older ones, whereas accumulation of noncollagenous protein was decreased in the latter.[183] Outcome after abdominal wound dehiscence may be worse in the elderly.[184]

Immune Function

There is abundant evidence that changes in immune function occur with advancing age and that these changes may predispose to infectious, neoplastic, and perhaps vascular disease.[185,186] The delayed-type hypersensitivity (DTH) response to intradermal challenge with common antigens can be used as a global measure of immune function.[186] For a normal response (i.e., erythema and induration), intact antigen processing and stimulation of lymphocytes, release of soluble mediators, and migration of macrophages to the injection site are necessary. The likelihood of diminished or absent DTH responses to common antigens increases after the eighth decade of life, and the probability of achieving primary sensitization to an antigen to which the individual had not previously been exposed is diminished after 70 years of age.[187,188] Aging-associated changes in cell-mediated and humoral immune responses have been reviewed in detail elsewhere.[185,186] In general, responses to foreign antigens are diminished and responses to autologous antigens may be increased. The limited information available on phagocytic responses suggests that polymorphonuclear leukocyte function may decrease with age.[186]

Assessment of Risks

"There is undoubtedly a basic flaw in characterizing a person as elderly simply upon the attainment of a particular chronological age, but no mechanism has been suggested which gives a more consistently reliable appraisal. . . ."[189] Advanced age is commonly used as a marker for altered physiologic function and medical status, and when other factors are not considered, it is clearly related to increased mortality during surgical illness (i.e., operation, trauma, and severe infection). Aging is associated with recognizable patterns of change in the structure and function of most organ systems and in integrated responses (see above), and the clinical presentation of specific pathological conditions is altered in the elderly. Such generalizations must be treated with caution, however, because of the heterogeneity of the elderly population: aging is a highly variable process both among individuals and among different organ systems within an individual. To provide optimal management for elderly patients, it is essential to recognize this variability and to carefully assess each organ system in each patient. Assessment of operative risk must rest on more specific and more strongly predictive criteria than age alone.

STUDIES OF AGING AND THE AGED

Of major importance in studies of aging and the aged is the distinction between the physiologic consequences of aging and the pathological effects of concomitant disease.[190] Screening tests used to identify a disease-free population must be sensitive but must not restrict the study population to unusually healthy older individuals. Although changes characteristic of so-called normal aging are generally predictable, there remains substantial heterogeneity within study groups.[191] Some investigators believe that many age-associated changes are attributable to habitual levels of physical activity, diet, lifestyle, and other psychosocial factors.[191] Accordingly, it has been proposed that individuals in the heterogeneous, disease-free, normal geriatric population should be classified into two groups: those who have aged successfully (i.e, who manifest little or no decline in the physiologic variable under study, in comparison with average levels in younger individuals) and those who have aged in the more usual, predicted manner (i.e., who manifest gradual declines in various physiologic functions). It must also be remembered that aging is a continuous process. For example, a 65-year-old person and an 85-year-old person, each in good health, could well be very different with respect to physiologic and functional status, even though they would often be grouped together into a single "elderly" category.

Two basic study designs are employed in clinical studies of aging. Cross-sectional studies are more easily carried out and less expensive but are subject to error and may not reflect true age-related changes. Elderly patients, when younger, may have been very different from the young patients with whom they are being compared; that is, changes may occur in the population as a whole over time. In addition, elderly individuals (particularly those older than 75 years) make up what may be thought of as a biologically superior group in that they have been selected by the very fact of their survival from a larger group, many of whose members have died.[115,190] Cross-sectional studies thus may demonstrate age differences rather than age changes.[192] Longitudinal studies require a stable, dedicated population observed over a prolonged period and are particularly sensitive to subtle alterations in methods. Among the most comprehensive and widely cited longitudinal studies is the Baltimore Longitudinal Study of Aging, which has been conducted using carefully screened, community-residing, independent adults.[192] A study design in which groups overlapping in age are studied for a limited number of years may be a useful compromise.

NATURE OF THE SURGICAL PROCEDURE

Operative mortality varies with the nature and magnitude of the surgical procedure: those procedures that cause the least tissue injury and physiologic perturbation, particularly those that are peripheral and require only local anesthesia, carry the lowest morbidity and mortality.[12,13,68,193,194] For example, transurethral resection of the prostate can be carried out with very little risk in the elderly,[195,196] as can elective inguinal hernia repair,[197,198] whereas the overall operative mortality for major abdominal, thoracic, vascular, and orthopedic procedures may be 10 percent or higher.[12,193-195]

Morbidity and mortality are invariably greater for emergency operations than for elective ones, presumably because of the greater physiologic disturbance caused by the condition requiring urgent treatment and the limited opportunity to assess and optimize the patient's general medical condition.[13,194,197-203] Mortality for emergency gastrointestinal procedures, for example, has been reported to be at least three times higher than mortality for elective procedures.[202,204]

Overall operative mortality in elderly patients is declining, according to comparisons of results from the past several decades.[8,12,193,195] This decline in mortality has been attributed to better preoperative preparation of patients and to improvements in anesthetic and postoperative management (including the widespread use of hemodynamic monitoring) and in surgical technique; however, different series may not be directly comparable in terms of patient selection and other variables. In addition, although published series can guide the assessment of relative risks, local results may differ substantially from published results, depending on such factors as caseload and indications for referral, the availability of various diagnostic and treatment facilities, and anesthetic, medical, and surgical expertise.

MEDICAL AND PHYSIOLOGIC STATUS

The mortality associated with surgery, trauma, bacteremia, septic shock, and multiple organ failure increases consistently with age,[193,200,205-208] as does the rate of complications associated with anesthesia.[199] Yet operative mortality remains strongly dependent on medical and physiologic status, which may in fact be a more powerful predictor of postoperative death than age is.[194,196,197,199,200,204,209] The American Society of Anesthesiologists Physical Status Scale is subjective but is nonetheless a useful predictor of operative mortality and anesthetic complications. Data from a series of 34,145 consecutive patients, although not current (being derived from patients operated on between 1965 and 1969), illustrate the strong correlation between ASA class and mortality in each age group.[200] Of particular importance in this series and more recent ones is the observation that operative mortality in generally fit elderly patients appears to be very low.[196,200,204] For example, in a study of 500 patients older than 80 years who underwent a range of major and minor procedures, postoperative mortality was less than one percent in ASA class 2 patients, four percent in ASA class 3 patients, and 25 percent in ASA class 4 patients.[196] Forty-seven patients underwent cholecystectomy and 27 underwent peripheral vascular surgery without any hospital mortality. Moreover, in a study of 224 surgical patients 90 years of age or older (of whom 85 percent were ASA class 3 or higher), 92 percent were discharged from the hospital and had a five-year survival rate similar to that derived from cohort life tables.[195] One investigator reported on five consecutive patients 100 years of age or older who underwent various major and minor procedures during a five-year period, including open reduction and fixation of hip fracture and cholecystectomy.[210] All five survived for one to two years afterward. The prolonged survival of such patients is in itself suggestive of an unusual level of physiologic function and reserve.

CAUSES OF POSTOPERATIVE MORTALITY

Conditions and events directly related to the primary surgical illness, such as carcinomatosis, bowel infarction, and ruptured abdominal aortic aneurysm, account for one third to two thirds of postoperative deaths in elderly patients.[12,195,196,203,211] It is not clear how many such deaths are potentially preventable. One study identified specific complications attributed to failure of technical aspects of the surgical procedure (e.g., anastomotic leak, intra-abdominal abscess, bleeding, and wound dehiscence), which led to 40 of 193 deaths after 4,050 operations on surgical patients 70 years of age or older.[12] Of the 4,050 operations, 78 percent were for indications related to a diagnosis of cancer, and malignant disease was considered the immediate cause of 48 of the 193 deaths. That elderly patients tolerate complications poorly is well recognized: a mortality of 69 percent has been reported in patients older than 65 years who required a second laparotomy for bleeding, infection, or suture line fault, and outcome after abdominal wound dehiscence may be worse in elderly patients.[184]

In one study, deaths were classified as those that occurred in nonviable patients (i.e., those in whom death could not have been prevented by surgical intervention, alterations in surgical intervention, or alterations in perioperative care) and those that occurred in potentially viable patients.[13] Of 505 patients 65 years of age or older admitted to a general surgical unit, 73 died: 55 in the nonviable group and 18 in the potentially viable group. The 15 deaths that occurred after operation in the potentially viable group were further classified as related to medical complications or surgical complications. Medical complications comprised pneumonia (four patients), pulmonary edema (three patients), myocardial infarction (two patients), and other causes (three patients), and surgical complications comprised anastomotic leak (one patient) and postoperative sepsis (two patients). Three potentially preventable deaths (attributable to ruptured aneurysm, peritonitis, and renal failure) occurred in patients who did not undergo operations. Patients with advanced malignancy, including those in whom no operation was performed, accounted for 38 of the 73 total deaths. The relatively large proportion of surgical deaths related to malignancy in the elderly has been noted in several series.

In several large unselected groups of elderly patients who underwent elective and emergency procedures, cardiovascular complications (myocardial infarction and congestive heart failure) were the major cause of postoperative death that was not directly related to the primary condition.[12,196,197] Other important potentially preventable causes of postoperative death in elderly patients include pulmonary embolus, pneumonia, and respiratory failure.[3,12,194-196,203,211,212] The increased mortality associated with the presence of coexisting diseases, such as diabetes mellitus and renal failure, is well recognized; it is apparent that such diseases have a greater impact on outcome than age per se does.[40,194,212-214] In a study of 7,292 surgical patients 70 years of age or older, age had little effect on outcome in patients who had no concomitant diseases or only one, and the observed relation between operative mortality and age in those who had more than one concomitant disease could be accounted for by the number of concomitant diseases.[214]

References

1. Smith OC: Advanced age as a contraindication to operation. Med Rec (New York) 72:642, 1907
2. Rowe JW, Minaker KL: Geriatric medicine. Handbook of the Biology of Aging, 2nd ed. Finch CE, Schneider EL, Eds. Van Nostrand Reinhold, New York, 1985, p 932
3. Puxty JA, Horan MA, Fox RA: Necropsies in the elderly. Lancet 1:1262, 1983
4. Tinetti ME, Speechley M: Prevention of falls among the elderly. N Engl J Med 320:1055, 1989
5. Edwards RT, Bransom CJ, Crosby DL, et al: Colorectal carcinoma in the elderly: a geriatric and surgical practice compared. Age Ageing 12:256, 1983
6. Brewer RJ, Golden GT, Hitch DC, et al: Abdominal pain: an analysis of 1,000 consecutive cases in a university hospital emergency room. Am J Surg 131:219, 1976

7. Albano WA, Zielinski CM, Organ CH: Is appendicitis in the aged really different? Geriatrics 30:81, 1975
8. Fenyö G: Acute abdominal disease in the elderly: experience from two series in Stockholm. Am J Surg 143:751, 1982
9. Goldman A, Exton-Smith AN, Francis G, et al: A pilot study of low body temperatures in old people admitted to hospital. J R Coll Physicians Lond 11:291, 1977
10. Irvin TT, Arnstein PM: Management of symptomatic gallstones in the elderly. Br J Surg 75:1163, 1988
11. Feldman AR, Kessler L, Myers MH, et al: The prevalence of cancer: estimates based on the Connecticut Tumor Registry. N Engl J Med 315:1394, 1986
12. Turnbull AD, Gundy E, Howland WS, et al: Surgical mortality among the elderly: an analysis of 4,050 operations (1970–1974). Clin Bull 8:139, 1978
13. Seymour DG, Pringle R: A new method of auditing surgical mortality rates: application to a group of elderly general surgical patients. Br Med J 284:1539, 1982
14. Watters JM: Special considerations in the elderly. Management of Trauma. Bessey PQ, Hoyt DB, Eds. WB Saunders (in press)
15. Sacco WJ, Copes WS, Bain LWJ, et al: Effect of preinjury illness on trauma patient survival outcome. J Trauma 35:538, 1993
16. Morris JA Jr, MacKenzie EJ, Edelstein SL: The effect of preexisting conditions on mortality in trauma patients. JAMA 263:1942, 1990
17. Finelli FC, Jonsson J, Champion HR, et al: A case control study for major trauma in geriatric patients. J Trauma 29:541, 1989
18. Baker SP, Spitz WU: Age effects and autopsy evidence of disease in fatally injured drivers. JAMA 214:1079, 1970
19. Rackoff NJ, Mourant RR: Driving performance of the elderly. Accid Anal & Prev 11:247, 1979
20. Planek TW, Fowler RC: Traffic accident problems and exposure characteristics of the aging driver. J Gerontology 26:224, 1971
21. Viano DC, Culver CC, Evans L, et al: Involvement of older drivers in multivehicle side-impact crashes. Accid Anal & Prev 22:177, 1990
22. Cushman LA, Good RG, Annechiarico RP, et al: Effect of safety belt usage on injury patterns of hospitalized and fatally injured drivers 55+. 34th Annual Proceedings. Scottsdale, Arizona: Association for the Advancement of Automotive Medicine, 1990, p 127
23. Dischinger PC, Cushing BM, Kerns TJ: Injury patterns associated with direction of impact: drivers admitted to trauma centers. J Trauma 35:454, 1993
24. McCoy GF, Johnstone RA, Duthie RB: Injury to the elderly in road traffic accidents. J Trauma 29:494, 1989
25. Allen JE, Schwab CW: Blunt chest trauma in the elderly. Am Surgeon 51:697, 1985
26. Richardson JD, Adams L, Flint LM: Selective management of flail chest and pulmonary contusion. Ann Surg 196:481, 1982
27. Riggs BL, Melton LJ: Involutional osteoporosis. N Engl J Med 314:1676, 1986
28. Linn BS: Age differences in the severity and outcome of burns. J Am Geriatr Soc 28:118, 1980
29. Osler T, Hales K, Baack B, et al: Trauma in the elderly. Am J Surg 156:537, 1988
30. Pellicane JV, Byrne K, DeMaria EJ: Preventable complications and death from multiple organ failure among geriatric trauma victims. J Trauma 33:440, 1992
31. Knudson MM, Lieberman J, Morris JA, et al: Mortality factors in geriatric blunt trauma patients. Arch Surg 129:448, 1994
32. Champion HR, Copes WS, Buyer D, et al: Major trauma in geriatric patients. Am J Public Health 79:1278, 1989
33. DeMaria EJ, Kenney PR, Merriam MA, et al: Aggressive trauma care benefits the elderly. J Trauma 27:1200, 1987
34. Carrillo EH, Richardson JD, Malias MA, et al: Long term outcome of blunt trauma care in the elderly. Surg Gynecol Obstet 176:559, 1993
35. Day RJ, Vinen J, Hewitt-Falls E: Major trauma outcomes in the elderly. Med J Australia 160:675, 1994
36. van Aalst JA, Morris JA Jr, Yates HK, et al: Severely injured geriatric patients return to independent living: a study of factors influencing function and independence. J Trauma 31:1096, 1991
37. Oreskovich MR, Howard JD, Copass MK, et al: Geriatric trauma: injury patterns and outcome. J Trauma 24:565, 1984
38. Koval KJ, Zuckerman JD: Functional recovery after fracture of the hip. J Bone Joint Surg 76A:751, 1994
39. Oreskovich M: Discussion of DeMaria EJ et al. J Trauma 27:1205, 1987
40. Goldman L, Caldera DL, Nussbaum SR, et al: Multifactorial index of cardiac risk in noncardiac surgical procedures. N Engl J Med 297:845, 1977
41. MacDonald JB: Presentation of acute myocardial infarction in the elderly: a review. Age Ageing 13:196, 1984
42. Von Knorring J: Postoperative myocardial infarction: a prospective study in a risk group of surgical patients. Surgery 90:55, 1981
43. Steen PA, Tinker JH, Tarhan S: Myocardial reinfarction after anesthesia and surgery. JAMA 239:2566, 1978
44. Rao TL, Jacobs KH, El-Etr AA: Reinfarction following anesthesia in patients with myocardial infarction. Anesthesiology 59:499, 1983
45. Mangano DT: Perioperative cardiac morbidity. Anesthesiology 72:153, 1990
46. Goldman L, Caldera DL: Risks of general anaesthesia and elective operation in the hypertensive patient. Anesthesiology 50:285, 1979
47. Goldman L, Caldera DL, Southwick FS, et al: Cardiac risk factors and complications in non-cardiac surgery. Medicine (Baltimore) 57:357, 1978
48. Törnebrandt K, Fletcher R: Pre-operative chest x-rays in elderly patients. Anaesthesia 37:901, 1982
49. Tisi GM: Preoperative evaluation of pulmonary function: validity, indications, and benefits. Am Rev Respir Dis 119:293, 1979
50. Gass GD, Olsen GN: Preoperative pulmonary function testing to predict postoperative morbidity and mortality. Chest 89:127, 1986
51. Milledge JS, Nunn JF: Criteria of fitness for anaesthesia in patients with chronic obstructive lung disease. Br Med J 3:670, 1975
52. Stein M, Koota JM, Simon M, et al: Pulmonary evaluation of surgical patients. JAMA 181:765, 1962
53. Nunn JF, Milledge JS, Chen D, et al: Respiratory criteria of fitness for surgery and anaesthesia. Anaesthesia 43:543, 1988
54. Rowe JW, Andres R, Tobin JD, et al: The effect of age on creatinine clearance in men: a cross-sectional and longitudinal study. J Gerontol 31:155, 1976
55. Garella S, Matarese RA: Renal effects of prostaglandins and clinical adverse effects of non-steroidal anti-inflammatory agents. Medicine (Baltimore) 63:165, 1984
56. Cruse PJE, Foord R: The epidemiology of wound infection: a 10-year prospective study of 62,939 wounds. Surg Clin North Am 60:27, 1980
57. Gilliss CL, Gortner SR, Hauck WW, et al: A randomized clinical trial of nursing care for recovery from cardiac surgery. Heart & Lung 22:125, 1993
58. Rozanski A, Bairey CN, Krantz DS, et al: Mental stress and the induction of silent myocardial ischemia in patients with coronary artery disease. N Engl J Med 318:1005, 1988
59. Roberts CS, Cox CE, Reintgen DS, et al: Influence of physician communication on newly diagnosed breast patients' psychological adjustment and decision-making. Cancer 74(1 Suppl):336, 1994
60. McClaran J, Tover-Berglas R, Franco ED: Long hospital stay & alternate level of care in elderly patients: does family make a difference? Can Fam Physician, in press
61. Mazur DJ, Merz JF: How age, outcome severity, and scale influence general medicine clinic patients' interpretations of verbal probability terms. J Gen Intern Med 9:295, 1994
62. Farnill D, Inglis S: Patients' desire for information about anaesthesia: Australian attitudes. Anaesthesia 49:162, 1994
63. Lonsdale M, Hutchison GL: Patients' desire for information about anaesthesia: Scottish and Canadian attitudes. Anaesthesia 46:410, 1991
64. Inglis S, Farnill D: The effect of providing preoperative statistical anaesthetic-risk information. Anaesth Intens Care 21:799, 1993
65. Lella J, Kaye M: Ethics and surgical practice with the elderly. Surgical Care of the Elderly. Meakins JL, McClaran JC, Eds. Year Book Medical Publishers, Chicago, 1988, p 50
66. Langslow A: Nursing and the law: who has the capacity to consent to surgery? Austr Nurs J 2:31, 1995
67. Markson LJ, Kern DC, Annas GJ, et al: Physician assessment of patient competence. J Am Geriatr Soc 42:1074, 1994
68. Roy RC: Anesthetic techniques for the elderly. American Society of Anesthesiologists 1988 Annual Refresher Course Lectures. 276:1, 1988
69. Sullivan DR, Siker ES: The pros and cons of regional anesthesia. Geriatric Anesthesia: Principles and Practice. Stephen CR, Assaf RA, Eds. Butterworth Publishers, Stoneham, Massachusetts, 1986, p 277
70. McLeskey CH: Principles of anesthetic management of elderly patients. Review Course Lectures (63rd Congress) 1989, p 144
71. Brandt MR, Korshin J, Hansen AP, et al: Influence of morphine anaesthesia on the endocrine-metabolic response to open-heart surgery. Acta Anaesthesiol Scand 22:400, 1978
72. George JM, Reier CE, Lanese RR, et al: Morphine anesthesia blocks cortisol and growth hormone response to surgical stress in humans. J Clin Endocrinol Metab 38:736, 1974
73. Taylor JW, Hander EW, Skreen R, et al: The effect of central nervous system narcosis on the sympathetic response to stress. J Surg Res 20:313, 1976
74. McKenzie PJ, Wishart HY, Dewar KM, et al: Comparison of the effects of spinal anaesthesia and general anaesthesia on postoperative oxygenation and perioperative mortality. Br J Anaesth 52:49, 1980
75. Hole A, Terjesen T, Breivik H: Epidural versus

general anaesthesia for total hip arthroplasty in elderly patients. Acta Anaesth Scand 24:279, 1980
76. Valentin N, Lomholt B, Jensen JS, et al: Spinal or general anaesthesia for surgery of the fractured hip? A prospective study of mortality in 578 patients. Br J Anaesth 58:284, 1986
77. Karhunen U, Jonn G: A comparison of memory function following local and general anaesthesia for extraction of senile cataract. Acta Anaesthesiol Scand 26:291, 1982
78. Riis J, Lomholt B, Haxholdt O, et al: Immediate and long-term mental recovery from general versus epidural anaesthesia in elderly patients. Acta Anaesthesiol Scand 27:44, 1983
79. Craig DB: Postoperative recovery of pulmonary function. Anesth Analg 60:46, 1981
80. Catley DM, Thornton C, Jordan C, et al: Pronounced, episodic oxygen desaturation in the postoperative period: its association with ventilatory pattern and analgesic regimen. Anesthesiology 63:20, 1985
81. Kehlet H, Brandt MR, Rem J: Role of neurogenic stimuli in mediating the endocrine-metabolic response to surgery. J Parenter Enteral Nutr 4:152, 1980
82. Wells PH, Kaplan JA: Optimal management of patients with ischemic heart disease for noncardiac surgery by complementary anesthesiologist and cardiologist interaction. Am Heart J 102:1029, 1981
83. Del Guercio LR, Cohn JD: Monitoring operative risk in the elderly. JAMA 243:1350, 1980
84. Schultz RJ, Whitfield GF, LaMura JJ, et al: The role of physiologic monitoring in patients with fractures of the hip. J Trauma 25:309, 1985
85. McDaniel DD, Stone JG, Faltas AN, et al: Catheter-induced pulmonary artery hemorrhage. J Thorac Cardiovasc Surg 82:1, 1981
86. Goldberg MJ, Roe CF: Temperature changes during anesthesia and operations. Arch Surg 93:365, 1966
87. Vaughan MS, Vaughan RW, Cork RC: Postoperative hypothermia in adults: relationship of age, anesthesia, and shivering to rewarming. Anesth Analg 60:746, 1981
88. Bay J, Nunn JF, Prys-Roberts C: Factors influencing arterial P_{O_2} during recovery from anaesthesia. Br J Anaesth 40:398, 1968
89. Roe CF, Goldberg MJ, Blair CS, et al: The influence of body temperature on early postoperative oxygen consumption. Surgery 60:85, 1966
90. Horvath SM, Spurr GB, Hutt BK, et al: Metabolic cost of shivering. J Appl Physiol 8:595, 1956
91. Latimer G, Dickman M, Day WC, et al: Ventilatory patterns and pulmonary complications after upper abdominal surgery determined by preoperative and postoperative computerized spirometry and blood gas analysis. Am J Surg 122:622, 1971
92. Ford G, Whitelaw W, Rosenal TW, et al: Diaphragm function after upper abdominal surgery in humans. Am Rev Respir Dis 127:431, 1983
93. Simonneau G, Vivien A, Sartene R, et al: Diaphragm dysfunction induced by upper abdominal surgery: role of postoperative pain. Am Rev Respir Dis 128:899, 1983
94. Chuter TA, Weissman C, Starker PM, et al: Effect of incentive spirometry on diaphragmatic function after surgery. Surgery 105:488, 1989
95. Rizzato G, Marrazzini L: Thoracoabdominal mechanics in elderly men. J Appl Physiol 28:457, 1970
96. Vaughan RW, Wise L: Postoperative arterial blood gas measurement in obese patients: effect of position on gas exchange. Ann Surg 182:705, 1975
97. Celli BR, Rodriguez KS, Snider GL: A controlled trial of intermittent positive pressure breathing, incentive spirometry, and deep breathing exercises in preventing pulmonary complications after abdominal surgery. Am Rev Respir Dis 130:12, 1984
98. Ford GT, Guenter CA: Toward prevention of postoperative pulmonary complications. Am Rev Respir Dis 130:4, 1984
99. Ball M, McQuay HJ, Moore RA, et al: Renal failure and the use of morphine in intensive care. Lancet 1:784, 1985
100. Bellville JW, Forrest WH Jr, Miller E, et al: Influence of age on pain relief from analgesics: a study of postoperative patients. JAMA 217:1835, 1971
101. Reidenberg MM, Levy M, Warner H, et al: Relationship between diazepam dose, plasma level, age, and central nervous system depression. Clin Pharmacol Ther 23:371, 1978
102. Wheatley RG, Somerville ID, Sapsford DJ, et al: Postoperative hypoxaemia: comparison of extradural, I.M., and patient-controlled opioid analgesia. Br J Anaesth 64:267, 1990
103. Dahl JB, Kehlet H: Non-steroidal anti-inflammatory drugs: rationale for use in severe postoperative pain. Br J Anaesth 66:703, 1991
104. Egbert AM, Parks LH, Short LM, et al: Randomized trial of postoperative patient-controlled analgesia vs intramuscular narcotics in frail elderly men. Arch Intern Med 150:1897, 1990
105. Smith AW, Berg K: The surgical ward. Surgical Care of the Elderly. Meakins JL, McClaran JC, Eds. Year Book Medical Publishers, Chicago, 1988, p 203
106. Young A: Exercise physiology in geriatric practice. Acta Med Scand 711(suppl):227, 1986
107. Chobanian AV, Lille RD, Tercyak A, et al: The metabolic and hemodynamic effects of prolonged bed rest in normal subjects. Circulation 49:551, 1974
108. Convertino V, Hung J, Goldwater D, et al: Cardiovascular responses to exercise in middle-aged men after 10 days of bed rest. Circulation 65:134, 1982
109. Sullivan MJ, Binkley PF, Unverferth DV, et al: Prevention of bedrest-induced physical deconditioning by daily dobutamine infusions. J Clin Invest 76:1632, 1985
110. King DS, Dalsky GP, Clutter WE, et al: Effects of lack of exercise on insulin secretion and action in trained subjects. Am J Physiol 254:E537, 1988
111. Allman RM: Pressure ulcers among the elderly. N Engl J Med 320:850, 1989
112. Vestal RE, Dawson GW: Pharmacology and aging. Handbook of the Biology of Aging, 2nd Ed. Finch CE, Schneider EL, Eds. Van Nostrand Reinhold, New York, 1985, p 744
113. Skoll SL, August RJ, Johnson GE: Drug prescribing for the elderly in Saskatchewan during 1976. Can Med Assoc J 121:1074, 1979
114. Aoki FY, Hildahl VK, Large GW, et al: Aging and heavy drug use: a prescription survey in Manitoba. Journal of Chronic Diseases 36:75, 1983
115. Brennan M, Gowdey CW: Adverse drug reactions: a review of fatalities reported in Ontario. Ontario Medical Review, August 23, 1989
116. Montamat SC, Cusack BJ, Vestal RE: Management of drug therapy in the elderly. N Engl J Med 321:303, 1989
117. Wynne HA, Cope LH, Mutch E, et al: The effect of age upon liver volume and apparent liver blood flow in healthy men. Hepatology 9:297, 1989
118. Vestal RE, Wood AJ, Shand DG: Reduced beta-adrenoceptor activity in the elderly. Clin Pharmacol Ther 26:181, 1979
119. Shepherd AM, Hewick DS, Moreland TA, et al: Age as a determinant of sensitivity to warfarin. Br J Clin Pharmacol 4:315, 1977
120. Miller PD, Krebs RA, Neal BJ, et al: Hypodipsia in geriatric patients. Am J Med 73:354, 1982
121. Phillips PA, Rolls BJ, Ledingham JG, et al: Reduced thirst after water deprivation in healthy elderly men. N Engl J Med 311:753, 1984
122. Helderman JH, Vestal RE, Rowe JW, et al: The response of arginine vasopressin to intravenous ethanol and hypertonic saline in man: the impact of aging. J Gerontol 33:39, 1978
123. Rowe JW, Robertson GL: Age-related failure of volume-pressure mediated vasopressin (AVP) release in man (abstr). Kidney Int 14:660, 1978
124. Crane MG, Harris JJ: Effect of aging on renin activity and aldosterone excretion. J Lab Clin Med 87:947, 1976
125. Saruta T, Suzuki A, Hayashi M, et al: Mechanism of age-related changes in renin and adrenocortical steroids. J Am Geriatr Soc 28:210, 1980
126. Kenney RA: Physiology of aging. Clin Geriatr Med 1:37, 1985
127. Rowe JW, Shock NW, DeFronzo RA: The influence of age on the renal response to water deprivation in man. Nephron 17:270, 1976
128. Epstein M, Hollenberg NK: Age as a determinant of renal sodium conservation in normal man. J Lab Clin Med 87:411, 1976
129. Rowe JW: Aging and renal function. Ann Rev Gerontol Geriatr 1:161, 1980
130. Adler S, Lindeman RD, Yiengst MJ, et al: Effect of acute acid loading on urinary acid excretion by the aging human kidney. J Lab Clin Med 72:278, 1968
131. Guyton AC: Textbook of Medical Physiology. WB Saunders Co, Philadelphia, 1986
132. Kronenberg RS, Drage CW: Attenuation of the ventilatory and heart rate responses to hypoxia and hypercapnia with aging in normal men. J Clin Invest 52:1812, 1973
133. Brischetto MJ, Millman RP, Peterson DD, et al: Effect of aging on ventilatory response to exercise and CO_2. J Appl Physiol 56:1143, 1984
134. Kenney RA: Physiology of aging. Clin Geriatr Med 1:37, 1985
135. Watters JM, Clancey SM, Moulton SB, et al: Impaired recovery of strength in older patients after major abdominal surgery. Ann Surg 218:380, 1993
136. Exton-Smith AN: Mineral metabolism. Handbook of the Physiology of Aging, 2nd ed. Finch CE, Schneider EL, Eds. Van Nostrand Reinhold, New York, 1985, p 511
137. Chernoff R, Lipschitz DA: Nutrition and aging. Modern Nutrition in Health and Disease, 7th ed. Shils ME, Young VR, Eds. Lea & Febiger, Philadelphia, 1988, p 982
138. DeBiasse MA, Wilmore DW: What is optimal nutritional support? New Horizons 2:122, 1994
139. Chandra RK: Effect of vitamin and trace-element supplementation on immune responses and infection in elderly subjects. Lancet 340:1124, 1992
140. Bastow MD, Rawlings J, Allison SP: Benefits of supplementary tube feeding after fractured neck of femur: a randomised controlled trial. Br Med J 287:1589, 1983
141. Delmi M, Rapin C-H, Bengoa J-M, et al: Dietary supplementation in elderly patients with fractured neck of the femur. Lancet 335:1013, 1990
142. Tkatch L, Rapin CH, Rizzoli R, et al: Benefits of oral protein supplementation in elderly patients with fracture of the proximal femur. J Am Coll

Nutr 11:519, 1992
143. Shock NW: Energy metabolism, caloric intake and physical activity in the aging. Symposium on Nutrition in Old Age. 10th Symposium of the Swedish Nutrition Foundation. Carlson LA, Ed. Almqvist and Wiksell, Uppsala, Sweden, 1972, p 12
144. Kirk SJ, Hurson M, Regan MC, et al: Arginine stimulates wound healing and immune function in elderly human beings. Surgery 114:155, 1993
145. Watters JM, Moulton SB, Clancey SM, et al: Aging exaggerates glucose intolerance following injury. J Trauma 37:786, 1994
146. Black PR, Brooks DC, Bessey PQ, et al: Mechanisms of insulin resistance following injury. Ann Surg 196:420, 1982
147. Buskirk ER: Health maintenance and longevity: exercise. Handbook of the Biology of Aging, 2nd ed. Finch CE, Schneider EL, Eds. Van Nostrand Reinhold, New York, 1985, p 894
148. Jeevanandam M, Holaday NJ, Shamos RF, et al: Acute IGF-1 deficiency in multiple trauma victims. Clin Nutr 11:352, 1992
149. Jeevanandam M, Ramias L, Shamos RF, et al: Decreased growth hormone levels in the catabolic phase of severe injury. Surgery 111:495, 1992
150. Cohn SH, Vartsky D, Yasumura S, et al: Compartmental body composition based on total-body nitrogen, potassium, and calcium. Am J Physiol 239:E524, 1980
151. Moore FD, Olesen KH, McMurrey JD, et al: The Body Cell Mass and Its Supporting Environment: Body Composition in Health and Disease. WB Saunders Co, Philadelphia, 1963
152. Larsson L, Grimby G, Karlsson J: Muscle strength and speed of movement in relation to age and muscle morphology. J Appl Physiol 46:451, 1979
153. Montoye HJ, Lamphear DE: Grip and arm strength in males and females, age 10 to 69. Research Quarterly 48:109, 1977
154. Wahba WM: Influence of aging on lung function: clinical significance of changes from age twenty. Anesth Analg 62:764, 1983
155. Skrobak-Kaczynski J, Andersen KL: The effect of a high level of habitual physical activity in the regulation of fatness during aging. Int Arch Occup Environ Health 36:41, 1975
156. Heath GW, Hagberg JM, Ehsani AA, et al: A physiological comparison of young and older endurance athletes. J Appl Physiol 51:634, 1981
157. DeVries HA: Physiological effects of an exercise training regimen upon men aged 52 to 88. J Gerontol 25:325, 1970
158. Sidney KH, Shephard RJ, Harrison JE: Endurance training and body composition of the elderly. Am J Clin Nutr 30:326, 1977
159. Larsson L: Physical training effects on muscle morphology in sedentary males at different ages. Med Sci Sports Exerc 14:203, 1982
160. Gribbin B, Pickering TG, Sleight P, et al: Effect of age and high blood pressure on baroreflex sensitivity in man. Circ Res 29:424, 1971
161. Collins KJ, Exton-Smith AN, James MH, et al: Functional changes in autonomic nervous responses with ageing. Age Ageing 9:17, 1980
162. Lakatta EG: Cardiovascular regulatory mechanisms in advanced age. Physiol Rev 73:413, 1993
163. Davies CT: The oxygen-transporting system in relation to age. Clin Sci 42:1, 1972
164. Strandell T: Circulatory studies on healthy old men: with special reference to the limitation of the maximal physical working capacity. Acta Med Scand 175:1, 1964
165. Brandfonbrener M, Landowne M, Shock NW: Changes in cardiac output with age. Circulation 12:557, 1955
166. Gerstenblith G, Fleg JL, Becker LC, et al: Maximum left ventricular filling rate in healthy individuals measured by gated blood pool scans. Circulation 68(III):101, 1983
167. Miyatake K, Okamoto M, Kinoshita N, et al: Augmentation of atrial contribution to left ventricular inflow with aging as assessed by intracardiac doppler flowmetry. Am J Cardiol 53:586, 1984
168. Davidson WR Jr, Fee EC: Influence of aging on pulmonary hemodynamics in a population free of coronary artery disease. Am J Cardiol 65:1454, 1990
169. Rodeheffer RJ, Gerstenblith G, Becker LC, et al: Exercise cardiac output is maintained with advancing age in healthy human subjects: cardiac dilatation and increased stroke volume compensate for a diminished heart rate. Circulation 69:203, 1984
170. Port S, Cobb FR, Coleman RE, et al: Effect of age on the response of the left ventricular ejection fraction to exercise. N Engl J Med 303:1133, 1980
171. Yin FCP, Raizes GS, Guarnieri T, et al: Age-associated decrease in ventricular response to haemodynamic stress during beta-adrenergic blockade. Br Heart J 40:1349, 1978
172. Stratton JR, Cerqueira MD, Schwartz RS, et al: Differences in cardiovascular responses to isoproterenol in relation to age and exercise training in healthy men. Circulation 86:504, 1992
173. Rich MW, Imburgia M: Inotropic response to dobutamine in elderly patients with decompensated congestive heart failure. Am J Cardiol 65:519, 1990
174. Dehn MM, Bruce RA: Longitudinal variations in maximal oxygen intake with age and activity. J Appl Physiol 33:805, 1972
175. Leenders KL, Perani D, Lammertsma AA, et al: Cerebral blood flow, blood volume, and oxygen utilization. Brain 113:27, 1990
176. Amery A, Bossaert H, Verstraete M: Muscle blood flow in normal and hypertensive subjects. Influence of age, exercise, and body position. Am Heart J 78:211, 1969
177. Lindbjerg IF: Diagnostic application of the 133xenon method in peripheral arterial disease. Scand J Clin Lab Invest 17:589, 1965
178. Tsuchida Y: Age-related changes in skin blood flow at four anatomic sites of the body in males studied by xenon-133. Plast Reconstr Surg 85:556, 1990
179. Collins KJ, Exton-Smith AN: Thermal homeostasis in old age. 1983 Henderson Award Lecture. J Am Geriatr Soc 31:519, 1983
180. Wagner JA, Robinson S, Marino RP: Age and temperature regulation of humans in neutral and cold environments. J Appl Physiol 37:562, 1974
181. Bastow MD, Rawlings J, Allison SP: Undernutrition, hypothermia, and injury in elderly women with fractured femur: an injury response to altered metabolism? Lancet 1:143, 1983
182. Allison SP: Some metabolic aspects of injury. The Scientific Basis for the Care of the Critically Ill. Little RA, Frayn KN, Eds. Manchester University Press, Manchester, 1986, p 169
183. Holt DR, Kirk SJ, Regan MC, et al: Effect of age on wound healing in healthy human beings. Surgery 112:293, 1992
184. White H, Cook J, Ward M: Abdominal wound dehiscence: a 10-year survey from a district general hospital. Ann R Coll Surg Engl 59:337, 1977
185. Hausman PB, Weksler ME: Changes in the immune response with age. Handbook of the Biology of Aging, 2nd ed. Finch CE, Schneider EL, Eds. Van Nostrand Reinhold, New York, 1985, p 414
186. Christou NV: Immune function and the aged surgical patient. Surgical Care of the Elderly. Meakins JL, McClaran JC, Eds. Year Book Medical Publishers, Chicago, 1988, p 149
187. Waldorf DS, Willkens RF, Decker JL: Impaired delayed hypersensitivity in an aging population. JAMA 203:831, 1968
188. Pietsch JB, Meakins JL, MacLean LD: The delayed hypersensitivity response: application in clinical surgery. Surgery 82:349, 1977
189. Brody JA, Brock DB: Epidemiologic and statistical characteristics of the United States elderly population. Handbook of the Biology of Aging, 2nd ed. Finch CE, Schneider EL, Eds. Van Nostrand Reinhold, New York, 1985, p 3
190. Bleich HL, Boro ES, Rowe JW: Clinical research on aging: strategies and directions. N Engl J Med 297:1332, 1977
191. Rowe JW, Kahn RL: Human aging: usual and successful. Science 237:143, 1987
192. Shock NW, Greulich RC, Andres R, et al: Normal Human Aging: The Baltimore Longitudinal Study of Aging. NIH Publication No. 84-2450. Superintendent of Documents, US Government Printing Office, Washington, DC, 1984
193. Ziffren SE: Comparison of mortality rates for various surgical operations according to age groups, 1951–1977. J Am Geriatr Soc 27:433, 1979
194. Palmberg S, Hirsjarvi E: Mortality in geriatric surgery: with special reference to the type of surgery, anaesthesia, complicating diseases, and prophylaxis of thrombosis. Gerontology 25:103, 1979
195. Warner MA, Hosking MP, Lobdell CM, et al: Surgical procedures among those greater than or equal to 90 years of age: a population-based study in Olmsted County, Minnesota, 1975–1985. Ann Surg 207:380, 1988
196. Djokovic JL, Hedley-Whyte J: Prediction of outcome of surgery and anesthesia in patients over 80. JAMA 242:2301, 1979
197. Nehme AE: Groin hernias in elderly patients: management and prognosis. Am J Surg 146:257, 1983
198. Tingwald GR, Cooperman M: Inguinal and femoral hernia repair in geriatric patients. Surg Gynecol Obstet 154:704, 1982
199. Tiret L, Desmonts JM, Hatton F, et al: Complications associated with anaesthesia: a prospective survey in France. Can Anaesth Soc J 33:336, 1986
200. Marx GF, Mateo CV, Orkin LR: Computer analysis of postanesthetic deaths. Anesthesiology 39:54, 1973
201. Vacanti CJ, Van Houten RJ, Hill RC: A statistical analysis of the relationship of physical status to postoperative mortality in 68,388 cases. Anesth Analg 49:564, 1970
202. Greenburg AG, Saik RP, Coyle JJ, et al: Mortality and gastrointestinal surgery in the aged: elective versus emergency procedures. Arch Surg 116:788, 1981
203. Williams JH, Collin J: Surgical care of patients over eighty: a predictable crisis at hand. Br J Surg 75:371, 1988
204. Boyd JB, Bradford B Jr, Watne AL: Operative risk factors of colon resection in the elderly. Ann Surg 192:743, 1980
205. Baker SP, O'Neill B, Haddon W Jr, et al: The injury severity score: a method for describing patients with multiple injuries and evaluating

emergency care. J Trauma 14:187, 1974
206. McCoy GF, Johnston RA, Duthie RB: Injury to the elderly in road traffic accidents. J Trauma 29:494, 1989
207. Weinstein MP, Murphy JR, Reller LB, et al: The clinical significance of positive blood cultures: a comprehensive analysis of 500 episodes of bacteremia and fungemia in adults: II. Clinical observations, with special reference to factors influencing prognosis. Rev Infect Dis 5:54, 1983
208. Knaus WA, Draper EA, Wagner DP, et al: Prognosis in acute organ-system failure. Ann Surg 202:685, 1985
209. Lewin I, Lerner AG, Green SH, et al: Physical class and physiologic status in the prediction of operative mortality in the aged sick. Ann Surg 174:217, 1971
210. Katlic MR: Surgery in centenarians. JAMA 253:3139, 1985
211. Blake R, Lynn J: Emergency abdominal surgery in the aged. Br J Surg 63:956, 1976
212. Denney JL, Denson JS: Risk of surgery in patients over 90. Geriatrics 27:115, 1972
213. Fowkes FG, Lunn JN, Farrow SC, et al: Epidemiology in anaesthesia: III. Mortality risk in patients with coexisting physical disease. Br J Anaesth 54:819, 1982
214. Andersen B, Genster H, Langberg K: Geriatric surgery in a community: a statistical analysis of 7,292 aged patients admitted to the surgical departments in a Danish County in the 10-year period 1952-1961. Acta Chir Scand 354(suppl):1, 1965
215. McClaran J: Preoperative assessment of the elderly patient. Current Surgical Therapy, Vol III. Cameron JL, Ed. BC Decker, Philadelphia, 1989, p 785
216. Mangione CM, Phillips RS, Lawrence MG, et al: Improved visual function and attenuation of declines in health-related quality of life after cataract extraction. Arch Ophthalmol 112:1419, 1994
217. Duggan MM, Woodson J, Scott TE, et al: Functional outcomes in limb salvage vascular surgery. Am J Surg 168:188, 1994
218. Comprehensive functional assessment for elderly patients. Health and Public Policy Committee, American College of Physicians. Ann Intern Med 109:70, 1988
219. Branch LG, Jette AM: The Framingham Disability Study: I. Social disability among the aging. Am J Public Health 71:1202, 1981
220. Rubenstein LV, Calkins DR, Young RT, et al: Improving patient function: a randomized trial of functional disability screening. Ann Intern Med 111:836, 1989
221. Branch LG, Katz S, Kniepmann K, et al: A prospective study of functional status among community elders. Am J Public Health 74:266, 1984
222. McClaran JC: Preoperative assessment: the geriatrician's viewpoint. Surgical Care of the Elderly. Meakins JL, McClaran JC, Eds. Year Book Medical Publishers, 1988, p 217
223. Goldstein S: The biology of aging. N Engl J Med 285:1120, 1971
224. Katz S: Assessing self-maintenance: activities of daily living, mobility, and instrumental activities of daily living. J Am Geriatr Soc 31:721, 1983
225. Katz S: The science of quality of life (editorial). Journal of Chronic Diseases 40:459, 1987
226. Dales RE, Dionne G, Leech JA, et al: Preoperative prediction of pulmonary complications following thoracic surgery. Chest 104:155, 1993
227. McLauchlan GJ, Anderson ID, Grant IS, et al: Outcome of patients with abdominal sepsis treated in an intensive care unit. Br J Surg 82:524, 1995
228. Haab F, Boccon-Gibod L, Delmas V, et al: Perineal versus retropubic radical prostatectomy for T1, T2 prostate cancer. Br J Urol 74:626, 1994
229. Oxman TE, Freeman DH Jr, Manheimer ED: Lack of social participation or religious strength and comfort as risk factors for death after cardiac surgery in the elderly. Psychosomatic Medicine 57:5, 1995
230. Bombardier C, Melfi CA, Paul J, et al: Comparison of a generic and a disease-specific measure of pain and physical function after knee replacement surgery. Med Care 33(4 Suppl):AS131, 1995
231. Shimamoto M, Yamazaki F, Nakamura T, et al: Aortic valve replacement in patients older than 75 years of age (Japanese). Nippon Kyobu Geka Gekkai Zasshi 42:2207, 1994
232. Jaeger AA, Hlatky MA, Paul SM, et al: Functional capacity after cardiac surgery in elderly patients. J Am Coll Cardiol 24:104, 1994
233. Weller SJ, Rossitch E Jr: Unilateral posterolateral decompression without stabilization for neurological palliation of symptomatic spinal metastasis in debilitated patients. J Neurosurg 82:739, 1995
234. Munin MC, Kwoh CK, Glynn N, et al: Predicting discharge outcome after elective hip and knee arthroplasty. Am J Phys Med Rehabil 74:294, 1995
235. Houry S, Amenabar J, Rezvani A, et al: Should patients over 80 years old be operated on for colorectal or gastric cancer? Hepatogastroenterology 41:521, 1994
236. Linn MW, Linn BS: The rapid disability rating scale: 2. J Am Geriatr Soc 30:378, 1982
237. Tinetti NE: Performance-oriented assessment of mobility problems in elderly patients. J Am Geriatr Soc 34:119, 1986
238. Multidimensional Functional Assessment: The OARS (Older Americans Retirement Survey) Methodology (a Manual), 2nd ed. Duke University Center for the Study of Aging and Human Development, Duke University Medical Center, Durham, North Carolina, 1978
239. Folstein MF, Folstein SE, McHugh PR: "Mini-Mental State": a practical method for grading the cognitive state of patients for the clinician. J Psychiatr Res 12:189, 1975
240. Spector WD, et al: The hierarchical relationship between activities of daily living and instrumental activities of daily living. Journal of Chronic Diseases 40:481, 1987
241. Katz S, Akpom CA: A measure of primary sociobiological functions. Int J Health Serv 6:493, 1976
242. Katz S, Akpom CA: Index of ADL. Med Care 14(suppl):116, 1976
243. Lawton MP, Brody EM: Assessment of older people: self-maintaining and instrumental activities of daily living. Gerontologist 9:179, 1969
244. Jay S, Ruddy J, Cullen RJ: Laryngectomy: the patient's view. J Laryngol Otol 105:934, 1991
245. Katz S, Ford AB, Moskowitz RW, et al: Studies of illness in the aged, the index of ADL: standardized measure of biological and psychosocial function. JAMA 185:914, 1963
246. Healey F: Does flooring type affect risk of injury in older in-patients? Nursing Times 90:40, Jul 1994
247. Landefeld CS, Palmer RM, Kresevic DM, et al: A randomized trial of care in a hospital medical unit especially designed to improve the functional outcomes of acutely ill older patients. N Engl J Med 332:1376, 1995
248. Kovach CR, Stearns SA: DSCUs: a study of behavior before and after residence. J Gerontol Nursing 20:33, Dec 1994
249. Hahn JE, Jones MR, Waszkiewicz M: Renovation of a semiprivate patient room. Bowman Center Geriatric Rehabilitation Unit. Nurs Clin North Am 30:97, 1995
250. Powell C, Mitchell-Pedersen L: Freedom from restraint: consequences of reducing physical restraints in the management of the elderly. Can Med Assoc J 141:561, 1989
251. Inouye SK, Acampora D, Miller RL, et al: The Yale Geriatric Care Program: a model of care to prevent functional decline in hospitalized elderly patients. J Am Geriatr Soc 41:1345, 1993
252. Inouye SK, Wagner DR, Acampora D, et al: A controlled trial of nursing-centered intervention in hospitalized elderly medical patients: the Yale Geriatric Care Program. J Am Geriatr Soc 41:1353, 1993
253. Margitic SE, Inouye SK, Thomas JL, et al: Hospital Outcomes Project for the Elderly (HOPE): rationale and design for a prospective pooled analysis. J Am Geriatr Soc 41:258, 1993
254. Solomon DH, Wagner DR, Marenberg ME, et al: Predictors of formal home health care use in elderly patients after hospitalization. J Am Geriatr Soc 41:961, 1993
255. Seals DR, Hagberg JM, Allen WK, et al: Glucose tolerance in young and older athletes and sedentary men. J Appl Physiol 56:1521, 1984
256. Soman VR, Koivisto VA, Deibert D, et al: Increased insulin sensitivity and insulin binding to monocytes after physical training. N Engl J Med 301:1200, 1979
257. Seals DR, Hagberg JM, Hurley BF, et al: Effects of endurance training on glucose tolerance and plasma lipid levels in older men and women. JAMA 252:645, 1984
258. Hagberg JM, Allen WK, Seals DR, et al: A hemodynamic comparison of young and older endurance athletes during exercise. J Appl Physiol 58:2041, 1985
259. Larson EB, Bruce RA: Health benefits in an aging society. Arch Intern Med 147:353, 1987
260. Morris JN, Everitt MG, Pollard R, et al: Vigorous exercise in leisure time: protection against coronary heart disease. Lancet 2:1207, 1980
261. Paffenbarger RS Jr, Hyde RT, Wing AL, et al: A natural history of athleticism and cardiovascular health. JAMA 252:491, 1984
262. Paffenbarger RS Jr, Hyde RT, Wing AL, et al: Physical activity, all-cause mortality, and longevity of college alumni. N Engl J Med 314:605, 1986
263. Pocock NA, Eisman JA, Yeates MG, et al: Physical fitness is a major determinant of femoral neck and lumbar spine bone mineral density. J Clin Invest 78:618, 1986
264. Chalmers J, Ho KC: Geographical variations in senile osteoporosis: the association with physical activity. J Bone Joint Surg [Br] 52:667, 1970
265. Bortz WM II: Disuse and aging. JAMA 248:1203, 1982
266. Lakatta EG: Heart and circulation. Handbook of the Biology of Aging, 2nd ed. Finch CE, Schneider EL, Adelman RC, et al, Eds. Van Nostrand Reinhold Co, New York, 1985, p 413
267. Seely JF: Renal function in the elderly. Surgical Care of the Elderly. Meakins JL, McClaran JC, Eds. Year Book Medical Publishers, Chicago, 1988

268. Shock NW: Energy metabolism, caloric intake and physical activity in the aging. 10th Symposium of the Swedish Nutrition Foundation. Carlson LA, Ed. Almqvist and Wiksell, Uppsala, Sweden, 1972

269. McGrandy RB, Barrows CH Jr, Spanias A, et al: Nutrient intakes and energy expenditure in men of different ages. J Gerontol 21:581, 1966

270. Lakatta EG: Cardiovascular reserve capacity in healthy older humans. Aging (Milano) 6:213, 1994

271. Lakatta EG: Heart and circulation. Handbook of the Biology of Aging, 3rd ed. Schneider EL, Rowe SW, Eds. Academic Press, San Diego, 1990, p 181

272. Kane RL, Ouslander JG, Abrass IB: Immobility. Essentials of Clinical Geriatrics, 2nd ed. McGraw-Hill Information Services Co, New York, 1989, p 213

273. Kane RL, Ouslander JG, Abrass IB: Drug therapy. Essentials of Clinical Geriatrics, 2nd ed. McGraw-Hill Information Services Co, New York, 1989, p 341

76 THE PEDIATRIC SURGICAL PATIENT

Arnold G. Coran, M.D.

Perioperative care of infants and children presents many management problems that differ significantly from those seen in adults.[1] This chapter is concerned with recognition and management of certain clinical problems that occur frequently in neonates, infants, and children, with special attention paid to seven areas: (1) monitoring, (2) shock, (3) fluid and electrolyte management, (4) infection and antibiotics, (5) ventilatory support, (6) nutritional support, and (7) trauma. More emphasis is placed on the special needs of neonates (i.e., babies younger than 28 days) and infants (i.e., babies 28 days to 1 year of age) because management of these patients diverges more from management of adults than does management of older children. Several special conditions for which pediatric management differs significantly from adult management (e.g., intestinal obstruction, respiratory distress, and abdominal pain) are discussed in more detail [see Sidebars Intestinal Obstruction in the Newborn, Respiratory Distress in the Newborn, Abdominal Pain, Analgesic Dosage Guidelines in Children, and Preparation of the Neonate with Emergency Surgical Problems].

Parameters to Monitor

It is only since the middle to late 1980s that the most advanced techniques for monitoring critically ill patients have been used in neonates, especially in premature and young infants, because of the technical difficulties involved.

TEMPERATURE

Temperature regulation is critical in neonates because in comparison with older children and adults, they have a large body surface area, little subcutaneous fat (and therefore poor thermal insulation), and reduced lean body mass (required for generating and retaining heat). Most of the heat loss from newborns occurs through radiation, convection, and evaporation; very little heat is lost through conduction. Although the role of evaporation in heat loss increases with increasing prematurity, radiation and convection account for the greater part of the heat lost. Incubators are manufactured so as to minimize radiation and convection by decreasing airflow across the skin and by providing a tightly regulated, thermally neutral environment.

Temperature is monitored by measuring both skin temperature and rectal temperature (core temperature); there is normally a 1.5° C difference between the two. Maintaining body temperature in neonates and young infants is critical both in the neonatal intensive care unit and in the operating room. In the neonatal ICU, temperature is regulated by placing the infant in an incubator or on a bed with an overhead radiant heater. In the OR, an overhead radiant heater is also used; however, the most effective way of maintaining body temperature is to keep the extremities of the infant wrapped or covered.

BODY WEIGHT

Measurement of body weight is especially helpful in evaluating neonates and young infants. Most acute changes in body weight result from changes in total body water; serial measurements of body weight are therefore useful guides to fluid replacement [see Fluid and Electrolyte Management, below]. In general, a 1 g loss of body weight is equivalent to a 1 ml loss of total body water. Serial measurements should be made every 8 to 12 hours and possibly more frequently in neonates. It is important to keep in mind that in their first day of life newborns undergo significant diuresis that reduces extracellular fluid (ECF) volume and total body water.

URINE OUTPUT

Urine flow is a very useful guide to fluid management in all age groups [see Fluid and Electrolyte Management, below]. Measurement of urine output requires accurate collections. In critically ill female infants and in all children, a urinary catheter should be inserted for accurate urine collections. I prefer not to catheterize male neonates and infants because of the risk of trauma to the small urethra; in these patients, properly secured collection bags will allow accurate measurement of urine output. An appropriate urine output is 1 to 2 ml/kg/hr with an osmolality of 250 to 300 mOsm/kg. In premature infants, the flow may have to be somewhat higher, and the osmolality may tend to be slightly lower.

CARDIAC FUNCTION

In critically ill patients, even in premature infants, heart rate and rhythm must be monitored by continuous electrocardiography. In addition, continuous measurements of arterial blood pressure are very helpful [see Table 1]. The standard technique of blood pressure measurement with a sphygmomanometer and a stethoscope has significant disadvantages in the pediatric age group, especially in neonates and infants, because it is so dependent on cuff size, which is highly variable among children. Palpation methods are even less reliable. Of all the noninvasive systems, the Doppler ultrasound technique is by far the most accurate. None of the noninvasive techniques can be used for continuous monitoring, however, nor are they as accurate as intra-arterial measurements. In very sick infants and

Table 1 Normal Values for Vital Signs in Children up to 10 Years of Age

Age (yr)	Pulse Rate (beats/min)	Blood Pressure (mm Hg)	Respirations (breaths/min)
0–1	120	80/40	40
1–5	100	100/60	30
5–10	80	120/80	20

children, direct intra-arterial pressure monitoring should be done via a percutaneous or direct cutdown approach to a peripheral artery. The radial artery is most commonly used,[2,3] but the posterior tibial artery and the dorsalis pedis artery can also be utilized if necessary. In neonates, the umbilical artery is easily accessible and can be used for arterial monitoring.

When there are no cardiac abnormalities, central venous pressure correlates roughly with blood volume. The central venous catheter can be inserted percutaneously into the subclavian or internal jugular vein in older children[4,5]; however, cutdown via the external jugular vein is preferred in neonates and infants.[6] If the external jugular vein cannot be used, the internal jugular vein, the facial vein, the basilic vein, and the proximal saphenous vein are acceptable substitutes. Because of the contamination associated with procedures in the groin, the saphenous vein is the least desirable route.

Swan-Ganz catheters are occasionally used in infants and children, even in newborns and premature neonates.[7-9] No. 5 catheters with triple lumens are available, as are No. 4 catheters with double lumens. The No. 4 catheter can be inserted into premature neonates weighing as little as 1,500 g. These catheters allow simultaneous measurement of right atrial pressure, pulmonary arterial pressure, and pulmonary arterial wedge pressure (PAWP). In addition, the No. 5 catheter can be obtained with a thermistor tip for continuous measurement of cardiac output with thermodilution techniques using small volumes of room-temperature standard infusates [see 89 Cardiopulmonary Monitoring].

PAWP is a good index of left atrial pressure. If there is no obstruction between the left atrium and the left ventricle, PAWP will reflect left ventricular end-diastolic pressure, which in turn is a measure of left ventricular volume. A low PAWP suggests that blood volume must be expanded for cardiac output to be adequate and for blood flow to improve [see Fluid and Electrolyte Management, below]. A high or normal PAWP in the face of hypotension suggests inadequate myocardial function.

OXYGENATION

Arterial Blood Gases

The umbilical artery can also be used for the collection of specimens for arterial blood gas monitoring. Serial measurement of arterial pH is extremely important in monitoring acid-base status. Metabolic alkalosis is related to electrolyte loss [see Fluid and Electrolyte Management, below], whereas metabolic acidosis is usually the result of poor tissue perfusion. Arterial oxygen tension (P_aO_2) and arterial carbon dioxide tension (P_aCO_2) are excellent measures of the adequacy of oxygenation and ventilation [see Ventilatory Support, below].

Pulse Oximetry

Although the standard and most effective way of monitoring oxygenation in any age group is to measure arterial blood gases, the introduction of pulse oximetry has revolutionized this type of monitoring. Pulse oximetry is based on the comparison of the light absorption properties of oxyhemoglobin with those of reduced hemoglobin. Its advantages are immediate availability of oxygen saturation data, minimal cost, the absence of any need for calibration, and the possibility of leaving the probe in place for several hours.

Shock

The two most common types of shock seen in infants, children, and adults are hypovolemic shock and septic shock; in infants and children, septic shock is the most common.[10] How newborns and infants respond to either type of shock is significantly different from how older children and adults respond. For example, in a neonate affected by profound shock, bradycardia is a common response, rather than tachycardia, which is more common in adults. Moreover, neonates, especially premature neonates, normally have a low blood pressure; consequently, the shock insult often does not evoke a further significant reduction of blood pressure. The hypovolemia caused by the shock results in decreased venous return, which lowers cardiac output; the low cardiac output leads to poor tissue perfusion and the development of lactic acidosis.

Septic shock is usually caused by gram-negative bacteria. Peritonitis resulting from intestinal perforation is a common cause of septic shock in neonates and infants; other causes are urinary tract infections, respiratory tract infections, and contaminated intravascular catheters. Although the pathophysiology of septic shock differs substantially from that of hypovolemic shock, in both states the stasis and pooling of blood in the capillary bed lead to reduction of the circulating blood volume.[11]

TREATMENT

The mainstay of treatment of hypovolemic shock is fluid and blood replacement [see Fluid and Electrolyte Management and Trauma, below]. In neonates, the hematocrit should be maintained at 45% to ensure adequate oxygen delivery. In many infants, hypovolemic shock is caused not by hemorrhage but by dehydration (e.g., from severe gastroenteritis). The subsequent dehydration is usually hypertonic because of the significant loss of hypotonic fluid. As a rule, much more water is lost than electrolytes, which results in serum sodium levels as high as 150 mEq/L. Emergency treatment involves infusion of hypotonic solutions of sodium chloride.

Because septic shock, like hypovolemic shock, is characterized by reduced circulating blood volume, initial therapy involves infusion of large volumes of colloid solutions. Most of the experimental and clinical data suggest that colloid solutions are preferable to crystalloid for treating septic shock, both in children and in adults. In addition, broad-spectrum antibiotics should always be administered. Agents that are effective against anaerobic bacteria, such as clindamycin, metronidazole, and chloramphenicol, must be included as well [see Table 2]. The use of corticosteroids to treat septic shock has been controversial since its introduction in 1964.[12-20] In experimental settings, pharmacologic doses of corticosteroids appear to increase cardiac output and decrease peripheral resistance.[21] Methylprednisolone, administered intravenously in a dosage of about 30 mg/kg every 6 hours, is used in critically ill infants or children in whom other methods of resuscitation have been unsuccessful.

If fluid infusion has achieved its maximal effects, as evidenced by a normal to elevated central venous pressure or PAWP, but hypotension persists, pharmacologic agents must be used to improve myocardial contractility. The agent of choice is dopamine, which is an alpha and beta agonist.[22-28] In low dosages (0.5 to 5.0 μg/kg/min), this agent activates specific dopamine receptors, causing vasodilatation of the renal and mesenteric arteries and, to a lesser extent, of the coronary and cerebral arteries. In higher dosages (5 to 10 μg/kg/ min), it increases myocardial contractility and thus cardiac output. Up to dosages of approximately 10 μg/kg/min, dopamine primarily exerts a beta-adrenergic effect. Above this point, it begins to exert alpha-adrenergic effects—namely, increases in peripheral resistance, which can have a detrimental effect on the course of septic shock. Dobutamine, which has primarily inotropic and vasodilatory effects, can be used instead of dopamine.

Fluid and Electrolyte Management

Fluid and electrolyte management of neonates and infants requires a thorough understanding of the body fluid compartment

```
┌─────────────────────────────────────────┐
│ Newborn presents with abdominal distention, │
│ failure to pass meconium, or bilious vomiting │
├─────────────────────────────────────────┤
│ Perform abdominal and rectal examination. │
│ Obtain x-ray of abdomen.                │
└─────────────────────────────────────────┘
```

Flowchart:

- **Double bubble is evident** → Diagnose duodenal atresia. → Transport baby to tertiary care facility with NG or orogastric tube in place and I.V. fluids running.

- **Several loops of distended bowel with air-fluid levels are evident** → Transport baby to tertiary care facility with NG or orogastric tube in place and I.V. fluids running. → Perform barium enema.
  - **Finding: microcolon** → Diagnose intestinal atresia.
  - **Finding: normal or slightly small colon** → Diagnose Hirschsprung disease.
  - **Other findings** → Diagnose malrotation, meconium ileus, necrotizing enterocolitis, imperforate anus.

Prepare for operation

Provide
- Fluids
- NG decompression
- Temperature control
- Antibiotics
- Vitamin K

Provide postoperative care:
- Postoperative fluids
- NG decompression and feeding
- Ambient temperature control

Treat postoperative complications

Shock: Administer fluids, pharmacologic agents, and ?corticosteroids.
Peritonitis: Operate; administer antibiotics and fluids.
Ileus/bowel dysfunction: Provide nutritional support.

Intestinal Obstruction in the Newborn

Abdominal distention, bilious vomiting, and failure to pass meconium are the cardinal symptoms and signs of mechanical intestinal obstruction in the newborn. Occasionally, nonsurgical problems such as congestive heart failure, sepsis, and respiratory distress can present a similar clinical picture; however, mechanical causes of intestinal obstruction should always be ruled out before a nonsurgical diagnosis is accepted.

Diagnosis

Congenital duodenal obstruction is usually manifested by bilious vomiting of early onset and only mild upper abdominal distention. With duodenal atresia, the classic x-ray finding is a double bubble, which represents air-fluid levels in the stomach and the duodenum. When this finding is absent, a barium enema should be performed. If the barium enema demonstrates a microcolon, intestinal atresia or stenosis is likely. If the enema yields normal results or reveals a slightly decreased caliber of the colon, total colonic aganglionosis (Hirschsprung disease) must be suspected; the diagnosis can be confirmed by demonstration of the absence of ganglion cells and the presence of hypertrophic nerves on rectal biopsy.

The differential diagnosis of intestinal obstruction in the newborn should also include meconium ileus, meconium plug syndrome, necrotizing enterocolitis, imperforate anus, malrotation and volvulus, and annular pancreas. Of all these conditions, malrotation with midgut volvulus is the one for which prompt diagnosis and treatment are most critical (because of the risk of necrosis of the entire small intestine). The diagnosis of malrotation is best made by means of an upper GI series.

Preoperative Care

All newborns should be given vitamin K I.V. or I.M. before operation because of the normally low levels of prothrombin present in all neonates.

Postoperative Care

Postoperative fluid and electrolyte requirements of infants are easily calculated. One may assume that maintenance fluid requirements are 100 ml/kg/24 hr and that third-space loss into the peritoneal cavity and the intestinal lumen is about half that volume. In general, the maintenance requirements and third-space losses—provided that the third-space losses are relatively small—can be replaced with 5% dextrose in 0.25 normal saline with supplemental potassium chloride at 3 mEq/kg/24 hr. If the third-space losses are large and prolonged, they are best replaced with 5% dextrose in lactated Ringer solution or with plasma. Gastric drainage should be replaced with 5% dextrose in 0.5 normal saline plus 30 mEq/L of potassium chloride.

If total parenteral nutrition (TPN) is required for 2 weeks or less, peripheral TPN is most appropriate; however, if TPN is required for longer than 2 weeks, a central venous Silastic catheter should be inserted.

When an infant on a ventilator becomes clinically stable, weaning should be started by simultaneously reducing the fractional concentration of oxygen in inspired gas (F_iO_2), the backup rate, and the peak inspiratory pressure (because most of the ventilators used on

(*continued*)

Intestinal Obstruction (continued)

infants are pressure controlled). Once the F_IO_2 is down to 21%, the backup rate is further reduced until the baby can be taken off the ventilator.

Postoperative Complications

PERITONITIS

Postoperative peritonitis is often difficult to diagnose in neonates. Tenderness can usually be elicited from the infant but not in every case. Cellulitis of the abdominal wall is a more useful sign. The best way of detecting free air on x-ray examination is with a cross-table lateral view; the free air is usually just under the abdominal wall. If peritonitis is present in the newborn, antibiotic coverage should be broad and should include ampicillin, an aminoglycoside, and metronidazole or clindamycin.

SEPTIC SHOCK

The development of septic shock in newborns can be very subtle and sudden. Because the blood pressure in newborns is normally low, the drop in blood pressure that follows the onset of septic shock may not be very significant. Possibly, a more helpful sign is the development of bradycardia. The initial therapy for septic shock in all age groups, and especially in neonates, is rapid I.V. infusion of colloid after broad-spectrum antibiotics have been administered and the surgical problem has been handled.

ILEUS AND BOWEL DYSFUNCTION

In many newborns, the ileostomy drainage is so high that they cannot tolerate enteral feeding and must have their intestinal tract put at complete rest with parenteral nutrition.

---

changes that occur before and after birth [see Figure 1].[29-34] During the first trimester, total body water accounts for 95% of body weight. This percentage falls to 80% by 32 weeks' gestation, to 78% at term, and to 75% by the end of the first postnatal week. Body water then decreases slowly over the next 1 to 2 years to 60% of total body weight. Similarly, extracellular fluid volume decreases from 60% of body weight during the second trimester to 45% at birth and eventually to 20% during the next 2 years. This normal physiologic process is interrupted in premature neonates, who must diurese excess fetal and postnatal total body water in a relatively short period after birth. This interruption has a significant effect on the fluid and electrolyte requirements of premature infants undergoing major surgery.[35] An expanded ECF volume in a premature infant is a potent stimulus for the release of prostaglandin E_2, which maintains the patency of a ductus arteriosus.[36-38]

Renal function is related to two physiologic processes: glomerular filtration and tubular excretion and reabsorption. In newborns, glomerular filtration rates are 25% of adult values, which are reached by 2 years of age. Likewise, renal concentrating ability is significantly reduced in both premature and full-term infants. A full-term infant can maximally concentrate urine to only 500 to 600 mOsm/kg (versus 1,200 mOsm/kg for an adult)[39,40]; a premature infant has even

Table 2 Antibiotic Dosages for Neonates

Antibiotic	Route of Administration	Dosage (mg/kg/day)			
		Body Weight < 2,000 g		Body Weight > 2,000 g	
		Age 0–7 days	Age > 7 days	Age 0–7 days	Age > 7 days
Amikacin	I.M., I.V.	15 div q. 12 hr	22.5 div q. 8 hr	20 div q. 12 hr	30 div q. 8 hr
Ampicillin	I.V., I.M.	50 div q. 12 hr	75 div q. 8 hr	75 div q. 8 hr	100 div q. 6 hr
Cefazolin	I.V., I.M.	40 div q. 12 hr	40 div q. 12 hr	40 div q. 12 hr	60 div q. 8 hr
Cefotaxime	I.V., I.M.	100 div q. 12 hr	150 div q. 8 hr	100 div q. 12 hr	150 div q. 8 hr
Ceftazidime	I.V., I.M.	100 div q. 12 hr	150 div q. 8 hr	100 div q. 12 hr	150 div q. 8 hr
Ceftriaxone	I.V., I.M.	50 once daily	50 once daily	50 once daily	75 once daily
Cephalothin	I.V.	40 div q. 12 hr	60 div q. 8 hr	60 div q. 8 hr	80 div q. 6 hr
Chloramphenicol	I.V., p.o.	25 once daily	25 once daily	25 once daily	50 div q. 12 hr
Clindamycin	I.V., I.M., p.o.	10 div q. 12 hr	15 div q. 8 hr	15 div q. 8 hr	20 div q. 6 hr
Erythromycin	p.o.	20 div q. 12 hr	30 div q. 8 hr	20 div q. 12 hr	30–40 div q. 8 hr
Gentamicin	I.M., I.V.	5 div q. 12 hr	7.5 div q. 8 hr	5 div q. 12 hr	7.5 div q. 8 hr
Kanamycin	I.M., I.V.	15 div q. 12 hr	22.5 div q. 8 hr	20 div q. 12 hr	30 div q. 8 hr
Methicillin	I.V., I.M.	50 div q. 12 hr	75 div q. 8 hr	75 div q. 8 hr	100 div q. 6 hr
Metronidazole	I.V., p.o.	15 div q. 12 hr	15 div q. 12 hr	15 div q. 12 hr	30 div q. 12 hr
Mezlocillin	I.V., I.M.	150 div q. 12 hr	225 div q. 8 hr	150 div q. 12 hr	225 div q. 8 hr
Oxacillin	I.V., I.M.	50 div q. 12 hr	100 div q. 8 hr	75 div q. 8 hr	150 div q. 6 hr
Nafcillin	I.V.	50 div q. 12 hr	75 div q. 8 hr	50 div q. 8 hr	75 div q. 6 hr
Netilmicin	I.M., I.V.	5 div q. 12 hr	7.5 div q. 8 hr	5 div q. 12 hr	7.5 div q. 8 hr
Penicillin G	I.V.	50,000 U div q. 12 hr	75,000 U div q. 8 hr	50,000 U div q. 8 hr	100,000 U div q. 6 hr
Penicillin G Benzathine	I.M.	50,000 U (one dose)	50,000 U (one dose)	50,000 U (one dose)	50,000 U (one dose)
Procaine		50,000 U once daily	50,000 U once daily	50,000 U once daily	50,000 U once daily
Ticarcillin	I.V., I.M.	150 div q. 12 hr	225 div q. 8 hr	225 div q. 8 hr	300 div q. 6 hr
Tobramycin	I.M., I.V.	4 div q. 12 hr	6 div q. 8 hr	4 div q. 12 hr	6 div q. 8 hr
Vancomycin	I.V.	30 div q. 12 hr	45 div q. 8 hr	30 div q. 12 hr	45 div q. 8 hr

```
                    Newborn presents with labored breathing
                                      |
                    ┌─────────────────┴─────────────────┐
              Passage of NG tube is difficult      NG tube passes easily
                          |
              ┌───────────┴───────────┐
        Newborn demonstrates   Newborn does not demonstrate
        excessive salivation   excessive salivation
                                      |
                    Perform chest x-ray, echocardiography, and other studies.
```

```
┌──────────────────────────┬──────────────────────────┬──────────────────────────┐
Tip of nasogastric tube is in  Loops of bowel are evident  Cystic areas are evident in
the chest; abdominal disten-   in left side of chest       left lower lobe of lung
tion is evident, with gas in
the small bowel

Diagnose esophageal atresia   Diagnose diaphragmatic      Diagnose cystic disease of
with tracheoesophageal fistula. hernia.                    the lung.

Transport baby to tertiary    Transport baby to tertiary   Transport baby to tertiary
care facility.                care facility.               care facility.
```

```
┌─────────────────┬─────────────────┐
Body weight ≥ 1.5 kg  Body weight < 1.5 kg   Resuscitate; correct acidosis

Prepare for operation.  Support until weight    If baby is stable, wait 24 hours
Give antibiotics and    ≥ 1.5 kg.               to 14 days until all ventilatory
vitamin K.              Suction the upper       parameters are normal and the
Suction.                esophageal pouch.       patient is extubated. If baby
                        Perform gastrostomy;    cannot be resuscitated with
                        provide parenteral      conventional, jet, high-frequency,
                        nutrition.              or oscillation ventilation, place
                                                on ECMO and repair hernia after
                                                baby is off ECMO.
```

Operate.
Postoperative supportive care includes monitoring, ventilatory support, and administration of fluids.

Respiratory Distress in the Newborn

Esophageal Atresia

In many obstetric units, a nasogastric or orogastric tube is routinely inserted immediately after birth to exclude an esophageal atresia. The most common form of esophageal atresia occurs in combination with a tracheoesophageal fistula; the proximal esophagus ends in a blind upper pouch, and there is a connection between the distal esophagus and the carina of the trachea.[150] Infants with this condition manifest significant respiratory distress within a few hours of birth as a result of salivary aspiration, gastroesophageal reflux of acid into the trachea through the distal fistula, and elevation of the diaphragm as a result of gastric distention with air from the tracheoesophageal fistula.

Diagnosis is confirmed when attempts to pass a nasogastric tube are unsuccessful and chest x-ray reveals the nasogastric tube curled in the esophageal pouch. Aspiration pneumonia should be looked for on the x-ray; its presence suggests that primary repair should be delayed. Echocardiography helps to identify associated cardiac anomalies and also demonstrates the location of the aortic arch. Esophageal anastomosis is most easily accomplished by means of thoracotomy opposite the side of the aortic arch.

PREOPERATIVE CARE

The related pathophysiologic processes must be corrected immediately to stabilize the baby for definitive repair. A sump catheter should be passed into the upper esophageal pouch; constant suction is necessary to prevent pneumonia. A gastrostomy tube (which is only placed if delayed primary repair is contemplated) relieves gastric distention and decreases acid reflux. The infant should be placed in an upright position to prevent gastric reflux.

Once the infant has been stabilized and major associated anomalies have been evaluated, primary repair can be carried out. In a small premature infant (< 1.5 kg) with esophageal atresia, however, it is best merely to perform a gastrostomy within 24 hours of birth and to treat the baby with gastrostomy drainage, sump suction of the upper esophageal pouch, and parenteral nutrition until the infant reaches a weight of 1.5 kg. This approach is better than an early division of the fistula retropleurally and a subsequent primary esophageal anastomosis transpleurally.

(continued)

Respiratory Distress (continued)

Diaphragmatic Hernia

Infants with congenital diaphragmatic hernia are usually quite sick at birth. They do not have difficulty swallowing their saliva; however, it may be difficult to pass a nasogastric tube into the stomach because the entire stomach may be in the chest. A plain x-ray will usually confirm the diagnosis of congenital diaphragmatic hernia.

These babies require immediate resuscitation with endotracheal intubation and sodium bicarbonate to correct acidosis. It should be noted that standard sodium bicarbonate solutions are extremely hypertonic and should be diluted before being administered, especially in neonates. Once the baby is relatively stable, it is best to wait 24 hours to as much as 14 days before operating to allow the pulmonary hypertension to decrease or disappear. If the baby cannot be resuscitated with conventional, jet, high-frequency, or oscillation ventilation, then he or she should be placed on extracorporeal membrane oxygenation (ECMO), and the hernia should be repaired after the baby is off ECMO.[151-153] In the OR, the intestines are reduced into the abdominal cavity, and the diaphragmatic defect is repaired. However, this operative procedure usually does not result in significant improvement. Often, the newborn's condition will improve during the first 12 hours postoperatively and then begin to deteriorate. If the baby fails to respond to vasodilators and inotropic agents, ECMO will be required postoperatively. Usually, ECMO permits survival of the infant under circumstances in which the mortality would be close to 100% were ECMO not available.

Cystic Disease of the Lung

Cystic lung disease, especially cystic adenomatoid malformation of the left lower lobe, can mimic diaphragmatic hernia both clinically and radiographically.[154,155] However, in contrast to a newborn with diaphragmatic hernia, a baby with cystic adenomatoid malformation will demonstrate the normal protuberance of a newborn's abdomen. If an infant with cystic adenomatoid malformation of the lungs manifests marked respiratory distress necessitating intubation and mechanical ventilation, it is preferable to perform an emergency lobectomy rather than subject the baby to a period of mechanical ventilation with the attendant risks of barotrauma and oxygen toxicity.

---

less concentrating ability (up to a maximum of 400 mOsm/kg). As a consequence, newborns tolerate dehydration poorly. Furthermore, the kidneys of newborns cannot excrete a water load as effectively as mature kidneys can. This phenomenon, combined with the low concentrating ability of the newborns' kidneys, makes fluid management very difficult. An initial fluid and electrolyte program for newborns and infants must replace the insensible water loss, the renal water loss, and the sodium and potassium losses.

INSENSIBLE WATER LOSS

Insensible water loss is a result of continuous loss of water from the respiratory tract and the skin.[41] In both full-term and premature infants, transepithelial water loss is the major component of insensible water loss.[42] The stratum corneum is the major barrier to the passive diffusion of water from the superficial capillaries of the skin to the epidermal surface. Premature infants have a less developed stratum corneum than full-term infants and therefore experience a greater diffusion of water through the epidermal surface and a greater insensible water loss through the skin. In full-term neonates, in an environment of thermal neutrality and a humidity of 50%, total insensible water loss is 12 ml/kg/24 hr, of which 7 ml is lost through the skin and 5 ml through the lungs. In full-term infants, overhead radiant heaters and phototherapy may increase insensible water loss from skin by 50%.[43-49] In premature infants, radiant heaters and phototherapy may increase insensible water loss from skin by 50% to 100%.

Full-term babies sweat at birth if body temperature exceeds 37.5° C (99.5° F); however, the amount of water they lose by this mechanism is quite small. Respiratory water loss accounts for about one third of total insensible water loss in full-term infants and is related to the volume of inspired air, respiratory rate, body temperature, and the humidity of the expired air.[50] Premature infants of less than 36 weeks' gestation do not sweat in the first few days of life. In these infants, especially those who are born after less than 32 weeks' gestation, the respiratory water loss is less than it is in full-term infants because the transepithelial water loss is greater.

Insensible water loss from the skin can be minimized by the use of incubators in the neonatal ICU and extremity coverings in the OR. Water loss from the lungs can be decreased by humidifying the inspired gases.

RENAL WATER REQUIREMENTS

The water required for excretion of the products of catabolism is based on the renal solute load, including any exogenous solute load,[51] and on the maximal renal concentrating ability. Therefore, the volume of fluid administered must allow excretion of the entire solute load at an osmolality of 250 mOsm/kg, a level achievable by even the smallest premature infant. The solute load of the newborn is approximately 15 mOsm/kg/24 hr during the first week of life if the infant receives only intravenous fluids; 17.5 mOsm/kg/24 hr during the second week of life if the infant is on partial oral intake; and 30 mOsm/kg/24 hr thereafter if the infant is maintained on formula. The amount of water required for excretion of these osmolar loads can be calculated by using the following formula:

$$\text{H}_2\text{O requirements (ml/kg/24 hr)} = \frac{\text{osmolality of solute load (mOsm/kg)}}{\text{osmolality of urine (mOsm/kg)}} \times 1{,}000$$

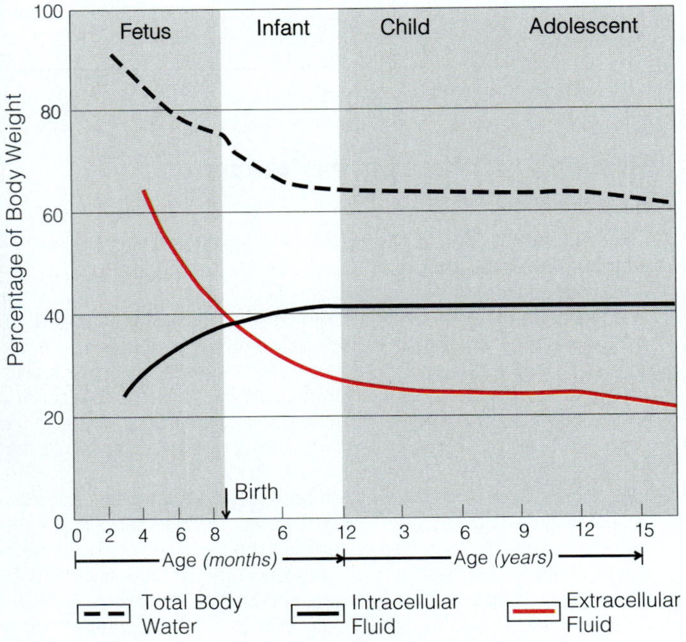

Figure 1 **Total body water (TBW) and extracellular fluid (ECF) decrease between fetal life and adulthood, and intracellular fluid (ICF) increases.**

> ### Abdominal Pain
>
> Abdominal pain in a pubertal female can have many different causes. Acute appendicitis is the most common cause; nevertheless, the differential diagnosis should also include perforated duodenal ulcer, Meckel diverticulum, ulcerative colitis, Crohn disease, ruptured ovarian cyst, pelvic inflammatory disease, pancreatitis, and, in much younger children, intussusception. The diagnosis of appendicitis is based on the presence of localizing physical findings in the right lower quadrant of the abdomen. Even if the history and laboratory data are not typical, the presence of localizing physical findings should allow one to make the diagnosis and to proceed with appropriate operation.
>
> If perforation of the appendix is suspected preoperatively, broad-spectrum antibiotics should be started, and the patient should be given I.V. crystalloid. There is no value in leaving a drain, even if pus is encountered in the peritoneal cavity, because it is impossible to drain the peritoneal cavity adequately. Instead, the cavity should be vigorously irrigated with saline. In most cases of perforated appendicitis, the wound can be closed primarily if irrigation has been adequate. Currently, many pediatric surgeons treat perforated appendicitis nonoperatively with I.V. antibiotics followed by laparoscopic interval appendectomy at 6 weeks.
>
> A pelvic abscess after operation for acute appendicitis typically develops between postoperative days 5 and 7. It is usually manifested by fever and elevation of the white blood cell count and not infrequently by diarrhea. In almost all cases, surgical drainage is not necessary, and treatment with I.V. antibiotics is sufficient.
>
> Very often, a teenager who exhibits the classic signs and symptoms of appendicitis turns out to have Crohn disease of the terminal ileum. This condition will be obvious at operation if the mesenteric fat is seen to be creeping up along the sides of the inflamed ileum. In the past, it was generally agreed that an appendectomy should not be performed under these circumstances because of the theoretical risk that a cecal fistula would develop. In fact, this reservation has not been shown to be well founded, and most surgeons now recommend appendectomy at the time of exploratory laparotomy. When the child has fully recovered from the operation, a definitive workup should be performed to ascertain the extent of the Crohn disease. The workup should include a small-bowel series and a colonoscopy with biopsy. If an enterocutaneous fistula should develop, TPN will be required for a prolonged period.
>
> **Patient between the ages of 5 and 14 presents with abdominal pain, fever, and leukocytosis**
>
> Establish preoperative diagnosis.
> Most likely diagnoses are
> - Appendicitis
> - Inflammatory bowel disease (ulcerative colitis, Crohn disease)
>
> Less likely diagnoses are
> - Perforated ulcer
> - Meckel diverticulum
> - Pelvic inflammatory disease
> - Pancreatitis
> - Intussusception
> - Ruptured ovarian cyst
>
> ↓
>
> Postoperative care includes general support, administration of fluids, and administration of antibiotics.
> Avoid complications:
> - Wound infection
> - Intra-abdominal abscess
> - Enterocutaneous fistula
> - Malnutrition

If the urine osmolality is 250 mOsm/kg, the renal water requirements are 60 ml/kg/24 hr during the first week of life, 72 ml/kg/24 hr during the second week of life, and 84 ml/kg/24 hr thereafter. This rate of fluid infusion will produce a urine output of approximately 2.5 ml/kg/hr. Renal water requirements are modified by a number of factors. An anabolic, growing infant has a lower solute load and therefore a lower water requirement. A certain amount of water is required for active growth, between 10 and 15 ml/kg/24 hr. On the other hand, if the infant has recently undergone an operation or is otherwise stressed, a catabolic state exists, and the solute load will increase. Tissue destruction secondary to trauma or surgery increases the solute load even further.

WATER LOSS FROM THE GASTROINTESTINAL TRACT

In general, water loss from the stool need not be considered in calculating water requirements; such water loss amounts to an expenditure of only 5 to 10 ml/100 kcal. Infants who are receiving nothing through the GI tract will have smaller losses than infants who are being fed orally. Short-bowel syndrome or significant diarrhea increases the stool water loss; phototherapy doubles stool water content. Measurable water and electrolyte losses from the GI tract or other sites should be replaced.

SODIUM REQUIREMENTS

The sodium requirements of full-term infants average 2 mEq/kg/24 hr; preterm infants older than 32 weeks in gestational age require 3 mEq/kg/24 hr; and babies who are of low gestational age or who are critically ill require 4 to 5 mEq/kg/24 hr. Conditions such as intestinal obstruction [see Sidebar Intestinal Obstruction in the Newborn] and peritonitis increase sodium loss and therefore increase the sodium requirements.

Although full-term infants can retain sodium as well as adults do in the face of a sodium deficit, they are unable to excrete excess sodium as effectively as adults. As a result, excessive infusion of intravenous sodium can rapidly result in hypernatremia. The problem is exaggerated in premature infants. Sodium excretion during the last half of gestation is significant but quickly drops off after birth in full-term infants. Premature neonates excrete large amounts of sodium to complete the normal intrauterine process of sodium excretion, but this ability appears to be fixed; premature infants are unable to respond to an excessive infusion of sodium by increasing sodium excretion, perhaps because of immaturity of the renal tubules or because of unresponsiveness of the renal tubules to aldosterone.

POTASSIUM REQUIREMENTS

Potassium requirements of infants are not well documented. The generally accepted requirements are 2 mEq/kg/24 hr after the first 2 to 3 days of life. The delay in administration has been recommended because of the concern about immature renal function in the first few days of life. In fact, however, potassium requirements are significant in the first few days of life, especially after a major operation, because in the catabolic state, protein breakdown leads to nitrogen loss in the urine and a concomitant potassium loss. Thus, potassium should be administered in the first 1 or 2 days of life after an operation once urine output is established.

Given all the considerations described, the initial fluid used for surgical management of the neonate and infant, both preoperatively and postoperatively, should be 5% or 10% dextrose in 0.2% saline at a dosage of approximately 100 to 150 ml/kg/24 hr [see Table 3].

ACID-BASE STATUS

Metabolic alkalosis caused by electrolyte loss, specifically chloride, may occur with prolonged gastric suction or vomiting and is usually easily corrected by replacement of the appropriate electrolytes (e.g., with potassium chloride). Metabolic acidosis, on the other hand, is usually the result of poor tissue perfusion and lactic acidosis. It is best corrected by treating the underlying cause of the poor perfusion and by temporarily administering buffers, such as sodium bicarbonate, which is usually done when the pH falls below 7.3. Standard sodium bicarbonate solutions are extremely hypertonic and should be diluted before being administered, especially in neonates. The dose can be calculated from the following formula:

$$\text{NaHCO}_3 \text{ dose (mmol)} = \frac{\text{base excess} \times \text{body weight (kg)}}{3}$$

Infection and Antibiotics

INFECTION IN NEONATES

Immediately after birth, bacterial colonization of the newborn begins.[52] This process begins with the skin and shortly thereafter involves the GI tract.[53,54] By 10 days of age, normal newborns have the common aerobic and anaerobic bacteria in their GI tract.[55] Neonates in ICUs undergo delayed colonization with a small number of pathogenic bacteria.[56,57] Normal barriers to invasive infection, especially the skin and GI tract, are underdeveloped in newborns.[58] The normal mucosal barrier to bacterial invasion in the neonatal ileum is defective,[59] which may explain the etiology of neonatal sepsis (see below) and possibly of necrotizing enterocolitis (NEC) as well. Postischemic reperfusion injury may give rise to NEC, in which case serum levels of several cytokines (e.g., tumor necrosis factor, interleukin-1 [IL-1], and IL-6) may rise. Enteral administration of nonabsorbable antibiotics and immunoglobulins may reduce the amount of bacterial translocation that occurs during NEC and may thereby lower the incidence of bacteremia and neonatal sepsis.[60]

Nor are normal host defense mechanisms completely developed at birth: full immunocompetence develops during the first few months of life. In premature infants, antibody levels are not high enough for adequate response to invasive sepsis. Normal full-term infants have adequate levels of IgG antibodies from their mothers, but lack of IgM antibodies, which include many opsonins, makes newborns susceptible to infection with gram-negative bacteria. Secretory IgA antibodies from the intestine do not reach effective levels until 3 weeks of age; they are passively acquired from colostrum in the first few days of life. Phagocytes in breast milk are another source of passive protection for the neonate.[61]

Usually, the first sign of a postoperative infection is fever, except in neonates, who rarely manifest temperature elevation. The usual sites of postoperative infection are the lungs, the surgical wound, the urinary tract, and I.V. catheter sites. The time of onset of postoperative wound infection is usually related to the pathogen involved. For example, wound infection within 48 hours after operation is usually caused by *Clostridium perfringens* or by β-hemolytic streptococcus.

Table 3 Daily Fluid Requirements for Neonates and Infants*

Weight	Volume
Premature < 1.5 kg	150 ml/kg
Neonates and infants 1.5–10 kg	100 ml/kg for first 10 kg
Infants and children 10–20 kg	1,000 ml + 50 ml/kg over 10 kg
Children > 20 kg	1,500 ml + 20 ml/kg over 20 kg

*Maintenance Na⁺ and K⁺ requirements range from 2 to 4 mEq/kg; solution can generally be given as 0.2% saline with 5% or 10% dextrose and K⁺ added.

Analgesic Dosage Guidelines in Children

Drug	Dosage	Comments
Mild Pain		
Acetaminophen	10–15 mg/kg p.o. q. 4 hr 15–20 mg/kg p.r. q. 4 hr	Wide margin of safety
Aspirin	10–15 mg/kg p.o.	For inflammatory disorders
Ibuprofen	3–10 mg/kg p.o. q. 6 hr	For inflammatory disorders
Moderate to Severe Pain*		
Codeine	0.5–1 mg/kg p.o. or I.M. q. 4 hr	
Morphine	0.06 mg/kg/hr continuous I.V. infusion (average effective rate) 0.02 mg/kg/hr (neonates) 0.07–0.1 mg/kg I.V. q. 2 hr 0.1–0.15 mg/kg I.M. q. 3–4 hr 0.2–0.6 mg/kg p.o. q. 4–6 hr	Slow-release preparations can be given two to three times a day
Methadone	0.1 mg/kg I.V. q. 4 hr, first 2 doses only, then 0.05 mg/kg I.V. q. 4–6 hr 0.1–0.2 mg/kg p.o. q. 6–12 hr	Careful titration is required
Fentanyl	0.5–1.5 μg/kg I.V. bolus for short procedures 1–2 μg/kg/hr I.V. continuous infusion	
Hydromorphone	⅕–¼ the comparable morphine dose	
Meperidine	8–10 times the comparable morphine dose	

*Continue acetaminophen, ibuprofen, or other NSAIDs as above if the oral route is available and there is no contraindication.

Staphylococcus aureus wound infection usually occurs between postoperative days 3 and 5. Wound infection from gram-negative bacteria, usually of enteric origin, occurs after postoperative day 5. An infected wound should be opened, packed, and treated with dressing changes until the wound has closed on its own. Intravenous and urinary catheters and endotracheal tubes are common sources of infection in neonates. *S. epidermidis* is the most common cause of infection from indwelling vascular catheters[62]; this type of infection calls for removal of the catheter and treatment with parenteral vancomycin if initial treatment with I.V. vancomycin through the catheter for 7 to 10 days is unsuccessful.[63]

Neonatal Sepsis

Neonatal sepsis is a systemic bacterial infection occurring during the first month of life.[64] Bloodstream invasion is always present. Meningitis develops in about 25% of cases. When overwhelming sepsis intervenes, shock occurs, accompanied by oliguria and coma [see Shock, Treatment, *above*]. Mortality averages about 50%.

Diagnosis of neonatal sepsis is often difficult because the clinical findings are subtle and include such symptoms as lethargy, poor feeding, hypothermia, ileus, hyperglycemia, and respiratory distress. Lab-

Preparation of the Neonate with Emergency Surgical Problems

In many communities, the general surgeon is frequently called to aid in diagnosis and initial care of the neonate with an apparent surgical problem. After preliminary tests to establish a diagnosis along with stabilization of the infant, the baby may be transported to a pediatric center that is specially equipped and staffed to study and treat the specific surgical problem.

The steps in the stabilization of a critically ill neonate before transport are similar to the ABCs of initial care in the adult. By the time the surgeon is consulted, the neonatologist or pediatrician may have accomplished initial stabilization and begun to prepare the baby for transfer. The surgeon may be needed to establish vascular access; in some cases, a peripheral venous cannula may be appropriate, but more often, central catheters are inserted via the umbilical vein or arteries. In the case of babies with omphalocele or gastroschisis, the I.V. line should be placed in the upper extremities or the neck. Appropriate fluids should be provided to prevent dehydration and to restore any fluid and electrolyte deficits. When required, a nasogastric or esophageal pouch suction tube should be placed and decompression initiated. This maneuver is extremely important if transport by air is considered because trapped gases will change with alterations in barometric pressure, and such changes may have particularly deleterious effects on infants with intestinal gas or with pneumothorax or pneumomediastinum.

Vitamin K should be given as the natural K oxide, phytonadione, in a dose of 1 mg I.V. or I.M. (the dose for babies who weigh less than 1,500 g is 0.5 mg). Appropriate antibiotics should also be administered. Finally, the infant should be wrapped and placed in an incubator or radiant warmer to stabilize and maintain normal body temperature.

Sophisticated transport teams with appropriate equipment and supplies frequently participate in moving these babies between hospitals. However, early stabilization and communication with the primary physician and transport team is essential to minimize potential risks and morbidity associated with patient transfer.

Steps in the preparation of the neonate with emergency surgical problems for interhospital transfer are as follows:

Diaphragmatic hernia
Insert NG or OG tube. Ventilation by face mask is contraindicated; if ventilation is required, intubate. Paralyze or anesthetize infant to assist ventilation until operation.

Esophageal atresia
Insert tube to aspirate secretions from pouch (use Replogle tube, if available). If possible, avoid mechanical ventilation; if intubation is required, use high-frequency, low-pressure ventilation to prevent distention and possible perforation of the stomach.

Congenital lobar emphysema
Support normal oxygenation.

Intestinal obstruction
Use nasogastric or orogastric suction. Verify I.V. lines.

Omphalocele/gastroschisis
Use nasogastric or orogastric suction. Cover sac with a nonadherent gauze, and take care not to rupture membrane; cover intestine with saline-soaked gauze. Place I.V. line in upper extremity or neck. Maintain hydration by increasing fluid administration to account for fluid lost from exposed bowel. Support bowel with dressings. Maintain body temperature.

Exstrophy of the bladder
Cover exposed bladder with a nonadherent dressing.

Meningomyelocele
Cover sac with a nonadherent dressing.

---

oratory studies are not very helpful in establishing the diagnosis. In fact, the white cell count is usually normal or low. Very often, the platelet count drops with the onset of sepsis and returns toward normal once the sepsis is under control.[65] When neonatal sepsis is suspected, cultures of blood, cerebrospinal fluid, and urine must be obtained immediately. Broad-spectrum antibiotics, including a penicillin and an aminoglycoside, should be started before the culture results have returned; the antibiotics can be adjusted when culture results become available [see Table 2]. Group B streptococcus and *Escherichia coli* account for the majority of cases of neonatal sepsis.[66] Anaerobic bacteria rarely cause neonatal sepsis unless the etiology is perforation of the GI tract with peritonitis.

ANTIBIOTICS

In general, the indications for antibiotic use in neonates, infants, and children are the same as those in adults [see 80 Antibiotics]. Peritonitis of gastrointestinal origin, for example, is treated with triple antibiotic therapy that includes a penicillin, an aminoglycoside, and clindamycin.[67] Intravenous metronidazole is an appropriate substitute for clindamycin as a potent antianaerobic agent. Some surgeons prefer to administer a third-generation cephalosporin (e.g., moxalactam, cefotaxime, or cefoperazone) instead of triple antibiotic therapy, but patients treated with cephalosporins alone are at risk for sepsis from cephalosporin-resistant *Pseudomonas aeruginosa* and enterococci.[68,69]

For clean-contaminated elective surgical procedures, such as elective colon operation,[70] the commonly used prophylactic systemic antibiotic regimen in infants and children is either a penicillin with an aminoglycoside or a third-generation cephalosporin; I tend to prefer the latter. The first dose is given just before the operation so that an adequate tissue level is achieved during the procedure. The antibiotics are continued for 24 hours postoperatively.

The side effects of antibiotics in neonates, infants, and children are similar to those seen in adults, with certain important exceptions. Sulfonamide administration is associated with an increased incidence of kernicterus in neonates, and chloramphenicol is associated with the so-called gray syndrome (in which the baby looks gray from drug toxicity); these agents should not be administered to newborns. Tetracyclines cause staining and hypoplasia of the enamel of developing teeth and thus should not be administered to children.

Serum levels of certain antibiotics, especially gentamicin, must be measured to ensure that therapeutic levels are achieved and toxic levels avoided. Patients in a septic state require higher doses of gentamicin to achieve therapeutic levels because they tend to metabolize the agent more rapidly than nonseptic patients. In septic patients, serum levels must be monitored carefully. It is important to remember that the gentamicin dosage schedule in neonates is 7.5 mg/kg/day in two divided doses given every 12 hours, whereas in adults it is 5 mg/kg/ day every 8 hours.

Almost every antibiotic has been implicated in pseudomembranous enterocolitis,[71] which probably develops from the overgrowth of *C. difficile* after antibiotic suppression of the normal colonic bacteria [see 81 Nosocomial Infection].[72] The clinical picture of severe diarrhea is probably secondary to the *C. difficile* toxin. Treatment consists of oral administration of vancomycin and withdrawal of the antibiotics that caused the syndrome.

Ventilatory Support

Respiratory failure is manifested by either poor oxygenation (hypoxemia) or inadequate ventilation; occasionally, a combination of the two exists. Hypoxemia, or low arterial oxygen tension, is a result either of an alveolar ventilation-perfusion imbalance or of impaired diffusion through the alveolar wall to the pulmonary capillary. Inadequate ventilation results from hypoventilation and leads to elevated arterial CO_2 tension. The hypoventilation may be secondary to depression of the respiratory center; abnormalities of central or peripheral nerves, muscles, or skeleton; ventilation-perfusion mismatch; or excessive CO_2 production. In managing acute respiratory failure, it is important to distinguish between inadequate ventilation and inadequate oxygenation. Mild hypoxemia can usually be treated adequately by increasing the oxygen content of air inspired via nasal cannulas, masks, hoods, and incubators. In general, higher concentrations of oxygen can be produced with cannulas or masks in infants and children than in adults because of the smaller tidal volumes required.[73] Humidification of the gas is important to avoid drying of the nasal and pharyngeal mucosa by otherwise desiccant gases.

If increasing the fraction of inspired oxygen (F_IO_2) is unsuccessful, the transpulmonary distending pressure must be increased, initially with a nasal cannula or prongs. If this measure is unsuccessful, an endotracheal tube should be inserted [see Table 4]. If airway pressure with an endotracheal tube is still inadequate, mechanical ventilation must be started. In critically ill neonates (particularly premature infants), pressure-controlled ventilators are more commonly used than volume-controlled ventilators [see 92 Use of the Mechanical Ventilator]. When the ventilator is properly set, tidal volumes average about 8 ml/kg body weight.

The initial approach to mechanical ventilation in the pediatric patient should be intermittent mandatory ventilation (IMV)—that is, unassisted, unrestricted spontaneous respirations supplemented at regular intervals with mechanical breaths. The mechanical minute ventilation should be adjusted so that normal arterial CO_2 tension and pH are achieved. The adequacy of the mechanical ventilation is monitored by intermittent determination of arterial blood gases obtained from an intra-arterial cannula or from arterialized capillary blood. When an infant on a ventilator becomes clinically stable, weaning should be started by decreasing the fixed ventilator breath rate slowly while maintaining a normal arterial CO_2 tension and pH and simultaneously reducing the F_IO_2, the backup rate, and the peak inspiratory pressure. Once the F_IO_2 is down to 21%, the backup rate and the peak inspiratory pressure are further reduced until the baby can be taken off the ventilator.

Other means of elevating airway pressure include continuous positive airway pressure (CPAP), intermittent positive pressure breathing (IPPB), and continuous positive pressure ventilation (CPPV). The principles of mechanical ventilation are much the same in children and adults [see 92 Use of the Mechanical Ventilator]. With CPAP, the patient breathes spontaneously through a gas delivery system into which the fresh gas flow exceeds or equals the patient's peak inspiratory flow rate. A valve maintains system pressure by eliminating exiting gas flow when a predetermined threshold is reached during exhalation. An alternative to CPAP is positive end-expiratory pressure (PEEP), in which a reservoir furnishes inspired volume. The reservoir is placed between the patient and the compressed gas source delivering low flow. A valve between the reservoir and the patient prevents exhaled gases from flowing toward the reservoir and prevents rebreathing.

There are four different techniques for delivering CPPV. The first is controlled ventilation. When a patient is unable to generate any voluntary respiratory effort, because of respiratory center depression, spinal cord respiratory muscle dysfunction, or neuromuscular blockade, for example, the mechanical ventilator must deliver the entire minute ventilation. To avoid atelectasis and to improve gas exchange, PEEP can be added to the system. The second technique is patient-initiated ventilation: a spontaneous respiratory effort by the patient signals the ventilator to initiate a mechanical inspiration. The tidal volume is preset; however, the respiratory rate is determined by the patient's spontaneous efforts. The third technique is supplemental ventilation, in which unrestricted and unassisted spontaneous ventilation is augmented by a mechanical ventilator. The respiratory rate and tidal volume are preset so that a specific minute ventilation is achieved, which will diminish as the spontaneous breathing of the patient improves. The fourth technique is pressure-controlled ventilation, in which a preset expiratory pressure above the patient's own expiratory pressure is maintained during spontaneous respiration.

Because mechanical ventilation decreases venous return, thereby also decreasing cardiac output, and because conventional mechanical ventilation is associated with barotrauma, high-frequency ventilation is often used for neonates and infants.[74] This type of ventilation can be delivered either as positive pressure ventilation through an endotracheal tube or as jet ventilation through a catheter. At present, oscillation ventilation is increasingly being used in neonates to reduce barotrauma.

Mechanical ventilation is associated with a number of other complications as well. Pneumothorax, pneumomediastinum, and subcutaneous emphysema can occur when the inspiratory pressures are high.[75] In addition, the presence of an endotracheal tube in the tracheobronchial tree can result in pulmonary infection.[76] All patients on mechanical ventilators should thus receive antibiotics; the appropriate agent can be determined by culture of tracheal secretions. Moreover, the endotracheal tube can injure the subglottic area, especially in premature infants, and result in subglottic stenosis. Finally, high concentrations of oxygen can result in oxygen toxicity to the lungs and eyes, which can produce bronchopulmonary dysplasia and retrolental fibroplasia in neonates, especially in premature neonates.

Nutritional Support

Whereas the nutritional requirements of children and teenagers do not differ significantly from those of adults [see 97 Nutritional Support], the requirements of infants do. Sick infants in need of nutritional support pose therapeutic problems that are different from and frequently more complex than those of their adult counterparts. Not only must the metabolic demands that a major illness or operation imposes on all patients be taken into account, but additionally, special consideration must be given to the unique characteristics of pediatric patients, such as smaller body size, rapid growth, highly variable fluid requirements, and, in newborns, the immaturity of certain organ systems. These characteristics, coupled with low caloric reserves in premature infants and sick children, make adequate nutritional intake particularly important. Consequently, infants whose nutritional needs are not met as a result of a functional or organic disorder of the GI tract can rapidly acquire protein-calorie malnutrition. That a problem indeed exists is clear from one nutritional survey in a pediatric referral center, which demonstrated that one third of hospitalized pediatric patients show evidence of acute malnutrition.[77] Even a relatively short period of inadequate nutrition an lead to decreased host resistance, increased infection, and poor

Table 4 Tracheal Tube Size by Age

Age of Patient	Internal Diameter of Tube (mm)
Premature	2.5
0–3 mo	3.0
3–7 mo	3.5
7–15 mo	4.0
15–24 mo	4.5
2–10 yr	(16 + age) ÷ 4
10–19 yr	6.0–8.0 cuffed

wound healing, which contribute appreciably to morbidity and mortality in infants and children with surgical disease.

NUTRITIONAL REQUIREMENTS

An infant's body contains more water than an adult's body (70% to 75% versus 60% to 65%); therefore, infants require more water per unit of body weight. Healthy infants consume water at a daily rate of 10% to 15% of body weight, in contrast to a rate of only 2% to 4% in adults. They retain only 0.5% to 3% of their fluid intake: about 50% is excreted through the kidneys, 3% to 10% is lost through the GI tract, and 40% to 50% is insensible loss.

Infants also have much higher caloric requirements than older children and adults [see Table 5], and these requirements are further increased by periods of active growth and extreme physical activity.[78-80] Major illness or surgical trauma raises caloric requirements even further: there is a 12% increase for each 1° of fever above 37° C (98.6° F), a 20% to 30% increase with a major operation, a 40% to 50% increase with severe sepsis, and a 50% to 100% increase with long-term growth failure. In general, calories should be provided in the proportions found in a well-balanced diet—that is, 50% carbohydrate, 35% fat, and 15% protein. Carbohydrates contain 3.4 kcal/g, fat contains 9.0 kcal/g, and protein contains 4.0 kcal/g.

Most of an infant's caloric requirements are supplied by carbohydrates. Much less glycogen can be stored in an infant's liver than in an adult's, however; for this reason, fats are the other major nonprotein calorie source in infants. One of the fatty acids, linoleic acid, an 18-carbon chain with two double bonds, cannot be synthesized by the human body. It must be supplied in the diet and is therefore an essential fatty acid. A deficiency of this fatty acid results in a dry, flaky, erythematous skin rash. To prevent this deficiency, a total of 2% to 4% of required kilocalories must be in the form of linoleic acid.

Protein needs of infants are based on the combined requirements for maintenance and growth. Protein constitutes 13% of an infant's body weight, compared with 20% of an adult's. Most of the increase in body protein occurs during the first year of life, which explains why protein requirements are highest in infancy and decrease with age. Of the 20 amino acids that have been identified, eight are essential in adults, but it is thought that nine are essential in infants and 11 are essential in premature infants [see Table 6].

In general, infants require more vitamins and minerals than adults. Increased amounts of calcium and phosphorus are particularly important because of the rapid growth rate of the infant's skeleton.

METABOLIC RESPONSE TO SURGERY

Nutritional management of the surgical patient is complicated by the patient's metabolic response to the stress and trauma of the operation, which in turn affects nutritional requirements and management. This metabolic response to surgery was well described in adults by Francis D. Moore in 1959.[81] Although it was initially thought that infants did not respond to this type of stress in the same way that adults did,[82] later studies confirmed that the response of infants was indeed the same as that of adults.[83-86] Metabolic response to surgery can be divided into four phases: (1) the adrenergic-corticoid phase, (2) the corticoid withdrawal phase, (3) the spontaneous anabolic phase, and (4) the fat gain phase. The length of each phase is directly related to the severity of the trauma: phase 1 usually lasts 2 to 4 days and phase 2 usually lasts 2 to 3 days, whereas the duration of phases 3 and 4 is variable.

During phase 1, which begins on induction of anesthesia, serum and urine levels of glucocorticoids and mineralocorticoids increase. At the same time, there is a significant rise in catecholamine levels and in the secretion of antidiuretic hormone (ADH). The increase in ADH results in early water retention that usually lasts for 36 to 72 hours. The increased secretion of glucocorticoids and mineralocorticoids—especially aldosterone—along with the body's unique response to trauma and surgery leads to increased protein breakdown and elevation of the urinary nitrogen level. The potassium-to-nitrogen ratio in the urine, which is usually 3 mEq of potassium for every gram of nitrogen excreted, increases in the early postoperative period to 6 mEq of potassium per gram of nitrogen excreted.

Phase 2 usually begins on postoperative day 4. In this phase, the adrenal steroid output begins to return to normal, sodium excretion increases, and potassium and nitrogen excretion in the urine decreases. The antidiuretic effect is usually over, and a water diuresis ensues.

In phase 3, protein synthesis begins, and the nitrogen balance changes from negative to positive and thus begins the anabolic phase of recovery. During this time, any weight gain that occurs is usually caused by synthesis of new protein.

In phase 4, most of the increase in body weight is related to accumulation of fat. It is important to remember that infants, because of the rapid growth of their skeletons, have a more severe negative phosphorus balance than adults. A normal adult has a nutritional requirement of 150 nonprotein kcal for every gram of nitrogen administered. Stress and trauma probably increase this requirement, but the precise extent of the increase under these conditions is not known. Infants probably require 230 nonprotein kcal for every gram of nitrogen administered after a major operation.[87] Although the response in neonates is similar to that in adults, the duration of each phase is significantly shorter in neonates (e.g., phase 1 lasts only 48 to 72 hours), and the negative nitrogen balance may be minimal because protein synthesis is diverted away from growth to tissue repair.

NUTRITIONAL ASSESSMENT

In many cases, a sick infant's history and overall appearance provide sufficient grounds for initiating nutritional support. For example, a preterm infant with respiratory distress who is small for his or her gestational age will clearly require parenteral nutrition, as will a newborn with gastroschisis. Physical variables that should be considered in nutritional assessment include weight, length, head circumference, chest circumference, and triceps skin-fold thickness. There are no blood tests sufficiently sensitive to reflect changes in the patient's nu-

Table 5 Kilocalorie and Protein Requirements for Infants and Children

Age (yr)	Kilocalories* (kcal/kg)	Protein (g/kg)
0–1	90–120	2.0–3.5
1–7	75–90	2.0–2.5
7–12	60–75	2.0
12–18	30–60	1.5
18	25–30	1.0

*These numbers represent volume administered when solutions of 1 kcal/ml are used.

Table 6 Essential Amino Acids

Threonine	Lysine	Histidine*
Leucine	Methionine	Tyrosine†
Isoleucine	Phenylalanine	Cystine†
Valine	Tryptophan	

*Essential only in infancy.
†May be essential in premature infants.

tritional status accurately; the serum albumin level is probably the most useful test, and it is both economical and readily obtainable. A serum albumin concentration of 2.8 to 3.5 g/dl indicates moderate malnutrition, and a concentration of less than 2.8 g/dl suggests severe malnutrition (except in newborns, in whom levels are normally low). The serum transferrin level is actually a more sensitive index of nutritional status than the serum albumin level because transferrin has a half-life of only 9 days, whereas albumin has a half-life of 20 days.

ENTERAL FEEDING

The type of nutritional support to be employed depends on the disease affecting the patient and the patient's status. From a physiologic standpoint, enteral feedings are preferable and are the first choice for patients whose GI tract is functioning adequately.[88] Breast milk or a standard infant formula is used for oral or tube feeding of infants younger than 1 year[89] [see Table 7]. A liquid diet of either blenderized food or liquid formula may be used for feeding older children who are unable or unwilling to eat. A number of nutritionally complete liquid formulas are commercially available [see Table 8]. Specialized formulas are available for use in patients who have lactose intolerance or protein sensitivity or who suffer from renal or hepatic failure.

POSTOPERATIVE FEEDING

Infants have more difficulty feeding during the early months of life, especially premature infants, in whom the complex physiology of sucking and swallowing is not yet fully developed. In addition, the work of feeding accounts for most of an infant's caloric expenditure in the early months, and the stressed infant tires easily. For this reason, gavage or gastrostomy tube feedings are generally employed for the early stages of postoperative feeding in infants. Feedings are begun after the resolution of postoperative ileus has been demonstrated by the passage of meconium or stool. Further evidence that the bowel is beginning to function is the disappearance of the bilious green color of the gastric aspirate and the decrease in volume of the aspirate from the nasogastric or gastrostomy tube. The average volume of gastric aspirate in neonates with unobstructed intestines is 50 ml/24 hr. The return of bowel sounds, a helpful sign in older children, is not as sensitive or reliable in determining the resolution of ileus in infants.

Feedings of small volumes of sugar water are given by mouth or by gastrostomy tube. The initial feeding is 10 to 15 ml every 2 to 3 hours, which is increased by 2 to 5 ml increments over the next 12 to 24 hours until the infant is ingesting 30 to 45 ml of sugar water every 3 hours. Administration of half-strength formula is then started, and the infant is fed a similar volume every 3 hours during the next 12 to 24 hours. When the infant is able to tolerate this regimen, the diet is changed to the same amount of full-strength formula. At this point, the nurse or the mother feeds the infant whatever amount the infant will tolerate.

It is almost axiomatic that infants tolerate increases in volume much more readily than increases in osmolarity; it is generally best to use diluted formulas (three-quarters strength, half strength, or quarter strength) and to increase the volume as necessary to supply the calories needed. Inability to tolerate increased osmolarity is usually manifested by diarrhea. Inability to tolerate increased volume is usually evidenced by vomiting or increased residuals in the gastrostomy or nasogastric tube. If a gastrostomy tube is in place in an infant or child, it is usually elevated 8 to 12 in. above the abdominal wall for 12 to 24 hours after bowel function first returns, and the volume and bile content of the gastric reflux are observed; clear color and diminished volume of gastric juice are often the best indications that the patient is ready for oral feeding. The next step is to clamp the tube for 3 hours and then to drain for 1 hour. If there is no significant drainage during the 1-hour period, the infant or child is ready for feeding. If the infant or child has difficulty digesting a standard or lactose-free formula, one of the formulas containing predigested components should be tried. When selecting a predigested formula, one must make sure that the osmolarity of the formulation is not too high.

Elemental or chemically defined diets require a minimum of digestive work and are free of residual bulk [see Table 9]; however, they are unpalatable and thus are usually given by tube. Constant infusion with a pump is the preferred method of administration. Because of the high osmolarity of these diets, bolus feeding induces nausea, cramps, and diarrhea (the dumping syndrome). Accordingly, feedings are started with quarter-strength or half-strength formula and are increased first in volume and then in concentration during a period of 3 to 4 days. Once the patient is able to tolerate formula in sufficiently high concentration and volume to meet nutritional needs, I.V. fluids are no longer required. Patients on elemental diets should be monitored in the same way as those receiving total parenteral nutrition (TPN). When administered by continuous drip through a feeding tube, elemental and chemical diets furnish roughly the same amounts of calories and protein that TPN does, at considerably lower cost.[90] Unfortunately, they are not as well tolerated in infants and neonates as they are in older children and adults and consequently are only infrequently employed in treating these very young patients. Two available forms of the elemental diet, Vivonex and Criticare, are the ones most often used. The ease of gastrointestinal absorption and minimal residue make elemental diets extremely useful as an intermediate step between parenteral nutrition and regular feedings.

TOTAL PARENTERAL NUTRITION

TPN is a well-balanced system of intravenous feeding that was developed to meet the needs of nutritionally compromised patients

Table 7 Composition of Infant Formulas

Formula	Kilocalories		Na (mEq/L)	K (mEq/L)	Ca (mg/L)	P (mg/L)	Fe (mg/L)	Osmolarity (mOsm/L)
	(kcal/oz)	(kcal/ml)						
Breast milk	20	0.67	7	14	340	162	1.5	100
Cow's milk	20	0.67	25	35	1,240	950	1	270
Enfamil	20	0.67	11	19	546	462	trace	285
Nutramigen	20	0.67	14	17	630	473	13	460
Portagen	20	0.67	14	21	630	473	13	210
Pregestimil	20	0.67	14	17	630	473	13	311
ProSobee	20	0.67	18	19	788	525	13	250
Similac 20	20	0.67	11	19	580	430	trace	285
S-M-A	20	0.67	7	15	400	200	12	250

Table 8 Formulas for Routine Infant Feeding

	Mature Human Milk	Enfamil with Iron	Pregestimil	Ross Carbohydrate Free*	Nursoy	Enfamil Premature	Whole Cow Milk†	Peptamen Junior
Protein‡	1.1	1.4	1.9	1.8	2.1	2.0	3.6	3.0
Casein	40%	40%	—	—	—	40%	82%	—
Whey	60%	60%	—	—	—	60%	18%	—
Soy	—	—	—	100%	100%	—	—	100%
Hydrolyzed casein	—	—	100%	—	—	—	—	—
Osmolarity (mOsm/kg H_2O)	300	270	320	70	296	260	290	260
Fat‡	3.9	3.5	2.7	3.7	3.6	3.4	3.7	3.9
Long-chain triglycerides	100%	100%	60%	100%	100%	60%	100%	40%
Medium-chain triglycerides	—	—	40%	—	—	40%	—	60%
Carbohydrate‡	7.2	7.3	9.0	0	6.9	7.4	4.8	13.8
Type	Lactose	Lactose	Partially hydrolyzed starch		Sucrose	Lactose, glucose polymer	Lactose	Maltodextrin, starch
Minerals (selected) (mg/L)								
Sodium§	150	180	315	320	200	260	520	460
Potassium‖	550	720	730	950	700	690	1,480	1,320
Calcium	340	520	630	710	600	400	1,220	1,080
Phosphorus	140	350	415	510	420	550	960	800
Iron	0.5	12	12.5	12	12	12	0.6	14
Energy (kcal/30 ml)	20	20	20		20	20		30
Indication			Malabsorption, hypoallergenic also for short bowel syndrome and biliary atresia	Carbohydrate intolerance (carbohydrate added as tolerated)	Lactose intolerance	For premature, up to full-term birth weight		For child with impaired GI function; 1 to 6 yr of age
Similar formulas		Similac Gerber Carnation	Nutramigen¶ Portagen Alimentum	3232 A	Isomil ProSobee I-Soyalac	Similac Special Care		

*Not a complete formula as provided by the manufacturer and contains no carbohydrates. Carbohydrate can be reintroduced as dextrose, up to 7 g/dl, and slowly changed from dextrose to sucrose.
†For comparison only. Whole cow milk should not be fed to infants until they are at least 6 mo of age and have developed renal maturity.
‡Values stated are percentages of weight per volume.
§To determine mEq/L, divide by 23.
‖To determine mEq/L, divide by 39.1.
¶Lacks medium-chain triglycerides.

who can neither accept nor assimilate foods given enterally. Experience in a large number of institutions confirms the lifesaving potential of TPN in infants and children with inadequate GI tract function. In 1944, Helfrick and Abelson reported the first successful use of TPN in an infant.[91] During the next 20 years, however, efforts to duplicate this achievement met with failure, largely because the peripheral veins were unable to tolerate the infusates. The venous endothelium was damaged by the high osmolality of the glucose solutions, but the high osmolality was necessary to provide sufficient calories for anabolism of the administered amino acids. The alternative, administration of large volumes of a dilute solution of glucose, was equally unsuccessful: it created a different set of complications, mostly related to increased fluid volume (e.g., pulmonary edema, peripheral edema, and congestive heart failure). In an effort to bypass these two alternatives, fat emulsions were administered. At first, this approach also failed, but eventually, after the introduction of Intralipid (soybean oil) in 1962, it proved successful.[92] Fat emulsions have a substantial advantage over glucose solutions in that they have both high caloric density and isotonicity; this advantage allows them to be infused into peripheral veins.[93-95] The most significant breakthrough in TPN, however, occurred in the late 1960s, when Dudrick and associates introduced the concept of TPN based on the infusion of a hypertonic solution of glucose into a central vein.[96,97] In the early years after this group's initial success, this approach to TPN began to be widely used in newborns with GI anomalies.[98,99] Since then, the technique has come to be applied to care of all age groups, with dramatic results [*see 97 Nutritional Support*].

There are essentially two approaches to I.V. nutrition in infants and children[100]: (1) central infusion of hypertonic glucose–amino acid solutions and (2) peripheral infusion of moderately hypertonic solutions of glucose and amino acids, along with a fat emulsion. Each of these techniques induces nitrogen retention and weight gain. In difficult cases, both may be required for an extended period.[101]

Indications

TPN is generally reserved for infants and children threatened by catabolic or nutritional deficits because feeding via the GI tract is either hazardous, inadequate, or impossible. In some instances—for

Table 9 Elemental Diets

	Vivonex High Nitrogen, Vivonex Standard Diet	Criticare HN
Form	Powder	Fluid
Carbohydrate	Glucose and glucose oligosaccharides	Maltodextrin, cornstarch, citrate
Fat	Safflower oil	Safflower oil
Protein	Crystalline amino acids	Casein hydrolysate supplemented by L-amino acids
Essential amino acids (%)	36.25	30.4
Nonessential amino acids (%)	63.75	69.56

example, cases of chronic nonspecific diarrhea—providing TPN and placing the GI tract at rest for a time are sufficient for cure. In others—for example, cases of inflammatory bowel disease—restoration and maintenance of adequate nutrition permit subsequent corrective operative procedures.

Parenteral nutrition is used in the treatment of a wide range of common conditions, including intestinal obstruction caused by congenital disorders; postoperative adhesions; peritonitis; intestinal fistulas; chronic nonspecific diarrhea; necrotizing enterocolitis; short-bowel syndrome; extensive burns; and abdominal neoplasms treated by surgery, chemotherapy, and radiation. Besides being used for nutritional repletion of malnourished children, I.V. nutrition may also be employed as prophylaxis when prolonged starvation is expected, as in cases of gastroschisis. In infants, TPN is indicated if nutrition is inadequate for 4 or 5 days. Older children and adults may tolerate a longer period of inadequate nutrition depending on their nutritional status before operation or at the onset of illness. The benefits of improved nutrition in reducing mortality and morbidity must be weighed against the risks of serious complications secondary to I.V. nutrition (see below), especially sepsis. TPN should not be used when enteral nutrition is possible.

Composition of TPN Solutions

Central vein infusions When administered through a central vein, the basic parenteral nutrition solution contains 25% glucose and 3.5% amino acids [*see Table 10*]. Electrolytes, trace elements, and vitamins are added in the amounts appropriate to the infant's weight. The final solution provides 1 kcal/ml. Infusion of 100 to 120 ml/kg/day of this solution provides the glucose, amino acids, and other nutrients that normal infants need for tissue growth and repair; the volume is lower in older children because their requirements are lower. Iron requirements are met through either blood transfusions or daily addition of 2 mg of iron-dextran to the solution. Linoleic acid, an essential fatty acid, is provided through weekly infusion of a commercial fat emulsion in amounts equivalent to 2% to 4% of the patient's daily caloric requirement. Protein is supplied in amounts not exceeding 3.5 g/kg/day. If fat is used as a nonprotein calorie source in the basic solution, it should account for no more than 50% of the daily calories. Furthermore, no more than 4 g/kg/day of fat should be infused into an infant and no more than 3 g/kg/day into an older child. Fat should be infused in small amounts (1 g/kg/day) initially and gradually raised to maximal levels during a period of 2 to 3 days.

Peripheral vein infusions When the basic parenteral nutrition solution is administered through a peripheral vein, it is made up of equal volumes of 4% amino acids and 20% glucose [*see Table 11*].

The final concentration of this solution is 2% amino acids and 10% glucose, which yields 0.48 kcal/ml. As with the central infusate, electrolytes, trace elements, and vitamins are added to the solution routinely. In neonates, 160 to 200 ml/kg/day is infused, providing 77 to 96 kcal/kg/day; in older children, the volume is reduced according to the caloric need. Unless contraindications are present, it is generally advantageous to use an I.V. fat emulsion as a major calorie source in the peripheral feeding regimen. As much as 4 g/kg/day of fat may be administered to infants and younger children; the nonlipid part of the solution is reduced by a corresponding caloric amount. This formula provides 102 to 121 kcal/kg/day, which is generally adequate for weight gain and growth. In older children, 3 g/kg/day of fat emulsion is given, with the glucose-protein solution supplying the remainder of the caloric needs. If a fat emulsion is not used, the infant's essential fatty acid requirements must be supplied by daily application of sunflower seed oil to the skin of the chest.

Whatever form of parenteral nutrition is used, one of the most important considerations is the ratio of nonprotein calories to grams of nitrogen, which should be somewhere between 150 and 300. This range is necessary to achieve the optimal utilization of the administered amino acids.

Administration

In central parenteral nutrition, hypertonic nutrient solutions are delivered through a central venous catheter to avoid peripheral venous inflammation and thrombosis. In infants, a venous cutdown is performed, and a pediatric silicone rubber (Broviac) catheter is passed through the external or internal jugular vein to the superior vena cava [*see Figure 2*]. This procedure is carried out in an operating room or, if necessary, a neonatal ICU, where adequate exposure, proper instruments, and intraoperative fluoroscopy are available and strict aseptic conditions can be maintained. The venous catheter is tunneled from the point of entry to the vein to a skin exit site 5 to 10

Table 10 Central Parenteral Nutrition in Infants*

Constituent	Amount (per kg/24 hr)
Glucose	15–30 g
Protein	2.0–4.0 g
Sodium	2.4 mEq
Potassium	2.4 mEq
Chloride	3–6 mEq
Magnesium	0.5–1.0 mEq
Calcium	0.5–3.0 mEq
Phosphate	0.5–1.0 mM
Trace elements†	0.1 ml (0.3 ml for neonates)
Multivitamin infusion (MVI)‡	1 vial (diluted to 3 ml)
Heparin	1.0 IU/ml
Glucose-protein volume	60–114 ml
Fat	1–4 g
10% fat emulsion volume	10–40 ml
Total volume	70–154 ml
Total kilocalories	70–154 kcal

*Each 1,000 ml of a standard solution is prepared by mixing 500 ml of 50% dextrose and water with 500 ml of 7% amino acids to give a final concentration of 25% dextrose and 3.5% amino acids. The appropriate amounts of electrolytes, vitamins, and trace elements are added according to the patient's weight.

†Each 0.1 ml of trace element solution (University of Michigan Pharmacy) contains zinc, 100 µg; copper, 20 µg; manganese, 10 µg; chromium, 0.2 µg; and selenium, 1.2 µg. Special neonatal trace element solution contains 300 µg of zinc in 0.3 ml and the same amounts of the other elements.

‡Each vial (diluted to 3 ml) of pediatric MVI (USV Pharmaceutical Corporation) contains vitamin A, 2,300 IU; vitamin D, 400 IU; ascorbic acid, 80 IU; thiamine (vitamin B_1), 1.2 mg; riboflavin (vitamin B_2), 1.4 mg; niacinamide, 17 mg; pyridoxine (vitamin B_6), 1 mg; dexpanthenol, 5 mg; vitamin E, 7 IU; folic acid, 140 µg; cyanocobalamin (vitamin B_{12}), 1 µg; phytonadione (vitamin K_1), 200 µg; and biotin, 20 µg.

Table 11 Peripheral Parenteral Nutrition with Fat in Infants*

Constituent	Amount (per kg/24 hr)
Glucose	15–20 g
Protein	2.0–4.0 g
Sodium	2–4 mEq
Potassium	2–4 mEq
Chloride	3–6 mEq
Magnesium	0.5–1.0 mEq
Calcium	0.5–3.0 mEq
Phosphate	0.5–1.0 mM
Trace elements [see Table 10][†]	0.1 ml (0.3 ml for neonates)
Multivitamin infusion (MVI) [see Table 10][‡]	1 vial (diluted to 3 ml)
Heparin	1.0 IU/ml
Glucose-protein volume	120–160 ml
Fat	4 g
10% fat emulsion volume	40 ml
Total volume	160–200 ml
Total kilocalories	102–121 kcal

*Each 1,000 ml of a standard solution is prepared by mixing 500 ml of 20% dextrose and water with 500 ml of 4% amino acids to give a final concentration of 10% dextrose and 2% amino acids. The appropriate amounts of electrolytes, vitamins, and trace elements are added according to the patient's weight.
[†]Each 0.5 ml of trace element solution (University of Michigan Pharmacy) contains zinc, 100 μg; copper, 20 μg; manganese, 10 μg; and chromium, 0.2 μg.
[‡]Each ml of MVI (USV Pharmaceutical Corporation) contains vitamin A, 2,000 IU; vitamin D, 200 IU; ascorbic acid, 100 IU; thiamine (vitamin B_1), 10 mg; riboflavin (vitamin B_2), 2 mg; niacinamide, 20 mg; pyridoxine (vitamin B_6), 3 mg; dexpanthenol, 5 mg; and vitamin E, 1 IU.

pass through a millipore filter, the filter is inserted into the line containing the amino acid solution at a point proximal to that at which the fat solution enters the nipple. The injection site usually must be changed every 2 to 3 days because of infiltration, which is usually bland and nonphlebitic. The same technique is used for peripheral parenteral nutrition without fat; however, the injection sites must be changed more frequently because of the greater tonicity of the infusate.

Monitoring

Infants receiving TPN must be carefully monitored. Essential clinical measurements include body weight (assessed daily), body length (weekly), head circumference (weekly), and intake and output volumes. Urinary glucose and acetone levels are monitored, initially with each voiding and then, after the patient is stable, once each nursing shift. Blood tests must be employed judiciously and sparingly in infants and children because of their small total blood volume. At the start of therapy and once a week thereafter, a complete blood count should be done, blood urea nitrogen should be measured, and

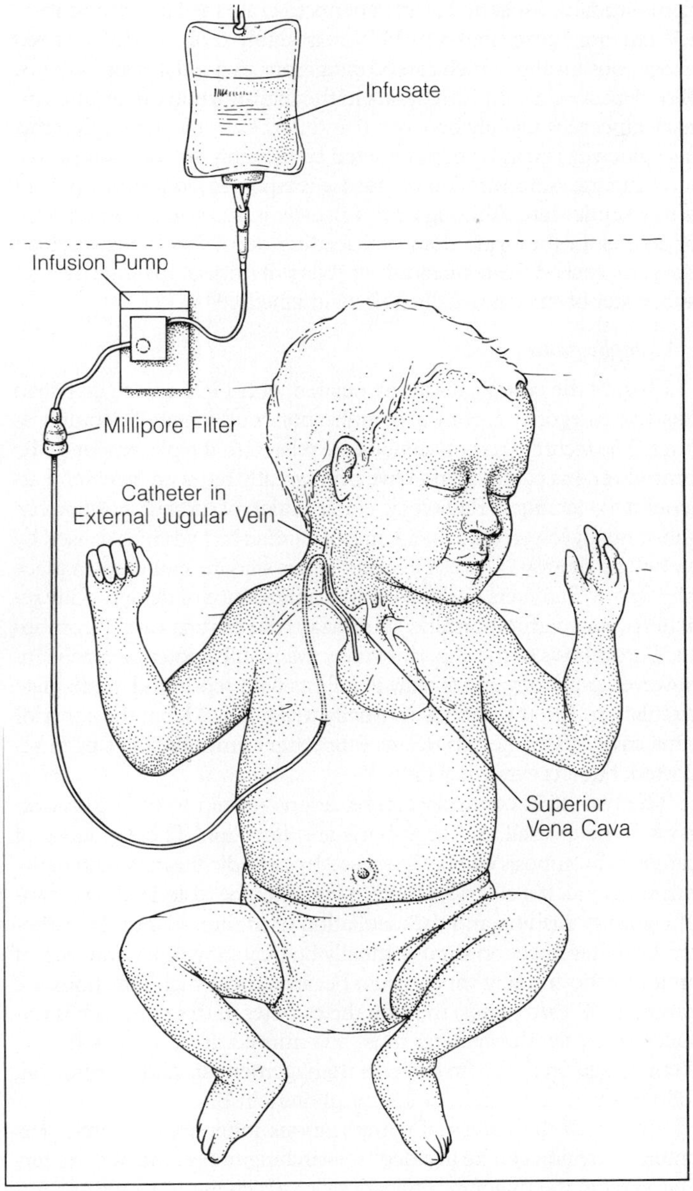

cm away, with the aim of minimizing the likelihood of bloodstream contamination from dressing changes at the skin exit site. The catheter is brought out on the chest wall, where it is easily accessible and not likely to be disrupted by an active patient. When no vein sites are available in the neck, the catheter may be placed in the external iliac vein via a cutdown on the greater saphenous vein and tunneled out on the abdominal wall.[102]

Central venous insertion by percutaneous subclavian vein puncture is often performed in older children and adults; the subclavian percutaneous technique has now been used in infants.[103] Every 48 hours, the dressing is changed aseptically, the skin is cleansed with an antiseptic, and povidone-iodine ointment is applied to the catheter skin junction to protect against bacterial and fungal infection. A millipore filter (0.22 μm) is placed in the line to remove particulate matter, such as calcium salts and microorganisms, that may have contaminated the solution. A calibrated burette is necessary for accurate monitoring of the volume delivered; it is used even when the solution is infused with a volumetric pump. To minimize the risk of infection, an alternate I.V. line should be utilized whenever possible for infusing drugs, measuring central venous pressure, sampling blood, and transfusing blood products. The infusate must be delivered at a uniform rate to ensure proper utilization of the glucose and amino acids. Currently, peripherally inserted central venous catheters (PICC lines) are increasingly being used to provide central venous parenteral nutrition to pediatric patients.

Peripheral parenteral nutrition with fat involves the insertion of a No. 21 or 23 needle into a peripheral vein (in infants, usually a scalp vein). The I.V. tubing from the bottle containing the glucose–amino acid solution is connected to the needle, and the tubing from the fat emulsion bottle is then inserted piggyback into the rubber nipple at the end of the tube from the first bottle. A calibrated burette is placed in each I.V. line, and the two bottles are infused for 24 hours with two separate constant-infusion pumps. Because the fat emulsion will not

Figure 2 Depicted is the preferred approach for central venous parenteral nutrition in infants.

serum levels of electrolytes, glucose, phosphorus, and albumin should be assessed. Serum levels of liver enzymes, bilirubin, and creatinine should be measured at the start of therapy and every 2 weeks thereafter [see Table 12].

Weight changes during TPN vary according to the patient's overall clinical status. During the first 2 weeks of therapy, significant weight gain is rarely seen in infants and children who are severely malnourished or in a septic state at the start of treatment; pathologic increases in metabolic demands, such as result from sepsis, produce a flatter growth curve. However, weight gains comparable to those seen in normal infants may be expected in patients who are not severely malnourished or in a septic state. The weight gains observed with the two I.V. nutrition techniques are comparable, averaging 15 to 25 g/day in the neonate and 0.5% of total body weight (kg)/day in older children. Greater weight gains may signal excessive fluid administration and fluid retention.

Urine output should be 1 ml/kg/hr or more, with the urine specific gravity falling between 1.005 and 1.015 in the absence of glucosuria. Positive nitrogen balance has been observed in almost all patients studied. Most pediatric patients tolerate the large amounts of I.V. glucose administered in TPN reasonably well and do not need exogenous insulin, which can be dangerous to neonates and infants. Blood glucose generally remains in the high-normal range, and urinary glucose is usually between 0 and 2+. As a rule, hyperglycemia and glucosuria can be counteracted by slowing the infusion rate or lowering the concentration of glucose temporarily, unless the patient is in a septic state. Although TPN usually induces greater excretion of solutes in the urine than oral feeding does, this increased load does not exceed the concentrating ability of normal kidneys. As a result, water balance is usually well maintained.[104,105]

Complications

Most of the complications associated with TPN can be classified into two categories: technical complications and metabolic complications. The technical complications are related to the placement of the central venous catheter and have been greatly reduced by careful attention to technique. Radiologic confirmation of catheter position has substantially lowered the incidence of cardiac arrhythmias caused by catheter irritation. The use of nonreactive silicone catheters in place of polyvinyl catheters has decreased the incidence of foreign-body reactions, vein perforation, and subclavian vein or vena caval thrombosis. Thrombosis of the superior vena cava is still a potential problem, however, especially in critically ill infants with sepsis and inadequate circulation. The thrombosis is usually well tolerated, but the superior vena cava syndrome can occur. Pulmonary embolism has been reported, but it is extremely rare.

The two most common complications related to the central venous catheter itself are thrombosis and infection. The incidence of catheter thrombosis can be decreased by periodic flushing with heparinized saline. If a clot does form, it can often be dislodged by means of vigorous flushing and the instillation of urokinase into the catheter. Catheter infection should initially be treated with I.V. infusion of an antibiotic (usually vancomycin because most such infections are caused by *S. epidermidis*) through the catheter. If this approach is unsuccessful, then the catheter must be removed. If *Candida* is the infecting organism, the first step in management should be removal, followed by 2 to 6 weeks of I.V. amphotericin B.

Almost all the technical complications inherent in central parenteral nutrition can be avoided by switching to peripheral parenteral nutrition, the major complications of which are phlebitis and superficial skin sloughing.

Almost every conceivable metabolic abnormality has been reported to occur during TPN [see Table 13]; the ones most frequently observed

Table 12 Blood Values Monitored Routinely during Total Parenteral Nutrition

Values Monitored at Start of Therapy and Weekly	Values Monitored at Start of Therapy and Every 2 Weeks	Values Monitored as Indicated
Na, K, Cl Urea Glucose Magnesium Calcium Phosphorus Albumin Hemoglobin Hematocrit White blood cell count Platelet count	AST Lactic dehydrogenase Alkaline phosphatase Bilirubin (direct/total) Creatinine	Copper Zinc Iron Ammonia Osmolarity pH

AST—aspartate aminotransferase

are hyperglycemia, hypoglycemia, hypocalcemia, hypercalcemia, hypophosphatemia, and hyperphosphatemia. As a rule, hyperglycemia is best treated by decreasing the I.V. glucose load rather than by administering insulin, especially in infants. Usually, metabolic complications can be prevented by careful attention to the nutrient content of the infusate. Now that trace element solutions are routinely administered at the beginning of therapy, deficiencies of copper and zinc are no longer seen. Likewise, routine administration of fat emulsions has eliminated the syndrome of fatty acid deficiency. Central infusion can lead to osmotic diuresis because of the high concentrations of glucose involved; premature infants, with their underdeveloped renal tubules, are most susceptible to this complication. Fluid overload in the form of pulmonary edema, peripheral edema, or congestive heart failure is rare, provided that patients are properly selected and monitored.[106] In patients with obstructed airways and compromised respiratory function, the large dextrose load provided by TPN can precipitate respiratory failure by increasing production of carbon dioxide, the elimination of which demands increased respiratory effort. If these patients are receiving ventilatory assistance, they may be difficult to wean. This complication may be resolved by decreasing the dextrose load and substituting fat calories for dextrose calories.[107]

Abnormalities in liver function, such as elevations in liver enzyme levels and serum bilirubin (both total and direct), often occur after 1 month of TPN, especially in neonates (premature neonates, in particular). These functional abnormalities result from cholestasis in the small bile ductules of the liver. If TPN is continued, the bilirubin levels, especially the direct fraction, will continue to rise, sometimes reaching 35 mg/dl (half of which is accounted for by the direct fraction). This process can result in cirrhosis and liver failure and ultimately in death. It appears that the cholestasis can be stopped and even reversed by increasing the enteral feedings, even in infants who are unable to tolerate large amounts of food given via the GI tract.[108]

Sepsis continues to be the major complication of central parenteral nutrition in infants and children. Long-term indwelling venous catheters are well-documented sources of bloodstream infection [see 81 Nosocomial Infection]. Organisms may enter the bloodstream along the catheter tract, via a contaminated I.V. solution, or may travel from a distant infected site and attach to the catheter, which serves as a foreign-body focus for bacterial growth. Placement of catheters under strict aseptic conditions, together with meticulous care of the catheter site with standardized dressing changes every other day, greatly reduces the incidence of septic complications.

Fever, leukocytosis, unexplained glucosuria, or any combination

Table 13 Potential Metabolic Complications Resulting from TPN

Electrolyte imbalance	Hyper/hyponatremia Hyper/hypokalemia Hyper/hypochloremia Hyper/hypocalcemia Hyper/hypomagnesemia Hyper/hypophosphatemia
Complications related to carbohydrate administration	Hyper/hypoglycemia Hyperosmolarity and associated osmotic diuresis with dehydration, leading to nonketotic hyperglycemic coma
Complications related to protein administration	Cholestatic jaundice Azotemia Hyperchloremic metabolic acidosis (with protein hydrolysate)
Complications related to lipid administration	Hyperlipidemia Alteration of pulmonary function Displacement of albumin-bonded bilirubin by plasma free fatty acid Overloading syndrome characterized by hyperlipidemia, fever, lethargy, liver damage, and coagulation disorders—reported in adults but rarely seen in children
Trace element deficiencies	Zinc Copper Chromium
Essential fatty acid deficiency	If lipids not used; manifested by skin rash

of these is often the first indication of catheter sepsis. Infection is confirmed by culturing microorganisms from blood obtained from the central vein through the venous line and from other venous sites. If no other site of sepsis is found, the catheter should be removed. In general, antibiotics should not be administered unless fever persists for longer than 24 hours after removal of the catheter or the patient exhibits a clinical septic response. Peripheral parenteral nutrition has the advantage of being free of most of the septic and technical complications inherent in central parenteral nutrition. In our study of 102 pediatric patients receiving peripheral parenteral nutrition, invasive sepsis was noted in none of the subjects being given fat and in only one of the infants and children not being given fat.

Complications of parenteral nutrition in infants and children are potentially numerous and frequent. Nevertheless, with careful patient selection, proper preparation of the solution, careful monitoring, and meticulous attention to technical details, the benefits of parenteral nutrition far outweigh the risks. Parenteral nutrition has been directly responsible for the survival of many infants and children who in the past would have died of malnutrition.

Special Problems

Infants with short-bowel syndrome pose an extremely difficult management problem. Great skill and patience are demanded of the surgeon, the pediatrician, the nutritionist, and the nurse. A full-term infant is born with approximately 200 cm of small intestine. Although the shortest intestinal length compatible with life has not been clearly defined, most pediatric surgeons agree that survival on oral alimentation is generally impossible when intestinal length is less than 25 to 30 cm with an intact ileocecal valve or less than 50 cm without an intact ileocecal valve. There are a few reports of infants surviving with shorter intestinal lengths, but they represent the exception rather than the rule.

Management of short-bowel syndrome is complex and not well defined. In most cases, treatment rests on a combination of parenteral nutrition, elemental diets, and predigested formulas. Regular feedings are gradually achieved during a period of several weeks to several months. Requirements for growth and development should be kept in mind at all times, and TPN with all of the necessary carbohydrate, fat, and protein calories should be provided continuously while various oral diets are being tried. The infant is gradually weaned from I.V. nutrition as the GI tract adapts to oral feedings. Because babies with short-bowel syndrome have very little tolerance for even moderately hypertonic diets, predigested formulas of high osmolarity must be administered in highly dilute form. The volume is increased gradually during a period of several days to weeks; only after sufficient volume is tolerated is the concentration slowly increased. As the infant grows, the intestine adapts by lengthening and by manifesting villous hypertrophy. It is not unusual for these infants to be hospitalized for several months to a year or even longer. During hospitalization, the infant's condition may improve or deteriorate markedly on several occasions, and it is very easy for parents and medical staff to become discouraged. Such discouragement is understandable, but it must be combated because it invariably results in decreased attention being paid to the critical details and imaginative approaches that are essential for the management of these patients. One of the most important elements of the treatment of infants with short-bowel syndrome is maintenance of high morale among the physicians, nutritionists, and nurses caring for them.

In some patients with short-bowel syndrome or inflammatory bowel disease, complete or partial parenteral nutrition may be required indefinitely. Such patients have benefited from programs designed to deliver parenteral nutrition at home. Although home parenteral nutrition has been used for several years in older children and adults [see 97 *Nutritional Support*], it has only now come to be successfully used in infants. The two main advantages of the program are (1) improved morale for the infant or child and the mother, as a result of placement in the home environment, and (2) significant reduction in cost, as a result of the patient's discharge from the hospital. It should be kept in mind, however, that considerable dedication on the part of the parents is necessary if complications are to be minimized.

Trauma

Whereas accidents are the third most common cause of death in the United States population as a whole, they are the single most common cause of death in children between 1 and 15 years of age.[109,110] Every year, about 20 million injuries occur in children, resulting in approximately 15,000 deaths and 100,000 cases of permanent disability. The consequences of permanent disability in this age group are obvious: these disabled children will place a burden on society for an additional 50 or 60 years after the accident. The first approach to be considered in managing pediatric trauma is clearly prevention; preventive efforts have in fact been gaining momentum, thanks in part to support from federal funds. These efforts have included greater emphasis on the use of pediatric restraint devices in automobiles, the wearing of crash helmets by bicycle and motorcycle riders, improvements in the design of space heaters, the use of fire-retardant material for children's clothes (as dictated by the Flammable Fabrics Act), the proper packing and labeling of poisons and medications, and the installation of proper fencing around swimming pools.

GENERAL PRINCIPLES OF CARE IN CHILDREN

Although the general principles of trauma care are essentially the same for children as for adults, there are several significant differences

Blunt Trauma in Children

Initial resuscitation of children suffering from blunt trauma is no different from that of their adult counterparts. It is important, however, to keep in mind that the vital signs of children are different: blood pressures are lower, and heart rates are higher.

If the child is hemodynamically stable, a nasogastric tube should be inserted early in the course of evaluation because of the high incidence of gastric dilatation after severe trauma in this age group. If severe head injury is present, physical examination of the abdomen is not very reliable. If auscultation of the lungs yields abnormal findings, an immediate portable chest x-ray is helpful for determining whether a pneumothorax is present before more complicated diagnostic studies are initiated. If hypotension is present, the first fluid to be infused should be lactated Ringer solution in a bolus of 20 ml/kg. Cervical spine x-rays should be obtained as well.

Once the child is hemodynamically stable and is receiving ventilatory support through an endotracheal tube, definitive evaluation of the intra-abdominal injuries can be performed. I prefer to assess such injuries with a total-body CT scan because I prefer to manage intra-abdominal solid visceral injuries nonoperatively. Nonoperative management of childhood liver and spleen injuries has been shown to be safe and effective in pediatric trauma centers throughout the world. CT scanning can accurately define injuries to the liver and spleen and precisely estimate the volume of fluid in the peritoneal cavity.

There arises the question of what to do if blood is detected in the peritoneal cavity. Given this finding in adults, most surgeons would proceed to laparotomy. In some cases, the bleeding may have stopped at the time of laparotomy. If the bleeding is restarted in an attempt to determine the extent of the injuries to the spleen, it may not be controllable with suture techniques. If a fractured spleen is discovered at the time of laparotomy, there should be a vigorous attempt to save the spleen with whatever technique is required. Sometimes, however, salvage is not possible, and a splenectomy must be carried out to control the bleeding. If the spleen had not been manipulated at the time of laparotomy, it probably would have healed on its own postoperatively. The risks of infection after splenectomy, especially in the child, are well known. They may be managed with administration of Pneumovax and the prophylactic use of oral penicillin.

It is not known how long it actually takes a fractured liver or spleen to heal. Usually, a CT scan at 3 months shows complete healing of these two organs. For that reason, I generally recommend abstinence from contact sports for 3 months after an injury.

Patient presents with history of blunt trauma
Perform physical examination.
Provide initial care:
- Airway
- Resuscitation

Perform initial tests:
- Chest x-ray
- Cervical spine x-rays
- CT scan

Perform laparotomy
Criteria for operation:
- Hemodynamic instability
- Intestinal perforation

Observe patient (in facility with pediatric ICU)
Criteria for operation:
- Development of hemodynamic instability after stabilization
- Continued unexplained blood loss
- Development of peritonitis

---

that must be taken into account in the care of pediatric accident victims.[111-116] For example, children do not react to trauma in the same way as adults. They often have difficulty in expressing pain and in articulating their complaints. They are often extremely frightened after an accident, and this fear may cause them to give misleading signals—for instance, by exhibiting signs of an acute abdomen even though no intra-abdominal injury has occurred. Children who experience stress often undergo developmental regression, typically accompanied by severe depression. All these psychological factors must be taken into account in treatment of a pediatric accident victim.

Another key difference between children and adults is that children are still growing. Postoperative metabolic management after any form of stress, whether it is a surgical procedure, trauma, or some other event, must take this difference into account. A small blood loss that is insignificant in an adult can result in marked hemodynamic changes in a small child. Moreover, water and heat loss can be far greater in small children than in older children and adults because of their greater surface area relative to their weight and their relative lack of insulating subcutaneous fat. Hypothermia aggravates acidosis and makes hemodynamic resuscitation much more difficult. Gastric dilatation, which can result in vomiting and pulmonary aspiration, is very common in young children after all forms of trauma. Finally, the nutritional requirements of injured children are greater than those of adults because children, as growing organisms, naturally have a high metabolic rate. Consequently, TPN often must be started earlier in a child than it would be in an adult in a comparable condition.

Not only are there significant physiologic and psychological differences between children and adults after trauma, there are also differences in accident pattern. Most childhood injuries result from blunt trauma [see Sidebar Blunt Trauma in Children], whereas in adults, blunt trauma is no more common than penetrating trauma.[117] More specifically, head trauma is far more common in children than in adults; in fact, it accounts for most of the morbidity and mortality in the pediatric population. After motor vehicle accidents, which are the major cause of trauma in both children and adults, the next most frequent causes of trauma in children are events that are less important causes in adults: falls, bicycle accidents, drownings, poisonings, and burns from fires. Child abuse and birth trauma are unique and important causes of trauma in children.

Pediatric accident victims must be treated in centers experienced in the care of traumatized children [see Table 14]. Such centers must have an emergency department with a section that is specifically set aside for the care of children and is staffed by nurses and physicians experienced in the management of pediatric trauma. They must have a hospital with a pediatric ICU that is also staffed with experienced medical and paramedical personnel. Finally, they must have a transportation system capable of rapidly transporting critically ill pediatric trauma victims both by air and by land or water.

EMERGENCY MANAGEMENT

As in emergency management of an adult, the first priority in emergency management of an injured child is to ensure and maintain an adequate airway. If the child has several injuries, the neck must be stabilized before assessment of the airway in case the cervical spine has been injured (although this type of injury rarely happens). Stabilization can be accomplished with a collar or with sandbags placed on either side of the neck. The airway must be cleared of regurgitated food, blood, or broken teeth. In some circumstances, it may be appropriate to try an oral airway; in general, however, it is best to proceed immediately to oral tracheal intubation [see Table 4]. While the necessary preparations are being made, the airway can be improved by pulling the chin forward, and oxygenation can be improved by administering oxygen through an oral or nasal cannula.

As a rule, uncuffed endotracheal tubes are used. The tube size can be estimated from the size of the child's fifth fingernail or from visual measurements [see Table 4]. It is rare that an emergency tracheostomy must be performed in a child in the ED, except when severe facial trauma is present, in which case it is preferable to insert a No. 14 plastic catheter through the cricothyroid membrane and then to proceed to the OR for a tracheostomy under controlled conditions if the patient is otherwise stable.[118] If respiration continues to be labored after an endotracheal tube has been placed, pneumothorax is a strong possibility. Unfortunately, pneumothorax is difficult to diagnose clinically in a young child because breath sounds are so easily transmitted; an immediate portable chest x-ray will help make the diagnosis. The first step in treatment of pneumothorax is the insertion of a plastic cannula into the chest. Later, under more elective conditions, a chest tube can be placed. Hyperventilation is a common response to stress in all age groups, especially in children, and it often results in rapid gastric dilatation, which can be managed easily with the insertion of a nasogastric tube.

Once respiration is under control, I.V. access must be established. Such access is often difficult to achieve when a needle is percutaneously placed into a peripheral vein in a child because the vein is small and becomes markedly vasoconstricted in the presence of hypovolemia. If a needle cannot be rapidly inserted into a peripheral vein, then a cutdown into the greater saphenous vein at the ankle should be performed. An alternative is to insert an interosseous needle into the tibia to begin fluid resuscitation.

Initially, superficial bleeding can be managed by simple pressure on the site of injury or laceration. Large scalp lacerations can lead to significant blood loss; therefore, it is important to place pressure on such lacerations early in the management of the traumatized child.

Almost all cases of shock in traumatized children following an accident are related to hemorrhage. Therefore, shock should be treated initially with relatively rapid infusion of 20 ml/kg of a crystalloid solution such as lactated Ringer solution or normal saline, to which should be added 2 mEq/kg of sodium bicarbonate to correct any acidosis that may be present. If shock continues, a second infusion of crystalloid should be given, followed by uncrossed O negative blood if there is no response. Once hemodynamic stability is established, a Foley catheter should be inserted, and insertion of a central venous line and an arterial catheter should be considered. A stable patient in whom operative intervention is not contemplated should be transferred to a pediatric ICU, where monitoring will be continued. In general, central venous pressure or, if a Swan-Ganz catheter has been inserted, PAWP should be maintained between 5 and 10 mm Hg.

ABDOMINAL TRAUMA

Abdominal trauma in children is usually blunt. Penetrating injuries occur in only about 20% of children who sustain trauma and are managed in essentially the same way in children as in adults [see III Trauma and Thermal Injury].

Children who sustain major trauma often suffer intra-abdominal injury. Because gastric dilatation and reflex ileus are far more common in children than in adults after a major injury, the initial clinical evaluation of the child's abdomen may be highly misleading. The early insertion of a nasogastric tube will decompress the stomach and allow more accurate physical examination of the abdomen. In addition, decompression of the stomach with a nasogastric tube will reduce the risk of aspiration pneumonitis. Once the child is stable

Table 14 Pediatric Trauma Score

	Coded Value
Size	
> 20 kg	+2
10–20 kg	+1
< 10 kg	−1
Airway	
Normal	+2
Maintainable	+1
Not maintainable	−1
Systolic Blood Pressure	
> 90 mm Hg	+2
50–90 mm Hg	+1
< 50 mm Hg	−1
In the absence of proper size BP cuff, assess BP by assigning these values:	
Pulse palpable at wrist	+2
Pulse palpable at groin	+1
Pulse not palpable	−1
Central Nervous System Status	
Awake	+2
Partially conscious or unconscious	+1
Comatose or decerebrate	−1
Open Wounds	
None	+2
Minor	+1
Major	−1
Skeletal Injury	
None	+2
Closed fracture	+1
Open/multiple fractures	−1
Score	−6 to +12
Scoring triage criterion for direct transport of the patient to a trauma center	< 9

from a hemodynamic and respiratory point of view, the abdomen should be carefully examined for external evidence of trauma, such as ecchymoses, abrasions, and tire tracks. The abdomen should then be carefully and gently palpated; the examiner should keep in mind that a frightened child will tend to tighten his or her rectus muscles in a way that gives a false impression of intra-abdominal injury. Serial abdominal examinations are essential.

Although peritoneal lavage is an acceptable diagnostic tool for the evaluation of a child with blunt abdominal trauma,[119-121] most pediatric surgeons now prefer to proceed directly to computed tomography of the abdomen, especially when the child has suffered from severe head injuries, which almost always require a CT scan for complete evaluation.[122] The CT scan is extremely accurate in the evaluation of liver and spleen injuries and in the determination of the amount of blood in the peritoneal cavity [see Figures 3 and 4]. The CT scan is also useful for detecting pneumoperitoneum resulting from perforation of the intestine.

Because hollow viscus injury is extremely uncommon in children after blunt abdominal trauma, nonoperative treatment is the accepted method of management for most liver and spleen injuries. Although associated fractures of the lower ribs are fairly common in adults with liver and spleen injuries, they are rare in children with such injuries.[123]

The initial plain film of the abdomen will often demonstrate medial and inferior displacement of the gastric bubble caused by an accumulation of blood under the left diaphragm. A CT scan will then accurately confirm the diagnosis of a splenic injury. CT scanning has the additional advantage of allowing postoperative follow-up of the healing of the splenic injury.[124,125] A major reason why nonoperative treatment is recommended for pediatric splenic injuries is that the risk of overwhelming postsplenectomy infection (OPSI) is far higher in children than in adults[126]; the younger the child, the higher the risk of OPSI. OPSI develops in 1.5% of splenectomized patients and carries a mortality of 25% to 50%.

The only type of liver trauma that necessitates surgery is that associated with injury to the hepatic veins or inferior vena cava.[127] Injury to these vascular structures is usually obvious: the patient will hemorrhage extensively into the peritoneal cavity or retroperitoneum and will be hemodynamically highly unstable, even after receiving massive transfusions.

Once a liver or spleen injury has been diagnosed, the child should immediately be transferred to a pediatric ICU staffed with experienced medical and paramedical personnel. The child should remain in the ICU for 2 or 3 days and on bed rest on the hospital ward for the rest of the week; however, some authorities currently advocate earlier discharge for patients with lesser splenic injuries. If hemodynamic instability persists despite significant transfusion of blood, exploratory laparotomy will be necessary.[128] Fortunately, this situation is extremely unusual; in fact, in our institution, we have never had to take a child to the OR for a liver or spleen injury after admission to the ICU.[129] If laparotomy is necessary, the liver and spleen should be repaired. Most liver lacerations can be simply debrided and drained, and most splenic lacerations, even lacerations through the hilum of the spleen, can be repaired with absorbable sutures.

Among the less common injuries to intra-abdominal organs that occur in children are perforation of the stomach when an accident has occurred shortly after eating and the stomach is distended; perforation of the small intestine and large intestine at points of fixation, such as the ligament of Treitz and the cecum; rupture of the left diaphragm; and damage to the duodenum and pancreas. Retroperitoneal perforation of the duodenum can result from blunt abdominal trauma; it is often suggested by the presence of air around the right kidney on a plain abdominal x-ray. Traumatic pancreatitis can be diagnosed by an elevation in serum amylase and lipase levels and by the presence of pancreatic edema on ultrasonography and CT scan. Obviously, perforations of the stomach, the intestine, and the duodenum call for exploratory laparotomy and, in most cases, simple suture repair of the laceration. Traumatic pancreatitis, on the other hand, can usually be managed nonoperatively with nasogastric decompression and I.V. fluids. Fracture of the pancreatic duct is usually secondary to compression of the pancreas against the vertebral column and is quite rare in children.[130] This injury necessitates exploratory laparotomy and distal pancreatectomy with suture closure of the proximal pancreatic duct; however, more recent experience indicates that it can often be successfully treated nonoperatively, though there is a risk that pseudocysts will subsequently develop. Intramural duodenal hematoma is relatively uncommon in children and is usually well managed by nasogastric decompression for about 10 days and institution of TPN.[131]

In the assessment of the child with abdominal trauma, the diagnosis of a pelvic fracture should be seriously considered. Pelvic fractures can result in significant bleeding into the retroperitoneum, in addition to injuries to the bladder and urethra.[132] The diagnosis can be confirmed by x-ray studies of the pelvis. In most cases, the fracture can be treated with bed rest, immobilization, and the replacement of blood loss.

Unless they have sustained head injuries, children with blunt multisystem injuries rarely die if they are alive when brought to an ED.

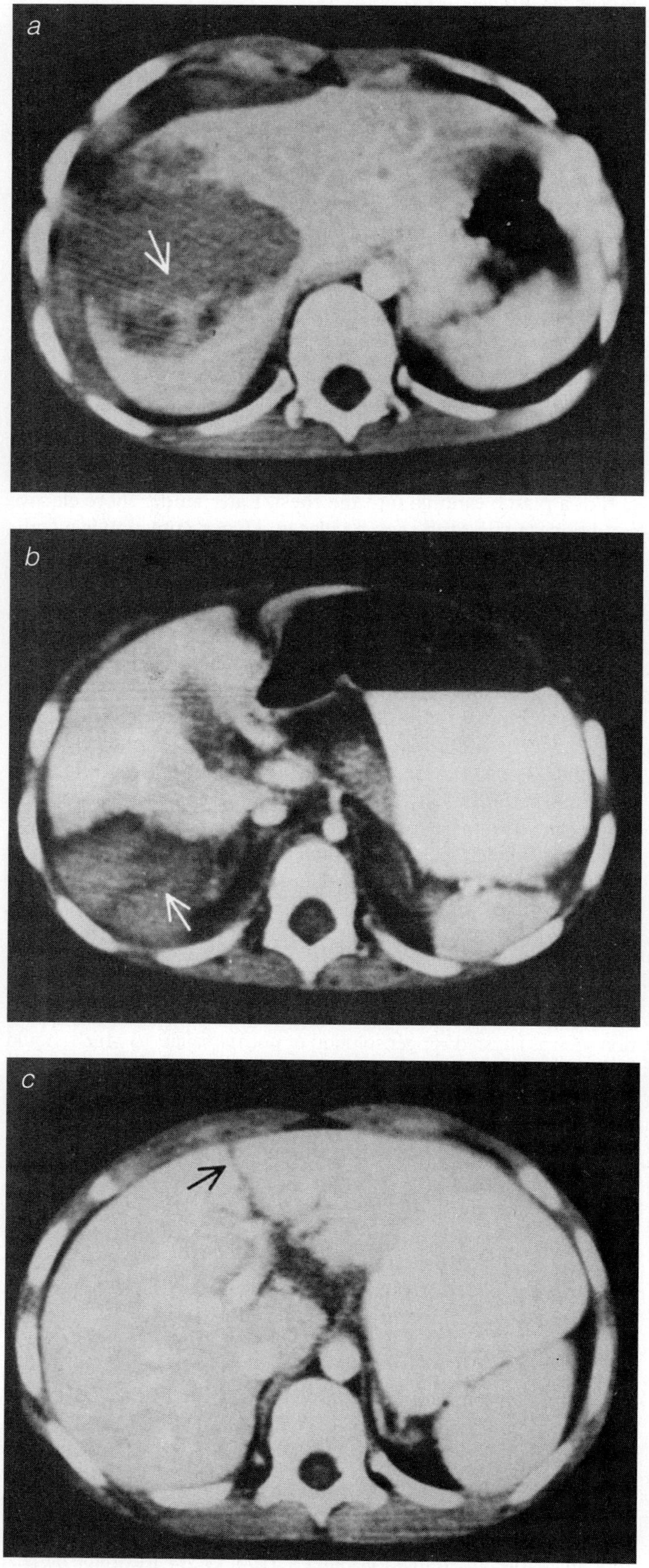

Figure 3 These three CT scans of children's livers were obtained after blunt abdominal trauma. In *a* and *b*, the areas of radiolucency in the right lobe of the liver (arrows) represent trauma to the liver. In *c*, note the crack at the level of the falciform ligament (arrow), with blood in the porta hepatis.

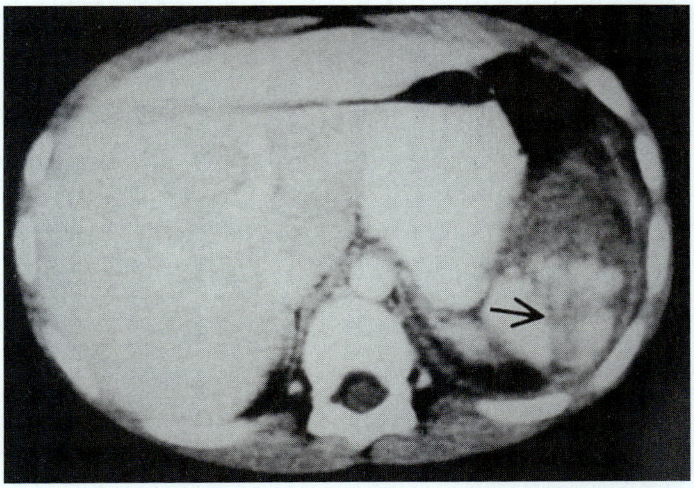

Figure 4 This CT scan was obtained after blunt abdominal trauma in a child. Note several large cracks in the spleen (arrow).

Care of these patients requires aggressive, coordinated efforts on the part of a multispecialty team under the direction of a pediatric surgeon. The evolution of specifically designated pediatric trauma centers around the country was one of the most important developments in the care of children to occur in the 1980s.

CHILD ABUSE

One of the unique varieties of pediatric trauma is child abuse or the battered-child syndrome. Although the exact incidence of child abuse is not known, it is thought that about 50,000 to 100,000 children are abused in the United States every year.[133] In most cases, the children come from a low socioeconomic background and their parents are very young.[112,114,134-136] The children tend to be younger than 2 years, except when sexual abuse is involved, in which case the average age is about 10 years. The abuse can take many different forms, such as physical or mental injury, nutritional or hygienic neglect, delayed or inadequate treatment of disease, sexual abuse, or verbal abuse. Clues to the diagnosis include a marked delay in seeking medical help on the part of the parents, poor hygiene in the child, and marked depression and lack of emotion in the child. The injuries most commonly seen are soft tissue injuries, burns, fractures, and head trauma. X-ray evidence of healing fractures of different ages, a finding described in 1946,[137] is strong evidence of child abuse. Visceral injuries, including liver fractures, splenic fractures, duodenal hematomas, and pancreatic fractures, also occur, although less frequently.

Once a physician suspects child abuse, he or she is both legally and ethically obliged to report the situation to the appropriate team in the hospital dealing with these problems. The typical hospital team usually includes a physician, a social worker, and a nurse. Prompt and full reporting often makes it more likely that the parents will receive positive counseling, which may well reduce their subsequent abuse of the child.

BIRTH TRAUMA

About 0.5% of all births result in trauma to the neonate; in general, larger infants are at greater risk.[138-140] However, routine use of prenatal ultrasonography has reduced the incidence of birth trauma because those infants ascertained to be at risk are now delivered by cesarean section. The injuries typically associated with birth trauma are fractures, nerve injuries, and visceral injuries to the liver, spleen, and adrenal glands.[141-143] Full-term infants are generally at greater risk than premature infants, and infants with preexisting anomalies, such as hydronephrotic kidneys, are at still greater risk.[144]

The fracture most commonly seen is that of the clavicle, usually caused by shoulder dystocia. Treatment is usually expectant because displacement is rare. Fractures in the humerus or the femur are less common and are often epiphyseal.

Peripheral facial nerve paralysis sometimes occurs, generally as a result of direct pressure against the infant's face from the mother's pelvis.[145] Complete recovery is usual by 1 year of age. Erb-Duchenne paralysis, or upper brachial plexus palsy, is usually secondary to shoulder dystocia or breech presentation. This injury results in lack of shoulder motion and winging of the scapula, with no evidence of motor or sensory dysfunction in the hand. The upper arm tends to be abducted, and the forearm cannot be supinated.[146] Klumpke's paralysis, or lower brachial plexus palsy, produces sensory deficits and an ipsilateral Horner's syndrome as a result of damage to the sympathetic fibers of the first thoracic root. In about 5% of cases of Erb-Duchenne paralysis, there is an associated phrenic nerve paralysis resulting in elevation of the ipsilateral diaphragm.

Hemoperitoneum can occur during birth as a result of fracture of the liver, the spleen, or the adrenal gland caused by direct pressure from the birth canal against the newborn's abdomen.[147,148] In these three instances, nonoperative management is appropriate. The baby should be stabilized with blood transfusions and observed. In almost all cases, the bleeding will stop, and no operative intervention will be required. Fracture of the kidneys is extremely rare but has been reported.

Direct birth trauma can disrupt some of the fibers of the sternocleidomastoid muscle, which leads to formation of a hematoma and eventually to a torticollis.[149] Passive and active exercises bring about complete recovery in most infants, although surgical correction is occasionally necessary if recognition of the condition is delayed for any reason.

Pharyngeal or cervical esophageal perforation can occur after a breech delivery, usually because the physician's finger was placed in the baby's mouth. This injury is usually well handled by placing a nasogastric tube, instituting I.V. antibiotics, and giving the baby nothing orally.

References

1. Coran AG: Perioperative care of the pediatric patient (pt 1). Surg Annu 23:31, 1991
2. Adams JM, Rudolph AJ: The use of indwelling radial artery catheters in neonates. Pediatrics 55:261, 1975
3. Barr PA, Sumners J, Wirtschafter D, et al: Percutaneous peripheral arterial cannulation in the neonate. Pediatrics 59(suppl 6):1058, 1977
4. Groff DB, Ahmed N: Subclavian vein catheterization in the infant. J Pediatr Surg 9:171, 1974
5. Hall D, Geefhuysen J: Percutaneous catheterization of the internal jugular vein in infants and children. J Pediatr Surg 12:719, 1977
6. James P: Central venous cannulation. J Pediatr Surg 13:107, 1977
7. Pollock MM, Reed TP, Holbrook PR, et al: Bedside pulmonary artery catheterization in pediatrics. J Pediatr 96:274, 1980
8. Todres ID, Crone RK, Rogers MC, et al: Swan-Ganz catheterization in the critically ill newborn. Crit Care Med 7:330, 1979
9. Wetxel RC, Rogers MC: Pediatric monitoring. Textbook of Critical Care. Shoemaker WC, Thompson WL, Holbrook PR, Eds. WB Saunders Co, Philadelphia, 1984, p 136
10. Wesley JR, Coran AG: Infants and children. Treatment of Shock: Principles and Practice, 2nd ed. Barrett J, Nyhus LM, Eds. Lea & Febiger, Philadelphia, 1986, p 211
11. Holcroft JW, Trunkey DD, Carpenter MA: Extravasation of albumin in tissues of normal and septic baboons and sheep. J Surg Res 26:341, 1979

12. Lillihei RC, Longerbeam JK, Boch JH, et al: The nature of irreversible shock: experimental and clinical observations. Ann Surg 160:682, 1964
13. Spink WW, Weil MH, Melby JC, et al: Clinical experience with corticoids in shock. Corticosteroids in the Treatment of Shock. Schumer W, Nyhus LM, Eds. University of Illinois Press, Urbana, 1970
14. Pierce CH, Briggs BT, Gutelius JR: Methylprednisolone and phenoxybenzamine in experimental cardiovascular dynamics and platelet function. Shock in Low Flow States. Forscher BK, Lillehei RC, Stubbs SS, Eds. Excerpta Medica, Amsterdam, 1972
15. Sambhi MP, Weil MH, Udhoji VN: Acute pharmacodynamic effects of glucocorticoids: cardiac output and related hemodynamic changes in normal subjects and patients in shock. Circulation 31:523, 1965
16. Thomas CS Jr, Brockman SK: The role of adrenal corticosteroid therapy in Escherichia coli endotoxin shock. Surg Gynecol Obstet 126:61, 1968
17. Hinshaw LB, Beller-Todd BK, Archer LT: Current management of the septic shock patient: experimental basis for treatment. Circ Shock 9:543, 1982
18. Schumer W: Steroids in the treatment of clinical septic shock. Ann Surg 184:333, 1976
19. Lucas CE, Ledgerwood AM: The cardiopulmonary response to massive doses of steroids in patients with septic shock. Arch Surg 119:537, 1984
20. Sprung CL, Caralis PV, Marcial EH, et al: The effects of high-dose corticosteroids in patients with septic shock: a prospective controlled study. N Engl J Med 311:1137, 1984
21. Connors RH, Coran AG, Drongowski RA, et al: Combined fluid and corticosteroid therapy in septic shock in puppies. World J Surg 7:661, 1983
22. Chatterjee K: Digitalis versus newer inotropic agents: which to use? Drug Ther 13:77, 1983
23. Goldberg LI: Cardiovascular and renal actions of dopamine: potential clinical applications. Pharmacol Rev 24:1, 1972
24. Goldberg LI: Dopamine—clinical uses of an endogenous catecholamine. N Engl J Med 291:707, 1974
25. Herbert P, Tinker J: Inotropic drugs in acute circulatory failure. Intensive Care Med 6:101, 1980
26. Latts JR, Goldberg LI: Dopamine in the management of shock. Drug Ther 4:25, 1979
27. Loeb HS, Winslow EBJ, Rahimtoola SH, et al: Acute hemodynamic effects of dopamine in patients in shock. Circulation 44:163, 1971
28. Rosenblum R, Tai AR, Lawson D: Dopamine in man: cardiorenal hemodynamics in normotensive patients with heart disease. J Pharmacol Exp Ther 183:256, 1972
29. Friis-Hansen B: The extracellular fluid volume in infants and children. Acta Paediatr 43:444, 1954
30. Friis-Hansen B: Changes in body water compartments during growth. Acta Paediatr [suppl] 207:1, 1957
31. Friis-Hansen B, Holiday M, Stapleton T, et al: Total body water in children. Pediatrics 7:321, 1951
32. Friis-Hansen B: Body water compartments in children: changes during growth and related changes in body composition. Pediatrics 28:169, 1961
33. Friis-Hansen B: Body composition during growth: in vivo measurements and biochemical data correlated to differential anatomical growth. Pediatrics 47:264, 1971
34. Friis-Hansen B: Water distribution in the foetus and newborn infant. Acta Paediatr Scand [Suppl] 305:7, 1983
35. Coran AG, Drongowski RA: Body fluid compartment changes following neonatal surgery. J Pediatr Surg 24:829, 1989
36. Bell EF, Warburton D, Stonestreet BS, et al: High-volume fluid intake predisposes premature infants to necrotising enterocolitis. Lancet 2:90, 1979
37. Stevenson JG: Fluid administration in the association of patent ductus arteriosus complicating respiratory distress syndrome. J Pediatr 90:257, 1977
38. Bell EF, Warburton D, Stonestreet BS, et al: Effect of fluid administration on the development of symptomatic patent ductus arteriosus and congestive heart failure in premature infants. N Engl J Med 302:598, 1980
39. Aperia A, Broberger O, Herin P, et al: Postnatal control of water and electrolyte homeostasis in pre-term and full-term infants. Acta Paediatr Scand [Suppl] 305:61, 1983
40. Aperia A, Broberger O, Thodenius K, et al: Renal control of sodium and fluid balance in newborn infants during intravenous maintenance therapy. Acta Paediatr Scand 64:725, 1975
41. Doyle LW, Sinclair JC: Insensible water loss in newborn infants. Clin Perinatol 9:453, 1982
42. Hammarlund K, Nilsson GE, Oberg PA, et al: Transepidermal water loss in newborn infants: I. Relation to ambient humidity and site of measurement and estimation of total transepidermal water loss. Acta Paediatr Scand 66:553, 1977
43. Baumgart S, Engle WD, Fox WW, et al: Radiant warmer power and body size as determinants of insensible water loss in the critically ill neonate. Pediatr Res 15:1495, 1981
44. Bell EF, Weinstein MR, Oh W: Heat balance in premature infants: comparative effects of convectively heated incubator and radiant warmer with and without plastic heat shield. J Pediatr 96:460, 1980
45. Engle WD, Baumgart S, Fox WW, et al: Effect of increased radiant warmer power output on state of hydration in the critically ill neonate. Crit Care Med 10:673, 1982
46. Oh W, Karecki H: Phototherapy and insensible water loss in the newborn infant. Am J Dis Child 124:230, 1972
47. Tan KI, Jacob E: Effect of phototherapy on neonatal fluid and electrolyte status. Acta Pediatr Hung 22:187, 1981
48. Bell EF, Neidich GA, Cashore WJ, et al: Combined effect of radiant warmer and phototherapy on insensible water loss in low-birth-weight infants. J Pediatr 94:810, 1979
49. Engel WD, Baumgart S, Schwartz JG, et al: Insensible water loss in the critically ill neonate: combined effect of radiant-warmer power and phototherapy. Am J Dis Child 135:516, 1981
50. Sosulski R, Polin RA, Baumgart S: Respiratory water loss and heat balance in intubated infants receiving humidified air. J Pediatr 103:307, 1983
51. Saigal S, Sinclair JC: Urine solute excretion in growing low-birth-weight infants. J Pediatr 90:934, 1977
52. Brook I, Barrett CT, Brinkman CR III, et al: Aerobic and anaerobic bacterial flora of the maternal cervix and newborn gastric fluid and conjunctiva: a prospective study. Pediatrics 63:451, 1979
53. Van Camp J, Drongowski RA, Gorman R, et al: Colonization of intestinal bacteria in the normal neonate: comparison between mouth and rectal swabs and small and large bowel specimens. Surg Forum 44:627, 1993
54. Van Camp J, Drongowski RA, Gorman R, et al: Colonization of intestinal bacteria in the normal neonate: comparison between mouth and rectal swabs and small and large bowel specimens. J Pediatr Surg 29:1366, 1994
55. Long SS, Swenson RM: Development of anaerobic fecal flora in healthy newborn infants. J Pediatr 91:298, 1977
56. Goldman DA, Leclair J, Macone A: Bacterial colonization of neonates admitted to an intensive care environment. J Pediatr 93:288, 1978
57. Lawrence G, Bates J, Gaul A: Pathogenesis of neonatal necrotising enterocolitis. Lancet 1:137, 1982
58. Van Camp J, Tomaselli V, Coran AG: Intestinal bacterial translocation in the newborn. Curr Opin Pediatr 6:327, 1994
59. Walker WA: Gastrointestinal host defense: importance of gut closure in control of macromolecular transport. Ciba Found Symp 70:201, 1979
60. Lelli JL Jr, Drongowski RA, Coran AG, et al: Hypoxia-induced bacterial translocation in the puppy. J Pediatr Surg 27:974, 1992
61. Barlow B, Santulli TV, Heird WC, et al: An experimental study of acute neonatal enterocolitis—the importance of breast milk. J Pediatr Surg 9:587, 1974
62. Noel GJ, Edelson PJ: Staphylococcus epidermidis bacteremia in neonates: further observations and the occurrence of focal infection. Pediatrics 74:832, 1984
63. Scherer LR, West KW, Weber TR, et al: Staphylococcus epidermidis sepsis in pediatric patients: clinical and therapeutic considerations. J Pediatr Surg 19:358, 1984
64. Siegel JD, McCracken GH: Sepsis neonatorum. N Engl J Med 304:642, 1981
65. Rowe MI, Buckner DM, Newmark S: The early diagnosis of gram-negative septicemia in the pediatric surgical patient. Ann Surg 182:280, 1975
66. Freedman RM, Ingram DL, Gross I, et al: A half century of neonatal sepsis at Yale: 1928–1978. Am J Dis Child 135:140, 1981
67. Bell MJ, Ternberg JL, Bower RJ: The microbial flora and antimicrobial therapy of neonatal peritonitis. J Pediatr Surg 15:569, 1980
68. Stone HH, Strom PR, Fabian TC, et al: Third-generation cephalosporins for polymicrobial surgical sepsis. Arch Surg 118:193, 1983
69. Fry DE: Third generation cephalosporin antibiotics in surgical practice. Am J Surg 151:306, 1986
70. Burke JF: The effective period of preventive antibiotic action in experimental incisions and dermal lesions. Surgery 50:161, 1961
71. Rifkin GD, Fekety RF, Silva J Jr, et al: Antibiotic-induced colitis: implication of a toxin neutralised by Clostridium sordellii antitoxin. Lancet 2:1103, 1977
72. Bartlett JG, Chang TW, Gurwith M, et al: Antibiotic-associated pseudomembranous colitis due to toxin-producing clostridia. N Engl J Med 298:531, 1978
73. Shapiro BA, Harrison RA, Trout CA: Clinical Application of Respiratory Care, 2nd ed. Year Book Medical Publishers, Chicago, 1979, p 139
74. Sjostrand U, Borg U, Eriksson I: Minor circulatory interference and improved alveolar gas distribution during continuous positive-pressure ventilation by means of high ventilatory frequency and ventilatory system of negligible compression volume (abstr). Excerpta Medica International Congress Series 452:516, 1978
75. Kirby RR, Downs JB, Civetta JM, et al: High level positive end expiratory pressure (PEEP) in acute respiratory insufficiency. Chest 67:156, 1975
76. Holzman BH, Scott GB: Control of infection and techniques of isolation in the pediatric intensive care unit. Pediatr Clin North Am 28:703, 1981
77. Merrit RJ, Suskind RM: Nutritional survey of hospitalized pediatric patients. Am J Clin Nutr 32:1320, 1979
78. Dechert R, Wesley J, Schafer L, et al: Comparison of oxygen consumption, carbon dioxide production, and resting energy expenditure in premature and full-term infants. J Pediatr Surg 20:792, 1985
79. Dechert RE, Wesley JR, Schafer LE, et al: A water-sealed indirect calorimeter for measurement of oxygen consumption (VO_2), carbon dioxide production (VCO_2), and energy expenditure in infants. JPEN J Parenter Enteral Nutr 12:256, 1988
80. Mendeloff E, Wesley JR, Dechert RE, et al: Comparison of measured resting energy expenditure (REE) versus estimated energy expenditure (EEE) in infants. JPEN J Parenter Enteral Nutr (in press)
81. Moore FD: Metabolic Care of the Surgical Patient. WB Saunders Co, Philadelphia, 1959
82. Rickham PP: The Metabolic Response to Neonatal Surgery. Harvard University Press, Cambridge, Mass, 1957
83. Knutrud O: The water and electrolyte metabolism in the newborn child after major surgery: with special reference to the potassium, phosphorus and magne-

sium metabolism. Norwegian Monographs on Medical Science, Oslo, 1965
84. Schmeling DJ, Coran AG: The hormonal and metabolic response to stress in the neonate. Pediatr Surg Int 5:307, 1990
85. Schmeling DJ, Coran AG: Hormonal and metabolic response to operative stress in the neonate. JPEN J Parenter Enteral Nutr 15:215, 1991
86. Coran AG, Pierro A, Schmeling DJ: Metabolism of the neonate requiring surgery. Principles of Perinatal and Neonatal Metabolism. Cowett RM, Ed. Springer-Verlag, New York, 1996, p 1131
87. Benner JW, Coran AG, Weintraub WH, et al: The importance of different calorie sources in the intravenous nutrition of infants and children. Surgery 86:429, 1979
88. Heymsfield SB, Bethel RA, Ansley JO, et al: Enteral hyperalimentation: an alternative to central venous hyperalimentation. Ann Intern Med 90:63, 1979
89. Johnson LR, Copeland EM, Dudrick SJ, et al: Structural and hormonal alterations in the gastrointestinal tract of parenterally fed rats. Gastroenterology 68:1177, 1975
90. Stephens RV, Randall HT: Use of the concentrated, balanced, liquid elemental diet for nutritional management of catabolic states. Ann Surg 170:642, 1969
91. Helfrick FW, Abelson NM: Intravenous feeding of a complete diet in a child: report of a case. J Pediatr 25:400, 1944
92. Lee HA: Parenteral Nutrition in Acute Metabolic Illness. Academic Press, Inc, San Diego, 1974, p 3
93. Coran AG: The long-term intravenous feeding of infants using peripheral veins. J Pediatr Surg 8:801, 1973
94. Coran AG: Total intravenous feeding of infants and children without the use of a central venous catheter. Ann Surg 179:445, 1974
95. Coran AG: Lipids. Intravenous Feeding of the Neonate. Yu VYH, MacMahon RA, Eds. Edward Arnold, Melbourne, 1992, p 50
96. Dudrick SJ, Wilmore DW, Vars HM, et al: Long-term total parenteral nutrition with growth, development, and positive nitrogen balance. Surgery 64:134, 1968
97. Dudrick SJ, Wilmore DW, Vars HM, et al: Can intravenous feeding as the sole means of nutrition support growth in the child and restore weight loss in an adult: an affirmative answer. Ann Surg 169:974, 1969
98. Filler RM, Eraklis AJ, Rubin VG, et al: Long-term parenteral nutrition in infants. N Engl J Med 281:589, 1969
99. Heird WC, Winters RW: Total parenteral nutrition: the state of the art. J Pediatr 86:2, 1975
100. Wesley JR, Coran AG: Intravenous nutrition for the pediatric patient. Semin Pediatr Surg 1:212, 1992
101. Coran AG, Drongowski RA: Studies on the toxicity and efficacy of a new amino acid solution in pediatric parenteral nutrition. JPEN J Parenter Enteral Nutr 11:368, 1987
102. Fonkalsrud EW, Berquist W, Burke M, et al: Long-term hyperalimentation in children through saphenous central venous catheterization. Am J Surg 143:209, 1982
103. Filston HC, Izant R Jr: The Surgical Neonate: Evaluation and Care. Appleton-Century-Crofts, East Norwalk, Connecticut, 1978, p 56
104. Polley TZ, Benner JW, Rhodin A, et al: Changes in total body water in infants receiving total intravenous nutrition. J Surg Res 26:555, 1979
105. Rhodin AGJ, Coran AG, Weintraub WH, et al: Total body water changes during high volume peripheral hyperalimentation. Surg Gynecol Obstet 148:196, 1979
106. Coran AG, Weintraub WH: Peripheral intravenous nutrition without fat in neonatal surgery. J Pediatr Surg 12:195, 1977
107. Askanazi J, Rosenbaum SH, Hyman AI, et al: Respiratory changes induced by the large glucose loads of total parenteral nutrition. JAMA 243:1444, 1980
108. Drongowski RA, Coran AG: An analysis of factors contributing to the development of total parenteral nutrition-induced cholestasis. JPEN J Parenter Enteral Nutr 13:586, 1989
109. Accident Facts. National Safety Council, Chicago, 1979
110. Accident Facts. National Safety Council, Chicago, 1982
111. Coran AG: Pediatric trauma. Pediatr Surg Int 5:301, 1990
112. Coran AG: Update: pediatric trauma. Compr Ther 17(10):16, 1991
113. Coran AG: Thoracic trauma. Pediatric Emergency Medicine. Reisdorff EJ, Roberts MR, Wiegenstein JG, Eds. WB Saunders Co, Philadelphia, 1992, p 881
114. Coran AG: Abdominal trauma. Pediatric Emergency Medicine. Reisdorff EJ, Roberts MR, Wiegenstein JG, Eds. WB Saunders Co, Philadelphia, 1992, p 886
115. Coran AG, Wesley JR: Shock in pediatric trauma. Pediatric Trauma: Proceedings of the Third National Conference. Coran AG, Harris BH, Eds. JB Lippincott Co, Philadelphia, 1990, p 29
116. Polley TZ Jr, Coran AG: Special problems in management of pediatric trauma. Crit Care Clin 2:775, 1986
117. Mayer T, Walker ML, Johnson DG, et al: Causes of morbidity and mortality in severe pediatric trauma. JAMA 245:719, 1981
118. O'Neill JA: Special pediatric emergencies. Emergency Care. Boswick JA, Ed. WB Saunders Co, Philadelphia, 1981, p 137
119. Drew R, Perry JF Jr, Fischer RP: The expediency of peritoneal lavage for blunt trauma in children. Surg Gynecol Obstet 145:885, 1977
120. DuPriest RW Jr, Rodriguez A, Shatney CH: Peritoneal lavage in children and adolescents with blunt abdominal trauma. Am Surg 48:460, 1982
121. Powell RW, Smith DE, Zarins CK, et al: Peritoneal lavage in children with blunt abdominal trauma. J Pediatr Surg 11:973, 1976
122. Karp MP, Cooney DR, Berger PE, et al: The role of computed tomography in the evaluation of blunt abdominal trauma in children. J Pediatr Surg 16:316, 1981
123. Eichelberger MR, Randolph JG: Thoracic trauma in children. Surg Clin North Am 61:1181, 1981
124. Cooney DR: Splenic and hepatic trauma in children. Surg Clin North Am 61:1165, 1981
125. Adler DD, Blane CE, Coran AG, et al: Splenic trauma in the pediatric patient: the integrated roles of ultrasound and computed tomography. Pediatrics 78:576, 1986
126. Francke EL, Neu HC: Postsplenectomy infection. Surg Clin North Am 61:135, 1981
127. Karp MP, Cooney DR, Pros GA, et al: The nonoperative management of pediatric hepatic trauma. J Pediatr Surg 18:512, 1983
128. Ein SH, Shandling B, Simpson JS, et al: Nonoperative management of traumatized spleen in children: how and why. J Pediatr Surg 13:117, 1978
129. Delius R, Frankel W, Coran AG: A comparison between operative and nonoperative management of blunt injuries to the liver and spleen in adult and pediatric patients. Surgery 106:788, 1989
130. Eichelberger MR, Hoelzer DJ, Koop CE: Acute pancreatitis: the difficulties of diagnosis and therapy. J Pediatr Surg 17:244, 1982
131. Touloukian RJ: Protocol for the nonoperative treatment of obstructing intramural duodenal hematoma during childhood. Am J Surg 145:330, 1983
132. Reichard SA, Helikson MA, Sorter N, et al: Pelvic fractures in children—review of 120 patients with a new look at general management. J Pediatr Surg 15:727, 1980
133. O'Neill JA, Rowe MI, Grosfeld JL, et al: Pediatric Surgery, 5th ed. CV Mosby, St. Louis, 1996, p 235
134. Holter JC, Friedman SB: Child abuse: early case finding in the emergency department. Pediatrics 42:128, 1968
135. O'Neill JA Jr, Meacham WF, Griffin JP, et al: Patterns of injury in the battered child syndrome. J Trauma 13:332, 1973
136. Rosenberg NM, Myers S, Shackleton N: Prediction of child abuse in an ambulatory setting. Pediatrics 70:879, 1982
137. Caffey J: Multiple fractures in the long bones of infants suffering from chronic subdural hematoma. AJR 56:163, 1946
138. Bauer O, Weidenback A, Thieme R: Die Knochernen Geburtsverletzungen des Neugeborenen. Münchener Medizinische Wochenschrift 109:998, 1967
139. Bianco AJ, Schlein AP, Kruss RL, et al: Birth fractures. Minn Med 55:471, 1972
140. Cohen AW, Otto SR: Obstetric clavicular fractures: a three-year analysis. J Reprod Med 25:119, 1980
141. Gordon M, Rich H, Deutschberger J, et al: The immediate and long-term outcome of obstetric birth trauma. Am J Obstet Gynecol 117:51, 1973
142. Abramson AH: Resuscitation of the Newborn Infant and Related Emergency Procedures in the Perinatal Center Special Care Nursery. CV Mosby Co, St Louis, 1973
143. Schwartz O, Cohn BD: Rupture of the normal spleen in the newborn, with survival. Surgery 59:1124, 1966
144. Tank ES, Davis R, Holt JF, et al: Mechanisms of trauma during breech delivery. Obstet Gynecol 38:761, 1971
145. Garza-Mercado R: Intrauterine depressed skull fractures of the newborn. Neurosurgery 10:694, 1982
146. Valman HB: Birth trauma. Br Med J 2:1566, 1979
147. Goodman JM: Liver trauma in the newborn: a case report. J Trauma 14:427, 1974
148. Monson DO, Raffensperger JG: Intraperitoneal hemorrhage secondary to liver laceration in a newborn. J Pediatr Surg 2:464, 1967
149. Sanerkin NG, Edwards P: Birth injury to the sternomastoid muscle. J Bone Joint Surg [Br] 48B:441, 1966
150. Manning PB, Morgan RA, Coran AG, et al: Fifty years' experience with esophageal atresia and tracheoesophageal fistula: beginning with Cameron Haight's first operation in 1935. Ann Surg 204:446, 1986
151. Bartlett RH, Gazzaniga AB, Toomasian J, et al: Extracorporeal membrane oxygenation (ECMO) in neonatal respiratory failure: 100 cases. Ann Surg 204:236, 1986
152. Stiemle CN, Meric F, Hirschl RB, et al: The effect of extracorporeal life support (ECLS) on survival when applied to all patients with congenital diaphragmatic hernia (CDH). J Pediatr Surg 29:997, 1994
153. Reickert CA, Hirschl RB, Schumacher R, et al: The effect of very delayed repair of congenital diaphragmatic hernia on survival and ECLS use. Surgery 120:766, 1996
154. Wesley JR, Heidelberger KP, DiPietro MA, et al: Diagnosis and management of congenital cystic disease of the lung in children. J Pediatr Surg 21:202, 1988
155. Coran AG: Congenital cystic disease of the tracheobronchial tree in infants and children: experience with 44 consecutive cases. Arch Surg 129:521, 1994

Acknowledgment

Figure 2 Carol Donner.

77 THE PREGNANT SURGICAL PATIENT

David C. Brooks, M.D., and Laura A. Sznyter, M.D.

Approach to Abdominal Pain in Pregnant Patients

There are approximately 3.6 million live births in the United States each year. Major complications are observed in 15% to 20% of pregnancies, but surgical complications are relatively uncommon, occurring in only 1% to 2% of pregnancies.[1,2] Surgical pathology in pregnant patients differs little from that seen in a similar nonpregnant population: pregnancy does not predispose women to many special problems, nor does it confer any significant protection from most acute surgical illnesses. Nevertheless, surgical treatment of a pregnant woman may be substantially more complicated than treatment of a similar nonpregnant patient, for several reasons. First, pregnancy induces a variety of mechanical, hormonal, and chemical alterations that may confuse and mislead even the most experienced surgeon [see Discussion, Physiologic Alterations in Pregnancy, below]. Second, a surgeon's natural inclination, when faced with a pregnant patient experiencing abdominal pain, is to temporize. This tendency, which generally arises from the misconception that surgical intervention may injure the fetus, is responsible for delays in diagnosis and ultimately for the unfavorable outcomes often associated with acute abdominal pathology in pregnant patients. Finally, and most important, a surgeon treating a pregnant woman is actually caring for two patients and has the same responsibility to both.

Initial Management

Initial management of any pregnant patient presenting with an acute abdomen or an acute surgical problem should include a thorough history and physical examination [see 14 Acute Abdominal Pain], with particular consideration given to historical aspects of the pregnancy, the expected date of delivery, and the presence of any pregnancy-related complications. Whenever possible, an obstetrician should be consulted and included in the decision-making process. Initial maneuvers should include placement of an intravenous line with the capacity to deliver ample amounts of fluid or blood, insertion of a nasogastric tube if significant vomiting is present, and performance of routine laboratory evaluations, such as a complete blood count, assessment of serum electrolyte levels, and urinalysis. If the pregnancy has passed the 26th week, a fetal monitor should be employed. Radiographic investigations should be kept to a minimum, although abdominal and pelvic ultrasonography may be especially useful not only in assessing the maternal pathology but also in evaluating the fetus.

Acute abdominal surgical problems must be dealt with immediately. Management of less acute problems, however, must take into account the stage of the pregnancy. The risk of spontaneous abortion at operation is highest during the first trimester. The optimal time for elective surgery is during the second trimester because the uterus is smaller at that time than it is in the third trimester and because the fetus can be maintained in a relatively stable condition during the administration of general anesthesia.

Specific Surgical Problems

TRAUMA

Although trauma is estimated to occur in approximately 6% to 7% of gestations, only 0.3% of pregnant women sustain traumatic injuries sufficiently severe to necessitate hospitalization.[3,4] Nevertheless, trauma remains the leading cause of maternal death.[5] Homicide is the most common cause of traumatic maternal death, followed by motor vehicle accidents, accidental injury, and suicide.[6] Major head injury and hemorrhagic shock account for most trauma-related deaths in pregnant women. Hepatic, splenic, and uterine injuries are common in high-speed motor vehicle accidents, but injuries to the GI tract, surprisingly, appear to be uncommon.[6] The more severe the injury to the mother, the greater the risk of injury to the fetus, although even minor injuries can pose a risk to the fetus. The most common cause of fetal death is abruptio placentae. Direct injury to the fetus as a result of blunt trauma is unusual because of the protective effects of the maternal abdominal wall and the uterus. Penetrating trauma, however, often results in direct fetal injury.

The physiologic alterations characteristic of pregnancy affect maternal responses to injury [see Discussion, Physiologic Alterations in Pregnancy, below]. The increased blood volume and enhanced cardiac output provide relative protection from minor hemodynamic alterations. One concern with advancing gestation is that the expansion of the gravid uterus can produce aortocaval compression, leading to supine hypotension. Left lateral displacement of the uterus is necessary to improve blood flow to both the mother and the fetus after the 20th week. The diaphragm is elevated in pregnant women, and this alteration leads to decreased functional residual capacity, increased tidal volume, and increased minute ventilation. These changes cause a chronic, compensated respiratory alkalosis and reduced blood buffering capacity.

Pregnancy is associated with decreased gastrointestinal motility and prolonged gastric emptying, which, in conjunction with relaxation of the lower esophageal sphincter, increase the risk of aspiration pneumonitis. Uterine distention displaces the bowel into the

Approach to Abdominal Pain in Pregnant Patients

Pregnant woman presents with acute abdomen

Obtain history, and perform physical examination.
Place I.V. line, and administer fluids as needed.
Insert nasogastric tube if significant vomiting is present.
Perform routine laboratory evaluations (e.g., CBC, serum electrolyte levels, urinalysis). Take into account normal changes in pregnancy.
Use fetal monitor after 26th week.
Use x-rays sparingly (only after first month); avoid radionuclide studies; employ abdominal and pelvic ultrasonography.

↓

Identify conditions that require immediate operation

↓

Condition requires immediate operation

Trauma

Management: proceed essentially as for nonpregnant patients. *Mother is first priority.* Stabilization of mother improves fetal survival. Determine gestational age, and perform external fetal monitoring as indicated. In the event of acute maternal decompensation, consider cesarean section.

Spontaneous visceral rupture

General signs and symptoms: intra-abdominal hemorrhage, shock, acute abdomen.

- Hepatic rupture: severe right upper quadrant pain; complication of preeclampsia
- Renal rupture: probably secondary to hydronephrosis
- Splenic rupture: occurs in conjunction with splenic artery aneurysm or capsular rupture, usually secondary to hypervolemia and splenomegaly
- Esophageal rupture: may be associated with excessive vomiting during pregnancy (hyperemesis gravidarum)
- Ruptured ectopic pregnancy

Note: in operation for hepatic rupture, cesarean section should be performed simultaneously.

Acute appendicitis

Signs and symptoms: nausea and vomiting (differentiate from morning sickness); pain higher and more lateral in pregnancy; fever not a prominent finding; leukocytosis shifted to left. Pain that lessens when patient is turned to left is most likely of adnexal or ovarian origin. Use graded, real-time ultrasonography.

Management: perform laparotomy; use transverse incision when diagnosis is certain; use low midline incision, right paramedian incision, or exploratory laparoscopy if diagnosis in doubt (to permit examination of peritoneum).

Intestinal obstruction

Signs and symptoms: nausea and vomiting; history of abdominal operation or adhesions. Rule out pseudo-obstruction.

Management: pass nasogastric tube; initiate fluid resuscitation and total parenteral nutrition, if needed. Begin operation as soon as possible. For large-bowel obstruction, perform sigmoidoscopy, resection of threatened bowel, and cecopexy.

Perforated duodenal ulcer

Management: plication of the perforation. Definitive ulcer operation should not be attempted. If patient is close to term, avoid cesarean section because of risk of uterine contamination.

Other conditions requiring urgent operation

Ectopic pregnancy
Ovarian torsion

Condition requires operation only if disease does not respond to medical management

Acute cholecystitis: presents with epigastric or upper right quadrant pain, nausea and vomiting, occasional radiation of pain to right scapula; use ultrasonography to visualize. Do not use HIDA scan. Manage nonoperatively during first and third trimesters (fluid resuscitation and antibiotics); during second trimester, perform cholecystectomy. Use intraoperative cholangiography.

Pancreatitis: presents with unremitting visceral pain that may radiate to the back and with raised amylase levels (2,000–3,000 IU). Operative intervention (preferably during second trimester) indicated by evidence of biliary obstruction but no evidence of stone passage or by failure of medical management.

Peptic ulcer disease: treatment is based on symptomatic relief. Prompt operative intervention is indicated in the event of perforated duodenal ulcer.

Inflammatory bowel disease: operative intervention is last resort if medical therapy ineffective. Indications for operation include abscess, fistula, or bowel obstruction (Crohn's disease) or toxic megacolon (ulcerative colitis).

upper abdomen; although this displacement protects the bowel from penetrating injury, it often interferes with peritoneal lavage. Uterine expansion also displaces the bladder into the abdomen, thereby increasing the risk of traumatic bladder injury. The upper urinary tract is generally spared from injury, however, because the gravid uterus shields the retroperitoneum from direct injury. It should be kept in mind that mild hydroureter is physiologic in pregnancy.

Uterine blood flow at term is approximately 500 ml/min; thus, pregnant women are at significant risk for extensive hemorrhage if the uterus is injured. The pregnant woman manifests a so-called physiologic anemia [see Discussion, Physiologic Alterations in Pregnancy, below]. Levels of all clotting factors except factors XI and XIII are elevated in pregnant women, and the risk of thrombosis is increased as a result.

In the first trimester, trauma generally poses little direct threat to fetal viability because the uterus is protected within the pelvis. Uncommon causes of early fetal loss include sepsis, shock, radiation exposure, pelvic fracture, and penetrating injury to the lower genital tract. In the second and third trimesters, however, when the uterus is located within the abdomen, penetrating trauma may result in direct fetal injury or rupture of the membranes. Blunt trauma may result in fetal injuries such as intracranial hemorrhage or disruption of the placenta. Nevertheless, fetal demise is rare and usually is secondary to maternal demise. When the mother survives, fetal death is generally related to abruptio placentae, complications of premature delivery, or direct penetrating injury to the fetus.

In the mother, blunt trauma (as in motor vehicle accidents) may cause multiple life-threatening injuries, including head trauma, intra-abdominal hemorrhage, pelvic fracture, and uteroplacental vascular injury. Hemorrhagic shock is a common feature. Pelvic fractures are a particular concern: because of the extensive vascular supply in this area, there is a significant risk of substantial hidden blood loss. Such fractures are associated with injuries to the maternal genitourinary system as well as with secondary fetal skull fractures. However, well-healed pelvic fractures rarely prohibit vaginal delivery. With penetrating abdominal trauma, the prognosis depends on which and how many organs are injured. Mortality from trauma is lower for pregnant women than for nonpregnant women with similar injuries, presumably because of the shielding effect of the uterus and the fetus.[7]

Management

Trauma is managed in essentially the same way in pregnant patients as in nonpregnant patients [see 2 Trauma Resuscitation]. It must be remembered, however, that the mother is the first priority: stabilization of the mother will improve both maternal and fetal survival. Initial measures include ensuring an adequate airway, maintaining fluid volume, and maximizing venous return by positioning the uterus away from the inferior vena cava when feasible. The expansion of intravascular fluid volume that occurs in pregnancy affects the amount of replacement fluid needed. In the third trimester, patients should receive 1.5 times the amount of fluid that would ordinarily be given to compensate for this effect. Use of military antishock trousers (MAST) may be attempted in certain extreme cases, although they have not been shown to be effective in pregnant patients and they could theoretically decrease maternal venous return by compressing the uterus on the inferior vena cava.

Prolonged supine positioning should be avoided to minimize the pressure of the uterus on the vena cava. Vasoconstrictive agents used for hemodynamic stabilization may lead to uteroplacental vasoconstriction and fetal compromise.

There are very few diagnostic procedures for which pregnancy is a contraindication. Radiographic investigation should be performed whenever necessary, without regard to the fetus, if the results are expected to affect management. It is usually possible to keep the total absorbed radiation dose below the level that is thought to increase teratogenic risk (i.e., 5 to 10 cGy) [see Table 1].[8] Plain films of the cervical spine provide useful information on head and neck injuries; computed tomographic (CT) scanning of the abdomen with contrast may offer the greatest amount of information on injuries to the retroperitoneum, the peritoneum, and the pelvis. Ultrasonography is now being used for acute trauma assessment in both pregnant and nonpregnant patients; the results to date have been good. Peritoneal lavage done in an open fashion through a supraumbilical incision may facilitate rapid assessment of intra-abdominal hemorrhage in cases of blunt trauma.[9] A Kleihauer-Betke test for fetal red blood cells in the maternal circulation will reveal any fetomaternal hemorrhage present. (Fetomaternal hemorrhage is the passage of fetal blood into the maternal vascular system; it occurs more frequently in pregnant women who have suffered traumatic injury than in those who have not, and it can lead to fetal anemia, arrhythmias, and fetal exsanguination.[10]) Rh_o (D) immune globulin and tetanus toxoid should be administered when indicated.

Early determination of gestational age is critical to further management decisions. External monitoring is indicated in viable gestations. Serial measurements of uterine fundal height may reveal concealed abruptio placentae. When appropriate, the patient should be evaluated for ruptured membranes. Cardiotocographic monitoring (after the 20th week of pregnancy) and ultrasonography (during the entire pregnancy) are important adjuncts for determining fetal status. Monitoring should be continued for 4 to 6 hours after stabilization.[11]

General principles of trauma management are applied when the need for laparotomy is under consideration. Each case, however, must be assessed individually when the need for concurrent hysterotomy is under consideration; fetal viability, gestational age, and the adequacy of surgical exploration are all important factors. Antibiotics should also be used according to usual indications. Patients undergoing an emergency cesarean section should receive a broad-spectrum antibiotic preoperatively.

Table 1 Radiation Dose Absorbed by Unshielded Gravid Uterus from Radiographic Studies Often Performed in Trauma Patients

Radiographic Study	Unshielded Uterine Dose (cGy)
Cervical spine	No detectable contribution
Chest (AP)	0.0003–0.0043
Pelvis (AP)	0.142–0.486
Abdomen (AP)	0.133–0.451
IVP	0.202–0.815
Full spine (AP)	0.154–0.527
Femur (AP)	0.0016–0.012
Humerus (AP)	<0.000001
Cystography	0.135–0.441
CT scan	
Head	< 0.05
Thorax	< 1
Upper abdomen	< 3
Cumulative dose (without CT scan)	0.768–2.736
Cumulative dose (with CT scan)	> 0.768–6.786

AP—anteroposterior   IVP—intravenous pyelography

In the event of acute maternal decompensation that does not respond to standard resuscitative measures, a cesarean section may be appropriate. In cases of particularly severe trauma, emergency operative resuscitation should be considered. If the patient is in cardiac arrest, thoracotomy and open chest massage, with concurrent cesarean section if the fetus is viable, have been recommended.[6] Cesarean section may increase maternal circulating volume. Occasionally, cardiopulmonary resuscitation (CPR) is more effective after the gravid uterus is emptied. There is also less risk of supine hypotension after cesarean section, although the associated surgical blood loss may exacerbate maternal instability. Timing is critical. If anoxia is limited to 4 to 6 minutes, the fetus generally will not be harmed. Therefore, any attempt to deliver the fetus should begin within 4 to 6 minutes after maternal cardiac arrest. If the fetus appears to be still viable after this period has passed, cesarean section should be performed; isolated cases of fetal salvage after prolonged maternal anoxia have been reported. CPR should be continued during and after the delivery because it may improve maternal status and survival.

Two caveats should be kept in mind: (1) cesarean section should not be performed in an unstable patient because of an anticipated cardiac arrest, and (2) if CPR is successful before surgical delivery is attempted, cesarean section should not be performed, because in utero resuscitation is likely.[12]

SPONTANEOUS VISCERAL RUPTURE

Spontaneous rupture of the liver during pregnancy is extremely uncommon, occurring no more frequently than one in 50,000 pregnancies and perhaps as infrequently as one in 250,000 pregnancies.[13] It is most commonly associated with preeclampsia or eclampsia but can also be brought on by abdominal trauma. Other events that increase intra-abdominal pressure, such as sudden coughing, sneezing, or unusually strong contractions, have also been implicated. Rupture may occur during the second or third trimester, during delivery, or even in the early postpartum period. Typically, patients present with severe right upper quadrant or substernal pain radiating to the back. Hypertension is frequently present, and the pain may precede the rupture by as much as a few days. A limited number of renal ruptures have been described in conjunction with hydronephrotic kidneys; they are thought to be secondary to the physiologic hydronephrosis seen in pregnancy. Splenic rupture is the most common nonobstetric cause of intra-abdominal hemorrhage during gestation. It usually occurs in conjunction with splenic artery aneurysms or spontaneous capsular rupture. In most cases, it is probably secondary to the increased blood volume and splenic enlargement seen toward the later part of pregnancy. Esophageal rupture has also been described, generally in association with heavy vomiting. Patients report sudden epigastric pain on vomiting that may radiate to the back and chest. X-rays may reveal air in the mediastinum. A barium meal will demonstrate the site of the rupture. Although esophageal rupture is not increased in pregnancy, it may be associated with the frequent nausea and vomiting seen with hyperemesis gravidarum. Ultrasonography, radionuclide scanning, and, ultimately, angiography may be helpful in diagnosing rupture of the liver, the kidney, or the spleen.

Management

Prompt institution of volume support is essential, followed by emergency surgery and correction of any coagulopathy. Operative management of hepatic rupture involves debridement of nonviable liver, hemostasis with electrocoagulation and a gelatin sponge, and adequate drainage. Cesarean section should be performed simultaneously, depending on the gestational age and the likelihood of fetal survival. This maneuver, when indicated, avoids labor and the attendant stress. Maternal mortality as high as 50% to 75% has been reported, even with prompt surgical intervention. Fetal mortality can be even higher, reaching nearly 80% in some series.[14] Renal rupture necessitates urgent operative exploration. Every effort should be made to salvage the ruptured kidney. Suspected splenic rupture necessitates immediate laparotomy and splenectomy. Esophageal rupture is treated with immediate repair through the left chest, if the injury is to the lower portion of the esophagus, or through the right chest, if the injury is to the upper portion.

ACUTE APPENDICITIS

Appendicitis is the surgical condition most commonly encountered during pregnancy, but pregnant women are at no greater risk than nonpregnant women.[15] The incidence is approximately one in 1,000 to 1,500 normal deliveries. The gestational changes that accompany pregnancy obscure the diagnosis and often make appendicitis more difficult to recognize. On the other hand, the natural history of appendicitis is not affected by the stage of pregnancy at the time of presentation.[16]

In most cases, appendicitis is not significantly harder to diagnose in pregnant women. Although many of the classic signs and symptoms commonly seen in the nonpregnant population may be absent in pregnant patients, the diagnosis can still be made in most cases if the surgeon is sufficiently thorough.[15,17] Pregnant women often overlook typical early signs of appendicitis, such as nausea and vomiting, because these signs are easily confused with preexisting dyspeptic complaints related to the pregnancy itself. During the first trimester, pregnant patients with acute appendicitis present with the usual early signs of nausea and vomiting and visceral discomfort progressing to peritoneal irritation in the right lower quadrant.[18] Fever is not a prominent finding. As the pregnancy progresses through the late first trimester and into the second, the signs and symptoms become less obvious. In the later part of the pregnancy, the uterus, because of its anatomic position between the abdominal wall and the inflamed appendix, may obscure typical rebound tenderness, spasm, and guarding. The location of the pain may be higher and more lateral because of displacement of the cecum and the appendix, particularly late in the third trimester, when the point of maximal tenderness may be in the right upper quadrant. A useful physical finding is Alder's sign. The point of maximal tenderness is identified while the patient is supine. The patient is then turned to her left; if the point of greatest pain shifts with the uterus, the etiology is generally adnexal or uterine.

Laboratory tests are of little diagnostic value. Because normal pregnancy is accompanied by a leukocytosis as high as 15,000 leukocytes/mm^3, the white cell count must be interpreted with care. The white cell differential is more useful than the absolute count; increased levels of band cells or immature forms suggest that the leukocytosis may be secondary to an infectious process. The urinalysis should be interpreted carefully because pyuria and hematuria are common. Bacteriuria, which occurs in about 10% of all pregnant women, raises the possibility that either pyelonephritis or cystitis is present.

In most circumstances, plain films of the abdomen are of little value in the evaluation of suspected appendicitis. Whenever possible, x-rays should be avoided in the early portion of the first trimester, but they can be performed during the second and third trimesters without risk to the fetus. The utility of x-rays of the abdomen in pregnant patients with uncomplicated abdominal pain, however, is questionable. On the other hand, ultrasonographic evaluation of the lower abdomen and pelvis can be of considerable value in pregnant patients.[19,20] Graded compression real-time ultrasonography has proved to be remarkably sensitive and specific in the evaluation of appendicitis, and it appears to have great potential for defining other acute surgical processes in pregnant women.

Differential Diagnosis

The condition most often confused with appendicitis is pyelonephritis. The two diseases may present remarkably similar clinical pictures, especially when pyelonephritis occurs on the right side. Because of the mechanical effects of the gravid uterus on the ureter, pyelonephritis is more common in pregnant women than in nonpregnant ones. Furthermore, urinalysis yields abnormal results—either pyuria or hematuria—in as many as 20% of patients with appendicitis as a result of extraluminal irritation of the ureter by the inflamed appendix.[16] A urine sample obtained by catheterization may be helpful. Nephrolithiasis can also be mistaken for appendicitis; it should be seriously considered whenever acute abdominal pain is present on the right side. Management of ureteral stones in pregnant patients presents a substantial challenge to both the surgeon and the urologist. Newer techniques, such as stents[21] and percutaneous nephrostomy tubes,[22] have been successful in obviating surgical intervention.

Torsion of an ovary or an ovarian cyst is also difficult to distinguish from appendicitis.[23] Although rare in pregnant patients, torsion of an ovarian cyst may occur in the early stages of the pregnancy. The physical examination is notable for pain in the right or left adnexa and the occasional presence of a tender mass. Pelvic ultrasonography will frequently detect the cyst. Treatment requires laparotomy. The differential diagnosis of acute abdominal pain in pregnancy should also include degenerating fibroid tumors, which can often be discovered by ultrasonography and physical examination.

Ectopic pregnancy may present as right lower quadrant pain. Typically, a patient will miss a period and then experience some degree of vaginal bleeding or spotting. Abdominal or pelvic pain as well as cervical motion tenderness is present, and a mass is often appreciated on pelvic examination. When ectopic pregnancy is suspected, serum human chorionic gonadotropin (HCG) radioimmunoassay should be performed, or urine HCG should be determined. When ectopic pregnancy is confirmed by laboratory tests, urgent laparotomy should be performed.

Other conditions that should be considered in the evaluation of pregnant women with right-sided abdominal pain are salpingitis, inflammatory bowel disease, cholecystitis, ovarian vein thrombosis, ruptured corpus luteum, rectus hematoma, round ligament pain, and adhesions. In certain cases, magnetic resonance imaging may be helpful in further delineating the source of pain.

Management

When there is evidence of appendicitis and no alternative diagnosis seems likely, laparotomy is warranted no matter what stage the pregnancy has reached.[24] The risk of the procedure to mother and child is minimal, but the risk of failing to recognize perforation and abscess formation is considerable. Mortality from these conditions can be as high as 1% for the mother and 10% to 33% for the fetus.[17,25,26] Although even satisfactory operation for appendicitis increases the risk of delivery within the week after surgery, decreases mean birth weight, and increases early (7-day) infant mortality, the risks involved in delayed diagnosis and therapy carry a significantly higher morbidity and mortality for both mother and child.[27] A negative laparotomy rate of 20% to 35% is acceptable in pregnant patients.[15,17,26]

Late in the pregnancy, or when the diagnosis is all but certain, a transverse muscle-splitting approach should be employed over the point of maximal tenderness. The patient should be turned 30° to the left to reduce pressure on the inferior vena cava and to facilitate exposure of the cecum. If there is significant doubt about whether the diagnosis is correct, a low midline incision, a right paramedian incision, or exploratory laparoscopy is recommended. If appendicitis is found at the time of laparotomy, no further investigation for other intra-abdominal processes should be performed; such investigation may disseminate the infectious process and lead to late pelvic or abdominal abscesses. If, however, appendicitis is not found, the surgeon should thoroughly examine the peritoneal contents on the right side of the abdomen, taking care to avoid exerting traction on the uterus, which might lead to preterm labor. Appendectomy is advisable to avoid later confusion. With the use of preoperative antibiotics, appendectomy can be safely performed at any stage of a pregnancy. Postoperative wound infection can be minimized if adequate attention is paid to aseptic technique and tissues are carefully and gently handled.

Laparoscopic appendectomy has not yet been prospectively evaluated during pregnancy, though early reports of its use in nonpregnant patient populations suggest that it is as safe and effective as a standard laparotomy. Laparoscopy during pregnancy is no more dangerous to either the mother or the fetus than laparotomy is.[28] Laparoscopic appendectomy is likely to find a place in the management of suspected appendicitis in the first and second trimesters.[16] Later in pregnancy, when the uterus is no longer confined within the pelvis and the lower abdomen, laparoscopic surgery is significantly more difficult.

INTESTINAL OBSTRUCTION

The incidence of bowel obstruction [see 17 *Intestinal Obstruction*] in pregnant patients is one in 2,500 to one in 3,500.[29] The most common cause of small-bowel obstruction during pregnancy is fibrous adhesions from previous abdominal surgery.[30] In addition, both volvulus and intussusception account for a significant number of bowel obstructions during gestation.[31] As the incidence of operative procedures and the average age of the mother at gestation have risen, the likelihood of adhesive obstruction has risen as well. This problem may be further exacerbated by the hypomotility or dysmotility known to occur during pregnancy.[32] Nonetheless, the need for laparotomy and lysis of adhesive bands during pregnancy is extremely low. With intestinal obstruction, the main concern is to ensure that diagnosis is not delayed. Accordingly, any pregnant patient presenting with nausea, vomiting, and a history of abdominal surgery should be presumed to have a small-bowel obstruction until it is proved otherwise.

Large-bowel obstruction is less common than small-bowel obstruction but can be seen more often as pregnancy progresses. The most common cause of large-bowel obstruction is cecal or sigmoid volvulus. Pseudo-obstruction, or Ogilvie's syndrome, has also been reported late in pregnancy or in the early puerperium.[33] Striking colonic dilatation without anatomic obstruction is apparent, with gas filling the entire length of the colon from cecum to rectum. The danger of cecal perforation is high when the maximum diameter of the cecum measures more than 12 cm.

Management

When the diagnosis of intestinal obstruction is considered, a nasogastric tube should be inserted, fluid resuscitation should be initiated, a Foley catheter should be placed, and a full battery of blood tests should be performed, including blood gas levels, electrolyte levels, and a complete blood count. Because of the leukocytosis known to occur in pregnancy, close attention should be paid to the differential blood count, with an eye to detecting any evidence of increasing acute-phase activity. Evaluation of the acid-base status may also be useful in assessing bowel viability. A flat-plate and an upright abdominal film may be useful. The risk of radiation exposure to the fetus must be weighed against the potential morbidity and mortality of a missed diagnosis.

Aggressive fluid resuscitation to ensure euvolemia and correction of electrolyte abnormalities must be instituted. If long-term nasogastric suction is anticipated, total parenteral nutrition should be considered. If conservative management does not lead to resolution, prompt operative intervention maximizes the chances of an excellent outcome for both fetus and mother. A vertical incision allows the best exposure. The entire bowel must be examined for points of obstruction and assessed for viability. Segments of necrotic bowel should be resected, and an ostomy should be fashioned if necessary.

Large-bowel obstruction is usually caused by volvulus. Sigmoid volvulus can usually be reduced by rigid or flexible sigmoidoscopy. Treatment of a recognized cecal volvulus involves prompt operative intervention, resection of any threatened bowel, and cecopexy to prevent recurrence.

Pseudo-obstruction should be managed initially with bowel rest, electrolyte replacement, and the placement of a rectal tube. If these conservative measures fail to reestablish normal peristaltic activity, colonoscopy and intraluminal aspiration of the gas-filled colon should be tried. This approach is effective in as many as 85% of cases; however, it should be undertaken only by a skilled endoscopist because the potential for iatrogenic perforation of the bowel is extremely high. If there is no change in the size of the colon after 72 hours, a cecostomy is indicated.

PERFORATED DUODENAL ULCER

Although rare, perforated duodenal ulcer has been reported.[34] When it occurs, it poses an extremely serious threat to both mother and fetus. There is no place for expectant, nonoperative therapy: prompt operative intervention is crucial. Surgical therapy should be directed at plication of the perforation, and no attempt should be made to perform a definitive ulcer operation. If the woman is close to term, the child should be delivered vaginally rather than by cesarean section because of the prohibitive risk of uterine contamination.

Conditions for Which Medical Management Should Be Attempted

ACUTE CHOLECYSTITIS

Acute cholecystitis is the second most common non-obstetric emergency in pregnant women. Symptomatic gallstone disease is far more common in women than in men because of the differential effects of the sex steroids on bile lipid composition and cholesterol saturation.[35] The difference in incidence begins at menarche, increases during the childbearing years, and decreases at menopause. The symptoms of gallstone disease generally become more pronounced after pregnancy, but they are not necessarily increased during gestation itself.

During the first and second trimesters, bile is more saturated with cholesterol. Cholesterol secretion increases, and the total bile acid pool grows. Chenodeoxycholic acid levels decrease in relation to cholic acid levels. Progesterone elevation produces decreases in smooth muscle activity that result in increased residual gallbladder volume and diminished gallbladder emptying. The further decrease in small-bowel motility that occurs secondary to progesterone elevation may alter enterohepatic circulation and decrease bile acid return to the liver.[36] These observations notwithstanding, cholecystectomy is rarely necessary in pregnant patients: it is undertaken once in every 20,000 to 40,000 pregnancies. The relative infrequency of symptomatic biliary disease is a function of the natural history of gallstones and the time required to precipitate sufficient stones to generate symptoms.[37]

The clinical signs and symptoms of cholecystitis are straightforward. Epigastric or right upper quadrant pain, nausea and vomiting, and occasional radiation of the pain into the right scapula are typical. The diagnosis can be accurately made by means of ultrasonography.[38] Radionuclide scans should be used sparingly, if at all, in pregnant patients.

Differential Diagnosis

The differential diagnosis of cholecystitis includes appendicitis (see above), pyelonephritis, acute pancreatitis, myocardial infarction, and peptic ulcer disease (see below). Significant hepatic syndromes can occur during pregnancy, such as intrahepatic cholestasis of pregnancy, acute fatty liver of pregnancy, infectious hepatitis, the hemolysis–elevated liver enzymes–low platelet count (HELLP) syndrome, and eclampsia.[39-41] These syndromes should be considered if the clinical signs and symptoms observed in a pregnant patient do not conform to the typical picture of gallstone disease.

Management

Management depends on the trimester of the pregnancy.[42] Initial management of cholecystitis is conservative, comprising intravenous hydration, administration of meperidine and antibiotics, and, if necessary, nasogastric decompression. This regimen is successful in two thirds of patients. If conservative management fails or if obstructive jaundice, gallstone pancreatitis, or peritonitis develops, operative intervention is indicated. Reports of modest-sized series demonstrate that cholecystectomy can be performed safely, without fetal loss. The introduction of improved diagnostic and tocolytic tools has improved the outlook significantly.[43,44] Intraoperative cholangiography can be used without problems in the second trimester; alternatively, intraoperative ultrasonography can be used to investigate the common bile duct.[45]

An option for the management of cholelithiasis during pregnancy is laparoscopic cholecystectomy [see 52 Laparoscopic Cholecystectomy]. Although initial reports and guidelines suggested that pregnancy was a contraindication to laparoscopic cholecystectomy, it has recently become clear that laparoscopic cholecystectomy can be performed safely and effectively through the end of the second trimester, at which point the gravid uterus has expanded beyond the confines of the pelvis and the lower abdomen. Once the uterus reaches this size, it is technically impossible to achieve adequate space for safe dissection of the gallbladder during laparoscopic cholecystectomy.[46-49]

Some surgeons, however, still harbor concerns about possible deleterious effects of laparoscopy on the pregnant patient and the fetus. The pneumoperitoneum can decrease venous return and cardiac output, resulting in decreased uterine blood flow and fetal hypoxia and acidosis.[50] The likelihood of fetal distress can be minimized by placing the patient in the left lateral decubitus position, rotating the operating table laterally, limiting the use of the reverse Trendelenburg's position, and keeping intra-abdominal pressure below 15 mm Hg. If fetal distress is detected intraoperatively by means of fetal monitoring, desufflation is indicated.[28]

PANCREATITIS

Pancreatitis is rare during pregnancy and is usually associated with gallstone disease.[51] As in the nonpregnant population, it is also associated with alcohol consumption; however, pancreatitis is less likely to occur today than formerly, probably because of the growing public awareness of the adverse effects of alcohol on the fetus. A few reports have linked pancreatitis with hypertriglyceridemia[52,53] as well as with thiazide administration[54] and hyperparathyroidism.[55] At present, there is little evidence to suggest that pregnancy itself is an etiologic mechanism in the development of pancreatitis.[56,57]

The signs and symptoms of pancreatitis in pregnant women are indistinguishable from those seen in the general population. The hallmark of the condition is diffuse abdominal pain combined with hyperamylasemia.[58] Amylase levels may approach 2,000 to 3,000 U/L and may be accompanied by lipase elevations.[59] The pain is an unremitting, deep visceral pain that is usually midabdominal but may radiate into the back. In addition to excruciating pain, typical clinical findings include hypotension, hypovolemia, and a rapid, thready pulse. The diagnosis can be established by measurement of serum amylase levels; the amylase-to-creatinine ratio is not helpful.[60] Ultrasonography should be undertaken with the aim of searching for evidence of cholelithiasis and choledocholithiasis. Visualization of the inflamed pancreatic head may be informative; however, this structure is often difficult to locate. Liver function tests should be performed, but the results should be interpreted with caution, in the light of the alkaline phosphatase elevation known to occur in normal pregnancy.

Management

Treatment should be aimed at correction of the hypovolemia that invariably accompanies pancreatitis.[61] The gut should be put at rest, and a nasogastric tube should be passed. Intramuscular administration of meperidine at a dosage of 50 to 75 mg every 3 to 4 hours provides adequate analgesia. Antibiotics should be reserved for treatment of a specific infectious complication. Calcium levels should be kept within the normal range. Arterial blood gases should be monitored as indicated.

Operative intervention should be reserved for patients with biliary obstruction in whom there is no evidence of stone passage. Efforts aimed at postponing operative intervention have been somewhat successful, though the recurrence rate approaches 50%. Early operative intervention has not been shown to improve fetal survival.[51] During the first trimester, loss of the fetus is common[42]; in the second, however, operative intervention has a good chance of yielding excellent results for both mother and fetus.[62] In patients with pancreatitis caused by extrahepatic biliary obstruction, endoscopic management has achieved excellent results. Endoscopic retrograde cholangiopancreatography (ERCP) and sphincterotomy [see 47 Gastrointestinal Endoscopy] can both be performed safely during pregnancy.[63] Although unusual, pseudocyst formation has been reported in pregnant women. It is managed conservatively, without operative intervention. Prolonged pancreatitis may necessitate lengthy periods of bowel rest. During extended periods without oral feeding, pregnant women should be maintained on total intravenous hyperalimentation.[64]

PEPTIC ULCER DISEASE

Because of the salutary effects of pregnancy on gastric acid production, peptic ulcer disease is extremely uncommon in pregnant women.[65] Elevated estrogen levels are believed to decrease gastric acidity during early pregnancy; in fact, some patients with known acid peptic disease show substantial symptomatic improvement during the course of gestation. Maternal gastrin production does not change during pregnancy, but histamine-stimulated acid output is lower. During the third trimester, however, maternal serum gastrin levels rise as a result of placental contribution, and symptomatic peptic ulcer disease may become more likely. During the late third trimester and the early postpartum period, basal and stimulated acid production return to normal.

The diagnosis is made in much the same way in pregnant patients as in nonpregnant ones, except that physicians treating pregnant women should rely more on clinical information and less on radiologic intervention. Intractable pain that is not relieved by the usual therapeutic interventions should prompt endoscopic evaluation.

Management

Treatment of peptic ulcer disease is based on symptomatic relief. Although there is no definite evidence linking H_2 receptor blockers with fetal abnormalities, these agents should be used cautiously in pregnant women. Sucralfate may be added to the antacid regimen as a supplement; it should have little effect on the fetus. Perforated duodenal ulcer must be treated surgically (see above).

INFLAMMATORY BOWEL DISEASE

Pregnancy does not affect either ulcerative colitis or Crohn's disease to any great degree, nor do these diseases affect the welfare of the fetus appreciably.[66-68] Active disease flare-ups are most common during the first trimester and during the early postpartum period.[69] In a recent review of pregnancies in patients with Crohn's disease, the outcome of the pregnancy was not adversely affected by the disease. Although patients with active disease at the time of conception or during pregnancy generally had poorer outcomes, neither pregnancy nor medical or surgical therapy affected the course of the disease.[70]

In addition to these frank forms of inflammatory bowel disease (IBD), ulcerative or granular proctitis may also occur in pregnancy. This poorly understood disorder is confined entirely to the distal 10 cm of the rectum. Endoscopically, the mucosa manifests multiple diffuse superficial ulcerations and friability. Bleeding is observed, ranging from spotting with defecation to measurable loss. Above the distal 12 to 15 cm of the rectum, the mucosa assumes a normal appearance. The disease is self-limited, almost never progressing to true IBD.

Management

Treatment of ulcerative colitis or Crohn's disease involves administration of sulfadiazine, steroids, or both.[71] Treatment with both of these agents is recommended.[72] Both steroids and sulfadiazine have been reported to cause congenital malformations in animal studies; however, because of the increased risk of fetal and maternal mortality in untreated cases of IBD, it is recommended that steroids and sulfadiazine be administered together as necessary to minimize the active effects of the disease.[73] If the disease does not respond to medical management, operative intervention may be undertaken, but only as a last resort. In patients with ulcerative colitis, the most common indication for operation is toxic megacolon, which, if left untreated, can cause significant infant and maternal mortality. In patients with Crohn's disease, the uncommon problems of abscess, fistula formation, and bowel obstruction may force operation; these conditions should be treated in the usual fashion. Greater reliance should be placed on fecal diversion in pregnant patients because of the increased risk of anastomotic dysfunction. Significant Crohn's activity may necessitate complete bowel rest and maintenance of nutrition by central intravenous feedings.[74,75]

Patients with ulcerative or granular proctitis should not receive systemic treatment with steroids or sulfadiazine because of the potential toxicity to the fetus. Steroid enemas or enemas concocted from an elixir preparation of sulfasalazine may be administered. Low-residue diets may help control particularly bothersome symptoms.

Discussion

Physiologic Alterations in Pregnancy

A variety of physiologic alterations occur during pregnancy. These include mechanical, hormonal, chemical, and hematologic changes [see Table 2] that are essential for the maintenance of pregnancy during the 40 weeks of gestation but that may also complicate the evaluation of abdominal problems in the pregnant patient.

MECHANICAL ALTERATIONS

The most obvious mechanical alteration in pregnancy is the effect of the expanding gravid uterus on the intra-abdominal contents and many of the retroperitoneal structures [see Figure 1]. This progressive expansion is of little importance during the first trimester, but it takes on increasing importance during the second and third trimesters. Although the effects are obvious for the most part, they are worth reiterating here.

The increasing mass of the uterus gradually displaces gut structures from the pelvis and the lower abdomen to the upper or middle abdomen. The appendix and cecum typically travel upward and laterally, so that McBurney's point may be located in the flank, as much as 6 to 8 cm cephalad to the anterior iliac spine. The importance of this change in the diagnosis of intra-abdominal pathology in pregnancy is clear.

The upward displacement of the uterus tends to expand the esophageal hiatus and promote incipient herniation of the stomach. In conjunction with the hormonal changes that occur in the lower esophageal sphincter, these changes can induce symptomatic reflux and regurgitation of gastric contents.

Compression of the rectosigmoid by the uterus late in pregnancy predisposes to constipation and obstipation. The pressure exerted by the pregnant uterus on the rectum increases the already elevated venous pressure in the pelvis and leads to an increased tendency to hemorrhoids, anorectal disease, and constipation.

In the retroperitoneum, the weight of the uterus tends to compress the ureters on both sides, but particularly on the right, possibly leading to stasis and mild hydronephrosis, as well as increased potential for stagnation and pyelonephritis. Furthermore, bladder capacity is decreased, which inevitably leads to functional frequency of urination. The pressure of the uterus on the retroperitoneal vascular structures predisposes to increased venous pressure in the pelvis and lower extremities. As a direct result, pregnant women are more prone to hemorrhoidal disease and varicosities of the lower extremities.

HORMONAL ALTERATIONS

It is not surprising that the tremendous physiologic elaboration of maternal hormones during gestation should have far-reaching effects. In addition to their effects on maternal and fetal growth and placental formation and maintenance, these hormones have effects at distant sites as well.

Estrogen levels in early pregnancy are similar to those seen in the postovulatory phase of the menstrual cycle. By the end of the first trimester, however, the contribution of placental estrogen is apparent. From that period through the remainder of the pregnancy, estrogen levels continue to rise. The role of estrogen in the maternal circulation is to control regional blood flow to the uterus and placenta as well as to stimulate changes in the breast, cervix, and vagina.

Progesterone levels follow a similar pattern. The initial low levels

Table 2 Chemical and Hematologic Alterations in Pregnant Patients[97]

Laboratory Test	Normal Values	
	Nonpregnant	Pregnant
Urinary acetone	Negative	Faint positive
Serum total protein (g/dl)	6.5–8.5	6.8
Serum albumin (g/dl)	3.5–5.0	2.5–4.5
Blood urea nitrogen (mg/dl)	10–25	5–15
Fasting blood glucose (mg/dl)	70–110	65–100
Two-hour postprandial blood glucose (mg/dl)	< 110	< 120 (plasma)
Serum calcium (mEq/L)	4.6–5.5	4.2–5.2
Serum phosphate (mg/dl)	2.5–4.8	2.3–4.6
Alkaline phosphatase (IU/L)	35–48	35–150
Cholesterol (mg/dl)	120–290	177–345
Triglycerides (mg/dl)	33–166	130–400
Serum folic acid (ng/ml)	5–21	4–14
Vitamin B_{12} (pg/ml)	430–1,025	Decreased
Hemoglobin (g/dl)	12	> 11
Hematocrit (%)	36	33
Serum iron (μg/dl)	> 50	> 60
TIBC (μg/dl)	250–400	300–600
% TIBC saturation	30	> 20
Serum zinc (μg/dl)	65–115	55–80
Urinary zinc (μg/dl)	200–450	200–450

TIBC—total iron-binding capacity

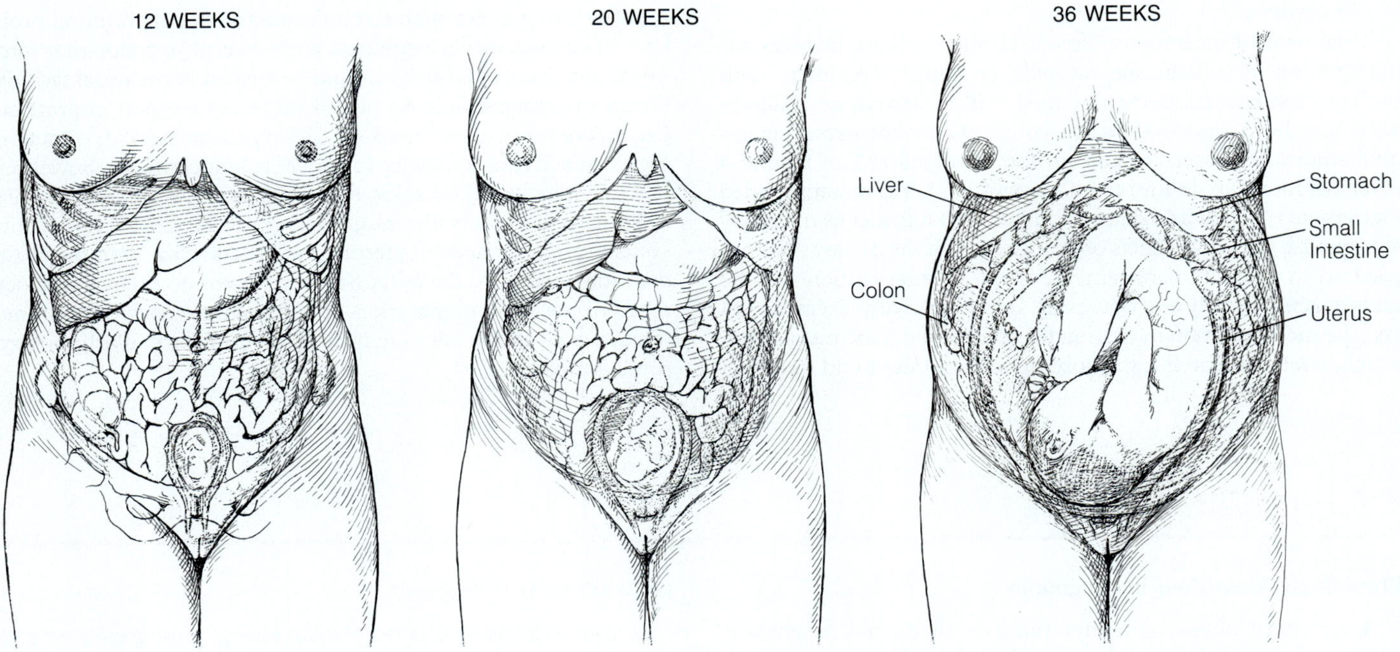

Figure 1 Enlargement of the uterus to accommodate the developing fetus shifts intra-abdominal contents superiorly and compresses retroperitoneal structures. These effects are particularly important during the second and third trimesters.

represent the contribution of the corpus luteum. Toward the end of the first trimester, the placenta increases its contribution, and progesterone levels continue to rise at a linear rate throughout the course of the pregnancy. The exact role of progesterone in the maternal circulation is not completely understood; however, its effects are thought to include maintenance of uterine stability and myometrial quiescence, diuresis that counterbalances the fluid retention observed in pregnancy, and modulation of maternal immune function in relation to the fetus.

HCG is produced by the syncytiotrophoblast at the onset of conception. The concentration rises rapidly, reaching its peak by the 10th week. Thereafter, it falls to significantly lower levels. Its role is to maintain the function of the corpus luteum during the early stages of pregnancy.

Carbohydrate metabolism is altered by the increased estrogen and progesterone levels in several ways. In early pregnancy, the increased levels of these hormones promote beta-cell hyperplasia and increased insulin secretion. This in turn leads to increased tissue glycogen storage, decreased central production, and decreased fasting glucose levels. In late pregnancy, however, the picture becomes more diabetogenic as human chorionic somatomammotropin and prolactin levels rise. Glucose tolerance decreases, hepatic stores are depleted, and hepatic gluconeogenesis increases. The presumed purpose of these alterations is to ensure adequate supplies of glucose and amino acids to the fetus.

Other possible effects of the elevated sex hormones have been proposed. Progesterone, which exerts a considerable inhibitory effect on smooth muscle in the uterus, also affects other smooth muscle sites. By decreasing the tone of the lower esophageal sphincter, it can facilitate reflux of gastric contents. By decreasing motility, it can induce gastroparesis, thereby further exacerbating esophageal dysfunction. This effect is offset, to some degree, by the decreased gastric acid secretion noted during gestation. Progesterone-induced smooth muscle inhibition decreases peristalsis in the colon. This effect, in conjunction with the mechanical effects of the gravid uterus, may lead to the typical obstipation seen in pregnancy. Estrogen and, to some degree, HCG can induce dyspepsia and gastric distress, which, in conjunction with the effects of progesterone, may be responsible for the typical picture of morning sickness.

CHEMICAL AND HEMATOLOGIC ALTERATIONS

Complete Blood Count

Mean hematocrit and hemoglobin level usually fall in a normal and uncomplicated pregnancy. These decreases are caused by an increase in plasma volume that may be as high as 45%. Although red blood cell volume also increases during pregnancy, this increase is lower than the increase in the plasma volume, which gives rise to a physiologic anemia of pregnancy. Toward the end of the first trimester, the hemoglobin concentration begins to decrease, becoming stationary toward the beginning of the second trimester. Anemia is not considered significant until the hemoglobin level has dropped below 10 g/dl. Specific anemias related to iron deficiency, folic acid deficiency, and inflammatory processes may also be present and should be treated in the appropriate fashion. Hemolytic anemias may be observed, in which case the underlying disease should be treated.

Normal pregnancies are also associated with a typical leukocytosis in the later stages and during labor. Elevation of the white blood cell count to levels as high as 16,000 to 17,000/mm^3 may not be considered abnormal unless there is evidence of a left shift. This important normal variant must be kept in mind in the evaluation of pregnant patients with acute operative pathology. The erythrocyte sedimentation rate is also elevated in pregnancy as a result of hepatic production of acute-phase reactants throughout gestation. It may not be possible to differentiate pathologic from nonpathologic processes reliably on the basis of serum determinations.

Urinalysis

Minimal pyuria and hematuria are not uncommon findings in late pregnancy. Bacteriuria is present in 10% or more of pregnant women. Glycosuria is a frequent finding during pregnancy as a result of central hormonal effects on resting glucose metabolism. The urine of pregnant women may also contain significant amounts of amino acids. Proteinuria is not cause for concern until levels higher than 300 mg/day are reached. Urine pH is typically somewhat more alkalotic than normal.

Serum Chemistries

The serum chemistries of pregnant patients undergo several important changes. Foremost is the elevation of serum alkaline phosphatase levels, which reflects not biliary tract disease but a normal process related to the release of alkaline phosphatase from the placenta. Liver transaminase activity is generally unaffected by pregnancy, and aspartate aminotransferase (AST) and alanine aminotransferase (ALT) values tend to remain normal. Although hepatic conjugation and excretion of bilirubin are diminished during pregnancy, these effects are not reflected in an elevated serum bilirubin level. Albumin levels may be decreased by as much as 1 g/dl during the later part of pregnancy; serum glucose is also decreased. These decreases are caused by concentration-driven uptake by the fetus and a variety of gestational hormones that produce an effect similar to starvation and may even lead to a degree of ketosis. When fed, pregnant women show impaired glucose disposal, which may lead to mild, transient hyperglycemia. Because of the physiologic increase in the glomerular filtration rate observed during pregnancy, blood urea nitrogen is decreased. In a similar fashion, serum creatinine levels are often decreased as well.

General Considerations in the Management of Pregnant Patients

RADIOLOGIC INVESTIGATION

All physicians know that radiation exposure in the first trimester poses a substantial risk to the fetus, but relatively few are aware that irradiation during the late second and the third trimester is usually well tolerated by the fetus. There is no evidence that exposure to less than 5 cGy is harmful. This does not mean that x-rays should be used routinely in the later part of pregnancy. Nevertheless, if significant management decisions must be made during this period and radiologic findings are likely to affect these decisions, then x-ray studies should be undertaken. In most cases, however, flat-plate, kidney-ureter-bladder (KUB), and upright films are of little diagnostic value. Furthermore, mammography will not obviate biopsy of a clinically suspicious breast lesion. Surgeons who are considering radiologic intervention in pregnant patients should therefore be sure to ask themselves, before proceeding, how much information they are likely to gain and how likely that information is to alter management.

LABORATORY TESTS

Serum and blood determinations pose no risk to the pregnant patient or the fetus. Unlike radiologic interventions, they may be used as often as is considered useful. It is essential to be aware of the variations in laboratory values typically seen in pregnancy [see Table 2]. Reliance on values normal for nonpregnant patients will lead to considerable diagnostic confusion [see Physiologic Alterations in Pregnancy, above].

ANALGESIA

Pain relief is an important consideration throughout pregnancy. It must be remembered, however, that at any stage of pregnancy, drug administration has the potential for teratogenic effects or fetal depression [see Table 3].

Minor pain or pain associated with chronic low-grade discomfort is readily controlled with acetaminophen or aspirin. Acetaminophen has a negligible effect on the fetus and is well tolerated at usual doses. Aspirin, however, can cause such problems as fetal or neonatal bleeding, placental bleeding, and coagulation defects. These effects are more critical toward the end of pregnancy. In addition, aspirin may act to prolong the pregnancy.[76]

Codeine can be given to control pain that exceeds the capabilities of the minor pain relievers and the nonsteroidal anti-inflammatory drugs (NSAIDs). It is relatively safe: codeine has the potential to depress neonatal respiration, but its teratogenic potential is low. On the whole, it is an adequate midrange analgesic.

Morphine and meperidine offer excellent relief of severe pain, but they pose a greater potential hazard to the fetus. If given for long periods (i.e., longer than 2 weeks), morphine may cause an infant to be small for its gestational age; if given close to term or delivery, it can lead to neonatal respiratory depression. Meperidine is not thought to be associated with small size for gestational age, but it does have the potential to induce respiratory depression.[77] Nevertheless, both morphine and meperidine are excellent analgesics and should be employed whenever necessary.

Operative Considerations in the Management of Pregnant Patients

Any operative procedure being considered during the first trimester should be postponed whenever possible because of the higher chance of abortion (reportedly about 12%) in this stage of pregnancy and, to a lesser degree, because of the teratogenic potential that all general anesthetics are believed (though not known) to have. Intra-abdominal operation is best performed during the second trimester. At this stage of the pregnancy, the fetus is relatively stable: major organ differentiation has occurred, and the fetus is simply awaiting further maturation. Moreover, because the pregnant woman's uterus has not yet displaced the other abdominal contents from their normal positions, exposure, retraction, and manipulation are far easier than they would be during the third trimester. Third-trimester operative procedures are complicated by the 40% risk premature labor and by the inherent problems generated by the expansion of the uterus.[43] Fetal vulnerability is diminished in the third trimester, but the relative fragility of the placental unit and the greater irritability of the uterus make operation more dangerous.

ANESTHESIA

Anesthesia for a major operation during pregnancy must be undertaken with the greatest possible caution and with the greatest possible attention to fetal and maternal safety—specifically, through use of close monitoring [see Fetal and Maternal Monitoring,

Light premedication with barbiturates will allay some of the natural fears that a pregnant woman undergoing an operative procedure is likely to feel. Amnestics should be used during general operative procedures.

The primary concern in anesthesia in pregnant patients is maintenance of both maternal and fetal safety. Although, to some extent, fetal safety is dependent on maternal safety, additional care must be taken to prevent teratogenesis in the early stages of pregnancy, to avoid asphyxia throughout the pregnancy, and to avoid premature labor during the late stages of pregnancy.

The choice of anesthetic technique depends largely on the procedure to be performed. When a choice is available, regional anesthesia (being the safest approach) is preferable. General anesthetics induce fetal depression, uterine relaxation, and possible fetal anomalies. Local anesthesia is generally quite safe and well

Table 3 Safety of Various Drugs Used during Pregnancy[98,99]

Drug (FDA Pregnancy Category)	Toxicity	Comments
Analgesics/tranquilizers		
Ibuprofen (B)	Risk of postpartum hemorrhage; premature patent ductus arteriosus closure; no teratogenic effects	Use with caution toward end of pregnancy
Meperidine (B)	Decreased neonatal respiration; CNS depression	Greatest risk near term
Morphine (C)	Small size for gestational age; respiratory depression; fetal death	Greatest risk near term
Codeine (C)	Possible congenital anomalies	Avoid in first trimester
Acetaminophen (B)	None known	Analgesic of choice
Aspirin (C)	Anticoagulation effect; fetal bleeding; possible prolongation of pregnancy; no teratogenesis known	Use with caution, especially toward end of pregnancy; not recommended for routine analgesia
Barbiturates (C)	Fetal addiction; neonatal bleeding; ?teratogenesis	Long-term administration not recommended
Diazepam (D)	?Cleft palate; ?heart defects; hypotonia; hypothermia; withdrawal symptoms	Long-term administration not recommended
Anesthetics		
Bupivacaine (C)	Bradycardia	Use with caution in late pregnancy
Lidocaine (B)	Bradycardia; CNS depression	Use with caution in late pregnancy
Halothane (C)	Uterine relaxation	Can cause abortion in early pregnancy
Nitrous oxide	?Teratogenesis in early pregnancy	Can be used in late pregnancy
Muscle relaxants (C)	Fetal curarization	Relatively safe; incidence of problems extremely low
Antibiotics		
Ampicillin (B)	None known	Safe
Aztreonam (B)	Not teratogenic in rodents	Safety in pregnancy unclear
Cephalosporins (B)	No embryocidal reports	Safe
Clindamycin (B)	None known	Safety in pregnancy unclear
Erythromycin, azithromycin (B)	Risk of cholestatic hepatitis; no reported congenital defects	Avoid in pregnancy
Fluoroquinolones (C)	Irreversible arthropathy in immature animals	Avoid in pregnancy
Gentamicin (C)	Possible 8th nerve toxicity; no reported congenital defects, neonatal ototoxicity, or nephrotoxicity	Avoid in pregnancy
Imipenem (C)	None known	Safety in pregnancy unclear
Metronidazole (B)	Carcinogenic in rodents; possibly teratogenic	Contraindicated in first trimester; use with caution thereafter
Nitrofurantoin (C)	Hemolytic anemia in newborns; no known teratogenic effects	Contraindicated at term
Penicillin G (B)	None known	Safe
Streptomycin (D)	8th cranial nerve abnormality	Contraindicated
Tetracycline (D)	Adverse effects on fetal teeth and bones; maternal hepatotoxicity; congenital defects	Contraindicated
Trimethoprim-sulfamethoxazole (C)	Hemolysis in G6PD-deficient patients; risk of kernicterus	Contraindicated at term
Vancomycin (C)	Potential fetal ototoxicity, nephrotoxicity	Avoid in pregnancy

ventilation should be avoided because of the physiologic effects of hypocapnia on regional blood flow. The hematocrit should be kept above 30%.

FETAL AND MATERNAL MONITORING

After the 26th week of fetal development, fetal heart rate monitoring should be continuously performed during general operative procedures whenever possible. This can be achieved with Doppler ultrasound scanning, which is done by placing a transducer on the maternal abdominal wall away from the operative site. An ultrasonic sound wave is directed at the fetus and records the motion of the fetal heart. For laparoscopic procedures, because the anterior abdominal wall is lifted away from the uterus, a transvaginal transducer is required for fetal monitoring.

The normal fetal heart rate ranges from 120 to 160 beats/min. Bradycardia is generally not associated with external stress; however, tachycardia is a common result of fetal hypoxia, infection (maternal or fetal), and drug administration, as well as of intrinsic fetal cardiac abnormalities.

Uterine activity can be monitored in the later part of pregnancy through use of a tocodynamometer. This instrument measures uterine muscular contractions and may aid in identifying early labor.

During procedures necessitating general anesthesia, maternal oxygen saturation should be continuously monitored by means of a transcutaneous oximeter. If this instrument is not available, arterial blood gas levels should be measured whenever there is any question about the adequacy of perfusion. Close attention should be paid to acid-base status so that any tendency to acidosis or alkalosis can be counteracted.

Liberal use of indwelling urinary catheters allows gross estimation of the adequacy of blood volume and splanchnic perfusion during general operative procedures. Moreover, if intra-abdominal operation is necessary after the 12th to 16th week, the bladder must be decompressed to allow adequate exposure in the pelvis and the lower abdomen.

OTHER CONSIDERATIONS

Because of the increased risk of aspiration in pregnant patients, nasogastric suction should be freely employed. The lower esophageal sphincter has less tone, and the potential for regurgitation is much higher. The stomach should be emptied before emergency procedures and continually decompressed during the operation and the early postoperative period.

Postoperative Considerations in the Management of Pregnant Patients

After the operation, continued close monitoring of the patient is essential. Observation of the fetal heart rate (with Doppler ultrasonography) and monitoring for signs of premature labor should be continued. The F_IO_2 should be maintained at a level sufficient to ensure adequate maternal and fetal oxygenation. Continued use of an indwelling urinary catheter in the early postoperative period allows simple monitoring of fluid status. Nasogastric tubes should not be removed until there is evidence of normal bowel function.

Breast Cancer

Carcinoma of the breast occurs in approximately one of every 5,000 pregnant women.[79] A new breast lesion in a pregnant woman should be treated without delay in accordance with the standard guidelines [see 13 Breast Complaints]. The mass may be a fibroadenoma, a lesion that is very common in young women and that tends to enlarge during pregnancy. It should first be aspirated to rule out the possibility that it is a cyst. If the mass disappears, follow-up via physical examination is appropriate; mammography is not advisable, because it may damage the fetus. If the mass does not resolve, a core biopsy or an open biopsy with local anesthesia should be performed, regardless of the stage of pregnancy. Strict attention to hemostasis and to ligature of obvious ductules is necessary to prevent postoperative hematoma or leakage of milk. Another common presentation is nipple discharge, which may signal a papilloma or duct ectasia and thus calls for biopsy.

Management of breast cancer is essentially the same in pregnant patients as in nonpregnant patients.[80,81] It has been suggested that the alterations in estrogen, progesterone, and prolactin levels during pregnancy may exacerbate preexisting breast carcinoma. There is increased lymphatic drainage during pregnancy, which may explain the increase in axillary node metastases. Nevertheless, when the statistics are corrected for age, size of lesion, and clinical stage, the prognosis is no worse for pregnant women with breast carcinoma than for nonpregnant women with the same condition.[82,83]

Termination of the pregnancy is of no benefit in the management of the tumor. If the woman is lactating when breast cancer is diagnosed, it is advisable to discontinue lactation by administering bromocriptine because prolactin may promote tumor growth.

Modified radical mastectomy [see 43 Breast Procedures] is the treatment of choice for breast cancer during pregnancy.[79] Breast conservation requires radiation therapy, which raises the issue of fetal exposure. No precise data on the effects of therapeutic radiation on the developing fetus are available,[84] nor is it known how effective radiation therapy is in pregnant and lactating women. For patients with stage III or IV breast cancer, termination of pregnancy may be considered to allow unrestricted treatment with chemotherapy and radiation. Teratogenic effects of cytotoxic agents have been described, but only in anecdotal reports.[85]

Inflammatory changes in the breast skin are generally caused by staphylococcal or streptococcal infections. They occur most frequently in the postpartum period but are also seen occasionally during pregnancy. If inflammation does not rapidly resolve after antibiotics are administered, drainage is indicated and biopsy should be considered.

Burns during Pregnancy

Thermal injury in pregnancy is an uncommon yet potentially lethal event for both the mother and the fetus. Of the roughly 75,000 patients who sustain significant burns each year,[86] approximately 7% are pregnant women.[87,88] Important variables affecting maternal survival include the depth of the thermal injury, the size of the burn, the anatomic location involved, the presence or absence of concurrent complicating medical problems, and the gestational age of the fetus at the time of maternal injury. Pregnancy itself does not exert a significant influence on maternal survival.[89]

Maternal mortality increases dramatically after burns larger than 40% of total body surface area (BSA). When thermal injury exceeds 80% of total BSA, maternal mortality approaches 100% [see Table 4].[90] Poor maternal-fetal outcome may be attributable to hypovolemia and prolonged fetal hypoxia resulting from underresuscitation of the mother.

Thermal injury raises prostaglandin levels and increases oxytocin release; these actions, in conjunction with hypovolemia, decreased uteroplacental perfusion, and hypoxia are believed to increase the risk of premature labor and delivery within 5 days of maternal thermal injury.[91] Fetal heart rate monitoring and an ultrasonographic biophysical profile are essential for assessment of fetal well-being when gestational age passes 24 weeks.

In a preterm fetus, attempts at tocolysis are indicated if there are no signs of fetal distress. Indomethacin, given for a short period (< 72 hours), has been recommended as a primary agent. Beta-adrenergic agents (which may cause hypotension, increased capillary permeability, and increased fluid requirements) and magnesium sulfate (which may cause vasodilatation and possibly electrolyte abnormalities) should be avoided until the patient is hemodynamically stable.

MANAGEMENT

Acute management of the burns in pregnant patients differs little from that in nonpregnant patients. Initial resuscitative efforts should include (1) fluid and electrolyte management; (2) ventilatory support as needed; (3) hemodynamic monitoring [see Table 5]; (4) antibiotic therapy; and (5) prompt, aggressive surgical intervention with eschar excision and skin grafting. Topical agents such as silver sulfadiazine may be used as necessary.

Skin contracture may be a long-term complication of serious abdominal burns. Usually, this scar tissue softens during pregnancy and thus poses little difficulty to the pregnant patient. Rarely, abdominal surgical release and skin grafting are required to accommodate the expanding uterus.[92]

Minor Surgical Problems of Pregnancy

The following conditions are the most common of the minor surgical problems that are known to occur during pregnancy [see Table 6].

HEARTBURN

Etiology

Heartburn is a common complaint of pregnancy that results in part from decreased lower esophageal sphincter pressure and regurgitation of stomach contents.[93] An alkaline reflux gastritis may in part be responsible because gastric acidity is decreased in pregnancy. Toward the later part of the pregnancy, 10% to 15% of pregnant women will also manifest severe reflux that is caused by a frank diaphragmatic hiatus hernia.

Treatment

Antacids containing aluminum hydroxide or magnesium hydroxide, such as Gelusil and Amphojel, should be taken one-half hour to 1 hour after meals.[73] Positional changes, such as elevation of the head of the bed and maintenance of an upright posture for several hours after meals, should be encouraged. Chewing gum or sucking on hard candies tends to increase esophageal motility and decrease reflux. In severe cases, sucralfate may be given to soothe and possibly to heal active gastritis and esophagitis. Metoclopramide has also been found to be efficacious in cases of heartburn that is refractory to oral antacids.

CONSTIPATION

Etiology

Increased levels of sex steroid hormones during pregnancy are thought to produce decreases in smooth muscle motility and subsequent functional decreases in bowel motility. Moreover, the pressure exerted by the expanded and displaced uterus on the bowel is thought to interfere with normal peristaltic activity.

Treatment

Stressing good bowel care and bowel training is helpful. Nonpharmacologic methods of increasing bowel activity, such as increasing the fiber and roughage in the diet to maximize stool bulk, are also useful. Foods with laxative properties, such as prunes, figs, apples, and citrus fruits, may facilitate stool passage. The patient should take

Table 4 Maternal and Perinatal Mortality after Maternal Burn Injuries[90]

Amount of Body Surface Area Injured (%)	Mortality (%)	
	Maternal	Perinatal
< 40	3	22
50	25	53
> 80	100	100

at least eight to 10 extra glasses of fluid a day; water is preferable, but non–caffeine-containing liquids are also acceptable. Increased exercise may help in the passage of stool. A bulk laxative, such as Metamucil, or a stool softener, such as Colace, should be prescribed, regardless of whether the natural roughage foods are effective.[73] Mild laxatives may be given when all other measures are inadequate. Small doses of milk of magnesia and similar osmotic reactive laxatives are useful. Small amounts of mineral oil may be cautiously administered; prolonged use of mineral oil can cause liver degeneration and interferes with the absorption of fat-soluble vitamins.

HEMORRHOIDS

Etiology

The development of hemorrhoids during pregnancy results from the decreased motility and tendency toward constipation that occur in all pregnancies. These changes lead to straining at stool, during which the shearing force generated in the rectal canal can exacerbate and intensify preexisting hemorrhoid disease. Furthermore, the weight and pressure of the uterus itself tends to decrease venous return and increase the amount of pooling in vascular structures in the lower pelvis.

Treatment

The best method of preventing hemorrhoids is to maintain adequate bowel function; when that is not feasible, the following general measures should be taken:

1. Warm sitz baths.
2. A local astringent, such as a Tucks pad or witch hazel.
3. Supine positioning with the legs elevated whenever possible.
4. Manual replacement of the hemorrhoids after each bowel movement, regardless of the pain incurred.
5. Astringent suppositories or creams, such as Anusol or Anusol HC.

Acutely thrombosed hemorrhoids should be incised with the patient under local anesthesia; the clot should be evacuated, astringent ointments applied, and bowel care resumed. Injection with scleros-

Table 5 Hemodynamic Values in Healthy Nonpregnant, Pregnant, and Postpartum Subjects[100,101]

Parameter	Nonpregnant	36–38 Weeks' Gestation*	Postpartum
Heart rate (beats/min)	60–100	83 ± 10	71 ± 10
Central venous pressure (mm Hg)	5–10	3.6 ± 2.5	3.7 ± 2.6
Mean pulmonary arterial pressure (mm Hg)	15–20	—	—
Pulmonary arterial wedge pressure (mm Hg)	6–12	7.5 ± 1.8	6.3 ± 2.1
Mean arterial pressure (mm Hg)	90–110	90.3 ± 5.8	86.4 ± 7.5
Cardiac output (L/min)	4.3–6.0	6.2 ± 1.0	4.3 ± 0.9
Stroke volume (ml/beat)	57–71	74.7	60.6
Systemic vascular resistance (dyne · cm · sec^{-5})	900–1,400	1,210 ± 266	1,530 ± 520
Pulmonary vascular resistance (dyne · cm · sec^{-5})	< 250	78 ± 22	119 ± 47

*Values in pregnant patients were determined with patient in left lateral decubitus position.

Table 6 Management of Minor Surgical Problems of Pregnancy

Problem	Management Approach
Heartburn	Give aluminum or magnesium hydroxide antacids Encourage positional changes—e.g., staying upright after meals for at least 1½ hr Chew gum or hard candies to increase motility Reserve sucralfate for refractory cases; use H_2 receptor blockers with caution
Constipation	Have patient drink at least 6–8 glasses of extra fluid daily Add Metamucil to diet: 1 tsp in water daily Add roughage and fiber to diet Have patient exercise regularly—e.g., walking 1–2 mi daily When all else fails, use laxatives such as milk of magnesia; mineral oil should be avoided
Hemorrhoids	Follow general preventive measures for constipation Have patient take sitz baths twice daily when hemorrhoids flare Use astringents for local perineal care Do not employ injection therapy Manually reduce prolapsing hemorrhoids after each bowel movement Prescribe Anusol, with or without cortisone Incise and extract acutely thrombosed piles Apply rubber bands to bleeding first- or second-degree hemorrhoids Operation is rarely indicated; if done, use spinal anesthesia
Varicose veins	Have patient increase exercise level Have patient elevate legs at rest for at least 1 hr twice daily Have patient use support stockings Ligate ulcerated or severely phlebitic veins If anticoagulation is required, use heparin intravenously
Deep vein thrombosis	Treat with intravenous heparin for 14 days Give heparin, 5,000–7,500 units three times daily subcutaneously, as maintenance therapy Do not use warfarin (because of potential teratogenicity)
Round ligament pain	Provide local heat and elastic support to the groin Alter patient position to reduce traction on ligament

ing agents is not advisable. The potential for submucosal abscess formation and pelvic sepsis, though small, makes the procedure extremely dangerous.

On rare occasions, hemorrhoid banding [see 59 *Anal Procedures*] may be indicated for excessive bleeding. It should be performed very carefully because of the potential for necrosis and infection. Banding should be done well above the underlying hemorrhoid to pull the mucosa into the canal.

VARICOSE VEINS

Etiology

Varicosities become a problem with successive pregnancies. They are generally a minor nuisance in the primipara but become more bothersome the more children a woman has. Thrombophlebitis is not uncommon, but embolism is a rare complication. Varicose veins develop in women who are predisposed to this problem as a result of weakness in the valvular structures in the veins. The increased stasis and venous pressure created by the expansion of the uterus leads to progressive enlargement and engorgement of the veins. Besides cosmetic problems, varicosities can cause muscle aching, swelling, and, in severe cases, ulceration.

Treatment

Increased exercise that includes regular walking and activity is suggested. Elevation of the legs at rest is advised; prolonged sitting is not. Support stockings and, in poor weather, support panty hose should be used. The stockings should be placed on the legs in the early morning, before substantial pooling has occurred. Injection therapy is contraindicated during pregnancy. Ligation of veins causing ulceration or phlebitis is recommended only in extreme cases. Administration of aspirin or other NSAIDs is also contraindicated. If anticoagulation is necessary, heparin should be given because it does not cause fetal damage and is fairly easily controlled.

DEEP VEIN THROMBOSIS

Etiology

Pregnant women are more prone to deep vein thrombosis (DVT) during the later stages of pregnancy and the early postpartum period, largely because of alterations in the normal blood coagulation system, such as increased levels of clotting factors and decreased fibrinolytic activity. These intrinsic factors may be exacerbated by the venous stasis and increased blood viscosity that occur during pregnancy. Although venous thrombosis is rare during pregnancy, recognition and management of the disorder [see 70 *Thromboembolic Problems*] are important to prevent the potentially life-threatening sequelae of pulmonary embolism.

Diagnosis

Leg swelling and prominent superficial veins are common in pregnancy and may delay the diagnosis of DVT. Phlebography is the most accurate, operator-independent study available for confirmation of DVT. Because the iliofemoral system is the most common site of DVT, it is crucial that it be well visualized; however, this may not be possible with the fetus shielded. Recent work suggests that the use of serial impedance plethysmography may be effective in diagnosing DVT while eliminating exposure of the fetus to radiation.[94] Doppler ultrasonography is relatively ineffective in predicting isolated pelvic thrombosis but may be attempted. Real-time B-mode ultrasonography is an extremely sensitive examination that is useful in detecting DVT. This technique achieves good visualization of venous thrombi within vessels; however, although clots in leg veins can be readily visualized, the technique is less specific above the inguinal ligament. Radioactive fibrinogen should not be used near term, because of the potential hazard to the fetal thyroid.

Treatment

When the diagnosis is made, continuous intravenous heparin therapy should be instituted at a dosage sufficient to maintain the partial thromboplastin time (PTT) at 1.5 to 2.0 times control for a period of 14 days. Subsequently, subcutaneous injections of heparin should be continued at a dosage of 5,000 to 7,500 units every 8 hours. Warfarin should not ordinarily be given for maintenance anticoagulation; it has teratogenic potential during the first trimester and may induce bleeding during the later part of pregnancy.[95] In patients who are at high risk for DVT because of previous episodes of DVT or bed rest, prophylactic intermittent subcutaneous administration of heparin should be begun in the 34th week of pregnancy and should continue through the first 4 to 6 weeks post partum.[96] When surgery is planned during pregnancy, patients should be fitted with graded compression boots beforehand and should continue to wear them until they are ambulating regularly. Ambulation should be begun on the night of the operation whenever possible.

ROUND LIGAMENT PAIN

Etiology

The general surgeon is occasionally asked to evaluate the pregnant woman in the late stages of her pregnancy with a possible inguinal hernia. Groin hernia in the pregnant patient is extremely uncommon because the expanded uterus acts as a shield against the abdominal wall, preventing incarceration or strangulation of bowel contents. Groin pain is generally caused by excessive traction on the round ligament, usually on the left, during the later part of pregnancy. As the uterus rotates and the patient's position changes, this pain can become quite severe.

Treatment

Local heat and abdominal support are the mainstays of treatment. Positional changes are necessary, and the patient should rest in the supine position.

References

1. Barron WM: The pregnant surgical patient: medical evaluation and management. Ann Intern Med 101:683, 1984
2. Munro A, Jones PF: Abdominal surgical emergencies in the puerperium. Br Med J 4:691, 1975
3. Lavin JP Jr, Polsky SS: Abdominal trauma during pregnancy. Clin Perinatol 10:423, 1983
4. Hoff WS, D'Amelio LF, Tinkoff GH, et al: Maternal predictors of fetal demise in trauma during pregnancy. Surg Gynecol Obstet 172:175, 1991
5. Fildes J, Reed L, Jones N, et al: Trauma: the leading cause of maternal death. J Trauma 32:643, 1992
6. Pearlman MD, Tintinalli JE, Lorenz RP: Blunt trauma during pregnancy. N Engl J Med 323:1609, 1990
7. Kuhlmann RS, Cruikshank DP: Maternal trauma during pregnancy. Clin Obstet Gynecol 37:274, 1994
8. Drost TF, Rosemurgy AS, Sherman HF, et al: Major trauma in pregnant women: maternal/fetal outcome. J Trauma 30:574, 1990
9. Sorensen VJ, Bivins BA, Obeid FN, et al: Management of general surgical emergencies in pregnancy. Am Surg 56:245, 1990
10. Goodwin TM, Breen MT: Pregnancy outcome and fetomaternal hemorrhage after noncatastrophic trauma. Am J Obstet Gynecol 162:665, 1990
11. Pearlman MD, Tintinalli JE, Lorenz RP: A prospective controlled study of outcome after trauma during pregnancy. Am J Obstet Gynecol 162:1502, 1990
12. Gonik B: Intensive care monitoring of the critically ill pregnant patient. Maternal-Fetal Medicine. Creasy RK, Resnik R, Eds. WB Saunders Co, Philadelphia, 1989, p 867
13. Ibrahim N, Payne E, Owen A: Spontaneous rupture of the liver in association with pregnancy. Br J Obstet Gynaecol 92:539, 1985
14. Henny CP, Lim AE, Brummelkamp WH, et al: A review of the importance of acute multidisciplinary treatment following spontaneous rupture of the liver capsule during pregnancy. Surg Gynecol Obstet 156:593, 1983
15. Babaknia A, Parsa H, Woodruff JD: Appendicitis during pregnancy. Obstet Gynecol 50:40, 1977
16. Tamir IL, Bongard FS, Klein SR: Acute appendicitis in the pregnant patient. Am J Surg 160:571, 1990
17. Masters K, Levine BA, Gaskill HV, et al: Diagnosing appendicitis during pregnancy. Am J Surg 148:768, 1984
18. Frisenda R, Roty AR Jr, Kilway JB, et al: Acute appendicitis during pregnancy. Am Surg 45:503, 1979
19. Adams DH, Fine C, Brooks DC: High-resolution real-time ultrasonography: a new tool in the diagnosis of acute appendicitis. Am J Surg 155:93, 1988
20. Anderson JM, Lee TG, Nagel N: Ultrasound diagnosis of nonobstetric disease during pregnancy. Obstet Gynecol 48:359, 1976
21. Loughlin KR, Bailey RB Jr: Internal ureteral stents for conservative management of ureteral calculi during pregnancy. N Engl J Med 315:1647, 1986
22. Kavoussi LR, Albala DM, Basler JW, et al: Percutaneous management of urolithiasis during pregnancy (pt 2). J Urol 148:1069, 1992
23. Novak ER, Lambrou CD, Woodruff JD: Ovarian tumors in pregnancy: an ovarian tumor registry review. Obstet Gynecol 46:401, 1975
24. McComb P, Laimon H: Appendicitis complicating pregnancy. Can J Surg 23:92, 1980
25. Horowitz MD, Gomez GA, Santiesteban R, et al: Acute appendicitis during pregnancy: diagnosis and management. Arch Surg 120:1362, 1985
26. Sharp HT: Gastrointestinal surgical conditions during pregnancy. Clin Obstet Gynecol 37:306, 1994
27. Mazze RI, Kallen B: Appendectomy during pregnancy: a Swedish registry study of 778 cases. Obstet Gynecol 77:835, 1991
28. Curet MJ, Allen D, Josloff RK, et al: Laparoscopy during pregnancy. Arch Surg 131:546, 1996
29. Kammerer WS: Nonobstetric surgery during pregnancy. Med Clin North Am 63:1157, 1979
30. Hill LM, Symmonds RE: Small bowel obstruction in pregnancy: a review and report of four cases. Obstet Gynecol 49:170, 1977
31. Perdue PW, Johnson HW, Stafford PW: Intestinal obstruction complicating pregnancy. Am J Surg 164:384, 1992
32. Milne B, Johnstone MS: Intestinal obstruction in pregnancy. Scot Med J 24:80, 1979
33. Shaxted EJ, Jukes R: Pseudo-obstruction of the bowel in pregnancy: case reports. Br J Obstet Gynaecol 86:411, 1979
34. Paul M, Tew WL, Holiday RL: Perforated peptic ulcer in pregnancy with survival of mother and child: case report and review of the literature. Can J Surg 19:427, 1976
35. Braverman DZ, Johnson ML, Kern F Jr: Effects of pregnancy and contraceptive steroids on gallbladder function. N Engl J Med 302:362, 1980
36. Kern F Jr, Everson GT, DeMark B, et al: Biliary lipids, bile acids, and gallbladder function in the human female: effects of pregnancy and the ovulatory cycle. J Clin Invest 68:1229, 1981
37. Glenn F, McSherry CK: Gallstones and pregnancy among 300 young women treated by cholecystectomy. Surg Gynecol Obstet 127:1067, 1968
38. Woodhouse DR, Haylen B: Gall bladder disease complicating pregnancy. Aust NZ J Obstet Gynaecol 25:233, 1985
39. Bynum TE: Hepatic and gastrointestinal disorders in pregnancy. Med Clin North Am 61:129, 1977
40. Cheng YS: Pregnancy in liver cirrhosis and/or portal hypertension. Am J Obstet Gynecol 128:812, 1977
41. Seymour CA, Chadwick VS: Liver and gastrointestinal function in pregnancy. Postgrad Med J 55:343, 1979
42. Hiatt JR, Hiatt JC, Williams RA, et al: Biliary disease in pregnancy: strategy for surgical management. Am J Surg 151:263, 1986
43. McKellar DP, Anderson CT, Boynton CJ, et al: Cholecystectomy during pregnancy without fetal loss. Surg Gynecol Obstet 174:465, 1992
44. Dixon NP, Faddis DM, Silberman H: Aggressive management of cholecystitis during pregnancy. Am J Surg 154:292, 1987
45. Machi J, Sigel B, McGarth EC, et al: Operative ultrasonography in the biliary tract during pregnancy. Surg Gynecol Obstet 160:119, 1985
46. Morrell DG, Mullins JR, Harrison PB: Laparoscopic cholecystectomy during pregnancy in symptomatic patients. Surgery 112:856, 1992
47. Soper NJ, Hunter JG, Petrie RH: Laparoscopic cholecystectomy during pregnancy. Surg Endosc 6:115, 1992
48. Weber AM, Bloom GP, Allen TR, et al: Laparoscopic cholecystectomy during pregnancy. Obstet Gynecol 78:958, 1991
49. Lanzafame RJ: Laparoscopic cholecystectomy during pregnancy. Surgery 118:627, 1995
50. Constantino GN, Vincent GJ, Mukalian GG, et al: Laparoscopic cholecystectomy in pregnancy. J Laparoendosc Surg 4:161, 1994
51. McKay AJ, O'Neill J, Imrie CW: Pancreatitis, pregnancy and gallstones. Br J Obstet Gynaecol 87:47, 1980
52. Glueck CJ, Christopher C, Mishkel MA, et al: Pancreatitis, familial hypertriglyceridemia, and pregnancy. Am J Obstet Gynecol 136:755, 1980
53. Lykkesfeldt G, Bock JE, Pedersen FD, et al: Excessive hypertriglyceridemia and pancreatitis in pregnancy: association with deficiency of lipoprotein lipase. Acta Obstet Gynecol Scand 60:79, 1981
54. Barnes CG: Medical Disorders in Obstetric Practice, 4th ed. Blackwell Scientific Publications, Oxford, England, 1974, p 145
55. Thomason JL, Sampson MB, Farb HF, et al: Pregnancy complicated by concurrent primary hyperparathyroidism and pancreatitis. Obstet Gynecol 57(suppl 6): 34S, 1981
56. Young KR: Acute pancreatitis in pregnancy: two case reports. Obstet Gynecol 60:653, 1982
57. Hasselgren PO: Acute pancreatitis in pregnancy: report of two cases. Acta Chir Scand 146:297, 1980
58. Jouppila P, Mokka R, Larmi TK: Acute pancreatitis in pregnancy. Surg Gynecol Obstet 139:879, 1974
59. Strickland DM, Hauth JC, Widish J, et al: Amylase and isoamylase activities in serum of pregnant women. Obstet Gynecol 63:389, 1984
60. DeVore GR, Bracken M, Berkowitz RL: The amylase/creatinine clearance ratio in normal pregnancy and pregnancies complicated by pancreatitis, hyperemesis gravidarum, and toxemia. Am J Obstet Gynecol 136:747, 1980

61. Dreiling DA, Bordalo O, Rosenberg V, et al: Pregnancy and pancreatitis. Am J Gastroenterol 64:23, 1975
62. Vonherzen J, Noe J, Goodlin R: Pancreatitis pseudocyst complicating pregnancy. Obstet Gynecol 45:588, 1975
63. Baillie J, Cairns SR, Putnam WS, et al: Endoscopic management of choledocholithiasis during pregnancy. Surg Gynecol Obstet 171:1, 1990
64. Gineston JL, Capron JP, Delcenserie R, et al: Prolonged total parenteral nutrition in a pregnant woman with acute pancreatitis. J Clin Gastroenterol 6:249, 1984
65. DeVore GR: Acute abdominal pain in the pregnant patient due to pancreatitis, acute appendicitis, cholecystitis, or PUD. Clin Perinatol 7:349, 1980
66. Vender RJ, Spiro HM: Inflammatory bowel disease and pregnancy. J Clin Gastroenterol 4:231, 1982
67. Nielsen OH, Andreasson B, Bondesen S, et al: Pregnancy in Crohn's disease. Scand J Gastroenterol 19:724, 1984
68. Mogadam M, Korelitz BI, Ahmed SW, et al: The course of inflammatory bowel disease during pregnancy and postpartum. Am J Gastroenterol 75:265, 1981
69. Baiocco PJ, Korelitz BI: The influence of inflammatory bowel disease and its treatment on pregnancy and fetal outcome. J Clin Gastroenterol 6:211, 1984
70. Woolfson K, Cohen Z, McLeod RS: Crohn's disease and pregnancy. Dis Colon Rectum 33:869, 1990
71. Warsof SL: Medical and surgical treatment of inflammatory bowel disease in pregnancy. Clin Obstet Gynecol 26:822, 1983
72. Mogadam M, Dobbins WO III, Korelitz BI, et al: Pregnancy in inflammatory bowel disease: effect of sulfasalazine and corticosteroids on fetal outcome. Gastroenterology 80:72, 1981
73. Witter FR, King TM, Blake DA: The effects of chronic gastrointestinal medication on the fetus and neonate. Obstet Gynecol 58(suppl 5):79S, 1981
74. Rivera-Alsina ME, Saldana LR, Stringer CA: Fetal growth sustained by parenteral nutrition in pregnancy. Obstet Gynecol 64:138, 1984
75. Jacobson LB, Clapp DH: Total parenteral nutrition in pregnancy complicated by Crohn's disease. JPEN 11:93, 1987
76. Niederhoff H, Zahradnik HP: Analgesics during pregnancy. Am J Med 75:117, 1983
77. Beeley L: Adverse effects of drugs in later pregnancy. Clin Obstet Gynaecol 8:275, 1981
78. Crawford JS, Lewis M: Nitrous oxide in early human pregnancy. Anesthesia 41:900, 1986
79. DiFronzo LA, O'Connell TX: Breast cancer in pregnancy and lactation. Surg Clin North Am 76:267, 1996
80. Anderson JM: Mammary cancers and pregnancy. Br Med J 1:1124, 1979
81. Barnavon Y, Wallack MK: Management of the pregnancy patient with carcinoma of the breast. Surg Gynecol Obstet 171:347, 1990
82. Demarsky LJ, Neishstadt EL: Breast cancer and pregnancy. Breast 7:17, 1980
83. King RM, Welch JS, Martin JL, et al: Carcinoma of the breast associated with pregnancy. Surg Gynecol Obstet 160:228, 1985
84. Miller R, Mulvihill S: Small head size after atomic radiation. Teratology 14:355, 1976
85. Garber JE: Long-term follow-up of children exposed in utero to antineoplastic agents. Semin Oncol 16:437, 1989
86. Smith BK, Rayburn WF, Feller I: Burns and pregnancy. Clin Perinatol 10:383, 1983
87. Amy BW, McManus WF, Goodwin CW, et al: Thermal injury in the pregnant patient. Surg Gynecol Obstet 161:209, 1985
88. Cheah SH, Sivanesaratnam V: Burns in pregnancy—maternal and fetal prognosis. Aust NZ J Obstet Gynaecol 29:143, 1989
89. Rode H, Millar AJ, Cywes S, et al: Thermal injury in pregnancy—the neglected tragedy. S Afr Med J 77:346, 1990
90. Gonik B: Intensive care monitoring of the critically ill pregnant patient. Maternal-Fetal Medicine: Principles and Practice, 3rd ed. Creasy RK, Resnick R, Eds. WB Saunders Co, Philadelphia, 1994
91. Rayburn W, Smith B, Feller I, et al: Major burns during pregnancy: effects on fetal well-being. Obstet Gynecol 63:392, 1984
92. Widgerow AD, Ford TD, Botha M: Burn contracture preventing uterine expansion. Ann Plast Surg 27:269, 1991
93. Hey VM, Cowley DJ, Ganguli PC, et al: Gastrooesophageal reflux in late pregnancy. Anaesthesia 32:372, 1977
94. Hull RD, Raskob GE, Carter CJ: Serial impedance plethysmography in pregnant patients with clinically suspected deep-vein thrombosis. Ann Intern Med 112:663, 1990
95. Ginsberg JS, Hirsh J: Anticoagulants during pregnancy. Annu Rev Med 40:79, 1989
96. Bolan JC: Thromboembolic complications of pregnancy. Clin Obstet Gynecol 26:913, 1983
97. MacBurney MM, Wilmore DW: Parenteral nutrition in pregnancy. Parenteral Nutrition. Rombeau JL, Caldwell M, Eds. WB Saunders Co, Philadelphia, 1986
98. Dashe JS, Gilstrap LC: Antibiotic use in pregnancy. Obstet Gynecol Clin North Am 24:617, 1997
99. Murray L, Seger D: Drug therapy during pregnancy and lactation. Emerg Med Clin North Am 12:129, 1994
100. Rosenthal MH: Intrapartum intensive care management of the cardiac patient. Clin Obstet Gynecol 24:789, 1981
101. Clark SL, Cotton DB, Lee W, et al: Central hemodynamic assessment of normal term pregnancy. Am J Obstet Gynecol 161:1439, 1989

Acknowledgment

Figure 1   Carol Donner.

78 CLINICAL AND LABORATORY DIAGNOSIS OF INFECTION

David C. Evans, M.D., and Jonathan L. Meakins, M.D., D.Sc.

Approach to Diagnosis of Surgical Infection

The presence of surgical infectious disease is determined clinically, usually with confirmation and microbiologic diagnosis provided by the laboratory. Identification of an infection is rarely incidental; usually, it is a response to a clinical *signal*. This signal is often fever but may be one of a number of other symptoms and signs or some combination thereof.

Most surgical infections are outpatient conditions that are easily diagnosed and treated. Infections in hospitalized patients, whether related to the primary surgical disease or resulting from surgical therapy, are less easily managed. The greatest challenges in diagnosis and treatment of surgical infections arise in the perioperative and postoperative periods.

Infection versus Sepsis

Before the advent of surgical critical care units, the definitions of a number of key concepts—infection, sepsis, bacteremia, septicemia, septic shock, endotoxemia—were either treated as interchangeable or, if not interchangeable, considered to be of interest primarily to academics with a research orientation. However, as diagnostic possibilities have expanded and our ability to resuscitate and support critically ill patients has improved, classic clinical problems have evolved into new and more complex problems that call for new definitions—especially for the fundamental concepts of infection and sepsis[1] [see Sidebar Definitions of Key Concepts]. The crucial point is that infection and sepsis are conceptually distinct: infection is a process, and sepsis is the response to that process. The response provides the clinical signals that lead to diagnosis of the initiating process. As a rule, infection, once diagnosed, is easily treated with antibiotics and drainage. It is the management of sepsis that is difficult [see 95 Multiple Organ Dysfunction Syndrome].

Normally Responsive versus Compromised or Complex Patients

The fact that signs and symptoms of infection in compromised or complex patients differ from those in normally responsive hosts has important diagnostic implications. The normally responsive patient, for whom the physician can obtain a history and perform a physical examination, responds to infection in the classic manner—that is, with fever, elevated white blood cell count, malaise, and other appropriate symptoms. If infection is severe, a normally responsive patient may become compromised. The compromised or complex patient is unable to meet inflammatory or infectious challenges in the normal manner [see 74 Non-AIDS Immunosuppression]. The clinical response to infection is altered in such a patient: the signals of infection differ from those in the normally responsive patient and often develop at a later stage of infection. A multitude of clinical conditions or physiologic states are represented by compromised or complex patients, who include elderly patients, patients who are immunosuppressed as a result of either disease or medications, patients with thermal injury or major trauma, patients receiving chemotherapy, patients receiving treatment for stable degrees of end-organ failure in intensive care units, and patients with more than one chronic disease. The prevalence of such patients in modern hospital surgical practice is increasing.

The normally responsive patient and the compromised or complex patient are merely extreme points on the clinical spectrum rather than categorically distinct populations.

General Approach to Clinical and Laboratory Diagnosis of Infection

The search for an infection is initiated in response to a clinical signal indicating a problem that requires resolution [see Table 1]. The

---

Definitions of Key Concepts

For the purposes of the present discussion, infection, bacteremia, sepsis, severe sepsis, and septic shock will be defined as follows[1]:

- Infection is a microbial phenomenon characterized by an inflammatory response to the presence of microorganisms or the invasion of normally sterile host tissue by these organisms.
- Bacteremia is the presence of viable bacteria in the blood.
- Sepsis is the systemic response to infection. This response is manifested by the occurrence of two or more of the following conditions as a result of infection: (a) temperature higher than 38° C or lower than 36° C, (b) heart rate greater than 90 beats/min, (c) respiratory rate greater than 20 breaths/min or arterial carbon dioxide tension less than 32 mm Hg, and (d) white blood cell count greater than 12,000/ mm³ or less than 4,000/mm³, or immature (band) forms accounting for more than 10% of the neutrophils present.
- Severe sepsis is sepsis associated with organ dysfunction, hypoperfusion, or hypotension. Hypoperfusion and perfusion abnormalities may include, but are not limited to, lactic acidosis, oliguria, or acute alteration of mental status.
- Septic shock is sepsis with hypotension, occurring despite adequate fluid resuscitation, along with the presence of perfusion abnormalities that may include, but are not limited to, lactic acidosis, oliguria, or acute alteration of mental status. Patients receiving inotropes or vasopressors may not be hypotensive at the time when perfusion abnormalities are measured.

Approach to Diagnosis of Surgical Infection

Clinical signals of infection in compromised or complex patients differ from those in normally responsive patients

The clinical signal is often fever but may be one of several other symptoms and signs or a combination thereof.

Infection in normally responsive patients usually presents with appropriate signals

Cardinal signs of inflammation are
- Redness • Heat • Pain • Swelling • Loss of function

Other appropriate signals include
- Fever (≥ 38° C) appearing after normal postoperative T° elevation has resolved
- ↑ WBC
- Infectious syndrome (manifested by failure to thrive, unexplained anorexia, and indefinably unsatisfactory clinical course)

Presence and location of infection (first suggested by clinical findings) are confirmed by directed laboratory assessment

---

Septic shock may be the first signal of infection

Manifestations include tachycardia; tachypnea; hypotension; warm, dry extremities; generalized flushing; other signs of a hyperdynamic, hypermetabolic state.

Diagnosis and therapy should proceed concurrently.

Empirical antibiotic therapy is always instituted before diagnosis is completed

Efficacy of empirical antibiotic therapy is assessed on the basis of the patient's clinical course; empirical antibiotic therapy is modified or discontinued accordingly.

General approach to diagnosis of infection

Begin with history and physical examination.

Perform laboratory assessment:
- Obtain Gram's stain and cultures of wound tissue, sputum, urine, and drainage effluent.
- Consider percutaneous aspiration and microbiologic examination of potentially infected fluid.
- Obtain WBC and blood chemistry measurements.
- Obtain chest x-ray; consider ultrasonography or CT scan of operative site.

In normally responsive patients, specific therapy is started on the basis of diagnosis

Infection in compromised or complex patients is often occult

Risk factors include
- Advanced age
- Thermal injury
- Major trauma
- Chemotherapy
- End-organ failure
- Presence of more than one chronic disease

Infection may be clinically manifested by
- Confusion
- Hypotension
- Ileus
- Water retention
- Gastric bleeding
- Delayed wound healing

Fever may or may not be present or related to infection.

Laboratory signs of occult infection include
- Renal, hepatic, or respiratory dysfunction
- Thrombocytopenia
- Hyperglycemia and insulin resistance
- Immune failure

Sepsis is mild to moderate

Empirical antibiotic therapy is sometimes instituted before diagnosis

Efficacy of empirical antibiotic therapy is assessed on the basis of the patient's clinical course; empirical antibiotic therapy is modified accordingly.

Sepsis is severe

Empirical antibiotic therapy is often instituted before diagnosis

Efficacy of empirical antibiotic therapy is assessed on the basis of the patient's clinical course; empirical antibiotic therapy is modified accordingly.

Presence and location of infection must be determined by laboratory tests, with clinical support

---

No infection present

Stop antibiotics. Maintain hemostasis and provide hemodynamic, nutritional, and physiologic support. Search for noninfectious causes of septic response. Support and wait.

Table 1 **Fundamental Approach to Diagnosis of Infection**

Recognize clinical signal and observe its characteristics:
  Nature
  Intensity
  Rapidity of development

Make best guess as to source and likely pathogen on the basis of
  History of surgical disease
  Physical examination
  Microbiologic examination of stained specimens
  Radiologic findings

Confirm presence of infection by means of
  Laboratory results
  Observation of clinical course
  Invasive procedures (e.g., paracentesis, thoracentesis, interventional radiology, operation)

---

signal represents the response of a patient to an infection and is a function of the patient's ability to react to the liberated stimuli and mediators and to generate a clinical response to the infectious process. All patients may exhibit one or more of these signals. Normally responsive patients tend to show the classic signals, whereas compromised or complex patients tend to show more subtle changes that often are first noted in the course of routine laboratory tests.

Simply stated, the proper approach to diagnosis in a patient with probable infection begins with a thorough history and physical examination followed by directed, specific laboratory tests. The details of the approach must be modified according to patient characteristics and the circumstances of presentation. For example, if a patient has undergone operation or is in the ICU, the list of possibilities to be considered must be modified, and the time allotted to diagnosis must be reduced.

Infection in Normally Responsive Patients

CARDINAL SIGNS OF INFLAMMATION

Rubor, calor, dolor, tumor, and functio laesa—that is, redness, heat, pain, swelling, and loss of function—have been considered the cardinal signs of inflammation since the times of Hippocrates and Galen. They remain the primary signals leading to medical consultation for outpatient surgical infections and for many of the infectious complications of operation. They represent the host response to infection and may signal the presence of infection even in cases in which the primary site of infection is a deeply situated organ or tissue. These cardinal signs are clinical manifestations of the infection and its accompanying inflammatory process; they either identify the process or guide the investigation. In the hospital setting, such signs, when present, are important clues to the existence of infection. Often, however, nosocomial infections are signaled in more subtle ways.

FEVER

Fever is the most important and the most common signal that an infectious process is present [see 98 Fever, Hyperpyrexia, and Hypothermia]. Postoperative fever is a normal part of the recovery process; understanding the typical febrile course is important in differentiating normal from pathologic fever. It is unusual for a sudden, very high fever to be the first signal of an infection. The infection usually begins to manifest itself with a prodrome, recognition of which speeds diagnosis and therapy. Investigation should be started when the patient's temperature reaches 38° C (100.4° F) rather than 40° C (104° F). Although this point may seem obvious, many of the crisis intervention measures required in managing fevers could be avoided if the significance of more modest temperature elevations were recognized more often.

A fever that appears after the normal postoperative temperature elevation has resolved must not be ignored. To simply wait for such a fever to go away is to court disaster. Complete physical examination of the patient and, in the absence of a diagnosis, directed laboratory tests, followed by reexamination as necessary, are required to determine the nature and severity of the problem.

MISCELLANEOUS SIGNALS

A variety of signals reflect a patient status between normal responsiveness and significant compromise. Many of these signals are soft; moreover, they can sometimes be attributed to patient anxiety, neurosis, or a wish to stay longer in the hospital. In the light of current changes in the hospital population (e.g., increased numbers of elderly patients and patients with multiple medical problems or degrees of organ dysfunction), however, these signals should be considered seriously because in compromised patients, each one can be a harbinger of infection.

Altered Heart Rate

A heart rate that is either too high or too low may signal an infection. On rare occasions, changes in rhythm in the elderly (e.g., paroxysmal atrial tachycardia, atrial flutter, or fibrillation) are indicators of an infectious process. An unexplained sustained increase in pulse rate should not be ignored.

Tachypnea

Tachypnea should be recognized as part of either the prodrome or the infectious syndrome itself. Because it may herald other important diagnoses—pulmonary embolus, for example—tachypnea should not be overlooked.

Pain

Pain that persists or is out of proportion to the expected response deserves attention. Infection is only one of the many possible causes of pain. Often, the pain is referred, and the painful area appears normal on examination. Pneumonia that presents with abdominal findings is a classic example, as is a subphrenic abscess that presents with shoulder-tip pain and a normal range of motion.

Confusion

Confusion may be the most common symptom of infection in the elderly; it is also an important signal in patients who had been well and fit. The physician's first response to confusion in an elderly patient in the postoperative period must be to seek a cause, not to order sedation.

Ileus

Ileus has many causes, some of which are not well understood. Prolonged ileus after abdominal operation—as well as almost any ileus after other operations—requires explanation. Infections at remote sites can produce ileus, as if the bowel were a target organ such as the kidney, liver, or lung. Wound infection and pneumonia are common examples of such infections.

THE INFECTIOUS SYNDROME

The normal response to infection includes what might be best described as a flulike syndrome: general malaise, headache, myalgias, fatigue, and loss of appetite. This syndrome is most often seen in outpatients or patients who have not undergone operation.

In hospitalized patients, particularly patients in the postoperative period, the infectious syndrome will be manifest in the form of failure to thrive, unexplained loss of appetite, and an indefinably unsatisfactory clinical course. These symptoms are so-called soft symptoms; that is, they are hard to recognize. In the current health care environment, characterized by adherence to the diagnosis-related group (DRG) system and growing pressure to shorten hospital stays, these symptoms are often not taken seriously.

Infection in Compromised or Complex Patients

The presence of fever remains a common signal of infection in the compromised or complex patient; however, it may be absent, or the patient's temperature may already be elevated as a result of other causes. Cardinal signs of infection, such as decubitus ulcers, may be present. More often, however, the infection is occult, and classic signals are unrelated to the infectious focus. In some very ill immunocompromised patients, findings that usually signal an infection may already be present. Slight changes in clinical status (such as very small temperature elevations, increased fluid requirements, confusion, or ileus) or changes in laboratory findings (such as an elevated white blood cell count, glucosuria, or hyperglycemia) should trigger investigation.

Patients in whom the first signal of an infectious process is organ dysfunction or failure are more ill than patients in whom high fever is the first signal; perhaps more important, however, is that they are a group whose diagnosis and management require more than standard clinical skills. Because the classic septic response may not be present, it is essential to be alert to the signs and symptoms of occult infection (see below). In these patients, the laboratory becomes increasingly important in diagnosing and understanding the evolution of the infection.

CLINICAL SIGNS AND SYMPTOMS OF OCCULT INFECTION

Subtle changes in temperature, mental status, pulse rate, or respiratory rate may signal occult infection, as may the development of pain or ileus.

Intermittent Hypotension and Septic Shock

Septic shock, an important signal of an unrecognized or occult focus of infection, is the original expression of multisystem failure, but it rarely occurs without warning. The prodrome often includes fever and, perhaps, one or two other signals. Intermittent hypotension is the most characteristic signal. It is not catastrophic and responds quickly to fluid resuscitation. Characteristically, it recurs, at which time it may again respond to fluids. Oliguria may accompany the hypotension. If this clinical picture is allowed to progress, the hypotension will lead to renal failure (see below), with a substantial amount of water retention. Septic shock will result if the infection is not identified, treated with antibiotics, and, if necessary, drained.

Both clinical assessment and laboratory studies are necessary to confirm the presence of septic shock, although florid septic shock is easily recognized on clinical examination alone [see 4 Shock]. Any or all of the following findings may be present in varying degrees in the patient with septic shock: tachycardia; tachypnea; hypotension; warm, dry extremities; generalized flushing; and other signs suggesting a hyperdynamic, hypermetabolic state. Swan-Ganz catheter measurements confirm high cardiac output and low peripheral resistance.

Gastric Hemorrhage

Gastric hemorrhage may be the presenting symptom for serious infection even if prophylactic measures against such hemorrhage have been taken. Gastric acidity and bleeding respond to drainage of an abscess. Hemorrhagic gastritis must be considered a signal of occult infection, which demands prompt diagnosis and treatment.

Delayed Wound Healing

The absence of wound healing can indicate the presence of a significant infection. Typically in such a case, wounds left for delayed primary closure or secondary closure do not exhibit the appropriate granulation tissue and appear pale, dry, and unhealthy. The development of good granulation tissue is a sign that infection is controlled.

LABORATORY SIGNS OF OCCULT INFECTION

Renal Failure

Renal failure is identified by elevations in serum creatinine and blood urea nitrogen (BUN) levels, which can be highly sensitive signals of developing infection. A still more sensitive indicator is an alteration in creatinine clearance, a laboratory test underutilized in the ICU. Such alterations are generally evident before changes in serum levels. Creatinine clearance should be measured at an early stage in high-risk patients. In the presence of shock, renal failure can develop suddenly. Otherwise, loss of renal function is insidious, but it can usually be identified if sought before oliguria or anuria develops. Resolution of infection is associated with return of function.

Hepatic and Respiratory Failure

Hepatic failure, primarily manifested as jaundice, and respiratory failure, initially presenting as a falling arterial oxygen tension and subsequently marked by a need for mechanical ventilation or by a change in the fraction of inspired oxygen (F_IO_2) requirements, can behave in the same way as renal failure (i.e., drainage and control of infection lead to restoration of function).

Thrombocytopenia

Thrombocytopenia may indicate serious infection, although it is not a common signal. If possible, its cause should be identified promptly.

Hyperglycemia and Insulin Resistance

Hyperglycemia and insulin resistance are often reliable signals of the presence of infection in diabetic patients as well as in nondiabetic patients. The degree of insulin resistance can reflect the severity of the infection as well as the effectiveness of infection control.

Immune Failure

Immune failure is discussed in detail elsewhere [see 74 Non-AIDS Immunosuppression]. Severe infection is immunosuppressive. The most clinically applicable assessment of immune failure at present is probably wound healing.

Evaluation for Presence of Infection

Essentially the same clinical and laboratory assessments are used to evaluate normally responsive and compromised or complex patients for the presence of infection. There is, however, a significant difference in emphasis. In normally responsive patients, the diagnosis of infection is usually made on clinical grounds with laboratory support, whereas in compromised or complex patients, the diagnosis is usually made on the basis of laboratory findings with clinical support.

The ICU patient presents a particular conundrum. Nosocomial infection is identified in an estimated 20% of such patients.[2] Despite the frequency with which it is suspected and reported, it is difficult to prove unequivocally. The perceived prevalence of nosocomial infection has created a strong predisposition toward instituting empirical antibiotic therapy in ICU patients; however, the global value of this action in terms of both patient outcome and the impact on the ecology of the ICU is unconfirmed and requires validation. The enormous inconsistencies in how infections are diagnosed have a tremendous effect on our ability to assess the efficacy of therapy for infection. The current approach to diagnosing infection in surgical patients, particularly those who are critically ill or compromised, is still in great need of clarification and standardization.[3] Until the issues are resolved, the clinician must be familiar with the strengths and limitations of a variety of current diagnostic methodologies and then exercise thoughtfulness and disciplined diligence. The likelihood that a particular patient is infected (i.e., the pretest probability) is as important in the decision to treat as the fulfillment of any particular constellation of diagnostic criteria.

HISTORY AND PHYSICAL EXAMINATION

The history should include all background diseases—such as diabetes, lung disease, cirrhosis, hepatitis, kidney disease necessitating dialysis, and previous important infections—as well as a hospitalization history that covers health status, surgical diagnosis and therapy, additional therapeutic interventions (including interventional radiology, monitoring devices, drains, and drugs), and other related variables.

In the early postoperative period (3 to 6 days after operation), the traditional causes of the signals of infection have their origin in the wound, intravascular lines, the urinary tract, and the lungs. Deep thrombophlebitis, with or without pulmonary embolism, may also give rise to the clinical picture of sepsis. The general physical examination is often unrewarding, but a number of specific examinations should be carefully performed, with emphasis given to (1) all wounds and operative sites, (2) all invasive monitoring or therapeutic devices and surrounding areas, (3) all drainage systems and surrounding tissue, with particular attention paid to the nature of the drainage and whether it has recently changed in character or volume (particularly if it has stopped), (4) the rectal examination (for pelvic or prostatic infection), (5) areas of potential decubitus ulcers, (6) the neck (for central nervous system infection), (7) intravascular lines, surrounding tissue, and proximal vessels, (8) the lungs, and (9) the legs. The physical examination is important as a guide for selecting specimens for microbiologic analysis, particularly when wounds or drainage has recently manifested significant changes. The decision to seek radiologic consultation may depend on the findings on physical examination.

BLOOD TESTS

After physical assessment, laboratory blood tests are routinely relied on to orient the surgeon toward or away from a clinical diagnosis of infection. Leukocytosis, particularly with an increase in band forms, is a usual but not constant marker for infection. The white blood cell (WBC) count is widely used to follow the response of infection to therapy and thus has been adopted as a surrogate indicator of the success or failure of therapy. Surprisingly, however, the documentation supporting this ubiquitous practice is sparse,[4,5] and the daily series of complete blood counts often ordered in conjunction with the initiation of antibiotic therapy usually tells the clinician little about a patient's clinical course that cannot be gleaned at the bedside.

In more complex surgical patients, other biochemical cues are used to varying degrees as means of assessing the likelihood of infection. In addition to thrombocytosis, thrombocytopenia, hyperglycemia, and metabolic acidosis, which commonly reflect the stress of severe infection, changes in the erythrocyte sedimentation rate (ESR) and blood levels of C-reactive protein (CRP), procalcitonin (PCT), interleukin-6 (IL-6), and tumor necrosis factor–α (TNF-α) have a significant association with the presence of clinical infection. Plasma CRP concentration, which has been extensively used in some European countries to monitor the evolution of infection, has been found to be significantly elevated in patients with pulmonary aspiration that has induced bacterial infection rather than sterile pneumonitis.[6] Some investigators have suggested that because CRP concentration appears to be particularly responsive to bacterial infection, it may be useful as a monitor of the efficacy of antibiotic use, thereby guiding discontinuance of treatment.[7] A host of cytokines, cellular adhesion molecules, oxidants, and other biomolecules known to participate in systemic inflammation from numerous causes are being extensively investigated to establish both diagnostic and therapeutic functions. As yet, however, no single mediator of systemic inflammation has been validated as a reliable clinical tool for surveillance of the progression of infection or the response of infection to treatment.

MICROBIOLOGIC STUDIES

As a rule, Gram's stains and cultures of wound tissue, sputum, urine, and drainage effluent are the most useful studies. In some cases, however, a battery of cultures of potential sites of infection may be the only feasible approach. Culture techniques are discussed more thoroughly elsewhere [see 79 Blood Cultures and Infection in the Patient with the Septic Response and 81 Nosocomial Infection]. The use of polymerase chain reaction technology to detect bacterial DNA is emerging as a potential alternative to microbiologic culture for determining the presence of infection. The accuracy of this methodology remains to be established, but the rapidity with which it yields results makes it highly promising as a potential guide to therapeutic intervention. Future developments are eagerly awaited.

RADIOLOGY

A chest x-ray is mandatory. Ultrasonographic examination of the operative site may be useful. The possibility of acalculous cholecystitis must be kept in mind [see 83 Infections in the Upper Abdomen: Biliary Tract, Pancreas, Liver, and Spleen]. Computed tomography of the operative site is often more useful than ultrasonography because the presence of wounds, dressings, and drainage tubes may obscure the findings on ultrasonography. In compromised or complex patients who have not recently undergone an operation, the medical and surgical history combined with the radiologic examination may be the only guide to the potential focus (e.g., ulcer, diverticulitis, cholecystitis or cholangitis, or obstructed ureter). Percutaneous aspiration of potentially infected fluid should be considered; the fluid should be microbiologically examined if possible.

Institution of Therapy

The response to infection must be thought of in terms of a continuum ranging from virtually no clinical expression in the immunosuppressed patient to full-blown septic shock. Sepsis, as defined earlier [see *Sidebar* Definitions of Key Concepts], represents a mild to moderate response occurring in normally responsive patients as well as in many compromised or complex patients. On the basis of the degree to which other clinical or laboratory signals manifest themselves, the clinician can evaluate the magnitude of the septic response and, therefore, its clinical gravity.

It is the magnitude of the septic response, as well as the nature and condition of the patient, that governs the clinician's use of specific or empirical therapy. The greater the degree of sepsis, the greater the clinical urgency of solving the two fundamental problems involved: resolution of the initiating process (i.e., treatment of the infection) and modulation of the response to that process (i.e., management of sepsis) [see *95 Multiple Organ Dysfunction Syndrome*]. The therapeutic approach to a given patient is based on the need for speed.

MILD TO MODERATE SEPSIS

The approach to treatment of infection in normally responsive and compromised patients with mild to moderate sepsis includes four steps: (1) if necessary, resuscitation and reestablishment of homeostasis and organ function, (2) diagnosis of the focus of infection by means of microbiologic culture and radiologic examination, (3) treatment with antibiotics, directed as specifically as possible at the presumed cause, and (4) drainage, which often amounts to definitive therapy. In compromised patients, empirical antibiotic therapy is often started before diagnosis and its efficacy gauged by the patient's clinical course [see *Discussion, below*].

Antibiotic treatment Antibiotic treatment must be directed against a likely cause, as determined by recent history (particularly procedures), past history, and physical examination. Examples of likely causes are (1) urinary manipulation, which indicates coverage against enterococci and gram-negative bacteria with ampicillin and an aminoglycoside, (2) colonic flora, which indicates coverage against anaerobes and aerobes, (3) vascular lines, which indicate coverage against gram-positive organisms, (4) cholangitis, which indicates coverage against aerobic gram-negative bacteria with ceftriaxone or an aminoglycoside, and (5) pneumonia, which indicates coverage against gram-positive and gram-negative aerobes.

Drainage The search for the focus of infection is important because drainage may resolve the entire problem. The clinical state can be changed dramatically by technical or mechanical management of pus behind an obstruction (e.g., in the biliary tree, urinary tract, or tracheobronchial tree) or of pus under pressure (e.g., an abscess), manipulation of a drain, or removal of a foreign body (e.g., an intravascular line or pacemaker). Prompt elimination of all foci of infection that can be drained or are operable is critical. Needle aspiration of peritoneal or pleural fluid may be very helpful. Wounds must be reevaluated constantly and the presence of pressure sores ruled out. Drainage can often be performed percutaneously (e.g., for pyelonephritis in an obstructed ureter or for subphrenic abscess) or endoscopically (e.g., for cholangitis).

SEVERE SEPSIS AND SEPTIC SHOCK

For assessment and management of severe sepsis and septic shock [see *Sidebar* Definitions of Key Concepts], the four steps in treatment—resuscitation, diagnosis of the infectious focus, antibiotic therapy, and drainage—must be performed concurrently. Specifically, I.V. administration of antibiotics must be initiated immediately, before the diagnostic process is completed, and the potentially drainable focus must be identified via physical examination or radiologic techniques. The choice of antibiotic depends on (1) what the likely source of infection is (e.g., a lung, a perforated viscus, or the biliary tract), (2) whether the infection is hospital acquired (in which case antibiotic resistance must be considered), and (3) whether the patient has previously received antibiotic therapy. No "shotgun" regimen can be universally recommended.

Case Study: Clinical Picture of Sepsis without Infection

Infection is a process; sepsis is the response.

The difficulty of managing the patient who manifests the septic response in the absence of infection is illustrated by the following case:

A 55-year-old insulin-dependent man with peripheral vascular disease presented with evidence of infection in both feet. Hydration and antibiotic therapy did not prevent progression of the infection, and within 18 hours, it was apparent that amputation would be required for source control. In the course of the operation, gas gangrene, more extensive than had been clinically suspected, was discovered. The initial below-the-knee amputations were eventually followed by a hip disarticulation on one side and a high above-the-knee amputation on the other. Over the 36-hour period during which the infectious process was being controlled, classic septic shock, renal failure, coma, and respiratory failure developed. There was no change in the patient's hyperdynamic and hypermetabolic state after the amputations. During the following 3 weeks, he required ventilator support and daily hemodialysis or hemofiltration; became jaundiced and more deeply comatose; received fluids in amounts significantly in excess of output to maintain blood volume; was hyperglycemic despite receiving regular insulin in dosages of 3 to 5 U/hr; and remained in a hyperdynamic state. Shortly after the last operation, an ileus developed, accompanied by gross fluid retention, which further increased the patient's girth.

This state of overt sepsis with hypermetabolism persisted while the wounds healed by primary closure, but no focus of infection could be found.

Antibiotic therapy was stopped 10 days after operation; the patient's clinical status did not change. Frequent searches were made to ensure that no infection had been overlooked. Suggestions—seriously put forward—to explore the patient's abdomen because "there must be something there" were not heeded. At the end of the third week, for no obvious reason, the patient started to urinate, his ileus resolved, and he was gradually weaned from the ventilator. His level of consciousness improved, the massive edema cleared, and the high cardiac output and low peripheral resistance resolved over a period of 72 hours. He was discharged from the surgical ICU 1 day later and from the hospital in 3 weeks. Some noninfectious process that had maintained this patient's persistent septic response had disappeared or had been turned off, and the result was rapid resolution of the septic state and recovery of health.

As noted, initial control of infection, though difficult, was achieved relatively early. Subsequent therapeutic efforts involved providing hemodynamic, metabolic, and physiologic support of the patient's failing organs and organ systems while waiting for the septic response to resolve. The real problem in this case was not the infection but the patient's unremitting septic response, which was initiated by the infection but maintained in its absence.

THE SYSTEMIC INFLAMMATORY RESPONSE IN THE ABSENCE OF INFECTION

In critically ill and traumatized ICU patients, it is not uncommon for clinical signs and symptoms indistinguishable from those of severe sepsis to arise or persist in the absence of any infection [see Sidebar Case Study: Clinical Picture of Sepsis without Infection]. Burn injury and pancreatitis are classic examples of conditions that can provoke such a response: both can give rise to a hyperdynamic, hypermetabolic clinical picture identical to that of sepsis or severe sepsis, even when no infection is present. Surgeons have learned, to their cost, not to give antibiotics unless there is evidence of infection. The instinctive reflex to do something must be held in check: "masterful inactivity" is the appropriate response until a specific source that can be controlled is identified.

Discussion

Approaches to Specific Infections in the Complex Surgical Patient

The following infections may occur in all surgical patients. They are, however, much more difficult to identify in complex surgical patients, such as those admitted to intensive care. Because the signals of infection are less specific and extremely difficult to interpret after injury or operation, the approach to diagnosing and treating infection must be cautious and disciplined.

SURGICAL SITE INFECTION

Surgical site infections include all infections occurring within the operative field, from the skin to the actual area of surgery.[8]

The patient history should address previous diseases as well as issues concerning the operation itself, such as classification, duration, difficulty, urgency, use of drains, other details of the procedure, time elapsed since the operation, and whether the patient was immunosuppressed, experienced trauma, or received chemotherapy. Physical examination should focus on the cardinal signs of infection and the absence or presence of a healing ridge.

Deeper infections tend to become apparent later in the postoperative course, often after a period in which the patient appears to be recovering, and are associated with a variety of signals, some of which can appear suddenly. The physical examination is often useless or misleading because of discomfort associated with the operation. Rectal examination is important because it may detect abscess formation or bleeding. Return of ileus after an abdominal operation is a significant clue to the presence of abdominal infection.

Culture is essential because use of the correct antibiotics is particularly vital in treatment of compromised or complex patients. Knowledge of the organism and its sensitivities is the key to identifying epidemic or multiresistant strains.

URINARY TRACT INFECTION

Nearly all patients admitted to the ICU have a urinary catheter in place; of these, it is estimated that about 20% progress to urinary tract infection (UTI).[2] Bacteria adhere to urinary catheter surfaces, where they promote growth of a so-called biofilm composed of microorganisms, bacterial glycocalices, Tamm-Horsfall protein, and urinary salts. Eradication of this infectious nidus is essentially impossible without catheter removal.[9] The standard criterion for the diagnosis of UTI (10^5 bacteria/ml) is difficult to apply in catheterized patients because antibiotic therapy without removal of the catheter and the source of bacteriuria would be ineffective. Furthermore, it is well established that urine cultures demonstrating as few as 10^1 or 10^2 bacteria/ml increase 1,000-fold within 1 to 2 days[10]; therefore, effectively any bacterial growth on a urine culture from a catheterized patient signals heavy colonization, if not infection.

More important than quantifying the degree of bacteriuria is determining whether there is any evidence of tissue invasion by urinary bacteria, which would present as pyelonephritis, cystitis, prostatitis, epididymitis, bacteremia, or systemic sepsis. The patient history should determine whether a Foley catheter was used and for how long; how, when, and why it was inserted; instrumentation (e.g., a so-called in-and-out catheter, cystoscopy, or transurethral resection of the prostate); and whether the patient has had any prior UTIs. The physical examination should ascertain whether there is any costovertebral angle tenderness or evidence of prostatic or epididymal tenderness.

Laboratory tests should include gross and microscopic urinalysis, urine culture, and sensitivity tests. Blood culture is important because it may substantiate the diagnosis, identify the bacteria present, and determine the degree of invasiveness of the infectious process.

VASCULAR CATHETER INFECTION

The most frequent sites of infection postoperatively are intravenous catheters, particularly peripheral ones. Diagnosis of peripheral catheter infection is simple and is made on clinical grounds. Diagnosis of central venous catheter (CVC) infection is more difficult. Because hospitalized patients are increasingly being supported by monitoring or therapeutic modalities that depend on vascular access (e.g., total parenteral nutrition and dialysis), line infections have become more common, with an incidence ranging from two to 30 infections per 1,000 central catheter days.[11] The combined pressures imposed by (1) the need to maintain vascular access in sicker and more complex patients and (2) the increasing predominance of gram-positive CVC infections observed since the late 1970s has led clinicians in many centers to administer empirical therapy without line removal to complex patients as a matter of course; some even advocate 10 to 21 days of vancomycin-based therapy. The problems associated with the latter approach—emerging vancomycin resistance, nephrotoxicity, and rash—are serious and relate specifically to the diagnostic strategy used to manage potential CVC infections. The distinction between contamination, colonization, and true infection is problematic; as a result, a number of diagnostic strategies have been advocated that are predicated more on practicality and cost-effectiveness than on microbiologic reality.

It is believed that CVC infection most commonly arises from invasion by skin microorganisms (*Staphylococcus aureus* or *Staphylococcus epidermidis* in about 80% of cases), which may manifest itself as exit-site purulence with or without local cellulitis, as a tunnel infection that may be clinically difficult to detect, or as catheter-related bloodstream infection (CR-BSI). Of these, CR-BSI, which complicates as many as 5% of line placements, is the most clinically important entity. It is strictly diagnosed by identification of the same microorganism (identical species and antibiogram) grown from both the catheter and a peripheral blood culture. The catheter may be cultured in one of several ways, the most common of which is the roll-plate method [see 81 Nosocomial Infection]. Because it is theoretically possible that this technique may fail to detect bacteria harbored within the catheter lumen, some authorities advocate the more sensitive sonication method, in which the catheter segment is immersed and agitated in a medium to produce a broth that contains bacteria from both the internal and the external surfaces of the line. This technique is both more costly and more time consuming, in that it requires quantitative cultures that are deemed positive only when more than 10^3 colony-forming units are detected. More often, blood drawn through the CVC or cultured from an exit-site exudate is compared with peripheral cultures, and thus there is no need to remove the line. If quantitative cultures are done, a line-blood culture showing five times more growth than the peripheral sample strongly suggests that the catheter is the source of the bacteremia; on its own, a line-blood culture is not sensitive or specific enough to be diagnostically useful.

PULMONARY INFECTION

Diagnosis and management of nosocomial pneumonia in surgical patients is addressed in detail elsewhere [see *103 Early Postoperative Pneumonia*]. The central issue is that there is no universal agreement as to how pneumonia—particularly ventilator-associated pneumonia—should be diagnosed. Of the innumerable diagnostic options, none can rely on demonstration of tissue invasion by microorganisms, as would be ideal: all are to some degree nonspecific, and any may be invoked to justify initiation of antibiotic therapy.[12] Randomized trials linking mode of diagnosis to therapeutic strategy and then to outcome are badly needed.[13]

SINUSITIS

All patients undergoing prolonged nasogastric intubation are predisposed to sinus infection. Previous facial trauma and a history of sinusitis are potential contributing factors as well. (Otitis and pharyngitis, which are not often considered, occur in much the same group of patients.) Because maxillary or frontal area tenderness is nonspecific in very ill surgical patients, the diagnosis is usually based on CT demonstration of sinus opacification or air-fluid levels. As a first step, sinus drainage should be reestablished by removal of an unnecessary nasogastric tube. When diagnosis seems urgent, many authorities advocate sinus aspiration for culture before empirical antibiotic therapy is begun.

PAROTITIS

Parotitis is an increasingly common clinical diagnosis in elderly patients. It is usually caused by *S. aureus* and diagnosed on the basis of the presence of the classic local signs of inflammation. Culture of Stensen's duct and blood culture are useful.

PROSTATITIS

Prostatitis (diagnosed by rectal examination) and epididymitis are clinical expressions of Foley catheter–related infection. The aid of prostatic massage is important in obtaining specimens for culture. It should be remembered that a blocked Foley catheter is the most common cause of hospital anuria. This obstruction can lead to devastating purulent cystitis and upper UTI.

PSEUDOMEMBRANOUS ENTEROCOLITIS

Antibiotic-associated pseudomembranous enterocolitis is diagnosed by performing proctosigmoidoscopy and obtaining specimens for serology and culture. *Clostridium difficile* is frequently identified as the causative pathogen. Although pseudomembranous colitis is rarely clinically impressive and is easy to overlook, it can be rapidly fatal. Initial appropriate antibiotic therapy is not always successful; therefore, reevaluation at the end of the treatment course is required.

The Systemic Inflammatory Response Syndrome: Terminology

The human body's physiologic response to systemic infection is well characterized and is often referred to as sepsis. As noted, however [see Infection versus Sepsis, *above*], infection and sepsis are distinct entities that do not always occur concurrently in seriously ill patients. The normal septic response to infection may, in fact, be completely absent in immunosuppressed patients. Most surgeons, for example, have encountered a patient receiving high doses of steroids who has a perforated intra-abdominal viscus and fecal peritonitis but whose leukocyte count, temperature, and blood pressure are all normal. Conversely, the septic response may be present in noninfected patients.[14,15] For example, patients with acute pancreatitis, tissue necrosis, or fractures may manifest physiologic and metabolic changes that are indistinguishable from those associated with bacteremia, even in the absence of infection. Animal studies have confirmed that a sepsislike syndrome can occur without microbial invasion of host tissues.[16]

Accordingly, several clinicians have used the term sepsis syndrome to refer to the group of signs, symptoms, and physiologic changes that result from a variety of sterile inflammatory processes as well as from systemic infection.[15,17] The problem with using the term in this way, however, is that it derives from a Greek word (*sepsis* "decay") that implies infection with microorganisms. The most recent edition of *Dorland's*[18] defines sepsis as "the presence in the blood or other tissues of pathogenic microorganisms or their toxins; the condition associated with such presence." It is therefore not surprising that application of the term sepsis syndrome to noninfectious settings has led to some confusion.[19,20]

Various attempts have been made to refine the terminology used to describe sepsis and related phenomena. The definitions of infection, bacteremia, sepsis, severe sepsis, and septic shock cited earlier [see Sidebar Definitions of Key Concepts] were derived from an August 1991 consensus conference held by the American College of Chest Physicians and the Society of Critical Care Medicine.[1] In addition to defining these commonly used terms, the conference participants proposed adoption of two new terms, systemic inflammatory response syndrome (SIRS) and multiple organ dysfunction syndrome (MODS), which were defined as follows:

1. SIRS is the systemic inflammatory response to a variety of severe clinical insults (either infectious or noninfectious). The response is manifested by two or more of the following conditions: (a) temperature higher than 38° C (100.4° F) or lower than 36° C (96.8° F), (b) heart rate greater than 90 beats/min, (c) respiratory rate greater than 20 breaths/min or arterial carbon dioxide tension less than 32 mm Hg, and (d) white blood cell count greater than 12,000/mm^3 or less than 4,000/mm^3, or immature (band) forms accounting for more than 10% of the neutrophils present.
2. MODS is the presence of altered organ function in an acutely ill patient such that homeostasis cannot be maintained without intervention. (This term was recommended as a replacement for multiorgan failure and multiple system organ failure [see *95 Multiple Organ Dysfunction Syndrome*].)

Clearly, SIRS includes all the signs, symptoms, and physiologic changes characteristic of the sepsis syndrome; however, use of the term SIRS avoids the idea that such manifestations are necessarily the product of infection. Both infectious and noninfectious insults may evoke SIRS. Sepsis may, in fact, be thought of as a special case of SIRS—SIRS associated with infection [see *Figure 1*]. The term sepsis syndrome, although very useful in guiding clinical thinking,

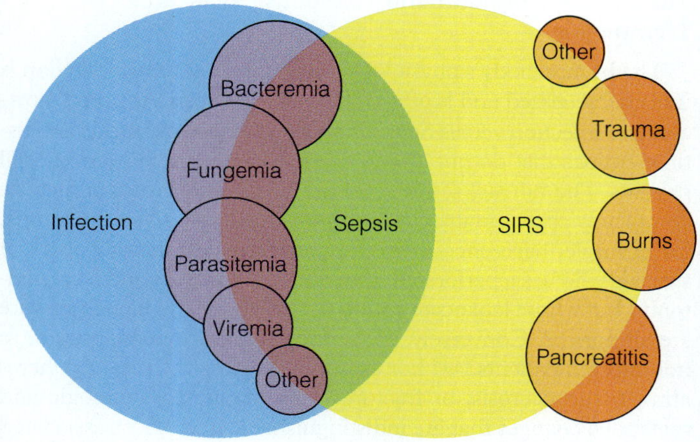

Figure 1 Depicted are the interrelations among infection, sepsis, and systemic inflammatory response syndrome (SIRS).

appears to be insufficiently precise for our current needs and probably should no longer be used. The term septicemia probably should not be used either.

The developing views expressed in this evolving terminology have clear therapeutic implications. There are two distinct problems to be faced: the initiating process and the systemic response. Treatment of the initiating process depends on the nature of the process (e.g., infection, trauma, burn, or pancreatitis). Treatment of the response—if indeed desirable—depends on the severity of the response; it should be thought of as independent of the initiating process.

Problems with Empirical Treatment of Infection

The frequent presence of SIRS in complex or critically ill surgical patients usually prompts a reflexive response to "pan culture" the patient if no credible source of infection is apparent. When permissive or loose diagnostic criteria for infection are invoked, the inevitable result is the commencement of empirical antibiotic therapy for suspected infection, which is often, by default, continued for days, if not weeks, pending definitive culture results. This strategy may seem reasonable and is undeniably difficult to resist, but it is potentially deleterious in many ways, and there are many sound objections to its reflexive use.[21] Empirical antibiotic therapy can obfuscate future cultures, predispose to the emergence of resistant organisms (which are associated with increased attributable mortality), promote derepression of homeostasis-maintaining endogenous flora, cause toxic reactions and secondary effects, alter the ecology of the unit in which it is used (as shown by the rising prevalence of methicillin-resistant *S. aureus* and vancomycin-resistant enterococci in both European and North American centers), and raise the cost of patient care. This widely used strategy is largely unvalidated.[4,5] It must be emphasized that the paramount principle of therapy for infection is treatment focused on appropriate microbiologic cultures in the context of strict diagnostic criteria for infection.

Many authorities espouse so-called streamlining of empirically begun broad-spectrum antibiotic therapy in response to microbiologic data once culture results are available; however, it is frequently difficult to discontinue antibiotics once they have been started. When strict diagnostic criteria for infection are not met or, more important, when antibiotic therapy based on nonmicrobiologic evidence of infection yields negligible results, strong consideration should be given to stopping the antibiotics, and an exhaustive effort should be made to identify and control any occult persistent cause of the inflammatory state. Of course, this is easier said than done. Moreover, positive cultures do not automatically confirm infection, and great discretion must be exercised in determining how the microbiologic information obtained should be used. For example, tracheal aspirates from intubated patients routinely reveal gram-negative flora, but this finding in no way confirms pneumonia. A single blood culture growing *S. epidermidis* is similarly difficult to interpret. Despite ubiquitous use in surgical patients, there is not a great deal of evidence in the clinical literature to substantiate the effectiveness of either empirical or streamlined antibiotic therapy. Further efforts must be made to find such evidence, if it exists, because this practice could theoretically exact a substantial cost from both the patient and the environment in which the patient is cared for. In the meantime, clinicians must approach the development of SIRS or other nonspecific signs of infection in their patients by predicating antimicrobial use on carefully formulated diagnostic criteria for the presence of infection; CDC consensus definitions of infection are a good starting point.

SOURCE CONTROL

In the past, as noted, the term sepsis was loosely used to describe any general systemic inflammatory state. Because such states often arose as a result of infection, it was assumed that antimicrobial therapy was generally appropriate in the management of the "septic" patient. Currently, however, sepsis should be defined exclusively as SIRS in a patient in whom a causative source of infection has been identified; in the absence of proven infection, the term SIRS should be used. This distinction is important because it encourages more discriminating management of this exceedingly common clinical situation.

In the same vein, so-called source control has been developed as a strategy for managing the "septic" patient. Like the term sepsis, the term source control traditionally connotes management of infection rather than, more generally, management of a cause of inflammation. Classically, source control consists of a three-pronged approach employing measures to (1) eradicate a focus of infection, (2) eliminate ongoing microbial contamination, and (3) render the local environment inhospitable to microbial growth and tissue invasion. Diligent source control has long been considered pivotal to successful management of sepsis. Although this traditional approach addresses the infectious causes of local or systemic inflammation very well in a great variety of clinical situations, it must not lead us to become dogmatic about or oversimplify our understanding of which processes are required to overcome infection and inflammation. Challenging convention, a surprising number of investigators have successfully managed many supposedly surgical conditions (e.g., appendicitis[22] and intra-abdominal abscess[23]) without intervention or by using only prolonged antibiotic therapy. Seasoned general surgeons know well that if acute cholecystitis is not operated on urgently, it may certainly harm the patient or cause recurring discomfort, but it may also resolve completely on its own. What actually constitutes adequate source control and how this can be measured are critical questions and are currently the subject of great debate. These questions become particularly problematic with respect to ICU patients, in whom SIRS is highly nonspecific.

It would seem rational to take our current understanding of SIRS as encompassing both infectious and noninfectious pathology and extrapolate it to the concept of source control. Indeed, as regards more complex surgical patients, it may be appropriate to broaden the definition of source control to include control of all causes of SIRS, not merely infectious ones. For example, debriding devitalized injured tissue, removing a rejected allograft, and resolving postoperative atelectasis are all important for successfully abating a systemic inflammatory state that might easily be mistaken for a manifestation of infection. Deemphasizing infection as the predominant cause of SIRS and withholding antibiotic therapy until stricter, more focused diagnostic criteria for infection are met should make treatment paradigms for managing difficult surgical patients, if not altogether more effective, at least more evaluable.

If one assumes that source control is in fact a therapeutic response to the presence of SIRS, one may then think of it as being either assisted or unassisted. This therapeutic response is initiated by the host, with either complete or partial success. Only in the latter instance should one assist the host's efforts at source control by providing antibiotics or taking surgical measures. This is by no means to suggest that one should not search diligently for a correctable cause of infection or inflammation but rather to suggest that when such an effort yields negligible results, one should consider the possibility that SIRS may be not only appropriate but desirable and may represent the patient's own adequate management of the underlying physiologic insult. Thus, in certain situations, source control may be best regarded as an endogenous or unassisted event. For instance, when fever, tachycardia, and leukocytosis are observed in a surgical patient who is coping well, antibiotics should not necessarily be given automatically. Indeed, such "default therapy" should be actively discouraged. (The reflexive and unnecessary use of antibiotic therapy to manage early acute cholangitis in an otherwise healthy person is a good example.) One should also keep in mind that some forms of injury or insult (e.g., some viral infections) not only are very well managed without intervention but may not even prompt a clinically evident systemic inflammatory response.

The notion that no intervention may be required is understandably difficult for many surgeons to embrace at the bedside. Nonetheless, extensive ongoing research elucidating the complex dynamic of circulating proinflammatory and counterinflammatory mediators (e.g., TNF-α, the interleukins, and a host of other cytokines) suggests that a poorly understood but highly sophisticated biologic apparatus exists for responding to injury and insult. Indeed, it is widely hypothesized (though yet unproved) that this systemic response can be manipulated to restore health in stressed or deteriorating surgical patients. The prospect of untangling the complex biology of systemic inflammation through advances in this field is truly engaging.

References

1. American College of Chest Physicians/Society of Critical Care Medicine Consensus Conference: Definitions for sepsis and organ failure and guidelines for the use of innovative therapies in sepsis. Crit Care Med 20:864, 1992
2. Vincent J, Bihari DJ, Suter PM, et al: The prevalence of nosocomial infection in intensive care units in Europe: results of the European Prevalence of Infection in Intensive Care (EPIC) Study. JAMA 274:639, 1995
3. Casadevall A: Crisis in infectious diseases: time for a new paradigm? Clin Infect Dis 32:790, 1996
4. Lennard ES, Mineshew BH, Dellinger EP, et al: Leukocytosis at termination of antibiotherapy: its importance for intra-abdominal sepsis. Arch Surg 115:918, 1980
5. Stone HH, Bourneuf AA, Stinson LD: Reliability of criteria for predicting recurrent sepsis. Arch Surg 120:17, 1985
6. Adnet F, Borron SW, Vicault E, et al: Value of C-reactive protein in the detection of bacterial contamination at the time of presentation in drug-induced aspiration pneumonia. Chest 112:466, 1997
7. Young B, Gleeson M, Cripps AW: C-reactive protein: a critical review. Pathology 23:118, 1991
8. The Society for Hospital Epidemiology of America, the Association for Practitioners in Infection Control, the Centers for Disease Control, the Surgical Infection Society: Consensus paper on the surveillance of surgical wound infections. Infect Control Hosp Epidemiol 13:599, 1992
9. Stamm WE, Hooton TM: Management of urinary tract infection in adults. N Engl J Med 329:1328, 1993
10. Stark RP, Maki DG: Bacteriuria in the catheterized patient: what quantitative level of bacteriuria is relevant? N Engl J Med 311:560, 1984
11. Bullard KM, Dunn DL: Diagnosis and treatment of bacteremia and intravascular catheter infections. Am J Surg 172(suppl 6A):13S, 1996
12. American Thoracic Society: Hospital-acquired pneumonia in adults: diagnosis, assessment of severity, initial antimicrobial therapy, and preventive strategies: a consensus statement. Am J Respir Crit Care Med 153:1711, 1995
13. Sterling TR, Ho EJ, Brehm WT, et al: Diagnosis and treatment of ventilator-associated pneumonia—impact on survival. Chest 110:1025, 1996
14. Marshall J, Sweeny D: Microbial infection and the septic response in critical surgical illness. Arch Surg 125:17, 1990
15. Meakins JL, Marshall JC: The gut as the motor of multiple system organ failure. Splanchnic Ischemia and Multiple Organ Failure. Marston A, Ed. Edward Arnold, London, 1989, p 339
16. Goris RJA, Boekhorst TAP, Nuytinck JKS, et al: Multiple organ failure: generalized autodestructive inflammation? Arch Surg 120:1109, 1985
17. Bone RC, Fisher CJ Jr, Clemmer TP, et al: Sepsis syndrome: a valid clinical entity. Crit Care Med 17:389, 1989
18. Dorland's Illustrated Medical Dictionary, 28th ed. Philadelphia, WB Saunders Co, 1994, p 1507
19. Bone RC: Let's agree on terminology: definitions of sepsis. Crit Care Med 19:973, 1991
20. Sibbald WJ, Marshall J, Christou N, et al: "Sepsis"—clarity of existing terminology . . . or more confusion? Crit Care Med 19:996, 1991
21. Timsit M, Misset B, Renaud B, et al: Effect of previous antimicrobial therapy on the accuracy of the main procedures used to diagnose nosocomial pneumonia in patients who are using mechanical ventilation. Chest 108:1036, 1997
22. Eriksson S, Granstrom L: Randomised controlled trial of appendectomy versus antibiotic therapy for acute appendicitis. Br J Surg 82:166, 1995
23. Montgomery RS, Wilson SE: Intraabdominal abscess: image-guided diagnosis and therapy. Clin Infect Dis 23:28, 1996

Acknowledgments

The authors wish to thank François Lemaire, Dominique Franco, A.P.H. McLean, and C. Brun-Buisson for their help and Fiorella Delcampe and Maria Betancourt for their secretarial assistance.

79 BLOOD CULTURES AND INFECTION IN THE PATIENT WITH THE SEPTIC RESPONSE

Donald E. Fry, M.D.

Approach to Blood Cultures in Patients with the Septic Response

It has been well established that infection and sepsis are distinct events [*see 78 Clinical and Laboratory Diagnosis of Infection* and Discussion, *below*]. Infection is local activation of the human inflammatory response secondary to local proliferation and invasion of tissue by microorganisms. When infection reaches a critical threshold of severity, the inflammatory response may be activated at a systemic level. Systemic activation of human inflammation is called the systemic inflammatory response syndrome (SIRS). When infection is the putative agent for SIRS, it is called sepsis.[1]

SIRS secondary to infection occurs when (1) whole microorganisms are disseminated from the primary site of infection, usually via the vascular or lymphatic system (e.g., bacteremia); (2) structural components of the cell wall (e.g., gram-negative endotoxin) or secreted exotoxins are systemically disseminated (e.g., toxic shock); or (3) normal autocrine and paracrine signals of inflammation at a local focus reach high systemic concentrations, and these proinflammatory signals (e.g., tumor necrosis factor [TNF]), through their exaggerated endocrine domain of action, activate SIRS.

Although biologic causes other than infection may precipitate SIRS and provoke a syndrome virtually identical to that resulting from invasive infection, infection is the most common cause of SIRS in acutely ill surgical patients. Effective management of infection in these patients requires recognition of the primary site of infection, control of the source of microbial contamination and dissemination (i.e., source control), characterization of the causative microorganism(s), drainage and debridement of inflammatory exudates and necrotic tissue at the primary site, and antibiotic therapy specific for the microbial pathogen.

Positive Blood Culture with Infection

A positive blood culture in a patient with the septic response serves to identify the putative cause of the infection. This identification not only permits institution of appropriate systemic antibiotic therapy [*see Figure 1*] but also facilitates assessment of potential primary sources of the infection because of the established associations between specific anatomic sites and specific microbial isolates. Although it is not always possible to identify the microorganism or microorganisms responsible for the septic response, organization of the discussion according to the proven or suspected pathogen that may be recovered in a blood culture is a convenient way of addressing treatment options.

GRAM-POSITIVE COCCI

Staphylococci

The identification of gram-positive organisms from a blood culture immediately arouses suspicion that a *Staphylococcus* species is the likely pathogen. Because staphylococci ordinarily colonize the skin and integument, infection from those sources must be considered responsible for the bacteremia.

In the surgical patient, a positive blood culture for staphylococci must be assumed to arise from an intravascular device until proved otherwise[2] [*see Table 1*]. Peripheral intravenous catheters, subclavian lines, Swan-Ganz catheters, systemic arterial lines, and even transvenous pacemaker wires are all documented sources for staphylococcal bacteremia [*see Table 2*]. All lines must be removed and their sites changed. The line and catheter tips should be cultured by semiquantitative methods[3] to document the role of the particular device in question [*see 81 Nosocomial Infection*]. Although this semiquantitative method uses a count of 15 colony-forming units as the threshold for a positive culture of the catheter, devices responsible for bacteremia will usually demonstrate a solid sheet of bacterial growth on the agar [*see Figure 2*]. Devices causing bacteremia must be removed. Treatment cannot consist of antibiotics alone.

Septic thrombophlebitis may occur at the site of a previously placed device even though the foreign body has been removed.[4,5] Pus within the vein becomes a source of persistent bacteremia until appropriate therapy is employed. Persistent evidence of gram-positive bacteremia after removal of all intravascular lines gives rise to a high index of suspicion for suppurative thrombophlebitis. Previous intravenous sites must be examined for evidence of pus; suspicious sites may even have to be explored with the patient under local anesthesia. When suppurative thrombophlebitis is identified, the entire length of septic vein must be surgically excised. Although many different species of bacteria may be responsible for suppurative thrombophlebitis, *S. aureus* is the most common.

Implantable synthetic prosthetic materials have become a major part of vascular, cardiac, and orthopedic surgery but may become sources of bacteremia secondary to infections resulting from intraoperative contamination. The synthetic implant should be considered the source of blood-borne infection when gram-positive organisms are identified in the blood of patients at risk. As the use of synthetic

Approach to Blood Cultures in Patients with the Septic Response

Patient has septic response

Perform blood culture to identify putative cause of infection.

Blood culture is positive

Common pathogens include
- Gram-positive cocci (staphylococci, streptococci)
- Gram-negative Enterobacteriaceae (*Escherichia coli, Klebsiella, Proteus, Serratia*)
- Anaerobes (*Bacteroides*, clostridia, certain streptococci)
- Fungi (*Candida*)

Attempt to determine whether there is a primary focus of infection.

Blood culture is negative

Attempt to determine whether there is a primary source of infection:
- Perform careful physical examination
- Order appropriate diagnostic studies for each anatomic area
- Aggressively culture suspicious fluids or exudates

Pay particular attention to
- Surgical site
- Insertion sites for monitoring and support devices

Infectious focus is identified

Initiate therapy as appropriate for pathogen identified [*see Figure 1*].

No infectious focus is identified

Presume GI microbial translocation. Likelihood of this diagnosis is increased by presence of "trilogy of translocation" in blood culture:
- Enterococcus
- *Staphylococcus epidermidis*
- *Candida*

Rule out intravascular device infection.
Continue to search for primary infectious focus.
Reinforce gut barrier function via
- Enteral nutritional support
- Patient mobilization
- Addition of glutamine and short-chain fatty acids to nutritional solution
- Possible alteration of antibiotic regimen

Infectious focus is identified

Drain primary focus mechanically.
Initiate empirical antibiotic therapy directed at suspected pathogens while culture and sensitivity data are pending.
Maintain constant vigilance for changing clinical findings, and observe response to empirical therapy carefully.

No infectious focus is identified

Consider noninfectious causes of septic response, such as
- Acute pancreatitis
- Aspiration pneumonitis
- Multiple trauma with extensive soft tissue damage
- Extracorporeal membrane oxygenation

Do not give antibiotics.
Provide supportive care:
- Fluids
- Ventilatory assistance

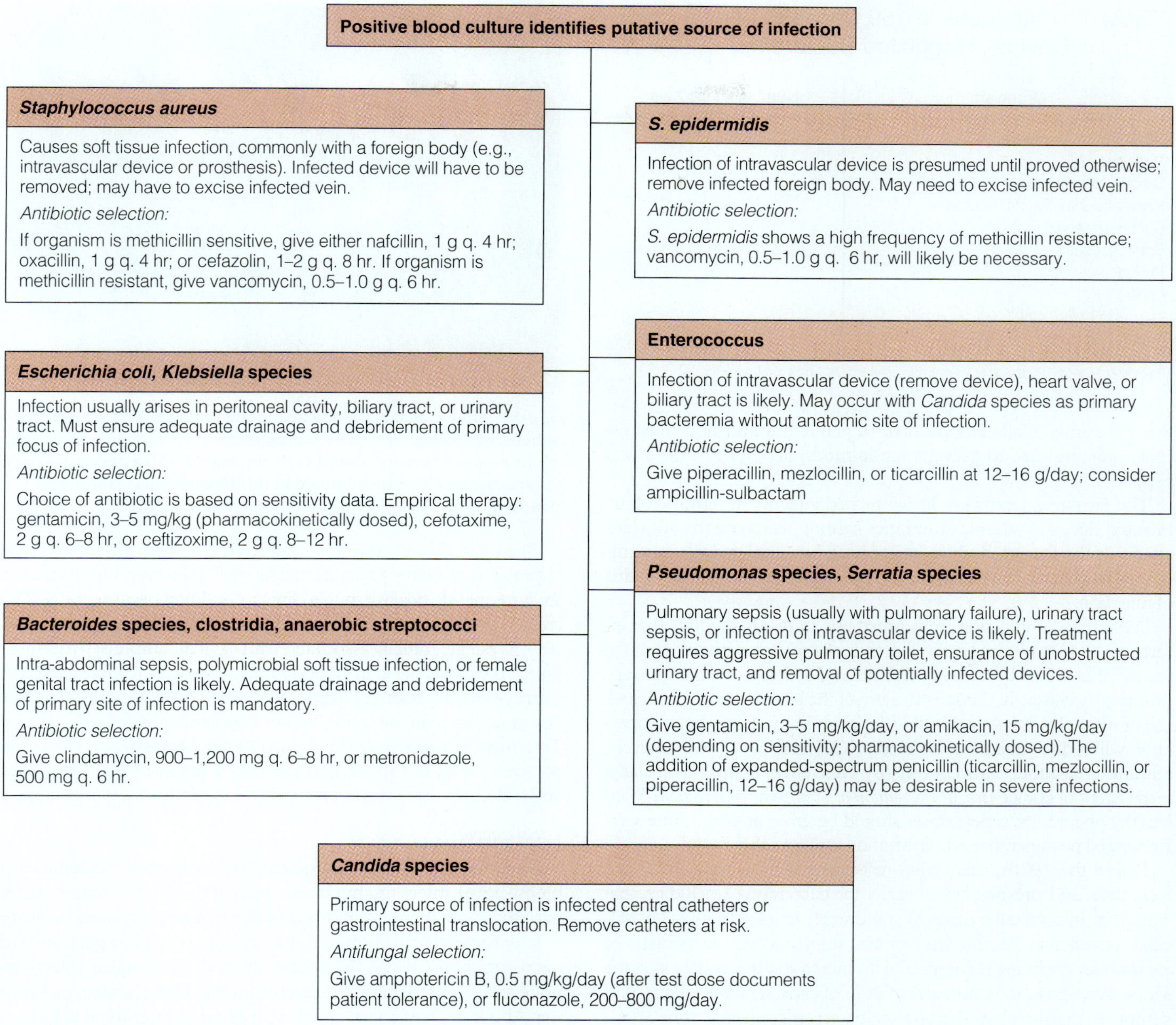

Positive blood culture identifies putative source of infection

Staphylococcus aureus

Causes soft tissue infection, commonly with a foreign body (e.g., intravascular device or prosthesis). Infected device will have to be removed; may have to excise infected vein.

Antibiotic selection:

If organism is methicillin sensitive, give either nafcillin, 1 g q. 4 hr; oxacillin, 1 g q. 4 hr; or cefazolin, 1–2 g q. 8 hr. If organism is methicillin resistant, give vancomycin, 0.5–1.0 g q. 6 hr.

Escherichia coli, Klebsiella species

Infection usually arises in peritoneal cavity, biliary tract, or urinary tract. Must ensure adequate drainage and debridement of primary focus of infection.

Antibiotic selection:

Choice of antibiotic is based on sensitivity data. Empirical therapy: gentamicin, 3–5 mg/kg (pharmacokinetically dosed), cefotaxime, 2 g q. 6–8 hr, or ceftizoxime, 2 g q. 8–12 hr.

Bacteroides species, clostridia, anaerobic streptococci

Intra-abdominal sepsis, polymicrobial soft tissue infection, or female genital tract infection is likely. Adequate drainage and debridement of primary site of infection is mandatory.

Antibiotic selection:

Give clindamycin, 900–1,200 mg q. 6–8 hr, or metronidazole, 500 mg q. 6 hr.

S. epidermidis

Infection of intravascular device is presumed until proved otherwise; remove infected foreign body. May need to excise infected vein.

Antibiotic selection:

S. epidermidis shows a high frequency of methicillin resistance; vancomycin, 0.5–1.0 g q. 6 hr, will likely be necessary.

Enterococcus

Infection of intravascular device (remove device), heart valve, or biliary tract is likely. May occur with *Candida* species as primary bacteremia without anatomic site of infection.

Antibiotic selection:

Give piperacillin, mezlocillin, or ticarcillin at 12–16 g/day; consider ampicillin-sulbactam

Pseudomonas species, Serratia species

Pulmonary sepsis (usually with pulmonary failure), urinary tract sepsis, or infection of intravascular device is likely. Treatment requires aggressive pulmonary toilet, ensurance of unobstructed urinary tract, and removal of potentially infected devices.

Antibiotic selection:

Give gentamicin, 3–5 mg/kg/day, or amikacin, 15 mg/kg/day (depending on sensitivity; pharmacokinetically dosed). The addition of expanded-spectrum penicillin (ticarcillin, mezlocillin, or piperacillin, 12–16 g/day) may be desirable in severe infections.

Candida species

Primary source of infection is infected central catheters or gastrointestinal translocation. Remove catheters at risk.

Antifungal selection:

Give amphotericin B, 0.5 mg/kg/day (after test dose documents patient tolerance), or fluconazole, 200–800 mg/day.

Figure 1 Identification of the putative cause of infection permits institution of appropriate antibiotic therapy.

devices increases, the delayed nature of some infections, particularly when *S. epidermidis* is the pathogen, is now being appreciated. These indolent infections are consequences of intraoperative contamination but may not be clinically evident for months to years after implantation. Because selected species of *S. epidermidis* produce a glycocalix "slime," culturing of the microorganism from the infected prosthesis can be very difficult even after removal of the prosthesis. Recovery of this microorganism from a blood culture is quite uncommon, because presentation of the infection occurs months after the primary operative procedure.[6]

Diagnosis of arterial graft, heart valve, and total-joint arthroplasty infections can be very difficult. Once infection has been established, however, prompt removal of the prosthesis is mandatory. Prosthesis removal is invariably associated with major morbidity because an active infection limits the reconstructive options available. Although antibiotic therapy alone will not eradicate the infection, it may prolong the decision to remove the prosthesis and result in arterial graft failure (e.g., thrombosis, pseudoaneurysm), cardiac valvular insufficiency, or extensive arthroplasty infection (e.g., extrusion, osteomyelitis).

S. epidermidis is being recognized as having a greater role in surgical infection than was previously appreciated.[7] Because *S. epidermidis* normally colonizes skin, it is also a potential contaminant in the blood culture process. The continued emphasis on technique in blood culture is important to minimize this potential artifact in diagnosis. A frequent cause of false positive cultures of this microorganism is use of the arterial line or the central venous catheter, instead of a separate and carefully prepared venipuncture site, for drawing of blood samples. When more than one culture shows *S. epidermidis* or when cultures taken at separate times show the same organism, however, the clinician must assume that the organism is participating in clinical infection.

Staphylococcal bacteremia is a preventable complication of indwelling devices and implants. Aseptic placement of intravascular devices cannot be compromised. Peripheral I.V. catheters should be changed routinely every 48 to 72 hours. Arterial lines that have been present for more than 72 hours are at considerable risk for being foci

Table 1 Pathogens in 159 Cases of Intravascular Device–Associated Bacteremia[119]

Organism	Number of Isolates
Staphylococcus aureus	78
S. epidermidis	33
Serratia marcescens	18
Klebsiella/Enterobacter species	16
Candida species	11
Enterococcus	8
Proteus species	6
Others	6
Total	176*

*The total exceeds 159 because of polymicrobial isolates in several patients.

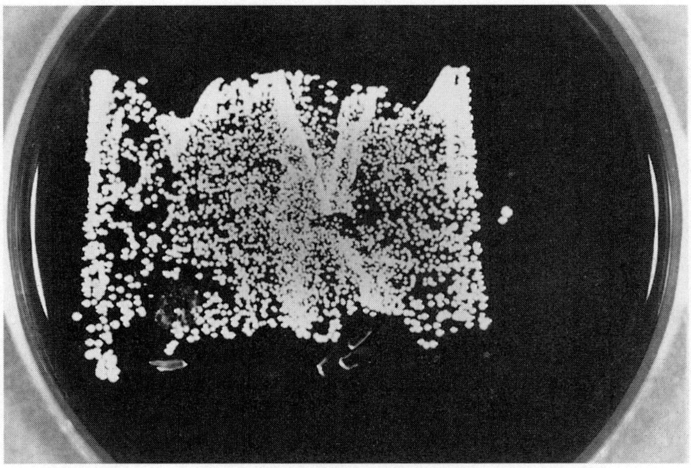

for bacteremia. Catheters devoted to parenteral nutrition must receive ongoing care to prevent septic morbidity [see 97 *Nutritional Support*].

The primary therapy for device-related infection is removal of the infected device. Systemic antibiotics cannot overcome the adjuvant effects of the foreign body in supporting bacterial growth. Antimicrobial therapy becomes adjunctive to removal of the primary nidus of infection.

Prevention of infection from prosthetic implants requires that efforts be made to minimize development of a microenvironment in the wound that favors bacterial proliferation. Meticulous technique, appropriate hemostasis, conservative use of the electrocautery, judicious use of suture ligatures, and antibiotics given immediately before operation will reduce infectious morbidity. Cefazolin, 1 g preoperatively, administered either intravenously (by preference) or intramuscularly, is the agent of choice [see 39 *Prevention of Postoperative Infection*]. With lengthy operations, repeat doses should be given at 4-hour intervals. Prolonged postoperative administration is of no value.

Before the 1970s, methicillin-resistant staphylococcal infections were rare, and presumptive therapy for bacteremia (including that caused by intravascular devices) could safely employ methicillin, nafcillin, or oxacillin. Methicillin-resistant staphylococci, particularly *S. epidermidis*, are being recognized with increasing frequency; in some series, they account for as many as 40% of clinical isolates. Thus, presumptive antimicrobial therapy for bacteremia arising from an intravascular or implantable device requires vancomycin, 0.5 to 1 g every 6 hours. When culture and sensitivity data are subsequently available, the antimicrobial choice may be modified. When methicillin-resistant species are not a concern, nafcillin, 1 g every 4 hours, is appropriate. Because of the risks of metastatic infectious complications from staphylococcal bacteremia, systemic antibiotics should be continued for a minimum of 7 days.

Table 2 Sites of Intravascular Device–Associated Bacteremia in 159 Patients[119]

Site	Number of Patients
Peripheral I.V. catheter	72
Central venous catheter	49
Arterial line	18
Subclavian dialysis catheter	12
Swan-Ganz catheter	4
Broviac catheter	3
Transvenous pacemaker wire	1

Figure 2 Illustrated is a blood agar plate 24 hours after an infected catheter has been cultured by semiquantitative technique. Although colony counts of greater than 15 are associated with a positive culture, the prolific growth noted in this illustration is commonly identified.

The toxic-shock syndrome, caused by *S. aureus*, gives the clinical impression of being a bacteremic illness.[8] However, blood cultures are infrequently positive in this clinical condition because the SIRS is created by the exotoxin produced by the microorganism, not by bacteremia per se. Initially associated with vaginal tampons, toxic-shock syndrome can be seen in any body cavity or open wound filled with gauze or other packing. Diagnosis of toxic shock requires a high index of suspicion in the septic, hypotensive patient with body packing. Treatment requires removal of the packing, aggressive systemic supportive care of the shock and associated organ-failure complexes, and systemic antibiotics appropriate for staphylococcal infection.

Streptococci

Streptococcal bacteremia occurs less often than staphylococcal blood-borne infection, but some areas of the United States are experiencing an apparent increase in these infections. Invasive group A streptococcal infection with bacteremia is seen in patients with necrotizing soft tissue infections, invasive pharyngeal infections, bone and joint infections, or severe and rapidly advancing pneumonia. About 20% of bacteremias with group A streptococci have no primary source of infection.[9]

Necrotizing soft tissue infection is the setting most likely to result in a positive blood culture of group A streptococci. These fulminant infections are seen after seemingly trivial cutaneous injuries but may also complicate chickenpox in children[10] and may even be seen as complications of elective surgery. The necrotizing infection is characterized by pain, tenderness, and induration around a wound that is out of proportion to the size or mechanism of the injury. The infection dissects along the fascial plane and can evolve from injury to a fatal illness in 24 hours. The diagnosis requires a high index of suspicion in a toxic patient with rapidly advancing cellulitis. The induration of the advancing infection, palpable in thin patients, differentiates this type of infection from clostridial gas gangrene. Although these infections are associated with the toxic-shock–like syndrome, patients with these infections—unlike those with true toxic shock—usually have blood cultures positive for group A streptococci.[8] Unfortunately, the positive blood culture is not available until the patient's fate has already been dictated by earlier clinical decisions.

Therapy requires aggressive debridement of the necrotic tissue, systemic antibiotic therapy, and systemic supportive therapy for the shock and organ-failure syndrome characteristic of severe infections. The antibiotic choice for these serious infections includes both penicillin, 12 to 24 million units/day, and clindamycin, 900 to 1,200 mg every 6 hours, in adult patients. The addition of clindamycin is thought to be important as an inhibitor of protein synthesis, reducing toxin production by the rapidly multiplying bacteria. Clindamycin is also useful because it is thought that large inocula of group A streptococci do not express penicillin-binding proteins.[11]

α-Hemolytic streptococcal bacteremia, well known in patients with endocarditis, is generally associated with this infection when blood cultures are positive for this organism. Echocardiographic confirmation of the diagnosis sets the stage for treatment with penicillin. Therapy is continued until there is conclusive evidence that the infection has been eradicated.

Other groups of streptococci identified by positive blood cultures usually occur in infections secondary to GI contamination. The group B streptococci are identified as bacteremic pathogens in neonates but are now being seen with somewhat greater frequency in adults. In adult bacteremia, the group D (nonenterococcal) streptococci are identified in circumstances similar to those associated with the group B pathogens. Gut-derived streptococcal pathogens are usually quite sensitive to the penicillins.

Enterococci

There continues to be debate concerning the true virulence and pathogenicity of the enterococcus when it is isolated as part of the polymicrobial microflora of a clinical exudate,[12,13] but no one would deny the need for antimicrobial chemotherapy when the organism is isolated in blood cultures. Mortalities in excess of 50% clearly underscore the severity of enterococcal bacteremia.[14]

The primary foci of infection in enterococcal bacteremia include intravascular devices and the biliary and gastrointestinal tracts. Enterococcal bacteremia ordinarily occurs in elderly or chronically ill patients who are being treated with broad-spectrum antibiotics. Cephalosporins in particular have been implicated as favoring enterococcal overgrowth.[15] The enterococcus is usually associated with other bacterial species at the primary site of intra-abdominal or soft tissue infection, and experimental observations suggest that a synergistic relation with other organisms may be part of its pathogenic expression.[16,17]

Therapy for enterococcal bacteremia requires definition of the primary focus of infection. When the enterococcus is a solitary isolate in blood, intravenous devices should be changed and semiquantitatively cultured. Potential biliary sources must be evaluated, with all available clinical data, including those from ultrasound examination of the gallbladder [see *83 Infection in the Upper Abdomen: Biliary Tract, Pancreas, Liver, and Spleen*], taken into account. Gangrenous, acalculous cholecystitis must be kept in mind because of the type of patient likely to have enterococcal bacteremia.[18] Intra-abdominal abscesses and serious soft tissue infections are customarily associated with polymicrobial isolates, which may include the enterococcus. The urinary tract, however, appears to be an infrequent cause of enterococcal bacteremia in the absence of anatomic obstruction to urine flow.

When the primary focus is identified, removal of the foreign body, drainage and debridement of infected material, and specific antibiotic therapy are indicated. Piperacillin, 12 to 16 g/day, is recommended. Ticarcillin and mezlocillin, 12 to 16 g/day, are alternatives. Although ampicillin appears to have nearly uniform activity against the enterococcus in vitro, the β-lactamase production of synergistic pathogens in the polymicrobial milieu raises serious questions about the effectiveness of this choice. The recent addition of sulbactam to ampicillin has improved enterococcal coverage in mixed infections.

In about 40% of patients with positive blood cultures for the enterococcus, no primary site of infection can be identified.[14] This observation has led to considerable speculation as to whether this organism is a marker of gastrointestinal bacterial translocation [see Positive Blood Culture without Infection, *below*] or whether the infection arises from a clinically obscure primary focus (e.g., infection at a catheter site).

The emergence of vancomycin-resistant enterococci has created considerable concern.[19] These nosocomial infections, like all enterococcal bacteremias and infections, occur in severely ill hospitalized patients and are associated with intensive care units using large amounts of vancomycin. Specific antibiotic therapy in these infections is highly problematic. Current recommendations are to start with an assessment of the sensitivity of the enterococcal isolate to the aminoglycosides.[20] If the isolate lacks a high level of resistance to aminoglycosides, then the choices for antibiotic treatment include (1) an aminoglycoside plus teicoplanin (if susceptible), (2) an aminoglycoside plus vancomycin (for a low level of resistance), (3) an aminoglycoside plus ampicillin plus vancomycin, and (4) an aminoglycoside plus ciprofloxacin plus rifampin (if susceptible). If the isolate is highly resistant to aminoglycosides, then antibiotic treatment may be (1) teicoplanin (if susceptible), (2) novobiocin plus a quinolone, (3) ampicillin plus a quinolone, or (4) ceftriaxone plus fosfomycin. In vitro susceptibility testing with the combination of quinupristin and dalfopristin has raised the hope that these agents will be of use in the management of vancomycin-resistant enterococcal infections.[21] Because vancomycin resistance is mediated by two separate genes, there is considerable concern in the academic community about transfer of these genes into staphylococci or other gram-positive organisms.

GRAM-NEGATIVE ENTEROBACTERIACEAE

The gram-negative Enterobacteriaceae represent a group of facultative bacteria that are associated with infections of the abdominal cavity, biliary tract, and genitourinary tract. Infections tend to be monomicrobial when the urinary and biliary tracts are involved[22,23] but are nearly always polymicrobial with peritonitis and intra-abdominal abscess.[24] The common gram-negative Enterobacteriaceae include *Escherichia coli*, *Klebsiella* species, *Enterobacter* species, and *Proteus* species. Because intra-abdominal infection is a polymicrobial process, bacteremia may involve one or more of the Enterobacteriaceae and may likewise occur with several different anaerobic enteric species. Thus, bacteremia with one of these organisms in patients with intra-abdominal infection represents only the tip of the iceberg, with a polymicrobial flora presumed to be present at the focus [see *82 Peritonitis and Intra-abdominal Abscesses and 83 Infection in the Upper Abdomen: Biliary Tract, Pancreas, Liver, and Spleen*].

In the surgical patient, eradication of gram-negative bacteremia requires identification of the primary focus because mechanical therapy is almost always necessary in addition to antibiotic treatment. The intra-abdominal compartment must be the primary consideration. Ultrasound examination of the biliary tract may be useful. Abdominal computed tomography is approximately 90% accurate in the definition of abscess. Urinary cultures may be useful but must be cautiously interpreted because a well-drained urinary tract is an improbable focus for bacteremia. *P. vulgaris* is a urease-producing organism, and its presence in patients with ileal conduits or staghorn calculi strongly favors a urinary tract source. Gram-negative bacteremia from hospital-acquired pneumonitis is always a possibility but is less common with the Enterobacteriaceae than with *Pseudomonas* or *Serratia* species. In general, bacteremia from nosocomial pneumonia is relatively uncommon in the surgical patient. *Klebsiella* and *Enterobacter* species are known pathogens for bacteremia from intravascular devices; appropriate cultures of the primary device are necessary to establish this potential source.

Mechanical treatment is necessary at the primary focus of infection. Defects in the gastrointestinal tract must be managed, pus drained, necrotic tissue debrided, urinary obstruction relieved, and infected catheters removed. Empirical exploration of the abdomen may be necessary in bacteremic patients in whom the likelihood of an intra-abdominal source is great, but CT of the abdominal compartment often eliminates the need for exploratory surgery.

Considerable latitude surrounds appropriate antibiotic therapy for gram-negative bacteremia, particularly when the bacteremia is secondary to intra-abdominal infection. When the infectious process responsible for the bacteremia is community-acquired, an expanded-spectrum β-lactam antibiotic is appropriate[25] [see Table 3]. Although anaerobic coverage is a necessary prerequisite in intra-abdominal infection, the expanded-spectrum β-lactam agents appear to have sufficient activity to provide equivalent results when compared with those combinations of drugs that might appear to have preferable anaerobic activity. Furthermore, single-agent treatment with the expanded-spectrum β-lactam antibiotics is less expensive than multiple-drug therapy and eliminates the toxicity and pharmacokinetic dosage complexities of the aminoglycoside alternatives.[26] Newer quinolone antibiotics with both gram-negative and anaerobic activity, as well as long elimination half-lives, may become additional choices for the treatment of bacteremia from intra-abdominal infection sites.[27]

Patients with bacteremia from hospital-acquired infections or infections that represent failures of prior antimicrobial therapy, however, will necessarily require therapy addressed to these more resistant isolates. Single antibiotics that may be chosen to cover hospital-acquired gram-negative bacteria include aminoglycosides, expanded-spectrum penicillins, ceftazidime, aztreonam, quinolones, and the carbapenems. Even though the bacteremic isolate may be sensitive to lesser drugs, a combination of an expanded-spectrum penicillin with an aminoglycoside is commonly chosen to cover potential pathogens [see Table 4] because of the synergism between these two types of agents. Culture and sensitivity data from the primary source of infection are particularly important to permit modification of drug therapy. Because

Table 3 Expanded-Spectrum β-Lactam Antibiotics Effective against Enterobacteriaceae

Drug	Half-life (hr)	Dose Interval (hr)	Total 24-Hr Dose (g)
Cephalosporins			
Cefoxitin	0.7–1.0	4–6	12–18
Cefotetan	3.5	12	2–4
Cefotaxime	1.0	6	8–12
Ceftizoxime	1.5	8	6
Ceftazidime	2.0	8	6
Ceftriaxone	6.5–8.0	12–24	2–4
Penicillins			
Ampicillin-sulbactam	1.0	6	12
Ticarcillin-clavulanate	1.0	4	18.6
Piperacillin-tazobactam	1.0	6	13.5
Monobactams			
Aztreonam	2.0	8	6
Carbapenems			
Imipenem-cilastatin	1.0	6	2–4
Meropenem	1.0	6	2–4

Table 4 Expanded-Spectrum Penicillins and Aminoglycosides Used in Combination Regimens in Treatment of Nosocomial Gram-Negative Bacteremia

Drug		Half-life (hr)	Total 24-Hr Dose
Penicillins	Ticarcillin	1.0	16–18 g
	Mezlocillin	1.0	16–18 g
	Piperacillin	1.0	12–18 g
Aminoglycosides*	Gentamicin	2.0	3–5 mg/kg
	Tobramycin	2.0	3–5 mg/kg
	Amikacin	2.0	15–20 mg/kg

*Dosing interval and total dose per day are variable and require pharmacokinetic dosing to avoid toxicity or underdosing.

the complex patient in the surgical ICU will have an expanded volume of distribution and an altered pattern of excretion of antibiotics,[26] it is essential that aminoglycoside therapy be pharmacokinetically dosed to minimize drug toxicity and ensure adequate therapy. Recently, there has been considerable interest in the use of single daily dosing of aminoglycosides for gram-negative hospital-acquired infections.[28] Because of limited data on the postoperative use of this strategy in surgical patients, it cannot be recommended.

Nosocomial bacteremia with gram-negative organisms is a significant complication in surgical patients [see 81 Nosocomial Infection]. The principal sites are usually the respiratory and urinary tracts and intravascular devices; the surgical wound is a common site for nosocomial infection but is only infrequently responsible for the septic response or bacteremia.

ANAEROBES

The refinements in anaerobic bacteriology since the early 1970s have resulted in an increased awareness of anaerobic pathogens in surgical infection. Anaerobes of particular significance to surgeons as bacteremic pathogens are principally colonizers of the human GI tract and the female genital tract. Oral or cutaneous anaerobes (e.g., diphtheroids) are rarely identified as bacteremic pathogens, although diphtheroids are commonly recognized skin contaminants of the blood-culturing process. *Bacteroides* species, anaerobic streptococci, and *Clostridium* species tend to be the more commonly identified anaerobic pathogens in blood.

Among all anaerobes, *Bacteroides* species, particularly *B. fragilis*, stand out as the preeminent pathogens. They are customarily identified in infections involving distal ileum or colonic contamination. Intra-abdominal infection must be considered the primary focus of *B. fragilis* bacteremia.[29] Soft tissue infections may also be the source of *Bacteroides* bacteremia, particularly in the presence of a polymicrobial infection or necrotic tissue and particularly in soft tissue infections of the perineum. In one series of patients with *B. fragilis* bacteremia, 80% required operative drainage and debridement as primary treatment.[29]

The selection of antimicrobial therapy for *B. fragilis* must be based on an understanding of the pathogenesis of anaerobic infections. Anaerobic infection in the abdomen and soft tissues is synergistic, wherein anaerobic and aerobic organisms mutually benefit from the polymicrobial environment. The aerobic species decrease the oxidation-reduction potential of the environment, which optimizes conditions for anaerobic proliferation. The anaerobe may then elaborate factors that accelerate the growth cycle of the aerobe, or it may shed a portion of its capsular polysaccharide into the environment and retard phagocytosis of all components of the infection.[30] The complexity of this synergistic relation may be further compounded by interactions between the enterococcus and either the gram-negative rod[16] or the anaerobic organism.[17]

Antimicrobial therapy must address both halves of the synergistic pair, with coverage of the aerobic Enterobacteriaceae species being a vitally important component of treatment for the anaerobe. Antibiotic therapy with the expanded-spectrum β-lactam antibiotics appears to provide adequate polymicrobial coverage in intra-abdominal infection. Clindamycin (900 to 1,200 mg every 6 to 8 hours) or metronidazole (500 mg every 6 hours) in combination with an aminoglycoside has been the traditional treatment but poses special problems (as identified earlier in this discussion). *B. fragilis* bacteremia arising from unusual sites (e.g., endocarditis) or bacteremia in the face of β-lactam antibiotic therapy calls for specific clindamycin or metronidazole therapy. It is of utmost importance that treatment of the patient with anaerobic bacteremia include complete drainage and debridement of the primary focus.

Peptostreptococci and, to a lesser degree, peptococci are anaerobic streptococcal species that may cause bacteremia from infection after gastrointestinal contamination. More commonly, their presence should arouse suspicion that bacteremia may be arising from the female genital tract. Puerperal sepsis and pelvic inflammatory disease may have either of these anaerobes as participants, with common gram-negative Enterobacteriaceae or enterococci, or both, being synergistic partners in the infection. *Bacteroides* species may similarly participate in these types of infections.

Bacteremia with anaerobic streptococci secondary to infection in the female genital tract mandates a search for a drainable primary focus. Puerperal sepsis may require dilatation and curettage to eliminate retained products of conception. Pfannenstiel flaps may become potential sources of wound infection that may cause bacteremia and thus necessitate drainage and debridement. Pelvic inflammatory disease may be complicated by tubo-ovarian abscess or extrauterine abscess within the pelvis that will have to be drained.

Appropriate antibiotic therapy for anaerobic streptococcal bacteremia remains unclear. Most anaerobic species likely to cause infection in the female genital tract are sensitive to penicillin, with *Bacteroides* species being a notable exception. Therapy with an anaerobe-specific agent (e.g., clindamycin or metronidazole) in combination with an aminoglycoside, however, appears to offer better clinical results in puerperal infection.[31] The role of the expanded-spectrum β-lactam agents remains poorly defined. Because enterococcus is commonly identified in infections involving the female genital tract, ampicillin is frequently added to the antibiotic regimen, but it is of unproven value.

Clostridium species are gram-positive anaerobic rods that may cause bacteremia in surgical patients. Relatively uncommon in blood cultures, the organism is ordinarily associated with clostridial myonecrosis or cellulitis. Usually, the fulminant nature of the infection is readily identifiable at the primary soft tissue focus, and blood culture is of little assistance in diagnosis. Therapy consists of radical debridement of the primary site of infection and aggressive administration of penicillin [*see 21 Soft Tissue Infection*].

Nonhistotoxic clostridial bacteremia has been identified with increased frequency. In a series of 47 patients with such bacteremia, only 25% had a focus of infection[32]; the remaining 75% had no clinically identifiable source. The patients in this latter group either were severely, chronically ill or were alcoholics; thus, the presence of a colonic anaerobe in blood may be evidence of primary bacteremia from the GI tract without a primary focus of infection, and nonhistotoxic clostridial bacteremia may be an expression of failed gastrointestinal barrier function rather than infection in the classic sense.

FUNGI

Fungemia in surgical patients has become a major problem since the early 1970s. *Candida* species have been the most common fungal organisms cultured from the blood in these patients. Candidemia is typically seen in a severely ill patient who has had or continues to have bacterial infection and is being treated with a prolonged course (more than 7 days) of broad-spectrum antibiotics.[33,34] Parenteral nutrition and corticosteroid therapy are associated with candidemia. The bacterial microflora becomes suppressed, and colonization by *Candida* organisms of the alimentary tract becomes the reservoir for dissemination.

Candidemia appears to occur principally via two mechanisms. In the first, indwelling catheters (particularly central lines) become colonized. Catheter removal and appropriate culture will document the process and likewise be effective treatment. The alternative mechanism of *Candida* dissemination, however, is gastrointestinal overgrowth with this fungal species, leading to impairment of host barrier function and resultant fungemia.[34] Although peritonitis and intra-abdominal abscess with *Candida* organisms have been identified,[35] translocation of the organisms across the gut barrier is the probable source of contamination.

Prevention of candidemia requires aseptic care of catheters and prompt catheter removal when fungemia is suspected or documented. A reduction in the spectrum and duration of systemic antibiotic therapy is probably the most important way of reducing fungal overgrowth and subsequent risk for dissemination. Oral nystatin, ketoconazole, and fluconazole have been recommended for prophylaxis in patients at risk for candidemia but remain unproven.

In the patient with established candidemia who has had all central lines removed, systemic chemotherapy with amphotericin B is recommended. A dosage of 0.5 to 1.0 mg/kg/day is suggested. The lower dosage (0.5 mg/kg/day) has been reported to be as effective as higher dosages but with reduced toxicity.[35] Fluconazole is a newer antifungal agent that has also been successful in the treatment of candidemia[36]; it is given in a dosage of 200 to as high as 800 mg/day. Because some resistance to fluconazole has been reported,[37] many feel that intravenous amphotericin B is the drug of choice for treatment of severe, life-threatening *Candida* infections. Although cessation of systemic antibiotic therapy has been recommended for the candidemic patient and is certainly desirable, more than 50% of these patients have synchronous bacteremia[33] [*see Table 5*], which compromises the decision to stop all antibiotics. Diagnosis and treatment of candidemia are discussed in detail elsewhere [*see 85 Fungal Infection*].

Positive Blood Culture without Infection

In the late 1950s, Jacob Fine proposed the theory that acute physiologic perturbations (e.g., hemorrhagic shock) could disrupt gastrointestinal barrier function to such a degree that bacteria and their cellular products could escape from the gut reservoir[38-40] and contribute to the patient's clinical illness. In other words, the septic response could be triggered by bacteria or their products (e.g., endotoxin) without infection, in the traditional sense of the term, being present. Although this theory was discredited in the 1960s in germ-free rat experiments,[41,42] it enjoyed a considerable resurgence in the late 1980s, as both experimental[43-47] and clinical[48,49] studies demonstrated that gastrointestinal microbial translocation appears to be a valid biologic event. Consequently, it has been proposed (although not universally accepted[50]) that a cohort of surgical patients

Table 5 Bacteria Identified in Blood Culture within 48 Hours of Positive Culture for *Candida* in 83 Patients[33]

Organism	Number of Isolates
Staphylococcus species	25
Enterococcus	25
Klebsiella species	22
Serratia species	20
Pseudomonas species	11
Bacteroides species	9
Enterobacter species	7
Proteus species	6
Escherichia coli	6
Miscellaneous	15
Total	146*

*Only 27 patients in the series did not have associated bacteria in blood culture. In the 56 patients with associated bacteria, the blood-borne infection was truly polymicrobial, with each patient averaging nearly three bacterial isolates in addition to the *Candida* organism.

may have the septic response secondary to microorganisms while lacking a primary focus of clinical infection.

MECHANISMS OF GUT BARRIER FUNCTION

For gastrointestinal microbial translocation to be a clinically relevant event, gut barrier function must be impaired. At its most distal site, the lumen of the human GI tract may contain as many as 10^{10} bacteria/g of colon contents. The biologic partition that prevents microbes from escaping from this reservoir is complex and consists of anatomic, physiologic, and immunologic mechanisms.

The physical barrier of the gut is constituted by a contiguous layer of enterocytes and colonocytes. An intercellular matrix exists between the cells. Both types of cell appear to obtain a large part of the nutrients they need directly from the gut lumen. Enterocytes have a specific nutrient requirement for glutamine,[51] and colonocytes require short-chain fatty acids.[52] Deficiencies of these critical nutrients lead to atrophy of the gut lining, which results in a defective physical barrier.

The surface of the gut mucosal cells is covered with the glycoprotein mucin,[53] which is an important component of the gut barrier. The mucin layer has a nonspecific retarding effect on bacterial adherence to mucosal cells. In addition, it has a nonspecific inhibitory effect on bacterial proliferation at the mucosal cell surface, thereby helping prevent invasion by luminal bacteria.

Secretory IgA also prevents the binding of bacteria to mucosal cells.[54] Presumably produced as nonspecific antibody from submucosal gut lymphocytes, IgA does not fix complement and does not have cytotoxic effects on bacteria. Rather, it is thought to bind to bacteria and impede their binding to the mucosal cell lining. The IgA concentration is highest at the mucosal cell surface.

The normal microflora that colonizes the GI lumen appears to make a significant contribution to normal gut barrier function. Anaerobic bacteria play a positive role by virtue of their species-specific adherence to mucosal cell-binding sites and their ability to prevent more noxious aerobic species from adhering to mucosal cells via competitive inhibition.[55,56] This positive role creates a real dilemma for clinicians attempting to formulate antimicrobial regimens for critically ill patients.

Normal gastrointestinal motility is perhaps the most important of the physiologic components of the gut barrier. Movement of luminal contents distally within the gut keeps luminal concentrations of bacteria relatively low in the proximal gut and reduces the risk of adherence and translocation. Conversely, there is considerable evidence to suggest that ileus and intestinal obstruction could be important factors in the so-called gut origin septic response.[57]

FACTORS THAT COMPROMISE BARRIER FUNCTION

In critically ill surgical patients, there are numerous associated clinical factors that compromise the various components of barrier function. Critical illness and injury lead to disordered gastrointestinal motility and ileus. Antibiotic therapy frequently covers the common aerobic and anaerobic members of the normal microflora, which results in overgrowth of the gut with resistant aerobic species. Parenteral nutrient solutions are characteristically deficient in glutamine and short-chain fatty acids, and sustained use of such solutions can cause atrophy of the mucosal barrier. IgA and mucin production may be compromised by the catabolic state typical of severe illness. In essence, all of the components of the gut barrier are potentially vulnerable; microbial translocation (and, subsequently, the systemic septic response) can result from impairment of any or all of them.

RECOGNITION AND MANAGEMENT OF MICROBIAL TRANSLOCATION

The clinical basis for the diagnosis of gastrointestinal microbial translocation is imprecise: there is no distinctive clinical marker of this event. Essentially, the diagnosis is one of exclusion. When all conventional infectious sources for a septic response have been excluded by careful clinical evaluation, microbial translocation is considered to be the cause. This clinical diagnosis is a treacherous one and can only be made presumptively. Even when the clinician is convinced that gastrointestinal microbial translocation is operative, he or she must remain vigilant and continue to search for infectious foci that may be driving the septic response.

Blood cultures that are positive for certain opportunistic microbes imply that gastrointestinal microbial translocation may be present. The so-called trilogy of translocation includes the enterococcus,[14] *S. epidermidis*,[7] and *Candida* species.[33,34,58] These three microbes are common overgrowth organisms after sustained courses of broad-spectrum antibiotic therapy and are commonly identified together in blood culture.[7,14,33] Obviously, when blood cultures are positive for these organisms, infectious sources must be ruled out, particularly bacteremia from intravascular devices.

Fundamental to the prevention and treatment of gastrointestinal microbial translocation is reinforcement of the gut barrier. Enteral rather than parenteral nutritional support is always recommended if the clinical circumstances permit.[59] Intraluminal nutrients are delivered directly to the mucosal cells and promote gastrointestinal motility[60]; moreover, they foster proliferation of a more normal intestinal microflora. Mobilization of the patient from the recumbent position likewise promotes gastrointestinal motility and is considered a critical feature of early fixation of long-bone fractures in multiple-trauma patients.[57,61] Immunonutritional regimens that are enhanced with glutamine, arginine, omega-3 fatty acids, and nucleotides have produced encouraging results in prospective clinical trials.[62]

Given what is known about the critical role of the normal gut microflora in the prevention of microbial translocation, it is important to reevaluate patterns of antibiotic use. Although anaerobes are pathogens that act synergistically with aerobes in intra-abdominal and soft tissue infection, in the gut lumen anaerobes are important components of the gut barrier.[63,64] Because anaerobes are seldom nosocomial pathogens, use of systemic antibiotics that cover anaerobes should be avoided in the ICU-acquired infection unless clearly necessary. Some authors have advocated selective gut decontamination (SGD), in which intraluminal antibiotics are employed to reduce aerobic colonization of the gut while preserving the anaerobic species.[65,66] Although SGD is popular in some areas, its value remains controversial.

Negative Blood Culture with Infection

A positive blood culture is generally accepted as proof that microbial dissemination has occurred and that this process is the stimulus for the septic response (although, as noted [see Positive Blood Culture without Infection, above], such an assumption is not always warranted). However, most patients who manifest the septic response secondary to severe infection do not have positive blood cultures. Thus, in these patients, it is the septic response, rather than the blood culture itself, that is the most useful clinical indicator of a systemic reaction to infection.

REASONS FOR NEGATIVE CULTURE

Patients with the septic response secondary to infection may have negative blood cultures for any of several reasons. First, the septic response may have been activated by disseminated microorganisms that are sensitive to concurrently administered antibiotic therapy. The patient may actually be bacteremic, but the presence of active antibiotic in the blood prevents bacterial growth in the culture. For certain antibiotics, there are laboratory methods for neutralizing the effects of their concurrent administration (e.g., penicillinase), but for most, this is not the case. Second, it may have been dissemination of bacterial cellular products rather than of whole, viable microorganisms that activated the septic response. Endotoxin is the most notable of the cellular products associated with the septic response. Third, the septic response may have been activated by systemic distribution of cytokine signals from an intense focus of infection (e.g., severe peritonitis), without bacteria or their products being disseminated from the primary site. Fourth, bacteremia is an episodic process, and blood culture a random event; thus, the culture sample may simply have been obtained at a time when the patient was temporarily nonbacteremic. The frequency of positive blood cultures in critically ill surgical patients in the ICU is so low, and the value of the occasional positive culture so minimal, that several authors have recommended discontinuing the practice of drawing blood samples from these patients.[67,68]

EVALUATION AND MANAGEMENT

Nonbacteremic patients who manifest the septic response must still be evaluated just as thoroughly as bacteremic patients would be, with the aim of ascertaining whether there is a primary source of infection. The lungs, the urinary tract, surgical or traumatic wounds, visceral compartments, and intravenous devices must all be sequentially evaluated. Careful physical examination, appropriate diagnostic studies for each anatomic area (e.g., CT scans for the abdomen), and aggressive culturing of suspicious fluids or exudates are indicated. Special emphasis must be placed on the surgical site and on sites where invasive monitoring devices (e.g., a Foley catheter) or support instruments (e.g., an endotracheal tube) have been introduced into the patient; these sites are frequently the source of the patient's problem. Nonbacteremic patients may indeed have the septic response without being infected [see Septic Response without Microorganisms, below], but this can be determined only after the patient has undergone systematic evaluation for a primary infectious focus.

Once a presumptive source of infection has been identified, the primary focus should be drained mechanically, and empirical antimicrobial therapy directed toward the anticipated pathogens should be initiated while culture and sensitivity data are pending. For intra-abdominal infections, the antibiotic regimen must cover both enteric aerobic and anaerobic bacteria. For postoperative pulmonary infection, it usually must cover the multiresistant gram-negative bacteria of the *Pseudomonas* and *Serratia* species[69,70] [see Table 6]. Postoperative urinary tract infections are usually caused by enteric aerobic gram-negative rods [see Table 7]. Intravascular device infections are generally attributable to staphylococci but are sometimes caused by gram-negative rods or even fungi.

In many cases, critically ill patients who have undergone operation have already received antibiotic therapy at some time during the course of their management. Culture and sensitivity information must therefore be continuously obtained because the pathogens found in complex ICU patients with the septic response will often be resistant to multiple conventional antibiotics.

Although in many cases the source of the infection and the attendant septic response is readily apparent, in many others the diagnosis

Table 6 Common Pathogens Identified in Severely Ill Surgical Patients with Postoperative Pneumonia

Cultured Pathogen	Number of Isolates	
	Rodriguez[69]	Fink[70]
Gram-negative		
Pseudomonas species	38 (22%)	70 (19.5%)
Haemophilus species	16 (9%)	53 (15%)
Enterobacter species	26 (15%)	32 (9%)
Klebsiella species	13 (7.5%)	38 (10.5%)
Escherichia coli	7 (4%)	24 (7%)
Acinetobacter species	12 (7%)	11 (3%)
Proteus species	10 (6%)	11 (3%)
Serratia species	14 (8%)	0
Others	0	46 (13%)
Gram-positive		
Staphylococcus aureus	37 (21%)	48 (13%)
Other	0	26 (7%)
Total	173	359

Table 7 Pathogens Cultured in 212 Postoperative Urinary Tract Infections That Occurred in 153 Surgical Patients[22]

Organism	Number of Isolates
Escherichia coli	56
Klebsiella species	38
Pseudomonas species	37
Proteus species	30
Enterobacter species	22
Enterococcus	22
Serratia species	16
Citrobacter species	10
Streptococcus species	9
Staphylococcus epidermidis	8
Providencia species	5
Candida species	3
Total	256*

*The total exceeds 212 because of polymicrobial isolates in a number of patients.

can only be presumptive. Constant vigilance for changing clinical findings and careful observation of the response to empirical therapy are essential. For example, if a postoperative patient with the septic response has a urinary tract culture that is positive for *E. coli* at 10^5 colony-forming units/ml, it does not necessarily follow that the urinary tract is the source of the patient's septic response. In my experience, a well-drained urinary tract is seldom the source of a septic response in a postoperative patient; other sources must be considered even when a positive urinary tract culture has been obtained.

The surgeon without a diagnosis is likely to find it difficult to handle either the infection or the septic response effectively; thus, continued intensive surveillance of these difficult patients is essential. The objective of management is to control, by mechanical and pharmacologic means, the primary infectious source or sources of the disseminated whole microorganisms, microbial cellular products, or inflammatory cytokines that are responsible for the clinical septic response. Unfortunately, this objective is not equally appropriate for all nonbacteremic septic patients: as is now well established, the septic response can be activated by processes other than clinical infection.

Septic Response without Microorganisms

Traditional assumptions notwithstanding, there is no necessary association between the activation of the septic response and the presence of infection. To underscore this point, some authors have advocated use of the term systemic inflammatory response syndrome to the exclusion of the term sepsis.[1] Nevertheless, the term sepsis is commonly used for SIRS that is secondary to infection [*see 78 Clinical and Laboratory Diagnosis of Infection*]. Any physiologic event that can trigger a severe local inflammatory response is potentially capable of activating the septic response.[71-73] In much the same way as in severe infection without bacteremia or dissemination of bacterial cellular products, extreme local tissue inflammation without a microbial component can cause the release of inflammatory cytokines into the circulation in sufficient quantities to evoke the septic response.

Several common clinical entities can trigger the systemic septic response. Of these, acute pancreatitis is perhaps the most notable. The clinical course of severe acute pancreatitis managed with aggressive volume resuscitation includes loss of peripheral vascular resistance, elevated cardiac output, elevated white blood cell counts, and fever. Indeed, Ranson's criteria reflect characteristics of systemic inflammation, including end-organ damage to the lungs, the liver, and the kidneys.[74] Patients with severe acute pancreatitis often clearly illustrate the rapid physiologic progression from the initiation of the septic response to multiorgan dysfunction [*see 95 Multiple Organ Dysfunction Syndrome*]. Other conditions that can activate the septic response are severe aspiration pneumonitis, which initially is a chemical event that evokes an intense inflammatory response, and multiple trauma with extensive soft tissue injury, necrosis at the injury site, and tissue hematoma. Even extracorporeal membrane oxygenation can be associated with acute activation of the complement cascade and a postoperative septic response leading to end-organ failure, without infection or bacteria being involved at all.

When the septic response occurs in a patient with one of these conditions, the clinician often becomes anxious about the possibility of infection and is tempted to initiate antimicrobial therapy, at the very least. The clinical manifestations of the septic response are essentially the same whether it is caused by infection or not. Accordingly, the diagnosis of the septic response secondary to sterile inflammation is one of suspicion and exclusion. The septic response caused by noninfectious inflammatory processes evolves rapidly after the biologic insult and is not associated with clinical evidence of infection at a specific anatomic site; it is this very response, rather than any infection, that is the fundamental problem to be dealt with in these patients. Obviously, then, antibiotic therapy will be ineffective in such cases, and specific treatment must be directed toward the septic response itself.

Effective supportive care is essential to the management of the septic response secondary to sterile inflammation. Volume support to maintain an adequate cardiac output and tissue perfusion is vital. The pulmonary microcirculation is the early target of the septic response; accordingly, support of systemic oxygenation with mechanical ventilation is commonly necessary.

A vexing problem associated with severe pancreatitis or aspiration pneumonia is that a number of separate stimuli capable of activating the septic response will present themselves during the course of protracted management. In a patient with severe pancreatitis, for example, the primary inflammatory focus gives rise to an initial septic response characterized by pulmonary failure. The patient is effectively resuscitated and appears clinically improved by the fourth or fifth day of hospitalization. By this point, however, an infectious focus, in the form of a pancreatic abscess, has often developed, and this focus evokes a second septic response. Multiple operations and prolonged antibiotic therapy then set the stage for gastrointestinal microbial translocation, which results in candidemia and a third septic response.

What is more, not only may a single condition give rise to multiple different stimuli for the elicitation of the septic response, but severely ill surgical patients may also have additional separate inciting causes (either sequentially or simultaneously) during the course of management, each of which may be associated with one or more septic stimuli. Indeed, a major challenge for the future—perhaps the major challenge—is better definition of clinical markers for specific stimuli of the septic response so that treatment can be better directed.

Discussion

Sepsis as Nonspecific Systemic Inflammatory Response

Infection has traditionally been viewed as a local inflammatory response within tissue that is initiated and perpetuated by microorganisms. It is generally agreed that the numerous elements of host defense are designed to both contain and eradicate the microbial provocateurs of this inflammatory process. It is also generally recognized that a threshold exists, the breaching of which results in the dissemination of the infectious process and the elicitation of a systemic inflammatory response. The precise point at which this threshold is passed has not been well defined clinically; however, the clinical expressions of this event are easily recognized [*see 78 Clinical and Laboratory Diagnosis of Infection*].

Characteristic systemic manifestations of infection include fever, leukocytosis, hyperglycemia, gastrointestinal ileus, and many other findings, depending on the acuteness and severity of the situation. Blood cultures may be positive (see above), and sophisticated laboratory analysis of peripheral blood may yield evidence of the presence of bacterial cell products, such as gram-negative bacterial endotoxin. In these clinical circumstances, patients are said to be septic, to have sepsis, or to have septicemia because the clinical response has been most closely identified with severe infection.[75]

There is considerable evidence to support the theory that the so-called septic patient has a generalized, systemic activation of the inflammatory cascade. The intricate inflammatory response to injury that is so salutary at the tissue level actually becomes a self-destructive process when activated at the systemic level.[76] Although these septic events have been associated most often with uncontrolled infection, it is now appreciated that the systemic inflammatory response is in fact a nonspecific host response in the same way that soft tissue inflammation is nonspecific. In other words, the septic response, despite its traditional association with severe infection, does not require infection or even the presence of microorganisms to be activated—hence the introduction of the term SIRS.[1]

We can now identify a changing perspective with respect to the stimuli of the septic response in the surgical intensive care unit. Current support technology permits sustained survival of critically ill and severely injured patients to a biologic point never before reached. As a result, the septic response may now be seen as a consequence of (1) microorganisms in the context of infection, (2) microorganisms in the absence of infection, and (3) inflammatory events not associated with either microorganisms or clinical infection.

Elements of the Septic Response

The septic response represents an evolution of multiple physiologic and metabolic changes. These changes do not constitute an either-or phenomenon but instead take place along an ever-changing continuum. Consequently, it is difficult to determine exactly when a patient ceases to manifest an appropriate stress response and begins to manifest a deleterious septic response.

The key physiologic elements of the septic response are (1) reduced peripheral vascular resistance, (2) hyperdynamic cardiac performance, and (3) narrowing of the arteriovenous oxygen content difference. The metabolic features of the septic response are quite complex but can be simplified into five main elements: (1) hypermetabolism, (2) accelerated hepatic gluconeogenesis, (3) accelerated hepatic ureagenesis, (4) increased urinary nitrogen loss, and (5) insulin resistance. These metabolic changes are discussed in greater detail elsewhere [see 96 Metabolic Response to Critical Illness].

Reduced peripheral vascular resistance—contrasting dramatically with the increased resistance associated with hypovolemia and cardiac failure—is the sine qua non of the septic response. (It must be emphasized that whereas resistance is reduced for the vascular system as a whole, this may not be the case for each individual tissue bed.) The loss of resistance is particularly interesting in the light of the elevated catecholamine concentrations that are simultaneously identified in these patients. The increases in catecholamine concentration reflect the counterregulatory metabolic milieu of the septic response.[77,78] The alpha-adrenergic effects of the catecholamines are obviously overridden by other peripheral mechanisms.

The systemic vasodilatation has been explained by several mechanisms, but it appears to be principally the result of nitric oxide from endothelial cells in the microcirculation.[79-82] Nitric oxide is a paracrine signal that mediates relaxation of vascular smooth muscle. Its synthesis and release are stimulated by several agonist agents, including endotoxin, bradykinin, and acetylcholine. While other mechanisms include prostacyclin and histamine as potential mediators of vasodilatation, at this time nitric oxide appears to be the principal one.

Hyperdynamic cardiac performance is the obligatory response of the left ventricle when peripheral vascular resistance declines. For cardiac output to increase, however, intravascular volume must be replenished, and the myocardium must possess sufficient physiologic reserve. Thus, elderly patients may not be able to meet the physiologic demands imposed by sepsis-induced afterload reduction, and such inability will result in the hypodynamic septic-shock state. Even in young, healthy patients, the sustained hyperdynamic state will ultimately lead to ventricular failure and low cardiac output.

Narrowing of the arteriovenous oxygen content difference in the hyperdynamic patient is perhaps the most important key to the critical mechanisms responsible for the septic response. Oxygen consumption is inadequate to meet the demands of hypermetabolism,[83,84] and lactate production is the result. When intravascular volume is fully expanded, further increases in cardiac output result in further narrowing of the arteriovenous oxygen content difference. The failure of peripheral oxygen utilization is fundamental to the septic process and underscores that the septic response is not a disease of inadequate myocardial performance until the very late stages in the natural history of the disease.

Natural History of the Septic Response

Studies from the late 1970s[85] provided an important classification system for the natural history of the septic response. This classification identifies exaggeration of the fundamental stress response as the basis for deterioration of the patient from a compensated state (i.e., the stress response) to a decompensated state (i.e., the septic response). The key element to be understood in the natural history of the septic response is the relation between cardiac output and peripheral vascular resistance [see Figure 3].

State A represents the normal adaptive stress response, the first-order response to biologic insults. Cardiac output is modestly elevated, and peripheral vascular resistance is modestly reduced. Systemic oxygen consumption is increased, but lactate concentration is not. This state reflects the postresuscitative physiology of the injured or postoperative patient. The hemodynamic profile progressively returns to normal over the ensuing several days, provided that there is no intercurrent insult (e.g., infection).

State B represents the exaggerated stress response and marks the transition to the beginning of biologic decompensation. Peripheral

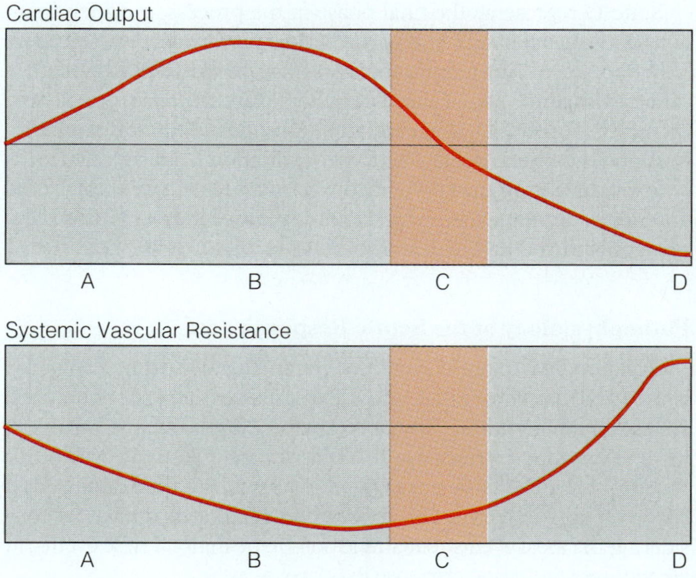

Figure 3 Illustrated is the relation of cardiac output to peripheral vascular resistance during the natural history of the septic response. The area indicated by the box is state C, reflecting the onset of clinical septic shock.

vascular resistance is profoundly reduced. A total peripheral vascular resistance lower than 800 dynes-sec/cm^5 is the commonly recognized threshold for the septic response; resistance may decline to 400 dynes-sec/cm^5 or even lower. The afterload reduction results in dramatic elevation of cardiac output. An acceptable arterial blood pressure can usually be sustained unless intrinsic myocardial disease or hypovolemia is present. The increased capacitance typical of state B necessitates considerable preload support, which often calls for aggressive fluid administration. Measurement of the pulmonary capillary wedge pressure is often necessary to facilitate the expansion of intravascular volume.

State B is also characterized by accumulation of lactate species in the blood before the evolution of frank clinical hypotension. Lactate concentrations in the blood reflect net lactate production in selected tissues minus lactate utilization in other tissues. Because not all tissues are necessarily affected equally by the septic response process, oxidation of lactate by selected well-perfused tissues may compensate for production of lactate by others. Lactic acidemia preceding lactic acidosis is usually seen in patients with sustained state B; compensatory mechanisms prevent acidosis until later in the process. These patients are actually in a state of shock, even though their arterial blood pressure is considered normal, because tissue oxygen utilization is clearly impaired.

State C heralds the beginning of septic shock as it has been traditionally defined—that is, as hypotension in a nonhypovolemic patient that is secondary to severe infection. State C patients fulfill this definition: they have mild to severe hypotension, with systolic arterial blood pressures lower than 80 mm Hg. In this setting, however, septic shock is secondary to the severe and exaggerated loss of peripheral vascular resistance; although cardiac output may be normal or slightly increased (8 to 10 L/min), it is insufficient to compensate for this loss.

State C patients are in so-called hot shock. They are warm to the touch and usually show evidence of diaphoresis. One has the clinical impression that the cutaneous tissues are well perfused, even though the arterial blood pressure is low. The loss of perfusion pressure acts synergistically with the peripheral defect in oxygen utilization to create a severe peripheral oxygen debt that is clearly reflected in the severe lactic acidosis seen in these patients.

State D represents the final phase in the process, in which frank congestive heart failure emerges. Cardiac performance is considerably depressed. Autonomic mechanisms override the vasodilatory influences seen in state C, and peripheral vascular resistance is now increased. In state D, low cardiac output, peripheral vasoconstriction, and peripheral defects in oxygen utilization work simultaneously to produce profound tissue hypoxemia and lactic acidosis. In the absence of dramatic therapeutic and supportive measures, this is the preagonal period before death.

Pathophysiology of the Septic Response

Fundamental to our current understanding of the septic response is the idea that its negative and destructive features are simply the systemic manifestations of what is otherwise a positive and beneficial local inflammatory response to tissue injury. The two types of response involve the same physiologic processes, but their domain and scope are very different. This crucial point can be illustrated by considering the local events that attend soft tissue injury. These events, in essence, are the septic response in microcosm.

LOCAL EVENTS

Soft tissue injury triggers a local inflammatory response that includes disruption of blood vessels, exposure of the collagen matrix, extravasation of red blood cells and plasma proteins, activation of the coagulation cascade, aggregation of platelets, and activation of the complement cascade via the alternative pathway.[86] It is likely that by-products of coagulation and complement activation, among other potential biochemical signals, are the stimuli to mast cells that initiate the first phases of the inflammatory response; the specific cleavage products of complement proteins C3, C4, and C5 (the soluble anaphylatoxins C3a, C4a, and C5a) are known to be the most potent stimuli of mast cell degranulation.[87-89] The production of bradykinin occurs from plasma protein precursors via the stimulation of activated factor XII from the coagulation cascade. Activation of these five initiators of inflammation (coagulation cascade, platelets, complement proteins, mast cells, and bradykinin) produces (1) local vasodilatation, increasing local flow but reducing flow velocity in the area of injury; (2) increased capillary permeability, resulting in extravasation of protein-rich plasma into the injured area, thereby initiating edema; and (3) generation of numerous inflammatory enzyme and protein cleavage products, which serve as chemoattractants.

Diffusion of the chemoattractant signals from the epicenter of injury begins the process of phagocytic infiltration of the injured area. Chemoattractants bind to specific receptor sites on vascular endothelial cells, initiating interaction between endothelial cells and intravascular neutrophils. Neutrophil "rolling" on the endothelial surface, initiated by surface selectin receptors, slows neutrophil transit velocity within the microcirculation and sets the stage for integrin interactions leading to margination of the neutrophil. The gradient of chemoattractant signals from the epicenter of the injury serves as a beacon, directing phagocytic diapedesis toward the site of injury and contamination. The severity of the injury, the extent of necrosis, and the degree of exogenous microbial contamination dictate the intensity of the summed chemoattractant signals that govern the rapidity and the quantity of neutrophil infiltration.

Approximately 24 hours after injury, macrophages infiltrate the area via the same mechanisms for margination and chemotaxis that mobilized the neutrophils. Macrophages orchestrate the severity of the inflammatory response. If necrotic tissue and foreign elements (e.g., bacteria) are minimally present in the area of injury, then the magnitude of the chemoattractant signal will be small, macrophages are minimally activated, and the neutrophils proceed with phagocytosis in an orderly fashion. If, however, bacterial contamination is severe and there is considerable necrotic tissue, then the amplitude of chemoattractant effects will be great, resulting in full activation of macrophages. The fully activated macrophage elaborates multiple proinflammatory cytokines with autocrine, paracrine, and endocrine functions.

One such cytokine, tumor necrosis factor, is itself capable of inducing full macrophage activation.[90] In addition, TNF serves as an activating signal from the macrophages to the neutrophils, causing the neutrophils to enter a state of accelerated and enhanced phagocytic activity and eliciting the extracellular release of reactive oxygen intermediates and lysosomal enzymes. The accelerated phagocytic activity, driven by the TNF and other proinflammatory signals from the macrophages, results in the death of the neutrophils and in the formation of pus. Suppuration at the epicenter of the injury is further enhanced when the TNF signal diffuses into the adjacent microcirculation, where marginated neutrophils, recruited into the inflammatory focus, are fully activated. Activation of these neutrophils, coupled with release of reactive oxygen intermediates and lysosomal enzymes, results in thrombosis of the adjacent microcirculation. This microcirculatory thrombosis is actually beneficial in that it prevents bacteria or their products from gaining systemic access. Indeed, the ultimate function of the inflammatory response is the containment and subsequent eradication of bacterial contaminants.

BLOOD CULTURES AND INFECTION — 1187

This microcirculatory arrest, in turn, leads to the formation of foci of necrotic tissue,[91] which evoke a local inflammatory response that eventually reactivates the septic response. A self-energized and futile cycle is created, in which an initial injury elicits a local response, the local response subsequently expands into a systemic response, and the systemic response finally generates tissue-level injuries that start up the whole process all over again [see Figure 4]. The progressive loss of microcirculatory units within the critical organ systems leads to multiorgan failure (now also known as multiple organ dysfunction syndrome) [see 95 Multiple Organ Dysfunction Syndrome] and ultimately to the death of the host.[92-94]

New Approaches to Management of the Septic Response

A clearer comprehension of the mechanisms involved in the evolution of the septic response and its end-organ effects should facilitate the development of new and better therapeutic regimens. On the basis of what is currently known, numerous new treatments have already been examined in experimental studies, and a few of them have been used on an investigational basis in humans [see 88 Immunomodulation]. These newer therapies have had three general areas of focus: (1) neutralization of stimuli that provoke the systemic inflammatory response, (2) inhibition or blockade of the initiator events of inflammation itself, or (3) inhibition or neutralization of effector mechanisms that are the consequence of activation of the systemic inflammatory response.

Efforts to neutralize or inhibit the provocative stimulation of SIRS have focused on bacterial endotoxin as the target. Antiendotoxin antibody has been given to septic patients in an attempt to neutralize the effects of a component of gram-negative bacteria that is a potent activator of the septic response. Although some clinical studies have found that certain groups of septic response patients benefit from administration of polyclonal sera[95-97] or the monoclonal antibody,[98,99] considerable controversy continues to surround this proposed treatment. Favorable reports focusing on beneficial effects in specific subpopulations of patients have not been validated by prospective studies addressed to these cohorts.[100,101] Because endotoxin is only one of numerous stimuli of the septic response, the use of the very expensive monoclonal antiendotoxin antibody in all septic response patients would be difficult to justify. It is unlikely that this treatment strategy will be generally adopted in clinical practice.

Numerous experimental studies have explored inhibition of initiators of inflammation: specifically, inhibition of coagulation and platelets,[103-105] bradykinin,[106] mast cells, and complement proteins.[108,109] Few have been put into prospective clinical trials. A prospective multicenter trial of a bradykinin antagonist failed to demonstrate any clinical benefit.

A third focus of investigation has been the inhibition of effector mechanisms or consequences of activation. Specific neutralization of TNF[111,112] or receptor effects of interleukin-1[113] were initially the most promising. However, clinical trials of both approaches have failed to demonstrate any meaningful benefit.[114-118] Other directions include antibodies to prevent neutrophil-endothelial interaction; platelet activating factor; neutralization of reactive oxygen species to prevent lipid peroxidation; inhibition of vasoactive derivatives; and strategies with dialysis, plasmapheresis, or hemofiltering cytokines or other adverse effectors. The theme is a constant one, in that experimental data look promising, but efforts to convert the experimental benefits into clinical results have consistently failed.

Shown is the self-energized cycle of tissue-level injury that causes the end-organ consequences of the septic response. Activation of the inflammatory cascade via several different stimuli results in neutrophil activation, which leads to autodestructive inflammation, tissue ischemia, tissue necrosis, and reactivation of the process.

SYSTEMIC EVENTS

The systemic septic response comprises the same sequence of events just described, except that the activation of the inflammatory cascade is generalized and lacks the clear directional focus that characterizes the local response. In severe infection, dissemination of bacteria and endotoxins leads to systemic activation of the initiator pathways of human inflammation. Systemic activation of coagulation, platelets, complement proteins, mast cells, and bradykinin results in generalized edema, systemic vasodilatation, and a generalized release of chemoattractant signals. Generalized neutrophil margination occurs. The up-regulation of the generalized inflammatory response results in full activation of marginated neutrophils. From their intravascular and perivascular position, the activated neutrophils subsequently release reactive oxygen intermediates and lysosomal enzymes. The resulting inflammatory injury to the microcirculation leads to aggregation of platelets, damage to the endothelial cells, and release of prostaglandin derivatives that promote vasoconstriction. The consequence of these events is a two-pronged injury comprising the biomechanical blockade caused by the inflammatory aggregate and the vasoconstriction caused by thromboxane A_2.

When an inflammatory focus is sufficiently severe (as, for example, in pancreatitis), it may release so much TNF that macrophages and neutrophils are activated within the circulation. In these circumstances, in situ macrophage cells, such as alveolar macrophages and Kupffer's cells, can be activated, and a generalized inflammatory response is the result. In this scenario, systemic dissemination of the pathogen or its cellular products may not be required for the systemic inflammatory response; instead, only the proinflammatory cytokine signal needs to be disseminated.

The current explosion in cytokine research has resulted in the identification of numerous new mediators of the inflammatory response. It is likely that still more will be recognized in the near future and that our understanding of the septic response will continue to evolve rapidly. At present, the major problem associated with mediator blockade or neutralization is that there are numerous redundant mechanisms at play in the human inflammatory response. Blockade of a single signal is unlikely to achieve the necessary physiologic effect. Furthermore, these chemical signals play a positive biologic role in the salutary local inflammatory response, which means that neutralization of the inflammatory response, could significantly impair host defense.

SIRS represents the biologic processes that are identified in every wound and in every infection. Surgical drainage of a severe soft tissue abscess down-regulation of the inflammatory signals. Intrinsic mechanisms for the inflammatory response are obvious when inflammation is no longer necessary. A clearer the natural counterinflammatory mechanisms will pathway to newer therapies for SIRS and its sequelae.

References

1. American College of Chest Physicians/Society of Critical Care Medicine Consensus Conference: Definitions for sepsis and organ failure and guidelines for the use of innovative therapies in sepsis. Crit Care Med 20:864, 1992
2. Fry DE, Fry RV, Borzotta AP: Nosocomial blood-borne infection secondary to intravascular devices. Am J Surg 167:268, 1994
3. Maki DG, Weise CE, Sarafin HW: A semiquantitative culture method for identifying intravenous-catheter–related infection. N Engl J Med 296:1305, 1977
4. JM, Pruitt BA Jr: Suppurative thrombophlebitis: iatrogenic disease. N Engl J Med 282:1452,
5. RN, Richardson JD, Fry DE: Catheter-septic thrombophlebitis. South Med J 75:
6. Bergamini TM, Kinney EV, et al: In situ vascular prostheses infected by bacteria. Surg 13:575, 1991
7. nor LB, Slotman GJ, et al: Staphy-sepsis in surgical patients. Arch
8. shock syndromes. Infect Dis 1996
9. Schwartz B, et al: Invasive tion in Ontario, Canada: ccal Study Group. N
10. terial complications Clin Infect Dis
11. et al: The eagulation, 102 ycin, erythro-l products, 107 of streptococ-ued into pro-al: Patho-of a promising fections. ion or alteration ions in the Infect tor blockade. promising ffects. failed coc-ections had let teractions; a to xygen inter va-ious eicos of heresis, or e is substance se, observation

19. mechanism and clinical relevance. Infect Dis Clin North Am 11:851, 1997
20. Landman D, Quale JM: Management of infection due to resistant enterococci: a review of therapeutic options. J Antimicrob Chemother 40:161, 1997
21. Collins LA, Malanoski GJ, Eliopoulos GM, et al: In vitro activity of RP 59500, an injectable streptogramin antibiotic, against vancomycin-resistant gram positive organisms. Antimicrob Agents Chemother 37:598, 1993
22. Asher EF, Oliver BG, Fry DE: Urinary tract infections in the surgical patient. Am Surg 54:466, 1988
23. Fry DE, Cox RA, Harbrecht PJ: Empyema of the gallbladder: a complication in the natural history of acute cholecystitis. Am J Surg 141:366, 1981
24. Mosdell DM, Morris DM, Voltura A, et al: Antibiotic treatment for surgical peritonitis. Ann Surg 214:543, 1991
25. Fry DE: Third generation cephalosporin antibiotics in surgical practice. Am J Surg 151:306, 1986
26. Niemiec PW Jr, Allo MD, Miller CF: Effect of altered volume of distribution on aminoglycoside levels in patients in surgical intensive care. Arch Surg 122:207, 1987
27. Brighty KE, Gootz TD: The chemistry and biological profile of trovafloxacin. J Antimicrob Chemother 39(suppl B):1, 1997
28. Koo J, Tight R, Rajkumar V, et al: Comparison of once-daily versus pharmacokinetic dosing of aminoglycosides in elderly patients. Am J Med 101:177, 1996
29. Fry DE, Garrison RN, Polk HC Jr: Clinical implications in bacteroides bacteremia. Surg Gynecol Obstet 149:189, 1979
30. Kasper DL, Hayes ME, Reinap BG, et al: Isolation and identification of encapsulated strains of *Bacteroides fragilis*. J Infect Dis 136:75, 1977
31. Ledger WJ, Kriewall TJ, Sweet RL, et al: The use of parenteral clindamycin in the treatment of obstetric-gynecologic patients with severe infections: a comparison of clindamycin-kanamycin with penicillin-kanamycin. Obstet Gynecol 43:490, 1974
32. Fry DE, Klamer TW, Garrison RN, et al: Atypical clostridial bacteremia. Surg Gynecol Obstet 153:28, 1981
33. Dyess DL, Garrison RN, Fry DE: *Candida* sepsis: implications of polymicrobial blood-borne infection. Arch Surg 120:345, 1985
34. Stone HH, Kolb LD, Currie CA, et al: *Candida* sepsis: pathogenesis and principles of treatment. Ann Surg 179:697, 1974
35. Solomkin JS, Flohr AB, Quie PG, et al: The role of *Candida* in intraperitoneal infections. Surgery 88:524, 1980
36. Rex JH, Bennett JE, Sugar AM, et al: A randomized trial comparing fluconazole with amphotericin B for the treatment of candidemia in patients without neutropenia. N Engl J Med 331:1325, 1994

37. Evans TG, Mayer J, Cohen ure in treatment of systemic 164:1232, 1991
38. Fine J, Frank ED, Ravin HA, et al tor in traumatic shock. N Engl J M
39. Ravin HA, Fine J: Biological implications endotoxins. Fed Proc 21:65, 1962
40. Schweinburg F, Fine J: Evidence for a lethal mia as the fundamental feature of irreversibility types of traumatic shock. J Exp Med 112:793
41. Zweifach BW: Hemorrhagic shock in germfree Ann NY Acad Sci 78:315, 1959
42. Zweifach BW, Gordon HA, Wagner M, et al: Irreversible hemorrhagic shock in germfree rats. J Exp Med 107:437, 1958
43. Maejima K, Deitch EA, Berg RD: Bacterial translocation from the gastrointestinal tracts of rats receiving thermal injury. Infect Immun 43:6, 1984
44. Baker JW, Deitch EA, Li M, et al: Hemorrhagic shock induces bacterial translocation from the gut. J Trauma 28:896, 1988
45. Deitch EA, Winterton J, Li M, et al: The gut as a portal of entry for bacteremia: role of protein malnutrition. Ann Surg 205:681, 1987
46. Deitch DE, Berg R, Specian R: Endotoxin promotes the translocation of bacteria from the gut. Arch Surg 122:185, 1987
47. Rush BF Jr, Sori AJ, Murphy TF, et al: Endotoxemia and bacteremia during hemorrhagic shock. Ann Surg 207:549, 1988
48. Deitch EA: Simple intestinal obstruction causes bacterial translocation in man. Arch Surg 124:699, 1989
49. Rush BF Jr, Redan JA, Flanagan JJ Jr, et al: Does bacteremia in hemorrhagic shock have clinical significance? A study in germ-free animals. Ann Surg 210:342, 1989
50. Lanser ME: An experimental phenomenon without clinical significance. Multiple System Organ Failure. Fry DE, Ed. Mosby–Year Book, Chicago, 1992, p 382
51. Wilmore DW, Smith RJ, O'Dwyer ST, et al: The gut: a central organ after surgical stress. Surgery 104:917, 1988
52. Roediger WE, Rae DA: Trophic effect of short chain fatty acids on mucosal handling of ions by the dysfunctioned colon. Br J Surg 69:23, 1982
53. McNabb PC, Tomasi TB: Host defense mechanisms at mucosal surfaces. Annu Rev Microbiol 35:477, 1981
54. Tomasi TB Jr, Bienenstock J: Secretory immunoglobulins. Adv Immunol 9:1, 1968
55. Savage DC, Dubos R, Schaedler RW: The gastrointestinal epithelium and its autochthonous bacterial flora. J Exp Med 127:67, 1968
56. Suegara N, Morotomi M, Watanabe T, et al: Behavior of the microflora in the rat stomach: adhesion of lactobacilli to the keratinized epithelial cells of the rat in vitro. Infect Immun 12:173, 1975

Border J, Hassett J, LaDuca J, et al: The gut origin septic states in blunt multiple trauma (ISS=40) in the ICU. Ann Surg 206:427, 1987

exander JW, Boyce ST, Babcock GF, et al: The pro- s of microbial translocation. Ann Surg 212:496,

re FA, Moore EE, Jones TN, et al: TEN versus following major abdominal trauma—reduced morbidity. J Trauma 29:916, 1989

zuki H, Trocki O, Dominioni L, et al: Mecha- prevention of postburn hypermetabolism bolism by early enteral feeding. Ann Surg 1984

LaDuca J, Hassett JM, et al: Blunt multiple S 36), femur traction, and the pulmonary ic state. Ann Surg 202:283, 1985

Minard G, Croce MA, et al: A random- onitrogenous enteral diets following se- an immune-enhancing diet (IED) re- mplications. Ann Surg 224:531, 1996

notion of the translocation of enteric gastrointestinal tracts of mice by oral enicillin, clindamycin, or metronida- n 33:854, 1981

rvenkov JI, Alexander JW, et al: Ef- l antibiotics on the translocation of burned guinea pigs. Burns 16:

onization resistance of the diges- nsequences and implications. her 10:263, 1982

A, Dunn DL, et al: Selective duces nosocomial infections ot mortality or organ failure e unit patients. Arch Surg

Klein SR: Are blood cul- tion of fever in periopera- 2:615, 1991

cacy of blood cultures in t. Surgery 120:752, 1996

Bitzer LG, et al: Pneu- s, and outcome in in- 7, 1991

derman MS, et al: a in hospitalized pa- andomized, double- s ciprofloxacin with Agents Chemother

er IP, et al: Multi- t bacteria: an ex- 7, 1986

, et al: System- hemodynamic Surg 123:316,

MC, et al: Fe- injury pro- hepatic dys-

l: Prognos- gement in t 139:69,

lti-organ itorial).

Multi- flam-

ined onse

in- ost

ry

80. Ignarro LJ: Biological actions and properties of en- dothelium-derived nitric oxide formed and released from artery and vein. Circ Res 65:1, 1989

81. Ignarro LJ: Biosynthesis and metabolism of endothe- lium-derived nitric oxide. Annu Rev Pharmacol Tox- icol 30:535, 1990

82. Vallance P, Collier J, Moncada S: Nitric oxide synthe- sised from L-arginine mediates endothelium depen- dent dilatation in human veins in vivo. Cardiovasc Res 23:1053, 1989

83. Siegel JH, Greenspan M, Del Guercio LRM: Abnor- mal vascular tone, defective oxygen transport and my- ocardial failure in human septic shock. Ann Surg 165:504, 1967

84. Siegel JH, Farrell EJ, Miller M, et al: Cardiorespirato- ry interactions as determinants of survival and the need for respiratory support in human shock states. J Trauma 13:602, 1973

85. Siegel JH, Cerra FB, Coleman B, et al: Physiological and metabolic correlations in human sepsis: invited commentary. Surgery 86:163, 1979

86. Pillemer L, Blum L, Lepow IH, et al: The properdin system and immunity: I. Demonstration and isola- tion of a new serum protein, properdin, and its role in immune phenomena. Science 120:279, 1954

87. Gorski JP, Hugli TE, Muller-Eberhard HJ: Charac- terization of human C4a anaphylatoxin. J Biol Chem 256:2707, 1981

88. da Silva WD, Eisele JW, Lepow IH: Complement as a mediator of inflammation: III. Purification of the ac- tivity with anaphylatoxin properties generated by in- teraction of the first four components of complement and its identification as a cleavage product of C'3. J Exp Med 126:1027, 1967

89. Shin HS, Snyderman R, Friedman E, et al: Chemo- tactic and anaphylatoxic fragment cleaved from the fifth component of guinea pig complement. Science 162:361, 1968

90. Beutler B, Cerami A: Cachectin: more than a tumor necrosis factor. N Engl J Med 316:379, 1987

91. Asher EF, Rowe RL, Garrison RN, et al: Experimen- tal bacteremia and hepatic nutrient blood flow. Circ Shock 20:43, 1986

92. Townsend MC, Hampton WW, Haybron DM, et al: Effective organ blood flow and bioenergy status in murine peritonitis. Surgery 100:205, 1986

93. Schirmer WJ, Townsend MC, Schirmer JM, et al: Galactose elimination kinetics in sepsis: correlations of hepatic blood flow with function. Arch Surg 122: 349, 1987

94. Haybron DM, Townsend MC, Hampton WW, et al: Alterations in renal perfusion and renal energy charge in murine peritonitis. Arch Surg 122:328, 1987

95. Lachman E, Pitsoe SB, Gaffin SL: Anti-lipopolysac- charide immunotherapy in management of septic shock of obstetric and gynaecological origin. Lancet 1:981, 1984

96. Baumgartner JD, Glauser MP, McCutchan JA, et al: Prevention of gram-negative shock and death in sur- gical patients by antibody to endotoxin core glyco- lipid. Lancet 2:59, 1985

97. Ziegler EJ, McCutchan JA, Fierer J, et al: Treatment of gram-negative bacteremia and shock with human antiserum to a mutant *Escherichia coli*. N Engl J Med 307:1225, 1982

98. Ziegler EJ, Fischer CJ, Sprung CL Jr, et al: Treatment of gram-negative bacteremia and septic shock with HA-1A human monoclonal antibody against endo- toxin: a randomized, double-blind, placebo-controlled trial. N Engl J Med 324:429, 1991

99. Greenman RL, Schein RMH, Martin MA, et al: A controlled clinical trial of E5 murine monoclonal IgM antibody to endotoxin in the treatment of gram- negative sepsis. JAMA 266:1097, 1991

100. McCloskey RV, Straube RC, Sanders C, et al: Treat- ment of septic shock with human monoclonal anti- body HA-1A: a randomized, double-blind, placebo- controlled trial. CHESS Trial Study Group. Ann Intern Med 121:1, 1994

101. Bone RC, Balk RA, Fein AM, et al: A second large controlled study of E5, a monoclonal antibody to en- dotoxin: results of a prospective, multicenter, random- ized, controlled trial. The E5 Sepsis Study Group. Crit Care Med 23:994, 1995

102. Jansen PM, Pixley RA, Brouwer M, et al: Inhibition of factor XII in septic baboons attenuates the activa- tion of complement and fibrinolytic system and re- duces the release of interleukin-6 and neutrophil elas- tase. Blood 87:2337, 1996

103. Hau T, Simmons RL: Heparin in the treatment of ex- perimental peritonitis. Ann Surg 187:294, 1978

104. O'Leary JP, Malik FS, Donahoe RP, et al: The effects of a minidose of heparin on peritonitis in rats. Surg Gynecol Obstet 148:571, 1979

105. Schirmer WJ, Schirmer JM, Naff GB, et al: Hepa- rin's effect on the natural history of sepsis in the rat (abstr). Circ Shock 21:363, 1987

106. Ridings PC, Blocher CR, Fisher BJ, et al: Beneficial effects of a bradykinin antagonist in a model of gram negative sepsis. J Trauma 39:81, 1995

107. Leeper-Woodford SK, Carey D, Byrne K, et al: Hista- mine receptor antagonists, cyclooxygenase blockade, and tumor necrosis factor curing acute septic insult. Shock 9:89, 1998

108. Jansen PM, Eisele B, de Jong IW, et al: Effect of C1 inhibition on inflammatory and physiologic re- sponse patterns in primates suffering from lethal sep- tic shock. J Immunol 160:475, 1998

109. Mohr M, Hopken U, Opperman M, et al: Effects of anti-C5a monoclonal antibodies on oxygen use in a porcine model of severe sepsis. Eur J Clin Invest 28: 227, 1998

110. Fein AM, Bernard GR, Criner GJ, et al: Treatment of severe systemic inflammatory response syndromes and sepsis with a novel bradykinin antagonist, deltibant (CP-0127): results of a randomized, double-blind, placebo-controlled trial. CP-1027 SIRS and Sepsis Study Group. JAMA 277:482, 1997

111. Beutler B, Milsark IW, Cerami AC: Passive immu- nization against cachectin/tumor necrosis factor pro- tects mice from lethal effect of endotoxin. Science 229:869, 1985

112. Tracey KJ, Fong Y, Hesse DG, et al: Anti-cachectin/ TNF monoclonal antibodies prevent septic shock during lethal bacteraemia. Nature 330:662, 1987

113. Wakabayashi G, Gelfand JA, Burke JF, et al: A spe- cific receptor antagonist for interleukin 1 prevents *Escherichia coli*-induced shock in rabbits. FASEB J 5:338, 1991

114. Abraham E, Wunderink R, Silverman H, et al: Ef- ficacy and safety of monoclonal antibody to human tumor necrosis factor alpha in patients with sepsis syndrome: a randomized, controlled, double-blind, multicenter clinical trial. JAMA 273:934, 1995

115. Cohen J, Carlet J: Intersept: an international, multi- center, placebo-controlled trial of monoclonal an- tibody to human tumor necrosis factor-alpha in pa- tients with sepsis. International Sepsis Trial Study Group. Crit Care Med 24:1431, 1996

116. Reinhart K, Wiegard-Lohnert C, Grimminger F, et al: Assessment of the safety and efficacy of the mono- clonal anti-tumor necrosis factor antibody-fragment, MAK 195F, in patients with sepsis and septic shock: a multicenter, randomized, placebo-controlled, dose- ranging study. Crit Care Med 24:733, 1996

117. Fisher CJ Jr, Dhainaut JF, Opal SM, et al: Recom- binant human interleukin 1 receptor antagonist in the treatment of patients with sepsis syndrome: re- sults from a randomized, double-blind, placebo-con- trolled trial. Phase III rhIL-1ra Sepsis Syndrome Study Group. JAMA 271:1836, 1994

118. Opal SM, Fisher CJ Jr, Dhainaut JF, et al: Confirming interleukin-1 receptor antagonist trial in severe sepsis: a phase III, randomized, double-blind, placebo-con- trolled, multicenter trial. The Interleukin-1 Receptor Antagonist Sepsis Investigation Group. Crit Care Med 25:1115, 1997

119. Fry DE, Fry RV, Borzotta AP: Nosocomial blood- borne infection secondary to intravascular devices. Am J Surg 167:268, 1994

80 ANTIBIOTICS

Nicolas V. Christou, M.D., Ph.D.

Antibiotic Therapy in Surgical Patients

Several important advances in antimicrobial therapy have been made since the early 1980s. Among these advances are (1) improved understanding of the microbiologic spectrum of so-called optimal therapy, (2) better application of pharmacokinetic principles to drug administration [see 107 Pharmacokinetics in Surgical Practice], (3) the development of several new classes of antibiotics, and (4) greater insight into the interplay among host resistance factors, microorganisms, and chemotherapy. Also, the wide range of antibiotics now available has made possible the tailoring of antibiotic therapy to various host factors and various infections.

General Principles of Antimicrobial Therapy

EMPIRICAL THERAPY

Surgeons often treat serious surgical infections without the benefit of microbiologic culture and sensitivity testing of the microbial pathogens. Even with the most rapid bacteriologic tests currently available, it may not be possible to identify a pathogen in less than 24 hours, and antimicrobial sensitivities can rarely be obtained in less than 48 to 72 hours. In seriously ill patients, treatment cannot be delayed for 2 to 3 days until these data become available. If therapy is to be successful, it must be started as soon as a life-threatening infection is diagnosed—or, in some patients, as soon as such an infection is suspected. Which antimicrobial agents are to be used depends on the suspected site of infection and on the organisms that are commonly pathogenic at this site. Therapy is initiated with an agent or combination of agents whose action is broad enough to cover all the suspected microbial pathogens. The application of such broad-spectrum antibiotic therapy in the absence of microbiologic confirmation is termed empirical therapy.

To make a rational decision regarding empirical therapy, the surgeon must be familiar with the organisms that are likely to be encountered when a particular infection (e.g., an intra-abdominal abscess) is suspected. Selection of the agent or agents is based on the history, the physical examination, where the infection was likely to have been acquired, the host defense status, the overall clinical severity of the infection, and the response of the host. Definitive therapy is initiated after the host response to the infection and to the empirical treatment has been monitored and the results from the microbiology laboratory—specifically, identification of the isolated organisms and the minimal inhibitory concentrations (MICs) of various antimicrobial agents—have been assessed. If the surgeon chooses an appropriate antimicrobial therapy, the patient will get well, will experience no adverse reactions, and will leave the hospital in a short time. In addition, the environment will not be harmed, and the cost of therapy will be low.

VARIABLES INFLUENCING TREATMENT

A surgeon planning a course of antimicrobial therapy must take into account a number of variables. One of these is efficacy, which is the ability of an agent to reach the site of the infection and to be active at that site. Therefore, knowledge of the absorption, distribution, and excretion characteristics of the agent is essential for selecting an agent and a method of administration [see 107 Pharmacokinetics in Surgical Practice].

Another variable is toxicity, which relates to immediate allergic-type reactions, idiosyncratic reactions that occur subsequently, and dose-dependent end-organ damage. It is vitally important to reduce the risks of treatment to the individual patient as much as possible, but it is also important to consider the broader effects of antimicrobial use. Indiscriminate use of antibiotics may produce microbial resistance that is peculiar to the institution, which increases the risk that other patients will be infected with these resistant organisms.

A third variable is cost, which involves much more than the price of a gram of the agent, the frequency with which doses are given, or the duration of treatment. The most expensive drug may be the most economical and logical choice if it shortens a hospital stay, allows outpatient treatment, or saves a life. Cost must be considered in relation to both efficacy and toxicity.

A fourth variable is dosage. Dosages for antimicrobial agents with a wide margin between therapeutic and toxic blood levels are usually standardized and independent of the adult patient's weight. Dosages for agents with a narrow margin between therapeutic and toxic blood levels (e.g., aminoglycosides), however, are calculated on the basis of body weight.

A fifth variable is route of administration. In patients with severe infections and in all compromised hosts, antimicrobial agents should be given parenterally because this approach is more likely to yield therapeutic blood levels and consequently higher tissue levels. Intravenous administration is also essential in patients who are hypotensive or in shock, because in such conditions, drug absorption from intramuscular sites is poor.

A sixth variable is the duration of antimicrobial treatment, which is dependent on the type and severity of infection, the host response, and the clinical course of the patient. Usually, the antibiotic is continued until the signs and symptoms of the infection resolve, which typically occurs within 5 to 14 days.

A final variable is whether single-agent therapy or multiagent therapy is indicated. In certain situations, administration of multiple agents is essential for optimal antimicrobial therapy.

Many patients who report a history of allergy to antibiotics are not genuinely allergic. Statements about allergic reactions can be neither taken for granted nor disregarded without risk of serious therapeutic consequences, not to mention legal problems. A carefully elicited history may reveal that the symptoms attributed to an allergic reaction are incompatible with such an interpretation. Skin testing with benzylpenicilloyl-polylysine and minor determinant antigens done just before a planned course of therapy with a penicillin, a penicillin derivative, or a cephalosporin may reveal a propensity to an immediate allergic reaction. Because skin testing itself is associated with some risk of reaction, it should be done only when the drug to be tested is clearly superior and is certain to be used if the test result is negative. A good deal of concern remains about possible cross-allergenicity between the penicillins and the cephalosporins. If the reaction is neither immediate nor severe, the patient usually will tolerate the antibiotic. There are numerous other in vivo interactions involving antimicrobials [see Table 1].

A number of antibiotics should be used with caution in pregnant women because they have significant toxic effects on the mother, the fetus, or both [see Table 2].

Laboratory Tests

Many laboratory tests, if used in the proper context, can guide selection of optimal antimicrobial therapy.

In vitro susceptibility tests are indicated when the susceptibility of an organism is not completely predictable or when certain other specific problems arise, such as the necessity of determining whether resistance has developed during the course of therapy. An organism is generally considered susceptible if the concentration of antimicrobial agent necessary to inhibit its growth is lower than that usually attainable in body fluids, particularly blood, cerebrospinal fluid, or urine. The results of these tests may vary from laboratory to laboratory, depending on the preparation of the antimicrobial agent, the size of the inoculum, the duration and temperature of incubation, the definition of inhibitory end points, and the characteristics of the medium used (especially its cation content and pH). For instance, a gentamicin susceptibility test performed at a pH of 7.4 may show considerable activity, but this result may not be clinically valid. The purulent fluid at the infection site may have a much lower pH, and aminoglycoside activity decreases with decreasing pH.

The disk diffusion method has been standardized by the National Committee for Clinical Laboratory Standards (NCCLS)[1] for in vitro susceptibility testing. Commercially available paper disks containing specific amounts of antimicrobial agents are placed on Mueller-Hinton agar plates that contain a standard bacterial inoculum. A zone of inhibition of bacterial growth develops around each active antibiotic after overnight incubation. The size of the zone determines the organism's susceptibility or resistance; prior studies have correlated zone sizes with MICs obtained through dilution tests. Arbitrary zone-size break points for susceptibility have been established by clinical and laboratory investigators on the basis of such additional factors as achievable serum levels, degree of protein binding, and toxicity. Worldwide, the standardized disk test is probably the most frequently used method for in vitro susceptibility testing, and results should be comparable from laboratory to laboratory. The organism must fall into one of three categories: susceptible, intermediate, or resistant.

The broth dilution method exposes an inoculum of bacteria to various concentrations of an antimicrobial agent during incubation. The MIC of an agent that inhibits growth can be determined, and this value can be correlated with blood, urine, or other body fluid levels of the antimicrobial agent. Moreover, those tubes that show inhibition of growth can be subcultured to an antimicrobial-free medium, and the minimal bactericidal concentration (MBC) can be determined. Unfortunately, this test is not well standardized at present, and its reproducibility is poor when it is subjected to intralaboratory and interlaboratory comparisons.[2]

The agar dilution method works in much the same way as the broth dilution method, except that it employs agar plates that contain various dilutions of antimicrobial agents, and as many as 36 organisms can be efficiently inoculated on each plate by means of a replicator device. The minimal inhibitory concentration is determined by reading inhibition of colony growth on the agar surface. Agar dilution has the advantage of producing MIC data efficiently in a laboratory that performs large numbers of tests daily.

In the serum bactericidal test (SBT), samples of the serum of the treated patient are obtained and incubated with the infecting organism in doubling dilutions with broth to determine the highest dilution that is bactericidal. (Not all antimicrobial agents exhibit bactericidal activity: some exhibit only bacteriostatic activity [see Table 3].) The drawing of serum specimens can be timed to coincide with anticipated peak and trough antimicrobial levels. In effect, this test indirectly assesses both the susceptibility of the organism and the serum concentration of the antimicrobial agent, as well as the interactions between serum and organism and serum and drug. The NCCLS has developed proposed guidelines for the SBT.[3] A comprehensive review of the technical and clinical considerations associated with the SBT has been provided.[4]

Antibiotic Therapy for Infections in Surgical Patients

The antimicrobial agents of choice for various infections (e.g., community-acquired pneumonia[5-8]) in adults are well established [see Table 4], as are their dosages in patients with normal renal function [see Table 5]. No attempt will be made to review all of that material in this discussion. Excellent reviews and practice guidelines have been published.[9,10]

Discussion

Penicillins

Although the original penicillins are still useful against specific bacteria, there are some infections in which both they and the penicillinase-resistant semisynthetic penicillins are ineffective because of the emergence of penicillinase-producing staphylococci and methicillin-resistant staphylococci. The penicillins can be classified by structure [see Figure 1], β-lactamase susceptibility, and spectrum of action. They have a number of adverse effects [see Table 6].

The action of the penicillins depends on the presence of a bacterial cell wall containing peptidoglycans that are accessible to the agent. In actively growing bacteria, interference with biosynthesis of the peptidoglycan structure—specifically, of

Table 1 In Vivo Drug Interactions Involving Antimicrobials[203,204]

Antimicrobial Agent	Interacting Drug	Adverse Effect	Proposed Mechanism
Aminoglycosides	Amphotericin B	↑ Nephrotoxicity	Synergism
	Ascorbic acid	↓ Antibacterial effect in urinary tract	Urinary acidification
	Bumetanide	↑ Ototoxicity	Additive actions
	Carbenicillin, ticarcillin	↓ Aminoglycoside effect	Inactivation of aminoglycosides by the penicillin at high concentrations
	Cephalosporins	↑ Nephrotoxicity	?
	Cisplatin	↑ Nephrotoxicity	?
	Curarelike drugs	↑ Neuromuscular blockade	Additive actions
	Cyclosporine	↑ Nephrotoxicity	Additive actions (monitoring of levels recommended)
	Digoxin	Probable ↓ digoxin effect with neomycin or gentamicin	↓ Absorption
	Ethacrynic acid	↑ Ototoxicity	Additive actions
	Furosemide	↑ Nephrotoxicity, ↑ ototoxicity	Additive actions
	Magnesium sulfate	Possible ↑ neuromuscular blockade	Additive actions
	Methotrexate	Possible ↑ methotrexate toxicity with kanamycin	?
		↓ Methotrexate effect with oral aminoglycosides	↓ Absorption
	Neuromuscular blocking agents	↑ Apnea, respiratory paralysis	?
	Nonsteroidal anti-inflammatory drugs	↑ Nephrotoxicity	Additive actions
	Polymyxins	↑ Nephrotoxicity, neuromuscular blockade	Additive actions
	Radiographic contrast agents	↑ Nephrotoxicity	Additive actions
Cephalosporins	Alcohol	Disulfiram-like effect with cefamandole, cefoperazone, and moxalactam	Probable inhibition of intermediary metabolism of alcohol
	Aminoglycosides	↑ Nephrotoxicity	?
	Oral anticoagulants	Possible ↑ anticoagulant effect with moxalactam, cefotetan, cefmetazole	?
	Aspirin, heparin	Possible ↑ risk of bleeding with moxalactam, cefotetan, cefmetazole	Additive actions
	Ethacrynic acid	↑ Nephrotoxicity	?
	Furosemide	↑ Nephrotoxicity	?
	Penicillins	Possible ↑ cefotaxime toxicity with azlocillin in azotemic patients	↓ Excretion
Chloramphenicol	Acetaminophen	Possible ↑ chloramphenicol toxicity	↓ Metabolism
	Oral anticoagulants	↑ Anticoagulant effect	Inhibition of microsomal enzymes
	Barbiturates	↑ Barbiturate effect	↓ Metabolism
		↓ Chloramphenicol effect	↑ Metabolism
	Cimetidine	Possible aplastic anemia (single case report)	?
	Etomidate	Prolonged anesthesia	↓ Metabolism
	Oral hypoglycemic agents	↑ Sulfonylurea-induced hypoglycemia	?
	Phenytoin	Possible ↑ chloramphenicol toxicity	?
		↑ Phenytoin toxicity	↓ Metabolism
Clindamycin	Neuromuscular blocking agents	↑ Neuromuscular blockade	Additive actions
	Theophylline	↓ Clindamycin levels, apnea, seizures	?
Erythromycin	Oral anticoagulants	↑ Anticoagulant effect	Possible ↓ metabolism
	Carbamazepine	↑ Carbamazepine toxicity	↓ Metabolism
	Corticosteroids	↑ Methylprednisolone effect and possible toxicity	↓ Excretion
	Cyclosporine	↑ Cyclosporine level	↓ Excretion
	Digoxin	↑ Digoxin effect	↑ Absorption
	Theophyllines	↑ Theophylline effect and toxicity	↓ Metabolism
Imipenem	Cyclosporine	↑ Cyclosporine levels, ↑ CNS effect	?
	Ganciclovir	↑ Seizures	?
Metronidazole	Alcohol	Nausea, cramps, headache, flushing	Possible inhibition of intermediary metabolism of alcohol
	Oral anticoagulants	↑ Anticoagulant effect	Inhibition of microsomal enzymes
	Cimetidine	Possible ↑ metronidazole toxicity	↓ Metabolism
	Ciprofloxacin	↑ Seizures	?
	Disulfiram	Organic brain syndrome	?
	Phenobarbital	↓ Phenobarbital clearance	?

(continued)

Table 1 (continued)

Antimicrobial Agent	Interacting Drug	Adverse Effect	Proposed Mechanism
Penicillins	Beta-adrenergic blockers	Possible ↓ atenolol effect with ampicillin	↓ Absorption
	Allopurinol	↑ Incidence of rashes with ampicillin	?
	Aminoglycosides	↓ Aminoglycoside effect with carbenicillin or ticarcillin at high concentrations	Aminoglycoside inactivation
	Oral anticoagulants	↓ Anticoagulant effect with nafcillin	↑ Metabolism
	Cephalosporins	Possible ↑ cefotaxime toxicity with azlocillin in azotemic patients	↓ Excretion
	Oral contraceptives	↓ Contraceptive effect with ampicillin	↓ Enterohepatic circulation of estrogen
	Lithium	Hypernatremia with ticarcillin	Large sodium load, ↓ renal excretion
	Methotrexate	Possible ↑ methotrexate toxicity	↓ Excretion
Polymyxins	Aminoglycosides	↑ Nephrotoxicity, ↑ neuromuscular blockade	Additive actions
	Neuromuscular blocking agents	↑ Neuromuscular blockade	Additive actions
Quinolones	Antacids	↓ Absorption of quinolones	Binding of aluminum and magnesium antacids to quinolones
	Oral anticoagulants	Possible ↑ anticoagulant effect	Possible alteration of hepatic metabolism; displacement from albumin binding site (warfarin)
	Caffeine	Exaggerated or prolonged effects of caffeine, ↑ half-life	?
	Cimetidine	↑ Quinolone levels	Competitive action
	Cyclosporine	Potentiation of cyclosporine nephrotoxicity	? (monitoring of levels recommended)
	Probenecid	↑ Quinolone levels	↓ Renal excretion
	Sucralfate	↑ Absorption of quinolones	pH changes
	Theophyllines	Possible ↑ theophylline levels, ↑ half-life	Possible alteration of hepatic metabolism
Sulfonamides	Oral anticoagulants	↑ Anticoagulant effect	Displacement from binding sites, decreased metabolism
	Cyclosporine	↓ Cyclosporine levels	?
	Digoxin	Possible ↓ digoxin effect with sulfasalazine	↓ Absorption
	Oral hypoglycemic agents	↑ Sulfonylurea-induced hypoglycemia	?
	Methotrexate	Possible ↑ methotrexate toxicity	Displacement from binding sites, ↓ renal clearance
	Phenytoin	↑ Phenytoin effect (except possibly with sulfisoxazole)	↓ Metabolism
	Monoamine oxidase inhibitors	Possible ↑ phenelzine toxicity	↓ Metabolism
	Pyrimethamine	↑ Hypersensitivity reaction, including fatalities, with sulfadoxine	?
	Thiopental sodium	↑ Thiopental sodium effect	↓ Albumin binding
Tetracyclines	Antacids	↓ Tetracycline effect	↓ Absorption
	Oral anticoagulants	↑ Anticoagulant effect	?
	Barbiturates	↓ Doxycycline effect	Induction of microsomal enzymes
	Bismuth subsalicylate	↓ Tetracycline effect	↓ Absorption
	Carbamazepine	↓ Doxycycline effect	Induction of microsomal enzymes
	Oral contraceptives	↓ Contraceptive effect	Possible ↓ enterohepatic circulation of estrogen
	Digoxin	↑ Digoxin effect	↑ Absorption
	Insulin	↑ Insulin effect	?
	Oral iron salts	↓ Tetracycline and iron effects	↓ Absorption of tetracycline and iron
	Lithium	↑ Lithium toxicity	↓ Renal excretion
	Phenytoin	↓ Doxycycline effect	Induction of microsomal enzymes
	Zinc sulfate	↓ Tetracycline effect	↓ Absorption
Trimethoprim	Amiloride, thiazides	Hyponatremia	Additive actions
	Oral anticoagulants	↑ Anticoagulant effect	↓ Metabolism
	Cyclosporine	↑ Nephrotoxicity	Synergism
	Mercaptopurine	↓ Antileukemic effect	?
	Digoxin	Possible ↑ effect	↓ Renal excretion
Trimethoprim-sulfamethoxazole	Oral anticoagulants	↑ Anticoagulant effect	↓ Metabolism

the cross-linkages between the peptide chains—prevents the bacterium from developing its normal structural firmness, and this lack of firmness leads to lysis. Enzymes located beneath the cell wall (transpeptidases and carboxypeptidases) are involved in synthesis of the cell wall. These penicillin-binding proteins are the sites at which β-lactam drugs bind.[11]

NATURAL PENICILLINS

Aqueous Crystalline Penicillin G

Aqueous crystalline penicillin G is used when a high serum concentration of the agent is required.[12] Its half-life is normally 30 minutes but may be as long as 10 hours in patients with

Table 2 Antibiotics in Pregnancy[203]

Drug	Major Toxic Potential		Pharmacology	
	Maternal	Fetal	Maternal Serum Levels	Excreted in Mother's Milk
Considered safe				
Cephalosporins	Allergies	None known	Decreased	Trace
Erythromycin base	Allergies, GI intolerance	None known	Decreased	Yes
Penicillins	Allergies	None known	Decreased	Trace
Use with caution				
Aminoglycosides	Ototoxicity, nephrotoxicity	Ototoxicity	Decreased	Yes
Clindamycin	Allergies, colitis	None known	Unchanged	Trace
Sulfonamides (contraindicated at term)	Allergies, crystalluria	Kernicterus (at term), hemolysis (G6PD deficiency)	Unchanged	Yes
Avoid if possible				
Metronidazole	Hypersensitivity, alcohol intolerance, neuropathy	None known (teratogenic in animals)	Probably unchanged	Yes
Contraindicated				
Chloramphenicol	Blood dyscrasias	Gray syndrome	Unchanged	Yes
Erythromycin estolate	Hepatotoxicity	None known	Decreased	Yes
Nalidixic acid	GI intolerance	Increased intracranial pressure	?	?
Nitrofurantoin	Allergies, neuropathy, GI intolerance	Hemolysis (G6PD deficiency)	Decreased	Trace
Norfloxacin	GI intolerance	Arthropathies in immature animals	?	?
Tetracyclines	Hepatotoxicity, renal failure	Tooth discoloration and dysplasia, impaired bone growth	Probably unchanged	Yes
Trimethoprim	Hypersensitivity	Teratogenicity	Unchanged	Yes

anuria. Approximately 50% of penicillin G is bound to plasma proteins. Penicillin G sodium contains approximately 2 mEq of sodium in each one million units. Therefore, the potassium salt of penicillin G should be used except in patients with renal insufficiency, who may not be able to tolerate the 1.7 mEq of potassium contained in each one million units. This agent is destroyed by gastric acid when given orally.

Penicillin G Benzathine

Penicillin G benzathine, 1.2 to 2.4 million units I.M., is used in the definitive management of certain infections, such as streptococcal sore throat, and as prophylaxis for several conditions, such as rheumatic fever, in which reinfection by β-hemolytic streptococci is a constant threat.

Penicillin G Procaine

Penicillin G procaine is used intramuscularly when a long-acting preparation is preferred and high blood levels are not required. It is indicated for treatment of pneumococcal pneumonia, uncomplicated cases of which are adequately treated by administration of one or two daily doses of 300,000 units, and for treatment of acute genitourinary gonorrhea, for which a dose of 4.8 million units is divided and injected at two sites and 1 g of probenecid is given orally before the injection.

Penicillin V

Because phenoxymethyl penicillin, or penicillin V, is resistant to gastric acid, it leads to higher serum concentrations when given orally than penicillin G does at similar doses. Penicillin V should not be substituted for parenterally administered penicillin G when such therapy is needed, but it can be given orally to treat mild infections of the throat, the respiratory tract, or soft tissue, in doses of 125 to 500 mg given four to six times daily.

PENICILLINASE-RESISTANT PENICILLINS

The semisynthetic penicillinase-resistant penicillins available for parenteral use are methicillin, oxacillin, and nafcillin; those available for oral use are oxacillin, nafcillin, cloxacillin, and dicloxacillin.

Methicillin

Methicillin is the least protein bound of this group (39%); nafcillin (90%), oxacillin (94%), cloxacillin (95%), and dicloxacillin (98%) all have higher rates of protein binding. Methicillin was the first of the semisynthetic penicillinase-resistant penicillins.[13] It must be administered parenterally and is usually given every 4 to 6 hours in a total daily dose of 100 to 300 mg/kg body weight.

Oxacillin and Nafcillin

Oxacillin seems to be as effective as methicillin against staphylococcal infections, and it causes interstitial nephritis less often. For

Table 3 Bactericidal and Bacteriostatic Agents[203]

Bactericidal Agents	Bacteriostatic Agents
Aminoglycosides*	Chloramphenicol
Aztreonam	Clindamycin
Bacitracin	Erythromycin
Cephalosporins	Sulfonamides
Imipenem	Tetracyclines
Penicillins	Trimethoprim
Polymyxins†	
Quinolones‡	
Vancomycin	

*Including streptomycin, neomycin, kanamycin, gentamicin, tobramycin, amikacin, and netilmicin.
†Including polymyxin B and colistimethate.
‡Including norfloxacin and ciprofloxacin.

parenteral use, oxacillin or nafcillin can be given in dosages of 100 to 300 mg/kg/day for children and up to 4 to 12 g/day for adults.

Cloxacillin and Dicloxacillin

One of the penicillinase-resistant penicillins or cefazolin (a first-generation cephalosporin) should be used as initial therapy for all cases of gram-positive coccal infections before identification and susceptibility testing. If laboratory data indicate that non–penicillinase-producing staphylococci (i.e., staphylococci that are susceptible to penicillin G) are the causative infectious agents, penicillin G is the agent of choice because it is more active against such organisms (i.e., it has a lower MIC), is less toxic, and costs less. If penicillinase-producing organisms are identified or suspected and oral therapy is desired, cloxacillin or dicloxacillin, 1 to 2 g/day, can be given.

AMINOPENICILLINS

Ampicillin

Ampicillin is active against a variety of bacteria, including many strains of *Escherichia coli*, *Proteus mirabilis*, *Salmonella*, *Shigella*, *Listeria*, and *Hemophilus influenzae*. Most strains of *Klebsiella* and all strains of *Pseudomonas aeruginosa* are resistant. The antienterococcal effect of ampicillin may be synergistically enhanced by concurrent administration of an aminoglycoside, which results in bactericidal activity.

Because it is stable in gastric juices, ampicillin is suitable for oral as well as parenteral use. When it is given orally, peak serum levels are reached in about 2 hours, but they seldom exceed 0.3 μg/ml. When it is given intramuscularly, peak serum levels are achieved in 1 hour, and they are both higher and more prolonged than the peak levels achieved after oral administration. About 10% of ampicillin is bound to plasma proteins. The recommended daily dose is 1 to 4 g; parenteral administration of up to 12 g/day is recommended for major systemic infections.

Amoxicillin

Amoxicillin is closely related to ampicillin, both in chemical structure and in spectrum of antibacterial activity.[14] Amoxicillin, however, is more completely absorbed than ampicillin is: approximately 70% of a dose of amoxicillin is absorbed, compared with approximately 50% of a dose of ampicillin. Consequently, the blood levels attainable with a given dose of amoxicillin are usually about twice those attainable with a comparable dose of ampicillin. Amoxicillin is at least as effective as ampicillin in the treatment of respiratory disorders that are caused by susceptible bacteria, including otitis media, sinusitis, and bronchitis.

CARBOXYPENICILLINS

Carbenicillin

Carbenicillin has an antibacterial range similar to that of ampicillin, with the added benefit of activity against certain strains of *P. aeruginosa*,[15] indole-positive *Proteus* species, and *Enterobacter* species.[16] Because carbenicillin is inactivated by penicillinase, penicillinase-producing *Staphylococcus aureus* is resistant to it. *Klebsiella* species are resistant to carbenicillin, as are many *Serratia* organisms. Carbenicillin is bactericidal and is recoverable from blood, urine, lymph, cerebrospinal fluid, and most body tissues. About 50% of the drug is bound to serum proteins.[17] For most gram-negative bacteremias, the MIC for carbenicillin is between 10 and 25 μg/ml; for *P. aeruginosa*, it is between 25 and 100 μg/ml.

Carbenicillin has been used to treat severe infections caused by *P. aeruginosa*, *Proteus* species, and other gram-negative bacteria that are susceptible to it. For systemic and soft tissue infections caused by *P. aeruginosa*, the dosage should be 400 to 500 mg/kg/day by continuous intravenous drip or in divided doses every 4 hours. The dosage should be reduced in patients with renal failure,[18] and close surveillance must be maintained for signs of bleeding. Currently, carbenicillin is used less often than it once was; it has been largely supplanted by ticarcillin and by the ureidopenicillins.

Ticarcillin

The antibacterial spectrum of ticarcillin is similar to that of carbenicillin; however, it is two to four times more active against *P. aeruginosa*. It is frequently preferred to carbenicillin in the treatment of serious gram-negative infections because of its greater potency and the lower incidence of adverse effects.[19] The primary use of ticarcillin is in the treatment of proven or suspected *Pseudomonas* infections. The recommended dosage is 16 to 24 g/day.

UREIDOPENICILLINS

Mezlocillin, Azlocillin, and Piperacillin

Mezlocillin, azlocillin, and piperacillin are semisynthetic penicillins derived from the ampicillin molecule with side-chain adaptations. The side chains of mezlocillin and azlocillin are acyl derivatives of a urea molecule—hence the term ureidopenicillins. The ureidopenicillins are generally bactericidal and act primarily by inhibiting cell wall synthesis in dividing bacteria. Pharmacokinetic studies show them to follow a first-order, two-compartment model. In comparison with the carboxypenicillins carbenicillin and ticarcillin, the ureidopenicillins exhibit less pronounced plasma protein binding, a shorter serum half-life, and a greater volume of distribution.[20-22] They are minimally metabolized (10%) and are primarily excreted in an active form by glomerular filtration and tubular secretion. Unlike carbenicillin and ticarcillin, the ureidopenicillins achieve high concentrations in bile because of increased biliary excretion.

In vitro, the ureidopenicillins are active against streptococci, enterococci, most Enterobacteriaceae, *Pseudomonas*, β-lactamase–negative staphylococci, *Neisseria*, and *Hemophilus*.[23-25] β-Lactamase–producing staphylococci and *H. influenzae* are resistant. The major advantage the ureidopenicillins have over other penicillins in clinical use is their increased activity against *P. aeruginosa* and *Klebsiella*.

The recommended dosages of the ureidopenicillins are 6 to 16 g/day for mild to moderate infections and 18 to 24 g/day for severe to life-threatening infections. Small doses may be given intramuscularly, but large doses must be given intravenously. The dosing interval is usually 4 to 6 hours.

An observed property of the ureidopenicillins that has given rise to some concern is their loss of activity as inoculum size increases; this is known as the inoculum effect. When the bacterial concentration is increased from 10^3 to 10^7 colony-forming units/ml, the MIC and the MBC increase substantially.[26,27] The inoculum effect has been consistently noted not only with *P. aeruginosa* but also with some strains of *E. coli*, *Klebsiella*, *Enterobacter*, and *Morganella*.

Monotherapy with mezlocillin or piperacillin has been efficacious in patients with pneumonia, bacteremia, osteomyelitis,

Table 4 Antimicrobial Drugs of Choice for Various Infections in Adults[203]

	Causative Organism	Drug of Choice	Alternative Drugs
Gram-Positive Cocci	*Staphylococcus aureus*		
	Methicillin-resistant[1]	Vancomycin,[2] with or without rifampin or gentamicin	Trimethoprim-sulfamethoxazole (TMP-SMX)[2] with or without rifampin,[2] a fluoroquinolone,[3] minocycline[4]
	Non–penicillinase-producing (uncommon)	Penicillin G[5] or penicillin V	A cephalosporin,[6] vancomycin,[7] clindamycin, imipenem, a fluoroquinolone[3]
	Penicillinase-producing (common)	Penicillinase-resistant penicillin[8]	A cephalosporin,[6] clindamycin, vancomycin,[7] imipenem,[9] ticarcillin-clavulanate, ampicillin-sulbactam, amoxicillin-clavulanate, piperacillin-tazobactam, a fluoroquinolone[3]
	S. epidermidis[10]	Vancomycin,[7] with or without rifampin[2] or gentamicin	A cephalosporin, a penicillinase-resistant penicillin, imipenem,[9] a fluoroquinolone[3]
	Anaerobic streptococcus (*Peptostreptococcus*)	Penicillin G[5]	Clindamycin, a cephalosporin,[6] vancomycin[7]
	Streptococcus bovis	Penicillin G[5,11]	A cephalosporin,[6] vancomycin[7]
	Enterococcus		
	Endocarditis or other serious infection	Penicillin or ampicillin, plus gentamicin[12] or streptomycin	Vancomycin,[7] with gentamicin or streptomycin; ampicillin-sulbactam with gentamicin or streptomycin, teicoplanin,[13] quinupristin/dalfopristin[14]
	Uncomplicated urinary tract infection	Ampicillin (or amoxicillin) or penicillin G	A fluoroquinolone[3] or nitrofurantoin[15]
	Groups A, G, and C streptococci	Penicillin G[5,16] or penicillin V	A cephalosporin,[6] vancomycin,[7] an erythromycin,[17] clindamycin, clarithromycin, azithromycin
	Group B streptococcus	Penicillin G[5,16] or ampicillin	A cephalosporin,[6] vancomycin,[7] an erythromycin
	S. pneumoniae (pneumococcus)	Penicillin G[5,16] or penicillin V	An erythromycin,[16,17] a cephalosporin,[6] chloramphenicol,[7,16] vancomycin[7,16] with or without rifampin, TMP-SMX, azithromycin, clarithromycin
	Viridans streptococcus	Penicillin G,[5,11] with or without gentamicin	A cephalosporin,[6] vancomycin[7]
Gram-Positive Bacilli	*Bacillus cereus, B. subtilis*	Vancomycin	Imipenem,[9] clindamycin
	B. anthracis	Penicillin G	A tetracycline, an erythromycin[2]
	Clostridium difficile	Vancomycin[18] or metronidazole[18]	Bacitracin
	C. perfringens	Penicillin G	Clindamycin, metronidazole, a tetracycline,[4] imipenem,[9] chloramphenicol[7]
	C. tetani	Penicillin G	A tetracycline[4]
	Corynebacterium diphtheriae	An erythromycin	Penicillin G
	Corynebacterium, JK group	Vancomycin	Penicillin G with gentamicin, an erythromycin
	Listeria monocytogenes	Ampicillin with or without gentamicin	TMP-SMX
	Propionibacterium	Penicillin G	Clindamycin, an erythromycin
Gram-Negative Cocci	*Moraxella* (formerly *Branhamella*) *catarrhalis*	TMP-SMX	Amoxicillin-clavulanate, an erythromycin, a tetracycline, cefuroxime, third-generation cephalosporins, clarithromycin, azithromycin, a fluoroquinolone[3]
	Neisseria gonorrhoeae[19]	Ceftriaxone[6]	Ampicillin or penicillin, spectinomycin,[20] cefotaxime,[5] a fluoroquinolone[3]
	N. meningitidis		
	Meningitis, bacteremia	Penicillin G	A third-generation cephalosporin,[6] TMP-SMX, chloramphenicol[7]
	Carrier state	Rifampin	Minocycline, ciprofloxacin
Enteric Gram-Negative Bacilli	*Bacteroides*		
	GI tract strains (*B. fragilis*)	Metronidazole	Clindamycin, cefoxitin, cefotetan, ceftizoxime, or cefmetazole; chloramphenicol[21]; imipenem[9]; ticarcillin–clavulanate; ampicillin-sulbactam, piperacillin-tazobactam
	Respiratory tract strains	Penicillin G or clindamycin	Cefoxitin,[6] cefotetan, metronidazole, chloramphenicol[7]
	Campylobacter fetus	Imipenem[9]	Gentamicin
	C. jejuni	A fluoroquinolone,[3] an erythromycin	A tetracycline,[4] gentamicin[7]
	Citrobacter	Gentamicin, a third-generation cephalosporin[6]	A fluoroquinolone,[3] imipenem,[9] tobramycin, chloramphenicol,[7] amikacin
	Enterobacter	Imipenem[9]	A third-generation cephalosporin[6]; for serious infections, use with ciprofloxacin or gentamicin; gentamicin, tobramycin, amikacin, a fluoroquinolone,[3] a carboxypenicillin or acylaminopenicillin,[22] aztreonam,[23] TMP-SMX, chloramphenicol[7]
	Escherichia coli[24]	Ampicillin, a cephalosporin,[6] a fluoroquinolone,[3] TMP-SMX[26]	Gentamicin,[25] tobramycin, amikacin, imipenem,[9] aztreonam,[23] chloramphenicol[7]
	Helicobacter pylori	Tetracycline with metronidazole and bismuth subsalicylate	Amoxicillin with metronidazole and bismuth subsalicylate; tetracycline with clarithromycin and bismuth subsalicylate; clarithromycin with omeprazole
	Klebsiella[24]	A cephalosporin[6]	Imipenem,[9] gentamicin,[25] tobramycin, amikacin, chloramphenicol,[7] TMP-SMX,[26] a carboxypenicillin or acylaminopenicillin,[22] amoxicillin-clavulanate, ampicillin-sulbactam, ticarcillin-clavulanate, piperacillin-tazobactam, aztreonam,[23] a fluoroquinolone[3]
	Proteus		
	mirabilis[24]	Ampicillin	A cephalosporin, gentamicin or tobramycin, chloramphenicol,[7] a carboxypenicillin or acylaminopenicillin,[22] imipenem,[9] TMP-SMX, aztreonam,[23] a fluoroquinolone[3]
	non-*mirabilis*,[24] including *P. vulgaris, Morganella morganii,* and *Providencia rettgeri*	A second- or third-generation cephalosporin[6]	Gentamicin, tobramycin, amikacin, a carboxypenicillin or acylaminopenicillin,[22] chloramphenicol,[7] imipenem,[9] aztreonam,[23] ampicillin-sulbactam, ticarcillin-clavulanate, piperacillin-tazobactam, amoxicillin-clavulanate, a fluoroquinolone[3]

Note: all superscript numbers refer to footnotes that follow table.

(continued)

Table 4 (continued)

	Causative Organism	Drug of Choice	Alternative Drugs
Enteric Gram-Negative Bacilli (continued)	*Providencia stuartii*	A second- or third-generation cephalosporin	An aminoglycoside, TMP-SMX,[26] imipenem,[9] aztreonam,[23] a carboxypenicillin or acylaminopenicillin,[22] a fluoroquinolone[3]
	Salmonella typhi	Ceftriaxone or a fluoroquinolone[3]	Chloramphenicol or ampicillin,[27] TMP-SMX
	Other *Salmonella* species	Ceftriaxone or cefotaxime or a fluoroquinolone[3]	Ampicillin or amoxicillin, TMP-SMX, chloramphenicol[7]
	Serratia	A third-generation cephalosporin	Gentamicin or amikacin, a carboxypenicillin or acylaminopenicillin,[22] chloramphenicol,[7] imipenem,[9] aztreonam, a fluoroquinolone[3]
	Shigella	A fluoroquinolone[3]	TMP-SMX, ampicillin, ceftriaxone, cefixime
Other Gram-Negative Bacilli	*Acinetobacter* (*Herellea*)	Imipenem[9]	Tobramycin, gentamicin, amikacin, doxycycline, minocycline, a carboxypenicillin or acylaminopenicillin,[22] TMP-SMX, a fluoroquinolone,[3] ceftazidime
	Aeromonas hydrophilia	TMP-SMX[2]	A fluoroquinolone,[3] gentamicin, tobramycin, imipenem[9]
	Bartonella henselae (cat-scratch disease)	Ciprofloxacin[3]	TMP-SMX, gentamicin; rifampin
	(bacillary angiomatosis)	An erythromycin	Doxycycline
	Brucella	A tetracycline, with gentamicin or streptomycin	Rifampin[2] with a tetracycline, chloramphenicol[7] with or without streptomycin, TMP-SMX[2] with or without gentamicin, a fluoroquinolone
	Eikenella corrodens	Ampicillin	An erythromycin, a tetracycline,[4] amoxicillin-clavulanate, ampicillin-sulbactam, ceftriaxone
	Francisella tularensis (tularemia)	Streptomycin	Gentamicin, a tetracycline,[4] chloramphenicol[7]
	Fusobacterium	Penicillin	Clindamycin, metronidazole, chloramphenicol,[7] cefoxitin
	Gardnerella (formerly *Hemophilus*) *vaginalis*	Metronidazole[2] (oral)	Intravaginal or oral clindamycin
	Hemophilus influenzae Bronchitis, otitis media	TMP-SMX	Ampicillin or amoxicillin; a tetracycline;[4] a sulfonamide with or without erythromycin; amoxicillin-clavulanate, cefuroxime axetil, ceftizoxime, clarithromycin, azithromycin, a fluoroquinolone,[3] cefamandole, cefprozil
	Meningitis, epiglottitis, life-threatening infections	Cefotaxime or ceftriaxone	Chloramphenicol[28]
	Legionella pneumophila (Legionnaires' disease)	Erythromycin	Rifampin,[29] TMP-SMX,[2] clarithromycin, a fluoroquinolone,[3] azithromycin
	L. micdadei	Erythromycin	Rifampin,[2] TMP-SMX[2]
	Pasteurella multocida	Penicillin G	A tetracycline,[4] a cephalosporin,[6] amoxicillin-clavulanate, ampicillin-sulbactam
	Calymmatobacterium granulomatis (granuloma inguinale)	A tetracycline[4]	Streptomycin, TMP-SMX, an erythromycin
	H. ducreyi (chancroid)	Ceftriaxone or erythromycin or azithromycin	A fluoroquinolone
	Pseudomonas aeruginosa Urinary tract infections	A fluoroquinolone[3]	Gentamicin or tobramycin; amikacin; ceftazidime[6] with or without gentamicin or tobramycin; imipenem[9]; aztreonam[23]; a carboxypenicillin or acylaminopenicillin[22]
	Other infections	Gentamicin or tobramycin with or without a carboxypenicillin or acylaminopenicillin,[22] ceftazidime, imipenem,[9] aztreonam[23] with or without gentamicin or tobramycin	Amikacin with or without a carboxypenicillin or acylaminopenicillin,[22] ciprofloxacin[7]
	P. cepacia	TMP-SMX	Chloramphenicol,[7] ceftazidime,[2] imipenem[2,9]
	Streptobacillus moniliformis (rat-bite fever)	Penicillin G	A tetracycline,[4] streptomycin
	Vibrio cholerae	A tetracycline[4]	TMP-SMX, a fluoroquinolone[3]
	V. vulnificus	A tetracycline[4]	Cefotaxime
	Agents of Vincent's stomatitis (trench mouth)	Penicillin G	A tetracycline,[4] an erythromycin
	Xanthomonas (formerly *Pseudomonas*) *maltophilia*	TMP-SMX	Minocycline, ceftazidime,[6] a fluoroquinolone[3]
	Yersinia enterocolitica	TMP-SMX[2]	A fluoroquinolone, gentamicin,[2] tobramycin,[2] amikacin, cefotaxime[2,6] or ceftizoxime[2,6]
	Y. pestis (plague)	Streptomycin	A tetracycline,[4] chloramphenicol,[7] gentamicin[2]
Acid-Fast Bacilli	*Mycobacterium avium* complex	Clarithromycin or azithromycin plus one or more of the following: ethambutol, rifabutin, ciprofloxacin, rifampin, clofazimine, amikacin	—
	M. fortuitum	Amikacin,[2] doxycycline,[2] or both	Rifampin,[2] cefoxitin, a sulfonamide
	M. kansasii	Isoniazid with rifampin, with or without ethambutol or streptomycin	Cycloserine, ethionamide, clarithromycin
	M. leprae	Dapsone[7] with rifampin, with or without clofazimine	Minocycline,[4] ofloxacin,[3] clarithromycin
	M. marinum (*balnei*)[30]	Minocycline	TMP-SMX, rifampin, ethambutol, clarithromycin, doxycycline
	M. tuberculosis[31]	Isoniazid with rifampin, and pyrazinamide with or without ethambutol or streptomycin	Ciprofloxacin or ofloxacin; third-line agent [see Subsection VIII]

Note: all superscript numbers refer to footnotes that follow table.

(continued)

Table 4 (continued)

	Causative Organism	Drug of Choice	Alternative Drugs
Actinomyces	Actinomyces israelii	Penicillin G	A tetracycline,[4] an erythromycin, clindamycin
	Nocardia	TMP-SMX	Minocycline, sulfisoxazole, imipenem,[9] amikacin,[2] cycloserine
Fungi	Aspergillus	Amphotericin B[7]	Itraconazole
	Blastomyces dermatitidis	Amphotericin B[7] or itraconazole	Ketoconazole
	Candida	Amphotericin B[7,32] or fluconazole	Ketoconazole, itraconazole, flucytosine,[33] nystatin (oral or topical), miconazole (topical),[34] clotrimazole (topical)
	Coccidioides immitis	Amphotericin B[7] or fluconazole	Ketoconazole, itraconazole
	Cryptococcus neoformans	Amphotericin B[7] with or without flucytosine[35]	Fluconazole, itraconazole
	Histoplasma capsulatum	Amphotericin B or itraconazole	Ketoconazole
	Phycomycetes (e.g., Mucor)	Amphotericin B	No dependable alternative
	Sporothrix schenckii (sporotrichosis)	Amphotericin B[7] or itraconazole	Saturated solution of potassium iodide[36]
Chlamydia	Chlamydia psittaci (psittacosis)	A tetracycline[4]	Chloramphenicol[7]
	C. trachomatis		
	Inclusion conjunctivitis	An erythromycin (oral or I.V.)	A sulfonamide (topical plus oral)
	Lymphogranuloma venereum	A tetracycline[4]	An erythromycin
	Pneumonia	An erythromycin	A sulfonamide
	Trachoma	Azithromycin	A tetracycline[4] (topical plus oral), a sulfonamide (topical plus oral)
	Urethritis or pelvic inflammatory disease	Doxycycline or azithromycin	Erythromycin, ofloxacin, sulfisoxazole, amoxicillin
	C. pneumoniae	An erythromycin or clarithromycin, a tetracycline	—
Mycoplasma	Mycoplasma pneumoniae	An erythromycin[37] or a tetracycline[4]	Clarithromycin, azithromycin
	Ureaplasma urealyticum	An erythromycin	A tetracycline,[4] clarithromycin
Rickettsia	Various rickettsial organisms Rocky Mountain spotted fever, epidemic and endemic (murine) typhus, rickettsial pox, Q fever, scrub typhus	A tetracycline[3]	Chloramphenicol,[7] a fluoroquinolone[3]
Spirochetes	Borrelia burgdorferi (Lyme disease)	Doxycycline or amoxicillin or ceftriaxone	Penicillin, an erythromycin, clarithromycin, azithromycin
	B. recurrentis (relapsing fever)	A tetracycline[4]	Penicillin G
	Leptospira	Penicillin G	A tetracycline,[4] an erythromycin
	Treponema pallidum	Penicillin G	A tetracycline,[4] an erythromycin, ceftriaxone
Viruses	Herpes simplex		
	Disseminated	Acyclovir	Vidarabine, foscarnet[2]
	Encephalitis	Acyclovir	Vidarabine
	Genital	Acyclovir	Vidarabine, foscarnet[2]
	Keratitis	Trifluridine (topical)	Idoxuridine (topical), vidarabine (topical)
	Neonatal	Acyclovir	Vidarabine
	HIV[38]	Therapeutic regimens are rapidly evolving	—
	Cytomegalovirus	Ganciclovir or foscarnet[2]	None
	Influenza A	Amantadine or rimantadine	No dependable alternative
	Respiratory syncytial virus	Ribavirin	None
	Varicella-zoster	Acyclovir	Foscarnet
	Hepatitis B or C	Interferon alfa-2b	None

1. Some strains of S. aureus and most strains of S. epidermidis are resistant to penicillinase-resistant penicillins; these strains are also resistant to cephalosporins.
2. Not approved for this indication by the FDA.
3. For most infections, ciprofloxacin or ofloxacin, either orally or I.V. For urinary tract infection, norfloxacin, lomafloxacin, or enoxacin can be used. None of these drugs is recommended for children.
4. Tetracycline is preferred for most uses. Doxycycline is the safest tetracycline for treatment of extrarenal infections in renal insufficiency. Tetracyclines should be avoided in pregnant women and in children younger than 8 yr.
5. Crystalline penicillin G is administered parenterally in serious infections. For less severe infections caused by pneumococci, group A streptococci, gonococci, or Treponema pallidum, procaine penicillin is administered I.M. once or twice daily. For mild infections caused by streptococci and pneumococci, oral penicillin V is preferable to oral penicillin G. Benzathine penicillin G is given I.M. (once monthly for the prophylaxis of rheumatic fever; a single injection for the treatment of group A streptococcal pharyngitis) when patient compliance for oral medication is questionable and for treatment of syphilis, in one to three doses at weekly intervals, depending on the stage of the disease.
6. Cephalosporins are sometimes used as alternatives to penicillin in patients with suspected penicillin allergy but not in patients with serious hypersensitivity (especially immediate anaphylactic or accelerated urticarial reactions). Patients allergic to penicillin may be hypersensitive to cephalosporins. Only third-generation cephalosporins are effective in bacterial meningitis.
7. In view of the occurrence of adverse reactions, this drug should be used only for serious infections and when less toxic drugs are ineffective.
8. For severe infections, I.V. nafcillin or oxacillin should be used. For mild infections, oral cloxacillin, dicloxacillin, or oxacillin may be employed. One to two percent of S. aureus strains are resistant to penicillinase-resistant penicillins (and usually to cephalosporins) but are susceptible to vancomycin. High doses of penicillin G, ampicillin, amoxicillin, carbenicillin, or ticarcillin do not overcome the clinical resistance of penicillinase-producing staphylococci to these drugs.
9. Imipenem is a β-lactam antibiotic that should be used with caution in patients who are allergic to penicillins and cephalosporins. Meropenem is a similar carbapenem.
10. In vitro sensitivity testing with cephalosporins or penicillins may be misleading because of heteroresistance and because these antibiotics may be bacteriostatic only. For serious infections, vancomycin is preferred (see text).
11. The combination of penicillin G with streptomycin for the first two weeks of treatment of endocarditis caused by viridans streptococci is preferred by some.
12. Various aminoglycosides have been used in synergistic combination with penicillin or vancomycin. Because of the appearance of enterococcal strains resistant to the synergistic action with streptomycin (but not gentamicin), gentamicin is preferred for use in the combination.
13. An investigational drug in the United States (Targocid—Hoechst Marion Roussel)
14. An investigational drug in the United States (Synercid—Rhône-Poulenc Rorer)
15. Contraindicated in pregnancy or in the presence of renal insufficiency.

(continued)

Table 4 (continued)

16. In patients with major allergy to penicillin, erythromycin is the alternative for respiratory tract infections; chloramphenicol is the preferred alternative for meningitis. Occasional strains of pneumococci have high-level resistance to penicillin and to most other antibiotics except vancomycin.
17. Some strains of pneumococci and group A streptococci are erythromycin resistant.
18. Antibiotics may be administered orally for antibiotic-associated pseudomembranous enterocolitis. Vancomycin has been the drug of choice, but metronidazole appears to be as effective and is much less expensive.
19. Large doses of penicillin G or ampicillin (or amoxicillin) may be required because some strains are resistant to these drugs. Penicillinase-producing gonococci, which are more resistant to penicillin, have appeared in the United States; spectinomycin is the treatment of choice for infections with such strains.
20. Rare strains of gonococci are resistant to spectinomycin; use cefoxitin, cefuroxime, cefotaxime, or TMP-SMX to treat these strains.
21. In CNS infection, metronidazole or chloramphenicol should be used.
22. The carboxypenicillins are carbenicillin and ticarcillin; the acylaminopenicillins are mezlocillin, azlocillin, and piperacillin. When one of these drugs is used for a severe infection, an aminoglycoside is often recommended as well.
23. Aztreonam is a β-lactam antibiotic; cross-sensitivity has not occurred, but use with caution in patients allergic to penicillins, cephalosporins, or imipenem.
24. An oral sulfonamide such as sulfisoxazole is often the initial therapy for an acute uncomplicated urinary tract infection, before the results of culture and susceptibility testing have been obtained. Alternatives include oral ampicillin or amoxicillin. Should the causative agent be a *Klebsiella* organism, an oral cephalosporin can be used; should it be a non-*mirabilis* *Proteus* organism, carbenicillin indanyl can be employed.
25. In severely ill patients, an aminoglycoside is combined with a cephalosporin.
26. Principally in treatment of uncomplicated urinary tract infections.
27. Ampicillin or amoxicillin may be effective in milder cases.
28. Some encapsulated *H. influenzae* (type b) strains and some unencapsulated strains are resistant to ampicillin, and rare strains are resistant to chloramphenicol. Chloramphenicol plus ampicillin (or chloramphenicol alone) should be used for initial treatment of meningitis or epiglottitis in children until the organism is identified and its susceptibility is determined. In adults with meningitis of unknown etiology and an indeterminate Gram's stain and in whom *H. influenzae* is suspected, chloramphenicol is added to ampicillin (or penicillin G) for the first 24 hours until the results of culture are available. Ampicillin is preferred when the infecting strain of *H. influenzae* is susceptible.
29. Not an FDA-approved use. Evidence for possible efficacy comes only from in vitro susceptibility testing and from treatment of infections in experimental animals. In both cases, *L. pneumophila* is highly susceptible to rifampin.
30. Most infections are self-limited without therapy.
31. Various combination treatments are available [*see Subsection VIII*].
32. I.V. amphotericin B is the drug of choice for systemic candidal infections. If in vitro synergism can be demonstrated with flucytosine, the combination may be indicated in therapy. For GI infections or oral thrush, oral nystatin may be adequate. Topical nystatin, miconazole, or clotrimazole is useful for skin or vaginal infections.
33. Some strains of *Candida* may be resistant to flucytosine, or resistance may develop during treatment. Bone marrow depression may be produced by flucytosine administration in the presence of renal insufficiency.
34. I.V. miconazole appears to have promise in treatment of coccidiodomycosis, particularly when amphotericin B has failed or cannot be tolerated. Its role in treatment of cryptococcal meningitis in patients who cannot tolerate amphotericin B is under study.
35. Combined therapy for cryptococcal meningitis with amphotericin B and flucytosine may provide more rapid sterilization of CSF. Combined therapy may decrease amphotericin B toxicity by allowing some dose reduction without loss in therapeutic effect.
36. For treatment of lymphocutaneous form only.
37. Erythromycin and tetracycline have been equally effective in the treatment of mycoplasmal pneumonia. Because of the initial clinical similarity between mycoplasmal pneumonia and some cases of Legionnaires' disease and because erythromycin is effective in both diseases, it is the drug of choice in patients presumed to have mycoplasmal pneumonia.
38. Guidelines for the treatment of HIV infections are evolving rapidly.

---

soft tissue infections, urinary tract infections, peritonitis, and pelvic infection.[28-31] These agents are usually well tolerated, but bacterial resistance may occur in 10% to 15% of patients. Their use has been limited by concerns about their increased sensitivity to β-lactamase, the inoculum effect, and their reduced bacteriolytic activity. To address the first concern, piperacillin has been given in combination with the β-lactamase inhibitor tazobactam [*see β-Lactamase Inhibitors, below*].

Cephalosporins

Cephalosporium acremonium was discovered in 1948. This fungus was found to produce cephalosporin C, from which cephalothin, the first cephalosporin to be introduced, was in turn derived. The basic cephalosporin structure consists of a dihydrothiazine ring fused to a β-lactam ring.

Various side chains have been substituted at the number 3 carbon position of the six-membered ring and at the acyl side chain of this basic cephalosporin nucleus. Changes at position 3 are thought to affect pharmacologic activity primarily. Several cephalosporins, including cefamandole, cefoperazone, moxalactam (not a true cephalosporin but a close relative with very similar characteristics), and ceftazidime, have a methyltetrazolethiol side chain at this position. This substitution results in effects similar to those of disulfiram: alcohol cannot be metabolized, and acetaldehyde accumulates in the blood, causing headache, nausea, flushing, and dizziness. Another side effect associated with this substitution is hypoprothrombinemia, which is usually reversible with pharmacologic doses of vitamin K.

Substitutions at the acyl side chain have led to differences in antibacterial spectrum and β-lactamase stability. The side chains substituted at this position interfere with proper stereotactic binding of the molecule to the β-lactamase active site, thus preventing degradation of the cephalosporin. Some of the side effects involving platelet aggregation that have been observed with the use of moxalactam can be traced to substitutions at this position.

For convenience, cephalosporins are divided into three groups, or generations, according to the nature and extent of their antibacterial spectra. More specifically, the division into generations is based on the number of gram-negative bacterial species against which each cephalosporin demonstrates clinical activity. For example, first-generation cephalosporins are active against three common gram-negative bacteria—*E. coli*, *Klebsiella pneumoniae*, and *P. mirabilis*—but they have a wider range of activity against gram-positive organisms than do second- and third-generation agents. It must be remembered, however, that although the members of each generation are sufficiently similar to be grouped together, they also are different from each other in a number of ways [*see Table 7*].

Three critical variables determine the antimicrobial activity of a cephalosporin: (1) ability to penetrate the outer cell wall of the bacterium, (2) ability to resist β-lactamase activity, and (3) ability to bind and inhibit the penicillin-binding protein enzymes (PBPs) that synthesize the bacterial cell wall. The membrane complexes in the outer cell wall of gram-positive bacteria do not block entry of cephalosporins, whereas those of gram-negative bacteria, especially *P. aeruginosa*, tend to resist cephalosporin penetration. As many as six PBPs can be found in gram-negative bacteria. Each cephalosporin binds best to a different PBP. PBPs 1, 2, and 3 are the most important. Binding to these target proteins results in inhibition of transpeptidation of glycopeptide polymers, the final step in bacterial cell wall synthesis. This action eventually triggers autolytic enzymes in susceptible bacteria, which leads to cell lysis. Because cephalosporins do not bind well to enterococcal PBPs, the MIC of cephalosporins for these bacteria is 64 to 128 times that of penicillin G and ampicillin.

FIRST-GENERATION CEPHALOSPORINS

First-generation cephalosporins have good activity against aerobic gram-positive cocci such as *S. aureus*, group B streptococci, and *Streptococcus pneumoniae*. In addition, they are effective against three aerobic gram-negative bacilli—*E. coli*, *K. pneumoniae*, and *P. mirabilis*—although even among these three, resistance is common, occurring in as many as 30% of cases. First-generation cephalosporins are also active against most anaerobic cocci and bacilli (other than *Bacteroides fragilis*). They have little or no activity against *Enterobacter*, *Serratia*, *Acinetobacter*, *Pseudomonas*, methicillin-resistant *S. aureus*, *S. epidermidis*, and enterococci. They are also inactive against *B. fragilis*, *Citrobacter*, *Listeria monocytogenes*, *Proteus* (except for *P. mirabilis*), and *Providencia*.

First-generation cephalosporins are used for infections caused by gram-positive cocci, such as skin infections and osteomyelitis, although penicillins are the agents of choice for all streptococcal infections and for infections proven by culture to be caused by susceptible staphylococci. First-generation cephalosporins are often combined with aminoglycosides to provide broad-spectrum coverage in patients with hospital-acquired pneumonias; however, this practice is falling out of favor because of the high incidence of resistance to first-generation agents observed in gram-positive organisms. The best use for first-generation cephalosporins is in surgical prophylaxis. For this application, cefazolin sodium is the preferred agent. In fact, cefazolin sodium is the most commonly used first-generation cephalosporin: it is on the drug formulary of more than 90% of United States hospitals.[32]

SECOND-GENERATION CEPHALOSPORINS

Second-generation cephalosporins possess the same spectrum of activity as the first-generation cephalosporins, with the addition of broader coverage of gram-negative organisms, including *H. influenzae*, *Enterobacter aerogenes*, and some *Neisseria* species. Fewer than 5% of *E. coli* and *Proteus* strains are resistant to second-generation cephalosporins. The activity of second-generation agents against *S. pyogenes* and *S. pneumoniae* is equal to that of the first-generation agents, but their activity against staphylococci is variable: the MIC ranges from 0.2 to 25 μg/ml. Of the second-generation agents, the most active against staphylococci is cefamandole, which has an MIC of 0.6 μg/ml for *S. aureus*. Cefotetan and cefoxitin have significant activity against *B. fragilis*. Cefoxitin is less active against *H. influenzae* and *E. aerogenes* than other second-generation cephalosporins are, but it is more active against *Serratia* species. Cefoxitin is resistant to destruction by β-lactamase and is the most potent cephalosporin against *B. fragilis*. For this reason, it is a useful primary agent in mixed infections,[33] which the rest of the second-generation cephalosporins, for the most part, are not. Cefoxitin by itself is effective in patients with community-acquired peritonitis who are unlikely to be infected with *Enterobacter* or *P. aeruginosa*.[34] Cefuroxime and cefamandole have been used with some success in empirical therapy for community-acquired pneumonia.[35] Cefuroxime axetil, an orally administered prodrug formulation of cefuroxime, is active in vitro against many gram-positive organisms and some gram-negative organisms. Its resistance to β-lactamase makes it useful for treating infections caused by β-lactamase–producing strains of *H. influenzae*, *Moraxella* (formerly *Branhamella*) *catarrhalis*, and *S. aureus*. Cefuroxime axetil provides good coverage against the Enterobacteriaceae and moderate coverage against non–*B. fragilis* anaerobes.[36]

Cefotetan, a cephamycin introduced in 1986, has a spectrum of activity very similar to that of cefoxitin.[37] It is as active as cefoxitin against *B. fragilis* but is less active against other strains in the *B. fragilis* group. Unlike cefoxitin, cefotetan is active against *H. influenzae*. Both cefoxitin and cefotetan are active against gonococci and many enteric gram-negative bacilli, but neither is effective against *Enterobacter*, *Pseudomonas*, and *Acinetobacter* species or enterococci. Cefotetan has proved effective and safe in a variety of clinical situations, including gynecologic infections and surgical prophylaxis.[38]

Cefprozil is a new oral agent whose spectrum of activity includes gram-positive and gram-negative pathogens. It has achieved good results in patients with pharyngitis or tonsillitis.[39]

Loracarbef is a new oral agent of the carbacephem class that is active in vitro against the common pathogens associated with skin infections, otitis media, sinusitis, bronchopulmonary infections, and urinary tract infections.[40] Its in vitro activity against these common outpatient pathogens is similar to that of other oral antimicrobials, such as cefaclor, cefuroxime axetil, cefixime, amoxicillin-clavulanate, and trimethoprim-sulfamethoxazole.

THIRD-GENERATION CEPHALOSPORINS

In the third-generation cephalosporins, activity against gram-positive cocci is replaced by broader gram-negative coverage. This development is illustrated by susceptibility testing done on *S. aureus*: the MIC of first-generation cephalosporins is 1 μg/ml, that of second-generation cephalosporins is 2 μg/ml, and that of third-generation cephalosporins is 3 μg/ml. Third-generation cephalosporins are more active against the enteric gram-negative bacilli covered by first- and second-generation cephalosporins. Their spectrum of activity includes *Serratia* and *Citrobacter*. They are also highly active against *H. influenzae* and *N. gonorrhoeae* and moderately active against *P. aeruginosa* and some anaerobes. At first, the third-generation cephalosporins seemed capable of providing the same spectrum of activity as the aminoglycosides but without their inherent toxicity; however, they have failed to gain wide popularity in the treatment of high-risk patients or patients with extensive infections. The reasons for this failure include their incomplete spectra of activity against the range of organisms likely to be encountered in polymicrobial infections, their unexpected agent-specific toxicity, their suboptimal pharmacokinetic properties, and their high propensity for inducing resistance.

Several new cephalosporins are under development. Cefixime, an orally absorbed iminomethoxyaminothiazolyl cephalosporin, inhibits 90% of *S. pneumoniae*, *H. influenzae*, and *H. parainfluenzae* strains, whether they produce β-lactamase or not, at concentrations of less than 0.25 mg/L. It inhibits 90% of *M. catarrhalis* strains at concentrations of less than 1 mg/L. With respect to in vitro activity, cefixime is generally superior to cefaclor and the other cephalosporins as well as to erythromycin and amoxicillin.[41]

Ceftibuten is an orally active third-generation cephalosporin that possesses increased potency against members of the Enterobacteriaceae.[42] Generally, it is about 16 times more active than cefuroxime, cefaclor, cephalexin, or amoxicillin-clavulanate; its activity is comparable to that of cefixime. Ceftibuten is ineffective against staphylococci and only partially effective against *S. pneumoniae*. *H. influenzae* and *Neisseria* species, however, are highly susceptible to this agent.

Cefepime is a new extended-spectrum parenteral cephalosporin that provides coverage against both gram-positive and gram-negative organisms, including *S. aureus* and *P. aeruginosa*. It has been used to treat patients with pneumonia, with results comparable to those obtained with ceftazidime.[43]

Antimicrobial Spectra of Activity

Enterobacteriaceae such as *E. coli*, *Klebsiella*, *Citrobacter diversus*, *Proteus* species, and *Morganella* are usually highly susceptible to third-generation cephalosporins; in general, *Enterobacter* species, *C. freundii*, *Serratia marcescens*, and *Providencia* species are less susceptible to third-generation cephalosporins, though there is a fair amount of variability among published reports. Frequently, no more than 50% of *P. aeruginosa* isolates are susceptible at cephalosporin levels of 16 μg/ml. For cephalosporins as a group, the MIC is generally 32 to 64 μg/ml for this organism. Cefoperazone tends to be more active against *P. aeruginosa* than are the other third-generation agents: some papers report an MIC of 8 to 16 μg/ml for carbenicillin-susceptible *P. aeruginosa* strains.[44-47] Isolates

Table 5 Antimicrobial Drug Dosages for Treatment of Bacterial Infections in Adults with Normal Renal Function[203]

Class of Agent	Specific Agent	Trade Names	Modest Infections*			
			Oral		Intramuscular	
			Daily Dose	Interval	Daily Dose	Interval
Penicillinase-susceptible penicillins	Penicillin G	—	0.8–3.2 million units	6 hr	1.2 million units	8 hr
	Penicillin G benzathine	Bicillin	—	—	1.2–2.4 million units	See fn. 1
	Penicillin G procaine	Crysticillin, Duracillin, etc.	—	—	0.6–4.8 million units	6–24 hr
	Penicillin V	Pen-Vee K, V-Cillin K, etc.	0.8–3.2 million units (0.5–2.0 g)	6 hr	—	—
Penicillinase-susceptible penicillins with activity against gram-negative bacilli	Amoxicillin	Amoxil, Larotid, etc.	750–1,500 mg	8 hr	—	—
	Ampicillin	Omnipen, Polycillin, etc.	1–4 g	6 hr	1–2 g	6 hr
	Azlocillin	Azlin	—	—	—	—
	Carbenicillin	Pyopen, Geopen	—	—	See fn. 2	See fn. 2
	Carbenicillin indanyl sodium	Geocillin	—	—	—	—
	Mezlocillin	Mezlin	—	—	—	—
	Piperacillin	Pipracil	—	—	See fn. 4	See fn. 4
	Ticarcillin	Ticar	—	—	See fn. 5	See fn.5
Penicillinase-resistant penicillins	Cloxacillin	Tegopen	1–3 g	6 hr	—	—
	Dicloxacillin	Dynapen, Pathocil	1–2 g	6 hr	—	—
	Methicillin	Celbenin, Staphcillin	—	—	4 g	6 hr
	Nafcillin	Nafcil, Unipen	2–4 g[6]	6 hr	2–3 g	4–6 hr
	Oxacillin	Bactocill, Prostaphlin	2–4 g	6 hr	1–2 g	6 hr
Penicillins with clavulanate	Amoxicillin-clavulanate	Augmentin	750–1,500 mg (amoxicillin)	8 hr	—	—
	Ticarcillin-clavulanate	Timentin	—	—	—	—
Cephalosporins	Cefaclor	Ceclor	750 mg–1.5 g	8 hr	—	—
	Cefadroxil	Duricef, Ultracef	500 mg–2g	12–24 hr	—	—
	Cefamandole	Mandol	—	—	2–4 g	6 hr
	Cefazolin	Ancef, Kefzol	—	—	750 mg–1.5 g	8 hr
	Cefonicid	Monocid	—	—	See fn. 8,9	See fn. 8,9
	Cefoperazone	Cefobid	—	—	See fn. 8,9	See fn. 8,9
	Ceforanide	Precef	—	—	See fn. 8,9	See fn. 8,9
	Cefotaxime	Claforan	—	—	See fn. 8,9	See fn. 8,9
	Cefotetan	Cefotan	—	—	See fn. 8,9	See fn. 8,9
	Cefoxitin	Mefoxin	—	—	2–4 g	6 hr
	Ceftazidime	Fortaz, Tazicef, Tazidime	—	—	See fn. 8,9	See fn. 8,9
	Ceftizoxime	Cefizox	—	—	See fn. 8,9	See fn. 8,9
	Ceftriaxone	Rocephin	—	—	See fn. 8,9	See fn. 8,9
	Cefuroxime	Kefurox, Zinacef	—	—	See fn. 8,9	See fn. 8,9
	Cephalexin	Keflex	1–4 g	6 hr	—	—
	Cephalothin	Keflin	—	—	2–3 g	6 hr
	Cephapirin	Cefadyl	—	—	2–3 g	6 hr
	Cephradine	Anspor, Velosef	1–4 g	6 hr	2 g	6 hr
Carbapenems	Imipenem-cilastatin	Primaxin	—	—	—	—
	Meropenem	Merrem	—	—	—	—
Monobactams	Aztreonam	Azactam	—	—	1–2 g	8–12 hr
Aminoglycosides	Amikacin	Amikin	—	—	—	—
	Gentamicin	Garamycin	—	—	3–5 mg/kg[12]	8 hr
	Kanamycin	Kantrex	—	—	—	—
	Neomycin	—	See fn. 16	See fn. 16	—	—
	Netilmicin	Netromycin	—	—	4–6 mg/kg[12,13]	8 hr
	Streptomycin	—	—	—	1–2 g	12 hr
	Tobramycin	Nebcin	—	—	3–5 mg/kg[12]	8 hr
Tetracyclines	Demeclocycline	Declomycin	600 mg	6 hr	—	—
	Doxycycline	Vibramycin, etc.	100–200 mg[18]	12 hr	—	—

Note: all superscript numbers refer to footnotes following table.
*Infections of the upper respiratory tract, soft tissues, etc.

(continued)

Table 5 (continued)

Uncomplicated Urinary Tract Infections		Major and Systemic Infections[†]			
Oral		Intramuscular		Intravenous	
Daily Dose	Interval	Daily Dose	Interval	Daily Dose	Interval
—	—	—	—	4–24 million units	2–4 hr
—	—	—	—	—	—
—	—	—	—	—	—
—	—	—	—	—	—
750–1,500 mg	8 hr	—	—	—	—
2–4 g	6 hr	—	—	4-12 g	2–4 hr
—	—	—	—	12–18 g	4 hr
—	—	—	—	30–40 g	3–4 hr
4–8 tablets[3]	6 hr	—	—	—	—
—	—	—	—	12–18 g	4 hr
—	—	See fn. 4	See fn. 4	12–18 g	4 hr
—	—	—	—	16–24 g	3–6 hr
—	—	—	—	—	—
—	—	—	—	—	—
—	—	—	—	6–12 g	4–6 hr
—	—	—	—	4–12 g	4–6 hr
—	—	—	—	4–12 g	4–6 hr
750 mg (amoxicillin)	8 hr	—	—	—	—
—	—	—	—	12–18 g (ticarcillin)	4–6 hr
750 mg–1.5 g	8 hr	—	—	—	—
500 mg–2 g	12–24 hr	—	—	—	—
—	—	—	—	4–12 g	2–4 hr
See fn. 7	See fn. 7	2–3 g	6–8 hr	2–6 g	6–8 hr
—	—	—	—	0.5–2.0 g	12–24 hr
—	—	—	—	2–12 g	6–8 hr
—	—	—	—	1–2 g	12 hr
—	—	—	—	2–12 g	4–6 hr
—	—	—	—	2–6 g	12 hr
—	—	—	—	4–12 g	4 hr
—	—	—	—	2–6 g	8–12 hr
—	—	—	—	2–6 g	8–12 hr
—	—	—	—	1–4 g	12–24 hr
—	—	—	—	3–6 g	6 hr
1–4 g	6 hr	—	—	—	—
—	—	—	—	4–12 g	2–4 hr
—	—	—	—	4–12 g	2–4 hr
2 g	6 hr	—	—	3–8 g	4–6 hr
—	—	—	—	1–4 g	6–8 hr
—	—	—	—	3 g	8 hr
—	—	—	—	3–8 g	6–8 hr
—	—	15 mg/kg[10]	8–12 hr	15 mg/kg[11]	8 hr
—	—	3–5 mg/kg	8 hr	3–5 mg/kg[13]	8 hr
—	—	15 mg/kg[14]	8–12 hr	15 mg/kg[15]	8 hr
—	—	—	—	—	—
—	—	4–6 mg/kg	8 hr	4–6 mg/kg[17]	8 hr
—	—	1–2 g	12 hr	—	—
—	—	3–5 mg/kg	8 hr	3–5 mg/kg[17]	8 hr
600 mg	6 hr	—	—	—	—
100–200 mg[18]	12 hr	—	—	100–200 mg[19]	12 hr

[†]Osteomyelitis, peritonitis, bacteremia, meningitis, endocarditis, etc.

(continued)

Table 5 (continued)

Class of Agent	Specific Agent	Trade Names	Modest Infections*			
			Oral		Intramuscular	
			Daily Dose	Interval	Daily Dose	Interval
Tetracyclines (continued)	Minocycline	Minocin	200 mg[20]	12 hr	—	—
	Oxytetracycline	Terramycin	1–2 g	6 hr	See fn. 22	See fn. 22
	Tetracycline	Achromycin, Panmycin, Sumycin, Tetracyn, etc.	1–2 g	6 hr	See fn. 22	See fn. 22
Erythromycins	Erythromycin	E-Mycin, Erythrocin, Ilotycin	1–2 g	6 hr	See fn. 22	See fn. 22
	Erythromycin estolate[24]	Ilosone	1–2 g	6 hr	—	—
Lincomycins	Clindamycin	Cleocin	600 mg–1.8 g	6 hr	600 mg–1.2 g	6–8 hr
	Lincomycin[25]	Lincocin	1.5–2.0 g	6–8 hr	600 mg–1.2 g	8–12 hr
Polymyxins	Colistimethate	Coly-Mycin M	—	—	—	—
	Polymyxin B	Aerosporin, etc.	—	—	—	—
Sulfonamides	Sulfadiazine	—	2–4 g[27]	6 hr	—	—
	Sulfisoxazole	Gantrisin	2–6 g[27]	6 hr	—	—
	Trimethoprim-sulfamethoxazole	Bactrim, Septra	4 tablets[28]	12 hr	—	—
Miscellaneous antibacterial agents	Chloramphenicol	Chloromycetin	1.5–3.0 g	6 hr	See fn. 29	See fn. 29
	Metronidazole	Flagyl	250 mg	8 hr	—	—
	Spectinomycin	Trobicin	—	—	2 g[31]	Single injection
	Trimethoprim	Proloprim, Trimpex	200 mg	12 hr	—	—
	Vancomycin	Vancocin	2 g[32]	6 hr	—	—
Quinolones	Ciprofloxacin[33]	Cipro	500 mg	12 hr	—	—
	Enoxacin	—	—	—	—	—
	Nalidixic acid	NegGram	—	—	—	—
	Norfloxacin	Noroxin	—	—	—	—
	Ofloxacin	—	—	—	—	—
	Perfloxacin	—	—	—	—	—

Note: all superscript numbers refer to footnotes following table.

*Infections of the upper respiratory tract, soft tissues, etc.

1. Benzathine penicillin G is used primarily in three circumstances. (1) Treatment of streptococcal pharyngitis in cases in which patient compliance is questionable (a single dose of 1.2 million units I.M.). (2) Prophylaxis of rheumatic fever recurrences (1.2–2.4 million units I.M. once monthly). (3) Treatment of syphilis: for primary, secondary, or early (< 1 yr) latent syphilis, a single dose of 2.4 million units I.M.; for late syphilis (late latent, cardiovascular, neurosyphilis, etc.), 2.4 million units I.M. weekly for three doses has been recommended, but many authorities now treat neurosyphilis with high-dose I.V. penicillin.

2. Parenteral carbenicillin is usually used in the treatment of serious infections caused by susceptible *Pseudomonas, Enterobacter,* and non-*mirabilis Proteus* strains and is given in maximal dosage (30–40 g I.V. daily). It is often used in synergistic combination with gentamicin or tobramycin for I.V. treatment of *Pseudomonas* infections. Occasionally, it is given in smaller dosages (1–2 g I.M. or I.V. q. 6 hr) to treat an uncomplicated urinary tract infection caused by the same organisms.

3. Each tablet of carbenicillin indanyl sodium is equivalent to 382 mg of carbenicillin (usual dosage is 1 or 2 tablets p.o., q.i.d.).

4. Piperacillin is most often used in the treatment of serious infections caused by susceptible *Pseudomonas, Klebsiella, Enterobacter,* and non-*mirabilis Proteus* strains; the agent is given in maximal dosage (12–18 g I.V. daily). It is commonly used in synergistic combination with tobramycin or gentamicin for treatment of *Pseudomonas* infections. Occasionally, it is given in smaller dosages (1.0–1.5 g I.M. or I.V. q. 6 hr) to treat an uncomplicated urinary tract infection caused by the same organisms.

5. Ticarcillin, piperacillin, mezlocillin, and azlocillin are usually used in the treatment of serious infections caused by susceptible *Pseudomonas,* and non-*mirabilis Proteus* strains and are given in maximal dosage (12–24 g I.V. daily). One of these agents is commonly used in synergistic combination with tobramycin or gentamicin for treatment of *Pseudomonas* infections. Occasionally, they are given in smaller dosages (1 g I.M. or I.V. q. 6 hr) to treat an uncomplicated urinary tract infection caused by the same organisms.

6. Nafcillin is not reliably absorbed by the oral route.

7. Cefazolin may be used in the treatment of acute uncomplicated urinary tract infections caused by susceptible gram-negative bacilli (*E. coli, P. mirabilis,* and *Klebsiella*). It is administered I.M. in a dosage of 2 g daily (given as aliquots q. 8 hr).

8. Although the second- and third-generation cephalosporins can be used for milder infections at the lower end of their recommended dosage range, these potent but expensive agents should generally be reserved for treatment of serious infections or for the treatment of resistant organisms when the alternative is a more toxic antimicrobial drug.

9. The I.M. route is acceptable for milder illnesses, but the I.V. route is recommended for serious infections, including bacteremias and meningitis. The range for the I.M. dosage is the same as that for the I.V. dosage.

10. Dosage must be reduced in the presence of renal insufficiency. The daily parenteral dose should not exceed 15 mg/kg, and the total daily amount administered should not exceed 1.5 g, regardless of the patient's weight.

11. The I.V. dose should be infused during a period of 30–60 min q. 8 hr.

12. For urinary tract infections caused by resistant organisms.

13. Dosage must be reduced in the presence of renal insufficiency. The I.V. dose should be administered for a period of 30–60 min q. 8 hr. In patients with meningitis caused by susceptible gram-negative bacilli, intrathecal gentamicin (5 mg for adults, 1–2 mg for infants) is often administered once daily along with parenteral gentamicin until CSF cultures are negative.

14. Dosage must be reduced in the presence of renal insufficiency. The daily parenteral dose should not exceed 15 mg/kg (daily dose should not exceed 1.5 g, regardless of the patient's weight); the total quantity administered in a therapeutic course should not exceed 15 g.

15. The I.V. route should be employed only when I.M. administration is not possible. The I.V. dose should be administered during a period of at least 60 min q. 8 hr.

16. There are no clinical indications for the parenteral administration of neomycin in view of its marked toxicity and the availability of safer alternative drugs. The drug is given p.o. or by nasogastric tube (4–6 g daily in 4 divided doses) to reduce the number of ammonia-forming bacteria in the intestine in the short-term treatment of acute hepatic coma. It is also given in a total daily dose of 2–3 g in long-term therapy for chronic hepatic encephalopathy or episodic hepatic coma. Nephrotoxicity and ototoxicity have followed prolonged high-dose therapy in hepatic coma, particularly in patients with some renal impairment. Neomycin is also used along with vigorous mechanical cleansing of the large bowel as preoperative prophylaxis for bowel surgery. In this situation, it is administered for 1–3 days preoperatively (40 mg/kg p.o. daily in 6 divided doses).

17. Dosage must be reduced in the presence of renal insufficiency. The I.V. dose should be administered during a period of 30–60 min q. 8 hr.

18. Usually administered as 100 mg p.o. q. 12 hr on the first day of treatment, followed by 50 mg q. 12 hr. For more difficult infections, the dosage may be continued at 100 mg q. 12 hr.

19. Usually administered as 100 mg I.V. q. 12 hr on the first day of treatment. Thereafter, it may be given as 50–100 mg I.V. q. 12 hr. Each I.V. dose should be given during a period of 1–4 hr.

20. Usually administered initially as 200 mg p.o., followed by 100 mg q. 12 hr.

21. Usually given initially as 200 mg I.V., followed by 100 mg q. 12 hr. Maximum dose in any 24-hr period is 400 mg.

22. I.M. administration is generally unsatisfactory because of poor absorption and local irritation.

23. In special circumstances, it may be given in higher doses but not in excess of 500 mg q. 6 hr.

24. Cholestatic hepatitis may develop as a hypersensitivity response to erythromycin estolate

(continued)

Table 5 (continued)

Uncomplicated Urinary Tract Infections		Major and Systemic Infections†			
Oral		Intramuscular		Intravenous	
Daily Dose	Interval	Daily Dose	Interval	Daily Dose	Interval
200 mg[20]	12 hr	—	—	200 mg[21]	12 hr
1–2 g	6 hr	—	—	—	—
1–2 g	6 hr	See fn. 22	See fn. 22	750 mg–1.0 g[23]	6–12 hr
—	—	See fn. 22	See fn. 22	2–4 g	6 hr
—	—	—	—	—	—
—	—	1.2–2.4 g	6–8 hr	1.8–3.0 g	6–8 hr
—	—	1.2–1.8 g	8 hr	1.8–3.0 g	8 hr
—	—	2.5–5.0 mg/kg[26]	6 hr	2.5–5.0 mg/kg	6 hr
—	—	1.5–2.5 mg/kg	6–8 hr	1.5–2.5 mg/kg	6–8 hr
2–4 g[27]	6 hr	—	—	—	—
2–6 g[27]	6 hr	—	—	100 mg/kg[27]	4–6 hr
4 tablets[28]	12 hr	—	—	8–12 mg/kg[28] (trimethoprim)	6 hr[28]
1.5–2.0 g[30]	6 hr	See fn. 29	See fn. 29	2–4 g	6 hr
—	—	—	—	30 mg/kg	6 hr
200 mg	12 hr	—	—	—	—
—	—	—	—	1–2 g	6–12 hr
500 mg–1 g	12 hr	1.5 g p.o.	12 hr	—	—
800 mg	12 hr	800 mg–1.2 g	12 hr	—	—
2–4 mg	6 hr	—	—	—	—
800 mg	12 hr	—	—	—	—
400 mg	24 hr	400–800 mg	24 hr	—	—
400–800 mg	24 hr	800 mg–1.2 g	24 hr	—	—

†Osteomyelitis, peritonitis, bacteremia, meningitis, endocarditis, etc.

but not to the other erythromycin preparations. For this reason, erythromycin base or erythromycin stearate is preferable.

25. Clindamycin has supplanted lincomycin in clinical usage.
26. Dosage usually is 2.5–3.5 mg/kg daily parenterally. Occasionally, the dosage required is as high as 5 mg/kg daily; at this level, paresthesias and more serious neurotoxicity and nephrotoxicity may be manifest in some patients.
27. A loading dose of one half the daily dose is given initially. In severe infections, the dosage of sulfonamide is adjusted to provide a blood level of 10–15 mg/dl. Sulfonamides must be used with caution in patients with renal insufficiency. Sulfisoxazole is the preferred sulfonamide.
28. Each tablet contains 80 mg trimethoprim and 400 mg sulfamethoxazole. Double-strength tablets are also available (usual dosage is 1 tablet q. 12 hr). Pediatric suspensions contain 40 mg trimethoprim and 200 mg sulfamethoxazole/5 ml. Trimethoprim-sulfamethoxazole has also been used in the treatment of typhoid fever in the same dosage as recommended for urinary tract infections. It has been used in a dosage of 4–8 standard tablets daily in the treatment of brucellosis. For pneumonia caused by *Pneumocystis carinii*, the oral dosage is 20 mg/kg trimethoprim and 100 mg/kg sulfamethoxazole/24 hr (equally divided doses q. 6 hr). The I.V. dosage of trimethoprim-sulfamethoxazole ranges from 8 mg/kg trimethoprim and 40 mg/kg sulfamethoxazole/24 hr to 20 mg/kg trimethoprim and 100 mg/kg sulfamethoxazole/24 hr.

The lower dosage range is used in the treatment of urinary tract infections that require parenteral antimicrobial therapy and in the treatment of shigellosis; the larger dosage is employed in the treatment of *P. carinii* pneumonia.

29. Chloramphenicol sodium succinate, the parenteral preparation, should only be used I.V. It is ineffective when administered I.M.
30. Chloramphenicol should not be used in the treatment of a urinary tract infection that could be managed with another, safer, effective antimicrobial.
31. The only approved indication for the use of spectinomycin is in the treatment of anogenital and urethral gonorrhea in a penicillin-allergic patient or when the infecting organism is highly penicillin resistant. In geographic areas where antibiotic-resistant gonococci are prevalent, treatment with 4 g of spectinomycin (2 g in each gluteal region) may be indicated.
32. Vancomycin is not absorbed through the GI tract. Its use orally is for treatment of staphylococcal enterocolitis or antibiotic-associated enterocolitis.
33. Ciprofloxacin has been used with success in a variety of serious systemic infections, including pneumonias and osteomyelitis. The use of oral antibiotics in seriously ill patients must be weighed against the much greater experience with parenteral therapy; in particular, oral therapy may not be effective in those patients who have adynamic ileus and therefore may not reliably absorb drugs from the GI tract.

of *L. monocytogenes, Acinetobacter* species, *P. cepacia, Xanthomonas maltophilia, P. putida,* and *P. fluorescens* are variably sensitive to the third-generation cephalosoporins[48-51]; consequently, these drugs should not be relied on clinically.

Combinations of third-generation cephalosporins with aminoglycosides often exert additive or synergistic effects against gram-negative bacilli in vitro,[52,53] but this phenomenon has been demonstrated only in infections in neutropenic patients; these effects may not be achievable in all patients with intra-abdominal infections.

Despite their resistance to β-lactamase hydrolysis, all third-generation cephalosporins are subject to an inoculum effect; that is, the MIC and MBC are significantly increased when larger bacterial inocula (more than 10^5 organisms/ml) are tested in vitro. This is particularly true with *S. marcescens* and *P. aeruginosa*.[54] The clinical relevance of this effect is not known, but it may explain the failure of certain β-lactam compounds against infections in which large numbers of organisms may be present (e.g., pleural effusion with empyema or large intra-abdominal abscesses).

One piece of information that may help determine which cephalosporin is most active against a known infecting organism is the kill ratio, which is the ratio obtained by dividing the highest achievable blood or tissue level of an antibiotic by its average MIC for the organism. A kill ratio of 2 or greater is considered predictive of the eradication of the organism and thus of clinical cure. The following example illustrates the significance of the kill ratio as well as the importance of understanding the pharmacokinetics of antibacterial agents.

The mean MIC of cephalothin for *S. aureus* is 0.5 µg/ml, and that of cefazolin is 1.0 µg/ml. The obvious conclusion would be that cephalothin is twice as active against *S. aureus* as cefazolin. In fact, the reverse is true if the achievable serum concentrations are considered and kill ratios are constructed. The maximum attainable serum level of cephalothin after a 2 g dose is about 100 µg/ml, and the maximum attainable serum level of cefazolin after a 1 g I.V. dose is about 200 µg/ml. Therefore, the kill ratio is 200 for both cephalothin and cefazolin, but cefazolin achieves this ratio with a 1 g dose, whereas cephalothin does so with a 2 g dose.

A final concern regarding the in vitro activity of third-generation cephalosporins is their ability to induce chromosomally mediated β-lactamases in a variety of gram-negative bacilli.[55] The clinical implications of β-lactamase induction are not entirely clear, but this process is probably responsible for the development of resistance to these agents and others during therapy. Organisms that have become resistant include some *Enterobacter* species, *S. marcescens*, and *P. aeruginosa*.

Pharmacokinetics

After intravenous administration, third-generation cephalosporins conform to an open, two-compartment model, characterized by an initial rapid distribution phase followed by a slower terminal elimination phase. Peak serum concentrations attained after a 2- to 30-minute intravenous infusion of 1 g are highest for cefoperazone and ceftriaxone.[56,57] Because these two agents are very highly bound to serum proteins, they possess small apparent distribution volumes that are roughly equivalent to the volume of the intravascular space. In contrast, the distribution volume of free ceftriaxone is large, approximately 17 L.[58]

The relatively long elimination half-lives of many of the newer β-lactam antibiotics make less frequent dosing possible. Most third-generation cephalosporins are primarily eliminated renally, with two exceptions: cefoperazone and ceftriaxone. Cefoperazone is primarily eliminated unchanged in the bile, and only about 25% of an administered dose is recovered in the urine after 24 hours.[59] Peak biliary concentrations of cefoperazone approach or exceed 2,000 µg/ml after a 2 g I.V. dose.[60] Because cefoperazone's elimination half-life is essentially unaltered in patients with renal failure and the drug is not appreciably hemodialyzed, there is no need to adjust the dosage in such patients. Fifty percent of an administered dose of ceftriaxone is eliminated in the bile; the rest is eliminated renally. Ceftriaxone elimination is decreased to a small extent in end-stage renal disease; however, because the drug is normally given every 12 to 24 hours, there is little accumulation and therefore no need to adjust the dose. Ceftriaxone is not appreciably hemodialyzed.[61] Cefotaxime's half-life increases only when creatinine clearance is less than 5 ml/min, and very little accumulation occurs.[62]

In general, third-generation cephalosporins penetrate most tissue and fluid compartments in amounts that, though variable, usually exceed the MIC for most susceptible pathogens. Sputum concentrations in the range of 0.3 to 6.0 µg/ml are attained with all the agents, and higher concentrations are found in purulent sputum. Ascitic fluid concentrations ranging from 2.4 µg/ml with ceftizoxime to greater than 60 µg/ml with cefoperazone are seen in patients with peritonitis.[63]

Concentrations in excess of the MIC for susceptible aerobic and anaerobic organisms (except for *B. fragilis*) are achieved in female genital tissue with all these agents.[64] Moxalactam achieves concentrations of 4 to 28 µg/g in the myometrium and 6 to 40 µg/g in the endometrium and has been used successfully against gynecologic infections involving *B. fragilis*. These compounds also appear to penetrate the prostate, the testes, the ureters, and renal tissue in significant amounts.[65] Therapeutic gallbladder wall concentrations can be obtained with each of these agents; they may be as high as 60 µg/g with cefoperazone. Bone-penetration studies reveal penetration with each of these agents.[66]

Clinical Utility

Many studies have compared third-generation cephalosporins in an effort to establish a superior drug or drug combination for life-threatening infections; most have found no statistically significant differences. It is important to remember that even if there is a difference in efficacy between two or more antibiotics, that difference may not be apparent if the study group is not large enough. For example, if one agent fails in 10% of patients and another in only 5%, a study group of 250 to 500 patients would be required to show a statistical difference.[67,68] Most comparative antibiotic trials, however, have reported on fewer than 60 patients and thus have not been able to pinpoint small differences in efficacy between antibiotics.[69] Many studies that find no difference between two regimens are in fact subject to this type of error.

Respiratory tract infections Nosocomial gram-negative bacillary pneumonia carries a high mortality.[70-72] It is difficult to establish a diagnosis of gram-negative pneumonia and equally difficult to assess clinical cure in a disease in which bacteria may not be eradicated because of the structural problems that predispose to development of the pneumonia. The frequency of cure with third-generation cephalosporins ranges from 65% to 100%. Two comparative trials have evaluated ceftizoxime against cefamandole in gram-negative bacillary pneumonia.[73,74] The dosages employed were 2 to 6 g/day for ceftizoxime and 4 to 8 g/day for cefamandole. The gram-negative organisms encountered were primarily *Klebsiella, E. coli, Serratia, Acinetobacter,* and *Proteus* species. The two drugs were equally effective; the few failures observed were mainly related to resistant organisms or undrained abscesses.

Cephalosporin activity against *P. aeruginosa* is extremely variable; ceftazidime and cefoperazone are the only agents that are truly effective. The activity of cephalosporins against organisms that are difficult to manage, such as *Enterobacter* species, *Citrobacter,* and *Serratia,* varies.[75] Small clinical and in vitro bacteriologic studies comparing cefotaxime, 2 g every 8 hours, with imipenem-cilastatin, 500 mg every 8 hours, have shown both drugs to have 85% efficacy.[76,77]

On theoretical grounds, the third-generation cephalosporins can be recommended as therapy for pneumonia caused by *Klebsiella, E. coli,* and *Serratia,* but they have not been unequiv-

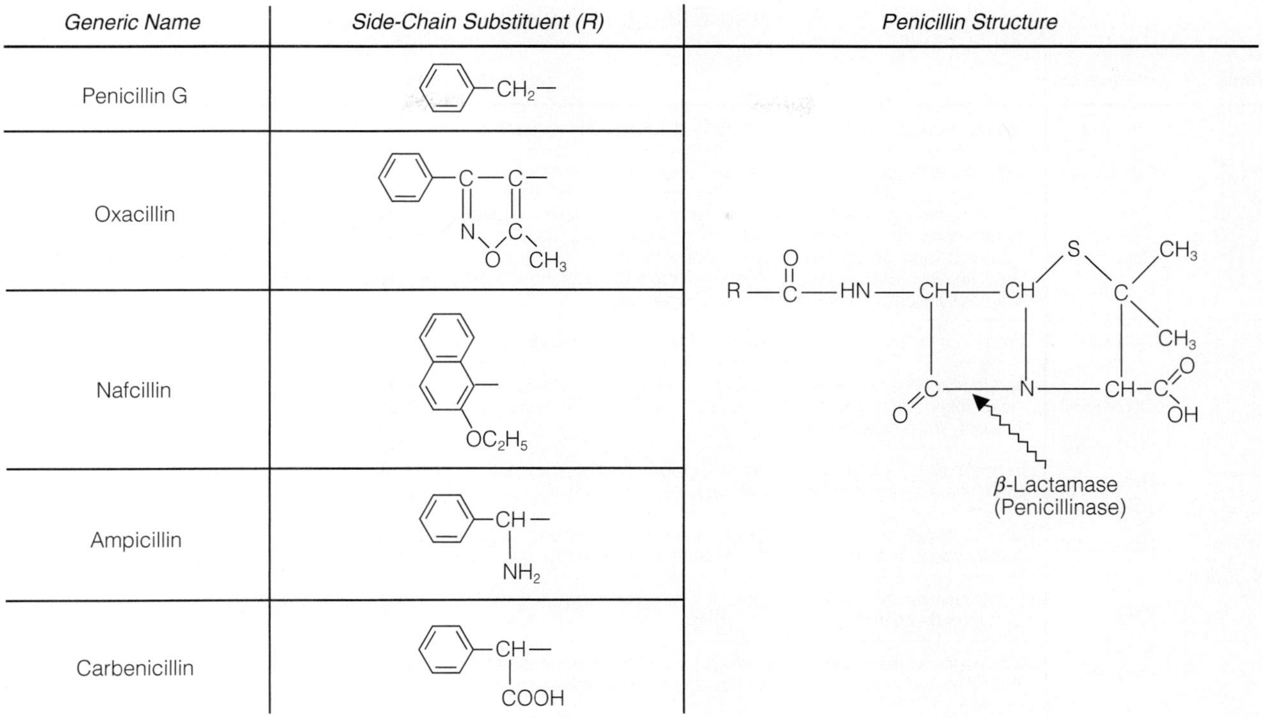

Generic Name	Side-Chain Substituent (R)	Penicillin Structure
Penicillin G	⌬–CH₂–	(see structure at right)
Oxacillin	phenyl-isoxazole-CH₃	
Nafcillin	naphthyl–OC₂H₅	
Ampicillin	⌬–CH(NH₂)–	
Carbenicillin	⌬–CH(COOH)–	

Figure 1 Various semisynthetic penicillins have been produced by modifying the structure of the side chain (R) attached to the penicillin nucleus (right). In this way, penicillins have been developed that lack some of the drawbacks of penicillin G, such as poor gastrointestinal absorption, limited spectrum of antibacterial activity, and inactivation by penicillinase-producing microorganisms; for example, oxacillin and nafcillin are resistant to inactivation by penicillinase. This bacterial enzyme (also termed β-lactamase) cleaves the β-lactam ring of penicillin to form an inactive product; the site of action of penicillinase is shown at right.

ocally shown to be superior to combinations of a first- or second-generation cephalosporin with an aminoglycoside. They probably should not be used alone in the treatment of *P. aeruginosa* infection; if they are used at all, they should be combined with an aminoglycoside. Another extremely important consideration bearing on the use of β-lactamase–stable agents to treat pneumonia is the inoculum effect. In respiratory tract infections, inocula are often as large as 10^9 colony-forming units/ml sputum. The development of resistance in *Enterobacter* species, *P. aeruginosa*, and occasionally *S. marcescens* has followed therapy with all of the third-generation cephalosporins[78,79]; this may be attributable, at least in part, to the inoculum effect.

Urinary tract infections The third-generation cephalosporins have been widely tested for use in treatment of complicated and uncomplicated urinary tract infections; however, orally administered drugs, such as trimethoprim-sulfamethoxazole or a quinolone, are preferable because they provide effective therapy at considerably less expense.

Intra-abdominal infections A therapeutic regimen for treatment of intra-abdominal infection should include agents that are active against *S. aureus*, enteric gram-negative bacilli, and anaerobes, including *B. fragilis*. The gold-standard regimen includes an aminoglycoside to cover the enteric gram-negative organisms and clindamycin or metronidazole to cover the anaerobes. Appropriate surgical control of the source of the intra-abdominal infection is of utmost importance in determining outcome; antibiotics play a necessary but secondary role.[80,81] The controversies regarding the pathogenicity of enterococci have been addressed by guidelines published by members of the Surgical Infection Society.[82] The third-generation cephalosporins have been proposed as candidates for single-agent therapy for infection in the abdominal cavity because their spectra of activity encompass both the aerobic gram-negative bacilli and some of the anaerobic isolates that cause infection in this region. No cephalosporin, of any generation, has been shown to have a clear advantage over an aminoglycoside-clindamycin combination in the treatment of intra-abdominal infections.

Interpretation of overall results in intra-abdominal infections is difficult because of the numerous variables involved, including the diversity of the possible infectious processes, the variable quality of the surgical technique employed, the variety of the patient characteristics observed, the possibility of one or more underlying diseases, and the differing doses of antibiotics used in individual studies.[83] Most third-generation cephalosporins do not cover anaerobes well and should be used in conjunction with an antianaerobic agent, such as clindamycin or metronidazole, for empirical therapy for serious intra-abdominal infections. A recent prospective, randomized, double-blind study[84] showed that cefoxitin was comparable in outcome (defined as survival) to imipenem; failure to cure infections was attributed to resistant organisms at the primary site in the cefoxitin arm of the trial.

Table 6 Adverse Effects of Selected Antibiotics[203]

Antibiotics	Frequency	Adverse Effects
Penicillins	Frequent	Rashes (more common with ampicillin); allergic reactions (rarely anaphylactic); diarrhea (most common with oral ampicillin)
	Occasional	Hemolytic anemia (with high parenteral doses); drug fever
	Rare	Myoclonic jerking and seizures (with high parenteral doses, especially in patients with renal insufficiency); interstitial nephritis; hemorrhagic cystitis (with methicillin); hyperkalemia with possible arrhythmias (with large doses of rapidly administered penicillin G); granulocytopenia; bleeding from platelet dysfunction (with high-dose I.V. therapy) or prolonged prothrombin time, or both; hepatitis (with semisynthetic penicillins such as oxacillin); sodium overload or hypokalemic alkalosis, or both (with high doses of carbenicillin); pseudomembranous colitis (with ampicillin)
Cephalosporins	Frequent	Thrombophlebitis with I.V. use; pain on I.M. injection; minor GI symptoms (particularly diarrhea)
	Occasional	Allergic reactions, including morbilliform and urticarial rashes, serum sickness, and anaphylaxis; drug fever and eosinophilia; reversible neutropenia and thrombocytopenia; pseudomembranous colitis; hemorrhagic diathesis (prolonged prothrombin time, primarily from moxalactam)
	Rare	Hemolytic anemia with direct Coombs'-positive reaction; transient rise in aspartate aminotransferase (AST) and alkaline phosphatase; interstitial pneumonitis; interstitial nephritis; disulfiram-like reaction with alcohol ingestion
Aminoglycosides	Occasional	Renal damage; rash (maculopapular); nausea and vomiting; ototoxicity (both auditory and vestibular to varying degrees—kanamycin effects more likely to be auditory; streptomycin and gentamicin effects more likely to be vestibular)
	Rare	Neuromuscular blockade and apnea (to be considered particularly in patients receiving succinylcholine or other blocking agents and in patients with myasthenia gravis)
Tetracyclines	Frequent	GI irritation (nausea, vomiting, diarrhea); inhibition of bone growth and discoloration and deformity of teeth in children younger than 8 yr and in neonates when the agent was administered after the first trimester of pregnancy; mucocutaneous candidiasis
	Occasional	Intestinal malabsorption; staphylococcal enterocolitis; pseudomembranous enterocolitis; photosensitivity (fever, sunburn reactions), most frequent with demeclocycline; negative nitrogen balance and increased azotemia with preexisting renal insufficiency (rarely with doxycycline); liver injury with large I.V. doses (> 1 g/day), especially when given to pregnant patients or to those with renal disease; prolongation of prothrombin time with extended use; vestibular reactions with minocycline; tooth discoloration in young adults with minocycline
	Rare	Allergic reactions; fixed drug eruptions; increased intracranial pressure (pseudotumor cerebri) in infants and extremely rarely in adults; Fanconi's syndrome after ingestion of outdated tetracycline; diabetes insipidus–like symptoms with demeclocycline
Erythromycin	Occasional	GI irritation (particularly epigastric distress); stomatitis; cholestatic hepatitis in adults treated with erythromycin estolate
	Rare	Allergic reactions with fever and rash (sometimes resembling Stevens-Johnson syndrome); reversible loss of hearing occurring after I.V. administration of 4 g/day; pseudomembranous colitis; potentiation of warfarin effect
Clindamycin	Frequent	Diarrhea; hypersensitivity reactions (maculopapular rashes)
	Occasional	Pseudomembranous colitis; nausea and vomiting
	Rare	Reversible neutropenia
Chloramphenicol	Occasional	Reversible anemia or leukopenia (dose-related toxic effect on bone marrow); gray syndrome in neonates; nausea, vomiting, diarrhea; glossitis; oropharyngeal candidiasis
	Rare	Aplastic anemia; rashes; drug fever; enterocolitis; neurotoxic reactions (with prolonged use: confusion, headache, peripheral neuritis, or optic neuritis)
Vancomycin	Occasional	Thrombophlebitis; chills and fever; ototoxicity (principally hearing loss with large doses or prolonged therapy, especially in patients with impaired renal function and in the elderly); nausea
	Rare	Nephrotoxicity; urticaria and other rashes; hypotension, which may be accompanied by paresthesias, pruritus, and upper-body rash (after rapid I.V. administration); neutropenia

ADVERSE EFFECTS

Cephalosporins are associated with a number of adverse side effects [see Table 6]. On the whole, however, third-generation cephalosporins are relatively nontoxic. The adverse reactions associated with their use are similar to those associated with use of other β-lactam compounds, such as local pain and irritation, hypersensitivity reactions, positive Coombs' reaction, leukopenia, thrombocytopenia, transient abnormalities in liver function enzymes, and gastrointestinal disturbances.[85,86] These reactions are usually mild and reversible, except in those rare patients who manifest life-threatening hypersensitivity reactions. Cephalosporins may be administered to most patients who are allergic to penicillin because only 5% to 15% of penicillin-allergic patients react adversely to cephalosporins.[87]

Aminoglycosides

Various aminoglycosides have been introduced into clinical practice since Waksman and colleagues discovered streptomycin more than 50 years ago. The aminoglycosides now available for clinical use worldwide are streptomycin, kanamycin, neomycin, gentamicin, tobramycin, amikacin, netilmicin, and sisomicin; dibekacin is not available in the United States, although it is marketed in other countries. Because of the formidable nephrotoxicity and ototoxicity associated with neomycin, it is available only for topical use, for oral treatment of hepatic encephalopathy, and for preoperative decontamination of the large bowel.

Aminoglycosides are composed of two or more amino sugars bound by glycosidic linkage to a central hexose (aminocyclitol)

Table 7 Properties of Cephalosporins[203]

	Specific Agent	Trade Names	Comment*
First Generation	**Oral**		
	Cefadroxil	Duricef, Ultracef	Longer half-life
	Cephalexin	Keflex	Most experience with this agent
	Cephradine	Anspor, Velosef	Properties are similar to those of cephalexin
	Parenteral		
	Cefazolin	Ancef, Kefzol	Longer half-life; well tolerated when given I.M.
	Cephapirin	Cefadyl	Properties are similar to those of other first-generation cephalosporins
	Cephradine	Anspor, Velosef	Properties are similar to those of other first-generation cephalosporins
Second Generation	**Oral**		
	Cefaclor	Ceclor	Moderately active against *Hemophilus influenzae*
	Cefprozil	Cefzil	Active against *H. influenzae*
	Cefuroxime axetil	Ceftin	Active against *H. influenzae*
	Loracarbef	Lorabid	A carbacephem with properties and spectrum similar to those of cefuroxime
	Parenteral		
	Cefamandole	Mandol	Active against *H. influenzae*; may cause bleeding
	Cefmetazole	Zefazone	Spectrum and half-life similar to cefoxitin; may cause bleeding
	Cefonicid	Monocid	Spectrum similar to that of cefamandole
	Ceforanide	Precef	Spectrum similar to that of cefamandole
	Cefotetan	Cefotan	Spectrum similar to that of cefoxitin; longer half-life than cefoxitin; may cause bleeding
	Cefoxitin	Mefoxin	Active against *Bacteroides fragilis, Serratia, Neisseria gonorrhoeae*
	Cefuroxime	Zinacef, Kefurox	Active against *H. influenzae*; only second-generation drug approved for meningitis (selected pathogens)
Third Generation	**Oral**		
	Cefixime	Suprax	More active against gram-negative bacilli, gonococci, *Moraxella catarrhalis*, and *H. influenzae* than other oral cephalosporins but much less active against *Staphylococcus aureus*; not active against *Pseudomonas*
	Cefpodoxime	Vantin	Similar to cefixime but more active against *S. aureus*
	Ceftibuten	Cedax	Similar to cefixime but has poor activity against pneumococci and staphylococci
	Parenteral		
	Cefepime	Maxipime	Active against most gram-positive cocci (except enterococci and methicillin-resistant staphylococci), *Neisseria, Hemophilus*, enteric gram-negative bacilli, and *Pseudomonas*
	Cefoperazone	Cefobid	Increased activity against *Pseudomonas aeruginosa* but less against Enterobacteriaceae; may cause bleeding
	Cefotaxime	Claforan	More active against gram-positive cocci
	Ceftazidime	Fortaz, Tazidime, Tazicef	Most active against *Pseudomonas*
	Ceftizoxime	Cefizox	Properties are similar to those of cefotaxime
	Ceftriaxone	Rocephin	Longer half-life; less active against *Pseudomonas, B. fragilis*

Note: detailed information about the various cephalosporins is covered in the text.
*Agents are being compared with other members of the same generation of cephalosporins.

nucleus. Their highly polar, polycationic structure contributes to their poor gastrointestinal absorption and their meager ability to penetrate the blood-brain barrier. They bind irreversibly to the 30S bacterial ribosome and interfere with protein synthesis. They must, however, penetrate the cell before ribosomal binding can occur. This crucial step is energy dependent and oxygen dependent and does not occur under anaerobic conditions. The uptake of aminoglycosides is facilitated by the presence of inhibitors of cell wall synthesis, such as β-lactam antibiotics or vancomycin.[88] Aminoglycosides also disturb calcium homeostasis and induce cell death as a result of efflux of potassium, sodium, and other essential bacterial constituents. Unlike most other antimicrobial agents that inhibit protein synthesis, aminoglycosides are bactericidal. Their bactericidal capacity is now thought to be attributable to their disruptive effect on calcium homeostasis.

All aminoglycosides share certain pharmacokinetic properties. Because they are poorly absorbed when given orally, adequate serum concentrations can be obtained only through parenteral administration. Protein binding is negligible,[89] and the volume of distribution approximates the volume of the extracellular space.[90] In adults with normal renal function, the aminoglycosides have a half-life of about 2 hours, but there is considerable variation from one individual to the next.[91] In patients with deteriorating renal function, their half-life increases, often exceeding 24 hours in patients with end-stage renal disease.[92] These prolonged half-lives are substantially shortened during hemodialysis[93]; the agents are much less efficiently removed by peritoneal dialysis.[94] The aminoglycosides do not penetrate the blood-brain barrier well, even in patients with meningeal inflammation.[95,96] Drug levels in pulmonary secretions are typically 20% to 40% of serum levels. Low concentrations of aminoglycosides in purulent fluids are probably related to local inactivation caused by DNA released from leukocytes[97] and by the low regional pH.

The aminoglycosides are rapidly excreted, primarily by glomerular filtration. Urine concentrations may be 100 times the serum level in patients with normal renal function. The aminoglycosides accumulate in the renal cortex; sensitive assay techniques can detect them in urine and serum for up to 10 days after cessation of therapy.

STREPTOMYCIN

Widespread resistance among Enterobacteriaceae has limited the usefulness of streptomycin. At present, streptomycin is almost always employed in combination with other antimicrobial agents. With penicillin or vancomycin, it is used to treat infective endocarditis caused by viridans streptococci or susceptible enterococcal streptococci. It may also be given in conjunction with other antituberculous drugs to treat mycobacterial diseases and in conjunction with tetracycline to treat brucellosis. Streptomycin is used alone in the treatment of tularemia and plague.

KANAMYCIN

Because of widespread resistance among Enterobacteriaceae and *P. aeruginosa*, kanamycin is rarely used today. It is occasionally used as a second-line agent in combination with other antibiotics in the treatment of tuberculosis.

NEOMYCIN

Neomycin is used primarily in oral bowel preparations [see *39 Prevention of Postoperative Infection*] and in local antiseptic ointments.

GENTAMICIN

Gentamicin continues to be the aminoglycoside of choice for serious hospital-acquired infections caused by Enterobacteriaceae and most strains of *P. aeruginosa* in institutions in which there is minimal background resistance to this agent (other *Pseudomonas* species are predictably resistant to aminoglycosides). Gentamicin is given with penicillin to treat enterococcal endocarditis and with vancomycin plus rifampin to treat prosthetic valve endocarditis caused by *S. epidermidis*. Finally, gentamicin together with antimicrobial agents active against *B. fragilis* is effective in the treatment of intra-abdominal infection.

TOBRAMYCIN

Tobramycin closely resembles gentamicin with respect to antimicrobial spectrum and pharmacokinetics. Tobramycin is more active against some strains of *Acinetobacter calcoaceticus* but less active against *S. marcescens*. Although tobramycin has slightly greater intrinsic activity against *P. aeruginosa*, most gentamicin-resistant strains of this organism are also resistant to tobramycin. The difference in nephrotoxicity between gentamicin and tobramycin is clinically insignificant.[98-100]

AMIKACIN

Amikacin is a semisynthetic derivative of kanamycin. Its major advantage is its resistance to aminoglycoside-modifying enzymes, the production of which is the principal mechanism of aminoglycoside resistance among bacteria. Amikacin may therefore be used against gentamicin-resistant organisms, and it is clearly the aminoglycoside of choice where gentamicin resistance is prevalent. Fortunately, no substantial increase in amikacin resistance has been noted, even in medical centers where it has been used extensively.[101]

NETILMICIN AND SISOMICIN

Netilmicin, a semisynthetic derivative of sisomicin, is not metabolized by most of the aminoglycoside-modifying enzymes and therefore is active against some strains of Enterobacteriaceae that are resistant to gentamicin and tobramycin; however, it is less active against *P. aeruginosa*. Animal studies suggest that netilmicin may be less nephrotoxic than other aminoglycosides,[99,102] and human studies suggest that it is somewhat less likely to exert toxic effects on cranial nerve VIII.[99] Sisomicin is more active than gentamicin against Enterobacteriaceae and *P. aeruginosa*, but the nephrotoxicity it has exhibited in animal studies exceeds that of other aminoglycosides.[103]

ADVERSE EFFECTS

Unlike β-lactam antibiotics, aminoglycosides have a narrow range between therapeutic and toxic levels and thus are prone to side effects [see *Table 6*]. Their ototoxicity is potentially more significant than their nephrotoxicity because it is often irreversible. Cochlear toxicity has been reported in 8% to 10% of patients and has been clinically evident in as many as 4% of patients treated with aminoglycosides for various infections.[104] Vestibular toxicity, as manifested by electronystagmographic changes, has been found in 5% to 10% of patients and has been clinically significant in 1% to 5%.[99] Vestibular toxicity is more frequently associated with streptomycin, gentamicin, and tobramycin, whereas auditory toxicity is more typical of kanamycin and amikacin. Ototoxicity and vestibular toxicity are difficult to monitor, particularly in hospitalized patients for whom formal audiometry and caloric testing may be cumbersome or uncomfortable. Because aminoglycoside-associated auditory toxicity generally affects the higher frequencies, early bedside detection is difficult. Toxic effects on cranial nerve VIII seem to be related to advanced age, prior aminoglycoside treatment, and excessive serum levels.

AMINOGLYCOSIDE PHARMACOKINETICS

Extremely active antibiotics, the aminoglycosides are clinically effective against many serious infections caused by gram-negative bacilli, and as patents have expired, these agents have become inexpensive. These advantages must be weighed against the potential renal and otovestibular toxicity of aminoglycosides. Peak aminoglycoside concentrations higher than 5 µg/ml are associated with improved survival in patients with gram-negative infections.[105,106] With gram-negative pulmonary infections, peak concentrations of 8 to 10 mg/ml are necessary because of poor penetration of aminoglycosides into the lungs.[107,108] It has been shown that a loading dose of gentamicin or tobramycin of 2 mg/kg lean body weight cannot guarantee adequate peak concentrations in acutely ill patients. The most likely explanation for the usually low peak serum concentrations of aminoglycosides in acutely ill patients is an expanded volume of distribution.[109-113] Dosage adjustments based on blood levels should be made as soon as possible after the beginning of therapy and after the steady state has been reached. The steady state is a level of drug accumulation in blood and tissue, after several doses have been given, at which input and output are in equilibrium [see *107 Pharmacokinetics in Surgical Practice*]. This state is reached after about five half-lives of the drug. It is essential to keep in mind that whenever the dosing regimen is changed, a new steady state is reached after about five half-lives.

Once-Daily Dosing of Aminoglycosides

Efforts to improve the toxic-to-therapeutic ratio of aminoglycosides include once-daily dose schedules and reevaluations of the recommended therapeutic ranges. In conventional administration of aminoglycosides to patients with normal renal function, divided doses are administered at 8- to 12-hour intervals. In an effort to improve efficacy and decrease toxicity and cost, once-daily regimens have been compared with conventional regimens. In most protocols, the total dose was equivalent in the single and divided-dose regimens. Two meta-analyses of such trials have concluded that once-daily dosing is as effective as divided dosing and has a lower risk of toxicity in patients with normal renal function.[114,115] Although most trials evaluated immunocompetent adults, similar trends were noted for children and for patients with febrile neutropenia. In elderly patients, however, the high peak serum concentrations that occur with once-daily dosing may increase the risk of nephrotoxicity,[116] probably because of diminished renal clearance. Once-daily dosing has not yet been studied adequately in pregnant women or in patients with renal dysfunction, burns, ascites, or endocarditis. There are several excellent reviews of the subject in the literature.[117,118]

Tetracyclines

The tetracyclines are close congeneric derivatives of the polycyclic substance naphthacenecarboxamide. They act against microorganisms by inhibiting protein synthesis; their site of action is the bacterial ribosome. At least two processes are necessary for the tetracyclines to gain access to the ribosomes of gram-negative microorganisms. The first is passive diffusion through hydrophilic pores in the outer cell membrane. The second is an energy-dependent active transport mechanism that pumps tetracyclines into the cell through the inner cytoplasmic membrane. Once inside the cell, the tetracyclines inhibit synthesis of protein by binding to the 30S ribosomes and preventing aminoacyl-transfer RNA (aminoacyl-tRNA) from gaining access to the messenger RNA–ribosome complex.

Resistance to the tetracyclines appears slowly and in a stepwise fashion and is mediated by plasmids. Plasmids impart resistance by coding for proteins that interfere with active transport of tetracycline through the cytoplasmic membrane. Microorganisms that acquire resistance to one tetracycline are usually resistant to the other tetracyclines as well.

At appropriate dosages, peak serum concentrations 1 hour after intravenous administration of tetracycline, doxycycline, or minocycline are typically 10 to 20 μg/ml. The newer semisynthetic tetracyclines—doxycycline, methacycline, and minocycline—have considerably longer serum half-lives than the older agents.

The tetracyclines bind to plasma proteins to varying degrees. Doxycycline, demeclocycline, and methacycline have the highest level of protein binding (80% to 95%). Minocycline and tetracycline exhibit an intermediate level of protein binding (65% to 75%). Oxytetracycline has the lowest level of protein binding (20% to 40%). Tetracyclines are metabolized by the liver and concentrated in the bile. Biliary concentrations of these agents are, on average, five to 10 times higher than concurrent plasma concentrations. The tetracyclines penetrate body tissues well and are capable of entering the CSF even in the absence of inflammation of the meninges. They readily cross the placental barrier, and relatively high concentrations are found in human milk.

Tetracyclines are useful in the treatment of sexually transmitted diseases, such as urethritis, endocervicitis, acute pelvic inflammatory disease, and rectal infections caused by *Chlamydia*. As a rule, doxycycline is used in combination with cefoxitin or another cephalosporin for treatment of patients with pelvic inflammatory infection. Tetracyclines are also effective for the treatment of other chlamydial infections, such as lymphogranuloma venereum, psittacosis, inclusion conjunctivitis, and trachoma. A tetracycline may also be used in the treatment of gonococcal infections in patients who are unable to tolerate penicillin G. Other sexually transmitted diseases that may be treated with tetracyclines are chancroid and granuloma inguinale.

A tetracycline or erythromycin is the agent of choice for the treatment of *Mycoplasma pneumoniae* infection. Tetracyclines are also effective against rickettsial infections, tularemia, and cholera; in patients unable to tolerate penicillin, they may be used to treat actinomycosis. Doxycycline is useful as prophylaxis against traveler's diarrhea caused by toxicogenic strains of *E. coli*. Unfortunately, the widespread use of tetracyclines as additives to livestock feed has resulted in increasing bacterial resistance to these agents.

Adverse effects of these agents are outlined elsewhere [*see Table 6*].

Macrolides

ERYTHROMYCIN

Erythromycin is a macrolide that contains a many-membered lactone ring to which one or more deoxy sugars are attached. Erythromycin and other macrolide antibiotics inhibit protein synthesis through reversible binding to the 50S ribosomal subunits of susceptible microorganisms.

Erythromycin is well absorbed from the GI tract. The presence of food in the stomach reduces absorption of the drug, except when it is in the estolate form.[119] Peak serum concentrations 4 hours after oral administration of 500 mg of the base, stearate, or ethylsuccinate are typically 1 to 2 μg/ml. Serum concentrations 1 hour after intravenous administration of 0.5 to 1.0 g are approximately 10 to 15 μg/ml. Erythromycin is excreted primarily in the bile; only 2% to 5% of a given dose is excreted in the urine. Concentrations in the bile may be more than 10 times those in plasma. Erythromycin diffuses readily into most tissues, except for the brain and the CSF.

Erythromycin is the agent of choice for the treatment of *M. pneumoniae* and *Legionella* infections. It is also effective against infections caused by group A β-hemolytic streptococci or *S. pneumoniae*. Accordingly, it is the agent of choice for the treatment of community-acquired pneumonia in nonimmunosuppressed patients who do not require hospitalization and who are allergic to penicillin.[120] In addition, erythromycin may be used to treat gonorrhea and syphilis in patients who are unable to tolerate penicillin G or tetracycline. The incidence of serious erythromycin-related adverse effects is low [*see Table 6*].

CLARITHROMYCIN AND AZITHROMYCIN

Clarithromycin and azithromycin are new semisynthetic macrolides that are structurally related to erythromycin. They inhibit protein synthesis in susceptible organisms by binding to the 50S ribosomal subunit. Alteration in this binding site confers simultaneous resistance to all macrolides. Clarithromycin and azithromycin are well absorbed and widely distributed, with excellent cellular and tissue penetration. Both agents have a broader spectrum of activity than erythromycin does; in addition, they have fewer gastrointestinal side effects (a major obstacle to compliance with erythromycin therapy).

Clarithromycin is several times more active against gram-positive organisms in vitro than erythromycin is, whereas azithromycin is two to four times less potent than erythromycin. Azithromycin has excellent in vitro activity against *H. influenzae*; clarithromycin, although less active against *H. influenzae* according to standard in vitro testing, is metabolized into an active compound with twice the in vitro activity of the parent drug. Both azithromycin and clarithromycin are equivalent to standard oral therapies for respiratory tract and soft tissue infections caused by susceptible organisms, including *S. aureus*, *S. pneumoniae*, *S. pyogenes*, *H. influenzae*, and *M. catarrhalis*.[121] Clarithromycin is more active in vitro against the atypical respiratory pathogens (e.g., *Legionella*), although insufficient in vivo data are available to demonstrate a clinical difference between azithromycin and clarithromycin. Azithromycin and clarithromycin also are active against some unexpected pathogens (e.g., *Borrelia burgdorferi*, *Toxoplasma gondii*, *Mycobacterium avium* complex, and *M. leprae*). At present, clarithromycin appears to be the more active of the two against atypical mycobacteria, giving new hope to surgeons faced with what has become a difficult group of infections to treat.

Superior pharmacodynamic properties distinguish these new macrolides from the prototypical macrolide, erythromycin. Azithromycin has a large volume of distribution, and although serum concentrations remain low, it concentrates readily within tissues, demonstrating a tissue half-life of approximately 3 days; a 5-day course of therapy will provide therapeutic tissue concentrations for at least 10 days. These properties allow novel dosing schemes. For instance, azithromycin can be given once daily for 5 days to treat respiratory tract and soft tissue infections, and administration of a single 1 g dose of azithromycin can effectively treat *Chlamydia trachomatis* genital infections; these more convenient dosing schedules improve patient compliance. Clarithromycin has a longer serum half-life and better tissue penetration than erythromycin and thus can be given twice daily to treat most common infections.

Currently, clarithromycin and azithromycin are approved for treatment of respiratory tract infections and skin infections, but they may also be of use in mycobacterial and *Toxoplasma* infections in patients with AIDS.[122]

Clindamycin

Clindamycin is a 7-deoxy-7-chloro derivative of lincomycin that consists of an amino acid attached to a sulfur-containing octose. Clindamycin binds exclusively to the 50S subunit of bacterial ribosomes and suppresses the synthesis of protein. Clindamycin, erythromycin, and chloramphenicol all act at the same site, and the binding of one of these antibiotics to the ribosome may inhibit the binding of the others. Plasmid-mediated resistance to clindamycin has been reported in *B. fragilis*; this may be caused by methylation of bacterial RNA found in the 50S ribosomal subunit.[123] Peak serum concentrations 1 hour after intravenous administration of a 600 mg dose are approximately 10 to 12 µg/ml. Clindamycin is metabolized by the liver and excreted in an inactive form in the urine. It readily penetrates most body tissues but not the CSF.[124]

Clindamycin is active against *B. fragilis* and other anaerobic microorganisms and is useful in the treatment of patients with intra-abdominal, pelvic, and pulmonary infections. It is associated with a modest number of adverse effects [see Table 6].

Chloramphenicol

Chloramphenicol is unique among antibiotics in that it contains a nitrobenzene moiety and is a derivative of dichloroacetic acid. Like clindamycin, it inhibits bacterial protein synthesis by binding reversibly to the 50S ribosomal subunit, thus keeping the amino acid–containing end of aminoacyl-tRNA from binding to the ribosome. Resistance to chloramphenicol is caused by a specific plasmid that causes production of acetyltransferase, which inactivates the drug.[125] Chloramphenicol is rapidly and completely absorbed from the GI tract, and absorption is not impaired by concomitant ingestion of food or administration of antacids. It is inactivated in the liver by glucuronyl transferase. It and its metabolites are excreted rapidly in the urine. About 80% to 90% of a dose is excreted in this way, about 5% to 10% of which is in the biologically active form. The drug penetrates well into all tissues, including the brain, and into the CSF and the aqueous humor.

Because of the risk of serious or fatal bone marrow toxicity, chloramphenicol should be used only against those infections for which the benefits of its use outweigh the risks of its potential toxicity. It still plays a major role in the treatment of typhoid fever, although plasmid-mediated resistance of *Salmonella typhi* to chloramphenicol has been reported. Chloramphenicol is effective therapy for bacterial meningitis and brain abscesses caused by susceptible microorganisms; in conjunction with penicillin, it is effective empirical therapy for brain abscesses. It is as effective as ampicillin against meningitis caused by susceptible strains of *H. influenzae*. It is active in vitro against most anaerobic bacteria, including *B. fragilis*. The most important toxic effect of chloramphenicol is bone marrow suppression [see Table 6].

Vancomycin

Vancomycin is a narrow-spectrum antibiotic derived from *Nocardia orientalis*. It was introduced in 1956, primarily because of its efficacy against resistant penicillinase-producing staphylococci (though it is also effective against other aerobic and anaerobic gram-positive organisms).[126,127] It became generally available before the semisynthetic bactericidal antistaphylococcal penicillins and cephalosporins were developed. These newer agents displaced vancomycin to a large extent, so that its main role became that of an alternative in situations in which the penicillins and cephalosporins could not be used.

Vancomycin exerts its bactericidal effect by inhibiting the biosynthesis of the major structural cell wall polymer, peptidoglycan, a complex glycopolypeptide with a molecular weight of about 1,500.[128] Vancomycin is about 55% protein bound. Its activity is not significantly affected by pH values between 6.5 and 8.0. It is poorly absorbed from the GI tract. Because patients invariably experience pain after intramuscular injections, parenteral administration is limited to the intravenous route. Vancomycin is primarily excreted by the kidneys; about 80% to 90% of the dose is eliminated in a 24-hour period. Its half-life is approximately 6 hours in patients with normal renal function. In anuric patients, the half-life may be prolonged to approximately 7 1/2 days.[129] Vancomycin is not removed by hemodialysis or peritoneal dialysis.

Vancomycin is mainly effective against gram-positive organisms. No cross-resistance has been demonstrated between vancomycin and other antibiotics, and resistance is uncommon. For streptococci, the MICs of vancomycin are uniformly low, but the MBCs vary: concentrations higher than 20 µg/ml are necessary for about one half of the viridans strains, and concentrations of 100 µg/ml or greater may be necessary to exert a bactericidal effect on the enterococci.

Vancomycin, given alone, is the agent of choice in the treatment of methicillin-resistant *S. aureus* infections.[130,131] Some strains of methicillin-resistant *S. aureus*, however, are resistant to vancomycin. If vancomycin therapy is ineffective against severe infections caused by such strains, the addition of an aminoglycoside, rifampin, or both should be considered. Several reports have indicated that vancomycin is not bactericidal for enterococci.[132] Vancomycin is indicated for other serious infections caused by organisms with multiple antibiotic resistance, such as

CSF shunt infections and prosthetic valve infection caused by *S. epidermidis* or *Corynebacterium diphtheriae*.[133] It is the agent of choice for infections caused by penicillin-resistant group JK corynebacteria[134] and is uniformly active against rare, multiply resistant strains of *S. pneumoniae*.[135] Given orally, vancomycin is also the agent of choice for *Clostridium difficile*–associated enterocolitis,[136] although less expensive agents, such as bacitracin[137] and metronidazole,[138] may be as effective.

The usual intravenous dosage of vancomycin in adults with normal renal function is 1 g every 12 hours; 500 mg every 6 hours is a commonly used alternative regimen. As with the aminoglycosides, therapy should be monitored carefully. The dosage of vancomycin must be decreased in patients who have impaired renal function. An initial dose of 15 mg/kg should be given regardless of the extent of renal impairment. When vancomycin is given in conjunction with an aminoglycoside, the dosage in adults should usually be no more than 0.5 g every 8 hours.

Anaphylactoid reactions to vancomycin have been reported since the earliest clinical trials. Such reactions can occur with the first dose; signs and symptoms range from mild pruritus to dramatic hypotension and cardiovascular arrest. The rapid intravenous infusion of vancomycin can cause a peculiar reaction consisting of pruritus; an erythematous or maculopapular rash involving the face, neck, and upper torso; and possible hypotension. This reaction has been referred to as the red neck or red man syndrome. It can often be prevented by slow infusion of the drug over a period of at least 60 minutes. When vancomycin is administered to patients with normal renal function or when therapy is monitored closely in patients with impaired renal function, the incidence of toxicity and side effects is low.[139] Highly purified preparations of vancomycin have been introduced,[140] but further clinical experience is necessary before it can be determined whether these new preparations cause fewer adverse reactions [*see Table 6*].

Metronidazole

Metronidazole was approved in 1959 for use as an antiparasitic agent against *Trichomonas vaginalis*; the drug later proved to be effective against the parasitic organisms *Entamoeba histolytica* and *Giardia lamblia*. In 1981, the FDA approved an intravenous preparation of metronidazole for the treatment of serious infections caused by anaerobic bacteria.[141] Orally administered metronidazole is excellent for treatment of pseudomembranous colitis caused by *C. difficile*. Metronidazole is also useful as part of preoperative prophylactic regimens for elective colorectal surgery. This agent, which appears to act by disrupting bacterial DNA and inhibiting nucleic acid synthesis,[142] is bactericidal against almost all anaerobic gram-negative bacilli, including *B. fragilis*, and against most *Clostridium* species. Although true anaerobic streptococci are generally susceptible to it, microaerophilic streptococci as well as *Actinomyces* and *Propionibacterium* species are often resistant.

Metronidazole is excellent for anaerobic infections of the abdomen and pelvis. For serious anaerobic infections, the drug is administered intravenously; a loading dose of 15 mg/kg is given, followed by 7.5 mg/kg every 6 hours until the patient is well enough to take an oral dosage of 7.5 mg/kg every 6 hours. The dosage need not be reduced in azotemic patients, but it should be reduced in patients with hepatic insufficiency. Because of its bactericidal action and excellent tissue penetration, intravenous metronidazole may be the treatment of choice for *B. fragilis* endocarditis and central nervous system infections, both of which are uncommon. When metronidazole is administered orally, it is well absorbed and is widely distributed in body tissues, including those of the CNS.

Side effects of metronidazole include dry mouth (associated with a metallic taste) and nausea. Concurrent use of alcohol may cause a reaction similar to that produced when alcohol is ingested after taking disulfiram. Neurologic symptoms, including peripheral neuropathy and encephalopathic reactions, and neutropenia are uncommon. Pancreatitis has been reported,[143] but alternative drugs are available.

Carbapenems

The carbapenems include the thienamycins, the olivanic acids, the carpetimycins, the asparenomycins, the pluracidomycins, and other natural and semisynthetic compounds. They are unique among antibiotics in that they have an extraordinary level of activity against commonly encountered anaerobes, such as *B. fragilis* and other *Bacteroides* species, while still possessing excellent activity against aerobic gram-positive and gram-negative organisms.

Structurally, the carbapenems resemble the penicillins in that they have a nucleus containing a β-lactam ring and a five-membered thiazolidine ring. In the carbapenems, however, there is a double bond between the carbon atoms at positions 2 and 3 of the thiazolidine ring, and carbon is substituted for sulfur at position 1. The carbapenems differ from each other primarily in the configurations of the side chains at positions 2 and 6 of the β-lactam ring. They vary with respect to their in vitro spectra of activity and their ability to resist, inhibit, and induce β-lactamases. Many of the carbapenems (e.g., thienamycin) are highly unstable in solution, and some (e.g., imipenem) are degraded by mammalian dehydropeptidases in vivo. A recent review[144] compared the two clinically available carbapenems, imipenem and meropenem.

IMIPENEM-CILASTATIN

Imipenem, the *N*-formimidoyl derivative of thienamycin, was the first commercially available carbapenem antibiotic to come out of the numerous innovative studies that have been done on β-lactam synthesis of penems and carbapenems.[145] It is extensively internalized and metabolized by the renal tubular epithelium. This results in rapid clearance of the agent and absence of active antibiotic in the urine. To circumvent this problem, an inhibitor of the enzyme mediating renal metabolism of imipenem (a dehydropeptidase) was developed. This inhibitor, known as cilastatin, has no documented toxicities, and it is now added to imipenem preparations by the manufacturer.

Imipenem has a broad antibacterial spectrum that includes both aerobes and anaerobes. This spectrum has not changed in the years since the agent was first tested. Early comparative studies showed that imipenem was as effective as cefazolin in the treatment of minor infections.[146] It has also been shown to be highly effective against most bacterial species likely to be encountered in intra-abdominal infections, including *B. fragilis*, most members of the Enterobacteriaceae (including *Enterobacter* species), *P. aeruginosa*, and *S. faecalis*.[147] Theoretically, because it is active against both aerobic and anaerobic organisms, imipenem would be ideally suited to treatment of gynecologic infections. At present, however, there is no convincing evidence that it is superior to the many other available agents, and as one investigator has noted, the frequency with which *Chlamydia* is found in gynecologic infections necessitates the use of an agent such as tetracycline in addition to the β-lactam.

A study comparing imipenem with the combination of clindamycin and gentamicin demonstrated no difference in efficacy but found that the incidence of nephrotoxicity was lower in patients receiving imipenem.[148]

Because of its broad antibacterial spectrum, imipenem has been promoted by its manufacturer as empirical therapy for many life-threatening infections. There are, however, a number of clinical situations in which it is not the first agent that should be considered—namely, community-acquired pneumonia, urinary tract infection, skin structure infection, and osteomyelitis. Imipenem is a useful alternative when toxicity would be a serious problem if an aminoglycoside were used. It can replace combination therapy in mixed infections.

A well-designed, controlled, prospective, randomized trial that compared imipenem therapy with acceptable aminoglycoside-based regimens supports the use of imipenem as monotherapy for intra-abdominal infections in which an enteric mixed flora is anticipated.[149] A total of 290 patients were enrolled in the study, 162 of whom were evaluable. Logistic regression was used to analyze outcome at the abdominal site of infection and mortality. When the analysis was restricted to the residual effect of treatment assignment, a significant improvement in outcome was found in the patients receiving imipenem ($P = 0.043$). The differences in outcome were explained by a higher failure rate for gram-negative infections in the patients receiving tobramycin and clindamycin ($P = 0.018$). This failure rate was reflected in the significantly higher incidence of fasciitis that necessitated reoperation and prosthetic fascial replacement. The study supports the view that imipenem-cilastatin therapy yields better outcomes at intra-abdominal sites of infection than regimens based on conventional dosages of aminoglycosides.

A second study compared broad-spectrum imipenem-cilastatin monotherapy with an aminoglycoside-based antibiotic regimen in the management of intra-abdominal infections.[150] In this study, patients treated with imipenem had fewer febrile episodes, fewer breakthrough bacteremias, less antibiotic resistance, less need for empirical change of drug, and a significantly shorter hospital stay. Imipenem appears to be a safe and efficacious alternative broad-spectrum antibiotic in the treatment of seriously ill patients with intra-abdominal infections.

The primary adverse effect of imipenem is potentiation of seizure disorders. Idiosyncratic reactions and diarrhea are less problematic.

MEROPENEM

Meropenem possesses the exceptional profile of activity typical of the carbapenems and even appears to have some in vitro advantages over imipenem.[151] Additional carbapenems under development include ALP-201 and LJC 10,627.

Carbapenems are among the antibiotics that exert a postantibiotic effect (PAE) against certain medically important bacteria: *S. aureus* (two strains), *P. aeruginosa* (four), *E. coli* (one), *S. marcescens* (one), *Morganella morganii* (one), and *Providencia stuartii* (one). (The PAE is the phenomenon in which bacteria are killed or inhibited from growing after the antibiotic has been eliminated.) The PAE is determined by comparing the serial colony counts of cultures recovering from exposure to drug concentrations at four times the MIC for 1.5 hours with those of control cultures not exposed to the drugs.

Monobactams

The monobactams are monocyclic β-lactam antibiotics that lack the thiazolidine ring found in penicillins and the dihydrothiazine ring found in cephalosporins. Although there are several monobactams under investigation, only aztreonam has been approved for clinical use in the United States. It has been evaluated in open and comparative studies against a number of agents currently used to treat infections.[152,153] It inhibits only aerobic gram-negative species. It can be administered two or three times daily. It is a poor hapten and has been successfully administered to small numbers of patients with proven allergy to penicillins and cephalosporins.[154]

Aztreonam has been shown to be effective against bacteremia caused by *E. coli*, *K. pneumoniae*, *P. mirabilis*, *S. marcescens*, *P. aeruginosa*, *Enterobacter* species, *Proteus* species, and *Providencia* species.[155,156] It has also been used, alone or in combination with clindamycin, to treat gram-negative aspiration pneumonia, with results comparable or superior to those obtained with an aminoglycoside-clindamycin combination.[157,158]

Aztreonam has been advocated as directed therapy to obviate more toxic drugs. It seems possible that aztreonam could replace aminoglycosides in many situations in which they are combined with other agents.

β-Lactamase Inhibitors

A novel approach to antibacterial chemotherapy is the use of β-lactamase inhibitors with β-lactam agents. Clavulanate has been combined with both amoxicillin and ticarcillin. Because neither clavulanate nor sulbactam inhibits the β-lactamases that function primarily as cephalosporinases in *Enterobacter*, *Serratia*, and *P. aeruginosa*, addition of clavulanate or sulbactam does not enhance ticarcillin's activity against *Pseudomonas*. The principal use of amoxicillin-clavulanate has been in the treatment of upper respiratory tract infections caused by β-lactamase–producing *H. influenzae* or *M. catarrhalis*. Ticarcillin-clavulanate has been used to treat pneumonia caused by *P. aeruginosa* and mixed β-lactamase–producing flora as well as intra-abdominal infections and gynecologic infections in which the infecting organisms often possess β-lactamases. In febrile neutropenic patients, its efficacy is comparable to that of other agents, but superinfections may be a problem.[159,160] Because some strains of *K. pneumoniae* are not adequately inhibited by ticarcillin-clavulanate, addition of an aminoglycoside would be appropriate in neutropenic patients. Sulbactam has also been combined with ampicillin.

Clavulanate, sulbactam, and tazobactam have all been combined with piperacillin in an attempt to enhance the agent's activity against β-lactamase–producing bacteria.[161,162] Tazobactam enhances the spectrum of action and potency of piperacillin to a greater extent than sulbactam does. Although piperacillin-clavulanate is more potent than piperacillin-tazobactam, the two combinations are effective against virtually the same spectrum of resistant β-lactamase–producing gram-negative organisms. Piperacillin-tazobactam is more potent than ticarcillin-clavulanate and is effective against a wider range of gram-negative enteric organisms. Combinations of piperacillin with tazobactam or clavulanate have a broader spectrum of activity than combinations of piperacillin with sulbactam against bacteria that produce characterized plasmid-mediated enzymes of clinical significance. In particular, piperacillin-tazobactam and piperacillin-clavulanate inhibit TEM-1, TEM-2, and SHV-1 β-lactamases, but piperacillin-sulbactam does not. In mice infected with β-lactamase–producing *E. coli, K. pneumoniae, P. mirabilis,* and *S. aureus,* both tazobactam and clavulanate have provided greater enhancement of the therapeutic efficacy of piperacillin than sulbactam has. Reviews of the TEM-type β-lactamases[163] and the piperacillin-tazobactam combinations[164] have been published.

Quinolones

The quinolones are promising agents for several reasons: their antimicrobial spectrum of activity is wide, some of them can be used both orally and parenterally, and their toxicity does not appear to be excessive.[165,166] The newer quinolones—ciprofloxacin, norfloxacin, enoxacin, pefloxacin, and ofloxacin—have excellent activity against most isolates of Enterobacteriaceae, including organisms resistant to aminoglycosides and cephalosporins. Worldwide, most isolates are inhibited by concentrations of 0.002 to 2 µg/ml; these concentrations are readily achievable at the usual dosages [see Table 5]. All five agents are highly active against *H. influenzae, N. gonorrhoeae,* and *M. catarrhalis.* All are effective against *P. aeruginosa* at achievable urine levels. In particular, ciprofloxacin inhibits 90% of isolates at a concentration of 1 µg/ml in most of the published studies. The quinolones are also strongly active against staphylococci, including methicillin-resistant isolates: 90% of isolates are inhibited by an ofloxacin or ciprofloxacin concentration of 1 µg/ml. In addition, they possess impressive activity against important intracellular pathogens, such as *Brucella* species, *Legionella* species, *C. trachomatis, M. pneumoniae,* and *M. tuberculosis.* They readily penetrate phagocytic cells.

The species that the quinolones may not be effective against are the streptococci, including *S. pneumoniae* and *S. faecalis*; anaerobic cocci and bacilli may also pose problems, depending on which agent is used. Some newly synthesized quinolones, which have not yet been administered to humans, do inhibit these organisms.[167]

Resistance to the quinolones as a result of single-step mutations occurs in fewer than 0.0000001% of cases and is at least 300 times rarer than comparable resistance to the older quinolone nalidixic acid. Nevertheless, repeated exposure of bacteria to any of the newer quinolones can result in the selection of resistant organisms.[168] Cross-resistance to all quinolones is usually observed, and resistance may extend to other classes of antibiotics, including β-lactam agents. Bacteria resistant to the newer quinolones (most often, *P. aeruginosa, S. marcescens,* and staphylococci) have been found in the sputum of cystic fibrosis patients, in chronic wounds, and occasionally in the lesions of urinary tract infections. Whether the use of combination therapy (see below) will decrease the development of resistance remains to be established.

Additional quinolones are currently under investigation; these include lomefloxacin, temafloxacin, rufloxacin, tosufloxacin, levofloxacin, and sporfloxacin.

PHARMACOKINETICS

All of the quinolones are well absorbed from the GI tract, even in elderly, debilitated, or critically ill patients; however, ofloxacin is absorbed better than ciprofloxacin, pefloxacin, or enoxacin.[169,170] The presence of food does not decrease absorption, but it delays attainment of peak serum concentrations. The quinolones are widely distributed to body tissues and fluids: the apparent volume of distribution is 90 to 110 L. Tissue concentrations (except in the brain, saliva, and bronchial secretions) are at least as high as serum concentrations. Excellent concentrations are achieved in the lungs, the bones, the prostate, the kidneys, and macrophages and leukocytes.[171]

The quinolones are metabolized to varying degrees: only about 5% of an ofloxacin dose is converted to metabolites, whereas pefloxacin is almost entirely metabolized. The metabolites are generally less active than the parent compounds and do not accumulate in tissues. All of the quinolones are excreted renally, primarily by tubular secretion. The concentrations attained in the urine far exceed the MICs for most urinary pathogens, even in the presence of renal insufficiency.[169,172] Nonrenal clearance helps compensate for decreased excretion in patients with renal dysfunction who are receiving a quinolone (except for those receiving ofloxacin)

CLINICAL UTILITY

Urinary Tract Infections

All of the quinolones have proved to be at least as effective as the traditional regimens of amoxicillin or trimethoprim-sulfamethoxazole in the treatment of uncomplicated and complicated urinary tract infections (UTIs).[173] Because of their higher cost and the possibility that resistance will develop, they are not recommended as therapy for simple cystitis. These agents may be used to treat complicated UTIs caused by multiresistant organisms, either as an alternative to or as follow-up to parenteral therapy. Their advantage lies in the possibility of achieving high urinary and intestinal concentrations, which decrease the likelihood of resistance and of reinfection or superinfection in bedridden patients.[169] In UTIs caused by *P. aeruginosa,* the fluoroquinolones have been proved effective, but resistant strains have emerged repeatedly.[173]

The quinolones have been used with some success in patients with renal failure[173]; however, dosages must be titrated properly. Concomitant use of antacids or phosphate binders that decrease intestinal absorption of the quinolones may adversely affect therapeutic outcome.

Acute and chronic prostatitis can also be treated with quinolones. Patients with chronic prostatitis, however, tend to relapse if the infecting organism is *P. aeruginosa* or *E. coli.* Still, the quinolones are at least as effective as the drugs used in the standard regimens.

Sexually Transmitted Diseases

All of the quinolones are effective as single-dose therapy for gonorrhea, including gonorrhea caused by penicillinase-producing strains.[174,175] They cannot, however, eradicate *Chlamydia* organisms.

Diarrheal Diseases

The quinolones are highly active against organisms that cause bacterial diarrhea: *Shigella* species, *Salmonella* species, toxicogenic *E. coli, Campylobacter* species, *Aeromonas* species, *Vibrio cholerae,* and *V. parahaemolyticus* are all eradicated by 48 hours of quinolone therapy.[169,176] *C. difficile,* however, is not inhibited and has caused colitis in rare instances. In addition, ciprofloxacin and norfloxacin have been effective in the carrier state of typhoid.

Skin and Skin Structure Infections

Many types of skin infections have been successfully treated with quinolones. Ofloxacin and ciprofloxacin are as effective as standard oral and parenteral regimens[171,177]; enoxacin appears to be somewhat less promising.[178]

Joint and Bone Infections

The main reason for testing the quinolones in joint and bone infections is that use of an oral agent eliminates the need to hospitalize patients for parenteral administration of antibiotics. Furthermore, because the quinolones have a long half-life and are well tolerated, compliance is likely to be high during the long treatment periods often necessary to cure these infections. To date, pefloxacin, ciprofloxacin, and ofloxacin have been studied.[179] The results achieved with these agents have been comparable to those achieved with parenteral regimens, but in many cases, follow-up has been too short or is still incomplete. As with skin infections, surgical intervention is often a valuable adjunct to antibiotic therapy.

Respiratory Infections

Ciprofloxacin, ofloxacin, enoxacin, and pefloxacin have been evaluated in the treatment of the acute exacerbation of chronic bronchitis.[180] Ofloxacin yields the best bacteriologic and clinical results because of its higher sputum concentration and its lower MIC for *S. pneumoniae*; ciprofloxacin yields the next best results. Even though some degree of success has been achieved with the quinolones, they remain second-line agents because of their limited activity against *S. pneumoniae*. This is true in patients with community-acquired pneumonia as well as in those with acutely exacerbated chronic bronchitis.

The problem of multiresistant organisms and the search for newer, more potent alternative treatments have led to growing interest in using quinolones as therapy for nosocomial pneumonia. Although further studies are necessary to define the potential role of the quinolones in this setting more clearly, the initial results are promising. These agents remain valid alternatives when resistance emerges or when follow-up oral therapy is indicated.[181]

The quinolones have also been used to treat pulmonary exacerbations in cystic fibrosis patients because they are highly active against the main causative organisms (*P. aeruginosa*, *S. aureus*, and *H. influenzae*) and can be given orally. The clinical improvement obtained after therapy with ciprofloxacin or ofloxacin is comparable to that obtained after parenteral antibiotic therapy.[169,171] However, *P. aeruginosa* is not eradicated from the sputum; in fact, a steady increase in MICs for this organism is a regular occurrence. This problem is also encountered with standard regimens. In either case, it can be minimized by avoiding prolonged therapy (longer than 4 to 8 weeks) and by alternating the agents used.

Intra-abdominal Infections

The fluoroquinolones currently available have modest activity against anaerobes. Newer fluoroquinolones with increased in vitro activity against anaerobes are under development. These include levofloxacin, clinafloxacin, sparfloxacin, trovafloxacin, grepafloxacin, and DU-6859[182]; trovafloxacin and grepafloxacin were recently approved for clinical use in the United States. A recent randomized, double-blind, multicenter trial comparing ciprofloxacin-metronidazole with imipenem-cilastatin for the treatment of complicated intra-abdominal infections demonstrated the efficacy of the quinolones.[183] Patients were randomized to I.V. ciprofloxacin-metronidazole, I.V. imipenem, or I.V. ciprofloxacin-metronidazole followed by oral ciprofloxacin-metronidazole when oral feeding was resumed. The results demonstrated statistical equivalence between I.V. ciprofloxacin-metronidazole and I.V. imipenem in both the intent-to-treat and valid populations. Conversion to oral therapy with ciprofloxacin appeared to be as effective as continued I.V. therapy in patients able to tolerate oral feedings. Of the new quinolones, those with extremely broad-spectrum in vitro coverage, such as clinafloxacin and trovafloxacin, have the potential for widespread use in intra-abdominal infections pending favorable outcomes of current phase III clinical trials. The excellent oral absorption of these agents permits I.V.-to-oral stepdown therapy, a promising practice that is likely to reduce costs and improve the quality of care of patients with intra-abdominal infections.[184]

ADVERSE EFFECTS

Adverse reactions to the quinolones are estimated to occur in 4% to 8% of cases.[185] Most such reactions are not severe: cessation of therapy has been necessary in only about 1% to 2% of patients, and in all cases, the reactions have been reversible. The most common adverse effects are gastrointestinal—namely, nausea, vomiting, and diarrhea. The next most common are central nervous system effects, which include dizziness, headache, insomnia, hallucinations, agitation, and seizures. (The last three have been attributed to coadministration of enoxacin and theophylline.) Other effects include skin rash, pruritus, photosensitivity (with ofloxacin and pefloxacin), and mild alterations in hematologic and biochemical laboratory values.

Complications of Antibiotic Therapy

Widespread resistance to antimicrobials has become a problem in the United States. This is especially evident in intensive care units. Organisms frequently encountered in ICUs include *P. aeruginosa*, *S. aureus*, *H. influenzae* (particularly in trauma victims), enterococci, *K. pneumoniae*, *Enterobacter* species, *Acinetobacter baumanii*, *E. coli*, and *Stenotrophomonas* (*Xanthomonas*) *maltophilia*. Although antibiotics have played a major role in the treatment of such infections, the pathogens have responded to the antibiotic challenge, developing resistance to all available antimicrobial agents to a greater or lesser degree. Specific mechanisms of resistance are evident in the reduced permeability of cell wall membranes, changes in the target sites of antimicrobial agents, enzymatic inactivation of antibiotics, and the development of pathways bypassing antimicrobial targets.[186]

Clinically significant resistance has been associated with some of the third-generation cephalosporins, such as ceftriaxone and ceftazidime, even in preclinical trials. These observations, based on reported in vivo use rather than on in vitro predictions, are extremely disconcerting.

Colonization and superinfection have long been recognized as potential complications of antimicrobial therapy. *Suprainfection*—a more descriptive term that refers to superinfection related to antibiotic therapy—must also be distinguished from colonization. Suprainfection connotes both clinical and bacteriologic evidence of a new infection, whereas colonization refers only to bacteriologic evidence of a new infection.[187,188]

The incidence of suprainfection with cephalosporin therapy is actually quite low (less than 5%); however, the organisms encountered are often more virulent and difficult to eradicate than the original infecting pathogen.[189] Commonly seen suprainfecting pathogens include *Enterobacter* species, *P. aeruginosa*, *S. aureus*, *Acinetobacter* species, enterococci, and *Candida* species. Because these organisms are generally multiresistant, therapy with antibiotic combinations, including aminoglycosides, is usually necessary.

There appear to be no significant differences among the cephalosporins with respect to the incidence of suprainfection or the types of suprainfecting pathogens found.

The most worrisome resistance is that of vancomycin-resistant enterococci (VRE). Risk factors for bloodstream infection with VRE are an increasing APACHE II (Acute Physiology and Chronic Health Evaluation II) score, treatment with vancomycin, or a diagnosis of hematologic malignancy. Thus, severe illness, underlying disease, and use of vancomycin are major risk factors for infection of the bloodstream with VRE.[190]

In the United States, more than 90% of strains of *S. aureus*, one of the most common disease-producing organisms in humans, are resistant to penicillin and other β-lactam antibiotics.[191] Before 1987, antibiotic-resistant strains of *S. pneumoniae* (pneumococci) were relatively rare in the United States, but recent reports document an alarming increase in pneumococcal infections resistant to commonly used antibiotics.[192] According to the National Centers for Disease Control and Prevention (CDC), the incidence of vancomycin-resistant enterococci in the United States increased 20 times from January 1989 to March 1993.[193] Enterococci are the most common cause of hospital-acquired infections, and vancomycin is often the weapon of last resort against these potentially deadly microbes.

Fueling the excessive use of broad-spectrum antimicrobial drugs is the lack of reliable tests that would permit physicians to discern when antimicrobial drugs are not needed. When antimicrobial therapy is needed, improved diagnostic tests would permit better targeting and thereby reduce the widespread administration of broad-spectrum drugs. Selective pressure exerted by widespread antimicrobial use is the driving force in the development of antibiotic resistance. The association between increased rates of antimicrobial use and resistance has been documented for nosocomial infections[194] and community-acquired infections in studies associating resistance patterns with rates of drug use on a regional or national basis.[195] Case-control studies have shown that antimicrobial use is a significant risk factor for infection with a resistant pathogen.[196] In 1988, the National Academy of Sciences/Institute of Medicine estimated that nearly half of the annual production of antibiotics is directed toward use in farm animals.[197]

Resistance to antimicrobial drugs is a global problem. Multi-drug-resistant pathogens travel not only locally but globally. Because of increased international travel and increased foreign trade in fresh-food products, the threat of global spread of antibiotic resistance is greater than ever. There is no national or global surveillance system for monitoring of antibiotic resistance in animals or humans. The most recent survey available, conducted in 1992, found that the United States spends less than $55,000 at the federal, state, and local levels for monitoring of antibiotic resistance in human pathogens.[198] National and international surveillance systems should be established, and basic research is needed to delineate the genetic and metabolic pathways, including essential regulatory factors, that determine virulence as well as antibiotic susceptibility or resistance in pathogens of human and veterinary importance.

The Future

In the war against bacterial disease, microbes have been on the offensive, and they can evade antibiotics in many ways. They have general pumps that remove several types of harmful compounds, including antibiotics, from the cell as well as pumps for specific antibodies. Bacteria can also produce enzymes that destroy or inactivate antibiotics, develop substitute proteins that are not targeted by the drugs, or change their cell wall proteins to keep drugs from getting in.[199] Researchers have recently reported work on nearly a dozen new antibiotics that show promise in controlling drug-resistant organisms. These antibiotics target protein synthesis (oxazolidinones, glycylcyclines, streptogramines, boxazomycins, and ketolides), cell wall formation (LY333328 and new β-lactams), or DNA replication (2-pyridone and new fluoroquinolones). Other antibiotics target tyrosine kinase inhibition[200] or lipid A.[201] More innovative approaches will use peptide antibiotics such as defensins and thionins, cepropins, indocidin, and bactenecin.[202] Most investigators working on these agents feel that the era of "classical antibiotics" is over and that novel approaches to bacterial resistance are needed if we are to win the battle of the microbes.

References

1. Jones RN: NCCLS regulatory guidelines. Antimicrobic Newsletter 1:5, 1984
2. Murray PR, Jorgensen JH: Quantitative susceptibility test methods in major United States medical centers. Antimicrob Agents Chemother 20:66, 1981
3. Reller LB: The serum bactericidal test. Rev Infect Dis 8:803, 1986
4. Weinstein MP, Stratton CW, Ackley A, et al: Multicenter collaborative evaluation of a standardized serum bactericidal test as a prognostic indicator in infective endocarditis. Am J Med 78:262, 1985
5. MacFarlane JT, Finch RG, Ward MJ, et al: Hospital study of adult community-acquired pneumonia. Lancet 2:255, 1982
6. Hausmann W, Karlish AJ: Staphylococcal pneumonias in adults. Br Med J 2:285, 1956
7. Feldman C, Kallenbach JM, Miller SD, et al: Community-acquired pneumonia due to penicillin-resistant pneumococci. N Engl J Med 313:615, 1985
8. Finegold SA: Aspiration pneumonia, lung abscess, and empyema. Respiratory Infections: Diagnosis and Management. Pennington JE, Ed. Raven Press, New York, 1983, p 191
9. Bohnan JA, Solomkin JS, Dellinger EP, et al: Guidelines for clinical care: anti-infective agents for intra-abdominal infection (a Surgical Infection Society policy statement). Arch Surg 127:83, 1992
10. Williams DN, Rehm SJ, Tice AD, et al: Practice guidelines for community-based parenteral anti-infective therapy. Clin Infect Dis 25:787, 1997
11. Tomasz A: From penicillin-binding proteins to the lysis and death of bacteria: a 1979 view. Rev Infect Dis 1:434, 1979
12. Wormer DC, Martin WJ, Nichold DR, et al: Concentrations in serum of procaine and crystalline penicillin G administered orally or parenterally. Antibiotics in Medicine 1:589, 1955
13. Gilbert DN, Sanford JP: Methicillin: critical appraisal after a decade of experience. Med Clin North Am 54:1113, 1970
14. Amoxicillin. Med Lett Drugs Ther 16:49, 1974
15. Bodey GP, Whitecar JP Jr, Middleman E, et al: Carbenicillin therapy for *Pseudomonas* infections. JAMA 218:62, 1971
16. Hoffman TA, Bullock WE: Carbenicillin therapy of *Pseudomonas* and other gram-negative bacillary infections. Ann Intern Med 73:165, 1970
17. Butler K, English AR, Ray VA, et al: Carbenicillin: chemistry and mode of action. J Infect Dis 122(suppl):S1, 1970
18. Hoffman TA, Cestero R, Bullock WE: Pharmacodynamics of carbenicillin in hepatic and renal failure. Ann Intern Med 73:173, 1970
19. Ticarcillin. Med Lett Drugs Ther 19:17, 1977
20. Tjandramaga TB, Mullie A, Verbesselt R, et al: Piperacillin: human pharmacokinetics after intravenous and intramuscular administration. Antimicrob Agents Chemother 14:829, 1978
21. Bergan T: Pharmacokinetics of mezlocillin in healthy volunteers. Antimicrob Agents Chemother 14:801, 1978
22. Bergan T, Brodwall EK, Wiik-Larsen E: Mezlocillin pharmacokinetics in patients with

normal and impaired renal functions. Antimicrob Agents Chemother 16:651, 1979

23. Gentry LO, Jemsek JG, Natelson EA: Effects of sodium piperacillin on platelet function in normal volunteers. Antimicrob Agents Chemother 19:532, 1981

24. Fu KP, Neu HC: Azlocillin and mezlocillin: new ureido penicillins. Antimicrob Agents Chemother 13:930, 1978

25. Bodey GP, Le Blanc B: Piperacillin: in vitro evaluation. Antimicrob Agents Chemother 14:78, 1978

26. White AR, Comber KR, Sutherland R: Comparative bactericidal effects of azlocillin and ticarcillin against Pseudomonas aeruginosa. Antimicrob Agents Chemother 18:182, 1980

27. Basker MJ, Edmondson RA, Sutherland R: Comparative antibacterial activity of azlocillin, mezlocillin, carbenicillin and ticarcillin and relative stability to beta-lactamases of Pseudomonas aeruginosa and Klebsiella aerogenes. Infection 7:67, 1979

28. Pancoast SJ, Jahre JA, Neu HC: Mezlocillin in the therapy of serious infections. Am J Med 67:747, 1979

29. Pancoast S, Prince AS, Francke EL, et al: Clinical evaluation of piperacillin therapy for infection. Arch Intern Med 141:1447, 1981

30. Winston DJ, Murphy W, Young LS, et al: Piperacillin therapy for serious bacterial infections. Am J Med 69:255, 1980

31. Ellis CJ, Geddes AM, Davey PG, et al: Mezlocillin and azlocillin: an evaluation of two new β-lactam antibiotics. J Antimicrob Chemother 5:517, 1979

32. Kunin CM, Chambers S: Responsibility of the infectious disease community for optimal use of antibiotics: views of the membership of the Infectious Diseases Society of America. Rev Infect Dis 7:547, 1985

33. Malangoni MA, Condon RE, Spiegel CA: Treatment of intra-abdominal infections is appropriate with single-agent or combination antibiotic therapy. Surgery 98:648, 1985

34. Tally FP, McGowan K, Kellum JM, et al: A randomized comparison of cefoxitin with or without amikacin and clindamycin plus amikacin in surgical sepsis. Ann Surg 193:318, 1981

35. Donowitz GR, Mandell GL: Empiric therapy for pneumonia. Rev Infect Dis 5(suppl):S40, 1983

36. Marx MA, Fant WK: Cefuroxime axetil. Drug Intell Clin Pharm 22:651, 1988

37. Cefotetan disodium (Cefotan). Med Lett Drugs Ther 28:70, 1986

38. Orr JW Jr, Varner RE, Kilgore LC, et al: Cefotetan versus cefoxitin as prophylaxis in hysterectomy. Am J Obstet Gynecol 154:960, 1986

39. McCarty JM, Renteria A: Treatment of pharyngitis and tonsillitis with cefprozil: review of three multicenter trials. Clin Infect Dis 14(suppl 2):S224, 1992

40. Doern G: In vitro activity of loracarbef and effects of susceptibility test methods. Am J Med 92:7S, 1992

41. Stefani S, Pellegrino MB, D'Amico G, et al: In vitro activity of a new broad-spectrum, beta-lactamase-stable oral cephalosporin, cefixime, in comparison with other drugs, against Haemophilus influenzae, Haemophilus parainfluenzae, Moraxella catarrhalis and Streptococcus pneumoniae. Chemotherapy 38:36, 1992

42. Wise R, Andrews JM, Ashby JP, et al: Ceftibuten: a new orally absorbed cephalosporin: in vitro activity against strains from the United Kingdom. Diagn Microbiol Infect Dis 14:45, 1991

43. Edelstein H, Chirurgi V, Oster S, et al: A randomized trial of cefepime (BMY-28142) and ceftazidime for the treatment of pneumonia. J Antimicrob Chemother 28:569, 1991

44. Reeves DS: In vitro activity of piperacillin and other microbials on 491 bacterial isolates. Arch Intern Med 142:2023, 1982

45. Hall WH, Opfer BJ, Gerding DN: Comparative activities of the oxa-β-lactam LY127935, cefotaxime, cefoperazone, cefamandole, and ticarcillin against multiply resistant gram-negative bacilli. Antimicrob Agents Chemother 17:273, 1980

46. Woolfrey BF, Fox JMK, Quall CO: Susceptibility of Pseudomonas aeruginosa to cefoperazone, cefotaxime, and moxalactam with special reference to isolates resistant to aminoglycosides, carbenicillin and ticarcillin. J Antimicrob Chemother 8:205, 1981

47. Magnussen CR, Sammartino MT, Ernest KD: Aminoglycoside-resistant gram-negative bacilli in a community hospital: comparative in vitro activity of cefotaxime, moxalactam, cefoperazone and piperacillin. Antimicrob Agents Chemother 22:154, 1982

48. Neu HC: The new beta-lactamase–stable cephalosporins. Ann Intern Med 97:408, 1982

49. Jones RN, Barry AL: Cefoperazone: a review of its antimicrobial spectrum, β-lactamase stability, enzyme inhibition, and other in vitro characteristics. Rev Infect Dis 5(suppl):S108, 1983

50. Carmine AA, Brogden RN, Heel RC, et al: Cefotaxime: a review of its antibacterial activity, pharmacological properties and therapeutic use. Drugs 25:223, 1983

51. Strandberg DA, Jorgensen JH, Drutz DJ: Activities of aztreonam and new cephalosporins against infrequently isolated gram-negative bacilli. Antimicrob Agents Chemother 24:282, 1983

52. Moellering RC Jr, Willey S, Eliopoulos GM: Synergism and antagonism of ceftizoxime and other new cephalosporins. J Antimicrob Chemother 10(suppl C):69, 1982

53. Watanakunakorn C: In vitro activity of ceftriaxone alone and in combination with gentamicin, tobramycin, and amikacin against Pseudomonas aeruginosa. Antimicrob Agents Chemother 24:305, 1983

54. Corrado ML, Landesman SH, Cherubin CE: Influence of inoculum size on activity of cefoperazone, cefotaxime, moxalactam, piperacillin, and N-formimidoyl thienamycin (MKO787) against Pseudomonas aeruginosa. Antimicrob Agents Chemother 18:893, 1980

55. Sanders CC, Sanders WE Jr: Emergence of resistance during therapy with the newer β-lactam antibiotics: role of inducible β-lactamases and implications for the future. Rev Infect Dis 5:639, 1983

56. Shimizu K: Cefoperazone: absorption, excretion, distribution, and metabolism. Clin Ther 3(special issue):60, 1980

57. Patel IH, Chen S, Parsonnet M, et al: Pharmacokinetics of ceftriaxone in humans. Antimicrob Agents Chemother 20:634, 1981

58. Stoeckel K, McNamara PJ, Brandt R, et al: Effects of concentration-dependent plasma protein binding on ceftriaxone kinetics. Clin Pharmacol Ther 29:650, 1981

59. Boscia JA, Korzeniowski OM, Snepar R, et al: Cefoperazone pharmacokinetics in normal subjects and patients with cirrhosis. Antimicrob Agents Chemother 23:385, 1983

60. Kemmerich B, Lode H, Borner K, et al: Biliary excretion and pharmacokinetics of cefoperazone in humans. J Antimicrob Chemother 12:27, 1983

61. Ti TY, Fortin L, Kreeft JH, et al: Kinetic disposition of intravenous ceftriaxone in normal subjects and patients with renal failure on hemodialysis or peritoneal dialysis. Antimicrob Agents Chemother 25:83, 1984

62. Wise R, Wright N, Wills PJ: Pharmacology of cefotaxime and its desacetyl metabolite in renal and hepatic disease. Antimicrob Agents Chemother 19:526, 1981

63. Wittmann DH, Schassan HH: Distribution of moxalactam in serum, bone, tissue fluid, and peritoneal fluid. Rev Infect Dis 4(suppl):S610, 1982

64. Saito Y, Kushima T, Seimori T, et al: Absorption and excretion of cefotaxime and its levels in uterine arterial blood, female internal genital organ tissue and pelvic cavity fluid. Jpn J Antibiot 34:481, 1981

65. Grabe M, Andersson KE, Forsgren A, et al: Concentrations of cefotaxime in serum, urine, and tissues of urological patients. Infection 9:154, 1981

66. Kosmidis J, Stathakis C, Mantopoulos K, et al: Clinical pharmacology of cefotaxime including penetration into bile, sputum, bone and cerebrospinal fluid. J Antimicrob Chemother 6(suppl A):147, 1980

67. Watts JM, McDonald PJ, Woods PJ: Clinical trials of antimicrobials in surgery. World J Surg 6:321, 1982

68. Solomkin JS, Meakins JL Jr, Allo MD, et al: Antibiotic trials in intra-abdominal infections: a critical evaluation of study design and outcome reporting. Ann Surg 200:29, 1984

69. Feinstein AR: Clinical Biostatistics. CV Mosby Co, St Louis, 1977

70. Phair JP, Bassaris HP, Williams JE, et al: Bacteremic pneumonia due to gram-negative bacilli. Arch Intern Med 143:2147, 1983

71. Gross PA, Neu HC, Aswapokee P, et al: Deaths from nosocomial infections: experience in a university hospital and a community hospital. Am J Med 68:219, 1980

72. Bryan CS, Reynolds KL: Bacteremic nosocomial pneumonia: analysis of 172 episodes from a single metropolitan area. Am Rev Respir Dis 129:668, 1984

73. Rodriguez J, Vazquez GJ, Bermudez RH, et al: A randomized clinical trial of ceftizoxime and cefamandole in the treatment of serious lower respiratory tract infections. J Antimicrob Chemother 10(suppl C):209, 1982

74. LeFrock JL, Molavi A, Lentnek AL, et al: Comparative study of ceftizoxime and cefamandole in the treatment of bronchopulmonary infections. J Antimicrob Chemother 10(suppl C):215, 1982

75. Neu HC: β-Lactam antibiotics: structural relationships affecting in vitro activity and pharmacologic properties. Rev Infect Dis 8(suppl 3):S237, 1986

76. Baumgartner JD, Glauser MP: Comparative study of imipenem in severe infections. J Antimicrob Chemother 12(suppl D):141, 1983

77. Stamboulian D, Argüello EA, Jasovich A, et al: Comparative clinical evaluation of imipenem/cilastatin vs. cefotaxime in treatment of severe bacterial infections. Rev Infect Dis 7:S458, 1985

78. Collatz E, Gutmann L, Williamson R, et al: Development of resistance to β-lactam antibiotics with special reference to third-generation cephalosporins. J Antimicrob Chemother 14(suppl B):13, 1984

79. Sanders CC, Sanders WE Jr: Microbial resistance to newer generation β-lactam antibiotics: clinical and laboratory implications. J Infect Dis 151:399, 1985

80. Nichols RL: Empiric antibiotic therapy for intraabdominal infections. Rev Infect Dis 5:S90, 1983

81. Lea AS, Feliciano DV, Gentry LO: Intra-abdominal infections: an update. J Antimicrob Chemother 9(suppl A):107, 1982

82. Barie PS, Christou NV, Dellinger EP, et al: Pathogenicity of the enterococcus in surgical infections. Ann Surg 212:155, 1990

High fever (> 38.9° C [102.02° F]) develops within 48 hr of operation
Consider:
• Atelectasis (suggested by decreased breath sounds or rales, or both, and by platelike densities or volume loss on x-ray): Manage via standard physical measures.
• Peritonitis from a leaking viscus (suggested by hemodynamic changes, diffuse abdominal tenderness, excessive early fluid requirements, and tachycardia): Treat with operative intervention and antibiotics.
• Invasive wound infection: Inspect wound and obtain Gram's stain of wound contents; treat with operative intervention and antibiotics.

Infection related to intravascular devices

Catheter-associated urinary tract infection

Remove catheter as soon as possible.
Symptomatic bacteriuria:
Give appropriate antibiotics on the basis of culture and sensitivity results.
Asymptomatic bacteriuria: Treat with appropriate antibiotic for 1 day after catheter removal. Culture urine 1 wk later; if bacteriuria persists, give appropriate antibiotics for 7 to 10 days.

Enteric infection

Consider antibiotic-associated colitis in any patient with diarrhea.
Severe cases: Identify mucosal changes immediately via endoscopy.
All cases: Culture stool for *Clostridium difficile* and assay for *C. difficile* toxin.
Severe diarrhea with systemic manifestations: Discontinue antibiotics. Give metronidazole (500 mg p.o., t.i.d.); if unresponsive to metronidazole, give vancomycin (125 mg p.o., q.i.d.).
Mild cases: Discontinue antibiotics.

Systemic symptoms suggest catheter-related septicemia

Peripheral catheters:
Remove and culture via semiquantitative technique.
Central venous catheters:
If local signs of infection are present, remove catheter and culture insertion site and catheter.
If local infection is not present:
• Consider placing a second catheter over a guide wire.
• Culture intracutaneous segment, or the intracutaneous segment and the distal tip, of first catheter semiquantitatively.

Infection is localized

Remove catheter promptly, and culture via semiquantitative technique. Place any new catheter in a different site.

Infection progresses to septic thrombophlebitis

Correct surgically.

Culture results are not available, or empirical treatment is required

Include antibiotic effective against methicillin-resistant *Staphylococcus aureus* (e.g., vancomycin) in therapy.

Culture results are positive

Give appropriate antibiotics. Remove any second catheter placed by guide wire; place any new catheter in a different site.

Culture results are negative

Second catheter may be left in place.

ing the probable cause. If tracheitis or bronchitis is suspected, it can be treated with a brief course of antibiotics.

Paranasal sinusitis is a potentially lethal nosocomial infection, especially in ICU patients with nasogastric or nasotracheal tubes in place.[15-20] In one report, it accounted for 5% of all nosocomial infections.[15] The diagnosis of paranasal sinusitis should be considered in any febrile postoperative patient with nasal tubes or with facial fractures. Purulent nasal drainage is an important clue but may not be present. Plain films can be diagnostic but are often difficult to interpret in these patients because of superimposition of tubes, preexisting injuries, and suboptimal portable films. Fluid, air-fluid levels, and mucosal thickening are more easily detected by computed tomography. Diagnosis ultimately requires demonstration of white blood cells and bacteria on Gram's stain of sinus aspirate as well as culture for identification and sensitivity testing.

In one study of 67 patients with craniofacial injuries who underwent prospective otoscopy three times a week, 11 patients experienced either serous or purulent otitis media and were all found to have purulent paranasal sinusitis as well. Eleven of 12 patients who were ultimately diagnosed as having purulent paranasal sinusitis had coexistent otitis media.[21]

The spectrum of causative bacteria of paranasal sinusitis is similar to that of nosocomial pneumonia. Treatment includes removal of all nasal tubes and administration of decongestants and antibiotics. Occasionally, sinus irrigation or drainage, or both, may be required. If empirical therapy must be initiated before specific culture results are known, the agents chosen should be effective against bacteria known to be present in sputum. The best method of prevention is to limit the number and the duration of use of nasal tubes.

Inflammation and infection of the nasopharyngeal mucosa can be significant in an ICU patient, although it is not often identified. Eustachian tube blockage, either from tubes or from inflammation, can be associated with either serous or infective otitis media. Prudent use of tubes is the most effective preventive measure. If clinical infection is recognized, tube removal and decongestants will usually provide adequate treatment.

Infection Related to Operative Site or Injury

SURGICAL SITE INFECTION

An infection of a surgical wound—that is, an incisional surgical site infection (SSI) [see 39 Prevention of Postoperative Infection]—traditionally reflects on a surgeon's care and skill and is the classic surgical nosocomial infection. Such infections are diagnosed primarily on the basis of local findings. Erythema, swelling, and drainage, as well as increasing local pain and tenderness in a site at which pain should be decreasing, all suggest infection. Fever and an elevated white blood cell count may or may not be present. An incisional SSI develops most commonly in the subcutaneous layer, although animal studies fail to explain this observation.[22] In an obese patient, however, a thick, overlying layer of uninfected tissue may obscure evidence of infection and thus delay diagnosis. Presentation may also be delayed if the infection begins in anatomic layers below fascial and muscular barriers, such as after a thoracotomy or an operation on the femur.

Whether an infection will occur in a wound is probably determined within the first few hours of wounding[23,24]; efforts to prevent wound infection are probably ineffective after this period.[25-29] The incidence of SSI is reduced with appropriate use of perioperative antibiotics [see 39 Prevention of Postoperative Infection].[30,31] However, there is no advantage to continuing prophylactic antibiotics beyond the perioperative period in response to fever or local wound erythema in the hope of preventing an overt SSI.[32,33]

The risk that an SSI will develop in an individual patient is best described by an index defined by the Centers for Disease Control and Prevention (CDC) in its National Nosocomial Infections Surveillance (NNIS) System. The index awards one point each for an American Society of Anesthesiologists (ASA) preoperative assessment score of 3, 4, or 5; an operation classified as either contaminated or dirty-infected; and an operation duration exceeding the 75th percentile for that procedure.[34,35] The CDC definitions for SSI have been agreed to by a consensus panel representing the CDC, the Society for Hospital Epidemiology of America, the Association for Practitioners in Infection Control, and the Surgical Infection Society.[35,36]

The primary treatment of an SSI is to open the wound. When an SSI is suspected, the patient should not be given antibiotics without the wound having been opened. In most cases, the infection is confined to the incision. If the infection is of a superficial wound and if no major systemic manifestations are present, antibiotic therapy is unnecessary. If the local reaction around an infected wound is severe or extensive, administration of antibiotics is advisable until the reaction subsides. In clean wounds that are away from the perineum and that are not associated with an operation that entered the bowel, the likely pathogens are *Staphylococcus aureus*, streptococcal species, or both of these. In such cases, treatment with cefazolin, 1 g I.V. every 8 hours, or oxacillin, 1 g I.V. every 6 hours, is satisfactory. By contrast, SSIs in the perineum and those that occur after operations on the bowel often involve mixed aerobic and anaerobic bacterial flora. If the infection is not very serious, it can be treated with cefoxitin, 1 g I.V. every 6 hours, or with cefotetan, 1 g I.V. every 12 hours. For more aggressive infections with evidence of tissue invasion or necrosis beyond the immediate wound or with severe systemic reaction, more comprehensive antibiotic treatment is indicated—that is, a third-generation cephalosporin; a quinolone combined with clindamycin or metronidazole; aztreonam combined with clindamycin; or imipenem-cilastatin, meropenem, piperacillin-tazobactam, or trovafloxacin alone. Infection of an abdominal incision may be a superficial manifestation of an underlying intra-abdominal abscess or of peritonitis.

Occasionally, infection is invasive and necrotizing. In surgical wounds, such infection is most common after a GI procedure in which the wound was exposed to colonic microflora and in which wound closure was difficult. Necrotizing infection is also more likely in a patient who is seriously ill or who has evidence of multiple organ failure. Such infection should be suspected if there is undermining of the wound edges, extensive fascial necrosis, distant signs of infection, or a marked systemic response. It requires aggressive operative debridement and administration of antibiotics [see 21 Soft Tissue Infection].

Clostridium species, which can cause life-threatening postoperative necrotizing SSI, can also cause routine postoperative incisional infection limited to the wound and without myonecrosis.[37] Such infection is marked by the absence of the systemic symptoms associated with clostridial myonecrosis and by the presence of intact white blood cells on Gram's stain of the wound contents. (Clostridial myonecrosis, on the other hand, is characterized by a Gram's stain that shows gram-positive rods but few or no white blood cells [see 21 Soft Tissue Infection].)

INTRA-ABDOMINAL INFECTION

Intra-abdominal infections—that is, organ/space SSIs—are a major cause of postoperative morbidity and mortality, particularly when diagnosis is delayed.[38,39] Suspected intra-abdominal organ/space SSI in a patient with fever or abdominal tenderness, or both, after an abdominal procedure or injury should not be treated with antibiotics alone; after a specific diagnosis, the appropriate operative or percutaneous procedure must be performed [see 82 Peritonitis and Intra-abdominal Abscesses].

EMPYEMA

Empyema, which may follow thoracotomy or chest trauma requiring tube thoracostomy, is a significant cause of posttraumatic infection.[40] Less commonly, empyema develops as a complication of pneumonia. Empyema should be suspected in any patient with systemic signs of infection, a pleural effusion, and no other obvious source of infection. Diagnosis requires thoracentesis of pleural fluid for Gram's stain and culture. The most common pathogen is *S. aureus*, although many other pathogens may be found. Initial treatment is by drainage with a chest tube and by administration of appropriate antibiotics based on the results of Gram's stain and culture. Because treatment is invasive, it should not be instituted until the diagnosis is confirmed. Cases that fail to resolve promptly and completely may ultimately require thoracoscopy or thoracotomy and decortication. Empyema after pulmonary resection or esophageal operation raises the possibility of a leaking bronchial closure or esophageal anastomosis. A leak is almost certain if an air-fluid level is present on chest x-ray. An esophageal leak requires repair or diversion.

STERNAL AND MEDIASTINAL INFECTION

Sternal and mediastinal infections are the most serious infectious complications of operations that involve a median sternotomy.[41-43] The risk that a superficial infection will spread to involve the sternum and mediastinum is high because there is little soft tissue between the skin and the sternum. Infection may also start deep to the sternum without early superficial evidence. Sternal instability is an important indication of sternal infection. Computed tomography of the chest is sensitive and specific for the diagnosis of sternal osteomyelitis and mediastinitis.[44] All such infections require operative debridement of the sternum and of affected mediastinal tissues. Some wounds can then be closed. Many wounds require closure of the mediastinal space by transposition of viable soft tissue. Pectoralis or rectus muscle flaps, omental flaps, or both are commonly used.[45]

POSTTRAUMATIC MENINGITIS

A basilar skull fracture with a cerebrospinal leak increases the risk of posttraumatic meningitis.[46] The most common pathogens are *Streptococcus pneumoniae*, *S. aureus*, other *Streptococcus* species, and *Haemophilus influenzae*, but any oropharyngeal organism can be responsible.[47] Since the association between trauma and meningitis was first reported in 1970,[46] the appropriate use of antibiotics in these patients has been debated. Some researchers advocate prophylactic administration of antibiotics until any CSF leak ceases,[48] whereas others advocate them for an arbitrary period after injury (usually 5 days); however, controlled studies have failed to support a specific protocol.[47] Furthermore, experience in other clinical settings suggests that prophylactic antibiotics would be as likely to promote the development of resistant oropharyngeal flora and subsequent meningitis as to prevent it.[49,50]

The ideal approach to patients with CSF rhinorrhea or otorrhea is to maintain a high index of suspicion for the development of meningitis. Fever not clearly attributable to another source or not immediately responsive to specific treatment for its presumed cause should prompt a lumbar puncture for examination and culture of spinal fluid. Lumbar puncture should also be performed to investigate headache, spinal pain or stiffness, or unexplained changes in mental status. Such an approach should result in a prompt diagnosis and permit early specific treatment of the responsible pathogen if meningitis is diagnosed.

OSTEOMYELITIS

Osteomyelitis is a relatively rare complication after elective orthopedic procedures. Its diagnosis and management are similar to those of infections involving other operative sites, but because the infection is deep and covered by muscular and fascial planes, diagnosis may be delayed. Nonunion of a fracture or loosening of a prosthesis may be the first sign of infection. Infection after open fractures is common; rates range from 5% to 50%.[51-55] The primary determinants of infection after open fracture are the degree of soft tissue damage surrounding the fracture and the surgeon's ability to stabilize the fracture fragments.[51,53,54] Other important factors include the patient's age and overall condition, the severity of other injuries, the interval between injury and definitive management, and the use of prophylactic antibiotics. Reports suggest that a brief course of perioperative antibiotics may prevent subsequent infection as effectively as a more prolonged course.[32,56]

Treatment of osteomyelitis may require repeated operative debridement, prolonged use of specific antibiotics, and fracture stabilization. Pathogens include *S. aureus* for all grades of open fracture and, increasingly, gram-negative bacteria (e.g., *Pseudomonas aeruginosa* and *Klebsiella* and *Enterobacter* species) for grade III fractures.[56]

Infection Associated with Intravascular Devices

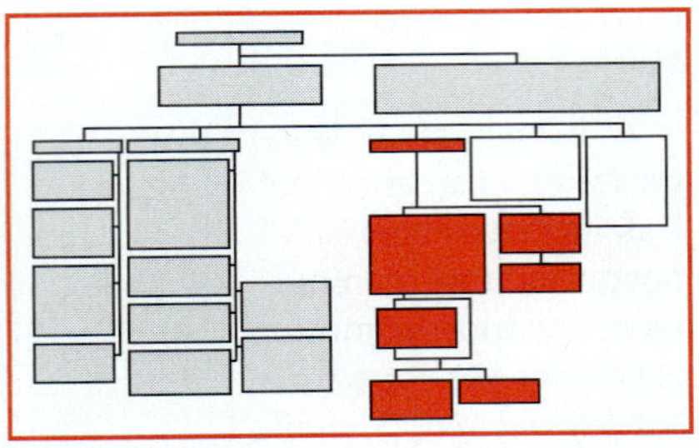

Every type and location of intravascular device has been associated with clinically significant nosocomial bloodstream infection. The incidence of infection is highest with central venous catheters used for monitoring purposes.[57,58]

It is important to specify the different definitions of catheter infection and catheter-related septicemia. Infection at the catheter site is commonly defined as the presence of lymphangitis, purulence, or at least two of the following: erythema, tenderness, increased warmth, and a palpable thrombosed vein. However, many cases of phlebitis with no evidence of bacterial infection present with erythema and with tenderness, a palpable thrombosed vein, or both.[59] Few or no premonitory signs occur before phlebitis is obvious, and the first evidence of as many as 45% of phlebitis cases appears more than 24 hours after catheter removal. If a functional catheter remains in place for 12 hours after the onset of phlebitis symptoms, the duration and severity of symptoms increase markedly.[60]

Catheter-related septicemia is characterized by (1) isolation of the same organism from the catheter and the blood, (2) clinical (or autopsy) and microbiologic data disclosing no other source of the septicemia, and (3) clinical features of bloodstream infection (e.g., fever and leukocytosis).[61] For indwelling, long-term central venous catheters (e.g., Hickman, Broviac, and Groshong), infections have been classified as exit-site and tunnel infections. Infections at the exit site are defined as the presence of erythema, tenderness, induration, or purulence within 2 cm of the skin around the exit site. They are presumably confined to the portion of the catheter external to the subcutaneous Dacron cuff. Tunnel infections are defined as the presence of the same signs along the subcutaneous tract, at a distance more than 2 cm from the tract.[62,63] The importance of this distinction is that many infections at the exit site are successfully treated with antibiotic therapy and local wound care, whereas tunnel infections usually require removal of the catheter.[62,63]

A semiquantitative technique for culturing intravascular catheters has been shown to distinguish between infection and contamination of the catheter and is more specific in the diagnosis of catheter-related septicemia than is broth culture of the catheter.[61,64,65] The catheter is removed from the patient after antiseptic cleansing of the insertion site to prevent contamination from surrounding skin. A 5 to 6 cm segment of the catheter is aseptically removed; transported to the laboratory in a dry, sterile tube; placed on the surface of an agar culture plate; and rolled at least four times across the surface of the plate [see Figure 1]. If the plate grows at least 15 colonies, the culture is positive. Most catheters associated with septicemia actually grow more than 1,000 colonies [see Figure 1]. For peripheral catheters, the entire catheter is cultured. For central catheters that are longer than 6 cm, either the intracutaneous segment or both the intracutaneous segment and the distal tip should be cultured [see Figure 2].

The most common source of bacteria involved in catheter infection is the skin around the insertion site.[66-69] When all catheter segments are studied, the intracutaneous segment almost always has a greater number of bacteria than the catheter tip.[69] Patients who have a skin colonization at the insertion site of greater than 10^3 colony-forming units per 25 cm^2 are 10 times more likely to have a catheter infection than those whose skin colonization was less. With the semiquantitative culture technique, 16% to 44% of catheters that have tested positive have been implicated as the source of septicemia.[61,65,70-74]

More recently, the catheter hub and lumen have been recognized as important routes of infection. These sites are not detected by roll-plate cultures but by sonication culture of catheter segments or by simultaneous cultures of blood drawn through the suspect catheter and from a distant site. Sonication cultures recovering more than 10^2 colonies, or catheter cultures more than five times the number recovered from distant sites, are sensitive and specific for catheter infection.[75-77]

For catheters that are only locally infected and not responsible for septicemia, removal is adequate treatment; the same is true for most catheters that cause septicemia. If the patient's temperature and WBC count return to normal within 24 hours after removal of the catheter and if local signs of inflammation at the catheter insertion site resolve within that period, antibiotics are not necessary.[78] However, if the patient continues to show clinical signs of bacteremia, a brief course of specific antibiotic therapy is indicated. Specific antibiotic therapy is also indicated if semiquantitative catheter

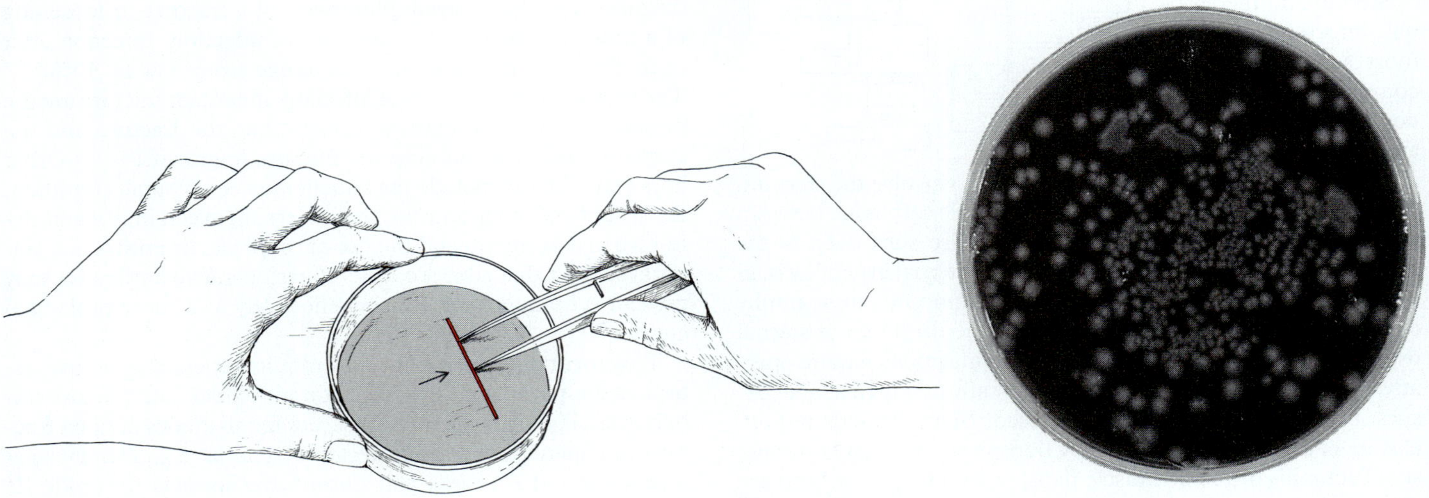

Figure 1 In a semiquantitative technique used to distinguish between infection and contamination of intravascular catheters, a 5 to 6 cm segment of the catheter is rolled at least four times across the surface of an agar culture plate (left). Typically, a positive culture grows far more than 15 colonies (right).

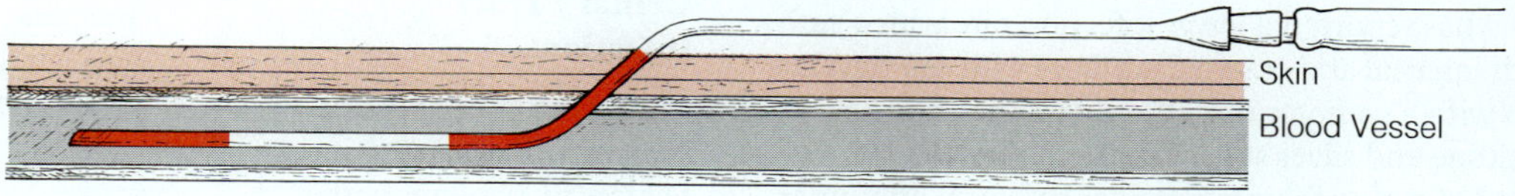

Figure 2 When a catheter is longer than 6 cm, either a 5 to 6 cm intracutaneous segment or both this segment and the distal 5 to 6 cm (red) can be cultured.

culture reveals a large number of *S. aureus* organisms in conjunction with systemic signs of infection. If empirical therapy for catheter-related septicemia is undertaken before culture and sensitivity results are available, the antibiotic regimen should include vancomycin or another antibiotic known to be effective against methicillin-resistant staphylococci, because coagulase-negative staphylococci are the most commonly implicated pathogens[57,78-80] and there is a high rate of methicillin resistance among these organisms. For patients with intravenous catheters and candidemia, the candidemia resolves an average of 3 days earlier if the catheters are removed at the time of diagnosis and initiation of antifungal therapy.[81]

In a small proportion of patients, local catheter-related infection may progress to a life-threatening condition characterized by the formation of microabscesses within the cannulated vein and by persistent bacteremia after catheter removal.[82,83] Septic thrombophlebitis can occur in a broad range of hospitalized patients and should be suspected when clinical signs of systemic sepsis, local signs of inflammation, and positive blood cultures persist after removal of the catheter. A surgical approach to the affected vein is required. When possible, the vein should be excised over the affected area and the wound left open. The presence of gross pus within the vein wall is not necessary for the diagnosis. The wall of the affected vein may simply appear thickened, with inflammation surrounding it and an edematous, pale thrombus enclosed within it.[83] Fungal peripheral thrombophlebitis may be especially difficult to diagnose because the local site often does not appear infected.[84] In the presence of continued candidemia without an obvious source, any palpably thrombosed vein near a site of present or previous catheterization must be suspected. Gram's stain and hematoxylin-eosin stain of the vein contents or the vein wall are relatively insensitive, whereas silver stain and culture are more sensitive.[84]

Even more rare is catheter-related septic central venous thrombosis. The diagnosis is made by the occurrence of (1) thrombosis of the internal jugular, subclavian, or brachiocephalic vein proved by venography or duplex Doppler examination; (2) central venous catheter infection with positive catheter tip culture and positive peripheral blood cultures; and (3) persistent bacteremia or candidemia after catheter removal.[85,86] Initial therapy consists of catheter removal, systemic antibiotics based on sensitivity testing and administered in a quantity and duration appropriate to treatment of endocarditis, and systemic anticoagulation during the same period. Surgical excision or drainage is reserved for failure of nonoperative measures.

Previous practice often required either complete change or exchange over a wire of both central and peripheral venous catheters at fixed intervals to reduce the risk of infection. Data from randomized, controlled, prospective trials do not demonstrate an advantage to this policy.[59,87] These trials demonstrate that the risk of infection is linear, increasing with the duration of intravenous catheterization, whether one or multiple catheters are used.

Current recommendations are to change catheters when infection is suspected, when the catheters are not working, or when they are not needed.[59,76,87-89] Clearly, any catheter that is a cause of septicemia must be removed, as should infected catheters that may not yet have caused septicemia. The practical problem is that not all infected catheters show external evidence of infection. In addition, catheter culture and the subsequent clinical course confirm infection in only a small proportion of patients with central venous catheters or pulmonary artery catheters who are suspected on clinical grounds of having septicemia.[90] Changing central venous catheters over a guide wire circumvents most of the mechanical complications associated with central venous catheterization, saves time, and is more comfortable for the patient.[91] However, if a culture of the first catheter is positive, the second catheter should be removed immediately, and any new catheter should be placed in a different location.[59,76,87-90]

Recommendations for changing central venous and pulmonary artery catheters are as follows:

1. Signs of inflammation, skin irritation, or purulence at the insertion site should prompt immediate removal of the catheter. Any new catheter should be inserted in a different site. In a patient with systemic signs of infection (fever, leukocytosis, malaise), culture of the insertion site or of the catheter, or both, is indicated to identify potential pathogens and to direct therapy. In a patient without systemic signs of infection, culture is not necessary.

2. If a patient with a catheter experiences systemic signs and symptoms of infection without a readily apparent source, the catheter should be removed even in the absence of inflammation at the insertion site. In this setting, however, approximately 75% of catheters are not infected, and a new catheter can be inserted at the same site over a guide wire placed through the first catheter.[90,92-98] However, a catheter exchange places the new catheter in the old subcutaneous tunnel, which would be the most likely origin of catheter infection. The first catheter should be cultured semiquantitatively. If the culture is negative (i.e., < 15 colonies), the second catheter can be left in place. If the culture is positive (i.e., ≥ 15 colonies), the second catheter should be removed immediately, and any new catheter should be placed at a different site.

Sterile technique is always required for catheter insertion. However, most authorities advocate a surgical approach to preparation of the insertion site, with the operator wearing gown, gloves, mask, and hat for the procedure, if one or more of the following risk factors are present[99,100]: (1) the location is central, (2) catheterization will probably be long term, (3) the patient is seriously ill, or (4) parenteral nutrition is to be employed.

Traditionally, central venous catheters have been inserted most commonly via either the subclavian or the internal jugular route. There is a well-demonstrated increase in infection risk when catheters are inserted by the jugular route instead of the subclavian.[74,89,101,102] There is a prejudice against the femoral route, but published data do not demonstrate a higher incidence of either infection or thrombotic complications when the femoral route is used instead of the internal jugular route,[101] and therefore, the femoral route can be used if other access routes are not available.

A recent approach to prevention of catheter infection is antibiotic bonding of the entire catheter surface. Two trials[103,104] have reported fewer catheter and bloodstream infections in patients with antimicrobial-bonded catheters than in patients with control catheters, and one trial[105] has reported a lower infection rate with a catheter coated on both internal and external surfaces with minocycline and rifampin than with a catheter coated only on the external surface with chlorhexidine and silver sulfadiazine.

The ideal method of caring for intravascular catheters after insertion is not firmly established. Sterile dressings of gauze and tape as well as a variety of commercially available transparent dressings have been advocated. The transparent dressings appear to save nursing time and permit the insertion site to be inspected without changing the dressing, but they promote bacterial growth on the underlying skin, as compared with gauze and tape dressings.[69,106-108] Transparent dressings have also been associated with an increased number of cases of catheter infections and catheter-related septicemia in patients with central venous catheters.[109] Thus, use of transparent dressings is not recommended, at least for central lines.

In addition, there is no firm evidence that the use of polyantibiotic ointments or iodophor ointments at the insertion site prevents infection, although these ointments have not been associated with an increase in infections with resistant organisms.[99] In some hospitals, catheter teams care for all parenteral nutrition lines with excellent results. Regular inspection of insertion sites and adherence to a specific protocol for catheter care can result in acceptably low infection rates.[76,110-113]

Catheters with two or three internal lumina have become widely available and are often sold in kits that include equipment for guide-wire insertion. These catheters are more convenient when a patient requires multiple lines for monitoring and for delivery of intravenous medications and parenteral nutrition. However, these multiple-lumen lines may be associated with a higher incidence of catheter-associated septicemia than are single-lumen catheters[114,115]; the data are inconclusive.[98,116] In one small study, the insertion of two single-lumen catheters did not result in a lower complication rate than that of one double-lumen catheter.[117] A catheter with multiple infusion ports is likely to be manipulated more often than a single-lumen catheter, but it is unclear whether the extra manipulation results in a higher infection rate. In situations in which one lumen would suffice, the temptation to insert a multiple-lumen line in case additional lumina are needed later should be resisted. One study showed that 53% of all triple-lumen lines observed had only one lumen being used,[114] indicating that multiple-lumen lines are often used unnecessarily.

When long-term use of catheters is required, insertion of a Silastic catheter with a subcutaneous Dacron cuff (e.g., Broviac, Hickman, or Groshong) is associated with the lowest rate of catheter-associated infection and the longest useful catheter life.[62] In the largest reported study of these catheters, the incidence of infection was only 0.14 infection per 100 catheter-days (range, 0.0 to 0.8).[62] The study also showed that double-lumen catheters did not have a higher rate of infection than single-lumen catheters, but the rate of catheter infections was increased 10-fold in patients who had catheter-related thrombosis.[62] The mean catheter life span in this report was greater than 120 days.

Very low infection rates and long catheter life are also reported with nontunneled Silastic catheters and with peripherally inserted central catheters (PICC).[76,118] The lowest infection rates are associated with totally implantable devices with subcutaneous reservoirs.[119]

Use of warfarin to prevent thrombosis may result in a reduced rate of catheter infection. A prospective trial found a clinically and statistically significant reduction in the incidence of catheter-associated thrombosis (from 38% to 10%) over 90 days with the administration of 1 mg of warfarin daily, beginning 3 days before catheter insertion.[120] Measured prothrombin times did not increase, and no bleeding complications occurred.

Urinary Tract Infection

The traditional definition of urinary tract infection in patients without urinary catheters specifies the presence of at least 10^5 organisms/ml, but this criterion is probably not appropriate for catheterized patients. Research has shown that of catheterized patients who have any detectable organisms in their urine (even $< 10^2$/ml), whose catheters remain in place, and who receive no specific antimicrobial therapy, 96% have organism counts higher than 10^5/ml within 3 days.[121] (By comparison, 27% of patients with sterile urine subsequently have colony counts higher than 10^5/ml before catheter removal.)

Although a catheter-associated urinary tract infection is a significant nosocomial infection with measurable morbidity and mortality [see Discussion, below], not all cases of bacteriuria should be treated with antibiotics. If a patient with bacteriuria is symptomatic, treatment should be initiated according to culture results and sensitivity testing. Although bacteriuria can sometimes be cleared without removal of the catheter, the risk of a new episode continues while the catheter is in place.[122] Ideally, the catheter should be removed as soon as possible. In one study, only 36% of untreated women with asymptomatic bacteriuria cleared their urine within 2 weeks of catheter removal, and 17% progressed to symptomatic bacteriuria. Patients treated with a single dose of trimethoprim-sulfamethoxazole cleared their urine in 81% of cases.[123] Thus, it is prudent to obtain a culture at the time of catheter removal and to treat any bacteriuria detected.

A condom catheter is often used in male patients in place of a urethral catheter when neurologic injury or incontinence mandates long-term drainage. Data concerning the ideal care of these devices and the true infection rate associated with their use are not clear. Urinary tract infection rates as low as 0% in 79 patients managed with condom catheter drainage[124] and as high as 53%[122] to 63%[125] have been reported. Severe noninfectious local complications such as ulceration and maceration of the penis also can occur.[124,125]

Because indwelling urinary catheters are a major source of nosocomial infection, they should be employed only when necessary and removed as soon as practicable. The most effective method of reducing infections among patients with urinary catheters is to use completely closed urinary drainage systems and to limit breaks in the closed system.[126] The incidence of new infections doubles on any day in which a closed urinary drainage system is opened.[127,128] Urine samples for culture should be aspirated with a needle and syringe from the lumen of the catheter after antiseptic cleansing of the catheter sampling port. The catheter junction should not be disconnected to obtain a specimen. The use of a preconnected and sealed catheter and drainage bag system has been shown to result in a 2.7-fold reduction in the rate of catheter-associated urinary tract infections and an adjusted risk ratio for death of 0.29.[129]

Antibiotic irrigation systems do not reduce infections, but they do increase the incidence of resistant organisms.[128] Systemic antibiotics have been shown to reduce infections to a modest degree in the first 4 days of catheterization, but they do so at the expense of an increase in resistant organisms. The rate of infection is increased in females as compared with males and in patients with critical illness as compared with those without critical illness.[127] Patients with nosocomial diarrhea and an indwelling bladder catheter have a ninefold higher risk of subsequent urinary tract infection than do patients with an indwelling bladder catheter who do not have diarrhea.[130]

Although most urinary tract infections acquired by hospitalized patients are assumed to be simple bladder infections, a poor correlation exists between the location of infection and the clinical symptoms.[131,132] Many patients with upper urinary tract infections do not have flank pain, fever, or other signs of systemic infection, and patients with a bladder infection may not have dysuria or suprapubic tenderness. Many patients with upper urinary tract infections are treated without the diagnosis ever being made. Systemic infection and associated bacteremia or complications such as intrarenal or perinephric abscesses occur more commonly in immunocompromised patients, such as those with urinary tract obstruction or diabetes.[133,134] In patients with a neurogenic bladder or indwelling bladder catheters, urinary sepsis may develop without symptoms referable to the urinary tract. However, symptoms of localized flank or low back pain, along with systemic signs, such as fever, rigors, sweats, and nausea, are relatively specific indicators of renal infection.[135]

If a patient has fever and bacteriuria during the postoperative period, the surgeon should carefully evaluate the patient to determine whether he or she has pyelonephritis or a postoperative intra-abdominal infectious complication. Pyelonephritis can be treated solely with antimicrobial therapy in most cases, whereas all postoperative intra-abdominal infectious complications require surgical intervention as well as antimicrobial therapy. No simple methods are available to distinguish between these diagnoses. The operating surgeon should carefully evaluate all of the patient's clinical signs and symptoms. A hospitalized patient with pyelonephritis should usually receive antimicrobial therapy for at least 14 days. An agent demonstrated to be effective against the causative organism by in vitro sensitivity testing should be used.[135] In a patient with severe signs of systemic response to infection or in any patient who does not respond promptly to treatment, an ultrasound examination, a renal scan, or an intravenous pyelogram should be done to rule out obstruction. If obstruction is found, it must be corrected. If the patient has an indwelling bladder catheter, the catheter should be removed, appropriate therapy started, and a new, clean catheter inserted.[135]

Enteric Infection

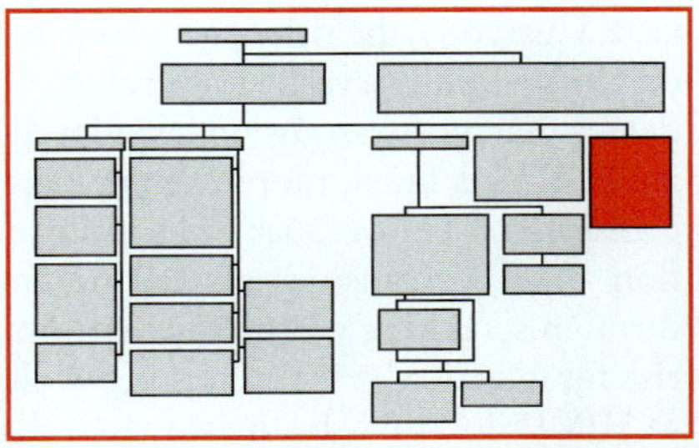

Any organism that can cause food-borne enteric infection in the community can do so in the hospital,[136] but cultures for routine enteric pathogens are not useful for patients who have been hospitalized for more than 3 days.[137] The most important nosocomial enteric disease to confront most surgeons is antibiotic-associated diarrhea, which can range from trivial, self-limited episodes of diarrhea to fulminant disease with systemic signs of sepsis, collapse, and death.

The first step in diagnosis is to consider antibiotic-associated colitis in any hospitalized patient with diarrhea. Mild cases may not be associated with any systemic signs or pathologic findings in the colon, and in the majority of mild episodes, there are no identifiable pathogens. More severe cases are marked by one or more of the following signs: nonspecific hyperemia, edema, granularity, or ulceration of colonic mucosa. The most severe cases are marked by pseudomembrane formation.

The single most efficient specimen for detection of *C. difficile*–associated diarrhea is a stool sample for cytotoxin determination, with a sensitivity of 70% to 100%. Sensitivity increases slightly (to 96%) if a sample is sent for stool culture as well, but if *C. difficile* is grown, the organism must still be tested for cytotoxin production, and this takes another day.[137,138] Rectal swab cultures, transported in anaerobic containers, are at least as sensitive as conventional stool cultures[139] but are not adequate to detect cytotoxin.[138] Although there is a potential for the development of polymerase chain reaction assays for the cytotoxin gene in stool, these are not available at present. Stool smears for detection of white blood cells are not helpful.[137,138] Endoscopy, for the detection of pseudomembranes, is indicated if the patient is seriously ill and a prompt diagnosis and initiation of specific treatment are desired. Empirical therapy until a specific pathogen is identified is appropriate in this circumstance.[138]

Severe and persistent cases of antibiotic-associated diarrhea are most commonly associated with the recovery of *C. difficile* by culture and of *C. difficile* toxin by tissue culture assay.[140,141] In more than 90% of patients who have pseudomembranous colitis, *C. difficile* toxin will be present on tissue culture assay. In antibiotic-associated diarrhea without pseudomembrane formation, positive toxin titers may be found in 70% of patients with signs of colitis and in 11% to 27% of patients without colitis.[140,142-145]

Pseudomembranes, present in about half of patients with *C. difficile*–associated diarrhea,[138] are elevated, whitish plaques that vary in size from a few millimeters to 1 to 2 cm and may coalesce and slough. Histologically, the plaques show epithelial debris, polymorphonuclear infiltrate, chronic inflammatory cells, and fibrin deposition.[141] The diagnosis of pseudomembrane formation is made by endoscopy [*see Figure 3*]. Most cases involve the rectum and the left colon, but as many as 25% may be missed by rigid sigmoidoscopy; by comparison, the false negative rate with flexible endoscopy is only 10%.[146] Although the great majority of cases involve only the colon, two fatal cases that primarily involved the ileum and the jejunum have been recorded.[147,148] The clinical picture of pseudomembranous colitis includes watery diarrhea in 90% to 95% of cases, with bloody diarrhea in the remaining cases. Abdominal cramps, leukocytosis, and elevated temperature are present in approximately 80% of cases.[140,141]

All commonly employed antibiotics have been implicated in cases of antibiotic-associated pseudomembranous colitis, including vancomycin[149-151] and antibiotics used for perioperative antibiotic prophylaxis, even in a single dose.[152] Treatment should include cessation of the offending antimicrobial agent, if possible, which in

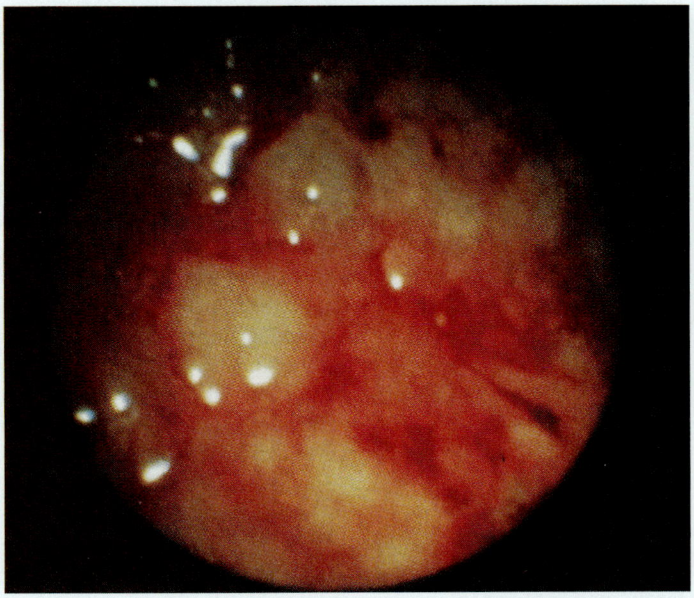

Figure 3 An endoscopic view of pseudomembrane formation is shown.

mild cases may be all that is necessary. In 23% of such cases, resolution occurs within 2 to 3 days of stopping the antibiotic therapy.[138]

A patient with systemic symptoms should also receive one of the agents with proven efficacy against the disease. The agent with which there has been the most recorded experience is vancomycin, but it is more expensive than the alternatives. The usual dosage is 500 mg/day orally in four divided doses. Metronidazole, 500 mg three or four times daily, or bacitracin, 20,000 to 25,000 units four times daily, is also effective.[138,153-155] The current recommendation is to begin therapy with metronidazole to reduce the risk of inducing vancomycin-resistant enterococci [see Pathogens, below].[138,156]

Relapses after treatment for *C. difficile* colitis are common, occurring in 5% to 30% of cases, perhaps because of persistence of the organism in spore form; 92% of these cases respond to a second course of treatment without relapse.[138] However, in one report, five of 11 patients who experienced relapse had new strains of *C. difficile*, distinct from the original strain, as determined by restriction endonuclease analysis.[157]

A profound ileus is sometimes associated with the severe form of the disease and may prevent the delivery of oral antibiotics to the site of infection. Limited experience suggests that parenteral metronidazole may be effective in these cases.[140] However, studies have reported several cases of unsuccessful intravenous metronidazole treatment of *C. difficile*–associated colitis and of the development of *C. difficile* colitis in patients receiving intravenous metronidazole alone or together with other antibiotics.[151,158-160] In the most severe cases, the clinical evolution resembles that of toxic colitis associated with inflammatory bowel disease, and the patient may require a colectomy if the disease is unresponsive to nonoperative management.[140,161] In as many as 5% of cases, colitis may present with acute abdominal pain and tenderness and leukocytosis without diarrhea.[162,163] If colitis is suspected because of previous antibiotic administration, sigmoidoscopy may facilitate the correct diagnosis and avert unnecessary abdominal exploration. Computed tomography may show thickening of the bowel wall, but findings of operative exploration are often unimpressive.[163] Extraintestinal infections have also been reported.[164]

Transfusion-Associated Infection

The transfusion of blood would seem to be an excellent method for transmitting blood-borne diseases; however, except for posttransfusion hepatitis, transmission of disease by blood transfusion is rare.[165,166] Transfusion-associated malaria is occasionally reported in North America but occurs quite infrequently. The primary method for preventing malaria transmission is careful screening of donors by history. A handful of cases of babesiosis, Chagas' disease, trypanosomiasis, and toxoplasmosis have been reported over many years but are rare as well.[165-167] In the early years of blood collection and transfusion, cases of syphilis related to blood transfusion were reported infrequently. The practice of refrigerating blood, which kills circulating spirochetes within 1 to 2 days, is probably responsible for the absence of transfusion-associated syphilis today. The last reported case occurred in 1969.[165] Unfortunately, refrigerating blood does not kill all potential pathogens. Bacterial pathogens that can survive blood storage and cause subsequent symptomatic infection include *Yersinia enterocolitica* and *Pseudomonas fluorescens*, the two most common isolates, as well as *P. putida* and *Campylobacter jejuni*. Bacterial sepsis is estimated to cause death after only one of six million transfused units.[168] *Yersinia* infection occurs after approximately one in 500,000 units transfused, and some type of bacterial contamination is found in approximately one of 1,700 pooled units of platelets.[169] When transfusion-associated bacteremia or endotoxemia is suspected, the residual blood product in the bag should be examined by a hematologic stain, and the blood in the bag and samples of the recipient's blood should be cultured.[170]

The most severe and frequently occurring disease transmitted by blood transfusion in North America is viral hepatitis [see 86 Viral Infection]. Since the development of a specific and sensitive test for detecting hepatitis B surface antigen (HBsAg), the incidence of posttransfusion hepatitis B has dropped, from 25% to 30% of all cases of transfusion-associated hepatitis to 5% to 10%. However, serologic tests for hepatitis B have not resulted in an overall decrease in posttransfusion hepatitis (PTH), because 80% to 90% of cases of PTH were caused by hepatitis C (HCV), previously labeled non-A, non-B (NANB) hepatitis. The risk of developing NANB was estimated to be approximately 7% for recipients of volunteer blood and 28% for recipients of commercial blood.[171,172]

Molecular biologic techniques have identified HCV as the cause of most cases of NANB, and diagnostic tests for antibody to HCV have been developed to screen blood.[173] In Taiwan, 58% of patients with chronic liver disease who do not have antibodies to hepatitis B have antibodies to hepatitis C.[174]

Although most cases of hepatitis C are asymptomatic and self-limited, fulminant cases with a fatal outcome have been reported. Moreover, up to one half of hepatitis C patients may show evidence of chronic liver disease, and for some of these, there will be biopsy evidence of cirrhosis many years later.[165,171,175] Detectable anti–hepatitis C antibodies are typically found 4 weeks after transfusion of an infectious unit of blood.[173] Of the patients who seroconvert, 54% are asymptomatic, but 77% progress to have chronic elevations of alanine aminotransferase (ALT). Those who develop chronic hepatitis usually remain seropositive, but up to 27% of patients who seroconvert have no detectable antibody at 1 year.[176,177] Tests for antibody to hepatitis C have been refined and are now almost 100% sensitive. However, specificity is much lower, and additional testing is necessary, particularly in low-risk populations, to confirm the diagnosis of hepatitis C infection.[173]

The spread of AIDS [see 87 Acquired Immunodeficiency Syndrome] has brought a new risk of transfusion-associated viral disease. Currently, the risk of acquiring transfusion-associated HIV is extremely low. It is vastly less likely to occur and accounts for fewer deaths than posttransfusion hepatitis. However, transfusion-associated AIDS is much more frightening to most patients and physicians than PTH because of its uniformly fatal prognosis. Prevention of HIV transmission during transfusion is accomplished through screening of potential donors to eliminate those at high risk for infection[178-180] and testing of all donated units for antibody to HIV.[179,180] It has been estimated that predonation screening is 98% effective in eliminating donation of positive units and that postdonation antibody testing is more than 95% effective, for a combined effectiveness of approximately 99.9%.[179] In aggregate, posttransfusion HIV infections were reduced by 76% between 1985 and 1988, a time during which the overall prevalence of the condition was increasing.[179] The continued concern about possible HIV transmission during transfusion arises from the so-called window of seronegativity between the time at which a potential donor becomes infected and the time at which the donor's antibody test becomes positive. An analysis of available data from most United States blood banks concluded that the risk of receiving a unit of blood that contained HIV but was negative for anti-HIV antibody in 1987 was approximately one in 153,000 on the basis of an average window of 8 weeks.[179] The incidence of positive units detected through postdonation screening decreased by more than 50% between 1985 and 1987.[179] The risk of transfusing infectious seronegative blood is assumed to be proportional to the number of seropositive units detected through antibody screening.

The risk of receiving seronegative blood was also estimated by a San Francisco group, which studied seronegative blood samples from 71,800 donations by culture and polymerase chain reaction techniques before 1991. They found a point estimate of the risk of one in 61,171, with an upper limit of the 95% confidence interval of one in 10,695.[181] Because this study was conducted in a population with a high prevalence of HIV infection, the risk is probably lower in regions with a lower prevalence. A subsequent study in five blood centers across the United States tested 2,318,356 units of blood from 586,507 donors during the years 1991 through 1993. They found that the risk of acquiring an HIV infection from a unit of blood was one in 493,000. The corresponding risk for acquiring HCV was one in 103,000 and, for HBV, one in 63,000. The aggregate risk of acquiring any virus was one in 34,000, and 88% of that risk came from HBV and HCV.[182] Because of donor screening, this risk is lower than the risk among a random sample of the population. Newer and more sensitive tests have the potential to reduce the risk another 27% to 72%.[182] In comparison, the risk of experiencing a fatal hemolytic transfusion reaction is one in 100,000.[180] Thus, a transfusion recipient is more likely to die of hepatitis B or C or a hemolytic reaction than of AIDS.

The mean incubation period for transfusion-associated AIDS is 23 months, with a range from 10 to 43 months; the interval to the development of antibody is 2 to 3 months after infection.[178] The clinical progression of the disease is similar to its occurrence in the traditional high-risk groups.[183] With transfusion-associated AIDS, as with post-transfusion hepatitis, the primary preventive response of the physician should be to limit unnecessary transfusion.[184] Analysis of transfusion practices in the United States between 1982 and 1988 reveals a decrease in the number of blood, platelet, and plasma transfusions after 1986; previously, the number of these transfusions increased each year. In addition, from 1982 to 1987, the number of autologous units donated increased from 30,000 to 397,000 a year. In 1987, autologous units accounted for 3% of all blood transfused.[185]

Discussion

Postoperative Fever

Many patients experience fever in the postoperative period without infection. In a prospective study of 871 general surgery patients, 213 (24%) had a documented infection or an unexplained fever in the postoperative period.[186] The most common occurrence was unexplained fever in 81 cases (38%), followed by wound infection in 55 (26%), urinary tract infection in 44 (21%), respiratory tract infection in 27 (13%), and other infections in 6 (3%). Of all unexplained fevers, 72% occurred in the first 2 days, and of all occurrences in the first 3 days, 67 (71%) of 95 were unexplained, with only 18 (27%) representing true infection. In another study, 73 (45%) of 162 patients experienced unexplained fever after general surgical or orthopedic procedures; 25% of the unexplained fevers were at least 38.3° C (101° F).[187]

At Harborview Medical Center, 316 (98%) of 322 patients who had laparotomy for penetrating trauma experienced a temperature of at least 37.5° C (99.5° F) orally during the first 5 days after operation. Of these patients, however, only 67 (21%) actually acquired any infection during a 30-day follow-up. Even for the 80 patients whose temperatures were as high as 39° C (102.2° F) orally, only 48% actually acquired an infection before discharge. Fever that persisted or began after postoperative day 4 was more likely to represent true infection. Similarly, an elevated WBC count was nonspecific during the first 5 postoperative days: 89% of all patients had a WBC count greater than 10,000/mm^3.[188,189]

Magnitude and Significance of Nosocomial Infection

An understanding of the prevalence of nosocomial infections and of the factors predisposing to their occurrence will help in prevention, diagnosis, and treatment. Since 1970, the National Nosocomial Infections Surveillance (NNIS) system[3] has collected and analyzed data on the frequency of nosocomial infections in a voluntary sample of 51 hospitals in the United States. Although more intensive studies suggest that the NNIS underestimates the true incidence of nosocomial infections by 30% to 40%,[4,190,191] the large number of cases studied during consecutive years provides a useful description of the most frequently encountered infections, their relative incidences, and the responsible pathogens.

INCIDENCE

In the 1986 NNIS report, 33.5 patients per 1,000 discharges had acquired a nosocomial infection. The incidence ranges from 46.7 per 1,000 surgical discharges to 13.3 per 1,000 pediatric discharges. Overall, the rate of infection is highest in large teaching hospitals and lowest in nonteaching hospitals. The higher incidence of infection among surgical patients is largely attributable to SSI. Across all services, urinary tract infection is the most common infection, accounting for 38.5% of all nosocomial infections, followed by lower respiratory tract infection (17.8%), surgical wound infection (16.6%), primary bacteremia (7.5%), and cutaneous infection (5.8%). All other categories combined account for 13.8% of nosocomial infections. The total incidence of nosocomial infection from all sites on surgical services ranged from 30.8 to 59.3 per 1,000 discharges. The risk that a surgical patient will acquire any infection varies according to the type of procedure performed as well as the patient's underlying risk.[192]

A more recent NNIS report, focusing on surgical patients, found that SSIs were the most common (37%, including 24% incisional and 13% organ/space), followed by urinary tract infections (27%), pneumonia (15%), primary bloodstream infections (7%), and all other sites combined (15%). Of the infected surgical patients, 17% had more than one nosocomial infection, and 9% of surgical patients with nosocomial infections subsequently died; nosocomial infections were reported to have caused or contributed to 60% of the deaths. Of infections related to death, 38% were pneumonia, 21% at the surgical site, and 20% primary bloodstream infections. The likelihood that a specific infection will be related to death varies with the type of infection [see Table 1].[192]

Urinary Tract Infection

With so many cases of bacteriuria occurring in catheterized patients, it would be easy to become complacent about the problem. Urinary tract catheterization is performed seven to eight million times a year in acute care hospitals in the United States.[193] Approximately 5% to 8% of catheterized, uninfected patients will acquire a urinary tract infection for each day of catheterization, leading to a cumulative infection rate of 40% to 50% after 10 days.[126,127] However, the great majority of catheterized patients with bacteriuria are asymp-

Table 1 Contribution of Nosocomial Infection to Death in Infected Surgical Patients Who Died[192]

Type of Nosocomial Infection	Probability That Infection Was Related to Death (%)
Organ/space surgical site infection	89
Primary bloodstream infection	79
Pneumonia	77
Other	48
Incisional surgical site infection	46
Urinary tract infection	22

tomatic.[115] It has been estimated that only 0.7% of catheterized patients will acquire a symptomatic infection and that 8% to 10% of patients will have bacteriuria after the catheter has been removed.[125]

In many of these patients, the bacteriuria will resolve without specific therapy after the catheter has been removed. However, a careful study of more than 1,458 patients has clearly demonstrated that mortality in catheterized patients who acquire bacteriuria is higher than in those who do not acquire it.[193] In this study, 9% of all catheterized patients acquired catheter-related urinary tract infection; this infection was associated with a threefold increase in deaths occurring during hospitalization, even after correction for other factors, such as age, severity of illness, hospital service, duration of catheterization, and renal function. In surgical patients between 50 and 70 years of age with normal renal function and without a fatal underlying disease, an increase in the death rate of 3% per patient per hospitalization was associated with the occurrence of a urinary tract infection. Of all deaths of catheterized patients, 14% were associated with a urinary tract infection.[193] By extrapolation, this mortality suggests that as many as 56,000 deaths a year in the United States may be related to catheter-acquired urinary tract infection.

Although the risk of bacteremia is small for any individual patient with bacteriuria, the large number of hospitalized patients with bacteriuria accounts for many bacteremic episodes. Urinary tract infection is the most commonly diagnosed source of gram-negative sepsis, and the rate of bacteremia secondary to urinary catheters is estimated to be between 0.7% and 2%.[194] In a case-matched study in 1978, a postoperative urinary tract infection was associated with a 2.4-day prolongation of hospital stay and an excess cost of more than $500.[195] One study revealed that 2.3% of postoperative patients with urinary tract infections were subsequently diagnosed as having a wound infection caused by the same organism responsible for the urinary tract infection. This finding accounted for 3.4% of the wound infections occurring during the study.[196]

Infection Associated with Intravascular Devices

Nosocomial infection associated with intravascular devices, which are placed for either monitoring or therapeutic purposes, assumed increasing importance during the 1970s and 1980s. As many as 8% of all venous cannulations are estimated to be complicated by catheter-related septicemia,[197] affecting approximately 23,000 patients in the United States each year.[60] Of all cases of nosocomial bacteremia occurring in NNIS hospitals between September 1984 and July 1986, 82% were associated with intravascular devices[198]: 27% were associated with parenteral nutrition catheters and 55% with other vascular access devices. With the semiquantitative culture technique for catheters, 16% to 44% of positive catheters have been implicated as the source of septicemia.[60,64,69-72] Reports from as early as 1963 called attention to the risk of serious systemic infections arising from peripheral intravenous catheters.[199-201] A study in 1971 documented the frequent occurrence of thrombophlebitis and sepsis 3 to 4 days after operation and the insertion of intravenous catheters.[202] For ICU patients with bloodstream infections associated with central venous catheters, the attributable mortality is 25% to 35%, and the excess cost for survivors is $23,000 to $33,000.[203]

In terms of infection risk, pulmonary artery catheters are no different from central venous catheters, except for their potential to cause right-sided heart lesions that could predispose to right-sided endocarditis.[204,205] Pulmonary artery catheters can be responsible for septicemia, and they require as much precaution during insertion and subsequent care as other central venous catheters.[72,204,206-210]

Arterial catheters, which are used for monitoring purposes in the ICU, have been thought to be less frequently associated with infection and septicemia than central venous catheters, but it is clear that life-threatening infections can originate with peripheral arterial lines.[211-213] In early studies of radial artery catheters in which nonquantitative culture techniques were employed, catheter contamination rates of 4% to 39% were recorded, but there were no cases of septicemia or clinical infection in 605 catheterizations.[214,215] In these studies, the majority of catheters were removed from patients within 3 days.

Two prospective studies of arterial catheters demonstrated that 18% to 35% of the lines were locally infected, as reflected in semiquantitative cultures of at least 15 colonies.[67,216] In one study, five cases of septicemia occurred, representing an overall incidence of 4% and an incidence of 23% among locally infected catheters.[216] The incidence of septicemia was increased in catheters that were inserted by cutdown rather than percutaneous puncture and in catheters with signs of local inflammation. In another, the clinical features of septicemia arising from an arterial catheter were indistinguishable from clinical features of episodes arising from a central venous line; 12% of all nosocomial bacteremias in the ICU originated from an arterial catheter. Clearly, arterial lines as well as venous lines must be considered in the examination of a patient for the source of fever or septicemia in the ICU.[72,209,213,216,217] Twelve cases of radial artery rupture after arterial line infection have been reported. All but one were associated with infection by *S. aureus*, and nearly all demonstrated systemic signs of infection for 2 or more days after catheter removal.[213] Although there is no published experience with the use of guide wires to change and culture arterial lines in relation to possible catheter-related infection, the technique can be applied with the same rationale used for central venous catheters.

PATHOGENS

In 1984, the NNIS reported on 26,965 infections. Of these cases, 64% were caused by single pathogens, 20% were caused by multiple pathogens, 6% had no pathogen identified on culture, and 10% were not cultured [see Figure 4]. Of the 84% in which a pathogen was identified, 86% were caused by aerobic bacteria, 2% by anaerobes, and 8% by fungi [see Figure 4 and Table 2]. Overall on the surgical services, the most common pathogen isolated was *Escherichia coli*, followed by *P. aeruginosa*, enterococci, *S. aureus*, *Enterobacter* species, *Klebsiella* species, coagulase-negative staphylococci, and *Proteus*, *Candida*, and *Serratia* species. These 10 types of pathogens accounted for 84% of all isolates. Gram-negative rods were most common in urinary tract infection and lower respiratory tract infection, although *S. aureus* was the second most common pathogen isolated in lower respiratory tract infection. *S. aureus* was the most common isolate from surgical wound infection, whereas coagulase-negative staphylococci, followed closely by *S. aureus*, were the pathogens most often responsible for primary bacteremia.

Nosocomial infections with resistant enterococci have become a

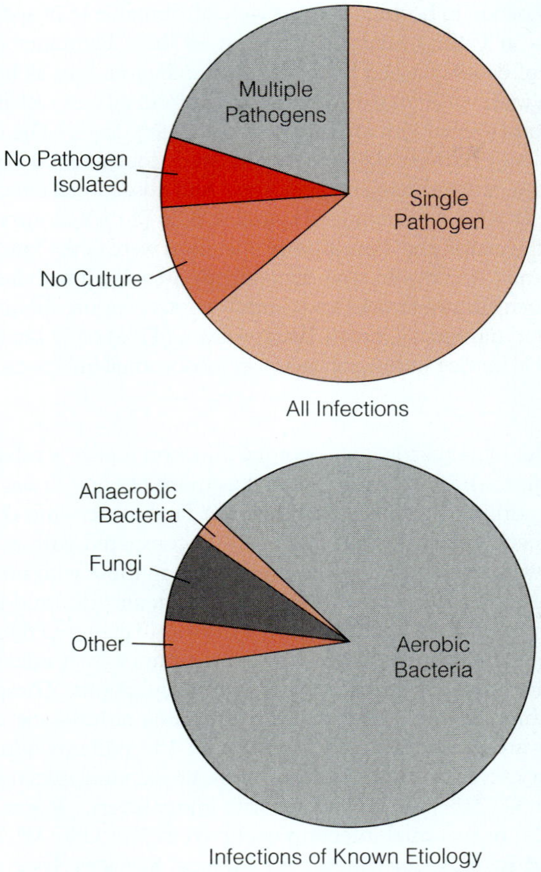

Figure 4 **Illustrated is a breakdown of the etiology of 26,965 nosocomial infections from the National Nosocomial Infections Surveillance System.**[3]

serious problem over the past 10 years. Enterococci were the third most common nosocomial bloodstream isolate reported by NNIS hospitals between 1990 and 1992.[218] The incidence of vancomycin-resistant enterococci (VRE) increased 26-fold between 1989 and 1993, from 0.3% to 7.9%, with a 34-fold rise in ICUs,[219] and the rate has continued to increase. These strains arise from endogenous flora of the patient, but nosocomial spread within the hospital environment is also an important route of spread.[219,220] The environment around infected patients is heavily contaminated with VRE, and gown and glove isolation techniques are required to stop transmission.[220] VRE are also highly resistant to other available antibiotics. Acquisition of VRE is significantly associated with prior hospitalization and with use of third-generation cephalosporins, vancomycin, or multiple antibiotics.[221,222] In one study, 16% of stool specimens submitted for testing for *C. difficile* toxin were colonized with VRE, and all surgical patients in that study had the same strain.[223]

High mortality can be associated with VRE infections. When the outcome of patients with VRE bacteremia was compared with the outcome of patients with bacteremia caused by vancomycin-sensitive enterococci (VSE), mortality was 2.3 times higher in those with VRE bacteremia, and 89% of patients with VRE bacteremia were colonized or infected with VRE at another site.[224] Prior treatment with third-generation cephalosporins is another risk factor for increased mortality.[218] Liver transplant patients with VRE bacteremia had a 92% higher mortality than comparable patients with VSE bacteremia, and those with VRE bacteremia also had a higher recurrence rate and greater need for invasive procedures.[225]

Current recommendations include decreased use, and possibly restricted use, of vancomycin as well as aggressive infection control measures whenever VRE are isolated in a hospitalized patient.[219] In particular, vancomycin should not be used as primary treatment for *C. difficile*–associated diarrhea and should be avoided for surgical prophylaxis unless the hospital has a specific MRSA problem or the patient cannot receive other appropriate antibiotics.

ENTERIC INFECTION

C. difficile is often found in patients with severe antibiotic-associated enteric infections. In one report, 691 (2%) of 32,757 consecutive postoperative patients experienced watery diarrhea significant enough to stimulate a request for *C. difficile* toxin assay.[226] Of this number, 75 (11% of patients with diarrhea) had a positive toxin assay. All cases were associated with antibiotic administration, and 94% of the patients had received a cephalosporin either alone or in combination with other antibiotics; 29% of these responded to cessation of antibiotics and supportive measures. The remainder were treated with vancomycin, metronidazole, or bacitracin. Six (14%) of the patients who required specific therapy relapsed after initial response to treatment and were subsequently cured with one or more additional courses of treatment. Two patients died, and the overall hospital stay for the remaining patients was prolonged on average by 50%.

Most patients with mild cases of antibiotic-associated diarrhea do not have either positive cultures for *C. difficile* or positive toxin assays, and the etiologic role of *C. difficile* is unclear. Many hospitalized patients without diarrhea also have *C. difficile* in the stool, with

Table 2 **Five Most Common Pathogens Isolated from Surgical Patients and Percentage of Total within Each Site**[3]

Infection Site	Organism	Isolates at That Site (%)
Urinary tract infection	*Escherichia coli*	29
	Pseudomonas aeruginosa	16
	Enterococci	13
	Proteus species	7
	Klebsiella species	7
Surgical wound infection	*Staphylococcus aureus*	19
	Enterococci	12
	E. coli	12
	P. aeruginosa	10
	Coagulase-negative staphylococci	8
Lower respiratory infection	*P. aeruginosa*	17
	S. aureus	12
	Enterobacter species	11
	Klebsiella species	11
	Serratia species	7
Bacteremia	Coagulase-negative staphylococci	14
	S. aureus	10
	Enterobacter species	9
	Enterococci	9
	Klebsiella species	8
Cutaneous infections	*S. aureus*	19
	P. aeruginosa	13
	Enterococci	11
	Coagulase-negative staphylococci	10
	E. coli	8

or without toxin production,[143,144,227] and the likelihood of isolating this pathogen increases with patients' increasing length of stay.[137] A nonpathogenic yeast, *Saccharomyces boulardii*, when administered by mouth to hospitalized patients receiving antibiotics, significantly reduced the occurrence of antibiotic-associated diarrhea without affecting the rate of acquisition of *C. difficile*.[143]

Approximately 3% of asymptomatic adults carry *C. difficile* in their stools, but 30% to 40% of healthy neonates may carry the organism. The rate of carriage declines after the age of 1 to 2 years. *C. difficile* can be spread in the hospital and has been isolated from 10% of inanimate objects in the environment of patients with *C. difficile* colonization, compared with 3% in hospital areas with no known cases.[228] In one report, this organism was recovered from the hands of 13% of medical personnel working in a ward with affected patients[228]; in another, it was recovered from 60% of personnel immediately after caring for an affected patient.[229] Soap-and-water washing was ineffective in preventing acquisition, but the combination of glove use and chlorhexidine washing was effective. In another medical center, clusters of new nosocomial *C. difficile* diarrhea were prevented by screening all patients with diarrhea by active surveillance (using culture to identify *C. difficile* infection) and by instituting isolation precautions and daily disinfection of infected patients' rooms.[230]

The incidence of *C. difficile* in the environment is increased when a patient has diarrhea, compared with stool carriage without diarrhea.[228,229] In one prospectively studied cohort of patients, 21% of patients without *C. difficile* in their stools on admission acquired the organism during hospitalization, and 37% of these patients developed diarrhea. No cases of colitis occurred.[228] Diarrhea was more common in patients who received antibiotics. The rate of acquisition of *C. difficile* was 73% higher if a patient had a roommate colonized with *C. difficile*.

COST

The cost of nosocomial infections, both in dollars and in morbidity, is high. According to one estimate, 8.7 million extra hospital days and $4.5 billion in hospital charges were attributable to nosocomial infections in United States hospitals in 1976.[231] Estimates of the number of deaths caused by nosocomial infections run as high as 58,000 a year; 9,700 of these deaths and 36% of all costs attributed to nosocomial infections are due to wound infections.[231] The actual numbers may be even higher.[9] Another study found that 63 of 200 consecutive patients dying in the hospital had nosocomial infections, of which 18 (29%) were judged causal and 26 (41%) contributory. Most of the causal and contributory infections were of the lower respiratory tract, and deaths were significantly associated with invasive devices such as intra-arterial and central venous pressure monitoring devices and nasogastric tubes. Twenty-seven (47%) of 57 deaths on the surgical service were associated with nosocomial infections.

RISK

The risk of acquiring a nosocomial infection is clearly related to the reason for hospitalization as well as to underlying disease.[9,232] Patients admitted to the hospital with a fatal underlying disease have a nosocomial infection rate of 24%, compared with 10% in patients with ultimately fatal disease and 2% in those with nonfatal disease. Among 100 consecutive trauma patients admitted to the ICU at Harborview Medical Center in 1986, 42 acquired 64 nosocomial infections, including 23 lower respiratory tract infections, 17 urinary tract infections, and 6 wound infections. These 100 ICU admissions and 101 consecutive trauma admissions to the general ward were examined together. Of 153 patients admitted with injury severity scores[233] of 25 or less, nosocomial infection occurred in 32 (21%). Of 48 patients with injury severity scores higher than 25, nosocomial infection occurred in 26 (54%).[189] At the Maryland Institute for Emergency Medical Services System, the rate of nosocomial infection was 16% in 1981 and 30% in 1979.[234,235] A statewide survey of hospitals in Virginia from 1978 to 1982 found that infections in ICU patients accounted for 25% of all cases of nosocomial infections, although fewer than 10% of the beds were in ICUs.[236]

References

1. Haley RW, Schaberg DR, Crossley KB, et al: Extra charges and prolongation of stay attributable to nosocomial infections: a prospective interhospital comparison. Am J Med 70:51, 1981
2. Haley RW, Schaberg DR, Von Allmen SD, et al: Estimating the extra charges and prolongation of hospitalization due to nosocomial infections: a comparison of methods. J Infect Dis 141:248, 1980
3. Horan TC, White JW, Jarvis WR, et al: Nosocomial infection surveillance, 1984. CDC Surveillance Summaries. MMWR Morb Mortal Wkly Rep 35:17SS, 1986
4. Haley RW, Culver DH, White JW, et al: The nationwide nosocomial infection rate: a new need for vital statistics. Am J Epidemiol 121:159, 1985
5. Haley RW, White JW, Culver DH, et al: The financial incentive for hospitals to prevent nosocomial infections under the prospective payment system: an empirical determination from a nationally representative sample. JAMA 257:1611, 1987
6. Haley RW, Culver DH, Morgan WM, et al: Increased recognition of infectious diseases in US hospitals through increased use of diagnostic tests, 1970 to 1976. Am J Epidemiol 121:168, 1985
7. Roberts J, Barnes W, Pennock M, et al: Diagnostic accuracy of fever as a measure of postoperative pulmonary complications. Heart Lung 17:166, 1988
8. Engoren M: Lack of association between atelectasis and fever. Chest 107:81, 1995
9. Gross PA, Neu HC, Aswapokee P, et al: Deaths from nosocomial infections: experience in a university hospital and a community hospital. Am J Med 68:219, 1980
10. Andrews CP, Coalson JJ, Smith JD, et al: Diagnosis of nosocomial bacterial pneumonia in acute, diffuse lung injury. Chest 80:254, 1981
11. Craven DE, Steger KA: Ventilator-associated bacterial pneumonia: challenges in diagnosis, treatment, and prevention. New Horizons 6:S30, 1998
12. Croce MA, Fabian TC, Schurr MJ, et al: Using bronchoalveolar lavage to distinguish nosocomial pneumonia from systemic inflammatory response syndrome: a prospective analysis. J Trauma 39:1134, 1995
13. Valles J, Artigas A, Rello J, et al: Continuous aspiration of subglottic secretions in preventing ventilator-associated pneumonia. Ann Intern Med 122:179, 1995
14. Fernandez-Crehuet R, Diaz-Molina C, de Irala J, et al: Nosocomial infection in an intensive-care unit: identification of risk factors. Infect Control Hosp Epidemiol 18:825, 1997
15. Caplan ES, Hoyt NJ: Nosocomial sinusitis. JAMA 247:639, 1982
16. O'Reilly MJ, Reddick EJ, Black W, et al: Sepsis from sinusitis in nasotracheally intubated patients: a diagnostic dilemma. Am J Surg 147:601, 1984
17. Deutschman CS, Wilton PB, Sinow J, et al: Paranasal sinusitis: a common complication of nasotracheal intubation in neurosurgical patients. Neurosurgery 17:296, 1985
18. Kronberg FG, Goodwin WJ Jr: Sinusitis in intensive care unit patients. Laryngoscope 95:936, 1985
19. Deutschman CS, Wilton P, Sinow J, et al: Paranasal sinusitis associated with nasotracheal intubation: a frequently unrecognized and treatable source of sepsis. Crit Care Med 14:111, 1986
20. Grindlinger GA, Niehoff J, Hughes SL, et al: Acute paranasal sinusitis related to nasotracheal intubation of head-injured patients. Crit Care Med 15:214, 1987
21. Christensen L, Schaffer S, Ross SE: Otitis media in adult trauma patients: incidence and clinical significance. J Trauma 31:1543, 1991
22. Roettinger W, Edgerton MT, Kurtz LD, et al: Role of inoculation site as a determinant of infections in soft tissue wounds. Am J Surg 126:354, 1973
23. Miles AA, Milles EM, Burke J: The value and duration of defence reactions of the skin to the primary lodgement of bacteria. Br J Exp Pathol 38:79, 1957
24. Burke JF, Miles AA: The sequence of vascular events

in early infective inflammation. J Pathol Bacteriol 76: 1, 1958
25. Burke JF: The effective period of preventive antibiotic action in experimental incisions and dermal lesions. Surgery 50:161, 1961
26. Alexander JW, Altemeier WA: Penicillin prophylaxis of experimental staphylococcal wound infections. Surg Gynecol Obstet 120:243, 1965
27. Edlich RF, Smith QT, Edgerton MT: Resistance of the surgical wound to antimicrobial prophylaxis and its mechanisms of development. Am J Surg 126:583, 1973
28. McKittrick LS, Wheelock FC: The routine use of antibiotics in elective abdominal surgery. Surg Gynecol Obstet 99:376, 1954
29. Barnes J, Pace WG, Trump DS, et al: Prophylactic postoperative antibiotics: a controlled study of 1007 cases. AMA Arch Surg 79:190, 1959
30. Dellinger EP, Gross PA, Barrett TL, et al: Quality standard for antimicrobial prophylaxis in surgical procedures. Clin Infect Dis 18:422, 1994
31. Page CP, Bohnen JMA, Fletcher JR, et al: Antimicrobial prophylaxis for surgical wounds: guidelines for clinical care. Arch Surg 128:79, 1993
32. Dellinger EP: Antibiotic prophylaxis in trauma: penetrating abdominal injuries and open fractures. Rev Infect Dis 13(suppl 10):S847, 1991
33. Fabian TC, Croce MA, Payne LW, et al: Duration of antibiotic therapy for penetrating abdominal trauma: a prospective trial. Surgery 112:788, 1992
34. Culver DH, Horan TC, Gaynes RP, et al: Surgical wound infection rates by wound class, operative procedure, and patient risk index: National Nosocomial Infections Surveillance System. Am J Med 91:152S, 1991
35. Consensus paper on the surveillance of surgical wound infections. The Society for Hospital Epidemiology of America, The Association for Practitioners in Infection Control, The Centers for Disease Control, The Surgical Infection Society. Infect Control Hosp Epidemiol 13:599, 1992
36. Horan TC, Gaynes RP, Martone WJ, et al: CDC definitions of nosocomial surgical site infections, 1992: a modification of CDC definitions of surgical wound infections. Am J Infect Control 20:271, 1992
37. MacLennan JD: The histotoxic clostridial infections of man. Bacteriologic Reviews 26:177, 1962
38. Pitcher WD, Musher DM: Critical importance of early diagnosis and treatment of intra-abdominal infection. Arch Surg 117:328, 1982
39. Bohnen J, Boulanger M, Meakins JL, et al: Prognosis in generalized peritonitis: relation to cause and risk factors. Arch Surg 118:285, 1983
40. Caplan ES, Hoyt NJ, Rodriguez A, et al: Empyema occurring in the multiply traumatized patient. J Trauma 24:785, 1984
41. Rutledge R, Applebaum RE, Kim BJ: Mediastinal infection after open heart surgery. Surgery 97:88, 1985
42. Fong IW, Baker CB, McKee DC: The value of prophylactic antibiotics in aorta-coronary bypass operations: a double-blind randomized trial. J Thorac Cardiovasc Surg 78:908, 1979
43. Milano CA, Kesler K, Archibald N, et al: Mediastinitis after coronary artery bypass graft surgery: risk factors and long-term survival. Circulation 92:2245, 1995
44. Gur E, Stern D, Weiss J, et al: Clinical-radiological evaluation of poststernotomy wound infection. Plast Reconstruct Surg 101:348, 1998
45. Pairolero PC, Arnold PG, Harris JB: Long-term results of pectoralis major muscle transposition for infected sternotomy wounds. Ann Surg 213:583, 1991
46. Hand WL, Sanford JP: Posttraumatic bacterial meningitis. Ann Intern Med 72:869, 1970
47. MacGee EE, Cauthen JC, Brackett CE: Meningitis following acute traumatic cerebrospinal fluid fistula. J Neurosurg 33:312, 1970

48. Leech PJ, Paterson A: Conservative and operative management for cerebrospinal-fluid leakage after closed head injury. Lancet 1:1013, 1973
49. Davis CH: Traumatic CSF fistula: investigation and treatment. Current Controversies in Neurosurgery. Morley TP, Ed. WB Saunders Co, Philadelphia, 1976, p 572
50. Petersdorf RG, Curtin JA, Hoeprich PD, et al: A study of antibiotic prophylaxis in unconscious patients. N Engl J Med 257:1001, 1957
51. Clancey GJ, Hansen ST: Open fractures of the tibia: a review of one hundred and two cases. J Bone Joint Surg [Am] 60:118, 1978
52. Chapman MW, Mahoney M: The role of early internal fixation in the management of open fractures. Clin Orthop 138:120, 1979
53. Gustilo RB, Mendoza RM, Williams DN: Problems in the management of type III (severe) open fractures: a new classification of type III open fractures. J Trauma 24:742, 1984
54. Gustilo RB, Anderson JT: Prevention of infection in the treatment of one thousand and twenty-five open fractures of long bones: retrospective and prospective analyses. J Bone Joint Surg [Am] 58:453, 1976
55. Rittmann WW, Schibli M, Matter P, et al: Open fractures: long-term results in 200 consecutive cases. Clin Orthop 138:132, 1979
56. Dellinger EP, Miller SD, Wertz MJ, et al: Risk of infection after open fracture of the arm or leg. Arch Surg 123:1320, 1988
57. Sattler FR, Foderaro JB, Aber RC: *Staphylococcus epidermidis* bacteremia associated with vascular catheters: an important cause of febrile morbidity in hospitalized patients. Infect Control 5:279, 1984
58. Rhame FS, Maki DG, Bennett JV: Intravenous cannula-associated infections. Hospital Infections. Bennett JV, Brachman PS, Eds. Little, Brown & Co, Boston, 1979, p 433
59. Bregenzer T, Conen D, Sakmann P, et al: Is routine replacement of peripheral venous catheters necessary? Arch Intern Med 158:151, 1998
60. Hershey CO, Tomford JW, McLaren CE, et al: The natural history of intravenous catheter-associated phlebitis. Arch Intern Med 144:1373, 1984
61. Maki DG, Weise CE, Sarafin HW: A semiquantitative culture method for identifying intravenous-catheter-related infection. N Engl J Med 296:1305, 1977
62. Press OW, Ramsey PG, Larson EB, et al: Hickman catheter infections in patients with malignancies. Medicine (Baltimore) 63:189, 1984
63. Clarke DE, Raffin TA: Infectious complications of indwelling long-term central venous catheters. Chest 97:966, 1990
64. Band JD, Alvarado CJ, Maki DG: A semiquantitative culture technic for identifying infection due to steel needles used for intravenous therapy. American Society of Clinical Pathologists 72:980, 1979
65. Maki DG, Jarrett F, Sarafin HW: A semiquantitative culture method for identification of catheter-related infection in the burn patient. J Surg Res 22:513, 1977
66. Maki DG, Cobb L, Garman JK, et al: An attachable silver-impregnated cuff for prevention of infection with central venous catheters: a prospective randomized multicenter trial. Am J Med 85:307, 1988
67. Conly JM, Grieves K, Peters B: A prospective, randomized study comparing transparent and dry gauze dressings for central venous catheters. J Infect Dis 159:310, 1989
68. Franceschi D, Gerding RL, Phillips G, et al: Risk factors associated with intravascular catheter infections in burned patients: a prospective randomized study. J Trauma 29:81, 1989
69. Pittet D, Lew PD, Auckenthaler R, et al: Bacterial spread as a pathogenic factor in catheter-related infections (abstr No. 26). Read before the 30th Interscience Conference on Antimicrobial Agents and Chemotherapy, October 21, 1990, Atlanta. American Society for Microbiology, Washington, D.C.

70. Moyer MA, Edwards LD, Farley L: Comparative culture methods on 101 intravenous catheters: routine, semiquantitative, and blood cultures. Arch Intern Med 143:66, 1983
71. Myers ML, Austin TW, Sibbald WJ: Pulmonary artery catheter infections: a prospective study. Ann Surg 201:237, 1985
72. Cooper GL, Hopkins CC: Rapid diagnosis of intravascular catheter-associated infection by direct Gram staining of catheter segments. N Engl J Med 312:1142, 1985
73. Singh S, Nelson N, Acosta I, et al: Catheter colonization and bacteremia with pulmonary and arterial catheters. Crit Care Med 10:736, 1982
74. Charalambos C, Swoboda SM, Dick J, et al: Risk factors and clinical impact of central line infections in the surgical intensive care unit. Arch Surg 133:1241, 1998
75. Raad I: Intravascular-catheter-related infections. Lancet 351:893, 1998
76. Guideline for prevention of intravascular device-related infections. Hospital Infection Control Practices Advisory Committee. Infect Control Hosp Epidemiol 17:438, 1996
77. Sherertz RJ, Heard SO, Raad II: Diagnosis of triple-lumen catheter infection: comparison of roll plate, sonication, and flushing methodologies. J Clin Microbiol 35:641, 1997
78. Sanders RA, Sheldon GF: Septic complications of total parenteral nutrition: a five year experience. Am J Surg 132:214, 1976
79. Freeman JB, Litton AA: Preponderance of gram-positive infections during parenteral alimentation. Surg Gynecol Obstet 139:905, 1974
80. Ponce de Leon S, Wenzel RP: Hospital-acquired bloodstream infections with *Staphylococcus epidermidis*. Am J Med 77:639, 1984
81. Rex JH, Bennett JE, Sugar AM, et al: Intravascular catheter exchange and duration of candidemia: NIAID Mycoses Study Group and the Candidemia Study Group. Clin Infect Dis 21:994, 1995
82. Stein JM, Pruitt BA: Suppurative thrombophlebitis: a lethal iatrogenic disease. N Engl J Med 282:1452, 1970
83. Munster AM: Septic thrombophlebitis: a surgical disorder. JAMA 230:1010, 1974
84. Hauser CJ, Bosco P, Davenport M, et al: Surgical management of fungal peripheral thrombophlebitis. Surgery 105:510, 1989
85. Kaufman J, Demas C, Stark K, et al: Catheter-related septic central venous thrombosis: current therapeutic options. West J Med 145:200, 1986
86. Strinden WD, Helgerson RB, Maki DG: *Candida* septic thrombosis of the great central veins associated with central catheters: clinical features and management. Ann Surg 202:653, 1985
87. Cobb DK, High KP, Sawyer RG, et al: A controlled trial of scheduled replacement of central venous and pulmonary-artery catheters. N Engl J Med 327:1062, 1992
88. Cook D, Randolph A, Kernerman P, et al: Central venous catheter replacement strategies: a systematic review of the literature. Crit Care Med 25:1417, 1997
89. Reed CR, Sessler CN, Glauser FL, et al: Central venous catheter infections: concepts and controversies. Intens Care Med 21:177, 1995
90. Pettigrew RA, Lang SD, Haydock DA, et al: Catheter-related sepsis in patients on intravenous nutrition: a prospective study of quantitative catheter cultures and guidewire changes for suspected sepsis. Br J Surg 72:52, 1985
91. Newsome HH, Armstrong CW, Mayhall GC, et al: Mechanical complications from insertion of subclavian venous feeding catheters: comparison of de novo percutaneous venipuncture to change of catheter over guidewire. J Parenter Enteral Nutr 8:560, 1984

92. Sitzmann JV, Townsend TR, Siler MC, et al: Septic and technical complications of central venous catheterization: a prospective study of 200 consecutive patients. Ann Surg 202:766, 1985
93. Hopkins S: Diagnosing bacterial complications of temporary central venous catheters. Clinical Consultations in Nutritional Support 2:14, 1982
94. Bozzetti F, Terno G, Bonfanti G, et al: Prevention and treatment of central venous catheter sepsis by exchange via a guidewire: a prospective controlled trial. Ann Surg 198:48, 1983
95. Maher MM, Brennan MF: Central venous catheter exchange using a guidewire. J Parenter Enteral Nutr 3:515, 1979
96. Powell C, Kulich P, Mandelbaum J, et al: Effect of frequent guidewire changes on triple-lumen catheter (TLC) sepsis. J Parenter Enteral Nutr 11:15S, 1987
97. Norwood S, Jenkins G: An evaluation of triple-lumen catheter infections using a guidewire exchange technique. J Trauma 30:706, 1990
98. Norwood S, Ruby A, Civetta J, et al: Catheter-related infections and associated septicemia. Chest 99:968, 1991
99. Williams WW: Infection control during parenteral nutrition therapy. J Parenter Enteral Nutr 9:735, 1985
100. Raad II, Hohn DC, Gilbreath BJ, et al: Prevention of central venous catheter-related infections by using maximal sterile barrier precautions during insertion. Infect Control Hosp Epidemiol 15:231, 1994
101. Collignon P, Soni N, Pearson I, et al: Sepsis associated with central vein catheters in critically ill patients. Intens Care Med 14:227, 1988
102. Richet H, Hubert B, Nitemberg G, et al: Prospective multicenter study of vascular-catheter-related complications and risk factors for positive central-catheter cultures in intensive care unit patients. J Clin Microbiol 28:2520, 1990
103. Central venous catheters coated with minocycline and rifampin for the prevention of catheter-related colonization and bloodstream infections: a randomized, double-blind trial. The Texas Medical Center Catheter Study Group. Ann Intern Med 127:267, 1997
104. Maki DG, Stolz SM, Wheeler S, et al: Prevention of central venous catheter-related bloodstream infection by use of an antiseptic-impregnated catheter: a randomized, controlled trial. Ann Intern Med 127:257, 1997
105. Darouiche RO, Raad II, Heard SO, et al: A comparison of two antimicrobial-impregnated central venous catheters. N Engl J Med 340:1, 1999
106. Powell C, Regan C, Fabri PJ, et al: Evaluation of op site catheter dressings for parenteral nutrition: a prospective, randomized study. J Parenter Enteral Nutr 6:43, 1982
107. Palidar PJ, Simonowitz DA, Oreskovich MR, et al: Use of op site as an occlusive dressing for total parenteral nutrition catheters. J Parenter Enteral Nutr 6:150, 1982
108. Maki DG, Band JD: A comparative study of polyantibiotic and iodophor ointments in prevention of vascular catheter–related infection. Am J Med 70:739, 1981
109. Hoffman KK, Weber DJ, Samsa GP, et al: Transparent polyurethane film as an intravenous catheter dressing: a meta-analysis of the infection risks. JAMA 267:2072, 1992
110. Forlaw L, Torosian MH: Central venous catheter care. Rombeau JL, Caldwell MD, Eds. Clinical Nutrition, Vol 2: Parenteral Nutrition. WB Saunders Co, Philadelphia, 1986, p 316
111. Ryan JA Jr, Abel RM, Abbott WM, et al: Catheter complications in total parenteral nutrition: a prospective study of 200 consecutive patients. N Engl J Med 290:757, 1974
112. Copeland EM, MacFayden BV Jr, Dudrick SJ: Prevention of microbial catheter contamination in patients receiving parenteral hyperalimentation. South Med J 67:303, 1974
113. Padberg FT Jr, Ruggiero J, Blackburn GL, et al: Central venous catheterization for parenteral nutrition. Ann Surg 193:264, 1981
114. Hilton E, Haslett TM, Borenstein MT, et al: Central catheter infections: single- versus triple-lumen catheters: influence of guidewires on infection rates when used for replacement of catheters. Am J Med 84:667, 1988
115. Pemberton LB, Lyman B, Lander V, et al: Sepsis from triple- vs single-lumen catheters during total parenteral nutrition in surgical or critically ill patients. Arch Surg 121:591, 1986
116. Miller JJ, Venus B, Mathru M: Comparison of the sterility of long-term central venous catheterization using single lumen, triple lumen, and pulmonary artery catheters. Crit Care Med 12:634, 1984
117. Powell C, Fabri PJ, Kudsk KA: Risk of infection accompanying the use of single-lumen vs. double-lumen subclavian catheters: a prospective randomized study. J Parenter Enteral Nutr 12:127, 1988
118. Raad I, Davis S, Becker M, et al: Low infection rate and long durability of nontunneled Silastic catheters: a safe and cost-effective alternative for long-term venous access. Arch Intern Med 153:1791, 1993
119. Groeger JS, Lucas AB, Thaler HT, et al: Infectious morbidity associated with long-term use of venous access devices in patients with cancer. Ann Intern Med 119:1168, 1993
120. Bern MM, Lokich JJ, Wallach SR, et al: Very low doses of warfarin can prevent thrombosis in central venous catheters: a prospective randomized trial. Ann Intern Med 112:423, 1990
121. Stark RP, Maki DG: Bacteriuria in the catheterized patient: what quantitative level of bacteriuria is relevant? N Engl J Med 311:560, 1984
122. Kunin CM: Genitourinary infections in the patient at risk: extrinsic risk factors. Am J Med 76:131, 1984
123. Harding GK, Nicolle LE, Ronald AR, et al: How long should catheter-acquired urinary tract infection in women be treated? A randomized controlled study. Ann Intern Med 114:713, 1991
124. Hirsh DD, Fainstein V, Musher DM: Do condom catheter collecting systems cause urinary tract infection? JAMA 242:340, 1979
125. Johnson ET: The condom catheter: urinary tract infection and other complications. South Med J 76:579, 1983
126. Kunin CM: Urinary tract infections. Hospital Infection. Bennett JV, Brachman PS, Eds. Little, Brown & Co, Boston, 1979, p 239
127. Garibaldi RA, Burke JP, Dickman ML, et al: Factors predisposing to bacteriuria during indwelling urethral catheterization. N Engl J Med 291:215, 1974
128. Warren JW, Platt R, Thomas RJ, et al: Antibiotic irrigation and catheter-associated urinary tract infections. N Engl J Med 299:570, 1978
129. Platt R, Polk BF, Murdock B, et al: Reduction of mortality associated with nosocomial urinary tract infection. Lancet 1:893, 1983
130. Lima NL, Guerrant RL, Kaiser DL, et al: A retrospective cohort study of nosocomial diarrhea as a risk factor for nosocomial infection. J Infect Dis 161:948, 1990
131. Jones SR, Smith JW, Sanford JP: Localization of urinary-tract infections by detection of antibody-coated bacteria in urine sediment. N Engl J Med 290:591, 1974
132. Latham RH, Stamm WE: Role of fimbriated *Escherichia coli* in urinary tract infections in adult women: correlation with localization studies. J Infect Dis 149:835, 1984
133. Anderson RU: Urinary tract infections in compromised hosts. Urol Clin North Am 13:727, 1986
134. Cattell WR: Urinary infections in adults—1985. Postgrad Med J 61:907, 1985
135. Stamm WE: Approach to the patient with urinary tract infection. Infectious Disease. Gorbach SL, Bartlett JG, Blacklow NR, Eds. WB Saunders Co, Philadelphia, 1992, p 788
136. DuPont HL: Infectious gastroenteritis. Hospital Infection. Bennett JV, Brachman PS, Eds. Little, Brown & Co, Boston, 1979, p 381
137. Hines J, Nachamkin I: Effective use of the clinical microbiology laboratory for diagnosing diarrheal diseases. Clin Infect Dis 23:1292, 1996
138. Gerding DN, Johnson S, Peterson LR, et al: *Clostridium difficile*-associated diarrhea and colitis. Infect Control Hosp Epidemiol 16:459, 1995
139. McFarland LV, Coyle MB, Kremer WH, et al: Rectal swab cultures for *Clostridium difficile* surveillance studies. J Clin Microbiol 25:2241, 1987
140. Bartlett JG: Antibiotic-associated colitis. Dis Mon 30:1, 1984
141. George WL: Antimicrobial agent–associated colitis and diarrhea: historical background and clinical aspects. Rev Infect Dis 6:S208, 1984
142. Grube BJ, Heimbach DM, Marvin JA: *Clostridium difficile* diarrhea in critically ill burned patients. Arch Surg 122:655, 1987
143. Bartlett JG, Moon N, Chang TW, et al: Role of *Clostridium difficile* in antibiotic-associated pseudomembranous colitis. Gastroenterology 75:778, 1978
144. Surawicz CM, Elmer GW, Speelman P, et al: Prevention of antibiotic-associated diarrhea by *Saccharomyces boulardii*: a prospective study. Gastroenterology 96:981, 1989
145. McFarland LV, Surawicz CM, Stamm WE: Risk factors for *Clostridium difficile* carriage and *C. difficile*-associated diarrhea in a cohort of hospitalized patients. J Infect Dis 162:678, 1990
146. Tedesco FJ, Corless JK, Brownstein RE: Rectal sparing in antibiotic-associated pseudomembranous colitis: a prospective study. Gastroenterology 83:1259, 1982
147. Dane TE, King EG: Fatal pseudomembranous enterocolitis following clindamycin therapy. Br J Surg 63:305, 1976
148. Cheung A, Tank RE, Dellinger EP: Antibiotic-associated enterocolitis involving the small bowel. Surgical Rounds 14:821, 1991
149. Hecht JR, Olinger EJ: *Clostridium difficile* colitis secondary to intravenous vancomycin. Dig Dis Sci 34:148, 1989
150. Miller SN, Ringler RP: Vancomycin-induced pseudomembranous colitis (letter). J Clin Gastroenterol 9:114, 1987
151. Oliva SL, Guglielmo BJ, Jacobs R, et al: Failure of intravenous vancomycin and intravenous metronidazole to prevent or treat antibiotic-associated pseudomembranous colitis (letter). J Infect Dis 159:1154, 1989
152. Freiman JP, Graham DJ, Green L: Pseudomembranous colitis associated with single-dose cephalosporin prophylaxis (letter). JAMA 262:902, 1989
153. Bartlett JG: Treatment of *Clostridium difficile* colitis (editorial). Gastroenterology 89:1192, 1985
154. Bartlett JG: Treatment of antibiotic-associated pseudomembranous colitis. Rev Infect Dis 6(suppl 1):S235, 1984
155. Young GP, Ward PB, Bayley N, et al: Antibiotic-associated colitis due to *Clostridium difficile*: double-blind comparison of vancomycin with bacitracin. Gastroenterology 89:1038, 1985
156. Recommendations for preventing the spread of vancomycin resistance. Hospital Infection Control Practices Advisory Committee. MMWR Morb Mortal Wkly Rep 44:1, 1995
157. Johnson S, Adelmann A, Clabots CR, et al: Recurrence of *Clostridium difficile* diarrhea not caused by the original infecting organism. J Infect Dis 159:340, 1989
158. Guzman R, Kirkpatrick J, Forward K, et al: Failure of parenteral metronidazole in the treatment of pseudomembranous colitis (letter). J Infect Dis 158:1146, 1988

159. Johnson S, Peterson LR, Gerding DN: Intravenous metronidazole and *Clostridium difficile*-associated diarrhea or colitis (letter). J Infect Dis 160:1087, 1989
160. Gerding DN, Olson MM, Johnson S, et al: *Clostridium difficile* diarrhea and colonization after treatment with abdominal infection regimens containing clindamycin or metronidazole. Am J Surg 159:212, 1990
161. Levine R, Peskin GW, Saik RP: Drug-induced colitis as a surgical disease. Arch Surg 111:987, 1976
162. Drapkin MS, Worthington MG, Chang TW, et al: *Clostridium difficile* colitis mimicking acute peritonitis. Arch Surg 120:1321, 1985
163. Chatila W, Manthous CA: *Clostridium difficile* causing sepsis and an acute abdomen in critically ill patients. Crit Care Med 23:1146, 1995
164. Byl B, Jacobs F, Struelens MJ, et al: Extraintestinal *Clostridium difficile* infections. Clin Infect Dis 22: 712, 1996
165. Kahn RA: Diseases transmitted by blood transfusion. Hum Pathol 14:241, 1983
166. Kahn RA, Barrios SDP: Diseases transmitted by blood transfusion. Transfusion Therapy: Principles and Procedures. Rutman RC, Miller WV, Eds. Aspen Publishers, Rockville, Maryland, 1985, p 311
167. Herwaldt BL, Kjemtrup AM, Conrad PA, et al: Transfusion-transmitted babesiosis in Washington State: first reported case caused by a WA1-type parasite. J Infect Dis 175:1259, 1997
168. Wagner SJ, Friedman LI, Dodd RY: Transfusion-associated bacterial sepsis. Clin Microbiol Rev 7:290, 1994
169. Red blood cell transfusions contaminated with *Yersinia enterocolitica*—United States, 1991-1996, and initiation of a national study to detect bacteria-associated transfusion reactions. MMWR Morb Mortal Wkly Rep 46:553, 1997
170. Update: *Yersinia enterocolitica* bacteremia and endotoxin shock associated with red blood cell transfusions—United States, 1991. MMWR Morb Mortal Wkly Rep 40:176, 1991
171. Shorey J: The current status of non-A, non-B viral hepatitis. Southwestern Internal Medicine Conference. Am J Med Sci 289:251, 1985
172. Aach RD, Kahn RA: Post-transfusion hepatitis: current perspectives. Ann Intern Med 92:539, 1980
173. Iwarson S, Norkrans G, Wejstal R: Hepatitis C: natural history of a unique infection. Clin Infect Dis 20:1361, 1995
174. Chen D-S, Kuo GC, Sung J-L, et al: Hepatitis C virus infection in an area hyperendemic for hepatitis B and chronic liver disease: the Taiwan experience. J Infect Dis 162:817, 1990
175. Koretz RL, Stone O, Mousa M, et al: Non-A, non-B posttransfusion hepatitis—a decade later. Gastroenterology 88:1251, 1985
176. Esteban JI, González A, Hernández JM, et al: Evaluation of antibodies to hepatitis C virus in a study of transfusion-associated hepatitis. N Engl J Med 323:110, 1990
177. Lee S-D, Hwang S-J, Lu R-H, et al: Antibodies to hepatitis C virus in prospectively followed patients with posttransfusion hepatitis. J Infect Dis 163:1354, 1991
178. Transfusion-associated human T-lymphotropic virus type III/lymphadenopathy-associated virus infection from a seronegative donor—Colorado. MMWR Morb Mortal Wkly Rep 35:389, 1986
179. Cumming PD, Wallace EL, Schorr JB, et al: Exposure of patients to human immunodeficiency virus through the transfusion of blood components that test antibody-negative. N Engl J Med 321:941, 1989
180. Menitove JE: Current risk of transfusion-associated human immunodeficiency virus infection. Arch Pathol Lab Med 114:330, 1990
181. Busch MP, Eble BE, Khayam-Bashi H, et al: Evaluation of screened blood donations for human immunodeficiency virus type 1 infection by culture and DNA amplification of pooled cells. N Engl J Med 325:1, 1991
182. Schreiber GB, Busch MP, Kleinman SH, et al: The risk of transfusion-transmitted viral infections: The Retrovirus Epidemiology Donor Study. N Engl J Med 334:1685, 1996
183. Curran JW, Lawrence DN, Jaffe H, et al: Acquired immunodeficiency syndrome (AIDS) associated with transfusions. N Engl J Med 310:69, 1984
184. Bove JR: Transfusion-associated AIDS—a cause for concern (editorial). N Engl J Med 310:115, 1984
185. Surgenor DMacN, Wallace EL, Hao SH: Collection and transfusion of blood in the United States, 1982-1988. N Engl J Med 322:1646, 1990
186. Garibaldi RA, Brodine S, Matsumiya S, et al: Evidence for the non-infectious etiology of early postoperative fever. Infect Control 6:273, 1985
187. Dykes MH: Unexplained postoperative fever: its value as a sign of halothane sensitization. JAMA 216:641, 1971
188. Dellinger EP, Wertz MJ, Oreskovich MR, et al: Specificity of fever and leukocytosis after laparotomy for penetrating abdominal trauma (abstr). J Trauma 23:633, 1983
189. Dellinger EP: Prevention and management of infections. Trauma, 2nd ed. Moore EE, Mattox KL, Feliciano DV, Eds. Appleton & Lange, Norwalk, 1988, p 231
190. Haley RW, Culver DH, White JW, et al: The efficacy of infection surveillance and control programs in preventing nosocomial infections in US hospitals. Am J Epidemiol 121:182, 1985
191. Haley RW, Hooton TM, Culver DH, et al: Nosocomial infections in US hospitals, 1975 to 1976: estimated frequency by selected characteristics of patients. Am J Med 70:947, 1981
192. Horan TC, Culver DH, Gaynes RP, et al: Nosocomial infections in surgical patients in the United States, January 1986-June 1992: National Nosocomial Infections Surveillance (NNIS) System. Infect Control Hosp Epidemiol 14:73, 1993
193. Platt R, Polk BF, Murdock B, et al: Mortality associated with nosocomial urinary tract infection. N Engl J Med 307:637, 1982
194. Stamm WE: Urinary tract infections. Hospital Infections, 4th ed. Bennett JV, Brachman PS, Eds. Lippincott-Raven, Philadelphia, 1998, p 477
195. Givens CD, Wenzel RP: Catheter-associated urinary tract infections in surgical patients: a controlled study on the excess morbidity and costs. J Urol 124:646, 1980
196. Krieger JN, Kaiser DL, Wenzel RP: Nosocomial urinary tract infections cause wound infections postoperatively in surgical patients. Surg Gynecol Obstet 156:313, 1983
197. Maki DG, Goldman A, Rhame FS: Infection control in intravenous therapy. Ann Intern Med 79:867, 1973
198. Dickinson GM, Bisno AL: Infections associated with indwelling devices: concepts of pathogenesis; infections associated with intravascular devices. Antimicrob Agents Chemother 33:597, 1989
199. Collins RN, Braun PA, Zinner SH, et al: Risk of local and systemic infections with polyethylene intravenous catheters: a prospective study of 213 catheterizations. N Engl J Med 279:340, 1968
200. Druskin MS, Siegel PD: Bacterial contamination of indwelling intravenous polyethylene catheters. JAMA 185:966, 1963
201. Bentley DW, Lepper MH: Septicemia related to indwelling venous catheter. JAMA 206:1749, 1968
202. Altemeier WA, McDonough JJ, Fullen WD: Third day surgical fever. Arch Surg 103:158, 1971
203. Pittet D, Hulliger S, Auckenthaler R: Intravascular device-related infections in critically ill patients. J Chemother 7(suppl 3):55, 1995
204. Elliott CG, Zimmerman GA, Clemmer TP: Complications of pulmonary artery catheterization in the care of critically ill patients: a prospective study. Chest 76:647, 1979
205. Rowley KM, Clubb KS, Walker Smith GJ, et al: Right-sided infective endocarditis as a consequence of flow-directed pulmonary-artery catheterization: a clinicopathological study of 55 autopsied patients. N Engl J Med 311:1152, 1984
206. Applefeld JJ, Caruthers TE, Reno DJ, et al: Assessment of the sterility of long-term cardiac catheterization using the thermodilution Swan-Ganz catheter. Chest 74:377, 1978
207. Hudson-Civetta JA, Civetta JM, Martinez OV, et al: Risk and detection of pulmonary artery catheter-related infection in septic surgical patients. Crit Care Med 15:29, 1987
208. Prachar H, Dittel M, Jobst C, et al: Bacterial contamination of pulmonary artery catheters. Intensive Care Med 4:79, 1978
209. Pinilla JC, Ross DF, Martin T, et al: Study of the incidence of intravascular catheter infection and associated septicemia in critically ill patients. Crit Care Med 11:21, 1983
210. Michel L, Marsh HM, McMichan JC, et al: Infection of pulmonary artery catheters in critically ill patients. JAMA 245:1032, 1981
211. Rose HD: Gas gangrene and *Clostridium perfringens* septicemia associated with the use of an indwelling radial artery catheter. Can Med Assoc J 121:1595, 1979
212. Meakins JL: Infection associated with radial artery catheters (editorial). Can Med Assoc J 121:1564, 1979
213. Arnow PM, Costas CO: Delayed rupture of the radial artery caused by catheter-related sepsis. Rev Infect Dis 10:1035, 1988
214. Gardner RM, Schwartz R, Wong HC, et al: Percutaneous indwelling radial-artery catheters for monitoring cardiovascular function: prospective study of the risk of thrombosis and infection. N Engl J Med 290:1227, 1974
215. Davis FM, Cornere B: Bacterial contamination of radial artery catheters. NZ Med J 89:128, 1979
216. Band JD, Maki DG: Infections caused by arterial catheters used for hemodynamic monitoring. Am J Med 67:735, 1979
217. Kaye W, Wheaton M, Potter-Bynoe G: Radial and pulmonary artery catheter-related sepsis (abstr). Crit Care Med 11:249, 1983
218. Stroud L, Edwards J, Danzing L, et al: Risk factors for mortality associated with enterococcal bloodstream infections. Infect Control Hosp Epidemiol 17:576, 1996
219. Recommendations for preventing the spread of vancomycin resistance: recommendations of the Hospital Infection Control Practices Advisory Committee (HICPAC). Centers for Disease Control and Prevention. MMWR Morb Mortal Wkly Rep 44(RR-12):1, 1995
220. Murray BE: What can we do about vancomycin-resistant enterococci? Clin Infect Dis 20:1134, 1995
221. Weinstein JW, Roe M, Towns M, et al: Resistant enterococci: a prospective study of prevalence, incidence, and factors associated with colonization in a university hospital. Infect Control Hosp Epidemiol 17:36, 1996
222. Tornieporth NG, Roberts RB, John J, et al: Risk factors associated with vancomycin-resistant *Enterococcus faecium* infection or colonization in 145 matched case patients and control patients. Clin Infect Dis 23:767, 1996
223. Rafferty ME, McCormick MI, Bopp LH, et al: Vancomycin-resistant enterococci in stool specimens submitted for *Clostridium difficile* cytotoxin assay. Infect Control Hosp Epidemiol 18:342, 1997
224. Edmond MB, Ober JF, Dawson JD, et al: Vancomycin-resistant enterococcal bacteremia: natural history and attributable mortality. Clin Infect Dis 23:1234, 1996

225. Linden PK, Pasculle AW, Manez R, et al: Differences in outcomes for patients with bacteremia due to vancomycin-resistant *Enterococcus faecium* or vancomycin-susceptible *E. faecium*. Clin Infect Dis 22:663, 1996
226. Rosenberg JM, Walker M, Welch JP, et al: *Clostridium difficile* colitis in surgical patients. Am J Surg 147:486, 1984
227. McFarland LV, Elmer GW, Stamm WE, et al: Correlation of immunoblot type, enterotoxin production, and cytotoxin production with clinical manifestations of *Clostridium difficile* infection in a cohort of hospitalized patients. Infect Immun 59:2456, 1991
228. Fekety R, Kim KH, Brown D, et al: Epidemiology of antibiotic-associated colitis: isolation of *Clostridium difficile* from the hospital environment. Am J Med 70:906, 1981
229. McFarland LV, Mulligan ME, Kwok RY, et al: Nosocomial acquisition of *Clostridium difficile* infection. N Engl J Med 320:204, 1989
230. Struelens MJ, Maas A, Nonhoff C, et al: Control of nosocomial transmission of *Clostridium difficile* based on sporadic case surveillance. Am J Med 91(suppl 3B):138S, 1991
231. Martone WJ, Jarvis WR, Edwards JR, et al: Incidence and nature of endemic and epidemic nosocomial infections. Hospital Infections, 4th ed. Bennett JV, Brachman PS, Eds. Lippincott-Raven, Philadelphia, 1998, p 461
232. Britt MR, Schleupner CJ, Matsumiya S: Severity of underlying disease as a predictor of nosocomial infection: utility in the control of nosocomial infection. JAMA 239:1047, 1978
233. Baker SP, O'Neill B, Haddon W Jr, et al: The injury severity score: a method for describing patients with multiple injuries and evaluating emergency care. J Trauma 14:187, 1974
234. Caplan ES, Hoyt N, Cowley RA: Changing patterns of nosocomial infections in severely traumatized patients. Am J Surg 45:204, 1979
235. Caplan ES, Hoyt N: Infection surveillance and control in the severely traumatized patient. Am J Med 70:638, 1981
236. Wenzel RP, Thompson RL, Landry SM, et al: Hospital-acquired infections in intensive care unit patients: an overview with emphasis on epidemics. Infect Control 4:371, 1983

Acknowledgments

Figures 1 and 2 Carol Donner.

Figure 4 Albert Miller.

82 PERITONITIS AND INTRA-ABDOMINAL ABSCESSES

Ori D. Rotstein, M.D., M.Sc., and Avery B. Nathens, M.D., Ph.D., M.P.H.

Approach to Peritonitis and Intra-abdominal Abscesses

There are two major manifestations of intra-abdominal infection: (1) peritonitis, or inflammation of the peritoneum, and (2) abscess formation, in which infection has become walled off from the remainder of the peritoneal cavity. Peritonitis has been classically divided into a primary form and a secondary form, which is by far the more common. In secondary peritonitis, peritoneal infection and inflammation are caused by visceral disruption that is a result of an intrinsic pathological condition or of external trauma. Because of its greater clinical importance, secondary peritonitis will receive somewhat greater emphasis than primary peritonitis.

Peritonitis

SECONDARY PERITONITIS

Secondary bacterial peritonitis is defined as peritoneal infection caused by perforation of a hollow viscus or transmural necrosis of the gastrointestinal tract. Excluding trauma, the common causes of generalized peritonitis include a perforated appendix, perforated duodenal ulcer, perforated sigmoid colon (caused by diverticulitis, volvulus, or cancer), strangulation obstruction of the small bowel, and postoperative peritonitis caused by anastomotic disruption.

Clinical Presentation and Diagnosis

The diagnosis of peritonitis is usually a clinical one. The predominant symptom is invariably abdominal pain. The onset of the pain may be acute or more insidious. The pain is often steady, severe, and aggravated by movement. The patient is frequently lying still in bed, either in the fetal position or supine with knees bent and head elevated. Both these maneuvers reduce the tension on the abdominal wall and thereby alleviate abdominal discomfort. Anorexia and nausea are often accompanying symptoms. Depending on the etiology of the peritonitis, a history of recent symptoms may be obtained from the patient.

The results of physical examination vary according to the cause and the extent of the peritonitis. Most patients, however, look unwell and are in acute distress. Body temperature is usually higher than 38° C (100.4° F), but in cases of severe septic shock, the patient may be hypothermic. Tachycardia and diminished pulse volume, indicative of hypovolemia, are common. Patients in septic shock may manifest high cardiac output and reduced peripheral resistance, as shown by bounding pulses with increased pulse pressure and warm extremities [*see 4 Shock*].

Abdominal tenderness is the hallmark of peritonitis. Patients with generalized peritonitis suffer diffuse tenderness. The point of maximum tenderness frequently overlies the diseased organ. Increased abdominal tone is initially from voluntary guarding by the patient and is subsequently a result of reflex muscular spasm. The abdomen is characteristically distended, and bowel sounds are usually absent, although an occasional bowel sound may be heard.

Localized peritonitis generally produces less extreme effects in the patient. The abdomen distant from the site of maximum tenderness may be soft and nontender, and bowel sounds are frequently present. Referred rebound tenderness may accurately pinpoint the site of maximal peritoneal irritation; the rectal examination, although an essential part of the physical examination, rarely pinpoints the origin of the peritonitis.

Laboratory data, particularly the presence of a leukocytosis greater than 11,000 cells/mm³ with a shift to the left, support the clinical diagnosis of peritonitis. Leukopenia is compatible with overwhelming sepsis. Blood chemistry is generally undisturbed but in severe cases may show evidence of dehydration with elevated blood urea nitrogen levels as well as metabolic acidosis. Urinalysis is essential to rule out urinary tract diseases, such as pyelonephritis and renal colic, which may mimic peritonitis. White and red blood cells are occasionally found in the urine of patients with peritonitis, but the presence of bacteria, white blood cell casts, and large numbers of erythrocytes in the urine should suggest a urinary tract source of the pain.

Plain abdominal x-rays may show evidence of ileus, with distended loops of large and small bowel, air-fluid levels, and free fluid in the peritoneal cavity. Upright films are useful for demonstrating free air under the diaphragm, an indication of a perforated viscus. Free air is evident in 80 percent of cases of perforated duodenal ulcer but occurs much less frequently after perforation of the appendix, the small bowel, or the sigmoid colon.

```
┌─────────────────────────────────────────────────────────────────────┐
│ Patient presents with abdominal pain; history and physical examination │
│ suggest peritonitis (signs may be equivocal in the elderly)         │
└─────────────────────────────────────────────────────────────────────┘
```

Patient is receiving peritoneal dialysis

Clinical signs are attenuated in these patients.
Diagnosis of peritonitis requires two or more of the following findings:
- Microorganisms in fluid
- Inflammatory cells in cloudy fluid
- Peritoneal irritation

Send fluid for culture, and initiate management

Drain peritoneal fluid; flush four times.
Start empirical antibiotics (cefazolin plus tobramycin; dwell time, 8 hr).

Initiate specific antibiotic therapy when culture results are available

Organisms are polymicrobial

GI perforation is probable.
Perform barium enema.
Consider laparotomy.

Organisms are monomicrobial

Continue antibiotics for at least 7 days.

Condition does not improve after 3 to 4 days

Reculture, and adjust antibiotics.
If *Pseudomonas* is present, consider catheter removal.

Condition resolves

If condition recurs, consider exit-site infection or tunnel infection.
Consider catheter removal.

Peritonitis is diffuse

Secondary peritonitis is present

In patients with cirrhosis or nephrotic syndrome, consider primary peritonitis and initiate diagnostic tests

Obtain abdominal views with radiocontrast.
Perform paracentesis; examine fluid for cell count, pH, and lactate level, and obtain Gram's stain and culture.

Fluid findings include elevated levels of polymorphonuclear leukocytes, reduced pH, and high lactate

Provide general supportive care and antibiotics.

Fluid findings include fecal material, bile, and polymicrobial infection

Condition resolves

Condition fails to resolve

1240

Approach to Peritonitis and Intra-abdominal Abscesses

Peritonitis is localized

Obtain abdominal x-rays.

Free air is seen on x-rays

No free air is seen on x-rays

Rule out nonoperative conditions (particularly cholecystitis, pancreatitis, diverticulitis, and non-GI causes) with clinical examination, laboratory tests (e.g., serum amylase, urinalysis), chest x-ray, ECG, and abdominal ultrasonography.

History is acute

History is chronic

Tender mass may be palpable.

Search for abscess

Perform ultrasonography.
Obtain CT scan.

**Drain abscess percutaneously
Administer antibiotics**

Abscess fails to resolve

Abscess resolves

Prepare patient for operation:
- Initiate fluid resuscitation, and monitor fluid status
- Initiate empirical antibiotics

Goals of operation:
- Eliminate source of contamination
- Reduce bacterial inoculum
- Prevent recurrent sepsis

Continue antibiotics until patient is afebrile for 48 hr, with a normal leukocyte count and band count < 3%.

Although the diagnosis of peritonitis is a clinical one, the history and physical examination may be either inconclusive with respect to the diagnosis or unreliable because of underlying patient factors, such as altered consciousness caused by head injury or toxic encephalopathy, paraplegia, the effects of immunosuppressive drugs, and, occasionally, advanced age. In these situations, several adjunctive diagnostic modalities can be helpful.

Imaging techniques may provide evidence of an inflammatory process within the peritoneal cavity. Ultrasonography is useful in equivocal cases of right lower quadrant pain, with specificity and sensitivity of 90 percent and 80 percent, respectively, for the diagnosis of appendicitis.[1] The ability of ultrasonography to detect less than 100 ml of fluid in the peritoneal cavity may support the diagnosis of peritonitis when the physical findings are equivocal.

Like ultrasonography, computed tomography is capable of detecting minute quantities of intraperitoneal fluid. In one prospective study, computed tomography provided a diagnosis in 95 percent of cases and altered the primary therapeutic strategy in 30 percent of patients.[2]

Diagnostic peritoneal lavage appears to be a safe and accurate method of determining the presence of peritonitis necessitating operation in these patients.[3,4] Several criteria for a positive lavage have been used, but the presence of more than 500 white blood cells/mm³ after a 1 L saline lavage appears to correlate best with the presence of intra-abdominal pathology. Gross pus, turbid fluid, bile, or a positive Gram's stain is a clear indication for laparotomy. In well-localized inflammatory processes or in patients who are unable to mount a significant white blood cell response, peritoneal lavage may produce false negative results. Nuclear scanning of the biliary tree with the technetium-99m–labeled iminodiacetic acid (IDA) family of compounds may also be useful for investigating right upper quadrant peritonitis in the critically ill patient in whom congestive hepatomegaly or pneumonia may mimic either calculous or acalculous cholecystitis.[5]

The laparoscope has become an important diagnostic tool, with laparoscopy providing a definitive diagnosis in more than 90 percent of cases.[6] Preoperative laparoscopy may lead to a significant modification of the therapeutic strategy in as many as 10 percent of patients.[7] The most common indication for laparoscopy is lower abdominal or pelvic pain in young women, particularly in the right iliac fossa, where the possibility of appendicitis versus tubo-ovarian processes complicates diagnosis.

In the majority of cases, the diagnosis of peritonitis is straightforward. The patient complains of abdominal pain and demonstrates evidence of peritoneal irritation on physical examination. Generally, the presence of peritonitis is an indication for early laparotomy and surgical repair. However, some disease entities, either intra-abdominal or extra-abdominal, mimic peritonitis but do not call for early surgery [see Table 1]. Many can be easily ruled out by clinical examination and laboratory tests (e.g., serum amylase level, urinalysis, electrocardiography, chest x-ray, and abdominal ultrasonography). Finally, it is worthwhile to remember a short list of diagnoses that occasionally escape consideration and can be rapidly fatal if overlooked. In patients with peritonitis, these include ruptured ectopic pregnancy and ruptured abdominal aortic aneurysm.

Table 1 **Common Nonsurgical Causes of Peritonitis**

INTRA-ABDOMINAL	EXTRA-ABDOMINAL

Gastrointestinal system
  Congestive hepatomegaly
  Pancreatitis
  Acute diverticulitis
  Acute cholecystitis
	Pulmonary system
	  Basilar pneumonia
	  Pulmonary embolus

Gynecologic system
  Pelvic inflammatory disease
  Ovarian pathology
    Torsion of a cyst
    Bleeding into a cyst
	Cardiac system
	  Myocardial infarction
	  Pericarditis

Urinary tract system
  Renal colic
  Pyelonephritis
  Cystitis
	Metabolic problems
	  Methanol poisoning
	  Addisonian crisis
	  Sickle cell disease

Management

Preoperative preparation The principal objectives in preparing patients with secondary peritonitis for operation are fluid resuscitation and the initiation of antibiotic therapy.

Fluid resuscitation entails the administration of fluids and the monitoring of fluid status. The extent of these measures depends very much on the patient's premorbid status and on the underlying disease process. Clearly, a teenager with acute appendicitis does not require the same preoperative resuscitation as an octogenarian with a perforated sigmoid volvulus. However, the principles are the same. All patients with peritonitis have some degree of hypovolemia. Adequate volumes of fluid should therefore be administered to restore blood volume. Adequacy of resuscitation may be assessed by monitoring blood pressure, central venous pressure, and urine output. In the elderly or critically ill patient, resuscitative measures must be directed by invasive monitoring techniques, including (1) arterial cannulation to measure blood pressure directly and to sample arterial blood for blood gas determination, (2) central venous monitoring, preferably with a Swan-Ganz catheter to measure pulmonary and left atrial pressures, and (3) measurement of urine output with an indwelling catheter. Fluid may be rapidly administered, even to elderly patients with limited cardiac reserve, if these monitoring techniques are used.

Antibiotic therapy should be initiated as soon as the clinical diagnosis of peritonitis is made, even before samples can be taken from the peritoneal cavity for aerobic and anaerobic culture. Although the initial antibiotic therapy is given on an empirical basis, the choice of antimicrobial agents should be based on the suspected offending organisms (see below) and on the ability of the antibiotics to achieve adequate levels in the peritoneal cavity. Fortunately, most antibiotics have this ability.

Table 2 Bacteria Causing Secondary Peritonitis

Aerobic bacteria	Anaerobic bacteria
Escherichia coli	*Bacteroides*
Streptococci	*B. fragilis*
Enterobacter, Klebsiella	Eubacteria
Enterococci	*Clostridium*
Proteus	Anaerobic streptococci

The spectrum of microorganisms inoculating the peritoneum after perforation of the gastrointestinal tract depends on the level of the perforation.[7] Upper gastrointestinal perforations usually release predominantly gram-positive organisms, which are sensitive to penicillins and cephalosporins. Patients who have been taking antacids or H_2-receptor blockers have greater numbers of facultative gram-negative bacilli in their stomachs before perforation.[8] Perforation of the distal small bowel or the colon results in the release of more than 500 bacterial species into the peritoneal cavity. It is noteworthy that many species are rapidly eliminated by host defenses or by the hostile environment. In established intraperitoneal sepsis, only a few species remain [see Table 2].[9-11] These infections are almost always polymicrobial, containing a mixture of aerobic and anaerobic bacteria.[9,11]

Several recent publications have reviewed antibiotic use in patients with peritonitis. It is worthwhile to summarize the recommendations for antibiotic selection [see Table 3].[12,13] Antimicrobial therapy for secondary peritonitis should include an agent or a combination of agents with activity against both aerobic and anaerobic bacteria. In particular, gram-negative enteric bacteria (e.g., *Escherichia coli*) and anaerobic bacteria (e.g., *Bacteroides fragilis*) should be the prime targets of antibiotic therapy. There are several single agents or combinations that fulfill these criteria. Both single-drug therapy with a broad-spectrum cephalosporin and combination therapy with agents effective against aerobes and anaerobes have proved effective for the treatment of patients presenting to the hospital with community-acquired peritonitis of mild to moderate severity. Several different agents [see Table 3] are available for use in patients with postoperative peritonitis or severe physiologic derangements related to the development of peritonitis. Aminoglycosides should be used with care in elderly patients and in patients with hypotension, renal dysfunction, or both.

The guidelines for determining the duration of antibiotic therapy in patients after operative management of peritonitis are derived from retrospective studies evaluating outcome after the discontinuance of antibiotic therapy. If a patient is afebrile and has a normal leukocyte count and a band count of less than three percent, then the chance of recurrent sepsis after discontinuance of antibiotic therapy is virtually zero.[14] On the other hand, if the patient's temperature or leukocyte count is elevated, the probability of recurrent sepsis ranges from 33 to 50 percent.[15]

Practically speaking, the presence of a normal leukocyte count and a normal rectal temperature for 48 hours should be considered adequate criteria for stopping antibiotics. In a recent trial using these criteria, antibiotics were discontinued at an average of eight days, which indicated that these criteria were usually met by about day 6.[16] Antibiotics have been discontinued as early as postoperative day 4 with this approach. Conversely, if leukocytosis or fever persists after postoperative day 7, a diligent search is initiated to locate the source of persistent sepsis. There are several clinical circumstances in which the duration of antibiotic therapy approximates that used for prophylaxis rather than that for treatment. These include simple acute appendicitis, necrotic small intestine without perforation, and traumatic enteric perforations operated on within 12 hours of injury.[12] The common feature of these diagnoses is the minimal degree of peritoneal soiling and inflammatory response present at the time of laparotomy. A preoperative dose of antibiotics followed by two doses within 24 hours of surgery is appropriate therapy for these conditions.

Operative management The goals of operative management of peritonitis are to eliminate the source of contamination, to reduce the bacterial inoculum, and to prevent recurrent or persistent infection.

In patients with generalized peritonitis, the incision of choice is a midline vertical incision, which provides access to the entire abdomen and is readily opened and closed. When peritonitis is localized, as in appendicitis, an incision directly over the site of inflammation may be adequate. The use of laparoscopy for the

Table 3 Antimicrobial Therapy for Intra-abdominal Infection[13]

	Monotherapy	Combination Therapy
Community-acquired infections of mild to moderate severity	Cefoxitin Cefotetan Cefmetazole Ampicillin-sulbactam Ticarcillin-clavulanate	Antianaerobe plus aminoglycoside
Severe infections (possibly resistant gram-negative organisms)	Carbapenem imipenem-cilastatin or meropenem Piperacillin-tazobactam	Antianaerobe plus third-generation cephalosporin or aminoglycoside Clindamycin plus aztreonam Ciprofloxacin plus metronidazole

Table 4 Surgical Options for Common Causes of Peritonitis[17]

Pathology	Options	Comments
Perforated duodenal ulcer	• Omental patch • Omental patch and vagotomy plus drainage (gastrojejunostomy or pyloroplasty)	• Definitive surgery may be considered when operation is performed early, there is minimal peritoneal soiling, and there is a history of chronic peptic ulcer disease • Bypass procedure rather than simple outlet drainage may be necessary if gastric outlet is obstructed
Perforated gastric ulcer	• Gastric resection, including ulcer with Billroth I or II anastomosis • Excision of ulcer with primary closure ± patch	• Resection is preferred when perforation occurs at the site of malignancy • A patch may be considered in an elderly or unstable patient or when perforation is in a difficult area (e.g., proximal stomach)
Small bowel infarction/perforation	• Resection of small bowel with primary anastomosis • Resection of small bowel with exteriorization of ends	• The need for primary anastomosis depends on the degree of peritoneal soiling, the magnitude of the inflammatory response, and patient status
Appendicitis	Appendectomy	Perform laparoscopic appendectomy if feasible [see text]
Large bowel perforation	• Resection with end colostomy (ileostomy) and mucous fistula or Hartmann's procedure • Defunctioning colostomy with drainage	• Resection is preferred, but defunctioning with drainage may be used if inflammation is too intense for safe resection • Anastomosis after resection for free perforation is generally considered unsafe; when resection encompasses peridiverticular abscess, anastomosis may be considered
Postoperative peritonitis	• Depends on underlying pathology: For anastomotic dehiscence, exteriorize ends when possible; use drain ± defunction if exteriorization not possible	• Reanastomosis or closure of anastomotic dehiscence is not likely to be successful
Cholecystitis ± perforation or pericholecystic abscess	• Laparoscopic cholecystectomy • Tube cholecystostomy	• Laparoscopy is more likely to be successful if performed earlier • Use tube cholecystostomy (operative) when resection is not possible; in the critically ill, consider percutaneous cholecystostomy

diagnosis and treatment of various pathological entities, such as acute appendicitis and acute cholecystitis, has modified this approach to a significant degree. Incisions are made away from the inflamed organ to provide better visualization of the operative field and to permit manipulation of the tissues from various angles.

The operative technique used to control contamination depends on the location and the nature of the pathological condition in the gastrointestinal tract [see Table 4].[17] In general, continued peritoneal soiling is controlled by closing, excluding, or resecting the perforated viscus. When feasible, resection of the diseased tissue appears to be the best option, preventing continued contamination from the source. One important exception to this principle occurs when the GI tract is disrupted by trauma. In cases of hollow-viscus injury, with minimal peritoneal contamination in a patient in stable condition with a limited number of associated injuries, primary closure of the viscus is optimal.[18-20] For an inflammatory process where the disease is expected to progress in the absence of a frank perforation (e.g., acute appendicitis or small bowel necrosis), resection is clearly preferred, because the underlying disease, if left in situ, will act as a focus of ongoing infection. Occasionally, self-limited inflammatory processes are unexpectedly discovered at laparotomy. Examples include acute Crohn's disease, an ischemic but viable loop of torsive small intestine, and acute phlegmonous pancreatitis. Under these circumstances, excision is not indicated, and treatment should address the underlying pathology.

Technical factors may also preclude resection of the diseased viscus. Perforation of extraperitoneal viscera such as the duodenum and the rectum is not routinely treated by excision, because of the technical difficulties of operating on these organs during acute inflammation. Similarly, extremely intense inflammatory changes may prevent safe excision of various organs that usually can be resected during acute inflammation. These include the gallbladder in cases of acute cholecystitis and a portion of the intraperitoneal GI tract in cases of acute perforated diverticulitis. For a pathological condition of the colon, control is usually accomplished by resecting the perforated segment of intestine, exteriorizing the proximal end as an end colostomy, and dealing with the distal end by creating a mucous fistula or oversewing it. The general principle is that a primary anastomosis in this location is at high risk for dehiscence and should be avoided.[21]

The risk associated with primary anastomosis of the small intestine after resection of a diseased segment is much lower. However, resection plus proximal and distal enterostomy may be appropriate if peritoneal soiling is particularly extensive or if the viability of the intestine is uncertain. Perforation of the duodenum because of peptic ulcer disease may be safely patched with a piece of omentum; a perforated gastric ulcer is either included in a distal gastric resection with subsequent gastroduodenal or gastrojejunal anastomosis or locally excised with primary closure. Appendicitis is treated by appendectomy.

Laparoscopy is a major advance in the diagnosis and management of the acute abdomen. Several reports demonstrate that laparoscopic cholecystectomy [see 52 Laparoscopic Cholecystectomy] is safe for the treatment of acute cholecystitis and can reduce the length of stay. There is little morbidity in patients treated successfully by the laparoscopic approach. The principal reason for conversion is the presence of extensive adhesions or inflammation, precluding safe identification and dissection within Calot's triangle.[22,23] This is more common in patients with gangrenous cholecystitis or empyema of the gallbladder.[24,25] Compared with delayed or even interval cholecystectomy, a laparoscopic approach appears to have a higher success rate if performed early in the course of the disease.[26,27] Trocar insertion may be safer via an open technique, reducing the likelihood of hollow-viscus injury in the presence of an ileus.

Laparoscopic appendectomy, a logical extension of diagnostic laparoscopy for lower abdominal pain, appears to be safe and can be performed with a low conversion rate. Conversions are often caused by a perforated appendix or an inflammatory mass.[28] For patients with nonperforated appendicitis, the duration of hospital stay and the return to work appear to be independent of the approach (open versus laparoscopic), but hospital costs are higher for laparoscopic surgery.[29-31] For complicated appendicitis, laparoscopic removal shortens the hospital stay. Laparoscopic management of perforated gastric and duodenal ulcers, recently reported, appears to be effective.[32]

The second major goal of operative management of peritonitis is to reduce the bacterial inoculum and to prevent recurrent or persistent sepsis. At operation, gross purulent exudates should be aspirated, and loculations in the pelvis, paracolic gutters, and subphrenic regions should be gently opened and debrided. An attempt should be made to remove particulate debris, such as fecal matter or barium sulfate, if present.

Although intraoperative peritoneal lavage has become a standard procedure during operation for peritonitis, its efficacy has not been well documented. Its major roles are to reduce the quantity of bacteria and to remove adjuvant substances. The fear that this procedure may disseminate bacteria is probably unfounded; experimental studies have demonstrated that dynamics in the peritoneum cause locally applied bacteria to spread rapidly throughout the peritoneal cavity even without irrigation. The risk of leaving collections of infected fluid undrained is probably greater than the risk of spreading a small inoculum of bacteria within the peritoneal cavity. However, because the fluid itself acts as an adjuvant to infection by impairing phagocytosis and leukocyte migration, it is imperative that all fluid collections be aspirated before the abdomen is closed.

It is impossible to drain the peritoneal cavity in patients with diffuse peritonitis. Therefore, the use of drains in these patients is not indicated unless (1) the drain is to be used for postoperative lavage, (2) the drain is placed in a well-defined abscess cavity, and (3) the drain is used to establish a controlled fistula. Drains left in situ are not innocuous: they may erode into the intestine or the blood vessels or provide external bacteria with an access route into the peritoneal cavity. Researchers have demonstrated that children in whom Penrose drains were placed at operation for perforated appendicitis averaged 3.7 more hospital days than those without drains.[33]

Abdominal wall closure is accomplished with a single fascial layer of either interrupted or running monofilament suture. We routinely use Prolene, although wire or nylon is also acceptable. In the elderly, malnourished, or immunocompromised patient, full-thickness abdominal wall retention sutures are used in addition to the fascial closure. Care should be taken not to tie these sutures too tightly, because abdominal distention and abdominal wall swelling may cause pressure necrosis at suture insertion sites and lead to stitch abscesses and spreading cellulitis.

Because the risk of wound infection associated with diffuse peritonitis is 20 percent or greater, wounds should be managed by delayed primary closure of the skin and subcutaneous tissues.[34] The wound is gently packed with saline-soaked gauze during operation, and the gauze is changed every eight hours for three to four days. At that time, if the wound appears clean, with a granulating base, the skin edges can be apposed with skin tapes or fine sutures. The practice of obtaining a biopsy specimen from the subcutaneous tissue and performing quantitative bacterial counts to determine whether the wound is safe to close is somewhat impractical and is rarely undertaken.[35] If any question exists about the wound, it can be left open and allowed to close secondarily. The technique of closure of the primary wound over suction catheters irrigated with antibiotics has not reduced wound infection rates in the abdomen.[36]

PRIMARY PERITONITIS

Primary peritonitis is defined as an infection of the peritoneal cavity in which there is no obvious source, such as a perforated viscus. This type of peritonitis occurs in both children and adults.

The incidence of primary peritonitis in children appears to be decreasing.[37] In the preantibiotic era, it accounted for 10 percent of acute abdominal emergencies; this incidence has been reduced to approximately one to two percent.[38,39] Children with nephrotic syndrome or postnecrotic cirrhosis appear to be at particularly high risk.[38] In adults, the presence of alcoholic cirrhosis and ascites is the most frequent underlying risk factor.[40] Primary peritonitis represents a significant source of morbidity and mortality in cirrhotic patients with ascites: it is present in 10 to 25 percent of these patients on hospital admission and accounts for as many as 30 percent of all infections in cirrhotic patients.[41,42] Cirrhotic ascites predisposes to infection because of reduced total protein and complement levels, which result in impaired bacterial opsonization.[43] Patients with systemic lupus erythematosus may also be subject to primary peritonitis or serositis; the latter mimics peritonitis and may necessitate operation.[44]

Causative organisms generally fall into two categories, depending on the patient's age. In children, the usual organisms are gram-positive cocci, such as *Streptococcus pneumoniae* and group A streptococci.[37,38] In cirrhotic patients, monomicrobial infections with enteric microorganisms, particularly *E. coli*, tend to predominate.[45] Anaerobes are rare, and in marked contrast to the frequency of polymicrobial infection in patients with secondary peritonitis, polymicrobial infection is present in fewer than 10 percent of cases. Immunocompromised patients are at risk for the development of primary peritonitis. In patients with the acquired immunodeficiency syndrome, *M. tuberculosis*, cytomegalovirus, and a variety of other opportunistic pathogens may cause primary peritonitis.[46]

Clinical Presentation and Diagnosis

In children, the clinical picture mimics that of secondary bacterial peritonitis with presenting signs and symptoms consisting of fever, nausea, vomiting, and abdominal pain. Abdominal examination reveals diffuse tenderness, rebound tenderness, guarding, and loss of bowel sounds. Primary peritonitis in patients with cirrhosis presents in a more subtle fashion. These patients may have a low-grade fever with minimal or no abdominal tenderness and peritonitis masked by evidence of hepatic decompensation, such as encephalopathy, hepatorenal syndrome, or increased accumulation of ascitic fluid. Tuberculous peritonitis is usually gradual in onset, with fever, night sweats, weight loss, and progressive abdominal distention. Abdominal examination may reveal some increased tone with mild diffuse discomfort on palpation. Classic signs of peritonitis are usually absent.

Primary peritonitis in children is rarely diagnosed preoperatively. Children presenting to the hospital with evidence of peritonitis usually undergo laparotomy with a provisional diagnosis of acute appendicitis. The diagnosis is made after a negative laparotomy, when gram-positive organisms are cultured from the peritoneal swabs.

In cirrhotic patients with evidence of peritonitis, a much more conservative approach is taken because of the high operative risk in these patients.[47] Two major diagnostic issues should be addressed in these patients, who frequently present with an atypical clinical picture. The first objective is to decide whether the patient has peritonitis so that treatment can be initiated. This is readily accomplished by diagnostic paracentesis. Fluid should be examined for the cell count and differential, pH, and levels of lactate, glucose, protein, and lactic dehydrogenase; Gram's stain and cultures should be performed as well. The most accurate method of culturing ascitic fluid is to inoculate 10 to 20 ml into an aerobic blood culture bottle and the same amount into an anaerobic bottle. Inoculation should be done at the bedside to enhance the sensitivity of the test.[48,49] Gram's stain of a centrifuged specimen of ascitic fluid, although helpful when positive, has a high false negative rate (60 to 80 percent).[40] Because an incubation period of 24 to 72 hours is necessary before peritonitis can be diagnosed microbiologically, it is optimal to rely on a few rapid tests to guide the initiation of therapy. In many studies,[50,51] an elevated neutrophil count ($> 250/mm^3$), a reduced pH (< 7.35), and an elevated lactate level (> 32 mg/dl) have been found to be highly predictive of the presence of peritonitis. One review of several studies concluded that evaluation of the neutrophil count in the ascitic fluid was the single best test for the detection of peritonitis and that elevation of this count was an indication for treatment.[52] An elevated neutrophil count in combination with an elevated arterial–ascitic fluid pH gradient (> 0.10) or a reduced ascitic fluid pH has a diagnostic accuracy of 91 to 97 percent.[50]

The diagnosis of peritonitis having been established, it is critical to determine whether the peritonitis is from perforation or inflammation of the gastrointestinal tract (i.e., secondary peritonitis) or spontaneous (i.e., primary peritonitis). It is difficult to distinguish these entities on the basis of clinical findings or the magnitude of the increase in the ascitic fluid neutrophil count. If the ascitic fluid is found to have a glucose level below 50 mg/dl, a lactic dehydrogenase level higher than the upper limit of the normal serum range, and a protein concentration higher than 1 g/dl, the likelihood of secondary peritonitis is significantly increased, and further investigation is warranted.[52] Plain abdominal x-rays should be taken, and Gastrografin studies should be done. Surgical intervention is indicated if (1) the ascitic fluid culture yields a mixed aerobic-anaerobic flora, (2) Gastrografin studies reveal leakage from the gastrointestinal tract, (3) free air is present on x-ray views of the abdomen, and (4) the patient fails to benefit from medical therapy. A repeat paracentesis 48 hours after initiation of therapy may be helpful because in primary peritonitis, the leukocyte count falls rapidly, whereas in secondary peritonitis, it remains stable or rises.[53] Obviously, if the fluid aspirate reveals gross feces, bile, or blood-tinged material, then a surgical course is indicated. However, this scenario is rare.

The diagnosis of tuberculous peritonitis is made by laparoscopy, with characteristic findings of a thickened peritoneum with miliary yellow-white tubercles.[54] In most cases, diagnosis can be based on the gross findings, supplemented by results of a laparoscopic peritoneal biopsy. Systemic antimicrobials directed against *M. tuberculosis* are indicated.

Management

Bacterial peritonitis caused by *S. pneumoniae* or group A streptococci should be treated with intravenous penicillin G. Single-drug therapy with cefotaxime is the preferred regimen for spontaneous bacterial peritonitis and is associated with less toxicity than aminoglycoside-containing regimens.[55] Antimicrobial therapy should be adjusted when the results of culture and sensitivity testing become available. There is no specific indication for peritoneal dialysis in these patients, because parenterally administered antibiotics achieve adequate levels in ascitic fluid.

The duration of therapy for spontaneous bacterial peritonitis is now better defined. Recurrent infection after the neutrophil count in the ascitic fluid falls below $250/mm^3$ is extremely rare.[56] In a randomized trial, five days of therapy was equal to 10 days with respect to mortality, cure rate, and recurrence rate.[57]

Prognosis Hospital mortality for cirrhotic patients in whom spontaneous bacterial peritonitis develops is approximately 50 percent[58]; most of the deaths are the result of liver failure. Furthermore, survivors of the initial episode of peritonitis are at high risk for recurrence (69 percent at one year) and have a significantly shorter survival than comparable cirrhotic patients in whom peritonitis does not develop.[59] This complication of cirrhosis may be the sign of a high-failure group that might benefit from liver transplantation.

Prevention of recurrent peritonitis may influence the outcome in this high-risk population. In one study, selective intestinal decontamination with oral norfloxacin, 400 mg a day, lowered the probability of recurrence from 68 percent to 20 percent at one year.[60] Overall mortality, however, was not altered; most patients died of liver failure and its complications. Other antimicrobials, including ciprofloxacin and trimethoprim-sulfamethoxazole, demonstrate comparable effects.[61,62] These data suggest that spontaneous bacterial peritonitis is a predictor of poor outcome caused by progressive liver failure rather than an independent cause of increased mortality.

PERITONITIS IN PERITONEAL DIALYSIS PATIENTS

Clinical Presentation and Diagnosis

The manifestations of peritonitis in patients on peritoneal dialysis include mild abdominal pain, low-grade fever, and mild abdominal tenderness. These manifestations tend to be variable, probably because the dialysate dilutes or removes some of the products of inflammation. One definition of peritonitis includes satisfaction of at least two of the following criteria: (1) the presence of microorganisms on Gram's stain or culture of the peritoneal effluent, (2) cloudy fluid with inflammatory cells (leukocyte count > $100/mm^3$, with at least 50 percent neutrophils), and (3) signs and symptoms of peritoneal inflammation.[63] Occasionally, although the effluent may be contaminated with microorganisms, there are no signs of clinical infection. These findings do not constitute an episode of peritonitis, and dialysis should be continued without antibiotic therapy.

Management

Selection of antimicrobial agents In cases of peritonitis, specific antimicrobial agents must be selected before culture results are available. Thus, treatment decisions are based on the most probable causative microorganisms. Normal skin commensals are the most common causative microbes, with staphylococcal species accounting for 45 to 60 percent of all peritonitis episodes. Two thirds of these are attributable to *Staphylococcus epidermidis* and one third to *S. aureus*. Gram-negative bacteria account for 20 to 35 percent; the remainder are caused by fungi, anaerobes, and mycobacterial species.[64]

The choice of antimicrobial agent or agents should reflect the fact that gram-positive or gram-negative microorganisms cause about 90 percent of episodes, and the choice should consider sensitivity patterns within the specific institution. In our institution, we take the following approach when peritonitis is suspected. Patients are instructed to drain the fluid in the abdomen completely and to put the effluent aside for culture and cell count. The next 2 L bag, containing 1 g of cefazolin (1.5 g if body weight exceeds 50 kg) and 40 mg of tobramycin (60 mg if body weight exceeds 50 kg), is allowed to dwell for eight hours. Three more 2 L exchanges, without antibiotics, are evenly spaced over the remainder of the 24-hour period. If the aminoglycoside is given once daily, aminoglycoside levels need not be monitored. Heparin (500 to 1,000 U) is added to each bag, and a two percent lidocaine solution is included if there is significant pain. The effluent is sent daily for cell counts and every other day for culture. The selection of an antibiotic depends on whether culture results are available. In centers where methicillin-resistant staphylococci are common, the empirical regimen should include 1 g of vancomycin (2 g if body weight exceeds 50 kg) instead of a cephalosporin. Because of its long half-life in patients with renal failure and its limited clearance by dialysis, vancomycin is administered once every seven days.[65]

Within three to four days of the initiation of therapy, clinical improvement as well as a decreased cell count in the dialysate should occur. The optimal length of therapy is not well established, varying from center to center and ranging from seven to 21 days. One approach is to continue treatment for seven days after the last positive culture is obtained. For some microorganisms, such as *Pseudomonas* or *Xanthomonas* species, antibiotic treatment should be continued for at least 21 days. If clinical improvement does not occur within four to five days, antibiotic selection should be reevaluated on the basis of culture results. If severe peritonitis persists, the dialysis cannula should be removed. Rapid resolution by catheter removal helps maintain a peritoneal membrane capable of efficient exchange.

Additional issues In addition to the standard treatment protocol, a few specific issues should be addressed. The first is the management of exit-site and tunnel infections. These infections rarely cause symptoms. Exit-site infections produce local inflammation and a purulent discharge. Tunnel infections are more difficult to diagnose, particularly if there is no accompanying exit-site infection. In about 50 percent of patients, these infections can be managed by daily cleansing of the exit site with a disinfectant, together with oral administration of antibiotics.

The next issue is catheter removal and replacement. Catheters should be removed (1) when there is a persistently infected exit site or tunnel tract, (2) when there are recurrent episodes of peritonitis caused by the same organism (i.e., when the catheter may be the source), or (3) when laparotomy is required for fecal peritonitis. Occasionally, when virulent organisms, such as *Pseudomonas* species or fungi, are the causative agents, antibiotic therapy may fail, and catheter removal is required to resolve the infection.[66] Catheters removed for exit-site infections can be replaced at a new site. However, catheters removed for recurrent or fecal peritonitis should not be replaced for two to three weeks to allow the peritonitis to resolve. Dialysis can be continued during this period with a temporary catheter placed at the time of removal or with hemodialysis. One study has advocated immediate replacement of a permanent cannula, thereby obviating hemodialysis[67]; this approach may be appropriate in certain circumstances. For example, patients with recurrent bouts of peritonitis in whom the most recent bout has been adequately treated are good candidates for catheter replacement during the same operation. However, catheter replacement is probably not indicated for more complex infections, such as those caused by *Pseudomonas* species, fungi, mycobacteria, and polymicrobial fecal flora.[65]

An obvious solution to the problem of catheter-related infection is prevention. Strict aseptic technique is the most important preventive measure. The Y-system "flush-before-fill," in which the patient flushes sections of the administration set and the catheter between exchanges, has been reported to reduce the infection rate markedly.[68] Oral antimicrobial prophylaxis with cephalexin has been shown to be ineffective.[69] Nasal carriage of *S. aureus* appears to be associated with an increased risk of infection at the exit site of the catheter.[70] One study[71] suggested that intranasal mupirocin markedly reduced *S. aureus* exit-site infection and peritonitis and lessened the rate of catheter loss; the recolonization rate was frequent, however, and retreatment was required periodically.

The management of patients whose peritoneal fluid cultures reveal multiple enteric organisms or anaerobic bacteria, or both, requires comment. If organisms appear during the first 24 to 48 hours after percutaneous insertion of a temporary catheter, laparotomy should be performed for closure of the presumed perforated segment of intestine and for reinsertion of the catheter. In patients on long-term dialysis, such underlying gastrointestinal pathological conditions as appendicitis, perforated diverticulitis, or a perforated duodenal ulcer are likely to be the cause. Hypaque studies of the gastrointestinal tract may help confirm the diagnosis and the need for operation. At our institution, a laparotomy is not performed when the contrast examination is normal, the patient shows clinical improvement on dialysis, and the effluent is rendered sterile by appropriate antibiotics. In one review, 10 episodes of peritonitis with multiple enteric organisms were treated in this manner.[72] Four patients had persisting abdominal pain and required laparotomy. Significant pathological conditions were found in all four, including perforating appendicitis, gangrenous cholecystitis, perforated sigmoid diverticulitis, and perforated cecum. No postoperative sequelae were reported. Of the remaining six patients, all responded to antibiotic therapy and did not require laparotomy. Presumably, these patients had walled-off perforations of the gastrointestinal tract that were adequately controlled by local mechanisms.

Intra-abdominal Abscess

Abscesses are well-defined collections of pus that are walled off from the rest of the peritoneal cavity by inflammatory adhesions, loops of intestine and their mesentery, the greater omentum, or other abdominal viscera. Abscesses may occur in the peritoneal cavity, either within or outside of abdominal viscera, as well as in the retroperitoneum.[73] Extravisceral abscesses arise in two situations: (1) after resolution of diffuse peritonitis in which a loculated area of infection persists and evolves into an abscess and (2) after perforation of a viscus or an anastomotic breakdown that is successfully walled off by peritoneal defense mechanisms. More than 80 percent of intra-abdominal abscesses occur in the postoperative period, the majority after pancreaticobiliary or colorectal surgery [see Table 5].[74,75] This pattern may reflect the technical difficulty of anastomoses in the former and the large bacterial load in the latter. Over 30 percent of abscesses are associated with clear evidence of an anastomotic leak.[75] By contrast, intra-abdominal abscesses unassociated with previous surgery are usually attributable to inflammatory processes with a small, localized perforation, as in appendicitis, diverticulitis, and Crohn's disease.[75,76] Visceral abscesses are most commonly caused by hematogenous or lymphatic spread of bacteria to the organ. Retroperitoneal abscesses may be caused by several mechanisms, including perforation of the gastrointestinal tract into the retroperitoneum and hematogenous or lymphatic spread of bacteria to retroperitoneal organs, particularly the inflamed pancreas.

Table 5 Incidence of Postoperative Abscess Formation in Relation to Site of Initial Operation[74]

Site of Operation	Incidence of Postoperative Abscess (%)
Pancreas and biliary tract	20
Colon	15
Stomach	9
Retroperitoneum	9
Trauma laparotomy	9
Duodenum	8
Appendix	6
Kidney and adrenal gland	5
Small intestine	4
Spleen	4
Liver	4
Vascular	2
Uterus and ovary	1
Others	11

CLINICAL PRESENTATION AND DIAGNOSIS

Diagnosis is based on clinical suspicion of an abscess and radiologic confirmation of this suspicion. Patients with intra-abdominal abscesses usually have local and systemic signs of inflammation. Characteristically, mild abdominal pain and localized tenderness exist in the region of the infection. Because of the presence of adherent omentum, bowel, or adjacent viscera, it is common to feel a diffuse, rather than a discrete, mass. The patient is usually febrile and anorexic and has a leukocytosis with a shift to the left. The clinical findings associated with an intra-abdominal abscess may be masked by the administration of antibiotics to the patient. However, as previously noted, in the face of antibiotic use, the presence of a fever or a leukocytosis with a band count higher than three percent, or both, is highly indicative of persistent sepsis and should lead to more intensive investigation of the patient's condition.[14,15]

The armamentarium of radiologic techniques available for the diagnosis of intra-abdominal sepsis is quite extensive.[77] Plain abdominal x-rays, though rarely diagnostic, frequently point to the need for further investigation. These x-ray findings may document loculated extraluminal gas collections or mottled soft tissue masses, either of which is indicative of abscess formation. More subtle signs include the presence of a localized ileus, a pleural effusion, and atelectasis. A limited contrast examination may be useful, particularly when left upper quadrant abnormalities are found on x-ray examination, to differentiate the stomach from an extraluminal mass or to detect a leak. This investigation may be particularly important after splenectomy, when fluid may collect in the left upper quadrant as the result of a gastric fistula developing from the greater curvature of the stomach. Suspicion of an abscess, based on either clinical or basic radiologic findings, should indicate the necessity for imaging techniques to confirm the diagnosis and to pinpoint the location of the abscess.

Ultrasonography and computed tomographic scanning are clearly the examinations of choice; studies comparing the various techniques of imaging an abscess usually suggest CT scanning to be the superior modality.[78,79] Our general approach is to suit the imaging technique to the patient. If the potential site of infection can be localized clinically, then ultrasonography is used to confirm clinical suspicions and to direct diagnostic aspiration of the collection. If the patient appears clinically septic but the site of the infection is not obvious or if the ultrasonographic examination is unsatisfactory, then we prefer to use CT scanning of the abdomen. Nuclear medicine techniques are rarely used in this setting.

MANAGEMENT

Three basic principles guide the management of intra-abdominal abscesses: (1) general patient care, (2) antibiotic administration, and (3) drainage of the abscess.

General Patient Care

Patients with intra-abdominal abscess show a spectrum of clinical presentations: they range from the relatively well with low-grade fever and leukocytosis to those with septic shock. Clearly, the initial management of all such patients should be tailored to their clinical picture. In general, these patients have some degree of intravascular volume depletion that calls for fluid resuscitation. Resuscitation should be monitored by observing vital signs, urine output, and mental status. In the critically ill patient, Swan-Ganz catheterization and invasive arterial monitoring are essential to direct initial resuscitation, particularly if administration of inotropic agents is necessary.

Hypoxemia may be present for several reasons. Atelectasis, basilar pneumonia, and pleural effusions may exist secondary to abdominal distention with elevation of the diaphragm as well as to subphrenic infectious processes.[80] In addition, advanced sepsis may result in increased alveolar-capillary permeability and the development of adult respiratory distress syndrome in the context of the multiple organ dysfunction syndrome (MODS).[81]

Nutritional support is important in the management of patients with intra-abdominal abscess. Patients in whom abscesses develop in the postoperative period are already at a nutritional disadvantage because they have usually spent seven to 10 days without adequate caloric intake. The marked catabolic response associated with sepsis further aggravates this problem.[82] Historically, total parenteral nutrition has been preferred in patients with intra-abdominal infection. Recent evidence, however, suggests that nutritional supplementation by the enteral route may reduce the incidence of infectious complications and improve the immune status of critically ill patients.[83,84] Furthermore, enteral feeding within 24 hours of laparotomy appears to be well tolerated in most patients. This approach may be used in patients with enterocutaneous fistulas if adequate drainage prevents further contamination of the peritoneal cavity.[85] Feeding is usually accomplished by passing a tube into the upper small intestine and using an enteral pump to administer the solution. Such a technique avoids the complications of vomiting and aspiration associated with gastroparesis. In patients for whom enteral feeding is not satisfactory, parenteral nutrition should be instituted. Total caloric requirements, optimal amino acid solutions, and lipid requirements are dealt with elsewhere [see 97 *Nutritional Support*].

Antibiotics

Antibiotic therapy should be directed against the microorganisms most likely to be recovered from the abscess, which almost always include a combination of aerobic and anaerobic bacteria.[86] As for secondary peritonitis, administration of antibiotic combinations or single agents that are active against both aerobes and anaerobes is generally considered the gold standard for the management of intra-abdominal infection [see Table 3].

It should be emphasized that general patient care and antibiotic therapy serve primarily as adjuncts to drainage of the abscess cavity. Antibiotics alone are unlikely to be effective for numerous reasons, including poor penetration of antibiotics into the abscess center, inactivation of antibiotics in the microenvironment of the infection (i.e., hypoxia and acidity), and inactivity of the drug against a large bacterial inoculum. Drainage of an abscess usually reverses these adverse conditions and increases the efficacy of the antibiotics.

Drainage

Drainage, either percutaneous or surgical, is the mainstay of the management of intra-abdominal abscess. The ability to perform either technique depends on precise localization of the infection by means of CT scanning or ultrasonography.

Percutaneous drainage has made a major contribution to the management of intra-abdominal abscess. It is the treatment of choice in the management of single, well-defined intra-abdominal abscesses. The management of the patient with a well-defined abscess amenable to drainage requires close collaboration between the radiologist and the surgeon. In essence, the problem is approached from a surgical viewpoint, except that percutaneous drainage is used [see Figure 1]. If the patient has not improved markedly by 48 hours after initial percutaneous drainage, he or she is returned to the radiology department for a repeat CT scan. A residual abscess will be percutaneously drained at this time. However, if there is residual infection that cannot be adequately drained or if no residual collection is found, then serious consideration should be given to performing

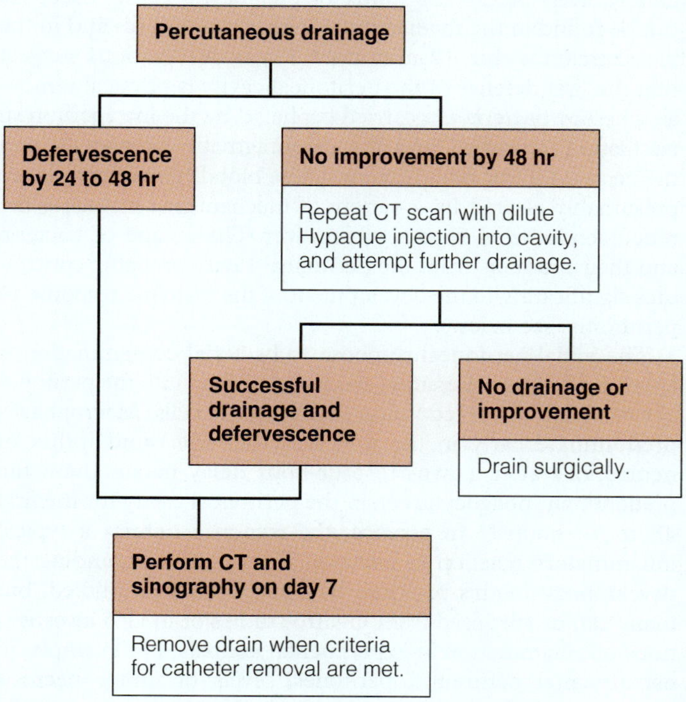

Figure 1 Algorithm outlines the management of intra-abdominal abscess by means of percutaneous drainage.

a formal laparotomy. Criteria for removal of the percutaneous catheter are (1) clinical resolution of sepsis as determined by the patient's well-being, temperature, and leukocyte count, (2) minimal drainage from the catheter, and (3) radiologic evidence of resolution of the abscess on sinogram or CT scan. The overall duration of drainage varies widely, ranging from four to 30 days. In general, prolonged periods of drainage are related to the presence of an enteric communication. Major complications of percutaneous drainage, which include hemorrhage, enteric fistula, and empyema, are relatively rare.

Improved localization techniques using either ultrasonography or CT scanning have also greatly simplified the surgical approach to the treatment of intra-abdominal abscess. Before the regular use of these techniques, a general abdominal exploration was usually performed for fear of missing multiple abscesses in the peritoneal cavity.[87] When the abscess can be located accurately by CT, a direct (often extraserous) approach to abscesses in the subphrenic, subhepatic, or pelvic region can be made, amounting to the surgical equivalent of percutaneous drainage. A general laparotomy under these circumstances is unnecessary and may lead to such complications as enteric fistula or bleeding. On the other hand, laparotomy is necessary when the abscesses are in the lesser sac or interloop or are multiple; the latter is particularly true in the early postoperative period. After evacuation of the abscess cavity, Penrose or soft sump drains should be left in situ. Criteria for removal of these drains are similar to those for removal of percutaneous drains.

Discussion

Host Response to Peritoneal Injury and Infection

LOCAL RESPONSE

After bacterial contamination of the peritoneal cavity, a complex series of events is initiated that, under ideal circumstances, effects complete eradication of invading bacteria. The three major defense mechanisms are (1) mechanical clearance of bacteria via the diaphragmatic lymphatics, (2) phagocytosis and destruction of suspended or adherent bacteria by phagocytic cells, and (3) sequestration and walling off of bacteria coupled with delayed clearance by phagocytic cells. The first two mechanisms act rapidly, usually within hours. When a pure suspension of bacteria is injected into the peritoneal cavity of an experimental animal, the bacteria begin to disappear immediately, even before the influx of phagocytic cells.[88] Bacteria can be found in the mediastinum within six minutes and in the bloodstream within 12 minutes.[89] These observations suggest that the first defense of the peritoneal cavity is physical removal, whereby bacteria are carried cephalad by the intraperitoneal circulation, absorbed into the diaphragmatic lymphatics, and then carried to the bloodstream. These blood-borne bacteria are presumably cleared by a variety of mechanisms, including the reticuloendothelial system of the liver. The escape of bacteria and their products from the peritoneal cavity probably contributes significantly to the development of the systemic response to peritonitis (see below).

The initial peritoneal response to bacterial contamination is characterized by hyperemia, exudation of fluid into the peritoneal cavity, and a marked influx of phagocytic cells. Macrophages predominate early in the infection, but the rapid influx of neutrophils after a two- to four-hour delay makes them the predominant phagocytic cell in the peritoneal cavity for the first 48 to 72 hours.[88] In essence, the response mimics a typical inflammatory reaction to bacteria. The events surrounding the development of this response have not been well studied, but many can be surmised from in vitro studies or in vivo investigations of inflammation in experimental animals. For example, in experimental peritonitis, peritoneal levels of tumor necrosis factor-α (TNF-α) and interleukin-1 (IL-1) increase rapidly after the initiation of infection.[90,91] Similarly, in humans with severe intra-abdominal infection, peritoneal levels of TNF-α, IL-1, and IL-6 are higher than levels measured simultaneously in plasma.[92,93] Lipopolysaccharide derived from gram-negative enteric bacteria is a particularly strong stimulus for production of many of these cytokines by peritoneal macrophages. Recent studies have reported that other cell types are important in the initiation of the local peritoneal response. Peritoneal mast cells appear to release preformed tumor necrosis factor early in the genesis of peritoneal inflammation and contribute significantly to recruiting neutrophils to the peritoneal cavity. The peritoneal mesothelial cells have also been shown to be potent producers of a range of cytokines and procoagulants. Given the strategic position of both of these cell types, their role in the initiation of the local response is undoubtedly important.[94,95] The combined effects of these cytokines from various sources clearly contribute to the inflammatory response observed during peritonitis [see 101 Cytokines and the Cellular Response to Injury and Infection].[96] In addition, generation of other inflammatory mediator molecules, such as leukotriene B_4, platelet-activating factor, and components of the complement cascade (e.g., C3a and C5a), further promotes the development of local inflammation.[97-99]

Finally, fibrin deposition appears to play an important role in walling off infection, not only by incorporating large numbers of bacteria within its interstices[100] but also by causing loops of intestine to adhere to each other and the omentum, thereby creating a physical barrier against dissemination. Fibrin deposition is initiated after the exudation of protein-rich fluid containing fibrinogen into the peritoneal cavity. The conversion of fibrinogen to fibrin is promoted by the release of tissue thromboplastin from both mesothelial cells and stimulated peritoneal macrophages.[101] Furthermore, a plasminogen activator, which is responsible for the activation of fibrinolytic enzymes and is normally present in the mesothelial and submesothelial cell membranes, disappears in the face of bacterial infection.[102]

In addition to favorable effects, peritoneal defenses against bacterial soilage have seemingly paradoxical effects on the overall well-being of the host. Early mechanical clearance via diaphragmatic lymphatics reduces bacterial numbers but also results in bacteremia, which, if massive, can result in death. The influx of large amounts of protein-rich exudate into the peritoneal cavity, though important in providing opsonins and enhancing phagocyte influx, also produces massive third-space fluid shifts, which may produce hypovolemic shock. In addition, there may be significant loss of albumin into the peritoneal cavity. Locally, fluid may impair bacterial opsonization by diluting opsonins and may reduce phagocytosis both by this mechanism and by altering the neutrophils' ability to reach the bacterium.[103] Furthermore, the deposition of fibrinous exudate provides a protected sanctuary in which bacteria may proliferate and thus leads to abscess formation.[104]

In a similarly paradoxical manner, part of the objective in the management of intra-abdominal infection is to treat specific areas where peritoneal defenses have been successful (e.g., by administering antibiotics to treat systemic infection resulting from lymphatic clearance and by removing fluid and fibrinous debris from the peritoneal cavity to prevent residual intra-abdominal sepsis).

SYSTEMIC RESPONSE

The systemic response to bacterial peritonitis mimics the body's response to trauma in general and includes the rapid release of catecholamines, increased secretion of adrenocortical hormones, and secretion of aldosterone and antidiuretic hormone. Of particular note, especially with respect to the management of bacterial peritonitis, are the hemodynamic and metabolic responses to intra-abdominal infection.

The hemodynamic alterations observed in patients with intra-abdominal infection have several causes. Hypovolemia induced by peritoneal inflammation is a major contributor to the picture. Diffuse peritonitis has been likened to a total burn surface of 50 percent in terms of its effects on fluid shifts. A contracted extracellular fluid volume caused by massive fluid shifts into the peritoneal tissues and cavity produces hypovolemic shock with a reduced cardiac index, elevated peripheral vascular resistance, and increased peripheral oxygen extraction.[105] Patients with fulminant peritonitis demonstrate the more classic septic picture after fluid resuscitation[106,107]: elevated cardiac output, reduced peripheral vascular resistance, and a narrowed arteriovenous O_2 difference. Hemodynamic studies in surgical patients with peritonitis have demonstrated combined abnormalities—that is, patients initially present with evidence of hypovolemia caused by peritoneal fluid losses, and only after resuscitation do they manifest the hyperdynamic picture associated with sepsis.[107] Because survival is generally better in patients with a profile of septic shock, it appears clear that aggressive fluid resuscitation is critical in the early management period [see 4 Shock].

As proposed for the local response to infection in the peritoneal cavity, the stimulated release of products of cells of the monocyte-macrophage lineage also appears to be responsible for the characteristic septic host response observed in patients with bacterial peritonitis. Intravenous infusion of TNF into experimental animals mimics the hemodynamic alteration and lactic acidosis that follow the administration of bacterial endotoxin.[108] Both TNF and IL-1 cause fever and neutrophilia,[108,109] and IL-6 initiates the acute-phase protein response characteristic of infection.[110]

A correlation between the magnitude of the cytokine response and outcome in infected patients has been demonstrated in several clinical studies. Higher levels of circulating TNF-α and IL-6 have been recorded in patients who later die with intra-abdominal infection.[111] Temporal analysis of this cytokine response in relation to the time of laparotomy confirms that peak TNF-α and IL-6 levels occur within two to four hours of skin incision.[112] The exaggerated cytokine response may occur as a result of mobilization of the infectious focus, with spilling of bacteria and bacterial products into the circulation. This phenomenon may account for the pronounced hemodynamic instability soon after laparotomy for intra-abdominal infection. Most recently, elevated levels of interleukin-10 have been documented in patients with intra-abdominal infection.[113] Unlike TNF-α, IL-10 has anti-inflammatory properties and may limit secretion of TNF-α by macrophages. This interleukin may provide an endogenous means to down-regulate an uncontrolled systemic inflammatory response.

The improved understanding of the cell biology of the host response to infection and inflammation has suggested potentially innovative approaches to the management of patients with intra-abdominal infection. Obviously, prevention of the adverse effects of cytokinemia would appear to represent a rational adjuvant treatment measure in these patients. In animal models, administration of anti-TNF antibody and antagonism with IL-1 receptor antagonists effectively prevents the end-organ dysfunction and the adverse hemodynamic and metabolic effects of endotoxin infusion. Before this approach is widely applied, however, consideration should be given to the beneficial effects of TNF and other cytokines in orchestrating the clearance of bacteria from the peritoneal cavity and the possible adverse effects of anticytokine therapy on this useful host response mechanism.

Management of Secondary Peritonitis—Controversies and New Concepts

ANTIBIOTICS

Research over the past three decades has created a body of knowledge forming the basis for rational recommendations for antimicrobial use in patients with intra-abdominal infection.[114-118] On the basis of this evidence, empirical antimicrobial therapy should be directed against *E. coli* and other common members of the Enterobacteriaceae as well as against the anaerobe *B. fragilis*. Guidelines have been proposed that define acceptable antimicrobial regimens for the treatment of intra-abdominal infections [see Table 3].[12,13] Decisions about a particular regimen should be tailored to the individual patient, taking into consideration the possibility of resistant organisms and the potential for adverse effects. Other considerations that may affect the choice of an antimicrobial regimen include its pharmacokinetic properties in the particular patient and its cost. The calculation of costs must include not only acquisition, which may be institution dependent, but also the costs of administration, monitoring, and management of toxicity.

Combination Regimens

The combination of an aminoglycoside and an antianaerobic agent (clindamycin or metronidazole) has, until recently, been considered the gold standard for treatment of patients with intra-abdominal infection. Aminoglycosides have broad coverage of gram-negative bacteria, are inexpensive, have a low incidence of inducing resistant microorganisms, and have been used extensively with great success in a large number of clinical trials. Aminoglycoside-based regimens have fallen into dis-

complications were noted even in the control group, which suggests that the patient group studied was not at high enough risk to warrant such aggressive therapy. This technique is extremely labor intensive, necessitates intensive care unit monitoring, and is potentially complicated by the development of enteric fistulas from erosion of the cannula. A well-performed prospective, randomized trial of postoperative peritoneal lavage in high-risk patients is required to determine the efficacy of the technique.

Over the past decade, the concept of planned relaparotomy (or staged abdominal repair [STAR]) and open management for severe peritonitis has been rejuvenated with the expectation that they might prevent recurrent intra-abdominal infection and associated morbidity. Planned relaparotomy refers to the practice of performing repeat operations at fixed intervals (usually 24 to 72 hours) regardless of the patient's clinical condition. In this way, the development of new abscesses is prevented, necrotic tissue is debrided, and enteric fistulas are recognized early. The difficulties arising from frequent exploration, with its forceful, repeated closure of the abdominal wall, have resulted in the development of the open abdomen approach, or laparostomy. Reported benefits of this technique include the conceptual advantage of treating the entire peritoneal cavity as one large abscess, with exteriorization permitting drainage. Other possible advantages include improved ventilation and renal perfusion [see Abdominal Compartment Syndrome, below]. In the open abdomen approach, the fascia is kept open with saline gauze packing. Complications of this technique include evisceration, massive fluid losses, spontaneous fistulas, and contamination of the open wound, as well as the necessity for mechanical ventilation. Moreover, an open abdomen does not necessarily eliminate the need for repeat abdominal exploration.

Complications associated with the open abdomen approach have resulted in popularization of a semiopen technique, in which temporary abdominal closure prevents evisceration yet allows easy reexploration of the peritoneal cavity. Towel clips and mesh composed of polypropylene (Marlex), polyglycolic acid (Dexon), or an expanded polytetrafluoroethylene patch (PTFE, Gore-Tex) have all been used for this purpose. One popular strategy involves the use of polypropylene with or without an insewn zipper or burr-like device (Velcro) to allow repeated and rapid access to the peritoneal cavity [see Figure 2].[146-148] Mesh prevents evisceration in the early postoperative period, reduces the risk of spontaneous fistulization, allows for drainage of fluid and pus through its interstices, and may function as an exit site for a stoma or drain. At reexploration, adhesions are lysed, and fibrinous exudates, fluid, and necrotic debris are removed. This procedure is continued daily until clinical evidence of sepsis has subsided and the abdominal cavity appears clean, as determined by the presence of healthy granulation tissue and adhesion formation. The mesh and zipper are then removed, and the wound is allowed to granulate and contract. A split-thickness skin graft may be used for coverage, although this is not absolutely necessary. Several complications have been associated with the use of mesh, including enteric fistulization, prolonged ventilation, and hernia formation.

Initial reports evaluating the use of planned relaparotomy were quite positive.

Two studies used the Acute Physiology and Chronic Health Evaluation II (APACHE II) stratification system to define underlying severity of illness.[148,149] In one, the Marlex mesh technique was applied to patients with diffuse nonlocalizing peritonitis.[149] The mortality in patients receiving a mesh at the time of reoperation for postoperative peritonitis was one third the rate predicted on the basis of APACHE II scores. Evaluation of the subgroups of APACHE II scores indicated that critically ill patients with scores higher than 25 had a mortality of 100 percent, whereas those with low scores already had a low mortality that was independent of treatment. These data suggest that patients with midrange APACHE II scores are the ones who may derive the greatest benefit from this approach—a finding that was confirmed in the second study mentioned.[148]

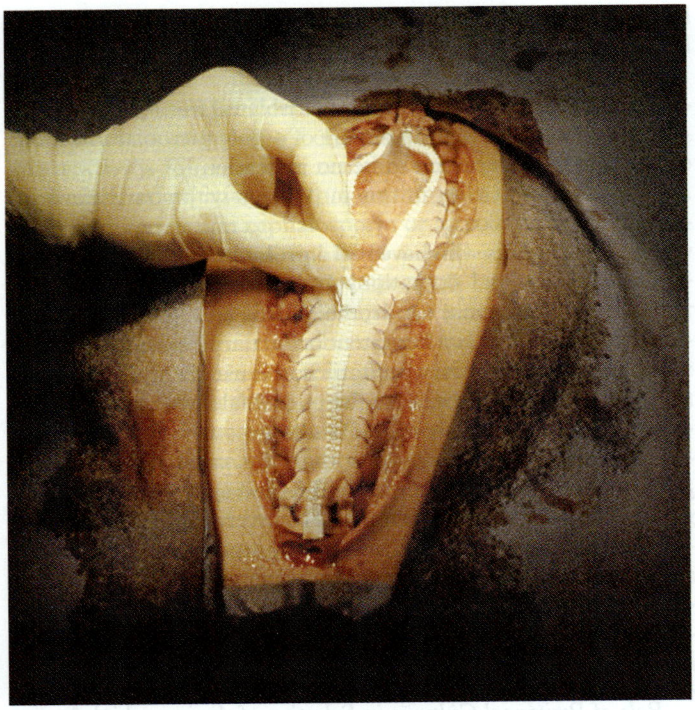

Figure 2 A plastic zipper sewn into a Marlex mesh is opened to gain access to the peritoneal cavity for repeated laparotomies.

More recent data have tempered the initial enthusiasm for planned relaparotomy. A case-control study matching patients managed with planned relaparotomy to patients managed with relaparotomy on demand (based on APACHE II score, age, cause of infection, site of origin of peritonitis, and the ability of the surgeon to securely eliminate the source of infection) found that patients managed by planned relaparotomy had higher rates of recurrent intra-abdominal sepsis, anastomotic leaks, and septicemia as well as worse organ dysfunction than those managed by relaparotomy on demand.[150] Further, the patients in the former group had a higher rate of unplanned laparotomies than their conventionally managed controls (21 percent versus eight percent), although this difference was not statistically significant. These data suggest that planned relaparotomy may not even obviate unplanned laparotomy. A review of the literature, compiling data on 642 patients in 22 series, concluded that there was insufficient evidence to support either open management or planned relaparotomy in patients with postoperative peritonitis.[151]

Because of the limited data supporting the efficacy of planned relaparotomy in the critically ill patient with severe peritonitis, our general approach is to tailor the need for subsequent laparotomy to the patient's clinical status (i.e., relaparotomy on demand). Absence of improvement or clinical deterioration requires either abdominal imaging studies or laparotomy, or both, depending on the clinical status of the patient. In certain situations, we find that planned relaparotomy may be useful. For example, it may be practical in patients in whom there is a large segment of bowel with marginal viability. These patients may best be served with a second operation that allows the bowel to demarcate, thus minimizing the length of bowel resected. Patients with necrotizing pancreatitis may also benefit from planned relaparotomy. Complete debridement may be precluded by extensive bleeding or a lack of demarcation of necrotic tissue. Under such circumstances, we recommend multiple limited operations rather than a single attempt at complete debridement.

PROGNOSIS OF SECONDARY PERITONITIS

The morbidity and mortality of intra-abdominal infection vary widely depending on the particular study quoted. Studies examining the efficacy of antibiotics in intra-abdominal infection tend to include patients within a defined age limit, with normal organ function, and with minimally deranged physiologic parameters.[152] As a result, these studies show a very favorable outcome for intra-abdominal infection, with a mortality in the range of three to five percent. Conversely, studies specifically designed to investigate mortality associated with intra-abdominal infection have yielded rates exceeding 20 percent.[153,154] This discrepancy is consistent with the fact that intra-abdominal infection is not a homogeneous disease but rather one that poses a high risk of complications for some patients and a low risk for others. The ability to stratify patients into these risk groups is of critical importance for several reasons. First, it allows us to predict which patients are at high risk. Second, the ability to identify high-risk patients will pinpoint the subgroup in which new and innovative techniques should be tried. Finally, stratification of patients into risk groups enhances our ability to interpret the results of studies examining new treatments. A clear example for surgeons is the importance of wound classification for identifying patients who will benefit from administration of prophylactic antibiotics [see 39 Prevention of Postoperative Infection].

Several scoring systems are currently available for accurate assessment of patient risk. Few of these methods adequately address the risk associated with intra-abdominal infection. One study approached classification from an anatomic standpoint: risk correlated well with the organ from which the peritonitis originated.[155] Peritonitis arising from duodenal or appendiceal pathology was associated with low mortality (about 10 percent), whereas peritonitis in the postoperative period was associated with high mortality (60 percent). A discriminant function equation, based on the patient's age, immunologic function (as measured by delayed-type hypersensitivity), and nutritional status (based on albumin level), has been developed.[156] It accurately predicted mortality after major operations, including those for intra-abdominal infection.

A surgical infection stratification system has been developed for patients with intra-abdominal infection.[154] In a five-center study, 178 patients with established intra-abdominal sepsis were found to have an overall mortality of 24 percent. When risk factors were analyzed independently, it was found that the patients who died were generally older, had higher acute physiology scores (APS, which measures the degree of deviation from normal in 34 routinely measured laboratory tests or physical findings), and tended to be diabetic, malnourished, or in shock on admission. Multivariate analysis determined that APS, malnutrition, and age were the most reliable predictors of outcome. A discriminant function based on these parameters could predict survival or death with an 84 percent accuracy. The APACHE II stratification system has now supplanted APS as a useful predictive score.[157] This system is based on the evaluation of 12 acute physiology parameters as well as an assessment of the patient's general state of health.[158]

In a recent multicenter trial evaluating outcome in patients with severe peritonitis (APACHE II score > 10), logistic regression analysis showed that a high APACHE II score, a low serum albumin level, and high New York Heart Association cardiac function status were significantly and independently associated with death.[159] Although the APACHE II system is used most often, recent evidence suggests that the APACHE II score may underestimate mortality risk in critically ill patients with intra-abdominal infection.[160] A slight improvement in the predictive value of the APACHE II system has been demonstrated when delayed-type hypersensitivity (DTH) scores were added to the discriminant analysis, reflecting the importance of host immune function in prognosis.[161]

Persistent or Tertiary Peritonitis

In most patients, the combination of appropriate antibiotic therapy, timely surgical intervention, and normal host defense mechanisms results in complete resolution of the infection and subsequent recovery. Even when infection persists, localization of the infection with resultant abscess formation limits the magnitude of the systemic response and permits straightforward management by means of either percutaneous or directed surgical drainage. Some patients, however, are unable to localize infection because of either impaired host defenses or overwhelming infection, and these individuals may go on to manifest persistent diffuse peritonitis, also called tertiary peritonitis. The clinical picture is one of occult infection, signaled by fever, leukocytosis, hyperdynamic cardiovascular parameters, and a general hypermetabolic state. The development of progressive dysfunction of one or more organ systems is a frequent concomitant finding.[131] In this patient population, mortality has been as high as 64 percent despite aggressive surgical and antibiotic therapy.[162]

Laparotomy often reveals poorly defined serosanguineous collections instead of discrete purulent abscesses. This probably indicates the host's inability to localize an infectious process, reflecting global immune dysfunction. Additional support for this hypothesis is provided by the flora associated with tertiary peritonitis. Peritoneal cultures yield organisms markedly different from those isolated in cases of community-acquired secondary peritonitis. Organisms traditionally thought to be of low virulence, such as enterococci, *Candida, S. epidermidis,* and *P. aeruginosa,* predominate.[131,162,163] Their presence may reflect selection by antibiotic pressures or the impaired systemic and local host defenses of MODS.

Early studies of multiorgan failure in patients with peritonitis

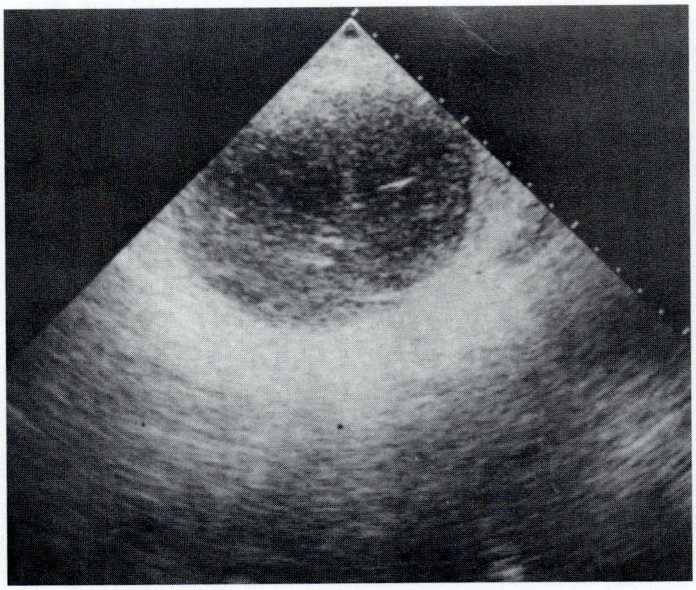

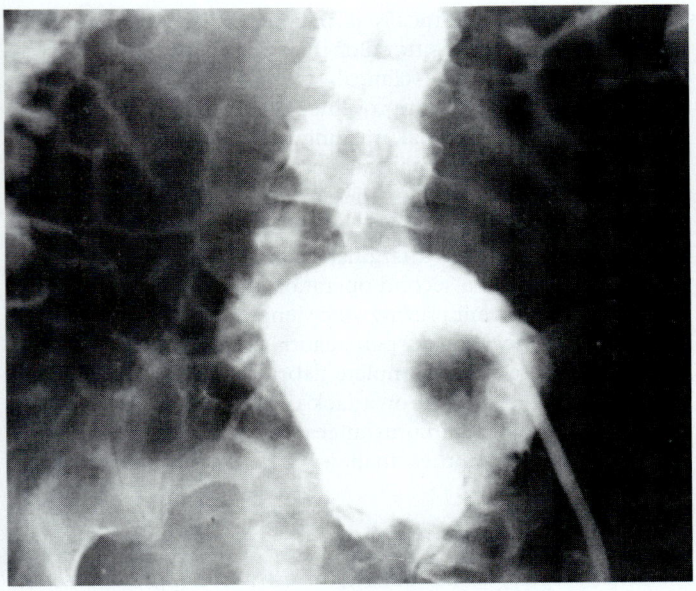

Figure 3 Ultrasonographic examination of the left lower quadrant demonstrates the presence of an abscess (left). An obvious mass was palpable at this site on clinical examination. Under ultrasonographic guidance, a pigtail catheter was placed percutaneously into the abscess. The cavity is well outlined after injection of a small amount of contrast material (right).

showed a strong association between organ failure and the presence of uncontrolled residual infection in the peritoneal cavity.[81] As a result, surgeons were encouraged, for a short time, to perform so-called blind laparotomy to look for undrained abscesses. However, comparison of preoperative CT scans with operative findings showed that significant radiologically occult infectious foci were uncommon and that even when such foci were encountered, MODS persisted despite surgical drainage.[132,164-166] Laparotomy is recommended only if imaging studies, blood cultures, or a change in clinical status is consistent with the presence of an undrained infection.

Given the postulated role of the GI tract in the development and perpetuation of MODS in these patients, selective decontamination of the GI tract, enteral feeding, and avoidance of H_2-receptor blockade represent worthwhile management strategies [see 95 Multiple Organ Dysfunction Syndrome].

ABDOMINAL COMPARTMENT SYNDROME

Markedly increased intra-abdominal pressures may develop in critically ill patients with intra-abdominal infection as a result of visceral edema, the accumulation of peritoneal fluid, and closure of an edematous, noncompliant abdominal wall. Intra-abdominal pressures may increase to the point that systemic hemodynamics, respiratory function, and renal function are compromised. This entity, referred to as the abdominal compartment syndrome, is characterized by hypotension and low cardiac output in the presence of elevated central filling pressures, high systemic vascular resistance, elevated peak airway pressures, and oliguria.[167,168] High intra-abdominal pressure impairs venous return and increases systemic vascular resistance. Elevation of the diaphragm increases intrathoracic pressure, impairing ventilation and artificially elevating central filling pressures.[169] Renal vein compression, coupled with a reduction in cardiac output and renal blood flow, may play a role in renal dysfunction associated with the syndrome. The syndrome may account for some of the adverse consequences of laparotomy for peritonitis that have previously been attributed to the release of proinflammatory mediators. The incidence of this syndrome is difficult to ascertain because intra-abdominal pressures are rarely measured.

The diagnosis should be suspected in patients with the clinical picture described above. Intra-abdominal pressure may be evaluated indirectly by measuring urinary bladder pressure.[168] Sterile saline (50 to 100 ml) is injected into the empty bladder through a Foley catheter. Tubing for the drainage bag is connected to the catheter, and once the catheter and proximal tubing are filled with saline, a clamp is placed on the tubing of the drainage bag distal to the culture aspiration port. A 16-gauge needle is inserted into the aspiration port and connected to a pressure transducer. The zero reference point is the symphysis pubis. Normal intra-abdominal pressure approximates atmospheric pressure. Clinically significant changes in hemodynamics occur with intra-abdominal pressures above 20 mm Hg, with severe alterations occurring when pressures exceed 40 mm Hg.

Management involves decompressive laparotomy with concomitant fluid resuscitation. Laparotomy usually results in prompt resolution of the hemodynamic alterations and a brisk diuresis. The abdominal wall should be closed without tension, usually with the fascia opened and a prosthesis used to prevent evisceration. Fascial closure may be attempted after the acute process has resolved and the likelihood of repeat laparotomies is remote.

Intra-abdominal Abscess—
Radiologic Diagnosis and Intervention

Ultrasonography and CT scanning have become the modalities of choice for the diagnosis of intra-abdominal abscess. Each has its own advantages and disadvantages. Ultrasonography is fast and inexpensive and delivers no radiation. It is also highly accurate in the appropriate setting [see Figure 3].[170] Furthermore, the availability of mobile machines permits bedside and intraoperative examination. Endoluminal probes allow transvaginal and transrectal visualization and potential drainage of deep pelvic abscesses.[171,172] The major disadvantages of ultrasonography are that it is extremely operator dependent, its images may be obscured by gas, and it is difficult to study patients with open wounds or drains. The last two problems are particularly relevant for the critically ill postoperative patient who has intestinal ileus and has had multiple operative interventions.

Computed tomography is the most accurate technique available for the diagnosis of intra-abdominal abscess.[110,173] The major advantage of CT is its ability to display, independent of the operator, both intraperitoneal and retroperitoneal structures with a high degree of resolution and accuracy [see Figure 4]. In addition, the presence of ileus, as well as of drains, dressings, or stomas, does not interfere with the performance of the test. The major disadvantages of CT scanning are its nonportability and the need for the patient to be cooperative and immobile. The accuracy of the scan is reduced in those patients whose GI tract is not opacified with contrast. Under these circumstances, the scans are limited in their ability to distinguish fluid-filled bowel loops from an abscess. Interloop abscesses, which represent approximately four percent of all abscesses, are also poorly visualized on CT scan.[77]

Two other imaging techniques for intra-abdominal infections involve the use of radionuclides: granulocytes are labeled with gallium-67 citrate or indium-111. Gallium has an affinity for iron-binding proteins (e.g., lactoferrin, ferritin, and bacterial siderophores) and is incorporated into abscesses by binding to lactoferrin present in leukocytes at the site of infection and by binding to bacterial surfaces.[174] The detection of an abscess is based on increased uptake outside of expected sites. One major drawback is that gallium is excreted in the colon and therefore accumulates in the stool. An enema to clear radiolabeled stool is frequently necessary to permit interpretation of the study. Other shortcomings of this technique include the false positive imaging of neoplasms and the 24- to 72-hour delay required between injection of the radionuclide and the scanning procedure.

Indium-111 in the form of the chelate indium In 111 oxyquinoline is used to label granulocytes drawn from the patient.[175,176] After labeling, the cells are reinjected into the

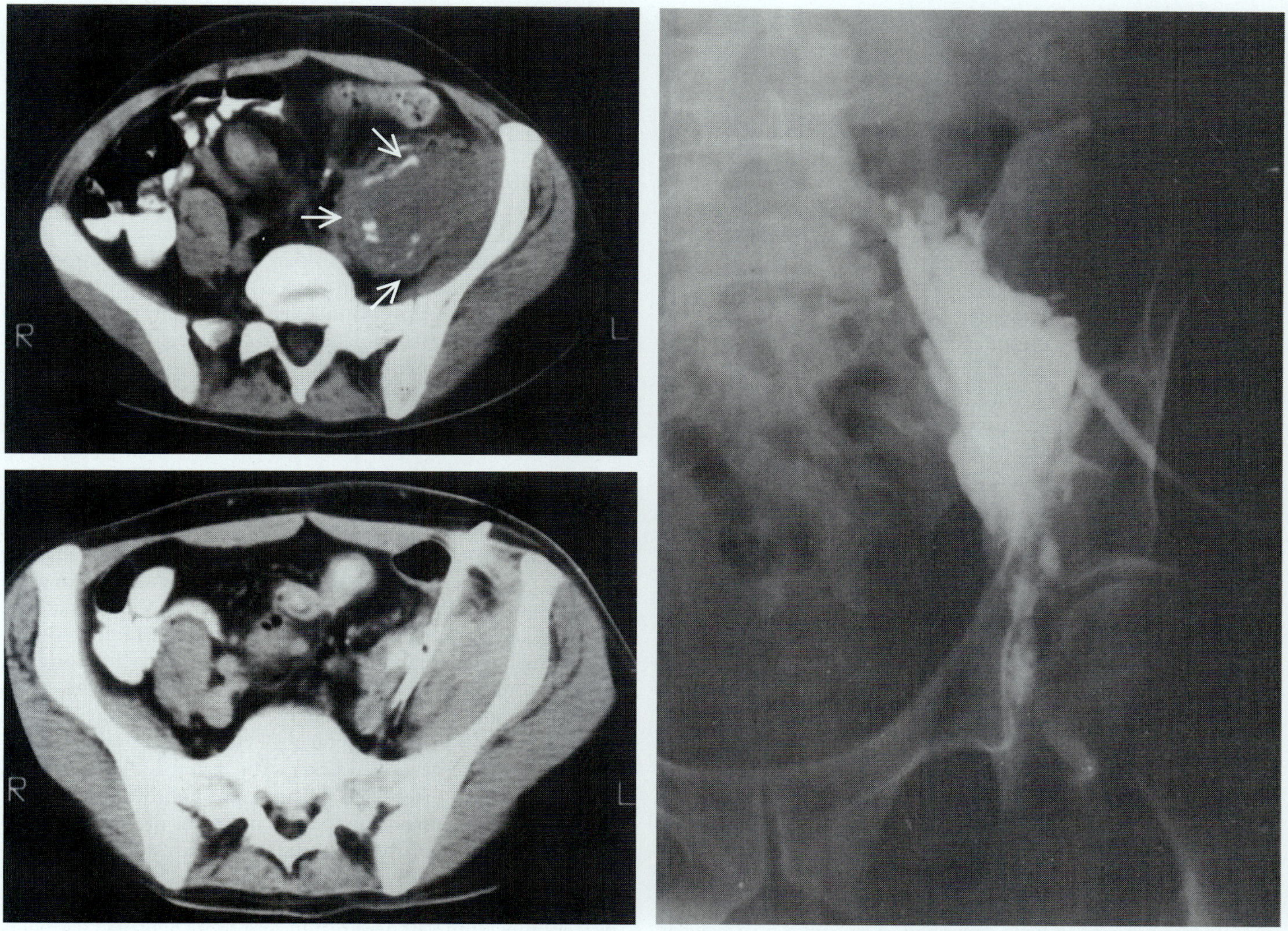

Figure 4 CT scan demonstrates a left psoas abscess (arrows) in a patient with Crohn's disease (top, left). After percutaneous insertion of a pigtail catheter, CT scan shows the catheter to be situated in the abscess (bottom, left). A small amount of contrast injected via the catheter illustrates the extent of the retroperitoneal abscess cavity (right).

Table 6 Probability of Success Using Percutaneous Drainage of Intra-abdominal Abscesses

Clinical Condition	Probability of Success		Reason for Failure
Single, well-defined bacterial abscess with no enteric communication	High	Curative	
Abscess with enteric communication (e.g., diverticular abscess or Crohn's disease abscess)	High	Palliative	Prolonged drainage or recurrence
Abscess with enteric communication	Medium	Curative	
Infected tumor mass	Medium	Palliative	Poor drainage
Fungal abscess	Low		Poor drainage
Infected hematoma	Low		Poor drainage
Early postoperative diffuse peritonitis (e.g., caused by anastomotic dehiscence or bile peritonitis)	Low		Inadequate drainage
Interloop abscess	Low		Difficult visualization using scanning techniques; inaccessibility

patient, and the patient is scanned with a gamma camera. Presumably, normal granulocytes will accumulate at the site of an acute infection. The major disadvantage of indium-111 scanning is the significant number of false negative results in patients with chronic infections, which are less likely to lead to accumulation of acute inflammatory cells.[176] In general, these two techniques do not add much to the diagnostic armamentarium for intra-abdominal infection.

The role of magnetic resonance imaging in the diagnosis of intra-abdominal abscesses requires further definition. Initial studies suggest potential advantages.[177] Surgical clips do not interfere with imaging, and intravenous contrast is not necessary to outline the abscess or distinguish it from adjacent structures. Use of the sagittal plane may provide improved anatomic definition of the pelvis. The extended time required for imaging, compared with the excellent sensitivity and specificity of computed tomography and ultrasonography, suggests only a minor role for MRI in the diagnosis of intra-abdominal infection. The use of spectroscopy to evaluate parameters such as tissue pH may ultimately help differentiate between various fluid collections, something that ultrasonography and CT cannot do.

Percutaneous drainage is now well accepted as a treatment option in the management of intra-abdominal abscess. The early studies established rigid criteria for the use of this technique, including the presence of unilocular abscess and a direct window to the collection from the skin without intervening bowel or solid viscera.[178,179] When percutaneous drainage was used in accordance with these criteria, the success rate ranged from 80 to 90 percent. As radiologists have become more skilled in the technique and surgeons more confident in its use, the indications for percutaneous drainage have expanded, albeit with a somewhat lower overall success rate.[180] Acceptable criteria now include multiple or loculated abscesses, abscesses in which there is enteric communication, and, occasionally, abscesses that are reached by traversing solid viscera (e.g., traversing the liver to drain lesser sac abscesses).[181]

Successful percutaneous drainage has been redefined and is now divided into two categories[182]: (1) curative success—the drainage provides complete cure without the need for subsequent operation—and (2) palliative success—the drainage improves the patient's status so that operative intervention may be safely performed (e.g., an abscess with enteric communication). Palliative success also includes the patient for whom cure is impossible, such as the patient with an unresectable, infected tumor mass. For nonvisceral abscesses, clinical scenarios can be categorized according to the probability of successful drainage [see Table 6]. At the Toronto Hospital, percutaneous drainage is not attempted in that group in which the probability of success is low, except under unusual circumstances.

No randomized, controlled studies have been done comparing percutaneous with surgical drainage of intra-abdominal abscesses. The classic mortality figure associated with surgical drainage of intra-abdominal abscesses has been in the range of 30 percent.[153] Studies advocating the use of percutaneous drainage have quoted mortality figures between 11 and 15 percent, which suggests an advantage to the approach. However, comparisons in noncontrolled studies demonstrate no gross differences in mortality, although the percutaneously drained patient may stay in the hospital a shorter time.[183,184] The surgical patients were generally sicker, which perhaps explains this difference.[184] It is likely that the apparent improvement in survival associated with the use of percutaneous drainage is related to the use of improved imaging modalities, which can facilitate early diagnosis. One series, in which abscesses were treated surgically after location with CT scanning, reported a 12 percent mortality.[173] These results and those achieved with percutaneous drainage strongly support the concept that early diagnosis and treatment of abscesses before MODS develops are critical in reducing the overall mortality associated with such infections.

References

1. Abu-Yousef MM, Bleicher JJ, Maher JW, et al: High-resolution sonography of acute appendicitis. AJR Am J Roentgenol 149:53, 1987
2. Taourel P, Baron MP, Pradel J, et al: Acute abdomen of unknown origin: impact of CT on diagnosis and management. Gastrointestinal Radiology 17:287, 1992
3. Lobbato V, Cioroiu M, LaRaja RD, et al: Peritoneal lavage as an aid to diagnosis of peritonitis in debilitated and elderly patients. Am Surg 51:508, 1985
4. Richardson JD, Flint LM, Polk HC Jr: Peritoneal lavage: a useful diagnostic adjunct for peritonitis. Surgery 94:826, 1983
5. Fink-Bennett D, Freitas JE, Ripley SD, et al: The sensitivity of hepatobiliary imaging and real-time ultrasonography in the detection of acute cholecystitis. Arch Surg 120:904, 1985
6. Navez B, d'Udekem Y, Cambier E, et al: Laparoscopy for management of nontraumatic acute abdomen. World J Surg 19:382, 1995
7. Drasar BS, Hill MJ: Human Intestinal Flora. Academic Press, London, 1974
8. Ruddell WSJ, Axon ATR, Findlay JM, et al: Effect of cimetidine on the gastric bacterial flora. Lancet 1:672, 1980
9. Stone HH, Kolb LD, Geheber CE: Incidence and significance of intraperitoneal anaerobic bacteria. Ann Surg 181:705, 1975
10. Gorbach SL, Thadepalli H, Norsen J: Anaerobic microorganisms in intraabdominal infections. Anaerobic Bacteria: Role in Disease. Balows A, DeHann RH, Dowell VR, et al, Eds. Charles C Thomas, Publisher, Springfield, Illinois, 1974, p 339
11. Lorber B, Swenson RM: The bacteriology of intra-abdominal infections. Surg Clin North Am 55:1349, 1975
12. Bohnen JMA, Solomkin JS, Dellinger EP, et al: Guidelines for clinical care: anti-infective agents for intra-abdominal infection—a Surgical Infection Society policy statement. Arch Surg 127:83, 1992
13. Nathens AB, Rotstein OD: Antimicrobial therapy for intra-abdominal infections. Am J Surg 172:1S, 1996
14. Stone HH, Bourneuf AA, Stinson LD: Reliability of criteria for predicting persistent or recurrent sepsis. Arch Surg 120:17, 1985
15. Lennard ES, Dellinger EP, Wertz MJ, et al: Implications of leukocytosis and fever at conclusion of antibiotic therapy for intra-abdominal sepsis. Ann Surg 195:19, 1982
16. Solomkin JS, Reinhart HH, Dellinger EP, et al: Results of a randomized trial comparing sequential intravenous/oral treatment with ciprofloxacin plus metronidazole to imipenem/cilastatin for intra-abdominal infections. Ann Surg 223:303, 1996
17. Nathens AB, Rotstein OD: Therapeutic options in peritonitis. Surg Clin North Am 74:677, 1994
18. Burch DM, Brock JC, Gevirtzman L, et al: The injured colon. Ann Surg 203:701, 1986
19. Stahl WM, Ivatury R: Small bowel injury. Common Problems in Trauma. Hurst JM, Ed. Year Book Medical Publishers, Chicago, 1987, p 314
20. George SM, Fabian TC, Mangiante EC: Colon trauma: further support for primary repair. Am J Surg 156:16, 1988
21. Shrock TR, Deveney CW, Dunphy JE: Factors contributing to leakage of colonic anastomoses. Ann Surg 177:513, 1973
22. Zucker KA, Flowers JL, Bailey RW, et al: Laparoscopic management of acute cholecystitis. Am J Surg 165:508, 1993
23. Rattner DW, Ferguson C, Warshaw AL: Factors associated with successful laparoscopic cholecystectomy for acute cholecystitis. Ann Surg 217:233, 1993
24. Cox MR, Wilson TG, Luck AJ, et al: Laparoscopic cholecystectomy for acute inflammation of the gallbladder. Ann Surg 218:630, 1993
25. Singer JA, McKeen RV: Laparoscopic cholecystectomy for acute or gangrenous cholecystitis. Am Surg 60:326, 1994
26. Koo KP, Thirlby RC: Laparoscopic surgery in acute cholecystitis. What is the optimal timing for surgery? Arch Surg 131:540, 1996
27. Lo CM, Liu CL, Lai EC, et al: Early versus delayed laparoscopic cholecystectomy for treatment of acute cholecystitis. Ann Surg 233:37, 1996
28. Scott-Conner CEH, Hall TJ, Anglin BL, et al: Laparoscopic appendectomy: initial experience in a teaching program. Ann Surg 215:660, 1992
29. McCahill LE, Pellegrini CA, Wiggins T, et al: A clinical outcome and cost analysis of laparoscopic versus open appendectomy. Am J Surg 171:533, 1996
30. Martin LC, Puente I, Sosa JL, et al: Open versus laparoscopic appendectomy: a prospective randomized comparison. Ann Surg 222:256, 1995
31. Tate JJ, Dawson JW, Chung SC, et al: Laparoscopic versus open appendectomy: prospective randomized trial. Lancet 342:633, 1993
32. Nathanson LK, Easter DW, Cuschierei A: Laparoscopic repair/peritoneal toilet of perforated duodenal ulcer. Surg Endosc 4:232, 1990
33. Haller JA Jr, Shaker IJ, Donahoo JS, et al: Peritoneal drainage versus non-drainage for generalized peritonitis from ruptured appendicitis in children. Ann Surg 177:595, 1973
34. Bernard HR, Cole WR: Wound infections following potentially contaminated operations. JAMA 184:290, 1963
35. Robson MC, Hegger JP: Delayed wound closures based on bacterial counts. J Surg Oncol 2:379, 1970
36. Farnell MB, Worthington-Self S, Mucha P Jr, et al: Closure of abdominal incisions with subcutaneous catheters: a prospective randomized trial. Arch Surg 121:641, 1986
37. Harken AH, Shochat SJ: Gram-positive peritonitis in children. Am J Surg 125:769, 1973
38. McDougal WS, Izant RJ Jr, Zollinger RM Jr: Primary peritonitis in infancy and childhood. Ann Surg 181:310, 1975
39. Golden GT, Shaw A: Primary peritonitis. Surg Gynecol Obstet 135:513, 1972
40. Conn HO, Fessel JM: Spontaneous bacterial peritonitis in cirrhosis: variations on a theme. Medicine (Baltimore) 50:161, 1971
41. Hoefs JC, Runyon BA: Spontaneous bacterial peritonitis. Dis Mon 31:1, 1985
42. Wyke RJ: Problems of bacterial infection in patients with liver disease. Gut 28:623, 1987
43. Akalin HE, Laleli Y, Telatar H: Bactericidal and opsonic activity of ascitic fluid from cirrhotic and noncirrhotic patients. J Infect Dis 147:1011, 1983
44. Shesol BF, Rosato EF, Rosato FE: Concomitant acute lupus erythematosus and primary pneumococcal peritonitis. Am J Gastroenterol 63:324, 1975
45. Correia JP, Conn HO: Spontaneous bacterial peritonitis in cirrhosis: endemic or epidemic? Med Clin North Am 59:963, 1975
46. Wilcox CM, Forsmark CE, Darragh TM, et al: Cytomegalovirus peritonitis in a patient with the acquired immunodeficiency syndrome. Dig Dis Sci 37:1288, 1992
47. Doberneck RC, Sterling WA Jr, Allison DC: Morbidity and mortality after operation in nonbleeding cirrhotic patients. Am J Surg 146:306, 1983
48. Runyon BA, Umland ET, Merlin T: Inoculation of blood culture bottles with ascitic fluid: improved detection of spontaneous bacterial peritonitis. Arch Intern Med 147:73, 1987
49. Runyon BA, Canawati HN, Akriviadis EA: Optimization of ascitic fluid culture technique. Gastroenterology 95:1351, 1988
50. Garcia-Tsao G, Conn HO, Lerner E: The diagnosis of bacterial peritonitis: comparison of pH, lactate concentration, and leukocyte count. Hepatology 5:91, 1985
51. Yang C-Y, Liaw Y-F, Chu C-M, et al: White count, pH and lactate in ascites in the diagnosis of spontaneous bacterial peritonitis. Hepatology 5:85, 1985
52. Hoefs JC: Diagnostic paracentesis: a potent clinical tool. Gastroenterology 98:230, 1990
53. Runyon BA, Hoefs JC: Spontaneous vs. secondary bacterial peritonitis: differentiation by response of ascitic fluid neutrophil count to antimicrobial therapy. Arch Intern Med 146:1563, 1986
54. Bhargava DK, Shriniwas, Chopra P, et al: Peritoneal tuberculosis: laparoscopic patterns and its diagnostic accuracy. Am J Gastroenterol 87:109, 1992
55. Felisart J, Rimola A, Arroyo V, et al: Cefotaxime is more effective than is ampicillin-tobramycin in cirrhotics with severe infections. Hepatology 5:457, 1985
56. Fong TL, Akriviadis EA, Runyon BA, et al: Polymorphonuclear cell count response and duration of antibiotic therapy in spontaneous bacterial peritonitis. Hepatology 9:423, 1989
57. Runyon BA, Antillon MR: Ascitic fluid pH and lactate: insensitive and nonspecific tests in detecting ascitic fluid infection. Hepatology 13:929, 1991
58. Gilbert JA, Kamath PS: Spontaneous bacterial peritonitis: an update. Mayo Clin Proc 70:365, 1995
59. Tito L, Rimola A, Llach J, et al: Recurrence of spontaneous bacterial peritonitis in cirrhosis: frequency and predictive factors. Hepatology 8:27, 1988
60. Gines P, Rimola A, Planas R, et al: Norfloxacin prevents spontaneous bacterial peritonitis recurrence in cirrhosis: results of a double-blind, placebo-controlled trial. Hepatology 12:716, 1990
61. Rolachon A, Cordier L, Bacq Y, et al: Ciprofloxacin and long term prevention of spontaneous bacterial peritonitis: results of a prospec-

tive controlled trial. Hepatology 22:1171, 1995
62. Singh N, Gayowski T, Yu VL, et al: Trimethoprim-sulfamethoxazole for the prevention of spontaneous bacterial peritonitis: a randomized trial. Ann Intern Med 122:595, 1995
63. Vas SI: Peritonitis during CAPD: a mixed bag. Perit Dial Bull 1:47, 1981
64. Bailie GR, Eisele G: Continuous ambulatory peritoneal dialysis: a review of its mechanics, advantages, complications, and areas of controversies. Ann Pharmacother 26:1409, 1992
65. Vas SI: Treatment of peritonitis. Perit Dial Int 14:S49, 1994
66. Bernardini J, Piraino B, Sorkin M: Analysis of continuous ambulatory peritoneal dialysis-related *Pseudomonas aeruginosa* infection. Am J Med 83:829, 1987
67. Paterson AD, Bishop MC, Morgan AG, et al: Removal and replacement of Tenckhoff catheter at a single operation: successful treatment of resistant peritonitis in continuous ambulatory peritoneal dialysis. Lancet 2:1245, 1986
68. Swartz R, Reynolds J, Lees P, et al: Disconnect during CAPD: retrospective experience with three different systems. Perit Dial Int 9:175, 1989
69. Low DE, Vas SI, Oreopoulos DG, et al: Prophylactic cephalexin ineffective in chronic ambulatory peritoneal dialysis (letter). Lancet 2:753, 1980
70. Luzar MA, Coles GA, Faller B, et al: *Staphylococcus aureus* nasal carriage and infection in patients on continuous ambulatory peritoneal dialysis. N Engl J Med 322:505, 1990
71. Perez-Fontan M, Garcia-Falcon T, Rosales M, et al: Treatment of *Staphylococcus aureus* nasal carriers in continuous ambulatory peritoneal dialysis with mupirocin: long-term results. Am J Kidney Dis 22:708, 1993
72. Spence PA, Mathews RE, Khanna R, et al: Indications for operation where peritonitis occurs in patients on chronic ambulatory peritoneal dialysis. Surg Gynecol Obstet 161:450, 1985
73. Altemeier WA, Culbertson WR, Shook CD: Intra-abdominal abscesses. Am J Surg 125:70, 1973
74. Levison MA, Zeigler D: Correlation of APACHE II score, drainage technique and outcome in postoperative intra-abdominal abscess. Surg Gynecol Obstet 172:89, 1991
75. Lambiase RE, Deyoe L, Cronan JJ, et al: Percutaneous drainage of 335 consecutive abscesses: results of primary drainage with 1-year follow-up. Radiology 184:167, 1992
76. Field TC, Pickleman J: Intra-abdominal abscess unassociated with prior operation. Arch Surg 120:821, 1985
77. Baker ME, Blinder RA, Rice RP: Diagnostic imaging of abdominal fluid collections and abscesses. CRC Crit Rev Diagn Imaging 25:233, 1986
78. Korobkin M, Callun PW, Filly RA, et al: Comparison of computed tomography, ultrasonography and gallium-67 scanning in the evaluation of suspected abdominal abscess. Radiology 129:89, 1978
79. Moir C, Robins RE: Role of ultrasonography, gallium scanning, and computerized tomography in the diagnosis of intraabdominal abscess. Am J Surg 143:582, 1982
80. Richardson JD, DeCamp MM, Garrison RN, et al: Pulmonary infection complicating intra-abdominal sepsis: clinical and experimental observations. Ann Surg 195:732, 1982
81. Polk HC Jr, Shields CL: Remote organ failure: a valid sign of occult intra-abdominal infection. Surgery 81:310, 1977
82. Wilmore DW, Aulick LH: Thermoregulatory responses and metabolism. Surgical Infectious Diseases. Simmons RL, Howard RJ, Eds. Appleton-Century-Crofts, East Norwalk, Connecticut, 1982, p 297
83. Moore F, Feliciano D, Andrassy R, et al: Early enteral feeding, compared with parenteral, reduces postoperative septic complications: the results of a meta-analysis. Ann Surg 216:172, 1992
84. Cerra F: Nutrient modulation of inflammatory and immune function. Am J Surg 161:230, 1991
85. Levy E, Frileux P, Cugnenc PH, et al: High-output external fistulae of the small bowel: management with continuous enteral nutrition. Br J Surg 76:676, 1989
86. Wang SMS, Wilson SE: Subphrenic abscess: the new epidemiology. Arch Surg 112:934, 1977
87. Halasz NA: Subphrenic abscesses: myths and facts. JAMA 214:724, 1970
88. Hau T, Hoffman R, Simmons RL: Mechanisms of the adjuvant effect of hemoglobin in experimental peritonitis: I. *In vivo* inhibition of peritoneal leukocytosis. Surgery 83:223, 1978
89. Steinberg B: Infections of the Peritoneum. Hoeber, New York, 1944
90. Bagby GJ, Plessala KJ, Wilson LA, et al: Divergent efficacy of antibody to tumor necrosis-alpha in intravascular and peritonitis models of sepsis. J Infect Dis 163:83, 1991
91. Astiz ME, Saha DC, Carpati CM, et al: Induction of endotoxin tolerance with monophosphoryl lipid A in peritonitis: importance of localized therapy. J Lab Clin Med 123:89, 1994
92. Holzheimer RE, Schein M, Wittmann DH: Inflammatory response in peritoneal exudate and plasma of patients undergoing planned relaparotomy for severe secondary peritonitis. Arch Surg 130:1314, 1995
93. Schein M, Wittmann DH, Holzheimer R, et al: Hypothesis: compartmentalization of cytokines in intra-abdominal infection. Surgery 119:694, 1996
94. Malaviya R, Ikeda T, Ross E, et al: Mast cell modulation of neutrophil influx and bacterial clearance at sites of infection through TNF-alpha. Nature 381:77, 1996
95. Topley N, Brown Z, Jorres A, et al: Human peritoneal mesothelial cells synthesize interleukin-8: synergistic induction by interleukin-1 beta and tumor necrosis factor-alpha. Am J Pathol 142:1876, 1993
96. West MA: Role of cytokines in leukocyte activation: phagocytic cells. Mechanisms of Leukocyte Activation: Current Topics in Membranes and Transport. Grinstein S, Rotstein OD, Eds. Academic Press, New York, 1990, p 537
97. Ford-Hutchinson AW: Leukotriene B_4 in inflammation. CRC Rev Immunol 10:1, 1990
98. Corderio RSB, Martins MA, Silva PMR: Proinflammatory activity of platelet-activating factor: pharmacological modulation and cellular involvement. Prog Biochem Pharmacol 22:156, 1988
99. Mason MJ, van Epps DE: In vivo neutrophil emigration in response to interleukin-1 and tumor necrosis factor-alpha. J Leukoc Biol 45:62, 1989
100. Dunn DL, Simmons RL: Fibrin in peritonitis: III. The mechanism of bacterial trapping by polymerizing fibrin. Surgery 92:513, 1982
101. Sinclair SB, Rotstein OD, Levy GA: Disparate mechanisms of induction of procoagulant activity by live and inactivated bacteria and viruses. Infect Immun 58:1821, 1990
102. Hau T, Payne WD, Simmons RL: Fibrinolytic activity of the peritoneum during experimental peritonitis. Surg Gynecol Obstet 148:415, 1979
103. Dunn DL, Barke RA, Ahrenholz DH, et al: The adjuvant effect of peritoneal fluid in experimental peritonitis: mechanism and clinical implications. Ann Surg 199:37, 1984
104. Ahrenholz DH, Simmons RL: Fibrin in peritonitis: I. Beneficial and adverse effects of fibrin in experimental *E. coli* peritonitis. Surgery 88:41, 1980
105. Beecher HK, Simeone FA, Burnett CH, et al: The internal state of the severely wounded man on entry to the most forward hospital. Surgery 22:672, 1947
106. Clowes GHA Jr, Vucinic M, Weidner MG: Circulatory and metabolic alterations associated with survival or death in peritonitis: clinical analysis of 25 cases. Ann Surg 163:866, 1966
107. MacLean LD, Mulligan WG, McLean APH, et al: Patterns of septic shock in man—a detailed study of 56 patients. Ann Surg 166:543, 1967
108. Tracey KJ, Beutler B, Lowry SF, et al: Shock and tissue injury induced by recombinant human cachectin. Science 234:470, 1986
109. Dinarello CA: Interleukin-1. Rev Infect Dis 6:51, 1984
110. Castell JV, Gomez-Lechon MJ, David M, et al: Interleukin-6 is a major regulator of acute phase protein synthesis in adult human hepatocytes. FEBS Lett 242:237, 1989
111. Holzheimer RG, Schein M, Wittmann DH: Inflammatory response in peritoneal exudate and plasma of patients undergoing planned relaparotomy for severe secondary peritonitis. Arch Surg 130:1314, 1995
112. Tang G-J, Kuo C-D, Yen T, et al: Perioperative plasma concentrations of tumor necrosis factor-alpha and interleukin-6 in infected patients. Crit Care Med 24:423, 1996
113. Galandiuk S, Gardner SA, Heinzelmann M: Constituent analysis may permit improved diagnosis of intra-abdominal abscess. Am J Surg 171:335, 1996
114. Rotstein OD, Pruett TL, Simmons RL: Mechanisms of microbial synergy in polymicrobial surgical infections. Rev Infect Dis 7:151, 1985
115. Berne TV, Yellin AW, Appleman MD, et al: Antibiotic management of surgically treated gangrenous or perforated appendicitis: comparison of gentamicin and clindamycin versus cefamandole versus cefoperazone. Am J Surg 144:8, 1982
116. Bartlett JG, Louie TJ, Gorbach SL, et al: Therapeutic efficacy of 29 antimicrobial regimens in experimental intraabdominal sepsis. Rev Infect Dis 3:535, 1981
117. Solomkin JS, Dellinger EP, Christou NV, et al: Results of a multicentre trial comparing imipenem/cilastatin to tobramycin/clindamycin for intra-abdominal infection. Ann Surg 212:581, 1990
118. Solomkin JS, Hemsell DL, Sweet R, et al: General guidelines for the evaluation of new anti-infective drugs for the treatment of intra-abdominal and pelvic infections. Clin Infect Dis 15:S33, 1992
119. Smith CR, Moore RD, Lietman PS: Studies of risk factors for aminoglycoside nephrotoxicity. Am J Kidney Dis 8:308, 1986
120. Niemiec PWJ, Allo MD, Miller CF: Effect of altered volume of distribution on aminoglycoside levels in patients in surgical intensive care. Arch Surg 122:207, 1987
121. Hollener LF, Bahnini J, De Manzini N, et al: A multicentric study of netilmicin once daily versus thrice daily in patients with appendicitis and other intra-abdominal infections. J Antimicrob Chemother 23:773, 1989

122. Prins JM, Buller HR, Kuijper EJ, et al: Once versus thrice daily gentamicin in patients with serious infections. Lancet 341:335, 1993
123. Gerding DN, Olson MM, Peterson LR, et al: *Clostridium difficile*-associated diarrhea and colitis in adults: a prospective case-controlled epidemiologic study. Arch Intern Med 146:95, 1986
124. Teasley DG, Gerding DN, Olson MM, et al: Prospective randomised trial of metronidazole versus vancomycin for the treatment of *Clostridium-difficile*-associated diarrhea and colitis. Lancet 2:1043, 1983
125. Christou NV, Turgeon P, Wassef R, et al: Management of intra-abdominal infection: the case for intraoperative cultures and comprehensive broad-spectrum antibiotic coverage. Arch Surg 131:1193, 1996
126. Cohn SM, Cohn KA, Rafferty MJ, et al: Enteric absorption of ciprofloxacin during the immediate postoperative period. J Antimicrob Chemother 36:717, 1995
127. Dougherty SH: Role of enterococcus in intra-abdominal sepsis. Am J Surg 148:308, 1984
128. Fry DE, Berberich S, Garrison RN: Bacterial synergism between the enterococcus and *Escherichia coli*. J Surg Res 38:475, 1985
129. Fass RJ, Scholand JF, Hodges GR, et al: Clindamycin in the treatment of serious anaerobic infections. Ann Intern Med 78:853, 1973
130. Barie PS, Christou NV, Dellinger EP, et al: Pathogenicity of the enterococcus in surgical infections. Ann Surg 212:155, 1990
131. Rotstein OD, Pruett TL, Simmons RL: Microbiologic features and treatment of persistent peritonitis in patients in the intensive care unit. Can J Surg 29:247, 1986
132. Marshall JC, Christou NV, Horn R, et al: The microbiology of multiple organ failure: the proximal gastrointestinal tract as an occult reservoir of pathogens. Arch Surg 123:309, 1988
133. Solomkin JS, Dougherty SH: The role of enterococci and *Candida* in intraabdominal infection. Topics in Intraabdominal Surgical Infection, Part 2. Simmons RL, Ed. Appleton-Century-Crofts, East Norwalk, Connecticut, 1984, p 17
134. Mosdell DM, Morris DM, Voltura A, et al: Antibiotic treatment for surgical peritonitis. Ann Surg 214:543, 1991
135. Dougherty SH, Saltzstein EC, et al: Perforated or gangrenous appendicitis treated with aminoglycosides. Arch Surg 124:1280, 1989
136. Hopkins JA, Lee JCH, Wilson SE: Susceptibility of intra-abdominal isolates at operation: a predictor of postoperative infection. Am J Surg 59:791, 1993
137. Hau T, Nishikawa R, Phangsab A: Irrigation of the peritoneal cavity and local antibiotics in the treatment of peritonitis. Surg Gynecol Obstet 156:25, 1983
138. Noon GP, Beall AC Jr, Jordon GL Jr, et al: Clinical evaluation of peritoneal irrigation with antibiotic solution. Surgery 62:73, 1967
139. Gerding DN, Hall WH, Schieri EA: Antibiotic concentrations in ascitic fluid of patients with ascites and bacterial peritonitis. Ann Intern Med 86:708, 1977
140. Sindelar WF, Mason GR: Intraperitoneal irrigation with povidone-iodine solution for presentation of intra-abdominal abscesses in the bacterially contaminated abdomen. Surg Gynecol Obstet 148:409, 1979
141. Pickard RG: Treatment of peritonitis with pre- and postoperative irrigation of the peritoneal cavity with noxythiolin solution. Br J Surg 59:642, 1972
142. Browne MK, MacKenzie M, Doyle PJ: A controlled trial of taurolin in established bacterial peritonitis. Surg Gynecol Obstet 146:721, 1978
143. Washington BC, Villalba MR, Lauter CB, et al: Cefamandole-erythromycin-heparin peritoneal irrigation: an adjunct to the surgical treatment of diffuse bacterial peritonitis. Surgery 94:576, 1983
144. Hallerback B, Andersson C, Englund N, et al: A prospective randomized study of continuous peritoneal lavage postoperatively in the treatment of purulent peritonitis. Surg Gynecol Obstet 163:433, 1986
145. Stephen M, Loewenthal J: Continuing peritoneal lavage in high-risk peritonitis. Surgery 85:603, 1979
146. Wittmann DH, Aprahamian C, Bergstein JM, et al: A burr-like device to facilitate temporary abdominal closure in planned multiple laparotomies. Eur J Surg 159:75, 1993
147. Bleichrodt RP, Simmermacher RKJ, van der Lei B, et al: Expanded polytetrafluoroethylene patch versus polypropylene mesh for the repair of contaminated defects of the abdominal wall. Surg Gynecol Obstet 176:18, 1993
148. Walsh GL, Chiasson P, Hedderich G, et al: The open abdomen: the Marlex mesh and zipper technique: a method of managing intraperitoneal infection. Surg Clin North Am 68:25, 1988
149. Garcia-Sabrido JL, Tallado JM, Christou NV, et al: Treatment of severe intra-abdominal sepsis and/or necrotic foci by an "open-abdomen" approach: zipper and zipper-mesh techniques. Arch Surg 123:152, 1988
150. Hau T, Ohmann C, Wolmershauser A, et al: Planned relaparotomy vs relaparotomy on demand in the treatment of intra-abdominal infections. Arch Surg 130:1193, 1995
151. Schein M, Hirshberg A, Hashmonai M: Current surgical management of severe intra-abdominal infection. Surgery 112:489, 1992
152. Solomkin JS, Meakins JL Jr, Allo MD, et al: Antibiotic trials in intraabdominal infections: a critical evaluation of study design and outcome reporting. Ann Surg 200:29, 1984
153. Fry DE, Garrison RN, Heitsch RC, et al: Determinants of death in patients with intraabdominal abscess. Surgery 88:517, 1980
154. Dellinger EP, Wertz MJ, Meakins JL, et al: Surgical infection stratification system for intra-abdominal infection: multicenter trial. Arch Surg 120:21, 1985
155. Bohnen J, Boulanger M, Meakins JL, et al: Prognosis in generalized peritonitis: relation to cause and risk factors. Arch Surg 118:285, 1983
156. Christou NV: Predicting septic related mortality of the individual surgical patient based on admission host-defence measurements. Can J Surg 29:424, 1986
157. Bohnen JMA, Mustard RA, Oxholm SE, et al: APACHE II score and abdominal sepsis: a prospective study. Arch Surg 123:225, 1988
158. Knaus WA, Draper EA, Wagner DP, et al: APACHE II: a severity of disease classification system. Crit Care Med 13:818, 1985
159. Christou NV, Barie PS, Dellinger EP, et al: Surgical Infection Society Intra-abdominal Infection Study: prospective evaluation of management techniques and outcome. Arch Surg 128:193, 1993
160. Cerra FB, Negro F, Abrams J: APACHE II score does not predict multiple organ failure or mortality in postoperative surgical patients. Arch Surg 125:519, 1990
161. Poenaru D, Christou NV: Clinical outcome of seriously ill surgical patients with intra-abdominal infection depends on both physiologic (APACHE II score) and immunologic (DTH score) alterations. Ann Surg 213:130, 1991
162. Nathens AB, Rotstein OD, Marshall JC: Tertiary peritonitis: clinical features of a complex nosocomial infection. Crit Care Med 21(suppl):S129, 1993
163. Sawyer RG, Rosenlof LK, Adams RB, et al: Peritonitis into the 1990's: changing pathogens and changing strategies in the critically ill. Am Surg 58:82, 1992
164. Norwood SN, Civetta JM: Abdominal CT scanning in critically ill surgical patients. Ann Surg 202:166, 1985
165. Nel CJC, Pretorius DJ, DeVaal JB: Re-operation of suspected intra-abdominal sepsis in the critically ill patient. S Afr J Surg 24:60, 1986
166. Wells CL, Maddaus MA, Simmons RL: Proposed mechanisms for the translocation of intestinal bacteria. Rev Infect Dis 10:958, 1988
167. Bendahan J, Coetzee CJ, Papagianopoulos C, et al: Abdominal compartment syndrome. J Trauma 38:152, 1995
168. Schein M, Wittmann DH, Aprahamian CC, et al: The abdominal compartment syndrome: the physiologic and clinical consequences of elevated intra-abdominal pressure. J Am Coll Surg 180:745, 1995
169. Cullen DJ, Coyle JP, Teplick R, et al: Cardiovascular, pulmonary, and renal effects of massively increased intra-abdominal pressure in critically ill patients. Crit Care Med 17:118, 1989
170. Taylor KJW, Wasson JFM, De Graaff C, et al: Accuracy of grey-scale ultrasound diagnosis of abdominal and pelvic abscesses in 220 patients. Lancet 1:83, 1978
171. van Sonnenberg E, D'Agostino HB, Casola G, et al: US-guided transvaginal drainage of pelvic abscesses and fluid collections. Radiology 181:53, 1991
172. Bennett JD, Kozak RI, Taylor BM, et al: Deep pelvic abscesses: transrectal drainage with radiologic guidance. Radiology 185:825, 1992
173. Saini S, Kellum JM, O'Leary MP, et al: Improved localization and survival in patients with intraabdominal abscesses. Am J Surg 145:136, 1983
174. Hoffer P: Gallium mechanisms. J Nucl Med 21:282, 1980
175. Dutcher JP, Schiffer CA, Johnston GS: Rapid migration of 111-indium-labelled granulocytes to sites of infection. N Engl J Med 304:586, 1981
176. Knochel JQ, Koehler PR, Lee TG, et al: Diagnosis of abdominal abscesses with computed tomography, ultrasound and 111-In leukocyte scans. Radiology 137:425, 1980
177. Wall SD, Fisher MR, Amparo EG, et al: Magnetic resonance imaging in the evaluation of abscesses. Am J Radiol 144:1217, 1985
178. Gerzof SG, Robbins AH, Johnson WC, et al: Percutaneous catheter drainage of abdominal abscesses: a five year experience. N Engl J Med 305:653, 1981
179. Haaga JR, Weinstein AJ: CT-guided percutaneous aspiration and drainage of abscesses. AJR Am J Roentgenol 135:1187, 1980
180. Gerzof SG, Johnson WC, Robbins AH, et al: Expanded criteria for percutaneous abscess drainage. Arch Surg 120:227, 1985
181. Mueller PR, Ferrucci JT Jr, Simeone JF, et al: Lesser sac abscesses and fluid collections: drainage by transhepatic approach. Radiology 155:615, 1985
182. Pruett TL, Rotstein OD, Crass J, et al:

Percutaneous aspiration and drainage for suspected abdominal infection. Surgery 96:731, 1984

183. Johnson WC, Gerzof SG, Robbins AH, et al: Treatment of abdominal abscesses: comparative evaluation of operative versus percutaneous catheter drainage guided by computed tomography or ultrasound. Ann Surg 194:510, 1981

184. Olak J, Christou NV, Stein LA, et al: Operative vs percutaneous drainage of intraabdominal abscesses: comparison of morbidity and mortality. Arch Surg 121:141, 1986

Acknowledgments

This work was supported by the Medical Research Council of Canada and the Physicians' Services Incorporated Foundation. The author wishes to thank Christina Wareham for preparation of the manuscript.

83 INFECTIONS IN THE UPPER ABDOMEN: BILIARY TRACT, PANCREAS, LIVER, AND SPLEEN

Jeffrey S. Barkun, M.D., and Ronald T. Lewis, M.B.B.S., M.Sc.

Approach to the Patient with Upper Abdominal Sepsis

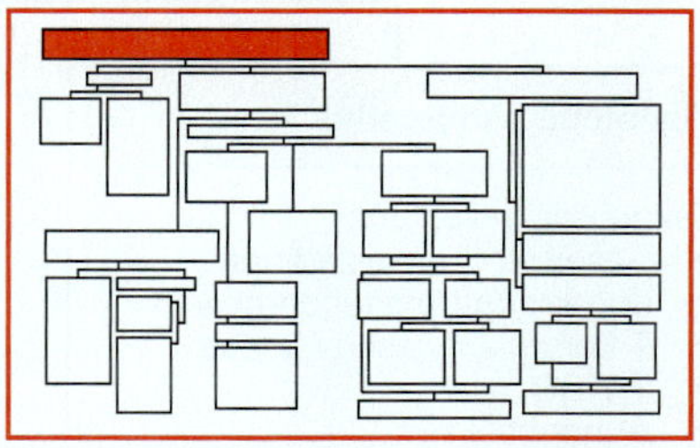

Biliary tract and pancreatic infection present as systemic sepsis or as infection localized in the upper abdomen. Typical findings include abdominal pain, a tender upper abdominal mass, fever and leukocytosis, and jaundice. Various combinations of these symptoms may occur, but it is convenient to consider three common clinical presentations; in each of these, one or two symptoms dominate: (1) upper abdominal pain and fever, (2) fever and jaundice, and (3) an upper abdominal mass and fever. These clinical findings signal the need for a battery of screening tests, which include a complete blood count; routine blood tests of liver function; determination of serum amylase level, prothrombin time, and partial thromboplastin time; blood culture; chest and abdominal x-rays; and an abdominal ultrasound examination. When considered together, the clinical findings and test results allow early differentiation of the three most common disease entities: acute cholecystitis, acute cholangitis, and acute pancreatitis.

Upper Abdominal Pain and Fever

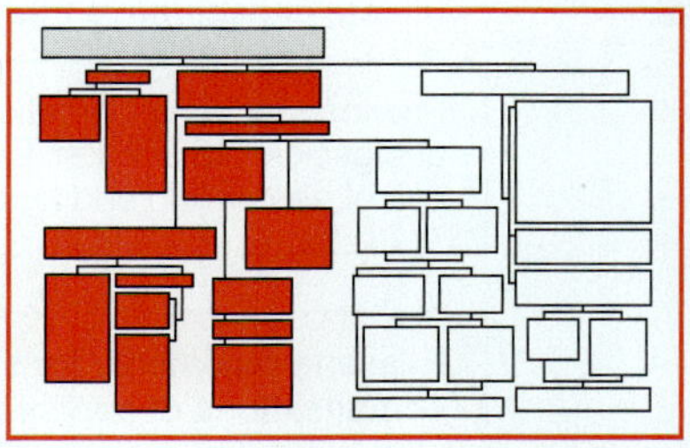

DIAGNOSIS

The patient with upper abdominal sepsis may present with epigastric or right upper quadrant pain and fever. Only two thirds of these patients admitted with a working diagnosis of acute cholecystitis have acute biliary inflammation.[1] In some patients, nonsurgical conditions such as pneumonia, acute hepatitis, familial Mediterranean fever, herpes zoster of intercostal nerves, and gastrointestinal disease can be distinguished clinically from biliary disease. The most important screening test for acute biliary infection is the abdominal ultrasound examination: an abnormal image of the gallbladder or bile ducts supports a biliary etiology [*see Figure 1*].

Diagnosis should include differentiation of acute cholecystitis, biliary colic, acute pancreatitis, and acute cholangitis because each of these entities requires specific management [*see Table 1*]. For example, the initial management of biliary colic and mild acute pancreatitis is usually nonoperative, whereas severe acute cholangitis and acute cholecystitis require surgical, endoscopic, or radiologic intervention (see below). The clinical features and blood test results are helpful but may be inconclusive. The abdominal ultrasonogram may provide specific clues. Stones appear in biliary colic [*see Figure 1*]; stones and thickening of the gallbladder wall, in acute cholecystitis; gallstones and dilatation of the common bile duct, in acute cholangitis; and pancreatic enlargement and sonolucency, in pancreatitis. A radionuclide excretion scan using technetium-99m–labeled HIDA differentiates acute cholecystitis from acute biliary colic if the common bile duct, but not the gallbladder, is visualized up to 4 hours after injection of the isotope.[2]

Differentiating acute pancreatitis from acute cholecystitis may be difficult. The serum amylase level lacks specificity,[3] but if the clinical

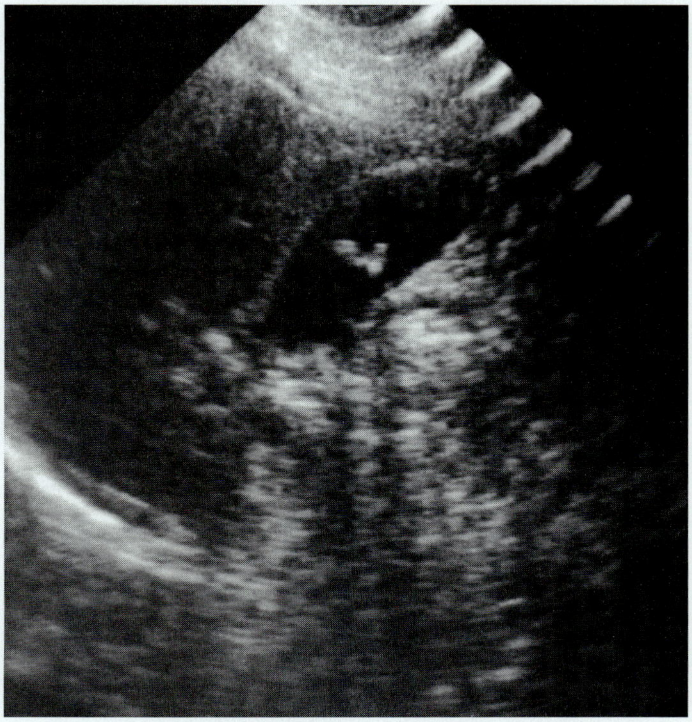

Figure 1 Abnormal abdominal ultrasound examination shows calculi in the gallbladder casting shadows on the underlying liver tissue.

Patient presents with one or more of the following: upper abdominal pain, fever, jaundice, upper abdominal mass

Order screening tests:
- Blood tests (CBC, liver function, serum amylase, PT, PTT, culture)
- Chest and abdominal x-rays
- Abdominal ultrasonography

Normal ultrasound image

No biliary tract disease
Consider acute MI, pleuritis, pneumonia, acute hepatitis, herpes zoster, or peptic ulcer. Provide appropriate care.

Nongallstone pancreatitis
Diagnosis supported by clinical findings, ↑ serum amylase, and normal HIDA scan.
Provide supportive care (e.g., I.V. fluids, narcotic analgesics, NG suction).
Evaluate repeatedly with CT scan for septic complications of pancreatitis.
Repeat ultrasonography to verify absence of gallstones.

Abnormal ultrasound image located in biliary tract (e.g., stones; distended, thick-walled, or shrunken gallbladder; distended common bile duct)

Perform HIDA scan when feasible if diagnosis is unclear.

Gallbladder is visualized on HIDA scan, or results are equivocal

Gallstone pancreatitis
Diagnostic indicators:
- Absence of localized right upper quadrant tenderness
- ↑ Serum amylase or lipase
- ↑ WBC
- Abnormal LFTs

Biliary colic
Diagnostic indicators:
- Stones in gallbladder
- WBC often normal
- LFTs occasionally abnormal

Treatment:
- Provide analgesics and fat-free diet
- Perform elective laparoscopic cholecystectomy

Initiate conservative treatment
Provide I.V. fluids, narcotic analgesics, NG suction. Consider use of gentamicin and ampicillin.

Evaluate repeatedly for septic complications of pancreatitis

Consider Ranson's signs in timing of operation

< 3 Ranson's signs: Perform cholecystectomy if pancreatitis is not settling or when settled.

≥ 3 Ranson's signs: If pancreatitis is not settling, perform ERCP and sphincterotomy. When pancreatitis settles, perform cholecystectomy.

Gallbladder is not visualized on HIDA scan
Diagnose acute cholecystitis, with right upper quadrant tenderness, abnormal LFTs, ? ↑ WBC, ? stones or gas in gallbladder.

Acute cholecystitis at high risk for perforation
Diagnostic indicators:
- Systemic toxicity
- Emphysematous cholecystitis
- Acalculous cholecystitis

Treatment:
- Give gentamicin and ampicillin or a single agent (e.g., piperacillin, ceftriaxone, or ciprofloxacin) for ≥ 5 days
- Perform urgent cholecystectomy
- Consider cholecystostomy

Ordinary acute cholecystitis

Good operative risk
Perform elective cholecystectomy. Give cefazolin on call.

Poor operative risk
Give gentamicin and ampicillin or a single agent (e.g., piperacillin, ceftriaxone, or ciprofloxacin) for ≥ 5 days. If antibiotics fail, perform percutaneous transhepatic cholecystostomy oroperation.

Approach to the Patient with Upper Abdominal Sepsis

Ultrasonography identifies mass not associated with biliary tree

Evaluate screening tests for WBC > 12,000/mm³, positive blood culture, and abnormal liver function

---

Liver mass

Perform serologic tests for *Entamoeba histolytica* and *Echinococcus*. Evaluate for history of travel to endemic areas. Perform GI evaluation.
Treat underlying cause:
- **Amebic abscess:** Give metronidazole for 10 days.
- **Echinococcal cyst with secondary infection:** Give gentamicin and ampicillin or single agent (e.g., ciprofloxacin). Perform definitive operation.
- **Pyogenic abscess:** Give gentamicin and metronidazole or single agent (e.g., imipenem or ticarcillin-clavulanate). Perform abdominal CT, followed by ERCP or PTC. Perform CT- or ultrasound-guided continuous percutaneous drainage or operative drainage.
- **Abscess secondary to inflammatory bowel disease:** Give gentamicin and metronidazole or single agent (e.g., imipenem or ticarcillin-clavulanate). Perform definitive operation, and drain abscess.
- **Cryptogenic abscess:** Give gentamicin and metronidazole or single agent (e.g., imipenem or ticarcillin-clavulanate). Perform continuous CT-guided closed drainage.

Splenic hypoechoic mass

Confirm splenic abscess via contrast-enhanced abdominal CT scan. Give gentamicin and cloxacillin. Perform percutaneous catheter drainage; consider splenectomy.

Pancreatic mass

Give imipenem.
Differentiate pancreatic abscess and pseudocyst from phlegmon via Ranson's signs and CT findings.

- **< 3 Ranson's signs and category A or B on CT:** Diagnose phlegmon; attempt nonoperative management first.
- **≥ 3 Ranson's signs and category C, D, or E on CT:** Suspect pancreatic abscess or infected pseudocyst. Confirm suspicion of abscess with fine-needle aspirate yielding pus cells and bacteria.

Perform urgent surgical debridement and sump drainage. Alternatively, consider open drainage or marsupialization. Perform ancillary procedures as indicated.

Acute cholangitis

Diagnostic indicators:
- Dilated biliary ducts on ultrasound
- Positive blood cultures
- Leukocytosis
- T° > 38.5° C
- Jaundice
- Abnormal LFTs

Biliary tract has undergone manipulation: Provide broad-spectrum antibiotic coverage (e.g., with imipenem or ticarcillin-clavulanate).

Biliary tract has not undergone manipulation: Give gentamicin and ampicillin. Alternatively, give a single agent (e.g., piperacillin, ceftriaxone, or ciprofloxacin).

Therapy is successful: Continue antibiotics for > 5 days. Perform abdominal CT scan, followed by ERCP or PTC. Perform definitive operation later.

Patient has serum bilirubin > 3 mg/dl, low BP, mental confusion, T° > 39.5° C: Perform emergency biliary decompression.

Previous cholecystectomy:
- Distal obstruction (dilated intrahepatic and extrahepatic biliary ducts on ultrasound): Perform ERCP and sphincterotomy.
- Proximal obstruction (dilated intrahepatic ducts): Perform PTC and PTBD.

No previous cholecystectomy:
- High operative risk: Evaluate via ERCP or PTC; perform endoscopic sphincterotomy or PTBD.
- Low operative risk: Perform urgent biliary exploration and appropriate drainage procedure.

Patients with cholangitis who remain in a septic state after biliary decompression should be evaluated for pyogenic liver abscess

Table 1 Diagnostic Indicators of
Upper Abdominal Pain and Fever

	Biliary Colic	Acute Cholecystitis	Acute Pancreatitis
Duration	Short: 40% < 1 hr	Persistent	Persistent
Pathogenesis	Visceral	Somatic	Retroperitoneal
Signs	Tender	Guarding and spasm	Guarding and spasm
Laboratory tests			
Liver function tests	Occasionally abnormal	Abnormal	Abnormal
Serum amylase	Normal	Normal or slightly increased	Increased
Leukocyte counts	Often normal	Increased	Increased

findings suggest acute pancreatitis, an elevated level of serum amylase clinches the diagnosis. In one study, the initial laboratory results in 100 patients with acute pancreatitis were compared with those in 100 patients with acute abdominal pain caused by acute cholecystitis, perforated peptic ulcer, or acute appendicitis.[4] The serum amylase concentrations were elevated in 95% of patients with acute pancreatitis but were normal in 95% of patients with acute abdominal pain of other causes. These concentrations peak within the first 48 hours and are almost always elevated in biliary pancreatitis[5]; in fact, a serum amylase concentration above 1,000 U/L strongly suggests a diagnosis of biliary pancreatitis.[6] Unless clinical findings and the results of biochemical tests and ultrasound are unequivocal, a contrast-enhanced spiral abdominal CT scan should be performed for establishment of the diagnosis and staging of acute pancreatitis. It has been suggested, however, that CT scanning should be reserved for patients with clinically suspected severe acute gallstone pancreatitis, on the grounds that the results would not change the recommended course of action in other patients.[7] Occasionally, a very mild pancreatitis may give rise to no findings on a CT scan, and the demonstration of a normal ^{99m}Tc-labeled HIDA scan may be helpful in differentiating this condition from acute cholecystitis.

Concurrent acute obstructive cholangitis must be considered in all patients with acute cholecystitis. Risk factors for acute cholangitis include advanced age, hypotension, a high serum bilirubin level, and a positive blood culture. Diagnostic indicators include a positive test for bilirubin in the urine, increased levels of the direct serum bilirubin, and increased alkaline phosphatase determinations. Positive blood cultures and a finding of dilated biliary ducts on the abdominal ultrasound examination usually confirm the diagnosis.

TREATMENT

Gallstone Pancreatitis

Standard therapy for gallstone pancreatitis includes intravenous fluids and narcotic analgesics. Nasogastric suction is useful in patients with severe pain or significant ileus but should not be used routinely.[8] The use of systemic antibiotics is controversial (see below); they are of benefit in the 10% to 34% of patients who have concomitant cholangitis.[9] Other treatments suggested previously have not proved useful when given in all cases of gallstone pancreatitis. These treatments include total parenteral nutrition and many pharmacologic agents, such as cimetidine, somatostatin, glucagon, and insulin.[10] Although continuous intraduodenal infusion of an elemental diet reduces exocrine pancreatic secretions in animal experiments,[11] enteral feeding is usually avoided in clinical treatment because premature feeding may cause a relapse of pancreatitis.[12]

In clinical practice, the need for further treatment depends on the severity of pancreatitis. The severity of the episode determines both the patient's risk of developing sepsis, which governs outcome, and the risk associated with early cholecystectomy [see 51 *Biliary Tract Procedures* and 52 *Laparoscopic Cholecystectomy*]. The clinical prognostic index developed by Ranson best defines the severity of pancreatitis [see Table 2]. In mild pancreatitis, one or two Ranson signs are present; in more severe pancreatitis, three to five signs are present; and in very severe pancreatitis, more than five signs are present. This distinction serves to stratify further treatment.

Mild pancreatitis usually subsides within 1 week of onset. Most surgeons defer cholecystectomy until then.[13] Urgent operation within 72 hours of admission may reveal acute cholecystitis in as many as 31% of patients.[14] It has also been suggested that urgent surgical decompression may prevent a relatively mild attack of pancreatitis from progressing to a lethal form.[15,16] An attack of acute gallstone pancreatitis is initiated by obstruction at the confluence of the lower end of the common bile duct and the pancreatic duct by a stone or by edema at the ampulla of Vater resulting from stone migration. These stones may be found and removed in 63% to 78% of patients who undergo operation within 72 hours of admission[14,15,17]; by contrast, they are present in only 3% to 33% of patients explored after the first week.[15,17-20] A randomized trial of the timing of surgery for gallstone pancreatitis showed that early surgery (within 48 hours after admission) was not associated with a significant increase in morbidity or mortality in patients with mild pancreatitis but did not change prognosis.[13]

Some surgeons have suggested that early endoscopic retrograde cholangiopancreatography (ERCP) and sphincterotomy [see 47 *Gastrointestinal Endoscopy*] is an alternative to surgery of the common bile duct in patients with mild pancreatitis.[21] However, randomized trials comparing endoscopic treatment with conservative treatment within the first 72 hours in patients with mild pancreatitis did not find that urgent endoscopic sphincterotomy improved outcome in this group of patients.[22,23] Other studies[24,25] found that delaying surgery beyond 6 weeks may lead to a 32% to 57% risk of recurrent pancreatitis. Therefore, cholecystectomy and cholangiography should be delayed only until just before patients are discharged from the hospital 5 to 15 days after the onset of symptoms. Laparoscopic cholecystectomy has facilitated this approach without prolonging hospital stay.

Severe pancreatitis Patients with three or more Ranson signs are at particular risk for pancreatic sepsis.[12] Repeated clinical and ra-

Table 2 Ranson's Early Objective Signs
of Severity of Acute Pancreatitis[4]

On Admission	After Initial 48 Hours
Age > 55 yr	Serum Ca^{2+} < 8 mg/dl
Glucose > 200 mg/dl	Arterial Po_2 < 60 mm Hg
WBC > 16,000/mm³	Base deficit > 4 mEq/L
LDH > 350 IU/L	BUN increase > 5 mg/dl
AST > 250 Sigma Frankel U/dl	Hematocrit fall > 10%
	Fluid sequestration > 6,000 ml

Note: < 3 signs = mild pancreatitis; ≥ 3 signs = severe pancreatitis.
AST—aspartate aminotransferase BUN—blood urea nitrogen Po_2—oxygen tension
WBC—white blood cell

diologic evaluation is required in these patients to ensure early detection of complications, because the outcome of an episode of pancreatitis depends on whether sepsis supervenes. When infection occurs, operative debridement and drainage are required [see Fever and Abdominal Mass, below]. Some surgeons have attempted to alter the course of severe disease by early operation. However, urgent operation is associated with a high mortality in patients with more than three Ranson signs.[13,17,19,26] To avoid the mortality associated with early operative intervention, some clinicians advocate early diagnosis by ERCP [see Figure 2] followed by biliary decompression by means of endoscopic sphincterotomy and stone extraction.[21] In a randomized trial comparing early ERCP and sphincterotomy to conservative therapy in patients with severe acute pancreatitis, ERCP and sphincterotomy decreased morbidity from 61% to 24% and lowered mortality from 18% to 4%.[22] The results of this trial, however, have been the subject of debate, and the success of this approach has been attributed by some authors to the treatment of a concomitant cholangitis rather than of the actual pancreatitis.[23] A well-conducted trial that excluded patients with concomitant cholangitis was published in 1997; unfortunately, this trial was unable to answer the question definitively, because too few patients with severe pancreatitis had been recruited.[27] Some authors have also argued that ERCP may also show pancreatic ductal disruption in some patients, and endoscopic placement of a pancreatic ductal stent may help reduce morbidity.[28]

Use of peritoneal lavage in early severe pancreatitis was advocated in one study[29] to decrease morbidity and mortality. Use of standard lavage over a 2-day period did not improve patient outcome, but use of peritoneal lavage for 7 days (long peritoneal lavage) provided some improvement in outcome.[30] Early use of antibiotics and selective decontamination have been proposed as means of reducing septic complications, but neither has convincingly or reproducibly been shown to improve prognosis.[31,32] More recently, investigators have made renewed attempts to modulate the initial systemic inflammatory response seen in early severe acute pancreatitis in such a way as to reduce the risk of subsequent infection and improve overall prognosis. Somatostatin has exhibited limited success in this regard,[33,34] but early reports on the use of lexipafant, an inhibitor of platelet-aggregating factor, have yielded promising results.[35]

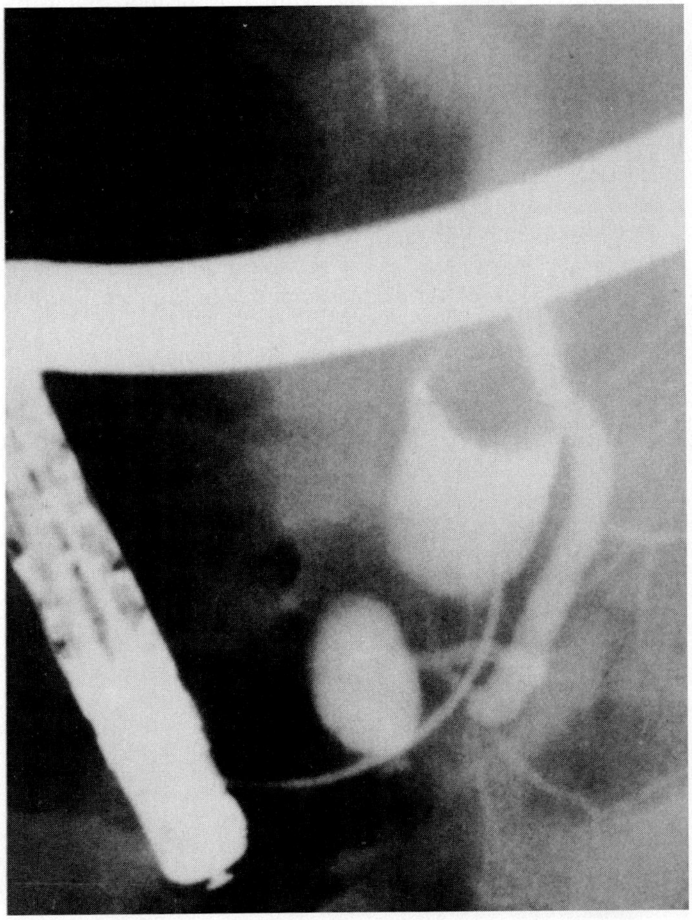

Acute Cholecystitis

The standard treatment of acute cholecystitis consists of intravenous fluid administration, analgesics, and cholecystectomy. Although the timing of operation is somewhat controversial in ordinary acute cholecystitis,[36] cholecystectomy should be performed at the earliest opportunity [see 51 Biliary Tract Procedures and 52 Laparoscopic Cholecystectomy]. This approach has been confirmed by a randomized trial comparing early to late laparoscopic cholecystectomy.[37] The delayed-surgery group demonstrated a greater need for conversion to open cholecystectomy (23% versus 11%) as well as a longer total hospital stay and convalescence. The administration of systemic antibiotics is not required; however, single-dose antibiotic prophylaxis, such as cefazolin, 2 g I.V., can be given at the start of operation to prevent postoperative wound infection and intra-abdominal infection.[38]

Some patients with acute cholecystitis are at high risk for gangrene and perforation of the gallbladder. It is crucial to identify these patients and perform cholecystectomy promptly because delay increases morbidity and mortality. The three risk factors for gangrene and perforation of the gallbladder in patients with acute cholecystitis are marked systemic toxicity, emphysematous cholecystitis, and acute acalculous cholecystitis.

In ordinary acute cholecystitis, body temperature averages 37.8°C (100.04°F) but is normal in 20% of patients.[39] By comparison, the risk of gangrene and perforation is reportedly higher in patients with marked systemic toxicity, which is manifested by a pulse rate greater than 120 beats/min, body temperature above 39°C (102.2°F), and a shift to the left of the differential white blood cell count, showing more than 90% polymorphonuclear leukocytes.[40] Unfortunately, findings of systemic toxicity are frequently absent in elderly patients.

Emphysematous cholecystitis is an uncommon and insidious variant of acute cholecystitis; it is characterized by gas in the gallbladder lumen, wall, or pericholecystic soft tissue and biliary ducts secondary to gas-forming bacteria. The key to diagnosis is the evidence of air on abdominal x-ray[41] [see Figure 3] or ultrasound examination. Three stages of emphysematous cholecystitis have been defined: (1) gas is seen only in the lumen of the gallbladder, (2) a ring of gas is identified in the wall of the gallbladder, and (3) gas is seen in the tissues adjacent to the wall.[42] Compared with ordinary acute cholecystitis, emphysematous cholecystitis is associated with a fivefold increase in the risk of gallbladder perforation as well as a 10-fold increase in mortality in patients younger than 60 years [see Table 3].[43]

Studies from the 1960s noted an increased risk of gangrene and perforation of the acutely inflamed gallbladder in patients with diabetes mellitus.[44,45] The mortality for acute cholecystitis was shown to be five to 10 times higher in patients with diabetes than in other patients. Later studies, however, did not show an increased mortality in patients with both diabetes and acute cholecystitis.[46,47] Nevertheless, one third of patients with emphysematous cholecystitis also have diabetes. This factor plus the current tendency to perform chole-

Figure 2 Endoscopic retrograde cholangiopancreatography shows distal common bile duct stone in acute pancreatitis. The papillotome has been placed through the sphincter of Oddi in preparation for endoscopic sphincterotomy.

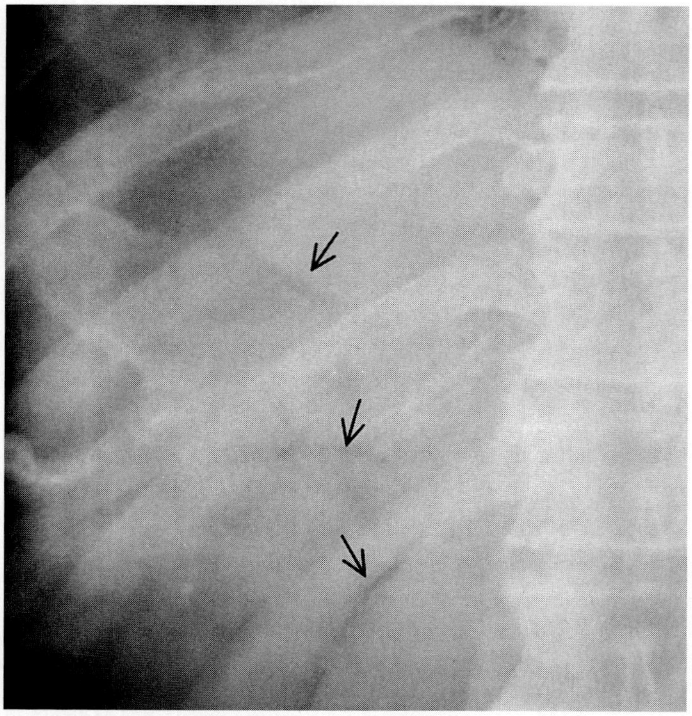

Figure 3 Air outlines the gallbladder and bile ducts in emphysematous cholecystitis.

Table 3 Comparison of Acute Cholecystitis and Emphysematous Cholecystitis

	Emphysematous Cholecystitis	Acute Cholecystitis
Gender	70% male	70% female
Stones	70%	90%
Bile culture positive	95%	66%
Clostridia found	46%	1.2%
Gangrenous gallbladder	75%	2.5%
Perforation of gallbladder	20%	4%
Mortality at age < 60 yr	15%	1.5%
Pathogenesis	Ischemia, obstruction	Obstruction

cystectomy early in most patients with acute cholecystitis may account for the disparity between previous studies and current reports.

Acute acalculous cholecystitis is another rare variant of acute cholecystitis, although its frequency has increased from the 1950s through the 1990s.[48] This disease was originally described as occurring after surgical treatment of unrelated disease[49]; however, it has since been identified in patients with multiple trauma,[50] prolonged critical illness,[51] and sepsis.[52] Predisposing factors include gallbladder ischemia (in patients with shock or trauma) and biliary stasis (in prolonged fasting, hyperalimentation, and sustained narcotics therapy). In addition, focal inflammation may cause biliary colonization[51] or may activate coagulation factor XII, thereby causing severe injury to the blood vessels in the gallbladder muscularis and serosa.[48] A high index of suspicion is necessary. Acute acalculous cholecystitis should be considered in any postoperative or acutely ill patient with upper abdominal pain and fever or with unexplained fever and leukocytosis. It is particularly common 2 to 4 weeks after injury. The diagnosis is confirmed by findings on abdominal ultrasound examination [see Figure 4][53] and 99mTc–labeled HIDA scanning coupled with infusion of cholecystokinin and morphine.[54-56]

Patients with acute cholecystitis who demonstrate systemic toxicity, emphysematous cholecystitis, or acalculous cholecystitis are at high risk for gallbladder gangrene and perforation and therefore require prompt and aggressive treatment. Intravenous antibiotic therapy with agents such as gentamicin, 1.5 mg/kg every 8 hours, and ampicillin, 1 g every 6 hours, should be given for a period of at least 5 days. In patients exhibiting renal failure, a single agent, such as ceftriaxone, piperacillin, or a quinolone (e.g., ciprofloxacin or ofloxacin) can be used.[57,58] Early cholecystectomy is the treatment of choice.

If perforation and gangrene are not suspected but medical illness poses a high risk of mortality from operation, nonoperative supportive therapy may suffice. If this fails, another treatment option is cholecystostomy. Unfortunately, mortality may be as high as 20% to 30% with the traditional surgical approach.[59] Percutaneous transhepatic cholecystostomy has therefore been recommended for these high-risk patients,[60] particularly for those at low risk for perforation of the gallbladder.[61] To determine the risk of gallbladder perforation, a risk score can be assigned to each of seven findings that may be present on the preoperative abdominal ultrasound examination: pericholecystic fluid, 7 points; distention of the gallbladder, 4 points; intraluminal membrane, 4 points; intraluminal debris, 3 points; round gallbladder, 3 points; sonolucent zone in the gallbladder wall, 2 points; and a thick gallbladder wall (> 3.5 mm), 1 point.[61] A patient with a total risk score of 12 or more points requires urgent cholecystectomy; one with a lower score who does not respond to conservative treatment may be treated with percutaneous transhepatic cholecystostomy. A 1997 review of 59 patients exhibiting the septic response who underwent successful percutaneous radiologic cholecystostomy defined predictors of a successful clinical outcome: localized right upper quadrant tenderness and gallstones, as well as gallstones and pericholecystic fluid on ultrasound examination.[62] Patients with more equivocal findings may derive greater benefit from more invasive techniques that can simultaneously be used for diagnostic purposes (e.g., laparoscopy, which can even be performed at the ICU bedside[63]).

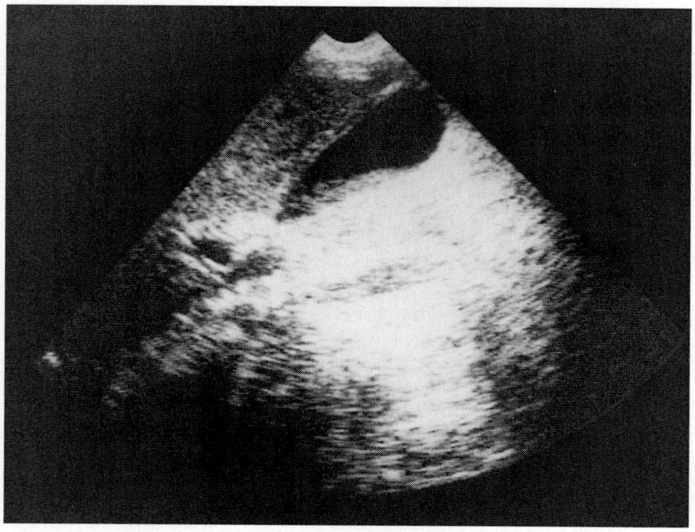

Figure 4 Abnormal abdominal ultrasound examination confirms diagnosis of acute acalculous cholecystitis. When this image is compared with that in Figure 1, the thickening of the gallbladder wall and intraluminal debris are obvious.

A few patients with acute cholecystitis will have concurrent acute cholangitis. Cholecystostomy is contraindicated in these patients because of its high mortality.[64] Adequate drainage of the common bile duct is required [see Fever and Jaundice, below].

Fever and Jaundice

DIAGNOSIS

If a patient presents with a temperature greater than 38.5°C (101.3°F) and jaundice [see 16 Jaundice], the possibility of acute cholangitis should be investigated. If cholangitis is present, laboratory studies will reveal leukocytosis, and blood cultures will often be positive. A finding of gallstones and dilated biliary ducts on abdominal ultrasound examination supports the diagnosis. Reynolds' pentad is present in the full-blown syndrome.[65] This syndrome includes upper abdominal pain, fever and chills, jaundice, hypotension, and mental confusion.

Most of the findings associated with acute cholangitis are mimicked in empyema of the gallbladder.[66] In this condition, acute cholecystitis is complicated by suppuration within the gallbladder, which then becomes the focus of generalized sepsis. The distended gallbladder may be palpable and tender. When jaundice is present in empyema of the gallbladder, it is less likely to be obstructive than jaundice in acute cholangitis. True empyema of the gallbladder is rare. A positive ^{99m}Tc–labeled HIDA scan clinches the diagnosis. Treatment includes administration of intravenous fluids, systemic antibiotic therapy, analgesics, and early cholecystectomy.

Acute cholecystitis is occasionally manifest as an acute nonobstructive cholangitis; in this condition, systemic toxicity and low-grade obstructive jaundice are caused by a diffuse intrahepatic process transported from the acutely inflamed gallbladder to the liver through the lymphatics.[67] In some patients, the inflammatory process extends to involve the common bile duct and is most pronounced in the region of the ampulla. The obstructive edema in this area accounts for a transient mild elevation of the serum bilirubin concentration to approximately 3 mg/dl and for an increase in the serum alkaline phosphatase level to the upper limit of normal. These patients are not usually sufficiently ill to warrant immediate exploration. The ^{99m}Tc–labeled HIDA scan confirms acute cholecystitis, and blood cultures are negative. These patients are treated for acute cholecystitis.

In some patients with jaundice and inflammation, a stone impacted in the cystic duct or Hartmann's pouch of the gallbladder may suggest choledocholithiasis, but preoperative diagnosis by ERCP shows an extrinsic compression of the duct known as Mirizzi's syndrome. Two types of Mirizzi's syndrome exist. In type I Mirizzi's syndrome, a stone impacted in the cystic duct or Hartmann's pouch compresses the common hepatic duct and causes inflammation, thereby leading to jaundice. Treatment of type I Mirizzi's syndrome consists of obliteration of the cystic duct and careful partial cholecystectomy, with the neck of the gallbladder left in place. In type II Mirizzi's syndrome, protrusion of the stone into the hepatic duct erodes the septum between the cystic duct and the hepatic duct and causes a cholecystocholedochal fistula. Treatment of type II Mirizzi's syndrome involves internal biliary drainage to the wall of the cholecystocholedochal defect, usually with a choledochojejunostomy [see 51 Biliary Tract Procedures], in addition to cholecystectomy.[68]

Patients with primary sclerosing cholangitis, especially those who have undergone internal or external biliary drainage, are at high risk for recurrent bouts of ascending cholangitis.[69,70] Primary sclerosing cholangitis predominantly affects young males, particularly those with chronic ulcerative colitis. The diagnosis is suggested by the dominant cholestatic biochemical profile—that is, elevation of the serum bilirubin concentration, the serum alkaline phosphatase level, and aspartate aminotransferase activity. Because of the concomitant hepatic scarring, ultrasonography may not reveal the presence of dilated intrahepatic ducts [see 16 Jaundice]. Definitive diagnosis requires visualization of the beaded appearance of the biliary tree by cholangiography. Cho-langiocarcinoma and secondary sclerosing cholangitis in patients with Caroli's disease or choledochal cysts may mimic these clinical, biochemical, and radiologic features, but this is an unusual occurrence and can be distinguished by careful follow-up of patients.

Patients with oriental cholangiohepatitis present with recurrent episodes of cholangitis. Subsequent intrahepatic duct scarring will be shown by cholangiography. Irreversible extrahepatic liver damage may result because of the overwhelming propensity of these patients to form calcium bilirubinate stones.[71]

TREATMENT OF ACUTE CHOLANGITIS

Once acute cholangitis is diagnosed, resuscitation is started with intravenous fluids and a combination of antibiotics, such as gentamicin, 1.5 mg/kg I.V. every 8 hours, and ampicillin, 1 g I.V. every 6 hours. Alternatively, a single agent may be used, such as mezlocillin, cefoperazone, or piperacillin,[57,72-75] particularly in patients with marked hyperbilirubinemia, in whom treatment with aminoglycosides may contribute to renal toxicity in up to 33% of cases.[76] These antibiotics are required to deal with the various aerobic bacteria: most frequently, *Escherichia coli*, *Klebsiella* species, and enterococci. Anaerobic bacteria may be isolated in 15% to 30% of patients and are particularly likely to be present in diabetics, the elderly, or patients who have previously undergone biliary manipulation [see Discussion, Bacteriology of Acute Biliary Infection, below]. In patients with indwelling catheters, *Enterobacter*, *Pseudomonas*, and *Candida* organisms are now being isolated with increasing frequency. Indications of high risk include a serum bilirubin concentration greater than 3 mg/dl.

Approximately 75% of patients with acute cholangitis will respond to conservative measures,[77] and supportive treatment is continued. Subsequent investigations may include computed tomography followed by ERCP or needle percutaneous transhepatic cholangiography (PTC) to investigate proximal duct obstruction.[78,79]

For the 25% of patients who do not respond to conservative treatment, early recognition may improve their prognosis. In one study, patients who did not respond immediately to antibiotics had a mortality of 62%, compared with a mortality of 1.5% in those who improved.[80] In another study, indicators of high risk were an arterial blood pH less than 7.4, a serum bilirubin concentration above 9 mmol/L, a blood platelet count below 150×10^9/L, and a serum albumin concentration less than 30 g/L.[81] These high-risk patients will often have systemic hypotension, mental confusion, or temperature above 39°C (102.2°F) or hypothermia. Occasionally, acute cholangitis is complicated by disseminated intravascular coagulation [see 5 Bleeding and Transfusion], which manifests itself as a tendency to bruise and bleed or merely as prolongation of the prothrombin time and the partial thromboplastin time, together with a fall in the blood platelet count. If disseminated intravascular coagulation is suspected, diagnosis should be confirmed and treatment started before biliary decompression.

Patients with refractory cholangitis who do not improve within 24 hours will require urgent biliary decompression.[82] Urgent biliary decompression has traditionally been accomplished via surgical exploration of the common bile duct and T-tube drainage [see 51 Biliary Tract Procedures]. Cholecystostomy is an inadequate and often fatal option.[64,83] T-tube insertion alone may be lifesaving in the desperately ill patient,[84] but definitive internal decompression by means of an operative drainage procedure may be preferable in less urgent cases. In patients treated by choledochoduodenostomy, blood cultures and liver function returned to normal more rapidly, hospital stay was reduced, and no infection or recurrent stones developed. By contrast, 10% of patients treated with T-tube drainage had recurrent choledocholithiasis during a follow-up period that ranged from 1 to 5 years. A large common bile duct diameter is recommended for choledochoduodenostomy.[85]

Unfortunately, surgical decompression in these critically ill patients can result in a mortality of 30% to 40%.[82,86-89] Furthermore, reoperation is required in one third of survivors because important diagnostic information is not available at the initial laparotomy. As a result, nonoperative methods of biliary decompression, including percutaneous transhepatic biliary drainage (PTBD) and endoscopic sphincterotomy, have gained favor. PTBD was originally developed for preoperative management of biliary obstruction without cholangitis[90] but has not been found to be beneficial in that setting. PTBD has been associated with several minor periprocedural complications as well as major complications, such as septicemia and bleeding.[91] However, the so-called skinny Chiba needle technique and the use of a small volume of contrast material to locate catheter placement have lowered the complication rate during original catheter placement to less than 10%.[92]

Although PTBD can reduce the mortality associated with initial biliary decompression, definitive operation is still required for many patients. Consequently, endoscopic sphincterotomy [see 47 Gastrointestinal Endoscopy] has been proposed as a definitive means of decompressing the biliary tree in patients with acute cholangitis [see Figure 5].[93] In a study of 82 patients with acute cholangitis caused by common bile duct calculi, early operation was employed in 28 patients, endoscopic sphincterotomy in 43, and antibiotic therapy alone in 11. Surgical mortality was 21% and morbidity 57%; by comparison, mortality for endoscopic sphincterotomy was 5% and morbidity 28%. A more recent study has confirmed these findings.[81] In patients whose gallbladder is still in place, endoscopic sphincterotomy may even be a reasonable long-term option in the absence of cholecystectomy. Of 23 patients whose gallbladders were left in situ,[93] only two required cholecystectomy in the follow-up period of 1 to 7 years: one for empyema of gallbladder and one for recurrent cholangitis. The final choice of the method of nonoperative drainage will of course depend on local practice and available resources, as well as the patient's biliary anatomy.

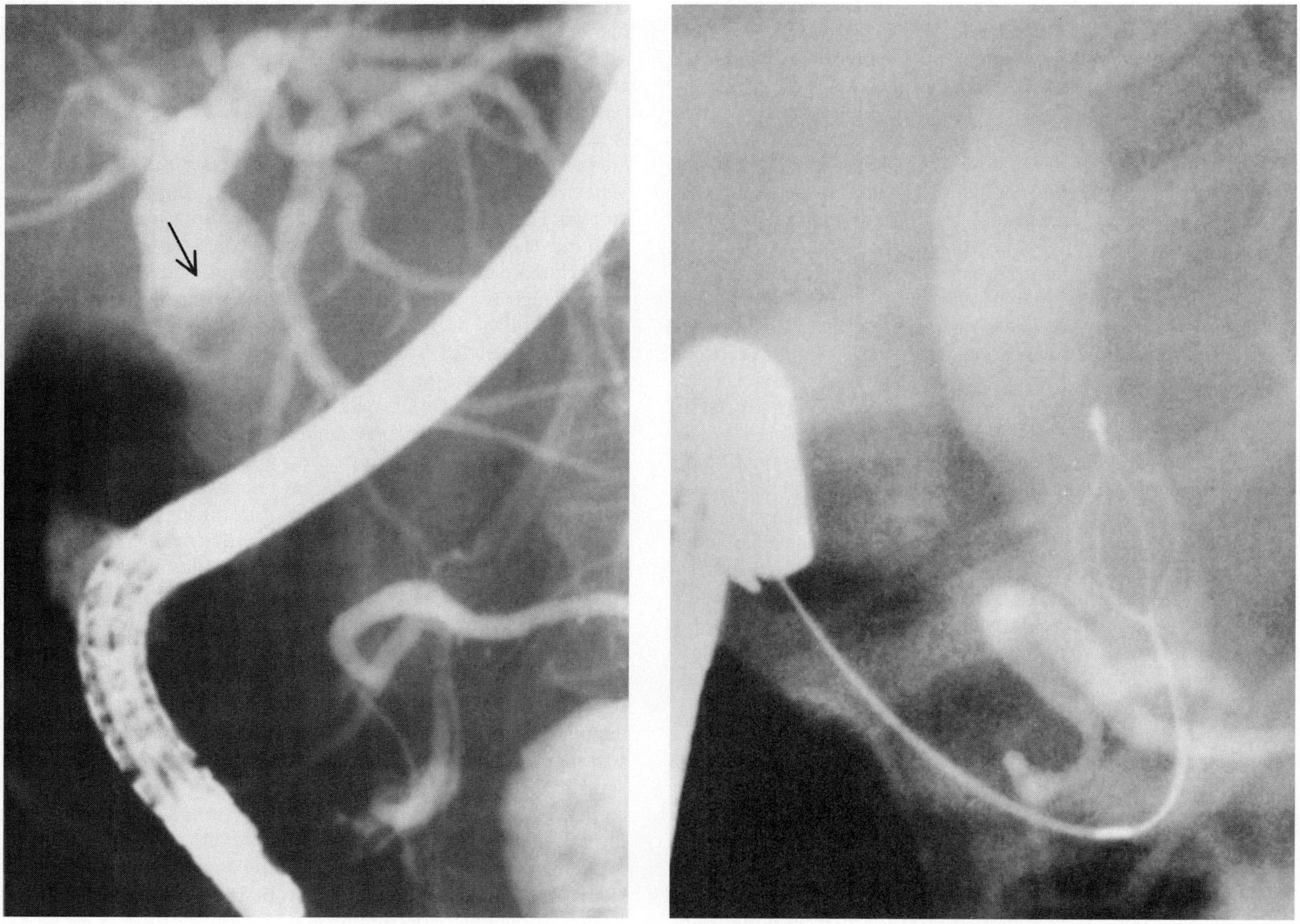

Figure 5 **Endoscopic sphincterotomy for acute biliary decompression in acute obstructive cholangitis is shown: at left, a stone is visible in the common hepatic duct, and the papillotome has been passed through the sphincter of Oddi; at right, the stone is held within a Dormia basket before extraction.**

Fever and Abdominal Mass

A third group of patients who have upper abdominal sepsis present with fever and an upper abdominal mass that is identified either by clinical signs or by imaging techniques. Even if the mass is only vaguely palpable, the mass effect will be clarified by ultrasound examination of the abdomen. If the abdominal ultrasound examination is technically unsatisfactory because of intestinal gas, contrast-enhanced computed tomography of the abdomen will facilitate the diagnosis. The differential diagnosis is aided by the location of the mass. A mass that is located in the right upper quadrant usually indicates acute cholecystitis, although the presence of a liver abscess must also be considered. A mass that is located in the epigastrium or in the left upper quadrant usually signals a pancreatic infection; in rare instances, a solitary splenic abscess will be found. Patients with an intra-abdominal abscess in the subphrenic space or an interloop abscess may also present in this manner [see 82 Peritonitis and Intra-abdominal Abscesses].

RIGHT UPPER QUADRANT MASS

Diagnosis

In the setting of acute upper abdominal sepsis, a tender mass in the right upper quadrant is most likely an enlarged inflamed gallbladder. The diagnosis and treatment of acute cholecystitis have been discussed [see Upper Abdominal Pain and Fever, *above*].

Occasionally, abdominal ultrasound examination will reveal a pyogenic liver abscess. The most common cause of this abscess is biliary tract obstruction (35% of cases) caused by gallstones or malignant disorders, and the ultrasound examination may reveal both the abscess and the dilated biliary ducts. Previously, the most common cause of pyogenic liver abscess was portal pyemia caused by diverticulitis, inflammatory bowel disease, or perforated appendicitis. It now accounts for 20% of cases. Even less common is hematogenous spread via the hepatic artery. Approximately 20% of hepatic abscesses are cryptogenic. Ultrasonographic imaging of the liver may demonstrate lesions as small as 2 cm in the liver substance.[94] CT scanning, however, is superior to ultrasonography for evaluating the presence of air and abscesses as small as 0.5 cm in diameter, especially near the hemidiaphragms.[95,96] Abdominal CT is also the diagnostic modality of choice in the postoperative patient.[97] Radionuclide scanning with ^{99m}Tc sulfur colloid or gallium-67 citrate complements ultrasonography or CT scan[98,99] but cannot identify abscesses less than 2 cm in diameter. ERCP and percutaneous transhepatic cholangiography are indicated only when gallstone or biliary malignancy is the potential source of the abscess. Most liver abscesses occur in the right lobe: 40% are 1.5 to 5 cm in diameter, 40% are 5 to 8 cm in diameter, and 20% are more than 8 cm in diameter.

No imaging technique can reliably differentiate pyogenic from amebic abscesses. The best indication of a parasitic infection is a history of travel to an endemic area, such as Mexico, Central America, or Southeast Asia. However, when a hepatic abscess is detected by an imaging technique, serologic tests should be performed to rule out active amebiasis or echinococcal infection. Examination of stool for amebae is insensitive; consequently, isoenzyme analysis, *Entamoeba histolytica*–specific antigen detection, or even PCR is preferred to confirm the diagnosis of amebiasis.[100] The diagnosis of echinococcal liver abscess can be confirmed by means of elevated indirect hemagglutination (IHA) titers (> 250).[101] In the late 1980s, a combination of tests that included IHA for *Echinococcus granulosus* and enzyme-linked immunosorbent assay (ELISA) using *E. multilocularis* antigen was shown to allow an 89% species-specific diagnosis of echinococcal disease.[102] Later work indicated that IgG ELISA and IHA were the best tests for follow-up after resection of the abscess. In patients with a favorable clinical outcome, the specific IgG level decreased toward the end of the first year; in some cases, a positive serologic result persisted beyond 6 years.[103] Diagnostic aspiration is indicated when a diagnosis of pyogenic or amebic abscess is in doubt, but not in echinococcal disease. Aspiration may also be beneficial in patients with left-sided abscesses and abscesses more than 10 cm in diameter. Chest x-ray will be abnormal in up to 50% of cases of amebic abscess; the plain abdominal x-ray may show calcification of an echinococcal cyst with secondary pyogenic infection.

It is essential to differentiate infected echinococcal cysts from pyogenic abscess: special precautions are required for drainage of echinococcal cysts because of the risk of spillage and anaphylaxis. Blood cultures are positive in up to 50% of patients with pyogenic abscess, particularly in those with multiple abscesses; in fact, the presence of *Streptococcus milleri* in the blood suggests a visceral abscess.[104]

Treatment

The preferred treatment of pyogenic abscess is closed continuous percutaneous drainage guided by CT or ultrasonography, provided that the technique is technically feasible and no other indication for laparotomy exists.[105] Use of more than one catheter may be required for complete drainage. An alternative treatment is repeated percutaneous needle aspiration, the results of which have been comparable to those of continuous drainage.[106] One advantage to repeated needle aspiration is the elimination of cumbersome, painful drainage tubes, which are prone to dislodgment. Further studies, however, will be required to establish the place of this modality in the treatment of pyogenic abscess.

The abscess cavity is followed up by serial imaging until it collapses, and the catheter can usually be removed 2 to 3 weeks later. In the English literature, continuous percutaneous drainage has been associated with a complication rate of 4% and a failure rate of 15%.[107] However, operative drainage is the treatment of choice in patients with an identified intra-abdominal focus of infection and in patients in whom percutaneous drainage is not feasible or has failed.[108] Operative drainage is a highly effective treatment option that is associated with low mortality and morbidity.[109] In some patients, a limited hepatic resection may be required to eliminate multiple abscesses, particularly when an underlying intrahepatic stricture is the source.[110,111]

Treatment of pyogenic liver abscess should include systemic antibiotic therapy. Approximately 70% of pyogenic liver abscesses yield polymicrobial isolates,[112] and 25% to 45% of the organisms are anaerobic.[113] Multiple anaerobic isolates suggest the colon as a source, whereas a single isolate of *E. coli* suggests a nidus in the biliary tree. Antibiotic treatment should include initial coverage of both aerobes and anaerobes with either a single agent or multiple agents. The need to cover enterococci has been debated, but these organisms are becoming increasingly important nosocomial pathogens. Antipseudomonal treatment, on the other hand, appears to be unnecessary when antibiotic coverage is chosen empirically; thus, there is less need for an aminoglycoside as part of a dual drug treatment regimen.[114] An acceptable initial treatment regimen is gentamicin, 1.5 mg/kg, and metronidazole, 500 mg I.V. every 8 hours; alternatively, a single broad-spectrum agent (e.g., ticarcillin-clavulanate or meropenem) may be given.

The duration of antibiotic therapy is controversial[115]; according to one set of guidelines, antibiotics should be continued for 3 to 4 weeks when the abscess has been excised, 4 to 8 weeks when a solitary abscess has been drained, and 6 to 8 weeks when multiple macroscopic abscesses have been drained.[116] Multiple microscopic abscesses require that the biliary source be treated by decompression.[89] The overall prognosis for multiple small hepatic abscesses is not as good as that for solitary abscesses, and the development of a pyogenic abscess in a patient with an underlying hepatobiliary or pancreatic malignancy has been identified as a preterminal event associated with a hospital mortality of 28% and survival of less than 6 months.[117]

Medical treatment is now the standard approach to management of the patient with amebic liver abscess. Administration of the antiprotozoal agent metronidazole, 750 mg orally three times a day for 10 days, is a highly effective regimen.[118] A favorable response to treatment occurs within 4 to 5 days, and a decrease in the size of the abscess is apparent within a week on ultrasonographic examination, although a small residual cavity may persist for as long as 2 years.[119] If the patient's condition does not improve, needle aspiration and culture are indicated. Secondary infection is treated as a pyogenic abscess. Otherwise, oral emetine, 65 mg/day, is added for up to 10 days. Symptomatic or secondarily infected echinococcal cysts are best treated by means of surgical excision or marsupialization. The use of oral anthelmintics such as mebendazole has met with limited success.[120]

EPIGASTRIC OR LEFT UPPER QUADRANT MASS

Diagnosis

When the mass is in the epigastrium or left upper quadrant, a pancreatic source is most likely. Prompt and accurate diagnosis is crucial because severe pancreatic infection is fatal if untreated. The key to successful treatment is early diagnosis of infected pancreatic necrosis, infected pseudocyst, and pancreatic abscess. A high index of suspicion is required to diagnose these three infectious processes and to differentiate them from pancreatic inflammatory mass or phlegmon,[12] in which pancreatic edema and inflammation are present without necrosis or infection.

Correct diagnosis and treatment of infected pancreatic necrosis, infected pseudocyst, and pancreatic abscess requires an understanding of pathophysiology. It is generally assumed that infected pancreatic necrosis develops by a transmural, transductal, lymphatic, or hematogenous infection of a necrotic region of the pancreas. Infection develops in 40% of cases of pancreatic necrosis, usually in the second or third week of acute pancreatitis.[121] Surgical debridement is required in these cases to prevent death. Pancreatic abscesses form by liquefaction of infected necrosis. They usually occur after the fifth week of pancreatitis, when the acute phase of disease has subsided.[122] Pancreatic abscesses are associated with a lower mortality than infected pancreatic necrosis. Like pancreatic abscesses, infected pancreatic collections and pseudocysts present late in the course of pancreatitis. They are associated with a lower mortality than pancreatic abscesses. Caused by infection in 13% of localized collections resulting from ductal blowout, infected pancreatic collections and pseudocysts may occur in the pancreas, in contiguous peripancreatic tissue, or in remote (extrapancreatic) tissue.

Clinical evaluation alone is generally insufficient to diagnose pancreatic infection. A clearly defined upper abdominal mass is palpable in only 50% to 75% of cases.[12] In most patients, the screening battery of tests reveals leukocytosis with leukocyte counts greater than 15,000/mm³. Blood cultures are positive in 50% of cases. However, the common clinical indicators of sepsis (i.e., fever, leukocytosis, and toxicity) only suggest infection. CT-guided percutaneous aspiration and Gram's stain[121] and culture[123] provide the best method of diagnosing pancreatic infection. In one study of 75 patients with clinical toxicity suggestive of pancreatic sepsis, infection was confirmed in only 40%.[124] In another study of 21 patients with pancreatic infection, only five had specific signs on abdominal CT scan.[125] The use of CT-guided diagnostic needle aspiration permitted correct diagnosis within 72 hours in two thirds of patients, and the mortality associated with operative intervention was 19%.

CT-guided needle aspiration, however, is only beneficial to the patient if pancreatic infection is suspected and if the technique is used early in the course of disease. The most important risk factors for pancreatic sepsis are clinical indicators of severe pancreatitis and findings on dynamic abdominal CT scan suggesting pancreatic necrosis.

Of the several methods of grading the severity of pancreatitis,[126-128] Ranson's method is the most widely used [see Table 2]. Pancreatic abscess occurs in 3% of patients with fewer than three signs, in 30% of patients with three to five signs, and in approximately 50% of patients with more than five signs.[12] To these criteria, Bank has added the clinical criterion of multisystem illness [see Table 4].[127] The presence of any one of these criteria indicates severe and potentially lethal disease. In patients with acute pancreatitis, shock and respiratory distress have been associated with mortalities of 88% and 71%, respectively[129]; furthermore, pancreatic abscess subsequently develops in 25% of patients with pancreatitis and shock.[130]

Comparison of these prognostic systems in acute pancreatitis shows that no system is more effective than another.[131] Their overall accuracy is 60% to 70%, but their correlation with pancreatic pathology is poor.[132] Nevertheless, it may be difficult to differentiate between pancreatic phlegmon, pseudocyst, and abscess.[130] In one study, the correct preoperative diagnosis of pancreatic abscess was made in only 44% of cases.[133]

Contrast-enhanced spiral abdominal CT scanning (dynamic pancreatography) helps to predict the severity of pancreatitis[134,135]; it has become an indispensable tool in the management of complicated pancreatitis. The finding of enhancement defects on abdominal CT distinguishes pancreatic necrosis from the inflammation and edema of pancreatic phlegmon; the site and size of major pancreatic collection or pseudocysts are clearly defined; and pancreatic abscess may be diagnosed by the presence of gas on the CT scan. CT scanning should, however, be repeated weekly in patients suspected of pancreatic infection because enhancement of the pancreas in a single examination does not rule out the presence of necrosis.[136]

Several laboratory markers of pancreatic necrosis have been investigated, such as serum methemalbumin,[137,138] serum ribonuclease,[139] and C-reactive protein.[140] Most of these markers are too insensitive for routine clinical practice. However, serum levels of

Table 4 **Clinical Criteria for Severity of Pancreatitis**[127]

Cardiac	Shock, tachycardia > 130 beats/min, arrhythmia, ECG changes
Pulmonary	Dyspnea, rales, P_{O_2} < 60 mm Hg, adult respiratory distress syndrome
Renal	Urine output < 50 ml/hr; rising blood urea nitrogen or creatinine, or both
Metabolic	Low or falling Ca^{2+}, pH, albumin
Hematologic	Falling hematocrit, diffuse intravascular coagulation (low platelets, split products)
Hemorrhagic pancreatitis	Signs or peritoneal tap findings
Tense distention	Severe ileus, fluid

Note: positive signs in one system or more indicate severe (potentially lethal) disease.

C-reactive protein above 10 mg/dl were reported to have 95% accuracy in predicting necrosis.[141]

Currently, the best indicators of infected pancreatic necrosis or abscess are a combination of Ranson's objective prognostic signs and dynamic abdominal CT scan findings.[142] In Ranson's series, the pancreatic findings on computed tomography have been graded in five categories [see Figure 6][142,143]: (a) normal, (b) pancreatic enlargement alone, (c) inflammation of the pancreas and peripancreatic fat, (d) one peripancreatic fluid collection, and (e) two or more peripancreatic fluid collections. Only category e was associated with a high incidence (61%) of pancreatic abscess. The number of objective prognostic signs present also predicted the incidence of abscess: fewer than three signs, 12.5%; three to five signs, 31.8%; and more than five signs, 80%. However, the value of this method was limited because only five of the 83 patients evaluated had more than five prognostic signs. By combining the objective prognostic signs with positive abdominal CT findings, the investigators identified 30 patients who had three or more objective signs and were graded as either category c, d, or e on abdominal CT scan; in these patients, the incidence of pancreatic abscess was 56.7%. By contrast, no patient with fewer than three prognostic signs and graded as category a or b on abdominal CT scan had a pancreatic abscess.

Treatment

Once pancreatic infection is diagnosed, supportive measures are initiated. These include nasogastric suction, withholding of oral feeding, meticulous attention to respiratory care and fluid and electrolyte balance, systemic antibiotic therapy, and nutritional support (see below). However, the key to successful treatment is surgical, interventional radiologic, or endoscopic drainage.

Sterile pancreatic necrosis is not an indication for surgical debridement. In one prospective study, 11 patients with demonstrated sterile pancreatic necrosis were all followed successfully with conservative treatment.[144] Once infected pancreatic necrosis is confirmed by Gram's stain or culture, surgical debridement is required to remove the infected slough because radiologic or endoscopic methods are not effective.

The choice of drainage technique is controversial. Many clinicians prefer operative debridement and sump drainage.[12,145] The mortality associated with operative debridement and sump drainage may range from 30% to 40%[146]; unfortunately, this technique may be associated with a 30% to 40% reoperation rate because of sepsis or gastrointestinal complications.[12,145,147]

To reduce the frequency of reoperation and to lower mortality, some clinicians have opted for open drainage or marsupialization of the infected pancreas.[148,149] Others have modified the method further by employing Marlex mesh and a zipper to facilitate repeated reexplorations in patients with severe intra-abdominal abscess.[150] A 1991 meta-analysis of published surgical studies on infected pancreatic necrosis since 1980 found statistically better results with debridement and lavage or debridement and open packing than with conventional debridement and sump drainage.[151] However, surgical treatment should be customized for each patient. In one study, open packing was used for massive necrosis (more than 100 g removed by debridement at operation or CT evidence of at least 50% pancreatic necrosis) or for extrapancreatic necrosis, whereas conventional debridement and sump drainage were used in other cases[143]; the overall mortality in this study was only 14%. Pancreatic abscess resulting from liquefaction of necrosis is also best treated by surgical drainage because residual necrosis may cause failure of treatment by percutaneous methods.[152] On the other hand, infected pancreatic fluid collections and pseudocysts can usually be treated by nonoperative methods. In one prospective study, percutaneous and surgical methods of drainage were equally successful in treating infected pancreatic fluid collections and pseudocysts.[153] Clinical findings rather than CT findings are the best indicators of the need for intervention, and nonoperative methods should be attempted before open surgery is planned.

In the past, debridement and sump drainage were accompanied by the triple ostomy technique, which comprises cholecystostomy, gastrostomy, and jejunostomy.[154] However, the role of these ancillary procedures is controversial. Cholecystostomy is now employed only if gallstones are detected. Evidence also suggests that intravenous hyperalimentation is preferable to jejunostomy feeding because early oral feeding appears to predispose to recrudescence of pancreatitis and eventual abscess formation, whereas prolonged restriction of oral feeding allows pancreatic inflammation to subside.[12]

Other operative procedures may be required to manage gastric or colonic complications. Gastric bleeding, gastric outlet obstruction, and gastric fistula requiring reoperation are relatively infrequent in this setting. By contrast, colonic necrosis and fistula formation are more common and occur either spontaneously or as a result of treatment. The usual site of involvement is the splenic flexure or upper descending colon. Treatment consists of colonic resection or diverting colostomy [see 57 Colorectal Procedures].

The role of systemic antibiotic therapy in the prophylaxis of pancreatic abscess is controversial. Experimental evidence suggests that antibiotics may sometimes decrease the severity of pancreatitis,[155] and endoscopic cannulation of the pancreatic duct has now yielded bacteria in pancreatic secretions of patients with acute pancreatitis.[156] In patients with pancreatic abscess, bacteriologic cultures are usually polymicrobial. The most common organisms are *E. coli*, enterococci, *K. pneumoniae*, *P. aeruginosa*, *Staphylococcus aureus*, *B. fragilis*, and *Clostridium perfringens*. The reported incidence of anaerobic infection is low (6%). As a result, broad-spectrum antibiotic therapy, such as gentamicin, 1.5 mg/kg I.V. every 8 hours, and clindamycin, 600 mg I.V. every 6 hours, is indicated. Intravenous monotherapy, such as imipenem, ticarcillin-clavulanate, or ciprofloxacin, which are effective against most pancreatic pathogens, is becoming increasingly popular. Of late, there has been a growing trend toward early use of prophylactic antibiotics in cases of pancreatic necrosis, even though there are no data that convincingly demonstrate a clinical benefit.[31] This trend may be partly responsible for the increasing prevalence of *Candida* species in pancreatitis-related sepsis. A 1996 report stated that *Candida* infection was detected in 21% of patients.[157]

Nutritional support of the patient with pancreatic abscess usually consists of total parenteral nutrition. In these patients, the metabolic demand is high, and glucose intolerance or hyperlipidemia may occur. Still, intravenous feeding is generally well tolerated. A 10-fold increase in mortality (2.5% versus 21%) has been reported in patients in whom a positive nitrogen balance had not been achieved.[158]

Splenic Abscess

Diagnosis Splenic abscess should be considered in patients who present with fever and a left upper quadrant mass, although it is rarely the cause of these symptoms. Most abscesses encountered by the clinician are solitary. Multiple abscesses are usually covert and are found at autopsy of patients who had disseminated malignancy, collagen vascular disease, or chronic debility.[159]

Because splenic abscess is rare, correct diagnosis requires a high index of suspicion. The main clue is the clinical setting: both bacteremia and local splenic disease are required to produce splenic abscess.[160] In the preantibiotic period, this combination was seen most

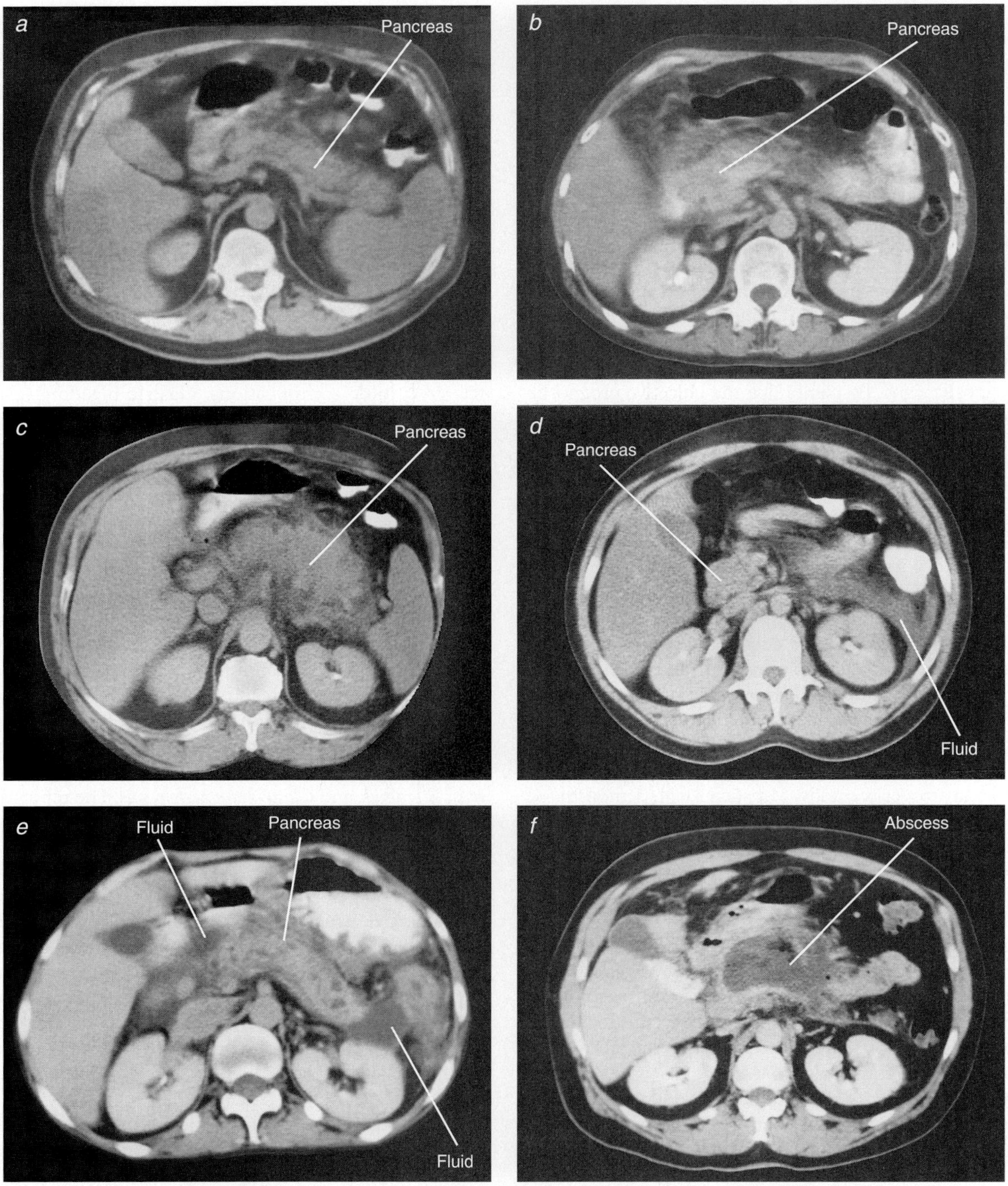

Figure 6 Pancreatic findings on CT scan have been graded by Ranson into five categories: grade A—normal pancreas (*a*); grade B—diffuse enlargement of the pancreas and nonhomogeneous density of the gland (*b*); grade C—diffuse enlargement of the pancreas associated with peripancreatic inflammation (*c*); grade D—high-density fluid collection in left anterior pararenal space (only the head of the pancreas is visualized at this level) (*d*); and grade E—diffuse enlargement of the pancreas with several intrapancreatic small fluid collections and poorly defined fluid collections adjacent to the tail and head of the pancreas (*e*). In the final CT scan of this series (*f*), a pancreatic abscess is demonstrated; a partially encapsulated fluid collection containing bubbles of air represents a large abscess.

frequently in patients with bacterial endocarditis[161] and typhoid.[162] Even today, 80% of splenic abscesses occur in patients in whom an infection is already evident elsewhere in the body[163]; splenic abscesses can also occur in patients with splenic infarcts, splenic hematomas, or local splenic disease caused by hemoglobinopathies.[164,165]

The diagnosis of splenic abscess may be supported by indirect radiologic signs, such as an elevated left hemidiaphragm or the finding of a left upper quadrant air-fluid level simulating the stomach. To clinch the diagnosis, an abdominal ultrasound examination or abdominal CT scan is required. The abdominal CT scan, enhanced by intravenous or oral contrast, is preferred [*see Figure 7*].[166] This technique provides a direct image of the spleen; abscesses appear as low-density areas that may contain gas.

Treatment Treatment of splenic abscess includes intravenous administration of antibiotics and splenectomy. The usual pathogen-

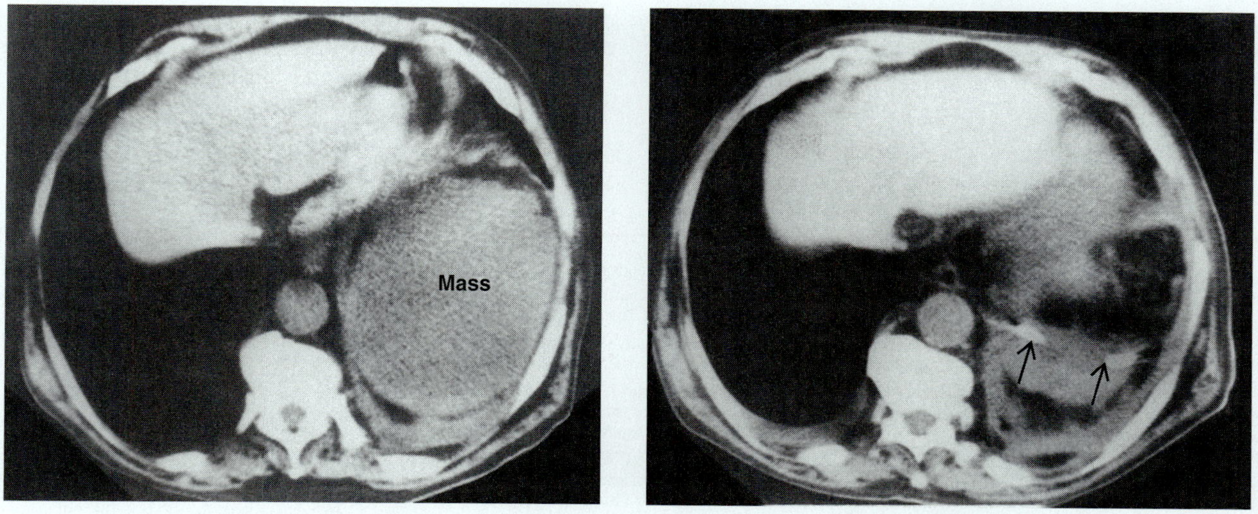

Figure 7 Abdominal CT scan, enhanced by contrast material, confirms diagnosis of splenic abscess.

ic organisms found are staphylococci and streptococci, although gram-negative bacilli and anaerobic bacteria may also be present. Cloxacillin, 1 g intravenously every 6 hours, and gentamicin, 1.5 mg/kg intravenously every 8 hours, should be given for a period of at least 5 days. When splenic abscesses are not drained, the mortality approaches 100%. In previous years, splenotomy was the preferred operative treatment of splenic abscess,[162-167] but splenectomy has since become the preferred method. Percutaneous catheter drainage is currently being performed with increasing frequency and appears to be as effective as operative drainage.[8,168-171]

Discussion

Pathophysiology of Acute Bacterial Cholangitis

Longmire's widely accepted classification of acute bacterial cholangitis consists of five categories—acute nonobstructive, acute nonsuppurative, acute suppurative, acute obstructive suppurative, and acute suppurative with intrahepatic abscess. It implies that the severity of disease parallels the degree of obstruction of biliary ducts.[171] This suggestion is well founded. In acute nonobstructive cholangitis associated with acute cholecystitis, infection ascends along the intrahepatic and extrahepatic lymphatics.[67] In obstructive cholangitis, the bile duct contains bacteria under pressure. When the pressure is at or above the normal secretion pressure (i.e., 200 mm Hg), bacteria pass into the lymphatic system. At a pressure greater than 250 mm Hg, bacteria may pass directly from the bile ductules through the spaces of Mall and Disse and into the hepatic sinusoids via cholangiovenous reflux.[172,173] One study confirmed the clinical significance of increasing ductal pressure by demonstrating a higher ductal pressure and a higher incidence of bacteremia in patients with proximal ductal obstruction, compared with those with distal malignant biliary obstruction.[174] However, no correlation exists between the degree of suppuration in the duct and the clinical or pathologic severity of obstructive cholangitis.[82,175] Therefore, the terms acute nonsuppurative cholangitis and acute suppurative cholangitis are purely descriptive and do not imply differing degrees of severity.

The source of bacteria in acute cholangitis is most often the duodenum. The ease with which organisms reflux from the duodenum is dependent on the degree of obstruction. Thus, in patients with malignant biliary obstruction, in whom obstruction is usually complete, bile culture is positive in only 10% to 15% of patients[176]; acute cholangitis is seldom spontaneous in this setting but often follows radiologic intervention.[177] By comparison, in patients with ductal stones or benign strictures, in whom biliary obstruction is often incomplete, bile cultures obtained on ERCP are positive in 64% to 87% of cases; in these patients, acute cholangitis occurs frequently, both spontaneously and after ductal manipulation.[178]

An alternative source of organisms in acute bacterial cholangitis is portal venous blood. In patients who have recurrent pyogenic cholangitis, which occurs frequently in the Far East, a 40% incidence of positive portal blood culture has been reported.[179] In studies in rats who have ligated bile ducts, bacteria were shown to be effectively transmitted to the bile ducts and liver through portal blood.[180] Finally, in nonobstructive cholangitis and acute cholecystitis, as well as in the early stages of obstructive cholangitis, infection ascends to the liver through the lymphatic system.

Bacteriology of Acute Biliary Infection

Most biliary infections are polymicrobial. The organisms most frequently cultured are *E. coli*, *Klebsiella* species, *Enterobacter* species, and enterococci.[83] Anaerobic bacteria are infrequently implicated in biliary infections. Peptostreptococci and clostridia are found occasionally; clostridia are especially common in patients with emphysematous cholecystitis.[43] Gram-negative anaerobic bacilli are rarely present in patients with biliary infection. In one study, only two of 28 patients with acute cholangitis had anaerobic bacteria in the bile; another investigator found anaerobic bacteria in 3% to 4% of cultures in similar patients.[181] However, a higher incidence of anaerobic bacteria has been reported in patients who have acute cholangitis and acute cholecystitis than in patients who have chronic cholecystitis and cholelithiasis.[182]

One investigator noted an increased incidence of anaerobic bacteria in biliary infection and suggested that *B. fragilis* may play a more important role in the polymicrobial flora of biliary tract infection than appreciated previously.[183] To date, these findings have been controversial. *Bacteroides* species are generally considered to be of limited importance in biliary tract infections, except in selected groups of patients. These patients include diabetics, the elderly,[184] and those with acute cholangitis who have previously undergone biliary operation[185,186]; in particular, malfunctioning biliary-intestinal anastomoses increase the risk of *Bacteroides* infection.[187]

References

1. Schofield PF, Hulton NR, Baildam AD: Is it acute cholecystitis? Ann R Coll Surg Engl 68:14, 1986
2. Weissmann HS, Frank MS, Bernstein LH, et al: Rapid and accurate diagnosis of acute cholecystitis with ^{99m}Tc-HIDA cholescintigraphy. AJR Am J Roentgenol 132: 523, 1979
3. Adams JT, Libertino JA, Schwartz SI: Significance of an elevated serum amylase. Surgery 63:877, 1968
4. Ranson JHC: Acute pancreatitis. Curr Probl Surg 16:1, 1979
5. Winslet M, Hall C, London NJ, et al: Relation of diagnostic serum amylase levels to etiology and severity of acute pancreatitis. Gut 33:982, 1992
6. Patti M, Pellegrini CA, Way LW: Serum amylase is useful in the differential diagnosis of acute abdominal pain. Gastroenterology 90:1580, 1986
7. Toosie A, Chang L, Renslo R, et al: Early computed tomography is rarely necessary in gallstone pancreatitis. Am Surg 63:904, 1997
8. Sarr MG, Sanfrey H, Cameron JL: Prospective, randomized trial of nasogastric suction in patients with acute pancreatitis. Surgery 100:500, 1986
9. Bradley EL III: Antibiotics in acute pancreatitis: current status and future direction. Am J Surg 158:472, 1989
10. Steinberg WM, Schlesselman SE: Treatment of acute pancreatitis: comparison of animal and human studies. Gastroenterology 93:1420, 1987
11. McArdle AH, Rosenberg M, Fried GM, et al: Pancreatic exocrine secretion in response to continuous and bolus feeding (abstr). Presented at the 19th Annual Meeting, Association for Academic Surgery, 1985, Cincinnati, Ohio
12. Ranson JH, Spencer FC: Prevention, diagnosis, and treatment of pancreatic abscess. Surgery 82:99, 1977
13. Kelly TR, Wagner DS: Gallstone pancreatitis: a prospective randomized trial of the timing of surgery. Surgery 104:600, 1988
14. Stone HH, Fabian TC, Dunlop WE: Gallstone pancreatitis: biliary tract pathology in relation to time of operation. Ann Surg 194:305, 1981
15. Acosta JM, Rossi R, Galli OMR, et al: Early surgery for acute gallstone pancreatitis: evaluation of a systematic approach. Surgery 83:367, 1978
16. Acosta JM, Pellegrini CA, Skinner DB: Etiology and pathogenesis of acute biliary pancreatitis. Surgery 88:118, 1980
17. Kelly TR: Gallstone pancreatitis: the timing of surgery. Surgery 88:345, 1980
18. Dixon JA, Hillam JD: Surgical treatment of biliary tract disease associated with acute pancreatitis. Am J Surg 120:371, 1970
19. Ranson JHC: The timing of biliary surgery in acute pancreatitis. Ann Surg 189:654, 1979
20. Paloyan D, Simonowitz D, Skinner DB: The timing of biliary tract operations in patients with pancreatitis associated with gallstones. Surg Gynecol Obstet 141:737, 1975
21. Neoptolemos JP, London N, Slater ND, et al: A prospective study of ERCP and endoscopic sphincterotomy in the diagnosis and treatment of acute pancreatitis: a rational and safe approach to management. Arch Surg 121:697, 1986
22. Neoptolemos JP, Carr-Locke DL, London NJ, et al: Controlled trial of urgent endoscopic retrograde cholangiopancreatography and endoscopic sphincterotomy versus conservative treatment for acute pancreatitis due to gallstones. Lancet 2:979, 1988
23. Fan S-T, Lai ECS, Mok FPT, et al: Early treatment of acute biliary pancreatitis by endoscopic papillotomy. N Engl J Med 328:228, 1993
24. Williamson RC: Early assessment of severity in acute pancreatitis. Gut 25:1331, 1984
25. Srinathan SK, Barkun JS, Mehta SN, et al: Evolving management of mild-to-moderate gallstone pancreatitis. J Gastrointest Surg 2:385, 1998
26. Osborne DH, Imrie CW, Carter DC: Biliary surgery in the same admission for gallstone-associated acute pancreatitis. Br J Surg 68:758, 1981
27. Foelsch UR, Nitsche R, Luedtke R, et al: Early endoscopic retrograde cholangiopancreatography was not beneficial in pancreatitis. N Engl J Med 336:237, 1997
28. Kozarek RA, Patterson DJ, Ball TJ, et al: Endoscopic placement of pancreatic stents and drains in the management of pancreatitis. Ann Surg 209:261, 1989
29. Stone HH, Fabian TC: Peritoneal dialysis in the treatment of acute alcoholic pancreatitis. Surg Gynecol Obstet 150:878, 1990
30. Ranson JHC, Berman RS: Long peritoneal lavage decreases pancreatic sepsis in acute pancreatitis. Ann Surg 211:708, 1990
31. Pedrezoli P, Bassi C, Vesentini S, et al: A randomized multicenter clinical trial of antibiotic prophylaxis of septic complications in acute necrotizing pancreatitis with imipenem. Surg Gynecol Obstet 176:483, 1993
32. Luiten EJ, Hop WC, Lange JF, et al: A controlled clinical trial of selective decontamination for the treatment of severe acute pancreatitis. Ann Surg 222:57, 1995
33. Fiedler F, Jauernig G, Keim V, et al: Octreotide treatment in patients with necrotizing pancreatitis and pulmonary failure. Intens Care Med 22:909, 1996
34. Paran H, Neufeld D, Mayo A, et al: Preliminary report of a prospective randomized study of octreotide in the treatment of severe acute pancreatitis. J Am Coll Surg 181:121, 1995
35. Kingsnorth AN, Galloway SW, Formela LJ: Randomized, double blind phase 2 trial of lexipafant, a platelet-activating factor antagonist, in human acute pancreatitis. Br J Surg 82:1414, 1995
36. Sianesi M, Ghirarduzzi A, Percudani M, et al: Cholecystectomy for acute cholecystitis: timing of operation, bacteriologic aspects, and postoperative course. Am J Surg 148:609, 1984
37. Lo CM, Liu CL, Fan ST, et al: Prospective randomized study of early versus delayed laparoscopic cholecystectomy for acute cholecystitis. Ann Surg 227:461, 1998
38. Lewis RT, Allan CM, Goodall RG, et al: A single preoperative dose of cefazolin prevents postoperative sepsis in high risk biliary surgery. Can J Surg 27:44, 1984
39. Eliason EL, Stevens LW: Acute cholecystitis. Surg Gynecol Obstet 78:98, 1944
40. Clifford WJ: Acute gangrenous cholecystitis. N Engl J Med 241:640, 1949
41. Hegner CF: Gaseous pericholecystitis with cholecystitis and cholelithiasis. Arch Surg 22:993, 1931
42. Jacob H, Appelman R, Stein HD: Emphysematous cholecystitis. Am J Gastroenterol 71:325, 1979
43. Mentzer RM, Golden GT, Chandler JG, et al: A comparative appraisal of emphysematous cholecystitis. Am J Surg 129:10, 1975
44. Turner RJ III, Becker WF, Coleman WO, et al: Acute cholecystitis in the diabetic. South Med J 62:228, 1969
45. Turrill FL, McCarron MM, Mikkelsen WP: Gallstones and diabetes: an ominous association. Am J Surg 102:184, 1961
46. Walsh DB, Eckhauser FE, Ramsburgh SR, et al: Risk associated with diabetes mellitus in patients undergoing gallbladder surgery. Surgery 91:254, 1982
47. Pickleman J: Controversies in biliary tract surgery. Can J Surg 29:429, 1986
48. Glenn F, Becker CG: Acute acalculous cholecystitis: an increasing entity. Ann Surg 195:131, 1982
49. Glenn F: Acute cholecystitis following the surgical treatment of unrelated disease. Ann Surg 126:411, 1947
50. Rice J, Williams HC, Flint LM, et al: Post-traumatic acalculous cholecystitis. South Med J 73:14, 1980
51. Long TN, Heimbach DM, Carrico CJ: Acalculous cholecystitis in critically ill patients. Am J Surg 136:31, 1978
52. Orlando R III, Gleason E, Drezner AD: Acute acalculous cholecystitis in the critically ill patient. Am J Surg 145:472, 1983
53. Deitch EA, Engel JM: Acute acalculous cholecystitis: ultrasonic diagnosis. Am J Surg 142:290, 1981
54. Weissmann HS, Berkowitz D, Fox MS, et al: The role of technetium-99m iminodiacetic acid (IDA) cholescintigraphy in acute acalculous cholecystitis. Radiology 146:177, 1983
55. Chen CC, Holder LE, Maunoury C, et al: Morphine augmentation increases gallbladder visualization in patients pretreated with cholecystokinin. J Nucl Med 38:644, 1997
56. Cabana MD, et al: Morphine-augmented hepatobiliary scintigraphy: a meta-analysis. Nucl Med Commun 16:1068, 1995
57. Karachalios GN, Nasiopoulou DD, Bourlinou PK, et al: Treatment of acute biliary tract infections with ofloxacin: a randomized, controlled clinical trial. Int J Clin Pharmacol Ther 34:555, 1996
58. Krajden S, Yaman M, Fuksa M, et al: Piperacillin versus cefazolin given perioperatively to high-risk patients who undergo open cholecystectomy: a double-blind, randomized trial. Can J Surg 36:245, 1993
59. Skillings JC, Kumal C, Hinshaw JR: Cholecystostomy: a place in modern biliary surgery? Am J Surg 139:865, 1980
60. Klimberg S, Hawkins I, Vogel SB: Percutaneous cholecystostomy for acute cholecystitis in high-risk patients. Am J Surg 153:125, 1987
61. Miyazaki K, Uchiyama A, Nakayama F: New approach to the timing of operative intervention for acute cholecystitis: use of ultrasound risk score (abstr). The 32nd World Congress of Surgery, Sydney, Australia, September 20–26, 1987
62. England RE, McDermott VG, Smith TP, et al: Percutaneous cholecystostomy: who responds? AJR Am J Roentgenol 168:1247, 1997
63. Orlando R 3rd, Crowell KL: Laparoscopy in the critically ill. Surg Endosc 11:1072, 1997
64. Gagic N, Frey CF: The results of cholecystostomy for the treatment of acute cholecystitis. Surg Gynecol Obstet 140:255, 1975
65. Reynolds BM, Dargan EL: Acute obstructive cholangitis: a distinct clinical syndrome. Ann Surg 150:299, 1959
66. DuPont HL, Spink WW: Infections due to gram-negative organisms: an analysis of 860 patients with bacteremia at the University of Minnesota Medical Center, 1958–1966. Medicine (Baltimore) 48:307, 1969
67. Glenn F: Anatomy and physiology of the liver and

biliary system and diseases of the gallbladder and bile ducts. Christopher's Textbook of Surgery, 6th ed. Davis L, Ed. WB Saunders Co, Philadelphia, 1956, p 722

68. Baer HU, Matthews JB, Schweizer WP, et al: Management of the Mirizzi syndrome and the surgical implications of cholecystocholedochal fistula. Br J Surg 77:743, 1990
69. Wiesner RH, Ludwig J, LaRusso NF, et al: Diagnosis and treatment of primary sclerosing cholangitis. Semin Liver Dis 5:241, 1985
70. Helzberg JH, Petersen JM, Boyer JL: Improved survival with primary sclerosing cholangitis: a review of clinicopathologic features and comparison of symptomatic and asymptomatic patients. Gastroenterology 92:1869, 1987
71. Nakayama F, Koga A: Hepatolithiasis: present status. World J Surg 8:9, 1984
72. Gerecht WB, Henry NK, Hoffman WW, et al: Prospective randomized comparison of mezlocillin therapy alone with combined ampicillin and gentamicin therapy for patients with cholangitis. Arch Intern Med 149:1279, 1989
73. Thompson JE Jr, Pitt HA, Doty JE, et al: Broad spectrum penicillin as an adequate therapy for acute cholangitis. Surg Gynecol Obstet 171:275, 1990
74. Thompson JN, Edwards WH, Winearls CE, et al: Renal impairment following biliary tract surgery. Br J Surg 74:843, 1987
75. Muller EL, Pitt HA, Thompson JE Jr, et al: Antibiotics in infections of the biliary tract. Surg Gynecol Obstet 165:285, 1987
76. Pitt HA, Postier RG, Cameron JL: Consequences of preoperative cholangitis and its treatment on the outcome of operation for choledocholithiasis. Surgery 94:447, 1983
77. Leung JW, Chung SC, Sung JJ, et al: Urgent endoscopic drainage for acute suppurative cholangitis. Lancet 1:1307, 1989
78. Elias E, Hamlyn AN, Jain S, et al: A randomized trial of percutaneous transhepatic cholangiography with the Chiba needle versus endoscopic retrograde cholangiography for bile duct visualization in jaundice. Gastroenterology 71:439, 1976
79. Pereiras R, Chiprut RO, Greenwald RA, et al: Percutaneous transhepatic cholangiography with the "skinny" needle: a rapid, simple, and accurate method in the diagnosis of cholestasis. Ann Intern Med 86:562, 1977
80. Gigot JF, Leese T, Derme T, et al: Acute cholangitis: multivariate analysis of risk factors. Ann Surg 209:435, 1989
81. Lai EC, Tam PC, Paterson IA, et al: Emergency surgery for severe acute cholangitis: the high risk patients. Ann Surg 211:55, 1990
82. Boey JH, Way LW: Acute cholangitis. Ann Surg 191:264, 1980
83. Saik RP, Greenburg AG, Peskin GW: Cholecystostomy hazard in acute cholangitis. JAMA 235:2412, 1976
84. Glenn F, Moody FG: Acute obstructive suppurative cholangitis. Surg Gynecol Obstet 113:265, 1961
85. Kraus MA, Wilson SD: Choledochoduodenostomy: importance of common duct size and occurrence of cholangitis. Arch Surg 115:1212, 1980
86. O'Connor MJ, Schwartz ML, McQuarrie DG, et al: Acute bacterial cholangitis: an analysis of clinical manifestation. Arch Surg 117:437, 1982
87. Thompson JE Jr, Tompkins RK, Longmire WP Jr: Factors in management of acute cholangitis. Ann Surg 195:137, 1982
88. Bismuth H, Kuntziger H, Corlette MB: Cholangitis with acute renal failure: priorities in therapeutics. Ann Surg 181:881, 1975
89. Cho SR, Turner MA: Hepatic abscesses due to suppurative cholangitis. South Med J 75:488, 1982
90. Ferrucci JT, Mueller PR, Harbin WP: Percutaneous transhepatic biliary drainage: technique, results and applications. Radiology 135:1, 1980
91. Mueller PR, vanSonnenberg E, Ferrucci JT Jr: Percutaneous biliary drainage: technical and catheter-related problems in 200 procedures. AJR 138:17, 1982
92. Gould RJ, Vogelzang RL, Neiman HL, et al: Percutaneous biliary drainage as an initial therapy in sepsis of the biliary tract. Surg Gynecol Obstet 160:523, 1985
93. Leese T, Neoptolemos JP, Baker AR, et al: Management of acute cholangitis and the impact of endoscopic sphincterotomy. Br J Surg 73:988, 1986
94. Richardson R, Norton LW, Eule J, et al: Accuracy of ultrasound in diagnosing abdominal masses. Arch Surg 110:933, 1975
95. Alfidi RJ, MacIntyre WJ, Haaga JR: The effects of biological motion on CT resolution. AJR 127:11, 1976
96. Saini S: Imaging of the hepatobiliary tract. N Engl J Med 336:1889, 1997
97. Bearcroft PW, Miles KA: Leucocyte scintigraphy or computed tomography for the febrile post-operative patient? Eur J Radiol 23:126, 1996
98. McAfee JG, Ause RG, Wagner HN: Diagnostic value of scintillation scanning of the liver: follow-up of 1,000 studies. Arch Intern Med 116:95, 1965
99. Lomas F, Dibos PE, Wagner HN: Increased specificity of liver scanning with the use of ^{67}gallium citrate. N Engl J Med 286:1323, 1972
100. Haque R, Ali JK, Akther S, et al: Comparison of PCR, isoenzyme analysis and antigen detection for diagnosis of E. histolytica infection. J Clin Microbiol 36:449, 1998
101. Moazam F, Nazir Z: Amebic liver abscess: spare the knife but save the child. J Pediatr Surg 33:119, 1998
102. Auer H, Picher O, Aspock H: Combined application of enzyme-linked immunosorbent assay (ELISA) and indirect haemagglutination test (IHA) as a useful tool for the diagnosis and post-operative surveillance of human alveolar and cystic echinococcosis. Zentralbl Bakteriol Mikrobiol Hyg 270:313, 1988
103. Force L, Torres JM, Carrillo A: Evaluation of eight serological tests in the diagnosis of human echinococcosis and follow-up. Clin Infect Dis 15:473, 1992
104. Moore-Gillon JC, Eykyn SJ, Phillips I: Microbiology of pyogenic liver abscess. Br Med J 283:819, 1981
105. Aeder MI, Wellman JL, Haaga JR: Role of surgical and percutaneous drainage in the treatment of abdominal abscesses. Arch Surg 118:273, 1983
106. Ch Yu S, Hg Lo R, Kan PS: Pyogenic liver abscess: treatment with needle aspiration. Clin Radiol 52:912, 1997
107. Gerzof SG, Johnson WC, Robbins AH, et al: Intrahepatic pyogenic abscesses: treatment by percutaneous drainage. Am J Surg 149:487, 1985
108. Seeto RK, Rockey DC: Pyogenic liver abscess: changes in etiology, management, and outcome. Medicine (Baltimore) 75:99, 1996
109. Herman P, Pugliese V, Montagnini AL, et al: Pyogenic liver abscess: the role of surgical treatment. Int Surg 82:98, 1997
110. Pitt HA, Zuidema GD: Factors influencing mortality in the treatment of pyogenic hepatic abscess. Surg Gynecol Obstet 140:228, 1975
111. Klatchko BA, Schwartz SI: Diagnostic and therapeutic approaches to pyogenic abscess of the liver. Surg Gynecol Obstet 168:332, 1989
112. Gyorffy EJ, Frey CF, Silva J Jr, et al: Pyogenic liver abscess: diagnostic and therapeutic strategies. Ann Surg 206:699, 1987
113. Sabbaj J, Sutter VL, Finegold SM: Anaerobic pyogenic liver abscess. Ann Intern Med 77:629, 1972
114. Bartlett JG: Intraabdominal sepsis. Med Clin North Am 79:599, 1995
115. Schein M, Wittmann DH, Lorenz W: Duration of antibiotic treatment in surgical infections of the abdomen. Forum statement: a plea for selective and controlled postoperative antibiotic administration. Eur J Surg Suppl 576:66, 1996
116. Rubin RH, Swartz MN, Malt R: Hepatic abscess: changes in clinical, bacteriologic and therapeutic aspects. Am J Med 57:601, 1974
117. Yeh TS, Jan YY, Jeng LB: Pyogenic liver abscesses in patients with malignant disease: a report of 52 cases treated at a single institution. Arch Surg 133:242, 1998
118. Cohen HG, Reynolds TB: Comparison of metronidazole and chloroquine for the treatment of amoebic liver abscess. Gastroenterology 69:35, 1975
119. Sheen IS, Chien CS, Lin DY, et al: Resolutions of liver abscesses: comparison of pyogenic and amebic liver abscess. Am J Trop Med Hyg 40:384, 1989
120. Most H: Treatment of parasitic infections of travelers and immigrants. N Engl J Med 310:298, 1984
121. Stiles GM, Byrne TV, Thommen VD, et al: Fine needle aspiration of pancreatic fluid collections. Am Surg 56:764, 1990
122. Bittner R, Block S, Buchler M, et al: Pancreatic abscess and infected pancreatic necrosis: different local septic complications in acute pancreatitis. Dig Dis Sci 32:1082, 1987
123. Beger HG, Bittner R, Block S, et al: Bacterial contamination of pancreatic necrosis: a prospective clinical study. Gastroenterology 91:433, 1986
124. Banks PA, Gerzof SG, Chong FK, et al: Bacteriologic status of necrotic tissue in necrotizing pancreatitis. Pancreas 5:330, 1990
125. Crass RA, Meyer AA, Jeffrey RB, et al: Pancreatic abscess: impact of computerized tomography on early diagnosis and surgery. Am J Surg 150:127, 1985
126. Ranson JHC, Rifkind KM, Roses DF, et al: Prognostic signs and the role of operative management in acute pancreatitis. Surg Gynecol Obstet 139:69, 1974
127. Bank S, Wise L, Gersten M: Risk factors in acute pancreatitis. Am J Gastroenterol 78:637, 1983
128. Imrie CW, Whyte AS: A prospective study of acute pancreatitis. Br J Surg 62:490, 1975
129. Satiani B, Stone HH: Predictability of present outcome and future recurrence in acute pancreatitis. Arch Surg 114:711, 1979
130. Kune GA, King R: The late complications of acute pancreatitis: pancreatic swelling, cyst and abscess. Med J Aust 1:1241, 1973
131. Demmy TL, Burch JM, Feliciano DV: Comparison of multiple-parameter prognostic systems in acute pancreatitis. Am J Surg 156:492, 1988
132. Nordback I, Pessi T, Auvinen O, et al: Determination of necrosis in necrotizing pancreatitis. Br J Surg 72:225, 1985
133. Becker JM, Pemberton JH, DiMagno EP, et al: Prognostic factors in pancreatic abscess. Surgery 96:455, 1984
134. Balthazar EJ, Freeny PC, van Sonnenberg E: Imaging and intervention in acute pancreatitis. Radiology 193:297, 1994
135. Balthazar EJ, Robinson DL, Megibow AJ: Acute pancreatitis: value of CT in establishing prognosis. Radiology 174:331, 1990
136. Maier W: Early objective diagnosis and staging of acute pancreatitis by contrast enhanced computed tomography. Acute Pancreatitis. Beger HG, Buchler M, Eds. Springer-Verlag, Berlin, 1987, p 132
137. Northam BE, Rowe DS, Winstone NE: Methaemalbumin in the differential diagnosis of acute haemorrhagic and oedematous pancreatitis. Lancet 1:348, 1963
138. Geokas MC, Rinderknecht H, Walberg CB, et al: Methaemalbumin in the diagnosis of acute hemorrhagic pancreatitis. Ann Intern Med 81:483, 1974
139. Warshaw AL, Lee KH: Serum ribonuclease elevations and pancreatic necrosis in acute pancreatitis. Surgery 86:227, 1979
140. Wilson C, Heads A, Shenkin A, et al: C-reactive protein, antiproteases and complement factors as objective markers of severity in acute pancreatitis. Br J Surg 76:177, 1989
141. Buchler M, Malfertheiner P, Schoetensack C, et al:

Sensitivity of antiproteases, complement factors and C-reactive protein in detecting pancreatic necrosis: results of a prospective clinical study. Int J Pancreatol 1:227, 1986

142. Ranson JHC, Balthazar E, Caccavale R, et al: Computed tomography and the prediction of pancreatic abscess in acute pancreatitis. Ann Surg 201:656, 1985
143. Stanten R, Frey CF: Comprehensive management of acute necrotizing pancreatitis and pancreatic abscess. Arch Surg 125:1269, 1990
144. Bradley EL III, Allen K: A prospective longitudinal study of observation versus surgical intervention in the management of necrotizing pancreatitis. Am J Surg 161:19, 1991
145. Aranha GV, Prinz RA, Greenlee HB: Pancreatic abscess: an unresolved surgical problem. Am J Surg 144:534, 1982
146. Warshaw AL: Pancreatic abscesses. N Engl J Med 287:1234, 1972
147. Frey CF, Lindenauer SM: Pancreatic abscess. Surg Gynecol Obstet 149:722, 1979
148. Bolooki H, Jaffe B, Gliedman ML: Pancreatic abscesses and lesser omental sac collections. Surg Gynecol Obstet 126:1301, 1968
149. Davidson ED, Bradley EL III: "Marsupialization" in the treatment of pancreatic abscess. Surgery 89:252, 1981
150. Hedderich GS, Wexler MJ, McLean APH, et al: The septic abdomen: open management with Marlex mesh and a zipper. Surgery 99:399, 1986
151. D'Egidio A, Schein M: Surgical strategies in the treatment of pancreatic necrosis and infection. Br J Surg 78:133, 1991
152. Rotman N, Mathieu D, Anglade MC, et al: Failure of percutaneous drainage of pancreatic abscesses complicating severe acute pancreatitis. Surg Gynecol Obstet 174:141, 1992
153. Lang EK, Paolini RM, Pottmeyer A: The efficacy of palliative and definitive percutaneous versus surgical drainage of pancreatic abscess and pseudocysts: a prospective study of 85 patients. South Med J 84:55, 1991
154. Lawson DW, Daggett WM, Civetta JM, et al: Surgical treatment of acute necrotizing pancreatitis. Ann Surg 172:605, 1970
155. Williams LF Jr, Byrne JJ: The role of bacteria in hemorrhagic pancreatitis. Surgery 64:967, 1968
156. Gregg JA: Detection of bacterial infection of the pancreatic ducts in patients with pancreatitis and pancreatic cancer during endoscopic cannulation of the pancreatic duct. Gastroenterology 73:1005, 1977
157. Farkas G, Marton J, Mandi Y: Surgical strategy and management of infected pancreatic necrosis. Br J Surg 80:980, 1996
158. Grant JP, James S, Grabowski V, et al: Total parenteral nutrition in pancreatic disease. Ann Surg 200:627, 1984
159. Lawhorne TW Jr, Zuidema GD: Splenic abscess. Surgery 79:686, 1976
160. Caldarera E: L'ascesso acuto della milza. Ann Ital Chir 16:953, 1937
161. Blumer G: Subacute bacterial endocarditis. Medicine (Baltimore) 2:105, 1923
162. Billings AE: Abscess of the spleen. Ann Surg 88:416, 1928
163. Chulay JD, Lankerani MR: Splenic abscess: report of 10 cases and review of the literature. Am J Med 61:513, 1976
164. Pickleman JR, Paloyan E, Block GE: The surgical significance of splenic abscess. Surgery 68:287, 1970
165. Parrish RA, Sherman HC: The surgical significance of splenic abscess. Am Surg 30:712, 1964
166. Johnson JD, Raff MJ, Drasin GF, et al: Radiology in the diagnosis of splenic abscess. Rev Infect Dis 7:10, 1985
167. Reid SE, Lang SJ: Abscess of the spleen. Am J Surg 88:912, 1954
168. Sones PJ: Percutaneous drainage of abdominal abscesses. AJR Am J Roentgenol 142:35, 1984
169. Teich S, Oliver G, Canter JW: The early diagnosis of splenic abscess. Am Surg 52:303, 1986
170. Berkman WA, Harris SA Jr, Bernardino ME: Nonsurgical drainage of splenic abscess. AJR Am J Roentgenol 141:395, 1983
171. Longmire WP: Suppurative cholangitis. Critical Surgical Illness. Hardy JD, Ed. WB Saunders Co, Philadelphia, 1971, p 400
172. Huang T, Bass JA, Williams RD: The significance of biliary pressure in cholangitis. Arch Surg 98:629, 1969
173. Stewart L, Pellegrini CA, Way LW: Cholangiovenous reflux pathways as defined by corrosion casing and scanning electron microscopy. Am J Surg 155:23, 1988
174. Lygidakis NJ, Brummelkamp WH: Bacteremia in relation to intrabiliary pressure in proximal versus distal malignant biliary obstruction. Acta Chir Scand 152:305, 1986
175. O'Connor MJ, Sumner HW, Schwartz ML: The clinical and pathologic correlations in mechanical biliary obstruction and acute cholangitis. Ann Surg 195:419, 1982
176. Flemma RJ, Flint LM, Osterhout S, et al: Bacteriologic studies of biliary tract infection. Ann Surg 166:563, 1967
177. Weissglas IS, Brown RA: Acute suppurative cholangitis secondary to malignant obstruction. Can J Surg 24:468, 1981
178. Elson CO, Hattori K, Blackstone MO: Polymicrobial sepsis following endoscopic retrograde cholangiopancreatography. Gastroenterology 69:507, 1975
179. Ong GB: A study of recurrent pyogenic cholangitis. Arch Surg 84:199, 1962
180. Jackaman FR, Triggs CM, Thomas V, et al: Experimental bacterial infection of the biliary tract. Br J Exp Pathol 61:369, 1980
181. Thompson JE, Tompkins RK, Longmire WP Jr: Factors in management of acute cholangitis. Ann Surg 195:137, 1982
182. Lewis RT, Goodall RG, Marien B, et al: Biliary bacteria, antibiotic use, and wound infection in surgery of the gallbladder and common bile duct. Arch Surg 122:44, 1987
183. Finegold SM: Anaerobes in biliary tract infection (editorial). Arch Intern Med 139:1338, 1979
184. Shimada K, Inamatsu T, Yamashiro M: Anaerobic bacteria in biliary disease in elderly patients. J Infect Dis 135:850, 1977
185. Shimada K, Noro T, Inamatsu T, et al: Bacteriology of acute obstructive suppurative cholangitis of the aged. J Clin Microbiol 14:522, 1981
186. Lee WJ, Chang KJ, Lee CS: Surgery in cholangitis: bacteriology and choice of antibiotic. Hepatogastroenterology 39:347, 1992
187. Bourgault AM, England DM, Rosenblatt JE, et al: Clinical characteristics of anaerobic bactibilia. Arch Intern Med 139:1346, 1979

Acknowledgments

Figures 2 through 5   Dr. L. Stein, Montreal, Quebec.

Figure 6   From "Computed Tomography and the Prediction of Pancreatic Abscess in Acute Pancreatitis," by J. H. C. Ranson, E. Balthazar, R. Caccavale, et al, in *Annals of Surgery* 201:656, 1985. Used by permission.

Figure 7   From "Nonsurgical Drainage of Splenic Abscess," by W. A. Berkman, S. A. Harris Jr., and M. E. Bernardino, in *American Journal of Roentgenology* 141:395, 1983. Used by permission.

84 HAND INFECTION

Thomas M. Sinclair, M.D., C.M., and H. Bruce Williams, M.D.

At the beginning of the 20th century, with the Industrial Revolution under way, hand injuries became extremely common, but most hand deformities or disabilities were still the result of minor injuries that became infected. Indeed, during the preantibiotic era, infection was responsible for 50% to 75% of hand deformities.[1] Kanavel's pioneering anatomic work on defining the fascial planes led to the development of a unique approach to the localization and proper surgical drainage of hand infections.[2] His principles of treating hand infections remain useful to this day.

Although antibiotics have greatly decreased the incidence of serious, life-threatening infections, minor hand infections are still responsible for considerable morbidity, numerous lost manpower hours, and substantial health care costs.[3] Accurate, prompt diagnosis is the first and most important step in the treatment of hand infections. The diagnosis is based on a clear understanding of the anatomy of the hand, a careful history and physical examination, a thorough knowledge of the organisms that are likely to be involved, and an informed awareness of the specific host factors that might alter the treatment plan (e.g., diabetes, intravenous drug abuse, and immunocompromised states).

Anatomy of the Hand

Almost all hand infections develop after the skin barrier has been violated in some manner. Because infectious organisms usually spread through specific anatomic fascial planes or compartments, it is often possible for the physician to predict how the infection will subsequently be disseminated throughout the hand. To this end, a brief review of the relevant anatomic structures in the hand should prove useful.

Tendon sheaths in the hand have double walls, made up of a visceral layer (epitenon) and a parietal layer. They are hollow structures that join at their proximal and distal ends.[4] In most hands, the sheaths of the index, long, and ring fingers extend from the palm at the midpalmar crease to just proximal to the distal interphalangeal joint [see Figure 1]. The flexor sheath of the little finger expands radially at the level of the midpalm to envelop the tendons of the ring, long, and index fingers and continues 2 cm proximal to the volar wrist crease. This expanded proximal portion of the sheath is commonly called the ulnar bursa. The thumb flexor sheath extends from 2 cm proximal to the volar wrist crease to the distal phalanx. The proximal half of this sheath is often called the radial bursa.[5,6] In 50% to 80% of patients, there is a communication between the radial bursa and the ulnar bursa, and this communication is responsible for the appearance of the so-called horseshoe abscess as a result of suppurative tenosynovitis of the little finger or the thumb[6] [see Management of Specific Common Hand Infections, Suppurative Flexor Tenosynovitis, *below*].

There are two major deep potential spaces within the hand [see Figure 1] whose function is to protect neurovascular structures and to permit the gliding of tendons within the hand.[5,7] The first potential space is the thenar space, which lies deep to the flexor tendons and extends from the third metacarpal bone toward the thumb to occupy the area of the thenar eminence. The dorsal boundary of this space is the adductor pollicis, and the volar boundary is the flexor tendon sheath of the index finger.[5,7,8] The second potential

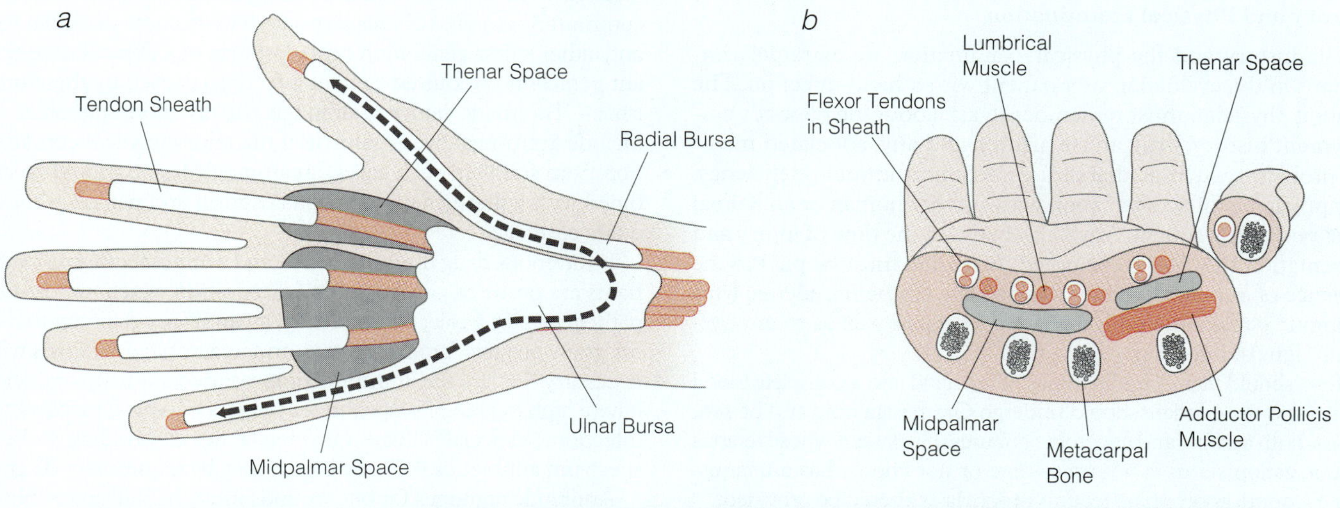

Figure 1 Depicted are the anatomic relations of the flexor sheaths, the bursae, and the deep spaces. The dashed arrow (*a*) represents the path of a horseshoe abscess, in which a communication exists between the radial bursa and the ulnar bursa. A cross-section of the hand through the palm (*b*) provides a different view of several of these structures. The midpalmar space and the thenar space are actually potential spaces in which infection can predictably spread.

Table 1 Causative Organisms and Appropriate Antibiotic Therapy for Specific Hand Infections

Infection	Causative Organisms	Antibiotic Therapy
Cellulitis/lymphangitis	Streptococci	First-generation cephalosporin or penicillin
Paronychia	*Staphylococcus aureus*	First-generation cephalosporin or penicillinase-resistant penicillin
Felon	*S. aureus*	First-generation cephalosporin or penicillinase-resistant penicillin
Suppurative flexor tenosynovitis	*S. aureus*, streptococci, gram-negative bacteria	First-generation cephalosporin and penicillin Consider aminoglycoside
Abscess in web space, thenar space, or midpalmar space	*S. aureus*, gram-negative bacteria, anaerobes	First-generation cephalosporin and penicillin Consider aminoglycoside
Human-bite wound infection	*S. aureus*, streptococci, *Eikenella corrodens*, anaerobes	First-generation cephalosporin and penicillin
Animal-bite wound infection	*Pasteurella*, *S. aureus*, viridans streptococci, anaerobes	First-generation cephalosporin and penicillin
Septic arthritis	*S. aureus*, streptococci, *Neisseria gonorrhoeae*, gram-negative bacteria	First-generation cephalosporin or penicillinase-resistant penicillin Consider aminoglycoside High-dose penicillin for gonococcal infection
Osteomyelitis	*S. aureus*, gram-negative bacteria, pseudomonads	First-generation cephalosporin or penicillinase-resistant penicillin Consider aminoglycoside Consider third-generation cephalosporin
Necrotizing fasciitis	Group A streptococci, mixed anaerobes (e.g., *Bacteroides*)	Penicillin with metronidazole and aminoglycoside Consider clindamycin and aminoglycoside

space is the midpalmar space, which extends from the third metacarpal bone to the hypothenar eminence. Its dorsal boundary consists of the metacarpal bones and the interosseous muscles, and its volar boundary is made up of the flexor tendons and the lumbrical muscles.[5,7,8]

Microorganisms usually enter these spaces either as a result of direct injury or by spreading from adjacent compartments such as tendon sheaths, joint spaces, or fascial planes. An infection that develops in one of these closed spaces can cause significant and rapid tissue necrosis; the inflammation and edema produce early venous congestion and subsequent local arterial compromise.

History and Physical Examination

The history and the physical examination are extremely important in the evaluation of a patient with a hand infection. The treating physician must remember to ask about the patient's employment history, drug abuse history, and any associated medical problems, such as diabetes or acquired immunodeficiency. Any possibility of an altercation with another human or an animal must be actively sought. Any delay between the time of injury and presentation should also be noted. Attention must be paid to the presence of puncture wounds, tenderness, erythema, edema, lymphangitic streaking, and lymphadenopathy as well as to any systemic signs of infection.

Tests should include radiographs of the hand and a complete blood count, and the exudate should undergo Gram's staining and be sent out for both aerobic and anaerobic cultures. If a patient whose tetanus immunization status is not up to date or not known has a tetanus-prone wound, appropriate tetanus prophylaxis should be provided.

Likely Pathogens

In the preantibiotic era, β-hemolytic streptococci were a common cause of rapidly spreading and often lethal hand infection. Since the advent of antibiotics, however, the situation has changed: at present, the principal bacterial pathogen in 50% to 80% of hand infections is *Staphylococcus aureus*.[9,10] Knowledge of the likely pathogen or pathogens is essential in planning antibiotic therapy for hand infections.

The mode of injury, the presentation of the infection, and the status of the host will all help identify the most likely causative organism. Cultures of the exudate and Gram's staining (see above) should be performed routinely before empirical antibiotic treatment is begun. Preliminary antibiotic therapy should be focused on the most likely causative organism [*see Table 1*] for the specific infection present (see below). In most home and industrial injuries, gram-positive organisms are the predominant pathogens. Because the majority of community-acquired *S. aureus* species have become penicillin resistant, either a first-generation cephalosporin or a penicillinase-resistant penicillin is required to treat infections caused by these organisms.[11] Traumatic injuries, although usually monomicrobial, may include gram-negative organisms if the injury involves contamination from soil.[12] In such cases, an aminoglycoside should be combined with a first-generation cephalosporin and penicillin for adequate coverage.

Intravenous drug users, diabetics, and immunocompromised patients are prone to polymicrobial infections in which opportunistic pathogens play a role; consequently, an antibiotic regimen that covers gram-positive, gram-negative, and anaerobic organisms will be necessary.[13-16] In the immunocompromised patient, one should have a high degree of suspicion for fungal or atypical mycobacterial infections, especially if the infection is not responding to broad-spectrum antibiotics.[13] Tissue biopsy may be required for diagnosis.

Antibiotic regimens for bite wounds must include anaerobic coverage. *Eikenella corrodens*, an anaerobic gram-negative rod, is isolated from a large number of human-bite wounds,[17,18] and *Pasteurella multocida*, a gram-negative facultative anaerobe, is often isolated from animal-bite wounds.[19,20] Both pathogens are highly sensitive to penicillin.

General Principles of Treatment

There are four general therapeutic principles that are fundamental to the treatment of hand infections: (1) appropriate antibiotic therapy, (2) adequate debridement and surgical drainage, (3) a period of immobilization and elevation, and (4) early remobilization.[18]

Administration of antibiotics is guided by the clinical situation and the suspected organism [see Likely Pathogens, above]. If an infection is still in the cellulitic phase with no suppuration, then a period of nonoperative treatment with antibiotics is indicated [see Table 1].

If there is no improvement after 24 to 48 hours of adequate antibiotic therapy or if suppuration is evident, surgical drainage is indicated. After adequate anesthesia has been induced, the extremity is elevated but not exsanguinated, and a tourniquet is applied. Incisions should be made in parallel with the neurovascular structures whenever possible but should never cross flexion crease lines at a perpendicular angle. It is essential that debridement of infected and necrotic tissue accompany surgical drainage of closed spaces. Abscesses are drained through an incision located over the point of maximal tenderness or fluctuance. It is best to leave incisions and contaminated wounds open so that they can drain and heal secondarily. Delayed primary closure can be considered once the infection has cleared and the wound is clean.

It is important to elevate and immobilize the hand. Splinting of the hand in the so-called safe position helps prevent joint stiffness, decrease pain, and prevent further spread of infection through muscle activity [see Figure 2]. Elevation of the hand above the level of the heart promotes drainage and alleviates edema and tenderness.

It is also important, however, that hand therapy and remobilization be started early, when pain, edema, and erythema begin to resolve. Early motion helps reduce morbidity by preventing joint stiffness and encouraging the patient to become actively involved with his or her treatment.[21]

Management of Specific Common Hand Infections

CELLULITIS AND LYMPHANGITIS

Cellulitis is a nonsuppurative inflammation of the connective tissue planes that is associated with pain, erythema, edema, and warmth in the involved region. Usually, a streptococcus is the responsible pathogen, but both aerobic and anaerobic organisms have been implicated.[4,15,16,22] Treatment involves administration of antibiotics and elevation and immobilization of the hand. If there is no improvement after 48 hours of adequate antibiotic therapy, then an abscess may be present that must be drained surgically.

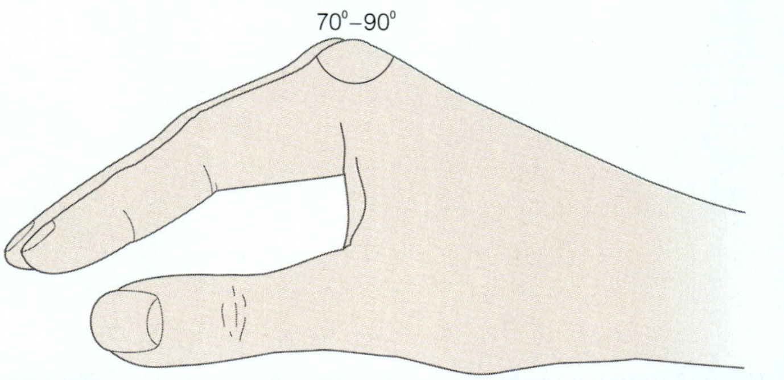

Figure 2 Shown is the proper hand position for splinting. The wrist is extended so that the slightly abducted thumb is in line with the axis of the radius. This safe position helps minimize joint stiffness, pain, and spread of infection.

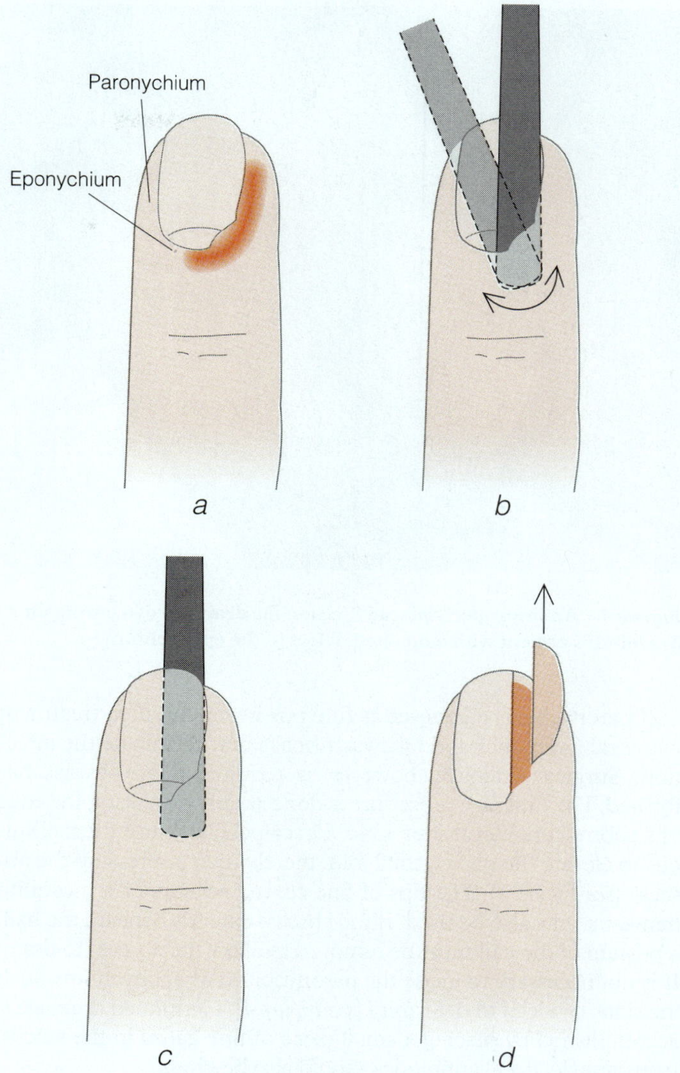

Figure 3 A paronychial infection can involve both the paronychium and the eponychium (*a*). The edge of a submucous elevator works well to lift the paronychium off the nail to facilitate abscess drainage (*b*). If the abscess has extended beneath the nail, the instrument should be gently pushed along the underside of the lateral portion of the nail to lift it off the nail bed (*c*). A small piece of the nail is then cut and removed to allow drainage (*d*).

Lymphangitis is an inflammation of the lymphatic pathways that is identified by red streaks extending along the dorsum of the hand and up the volar or dorsal aspect of the forearm. It is generally caused by streptococci. Treatment with appropriate antibiotics and elevation and splinting of the extremity usually lead to rapid improvement.[18,23]

PARONYCHIA

The thin layer of tissue extending onto the dorsum of the nail is called the paronychium laterally and the eponychium proximally [see Figure 3]. A paronychia is a subcuticular abscess in the paronychial fold. It must be distinguished from herpetic whitlow, which is a viral infection of the digit, because the two conditions are treated very differently [see Management of Specific Uncommon Hand Infections, Viral Infections, *below*]. A paronychia usually results from nail biting, manicures, or hangnails and is most commonly caused by *S. aureus*.[3,6,7,18,23] Local pain and swelling develop, but the infection may also spread proximally under the nail to involve the nail bed.

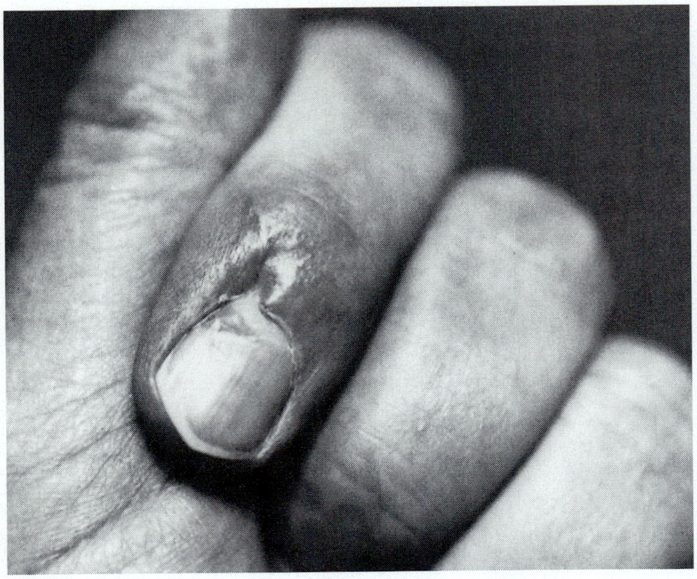

Figure 4 An improperly placed incision for drainage of a paronychia has left this patient with a notched defect in the eponychium.

If paronychia is diagnosed before pus is present, then treatment with oral antibiotics and lukewarm soaks may terminate the infection. Surgical drainage, however, is required if an abscess has formed. The drainage procedure is done simply by placing the edge of a submucous elevator or a No. 11 scalpel blade into the nail sulcus to elevate the paronychial fold, thereby decompressing the abscess [*see Figure 3*]. The tips of fine curved scissors or a mosquito hemostat may also be used. If the abscess extends beneath the nail, a portion of the nail must be removed to allow the abscess to drain. It is not necessary to incise the paronychium or eponychium; such incisions can lead to deformity [*see Figure 4*]. Continued drainage is accomplished by placing a small piece of fine gauze in the sulcus. Antistaphylococcal antibiotics should also be given.

Chronic paronychia is a different disease process and is commonly seen in persons whose hands are chronically exposed to moisture, such as cleaners, dishwashers, and swimmers. The nail fold becomes tender, swollen, and erythematous and pulls away from the nail. Repeated exacerbations are the rule and are difficult to treat.[3,7] Fungal organisms are commonly implicated in this condition. Appropriate treatment of chronic paronychia involves avoidance of chronic exposure to moisture and, sometimes, packing the nail fold with antifungal agents or surgically removing a crescent-shaped piece of skin parallel to the eponychium to promote drainage.[18]

FELON

A felon is a subcutaneous infection of the pulp space of the distal phalanx, but it is considered a closed-space infection because of the multiple septa that divide the pulp into fascial compartments[5] [*see Figure 5*]. An abscess forms in the pulp space, usually as a result of a penetrating injury. The organism most commonly implicated in the infection is *S. aureus*. The fingertip becomes painful, erythematous, and swollen. Since a felon is a closed-space infection, early treatment is advocated before increased pressure causes tissue necrosis. An untreated felon can lead to osteomyelitis of the distal phalanx, suppurative flexor tenosynovitis (see below), or skin necrosis.

Of the many incisions that have been used for drainage, the high lateral incision or the palmar longitudinal incision is recommended[3,8,24,25] [*see Figure 5*]. When the latter is used, care must be taken not to cross the flexion crease. A loose gauze packing and frequent lukewarm soaks help keep the wound draining. The patient should be instructed to elevate the hand so as to reduce the pain and swelling. An oral antistaphylococcal antibiotic (e.g., a penicillinase-resistant penicillin or a first-generation cephalosporin) should also be given.

SUPPURATIVE FLEXOR TENOSYNOVITIS

Pyogenic flexor tenosynovitis is an infection of the closed synovial flexor tendon sheaths [*see Figure 6*]. Although pyogenic flexor tenosynovitis is not as common as it once was, it is still potentially devastating. Penetrating trauma is the usual mode of entry; *S. aureus* is the most common pathogen, followed by streptococci and pseudomonads.[6] There are four cardinal signs associated with these tendon sheath infections: (1) fusiform swelling of the entire finger, (2) semiflexed resting position of the finger, (3) excessive tenderness along the entire sheath, and (4) excruciating pain along the entire sheath on passive extension of the digit. The last sign is the most important because the first three may be seen in other finger infections that do not involve the sheaths.[25,26]

If the diagnosis is made early in the disease process, nonoperative treatment is indicated: I.V. administration of high doses of a broad-spectrum cephalosporin, immobilization, and elevation. Because ongoing infection can lead to tendon necrosis or proximal spread, surgical treatment is indicated if improvement is not seen after 24 hours of conservative management. Suppurative tenosynovitis of the little finger or thumb can develop into a horseshoe abscess if the infection spreads proximally and there is a communication between the radial bursa and the ulnar bursa[5,8,26] [*see Figure 7*]. An ulnar bursa infection should be drained through an incision along the radial aspect of the hypothenar eminence and a proximal incision on the ulnar aspect of the wrist[5,7] [*see Figure 8*]. The radial bursa is opened with both a thenar crease incision and a longitudinal incision on the proximal radial aspect of the wrist.

The closed flexor tendon sheath irrigation technique is a popular method of drainage that lacks the disadvantages associated with an extensive digital incision.[26] Incisions are made at the proximal and distal levels of the sheath [*see Figure 9*]. After the fluid is cultured, a 16- or 18-gauge catheter is placed within the proximal portion of the sheath and sutured in place. Another catheter or a small rubber drain is placed in the distal end of the sheath to form a patent irriga-

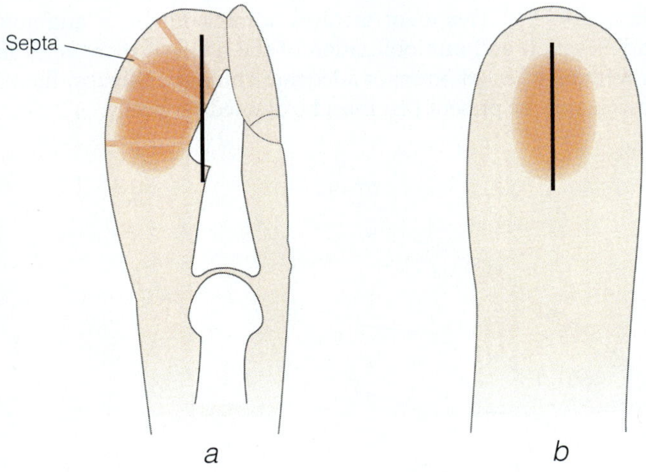

Figure 5 A felon can be drained through a high lateral incision with blunt dissection carried into the closed spaces defined by the septa in the finger pulp (*a*). An alternative method of drainage is through a palmar longitudinal incision that must not cross the distal flexion crease (*b*).

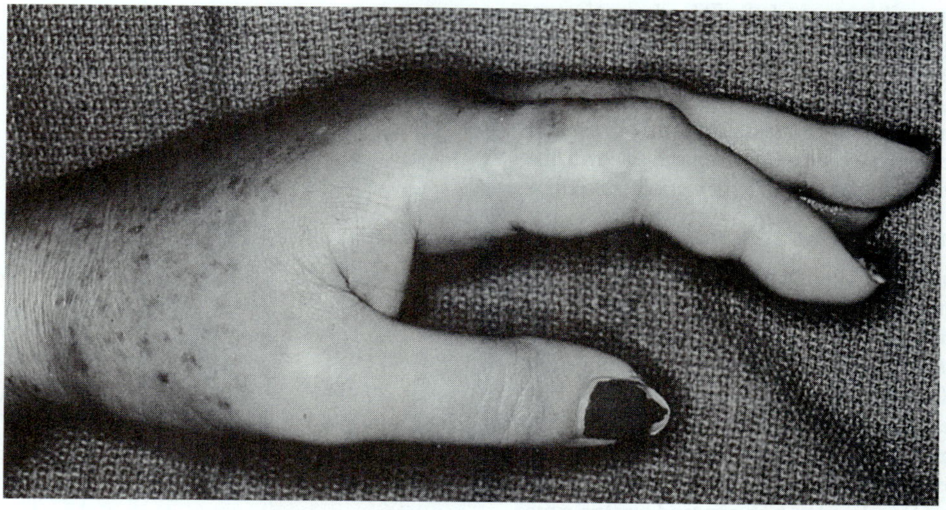

Figure 6 This patient has suppurative flexor tenosynovitis of the index finger caused by a puncture wound. Note the fusiform swelling and the classic semiflexed resting position of the finger.

tion system. The hand is then placed in a bulky dressing, and the sheath is irrigated every 2 hours with 50 ml of saline. In 48 to 72 hours, if the tenderness is gone, the catheter can be removed and hand therapy with mobilization can begin.

WEB SPACE INFECTION

A subcutaneous infection of the web between the digits is most commonly caused by a puncture or by extension of a palmar blister or callus that becomes secondarily infected.[18,27] Because the skin adheres to the underlying fascia, pus can track dorsally to produce a secondary abscess on the dorsum of the hand. An infection of this sort is called a collar button abscess because of its hourglass appearance.[27] Both a palmar and a dorsal incision are required to drain these abscesses [see Figure 10]. Drains should be used to keep the wound open until no more purulent material is forthcoming.

An unusual type of web space infection is that known as barber's hand. Cellulitis, an abscess, or an epithelialized fistulous tract can develop between the fingers of barbers as a result of hairs that have penetrated the skin of the web space.[28] Usually, a pinpoint opening with a protruding hair is noted in the web space, and occasionally, a localized cyst may develop. Treatment primarily consists of removal of the offending hair and, if cellulitis is present, administration of antibiotics. Abscess drainage may be required. Once the cellulitis has resolved, the cyst and the fistulous tract should be excised.

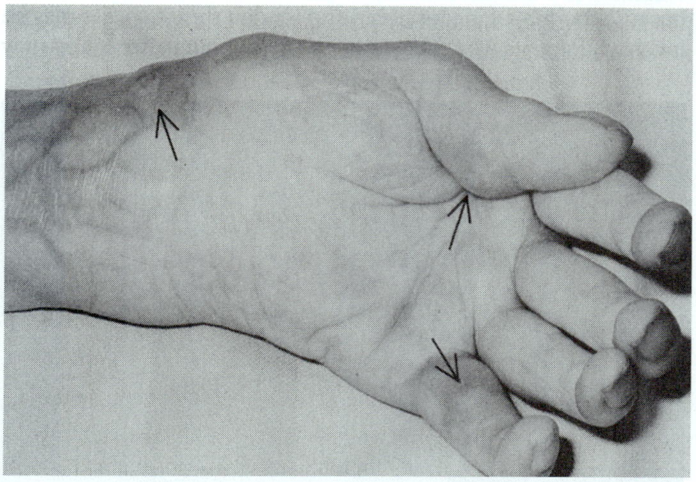

THENAR SPACE INFECTION

The thenar space is vulnerable to infection resulting from puncture wounds or from contiguous spread of flexor tendon sheath infections. Clinically, thenar space infections present as a swollen thenar eminence with the thumb abducted [see Figure 11]. Passive adduction of the thumb causes significant pain. Pus in the thenar space can spread dorsally around the adductor pollicis to produce swelling on the dorsum of the hand.[18,27] Again, both a palmar incision and a dorsal incision may be necessary for adequate drainage of these infections. The palmar incision parallels the thenar crease, and the dorsal incision extends longitudinally along the border of the first dorsal interosseous muscle. Catheters may be left in place for irrigation with saline.

MIDPALMAR SPACE INFECTION

Like thenar space infections, midpalmar space infections result from penetrating trauma or from spread of sheath infections of the overlying long and ring fingers. Infection may spread to the dorsal subcutaneous space to cause impressive swelling. Infections in the midpalmar space can be drained through a transverse incision located near the distal palmar crease[27] [see Figure 10].

BITE WOUND INFECTION

Dogs and cats are responsible for the majority of bites to the human hand. Although rabies is uncommon in domestic dogs and cats, it is essential to verify the rabies immunization status of any dog or cat that bites a human; if this is impossible, the animal must be observed for signs of rabies. Both dogs and cats harbor a variety of organisms in their saliva, including *S. aureus,* viridans streptococci, and *P. multocida*.[19,23,29,30] *Pasteurella* is isolated from 50% of dog-bite wounds and 75% of cat-bite wounds.[20] Cat bites are usually more severe than dog bites because cats' sharp teeth can penetrate farther into the tissue, making the wound more difficult to clean.[29] When

Figure 7 A horseshoe abscess has developed in this 73-year-old patient with rheumatoid arthritis who is receiving long-term steroid therapy. The arrows show the abscess "pointing" over the flexor tenosynovial sheaths of the thumb and the little finger as well as over the radial bursa. Despite aggressive surgical drainage, the patient died of overwhelming sepsis.

The infection progresses rapidly and is usually associated with signs of systemic toxicity. Treatment involves fluid resuscitation, immediate debridement of all involved tissue, and high-dose I.V. penicillin. Hyperbaric oxygen therapy may also have a role in the treatment of these serious infections.

VIRAL INFECTIONS

The virus most commonly associated with infection of the hand is herpes simplex virus, which causes a cyclic infection of the skin.[18] The virus is spread by direct contact or autoinoculation.[36,37] In the hand, herpetic whitlow presents as a painful localized swelling of the distal phalanx coupled with the appearance of clear vesicles[38] [see Figure 13]. The most important aspect of diagnosis of this infection is to recognize it and distinguish it from a felon or paronychia; with herpetic whitlow, surgical drainage is contraindicated because it can lead to viral dissemination. The appearance of vesicles is virtually pathognomonic of a herpetic infection; however, the diagnosis can be confirmed by means of a relatively simple and rapid immunofluorescent diagnostic test. Scrapings from the bases of the vesicles are placed on a glass slide, which is then fixed with a fluorescein-labeled monoclonal antibody that is specific for the herpes simplex virus. The diagnosis is made if the preparation fluoresces when exposed to ultraviolet light.

The infection is self-limited but may take up to 4 weeks to disappear. Simple unroofing of the vesicles may help relieve the pain.[36] Over the first 2 weeks, the vesicles coalesce to form an ulcer, which gradually resolves. Acyclovir is generally not necessary except for immunocompromised patients, in whom it may decrease morbidity and may actually be needed to cure the infection.[15]

MYCOBACTERIAL INFECTIONS

Mycobacterium tuberculosis infections are rare in the hand but may be seen in immunocompromised patients[15] or in patients who live in areas where tuberculosis is very prevalent. The ubiquitous atypical mycobacteria, however, are being identified more frequently in hand infections, and in fact, approximately 75% of all atypical mycobacterial infections involve the hand. *M. marinum* is the most common pathogen.[18] This organism inhabits freshwater and saltwater environments; accordingly, inoculation is usually the result of penetrating trauma (e.g., fish bites) or scrapes from boat docks, fish tanks, or swimming pools.[39,40] Diagnosis of mycobacterial infections in the hand is difficult and depends on a high degree of suspicion. Cultures and tissue biopsy are usually required. Histologic evidence of granulomas or smears showing acid-fast bacilli also help verify the diagnosis.

Most mycobacterial skin lesions are self-limited; however, deeper infections involving the tendon sheath, the bursae, the joints, or bone call for surgical debridement and long-term administration of oral antituberculous antibiotics, such as isoniazid, ethambutol, and rifampin. Minocycline has also been shown to be effective in the treatment of *M. marinum* infections.[39,40] Antibiotic treatment usually must be continued for anywhere from 3 months to a year.

Other atypical mycobacterial organisms involved in hand infections include *M. kansasii*, *M. fortuitum*, and *M. chelonei*.

FUNGAL INFECTIONS

Fungal infections should always be considered in the differential diagnosis of chronic nail and skin lesions. *Trichophyton rubrum* is the most common pathogen, causing tinea of the skin and infections of the fingernails (onychomycosis).[41] Treatment involves removal of the nail and topical administration of fungicides.

Fungal infections involving the subcutaneous tissues or the closed spaces of the hand are relatively uncommon but are difficult to treat when present. Sporotrichosis is a lymphocutaneous infection caused by *Sporothrix schenckii*,[18,41] an organism that is found in soil and plant material. A chronic granulomatous infection develops and then ulcerates. A chain of nodules or ulcers develops and ascends the arm along the course of the lymphatic vessels. The lesions heal spontaneously but will recur unless they are treated with oral potassium iodide. Deep histoplasmosis, blastomycosis, or coccidioidomycosis can cause tenosynovitis, septic arthritis, or osteomyelitis. These conditions may be seen in immunocompromised surgical patients; surgical debridement and intravenous administration of amphotericin B are required.

Conclusion

In summary, hand infections should be treated with the utmost respect. The key to successful management of these infections is accurate diagnosis and prompt treatment. Appropriate tetanus prophylaxis must be provided, when indicated, in cases of penetrating injury. Many hand infections, if diagnosed early, can be treated with antibiotic therapy and elevation and immobilization of the hand. In the case of an established infection characterized by suppuration or involvement of a closed space, prompt surgical drainage and debridement are required in addition to the steps just mentioned. Once the infection has resolved, hand therapy and remobilization are essential. If these principles are followed, rapid and complete recovery can be achieved, with minimal morbidity.

References

1. Mock HE: Treatment of hand infections from an economic viewpoint: based on a study of 1600 cases. Surg Gynecol Obstet 21:481, 1915
2. Kanavel AB: An anatomical, experimental, and clinical study of acute phlegmons of the hand. Surg Gynecol Obstet 1:221, 1905
3. Canales FL, Newmeyer WL 3rd, Kilgore ES Jr: The treatment of felons and paronychias. Hand Clin 5:515, 1989
4. Neviaser RJ: Tenosynovitis. Hand Clin 5:525, 1989
5. Lampe EW: Surgical anatomy of the hand: with special reference to infections and trauma. Clin Symp 40(3):1, 1989
6. Siegel DB, Gelberman RH: Infections of the hand. Orthop Clin North Am 19:779, 1988
7. McGrath MH: Infections of the hand. Plastic Surgery, Vol 8: The Hand. McCarthy JG, Ed. WB Saunders Co, Philadelphia, 1990
8. Neviaser RJ: Infections. Operative Hand Surgery, 2nd ed. Green DP, Ed. Churchill Livingstone, New York, 1988, p 1027
9. Carter SJ, Mersheimer WL: Infections of the hand. Orthop Clin North Am 1:445, 1970
10. Mann RJ: Infections of the Hand. Lea & Febiger, Philadelphia, 1988
11. Spiegel JD, Szabo RM: A protocol for the treatment of severe infections of the hand. J Hand Surg 13:254, 1988
12. Fitzgerald RH Jr, Cooney WP 3rd, Washington JA 2nd, et al: Bacterial colonization of mutilating hand injuries and its treatment. J Hand Surg 2:85, 1977
13. Jones NF, Conklin WT, Albo VC: Primary invasive aspergillosis of the hand. J Hand Surg 11:425, 1986
14. Dhaliwal AS, Garnes AL: Tenosynovitis in drug addicts. J Hand Surg 7:626, 1982
15. Glickel SZ: Hand infections in patients with acquired immunodeficiency syndrome. J Hand Surg 13:770, 1988
16. Mann RJ, Peacock JM: Hand infections in patients with diabetes mellitus. J Trauma 17:376, 1977
17. Faciszewski T, Coleman DA: Human bite wounds. Hand Clin 5:561, 1989
18. Hausman MR, Lisser SP: Hand infections. Orthop Clin North Am 23:171, 1992
19. Arons MS, Fernando L, Polayes IM: *Pasteurella multocida*—the major cause of hand infections following domestic animal bites. J Hand Surg 7:47, 1982
20. Lucas GL, Bartlett DH: *Pasteurella multocida* infection in the hand. Plast Reconstr Surg 67:49, 1981

21. Mancini LH, Fort LK: Rehabilitation of the infected hand. Hand Clin 5:635, 1989
22. Burton RI: The hand. Principles of Surgery, 4th ed. Schwartz SI, Ed. McGraw-Hill, New York, 1984, p 2061
23. Kilgore ES Jr: Hand infections. J Hand Surg 8:723, 1983
24. Kilgore ES Jr, Brown LG, Newmeyer WL, et al: Treatment of felons. Am J Surg 130:194, 1975
25. American Society for Surgery of the Hand: The Hand: Primary Care of Common Problems. ASSH, Aurora, Colorado, 1985
26. Neviaser RJ: Closed tendon sheath irrigation for pyogenic flexor tenosynovitis. J Hand Surg 3:462, 1978
27. Burkhalter WE: Deep space infections. Hand Clin 5:553, 1989
28. Cahill JM: Special infections of the hand. Hand Surgery. Flynn JE, Ed. Williams & Wilkins, Baltimore, 1966, p 832
29. Snyder CC: Animal bite wounds. Hand Clin 5:571, 1989
30. Goldstein EJ, Citron DM, Wield B, et al: Bacteriology of human and animal bite wounds. J Clin Microbiol 8:667, 1978
31. Chuinard RG, D'Ambrosia RD: Human bite infections of the hand. J Bone Joint Surg [Am] 59:416, 1977
32. Mann RJ, Hoffield TA, Farmer CB: Human bites of the hand: twenty years of experience. J Hand Surg 2:97, 1977
33. Dreyfuss UY, Singer M: Human bites of the hand: a study of one hundred six patients. J Hand Surg 10:884, 1985
34. Freeland AE, Senter BS: Septic arthritis and osteomyelitis. Hand Clin 5:533, 1989
35. Schecter W, Meyer A, Schecter G, et al: Necrotizing fasciitis of the upper extremity. J Hand Surg 7:15, 1982
36. Polayes I, Arons M: The treatment of herpetic whitlow—a new surgical concept. Plast Reconstr Surg 65:811, 1980
37. Fowler JR: Viral infections. Hand Clin 5:613, 1989
38. Louis DS, Silva J Jr: Herpetic whitlow: herpetic infections of the digits. J Hand Surg 4:90, 1979
39. Hurst LC, Amadio PC, Badalamente MA, et al: *Mycobacterium marinum* infections of the hand. J Hand Surg 12:428, 1987
40. Gunther SF, Levy CS: Mycobacterial infections. Hand Clin 5:591, 1989
41. Hitchcock TF, Amadio PC: Fungal infections. Hand Clin 5:599, 1989

Recommended Reading

Burton RI, Rockwell WB: Hand. Principles of Surgery, 6th ed. Schwartz SI, Shires GT, Spencer FC, Eds. McGraw-Hill, New York, 1994, p 2001

Dunn DL: Infection. Surgery: Scientific Principles and Practice, 2nd ed. Greenfield LJ, Mulholland MW, Oldham KT, et al, Eds. Philadelphia, Lippincott-Raven Publishers, 1997, p 173

Acknowledgments

Figures 1 through 3, 5, 8 through 10, and 12 Tom Moore. Adapted from original drawings by Jennifer Morrison, Audiovisual Department, Montreal Children's Hospital.

Figures 6 and 7 Supplied by H. Brown, M.D., Division of Plastic and Reconstructive Surgery, Montreal General Hospital.

Figure 11 Supplied by C. L. Kerrigan, M.D., Division of Plastic and Reconstructive Surgery, Royal Victoria Hospital, Montreal.

Figure 13 Supplied by B. Moroz, M.D., Department of Dermatology, Montreal Children's Hospital.

85 FUNGAL INFECTION

Elias J. Anaissie, M.D., Bishara B. Albair, M.D., and Joseph S. Solomkin, M.D.

Approach to the Surgical Patient at Risk for Candidiasis

The infectious diseases that are most commonly encountered by surgeons are acute events in which fever, leukocytosis, and localized signs of inflammation develop in a reasonably healthy host. In this clinical situation, the presence of microorganisms in such normally sterile foci as blood and intra-abdominal sites indicates an infection and the need for antimicrobial chemotherapy.

The clinical setting in which *Candida* species are isolated from various body sites is generally much different. Patients harboring *Candida* infections frequently have had antecedent infections that were treated with antibacterial agents, have received therapy that suppressed their immunologic responses,[1] or have undergone extensive surgery or several operations, especially on the gastrointestinal tract. Such patients are generally long-term residents in acute care hospitals. Previous operative intervention may have left surgical wounds or drainage tracts. These circumstances favor colonization by various opportunistic pathogens, with the resultant risk of overgrowth or invasion by normal enteric microorganisms such as *Candida* species. In this setting, the elements that characterize most infectious processes (i.e., an acute change from wellness to illness and isolation of microorganisms from ordinarily sterile sites) no longer have great diagnostic value.

The problem of defining indications for administration of antifungal therapy in surgical patients is compounded by the limited data available, the difficulty of establishing a diagnosis, and the small number of effective antifungal agents. Although amphotericin B is currently the standard antifungal agent, fluconazole, a newer triazole antifungal that is generally well tolerated, appears to be effective in the treatment of serious *Candida* infections in surgical patients.

Noncandidal fungal infections, although still rare in surgical patients, may cause morbidity and mortality. Because infections such as aspergillosis and mucormycosis may be refractory to standard antifungal therapy, there is an urgent need to define the role of novel antifungal agents in surgical patients.

This chapter summarizes the current understanding of fungal infections, particularly candidiasis, in nonneutropenic surgical patients and provides recommendations for prophylaxis and therapy.

Magnitude of the Problem in the Surgical Patient

Whereas the high mortality associated with bacterial infections in surgical patients has been reduced by the early administration of antibacterial therapy, the incidence of fungal infections, particularly with *Candida* species, has dramatically increased.[2] In a 1984 nationwide survey of medical and surgical patients, *Candida* species were the eighth most common cause of nosocomial bloodstream infection.[3] In a similar survey conducted between October 1986 and December 1990, *Candida* species became the fourth leading cause of nosocomial bloodstream infection, preceded only by coagulase-negative-staphylococci, *Staphylococcus aureus*, and enterococci.[3] According to the National Nosocomial Infections Surveillance (NNIS) system, the percentage of nosocomial infections caused by *C. albicans* increased from 2% in 1980 to an average of 5% over the 4-year period from 1986 through 1989.[4] Data from NNIS hospitals also show that between 1980 and 1989, the incidence of primary bloodstream infections attributable to *Candida* species increased by 487% in large teaching hospitals and by 219% in small (< 200 bed) hospitals.[5] In addition, the NNIS system reported that the rate of nosocomial fungal infection increased from 2.0 to 3.8 infections per 1,000 patients discharged between 1980 and 1990.[6] Current data from the SCOPE (Surveillance and Control of Pathogens of Epidemiologic Importance) system confirm that *Candida* species were the fourth leading cause of bloodstream infection.[7] These data are supported by the Surveillance Network–USA, which compiles information from more than 100 laboratories in the United States. Fungi including *Candida* species were isolated from 17% of 10,038 patients included in a European study of the prevalence of infection in patients in intensive care units.[8]

The most marked increase in candidiasis occurred in surgical patients, particularly in burn and trauma patients followed by cardiac surgery patients and general surgery patients. *Candida* species now account for 78% of all nosocomial fungal infections.[6]

Nosocomial bloodstream infections caused by *Candida* species are an independent predictor of risk of mortality (38% mortality directly attributable to candidiasis) and prolonged hospital stay (30 additional days in comparison with controls).[1] In a more recent prospective study, *Candida* species were the only microorganisms that independently influenced the outcome of nosocomial primary infections of the bloodstream (odds ratio for mortality, 1.84; 95% confidence interval [CI]) and were associated with the highest mortalities (35% at 28 days and 69% at discharge).[9] In properly conducted multivariate analyses, the most important prognostic factors in patients with hematogenous candidiasis include older age, poor performance status (on Acute Physiology and Chronic Health Evaluation [APACHE] or other measures), the presence and persistence of neutropenia, and dissemination of the infection to noncontiguous organs. Central venous catheter retention appears to play a minimal role.[8,10]

Definitions of Hematogenous *Candida* Infection Syndromes

In this chapter, the general term hematogenous candidiasis is used to identify all infections involving the bloodstream. Hence,

Identify patient at risk for *Candida* infection

Major risk factors include
- Previous bacterial infection and therapy with multiple antibiotics.
- Isolation of *Candida* from ≥ 2 sites.
- Disruption of the intestinal mucosal barrier (total parenteral nutrition, severe diarrhea, colitis, major operation, trauma, or extensive burns).
- Immunosuppression (neutropenia, cancer, organ transplantation, hemodialysis, or extensive burns).

Other risk factors include
- Tunneled central venous catheters • Urinary catheters • Prematurity • Heroin addiction.

Initiate studies to diagnose candidiasis

Obtain cultures of sputum, oropharynx, stool, urine, drain sites, and blood.

Obtain 2 sets of blood cultures daily for 2 days (or longer if the patient remains febrile).

Consider serologic tests and histologic analyses (see text).

Look for findings that may signal hematogenous candidiasis:
- Endophthalmitis • Suppurative thrombophlebitis • High-grade candiduria without instrumentation of the bladder or the renal pelvis.

Exclude other possible causes of persistent fever.

Blood cultures are positive for *Candida*, or clinical or laboratory signal of potential hematogenous candidiasis is present

---

Patient is hemodynamically stable, does not have high-grade candidemia, and does not appear to have organ infection

Remove all venous catheters.   *or*

Leave venous catheter in place initially, and consider removal if clinical condition deteriorates or does not improve after 2 days of therapy.

Patient is infected or colonized by *C. albicans*, *C. tropicalis*, *C. parapsilosis*, or other germ tube–positive candidal organism

Give fluconazole, 600–800 mg/day I.V. for 2–3 days, then, if possible, lower dosage to 400 mg/day p.o.

Treat for 7–10 days (patient should be free of signs and symptoms of infection for 5 days before treatment is ended).

Patient is infected or colonized by *C. krusei*, *C. glabrata*, or *C. lusitaniae*

Give amphotericin B, 0.5–0.7 mg/kg/day. (Consider adding flucytosine, 25 mg/kg/day p.o. in 2 divided doses, for *C. glabrata* and *C. lusitaniae*.)

Treat for 5–7 days (patient should be free of signs and symptoms of infection for 5 days before treatment is ended).

Approach to the Surgical Patient at Risk for Candidiasis

Blood cultures are negative for *Candida*, and no clinical or laboratory signal of potential hematogenous candidiasis is present, but *Candida* is isolated from ≥ 2 remote sites (≥ 1 site for *C. tropicalis*)

Give fluconazole, 400 mg/day I.V. for 2–3 days, then 400 mg/day p.o. If patient is colonized by *C. krusei*, *C. glabrata*, or *C. lusitaniae*, give amphotericin B, 0.5 mg/kg/day. (Consider adding flucytosine, 25 mg/kg/day p.o. in 2 divided doses, for *C. glabrata* and *C. lusitaniae*.)

Treat for 7–10 days (patient should be free of signs and symptoms of infection for 5 days before treatment is ended).

Blood cultures are negative for *Candida*, no clinical or laboratory signal of potential hematogenous candidiasis is found, and *Candida* is isolated from ≤ 1 remote site (0 sites for *C. tropicalis*)

Continue surveillance cultures weekly.

Patient is hemodynamically unstable, has high-grade candidemia, or shows evidence of organ infection

Remove all venous catheters.
Treat any associated syndromes of hematogenous candidiasis (e.g., endophthalmitis, pericarditis, suppurative thrombophlebitis, endocarditis).

Patient is infected or colonized by *C. albicans*, *C. tropicalis*, *C. parapsilosis*, or other germ tube–positive candidal organism

Give fluconazole, 800 mg/day I.V. (Consider adding flucytosine, 25 mg/kg/day p.o. in 2 divided doses. Also consider adding G-CSF, 300 µg/day.)

Treat for 10–14 days after disappearance of all signs and symptoms of infection.

Patient is infected or colonized by *C. krusei*, *C. glabrata*, or *C. lusitaniae*

Give amphotericin B, 0.7–1.0 mg/kg/day I.V. (Consider adding flucytosine, 25 mg/kg/day p.o. in 2 divided doses. Also consider adding G-CSF, 300 µg/day).

Treat for 10–14 days after disappearance of all signs and symptoms of infection.

hematogenous candidiasis refers to candidemia, disseminated candidiasis, or both.

CANDIDEMIA

Candidemia is defined as the isolation of any pathogenic species of *Candida* from at least one blood culture specimen. The recovery of *Candida* species from the bloodstream can be a significant observation in the absence of clinical signs and symptoms, especially if the patient is debilitated or uremic or is receiving adrenal corticosteroid therapy.

CATHETER-ASSOCIATED CANDIDEMIA

Catheter-associated candidemia is candidemia that occurs in a patient with an intravascular catheter and no other obvious origin of infection after careful clinical and laboratory evaluation. Several procedures have been developed to aid in the diagnosis of catheter-associated candidemia. If the catheter is removed, a quantitative culture of the tip should recover at least 15 colony-forming units (CFU) of the same *Candida* species as that found in blood culture by the roll-plate technique (or at least 100 CFU of the same *Candida* species as that found in blood culture by the sonication technique). If the catheter is not removed, a quantitative blood culture collected through a central catheter should contain at least a 10-fold greater concentration of *Candida* species than a simultaneously collected quantitative peripheral blood culture. Routine catheter tip cultures appear to be of no value.

ACUTE DISSEMINATED CANDIDIASIS

Patients who have several noncontiguous organs infected by *Candida* species have a disseminated infection acquired through hematogenous spread. For diagnosis, the organism must be identified by histologic analysis, culture of tissue samples obtained from at least one internal organ, or both; the patient should have radiographic, pathologic, or cultural evidence of infection in at least one other organ. Candidemia associated with *Candida* skin lesions or endophthalmitis consistent with a diagnosis of *Candida* infection also indicates a diagnosis of disseminated candidiasis.[11]

CHRONIC DISSEMINATED CANDIDIASIS

Chronic disseminated candidiasis, a chronic form of disseminated infection that is also known as hepatosplenic candidiasis, occurs in cancer patients who have been afflicted with protracted neutropenia.[12] This form of hematogenous candidiasis has not yet been described in the nonneutropenic surgical patient.

Characteristics of Surgical Patients at Risk for Candidiasis

Fungal translocation that leads to hematogenous candidiasis is believed to be promoted by (1) colonization of the GI tract by *Candida* species, (2) physical disruption of the intestinal mucosal barrier, and (3) immunosuppression of the host leading to dissemination of the infection in the bloodstream and other organs [see Discussion, *below*].

Other important risk factors for hematogenous candidiasis include malignancies,[13] neutropenia and immunosuppressive therapy,[14] use of urinary catheters and diarrhea, prematurity,[15] heroin addiction,[16] abdominal surgery,[17] organ transplantation,[18] and extensive burns.[19]

The reported frequency of hematogenous candidiasis in burn patients ranges from 2% to 14%, depending on the reporting center and the study period.[19-21] Colonization by *Candida* species, hematogenous dissemination, and mortality caused by *Candida* infections have been found to correlate with the amount of body surface area burned and with the extent of full-thickness burn.

The pathogenesis, the incidence, and the microbial etiology of fungal infection vary in different groups of transplant recipients, depending on the organ transplanted, the donor source, the type of surgical procedure performed, and the recipient's age and general condition at the time of the procedure; other influential factors are the conditioning regimen, the type and duration of immunosuppressive therapy, and the presence or absence of organ rejection and graft versus host disease. In heart transplant recipients, for example, *Aspergillus* infection is a major problem, whereas in other organ transplant recipients, most fungal infections are attributable to *Candida*.[22] The infection is usually located at the site of the operation (e.g., an intra-abdominal abscess in liver[18] or pancreas[23] transplantation, the mediastinum or the lungs in heart[24] or heart-lung[25] transplantation, and the urinary tract in kidney[26] transplantation); however, dissemination from the primary site is common.

The central venous catheter has been reported as a risk factor in some studies but not in others,[10] particularly with *Candida parapsilosis*. This species, which may become part of the biofilm of intravascular catheters, may not respond to antifungal agents. Alternatively, *Candida* colonization of the catheter may result from gut-derived hematogenous seeding.[27,28]

Laboratory and Clinical Assessment of Candidiasis

CULTURES

The workup of the surgical patient suspected of having hematogenous candidiasis begins with a complete set of cultures of sputum, oropharynx, stool, urine, all drain sites, and blood [see Table 1]. Candidiasis rarely develops in patients whose cultures show no evidence of *Candida* at some site. Obtaining more than six sets of blood cultures has little value, and there is no evidence to support arterial cultures.

The incidence of positive antemortem blood cultures in patients found to have candidiasis at autopsy is about 30% to 50%, possibly as a result of concomitant bacteremia, which may decrease the recovery of *Candida* species from the bloodstream. Because *Candida* species grow poorly under anaerobic conditions, venting the blood culture bottles is thought to improve the yield. The use of biphasic media also improves recovery of *Candida* species from the blood. Improved sensitivity and time to positivity of fungal blood cultures has been achieved with the development of new media, including biphasic media, automated radiometric and nonradiometric systems, and the lysis-centrifugation technique, a system that allows estimation of the number of *Candida* CFU/ml blood).[29] Commercial applications of these techniques include the BACTEC high-blood-volume fungal media system and the BacT/Alert system, both having comparable sensitivity to lysis-centrifugation. There is little evidence, however, that use of these newer methods provides a clinical advantage in the management of patients with hematogenous candidiasis. In a study by Berenguer and colleagues, the sensitivity of the lysis-centrifugation method increased with increasing numbers of involved organs but was still only 58% overall.[30]

Table 1 Clinical Presentation and Diagnostic Methods for Common Fungal Infections[139]

Host Fungus	Major Clinical Presentations	Diagnostic Methods
Normal host		
Aspergillus	Allergic bronchopulmonary	Serum IgE, precipitins
Blastomyces	Acute pneumonitis: chronic lung or skin	Culture, tissue
Candida	Vaginitis, thrush, candidemia, I.V. catheter	Culture/smear
Coccidioides	Acute pneumonitis, chronic cavitary, pulmonary nodule	Precipitins, complement fixation, culture
Cryptococcus	Pulmonary, meningitis	Culture, latex agglutination
Histoplasma	Acute pulmonary, progressive dissemination in infants and elderly, chronic cavitary in chronic airway obstruction	Culture, antigen detection
Compromised host		
Diabetes mellitus		
Candida	Disseminated, pyelonephritis, vaginitis	Culture/smear
Torulopsis	Pyelonephritis	Culture
Zygomycetes	Rhinocerebral, paranasal, pulmonary, gastrointestinal, cutaneous	Culture, tissue
Malignancy or corticosteroids		
Aspergillus	Invasive/lung, sinuses, disseminated	Culture, tissue
Candida	Fungemia, acute and chronic disseminated candidiasis	Culture, tissue
Coccidioides	Disseminated	Culture, precipitins, complement fixation
Cryptococcus	Pulmonary, meningeal, disseminated	Culture, latex agglutination, India ink preparation
Dematiaceous fungi	Lung, sinuses, brain, disseminated	Culture, tissue
Fusarium	Lung, sinuses, cellulitis at site of onychomycosis, disseminated	Culture, tissue
Histoplasma	Progressive disseminated	Culture, antigen detection
Torulopsis	Disseminated	Culture, tissue
Trichosporon	Disseminated	Culture, tissue
Zygomycetes	Rhinocerebral, paranasal, pulmonary, gastrointestinal, cutaneous, disseminated	Culture, tissue
Extensive surgery and previous antibiotic therapy		
Candida	Vaginitis, thrush, esophagitis, disseminated	Culture, tissue
Torulopsis	Disseminated	Culture

A rapid and inexpensive test is the germ tube test that can distinguish *C. albicans* (positive test) from other *Candida* species. More than 90% of *C. albicans* isolates produce germ tubes when incubated in serum for 2 to 3 hours at 37° C.

Several new culture media allow the rapid identification of *C. albicans*. These include Albicans ID (bioMerieux, France), CandiSelect (Sanofi Diagnostics Pasteur, France), CHROMagar *Candida* (Becton Dickinson, USA), Fluoroplate *Candida* (Merck, Germany), Fongiscreen 4H (Sanofi Diagnostics Pasteur), and Murex *Candida albicans* (Murex Diagnostics, USA). CHROMagar and Fongiscreen 4H are also used for detection of other *Candida* species, including *C. glabrata*, *C. tropicalis*, and *C. krusei*. A recent study of 485 isolates (350 of *C. albicans* and 135 of other candidal species) evaluated the presumptive identification of *C. albicans* by comparing results of the germ-tube test to results of these six commercial tests. For *C. albicans,* the sensitivity and specificity of all six tests were greater than 97%. The sensitivity and specificity of the two tests that allow presumptive identification of other candidal species (CHROMagar *Candida* and Fongiscreen 4H) were lower, especially for *C. glabrata* and *C. tropicalis*.

Positive cultures from nonsterile sites (sputum, urine, and wound drainage) need to be interpreted with caution because of the frequent occurrence of *Candida* as a normal commensal of humans. Such cultures are useful mainly as an indication of colonization and, consequently, of the risk of infection in the appropriate setting.

ANTIBODY DETECTION

Previous studies have reported the use of incompletely characterized antigenic extracts of *C. albicans* to detect anticandidal antibodies in human sera. Difficulties with consistent production of uniform materials[31] have limited the usefulness of these tests. A variety of detection technologies (enzyme-linked immunosorbent assay [ELISA], immunodiffusion, and latex agglutination) have been used in attempts to detect antibodies directed toward defined purified antigen, but the sensitivity and specificity of these methods are low.[32] Methods using newly described antigens appear more promising.[33]

ANTIGEN DETECTION AND POLYMERASE CHAIN REACTION

Mannan, a polysaccharide component of the *Candida* cell wall, has the disadvantages of a short serum half-life and binding by antimannan antibody.[34] Although mannan can be detected by several methods,[35] complicated techniques are required to dissociate the mannan-antibody complex.[36] The sensitivity of mannan detection is approximately 70%.

A simple test available commercially (CAND-TEC *Candida* detection system, manufactured by Ramco Laboratories, USA) relies on the detection of a heat-labile antigen; however, its low sensitivity (as low as 19%) and specificity have limited its clinical use.[37] An antigen studied more recently is an immunodominant 48 kd cytoplasmic protein, *Candida* enolase. Because it is thought that cytoplasmic antigens are released during invasive infection, detection of this antigen may be able to distinguish between colonization and invasive infection.[33] A sensitivity of 54% was demonstrated in a study of 24 patients with invasive candidiasis,[38] but the sensitivity increases to 75% with the use of multiple samples. A sensitivity of 65% and a specificity of 97% were shown in a study assessing multiple samples.[39] Unfortunately, this test is not commercially available.

A commercial kit (Bichro-latex albicans) using monoclonal antibodies against cell wall extracts of *C. albicans* mannoprotein appears to have high sensitivity and specificity for *C. albicans*.[40]

Another antigen studied is (1-3)-β-D-glucan, an important cell wall constituent of fungi that is not shared with bacteria. Studies of this assay, which indicates the presence of fungi but does not identify the genus causing infection, have been promising in patients with fungal colonization. In these patients, its concentration remains lower than 20 pg/ml.

Amplification of the DNA of *Candida* species appears to be a quick and specific diagnostic tool. Although multiple approaches have been pursued,[41-43] several limitations need to be overcome before this method can be used routinely.[44]

METABOLITES

Systems based on the detection of D-arabinitol and mannose release by the fungus have been proposed,[45] but only those detecting D-arabinitol have been extensively developed. D-Arabinitol, a pentose produced by all of the major *Candida* species except *C. krusei* and *C. glabrata*, is excreted by the kidneys in the same rate as creatinine, and the ratio of D-arabinitol to creatinine must be used to interpret any observed concentration of D-arabinitol. Gas-liquid chromatographic as well as enzymatic methods are available for the detection of D-arabinitol, but gas-liquid chromatography is both technically demanding and expensive; it has been replaced by the recently developed enzymatic assay system. The sensitivity of the serum D-arabinitol–creatinine ratio for the diagnosis of invasive candidiasis, reported in the range of 40% to 83%, rises with repeated sampling.[46] Sensitivity is highest in patients with fungemia (74% to 83%) and lowest in patients with tissue-invasive *Candida* infections (40% to 44%). The magnitude of the D-arabinitol–creatinine ratio is strongly related to the degree of tissue invasion.[28,46] Although this assay may produce false positive results in some patients, it offers the promise of earlier detection of invasive candidiasis.[46]

Mannose, the other metabolite of *Candida* species that has been studied, can be detected only by a complicated gas-liquid chromatographic system. Initial estimates of its sensitivity (39%) have limited interest in this technique.[45]

HISTOLOGIC ANALYSES

Fungal smears are relatively insensitive methods of diagnosing candidiasis in otherwise sterile sites (e.g., joint fluid, peritoneal fluid, vitreous humor, or cerebrospinal fluid). Centrifugation of these fluids and examination of the sediment may improve the diagnostic yield. Conventional fungal stains, such as hematoxylin-eosin, periodic acid–Schiff (PAS), and Gomori methenamine-silver (GMS), are useful. The most sensitive stain is calcofluor white, but unfortunately, it requires fluorescent microscopy. Deep tissue biopsy provides a definitive diagnosis of candidiasis.

CLINICAL DIAGNOSIS

Hematogenous candidiasis has no characteristic clinical picture. Three clinical findings that may lead to an early diagnosis of hematogenous candidiasis in the surgical patient are candidal endophthalmitis, suppurative phlebitis, and candiduria in the absence of bladder instrumentation. A careful eye examination to identify the presence of candidal infection should be performed while the results of cultures of various sites are being awaited, and a repeat examination should be performed after therapy for proven candidemia. Candidal endophthalmitis may remain asymptomatic until late in the course of infection.

The presence of peripheral suppurative phlebitis that fails to yield bacteria or does not respond to antibacterial agents may be an early clue to the presence of hematogenous candidiasis. Gentle squeezing of the venous catheter exit site may express pus that yields *Candida* species on a smear or culture. Surgical excision of the infected vein usually reveals *Candida* infection in its lumen.

The presence of high-grade candiduria in surgical patients who have not had instrumentation of the renal pelvis or the bladder suggests hematogenous candidiasis and should prompt a workup for this infection. In this setting, candiduria may result from seeding of or filtering through the kidney.

Fever may be the only sign of infection but may be absent in patients who are receiving corticosteroids. Occasionally, a patient with hematogenous candidiasis presents with the systemic inflammatory response syndrome (SIRS) or septic shock. The diagnosis should be seriously considered in high-risk patients who are persistently febrile. Because of the high mortality associated with this infection, empirical antifungal therapy is recommended for early treatment of a clinical occult fungal infection or for the prevention of new fungal infections.

Management of Hematogenous Candidiasis

CANDIDEMIA AND ACUTE DISSEMINATED CANDIDIASIS

During the 1960s and the 1970s, the standard approach to managing candidemia was to classify patients according to degree of risk of disseminated candidiasis and to withhold antifungal treatment from those in whom dissemination appeared to be unlikely. This approach was based on unawareness of the magnitude of the problem in surgical patients and on acute awareness of the toxicities of amphotericin B, which was the only systemic antifungal agent available at the time; eventually, this type of management was found to be associated with a substantial mortality and a high incidence of long-term sequelae (e.g., deep-seated candidiasis presenting with endophthalmitis or other organ infection).[1] Consequently, it is now common practice to treat all candidemic patients except those who are afebrile, asymptomatic, or at low risk for disseminated candidiasis [see Table 2].

Candidates for empirical antifungal therapy are at high risk for candidiasis, colonized by *Candida* species (at one or more sites for *C. tropicalis* or at two or more for other candidal species), and unresponsive to broad-spectrum antibiotics in the absence of any other cause for their fever. Unresponsive patients may be characterized by rapid clinical deterioration, particularly if there is evidence of physical disruption of the intestinal mucosal barrier or immunosuppression.

The role of amphotericin B in the treatment of hematogenous candidiasis in surgical patients has been difficult to determine—first, because most of the studies that evaluated amphotericin B were retrospective trials with small sample sizes, and second, because few of the studies defined hematogenous candidiasis in the same way. In one study, treatment with amphotericin B had no effect on overall outcome in a mixed population of patients; however, the timing of therapy and the dose administered were not clearly stated.[47] In general, mortality was lower in patients who re-

Table 2 Antimicrobial Agents of Choice for Candidal Infections*

Infection	Agent of Choice	Alternative Agents	Comments
Hematogenous			
Candidemia and acute disseminated candidiasis	Fluconazole, or amphotericin B ± flucytosine	Lipid formulations of amphotericin B	Fluconazole should be given for *C. albicans*, amphotericin for all other *Candida* species; a 2-drug regimen should be given to hemodynamically unstable patients with persistent high-grade fungemia
Candida endophthalmitis	Fluconazole	Amphotericin B + flucytosine	Patients with vitral involvement require vitrectomy in addition to antifungal therapy
Suppurative phlebitis	Fluconazole + flucytosine	Amphotericin B + flucytosine	The central venous catheter should be removed and the infected vein excised
Endocarditis	Amphotericin B + flucytosine	—	Surgical replacement or repair of valves is essential to prevent death from embolization or cardiac failure; oral fluconazole should be given after successful completion of a prolonged course of amphotericin B therapy
Pericarditis	Amphotericin B	Fluconazole	—
Prosthetic device–related infection	Fluconazole or amphotericin B	—	Removal of device is required for successful therapy
Arthritis	Fluconazole	—	—
Osteomyelitis	Amphotericin B	Fluconazole	Surgical drainage of pus is required
Meningitis	Amphotericin B + flucytosine	Fluconazole + flucytosine	—
Nonhematogenous			
Oropharyngeal			
Otherwise normal host	Nystatin	Ketoconazole, fluconazole, clotrimazole troches	—
Patients at risk for hematogenous infection (e.g., cancer patients, surgical patients)	Fluconazole	Ketoconazole	—
Deep candidiasis			
Esophagitis and GI candidiasis	Fluconazole	Amphotericin B	Amphotericin B should be reserved for cases of fluconazole failure without endoscopic evidence of other causes of disease
Peritonitis and intra-abdominal	Fluconazole	Amphotericin B	—
Wound	Fluconazole	Amphotericin B	Antifungal therapy should be given to patients who do not respond to antibacterial therapy
Urinary tract			
Cystitis	Fluconazole	Amphotericin B	Fluconazole is preferable because of its high drug concentration in urine and because it is better tolerated
Pyelitis			
Without papillitis	Fluconazole	—	—
With papillitis	Fluconazole + flucytosine	Amphotericin B	—
Pyelonephritis	Fluconazole + flucytosine	Amphotericin B	—

*Therapy is individualized on the basis of the patient's clinical condition and the infecting species.

ceived amphotericin B than in those who did not.[48] Significant amphotericin B–related nephrotoxicity may occur.

The discovery of the azole antifungal agents has changed the management of *Candida* infections. The first two azoles, clotrimazole and miconazole, were not, however, suitable for systemic use. As for ketoconazole, the lack of a parenteral formulation and the erratic bioavailability of the drug in patients receiving H_2 receptor blockers or antacids have limited its use in the treatment of hematogenous candidiasis in surgical patients.

Fluconazole is a well-tolerated triazole with good activity in hematogenous candidiasis. Data available from several clinical trials suggest that the drug is as effective as and better tolerated than amphotericin B. Overall, four comparative studies have been completed in various patient populations. Two were randomized,[49,50] one was prospective observational,[51] and one used matched cohorts.[50] Fluconazole dosages ranged from 200 to 800 mg/day, given orally or intravenously, while intravenous amphotericin B was given at doses of 0.3 to 1.2 mg/kg.

The first prospective, randomized study of fluconazole included 40 surgical patients with hematogenous candidiasis, of whom 20 received 300 mg/day of fluconazole and 20 received 0.5 mg/kg/day of amphotericin B plus flucytosine.[52] There were no significant differences in outcome between the two study groups.

A matched-pair study compared the outcomes of 45 candidemic cancer patients who were treated with fluconazole with the outcomes of 45 candidemic cancer patients who were treated with amphotericin B[53]; in several of the 90 patients, hematogenous candidiasis had developed after operation. This study demonstrated that fluconazole was as effective as and better tolerated than amphotericin B. In one prospective, randomized multicenter study, 164 patients with documented or presumed invasive candidiasis received either amphotericin B, 0.7 mg/kg/day, or fluconazole, 400 mg/day.[50] The response rate for fluconazole (62%) was virtually identical to that for amphotericin B (63%), and fluconazole was better tolerated. In another prospective, randomized multicenter study, 206 nonimmunocompromised candidemic patients received either amphotericin B or fluconazole.[49] Once again, the two drugs were comparable in their efficacy, and fluconazole had a better safety profile.

Newer therapeutic options have now become available with the advent of the lipid-associated formulations of amphotericin B, which are less nephrotoxic than the parent compound.[54] Thus far, three lipid products of amphotericin B have been marketed in Europe or the United States: Abelcet (amphotericin B lipid complex), Amphocil (amphotericin B colloidal dispersion), and AmBisome (liposomal amphotericin B). A prospective, randomized trial has shown that Abelcet is as efficacious as conventional amphotericin B in hematogenous candidiasis.[55]

All patients with candidemia should receive antifungal therapy. We recommend the administration of fluconazole, 600 to 800 mg/day I.V. for 3 days, particularly if the infecting organism is known to be or is likely to be *C. albicans*. If the patient responds rapidly to this regimen, the dosage may be decreased to 400 mg/day and administered orally. For patients with hematogenous candidiasis who are known to be colonized by *C. glabrata*, *C. krusei*, or *C. lusitaniae*, amphotericin B, 0.5 to 0.7 mg/kg/day, should remain the treatment of choice. For patients who are hemodynamically unstable and for those who have high-grade persistent fungemia, we recommend a two-drug antifungal regimen: the combination of fluconazole and flucytosine or the combination of amphotericin B and flucytosine, depending on the infecting strain.

Clinical data on the effect of itraconazole in hematogenous candidiasis are scant. Given that itraconazole has limited bioavailability in the presence of antacids and H_2 receptor blockers, it should not be used to treat hematogenous candidiasis in the critically ill. However, an I.V. formulation of itraconazole is now available, and it is possible that this formulation may prove effective in patients with hematogenous candidiasis.

Liposomal formulations of amphotericin B offer new therapeutic alternatives. Their substantial cost limits their routine use, but they are appropriate if the patient has renal failure and is infected with an azole-resistant strain. Of the three available formulations, AmBisome is the best tolerated and yields the highest blood levels of amphotericin B.

The duration of therapy depends on the extent and severity of the infection. Therapy can be limited to 7 to 10 days for patients with low-grade fungemia and no evidence of organ involvement or hemodynamic instability. Patients with high-grade fungemia and evidence of organ involvement or hemodynamic instability need to receive antifungal therapy for 10 to 14 days after resolution of all signs and symptoms of infection.

Catheter Management

Controversy remains concerning the role of central venous lines in patients' outcome in hematogenous candidiasis. According to Nguyen and colleagues,[51] patients with catheter-related candidemia had a more favorable prognosis than patients with candidemia from other sources, but the prognosis was worse in patients whose catheters were retained. In contrast, studies by Carroll and colleagues, Nucci and coworkers,[56] and Anaissie and associates[10] failed to show a major role for retention of central venous catheters in the outcome of hematogenous candidiasis. The study by Anaissie and associates[10] examined the impact of catheter management on outcome in 416 cancer patients with candidemia who had an indwelling catheter at the time of candidal infection. Catheter exchange within 0, 2, or 4 days of the first positive blood culture had no significant effect on outcome. A second analysis, performed in a subset of 363 patients who had a central venous catheter in place and received antifungal therapy, revealed that catheter exchange was associated with improved outcome (80% versus 54%; $P < 0.001$). However, the subset in which the catheter was not exchanged had higher APACHE III scores and were more likely to be neutropenic. By multivariate analysis, catheter retention was not found to significantly affect outcome.

In one study in noncancer patients, Rex and colleagues[57] showed that replacement of all vascular catheters shortened the duration of candidemia from 5.6 days to 2.6 days. This finding suggests that catheters may play a role in perpetuating infection in nonneutropenic patients. In neutropenic patients, however, the primary source of candidemia is usually the GI tract, not the intravenous catheter, and other factors (e.g., the severity of disease, visceral dissemination, and neutrophil recovery) appear to have more impact on the outcome of neutropenic patients with candidemia.

Given the available data, we recommend that physicians consider the removal of all intravascular catheters in inpatients who have candidemia with persistent fever, persistent or high-grade fungemia, or *C. parapsilosis* (which is more likely to be catheter related than infection with other *Candida* species).

Cytokine Therapy for Opportunistic Infections

Polymorphonuclear leukocytes and macrophages are the predominant host defense against candidal infections. Candidal antigens induce lymphocyte proliferation and cytokine synthesis (interferon gamma and tumor necrosis factor); tumor necrosis factor enhances the candidacidal activity of phagocytes,[58] probably through increased production of reactive oxygen radicals. Another mechanism by which interferon gamma may augment host defenses against candidal infections is modulation of endothelial cell phagocytosis of *C. albicans*.[59] Granulocyte colony-stimulating factor (G-CSF) and granulocyte-macrophage colony-stimulating factor (GM-CSF) activate phagocytic cells to restrict the growth of *C. albicans*.[60]

Recently, a multicenter, double-blind, randomized phase II trial examined the activity of G-CSF in combination with fluconazole for treatment of hematogenous candidiasis in nonneutropenic patients. Preliminary analysis (Kullberg BJ and associates, unpublished report, 2000) indicated that an increase in the number of circulating neutrophils strongly correlates with accelerated clearance of bloodstream infection and reduced mortality. Additional data are needed to confirm these findings.

Antifungal Prophylaxis

Prophylaxis may be considered in surgical patients at high risk for invasive candidiasis. To date, there have been few trials of antifungal prophylaxis, whether as part of selective bowel decontamination[61] or in the form of low-dose amphotericin B[62] or liposomal formulations of amphotericin B in surgical transplant recipients.[63]

Fluconazole prophylaxis has been shown to reduce the rate of superficial and systemic fungal infections in cancer patients undergoing chemotherapy (with or without bone marrow transplantation)[64,65] and oropharyngeal and esophageal candidiasis in patients infected with HIV.[66] A recent double-blind randomized trial showed that intravenous fluconazole prophylaxis was effective in preventing candidal colonization and invasive intra-abdominal candidal infections in high-risk surgical patients.[67]

A retrospective study in burn patients reported that topical nystatin in the wound dressing was associated with a significant decrease in yeast acquisitions in burn wounds and fungemia but with an increase in colonization and fungemia caused by nystatin-resistant, amphotericin B–susceptible *C. rugosa*.[68]

Invasive fungal infection is one of the most important causes of mortality in organ transplant recipients.[69] Antifungal prophylaxis has been recommended in organ transplant recipients undergoing immunosuppressive therapy, but there is controversy about which drug is most effective and least toxic. Some physicians use fluconazole prophylactically in organ transplant recipients, but others recommend itraconazole or liposomal amphotericin B.[1,70,71]

ORGAN INFECTIONS

Candida *Endophthalmitis*

The diagnosis of candidal endophthalmitis usually implies hematogenous spread to multiple organs and the need for systemic antifungal therapy. Patients with chorioretinitis alone respond better to drug therapy alone than do those with vitreal involvement. Because antifungal drugs do not penetrate the vitreous body as well as the other ocular compartments,[72] patients with vitreal involvement require early vitrectomy in addition to antifungal therapy. Fluconazole is currently the drug of choice because of its proven efficacy and its higher concentration (20% to 70% of the corresponding plasma level) in ocular tissue, including the vitreous body.[73] Thus, we recommend 800 mg/day of fluconazole until a major response is observed, at which time it may be possible to reduce the dose to 400 mg/day. Although endophthalmitis due to *C. albicans* is commonly seen, recent series have reported on the importance of endophthalmitis caused by other candidal species. If the infecting organism (especially *C. krusei*) is potentially resistant to fluconazole, the recommended therapy is amphotericin B, 0.7 to 1.0 mg/kg/day I.V., preferably in conjunction with flucytosine.[74] Intravitreal injection of amphotericin B is recommended for vitreal infections.

The optimal duration of therapy for endogenous endophthalmitis is unknown, but we recommend that treatment be continued for at least 10 to 14 days after complete resolution of all signs and symptoms of infection. Ophthalmologic consultation is critical in establishing the diagnosis, assessing the patient's response to therapy, detecting complications, and determining whether early vitrectomy is indicated to prevent loss of sight.[75]

Suppurative Thrombophlebitis

A rare but serious consequence of hematogenous candidemia is suppurative thrombophlebitis, which results from infection of a vessel traumatized by prolonged catheterization. Endothelial disruption exposes the basement membrane and leads to thrombus formation and propagation. Suppurative thrombophlebitis is particularly serious because intravascular infection results in a persistent high-density fungemia. Management of this disease consists of high-dose antifungal therapy, removal of the central venous catheter, and excision of the infected vein, when possible.[76] Typically, blood cultures remain positive for several days; sometimes, they remain positive for as long as 3 to 4 weeks despite appropriate antifungal therapy, if the infected vein is not excised.

Endocarditis

Hematogenous candidiasis may also lead to the establishment of endocarditis, particularly in patients with a prosthetic heart valve or with a previously damaged native valve. Intravenous drug abuse and central intravenous catheterization appear to be predisposing factors. Candidal endocarditis after permanent pacemaker implantation has also been reported. The clinical picture is similar in many respects to that of bacterial endocarditis, although embolic phenomena have been more commonly associated with fungal endocarditis. Transesophageal echocardiography is more sensitive than transthoracic echocardiography in detecting candidal vegetation. Mortality due to *Candida* prosthetic valve endocarditis (PVE) is high, especially when complicated by congestive heart failure and persistent fungemia. For uncomplicated PVE, the mortality for patients receiving antifungal therapy alone (40%) is no worse than that for patients receiving combined medical and surgical therapy (33%).

Candidal endocarditis is very difficult to treat. Surgical replacement or repair of valves is essential to prevent death from embolization or cardiac failure in patients with complicated PVE. Amphotericin B, with or without flucytosine, has been the therapy of choice; however, neither the optimal dosage nor the optimal duration of therapy has been determined. There is anecdotal information on the successful use of fluconazole in this setting, primarily as long-term suppressive therapy after the initial administration of amphotericin B.[73,77] Because of the high risk of late relapse, long-term maintenance therapy with oral fluconazole should be begun after successful completion of a prolonged course of amphotericin B.

Pericarditis

Candidal pericarditis is a very rare complication of hematogenous candidiasis. The surgical patients at risk for purulent pericarditis caused by *Candida* species are those who have undergone a cardiac operation, those who have a malignancy and whose host defenses are impaired, and those who have a debilitating chronic disease.[78] High-dose amphotericin B therapy, with or without surgical drainage, is recommended in these cases.

Arthritis

Joint infections with *Candida* species have resulted from hematogenous spread from inadvertent direct inoculation during joint procedures or intra-articular injection of corticosteroids. These infections typically involve a single joint, most frequently the knee, and tend to occur in patients with rheumatoid arthritis or prosthetic joint devices.[79] Local symptoms of pain on weight bearing or on full extension may be present. Diagnosis is best achieved by visualizing or growing the organisms from the joint fluid. Early diagnosis and systemic antifungal therapy are important to prevent destruction of the cartilage or loosening of the prosthesis. Successful treatment with fluconazole has been reported in several patients with fungal arthritis.[80] We recommend a dose of 400 to 800 mg/day for 6 months. Fluconazole can be used in acute therapy, alone or in combination with surgery, as well as in long-term suppressive therapy in patients at risk for recurrence or those who cannot undergo surgical debridement.

Osteomyelitis

Except for sternal infections complicating median sternotomy, most cases of candidal osteomyelitis have followed hematogenous spread. Vertebral body involvement is common. Back pain and fever may be followed by radiculopathy. Surgical drainage of pus is essential for a good response; however, surgical debridement of bony lesions may not be needed. Although amphotericin B has been the standard drug of choice, fluconazole offers an alternative in the treatment of these cases.[81]

Meningitis

Candidal meningitis may follow hematogenous spread or be a complication of neurosurgery or the implantation of ventriculoperitoneal shunts.[82] The infection is insidious and may remain undiagnosed. Most patients have recently received antibacterial agents, and half have had antecedent bacterial meningitis. The overall mortality is around 10%. The standard therapy is amphotericin B with flucytosine. The combination of high-dose fluconazole (800 mg/day) and flucytosine (50 mg/kg/day) is a particularly attractive approach because of the high CSF concentrations achieved with both agents. Removal of the infected shunts is recommended when possible.[51,82] The duration of treatment should be based on clinical response and culture results.

Nonhematogenous Candidiasis

SUPERFICIAL INFECTION

Oral candidiasis (thrush) appears as a whitish, patchy pseudomembrane covering an inflamed oropharynx and commonly involves the tongue, the hard and soft palates, and the tonsillar pillars. Controlled trials have documented the efficacy of nystatin suspension, clotrimazole troches, oral ketoconazole, fluconazole, or itraconazole in eradicating the clinical symptoms of oral candidiasis.[83,84]

Nystatin should be given as a 10 to 30 ml suspension five times daily, and the patient should be instructed to swish it around the mouth before swallowing; alternatively, the patient may take one or two troches five times daily. Clotrimazole troches are given five times daily as a 10 mg troche that should be held in the mouth until dissolved. In surgical patients at risk for hematogenous infection, systemic therapy with ketoconazole (200 to 400 mg once daily), itraconazole (100 to 200 mg/day), or fluconazole (100 mg once daily) is preferred.[85] Antifungal therapy should be administered for 1 week, except for fluconazole therapy, which is likely to be effective when given for 2 or 3 days.

DEEP CANDIDIASIS

Esophagitis and Gastrointestinal Candidiasis

Superficial candidiasis involving only mucosal surfaces used to be a common finding at autopsy in surgical patients who had a protracted hospital stay characterized by recurrent sepsis. Such lesions may arise at any site in the GI tract but appear most commonly in the esophagus and the small bowel and may progress to hematogenous infection [see Figure 1].

In a minority of patients, the pathology of infection of the lower GI tract by *Candida* species may change from diarrhea without demonstrable tissue invasion to direct penetration into the submucosa, which eventually leads to pseudomembranous enterocolitis. Direct vascular invasion through the bowel wall has been reported only in patients receiving immunosuppressive chemotherapy.[86] These patients may have extensive involvement of the GI tract from mouth to anus. Nonneutropenic surgical patients exhibit more localized involvement.

The preferred therapy for esophageal candidiasis is fluconazole or itraconazole, 200 mg daily. In patients who remain symptomatic after 5 days of therapy, endoscopy is needed to rule out other causes of esophagitis. If endoscopy proves that esophagitis is caused by candidal infection, low-dose amphotericin B (0.4 mg/kg/day) should be administered. Therapy for esophageal candidiasis should be continued for at least 4 days after symptoms resolve; immunosuppressed patients generally require more extended therapy to prevent relapse.

Because stool cultures do not differentiate between colonization and infection, candidiasis in the lower gastrointestinal tract is usually a postmortem diagnosis; hence, there are no reliable criteria governing when and how to treat this condition. It has been reported, however, that patients who have diarrhea that can only be caused by heavy colonization with *Candida* species may respond dramatically to 2 to 4 days of nystatin therapy.[87]

Peritonitis and Intra-abdominal Abscess

Perhaps the most controversial aspect of *Candida* infectious syndromes in surgical patients is whether specific systemic therapy is required to eradicate the infection within intra-abdominal abscesses, peritoneal fluid, or fistula drainage. *Candida* is frequently cultured from intra-abdominal infectious foci but should be considered a serious threat only in high-risk patients. Four risk factors for intra-abdominal candidiasis are gastrointestinal perforations, anastomotic leakage, surgery for acute pancreatitis, and splenectomy.[88]

Patients with peritonitis and intra-abdominal abscesses should receive systemic antifungal therapy, usually in combination with antibacterial therapy, given that these infections are almost always polymicrobial in origin. The risk of dissemination is increased by both the recurrence of intra-abdominal infections and the presence of extensive areas of communication between the abdominal cavity and the external environment via either fistulas or drain tracts.

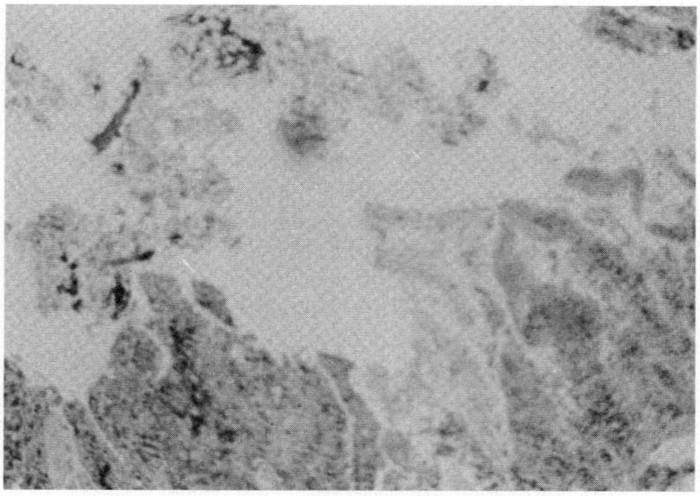

Figure 1 Superficial candidiasis may be found at all levels of the GI tract. Here, the esophagus of a patient found at autopsy to have disseminated candidiasis shows disrupted epithelium, submucosal inflammation, and the presence of yeast in the submucosa.

On rare occasions, candidal peritonitis occurs after long-term ambulatory peritoneal dialysis. In such cases, the infection tends to remain localized and to manifest with low-grade fever and abdominal pain and tenderness. The peritoneal dialysate is usually cloudy and contains more than 100 neutrophils/mm³. Therapy consists of systemic antifungal therapy and removal of the peritoneal catheter. The abdominal pain caused by the addition of amphotericin B to the dialysate has raised concern that chemical peritonitis might give rise to adhesions and thus impair the efficacy of dialysis.

Because fluconazole is very safe and is capable of reaching high concentrations in peritoneal fluid, it is likely to be useful in the management of candidal peritonitis.[89] Fluconazole should be given at a dosage of 100 to 200 mg/day orally for 2 to 6 weeks. Immediate removal of the peritoneal catheter has been recommended. In one study, however, seven of nine patients treated with oral flucytosine responded to therapy without catheter removal.[90]

A prospective, randomized study in patients on continuous ambulatory dialysis found that successful prophylaxis for *Candida* peritonitis was achieved with oral nystatin (tablets containing 500,000 units given four times a day).[91]

Occasionally, *Candida* species may cause cholangitis, biliary tract disease, pancreatic abscess, or liver abscess. This problem is increasingly found in patients with percutaneously placed drainage catheters for malignancy. Such patients must be given systemic therapy for clinical evidence of infection, including candidemia, and the drainage catheter must be changed. Diverticulitis complicated by candidal pylephlebitis has also been reported.

Wound Infections

The diagnosis and treatment of candidal wound infections are problematic. Recovering *Candida* species from drains and wounds does not necessarily mean that this organism is causing tissue infection. Colonization of wounds by *Candida* species should not compel physicians to use systemic antifungal therapy. However, such therapy should be administered to those patients whose wound infections do not respond to appropriate antibacterial therapy, particularly if one *Candida* species is repeatedly isolated from the site and the patient is at high risk for hematogenous infection. Antifungal therapy should be administered to prevent the establishment of Candida osteomyelitis when sternal wound cultures obtained after coronary artery bypass surgery yield Candida species.

Urinary Tract and Genital Candidiasis

The recovery of Candida species from the urinary tract most commonly results from contamination from the perirectal or the genital area or from colonization of the bladder, which is usually seen in patients who have undergone prolonged catheterization or who have diabetes mellitus or another disease that leads to incomplete bladder emptying. In addition, Candida species usually colonize ileal conduits. Persistent candiduria in the surgical intensive care unit may, however, be an early marker of disseminated infection in critically ill high-risk patients.[92] In a study of 91 pediatric ICU patients who were clinically suspected of having disseminated candidiasis, the isolation of candidal species other than C. albicans from the urine was a better indicator of candidemia than was isolation of C. albicans; 60% of the patients whose urine contained candidal species other than C. albicans had candidemia, versus 33.3% of the patients whose urine contained C. albicans.[93]

Alkalization of the urine with oral potassium-sodium hydrogen citrate is a simple and effective method of treating candiduria in patients with an indwelling catheter.[94] Replacing or removing the bladder catheter is preferable. If Candida colonization persists, particularly if the patient has a risk factor for cystitis (e.g., diabetes mellitus or a disease that leads to incomplete bladder emptying) or for hematogenous dissemination (e.g., immunosuppression or manipulation of the genitourinary system), antifungal therapy should be considered. Amphotericin B bladder irrigation provides only temporary clearance of funguria, and systemic agents (a single I.V. dose of amphotericin B or a 5-day course of oral fluconazole) are usually needed.

The spectrum of urinary tract infection by Candida species includes cystitis, pyelitis (i.e., infection of the renal pelvis), fungus ball of the ureter, and renal abscesses. The diagnosis of cystitis is based on the presence of symptoms of cystitis, diffuse erythema or fungal plaques on cystoscopy, candiduria, and pyuria. Candida cystitis warrants therapy. If a triple-lumen catheter is in place, bladder irrigation with amphotericin B, 50 mg/L/day for 2 days, may be tried. Fluconazole, 200 mg once daily, is a more attractive approach because of the convenience, lower cost, and very high drug concentrations achieved in the urine.[95] Flucytosine is excreted in the urine in high concentrations and may be particularly useful against C. glabrata infection.

The management of pyelitis depends on whether the renal papillae are invaded or the ureter is obstructed with a fungus ball. Patients with no papillitis and an open ureter usually respond to irrigation with amphotericin B through a ureteral or percutaneous catheter. If papillitis is present, systemic antifungal therapy with fluconazole, 400 mg daily, is recommended. If fungus balls are present, surgical removal should be considered in addition to treatment with antifungal agents.

Hematogenous infections of the kidneys leading to multiple renal abscesses are treated as instances of hematogenous candidiasis. However, because both fluconazole and flucytosine are well tolerated, have good tissue diffusion, and are excreted in the urine in high concentrations, it is reasonable to assume that the combination of these two agents represents the therapy of choice for candidiasis that involves renal parenchyma.

Surgical patients are also at risk for vulvovaginal candidiasis. The diagnosis is based on the clinical findings and on the presence of pseudohyphae on a fungal smear. Various antifungal agents, including oral azoles and topical medications (suppositories, creams, and vaginal tablets) are effective in more than 80% of uncomplicated infections. Oral agents include fluconazole (150 mg in a single dose), ketoconazole (400 mg daily for 5 days), and itraconazole (200 mg in a single dose). However, women with four or more episodes of vulvovaginal candidiasis during a 12-month period and women with acute severe attacks of candidal vaginitis are less likely to respond to conventional therapy. Preventive measures include control of host factors such as diabetes mellitus, antifungal prophylaxis during the use of antibiotics and under other high-risk conditions, and the avoidance of systematic corticosteroids, oral contraceptives, and antibiotics if possible. Therapy with oral fluconazole, itraconazole, or ketoconazole is recommended for approximately 14 days to ensure clinical remission and negative fungal culture, followed by a maintenance regimen of fluconazole (150 mg once weekly for 6 months). Recurrence of vulvovaginal candidiasis is common, occurring in 30% to 40% of patients after cessation of the maintenance regime.[96]

Other Fungal Infections

ASPERGILLOSIS

Aspergillosis, a rare infection in the surgical patient, usually occurs in those who are markedly immunosuppressed after undergoing chemotherapy with cytotoxic agents or adrenal corticosteroids. Most cases of nosocomial aspergillosis are acquired via airborne transmission.[13,97] Colonization of the respiratory tract is followed by invasive disease if these predisposing factors are present. Sources of airborne fungi in microepidemics frequently are associated with construction within the hospital or at adjacent sites. Other modes of transmission of aspergillosis have been reported, including infections associated with foreign bodies, catheters, and bandages.

Acute invasive pulmonary aspergillosis is the most common form of Aspergillus infection in immunocompromised surgical patients. The organisms tend to invade blood vessels and cause thrombosis and infarction of the surrounding tissues. The infection may manifest itself in the form of acute vascular events such as pulmonary embolus or, more rarely, myocardial infarction, cerebral hemorrhage, or Budd-Chiari syndrome. Pulmonary Aspergillus infections include necrotizing bronchopneumonia and hemorrhagic pulmonary infarction, each accounting for about one third of these infections. Pulmonary aspergillosis may extend to contiguous organs or be disseminated. The rhinocerebral form of aspergillosis occurs less often than pulmonary infection. It originates in the sinuses and progresses through soft tissues, cartilage, and bone, causing lesions in the palate and the nose. Occasionally, the infection progresses through the base of the skull and involves the brain.

Diagnosis of Aspergillus infection is difficult and relies on identifying the organism in culture or histopathologic specimens.[13] The recovery of Aspergillus species from the respiratory tract culture of a surgical patient should be considered to represent contamination or colonization unless the patient is symptomatic and severely immunosuppressed. The standard therapy is high-dose amphotericin B (1 mg/kg/day) for a minimum of 2 g.[98] The addition of flucytosine may be useful. Liposomal formulations of amphotericin B and itraconazole offer additional treatment alternatives; at present, however, clinical experience with these new antifungal agents in patients with aspergillosis is limited.

ZYGOMYCOSIS (MUCORMYCOSIS)

Agents of zygomycosis have caused nosocomial infections in the surgical patient. The reservoir, the mode of transmission, the pathogenesis, and the clinical presentations are similar to those of *Aspergillus* species. In the surgical patient, the major risk factors include diabetic ketoacidosis, immunosuppression after cytotoxic chemotherapy, adrenocorticosteroid therapy, organ transplantation, skin damage (e.g., from adhesive tape, an arm board, or severe burns), and a prolonged postoperative stay.[99] Zygomycotic infections include rhinocerebral, paranasal, pulmonary, gastrointestinal, cutaneous, and, very rarely, disseminated disease.

Appropriate management of zygomycosis consists of extensive surgical debridement of infected areas, rapid correction of the underlying disease, and high-dose amphotericin B therapy up to a total dose of 2 to 3 g.

EMERGING PATHOGENS

Fungi such as *Fusarium* species, *Curvularia* species, *Alternaria* species, and *Trichosporon beigelii* were once thought to represent contamination or harmless colonization when isolated from tissue specimens. These and other newly recognized fungi have since been clearly shown to be potentially serious pathogens in immunosuppressed surgical patients.[100] In such patients, the recovery of any fungus from any site should prompt an evaluation by an infectious disease specialist to determine the clinical significance of the isolate.

Systemic Antifungal Agents

AMPHOTERICIN B

Amphotericin B is structurally similar to membrane sterols, and its major mechanism of action is believed to be through interaction with membrane sterols and creation of pores in the fungal outer membrane. The clinical usefulness of amphotericin B is believed to be attributable to the greater affinity of amphotericin B for ergosterol (found in fungal cell membranes) than for cholesterol (the principal sterol found in mammalian cell membranes). Oxidation-dependent amphotericin B-induced stimulation of macrophages is another proposed mechanism of action.[101] Most species of fungi that cause human infections are susceptible to amphotericin B.

Amphotericin B is supplied as a sterile lyophilized powder in vials containing 50 mg of amphotericin B, deoxycholate, and buffer. The contents are then diluted in 5% dextrose in water at a concentration of 10 mg/dl. Less precipitation occurs in saline solutions. The agent is stable at room temperature for 24 hours and is not sensitive to light. An acute infusion-related reaction, consisting of fever, hypotension, and tachycardia, occurs in about 20% of patients.[90] Premedication with acetaminophen may blunt this response. If this approach is unsuccessful, premedication with meperidine (25 to 50 mg I.V.) or hydrocortisone (25 to 50 mg I.V.) is recommended. Hypotension, hypertension, hypothermia, and bradycardia are other reported infusion-related toxic effects of amphotericin B deoxycholate. Ventricular arrhythmias have been associated with rapid infusion of amphotericin B deoxycholate and with administration of the agent to patients with severe hypokalemia or renal failure. Through inhibition of erythropoietic production secondary to nephrotoxicity, amphotericin B suppresses the production of red blood cells, causing a normocytic, normochromic anemia.

Common practice is to give a 1 mg test dose and observe the patient for 1 hour in the hope of identifying patients at risk for severe acute reactions. The full dose of the drug (0.6 to1 mg/kg/day) is then infused over a period of 4 to 6 hours, although there is evidence to suggest that much shorter infusion times (e.g., 1 hour in patients with adequate cardiopulmonary and renal function) may be acceptable. The total dose depends on the extent of the infection and the patient's condition. Patients must be monitored carefully during the first day of therapy. The infusion should be discontinued if the patient becomes hemodynamically unstable.

If acute reactions limit the amount of drug that can be infused, patients are premedicated with hydrocortisone, 25 to 50 mg I.V., either alone or in combination with meperidine, 25 to 50 mg I.V., 30 minutes before amphotericin B infusion is begun.

The distribution of the drug after I.V. infusion does not directly correlate with the daily dose. This finding is consistent with the unusual pharmacokinetics of amphotericin B. The initial serum half-life of the drug is about 24 hours, and the terminal half-life is about 15 days.

Renal toxicity and hypokalemia are the primary toxicities of amphotericin B [*see Table 3*]. Amphotericin B-induced nephrotoxicity may be glomerular, characterized by a decrease in glomerular filtration rate and renal blood flow, or tubular, with urinary casts, hypokalemia, hypomagnesemia, renal tubular acidosis, and nephrocalcinosis).[102] All of these abnormalities occur to varying degrees in almost all patients receiving the drug. In most patients, renal dysfunction gradually resolves after discontinuance of therapy. Amphotericin B nephrotoxicity may be minimized by avoiding other agents with synergistic nephrotoxicity (e.g., aminoglycosides, vancomycin, cisplatin, and cyclosporine) and by the administration of sodium supplementation. The latter approach consists of I.V. infusion of 500 ml of 0.9% saline solution 30 minutes before the administration of amphotericin B and a second infusion of the same amount of saline after the amphotericin B infusion is completed.

If the serum creatinine level exceeds 3.5 mg/dl, amphotericin B should be discontinued and the serum creatinine level monitored twice weekly. Administration of amphotericin B may be resumed at 50% to 75% of the original dosage when the serum creatinine level falls below 3 mg/dl.

The combined use of amphotericin B deoxycholate and other nephrotoxic agents, such as cyclosporine, aminoglycosides, and foscarnet, may result in synergistic nephrotoxicity.[103] Less nephrotoxic lipid formulations of amphotericin B include amphotericin B lipid complex (Abelcet), amphotericin B colloidal dispersion (Amphotec), and liposomal amphotericin B (AmBisome). These preparations differ in the amount of amphotericin B and the type of lipid used as well as in the physical form, pharmacokinetics, and toxicities. Of the three formulations, AmBisome is the one that is best tolerated.

FLUCYTOSINE

Flucytosine can be useful for the treatment of hematogenous candidiasis; however, a high failure rate and secondary emergence of resistance have been reported when flucytosine was used alone, and serious concerns exist regarding its myelosuppressive potential. A review of the literature on the activity of flucytosine in acute disseminated candidiasis and candidemia indicates a good response rate.

The standard dosage for flucytosine is 37.5 mg/kg every 6 hours. On the basis of the pharmacokinetics of flucytosine and the in vitro susceptibility of *Candida* species to the drug, much lower dosages of flucytosine (e.g., 12.5 mg/kg every 12 hours) would probably maintain serum and tissue levels significantly above the minimal inhibitory concentration (MIC) needed for most susceptible strains throughout therapy. For example, giving 25 mg/kg/day at 12-hour intervals would result in peak and trough serum levels of about 25 and 5 µg/ml, respectively, given a steady state and normal kidney function in a 70 kg patient. Because the MIC of flucytosine for most susceptible *Candida* species is usually 1 µg/ml or less, such a dosage schedule will constitute

Table 3 Antifungal Chemotherapy[140]

Drug	Indications	Route of Administration	Major Side Effects
Amphotericin B	Hematogenous and deep-seated candidiasis; aspergillosis; blastomycosis; coccidioidomycosis; histoplasmosis; cryptococcosis	Intravenous, intrathecal	Anemia, headache, chills, fever, nausea, renal dysfunction, hypotension, tachypnea, hypokalemia, phlebitis
Clotrimazole	Oropharyngeal candidiasis	Oral	—
Flucytosine	Candidiasis (septicemia, endocarditis, and urinary tract infections); cryptococcosis	Oral	Leukopenia, thrombocytopenia, liver dysfunction, diarrhea
Fluconazole	Oropharyngeal and esophageal candidiasis; hematogenous candidal infection; other candidal infections (e.g., urinary tract infections, peritonitis); meningeal coccidioidomycosis; cryptococcosis	Oral, intravenous	Nausea and vomiting, skin rash, liver dysfunction
Itraconazole	Histoplasmosis; blastomycosis; aspergillosis	Oral	Nausea, vomiting, liver dysfunction
Ketoconazole	Candidiasis (chronic mucocutaneous candidiasis or oropharyngeal candidiasis); candiduria; blastomycosis; coccidioidomycosis; histoplasmosis; chromomycosis; paracoccidioidomycosis	Oral	Hepatotoxicity, nausea or vomiting, occasional suppression of adrenal function

appropriate therapy, given that the drug is used in combination with other antifungals. This approach may decrease the myelosuppressive potential that the drug usually exhibits at levels of 100 µg/ml, and it may lead to the drug's wider use.

Peak serum concentrations should be monitored and the dosage adjusted so as to maintain a peak level of about 25 µg/ml. Flucytosine is removed by hemodialysis and peritoneal dialysis. Patients undergoing hemodialysis should receive a 37.5 mg/kg dose of flucytosine after each dialysis session unless their initial peak serum concentration is higher than 25 µg/ml or their postdialysis concentration is higher than 10 µg/ml. Patients undergoing peritoneal dialysis should receive a single 37.5 mg/kg dose daily.

FLUCONAZOLE

The mechanism of action of fluconazole is preferential inhibition of cytochrome P-450 enzymes in fungal organisms. Fluconazole is active against several *Candida* species, including *C. tropicalis*. *C. krusei*, however, is highly resistant to this agent.[90] Fluconazole also does not appear to have good clinical activity against *Aspergillus* species. Fluconazole is available in either an oral form or an I.V. form, both of which are rapidly and almost completely absorbed from the GI tract. The serum concentrations after oral administration are almost identical to those achieved when the drug is administered intravenously. A major advantage of fluconazole over ketoconazole is its high degree of GI absorption, which is not affected by gastric acidity or the presence of food. Steady-state serum concentrations of fluconazole are obtained within 5 to 10 days. An initial loading dose that is twice the usual daily dose is recommended. Fluconazole is distributed evenly in body tissues, penetrates into the vitreous humor and the aqueous humor of the eye, and crosses the blood-brain barrier. The drug is excreted largely unchanged in the urine, with only minimal liver metabolism. Consequently, dosage schedules must be adjusted in patients with renal impairment. Hemodialysis significantly reduces the serum concentrations, and the drug appears also to be removed by peritoneal dialysis. A standard dose should be given after each course of dialysis.

The toxicities of fluconazole are similar to those of other azoles and include nausea and vomiting in about 2% of patients, as well as headache, fatigue, abdominal pain, and diarrhea[104]; exfoliative dermatitis also occurs, but very rarely. Transient abnormalities of liver function have been observed in 3% of patients receiving fluconazole. In addition, fatal hepatic necrosis developed in two patients who were receiving fluconazole, but it was unclear whether the agent played a causal role in this event. No significant hormonal abnormalities have been reported after administration of fluconazole.

Because fluconazole interacts with warfarin, phenytoin, and cyclosporine when given in a daily dose of 200 mg or more,[104] serum concentrations of these agents should be monitored.

ITRACONAZOLE

Itraconazole is the only available azole that has substantial activity against *Aspergillus* species. It exists in an oral capsule formulation, the bioavailability of which is approximately 55%. Absorption is enhanced by the presence of food in the stomach but is significantly reduced by the presence of antacids or H_2 receptor blockers. A new solution, which has significantly higher bioavailability, may not be well tolerated by patients. When erratic absorption is of concern, use of the I.V. formulation is recommended. The serum elimination half-life, 15 to 25 hours, increases to 34 to 42 hours after weeks of administration and with increasing itraconazole doses.

Metabolized by the liver, itraconazole is excreted as metabolites primarily in the feces (54%) and urine (35%). A hepatic metabolite, hydroxyitraconazole, has an antifungal spectrum similar to that of the parent compound. Because itraconazole is metabolized to a large degree in the liver, the dosage must be adjusted in patients with hepatic failure; however, its pharmacokinetics are not affected by renal impairment or hemodialysis. Serum concentrations of digoxin may increase when this agent is given with itraconazole,[105] and the metabolism of itraconazole may be accelerated when drugs that induce hepatic enzymes are given simultaneously.[106] Serum concentrations of itraconazole should therefore be measured in patients with invasive infections.

Itraconazole is generally well tolerated in dosages of up to 400 mg/day. The most common side effects are nausea, vomiting, diarrhea, and abdominal discomfort. Headaches, rash, pruritus, and dizziness occasionally occur. At higher doses, a mineralocorticoid excess syndrome (hypokalemia, hypertension, and edema) has been described, and hypokalemia develops in as many as 6% of patients who take 400 mg/day for several months.[107]

Itraconazole is available in 100 mg capsules and oral suspension (10 mg/ml). Because itraconazole may be teratogenic, it should be avoided in pregnant patients. A large number of drug interactions occur with itraconazole, many related to inhibition of the cytochrome P-450 enzyme system. Care should be taken in prescribing itraconazole with these agents. Itraconazole is currently approved for the treatment of blastomycosis, histoplasmosis, and aspergillosis but is also effective for the treatment of candidiasis and cryptococcosis.

KETOCONAZOLE

Ketoconazole is effective against yeast infections of the skin and the mucous membranes; however, it should not be used to treat hemato-

Table 4 Characteristics of Currently Available Azoles*[139]

	Ketoconazole	Fluconazole	Itraconazole
Spectrum	Narrow	Expanded	Expanded
Route(s) of administration	Oral	Oral, intravenous	Oral
Bioavailability	Erratic, requires gastric acidity	Excellent	Erratic, requires gastric acidity
Plasma half-life (hr)	6–9	30	20–40
Hepatotoxicity	Occasional	Occasional	Occasional
Gastrointestinal intolerance	Frequent	Occasional	Occasional
CSF penetration	No	Yes	No
Renal excretion	No	Yes	No
Interaction with other drugs	Frequent	Occasional	Frequent

*Intravenous miconazole is also available but offers no advantage over the currently available azoles.

genous candidiasis. Ketoconazole is not available in an intravenous form, and the serum levels it is capable of reaching depend largely on gastric acidity [see Table 4]. The same adverse events and drug-drug interactions observed with itraconazole occur with ketoconazole.

SPECIAL CONSIDERATIONS IN ORGAN TRANSPLANT RECIPIENTS

Intravenous amphotericin B (0.4 to 0.8 mg/kg/day) has been the mainstay of treatment in organ transplant recipients, but concerns have been expressed about increased nephrotoxicity, particularly in patients receiving cyclosporine or tacrolimus. The lipid formulations of amphotericin B (1 to 3 mg/kg/day) are less nephrotoxic, particularly liposomal amphotericin B (AmBisome). Fluconazole has a minimal effect on hepatic microsomal enzymes in comparison with ketoconazole and itraconazole and therefore is the drug of choice in organ transplant recipients who have candidiasis caused by fluconazole-susceptible strains.

Conclusion

Continued progress in supportive care, including the development of antibiotics with increasingly broad spectra of activity, has resulted in an increased incidence of fungal infections, particularly candidiasis. Because of the inadequacy of the available knowledge base, we do not fully understand the pathophysiology of these infections in surgical patients, nor can we be certain precisely when prophylaxis and therapy should be administered.

Despite these limitations, there is now sufficient information available to justify an aggressive therapeutic approach to suspected *Candida* infections. Now that less toxic agents are available (the newer triazoles, particularly fluconazole, and the lipid formulations of amphotericin B), the clinical approach to presumed fungal infections in surgical patients has been made far simpler.

Discussion

Microbiologic Characteristics of Pathogenic *Candida* Species

Candida species multiply by producing buds from ovoid yeast cells. They are differentiated from other yeasts (e.g., *Saccharomyces* species) by their ability to produce pseudohyphae on certain media and, in the case of *C. albicans*, true hyphae in serum [see Figure 2].

VIRULENCE FACTORS

Four virulence factors have been demonstrated for *Candida* species: adherence to mucosal epithelial cells; secretion of proteinases, which degrade connective tissue proteins, thereby allowing yeast to enter beyond connective tissue barriers; ambient pH[108]; and resistance to oxidative killing by neutrophils.

For *Candida* species to disseminate, the organisms must be able to adhere to the vascular system (i.e., endothelium, the basement membrane, or both), an ability that is probably receptor mediated.[109] In vitro, however, *Candida* adheres more avidly to the subendothelial extracellular matrix than to endothelial cells. This finding may explain the increased risk of hematogenous candidiasis in patients receiving cytotoxic chemotherapy. Such therapy causes denudation of endothelium and consequent exposure of the basement membrane, to which *Candida* then readily adheres.

Genetic studies have evaluated the role of various virulence factors for *Candida* species, including ambient pH,[108] adherence mechanisms, and enzyme production. Mechanisms by which *Candida* species lose virulence include the following: gene dysregulation, stopping the switch from budding yeast to filamentous form; disruption of a gene that results in decreased hyphal growth, adherence, and virulence[110]; deficiency of *C. albicans* in mannosyl transferase, resulting in decreased adherence and virulence; and deletion of the gene that encodes the production of phospholipase leading to decreased cell wall penetration.

CHANGING MICROBIOLOGIC SPECTRUM OF *CANDIDA*

Although there are more than 100 described species of *Candida*, only four are commonly associated with infection: *C. albicans, C. tropi-*

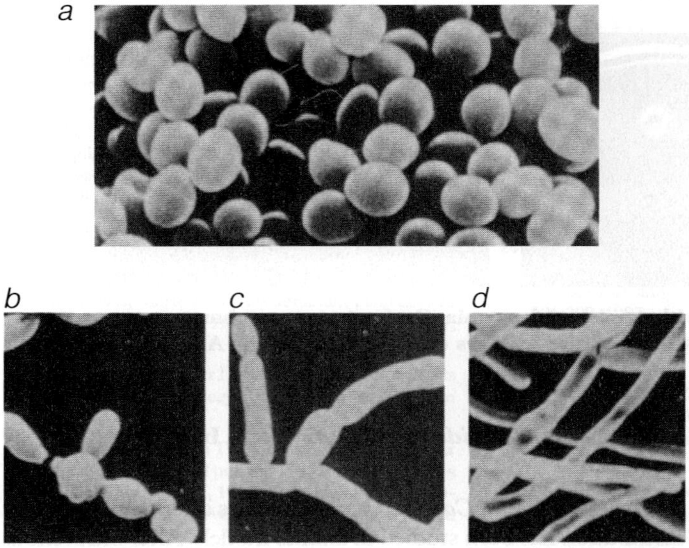

Figure 2 *Candida* takes several forms as it grows. A blastospore is a unicellular form (*a*). Blastospores divide by budding, a process in which new cellular material grows from a site on the blastospore (*b*). Nuclear division then occurs, and a septum forms between the two new cells. A hypha is a long tube of several cells divided by septa (*c*). A mycelium is a cellular aggregate that includes a hypha and its branches (*d*). A pseudohypha differs from a true hypha in that it is composed of morphologically distinct, elongated blastospores.

calis, *C. parapsilosis,* and *C. glabrata.*[10] Of these, *C. albicans* has been isolated from more than 60% of candidal infections; the other three major species are seen at rates varying from 5% to 20%. Mucosal colonization by *C. tropicalis,* a virulent organism, frequently leads to invasive infection. *C. glabrata* and *C. parapsilosis* appear to be relatively less virulent,[111] and the latter typically causes infection in association with prosthetic materials (e.g., catheters) or glucose-rich intravenous solutions.[10] Finally, *C. krusei* and *C. lusitaniae* rarely cause disease, being isolated from fewer than 1% of cultures.[10] The epidemiology of candidiasis has changed, with reduced rates of *C. albicans* in favor of other candidal species—in particular, *C. glabrata* and *C. krusei*.[112] This change is important because *C. krusei* and several strains of *C. glabrata* are highly resistant to the triazoles such as fluconazole and itraconazole.[10,112]

A study by the NNIS group evaluated 1,579 bloodstream isolates of *Candida* species obtained from more than 50 hospitals in the United States over a 7-year period (1992–1998) to detect trends in species distribution and susceptibility to fluconazole. *C. albicans* accounted for 52% of isolates, followed by *C. glabrata* (18%), *C. parapsilosis* (15%), *C. tropicalis* (11%), and *C. krusei* (2%). Since 1995, *C. glabrata* has been more prevalent than *C. parapsilosis*. The susceptibility of all *Candida* species to fluconazole has remained stable.[113]

Pathogenesis of Candidiasis in the Surgical Patient

COLONIZATION OF THE GUT BY *CANDIDA* SPECIES

That colonization is a necessary prelude to infection is supported by studies demonstrating (1) that 95% of neutropenic patients and 84% of nonneutropenic patients were infected with the same strains that had previously colonized them and (2) that infection was significantly less likely to develop in patients who were not colonized.[114,115] In a study investigating the sequence of colonization and candidemia in nonneutropenic patients, Voss and colleagues[114] found that the strains recovered from the initial colonized or infected site and from the bloodstream were identical in patients with disseminated candidiasis; furthermore, nearly every patient was infected with a distinct or unique *Candida* strain. In another study, positive surveillance cultures were found to be highly predictive of systemic infection, whereas negative surveillance cultures correlated with a low risk of candidal dissemination.[116] Clinical studies of antifungal prophylaxis in neutropenic cancer patients have also suggested that antifungal regimens effectively prevent hematogenous infection when they can eliminate or reduce colonization by *Candida.*[117]

The density of colonization appears to be predictive of the risk of hematogenous candidiasis. In two large series of neutropenic cancer patients, hematogenous candidiasis almost never developed in noncolonized patients, compared with an infection rate of more than 30% in patients with multiple colonized sites.[115,118] In a study of patients with acute lymphocytic leukemia, a relatively high concentration of *Candida* organisms in the stools was found to be a significant risk factor for hematogenous candidiasis.[119] In 40 infants of very low birth weight, a value of 8×10^6 *Candida* CFU/g stool was established as a threshold, beyond which GI symptoms (attributed to *Candida*) developed in 50% of the infants and a systemic septic response in 28.5% during 1 to 3 weeks of heavy colonization.[120] In a prospective study of patients admitted to surgical and neonatal intensive care units, Pittet and coworkers demonstrated that the intensity of *Candida* colonization (as determined by a *Candida* colonization index) was significantly higher in patients who subsequently became infected than in those who did not.[121] Other case-control studies have demonstrated that colonization by *Candida* species at various body sites and exposure to several antibiotics were independent risk factors for candidemia.[122]

The normal endogenous intestinal flora inhibits GI colonization and overgrowth by potentially pathogenic bacteria and fungi by forming what may be thought of as living wallpaper in the large intestine. Suppression of endogenous microflora as a consequence of antimicrobial administration[123] may permit overgrowth of pathogenic strains in the GI tract and selection of resistant strains, which may result in enterocolitis, systemic infection, or the septic response.

PHYSICAL DISRUPTION OF THE INTESTINAL MUCOSAL BARRIER

In humans, as well as in animals, the GI tract is considered to be the most important portal of entry for microorganisms, including yeasts, into the bloodstream. The passage of endogenous fungi from the GI tract to extraintestinal sites can be referred to as fungal translocation (by analogy with bacterial translocation).

Although yeast cells have no intrinsic motility, they are able to translocate from the intestinal lumen within a few hours of ingestion. In a study conducted in the 1960s, two nonpathogenic yeasts were surgically instilled into the rat duodenum and were recovered from the cisterna chyli within 4 hours.[124] Even in the absence of disease, any marked increase in the intestinal population of *Candida* can lead to fungal translocation and subsequent hematogenous infection. That candidal species can translocate from the gut to the bloodstream was demonstrated in a study in which signs and symptoms of sepsis developed in a healthy volunteer 2 hours after ingestion of a suspension containing 10^{12} *C. albicans* organisms, and blood cultures taken 3 and 6 hours after ingestion were positive for *Candida.*[125] In addition, autopsy studies conducted in patients with hematogenous candidiasis found involvement of the GI tract and submucosal invasion in almost all patients.[86]

Microbial translocation has been demonstrated in several animal models and has been shown to be enhanced by several factors, including fasting, which induces complex changes in host defenses, and protein deficiency, which results in intestinal microbial overgrowth, increased intestinal absorption of intact proteins, and decreased intracellular killing of bacteria and fungi. In one study involving *C. albicans,* volatile fatty acids and secondary bile salts

61. Gorensek MJ, Carey WD, Washington JA 2nd, et al: Selective bowel decontamination with quinolones and nystatin reduces gram-negative and fungal infections in orthotopic liver transplant recipients. Cleve Clin J Med 60:139, 1993
62. Mora NP, Cofer JB, Solomon H, et al: Analysis of severe infections (INF) after 180 consecutive liver transplants: the impact of amphotericin B prophylaxis for reducing the incidence and severity of fungal infections. Transplant Proc 23:1528, 1991
63. Tollemar J, Ringden O, Andersson S, et al: Randomized double-blind study of liposomal amphotericin B (AmBisome) prophylaxis of invasive fungal infections in bone marrow transplant recipients. Bone Marrow Transplant 12:577, 1993
64. Slavin MA, Osborne B, Adams R, et al: Efficacy and safety of fluconazole prophylaxis for fungal infections after bone marrow transplantation—a prospective, randomized, double-blind study. J Infect Dis 171:1545, 1995
65. Rotstein C, Bow EJ, Laverdiere M, et al: Randomized placebo-controlled trial of fluconazole prophylaxis for neutropenic cancer patients: benefit based on purpose and intensity of cytotoxic therapy. The Canadian Fluconazole Prophylaxis Study Group. Clin Infect Dis 28:331, 1999
66. Powderly WG, Finkelstein D, Feinberg J, et al: A randomized trial comparing fluconazole with clotrimazole troches for the prevention of fungal infections in patients with advanced human immunodeficiency virus infection. NIAID AIDS Clinical Trials Group. N Engl J Med 332:700, 1995
67. Eggimann P, Francioli P, Bille J, et al: Fluconazole prophylaxis prevents intra-abdominal candidiasis in high-risk surgical patients. Crit Care Med 27:1066, 1999
68. Dube MP, Heseltine PN, Rinaldi MG, et al: Fungemia and colonization with nystatin-resistant Candida rugosa in a burn unit. Clin Infect Dis 18:77, 1994
69. Torbenson M, Wang J, Nichols L, et al: Causes of death in autopsied liver transplantation patients. Mod Pathol 11:37, 1998
70. Lumbreras C, Cuervas-Mons V, Jara P, et al: Randomized trial of fluconazole versus nystatin for the prophylaxis of Candida infection following liver transplantation. J Infect Dis 174:583, 1996
71. Lorf T, Braun F, Ruchel R, et al: Systemic mycoses during prophylactical use of liposomal amphotericin B (AmBisome) after liver transplantation. Mycoses 42:47, 1999
72. Savani DV, Perfect JR, Cobo LM, et al: Penetration of new azole compounds into the eye and efficacy in experimental Candida endophthalmitis. Antimicrob Agents Chemother 31:6, 1987
73. Venditti M, De Bernardis F, Micozzi A, et al: Fluconazole treatment of catheter-related right-sided endocarditis caused by Candida albicans and associated with endophthalmitis and folliculitis. Clin Infect Dis 14:422, 1992
74. Moyer DV, Edwards JE Jr: *Candida* endophthalmitis and central nervous system infection. Candidiasis: Pathogenesis, Diagnosis, and Treatment. Bodey GP, Ed. Raven Press, New York, 1993, p 331
75. Martinez-Vazquez C, Fernandez-Ulloa J, Bordon J, et al: Candida albicans endophthalmitis in brown heroin addicts: response to early vitrectomy preceded and followed by antifungal therapy. Clin Infect Dis 27:1130, 1998
76. Yackee JM, Topiel MS, Simon GL: Septic phlebitis caused by Candida albicans and diagnosed by needle aspiration. South Med J 78:1262, 1985
77. Czwerwiec FS, Bilsker MS, Kamerman ML, et al: Long-term survival after fluconazole therapy of candidal prosthetic valve endocarditis. Am J Med 94:545, 1993
78. Kraus WE, Valenstein PN, Corey GR: Purulent pericarditis caused by Candida: report of three cases and identification of high-risk populations as an aid to early diagnosis. Rev Infect Dis 10:34, 1988
79. Cuende E, Barbadillo C, E-Mazzuchelli R, et al: Candida arthritis in adult patients who are not intravenous drug addicts: report of three cases and review of the literature. Semin Arthritis Rheum 22:224, 1993
80. Penk A, Pittrow L: [Status of fluconazole in the therapy of endogenous Candida endophthalmitis]. Mycoses 41(suppl 2):41, 1998
81. Tang C: Successful treatment of Candida albicans osteomyelitis with fluconazole. J Infect 26:89, 1993
82. Shapiro S, Javed T, Mealey J Jr: Candida albicans shunt infection. Pediatr Neurosci 15:125, 1989
83. Mascarenas CA, Hardin TC, Pennick GJ, et al: Treatment of thrush with itraconazole solution: evidence for topical effect. Clin Infect Dis 26:1242, 1998
84. Crutchfield CE 3rd, Lewis EJ: The successful treatment of oral candidiasis (thrush) in a pediatric patient using itraconazole (letter). Pediatr Dermatol 14:246, 1997
85. Tunkel AR, Thomas CY, Wispelwey B: Candida prosthetic arthritis: report of a case treated with fluconazole and review of the literature. Am J Med 94:100, 1993
86. Walsh TJ, Merz WG: Pathologic features in the human alimentary tract associated with invasiveness of Candida tropicalis. Am J Clin Pathol 85:498, 1986
87. Gupta TP, Ehrinpreis MN: Candida-associated diarrhea in hospitalized patients. Gastroenterology 98:780, 1990
88. Calandra T, Bille J, Schneider R, et al: Clinical significance of Candida isolated from peritoneum in surgical patients. Lancet 2:1437, 1989
89. Corbella X, Sirvent JM, Carratala J: Fluconazole treatment without catheter removal in Candida albicans peritonitis complicating peritoneal dialysis. Am J Med 90:277, 1991
90. Eisenberg ES, Leviton I, Soeiro R: Fungal peritonitis in patients receiving peritoneal dialysis: experience with 11 patients and review of the literature [published erratum appears in Rev Infect Dis 8:839, 1986]. Rev Infect Dis 8:309, 1986
91. Lo WK, Chan CY, Cheng SW, et al: A prospective randomized control study of oral nystatin prophylaxis for Candida peritonitis complicating continuous ambulatory peritoneal dialysis. Am J Kidney Dis 28:549, 1996
92. Huang CT, Leu HS: Candiduria as an early marker of disseminated infection in critically ill surgical patients (letter; comment). J Trauma 39:616, 1995
93. Chakrabarti A, Reddy TC, Singhi S: Does candiduria predict candidaemia? Ind J Med Res 106:513, 1997
94. Strassner C, Friesen A: [Therapy of candiduria by alkalinization of urine: oral treatment with potassium-sodium-hydrogen citrate]. Fortschr Med 113:359, 1995
95. Tacker JR: Successful use of fluconazole for treatment of urinary tract fungal infections. J Urol 148:1917, 1992
96. Sobel JD: Recurrent vulvovaginal candidiasis: a prospective study of the efficacy of maintenance ketoconazole therapy. N Engl J Med 315:1455, 1986
97. Walsh TJ, Dixon DM: Nosocomial aspergillosis, environmental microbiology, hospital epidemiology, diagnosis and treatment. Eur J Epidemiol 5:131, 1989
98. Denning DW, Stevens DA: Antifungal and surgical treatment of invasive aspergillosis: review of 2,121 published cases [published erratum appears in Rev Infect Dis 13:345, 1991]. Rev Infect Dis 12:1147, 1990
99. Anaissie E, Bodey GP: Nosocomial fungal infections: old problems and new challenges. Infect Dis Clin North Am 3:867, 1989
100. Anaissie E, Bodey GP, Kantarjian H, et al: New spectrum of fungal infections in patients with cancer. Rev Infect Dis 11:369, 1989
101. Sokol-Anderson ML, Brajtburg J, Medoff G: Amphotericin B-induced oxidative damage and killing of Candida albicans. J Infect Dis 154:76, 1986
102. Burgess JL, Birchall R: Nephrotoxicity of amphotericin B, with emphasis on changes in tubular function. Am J Med 53:77, 1972
103. Kennedy MS, Deeg HJ, Siegel M, et al: Acute renal toxicity with combined use of amphotericin B and cyclosporine after marrow transplantation. Transplantation 35:211, 1983
104. Zervos M, Meunier F: Fluconazole (Diflucan): a review. Int J Antimicrob Agents 3:147, 1993
105. McClean KL, Sheehan GJ: Interaction between itraconazole and digoxin (letter; comment). Clin Infect Dis 18:259, 1994
106. Drayton J, Dickinson G, Rinaldi MG: Coadministration of rifampin and itraconazole leads to undetectable levels of serum itraconazole (letter). Clin Infect Dis 18:266, 1994
107. Tucker RM, Haq Y, Denning DW, et al: Adverse events associated with itraconazole in 189 patients on chronic therapy. J Antimicrob Chemother 26:561, 1990
108. De Bernardis F, Muhlschlegel FA, Cassone A, et al: The pH of the host niche controls gene expression in and virulence of Candida albicans. Infect Immun 66:3317, 1998
109. Klotz SA: Fungal adherence to the vascular compartment: a critical step in the pathogenesis of disseminated candidiasis. Clin Infect Dis 14:340, 1992
110. Gale CA, Bendel CM, McClellan M, et al: Linkage of adhesion, filamentous growth, and virulence in Candida albicans to a single gene, INT1. Science 279:1355, 1998
111. Lecciones JA, Lee JW, Navarro EE, et al: Vascular catheter-associated fungemia in patients with cancer: analysis of 155 episodes. Clin Infect Dis 14:875, 1992
112. Abi-Said D, Anaissie E, Uzun O, et al: The epidemiology of hematogenous candidiasis caused by different Candida species [published erratum appears in Clin Infect Dis 25:352, 1997]. Clin Infect Dis 24:1122, 1997
113. Pfaller MA, Messer SA, Hollis RJ, et al: Trends in species distribution and susceptibility to fluconazole among blood stream isolates of Candida species in the United States. Diagn Microbiol Infect Dis 33:217, 1999
114. Voss A, Hollis RJ, Pfaller MA, et al: Investigation of the sequence of colonization and candidemia in nonneutropenic patients. J Clin Microbiol 32:975, 1994
115. Martino P, Girmenia C, Venditti M, et al: Candida colonization and systemic infection in neutropenic patients: a retrospective study. Cancer 64:2030, 1989
116. Pfaller M, Cabezudo I, Koontz F, et al: Predictive value of surveillance cultures for systemic infection due to Candida species. Eur J Clin Microbiol Infect Dis 6:628, 1987
117. Uzun O, Anaissie EJ: Antifungal prophylaxis in patients with hematologic malignancies: a reappraisal. Blood 86:2063, 1995
118. Martino P, Girmenia C, Micozzi A, et al: Fungemia in patients with leukemia. Am J Med Sci 306:225, 1993
119. Richet HM, Andremont A, Tancrede C, et al: Risk factors for candidemia in patients with acute lymphocytic leukemia. Rev Infect Dis 13:211, 1991
120. Pappu-Katikaneni LD, Rao KP, Banister E: Gastrointestinal colonization with yeast species and Candida septicemia in very low birth weight infants.

Mycoses 33:20, 1990
121. Pittet D, Monod M, Suter PM, et al: Candida colonization and subsequent infections in critically ill surgical patients. Ann Surg 220:751, 1994
122. Wey SB, Mori M, Pfaller MA, et al: Risk factors for hospital-acquired candidemia: a matched case-control study. Arch Intern Med 149:2349, 1989
123. Giuliano M, Barza M, Jacobus NV, et al: Effect of broad-spectrum parenteral antibiotics on composition of intestinal microflora of humans. Antimicrob Agents Chemother 31:202, 1987
124. Wolochow H, Hildebrand GJ, Lamanna C: Translocation of microorganisms across the intestinal wall of the rat: effect of microbial size and concentration. J Infect Dis 116:523, 1966
125. Krause W, Matheis H, Wulf K: Fungaemia and funguria after oral administration of Candida albicans. Lancet 1:598, 1969
126. Kennedy MJ, Volz PA: Ecology of Candida albicans gut colonization: inhibition of Candida adhesion, colonization, and dissemination from the gastrointestinal tract by bacterial antagonism. Infect Immun 49:654, 1985
127. Deitch EA, Sittig K, Li M, et al: Obstructive jaundice promotes bacterial translocation from the gut. Am J Surg 159:79, 1990
128. Gianotti L, Alexander JW, Fukushima R, et al: Translocation of *Candida albicans* is related to the blood flow of individual intestinal villi. Circ Shock 40:250, 1993
129. Alexander JW, Boyce ST, Babcock JF, et al: The process of microbial translocation. Ann Surg 212:496, 1990
130. Pappo I, Polacheck I, Zmora O, et al: Altered gut barrier function to Candida during parenteral nutrition. Nutrition 10:151, 1994
131. Hennessey PJ, Black CT, Andrassy RJ: Nonenzymatic glycosylation of immunoglobulin G impairs complement fixation. JPEN J Parenter Enteral Nutr 15:60, 1991
132. Gogos CA, Kalfarentzos FE, Zoumbos NC: Effect of different types of total parenteral nutrition on T-lymphocyte subpopulations and NK cells. Am J Clin Nutr 51:119, 1990
133. Gogos CA, Kalfarentzos F: Total parenteral nutrition and immune system activity: a review. Nutrition 11:339, 1995
134. Shou J, Lappin J, Minnard EA, et al: Total parenteral nutrition, bacterial translocation, and host immune function. Am J Surg 167:145, 1994
135. Parker JC Jr, McCloskey JJ, Lee RS: Human cerebral candidosis—a postmortem evaluation of 19 patients. Hum Pathol 12:23, 1981
136. Parker JC Jr: The potentially lethal problem of cardiac candidosis. Am J Clin Pathol 73:356, 1980
137. Haron E, Vartivarian S, Anaissie E, et al: Primary Candida pneumonia: experience at a large cancer center and review of the literature. Medicine (Baltimore) 72:137, 1993
138. Gaines JD, Remington JS: Disseminated candidiasis in the surgical patient. Surgery 72:730, 1972
139. Greenburg SB: Fungal and viral infections. Critical Care, 2nd ed. Civetta JM, Taylor RW, Kirby RR, Eds. JB Lippincott Co, Philadelphia, 1993, p 1055
140. Medoff G, Kobayashi GS: Systemic fungal infections: an overview. Hosp Pract 26(2):41, 1991

86 VIRAL INFECTION

Jennifer W. Janelle, M.D., and Richard J. Howard, M.D., Ph.D.

Approach to Viral Exposure

Compared with primary care physicians, such as internists, family physicians, and pediatricians, surgeons are seldom called on to treat viral infections. Viral infections nonetheless deserve the attention of surgeons because these infections can cause illness in patients after operation, albeit infrequently, and can spread to the hospital staff. Some viral infections (e.g., infections with the hepatitis viruses, HIV, and cytomegalovirus [CMV]) can result from administration of blood or blood products or can be transmitted to hospital personnel through needle-stick injury. Viral infections can also result from organ transplantation or trauma (e.g., rabies, which is transmitted by the bite of an infected animal). Some viruses, especially the herpesviruses, frequently infect immunosuppressed patients, in whom the viruses can cause severe illness and even death. In many surgical practices, there are increasing numbers of immunosuppressed patients, including organ transplant recipients; patients with cancer; patients receiving cancer chemotherapy, steroids, and other immunosuppressive drugs; the elderly; and the malnourished. Some viral infections can cause neoplastic disease for which operation may become necessary. Examples are hepatitis B virus (HBV) and hepatitis C virus (HCV), which are implicated in the etiology of hepatocellular carcinoma; Epstein-Barr virus (EBV), which can cause a lethal lymphoproliferative disorder in immunosuppressed patients; and human T cell lymphotropic virus type I (HTLV-I), which can induce a T cell leukemia. Viral infections very likely can cause other neoplasms as well.

Prevention of Transmission of HIV, Hepatitis B Virus, and Hepatitis C Virus

TRANSMISSION FROM PATIENTS TO HEALTH CARE WORKERS

The Centers for Disease Control and Prevention (CDC) has published extensive recommendations for preventing transmission of HIV, the etiologic agent of AIDS.[1-5] Applicable to clinical and laboratory staffs,[3,4] to workers in health care settings [see Table 1][1] and in other occupational settings,[1] and to health care workers performing invasive procedures,[1-5] these precautions are appropriate for preventing transmission not only of HIV but also of other blood-borne viruses, including HBV and HCV. The recommendations share the objective of minimizing exposure of personnel to blood and body secretions from infected patients, whether through needle-stick injury or through contamination of mucous membranes or open cuts.

Despite the apparently low risk of such exposure, the CDC recommends enforcement of these as well as other standard infection control precautions, regardless of whether health care workers or patients are known to be infected with HIV or HBV. The CDC has taken the position that blood and body fluid precautions should be used consistently for all patients because medical history and physical examination cannot reliably identify all patients infected with HIV or other blood-borne pathogens and because in emergencies there may be no time for serologic testing. If these universal precautions are implemented, as the CDC recommends,[1-5] no additional precautions should be necessary for patients known to be infected with HIV.

The CDC does not recommend routine HIV serologic testing for all patients.[1-5] HIV serologic testing of patients is recommended for management of health care workers who sustain parenteral or mucous membrane exposure to blood or other body fluids, for patient diagnosis and treatment, and for counseling associated with efforts to prevent and control HIV transmission in the community.[1-5]

Nevertheless, some hospitals and physicians are likely to perform serologic testing of patients if it is possible that health care workers will be exposed to the patients' blood or other body fluids, as would be the case with patients undergoing major operative procedures or receiving treatment in intensive care units. Those who favor routine preoperative testing of patients undergoing invasive procedures maintain that precautions are more likely to be followed and additional steps taken to lower the likelihood of virus transmission from patients to health care workers when it is known which patients are HIV positive.[6,7] If such policies are adopted, the CDC advocates certain principles: (1) obtain consent for testing, (2) inform patients of results and provide counseling to seropositive patients, (3) ensure confidentiality, (4) ensure that seropositive patients will not receive compromised care, and (5) prospectively evaluate the efficacy of the program in reducing the incidence of exposure of health care workers to blood or body fluids of patients who are infected with HIV.

Although possible acquisition of HIV infection is the major concern for any health care worker who is exposed to blood products in the workplace, acquisition of viral hepatitis is actually much more likely. From a single needle-stick exposure, the estimated average risk of HIV transmission is 0.3%, whereas that of HCV transmission ranges from 0% to 10%.[8] The risk that HBV will be transmitted from a single needle-stick exposure varies according to the hepatitis B e antigen (HBeAg) status of the source patient, ranging from 1% to 6% for HBeAg-negative patients to 22% to 40% for HBeAg-positive patients.[9-11] That health care workers are at increased risk for hepatitis B is indicated by the seroprevalence of HBV in this population, which is two to four times that in the general United States population (6% to 15% versus < 5%).[9,12] This seroprevalence is expected to decrease with the availability of the hepatitis B vaccine and the mandate from the Occupational Safety

Human immunodeficiency virus (HIV)

Health care worker is exposed to any patient's blood or body secretions by a needle stick or by a splash in the eye or mouth

The health care worker should be counseled about the risk of HIV infection and should follow U.S. Public Health Service recommendations for preventing HIV transmission.

Patient is judged on clinical and epidemiologic grounds to be a likely source of HIV infection

Ask the patient to consent to serologic testing for HIV.

Patient refuses to be tested

Follow state and local laws regarding testing for a nonconsenting patient's HIV source status.

Patient is seropositive

Evaluate the health care worker for clinical or serologic evidence of HIV infection as soon as possible after the exposure. Consider prophylaxis:
Low to moderate risk: AZT plus 3TC.
High risk: AZT plus 3TC plus indinavir.

Patient is seronegative and has no other evidence of HIV infection

No further follow-up of the health care worker is necessary.

Patient is seronegative but has engaged in high-risk behaviors

Perform baseline HIV testing of the health care worker. Repeat test 3 months and 6 months after exposure.

Health care worker is seronegative

Repeat serologic testing 6 wk and 3, 6, 12 mo after exposure.

Rabies

All bites and wounds should be immediately and thoroughly cleansed with soap and water.

Bite of domestic animal (dog or cat)

- **Animal is healthy at time of attack** — Observe the animal for 10 days. If the animal shows signs of rabies, proceed with treatment.
- **Animal shows signs of rabies**
- **Animal escapes** — Consult with public health officials to determine need for treatment.

Bite of wild animal (skunk, bat, fox, coyote, raccoon, bobcat, or other carnivore)

Regard as rabid unless proved negative by laboratory tests.

Bite of another animal (e.g., livestock)

Consult with public health officials to determine need for treatment.

Give the exposed person RIG (20 IU/kg). If anatomically feasible, infiltrate the full dose around the wounds. Infiltrate any remaining RIG I.M. at a site distant from that of vaccine administration. Also, administer 1.0 ml of HDCV into the deltoid muscle or, in children, the upper thigh on days 0, 3, 7, 14, and 28. If the animal is available, kill it and immediately examine its brain tissue for the presence of rabies by using fluorescent antibody tests. If the tests are negative, discontinue HDCV.

Approach to Viral Exposure

Hepatitis B

- **Chronic exposure**
  Health care workers and other groups at risk for exposure to hepatitis B should receive the HB vaccine series before exposure.

- **Acute exposure**

  - **Source of exposure is HBsAg-positive**

    - **Exposed person has never been vaccinated**
      Give a single dose of HBIG. Initiate the HB vaccine series.

    - **Exposed person previously vaccinated with HB vaccine**
      Known responder: Test for anti-HBs. If adequate, no treatment is needed. If inadequate, give one booster dose.
      Known nonresponder: Give two doses of HBIG, or give one dose of HBIG and initiate revaccination.
      Responder unknown: Test for anti-HBs. If adequate, no treatment is needed. If inadequate, give one dose of HBIG plus an HB vaccine booster dose.

  - **Source of exposure is HBsAg-negative**
    No treatment is needed unless the exposed person has never received the HB vaccine series, in which case it should be initiated.

  - **HBsAg status of source of exposure is unknown**
    If source is known to be at high risk, act as if source is HBsAg-positive.

    - **Exposed person previously received HB vaccine series**
      Known responder: No treatment is needed.
      Known nonresponder: If the source is at high risk for HB virus infection, consider proceeding as if source had been proved positive for HB_sAg.
      Responder unknown: Test for anti-HB_s. If adequate, no treatment is needed. If inadequate, give one dose of HBIG plus an HB vaccine booster dose.

    - **Exposed person has never been vaccinated**
      Initiate the HB vaccine series.

Hepatitis C

Perform serologic testing for ALT and HCV antibody at time of exposure and again at 6 months. If anti-HCV is detected, confirmatory testing with recombinant immunoblot is indicated. HCV immunoglobulin is no longer recommended.

> **Table 1** Precautions to Prevent Transmission of HIV[1]
>
> **Universal Precautions**
>
> 1. All health care workers should use appropriate barrier precautions routinely to prevent skin and mucous membrane exposure when contact with blood or other body fluids of any patient is anticipated. Gloves should be worn for touching blood and body fluids, mucous membranes, or nonintact skin of all patients; for handling items or surfaces soiled with blood or body fluids; and for performing venipuncture and other vascular-access procedures. Gloves should be changed after contact with each patient. During procedures that are likely to generate aerosolized droplets of blood or other body fluids, masks and protective eyewear or face shields should be worn to prevent exposure of mucous membranes of the mouth, nose, and eyes. Gowns or aprons should be worn during procedures that are likely to generate splashes of blood or other body fluids.
> 2. Hands and other skin surfaces should be washed immediately and thoroughly if contaminated with blood or other body fluids. Hands should be washed immediately after gloves are removed.
> 3. All health care workers should take precautions to prevent injuries caused by needles, scalpels, and other sharp instruments or devices during procedures; when cleaning used instruments; during disposal of used needles; and when handling sharp instruments after procedures. To prevent needle-stick injuries, needles should not be recapped, purposely bent or broken by hand, removed from disposable syringes, or otherwise manipulated by hand. After they are used, disposable syringes and needles, scalpel blades, and other sharp items should be placed in puncture-resistant containers for disposal; the puncture-resistant containers should be located as close as practical to the area of use. Large-bore reusable needles should be placed in a puncture-resistant container for transport to the reprocessing area.
> 4. Although saliva has not been implicated in HIV transmission, to minimize the need for emergency mouth-to-mouth resuscitation, mouthpieces, resuscitation bags, or other ventilation devices should be available for use in areas in which the need for resuscitation is predictable.
> 5. Health care workers who have exudative lesions or weeping dermatitis should refrain from all direct patient care and from handling patient care equipment until the condition resolves.
> 6. Pregnant health care workers are not known to be at greater risk for contracting HIV infection than health care workers who are not pregnant; however, if a health care worker acquires HIV infection during pregnancy, the infant is at risk for infection resulting from perinatal transmission. Because of this risk, pregnant health care workers should be especially familiar with and strictly adhere to precautions to minimize the risk of HIV transmission.
>
> **Additional Precautions for Invasive Procedures**
>
> 1. All health care workers who participate in invasive procedures must use appropriate barrier precautions routinely to prevent skin and mucous membrane contact with blood and other body fluids of all patients. Gloves and surgical masks must be worn for all invasive procedures. Protective eyewear or face shields should be worn for procedures that commonly result in the generation of aerosolized droplets, splashing of blood or other body fluids, or the generation of bone chips. Gowns or aprons made of materials that provide an effective barrier should be worn during invasive procedures that are likely to result in the splashing of blood or other body fluids. All health care workers who perform or assist in vaginal or cesarean deliveries should wear gloves and gowns when handling the placenta or the infant until blood and amniotic fluid have been removed from the infant's skin and should wear gloves during postdelivery care of the umbilical cord.
> 2. If a glove is torn or a needle-stick or other injury occurs, the glove should be removed and a new glove used as promptly as patient safety permits; the needle or instrument involved in the incident should also be removed from the sterile field. In the event of an injury, postexposure evaluation should be sought as soon as possible.

& Health Administration (OSHA) directing that all health care workers potentially exposed to blood or other potentially infectious material either be offered hepatitis B vaccine free of charge, demonstrate immunity to hepatitis B, or formally decline vaccination.[13] That vaccination has been effective in decreasing the incidence of hepatitis B in health care workers is shown by the decrease in infection rates from 174/100,000 in 1982 to 17/100,000 in 1995.[14] Most series have not found the seroprevalence of HCV to be higher in health care worker groups at risk than in the general population.[14] That hepatitis B and hepatitis C are much more common than HIV in health care workers is a strong argument for using universal precautions in all patients.

One reason why hepatitis B is so much more transmissible than HIV is the greater number of virus particles in the blood of hepatitis B carriers. These persons have blood concentrations of 10^8 to 10^9 virus particles/ml, compared with 10^2 to 10^4/ml for persons with HIV infection and 10^6/ml for persons with HCV infection.

The extensive guidelines that have been established by the CDC for the care of patients with HBV infection[4,15-17] also apply to patients with HIV infection. Patients known to have hepatitis B, hepatitis C, or AIDS need not be put in a private room unless they are fecally incontinent or are shedding virus in body fluids. Health care workers should wear gloves and gowns when they have contact with or may have contact with a patient's blood, feces, or other body fluids. Needles used for drawing blood should be disposed of with special care: they must not be reused, recapped, or removed from the syringe. Hands must be washed before and after direct contact with the patient or with items that have been in contact with the patient's blood, feces, or body fluids.

Published recommendations also provide guidelines for health care workers who are not directly involved in patient care (e.g., housekeeping personnel, kitchen staff, and laundry workers).[1-7] No additional precautions are necessary for these individuals because their risk of acquiring HIV, HCV, or HBV is so low; in fact, transmission to them has not been documented. However, staff should be educated about appropriate procedures. Workers should wear gloves when handling blood and body fluids of all patients and should wear masks in areas where blood may spatter (e.g., the dialysis unit or the obstetrics unit).

TRANSMISSION FROM HEALTH CARE WORKERS TO PATIENTS

To date, there have been only two reports of HIV transmission from infected health care workers to patients. In one report, DNA sequence analysis linked a Florida dentist with AIDS to HIV infection in six of his patients.[18] In the other, an orthopedic surgeon in France may have transmitted HIV to one of his patients in the course of an operation.[19] Despite extensive investigation, no break in infection control precautions was documented in either case, nor was any clear-cut means of transmission identified.

HBV transmission from health care workers to patients is known to occur. Nineteen case reports have documented physician-to-patient transmission.[20-32] Eighteen of the 19 physicians were surgeons; seven of the surgeons were gynecologists, three were cardiac surgeons, and one was an orthopedic surgeon. All of the physicians were positive for HBeAg. Three of the gynecologists made a practice of handling needle tips. Of the 135 patients studied, 121 had clinical hepatitis B, and 14 had only serologic evidence of infection. Forty-one of the 135 patients were accounted for by the only nonsurgeon, a family practitioner from rural Switzerland. There are many additional cases of HBV having been transmitted by dentists and oral surgeons. In addition, three patients' relatives, two members of a surgeon's family, and one laboratory technician became infected.

In five studies, patients of 16 health care workers (including two surgeons) who were positive for hepatitis B surface antigen (HBsAg) were prospectively followed for evidence of hepatitis.[33-37] A total of 784 patients were followed and were compared with 656 patients cared for by health care workers who were HBsAg negative. None of the patients acquired overt hepatitis or became seropositive for HBsAg. Eight (1.02%) of the 784 patients cared for by HBsAg-positive health care workers developed antibody to HBsAg (anti-HBs), but so did six (0.91%) of the 656 patients cared for by health care workers who were negative for HBsAg. These reports suggest that the likelihood of infected surgeons' or other health care workers' transmitting HIV or HBV to their patients is extremely low. Chronic carriers of HBsAg who are seronegative for HBeAg are much less likely to transmit HBV than persons who are HBeAg positive.

Before the cases of transmission of HIV from the dentist to six of his patients were reported, the CDC had not taken a position on whether HBV- or HIV-infected surgeons should be allowed to continue practicing medicine. After these cases were reported, the CDC held meetings of health care professionals and other interested parties and published its recommendations on July 12, 1991.[38] These recommendations called for physicians not to perform "exposure-prone invasive procedures" unless they sought counsel from an expert review panel and were advised under what circumstances, if any, they might be allowed to continue to perform these procedures. Physicians would have to notify prospective patients of their seropositivity. These recommendations were strongly resisted by the medical community because at that time, only one health care worker, the dentist, had been implicated in transmitting HIV to his patients, no mechanism of transmission had been elucidated, no other patients had HIV transmitted by a health care worker, and invasive procedures that were "exposure prone" (exposing the patient to blood of the health care worker) were impossible to define. After subsequent meetings, the CDC abandoned its attempts to define exposure-prone procedures but did not alter its recommendations. Rather, it left it up to the states to define exposure-prone procedures. Subsequently, the President's Commission on AIDS recommended that HIV-infected health care workers should not have to curtail their practices or inform their patients of their infection.

Transmission of HCV from health care workers to patients has been reported. In one such case, a cardiac surgeon transmitted HCV to at least five patients during valve replacement surgery.[39] In another, an anesthesiologist in Spain may have infected more than 217 patients by first injecting himself with narcotics, then giving the remainder of the drugs to his patients.[40] At present, no recommendations exist for restricting the professional activities of health care workers with HCV infection.

Management of Viral Exposure

HIV

The CDC has issued recommendations for the management of potential exposure of health care workers to HIV.[1,4,41] If a health care worker is exposed by a needle stick or by a splash in the eye or mouth to any patient's blood or other body fluids, and the HIV serostatus of the patient is unknown, the patient should be informed of the incident and, if consent is obtained, tested for serologic evidence of HIV infection. If consent cannot be obtained, procedures for testing the patient should be followed in accordance with state and local laws. Testing of needles or other sharp instruments associated with exposure to HIV is not recommended, because it is unclear whether the test results would be reliable and how they should be interpreted.[41]

Health care workers exposed to HIV should be evaluated for susceptibility to blood-borne infection with baseline testing, including testing for HIV antibody. If the patient who is the source of exposure is seronegative and exhibits no clinical evidence of AIDS or symptoms of HIV infection, further follow-up of the health care worker is usually unnecessary.[41] If the source patient is seropositive or is seronegative but has engaged in high-risk behaviors, baseline and follow-up HIV-antibody testing of the health care worker at 6 weeks, 3 months, and 6 months after exposure should be considered.[41] Seroconversion usually occurs within 6 to 12 weeks of exposure; infrequently, it occurs considerably later. Three cases of delayed HIV seroconversion among health care workers have been reported.[42-44] In all three patients, an HIV antibody test yielded negative results at 6 months but positive results at some point during the following 1 to 7 months. In two cases, coinfection with HCV had occurred and took an unusually severe course. At present, it is unclear whether coinfection with these two viruses directly influences the timing or severity of either infection, but most experts recommend close monitoring for up to 1 year for health care workers exposed to both viruses in whom serologic evidence of HCV infection develops.

Treatment of the exposed health care worker should begin with careful washing of the exposure site with soap and water. Mucous membranes should be flushed with water. There is no evidence that either expressing fluid by squeezing the wound or applying antiseptics is beneficial, though antiseptics are not contraindicated. The use of caustic agents (e.g., bleach) is not recommended.

Any health care worker concerned about exposure to HIV should receive follow-up counseling regarding the risk of HIV transmission, postexposure testing, and medical evaluation, regardless of whether postexposure prophylaxis is given. HIV antibody testing should be performed at specified intervals for at least 6 months after the exposure (e.g., at 6 weeks, 3 months, and 6 months). The risk of HIV transmission is believed to depend on several factors: how much blood is involved in the exposure, whether the blood came from a source patient with terminal AIDS (thought to be attributable to the presence of large quantities of HIV), whether any host factors are present that might affect transmissibility (e.g., abnormal CD4 receptors for HIV), and whether the source patient carries any aggressive HIV viral mutants (e.g., syncytia-inducing strains). Factors indicating exposure to a large quantity of the source patient's blood (and thus a high risk of HIV transmission) include a device visibly contaminated with the patient's blood, a procedure that involved a needle placed directly in a vein or artery, and a deep injury.[45]

During the follow-up period, especially the first 6 to 12 weeks, exposed health care workers should follow the U.S. Public Health Service recommendations for preventing further transmission of HIV.[1-4] These recommendations include refraining from blood, semen, or organ donation and either abstaining from sexual intercourse or using measures to prevent HIV transmission during intercourse.[46]

The circumstances of the exposure should be recorded in the worker's confidential medical record and should include the following:

Table 2 Recommendations for Hepatitis B Prophylaxis after Percutaneous or Permucosal Exposure[15]

Hepatitis B Vaccination Status of Exposed Person	HBsAg Status of Source of Exposure		
	HBsAg-Positive	HBsAg-Negative	Untested or Unknown
Unvaccinated	Give single dose of HBIG Initiate HB vaccine series	Initiate HB vaccine series	Initiate HB vaccine series
Previously vaccinated Known responder	Test exposed person for anti-HBs If anti-HBs levels are adequate,* no treatment is needed; if they are inadequate, give an HB vaccine booster dose	No treatment is needed	No treatment is needed
Known nonresponder	*No response to three-dose vaccine series:* give two doses of HBIG or one dose of HBIG plus revaccination *No response to three-dose vaccine series plus revaccination:* give one dose of HBIG as soon as possible and a second dose 1 mo later	No treatment is needed	If source is at high risk for hepatitis B infection, consider proceeding as if source had been demonstrated to be HBsAg-positive
Response unknown	Test exposed person for anti-HBs If anti-HBs levels are adequate,* no treatment is needed; if they are inadequate, give one dose of HBIG plus an HB vaccine booster dose	No treatment is needed	Test exposed person for anti-HBs If anti-HBs levels are adequate,* no treatment is needed; if they are inadequate, initiate revaccination

*An adequate anti-HBs level is ≥ 10 mIU/ml, which is approximately equivalent to 10 sample ratio units (SRU) on radioimmunoassay or a positive result on enzyme immunoassay.

1. The date and time of the exposure.
2. Details of the exposure, including (a) where and how the exposure occurred, (b) the type and amount of fluid or other material involved, and (c) the severity of the exposure (for a percutaneous exposure, this would include the depth of injury and whether fluid was injected; for a skin or mucous membrane exposure, it would include the extent and duration of contact and the condition of the skin—chapped, abraded, or intact).
3. A description of the source of the exposure, including (if known) whether the source material contained HIV or other blood-borne pathogens, whether the source was HIV positive, the stages of any diseases present, whether the patient had previously received antiretroviral therapy, and the viral load.
4. Details about counseling, postexposure management, and follow-up.[41]

The data currently available on primary HIV infection indicate that systemic infection does not occur immediately. There may be a brief window of opportunity during which postexposure antiretroviral therapy may modify viral replication. Findings from animal and human studies provide indirect evidence of the efficacy of antiretroviral drugs in postexposure prophylaxis. The majority of these studies included zidovudine (AZT); consequently, all postexposure prophylaxis regimens now in use include AZT. Combination treatment regimens using nucleoside reverse transcriptase inhibitors and protease inhibitors have proved effective. Accordingly, most experts now recommend dual therapy with two nucleosides (zidovudine and lamivudine) for low- to moderate-risk exposures. For high-risk exposures, most experts would add a protease inhibitor (usually either indinavir or nelfinavir) to the two nucleoside reverse transcriptase inhibitors. These medications should be started as soon as possible after the exposure (within hours rather than days) and should be continued for 4 weeks.

An important component of postexposure care is encouraging and facilitating compliance with the lengthy course of medication. Therefore, careful consideration must be given to the toxicity profiles of the antiretroviral agents chosen. All of these agents have been associated with side effects, include GI (e.g., nausea or diarrhea), hematologic, endocrine (e.g., diabetes), and urologic effects (e.g., nephrolithiasis with indinavir). According to some early data, 50% to 90% of health care workers receiving combination regimens for postexposure prophylaxis (e.g., zidovudine plus 3TC, with or without a protease inhibitor) reported one or more subjective side effects that were substantial enough to cause 24% to 36% of the workers to discontinue postexposure prophylaxis.[47-49]

Whether antiretroviral agents should be chosen for postexposure prophylaxis on the basis of the resistance patterns of the source patient's HIV remains unclear. Transmission of resistant strains has been reported[50-52]; however, in the perinatal clinical trial that studied vertical transmission of HIV, zidovudine prevented perinatal transmission despite genotypic resistance of HIV to zidovudine in the mother.[53] Further study of the significance of genotypic resistance is necessary before definitive recommendations can be made.

HEPATITIS B

Both passive immunization with hepatitis B immune globulin (HBIG) and active immunization with hepatitis B vaccine (HB vaccine) are currently available for prophylaxis against hepatitis B [see Table 2].

Passive Immunoprophylaxis

HBIG is prepared by Cohn ethanol fractionation from plasma selected to contain a high titer of anti-HBs; this process inactivates and eliminates HIV from the final product. In the United States, HBIG has an anti-HBs titer of at least 1:100,000 by radioimmunoassay.[54] HBIG provides temporary, passive protection. It is indicated after low-volume percutaneous or mucous membrane exposure to HBV; it is not effective for high-

Table 3 Candidates for Hepatitis B Vaccine[15]

Preexposure vaccination	Persons with occupational risk (e.g., health care workers, public safety workers)
	Clients and staffs of institutions for the developmentally disabled
	Hemodialysis patients
	Sexually active homosexual men
	Users of illicit injectable drugs
	Recipients of certain blood products (e.g., patients with clotting disorders who receive clotting factor concentrates)
	Household and sexual contacts of HBV carriers
	Adoptees from countries of high HBV endemicity
	Other contacts of HBV carriers (vaccination is usually not required unless there are special circumstances, such as biting or scratching, or medical conditions, such as severe skin disease, that facilitate transmission)
	Populations with high endemicity of HBV infection (e.g., Alaskan natives, Pacific islanders, and refugees from HBV-endemic areas)
	Inmates of long-term correctional facilities
	Sexually active heterosexual persons with multiple sexual partners
	International travelers who spend more than 6 mo in HBV-endemic areas and have close contact with the local population
	All infants born in the United States
	Adolescents 11 to 12 years old who have not previously been vaccinated
Postexposure vaccination	Perinatal exposure (infants born to HBsAg-positive mothers)
	Acute exposure to blood that contains (or might contain) HBsAg
	Sexual partners of persons with acute HBV infections
	Household contacts of persons with acute HBV infections (infants and older persons who have had identifiable blood exposure to the index patient)

volume exposure (e.g., blood transfusion). The recommended dose of HBIG for adults is 0.06 ml/kg I.M. Passive prophylaxis with HBIG should begin as soon as possible after exposure—ideally, within 24 hours.[54]

Active Immunoprophylaxis

Two types of HB vaccine are currently licensed in the United States, plasma-derived vaccine (Heptavax-B) and recombinant vaccine (Recombivax HB and Engerix-B). Heptavax-B contains alum-adsorbed 22 nm HBsAg particles purified from human plasma and processed to inactivate the infectivity of HBV and other viruses. Plasma-derived vaccine is no longer being produced in the United States, but similar vaccines are produced and used in China and other countries. In the United States, use of Heptavax-B is limited to persons allergic to yeast. Recombivax HB and Engerix-B are prepared by recombinant DNA technology in common baker's (or brewer's) yeast, *Saccharomyces cerevisiae*.

For primary vaccination, three I.M. injections (into the deltoid muscle in adults and children and into the anterolateral thigh muscle in infants and neonates) are given, with the second and third doses 1 and 6 months after the first dose.[54] The dose for Heptavax-B and Engerix-B is 20 µg (volume, 1.0 ml) for persons older than 11 years, and that for Recombivax HB is 10 µg (1.0 ml) for persons older than 19 years and 5 µg (0.5 ml) for persons 11 to 18 years of age. For immunologically impaired patients, including hemodialysis patients, the dose is 40 µg for all three vaccines. For postexposure prophylaxis with Engerix-B, a regimen of four doses given soon after exposure and 1, 2, and 12 months afterward has been approved.

HB vaccine is more than 90% effective at preventing infection or clinical hepatitis in susceptible persons. Protection is virtually complete in persons who develop adequate antibody. Routine testing for immunity after vaccination is not recommended, but testing should be considered for persons at occupational risk who require postexposure prophylaxis for needle-stick exposure.

Between 30% and 50% of persons who have been vaccinated will cease to have detectable antibody levels within 7 years, but protection against infection and clinical disease appears to persist.[54,55] The need for booster doses has not been established. Revaccination of individuals who do not respond to the primary series will produce adequate antibody in 15% to 25% of cases after one additional dose and in 30% to 50% after three additional doses.[56]

Although effective HB vaccines have been available since 1982, the incidence of hepatitis B in the United States continued to increase in the first decade of HB vaccine use. In 1991, the Advisory Committee for Immunization Practices (ACIP), citing the safety of the vaccine and the evidence of continuing spread of HBV, recommended universal vaccination of all infants born in the United States.[57]

Recommendations for Exposure to Blood That Contains (or May Contain) HBsAg

Acute exposure The U.S. Public Health Service has provided recommendations for hepatitis B prophylaxis after accidental percutaneous, mucous membrane, or ocular exposure to blood that contains (or may contain) HBsAg [see Table 2].[43] These recommendations are based on consideration of several factors: (1) whether the source of the blood is available, (2) the HBsAg status of the source, and (3) the hepatitis B vaccination and vaccination-response status of the exposed person. After exposure, a blood sample should be obtained from the person who was the source of the exposure and should be tested for HBsAg. The hepatitis B vaccination status and the anti-HBs response status (if known) of the exposed person should be reviewed. Because passive administration of antibody with HBIG does not inhibit the active antibody response to HB vaccine, the two can be given simultaneously

Chronic exposure The U.S. Public Health Service recommends that persons who are at risk for exposure to HBV receive the HB vaccine series [see Table 3].[54] Health care workers who are at increased risk for acquiring hepatitis B include all physicians (especially surgeons), dentists, and laboratory and support personnel, such as nurses and technicians who work in the operating room or who have contact with infected patients, blood or blood products, or excreta. Because of their frequent exposure to blood and their high risk of hepatitis B, all surgeons should receive HB vaccine. As of 1994, however, only 50% of surgeons had been vaccinated, despite the proven efficacy and safety of the vaccine and surgeons' increased risk of exposure.[58] Hospital personnel who do not have frequent contact with blood or blood products (e.g., the janitorial, laundry, and kitchen staffs) need not be vaccinated.

Screening of personnel and patients for anti-HBs before vaccination is indicated only for individuals in high-risk groups; it has not been found to be cost-effective outside these groups.

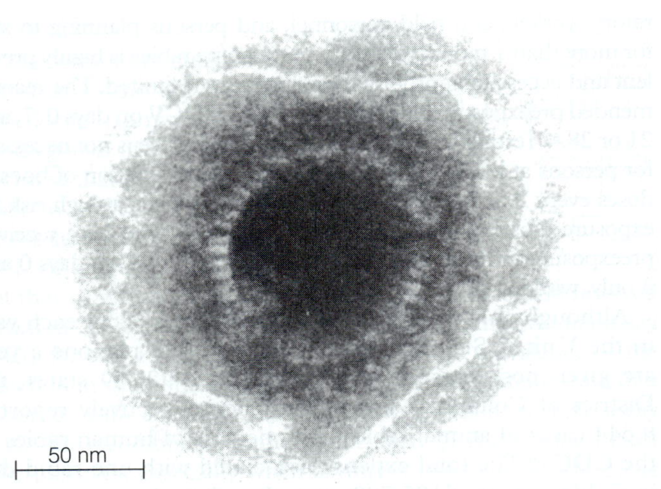

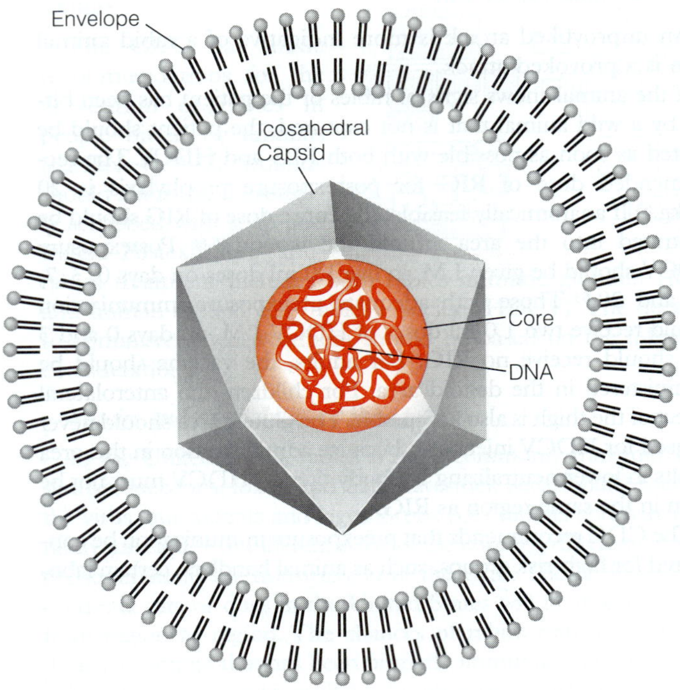

Figure 1 The capsomers and the irregularly shaped surrounding envelope of a cytomegalovirus are highlighted by negative staining with uranyl acetate (above). A typical herpesvirus (right) consists of a central core containing DNA; an icosahedral capsid, a surrounding layer of protein made up of 162 individual capsomers; and an envelope, a membrane coat acquired when the virus buds from the nuclear membrane of the host cell.

For most acute primary infections, serum obtained during late recovery or after recovery (convalescent serum) has an increased antibody titer, compared with serum obtained early in the course of the disease (acute serum). Most tests are performed on an initial serum dilution of 1:2 or 1:10 and on serial twofold dilutions thereafter. A fourfold increase in titer (indicated by reactivity of a two-tube dilution) usually represents a significant increase in antibody response and is considered to constitute seroconversion. An immunocompromised host may occasionally fail to mount an antibody response.

Some viruses are so common that patients may already have antibody titers when the disease is first suspected. Herpesviruses are ubiquitous and are present in many healthy people in latent form. At the onset of herpesvirus infections, patients may already have the corresponding antibody. Nevertheless, their antibody titer will almost always increase significantly after recovery.

A variety of serologic tests are available in the clinical laboratory: complement fixation, radioimmunoassay, enzyme-linked immunosorbent assay (ELISA), immunofluorescence, immune precipitation, immune blotting, latex agglutination, virus neutralization, indirect hemagglutination, immune adherence hemagglutination, and hemagglutination inhibition. None of these serologic tests is appropriate for identification of all viruses.

ISOLATION OF VIRUS

The isolation of virus requires appropriate specimen collection and inoculation into animals or onto appropriate cell lines. Blood sent for virus isolation should be unclotted because some viruses, such as herpesviruses, are found primarily in lymphocytes. If cell-associated viruses are suspected, lymphocytes should be inoculated directly onto target cells. Several types of cells are available for growing viruses, and no single cell line is appropriate for all of them. Therefore, it is helpful to the laboratory to know which virus the clinician suspects.

Viruses that grow in cell monolayers in tissue culture have cytopathic effects that can be recognized under the microscope (e.g., rounding, transformation, or death) [*see Figure 2*]. Some viruses, such as rubella, produce no direct cytopathic effects but can be detected because they inhibit the cytopathic effects of a second test virus. This phenomenon is called viral interference. Other viruses (e.g., myxoviruses) cause changes in the cell membrane so that red blood cells adhere to the cell surface (hemadsorption). The identity of isolated viruses can be confirmed by use of specific antisera that are known to inhibit viral growth.

Tissue suspected of containing an encephalitis or other neurotropic virus can be minced and the extract injected intracerebrally into an infant mouse. If the mouse dies and bacteria cannot be cultured from the brain, the injected material presumably contained such a virus. If antiserum of known specificity neutralizes the virus, the specificity of the antiserum indicates the specific identity of the virus. The criterion for neutralization is that inoculation of neutralized virus will not kill the mouse.

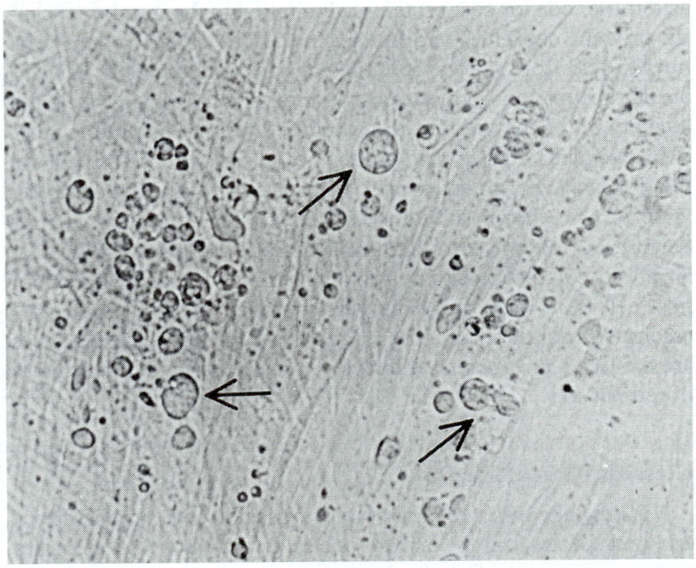

Figure 2 Cells infected with cytomegalovirus become large and round (arrows). Note the uniform appearance of adjacent uninfected cells.

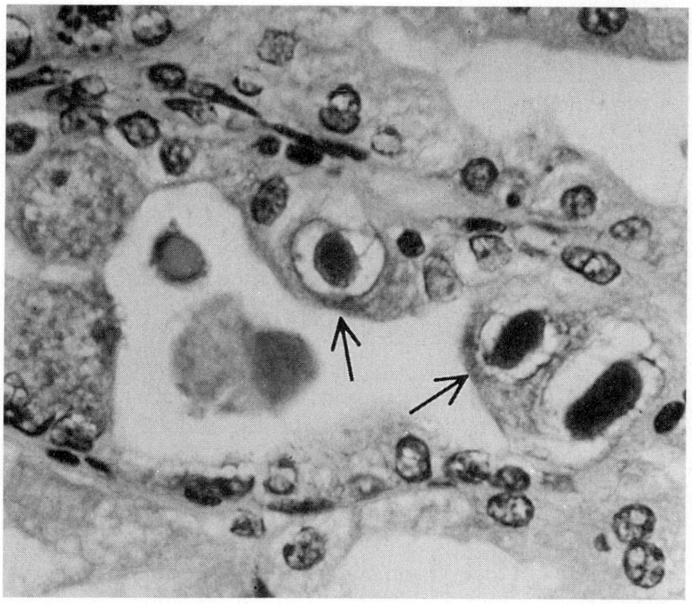

Figure 3 Kidney biopsy shows cytomegalovirus-infected tubular epithelial cells (arrows). In such cells, a dark intranuclear inclusion is surrounded by a clear halo. Inclusions usually indicate sites of previous or current viral replication.

HISTOLOGIC EXAMINATION

Histologic examination of biopsy and autopsy tissues may demonstrate changes that are typical of certain viruses. Members of the herpesvirus group can be characterized by intranuclear inclusions surrounded by a clear halo [see Figure 3]. RNA viruses usually produce inclusions in the cytoplasm; for instance, dark-staining intracytoplasmic inclusions in the brain tissue of animals or patients are diagnostic of rabies infection and are called Negri bodies. Inclusion bodies are either masses of closely packed virus particles or remnants of prior virus replication.

DETECTION OF VIRAL ANTIGENS

Viral antigens can be detected in tissues by techniques employing their corresponding antibodies. If virus is present, these antigens may be visible microscopically under ultraviolet light either by direct immunofluorescence (i.e., in tissue sections stained with fluorescein-labeled antiviral antibody) or by indirect immunofluorescence (i.e., in tissue sections exposed first to antiviral antibody and then to fluorescein-labeled anti–γ-globulin antibody). Fluorescence microscopy requires specimens that are fresh frozen (preferably in liquid nitrogen). Immunofluorescence staining of cells in tissue culture can detect viral antigens before cytopathic effects are evident. Viral antigens in formalin-fixed tissue can be identified by immunohistochemical microscopy (e.g., using peroxidase-labeled antibodies).

DETECTION OF VIRAL NUCLEIC ACID

Viral nucleic acids can be detected in body fluids and tissues at virus concentrations too low to be detected by other means. The PCR permits amplification of even a small number of copies of viral nucleic acid. In theory, even a single copy of a specific DNA can be detected by PCR. Before PCR is performed, DNA can be synthesized from viral RNA by means of reverse transcriptase. The PCR product can be detected by gel electrophoresis and compared with known viral DNA. This test is currently being used to diagnose CMV infection and is more sensitive than current serologic testing for HCV. Nucleic acid hybridization can detect viral nucleic acid in tissue specimens. Epstein-Barr virus genomes can be detected in this way in EBV-related cancers and lymphoproliferative disorders.

ELECTRON MICROSCOPY

Although seldom used routinely, electron microscopy allows rapid identification (in a matter of hours) of viruses in body fluids, tissues, and tissue extracts. Identification of viruses in body fluids and tissue extracts by this method is easier if the samples are first concentrated by ultracentrifugation, evaporation, or ultrafiltration. HBV has been observed in specimens from hepatitis patients only after ultracentrifugation.

Epidemiology of Viral Infections of Interest to Surgeons

Viral infections are spread to humans via several patterns of transmission: (1) direct transmission from humans with symptomatic infection (e.g., HBV, HCV herpesviruses, and HIV), (2) transmission from asymptomatic human carriers (e.g., HBV, HCV, HIV, and varicella-zoster virus), (3) transmission from arthropods (e.g., encephalitis and dengue viruses), and (4) transmission from other animals (e.g., rabies virus).

Viral infections are common in immunosuppressed patients in general and especially in recipients of organ transplants, who must take immunosuppressive drugs to prevent rejection. The overwhelming majority of these infections are caused by members of the herpesvirus family (e.g., CMV, herpes simplex viruses, varicella-zoster virus, and EBV); infections with HBV and with papovaviruses (e.g., human papillomavirus, which causes warts, and BK virus) are also frequent.

Because surgical patients are frequently given transfusions of blood or blood products and because hospital staff often incur accidental needle-stick injury, viruses that can be transmitted by these routes are of prime interest to surgeons and their patients. Examples of such viruses are HBV, hepatitis D, HCV, HIV, HTLV-I, and the herpesviruses, including EBV and CMV. These viruses can also be transmitted by organ transplantation either from the cells of the organ itself (e.g., HBV in liver cells or CMV in kidney cells) or from blood that has not been completely removed from the organ. Changes in donor acceptance and screening policies over time have increased the safety of the blood supply and should continue to do so in the future [see Table 5].[71]

HIV

Two serotypes of HIV, HIV-1 and HIV-2, have been identified. Both can cause AIDS. HIV-1 accounts for virtually all cases of AIDS in the United States and equatorial Africa. HIV-2 is found almost exclusively in West Africa; only a few cases of HIV-2 infection have occurred in the United States.

Because AIDS patients are immunodepressed, they are susceptible to opportunistic infections and neoplasms, especially non-Hodgkin lymphoma, *Pneumocystis carinii* pneumonia, and Kaposi sarcoma. AIDS is most prevalent in the United States among male homosexuals, abusers of I.V. drugs, and hemophiliacs. Since the implementation of testing for blood-borne HIV and the near-elimination of HIV from blood products, the incidence of HIV infection in the hemophiliac population has diminished markedly; however, in recent years, the incidence in the heterosexual population has been increasing rapidly.

HIV can be transmitted by transfusion of whole blood, packed red cells, plasma, factor VIII concentrates, factor IX concentrates, and platelets. The likelihood that a person will become infected with HIV after receiving a single-donor blood product that tests

Table 5 Changes in Donor Acceptance and Screening Policies Instituted to Reduce the Risk of Transmitting Infectious Diseases[71]

Policy	Implementation Date
Screening for HBsAg	July 1972
Voluntary exclusion of persons at high risk for AIDS	March 1983
Redefinition of high-risk behavior to include men who have had sex with more than one man since 1979	December 1984
Testing for antibody to HIV-1	Spring 1985
Redefinition of high-risk behavior to include any man who has had sex with another man since 1977	September 1985
Implementation of a mechanism to allow donors to indicate confidentially that their donations should not be used for transfusion	October 1986
Testing for alanine aminotransferase (ALT, formerly SGPT)	Winter 1986–1987
Testing for anti-HBc	Spring 1987
Testing for antibody to HTLV-1	January 1990
Testing for antibody to HCV	May 1990
Testing for antibody to HIV-2	April 1992
Testing for HIV-1 antigen	March 1996

positive for HIV approaches 100%.[72-73] Before the advent of serologic testing for HIV in 1985, 0.04% of 1,200,000 blood donations in the United States were estimated to be HIV positive.[74] AIDS has developed in more than 8,500 recipients of blood transfusions, blood components, or transplanted organs or tissue.

Federal regulations now require that all prospective blood and plasma donors be screened for antibody to HIV by ELISA. Because this test yields a low rate of false positive results, assay by the more sensitive Western blot electrophoresis is always used to confirm positive ELISA results. Routine testing of blood donors has greatly reduced HIV transmission via blood transfusions, but infection can still occur if the donor has been infected with HIV but has not yet developed antibody.[75] The risk of HIV transmission via transfusion of screened blood that is negative for HIV is estimated to be one in 200,000 to one in 2,000,000 per unit transfused in the United States.[76] Antibody to HIV usually develops within 4 weeks to 6 months of HIV infection.[77] From the time of infection until the appearance of antibody, infected individuals will test negative by ELISA or Western blot, and their blood might still be used for transfusion.

HIV and AIDS can also be transmitted by organ transplantation.[78] So far, only a small number of patients have been found to be infected in this way, but more will undoubtedly be reported. These patients received transplants before HIV testing of potential donors became possible. All prospective organ and tissue donors now should be tested for HIV infection and other blood-borne viral infections.

HIV infection is also a potential problem in health care workers, who are exposed to a large and growing population of AIDS patients. In the United States, an estimated 1.0 to 1.5 million people are infected with HIV but as yet have no symptoms. HIV transmission from blood, tissue, or other body fluids can occur in the health care setting as a result of percutaneous injury (e.g., from needles or other sharp objects), contamination of mucous membranes or nonintact skin (e.g., skin that is chapped, abraded, or affected by dermatitis), prolonged contact with intact skin, or contamination involving an extensive area.[79] HIV infection may be contracted through a variety of sources including blood, semen, vaginal secretions, visibly bloody fluids, and a number of other fluids for which the precise risk of transmission is undetermined (e.g., cerebrospinal, synovial, pleural, peritoneal, pericardial, and amniotic fluid). Infection may also be contracted from concentrated HIV used in research settings.[79] The results of multiple prospective studies quantifying transmission risk associated with a discrete occupational HIV exposure indicate that the average risk of HIV transmission associated with needle punctures or similar percutaneous injuries is approximately 0.3%. The estimated risk of transmission from mucocutaneous exposure to HIV-contaminated material is 0.03%. As of December 1999, the CDC had received reports of 56 U.S. health care workers in whom documented HIV seroconversion was temporally related to occupational HIV exposure. Of these 56, 48 had percutaneous exposures, five mucocutaneous exposures, two both percutaneous and mucous membrane exposures, and one an unknown route of exposure.[80] Another 138 possible cases of occupational HIV transmission—six involving surgeons—have been reported in persons with no risk factors for HIV transmission other than workplace exposure; however, seroconversion after a specific exposure was not documented. There may be other health care workers who also have acquired HIV infection from needle-stick or mucous membrane exposure but have not been reported, either because they and their patients have not been tested or because they have other risk factors for HIV infection

The concentration of virus in the blood or serum of antigen-positive individuals is several orders of magnitude less for HIV than for HBV. The number of needle-stick exposures to HIV that have actually led to a positive test result for HIV has been extremely small, whereas hepatitis B occurs in as many as 40% of health care workers exposed to the virus by needle-stick injury. Despite this relatively low infectiousness, AIDS is much more feared than hepatitis B because AIDS is often fatal. Although hepatitis B is usually not fatal and is often of short duration, several health care workers die of hospital-acquired hepatitis B and hepatitis C each year.

Hepatitis

Several viruses can cause hepatitis. Hepatitis A virus (HAV) and HBV cause what were formerly known as infectious hepatitis and serum hepatitis, respectively. HCV is the major cause of parenterally transmitted non-A, non-B hepatitis. Hepatitis E virus is a common cause of epidemic non-A, non-B hepatitis, which is chiefly found in developing countries in Africa and Asia. Hepatitis D virus (HDV, formerly called the delta agent) is defective or incomplete and is pathogenic only in the presence of HBV. The hepatitis viruses are the most common infectious agents to which hospital personnel may be exposed. Herpesviruses can also cause serious and sometimes fatal hepatitis, especially in severely immunocompromised patients, such as recipients of organ or bone marrow transplants and patients receiving intensive chemotherapy for cancer.

HEPATITIS A

HAV is a small (27 nm), single-stranded RNA virus belonging to the enterovirus subgroup of picornaviruses. Its almost exclusive transmission by the fecal-oral route is enhanced by poor personal hygiene, poor sanitary conditions, and crowding. Transmission can be contained by careful hand washing and the isolation of excretions. Unlike other types of viral hepatitis, hepatitis A is rarely transmitted by blood, blood products, or needle sticks and is rarely transmitted among hemodialysis patients, health care workers, and I.V. drug abusers. The infrequent parenteral transmission of HAV is attributed in part to its lack of an asymptomatic carrier state. Hepatitis A can be transmitted percutaneously only during a brief period of viremia before the onset of symptoms and jaundice. The chance that an infected person will donate blood during this short period is small; also, patients are usually outside the hospital during this period.

HEPATITIS B

HBV is a member of the Hepadnaviridae family of DNA viruses. It is most prevalent in the Far East, the Middle East, Africa, and parts of South America, where as many as 15% of the general population are chronic carriers. Worldwide, the most common mode of transmission is from mother to child during the perinatal period. In the United States, however, sexual or parenteral transmission has been implicated in most infections. The high-risk groups for chronic HBV infection in the United States include I.V. drug users, men who have sex with men, other individuals with multiple sexual partners, household contacts and sexual partners of HBV carriers, health care workers, patients on long-term hemodialysis, and organ transplant recipients.[81]

Clinical Course

The clinical course of hepatitis B is extremely variable: infection ranges from the completely asymptomatic to the rapidly fatal. The incubation period averages 75 days but can last from 40 to 180 days. Exposure to HBV has five potential outcomes: (1) no infection occurs; (2) acute hepatitis develops, followed by clearance of infection; (3) acute fulminant infection develops, leading to hepatic necrosis and death; (4) acute hepatitis develops without clearance of infection, and a chronic carrier state ensues; and (5) no acute illness develops, but a chronic carrier state ensues.

Approximately 55% of adults infected with HBV have no symptoms despite serologic documentation of infection (see below), which explains why blood donors who seem to be in good health are capable of transmitting the virus. Other individuals infected with HBV may have such mild symptoms (e.g., slight malaise, fatigability, and loss of appetite) that they do not seek medical attention.

Approximately 45% of people infected with HBV experience typical acute, icteric hepatitis, which is characterized by fatigue, anorexia, nausea, vomiting, and hepatomegaly. In approximately 1% of adults infected with HBV, acute fulminant hepatitis develops. This condition is characterized by progressive hepatocellular destruction, encephalopathy, and deepening coma. Fulminant hepatitis causes death in approximately 80% of affected adults and 30% of affected children.

In approximately 5% to 10% of hepatitis B cases, the infection becomes chronic. Patients with chronic hepatitis may be asymptomatic or may have clinical and histologic evidence of the disease, as well as persistently elevated levels of serum aminotransferases [see Figure 4]. With time, many patients pass to an asymptomatic carrier state, and serum aminotransferase levels fall. The duration of the asymptomatic carrier state appears to be indefinite. Chronic HBV infection can result in hepatocellular carcinoma, which is especially common in China, Southeast Asia, and sub-Saharan Africa.

Because most patients remain asymptomatic until the development of end-stage liver disease, there are no specific clinical findings that are indicative of chronic HBV infection. There are, however, several clinical syndromes linked to HBV infection that may provide a clue to the presence of chronic HBV infection. These syndromes include polyarteritis nodosa, membranous or membranoproliferative glomerulonephritis, leukocytoclastic vasculitis, erythema nodosum, arthritis, and serum sickness.

Antigens

HBV has a diameter of 42 nm and contains circular, double-stranded DNA. The protein coat on its outer surface is termed hepatitis B surface antigen. HBsAg is made in quantities greatly exceeding the amount required to coat the nucleic acid. The excess surface antigen appears in the serum as spheres 22 nm in diameter or tubules of the same diameter and of varying length. These spheres and tubules contain no nucleic acid and hence are not infectious. They may persist in the serum for prolonged periods, even for life, and in great quantities, up to 10^{12} to 10^{14} surface antigen particles (500 µg protein) per milliliter.[82]

The hepatitis B virus also has a nucleocapsid core, the outside of which contains the hepatitis B core antigen (HBcAg). HBcAg is not detected in hepatitis B during acute infection, because its antigenic determinants are hidden by the outer surface antigen of the intact virion.

Inside the hepatitis B nucleocapsid is a DNA-dependent DNA polymerase and the hepatitis B e antigen, which is thought to be either an internal component or a degradation product of the core antigen. HBeAg is found only in the serum of individuals whose serum also contains HBsAg, and it appears in the serum of virtually all patients early in the course of HBV infection. The presence of HBeAg in serum is indicative of the presence of large numbers of circulating intact virions: serum containing HBeAg is estimated to be one million times more infectious than serum containing HBsAg but not HBeAg.

Serology

HBsAg can be detected in the serum within a few weeks of viral exposure [see Figure 5]. It usually persists throughout the symptomatic period and does not disappear until after recovery. Anti-HBs appears shortly after the disappearance of HBsAg [see Table 6]. During this window period, neither HBsAg nor anti-HBs is detectable [see Table 7]. Anti-HBs persists for years and is associated with immunity to reinfection. HBV can be differentiated into eight serotypes on the basis of determinants of the surface antigen.

Hepatitis B core antigen (HBcAg) is not found free in the serum, but antibody to HBcAg (anti-HBc) becomes detectable at an early stage in the course of acute infections, 1 to 2 weeks after the appearance of HBsAg. Titers of anti-HBc fall after the disappearance of HBsAg but persist for life. In patients with chronic hepatitis B, HBsAg remains detectable indefinitely, and titers of anti-HBc remain high. Years after infection, titers of anti-HBs may have fallen to undetectable levels, and anti-HBc may be the only marker of previous infection. HBeAg is detectable immediately after the appearance of HBsAg. Antibody to HBeAg (anti-HBe) appears just after HBeAg becomes undetectable (usually before the disappearance of HBsAg) and persists for 1 to 2 years [see Figure 5].

HEPATITIS D

HDV is a defective, 35 to 37 nm RNA virus that can infect only persons who are also infected with HBV, because it uses HBsAg for its structural protein shell. HDV is found worldwide and is especially prevalent in the Amazon basin, central Africa, southern Italy, and the Middle East.[83] HDV infection is less common in the United States and Western Europe, where it is generally associat-

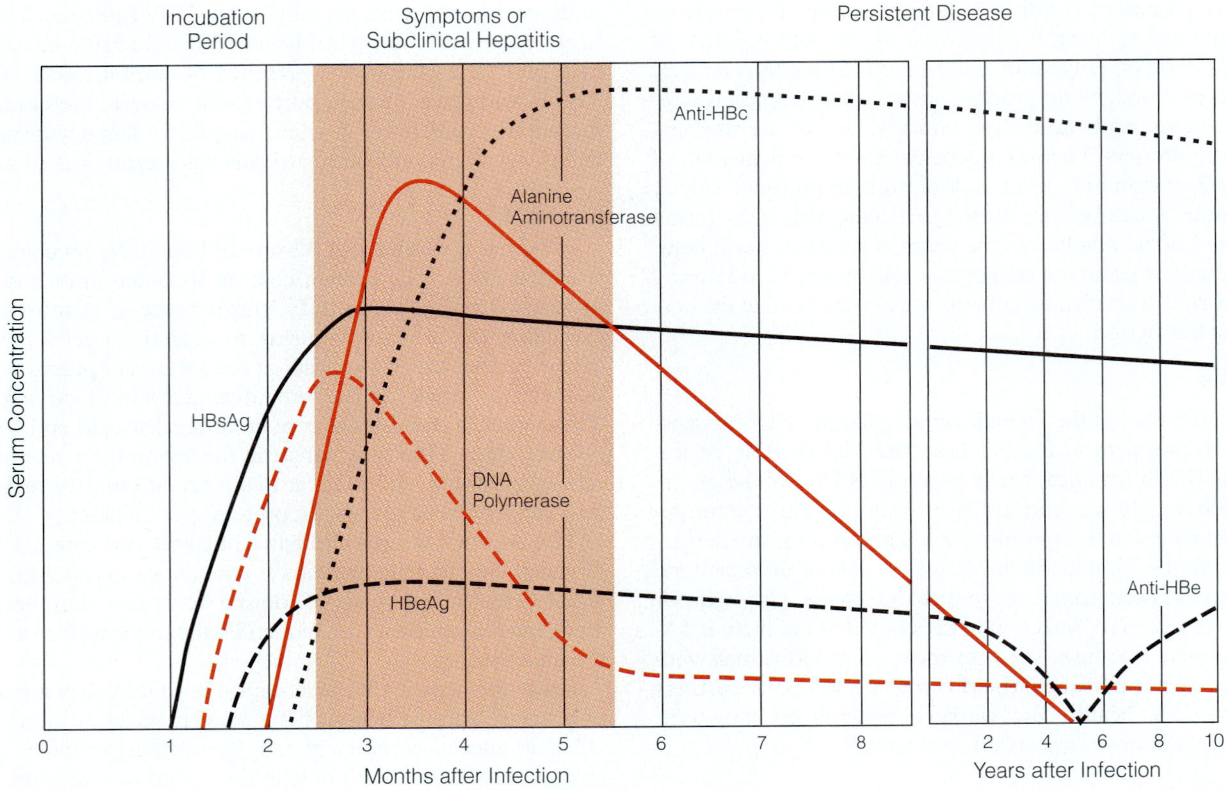

Figure 4 Schematic shows virologic, clinical, and serologic events of a hepatitis B infection that becomes persistent.

ed with parenteral blood exposure, typically in the setting of I.V. drug abuse or multiple transfusions.

Clinically, hepatitis D is found only in association with acute or chronic hepatitis B, and it cannot last longer than hepatitis B does. Depending on the state of the HBV infection, HDV infection appears either as a coinfection or a superinfection. Coinfection occurs when acute HDV infection and acute HBV infection are present simultaneously; superinfection occurs when acute HDV infection is superimposed on chronic HBV infection. Coinfection with HDV is associated with fulminant hepatitis and a mortality of 2% to 20%.[84] Fewer than 5% of cases of coinfection progress to chronic hepatitis D. In contrast, superinfection with HDV results in chronic HDV hepatitis, often with cirrhosis, in more than 70% of cases. The clinical and biochemical features of HDV infection resemble those of HBV infection alone. Chronic active hepatitis B progresses faster when hepatitis D is also present. Chronic HDV infection is more likely to result in severe morbidity and mortality than chronic HBV or HCV infection alone.

Diagnosis of acute HDV infection may be difficult: HDAg appears in the circulation only briefly and often goes undetected. Antibody to HDAg (anti-HD) of the IgM class subsequently appears in serum in low titers. Because no anti-HD IgG response occurs, no serologic marker of previous HDV infection may remain after recovery. Chronic HDV infection is easier to diagnose: high titers of anti-HD in the serum indicate ongoing HDV infection, and HDV antigen is detectable in the liver by means of immunohistochemical techniques. Moreover, IgM anti-HD remains detectable in serum.[83]

NON-A, NON-B HEPATITIS: HEPATITIS E AND HEPATITIS C

Non-A, non-B hepatitis is divided into two varieties, an epidemic form (hepatitis E) and a parenterally transmitted form (hepatitis C).[85] Hepatitis E is an acute, self-limited disease whose clinical features are similar to those of other types of hepatitis. Hepatitis E virus (HEV) is prevalent in the developing world, where it is spread by the fecal-oral route and has been associated with large outbreaks as well as sporadic cases. Outbreaks have been linked to contaminated water supplies. No cases of HEV infection acquired in the United States have been reported to date, but HEV acquisition has been reported in international travelers.

Hepatitis C is the most common cause of nonalcoholic liver disease in the United States. HCV is an RNA virus of the flavivirus family. It can be transmitted through parenteral exposure (usually in the setting of I.V. drug abuse), sexual contact, or the sharing of a household with an HCV-infected person; however, some persons with HCV infection have none of these risk factors, and there may be other means of transmission that have yet to be elucidated. Before the advent of antibody testing, HCV infection accounted for the majority (75% to 95%) of cases of posttransfusion hepatitis.[83] Since the spring of 1990, when a serologic test for HCV became available, all transfused blood has been screened for HCV, and the incidence of transfusion-associated hepatitis C has fallen precipitously. At present, however, I.V. drug use still accounts for a large proportion (60%) of HCV transmission in the United States.[59]

The presence of anti-HCV IgG appears not to be protective: blood donors with anti-HCV antibody can transmit hepatitis.[62] Surveys of HCV seropositivity indicate that 0.2% to 0.6% of volunteer blood donors carry anti-HCV IgG,[83] and the prevalence may be much higher among high-risk populations (e.g., residents of large inner-city communities). The prevalence of anti-HCV IgG is high among I.V. drug users, hemodialysis patients, and hemophiliacs.

Clinical Manifestations

The incubation period of hepatitis C averages 7 to 8 weeks in length but may be as short as 2 weeks or as long as 15. The clini-

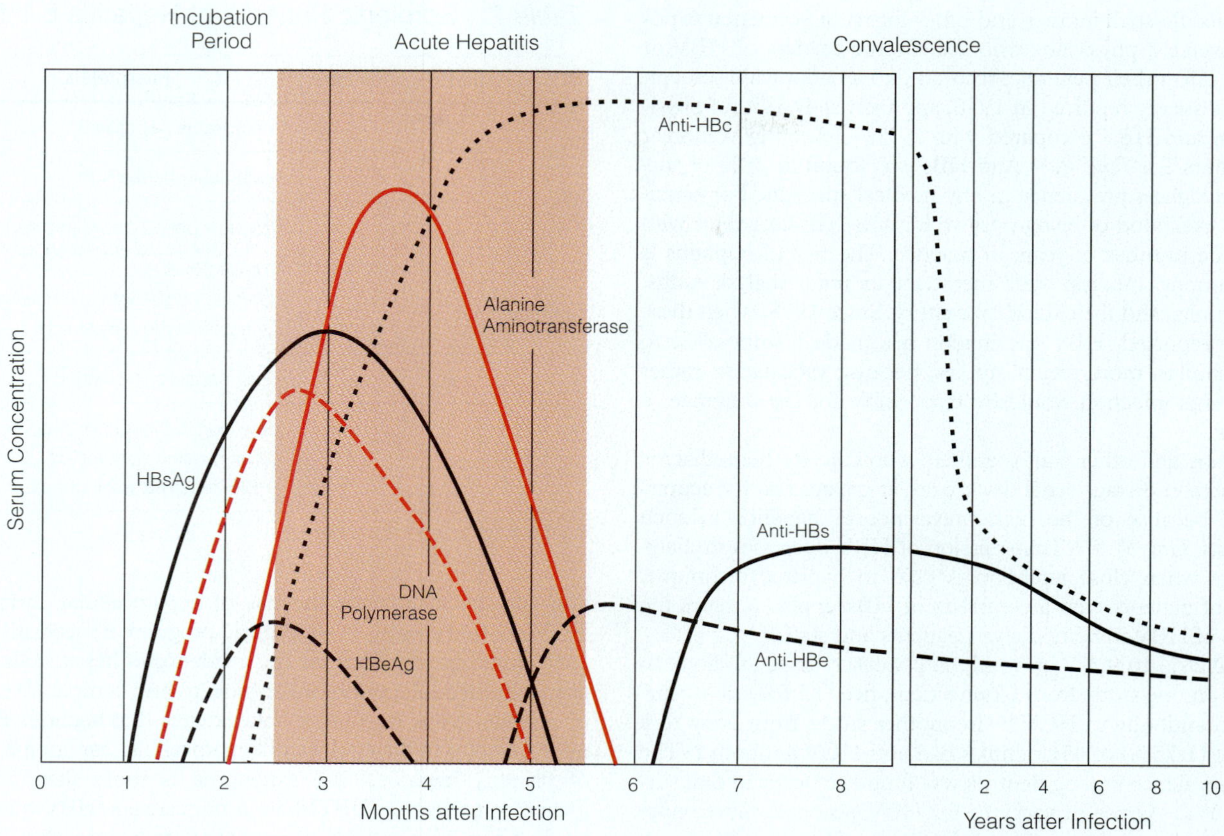

Figure 5 Schematic shows virologic, clinical, and serologic events during acute hepatitis B infection.

cal manifestations and biochemical alterations associated with acute hepatitis C are similar to but milder than those associated with hepatitis B. Serum aminotransferase levels can fluctuate widely; the peak levels are lower than those seen in hepatitis B (10 to 20 times normal as opposed to 20 to 50 times normal). Only about 25% of cases of acute HCV infection are icteric, and the mortality for acute infection is about 1%. Most patients have no acute illness suggestive of HCV infection. Antibody is not always present early in infection, and there are no clinically available assays for detecting IgM antibody to HCV. Thanks to improvements in the immunodetection of HCV, however, the interval before anti-HCV can be detected has decreased from the 6 to 12 months required with the first-generation tests to 8 to 12 weeks with the second-generation assays.[83]

The most striking feature of HCV infection is its tendency to become chronic in as many as 50% to 75% of cases. One study found that even among the 1% to 10% of individuals with HCV whose bloodstreams had been cleared of HCV according to RT-PCR assay, as many as 90% still had HCV in the liver.[86] It is estimated that in the United States, nearly four million people are seropositive for HCV, and more than 30% of liver transplantations are performed to treat end-stage liver disease related to chronic HCV infection. The presence of anti-HCV IgG does not distinguish acute from chronic hepatitis. Within 10 years, cirrhosis may develop in as many as 20% to 25% of patients with active hepatitis[87]; accordingly, these patients must be followed up carefully.

Chronic active hepatitis is characterized by elevated serum aminotransferase levels; however, other test results remain normal, and the patient is usually asymptomatic until end-stage liver disease develops. Liver biopsy shows inflammation around the portal triads. Recombinant interferons have been used to treat chronic HCV infection, with mixed results: frequently, there is little response to treatment, or viremia returns after treatment. The combination of interferon with ribavirin has shown promise, however. Interferon treatment is generally reserved for patients who have chronic HCV infection and show evidence of active necroinflammatory liver disease with persistent ALT elevations.

HEPATITIS IN HOSPITAL PERSONNEL

Patients with hepatitis can infect hospital personnel with the

Table 6 Serologic Markers of Hepatitis B Infection

HBsAg	Present in acute and chronic infection Indicator that person is infectious
Anti-HBs	Appears 2 to 16 wk after HBsAg disappears from the serum Persists for years Confers immunity
HBcAg	Not present in the serum Found in the hepatocyte
Anti-HBc	Appears in serum with or shortly after HBsAg Persists for years May be only indicator of hepatitis B infection
HBeAg	Appears in the early acute phase Indicates serum is highly infectious Persistence beyond 10 wk suggests progression to chronic carrier state
Anti-HBe	Good prognosis for resolution of infection

virus via needle-stick injuries and other forms of accidental exposure. Conversely, physicians who are chronic carriers of HBV or HCV can infect their patients. According to a nationwide seroepidemiologic survey reported in 1978, approximately 19% of physicians have anti-HBs, compared with 3.5% of healthy volunteer blood donors [see Table 8].[88] Anti-HBs was found in 28% of surgeons, the highest prevalence in any medical specialty. For physicians, the likelihood of being positive for anti-HBs correlates with age and the number of years in practice. The risk of hepatitis is greatest among medical staff members in renal dialysis units, oncology units, and the clinical laboratory. Since 1978, when these data were reported, HBV vaccination has made it impossible to perform similar, more recent studies, because vaccination rather than previous infection would be responsible for the presence of antibodies.

Physicians and other staff members who care for hemodialysis patients with end-stage renal disease are at greater risk for acquiring HBV because of the high prevalence of hepatitis in such patients [see Table 9].[89,90] Transmission of HBV decreases in dialysis centers when close attention is paid to hygienic technique. Isolation of patients who are carriers of HBsAg also reduces the incidence of HBV in hemodialysis patients and staff.[91]

From 0.28% to 9.3% of health care workers have antibody to HCV.[92-94] In one study from Connecticut, five (12.5%) of 40 surgeons had antibody to HCV.[92] In another study, from New York City, eight (1.75%) of 456 dentists had anti-HCV antibody.[93] The highest prevalence among dentists was found to occur in oral surgeons (9.3%). As use of vaccines for HBV becomes more widespread [see Management of Viral Exposure, Hepatitis B, above], HCV may come to predominate over HBV as the cause of the rare cases of hepatitis transmitted from hospital personnel to patients.

EPIDEMIOLOGY OF POSTTRANSFUSION HEPATITIS

Both HBV and HCV can be transmitted by percutaneous and other routes.[89] Rare cases of hepatitis have been attributed to the infusion of immune globulin, although its preparation by ethanol fractionization normally destroys hepatitis virus (as well as HIV). Albumin is pasteurized by heating at 60° C for 10 hours, which destroys hepatitis virus.

Because of the current criteria for acceptable blood donors, elimination of payment for blood donation, and serologic testing for HBV and HCV, the risk of contracting hepatitis B from a blood transfusion is now much lower than it once was. In the United States, it is now rare for either HBV or HCV to be transmitted via blood transfusion. According to the latest estimates available, the risk of HCV transmission via this route is approximately 1/103,000 (95% CI, 28,000 to 288,000), and that of HBV transmission is 1/63,000 (95% CI, 31,000 to 147,000).[95]

HDV can also be passed by transfusion. In a study of 262 patients who had posttransfusion hepatitis and whose serum was positive for HBsAg, anti-HD was found in nine patients.[96] HDV can be detected in 24% of HBsAg-positive drug abusers and in approximately 50% of HBsAg-positive hemophiliacs.

LONG-TERM EFFECTS OF CHRONIC HEPATITIS

Chronic hepatitis can lead to problems requiring surgical intervention. It can cause cirrhosis, which in turn can cause portal hypertension and bleeding varices that necessitate portal systemic shunting. In addition, HBV and HCV predispose to hepatocellular carcinoma, the most prevalent visceral cancer in the world. The condition is especially prevalent in China, Southeast Asia, and sub-Saharan Africa. It is estimated that 25% of chronically infected persons die of cirrhosis or hepatocellular carcinoma.[97] HBV coinfection appears to increase the risk of hepatocellular carcinoma in HCV-infected persons. A widespread program of vaccination against HBV could greatly decrease the incidence of hepatocellular carcinoma. Epidemiology, molecular biology, and comparative pathology provide strong circumstantial evidence that hepatitis B is a significant factor in the etiology of hepatocellular carcinoma. The risk of primary hepatocellular carcinoma is more than 250 times greater in carriers of HBV than in noncarriers. HBV markers can be found in 80% to 90% of patients with hepatocellular carcinoma. Perhaps the best epidemiologic data indicating that hepatitis B precedes hepatocellular carcinoma were obtained in Taiwan from male civil servants between 40 and 60 years of age.[98] Approximately 3,500 HBsAg carriers were matched by age and place of birth (either mainland China or Taiwan) to 3,000 HBsAg-negative men, who served as control subjects. An additional group of 16,000 HBsAg-negative men between 40 and 60 years of age served as unmatched control subjects. After subjects were followed for 2 to 4 years, 50 cases of hepatocellular carcinoma were found, all but one of which occurred in chronic HBsAg carriers.

HCV is also associated with chronic infection in a high percentage (approximately 50%) of cases. In many countries, chronic HBV infection remains the leading factor in the development of hepatocellular carcinoma, whereas in Japan, Korea, and southern Europe, 50% to 75% of cases of hepatocellular carcinoma are

Table 7 Serologic Patterns of Hepatitis B Infection

HBsAg	Anti-HBs	Anti-HBe	Interpretation
+	–	–	Early acute hepatitis B
+	–	+	Late acute hepatitis B
–	–	+	Window period between disappearance of HBsAg and appearance of anti-HBs *or* Chronic carrier with low HBsAg level *or* Infection in the remote past
–	+	+	Past hepatitis B infection
–	+	–	Infection in the remote past *or* Immunization with hepatitis B vaccine *or* HBIG received within the past 1 to 2 mo

+ = detectable   – = not detectable

Table 8 Frequency of Antibody to Hepatitis B Surface Antigen (Anti-HBs) by Physician Specialty[88]

Specialty	Number of Patients Tested	Positive Results (%)
Surgery	176	50 (28)
Pathology	37	10 (27)
Pediatrics	63	13 (21)
Internal medicine	259	46 (18)
Anesthesiology	59	10 (17)
Obstetrics-gynecology	63	10 (16)
Family practice	341	54 (16)
Nonpatient care	25	1 (4)
All others combined	169	26 (15)
Total	1,192	220 (18.5)

Table 9 Prevalence of Hepatitis B Virus (HBV) Serologic Markers in Various Populations[90]

Population		Prevalence of Serologic Markers of HBV Infection (%)	
		HBsAg	All Markers
High risk	Immigrants or refugees from areas where HBV is highly endemic	13	70–85
	Clients in institutions for the mentally retarded	10–20	35–80
	Users of illicit parenteral drugs	7	60–80
	Homosexually active men	6	35–80
	Household contacts of HBV carriers	3–6	30–60
	Hemodialysis patients	3–10	20–80
Intermediate risk	Health care workers with frequent blood contact	1–2	15–30
	Prisoners (male)	1–8	10–80
	Staffs of institutions for the mentally retarded	1	10–25
Low risk	Health care workers with no or infrequent blood contact	0.3	3–10
	Healthy adults (first-time volunteer blood donors)	0.3	3–5

associated with chronic HCV infection.[99] In Japan, mortality from hepatocellular carcinoma increased approximately twofold in the 1980s, a change that may be attributable to a higher incidence of HCV-associated liver cancer.[100]

Herpesviruses

CYTOMEGALOVIRUS

CMV is a member of the B herpesvirus family and is the largest virus known to infect humans. In some U.S. cities, the seroprevalence of CMV is 60% to 70%. Like other members of the herpesvirus family, CMV is capable of remaining within its host in a latent state, probably by down-regulating cell surface markers (e.g., HLA-1) and thus avoiding immune destruction. Latent CMV has been found in circulating mononuclear cells, polymorphonuclear cells, vascular endothelium, renal epithelial tissue, and pulmonary secretions. The virus may become reactivated in the setting of immunodeficiency, such as may arise with HIV infection, transplantation, or significant stress from operations or injuries. In nonimmunocompromised patients, CMV typically causes a self-limited mononucleosis-like syndrome characterized by fever and mild hepatic transaminase abnormalities. In immunocompromised patients, however, CMV infection can be much more severe and even potentially life threatening, causing myelosuppression, pneumonitis, colitis, and retinopathy.

Posttransfusion Cytomegalovirus Infection (Posttransfusion or Postperfusion Syndrome)

The transmission of CMV by extracorporeal perfusion is responsible for the occasional development of a syndrome similar to mononucleosis in patients who have undergone open-heart operation. The syndrome characteristically appears 3 to 5 weeks after operation; its features are splenomegaly, fever, atypical lymphocytosis, and, occasionally, hepatomegaly, erythematous rash, and eosinophilia.[89] CMV can be isolated from the blood of virtually all patients with the typical posttransfusion syndrome and from the urine of half of these patients.[89] The condition is nonfatal and self-limited, but it may result in prolonged hospitalization and a long, expensive search for the source of fever. Although uncommon in adults 30 years of age and older, the syndrome can occur in as many as 10% of susceptible children and adults younger than 30 years.

This syndrome can also occur in patients who receive transfusions but who do not undergo open-heart operation. Occasional cases that develop postoperatively in patients who did not receive transfusions are thought to be the result of reactivation of latent infection. EBV can sometimes cause the syndrome.

The incidence of posttransfusion CMV infection is related to the kind of blood or blood product transfused. CMV is highly cell associated and is transmitted with leukocytes, which may be present in transfusions of packed red blood cells, platelets, or white blood cells; transmission from transfusion of fresh frozen plasma or cryoprecipitate has not been documented.[14] Therefore, efforts to decrease the number of white blood cells in the transfused blood would be expected to decrease the rate of transfusion-associated CMV infection. Approximately 50% of patients who receive whole blood seroconvert to CMV, whereas only 10% of those who receive washed packed red blood cells seroconvert. The risk of seroconversion to CMV is between 12% and 100% when whole blood, either fresh or stored, is transfused.[101] In one study, transfusion of frozen deglycerolized red blood cells resulted in seroconversion in only 3% of patients,[89] whereas in another, seroconversion occurred in 58% of 36 leukemic patients transfused with lymphocytes.[102]

The risk of posttransfusion CMV infection is also related to the volume of blood received. In one study, 7% of patients receiving a single unit of whole blood seroconverted, whereas anti-CMV antibody titers rose in 21% of patients receiving more than one unit.[103] The risk of infection per unit of blood transfused is estimated to range between 2.7% and 12%.[104]

Preexisting antibody to CMV does not protect transfusion recipients against reinfection. After transfusion of whole blood, titers of antibody to CMV will increase in 10% of recipients (an indication of reinfection) and in 19% of patients who did not have antibody to CMV before transfusion (an indication of infection). Whereas a seronegative recipient of CMV-positive blood has a 21% chance of seroconversion, the risk of seroconversion from the receipt of one unit of CMV-negative blood is only 2%.[89] However, the sensitivity of the serologic test for CMV is such that even when blood that tests seronegative is used, there is still a residual 0% to 6% risk of CMV transmission.[105]

Because so many patients receive blood transfusions during operation, it is understandable that evidence of posttransfusion CMV infection has been found in many patients postoperatively (e.g., after gynecologic surgery, cholecystectomy, appendectomy, lumbosacral fusion, splenectomy, and transplantation). It has also been found in surgical patients who are victims of trauma or burns.

However, it is surprising that infection with CMV, a ubiquitous virus, does not occur more frequently after transfusion. Between 30% and 54% of the adult population in the United States have antibody to CMV, an indication of previous infection.[89] Because infection with the virus is probably lifelong, a significant proportion of blood donors harbor the virus. The prevalence of antibody to CMV is 25% in units of blood from donors between 18 and 23 years of age and increases to 89% in blood from donors older than 60 years. The overall prevalence of seropositive blood donors is between 30% and 70%.

Cytomegalovirus in Transplant Recipients

CMV infection occurs not only in patients who have received blood transfusions but also in those who have suffered trauma, those receiving immunosuppressive therapy, and those with neoplastic disease. The groups at highest risk for CMV infection are probably recipients of organ transplants and of bone marrow transplants.[106-108] Numerous studies have documented the high incidence of CMV infection after organ transplantation: the rates range from 26% to 100%.[89,109,110] Primary CMV infection occurs in patients who do not have antibody to CMV before receiving transplants. Infections are considered to be reactivated if they occur in patients who did have antibody to CMV before receiving transplants. Rates of infection in patients receiving cardiac or bone marrow transplants are similar to those in patients receiving kidney transplants.

The high incidence of CMV infections after transplantation was recognized in the early days of such procedures. At autopsy of patients who died after renal transplantation, the intranuclear inclusions typical of CMV were found in tissue from the lungs, the parotid glands, the lymph nodes, the liver, the pancreas, the parathyroid, and the brain. CMV has been cultured repeatedly from the urine of transplant recipients, and the frequency of seroconversion among them has been high.

Likely sources of the virus are blood, because fresh blood can transmit CMV, and the organ transplant itself, because CMV can grow in renal tubular epithelial cells and can be transmitted as a latent virus. In several studies, recipients of kidney transplants had a much higher incidence of CMV infection when the donors had antibody to CMV than when the donors did not. In one study, 57% of recipients of kidneys from seropositive donors acquired CMV infection after transplantation, compared with 8% of recipients of kidneys from seronegative donors.[111] Even patients who have antibody to CMV can acquire new CMV infections as a result of transfusion or transplantation because there is more than one antigenic variety of the virus. Also, CMV that is latent in many patients who have antibody before transplantation may be reactivated after transplantation by host versus graft reactions, corticosteroids, or other immunosuppressive drugs. Hospital personnel, family members, and the environment play very small roles in transmission of CMV to transplant recipients.

Several systematic studies have demonstrated that CMV causes clinical illness in renal transplant recipients. In four studies, clinical illness developed in 83% of 76 patients with primary infection, compared with 44% of 268 patients with reactivation of a previous infection.[89,109,110]

Recipients of renal transplants in whom CMV causes clinical illness most commonly present with fever. Fever occurs in 95% of patients with CMV infection and may be prolonged. Patients with CMV infection also frequently present with anorexia, arthralgias, and leukopenia. Other clinical features of the disease are diffuse pulmonary infiltrates, pancreatitis, transplant malfunction, and systemic bacterial and fungal superinfections. Invasion of the GI tract by CMV may cause gastritis and ulcers in both the duodenum and the colon, which in turn may lead to hemorrhage and perforation. Biopsies demonstrate CMV inclusions at the base of the ulcers. The virus appears to invade the vascular endothelium, and bleeding is possibly a result of vascular occlusion and ischemic necrosis of the overlying tissue.

Lethal CMV disease is characterized by the presence of most of the features listed above. Liver dysfunction is found in 100% of patients with lethal disease but in only 50% to 75% of patients with mild or moderate infection, and CMV viremia occurs in 46% to 48% of patients with severe CMV infection but in only 26% to 28% of patients with mild to moderate infection. Leukopenia and the presence of atypical leukocytes also correlate with the severity of the disease. CMV infection after renal transplantation is also associated with pneumonia, hepatitis, encephalitis, and retinitis.

Whether or not CMV infection causes or leads to graft rejection is uncertain. Both the highest incidence of CMV infection (> 80%)[89,109,110] and the highest incidence of graft rejection occur within the first 3 months after transplantation. In several studies, young patients and recipients of second kidney transplants were at higher risk for graft loss if they had CMV than if they did not.[89,109,110] In most studies, however, it is extremely difficult to demonstrate a relation between CMV infection and graft rejection.

Of the multiple factors affecting the risk of CMV infection in transplant recipients, the most important are (1) the familial relation and HLA matching between the kidney donor and the recipient and (2) the CMV serology of both the donor and the recipient. The presence of antibody in transplant recipients before transplantation seems to offer a small amount of protection against fever caused by CMV but does not protect against more serious consequences of the infection, such as leukopenia, graft failure, and death.

CMV infection is also a major problem in liver, heart, and bone marrow transplant recipients.[106,108] In liver transplant recipients, CMV is a cause of hepatitis and liver dysfunction that can be confused with rejection or other causes of liver malfunction,[106] and it can lead to lethal infection. CMV pneumonitis in bone marrow transplant recipients is the most common life-threatening infectious complication after transplantation. The severity of infection in bone marrow transplant recipients may be attributable to the higher incidence of host versus graft disease in patients with CMV pneumonitis (82%) than in those without CMV pneumonitis (27%).[112]

Prevention and Treatment of Cytomegalovirus Infection

Several methods have been proposed to reduce the incidence of CMV infection after transfusion or transplantation. One method is to eliminate as many white blood cells as possible from transfused blood because CMV is almost certainly transmitted solely through these cells. From 90% to 100% of viable leukocytes in blood have been removed from frozen deglycerolized erythrocytes. In one study, transfusion of 24 hemodialyzed patients with leukocyte-free red blood cells from frozen deglycerolized blood prevented subsequent CMV infection.[104]

Another approach is to transfuse blood only from CMV-negative donors. Because the majority of posttransfusion CMV infections are asymptomatic, however, the increased cost of performing serologic tests on all donated units might be difficult to justify.

Storage of blood to reduce infectiousness of CMV is another approach, but storage from 48 to 72 hours does not significantly reduce transmission of CMV infection. Irradiating the blood to render the CMV noninfectious is unacceptable because it causes cell transformation in vitro. Furthermore, in one study, administration of leukocytes previously exposed to 1,500 cGy (1,500 rads) of gamma radiation resulted in an increased incidence of CMV infection among recipients of these cells.[102]

Because the incidence of CMV infection is higher in patients who receive kidney transplants from seropositive donors, some centers do not transplant kidneys from seropositive donors into seronegative recipients. However, no published reports indicate that this practice leads to a significant alteration in the outcome of renal transplantation with respect to graft rejection. Moreover, excluding kidneys from seropositive donors makes it more difficult to find kidneys for seronegative recipients.

Many attempts have been made to develop a CMV vaccine for administration before viral exposure by multiple passages of the virus in tissue culture. Two such vaccines have been used in clinical trials, one prepared from the AD169 strain and the other from the Towne 125 strain of the virus. Immunization with these vaccines can elicit both serum antibody and cell-mediated immunity. In one trial, the vaccine prepared from the Towne 125 strain lowered the incidence of clinical disease but not of infection, and the disease tended to be less severe in vaccinated patients than in control subjects who received placebo.[113]

Human IG has been administered after transfusion or transplantation in attempts to prevent associated CMV infection. In one study, it reduced life-threatening infection to a less severe form in most patients, but in other studies, not surprisingly, it provided no consistent benefit.[114-117] In patients who are already seropositive, the virus is latent inside their cells, where it is probably not accessible to serum antibody. Patients with primary infections may not benefit from antibody treatment, because herpesviruses seem to transfer from cell to cell without ever existing free in serum. Even CMV hyperimmune globulin has no clear benefit in patients with clinical CMV infection.[118] It may, however, help control severe infections, such as those seen in bone marrow transplant recipients.

Several antiviral agents have been used in attempts to reduce the incidence or lessen the effect of CMV infection. Among these agents are interferon, transfer factor, immune globulin, and nucleoside derivatives, such as cytarabine, vidarabine, and acyclovir (see below). Immune globulins, acyclovir, and ganciclovir are effective at preventing CMV infection in transplant recipients.[109,110,114,119,120] Ganciclovir and foscarnet are active against CMV in vitro. Ganciclovir is currently being used to treat CMV and is the most effective agent in organ transplant recipients (see below).[109,110,119-121]

EPSTEIN-BARR VIRUS

EBV is the herpesvirus responsible for infectious mononucleosis. It can be found in B cells in peripheral blood of infected patients and in tumor cells of patients with Burkitt lymphoma and nasopharyngeal carcinoma. It remains in a latent form in an infected host for years, probably for life. Most posttransfusion EBV infections are asymptomatic. Seroconversion to EBV will develop in approximately 8% of recipients transfused with between two and 14 units of blood. In as many as 5% of patients with preexisting antibody to EBV, significant elevations of antibody titers may develop, beginning 2 weeks after transfusion. These elevations indicate either reinfection or reactivation of a latent infection.[89] Because EBV is associated with cells and does not exist free in serum to any great extent, antibody to EBV in either donors or recipients is unlikely to provide substantial protection against infection resulting from blood transfusions or organ transplants. Among transfused patients who do not have preexisting antibody to EBV, the prevalence of EBV infection can reach 33% to 46%. In these patients, the absence of preexisting antibody presumably rules out reactivation of latent EBV infection as the source of infection.

EBV occurs worldwide. In the United States, nearly all adults and as many as 65% of persons of all ages have antibody to EBV. Infection is thought to occur in infancy, and as many as 17% of infants have antibody to EBV. By 5 years of age, 72% of children have antibody to EBV, and the prevalence in adults is similar.[122] Thus, the majority of blood donors in the United States have been previously infected with EBV and probably have latent virus in their leukocytes. Although it is clear that EBV can be transmitted by blood when the transfusion occurs within 3 days of donation, it is not known whether blood stored for longer periods can transmit the virus. Because EBV is predominantly intracellular, plasma and its derivatives do not transmit the virus.

The diagnosis of EBV infection is made serologically. Tests both for IgM antibody to capsid antigens and for IgG antibody to the early antigens of EBV or tests of serial samples for IgG antibody to capsid antigens must be used. The heterophil antibody test (the Paul-Bunnell test) and a rapid slide test that is equivalent (the monospot test) are also used in most clinical studies to screen for EBV infection before more specific diagnostic tests are performed.

In cases of posttransfusion infection, IgG antibody to EBV can be detected at least 10 days before the onset of symptoms, and EBV can be cultured from circulating lymphocytes 11 days before the onset of symptoms. In patients with acute infection, EBV is found in approximately three of every 10^4 peripheral blood lymphocytes.[123] In contrast, all recovered persons with antibodies to EBV are thought to have the virus in one of every 10^7 circulating lymphocytes.

EBV is strongly implicated in the etiology of a posttransplantation lymphoproliferative disorder (PTLD).[89,124,125] EBV has been isolated from the tissues of most cases of PTLD, but not all.[126,127] Non–EBV-related cases of PTLD typically occur later after transplantation, and their etiology has not been elucidated.

PTLD comprises three general clinical presentations: (1) a mononucleosis-like syndrome involving the tonsils and the peripheral lymph nodes, (2) a diffuse polymorphous B-cell infiltration in many visceral organs, and (3) localized extranodal tumors in the GI tract, the neck, the thorax, or other parts of the body. Patients whose disease is limited to a single organ or to lymph nodes often respond to a reduction in immunosuppression or antiviral therapy; however, once the infection becomes widespread, the disease progresses rapidly and is fatal in more than 75% of cases.[128] In solid organ transplant recipients, PTLD may be limited to the allograft. There is some evidence to suggest that PTLD may have organ-specific features that promote lymphoproliferation: allograft involvement has been reported in 17% of renal transplant recipients, 8.6% of liver transplant recipients, and as many as 60% to 80% of lung or intestinal transplant recipients.[128]

The persons at highest risk for PTLD are EBV-seronegative persons receiving EBV-positive organs or bone marrow. Most infections occur within the first 4 months after transplantation.[129] Several specific risk factors for the development of PTLD have been identified: a seropositive graft in a seronegative recipient, certain types of organ allografts (with intestinal transplants carrying the highest risk), any type of immunosuppression that blunts cellular immunity to EBV (with risk increasing as immunosuppression becomes more pronounced), and the presence of other infections (CMV in particular).

The optimal treatment of lymphoproliferative disorders remains unclear. Some early EBV-associated lymphoproliferative disorders in solid organ transplant recipients have regressed completely after reduction of immunosuppression.[130,131] Early PTLD may respond to antiviral therapy with acyclovir or ganciclovir, which may prevent infection of resting B cells, but such therapy is less likely to be effective in the face of high concentrations of latently infected circulating or tissue-invasive B cells. Some investigators also report resolution of PTLD after treatment with interferon alfa.[132,133]

Transmission of EBV can occur simultaneously with transmission of CMV or hepatitis virus. Although hepatitis accompanies EBV infections in sporadic cases, EBV alone has not been documented as a cause of posttransfusion hepatitis.

HERPES SIMPLEX VIRUS

Infection or reactivation of infection with herpes simplex virus type 1 (HSV-1) follows renal transplantation in 50% to 75% of patients, most often within 30 days after transplantation. Reactivation of infection is more common than primary infection: only 14% of patients who are seronegative before transplantation become infected, but infection is reactivated in 64% of patients who were already seropositive before transplantation.

Most cases of HSV-1 infection after transplantation are clinically inapparent and are indicated only by a significant rise in titer of antibody to the virus. The most prevalent clinical manifestation is herpes labialis, that is, fever blisters affecting not only the lips but also the mucous membranes of the oral cavity and the skin of the head and neck. Although these lesions are painful and may make eating, drinking, and taking oral medications difficult, they are usually self-limited and heal without treatment or reduction of immunosuppression. However, HSV-1 infection can take a much more malignant course, disseminating to cause pneumonitis, fulminant hepatitis, upper GI hemorrhage, encephalitis, aseptic meningitis, and death.

VARICELLA-ZOSTER VIRUS

Varicella-zoster virus (VZV), another herpesvirus, is the etiologic agent of herpes zoster and chicken pox. This virus resides in the dorsal root ganglia of adults who had primary varicella infection in childhood. Herpes zoster is more common in organ transplant recipients, in patients with cancer (especially those who have leukemia or lymphomas), in burn patients, and in patients receiving immunosuppressive drugs. Serologic evidence of VZV infection occurs in 8% to 16% of renal transplant recipients. The lesions of herpes zoster become evident 12 to 511 days after organ transplantation.

In children or adults who have not already had chicken pox and occasionally even in children who have, VZV can cause disseminated chicken pox in many organs, which may be fatal.

AGENTS EFFECTIVE AGAINST HERPESVIRUSES

Because the essential synthetic activities of viruses depend on the metabolic machinery of their host, it has been difficult to devise specific antiviral agents that interfere with viral replication but are not harmful to host cells.[134,135] Many antiviral agents are too toxic to be used clinically. In contrast, antibacterial agents that are both toxic to bacteria and safe for human cells are easier to design because the structure and metabolic machinery of bacteria are distinct from those of host cells.

Although intracellular processes unique to viral replication have been identified and specifically targeted for chemotherapeutic attack, very few agents have been effective against human viruses. Among these is amantadine, which is used for both prophylaxis and treatment of influenza A. Agents that were found to be effective for prophylaxis against smallpox, such as methisazone, now have no use, because the disease has been eradicated.

There are few effective chemotherapeutic agents for hepatitis or most of the other major viral diseases that concern surgeons, but several agents have been used for the treatment of herpesvirus infections, especially in immunosuppressed patients [see Table 10]. These agents, derivatives of purines and pyrimidines, interfere with viral nucleic acid synthesis.

Acyclovir and Valacyclovir

Acyclovir (acycloguanosine) is a nucleoside derivative that is used to treat herpesvirus infections, especially herpes simplex and varicella-zoster infections in immunocompromised hosts. Valacyclovir is the L-valyl ester prodrug of acyclovir. In cases of mucocutaneous herpes simplex and herpes zoster, acyclovir can shorten the period of virus shedding, decrease pain, and promote more rapid scabbing and healing of lesions. Acyclovir is also the drug of choice for encephalitis caused by herpes simplex, but it is not effective in patients with established neurologic damage resulting from herpes simplex or varicella-zoster infections or in patients infected with CMV. Acyclovir inhibits the replication of EBV in actively replicating cells but does not affect latent or persistent infection.

The total daily dose of acyclovir is 10 to 25 mg/kg, given by I.V. infusion lasting 60 minutes. The recommended length of parenteral acyclovir therapy ranges from 5 to 10 days, depending on the indication. A major side effect of such therapy is phlebitis at the injection site; rash, leukopenia, and neurotoxicity may also occur. Acyclovir applied topically as a 5% ointment is effective in immunocompromised patients for the treatment of limited cutaneous herpes infections and in patients with normal immunity for the treatment of initial episodes (but not recurrent episodes) of genital herpes simplex infection. Oral acyclovir seems to be effective as prophylaxis against reactivated herpes simplex infection in recipients of bone marrow transplants and in patients immunosuppressed as a result of HIV infection.

Penciclovir and Famciclovir

Penciclovir is a nucleoside analogue that is similar to acyclovir with respect to spectrum of activity and potency against herpesviruses. Famciclovir is the diacetyl ester of penciclovir. Penciclovir requires thymidine kinase (TK) for phosphorylation and thus is inactive against thymidine kinase–deficient strains of HSV or VZV; however, it may be active against some TK-altered or polymerase mutants that are resistant to acyclovir as well as against some foscarnet-resistant HSV isolates. In experimental settings, topical, parenteral, and oral penciclovir and oral famciclovir have been effective against HSV infection.

Vidarabine

Vidarabine (ara-A) is effective against herpes simplex and varicella-zoster viruses as well as poxviruses, oncornaviruses, and rhabdoviruses. It is used mostly to combat herpesvirus infections in immunosuppressed patients. In these patients, vidarabine accelerates healing of cutaneous herpes zoster, decreases its rates of cutaneous dissemination and of visceral complications, and shortens the duration of postherpetic neuralgia. For systemic use, a daily dose of 10 to 15 mg/kg of vidarabine is administered I.V. over a period of 12 hours. The duration of therapy for herpes zoster is

Table 10 Antiviral Therapy of Clinical Benefit

Virus	Condition	Regimen
Herpes simplex virus	Keratitis	3% Acyclovir ointment *or* 1% Trifluridine solution *or* 3% Vidarabine ointment *or* 0.5% IDU ointment or 0.1% IDU drops
	Herpes labialis	Treatment usually not indicated; may use 1% penciclovir cream or topical acyclovir q. 2 hr while patient is awake for 4 days
	Genital herpes Primary	Acyclovir, 200 mg p.o. 5 times daily or 400 mg p.o., t.i.d., for 10 days, *or* Valacyclovir, 500 mg–1 g p.o., b.i.d., for 10–14 days, *or* Famciclovir, 250 mg p.o., t.i.d., for 10 days*
	Recurrent	Acyclovir, 200 mg p.o. 5 times daily or 400 mg p.o., t.i.d., for 5 days, *or* Valacyclovir, 500 mg p.o., b.i.d., for 5 days, *or* Famciclovir, 125 mg p.o., b.i.d., for 5 days
	Prophylaxis	Acyclovir, 400 mg p.o., b.i.d., *or* Valacyclovir, 500 mg–1 g p.o., q.d., *or* Famciclovir, 250 mg p.o., b.i.d.
	Encephalitis	Acyclovir, 10 mg/kg t.i.d. I.V. for 14–21 days
	Neonatal HSV	Acyclovir, 10 mg/kg I.V. q. 8 hr for 10–21 days (20 mg/kg I.V. q. 8 hr if neonate is premature)
	Immunocompromised host	Acyclovir, 5 mg/kg I.V. q. 8 hr for 7 days or 400 mg p.o. 5 times daily for 14–21 days, *or* Famciclovir, 500 mg p.o., b.i.d., for 7 days,* *or* Valacyclovir, 1 g p.o., t.i.d., for 7 days*

Varicella-zoster virus	Immunocompetent host
	   Eye infections
	   Shingles
		3% Acyclovir ointment
		 Acyclovir, 800 mg p.o. 5 times daily for 7–10 days, *or*
		 Valacyclovir, 1 g p.o., t.i.d., for 7–10 days, *or*
		 Famciclovir, 500 mg p.o., t.i.d., for 7–10 days

	Immunocompromised host	Acyclovir, 10–12 mg/kg I.V. q. 8 hr for 7 days (500 mg/m²)
Cytomegalovirus	Immunocompromised host Retinitis	Ganciclovir, 5 mg/kg I.V. q. 12 hr for 14–21 days,† *or* Foscarnet, 90 mg/kg (adjusted for renal function) I.V. q. 12 hr for 14–21 days, *or* Cidofovir, 5 mg/kg I.V. weekly for 2 weeks, then every other week
	CMV pneumonia	Ganciclovir, 2.5 mg/kg I.V. q.d. for 20 days

*Not approved by the FDA for this indication.
†An intraocular insert is also available.

5 days. Side effects include anorexia, weight loss, nausea, vomiting, weakness, anemia, leukopenia, thrombocytopenia, tremors, and thrombophlebitis at the site of administration.

Idoxuridine

Idoxuridine (5-iodo-2′-deoxyuridine) (IUdR, IDU) was the first clinically effective antiviral nucleoside. It is a halogenated pyrimidine that resembles thymidine in structure. Topical application of either a 0.1% solution or a 0.5% ointment of idoxuridine is effective treatment of herpes simplex keratitis but not of recurrent herpes labialis or localized zoster. In the United States, IDU is approved only for topical treatment of HSV keratitis. When combined with dimethyl sulfoxide (DMSO), IDU is active against herpes zoster and recurrent or primary genital HSV infection. In Europe, IDU is available in combination with DMSO for the treatment of herpes labialis, herpes genitalis, and herpes zoster.

Ganciclovir

Ganciclovir (DHPG, 2′-NDG, or BIOLF-62) is an acyclic nucleoside structurally related to acyclovir but with greater activity against CMV in vitro and in vivo. It is effective in treating CMV disease in transplant recipients and AIDS patients. The usual total daily dose of ganciclovir is 7.5 to 10 mg/kg, given in two or three divided doses. The dosage should be adjusted if the patient has decreased renal function. Myelosuppression is the principal dose-limiting toxic side effect.

Foscarnet

Foscarnet (trisodium phosphonoformate) is a pyrophosphate derivative that inhibits herpesvirus DNA polymerases and retroviral reverse transcriptases.[134-136] In the United States, it has been used for the prevention and treatment of CMV retinitis in patients with AIDS. For patients who have received renal or bone marrow transplants, foscarnet is given in a bolus injection of 9 mg/kg followed by infusion of 0.015 to 0.090 mg/kg/min I.V. for 7 days. Foscarnet is also used to treat acyclovir-resistant HSV infection. The major toxicity associated with foscarnet is nephrotoxicity; CNS side effects (e.g., headache, tremor, irritability, and seizures) can also occur.

Viral Infections from Animal and Human Bites

Surgeons are frequently called on to treat patients who have been bitten by either an animal or another person. Such bites can transmit several viruses and other infections. Certainly, rabies is the most feared viral infection transmitted in this way. Viruses that are found in saliva, such as HBV, herpesviruses, and possibly HIV, can be transmitted by a human bite, although such cases are most likely rare.

From zero to five cases of human rabies occur each year in the United States. Animal rabies is widespread and is found in every state except Hawaii. In 1992, more than 8,600 cases of animal rabies were reported to the CDC by 49 states, the District of Columbia, and Puerto Rico. The great majority of cases occur in wild animals.[69] Before 1950, more than 8,000 cases of rabies in dogs were reported each year in the United States; the number is now fewer than 150 a year.

Rabies proceeds from a prodrome of fever, malaise, and headache, to hyperactivity and diffuse cerebral dysfunction, and then to coma and death. From 5% to 20% of patients may also show progressive paralysis. Occasionally, there is no history of an animal bite. Diagnosis can be confirmed by culture of saliva, cerebrospinal fluid, or brain tissue; demonstration of rabies antigen in the cornea or skin; or measurement of serum antibody to rabies virus. At postmortem examination, typical intracytoplasmic inclusions (Negri bodies) can be seen in the brain cells.

Although the number of cases of human rabies is small, the disease is an important problem because of the large number of animal bites that occur each year. Surgeons may have to consider rabies prophylaxis in patients whom they treat for bite injuries [see Management of Viral Exposure, Rabies, *above*, and 8 Acute Wound Care]. Also, two fatal cases of rabies have occurred in recipients of corneal transplants from a patient whose cause of death was later found to be rabies.[137]

References

1. Recommendations for prevention of HIV transmission in health-care settings. MMWR Morb Mortal Wkly Rep 36(suppl 2):1S, 1987
2. Recommendations for preventing transmission of infection with human T-lymphocyte type III/lymphadenopathy-associated virus in the workplace. MMWR Morb Mortal Wkly Rep 34:681, 1985
3. Update: universal precautions for prevention of transmission of human immunodeficiency virus, hepatitis B virus, and other blood-borne pathogens in health-care settings. MMWR Morb Mortal Wkly Rep 37:377, 1988
4. Guidelines for prevention of transmission of human immunodeficiency virus and hepatitis B virus to health-care and public-safety workers. MMWR Morb Mortal Wkly Rep 38(suppl 6):1, 1989
5. Recommendations for HIV testing services for inpatients and outpatients in acute-care hospital settings and technical guidance on HIV counseling. MMWR Morb Mortal Wkly Rep 42(RR-2):1, 1993
6. Rhame F, Maki D: The case for wider use of testing for HIV infection. N Engl J Med 320:1248, 1989
7. Telford GL, Quebbeman EJ, Condon RE: A protocol to reduce risk of contracting AIDS and other blood-borne disease in the OR. Surg Rounds 10:30, 1987
8. Recommendations for follow up of health care workers after occupational exposure to hepatitis C. MMWR Morb Mortal Wkly Rep 46:603, 1997
9. Mast EE, Alter MJ: Prevention of hepatitis B virus infection among health-care workers. Hepatitis B Vaccines in Clinical Practice. Ellis RW, Ed. Marcel Dekker, New York, 1993, p 295
10. Werner BG, Grady GF: Accidental hepatitis B-surface-antigen-positive inoculations: use of e antigen to estimate infectivity. Ann Intern Med 97:367, 1982
11. Gerberding JL: Management of occupational exposures to blood-borne viruses. N Engl J Med 125:917, 1996
12. Sepkowitz KA: Occupationally acquired infections in health care workers (part II). Ann Intern Med 125:917, 1996
13. Department of Labor, OSHA: Occupational exposure to blood-borne pathogens. Final rule. Fed Regist 56:64175, 1991
14. Sepkowitz KA: Nosocomial hepatitis and other infections transmitted by blood and blood products. Principles and Practice of Infectious Disease, 5th ed. Mandell GL, Bennet JE, Dolin R, Eds. Churchill Livingstone, Philadelphia, 2000, p 3039
15. Protection against viral hepatitis: recommendations of the Immunization Practices Advisory Committee (ACIP). MMWR Morb Mortal Wkly Rep 39 (RR-2):1, 1990
16. Syndman DR, Bryan JA, Dixon RE: Prevention of nosocomial viral hepatitis, type B (hepatitis B). Ann Intern Med 83:838, 1975
17. Favero MS, Maynard JE, Leger RT, et al: Guidelines for the care of patients hospitalized with viral hepatitis. Ann Intern Med 91:872, 1979
18. Ciesielski C, Marianos D, Ou C-Y, et al: Transmission of human immunodeficiency virus in a dental practice. Ann Intern Med 116:798, 1992
19. Lot F, Seguier J, Fegeus S, et al: Probable transmission of HIV from an orthopedic surgeon to a patient in France. Ann Intern Med 130:1, 1999
20. Welch J, Webster M, Tilzey A, et al: Hepatitis B infections after gynecological surgery. Lancet 1:205, 1989
21. Lettau LA, Smith JD, Williams D, et al: Transmission of hepatitis B with resultant restriction of surgical practice. JAMA 255:934, 1986
22. Communicable Disease Surveillance Centre: Acute hepatitis B associated with gynaecological surgery. Lancet 1:1, 1980
23. Carl M, Frances DP, Blakey DL, et al: Interruption of hepatitis B transmission by modification of a gynaecologist's surgical technique. Lancet 1:731, 1982
24. Coutinho RA, Albrecht-van Lent P, Stoutjesdijk L, et al: Hepatitis B from doctors (letter). Lancet 1:345, 1982
25. Grob PJ, Bischof B, Naeff F: Cluster of hepatitis B transmitted by a physician. Lancet 2:1218, 1981
26. Meyers JD, Stamm WE, Kerr MM, et al: Lack of transmission of hepatitis B after surgical exposure. JAMA 240:1725, 1978
27. Haerem JW, Siebke JC, Ulstrup J, et al: HBsAg transmission from a cardiac surgeon incubating hepatitis B resulting in chronic antigenemia in four patients. Acta Med Scand 210:389, 1981
28. Acute hepatitis B following gynecological surgery. J Hosp Infect 9:34, 1987
29. Polakoff S: Acute hepatitis B in patients in Britain related to previous operations and dental treatment. Br J Med 293:33, 1986
30. Heptonstall J: Outbreaks of hepatitis B virus infection associated with infected surgical staff. Communicable Disease Report 1:R81, 1991
31. Surgeons who are hepatitis B carriers. BMJ 303:184, 1991
32. Jones D: Hepatitis leaves Halifax surgeon an operating room outcast. Can Med Assoc J 145:1345, 1991
33. Alter HJ, Chalmers TC, Freeman BM, et al: Healthcare workers positive for hepatitis B surface antigen: are their contacts at risk? N Engl J Med 292:454, 1975
34. Williams SV, Pattison CP, Berquist KR: Dental infection with hepatitis B. JAMA 232:1231, 1975
35. Gerber MA, Lewin EB, Gerety RJ, et al: The lack of nurse-infant transmission of type B hepatitis in a special care nursery. J Pediatr 91:120, 1977
36. LaBrecque DR, Dhand AK: The risk of hepatitis B transmission from staff to patients in hemodialysis units—an overrated problem? Hepatology 1:398, 1981
37. LaBrecque DR, Muhs JM, Lutwick LI, et al: The risk of hepatitis B transmission from health care workers to patients in a hospital setting—a prospective study. Hepatology 6:205, 1986
38. Recommendations for preventing transmission of human immunodeficiency virus and hepatitis B virus to patients during exposure-prone invasive procedures. MMWR Morb Mortal Wkly Rep 40(RR-8), 1991
39. Esteban JI, Gomez J, Martell M, et al: Transmission of hepatitis C by a cardiac surgeon. N Engl J Med 334:555, 1996
40. Bosch H: Hepatitis C outbreak astounds Spain. Lancet 352:1415, 1998
41. Public Health Service guidelines for the management of health-care worker exposures to HIV and recommendations for post-exposure prophylaxis. MMWR Morb Mortal Wkly Rep 47:1, 1998
42. Chiarello LA, Gerberding JL: Human immunodeficiency virus in health care settings. Principles and Practice of Infectious Disease, 5th ed. Mandell GL, Bennett JE, Dolin R, Eds. Churchill Livingstone, Philadelphia, 2000, p 3052
43. Ciesielski CA, Metler RP: Duration of time between exposure and seroconversion in healthcare workers

with occupationally acquired infection with human immunodeficiency virus. Am J Med 102(suppl 5B):S115, 1997

44. Busch MP, Satten GA: Time course of viremia and antibody seroconversion following human immunodeficiency virus exposure. Am J Med 102(suppl 5B):S117, 1997

45. Cardo DM, Culver DH, Ciesielski CA, et al: A case-control study of HIV seroconversion in healthcare workers after percutaneous exposure. N Engl J Med 337:1485, 1997

46. Public Health Service Statement on management of occupational exposure to human immunodeficiency virus, including considerations regarding zidovudine postexposure use. MMWR Morb Mortal Wkly Rep 39 (RR-1):1, 1990

47. Wang SA, the HIV PEP Registry Group: Human immunodeficiency virus (HIV) postexposure prophylaxis (PEP) following occupational HIV exposure: findings from the HIV PEP Registry (abstract 482). Program and abstracts of the 35th Annual Meeting of the Infectious Diseases Society of America, Alexandria, Virginia, Sept 13–16, 1997, p 161

48. Steger KA, Swotinsky R, Snyder S, et al: Recent experience with post-exposure prophylaxis (PEP) with combination antiretrovirals for occupational exposure (OE) to HIV (abstract 480). Program and abstracts of the 35th Annual Meeting of the Infectious Diseases Society of America, Alexandria, Virginia, Sept 13–16, 1997, p 161

49. Beekmann R, Fahrner R, Nelson L, et al: Combination post-exposure prophylaxis (PEP): a prospective study of HIV-exposed health care workers (HCW) (abstract 481). Program and abstracts of the 35th Annual Meeting of the Infectious Diseases Society of America, Alexandria, Virginia, Sept 13–16, 1997, p 161

50. Imrie A, Beveridge A, Genn W, et al: Transmission of human immunodeficiency virus type 1 resistant to nevirapine and zidovudine. J Infect Dis 175:1502, 1997

51. Veenstra J, Schuurman R, Cornelissen M, et al: Transmission of zidovudine-resistant human immunodeficiency virus type 1 variants following deliberate injection of blood from a patient with AIDS: characteristics and natural history of the virus. Clin Infect Dis 21:556-60, 1995

52. Fitzgibbon JE, Gaur S, Frenkel LD, et al: Transmission from one child to another of human immunodeficiency virus type 1 with a zidovudine-resistance mutation. N Engl J Med 329:1835, 1993

53. Coombs RW, Shapiro DE, Eastman PS, et al: Maternal viral genotypic zidovudine (ZDV) resistance and infrequent failure of ZDV therapy to prevent perinatal transmission (abstract 17). Program and abstracts of the 35th Annual Meeting of the Infectious Diseases Society of America, Alexandria, Virginia, Sept 13–16, 1997, p 74

54. Protection against viral hepatitis. Recommendations of the Immunization Practices Advisory Committee (ACIP). MMWR Morb Mortal Wkly Rep 39(RR-2):1, 1990

55. Hadler SC: Are booster doses of hepatitis B vaccine necessary? Ann Intern Med 108:457, 1988

56. Hadler SC, Francis DP, Maynard JE, et al: Long-term immunogenicity and efficacy of hepatitis B vaccine in homosexual men. N Engl J Med 315:209, 1986

57. Hepatitis B virus: A comprehensive strategy for eliminating transmission in the United States through universal childhood vaccination. Advisory Committee for Immunization Practices. MMWR Morb Mortal Wkly Rep 40:PR-13, 1991

58. Barie PS, Dellinger EP, Dougherty SH, et al: Assessment of hepatitis B virus immunization status among North American surgeons. Arch Surg 129:27, 1994

59. Recommendations for prevention and control of hepatitis C virus (HCV) infection and HCV-related chronic disease. MMWR Morb Mortal Wkly Rep 47(RR-19):1, 1998

60. Noguchi S, Sata M, Suzuki H, et al: Early therapy with interferon for acute hepatitis C acquired through the needlestick. Clin Infect Dis 24:992, 1997

61. Vogen W, Graziadei I, Umlauft F, et al: High-dose interferon-α_{2b} treatment prevents chronicity in acute hepatitis C: a pilot study. Dig Dis Sci 41(suppl 12):81S, 1996

62. Ohnishi K, Nomura F, Nakano M: Interferon therapy for acute posttransfusion non-A, non-B hepatitis: response with respect to anti-hepatitis C virus antibody status. Am J Gastroenterol 86:1041, 1991

63. Rabies prevention—United States, 1991: recommendations of the Immunization Practices Advisory Committee (ACIP). MMWR Morb Mortal Wkly Rep 40:1, 1991

64. Fishbein DB, Robinson LE: Rabies. N Engl J Med 329:1632, 1993

65. Rabies prevention—United States, 1999: recommendations of the Immunization Practices Advisory Committee (ACIP). MMWR Morb Mortal Wkly Rep 48(RR-1):1, 1999

66. WHO Recommendations on Rabies Post-exposure Treatment and the Correct Technique of Intradermal Immunization against Rabies. World Health Organization, Geneva, 1997

67. Rabies prevention: supplementary statement on the preexposure use of human diploid cell rabies vaccine by the intradermal route. MMWR Morb Mortal Wkly Rep 35:767, 1986

68. Bleck TP, Rupprecht CE: Rabies virus. Principles and Practice of Infectious Disease, 5th ed. Mandell GL, Bennett JE, Dolin R, Eds. Churchill Livingstone, Philadelphia, 2000, p 1811

69. Krebs JW, Strine TW, Childs JF: Rabies surveillance in the United States during 1992. J Am Vet Med Assoc 203:1718, 1993

70. The cost of one rabid dog—California. MMWR Morb Mortal Wkly Rep 30:527, 1981

71. Bove JR: Transfusion-associated hepatitis and AIDS: what is the risk? N Engl J Med 317:242, 1987

72. Donegan E, Stuart M, Niland JC, et al: Infection with the human immunodeficiency virus type 1 (HIV1) among recipients of antibody-positive blood donations. Ann Intern Med 113:733, 1990

73. Ward JW, Deppe DA, Samson S, et al: Risk of human immunodeficiency virus infection from blood donors who later developed the acquired immunodeficiency syndrome. Ann Intern Med 106:61, 1987

74. Ward JW, Grindon AJ, Feorino PM, et al: Laboratory and epidemiologic evaluation of an enzyme immunoassay for antibodies to HTLV-III. JAMA 256:357, 1986

75. Ward JW, Holmberg AD, Allen JR, et al: Transmission of human immunodeficiency virus (HIV) by blood transfusions screened as negative for HIV antibody. N Engl J Med 318:473, 1988

76. Schreiber GB, Bush MP, Kleinman SH, et al: The risk of transfusion-transmitted viral infections: the retrovirus epidemiology donor study. N Engl J Med 334:1685, 1996

77. Horsburgh BR Jr, Ou C-Y, Jason J, et al: Duration of human immunodeficiency virus infection before detection of antibody. Lancet 2:637, 1989

78. Erice A, Rhame FS, Heussner RC, et al: Human immunodeficiency virus infection in patients with solid-organ transplants: report of five cases and review. Rev Infect Dis 13:537, 1991

79. Public Health Service guidelines for the management of health-care worker exposures to HIV and recommendations for post-exposure prophylaxis. MMWR Morb Mortal Wkly Rep 47:1, 1998

80. Guidelines for national human immunodeficiency virus case surveillance, including monitoring for human immunodeficiency virus infection and acquired immunodeficiency syndrome. MMWR Morb Mortal Wkly Rep 48(RR-13):1, 1999

81. Alter M, Mast E: The epidemiology of hepatitis in the United States. Gastroenterol Clin North Am 23:437, 1994

82. Kim CY, Tilles JG: Purification and biophysical characterization of the hepatitis B antigen. J Clin Invest 52:1176, 1973

83. Kawai H, Feinstone SM: Acute viral hepatitis. Principles and Practice of Infectious Diseases, 5th ed. Mandell GL, Bennett JE, Dolin R, Eds. Churchill Livingstone, Philadelphia, 2000, p 1279

84. Omata M: Treatment of chronic hepatitis B infection. N Engl J Med 339:114, 1998

85. Kuo G, Choo Q-L, Alter HJ, et al: An assay for circulating antibodies to a major etiologic virus of non-A, non-B hepatitis. Science 244:362, 1989

86. Hayden GH, Jarvis LM, Blair CS, et al: Clinical significance of intrahepatic hepatitis C virus levels in patients with chronic HCV infection. Gut 42:570, 1998

87. Koretz RL, Stone O, Gitnick GL: The long-term course of non-A, non-B post-transfusion hepatitis. Gastroenterology 79:893, 1980

88. Denes AE, Smith JL, Maynard JE, et al: Hepatitis B infections in physicians: results of a nationwide seroepidemiologic survey. JAMA 239:210, 1978

89. Howard RJ: Viral infections in surgery. Problems in General Surgery 1:522, 1984

90. Recommendations for protection against viral hepatitis. MMWR Morb Mortal Wkly Rep 34:313, 1985

91. Valent WM, Wehrle PP: Selected viruses of nosocomial importance. Hospital Infections, 2nd ed. Bennett JV, Brachman PS, Eds. Little, Brown & Company, Boston, 1986, p 531

92. Cooper BW, Krusell A, Tilton RC, et al: Seroprevalence of antibodies to hepatitis C virus in high-risk hospital personnel. Infect Control Hosp Epidemiol 13:82, 1992

93. Klein RS, Freeman K, Taylor PE, et al: Occupational risk for hepatitis C virus infection among New York City dentists. Lancet 338:1539, 1991

94. Zuckerman J, Clewley G, Griffiths P, et al: Prevalence of hepatitis C antibodies in clinical health-care workers. Lancet 343:1618, 1994

95. Schreiber GB, Busch MP, Kleinman SH, et al: The risk of transfusion-transmitted viral infections. N Engl J Med 334:1685, 1996

96. Rosina F, Saracco G, Rizzetto M: Risk of posttransfusion infection with hepatitis delta virus: a multicenter study. N Engl J Med 312:1488, 1985

97. Friedman LS, Dienstag JL: Recent developments in viral hepatitis. Dis Mon 32:320, 1986

98. Beasley PR, Lin CC: Hepatoma risk among HBsAg carriers. Am J Epidemiol 108:247, 1978

99. Edamoto Y, Tani M, Durata T, et al: Hepatitis C and B virus infections in hepatocellular carcinoma—analysis of direct detection of viral genome in paraffin embedded tissues. Cancer 77:1787, 1996

100. Kiyosawa K, Furuta S: Hepatitis C virus and hepatocellular carcinoma. Curr Stud Hematol Blood Transfus 61:98, 1994

101. Rook AH, Quinnan GV Jr: Cytomegalovirus infections following blood transfusions. Infectious Complications of Blood Transfusion. Tabor E, Ed. Academic Press, San Diego, 1982, p 45

102. Winston DJ, Ho WG, Howell CL, et al: Cytomegalovirus infections associated with leukocyte transfusions. Ann Intern Med 93:671, 1980

103. Prince AM, Szmuness W, Millins SJ, et al: A serological study of cytomegalovirus infections associated with blood transfusions. N Engl J Med 284:1125, 1971

104. Tolkoff-Rubin NE, Rubin RH, Keller EE, et al: Cytomegalovirus infection in dialysis patients and personnel. Ann Intern Med 89:625, 1978

105. Bowden RA: Transfusion-transmitted cytomegalovirus infection. Hematol Oncol Clin North Am 9:155, 1995

106. Paya CV, Hermans PE, Wiesner RH, et al: Cytomegalovirus hepatitis in liver transplantation: prospective analysis of 93 consecutive orthotopic liver transplantations. J Infect Dis 160:752, 1988

107. Barkholt LM, Ericzon BG, Ehrnst A, et al: Cytomegalovirus infections in liver transplant patients: incidence and outcome. Transplant Proc 22:235, 1990
108. Englehard D, Or R, Strauss N, et al: Cytomegalovirus infection and disease after T cell depleted allogeneic bone marrow transplantation for malignant hematologic disease. Transplant Proc 21:3101, 1989
109. Griffiths PD: Current management of cytomegalovirus disease. J Med Virol (suppl 1):106, 1993
110. Farrusia E, Schwab TR: Management and prevention of cytomegalovirus infection after renal transplantation. Mayo Clin Proc 67:879, 1992
111. Ho M, Suwansirikul S, Dowling JN, et al: The transplanted kidney as a source of cytomegalovirus infection. N Engl J Med 293:1109, 1975
112. Myers JD, Fluornoy N, Thomas ED: Risk factors for cytomegalovirus infection after human marrow transplantation. J Infect Dis 153:478, 1986
113. Balfour HH Jr, Sachs GW, Welo P, et al: Cytomegalovirus vaccine in renal transplant candidates: progress report of a randomized, placebo-controlled, double-blind trial. Birth Defects 20:289, 1984
114. Snydman DR, Werner BG, Heinze-Lacey B, et al: Use of cytomegalovirus immune globulin to prevent cytomegalovirus disease in renal-transplant recipients. N Engl J Med 317:1049, 1987
115. Martin M: Antiviral prophylaxis for CMV infection in liver transplantation. Transplant Proc 25(suppl 4):10, 1993
116. Steinmuller DR, Novick AC, Streem SB, et al: Intravenous immunoglobulin infusions for the prophylaxis of secondary cytomegalovirus infection. Transplant 49:68, 1990
117. Kasiske BL, Heim-Duthoy KL, Tortorice KL: Polyvalent immune globulin and cytomegalovirus infection after renal transplantation. Arch Intern Med 149:2733, 1989
118. Lautenschlager I, Ahonen J, Eklund B, et al: Hyperimmune globulin therapy of clinical cytomegalovirus infection in renal allograft recipients. Scand J Infect Dis 21:139, 1989
119. Balfour HH Jr: Prevention of cytomegalovirus disease in renal allograft recipients. Scand J Infect Dis Suppl 80:88, 1991
120. Snydman DR, Rubin RH, Werner BG: New developments in cytomegalovirus prevention and management. Am J Kidney Dis 21:217, 1993
121. Emanuel D: Treatment of cytomegalovirus disease. Semin Hematol 27(suppl 1):22, 1990
122. Tabor E: Epstein-Barr virus and blood transfusion. Infectious Complications of Blood Transfusion. Tabor E, Ed. Academic Press, San Diego, 1982, p 65
123. Rocchi G, de Felici A, Ragona G, et al: Quantitative evaluation of Epstein-Barr-virus-infected mononuclear peripheral blood leukocytes in infectious mononucleosis. N Engl J Med 296:132, 1977
124. Armitage JM, Kormos RL, Stuart RS, et al: Posttransplant lymphoproliferative disease in thoracic organ transplant patients: ten years of cyclosporine-based immunosuppression. J Heart Lung Transplant 10:877, 1991
125. Lager DJ, Burgart LJ, Slagel DD: Epstein-Barr virus detection in sequential biopsies from patients with a posttransplant lymphoproliferative disorder. Mod Pathol 6:42, 1993
126. Dotti G, Fiocchi R, Motta T, et al: Epstein-Barr virus-negative lymphoproliferative disorders in long-term survivors after heart, kidney, and liver transplant. Transplantation 69:827, 2000
127. Leblond V, Davi F, Charlotte F, et al: Posttransplant lymphoproliferative disorders not associated with Epstein-Barr virus: a distinct entity? J Clin Oncol 16:2052, 1998
128. Preiksaitis JK, Cockfield AM: Epstein-Barr virus and lymphoproliferative disorders after transplantation. Transplant Infections. Bowden RA, Ljungman P, Paya CV, Eds. Lippincott-Raven Publishers, Philadelphia, 1998, p 245
129. Breinig MK, Zitelli B, Ho M: Epstein-Barr virus, cytomegalovirus and other viral infections in children after liver transplantation. J Infect Dis 156:273, 1987
130. Starzl TE, Porter KA, Iwatsuki SK, et al: Reversibility of lymphomas and lymphoproliferative lesions developing under cyclosporine-steroid therapy. Lancet 1:583, 1984
131. Hanto DW, Frizzera G, Gajl-Peczalska KJ, et al: Epstein-Barr virus, immunodeficiency, and B cell lymphoproliferation. Transplantation 39:461, 1985
132. Shapiro RS, McClain K, Frizzera G, et al: Epstein-Barr virus associated B cell lymphoproliferative disorders following bone marrow transplantation. Blood 71:1234, 1988
133. Benkerru M, Durandy A, Fischer A: Therapy for transplant-related lymphoproliferative diseases. Hematol Oncol Clin North Am 7:467, 1993
134. Keating MR: Antiviral agents. Mayo Clin Proc 67:160, 1992
135. de Clercq E: Antivirals for the treatment of herpesvirus infections. J Antimicrob Chemother 32(suppl A):121, 1993
136. Oberg B: Antiviral effects of phosphonoformate (PFA, foscarnet sodium). Pharmacol Ther 40:213, 1989
137. Houff SA, Burton RC, Wilson RW, et al: Human-to-human transmission of rabies virus by corneal transplant. N Engl J Med 300:603, 1979

Acknowledgments

Figure 1 Micrograph courtesy of F. K. Lee, A. J. Nahmias, and S. Stagno, Emory University. Drawing by George V. Kelvin.

Figures 4 and 5 Albert Miller.

87 ACQUIRED IMMUNODEFICIENCY SYNDROME

John Mihran Davis, M.D.

Approach to Human Immunodeficiency Virus Infection

No immediate end to the epidemic of acquired immunodeficiency syndrome (AIDS) is in sight. Because surgeons will be increasingly involved with AIDS patients, it is important for them to become familiar with the basic principles of the disease process. All operating room personnel need to take great care in handling tissue, all sharp instruments, and body secretions. Although it is hoped that a cure for human immunodeficiency virus (HIV) infection will be found soon, the likelihood of this is small.

CDC Classification of HIV Infection

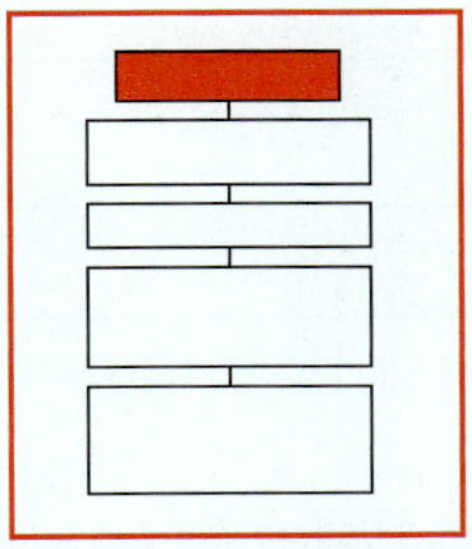

The Centers for Disease Control and Prevention (CDC) has devised a classification system that includes all individuals with HIV infection, the cause of AIDS.[1] Four groups are defined. They are mutually exclusive and hierarchical in that patients classified into a particular group should not be reclassified into a preceding group if clinical findings resolve. A given patient does not necessarily pass through all four groups. This classification is based on data accumulated during the clinical application of serum antibody testing for HIV. Before the availability of such antibody testing, national reporting was considered appropriate only for patients with AIDS (i.e., severely immunosuppressed patients with opportunistic infection or secondary malignancy).[2] It is now evident that AIDS patients represent only a fraction of a larger group of HIV-infected individuals [see Figure 1], although the fraction has increased over the past decade and is expected to increase further.

Within most groups considered to be at risk for infection, the incidence of HIV positivity is quite high but varies depending on the region of the country. The HIV seropositivity rate in homosexual and bisexual men ranges from 10 to 70 percent and averages 25 percent. Among intravenous drug abusers in New York, northern New Jersey, and Puerto Rico, the rate of seropositivity approaches 60 percent. In contrast, in other areas of the United States, the rate of seropositivity for intravenous drug abusers is about five percent. Among hemophiliacs, the HIV seropositivity rate varies depending on the patient's need for blood products: 35 percent of hemophiliacs with the less severe hemophilia B are seropositive for HIV, whereas 70 percent of those with hemophilia A are seropositive. Sexual partners of intravenous drug abusers, bisexuals, and hemophiliacs have an HIV-positive rate of approximately five percent.[3]

Although the natural history of AIDS has been well studied during the past several years, the prognosis for HIV-infected patients who do not have opportunistic infections or secondary cancers is still not well defined. The availability and widespread use of antibody testing should allow further understanding of the natural history of HIV infection.

GROUP I—THE ACUTE SYNDROME

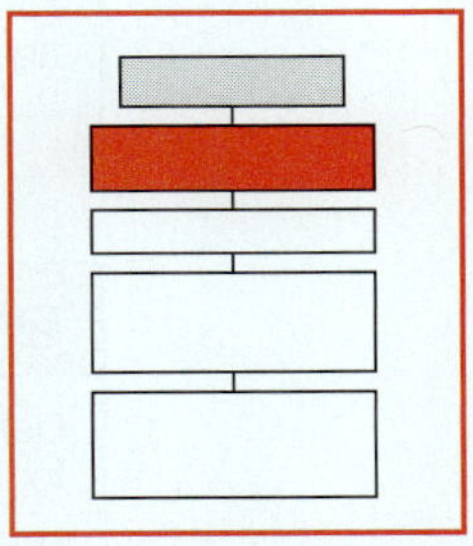

The acute syndrome that occurs in some patients after HIV infection is an acute viral illness, similar in nature to an episode of mononucleosis.[4] Patients in this group are reclassified into one of the other three groups (see below) once their acute symptoms resolve. For surgeons and other health care workers, the major significance of patients with the acute syndrome is the risk these patients pose of transmitting HIV infection. Although some studies document that the antibody response to HIV may not appear for more than one year after exposure to the virus, detectable antibodies usually appear in six to eight weeks.[5-7] It is during the initial six weeks of infection that a patient with a negative antibody may unknowingly transmit the virus.

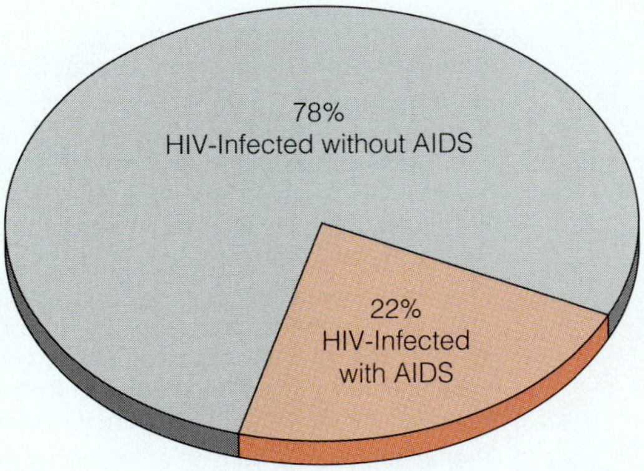

Figure 1 Shown is the percent of HIV-infected individuals in the United States with AIDS in 1992.[85]

Approach to Human Immunodeficiency Virus Infection

CDC classification of HIV infection

The four groups defined are mutually exclusive and hierarchical in that patients classified into a particular group should not be reclassified into a preceding group if clinical findings resolve. A given patient does not necessarily pass through all four groups.

Group I—the acute syndrome

In some individuals, HIV infection may cause an acute viral illness similar to mononucleosis. Such patients may not have detectable serum antibodies to HIV. Test symptomatic individuals who belong to one of the AIDS risk groups for HIV antibodies at the onset of symptoms and then every 3 mo for a year or until seroconversion. To detect HIV antibodies, first test serum by enzyme-linked immunosorbent assay; positive results must be confirmed by Western blot assay.

Group I patients are reclassified into one of the other three groups once their acute symptoms resolve.

Group II—the asymptomatic carrier

A large number of asymptomatic carriers are expected to undergo operation unrelated to their HIV infection. Screening of all potential surgical patients is controversial; adoption of universal precautions against HIV transmission is more appropriate.

Group III—persistent generalized lymphadenopathy

Definition is palpable lymphadenopathy > 1 cm in diameter in at least two extrainguinal sites persisting for longer than 3 mo.

Lymph node biopsy provides prognostic information:
- Explosive follicular hyperplasia, either alone or in a mixed pattern with follicular involution, suggests a prolonged clinical course, even in the presence of Kaposi's sarcoma
- Follicular involution alone is associated with opportunistic infection, Kaposi's sarcoma, lymphoma, and survival time < 1 yr
- Lymphocyte depletion represents end-stage disease

Prognosis is also closely correlated with the number of circulating helper T cells. Currently, the only indication for lymph node biopsy is to rule out a *treatable* lymphoma; however, it may be used to confirm the presence of ongoing infection.

Group IV—other human immunodeficiency virus diseases

Included are patients meeting the CDC definition of AIDS:
- Patients with at least one of 12 specified secondary infections (e.g., *Pneumocystis carinii* pneumonia) with no explanation other than HIV infection
- Patients with at least one of three secondary cancers known to be associated with HIV infection (e.g., Kaposi's sarcoma)

Surgical interventions that may be suitable for possible complications of AIDS are
- Biliary surgery for acute cholecystitis or acute cholangitis
- Resection, bypass, or colostomy for acute GI perforation or obstruction
- Splenectomy for splenomegaly or thrombocytopenia
- Indwelling central venous catheterization for drug therapy or venous access

Protect the patient from other infections by proper sterilization or disinfection of instruments and equipment.

Because acute HIV infection is possible in any symptomatic patient who is involved in high-risk behavior, antibody testing should be done at the onset of symptoms, at six weeks, and then every three months for a year or until the patient seroconverts.

Since the outbreak of the AIDS virus, the composition of AIDS patients has gradually shifted. In 1986, 90 percent of patients with AIDS were homosexual men, bisexual men, or intravenous drug abusers. The remaining 10 percent included hemophiliacs, recipients of HIV-contaminated blood, and sex partners of persons in high-risk groups. By 1995, the percentage of AIDS patients who were homosexual men had declined significantly, from 65 percent to 45 percent, and the incidence of perinatal and heterosexual transmission of HIV had increased from one percent to 11 percent.[8,9] A significant number of instances of heterosexual transmission occur among young inner-city adults and are related to the use of crack cocaine, which seems to promote high-risk sexual behavior.[10]

Detection of HIV Infection

Two tests for determining if a patient is infected with HIV are commercially available: the enzyme-linked immunosorbent assay (ELISA) and the Western blot assay. Both tests are designed to detect the presence of HIV antibody in serum. The ELISA test uses antigenic material that is adsorbed onto wells in plastic dishes. The wells are then exposed to serum from the patient who is being tested. After the test serum has reacted with the antigen, the wells are washed and then incubated with an antibody to human immunoglobulin. Before application to the wells, the antibody is linked to an enzyme that can be detected by a colorimetric reaction when exposed to the appropriate substrate. The intensity of color that is ultimately produced is directly related to the concentration of HIV antibody in the patient's blood. The ELISA test is considered very sensitive (i.e., its false negative rate is low), but its false positive rate is high. The weakness of the ELISA test is that some individuals have antibodies that react with HIV antigens but are not specific for HIV.

The Western blot assay is considered a more specific test but has a high false negative rate. It is therefore used most effectively in confirming ELISA results; it is not a good screening test. In Western blotting, antigenic HIV particles are separated by electrophoresis and then allowed to react with serum from the patient. Antigen-antibody complexes form and are subsequently identified by tagging with radiolabeled staphylococcal A protein, which has a high affinity for antigen-antibody complexes. This test is almost 100 percent positive in HIV-infected patients whose blood shows a positive ELISA reaction. Results of both the ELISA test and the Western blot assay must be positive in an individual before HIV infection can be confirmed. However, most blood banks will not use blood that has demonstrated a positive ELISA reaction, even if HIV antibody was not detected by Western blotting.[11]

On August 8, 1995, the Food and Drug Administration recommended that all blood donated for transfusion be screened for the p24 antigen (the core structural protein of HIV) to reduce the risk of administering HIV-contaminated blood.[12] With the current test for HIV, there is a so-called window period of 25 days between infection and seroconversion. It has been estimated that since 1985, when all banked blood was tested for HIV, 35 patients have contracted HIV infection because the donor blood was collected from an HIV-infected individual during this window period.[13,14]

The p24 antigen is present in blood as soon as the virus begins to replicate, typically about two to three weeks after infection. Thus, the window period can be reduced by six days if the assay for this antigen is added to routine screening for HIV antibody. As the host begins to make virus-specific antibody to HIV, the p24 antigen is either cleared or neutralized, so that in an HIV-infected patient, the assay eventually yields negative results. For this reason, the p24 antigen assay is useful primarily as a screening test for blood, and it must be combined with a neutralization assay. In selected patients, the p24 antigen assay may be a helpful clinical tool. Additional laboratory tests that may help in the diagnosis of patients who are believed to have HIV infection but in whom HIV antibody screening yields negative results include DNA polymerase chain reaction (PCR), antigen testing after immune complex disruption, and reverse transcriptase PCR.[14]

GROUP II—
THE ASYMPTOMATIC CARRIER

The asymptomatic carrier is the second major category of patients with HIV infection. The growing numbers of patients with heterosexually or perinatally transmitted disease [see Figure 2] has been well established by continued CDC monitoring. The evidence that military recruits and candidates for the Job Corps have HIV seroprevalence rates similar to the national average is significant because these groups are composed primarily of heterosexual sexually active teenagers.[15,16] Although the need for educational programs to reach this group of potential AIDS victims is clear, the approach has been controversial.

A 1992 analysis of hospitalized patients revealed an even higher incidence of HIV seroprevalence in this patient population (4.7 percent) than in the population at large. Because only one third of those patients with HIV seroreactivity were aware of their condition, a large population of patients were unable to benefit from antiretroviral therapy.[17] These data stress the need for routine voluntary testing and emphasize the importance of the use of universal precautions for protecting all health workers in the hospital environment.

GROUP III—PERSISTENT GENERALIZED LYMPHADENOPATHY

Another group of HIV-infected patients defined by the CDC comprises those with persistent generalized lymphadenopathy, that is, palpable lymphadenopathy measuring greater than 1 cm in diameter in at least two extrainguinal sites and persisting for longer than three months. Before the availability of HIV antibody testing, the relation of this lymphadenopathy to systemic manifestations of immunosuppression (systemic symptoms, neurologic symptoms, secondary infections, or cancers) was not known. It is now clear that lymphadenopathy is part of the general clinical spectrum associated with HIV infection, and opportunistic infection, Kaposi's sarcoma, or large cell lymphoma will develop in some, if not all, lymphadenopathy

GROUP IV—OTHER HIV DISEASES

Patients whose clinical problems place them in group IV have more generalized and serious symptoms than patients in the first three disease groups. Not all patients in this group, however, fulfill the current definition of AIDS as used by the CDC for national reporting. Only those patients in category C-1 and subgroup D are classified as AIDS patients. The subgroups and categories of group IV are defined as follows[1]:

Subgroup A—constitutional disease. One or more of the following with no explanation other than HIV infection: fever persisting for more than one month, involuntary weight loss amounting to more than 10 percent of baseline weight, and diarrhea persisting for more than one month.

Subgroup B—neurologic disease. One or more of the following with no explanation other than HIV infection: dementia, myelopathy, and peripheral neuropathy.

Subgroup C—secondary infectious disease. An opportunistic infection that indicates a defect in cell-mediated immunity with no explanation other than HIV infection. These infectious diseases are subdivided into two categories. Category C-1 includes patients with symptomatic or invasive disease stemming from one or more of the 12 specified secondary infectious diseases listed in the CDC surveillance definition of AIDS: *Pneumocystis carinii* pneumonia (PCP), chronic cryptosporidiosis, toxoplasmosis, extraintestinal strongyloidiasis, isosporiasis, candidiasis (esophageal, bronchial, or pulmonary), cryptococcosis, histoplasmosis, mycobacterial infection with *Mycobacterium avium-intracellulare* or *M. kansasii*, cytomegalovirus infection, chronic mucocutaneous or disseminated herpes simplex virus infection, and progressive multifocal leukoencephalopathy. Category C-2 includes patients with symptomatic or invasive disease arising from six other specified secondary infectious diseases: oral hairy leukoplakia, multidermatomal herpes zoster, recurrent *Salmonella* bacteremia, nocardiosis, tuberculosis, and oral candidiasis (thrush).

Subgroup D—secondary cancers. The diagnosis of one or more of the kinds of cancers known to be associated with HIV infection and included as part of the CDC surveillance definition of AIDS: Kaposi's sarcoma, non-Hodgkin's lymphoma (small noncleaved cell lymphoma or immunoblastic sarcoma), and primary lymphoma of the brain.

Subgroup E—other conditions in HIV infection. The presence of unclassifiable clinical findings or diseases, such as chronic lymphoid interstitial pneumonitis, that may be attributed to HIV infection or may indicate a defect in cell-mediated immunity. Also included are those patients whose signs or symptoms could be attributed either to HIV infection or to another coexisting disease not classified elsewhere and those patients with other clinical illnesses, the course or management of which may be complicated or altered by HIV infection.

Surgical Interventions

The treatment of patients with AIDS involves multimodality therapy and consultation with oncology and infectious disease specialists. It is beyond the scope of this discussion to describe the specific therapeutic approaches to the complications of HIV infections; however, three principal problems must be addressed when a cure for these infections is considered. First, the opportunistic infection or secondary malignant disorder must be treated; second, the underlying immunodeficiency must be corrected; and finally, the cause of the problem, the HIV infection, must be eradicated from the host. Although there has been some progress in treating patients with HIV infections, no fast or simple cures are expected in the near future. The role of surgeons in the management of these chronically ill, and sometimes critically ill, patients includes performing diagnostic biopsies, giving supportive care, and managing complications of malignant or infectious processes. These complications include a number of nonsurgical gastrointestinal problems, such as so-called gay bowel syndrome, gonococcal proctitis, and a fulminant watery diarrhea caused by *Cryptosporidium*.[25,26] A growing number of studies have documented the strange surgical complications caused by the opportunistic infections and secondary cancers that plague the AIDS patient.

Cryptosporidiosis and cytomegalovirus infection of the biliary tree have been reported to cause acute cholecystitis and acute cholangitis, necessitating emergency surgical intervention.[27] It is suggested that choledochoenteric bypass provides the best palliation in these patients. It is not known, however, whether the biliary tree is ever cleared of the infectious pathogens. *Candida* infection and Kaposi's sarcoma have also caused cholangitis, necessitating bypass operation.[28]

Acute perforations of the gastrointestinal tract from cytomegalovirus infection, cryptosporidiosis, and candidiasis, as well as from necrotic lymphoma, have been reported.[18,29,30] Obstruction of the gastrointestinal tract caused by Kaposi's sarcoma or lymphoma may also be an indication for resection, bypass, or colostomy. One study of AIDS patients who required abdominal operation described four distinct clinical syndromes that called for surgical intervention: (1) peritonitis secondary to cytomegalovirus enterocolitis and perforation, (2) non-Hodgkin's lymphoma of the gastrointestinal tract (usually the terminal ileum), presenting as obstruction or bleeding, (3) Kaposi's sarcoma of the gastrointestinal tract, and (4) mycobacterial infection of the retroperitoneum or the spleen.[31]

The role of splenectomy in patients with marked splenomegaly or with thrombocytopenia must be individualized. Thrombocytopenia occurs in AIDS patients as a result of the circulating immune complex deposition on platelets rather than as a result of a specific antiplatelet antibody.[32,33] Splenectomy has been a very successful means of managing some of these patients. Occasionally, patients in subgroup A (see above) who have debilitating fevers associated with significantly enlarged spleens experience dramatic palliation after splenectomy. In patients with massive splenomegaly and fever, simple splenomegaly is sometimes difficult to distinguish from abscess or parenchymal necrosis. In addition, splenectomy may be indicated in instances in which there is merely a likelihood of injury and in those in which a large spleen compresses the stomach, thereby contributing to the patient's malnutrition.

A request frequently directed to the general surgeon from the primary care physician, the infectious disease consultant, or the hematologist caring for an AIDS patient is for placement of an indwelling central catheter. Long-term venous access for treating fungal infections or, occasionally, for nutritional support in patients with debilitating diarrheal syndromes can significantly enhance the delivery of care to these patients. However, line placement often occurs when the patient is febrile, as a result of either the underlying infectious problem or treatment with amphotericin B. Therefore, the surgeon should keep a close watch postoperatively to ensure that fevers are not related to an infected catheter [see 81 Nosocomial Infection].

Protection from Common Infections

Although AIDS patients with general surgical complications are quite ill, morbidity and mortality from surgical intervention usually result from progression of the disease rather than from common pathogenic bacteria: infectious complications in AIDS patients are usually caused by opportunistic organisms associated with severe immunosuppression. The incidence of the perioperative infections seen in the general population as complications of abdominal operation, such as infections with gram-negative anaerobes and aerobes, is not increased in the AIDS patient postoperatively.[26-29] A study that prospectively evaluated infection rates in almost 100 AIDS patients who had clean operative procedures (lymph node biopsies) found that bacterial infection occurred at a rate approaching one percent.[34] This rate is comparable to that in the population at large. Additional clinical studies have confirmed these findings.[28] These data support research showing little or no change in neutrophil function despite significant alterations in lymphocyte and macrophage responsiveness.

It is also quite evident that the organisms that often infect an AIDS patient have, in the past, not been very contagious. A key question for surgeons, operating room committees, infection control committees, and clinicians involved with endoscopy is how to effectively clean instruments, equipment, or other inanimate objects to be used with AIDS patients. Agents that are effective against mycobacteria, the most resistant group of organisms, are also the agents considered most effective against other bacterial and viral pathogens.[35] (A complete list of agents and their efficacies can be obtained from the Disinfectants Branch, Office of Pesticides, United States Environmental Protection Agency, 401 M Street, S.W., Washington, DC 20460.)

Agents are classified according to whether they are to be used for sterilization, disinfection, or antisepsis.[36] Agents that sterilize inanimate objects kill all microbial organisms as well as bacterial endospores. Disinfectants are not quite as effective in that they are not capable of killing bacterial spores. In many cases, an agent may serve as a disinfectant when placed in contact for a short time with the object requiring cleansing. The same agent may be capable of sterilizing surgical instruments when exposed to them for longer periods. Disinfectants are subclassified as having high-level, intermediate-level, and low-level germicidal activity. High-level agents are effective against bacterial spores. Intermediate-level disinfectants are less effective against spores but are mycobactericidal. Low-level disinfectants do not kill mycobacteria and some fungi. Antiseptic agents are used on tissue and therefore must be less toxic than sterilants or disinfectants.

According to the current recommendations from the CDC, agents classified by the United States Environmental Protection Agency as sterilants can be used for sterilization or high-level disinfection, depending on contact time. All instruments entering the bloodstream or other sterile tissues should be sterilized before use. Instruments that contact mucosal surfaces, such as endoscopes, should receive high-level disinfection, which can be achieved with solutions of glutaraldehyde (two percent), hydrogen peroxide (three to six percent), or formaldehyde (one to eight percent).

Prevention of HIV Transmission

RISKS TO PATIENTS

Transfusions

All fresh whole blood, packed red blood cells, platelets, plasma (not Plasmanate), cryoprecipitate, and leukocytes can carry HIV. In addition, clotting factor concentrates may also carry the virus. Some preparations of γ-globulin can temporarily cause a false positive ELISA test for HIV, but they do not contain the virus or transmit it to recipients. Albumin and plasma extracts (Plasmanate), although prepared from whole blood, do not carry HIV, hepatitis B virus (HBV), or hepatitis C virus, because the process by which they are purified inactivates the virus particles. Since adequate antibody testing has become available, the incidence of undetected HIV in transfused blood has been extremely low.

To minimize the risk of HIV being transmitted by transfusion, patients have increasingly requested the use of predeposited autologous blood or blood donated by family members or friends. Although this approach was originally discouraged by some blood bank administrators,[37] both directed donations and predeposited autologous blood storage have become widely accepted [see 5 Bleeding and Transfusion]. Analysis of the incidence of HIV seropositivity in directed donation programs has not established that these programs pose any greater risk of transmitting HIV; however, directed donations are more costly.

Intraoperative blood salvage in trauma or emergency cases is a reasonable alternative to blood transfusion. At present, however, such collection methods are very costly because of the need to maintain trained personnel to run the equipment.

Transplantation

Because it has been shown that HIV can be present in semen, blood, urine, tears, breast milk, cerebrospinal fluid, and saliva and because it is suspected that HIV can be present in all secretions and excretions as well as all body tissues,[38] potential donors of tissue for transplantation must be tested for serum antibodies to HIV to prevent inadvertent transfer of the virus. (The risk of transmitting the virus by artificial insemination has also been documented and should be considered whenever artificial insemination is planned.[39])

Transmission from Surgical Personnel

Whenever a surgeon who is an asymptomatic carrier of the human immunodeficiency virus performs an operation, there is a risk that he or she will transmit the virus to the patient. This risk is well known to the public and consequently has become a potential medicolegal issue.[40] The question of whether HIV-infected surgeons should cease operating is surrounded by controversy. Because there have been no documented instances of transmission of the virus from a surgeon to a patient, the Centers for Disease Control and Prevention has not recommended that surgeons who are seropositive for human immunodeficiency virus refrain from performing surgery.[41] The report from a few years ago of HIV transmission to five patients from an HIV-positive dentist rekindled debate and prompted the CDC to reassess its policy. Recent court decisions have further confused the situation. In New York State, a case was brought by an HIV-positive pharmacist against a hospital that denied him a job because it feared he could possibly spread HIV while preparing intravenous solutions. After a year of testimony and 17 expert witnesses, the court found that the pharmacist should not be restrained from performing his clinical duties. In neighboring New Jersey, a hospital permitted an ENT surgeon who had AIDS to continue to practice, provided that he inform his patients of his disease. The doctor sued his hospital for discrimination. In this case, the judge ruled that patients have the right to know whether their doctor is HIV positive. What impact these decisions may have on national policy is currently unclear.

The issue of HBV transmission provides a noteworthy counterpoint. In a well-documented report involving a nonimmunized cardiac surgeon who acquired HBV infection in the workplace, transmission of the virus occurred in 19 (13 percent) of 122 patients on whom the surgeon operated over a 12-month period.[42] The surgeon was positive for hepatitis B e antigen (HB_eAg), and sweat from inside his glove was found to contain both the antigen and HBV DNA. No deficiencies were found in the surgeon's infection control practice by the CDC, which suggested that the virus may have spread through microperforations in his gloves. This case did not receive the same publicity that cases of HIV transmission have received in the lay press. However, its significance is clear: contact between health care workers who are HBV (HB_eAg) positive and patients should be restricted.

RISKS TO HEALTH CARE WORKERS

Asymptomatic HIV carriers present a potential threat to health care workers, especially to surgeons who may be operating on them. Such carriers may not know that they have the virus or have been exposed to it. The number of asymptomatic HIV carriers in the United States is estimated to be between one million and two million. For this reason, surgeons in the operating room as well as all others in the hospital environment should exercise extreme caution to prevent injury by sharp instruments. The threat of HIV transmission is significant because it results in a uniformly fatal outcome for all individuals in whom an opportunistic infection or secondary malignant disorder develops.

Although the risk of transmission of HIV in the operating room is very low, the documented incidence of tuberculosis in AIDS patients is of great concern, especially to health care workers involved in the care of AIDS patients.[43] After a 30-year decline in the incidence of tuberculosis, the incidence has steadily risen approximately 20 percent a year since 1984. This increase is thought to be due in part to the AIDS epidemic. Of greater concern is the very high percentage of patients who have multiple drug–resistant tuberculosis (MDR-Tb). Approximately 30 percent of AIDS patients infected with tuberculosis have MDR-Tb, and these patients require prolonged antitubercular therapy and have an extremely high case mortality. A significant risk of transmission to health care workers has clearly been established.[44] AIDS patients, the homeless, prison inmates, and indigent patient populations with pulmonary symptoms need to be adequately screened, especially before undergoing surgery.

The CDC now recommends that all precautions to prevent HIV transmission be taken with all patients, not only those known to be infected with HIV or at high risk for such infection [see 86 Viral Infection].[45-48] It is important that any hospital personnel who come in contact with patients, with their tissues, or with their blood, body fluids, or excreta know of the potential risk in handling materials from these patients and take appropriate precautions. Patients in high-risk groups should be placed on enteric precautions to protect health care workers not only from HIV infection but also from hepatitis B infection (up to 80 percent of such patients are hepatitis B carriers). As part of any operative procedure on HIV-infected patients, all operating room, nursing, and anesthesia personnel, as well as employees of surgical pathology laboratories and any other laboratories, should employ universal precautions. Employees in ancillary areas, such as housekeeping and dietary services, and the venipuncture team need to be trained in the use of universal precautions.

Exposure to the virus in the workplace is considered to be preventable in many cases.[49] Most injuries result from carelessness in handling sharp objects, such as needles [see Table 1]. Self-inflicted puncture incurred in the course of recapping used needles is the most common cause of inadvertent exposure to the human immunodeficiency virus. Consequently, the most important rule to follow when handling used needles is to discard them—uncapped—in a container that is large enough to accommodate the attached syringe. Tissue specimens, wastes, soiled linen, blood samples, and sharp objects (e.g., surgical instruments, needles, and glassware) must be handled with extreme care. Dressings and other disposable materials should be discarded in specially marked containers and not with the regular hospital refuse.

The use of double gloves has been shown to minimize the possibility of contact with patient blood through small defects in the gloves, and it reduces the likelihood of blood contact with skin when a glove puncture occurs.[50,51]

The following are some additional precautions health care workers should take when handling any potentially infectious materials.

Table 1 Preventable Exposures to HIV among Health Care Workers*[49]

Circumstances of Preventable Exposure	Number of Health Care Workers (% of 938 Exposed Health Care Workers)
Recapping of needle	152 (16%)
Injury from improper disposal of needle or sharp object	119 (13%)
Contamination of open wound	93 (10%)
Use of needle-cutting device	9 (1%)
Total preventable exposures	373 (40%)

*The total sample under surveillance consisted of 938 health care workers exposed to blood or other body fluids of a patient with AIDS or an AIDS-related illness.

1. Wear gloves when handling body fluids.
2. Wear a gown to prevent contamination of clothing.
3. Wash hands after contact with body fluids.
4. Place fluid from a potentially contaminated host in two impervious containers.
5. Clean spills with either a 1:10 dilution of 5.25 percent sodium hypochlorite in water or with some other type of sterilant.
6. Wear masks and protective eyeglasses when there is a possibility of aerosolization of material.

Even health care workers who do not have exfoliative dermatitis or an open wound should wear gloves during patient care. Evidence suggests that the affinity of HIV for Langerhans cells may permit the virus to invade a host through intact skin or mucous membranes.[52]

Discussion

Epidemiology

AIDS

In June 1981, the CDC published a report of *P. carinii* pneumonia in a unique cohort of five previously healthy homosexual males living in Los Angeles.[53] At that time, the CDC was the sole distributor of pentamidine, the only treatment for this rare pulmonary infection. PCP traditionally was seen only in severely immunosuppressed patients who were receiving chemotherapy for disseminated cancer. Even in this select group, PCP was rare, and *P. carinii* was not considered pathogenic in otherwise healthy adults. The sudden increased demand for pentamidine in one geographic area raised the prospect of a new disease process. In July 1981, the CDC reported a group of young homosexual males with Kaposi's sarcoma.[54] Kaposi's sarcoma, like PCP, was a rare lesion not commonly seen in young, healthy adults. Many of these patients also had severe infections caused by organisms associated with immunodeficiency (PCP, toxoplasmosis, candidiasis, cryptococcosis, and cytomegalovirus infections). These two accounts represent the first recognition that AIDS was a new disease complex, although it is believed that infection by the causative agent must have occurred at least three to four years earlier. The cause of the severely depressed immune function in these individuals, who were not otherwise at risk for opportunistic infection, was controversial until late 1983 and early 1984, when two independent laboratories isolated similar retroviruses in patients with the syndrome of acquired immunodeficiency.[55,56] These retroviruses, formerly known as human T cell lymphotropic virus type III (HTLV-III) and lymphadenopathy-associated virus (LAV), are now recognized to be the same virus, which has been renamed human immunodeficiency virus.

Since 1981, the number of AIDS victims has increased. All individuals in whom clinical manifestations of the disease, such as Kaposi's sarcoma, lymphoma, or opportunistic infections, have developed either have died or are expected to die as a result.[57] In September 1987, the definition of AIDS was expanded to include symptomatic, HIV-infected patients who were suspected of having an opportunistic infection. This new definition precipitated a misleading sudden increase in the number of new cases.[58]

Since 1986, the percentage of homosexual or bisexual AIDS patients has steadily declined, and the percentage of AIDS patients who are intravenous drug abusers or heterosexual has increased [see Figure 2].

TRANSFUSION-ASSOCIATED HIV TRANSMISSION

Although currently administered blood transfusions are very safe, a vast number of patients who received blood between 1977 and April 1985 may have received HIV-infected blood. This eight-year period is when blood was most likely to have been unknowingly contaminated. The New York Blood Center studied stored blood samples from a group of 600,000 individuals who received blood transfusions during this eight-year period and who consequently were at risk for receiving HIV-contaminated blood. It was estimated that only 418 of these former patients received infected transfusions. On the basis of these data, the risk of any one unit of blood being HIV-infected was 0.01 percent during the years 1977 to 1980, 0.02 percent for 1981 to 1982, and 0.03 percent for 1984 to 1985. The risk of becoming infected equals the number of units transfused multiplied by the risk for each time period. Thus, it is evident that even during the maximal risk period, blood transfusions were remarkably safe.

Since May 1985, all blood for clinical use has been screened for antibody to HIV, and only anecdotal cases of contaminated blood have since been reported to the CDC. It is currently estimated that the risk of receiving a unit of blood that is contaminated with HIV is one in 150,000 (< 0.0007 percent).[59]

The first transmission of HIV from a blood donor since antibody testing became available for use in blood banking occurred when a seronegative but recently infected victim donated blood.[60] In two patients—one receiving a unit of platelet-poor packed red blood cells and the other a unit of platelets, both of which were isolated from the infected donor—positive titers of HIV antibodies developed after transfusion. The new p24 antigen assay (see above) should help detect such donors.

Pathogenesis of HIV Infection

HIV is an oncovirus belonging to the retrovirus family. The potential of retroviruses to cause neoplasia was first recognized in 1911 by the American pathologist Rous, who associated them with certain malignant disorders in animals.[61] Human T cell lymphotropic virus type I (HTLV-I), which is a retrovirus that is related to HIV, has been identified as causing leukemia in humans.[62]

One of the characteristic features of retroviruses such as HIV is the presence of an enzyme called reverse transcriptase. This enzyme allows the virus to transcribe viral RNA to DNA. The virus can synthesize double-stranded DNA from single-stranded DNA that has been liberated from the RNA-DNA hybrid. This double-stranded DNA inserts itself into the host's nucleus and serves as a template for viral replication. Thus, whenever the infected host cell divides, new HIV particles are also reproduced. HIV has been isolated in many cell types, but it is thought that the helper T cell is the cell that is most frequently infected. The virus resides in the nucleus of these cells, and it is believed that when the cell is activated by some secondary infection, the virus is replicated, resulting in the dissemination of mature virions. During this process, the virus also kills the cell in which it was residing. The length of time between HIV infection and the development of AIDS (i.e., the manifestation of opportunistic infections or secondary cancers) is not known, but data from patients in the risk groups for AIDS suggest that the latency period is approximately five years.

This estimate of latency period is probably misleading because patients in the high-risk groups are more frequently exposed to other infectious challenges, and exposure to various microbes activates the T cells that harbor HIV. Frequent and repetitive activation of the immune system disseminates the virus throughout the host and significantly impairs cellular immunity. Thus, the latency period of HIV infection will probably be longer in members of the general population than has been previously documented in members of high-risk groups. The reason is the lower incidence of concomitant infectious problems in members of the general population.

Table 2 Health Care Workers with Documented or Suspected HIV Infection[9]

	Number of Health Care Workers	
	With Documented HIV (%)*	With Suspected HIV (%)†
Dental	0	7 (7%)
Mortician	0	3 (3%)
Emergency medical team/paramedic	0	9 (9%)
Health aide	1 (2%)	12 (12%)
Housekeeper	1 (2%)	7 (7%)
Laboratory technician	18 (37%)	15 (15%)
Nurse	19 (39%)	24 (24%)
Physician		
Surgeon	0	4 (4%)
Nonsurgeon	6 (12%)	10 (10%)
Respiratory therapist	1 (2%)	2 (2%)
Surgical technician	2 (4%)	1 (1%)
Other	1 (2%)	8 (8%)
Total	49	102

*Evidence of seroconversion after occupational exposure to HIV.
†HIV seropositivity in health care workers with occupational exposure to HIV who do not have behavioral or transfusion risks for HIV infection.

Risks to Surgeons

HIV TRANSMISSION

The risk to a surgeon of acquiring an HIV infection while treating a patient who has undetected AIDS is quite low.[41,49] The CDC initially evaluated nearly 1,500 health care workers who cared for AIDS victims. Serum samples were taken from these workers when they first began to work with immunocompromised patients and were stored in anticipation of a test for HIV. Of these workers, 666 were exposed to HIV through needle sticks or through cuts from sharp instruments. When tests were performed on these exposed individuals, none were found to have seroconverted after their exposure to HIV. However, two health care workers who had had no baseline blood sample drawn did show a positive antibody test after an injury. Because they did not belong to a known risk group for AIDS, they were believed to have generated antibody to HIV as a result of exposure in the workplace. On the basis of this study, the risk to a health care worker of acquiring HIV infection after an accidental needle-stick exposure was concluded to be 2 divided by 666, or 0.3 percent. A follow-up study found the rate of infection to be 0.5 percent.[63] Subsequent surveillance of health care workers identified 151 individuals who acquired HIV infection in the workplace [see Table 2]; 49 had proven seroconversion and 102 were HIV-positive, with no HIV-negative baseline serum sample.

A serosurvey of 770 surgeons practicing in two inner-city areas, where more than 3,000 cases of AIDS have been reported, was recently conducted by the CDC.[64] Accompanying the assay for HIV, HBV, and HCV was a questionnaire designed to elucidate the various practice patterns of the surgeons tested. One (0.13 percent) of the 770 surgeons was HIV positive; he had practiced for more than 25 years and performed more than 300 operations in the past year. The study did not specify how the surgeon acquired HIV, except to note that he did not participate in high-risk behavior. To date, there has been no documented seroconversion in OR personnel after a solid-bore needle injury in the operating room.

Transmission via skin contact with body fluids was documented in the case of a woman whose infant had received multiple transfusions, one of which was from an HIV-infected donor. The baby had received the contaminated transfusion at three months of age. The presence of HIV antibody in the mother was not determined until one year later, at which time an ELISA result was positive. The mother was closely involved with the baby's care and took no precautions against contact with the child's blood and body fluids. Seventeen months after the child received the infected blood transfusion, the mother seroconverted. No other risk factors accounted for the change in the mother's HIV antibody titer.[65]

Exposure to blood in the operating room has been of great concern to all operating room personnel since the AIDS epidemic began. The average practicing surgeon has 30 parenteral exposures to blood a year.[66] The fact that hollow-bore needles carry more blood than solid-bore needles may be the reason transmission in the operating room has not yet occurred. Four studies from the early 1990s established a blood-skin exposure rate of approximately 20 percent and a parenteral exposure rate of approximately four percent.[51,67-69] Long operative procedures requiring transfusions are most likely to be associated with blood exposure. Procedures that pose a high risk of exposure to blood are cardiac surgery; obstetrics, especially cesarean sections; trauma surgery; and emergency surgery. Special care must be taken to minimize exposure in these procedures; eye protection and use of double gloves are two barrier precaution measures that can reduce the likelihood of surgeon-patient blood contact.

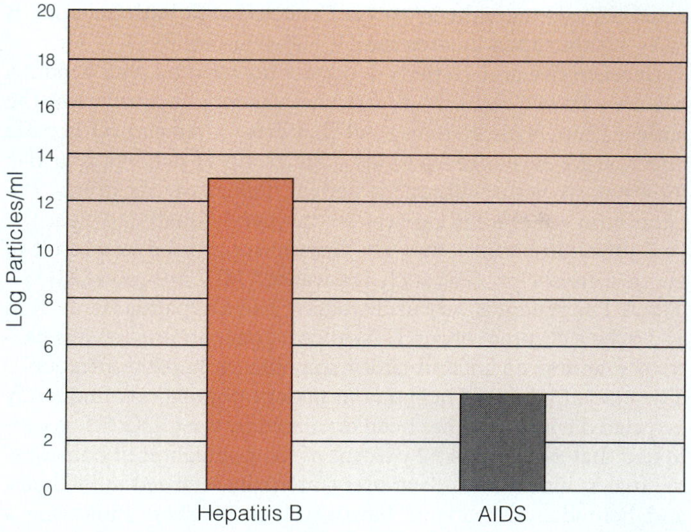

Figure 7 The numbers of infectious viral particles per milliliter of blood in patients with active hepatitis B infections and in AIDS patients are compared.[70]

Transmission of HIV to hospital workers is uncommon when compared with transmission of hepatitis B virus because of the relatively low concentration of HIV in the blood of AIDS patients [see Figure 7]. The concentration of virus particles is estimated to be 10^4 particles/ml in an AIDS patient, whereas it is 10^{13} particles/ml in a patient who has an active hepatitis B infection.[70]

Although HIV transmission is uncommon in the hospital environment, the risk to surgeons is very real. Unprotected anal intercourse is considered to be high-risk behavior, with a transmission rate of 0.4 percent (one in 250), and is discouraged by health officials.[71] The 0.5 percent (one in 200) risk of acquiring HIV infection through a needle stick is comparable.[72] Three independent factors are important in determining a surgeon's risk of acquiring HIV infection: (1) the number of needle sticks or punctures contaminated with the patient's body fluids, (2) the percent of HIV-infected patients in the surgeon's patient population, and (3) the number of years a surgeon is at risk for acquiring an HIV infection. If the risk of HIV transmission by a contaminated needle is 0.5 percent, the HIV-infected population is 10 percent, the number of needle sticks averages 30 a year, and a practicing surgeon has 40 years of exposure, then the lifetime risk of acquiring AIDS is 60 percent![73]

If a health care worker is injured by a sharp object contaminated by exposure to fluid or tissue from an HIV-positive patient, a series of blood samples should be drawn at the time of injury and again at six weeks, three months, six months, and 12 months after the injury to determine whether HIV infection has occurred.

Although administration of antiretroviral therapy is recommended,[74] to date no prospective trials have been performed to confirm its effectiveness in humans. In 1996, a retrospective case-control study was published that supported the use of zidovudine.[75] The current recommendations for prophylaxis after a needle-stick injury are based on the amount of blood in the inoculum and on the likelihood that the source patient has a high HIV titer.[76] (In general, terminally ill HIV-infected patients have high HIV titers because the virus is rapidly replicating and destroying host cells.) The injuries associated with the highest degree of risk are those in which a health care worker is injured by a hollow-bore needle containing blood from a terminally ill HIV-infected patient. The injuries associated with the next highest degree of risk are those involving *either* a large inoculum (e.g., from a hollow-bore needle) *or* parenteral exposure to blood from a patient with a high HIV titer (e.g., a terminally ill HIV-infected patient). For all of these high-risk injuries, the recommended approach is a four-week course of treatment with a combination of zidovudine, lamivudine (3TC), and indinavir (IND). If the injury was from a solid-bore needle or the source patient is asymptomatic, zidovudine alone is offered. In these lower-risk situations, the risk of drug

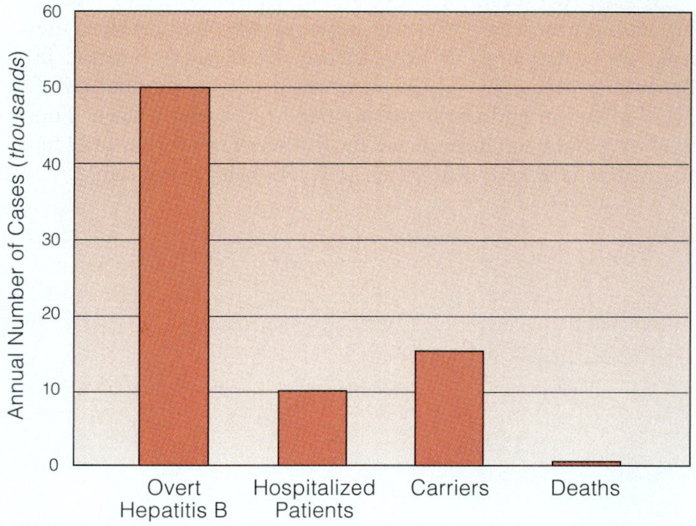

Figure 8 The annual incidence of hepatitis B infection in the United States is 200,000 cases. Various subgroups of hepatitis B patients are shown.[77]

Table 3 Prevalence of Hepatitis B Virus (HBV) Serologic Markers in Various Populations[87]

Population	Maximum Expected Prevalence of Serologic Markers of HBV Infection (%)
High risk	
Immigrants or refugees from areas where HBV is highly endemic	85
Clients in institutions for the mentally retarded	80
Users of illicit parenteral drugs	80
Homosexually or bisexually active men	80
Individuals who have household contact with HBV carriers	60
Hemodialysis patients	80
Intermediate risk	
Staff of institutions for the mentally retarded	25
Health care workers who have frequent contact with blood	30

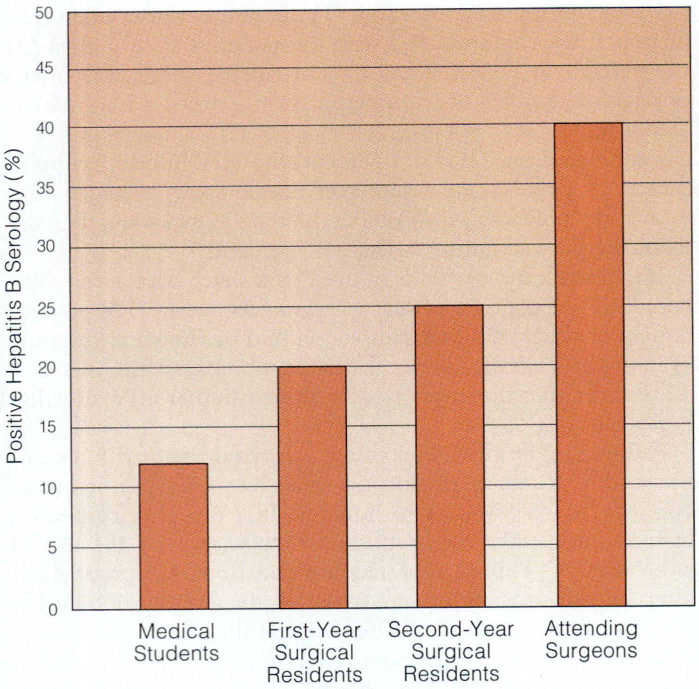

Figure 9 The prevalence of positive serology for hepatitis B increases among individuals in successive stages of a surgical career.[83]

toxicity must be carefully weighed against the benefits of protection against HIV transmission.

HEPATITIS TRANSMISSION

The primary health risk to surgeons caring for immunocompromised patients is that of acquiring hepatitis B or hepatitis C (non-A, non-B hepatitis). The epidemiology of hepatitis B has been well studied because there are numerous antigen and antibody markers of the virus in the blood of chronic carriers. On the basis of data from assays of these markers, it is estimated that more than 200,000 Americans acquire new hepatitis B infections each year.[77] Of these individuals, 25 percent will have symptoms of hepatitis. Five percent of the 200,000 will require hospitalization for their acute illness, and fulminant hepatitis that is fatal will develop in one to two percent of these hospitalized patients [see Figure 8]. The hepatitis D virus has been identified as causing an additional risk of death in patients with acute hepatitis, and individuals who are infected with both hepatitis B virus and hepatitis D virus have a higher mortality.[78]

Between five and 10 percent of patients infected with hepatitis become chronic carriers—that is, they do not effectively clear the antigen from their systems, and they have a subclinical hepatic infection for prolonged periods. This group of patients is at risk for cirrhosis with subsequent hepatic failure or hepatoma. Patients who are chronic carriers are frequently unable to clear the viral infection because they are immunosuppressed as a result of another disease process, such as advanced HIV infection (AIDS). The AIDS patient is very likely to have had a hepatitis B infection and to be a chronic carrier. HIV-infected patients are also less likely to manifest an inflammatory response to hepatic infection.[79] The epidemiology of hepatitis in patient populations frequently associated with AIDS has been evaluated by the CDC.[80] It is estimated that as many as 80 percent of the population of homosexual males, intravenous drug users, mentally retarded individuals, and hemodialysis patients have serologic markers indicating a prior hepatitis B infection. Household contact or sexual relations with these high-risk individuals also involves a significant risk of acquiring hepatitis B virus infection [see Table 3]. It is estimated that up to 60 percent of these contacts have positive serology for the hepatitis B virus.

Exposure to hepatitis carriers is a risk for health care workers, particularly for those who work with blood products [see 86 Viral Infection]. Physicians involved with direct patient care are at especially high risk.[81] Those in administrative situations who do not have clinical contact with patients have a relatively low risk of acquiring hepatitis, whereas surgeons, particularly cardiac surgeons and transplant surgeons, are at especially high risk. The risk of hepatitis infection also increases with age.[82,83] The incidence of positive hepatitis serology is between 12 and 13 percent in students in their last year of medical school, nearly 20 percent in surgical residents at the end of their first year, and about 25 percent in surgical residents after the second year. During the course of a senior surgeon's career, the risk of having hepatitis approaches 50 percent [see Figure 9]. These risks are exceedingly high and emphasize the importance of widespread use of the hepatitis B vaccine [see 86 Viral Infection].

At least two recent studies have shown that there are numerous nonimmunized practicing surgeons who had finished medical school, training, or both before the hepatitis vaccine first became available.[64,84] These surgeons are at substantial risk for HBV infection and consequently need to be immunized. Those who have not been immunized for five years or more should have their titers checked; if titers are low, a booster is advisable.

References

1. Classification system for human T-lymphotropic virus type III/lymphadenopathy-associated virus infections. MMWR 35:335, 1986
2. Update on Kaposi's sarcoma and opportunistic infections in previously healthy persons—United States. MMWR 31:294, 1982
3. Human immunodeficiency virus infection in the United States: a review of current knowledge. MMWR 36(suppl 6):1, 1987
4. Ho DD, Sarngadharan MG, Resnick L, et al: Primary human T-lymphotropic virus type III infection. Ann Intern Med 103:880, 1985
5. Wantzin GR, Lindhardt BO, Weismann K, et al: Acute HTLV III infection associated with exanthema, diagnosed by seroconversion. Br J Dermatol 115:601, 1986
6. Marlink RG, Allan JS, McLane MF, et al: Low sensitivity of ELISA testing in early HIV infection. N Engl J Med 315:1549, 1986
7. Imagawa DT, Lee MH, Wolinsky SM, et al: Human immunodeficiency virus type 1 infection in homosexual men who remain seronegative for prolonged periods. N Engl J Med 320:1458, 1989
8. Update: acquired immunodeficiency syndrome—U.S. MMWR 35:17, 1986
9. HIV/AIDS Surveillance Report, volume 7, No. 2, year-end edition 1995. US Department of Health and Human Services, Public Health Service, Centers for Disease Control and Prevention, National Center for HIV, STD, TB
10. Brown BR, Irwin KL, Faruque S, et al: Intersecting epidemics—crack cocaine use and HIV infection among inner city young adults. N Engl J Med 331:1422, 1994
11. Barnes DM: Keeping the AIDS virus out of blood supply. Science 233:514, 1986
12. Recommendations for donor screening with a licensed test for HIV-1 antigen. US Department of Health and Human Services, Public Health Service, Food and Drug Administration, Center for Biologics Evaluation and Research, Rockville, Maryland, 1995
13. US Public Health Service guidelines for testing and counseling blood and plasma donors for human immunodeficiency virus type I antigen. MMWR 45(R-22):1, 1996
14. Persistent lack of detectable HIV-1 antibody in a person with HIV infections—Utah, 1995. MMWR 45:182, 1996
15. Human T-lymphotropic virus type III/lymphadenopathy-associated virus antibody prevalence in U.S. military recruit applicants. MMWR 35:421, 1986
16. St. Louis ME, Conway GA, Hayman CR, et al: Human immunodeficiency virus infection in disadvantaged adolescents: findings from the US Job Corps. JAMA 266:2387, 1991
17. Janssen RS, St. Louis ME, Satten GA, et al: HIV infection among patients in U.S. acute care hospitals: strategies for the counseling and testing of the hospital patients. N Engl J Med 327:445, 1992
18. Nugent P, O'Connell TX: The surgeon's role in treating acquired immunodeficiency syndrome. Arch Surg 121:1117, 1986
19. Kaplan JE, Spira TJ, Fishbein DB, et al: Lymphadenopathy syndrome in homosexual men: evidence for continuing risk of developing the acquired immunodeficiency virus. JAMA 257:335, 1987
20. Goedert JJ, Biggar RJ, Melbye M, et al: Effect of T4 count and cofactors on the incidence of AIDS in homosexual men infected with human immunodeficiency virus. JAMA 257:331, 1987
21. Redfield RR, Burke DS: HIV infection: the clinical picture. Sci Am 259(October):90, 1988
22. Redfield RR, Wright DC, Tramont EC: The Walter Reed staging classification for HTLV-III/LAV infection. N Engl J Med 314:131, 1986
23. Fernandez R, Mouradian J, Metroka C, et al: The prognostic value of histopathology in persistent generalized lymphadenopathy in homosexual men. N Engl J Med 309:185, 1983
24. Davis JM, Chadburn A, Mouradian JA: Lymph node biopsy in patients with human immunodeficiency virus infections. Arch Surg 123:1349, 1988
25. Rubin RH: Acquired immunodeficiency syndrome. Scientific American Medicine, Section 7, Subsection XI. Rubenstein E, Federman DD, Eds. Scientific American, Inc, New York, 1990
26. Karchmer AW: Sexually transmitted diseases. Scientific American Medicine, Section 7, Subsection XXII. Rubenstein E, Federman DD, Eds. Scientific American, Inc, New York, 1990
27. Margulis SJ, Honig CL, Soave R, et al: Biliary tract obstruction in the acquired immunodeficiency syndrome. Ann Intern Med 105:207, 1986
28. Robinson G, Wilson SE, Williams RA: Surgery in patients with acquired immunodeficiency syndrome. Arch Surg 122:170, 1987
29. Barone JE, Gingold BS, Arvantis ML, et al: Abdominal pain in patients with acquired immunodeficiency syndrome. Ann Surg 204:619, 1986
30. Potter DA, Danforth DN, Macher AM, et al: Evaluation of abdominal pain in the AIDS patient. Ann Surg 199:332, 1984
31. Wilson SE, Robinson G, Williams RA, et al: Acquired immune deficiency syndrome (AIDS): indications for abdominal surgery, pathology, and outcome. Ann Surg 210:428, 1989
32. Morris L, Distenfeld A, Amorosi E, et al: Autoimmune thrombocytopenic purpura in homosexual men. Ann Intern Med 96:714, 1982
33. Walsh CM, Nardi MA, Karpatkin S: On the mechanism of thrombocytopenic purpura in sexually active homosexual men. N Engl J Med 311:635, 1984
34. Davis JM, Mouradian J, Fernandez R, et al: Acquired immune deficiency syndrome—a surgical perspective. Arch Surg 119:90, 1984
35. Favero MS: Sterilization, disinfection, and antisepsis in the hospital. Manual of Clinical Microbiology, 4th ed. Lenette EH, Balows A, Hausler W, et al, Eds. American Society for Microbiology, Washington, DC, 1985, p 129
36. Jawetz E, Melnick JL, Adelberg EA: Antimicrobial chemotherapy. Review of Medical Microbiology, 15th ed. Lange Medical Publications, Los Altos, California, 1982, p 117
37. Moore SB: AIDS, blood transfusions, and directed donations. N Engl J Med 314:1454, 1986
38. Ho DD, Byington RE, Schooley RT, et al: Infrequency of isolation of HTLV-III virus from saliva in AIDS. N Engl J Med 313:1606, 1985
39. Morgan J, Nolan J: Risks of AIDS with artificial insemination. N Engl J Med 314:386, 1986
40. Gerbert B, Maguire BT, Hulley SB, et al: Physicians and acquired immunodeficiency syndrome: what patients think about human immunodeficiency virus in medical practice. JAMA 262:1969, 1989
41. Summary: recommendations for preventing transmission of infection with human T-lymphotropic virus type III/lymphadenopathy-associated virus in the workplace. MMWR 34:681, 1985
42. Harpaz R, Von Seidlein L, Averhoff FM, et al: Transmission of hepatitis B virus to multiple patients from a surgeon without evidence of inadequate infection control. N Engl J Med 334:549, 1996
43. National action plan to combat multidrug-resistant tuberculosis. MMWR 41(RR-11):1, 1992
44. Beck-Sague C, Dooley SW, Hutton MD, et al: Hospital outbreak of multidrug-resistant *Mycobacterium tuberculosis* infections. JAMA 268:1280, 1992
45. Recommendations for prevention of HIV transmission in health-care settings. MMWR 36(suppl 2S):1, 1987
46. Update: Universal precautions for prevention of transmission of human immunodeficiency virus, hepatitis B virus, and other bloodborne pathogens in health-care settings. MMWR 37:377, 1988
47. Guidelines for prevention of transmission of human immunodeficiency virus and hepatitis B virus to health-care and public-safety workers. MMWR 38(suppl S-6):1, 1989
48. Recommendations for preventing transmission of HIV and HBV to patients during exposure-prone invasive procedures. MMWR 40(suppl RR-8):1, 1991
49. McCray E: Occupational risk of the acquired immunodeficiency syndrome among health care workers. N Engl J Med 314:1127, 1986
50. Genberding JL, Littel C, Tarkington A, et al: Risk of exposure of surgical personnel to patients' blood during surgery at San Francisco General Hospital. N Engl J Med 322:1788, 1990
51. Quebbeman EJ, Telford GL, Wadsworth K, et al: Double gloving: protecting surgeons from blood contamination in the operating room. Arch Surg 127:213, 1992
52. Braathen LR, Ramirez G, Kunze RO, et al: Langerhans cells as primary target cells for HIV infection (letter). Lancet 2:1094, 1987
53. *Pneumocystis* pneumonia—Los Angeles. MMWR 30:250, 1981
54. Kaposi's sarcoma and *Pneumocystis* pneumonia among homosexual men—New York City and California. MMWR 30:305, 1981
55. Barré-Sinoussi F, Chermann JC, Rey F, et al: Isolation of a T-lymphotropic retrovirus from a patient at risk for acquired immune deficiency syndrome (AIDS). Science 220:868, 1983
56. Popovic M, Sarngadharan MG, Reed E, et al: Detection, isolation, and continuous production of cytopathic retroviruses (HTLV-III) from patients with AIDS and pre-AIDS. Science 224:497, 1984
57. Institute of Medicine & National Academy of Sciences: Mobilizing against AIDS: The Unfinished Story of a Virus. Harvard University Press, Cambridge, Massachusetts, 1986
58. Update: acquired immunodeficiency syndrome—United States, 1981–1988. MMWR 38:229, 1989
59. Cumming PD, Wallace EL, Schorr JB, et al: Exposure of patients to human immunodeficiency virus through the transfusion of blood components that test antibody-negative. N Engl J Med 321:941, 1989
60. Transfusion-associated human T-lymphotropic virus type III/lymphadenopathy-associated virus infection from a seronegative donor—Colorado. MMWR 35:389, 1986
61. Rous T: Transmission of a malignant growth by means of a cell-free filtrate. JAMA 56:198, 1911
62. Robert-Guroff M, Nakao Y, Notake K, et al: Natural antibodies to human retrovirus HTLV in a cluster of Japanese patients with adult T-cell leukemia. Science 215:975, 1982
63. Marcus R, The CDC Cooperative Needlestick Surveillance Group: Surveillance of health care workers exposed to blood from patients infected with the human immunodeficiency virus. N Engl J Med 319:1118, 1988
64. Panlilio AL, Shapiro CN, Schable CA: Serosurvey of HIV, HBV, HCV infection among hospital-based surgeons. J Am Coll Surg 180:16, 1995
65. Apparent transmission of human T-lymphotropic virus type III/lymphadenopathy-associated virus from a child to a mother providing health care. MMWR 35:76, 1986
66. Howard RJ: Human immunodeficiency virus testing and the risk to the surgeon of acquiring HIV. Surg Gynecol Obstet 171:22, 1990

67. Popejoy SL, Fry DE: Blood contact and exposure in the operating room. Surg Gynecol Obstet 172:480, 1991
68. Panlilio AL, Foy DR, Edwards JR, et al: Blood contacts during surgical procedures. JAMA 265:1533, 1991
69. Tokars JI, Bell DM, Culver DH: Percutaneous injuries during surgical procedures. JAMA 267:2899, 1992
70. Levy JA, Kaminsky LS, Morrow JW, et al: Infection by the retrovirus associated with the acquired immunodeficiency syndrome: clinical, biological, and molecular features. Ann Intern Med 103:694, 1985
71. Lorian V: AIDS, anal sex, and heterosexuals (letter). Lancet 1:1111, 1988
72. Update: acquired immunodeficiency syndrome and human immunodeficiency virus infection among health-care workers. MMWR 37:229, 1988
73. Hagen MD, Meyer KB, Kopelman RI, et al: Human immunodeficiency virus infection in health care workers: a method for estimating individual occupational risk. Arch Intern Med 149:1541, 1989
74. Henderson DK, Gerberding JL: Prophylactic zidovudine after occupational exposure to the human immunodeficiency virus: an interim analysis. J Infect Dis 160:321, 1989
75. Case-control study of HIV seroconversion in health-care workers after percutaneous exposure to HIV-infected blood—France, United Kingdom, and United States, January 1988–August 1994. MMWR 44:929, 1996
76. Update: provisional Public Health Service recommendations for chemoprophylaxis after occupational exposure to HIV. MMWR 45:468, 1996
77. Alter HJ: The evolution, implications, and applications of the hepatitis B vaccine (editorial). JAMA 247:2272, 1982
78. Govindarajan S, Chin KP, Redeker AG, et al: Fulminant B virus hepatitis: role of delta agent. Gastroenterology 86:1417, 1984
79. Perrillo RB, Regenstein FG, Roodman ST: Chronic hepatitis B in asymptomatic homosexual men with antibody to human immunodeficiency virus. Ann Intern Med 105:382, 1986
80. Recommendation of the Immunization Practices Advisory Committee (ACIP): Recommendations for protection against viral hepatitis. MMWR 34:313, 1985
81. Denes AE, Smith JL, Maynard JE, et al: Hepatitis B infection in physicians: results of a nationwide seroepidemiologic survey. JAMA 239:210, 1978
82. Lemmer JH: Hepatitis B as an occupational disease of surgeons. Surg Gynecol Obstet 159:91, 1984
83. Parry MF, Brown AE, Dobbs LG: The epidemiology of hepatitis B infection in housestaff. Infection 6:204, 1978
84. Barie PS, Dellinger P, Dougherty SH, et al: Assessment of HBV immunization status among North American surgeons. Arch Surg 129:27, 1994
85. Mann J, Tarontola D, Netter T: AIDS in the World. Harvard University Press, Cambridge, Mass, 1992.
86. Update: acquired immunodeficiency syndrome—United States, 1991. MMWR 41:463, 1992
87. Surveillance for occupationally acquired HIV infection—United States, 1981–1992. MMWR 41:823, 1992.

Acknowledgments

Figures 1 and 2   Tom Moore.

Figures 3 through 6   Micrographs courtesy of Dr. Janet Mouradian, Department of Pathology, Cornell University Medical College, New York.

Figures 7 through 9   Albert Miller.

88 IMMUNOMODULATION

David L. Dunn, M.D., Ph.D.

Host Defenses against Infection

The mammalian host exists in a state of equilibrium with microbes in the external environment and the internal milieu. Invasion by these potential pathogens occurs frequently but is countered by a series of host defenses that act to prevent infection and maintain host vitality. Although these defenses are extremely effective in preventing microbial incursion, they are imperfect. Isolated failure of even a single component of host defense can result in severe infection, and global failure frequently results in death.

In surgical patients, host defenses can be depressed as a result of (1) the surgical procedure itself or an injurious event (e.g., polytrauma or thermal injury) and (2) underlying disease states (e.g., malnutrition, advanced age, diabetes mellitus, or renal failure). Blood loss, tissue trauma, microbial contamination, and other inciting events that occur during an operation clearly predispose surgical patients to infection. In addition, the commonplace use of immunosuppressive agents in transplant patients and chemotherapeutic agents in patients with malignancy or autoimmune disease has led to increasing recognition that infection is particularly detrimental in immunocompromised patients. This recognition, in turn, has led to attempts to selectively suppress cellular immunity without globally influencing host defenses and to augment specific components of host defense in both normal and immunosuppressed patients. The purpose of such interventions is either (1) to prevent microbial invasion and subsequent infection or (2) to allow incipient or established infection to be more readily contained and eradicated, particularly in the immunocompromised or critically ill patient.

Because the immune status of the host is so closely linked to the occurrence of infection, an understanding of the potential therapeutic applications of immunomodulation depends on an understanding of the various types of host defenses against microbial incursion.

BARRIERS

The most basic host defenses are physical or physicochemical barriers (e.g., the integument and epithelialized mucous membranes) that separate the host from microorganisms in the external environment or separate sterile body compartments from compartments that communicate with the external environment and possess an autochthonous microflora. There are also a number of ancillary defenses that act in concert with the physical barriers [see Figure 1]. For example, secretion of fatty acids from sebaceous glands in the skin reduces the proliferation of skin microflora; mucus secretion and ciliary motion enable the respiratory tract epithelium to trap and extrude microbes; and stomach acidity kills ingested microorganisms.

The resident microflora also acts as a barrier to microbial invasion by preventing virulent noncommensal microorganisms from adhering at the level of the epithelial barrier, a phenomenon termed colonization resistance. Within the intestinal tract, anaerobic bacteria appear to be principally responsible for colonization resistance, and a reduction in the quantity of anaerobes may predispose to infection by gram-negative aerobes.[1] Thus, the gut barrier comprises not only the intestinal wall itself but also resident microbes contained within a thick layer of mucus. Bacterial translocation to the adjacent mesenteric lymph nodes, to the liver, or to the systemic circulation may occur in response to a wide variety of stimuli (e.g., hemorrhagic shock or thermal injury) in animal models; this process may play a causal role in the development of the multiple organ dysfunction syndrome (MODS) in humans [see 95 Multiple Organ Dysfunction Syndrome]. Endotoxin (or lipopolysaccharide [LPS]) produced by gram-negative bacteria may also be able to escape the confines of the gut and enter the portal circulation, particularly after severe injury. This process may trigger activation of Kupffer's cells within the liver, causing hepatocyte dysfunction. The clinical relevance of these observations, however, remains unclear.

Complete breakdown of any physical barrier as a result of necrosis or traumatic penetration facilitates the entry of environmental microorganisms, autochthonous epithelial microorganisms, or both into the adjoining sterile body compartment. Thus, it is not surprising that patients with skin lacerations or certain types of surgical wounds may become infected with the most common skin organisms—that is, gram-positive bacteria such as *Staphylococcus aureus*—whereas patients with penetrating abdominal injury or perforation of the colon may become infected both with aerobes such as *Escherichia coli* and with anaerobes such as *Bacteroides fragilis*. That so few wounds actually become infected, despite the plethora of contaminating microbes, is a tribute to the effectiveness of normal mammalian host defenses.

HUMORAL IMMUNITY

Microbes that penetrate the physical barriers of the host encounter several different host defenses, which frequently act in concert to contain and eradicate infection. One such defense is humoral immunity. Antibodies (primarily IgG and IgM in body fluids and secretory IgA at mucosal interfaces) bind to microorganisms (to inhibit microbial growth) or microbial toxins (to inhibit toxicity). The binding of IgM and most subclasses of IgG to antigens causes a conformational change in the heavy-chain region that exposes complement binding sites, thereby activating the classic complement pathway. Alternative pathway activation is largely independent of IgG; complement components of this pathway are capable of binding to microbial cell walls directly. Once the complement cascade is activated, whether via the classical pathway or via the alternative pathway, inflammatory complement breakdown products (C3a, C5a, and C5b67) are released that enhance vascular permeability and stimulate an influx of leukocytes to the infected site. Activation of the common terminal sequence of the two complement systems (C5b–C9) produces extremely effective microbial lysis and killing. Previous exposure to a specific microbial antigen may lead to enhanced production of high-affinity antibody by plasma cells—the so-called second-set phenomenon.

CELL-MEDIATED IMMUNITY

Cell-mediated immunity, in the form of activation of macrophages, polymorphonuclear leukocytes (PMNs), and T cells, func-

IL-6 is a glycoprotein that is produced by macrophages and fibroblasts in response to the presence of viruses, bacteria, endotoxin, and other cytokines (e.g., TNF-α and IL-1β). Elevated levels of IL-6 have been demonstrated during many different types of infections, including those caused by gram-negative and gram-positive bacterial organisms. IL-6 induces B cell differentiation, increases synthesis of acute-phase serum proteins by the liver, and is capable of provoking fever. It is noteworthy that anti–IL-6 antibodies protect against either lethal gram-negative bacterial infection or TNF-α challenge.[18,28-31]

IL-8 (formerly neutrophil-activating peptide–1, or NAP-1) is produced by macrophages and other cell types (e.g., lymphocytes and endothelial cells) in response to endotoxin, TNF-α, and IL-1. IL-8 is a potent PMN activator and chemoattractant, eliciting release of storage granules, induction of directed migration, and production of superoxide and hydrogen peroxide. Even though elevated levels of IL-8 have been observed during sepsis and can be demonstrated in primates after administration of endotoxin or IL-1, administration of IL-8 does not lead to secretion of other cytokines or to deleterious effects similar to those associated with sepsis. Direct injection of IL-8 into primates elicits several effects related solely to the cytokine's action on PMNs (e.g., neutrophilia and margination).[19,32]

Interferon Gamma

IFN-γ is a glycoprotein cytokine that is mainly produced by lymphocytes. Endotoxin also stimulates synthesis and secretion of IFN-γ in vitro and in vivo, and in the latter setting, IFN-γ appears to provoke activation of monocytes and PMNs. The evidence that IFN-γ plays an important role during sepsis is as follows[15,33,34]:

1. Elevated levels of IFN-γ have been observed after the inception of experimental gram-negative bacterial sepsis and after endotoxin challenge.
2. Administration of IFN-γ during experimental sepsis increases mortality.
3. Administration of anti–IFN-γ antibody protects mice from endotoxic shock or the generalized Shwartzman reaction.

Modulation of Host Defenses: Potential Areas of Intervention

SURGICAL INTERVENTION

Eradication of the source of infection—via surgical debridement of infected necrotic tissue, surgical or percutaneous drainage of infected abscesses, or removal of an infected intravenous catheter—is the primary precept of therapy for infected surgical patients. This simple principle of appropriate source control has been known to surgeons for many years and should be employed in virtually every infected individual. It is presumed that source control is capable of exerting salutary effects on depressed host defenses in infected, critically ill patients and that surgical drainage of infection is beneficial to the host, though this hypothesis has not been precisely tested. The phenomenon has been extensively reviewed, however, and ancillary supporting data are available. Specifically, removal of inflammatory foci caused by infection improves neutrophil chemotaxis and reduces anergy.[35] In addition, it is known that the anergic state is associated with higher rates of complications (particularly infectious complications). Thus, it seems highly probable that severe infection is associated with depression of host defenses and that surgical intervention acts as an immunomodulatory agent to abrogate this effect. Unfortunately, it is extremely difficult to test the effect of surgery as an independent variable because of variations that occur in clinical practice and because of the plethora of other variables that can be identified in the clinical setting.

The search for and the eradication of primary and secondary sources of infection in patients exhibiting the septic response are critical components of immunomodulation because in the absence of source control, host defenses that initially remain intact may later fail and secondary superinfections may ensue. Without adequate debridement or drainage, antibiotic therapy will not be of much value in the vast majority of cases, nor will immunotherapy. Thus, immunotherapy should be considered adjunctive therapy to be used in concert with other, routine therapeutic modalities.

IMMUNOTHERAPY

Host defenses can be thought of as having a set point—that is, a normal state of activity that promotes health, prevents infection, and does not facilitate excessive internal host mediator reactions. Immunotherapy involves restoring host defenses to this set point or selectively modifying them in a salutary fashion. Such therapy takes three general forms [see Table 1]:

1. Immunostimulation, in which an agent is administered that exerts secondary effects on one or more components of host defenses, either returning them to normal in an immunosuppressed individual or enhancing their activity in an individual with normal immune response who may be subjected to a common but serious infection (e.g., tetanus) or who may be undergoing a form of therapy (e.g., a prolonged operation or cancer chemotherapy) that would predispose to severe, potentially lethal infection.
2. Immunorepletion, in which a critical component of host defenses that is lacking or present only in low levels is administered.
3. Immunoabrogation, in which an agent is administered that specifically inhibits a portion of the activated defense response that exerts deleterious effects on the host.

Unfortunately, immunotherapy has not yet come into widespread use for the treatment of infection in the clinical setting. There are several reasons why this is so. First, it is currently difficult or impossible to rapidly and precisely detect microbes or microbial toxins that provoke the host septic response—more specifically, to detect them before they trigger any of the deleterious aspects of host defenses. Second, the host response itself is still imprecisely charac-

Table 1 Forms of Immunotherapy

Immunostimulation	Administration of biologic response modifiers Nutritional support Selective gut decontamination Vaccination
Immunorepletion	Administration of antiendotoxin antibody Administration of anti-CMV antibody Administration of BPI
Immunoabrogation	Cytokine antagonism PAF antagonism Inhibition of PGE_2 synthesis Leukocyte receptor antagonism

BPI—bactericidal/permeability-increasing protein CMV—cytomegalovirus
PAF—platelet-activating factor PGE_2—prostaglandin E_2

terized, particularly with regard to how the various mediator systems interact and how the activity of host defenses at sites in close proximity to infection (i.e., the local cellular and tissue level) differs from that at sites distant from the infection (i.e., the systemic level). Third, any attempt to manipulate host defenses must carefully balance the beneficial effects associated with low-level activation (tolerance or resistance to infection) against the adverse effects associated with extreme activation [see Host Defenses against Infection, Cytokine Activity, above]. For example, with most agents that stimulate host defenses (e.g., biologic response modifiers), increasing efficacy is accompanied by increasingly significant toxicity.

Of all the future advances that might increase the clinical utility of immunotherapy, perhaps the most significant would be the ability to detect infection and identify the responsible microorganisms promptly and precisely, coupled with the ability to simultaneously measure the overall status of each host defense compartment (barriers, humoral immunity, cell-mediated immunity, and cytokine activity) both regionally and systemically. At present, we cannot effectively measure the level of activity of each of the various host defense compartments and therefore cannot invariably predict which patients will become infected or manifest mediator-provoked adverse sequelae. Recently, however, several seminal studies have indicated that such prediction may eventually become possible.[6,7] Only through quantitation of host defenses and early identification of specific pathogens or toxins is precise targeting of specific forms of immunotherapy achievable.

In fact, without such precise knowledge, immunomodulation may be detrimental to the host. Obviously, prophylactic manipulation of the immune response before the infectious insult occurs would be ideal, but alteration of cytokine regulation itself may cause adverse effects whether it is done before or after the insult. For instance, whereas suppression of TNF-α secretion at the systemic level may prevent various deleterious aspects of the septic response, it may also simultaneously abrogate TNF-α–mediated local stimulation of host defenses, thereby leading to loss of local control of infection. Similarly, immunostimulation of macrophage activity may enhance local control of infection but at the same time may provoke toxic systemic effects. For these and other reasons, the areas in which immunotherapy is currently being implemented, though intriguing, are limited in number.

Immunostimulation

BIOLOGIC RESPONSE MODIFIERS

A large number of biologic response modifiers have been examined experimentally and clinically [see Table 2]. The majority of these agents are of microbial origin: bacterial cell wall products (e.g., mycobacterial muramyl dipeptide); crude preparations of killed bacterial cells (e.g., *Corynebacterium parvum*); viable, relatively nonpathogenic bacteria (e.g., bacillus Calmette-Guérin); and fungal cell wall products (e.g., zymosan and its active component glucan, derived from *Saccharomyces cerevisiae*).[36-38] They typically act by activating macrophages nonspecifically, thereby conferring the ability to resist a wide variety of subsequent challenges from many different types of microorganisms. Whereas all of these agents have improved survival in certain types of experimental infection, to date there is only preliminary evidence of protective effects in the clinical setting.[39,40]

Agents from other sources also act as biologic response modifiers. The anthelmintic agent levamisole, for example, exhibits immunostimulatory properties. It has been shown to improve survival in experimental infections, and in the only clinical infection trial levamisole has received, it improved outcome in a small group of patients with intra-abdominal and other forms of surgical sepsis.[41] Unfortunately, levamisole has not been tested further as an immunostimulant.

Table 2 Biologic Response Modifiers

Muramyl dipeptide	Endotoxin
Corynebacterium parvum	Endotoxin derivatives
Bacillus Calmette-Guérin	Monophosphoryl lipid A
Zymosan	Lipid X
Glucan	SDZ MRL 953
Levamisole	Cytokines
RU 41 740	TNF-α
CP-46,665	IL-1
Thymopentin	IL-2
Colony-stimulating factors	IL-12
G-CSF	IFN-γ
M-CSF	
GM-CSF	
IL-3	

Two synthetic nonspecific macrophage immunostimulants, RU 41 740 and CP-46,665, have had a protective effect in animal models of infection.[42,43] Thymopentin, a pentapeptide consisting of the active moiety of a thymic hormone, has been administered to animals and to humans about to undergo cardiac surgery and has reduced postoperative anergy.[42,44-46] In clinical trials, however, administration of thymopentin did not reduce infectious complications and infection-related mortality, though the incidence of these complications was very low in both control groups and treatment groups.[45,46] Further testing is certainly warranted.

Finally, colony-stimulating factors (CSFs), small peptides that increase the rate of maturation and release of bone marrow cells, can act as immunostimulants. Four types of colony-stimulating factor—granulocyte CSF (G-CSF), macrophage CSF (M-CSF), granulocyte-macrophage CSF (GM-CSF), and IL-3—have been identified, and recombinant forms are available. Administration of these factors has improved survival during certain types of experimental sepsis.[47] Preliminary clinical trials are providing tantalizing data indicating the utility of CSFs in reversing neutropenia in patients who have hematologic malignancies or AIDS or who have undergone bone marrow transplantation, an event that is associated with a high predisposition to serious infection.[48]

Endotoxin and Derivatives

Although endotoxin is capable of provoking macrophage stimulation, in minute amounts it acts as an immunostimulant by inducing so-called host tolerance. This phenomenon occurs before antibody production begins and is characterized by resistance to a normally lethal dose of endotoxin within 12 to 48 hours after an initial sublethal endotoxin injection. It is interesting that TNF-α has similar effects: administration of small amounts results in tolerance to a normally lethal dose of TNF-α or LPS or to a bacteremic insult occurring 24 hours after the initial administration of TNF-α. Intriguing evidence indicates that cellular inhibition of production of TNF-α messenger RNA (mRNA) by macrophages and decreased cellular sensitivity to the effects of TNF-α itself may be responsible for both endotoxin tolerance and TNF-α tolerance.[49,50] These findings provide additional support for the contention that TNF-α and other cytokines are extremely important regulators of the local host milieu and the set point of host defenses, promoting salutary effects in all but the most extreme circumstances (e.g., during bacteremia and endotoxemia). Although the clinical implications of endotoxin tolerance have yet to be established, animal studies suggest that administration of sublethal doses of LPS, nontoxic LPS derivatives, or TNF-α may be beneficial during gram-negative bacterial sepsis.[51]

Because the toxicity of endotoxin precludes its direct administration to humans, an investigative effort has been mounted to determine whether nontoxic derivatives of the toxic lipid A portion of the LPS molecule might function as immunostimulants. Several such lipid A analogues have been isolated. Monophosphoryl lipid A, which is produced by acid hydrolysis of bacterial LPS, has been extensively studied and is less toxic and less pyrogenic than LPS. Lipid X (2,3-diacylglucosamine-1-phosphate) and SDZ MRL 953 are both monosaccharides that are similar to a portion of lipid A. Lipid X is a biosynthetic precursor of lipid A that provokes cytokine secretion by macrophages but is less toxic than either lipid A or endotoxin in vivo. It competitively inhibits endotoxin-induced procoagulant macrophage activity, PMN activation, platelet aggregation, serotonin secretion, and the mitogenetic response of murine splenocytes. Similarly, SDZ MRL 953 is less toxic and less pyrogenic than lipid A or endotoxin. Pretreatment with each of these compounds has been demonstrated to provide protection against lethal gram-negative bacterial or endotoxin challenge in several animal species. Evidence that pretreatment with a lipid A analogue provides protection in experimental models of gram-positive bacterial, fungal, and viral infection indicates that these compounds may indeed function as immunostimulants.[51-53] Unfortunately, each of these compounds retains some degree of toxicity. For this reason, clinical trials have not yet been implemented.

Cytokines

In animal studies, several investigators have found that administration of IL-1, IL-2, IL-12, or IFN-γ also may enhance host responses and survival during experimental gram-negative bacterial infection, indicating that the level of macrophage activation and the ability of the host to respond to cytokine secretion may be of critical importance. Administration of low doses of recombinant IL-1 to either normal or granulocytopenic mice has been associated with accelerated improvement in neutrophil counts and with increased survival during experimental *E. coli* infection or endotoxemia. In normal animals and in C3H/HeJ endotoxin-resistant mice, IL-1 induces profound neutrophilia.[54] IL-2 is a glycoprotein cytokine produced by lymphocytes that enhances natural killer cell activity and the generation of cytotoxic T cells; impaired production of this cytokine has been associated with increased susceptibility to infection in mice. Several studies also indicate that intraperitoneal administration of IL-2 can enhance survival during experimental gram-negative peritoneal infection.[55,56] In these studies, the greatest reduction in mortality was achieved by means of prophylactic administration of IL-2 at the site of infection, which supports the view that IL-2 acts by stimulating local host defenses.

IFN-γ also appears to be an immunostimulant under certain conditions: it has been shown to reduce mortality from experimental bacterial infection after trauma and to reduce the number and size of intra-abdominal abscesses after hemorrhagic shock.[57,58] Clinical data indicate that administration of IFN-γ reverses trauma-induced diminution of macrophage expression of MHC class II HLA-DR antigen, a critical component of antigen presentation and cellular host defenses.[10,59] A multicenter, randomized, double-blind, placebo-controlled trial was performed to assess the efficacy of IFN-γ in reducing infection rate and mortality in severely injured patients.[60] The 416 patients enrolled received either IFN-γ, 100 μg subcutaneously once daily for 21 days, or placebo. Although the infection rates were similar in the two groups, infection-related mortality was significantly lower in the IFN-γ treatment group than in the placebo group (3% versus 9%; $P < 0.05$).

Administration of IL-12 leads to enhanced resistance to infection in experimental animal models. Intriguingly, this effect may be attributable to IL-12's capacity for stimulating endogenous secretion of IFN-γ.[61]

Even though endotoxin, TNF-α, IL-1, IL-2, and IFN-γ (though not IL-6 or IL-8) achieve effective immunostimulation in animal models in which dosage adjustments can be readily accomplished, their toxicity makes it unlikely that they will be clinically useful in combating infection. Of particular concern is the possibility that administration of these agents could activate components of the host septic response that would augment the systemic adverse effects that occur during serious infection.

NUTRITIONAL SUPPORT

Severe infection is characterized by enhanced gluconeogenesis, ketone body formation, and disordered oxidative metabolism that leads to reduced production of branched-chain amino acids and increased synthesis of aromatic amino acids; these processes typically occur despite adequate provision of metabolic substrates. In most patients with the sepsis syndrome, metabolic control becomes disordered at the tissue level, and in some individuals, these metabolic derangements lead to progressive and sequential failure of one or more organs and eventually to death [*see 95 Multiple Organ Dysfunction Syndrome*]. Not surprisingly, metabolic support in the form of enteral or parenteral nutrition has become part of the standard armamentarium in the treatment of such patients [*see 97 Nutritional Support*]. Such metabolic support clearly exerts salutary effects on morbidity and mortality when used in conjunction with other standard treatment measures, such as debridement and drainage, fluid resuscitation, hemodynamic monitoring, and antibiotic therapy.[62] It is noteworthy, however, that a 7- to 15-day course of preoperative parenteral nutrition appears to decrease the incidence of noninfectious complications only in severely malnourished patients.[63]

Accumulating evidence indicates that provision of certain compounds may exert beneficial effects on the host response to infection by improving substrate metabolism. For example, administration of branched-chain amino acids may provide nutritional repletion, thereby facilitating the normal activity of a variety of metabolic pathways, including those within cells and tissues that are critical to the salutary aspects of the septic response.[62] Nutritional support appears to exert more direct immunoenhancing effects as well. For example, enteral nutrition may enhance gut barrier function, perhaps thereby decreasing bacterial translocation.[64] There is also some evidence that parenteral nutrition in humans results in a substantially greater host cytokine response to endotoxin administration than enteral feeding does.[65]

A number of nutritional compounds may act as immunostimulants, reversing the immunosuppression associated with severe trauma or a major operative event.[66,67] Glutamine is thought to act by stimulating gut enterocyte activity, perhaps thereby enhancing barrier function[66] [*see 97 Nutritional Support*]. Arginine appears to enhance a variety of T cell responses, an effect that has been associated with improved survival in animal models of sepsis.[68] Increased ingestion of omega-3 fatty acids, which are found in abundance in linseed and fish oils, is associated with diminished cytokine responses, presumably because their metabolism does not facilitate the synthesis of potentially immunosuppressive metabolites, such as prostaglandin E_2 (PGE_2) [see 100 Eicosanoids in Surgery]. In animal models of infection, however, use of these various compounds has not had uniformly beneficial effects.[69-71] It is difficult to differentiate their primary effects on host defenses from their secondary effects.

SELECTIVE GUT DECONTAMINATION

In patients with underlying hematologic malignant disorders who become neutropenic, microbial translocation appears to be causally linked with the occurrence of the sepsis syndrome and increased morbidity and mortality. The evidence for this contention is as follows[72,73]:

1. These patients exhibit bacteremia caused by facultative gram-negative aerobes such as *E. coli, Klebsiella pneumoniae,* and *Pseudomonas aeruginosa,* and the same biotypes or serotypes of these organisms can be identified in the intestinal microflora before and at the time of the septic event.
2. Selective gut decontamination (SGD)—that is, administration of oral antimicrobial agents that kill these aerobes and yeasts while sparing the anaerobic microflora—reduces the incidence of bacteremia.

In seriously ill surgical patients, however, the evidence for such a causal relation is considerably less compelling. The line of reasoning that gram-negative enteric bacilli might translocate to the liver and trigger mediator-induced injury is extremely attractive for two reasons: first, the liver is frequently the first organ to fail during MODS, and second, escape of bacteria from hepatic defenses could explain the occurrence of episodes of gram-negative bacterial sepsis without a defined local source. This hypothesis, however, has not been substantiated by clinical trials of SGD in ICU patients: although reductions in overall infectious episodes have been demonstrated, no clear-cut reductions in mortality have been documented.[74-76] In one study, SGD reduced the incidence of gram-negative infection, but other types of infection continued to occur, and overall morbidity and mortality were unaffected.[77] Recently, investigation of this problem has been returned to the laboratory, where several researchers have been unable to correlate translocation with the effects of SGD.[78]

VACCINATION

Vaccination may invoke humoral immunity, cell-mediated immunity, or both, depending on the immunogen used. It is useful for dealing with pathogens that possess limited antigenic diversity, particularly when employed before the septic event. For vaccination to be effective, three criteria must be met:

1. A suitable antigenic form of the pathogen or the critical antigenic determinants of the pathogen must be available; administration of the antigen must not produce the disease itself and must not lead to significant toxicity.
2. The vaccine must provoke a protective host defense response that prevents disease.
3. If the pathogen exhibits little or no antigenic diversity, a univalent vaccine can be used. If, however, the pathogen or group of pathogens has considerable antigenic diversity, either a polyvalent vaccine must be used or common antigen structures must be identified and used as targets for development of protective immunity.

Vaccination has effectively prevented many viral diseases (e.g., measles, mumps, rubella, smallpox, polio, hepatitis B, rabies, yellow fever, and influenza) as well as a number of bacterial infections (e.g., whooping cough, diphtheria, and tetanus, caused by toxins produced by *Bordetella pertussis, C. diphtheriae,* and *Clostridium tetani,* respectively). In one study of patients who had undergone splenectomy or who had impaired splenic function as a result of sickle cell anemia or another similar disease, immunization with a polyvalent pneumococcal vaccine consisting of the primary antigens of 23 different strains of *Streptococcus pneumoniae* reduced the rate of infection and severe sepsis caused by this organism.[79] In another study, vaccination with *Hemophilus influenzae* type b polysaccharide vaccine protected high-risk pediatric populations against disease caused by this organism.[80] Vaccination also has been effective against hepatitis A virus, *Salmonella typhi, S. paratyphi* A, *Vibrio cholerae, Neisseria meningitidis, Mycobacterium tuberculosis, Yersinia pestis, Francisella tularensis,* and rickettsiae such as *Rickettsia prowazekii.*

Initial clinical trials with *Pseudomonas* vaccines employed endotoxin-based preparations that provided varying degrees of protection but had significant local and systemic toxic effects.[81,82] Other vaccines have been developed that are directed against *Pseudomonas* cell wall components other than endotoxin (e.g., exopolysaccharide, pili, and flagella), though none have yet been shown to have salutary clinical effects. Preparations in which the nontoxic O-antigen polysaccharide region of endotoxin from common serotypes of *E. coli, Klebsiella* species, or *Pseudomonas* species has been linked to exotoxin A from *P. aeruginosa* or to cholera toxin also have been evaluated as vaccines. Numerous investigations are now under way that are aimed at developing effective vaccines against HIV, hepatitis C virus, and cytomegalovirus (CMV). Vaccination with an attenuated Towne strain of CMV has been used in solid-organ transplant patients but has met with little success,[83] probably because of the reduced ability of immunosuppressed patients to mount a protective antibody response. A new biotechnologic approach to vaccination involves the identification, isolation, and cloning of the viral genetic sequences that are responsible for critical expression of viral antigens that provoke a host response; the insertion of these genes into a nonpathogenic carrier virus or liposomes; and, finally, the administration of the immunogenic, nonpathogenic vaccine. Immunoadjuvants that will bolster the response to vaccination are now being intensively investigated as well.

Immunorepletion

ANTIENDOTOXIN ANTIBODY

Gram-negative bacterial sepsis is a lethal disease process that produces substantial morbidity and mortality in both normal patients (mortality, 10% to 20%) and immunocompromised patients (mortality, > 30%).[11,84-87] The incidence of gram-negative bacteremia and the mortality from gram-negative bacterial sepsis have remained relatively constant since the early 1980s, despite advances in routine therapeutic intervention, the use of antimicrobial agents, aggressive hemodynamic monitoring, fluid resuscitation, and metabolic support. Because endotoxin may be responsible for toxicity both directly and indirectly (through activation of host mediator systems), the possibility that antibody directed against this portion of the gram-negative bacterial outer membrane could reduce mortality during sepsis has received a great deal of study. This form of immunotherapy is extremely attractive in that it could theoretically prevent the action of endotoxin at an extremely proximal point in the host response, thereby blunting the effects of endotoxin on macrophage cytokine release. In addition, antiendotoxin antibody could be administered either prophylactically or during the course of incipient or established sepsis. Developments in this field have been hampered, however, by endotoxin's inherent toxicity, which precludes its use as a primary immunogen in humans, and by the extreme immunologic heterogeneity of the causative microorganisms.

Gram-negative bacterial endotoxin, or LPS, is composed of three regions: (1) lipid A, consisting of diphosphorylated diglucosamine with a high degree of substitution with ester-linked fatty acids whose carbon chains are 14 to 16 carbon atoms in length; (2) O-antigen polysaccharide, a series of repeating units generally consisting of four to six sugar residues in a combination that is different for each strain of gram-negative microorganism; and (3) the core region, consisting of 10 to 12 saccharides that link O-antigen polysaccharide with lipid A [see Figure 3]. The lipid A region is the toxic portion of the endotoxin molecule; injection of lipid A reproduces the majority of the pathophysiologic alterations that occur after administration of purified endotoxin. The core region of LPS is further divided into three portions—outer, intermediate, and deep (inner).[11,88] The deep core/lipid A (DCLA) region of LPS is biochemically and immunologically highly conserved across a wide variety of gram-negative microorganisms. For this reason, as well as because it represents the toxic moiety of LPS, the DCLA region is an ideal candidate for a target antigen against which a specific antibody can be directed.

Experimental Data

Two studies from the 1960s found passive transfer of type-specific (anti–O-antigen polysaccharide) polyclonal antiserum to be highly protective during experimental gram-negative bacterial sepsis. These studies did not define the identity of the protective component, and protection was not cross-reactive, being limited to the primary immunogen. Subsequent studies with purified polyclonal antibody established that antibody was indeed the active agent. Investigative work using polyclonal anticore antibodies, however, provided conflicting information concerning protective capacity during experimental gram-negative bacterial sepsis and endotoxemia. These initial studies were hindered by the unavailability of monospecific, purified antibody reagents, which meant that nonspecific effects could not be excluded.[89-92]

Subsequent experimental studies using murine monoclonal antibodies (MoAbs) more clearly defined the role of antibody in binding to LPS and providing protection against either endotoxin or bacterial challenge. Murine MoAbs directed against the O-antigen polysaccharide region of *E. coli* 0111:B4 LPS reacted specifically against the O-antigen polysaccharide and provided potent, albeit serotype-specific (i.e., non–cross-reactive), protection against either an endotoxin challenge or a gram-negative bacterial challenge in vivo.[93,94] It was subsequently demonstrated that anti–O-antigen polysaccharide MoAbs, of either the IgG class or the IgM class, that possessed similar but not identical specificity provided a similar degree of protection.[95]

Thereafter, other investigators developed MoAbs directed against various portions of the core region as well as against lipid A.[96-103] MoAbs directed against the DCLA region appear to be the most cross-reactive, though unique binding determinants appear to exist

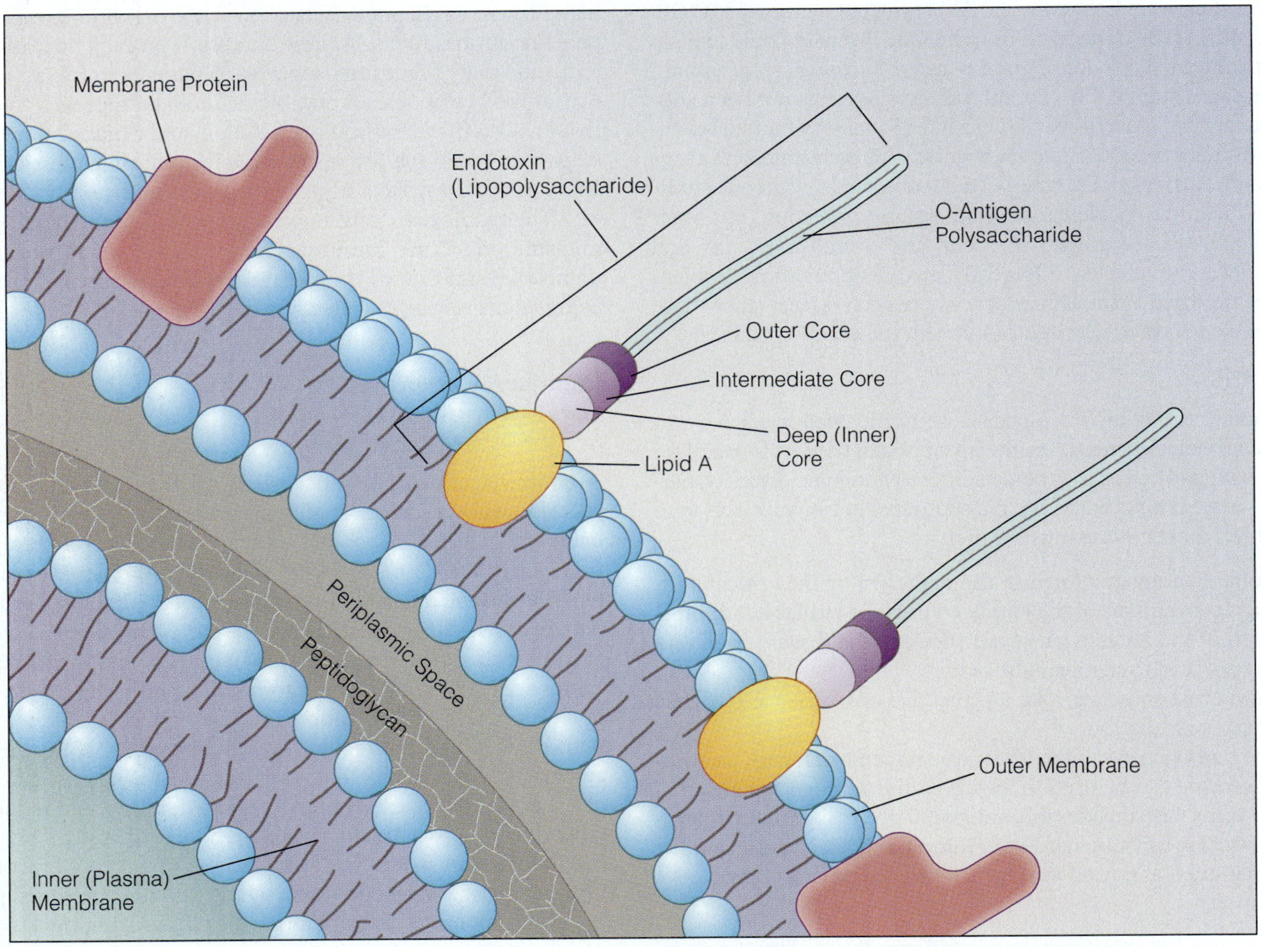

Figure 3 Shown are the structure of gram-negative bacterial endotoxin (lipopolysaccharide [LPS]) and its position in the outer bacterial membrane.

within this region.[98-103] In one study, a single anti-DCLA MoAb enhanced survival during endotoxemia and gram-negative bacteremia or peritonitis.[96,98] In another, an anti–O-antigen polysaccharide MoAb was compared with an anticore MoAb and found to be more protective, though lacking cross-reactivity.[102] Initial studies provided conflicting data regarding the degree to which DCLA determinants are exposed on the surface of intact microorganisms, and some studies indicated that binding may depend on the manner in which bacterial antigen was prepared and the growth phase of the culture. Western immunotransblot analysis has been used to examine the precise epitope binding sites of antiendotoxin MoAbs and has indicated that some, but not all, core epitopes are available for binding on intact LPS molecules.[99,102,103]

There is preliminary evidence that antiendotoxin MoAbs abrogate cytokine secretion at several different levels and that this phenomenon is associated with reduced mortality in experimental animal models of sepsis.[104-107]

Clinical Trials

Initial studies of gram-negative bacterial infection in humans revealed that elevated anti–O-antigen polysaccharide antibody titers were correlated with a favorable outcome and that elevated anti–deep core antibody titers tended to be associated with enhanced survival, regardless of the actual infecting gram-negative organism.[108] Subsequently, several investigators showed that survival was correlated with both the initial presence of endogenous anticore antibodies and their subsequent appearance during gram-negative bacterial infection, which suggests that naturally occurring cross-reactive antibody is an important facet of host defense in humans.[109] Supporting studies indicated that premature infants exhibit low levels of anticore antibodies and that these levels of these antibodies rise until the individual reaches 15 years of age, at which time adult levels are achieved.[110] A 1995 clinical study confirmed and expanded on these findings.[111]

A number of clinical trials have examined the effects of immunorepletion with polyclonal antiendotoxin antibody on either treatment of serious gram-negative bacterial sepsis and shock or prevention of such infection in high-risk patients. In 1982, investigators developed a human polyclonal antiserum preparation directed against *E. coli* J5—a mutant organism that expresses the intermediate core region of LPS extensively on its cell surface—by immunizing normal human volunteers with a heat-killed vaccine derived from the organism. They performed a well-controlled, randomized, double-blind study in which a single unit of either the immune serum or a preimmune control serum was administered to 212 critically ill patients with presumed gram-negative bacterial sepsis; the outcome parameter was death from gram-negative bacteremia or from causes directly attributable to bacteremia.[112] Mortality associated with gram-negative bacteremia was lower in those patients who received human anti–*E. coli* J5 antiserum than in those given preimmune serum (22% versus 39%; $P < 0.05$), and mortality was reduced in those patients with clinical evidence of shock, with or without positive blood cultures (44% versus 77%; $P < 0.01$).

In a separate clinical trial, either an anti–*E. coli* J5 antiserum preparation or a control serum was administered to 100 patients at the onset of neutropenia.[113] Anti–*E. coli* J5 antiserum failed to prevent gram-negative bacteremia or febrile episodes or to reduce mortality. In a subsequent trial, either an anti–*E. coli* J5 plasma preparation or a control plasma was administered to 262 surgical patients deemed to be at high risk for gram-negative bacterial sepsis and shock.[114] The incidence of shock and the mortality were lower in patients receiving the anti–*E. coli* J5 antiserum than in those receiving the control serum (5% versus 11% and 2% versus 7%, respectively; $P < 0.05$), results that support the findings of the earlier study. Several other recent clinical trials, however, did not find similar antibody preparations to have a beneficial effect in patients with sepsis and organ dysfunction, in children with severe infectious purpura, or in patients at high risk for postoperative infection.[115-117]

Many of these studies had inconclusive results, for a variety of reasons. In some, protective capacity was not demonstrated. In others, protective capacity was equivocally demonstrated, either because too few patients were enrolled for the findings to have a high degree of statistical significance or because the study design was flawed.[112-118] Furthermore, even in those two trials in which antiendotoxin antibody was shown to have protective capacity, the polyclonal nature of the preparations made it impossible to determine whether antibody was the protective factor. The inconclusiveness of these study outcomes provided the impetus for the development of antiendotoxin MoAbs, which were extensively studied in a series of trials.

Four multicenter, double-blind, randomized clinical trials evaluated the effect of cross-reactive anti–lipid A IgM MoAbs in patients with a presumptive diagnosis of gram-negative bacterial sepsis [see Table 3]. In these trials, routine resuscitative and supportive measures, including fluid resuscitation, administration of vasopressors, and antibiotic therapy, were implemented or continued, and patients were followed for at least 28 to 30 days or until death. In one trial, an E5 murine MoAb, 2 mg/kg I.V. twice daily, was compared with placebo in a group of 486 septic patients.[119] Although administration of the E5 MoAb did not significantly affect survival in this group as a whole (40% mortality for the E5 group versus 41% for the placebo group; $P = $ NS), it did enhance survival in a subgroup of 137 patients who were not in shock at the time of entry into the study (30% mortality for those receiving the E5 MoAb

Table 3 Results of Clinical Trials Using MoAbs to Treat Sepsis

MoAb	N	Regimen	Mortality (%)	Results
E5[117]	468	E5 Placebo	40 41	Decreased mortality in E5-treated patients with gram-negative bacterial sepsis who were not in shock at study entry
E5[118]	530	E5 Placebo	30 26	Enhanced resolution of organ failure in E5-treated patients with gram-negative sepsis
HA-1A[119]	543	HA-1A Placebo	39 43	Decreased mortality in HA-1A–treated patients with gram-negative bacteremia as well as in a subset within this group of patients who were in shock at study entry
HA-1A[120]	2,199	HA-1A Placebo	33 32	—

versus 43% for those receiving placebo; $P < 0.05$). In another trial, however, E5 MoAb therapy yielded no salutary effects in a study group consisting of a total of 831 patients with known or suspected gram-negative sepsis, clinical evidence of sepsis, or signs of end-organ dysfunction.[120] Even among the 530 patients in whom gram-negative sepsis developed, the 30-day mortality was 30% for those receiving E5 and 26% for those receiving placebo; however, within this subgroup, resolution of organ failure was enhanced in those treated with E5.

A similar trial compared a single 100 mg I.V. dose of an MoAb derived from a human murine heteromyeloma (HA-1A) with placebo in a population of 543 patients.[121] Overall survival was similar in the two groups (39% mortality for the HA-1A group versus 43% for the placebo group; $P = NS$). Among the 197 patients in whom gram-negative bacteremia actually developed, 63% of those receiving HA-1A survived for 28 days, compared with 48% of those receiving placebo ($P < 0.05$); among the 101 patients in whom septic shock developed, 33% of those receiving HA-1A died, whereas 57% of those receiving placebo died ($P < 0.05$).

A second randomized, double-blind multicenter trial was initiated to study the effect of HA-1A using only 14-day mortality as an end point.[122] A total of 2,199 patients were enrolled in the study. No salutary effect of HA-1A was demonstrated: mortality was 32% in the treatment group versus 33% in the control group ($P = 0.864$). In fact, mortality for patients without gram-negative bacteremia was higher in the treatment group than in the control group (37% versus 41%; $P = 0.073$), and as a result of this finding, the trial was halted.

Taken together, these trials yielded three significant findings: (1) the current mortality from the sepsis syndrome remains approximately 30% to 40%; (2) despite similar initial clinical presentations, more than 60% of patients with this syndrome did not in fact have gram-negative bacterial sepsis but instead had gram-positive bacterial or fungal infections; and (3) neither E5 nor HA-1A was efficacious. Since these studies were published, concerns have arisen regarding the binding specificity and in vivo efficacy of these two MoAbs. Analysis of experimental data indicates that HA-1A may bind in vitro not only to lipid A but also to irrelevant substances such as gram-positive bacterial and fungal antigens, as well as to unrelated lipids.[123-125] In addition, testing of both HA-1A and E5 in experimental animal models of gram-negative bacterial sepsis indicates that these agents lack substantial biologic activity. It appears highly likely, therefore, that the large-scale clinical trials published to date have tested antiendotoxin antibody preparations that do not exhibit suitable in vitro or in vivo activity. The disappointing results of these trials may be attributable to the poor activity of the reagents studied and the inability to identify endotoxemic patients with sufficient accuracy rather than to any lack of validity on the part of this therapeutic approach. It remains to be seen whether additional antiendotoxin MoAbs that possess suitable activity will be studied in the clinical setting.

NEW POTENTIAL ANTIENDOTOXIN REAGENTS

There are a number of new biologic antiendotoxin reagents that are undergoing experimental and preliminary clinical testing. For example, there exist three naturally occurring host defense proteins—bactericidal/permeability-increasing protein (BPI), Limulus antilipopolysaccharide factor (LALF), and LPS-binding protein (LBP)—all of which appear to bind endotoxin. Each of these proteins has a region within the amino (N) terminus that appears to be responsible for LPS binding, and the DNA sequences encoding these three binding regions demonstrate considerable homology. The specificity of these substances for LPS appears to result from the high affinity of the binding regions for the lipid A region of LPS. This affinity involves both charge and hydrophobic interactions. For example, the N-terminal portion of the 55 kd BPI molecule is positively charged and thus has a strong electrostatic attraction to the anionic sites in the core region of LPS. In addition, hydrophobic stretches in the N-terminal region of BPI assume a β-sheet configuration and appear to interact with the lipid A moiety of LPS.

BPI is produced within polymorphonuclear leukocyte azurophilic granules. It is bifunctional, acting specifically against gram-negative bacteria to cause (1) bacterial killing and lysis and (2) endotoxin neutralization; separate portions of the molecule are responsible for these different activities. LBP possesses similar activity, binding to and forming a complex with LPS; this complex, in turn, binds to the CD14 receptor found on macrophages and other cell types. LBP also appears to be a bifunctional compound, possessing (1) the ability to bind to LPS and (2) the ability to augment LPS-induced TNF-α secretion by macrophages in vitro. LBP probably acts similarly in vivo, at least in the presence of small amounts of LPS.

Both BPI and a portion of the molecule that encompasses the endotoxin-binding domain (BPI_{23}) demonstrate considerable activity in vitro and exhibit protective capacity in experimental animal models of endotoxemia and gram-negative bacterial infection.[126-128] Investigations are under way to more precisely define the characteristics of the region that accounts for LPS binding. For example, 27-amino-acid peptides generated on the basis of the common regions of BPI, LALF, and LBP apparently possess considerable endotoxin-neutralizing capacity, reduce cytokine levels in vitro and in vivo, and provide in vivo protective capacity.[129] In addition, the CD14 receptor may be shed, and the soluble form (sCD14) may act as an endotoxin antagonist by blocking the interaction of the LPS-LBP complex with the cell-bound CD14 receptor, thereby inhibiting cytokine secretion.[130]

Chemical analogues of lipid A that may be capable both of abrogating the effects of lipid A and of acting as immunostimulants are also being examined. Anti-DCLA anti-idiotypic MoAbs have been developed in an attempt to block the interaction of LPS with the macrophage cellular receptors that trigger cytokine synthesis and secretion. These MoAbs have been shown to bind specifically to the original anti-DCLA MoAb and to inhibit TNF-α–induced endotoxic activity in vitro. Polymyxin B is an antibiotic that binds stoichiometrically to lipid A, thereby neutralizing endotoxin. It is quite toxic when administered parenterally. It has been immobilized to a solid fiber matrix, and ex vivo hemoperfusion has been used to remove endotoxin without systemic toxicity. The effect of taurolidine, an amino acid derivative with antiendotoxic properties, was tested in a randomized, controlled trial involving 100 patients with the sepsis syndrome.[131] Only 12% of the patients had gram-negative bacterial sepsis, however, and no reduction in mortality was observed in the patients who received the drug. Thus, the activity of these reagents in the clinical setting remains to be demonstrated.

OTHER AGENTS

Other forms of immunorepletion that have been used in attempts to reduce sepsis-related mortality include the administration of leukocytes and the administration of fibronectin, neither of which has been demonstrated to be efficacious. Immunorepletion has been successful, however, in preventing CMV disease after solid-organ or bone marrow transplantation, particularly in recipients who have not been exposed to CMV and who receive tissue from an individual who has serologic evidence of previous CMV infection. In one study, for example, prophylactic administration of a CMV immunoglobulin preparation to CMV-seronegative renal transplant recipients reduced the incidence of CMV disease, though it did not affect viral shedding and seroconversion rates.[132] Because CMV disease is associated with a significant reduction in allograft and patient survival, this form of prophylaxis (or equivalent therapy, in the form of administration of antiviral agents such as ganciclovir) is being widely used.[133] Highly active immunoglobulin preparations also are available to prevent—and, in some cases, to treat—disease caused by toxins produced by *C. botulinum*, *C. tetani*, and *C. diphtheriae*, as well as by hepatitis A and B viruses, measles virus, rabies virus, and varicella-zoster virus; however, surgeons rarely encounter infections caused by these pathogens.

Immunoabrogation

Given the plethora of physiologic alterations that occur after a septic insult, it is not surprising that confusion exists regarding the relative importance of the various contributions different mediators make to host mortality. Of particular interest in this regard is a body of experimental data indicating that some of the sequelae of the septic response may be abrogated by administering (1) agents (e.g., MoAbs) that inhibit the effects of certain cytokines or platelet-activating factor (PAF), (2) agents that inhibit PGE_2 synthesis, or (3) MoAbs that bind directly to PMN adherence proteins such as CD18 (thereby preventing leukocyte margination).

CYTOKINE ANTAGONISM

Several groups of investigators have demonstrated that treatment of mice or rabbits with polyclonal anti–TNF-α antiserum before endotoxin injection confers protection against a lethal gram-negative bacterial or endotoxin challenge, but not during experimental peritonitis. Anti–TNF-α antibodies have also proved to be protective in both murine and primate models of *E. coli* bacteremia.[26] Two preliminary clinical studies indicated that administration of a murine anti–human TNF-α MoAb may have salutary effects during septic shock. Anti–TNF-α MoAbs do not completely abrogate TNF-α–related sequelae: the febrile response, stress hormone production, hypoglycemia, and neutrophil activation still occur to some degree.

Two later clinical trials examined the effect of several different anti–TNF-α MoAbs on sepsis-related mortality [*see Table 4*]. An initial randomized study of this type of reagent involved 80 patients with the sepsis syndrome who were given two doses of either placebo or anti–TNF-α MoAb; one subgroup of the treatment group received 0.1 mg/kg doses, another 1.0 mg/kg doses, and the third 10 mg/kg doses.[134] Overall, treated patients did not derive any observable survival benefit; however, the subgroup of patients who received the highest dose of anti–TNF-α MoAb and exhibited high circulating levels of TNF-α appeared to derive some benefit from this form of therapy.

The effects of anti–TNF-α MoAb were then examined in a randomized, double-blind, placebo-controlled multicenter clinical trial involving 971 patients with the sepsis syndrome.[135] At the time of identification of the syndrome and entry into the study, patients were stratified into shock and nonshock groups and then were randomly selected to receive a single dose of placebo, a single 7.5 mg/kg dose of anti–TNF-α MoAb, or a single 15.0 mg/kg dose of

Table 4 Results of Clinical Trials Using Cytokine Antagonists to Treat Sepsis Syndrome

Cytokine Antagonist	N	Regimen	Mortality (%)	Results
BAYx1351[133]	971	BAYx1351, 7.5 mg/kg BAYx1351, 15.0 mg/kg Placebo	37.7 37.8 45.6	—
BAYx1351[134]	533	BAYx1351, 3.0 mg/kg BAYx1351, 15.0 mg/kg Placebo	39.5 31.5 42.4	More rapid reversal of shock in surviving BAYx1351-treated patients, as well as a delay in the time at which initial organ failure developed
MAK 195F[135]	122	MAK 195F, 0.1 mg/kg MAK 195F, 0.3 mg/kg MAK 195F, 1.0 mg/kg Placebo	56 47 38 41	Decreased mortality in MAK 195F–treated patients with baseline IL-6 > 1,000 pg/ml
TNFR:Fc[136]	141	TNFR:Fc, 0.15 mg/kg TNFR:Fc, 0.45 mg/kg TNFR:Fc, 1.50 mg/kg Placebo	30 48 53 30	Increased mortality in patients who received high-dose TNFR:Fc
TNFR:Fc[137]	498	TNFR:Fc, 0.008 mg/kg TNFR:Fc, 0.042 mg/kg TNFR:Fc, 0.083 mg/kg Placebo	—* 37 33 39	Trend toward increased survival in treated patients with severe sepsis and early septic shock
IL-1ra[141]	99	IL-1ra, 17 mg/hr IL-1ra, 67 mg/hr IL-1ra, 133 mg/hr Placebo	32 25 16 44	Dose-related efficacy of IL-1ra
IL-1ra[142]	893	IL-1ra, 1.0 mg/kg/hr IL-1ra, 2.0 mg/kg/hr Placebo	31 29 34	Increased survival times in IL-1ra–treated patients with failure of one or more organs, > 24% predicted mortality at study entry, or both
IL-1ra[143]	696	IL-1ra, 2.0 mg/kg/hr Placebo	33.1 36.4	—

*This arm of the study was discontinued.

the MoAb. Although both MoAb doses reduced mortality at 3 days after study entry in the 478 patients in the shock group (27.5% mortality with placebo, 14.1% with the 7.5 mg/kg dose, and 15.4% with the 15.0 mg/kg dose; $P \leq 0.01$), neither dose had a significant effect on mortality at 28 days (45.6% mortality with placebo, 37.7% with the 7.5 mg/kg dose, and 37.8% with the 15.0 mg/kg dose), and no salutary effects were observed in the study group encompassing all patients and the group encompassing patients who were not in shock when they were enrolled in the study.

Subsequently, two additional multicenter clinical trials were performed. One examined the effect of an infusion of either placebo or the anti–TNF-α MoAb BAYx1351 (in a dose of 3.0 mg/kg or 15.0 mg/kg) on sepsis-related parameters and mortality in 533 patients with the sepsis syndrome.[136] There were no significant differences in 28-day mortality among the three groups (42.4% mortality with placebo, 39.5% with the 3.0 mg/kg dose, and 31.5% with the 15.0 mg/kg dose). There was, however, some indication that in the surviving patients who were treated with anti–TNF-α MoAb, shock was reversed more rapidly and the onset of initial organ failure was delayed.

In another trial, the effect of the anti-TNF MoAb fragment MAK 195F on similar parameters was examined in 122 patients.[137] Patients with the sepsis syndrome received either placebo or MAK 195F (in doses of 0.1 mg/kg, 0.3 mg/kg, or 1.0 mg/kg) at 8-hour intervals over 3 days. Although no overall differences in mortality were observed among these four groups, the subset of patients whose serum IL-6 concentration was higher than 1,000 pg/ml did appear to exhibit reduced mortality; the effect was particularly noticeable in the high-dose treatment subgroup. This finding is concordant with clinical data that seem to indicate that IL-6 is an important indicator of sepsis-related mortality; however, it has yet to be substantiated.

The in vitro effects of TNF also are diminished in the presence of TNF-binding protein (TNF-BP), a naturally occurring compound that is secreted in small quantities during infection. TNF-BP appears to be a soluble form of the TNF-α receptor (TNFR); it may be secreted as part of a regulatory response to an increase in TNF-α levels. TNF-BP is difficult to test in vivo, because of the lack of a biologically active, stable form. However, this problem has been circumvented through the production of a cloned chimeric molecule consisting of TNF-BP plus the heavy chain of IgG (TNFR:Fc). Administration of this stable hybrid compound has demonstrated significant protective capacity during murine endotoxemia.[138,139]

Discouraging results were obtained in a randomized phase II study in which 141 patients with the sepsis syndrome received either placebo or a single infusion of one of three different doses (0.15 mg/kg, 0.45 mg/kg, or 1.50 mg/kg) of a bioengineered fusion protein (TNFR:Fc) consisting of two tumor necrosis factor p80 receptors coupled to the Fc portion of human IgG.[140] Mortality was substantially higher in the high-dose treatment subgroup than in the placebo group. Unfortunately, it remains unclear whether this result was attributable to an effect of therapy (e.g., extensive suppression of TNF-α rendering local host defenses inactive, thereby facilitating infection) or to an imbalance of seriously ill patients within groups. However, a more recent study, involving 498 patients, demonstrated that TNFR:Fc may be capable of reducing mortality during the sepsis syndrome.[141] Patients received either placebo or one of three doses of TNFR:Fc (0.008 mg/kg, 0.042 mg/kg, or 0.083 mg/kg). Because no effect was demonstrated among patients receiving the lowest dose at the time of a planned interim analysis, this arm of the study was discontinued. Although there was no overall diminution in 28-day mortality among the treated patients (39% mortality with placebo, 37% with the 0.042 mg/kg dose, and 33% with the 0.083 mg/kg dose), the subset of patients who experienced severe sepsis and early septic shock did appear to benefit from TNFR:Fc therapy (36% mortality with placebo, 37% with the 0.042 mg/kg dose, and 23% with the 0.083 mg/kg dose).

Finally, preliminary clinical evidence indicates that pentoxifylline, a methylxanthine derivative, is capable of diminishing TNF-α levels in patients exhibiting the septic response, though its effect on sepsis-related mortality has yet to be determined.[142]

Similar experimental work has indicated that blockade of IL-1 activity with an IL-1ra is associated with significant in vivo protective effects. IL-1ra is a 17 kd protein that exhibits a high degree of structural homology with both IL-1α and IL-1β. It appears to bind directly to IL-1 cell surface receptors without causing cellular activation and IL-1 secretion. Intravenous administration of IL-1ra has reduced mortality from experimental gram-negative bacterial and endotoxic shock in rabbits, from endotoxic shock in mice, and from gram-negative bacterial shock in newborn rats and has reduced PMN-mediated acute pulmonary inflammation in rats.[27] In both in vitro and in vivo systems, a large excess of IL-1ra is required to interdict the effects of IL-1.

The effects of IL-1ra initially were examined in a prospective, open-label, placebo-controlled, multicenter phase II clinical trial [see Table 4].[143] Ninety-nine patients with the sepsis syndrome received either placebo or a 100 mg loading dose of IL-1ra, then were given placebo or IL-1ra (in a dosage of 17 mg/hr, 67 mg/hr, or 133 mg/hr) by infusion over a 72-hour period. IL-1ra treatment reduced 28-day mortality in a dose-dependent fashion (44% mortality with placebo, 32% with the 17 mg/hr dosage, 25% with the 67 mg/hr dosage, and 16% with the 133 mg/hr dosage; $P = 0.015$).

Subsequently, a randomized, double-blind, placebo-controlled, multicenter, multinational clinical trial involving 893 patients with the sepsis syndrome was performed to substantiate the effects of this agent.[144] Much as in the initial anti–TNF-α MoAb trial, patients received a 100 mg loading dose, then were given either placebo or IL-1ra (in a dosage of 1.0 mg/kg/hr or 2.0 mg/kg/hr) by infusion over a period of 72 hours. The patients were divided as follows: 302 received placebo; 298 received the lower dosage of IL-1ra; and 293 received the higher dosage. Neither dosage of IL-1ra improved 28-day survival in comparison with placebo (34% mortality with placebo, 31% with the 1.0 mg/kg/hr dosage, and 29% with the 2.0 mg/kg/hr dosage; $P = 0.22$). Secondary and retrospective data analysis indicated, however, that survival time was increased in patients who experienced failure of one or more organs or whose predicted risk of mortality was greater than 24% at the time of study entry ($P \leq 0.005$). Thus, despite the promising results of the initial clinical trial, the second, larger clinical trial failed to substantiate any overall benefit from IL-1ra therapy in the treatment of the sepsis syndrome, though the potential for efficacy in the above-mentioned subgroups was intriguing.

Thereafter, another randomized, double-blind, placebo-controlled phase III trial, involving 696 patients, was performed to study the effect of IL-1ra therapy in patients with severe sepsis.[145] Patients received either placebo or an initial 100 mg bolus of IL-ra, followed by a continuous infusion of either placebo or IL-1ra, 2.0 mg/kg/hr, respectively. This study was terminated prematurely after an interim analysis demonstrated lack of efficacy: 28-day mortality was 36.4% in the placebo group and 33.1% in the IL-1ra therapy group ($P = 0.36$).

Although the time course of macrophage cytokine secretion has been delineated, the precise manner in which each cytokine acts to cause secretion of other cytokines has not been established unequivocally. Of interest are the observations that although administration of anti–TNF-α MoAb abrogates the increase in serum levels of IL-6, IL-1ra does not significantly alter TNF-α levels during experimental gram-negative bacterial sepsis. In addition, even though IL-6 appears not to have significant toxic effects, administration of anti–IL-6 MoAbs has improved survival after experimental TNF-α or gram-negative bacterial challenges.[30,31] Although these data suggest that both TNF-α and IL-1 are significant proximal mediators of certain aspects of the septic response, they also point out the complexity of the host cytokine response. It may be that prevention of the interaction of endotoxin with effector cells, abrogation of the effects of one or more cytokines (as well as those of other mediators), or both are required to eliminate the full spectrum of deleterious effects observed during serious infection.

PLATELET-ACTIVATING FACTOR ANTAGONISM

Platelet-activating factor is a phospholipase A_2–sensitive phospholipid that is released from basophilic leukocytes via an IgE-dependent process. Intravenous administration of PAF or certain of its congeners provokes some of the manifestations of gram-negative bacterial sepsis and endotoxemia (hypotension, increased vascular permeability, thrombocytopenia, neutropenia, and death). These effects are highly dependent on the animal species tested and the route of administration, and their pathophysiology is highly dependent on rapid intravascular platelet aggregation and neutrophil margination. Data obtained from animal models also indicate that PAF levels are elevated during endotoxic and other types of shock. A number of agents (e.g., calcium channel blockers and adrenergic agonists) inhibit the effects of PAF, and several specific PAF antagonists (e.g., BM-14-440, A23187, SRI 63-072, and WEB 2086) have been synthesized. PAF receptors exist on platelets and neutrophils, and PAF antagonists appear to block the interaction between these receptors and PAF. PAF antagonists have lowered mortality in animal models of sepsis, and in vitro data support the contention that PAF amplifies the cellular response to LPS, enhancing the release of IL-1 and TNF-α.

The effect of the PAF-receptor antagonist BN 52021 was tested in a multicenter, prospective, randomized, placebo-controlled, double-blind, phase III clinical trial involving 262 patients with the sepsis syndrome.[146] Patients received either placebo or BN 52021, 120 mg, every 12 hours for 4 days; the resulting 28-day mortalities were 51% and 42%, respectively ($P = 0.17$). Retrospective analysis indicated that administration of BN 52021 led to a significant reduction in 28-day mortality among the 120 patients in whom the sepsis syndrome developed as a result of gram-negative bacterial infection (57% mortality with placebo and 33% with BN 52021; $P = 0.01$), particularly if patients were in shock at the time of study entry (65% mortality with placebo and 37% with BN 52021; $P = 0.01$). The results of this trial have yet to be confirmed.

INHIBITION OF PGE_2 SYNTHESIS

Considerable data obtained from animal models of infection and studies of trauma in humans indicate that secretion of prostaglandins by macrophages produces suppression of a variety of host defense components. Specifically, decreases in PMN and T cell activity, immunoglobulin secretion, and IL-2 secretion have been observed. The knowledge that PGE_2 is produced via the cyclooxygenase pathway of eicosanoid synthesis [see 100 Eicosanoids in Surgery] has led to attempts to block its effect through the use of certain nonsteroidal anti-inflammatory drugs, which inhibit cyclooxygenase and thereby diminish PGE_2 production.

Administration of cyclooxygenase inhibitors has been examined in vitro and in animal models of trauma and infection (in both of which settings PGE_2 synthesis occurs) and has been associated with beneficial effects. In one study, administration of indomethacin reduced postoperative anergy in individuals undergoing gastrectomy or aortic vascular surgery. Although improvements were noted with respect to depressed IL-2 synthesis and anergy, no statistical decrease in the rate of infectious complications was observed.

LEUKOCYTE RECEPTOR ANTAGONISM

The CD11/CD18 leukocyte integrin complex, which is present on lymphocytes, macrophages, killer T cells, and PMNs, mediates adhesion of leukocytes to cellular targets and noncellular surfaces. PMN margination and adhesion lead to the release of lysosomal enzymes with ensuing tissue destruction and deleterious systemic effects. Three forms of CD11 exist—CD11a, CD11b, and CD11c. Each of these combines with CD18 to form a heterodimer: CD11a/CD18 (also known as LFA-1) is found on all leukocytes, whereas CD11b/CD18 (also known as complement receptor 3 [CR3], Mac-1, or Mol-1) and CD11c/CD18 (also known as p150,95) are found on the cell surface of phagocytic leukocytes. The CD11/CD18 complex binds both intact gram-negative bacteria and LPS and appears to facilitate opsonization. There is also some evidence that this integrin complex may regulate TNF-α secretion.

Several murine MoAbs have been developed that recognize a CD11/CD18 complex. Administration of these MoAbs has prevented neutropenia and alveolar capillary membrane injury in response to administration of viable P. aeruginosa to pigs.[147] A study indicating that pretreatment with anti-CD18 MoAb increased the incidence and severity of subcutaneous abscesses caused by S. aureus generated some concern over the potentially detrimental effects of this antibody on local host defenses and containment of infection at the tissue level.[148] A subsequent experimental study, however, demonstrated that administration of anti-CD18 MoAb was not associated with increased mortality in a rabbit model of intra-abdominal sepsis.[149] Clinical testing of this antibody is currently being considered.

Summary and Recommendations

Our understanding of host defenses may be incomplete, but studies have identified those critical components that, although they provide crucial protection against infection, nonetheless may also exert deleterious effects. Improvements in our ability to identify pathogens and microbial toxins rapidly and precisely and to measure the activation state of host defenses accurately, coupled with a clearer comprehension of the interactions among various components of host defenses during health and disease, may allow us to employ immunotherapeutic intervention effectively in surgical patients in the near future. It seems obvious (1) that interventions targeting specific bacterial pathogens or toxins will be futile if the host septic response is caused by pathogens against which the reagent has no efficacy and (2) that abrogation of certain components of the host response itself may depend on precise measurement of the status of host defenses in many, if not most, clinical situations. The importance of these precepts is illustrated by the initial clinical trials in which antiendotoxin antibody was administered to patients exhibiting the septic response; although the results were promising, nearly two thirds of the patients studied proved not to have gram-negative bacterial sepsis and thus received no benefit from this form of intervention. Similarly, clinical trials involving the administration of cytokine antagonists have, to date, yielded no evidence that this approach is effective against the sepsis syndrome. This disappointing finding is probably the result of our current inability to identify those subgroups of patients who will benefit from such therapy. We may well eventually find, for example, that anti–TNF-α MoAb should be administered solely to patients with highly elevated TNF-α levels. Experimental studies and clinical trials in the area of immunomodulation have provided a great deal of new information, with the result that new, highly promising reagents (e.g., BPI and IL-12) are being examined experimentally and, it is to be hoped, will be tested in the clinical setting as well.

References

1. Dunn D: Autochthonous microflora of the gastrointestinal tract. Perspect Colon Rectal Surg 2:105, 1990
2. Dunn DL, Barke RA, Knight NB, et al: Role of resident macrophages, peripheral neutrophils, and translymphatic absorption in bacterial clearance from the peritoneal cavity. Infect Immun 49:257, 1985
3. Christou NV, Rode H, Larsen D, et al: The walk-in anergic patient: how best to assess the risk of sepsis following elective surgery. Ann Surg 199:438, 1984
4. O'Gorman RB, Feliciano DV, Matthews KS, et al: Correlation of immunologic and nutritional status with infectious complications after major abdominal trauma. Surgery 99:549, 1986
5. Schackert HK, Betzler M, Zimmermann GF, et al: The predictive role of delayed cutaneous hypersensitivity testing in postoperative complications. Surg Gynecol Obstet 162:563, 1986
6. Christou NV, Tellado-Rodriguez J, Chartrand L, et al: Estimating mortality risk in preoperative patients using immunologic, nutritional, and acute-phase response variables. Ann Surg 210:69, 1989
7. Poenaru D, Christou NV: Clinical outcome of seriously ill surgical patients with intra-abdominal infection depends on both physiologic (APACHE II score) and immunologic (DTH score) alterations. Ann Surg 213:130, 1991
8. Pietsch JB, Meakins JL, MacLean LD: The delayed hypersensitivity response: application in clinical surgery. Surgery 82:349, 1977
9. Nohr CW, Christou NV, Rode H, et al: In vivo and in vitro humoral immunity in surgical patients. Ann Surg 200:373, 1984
10. Polk HC Jr, George CD, Wellhausen SR, et al: A systematic study of host defense processes in badly injured patients. Ann Surg 204:282, 1986
11. Burd RS, Cody CS, Dunn DL: Immunotherapy of Gram-Negative Bacterial Sepsis. R.G. Landes Co, Austin, Texas, 1992
12. Suffredini AF, Fromm RE, Parker MM, et al: The cardiovascular response of normal humans to the administration of endotoxin. N Engl J Med 321:280, 1989
13. Fong Y, Moldawer L, Shires GT, et al: The biologic characteristics of cytokines and their implication in surgical injury. Surg Gynecol Obstet 170:363, 1990
14. Michie HR, Spriggs DR, Manogue KR, et al: Tumor necrosis factor and endotoxin induce similar metabolic responses in human beings. Surgery 104:280, 1988
15. Hesse DG, Tracey KJ, Fong Y, et al: Cytokine appearance in human endotoxemia and primate bacteremia. Surg Gynecol Obstet 166:147, 1988
16. Mayoral JL, Schweich CJ, Dunn DL: Decreased tumor necrosis factor production during the initial stages of infection correlates with survival during murine gram-negative sepsis. Arch Surg 125:24, 1990
17. Fong Y, Lowry SF: Tumor necrosis factor in the pathophysiology of infection and sepsis. Clin Immunol Immunopathol 55:157, 1990
18. Helfgott D, Clarick R, May L, et al: Interferon-β_2/interleukin-6 in plasma and body fluids during acute bacterial infection. Ann NY Acad Sci 557:562, 1988
19. Van Zee KJ, DeForge LE, Fischer E, et al: IL-8 in septic shock, endotoxemia, and after IL-1 administration. J Immunol 146:3478, 1991
20. Michie HR, Manogue KR, Spriggs DR, et al: Detection of circulating tumor necrosis factor after endotoxin administration. N Engl J Med 318:1481, 1988
21. Cannon JG, Tompkins RG, Gelfand JA, et al: Circulating interleukin-1 and tumor necrosis factor in septic shock and experimental endotoxin fever. J Infect Dis 161:79, 1990
22. Fong Y, Moldawer LL, Marano M, et al: Endotoxemia elicits increased circulating β_2-IFN/IL-6 in man. J Immunol 142:2321, 1989
23. Martich GD, Danner RL, Ceska M, et al: Detection of interleukin 8 and tumor necrosis factor in normal humans after intravenous endotoxin: the effect of antiinflammatory agents. J Exp Med 173:1021, 1991
24. Tracey KJ, Beutler B, Lowry SF, et al: Shock and tissue injury induced by recombinant human cachectin. Science 234:470, 1986
25. Beutler B, Milsark IW, Cerami AC: Passive immunization against cachectin/tumor necrosis factor protects mice from lethal effect of endotoxin. Science 229:869, 1985
26. Tracey KJ, Fong Y, Hesse DG, et al: Anti-cachectin/TNF monoclonal antibodies prevent septic shock during lethal bacteraemia. Nature 330:662, 1987
27. Ohlsson K, Björk P, Bergenfeldt M, et al: Interleukin-1 receptor antagonist reduces mortality from endotoxin shock. Nature 348:550, 1990
28. Bauer J: Interleukin-6 and its receptor during homeostasis, inflammation, and tumor growth. Klin Wochenschr 67:697, 1989
29. Kishimoto T: The biology of interleukin-6. Blood 74:1, 1989
30. Starnes HF Jr, Pearce MK, Tewari A, et al: Anti–IL-6 monoclonal antibodies protect against lethal *Escherichia coli* infection and lethal tumor necrosis factor-α challenge in mice. J Immunol 145:4185, 1990
31. Yim J, Tewari A, Pearce M: Monoclonal antibody against murine interleukin-6 prevents lethal effects of *Escherichia coli* sepsis and tumor necrosis factor challenge in mice. Surg Forum 41:114, 1990
32. Van Zee KJ, Fischer E, Hawes AS, et al: Effects of intravenous IL-8 administration in nonhuman primates. J Immunol 148:1746, 1992
33. Heremans H, Van Damme J, Dillen C, et al: Interferon-γ, a mediator of lethal lipopolysaccharide-induced Shwartzman-like shock reactions in mice. J Exp Med 171:1853, 1990
34. Billiau A, Heremans H, Vandekerckhove F, et al: Anti–interferon-γ antibody protects mice against the generalized Shwartzman reaction. Eur J Immunol 17:1851, 1987
35. Meakins JL: Surgeons, surgery, and immunomodulation. Arch Surg 126:494, 1991
36. Polk HC Jr, Galland RB, Ausobsky JR: Nonspecific enhancement of resistance to bacterial infection: evidence of an effect supplemental to antibiotics. Ann Surg 196:436, 1982
37. Williams DL, Sherwood ER, Browder IW, et al: Effect of glucan on neutrophil dynamics and immune function in *Escherichia coli* peritonitis. J Surg Res 44:54, 1988
38. Cisneros RL, Gibson FC 3rd, Tzianabos AO: Passive transfer of poly-(1-6)-beta-glucotriosyl-(1-3)-beta-glucopyranose glucan protection against lethal infection in an animal model of intra-abdominal sepsis. Infect Immun 64:2201, 1996
39. de Felippe J Jr, da Rocha e Silva M Jr, Maciel FMB, et al: Infection prevention in patients with severe multiple trauma with the immunomodulator beta 1-3 polyglucose (glucan). Surg Gynecol Obstet 177:383, 1993
40. Babineau TJ, Marcello P, Swails W, et al: Randomized phase I/II trial of a macrophage-specific immunomodulator (PPG-glucan) in high-risk surgical patients. Ann Surg 220:559, 1994
41. Meakins JL, Christou NV, Shizgal HM, et al: Therapeutic approaches to anergy in surgical patients. Ann Surg 190:286, 1979
42. Waymack JP, Miskell P, Gonce SJ, et al: Effect of two new immunomodulators on normal and burn injury neutrophils and macrophages. J Burn Care Rehabil 8:9, 1987
43. Christou NV, Zakaluzny I, Marshall JC, et al: The effect of the immunomodulator RU 41,740 (biostim) on the specific and nonspecific immunosuppression induced by thermal injury or protein deprivation. Arch Surg 123:207, 1988
44. Ogle CK, Ogle JD, Keynton L, et al: The effect of TP-5 on the production of C3, PGE_2, and TXB_2 by macrophages obtained from burned guinea pigs. J Burn Care Rehabil 10:146, 1989
45. Waymack JP, Jenkins M, Warden GD, et al: A prospective study of thymopentin in severely burned patients. Surg Gynecol Obstet 164:423, 1987
46. Faist E, Markewitz A, Fuchs D, et al: Immunomodulatory therapy with thymopentin and indomethacin: successful restoration of interleukin-2 synthesis in patients undergoing major surgery. Ann Surg 214:264, 1991
47. O'Reilly M, Silver GM, Greenhalgh DG, et al: Treatment of intra-abdominal infection with granulocyte colony-stimulating factor. J Trauma 33:679, 1992
48. Frumkin LR: Role of granulocyte colony-stimulating factor and granulocyte-macrophage colony-stimulating factor in the treatment of patients with HIV infection. Curr Opin Hematol 4:200, 1997
49. Sanchez-Cantu L, Rode HN, Christou NV: Endotoxin tolerance is associated with reduced secretion of tumor necrosis factor. Arch Surg 124:1432, 1989
50. Sheppard BC, Fraker DL, Norton JA: Prevention and treatment of endotoxin and sepsis lethality with recombinant human tumor necrosis factor. Surgery 106:156, 1989
51. Henricson BE, Benjamin WR, Vogel SN: Differential cytokine induction by doses of lipopolysaccharide and monophosphoryl lipid A that result in equivalent early endotoxin tolerance. Infect Immun 58:2429, 1990
52. Proctor RA: Lipid A precursors protect against endotoxin challenge. Adv Exp Med Biol 256:641, 1990
53. Rudbach JA, Cantrell JL, Ulrich JT, et al: Immunotherapy with bacterial endotoxins. Adv Exp Med Biol 256:665, 1990
54. McIntyre KW, Unowsky J, DeLorenzo W, et al: Enhancement of antibacterial resistance of neutropenic, bone marrow-suppressed mice by interleukin-1α. Infect Immun 57:48, 1989
55. Weyand C, Goronzy J, Fathman CG, et al: Administration in vivo of recombinant interleukin 2 protects mice against septic death. J Clin Invest 79:1756, 1987
56. Chong KT: Prophylactic administration of interleukin-2 protects mice from lethal challenge with gram-negative bacteria. Infect Immun 55:668, 1987
57. Livingston DH, Malangoni MA: Interferon-γ restores immune competence after hemorrhagic shock. J Surg Res 45:37, 1988

58. Malangoni MA, Livingston DH, Sonnenfeld G, et al: Interferon gamma and tumor necrosis factor alpha: use in gram-negative infection after shock. Arch Surg 125:444, 1990
59. Polk HC, Cheadle WG, Livingston DH, et al: A randomized prospective clinical trial to determine the efficacy of interferon-γ in severely injured patients. Am J Surg 163:191, 1992
60. Dries DJ, Jurkovich GJ, Maier RV, et al: Effect of interferon gamma on infection-related death in patients with severe injuries: a randomized, double-blind, placebo-controlled trial. Arch Surg 129:1031, 1994
61. Gately MK, Mulqueen MJ: Interleukin-12: potential clinical applications in the treatment and prevention of infectious diseases. Drugs 52:18, 1996
62. Cerra FB, Mazuski JE, Chute E, et al: Branched chain metabolic support: a prospective, randomized, double-blind trial in surgical stress. Ann Surg 199:286, 1984
63. Perioperative total parenteral nutrition in surgical patients. The Veterans Affairs Total Parenteral Nutrition Cooperative Study Group. N Engl J Med 325:525, 1991
64. Inoue S, Epstein MD, Alexander JW, et al: Prevention of yeast translocation across the gut by a single enteral feeding after burn injury. J Parenter Enteral Nutr 13:565, 1989
65. Fong YM, Marano MA, Barber A, et al: Total parenteral nutrition and bowel rest modify the metabolic response to endotoxin in humans. Ann Surg 210:449, 1989
66. Alexander JW, Peck MD: Future prospects for adjunctive therapy: pharmacologic and nutritional approaches to immune system modulation. Crit Care Med 18(suppl):S159, 1990
67. Peck MD, Alexander JW, Gonce SJ, et al: Low protein diets improve survival from peritonitis in guinea pigs. Ann Surg 209:448, 1989
68. Gonce SJ, Peck MD, Alexander JW, et al: Arginine supplementation and its effect on established peritonitis in guinea pigs. J Parenter Enteral Nutr 14:237, 1990
69. Alexander JW, Saito H, Trocki O, et al: The importance of lipid type in the diet after burn injury. Ann Surg 204:1, 1986
70. Gottschlich MM, Jenkins M, Warden GD, et al: Differential effects of three enteral dietary regimens on selected outcome variables in burn patients. J Parenter Enteral Nutr 14:225, 1990
71. Endres S, Ghorbani R, Kelley VE, et al: The effect of dietary supplementation with n-3 polyunsaturated fatty acids on the synthesis of interleukin-1 and tumor necrosis factor by mononuclear cells. N Engl J Med 320:265, 1989
72. Tancrede CH, Andremont AO: Bacterial translocation and gram-negative bacteremia in patients with hematological malignancies. J Infect Dis 152:99, 1985
73. Guiot HF, Helmig-Schurter AV, van der Meer JW, et al: Selective antimicrobial modulation of the intestinal microbial flora for infection prevention in patients with hematologic malignancies: evaluation of clinical efficacy and the value of surveillance cultures. Scand J Infect Dis 18:153, 1986
74. Ledingham IM, Alcock SR, Eastaway AT, et al: Triple regimen of selective decontamination of the digestive tract, systemic cefotaxime, and microbiological surveillance for prevention of acquired infection in intensive care. Lancet 1:785, 1988
75. Ulrich C, Harinck-de Weerd JE, Bakker NC, et al: Selective decontamination of the digestive tract with norfloxacin in the prevention of ICU-acquired infections: a prospective randomized study. Intensive Care Med 15:424, 1989
76. Tetteroo GW, Wagenvoort JH, Castelein A, et al: Selective decontamination to reduce gram-negative colonisation and infections after oesophageal resection. Lancet 335:704, 1990
77. Cerra FB, Maddaus MA, Dunn DL, et al: Selective gut decontamination reduces nosocomial infections and length of stay but not mortality or organ failure in surgical intensive care unit patients. Arch Surg 127:163, 1992
78. Goris RJ, van Bebber IP, Mollen RM, et al: Does selective decontamination of the gastrointestinal tract prevent multiple organ failure? An experimental study. Arch Surg 126:561, 1991
79. Gable CB, Holzer SS, Engelhart L, et al: Pneumococcal vaccine: efficacy and associated cost savings. JAMA 264:2910, 1990
80. FDA workshop on *Haemophilus* b polysaccharide vaccine—a preliminary report. MMWR 36:529, 1987
81. Alexander JW, Fisher MW, MacMillan BG, et al: Prevention of invasive *Pseudomonas* infection in burns with a new vaccine. Arch Surg 99:249, 1969
82. Young LS, Meyer RD, Armstrong D: *Pseudomonas aeruginosa* vaccine in cancer patients. Ann Intern Med 79:518, 1973
83. Marker SC, Howard RJ, Simmons RL, et al: Cytomegalovirus infection: a quantitative prospective study of three hundred twenty consecutive renal transplants. Surgery 89:660, 1981
84. Dunn DL: Immunotherapeutic advances in the treatment of gram-negative bacterial sepsis. World J Surg 11:233, 1987
85. Dunn DL: Vaccines and antibody immunotherapy in surgical patients. Am J Surg 153:409, 1987
86. Kreger BE, Craven DE, McCabe WR: Gram-negative bacteremia: IV. Re-evaluation of clinical features and treatment in 612 patients. Am J Med 68:344, 1980
87. Bryan CS, Reynolds KL, Brenner ER: Analysis of 1,186 episodes of gram-negative bacteremia in nonuniversity hospitals: the effects of antimicrobial therapy. Rev Infect Dis 5:629, 1983
88. Cody CS, Dunn DL: Endotoxins in septic shock. CRC Handbook on Mediators in Septic Shock. Neugebauer E, Holaday J, Eds. CRC Press, Inc, Boca Raton, Florida (in press)
89. Dunn DL, Ferguson RM: Immunotherapy of gram-negative bacterial sepsis: enhanced survival in a guinea pig model by use of rabbit antiserum to *Escherichia coli* J5. Surgery 92:212, 1982
90. Johns M, Skehill A, McCabe WR: Immunization with rough mutants of *Salmonella minnesota*: IV. Protection by antisera to O and rough antigens against endotoxin. J Infect Dis 147:57, 1983
91. Dunn DL, Mach PA, Condie RM, et al: Anticore endotoxin F(ab')$_2$ equine immunoglobulin fragments protect against lethal effects of gram-negative bacterial sepsis. Surgery 96:440, 1984
92. McCabe WR, DeMaria A Jr, Berberich H, et al: Immunization with rough mutants of *Salmonella minnesota*: protective activity of IgM and IgG antibody to the R595 (Re chemotype) mutant. J Infect Dis 158:291, 1988
93. Kirkland TN, Ziegler EJ: An immunoprotective monoclonal antibody to lipopolysaccharide. J Immunol 132:2590, 1984
94. Dunn DL, Bogard WC, Cerra FB: Enhanced survival during murine gram-negative sepsis by use of a murine monoclonal antibody. Arch Surg 120:50, 1985
95. Dunn DL: Antibody immunotherapy of gram-negative bacterial sepsis in an immunosuppressed animal model. Transplantation 45:424, 1988
96. Dunn D, Mach P, Cerra F: Monoclonal antibodies protect against lethal effects of gram-negative sepsis. Surg Forum 14:142, 1983
97. Mutharia LM, Crockford G, Bogard WC Jr, et al: Monoclonal antibodies specific for *Escherichia coli* J5 lipopolysaccharide: cross-reaction with other gram-negative bacterial species. Infect Immun 45:631, 1984
98. Dunn DL, Bogard WC Jr, Cerra FB: Efficacy of type-specific and cross-reactive murine monoclonal antibodies directed against endotoxin during experimental sepsis. Surgery 98:283, 1985
99. Dunn DL, Ewald DC, Chandan N, et al: Immunotherapy of gram-negative bacterial sepsis: a single murine monoclonal antibody provides cross-genera protection. Arch Surg 121:58, 1986
100. Bogard WC Jr, Dunn DL, Abernethy K, et al: Isolation and characterization of murine monoclonal antibodies specific for gram-negative bacterial lipopolysaccharide: association of cross-genus reactivity with lipid A specificity. Infect Immun 55:899, 1987
101. Dunn DL, Priest BP, Condie RM: Protective capacity of polyclonal and monoclonal antibodies directed against endotoxin during experimental sepsis. Arch Surg 123:1389, 1988
102. Priest BP, Brinson DN, Schroeder DA, et al: Treatment of experimental gram-negative bacterial sepsis with murine monoclonal antibodies directed against lipopolysaccharide. Surgery 106:147, 1989
103. Pollack M, Chia JK, Koles NL, et al: Specificity and cross-reactivity of monoclonal antibodies reactive with the core and lipid A regions of bacterial lipopolysaccharide. J Infect Dis 159:168, 1989
104. Priest B, Bankey P, Cerra F, et al: An immunoprotective antibody directed against lipopolysaccharide inhibits tumor necrosis factor production in vitro. Surg Forum 39:29, 1988
105. Baumgartner JD, Heumann D, Gerain J, et al: Association between protective efficacy of anti-lipopolysaccharide (LPS) antibodies and suppression of LPS-induced tumor necrosis factor-α and interleukin 6: comparison of O side chain-specific antibodies with core LPS antibodies. J Exp Med 171:889, 1990
106. Mayoral JL, Schweich CJ, Dunn DL: Decreased tumor necrosis factor production during the initial stages of infection correlates with survival during murine gram-negative sepsis. Arch Surg 125:24, 1990
107. Mayoral JL, Dunn DL: Cross-reactive murine monoclonal antibodies directed against the core/lipid A region of endotoxin inhibit production of tumor necrosis factor. J Surg Res 49:287, 1990
108. Zinner SH, McCabe WR: Effects of IgM and IgG antibody in patients with bacteremia due to gram-negative bacilli. J Infect Dis 133:37, 1976
109. Nys M, Joassin L, Somzee A, et al: Enzyme-linked immunosorbent assay for immunoglobulin G subclass antibodies specific for enterobacterial Re core glycolipid in healthy individuals and in patients infected by gram-negative bacteria. J Clin Microbiol 26:857, 1988
110. Law BJ, Marks MI: Age-related prevalence of human serum IgG and IgM antibody to the core glycolipid of *Escherichia coli* strain J5, as measured by ELISA. J Infect Dis 151:988, 1985
111. Goldie AS, Fearon KCH, Ross JA, et al: Natural cytokine antagonists and endogenous antiendotoxin core antibodies in sepsis syndrome. JAMA 274:172, 1995
112. Ziegler EJ, McCutchan JA, Fierer J, et al: Treatment of gram-negative bacteremia and shock with human antiserum to a mutant *Escherichia coli*. N Engl J Med 307:1225, 1982
113. McCutchan JA, Wolf JL, Ziegler EJ, et al: Ineffectiveness of single-dose human antiserum to core glycolipid (*E. coli* J5) for prophylaxis of bacteremic, gram-negative infections in patients with prolonged neutropenia. Schweiz Med Wochenschr Suppl 14:40, 1983
114. Baumgartner JD, Glauser MP, McCutchan JA, et al: Prevention of gram-negative shock and death in surgical patients by antibody to endotoxin core glycolipid. Lancet 2:59, 1985
115. Lachman E, Pitsoe S, Gaffin SL: Anti-lipopolysaccharide immunotherapy in management of septic shock of obstetric and gynaecological origin. Lancet 1:981, 1984
116. Aitchison JM, Arbuckle DD: Anti-endotoxin in the treatment of severe surgical septic shock: results of a randomized double-blind trial. S Afr Med J 68:787, 1985
117. Calandra T, Glauser MP, Schellekens J, et al: Treat-

ment of gram-negative septic shock with human IgG antibody to *Escherichia coli* J5: a prospective, double-blind, randomized trial. J Infect Dis 158:312, 1988

118. Cometta A, Baumgartner JD, Lee ML, et al: Prophylactic intravenous administration of standard immune globulin as compared with core-lipopolysaccharide immune globulin in patients at high risk of postsurgical infection. N Engl J Med 327:234, 1992

119. Greenman RL, Schein RM, Martin MA, et al: A controlled clinical trial of E5 murine monoclonal IgM antibody to endotoxin in the treatment of gram-negative sepsis. The XOMA Sepsis Study Group. JAMA 266:1097, 1991

120. Bone RC, Balk RA, Rein AM, et al: A second large controlled clinical study of E5, a monoclonal antibody to endotoxin: results of a prospective, multicenter, randomized, controlled trial. Crit Care Med 23:994, 1995

121. Ziegler EJ, Fisher CJ Jr, Sprung CL, et al: Treatment of gram-negative bacteremia and septic shock with HA-IA human monoclonal antibody against endotoxin: a randomized, double-blind, placebo-controlled trial. The HA-1A Sepsis Study Group. N Engl J Med 324:429, 1991

122. McCloskey RV, Straube RC, Sanders C, et al: Treatment of septic shock with human monoclonal antibody HA-1A: a randomized, double blind, placebo-controlled trial. Ann Intern Med 121:1, 1994

123. Baumgartner JD: Immunotherapy with antibodies to core lipopolysaccharide: a critical appraisal. Infect Dis Clin North Am 5:915, 1991

124. Fujihara Y, Lei MG, Morrison DC: Characterization of specific binding of a human immunoglobulin M monoclonal antibody to lipopolysaccharide and its lipid A domain. Infect Immun 61:910, 1993

125. Warren HS, Amato SF, Fitting C, et al: Assessment of ability of murine and human anti-lipid A monoclonal antibodies to bind and neutralize lipopolysaccharide. J Exp Med 177:89, 1993

126. Rogy MA, Moldawer LL, Oldenburg SA, et al: Antiendotoxin therapy in primate bacteremia with HA-1A and BPI. Ann Surg 220:77, 1994

127. Fisher CJ, Marra MN, Palardy JE, et al: Human neutrophil bactericidal/permeability-increasing protein reduces mortality rate from endotoxin challenge: a placebo-controlled study. Crit Care Med 22:553, 1994

128. Lin Y, Leach WJ, Ammons WS: Synergistic effect of a recombinant N-terminal fragment of bactericidal/permeability-increasing protein and cefamandole in treatment of rabbit gram-negative sepsis. Antimicrob Agents Chemother 40:65, 1996

129. Battafarano RJ, Dahlberg PS, Ratz CA, et al: Peptide derivatives of three distinct lipopolysaccharide binding proteins inhibit lipopolysaccharide-induced tumor necrosis factor-α secretion *in vitro*. Surgery 118:318, 1995

130. Tobias PS, Soldau K, Gegner JA, et al: Lipopolysaccharide binding protein-mediated complexation of lipopolysaccharide with soluble CD14. J Biol Chem 270:10482, 1995

131. Willatts SM, Radford S, Leitermann M: Effect of the antiendotoxin agent, taurolidine, in the treatment of sepsis syndrome: a placebo-controlled, double-blind trial. Crit Care Med 23:1033, 1995

132. Snydman DR, Werner BG, Heinze-Lacey B: Use of cytomegalovirus immune globulin to prevent cytomegalovirus disease in renal-transplant recipients. N Engl J Med 317:1049, 1987

133. Dunn DL, Gillingham KJ, Kramer MA, et al: A prospective randomized study of acyclovir versus ganciclovir plus human immune globulin prophylaxis of cytomegalovirus infection after solid organ transplantation. Transplantation 57:876, 1994

134. Fisher CJ, Opal SM, Dhainaut JF, et al: Influence of an anti-tumor necrosis factor monoclonal antibody on cytokine levels in patients with sepsis. Crit Care Med 21:318, 1993

135. Abraham E, Wunderink R, Silverman H, et al: Efficacy and safety of monoclonal antibody to human tumor necrosis factor α in patients with sepsis syndrome. TNF-α MAb Sepsis Study Group. JAMA 273:9341, 1995

136. Cohen J, Carlet J: INTERSEPT: an international, multicenter, placebo-controlled trial of monoclonal antibody to human tumor necrosis factor-α in patients with sepsis. Crit Care Med 24:1431, 1996

137. Reinhart K, Wiegand-Lohnert C, Grimminger F, et al: Assessment of the safety and efficacy of the monoclonal anti-tumor necrosis factor antibody-fragment, MAK 195F, in patients with sepsis and septic shock: a multicenter, randomized, placebo-controlled, dose-ranging study. Crit Care Med 24:733, 1996

138. Peppel K, Crawford D, Beutler B: A tumor necrosis factor (TNF) receptor–IgG heavy chain chimeric protein as a bivalent antagonist of TNF activity. J Exp Med 174:1483, 1991

139. Ashkenazi A, Marsters SA, Capon DJ, et al: Protection against endotoxin shock by a tumor necrosis factor receptor immunoadhesin. Proc Natl Acad Sci USA 88:10535, 1991

140. Fisher CJ Jr, Agosti JM, Opal SM, et al: Treatment of septic shock with the tumor necrosis factor receptor:Fc fusion protein. The Soluble TNF Receptor Sepsis Study Group. N Engl J Med 334:1697, 1996

141. Abraham E, Glauser MP, Butler T, et al: A p55 tumor necrosis factor receptor fusion protein in the treatment of patients with severe sepsis and septic shock: a randomized controlled multicenter trial. Ro 45-2081 Study Group. JAMA 277:1531, 1997

142. Effects of pentoxifylline on circulating cytokine concentrations and hemodynamics in patients with septic shock: results from a double-blind, randomized, placebo controlled study. Crit Care Med 24:207, 1996

143. Fisher CJ, Slotman GJ, Opal SM, et al: Initial evaluation of human recombinant interleukin-1 receptor antagonist in the treatment of sepsis syndrome: a randomized, open-label, placebo-controlled multicenter trial. Crit Care Med 22:12, 1994

144. Fisher CJ, Dhainaut JFA, Opal SM, et al: Recombinant human interleukin 1 receptor antagonist in the treatment of patients with sepsis syndrome: results from a randomized, double-blind, placebo-controlled trial. JAMA 271:1836, 1994

145. Opal SM, Fisher CJ Jr, Dhainaut JF, et al: Confirmatory interleukin-1 receptor antagonist trial in severe sepsis: a phase III, randomized, double-blind, placebo-controlled, multicenter trial. Crit Care Med 25:1115, 1997

146. Dhainaut JF, Tenaillon A, Tulzo YL, et al: Platelet-activating factor receptor antagonist BN 52021 in the treatment of severe sepsis: a randomized, double-blind, placebo-controlled, multicenter clinical trial. Crit Care Med 22:1720, 1994

147. Walsh CJ, Carey PD, Cook DJ, et al: Anti-CD18 antibody attenuates neutropenia and alveolar capillary-membrane injury during gram-negative sepsis. Surgery 110:205, 1991

148. Sharar SR, Winn RK, Murry CE, et al: A CD18 monoclonal antibody increases the incidence and severity of subcutaneous abscess formation after high-dose *Staphylococcus aureus* injection in rabbits. Surgery 110:213, 1991

149. Mileski WJ, Winn RK, Harlan JM, et al: Transient inhibition of neutrophil adherence with the anti-CD18 monoclonal antibody 60.3 does not increase mortality rates in abdominal sepsis. Surgery 109:497, 1991

Acknowledgments

The author would like to thank Ms. Laci Aase and Ms. Lynnette Evans for their assistance in preparing the manuscript.

Figures 1 and 2   Lynn O'Kelley.

Figure 3   Tom Moore.

VII CARE IN THE ICU

89 CARDIOPULMONARY MONITORING

Jerome H. Abrams, M.D., Frank Cerra, M.D., and James W. Holcroft, M.D.

Indications for and Uses of ICU Monitoring Equipment

Monitoring of cardiopulmonary variables is frequently necessary in critically ill surgical patients. Specific indications for each of the monitoring devices are discussed elsewhere in the text. This discussion will concentrate on how to insert and use monitoring devices and how to interpret data obtained from them. Not all of the measurements available from these devices are provided in continuous readouts; some of the measurements made possible by the technology, such as blood gas analysis or determination of cardiac indices, require interventions or calculations by nurses or physicians [see Table 1]. Newer devices, such as pulse oximeters, are capable not only of providing information noninvasively but of doing so continuously. These sorts of devices will be used more and more as problems with calibration and reliability are solved.

Systemic Arterial Catheters

INDICATIONS FOR INSERTION

The information obtained from systemic arterial catheters includes measurements of systemic arterial pressure and blood gases [see Sidebar Insertion of Systemic Arterial Catheters]. Indications for insertion of such a catheter include the need for frequent or continuous monitoring of these parameters. Recognition of these needs requires clinical judgment. In general, if it is necessary to measure blood gases more often than three times a day, it is best to insert a catheter. Additionally, the possibility of sudden hemorrhage, the presence of sepsis, the need for titration of vasoactive drugs, or the need for administration of cardiotonic agents each dictates that such a catheter be inserted.

COMPLICATIONS ASSOCIATED WITH SYSTEMIC ARTERIAL CATHETERS

Line sepsis is probably the single most serious problem associated with any indwelling vascular device.[1] Infection rates with systemic arterial catheters are much lower than those with central venous or pulmonary arterial catheters, but even systemic arterial catheters must be protected from possible contamination. Diagnosis and treatment of infection arising from such catheters are described elsewhere [see 79 Blood Cultures and Infection in the Patient with the Septic Response and 81 Nosocomial Infection].

Thrombosis associated with insertion and maintenance of indwelling arterial catheters can lead to ischemia and even necrosis distal to the site of insertion. The risk of thrombosis is minimized by inserting the catheter in arteries with abundant collateral circulation. Thus, the radial artery is safer to use than the brachial artery, and the dorsalis pedis is safer than the femoral artery. The risk of thrombosis can also be reduced by continuous infusion of a dilute heparin solution through the catheter. If concern about heparin-induced thrombocytopenia arises, the heparin can be removed with only a minimal increase in the likelihood of catheter thrombosis. Flushing of the catheter must be done carefully with volumes of fluid no larger than 2 ml. Rapid infusion of large amounts of solution through radial artery catheters in particular can lead to retrograde flow and embolization to the brain of particulate matter or air.

MEASUREMENT OF SYSTEMIC ARTERIAL PRESSURE

Pressures obtained from systemic arterial catheters include the systolic, diastolic, and mean pressures. The mean pressure can be approximated as the diastolic pressure plus one third of the pulse pressure, the pulse pressure being defined as the systolic pressure minus the diastolic. Exact measurements of the mean pressure require computer analysis of the pressure waveform. Many pressure monitors perform such analysis, and the mean pressure can be taken from the digital readout on the oscilloscope screen. The mean pressure is the most accurate of the systemic arterial pressures obtained from the catheter and should be used for governing patient decisions [see Figure 1].

There are three reasons why the mean pressure should be used.[2] First, the systolic and diastolic pressures measured at the transducer will frequently be different from the systolic and diastolic pressures in the artery itself because the stiffness and resistance of the catheter and the rest of the measuring system can differ substantially from the stiffness and resistance of the vascular system. Second, movement of the catheter within the vessel can produce transient falls in measured hydrostatic pressures. Third, the systolic and diastolic pressures in the radial artery or in any distal artery will be higher and lower, respectively, than the systolic and diastolic pressures in the ascending aorta. The mean pressures in the distal artery and the ascending aorta will be the same, however.

1365

Indications for and Uses of ICU Monitoring Equipment

Monitoring of cardiopulmonary parameters is required to optimize O_2 consumption, nitrogen balance, and metabolic status

Systemic arterial catheters

Indications:
- Need for frequent or continuous monitoring of systemic arterial pressure and blood gases
- Possibility of sudden hemorrhage
- Presence of sepsis
- Need for titration of vasoactive drugs
- Need for administration of cardiotonic agents

Central venous catheters

Useful for monitoring only when it is certain that the cardiovascular abnormality is confined to the right side of the heart.

Systemic arterial pressures

Mean pressure taken from the monitor's digital readout is more accurate than systolic or diastolic pressure.

Consider effects of the following:
- Mismatch between measuring system and patient's vasculature
- Catheter whip
- Distance of measuring site from the heart

Systemic arterial blood gases

Values that may be obtained include the following:
- Partial pressure of O_2
- Partial pressure of CO_2
- Hydrogen ion concentration (pH)
- O_2 saturation
- O_2 content

Central venous pressure

Pulmonary arterial pressure

Monitoring of cardiopulmonary parameters is required to optimize O_2 consumption, nitrogen balance, and metabolic status

Values that may be derived from measurements obtained by monitoring devices include cardiac output, stroke volume, left ventricular and right ventricular end-diastolic volumes, left ventricular and right ventricular end-systolic volumes, left ventricular and right ventricular end-systolic unstressed volumes, left ventricular and right ventricular end-systolic pressures, vascular resistances, aortic root and pulmonary arterial end-systolic pressure-volume relations, left ventricular and right ventricular end-systolic pressure-volume relations, power, O_2 transport, O_2 return, O_2 consumption, sodium bicarbonate concentration, shunt fractions, and A-aD_{O_2} gradients

Pulmonary arterial catheters

Indicated to monitor central venous pressure, pulmonary arterial pressure, PAWP, cardiac output, right ventricular end-diastolic volume, and mixed venous gases in the following:
- Patients with severe cardiopulmonary derangements
- Patients at high risk for intraoperative or postoperative development of cardiopulmonary problems
- Patients undergoing procedures associated with large volume requirements or fluid shifts

Other monitoring techniques

It is possible to monitor the following values continuously:
- Arterial O_2 saturation (by means of pulse oximetry)
- P_aO_2 (by means of transcutaneous or conjunctival devices)
- Perfusion (by means of devices that measure skin temperature)
- Mixed venous O_2 saturation (by means of special pulmonary arterial catheters)
- End-expiratory CO_2 tension (by means of ventilatory monitoring devices)

Pulmonary arterial wedge pressure

PAWP correlates well with mean left atrial pressure and reflects pulmonary microvascular hydrostatic pressure. In the absence of mitral valve disease, PAWP correlates with LVEDP.

Cardiac output

Value is obtained by making 3 injections of cool solution at a consistent point in the ventilatory cycle. The thermistor in the catheter measures the T° drop in the pulmonary artery as the cool blood flows past; the monitor provides a digital readout.

Right ventricular end-diastolic volume

Measurement requires use of a cold injectate and a fast-response thermistor. Level is accurate if patient has a regular heart rate <140 beats/min. Echocardiography can determine if end-diastolic volume in the right ventricle is similar to that in the left.

Mixed venous blood gases

Use $P{CO_2}$ level to confirm a good specimen.

O_2 saturation is the most reliable measurement obtained from mixed venous blood.

Table 1 Normal Values Obtained from Commonly Used Monitors*

Parameters	Sources for Measurement or Calculations	Values Not Indexed or Indexed to Body Surface Area	Values in Subjects of Different Weights†					Units
			Formulas Used to Calculate Values‡	Subject Weight				
				45 kg	60 kg	75 kg	90 kg	
Heart rate (HR)§	Electrocardiogram	60 beats/min	$167 \div wt^{0.25}$	64	60	57	54	beats/min
Cardiac output (CO)	Swan-Ganz catheter	$3.5 \, L \cdot min^{-1} \cdot m^{-2}$	$0.28 \cdot wt^{0.75}$	4.9	6.0	7.1	8.2	L/min
Stroke volume (SV)§	CO ÷ HR	59 ml/m²	$1.67 \cdot wt$	75	100	125	150	ml
Left ventricular end-diastolic volume (LVEDV)	See text	88 ml/m²	$2.50 \cdot wt$	113	150	188	225	ml
Right ventricular end-diastolic volume (RVEDV)	Swan-Ganz catheter	88 ml/m²	$2.50 \cdot wt$	113	150	188	225	ml
Left ventricular end-systolic volume (LVESV)§	LVEDV − SV	29 ml/m²	$0.83 \cdot wt$	37	50	62	75	ml
Right ventricular end-systolic volume (RVESV)	RVEDV − SV	29 ml/m²	$0.83 \cdot wt$	37	50	62	75	ml
Left ventricular end-systolic unstressed volume (LV V_0)	See text	4 ml/m²	$0.10 \cdot wt$	5	6	8	9	ml
Right ventricular end-systolic unstressed volume (RV V_0)	See text	4 ml/m²	$0.10 \cdot wt$	5	6	8	9	ml
Mean systemic arterial pressure (MAP)	Arterial catheter	90 mm Hg	—	90	90	90	90	mm Hg
Mean pulmonary arterial pressure (MPAP)	Swan-Ganz catheter	15 mm Hg	—	15	15	15	15	mm Hg
Left ventricular end-systolic pressure (LVESP)	See text	100 mm Hg	—	100	100	100	100	mm Hg
Right ventricular end-systolic pressure (RVESP)	See text	20 mm Hg	—	20	20	20	20	mm Hg
Pulmonary arterial wedge pressure (PAWP)	Swan-Ganz catheter	5 mm Hg	—	5	5	5	5	mm Hg
Central venous pressure (CVP)	Swan-Ganz catheter	2 mm Hg	—	2	2	2	2	mm Hg
Systemic vascular resistance	(MAP − CVP) ÷ CO	$25 \, mm \, Hg \cdot L^{-1} \cdot min \cdot m^2$	$314 \div wt^{0.75}$	18.1	14.6	12.3	10.7	$mm \, Hg \cdot L^{-1} \cdot min$
Pulmonary vascular resistance	(MPAP − PAWP) ÷ CO	$2.9 \, mm \, Hg \cdot L^{-1} \cdot min \cdot m^2$	$35.7 \div wt^{0.75}$	2.1	1.7	1.4	1.2	$mm \, Hg \cdot L^{-1} \cdot min$
Aortic root end-systolic pressure-volume relation§	LVESP ÷ SV	$1.7 \, mm \, Hg \cdot ml^{-1} \cdot m^2$	$59.9 \div wt$	1.3	1.0	0.8	0.7	mm Hg/ml
Pulmonary arterial end-systolic pressure volume relation§	RVESP ÷ SV	$0.34 \, mm \, Hg \cdot ml^{-1} \cdot m^2$	$12 \div wt$	0.27	0.20	0.16	0.13	mm Hg/ml
Left ventricular end-systolic pressure-volume relation	LVESP ÷ (LVESV − V_0)	$4.0 \, mm \, Hg \cdot ml^{-1} \cdot m^2$	$137 \div wt$	3.0	2.3	1.8	1.5	mm Hg/ml

(continued)

Table 1 (continued)

Parameters	Sources for Measurement or Calculations	Values Not Indexed or Indexed to Body Surface Area	Values in Subjects of Different Weights[†]					Units
			Formulas Used to Calculate Values[‡]	Subject Weight				
				45 kg	60 kg	75 kg	90 kg	
Right ventricular end-systolic pressure-volume relation	$RVESP \div (RVESV - V_0)$	0.24 mm Hg $\cdot$ ml^{-1} $\cdot$ m^2	$27.4 \div wt$	0.61	0.46	0.37	0.30	mm Hg/ml
Total power delivered into aorta	$LVESP \cdot CO$	350 mm Hg $\cdot$ L $\cdot$ ml^{-1} $\cdot$ m^{-2}	$28 \cdot wt^{0.75}$	490	600	710	820	mm Hg $\cdot$ L $\cdot$ min^{-1}
Steady-flow aortic power	$MAP \cdot CO$	315 mm Hg $\cdot$ L $\cdot$ ml^{-1} $\cdot$ m^{-2}	$25.2 \cdot wt^{0.75}$	440	540	640	740	mm Hg $\cdot$ L $\cdot$ min^{-1}
Power dissipated in microvasculature	$(MAP - CVP) \cdot CO$	308 mm Hg $\cdot$ L $\cdot$ ml^{-1} $\cdot$ m^{-2}	$24.6 \cdot wt^{0.75}$	427	530	627	719	mm Hg $\cdot$ L $\cdot$ min^{-1}
Power used to fill right heart	$CVP \cdot CO$	7 mm Hg $\cdot$ L $\cdot$ ml^{-1} $\cdot$ m^{-2}	$0.56 \cdot wt^{0.75}$	10	12	14	16	mm Hg $\cdot$ L $\cdot$ min^{-1}
Oscillatory power	$(LVESP - MAP) \cdot CO$	35 mm Hg $\cdot$ L $\cdot$ ml^{-1} $\cdot$ m^{-2}	$2.80 \cdot wt^{0.75}$	49	60	71	82	mm Hg $\cdot$ L $\cdot$ min^{-1}
Total power delivered into pulmonary artery	$RVESP \cdot CO$	70 mm Hg $\cdot$ L $\cdot$ ml^{-1} $\cdot$ m^{-2}	$5.6 \cdot wt^{0.75}$	97	121	143	164	mm Hg $\cdot$ L $\cdot$ min^{-1}
Steady-flow pulmonary arterial power	$MPAP \cdot CO$	53 mm Hg $\cdot$ L $\cdot$ ml^{-1} $\cdot$ m^{-2}	$4.2 \cdot wt^{0.75}$	73	91	107	123	mm Hg $\cdot$ L $\cdot$ min^{-1}
Power dissipated in microvasculature	$(MPAP - PAWP) \cdot CO$	35 mm Hg $\cdot$ L $\cdot$ ml^{-1} $\cdot$ m^{-2}	$2.8 \cdot wt^{0.75}$	49	60	71	82	mm Hg $\cdot$ L $\cdot$ min^{-1}
Power used to fill left heart	$PAWP \cdot CO$	18 mm Hg $\cdot$ L $\cdot$ ml^{-1} $\cdot$ m^{-2}	$1.4 \cdot wt^{0.75}$	24	30	36	41	mm Hg $\cdot$ L $\cdot$ min^{-1}
Oscillatory power	$(RVESP - MPAP) \cdot CO$	18 mm Hg $\cdot$ L $\cdot$ ml^{-1} $\cdot$ m^{-2}	$1.4 \cdot wt^{0.75}$	24	30	36	41	mm Hg $\cdot$ L $\cdot$ min^{-1}
Systemic arterial O_2 tension (P_aO_2)[‖]	O_2 electrode	70–97 mm Hg	—	70–97	70–97	70–97	70–97	mm Hg
Mixed venous O_2 tension ($P_{mv}O_2$)[¶]	O_2 electrode	37–47 mm Hg	—	37–47	37–47	37–47	37–47	mm Hg
Arterial O_2 saturation (S_aO_2)[‖]	Co-oximeter	93%–97%	—	93%–97%	93%–97%	93%–97%	93%–97%	—
Mixed venous O_2 tension ($S_{mv}O_2$)[¶]	Co-oximeter	73%–80%	—	73%–80%	73%–80%	73%–80%	73%–80%	—
Arterial CO_2 tension	CO_2 electrode	40 mm Hg	—	40	40	40	40	mm Hg
Mixed venous CO_2 tension	CO_2 electrode	45 mm Hg	—	45	45	45	45	mm Hg
Arterial pH	pH electrode	7.40	—	7.40	7.40	7.40	7.40	—
Mixed venous pH	pH electrode	7.35	—	7.35	7.35	7.35	7.35	—
Arterial venous O_2 content difference	$1.39 \cdot [Hb] \cdot (S_aO_2 - S_{mv}O_2)$	3.6 ml O_2/dl	—	3.6	3.6	3.6	3.6	ml O_2/dl
O_2 consumption	$1.39 \cdot [Hb] \cdot (S_aO_2 - S_{mv}O_2) \cdot CO$	126 ml O_2 $\cdot$ min^{-1} $\cdot$ m^{-2}	$10 \cdot wt^{0.75}$	174	216	255	292	ml O_2/min

*Mean values in young 60 kg subject in good condition, height 169 cm, body surface area 1.70 m², in a supine position, fasting, and breathing spontaneously; thermoneutral environment. Range of normal, approximately ± 25% of values listed.

†Values for subjects of different weights calculated taking into account fractal distributions of nutrient blood vessels and minimization of energy distribution to metabolizing organs.[29]

‡All weights in kg.

§Resting HR in a poorly conditioned subject is faster than that in a well-conditioned subject by a factor of approximately 1.2; however, resting CO is the same. As a consequence, resting SV is smaller and parameters that depend on SV differ from those in a well-conditioned person.

‖P_aO_2 and S_aO_2 decrease with age: 98 mm Hg (97% saturation) is normal for a person 20 yr of age, and 75 mm Hg (95% saturation) for a person 70 yr of age.

¶$P_{mv}O_2$ and $S_{mv}O_2$ depend on [Hb], arterial O_2 content, cardiac output, and O_2 consumption. For a 60 kg person with an arterial saturation of 97%, a cardiac output of 6 L/min, and an O_2 consumption of 216 ml O_2/min, [Hb] of 11, 13, and 15 g/dl will result in $S_{mv}O_2$ of 73% (37 mm Hg), 77% (43 mm Hg), and 80% (47 mm Hg), respectively.

Matching the Measuring System to the Patient's Vasculature

The systolic and diastolic pressures depend not only on the true pressures in the patient's vascular system but also on the nature of the equipment used to measure those pressures.[2,3] If the catheter-tubing-transducer system is excessively stiff in comparison with the stiffness of the vasculature, the systolic and diastolic pressures will be exaggerated: the systolic pressure at the transducer will be higher than the true systolic pressure, and the diastolic pressure will be lower than the true diastolic pressure. Conversely, if the measuring system is more compliant than the patient's vasculature, the systolic and diastolic pressures will be damped: the systolic pressure measured at the transducer will be lower than the true systolic, and the diastolic pressure will be greater than the true diastolic. Damping will also be introduced if the vascular catheter is obstructed by a blood clot or if the tube is too narrow or too long or has a kink in it.

The accuracy of systolic and diastolic pressures at the transducer can be assessed by the so-called snap test [*see Figure 2*].[3] This test consists of infusing a square wave of pressure into the catheter-tubing-transducer system by pulling on the tab that allows influx of fluid from the high-pressure bag used to keep the tubing-catheter system patent. The tab is then snapped shut, and the pressure in the system returns abruptly to baseline levels. If the catheter-tubing-transducer system is adequately matched to the patient's vasculature, this abrupt return to baseline pressures will occur smoothly and with no interruption of the arterial pressure tracing.

If the measuring system is too stiff, the snap will result in hyperresonance and overshooting of the pressure recording on the oscilloscope screen. If the measuring system is too compliant or if the catheter or tubing is obstructed, sudden release of the tab will lead to a slow and slurred descent toward the baseline.

The catheter-tubing-transducer system should be set up so that it is hyperresonant. The stiffest possible tubing should be obtained from the manufacturer, and the tubing should be kept at the shortest length consonant with patient care. If the system introduces excessive resonance, it can be damped with commercially available devices. It is not possible to compensate for systems that are too compliant.

Systolic and diastolic pressure measurements from the transducer cannot be relied on unless the snap test indicates that the measuring system and the patient's vasculature are adequately matched.

Catheter Whip

Systolic and diastolic pressures are also not to be trusted if the intravascular catheter moves around in the vascular lumen as the heart beats[2] [*see Figure 3*]. This movement, called catheter whip or catheter fling, is usually not a problem if the systemic arterial pressure is being measured by a catheter in the radial artery—such catheters cannot move around very much. When measurements are made by catheters in larger arteries, however, such as the femoral, catheter whip can introduce errors of 20 mm Hg or more in measurements of arterial pressures. Again, mean measurements are more accurate than systolic or diastolic measurements. Often, distortion introduced by a hyperresonant measuring system looks very much like catheter whip, and the two causes of distortion cannot be distinguished from each other. If this is the case, a device can be added to the catheter-tubing-transducer system to eliminate hyperresonance. Distortions that remain must be the result of catheter whip.

Pressure Differences at Varying Distances from the Heart

Systolic and, to a lesser extent, diastolic pressures in distal arteries are usually exaggerated with respect to central arterial or aortic pressures.[2,4] Systolic pressures in the radial artery tend to be higher than those in the brachial, which in turn tend to be higher than those in the aorta. The diastolic pressures tend to be slightly lower in the radial artery. These effects are caused by pulse wave reflection[5] [*see Figure 4*]. In normal persons younger than 50 years, the peak systolic pressure in the aortic root is approximately 20 mm Hg less than the systolic pressure in the radial artery; in normal persons 50 years of age and older, the peak systolic pressure in the aortic root is approximately 10 mm Hg less than the systolic pressure in the radial artery.[4] Once again, however, the mean pressures in the smaller arteries are close to the mean pressures in the larger ones.

Thus, measurements of systolic and diastolic pressures, even by catheter-transducer systems, can be suspect for three reasons: mismatched measuring systems, catheter whip, and true differences in systolic and diastolic pressures in arteries at different distances from the heart. It is always safe to use the mean pressure. With appropriate precautions—such as performing the snap test and making allowances for pulse wave amplification as the pressure wave advances distally—it is possible to use the systolic pressure in a peripheral artery to calculate back to the systolic pressure in the aortic root.

Insertion of Systemic Arterial Catheters

Systemic arterial lines are generally placed in one of four major vessels: radial artery, brachial artery, femoral artery, or dorsalis pedis artery.

When using the radial artery, the clinician should perform an Allen test before catheter placement. In the Allen test, the fist is clenched or the arm elevated to drain blood from the hand. Both the ulnar and radial arteries are compressed by the clinician. The fist is released or the arm lowered, and the ulnar artery is released. A blush of the hand indicates a patent palmar arch that is supplied by the ulnar artery. If occlusion of the radial artery were to occur, the ulnar artery should then be able to provide adequate blood supply to the hand. Although very few patients have inadequate palmar arch collateral, some groups are at risk for necrosis of the hand if the radial artery is occluded. These patients include those with arteritis, diabetes, low-flow states, and hypercoagulable states. Once evidence of ulnar flow through the palmar arch is established, the area is prepared with antiseptic solution and draped in sterile fashion. The catheter is then placed into the arterial lumen percutaneously, using sterile technique. The dorsalis pedis artery may be used as an alternative to the radial artery.

Use of the brachial artery is associated with a higher likelihood of complication. The brachial artery lies between the bicipital tendon and median nerve at the antecubital fossa. Nerve injury as the result of catheter placement is more likely. If thrombosis occurs, circulation to the hand and arm may be severely compromised; in patients with diabetes, upper extremity vascular disease may be sufficiently advanced that partial loss of the hand may occur.

In patients who are restricted to bed, femoral arterial lines have a low complication rate and may be the most satisfactory choice. The femoral artery is usually superficial and easy to palpate. Disadvantages of the femoral site include difficulty in controlling bleeding near the genital region should such bleeding occur, impairment of mobility, and vascular compromise caused by thrombosis of the femoral artery or embolization from the catheter.

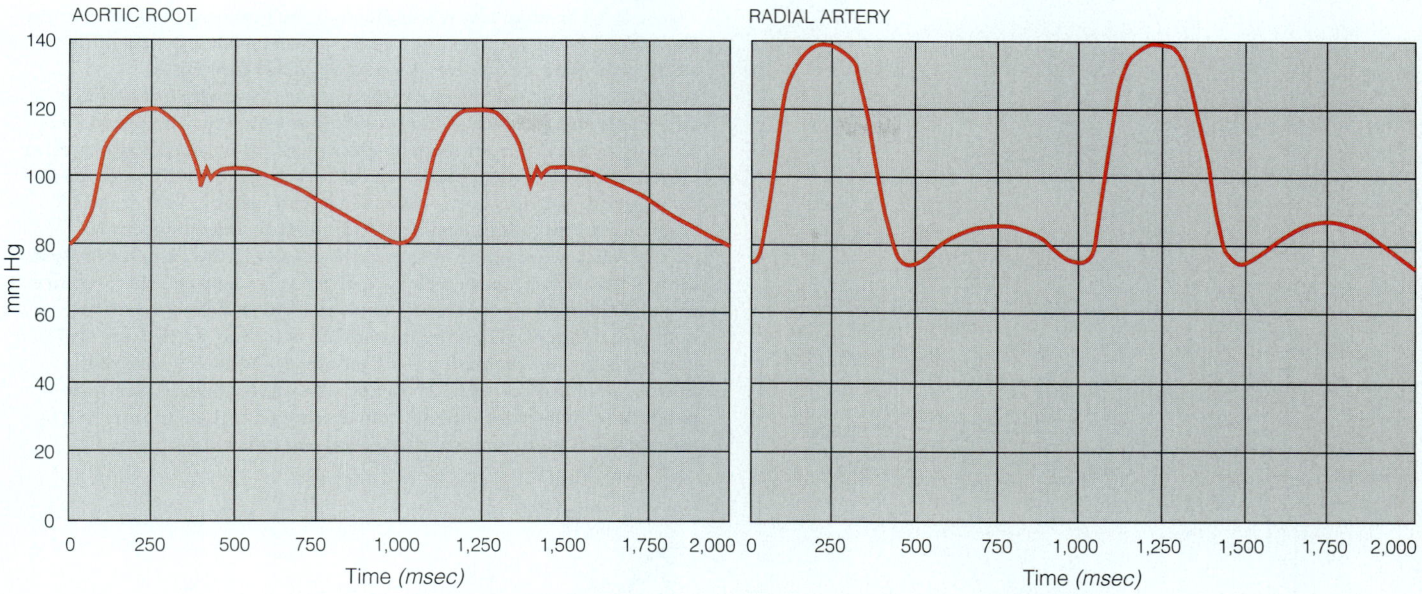

Figure 1 The mean pressure is defined as the area under a pressure tracing over an entire cycle divided by the time needed to produce that cycle. A pressure wave in the ascending aorta with a blood pressure of 120/80 mm Hg will have the same mean pressure as a pressure wave in the radial artery of the same patient, even though the radial artery pressure might be 140/75 mm Hg, because the systolic pressure in the radial artery is usually inscribed more rapidly than the systolic pressure in the aorta. The areas underneath the aortic pressure and radial artery pressure curves are identical. A useful but not infallible approximation of the mean pressure is to take the diastolic pressure plus one third of the difference between the systolic and diastolic pressures. In these examples, this formula would not work. The mean aortic pressure would be approximated at 93 mm Hg, whereas the mean radial artery pressure would be approximated at 97 mm Hg. Such results would be impossible: if the mean pressure in the radial artery actually were greater than the mean pressure in the aorta, blood would flow backward. This confusion is avoided by actually measuring the area under the curve and calculating the mean pressure exactly. Computer circuits in most pressure-monitoring systems make exact calculations of the mean pressure. Thus, the mean pressure taken from the digital readout of the pressure monitor is the single most accurate indicator of the actual pressure being measured and should be used for measurements of systemic arterial pressure.

MEASUREMENTS OBTAINED FROM SYSTEMIC ARTERIAL BLOOD

An indwelling systemic arterial catheter allows measurement of systemic arterial blood gases (i.e., the partial pressures of both oxygen [Po_2] and carbon dioxide [Pco_2] and the hydrogen ion concentration, which is expressed as the pH), oxygen saturation, and oxygen content. The partial pressure of oxygen or CO_2 refers to the pressure exerted by those gases dissolved in the plasma. Partial pressures are relatively easy and inexpensive to measure, and they are the most commonly used measurements of oxygen and CO_2 levels in the blood.

The partial pressure of oxygen may not provide sufficient information, however, because it is not linearly proportional to the total amount of oxygen in the blood: most of the blood's oxygen is not dissolved in the plasma but is combined with hemoglobin molecules and exerts no pressure whatsoever.[1] Of more consequence is the oxygen saturation. This term refers to the fraction of hemoglobin occupied by oxygen. The saturation can be approximated from measurements of blood Po_2, pH, Pco_2, and temperature. These calculations are typically made by computer in the blood gas laboratory, and the approximated saturation value is returned by the laboratory along with the measured values of partial pressures and pH. Oxygen saturation can also be measured directly through use of a co-oximeter. This device is simple to use and inexpensive, and it gives a more accurate value because it makes a direct measure of the saturation. It does require another several milliliters of blood, however, and therefore adds to the amount of blood required of the patient.

But the greatest significance of the oxygen saturation measurement lies in its role in yielding values for oxygen content. The content shows the concentration of oxygen in the blood, and it is this value that counts. It literally refers to the amount of oxygen contained in a given volume of blood and is typically expressed as a volume percent or as milliliters of oxygen dissolved in 100 ml of blood. The oxygen content is a measure of all the oxygen in the blood, including oxygen attached to the hemoglobin molecule and oxygen dissolved in the plasma.

The amount of oxygen dissolved in plasma is small compared with the amount that is bound to hemoglobin. As long as the Po_2 is less than about 100 mm Hg, the contribution of the oxygen in the plasma to the total oxygen content need not be considered, assuming that the hemoglobin concentration is at least 7 g/dl. Neglecting to count the oxygen dissolved in the plasma makes calculation of oxygen content simple: the oxygen content is approximately 1.39 multiplied by the hemoglobin concentration multiplied by the oxygen saturation (So_2):

$$O_2 \text{ content} = 1.39 \times [Hb] \times So_2$$

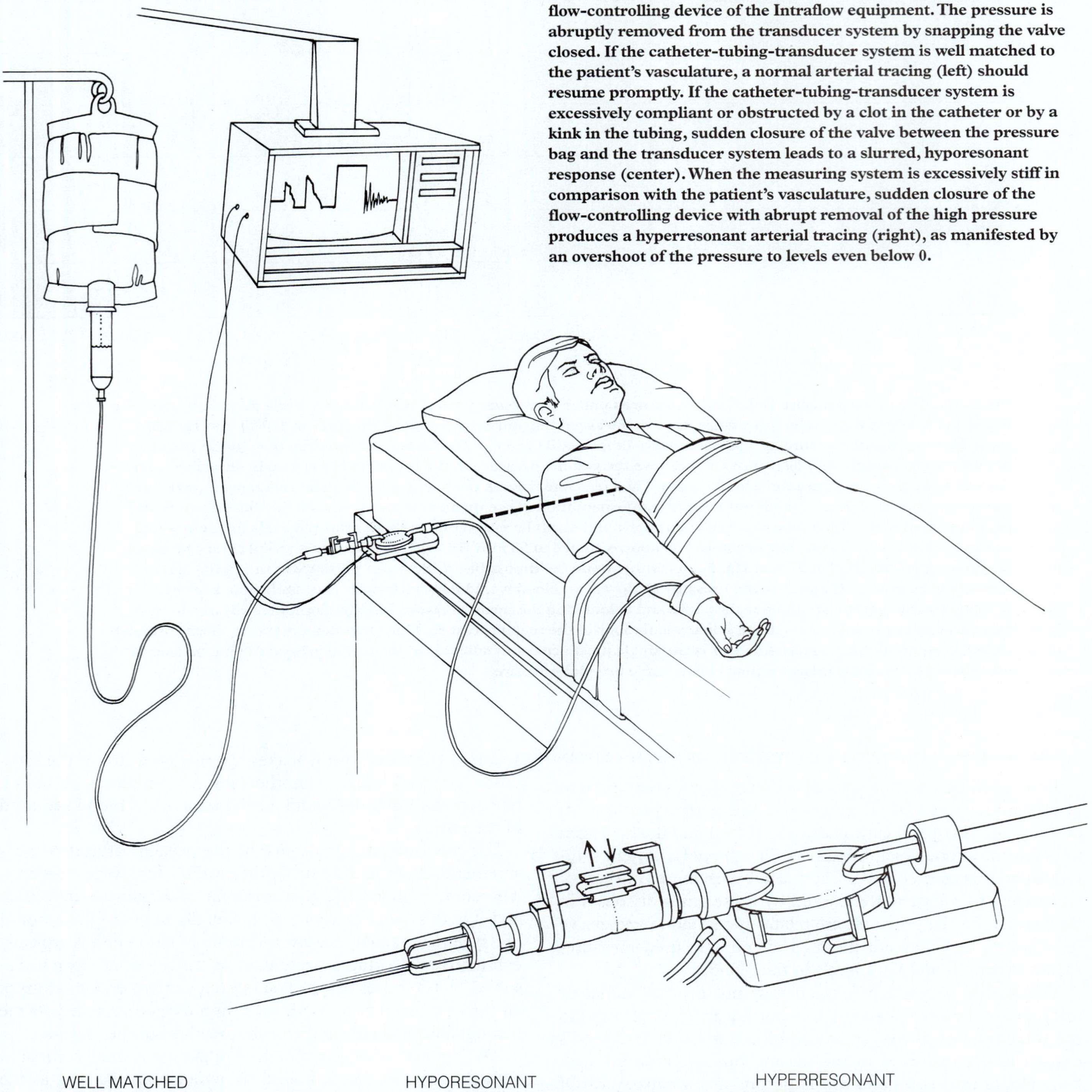

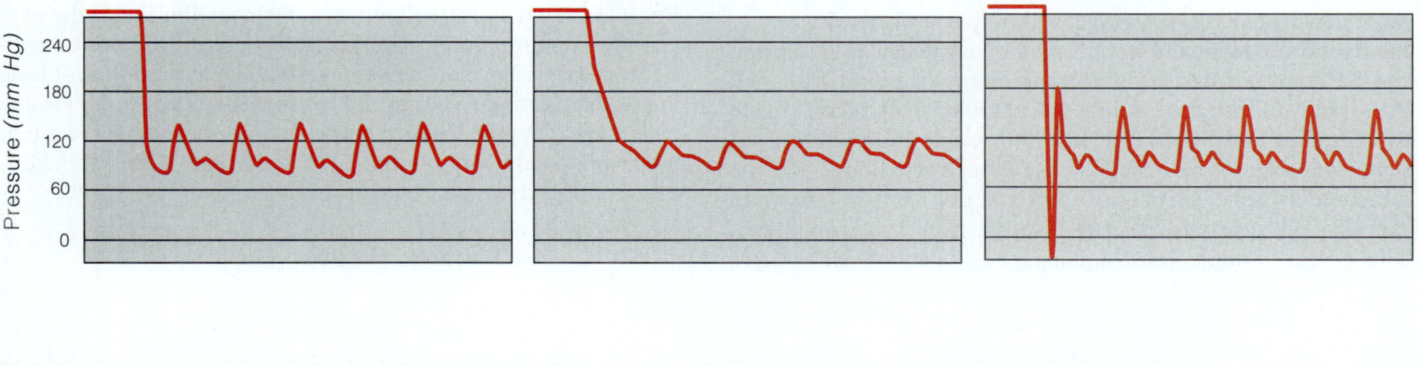

Figure 2 The snap test will indicate if the pressure measured at the transducer is the same as the pressure measured at the tip of the catheter in the vasculature. A pressure of 250 mm Hg is superimposed on the pressure-measuring system by opening the flow-controlling device of the Intraflow equipment. The pressure is abruptly removed from the transducer system by snapping the valve closed. If the catheter-tubing-transducer system is well matched to the patient's vasculature, a normal arterial tracing (left) should resume promptly. If the catheter-tubing-transducer system is excessively compliant or obstructed by a clot in the catheter or by a kink in the tubing, sudden closure of the valve between the pressure bag and the transducer system leads to a slurred, hyporesonant response (center). When the measuring system is excessively stiff in comparison with the patient's vasculature, sudden closure of the flow-controlling device with abrupt removal of the high pressure produces a hyperresonant arterial tracing (right), as manifested by an overshoot of the pressure to levels even below 0.

WELL MATCHED HYPORESONANT HYPERRESONANT

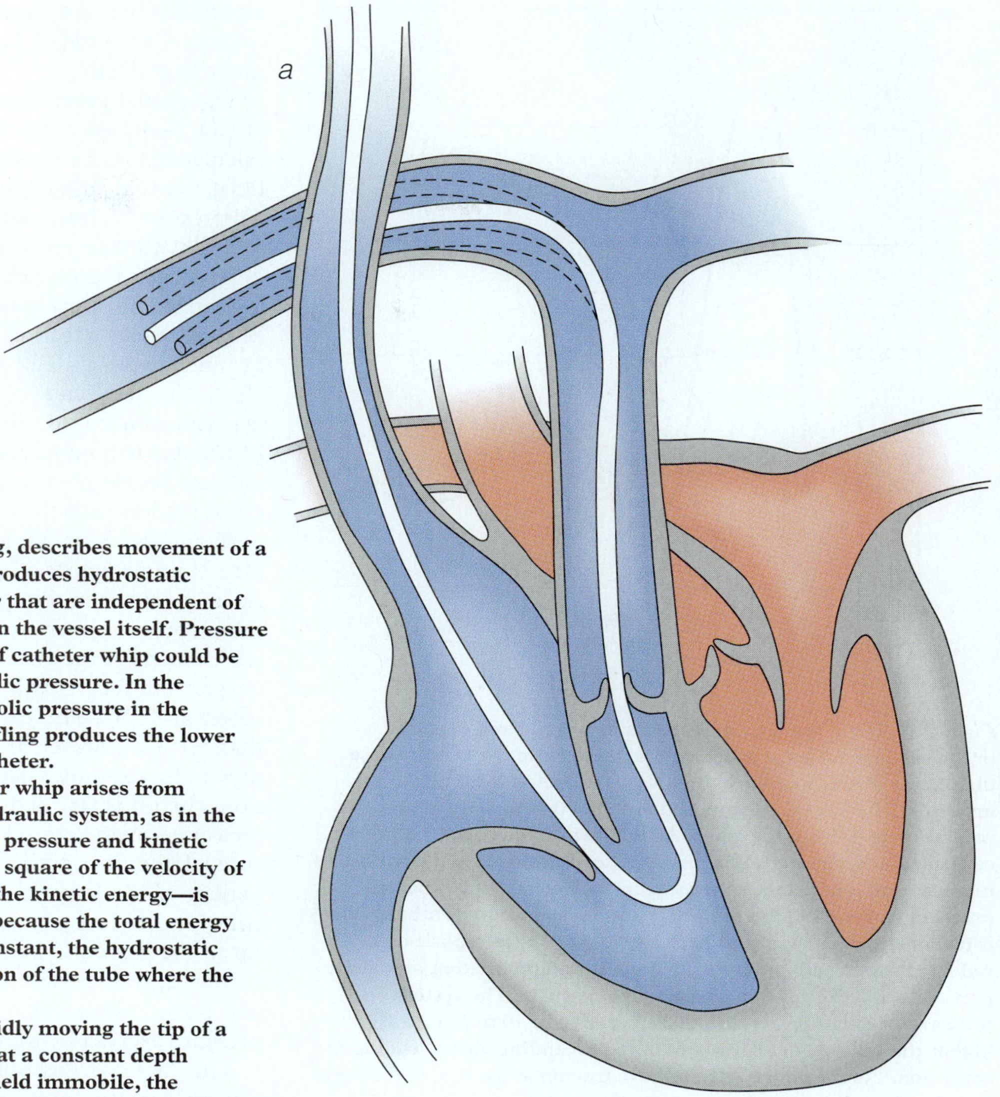

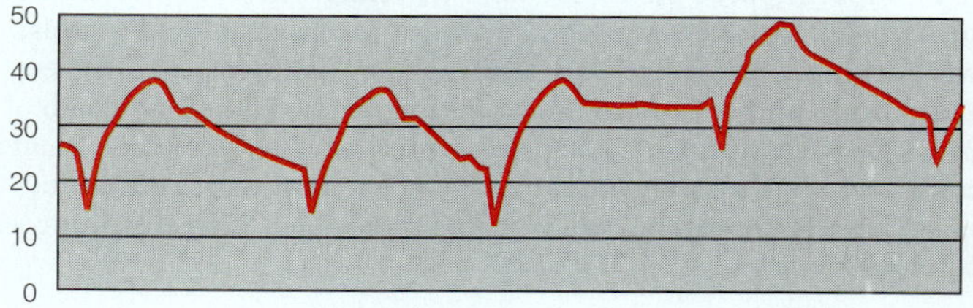

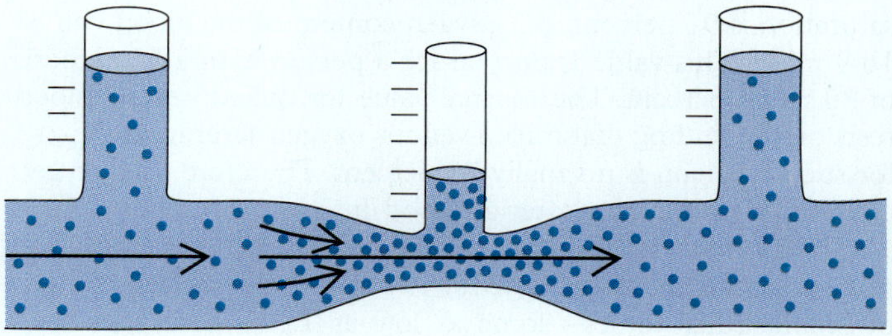

Figure 3 Catheter whip, or catheter fling, describes movement of a catheter within the vasculature (*a*) that produces hydrostatic pressure changes at the tip of the catheter that are independent of any changes in hydrostatic pressure within the vessel itself. Pressure drops during diastole that are the result of catheter whip could be falsely interpreted as true vascular diastolic pressure. In the pressure tracing shown (*b*), the true diastolic pressure in the pulmonary artery is 24 mm Hg; catheter fling produces the lower pressure of 12 mm Hg at the tip of the catheter.

The pressure drop produced by catheter whip arises from Bernoulli's principle: total energy in a hydraulic system, as in the vascular system, is the sum of hydrostatic pressure and kinetic energy. The kinetic energy depends on the square of the velocity of the fluid. Because the velocity—and thus the kinetic energy—is greater the narrower the system (*c*), and because the total energy measured at any point in the system is constant, the hydrostatic pressure must be less in the narrow portion of the tube where the velocity of flow is higher.

Catheter whip can be simulated by rapidly moving the tip of a fluid-filled catheter through a water bath at a constant depth beneath the surface. If the catheter were held immobile, the hydrostatic pressure would be seen to be constant at a given depth in the bath. The kinetic energy, however, increases as the catheter moves through the water because the more rapidly the catheter moves, the greater is the velocity of the fluid past the tip and the greater the kinetic energy component; the greater the kinetic energy, the lower the hydrostatic pressure as measured at the tip. Similarly, if a femoral or pulmonary arterial catheter moves within the vasculature as the heart beats, the velocity of blood across its orifice will increase; as the velocity increases and the kinetic energy increases, the hydrostatic pressure as measured at the tip will fall. This transient decrease in hydrostatic pressure at the tip of the catheter (as seen in the tracing) does not reflect the true hydrostatic pressure in the artery.

The radial artery catheter is best for determining the total energy in the blood flow. The catheter will not whip, because the artery is small and the catheter has no room to move about, and there will be no kinetic energy component in the blood, because the radial artery catheter is end-on (i.e., it faces into the direction of the flow) and thus the velocity of the blood as it runs into the end of the catheter is zero. Therefore, the hydrostatic pressure will represent the total energy of the blood at that point of the vasculature. A catheter placed in the ascending aorta will be buffeted by the rapidly accelerating blood in the aorta, and catheter whip will be introduced. A pulmonary arterial catheter potentially has both the problem of catheter whip and the problem that it measures pressure in the direction of flow rather than end-on.

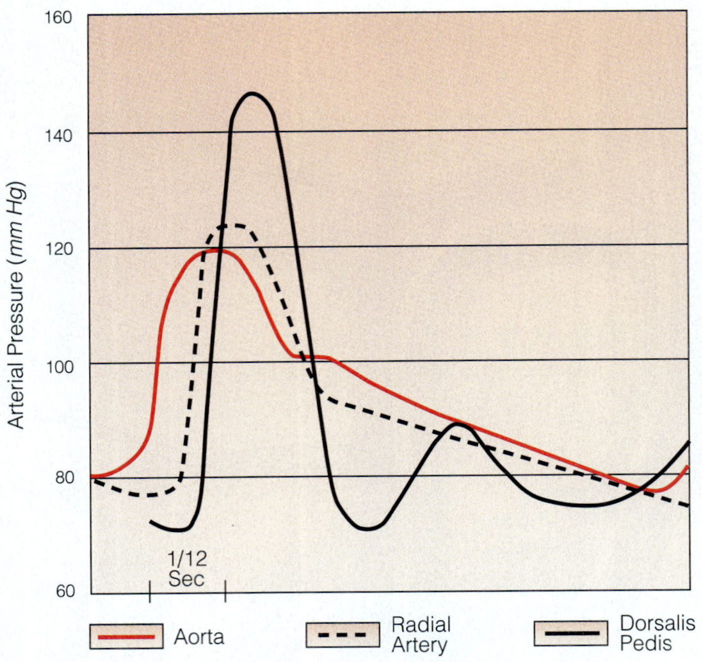

Figure 4 There are true differences in systolic and diastolic pressures in arteries at different distances from the heart. These differences result when pressure waves reflected from distal arteriolar sites are superimposed onto the forward-traveling pressure waves from the aorta. As the measuring point (i.e., the catheter) moves closer to the distal reflecting site, systolic pressures increase and diastolic pressures decrease because the reflected pressure waves from the periphery return sooner to a catheter that is placed distally. The result of this in-phase superimposition of reflected waves onto anterograde waves is augmentation of systolic pressures and diminution of diastolic pressures. The systolic pressure in the radial artery, therefore, can be 10 to 20 mm Hg higher than the systolic pressure in the ascending aorta, leading to confusion. Furthermore, the pressure tracing at the root of the aorta is wider than the pressure tracing in the radial artery because reflected waves are returning from the periphery at different times; their effect is thus distributed over a larger portion of the cardiac cycle, and the pressure wave in the aorta is broad. The pressure wave in the radial artery is narrow because the reflected waves tend to be superimposed on the forward-traveling waves, in phase. The mean pressures, however, will be almost the same in both vessels, with the mean pressure in the radial artery being just slightly less than the mean pressure in the ascending aorta. Use of the mean pressure will eliminate inaccuracies introduced by catheter-vascular mismatching and confusion introduced by pulse wave reflection; inspection of the tracing will usually reveal aberrations introduced by catheter whip.

Thus, if the hemoglobin concentration is 12.5 and the oxygen saturation is 97 percent, the oxygen content of the blood will be 16.9 ml/dl. This value is normal for a person with a hematocrit of 38 to 39 percent. The normal value for mixed venous blood rests on the finding that mixed venous oxygen saturation ($S_{mv}O_2$) for such a person is normally 75 percent. Therefore, the oxygen content of pulmonary arterial blood in this example is 1.39 × 12.5 × 75 percent, or 13 ml/dl. Although 1.39 is probably the most accurate figure available for calculating the oxygen content of blood, other values—some as low as 1.33—have also been reported. Thus, for purposes of simplification, one may use a value of 4/3 instead of 1.39. The value of 4/3 makes calculations easier to perform.

The partial pressure of carbon dioxide indicates the amount of CO_2 dissolved in the plasma. Carbon dioxide content can be calculated, but it seldom is because within physiologic ranges of P_{CO_2}, the CO_2 in the blood is almost linearly related to the partial pressure.[6] Thus, measurements of carbon dioxide are easier to deal with than measurements of oxygen levels.

Hydrogen ion concentration is usually expressed as pH and is obtained by direct measurement with ion-sensitive electrodes. Measurements of serum lactate can also be used to identify and quantitate acidosis. The arterial blood reflects whole body metabolism. Normal lactate concentrations are less than 2 mmol/L. In hypermetabolic critically ill patients, lactate concentrations can be elevated to 3 mmol/L or greater; values greater than 8 mmol/L indicate severe metabolic acidosis. Normal lactate-to-pyruvate ratios are less than 20.

Blood that is drawn for blood gas determinations should be placed immediately on ice to inhibit oxygen consumption by the neutrophils in the specimen. The blood, when measured in the blood gas apparatus, will be rewarmed to 37° C by a heating element in the cuvette. Thus, values for partial pressure of oxygen and for pH will be obtained by the laboratory with the blood at 37° C. The patient's blood may be warmer or colder than 37° C, however. If the patient's blood is 35° C when it is drawn, for example, some of the oxygen will come out of solution when it is warmed up to 37° C. Thus, the partial pressure measured by the apparatus will be higher than the partial pressure of the gas in the blood when it was circulating in the patient at the lower temperature. One way to remember this concept is to imagine a glass of cool beer as it gradually warms up to the surrounding room temperature. As the beer warms, carbon dioxide dissolved in the liquid will come out of solution and form bubbles; that is, as the liquid warms up, the partial pressure exerted by the gas will increase.

The physician and nurse caring for the patient need not make this temperature correction themselves. The blood gas laboratory typically will report temperature-corrected values for the partial pressures and pH if the patient's temperature is supplied to the laboratory along with the specimen.[7]

An increasing number of clinicians, however, no longer make temperature corrections for blood gases.[8] This technique has been termed the alpha-stat method for managing blood gas abnormalities in hypothermic or hyperthermic patients. It is thought to induce fewer abnormalities in acid-base balance when the patient's temperature returns to normal [*see 7 Life-Threatening Acid-Base Disorders*].

Central Venous Catheters

INDICATIONS FOR INSERTION

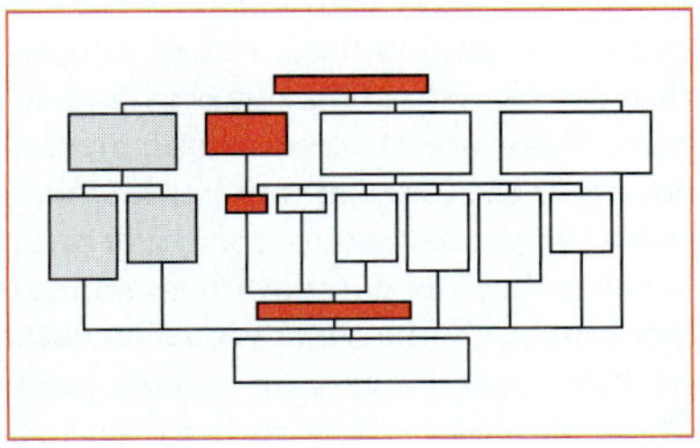

There are several indications for placement of central venous catheters[1] [*see Sidebar* Insertion of Central Venous Catheters]. Administration of parenteral nutrition requires a suitably placed central venous catheter [see 97 Nutritional Support]. In addition, prolonged administration of antibiotics or chemotherapeutic regimens may require central venous access. Central venous pressure (CVP), or right atrial pressure, is used to aid in the assessment of right-sided heart function. When combined with variables obtained from placement of a pulmonary arterial catheter, the measurement of right atrial pressure can be used to calculate pulmonary vascular resistance. Right-sided heart function, especially in critically ill patients, is a poor predictor of left-sided heart function.

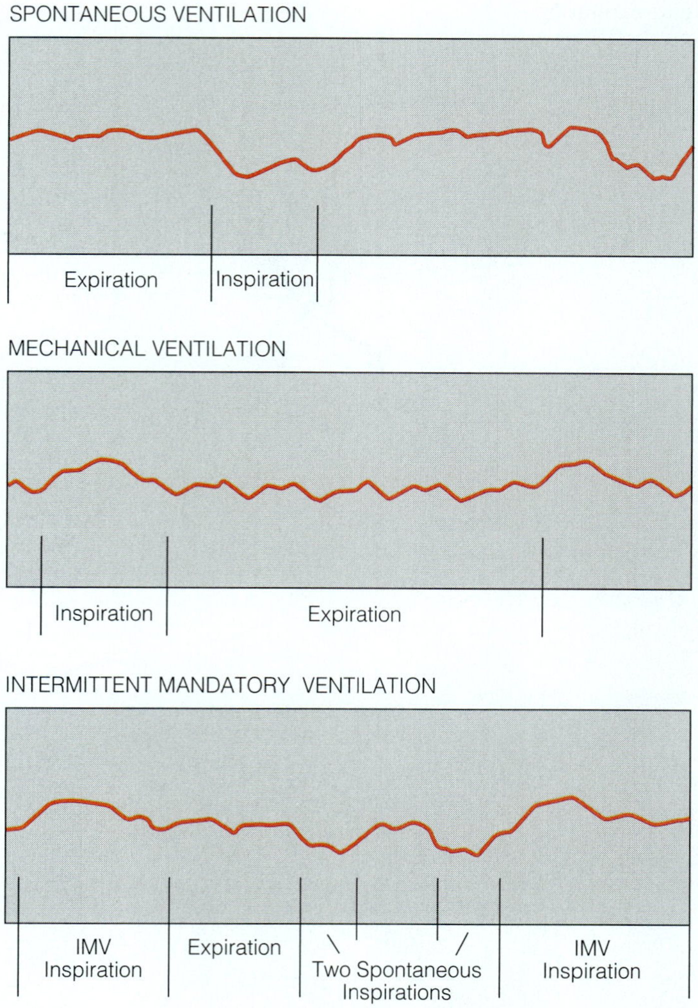

Insertion of Central Venous Catheters

Several sites of central venous access are commonly used: internal jugular [see Figure 6], subclavian, and external jugular veins and subcutaneous veins in the antecubital fossa or arm. A determination of whether to use the internal jugular or the subclavian approach must take several considerations into account. The right internal jugular has the lowest overall complication rate. The right side also provides a straight course to the right atrium. When the internal jugular approach is used, injury to the carotid artery is possible, but the carotid artery is also more easily palpated than the subclavian artery. On the left side, the thoracic duct is at risk for injury. The potential for nerve damage is greater with use of the internal jugular vein. The subclavian approach is generally more comfortable for the patient.

When the subclavian approach is used, the patient is placed in the supine position and Trendelenburg's position. The subclavicular area is prepared and draped in sterile fashion. Local anesthesia is obtained along the inferior portion of the clavicle. A 21-gauge needle is used to locate the subclavian vein. The needle is directed perpendicular to the sagittal plane and parallel to the coronal plane. The skin is entered, and the clavicle is followed inferiorly. Contact with the underside of the clavicle is essential. The subclavian vein is between the clavicle and first rib. When blood is aspirated, a guide wire is placed through the needle. The needle is then removed and the catheter placed over the guide wire. A chest x-ray is obtained to verify satisfactory positioning of the catheter. The subclavian approach to central venous catheterization is illustrated elsewhere [see 97 Nutritional Support].

The external jugular approach is associated with a risk of subclavian vein injury when a relatively stiff catheter is used. Catheters placed in the external jugular vein are more frequently used as peripheral lines than as central venous lines.

The long arm approach has a high incidence of thrombophlebitis but may be satisfactory for 48 to 72 hours. In the long arm approach, the antecubital fossa is prepared and draped in sterile fashion. The basilic vein is percutaneously entered and the catheter advanced. On average, 50 cm of catheter must be inserted from the left antecubital vein to reach the right atrium [see Table 2]. A chest x-ray is obtained to verify satisfactory placement of the catheter.

Figure 5 **End-expiratory pressure is relatively independent of the patient's ventilatory status and thus is most representative of the patient's vascular volume. For example, in a patient breathing spontaneously (top), central venous pressure (or, equivalently, right atrial pressure) falls as the lungs pull away from the intrathoracic great veins and right atrium. In these patients, the end-expiratory pressure is the highest pressure measured during the ventilatory cycle. During mechanical ventilation (middle), the lungs are pushed against the outside of the heart and great veins; intracavitary and intravascular pressures are thereby increased during inspiration, and the end-expiratory pressure is the lowest pressure measured during the ventilatory cycle. During intermittent mandatory ventilation (bottom), the machine-generated breaths produce increases in the CVP and spontaneous breaths produce decreases; the end-expiratory pressure is the plateau pressure between the two extremes.**

COMPLICATIONS ASSOCIATED WITH CENTRAL VENOUS CATHETERS

Percutaneous puncture of central veins, through either a jugular or a subclavian approach, can lead to several complications, some of which are immediately life threatening.[1] Penetration of the parietal pleura can produce a pneumothorax. This complication occurs in approximately six percent of cases. Puncture of the subclavian artery can lead to exsanguination into the pleural cavity. Intrapleural infusion of administered hyperalimentation can occur with improper catheter placement. The brachial plexus lies near the large veins that are commonly catheterized. Puncture of one of the major trunks or divisions can permanently impair the extremity. Puncture of the trachea, esophagus, or lung during catheter insertion can lead to subcutaneous emphysema. Puncture of the internal jugular vein on the left side can damage the thoracic duct and lead to a chylothorax. Improper use of the introducing needle can result in shearing of the catheter and catheter emboli. These complications will occur occasionally no matter how experienced the person performing the procedure; the goal is to keep the incidence of such complications to a minimum. All are results of technical errors, and as with all technical errors associated with procedures, prevention requires knowledge of anatomy and gentleness in performing the procedure.

MEASUREMENT OF CENTRAL VENOUS PRESSURE

Ideally, central venous pressures are measured with a transducer rather than with a manometer. It may be necessary to use manometers while waiting for the required equipment to be set up or when working in areas of the hospital where monitors are not available. It is preferable, however, to place the patient in a unit with the appropriate monitoring devices.

Central venous pressure measurements are usually made at end-expiration and are best obtained by direct observation of the pressure tracing on the oscilloscope screen. In some monitoring systems, digital readouts of the central venous pressure represent the mean pressure averaged over several ventilatory cycles; in other monitoring units, the digital readouts make an attempt to give the end-expiratory values. In the case of arterial pressures, mean pressure averaging is desirable [see Systemic Arterial Catheters, Measurement of Systemic Arterial Pressure, *above*]; in the case of central venous pressures, however, such averaging will usually result in values that are higher than those attained at end-expiration.

The end-expiratory pressure is often the most representative of the patient's vascular volume because it is relatively independent of the patient's ventilatory status. During spontaneous inspiration, as the lungs pull away from the great veins and cardiac chambers, the intracardiac pressures fall. Thus, the end-expiratory pressure is typically the highest pressure recorded on the oscilloscope. In contrast, during mechanical ventilation, insufflation of the lungs compresses the cardiac chambers, thereby increasing intracardiac pressures, and the end-expiratory pressure is typically the lowest pressure recorded. Intermittent mandatory ventilation produces both augmented vascular pressures when the ventilator gives a mechanical breath and lowered intracardiac pressures when the patient takes a spontaneous breath. In this case, the end-expiratory pressure is typically the plateau that develops between the two extremes [see Figure 5].

During inspiration, large tidal volumes or rapid inspiratory flow rates can produce peak intracardiac pressures that exceed end-expiratory values by as much as 10 mm Hg. If end-expiratory values are used, these effects are eliminated. Some physicians try to minimize the effects of positive-pressure ventilation on interpretation of pressure tracings by taking the patient off the ventilator while making the measurements. This maneuver makes it easier to interpret the pressures, but it has the disadvantage that the most significant pressures are those that exist when the patient is being ventilated. Removing the critically ill patient from the ventilator produces a condition that no longer represents accurate values.

Although most physicians use the end-expiratory pressures with the patient on the ventilator as the values on which to base clinical decisions, some physicians have switched to the use of digital readouts. The advantage of the digital readouts is that the readings are independent of the nurse or physician. Attempting to read end-expiratory pressure tracings can sometimes be difficult even for the most experienced clinician or nurse,[9,10] and digital readouts eliminate this element of potential variability.

Zeroing of the transducer or manometer must be done precisely. Small errors in positioning of the transducer can lead to large errors in measurement. Most intensive care units use the midaxillary line as the zero level for vascular pressures.

Pulmonary Arterial Catheters

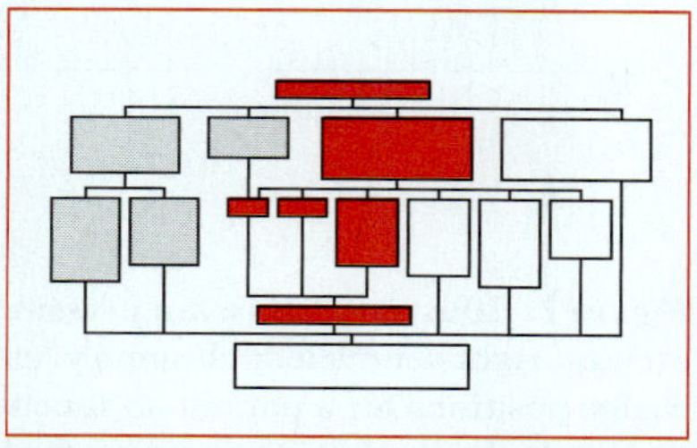

INDICATIONS FOR INSERTION

Use of pulmonary arterial catheters (Swan-Ganz catheters) is indicated in patients with any severe cardiopulmonary derangement[11] [see Sidebar Insertion of Pulmonary Arterial Catheters]. For example, when myocardial function is compromised in myocardial failure or myocardial infarction, the catheter can provide crucial information on the efficacy of pharmacological support and can aid in the diagnosis of abnormalities such as pericardial tamponade and acute mitral regurgitation.

Hypovolemic shock that does not respond readily to volume administration is another indication for insertion of a pulmonary arterial catheter; the catheter may reveal abnormalities of myocardial function or of the pulmonary or systemic vasculature that require specific interventions in addition to volume loading. Similarly, pulmonary arterial monitoring is frequently required in patients with sepsis who have inadequate urine output or who are hypotensive; the information provided by the catheter about the adequacy of oxygen consumption and of pharmacological support is of great value.

Pulmonary disorders, especially those that carry a high risk of associated myocardial dysfunction, are another indication. For example, pulmonary edema may be caused by elevated left atrial and pulmonary microvascular hydrostatic pressures or by endothelial disruption, which in turn may reflect inadequately resuscitated shock. (In the first example, treatment of the pulmonary failure would require diuresis; in the case of increased microvascular permeability, the treatment may require more aggressive fluid resuscitation.)

Figure 6 For central venous access via the internal jugular vein, first place the patient in the supine position. Clear all objects from the head of the bed, pull the bed away from the wall to gain access to the head of the bed, and remove the headboard. Adjust the bed to a comfortable height for working, and place the patient in Trendelenburg's position (10° to 20°) to prevent air emboli and to produce venous distention. Have the patient turn his or her head 90° away from the side of venipuncture. The right side is preferred for two reasons: first, because it provides direct access to the superior vena cava, and second, because injury to the thoracic duct is avoided. Put on mask and hat, wash hands, and put on gown and gloves. Prep and drape the patient.

Identify the triangle formed by the two heads of the sternocleidomastoid muscle. The apex of the triangle is more apparent if the patient is able to lift his or her head. Infiltrate local anesthetic into the skin and underlying soft tissue along the proposed path of the introducer needle. Generally, this path will run from the apex of the triangle to the nipple of the opposite breast. Aspirate before infiltration to avoid intravascular injection.

The internal jugular vein is then located in the coronal plane posterior to the sternocleidomastoid and above the first rib insertion of the scalenus anticus muscle. Either the lateral or the central approach should be used. The initial efforts at finding the internal jugular vein should be done parallel to the coronal plane, with the needle directed toward the nipple of the opposite breast, and at an angle of 30° to the sagittal plane (*a*, *b*, and *c*). All attempts at finding the internal jugular vein should be made with an 18-gauge or smaller needle. The operator should be aware of the carotid artery, which is located medially to the vein.

Once the vein is located, enlarge the skin wound at the puncture site. If the finder needle is of a diameter too small for the guide wire, one must use the appropriate size introducer needle to cannulate the internal jugular vein. The finder needle may be left in place to serve as a guide, or it may be removed. Once the internal jugular vein is cannulated, insert the guide wire (*d*). The guide wire must thread easily. When the guide wire has been inserted a generous length, remove the introducer needle, holding the guide wire in place. Insert a dilator and then the catheter (*e*). Firm pressure can be maintained on these objects during insertion as long as the guide wire maintains free movement in the lumen. Insert the catheter to an appropriate length. Remove the wire and the dilator. Aspirate blood, flush the catheter with heparinized saline, and place Luer-lock caps on all ports. Suture the catheter in place, and apply sterile dressings. A chest x-ray should be obtained to verify placement and to rule out pneumothorax.

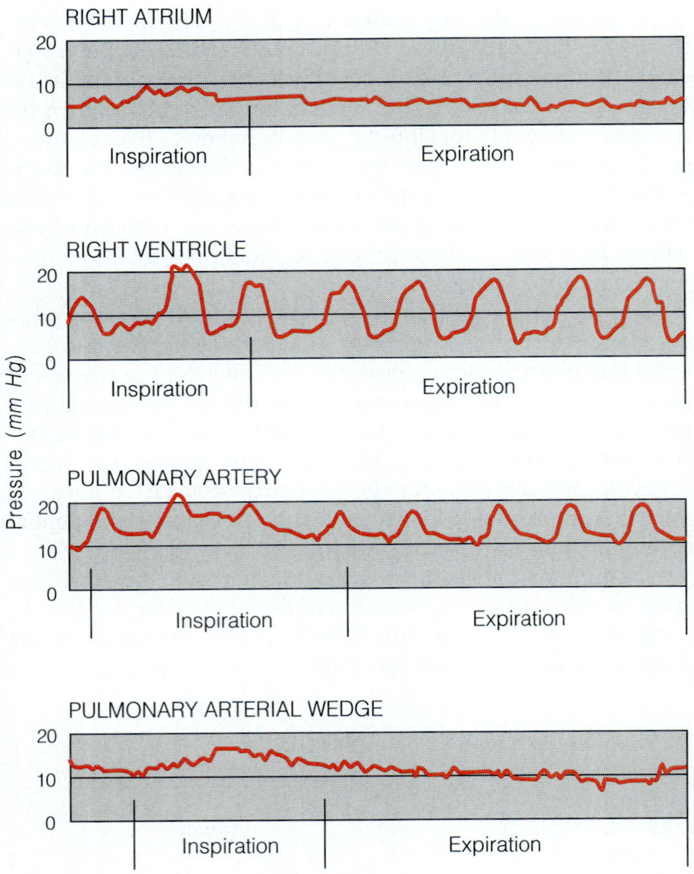

Figure 7 Illustrated here are pressure tracings in the right atrium, right ventricle, pulmonary artery, and pulmonary arterial wedge positions for a patient on mechanical ventilation. Note the gradually increasing pressure during diastole and the low mean diastolic pressure in the right ventricle. The pulmonary arterial tracing is characterized by a relatively high mean diastolic pressure and decreasing pressures during diastole. The pressure in the pulmonary arterial wedge position is characterized by a damped waveform, compared with the pulmonary arterial pressure. More important, the wedge pressure is easily converted to a pulmonary arterial pressure by deflation of the balloon.

Pulmonary arterial catheters may also be indicated for patients with good cardiopulmonary function who are undergoing procedures associated with large volume requirements and fluid shifts (e.g., procedures on the abdominal aorta), as well as for patients who will undergo elective procedures and who either have underlying myocardial or pulmonary disease or are at high risk for intraoperative or postoperative development of cardiopulmonary problems. A pulmonary arterial catheter is indicated if the patient has failure of two organs that might have different priorities with respect to fluid administration: a patient with both pulmonary failure and oliguria might benefit from fluid restriction, to reduce pulmonary microvascular hydrostatic pressures; on the other hand, that patient's kidneys might require fluid administration. A patient with a head injury and oliguria poses the same problem. The catheter, by giving precise information about the cardiovascular system, can greatly simplify the management of such complicated patients.

COMPLICATIONS ASSOCIATED WITH SWAN-GANZ CATHETERS

Complications of Swan-Ganz catheter insertion include those associated with central venous puncture [*see* Central Venous Catheters, Complications Associated with Central Venous Catheters, *above*] and others that are unique to the long intra-

Insertion of Pulmonary Arterial Catheters

Sites of access that are commonly used for insertion of a Swan-Ganz catheter include the right internal jugular and the subclavian veins. Before the catheter is placed, all lines are flushed and the balloon is tested and verified to be functional. Swan-Ganz catheters are typically placed without fluoroscopic equipment; passage relies on correct interpretation of pressures as the catheter passes through the cardiac chambers and into the pulmonary artery. The catheter is placed through an introducer and advanced under constant pressure monitoring [*see Figure 7*]. When respiratory excursion is seen, the balloon is inflated, and the catheter is advanced until a right atrial tracing is encountered. The catheter is then advanced to the right ventricle. Entry into the right ventricle is usually obvious because right ventricular pressure tracings show pressure excursions that far exceed any seen in tracings from the superior vena cava or the right atrium. The right ventricular pressure tracing is also characterized by an increase in pressure during diastole. The catheter should then be drawn gently back into the right atrium with the balloon inflated. The balloon will be felt to tug on the tricuspid valve as the catheter passes between the two chambers. The precise position of the tricuspid valve then becomes known, and the catheter should be reinserted into the right ventricle and advanced into the pulmonary artery with the insertion of only a few more centimeters of catheter. The pulmonary arterial tracing is characterized by a gradually decreasing pressure during diastole and by a mean diastolic pressure that is greater than the mean right ventricular diastolic pressure. Once entry into the pulmonary artery is confirmed, the catheter should be advanced until a wedge tracing is obtained; the wedge tracing is usually easily recognized by damping of the pressure tracing. The balloon should then be deflated; deflation should produce a full pulmonary arterial excursion. Reinflation of the balloon should reproduce the wedge reading.

Mechanical ventilation exerts an influence on pressure tracings that can lead to misinterpretations. In patients on mechanical ventilation, the right ventricular diastolic pressure may be higher than the pulmonary arterial diastolic pressure during expiration. Looking only at a diastolic pressure, without coordinating the reading with the phase of the ventilator cycle, can be very confusing [*see Figure 8*].

One of the difficulties that may be encountered during insertion of a pulmonary arterial catheter is curling of the catheter in the right atrium. It is important to remember that once the catheter passes the tricuspid valve, it should enter the pulmonary artery with passage of just a few more centimeters [*see Table 2*]. If a pulmonary arterial tracing is not obtained with insertion of an additional 10 cm of catheter, the catheter must be curling in the right ventricle. Another difficulty is entrapment of the end of the catheter in the muscular trabeculae of the right ventricle; the resultant damped tracing can closely resemble a pulmonary arterial wedge tracing [*see Figure 9*]. Entrapment can be avoided by verifying that the catheter has entered the pulmonary artery before advancing more tubing. Lastly, arrhythmias can develop during passage of the pulmonary arterial catheter, particularly while the end of the catheter is in the right ventricle. The risk of arrhythmias is minimized by keeping the balloon inflated as the catheter passes through the ventricle and, when appropriate, with administration of prophylactic doses of lidocaine during insertion.

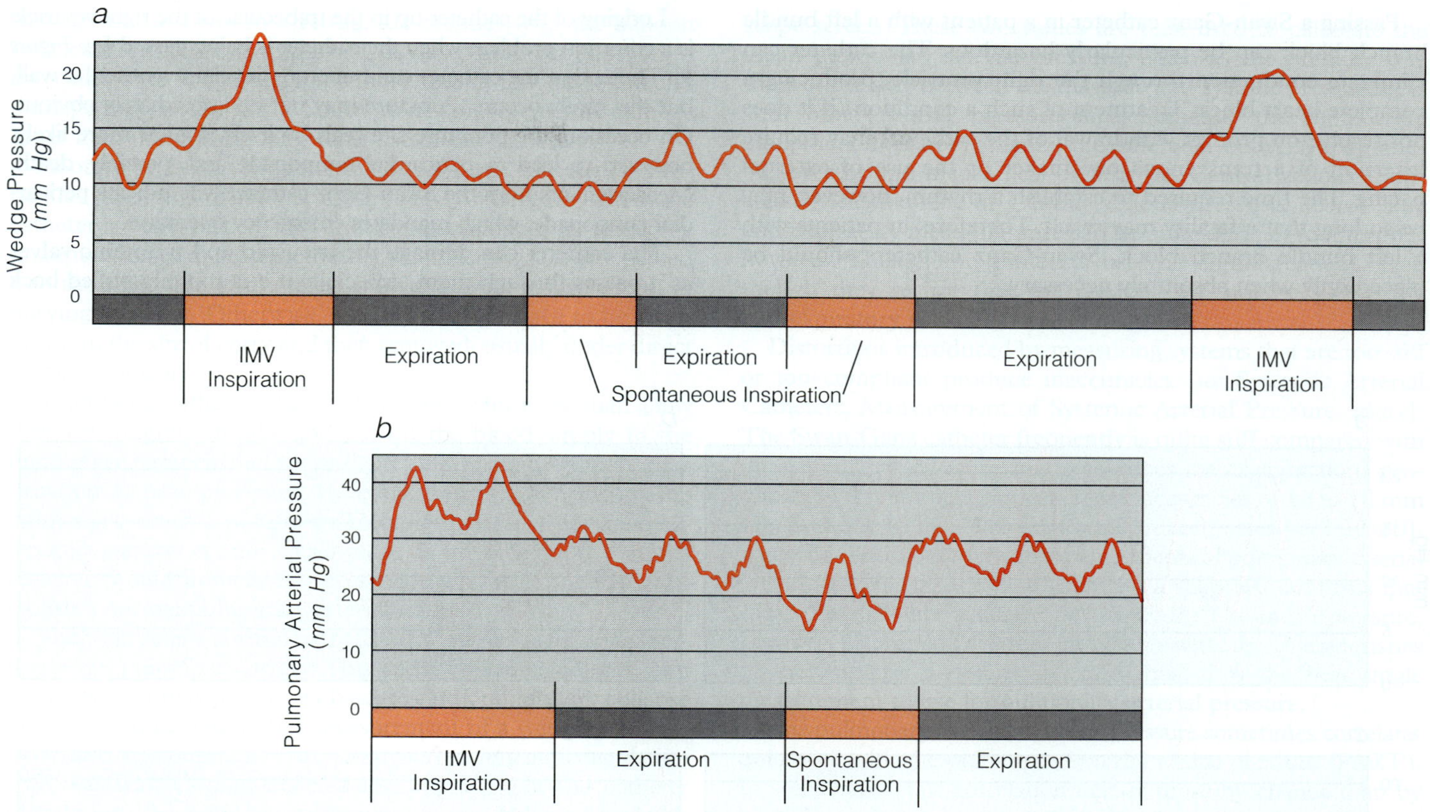

Figure 8 Mechanical ventilation can generate wide swings in pressure and make it difficult to assign a value to wedge or pulmonary arterial pressures. When the wedge tracing shown here (*a*) was obtained, the patient was on intermittent mandatory ventilation (IMV). The mechanical breaths generated pressure peaks of more than 20 mm Hg; spontaneous inspiratory efforts by the patient developed trough pressure readings of 8 mm Hg. The correct value, which should be taken at the plateau between the machine and spontaneous breaths, in this patient is 12 mm Hg. Similar difficulties arise with interpretation of pulmonary arterial pressure (*b*). Wide swings in pressure between systole and diastole in the pulmonary artery compound the problem even more. The mean pressure is somewhere between the two extremes; during the IMV inspiration shown here, the mean pressure is between 32 and 43 mm Hg. Approximating the mean pressure as the diastolic pressure plus one third of the pulse pressure would give a value of 36 mm Hg. During the spontaneous inspiration, the mean pressure is between 15 and 28 mm Hg; approximating the mean pressure would give a value of 19 mm Hg. The ideal is to read the mean pressure during expiration, toward the end of the expiratory cycle, but this can be a challenge for even the most experienced ICU nurse. Here, the mean pressure during expiration is between 23 and 31 mm Hg; the approximated mean pressure is 26 mm Hg.

vascular device.[1] These complications include ventricular arrhythmias, ventricular rupture, valvular damage on the right side of the heart, intracardiac knotting of the catheter, and pulmonary infarction induced by permanent wedging of the catheter in the distal pulmonary vasculature. It is necessary that pressures be interpreted correctly as the catheter passes through the cardiac chambers [*see Figure 7*].

Ventricular arrhythmias are relatively common during passage of the catheter, particularly in patients who have suffered recent myocardial infarctions and in those with an irritable myocardium as indicated by a preexisting arrhythmia or conduction defect. Some of these patients are best served by prophylactic administration of lidocaine. In rare instances, aggressive treatment of such arrhythmias may be required. Usually, the arrhythmia will subside when the end of the catheter finally passes through the ventricle and enters the pulmonary artery; sometimes, however, the arrhythmia can be ablated only by completely removing the catheter. The balloon on the end of the catheter should be kept inflated during passage to cushion the tip and minimize myocardial irritability.

Table 2 Distances between Catheter Insertion Sites and the Right Atrium

Insertion Site	Distance to Right Atrium*
Internal jugular subclavian vein	15 cm
Right antecubital vein	40 cm
Left antecubital vein	50 cm
Femoral vein	30 cm

*Add 15 cm to obtain distance to main pulmonary artery.

cular pressure is between the mean pulmonary arterial pressure and the left atrial (or wedge) pressure. If the wedge pressure is high, the pulmonary microvascular pressure must also be high. A high PAWP ($\geq$ 25 mm Hg) will always be associated with microvascular pressures that will generate at least some interstitial pulmonary edema, even if the microvascular endothelium is intact. If the endothelium is disrupted, as in sepsis, pulmonary edema can be produced even with wedge pressures in the mid-teens. In this setting, the pulmonary microvascular leak is the result of injury to the microvasculature rather than of ventricular dysfunction and high left atrial pressures.

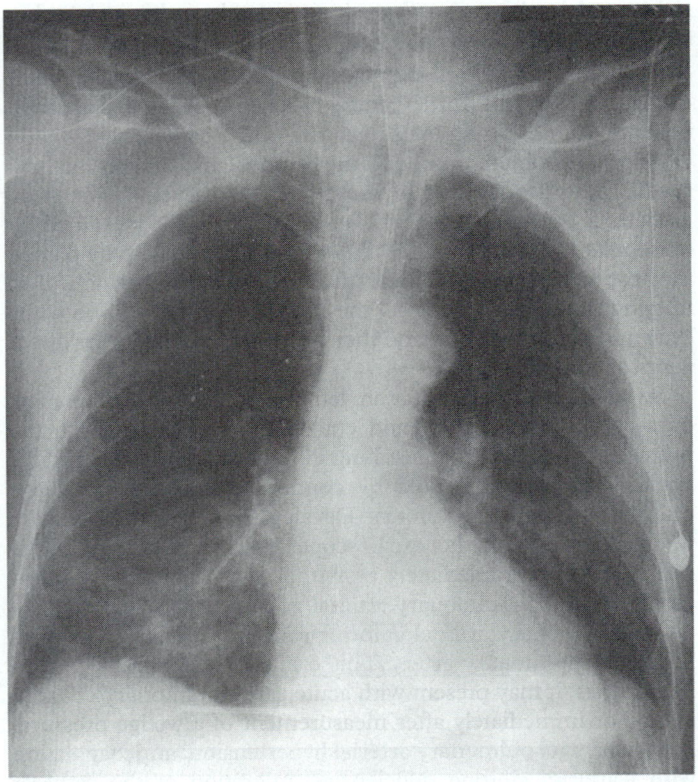

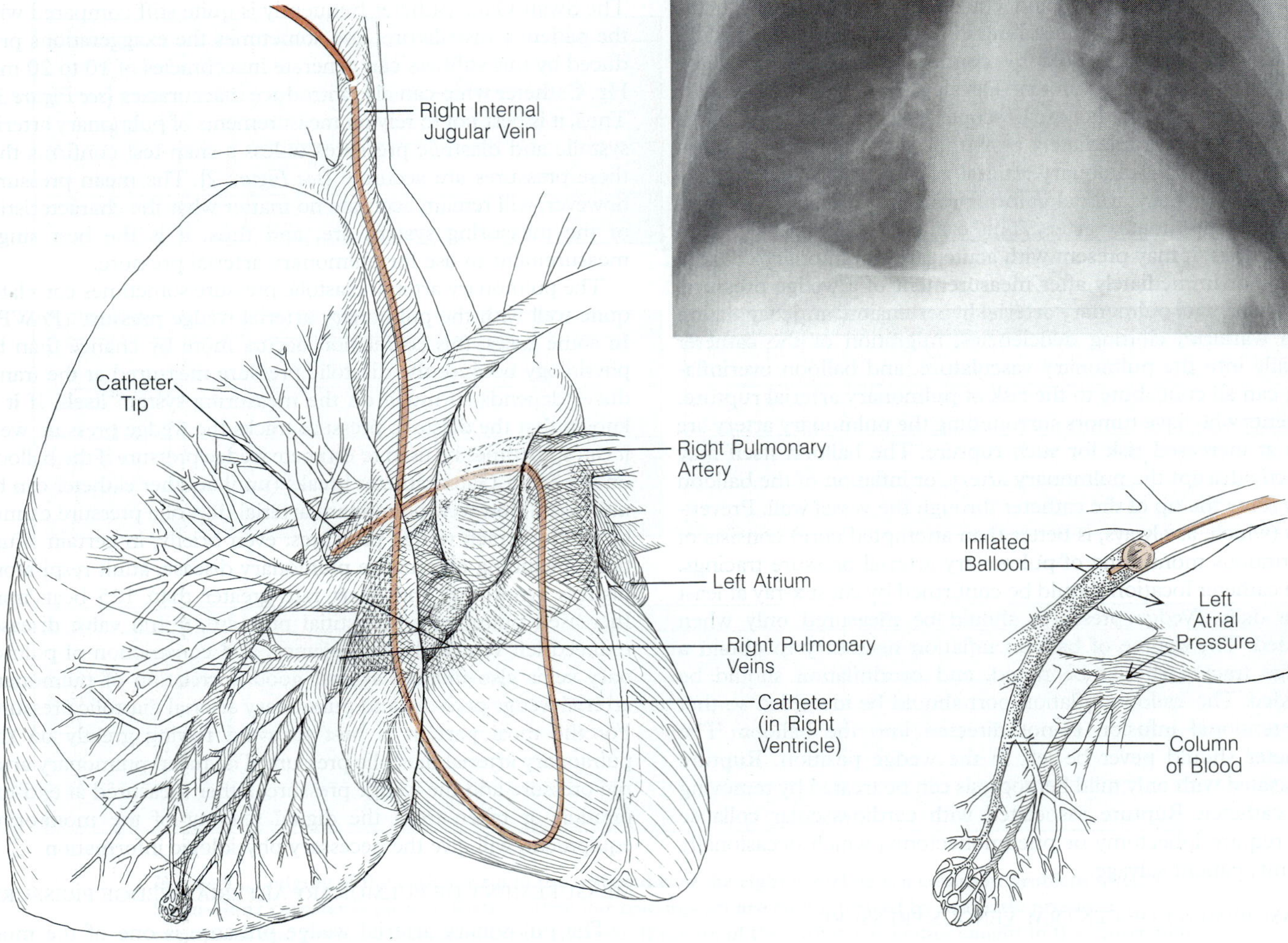

Figure 10 The pulmonary arterial catheter measures pressure in the pulmonary artery when the balloon is deflated. Because flow in the vascular system generates a pressure drop as the blood passes through the microvasculature, the pressure from the pulmonary artery to the left atrium gradually falls. When the balloon is inflated, flow in the vasculature distal to the tip is eliminated; therefore, there is no pressure drop. Because there is no pressure drop and because there are no valves between the left atrium and the pulmonary artery, the pressure in the pulmonary artery distal to the point of occlusion must equal the pressure in the left atrium, provided that there is an open column of blood between the end of the catheter and the left atrium. That is, pulmonary arterial wedge pressure will equal left atrial pressure as long as the catheter is in a dependent portion of the lung with a vasculature that remains open during ventilation. Because the catheter is flow directed, it usually will end up in such a dependent, well-perfused area. This is not a certainty, however. If inflated alveoli occlude the microvasculature, wedge pressure will equal alveolar pressure. This inaccuracy cannot be easily detected. Verification that the catheter is in the dependent portion of the lung requires a cross-table lateral chest x-ray. We do not routinely obtain these x-rays unless the wedge pressures are absolutely critical for treatment and unless the reliability of the wedge pressure tracing is suspect. Suspicion usually arises when excessively wide pressure swings are evident as the lungs are inflated and deflated.

Although the wedge pressure gives indirect information about the microvascular pressure, the two pressures are not the same. The term pulmonary capillary wedge pressure is misleading and should probably be discarded.

Cardiac output is affected by preload, which can be quantified as left ventricular end-diastolic volume (LVEDV), as reflected by the Frank-Starling curve or by pressure-volume loops. Changes in preload are reflected by changes in LVEDV. It is frequently assumed that PAWP, which reflects changes in left ventricular end-diastolic pressure, is also a reliable monitor of LVEDV and that PAWP can be used to judge the adequacy of preload and to make the diagnosis of cardiac failure and volume overload. Pressure is not equivalent to volume. Starling's law of the heart states that ventricular contraction depends on the myocardial fiber length that precedes the next contraction. That length is determined largely by LVEDV. Measurement of pressure (e.g., PAWP or right atrial pressure) does not necessarily reflect end-diastolic volume, because of diastolic ventricular compliance. A high intracavitary pressure in a ventricle with small diastolic compliance may be associated with a small end-diastolic volume. Similarly, a low intracavitary pressure in a ventricle with a large diastolic compliance may be associated with a large end-diastolic volume.

Because of the pressure-volume relation, in many clinical settings PAWP may not differentiate changes or problems in left ventricular contractility from those in left ventricular compliance.[12] A bedside echocardiogram may contribute to more effective management of the patient in these settings. As an index of blood volume, the PAWP may be neither very sensitive nor very specific. Ventricular compliance can be estimated at the bedside by administering a fluid bolus, usually 250 ml, and monitoring the rate of change of filling pressure [see 4 Shock]. A rapid increase suggests that there is a stiff ventricle during diastole. Diastolic myocardial compliance is reduced by ischemia, septic or hypovolemic shock, pericardial effusion, inotropic support, and positive end-expiratory pressure (PEEP).[14-16] On the other hand, afterload reduction, cardiomyopathy, malnutrition, and a reduction of inotropic support usually increase myocardial compliance.

If the catheter is located in lung zones where alveolar pressure is greater than arterial pressure (zone I) or venous pressure (zones I and II), PAWP may reflect airway pressure and not left atrial pressure (LAP). In this situation, the fundamental assumption of PAWP measurement is not met.

In zone III (the dependent portion of the lung), in which both arterial and venous pressures exceed alveolar pressure, there is continuous flow, and PAWP correlates with LAP. Most of the lung enters zone III when the patient is supine, and most pulmonary arterial catheters will preferentially float into zone III. It has been shown that if the tip of the catheter is at or below the level of the left atrium, the conditions in zone III exist even if positive end-expiratory pressures are as high as 30 cm H_2O, provided that there is no embolic obstruction. On occasion, if accuracy of left atrial pressure measurement is absolutely essential for patient care, a cross-table lateral film should be obtained to confirm the location of the catheter tip relative to the left atrium [see Figure 10]. If the tip is above the atrium, the catheter should be repositioned. A damped tracing, the need for balloon overinflation to produce a wedged reading, and wide pressure changes on respiration should all call into question the reliability of the measurement.

MEASUREMENT OF CARDIAC OUTPUT

Today, pulmonary arterial catheters are almost always equipped to measure cardiac output by means of thermodilution. The outputs are obtained by injecting a solution that is colder than blood through the right atrial port of the catheter and measuring the resultant temperature drop in the pulmonary artery as the cool blood flows past the thermistor. Commercially available computers calculate the cardiac output on the basis of indicator dilution theory [see Figure 11]. Flow into the cardiovascular system is calculated on the basis of the amount of cold solution injected proximally, the temperature of that solution compared with the baseline temperature of the blood, the physical characteristics of the solution that determine its cold capacity, and the area inscribed under the thermodilution curve. Cardiac output computers allow calibration for varying amounts and temperatures of injectates. The computer finds the area under the thermodilution curve and gives a digital readout of the cardiac output, usually in liters per minute. Either room-temperature or ice-cold solutions may be used as the thermal indicators. The important point is to know the exact temperature of the injectate because the temperature is necessary for accurate computer calculation of output. The advantages of room-temperature injections include simplicity and little variation in the injectate temperature. Ice-cold injections generate a large signal-to-noise ratio because the magnitude of the pulmonary arterial temperature changes increases as the temperature of the injectate decreases. Ventilation affects flow into and out of the right ventricle, and the pulmonary arterial temperature changes as a function of insufflation of the lungs. Therefore, three injections should be made for each determination of cardiac output. The injections should be made at a consistent point in the ventilatory cycle, typically at end-expiration.[17] The three values should be within 15 percent of one another; otherwise, the series should be repeated.

Methods have been developed to measure cardiac output without placement of invasive pulmonary arterial catheters. The direct Fick method is best used in awake, alert patients.[18] Transthoracic electrical impedance requires placement of electrodes, which may interfere with surgical procedures.[19] Doppler ultrasonography probes have been placed at the suprasternal notch and the esophagus for continuous cardiac output determination.[20,21] The suprasternal notch probe requires an estimate of the diameter of the ascending aorta. The esophageal Doppler probe measures the blood velocity in the descending aorta distal to the origins of the aortic arch vessels. Measurement of cardiac output in the descending aorta requires ascending aortic velocity calibration, which is obtained by a suprasternal notch probe. Expired gas analysis has also been used to obtain cardiac output. These methods are currently under clinical evaluation.[22-24]

MEASUREMENT OF RIGHT VENTRICULAR END-DIASTOLIC VOLUME

The introduction of fast-response thermistors has allowed development of thermodilution pulmonary arterial catheters for measurement of right ventricular end-diastolic volume.[25,26] Such measurements require use of a cold injectant. They have proved to be accurate as long as the patient has a

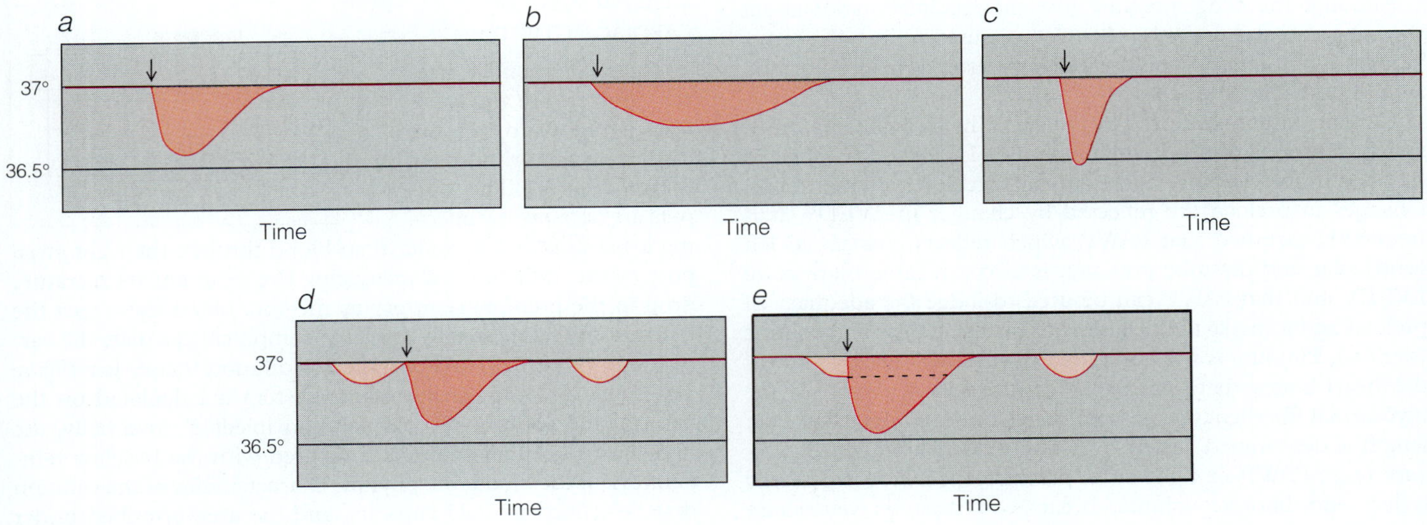

Figure 11 In the normal thermodilution curve shown here (*a*), the baseline pulmonary arterial temperature is 37° C; when a cold solution is injected to measure cardiac output (arrow), the temperature may fall to a low of 36.6° C as the cooled blood flows past the thermistor. When cardiac output is low (*b*), the cooled blood flows sluggishly past the end of the thermistor. The temperature drop in the blood might be to 36.7° C, but the cooled blood stagnates near the thermistor, and the blood at that portion of the pulmonary artery remains cool for a long time. Because the cardiac output is calculated as the inverse of the area, the output is recorded as a smaller number. By contrast, a supranormal cardiac output (*c*) pushes the pulse of cool blood rapidly past the thermistor. The result is a transiently low pulmonary arterial temperature. The area under the curve, however, is smaller than normal because the fall in temperature is brief; this small area leads to a calculation of a high cardiac output. These examples assume a stable temperature for pulmonary arterial blood, however, which is usually not the case. Pulmonary arterial blood temperature can vary during the ventilatory cycle by as much as several hundredths of a degree as a result of sequential and cyclic return of blood from different parts of the body. (The cyclic dips in temperature are represented here by the lightly shaded areas in *d* and *e*.) During inspiration, elastic recoil in the venules and small veins of the nonsplanchnic part of the body pushes the cool blood from the extremities back to the right atrium; relatively little blood returns from the hepatic veins as the diaphragm pushes down on the liver and kinks those vessels. During expiration, the diaphragm and liver rise, and the accumulated warm blood in the liver is discharged into the inferior vena cava as the hepatic veins open up and the liver reassumes its normal anatomic position. This cyclic return of blood to the right atrium leads to temperature changes in the blood in that chamber. This fact becomes important in the timing of the three injections for cardiac output determinations. If an injection is superimposed onto the baseline high temperature (*d*), the computer will detect a relatively small area under the curve. If an injection is superimposed onto a dip in the pulmonary arterial temperature (*e*), however, the computer will detect a larger area because it will be using the temperature of 37° C for its baseline. (The excess area is that above the broken line.) The only way to eliminate the variability introduced by ventilation-dependent changes in baseline pulmonary arterial temperature is to make each of the three injections at the same point in the ventilatory cycle. We make all of our injections at end-expiration.

regular heart rate of less than 140 beats/min. Right ventricular end-diastolic volume does not necessarily reflect left ventricular end-diastolic volume, but transesophageal or transthoracic echocardiography can determine whether the end-diastolic volume in the ventricles is similar. If so, measurement of the right ventricular volume can be used for estimates of the left.

The availability of the right ventricular end-diastolic volume can be very useful for patient management. Many patients with severe lung disease induced by critical illness have right-sided ventricular dysfunction. Knowledge of the end-diastolic volume can facilitate decisions about whether to volume load or diurese, whether to attempt pulmonary vasodilatation, or whether to use inotropic agents.

MEASUREMENT OF MIXED VENOUS GASES

Mixed venous, or pulmonary arterial, blood can be obtained from the end of the Swan-Ganz catheter for measurement of mixed venous gases. Mixed venous blood, by definition, is blood that represents a mixture of all blood returned from all organs of the body. Venous blood from the heart is returned to the right atrium through the coronary sinus. This blood is markedly desaturated (the heart, after all, is a working muscle). Blood in the right ventricle or in the pulmonary artery will be truly mixed venous blood because it includes the blood from the heart as well as the blood from the rest of the body. Measurements of gases in blood from the superior vena cava may be falsely elevated because that sample will not include the blood from the heart. Measurements of gases in blood obtained from the right atrium may be falsely low if the catheter tip is placed near the coronary sinus.

The residual blood in the catheter should be removed before the specimen is obtained for measurements of mixed venous gases. If the blood sample is withdrawn too forcefully, the pulmonary artery may collapse around the end of the catheter, and the blood will have been drawn in a retrograde manner past ventilated alveoli [*see Figure 12*]. The result, a specimen with very high oxygen levels, does not reflect desaturated pulmonary arterial blood. The possibility that blood has been drawn in a retrograde fashion can be checked by measuring the P_{CO_2} in the specimen. The P_{CO_2} in true pulmonary arterial blood is typically 5 mm Hg higher than the P_{CO_2} in a simultaneously drawn specimen of systemic arterial blood.[6] Blood drawn back past ventilated alveoli will have a very low P_{CO_2}. If the P_{CO_2} in the specimen is equal to or less than that in systemic arterial blood, the specimen should be discarded. Another specimen should be obtained by drawing back on the syringe more slowly. One should rely on measurements of oxygen saturation of the specimen (by co-oximetry) rather than on the P_{O_2}. The mixed venous partial pressure of oxygen and the oxygen saturation lie on the steep portion of the oxyhemoglobin dissociation curve. A minor error in measurement of partial pressure can result in a major error in calculation of the saturation [see 7 Life-Threatening Acid-Base Disorders].

In certain situations, it may be worthwhile to monitor $S_{mv}O_2$ continuously with a specially equipped pulmonary arterial catheter. An oximeter attached to the tip of a pulmonary arterial catheter can measure the $S_{mv}O_2$ by means of spectrophotometry. Continuous measurement of this variable is useful because abrupt drops in $S_{mv}O_2$ usually indicate that something is amiss. The heart extracts much of the oxygen delivered to it. If the blood returning from the heart and the rest of the body is markedly desaturated, it is likely that not enough blood is being transported to the heart. The $S_{mv}O_2$ falls if the heart suddenly delivers less oxygen to the tissues (e.g., if the cardiac index decreases rapidly or if the hemoglobin concentration or arterial oxygen saturation [S_aO_2] drops rapidly) or if the body suddenly demands increased amounts of oxygen (as with the onset of a hypermetabolic septic state or with the onset of shivering).

However, although a low $S_{mv}O_2$ is a warning signal, a normal or high value provides no assurances, because normal or high values do not necessarily reflect satisfactory cardiopulmonary status or adequate oxygen for metabolic demands. In low-output septic shock, for example, well-oxygenated blood is returned to the heart because blood is functionally shunted away from the tissues. High $S_{mv}O_2$ in patients with low-output sepsis do not

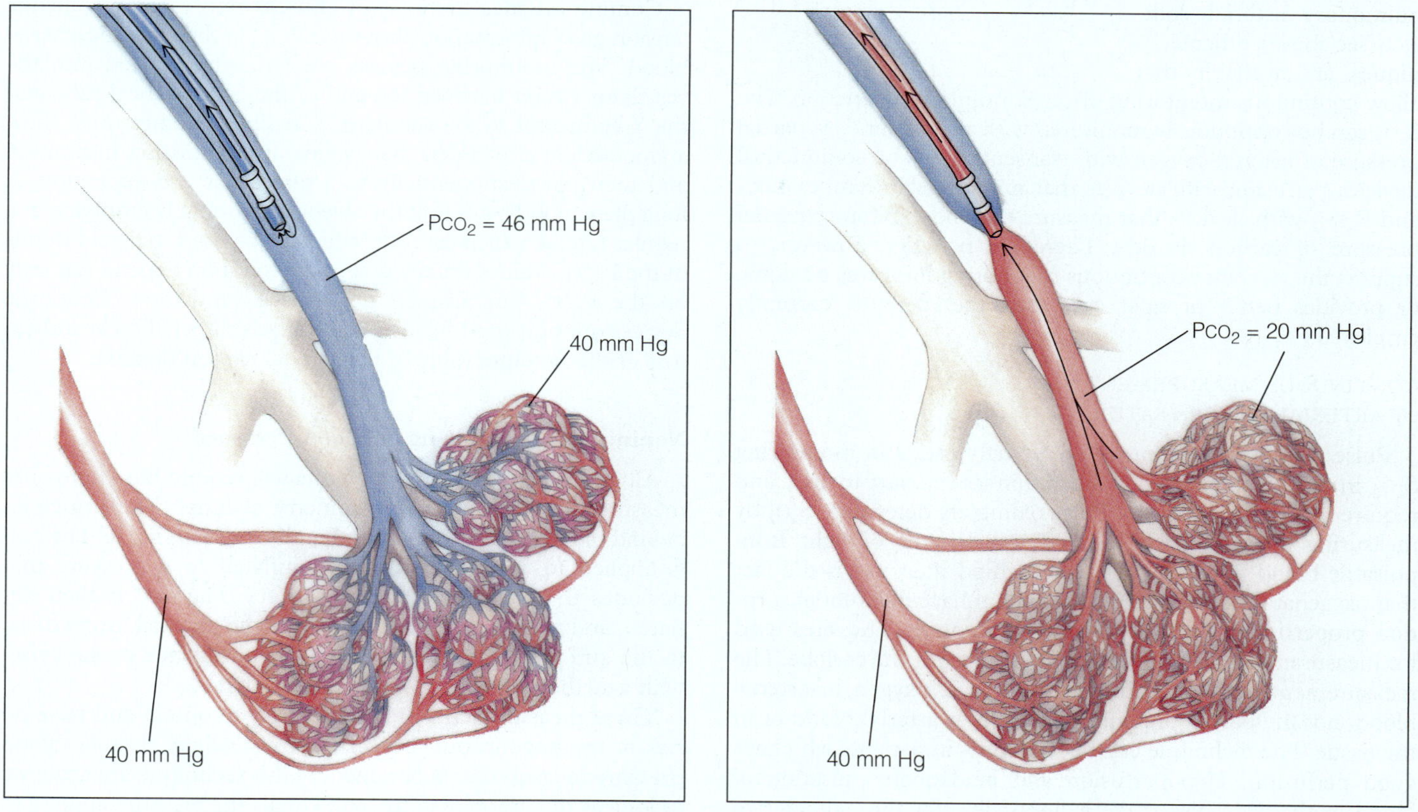

Figure 12 The Swan-Ganz catheter allows collection of mixed venous blood for measurement of mixed venous oxygen saturation and content (left). If blood from the pulmonary artery is withdrawn through the catheter too forcefully, however, arterial walls can collapse around the tip of the catheter (right). The blood that is withdrawn for sampling will in that case consist of blood from the distal pulmonary vasculature that has been pulled back past ventilated alveoli. To determine whether pullback of blood through the catheter has led to retrograde flow (right), the partial pressure of carbon dioxide in the sample can be checked. P_{CO_2} in mixed venous blood is typically about 5 mm Hg greater than P_{CO_2} in systemic arterial blood. If the arterial walls have collapsed around the catheter, the sample will consist of blood from which much of the CO_2 will already have been excreted into the ventilated alveoli, and the recovered blood will have a P_{CO_2} that may be as much as 20 mm Hg lower than that of simultaneously obtained arterial blood. Specimens of this sort should be discarded and new specimens obtained.

indicate that these patients' metabolic needs are being met; rather, the high values result from deranged peripheral metabolic processes with futile metabolic cycling. Cirrhotic patients, who have functional arteriovenous shunts, are another group in whom $S_{mv}O_2$ is generated in the presence of inadequate metabolic activity.

Catheters are available for continuous measurement of $S_{mv}O_2$. They can be difficult to keep calibrated and require some nursing time for maintenance. Nevertheless, they can be useful in selected patients if physicians or nurses are familiar with the potential drift of the calibration. If the $S_{mv}O_2$ drops, measurements should be made of the cardiac index, hemoglobin concentration, systemic S_aO_2, oxygen consumption, and other indicators of overall cardiopulmonary function. Therapy should be directed as indicated by these measurements.

Continuous Monitoring Techniques

In addition to continuous measurement of $S_{mv}O_2$ with a specially equipped pulmonary arterial catheter (see above), other techniques are available that allow continuous monitoring of cardiopulmonary function. The S_aO_2 can be continuously monitored with pulse oximetry, partial pressure of arterial oxygen with transcutaneous or conjunctival devices, perfusion with devices that measure skin temperature, and P_aCO_2 with devices that measure the end-expiratory partial pressure of carbon dioxide. There are no data, however, to support the view that continuous monitoring improves outcome or provides better or safer care than the methods currently employed.

CONTINUOUS MEASUREMENT OF ARTERIAL OXYGEN SATURATION

Pulse oximeters have proved extremely useful in monitoring S_aO_2 in ICU patients. They are noninvasive, easy to use, and require minimal calibration. Pulse oximeters determine S_aO_2 by measuring absorption of selected wavelengths of light from pulsatile blood flow. The principle behind their use is the fact that oxygenated and reduced hemoglobin have different absorption properties for light of known wavelengths. The sites used for measurement are the nail bed on a finger or the earlobe. The measurement obtained is the saturation of oxygen in arterial blood, not the partial pressure of oxygen in arterial blood or in the tissue. The technique can be used only in patients who have good perfusion. Hypoperfusion and inadequate pulsation of blood in the arterioles make it impossible for the oximeter to distinguish between arteriolar and venular blood.

CONTINUOUS MEASUREMENT OF TISSUE OXYGEN TENSION

PO_2 in the tissues can be determined by monitoring conjunctival or cutaneous tissues. Conjunctival oxygen tension is measured by a small oxygen sensor placed directly on the conjunctiva. The device is safe, and it does reflect changes in oxygen delivery to the tissue. It is not commonly used in most ICUs. Transcutaneous oxygen tension can be determined by placing a polarographic surface oxygen electrode directly on heated skin (heating the skin results in arterialized cutaneous tissue); tissue oxygen tension is measured beneath this surface electrode. This value correlates well with P_aO_2 if local tissue perfusion is good.

A decrease in S_aO_2 measured by pulse oximetry or a decrease in tissue oxygen tension measured by conjunctival or transcutaneous devices should prompt a search for evidence of cardiac or pulmonary impairment, such as decreases in cardiac index, hemoglobin concentration, and S_aO_2 or increases in peripheral oxygen consumption.

CONTINUOUS MEASUREMENT OF SKIN TEMPERATURE

Skin temperature can be monitored on the toe or thumb with noninvasive devices, but accurate measurements are difficult to obtain unless there is good control of ambient temperatures in the ICU. Skin temperature, however, is a sensitive indicator of poor perfusion: a gradient of less than 2° C between the skin temperature and the ambient temperature indicates critically low perfusion. Fluid loading or pharmacological support should increase skin perfusion and increase the gradient, so that the skin is substantially warmer than the environment.

CONTINUOUS MEASUREMENT OF END-EXPIRATORY CARBON DIOXIDE TENSION

Continuous measurement of end-expiratory carbon dioxide tension gives information about the PCO_2 in the systemic arterial blood. The monitoring devices are typically inserted into the ventilator circuit between the end of the endotracheal tube and the Y connector to the ventilator. Credible readings must show a smooth curve of PCO_2 that begins at zero during inspiration and then rises exponentially to a plateau at end-expiration. A long plateau indicates that the alveoli are probably emptying at a regular rate, in which case the value can be used to detect trends in the P_aCO_2. Values obtained at end-expiration depend not only on the P_aCO_2 but also on dead-space ventilation. Thus, the devices are best used for detecting trends rather than as indicators of the absolute value of the arterial carbon dioxide.

Noninvasive Monitoring of Blood Pressure

All patients in intensive care units will require blood pressure measurement by sphygmomanometry at times. The principles behind blood pressure measurement by cuff are simple. The cuff is applied to the upper arm and inflated to a pressure that occludes the underlying brachial artery. The cuff is then deflated, and resumption of blood flow in the brachial artery distal to the cuff is detected by listening for turbulence in the vessel with a stethoscope or with a Doppler flowmeter.

These measurements are usually easy to obtain and pose no risk to the patient, but they can be misleading. Systolic blood pressure measurements obtained by this technique are accurate as long as the pressure in the cuff equals the pressure applied to the inside of the artery. These pressures will usually be equal, except in diabetic patients who have calcified brachial arteries and in obese patients, in whom the subcutaneous fat between the cuff and the artery can dissipate any pressure applied externally, especially if the cuff is narrow with respect to the diameter of the arm. In both diabetic and obese patients, the systolic pressure indicated by the cuff method will be higher than the true intravascular systolic pressure. In all patients, measurement of diastolic pressures by the cuff method poses even greater problems. As the cuff is deflated, the sounds change character and then cease altogether. The diastolic pressure is now taken at the level at which the sound disappears. The sounds, however, can be so hard to detect that it becomes difficult to make this determination accurately.

The measurements obtained by this method reflect the pressure in the portion of the arterial system that is underneath the cuff. Using a Doppler device over the radial artery with the cuff over the brachial artery gives a measure of systolic pressure in the arm, not at the wrist.

Doppler devices give no measure of diastolic pressures; they can help only with measurements of systolic pressure in patients who have soft sounds in their brachial arteries that are difficult to hear with the stethoscope. Other devices that facilitate the measurement of blood pressure by cuff suffer from similar limitations. Some of these devices have Doppler probes incorporated into the cuff apparatus. These can automatically record systolic pressures, but they have the same limitations as hand-held Doppler devices. Other automatic devices sense pulsatility in volume changes in the arm as the cuff is deflated. These can work well in euvolemic patients, but they frequently fail in the presence of hypovolemia.

The inability to measure any pressures accurately in obese patients or in patients with calcified vessels, the uncertainty associated with measurements of diastolic pressure in all patients, and the inability of Doppler measurements to give any indication of diastolic pressures under any circumstances all make cuff measurements of arterial pressure less than ideal in critically ill patients. Most patients in an intensive care unit will benefit from the use of intra-arterial catheters for measurement of blood pressure, at least for some of their time in the ICU.

Derived Values

The measurements obtained from the devices described above allow calculation of derived values, which include cardiac output, stroke volume, left ventricular and right ventricular end-diastolic volumes, left ventricular and right ventricular end-systolic volumes, left ventricular and right ventricular end-systolic unstressed volumes, left ventricular and right ventricular end-systolic pressures, vascular resistances, aortic root and pulmonary arterial end-systolic pressure-volume relations, left ventricular and right ventricular end-systolic pressure-volume relations, power, oxygen transport, oxygen return, oxygen consumption, and bicarbonate concentration [see Table 1]. Values can also be derived for shunt fractions and alveolar-arterial oxygen gradients, both of which are discussed elsewhere [see 91 Pulmonary Dysfunction].

CARDIAC OUTPUT

The cardiac output computers that are used with thermodilution Swan-Ganz catheters typically report flow in terms of liters per minute. This value is important because it indicates the absolute volume flow, but it can be misleading unless the patient's size is taken into account. This problem can be overcome by dividing output by body surface area to calculate the cardiac index (CI), which is expressed in terms of liters per minute per square meter, or by dividing output by the patient's weight, which gives the output as milliliters of blood flow per kilogram per minute.

Body surface area is typically calculated from a nomogram.[27] The weight used in the nomogram can be the patient's weight at the time of cardiac output measurements, premorbid weight, or ideal weight. The patient's weight during the critical illness is the least representative of the patient's metabolically active mass as a result of illness-associated water accumulation. The premorbid weight has an advantage in that it avoids the problem of water accumulation. The ideal weight has the added advantage that it emphasizes the portion of the body that is most metabolically active and deemphasizes the role played by fat.[28]

Alternatively, one can use values that take into account the fractal distribution of the nutritive arterial network and the consequences of minimizing the energy requirements of the cardiovascular system.[29] The values for a 60 kg well-conditioned woman are easy to remember and can be adjusted to subjects of different weights [see Table 1].

STROKE VOLUME

The stroke volume is calculated by dividing the cardiac output by the heart rate. The value can be expressed as milliliters, or it can be indexed to the body surface area or to the patient's weight [see Table 1].

LEFT VENTRICULAR AND RIGHT VENTRICULAR END-DIASTOLIC VOLUMES

The ventricular end-diastolic volumes can be estimated from the filling pressures, though one must take into account that filling pressures reflect only intracavitary pressures. A pulmonary arterial catheter equipped to measure right ventricular end-diastolic volume can be very useful in patients who are thought to have decreased diastolic compliance or compression of the heart caused by mechanical ventilation or a raised diaphragm.[30] The left ventricular end-diastolic volume can be estimated by means of transesophageal echocardiography. These values can be indexed either to the body surface area or to the body weight [see Table 1].

LEFT VENTRICULAR AND RIGHT VENTRICULAR END-SYSTOLIC VOLUMES

End-systolic volumes can be obtained by subtracting the stroke volume from the end-diastolic volumes [see Table 1].

LEFT VENTRICULAR AND RIGHT VENTRICULAR END-SYSTOLIC UNSTRESSED VOLUMES

The term end-systolic unstressed volume refers to the volume that a ventricle would assume if all of its blood were removed with the ventricle in a fully contracted state.[31] These unstressed volumes cannot be measured routinely in the ICU. For the great majority of patients, unstressed volumes are quite small, on the order of 5 ml/m². In severe congestive heart failure, however, values can increase to as much as 40 ml/m².[32]

LEFT VENTRICULAR AND RIGHT VENTRICULAR END-SYSTOLIC PRESSURES

The left ventricular end-systolic pressure can be estimated by multiplying the aortic root systolic pressure by 0.9.[33] The aortic root systolic pressure can be obtained in patients younger than 50 years by subtracting 20 mm Hg from the radial artery systolic pressure and in patients 50 years of age or older by subtracting 10 mm Hg from the radial artery systolic pressure.[34] The right ventricular end-systolic pressure can be obtained by multiplying the pulmonary arterial systolic pressure by 0.9.

For calculation of both the left ventricular and right ventricular end-systolic pressures, it is important that measurements of the arterial pressure be as accurate as possible. A snap test should be performed to ensure that the stiffness and resistance of the measuring system reasonably approximate the stiffness and resistance of the vasculature being interrogated.

VASCULAR RESISTANCES

Pressure across a resistance equals the flow across the resistance multiplied by the resistance itself. This equation can be used to solve for the systemic vascular resistance: the cardiac index (representing the flow) is divided into the difference between the mean aortic pressure and the right atrial pressure. Pulmonary vascular resistance equals the CI divided into the difference between the mean pulmonary arterial and pulmonary arterial wedge pressures.

The advantage of dividing by cardiac indices rather than by cardiac outputs is that the values obtained are relatively independent of the patient's size.[5] For example, small and large patients tend to have equivalent pressures throughout their vascular spaces. Dividing by the CI will give equivalent values for the vascular resistances. If cardiac outputs are used as the denominator, quite different values will be obtained for the resistances, complicating assessment of individual values.

Units used for expression of vascular resistances vary from hospital to hospital. It is simplest, and also perfectly acceptable scientifically, to express the resistances in arbitrary units. We prefer mm Hg $\cdot$ L^{-1} $\cdot$ min $\cdot$ m^2. That is, we divide the difference in pressure by the CI, using the body surface area calculated on the basis of the patient's ideal weight, and use the number so obtained without making any further corrections [see Table 1]. Some prefer to multiply this raw number by 80 to convert the resistances to units in the centimeter-gram-second (CGS) system.

The pulmonary vascular resistance index is more difficult to measure than the systemic vascular resistance index. It is also more likely to change under different conditions. The pulmonary vascular resistance depends on the difference between two relatively small numbers: the mean pulmonary arterial pressure and the PAWP. A slight error in the measurement of either of these pressures can result in a large error in the calculated resistance. Furthermore, the pulmonary arterial pressure and, to a lesser extent, the wedge pressure vary tremendously with phases of ventilation. In patients on mechanical ventilation, swings in pulmonary arterial pressure can exceed 20 mm Hg. It can be difficult for even the most experienced ICU nurse to obtain accurate end-expiration measurements of these pressures. Furthermore, the mode of ventilation can substantially affect the pulmonary vascular resistance index. Hyperinflation of the lungs with mechanical ventilation can compress the intra-alveolar vasculature and increase the pulmonary vascular resistance index.

The variability of the pulmonary vascular resistance makes it difficult to state a specific normal value. Consequently, although we rely heavily on systemic vascular resistance indices to govern care of the patient, pulmonary vascular resistance is less heavily weighted.

AORTIC ROOT AND PULMONARY ARTERIAL END-SYSTOLIC PRESSURE-VOLUME RELATIONS

The aortic root end-systolic pressure-volume relation can be calculated by dividing the left ventricular end-systolic pressure by the stroke volume.[35] The pulmonary arterial end-systolic pressure-volume relation can be determined by dividing the right ventricular end-systolic pressure by the stroke volume. This relation gives a good approximation of the input impedance [see Table 1]. Input impedance reflects the total hindrance that a ventricle faces when it ejects its pulsatile load into a vasculature that has both compliant and resistive elements.[5,36,37]

LEFT VENTRICULAR AND RIGHT VENTRICULAR END-SYSTOLIC PRESSURE-VOLUME RELATIONS

The left ventricular end-systolic pressure-volume relation can be determined by subtracting the left ventricular end-systolic unstressed volume from the left ventricular end-systolic volume and dividing the difference into the left ventricular end-systolic pressure [see Table 1].[30,31] The right ventricular end-systolic pressure-volume relation can be determined in a similar manner. These relations give a good indication of the contractile state of the ventricles.

POWER

The total power delivered into the aorta can be calculated as the left ventricular end-systolic pressure multiplied by the cardiac output, indexed appropriately.[32] The steady-flow aortic power is the mean arterial pressure multiplied by the cardiac output. The oscillatory power is the difference between the total power and the steady-flow power. Of the steady-flow power, a great majority is dissipated as heat in the microvasculature; the amount of heat dissipated can be calculated as the mean arterial pressure minus the central venous pressure multiplied by the cardiac output. The remainder of the steady-flow power fills the right atrium and right ventricle during diastole; this value can be calculated as the central venous pressure multiplied by the cardiac output. Similar formulas [see Table 1] can be used to calculate the power delivered by the right side of the heart into the pulmonary vasculature.

Power calculations are useful; they quantify the energy available for delivery of nutrients to tissues and for delivery of energy to the contralateral heart.

OXYGEN TRANSPORT

Oxygen transport—the amount of oxygen delivered by the heart to the tissues—is calculated by multiplying the cardiac index by the systemic arterial oxygen content (C_aO_2).[1] The calculation is simple, although care must be taken to obtain the correct units. Cardiac indices are typically expressed as liters of blood $\cdot$ min^{-1} $\cdot$ m^{-2}. Oxygen content is usually expressed as ml O_2/100 ml of blood. Multiplying liters of blood $\cdot$ min^{-1} $\cdot$ m^{-2} by milliliters of blood $\cdot$ min^{-1} introduces a factor of 10 (from division of the unit of 100 ml of blood used for expression of oxygen content into the liters of blood used for expression of CI).

For example, in a patient with a normal CI of 3.6 L $\cdot$ min^{-1} $\cdot$ m^{-2}, a normal hemoglobin concentration of 12.5 g/dl, and a normal S_aO_2 of close to 100 percent, normal oxygen transport is 607 ml O_2 $\cdot$ min^{-1} $\cdot$ m^{-2}.

$$\begin{aligned}
O_2 \text{ transport} &= \text{cardiac index} \times \text{arterial } O_2 \text{ content} \\
&= 36 \text{ dl blood} \cdot \text{min}^{-1} \cdot \text{m}^{-2} \times 1.39 \times 12.5 \times 97\% \\
&= 36 \text{ dl blood} \cdot \text{min}^{-1} \cdot \text{m}^{-2} \times 16.9 \text{ ml } O_2/\text{dl blood} \\
&= 607 \text{ ml } O_2 \cdot \text{min}^{-1} \cdot \text{m}^{-2}
\end{aligned}$$

A decrease in CI, the hemoglobin concentration, or S_aO_2 will decrease oxygen transport.

OXYGEN RETURN

The amount of oxygen returned to the heart can be calculated by multiplying the CI by the mixed venous oxygen content ($C_{mv}O_2$). For a normal CI of 3.6 L · min^{-1} · m^{-2}, with a hemoglobin concentration of 12.5 g/dl and an $S_{mv}O_2$ of 75 percent (for a $C_{mv}O_2$ of 13.0 ml/dl), the oxygen return to the heart will be 470 ml O_2 · min^{-1} · m^{-2}.

OXYGEN CONSUMPTION

Oxygen consumption is the difference between oxygen delivered by the heart and oxygen returned to the heart. The formula thus becomes CI multiplied by the difference between the oxygen content in the systemic arterial blood and the oxygen content in the mixed venous blood.

$$\text{Oxygen consumption} = CI \times (C_aO_2 - C_{mv}O_2)$$

Normal oxygen consumption, then, is 140 ml O_2 · min^{-1} · m^{-2} because

$$36 \text{ dl blood} \cdot \text{min}^{-1} \cdot \text{m}^{-2} \times (16.9 - 13.0) \text{ ml } O_2/\text{dl blood}$$
$$= 140 \text{ ml } O_2 \cdot \text{min}^{-1} \cdot \text{m}^{-2}$$

The values given in the examples above are average values only. It is probably easiest to memorize a single normal value, however, rather than ranges of values. As long as the physician recognizes that, for example, an oxygen consumption calculated to be 120 ml · min^{-1} · m^{-2} is close to the average of 140, no harm will be done. An oxygen consumption of 100 ml · min^{-1} · m^{-2}, however, is clearly abnormally low. A value this low should prompt investigation to detect a low CI, a low hemoglobin concentration, or a low C_aO_2 and to correct the abnormality.

BICARBONATE CONCENTRATION

The calculated value for bicarbonate concentration is obtained from measurements of the P_{CO_2} and the hydrogen ion concentration of the blood by using the Henderson-Hasselbalch equation [see 7 Life-Threatening Acid-Base Disorders]. The advantage of this equation is its familiarity; its disadvantage is that it involves the use of logarithms.

It is possible, however, to estimate bicarbonate concentration without using logarithms. The formula is as follows:

$$[HCO_3^-] = 24 \times P_{CO_2} \div [H^+]$$

The formula will give a value for bicarbonate concentration in mmol/L. The P_{CO_2} should be expressed as mm Hg; the hydrogen ion concentration, however, has to be expressed as nmol/L [see Table 3]. Note that most of the values can be obtained by multiplying the preceding value by 0.8. A pH of 7.0 corresponds to a hydrogen ion concentration of 100 nmol/L; a pH of 7.1 corresponds to a hydrogen ion concentration of 80 nmol/L.

Thus, for example, if the P_{CO_2} is 40 mm Hg and the hydrogen ion concentration is 80 nmol/L, the bicarbonate concentration is 12 mmol/L. This bicarbonate concentration closely approximates the actual concentration of bicarbonate in the arterial blood. The value obtained from the clinical laboratories for a venous blood specimen includes all of the compounds involved with dissociation of carbonic acid, including carbonic acid itself, bicarbonate, and carbon dioxide. Thus, the bicarbonate calculated from the blood gases gives a value for a specific compound and is usually of more use than values obtained from the laboratories for a venous specimen.

Table 3 Conversion of pH to Hydrogen Ion Concentration

pH		Hydrogen Ion Concentration (nmol/L)
7.0		100
7.1	100 × 0.8 =	80
7.2	80 × 0.8 =	64
7.3	63 × 0.8 ≈	50
7.4	50 × 0.8 =	40
7.5	40 × 0.8 =	32
7.6	32 × 0.8 ≈	25

Note: values not indicated in the table can be derived by interpolation. For example, a pH of 7.35 corresponds to a hydrogen ion concentration of approximately 45.

INFLUENCE OF AGE AND OTHER VARIABLES

The values given in the example [see Table 1] are for a young patient in normal cardiovascular condition under resting circumstances in a supine position. However, several variables can affect these values, including the patient's age, cardiovascular condition, positioning, consumption of a large meal, mechanical ventilation, and thermal stress.

Age does not affect the resting heart rate, cardiac output, stroke volume, or ventricular end-diastolic volumes [see 75 The Elderly Surgical Patient]. Increased age is associated, however, with increases in ventricular end-systolic pressure and mean and systolic pressures in both the pulmonary and systemic arterial circulations.[38]

The achieving of good cardiovascular condition results in a slower resting heart rate, a larger stroke volume, and larger ventricular end-diastolic volumes.[39] Conditioning does not influence the resting cardiac output or, in an otherwise normal individual, the resting blood pressures.

Assumption of an upright position does not affect the resting heart rate, but it does decrease the cardiac output and the stroke volume by approximately 25 percent.[40]

Consumption of a large meal can slightly increase the cardiac output and oxygen consumption values. Institution of mechanical ventilation can decrease the oxygen consumption by approximately 10 percent. The effects of mechanical ventilation on the other parameters vary depending on the intravascular volume status of the patient. As a rule, mechanical ventilation with tidal volumes of 10 ml/kg decreases the ventricular end-diastolic volumes, the stroke volume, and the cardiac output. These effects can be partially reversed by the infusion of fluid to return the ventricular end-diastolic volumes back toward normal.

Any environment that poses a thermal stress on the patient can influence the values obtained. If the environment is cold enough to produce shivering, oxygen consumption and cardiac output can rise to levels several times greater than those of a normal person. Hypothermia in the absence of shivering decreases the oxygen consumption and the cardiac output. Extreme hypothermia can decrease these values to as low as one fourth of normothermic values. Hyperthermia or systemic inflammation can increase oxygen consumption and cardiac output to values as high as twice those of a normothermic or uninjured or noninfected person, but no higher [see 96 Metabolic Response to Critical Illness].

References

1. Cerra FB: Manual of Critical Care. CV Mosby Co, St Louis, 1987
2. Kofke WA, Levy JH: Postoperative Critical Care Procedures of the Massachusetts General Hospital. Little, Brown & Co, Boston, 1986
3. Gardner RM: Direct blood pressure measurement—dynamic response requirements. Anesthesiology 54:227, 1981
4. Karamanoglu M, O'Rourke MF, Avolio AP, et al: An analysis of the relationship between central aortic and peripheral upper limb pressure waves in man. Eur Heart J 14:160, 1993
5. O'Rourke MF: Vascular impedance in studies of arterial and cardiac function. Physiol Rev 62:570, 1982
6. Klocke RA: Carbon dioxide transport. Handbook of Physiology, Sect 3, Vol 4. American Physiological Society, Bethesda, Maryland, 1987, p 173
7. Andritsch RF, Muravchick S, Gold MI: Temperature correction of arterial blood-gas parameters: a comparative review of methodology. Anesthesiology 55:311, 1981
8. Swain JA: Hypothermia and blood pH: a review. Arch Intern Med 148:1643, 1988
9. Morris AH, Chapman RH, Gardner RM: Frequency of wedge pressure errors in the ICU. Crit Care Med 13:705, 1985
10. Komadina KH, Schenk DA, LaVeau P, et al: Interobserver variability in the interpretation of pulmonary artery catheter pressure tracings. Chest 100:1647, 1991
11. Celoria G, Steingrub JS, Vickers-Lahti M, et al: Clinical assessment of hemodynamic values in two surgical intensive care units. Arch Surg 125:1036, 1990
12. O'Quin R, Marini JJ: Pulmonary artery occlusion pressure: clinical physiology, measurement, and interpretation. Am Rev Respir Dis 128:319, 1983
13. Raper R, Sibbald WJ: Misled by the wedge? the Swan-Ganz catheter and left ventricular preload. Chest 89:427, 1986
14. Alyono D, Ring WS, Chao RYN, et al: Characteristics of ventricular function in severe hemorrhagic shock. Surgery 94:250, 1983
15. Grossman W: Diastolic dysfunction in congestive heart failure. N Engl J Med 325:1557, 1991
16. Natanson C, Fink MP, Ballantyne HK, et al: Gram-negative bacteremia produces both severe systolic and diastolic cardiac dysfunction in a canine model that simulates human septic shock. J Clin Invest 78:259, 1986
17. Stevens JH, Raffin TA, Mihm FG, et al: Thermodilution cardiac output measurement: effects of the respiratory cycle on its reproducibility. JAMA 253:2240, 1985
18. Selzer A, Sudrann RB: Reliability of the determination of cardiac output in man by means of the Fick principle. Circ Res 6:485, 1958
19. Porter JM, Swain ID: Measurement of cardiac output by electrical impedance plethysmography. J Biomed Eng 9:222, 1987
20. Huntsman LL, Stewart DK, Barnes SR, et al: Noninvasive Doppler determination of cardiac output in man. Circulation 67:593, 1983
21. Mark JB, Steinbrook RA, Gugino LD, et al: Continuous noninvasive monitoring of cardiac output with esophageal Doppler ultrasound during cardiac surgery. Anesth Analg 65:1013, 1986
22. Kety SS: Theory and applications of the exchange of inert gas in the lungs and tissues. Pharmacol Rev 3:1, 1951
23. Homer LD, Denysyk B: Estimation of cardiac output by analysis of respiratory gas exchange. J Appl Physiol 39:159, 1975
24. Capek JM, Roy RJ: Noninvasive measurement of cardiac output using partial CO_2 rebreathing. IEEE Trans Biomed Eng 35:633, 1988
25. Diebel LN, Wilson RF, Tagett MG, et al: End-diastolic volume: a better indicator of preload in the critically ill. Arch Surg 127:817, 1992
26. Diebel L, Wilson RF, Heins J, et al: End-diastolic volume versus pulmonary artery wedge pressure in evaluating cardiac preload in trauma patients. J Trauma 37:950, 1994
27. Du Bois EF: The estimation of the surface area of the body. Basal Metabolism in Health and Disease, 3rd ed. Lea & Febiger, Philadelphia, 1936, p 125
28. Feldschuh J, Enson Y: Prediction of the normal blood volume: relation of blood volume to body habitus. Circulation 56:605, 1977
29. West GB, Brown JH, Enquist BJ: A general model for the origin of allometric scaling laws in biology. Science 276(5309):122, 1997
30. Guazzi M, Polese A, Magrini F, et al: Negative influences of ascites on the cardiac function of cirrhotic patients. Am J Med 59:165, 1975
31. Sagawa K: The end-systolic pressure-volume relation of the ventricle: definition, modifications and clinical use (editorial). Circulation 63:1223, 1981
32. Asanoi H, Sasayama S, Kameyama T: Ventriculoarterial coupling in normal and failing heart in humans. Circ Res 65:483, 1989
33. Kelly R, Fitchett D: Noninvasive determination of aortic input impedance and external left ventricular power output: a validation and repeatability study of a new technique. J Am Coll Cardiol 20:952, 1992
34. Kelly R, Hayward C, Avolio A, et al: Noninvasive determination of age-related changes in the human arterial pulse. Circulation 80:1652, 1989
35. Kelly RP, Ting C-T, Yang T-M, et al: Effective arterial elastance as index of arterial vascular load in humans. Circulation 86:513, 1992
36. O'Rourke MF, Kelly RP: Wave reflection in the systemic circulation and its implications in ventricular function. J Hypertens 11:327, 1993
37. Piene H: Pulmonary arterial impedance and right ventricular function. Physiol Rev 66:606, 1986
38. Avolio AP, Chen S-G, Wang R-P, et al: Effects of aging on changing arterial compliance and left ventricular load in a northern Chinese urban community. Circulation 68:50, 1983
39. Ogawa T, Spina RJ, Martin WH III, et al: Effects of aging, sex, and physical training on cardiovascular responses to exercise. Circulation 86:494, 1992
40. Bevegård S, Holmgren A, Jonsson B: The effect of body position on the circulation at rest and during exercise, with special reference to the influence on the stroke volume. Acta Physiol Scand 49:279, 1960

Acknowledgments

Figure 1   Albert Miller.

Figure 2   Top, Dana Burns-Pizer; bottom, Albert Miller.

Figure 3   Top and bottom, Dana Burns-Pizer; center, Albert Miller.

Figures 4 and 5   Albert Miller.

Figure 6   Carol Donner.

Figures 7 through 9   Albert Miller.

Figure 10   Carol Donner.

Figure 11   Albert Miller.

Figure 12   Dana Burns-Pizer.

90 SUPPORT OF THE FAILING HEART

Charles L. Rice, M.D., and R. John Solaro, Ph.D.

Approach to the Failing Heart

The sole purpose of the heart's electrical and mechanical activity is to provide adequate organ perfusion. When there is evidence of inadequate perfusion of more than one organ, cardiac function must be evaluated. The classic manifestations of shock, which are discussed elsewhere [*see 4 Shock*], are one indication of inadequate perfusion. The failing heart may also show evidence of left-sided heart failure (pulmonary edema), right-sided heart failure (peripheral edema, hepatic congestion, and distended neck veins), or both.

The principal determinants of cardiac output are preload (the volume presented to the heart), afterload (the resistance against which the heart must pump), and the inotropic state (the extent to which cells can contract against the preload). When a patient with circulatory instability is encountered, the first step must always be to verify that the patient's intravascular volume is adequate [*see 4 Shock*]. Measurement of the central venous pressure (CVP) is useful for this determination. If the CVP is low and the patient is hypotensive, volume replacement is the therapy of choice. If the CVP is high and the patient is hypotensive, insertion of a thermodilution Swan-Ganz catheter and measurement of the pulmonary arterial occlusion pressure (PAOP) and cardiac output are crucial [*see 89 Cardiopulmonary Monitoring*].

If the PAOP and the cardiac index are both elevated, the patient has most likely been overresuscitated. Volume infusion should be dramatically slowed. Patients who have pulmonary edema should also receive furosemide in a dose of 20 to 40 mg intravenously. Although there is a temptation to provide catecholamines (e.g., norepinephrine) to profoundly hypotensive patients in this situation, there is no evidence that this therapy is beneficial.

If the PAOP is low but the cardiac index is high, consider as underlying causes sepsis, anaphylaxis, and hepatic or autonomic dysfunction.

If the pulmonary arterial occlusion pressure and the cardiac index are both low, administer lactated Ringer's solution to raise the occlusion pressure by 3 to 5 mm Hg. Remeasure the cardiac index; if it is improving, continue volume resuscitation until the patient stabilizes.

If the PAOP is high and the cardiac index is low, the decision whether to administer an inotropic agent or an afterload-reducing agent is based on the adequacy of systemic arterial pressure. If the patient is normotensive, systemic vascular resistance is elevated, and afterload reduction can be employed.

There is no single, all-purpose cardiotonic agent that will meet every clinical situation. It is possible, however, to choose an agent or, occasionally, a combination of agents that best meets the patient's needs.

Afterload-Reducing Agents

SODIUM NITROPRUSSIDE

Sodium nitroprusside is valuable for reducing afterload. It is usually prepared by adding a 50 mg vial to 500 ml of five percent dextrose in water, for a final concentration of 100 µg/ml. Sodium nitroprusside's onset of action is rapid (usually one to two minutes), and its effect disappears almost immediately once the infusion is stopped. Resistance, tolerance, and tachyphylaxis are rare.[1] The infusion is begun at 0.5 µg/kg/min and titrated in 0.5 µg increments until the desired effect is achieved. Ideally, the reduction in systemic vascular resistance should result in improved cardiac output, so that the net effect on systemic arterial pressure should be minimal. It is advisable, however, to prevent the systolic blood pressure from falling below 80 mm Hg. Sodium nitroprusside administration also causes venous pooling, which, along with the unloading of the left ventricle, generally results in a lowered PAOP.

When sodium nitroprusside, which contains ferrous ion, reacts with sulfhydryl-containing compounds in erythrocytes, cyanide is produced. In the liver, cyanide is converted to less toxic thiocyanate, which is then excreted by the kidneys. Toxicity is caused by poisoning of the cytochrome system and occurs when the rate of cyanide production exceeds the rate of conversion to thiocyanate. Toxic reactions most often occur when the rate of sodium nitroprusside infusion exceeds 10 µg/kg/min or when administration is continued at lower rates for several days. The first manifestation of cyanide toxicity is usually a reduction in oxygen consumption over the course of a few hours. Although

Approach to the Failing Heart

Patient is hemodynamically unstable:
- MAP < 65 mm Hg
- Urine output < 0.5 ml/kg/hr
- Evidence of inadequate organ perfusion
- CNS status confused or comatose

Measure central venous pressure.

CVP < 12 mm Hg; pulmonary edema is absent

Give volume (e.g., lactated Ringer's solution or blood) until CVP increases to 12 mm Hg or until organ perfusion improves at a lower CVP.

CVP > 12 mm Hg

Insert thermodilution Swan-Ganz catheter; measure PAOP and cardiac index.

PAOP > 15 mm Hg; CI > 3 L/min/m²

Decrease volume infusion; give furosemide, 20–40 mg I.V., if pulmonary edema is present.

PAOP < 5 mm Hg; CI > 3 L/min/m²

No evidence of heart disease. Consider sepsis, anaphylaxis, and hepatic or autonomic dysfunction.

PAOP < 5 mm Hg; CI < 2 L/min/m²

Give volume (e.g., lactated Ringer's solution) to raise PAOP by 3–5 mm Hg. Remeasure CI.

PAOP > 15 mm Hg; CI < 2 L/min/m²

Measure blood pressure and calculate systemic vascular resistance.

CI improves

Continue volume resuscitation until patient is hemodynamically stable.

PAOP rises; CI remains low (< 2 L/min/m²)

Measure blood pressure and calculate systemic vascular resistance.

Patient is normotensive or hypertensive (SVR high)

Start afterload reduction: give sodium nitroprusside, 0.5 μg/kg/min I.V. to start; then increase until CI increases; maintain systolic BP > 80 mm Hg. During sodium nitroprusside administration, continuous arterial pressure monitoring is strongly recommended.

Patient is hypotensive, or afterload reduction has not increased CI

Give an inotropic agent, such as dobutamine, 5 μg/kg/min I.V. Increase up to 15 μg/kg/min until CI becomes adequate for organ perfusion or until ventricular ectopy develops.

No response

Give amrinone, 0.75 mg/kg over 3–5 min; then begin maintenance infusion, 5–10 μg/kg/min. (Loading dose may be omitted if BP is tenuous.)

No response

Consider intra-aortic balloon counterpulsation.

this reduction in oxygen consumption is not clinically apparent, it may be signaled by an otherwise unexplained rise in mixed venous oxygen tension or saturation or by a decrease in the calculated oxygen consumption. Treatment must be rapid to be effective and consists of administration of sodium nitrite (10 ml of a three percent solution). Sodium nitrite converts hemoglobin to methemoglobin, and the ferric ion in methemoglobin competes with the ferric ion in cytochrome for the cyanide ion. Methemoglobin is then reduced by the prompt administration (after administration of sodium nitrite) of methylene blue (1 mg/kg over five minutes), which induces the enzyme methemoglobin reductase. Thiocyanate is generally well tolerated up to levels of 10 mg/dl, but higher levels of thiiocyanate may necessitate hemodialysis.

NITROGLYCERIN

In patients in whom both preload and afterload are elevated (and especially in those with accompanying pulmonary edema), consideration should be given to the administration of nitroglycerin, a potent dilator of arteriolar and venous smooth muscle.[2] At lower concentrations (5 to 15 µg/min), the venous effect predominates, so that the principal effect is on preload. Infusion should be started at 5 µg/min and titrated to effect. The maximum rate is generally about 300 µg/min. Because nitroglycerin (like sodium nitroprusside) is a potent vasodilator, intravenous use requires monitoring of filling pressures, arterial pressure, and cardiac output; the principal adverse effects of administration are related to a too rapid reduction in these parameters. Should adverse effects occur, a reduction in dosage (or a temporary cessation of the infusion) results in rapid reversal.

GANGLIONIC BLOCKING AGENTS

Arterial pressure can be reduced by blockade of the autonomic ganglia responsible for maintenance of arteriolar tone.[3] The most important ganglionic blocking agent is trimethaphan camsylate. Although this drug has been used for rapid reduction in arterial pressure, it also reduces myocardial contractility. This property makes it useful for the control of hypertension in patients with acute aortic dissection but limits its value in the management of a failing heart. An additional disadvantage is the abrupt onset of tachyphylaxis. Trimethaphan may occasionally be useful, however, in those few patients who are resistant to sodium nitroprusside. It is generally administered at a rate of 0.3 to 3.0 mg/min.

ANGIOTENSIN-CONVERTING ENZYME INHIBITORS

Angiotensin-converting enzyme (ACE) is responsible for the conversion of angiotensin I to angiotensin II. Angiotensin II is a potent vasoconstrictor; in addition, it stimulates aldosterone secretion by the adrenal cortex. In a patient with congestive heart failure, therefore, inhibition of ACE has therapeutic benefit.

A recent study in patients with severe congestive heart failure and mitral regurgitation examined the effect of enalaprilat.[4] Afterload reduction was prompt and sustained, with improved cardiac index and decreased mitral regurgitation in the most severely ill patients. Enalaprilat is administered in a dosage of 1.25 mg I.V. every six hours (the dosage is lowered in patients with renal failure). Hypotension may occasionally result but is usually mild and self-limited.

ACE inhibitors are now an important adjunct in the management of patients with congestive heart failure, and initiation of treatment in the intensive care unit appears to be both safe and effective.

Inotropic Agents

If the patient is hypotensive or if afterload reduction has not resulted in increased cardiac output, an inotropic agent should be administered. This class of agents has been the subject of intense research activity during the 1980s and 1990s, with the development of a number of new agents and a better understanding of some of the older ones.[5,6]

CATECHOLAMINES

Catecholamines act on the heart by stimulating beta receptors; they act on the peripheral vasculature by activating alpha$_1$- and beta$_2$-adrenergic receptors, as well as D$_1$ and D$_2$ dopamine receptors [see Table 1]. The effects of these adrenergic agonists

Table 1 Cardiovascular Effects of Adrenergic Stimulation

Receptor Site	Heart	Systemic Arteries	Pulmonary Arteries	Veins
Alpha$_1$	0	↑Constriction (+++)*	↑Constriction (+)	↑Constriction (++)
Beta$_1$	↑Rate (++) ↑Contractility (+++) ↑Atrioventricular conduction (+++)	0	Constriction†	0
Beta$_2$	?↑Rate ?↑Contractility	Dilatation (++)	Dilatation (+)	Dilatation (++)
D$_1$ dopamine	0	Dilatation (++)	Dilatation (++)	0
D$_2$ dopamine	↓Rate‡	Dilatation†	?	?

*Plus symbols (+) indicate relative potency of effect.
†Indirect effect: mediated by increased renin secretion in the kidneys.
‡Indirect effect: inhibition of norepinephrine.

Table 2 Receptor Types Stimulated by Adrenergic Agonists

Agonist	Alpha$_1$	Beta$_1$	Beta$_2$	D$_1$ Dopamine	D$_2$ Dopamine
Epinephrine	++++*	+++	++	0	0
Norepinephrine	+++	+++	0	0	0
Isoproterenol	0	++++	++++	0	0
Dopamine†	++	+++	0	++++	++++
Dobutamine	0	++++	++	0	0
Ibopamine	+	+	+	++	++
Fenoldopam	0	0	0	++	0
Dopexamine	0	+	++++	+++	+++
Propylbutyldopamine	+	0	0	++	++++

*Plus symbols (+) indicate relative degree of stimulation.
†The action of dopamine is dose dependent.

vary according to their relative selectivity for specific receptors [*see Table 2*].

Dobutamine

Dobutamine, a synthetic sympathomimetic amine, is a potent inotropic agent that has less tendency to produce tachycardia or arrhythmias than does dopamine.[7,8] Dobutamine does have some peripheral vasodilating effects, but they are generally seen only at higher infusion rates (> 20 µg/kg/min). Ordinarily, an infusion rate of 5 to 15 µg/kg/min is sufficient to achieve the maximum inotropic effect. Infusion rates in excess of 15 µg/kg/min are likely to be accompanied by arrhythmias because of increased myocardial oxygen consumption.[9]

Dopamine

Dopamine is a naturally occurring precursor of epinephrine and norepinephrine that has several pharmacological effects, including increased heart rate, increased contractility, and peripheral vasoconstriction. Its effect on renal perfusion is controversial.[10] In general, it is of greatest use in those situations in which arterial pressure is insufficient to perfuse the brain, heart, or kidneys. It is given by continuous infusion; rates lower than 8 µg/kg/min are associated with maximum inotropic effect. At higher infusion rates, the peripheral vasoconstrictive effect predominates, increasing afterload and myocardial oxygen consumption. Dopamine is therefore less useful at these high doses when the predominant effect sought is inotropic support.

Dopexamine

Dopexamine, another synthetic inotropic agent, stimulates beta$_2$-adrenergic receptors and D$_1$ and D$_2$ dopamine receptors, producing both inotropic and vasodilating effects. Unlike dopamine, dopexamine does not stimulate alpha$_1$ receptors. In a study from Europe of patients who had undergone coronary artery bypass surgery, administration of dopexamine resulted in increased cardiac output (as a consequence of increased heart rate rather than increased stroke volume).[11] Systemic vascular resistance was unchanged. This study and others suggest that dosages higher than 5 µg/kg/min offer no additional benefit. Dopexamine for this use has not yet been approved by the Food and Drug Administration.

Epinephrine

Epinephrine was discovered in 1895. It is a naturally occurring, extremely potent alpha- and beta-adrenergic agonist. When administered intravenously, it produces a dose-dependent increase in both systolic and diastolic blood pressure, although systolic pressure is generally increased more than diastolic pressure. These increases in pressure are caused by the increases in heart rate and myocardial contractility (beta$_1$ effects) and an increase in peripheral vasoconstriction (an alpha$_1$ effect). Because of these increases in both peripheral vasoconstriction and heart rate, myocardial oxygen consumption is dramatically increased, and arrhythmias are common, limiting the usefulness of epinephrine for supporting the failing heart. If the patient is unresponsive to more selective agents, however, and particularly if the patient has profound hypotension, epinephrine may be of some limited value. It is titrated intravenously at a rate of 0.01 mg/kg/min, but the clinician must be alert to the development of malignant ventricular arrhythmias and severe hypertension (which will be short-lived).

Norepinephrine

Norepinephrine, also known as levarterenol, is a potent alpha$_1$- and beta$_1$-adrenergic agonist but a much weaker beta$_2$ agonist. Thus, its most pronounced effects are on peripheral vascular resistance. Norepinephrine may elevate blood pressure, but it usually causes cardiac output to fall. Its primary value, therefore, is in support of mean arterial pressure in a patient whose cardiac output is increased but whose blood pressure is too low to perfuse the pressure-dependent vascular beds in the heart, brain, and kidneys. Such situations are uncommon.

Isoproterenol

Isoproterenol is a powerful beta agonist that has virtually no effect on alpha receptors. When administered intravenously, therefore, it produces both peripheral vasodilatation (a $beta_2$ effect) and increases in heart rate and myocardial contractility ($beta_1$ effects). Although it is of some immediate benefit for complete heart block, its usefulness as an inotropic agent is outweighed by its arrhythmogenic potential; arrhythmia results from increased myocardial oxygen consumption that greatly exceeds increased cardiac output.

Mephentermine, Metaraminol, and Phenylephrine

Mephentermine, metaraminol, and phenylephrine all primarily produce peripheral vasoconstriction. None has any useful role in support of the failing heart, and all have potential for greatly increasing myocardial ischemia because of their effect on afterload.

PHOSPHODIESTERASE INHIBITORS

Amrinone

Amrinone is representative of a class of agents known as phosphodiesterase inhibitors.[12] Although its mechanism of action is not yet fully understood, it appears to inhibit the breakdown of intracellular cyclic adenosine monophosphate (cAMP).[13] Given intravenously, amrinone increases cardiac output and reduces afterload and preload.[14] It does not usually cause tachycardia or arrhythmias except when administered at higher doses. For these reasons, it is extremely useful in the acute management of refractory congestive heart failure. The recommended loading dose of amrinone is 0.75 mg/kg over three to five minutes, followed by continuous maintenance infusion of 5 to 10 µg/kg/min. Care must be taken when therapy with amrinone is initiated, however, because it is a potent vasodilator and patients frequently become profoundly hypotensive. In our experience, merely beginning with the maintenance infusion and titrating to effect appears to yield satisfactory results. Because the half-life of the drug is brief, stopping the infusion in the event of profound hypotension usually results in a return of blood pressure to preinfusion levels. Administration can then be resumed if the loading dose is omitted and the infusion rate is decreased. Amrinone is less useful for long-term therapy because of gastrointestinal side effects and thrombocytopenia. A few patients appear to benefit from the combination of dobutamine and amrinone.

Milrinone

Milrinone is related to amrinone, and its mechanism of action is similar.[15] It is approximately 20 times more potent in its inotropic effects than amrinone and has fewer side effects. Milrinone also has arteriolar and venous dilator activity. It is administered in an initial loading dose of 50 µg/kg over 10 minutes, followed by a maintenance infusion of 0.375 to 0.75 µg/kg/min. In one study comparing milrinone with dobutamine in patients with severe congestive heart failure, milrinone produced a sustained decline in PAOP and a prolonged improvement in stroke volume.[16] Dobutamine, on the other hand, resulted in tachycardia in 25 percent of patients, and increases in stroke volume disappeared after about 12 hours. This study suggests that milrinone may be of value in some patients with severe congestive heart failure who are unresponsive to or intolerant of dobutamine.

Enoximone

Enoximone is another phosphodiesterase inhibitor, with actions similar to those of milrinone and amrinone, although at least one study suggests that it may be a more potent inotropic agent.[17] A study that evaluated the combination therapy of moderate-dose dobutamine and enoximone in patients with severe congestive heart failure demonstrated that such therapy produced synergistic effects that outweighed the benefits of either drug used alone.[18] Enoximone has not yet been approved by the FDA for clinical use.

CALCIUM SENSITIZERS

Another class of inotropic agents, calcium sensitizers, or inodilators, both inhibits phosphodiesterase activity and acts directly on the cardiac myofilaments to increase their responsiveness to calcium.[19] The phosphodiesterase inhibitory activity is associated with smooth muscle relaxation. One example of this class of agents is pimobendan, which is in clinical use in Japan and is undergoing clinical trials in the United States. Another example is MCI-154, an agent being developed in Japan. Both of these agents increase cardiac contraction to the same extent as isoproterenol, but they cause only a minimal increase in the amount of calcium released during a cardiac cycle. Pimobendan and MCI-154 also increase the calcium-binding affinity of troponin C, the myofilament calcium receptor, and both are thought to reduce the energy cost of nonmechanical work.

COLFORSIN

Another agent under study is colforsin (forskolin), which directly activates the catalytic unit of adenylate cyclase. It also reduces cardiac afterload and produces venous pooling, thereby decreasing preload. In one study comparing colforsin with dobutamine and sodium nitroprusside in patients with severe congestive cardiomyopathy, patients treated with colforsin demonstrated a 70 percent increase in stroke volume—greater than the increases seen with either dobutamine or nitroprusside.[20] The drug has not yet been approved for this use by the FDA, but further studies are under way.[21]

CALCIUM

The calcium ion plays a central role in the development of contractile force in all muscles, including the heart. Although calcium administration has been widely employed for inadequate myocardial function, clinical improvement is relatively rare.[22] Moreover, because calcium administration increases arteriolar vasoconstriction, local ischemia and increased afterload may result from its use. In addition, excessive influx of calcium into myocardial cells results in muscle necrosis.[23] Routine administration of calcium in cardiopulmonary resuscitation is therefore no longer recommended.[24]

filaments, bind to actin, and, in a reaction powered by the splitting of adenosine triphosphate (ATP) into adenosine diphosphate and inorganic phosphage, tilt and impel the thin filaments toward the center of the sarcomere [see Figures 1 and 2]. The force generated is directly proportional to the number of cross-bridges reacting with the thin filaments.

In diastole, intracellular calcium is very low, and the actin cross-bridge reaction is blocked by the position of tropomyosin on the thin filament. Tropomyosin is held in this blocking position by the action of components of the troponin complex. When no calcium is bound, troponin C binds weakly to the thin filament, whereas the inhibitory protein troponin I binds strongly to actin and the tropomyosin-binding protein troponin T binds strongly to tropomyosin. These strong bonds are weakened when calcium binds to troponin C to promote a tight binding between troponin C and troponin I and between troponin C and troponin T.

The contractile state of the heart can be understood in terms of the myofilament activation by calcium. The binding of calcium to troponin C activates one functional unit that consists of a cross-bridge, actin, tropomyosin, and troponin in a ratio of 1:7:1:1. In basal inotropic states, enough calcium is released to the myofilaments to activate about 20 percent of the cross-bridges. Thus, there is a reserve of cross-bridges that can be recruited to participate in the contraction. This recruitment can happen in two ways: by the release of more calcium or by a change in the responsiveness of myofilaments to a given level of calcium.

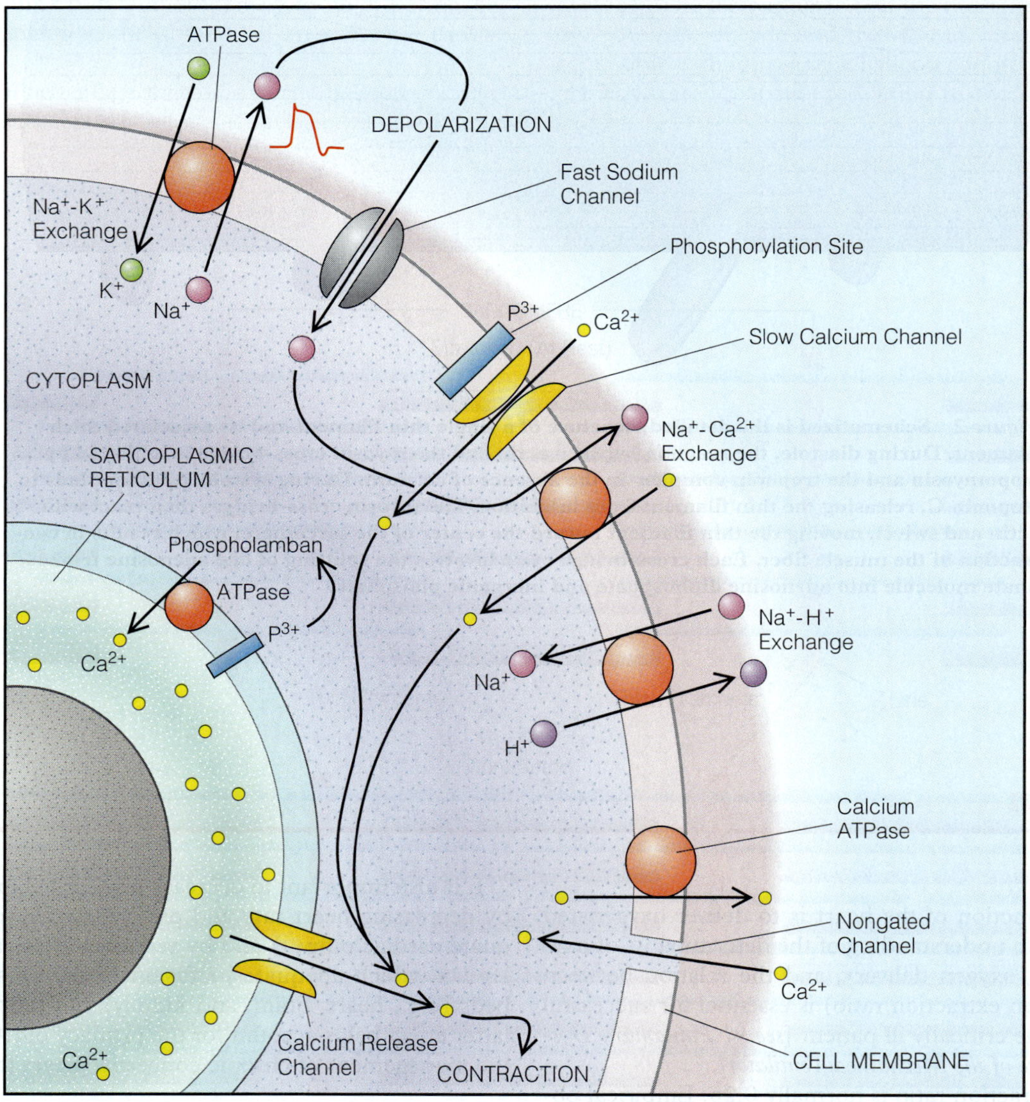

Figure 3 Ionic flux occurs via several pathways across the cell membrane and from within the sarcoplasmic reticulum. When the cell membrane is depolarized, calcium and sodium move into the cytoplasm. Sodium is exchanged for calcium, and additional calcium is released into the myofilament space from the sarcoplasmic reticulum, which provides ample amounts of calcium for binding with troponin. During repolarization, the process is reversed.

Calcium entry into and exit from the myofilaments occur across the cell surface membrane and across an internal, enclosed membrane network, the sarcoplasmic reticulum [see Figure 3]. During systole, calcium entry into the myofilament space from the interstitial space occurs via (1) voltage-sensitive channels (L-type channels), (2) a voltage-sensitive sodium-calcium exchange protein, and (3) nongated calcium channels. Calcium entry into the myofilament space from storage sites in the sarcoplasmic reticulum compartment occurs through a calcium-release channel that is gated by calcium. Depolarization of myocardial cells results in the opening of fast sodium channels. As the cell depolarizes, calcium channels open, the sodium-calcium exchanger reverses, and there is a relatively small and rapid net movement of calcium into the cell. These calcium ions gate the calcium-release channels of the sarcoplasmic reticulum, resulting in a relatively large release of calcium, which binds to troponin C and activates the myofilaments. Extrusion of calcium from the myofilament space during relaxation occurs primarily via a calcium–adenosine triphosphatase (ATPase) pump in the sarcoplasmic reticulum membrane but also through the sodium-calcium exchanger and through a surface-membrane calcium-ATPase pump.

Transmembrane ionic channels governing sodium movement play an important, albeit indirect, role in calcium homeostasis; these channels are (1) the fast sodium channel, (2) the Na^+-K^+-ATPase pump, which exchanges intracellular sodium for extracellular potassium, and (3) a sodium-hydrogen exchange protein. Thus, one of the more important mechanisms for increasing intracellular calcium is linked to the concentration of intracellular sodium. It follows that any process that increases intracellular sodium will act indirectly to increase intracellular calcium.

Cyclic adenosine monophosphate is a critically important intracellular regulator of calcium transport.[28] It is generated by the enzyme adenylate cyclase,[29] which is located in the cell membrane, and it is metabolized by a variety of phosphodiesterases. Increases in the intracellular level of cAMP result in enhanced movement of calcium through the slow channels and an increase in calcium that is stored in the sarcoplasmic reticulum.

INOTROPIC AGENTS

It should be apparent from this sequence of events that three of the most important variables governing myocardial contraction are the availability of intracellular calcium (to permit actin-myosin interaction), the response of the myofilaments to calcium, and the availability of ATP (to provide energy for both contraction and relaxation). Inotropic agents exert their actions primarily by increasing the intracellular calcium concentration.[5] This increase may result from an inhibition of Na^+-K^+ ATPase, which increases the level of intracellular sodium and, hence, exchange for calcium. Most investigators think that this mechanism underlies the activity of the cardiac glycosides.[25] This indirect effect of cardiac glycosides on the calcium level may explain their relative lack of potency.

A second mechanism that increases the intracellular calcium level is the stimulation of cAMP production by beta agonists. Agents such as isoproterenol, epinephrine, dopamine, and dobutamine bind to the $beta_1$ receptor, which is coupled to adenylate cyclase, an enzyme that mediates cAMP production. Levels of cAMP rise to activate kinases that phosphorylate the calcium channels (promoting their open state) and phospholamban, a protein that regulates calcium pumping by the sarcoplasmic reticulum ATPase. Both of these phosphorylations increase calcium entry into the myofilament space.

A third mechanism that increases intracellular calcium concentration is inhibition of phosphodiesterase, which degrades cAMP. Like adenylate cyclase stimulation, phosphodiesterase inhibition increases the intracellular calcium level and, hence, results in increased contractile force. This mechanism is thought to underlie the action of newer inotropic agents, such as amrinone, milrinone, and enoximone. Some of these agents may also enhance myofilament response to calcium.

PRELOAD

Within limits, the contractility of the myocardium varies directly with resting muscle length. In the intact heart, resting length is primarily dependent on end-diastolic volume, which is generally related to end-diastolic pressure. The relation between resting muscle length and the tension developed by contracting heart muscle is referred to as the Frank-Starling relation and is widely employed in clinical practice. When using this relation, however, it is essential to remember that measurement of left ventricular end-diastolic volume (LVEDV) is difficult and that the most widely used index—PAOP—is subject to a number of assumptions and confounding factors.[1] Notable among these factors are the influences of increased airway pressure, myocardial ischemia, and mitral valve disease on PAOP measurement and interpretation. These conditions may make PAOP high when LVEDV is low. Hence, in clinical practice, Frank-Starling curves must be interpreted with great caution.[30]

AFTERLOAD

The resistance against which the ventricle must pump is reflected primarily by the mean arterial pressure. Laplace's law states that the wall tension of a cylinder is directly proportional to the radius and to the pressure supported by the wall. Hence, left ventricular afterload increases with enlargement of the left ventricle (which increases the radius) and with increasing mean arterial pressure. Because wall tension, along with heart rate, is a prime determinant of myocardial oxygen consumption, it follows that reduction in afterload will beneficially decrease work done by the ischemic heart. This provides the rationale for afterload-reduction therapy for both acute and chronic heart failure.

References

1. Rudd P, Blaschke TF: Anti-hypertensive agents and the drug therapy of hypertension. The Pharmacologic Basis of Therapeutics, 7th ed. Gilman AG, Goodman LS, Roll TW, et al, Eds. Macmillan Publishing Co, New York, 1985, p 784
2. Leier CV, Bambach D, Thompson MJ, et al: Central and regional hemodynamic effects of intravenous isosorbide dinitrate, nitroglycerin and nitroprusside in patients with congestive heart failure. Am J Cardiol 48:1115, 1981
3. Salem MR: Therapeutic uses of ganglionic blocking drugs. Int Anesthesiol Clin 16:171, 1978
4. Varriale P, David W, Chryssos BE: Hemodynamic response to intravenous enalaprilat in patients with severe congestive heart failure and mitral regurgitation. Clin Cardiol 16:235, 1993
5. Collucci WS, Wright RF, Braunwald E: New positive inotropic agents in the treatment of congestive heart failure: mechanisms of action and recent clinical development (pt 1). N Engl J Med 314:290, 1986
6. Leier CV: General overview and update of positive inotropic therapy. Am J Med 81(suppl 4C):40, 1986
7. Leier CV, Unverferth DV: Drugs five years later: dobutamine. Ann Intern Med 99:490, 1983
8. Gray R, Shah PK, Singh B, et al: Low cardiac output states after open heart surgery: comparative effects of dobutamine, dopamine, and norepinephrine plus phentolamine. Chest 80:16, 1981
9. Monrad ES, Baim DS, Smith HS, et al: Milrinone, dobutamine, and nitroprusside: comparative effects on hemodynamics and myocardial energetics in patients with severe congestive heart failure. Circulation 73(suppl 3):168, 1986
10. Goldberg LI: Dopamine: clinical uses of an endogenous catecholamine. N Engl J Med 291:707, 1974
11. Friedel N, Wenzel R, Matheis G, et al: Haemodynamic effects of different doses of dopexamine hydrochloride in low cardiac output states following cardiac surgery. Eur Heart J 13:1271, 1992
12. Benotti JR, Grossman W, Braunwald E, et al: Hemodynamic assessment of amrinone: a new inotropic agent. N Engl J Med 299:1373, 1978
13. Endoh M, Yamashita S, Taira N: Positive inotropic effect of amrinone in relation to cyclic nucleotide metabolism in the canine ventricular muscle. J Pharmacol Exp Ther 221:775, 1982
14. Silke B, Verma SP, Midtbo KA, et al: Comparative hemodynamic dose-response effects of dobutamine and amrinone in left ventricular failure complicating acute myocardial infarction. J Cardiovasc Pharmacol 9:19, 1987
15. Earl CQ, Linden J, Weglicki WB: Biochemical mechanisms for the inotropic effect of the cardiotonic drug milrinone. J Cardiovasc Pharmacol 8:864, 1986
16. Mager G, Klocke RK, Kux A, et al: Phosphodiesterase III inhibition or adrenoreceptor stimulation: milrinone as an alternative to dobutamine in the treatment of severe heart failure. Am Heart J 121:1974, 1991
17. Installe E, De Coster P, Gonzalez M, et al: Comparison between the positive inotropic effects of enoximone, a cardiac phosphodiesterase III inhibitor, and dobutamine in patients with moderate to severe congestive heart failure. Eur Heart J 12:985, 1991
18. Thuillez C, Richard C, Teboul JL, et al: Arterial hemodynamics and cardiac effects of enoximone, dobutamine, and their combination in severe heart failure. Am Heart J 125:799, 1993
19. Rüegg JC, Solaro RJ: Calcium-sensitizing positive inotropic drugs. Heart Failure: Basic and Clinical Aspects. Gwathmey JK, Briggs GM, Allen PD, Eds. Marcel Dekker, New York, 1993, p 457
20. Baumann G, Felix S, Sattelberger U, et al: Cardiovascular effects of forskolin (HL 362) in patients with idiopathic congestive cardiomyopathy: a comparative study with dobutamine and sodium nitroprusside. J Cardiovasc Pharmacol 16:93, 1990
21. Mulieri LA, Leavitt BJ, Martin BJ, et al: Myocardial force-frequency defect in mitral regurgitation heart failure is reversed by forskolin. Circulation 88:2700, 1993
22. Hughes WG, Ruedy JR: Should calcium be used in cardiac arrest? Am J Med 81:285, 1986
23. Winegar CD, White BC: Physiology of resuscitation. Emerg Med Clin North Am 1:479, 1983
24. National Conference on Cardiopulmonary Resuscitation (CPR) and Emergency Cardiac Care (ECC) standards and guidelines for cardiopulmonary resuscitation (CPR) and emergency cardiac care (ECC): III. Adult advanced cardiac life support. JAMA 255:2933, 1986
25. Noble D: Mechanism of action of therapeutic levels of cardiac glycosides. Cardiovasc Res 14:495, 1980
26. Bregman D, Kaskel P: Intra-aortic balloon counterpulsation in refractory shock. Trauma: Emergency Surgery and Critical Care. Siegel JH, Ed. Churchill Livingstone, New York, 1987, p 331
27. Naunheim KS, Swartz MT, Pennington DG, et al: Intraaortic balloon pumping in patients requiring cardiac operations: risk analysis and long-term follow-up. J Thorac Cardiovasc Surg 104:1654, 1992
28. Osterrieder W, Brum G, Hescheler J, et al: Injection of subunits of cyclic AMP–dependent protein kinase into cardiac myocytes modulates Ca^{2+} current. Nature 298:576, 1982
29. Katz AM: Cyclic adenosine monophosphate effects on the myocardium: a man who blows hot and cold with one breath. J Am Coll Cardiol 2:143, 1983
30. Hansen RM, Viquerat CE, Matthay MA, et al: Poor correlation between pulmonary arterial wedge pressure and left ventricular end-diastolic volume after coronary artery bypass graft surgery. Anesthesiology 64:764, 1986

Acknowledgment

Figures 1, 2, and 3   Tom Moore.

91 PULMONARY DYSFUNCTION

Robert H. Demling, M.D.

Approach to Management of Pulmonary Dysfunction

Respiratory injury in surgical patients is usually acute in onset and is associated with a number of different primary diseases. Although some surgical patients with respiratory dysfunction have a history of chronic lung disease, most had normal pulmonary function before the onset of the surgical disease. The initial etiology of respiratory injury varies according to the disease involved, but the final physiologic and clinical manifestations are remarkably constant. Treatment modalities for a wide variety of respiratory syndromes are also relatively constant.

Each of the disease states that will be described can induce moderate to severe pulmonary dysfunction. The diagnosis of acute respiratory failure, which by definition usually necessitates mechanical ventilatory support, is based on the magnitude of the pulmonary abnormalities. Certain diagnostic criteria have been established [see Table 1]. It is not necessary, however, that all the criteria be met before the diagnosis is made or before endotracheal intubation and mechanical ventilation are instituted.

Initial Support Measures

ENDOTRACHEAL INTUBATION

There are four indications for controlling the airway by endotracheal intubation (the so-called rule of four P's): (1) impaired airway patency, (2) inadequate airway protection, (3) inadequate pulmonary toilet, and (4) requirement for positive pressure ventilation. Each of these is an absolute indication for intubation. Current and anticipated problems that may affect airway patency must be considered; for example, with direct injury from trauma or burns, one must anticipate mucosal edema or external compression by edema or hemorrhage. The objective is to secure the airway before the anticipated problem occurs. The adequacy of airway protection—in particular, protection from aspiration—depends on neurologic status as well as on the structural integrity of the larynx and the ability of the epiglottis to protect the airway. Pulmonary toilet is the clearance of secretions to avoid airway obstruction, atelectasis, and infection. If coughing is inadequate, direct airway access must be obtained for suctioning. Patients with an adequate cough but with voluminous secretions (e.g., those with inhalation injury) may also require intubation to avoid the fatigue attendant on the increased work of breathing. The tube selected should be of sufficient size (7 mm internal diameter or wider) to allow adequate suctioning while minimizing airflow resistance; the larger the diameter of the tube, the less the resistance to airflow. Positive pressure ventilation, which is indicated when spontaneous ventilation is inadequate, can be provided by continuous positive airway pressure (CPAP) with spontaneous breathing or by mechanical ventilation with or without positive end-expiratory pressure (PEEP).

Choice of Intubation Route

The choice of intubation route depends on the presence or absence of spontaneous breathing, on the skill of the physician, and on circumstances that may favor a particular approach [see Table 2]. In general, the initial choice is between nasal and oral routes. Endotracheal tubes provide adequate airway access and can be safely left in place for three to four weeks, after which patients requiring continued airway access should undergo tracheostomy. Patients with facial and neck injuries and those with copious airway secretions and large particulate debris (as seen in severe necrotizing inhalation injury) do better when

Table 1 Criteria for Diagnosis of Acute Respiratory Failure

Parameter	Normal Range	Respiratory Failure
Respiratory rate	12–20	> 35
Vital capacity (ml/kg body wt)*	65–75	< 15
FEV_1 (ml/kg body wt)*	50–60	≤ 10
Inspiratory force (cm H_2O)	–(75–100)	≥ –25
Compliance (ml/cm H_2O)	100	< 20
P_aO_2 (mm Hg)	80–95 (room air)	< 70
A-aDO_2 (mm Hg) (F_IO_2 = 1.0)	25–65	> 450
$\dot{Q}_S/\dot{Q}_T$ (%)	5–8	> 20
P_aCO_2 (mm Hg)	35–45	> 55†
V_D/V_T	0.2–0.3	> 0.60

*Ideal body weight should be used.
†Chronic lung disease constitutes the exception.

FEV_1—forced expiratory volume in one second P_aO_2—partial pressure of oxygen in arterial blood A-aDO_2—alveolar-arterial oxygen gradient F_IO_2—fraction of inspired oxygen $\dot{Q}_S/\dot{Q}_T$—shunt fraction P_aCO_2—partial pressure of carbon dioxide in arterial blood V_D/V_T—ratio of dead space to tidal volume

Approach to Management of Pulmonary Dysfunction

Clinical symptoms of pulmonary dysfunction include
- Dyspnea
- Tachypnea
- Cyanosis
- Suprasternal and intercostal retractions
- Altered mental state
- Tachycardia and hypotension or hypertension

↓

Order pulmonary function studies

Clinical and laboratory evaluation includes
- Measurement of arterial blood gases
- Chest x-rays
- Bronchoscopy
- Ventilation-perfusion scans
- Pulmonary function tests
- Microbial surveillance

↓

Absolute indications for intubation are
- Impaired airway patency
- Inadequate airway protection
- Inadequate pulmonary toilet
- Requirement for positive pressure ventilation

Cardiogenic pulmonary edema

Treat hypoxemia.
Measure pulmonary arterial pressures and cardiac output.
Administer dopamine or dobutamine if cardiac output is low.
Consider administration of furosemide.
Consider sodium nitroprusside for afterload reduction.

ARDS

Treat hypoxemia and hypercapnia.
Measure pulmonary arterial pressures and cardiac output.
Maintain PAWP below 15–18 mm Hg with infusion of crystalloid or red blood cells, if possible.
Give dopamine or dobutamine to maintain cardiac output.

Atelectasis

Treat hypoxemia.
Maintain airway toilet, with tracheal suctioning.
Order incentive spirometry.
Ensure airway humidification.
Relieve chest wall pain.
Evacuate pleural cavity.

Pulmonary embolism

Treat hypoxemia and hypercapnia.
If ventilation-perfusion lung scan shows defects, confirm with pulmonary angiogram.
Administer heparin in an initial bolus of 10,000 U, followed by 1,000 U/hr to maintain PTT at 1.5 times normal.
Consider caval interruption in selected patients.

Acid aspiration	**Lung contusion**	**Bacterial pneumonia**
Treat hypoxemia. Perform laryngoscopy or bronchoscopy, or both, for verification and removal of aspirated contents. Maintenance of intravascular volume may require pulmonary arterial monitoring. Administer bronchodilators for small airway obstruction.	Treat hypoxemia. Careful fluid management is indicated. Relieve chest wall pain. Monitor arterial blood gases to assess need for ventilatory support.	Treat hypoxemia. Order Gram's stain of sputum and antibiotic susceptibility testing. Maintain meticulous pulmonary toilet. Guide antibiotic therapy by surveillance and diagnostic cultures.

Impaired neuromuscular function

Treat hypoxemia.
Control pain from rib or muscle injury. Bilateral multiple fractures call for ventilatory assistance.
Maintain some degree of muscle work to prevent atrophy, taking care not to fatigue patient.
Optimize nutritional status.
Avoid overinflation of lung and distention of abdomen.
Avoid prolonged neuromuscular blockade.

Table 2 — Choice of Intubation Route

Route	Advantages	Disadvantages
Nasotracheal	Tube can be inserted blindly Can be performed with the neck in neutral position More comfortable Easily secured Allows better oral hygiene	Spontaneous breathing required for placement Diameter of tube limited by size of nares Longer tube required Pulmonary toilet diminished Nasal hemorrhage or sinusitis possible Tracheal damage possible
Orotracheal	Tube more easily inserted by less experienced personnel Tube can be wider and shorter, thereby allowing better pulmonary toilet	Neck hyperextension usually required Less comfortable Less easily secured Tracheal damage possible
Tracheotomy (cricothyrotomy)	Wide, short tube allows better pulmonary toilet More comfortable Tube can remain inserted for a very long time	Operative complications More experienced personnel required for safe and expedient placement Tracheal damage possible

tracheostomy is performed sooner [see 3 Burn Care in the Immediate Resuscitation Period, 24 Injuries to the Face and Jaw, and 25 Injuries to the Neck].

DEFINING MECHANICAL VENTILATION

Mechanical ventilation is largely defined as positive pressure ventilation. Positive pressure increases intra-alveolar pressure relative to pleural pressure, leading to lung expansion and in turn to expansion of the chest wall.[1] This approach makes possible adequate ventilation in the presence of major impairments in ventilatory mechanics involving either the lung or the chest wall. Lung volume can be maintained despite increased airway resistance and decreased lung compliance. Collapsed lung tissue can be reexpanded, which decreases the shunt fraction and improves arterial oxygen tension (P_aO_2).

The necessary increase in mean airway pressure can also produce complications [see Table 3]. The normal ventilation-to-perfusion ratio of spontaneous breathing can be disrupted, which leads to overexpansion and resultant regional hypoperfusion. Transmission of positive airway pressure to mediastinal structures and the pulmonary vasculature can cause a decrease in venous return and an increase in pulmonary vascular resistance, both of which can impair cardiac output and oxygen delivery.[2] The more compliant the lung or the less compliant the chest wall, the greater will be the transmission of the positive airway pressure to the mediastinum. The concomitant decrease in cardiac output can in large part be overcome by volume loading. Barotrauma will occur from high airway pressure, with the potential for alveolar disruption.

Ventilators can be classified as pressure cycled or volume cycled. With a pressure-cycled ventilator, inspiration is determined by a preset inspiratory pressure. With a volume-cycled ventilator, the inspiratory volume is preset. Volume-cycled ventilators are generally preferred in the intensive care unit because they maintain a relatively constant tidal volume and minute ventilation when changes in compliance or resistance occur. Procedures for initiating and maintaining positive pressure ventilation are described in detail elsewhere [see 92 Use of the Mechanical Ventilator].

Table 3 — Nonpulmonary Side Effects of Mechanical Ventilation[25]

Cardiac effects
- Impairment of preload attributable to decrease in venous return
- Increase in right ventricle size and decrease in left ventricle size as a result of right-to-left septal shift
- Support of the failing ventricle by the surrounding positive pressure and by reduction of preload and afterload
- Decrease in systemic oxygen demand through decreased work of breathing and increased sedation

Renal effects
- Decrease in renal blood flow comparable to overall decrease in cardiac output
- Redistribution of blood flow from cortical to medullary areas (thought to be the result of increased renal vein pressure), leading to decreased filtration rate and urine output
- Increase in antidiuretic hormone resulting from increased intrathoracic pressure and a neural reflex initiated by the pressure-distorted atrial wall
- Increase in plasma renin activity

Clinical Recognition of Pulmonary Dysfunction

CARDIOGENIC PULMONARY EDEMA

Cardiogenic, or high-pressure, pulmonary edema can be detected clinically through measurement of arterial blood gas pressures and invasive hemodynamic monitoring.[3] The interstitial edema that precedes any alveolar edema is generally manifested by dyspnea, tachypnea, mild hypoxemia, diffuse bilateral rhonchi, and wheezing (cardiac asthma). Signs of hypervolemia or congestive failure, such as distended neck veins and peripheral edema, are evident. Pulmonary arterial wedge pressure (PAWP) is usually high, about 25 mm Hg.[4] Radiographic signs of cardiogenic pulmonary edema include bronchovascular fluid cuffs (reflecting the interstitial edema), redistribution of blood flow to nondependent areas, cardiomegaly, and pleural effusions [see Table 4].[5]

Alveolar flooding, which ensues if interstitial edema progresses, dramatically accentuates lung dysfunction and hypoxemia. Diffuse rales become evident, and lung compliance and functional residual capacity (FRC) decrease. X-ray findings include evidence of interstitial edema followed by diffuse parenchymal involvement (usually greater in the bases).

The primary causes of interstitial edema are volume overload and left-sided heart failure resulting from myocardial ischemia or infarction. Frequently, elements of both causes are responsible, because a normal heart and normal kidneys can usually compensate for excessive fluid administration. Elevated pulmonary capillary hydrostatic pressure (P_{cap}) leads to increased fluid transport from the capillaries to the lung interstitium because of an imbalance of Starling forces. If the pumping capability of the lymphatics is overwhelmed, the excess fluid migrates beyond the lymphatic openings in the peripheral lung toward the loose interstitium around the larger airways and vessels. A decrease in the oncotic gradient between plasma and interstitium resulting from severe hypoproteinemia accentuates the edema.

Interstitial edema leads to external compression of the bronchovascular structures in the loose interstitial space, increasing airway resistance and vascular resistance. Increased vascular resistance redistributes blood flow away from areas of edema, resulting in ventilation-perfusion ($\dot{V}/\dot{Q}$) mismatch.

Alveolar flooding occurs when the interstitial space, including the septum, has expanded and interstitial pressure has increased to such a degree that alveolar cell apposition is disrupted and edema fluid enters the alveolar compartment. Each alveolus fills completely, and surfactant action is impaired. A fluid-filled alveolus is incapable of gas exchange, even when the fraction of inspired oxygen (F_IO_2) is increased. Positive end-expiratory pressure redistributes the contained water in a layer along the alveolus and allows oxygen to cross, although the alveolar-arterial oxygen gradient (A-aDo_2) is still significantly increased. A diffusion abnormality, however, is much more easily managed in this situation than is a complete shunt of blood past a totally fluid-filled alveolus, because the former can be partly corrected by administering oxygen to increase alveolar oxygen tension.

Cardiogenic edema resolves relatively rapidly once volume overload is corrected and capillary hydrostatic pressure decreases. Typically, there is improvement within 24 hours. Water is transported back into the interstitium and also is cleared through the airway. Edema fluid is a transudate rather than an exudate, so there is relatively little protein to remove. Excess water in the loose interstitium around the hilum has less effect on lung function, but it takes as long as several days to clear because its reabsorption rate is fairly slow. Consequently, chest films will continue to show evidence of interstitial edema for 24 to 48 hours after correction of the etiologic process and restoration of adequate gas exchange.

Table 4 Radiographic Manifestations of Pulmonary Edema[25]

Cardiogenic (High-Pressure) Pulmonary Edema	Low-Pressure Pulmonary Edema (as Seen in ARDS)
Redistribution of blood flow away from dependent lung	Normal vascular pattern
Bronchovascular fluid cuffs	Few to no fluid cuffs, but frequent air bronchograms
Increased septal (Kerley B) lines	Absence of septal lines
Cardiomegaly	Normal heart size
Pleural effusions	Infrequent effusions

ARDS—acute respiratory distress syndrome

Treatment

Young patients with high-pressure pulmonary edema caused by obvious fluid overload can be treated safely with only fluid restriction, diuretic therapy, or both. In surgical patients with underlying cardiopulmonary or renal disease, flow-directed pulmonary arterial catheters [see 89 Cardiopulmonary Monitoring] are necessary to distinguish high-pressure from low-pressure pulmonary edema; high-pressure edema is confirmed by PAWP greater than 20 to 25 mm Hg. Hypoxemia and hypercapnia are treated with oxygen administration or ventilatory support [see 92 Use of the Mechanical Ventilator]. Low cardiac output is restored to normal by administration of dopamine or dobutamine, beginning at 3 to 5 µg/kg/min and increasing as needed. Dobutamine is preferred in patients with a PAWP in excess of 20 mm Hg, tachycardia, or high systemic vascular resistance. Left atrial pressure is reduced by administration of a loop diuretic; furosemide is the drug of choice because it induces immediate venodilation in addition to diuresis. Low-dose dopamine (1 to 3 µg/kg/min) can be added to higher dosages of dobutamine to improve renal blood flow selectively and allow a more effective diuresis. In patients with high systemic vascular resistance, afterload should be reduced by administration of sodium nitroprusside. Patients who have coronary insufficiency and a high PAWP may benefit from intravenous nitroglycerin. Fluid administration must be appropriately monitored to avoid hypervolemia.

ACUTE RESPIRATORY DISTRESS SYNDROME

The term acute respiratory distress syndrome (ARDS) refers to the clinical manifestations of a number of indirect lung injury states characterized by dyspnea, severe hypoxemia, decreased lung compliance, and radiographic evidence of diffuse bilateral pulmonary infiltrates.[6,7] Pulmonary edema in the presence of a normal PAWP (i.e., low-pressure pulmonary edema) is also characteristic [see Table 5]. The lung damage is the result

Table 5 Identifying Characteristics of Cardiogenic and Low-Pressure Pulmonary Edema[25]

Cardiogenic (High-Pressure) Pulmonary Edema	Low-Pressure Pulmonary Edema
Initiated by local process: increased pulmonary capillary hydrostatic pressure	Initiated by distant focus, usually inflammation or infection
PAWP > 25 mm Hg	PAWP normal, usually 10–15 mm Hg
Low-protein edema	High-protein edema
Good correlation between increased water and increased shunt	Poor correlation between increased water and increased shunt: an indication other factors involved in shunt
Parenchymal involvement a later finding; interstitium involved first	Parenchymal involvement an early finding
Rapid resolution (24–48 hr)	Slow resolution (4–7 days)

of a systemic process, such as tissue damage, infection, or inflammation, rather than of a direct lung injury [see Table 6]. There are probably several distinct ARDS states, each with a different cause. The common practice of referring to ARDS as a single entity has probably been more confusing than helpful.

Although the various pathophysiologies are complex and the etiologies numerous, the presenting signs and symptoms for the ARDS states are nearly identical. They can be divided into three phases [see Table 7].

The first phase is characterized by dyspnea, tachypnea, relatively normal P_aO_2, and hyperventilation-induced respiratory alkalosis. Physical and x-ray examination reveal no significant lung findings. This prodrome is mediator induced.

The second phase usually begins within 12 to 24 hours of the onset of the early symptoms and is characterized by physiologic and pathological evidence of lung injury. Hypoxemia, accompanied by continuing dyspnea, is evident. The hypoxemia is typically refractory to an increase in F_IO_2, which indicates increased shunting. The degree of the shunt, however, is not directly correlated with the extent of the increase in alveolar and interstitial water content, as it is in cardiogenic edema. Auscultatory findings consist mostly of signs of early patchy consolidation rather than the rales heard with a strictly water-induced process. Radiographic evidence of scattered and heterogeneous early infiltrates appears initially in dependent lung fields; there is little evidence of loose interstitial fluid collection (i.e., cuffing) unless high-pressure edema is also present. Pathological changes include bilateral interstitial inflammation, with some intra-alveolar exudate containing water, protein, and blood. The interstitial and alveolar changes lead to a restrictive type of lung dysfunction that progressively impairs lung expansion; in this phase, modest decreases in dynamic and static compliance and FRC occur. A significant portion of the ventilatory impairment is unrelated to water; mediator-induced bronchoconstriction is the probable cause. In many cases, ARDS resolves in this phase if the initiating condition is controlled.

Progression to the third phase is manifested by the onset of acute respiratory failure necessitating mechanical ventilation. The lungs become more diffusely involved and stiffer. The shunt fraction increases as a result of patchy atelectasis and focal alveolar consolidation. The increasing thickness of the alveolar capillary membrane contributes to impaired diffusion. Redistribution of blood flow, together with vascular occlusion by microemboli or local thromboses, brings about an increase in physiologic dead space, which reduces alveolar ventilation and leads to a slow rise in arterial carbon dioxide tension (P_aCO_2) if a compensatory increase in minute ventilation is not initiated. Pulmonary arterial hypertension is usually seen. It is mediator induced; the likely agents are cytokines that activate the vasoconstrictors thromboxane A_2, leukotrienes C_4 and D_4, and serotonin.[8] These agents are produced and released by white cells and platelets. Thromboxane is also produced by the lung tissue itself. The hypertension can be exacerbated by hypoxic pulmonary vasoconstriction or by increased pulmonary blood flow, as is seen in systemic inflammatory response syndrome (SIRS). A hyperdynamic state frequently evolves: cardiac output is increased, but lactic acidosis develops because the tissues are unable to increase extraction of oxygen from hemoglobin in response to increased oxygen requirements. This impairment is characteristic of the septic syndrome of ARDS and may be related to impaired metabolic function of the lung, which normally removes vasodilating agents from the blood. These agents may cause the decrease in systemic vascular resistance (SVR) that occurs, producing maldistribution of blood flow to the tissues. The increasing cardiac output required to maintain adequate tissue oxygenation may accentuate the degree of pulmonary hypertension and the magnitude of the shunt.

If ARDS persists for more than seven days, the pathological manifestations begin to change from those typical of acute inflammation to those typical of mononuclear cell infiltration with interstitial fibrosis. In addition, areas of lung infection become evident as a result of impaired bacterial clearance or the presence of an endotracheal tube. The physiologic response consists of a gradual, progressive impairment of both gas exchange and ventilation. At this point, the process is no longer easily reversible. Areas of the lung become relatively acellular and are replaced by fibrous tissue.

The mechanism of the acute injury process has not been completely defined, but the initiating event is an injury to the circulatory side of the alveolar capillary membrane. Increased pulmonary vascular permeability is characteristic. The result is that protein-rich fluid crosses into the interstitial space. The

Table 6 Causes of ARDS

Disseminated intravascular coagulation
CNS injury (neurogenic pulmonary edema)
Drug reaction
Septic response
Fat embolism
Massive blood transfusion
Oxygen toxicity
Splanchnic ischemia
Tissue trauma
Barotrauma
Pancreatitis

mechanism of injury appears to be neutrophil margination in the lung vessels, followed by activation and release of a number of neutrophil-derived factors (e.g., oxygen radicals and proteases) toxic to the endothelial cells, the alveolar cells, and the interstitium. Intracapillary accumulation of neutrophils, platelets, and fibrin is evident at an early stage of the disease, and biochemical changes appear in lung tissue that are compatible with damage by neutrophil-derived factors.

An interstitial inflammatory reaction, accompanied by neutrophil and macrophage infiltration, is also evident. There is early accumulation of fluid and exudate in the alveoli without any preceding fluid filling of the perihilar loose interstitial space. These findings indicate that an alteration in the interstitium itself—probably involving basement membrane fibronectin and gel components, especially hyaluronic acid—disrupts this normal protective mechanism and facilitates fluid accumulation in the lung parenchyma.

The alveoli are found to contain not only fluid but also inspissated protein in the form of hyaline membranes. The increased protein must be cleared by macrophages. Surfactant production is altered, and there is an increased tendency toward alveolar collapse. Initially, this process of alveolar fluid collection and collapse appears to affect the dependent areas of the lung. The presence of alveolar protein, coupled with the initial neutrophil sequestration and activation, produces an inflammatory process in the lung that can lead to further inflammation and lung injury as chemotactic agents are released from injured tissue. Macrophages are a likely source of the mediators that exacerbate the inflammation. In addition, macrophage-derived factors can enhance the growth of the local fibroblast population and collagen deposition, resulting in an injury that is not readily reversible.

Treatment

Initial treatment of ARDS is aimed at removing the source of the lung injury. Overhydration should be avoided because it accentuates the edema. In the second phase, there is evidence of hypoxia. The hemoglobin oxygen saturation should be kept above 90 percent with supplementary oxygen.

If ARDS progresses rapidly toward acute respiratory failure, endotracheal intubation and positive pressure ventilation are needed.[1] Continued readjustment of ventilatory support is required to minimize the risks of oxygen toxicity and barotrauma. An F_IO_2 of 0.5 or less is preferred. Tidal volume may have to be decreased if the need for PEEP increases, to avoid marked increases in peak inspiratory and mean airway pressures.

Blood volume and electrolyte balance should be carefully maintained with blood, colloid, and crystalloid to replace losses. Early placement of a pulmonary arterial catheter is advantageous; clinical assessment of volume status is often misleading. Even small increases in capillary hydrostatic pressure can produce rapid progression of the edema because the permeability of lung capillaries is increased. Aggressive diuresis may improve P_aO_2 but can decrease tissue perfusion, producing inadequate oxygen delivery and lactic acidosis. Factors that increase oxygen demand—which include pain, anxiety, excessive muscle activity, and hyperthermia—should be minimized. Inotropic support may be needed to meet tissue oxygen demands. The beta agonists dopamine and dobutamine are the agents of choice.

Adequate nutritional support is also essential to meet the increased metabolic demands, which include increased work of breathing. On the basis of animal studies, the provision of increased quantities of antioxidants—vitamin C, 1 g/day; vitamin E, 500 to 1,000 IU/day; and glutamine, 30 g/day—has been recommended even though there are few hard data on the efficacy of this practice in humans. Close monitoring for nosocomial pneumonia is necessary because local lung and systemic immune defenses are impaired in ARDS. Appropriate antibiotic therapy for any lung infection must be initiated early to avoid progression of acute ARDS to chronic inflammation and fibrosis. In selected cases, instillation of nitric oxide through the ventilator has decreased pulmonary arterial hypertension to some extent: aerosolized surfactant has not been proved to be of benefit in adults with ARDS, as it has in infants.

ATELECTASIS

Atelectasis is the collapse of previously inflated lung tissue and the consequent collapse of alveoli [see Table 8]. If infection supervenes, inflammatory exudate and necrotic debris may obstruct larger bronchi, causing significant parenchymal collapse and consolidation.

Atelectasis in surgical patients is most often associated with a recent surgical procedure that results in a pain-induced decrease in respiratory excursion or with direct lung injury. As with any variety of pulmonary dysfunction, dyspnea, tachypnea, and tachycardia are prominent clinical features of alveolar collapse, especially when it occurs acutely. The response appears to be mediated in part by vagal stretch receptors in the lung. This mechanism may be responsible for the cough associated with atelectasis, which is usually nonproductive. Fever is almost always present and is often unrelated to concomitant infection. When the collapsed lung tissue reinflates, the fever promptly

Table 7 Clinical Presentation of ARDS

Prodrome
  Tachypnea
  Dyspnea, but no cyanosis
  Auscultation normal
  Chest x-ray usually normal

Onset of parenchymal changes
  Tachypnea
  Dyspnea
  Tachycardia
  Mild cyanosis
  Auscultation: few coarse rales
  Chest x-ray: early patchy infiltrates, usually in lower lung fields

Progression to respiratory failure
  Tachypnea
  Tachycardia
  Cyanosis
  Auscultation: diffuse rhonchi, signs of consolidation
  Chest x-ray: diffuse parenchymal infiltrates, air bronchograms, decreased lung volumes

ACID ASPIRATION

Aspiration of gastric contents is a major cause of pulmonary problems and subsequent mortality in surgical patients. About 50 percent of patients who aspirate gastric contents acquire pneumonia, and half of these die.[11,12] The volume and character of the aspirate dictate the degree of injury. Large particulate debris causes initial airway obstruction. However, a more important determinant of the magnitude of injury is the gastric pH. A pH of less than 3 induces the most severe injuries.

There are three main causes of aspiration [see Table 10]. The most common cause is impairment of laryngeal competence and glottic closure. This is usually caused by neurologic dysfunction, resulting either from drug use or from primary neurologic disease. The second major cause is increased gastric fluid volume or pressure, such as results from gastric outlet obstruction or poorly tolerated tube feedings. The third major cause is increased ease of passage of gastric contents up the esophagus, such as results from hiatal hernia.

The clinical presentation and pathogenesis of the acid aspiration syndrome can be divided into four sequential processes [see Table 11]. The first process is airway obstruction caused by particulate debris in the aspiration fluid. Immediately after aspiration, conscious, alert patients usually cough and expel particulate material; more obtunded patients begin to show symptoms of major airway obstruction. If the aspirated material is liquid, the acute incident may pass unnoticed. If the obstruction is extensive, however, it can itself be fatal. Obstruction atelectasis, accompanied by shunt formation and hypoxemia, occurs if the debris is not rapidly removed. Hypoventilation and hypercapnia can also ensue.

The second process in the acid aspiration syndrome is the direct airway injury caused by the acid. Within several hours after aspiration, the acid aspirate produces a chemical burn in the airway. Dyspnea, wheezing, and rhonchi are present, as with other types of burns. There is fluid loss (often massive) into the injured areas that leads to hypovolemia and compromised peripheral perfusion. The airway is severely irritated, and bronchoconstriction and bronchorrhea become apparent. In addition, the mucociliary activity of the airways is markedly impaired, which slows clearance of particles and mucus. The alveoli may also suffer direct injury if exposed to large volumes of a low-pH aspirate; edema and patchy atelectasis are the immediate results, and mortality is particularly high if this occurs. Dynamic compliance, static compliance, and functional residual capacity fall, and work of breathing and $\dot{V}/\dot{Q}$ mismatch increase.

The third process in the acid aspiration syndrome, which develops over the next 18 to 24 hours, is an inflammatory reaction to the chemical injury. Beginning several hours after aspiration, an intense leukocyte and platelet infiltration into the microvessels and airways of the injured lung is accompanied by increased release of vasoactive prostaglandins and leukotrienes. Platelets in the pulmonary vasculature release serotonin. Oxygen radicals and lysosomal enzymes from inflammatory cells promote thromboses and increase the permeability of the microvessels to protein. Degeneration of the alveolar epithelium leads to decreased surfactant production, and oxygen radicals alter the surfactant already formed, promoting alveolar collapse and flooding. Pulmonary edema and atelectasis result in increased shunting and hypoxemia, whereas microvascular thrombosis and vasoconstriction increase physiologic dead space and impair removal of carbon dioxide. The work of breathing is markedly raised as a consequence of decreased dynamic compliance (caused by increased airway resistance), decreased static compliance (caused by lung edema), and surfactant denaturation. Hypovolemia may occur as a result of loss of protein-rich fluid

Table 10 Causes of Acid Aspiration[25]

- Impaired laryngeal competence (glottic closure)
  - Neurologic impairment (e.g., head injury)
  - Drugs (e.g., narcotics, alcohol, sedatives)
  - Anesthesia
  - Laryngeal fracture
  - Laryngeal burn
- Increased gastric fluid volume or pressure
  - Bowel obstruction
  - Gastric atony
  - Recent meal
  - Poorly tolerated tube feedings
- Increased regurgitation
  - Impaired gastroesophageal junction
  - Hiatal hernia
  - Large-bore nasogastric tube

Table 11 Clinical Presentation of Acid Aspiration

- Mechanical effects of aspirate (immediately after aspiration)
  - Dyspnea
  - Tachypnea
  - Cyanosis (sometimes)
  - Chest wall retractions
  - Noisy respirations
  - Evidence of gastric aspiration in oropharynx
  - X-ray: progressing local infiltrate
- Response to chemical injury (within first several hours)
  - Continued dyspnea
  - Increasing sputum production
  - Wheezing, rhonchi on involved side
  - X-ray: progressing local infiltrate
- Response to inflammatory reaction (within first few days)
  - Increased dyspnea
  - Increased tachycardia
  - Evidence of decreased blood volume
  - More diffuse wheezing, rhonchi, rales
  - X-ray: beginning consolidation; extension of infiltrate beyond point seen on initial x-rays
- Infection (potential complication)
  - Clinical course of bacterial pneumonia

into the lung. This increases the physiologic dead space further because more of the lung is underperfused.

The fourth process in the acid aspiration syndrome is infection, which causes additional inflammation and tissue damage. The clinical course is that of bacterial pneumonia. The entire spectrum of bacterial infection may be found, depending on whether the normal flora has been eliminated early with prophylactic antibiotics and whether the more resistant hospital strains of bacteria have colonized the injury site.

Treatment

Treatment of the early phase of aspiration consists of rapid removal of any mechanical debris or gastric fluid from the upper airway. Endotracheal intubation is indicated if the patient cannot protect the airway. A nasogastric tube should be placed and the stomach evacuated to prevent a subsequent episode. Gas exchange is restored with oxygen administration and correction of hypoventilation.

Treatment during the next few hours consists of pulmonary support. Blood gas monitoring is necessary. A chest x-ray should be obtained to assess distal airway obstruction. If obstruction is evident, fiberoptic bronchoscopy is indicated to remove the obstructive debris. In the early stage, bronchospasm contributes to airway resistance; thus, bronchodilators can improve ventilatory function. Steroids have not proved advantageous.

If the injury progresses to an intense inflammatory process, treatment becomes that of acute respiratory failure, which includes positive pressure ventilation. The combined loss of fluid and protein into the lung can lead to hypovolemia, and it is essential to maintain normal volume status. Because hypervolemia will accentuate the lung edema, a pulmonary arterial catheter is indicated to optimize volume replacement. Inotropic support, preferably with a beta agonist, can help maintain tissue perfusion and oxygen delivery while minimizing edema-induced complications [*see 90 Support of the Failing Heart*]. The lung infection stage should be managed in the same way as nosocomial pneumonia would be.

PULMONARY INJURY FROM BLUNT CHEST TRAUMA (LUNG CONTUSION)

Blunt chest trauma is a common cause of pulmonary injury. There are often at least two components to the injury: impaired chest wall function and direct parenchymal disruption, or lung contusion.[13]

The clinical presentation ranges from modest tachypnea with blood-tinged secretions to labored respiration, cyanosis, and hemoptysis. Diffuse coarse rales are most marked in the areas of injury. In more severe injuries, evidence of consolidation is present. Some symptoms of impaired lung function are often present initially. Symptoms often worsen during the following 48 hours, particularly if there is an element of volume overload during resuscitation, which aggravates extravasation of fluid. The initial chest x-ray usually demonstrates localized parenchymal infiltrates that become progressively more opaque during the following 24 to 48 hours. Computed tomographic scanning of the chest can better define the magnitude of injury. Compared with chest x-ray, CT scanning has a higher degree of sensitivity in assessing the extent of lung parenchymal injury.

A major mechanism of trauma-induced lung dysfunction is direct damage to the underlying lung tissue. Disruption of alveolar capillary integrity results in local bronchoalveolar hemorrhage. The extent to which gas exchange is impaired depends on the amount of lung parenchyma involved and on the degree of concomitant chest wall injury. Progression of tissue damage during the first 24 to 48 hours usually stems initially from continued parenchymal bleeding and later from lysis of red cells and proteins. Bronchiolar plugging with blood initially elevates the shunt fraction and gives rise to significant hypoxemia; the disrupted parenchyma remains partially perfused. With the lysis of the localized parenchymal hemorrhage and the onset of inflammation in the damaged parenchyma, a more dense consolidation develops, and neighboring lung tissue becomes involved. Lung compliance decreases, further reducing the FRC and exacerbating the atelectasis. This process increases shunting and hypoxemia. Redistribution of ventilation and blood flow increases the $\dot{V}/\dot{Q}$ mismatch. Compliance continues to decrease, and the work of breathing increases.

An intrapleural process such as hemothorax can produce compressive atelectasis on the involved side. This compression is readily corrected by the removal of blood.

Disruption of chest wall function ranges from flail chest to chest wall splinting resulting from a single rib fracture. Much of the lung dysfunction that follows chest wall injury results from hypoventilation induced by pain. The main exception is severe flail chest, in which it is impossible to generate sufficient transpulmonary pressure for lung expansion. Inability to expand the chest wall—whether from pain or from flail chest—results in hypoventilation, decreased FRC, focal alveolar collapse, and, finally, hypoxemia with hypercapnia. In addition, the inability to clear mucus and bacteria with an effective cough leads to obstruction of airways and secondary infection. Mortality is correlated with the amount of lung directly damaged and the magnitude of the associated injuries.

Treatment

Initial treatment of chest trauma during resuscitation consists of correction or control of immediately life-threatening problems such as airway obstruction, tension pneumothorax, hemothorax, hypovolemia, myocardial contusion, and flail chest [*see 22 Emergency Department Evaluation of the Patient with Multiple Injuries*]. In addition, sufficient analgesia to permit an adequate respiratory effort and coughing is necessary. Positive pressure ventilation may be needed early if the chest wall is too unstable to maintain alveolar ventilation. A moderate flail segment can usually be managed without mechanical positive pressure ventilation. Continuous positive airway pressure can be delivered by mask if positive pressure is required. Initial fluid resuscitation must be carefully monitored to prevent overhydration, in particular administration of excessive crystalloid. Pulmonary arterial and peripheral arterial catheters are indicated in potentially severe cases.

Adequate treatment after resuscitation is critical to prevent acute respiratory failure. Good pulmonary toilet, including maintenance of an adequate cough, and avoidance of overhydration are crucial. During this period, lung compliance continues to decrease as contused and neighboring lung areas become inflamed. The increased work of breathing often augments the chest wall pain. Pain control is essential to pul-

Table 13 Gas Exchange Parameters

Parameter	Abbreviation	Derivation	Normal Value
Partial pressure of oxygen in arterial blood	P_aO_2	Direct measurement	Varies with age: 80–95 mm Hg (room air)
Partial pressure of carbon dioxide in the alveolus	P_ACO_2	Direct measurement	40 mm Hg
Partial pressure of carbon dioxide in arterial blood	P_aCO_2	Direct measurement	35–45 mm Hg
Partial pressure of oxygen in mixed venous blood	$P_{mv}O_2$	Direct measurement	Varies with $\dot{V}O_2$: 40–45 mm Hg
Partial pressure of carbon dioxide in mixed venous blood	$P_{mv}CO_2$	Direct measurement	44–51 mm Hg
Partial pressure of oxygen in the alveolus	P_AO_2	$[P_B - P_{H_2O} \times F_IO_2] - \dfrac{P_aCO_2}{0.8}$	Depends on P_B and F_IO_2: 95–110 mm Hg (room air), 630–670 mm Hg ($F_IO_2 = 1.0$)
Alveolar-arterial oxygen gradient	A-aDO_2	$P_AO_2 - P_aO_2$	25–65 mm Hg ($F_IO_2 = 1.0$)
Oxygen saturation of arterial hemoglobin	S_aO_2	Direct measurement	94%–95% (room air)
Oxygen saturation of mixed venous hemoglobin	$S_{mv}O_2$	Direct measurement	Varies with $\dot{V}O_2$: 75% by oximeter (room air)
Shunt fraction	$\dot{Q}_S/\dot{Q}_T$	$\dfrac{C_cO_2 - C_aO_2}{C_cO_2 - C_{mv}O_2}$	5%–8%

P_B—barometric pressure P_{H_2O}—water vapor pressure F_IO_2—fraction of inspired oxygen C_cO_2—oxygen content of pulmonary capillary blood $\dot{V}O_2$—oxygen consumption

---

Several of the terms used to describe oxygen exchange are discussed below [see Table 13].

P_aO_2 is a measure of the amount of oxygen dissolved in plasma; it is expressed in mm Hg. Because supplementary oxygen is often given to surgical patients, P_aO_2 by itself often is not a sensitive indicator of the adequacy of oxygen exchange.

Alveolar oxygen tension (P_AO_2) is the amount of oxygen in the alveolus. It is calculated by the alveolar air equation:

$$P_AO_2 = [(P_B - P_{H_2O}) \times F_IO_2] - \dfrac{P_aCO_2}{0.8}$$

where P_B is barometric pressure and P_{H_2O} is the partial pressure of water vapor (normally 45 to 48 mm Hg). The transfer of oxygen from inspired alveolar air across the alveolar capillary membrane to blood occurs by simple passive diffusion down a concentration gradient; no active mechanism is involved. P_AO_2 is normally 95 to 110 mm Hg, and P_aO_2 is normally 80 to 95 mm Hg.

A-aDO_2 is the average oxygen gradient across the alveolar capillary membrane. The higher the gradient necessary for adequate transfer of oxygen, the more abnormal the exchange process is. The gradient is typically 10 to 25 mm Hg.

Hemoglobin, with its high affinity for oxygen, acts as a sponge for the oxygen crossing from the alveolus. Normally, this process is in equilibrium with the P_aO_2; a P_aO_2 of 90 mm Hg yields an S_aO_2 of over 95 percent.

The P_{50} is the oxygen tension at which 50 percent of the hemoglobin is saturated with oxygen. At a pH of 7.4 and a temperature of 37°C, the P_{50} is 26 ± 2 mm Hg. The P_{50} increases—that is, the oxygen-hemoglobin dissociation curve shifts to the right—with a decrease in pH, an increase in temperature, or an increase in 2,3-diphosphoglycerate (2,3-DPG). This shift is advantageous to cells in need of additional oxygen because it increases oxygen unloading at the tissue level. A decrease in P_{50}—that is, a left shift—occurs with alkalosis, decreased temperature, or decreased 2,3-DPG. Less oxygen is unloaded from the hemoglobin at a given PO_2, which can be detrimental if oxygen delivery is marginal.

Pulmonary shunt fraction ($\dot{Q}_S/\dot{Q}_T$) is defined as the portion of the cardiac output ($\dot{Q}_T$) that perfuses unventilated alveoli ($\dot{Q}_S$). It measures the percentage of the cardiac output that returns to the left side of the heart unoxygenated. This process is also referred to as pulmonary venous admixture. Normal anatomic shunt flow through bronchial vessels and thebesian veins is about three to five percent of total pulmonary blood flow.

The shunt fraction can be measured with the patient breathing either 100 percent oxygen or a lesser concentration. Although an F_IO_2 of 1.0 simplifies the calculation, it is essential to recognize that an F_IO_2 of 1.0 can lead to absorption atelectasis and may itself impair oxygen exchange.

The shunt fraction is calculated as follows:

$$\dot{Q}_S/\dot{Q}_T = \dfrac{C_cO_2 - C_aO_2}{C_cO_2 - C_{mv}O_2}$$

where C_cO_2 is the oxygen content of pulmonary capillary blood. Because pulmonary capillary blood is inaccessible to direct measurement, C_cO_2 is assumed to be the oxygen content that arterial blood would have if it were fully equilibrated with alveolar air. The P_AO_2 in patients receiving 100 percent oxygen is always greater than 150 mm Hg; consequently, the pulmonary capillary blood can be assumed to be fully saturated.

CARBON DIOXIDE REMOVAL

Carbon dioxide production depends on the metabolic activity of the cells. It averages about 200 ml/min (120 ml/min/m²) in a healthy adult. Carbon dioxide is highly soluble and readily diffuses across cell membranes and into fluid compartments. It is removed by the same process of diffusion that governs oxygen exchange and by the weak buffer system. Carbon dioxide exists in a so-called open system: it is continually produced at the cellular level and removed via the lungs. A carbon dioxide gradient is maintained between the cell and plasma. As carbon dioxide enters the plasma, most of it (70 to 90 percent) is soaked up by red cells in the form of bicarbonate and then combines with hemoglobin or forms carbamino compounds.

Bound carbon dioxide equilibrates with a small amount of the gas dissolved in plasma at a given partial pressure (P_{CO_2}). The dissolved amount is calculated as follows:

$$CO_2 \text{ dissolved in plasma} = 0.03 \times P_{CO_2}$$

A second gradient exists between plasma and alveolar gas space, because ambient air contains essentially no carbon dioxide. This gradient drives carbon dioxide from the blood until the mixed venous P_{CO_2} equilibrates with the alveolar P_{CO_2}. As plasma P_{CO_2} falls, carbon dioxide unloads from red cells. The mixed venous carbon dioxide tension, which is usually 44 to 51 mm Hg, equilibrates with the alveolar carbon dioxide tension to reach a pressure of about 40 mm Hg at end inspiration (end-tidal P_ACO_2). If the P_ACO_2 is either lower or higher than 40 mm Hg, the P_ACO_2 equilibrates with this new value, which results in hypocapnia or hypercapnia. Thus, the adequacy of ventilatory mechanisms for removal of carbon dioxide dictates the plasma content of the gas. Approximately 24,000 mEq of acid is cleared daily through the lung in the form of carbon dioxide. Any impairment of carbon dioxide removal will have major effects on blood and tissue pH.

Carbon dioxide removal is dependent on adequate exchange of alveolar air [see Mechanics of Ventilation, below]. Elevation of P_aCO_2 indicates inadequate ventilation. Sometimes, a normal P_aCO_2 can be maintained by compensatory hyperventilation, even in the presence of significant lung failure. This is possible because blood from hyperventilated areas low in carbon dioxide mixes with blood from hypoventilated areas high in carbon dioxide. In contrast, low oxygen content in a hypoventilated area cannot be compensated for by regional hyperventilation.

Normal arterial pH is between 7.37 and 7.43. If the pH is less than 7.37, the patient has an acidosis. If the pH is greater than 7.43, the patient has an alkalosis. The normal P_aCO_2 is 37 to 43 mm Hg. If P_aCO_2 is greater than 43 mm Hg, there is a respiratory acidosis. If P_aCO_2 is less than 37 mm Hg, there is a respiratory alkalosis. The normal bicarbonate (measured as CO_2 content) is 22 to 28 mEq/L. If the bicarbonate is less than 22 mEq/L, there is a metabolic acidosis. If the bicarbonate is greater than 28 mEq/L, there is a metabolic alkalosis.

MECHANICS OF VENTILATION

Movement of air into and out of the lungs, or ventilation, involves three main processes: (1) the stimulus to breathe, (2) maintenance of open alveoli, and (3) mechanical motion of the lungs.

The Stimulus to Breathe

The stimuli for maintaining adequate alveolar ventilation ($\dot{V}_A$) are the P_aO_2 detected by chemoreceptors in the carotid body and aortic arch and the pH sensed by the central chemoreceptors in the brain stem. The pH is altered by dissolved carbon dioxide, which rapidly crosses the blood-brain barrier, whereas plasma buffers such as bicarbonate cannot. Small changes in blood carbon dioxide levels, therefore, yield significant changes in pH at the receptors. A decrease in pH (caused by increased carbon dioxide levels) is a strong stimulus to increase ventilation; conversely, an increase in pH sharply decreases the ventilatory drive. A decrease in P_aO_2 initiates a comparable increase in alveolar ventilation via the carotid body and aortic arch chemoreceptors. In the case of combined hypoxemia and hypercapnia, which occurs in some chronic forms of lung dysfunction, hypoxemia becomes the dominant stimulus.

Maintenance of Open Alveoli

The lung has a continual tendency to collapse, for two reasons. First, the elasticity of the interstitial connective tissue helps to deflate the lung. Interstitial elasticity accounts for about one third of the lung's total elastic recoil. Second, there is considerable surface tension in the thin fluid layer that lines the alveolar walls and protects alveolar cells from direct contact with air. The intermolecular forces in the surface fluid tend to reduce the surface area of the alveoli, and these forces increase as the radius of curvature, or the alveolar volume, decreases.

Surfactant—a mixture of phospholipids—reduces surface tension more effectively as alveolar size decreases, which helps counteract the increased surface tension at low lung volumes. Because surfactant has a half-life of about 48 hours, impairment of its production by type II alveolar cells may not be evident for several days after an injury. If surfactant is denatured, however—as may occur in alveolar edema or with local release of inflammatory mediators—alveoli become immediately unstable. Alveolar surface tension accounts for about two thirds of the lung's total elastic recoil.

Lung Movement

In the face of the tendency of the lungs to collapse, active chest wall work is needed to inflate the lungs. Muscle activity must expand the chest wall and contract the diaphragm to expand the lung effectively during spontaneous ventilation.

Several important terms used to describe the mechanics of ventilation are discussed below [see Table 14].

Physiologic dead space (V_D) is that portion of the tidal volume (V_T) that is not involved in exchanging gas with pulmonary blood. A portion of the V_D is anatomic dead space, made up of structures such as the trachea and the large airways; it amounts to about 150 ml in adults. The remainder, which is called alveolar dead space, is made up of nonperfused ventilated alveoli, such as result from embolic occlusion. The ratio of dead space to tidal volume (V_D/V_T) is normally 0.2 to 0.3. It is calculated as follows:

$$V_D/V_T = \frac{P_aCO_2 - P_ECO_2}{P_aCO_2}$$

where P_ECO_2 is the mean expired carbon dioxide tension. The V_D/V_T ratio varies with changes in either anatomic or alveolar dead space or in tidal volume; however, because it measures only total dead space, it does not distinguish changes in anatomic V_D from changes in alveolar V_D.

Minute ventilation ($\dot{V}_E$) is simply the amount of air moved into or out of the lungs in a minute. The normal resting value is usually about 5 to 8 L/min. This value includes ventilation of alveoli and dead space.

Alveolar minute ventilation ($\dot{V}_A$) is a measure of the amount of air being exchanged in the alveoli. It is determined by subtracting the calculated V_D from the V_T and multiplying the result by the respiratory rate.

Inspiratory force (IF) is the transpulmonary pressure generated during an inspiratory effort. The maximum inspiratory pressure is measured again st a completely occluded airway over about 10 seconds. This measurement does not require the cooperation of the patient and thus is particularly useful in unconscious or anesthetized patients. The inspiratory force usually required to generate a vital capacity of 15 ml/kg is at least −25 cm H_2O.

Vital capacity (V_C) is defined as the lung volume generated by a maximal expiration after a maximal inspiration. It is nor-

Table 14 **Ventilation Parameters**

Parameter	Abbreviation	Derivation	Normal Value
Tidal volume	V_T	Direct measurement	4–5 ml/kg
Vital capacity	V_C	Direct measurement	65–75 ml/kg
Functional residual capacity	FRC	Direct measurement	2,000–2,600 ml
Inspiratory force	IF	Direct measurement	–(75–100) cm H_2O
Dead space to tidal volume ratio	V_D/V_T	$\dfrac{P_aCO_2 - P_ECO_2}{P_aCO_2}$	0.2–0.3
Effective dynamic compliance	C_{dyn}	$V_T/(PIP - PEEP)$	Mechanical ventilation: 60–80 ml/cm H_2O
Static compliance	C_{stat}	$V_T/(\text{plateau pressure} - PEEP)$	Mechanical ventilation: 80–100 ml/cm H_2O

P_ECO_2—mean expired carbon dioxide tension   PIP—peak inspiratory pressure   PEEP—positive end-expiratory pressure

mally about 65 to 75 ml/kg. A vital capacity of less than 15 ml/kg is an indication for mechanical ventilatory assistance; at this level, alveolar volume is insufficient to prevent collapse.

Functional residual capacity (FRC) is the volume of gas left in the lung after normal expiration, which, in conjunction with surfactant, helps keep alveoli patent. FRC is decreased in patients with pulmonary insufficiency, resulting in atelectasis and impaired gas exchange. PEEP increases FRC.

Lung compliance is defined as the change in lung volume per unit of transpulmonary pressure. Lung compliance actually measures the combined performance of the lung parenchyma and the chest wall. During spontaneous ventilation, it is normally about 200 ml/cm H_2O. During mechanical ventilation, compliance is normally closer to 60 to 80 ml/cm H_2O, because the chest wall is expanded by the lung inflation rather than actively assisting in this process.

Dynamic compliance (C_{dyn}) refers to lung expansibility during air movement. It is measured during inspiration at the peak transpulmonary pressure. It is determined as follows:

$$C_{dyn} = V_T/\text{peak transpulmonary pressure}$$

When mechanical ventilation is employed, C_{dyn} is calculated differently:

$$C_{dyn} = V_T/PIP - PEEP$$

where PIP is peak inspiratory pressure. The C_{dyn} reflects lung and chest wall expansibility in addition to resistance to airflow in the airway, including ventilator tubing.

Static compliance (C_{stat}) is a measure of the recoil properties of the lung and chest wall or the ability of the system to stay inflated. C_{stat} is measured when there is no flow, at the end of inspiration. The inspiratory volume is held in the lung by an end-inspiratory pause or plateau; the transpulmonary pressure measured at this point is the plateau pressure. The C_{stat} is calculated as follows:

$$C_{stat} = V_T/\text{plateau pressure} - PEEP$$

Decreased static compliance can reflect alveolar collapse, as occurs with surfactant denaturation or pulmonary edema.

Work of breathing is an important parameter in ventilation. Normally, less than five percent of total oxygen consumption is used for the work of breathing. An increase in dead space or shunt or a decrease in compliance can markedly increase the work load. If the increased oxygen demand cannot be met or muscle fatigue occurs, respiratory distress will ensue. Work of breathing can be assessed by monitoring changes in oxygen consumption that result from changes in ventilatory effort, such as are seen in the process of weaning.

PULMONARY CIRCULATORY FUNCTION

The integrity of pulmonary circulatory function is essential to adequate gas exchange and tissue oxygenation. This function can be described in terms of (1) pulmonary blood flow, (2) blood volume and surface area, (3) vascular pressure and resistance, and (4) vascular permeability properties.

Pulmonary Blood Flow

Blood flow, or cardiac output, is a major component of lung oxygen exchange and systemic oxygen delivery. Low blood flow through ventilated lungs may actually improve the arterial oxygen tension and saturation because the increased lung transit time allows more oxygen loading; however, oxygen delivery will be inadequate. This illustrates the importance of assessing lung oxygen exchange and systemic oxygen delivery when evaluating a patient's physiologic status.

Blood flow must be present if gas exchange is to occur. Pulmonary blood flow can be divided into three lung zones as follows:

Zone I: alveolar pressure > mean PAP > venous pressure
Zone II: mean PAP > alveolar pressure > venous pressure
Zone III: mean PAP > venous pressure > alveolar pressure

where PAP is pulmonary arterial pressure. In zone I, alveolar pressure exceeds vascular pressure, resulting in cessation of flow and creation of dead space. In zone III, both PAP and pulmonary venous pressure exceed alveolar pressure, resulting in continual pulmonary blood flow. This zone accounts for most of a healthy lung.

Blood Volume and Surface Area

Blood volume in the pulmonary capillary bed depends on total body blood volume and vascular pressures and resistances. Capillary volume determines the vascular surface area available for gas exchange.

Vascular Pressure and Resistance

PAP is monitored through a Swan-Ganz catheter. A normal mean PAP is 12 to 16 mm Hg. Acute increases in PAP can be caused by several disease processes, including (1) an increase in pulmonary venous pressure, (2) increased pulmonary vascular tone caused by circulating mediators (for instance, in SIRS), (3) pulmonary emboli, with obstruction of flow, (4) hypoxia-induced vasoconstriction, and (5) positive airway pressure.

Pulmonary vascular tone is regulated by the autonomic nervous system and by many inflammatory vasoconstrictors and vasodilators. An elevated PAP increases the afterload to the right side of the heart, thereby increasing right-sided heart work. An acute increase in mean PAP to greater than 30 mm Hg can lead to right-sided heart dilatation, right-to-left shift of the ventricular septum, and subsequent impairment of left-sided heart function. The increased PAP may have little effect on capillary hydrostatic pressure if arterial resistance is increased as a result of smooth muscle constriction. This process can protect the lung from pulmonary edema.

Monitoring of capillary hydrostatic pressure is important because a significant increase can lead to pulmonary congestion and edema as a result of an imbalance of Starling forces. When the PAWP is about 20 mm Hg, there is usually radiographic evidence of pulmonary congestion, hilar engorgement, and other abnormalities. When PAWP exceeds 30 mm Hg, pulmonary edema is usually present.

Vascular Permeability

The rate at which fluid crosses the capillary membrane from plasma to interstitium is dictated by the Starling equation:

$$\dot{Q}_f = K_f[(P_{cap} - P_i) - \sigma(COP_{cap} - COP_i)]$$

where $\dot{Q}_f$ is the rate of fluid filtration, K_f is the filtration coefficient describing the ease of water transfer across the capillary membrane and through the interstitium, P_i is interstitial hydrostatic pressure, σ is the reflection coefficient describing the ability of the capillary membrane and interstitium to prevent protein crossing, and COP_{cap} and COP_i are the capillary and interstitial colloid osmotic (oncotic) pressures generated by proteins. The importance of oncotic pressure is reflected in the difference between plasma and interstitial values, which favors intravascular fluid retention. Interstitial protein content is normally about half that of plasma. Changes in the interstitial oncotic pressure can partially compensate for acute changes in the plasma forces. This compensatory capacity, however, depends on the ability of the pulmonary lymphatics to remove any increased fluid and protein from the interstitium and on the presence of relatively normal capillary permeability. An increase in capillary hydrostatic pressure forces more fluid but not more protein across the membrane; the result is a decrease in COP_i and an increase in the difference between COP_{cap} and COP_i. The increase in the oncotic gradient, which enhances intravascular fluid retention, counteracts the increase in P_{cap} pressure and minimizes the net increase in the rate of fluid filtration.

A decrease in plasma oncotic pressure, such as may occur in hypoproteinemia, transiently decreases the oncotic gradient. The COP_i also falls, however, and this compensatory mechanism can restore the oncotic gradient for decreases in plasma protein of as much as 40 percent. Greater decreases narrow the oncotic gradient because COP_i, normally about 15 mm Hg, can only decrease to 3 to 5 mm Hg.

The intact alveolar membrane is completely impermeable to protein. Under normal circumstances, water also cannot cross into the alveolus because of the surface tension properties of the alveolar membrane. Disruption of this membrane leads to alveolar flooding.

PULMONARY DEFENSE MECHANISMS

The normal lung is kept free of bacteria by a highly efficient system of bacterial and particle clearance. Alveolar clearance is provided by alveolar macrophages, which ingest the particles and either digest them or carry them along the ciliated bronchioles to the oropharynx. Particles or bacteria that are not eliminated, either because the macrophage defenses have been overwhelmed or because ciliary clearance has been impaired, initiate an inflammatory response that is signaled by the migration of neutrophils into the area. Tracheobronchial clearance is accomplished through the mucociliary action of the lining cells. The continued beating motion of the cilia moves a film of mucus containing entrapped particles, bacteria, and white cells from bronchioles to the oropharynx.

Impairment of clearance predisposes to pulmonary infection, particularly if organisms gain access to the lungs by way of a foreign body (e.g., a suction catheter or an endotracheal tube) or, less commonly, by the hematogenous route. Airway collapse impairs clearance of bacteria and mucus from the distal segments of the lung. Increased mucus production or impaired mucus clearance further aggravates the obstructing process. Increased alveolar or interstitial fluid allows an infectious process to spread more rapidly by impairing the walling off and clearance of the organisms by local defenses.

PULMONARY METABOLIC FUNCTION

Pulmonary endothelial cells are active in metabolizing biogenic amines, peptides, and prostaglandins. The lung is an important site for degradation of serotonin and, to a lesser degree, of norepinephrine. Metabolism of serotonin occurs in all pulmonary vessels. This function is impaired after hyperbaric oxygen injury, which results in increasing levels of serotonin in the blood.

Of greater importance is the role of the lung in peptide metabolism, in particular the degradation of bradykinin and the conversion of angiotensin I to angiotensin II. A single enzyme system in the lung is the major site of both these activities. Thus, extraction of the most potent vasodilator in the body, bradykinin, and activation of the most potent vasoconstrictor, angiotensin II, both take place in the lung. Patients with ARDS have decreased levels of angiotensin-converting enzyme; this may explain the systemic hypotension that can accompany ARDS. Cardiopulmonary bypass, in which the lung is excluded from the circulation, increases levels of endogenous bradykinin, providing further evidence of the nonrespiratory function of the lung. The lung is the major site of breakdown of prostaglandins of the E and F series as well as a major site of synthesis of these prostaglandins and prostacyclin. Alterations in this system may potentiate respiratory failure and failure of other organ systems.

General Pulmonary Abnormalities in Surgical Patients

Eight common pathophysiological mechanisms impair gas exchange and ventilation: (1) impaired diffusion, (2) $\dot{V}/\dot{Q}$ mismatch, (3) alveolar hypoventilation, (4) increased pulmonary shunt, (5) decreased oxygen delivery, (6) pulmonary hypertension, (7) decreased hypoxic pulmonary vasoconstriction, and (8) atelectasis. The last of these has already been discussed from a

Table 15 Causes of Hypoxia

Decreased oxygen tension in arterial blood (hypoxemia)
  Impaired diffusion
  V̇/Q̇ mismatch
  Alveolar hypoventilation
  Increased pulmonary shunt
Decreased oxygen content in arterial blood
  Decreased hemoglobin content
  Decreased arterial oxygen tension
  Carbon monoxide poisoning
  Methemoglobinemia
Decreased cardiac output
  Myocardial depression
  Decreased coronary perfusion
  Increased peripheral vascular resistance
  Increased pulmonary vascular resistance
  Cardiac arrhythmia
  Decreased circulating blood volume

clinical standpoint [see Clinical Recognition of Pulmonary Dysfunction, Atelectasis, above].

The end results of impaired gas exchange are hypoxia and hypercapnia. Hypoxia is the delivery of a less than adequate amount of oxygen to the tissues; hypercapnia is an excess of carbon dioxide in the blood. Hypoxemia is a lower than normal P_aO_2, which alters the amount of oxygen carried on hemoglobin. The components of oxygen delivery include S_aO_2, hemoglobin content, and cardiac output. Of these, the lung is directly responsible only for the first. The other two components are the responsibility of the vascular system [see Table 15]. The first four pathophysiological mechanisms discussed below—impaired diffusion, V̇/Q̇ mismatch, alveolar hypoventilation, and increased pulmonary shunt—constitute the principal abnormalities in the pulmonary component of oxygen delivery.

IMPAIRED DIFFUSION

Diffusion capacity refers to the volume of a gas that crosses a membrane per unit time per unit of partial pressure gradient. Diffusion capacity is determined by three variables: (1) the solubility of the gas in the membrane, (2) the surface area of the membrane, and (3) the thickness of the membrane. In the lung, both oxygen and carbon dioxide are readily soluble in the barrier that separates blood from alveolar air, and they rapidly equilibrate across this membrane. Thus, any changes in their diffusion capacity stem from changes in membrane surface area or thickness.

Diffusion abnormalities increase the alveolar-arterial oxygen gradient. If P_aO_2 falls below 70 mm Hg, arterial oxygen saturation and oxygen content decrease significantly. A modest diffusion impairment may not be clearly evident when the blood transit time through the lung is normal or even somewhat slower than normal, because oxygen readily crosses the membrane. The same diffusion abnormality becomes more evident, however, as cardiac output increases and the time available for oxygen exchange decreases, as occurs in the hyperdynamic septic state or during exercise. Increasing F_IO_2 raises P_aO_2 when the problem is abnormal membrane thickness. Hypoxemia induced by diffusion impairment is, therefore, correctable through the use of exogenous oxygen. Pulmonary function tests for diffusion capacity cannot, however, distinguish increased membrane thickness from decreased surface area.

VENTILATION-PERFUSION MISMATCH

Gas exchange would be optimal if ventilation and perfusion (capillary blood flow) were perfectly matched and completely uniform—that is, if the V̇/Q̇ ratio were 1.0. In the normal lung, however, there is some mismatch, and the average V̇/Q̇ ratio is about 0.8. There are several reasons for this. The shape of the thoracic cavity and the descent of the diaphragm result in greater lung expansion in the lower lobes than in the upper lobes. Blood flow is also more prominent in the dependent lung during spontaneous ventilation; this area is in zone III, in which both PAP and venous pressure exceed alveolar pressure. Blood flow also varies with body position and with changes in ventilatory volume.

When positive pressure ventilation is used, some lung areas may be overexpanded while obstructed or stiff areas remain hypoventilated. An increase in alveolar pressure can substantially alter blood flow by changing an area of the lung from zone III to zone I or II. In addition, local blood flow through hyperinflated areas of lung is retarded by compression of the loose interstitium through which the blood vessels travel on their way to forming the capillary bed; local pulmonary vascular resistance increases, and blood flow is redistributed to hypoventilated areas, where resistance is lower.

Pathological conditions can substantially increase V̇/Q̇ mismatch and severely impair gas exchange. An acute reduction in blood flow resulting from embolic occlusion or more chronic obliteration of the lung vasculature by processes such as emphysema yields a V̇/Q̇ ratio greater than 1.0. The relative increase in V̇/Q̇ ratio does not, however, improve S_aO_2 if oxygen exchange is already reasonably good. Much of the ventilation is therefore wasted. A ventilated area through which there is no perfusion contributes to dead space [see Table 16].

Alternatively, ventilation may be reduced in areas with normal or increased perfusion. This occurs in conditions such as focal atelectasis and edema and in chronic processes that destroy the alveolar architecture (e.g., emphysema). The result is a very low V̇/Q̇ ratio. Not enough alveolar oxygen is available to oxygenate the excessive amount of blood perfusing the area, especially if the patient is breathing room air. Consequently, S_aO_2 and P_aO_2 are reduced. This impairment cannot be compensated for by an increased V̇/Q̇ ratio in another part of the same lung. As with diffusion abnormalities, however, much of the impaired oxygen exchange in a low V̇/Q̇ area can be corrected by increasing F_IO_2, which makes

Table 16 Causes of Increased Dead Space[25]

Vascular destruction
Vascular obstruction by emboli or thrombi
Hypovolemia leading to impaired perfusion in nondependent lung areas
Regional lung hypoperfusion resulting from increased airway pressure

additional alveolar oxygen available. If an alveolus has no ventilation, no gas exchange will occur, regardless of the F_IO_2 [see Increased Shunt, below].

Carbon dioxide is removed in proportion to the degree of alveolar ventilation. The carbon dioxide dissociation curve is linear, and unlike the oxygen-hemoglobin dissociation curve, it does not plateau. Therefore, the greater the ventilation of perfused areas, the greater the removal of carbon dioxide. Actually, hyperventilation, which often follows hypoxemia, can increase elimination of carbon dioxide and give rise to hypocapnia.

The lung normally compensates for acute decreases in regional ventilation by decreasing pulmonary blood flow to these areas. The active vasoconstriction initiated by local alveolar hypoxia is known as hypoxic pulmonary vasoconstriction [see Decreased Hypoxic Pulmonary Vasoconstriction, below]. This protective mechanism is impaired by vasodilators given exogenously or produced locally by inflammation or by the septic response. Moreover, it may begin to fail if it is chronically activated, as it is in emphysema. The failure of hypoxic pulmonary vasoconstriction increases both $\dot{V}/\dot{Q}$ mismatch and the shunt fraction. If both alveoli and capillaries are destroyed—as, for example, in necrotizing pneumonia—total ventilation-perfusion matching remains relatively normal; gas exchange is impaired only if a large portion of the alveolar capillary exchange system is destroyed.

ALVEOLAR HYPOVENTILATION

Alveolar hypoventilation, or decreased alveolar minute ventilation, can be considered a specific form of alveolar minute ventilation mismatch. It is caused by impairment of CNS respiratory center activity or by physical impairment of ventilation [see Table 17]. Alveolar hypoventilation produces hypoxia and hypercapnia because neither gas is adequately exchanged. In alveoli with at least some ventilation, exogenous administration of oxygen increases the P_AO_2 and may maintain sufficient oxygen content and gas exchange. The P_ACO_2, however, will increase relatively rapidly, resulting in a concomitant increase in P_aCO_2, or respiratory acidosis. The P_aCO_2 in blood leaving an alveolus is equal to the end-inspiratory P_ACO_2 of that alveolus.

Total minute ventilation is often normal, but alveolar ventilation may decrease if the V_D/V_T ratio is greater than its normal value of 0.2 to 0.3. This can occur even in the absence of lung parenchymal injury. The ratio increases with shallow breathing because the anatomic dead space stays constant (100 to 150 ml) while the V_T decreases. When V_T is inadequate, FRC is reduced as well. Airway collapse and atelectasis result if FRC falls below the closing volume.

Physical Impairment

Upper airway obstruction A significant impairment in upper airway patency as a result of anatomic distortion—e.g., posterior tongue displacement or oropharyngeal edema—will lead to hypoventilation. Depression of CNS activity increases the potential for anatomic distortion and airway obstruction.

Impaired respiratory muscle function Considerable inspiratory force, in excess of −25 cm H_2O, is needed to produce an adequate spontaneous tidal volume and vital capacity. Any impairment of chest wall or diaphragmatic muscle function that prevents the generation of an adequate transpulmonary pressure will result in hypoventilation. A number of drugs, including muscle relaxants used intraoperatively and antibiotics such as neomycin, can produce such an impairment. Neurologic disorders that alter neuromuscular function or abdominal distention that limits excursion of the diaphragm will also impair respiratory activity.

Temporary paralysis caused by spinal anesthetic or more prolonged paralysis caused by trauma are additional causes of hypoventilation. Pain, either from direct muscle trauma, pleural irritation, or neuralgia, is a major cause of impaired respiratory muscle function in surgical patients.

Chest wall instability Multiple rib fractures, particularly those in more than one place that give rise to a flail segment, can substantially impair chest wall activity. Much of the impairment is the result of pain. With bilateral flail chest, ventilatory assistance is usually necessary.

Stiff lung Impaired lung expansion can result from a restrictive lung process, such as pneumonia, edema, or interstitial fibrosis (which causes decreased static compliance) or severe bronchospasm (which causes decreased dynamic compliance). Even very high transpulmonary pressures may be insufficient to expand a lung with poor compliance. A moderate impairment in compliance, as occurs with lung edema, may produce hypoventilation if the increased work of breathing causes oxygen demand to exceed oxygen transport to the respiratory muscles, resulting in fatigue [see Table 18].

INCREASED SHUNT

An increase in the shunt fraction lowers arterial oxygen tension and saturation because nonoxygenated blood from the shunt mixes with oxygenated blood from ventilated lung regions. Because the oxygen saturation of oxygenated blood normally approaches 100 percent, no satisfactory compensation can be made for the low oxygen saturation of the shunted blood. Raising the F_IO_2 will not improve oxygen exchange in the shunt area, because there is no ventilation. A shunt fraction of 15 percent or greater produces severe hypoxemia and tissue hypoxia. An increased anatomic shunt can result from a traumatic pulmonary arteriovenous fistula or a large vascular intrapulmonary tumor; however, this is rarely the case. Most often, increased venous admixture stems from functional or physiologic shunts created by alveolar collapse, edema, or consolidation.

DECREASED OXYGEN DELIVERY

A decrease in oxygen delivery, the product of cardiac output and arterial oxygen content, results in tissue hypoxia, even if

Table 17 Causes of Hypoventilation[25]

Impairment of CNS respiratory center activity
   Cerebral trauma
   Anesthesia, narcotics, sedatives
   Excessively high P_aCO_2

Physical impairment of ventilation (impaired lung expansion)
   Upper airway obstruction
   Muscular impairment: neuromuscular disease, drug-induced weakness, abdominal distention, pain
   Chest wall instability: rib fractures, flail chest
   Stiff lung parenchyma: edema, fibrosis, ARDS

92 USE OF THE MECHANICAL VENTILATOR

Robert H. Bartlett, M.D.

Approach to Mechanical Ventilation

An essential concept in mechanical ventilation is the distinction between two key processes, ventilation and oxygenation. The primary purpose of ventilation is to excrete carbon dioxide. The minute ventilation ($\dot{V}_E$) is the total amount of gas exhaled per minute, computed as the product of the rate and the tidal volume (V_T). Approximately two thirds of the minute ventilation reaches the alveoli and promotes gas exchange (alveolar ventilation, or $\dot{V}_A$); the remaining third moves in and out of the conducting airways and nonperfused alveoli (the dead space ventilation, or $\dot{V}_D$). Thus, the ratio of dead space to tidal volume (V_D/V_T) is normally 0.33. The efficiency of carbon dioxide excretion is directly related to the amount of alveolar ventilation. During spontaneous breathing, the minute ventilation is regulated by the respiratory center; during mechanical ventilation, the operator uses a mechanical ventilator to excrete enough CO_2 to maintain the partial arterial pressure of CO_2 (P_aCO_2) at 40 mm Hg. Ventilation is monitored by measuring P_aCO_2.

Oxygenation, on the other hand, refers to the equilibrium of oxygen in the pulmonary capillary blood and oxygen in inflated alveoli. The partial pressure of oxygen (PO_2) gradient between alveolus and capillary favors transfer of oxygen into blood because alveolar PO_2 is maintained by ventilation or by provision of supplemental oxygen to the airway. Hence, oxygenation depends less on good alveolar ventilation than on the appropriate matching of pulmonary blood flow to well-inflated alveoli, a process that can be affected by patient position, altered airway pressure, pulmonary parenchymal disease, or small airway disease. The efficiency of this ventilation-perfusion matching, and therefore of oxygenation, can be evaluated by measuring the PO_2 in arterial blood (P_aO_2) at a known value for the fraction, or concentration, of inspired oxygen (F_IO_2).

Mechanical ventilators are designed to provide ventilation by regulating tidal volume, rate, and inspiratory flow, thereby controlling CO_2 excretion. Because they can also regulate airway pressure and F_IO_2, they offer some control over oxygenation as well. In either case, proper use of a mechanical ventilator necessitates a solid understanding of normal and abnormal pulmonary mechanics, gas exchange, and the relation between systemic oxygen delivery and consumption. Most mechanical ventilators allow the operator to monitor at least some of these variables. In practice, a mechanical ventilator is employed differently depending on whether the main goal is adequate ventilation or adequate oxygenation. Therefore, these two aspects of ventilator use will be discussed separately.

Basic Mechanical Ventilation

VENTILATION

For basic mechanical ventilation, the rate should initially be set at 10/min and the tidal volume at 10 ml/kg, provided that the inspiratory plateau pressure (P_{plat}) is less than 30 cm H_2O; if P_{plat} is higher than 30 cm H_2O, smaller tidal volumes, such as 6 ml/kg, are appropriate. This setting will yield a minute ventilation of 100 ml/kg/min. If the V_D/V_T ratio is nearly normal, the alveolar ventilation produced (approximately 4 L/min) will be sufficient to eliminate all the metabolically produced CO_2 and to maintain the P_aCO_2 at about 40 mm Hg. If the patient's brain stem function is normal, the mechanical ventilator should be set on the assist mode, which allows the patient to adjust his or her own respiratory rate to keep the P_aCO_2 within normal limits. As a safeguard, a controlled backup rate is set below the patient's assist rate in case spontaneous effort ceases.

OXYGENATION

For basic oxygenation, the F_IO_2 should initially be set at 0.5. This level is not damaging to the alveoli and does not deplete nitrogen levels from the alveoli. If the pulmonary parenchyma and ventilation-perfusion relations are normal, P_aO_2 will be unnecessarily elevated, and the F_IO_2 should be turned down until the saturation and PO_2 are in the normal range. The positive end-expiratory pressure (PEEP) should be set at +5 cm H_2O. This value is high enough to maintain inflation of some alveoli that would close at end expiration at lower pressures yet low enough not to induce any deleterious effects. The peak inspiratory pressure (PIP), which is always measured after a short inspiratory hold or plateau, is determined by the tidal volume, inspiratory gas flow, and compliance of the lung. If the compliance is relatively normal, the ventilator settings described will lead to a P_{plat} of 20 cm H_2O. The high airway pressure cutoff and alarm should be set at 40 cm H_2O. These settings will result in a mean airway pressure of between 5 and 10 cm H_2O, with the exact lev-

CO_2

Worsening ↑

Respiratory rate, 30/min	Tidal volume, 15 ml/kg
Efficiency of ventilation decreases as rate increases.	Rarely indicated. Consider alternatives (see text).

Respiratory rate, 15/min	Tidal volume, 12 ml/kg
Adjust the rate before tidal volume to lower P_aCO_2.	Increasing tidal volume will increase airway pressure.

Start →

Respiratory rate, 10/min   **Tidal volume, 10 ml/kg**

Improving ↓

Spontaneous respiratory rate < 25/min

Tidal volume >5 ml/kg; vital capacity > 10 ml/kg; minute ventilation < 120 ml/kg/min

Weaning process

Effort (%) vs Time (minutes): Mechanical Ventilation transitioning to Spontaneous Breathing over 0–30 minutes

Simultaneous monitors of the weaning process

After 30 minutes, respiratory rate < 20/min and pulse rate < 100/min	After 30 minutes, respiratory rate > 25/min and pulse rate < 120/min

$P_aCO_2 \leq 40$ mm Hg and $P_aCO_2 \geq 60$ mm Hg	$P_aCO_2 > 40$ mm Hg and $P_aCO_2 < 60$ mm Hg

Extubate and remove patient from ventilator

Institute postventilation prophylaxis:
- Institute deep breathing or IPPB
- Clear secretions
- Avoid aspirations

Resume mechanical ventilation

Follow procedures for difficult weaning:
- CPAP or IMV trial
- Tracheostomy
- Bronchoscopy
- Nutritional assessment and therapy

O_2

PEEP > 15 cm H_2O
Decrease tidal volume to avoid high peak and mean pressures.

F_IO_2, 1.0
Rarely indicated. Maximize hemoglobin and cardiac output. Decrease $\dot{V}O_2$.

Peak inspiratory pressure, 35 cm H_2O; PEEP, 10 cm H_2O
PEEP testing indicated at 10 cm H_2O or above.

F_IO_2, 0.6
Use lowest F_IO_2 to keep arterial saturation > 95%.

Peak inspiratory pressure, 30 cm H_2O; PEEP, 5 cm H_2O
Measure peak inspiratory pressure after a short inspiratory hold.

F_IO_2, 0.5
Will not damage alveoli or deplete nitrogen.

Airway pressure
Best-effort inspiratory force > 20 cm H_2O.

F_IO_2 < 0.4
To maintain P_aO_2 > 60 mm Hg.

← Start

Worsening ↑ ↓ Improving

Approach to Mechanical Ventilation

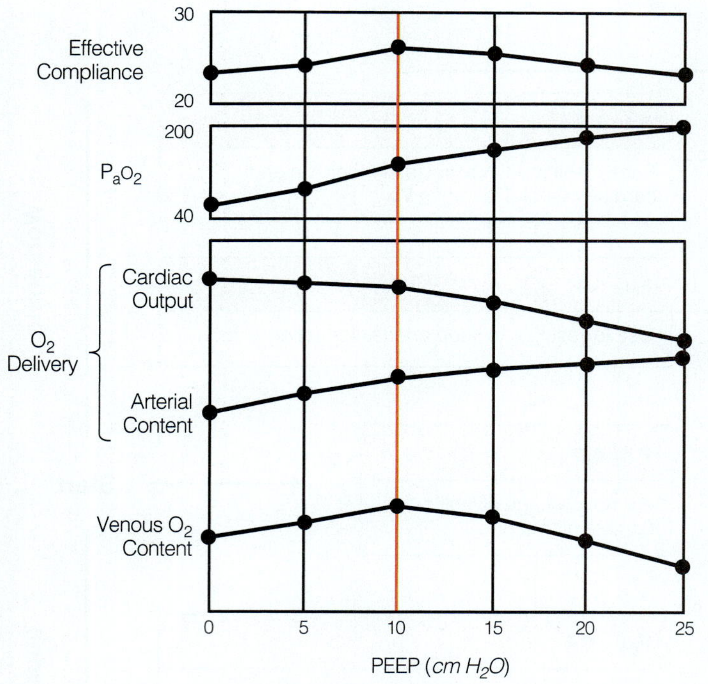

Figure 1 Shown are measurements for determining the optimal PEEP. The objective is to maximize the oxygen delivery:oxygen consumption ratio, which is measured by mixed venous saturation. Here, the best PEEP is 10 cm H_2O, even though the P_aO_2 and the arterial oxygen content are higher at higher levels of PEEP.

el depending on the respiratory rate, the inspiratory gas flow rate, and the amount of spontaneous inspiratory effort generated by the patient. The patient's inspiratory effort will appear as negative pressure measured at the airway, but such effort is beneficial rather than deleterious.

After the patient has been started on a course of mechanical ventilation, ventilation and oxygenation must be assessed, usually by measuring P_aCO_2 and P_aO_2. Adjustments are then made on the basis of this assessment [*see Figure 1*]. If P_aCO_2 and P_aO_2 are normal and if the patient is to remain on mechanical ventilation for pulmonary prophylaxis or because of CNS depression, these settings are maintained until it is time to wean the patient from ventilation [*see* Weaning from Mechanical Ventilation, *below*]. If the settings do not provide adequate gas exchange or if the patient's condition worsens, further adjustments are required.

Worsening Respiratory Status

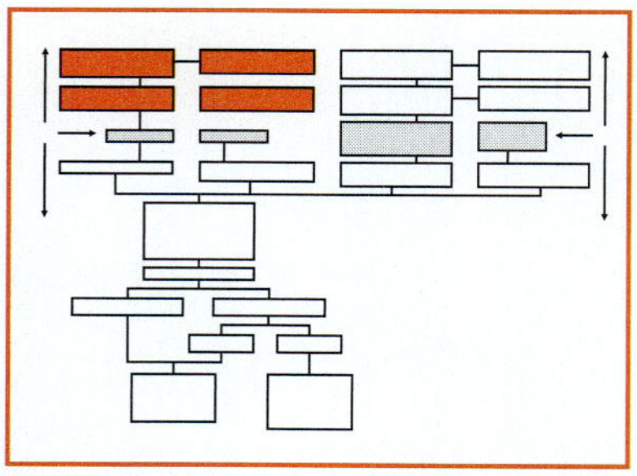

VENTILATION

If the P_aCO_2 is elevated despite a minute ventilation of 100 ml/kg/min, either the metabolically produced carbon dioxide is inappropriately high or the alveolar ventilation is an inappropriately low percentage of the tidal volume, or both. To increase ventilation, the first step should be to increase the respiratory rate (stepwise) to 20/min. (Increasing the respiratory rate raises the mean airway pressure and may necessitate administration of fluid volume to maintain hemodynamic stability; however, because increasing the tidal volume elevates the P_{plat}, possibly leading to barotrauma, the respiratory rate must be changed first.) The volume of CO_2 excreted is easily measured by collecting and analyzing exhaled gas. If it is greater than normal (130 ml/m²/min), CO_2 production can be decreased by reducing muscular activity or seizures, controlling hypermetabolic states (if possible), and minimizing the exogenous carbohydrate load.

If the P_aCO_2 has still not returned to normal after these measures have been taken, the respiratory rate can be increased to 25/min or higher, although it should be kept in mind that the efficiency of ventilation decreases as the respiratory rate increases (i.e., the percentage of minute ventilation that becomes alveolar ventilation decreases as the respiratory rate increases because there may be inadequate time for alveolar emptying during expiration and because the dead space remains unchanged). A tidal volume greater than 15 ml/kg is rarely necessary unless there is a major air leak. A minute ventilation higher than 300 ml/kg/min indicates major metabolic or respiratory dysfunction. The pressures required to generate this amount of ventilation are harmful to the lungs and adversely affect hemodynamic status. If the P_aCO_2 is higher than 40 mm Hg despite a respiratory rate of 20 to 25/min, a P_{plat} of 35 cm H_2O, and a minute ventilation of 250 to 300 ml/kg/min, alternatives should be seriously considered, such as allowing the patient to equilibrate at an abnormally high P_aCO_2, inducing paralysis to decrease muscular activity and CO_2 production, or instituting extracorporeal circulation through a membrane oxygenator to remove CO_2 [*see* Fighting the Ventilator, Permissive Hypercapnia, *and* Extracorporeal Life Support, *below*].

OXYGENATION

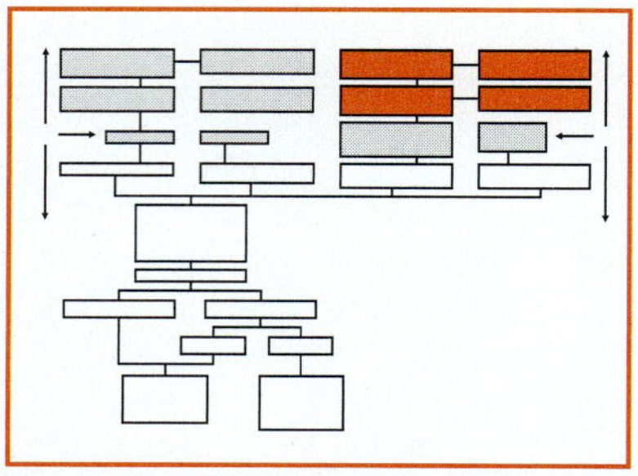

If the initial ventilator settings are not adequate to oxygenate the patient's arterial blood, then some areas in the lung are perfused but not inflated (i.e., right-to-left shunting). To enhance oxygenation, the first step is to raise the PEEP to 10 cm H_2O, in the hope of maintaining or improving alveolar inflation. It is wise to decrease tidal volume and to increase the respiratory rate at the same time, to avoid raising the P_{plat}. The P_{plat} should not exceed 45 cm H_2O. Even with these changes in ventilation, the mean airway pressure may increase to the point at which it interferes with venous return. Whenever the PEEP is raised above 5 cm H_2O, the balance between systemic oxygen delivery and oxygen consumption should be evaluated because increasing the mean airway pressure may raise the P_{O_2} but may actually decrease systemic oxygen delivery by decreasing cardiac output.

Several measurements are necessary for determining the optimal PEEP level [*see Figure 1*]. Effective lung compliance is the simplest measurement, but optimal lung compliance does not always correlate with optimal oxygen delivery. The best measurement is that of venous oxygen content, which is approximated as mixed venous oxyhemoglobin saturation. This measurement requires samples of blood from the pulmonary artery or, better yet, a continuous indwelling catheter to monitor venous saturation. Obviously, therefore, a pulmonary arterial catheter should be inserted whenever PEEP levels higher than 5 cm H_2O are necessary for ensuring adequate oxygenation. Venous saturation measures the ratio of systemic oxygen delivery to oxygen consumption. This ratio is normally 4, which corresponds to a mixed venous saturation of 75%, when arterial saturation is near 100%. (That is, normally 25% of the oxygen delivered to tissues is extracted and utilized.) Consequently, PEEP testing is best done by gradually increasing the

PEEP level until either oxygenation is sufficient to saturate arterial blood or mixed venous saturation drops below 70%, whichever comes first.

PEEP does not cause inflation of collapsed alveoli but only holds open alveolar units that would collapse at a lower airway pressure. Inflation can be facilitated by prolonging inspiration, which can be achieved by using a slower inspiratory flow rate, an inspiratory hold or plateau (0.5 to 1.0 second), or a designated pressure for a specific time (pressure-controlled ventilation). All of these maneuvers will increase the mean airway pressure and the inspiration-expiration ratio (I/E), which may limit venous return, thereby interfering with oxygen delivery. Venous saturation monitoring is the best way to titrate inspiratory pressure maneuvers.

AVOIDING LUNG INJURY

Positive airway pressure and oxygen are lifesaving when delivered in moderation but can damage the lungs when delivered in excess. An F_IO_2 of 0.6 and a peak airway pressure of 30 cm H_2O can be used for days or weeks if necessary without deleterious effects. Because oxygen and pressure are delivered only to inflated alveoli, the most normal area of the lung is subjected to injury when higher levels are used. Thus, excessive positive pressure and oxygen can contribute to the pathogenesis of progressive pulmonary failure in ventilated patients. Moreover, pressure above 40 cm H_2O simply causes overdistention of the inflated alveoli and decreases the efficiency of ventilation [see Discussion, below]. An F_IO_2 above 0.6 has a minimal effect on oxygenation when the major problem is transpulmonary shunt. For these reasons, before P_{plat} is raised above 40 cm H_2O or F_IO_2 is raised above 0.6, all other variables of systemic oxygen delivery should be considered [see Table 1].

If oxygenation remains inadequate at these higher airway pressures, then F_IO_2 can be increased to 0.6 or higher, although it should be noted that if the problem is a major transpulmonary shunt, major increases in F_IO_2 will have little effect on P_aO_2. High concentrations of oxygen in the airway should generally be avoided, primarily because of the resultant depletion of nitrogen, which helps maintain inflation of the alveoli. Only very rarely is it necessary to raise F_IO_2 above 0.6; usually, it is preferable to increase the PEEP instead while progressively decreasing tidal volume and supporting blood volume. PEEP is used to improve ventilation-perfusion matching; prone positioning and diuresis may be even more effective [see Discussion, below].

The goal in severe respiratory failure is to optimize oxygen delivery, not P_aO_2. Measures to be taken include administering red blood cells until a normal hemoglobin concentration (13 to 15 g/dl) is reached, increasing cardiac output by means of volume loading, decreasing systemic oxygen consumption by means of sedation or paralysis, and treating the cause of hypermetabolism (usually infection). The relation between systemic oxygen delivery and oxygen consumption can be monitored by measuring mixed venous saturation. If it is considered necessary to use high airway pressure and 100% oxygen, the variables of oxygen delivery should be set as just described. The F_IO_2 should then be decreased until venous saturation falls to 65% to 70%. If arterial saturation is less than 90% despite an F_IO_2 of 1.0, PEEP of more than 10 cm H_2O, and a hemoglobin of more than 13 g/dl, the next measures to be taken should be (1) to induce paralysis to decrease oxygen consumption, (2) to allow the patient to equilibrate at an abnormally low arterial oxygen saturation (S_aO_2), or (3) to institute extracorporeal circulation through a membrane oxygenator to deliver oxygen.

Improving Respiratory Status

VENTILATION

Patients whose respiratory status is improving should be alert enough to regulate their own respiratory rate with the ventilator in the assist mode. Tidal volume is maintained at 10 ml/kg until the patient is ready for weaning. (As noted, if P_{plat} is greater than 30 cm H_2O, a smaller tidal volume is appropriate.) When respiratory status is improving, the ventilator should remain in the assist mode rather than in the controlled mechanical ventilation (CMV) mode because the patient can adjust his or her respiratory rate to maintain a normal P_aCO_2.

Table 1 Interventions to Optimize the Ratio of Oxygen Delivery to Oxygen Consumption in Patients with Impaired Oxygenation

Intervention	Benefits	Risk
Increase O_2 content		
↑ F_IO_2 to above 0.6	0.3 ml O_2/dl for each 100 mm Hg P_aO_2 after full saturation	O_2 toxicity to lung Less nitrogen in alveoli
↑ Hemoglobin (Hb) to normal	1.36 ml O_2/dl for each g HbO_2/dl	Transfusion risk (viral infection)
Increase cardiac output		
↑ Blood volume to pulmonary capillary wedge pressure of 15–20 mm Hg	200 ml $\dot{D}O_2$ increase for each L/min increase in cardiac output*	Transfusion risk ↑ Pulmonary hydrostatic pressure
Administer inotropic drugs to achieve $S_{\bar{v}}O_2$ 75%–80%	200 ml $\dot{D}O_2$ increase for each L/min increase in cardiac output*	Increased $\dot{V}O_2$ and $\dot{V}CO_2$ with catecholamines Tachycardia
Administer vasodilator drugs to achieve $S_{\bar{v}}O_2$ 75%–80%	200 ml $\dot{D}O_2$ increase for each L/min increase in cardiac output*	Hypotension Variable regional blood flow
Decrease O_2 consumption		
Drain and treat infection	Eliminate stimulus to metabolism	None
Patient paralysis	10%–15% decrease in $\dot{V}O_2$ and $\dot{V}CO_2$	Weakness, atrophy, need for positional changes, difficult patient examination
↓ Body temperature	7% decrease in $\dot{V}O_2$ and $\dot{V}CO_2$ for each 1° C increase in body temperature	Requires patient paralysis, coagulopathy

*Hb = 15 g/dl; S_aO_2 = 100%.

OXYGENATION

The F_IO_2 should be decreased to a concentration (0.4 or 0.3) that ensures an arterial saturation higher than 90% (equivalent to a P_aO_2 higher than 60 mm Hg). Keeping the F_IO_2 in this range will lead to increased arterial oxygenation, which serves as a slight safety buffer during suctioning or disconnection. The PEEP can be reduced to 0, although there is a theoretical advantage to maintaining a low level of PEEP as long as the patient is intubated.

WEANING PARAMETERS

When the patient can maintain satisfactory gas exchange at the ventilator settings just given, the next step is to determine whether the patient is ready for extubation. Accordingly, the patient's ability to ventilate is measured during spontaneous breathing a few minutes after the removal of mechanical support. The findings that generally indicate that weaning and extubation can be carried out successfully are (1) a spontaneous respiratory rate lower than 25/min, (2) a tidal volume greater than 5 ml/kg, (3) a vital capacity greater than 10 ml/kg, (4) a minute ventilation less than 120 ml/kg/min, and (5) an inspiratory pressure that is more negative than –20 cm H_2O. If the patient meets these parameters and if arterial oxygenation is satisfactory at an F_IO_2 of 0.4 or less, then pulmonary mechanics and gas exchange are probably close enough to normal to permit extubation and spontaneous breathing. It should be kept in mind that these measurements are made while the patient is breathing through a long, narrow endotracheal or tracheostomy tube, which causes significant resistance and increases the work of breathing. Therefore, the results will be even better when the patient is extubated and breathing through his or her own airway. If metabolic alkalosis is present, it should be corrected before weaning is attempted. The one variable that cannot be measured with this amount of testing is the endurance of the patient's respiratory efforts. Measurement of endurance is, in essence, the weaning process.

Weaning from Mechanical Ventilation

In the weaning process, the work of breathing that had been the task of the mechanical ventilator is reassumed by the respiratory muscles of the patient. When the results of respiratory testing indicate that the patient can be weaned from the ventilator, a trial of spontaneous breathing is indicated. During this trial, supplemental humidified oxygen is supplied by way of the endotracheal tube. The balloon is deflated to allow some breathing around the tube and to minimize airway resistance. The patient should be sitting upright. The transition from mechanical support to spontaneous breathing should be swift: the mechanical ventilator should be either turned down rapidly or simply disconnected [see Figure 2]. In addition, the gas supply to the endotracheal tube must be free-flowing; at no point in the trial should the patient have to trigger a demand valve on the ventilator. Most ventilators do not supply a free flow of gas in the continuous positive airway pressure (CPAP) or intermittent mandatory ventilation (IMV) mode but require patient effort to trigger gas flow. The purpose of the spontaneous breathing trial is to determine the endurance of the patient. If it is obvious that the patient can make a strong respiratory effort and is fully alert and awake, he or she can be extubated without further testing after a few minutes of spontaneous breathing.

The simplest way to monitor a spontaneous breathing trial is to watch respiratory rate and pulse rate. If, after 5 to 30 minutes of spontaneous breathing, the respiratory rate is lower than 25/min, the patient will probably be able to sustain an adequate minute ventilation when extubated. If the pulse rate is less than 120/min, the work of breathing is probably not excessive. If the respiratory rate is lower than 20/min and the pulse rate less than 100/min, the patient can be extubated without any further measurements being made. If, however, the pulse rate and respiratory rate are moderately elevated, the P_aCO_2 and P_aO_2 should be measured; if the P_aCO_2 is 40 mm Hg or lower and the P_aO_2 is 60 mm Hg or higher, the patient may be extubated. Postventilation prophylactic maneuvers, to be discussed later [see Postventilation Prophylaxis, below], are indicated. If the results of these four measurements indicate that the trial of spontaneous breathing has failed, mechanical ventilation is resumed to improve the patient's respiratory status before weaning is tried again.

The weaning process should never take more than an hour. If the indicators for weaning are present, the trial of spontaneous breathing is usually successful, and the patient should be extubated. If the indicators are not present, mechanical support should not be gradually decreased—for example, over a period of hours or days—except under strictly controlled conditions.

Difficult Weaning

There are a number of reasons why patients may remain ventilator dependent. If the patient has chronic lung disease that predated the acute event, it may be necessary to wean from the ventilator at a level of P_aCO_2 corresponding to compensated respiratory acidosis. If chronic bronchitis, acute resolving pneumonitis, or injury to the respiratory epithelium is present, bronchoscopy is indicated to examine the airway and clear any inspissated secretions. If the patient has lower-lobe infiltrates (as is commonly the case following a prolonged period of ventilation and supine position), vigorous chest physical therapy and postural drainage are indicated.

VENTILATION

Hypoventilation with gradual CO_2 accumulation is the most common finding in patients who are difficult to wean from mechanical ventilation. Hypermetabolism with increased CO_2 load is a common cause of this problem. Patients who have barely enough respiratory endurance to excrete a normal amount of carbon dioxide cannot maintain the extra ventilation necessary for sustained hyperventilation. Often, muscular weakness is the problem, particularly when compliance is decreased by the acute lung disease that requires extra work with every breath.

In addition to the general measures listed (see above), the first step in a patient in whom attempts at weaning have failed is to do a tracheostomy. This procedure not only minimizes the rebreathing space but also eliminates the urgency and potential risk of extubation, thereby greatly facilitating the weaning process. When the tracheostomy is in place and all the general measures have been carried out, progressive breathing exercises are begun. The type of progressive breathing exercise depends to some extent on the type of mechanical ventilator available. The tidal volume should remain greater than 5 ml/kg while the inspiratory work gradually shifts from the ventilator to the patient. The pressure-support mode on newer ventilators is ideal for this purpose, or a pressure-controlled mode can be

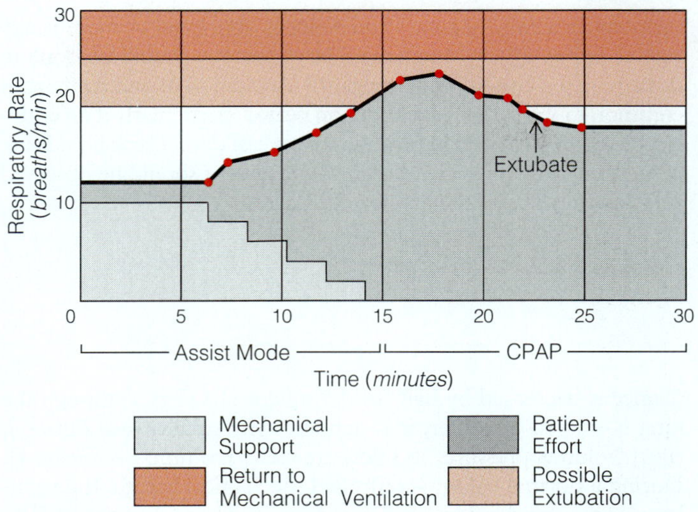

Figure 2 For most patients, ventilator weaning consists of a brief trial of spontaneous breathing in which pulse and respiratory rates are measured. Mechanical support is decreased until the patient can breathe spontaneously (with or without continuous positive airway pressure [CPAP]), and the respiratory rate is measured every few minutes to determine whether the patient can be extubated. If the respiratory rate is consistently below 20/min and the pulse rate is less than 100/min, the patient can be extubated without the need for further measurements; if it is consistently above 30/min, the patient must be returned to the ventilator; and if it is between 25/min and 30/min, measure P_{CO_2} and P_{O_2} to determine whether another trial of mechanical ventilation is needed.

used. In pressure-controlled or pressure-support ventilation, the peak airway pressure is decreased (typically, 2 cm H_2O/15 min) as long as the respiratory rate is lower than 25/min and the tidal volume is adequate. When the peak airway pressure is 5 to 10 cm H_2O for several hours, the patient can be extubated or can be managed with only humidified air to the tracheostomy [*see Table 2*].

Some volume ventilators do not allow pressure-controlled weaning and instead decrease the rate of volume-controlled breaths. The patient is expected to sustain normal minute ventilation by spontaneous nonassisted breaths. This so-called intermittent mandatory ventilation weaning technique often leads to rapid, shallow breathing and exhaustion in patients [*see Table 2*]. Periods of totally spontaneous breathing should be alternated with assist-mode volume ventilation if pressure-controlled weaning is not possible.

OXYGENATION

Oxygenation is rarely a problem with the hard-to-wean patient because supplemental inspired oxygen (30% to 40%) can counter the hypoventilation that makes weaning difficult. As mentioned earlier [*see* Worsening Respiratory Status, Oxygenation, *above*], other components of the oxygen delivery system (hemoglobin and cardiac output) should be optimized because the patient may have to be weaned at a lower than normal P_aO_2.

NUTRITION AND METABOLISM

A common cause of weaning failure is hypermetabolism caused by occult infection, which manifests itself as increased oxygen consumption ($\dot{V}O_2$) and CO_2 production ($\dot{V}CO_2$). The underlying cause should be treated before weaning is attempted again. Good nutrition is essential for respiratory muscle strength and endurance [*see 97 Nutritional Support*]. If a patient is chronically nutritionally depleted, enteral or parenteral feeding to improve muscular strength may be necessary before the patient can be weaned from the ventilator. On the other hand, if carbohydrates are given in amounts exceeding energy expenditure, lipogenesis occurs, which leads to excess CO_2 production. The appropriate nutritional manipulations to avoid this problem depend on direct measurement of $\dot{V}O_2$ and $\dot{V}CO_2$ and calculation of the respiratory quotient. As mentioned earlier [*see* Improving Respiratory Status, Weaning Parameters, *above*], it is important to correct metabolic alkalosis.

Postventilation Prophylaxis

The recently extubated patient is at risk for respiratory failure and consequently should be watched carefully. Airway secretions, stimulated by the chronic indwelling tube, may be thick and difficult to clear. The airway should be carefully lavaged and suctioned before the tube is removed. Direct endotracheal suctioning should be avoided in the period just after removal of the tube because of the risk of hypoxia, vagal stimulation, and vocal cord edema. Postural drainage combined with appropriate airway humidification is a better way of draining airway secretions. The patient should be encouraged to do deep breathing exercises hourly for a few days after extubation, aided, if desired, by an incentive spirometer. If the patient cannot or will not take spontaneous deep breaths, a mechanical ventilator fitted with a mouthpiece should be used every hour or two to ensure periodic maximal inflation (a procedure known as intermittent positive pressure breathing, or IPPB). During IPPB, the ventilator should be used as described in this

Table 2 Methods of Progressive Breathing Exercise in Patients Who Are Difficult to Wean from Mechanical Ventilation

Method	Benefit	Risk
Intermittent mandatory ventilation (IMV)	Commonly available Assisted breath V_T not dependent on compliance	Rapid, shallow breaths may be exhausting Unassisted breaths may require demand valve trigger
Pressure-controlled ventilation	Commonly available V_T supported during each breath	V_T varies with compliance
Pressure support (flow-controlled)	Best support of V_T during each breath	V_T varies with compliance Not commonly available
Pressure support with IMV	V_T supported during each breath IMV not dependent on compliance	IMV may slow the weaning process Not commonly available
Spontaneous-breathing trials	Easy to quantitate status and progress Not dependent on demand valve trigger Universally available	Rapid, shallow breaths may be exhausting

chapter, except that periodic maximal inflation (to a PIP of 30 to 40 cm H_2O) is used to ensure maximal alveolar filling. Even if only a few assisted deep breaths are taken every few hours, inflation will be sufficient to prevent atelectasis. Another option is the use of continuous positive airway pressure by mask or nasal catheter.

The vocal cords will be edematous and may be chronically damaged or dislocated. Aerosolized racemic epinephrine helps to minimize upper airway edema. If the voice is abnormal or there is any sign of upper airway obstruction, laryngoscopy should be done to determine the condition of the glottis. Aspiration of oral contents is common in the early postextubation period, particularly if an endotracheal tube has been in position for several days. Thick liquids are easier to swallow than clear liquids. The patient should be observed very carefully during the first few feedings.

Discussion

Pulmonary Physiology and Mechanical Ventilation

PULMONARY MECHANICS

The interrelations of gas volumes and pressures that are an integral part of ventilation are collectively referred to as pulmonary mechanics and are more fully described elsewhere [see 91 Pulmonary Dysfunction]. The use of a mechanical ventilator is an exercise in pulmonary mechanics, which may be illustrated by comparing the compliance curve for a normal lung with that for an atelectatic or edematous lung [see Figure 3]. The standard compliance, or volume-pressure, curve is obtained by measuring volume and pressure at stages of lung deflation after total inflation. Total lung compliance, normalized for patient size, is approximately 1 ml/cm H_2O/kg. A comparison of volume-pressure curves for normal lungs from three different patients shows the effect of patient size [see Figure 3, left]. In fact, the curves would be the same if normalized for patient size. If the lung volume is decreased by half (as a result of pneumonectomy or main bronchus occlusion, for example), the compliance is decreased by half (to 0.5 ml/cm H_2O/kg). Although the lung is said to be stiffer, it is actually only smaller [see Figure 3, right]. Volume, pressure, and flow are related in time [see Figure 4]. During a normal volume-controlled mechanical breath, the ventilator generates gas flow until the desired volume is reached. The pressure is then simply measured. In this example [see Figure 4], a short 1-second inspiratory hold is applied to show the difference between plateau pressure, which is equilibrated with alveoli, and peak inspiratory pressure, which is slightly higher because of airflow resistance in the tubing.

In acute respiratory failure, the cause of decreased compliance is almost always associated with a decrease in the functional residual capacity (FRC). In the example cited earlier [see Figure 3, right], normal tidal breathing from volume A to volume B would result with 10 cm of inflating pressure. During atelectasis, the decreased FRC (point C) represents the lost alveoli that are either collapsed or filled with fluid but are still perfused with blood. Tidal breathing (to volume D) requires higher pressure. Because the compliance curve is

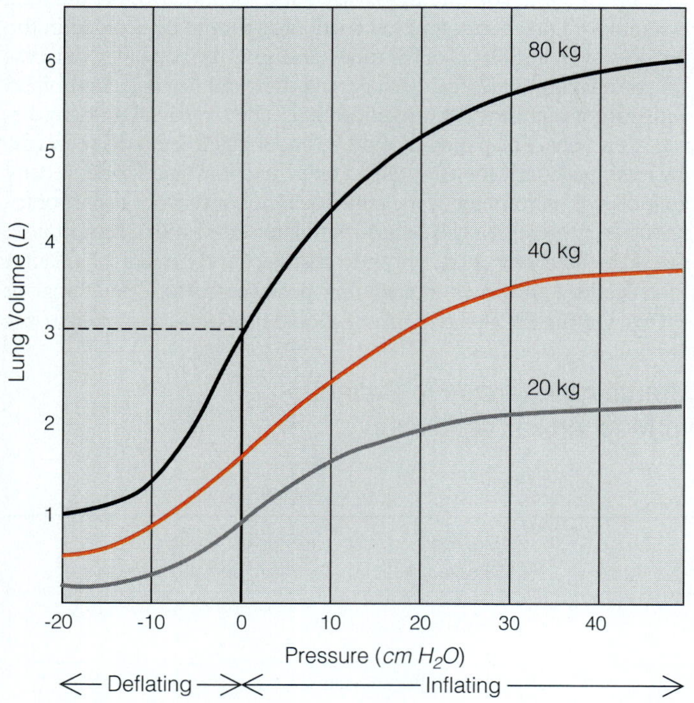

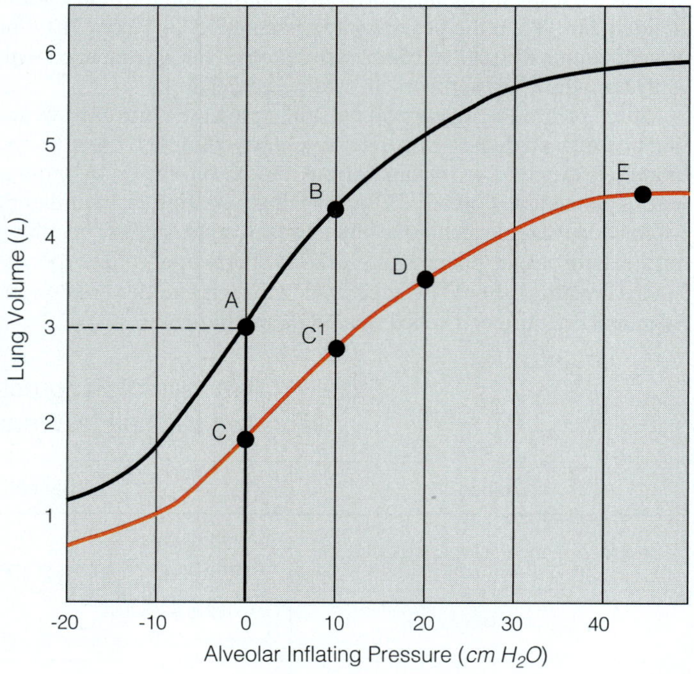

Figure 3 Depicted are pulmonary mechanics involved in mechanical ventilation. At left are compliance curves for a child weighing 20 kg, an adult weighing 40 kg, and an adult weighing 80 kg, all with normal lungs. The dotted line identifies FRC for the person weighing 80 kg. Functional residual capacity (FRC), total lung capacity, and compliance, which are proportional to patient size, must be normalized to patient weight to permit comparisons with other normal persons and between patients. At right are compliance curves for a patient weighing 80 kg who has normal lungs (upper curve) (compliance, 1 ml/cm H_2O/kg) and the same patient with major atelectasis (lower curve). The mechanics are altered in atelectasis because a smaller lung volume is available for inflation.

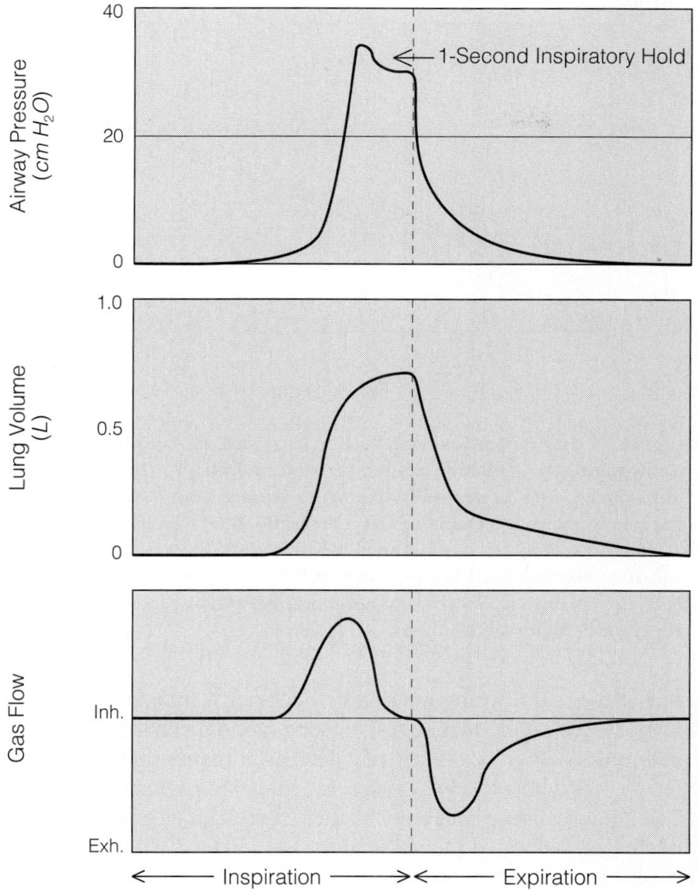

Figure 4 Shown are airway pressure, lung volume, and gas flow during a normal volume-controlled mechanical breath. The ventilator generates gas flow until the desired lung volume is reached, and the airway pressure is simply measured. A 1-second inspiratory hold shows the difference between peak inspiratory and plateau pressures. Dotted line separates inspiration from expiration.

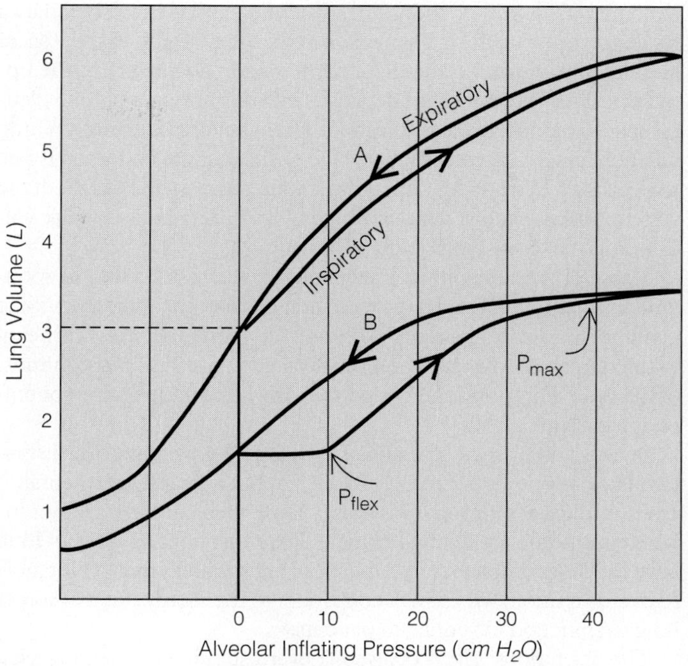

Figure 5 In a patient with normal lungs (black line), the inspiratory volume/pressure curve is very close to the expiratory curve. In a patient with severe parenchymal disease (red line), the inspiratory volume/pressure curve may be nearly flat until enough pressure is exerted to open edematous and collapsed airways and alveoli. As illustrated here, this event (identified as P_{flex}) occurs at 10 cm H_2O. The functional lung is fully inflated at 40 cm H_2O (the curve becomes flat at P_{max}). There is a substantial gap between the deflation curve and the inflation curve.

shifted to the right, much higher pressures are required to achieve the same level of inflation. To inflate the lung to point E, for example, a pressure of 40 cm H_2O would be necessary.

The best way of managing ventilation in these circumstances is to maintain positive end-expiratory pressure at 10 cm H_2O (point C^1 in Figure 3, right) and ventilate to point D with tidal breathing. The PEEP is set at this level to maintain the inflation of alveoli that might close at lower end-expiratory pressures; the volume of pressure used for tidal ventilation is safe and adequate for normal gas exchange.

In normal lungs, the inspiratory limb of the volume/pressure curve is almost the same as the expiratory limb. In severe respiratory failure, variable inspiratory inflation of the lung results in a significant difference between the inflation and deflation limbs, which can be useful in ventilation management [*see Figure 5*]. Collapsed small airways "pop" open at a critical inflating pressure, resulting in an inflation point early in inhalation (P_{flex}). The volume plateaus when all available alveoli are inflated (P_{max}). The P_{flex} and P_{max} are not always well defined, but when they are, it is reasonable to set PEEP above P_{flex} and to set P_{plat} at P_{max}.

Several measurements must be taken to determine whether positive airway pressure is recruiting collapsed alveoli or simply distending normal alveoli [*see Figure 6*]. The signs that collapsed alveoli are being reinflated are (1) improved normalized compliance, (2) decreased dead space ventilation, (3) unaffected cardiac output, and (4) improved oxygenation and decreased shunt at the same ventilator settings. These signs must be kept in mind during management of a patient on a mechanical ventilator.

The effect of the abdominal viscera on pulmonary mechanics is significant. Most data on patients and normal subjects were obtained from individuals in the sitting position, yet most patients on mechanical ventilation are in the supine position. Even in normal subjects, the functional residual capacity is decreased by 25% when measured with the subjects in the supine position. This effect is exaggerated in

Distention	Positive Airway Pressure	Recruitment
↓ Compliance	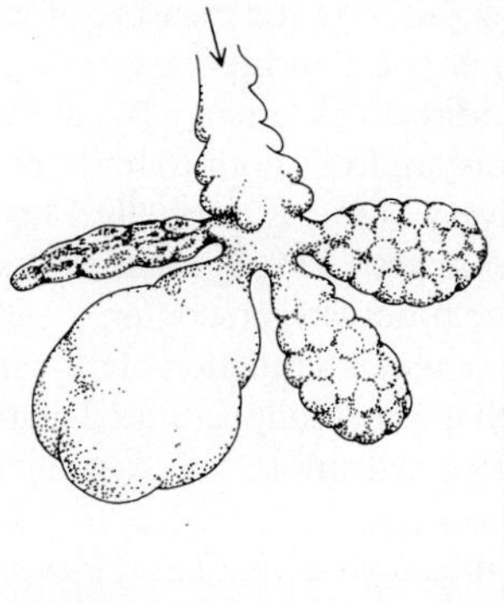	↑ Compliance
↑ V_D/V_T		↓ V_D/V_T
↓ Cardiac Output		→ Cardiac Output
→ Shunt		↓↓ Shunt
↑ Air Leak		→ Air Leak

Figure 6 The results of serial measurements of compliance, dead space ventilation, cardiac output, oxygenation, shunting, and air-leak risks indicate whether positive airway pressure is recruiting collapsed alveoli or simply distending normal alveoli.

patients with ascites or abdominal distention and is exacerbated by a weak inspiratory effort. The reason is that the weight of the viscera literally pulls down on the diaphragm when patients are in the upright position, creates slight negative (inflating) pressure in the pleural space, and facilitates inspiration. These beneficial effects on lung inflation are even greater in the prone position, if the abdomen is free to expand. When patients are in the supine position, the weight of the viscera pushes against the diaphragm, which decreases alveolar volume and makes inspiration more difficult.[1]

These principles apply to mechanical ventilation as well as spontaneous breathing. Unless unstable hemodynamics make the supine position necessary, patients who are on ventilators (or are being weaned from ventilators) should be placed in a sitting position most of the time. This positioning is particularly important during spontaneous-breathing trials.

Because high airway pressure can cause lung damage, overdistention [see Figure 6] is not merely inefficient but actually detrimental.[2-4] Even in diffuse pulmonary disease, some areas of lung are not inflated and some are nearly normal.[5] The most normal areas of lung have the best compliance and therefore are the areas most vulnerable to overdistention, which may contribute to the steady progression of lung dysfunction in ventilated patients.[6]

The deleterious effects of alveolar overdistention on the lung itself have been demonstrated in many laboratory studies.[2,4] It has been suggested that the resulting lung injury can trigger the multiple organ dysfunction syndrome. Recent prospective randomized clinical studies by Amato and associates[7] and the Acute Respiratory Distress Syndrome Network of the National Institutes of Health[8] confirm the risks of overdistention injury; moreover, these studies report improved survival and decreased organ failure when overdistention is avoided during either pressure-limited[7] or volume-limited[8] modes of mechanical ventilation. The point at which inflation becomes overdistention has not been precisely determined; however, using end-inspiratory P_{plat} as an indicator of alveolar distention, one would be wise to keep P_{plat} below 40 cm H_2O (some would say 30 cm H_2O) during any mode of mechanical ventilation.[9] In patients with decreased FRC and diminished compliance, limiting P_{plat} in this fashion will result in hypoventilation, which in turn will result in hypercapnia. The physiologic risks of respiratory acidosis are minimal in comparison with the risks of alveolar overdistention. Therefore, it is safer to avoid overdistention injury and tolerate respiratory acidosis (so-called permissive hypercapnia[10]).

OXYGEN KINETICS

Oxygen consumption ($\dot{V}O_2$) is normally 3 ml/kg/min (120 ml/m²/min) at rest and is moderately elevated (as high as 6 ml/kg/min) by catecholamines or sepsis. $\dot{V}O_2$, the measure of metabolic rate, is converted to resting energy expenditure expressed in calories through the arithmetic of indirect calorimetry (5 cal for each liter of $\dot{V}O_2$). $\dot{V}O_2$ at rest stays constant from hour to hour, even in critically ill patients. Oxygen delivery ($\dot{D}O_2$) is normally 12 to 15 ml/kg/min (480 to 600 ml/m²/min) at rest. $\dot{D}O_2$ is measured as cardiac output in deciliters per minute times oxygen content (milliliters of oxygen per deciliter). Oxygen content is a function of the saturation and amount of hemoglobin; each gram of fully saturated hemoglobin carries 1.36 ml of oxygen. A very small amount of oxygen is dissolved in plasma, which is measured as P_aO_2.

In patients on a mechanical ventilator, F_IO_2 and pressure are manipulated to optimize oxygen content and delivery without causing injury to the lung. When $\dot{V}O_2$ is increased, as in sepsis or hypermetabolism, $\dot{D}O_2$ increases through an automatic increase in cardiac output until the ratio between $\dot{D}O_2$ and $\dot{V}O_2$ ($\dot{D}O_2/\dot{V}O_2$) is reestablished at 5:1 [see Figure 7]. A compensatory increase in cardiac output also occurs during anemia or hypoxia to maintain a normal $\dot{D}O_2/\dot{V}O_2$. When $\dot{D}O_2$ changes, no corresponding change in $\dot{V}O_2$ occurs unless $\dot{D}O_2/\dot{V}O_2$ is severely decreased to less than 2:1. When $\dot{D}O_2$ is less than twice $\dot{V}O_2$, anaerobic metabolism occurs, $\dot{V}O_2$ falls, and hemodynamic instability results. These changes occur at both normal and elevated metabolic rates [see Figure 7].[11,12] Although it has been reported that pathologic supply dependency occurs in patients with the acute respiratory distress syndrome,[13,14] this is an artifact,[15] and normal oxygen kinetics exist, even in hypermetabolic conditions.[16] $\dot{D}O_2$ is optimal when it is four to five times greater than $\dot{V}O_2$. Although this point could be determined by repeated measurements of $\dot{V}O_2$, oxygen content, and cardiac output, a simpler way exists.

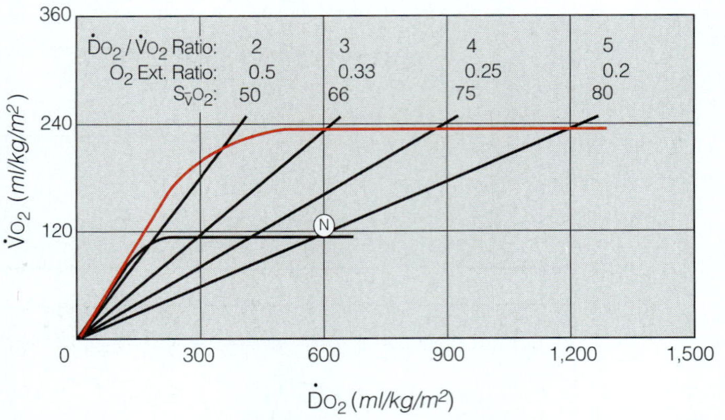

When arterial blood is nearly 100% saturated, the mixed venous oxygen saturation ($S_{\bar{v}}O_2$) directly reflects $\dot{D}O_2/\dot{V}O_2$, regardless of the metabolic rate. For example, if $\dot{D}O_2$ is three times $\dot{V}O_2$, the $S_{\bar{v}}O_2$ will be 66% [see Figure 7]. This variable can be measured in samples of pulmonary arterial blood or by continuous use of a fiberoptic catheter.[17,18] When $\dot{D}O_2$ is adequate, $\dot{V}O_2$ at rest stays constant. Thus, any change in $S_{\bar{v}}O_2$ over minutes or hours directly reflects changes in $\dot{D}O_2$. This phenomenon is used to adjust F_IO_2, PEEP, I/E, and mean airway pressure, in addition to inotropic drug dosages, blood volume, and blood transfusion. The ventilator should be set at the lowest settings that maintain $S_{\bar{v}}O_2$ above 70%.

$S_{\bar{v}}O_2$ does not show the cause of a problem, only whether $\dot{D}O_2/\dot{V}O_2$ is abnormal. If $S_{\bar{v}}O_2$ is abnormally high, the delivery may be higher than necessary (e.g., as in the case of arteriovenous shunt), or the $\dot{V}O_2$ may be decreased at the cellular level (e.g., as in the case of endotoxin affecting cellular enzymes). If $S_{\bar{v}}O_2$ is abnormally low, the delivery might be lower than necessary (e.g., low cardiac output), or the $\dot{V}O_2$ might be elevated above the level at which delivery can compensate (e.g., exercise in a patient with a fixed-rate pacemaker). All of these factors must be taken into account when using $S_{\bar{v}}O_2$ to regulate the mechanical ventilator. The principles of the physiology of oxygen kinetics become particularly important in patients with severe respiratory failure when their pressure and F_IO_2 requirements approach the limits of safety. When $\dot{D}O_2/\dot{V}O_2$ is low, it is better to raise oxygen content by transfusion or decrease $\dot{V}O_2$ by sedation than to use 100% oxygen or very high pressure [see Table 1].

Figure 7 In mechanical ventilation, F_IO_2 and airway pressure are manipulated to optimize oxygen content and $\dot{D}O_2$ so that the lung is not injured. $\dot{D}O_2$ is normally five times greater than $\dot{V}O_2$. Shown are the relationships between the $\dot{D}O_2/\dot{V}O_2$ ratio, the O_2 extraction (Ext.) ratio, and the $S_{\bar{v}}O_2$ when arterial blood is 100% saturated. Gas volumes are standard temperature (0° C) and pressure (760 mm Hg), dry. N indicates values in a normal person at rest; the red line represents hypermetabolism.

VENTILATION-PERFUSION MATCHING

In surgical patients with pulmonary failure, the lung is usually characterized by areas of congestion and atelectasis (low ventilation-perfusion matching [$\dot{V}/\dot{Q}$], or a shuntlike effect) and areas of normal inflation (high $\dot{V}/\dot{Q}$). When blood shunts through lung areas with low $\dot{V}/\dot{Q}$, arterial hypoxemia and hypercapnia result. Hyperventilation of lung areas with high $\dot{V}/\dot{Q}$ will normalize P_aCO_2 but will not improve oxygenation. Improving oxygenation depends on matching blood flow to inflated ventilated alveoli. This matching can be done in three ways: (1) reinflating alveoli by positive airway pressure, (2) reinflating alveoli by decreasing pulmonary interstitial edema, or (3) diverting blood flow to lung areas with high $\dot{V}/\dot{Q}$. The role of peak inspiratory pressure in opening alveoli and of PEEP in holding alveoli open has been discussed [see Pulmonary Mechanics, above]. Decreasing lung extravascular water is accomplished by diuresis, reduction of left atrial pressure, and postural drainage. The edematous lung is heavy, and dependent alveoli are compressed by the weight of the lung, which is why consolidation occurs in dependent areas in acute respiratory distress syndrome.[19] Decreasing edema minimizes compression, which results in improved lung function[20] and improved survival in patients with the acute respiratory distress syndrome.[21]

Turning the patient so that lung areas with high $\dot{V}/\dot{Q}$ are dependent (usually the prone position) usually improves oxygenation immediately by diverting blood flow to the inflated lung areas and decreasing the blood flow in the consolidated lung areas.[22] When patients are in the prone position for several hours, the effects of lung weight are reversed, so that consolidated areas of the lung may become reinflated, resulting in improved oxygenation even when the patient is returned to the supine position.[23] Of these three maneuvers, diuresis and positioning are usually safer and more effective than airway pressure manipulation.

Types and Features of Mechanical Ventilators

At least 20 makes and models of mechanical ventilators are used in North America today. Almost all the ventilators used in operating rooms, recovery rooms, and intensive care units are volume-controlled ventilators. With a device of this type, the operator sets the tidal volume, the respiratory rate, and the inspiratory gas flow, and the ventilator will keep delivering the set volume of gas regardless of the airway pressure (unless a pressure cutoff is set). In a pressure-controlled ventilator, however, the operator selects the respiratory rate, the inspiratory gas flow, and the peak airway pressure, and the ventilator delivers inspired gas until the desired pressure is reached. The tidal volume is measured. Most ICU ventilators can be used in the volume- or pressure-controlled mode or in combinations of the two.

Ventilators come with an extensive array of knobs, gauges, controls, electronic microprocessors, digital displays, and instruction books. Although the features and accoutrements of mechanical ventilators can be intimidating, the functions and controls are actually quite simple. All ventilators have certain basic controls and monitors [see Table 3]. They all are capable of delivering gas of known composition and volume at a given flow rate and of measuring and controlling the pressure at various phases of the respiratory cycle.

Different ventilators accomplish gas delivery in different ways, such as by employing a motor-driven piston, by metering in a quantity of gas supplied to the ventilator under very high pressure, or by keeping a constant reservoir of gas under moderate pressure. Measurement of airway pressure, gas volume, inspiratory effort, F_IO_2, and other parameters is also accomplished in a variety of different ways. A surgeon caring for ventilator patients should know what ventilator is used in his or her hospital and how these variables are controlled in that specific ventilator. Circuit diagrams and descriptions of how each make and model of ventilator functions are available from the hospital respiratory therapy department, from the manufacturer, and in the literature. Extensive and excellent descriptions of specific mechanical ventilators have been published by Mushin and Rendell-Baker,[24] Kirby and colleagues,[25] and Burton and associates.[26] Surgeons should familiarize themselves with the available documentation and descriptions so that they can better understand the limitations of the equipment they use as well as alert themselves and others to possible malfunctions.

The primary controls for tidal volume, rate, and F_IO_2 are straightforward. The end-expiratory airway pressure control, or PEEP control, provides graduated occlusion of the expiratory system, thereby regulating positive end-expiratory pressure. There is also a primary control for maximum inspiratory pressure, which is set by the operator. If this pressure is reached, an alarm sounds and inflation stops, so that the preset volume is not reached. These simple primary controls allow regulation of all the components of routine mechanical ventilation.

There is also a set of secondary controls for fine-tuning the mechanical ventilator. These controls vary the flow (and therefore the pressure) during the inflation phase of the ventilator. The most important of them is the inspiratory flow rate control. If the tidal volume is delivered at a low flow rate, the time of inspiration will be long, the pressure accumulation will be gradual and minimal, and ventilation will be smoother, but the patient may feel dyspneic. If the flow rate of gas is high, however, the inspiratory time will be short, the peak inspiratory pressure will be reached abruptly, the mean airway pressure will be increased, the high-pressure cutoff will be reached more often, and the blast of ventilating gas may stimulate coughing. Because the respiratory rate is set per minute, a higher inspiratory flow rate will shorten inspiration and result in a lower I/E. A short inspiratory phase with a low I/E favors expiration and CO_2

Table 3 Controls and Monitors on a Volume-Controlled Ventilator

Controls	Monitors and Alarms
Primary controls	
F_IO_2	
Tidal volume (minute volume)	Tidal volume
Respiratory rate	Respiratory rate
Positive end-expiratory pressure (PEEP)	PEEP
Maximum inspiratory pressure	PIP
	Mean airway pressure
	Apnea or disconnect
Secondary controls	
Inspiratory flow rate	
Inspiratory flow wave pattern	Inspiratory time, I/E
Inspiratory hold	
Sigh rate, volume, and maximum pressure	Sigh PIP
Trigger sensitivity for assist and IMV models	
Modes of Ventilation	
Controlled mechanical ventilation (CMV)	
Assist control (AC)	
Intermittent mandatory ventilation (IMV)	
Synchronized IMV	
Continuous positive airway pressure (CPAP)	
Pressure-controlled ventilation (PCV)	
Pressure-controlled inverse-ratio ventilation (PC-IRV)	
Pressure support (PS)	

excretion, whereas a long inspiration with a high I/E favors inflation and oxygenation. When a patient with normal lungs is undergoing mechanical ventilation, the inspiratory flow rate should be adjusted so that the patient is comfortable and I/E is close to normal (1:3). This is best done by examining the patient while adjusting the inspiratory flow rate. Often, high mean airway pressures can be decreased significantly simply by decreasing the inspiratory flow rate. When a patient with poor oxygenation is undergoing mechanical ventilation, the time spent during inflation should be increased. I/E can be increased until CO_2 excretion is inadequate. This unusual pattern of breathing is uncomfortable and often requires sedation.

Most ventilators provide an inspiratory flow wave pattern control, which varies the pattern of gas flow from sine wave to square wave to various combinations of waves. The normal inspiratory flow pattern is essentially a sine wave, which is usually the best pattern for mechanical ventilation. Most modern ventilators also provide a control for timed inspiratory hold, or plateau pressure. This setting occludes the expiratory circuit for 1 or 2 seconds. There are two reasons for using the inspiratory hold control: (1) to allow pressures throughout the system to equilibrate so that effective compliance (exhaled volume divided by plateau pressure as measured on the ventilator gauge) can be measured and (2) to simulate a forced sustained inspiration to reinflate collapsed alveoli (a procedure to be distinguished from an automatic sigh [see Modes of Ventilation, below]). As a rule, ventilators deliver gas only during the inflation phase of the respiratory cycle, but some provide continuous gas flow, which is a significant advantage in the CPAP and IMV modes of ventilation.

Humidification is an essential part of mechanical ventilation. The inspired gas is usually humidified by passing it over water warmed to 37° C. A chamber for nebulizing drugs may be included in the inspiratory circuit; it is powered by a gas line separate from the ventilator.

Modes of Ventilation

Ventilators always have at least two and sometimes as many as six modes of ventilation. Each mode of ventilation is characterized by what starts the gas flow (time- or effort-triggered) and what stops the gas flow (volume-controlled, pressure-time–controlled, or flow-controlled; or volume-limited, pressure-time–limited, or flow-limited) [see Figure 8]. In the controlled mechanical ventilation mode, the ventilator is time-triggered and either volume-limited or pressure-limited, and it functions exactly as determined by the primary controls, regardless of what the patient does. This mode is appropriate for a patient who is under anesthesia, paralyzed, heavily sedated, or suffering from brain stem injury.

In the assist-control mode, the ventilator is effort-triggered and either volume-controlled or pressure-controlled and delivers the V_T and F_IO_2 determined by the primary controls whenever the patient initiates a spontaneous breath. A control or backup rate is specified so that the ventilator will automatically deliver the tidal volume if the pa-

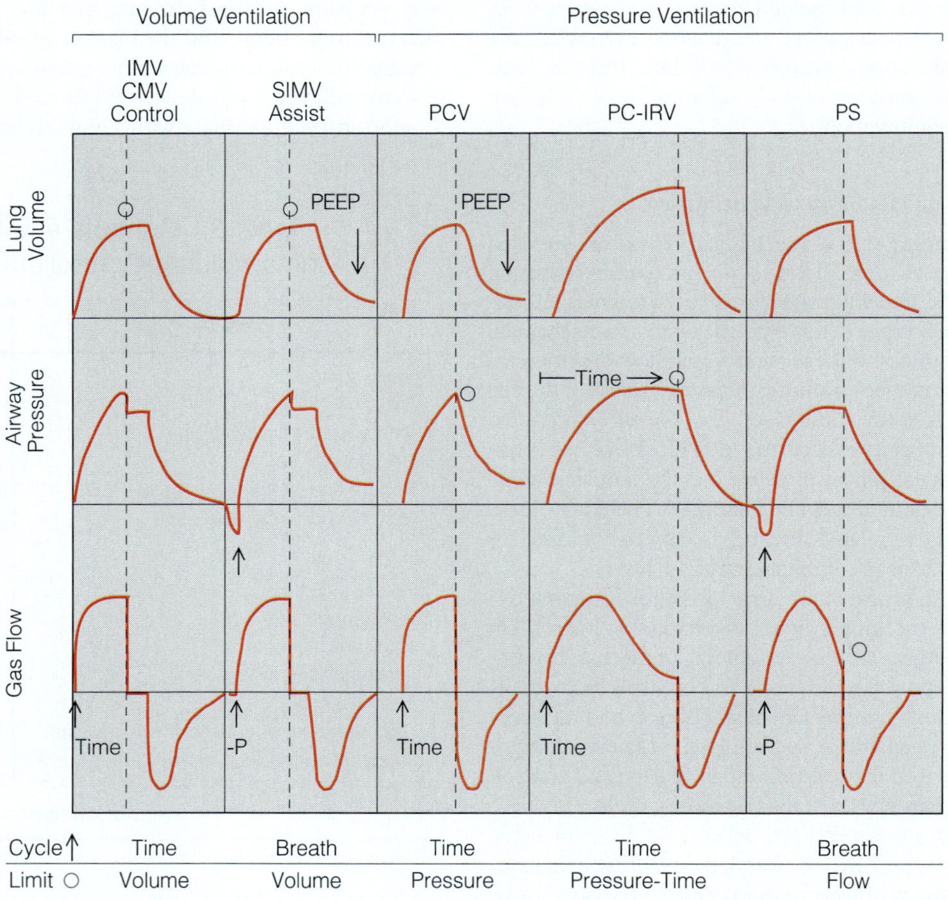

Figure 8 Shown are lung volume, airway pressure, gas flow, and the inspiration-expiration ratio (I/E) during commonly used modes of mechanical ventilation. The event that starts the gas flow is the cycle (↑), and the event that stops the gas flow is the limiting factor (○). The cessation of gas flow is shown by the dotted lines. Time and negative pressure (-P) may be responsible for cycling or limiting gas flow, as indicated. PEEP is shown in two modes of ventilation as examples of the effect of that maneuver.

tient does not initiate a spontaneous breath within an appropriate period. The control rate is usually set at approximately half the spontaneous rate. The ventilator is triggered to deliver an assisted breath when the pressure in the airway is decreased by the patient's inspiratory effort. When the assist-control mode is used, the sensitivity of this trigger mechanism should be adjusted. If the setting is too sensitive, a ventilator inflation may be triggered simply by the pressure drop during expiration. If the adjustment is not sensitive enough, the patient may be unable to generate enough pressure to trigger the ventilator.

Because of the relatively poor pressure transmission through the gas in the system, the negative deflection on the ventilator pressure gauge is not nearly as great as the negative pressure actually generated in the pleural space by inspiratory effort. Whenever possible, therefore, the patient's inspiratory pressure should be measured at the airway. The sensitivity control should be adjusted so that the mechanical breath is delivered with the minimum of effort by the patient. It must be readjusted whenever the PEEP level is changed. The assist mode greatly simplifies the monitoring and management of mechanical ventilation. It is the preferred mode in any patient with a normally functioning brain stem and respiratory center.

In the intermittent mandatory ventilation mode, time-triggered controlled mechanical ventilation occurs at the rate and volume determined by the primary controls (time-triggered and either volume-limited or pressure-limited), and additional inspired gas is made available if the patient generates a spontaneous inspiration. (The latter feature distinguishes IMV from CMV, in which no gas flows if the patient makes an inspiratory effort.) The volume of gas provided during the spontaneous effort is proportional to the patient's effort and is usually small. IMV was originally designed to be used with a continuous high-volume gas flow and PEEP (requiring minimal effort by the patient for spontaneous breaths) supplemented by intermittent mechanical breaths at a rate and volume sufficient to maintain CO_2 clearance.[27] The Emerson ventilator functions in this fashion, but most other mechanical ventilators have a type of pseudo-IMV, in which gas is delivered only when a demand valve is activated by the inspiratory effort. This method requires considerable work by the patient[28] and can lead to progressive exhaustion of respiratory muscles rather than the mild exercise desired. Synchronized IMV (SIMV) is simply a modification of IMV in which the controlled ventilation V_T is delivered at the time of spontaneous inspiratory effort (i.e., effort-triggered).

In the continuous positive airway pressure mode, breathing is entirely spontaneous, with expiratory pressure controlled by the PEEP control [see Figure 9]. This mode corresponds to the period of spontaneous breathing with IMV as described earlier and is subject to the same variables and criticisms. The CPAP mode should be used in conjunction with a continuous-flow and reservoir system. Because in most ventilators the CPAP mode requires the patient to trigger a demand valve during inspiration rather than supplying continuous flow of gas, this mode may at times be more exhausting than helpful. A variation of CPAP is so-called pressure-release ventilation, in which CPAP is applied and then released to a controlled PEEP level at intervals.

Pressure support is a time- or effort-triggered, flow-limited mode of ventilation.[29] Rapid gas flow is initiated by effort or a timer and continues until a preset pressure is reached. Gas flow continues at a slower rate, and pressure is maintained until the flow rate is only a fraction of the initial flow rate (typically 25%). This has the effect of an inspiratory hold but continues to supply gas during the inspiratory hold, which results in a relatively large tidal volume at moderate pressure. If the patient generates inspiratory effort during the pressure-support breath, an even higher tidal volume will result, making pressure support a valuable method of weaning. The same principle applies to the pressure-limited mode, without the inspiratory hold.

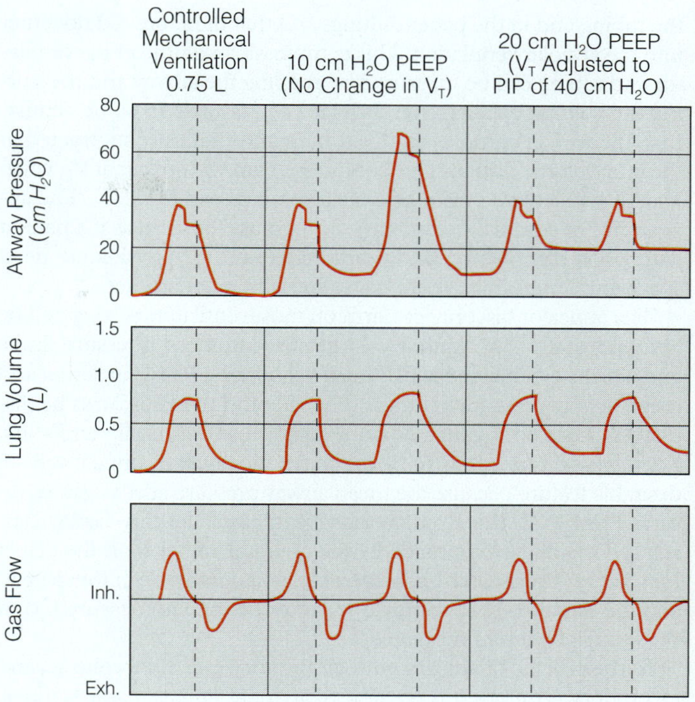

Figure 9 Shown is the effect of positive end-expiratory pressure (PEEP) during five breaths. PEEP is added after the second breath, so the third breath, with the same lung volume, results in unacceptably high peak inspiratory pressure (PIP). The lung volume is decreased until PIP is 40 cm H_2O, as shown in breaths four and five. The dotted vertical line separates inspiration from expiration.

Most ventilators have a control for automatic sighs. (It would be more accurate to call these automatic yawns because sighs are expiratory maneuvers.) In the sigh mode, the ventilator delivers a large V_T (typically 15 to 25 ml/kg) at regular intervals (usually several times each hour). This setting ensures regular maximal inflation, thereby simulating the normal physiologic pattern of breathing, in which total lung capacity is reached six times each hour. A separate high-pressure limit and alarm is provided for the sighs. Although the amount of gas contained in a sigh is considerably larger than the normal V_T, it is delivered at the same inspiratory flow rate; consequently, the inspiratory time will be two or three times longer than normal. This system is a more effective means of achieving maximal alveolar inflation than the inspiratory hold described earlier [see Types and Features of Mechanical Ventilators, *above*], in which a normal-sized tidal volume is simply held at pressure for a second or two. When PEEP is maintained above 5 cm H_2O and P_{plat} is close to 30 cm H_2O, the sigh mechanism is not necessary and may even lead to dangerously high airway pressures; however, when PEEP is 5 cm H_2O or lower and the tidal volume is controlled in the normal range, periodic sighs should be used to maintain alveolar inflation. Overdistention may be avoided by limiting P_{plat} to 40 cm H_2O or lower.

Monitors and Alarms

Most ventilators are equipped with a device to measure exhaled volume, usually by integrating a measurement of flow with time. The exhaled volume can be displayed either breath by breath or as minute ventilation. It should correspond to the preset inspired volume; if it does not, an air leak exists, and the volume of the leak can be calculated by simple subtraction. It should be remembered that a considerable part of the exhaled volume is gas that was compressed in the tubing and in the patient's lungs and that therefore did not enter into the alveolar ventilation. This compression volume in the ventilator and tubing can be measured by capping the airway and measuring the volume exhaled over a range of pressures. In some ventilators, the tubing compression volume is automatically subtracted in the final volume display. This compressed gas will appear as V_D when V_D/V_T is calculated from arterial and mixed expired CO_2. The appearance of compression volume as $\dot{V}_D$ makes it seem as if a patient with poor compliance has a large anatomic or physiologic dead space, but it is nothing more than a measurement artifact.

The apnea or disconnect alarm on most ventilators is triggered by an abnormally low expired volume measurement. Pressure limits and alarms can be set for PIP in all ventilators, PEEP in some, and mean airway pressure in others. The PIP and the PEEP can be displayed either on a gauge or on a digital readout in all ventilators. Some ventilators can display the mean airway pressure as well—a desirable feature because the mean airway pressure affects venous return. The F_IO_2 is displayed on most ventilators, but this display usually reflects the setting made by the operator rather than the actual F_IO_2 value. There can be considerable variation between the desired and the actual F_IO_2, so some device must be used to measure F_IO_2 if the ventilator cannot measure it.

In the process of adjusting the respiratory rate, tidal volume, and inspiratory flow rate, it is possible to arrive at unreasonable settings. Most ventilators have an alarm system to notify the operator. Usually, this alarm system will be triggered if I/E exceeds 2:1.

Some of the newer ventilators can calculate and display effective compliance, flow-volume loops, or volume-pressure curves. In the near future, mechanical ventilators will include apparatus to measure oxygen consumption, CO_2 production, respiratory quotient, and work of breathing. These measurements, combined with measurements of arterial and venous oxyhemoglobin saturation, will allow ventilators to display oxygen delivery-consumption ratios, cardiac output, and other hemodynamic variables, as well as energy expenditure expressed in calories. The same generation of ventilators will be able to regulate minute ventilation on the basis of CO_2 load and to regulate airway pressure and F_IO_2 on the basis of oxygenation. These devices will appear to be even more complex than today's ventilators, but they will have the same basic functions and features.

In addition to monitors built into the ventilator, some other patient monitors are used to manage mechanical ventilation. The use of the pulmonary arterial catheter and mixed venous oximetry has already been discussed [see Worsening Respiratory Status, Oxygenation, above]. An arterial catheter is helpful because of the frequency of arterial blood gas measurement. Pulse oximeters measure arterial saturation in capillary blood by ignoring the nonpulsatile venous phase. These instruments have become invaluable for both safety and management monitoring. Transcutaneous, corneal, and tissue gas sensors have not gained general acceptance, because they drift and require frequent recalibration. End-tidal CO_2 monitoring at the airway generally corresponds to P_aCO_2. End-tidal CO_2 is the same as P_aCO_2 when lung function is normal, and it is less than P_aCO_2 when real or apparent dead space (compression volume) is elevated. End-tidal CO_2 is particularly helpful during weaning.

Learning to Use a Mechanical Ventilator

Every surgeon who is responsible for ventilator patients should understand the mechanical ventilators at his or her hospital and should be able to set all the controls and make any necessary adjustments, even if such tasks are traditionally done by nurses or respiratory therapists. The best way for a surgeon to learn to use a mechanical ventilator is first to regulate the primary control settings by using a rubber-bag test lung, then to regulate the secondary controls and select the modes of ventilation while acting as the patient (easily accomplished by attaching a mouthpiece to the ventilator tubing and applying a noseclip). Whenever a new ventilator is introduced into the ICU, each surgeon who will use the ventilator should go through a detailed self-instruction routine [see Table 4]. It is well worth the cost of an extra set of sterile ventilator tubing.

Writing Ventilator Orders

Mechanical ventilators are generally operated by nurses and respiratory therapists under a set of orders from the responsible physician [see Table 5]. These orders may range from very specific directions to broad guidelines, depending on the experience and ability of the ICU personnel; however, the orders should always include a statement of the goals of mechanical ventilation and specify the system to be used to determine how well those goals have been achieved. For example, in an ICU in which ventilators are routinely used, it may be sufficient merely to say: "Measure arterial saturation and P_aCO_2 every 4 hours. Maintain P_aCO_2 between 35 and 45 mm Hg with rate and tidal volume, and maintain arterial saturation of more than 95% by using F_IO_2 less than 0.6 and PEEP less than 6." Conversely, if mechanical ventilators are not used routinely, or if a nurse or respiratory therapist on a given shift is not comfortable with such responsibility, it is advisable to specify the exact mode, the primary control and secondary control settings, and the monitoring alarm systems that are to be used.

Related Topics

FIGHTING THE VENTILATOR

Fighting the ventilator means that the patient is dyspneic and trying to breathe out while the ventilator is inflating. Usually, this situation can be handled by placing the ventilator in the assist mode

---

Table 4   **Self-Instruction Routine for Ventilator Training**

1. Set: F_IO_2, V_T, rate, PEEP, PIP.
2. Set mode: CMV.
3. Set ranges for alarms: V_T, rate, PIP, PEEP.
4. Attach test lung (rubber bag), and ventilate.
5. Measure: V_T, rate, minute volume, PIP, PEEP, effective compliance.
6. Limit the bag to simulate poor compliance. Readjust ventilator, and repeat measurements.
7. Set primary controls to ventilate yourself. Rate = 16/min.
8. With a mouthpiece and a noseclip, ventilate yourself. Relax until you are on controlled ventilation. Then, adjust V_T (5–20 ml/kg) and PEEP (0–10 cm H_2O) to get the feel, and observe the measurements. Try the sigh mode.
9. At baseline settings, resist inspiration, cough, and try to hyperventilate. How does it feel? Do the monitors and alarms work?
10. At baseline settings, turn to the AC mode. Rate = 0/min. Adjust the sensitivity from low to high.
11. In the AC mode, adjust the inspiratory flow rate and pattern. Which I/E feels comfortable?
12. Reset mode to IMV, then CPAP. How much work does it take to initiate a breath?
13. Repeat steps 10–12, but using an endotracheal tube instead of a mouthpiece in your mouth. What are the effects of the added resistance?

Table 5 Sample Orders for Ventilator Patients

1. Objectives (range of acceptable values)
   A. Arterial blood oxygenation
      Hemoglobin saturation _____ to _____
      or
      P_aO_2 _____ to _____
   B. Arterial carbon dioxide (P_aco_2) _____ to _____
2. Standard respiratory care for all ventilator patients
   A. Alternating lateral and sitting positions, never supine.
   B. 100% airway humidity at 35°–37° C.
   C. Airway irrigation and suctioning every 8 hours, more frequently as required.
   D. Percussion and chest physical therapy every 8 hours, more frequently as required.
   E. Deflation of cuffed tubes every 8 hours (before suctioning) and reinflation with the minimum volume necessary to achieve the required peak inspiratory pressure.
   F. Continuous monitoring of V_T and airway pressure.
   G. Mouth care every other hour (for patients with endotracheal tubes).
   H. Tracheal stoma care every other hour for patients with tracheostomy tubes.
3. Ventilator settings: Mode _____
   F_IO_2 _____
   V_T or PIP _____ Rate _____ PEEP _____
   Alarm limits: V_T _____ Rate _____ P_{plat} _____
   Other: _____
4. Monitoring frequency
   Arterial blood gases _____
   Venous blood gases _____
   Compliance _____
   Weaning parameters _____
   Chest x-ray _____

and increasing the inspiratory flow and tidal volume until respiratory alkalosis occurs and breathing slows, and then backing off to more comfortable settings. Mild sedation of the patient may be necessary, particularly if he or she is disoriented or extremely anxious. Almost never is it necessary or indicated to paralyze a patient to achieve mechanical ventilation. (There are, however, some specific indications for paralysis, such as tetanus, seizures, delirium tremens, and major ventilatory failure [*see* Worsening Respiratory Status, *above*].)

VENTILATION OF INFANTS AND CHILDREN

Although this discussion has been concerned solely with mechanical ventilation for adults, the principles underlying pulmonary mechanics, gas exchange, monitoring and alarms, and modes of ventilation all apply to pediatric patients as well. In children older than 2 years, volume-controlled ventilators can be used according to the guidelines given here for adults. Pressure-limited continuous-flow ventilators are generally preferred in infants. Techniques for neonatal ventilation are well described in standard texts [*see 76 The Pediatric Surgical Patient*].[30,31]

INTERMITTENT POSITIVE PRESSURE BREATHING

Intermittent positive pressure breathing is nothing more than mechanical ventilation through a mouthpiece rather than through direct tracheal access. All of the relevant variables can be monitored and controlled when a mouthpiece rather than an endotracheal tube is used, and any of the modes can be selected. Intermittent positive pressure breathing is a useful technique in patients who have borderline pulmonary function or minimal reserve.[32] When it is employed, the ventilator is placed at the bedside and set in the assist mode with a backup rate of zero, and all the primary and secondary controls are adjusted to the appropriate settings. The patient is taught to use the ventilator and is allowed to pick up the mouthpiece for mechanical assistance at will. He or she is encouraged to use the ventilator at least every hour while awake, to prevent or treat atelectasis.[33] This variety of mechanical ventilation differs considerably from intermittent positive pressure breathing provided by a nurse or respiratory therapist every 6 or 8 hours, which is useful for delivering nebulized drugs and for encouraging the patient to think about deep breathing but is usually ineffective unless the mechanical support is provided more frequently.

BRONCHOSCOPY

Bronchoscopy with flexible fiberoptic instruments is an essential adjunct to the management of mechanical ventilation. Introducing the instrument through a sphincter adapter allows bronchoscopy to be performed during ventilation but increases the resistance to gas flow through the airway. Therefore, ventilator adjustments are necessary to maintain adequate gas exchange. The inspiratory flow rate and peak inspiratory pressure must be increased significantly to maintain inspired tidal volume. This clinical setting is the one exception to the PIP limit of 40 cm H_2O; an inspiratory pressure of 50 to 80 cm H_2O may be required. This pressure level, required to overcome airway resistance, is not injurious to the lung. Distal pressure is low, and overdistention will not occur. Expiration is also limited by the increased resistance. More time will be required for exhalation, and PEEP should be decreased. Without these changes, exhalation of each breath will be incomplete, resulting in auto-PEEP [*see* Auto-PEEP, *below*] and CO_2 retention. Obviously, ventilator settings must be adjusted carefully to facilitate bronchoscopy.

Conversely, bronchoscopy is used to facilitate mechanical ventilation. Airway placement and positioning, evaluation of tracheal injury and bronchial patency, identification of sources of bleeding and mucus production, tissue level diagnoses, and selective lobar study and treatment all require bronchoscopy. A surgeon who is managing mechanical ventilation should be proficient in performing this procedure.[34]

AUTO-PEEP

When exhalation is incomplete, the functional residual capacity is increased, airway pressure increases, and alveoli are more inflated than they would be if exhalation continued to the point of equilibration with atmospheric pressure. This phenomenon can be exploited by using PEEP to limit exhalation and maintain alveolar inflation. If bronchial or prosthetic airway resistance is increased or if the time for exhalation is short, incomplete exhalation can occur regardless of externally regulated PEEP. If this process continues during many breaths, alveolar volume increases in association with increased alveolar pressure; this process has been referred to as auto-PEEP.[35] This phenomenon also occurs in asthma, with the same physiologic consequences of CO_2 retention and capillary obstruction. Auto-PEEP occurs during mechanical ventilation as a result of the ventilator settings, sometimes combined with bronchospasm. It can be measured by placement of a catheter-transducer system into the trachea or esophagus. Auto-PEEP should be suspected if CO_2 clearance is impaired and is paradoxically worsened by increasing respiratory rate (i.e., shortening exhalation time). If auto-PEEP is suspected, the respiratory rate or tidal volume, or both, should be decreased. If CO_2 clearance is enhanced by this maneuver, ventilator settings are readjusted to permit full exhalation or to control exhalation solely by the external PEEP valve.

Special Techniques for Patients with Severe Respiratory Failure

When the principles outlined above are used, most surgical patients can be managed without difficulty. However, a small percentage of patients with pneumonitis, aspiration, contusion, or the acute respiratory distress syndrome will develop such a large shunt, air leak, or alveolar damage that conventional mechanical ventilation is inadequate. The mortality associated with severe respiratory failure, defined as a shunt persistently over 30% despite and after all appropriate therapy, is 60% to 90%.[36-39] The following innovative approaches have been recommended for these patients.

NONVENTILATORY TREATMENT

Oxygenation can often be improved by placing the patient in the full lateral or prone position.[40] This positioning diverts blood flow to the anterior lung, which is usually the most inflated part of the lung, and promotes reinflation of the posterior lung. Oxygen delivery should be optimized by use of transfusion to achieve a normal hematocrit[41] and administration of inotropes (with the caveat that catecholamines increase $\dot{V}O_2$ and $\dot{V}CO_2$).[42] When the hematocrit and cardiac output are normal, an arterial saturation of 80% to 90% is well tolerated.

PERMISSIVE HYPERCAPNIA

Even in patients with severe lung disease, a normal P_aCO_2 can be maintained at 40 mm Hg by hyperventilation. Indeed, in patients with atelectasis and consolidation, a small portion of the lung is hyperventilated to maintain normocapnia while hypoxia is treated with attempted reinflation. However, because this intervention causes overdistention and induced tissue alkalosis in the most normal and compliant area of the lung, it can damage the lung in a very short time.[43] The risk of hypercapnia is minimal, particularly when it is compared with the risk of hyperventilation-induced lung damage. Therefore, ventilation should be limited to safe levels (plateau pressure below 40 cm) to avoid lung injury. This limitation may result in a P_aCO_2 as high as 80 mm Hg, but the resulting acidosis can be buffered with bicarbonate or TRIS buffer and no deleterious effects result. This approach has been used for many years in the management of asthma[44] and neonatal respiratory failure[45] but has rarely been used in acute adult respiratory failure. Recommendations to strictly limit peak airway pressure[46,47] were generally ignored in favor of normocapnia. In the early 1990s, this approach, named permissive hypercapnia, was advocated in patients with adult respiratory failure.[10] Critical care practitioners recognized the dangers of hyperventilation and began regulating mechanical ventilator peak pressure. Although transient hypercapnia may result, that is a small price to pay for ultimate lung recovery.

PRESSURE-LIMITATION (LOW-STRETCH) VENTILATION

The rationale for limiting overdistention (high pressure, high volume, or high stretch) was defined by Gattinoni and colleagues[5] and demonstrated by Hickling and coworkers.[6,10] Several recent prospective, randomized studies have shown a significant survival advantage to so-called low-stretch modes of ventilation.[7,8] Other studies have shown no advantage,[48] but the differences can be explained by the number of patients in the various treatment groups who were actually ventilated with damaging pressure. Ranieri and colleagues demonstrated that high-stretch ventilation was associated with increased plasma levels of inflammatory cytokines.[49] Amato and coworkers[7] advocate that the high-stretch limit be combined with PEEP adjustment based on P_{flex} (the so-called open-lung approach), a combination providing survival advantage.

HIGH-FREQUENCY OR OSCILLATION VENTILATION

High-frequency ventilation (HFV) is an intriguing technique in which oxygenation is achieved by continuous positive airway pressure with supplemental oxygen, and ventilation is achieved by shaking the airway—that is, by supplying a very small tidal volume (≤ 100 ml) at a very rapid rate (200 to 2,000/min) by means of a jet of gas, a piston, or a loudspeaker. This unusual airway pressure manipulation enhances CO_2 diffusion and induces excretion of a normal metabolic load of CO_2 without conventional tidal ventilation. Reports on HFV in adults indicate that the mean airway pressure is lower than with CMV and that barotrauma and air leaks are less frequent, but the duration of ventilation and the outcome in ventilated patients are about the same.[50,51] There are, however, anecdotal cases of spectacular recovery with HFV despite the apparent failure of conventional mechanical ventilation, suggesting that the development of this technique should be watched carefully.

PRESSURE-CONTROLLED INVERSE-RATIO VENTILATION

If one objective of mechanical ventilation is to inflate collapsed alveoli, inspiration can be prolonged until I/E (normally 1:3 or 1:4) reaches or, in certain cases, exceeds 1:1 (inverse). As long as there is adequate time during expiration for CO_2 clearance and as long as the effects of elevated mean airway pressure are taken into account, pressure-controlled inverse-ratio ventilation is an effective mode of mechanical ventilation. Because it requires total control of the breathing patterns, the patient must be heavily sedated. Pressure-controlled ventilation and pressure-controlled inverse-ratio ventilation are standard techniques in neonatal ventilation.

TRACHEAL INSUFFLATION

During mechanical ventilation, the major bronchi, trachea, and endotracheal airway make up the anatomic dead space. At the end of exhalation, this dead space is filled with alveolar gas that contains carbon dioxide. Under normal conditions, this CO_2 is rapidly diluted with fresh air, which creates a suitable gradient for CO_2 excretion. However, when V_D/V_T is more than 50%, reequilibration at a higher level of blood CO_2 may ultimately occur. This effect is not necessarily deleterious [see Permissive Hypercapnia, above]. However, preferably, a normal P_aCO_2 should be maintained as long as hyperventilation is avoided. CO_2 clearance can be facilitated by the insufflation of ventilating gas near the level of the carina through a small catheter. This maneuver, known as tracheal insufflation, removes CO_2 from the major airway. This removal lowers V_D/V_T and allows CO_2 clearance without overdistention and hyperventilation. When the gas flow is mechanically directed out of the airway, a Bernoulli effect results, which facilitates CO_2 clearance from the distal airways and alveoli.[52] This technique has been studied in detail by Kolobow, who refers to it as intratracheal pulmonary ventilation. This technique can be used in conjunction with conventional mechanical ventilation or as the sole source of ventilating gas. Of course, intratracheal pulmonary ventilation holds the greatest promise for patients whose conducting airways constitute a large fraction of the tidal volume, specifically newborn infants. This technique is now entering clinical trials.[53]

EXTRACORPOREAL LIFE SUPPORT

Extracorporeal membrane oxygenation (ECMO) is the use of a modified heart-lung machine for days or weeks to support gas exchange while resting the diseased lung.[54] This technique has the advantage of avoiding the oxygen toxicity and barotrauma that may accompany mechanical ventilation in severe respiratory failure. It has become standard treatment in the management of severe respiratory failure in newborn infants [see 76 The Pediatric Surgical Patient].[55] In patients with adult respiratory failure considered moribund, 50% survival with extracorporeal life support (ECLS) has been reported from several centers.[56,57] In adult patients, venovenous blood access is generally used for patients with adequate cardiovascular function; venoarterial access is used when cardiac failure coexists.

ECLS might be considered when the risk of mortality with continuing conventional ventilation is more than 90% and the primary process is reversible. Thus, the specific indications in most ECMO centers are a transpulmonary shunt over 30% and compliance less than 0.5 ml/cm H_2O/kg after and despite optimal therapy. The contraindications to ECLS are advanced age, malignancy or brain damage, and mechanical ventilation longer than 5 to 7 days. ECLS can play a significant role in the management of severe respiratory failure in adults.[58] However, ECLS is complex and requires a well-trained team.

Summary

Management of mechanical ventilation is an exercise in applied pulmonary mechanics, just as the management of respiratory failure is an exercise in the full spectrum of applied pulmonary physiology. CO_2 clearance and oxygenation should be considered and managed as distinctly separate processes, although they are obviously interrelated. CO_2 clearance is the result of breathing and is thus the goal in mechanical ventilation. Although it is almost always possible to maintain normal P_aCO_2 by hyperventilation, a peak airway pressure greater than 40 cm H_2O injures the lung and should be avoided. Maintaining and improving oxygenation is a process of matching pulmonary blood flow to inflated alveoli, which should be done by positioning, diuresis, and optimization of hemoglobin concentration and cardiac output. Although oxygenation can be facilitated by increased F_IO_2 and PEEP, these methods of treatment, like hyperventilation, do more harm than good when applied in excess. The goal of mechanical ventilation is to provide adequate gas exchange without damaging the lung.

References

1. Agostoni E, Mead J: Statics of the respiratory system. Handbook of Physiology, Vol 1. American Physiological Society, Washington, DC, 1964, Sect 3, p 387
2. Kolobow T, Moretti MP, Fumagalli R, et al: Severe impairment in lung function induced by high peak airway pressure during mechanical ventilation. Am Rev Respir Dis 135:312, 1987
3. Bowton DL, Kong DL: High tidal volume ventilation produces increased lung water in oleic acid–injured rabbit lungs. Crit Care Med 17:908, 1989
4. Dreyfuss D, Soler P, Basset G, et al: High inflation pressure pulmonary edema: respective effects of high airway pressure, high tidal volume, and positive end-expiratory pressure. Am Rev Respir Dis 137:1159, 1988
5. Gattinoni L, Pesenti A, Torresin A, et al: Adult respiratory distress syndrome profiles by computed tomography. J Thorac Imaging 1:25, 1986
6. Hickling KG: Ventilatory management of ARDS: can it affect the outcome? Intensive Care Med 16:219, 1990
7. Amato MB, Barbas CS, Medeiros DM, et al: Effect of a protective-ventilation strategy on mortality in the acute respiratory distress syndrome. N Engl J Med 338:347, 1998
8. Ventilation with lower tidal volumes as compared with traditional tidal volumes for acute lung injury and the acute respiratory distress syndrome. The Acute Respiratory Distress Syndrome Network. N Engl J Med 342:1301, 2000
9. Lee PC, Helsmoortel CM, Cohn SM, et al: Are low tidal volumes safe? Chest 97:430, 1990
10. Hickling KG, Henderson SJ, Jackson R: Low mortality associated with low volume pressure limited ventilation with permissive hypercapnia in severe adult respiratory distress syndrome. Intensive Care Med 16:372, 1990
11. Cilley RE, Polley TZ Jr, Zwischenberger JB, et al: Independent measurement of oxygen consumption and oxygen delivery. J Surg Res 47:242, 1989
12. Hirschl RB, Heiss KF, Cilley RE, et al: Oxygen kinetics in experimental sepsis. Surgery 112:37, 1992
13. Danek SJ, Lynch JP, Weg JG, et al: The dependence of oxygen uptake on oxygen delivery in the adult respiratory distress syndrome. Am Rev Respir Dis 122:387, 1980
14. Gutierrez G, Pohil RJ: Oxygen consumption is linearly related to O_2 supply in critically ill patients. J Crit Care 1:45, 1986
15. Bartlett RH, Dechert RE: Oxygen kinetics: pitfalls in clinical research (editorial). J Crit Care 5:77, 1990
16. Vermeij CG, Feenstra BW, Bruining HA: Oxygen delivery and oxygen uptake in postoperative and septic patients. Chest 98:415, 1990
17. Zwischenberger JB, Cilley RE, Kirsh MM, et al: Does continuous monitoring of mixed venous oxygen saturation accurately reflect oxygen delivery and oxygen consumption following coronary artery bypass grafting? Surg Forum 37:66, 1986
18. Rashkin MC, Bosken C, Baughman RP: Oxygen delivery in critically ill patients: relationship to blood lactate and survival. Chest 87:580, 1985
19. Gattinoni L, Mascheroni D, Turresin A, et al: Morphological response to positive end expiratory pressure in acute respiratory failure: computerized tomography study. Intensive Care Med 12:137, 1986
20. Ali J, Duke K: Colloid osmotic pressure in pulmonary edema clearance with furosemide. Chest 92:540, 1987
21. Simmons RS, Berdine GG, Seidenfeld JJ, et al: Fluid balance and the adult respiratory distress syndrome. Am Rev Respir Dis 135:924, 1987
22. Langer M, Mascheroni D, Marcolin R, et al: The prone position in ARDS patients. Chest 94:103, 1988
23. Gattinoni L, Presenti A: Computed tomography scanning in acute respiratory failure. Adult Respiratory Distress Syndrome. Zapol WM, Lemaire F, Eds. Marcel Dekker, New York, 1991, p 199
24. Mushin WW, Rendell-Baker L, Thompson DW, et al: Automatic Ventilation of the Lungs. Blackwell Scientific Publishers, Oxford, 1980
25. Kirby RR, Smith RA, Desautels DA: Mechanical Ventilation. Churchill Livingstone, New York, 1985
26. Burton GG, Hodgkin JE, Ward JJ: Respiratory Care, 3rd ed. JB Lippincott Co, Philadelphia, 1991
27. Downs JB, Mitchell LA: Intermittent mandatory ventilation following cardiopulmonary bypass (abstr). Crit Care Med 2:39, 1974
28. Marini JJ, Rodriguez RM, Lamb V: The inspiratory workload of patient-initiated mechanical ventilation. Am Rev Respir Dis 134:902, 1986
29. MacIntyre N, Nishimura M, Usada Y, et al: The Nagoya conference on system design and patient-ventilator interactions during pressure support ventilation. Chest 97:1463, 1990
30. Gille JP: Neonatal and Adult Respiratory Failure. Elsevier, Paris, 1989
31. Levin DL, Moriss FC: Essentials of Pediatric Intensive Care. Quality Medical Publishing, St. Louis, 1990
32. Anderson HL III, Bartlett RH: Respiratory Care of the Surgical Patient. Respiratory Care, 3rd ed. JB Lippincott Co, Philadelphia, 1991, p 821
33. Bartlett RH: Respiratory therapy to prevent postoperative pulmonary complications. Respiratory Intensive Care. Pierson DJ, Ed. Daedalus Enterprises, Dallas, 1986, p 369
34. Bartlett RH: Bronchoscopy in surgical patients. Surgical Endoscopy. Dent TL, Strodel WE, Turcotte JG, Eds. Year Book Medical Publishers, Inc, Chicago, 1985
35. Blanch L, Fernandez R, Artigas A: The effect of auto-positive end-expiratory pressure on the arterial end-tidal carbon dioxide pressure gradient and expired carbon dioxide slope in critically ill patients during total ventilatory support. J Crit Care 6:202, 1991
36. Zapol WM, Snider MT, Hill JD, et al: Extracorporeal membrane oxygenation in severe acute respiratory failure: a randomized prospective study. JAMA 242:2193, 1979
37. Bartlett RH, Morris AH, Fairley HB, et al: A prospective study of acute hypoxic respiratory failure. Chest 89:684, 1986
38. Gillespie DJ, Marsh HMM, Divertie MB, et al: Clinical outcome of respiratory failure in patients requiring prolonged (> 24 hours) mechanical ventilation. Chest 90:364, 1986
39. Zapol WM, Frikker MJ, Pontoppidan H, et al: The adult respiratory distress syndrome at Massachusetts General Hospital. Adult Respiratory Distress Syndrome. Zapol WM, Lemaire F, Eds. Marcel Dekker, New York, 1991
40. Maunder RJ, Shuman UP, McHugh JW, et al: Preservation of normal lung regions in the adult respiratory distress syndrome: analysis by computed tomography. JAMA 255:2463, 1986
41. Bryan-Brown CW, Gutierrez G: O_2 transport and tissue oxygenation in the critically ill. Clinical Aspects of O_2 Transport and Tissue Oxygenation. Rinhart K, Eyrich K, Eds. Springer-Verlag, Berlin, 1989
42. Ruttimann Y, Chiolero R, Jequier E, et al: Effects of dopamine on total oxygen consumption and oxygen delivery in healthy men. Am J Physiol 257:E541, 1989
43. Gattinoni L, Mascheroni D, Basilico E, et al: Volume/pressure curve of total respiratory system in paralyzed

patients: artefacts and correction factors. Intensive Care Med 13:19, 1987
44. Williams TJ, Tuxen DV, Scheinkestel CD, et al: Risk factors for morbidity in mechanically ventilated patients with acute severe asthma. Am Rev Respir Dis 146:607, 1992
45. Wung JT, James LS, Kilchevsky E, et al: Management of infants with severe respiratory failure and persistence of the fetal circulation, without hyperventilation. Pediatrics 76:488, 1985
46. Eriksen J, Andersen J, Rasmussen JP, et al: Effects of ventilation with large tidal volumes or positive end-expiratory pressure on cardiorespiratory function in anesthetized obese patients. Acta Anaesthesiol Scand 22:241, 1978
47. Bendixen HH, Hedley-White J, Laver MB: Impaired oxygenation in surgical patients during general anesthesia with controlled ventilation. N Engl J Med 269:991, 1963
48. Stewart TE, Meade MO, Cook DJ, et al: Evaluation of a ventilation strategy to prevent barotrauma in patients at high risk for acute respiratory distress syndrome. N Engl J Med 338:355, 1998
49. Ranieri VM, Suter PM, Tortorella C, et al: Effect of mechanical ventilation on inflammatory mediators in patients with acute respiratory distress syndrome: a randomized controlled trial. JAMA 282:54, 1999
50. Hurst JM, Branson RD, Davis K Jr, et al: Comparison of conventional mechanical ventilation and high-frequency ventilation: a prospective, randomized trial in patients with respiratory failure. Ann Surg 211:486, 1990
51. Carlon GC, Guy Y, Groeger JS, et al: Early prediction of outcome of respiratory failure: comparison of high-frequency jet ventilation and volume-cycled ventilation. Chest 86:194, 1984
52. Lehnert BE, Oberdorster G, Slutsky AS: Constant-flow ventilation of apneic dogs. J Appl Physiol 53:483, 1982
53. Wilson JM, Thompson JR, Schnitzer JJ, et al: Intratracheal pulmonary ventilation: human case report. Presented at 3rd Annual Extracorporeal Life Support Organization Meeting, Ann Arbor, Michigan, September 1991
54. Gattinoni L, Pesenti A, Mascheroni D, et al: Low-frequency positive-pressure ventilation with extracorporeal CO_2 removal in severe acute respiratory failure. JAMA 256:881, 1986
55. Stolar CJ, Snedecor SM, Bartlett RH: Extracorporeal membrane oxygenation and neonatal respiratory failure: experience from the extracorporeal life support organization. J Pediatr Surg 26:563, 1991
56. Kolla S, Awad SA, Rich PB, et al: Extracorporeal life support for 100 adult patients with severe respiratory failure. Ann Surg 226:544, 1997
57. Lewandowski K, Lewandowski M, Pappert D, et al: Outcome and follow-up of adults following extracorporeal life support. ECMO: Extracorporeal Cardiopulmonary Support in Critical Care. Zwischenberger JB, Bartlett RH, Eds. ELSO, Ann Arbor, Michigan, 1995
58. Bartlett RH: Management of ECLS in adult respiratory failure. ECMO: Extracorporeal Cardiopulmonary Support in Critical Care. Zwischenberger JB, Bartlett RH, Eds. ELSO, Ann Arbor, Michigan, 1995

Acknowledgments

Figure 1   Albert Miller.

Figures 2, 4, and 7 through 9   Talar Agasyan.

Figures 3 and 5   Marcia Kammerer.

Figure 6   Dana Burns-Pizer.

93 ACUTE RENAL FAILURE

Anthony Meyer, M.D., Ph.D.

Acute Renal Failure: Prevention, Early Diagnosis, and Treatment

The body responds to injury by attempting to reestablish the homeostatic state that permits normal function. Normal renal function provides a mechanism for eliminating toxic metabolites and maintaining homeostasis of fluid and electrolytes. Acute deterioration of renal function usually presents clinically as a decrease in urine output or a significant rise in serum creatinine. Fortunately, most patients in whom acute renal dysfunction develops do not progress to acute renal failure. However, acute renal failure remains a complex problem associated with a high mortality in surgical patients. Most of the renal failure encountered in contemporary surgical care is not single-organ failure; rather, it occurs in the context of the simultaneous dysfunction or failure of several organ systems.

Acute renal dysfunction is approached clinically from the presenting problems of oliguria or rising serum creatinine. Evaluation of renal dysfunction generally takes into account prerenal, renal parenchymal, and postrenal mechanisms of dysfunction [see Table 1].[1] In some patients, more than one cause of renal dysfunction may be present, and it is important to consider all possible mechanisms. The goals in management of acute renal failure are prevention and early diagnosis to limit renal damage and to maintain adequate residual function.

Recognition of Acute Renal Dysfunction

ACUTE OLIGURIA

Acute renal dysfunction may be signaled by the acute onset of oliguria, which is defined as a urine output of less than 0.5 ml/kg/hr or 400 ml/24 hr in an adult and less than 1.0 ml/kg/hr in a child weighing less than 10 kg.[2-5] A patient may progress to or even present with anuria, defined as a urine output of less than 100 ml/24 hr. Acutely decreased urine output most often is the result of a fall in renal perfusion from diminished circulating blood volume [see Clinical Assessment of Perfusion Status and Urinary Tract, *below*]. A Foley catheter should be placed in acutely oliguric patients to follow urine output closely and to evaluate the effects of treatment. Efforts should be made to determine the cause of the oliguria and to reestablish adequate urine output. Oliguria has many causes, and most patients who present with oliguria do not have acute renal failure.

INCREASED SERUM CREATININE

Creatinine, a product of amino acid metabolism, is cleared by the kidneys principally by glomerular filtration, although a limited amount of creatinine is secreted into the tubular fluid. A serum creatinine level of 1.2 mg/dl or less is considered normal. A rising serum creatinine level implies decreased renal clearance; an increase of 1 mg/dl over normal or baseline levels indicates a 50 percent decrease in the glomerular filtration rate (GFR). The serum creatinine can rise acutely even with normal urine output, and thus, it is another marker of acute renal dysfunction.

As with oliguria, most patients who present with a rising serum creatinine level do not have acute renal failure. However, an increase of more than 1 mg/dl above normal or baseline levels should be investigated and appropriate preventive and therapeutic measures taken. An increase of more than 2 mg/dl/day, even in the presence of anuria, suggests a rapid rate of protein breakdown, such as might occur in the presence of ischemic muscle or a resolving hematoma.[6] Furthermore, a blood urea nitrogen (BUN) to creatinine ratio higher than 10:1 suggests that dehydration is the cause of the rising creatinine.[7]

Clinical Assessment of Perfusion Status and Urinary Tract

Laboratory tests and imaging procedures do not replace physical examination as the first step in evaluating acute renal dysfunction. If a patient presents with acute oliguria or a rising serum creatinine level, a clinical examination is necessary to assess the patient's perfusion status and to rule out urinary tract obstruction as a cause of renal dysfunction. Signs of hypovolemia, congestive heart failure, poor peripheral perfusion, and urinary tract obstruction should be sought.

Decreased renal perfusion is the most common cause of acute renal dysfunction in surgical patients[8-10] and is usually the result of decreased intravascular volume, as signaled by flat neck veins, tachycardia, diminished jugular pulse, and other signs of hypovolemia [see *4 Shock*]. Perfusion can be estimated clinically on the basis of skin color, temperature, and capillary refill. It is important to remember, however, that although patients who have systemic infections, exhibit the systemic inflammatory response syndrome (SIRS), have been burned, or have recently undergone a major surgical procedure

```
┌─────────────────────────────────┐     ┌─────────────────────────────────┐
│ Patient becomes oliguric        │     │ Serum creatinine rises          │
├─────────────────────────────────┤     ├─────────────────────────────────┤
│ Urine output < 0.5 ml/kg/hr in  │     │ Creatinine rises 1.0 mg/dl over │
│ an adult or < 1 ml/kg/hr in a   │     │ normal or baseline.             │
│ child weighing < 10 kg.         │     │                                 │
└─────────────────────────────────┘     └─────────────────────────────────┘
```

Clinically assess perfusion status and urinary tract

Evaluate peripheral perfusion and estimate adequacy of intravascular volume. Consider a renal perfusion scan if damage to renal artery is a possibility. Look for bladder distention; closely monitor urine output.

Administer I.V. fluid challenge

Administer 10% of circulating volume as isotonic bolus, and reassess urine output and creatinine level (unless patient has intravascular overload).
If the patient has intravascular overload or normal urine output despite rising creatinine, do not give fluid challenge.

Renal function returns to normal

Continue to monitor urine output and serum creatinine level.

Prerenal dysfunction (urine sodium < 20 mEq/L or FE_{Na} < 1)

Expand intravascular volume if necessary. Improve renal blood flow; if intravascular volume is adequate, consider dopamine, 2–5 μg/kg/min. Monitor CVP or PAOP. If acute renal arterial problems are present, emergency operation and revascularization may be necessary.

Renal parenchymal dysfunction (no obstruction; urine sodium > 40 mEq/L or FE_{Na} > 3)

Stop nephrotoxic drugs if possible. Avoid using contrast agents if possible. Maintain renal perfusion. Assess tubular function. Evaluate for SIADH and hepatorenal syndrome.

Renal function returns to normal

Continue monitoring. Avoid nephrotoxic agents.

Acute Renal Failure: Prevention, Early Diagnosis, and Treatment

Evaluate renal dysfunction or failure

Assess
- Intravascular fluid volume (i.e., CVP or PAOP).
- Perfusion (i.e., cardiac output or mixed venous O_2 saturation).
- Tubular function (i.e., urine and plasma electrolyte levels, urinalysis). Calculate fractional excretion of sodium:

$$FE_{Na} = \frac{U_{Na}/P_{Na}}{U_{Cr}/P_{Cr}} \times 100$$

- Collecting system (i.e., ultrasonography or IVP). Review all recent and present medications. Stop nephrotoxic drugs if possible, and adjust all drug dosages as necessary.

Mixed prerenal and renal parenchymal dysfunction (urine sodium > 20 mEq/L but < 40 mEq/L and FE_{Na} > 1 but < 3)

Expand intravascular volume. Stop nephrotoxic drugs if possible. Monitor CVP, PAOP, and urine electrolyte concentrations.

Postrenal dysfunction (obstruction of urinary system)

Drain obstructed area:
- Bladder: use Foley catheter or suprapubic tube
- Ureter: use nephrostomy tube

Renal dysfunction progresses

Monitor and adjust medications and fluids. Maintain general supportive care.
Provide renal replacement therapy via hemodialysis, acute continuous hemodiafiltration, or plasma ultrafiltration.

renal parenchymal, or postrenal origin. In addition, although urinalysis and determination of urine sodium concentration and the fractional excretion of sodium can help identify the cause of acute renal failure, they do not indicate its severity. These studies can be supplemented by periodic measurements of creatinine clearance or free water clearance, which can be used to estimate the severity of acute renal failure and to assess the patient's clinical course. Normal creatinine clearance is greater than 100 ml/min; however, this value decreases by nearly half by 70 years of age.

Management

ACUTE DYSFUNCTION FROM PRERENAL CAUSES

Prerenal causes of acute renal dysfunction include those that diminish blood flow; hence, management is designed to improve renal blood flow. Intravascular volume is expanded to guarantee adequate preload. Central venous pressure or PAOP should be monitored to avoid excess fluid administration.

If cardiac dysfunction is present, inotropic support may be useful. It is important not to use agents with alpha-adrenergic activity, because although these agents increase blood pressure, their vasoconstrictive effect on renal arteries leads to reduced renal blood flow.[15] Selective renal artery vasodilatation can be achieved with low dosages of dopamine (2 to 5 µg/kg/min).[15] The contribution of this effect may be trivial or very significant, depending on the patient and coexisting problems. Administration of dopamine can be useful adjunctive therapy, however, and may be tried in patients who do not respond to simple fluid boluses [see Discussion, Treatment of Developing Acute Renal Failure, below].

If acute renal arterial problems are present, emergency operation and revascularization may be required. In cases of documented abdominal compartment syndrome, the abdomen may have to be reclosed with a prosthetic patch in the fascia to reduce the transmission of external pressure to the kidneys.

If prerenal mechanisms do not appear to be the cause of acute renal dysfunction, it is nevertheless important to maintain adequate renal blood flow to minimize injury and facilitate recovery.

ACUTE DYSFUNCTION FROM RENAL PARENCHYMAL CAUSES

Renal parenchyma can be affected or damaged by many substances and mechanisms. Initial attention in patients with renal parenchymal disorders should be directed at stopping the injury. Nephrotoxic drugs, such as aminoglycosides, other antibiotics, and nonsteroidal anti-inflammatory medications, should be discontinued and nonnephrotoxic drugs substituted. The use of radiographic contrast agents should be avoided; if this is not possible, a nonionic agent should be used. It is important to limit the amount of contrast medium given and to ensure that the patient's intravascular volume is adequate before administration begins. Clearance of circulating myoglobin and hemoglobin should be increased by encouraging diuresis with crystalloid solution infusion. Osmotic agents and urine alkalinization have been used to treat myoglobinuria, but they are no substitute for diuresis of at least 100 ml/hr until the urine is clear. Again, maintenance of renal perfusion is essential.[16]

In patients in whom the serum creatinine level is normal but the urine sodium level is greater than 40 mEq/L and the serum sodium level is normal or low, oliguria may reflect the syndrome of inappropriate antidiuretic hormone secretion (SIADH). SIADH is treated by water restriction and, if necessary, administration of diuretics. In patients who have a history of chronic or acute liver disorders, the combination of persistent oliguria, rising serum creatinine levels, low urine sodium levels, low serum sodium levels, and normal intravascular volume should suggest the hepatorenal syndrome [see 94 Hepatic Failure]. There are two findings by which this syndrome can be distinguished from prerenal causes of renal failure: (1) urine output does not increase in response to fluid challenge and (2) the ratio of urine creatinine to plasma creatinine is higher than 30:1 (this ratio is lower than 30:1 when prerenal causes are present).[17] There is no proven treatment for hepatorenal syndrome. Peritoneovenous shunts have been used but are of unproven efficacy. Liver transplantation is sometimes lifesaving.[17]

Renal dysfunction from parenchymal causes often takes longer to resolve and has a less predictable course than renal dysfunction from prerenal or postrenal causes. Identification of the specific injurious agent may not be possible. Any patient who is receiving nephrotoxic substances or who has been exposed to such substances should be monitored closely to permit early diagnosis of renal dysfunction and to limit damage. Daily measurement of serum levels of nephrotoxic drugs and adjustment of dosage are indicated in patients in whom these drugs cannot be substituted.

ACUTE DYSFUNCTION FROM A MIXTURE OF PRERENAL AND RENAL PARENCHYMAL CAUSES

Some patients exhibit a mixed pattern of renal dysfunction, in which the mechanism is not obviously prerenal or renal parenchymal. Such patients typically have oliguria or an elevated serum creatinine concentration. The urine sodium concentration is usually between 20 and 40 mEq/L, and the FE_{Na} is usually between 1 and 3. Several potential causes of dysfunction may be present, including diminished renal perfusion and exposure to nephrotoxic agents, and there may be some degree of baseline renal dysfunction. The administration of diuretics or osmotic agents may also lead to this mixed pattern through their effects on renal electrolytes.

Treatment of renal dysfunction of mixed origin is generally based on increasing intravascular volume. Unless the patient is known to have intravascular fluid overload, a fluid bolus should be given, and the I.V. fluid infusion rate should be increased. Edema in itself is not a sufficient reason to withhold further fluid challenge: it may be extravascular, rendering the patient paradoxically hypervolemic. Again, all nephrotoxic drugs should be discontinued to prevent any further injury to the renal parenchyma. The patient's CVP or PAOP should be monitored to ensure that intravascular volume is not pushed to a high level. Continued monitoring of urine electrolyte concentrations should be undertaken to detect any further deterioration of renal function.

ACUTE DYSFUNCTION FROM POSTRENAL CAUSES

Treatment of obstructive lesions that produce acute renal dysfunction is relatively straightforward. Decompression of the obstructed area will usually correct the problem and permit return of all or some degree of renal function. Obstruction lesions that are complicated by urosepsis may be associated with more prolonged renal dysfunction.

The bladder can be successfully drained by means of a Foley or suprapubic catheter. Continued monitoring of urine output is then possible. If ureteral obstruction is present, nephrostomy tubes can be placed percutaneously.

Return to Normal Renal Function

Successful management of acute renal dysfunction will correct oliguria and serum creatinine levels. However, continued monitoring of renal function is necessary until there appears to be no further risk, particularly if other medical problems necessitate ongoing treatment. Documentation of the acute renal dysfunction is important because it may help prevent recurrent problems in the future. Drug selection should be carefully reviewed with an eye to avoiding nephrotoxic agents, if possible. If nephrotoxic drugs must be used, the serum levels of the drugs and parameters of renal function, such as serum creatinine, must be followed closely.

Progressive Renal Dysfunction

Attempts to maintain renal blood flow and preserve urine output are important even in the presence of advancing renal failure.[18] Nonoliguric renal failure has a better prognosis than oliguric or anuric renal failure. Adequate hydration remains the principal method for sustaining urine output. Inotropic agents may have a positive influence in some patients but are not recommended as routine treatment. Attempts to preserve urine output and convert oliguric to nonoliguric renal failure by administering diuretics[19,20] have been unsuccessful; these attempts appear to identify only patients with the least severe renal dysfunction (i.e., those with enough residual renal function to respond to the diuretics). Furthermore, diuretics confer no long-term benefit in the treatment of acute renal failure.

If renal function deteriorates, medication doses and dosing intervals must be adjusted. Adjustments for drugs not listed should be based on product information from the manufacturer or on the recommendations of a pharmacologist. The principles to be considered in adjustment of drug dosage in patients with renal failure are (1) the desired concentration, (2) the volume distribution of the drug, and (3) the mechanism and rate of metabolism or excretion. Drug levels should be checked frequently as renal function changes; fluid and electrolyte therapy should also be adjusted.

The patient should continue to receive general supportive care. Adequate nutrition appears to be important for recovery from renal failure.[21,22]

RENAL REPLACEMENT THERAPY

Patients who have symptomatic fluid overload associated with congestive heart failure, encephalopathy, or acid-base and electrolyte disorders may require some degree of artificial renal support. Dialysis is necessary to correct encephalopathy or metabolic disorders. Acute continuous hemodiafiltration is an excellent option in critically ill patients, who often are too hemodynamically labile to tolerate standard hemodialysis.[23-25] Early dialysis in acute renal failure is associated with improved survival.[3,26] Absolute values of BUN and creatinine are not indicators for dialysis.

Patients who have fluid overload but no other need for dialysis can be treated with plasma ultrafiltration, which permits clearance of fluid and plasma solutes.[27-29] The process can also be very useful in patients who are too hemodynamically unstable to dialyze,[30] and it can be done with the patient's own perfusion pressure or with pump assist.

Treatment of patients requiring dialysis or other renal replacement therapy should be directed at returning renal function to normal levels or at least to levels that eliminate the need for renal support. Free water clearance or creatinine clearance should be monitored. Improvement in these urinary clearance measurements may signal a return to normal or baseline renal function. It is important to remember that baseline renal function in the elderly is usually less than half of normal.[31]

For patients who do progress to renal failure, recovery depends on age, cause of renal failure, and urine output during the time of renal dysfunction. Young patients and those who maintain adequate urine output despite acute renal failure have a significantly better prognosis.[32] Mortality in patients with severe acute renal failure has remained unchanged despite improved dialysis and other advances.[23,33] Mortality for acute renal failure ranges from 30 to 80 percent but varies with comorbid factors; it is highest in patients with multiorgan failure from infection or SIRS.[34] If patients do survive, they have a 25 to 30 percent chance of complete recovery of renal function and a 40 to 50 percent chance of partial recovery.[33]

Death related to renal failure is most often caused by infectious complications. Pneumonia is the most common fatal infection, although peritonitis and urinary infection may lead to sepsis and death. Bleeding complications caused by uremia may also contribute to death in these patients.

Discussion

Perspective on Acute Renal Failure

The incidence of acute renal failure has decreased since the mid-1940s; however, mortality among patients who have renal failure severe enough to necessitate dialysis has not been improved.[33,35-37] This lack of improvement appears to be related to the increasing percentage of patients who experience acute renal failure as one manifestation of multiorgan failure. Mortality from acute renal failure without multiorgan dysfunction is eight to 30 percent, whereas mortality from renal failure that is associated with sepsis or multiorgan failure is 70 to 80 percent.[38-40]

Groups of patients at risk for acute renal failure can be identified, but the specific degree of risk for an individual patient cannot be calculated. Patients with burns, severe injury, prolonged periods of hypoperfusion, or cardiopulmonary bypass are at significantly higher risk for acute renal failure than routine surgical patients.[41-43] Other than relative amount of injury or ischemia, the variables that correlate with renal failure are older age and a history of limited renal function.[44]

It is well accepted that the fundamental goal in the management of acute renal failure is prevention, or at least limitation of its severity.[45,46] Attention to the cause or causes of acute renal dysfunction and to the mechanisms involved often permits correction of the problem before progression to actual renal failure occurs.[7,47] If acute renal dysfunction and failure are to be managed by prevention, early diagnosis, and correction, it is necessary to understand renal pathophysiology.

Normal Renal Physiology

Understanding of both normal and altered renal physiology is greatly aided by familiarity with the anatomy of the nephron and with the sites of action of the hormones essential to normal renal function [see Figure 1]. Anatomic or functional injury to a sufficient number of nephrons can lead to measurable renal dysfunction and ultimately to renal failure. Renal function can be analyzed in terms of blood flow, glomerular filtration, and tubular reabsorption and secretion.

Blood flow to the kidneys is determined by cardiac output and renal vascular resistance. Renal vascular resistance is principally controlled at the arteriolar level. If renal perfusion pressure falls, the efferent arterioles constrict to maintain glomerular filtration pressure despite decreased flow. If the systemic systolic pressure falls below 70 mm Hg, this mechanism fails and the afferent arterioles constrict,[1] leading to a rapid decrease in glomerular filtration and consequently to a decrease in urine output.

This system is controlled by several hormonal and mediator systems that act at various sites in the nephron. The renin-angiotensin mechanism is important for the control of arteriolar resistance.[48,49] When renal perfusion pressure falls, secretion of renin by the juxtaglomerular apparatus increases; this increased renin secretion leads to increased production of angiotensin I, which is converted to angiotensin II, a powerful vasoconstrictor. Angiotensin II increases peripheral vascular resistance and raises both blood pressure and renal perfusion pressure.

Nitric oxide and prostaglandins have been found to be important mediators of blood flow to different areas of the kidney[50-52] and may exert some control over renin release through a feedback mechanism. Catecholamines,[53] ATP-MgCl$_2$,[54] and calcium[55,56] have also been found to participate in the control of renal blood flow. Adequate blood flow largely controls glomerular filtration and is essential for normal renal function.

Glomerular filtration is determined by the hydrostatic pressure in the afferent arteriole and by the filtration coefficient, K_f. The glomerular filtration rate is an important variable but is not easily measured[57]; it is usually approximated by calculations based on creatinine clearance (C_{Cr}) or free water clearance (C_{H_2O}). These clearance values (expressed in ml/min) can be calculated by the following formulas:

$$C_{Cr} = V \times \frac{U_{Cr}}{P_{Cr}}$$

$$C_{H_2O} = V - C_{osm} = V - \left(V \times \frac{U_{osm}}{P_{osm}}\right)$$

in which V is urine volume (ml/min), C_{osm} is osmolar clearance, U_{osm} is urine osmolality (mOsm/L), and P_{osm} is plasma osmolality (mOsm/L).

These calculations are usually indexed to a standard patient size (1.73 m^2 body surface area) by multiplying each calculated clearance by 1.73/patient's estimated body surface area. The creatinine clearance provides a good estimate of the glomerular filtration rate. A positive C_{H_2O} measures net water excretion; a negative C_{H_2O} measures water retention. A change in free water clearance into the range of ± 0.15 ml/min precedes a rise in creatinine by 24 to 48 hours. Free water clearance is not routinely measured, however, and does not usually establish the diagnosis of renal dysfunction. Rather, renal dysfunction is signaled clinically by the onset of oliguria or a rising serum creatinine level.

Most physicians use the serum creatinine level as an indicator of GFR because it is the simplest to determine. However, a small fraction of creatinine is secreted into the renal tubular fluid. The serum creatinine level becomes a less accurate measure of GFR as the relative component of creatinine clearance from GFR decreases.[58] Furthermore, medications such as cimetidine and the cephalosporin antibiotics can be measured as creatinine in laboratory tests and thus can give a falsely elevated measure of GFR.[59-61] Despite its limitations, however, measurement of serum creatinine levels continues to be the mainstay of assessing GFR and renal clearance.

The principal functions of the renal tubules are reabsorption of sodium and reabsorption of water.[62] Sodium reabsorption occurs in the distal tubule and is controlled primarily by aldosterone.[63] Water absorption occurs predominantly in the collecting tubule and is regulated by antidiuretic hormone (ADH), which is also known as vasopressin.[64] In addition, atrial natriuretic factor appears to affect tubular cells and the renal vasculature.[65] Hypovolemia and hypotension cause increased production of these hormones, which act to increase tubular reabsorption in an attempt to maintain intravascular volume.

Pathophysiology of Acute Renal Failure: Cellular and Molecular Changes

PRERENAL PATHOPHYSIOLOGY

Prerenal causes of acute renal failure are principally associated with inadequate blood flow and altered hemodynamics[66] and account for 50 to 90 percent of the cases of acute renal failure, with the exact distribution somewhat varied.[67,68] Impaired blood flow to the kidneys is the result of hypovolemia in most cases and of depressed myocardial function in a small percentage of patients with an acute cardiac insult or chronic cardiac dysfunction. Renal injury from inadequate perfusion can be exacerbated if low arterial oxygen saturation further impairs oxygen delivery.[69]

The decreased arterial and arteriolar pressures associated with hypovolemia cause production of ADH and aldosterone to increase; the reabsorption of sodium and water is thereby in-

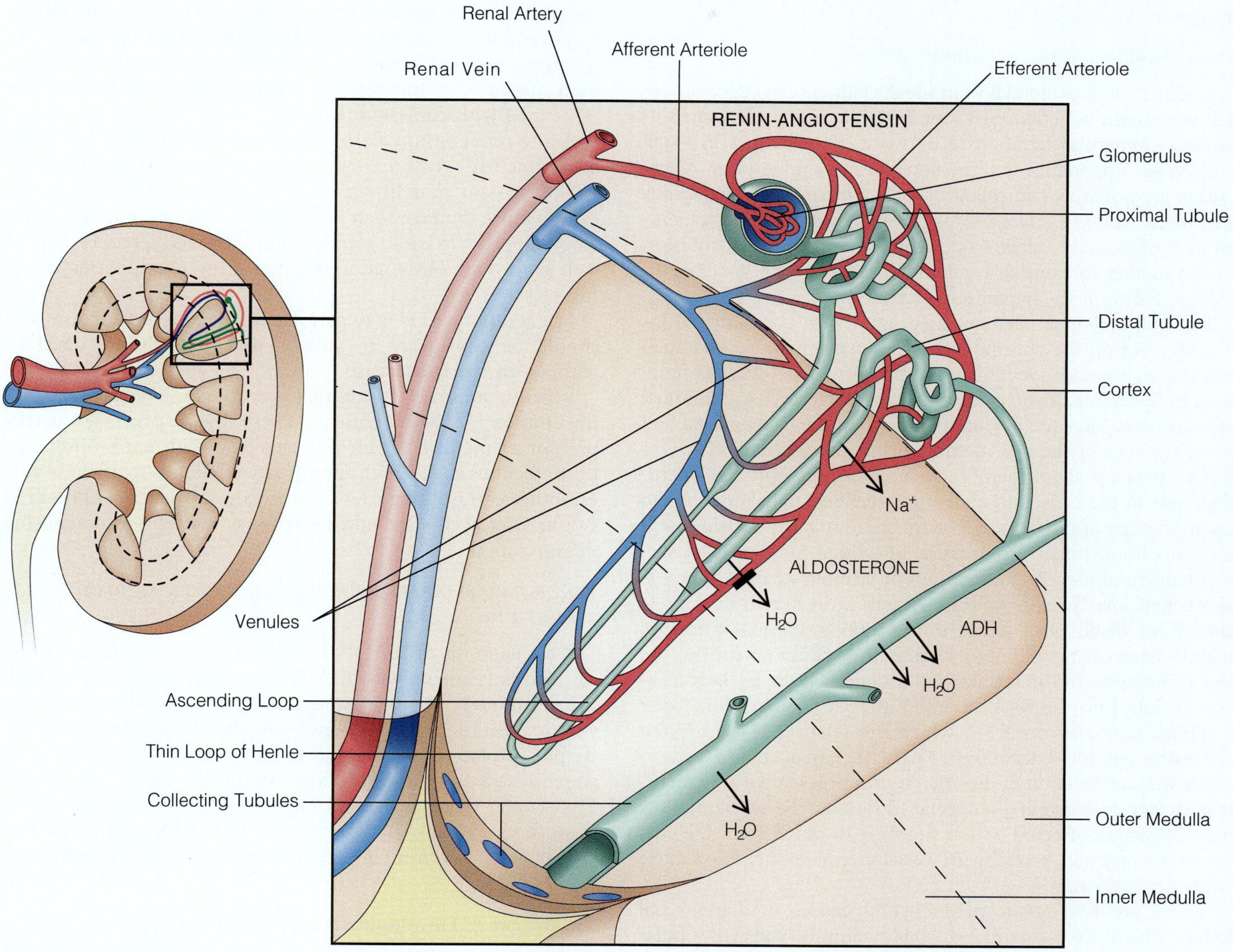

Figure 1 Depicted are the major anatomic features of a juxtamedullary nephron, its blood supply, and the sites of action of the renin-angiotensin system, aldosterone, and ADH. The renin-angiotensin system controls resistance in the renal arterioles, primarily the efferent arteriole. By constricting the efferent arteriole, angiotensin can increase the glomerular pressure, thereby helping to maintain a relatively constant glomerular filtration rate even in the face of low arterial pressure. Aldosterone affects sodium reabsorption in the late distal tubule and the collecting duct. When aldosterone is present in large amounts, virtually all of the sodium is reabsorbed, and almost none is excreted. In the absence of aldosterone, however, substantial quantities of sodium are not reabsorbed and are excreted in the urine. ADH affects the permeability of the epithelium of the collecting duct. When ADH is absent, the collecting duct is almost totally impermeable to water. When it is present in substantial concentrations, however, the collecting duct becomes highly permeable to water; this increased permeability, coupled with the hyperosmolality of the medullary interstitial fluid, results in rapid reabsorption of water from the collecting duct.

creased as well. If the systemic systolic pressure falls below 70 mm Hg, afferent arterioles constrict, decreasing the GFR further.[70] This decrease in glomerular filtration leads to increased sodium reabsorption and concentrated urine, eventually resulting in the urine characteristics associated with a prerenal cause of renal dysfunction—namely, low urine sodium levels, low fractional excretion of sodium, and high urine specific gravity.

Renal blood flow can also be impaired by high intra-abdominal pressure, which seems to decrease renal blood flow.[71,72] Prompt correction of increased intra-abdominal pressure appears to correct developing renal failure, possibly because of improved renal blood flow.

RENAL PARENCHYMAL PATHOPHYSIOLOGY

Redistribution of blood flow inside the kidneys can occur as a result of systemic infection, SIRS, or the hepatorenal syndrome,[17,52] causing glomerular filtration to decrease. The changes in small renal vessel impedance that mediate intrarenal blood flow distribution are probably controlled by local release of prostaglandins and nitric oxide.[52,73] The use of prostaglandin inhibitors or inhibitors of inducible nitric oxide synthase, however, has not been shown to alter function or outcome in patients with systemic infection, SIRS, or the hepatorenal syndrome.

Pathophysiological changes associated with parenchymal injury depend on the specific cause of renal injury. Several such changes may occur concomitantly. Impairment of tubular function by ischemia, toxic substances, or increased intraluminal pressure may alter the normal polarity between the luminal and basal surfaces of the cell membranes of the tubular cells. This loss of polarity alters membrane function, disrupts the microfilaments in the cells, and causes intercellular tight junctions to open, thereby affecting transport of sodium and potassium and inducing fluid shifts.[74] Progression of tubular functional impairment eventually leads to alterations in ultrafiltrate flow by several mechanisms. Swelling of tubular cells or increased back pressure from distal obstruction raises tubular luminal pressure, thereby decreasing glomerular filtration. Simultaneously, the loss of integrity of the tubular cell junctions leads to back-leakage of fluid into the renal interstitium.[75,76] Tubular glomerular feedback may also occur, in which the relatively high sodium concentration at the distal tubule near the macula densa leads to reflex vasoconstriction of the afferent arterioles and consequently a further decrease in glomerular filtration.[77] Renal blood flow may be further affected by the shunting of blood from the cortex to the medulla, probably in association with increased nitric oxide production.

There are two major parenchymal causes of acute renal failure. The first is ischemia, which is a common cause of tubular injury. The medullary thick ascending limb of the loop of Henle and the pars recta of the proximal tubule are the segments of the nephron most sensitive to ischemia.[78] Tubular cells can be identified in the urine of patients with this form of renal injury, which is sometimes called acute tubular necrosis. The term is not an accurate pathological description of this form of renal injury but continues to be used, frequently to describe any renal parenchymal cause of acute renal failure.

Toxic injury to renal cells is the other major parenchymal cause of acute renal failure. Many compounds are toxic to renal tissue; the most commonly encountered are aminoglycosides, ionic radiographic contrast media, myoglobin, hemoglobin, cyclosporine,[79] and nonsteroidal anti-inflammatory drugs.

Aminoglycosides appear to have toxic effects on tubular cells.[80] The extent of toxicity is related primarily to the trough levels of these antibiotics. Close monitoring of levels of these drugs is essential, especially in burn patients, in whom clearance of aminoglycosides and other drugs is increased and who therefore require higher doses to achieve therapeutic levels.[81] Aminoglycosides also appear to decrease renal blood flow independently of cardiac output.[82]

Intravenous ionic radiographic contrast media have been demonstrated to cause acute renal parenchymal injury.[83-85] The toxicity is potentiated by decreased renal perfusion. Nonionic contrast material appears to have less renal toxicity and may be an alternative for patients with borderline renal function. Pretreatment with 0.5 N saline has been shown to be more effective than mannitol or furosemide in preventing renal dysfunction associated with contrast media.[20]

Acute renal failure from myoglobinuria was first described in victims with crush injury and myonecrosis. Myoglobin is an 18 kd protein that filters easily through the glomeruli and causes more damage than hemoglobin, a 67 kd protein. Myoglobin appears to cause tubular injury through direct toxicity as well as through obstruction resulting from precipitation in the tubule.[86,87]

Many other toxins may play a role in acute renal failure and should be considered if parenchymal renal failure develops without an apparent cause.[75]

Inflammatory and vasculitic causes of acute renal failure are uncommon in surgical patients. These disease processes usually present as medical problems associated with autoimmune or postinfectious states. Still, appropriate workup is required to rule out other contributing causes or processes. Identification of red cell or white cell casts and proteinuria is useful in diagnosing inflammation.

SYNDROME OF INAPPROPRIATE ANTIDIURETIC HORMONE SECRETION

The diagnosis of SIADH is made by excluding other causes of oliguria. Patients with SIADH have low urine output, high urine sodium levels, and low serum sodium levels. Furthermore, serum creatinine levels do not usually rise in these patients, despite prolonged borderline oliguria. Treatment consists of water restriction, although some patients require diuretics.[88] Hypertonic saline is infused only if the patient appears to be symptomatic from hyponatremia. SIADH usually resolves spontaneously with no injurious consequences to the kidneys.

Treatment of Developing Acute Renal Failure

If prevention fails, treatment of developing acute renal failure is directed at preserving remaining renal function and limiting further damage[18,89] by increasing blood flow and urine output and decreasing tubular cell injury.

Adequate renal blood flow is essential in treating renal injury from all causes and is usually successfully achieved by volume infusion. In patients with normal cardiac and respiratory function, fluid administration can probably be guided with only a central venous line. Although inotropes can increase cardiac output and low-dose dopamine can increase renal blood flow, use of these agents has not been shown to affect the incidence or outcome of acute renal failure.[90,91] Even the combination of inotropes and diuretics has not been shown to have any effect.[92]

Despite this lack of proven efficacy, dopamine (2 to 5 µg/kg/min) should be considered if urine output does not respond to intravascular volume expansion.

Urine output should be maintained in patients with developing acute renal failure to ensure filtration; in addition, adequate urine output implies adequate blood flow. Patients with nonoliguric renal failure have a much better prognosis than patients whose renal failure is associated with oliguria.[93] Many physicians will attempt to convert oliguric to nonoliguric renal failure. It is unclear whether the increase in urine output upon treatment is an actual conversion or simply a means of identifying the patients with the most residual renal function. Attempts to increase urine output in acute renal failure have often involved administration of diuretics. Many studies have found that diuretics do increase GFR and urine output.[94,95] There have been no differences in outcome, however, between patients who received diuretics and those who did not; this result is most notable in prospective randomized trials.[86,96] Response to furosemide appears to have only prognostic value in acute renal failure.[38,96] There are also potential problems with high-dose diuretics, including ototoxicity.[97] Nevertheless, diuretics still are commonly used to treat developing acute renal failure.[3]

Decreasing tubular injury is an attractive concept. Mannitol has been found to shrink tubular cells, but like diuretics, it does not affect patient outcome.[94] The use of calcium channel blockers to limit tubular cell damage may have some clinical benefit.[98,99] The use of agents that modify nitric oxide production may provide a means of treating evolving renal failure. Other molecular therapies for renal failure, including the use of epidermal growth factor, are under investigation.[100] Elimination of nephrotoxic substances and maintenance of perfusion are currently the only effective methods for decreasing tubular injury.

Differential Diagnosis of Acute Renal Failure

Because prevention and limitation of renal injury are the goals in the management of acute renal failure, early diagnosis is essential. However, determination of which patients with oliguria or elevated serum creatinine levels will progress to acute renal failure and differentiation among the causes of their renal dysfunction remain difficult.

A measurable change in free water clearance into the range of ± 0.17 ml/min/1.73 m² body surface area or a creatinine clearance of 30 ml/min/1.73 m² body surface area indicates acute renal failure.[13] These calculated clearances do not identify the cause of acute renal failure, however. Identification of the cause is best accomplished through physical examination, review of the history and of treatment, urinalysis, and measurement of urine and plasma sodium and creatinine levels. The most reliable means of differentiating prerenal from other causes of acute renal failure are measurement of urine sodium levels and calculation of the fractional excretion of sodium.[12] The renal failure index (RFI) is another means of distinguishing prerenal causes and is defined as follows:

$$RFI = \frac{U_{Na}}{U_{Cr}/P_{Cr}} \times 100$$

This formula is similar to that for the fractional excretion of sodium:

$$FE_{Na} = \frac{U_{Na}/P_{Na}}{U_{Cr}/P_{Cr}} \times 100$$

Although the RFI is used by some nephrologists, it is not superior to FE_{Na} in discriminating between prerenal and renal parenchymal causes of acute renal failure.[68] The usefulness of FE_{Na} in diagnosing acute renal failure has been challenged by some reports[101,102]; however, these reports failed to measure FE_{Na} at the same period in the course of acute renal failure.[103] Furthermore, complaints that FE_{Na} is not predictive are not well founded, because the calculation is not intended to be a predictor but rather a tool for distinguishing prerenal from renal parenchymal causes of acute renal failure.[1,3,44,104]

Other tests to distinguish the causes of acute renal failure are of limited value, except in identifying possible parenchymal disorders. The presence of red cell and white cell casts may indicate vasculitic or inflammatory causes. Identification of tubular cells in the urine, either microscopically or by detection of surface antigen, suggests a postischemic cause, but these markers are not specific.

Measurement of urine electrolyte concentrations (e.g., chloride and bicarbonate), measurement of the products of inflammation (e.g., complement components), and renal biopsy are useful in assessing chronic renal problems; however, these determinations add little to the diagnosis and treatment of acute renal failure.

References

1. Farber MD, Kupin WL, Krishna GG, et al: The differential diagnosis of acute renal failure. Acute Renal Failure, 3rd ed. Lazarus JM, Brenner BM, Eds. WB Saunders Co, Philadelphia, 1993, p 133
2. Engle WD: Evaluation of renal function and acute renal failure in the neonate. Pediatr Clin North Am 33:129, 1986
3. Tilney NL, Lazarus JM: Acute renal failure in surgical patients: causes, clinical patterns, and care. Surg Clin North Am 63:357, 1983
4. Narayanan S: Renal biochemistry and physiology: pathophysiology and analytical perspectives. Adv Clin Chem 29:121, 1992
5. Espinel CH: Diagnosis of acute and chronic renal failure. Clin Lab Med 13:89, 1993
6. Baek SM, Makabali GG, Shoemaker WC: Clinical determinants of survival from postoperative renal failure. Surg Gynecol Obstet 140:685, 1975
7. Blachley JD, Henrich WL: The diagnosis and management of acute renal failure. Seminars in Nephrology 1:11, 1981
8. Finn WF, Arendshorst WJ, Gottschalk CW: Pathogenesis of oliguria in acute renal failure. Circ Res 36:675, 1975
9. Burnier M, Schrier RW: Pathogenesis of acute renal failure. Adv Exp Med Biol 212:3, 1987
10. Fishchereder M, Trick W, Nath KA: Therapeutic strategies in the prevention of acute renal failure. Semin Nephrol 14:41, 1994
11. Link D, Leff RG, Hildel J, et al: The use of percutaneous nephrostomy in 42 patients. J Urol 122:9, 1979
12. Miller TR, Anderson RJ, Linas SL: Urinary diagnostic indices in acute renal failure: a prospective study. Ann Intern Med 89:47, 1978
13. Brown R, Babcock R, Talbert J, et al: Renal function in critically ill postoperative patients: sequential assessment of creatinine osmolar and free water clearance. Crit Care Med 8:68, 1980

14. Kellen M, Aronson S, Roizen MF, et al: Predictive and diagnostic tests of renal failure: a review. Anesth Analg 78:134, 1994
15. Goldberg LI: Cardiovascular and renal actions of dopamine: potential clinical applications. Pharmacol Rev 24:1, 1972
16. Ron D, Taitelman U, Michaelson M, et al: Prevention of acute renal failure in traumatic rhabdomyolysis. Arch Intern Med 144:277, 1984
17. Laffi G, LaVilla G, Gentilini P: Pathogenesis and management of the hepatorenal syndrome. Semin Liver Dis 14:71, 1994
18. Finn WF: Enhanced recovery from postischemic acute renal failure: micropuncture studies in the rat. Circ Res 46:440, 1980
19. Russo D, Memoli B, Andreucci VE: The place of loop diuretics in the treatment of acute and chronic renal failure. Clin Nephrol 28(suppl 1):S69, 1992
20. Solomon R, Werner C, Mann D, et al: Effects of saline, mannitol and furosemide on acute decreases in renal function induced by radiocontrast agents. N Engl J Med 331:1416, 1994
21. Compher C, Mullen JL, Barker CF: Nutritional support in renal failure. Surg Clin North Am 71:597, 1991
22. Abel RM: Nutritional support in the patient with acute renal failure. J Am Coll Nutr 2:33, 1983
23. Bellomo R, Boyce N: Acute continuous hemodiafiltration: a prospective study of 110 patients and a review of the literature. Am J Kidney Dis 21:508, 1993
24. Kierdorf H: Continuous versus intermittent treatment: clinical results in acute renal failure. Contrib Nephrol 93:1, 1991
25. Ronco C: Continuous renal replacement therapies for the treatment of acute renal failure in intensive care patients. Clin Nephrol 40:187, 1993
26. Conger JD: Management of acute renal failure. Principles and Practice of Nephrology. Jacobson HR, Striker GE, Klahr S, Eds. BC Decker, Philadelphia, 1991, p 666
27. Reichow W, Koehler H, Dietrich K, et al: Continuous arterio-venous hemofiltration for the treatment of acute renal failure in septic shock. Prog Clin Biol Res 236B:235, 1987
28. Golper TA: Continuous arteriovenous hemofiltration in acute renal failure. Am J Kidney Dis 6:373, 1985
29. Lauer A, Saccaggi A, Ronco C, et al: Continuous arteriovenous hemofiltration in the critically ill patient: clinical use and operational characteristics. Ann Intern Med 99:455, 1983
30. Mault JR, Dechert RE, Lees P, et al: Continuous arteriovenous filtration: an effective treatment for surgical acute renal failure. Surgery 101:478, 1987
31. Kafety K: Renal impairment in the elderly: a review. J R Soc Med 76:398, 1983
32. Cioffi WG, Ashikaga T, Gamelli RL: Probability of surviving postoperative acute renal failure: development of a prognostic index. Ann Surg 200:205, 1984
33. Finn WF: Recovery from acute renal failure. Acute Renal Failure. Brenner BM, Lazarus JM, Eds. WB Saunders Co, Philadelphia, 1983
34. Milligan SL, Luft FC, McMurray SD, et al: Intra-abdominal infection and acute renal failure. Arch Surg 113:467, 1978
35. Eliahou HF: Acute renal failure revisited: the full circle in ARF mortality. Trans Am Soc Artif Intern Organs 30:700, 1984
36. Linton AL: Acute renal failure: a continuing enigma. Renal Failure 10:3, 1987
37. Chew SL, Lins RL, Daelemans R, et al: Outcome in acute renal failure. Nephrol Dial Transplant 8:101, 1993
38. Cameron JS: Acute renal failure in the intensive care unit today. Intensive Care Med 12:64, 1986
39. Wardle N: Acute renal failure in the 1980s: the importance of septic shock and of endotoxaemia. Nephron 30:193, 1982
40. Routh GS, Briggs JD, Mone JG, et al: Survival from acute renal failure with and without multiple organ dysfunction. Postgrad Med J 56:244, 1980
41. Tilney NL, Bailey GL, Morgan AP: Sequential system failure after rupture of abdominal aortic aneurysms: an unsolved problem in postoperative care. Ann Surg 178:117, 1973
42. Abel RM, Buckley MJ, Austen WG, et al: Etiology, incidence, and prognosis of renal failure following cardiac operations: results of a prospective analysis of 500 consecutive patients. J Thorac Cardiovasc Surg 71:323, 1976
43. Kron IL, Joob AW, Van Meter C: Acute renal failure in the cardiovascular surgical patient. Ann Thorac Surg 39:590, 1985
44. Danielson RA: Differential diagnosis and treatment of oliguria in post-traumatic and post-operative patients. Surg Clin North Am 55:697, 1975
45. Burnier M, Schrier RW: Protection from acute renal failure. Adv Exp Med Biol 212:275, 1987
46. Better OS, Rubenstein I, Winaver J: Recent insights into the pathogenesis and early management of the crush syndrome. Semin Nephrol 12:217, 1992
47. Schrier RW: Acute renal failure. JAMA 247:2518, 1982
48. Wilkes BM, Mailloux LU: Acute renal failure: pathogenesis and prevention. Am J Med 80:1129, 1986
49. Henrich WL, Anderson RJ, Berns AS, et al: The role of renal nerves and prostaglandins in control of renal hemodynamics and plasma renin activity during hypotensive hemorrhage in the dog. J Clin Invest 61:744, 1978
50. Dunn MJ, Hood VL: Prostaglandins and the kidney. Am J Physiol 233:169, 1977
51. Torres VE, Romero JC, Strong CS, et al: Renal prostaglandin E during acute renal failure. Prostaglandins 8:353, 1974
52. Garrison RN, Wilson MA, Matheson PJ, et al: Nitric oxide mediates redistribution of intrarenal blood flow during bacteremia. J Trauma 39:90, 1995
53. Henrich WL, Pettinger WA, Cronin RE: The influence of circulating catecholamines and prostaglandins on canine renal blood flow during hemorrhage. Circ Res 48:424, 1981
54. Garvin PJ, Jellinek M, Morgan R, et al: Renal cortical levels of adenosine triphosphate: restoration after prolonged ischemia by in situ perfusion of ATP-$MgCl_2$. Arch Surg 116:221, 1981
55. Humes HD: Role of calcium in pathogenesis of acute renal failure. Am J Physiol 250:F579, 1986
56. Rasmussen H, Kojima I, Apfeldorf W, et al: Cellular mechanism of hormone action in the kidney: messenger function of calcium and cyclic AMP. Kidney Int 29:90, 1986
57. Gates GF: Glomerular filtration rate: estimation from fractional renal accumulation of 99mTc-DTPA (stannous). AJR 138:565, 1982
58. Carrie BJ, Golbetz HV, Michaels AS, et al: Creatinine: an inadequate filtration marker in glomerular diseases. Am J Med 69:177, 1980
59. Larsson R, Bodemar G, Kagedal B, et al: The effects of cimetidine (Tagamet) on renal function in patients with renal failure. Acta Med Scand 208:27, 1980
60. Guay DR, Meatherall RC, Macaulay PA: Interference of selected second- and third-generation cephalosporins with creatinine determination. Am J Hosp Pharm 40:435, 1983
61. Nanji AA, Campbell DJ: Falsely-elevated serum creatinine values in diabetic ketoacidosis: clinical implications. Clin Biochem 14:91, 1981
62. Cronin RE, de Torrente A, Miller PD, et al: Pathogenic mechanisms in early norepinephrine-induced acute renal failure: functional and histological correlates of protection. Kidney Int 14:115, 1978
63. Morel F, Doucet A: Hormonal control of kidney functions at the cell level. Physiol Rev 66:377, 1986
64. Jard S, Butlen D, Cantau B, et al: The mechanisms of action of antidiuretic hormone. Adv Nephrol 13:163, 1984
65. Capasso G, Anastasio P, Giordano D, et al: Atrial natriuretic factor increases glomerular filtration rate in the experimental acute renal failure induced by cisplatin. Adv Exp Med Biol 212:285, 1987
66. Myers BD, Moran SM: Hemodynamically mediated acute renal failure. N Engl J Med 314:97, 1986
67. Levinsky NG: Pathophysiology of acute renal failure. N Engl J Med 296:1453, 1977
68. Oken DE: On the differential diagnosis of acute renal failure. Am J Med 71:916, 1981
69. Jones DP: Renal metabolism during normoxia, hypoxia, and ischemic injury. Annu Rev Physiol 48:33, 1986
70. Adams PL, Adams FF, Bell PD, et al: Impaired renal blood flow autoregulation in ischemic acute renal failure. Kidney Int 18:68, 1980
71. Harman PK, Kron IL, McLachlan HD, et al: Elevated intra-abdominal pressure and renal function. Ann Surg 196:594, 1982
72. Kron IL, Harman PK, Nolan SP: The measurement of intra-abdominal pressure as a criterion for abdominal re-exploration. Ann Surg 199:28, 1984
73. Epstein M, Lifschitz M, Ramachandran M, et al: Characterization of renal prostaglandin E responsiveness in decompensated cirrhosis: implications for renal sodium handling. Clin Sci 63:555, 1982
74. Molitoris BA: New insights into the cell biology of ischemic acute renal failure. J Am Soc Nephrol 1:1263, 1991
75. Stein JH: Acute renal failure: lessons from pathophysiology. West J Med 156:176, 1992
76. Hohenfellner M, Thuroff JW, Thurau K: Cellular changes in acute renal failure: functional and therapeutic consequences. Eur Urol 22:265, 1992
77. Braam B, Mitchell KD, Koomans HA, et al: Relevance of the tubuloglomerular feedback mechanism in pathophysiology. J Am Soc Nephrol 4:1257, 1993
78. Brezis M, Rosen S, Silva P, et al: Renal ischemia: a new perspective. Kidney Int 26:375, 1984
79. Myers BD: Cyclosporine nephrotoxicity. Kidney Int 30:964, 1986
80. Matzke GR, Lucarotti RL, Shapiro HS: Controlled comparison of gentamicin and tobramycin nephrotoxicity. Am J Nephrol 3:11, 1983
81. Loirat P, Rohan J, Baillet A, et al: Increased glomerular filtration rate in patients with major burns and its effect on the pharmacokinetics of tobramycin. N Engl J Med 299:915, 1978
82. Bayliss C: The mechanism of the decline in glomerular filtration rate in agent induced acute renal failure in the rat. J Antimicrob Chemother 6:381, 1980
83. Byrd L, Sherman RL: Radiocontrast-induced acute renal failure: clinical and pathophysiologic review. Medicine (Baltimore) 58:270, 1979
84. Mudge GH: Nephrotoxicity of urographic radiocontrast drugs. Kidney Int 18:540, 1980
85. D'Elia JA, Gleason RE, Alday M, et al: Nephrotoxicity from angiographic contrast material: a prospective study. Am J Med 72:719, 1982
86. Eneas JF, Schoenfeld PY, Humphreys MH: The effect of infusion of mannitol-sodium bicarbonate on the clinical course of myoglobinuria. Arch Intern Med 139:801, 1979
87. Braun SR, Weiss FR, Keller AI, et al: Evaluation of the renal toxicity of hemoproteins and their derivatives: a role in the genesis of acute tubular necrosis. J Exp Med 131:443, 1970

88. Rose BD: Syndrome of inappropriate ADH secretion (SIADH). Clinical Physiology of Acid-Base and Electrolyte Disorders, 2nd ed. McGraw-Hill Book Co, New York, 1984
89. Gaudio KM, Siegel NJ: Pathogenesis and treatment of acute renal failure. Pediatr Clin North Am 34:771, 1987
90. Parker S, Carlon GC, Isaacs M, et al: Dopamine administration in oliguria and oliguric renal failure. Crit Care Med 9:630, 1981
91. Duke GJ, Bensten AD: Dopamine and renal salvage in the critically ill patient. Anaesth Intensive Care 20:277, 1992
92. Graziani G, Cantaluppi A, Casati S, et al: Dopamine and frusemide in oliguric acute renal failure. Nephron 37:39, 1984
93. Hou SH, Bushinsky DA, Wish JB, et al: Hospital-acquired renal insufficiency: a prospective study. Am J Med 74:243, 1983
94. Warren SE, Blantz RC: Mannitol. Arch Intern Med 141:493, 1981
95. Cantarovich F, Galli C, Benedetti L, et al: High dose frusemide in established acute renal failure. Br Med J 4:449, 1973
96. Brown CB, Ogg CS, Cameron JS: High dose frusemide in acute renal failure: a controlled clinical trial. Clin Nephrol 15:90, 1981
97. Gallagher KL, Jones JK: Furosemide-induced ototoxicity. Ann Intern Med 91:744, 1979
98. Schrier RW: Role of calcium channel blockers in protection against experimental renal injury. Am J Med 90:21S, 1991
99. Wetzels JF, Burker JF, Schrier RW: Calcium channel blockers: protective effects in ischemic acute renal failure. Renal Failure 14:327, 1992
100. Humes HD: Potential molecular therapy for acute renal failure. Cleve Clin J Med 60:166, 1993
101. Pru C, Kjellstrand CM: The FE_{Na} test is of no value in acute renal failure. Nephron 36:20, 1984
102. Saha H, Mustonen J, Helin H, et al: Limited value of the fractional excretion of sodium test in the diagnosis of acute renal failure. Nephrol Dial Transplant 2:79, 1987
103. Brosius FC, Lau K: Low fractional excretion of sodium in acute renal failure: role of timing of the test and ischemia. Am J Nephrol 6:450, 1986
104. Lucas CE: The renal response to acute injury and sepsis. Surg Clin North Am 56:953, 1976

Acknowledgment

Figure 1   Dana Burns.

94 HEPATIC FAILURE

Walid S. Arnaout, M.D., and Achilles A. Demetriou, M.D., Ph.D.

Approach to the Patient with Liver Failure

Hepatic failure and cirrhosis continue to be major causes of morbidity and mortality among critically ill patients. Since the beginning of the 1980s, several advances have been made in the management of hepatic failure. Newer diagnostic techniques and therapeutic modalities have been introduced that have led to significantly better overall outcomes. In addition to improved medical therapy, liver transplantation has proved to be effective in treating end-stage liver disease and liver failure, regardless of etiology.

In what follows, we outline general management guidelines for hepatic failure and its complications. We also discuss the role of artificial liver support and its potential use in managing hepatic failure.

Patient Evaluation

RISK FACTORS AND WORKUP

Liver disease is usually suspected on the basis of several risk factors, including a history of alcohol or I.V. drug abuse. Receipt of a blood transfusion before 1992 raises the index of suspicion for viral hepatitis, hepatitis C virus (HCV) infection in particular.[1-3] Other risk factors for liver disease are tattoos, sexual promiscuity, and snorting cocaine. Rare risk factors include a family history of certain liver diseases and exposure to various toxins and chemicals (e.g., aflatoxin and carbon tetrachloride).

Evaluation of patients with suspected liver disease is often complex and typically requires an extensive workup—including a detailed history and physical examination as well as various diagnostic studies—to establish the diagnosis and confirm the underlying cause. The laboratory data usually required include a complete blood count, a platelet count, liver function tests, a prothrombin time (PT), and serum albumin and cholesterol levels. In addition, imaging studies (e.g., abdominal ultrasonography, computed tomography, or magnetic resonance imaging) may be indicated. These studies usually demonstrate anatomic and structural abnormalities in the liver parenchyma, the biliary tree, or the vascular system. Occasionally, a liver biopsy is required to establish or confirm the diagnosis of liver disease.

Liver disease commonly gives rise to several manifestations that are easily recognized by most health care workers: jaundice [*see 16 Jaundice*], muscle wasting, malnutrition, ascites, lower-extremity edema, and varying degrees of hepatic encephalopathy. Common findings on physical examination of patients with liver disease include bitemporal muscle wasting, vascular spiders, abdominal wall collaterals, caput medusae, palmar erythema, and clubbing. Umbilical and inguinal hernias are frequently noted in patients with tense ascites. Bilateral gynecomastia and testicular atrophy are often seen in male patients.

PRIMARY VERSUS SECONDARY HEPATIC FAILURE

Hepatic failure is generally classified as either primary or secondary, depending on the underlying cause. Primary hepatic failure derives from underlying liver disease, whereas secondary hepatic failure is caused by various underlying conditions unrelated to the liver. Most patients with primary hepatic failure have a history of preexisting liver disease and possibly of cirrhosis, generally presenting with one or more complications of chronic liver disease (e.g., GI bleeding, hepatic encephalopathy, spontaneous bacterial peritonitis, or renal failure). A subgroup of patients, however, exhibit hepatic failure secondary to acute exacerbation of the preexisting liver disease (e.g., acute reactivation of hepatitis B, acute decompensated Wilson disease, or autoimmune hepatitis). In another subgroup, primary hepatic failure develops acutely among patients who have no preexisting liver disease and no known risk factors (so-called acute or fulminant hepatic failure). These patients present with massive liver necrosis, jaundice, and profound coagulopathy and often go on to experience deep coma and cerebral edema, which may lead to irreversible brain damage and death. Acute liver failure can be associated with severe multisystem organ involvement, as in the acute respiratory distress syndrome (ARDS) or the multiple organ dysfunction syndrome (MODS), which makes diagnosis difficult. (This may also be the case with chronic liver disease, but to a lesser degree.)

Secondary liver failure is seen among critically ill patients admitted to the ICU for management of a non–liver-related illness. It is usually manifested by cholestatic jaundice, impaired synthetic activity, varying degrees of hepatocellular damage, and altered mental status. Hepatic insufficiency is common in patients with life-threatening injuries, severe systemic infection, or ARDS. These patients usually have no preexisting liver disease: their liver dysfunction is simply a reflection of their overall critical condition. The extent of the liver dysfunction in such cases usually depends on the severity of the underlying nonhepatic disease; in general, it tends to lessen as the causative problem is controlled or resolved. Failure to control the primary underlying condition leads to progressive MODS and death.

Management of secondary hepatic failure typically involves treating underlying nonhepatic disorders. Accordingly, we focus here on management of acute and chronic primary hepatic failure, which by definition involves treating hepatic disease and its associated complications.

Approach to the Patient with Liver Failure

Patient has signs of liver disease or known risk factors

Perform extensive workup: history, physical examination, laboratory tests, and imaging studies as needed. Liver biopsy is occasionally required.

Distinguish primary from secondary hepatic failure.

Primary hepatic failure

Acute liver failure

Determine etiology—viral, drug-induced, toxin-induced, or other—and treat accordingly.

Begin medical management of complications.

Concurrently, assess prognosis by means of King's College criteria.

Cerebral edema

Initiate invasive ICP monitoring.
Manage elevated ICP.

Extrahepatic complications

Treat fluid, electrolyte, and nutritional abnormalities; renal failure; pulmonary complications; infectious complications; and coagulopathy and bleeding.

Good prognosis with medical management

Continue medical therapy.

Poor prognosis with medical management

Medical management succeeds

Medical management fails

Consider emergency OLT if not contraindicated.

Treat toxic liver syndrome with total hepatectomy and end-to-side portacaval shunt, followed by OLT.

Consider use of BAL support system.

Transplantation is contraindicated

Manage medically.

No contraindications to transplantation are present

Secondary hepatic failure

Treat underlying nonhepatic cause.

Chronic liver disease

Determine etiology [see Table 4], and treat accordingly.
Begin medical management of complications.

Portal hypertension

Treat complications of PHT:
- Variceal bleeding
- Ascites: restrict sodium and give diuretics. If medical management fails, perform LVP or use a shunt (peritoneovenous or TIPS).

Hepatic encephalopathy

Control precipitating factors, and control ammonia levels with lactulose or antibiotics.

Renal failure

Treat HRS, ATN, RTA, and drug-induced interstitial nephritis.
Correct underlying causes. Manage fluids and electrolytes carefully.

Malnutrition

Give glucose with fat emulsion.
Use enteral feeding unless contraindicated.

Coagulopathy and bleeding

Identify hemostatic defect.
Give FFP, cryoprecipitate, prothrombin complex concentrates, platelets, AT-III concentrate, or antifibrinolytic agents as appropriate.

Medical management is unsatisfactory, and no contraindications to transplantation are present

Medical management is satisfactory, or transplantation is contraindicated

Manage medically.

Perform OLT when donor organ is available. Consider use of BAL support system while awaiting organ.

Acute Liver Failure

In the United States, acute liver failure (ALF) affects approximately 5,000 persons each year. The definition of ALF depends on the temporal relation between the initial onset of illness and the manifestation of jaundice, encephalopathy, and coagulopathy. The classic definition of Trey and Davidson is based on massive liver necrosis associated with encephalopathy developing within 8 weeks of the onset of illness.[4] In most cases, however, it is difficult to determine the precise time of onset of the disease process and thus the exact time elapsed before the establishment of hepatic failure. Recognizing that clinical findings and prognosis varied depending on the interval between onset of jaundice and encephalopathy, Bernuau and coworkers defined fulminant hepatic failure (FHF) as ALF complicated by encephalopathy developing within 2 weeks of the onset of jaundice and defined subfulminant hepatic failure (SFHF) as ALF complicated by encephalopathy developing 2 to 12 weeks after onset of jaundice.[5]

Differences in nomenclature and classification notwithstanding, the defining characteristic of ALF is the absence of known preexisting liver disease. We use the term FHF more or less interchangeably with ALF as defined by Trey and Davidson.

ETIOLOGY

The causes of FHF may be classified into four major groups: viral, drug-induced, toxin-induced, and miscellaneous. In one multicenter study, acetaminophen-induced FHF toxicity was found to be the most common variety (20%), followed by FHF of indeterminate etiology (15%).[6]

Viral Hepatitis

Hepatitis A The incidence of FHF and SFHF in hepatitis A virus (HAV) infection is very low (< 0.01%).[5] Young patients with HAV infection rarely manifest FHF, and their chances of survival with medical therapy are relatively good (40% to 60%). About 10% of patients experience relapses, usually within 2 to 3 months after an initial clinical improvement. Relapse is signaled by an increase in serum transaminase and bilirubin levels and the reappearance of virus in the stool. If encephalopathy occurs during this period, the outcome is poor.[7]

Hepatitis B ALF related to hepatitis B virus (HBV) accounts for fewer than 1% of HBV infections but is the most common form of viral-induced FHF.[6,8] Like HAV infection, HBV infection leads to FHF more often than to SFHF. Hepatitis B surface antigen (HBsAg) and HBV DNA may be absent in some cases of FHF secondary to HBV infection.[9] These findings indicate that in certain FHF patients, an enhanced immune response prevents further HBV replication and results in more rapid clearance of HBsAg. The survival rate for patients who are HBsAg-positive on presentation (17%) is much lower than that for patients who are HBsAg-negative (47%).[5] Clearance of HBsAg and HBV DNA results in better survival rates as well as lower recurrence rates after emergency liver transplantation.[10]

Hepatitis D Hepatitis D virus (HDV, also referred to as the delta agent) is a defective virus that uses HBsAg as its envelope protein. HDV RNA is detected in only 10% of patients with fulminant hepatitis D.[11] HDV infection can be either a coinfection, in conjunction with HBV infection, or a superinfection in patients with previous HBV infection [see 86 Viral Infection].[12] Among patients with FHF, HDV coinfection is more common than superinfection; however, HDV superinfection is associated with a higher mortality than HDV coinfection (72% versus 52%) and more often predisposes to chronic liver disease (54% versus 31%).[13]

Hepatitis C and hepatitis of indeterminate etiology Previously, FHF of indeterminate etiology was attributed to non-A, non-B viral hepatitis. It is now clear that some such cases are caused by hepatitis C virus (HCV) infection, though the precise extent to which HCV infection contributes to this indeterminate group is unclear. Unlike HAV and HBV infection, HCV infection is more likely to cause SFHF than FHF. Despite the availability of advanced serologic testing, there are still many cases of FHF and SFHF whose cause cannot be determined.[14,15] These patients are placed into a non-A, non-B, non-C (NANBNC) category, implying a viral etiology. A more accurate designation for this category would be "of indeterminate etiology," in that the true cause is unknown and may not, in fact, be undiagnosed viral hepatitis.

Drugs

Drug toxicity accounts for 35% of all cases of FHF and SFHF and usually runs a subfulminant course.[6] Drug ingestion causes hepatic injury in fewer than 1% of patients, about 20% of whom manifest FHF or SFHF. Increasing the total drug dose, simultaneously ingesting other drugs that induce or inhibit hepatic enzymes, and continuing drug administration after the onset of liver disease all increase the risk of hepatic failure.[5] Acetaminophen toxicity is the most common cause of drug-induced hepatic failure. The prognosis for FHF caused by acetaminophen is usually better than that for FHF caused by other drugs (e.g., isoniazid, psychotropic drugs, antihistamines, and nonsteroidal anti-inflammatory drugs [NSAIDs]).[16] Halothane-induced FHF occurs within 2 weeks of general anesthesia and carries a high mortality.[17]

Toxins

Most cases of toxin-induced FHF involve mushroom poisoning or exposure to industrial hydrocarbons. In mushroom poisoning, the active agents are heat-stable and are not destroyed by cooking. Liver damage from mushroom toxins is delayed and is usually preceded by several days of vomiting and diarrhea. Mortality is high: up to 22% in one series.[18] Emergency liver transplantation is sometimes successful.[19]

Industrial hydrocarbons (e.g., carbon tetrachloride and trichloroethylene) are rare causes of FHF. In developing nations, aflatoxin and herbal medicines have been implicated as causes of FHF.

Miscellaneous Conditions

Wilson disease may present as FHF or SFHF with intravascular hemolysis and renal failure.[20,21] A family history of hepatic and neurologic disease, the presence of Kayser-Fleischer rings, and low serum ceruloplasmin levels help establish the diagnosis. Acute decompensated Wilson disease carries a high mortality and is therefore an indication for emergency liver transplantation.[22]

Acute fatty liver of pregnancy is a rare cause of FHF that carries a high mortality for both mother and infant. Delivery of the fetus results in regression of the microvesicular steatosis and abnormal liver test results for the mother. The risk of FHF is increased with misdiagnosis and continuation of pregnancy. Liver transplantation has been successfully performed.[23]

Several other conditions and disease processes are known to cause ALF in both adults and children [see Table 1].

ASSESSMENT OF PROGNOSIS

Several prognostic criteria and indicators have been proposed for

Table 1 Etiology of Acute Liver Failure

Infectious
  Viral: hepatitis A, B, C, D, and E and hepatitis of indeterminate etiology; infection by herpes simplex virus, cytomegalovirus, Epstein-Barr virus, or adenovirus
  Bacterial: Q fever
  Parasitic: amebiasis
Drugs
Toxins
  Mushrooms: *Amanita phalloides, verna,* and *virosa; Lepiota* species
  Bacillus cereus
  Hydrocarbons: carbon tetrachloride, trichloroethylene, 2-nitropropane, chloroform
  Copper
  Aflatoxin
  Yellow phosphorus
Miscellaneous conditions
  Wilson disease
  Acute fatty liver of pregnancy
  Reye syndrome
  Hypoxic liver cell necrosis
  Hypothermia or hyperthermia
  Budd-Chiari syndrome
  Veno-occlusive disease of the liver
  Autoimmune hepatitis
  Massive malignant infiltration of the liver
  Partial hepatectomy
  Liver transplantation
  Postjejunoileal bypass
  Galactosemia
  Hereditary fructose intolerance
  Tyrosinemia
  Erythropoietic protoporphyria
  Irradiation
  α_1-Antitrypsin deficiency
  Niemann-Pick disease
  Neonatal hemochromatosis
  Cardiac tamponade
  Right ventricular failure
  Circulatory shock
  Tuberculosis

predicting outcome after optimal medical management of FHF. The two main factors determining the likelihood of survival are (1) the extent of liver necrosis and (2) the potential for hepatocyte regeneration. In a 1989 study, investigators at King's College Hospital in London compiled a set of indicators for predicting a poor outcome after medical therapy and hence the need for emergency liver transplantation.[24] Underlying etiology was the single most important predictive variable. Therefore, patients were divided into two groups, one comprising all cases of acetaminophen-induced FHF and the other all cases of FHF from other causes. Age, degree of encephalopathy, serum pH, PT, interval to onset of encephalopathy, and admission serum creatinine and bilirubin levels also proved to be significant variables [see Table 2]. Patients who met the criteria in either group had a 95% chance of dying with medical therapy alone and were identified as candidates for emergency liver transplantation.

The major strength of the King's College study is that it based patient assessment on parameters that are easily obtained within a few hours of admission to the emergency department. This approach to assessment facilitates early referral of patients with a poor prognosis to a specialized liver unit for evaluation for transplantation. In another study, plasma factor V level and age were found to be independent predictors of survival.[25] The criteria for liver transplantation were the presence of hepatic encephalopathy (stage III or IV) and a factor V level either less than 20% of normal in patients younger than 30 years or less than 30% of normal in patients older than 30 years.

In addition to biochemical and synthetic activities, assessment of the residual functional reserve of the liver has been studied as an indicator of prognosis. The ratio of acetoacetate to β-hydroxybutyrate in an arterial blood sample (also known as the arterial ketone body ratio [AKBR]) is thought to reflect hepatic energy status.[26] Galactose clearance reflects both residual liver mass and hepatic blood flow.[27] This test has long been considered a standard test of liver functional reserve, and newer tests are routinely compared to it. At present, functional assessment tools are not routinely used in patient assessment.

The wide variety of potential prognostic indicators for FHF notwithstanding, the King's College criteria are still the most widely used. These criteria have been validated in several large series and are currently considered the gold standard for predicting outcome in FHF patients undergoing medical management.

At our center, we apply the King's College criteria at admission to predict the likely outcome with medical therapy. Once the initial assessment is completed, the decision for or against emergency evaluation for liver transplantation is made. Evaluation, if indicated, is usually completed within 12 to 24 hours. The evaluation is similar to that of patients with chronic liver disease [see Chronic Liver Disease, below], with a few exceptions. In particular, patients with FHF usually do not have preexisting liver disease; thus, it is vital that the evaluation [see Table 3] reveal the probable cause of liver failure. Unlike chronic liver disease, FHF is associated with cerebral edema and elevated intracranial pressure (ICP), which is the leading cause of death among these patients. Therefore, an extensive neurologic evaluation should be completed before a patient is listed for transplantation. Serial neurologic assessment is necessary to rule out irreversible brain damage and brain-stem herniation; however, previous sedation often makes this step very difficult.

Table 2 King's College Hospital Prognostic Criteria Predicting Poor Outcome for Patients with FHF

Acetaminophen-induced FHF	pH < 7.30 (irrespective of grade of encephalopathy) *or* All of the following: PT > 100 sec (INR > 6.5) Serum creatinine > 3.4 g/dl Stage III or IV hepatic encephalopathy
Non–acetaminophen-induced FHF	PT > 100 sec (INR > 6.5) (irrespective of grade of encephalopathy) *or* Any three of the following (irrespective of grade of encephalopathy): Age < 10 or > 40 yr Etiology: non-A, non-B hepatitis, halothane hepatitis, drug toxicity Duration of jaundice to encephalopathy > 7 days PT 50 sec (INR > 3.5) Serum bilirubin > 17.5 g/dl

FHF—fulminant hepatic failure   INR—international normalized ratio
PT—prothrombin time

TREATMENT OF COMPLICATIONS

Cerebral Edema

Cerebral edema is one of the hallmarks of FHF, and its presence significantly influences management and outcome. Autopsy studies indicate that cerebral edema is present in 80% of patients who die of FHF.[28,29] It occurs in advanced stages of FHF and can be recognized by clinical, radiologic, or invasive means. Clinical findings include decerebrate posturing, myoclonus, spastic rigidity, seizure activity, systemic hypertension, bradycardia, hyperventilation, and mydriasis with diminished pupillary response. These findings initially are paroxysmal but later become persistent. Papilledema is a late finding and often does not occur at all, even in the advanced stages of the disease.[30] Noninvasive diagnostic modalities (e.g., CT scanning, electroencephalographic monitoring, and transcranial Doppler flow measurement) have not proved helpful for early detection and management of cerebral edema.[31,32] CT scanning of the brain is not a sensitive test for detecting early cerebral edema: 25% to 30% of patients with high ICP exhibit no radiographic changes.[33] It is, however, useful for ruling out intracranial bleeding.

Currently, ICP monitoring is the best means of monitoring intracranial hypertension and is recommended for guiding treatment in patients with stage III or IV encephalopathy. ICP can be measured by using epidural, subdural, or intraventricular catheters. Although epidural catheters are slightly less sensitive to ICP changes, they have the lowest complication rate (3.8%) and lowest rate of fatal hemorrhage (1%).[34] Despite a slightly higher complication rate, we prefer subdural catheters: in our view, they offer more reliable ICP monitoring. Institution of ICP monitoring necessitates aggressive treatment of any concomitant coagulopathy. Fresh frozen plasma (FFP) infusions are given to bring the PT below 25 seconds, and platelet transfusions are indicated if the patient has severe thrombocytopenia (platelet count < 50,000/mm³). Once ICP monitoring is established, bolus administration of FFP is repeated as needed to keep the prothrombin time low (international normalized ratio [INR] ≤ 5) so as to reduce the risk of intracranial bleeding.

The goal of invasive monitoring is to keep ICP below 15 mm Hg while keeping cerebral perfusion pressure (CPP), which is a better predictor of outcome, above 50 mm Hg. CPP is calculated by subtracting ICP from mean arterial pressure (MAP) [see 9 Coma, Seizures, Cognitive Impairment, and Brain Death]. ICP monitoring allows early detection of cerebral edema and hence early introduction of aggressive management. To date, no randomized, controlled trials have addressed the effect of either high ICP or low CPP on outcome after liver transplantation; however, it appears that the persistence of either an ICP higher than 25 mm Hg or a CPP lower than 40 mm Hg for more than 2 hours is associated with an increased risk of irreversible brain damage and a poor outcome.[35,36]

Management of elevated ICP involves hyperventilation, minimization of external stimuli, deep sedation, elevation of the head, maintenance of hemodynamic stability, and infusion of mannitol. Patients are usually sedated with a short-acting agent (e.g., fentanyl) in small boluses before operation, nasotracheal suction, venipuncture, or line placement. Mechanical hyperventilation lowers ICP by lowering arterial carbon dioxide tension (P_aCO_2) to 25 to 30 mm Hg, thereby maximizing cerebral vascular constriction and reducing blood flow. This vascular effect diminishes progressively after 6 hours of therapy, though a clinical response is apparent for days. As many as 80% of patients without renal failure respond to mannitol infusions.[37] Serum osmolality should be measured frequently and maintained at 300 to 320 mOsm/L. Mannitol should be withheld if osmolality reaches or exceeds 320 mOsm/L, if renal failure occurs, or if oliguria and rising serum osmolality develop simultaneously. Repeated administration of mannitol may reverse the osmotic gradient. Mannitol should be discontinued if ICP does not respond after the first few boluses.

Patients who do not respond to conventional therapy may be placed in a barbiturate coma. Thiopental infusion decreases cerebral metabolic activity, lowers CNS oxygen demand, and protects the brain from ischemic injury secondary to decreased cerebral blood flow. In one retrospective, nonrandomized study, it lowered ICP and reduced mortality from FHF.[38] In our experience, however, the effect of thiopental infusion on ICP is transient and unpredictable.

Other Complications

In addition to cerebral edema and increased ICP, MODS and a variety of life-threatening complications are associated with FHF. Most of these complications are similar to those seen in chronic liver disease [see Chronic Liver Disease, Treatment of Complications, below]; however, the following complications are seen with particular frequency in FHF.

Table 3 **Liver Transplant Evaluation and Workup for FHF Patients**

Laboratory workup
  CBC and differential count
  Chemistry panel
  Coagulation profile
  24-hr creatinine clearance
  Urinalysis
  Arterial blood gases
  ANA, AMA, ceruloplasmin, urinary copper, α_1-antitrypsin
  AFP
  RPR
  Thyroid function tests
  Alcohol and drug toxicology screen
Viral serologies
  Hepatitis A virus (IgM, IgG)
  Hepatitis B virus (HBsAg, HBcAb, HBeAg, HBV DNA)
  Hepatitis C virus (HCV antibody, HCV RNA-PCR)
  Cytomegalovirus
  Epstein-Barr virus
  HIV
Cultures
  Bacterial, fungal, and viral cultures
  Blood
  Sputum
  Urine
  Ascites
12-lead ECG
Chest x-ray
Pulmonary function tests
Abdominal Doppler ultrasonography
CT scans of head

AFP—α-fetoprotein   AMA—antimitochondrial antibody   ANA—antinuclear antibody   RPR—rapid plasma reagent

Fluid, electrolyte, and nutritional abnormalities Euvolemia must be maintained to prevent fluid overload, pulmonary edema, and dehydration; extreme fluid shifts should be avoided. The presence of cerebral edema and intracranial hypertension calls for careful fluid administration so as not to expand the intravascular space or exacerbate the edema. Electrolyte and acid-base imbalances are frequent in FHF patients and should be managed appropriately. Hyperkalemia may be multifactorial; usually, it is secondary to liver necrosis, massive transfusion, acid-base imbalance, or renal failure. Acidosis results from increased lactic acid production and decreased handling of lactate by the failing liver. Compensatory respiratory alkalosis develops initially, but if encephalopathy progresses, respiratory acidosis may result. Sodium or potassium bicarbonate infusions should be administered in cases of severe acidosis. Acetate provides twice the bicarbonate load and is metabolized outside the liver; thus, if sodium and potassium intake is severely restricted, continuous infusion of acetate salts may be useful.

Initially, amino acids should be withheld to prevent excessive nitrogen loading; later, limited nitrogen supplementation (70 to 80 g protein/day) may be provided. Most patients present with severe hypoglycemia, which can be fatal and warrants aggressive therapy. Hypoglycemia should be corrected rapidly by infusion of a 50% dextrose solution, followed by continuous infusion of a more dilute solution at a rate of 4 mg/kg/min. A 10% solution is usually adequate; however, higher concentrations should be considered in patients whose hypoglycemia persists or whose fluid intake is restricted. Caloric supplementation has not been extensively studied in FHF.

Renal failure Renal failure occurs in as many as 55% of FHF patients. Functional renal failure is the most common cause of renal failure in this population. However, acute tubular necrosis is more common in these patients than in those with chronic liver disease and cirrhosis.[39] This is especially true in patients who have not been resuscitated adequately, who have experienced prolonged hypotension, or who have ingested hepatotoxins that are also nephrotoxic (e.g., acetaminophen).

Adequate urine volume can be maintained by means of judicious volume expansion, administration of loop diuretics, or both, along with infusion of renal doses of dopamine. Depleted intravascular volume may be managed by giving blood products, volume expanders, or both. Because the plasma albumin level is invariably low, salt-poor albumin solutions may be preferable to carbohydrate-based volume expanders. If oliguria is present—especially if mannitol is administered to treat ICP—hemodialysis or hemofiltration may be needed to maintain optimal fluid volume.

Pulmonary complications Pulmonary complications—especially pulmonary edema, aspiration pneumonia, and ARDS—are common in FHF patients.[40] Pulmonary edema is seen in as many as 40% of cases. Supplemental oxygen and mechanical ventilation are always indicated. Sedative and paralytic agents may be required to ensure tolerance of ventilation; however, they should be used sparingly because they may hinder neurologic evaluation. Aspiration pneumonia should be treated aggressively because it is a potential contraindication to transplantation.

Infectious complications Infection poses a serious threat to FHF patients both by placing them at risk for sepsis and by constituting a contraindication to liver transplantation. Immunologic defects observed in this setting include impaired opsonization, impaired chemotaxis, impaired neutrophil and Kupffer cell function, and complement deficiency.[41,42] Bacterial infection, usually deriving from the respiratory or urinary tract or from a central venous catheter, occurs in more than 80% of cases. In one study, bacteremia was documented in 25% of patients, with staphylococci, streptococci, and gram-negative rods the most common pathogens.[43] Because most FHF patients have percutaneous lines and indwelling catheters in place, iatrogenic sources must always be considered. Fungal infection is less common than bacterial infection in this setting; however, one series found a significant incidence of fungal infections, with *Candida albicans* cultured in 33% of the patients studied.[44] The majority of these patients had renal failure and had been treated with antibiotics for longer than 5 days.

The high prevalence of infection notwithstanding, we do not advocate antibiotic prophylaxis in this population unless there is a strong suspicion of active infection or an ICP monitor is in place. However, our decision threshold for starting antibiotics is low, given that the usual clinical presentations (e.g., fever and leukocytosis) may be absent in as many as 30% of FHF patients.[43] Surveillance cultures for bacteria and fungi must be obtained at frequent intervals from blood (peripheral and central lines), urine, sputum, and open wounds. If ascites is present, the ascitic fluid should be cultured. In addition, chest x-rays should be obtained to identify developing infiltrates. Administration of broad-spectrum antibiotics should be initiated at the first sign of infection; as soon as an organism is identified, coverage may be focused more narrowly. Initiation of antifungal therapy with either amphotericin B or another agent should be considered either if fungal culture is positive or if fever persists beyond 5 days while the patient is receiving antibiotics—especially if renal failure is present. The duration of antimicrobial therapy should be individualized for each patient. Follow-up cultures are recommended if a specific organism is isolated.

Coagulopathy and bleeding Bleeding is a frequent complication of FHF, typically resulting from massive liver necrosis, impaired hepatic synthesis of clotting factors, and platelet dysfunction. All clotting factors synthesized by the liver (i.e., factors II, V, VII, IX, and X) exhibit depressed plasma activity in FHF. Factor II, with a half-life of 2 hours, is the first to be depleted with hepatocellular dysfunction and also the first to be repleted with hepatocellular recovery. The PT is invariably prolonged, reflecting a generalized clotting factor deficiency; it is used as one of the criteria for determining the chances of spontaneous recovery. At some centers, FFP transfusion is withheld and the PT is followed carefully to determine upward or downward trends in the course of the disease and hence the likelihood of spontaneous recovery or need for transplantation (unless the PT > 25 seconds or the INR > 5, especially if an ICP monitor is in place). Intracranial bleeding and its neurologic sequelae are the most devastating complications of coagulopathy in FHF patients.

Thrombocytopenia and abnormalities of platelet function are also common in FHF. Acute splenomegaly, consumptive coagulopathy, and bone marrow suppression all contribute to the development of thrombocytopenia. Conversely, clearance of older platelets from the blood by the reticuloendothelial system is hindered, which results in an older, less effective platelet pool. In one study, a mean platelet count of 50,000/mm^3 was associated with a higher incidence of GI hemorrhage.[45] Our current practice is to give platelets to patients who either are thrombocytopenic (platelet count < 50,000/mm^3) or are actively bleeding.

OUTCOME OF MEDICAL THERAPY

Because of the complexity of the underlying disease, medical management of FHF requires a multidisciplinary approach. Hemodynamic and respiratory support and prevention and treatment of cerebral edema are major goals. Complications of liver failure must be treated aggressively to prevent sepsis, ARDS, and MODS, which is the second most common cause of death in these patients if they survive the first few days. As noted [see Assessment of Prognosis, above], liver transplant evaluation must be carried out simultaneously with aggressive ICU care, and the patient's chances of spontaneous recovery must be assessed. In addition to determining the King's College prognostic score at admission, we follow the general trend in the clinical course with respect to the development of encephalopathy, ICP elevation, coagulopathy, metabolic acidosis, and renal failure. The decision whether to continue with medical therapy or to perform liver transplantation must be made whenever a donor liver becomes available. In general, patients who appear to be deteriorating rapidly and who have no contraindications to liver transplantation should undergo emergency liver transplantation. Similarly, patients whose synthetic function does not improve within the first 48 to 72 hours should be considered for liver transplantation: the risk of complications and death from MODS if transplantation is not done outweighs the risk attendant on the procedure.

Toxic Liver Syndrome

Even with a multidisciplinary, comprehensive approach to therapy, a few patients with FHF go on to manifest the so-called toxic liver syndrome, characterized by severe intracranial hypertension, profound lactic acidosis, hemodynamic instability, and MODS. It has been suggested that removal of the necrotic liver might improve the hemodynamic status of these patients and lower their ICP. In such extreme cases, a two-stage procedure has been performed: total hepatectomy with an end-to-side portacaval shunt, followed by liver transplantation when an allograft becomes available. In one large series,[46,47] 32 adult patients with toxic liver syndrome underwent total hepatectomy with a portacaval shunt. The patients were anhepatic for several hours (range, 6.5 to 41.4). Whereas 13 patients showed no signs of improvement after hepatectomy and soon died of MODS, 19 became more stable and underwent the full procedure. Only seven patients were alive at 46 months.

In the early 1990s, we used this approach to treat an 18-year-old female patient with uncontrollable cerebral edema secondary to FHF; she underwent total hepatectomy with a portacaval shunt, followed by orthotopic liver transplantation (OLT) 14 hours later.[48] During the anhepatic period, she was supported with the help of a bioartificial liver (BAL) [see Discussion, Bioartifical Liver Support System, below]. With artificial liver support, the severe neurologic dysfunction was reversed, ICP was normalized, and the serum ammonia level was reduced. The patient recovered completely, with no neurologic deficits. We subsequently used the same approach with another FHF patient in our unit, also successfully (unpublished data). It appears that for highly selected patients exhibiting severe toxic metabolic derangement and uncontrollable intracranial hypertension, total hepatectomy with a portacaval shunt—preferably accompanied by some form of artificial liver support—followed by OLT may be considered as a desperate salvage measure.

LIVER TRANSPLANTATION

With the introduction of OLT as a treatment modality for FHF patients, overall patient survival has improved from less than 20% to greater than 60%.[49,50] As more experience was gained with OLT, it became apparent that optimal patient selection is essential for successful outcome. FHF patients must be considered for OLT before irreversible brain injury, MODS, and sepsis develop. Patient selection should be based on a clear understanding of the natural history of the disease as well as of the underlying etiology and the likelihood of spontaneous recovery without transplantation. One of the most difficult aspects of the management of these patients is the lack of reliable prognostic indicators or criteria predicting outcome. In our experience, the King's College criteria are less sensitive and specific in determining prognosis for patients with acetaminophen-induced FHF than for patients with FHF from other causes (71% and 78% versus 96% and 100%).[51]

As a result of these imperfectly reliable criteria, a small number of patients who either might have recovered spontaneously or might have sustained irreversible brain damage undergo unnecessary or unwarranted liver transplantation. Given the severe shortage of organ donors as well as the cost and medical consequences of liver transplantation and a commitment to lifelong immunosuppression, this is a significant problem.

Chronic Liver Disease

Chronic liver disease usually develops as a result of long-standing, ongoing injury to one or more components of the liver, including the liver parenchyma, the biliary tree, and the hepatic and biliary blood vessels. The repeated injury and the ensuing repair usually result in deposition of excessive amount of extracellular matrix (ECM), with or without accompanying inflammation. As the disease process progresses, excess ECM forms connective tissue bridges linking portal and central areas (so-called bridging fibrosis), which eventually lead to the formation of dense collagen bands enclosing nodules of hepatocytes—that is, to cirrhosis. Cirrhosis is an irreversible state that gives rise to significant physiologic impairment, including poor exchange of nutrients and metabolites between sinusoidal blood and hepatocytes. Eventually, the lobular architecture becomes distorted and blood flow altered, leading to portal hypertension and its numerous complications. In addition to portal hypertension, repeated parenchymal injury results in the loss of a large number of functioning hepatocytes and subsequently in hepatic failure.

ETIOLOGY

Like ALF, chronic liver disease is usually classified into various categories on the basis of the underlying causative process [see Table 4].

TREATMENT OF COMPLICATIONS

Chronic liver disease may be associated with a variety of complications, depending on the nature and extent of hepatocyte injury and regeneration. Most patients with chronic liver disease and possible cirrhosis are well compensated, maintain a relatively normal functional status, and remain essentially undiagnosed; however, a small percentage eventually become symptomatic. Hepatic failure secondary to cirrhosis is not an all-or-none phenomenon: patients may lose one or more specific liver functions while retaining the remainder. In addition to the hepatic effects, cirrhosis and hepatic failure can exert a wide range of extrahepatic effects that involve virtually every organ system, leading to MODS and death in most cases if appropriate therapy is not instituted promptly. Consequently, treatment of cirrhosis and chronic hepatic failure must focus on treating both the underlying primary disease and all of its extrahepatic manifestations and complications.

Table 4 Etiology of Chronic Liver Disease

Alcoholic liver disease (exclude acute alcoholic hepatitis)
Viral hepatitis
    Hepatitis B virus
    Hepatitis C virus
Biliary cirrhosis
    Primary biliary cirrhosis
    Primary sclerosing cholangitis
    Secondary sclerosing cholangitis
    Biliary atresia
Autoimmune hepatitis
Metabolic abnormalities
    Wilson disease
    α_1-Antitrypsin deficiency
    Hemochromatosis
    Inborn errors of metabolism
Cryptogenic cirrhosis
Miscellaneous
    Vascular anomalies (Budd-Chiari syndrome)
    Toxin- or drug-induced
    Inborn errors of metabolism
    Other

Portal Hypertension

In the majority of patients with chronic liver disease and cirrhosis, portal hypertension (PHT) develops as a result of increased resistance to portal venous blood flow within the liver. PHT is defined as portal venous pressure higher than 12 mm Hg or a hepatic wedge venous pressure that exceeds the inferior vena cava pressure by more than 5 mm Hg. It is classified as prehepatic, hepatic, or posthepatic according to the anatomic site of increased portal venous resistance [*see Table 5*]. Hepatic PHT is further classified according to the functional relationship to the hepatic sinusoids. Sinusoidal obstruction is more frequently seen with postnecrotic cirrhosis (e.g., from HCV and HBV infection), whereas postsinusoidal obstruction is more common with alcoholic cirrhosis. Prehepatic and posthepatic causes of PHT are less often encountered in patients with cirrhosis; however, efforts should always be made to rule out such causes, because these conditions all require different therapeutic approaches.

PHT is associated with numerous complications, most of which are life-threatening if not diagnosed and treated promptly [*see Table 6*]. Generally, these complications result from adaptive physiologic responses to elevated portal venous pressure, which lead to the development of collateral vessels or shunts to decompress the portal venous system. The absence of valves within the portal venous system allows retrograde portal blood flow into the splenic and mesenteric circulation and rerouting of blood into the systemic circulation through newly formed collaterals. Several portosystemic venous collateral networks have been identified within the GI tract, the peritoneal cavity, the chest, the retroperitoneum, and subcutaneous tissue. Patients with cirrhosis frequently have one or more areas of collateral formation.

Variceal bleeding The most dramatic and catastrophic complication of PHT is bleeding from esophageal and gastric varices. Prompt diagnosis and management are vital. Since the early 1990s, management of variceal bleeding has evolved significantly, thanks to the advent of novel endoscopic therapies and nonoperative portosystemic shunt procedures.

Although the esophagus and the stomach are the most common sites of bleeding varices, other sites within the GI tract may be involved as well, including the duodenum, the jejunum, the rectum, and ileostomy and colostomy sites [*see Table 7*]. The diagnosis and management of gastrointestinal bleeding associated with varices are discussed in more detail elsewhere in this text [*see 18 Upper Gastrointestinal Bleeding*].

Ascites Ascites—that is, leakage of lymph fluid into the peritoneal cavity—is one of the principal clinical manifestations of cirrhosis and PHT. Its appearance is indicative of advanced liver disease and is associated with a poor prognosis.[52] It is believed that increased hepatic sinusoidal pressure results in increased formation of lymph and causes hepatic lymph to weep from Glisson's capsule into the peritoneal cavity. As ascitic fluid accumulates, patients exhibit increasing abdominal distention, which causes abdominal pain, decreased appetite, dyspnea, and, occasionally, pleural effusion (so-called hepatic hydrothorax). Umbilical and inguinal hernias are common in patients with tense ascites.

Evaluation. Hepatic ascites should be distinguished from other types of ascites (e.g., chylous, malignant, or cardiac). All patients with ascites should undergo diagnostic paracentesis to characterize the fluid and rule out bacterial peritonitis (see below). In addition, therapeutic large-volume paracentesis (LVP) is indicated for patients who are symptomatic as a result of the large volume of ascitic fluid.

Ascitic fluid analysis should include a white blood cell count and a differential count, Gram stain and cultures, and measurement of total protein, albumin, glucose, lactic dehydrogenase (LDH), and

Table 5 Etiology of Portal Hypertension

Prehepatic obstruction
    Splenic vein thrombosis
    Portal vein thrombosis
    Partial nodular transformation
Hepatic obstruction
    Presinusoidal
        Idiopathic portal hypertension
        Schistosomiasis
        Congenital hepatic fibrosis
        Sarcoidosis
    Sinusoidal
        Nodular regenerative hyperplasia
        Most forms of cirrhosis
        Viral hepatitis
        Acute alcoholic hepatitis
    Postsinusoidal
        Alcoholic cirrhosis
        Veno-occlusive disease
Posthepatic obstruction
    Budd-Chiari syndrome
    IVC web
    Right-sided congestive heart failure/tricuspid valve insufficiency
    Constrictive pericarditis

IVC—inferior vena cava

Table 6 **Complications of Portal Hypertension**

Variceal bleeding
Portal hypertensive gastropathy
Ascites
    Spontaneous bacterial peritonitis
Spontaneous shunts
Encephalopathy
Hypersplenism

amylase concentrations. In addition, the serum albumin level should be measured at the same time so that the serum-ascites albumin gradient (SAAG) may be determined; this value has been shown to correlate directly with portal pressure.[53,54] Portal hypertensive ascitic fluid is characterized by a low albumin content, with a SAAG greater than 1.1 g/dl; non–portal hypertensive ascites fluid is characterized by a SAAG less than 1.1 g/dl.[55]

Spontaneous bacterial peritonitis. An elevated WBC count in the ascitic fluid provides immediate information about possible bacterial infection. Cell counts higher than 500/mm^3 suggest bacterial peritonitis, especially when the absolute neutrophil count exceeds 250/mm^3.[56] More than 20% of cirrhotic patients with ascites eventually manifest bacterial peritonitis—an occurrence known as spontaneous bacterial peritonitis (SBP). Patients with a low total protein level in their ascitic fluid (< 1.5 g/dl) appear to be at highest risk as a result of the reduced complement level and opsonic activity in the fluid. SBP should be considered in any cirrhotic patient with fever, abdominal pain, or worsening encephalopathy or renal function. Ascitic fluid analysis [*see Table 8*] allows SBP to be distinguished from secondary bacterial peritonitis, which develops as a consequence of an intra-abdominal abscess or a perforated viscus.

Once the diagnosis is made, empirical antibiotic therapy is employed until the final culture result becomes available. At present, cefotaxime (or a similar third-generation cephalosporin) is considered the treatment of choice. A dosage of 1 to 2 g I.V. every 6 to 8 hours (depending on renal function) is optimal. Therapy is continued for 14 days. The response to therapy should be monitored by repeating the paracentesis within 48 hours. Ciprofloxacin, either 200 mg I.V. every 12 hours for 7 days or 200 mg I.V. every 12 hours for 2 days followed by 500 mg orally every 12 hours for 5 days, has been shown to be effective as well.[57]

Currently, it is recommended that antibiotic prophylaxis for SBP (norfloxacin, 400 mg/day) be given only to patients with active GI bleeding and low protein levels in their ascitic fluid or to those who have had SBP before and are awaiting liver transplantation.[58] There is no good evidence to support antibiotic prophylaxis in patients whose ascitic fluid protein levels are low and who have never had SBP. Like ascites, SBP carries a grave prognosis: estimated 1-year survival is less than 50% without liver transplantation.[59,60]

Table 7 **Ectopic Sites for Variceal Bleeding**

Site	Frequency
Duodenum	17%
Jejunum and ileum	18%
Colon	15%
Rectum	9%
Ileostomy or colostomy	27%
Miscellaneous	14%

Medical management. Sodium retention is the pathophysiologic hallmark of ascites in cirrhotic patients, and the rate of fluid accumulation is directly related to the amount of sodium retained. Many patients excrete sodium at rates lower than 10 mmol/day, in which case even a modest sodium intake results in a positive sodium balance and continued accumulation of ascitic fluid. Therefore, to achieve effective control of ascites, dietary intake of sodium should be restricted to 1 to 2 g/day (43 to 87 mmol/day). With simple bed rest and salt restriction, ascites can be controlled in about 20% of patients.[61]

In addition to salt retention, patients with cirrhosis exhibit impaired free water excretion, which may cause hyponatremia. This state appears to be partially attributable to excessive secretion of antidiuretic hormone (ADH) caused by a reduced effective plasma volume. Water intake need not be restricted in all patients with ascites, because many will not become seriously hyponatremic. Water intake should be restricted (to 1.0 to 1.5 L/day) only in patients who become hyponatremic (serum sodium level < 130 mmol/L) and in those who continue to gain weight despite severe sodium restriction and diuretic therapy. Hyponatremia is associated with a variety of neurologic symptoms resembling those of hepatic encephalopathy. Severe hyponatremia (serum sodium < 120 mmol/L), on the other hand, is associated with seizure activity and should be corrected judiciously. Given the risk of the development of demyelinating lesions associated with rapid changes in the serum sodium concentration, it is recommended that correction of serum sodium—mainly by free water restriction to a serum sodium level between 120 and 130 mmol/L—be carried out gradually.

Diuretic therapy remains the cornerstone of management of cirrhotic ascites; however, it should be monitored carefully to ensure that intravascular volume depletion, development of prerenal azotemia, and electrolyte imbalances do not occur. The peritoneum can absorb no more than 700 to 900 ml of ascitic fluid a day; accordingly, vigorous diuresis in excess of this amount (in the absence of peripheral edema) results in intravascular volume depletion and renal failure.

The two groups of diuretic agents most commonly used to treat ascites are distal tubular–acting agents (e.g., spironolactone) and loop diuretics (e.g., furosemide). Spironolactone inhibits sodium reabsorption in the distal tubules by blocking the effect of serum aldosterone, which is usually elevated in patients with cirrhosis. A spironolactone dosage of 150 to 300 mg/day is sufficient for achieving effective natriuresis in many patients; however, larger dosages (up to 500 to 600 mg/day) may be preferable in certain patients with markedly elevated serum aldosterone concentrations. Adverse effects of spironolactone therapy include hyperkalemia and hyperchloremic acidosis. Tender gynecomastia is also an important side effect; if gynecomastia occurs, amiloride (20 to 40 mg/day) is a good alternative to spironolactone.

Furosemide therapy is usually started if the desired diuresis is not achieved with spironolactone or if the urinary sodium-potassium ratio is less than 1. A typical starting dosage is 40 to 80 mg/day, which is gradually increased until adequate diuresis is achieved. Because furosemide causes loss of urinary sodium and potassium, its use may lead to hypokalemia and metabolic alkalosis.

Surgical management. Despite large doses of diuretics, some patients become refractory to medical therapy and manifest tense ascites. Abdominal paracentesis is a safe and effective alternative to diuretic therapy and is currently used in patients with poor renal function who cannot tolerate aggressive diuresis and intravascular volume depletion. Most patients tolerate removal of large amounts of ascitic fluid (5 to 10 L) without significant adverse hemodynamic effects.[62] Albumin replacement (7 to 9 g/L) with LVP has been asso-

Table 8 Differentiation of Spontaneous Bacterial Peritonitis from Secondary Bacterial Peritonitis through Analysis of Ascitic Fluid

Fluid Assay	Spontaneous Bacterial Peritonitis	Secondary Bacterial Peritonitis
WBC (cells/mm^3)	> 500	> 500
Total protein (g/dl)	< 1.0	> 1.0
Glucose (mg/dl)	> 50	< 50
Lactic dehydrogenase (U/L)	< 225	> 225
Gram stain	Monomicrobial	Polymicrobial

ciated with a significantly lower rate of complications (e.g., hyponatremia, encephalopathy, and renal insufficiency) and is recommended when repeated LVP is indicated.[63]

In performing paracentesis, one should avoid surgical scars and obvious large subcutaneous collaterals. In general, a point 1 to 2 cm below the umbilicus along the midline is an optimal site in patients with no previous surgical incisions. Ultrasonographic guidance is usually necessary for localization when the amount of fluid present is small and when the fluid is loculated because of earlier episodes of peritonitis or previous surgical procedures.

The most common complications of LVP are bleeding, peritonitis, perforated viscus, and intra-abdominal abscess. Other complications (e.g., renal failure and cardiovascular instability) are less common and can usually be prevented by means of albumin and colloid replacement and intravascular volume expansion.

A few patients with ascites either become refractory to medical therapy or have contraindications to diuretic therapy or LVP. The usual practice has been to treat these patients with a peritoneovenous shunt through which the ascitic fluid can be reinfused into the systemic circulation, so that effective plasma volume is not reduced. The early enthusiasm for these shunts and their potential advantages notwithstanding, it is clear that there are a number of major complications limiting their use—in particular, early shunt occlusion, disseminated intravascular coagulation (DIC), sepsis, and central venous thrombosis. These complications occur with widely varying degrees of frequency; overall, however, it is estimated that about half of all shunted patients die within 1 year of the operation.[64,65]

If ascites develops as a result of PHT, it is logical to assume that reduction of the portal pressure might relieve the stimulus for ascites and control its formation. Earlier experience with the side-to-side portacaval shunt showed that this approach effectively controlled ascites; however, about one third of the patients died of postoperative complications and liver failure.[66] More recently, the transjugular intrahepatic portosystemic shunt (TIPS) has proved effective in correcting portal hypertension and controlling acute variceal bleeding while carrying low morbidity and mortality.[67]

These results have led to increasing use of TIPS to manage refractory ascites. In most patients, ascites can be completely or partially controlled with TIPS.[68,69] Approximately two thirds of patients with refractory ascites exhibit significantly reduced fluid accumulation and improved renal function. There are, however, a number of complications. Some of these complications are technical (e.g., bleeding from the liver capsule caused by inadvertent puncture, hemobilia, contrast-induced renal failure, and stent malposition or migration). The most significant nontechnical complications associated with the use of TIPS are an increased incidence of encephalopathy (seen in about 25% to 30% of patients),[70,71] hemolysis, and worsening jaundice.[72]

Stenosis or occlusion of the shunt that necessitates shunt revision is so frequent that it is considered the norm rather than a complication: in most series, 1-year patency rates range from 27% to 57%.[73] No long-term follow-up data are available; however, in one study, the overall survival rate was lower among patients who underwent TIPS placement than among those who received repeated LVP.[74] These data suggest that whereas TIPS is superior to LVP in controlling refractory ascites, it confers no survival advantage, and most patients will die of other complications of cirrhosis.

Hepatic Encephalopathy

Hepatic encephalopathy is a complex neuropsychiatric syndrome that arises in patients with severe hepatic insufficiency and cirrhosis. It is characterized by progressive alteration of cognitive function and coordination and depression of consciousness, leading to deep coma. Hepatic encephalopathy takes two main forms: (1) acute encephalopathy associated with FHF and (2) portosystemic encephalopathy (PSE) associated with cirrhosis and portosystemic shunts. It is classified into four stages according to the severity and extent of CNS impairment [see Table 9].

For accurate diagnosis of hepatic encephalopathy, all other disorders that affect cerebral function—including fluid and electrolyte abnormalities, hypoglycemia, azotemia, metabolic acidosis or alkalosis, hypoxia, and plasma hyperosmolality—must be recognized and corrected. Sedatives and paralytic agents should be avoided during the initial assessment period if possible; if sedation or paralysis is required, the combination of poor hepatic function with the shunting of blood away from the liver may greatly lengthen drug elimination, thereby complicating patient assessment.

Management of PSE begins with treatment and reversal of all potential precipitating factors: sedatives and other drugs with CNS effects should be discontinued, fluid and electrolyte abnormalities should be corrected, GI bleeding should be controlled, and underlying infectious states (especially SBP) should be treated. Early elective tracheal intubation and airway protection may be necessary in patients with stage III or IV encephalopathy because of the high risk of aspiration and subsequent pneumonia.

The classic therapeutic objectives in the management of hepatic

Table 9 Grading of Hepatic Encephalopathy

Encephalopathy Stage	Neurologic Changes
Stage I	Mild confusion, euphoria or depression, decreased attention span, slowing of ability to perform mental tasks, irritability, disorder of sleep pattern
Stage II	Drowsiness, lethargy, gross deficit in ability to perform mental tasks, obvious personality changes, inappropriate behavior, intermittent and short-lived disorientation
Stage III	Somnolent but arousable, unable to perform mental tasks, disorientation with respect to time or place, marked confusion, amnesia, occasional fits of rage, speech present but incomprehensible
Stage IV	Coma

encephalopathy are (1) to minimize ammonia formation and (2) to augment ammonia elimination [see Discussion, Mechanism of Hepatic Encephalopathy, below]. Lactulose and certain antibiotics are commonly employed to achieve these ends. Lactulose is a synthetic disaccharide cathartic that can be delivered orally, through a nasogastric tube, or via a high enema and can be administered early in the course of the disease. The dosage should begin at 25 g/day and then be titrated to a level at which the patient can produce three or four loose bowel movements a day. Lactulose is neither absorbed nor metabolized in the upper GI tract. When it reaches the colon, the ensuing bacterial degradation acidifies the luminal contents and causes an intraluminal osmotic shift. The more acid environment that results inhibits coliform bacterial growth, thereby reducing ammonia production. Additionally, the low intraluminal gut pH causes ammonia to be converted to ammonium ions, which do not enter the bloodstream easily. Finally, the cathartic action of lactulose clears ammonium ions from the bowel. Aggressive lactulose therapy may induce volume depletion and electrolyte imbalances; metabolic acidosis is a rare occurrence.

Neomycin, an agent commonly used for bowel preparation, alters gut flora, especially *Escherichia coli* and other urease-producing organisms, and thereby causes production of ammonia to fall. Only about 1% of a neomycin dose is absorbed systemically; because of possible ototoxicity and nephrotoxicity, special care should be taken if it is administered on a continuous basis.[75] Other oral antibiotics used to treat hepatic encephalopathy are polymyxin B, metronidazole, and vancomycin; they affect gut flora in much the same fashion as neomycin.

Aromatic amino acids (AAAs) are known neurotransmitter precursors, and it has been suggested that their products interfere with the activity of true neurotransmitters. It has also been shown that the ratio of branched-chain amino acids (BCAAs) to AAAs in plasma decreases steeply with encephalopathy. Because AAAs and BCAAs compete for the same blood-brain barrier carrier transport sites, the relative paucity of BCAAs leads to increased cerebral uptake of AAAs, which in turn promotes synthesis of false neurotransmitters that then compete with the endogenous transmitters dopamine and norepinephrine.[76] Parenteral administration of BCAA-enriched formulas to patients with hepatic encephalopathy has been advocated, but it has not proved beneficial in comparison with administration of conventional parenteral amino acid solutions.[77]

Renal Failure

Liver disease and cirrhosis are commonly associated with functional renal failure—that is, impaired renal function in the absence of significant underlying renal pathology. The most common functional renal abnormality in cirrhotic patients is a condition known as hepatorenal syndrome (HRS). HRS is defined as a reversible state of renal failure characterized by azotemia, oliguria (< 500 ml/day), low urinary sodium excretion (< 10 mEq/L), and an increased urine-plasma osmolality ratio (U/P > 1.0) in the absence of urinary sedimentation. HRS occurs in 18% to 55% of cirrhotic patients with ascites and is characterized by intense renal vasoconstriction, a decreased glomerular filtration rate (GFR), preserved tubular function, and normal renal histology.[39,78] Although the exact etiology of HRS is not known, the evidence currently available suggests that it is multifactorial, involving systemic vasodilatation and reduced effective plasma volume along with increased activity of the renin-angiotensin-aldosterone system, which causes further reduction of the GFR. On clinical grounds,

Table 10 Differentiation of Hepatorenal Syndrome from Acute Tubular Necrosis

Criteria	Hepatorenal Syndrome	Acute Tubular Necrosis
Underlying liver disease	Advanced liver damage with jaundice and impaired synthetic function	Mild or severe liver disease
Precipitant	GI bleeding, diuretics, paracentesis, sepsis, or none	Shock, nephrotoxins, sepsis
Onset	Days to weeks	Hours to days
Urinalysis	Renal epithelial cells with or without pigmented granular cells	Pigmented granular casts with or without RBCs, WBCs
Urinary sodium concentration	< 10 mEq/L	> 10 mEq/L
Urinary osmolarity	> Serum osmolarity	Isotonic
Urinary volume	Oliguric	Variable
Course	Progressive, unremitting	Deterioration followed by improved renal function

HRS has been classified into two types: (1) type 1 HRS, in which renal failure is rapidly progressive, as defined by a doubling of the initial serum creatinine level to a value higher than 2.5 mg/dl or a 50% reduction in the initial creatinine clearance to a value lower than 20 ml/min in less than 2 weeks; and (2) type 2 HRS, in which renal failure takes a slower, more gradual course.

The prognosis for patients with HRS is poor: to date, all therapeutic approaches have proved unsuccessful. Pharmacologic therapy has consisted of correcting effective volume status and attempting to reverse renal vasoconstriction through I.V. administration of vasodilators (e.g., dopamine, misoprostol, and aminophylline) or drugs that inhibit the synthesis or the effects of endogenous vasoconstrictors (e.g., captopril and thromboxane inhibitors). These approaches have not yielded any effective and reproducible improvements in renal hemodynamics and renal function. Several investigators, however, have reported improved renal function after OLT.[79]

Subsequently, a newer approach to the management of HRS was introduced that aimed at correcting the primary underlying defect (i.e., systemic vasodilatation) instead of the secondary renal vasoconstriction. Two classes of drugs have been investigated, either individually or in various combinations: (1) agents that inhibit the effects of endogenous systemic vasodilators (e.g., prostacyclin, nitric oxide, and glucagon) and (2) agents that cause systemic vasoconstriction (e.g., ornipressin and terlipressin). In one small series of patients with type 1 HRS, a combination of an oral β-adrenergic drug with midodrine and octreotide led to improved renal function and better long-term outcome.[80]

Besides functional renal failure, various types of nonfunctional, or organic, renal failure (e.g., acute tubular necrosis [ATN], renal tubular acidosis [RTA], and drug-induced interstitial nephritis) may occur in patients with cirrhosis. ATN is especially common among patients with chronic liver disease or FHF and is usually seen in patients who are poorly resuscitated, have experienced prolonged hypotension, have undergone severe septic episodes, or have ingested hepatotoxins that are also nephrotoxic (e.g., acetaminophen). ATN is characterized by an abrupt rise in blood urea nitrogen (BUN) and serum creatinine levels accompanied by oliguria or anuria. Unlike HRS, ATN leads to impairment of the concentrating ability of the tubular system and to excessive urinary sodium excretion; accordingly, a urine sodium concentration higher than 10 mEq/L has been proposed as a diagnostic criterion for ATN in cirrhotic patients [see Table 10]. RTA is commonly seen in patients with primary biliary cirrhosis (PBC), autoimmune liver disease, and alcoholic cirrhosis. It is characterized by an inability of the renal tubules to acidify the urine in the presence of a normal GFR.

Management of renal failure is usually aimed at correcting the underlying precipitating causes. In patients with ascites, who experience ongoing loss of fluid and protein into the peritoneum, it is important to maintain an adequate intravascular volume. If intravascular volume is depleted, blood components, volume expanders, or both should be given. Given that the plasma albumin level is invariably low in these patients, salt-poor albumin solutions may be preferable to carbohydrate-based volume expanders. Albumin replacement has been effectively used for volume expansion after LVP.[63]

Because of the complex interaction between the liver and the kidneys, fluid and electrolyte management often proves exceptionally challenging. In particular, it is difficult to estimate the actual intravascular volume, which is depleted in most cirrhotic patients even though total body fluid volume is higher than normal. Sodium retention and free water retention are the two most common abnormalities of renal function that lead to ascites and dilutional hyponatremia. Typically, sodium retention is an early manifestation, whereas water retention and renal failure are late findings. Nephrotoxic drugs and I.V. contrast agents should be avoided, and dosages of antibiotics and other medications should be adjusted appropriately.

Hypernatremia and metabolic acidosis can develop secondary to excessive lactulose therapy and dehydration and cause renal function to deteriorate. Hypokalemia is also common; it develops secondary to increased serum aldosterone concentration, which leads to excessive excretion of potassium in exchange for sodium. Once renal failure develops, hyperkalemia, hypercalcemia, and hyperphosphatemia become significant problems, often necessitating dialysis.

Malnutrition

Most cirrhotic patients present with depleted glycogen stores, severe protein-calorie malnutrition, and wasting. Impaired hepatic synthetic activity, causing a deficiency of both visceral and structural proteins, is one of the hallmarks of advanced liver disease. In addition, poor appetite, tense ascites, abdominal pain, and excessive loss of protein through repeated LVP and overall increased energy expenditure tend to exacerbate malnutrition.

Excessive protein administration can induce hepatic encephalopathy; accordingly, protein intake should be limited to 1 to 1.2 g/kg/day. Glucose is the main energy source given to malnourished cirrhotic patients; however, its use is not without complications, in that these patients typically exhibit glucose intolerance. Lipid emulsion can be safely administered to most patients with liver failure and should be withheld only from patients with overt coma.[81] It is generally agreed that the ideal energy source should consist of a mixture of glucose and fat emulsion. Approximately 30% to 40% of all nonprotein calories can be provided in the form of fat. The total energy requirement should be in the range of 25 to 35 kcal/kg/day.

As noted [see Hepatic Encephalopathy, above], although AAAs have been implicated in the pathogenesis of hepatic encephalopathy, administration of BCAA solutions has not proved helpful, and the evidence does not support their routine use.[77,82]

In general, the potential risks and complications associated with total parenteral nutrition (TPN) outweigh the benefits in patients with a functioning GI tract. When properly administered, enteral nutrition is safer, more physiologically correct, and significantly more cost-effective than TPN. It should therefore be considered the first choice for nutritional support in most patients with chronic liver disease unless a contraindication to enteral feeding is present.

Coagulopathy and Nonvariceal Bleeding

The spectrum of coagulation disorders in patients with liver disease varies from minor localized bleeding to massive life-threatening hemorrhage. Abnormal bleeding may be spontaneous in some patients, but it is more often the result of a hemostatic challenge (e.g., surgical wounds or procedures, gastritis, portal hypertensive gastropathy, gastric or duodenal ulcers, or ruptured varices). The underlying anatomic lesion is believed to be as responsible for bleeding as the hemostatic defect is; accordingly, therapy should be directed at correcting both.

Although most bleeding episodes are secondary to decreased synthesis of clotting factors, other causes of bleeding (e.g., defective or dysfunctional factor synthesis and increased consumption of clotting components) must always be ruled out [see 5 Bleeding and Transfusion]. In most patients, the decreased levels of clotting factors parallel the progressive loss of parenchymal cell function. Usually, the levels of the vitamin K–dependent factors (i.e., prothrombin, factor VII, factor IX, factor X, protein S, and protein C) fall first, followed by the levels of other factors as cirrhosis progresses. Factor V is synthesized independently of vitamin K availability, and its concentration is of special interest because the plasma factor V level seems to be a predictor of the extent of liver cell damage. Impaired synthesis of coagulation proteins also has an impact on antithrombin III (AT-III), protein C inhibitor, plasminogen, and α_2-antiplasmin as well as on several other inhibitors and activators of both the extrinsic coagulation pathway and the intrinsic pathway. The combination of decreased factor levels and impaired synthesis of coagulation proteins explains the prolongation of the PT, the activated partial thromboplastin time (aPTT), and the thrombin clotting time (TCT) in these patients.[83,84]

Given the complexity of hemostasis in cirrhotic patients, accurate diagnosis of a bleeding disorder is often hard to achieve. Several disorders and abnormalities may be present simultaneously, and one or more parameters of hemostasis and coagulation may be impaired. Therefore, any effective treatment approach should be broad-based and aimed at correcting several deficiencies or abnormalities at once. FFP contains all of the components of the clotting and fibrinolytic systems but lacks platelets. In most cases, transfusion of 6 to 8 units of FFP suffices to correct severe clotting factor defects; however, the excess volume may not be well tolerated. Cryoprecipitate, the precipitate formed when FFP is thawed at 4°C, is rich in factor VIII, von Willebrand factor, and fibrinogen but lacks the vitamin K–dependent factors. Therefore, it should be given only when the fibrinogen level is lower than 100 mg/dl. Prothrombin complex concentrates contain only the vitamin K–dependent factors and proteins, and their use can provoke serious thromboembolic complications, including disseminated intravascular coagulation (DIC). Therefore, their potential utility must be weighed carefully against the risk that thrombotic events may develop.[85]

Other major disorders of hemostasis in patients with chronic liver disease and cirrhosis involve platelets and are manifested as thrombocytopenia, abnormal platelet function (thrombocytopathy), or both. In most cases, thrombocytopenia is related to splenomegaly and hypersplenism (a common feature of PHT). Abnormal platelet function is attributed to many causes, including intrinsic platelet defects and abnormal interaction among platelets, endothelial surfaces, and clotting factors. It is manifested by a prolonged bleeding time, impaired platelet aggregation, and reduced adhesiveness. Some authorities attribute the inhibition of platelet aggregation to fibrin degradation products (FDPs); however, the FDP levels noted in the plasma of cirrhotic patients are not sufficient to impair platelet aggregation, nor do they correlate with the observed reductions in platelet aggregation.[86]

Platelets should be transfused whenever a patient with either a quantitative or a qualitative defect experiences active bleeding. A normal response is a rise of 10,000/mm³ with each unit transfused; however, in cases of hypersplenism and accelerated consumption, such a response is rare. Transfusion should be continued until all serious bleeding has ceased, with the therapeutic goal being the maintenance of a platelet count near 50,000/mm³. Platelet transfusion is also indicated before any surgical or invasive procedure (e.g., paracentesis or liver biopsy). Indications for prophylactic platelet transfusion are less clear, and any potential gains must be balanced against potential side effects and development of antibodies. Most patients with advanced cirrhosis and liver failure have platelet counts lower than 100,000/mm³; however, prophylactic platelet transfusion is usually not recommended until the count falls below 15,000 to 20,000/mm³, at which point the risk of spontaneous bleeding is considerably increased.

Another feature of severe liver disease is increased fibrinolytic activity, which may be either primary or secondary to DIC.[87] The exact causes of primary fibrinolysis and DIC remain unclear. Primary fibrinolysis appears to derive from increased activity of tissue plasminogen activator and decreased levels of α_2-antiplasmin.[88] DIC is believed to be triggered by the release of thromboplastic substances into the circulation as a consequence of liver cell damage or necrosis and by poor clearance of circulating activated tissue and clotting factors and FDPs by a defective reticuloendothelial system. Accelerated fibrinolysis is manifested by reductions in the whole blood clot lysis time and the euglobulin clot lysis time as well as by elevated levels of fibrinolysis products (e.g., FDPs and D-dimer). Although enhanced fibrinolysis is relatively common in patients with cirrhosis, most of the characteristic abnormalities can occur after many types of physiologic stress and are not necessarily accompanied by a bleeding tendency.

At present, no satisfactory method of managing DIC is available. An extensive workup must be completed to rule out underlying causes (e.g., sepsis, ARDS, and MODS). FFP, platelet concentrates, and, possibly, low-dose heparin (200 to 800 U/hr) may be given. AT-III concentrate has been used in an attempt to inhibit the action of thrombin, thereby decreasing procoagulant consumption, restoring normal levels of factors, and improving hemostasis. Clinical experience with AT-III therapy in this setting has been limited to a few case reports and a few small series; however, there is some evidence to suggest that AT-III may reduce the hemostatic abnormalities and help control bleeding.[89]

Antifibrinolytic agents (e.g., ε-aminocaproic acid and tranexamic acid) impede fibrinolysis and thus may be useful for treating bleeding in patients who have liver disease and show evidence of fibrinolysis.[90] In patients with DIC, however, administration of antifibrinolytic agents is contraindicated because of the potential for thrombotic complications. D-dimer levels should be determined to rule out DIC before use of these medications is considered. Because DIC is difficult to rule out in patients with liver disease, the use of antifibrinolytic agents in liver disease is limited.

LIVER TRANSPLANTATION

The standard indications for liver transplantation are well documented[91]: they include PHT, poor hepatic synthetic function, hepatic encephalopathy, progressive jaundice, severe malnutrition, and excessive fatigue. As noted [see Treatment of Complications, above], PHT is manifested by variceal bleeding, hypersplenism, thrombocytopenia, ascites, hepatic hydrothorax, and SBP. Poor synthetic function is usually manifested by a prolonged PT and low serum albumin and cholesterol levels. In general, any concurrent medical or psychosocial condition that prohibits a major surgical procedure or subsequent immunosuppression constitutes a contraindication to liver transplantation [see Table 11].

The United Network for Organ Sharing (UNOS) currently regulates organ allocation to transplant candidates. In January 1988, minimal listing criteria for liver transplantation were implemented.[92] These criteria are based on the Child-Turcotte-Pugh (CTP) scoring system [see Table 12], which includes five parameters: serum albumin

Table 11 Contraindications to Liver Transplantation

Absolute contraindications	Severe, irreversible brain damage
	HIV infection
	Extrahepatic malignancy
	Uncontrolled sepsis
	Severe pulmonary hypertension and advanced cardiopulmonary disease
	Active substance abuse or major psychosocial problems
	Extrahepatic portal vein thrombosis in patients with hepatocellular carcinoma
Relative contraindications	Elevated ICP or reduced CPP (in patients with FHF)
	Multiple organ dysfunction syndrome
	Hemodynamic instability
	Advanced age
	Portal vein thrombosis (except when secondary to hepatocellular carcinoma)

CPP—cerebral perfusion pressure   ICP—intracranial pressure

Table 12 Child-Turcotte-Pugh Scoring System

Points	1	2	3
Encephalopathy	None	Stage I or II	Stage III or IV
Ascites	Absent	Slight (or controlled by diuretics)	Moderate despite diuretic treatment
Bilirubin (mg/dl)	< 2	2–3	> 3
Patients with PBC or PSC	< 4	4–6	> 6
Albumin (g/L)	> 3.5	2.8–3.5	< 2.8
PT (prolonged sec)	< 4	4–6	> 6
INR	< 1.7	1.7–2.3	> 2.3

PBC—primary biliary cirrhosis   PSC—primary sclerosing cholangitis

and bilirubin levels, PT, ascites, and hepatic encephalopathy. To be listed for liver transplantation, a patient must have a CTP score of 7 or higher. In addition to the general listing criteria, various disease-specific criteria were developed for patients with alcoholic liver disease, patients with cholestatic liver disease (e.g., PBC or primary sclerosing cholangitis), and patients with hepatocellular carcinoma.

Discussion

Mechanisms of Hepatic Encephalopathy

The association between liver disease and altered mental status and consciousness has been recognized for centuries, but the exact underlying mechanisms remain unknown. It appears that this syndrome has a multifactorial etiology and is associated with a number of complex changes, which are manifested collectively as hepatic encephalopathy. It is generally believed that hepatocerebral dysfunction is caused by accumulation of cerebral toxins as a result of low hepatic clearance.[93]

Of all the physiologic factors thought to contribute to the development of encephalopathy, the best known is ammonia. Arterial ammonia levels are frequently elevated in persons with hepatic encephalopathy; however, the clinical severity of hepatic encephalopathy correlates poorly with the degree to which the ammonia level is elevated.[94] The precise contribution of ammonia to hepatic encephalopathy remains unclear; however, ammonia is known to inhibit the uptake of glutamate into the astrocytes, thereby causing a rise in the extracellular glutamate level that appears to downregulate the postsynaptic glutamate receptors, resulting in decreased neuronal excitation.[95]

Endogenous or exogenously ingested benzodiazepines may also play a role in the etiology of acute and chronic hepatic encephalopathy by interacting with the high-affinity γ-aminobutyric acid (GABA)–benzodiazepine receptor complexes. These substances are known to enhance inhibitory GABA-ergic tone. Animal studies suggest that the gut flora may contribute benzodiazepine ligand activity[96] as well as increased benzodiazepine receptor agonist activity.[97] Clinical studies of FHF patients show increased benzodiazepine receptor ligands with enhanced GABA-ergic tone in all stages of encephalopathy.[98] Ammonia-induced activation of peripheral-type benzodiazepine receptors on astrocytes may cause the release of neurosteroids that enhance GABA-ergic neurotransmission. Hence, neurosteroids may potentate the inhibitory actions of GABA at the receptor level as well as lengthen the period during which the GABA ligand remains in the synaptic cleft. Ammonia also acts directly to potentiate GABA-ergic tone by enhancing the affinity of GABA for GABA-A receptors.[99]

Despite these seemingly compelling findings, there is no apparent correlation between benzodiazepine ligand activity and clinical stage of encephalopathy, nor is ligand elevation a consistent finding in all patients. Furthermore, clinical and animal studies in which a benzodiazepine receptor antagonist has been administered have not shown consistent effects. The anecdotal success of flumazenil, the principal benzodiazepine antagonist, has been ascribed to the antagonism of benzodiazepines ingested by patients. Support for the concept of so-called endogenous benzodiazepines arising from the intestine can be found in a number of sources, including studies of dogs with congenital portacaval shunts, which document ligand activity in stool samples.[100] Whether there is a causal relation to hepatic encephalopathy or whether this is merely a case of associated phenomena remains to be determined. Whatever the contribution of benzodiazepines to the pathophysiology of acute hepatic encephalopathy and cerebral edema, it appears likely that other mechanisms are involved.

Bioartificial Liver Support System

Despite the best management efforts, the morbidity and mortality associated with ALF remain exceptionally high. For most severe cases, liver transplantation is still the only effective therapeutic modality. Unfortunately, because of the severe organ donor shortage, the waiting period for transplantation is long, and patients consequently are at risk for the development of irreversible complications or contraindications to liver transplantation while awaiting a donor. In an effort to mitigate this problem, investigators have studied various artificial liver support systems designed to provide full metabolic, hemodynamic, and physiologic support until either the native liver regenerates or a liver becomes available for transplantation. From the 1970s to the 1990s, most therapeutic attempts focused primarily on detoxifying plasma. All such attempts either failed or had no significant impact on survival.[101]

The ongoing severe organ shortage has led several investigators to develop and test a number of xenogeneic-based liver support systems employing whole-organ perfusion or isolated hepatocytes. At our institution, we developed and tested a hybrid bioartificial liver (BAL) support system employing isolated porcine hepatocytes in an extracorporeal perfusion circuit. We subsequently initiated a clinical trial addressing the use of this system in patients with severe ALF as a bridge to either transplantation or spontaneous recovery.[102-104]

CLINICAL TRIAL

Study Design

Hepatocytes Methods of porcine hepatocyte isolation, purification, attachment to a collagen-coated matrix, cryopreservation,

Table 13 Neurologic Effects of BAL Treatment

Study Group	Results		
	Pre-BAL	Post-BAL	P
Group I			
ICP (mm Hg)	17.0 ± 1.5	10.9 ± 1.0	< 0.0002
CPP (mm Hg)	70 ± 2	75 ± 2	< 0.04
GCS	6.8 ± 0.4	7.4 ± 0.4	< 0.01
CLOCS	24.7 ± 1.2	32.0 ± 1.1	< 0.000001
Group II			
GCS	5.0 ± 1.1	7.0 ± 1.4	< 0.2
CLOCS	29.7 ± 7.4	31.7 ± 7.9	< 0.5
Group III			
ICP (mm Hg)	12.3 ± 0.9	14.0 ± 1.5	< 0.4
CPP (mm Hg)	85 ± 1	98 ± 8	< 0.3
GCS	8.2 ± 0.7	8.4 ± 0.7	< 0.4
CLOCS	29.7 ± 2.3	34.0 ± 1.7	< 0.001

BAL—bioartificial liver   CLOCS—Comprehensive Level of Consciousness score
CPP—cerebral perfusion pressure   GCS—Glasgow Coma Scale   ICP—intracranial pressure

Table 14 Metabolic Effects of BAL Treatment

Study Group	Results		
	Pre-BAL	Post-BAL	P
Group I			
AST (U/L)	1,255 ± 261	879 ± 148	< 0.002
ALT (U/L)	1,075 ± 184	674 ± 120	< 0.000005
Total bilirubin (mg/dl)	17.9 ± 1.5	14.6 ± 1.2	< 0.000001
Glucose (mg/dl)	126 ± 5	175 ± 7	< 0.0000006
Ammonia (μmol/L)	160 ± 8	134 ± 6	< 0.0002
Lactate (mmol/L)	4.4 ± 0.7	4.2 ± 0.6	< 0.2
Albumin (g/dl)	3.12 ± 0.08	2.6 ± 0.1	< 0.0000006
Creatinine (mg/dl)	1.5 ± 0.2	1.1 ± 0.1	< 0.000001
Group II			
AST (U/L)	5,661 ± 2,613	2,821 ± 1,291	< 0.1
ALT (U/L)	2,139 ± 704	1,633 ± 544	< 0.05
Total bilirubin (mg/dl)	19.1 ± 2.2	14.7 ± 1.7	< 0.009
Glucose (mg/dl)	117 ± 26	144 ± 24	< 0.06
Ammonia (μmol/L)	81 ± 9	91 ± 13	< 0.03
Lactate (mmol/L)	13.1 ± 2.9	13.2 ± 2.2	< 0.9
Albumin (g/dl)	3.7 ± 0.3	2.7 ± 0.1	< 0.01
Creatinine (mg/dl)	1.6 ± 0.3	1.6 ± 0.3	< 1.0
Group III			
AST (U/L)	692 ± 374	723 ± 409	< 0.5
ALT (U/L)	349 ± 126	281 ± 114	< 0.06
Total bilirubin (mg/dl)	26.0 ± 2.7	21.6 ± 2.2	< 0.000003
Glucose (mg/dl)	141 ± 9	171 ± 11	< 0.001
Ammonia (μmol/L)	173 ± 31	131 ± 15	< 0.08
Lactate (mmol/L)	5.7 ± 1.1	5.6 ± 0.9	< 0.9
Albumin (g/dl)	3.0 ± 0.1	2.6 ± 0.1	< 0.00003
Creatinine (mg/dl)	2.8 ± 0.3	2.2 ± 0.2	< 0.00002

ALT—alanine aminotransferase   AST—aspartate aminotransferase   BAL—bioartificial liver

and storage were developed. Five to seven billion fresh or cryopreserved hepatocytes (70% to 90% viability) were used for each patient treatment.[103,104]

System characteristics   The system was standardized and subsequently modified and is currently manufactured as the HepatAssist 2000 (Circe Biomedical, Inc., Lexington, Massachusetts). The main components are (1) a plasmapheresis unit, (2) an activated cellulose-coated charcoal column, (3) an oxygenator, (4) a blood warmer, and (5) a hollow-fiber module containing isolated microcarrier-attached porcine hepatocytes. The module consists of (a) an intracapillary chamber made of several porous, hollow 0.2 μm fibers through which plasma flows and (b) an extracapillary chamber surrounding the hollow fibers, where the microcarrier-attached hepatocytes are suspended. Plasma circulates through the fibers at a rate of 400 ml/min, with free exchange of macromolecules across the surface of the fibers driven by a transmembrane pressure gradient. When plasma and blood cells return from the BAL, they are reconstituted and returned to the patient via the double-lumen venous dialysis catheter.

Patient population   Three groups of patients were enrolled in the phase 1 trial. Group I patients (N = 24) had no previous history of liver disease, fulfilled all the diagnostic criteria of FHF, and were candidates for OLT at the time of admission. Group II patients (N = 3) had undergone OLT and exhibited primary nonfunction (PNF) of the transplanted liver in the immediate postoperative period with rapid deterioration. Group III patients (N = 10) presented with acute exacerbation of known underlying chronic liver disease and were not candidates for OLT at the time of study enrollment. Patients were enrolled in the study when stage III or IV encephalopathy developed in the course of optimal standard medical therapy.

Results

Of the 24 group I patients, 18 were candidates for OLT. Five additional patients with FHF secondary to acetaminophen toxicity who were treated with the BAL support system recovered fully without the need for liver transplantation. One patient with FHF secondary to heatstroke received BAL treatment while awaiting OLT; he died as a result of MODS after 21 days. All 18 OLT candidates in group I and all three patients in group II were successfully bridged to transplantation, experienced full neurologic and functional recovery, and were discharged from the hospital. Patients in group III experienced transient clinical improvement after BAL treatment. Two patients recovered enough native liver function to survive; they subsequently became candidates for OLT and underwent the procedure successfully. The remaining eight patients died 1 to 21 days (mean, 7.1 days) after their last BAL treatment as a result of variceal bleeding, sepsis, or MODS.

Treatment with the BAL support system gave rise to several neurologic and metabolic effects that were seen in all three groups of patients. Of these, the neurologic changes were the most dramatic. Patients with FHF (group I) exhibited remarkable neurologic improvement after BAL treatment, with the reversal of decerebrate posturing states, anisocoria, and sluggish pupillary reflexes. Both responsiveness to external stimuli and brain-stem function improved, as shown by a higher comprehensive level of consciousness score. There was a significant reduction in ICP with a concomitant increase in CPP; these changes were most dramatic in patients with ICP levels higher than 25 mm Hg [*see Table 13*]. In patients with PNF (group II), the impact of BAL treatment on neurologic status was difficult to assess because heavy sedation was used in the postanesthetic period; however, transient neurologic improvements were noted after BAL treatment, manifested primarily by increased responsiveness.

Additional metabolic effects of BAL treatment on liver function included improvements in renal function and hematologic and coagulation parameters [*see Table 14*]. There was a significant ($P < 0.01$) increase in the plasma BCAA-AAA ratio in plasma, which may be one of many possible reasons for the observed mitigation of encephalopathy. This increase was primarily due to a reduction in AAA levels.

References

1. Kotwal GJ, Baroudy BM, Kuramoto IK, et al: Detection of acute hepatitis C virus infection by ELISA using a synthetic peptide comprising a structural epitope. Proc Natl Acad Sci USA 89:4486, 1992
2. Polito AJ, DiNello RK, Quan S, et al: New generation RIBA hepatitis C strip immunoblot assays. Ann Biol Clin (Paris) 50:329, 1992
3. Bukh J, Purcell RH, Miller RH: Importance of primer selection for the detection of hepatitis C virus RNA with the polymerase chain reaction assay. Proc Natl Acad Sci USA 89:187, 1992
4. Trey C, Davidson CS: The management of fulminant hepatic failure. Prog Liver Dis 3:282, 1970
5. Bernuau J, Rueff B, Benhamou JP: Fulminant and subfulminant liver failure: definitions and causes. Semin Liver Dis 6:97, 1986
6. Schiodt FV, Atillasoy E, Shakil AO, et al: Etiology and outcome for 295 patients with acute liver failure in the United States. Liver Transpl Surg 5:29, 1999
7. Ritt DJ, Whelan G, Werner DJ, et al: Acute hepatic

necrosis with stupor or coma: an analysis of thirty-one patients. Medicine (Baltimore) 48:151, 1969
8. Lettau LA, McCarthy JG, Smith MH, et al: Outbreak of severe hepatitis due to delta and hepatitis B viruses in parenteral drug abusers and their contacts. N Engl J Med 317:1256, 1987
9. Gimson AE, Tedder RS, White YS, et al: Serological markers in fulminant hepatitis B. Gut 24:615, 1983
10. Samuel D, Bismuth A, Mathieu D, et al: Passive immunoprophylaxis after liver transplantation in HBsAg-positive patients. Lancet 337:813, 1991
11. Govindarajan S, Chin KP, Redeker AG, et al: Fulminant B viral hepatitis: role of delta agent. Gastroenterology 86:1417, 1984
12. Smedile A, Farci P, Verme G, et al: Influence of delta infection on severity of hepatitis B. Lancet 2:945, 1982
13. Lichtenstein DR, Makadon HJ, Chopra S: Fulminant hepatitis B and delta virus coinfection in AIDS. Am J Gastroenterol 87:1643, 1992
14. Rakela J, Lange SM, Ludwig J, et al: Fulminant hepatitis: Mayo Clinic experience with 34 cases. Mayo Clin Proc 60:289, 1985
15. Castells A, Salmeron JM, Navasa M, et al: Liver transplantation for acute liver failure: analysis of applicability. Gastroenterology 105:532, 1993
16. Zimmerman HJ: Update of hepatotoxicity due to classes of drugs in common clinical use: non-steroidal drugs, anti-inflammatory drugs, antibiotics, antihypertensives, and cardiac and psychotropic agents. Semin Liver Dis 10:322, 1990
17. Carney FM, Van Dyke RA: Halothane hepatitis: a critical review. Anesth Analg 51:135, 1972
18. Floersheim GL: Treatment of human amatoxin mushroom poisoning. Myths and advances in therapy. Med Toxicol 2:1, 1987
19. Klein AS, Hart J, Brems JJ, et al: Amanita poisoning: treatment and the role of liver transplantation. Am J Med 86:187, 1989
20. Rector WG Jr, Uchida T, Kanel GC, et al: Fulminant hepatic and renal failure complicating Wilson's disease. Liver 4:341, 1984
21. McCullough AJ, Fleming CR, Thistle JL, et al: Diagnosis of Wilson's disease presenting as fulminant hepatic failure. Gastroenterology 84:161, 1983
22. Stremmel W, Meyerrose KW, Niederau C, et al: Wilson disease: clinical presentation, treatment, and survival. Ann Intern Med 115:720, 1991
23. Amon E, Allen SR, Petrie RH, et al: Acute fatty liver of pregnancy associated with preeclampsia: management of hepatic failure with postpartum liver transplantation. Am J Perinatol 8:278, 1991
24. O'Grady JG, Alexander GJ, Hayllar KM, et al: Early indicators of prognosis in fulminant hepatic failure. Gastroenterology 97:439, 1989
25. Bernuau J, Goudeau A, Poynard T, et al: Multivariate analysis of prognostic factors in fulminant hepatitis B. Hepatology 6:648, 1986
26. Saibara T, Onishi S, Sone J, et al: Arterial ketone body ratio as a possible indicator for liver transplantation in fulminant hepatic failure. Transplantation 51:782, 1991
27. Ranek L, Andreasen PB, Tygstrup N: Galactose elimination capacity as a prognostic index in patients with fulminant liver failure. Gut 17:959, 1976
28. Ware AJ, D'Agostino AN, Combes B: Cerebral edema: a major complication of massive hepatic necrosis. Gastroenterology 61:877, 1971
29. Silk DB, Trewby PN, Chase RA, et al: Treatment of fulminant hepatic failure by polyacrylonitrile-membrane haemodialysis. Lancet 2:1, 1977
30. Lidofsky SD: Fulminant hepatic failure. Crit Care Clin 11:415, 1995
31. Wijdicks EF, Plevak DJ, Rakela J, et al: Clinical and radiologic features of cerebral edema in fulminant hepatic failure. Mayo Clin Proc 70:119, 1995
32. Sidi A, Mahla ME: Noninvasive monitoring of cerebral perfusion by transcranial Doppler during fulminant hepatic failure and liver transplantation. Anesth Analg 80:194, 1995
33. Munoz SJ, Robinson M, Northrup B, et al: Elevated intracranial pressure and computed tomography of the brain in fulminant hepatocellular failure. Hepatology 13:209, 1991
34. Blei AT, Olafsson S, Webster S, et al: Complications of intracranial pressure monitoring in fulminant hepatic failure. Lancet 341:157, 1993
35. Aldersley MA, Juniper M, Richardson P, et al: Inability of intracranial pressure monitoring to select patients with acute liver failure for transplantation (abstract). Hepatology 22:208A, 1995
36. Davies MH, Mutimer D, Lowes J, et al: Recovery despite impaired cerebral perfusion in fulminant hepatic failure. Lancet 343:1329, 1994
37. Canalese J, Gimson AE, Davis C, et al: Controlled trial of dexamethasone and mannitol for the cerebral oedema of fulminant hepatic failure. Gut 23:625, 1982
38. Forbes A, Alexander GJ, O'Grady JG, et al: Thiopental infusion in the treatment of intracranial hypertension complicating fulminant hepatic failure. Hepatology 10:306, 1989
39. Ring-Larsen H, Palazzo U: Renal failure in fulminant hepatic failure and terminal cirrhosis: a comparison between incidence, types, and prognosis. Gut 22:585, 1981
40. Trewby PN, Warren R, Contini S, et al: Incidence and pathophysiology of pulmonary edema in fulminant hepatic failure. Gastroenterology 74(5 pt 1):859, 1978
41. Bailey RJ, Woolf IL, Cullens H, et al: Metabolic inhibition of polymorphonuclear leucocytes in fulminant hepatic failure. Lancet 1:1162, 1976
42. Imawari M, Hughes RD, Gove CD, et al: Fibronectin and Kupffer cell function in fulminant hepatic failure. Dig Dis Sci 30:1028, 1985
43. Rolando N, Harvey F, Brahm J, et al: Prospective study of bacterial infection in acute liver failure: an analysis of fifty patients. Hepatology 11:49, 1990
44. Rolando N, Harvey F, Brahm J, et al: Fungal infection: a common, unrecognised complication of acute liver failure. J Hepatol 12:1, 1991
45. O'Grady JG, Langley PG, Isola LM, et al: Coagulopathy of fulminant hepatic failure. Semin Liver Dis 6:159, 1986
46. Ringe B, Pichlmayr R, Lubbe N, et al: Total hepatectomy as temporary approach to acute hepatic or primary graft failure. Transplant Proc 20(1 suppl 1):552, 1988
47. Ringe B, Lubbe N, Kuse E, et al: Management of emergencies before and after liver transplantation by early total hepatectomy. Transplant Proc 25(1 pt 2): 1090, 1993
48. Rozga J, Podesta L, LePage E, et al: Control of cerebral oedema by total hepatectomy and extracorporeal liver support in fulminant hepatic failure. Lancet 342: 898, 1993
49. Ascher NL, Lake JR, Emond JC, et al: Liver transplantation for fulminant hepatic failure. Arch Surg 128:677, 1993
50. Emond JC, Aran PP, Whitington PF, et al: Liver transplantation in the management of fulminant hepatic failure. Gastroenterology 96:1583, 1989
51. Choi W-C, Arnaout WS, Villamil FG, et al: Comparison of the applicability of two prognostic indicator scores in patients with fulminant hepatic failure (abstract). Gastroenterology 118(suppl 2, pt 1):A896, 2000
52. Powell WJ, Jr., Klatskin G: Duration of survival in patients with Laennec's cirrhosis: influence of alcohol withdrawal, and possible effects of recent changes in general management of the disease. Am J Med 44: 406, 1968
53. Pare P, Talbot J, Hoefs JC: Serum-ascites albumin concentration gradient: a physiologic approach to the differential diagnosis of ascites. Gastroenterology 85: 240, 1983
54. Runyon BA: Paracentesis and ascitic fluid analysis. Textbook of Gastroenterology. Yamada T, Alpers D, Owyang C, et al, Eds. JB Lippincott Co, New York, 1991, p 2455
55. Runyon BA, Montano AA, Akriviadis EA, et al: The serum-ascites albumin gradient is superior to the exudate-transudate concept in the differential diagnosis of ascites. Ann Intern Med 117:215, 1992
56. Akriviadis EA, Runyon BA: Utility of an algorithm in differentiating spontaneous from secondary bacterial peritonitis. Gastroenterology 98:127, 1990
57. Terg R, Cobas S, Fassio E, et al: Oral ciprofloxacin after a short course of intravenous ciprofloxacin in the treatment of spontaneous bacterial peritonitis: results of a multicenter, randomized study. J Hepatol 33:504, 2000
58. Gines P, Rimola A, Planas R, et al: Norfloxacin prevents spontaneous bacterial peritonitis recurrence in cirrhosis: results of a double-blind, placebo-controlled trial. Hepatology 12(4 pt 1):716, 1990
59. Hoefs JC, Canawati HN, Sapico FL, et al: Spontaneous bacterial peritonitis. Hepatology 2:399, 1982
60. Mihas AA, Toussaint J, Hsu HS, et al: Spontaneous bacterial peritonitis in cirrhosis: clinical and laboratory features, survival and prognostic indicators. Hepatogastroenterology 39:520, 1992
61. Gregory PB, Broekelschen PH, Hill MD, et al: Complications of diuresis in the alcoholic patient with ascites: a controlled trial. Gastroenterology 73:534, 1977
62. Tito L, Gines P, Arroyo V, et al: Total paracentesis associated with intravenous albumin management of patients with cirrhosis and ascites. Gastroenterology 98:146, 1990
63. Gines P, Tito L, Arroyo V, et al: Randomized comparative study of therapeutic paracentesis with and without intravenous albumin in cirrhosis. Gastroenterology 94:1493, 1988
64. Bernhoft RA, Pellegrini CA, Way LW: Peritoneovenous shunt for refractory ascites: operative complications and long-term results. Arch Surg 117:631, 1982
65. Greig PD, Langer B, Blendis LM, et al: Complications after peritoneovenous shunting for ascites. Am J Surg 139:125, 1980
66. Welch HF: Prognosis after surgical treatment of ascites: results of side-to-side shunt in 40 patients. Surgery 56:75, 1964;
67. Burroughs AK, Patch D: Transjugular intrahepatic portosystemic shunt. Semin Liver Dis 19:457, 1999
68. Ochs A, Rossle M, Haag K, et al:. The transjugular intrahepatic portosystemic stent-shunt procedure for refractory ascites [published erratum appears in N Engl J Med 332:1587, 1995]. N Engl J Med 332: 1192, 1995
69. Trotter JF, Suhocki PV, Rockey DC: Transjugular intrahepatic portosystemic shunt (TIPS) in patients with refractory ascites: effect on body weight and Child-Pugh score. Am J Gastroenterol 93:1891, 1998
70. Rossle M: [Transjugular intrahepatic portasystemic shunt (TIPS)—indications and outcome]. Z Gastroenterol 35:505, 1997
71. Jalan R, Forrest EH, Stanley AJ, et al: A randomized trial comparing transjugular intrahepatic portosystemic stent-shunt with variceal band ligation in the prevention of rebleeding from esophageal varices. Hepatology 26:1115, 1997
72. Rouillard SS, Bass NM, Roberts JP, et al: Severe hyperbilirubinemia after creation of transjugular intrahepatic portosystemic shunts: natural history and predictors of outcome. Ann Intern Med 128:374, 1998
73. Sterling KM, Darcy MD: Stenosis of transjugular intrahepatic portosystemic shunts: presentation and management. AJR Am J Roentgenol 168:239, 1997
74. Lebrec D, Giuily N, Hadengue A, et al: Transjugular intrahepatic portosystemic shunts: comparison with paracentesis in patients with cirrhosis and refractory ascites: a randomized trial. French Group of Clinicians and a Group of Biologists. J Hepatol 25:135, 1996
75. Berk DP, Chalmers T: Deafness complicating antibiotic therapy of hepatic encephalopathy. Ann Intern Med 73:393, 1970

76. Soeters PB, Fischer JE: Insulin, glucagon, aminoacid imbalance, and hepatic encephalopathy. Lancet 2:880, 1976
77. DerSimonian R: Parenteral nutrition with branched-chain amino acids in hepatic encephalopathy: meta analysis. Hepatology 11:1083, 1990
78. Gines A, Escorsell A, Gines P, et al: Incidence, predictive factors, and prognosis of the hepatorenal syndrome in cirrhosis with ascites. Gastroenterology 105:229, 1993
79. Gonwa TA, Goldstein M, Holman M, et al: Orthotopic liver transplantation and renal function: outcome of hepatorenal syndrome and trial of verapamil for renal protection in nonhepatorenal syndrome. Transplant Proc 25:1891, 1993
80. Angeli P, Volpin R, Gerunda G, et al: Reversal of type 1 hepatorenal syndrome with the administration of midodrine and octreotide. Hepatology 29:1690, 1999
81. Nagayama M, Takai T, Okuno M, et al: Fat emulsion in surgical patients with liver disorders. J Surg Res 47:59, 1989
82. Gluud C: Branched-chain amino acids for hepatic encephalopathy? Hepatology 13:812, 1991
83. Mammen EF: Coagulopathies of liver disease. Clin Lab Med 14:769, 1994
84. Mammen EF: Coagulation defects in liver disease. Med Clin North Am 78:545, 1994
85. Mannucci PM, Franchi F, Dioguardi N: Correction of abnormal coagulation in chronic liver disease by combined use of fresh-frozen plasma and prothrombin complex concentrates. Lancet 2:542, 1976
86. Ballard HS, Marcus AJ: Platelet aggregation in portal cirrhosis. Arch Intern Med 136:316, 1976
87. Brophy MT, Fiore L, Deykin D: Hemostasis. Hepatology: A Textbook of Liver Disease. Zakim D, Boyer T, Eds. WB Saunders Co, Philadelphia, 1996, p 691
88. Hersch SL, Kunelis T, Francis RB Jr: The pathogenesis of accelerated fibrinolysis in liver cirrhosis: a critical role for tissue plasminogen activator inhibitor. Blood 69:1315, 1987
89. Riewald M, Riess H: Treatment options for clinically recognized disseminated intravascular coagulation. Semin Thromb Hemost 24:53, 1998
90. Bismuth H, Samuel D, Castaing D, et al: Liver transplantation in Europe for patients with acute liver failure. Semin Liver Dis 16:415, 1996
91. Rosen HR, Shackleton CR, Martin P: Indications for and timing of liver transplantation. Med Clin North Am 80:1069, 1996
92. Lucey MR, Brown KA, Everson GT, et al: Minimal criteria for placement of adults on the liver transplant waiting list: a report of a national conference organized by the American Society of Transplant Physicians and the American Association for the Study of Liver Diseases. Liver Transpl Surg 3:628, 1997
93. Butterworth RF: The neurobiology of hepatic encephalopathy. Semin Liver Dis 16:235, 1996
94. Ferenci P, Puspok A, Steindl P: Current concepts in the pathophysiology of hepatic encephalopathy. Eur J Clin Invest 22:573, 1992
95. Maddison JE, Watson WE, Dodd PR, et al: Alterations in cortical [3H]kainate and alpha-[3H]amino-3-hydroxy-5-methyl-4-isoxazolepropionic acid binding in a spontaneous canine model of chronic hepatic encephalopathy. J Neurochem 56:1881, 1991
96. Yurdaydin C, Walsh TJ, Engler HD, et al: Gut bacteria provide precursors of benzodiazepine receptor ligands in a rat model of hepatic encephalopathy. Brain Res 679:42, 1995
97. Jones EA, Basile AS, Skolnick P: Hepatic encephalopathy, GABA-ergic neurotransmission and benzodiazepine receptor ligands. Adv Exp Med Biol 272:121, 1990
98. Basile AS, Harrison PM, Hughes RD, et al: Relationship between plasma benzodiazepine receptor ligand concentrations and severity of hepatic encephalopathy. Hepatology 19:112, 1994
99. Takahashi K, Kameda H, Kataoka M, et al: Ammonia potentiates GABAA response in dissociated rat cortical neurons. Neurosci Lett 151:51, 1993
100. Aronson LR, Gacad RC, Kaminsky-Russ K, et al: Endogenous benzodiazepine activity in the peripheral and portal blood of dogs with congenital portosystemic shunts. Vet Surg 26:189, 1997
101. Demetriou AA, Watanabe F: Support of the Acutely Failing Liver, 2nd ed. RG Landes Co, Austin, Texas, 2000.
102. Rozga J, Holzman MD, Ro MS, et al: Development of a hybrid bioartificial liver. Ann Surg 217:502, 1993
103. Watanabe FD, Mullon CJ, Hewitt WR, et al: Clinical experience with a bioartificial liver in the treatment of severe liver failure: a phase I clinical trial. Ann Surg 225:484, 1997
104. Watanabe FD, Arnaout WS, Ting P, et al: Artificial liver. Transplant Proc 31:373, 1999

95 MULTIPLE ORGAN DYSFUNCTION SYNDROME

John C. Marshall, M.D., and *Avery B. Nathens*, M.D., Ph.D., M.P.H.

Approach to Multiple Organ Dysfunction Syndrome

Recognition of the Susceptible Patient

The phenomenon of multiple organ dysfunction syndrome (MODS) is characterized by the progressive but potentially reversible physiologic dysfunction of two or more organs or organ systems that arises after resuscitation from an acute life-threatening event. Formerly known as progressive systems failure,[1] multiple organ failure,[2] and multiple organ systems failure,[3] the phenomenon was designated multiple organ dysfunction syndrome by a 1991 consensus conference of the American College of Chest Physicians (ACCP) and the Society of Critical Care Medicine (SCCM). This designation is meant to emphasize that certain dynamic alterations in physiologic function in the critically ill patient may constitute a clinical syndrome with common pathophysiological underpinnings.[4] However, MODS may be less a syndrome than a paradigm—an approach to the care of the critically ill patient that emphasizes intensive monitoring and support of organ system function, specific therapies for isolated disease processes, and prevention or minimization of physiologic derangements resulting from ICU interventions.

MODS evolves in the wake of a profound disruption of systemic homeostasis.[5] Classic MODS is seen in patients with overwhelming infection, multiple injuries, or massive ischemia, but the syndrome has a number of risk factors, some of which overlap [see Table 1].

The hallmark of MODS is the involvement of organs or organ systems remote from the site of the original insult in a dynamic process that ranges in severity from mild, transient dysfunction to frank, irreversible organ system failure. Disruption of normal homeostasis causes altered patterns of organ system interaction; the fundamental problem in the clinical approach to MODS is that attempts to support one organ or organ system may aggravate dysfunction in another. Although preexisting abnormalities of organ system function—such as those that occur in diabetes, chronic renal failure, and hepatic failure—also contribute to adverse outcomes in critical illness, MODS is considered to be an acute and potentially reversible process rather than a manifestation of chronic and irreversible disease.

Prevention

Any patient with acute physiologic instability from a variety of diagnoses [see Table 1] is at risk for MODS. Varying degrees of organ system dysfunction may be present at the time of ICU admission—depending on the severity of the process and the duration of its evolution—and these derangements have an important impact on prognosis.[6] The cornerstone of care for ICU patients with minimal organ dysfunction is the prevention of MODS through the support of optimal systemic physiologic function in circumstances in which an acute insult has altered patterns of normal homeostasis. In general, such prevention consists of the provision of the highest-quality clinical care. This objective has three discrete elements: hemodynamic support, metabolic support, and immunologic support. In each case, optimal care involves both physiologic intervention and appropriate monitoring to direct that intervention.

HEMODYNAMIC SUPPORT

Optimal hemodynamic homeostasis is achieved when oxygen delivery to tissues and use of oxygen by tissues are maximized and when anaerobic metabolism is prevented.

Oxygen delivery ($\dot{D}o_2$) is a function of three variables: the hemoglobin level, the oxygen saturation, and the cardiac output. In cases of mild or moderate surgical stress, oxygen demands are not substantially altered, myocardial function remains intact, and microvascular permeability remains normal. Adequate $\dot{D}o_2$ can thus be assumed if the pulse rate, blood pressure, urine output, and central venous pressure (CVP) remain normal.

In a normal person, oxygen consumption (calculated as the product of the cardiac output and the arteriovenous gradient in oxygen content) remains constant despite changes in $\dot{D}o_2$, until oxygen delivery reaches a critically low level, at which point oxygen consumption is said to be supply dependent. In a patient at

Recognize the susceptible patient

Patients at high risk for multiple organ dysfunction syndrome (MODS) are those who have experienced a profound disruption of systemic homeostasis resulting from one or more of the following:

- Overwhelming infection
- Sterile inflammation
- Massive injury
- Massive ischemia
- Immune system activation
- Intoxication
- Iatrogenic factors
- Idiopathic factors

Minimal organ dysfunction

Prevent progression to MODS by optimizing support of hemodynamic, metabolic, and immunologic function.

Hemodynamic support

Maximize O_2 delivery to tissues by the following measures:

- Fluid replacement therapy
- Inotropic agents
- Vasoactive agents
- Mechanical ventilation

Metabolic support

Reverse catabolic state with early, definitive surgical therapy, including the following:

- Debridement of devitalized tissue
- Burn wound excision and grafting
- Rigid fixation of long bone fractures

Provide early, aggressive nutritional support, by the enteral route if possible. If gut function is inadequate, total parenteral nutrition should be employed until gut function returns.

Immunologic support

Prevent nosocomial infection, eradicate established infection, and minimize the effects of injurious host defense responses by such measures as the following:

- Timely and appropriate surgical intervention
- Limiting the breach of mucosal defenses
- Avoidance of antacids for stress ulcer prophylaxis
- Selective, targeted use of systemic antibiotics

Organ function is restored

Patient survives. Discharge patient from ICU.

Organ function deteriorates

Approach to Multiple Organ Dysfunction Syndrome

Significant organ dysfunction

Characterize the physiologic derangement and institute supportive therapy.

Single organ dysfunction

Search for correctable causes, including the following:
- Exacerbation of preexisting chronic disease
- Complications from invasive devices and medications
- Local complications (e.g., fluid overload, pneumothorax, biliary tract obstruction)
- Local pathology (e.g., myocardial infarction, pulmonary embolism, pneumonia)

Multiple organ dysfunction

Search for correctable causes, including the following:
- Occult infection
- Missed injuries
- Adverse effects of medical therapy (e.g., transfusions, total parenteral nutrition)

Modify supportive care

Minimize adverse consequences of supportive care through the use of techniques such as pressure-limited ventilation and continuous hemodialysis. Manage infectious complications with local measures and sparing use of antimicrobial agents. Evaluate need for antibiotic therapy or surgical intervention.

Antibiotic therapy

- Sparing use of empirical antibiotic therapy
- Microbiological diagnosis can almost always be made in MODS
- If organism cannot be isolated, discontinue antibiotics and repeat cultures

Surgical intervention

Prepare the patient for operation through the following measures:
- Preoperative optimization of physiologic function
- Safe, well-organized transport to the operating room
- Surgical intervention in the ICU when appropriate and feasible

Reevaluate clinical status

MODS resolves, and patient's condition improves

Transfer patient from ICU.

MODS persists, and patient's condition deteriorates or fails to improve despite support and in the absence of correctable underlying disease

Probability of death is overwhelming. Consider withdrawal of life support.

organisms.[50] Therefore, use of antimicrobial agents in critically ill patients must be selective and targeted, and the use of broad-spectrum empirical therapy should be minimized by regular reviews of culture and sensitivity results and through restrictions on antibiotic prescription practices.

Although it is generally believed that nosocomial infections in critically ill patients arise from endogenous reservoirs, patient-to-patient and environment-to-patient spreads of pathogens also occur. Certain organisms—particularly *Acinetobacter*, *Xanthomonas*, and *Legionella*—are transmitted through aqueous sources in the ICU, and the isolation of such organisms from critically ill patients is evidence of a potential problem in environmental infection control. Hand washing is an important but underutilized mode of infection prevention in the ICU [*see 108 Infection Control in Surgical Practice*]. There is no clear evidence that protective isolation of critically ill patients warrants the increased costs and increased demands on nursing staff.

Untreated infection is both a cause of impaired immunologic responsiveness and a potent stimulus of the inflammatory and cytokine responses that figure centrally in the pathogenesis of MODS. Early fixation of fractures not only attenuates hypermetabolism but also reduces infectious complications.[30]

The role of immunomodulation in the prevention of MODS is undefined. Nonspecific immunomodulatory techniques have aroused considerable theoretical interest; however, there are as yet no convincing data to support the use of these techniques in clinical situations. Moreover, attempts to enhance host immunity by pharmacological means may actually augment morbidity by amplifying the detrimental consequences of the cytokine response.[51] To date, studies of immunomodulation using specific immunotherapy directed against endotoxin[52-54] and other strategies designed to moderate the proinflammatory cytokine response[55,56] have yielded generally disappointing results. Although improved techniques for identifying the patient populations that may benefit from such interventions will likely establish a role for these strategies, it is clear that timely and appropriate surgical intervention remains the most potent form of immunotherapy currently available to the surgeon[57] [*see 88 Immunomodulation*].

Definitions of Organ System Dysfunctions

No consensus has yet been reached on how best to characterize MODS according to the dysfunctioning organ systems, the descriptors that optimally reflect dysfunction within a given organ system, or the degree of abnormality that constitutes the dysfunction or failure of a particular organ system. Nonetheless, it would appear that such a consensus may not be far off.

A systematic review of the published literature from 1969 through 1993 identified 30 clinical studies of 20 or more patients with MODS that provided explicit criteria for organ failure or dysfunction.[58] Although criteria varied significantly among the studies, seven organ systems were cited in over half of the published reports: the respiratory system (all 30 reports), the renal system (29 reports), the hepatic system (27 reports), the cardiovascular system (25 reports), the hematologic system (23 reports), the GI system (22 reports), and the central nervous system (18 reports). Both a recent European consensus conference and two North American collaborations[59] define MODS by the above systems, eliminating the GI system because of the declining incidence of stress-related upper GI bleeding and the lack of satisfactory descriptors of GI dysfunction. The available scoring systems have many similarities [*see Table 2*], and it is likely that a wider consensus on the description of clinical MODS will emerge over the next few years.

RESPIRATORY DYSFUNCTION

The adult respiratory distress syndrome (ARDS) is the prototypical expression of respiratory dysfunction in MODS.[60] In its mildest form, respiratory dysfunction is characterized by tachypnea, hypocapnia, and hypoxemia. As the injury evolves, a combination of worsening hypoxemia and an increase in the work of breathing necessitates mechanical ventilatory support [*see 91 Pulmonary Dysfunction and 92 Use of the Mechanical Ventilator*].

Increased capillary permeability is the earliest pathological event in ARDS.[61] Respiratory impairment is reflected in a reduction in functional lung capacity and results from both the increased distance across which oxygen must pass from the alveolus to the capillaries and the decreased compliance of the edematous lung.[62] As the acute inflammatory process resolves, further lung injury results from the process of repair, which involves fibrosis and deposition of hyaline material.[63]

Lung involvement in ARDS is inhomogeneous: areas of functional and aerated alveoli are interspersed between areas of nonfunctional alveoli.[64] Pathological examination of an involved lung reveals injury to alveolar epithelial cells and capillary endothelial cells, with plugging of the alveoli by proteinaceous fluid containing inflammatory cells and cell fragments. Deposition of hyaline material is seen in the alveolar ducts.[65] The aerated lung units that remain appear to have normal gas-tissue ratios and well-preserved mechanical and gas-exchanging properties.

Physiologic impairment of the respiratory system is reflected by a reduced arterial oxygen tension (P_aO_2). Normalization of the P_aO_2 often requires the institution of mechanical ventilation with an adequate value for the fraction of inspired oxygen (F_IO_2) [*see 92 Use of the Mechanical Ventilator*]. The ratio of P_aO_2 to F_IO_2 is an objective measurement of the degree to which oxygenation is impaired and is probably the best available measurement of respiratory dysfunction.[66]

RENAL DYSFUNCTION

Acute renal failure emerged as a significant clinical problem during World War II, but supportive therapy, in the form of dialysis, did not become available until the 1950s. Clinical or subclinical evidence of renal dysfunction is common in MODS. Early-onset renal dysfunction typically results from hypotension. The etiology of late-onset renal failure is multifactorial and includes both prerenal factors (e.g., decreased cardiac output, hypovolemia) and the cumulative effects of nephrotoxic agents, such as medications and radiocontrast

Table 2 Recognition and Assessment of Organ System Dysfunctions[59,179,264,285,286]

Organ System	Indicators of Dysfunction	Degree of Dysfunction				
		None (0)*	Minimal (1)*	Mild (2)*	Moderate (3)*	Severe (4)*
Respiratory	P_aO_2/F_IO_2 ratio	> 300[†] > 400[‡]	226–300[†] 300–400[‡]	151–225[†] 200–300[‡]	76–150[†] 100–200[‡]	≤ 75[†] < 100[‡]
	Duration of mechanical ventilation	—	—	> 48 hr	> 72 hr	> 72 hr (PEEP > 10 or F_IO_2 > 0.50)
Renal	Creatinine level	≤ 100 µmol/L	101–200 µmol/L	201–350 µmol/L	351–500 µmol/L	> 500 µmol/L
	Urine output	—	—	—	< 500 ml/day	< 200 ml/day
	Need for dialysis	—	—	—	—	Dialysis
Neurologic	Glasgow Coma Scale score	Glasgow Coma Scale score, 15	Glasgow Coma Scale score, 13–14	Glasgow Coma Scale score, 10–12	Glasgow Coma Scale score, 7–9	Glasgow Coma Scale score, ≤ 6
Hepatic	Bilirubin	≤ 20 µmol/L[†] < 20 µmol/L[‡]	21–60 µmol/L[†] 20–32 µmol/L[‡]	61–120 µmol/L[†] 33–101 µmol/L[‡]	121–240 µmol/L[†] 162–204 µmol/L[‡]	> 240 µmol/L[†] > 204 µmol/L[‡]
	Albumin	—	—	< 28 mg/dl	< 23 mg/dl	< 19 mg/dl
	AST	—	< 25 U/L	—	25–50 U/L	> 50 U/L
Cardiovascular	Systolic blood pressure	> 90 mm Hg	71–90 mm Hg (fluid responsive)	61–70 mm Hg (not fluid responsive)	51–60 mm Hg	≤ 50 mm Hg
	pH	—	—	—	≤ 7.3	≤ 7.2
	Inotropic agent dosages	—	—	Dopamine < 5 µg/kg/min or Any dose of dobutamine	Dopamine > 5 µg/kg/min or Epinephrine < 0.1 µg/kg/min or Norepinephrine < 0.1 µg/kg/min	Dopamine > 15 µg/kg/min or Epinephrine > 0.1 µg/kg/min or Norepinephrine > 0.1 µg/kg/min
	Heart rate × CVP / MAP	< 10.0	10.1–15.0	15.1–20.0	20.1–30.0	> 30.0
Hematologic	Platelet count	> 120,000/mm³	81,000–120,000/mm³	51,000–80,000/mm³	21,000–50,000/mm³	≤ 20,000/mm³
	Leukocyte count	—	—	—	> 30,000/mm³	> 60,000/mm³ or < 2,500/mm³
Gastrointestinal	Enteral nutrition	—	—	Mild intolerance	Moderate intolerance	Severe intolerance
	Stress ulcer bleeding	None	None	None	Stress bleeding	> 2 U/day
Metabolic	Insulin requirements	None	None	> 1 U/hr	2–4 U/hr	> 4 U/hr

*Multiple organ dysfunction syndrome (MODS) score.
[†]Data from reference 59.
[‡]Data from references 285 and 286.
AST—aspartate aminotransferase F_IO_2—fraction of inspired oxygen MAP—mean systemic arterial pressure P_aO_2—arterial oxygen tension
PEEP—positive end-expiratory pressure CVP—central venous pressure

material.[67] Histologic studies show acute tubular necrosis with disruption of the basement membrane, patchy necrosis of the tubules, interstitial edema, and tubular casts; these changes correlate poorly with functional impairment[68] [*see* 93 *Acute Renal Failure*].

Renal dysfunction in the multiple organ dysfunction syndrome is reflected biochemically by an increasing serum creatinine level. The creatinine clearance provides a sensitive reflection of early subclinical renal dysfunction[69] but is probably too sensitive to be of use in the evaluation of established dysfunction.

HEPATIC DYSFUNCTION

Hepatic dysfunction in critical illness was first described during World War II[70] and occurs in up to 54 percent of patients admitted to an ICU[71] [*see* 94 *Hepatic Failure*]. Two clinical syndromes have been described: ischemic hepatitis and ICU jaundice. Ischemic hepatitis, or shock liver, characteristically follows an episode of hypotension. Early elevations of aminotransferase levels are striking and may be associated with an increased prothrombin time and hypoglycemia; centrilobular necrosis is evident histologically. Successful resuscitation of the shock state results in rapid normalization of the biochemical abnormalities.[71] ICU jaundice, which is more common than ischemic hepatitis, typically evolves many days after the inciting physiologic insult. Conjugated hyperbilirubinemia is a prominent feature, whereas elevation of aminotransferase levels and prothrombin time are less pronounced.[72] Histologic features include intrahepatic cholestasis, steatosis, and Kupffer cell hyperplasia.[73] The pathogenesis is multifactorial and includes ongoing hepatic ischemia, TPN-induced cholestasis, and drug toxicity.

CARDIOVASCULAR DYSFUNCTION

Both peripheral vascular and myocardial function are altered in MODS. Characteristic changes in the peripheral vasculature include a reduction in vascular resistance and an increase in microvascular permeability, resulting in a hyperdynamic circulatory profile and peripheral edema. The reduction in systemic vascular resistance results in an increase in cardiac index; however, this increase may be insufficient to maintain an adequate mean arterial pressure because of intrinsic impairment of myocardial contractility. Cardiovascular dysfunction in MODS is evident clinically as hypotension that is refractory to volume challenge (necessitating inotropic and vasopressive support), tachydysrhythmias, and peripheral edema. Biventricular dilatation with a reduction in right and left ventricular ejection fractions is apparent.[74] Right ventricular dysfunction is particularly prominent, perhaps as a consequence of increased pulmonary vascular resistance secondary to concomitant lung injury.[75,76]

The mechanisms of altered myocardial function in MODS are incompletely characterized, though the myocardial depressant effects of circulating cytokines,[77] potentially mediated through the local release of nitric oxide,[78] appear to play an important role.

NEUROLOGIC DYSFUNCTION

Abnormalities of both central and peripheral nervous system function have been described in critical illness. CNS dysfunction occurs in up to 70 percent of critically ill patients, typically presenting as alterations in level of consciousness without localizing signs.[79] Its pathophysiology is poorly understood; postulated mechanisms include the direct effects of proinflammatory mediators on cerebral function, the development of vasogenic cerebral edema, areas of infarction related to hypotension, and alterations in the blood-brain barrier that result in changes in the composition of the interstitial fluid.[80] The electroencephalogram typically shows one of four patterns indicating increasingly abnormal activity: diffuse theta wave rhythms, intermittent rhythmic delta waves, triphasic delta waves, and suppression or burst-suppression patterns.[80]

The peripheral nervous system dysfunction of MODS, also known as critical illness polyneuropathy, affects up to 70 percent of critically ill patients.[81] The clinical presentation of peripheral neuropathy in the critically ill patient is subtle. It may present as failure to wean a patient from mechanical ventilation.[82] Other manifestations include weakness of the limbs or absent deep tendon reflexes, with relative sparing of the cranial nerves, resulting in weak or absent limb movements with preservation of facial grimacing in response to painful stimuli. Like the encephalopathy of MODS, the pathophysiology of peripheral neuropathy remains speculative; however, endoneural edema and axonal hypoxia have been implicated.[83]

HEMATOLOGIC DYSFUNCTION

The most common hematologic abnormality of critical illness is thrombocytopenia, which occurs in approximately 20 percent of ICU admissions.[84] Causes include increased consumption, intravascular sequestration, and impaired thrombopoiesis secondary to suppression of bone marrow function.[85] In addition, heparin-induced thrombocytopenia resulting from antibodies to complexes of heparin and platelet factor 4 develops in up to 10 percent of patients receiving heparin.[86] Prolongation of the prothrombin time and the partial thromboplastin time occurs less frequently. The most fulminant expression of hematologic dysfunction in MODS is disseminated intravascular coagulation (DIC), which is characterized by derangements in platelet numbers and clotting times and the presence in plasma of fibrin degradation products.[87]

Anemia is common in critical illness and arises not only as a result of diagnostic blood draws but also as a manifestation of the acute-phase response mediated in part by interleukin-1 (IL-1).[88] Transient leukopenia is a classic manifestation of early endotoxemia[89]; more commonly, the leukocyte count in MODS is elevated as a manifestation of a systemic septic response. Lymphopenia is common, though the cause is unknown.

GASTROINTESTINAL DYSFUNCTION

Upper GI hemorrhage after burn injury was first described by Curling in 1842.[90] Until recently, stress GI bleeding was a common problem, occurring in up to a quarter of all ICU admissions.[91] Improved techniques of resuscitation and hemodynamic support, earlier diagnosis of infection, and the widespread use of stress ulcer prophylaxis have contributed to a reduction in the frequency of this complication; through such measures, rates of clinically important bleeding in the contemporary ICU have dropped below four percent.[45] Other manifestations of GI dysfunction in MODS include ileus and intolerance of enteral feeding,[92] pancreatitis,[93] and acalculous cholecystitis.[94] Splanchnic hypoperfusion with mucosal acidosis is a pathological feature common to all of these.[95]

OTHER ORGAN SYSTEM DYSFUNCTION

Hyperglycemia with insulin resistance is the most common manifestation of endocrine dysfunction in critical illness.[96] The sick euthyroid syndrome, which is characterized by reductions in serum T_3 with or without an increase in reverse T_3 levels and a normal T_4 level, is another expression of endocrine dysfunction in the critically ill; thyrotropin levels are reduced, and the magnitude of the reduction correlates with the severity of illness.[97] Abnormalities of adrenal function have also been reported.[98,99]

Immunologic dysfunction can be evaluated by means of delayed hypersensitivity skin-testing[100]; responses of critically ill patients are characteristically suppressed.[101,102] Documentation of the full spectrum of immune derangements in critical illness requires more complex technology than is available in the average ICU; however, the development of ICU-acquired infection with endemic ICU pathogens of low intrinsic virulence, such as *Candida*, coagulase-negative staphylococci, and enterococci, can be considered a surrogate marker of immune dysfunction in MODS.[102]

Abnormalities of wound healing represent an expression of MODS. Common manifestations of impaired wound healing include the failure of an open wound to develop satisfactory granulation tissue and the development of decubitus ulcers.

Evaluation of the Patient with Organ Dysfunction

SINGLE-ORGAN DYSFUNCTION

Single-organ dysfunction strongly suggests local pathology and should trigger a search for potentially correctable causes in the affected organ system. Isolated organ dysfunction may arise as a result of preexisting chronic disease or may reflect a local problem, such as fluid overload, atelectasis, biliary tract obstruction, or increased intracranial pressure. Complications related to invasive devices and adverse effects of medication are common causes of single-organ dysfunction; the diagnosis is often presumptive, established on the basis of improvement after discontinuance of the agent or removal of the device. Finally, single organ dysfunction may indicate acute organ injury such as a myocardial infarction, pulmonary embolism, or pneumonia. Because the prognosis of single-organ dysfunction is relatively good—even in cases of profound functional deficit—consideration of heroic supportive measures is justified.[103]

Search for Correctable Causes

Deteriorating function in a single organ system should prompt an evaluation to detect potentially reversible problems. Respiratory dysfunction may occur as a result of complications such as fluid overload, pneumonia, pleural effusion, pneumothorax, or pulmonary embolism. Hypotension can be caused by hypovolemia or overly aggressive diuresis. Central venous and pulmonary arterial catheters may induce tachyarrhythmias as a result of mechanical irritation of the conducting system. Renal dysfunction may reflect inadequate intravascular volume or the nephrotoxic effects of medications (e.g., acute tubular necrosis caused by aminoglycosides and interstitial nephritis caused by penicillins and cephalosporins). Occasionally, renal dysfunction arises from a postrenal cause, such as ureteral obstruction or blockage of a Foley catheter.

Medications are important causes of liver dysfunction in the critically ill patient. Erythromycin, ketoconazole, and haloperidol can induce cholestatic liver injury.[104] Thrombocytopenia is an important adverse effect of a number of medications, including heparin flushes used to maintain the patency of arterial lines.[105] A decreased level of consciousness is usually the result of the poorly characterized metabolic encephalopathy of critical illness; however, it is necessary to rule out other causes, such as meningitis, encephalitis, brain abscess, and subdural empyema. Excessive or prolonged use of narcotics or sedative-hypnotics may lead to prolonged alterations in level of consciousness, particularly when hepatic or renal function is impaired. Nondepolarizing muscle relaxants, such as vecuronium, may cause prolonged neuromuscular blockade and persistent peripheral nerve dysfunction.[106]

MULTIPLE ORGAN DYSFUNCTION

Some authors have described a characteristic temporal sequence to the evolution of MODS[3,59] [see Table 3]; however, the clinical course tends to be highly variable. The specific pattern of dysfunction is much less important than the course of the evolving syndrome. Resolution of dysfunction suggests an appropriate response to specific and supportive therapy. Worsening of dysfunction, on the other hand, should prompt a search for potentially correctable causes and a reevaluation of the specific methods of supportive care being used. Not infrequently, a readily treatable cause of evolving MODS is found; often, however, no cause will be evident. In cases with an unknown cause, the objective of therapy is to optimize supportive measures to limit iatrogenic injury until the patient recovers or, alternatively, until a considered decision is made regarding the futility of continued active care.

Search for Correctable Causes

Occult infection Uncontrolled infection, particularly that arising in the abdomen, is an important risk factor for MODS[2,3,107,108]; the development of otherwise unexplained organ dysfunction should trigger a careful search for an occult intra-abdominal focus.[109] However, MODS also develops in patients with pneumonia[109] and other life-threatening infections, and it can evolve in patients in whom no significant focus of infection can be identified.[102,110]

When MODS develops in the postoperative surgical patient, a careful search for infection must be undertaken, concentrating in particular on the operative site. With appropriate attention to the clinical possibilities, aided by ultrasonography and CT scanning, the presence or absence of significant intra-abdominal pathology can usually be established. Local wound exploration can suggest the possibility of occult intra-abdominal injury through the demonstration of impaired wound heal-

Table 3 Temporal Evolution of MODS[3,59]

System	Time from ICU Admission to Onset of Significant Dysfunction (days)
Respiratory	2
Hematologic	3
Central Nervous	4
Cardiovascular	4
Hepatic	5–6
Renal	4–11
Gastrointestinal	10

ing or fascial dehiscence or through the isolation of typical intestinal microflora from a wound infection. The diagnosis of pneumonia in intubated ICU patients is notoriously difficult[111]; however, the use of quantitative techniques, such as protected specimen brush bronchoscopy[112] and bronchoalveolar lavage,[113] can establish or rule out this diagnosis with confidence in most cases.[114]

Urinary tract infections or device-related bacteremias are rarely the cause of MODS, though they commonly develop in patients with significant organ dysfunction.[102] Disseminated candidiasis, however, may present as deteriorating organ dysfunction in critically ill patients.

Iatrogenic factors MODS can be considered the quintessential iatrogenic disorder, reflecting both the successes and the shortcomings of contemporary ICU practice. MODS has developed only because advances in supportive care have permitted the prolonged survival of critically ill patients who once would have died; however, several iatrogenic factors that figure prominently in its expression are potentially avoidable.[21]

Technical and judgmental errors often set the stage for the development of MODS.[32,115,116] Whenever a patient manifests unexplained organ failure in the postoperative period, the surgeon must consider the possibility of an iatrogenic complication—for example, a missed intestinal perforation in a trauma victim, a leak from a tenuous anastomosis, or left colon ischemia after aneurysmectomy.

Many of the therapeutic interventions that are mainstays of ICU care have the potential to induce organ dysfunction. Oxygen in high concentrations can produce pulmonary damage, probably as a result of the generation of toxic oxygen intermediates[117] [see 99 Reactive Oxygen Metabolites], and mechanical ventilation can induce barotrauma, particularly when high peak airway pressures are generated[118] [see 92 Use of the Mechanical Ventilator]. Ventilatory strategies designed to limit airway pressure and maintain F_IO_2 at the lowest level compatible with an adequate arterial oxygen saturation are preferable in the management of patients with acute lung injury.

Blood transfusion has been implicated in the development of organ dysfunction, an effect that occurs independent of the effects of shock, blood loss, and fluid resuscitation.[119] Both to reduce the risk of blood-borne diseases and to minimize the potential for aggravating organ dysfunction, transfusion should probably be withheld if the hemoglobin level is greater than 8 g/dl unless a critical need for enhanced oxygen delivery exists. The optimal target for transfusion of critically ill patients is unknown.[120] The age of the blood administered may be an underappreciated factor in defining optimal transfusion strategies: Marik and Sibbald demonstrated in 1993 that the effects of blood transfusion on splanchnic blood flow as measured by a gastric tonometer depended on the age of the blood administered and that the use of blood more than 12 days old had an adverse impact on oxygen delivery.[121]

Total parenteral nutrition can also contribute to organ dysfunction. TPN-associated alterations in hepatic function with intrahepatic cholestasis and fatty infiltration are relatively common and are manifested by elevated aminotransferase and alkaline phosphatase levels.[122] TPN may also give rise to glucose intolerance and can aggravate ventilatory impairment because of increased CO_2 production. In patients with borderline pulmonary function, this additional CO_2 production may prevent weaning from ventilatory support.[123] Animal studies demonstrate that TPN is associated with a loss of gut barrier function and increased rates of bacterial translocation[124]—an observation that may explain the increased risk of infectious complications in trauma patients maintained on TPN.[125] It has even been proposed that deliberate limitation of nutritional support may be beneficial for critically ill patients,[126] though the merits of this approach are unproved.

Prophylactic control of gastric pH to prevent stress ulceration leads to gastric overgrowth with gram-negative organisms and appears to increase rates of nosocomial pneumonia.[46] Gastric colonization with common ICU pathogens is frequent and is significantly correlated with the development of invasive infection at multiple sites, including the lungs, the urinary tract, and the blood.[127] Whether the severity of MODS can be reduced through suppression of pathological colonization with topical antibiotics,[47] acidification of enteral feeds,[49] or the use of cytoprotective agents for stress ulcer prophylaxis[128] remains unresolved. A recent epidemiological study suggests that stress ulcer prophylaxis can be safely omitted from the regimen of most ICU patients[45] [see Prevention, Immunologic Support, above].

Support of the Patient with MODS

MODS is a complication to be prevented rather than a disease to be treated. Unfortunately, even with optimal attention to preventive measures and a careful search for treatable complications, progressive and refractory MODS presents the intensivist with a significant challenge: to support the patient during a period of otherwise lethal organ system dysfunction without causing further injury in the process. Detailed approaches to organ-specific supportive care are outlined elsewhere in this text. Selected approaches to supportive care that may minimize some of the adverse consequences of MODS are discussed below.

RESPIRATORY SUPPORT

In patients with MODS, the immediate challenge of respiratory support is to maintain an adequate arterial oxygen saturation and allow for the elimination of CO_2—particularly in the patient with renal dysfunction—without inducing lung injury from hyperoxia or barotrauma. Oxygenation can be optimized through the judicious use of positive end-expiratory pressure, a maneuver that may in addition decrease accumulation of interstitial fluid and minimize ventilator-associated lung injury.[118] Ventilation with large tidal volumes and high peak inspiratory pressures contributes to lung injury, and as a result, ventilatory strategies that limit airway pressures are being used more widely. Pressure-controlled ventilatory techniques limit peak airway pressures to a maximum predetermined level, optimizing gas exchange by inverting the inspiration:expiration (I:E) ratio (i.e., reducing the I:E ratio from a normal value of 1:2 to a value of 1:1 or less) and by changing the shape of the inspiratory flow curve (normally square) to one in which flow is initially rapid, then decelerates[129] [see 92 Use of the Mechanical Ventilator]. Peak airway pressure can also be limited by the use of low tidal volumes. Although oxygenation can be maintained with low tidal volumes, ventilation is jeopardized and CO_2 levels rise; as a result, this approach is known as permissive hypercapnia. As long as renal compensatory mechanisms are intact, acidosis is usually not life-threatening, despite levels of P_aCO_2 in excess of 100 mm Hg, and mortality may be improved, even in patients with established organ failure.[130] Another strategy developed to optimize ventilation while minimizing both peak airway pressures and the hemodynamic consequences of positive pressure ventilation is the technique of airway pressure–release ventilation, in which airway pressures are maintained at a continuous positive baseline level and intermittently decreased or released to permit gas exchange in the lung.[131]

Inhaled nitric oxide, a potent vasodilator, is selectively delivered to ventilated lung segments and has shown some preliminary promise as a means of reducing pulmonary arterial pressures and $\dot{V}/\dot{Q}$ mismatch in patients with acute lung injury.[132] The benefits of nitric oxide administration are still largely anecdotal, and properly designed clinical trials will be needed to define its role in the management of ARDS. Extracorporeal lung support by means of extracorporeal membrane oxygenation or extracorporeal CO_2 removal can be lifesaving in patients with isolated severe respiratory failure that has been refractory to all other forms of respiratory support.[103] However, these techniques are resource intensive and have not been shown to improve outcome in clinical trials comparing them with conventional mechanical ventilation.[133,134]

CARDIOVASCULAR SUPPORT

Recent reports suggest that after ICU admission, a patient's prognosis is improved if $\dot{D}o_2$ is increased to supraphysiologic levels (in excess of 600 ml/min/m², compared with a normal value of approximately 450 ml/min/m²).[9,135,136] However, a cautionary note has been sounded by the results of a recent prospective, randomized study that demonstrated an *increase* in mortality and a worsening of organ dysfunction when attempts were made to drive $\dot{D}o_2$ to supranormal levels with dobutamine[137]; therefore, an alternative interpretation has been offered—that the *ability* to raise $\dot{D}o_2$ to supranormal levels identifies a subgroup of patients with a more favorable prognosis.[135,138]

Fluid administration is the mainstay of cardiovascular support of the critically ill. However, it too carries a potential cost in aggravating the dysfunction of other organ systems, and a recent randomized study has suggested that intentional under-resuscitation of patients with penetrating chest trauma may improve outcome.[139] The potential reasons for this are speculative. The critically ill patient receives massive volumes of fluid as a result of a generalized reduction in peripheral vascular resistance, an increase in vascular permeability, and an increase in the level of preload required for optimal cardiac function. Excessive interstitial fluid contributes to impairment of pulmonary gas exchange and increases the distance across which oxygen must diffuse in the tissues. Cerebral edema may contribute to worsening of injury in head-injured patients and to alterations in neurologic function in critically ill patients.

RENAL SUPPORT

Dopamine is commonly employed at low dosages (1 to 3 μg/kg/min) to minimize renal dysfunction. Dopamine increases renal blood flow directly via effects on D_1 and D_2 dopamine receptors in the renal vasculature[140,141] and, indirectly, by increasing the cardiac index. In addition, diuresis may occur as a result of a direct renal tubular effect.[142] However, a recent clinical trial questioned the role of dopamine as a renal protective agent and suggested that dobutamine has a greater beneficial effect on creatinine clearance, with a lower incidence of side effects, especially tachyarrhythmias.[143]

Conventional intermittent hemodialysis is difficult when cardiovascular instability is present. Continuous renal replacement therapies—in particular, continuous arteriovenous hemodialysis (CAVHD) and continuous venovenous hemodialysis—have proved valuable in the management of these patients and may improve clinical outcomes.[144,145] Complications result from the need for vascular access; such complications include limb ischemia, hemorrhage, and arteriovenous fistula formation.[146] In addition to the conventional benefits of such therapy, hemodialysis may increase the elimination of a number of low-molecular-weight proinflammatory mediators.[147,148]

SUPPORT OF OTHER ORGANS

Techniques for support of hepatic and GI function are not well defined. Early enteral nutritional support is desirable and has been associated with a reduction in infectious complications after multiple trauma.[125,149,150] At least one report, however, suggests that enteral nutrition does not prevent the development of organ dysfunction in patients with persistent hypermetabolism.[151] Techniques for bioartificial liver support have been developed but remain experimental.[152]

Support of hematologic function is largely confined to replacement of cellular elements (e.g., red blood cells and platelets) and coagulation factors (using plasma or concentrates such as cryoprecipitate). Neurologic support is limited to the correction of metabolic abnormalities.

MODS AND ICU-ACQUIRED INFECTION

Just as uncontrolled infection is an important predisposing factor for the development of MODS, so is the reverse equally true. Patients with MODS are at significantly increased risk for the development of ICU-acquired infection, and the incidence increases as the severity of MODS increases.[102] Several series have documented a shift in the most common infecting species of microbial flora in ICU-acquired infection from enteric gram-negative organisms to *Staphylococcus epidermidis, Candida, Pseudomonas,* and enterococci.[102,153] There are two important reasons for this: (1) these organisms are the most common causes of proximal gastrointestinal colonization in critically ill patients[127] and (2) they are resistant to the antibiotics commonly used in the empirical treatment of nosocomial infection.

ICU-acquired infections develop in those patients at greatest risk for ICU mortality; however, it is unclear the extent to which the infections themselves contribute to that risk.[154-156] ICU-acquired infections are rarely true disseminated infections; more often, they are localized processes occurring as a consequence of a contaminated intravenous line or urinary catheter, in which case removal of the contaminated device is the appropriate therapy, rather than administration of systemic antibiotics.

CRITICAL DECISIONS IN THERAPY

Progression of MODS in a patient who is receiving apparently optimal ICU support is a relatively common occurrence that presents the clinician with a series of diagnostic and therapeutic dilemmas.

Infection is a common trigger of MODS, and the temptation to initiate empirical anti-infectious therapy is great, but as a rule, such an approach should be resisted. Antibiotics are a double-edged sword in critically ill patients with MODS. Although antibiotics eliminate susceptible microorganisms, they disrupt the normal indigenous flora and set the stage for superinfection with resistant microorganisms. Empirical broad-spectrum antibiotic therapy for suspected nosocomial infection has never been demonstrated to improve outcome; indeed, there are grounds for concluding that this practice may be harmful. Previous broad-spectrum antimicrobial therapy is an independent risk factor for death from nosocomial pneumonia[157] and for nosocomial infection with *Candida*.[158] Clinical manifestations of sepsis in critically ill patients frequently arise from noninfectious causes.[154,159] With techniques currently available, a microbiological diagnosis can almost always be made when an infection severe enough to induce organ dysfunction is present. When an organism cannot be isolated, it is safer to discontinue antibiotics and repeat cultures than to escalate empirical antibiotic therapy.

Empirical therapy with corticosteroids is less common today than it once was, largely as a result of two well-designed clinical trials that failed to demonstrate benefit for the use of high-dose corticosteroid therapy in patients with septic shock.[160,161]

The association of organ dysfunction with occult intra-abdominal infection[109,110] stimulated a period of enthusiasm for the practice of blind laparotomy, or laparotomy undertaken to identify and treat an intra-abdominal infectious focus in the absence of radiographic evidence that such a focus is present.[162,163] However, the role of blind, or nondirected, laparotomy in the ICU patient with worsening organ dysfunction has been controversial. Proponents of nondirected laparotomy have argued that the rate of positive findings may be as high as 60 percent,[164] whereas skeptics point out that even when correctable pathology is encountered, the ultimate prognosis remains poor.[165,166] We believe that evolving organ dysfunction in itself is rarely an indication for abdominal exploration and that the decision to operate must be made on the basis of careful analysis of the clinical circumstances, guided by appropriate radiologic investigations. With improvements in ultrasonography and CT scanning, missed intra-abdominal abscesses have become distinctly uncommon. Ultrasonography and CT scanning are less reliable for the diagnosis of anastomotic leaks with minimal spillage or of gut ischemia. Anastomotic leaks can frequently be delineated using water-soluble contrast studies; however, if the clinical concern is ischemic bowel, an aggressive surgical approach is indicated. Diagnostic peritoneal lavage may have a role to play in the abdominal evaluation of critically ill patients, yielding purulent fluid or bowel contents in cases of GI perforation and bloody fluid in cases of advanced gut ischemia [see 2 Trauma Resuscitation]. It goes without saying that conventional physical findings of peritonitis—particularly in the nonoperated abdomen—may be the sole indication for surgical exploration. Moreover, in the case of the complicated postoperative patient transferred from another institution because of worsening organ dysfunction, we have adopted the philosophy that laparotomy is a legitimate component of the admission physical examination.

Preparation of the Critically Ill Patient for Operation

Operative intervention is frequently required in the critically ill surgical patient: in our surgical ICU, approximately 10 percent of patients undergo an operative procedure during their ICU stay. Immediate operative intervention is occasionally required to control life-threatening hemorrhage or hemodynamic instability. More typically, however, intervention is undertaken either urgently (e.g., to drain an abscess or resect an ischemic bowel) or electively (e.g., to create a tracheostomy or feeding jejunostomy).[167] The logistical challenges involved in preparing critically ill patients for operation and transporting them to the operating room can be significant (see below). The decision to operate, however, is not synonymous with the decision to transport; it has become increasingly appropriate to consider the ICU as an extension of the operating room and to perform procedures of moderate complexity within the ICU setting.

OPTIMIZATION OF THE PATIENT

Operative intervention carries the risk of transient deterioration, and it is therefore critical that physiologic function be optimized before the surgical procedure. Intraoperative gas exchange may deteriorate as a result of inhibition of hypoxic pulmonary vasoconstriction—an effect of many volatile anesthetics.[168] Cardiac output may be jeopardized by the vasodilatory and myocardial depressant effects of anesthesia—effects that may be compounded by intraoperative blood and fluid loss. Moreover, evaluation of the patient while under operative drapes can be difficult, and the diagnosis of potentially life-threatening complications may be delayed. For this reason, it may be prudent to perform bilateral tube thoracostomies to prevent the development of tension pneumothorax when the patient requires high ventilatory pressures. Preoperative correction of electrolyte abnormalities and coagulopathies will also render the operative procedure safer [see 6 Life-Threatening Electrolyte Abnormalities].

TRANSPORT TO THE OPERATING ROOM

Transport between the ICU and the operating room is potentially dangerous for critically ill patients: significant per-

Table 4 Prognosis in MODS[3,6,177,178]

Number of Failing Systems	Mortality (%)
0	3
1	30
2	50–60
3	85–100
4	72–100
5	100

turbations in cardiovascular and respiratory status occur in more than 10 percent of such transports.[169,170] The most common problems are hypoxemia, hypotension, and arrhythmias, often as a result of migration of the endotracheal tube and mishaps associated with drug infusion pumps. Such problems are generally preventable if the transport is adequately planned and organized.

Placement of monitoring devices, such as arterial lines and pulmonary arterial catheters, should be undertaken in the ICU before transport both to facilitate monitoring during the transport phase and to permit optimization of preoperative therapy. Portable monitors permit a continuous display of heart rate, blood pressure, and So_2 during transport and should be used routinely. Planning of the transport must take into account the unexpected. For example, it is always wise to bring an extra tank of oxygen in the event of an elevator malfunction as well as adequate fluids and drugs to cover an unanticipated delay between the ICU and the operating theater. Battery-operated devices must be adequately charged to ensure uninterrupted operation.

Transfers of the patient from the ICU bed to a transport stretcher and from the stretcher to the operating room table carry the risk of inadvertent dislodgment of endotracheal tubes and vascular lines. One member of the operating team—usually the anesthetist—must assume responsibility for the integrity of these devices while the patient is being moved.

SURGICAL INTERVENTIONS IN THE ICU

The risks associated with patient transport and the delays in arranging timely intervention can be eliminated by performing certain surgical procedures in the intensive care unit. The operating room has the advantage of better lighting and equipment and the availability of skilled anesthetic and nursing support; however, it is often possible to duplicate these conditions in the intensive care unit. The advantages of the operating room environment from an infection control perspective are negligible.

Tracheostomy is readily performed at the bedside in the ICU, with complication rates comparable to those in the operating room.[171-173] A greater risk of complications exists for patients with preexisting coagulopathy, morbidly obese persons, nonintubated patients, and patients with abnormal neck anatomy (e.g., those in whom the cricoid cartilage is not palpable above the sternal notch during neck extension); such patients are probably managed more safely in the operating room setting.[171] Loss of control of the airway in critically ill patients can be fatal; thus, elective bedside tracheostomies should be performed only by skilled personnel capable of dealing with any such complications. Several reports have documented the ease and relative safety of bedside percutaneous tracheostomy, though the risks and contraindications remain to be defined.[174,175] Zipper laparotomy for poorly controlled intra-abdominal infection is readily performed in the ICU,[176] as are gastrostomy, jejunostomy, open-lung biopsy, and exploratory laparotomy.

Prognosis of MODS

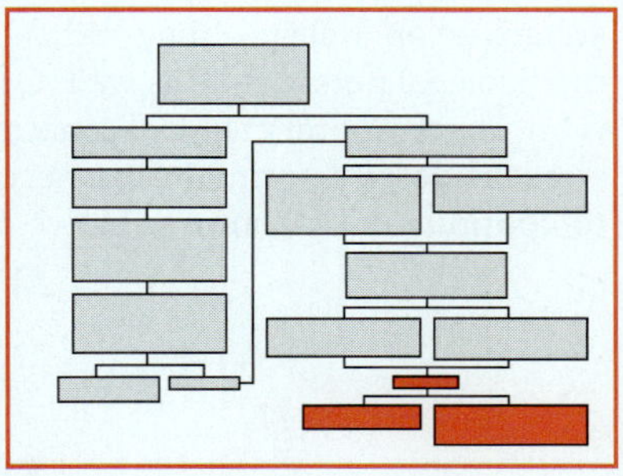

The prognosis of MODS is directly related to the severity of the underlying organ dysfunction, which can be expressed either as the number of failing systems[3,6,177,178] [see Table 4] or as the global severity of dysfunction as determined by an organ dysfunction score[59,179] [see Figure 1]. It must be emphasized, however, that prognostic indicators reflect the expected outcome for a group of patients and are of limited use in making decisions about the care of an individual patient. Moreover, these indicators reflect standards of critical care prevalent at a particular time and in a particular clinical setting. For instance, although in 1976 patients with pancreatitis and six or more positive indicators (according to Ranson's criteria[180]) had a mortality of 100 percent, a significant

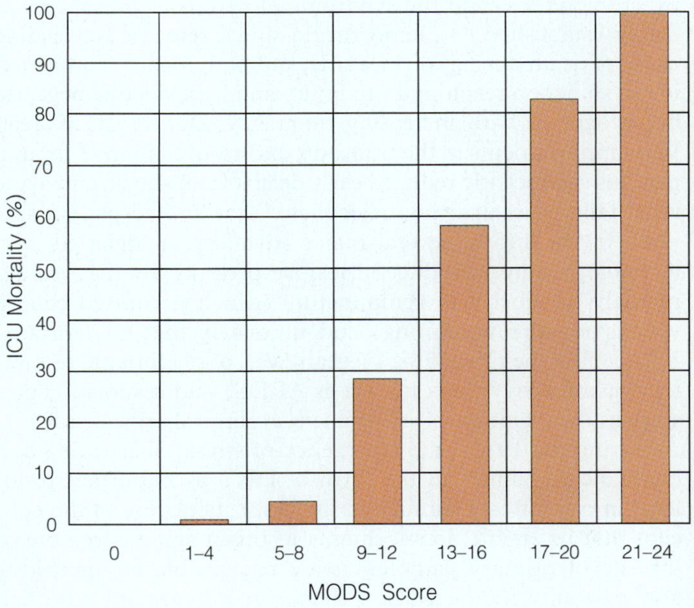

Figure 1 Mortality increases as the overall degree of organ system dysfunction, reflected in the MODS score, increases. To calculate a MODS score, dysfunction in each of six different organ systems (renal, hematologic, cardiovascular, hepatic, respiratory, and central nervous systems) is first separately assigned a score from 0 to 4 [see Table 2]. The worst scores for each of the six systems over the length of the ICU stay are then totaled to produce the MODS score.[59]

number of such patients now survive.[181]

Organ dysfunction in MODS is potentially recoverable when the factors responsible for the persistence or progression of the syndrome can be reversed. Identifying these factors, treating them appropriately, and providing optimal physiologic support can prove a daunting challenge, and it is often advisable to consider seeking independent advice or transporting the patient to a center that has the clinical expertise and facilities to manage the multidisciplinary problems faced by patients with MODS. Given that MODS not uncommonly evolves as a consequence of medical misadventure, early consultation or referral may be a sound philosophy from a medicolegal perspective as well. On the other hand, it is a common contemporary ICU scenario that MODS evolves and worsens despite optimal care, necessitating a decision whether to continue or discontinue active care.

WITHDRAWAL OF LIFE SUPPORT

The most common mode of death for the patient with advanced MODS is the limiting or withdrawal of life support in the face of a persistent failure to respond to full, aggressive ICU care. Such decisions are complex, and it is clear that there is considerable divergence of professional approach regarding the decision to withdraw life support.[182] Factors that must be taken into consideration include the nature of the underlying disease, the premorbid health of the patient, the wishes of the patient and family regarding long-term ICU care, the ultimate prospects for independent existence, and the presence of active problems amenable to medical therapy. Although such deliberations are difficult for medical staff and family alike, proper consideration for the expectations of all involved can facilitate a decision to discontinue active therapy in an atmosphere that is dignified and humane rather than adversarial.

Discussion

Evolution of MODS

The evolution of MODS has been an inevitable consequence of advances in the management of multiply traumatized and critically ill patients.[1] Prolongation of survival of the most severely ill patients has led to the emergence of a new spectrum of problems resulting not from the underlying disease process itself but from the host response to that process and from the measures required to sustain vital organ system function.

Blood transfusions were first used extensively during World War I[183]; however, it was not until 1930 that the connection between blood loss and the syndrome of hemorrhagic shock was firmly established.[184] Hemorrhagic shock remained a leading cause of death during World War II, and both renal[185] and hepatic[70] dysfunction resulting from injury and hypovolemia began to be recognized with increasing frequency. During the Korean War, improvements in the transport and resuscitation of injured patients significantly reduced early deaths from shock, and acute renal failure became the major factor that limited patient survival. In the 1950s, several major advances in organ-support technology were introduced: positive pressure ventilation, hemodialysis, subclavian venipuncture (which permitted central venous pressure monitoring), and, ultimately, the first dedicated ICUs.[186] By the time of the Vietnam War, posttraumatic respiratory insufficiency (now known as ARDS) had assumed center stage as the major unsolved problem in surgical critical care.

During the 1960s, the emergence of stress GI bleeding and hematologic failure (in the form of DIC) as important problems in patient care stimulated the first articulation of the concept that reversible derangements in organ systems remote to the site of primary pathology were responsible for morbidity and mortality in the ICU.[187] Baue, in a landmark editorial, coined the term "multiple, progressive, or sequential systems failure"[1] and established this as the dominant paradigm of critical care. Clinical reports used a variety of terms to describe this new syndrome: multiple organ failure,[2] multiple system organ failure,[3] multiple organ system failure,[93] nonbacteremic clinical sepsis,[107] and the hypermetabolism organ failure complex.[188] The 1991 ACCP-SCCM consensus conference proposed the designation MODS to reflect the contemporary view that it is a clinical syndrome with common pathological and prognostic implications.[4]

Changes in microbial ecology and in the clinical management of infection in hospitalized patients paralleled advances in ICU therapy. In the 1940s and 1950s, the widespread use of antibiotics in hospitalized patients produced a shift in the cause of microbial infections from primarily exogenous to primarily endogenous species. However, the overall prevalence of infection remained unchanged.[189] By the 1960s, gram-negative species replaced pneumococci and streptococci as the leading causes of lethal bacterial infection.[190] Studies of the systemic effects of gram-negative bacteremia gave rise to important advances in the hemodynamic management of critically ill patients, with the result that florid septic shock is seen less frequently today. In its place has emerged a more indolent syndrome of recurrent infection with organisms of relatively low pathogenicity: *S. epidermidis*, *Candida*, and enterococci.

As MODS has evolved, awareness has grown of the central role played by endogenous host factors in the syndrome's pathogenesis. Studies of host defenses in critical illness demonstrate that immune responses are altered and suggest that the critically ill patient should be considered an immunocompromised host.[101,191] More recently, it has been suggested that overactivity, rather than failure, of host defense is responsible for the morbidity of critical illness.[154,192] These notions are by no means contradictory; both, in fact, reflect the complexities of the interactions of infection and the host inflammatory response.

Evolving Terminology

The earliest descriptions of MODS emphasized its intimate association with infection[3,108,109,187] and uncontrolled inflammation.[179] Advances in the understanding of the biology of the host inflammatory response have rendered obsolete much of the terminology classically used to describe these processes[193] and have triggered a vigorous debate on optimal phraseology.[194,195] These debates are much more than semantic quibbles, for terminology reflects a model of biology for the guidance of therapy. Moreover, the inflammatory response is clearly a biologic double-edged sword, with the potential both to benefit and to harm the host; therefore, it is critical that therapeutic decisions be based on an adequate evaluation of the precise nature of the physiologic process.

In an attempt to reconcile terminology with a contemporary understanding of biology, the 1991 ACCP-SCCM consensus conference proposed that a new term, the systemic inflammatory response syndrome (SIRS), should be used to describe the clinical syndrome of disseminated inflammation, independent of its cause [see 78 Clinical and Laboratory Diagnosis of Infection]. SIRS is a clinical syndrome whose differential diagnosis includes autoimmune disease, drug reactions, sterile inflammation in pancreatitis, and a variety of other disorders associated with activation of an inflammatory response. Under the new definitions, sepsis describes the development of SIRS as a consequence of infection, whereas infection denotes the invasion of normally sterile tissues by bacteria or their toxins, independent of the response evoked in the host.

By this model, MODS develops not because of uncontrolled infection but as a consequence of SIRS. In other words, if SIRS represents an appropriate adaptive response to disruptions of homeostasis, MODS is the maladaptive consequence of that systemic response.

Theories of Pathogenesis

Although the epidemiological association between organ dysfunction and SIRS is strong, no compelling pathogenetic model has yet been determined to account for the evolution of MODS, nor is it even known whether the clinical syndrome reflects a single pathological process. A number of overlapping theories have been advanced,[196] the most compelling of which interpret MODS as a dynamic process—the outcome of the interaction between an acute stimulus and the host response to that stimulus.

INFECTION AND THE HOST SEPTIC RESPONSE

Cellular Mechanisms

Activated host immune cells—particularly neutrophils and macrophages—have been shown to produce tissue injury similar to that produced by MODS in both clinical studies and animal models.

Neutrophils are critical effectors of local inflammatory responses, and it is postulated that they play a role in the pathological organ injury of MODS.[197-200] Experimental studies demonstrate a critical role for neutrophils in acute injury to the lung,[201,202] gut,[203,204] and liver,[205,206] as well as in the pathogenesis of increased vascular permeability in a variety of acute models of injury and infection.[207-209] Descriptive clinical studies have shown neutrophils from patients with SIRS to be activated[210-212] and, more specifically, have shown increased activation of neutrophils that have passed through the lung in patients with acute lung injury.[213] Similarly, experimental interventions to deplete neutrophils or to block their interactions with endothelial cells have resulted in attenuation of organ injury.[199,201,209] It has been recognized, however, that neutrophils alone cannot account for the development of clinical MODS, because although neutrophil depletion has reduced lung injury in a variety of experimental models, the phenomenon of ARDS is still seen in neutropenic patients.[214]

Circulating monocytes and fixed-tissue macrophages are also recognized to be key cellular mediators of tissue injury,[215] largely on the basis of their ability to release virtually all of the endogenous mediator molecules that have been implicated in tissue injury in acute injury and infection.[216] Macrophages exert an important regulatory influence, modulating the expression of lymphocyte-mediated immunity[217] and releasing substances, such as IL-8, that serve as potent chemoattractants for neutrophils.[218] Through the expression of cellular procoagulants, activated macrophages can initiate intravascular coagulation and fibrin deposition.[219] Endotoxin-activated hepatic Kupffer cells modulate hepatocyte protein synthesis in vitro[220]; activation of these cells in vivo can reproduce the hypermetabolic state[221] and immunologic abnormalities[222] characteristic of critical illness. In experimental animals, Kupffer cell blockade reduces mortality in endotoxemia[223] but increases mortality in peritonitis induced by cecal ligation and puncture.[224]

Humoral Mediators

A large number of inflammatory mediators of host origin can reproduce manifestations of MODS when administered to experimental animals. Tumor necrosis factor (TNF),[225,226] IL-1,[227,228] and platelet-activating factor (PAF)[229] are among the most extensively studied of these, and strategies to alter their activities have undergone clinical trials (see below). Experimental studies have shown that diffuse organ injury can be induced not only by the excess activation of proinflammatory mediators but also by the deficiency of counterinflammatory mediators, such as transforming growth factor–β (TGF-β)[230] and IL-10.[231] These and other host-derived mediators are discussed in greater detail elsewhere [see 101 Cytokines and the Cellular Response to Injury and Infection].

Cytokines and other inflammatory mediators exert their most important activities locally within the microenvironment of inflammation, and there is considerable variability in circulating cytokine levels from one patient to the next.[232,233] Levels of inflammatory mediators in the systemic circulation correlate poorly with clinical status and outcome. IL-6[234,235] and IL-8[236-238] appear to be the most reliable markers of the activation of a systemic inflammatory response.

THE MICROVASCULATURE

Microvascular Injury

Autopsies of MODS patients show diffuse microvascular thrombosis with neutrophil sequestration,[239] pointing to a pathogenetic role for the microvasculature. Neutrophils and monocytes accumulate in sites of inflammation through a series of interactions with microvascular endothelial cells. These interactions are mediated by complementary adhesion molecules expressed on the circulating inflammatory cells and on the endothelium.[240,241] Bacterial products and host inflammatory cytokines up-regulate endothelial adhesion molecules. Moreover, activated endothelial cells lose their anticoagulant properties and express tissue factors, and as a consequence, the extrinsic coagulation pathway is activated.[242] Tissue injury results from both the local release of cytodestructive products from neutrophils and monocytes and ischemia secondary to

Table 5 Divergent Effects of Cytokine Manipulation in Animal Models

Mediator	Administration Augments Survival	Blockade Augments Survival
Tumor necrosis factor	Pretreatment before cecal ligation and puncture *Listeria* infection	Endotoxemia Gram-negative bacteremia *Staphylococcus aureus* enterotoxin administration
Interleukin-1 (IL-1)	*Escherichia coli* peritonitis *Klebsiella* infection	*E. coli* bacteremia *Klebsiella* (when IL-1 is given at low dose for short course)
Interleukin-10	Endotoxemia	*Candida albicans* infection *Listeria* infection
Interferon gamma	*Listeria* infection	Endotoxemia

microvascular thrombosis. Animal studies have demonstrated that remote organ injury both in thermal injury[243] and in gram-negative infection[244] can be attenuated by pretreatment with monoclonal antibodies directed against adhesion molecules.

Reperfusion Injury

After short, nonlethal periods of ischemia, tissue injury evolves as a result of events that occur during reperfusion—in particular, the generation of reactive oxygen species.[245] Free radical–mediated tissue injury results from damage to the plasma membrane, oxidation of critical intracellular proteins, adenosine triphosphate depletion, and DNA strand breakage[246]; in addition, oxidative stress can induce programmed cell death, or apoptosis.[247] Oxygen free radicals contribute to further local injury by triggering the expression of endothelial adhesion molecules[248,249] and the release of the neutrophil chemoattractant PAF.[250] This local injury results in intravascular thrombosis and increased capillary permeability. In addition, ischemia-reperfusion injury to the intestine or to a limb can induce remote organ injury in the lung.[203,251]

THE GUT HYPOTHESIS

MODS sometimes evolves in patients in whom no obvious focus of infection or ischemia is clinically evident[102] and persists despite apparently adequate management of identifiable foci.[166] It was for this reason that a number of authors, building on concepts articulated nearly a half century ago,[252,253] proposed that the GI tract may sometimes serve as an unseen motor of MODS.[36,151,198,254] This involvement of the GI tract may arise from the gut's role as both an occult microbial reservoir and a potent immunoregulatory organ whose normal function is to maintain a tonic counterinflammatory influence on immunologic activation.

The normal GI tract harbors in excess of 400 discrete microbial species whose ecological balance is maintained by competition for nutrients and mucosal binding sites.[255] Pathological colonization of the oropharynx[256] and the proximal GI tract[127,257,258] develops rapidly in the critically ill patient and predisposes to nosocomial infection with the same organism.[127] Such infections may develop as a result of subclinical aspiration[44,259] but may also arise as a consequence of the passage of viable bacteria through the wall of the gut, a phenomenon termed bacterial translocation. Bacterial translocation is readily observed in the experimental animal in response to the same insults that predispose to MODS: trauma, hemorrhage, burn injury, pancreatitis, intra-abdominal infection, and endotoxemia.[260] Evidence that translocation occurs as a clinically relevant phenomenon in humans is largely circumstantial[261-263] and occasionally contradictory.[264] Endotoxin presumably of gut origin has been detected in the plasma of patients after thermal injury[265] and repair of ruptured aortic aneurysms[266]; however, its significance, too, is controversial.

Under normal circumstances, the extensive immunologic tissues of the gut and liver blunt the expression of the immune response[267]; this influence may be impaired in critical illness, permitting the expression of a systemic inflammatory response. Intestinal epithelial cells dampen the release of TNF by macrophages in response to endotoxin, but they lose this suppressive activity in a hypoxic environment.[268] Levels of TNF and IL-6 are elevated in portal venous blood from animals subjected to hemorrhagic shock,[269] and elevated systemic TNF levels are observed within minutes of intestinal reperfusion after an ischemic insult.[270] Elevated portal venous levels of TNF have been seen in humans after aortic aneurysm repair.[271] Portal endotoxemia with resultant Kupffer cell activation triggers the release of potent immunosuppressive activity from alveolar and splenic macrophages[272]; conversely, Kupffer cell blockade lessens the clinical manifestations and reduces the mortality of systemic inflammation.[273]

THE TWO-HIT HYPOTHESIS

A complementary hypothesis of MODS pathogenesis suggests that an acute insult, such as infection or trauma, serves to prime the host in such a way that a second, relatively trivial, insult produces a markedly exaggerated host response.[197,274] Such a model would explain the apparent differences between MODS that develops early after trauma and MODS that occurs later[178]; like other theories of MODS, however, this hypothesis remains unproved.

Experimental Therapies

MANIPULATION OF INFLAMMATORY MEDIATORS

The administration or blockade of a number of the putative mediators of the systemic inflammatory response can improve survival in a variety of animal models of acute infectious challenge [see *101 Cytokines and the Cellular Response to Injury and Infection*]. However, attempts to apply insights derived from these studies to the care of critically ill patients have proved disappointing.

Nonspecific blockade of systemic inflammation with the use of high-dose corticosteroids has been evaluated in two clinical trials, both of which failed to demonstrate clinical efficacy.[161,162] A phase II clinical study of IL-1 receptor antagonist, a naturally occurring antagonist of IL-1, showed great promise,[275] but this promise failed to be realized in a subsequent double-blind, multicenter trial.[55] A number of phase II trials evaluating monoclonal antibodies to TNF have been undertaken; however, clinical benefit has been evident primarily in retrospective subgroup analyses, and a trial employing soluble TNF receptors has suggested that experimental manipulation may actually increase mortality.[56] At least two large phase III studies of anti-TNF monoclonal antibodies are in progress. Finally, one phase III trial of an antagonist to PAF has shown a significant reduction in mortality in a subgroup of patients with gram-negative infection and shock.[276]

Although efficacy has been suggested in retrospective subgroup analyses, no overall benefit has yet been documented in the use of mediator-targeted therapy in the management of critically ill patients at risk for MODS. There are many potential explanations for the apparent failure of these strategies. Entry criteria defined for the original corticosteroid trials identify a group of patients at significant risk for mortality,[277] but this population is highly heterogeneous with regard to the underlying clinical diagnoses and mediator profiles, and a significant percentage of these patients ultimately prove to be uninfected.[234] Moreover, the population is also heterogeneous in regard to its risk of ICU mortality.[278,279] Dosing intervals have been arbitrary, and the validity of using 28-day mortality as an outcome measure has been questioned.[280] Finally, animal studies demonstrate striking differences in the effects of antagonism of specific mediators, depending on the model used [*see Table 5*]. In general, strategies that improve survival in animal endotoxemia models have the opposite effect in models in which the problem is uncontrolled infection. Which model is most relevant to the critically ill patient with MODS is unknown, and at present, the potential for harm appears to be as great as the potential for benefit.

EXTRACORPOREAL TECHNIQUES

Another experimental strategy for the management of MODS has been to attempt to remove circulating mediators without identifying which ones may be present. Preliminary studies have suggested that CAVHD may remove mediators such as PAF.[148] Similarly, case reports have demonstrated the potential utility of plasma exchange in the management of patients with MODS.[281-283] Another experimental strategy has been the extracorporeal adsorption of circulating endotoxin to polymyxin B–coated filters.[284] Evaluation of potential roles for these approaches awaits the results of larger clinical trials.

Conclusion

MODS is a complex phenomenon, the course of which is determined by the dynamic interplay of the inciting event, the host response to that stimulus, and the consequences of ICU supportive care. As an outcome in critical illness, MODS is a relatively homogeneous process, with predictable patterns of organ dysfunction and characteristic patterns of organ injury; however, the disease processes leading to this outcome are highly heterogeneous. Considerable progress has been made in understanding the pathogenesis of the syndrome; increasingly, it appears that the mediators of MODS are endogenous products of the host response rather than the exogenous stimuli that evoke that response. At present, however, it is unclear whether MODS is the outcome of a single process of mediator activation or whether there are multiple pathways to the same outcome. Indeed, it remains to be determined whether the final outcome reflects variable expression of a single pathogenetic process or similar expression of a number of biologically diverse processes.

An increased understanding of the role of cytokines has stimulated research interest in the potential benefits of mediator manipulation therapies. However, there are as yet no data to justify the use of cytokine modulators outside of the context of clinical trials.

Ultimately, the most successful approaches to the multiple organ dysfunction syndrome have been those focusing on prevention by the application of time-honored surgical principles: aggressive resuscitation, timely operative intervention, adequate drainage of infection and debridement of devitalized tissue, and sound surgical judgment.

References

1. Baue AE: Multiple, progressive, or sequential systems failure: a syndrome of the 1970s. Arch Surg 110:779, 1975
2. Eiseman B, Beart R, Norton L: Multiple organ failure. Surg Gynecol Obstet 144:323, 1977
3. Fry DE, Pearlstein L, Fulton RL, et al: Multiple system organ failure: the role of uncontrolled infection. Arch Surg 115:136, 1980
4. Bone RC, Balk RA, Cerra FB, et al: Definitions for sepsis and organ failure and guidelines for the use of innovative therapies in sepsis. Chest 101:1644, 1992
5. Tran DD, Cuesta MA, Van Leeuwen PAM, et al: Risk factors for multiple organ system failure and death in critically injured patients. Surgery 114:21, 1993
6. Knaus WA, Draper EA, Wagner DP, et al: Prognosis in acute organ-system failure. Ann Surg 202:685, 1985
7. Shoemaker WC: Relation of oxygen transport patterns to the pathophysiology and therapy of shock states. Intensive Care Med 13:230, 1987
8. Phang PT, Cunningham KF, Ronco JJ, et al: Mathematical coupling explains dependence of oxygen consumption on oxygen delivery in ARDS. Am J Respir Crit Care Med 150:318, 1994
9. Shoemaker WC, Appel PL, Kram HB, et al: Prospective trial of supranormal values of survivors as therapeutic goals in high risk surgical patients. Chest 94:1176, 1988
10. Parrillo JE, Parker MM, Natanson C, et al: Septic shock in humans: advances in the understanding of pathogenesis, cardiovascular dysfunction, and therapy. Ann Intern Med 113:227, 1990
11. Moncada S, Higgs A: The L-arginine nitric oxide pathway. N Engl J Med 329:2002, 1994
12. Kreuzfelder E, Joka T, Keinecke H, et al: Adult respiratory distress syndrome as a specific manifestation of a general permeability defect in trauma patients. Am Rev Respir Dis 137:95, 1988
13. Fleck A, Hawker F, Wallace PI, et al: Increased vascular permeability: a major cause of hypoalbuminaemia in disease and injury. Lancet 1:781, 1985
14. Hurd TC, Dasmahpatra KS, Rush BF: Red cell deformability in human end experimental sepsis. Arch Surg 123:217, 1988

15. Astiz ME, Galera-Santiago A, Rackow EC: Intravascular volume and fluid therapy for severe sepsis. New Horiz 1:127, 1993
16. Mizock BA, Falk JL: Lactic acidosis in critical illness. Crit Care Med 20:80, 1992
17. Antonsson JB, Boyle CC III, Kruithoff KL, et al: Validation of tonometric measurement of gut intramural pH during endotoxemia and mesenteric occlusion in pigs. Am J Physiol Gastrointest Liver Physiol 259:G519, 1990
18. Gutierrez G, Palizas F, Doglio G, et al: Gastric intramucosal pH as a therapeutic index of tissue oxygenation in critically ill patients. Lancet 339:195, 1992
19. Marik PE: Gastric intramucosal pH: a better predictor of multiorgan dysfunction syndrome and death than oxygen-derived variables in patients with sepsis. Chest 104:225, 1993
20. Boyd O, MacKay CJ, Lamb G, et al: Comparison of clinical information gained from routine blood gas analysis and from gastric tonometry for intramural pH. Lancet 341:142, 1993
21. Beal AL, Cerra FB: Multiple organ failure syndrome in the 1990's: systemic inflammatory response and organ dysfunction. JAMA 271:226, 1994
22. Beylot M, Chassard D, Chambrier C, et al: Metabolic effects of a D-beta-hydroxybutyrate infusion in septic patients: inhibition of lipolysis and glucose production but not leucine oxidation. Crit Care Med 22:1091, 1994
23. Bessey PQ, Lowe KA: Early hormonal changes affect the catabolic response to trauma. Ann Surg 218:476, 1993
24. Sganga G, Siegel JH, Brown G, et al: Reprioritization of hepatic plasma protein release in trauma and sepsis. Arch Surg 120:187, 1985
25. Ozawa K, Aoyama H, Yasuda K, et al: Metabolic abnormalities associated with postoperative organ failure: a redox theory. Arch Surg 118:1245, 1983
26. Heideman M, Saravis C, Clowes GHA: Effect of nonviable tissue and abscesses on complement depletion and the development of bacteremia. J Trauma 22:527, 1982
27. Herndon DN, Barrow RE, Rutan RL, et al: A comparison of conservative versus early excisional therapy in severe burn patients. Ann Surg 209:547, 1989
28. Cryer HG, Anigian GM, Miller FB, et al: Effects of early tangential excision and grafting on survival after burn injury. Surg Gynecol Obstet 173:449, 1991
29. Johnson KD, Cadambi A, Seibert B: Incidence of adult respiratory distress syndrome in patients with multiple musculoskeletal injuries: effect of early operative stabilization of fractures. J Trauma 25:375, 1985
30. Seibel R, LaDuca J, Hassett JM, et al: Blunt multiple trauma (ISS 36), femur traction, and the pulmonary failure-septic state. Ann Surg 202:283, 1985
31. Goris RJA: Prevention of ARDS and MOF by prophylactic mechanical ventilation and early fracture stabilization. Prog Clin Biol Res 236B:163, 1987
32. Henao FJ, Daes JE, Dennis RJ: Risk factors for multiorgan failure: a case control study. J Trauma 31:74, 1991
33. Moore FA, Feliciano DV, Andrassy RJ, et al: Early enteral feeding, compared with parenteral, reduces postoperative septic complications: the results of a meta-analysis. Ann Surg 216:172, 1992
34. Cerra FB, Shronts EP, Konstantinides NN, et al: Enteral feeding in sepsis: a prospective, randomized, double-blind trial. Surgery 98:632, 1985
35. Bower RH, Muggia-Sullam M, Vallgren S, et al: Branched chain amino acid–enriched solutions in the septic patient: a randomized prospective trial. Ann Surg 203:13, 1985
36. Wilmore DW, Smith RJ, O'Dwyer ST, et al: The gut: a central organ after surgical stress. Surgery 104:917, 1988
37. Tremel H, Kienle B, Weilemann LS, et al: Glutamine dipeptide-supplemented parenteral nutrition maintains intestinal function in the critically ill. Gastroenterology 107:1595, 1994
38. Bower RH, Cerra FB, Bershadsky B, et al: Early enteral administration of a formula supplemented with arginine, nucleotides, and fish oil in intensive care patients: results of a multicentre prospective, randomized, clinical trial. Crit Care Med 23:436, 1995
39. Nathens AB, Chu PTY, Marshall JC: Nosocomial infection in the surgical intensive care unit. Infect Dis Clin North Am 6:657, 1992
40. Craven DE, Kunches LM, Lichtenberg DA, et al: Nosocomial infection and fatality in medical and surgical intensive care unit patients. Arch Intern Med 148:1161, 1988
41. Nishijima MK, Takezawa J, Hosotsubo KK, et al: Serial changes in cellular immunity of septic patients with multiple organ-system failure. Crit Care Med 14:87, 1986
42. Maki DG: Risk factors for nosocomial infection in intensive care: devices vs nature and goals for the next decade. Arch Intern Med 149:30, 1989
43. Maki DG, Ringer M, Alvarado CJ: Prospective randomized trial of povidone iodine, alcohol, and chlorhexidine for prevention of infection associated with central venous and arterial catheters. Lancet 338:339, 1991
44. Du Moulin GC, Paterson DG, Hedley-Whyte J, et al: Aspiration of gastric bacteria in antacid-treated patients: a frequent cause of postoperative colonisation of the airway. Lancet 1:242, 1982
45. Cook DJ, Fuller H, Guyatt GH, et al: Risk factors for gastrointestinal bleeding in critically ill patients. N Engl J Med 330:377, 1994
46. Cook DJ, Laine LA, Guyatt GH, et al: Nosocomial pneumonia and the role of gastric pH: a meta-analysis. Chest 100:7, 1991
47. Meta-analysis of randomised controlled trials of selective decontamination of the digestive tract. Selective Decontamination of the Digestive Tract Trialists' Collaborative Group. BMJ 307:525, 1993
48. Meagher LC, Savill JS, Baker A, et al: Phagocytosis of apoptotic neutrophils does not induce macrophage release of thromboxane B_2. J Leukocyte Biol 52:269, 1992
49. Heyland D, Bradley C, Mandell LA: Effect of acidified enteral feedings on gastric colonization in the critically ill patient. Crit Care Med 20:1388, 1992
50. Van Der Waaij D: The ecology of the human intestine and its consequences for overgrowth by pathogens such as *Clostridium difficile*. Annu Rev Microbiol 43:69, 1989
51. Natanson C, Hoffman WD, Suffredini AF, et al: Selected treatment strategies for septic shock based on proposed mechanisms of pathogenesis. Ann Intern Med 120:771, 1994
52. Greenman RL, Schein RMH, Martin MA, et al: A controlled clinical trial of E5 murine monoclonal IgM antibody to endotoxin in the treatment of gram-negative sepsis. JAMA 266:1097, 1991
53. Ziegler EJ, Fisher CJ Jr, Sprung CL, et al: Treatment of gram-negative bacteremia and septic shock with HA-1A human monoclonal antibody against endotoxin: a randomized, double-blind, placebo-controlled trial. N Engl J Med 324:429, 1991
54. McCloskey RV, Straube RC, Sanders C, et al: Treatment of septic shock with human monoclonal antibody HA-1A: a randomized double-blind, placebo-controlled trial. Ann Intern Med 121:1, 1994
55. Fisher CJ, Dhainaut J-FA, Opal SM, et al: Recombinant human interleukin 1 receptor antagonist in the treatment of patients with sepsis syndrome: results from a randomized, double-blind, placebo-controlled trial. JAMA 271:1836, 1994
56. Dhainaut JF, Mira JP, Brunet F: Investigational therapy of sepsis: anti-TNF, IL-1ra, anti-PAF, and G-CSF. Clinical Trials for the Treatment of Sepsis. Sibbald WJ, Vincent J-L, Eds. Springer-Verlag, New York, 1995, p 267
57. Meakins JL: Surgeons, surgery, and immunomodulation. Arch Surg 126:494, 1991
58. Marshall JC: Multiple organ dysfunction syndrome (MODS). Clinical Trials for the Treatment of Sepsis. Sibbald WJ, Vincent J-L, Eds. Springer-Verlag, New York, 1995, p 122
59. Marshall JC, Cook DJ, Christou NV, et al: The multiple organ dysfunction score: a reliable descriptor of a complex clinical outcome. Crit Care Med 23:1638, 1995
60. Bone RC, Balk R, Slotman G, et al: Adult respiratory distress syndrome: sequence and importance of development of multiple organ failure. Chest 101:320, 1992
61. Sibbald WJ, Short AK, Warshawski FJ, et al: Thermal dye measurements of extravascular lung water in critically ill patients: intravascular Starling forces and extravascular lung water in the adult respiratory distress syndrome. Chest 87:585, 1985
62. Marini JJ: New options for the ventilatory management of acute lung injury. New Horiz 1:489, 1993
63. Clark RA: The commonality of cutaneous wound repair and lung injury. Chest 99(suppl):57S, 1991
64. Gattinoni L, Pesenti A, Bombino M: Relationships between lung computed tomographic density, gas exchange, and PEEP in acute respiratory failure. Anesthesiology 69:824, 1988
65. Pietra GG, Ruttner JR, Wust W, et al: The lung after trauma and shock: fine structure of the alveolar capillary barrier in 23 autopsies. J Trauma 21:454, 1981
66. Murray JF, Matthay MA, Luce JM, et al: An expanded definition of the adult respiratory distress syndrome. Am Rev Respir Dis 138:720, 1988
67. Morris JA Jr, Mucha P Jr, Ross SE, et al: Acute posttraumatic renal failure: a multicenter perspective. J Trauma 31:1584, 1991
68. Tilney NL, Lazarus JM: Acute renal failure in surgical patients: causes, clinical patterns and care. Surg Clin North Am 63:357, 1983
69. Wilson RF, Soullier G, Antonenko D: Creatinine clearance in critically ill surgical patients. Arch Surg 114:461, 1979
70. Bywaters EGL: Anatomical changes in the liver after trauma. Clin Sci 6:19, 1946
71. Hawker F: Liver dysfunction in critical illness. Anaesth Intens Care 19:165, 1991
72. Schwartz DB, Bone RC, Balk RA, et al: Hepatic dysfunction in the adult respiratory distress syn-

drome. Chest 95:871, 1989
73. Nunes G, Blaisdell FW, Margaretten W: Mechanism of hepatic dysfunction following shock and trauma. Arch Surg 100:546, 1970
74. Parker MM, Shelhamer JH, Bacharach SL, et al: Profound but reversible myocardial depression in patients with septic shock. Ann Intern Med 100:483, 1984
75. Redl G, Germann P, Plattner H, et al: Right ventricular function in early septic shock states. Intensive Care Med 19:3, 1993
76. Vincent JL, Gris P, Coffernils M, et al: Myocardial depression characterizes the fatal course of septic shock. Surgery 111:660, 1992
77. Vincent J, Bakker J, Marecaux G, et al: Administration of anti-TNF antibody improves left ventricular function in septic shock patients. Chest 101:810, 1992
78. Finkel MS, Oddis CV, Jacob TD, et al: Negative inotropic effect of cytokines on the heart mediated by nitric oxide. Science 257:387, 1992
79. Young GB, Bolton CF, Austin TW, et al: The encephalopathy associated with septic illness. Clin Invest Med 13:297, 1990
80. Bolton CF, Young GB, Zochodne DW: The neurological complications of sepsis. Ann Neurol 33:94, 1993
81. Witt NJ, Zochodne DW, Bolton CF, et al: Peripheral nerve function in sepsis and multiple organ failure. Chest 99:176, 1991
82. Coronel B, Mercatello A, Couturier J-C, et al: Polyneuropathy: potential cause of difficult weaning. Crit Care Med 18:486, 1990
83. Bolton CF: Neuromuscular complications of sepsis. Intensive Care Med 19(suppl 2):S58, 1993
84. Baughmann RP, Lower EE, Flessa HC, et al: Thrombocytopenia in the intensive care unit. Chest 104:1243, 1993
85. Sigurdsson G, Christenson J, El-Rakshy M, et al: Intestinal platelet trapping after traumatic and septic shock: an early sign of sepsis and multiorgan failure in critically ill patients? Crit Care Med 20:458, 1992
86. Aster RH: Heparin-induced thrombocytopenia and thrombosis. N Engl J Med 332:1374, 1995
87. Ten Cate H, Brandjes DP, Wolters HJ, et al: Disseminated intravascular coagulation: pathophysiology, diagnosis, and treatment. New Horiz 1:312, 1993
88. Dinarello CA: Interleukin-1 and the pathogenesis of the acute phase response. N Engl J Med 311:1413, 1984
89. Suffredini AF: Endotoxin administration to humans: a model of inflammatory responses relevant to sepsis. Mediators of Sepsis. Lamy M, Thijs LG, Eds. Springer-Verlag, New York, 1992, p 13
90. Curling TB: On acute ulceration of the duodenum in cases of burns. Medical-Chirurgical Transactions of London 25:260, 1842
91. Cook DJ, Witt LG, Cook RJ, et al: Stress ulcer prophylaxis in the critically ill: a meta-analysis. Am J Med 91:519, 1991
92. Chang RWS, Jacobs S, Lee B: Gastrointestinal dysfunction among intensive care unit patients. Crit Care Med 15:909, 1987
93. Bell RC, Coalson JJ, Smith JD, et al: Multiple organ system failure and infection in adult respiratory distress syndrome. Ann Intern Med 99:293, 1983
94. Glenn F, Becker CG: Acute acalculous cholecystitis: an increasing entity. Ann Surg 195:131, 1982
95. Fiddian-Green RG: Should measurements of tissue pH and Po_2 be included in the routine monitoring of intensive care unit patients? Crit Care Med 19:141, 1991
96. Black PR, Brooks DC, Bessey PQ, et al: Mechanisms of insulin resistance following injury. Ann Surg 196:420, 1982
97. Rothwell PM, Udwadia ZF, Lawler PG: Thyrotropin concentration predicts outcome in critical illness. Anaesthesia 48:373, 1993
98. Rothwell PM, Lawler PG: Prediction of outcome in intensive care patients using endocrine parameters. Crit Care Med 23:78, 1995
99. Baldwin WA, Allo M: Occult hypoadrenalism in critically ill patients. Arch Surg 128:673, 1993
100. Christou NV, Boisvert G, Broadhead M, et al: Two techniques of measurement of the delayed hypersensitivity skin test response for the assessment of host resistance. World J Surg 9:798, 1985
101. Meakins JL, Pietsch JB, Bubenick O, et al: Delayed hypersensitivity: indicator of acquired failure of host defenses in sepsis and trauma. Ann Surg 186:241, 1977
102. Marshall JC, Christou NV, Horn R, et al: The microbiology of multiple organ failure: the proximal GI tract as an occult reservoir of pathogens. Arch Surg 123:309, 1988
103. Egan TM, Duffin J, Glynn MFX, et al: Ten-year experience with extracorporeal membrane oxygenation for severe respiratory failure. Chest 94:681, 1988
104. Zimmerman HJ, Maddrey WC: Toxic and drug-induced hepatitis. Diseases of the Liver. Schiff L, Schiff ER, Eds. JB Lippincott, Philadelphia, 1987, p 591
105. Cines DB, Kaywin P, Bina M, et al: Heparin-associated thrombocytopenia. N Engl J Med 303:788, 1980
106. Segredo V, Caldwell JE, Matthay MA, et al: Persistent paralysis in critically ill patients after long-term administration of vecuronium. N Engl J Med 327:524, 1992
107. Fry DE, Garrison RN, Heitsch RC, et al: Determinants of death in patients with intraabdominal abscess. Surgery 88:517, 1980
108. Skillman JJ, Bushnell LS, Goldman H, et al: Respiratory failure, hypotension, sepsis, and jaundice: a clinical syndrome associated with lethal hemorrhage and acute stress ulceration in the stomach. Am J Surg 117:523, 1969
109. Polk HC, Shields CL: Remote organ failure: a valid sign of occult intraabdominal infection. Surgery 81:310, 1977
110. Meakins JL, Wicklund B, Forse RA, et al: The surgical intensive care unit: current concepts in infection. Surg Clin North Am 60:117, 1980
111. Tobin MJ, Grenvik A: Nosocomial lung infection and its diagnosis. Crit Care Med 12:191, 1984
112. Chastre J, Fagon JY, Soler P, et al: Diagnosis of nosocomial bacterial pneumonia in intubated patients undergoing ventilation: comparison of the usefulness of bronchoalveolar lavage and protected specimen brush. Am J Med 85:499, 1988
113. Johanson WG, Seidenfeld JJ, Gomez P, et al: Bacteriologic diagnosis of nosocomial pneumonia following prolonged mechanical ventilation. Am Rev Respir Dis 137:259, 1988
114. Meduri GU, Chastre J: The standardization of bronchoscopic techniques for ventilator-associated pneumonia. Chest 102:557S, 1992
115. Muckart DJ, Thomson SR: Undetected injuries: a preventable cause of increased morbidity and mortality. Am J Surg 162:457, 1991
116. Davis JW, Hoyt DB, McArdle MS, et al: The significance of critical care errors in causing preventable death in trauma patients in a trauma system. J Trauma 31:813, 1991
117. Deneke SM, Fanburg BL: Normobaric oxygen toxicity of the lung. N Engl J Med 303:76, 1980
118. Parker JC, Hernandez LA, Peevy KJ: Mechanisms of ventilator induced lung injury. Crit Care Med 21:131, 1993
119. Maetani S, Nishikawa T, Tobe T, et al: Role of blood transfusion in organ system failure following major abdominal surgery. Ann Surg 203:275, 1986
120. Hebert PC, Wells G, Marshall J, et al: Transfusion requirements in critical care: a pilot study. JAMA 273:1439, 1995
121. Marik PE, Sibbald WJ: Effect of stored blood transfusion on oxygen delivery in patients with sepsis. JAMA 269:3024, 1993
122. Grant JP, Cox CE, Kleinman LM, et al: Serum hepatic enzyme and bilirubin elevations during parenteral nutrition. Surg Gynecol Obstet 145:2398, 1977
123. Askanazi J, Rosenbaum SH, Hyman AI, et al: Respiratory changes induced by the large glucose loads of total parenteral nutrition. JAMA 243:1444, 1980
124. Alverdy JC, Aoys E, Moss GS: Total parenteral nutrition promotes bacterial translocation from the gut. Surgery 104:185, 1988
125. Moore FA, Moore EE, Jones TN, et al: TEN versus TPN following major abdominal trauma—reduced septic morbidity. J Trauma 29:916, 1989
126. Zaloga GP, Roberts P: Permissive underfeeding. New Horiz 2:257, 1994
127. Marshall JC, Christou NV, Meakins JL: The gastrointestinal tract: the "undrained abscess" of multiple organ failure. Ann Surg 218:111, 1993
128. Driks MR, Craven DE, Celli BR, et al: Nosocomial pneumonia in intubated patients given sucralfate as compared with antacids or histamine type 2 blockers: the role of gastric colonization. N Engl J Med 317:1376, 1987
129. Munoz J, Guerrero JE, Escalante JL, et al: Pressure-controlled ventilation versus controlled mechanical ventilation with decelerating inspiratory flow. Crit Care Med 21:1143, 1993
130. Hickling KG, Walsh J, Henderson S, et al: Low mortality rate in adult respiratory distress syndrome using low-volume, pressure-limited ventilation with permissive hypercapnia: a prospective study. Crit Care Med 22:1568, 1994
131. Räsänen J, Cane RD, Downs JB, et al: Airway pressure release ventilation during acute lung injury: a prospective multicenter trial. Crit Care Med 19:1234, 1991
132. Rossaint R, Falke KJ, Lopez F, et al: Inhaled nitric oxide for the adult respiratory distress syndrome. N Engl J Med 328:399, 1993
133. Zapol WM, Snider MT, Hill JD, et al: Extracorporeal membrane oxygenation in severe acute respiratory failure. JAMA 242:2193, 1979
134. Morris AH, Wallace CJ, Menlovet RL, et al: Randomized clinical trial of pressure-controlled inverse ratio ventilation and extracorporeal CO_2 removal for adult respiratory distress syndrome. Am J Respir Crit Care Med 149:295, 1994
135. Yu M, Levy MM, Smith P, et al: Effect of maximizing oxygen delivery on morbidity and mortality rates in critically ill patients: a prospective, randomized, controlled study. Crit Care Med 21:830, 1993
136. Tuchschmidt J, Fried J, Astiz M, et al: Elevation of cardiac output and oxygen delivery improves

outcome in septic shock. Chest 102:216, 1992
137. Hayes MA, Timmins AC, Yau EHS, et al: Elevation of systemic oxygen delivery in the treatment of critically ill patients. N Engl J Med 330:1717, 1994
138. Hayes MA, Yau EHS, Timmins AC, et al: Response of critically ill patients to treatment aimed at achieving supranormal oxygen delivery and consumption: relationship to outcome. Chest 103:886, 1993
139. Bickell WH, Wall MJ Jr, Pepe PE, et al: Immediate versus delayed fluid resuscitation for hypotensive patients with penetrating torso injuries. N Engl J Med 331:1105, 1994
140. McDonald RH, Goldberg LI, McNay JL, et al: Effects of dopamine in man: augmentation of sodium excretion, glomerular filtration rate, and renal plasma flow. J Clin Invest 45:733, 1973
141. Duke GJ, Bersten AD: Dopamine and renal salvage in the critically ill patient. Anaesth Intens Care 20:277, 1992
142. Krishna GG, Danivitch GM, Beck FWJ, et al: Dopaminergic mediation of the natriuretic response to volume expansion. J Lab Clin Med 105:214, 1985
143. Duke GJ, Briedis JH, Weaver RA: Renal support in critically ill patients: low dose dopamine or low dose dobutamine. Crit Care Med 22:1919, 1994
144. Hirasawa H, Sugai T, Ohtake Y, et al: Continuous hemofiltration and hemodiafiltration in the management of multiple organ failure. Contrib Nephrol 93:42, 1991
145. McDonald BR, Mehta RL: Decreased mortality in patients with acute renal failure undergoing continuous arteriovenous hemodialysis. Contrib Nephrol 93:51, 1991
146. Ronco C: Continuous renal replacement therapies for the treatment of acute renal failure in intensive care patients. Clin Nephrol 40:187, 1993
147. Tonneson E, Hansen MB, Hohndorf K, et al: Cytokines in plasma and ultrafiltrate during continuous arteriovenous haemofiltration. Anaesth Intens Care 21:752, 1993
148. Ronco C, Tetta C, Lupi A, et al: Removal of platelet-activating factor in experimental continuous arteriovenous hemofiltration. Crit Care Med 23:99, 1995
149. Kudsk KA, Croce MA, Fabian TC, et al: Enteral versus parenteral feeding. Ann Surg 215:503, 1992
150. Border JR, Hassett J, LaDuca J, et al: The gut origin septic states in blunt multiple trauma (ISS = 40) in the ICU. Ann Surg 206:427, 1985
151. Cerra FB, McPherson JP, Konstantinides FN, et al: Enteral nutrition does not prevent multiple organ failure syndrome (MOFS) after sepsis. Surgery 104:727, 1988
152. Rozga J, Podesta L, LePage E, et al: A bioartificial liver to treat severe acute liver failure. Ann Surg 219:538, 1994
153. Rotstein OD, Pruett TL, Simmons RL: Microbiologic features and treatment of persistent peritonitis in patients in the intensive care unit. Can J Surg 29:247, 1986
154. Marshall JC, Sweeney D: Microbial infection and the septic response in critical surgical illness: sepsis, not infection, determines outcome. Arch Surg 125:17, 1990
155. Poole GV, Muakkassa FF, Griswold JA: Pneumonia, selective decontamination, and multiple organ failure. Surgery 111:1, 1992
156. Poole GV, Muakkassa FF, Griswold JA: The role of infection in outcome of multiple organ failure. Am Surg 59:727, 1993
157. Rello J, Ausina V, Ricart M, et al: Impact of previous antimicrobial therapy on the etiology and outcome of ventilator associated pneumonia. Chest 104:1230, 1993
158. Wey SB, Mori M, Pfaller MA, et al: Risk factors for hospital acquired *Candidemia*: a matched case control study. Arch Intern Med 149:2349, 1989
159. Rangel-Frausto MS, Pittet D, Costigan M, et al: The natural history of the systemic inflammatory response syndrome. JAMA 273:117, 1995
160. Bone RC, Fisher CJ, Clemmer TP, et al: A controlled clinical trial of high dose methylprednisolone in the treatment of severe sepsis and septic shock. N Engl J Med 317:654, 1987
161. Effect of high dose glucocorticoid therapy on mortality in patients with clinical signs of systemic sepsis. The Veterans Administration Systemic Sepsis Cooperative Study Group. N Engl J Med 317:659, 1987
162. Ferraris VA: Exploratory laparotomy for potential abdominal sepsis in patients with multiple organ failure. Arch Surg 118:1130, 1983
163. Hinsdale JG, Jaffe BM: Re-operation for intraabdominal sepsis: indications and results in modern critical care setting. Ann Surg 199:31, 1984
164. Sutherland RF, Temple WJ, Snodgrass T, et al: Predicting the outcome of exploratory laparotomy in the ICU patients with sepsis or organ failure. J Trauma 29:152, 1989
165. Norton LW: Does drainage of intraabdominal pus reverse multiple organ failure? Am J Surg 149:347, 1985
166. Bunt TJ: Non-directed relaparotomy for intraabdominal sepsis: a futile procedure. Am Surg 52:294, 1986
167. Wolfe BM, Moore PG: Preparation of the intensive care patient for major surgery. World J Surg 17:184, 1993
168. Marshall C, Lindgren L, Marshall BE: Effects of halothane, enflurane, and isoflurane on hypoxic pulmonary vasoconstriction in rat lungs in vitro. Anesthesiology 60:304, 1984
169. Venkataraman ST, Orr RA: Intrahospital transport of critically ill patients. Crit Care Clin 8:525, 1992
170. Insel J, Weissman C, Kemper M, et al: Cardiovascular changes during transport of critically ill and postoperative patients. Crit Care Med 14:539, 1986
171. Futren ND, Dutcher PO, Roberst JK: The safety and efficacy of bedside tracheotomy. Otolaryngol Head Neck Surg 109:707, 1993
172. Goldstein SI, Breda SD, Schneider KL: Surgical complications of bedside tracheotomy in an otolaryngology residency program. Laryngoscope 97:1407, 1987
173. Dayal VS, el Masri W: Tracheotomy in the intensive care setting. Laryngoscope 96:58, 1986
174. Friedman Y, Mayer AD: Bedside tracheotomy in critically ill patients. Chest 104:532, 1993
175. Moore FA, Haenel JB, Moore EE, et al: Percutaneous tracheostomy after trauma and critical illness. J Trauma 32:133, 1992
176. Garcia-Sabrido JL, Tellado JM, Christou NV, et al: Treatment of severe intra-abdominal sepsis and/or necrotic foci by an "open abdomen" approach. Arch Surg 123:152, 1988
177. Faist E, Baue AE, Dittmer H, et al: Multiple organ failure in polytrauma patients. J Trauma 23:775, 1983
178. Pine RW, Wertz MJ, Lennard ES, et al: Determinants of organ malfunction or death in patients with intra-abdominal sepsis: a discriminant analysis. Arch Surg 118:242, 1983
179. Goris RJ, te Boekhorst TP, Nuytinck JK, et al: Multiple-organ failure: generalized autodestructive inflammation? Arch Surg 120:1109, 1985
180. Ranson JHC, Rifkind KM, Turner JW: Prognostic signs and nonoperative peritoneal lavage in acute pancreatitis. Surg Gynecol Obstet 143:209, 1976
181. Ranson JHC, Berman RS: Long peritoneal lavage decreases pancreatic sepsis in acute pancreatitis. Ann Surg 211:708, 1990
182. Cook DJ, Guyatt GH, Jaeschke R, et al: Determinants in Canadian health care workers of the decision to withdraw life support from the critically ill. JAMA 273:703, 1995
183. The Rise of Surgery: From Empiric Craft to Scientific Discipline. Wangensteen OH, Wangensteen SD. University of Minnesota Press, Minneapolis, 1979
184. Blalock A: Experimental shock: the cause of the low blood pressure produced by muscle injury. Arch Surg 20:959, 1930
185. Bywaters EGL, Beall O: Crush injuries with impairment of renal function. Br Med J 1:427, 1941
186. Safar P, DeKornfeld T, Pearson J, et al: Intensive care unit. Anesthesia 16:275, 1961
187. Burke JF, Pontoppidan H, Welch CE: High output respiratory failure: an important cause of death ascribed to peritonitis or ileus. Ann Surg 158:581, 1963
188. Cerra FB: The hypermetabolism organ failure complex. World J Surg 11:173, 1987
189. Rogers DE: The changing pattern of life-threatening microbial disease. N Engl J Med 261:677, 1959
190. McCabe WR, Jackson GG: Gram negative bacteremia: I. Etiology and ecology. Arch Intern Med 110:847, 1962
191. MacLean LD, Meakins JL, Taguchi K, et al: Host resistance in sepsis and trauma. Ann Surg 182:207, 1975
192. Tellado JM, Giannias B, Kapadia B, et al: Anergic patients before elective surgery have enhanced nonspecific host-defense capacity. Arch Surg 125:49, 1990
193. Bone RC: Let's agree on terminology: definitions of sepsis. Crit Care Med 19:973, 1991
194. Sibbald WJ, Marshall JC, Christou NV, et al: "Sepsis"—clarity of existing terminology . . . or more confusion? Crit Care Med 19:996, 1991
195. Sprung CL: Definitions of sepsis: have we reached a consensus? Crit Care Med 19:849, 1991
196. Deitch EA: Multiple organ failure: pathophysiology and potential future therapy. Ann Surg 216:117, 1992
197. Carrico CJ, Meakins JL, Marshall JC, et al: Multiple-organ–failure syndrome. Arch Surg 121:196, 1986
198. Anderson BO, Brown JM, Harken AH: Mechanisms of neutrophil-mediated tissue injury. J Surg Res 51:170, 1991
199. Bone RC: Inhibitors of complement and neutrophils: a critical evaluation of their role in the treatment of sepsis. Crit Care Med 20:891, 1992
200. Smith JA: Neutrophils, host defense, and inflammation: a double-edged sword. J Leukocyte Biol 56:672, 1994
201. Mallick AA, Ishizaka A, Stephens KE, et al: Multiple organ damage caused by tumor necrosis factor and prevented by prior neutrophil depletion. Chest 95:1114, 1989
202. Schmeling DJ, Caty MG, Oldham KT, et al:

Evidence for neutrophil-related acute lung injury after intestinal ischemia reperfusion. Surgery 106:195, 1989
203. Schoenberg MH, Poch B, Younes M, et al: Involvement of neutrophils in postischaemic damage to the small intestine. Gut 32:905, 1991
204. Simpson R, Alon R, Kobzik L, et al: Neutrophil and nonneutrophil mediated injury in intestinal ischemia reperfusion. Ann Surg 218:444, 1993
205. Holman JM, Saba TM: Hepatocyte injury during postopertive sepsis: activated neutrophils as potential mediators. J Leukocyte Biol 43:193, 1988
206. Langdale LA, Flaherty LC, Liggitt HD, et al: Neutrophils contribute to hepatic ischemia reperfusion injury by a CD18 independent mechanism. J Leukocyte Biol 53:511, 1993
207. Sekiya S, Yamashita T, Sendo F: Suppression of late phase enhanced vascular permeability in rats by selective depletion of neutrophils with a monoclonal antibody. J Leukocyte Biol 48:258, 1990
208. Welbourn R, Goldman G, Kobzik L, et al: Interleukin-2 induces early multisystem organ edema mediated by neutrophils. Ann Surg 214:181, 1991
209. Mileski WJ, Winn RK, Vedder NB, et al: Inhibition of CD18-dependent neutrophil adherence reduces organ injury after hemorrhagic shock in primates. Surgery 108:206, 1990
210. Trautinger F, Hammerle AF, Pöschl HG, et al: Respiratory burst capability of polymorphonuclear neutrophils and TNF: serum levels in relationship to the development of septic syndrome in critically ill patients. J Leukocyte Biol 49:449, 1991
211. Tellado JM, Christou NV: Critically ill anergic patients demonstrate polymorphonuclear neutrophil activation in the intravascular compartment with decreased cell delivery to inflammatory foci. J Leukocyte Biol 50:547, 1991
212. Fasano MB, Cousart S, Neal S, et al: Increased expression of the interleukin 1 receptor on blood neutrophils of humans with the sepsis syndrome. J Clin Invest 88:1452, 1991
213. Nahum A, Chamberlin W, Sznajder JI: Differential activation of mixed venous and arterial neutrophils in patients with sepsis syndrome and acute lung injury. Am Rev Respir Dis 143:1083, 1991
214. Ognibene FP, Martin SE, Parker MM: Adult respiratory distress syndrome in patients with severe neutropenia. N Engl J Med 315:547, 1986
215. Border JR: Hypothesis: sepsis, multiple organ failure, and the macrophage. Arch Surg 123:285, 1988
216. Nathan CF: Secretory products of macrophages. J Clin Invest 79:319, 1987
217. Pierce CW: Macrophages: modulators of immunity. Am J Pathol 98:10, 1980
218. Rankin JA, Sylvester I, Smith S, et al: Macrophages cultured in vitro release leukotriene B$_4$ and neutrophil attractant/activation protein (interleukin 8) sequentially in response to stimulation with lipopolysaccharide and zymosan. J Clin Invest 86:1556, 1991
219. Kucey DS, Kubicki EI, Rotstein OD: Platelet activating factor primes endotoxin stimulated macrophage procoagulant activity. J Surg Res 50:436, 1991
220. Keller GA, West MA, Cerra FB, et al: Macrophage mediated modulation of hepatic failure in multiple system failure. J Surg Res 39:555, 1985
221. Arita H, Ogle CK, Alexander JW, et al: Induction of hypermetabolism in guinea pigs by endotoxin infused through the portal vein. Arch Surg 123:1420, 1988
222. Marshall JC, Lee C, Meakins JL, et al: Kupffer cell modulation of the systemic immune response. Arch Surg 122:191, 1987
223. Iimuro Y, Yamamoto M, Kohno H, et al: Blockade of liver macrophages by gadolinium chloride reduces lethality in endotoxemic rats: analysis of mechanisms of lethality in endotoxemia. J Leukocyte Biol 55:723, 1994
224. Callery MP, Kamei T, Flye MW: Kupffer cell blockade increases mortality during intra-abdominal sepsis despite improving systemic immunity. Arch Surg 125:36, 1990
225. Tracey KJ, Fong Y, Hesse DG, et al: Anti-cachectin/TNF monoclonal antibodies prevent septic shock during lethal bacteraemia. Nature 330:662, 1987
226. Beutler B, Cerami A: Cachectin: more than a tumor necrosis factor. N Engl J Med 316:379, 1987
227. Okusawa S, Gelfand JA, Ikejima T, et al: Interleukin 1 induces a shock-like state in rabbits: synergism with tumour necrosis factor and the effect of cyclooxygenase inhibition. J Clin Invest 81:1162, 1988
228. Arend WP: Interleukin-1 receptor antagonist: a new member of the interleukin-1 family. J Clin Invest 88:1445, 1991
229. Anderson BO, Bensard DD, Harken AH: The role of platelet activating factor and its antagonists in shock, sepsis, and multiple organ failure. Surg Gynecol Obstet 172:415, 1991
230. Rabinovici R, Yue T, Farhat M, et al: Platelet activating factor (PAF) and tumor necrosis factor-α (TNF-α) interactions in endotoxemic shock: studies with BN 50739, a novel (PAF) antagonist. J Pharmacol Exp Ther 255:256, 1990
231. Kuhn R, Lohler J, Rennick D, et al: Interleukin-10 deficient mice develop chronic enterocolitis. Cell 75:263, 1993
232. Donnelly TJ, Meade P, Jagels M, et al: Cytokine, complement, and endotoxin profiles associated with the development of the adult respiratory distress syndrome after severe injury. Crit Care Med 22:768, 1994
233. Casey LC, Balk RA, Bone RC: Plasma cytokines and endotoxin levels correlate with survival in patients with the sepsis syndrome. Ann Intern Med 119:771, 1993
234. Hack CE, De Groot E, Felt-Bersma RJF, et al: Increased plasma levels of interleukin-6 in sepsis. Blood 74:1704, 1989
235. Damas P, Ledoux D, Nys M, et al: Cytokine serum level during severe sepsis in human IL-6 as a marker of severity. Ann Surg 215:356, 1992
236. Hack CE, Hart M, Strack van Schijndel RJM, et al: Interleukin-8 in sepsis: relation to shock and inflammatory mediators. Infect Immun 60:2835, 1992
237. Chollet-Martin S, Montravers P, Gibert C, et al: High levels of interleukin-8 in the blood and alveolar spaces of patients with pneumonia and adult respiratory distress syndrome. Infect Immun 61:4553, 1993
238. Marty C, Misset B, Tamion F, et al: Circulating interleukin-8 concentrations in patients with multiple organ failure of septic and nonseptic origin. Crit Care Med 22:673, 1994
239. Nuytinck HKS, Offermans X, Kubat K, et al: Whole-body inflammation in trauma patients. Arch Surg 123:1519, 1988
240. Carlos TM, Harlan JM: Leukocyte-endothelial adhesion molecules. Blood 84:2068, 1995
241. Talbott GA, Sharar SR, Harlan JM, et al: Leukocyte-endothelial interactions and organ injury: the role of adhesion molecules. New Horiz 2:545, 1994
242. Pober JS, Cotran RS: Cytokines and endothelial cell biology. Physiol Rev 70:427, 1990
243. Mulligan MS, Till GO, Smith CW, et al: Role of leukocyte adhesion molecules in lung and dermal vascular injury after thermal trauma of skin. Am J Pathol 144:1008, 1994
244. Walsh CJ, Carey PD, Cook DJ, et al: Anti-CD18 antibody attenuates neutropenia and alveolar capillary-membrane injury during gram-negative sepsis. Surgery 110:205, 1991
245. Weixiong H, Aneman A, Nilsson U, et al: Quantification of tissue damage in the feline small intestine during ischemia-reperfusion: the importance of free radicals. Acta Physiol Scand 150:241, 1994
246. Kehrer JP: Free radicals as mediators of tissue injury and disease. Crit Rev Toxicol 23:21, 1993
247. Buttke TM, Sandstrom PA: Oxidative stress as a mediator of apoptosis. Immunol Today 15:7, 1994
248. Patel KD, Zimmerman GA, Prescott SM, et al: Oxygen radicals induce human endothelial cells to express GMP-140 and bind neutrophils. J Cell Biol 112:749, 1991
249. Lo SK, Janakidevi K, Lai L, et al: Hydrogen peroxide-induced increase in endothelial adhesiveness is dependent on ICAM-1 activation. Am J Physiol 264:L406, 1993
250. Lewis MS, Whatley P, Cain TM, et al: Hydrogen peroxide stimulates the synthesis of platelet-activating factor by endothelial and induces endothelial cell–dependent neutrophil adhesion. J Clin Invest 82:2045, 1988
251. Anner H, Kaufman RP, Kobzik L, et al: Pulmonary hypertension and leukosequestration after lower torso ischemia. Ann Surg 206:642, 1987
252. Lillehei RC: The intestinal factor in irreversible hemorrhagic shock. Surgery 42:1043, 1957
253. Fine J, Frank ED, Ravin HA, et al: The bacterial factor in traumatic shock. N Engl J Med 260:214, 1959
254. Deitch EA: The role of intestinal barrier failure and bacterial translocation in the development of systemic infection and multiple organ failure. Arch Surg 125:403, 1990
255. Lee A: Neglected niches: the microbial ecology of the gastrointestinal tract. Adv Microbial Ecol 8:115, 1985
256. Johanson WG, Pierce AK, Sanford JP: Changing pharyngeal bacterial flora of hospitalized patients. N Engl J Med 281:1137, 1969
257. Garvey BM, McCambley JA, Tuxen DV: Effects of gastric alkalization on bacterial colonization in critically ill patients. Crit Care Med 17:211, 1989
258. Hillman KM, Riordan T, O'Farrell SM, et al: Colonization of the gastric contents in critically ill patients. Crit Care Med 10:444, 1982
259. Craven DE, Driks MR: Nosocomial pneumonia in the intubated patient. Semin Respir Infect 2:20, 1987
260. Wells CL, Maddaus MA, Simmons RL: Proposed mechanisms for the translocation of intestinal bacteria. Rev Infect Dis 10:958, 1988
261. Krause W, Matheis H, Wulf K: Fungaemia and funguria after oral administration of *Candida albicans*. Lancet 1:598, 1969
262. Fiddian-Green RG, Gantz NM: Transient episodes of sigmoid ischemia and their relation to infection from intestinal organisms after

262. ...abdominal aortic operations. Crit Care Med 15:835, 1987
263. Levy J, Van Laethem Y, Verhaegen G, et al: Contaminated enteral nutrition solutions as a cause of nosocomial bloodstream infection: a study using plasmid fingerprinting. J Parenter Enteral Nutr 13:228, 1989
264. Moore FA, Moore EE, Poggetti R, et al: Gut bacterial translocation via the portal vein: a clinical perspective with major torso trauma. J Trauma 31:629, 1991
265. Winchurch RA, Thupari JN, Munster AM: Endotoxemia in burn patients: levels of circulating endotoxins are related to burn size. Surgery 102:808, 1987
266. Roumen RM, Hendriks T, van der Jongekrijg J, et al: Cytokine patterns in patients after major vascular surgery, hemorrhagic shock, and severe blunt trauma: relation with subsequent adult respiratory distress syndrome and multiple organ failure. Ann Surg 218:769, 1993
267. Tomasi TB: Oral tolerance. Transplantation 29:353, 1980
268. Nathens AB, Rotstein OD, Dackiw A, et al: Intestinal epithelial cells downregulate macrophage TNF production: a mechanism for immune regulation in the gut-associated lymphoid tissues. Surgery 118:343, 1995
269. Deitch EA, Xu D, Franko L, et al: Evidence favoring the role of the gut as a cytokine generating organ in rats subjected to hemorrhagic shock. Shock 1:141, 1994
270. Caty MG, Guice KS, Oldham KT, et al: Evidence for tumor necrosis factor induced pulmonary microvascular injury after intestinal ischemia-reperfusion injury. Ann Surg 212:694, 1990
271. Cabie A, Farkas JC, Fitting C, et al: High levels of portal TNF-alpha during abdominal aortic surgery in man. Cytokine 5:448, 1993
272. Marshall JC, Ribeiro MB, Chu PTY, et al: Portal endotoxemia stimulates the release of an immunosuppressive factor from alveolar and splenic macrophages. J Surg Res 55:14, 1993
273. Nieuwenhuijzen GAP, Haskel Y, Lu Q, et al: Macrophage elimination increases bacterial translocation and gut origin septicemia but attenuates symptoms and mortality rate in a model of systemic inflammation. Ann Surg 218:791, 1993
274. Moore FA, Moore EE: Evolving concepts in the pathogenesis of postinjury multiple organ failure. Surg Clin North Am 75:257, 1995
275. Fisher CJ, Slotman GJ, Opal SM, et al: Initial evaluation of human recombinant interleukin-1 receptor antagonist in the treatment of sepsis syndrome: a randomized, open-label, placebo-controlled multicenter trial. Crit Care Med 22:12, 1994
276. Dhainaut J-FA, Tenaillon A, Le Tulzo Y, et al: Platelet-activating factor receptor antagonist BN 52021 in the treatment of severe sepsis: a randomized, double-blind, placebo-controlled, multicenter clinical trial. Crit Care Med 22:1720, 1994
277. Bone RC, Fisher CJ, Clemmer TP, et al: Sepsis syndrome: a valid clinical entity. Crit Care Med 17:389, 1989
278. Knaus WA, Harrell F, Fisher CJ, et al: The clinical evaluation of new drugs for sepsis: a prospective study design based on survival analysis. JAMA 270:1233, 1993
279. Le Gall J-R, Lemeshow S, Leleu G, et al: Customized probability models for early severe sepsis in adult intensive care patients. JAMA 273:644, 1995
280. Petros AJ, Marshall JC, van Saene HKF: Should morbidity replace mortality as an endpoint for clinical trials in intensive care? Lancet 345:369, 1995
281. McClelland P, Williams PS, Yaqoob M, et al: Multiple organ failure: role for plasma exchange? Intensive Care Med 16:100, 1990
282. Ahren B, Evander A, Hammarstrom L-E, et al: Plasmapheresis and hemodialysis in a case of septic cholangitis complicated by hepatic and renal failure. Acta Chir Scand 154:157, 1988
283. Barzilay E, Kessler D, Berlot G, et al: Use of extracorporeal supportive techniques as additional treatment for septic-induced multiple organ failure patients. Crit Care Med 17:634, 1989
284. Aoki H, Kodama M, Tani T, et al: Treatment of sepsis by extracorporeal elimination of endotoxin using polymyxin B-immobilized fiber. Am J Surg 167:412, 1994
285. Vincent J-L, Moreno R, Takala J, et al: The SOFA (sepsis-related organ failure assessment) score to describe organ dysfunction/failure. Intensive Care Med 22:707, 1996
286. Bernard GR, Doig BG, Hudson G, et al: Quantification of organ failure for clinical trials and clinical practice. Am J Respir Crit Care Med 151:A323, 1995

Acknowledgment

Figure 1 Marcia Kammerer.

96 METABOLIC RESPONSE TO CRITICAL ILLNESS

Palmer Q. Bessey, M.D.

Metabolic Responses in Surgical Patients

Debility commonly accompanies surgical illness. It occurs in varying degrees after elective operations, major trauma, burns, infections, and other critical illnesses. Debility is caused by a variety of factors, including specific biochemical and physiologic alterations that usually occur in response to injury and disease, especially those that persist for a long time. Some aspects of surgical care that are common to almost all patients can also cause debility. This discussion will review these clinical factors and metabolic responses in critically ill surgical patients and will indicate how the clinician can manage them so as to minimize patient debility.

The metabolic responses to critical illness have been studied in a variety of critically ill patients, especially those with trauma, burns, or sepsis. The responses are often grouped into phases on the basis of their temporal relation to the injury or insult. The so-called ebb phase, which is the early phase of the injury response, is characterized by (1) an elevated blood glucose level, (2) normal glucose production, (3) elevated free fatty acid levels, (4) a low insulin concentration, (5) elevated levels of catecholamines and glucagon, (6) an elevated blood lactate level, (7) depressed oxygen consumption, (8) below-normal cardiac output, and (9) below-normal core temperature.[1] The subsequent phase, the so-called flow phase, is characterized by (1) a normal or slightly elevated blood glucose level, (2) increased glucose production, (3) normal or slightly elevated free fatty acid levels, with flux increased, (4) a normal or elevated insulin concentration, (5) high normal or elevated levels of catecholamine and an elevated glucagon level, (6) a normal blood lactate level, (7) elevated oxygen consumption, (8) increased cardiac output, and (9) elevated core temperature.[1]

The ebb phase is dominated by cardiovascular instability, alterations in circulating blood volume, impairment of oxygen transport, and heightened autonomic activity. Emergency support of cardiopulmonary performance is the paramount therapeutic concern. Shock [*see 4 Shock*] is the prototypical clinical manifestation of the ebb phase. After effective resuscitation has been accomplished and restoration of satisfactory oxygen transport has been achieved, the flow phase comes into play. These responses are marked by hyperdynamic circulatory changes, signs of inflammation, glucose intolerance, and muscle wasting. Surgical patients in the ICU usually exhibit these clinical features; these patients and the clinical challenge they pose are the focus of this chapter.

When wounds are closed and infection has resolved, repletion of lean tissue and fat stores and restoration of strength and stamina can begin. This final, anabolic phase often begins near the time of hospital discharge and may persist for months before the patient fully recovers.

Features of Critical Illness That Can Cause Debility

THE WOUND

The surgical wound is not only a site of tissue disruption but also a site of inflammation and repair [*see 8 Acute Wound Care*]. After resuscitation, the surgeon's principal task is to expedite and promote wound healing and restore tissue integrity. Because the wound is often the proximate cause of patient debility, providing optimal wound care amounts to providing the best patient care.

Wounds with necrotic or devitalized tissue (e.g., from ischemic necrosis, gangrene, or burns), foreign debris, or grossly contaminated material do not heal readily, if they heal at all. Necrotic tissue and eschar (slough) must be debrided, usually surgically, although application of enzymatic agents to wounds has also been effective in some cases. Foreign material must be removed by either hydrotherapy or debridement. Pus must be drained or removed by irrigation and dressing changes. Contaminated wounds are left open so that they can be repeatedly examined and further necrotic material can be removed. Open wounds should be covered with a dressing to prevent drying (i.e., tissue oxidation) and further tissue slough, to reduce bacterial contamination, and to prevent further mechanical injury. Unfortunately, none of the currently available dressing materials achieve all of these goals. Once it becomes apparent that the wound tissues are viable and uninfected, the wound should be closed primarily if possible or with a skin graft.

The cellular processes involved in wound healing are critically dependent on adequate perfusion and delivery of oxygen, glucose, and other essential nutrients. Inadequate perfusion may result in relative tissue ischemia and delay wound healing. A principal responsibility of the clinician is therefore to ensure adequate tissue perfusion during the entire period of wound healing. For instance, resuscitation from shock should be continued after blood pressure is stabilized and until there is clinical evidence of adequate flow—usually associated with warm extremities, pink nail beds, brisk capillary refilling, full peripheral pulses, urine output greater than 0.5 ml/kg/hr (50 to 70 ml/hr in adults), clear sensorium, and improving metabolic acidosis. Adequate oxygenation must also be ensured. Occasionally, invasive monitoring of cardiopulmonary performance and tissue oxygenation as well as pharmacologic support may be required to ensure adequate perfusion and oxygen delivery.

Contused tissue, fractures, tissues surrounding an abscess or site of infection, inflammatory sites such as the pancreas in pancreatitis or the lung in acute respiratory distress syndrome (ARDS)—in fact, any mass of inflammatory tissue—can be considered to constitute the patient's wound because resolution of those focal sites of inflammation depends on the same basic cellular processes as does healing of an external wound.

Patients with a large total mass of inflammatory tissue—large wounds—usually are critically ill and clearly manifest most of the metabolic responses associated with critical illness [see Metabolic Responses That Can Cause Debility, below]. In contrast, patients with small wounds do not appear critically ill and are not significantly debilitated. Although elective operations result in wounds, the incisions are made under sterile, controlled conditions; there is minimal direct tissue injury, little contamination, no shock, and limited net loss of blood and fluid. The incisions are closed primarily and most often heal expeditiously. With the proliferation of minimally invasive surgical techniques in the past several years, operative incisions are now even more limited, patients recover more rapidly, and the resultant debility is minimal—often little more than a transient indisposition.

PAIN

Virtually all surgical patients experience some pain. Pain usually occurs in association with an incision or with a wound resulting from fracture, burn, contusion, or another type of injury. In addition to creating an unpleasant subjective experience, pain often limits physical activities, such as turning in bed, deep breathing, coughing, and walking, and thereby directly interferes with recovery. A variety of techniques are available for pain management. However, each approach has side effects, the potential for abuse, or other features that limit its application.

Acute pain has traditionally been managed by intermittent parenteral administration of narcotic analgesics when requested by the patient or when the nurse perceives the patient to be in pain. The intravenous route is now preferred, because it does not require a painful injection and avoids potential uptake abnormalities. Intravenous analgesics have a short duration of action and must be given frequently to maintain good, sustained pain control; the dose also must be relatively small to minimize the side effects of sedation and impaired gastric motility. Thus, this approach to pain control is relatively labor intensive. Theoretically, this approach can prevent overuse of narcotics; in practice, it often results in inconsistent pain control and underdosing.

Continuous infusion of narcotic analgesics provides more consistent pain control and is common in the ICU. The dose should be adjusted upward before painful procedures but otherwise should be kept as low as possible to avoid ileus and prolonged sedation. Patient-controlled analgesia (PCA) is an extension of this approach. The patient controls a pump that administers a prescribed dose of the agent when activated; the clinician determines the amount of drug in each dose and the total dose permissible in a given period. This technique has been well accepted by patients who are awake and alert and are capable of controlling the system. One benefit is that the total amount of drug administered for pain relief is usually less than is given in a conventional as-needed dosing schedule.[2]

Administration of local anesthetics or narcotics into the epidural space may provide effective local pain relief without the sedating effects of parenteral narcotics. In addition, epidural anesthetics (but not opioids) reduce postoperative ileus.[3] Effective epidural analgesia can be maintained for several days and may have a beneficial effect on pulmonary function in patients with rib fractures or truncal wounds.[4] This technique requires placement of a catheter in the epidural space.

Patients must be monitored closely, and the dosage schedule must be individualized. This technique is best suited to patients who will be relatively inactive for 24 to 36 hours postoperatively and who can be observed closely, such as patients in the ICU.

INFLAMMATION

Elevation of body temperature above normal, leukocytosis, and other signs of inflammation are common features of critical surgical illness and should be expected. The extent of temperature elevation is generally proportional to the severity of illness. In a patient with a major burn—an extreme example of critical surgical illness—body temperature may be as high as 39° C (102.2° F). The leukocyte count is also typically elevated and may be as high as 20,000 cells/ mm^3 during satisfactory recovery. A normal or subnormal body temperature or white blood cell count is atypical and may indicate sepsis, drug-induced leukopenia, or limited physiologic reserve. For example, a critically ill elderly patient with a major injury or infection may be afebrile and have a white blood cell count in the normal range.

Fever, however, is also a cardinal sign of infection. It may be difficult to distinguish between a typical postoperative or posttraumatic fever and a fever caused by invasive infection. An acute elevation in rectal temperature of 1.0° to 1.5° C (1.8° to 2.7° F) that occurs within a short period or a rectal temperature higher than 38.5° C (101.3° F) should be considered indicative of infection and should be investigated thoroughly. Sputum, urine, and blood cultures should be obtained, and all wounds should be inspected carefully for signs of inflammation or infection. Devices commonly associated with nosocomial infection—intravenous cannulas, urinary catheters, and endotracheal tubes—should be removed as soon as feasible or else changed (see below).

Because inflammation is such a prominent feature of all critical illness, including that in patients with serious infectious complications of chronic diseases, several clinical syndromes have been defined in an effort to stratify patients according to the severity of their inflammatory responses [see Table 1].[5] These syndromes are associated with increased mortality, even in the absence of documented infection.[6] In the remainder of this chapter, I will refer repeatedly to the metabolic responses to critical illness; this term incorporates these inflammatory syndromes and more besides, and its use permits a more comprehensive discussion.

Mild elevation of body temperature is usually well tolerated and requires no specific treatment. However, a higher fever may impose significant stress on the patient, as indicated by pronounced tachycardia, tachypnea, malaise, and, occasionally, restlessness. Thus, a body temperature higher than 39° C (102.2° F) is usually treated with antipyretics (acetaminophen, aspirin, indomethacin, or ibuprofen).

The fever experienced by critically ill patients is an upward adjustment of the thermoregulatory center in the brain, the central thermostat [see 98 Fever, Hyperpyrexia, and Hypothermia]. A consequence of this adjustment is that the patient usually prefers a warmer environmental temperature than do normal individuals. An ambient temperature in the hospital that is comfortable for the staff is often perceived as cool by the patient, who must generate extra heat to maintain the adjusted body temperature. Thus, patient areas of the

sion]. The syndrome of multiorgan failure and sepsis that may develop in association with the metabolic responses to critical illness is often the final route to death [see 95 Multiple Organ Dysfunction Syndrome]. Thus, in some ways, certain metabolic responses seem maladaptive in that they retard recovery and lead to organ failure and death.

An improved understanding of the metabolic responses to critical illness may benefit patients in two ways. First, it may facilitate the development of improved supportive therapies. Much of current critical care practice is based on our understanding of these processes and has been designed to support them. Second, a better understanding of the mechanisms underlying the metabolic responses to critical illness may lead to strategies for altering the responses in such a way that those features that are beneficial and promote recovery are stimulated and those features that are debilitating or lead to organ system dysfunction are suppressed or limited.

Integrated Metabolic Response to Critical Illness

The metabolic responses to injury and critical illness occur simultaneously. They primarily involve the liver, skeletal muscle, the gut, the kidneys, and the wound or focus of inflammation [see Figure 3]. The heart also plays a major role by providing the motive force for the high rate of blood flow that is required to support increased exchange of nutrients and other substances between organs. The central and autonomic nervous systems and endocrine tissues are mainly involved in regulation of the responses.

The wound, which may include one or more foci of infection and other sites of inflammation in addition to external injuries, plays a principal role. It acts as a large arteriovenous shunt, robbing the host of blood supply and demanding increased cardiovascular work. The wound also induces and controls profound metabolic changes, which subside as the wound heals. Tissues are broken down, presumably to provide substrates for a variety of synthetic and energy-producing processes. The cost to the patient is increased metabolic work, elevated energy requirements, erosion of lean body tissue, and debility.

The healing wound is a site of intense metabolic activity. Dissolution and removal of necrotic tissue, containment and killing of bacteria, collagen synthesis and wound repair, cellular proliferation, and restoration of tissue integrity occur, often simultaneously. These processes require energy and a variety of substrates, particularly amino acids for protein synthesis. The microenvironment of a wound is often relatively hypoxic. However, inflammatory cells have a marked capacity for glycolytic metabolism,[15] in which adenosine triphosphate (ATP) can be generated without the consumption of oxygen. This capacity persists even when oxygen delivery is sufficient. Glucose is thus the principal fuel for the healing wound. It is metabolized to lactate, which is then released into the circulation for transport to the liver.

The liver produces the additional glucose that is required by the wound. It is capable of manufacturing glucose from lactate. In this manner, glucose is recycled between the liver and the wound, and there is no net gain or loss of carbon atoms. The liver also synthesizes glucose from amino acids, principally alanine, which comes from both skeletal muscle and the gut. This mechanism is termed gluconeogenesis. The nitrogen contained in the amino acids is converted to urea and excreted. The liver also synthesizes a variety of circulating proteins in response to inflammation and infection (so-called acute-phase proteins). All of these synthetic processes require energy, produced in part by fat oxidation, and therefore contribute to a general increase in energy utilization, heat production, and metabolic rate.

Skeletal muscle protein breaks down at an accelerated rate after injury and critical illness, releasing a variety of substances into the circulation, including creatine and creatinine, 3-methylhistidine, potassium, magnesium, and amino acids. The amino acids serve as precursors for protein synthesis in the wound and in the liver. The released amino acids do not reflect a simple dissolution of protein. Rather, alanine and glutamine are disproportionately released. Alanine can be readily converted to glucose in the liver. Glutamine serves both as a fuel—especially for the gut and for rapidly proliferating cells, including inflammatory cells and fibroblasts—and as a precursor for renal ammonia production, which is an important mechanism for neutralizing excreted acid loads.

Although muscle tissue in healthy persons is usually quite sensitive to insulin and commonly serves as a site of glucose storage, muscle is resistant to insulin after injury or critical illness, and its capacity for glucose storage is reduced significantly. This response contributes to glucose intolerance and helps direct glucose to the healing wound.

The gut was long considered to be essentially inactive during convalescence, but it now appears to play a central role in the metabolic response to critical illness [see 97 Nutritional Support]. During critical illness, the gut utilizes glutamine as its principal fuel, converting glutamine to alanine, which is transported to the liver by the portal circulation. More important, perhaps, the gut can be a portal of entry for bacteria and bacterial toxins, which can worsen or perpetuate critical illness [see 95 Multiple Organ Dysfunction Syndrome and 82 Peritonitis and Intra-abdominal Abscesses].

The kidneys also contribute to the generalized increase in physiologic work and energy requirements that accompanies critical illness. The kidneys must excrete an increased solute load consisting of urea, potassium, magnesium, weak acids, and other intracellular constituents. In addition, many drugs and their metabolites depend on renal excretion. Production of ammonia from glutamine may be increased to neutralize acid loads. Many of these processes require energy.

All of these regional metabolic processes occur simultaneously. The net integrated metabolic response is evident clinically as increased energy expenditure and heat production, fever, accelerated nitrogen excretion and muscle wasting, and glucose intolerance. The wound appears to exert a controlling influence on the intensity and duration of the responses to critical illness or injury: the intensity is proportional to the size of the wound or the mass of inflammatory tissue. The larger the wound, the more intense the metabolic responses. As the wound heals and as inflammation subsides, the heightened metabolic demands abate. Expeditious wound closure and definitive treatment of infection are the most effective forms of anticatabolic therapy.

Hypermetabolism

Because humans maintain fairly constant body temperature, the heat generated by the body is equal to the heat lost in biochemical and physiologic processes and is an indicator of overall metabolic activity. This heat ultimately results from the oxidation of organic fuels. The rate of heat production, or metabolic rate (MR), is therefore related to $\dot{V}O_2$ and $\dot{V}CO_2$. It may be measured directly by means of direct calorimetry, or it may be calculated from measurements of $\dot{V}O_2$, $\dot{V}CO_2$, and body surface area (BSA) by means of indirect calorimetry:

$$MR\ (kcal/m^2/hr) = \frac{[(3.9 \times \dot{V}O_2\ [L/min]) + (1.1 \times \dot{V}CO_2\ [L/min])] \times 60\ (min/hr)}{BSA\ (m^2)}$$

A third term, $-3.3 \times$ urea nitrogen loss (g/time), is sometimes added to account for the heat produced by urea formation. However, it is usually a small factor, adjusting MR by only 2% to 3%.[16]

Values determined by direct and indirect calorimetry under steady-

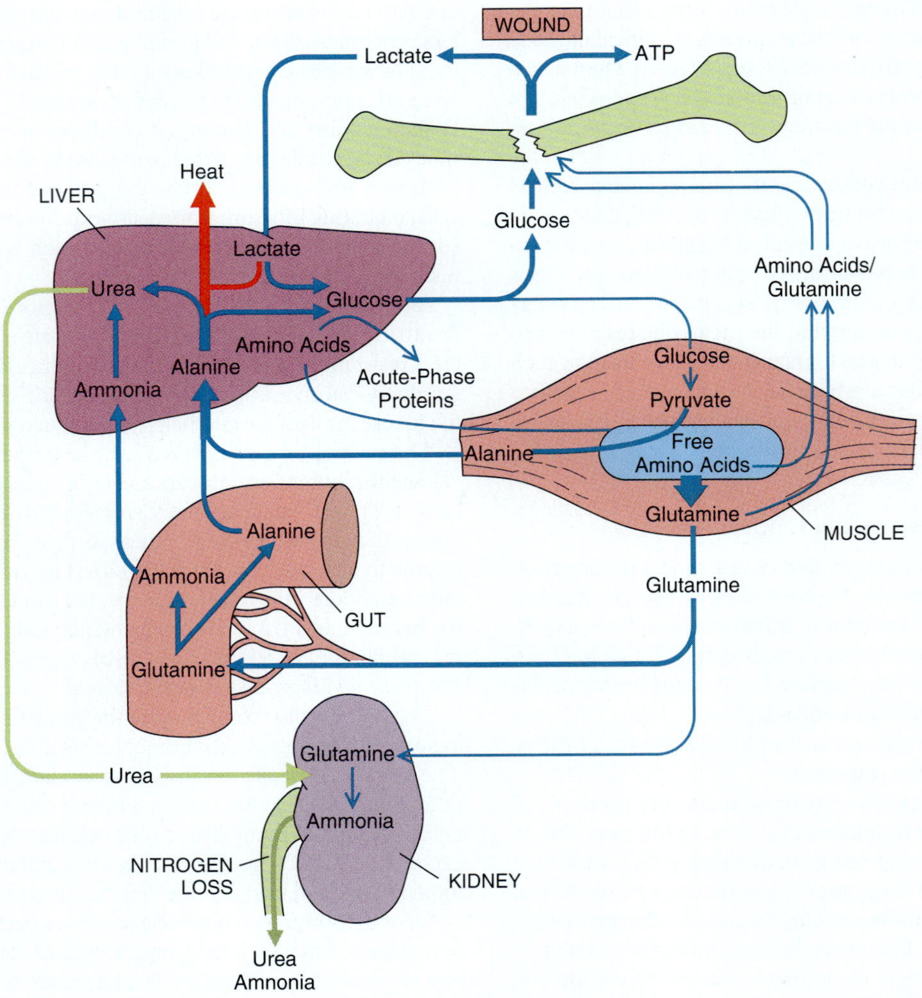

Figure 3 The metabolic response to critical illness includes characteristic alterations in the exchange of substrates between organs. Presumably, these responses occur in support of the healing wound and are facilitated by a hyperdynamic circulation. The wound requires glucose (and probably glutamine) as a primary respiratory fuel. Glucose is converted to lactate; this conversion can occur in an aerobic environment. Lactate is transported to the liver for conversion back into glucose. The recycling of lactate to glucose is a major pathway that requires the input of energy and thereby contributes to increased energy utilization. Most of the glucose required for the healing wound (i.e., inflammatory tissue) is produced by the liver, not only from lactate but also from alanine and other glucogenic amino acids. These reactions require energy and also result in the formation of urea. Muscle is the major source of amino acids, which are used for protein synthesis both in the wound and in the liver. The most abundant amino acids released from muscle are alanine and glutamine. Glutamine serves as a primary fuel for the gut, producing ammonia and other products (e.g., alanine) that are processed by the liver. In addition, glutamine may help buffer filtered acid loads in the kidneys by the formation of ammonia. These metabolic processes contribute to the hypermetabolism, hyperdynamic circulation, increased nitrogen loss, and glucose intolerance that are clinically evident in critically ill patients.

state conditions are comparable.[17] When metabolic rates of normal individuals are determined under controlled basal conditions, the values are reproducible and predictable (± 12%) on the basis of age, sex, and body size.[18] When metabolic rates of critically ill patients with satisfactory hemodynamic function are determined under similar conditions, the rates are greater than predicted. Thus, patients are said to be hypermetabolic.

The degree of hypermetabolism is proportional to the severity of illness. This phenomenon was most dramatically demonstrated in careful studies of burn patients performed in the 1970s.[19] The increase in resting metabolic rate was proportional to the extent of tissue injury—that is, to the amount of the BSA that was burned. Hypermetabolism has also been demonstrated in a variety of other critically ill patients, but it has usually been less severe than that seen in patients with major burns.[20] In the burn patients, moreover, there was a limit to the hypermetabolism: metabolic rates of patients with extensive burns were little different from those of patients with burns covering 50% to 60% of BSA.

These observations suggest that there is a limit to the metabolic activity that patients can support in response to critical illness. The difference between this limit and the magnitude of the patient's actual responses defines physiologic reserve [*see Figure 4*]. Physiologic reserve is presumably also affected by the patient's age and state of health before the critical illness. It reflects the patient's ability to meet additional complicating stresses, such as infection, volume loss, pain, anxiety, and cold ambient temperatures. For example, when patients are exposed to progressively colder ambient temperatures, the metabolic rate generally increases. However, when a group of patients with very large burns were exposed to cold temperatures, their already high metabolic rates did not increase but actually fell.[19] None of these patients survived the injury, presumably because of inability to respond to new stresses. In another group of burn patients, the inability to increase metabolic rate to facilitate rewarming after skin grafting procedures also identified nonsurvivors.[21] When patients are cared for in a warm environment, hypermetabolism is reduced and physiologic reserve is increased.

Hypermetabolism refers to an increase in total body oxidative metabolism that is manifested by increases in total body $\dot{V}O_2$, cardiac output, and MR. Regional $\dot{V}O_2$ is generally increased throughout most tissue beds, but regional blood flow is not. The additional total body flow is directed largely to the wound or site of inflammation and to the splanchnic circulation, and it appears to supply the wound with increased amounts of glucose and other nutrients. In studies of patients who had sustained a large burn on one leg and no burn on the other, Wilmore and colleagues found that $\dot{V}O_2$ of both limbs was increased in proportion to the total BSA burned and represented a fairly constant 6% of total body $\dot{V}O_2$.[22] However, blood flow to the injured extremity was approximately twice that to the uninjured limb. Blood flow was proportional to the extent of the local injury and was directed to the surface wound.[23]

Oxygen consumption by the splanchnic and renal circulations also increases in proportion to total body $\dot{V}O_2$ and hence in proportion to total body injury.[24] Splanchnic flow increases in proportion to total body flow (cardiac output), and together with the blood flow to the wound, it accounts for a large part of the increase in cardiac output in critically ill patients.[25] The increase in renal blood flow correlates with solute load rather than with $\dot{V}O_2$. From these and other studies, it is possible to calculate how oxygen consumption and cardiac output are partitioned among different vascular beds.[26]

Altered Temperature Regulation

Body temperature is determined by the balance between heat production and heat loss [see 98 Fever, Hyperpyrexia, and Hypothermia]. It is normally closely regulated and maintained within a narrow range. Critically ill patients typically have an elevated body temperature, even in the absence of clinical infection.[27] Heat production, as measured by metabolic rate, is increased in the critically ill patient. Heat loss may also be elevated in these patients.

It was once thought that increased evaporative heat loss was the driving force for hypermetabolism, at least in burn patients.[28,29] Barr and associates tested this assumption.[30] Although patients treated in warm, dry air showed substantially increased evaporation of water from the burn wound and more rapid drying of the wound surfaces than did patients exposed to normal ward conditions, they had reduced hypermetabolism and a smaller degree of weight loss.

Several other studies have examined the relation between thermoregulatory factors (evaporative heat loss and ambient temperature) and hypermetabolism. For example, the metabolic rates of burn patients were determined at several ambient temperatures, ranging from 19° to 33° C (66.2° to 91.4° F) [see Table 3].[31] Metabolic rate decreased as ambient temperature was increased, but core temperature remained elevated at all ambient temperatures, indicating that thermoregulation in these patients occurred in relation to an elevated central reference temperature. When febrile burn patients in another study were allowed to set the ambient temperature to achieve thermal comfort, they invariably preferred higher than normal temperatures, in the range of 30° to 33° C (86.0° to 91.4° F).[32] The patients' unburned skin remained relatively vasoconstricted at the higher temperatures as an additional way of maintaining the febrile state. However, even under these conditions of thermal comfort, the patients continued to maintain elevated metabolic rates. Thus, although thermoregulatory factors may influence hypermetabolism, the increased rate of heat production appears to be determined primarily by metabolic factors. Hypermetabolism is temperature sensitive but not temperature dependent.

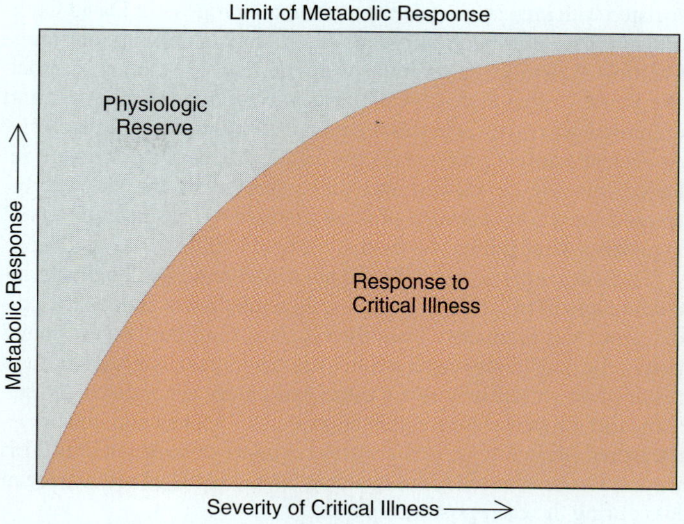

Altered Protein Metabolism

MUSCLE WASTING, NITROGEN LOSS, AND ACCELERATED PROTEIN BREAKDOWN

One of the most striking features of the metabolic response to critical illness is the marked degree of muscle wasting. This atrophy is as-

Figure 4 The intensity of the metabolic response to critical surgical illness increases as a function of the severity of illness. In patients with extremely severe critical illness (e.g., patients with burns covering 60% of the body surface area), responses are near maximal, and physiologic reserves, with which patients respond to additional stressors (e.g., infection, hemorrhage, or cold exposure), are limited. Patients may also have limited physiologic reserves because of preexisting disease, starvation, or advanced age. Therapies that attenuate the stressors of critical surgical illness improve physiologic reserve.

Table 3 Effect of Ambient Temperature on Metabolic Rate and on Core and Skin Temperatures

Ambient Temperature (°C)	N	Core Temperature (°C)	Skin Temperature (°C)	Metabolic Rate (kcal/m²/hr)
Normal subjects				
21	3	36.7	30.0	41.2
25	4	36.8	31.4	35.6
33	4	36.8	34.2	36.3
Burn patients (45% TBS)				
21	9	38.1	32.1	83.7
25	20	38.5	33.1	63.5
33	20	38.0	36.2	62.0

sociated with increased urinary excretion of nitrogen. Sir David Cuthbertson first described this phenomenon in patients with long-bone fractures.[27] Similar observations were made by Howard and associates in the United States.[33] Cuthbertson concluded that injured and uninjured skeletal muscle was the source of the excreted nitrogen.[34,35] As skeletal muscle protein is degraded, a variety of markers are released into the circulation and then excreted by the kidneys. Increased excretion of several of these markers[36,37] has been observed in patients with trauma,[36,38] burns,[39] and infections.[40]

There are other sources of nitrogen loss in critically ill patients, including loss of tissue from slough or excision, loss of blood and exudate, and loss of mucosa from the GI tract. Cuthbertson estimated that in the first 10 days after a burn, the amounts of nitrogen lost as a result of direct tissue injury, wound exudation, generalized catabolism, and atrophy were roughly equivalent.[41] Moore and coworkers measured nitrogen loss in the wound exudate of burn patients. This wound loss accounted for as much as 20% to 30% of total nitrogen loss during the early postburn period.[42]

The time course of nitrogen excretion during critical illness is distinctive. Cuthbertson observed that nitrogen excretion peaked several days after injury and gradually returned to normal during a period of several weeks.[34] The pattern was similar to that of increased oxygen consumption. Thus, both hypermetabolism and muscle proteolysis peak shortly after the onset of critical illness and gradually return to normal as recovery proceeds. This too appears to be a characteristic feature of the metabolic responses to critical illness [see Figure 2].[43-45]

Protein turnover is an indicator of overall protein metabolic activity. It is determined through use of tracers. Both extracellular and intracellular amino acids are considered part of a free amino acid pool. Nitrogen is added to this pool by nitrogen intake (diet) and by protein breakdown. Nitrogen is removed by protein synthesis and by conversion to urea. When a small quantity of a labeled amino acid is infused, the rate of appearance of nitrogen in the free amino acid pool can be determined. Under steady-state conditions, this appearance rate represents protein turnover and matches protein disappearance.[46] During critical illness, protein turnover is increased.[47] When nitrogen turnover data are combined with measurements of nitrogen intake and loss, rates of total body protein synthesis and catabolism can be estimated. These estimates indicate that protein catabolism is increased in critically ill patients.[48] Synthesis rates remain normal during fasting but increase to approach or match catabolic rates when feeding is adequate. Thus, the increase in net nitrogen loss during critical illness appears to result from an increase in protein breakdown. Decreased protein synthesis is less of a factor as long as nutritional intake is satisfactory [see Table 4].

ALTERED AMINO ACID METABOLISM

Protein synthesis and breakdown are processes that occur in cells and involve intracellular amino acids. It has been estimated that skeletal muscle contains as much as 80% of the free amino acid pool.[49] Intracellular concentrations of free amino acids in skeletal muscle are approximately 30 times greater than plasma concentrations of free amino acids.[50] Thus, the total muscle mass of a 70 kg man contains approximately 87 g of free amino acids in the intracellular water, whereas the extracellular pool contains only 1.2 g.

The relative amounts of individual free amino acids in cells differ from the proportions found in protein. Glutamine, a nonessential amino acid, accounts for only about 5% to 6% of protein, but it is the most abundant intracellular free amino acid, accounting for about 60% of the total intracellular free amino acid pool. In contrast, the eight essential amino acids together account for only 8.4% of the intracellular pool. The intracellular concentration of glutamine decreases under many catabolic conditions, including starvation, inactivity,[51] elective operation,[52] trauma,[53] and sepsis.[54] This decrease occurs early in the course of the acute illness, persists until late in convalescence, and appears to be related to the severity of illness.[55,56] The intracellular concentrations of phenylalanine, tyrosine, alanine, and the branched-chain amino acids (BCAAs)—leucine, isoleucine, and valine—typically increase after trauma and infection.[51,54] These levels return to normal during convalescence, usually before glutamine levels do.

Table 4 Alterations in Rates of Protein Synthesis and Catabolism That May Affect Hospitalized Patients

	Synthesis	Catabolism
Normal—starvation	↓	0
Normal—fed, bed rest	↓	0
Elective surgical procedure	↓	0
Injury/sepsis—I.V. dextrose	↑↑	↑↑↑
Injury/sepsis—fed	↑↑↑	↑↑↑

↓—decrease ↑—increase 0—no change

Plasma concentrations of free amino acids generally decrease after operation, injury, or infection, largely because of a fall in the concentrations of the nonessential amino acids. Changes in extracellular concentrations of specific amino acids have been inconsistent between studies, presumably as a reflection of differences in patient selection, analytic methods, or treatment.[54]

The ECF compartment is important for amino acid transport between organs and between regions of the body. Aulick and Wilmore calculated amino acid release rates from peripheral tissues of burn patients on the basis of measurements of leg blood flow and of femoral arterial and venous plasma concentrations of 10 amino acids.[57] The net release of amino acid nitrogen was five times greater in burn patients than in control subjects. Alanine was the only amino acid whose release rate was significantly elevated (glutamine concentration was not determined). Alanine release was related to total burn size (injury severity) and to total body $\dot{V}O_2$. In related studies, the accelerated peripheral amino acid release was matched by increased uptake across the splanchnic bed.[24] Alanine uptake was three to four times control values. This increased release of amino acids from the periphery and transport to splanchnic tissues appears to be another characteristic metabolic response to critical burn injury.

Garber and colleagues observed that glutamine and alanine together constituted as much as 70% of the amino acids released from skeletal muscle in vitro.[58] Furthermore, the release rates of alanine and glutamine reflected the net rates of formation from other amino acids.[59] Thus, during critical illness, skeletal muscle protein is broken down into amino acids that are largely converted to glutamine and alanine, which are then released into the ECF for transport. Although all amino acids are required for protein synthesis at remote locations, glutamine and alanine are the major nitrogen carriers from muscle. These two amino acids have other roles as well. Alanine is a precursor of glucose production in the liver. In that process, urea is also formed and subsequently excreted by the kidneys. Although there may be some minor recycling of urea nitrogen under certain conditions,[60] formation of urea is the final step in the loss of body protein, representing an irreversible loss of nitrogen.

Glutamine is a precursor for production of ammonia in the kidneys, an important buffering mechanism for excreted acid loads. Increased breakdown of intracellular constituents could result in such an acid load, and ammonia excretion is often increased after injury.

Intracellular skeletal muscle glutamine may be an important determinant of net skeletal muscle protein breakdown.[61,62] After a standard operation in an animal model, net amino acid efflux from the hindquarter was increased as the glutamine concentration fell. However, if the intracellular glutamine concentration was maintained by the provision of exogenous glutamine, net efflux was reduced.

Glutamine also appears to be an important respiratory fuel for rapidly dividing cells. Glutamine can be converted to glutamate and then to α-ketoglutarate for participation in the citric acid cycle. The nitrogen of glutamine is used to form ammonia, alanine, and citrulline.[63] This process occurs in colonocytes, enterocytes, fibroblasts, and, possibly, inflammatory cells such as macrophages. Phagocytic cells are found in fixed locations in the GI tract, such as Peyer's patches and other regions containing Kupffer's cells, as well as in the wound, at other sites of inflammation, and in the bone marrow. Windmueller measured the nutrient requirements of the rat intestine using an isolated, perfused segment of small bowel.[63] The intestinal segment extracted large amounts of glutamine from the recirculated perfusate. Souba and Wilmore measured amino acid uptake by the gut in conscious animals and demonstrated that the consumption of glutamine by the gut was significantly increased after celiotomy, even though the circulating glutamine concentration was reduced (i.e., glutamine was actively taken up by the intestine).[64]

Dissolution of skeletal muscle protein during critical illness seems to serve many purposes. First, it provides amino acids to support protein synthesis at remote sites such as the wound, other inflammatory foci, and the liver. Proteolysis also provides amino acid precursors for glucose production by the liver and for production of ammonia in the kidneys. Finally, it provides glutamine, which appears to be a specific fuel for the gut and possibly for other tissues with rapid cell turnover, such as the wound, bone marrow, and fixed macrophages of the GI tract. This mobilization of amino acids from muscle protein, however, leads to an irretrievable loss of nitrogen in the form of urea, ammonia, creatinine, uric acid, and other compounds. The cost to the patient is rapid erosion of muscle mass and debility.

Altered Carbohydrate Metabolism

ACCELERATED ENDOGENOUS GLUCOSE PRODUCTION

The liver normally produces sufficient glucose to permit maintenance of the blood glucose concentration within narrow limits, even during periods of fasting. During critical illness, the rate of endogenous glucose production is increased.[24,65,66] Increased basal glucose production is matched by an increase in glucose uptake, so that glucose levels remain relatively stable. Thus, the mass flow, or turnover, of glucose is increased. In studies of patients with burns, glucose turnover was related to total body $\dot{V}O_2$ and thus to the size of the burn (i.e., to injury severity).[67] Regional uptake was closely related to regional blood flow and regional lactate release but not to regional $\dot{V}O_2$. Thus, glucose was directed by the circulation to the wound, where it was taken up and converted via glycolysis to lactate, even in the presence of adequate or increased oxygen delivery.

The liver produces glucose by a variety of mechanisms. Hydrolysis of hepatic glycogen mobilizes glucose rapidly to serve as an energy source in times of acute need. This mechanism is most important immediately after injury and during acute stress states, such as shock, fever, pain, and anxiety (ebb-phase responses). Glycogen reserves are limited, however, and glycogen is not the major source of hepatic glucose production during recovery from critical illness.

Glucose can also be formed from lactate and from alanine.[68] The conversion of lactate to glucose occurs via the Cori cycle in the liver. Lactate is formed from pyruvate, which is the end product of glycolysis. In critically ill patients with adequate oxygen delivery, the wound is a major source of lactate. Adenosine triphosphate (ATP) is formed during glycolysis and provides energy for the wound, but ATP is required to convert lactate back to glucose. The increased mass flow of glucose serves as a fuel for the healing wound. It may also reflect an inefficient biochemical cycle that requires energy but in which there is no net gain or loss of substrate. Accelerated glucose cycling has been documented both in burn patients and in blunt trauma patients.[69,70] The purpose of these so-called futile cycles is not clear. Because they result in the net generation of heat, they presumably contribute to hypermetabolism. That overall conversion requires net input of ATP and is thus another energy drain for the patient.

GLUCOSE INTOLERANCE AND INSULIN RESISTANCE

When glucose is administered to critically ill patients, hyperglycemia is often the result. Glucose tolerance tests typically yield abnormal results after injury.[71] During shock, immediately after injury or operation, and in the course of ebb-phase responses, the insulin response to hyperglycemia may be blunted. During the flow phase, however, after resuscitation and stabilization, the insulin response to glucose is normal or even exaggerated.[72,73] Both glucose and insulin levels are greater in trauma patients than in control subjects [see Table 5], and the increase in the insulin level is proportionally greater than the rise in glucose.

Black and associates maintained a fixed level of hyperglycemia in patients recovering from trauma by adjusting a glucose infusion on the basis of bedside glucose readings and a negative-feedback algorithm.[74] Because the glucose concentration was at steady state, the glucose infusion rate reflected the rate of total body glucose uptake or disposal. Control subjects demonstrated continuously increasing glucose disposal over time; the glucose infusion rate was increased repeatedly to maintain fixed hyperglycemia. Glucose disposal was closely related to insulin concentration, which increased steadily during the 2-hour study. In contrast, glucose disposal in trauma patients was markedly lower than in control subjects, and it did not increase appreciably over time. The insulin concentrations did, however, increase throughout the study and were always greater than corresponding control values. The trauma patients were therefore less responsive (i.e., were resistant) to insulin.

These investigators also infused insulin into trauma patients and control subjects to maintain specific fixed levels of hyperinsulinemia. During these infusions, the glucose concentration was maintained at basal values (i.e., euglycemia). The glucose infusion rate again reflected total body glucose disposal, which was a function of tissue responsiveness to the insulin level. At all insulin levels, glucose disposal was lower in trauma patients than in control subjects. These studies quantitated posttraumatic insulin resistance and suggested that this response was caused by a postreceptor defect. In similar conditions, Brooks and associates demonstrated reduced forearm glucose uptake, indicating that peripheral tissue—principally skeletal muscle—was a major site of insulin resistance[75] [see Table 6].

Table 5 Basal Glucose and Insulin Concentrations*

	N	Plasma Glucose (mg/dl)	Serum Insulin (μU/ml)
Normal subjects	49	98 ± 1	12 ± 1
Trauma patients	19	104 ± 2	17 ± 2
P		< 0.02	< 0.01

*Mean ± SEM.

Lowe, D. C. Blake; unpublished data). Thus, the interacting effects of multiple hormones and the changing relationships among them over time appear to be capable of inducing, at least qualitatively, most of the metabolic responses to critical illness.

Several investigators have attempted to modulate the catabolic responses of critical illness by altering the endocrine environment. For example, Hulton and colleagues monitored hind-leg amino acid efflux after abdominal operation in an animal model.[99] The accelerated efflux of skeletal muscle amino acids observed postoperatively was attenuated by complete alpha- and beta-adrenergic blockade or by thoracic epidural anesthesia. Both pharmacologic techniques are known to attenuate the hormonal response to operative stress. Brandt and coworkers measured hormonal and protein catabolic responses after abdominal hysterectomy.[100] In the patients who underwent epidural anesthesia, concentrations of cortisol and catecholamines were lower and nitrogen loss was less than in patients who received general anesthesia alone. Tsuji and associates reported similar findings.[101] Subsequent studies have shown that perioperative management of patients with high thoracic epidural analgesia and intravenous somatostatin and etomidate to inhibit elaboration of glucagon and cortisol prevents the typical postoperative increases in amino acid clearance and urea synthesis.[102]

In summary, the altered endocrine environment characteristically associated with critical illness appears to play a major role in mediating the metabolic responses observed in critically ill surgical patients. Simple alteration of the hormonal environment in healthy individuals is capable of inducing many of these metabolic changes; however, the magnitude of these changes is generally less than that observed in critically ill patients. Blunting of the hormonal changes after operation or injury can modulate the catabolic responses.

CYTOKINES

A number of cell types appear in a healing wound soon after injury.[103] These cells are actively involved in angiogenesis, production and remodeling of collagen, scavenging of necrotic debris, and engulfment and killing of bacteria. Many of them release substances that influence cellular proliferation, development, and function and so regulate local inflammation and wound healing. These substances, collectively known as cytokines, can be produced by and interact with a wide variety of cells in addition to inflammatory cells and appear to be major mediators of multiple cellular responses to injury and infection [see 101 Cytokines and the Cellular Response to Injury and Infection].

Certain of the cytokines primarily stimulate inflammatory responses; these are known as proinflammatory cytokines. There are also anti-inflammatory cytokines, which retard inflammatory processes. In addition, specific receptor antagonists have been identified that interfere with the interaction between a cytokine and its cellular receptor. Finally, there are specific soluble receptors, unassociated with a cell, that can effectively neutralize the cytokine before it interacts with a target cell. Both proinflammatory and anti-inflammatory mechanisms may be stimulated together in acute illness.[104] The balance and interactions between them determine the course of the inflammatory process.

The major proinflammatory cytokines, tumor necrosis factor (TNF), interleukin-1 (IL-1), and IL-6, are closely related in that they are elaborated in a characteristic pattern (or cascade) in response to an inflammatory stimulus, such as trauma[105] or endotoxin.[106] TNF appears first, followed by IL-1 and then IL-6. The elaboration of TNF and IL-1 is relatively brief, but IL-6 persists longer.

Cytokines appear to play a dominant role in regulating cell recruitment, proliferation, development, and other cellular events that occur in the wound, but how and to what extent they exert systemic effects and modulate the metabolic responses to critical illness is less clear. One conceptual model proposes that when local cytokine production is particularly abundant, owing to extensive wounds or uncontrolled infection, certain cytokines spill over into the circulation and then affect tissues at distant sites [see Figure 5]. Although elevated circulating cytokine levels have been detected in critically ill patients, only IL-6 has been consistently associated with severe illness and outcome.[107,108]

Several investigations have sought to determine the metabolic effect of the proinflammatory cytokines. TNF can initiate the cytokine cascade, ultimately producing fever, leukocytosis, and other signs and symptoms of critical illness.[109] To characterize the role of TNF in proteolysis associated with endotoxin or sepsis, Michie and coworkers analyzed the responses of both animals and humans during prolonged infusions of TNF.[110] Negative nitrogen balance was related to the onset of anorexia and reduced food intake and not to the development of hypermetabolism. Mealy and associates performed adrenalectomies and abrogated the increase in nitrogen loss associated with TNF infusion.[111] Hall-Angeras and colleagues found that a steroid antagonist prevented the increase in myofibrillar protein breakdown usually seen in an animal model of intra-abdominal sepsis.[112] These observations suggest that even though TNF may be a major initiating signal for a variety of cellular events in critical illness, other mediators are required for the full development of the metabolic responses to injury and infection.

IL-1 was one of the first fever-producing cytokines, or pyrogens, to be identified.[113,114] Early in vitro studies appeared to present conflicting findings,[115-117] but the preponderance of the data currently available indicate that IL-1 can increase proteolysis, especially in intact animals. For example, Zamir and colleagues measured increased muscle protein breakdown in vitro after administration of IL-1 to intact animals.[118] In another study, they were able to reduce but not prevent the increased proteolysis that followed endotoxin administration by pretreating animals with IL-1 receptor antagonist (IL-1ra).[119]

To characterize the metabolic effects of IL-1 in vivo, Watters and associates gave daily intramuscular injections of etiocholanolone to normal individuals.[120] (This steroid stimulates the development of an inflammatory focus and the production of IL-1.) The subjects manifested an acute-phase response: fever, leukocytosis, increased concentrations of acute-phase proteins, and hypoferremia. They were not hypermetabolic, however, and they remained in nitrogen equilibrium when fed a standard diet. The concentrations of catabolic hormones were not affected by this treatment. When hydrocortisone, glucagon, and epinephrine were administered in conjunction with etiocholanolone, however, both inflammatory and metabolic responses were observed.[121] These healthy subjects exhibited the same clinical features as did patients with infection. These findings suggested that both endocrine and cytokine mechanisms influence the responses to critical illness.

IL-6 can induce many of the components of the acute-phase response[122] and may be measured in the blood of patients experiencing trauma,[123] sepsis,[124] pancreatitis,[125] or other critical illnesses (e.g., myocardial infarction).[126] Mateo and associates identified IL-6 in wound fluid from both animals and humans, and they found that the capacity of wound macrophages to produce IL-6 increased with time.[127] Thus, IL-6 might be one mechanism by which the wound influences critical illness. Persistent measurable levels of IL-6 have been related to mortality in both trauma[107] and burn[108] patients.

Stouthard and associates infused recombinant IL-6 (rIL-6) into uninjured cancer patients for 4 hours, then measured glucose and lipid kinetics, metabolic rate, and hormonal profiles during the infusion and during a saline control infusion.[128] IL-6–induced hypermetabolism and energy expenditure increased by 25%. Glucose production, lipolysis, and fatty acid oxidation also increased. Glucose clearance was also increased; serum glucose concentrations were not significantly affected by IL-6 infusion. Tsigos and colleagues administered increasing doses of IL-6 subcutaneously to healthy subjects and demonstrated a dose-response relationship between IL-6 dose and circulating level and glucose concentration.[129] In both of these studies, IL-6 also induced elevations in circulating stress hormone levels.

IL-6 also affects protein metabolism. Transgenic mice that overexpress IL-6 exhibit retarded growth and muscle atrophy. These observations have been correlated with reduced circulating concentrations of insulinlike growth factor–1 (IGF-1).[130] In another report, a specific IL-6 receptor antibody administered to the young IL-6 transgenic mice restored muscle growth to normal.[131] The muscle atrophy in these studies was associated with an increase in the synthesis and activity of several enzymes that catalyze muscle protein breakdown, and these changes too were blocked by IL-6 receptor antibody. The effects of IL-6 on long-term protein accretion in humans have not yet been elucidated, but severely burned children who survive after a long period of critical illness often experience growth retardation.[132]

Both endocrine and inflammatory mediators affect metabolic responses in critically ill patients. In fact, the two systems are closely linked—perhaps inseparably—and probably influence each other.[121] For example, Bornstein and colleagues identified IL-6 messenger RNA (mRNA) expression in the steroid-producing cells of the adrenal gland, which were located not only in the cortex but also in the medulla, adjacent to catecholamine-producing cells.[133] In a subsequent study, they detected IL-6 and IL-6 receptor expression in adrenal cell cultures, both with macrophages present and with macrophages absent.[134] They also found that IL-6 stimulated release of steroid hormones, aldosterone, cortisol, and androgens in vitro in a dose-dependent manner; however, these effects developed over a period of 24 hours. These findings indicate not only that IL-6 exerts autocrine and paracrine effects on adrenal cellular synthetic function but also that it is probably involved in the long-term regulation of adrenal steroidogenesis rather than being responsible for acute changes in adrenal function.

On the other hand, glucocorticoids have long been known to exert anti-inflammatory effects. They interfere with the proliferation and function of leukocytes and other immune cells, and they inhibit the synthesis and cellular action of cytokines and other molecules important for cellular responses.[135] In a clinical study, Barber and colleagues demonstrated that glucocorticoid administration led to a dose- and time-dependent reduction in TNF production and symptoms in response to endotoxin.[136]

Cytokines and hormones may also affect metabolic responses at the end-organ level via different mechanisms. For example, skeletal muscle protein breakdown can occur via any of at least four intracellular proteolytic systems.[137] One of the major pathways affecting myofibrillar proteins is energy dependent (i.e., ATP-dependent) and involves the cytosolic peptide cofactor ubiquitin. In animals, glucocorticoids stimulate an ATP-dependent proteolytic system and increase the expression of ubiquitin.[138] Zamir and colleagues administered a glucocorticoid antagonist to rats with intraperitoneal sepsis and demonstrated that it reduced but did not eliminate the increased muscle proteolysis.[118] In a subsequent study, they induced accelerated skeletal muscle proteolysis by injecting IL-1 intraperitoneally.[119] Previous adrenalectomy, which eliminated glucocorticoid elaboration, had little effect on the proteolysis observed.[139] These observations suggest that both glucocorticoid-dependent and glucocorticoid-independent proteolytic mechanisms can be activated during critical illness.

Role of the Central Nervous System

The CNS plays a major role in the regulation of the metabolic response to critical illness. Hume and Egdahl were among the first to demonstrate its role in mediating early responses to injury.[140] They measured the rise in 17-hydroxycorticosteroids in adrenal venous

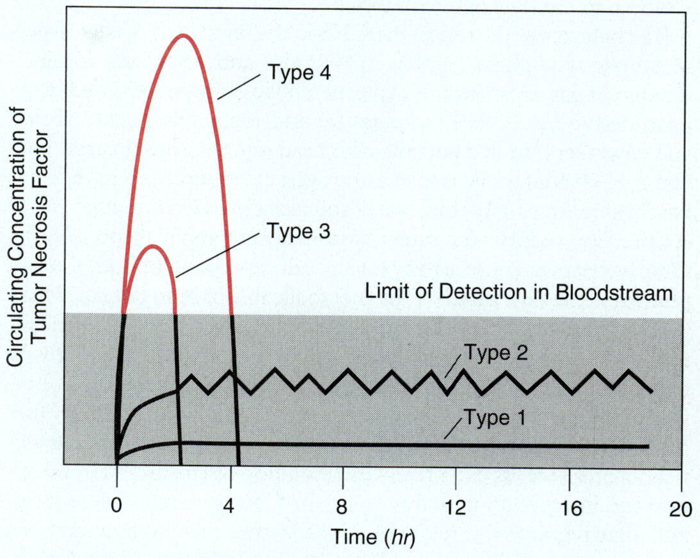

Figure 5 Different infectious states are likely to be associated with different patterns of cytokine release into the circulation.[232] Type 1 in this figure could be considered to represent localized cellulitis, such as might be present at an infected intravenous catheter infusion site. Generation of tumor necrosis factor (TNF) and other cytokines occurs locally to produce local responses that aid host defense and tissue repair. Overspill into the circulation is minimal.

The second type might represent the responses ensuing from appendiceal abscess. There is local generation of cytokines, and as bacteria or their endotoxins leak into the circulation, circulating mononuclear cells also elaborate cytokines and give rise to moderate systemic responses. The low level of persistent endotoxemia is reflected in the cytokine response. Because only a small number of cytokine-producing cells are stimulated at any one time, the responses of these cells, although of long duration, are not strong enough to be detectable in the bloodstream. However, this signal is sufficient to generate systemic manifestations of the localized infection.

A third type of infection might be one that follows manipulation of a catheter in the biliary tree or urinary bladder to resolve an obstruction. A few cytokine-producing cells simultaneously elaborate TNF to produce a high-amplitude signal. Because the endotoxemia is transient, both the signal and the host responses are short-lived. Clinical features include a brief episode of hyperpyrexia with rigors and severe symptoms, but the cytokine response is too short and of insufficient amplitude to give rise to life-threatening, irreversible host alterations.

A fourth type of infection might be precipitated by sudden dehiscence of a colonic anastomosis or by meningococcal septicemia. An acute, massive entry of endotoxins into the circulation stimulates virtually every cytokine-producing cell in the body. A very high amplitude signal occurs, but its duration is short, despite the host's continuing exposure to endotoxin. The short duration of the strong signal is caused by the quick disappearance of cytokines from the circulation; their half-life is short, and the cytokine-producing cells become refractory after their simultaneous explosive response to the initial, lethal signal. This high-amplitude signal is misinterpreted by the host, causing the entire body to behave as if it were a massive wound. The entire vascular tree shows increased permeability and vasodilatation, resulting in the clinical state of irreversible shock. These situations have been reversed or prevented by the use of TNF antibodies in animals and occasionally by the use of plasmapheresis in humans.

blood in response to a burn to the lower limb of an animal under anesthesia. The limb was almost completely separated from the body, so that the only connections between the limb and the rest of the animal were the femoral vessels and the sciatic nerve. The prompt rise in the venous adrenocorticoid concentration after the burn could be prevented by sectioning of the sciatic nerve or of any portion of the CNS up to the level of the midbrain.

To characterize the role of the CNS in the regulation of later hypermetabolic flow-phase responses, Wilmore and associates administered inert gas anesthesia to hypermetabolic burn patients and demonstrated reduced core temperature and metabolic rates.[141] Fried and coworkers studied patients with head injuries during barbiturate coma.[142,143] Metabolic rate and nitrogen excretion were reduced to basal values during barbiturate administration. Given that its global suppression reduces the intensity of hypermetabolic responses, the CNS appears to be necessary for the full expression of both the ebb phase and the flow phase of the metabolic response to critical illness.

The CNS has long been considered part of a neuroendocrine reflex arc,[144] a view that has proved useful for explicating underlying regulatory mechanisms. According to this concept, there must be afferent input whereby (1) the body is alerted to an injury or any other threat to its integrity and (2) the wound or inflammatory focus signals its presence, its extent, and its resolution or closure. After reception and interpretation of this input, the CNS generates efferent signals that regulate the regional and systemic metabolic alterations observed clinically. This model is most obviously relevant to the early phase of the response to critical illness (the ebb phase). The hypothalamus, the peripheral and spinal neural pathways, and the adrenals all participate in the classic fright-fight-flight syndrome. Pain, hypovolemia, acidosis, and hypoxia stimulate neural afferent signals to the CNS. The importance of these neural pathways in transmitting afferent signals to the CNS during hypermetabolism is less clear. For example, when lidocaine was applied to burn wounds to anesthetize them, no decrease in hypermetabolism was observed.[145]

Recent investigations have begun to elucidate the role the CNS may play in a variety of immunologic and inflammatory responses.[146] Early studies demonstrated that a small amount of IL-1 injected intrathecally elicited the same increase in body temperature as a much larger dose administered intravenously. This suggested that IL-1 could act centrally and that it might function as an afferent signal from the wound to the CNS.[147] Demonstration of IL-1 immunoreactivity in the hypothalamus of humans lent weight to this suggestion.[148] Later studies, however, showed that astrocytes and microglia could express cytokines and cytokine receptors themselves.[149,150] In addition, these cells increased expression of IL-1 and IL-6 in vitro in response to hypoxia or endotoxin in vitro,[151,152] and systemic administration of endotoxin to intact animals increased cytokine expression in the CNS.[153,154]

Hill and colleagues used an animal model to assess the metabolic effects of IL-1 continuously infused either subcutaneously or into the lateral ventricle for 6 days.[155] Subcutaneous IL-1 was given in different doses, which induced fever, anorexia, increased protein catabolism, and weight loss in a dose-dependent manner. Intracerebroventricular (ICV) IL-1 evoked qualitatively similar responses. Subcutaneous IL-1, however, resulted in a greater leukocytosis and a more pronounced acute-phase response than did ICV IL-1, even though the other systemic alterations were quantitatively similar. Thus, IL-1 produced in the CNS may not have the same physiologic consequences as IL-1 produced in other anatomic sites.

In another study, Hill and colleagues pair-fed control animals with animals receiving ICV IL-1.[156] They observed that the pair-fed animals also lost weight, but the weight loss was significantly less severe than in the animals receiving ICV IL-1. Long-term ICV IL-1 infusion also caused increased adrenal gland weight and corticosteroid levels in comparison with values in both pair-fed and chow-fed controls. The ICV IL-1–induced catabolic changes were not, however, attenuated by previous adrenalectomy. This finding indicates that the protein-catabolic effects induced by ICV IL-1 may involve not only glucocorticoid-dependent ATP-ubiquitin proteolysis but also systems that are independent of glucocorticoids. Such a conclusion is consistent with the finding by Zamir and associates that intraperitoneal IL-1 increased total and myofibrillar proteolysis in both adrenalectomized animals and sham controls.[139] Thus, the CNS may be able to influence metabolic responses via both endocrine pathways and other mechanisms that do not involve endocrine activation.

Elaboration of IL-6 typically follows elaboration of IL-1, and IL-6 is a potent activator of corticosteroid synthesis and release.[106,157] Long-term IL-1 infusion leads to increased muscle protein breakdown and nitrogen loss over and above what is attributable to reduced food intake, and it results in elevated circulating levels of IL-6.[158] When Hill and associates infused IL-6 into the CSF of rats, it had no effect, unlike ICV IL-1.[156] Reyes and Coe followed the appearance of IL-6 in CSF in primates after intravenous injection of IL-1α, IL-1β, and IL-6.[159] All three cytokines raised the circulating levels of IL-6, IL-1ra, and cortisol, but only IL-1β raised the CSF level of IL-6. Furthermore, IL-6 appeared in CSF from the lumbar region 2 hours after it peaked in CSF from the cervical region. These data suggest that the IL-6 in the CSF after the appearance of IL-1 in the periphery is elaborated by the brain.

Romero and colleagues gave an ICV injection of IL-1β to rats and measured IL-6 concentrations in CSF and in blood from the superior sagittal sinus and the aorta.[160] IL-6 was elevated in all three compartments, and the concentration gradient between the sagittal sinus and the aorta was widened in comparison with the control value. Both adrenergic pathways and adrenal activation are known to be stimulated by IL-1 administration; but the changes observed were not affected by sympathetic blockade, and ICV corticotropin-releasing hormone did not result in alterations in IL-6 levels in CSF or in blood. The investigators concluded that the IL-6 that appeared in both the CSF and the blood was derived from the brain.

Recent neurophysiologic research is also providing insights into the effects of injury and inflammation on nerve function. Numerous compounds elaborated by platelets, neutrophils, and other inflammatory cells can alter the phenotype of neurons, affecting their growth, function, and electrical properties[161]; IL-6 is one of these. The complex of IL-6 and its receptor can activate specific neuronal signal transduction systems on sensory neurons and so affect gene expression and protein synthesis.[162] Sensory nerve injury induces the expression of IL-6 and IL-6 receptor in more central neurons, and this seems to promote nerve repair.[163] Niijima gave varying doses of IL-1β to rats by portal vein injection.[164] He observed a dose-dependent increase in the afferent activity of the haptic branch of the vagus nerve. He also detected efferent signals in autonomic nerves to the spleen and thymus after intraportal administration of IL-1. Because these signals were eliminated by vagotomy, they appeared to be the result of reflex activation. These findings suggest that there are sensors in the hepatoportal system that can detect IL-1 and other inflammatory mediators and generate neural afferent activity, stimulating the brain to generate signals that affect host defense and other responses.

Thus, the CNS is intimately involved in the regulation of the metabolic response to critical illness. Not only pain, acidosis, hypoxia, and hypovolemia but also cytokines and other substances produced by inflammatory cells may generate afferent signals to the CNS through a variety of mechanisms. Some signals may elicit a rapid effector response, whereas others appear to induce mechanisms that result in delayed and more prolonged end-organ functional alterations. The CNS affects both metabolic and inflammatory processes, and it may do so in multiple complementary but largely independent ways. Activation of the hypothalamic-pituitary-adrenal axis is one of these mechanisms, but the CNS also appears to be able to induce catabolic responses without this intervention. The CNS may even be a source of mediators that are released into the circulation for systemic distribution, thus acting as an endocrine organ.

An early theory of how cytokines produced in wounds or other sites of inflammation might affect metabolic responses was that they spilled over into the circulation to be transported to other organs, including the brain, where they constituted an afferent signal. Some of the data now available suggest that there may also be much more direct lines of communication between a wound and the CNS, so that cytokines and other substances in the wound environment might stimulate specific neural afferent activity that could then elicit highly specific effector signals and end-organ responses. By this view, the CNS may support multiple streams of information and thus regulate physiologic processes in several coordinated and comprehensive ways. We have long tended to think of the nervous system as little more than a number of telegraph lines and a central switching station; however, a better metaphor might be a fiberoptic cable network, which is capable of transmitting television programming, computer data, and telephone and fax transmissions to and from multiple users simultaneously.

Role of the Gut

Although the idea that endotoxin absorbed from the gut lumen during shock states might result in irreversible critical illness was first proposed nearly 40 years ago,[165,166] most clinicians continued to think that the gut was inert after operation and injury until relatively recently. Now, however, it is generally recognized that the gut plays an important role in augmenting or perpetuating the response to critical illness.[167]

Gram-negative pathogens are the predominant infectious organisms in the ICU, and the gut appears to be a major source of contamination. The gut lumen forms a large reservoir for gram-negative enteric bacteria, but the normal GI mucosa protects the host from intraluminal bacteria and their toxins. The maintenance of tight intracellular junctions between epithelial cells prevents the transepithelial migration of bacteria.[168] The GI tract is also richly supplied with macrophages and fixed immune cells. The elaboration of surface immunoglobulins (e.g., IgA) aids in the recognition of foreign antigens.[169] Finally, the liver and the spleen serve as backup systems for trapping bacteria and neutralizing absorbed toxins. The combination of an intact gut mucosa and a normally functioning immune system provides maximal barrier function. Even in immunosuppressed states, the mucosa can still maintain an effective barrier to infection. This suggests that cell-mediated immunity is secondary in importance to an intact intestinal epithelial lining.

When the barrier function of the GI epithelium is impaired, intraluminal bacteria and toxins can invade the host. In one set of experiments in rabbits, fatal endotoxic shock was observed after temporary occlusion of the superior mesenteric artery or a 30% scald burn[170]; however, if the enteric flora was reduced, the animals did not die. Endotoxemia has been observed in patients with a variety of critical illnesses.[166] Wellmann and associates reported that whole gut lavage with saline reduced the concentration of circulating endotoxin and improved the clinical outcome in a large group of patients with inflammatory bowel disease that was unresponsive to medical therapy.[171] Moreover, bacteremia in portal blood has been observed at the time of operation in as many as 30% of patients with noninflammatory bowel disease.[172] Ambrose and associates cultured both intestinal serosa and mesenteric lymph nodes during abdominal operation.[173] In patients without inflammatory bowel disease, the incidence of positive cultures was low, but in patients with Crohn's disease, the incidence increased markedly, to approximately 30%.

Bacterial translocation is the migration of bacteria across the bowel wall to invade the host. In a review of the available animal and human data on this process, Berg identified three conditions that appear to promote translocation: altered permeability of the intestinal mucosa, decreased host defenses, and an increased number of bacteria within the intestinal lumen.[174] Deitch and colleagues observed this phenomenon in animals after a variety of insults, including burns,[175] hemorrhagic shock,[176] and endotoxin administration.[170] Malnutrition alone did not lead to translocation, but it made the gut barrier more susceptible to endotoxin.[177]

The extent of bacterial translocation in critically ill patients is not well defined. Moore and colleagues obtained both portal venous and systemic venous blood cultures in patients at risk for multiorgan failure after laparotomy for severe trauma.[178] Only 2% of cultures were positive in the first 5 days, which suggests that translocation of bacteria in sufficient quantities to cause portal vein bacteremia is not a major determinant of organ failure soon after injury.

More recent studies have focused on the gut as a source of cytokines. Even the normal gut contains a large number of intestinal lymphocytes that elaborate proinflammatory cytokines, and these are counteracted by expression of anti-inflammatory cytokines in a state of so-called controlled inflammation.[179] Guy-Grand and colleagues detected measurable levels of TNF, IL-6, and interferon gamma in proximal small bowel secretions in humans.[180] The presence of bacterial overgrowth, especially colonic-type bacteria, however, was associated with increased IL-6 concentrations. Wyble and associates investigated the cytokine response to intestinal ischemia-reperfusion in ex vivo perfused segments of human intestine.[181] Concentrations of TNF and IL-1 increased in the venous effluent after reperfusion. The investigators subsequently exposed cultured human endothelial cells to physiologic concentrations of TNF and IL-1 that were lower than those observed after ischemia-reperfusion. The cytokines up-regulated expression of E-selectin and intercellular adhesion molecule–1 (ICAM-1), which are thought to mediate the adhesion of neutrophils in the microcirculation and their transmigration across the capillary membrane into tissue, thus initiating tissue inflammation.

Mainous and colleagues produced sterile peritonitis with both a nonlethal and a median lethal dose (LD_{50}) of zymosan.[182] They detected increased IL-6 and TNF in both blood and lymph, but these changes did not correlate with zymosan dose or with bacterial translocation. Thus, the gut appears capable of producing cytokines in response to an inflammatory insult, and this may occur even in the absence of bacterial translocation.

Mochizuki and associates were among the first to demonstrate the importance of enteral feedings in maintaining gut mucosal integrity and modulating catabolic responses in critical illness.[183] They measured intestinal mucosal weight and several metabolic parameters in experimental animals after a standard burn injury. In one group of animals, feedings were delivered through a gastrostomy tube and were begun soon after the burn injury, whereas in a second group, feedings were oral and were begun after a 72-hour fast. Mucosal weight was preserved in the first group but reduced in the second group. In the animals that fasted, postburn hypermetabolism developed, but this response was attenuated in the ones that received early enteral feedings. Intravenous feeding did not preserve mucosal mass or modify postburn metabolic responses.[184] In an early clinical study, Alexander and colleagues documented improved survival in children with burns who were nourished enterally.[185] Furthermore, Border and associates found that the provision of enteral protein was one of only two factors statistically associated with improved survival in a large group of severely injured patients.[186]

Ogle and colleagues extended these observations by comparing intestinal and splenic cytokine expression in animals nourished by parenteral nutrition but allowed no oral intake with cytokine expression in control animals allowed food ad libitum.[187] After 7 days of infusion, mRNA expression for IL-1, IL-6, and TNF was increased in the intestine and decreased in the spleen. Lyoumi and associates also reported that protein malnutrition alone enhances intestinal IL-6 expression and acute-phase responses.[188] These findings suggest that augmented intestinal cytokine production is responsible, in part, for the earlier clinical observations that bowel rest or inadequate enteral protein amplifies the responses to critical illness and may adversely affect outcome.

The presence of food in the gut lumen is known to be a major stimulus for mucosal cell growth. Mucosal atrophy is observed in the absence of enteral nutrition (as occurs during starvation[189] or periods of parenteral nutrition[190]) and in defunctionalized intestinal segments.[191] Enteral feeding not only provides nutrients but also stimulates the elaboration of trophic hormones for the intestinal mucosa.[192,193] In addition to luminal bulk, specific nutrients (e.g., glutamine and butyrate) are important for the growth of gut mucosa. Glutamine is a major respiratory fuel for the gut, especially during critical illness (see above). Colonocytes also utilize butyrate, a short-chain fatty acid that is produced by bacterial fermentation of polysaccharides in the colonic lumen. In solution, glutamine decomposes into toxic substances; it is therefore not included in any commercially available parenteral amino acid solutions or in most enteral nutrition products. When glutamine was added to parenteral nutrition in place of other nonessential amino acids, however, increased mucosal cellularity was observed in the jejunum, ileum, and colon in an animal model.[194,195] In other studies, the toxic effects of methotrexate were alleviated and mucosal cellularity and nitrogen balance improved when parenteral solutions containing glutamine were used.[196]

If these study results correlate with any specific clinical situation, it might be that of a patient with abdominal and skeletal trauma in the ICU who is recovering from shock and is on bowel rest. Bowel rest frequently is associated with intraluminal bacterial overgrowth. This association, coupled with reperfusion of the gut during resuscitation and the presence of peritoneal inflammation, could contribute to increased intestinal production of proinflammatory cytokines. The gut may function, therefore, as an additional inflammatory focus and, in conjunction with the peripheral wounds, may act to stimulate systemic responses. The release of glutamine from muscle can support epithelial proliferation. If the initial injuries are limited, normal GI function soon returns, with the result that the intensity of the systemic inflammatory responses is reduced and the patient recovers. If, however, the insult is massive, if there is a prolonged period of reduced enteral nutrition, or if the supply of glutamine is insufficient to support mucosal cell growth, then recovery of mucosal integrity may be delayed, and the gut could continue to be an inflammatory focus, exacerbating and perpetuating the patient's catabolic responses.

Endotoxin, Bacteria, Inflammation, and Organ Failure

Endotoxin is a lipopolysaccharide component of bacterial cell walls that can reproduce the syndrome of sepsis and shock when given to animals or humans[197] [see 88 Immunomodulation]. The presence of endotoxin is considered a major determinant of the clinical sequelae of bacterial infection. A low continuous dose of endotoxin in animals produces a hypermetabolic state that exhibits all of the features of the response to critical illness.[198]

Revhaug and associates administered Escherichia coli endotoxin to normal individuals under controlled conditions of activity and diet and compared the metabolic responses with those of subjects given only saline.[199] About 2 to 4 hours after administration of endotoxin, the subjects experienced headache, chills, malaise, nausea, fever, tachycardia, and an increased respiratory rate. In these and subsequent studies, endotoxin injection was also associated with leukocytosis, mild glucose intolerance, an increased metabolic rate, and elevated concentrations of adrenocorticotropic hormone, cortisol, catecholamines, and growth hormone.

Michie and colleagues found that the symptoms that followed a single dose of endotoxin in normal subjects were preceded by an abrupt and transient rise in circulating TNF concentration.[200] The symptoms developing after endotoxin injection were similar to those developing during TNF infusion, but they appeared 60 to 90 minutes after injection, in contrast with the appearance of symptoms 30 minutes after the start of TNF infusion.[109] In these studies, IL-1 was not detected, but Fong and associates detected both a peak rise in TNF and a later peak of IL-1 after administration of a lethal dose of bacteria in primates.[201] In those studies, death was prevented by an anti-TNF antibody. Thus, TNF is the first in a characteristic cascade of cytokines that mediate the physiologic responses to endotoxin.

Circulating endotoxin can be detected in patients who have experienced trauma[107] or burns[108] and even in those who have undergone cardiopulmonary bypass.[202] In healthy persons, repeated doses of endotoxin result in tolerance. In injured or critically ill patients, however, the responses to sustained or repeated doses of endotoxin have not been well characterized.

O'Dwyer and associates measured intestinal permeability in healthy human volunteers after a single dose of E. coli endotoxin or saline.[203] Lactulose and mannitol were administered orally as markers of intestinal permeability. (Lactulose is not absorbed to any significant extent under normal conditions.) After endotoxin administration, the urinary excretion of lactulose was increased almost twofold, which indicated that intestinal permeability was markedly altered. This change was closely associated with increases in norepinephrine and cortisol levels, which suggested that these hormonal changes or other systemic responses induced by endotoxin were responsible for the change in permeability. If alteration of the gut barrier led to increased absorption of endotoxin, that could be another mechanism by which the systemic responses to critical illness were amplified and perpetuated.

Patients with infectious disease (e.g., typhoid fever or malaria)[204,205] manifest many of the clinical features observed in critically ill surgical patients; however, these phenomena are less intense in patients with infectious disease. Surgical patients with uninfected wounds also usually manifest relatively mild responses to injury; those with infected wounds exhibit the most intense metabolic alterations. The infection may be associated with the wound (e.g., surgical site infection, mature abscess, or ARDS and pulmonary sepsis), or it may be remote (e.g., pneumonia in a patient with multiple fractures). Peak catabolic responses in surgical patients often occur several days after operation or injury. This period corresponds to the development of the cellular phase of wound healing[103] and to colonization of the wound or another site.

Aulick and colleagues examined the possible contribution of bacteria or bacterial products to the metabolic response to injury in animals.[206] They measured $\dot{V}O_2$ and core temperature in animals for up to 3 weeks after a standard scald burn. Some of the wounds were seeded with bacteria (virulent and nonvirulent Pseudomonas aeruginosa and Staphylococcus epidermidis), and some of the infected wounds were treated with topical antibacterial agents. The use of topical antibiotics was associated with a reduction in hypermetabolism. In addition, in animals that became bacteremic, the degree of hypermetabolism was at least twice that in nonbacteremic animals. The metabolic effects of infection thus appear to be proportional to the severity and invasiveness of the infection. In analogous studies, Wilmore and associates examined burn patients with and without bacteremia.[24] Although total body $\dot{V}O_2$ and cardiac index were already elevated, the onset of bacteremia resulted in further increases in these parameters. In addition, hepatic glucose production and splanchnic uptake of lactate and alanine were significantly increased in patients with systemic infection. Hypermetabolism decreased, however, once organ failure occurred.

Bacteria are ubiquitous in both health and critical illness. The mechanisms by which bacteria become infective and invade host tissues and produce physiologic responses are only beginning to be elucidated. In part, these involve intracellular regulatory systems that respond to complex reciprocal interactions with the host and that can modify bacterial virulence. Guo and associates investigated the dual peptide system PhoP-PhoQ in *Salmonella*.[207] PhoP-PhoQ regulates genes required for the synthesis of lipid A, the active component of endotoxin. It is capable of modifying the structure of lipid A, and this structurally modified lipid A can affect the expression both of adhesion molecules by host endothelial cells and of TNF by neighboring monocytes. This capability may be a mechanism by which bacteria can not only increase their chances of survival in host tissues but also affect the character or intensity of host inflammatory responses to the infection. PhoP-PhoQ and other intracellular systems respond to characteristics of the host environment, such as pH, Po_2, and ionic composition.[208] Thus, the condition of the patient may influence the virulence characteristics of resident bacteria, and these characteristics, in turn, may modulate the patient's responses to critical illness.

The cellular response to localized injury or other inflammatory stimuli initially consists of the recruitment and proliferation of neutrophils. This process appears to be mediated in part by the expression of adhesion molecules by endothelial cells. These molecules capture passing circulating neutrophils and facilitate their passage through the capillary wall.[209] Neutrophils, macrophages, and other inflammatory cells have the capacity to engulf and dispose of necrotic debris and to kill bacteria. These same properties also make them potentially toxic to normal cells. Neutrophil infiltration of specific organs, such as the lung, appears to be a first step in the development of organ failure after shock, endotoxin, and other insults.[210] This finding suggests that neutrophils activated by potent inflammatory stimuli can invade unaffected tissues and so contribute to organ dysfunction in critically ill patients.

Not surprisingly, anti-inflammatory mechanisms exist to limit the intensity and toxicity of inflammatory processes. One such mechanism is apoptosis, or programmed cell death, which is thought to participate in the clearing of inflammatory cells as the wound heals and the inflammatory process subsides. Biffl and colleagues demonstrated that IL-6 inhibited apoptosis in human neutrophils in vitro.[211] They proposed that circulating IL-6 in critically ill patients retarded neutrophil apoptosis and thus enhanced and prolonged the toxic effects of the neutrophils. This could be another mechanism by which the responses to critical illness could be prolonged and lead to worsening organ failure and death.

Manipulating the Response to Critical Illness

The metabolic response to critical illness has survival value. Young patients are able to mount more intense hypermetabolic responses than elderly persons and in general have higher survival rates. However, these responses are debilitating in all patients and may be associated with organ failure and death. Many have sought to develop therapeutic strategies that would reduce the debilitating aspects of these responses, accelerate recovery, or both.

The endocrine response to injury or operation has been attenuated by adrenergic blockade or regional anesthesia (see above). These maneuvers are associated with an improved postoperative nitrogen balance[100,101] and decreased muscle protein breakdown.[99] Herndon and colleagues reported that continuous administration of propranolol to children with burns reduced cardiac work without adversely affecting mortality, postburn course, or wound healing.[212] This technique may benefit elderly, critically ill patients with limited cardiovascular reserve.

Several studies have evaluated the effectiveness of combined neural and humoral blockade in inhibiting the metabolic responses to operative injury. Schulze and associates compared the responses of patients receiving morphine and acetaminophen for pain control after colonic surgery with those of patients managed with methylprednisolone pretreatment, thoracic epidural analgesia, intrathecal anesthesia, and intravenous indomethacin.[213] In the patients receiving combined therapy, postoperative pain and fever were prevented, pulmonary function was improved, and fatigue was reduced. Synthesis of acute-phase proteins and IL-6 was reduced. Similarly, Heindorff and coworkers prevented the typical increases in amino acid clearance and urea synthesis with a combination of intravenous somatostatin and etomidate (to inhibit the elevation of glucagon and cortisol levels) and high thoracic epidural analgesia (to provide neural blockade).[102]

Advances in cell and molecular biology have led to an extraordinary expansion of knowledge about the mechanisms involved in the many local and systemic responses to injury, sepsis, and other critical illness. Developments in technology have also led to the formulation of novel strategies for inhibiting various components of these responses that were thought to be particularly deleterious. Thus, antibodies to endotoxin, IL-1, and TNF were developed and studied in clinical trials, along with receptor antagonists and other compounds designed to interfere with systemic inflammatory responses. None of these demonstrated clinical benefit in controlled trials.[214] Given that the regulatory mechanisms are highly complex and that the same ones that may be harmful in some cases promote recovery in others, it is not surprising that blockade of one component of the response might offer no net benefit.

An alternative strategic approach is to enhance or accelerate those components of the response to critical illness that seem to be primarily restorative and lead to wound healing and recovery.

Nutritional support of critically ill patients is important both for promoting protein synthesis and other anabolic processes essential to recovery and for reducing the net drain on the patient's fuel and protein stores. Enteral nutrition is preferred, but the availability of effective intravenous techniques allows the clinician to provide appropriate nutrition to virtually all patients. Exercise and mobility have clear anticatabolic effects and should be initiated as early as is practicable.

Previously, provision of glutamine to critically ill patients had not been possible; glutamine had not been included in most commercial nutrient preparations because of its instability in aqueous solutions. When added to standard TPN, however, glutamine can promote nitrogen retention in postoperative patients.[215] Ziegler and associates demonstrated that glutamine-supplemented TPN improved nitrogen balance, diminished clinical infection, and shortened hospital stay in a group of critically ill patients recovering from bone marrow transplantation.[216] Enteral preparations enriched with glutamine are now commercially available.

Kudsk and associates randomly selected patients with moderately severe injuries to receive either an enteral formulation enriched with glutamine, arginine, omega-3 fatty acids, and nucleotides or a standard formula that provided an isonitrogenous, isocaloric diet.[217] In both cases, protein content was moderately high (2 g/kg/day). Infectious complications in patients surviving to recovery were less frequent in those receiving the enhanced formula than in those receiving the standard diet.

Growth hormone is an anabolic hormone capable of improving nitrogen balance. Human growth hormone can be synthesized with recombinant technology, and recombinant growth hormone is safer and more readily available than an animal preparation. When administered to normal subjects, growth hormone improves nitrogen balance, even if caloric intake is less than energy expenditure.[218] Jiang and associates administered growth hormone and hypocaloric parenteral nutrition perioperatively to patients undergoing elective abdominal operations.[219] They monitored a variety of metabolic parameters and compared the results with those from a control group of patients receiving parenteral nutrition alone. Growth hormone markedly reduced cumulative nitrogen loss. Although both groups of patients lost weight, those receiving growth hormone lost less. Bioelectric impedance data indicated that most of the weight lost by patients receiving growth hormone came from fat mass and not from the muscle compartment. Growth hormone also preserved muscle strength.

Herndon and colleagues administered growth hormone to severely burned children in a randomized trial.[220] Growth hormone accelerated donor site healing, allowing earlier reharvesting of skin. As a result, the time between skin graft procedures and the total length of time required for the children's recovery were both reduced. Knox and associates gave growth hormone to a group of severely burned adults and compared their outcome with that of a similar group of patients cared for without growth hormone in the immediately preceding years[221]; mortality was lower in the growth hormone group.

Two large multi-institutional randomized trials were recently conducted in Europe in which the efficacy of growth hormone was evaluated in a variety of critically ill patients, including trauma patients, patients who had undergone cardiac procedures, and patients with other acute surgical illnesses. In all, more than 500 patients were enrolled. The two studies obtained very similar results. The combined mortality of the patients receiving growth hormone was 42%, more than twice the 18% mortality in the control subjects. Although the reasons for this adverse outcome have not yet been elucidated, the manufacturer of the recombinant product issued a safety statement recommending that recombinant growth hormone not be used in catabolic patients.[222]

Although there has been good experience with growth hormone in burn patients and other surgical patients in some centers, the widespread use of growth hormone cannot be recommended at present. Certain anabolic steroids, such as oxandrolone, are available and have a good margin of safety. These may also promote nitrogen retention and accelerate recovery. Oxandrolone, combined with a high-protein diet (2 mg/kg/day), promoted weight gain and functional improvement in a randomized study of burn patients who had recovered sufficiently to enter a rehabilitation program.[223] Controlled data in critically ill patients, however, are not yet available.

Insulin attenuates cortisol-induced breakdown of skeletal muscle protein in vitro.[224] Inculet and associates demonstrated improved nitrogen utilization in patients receiving TPN and insulin after operation.[225] The apparent mild beneficial effects of TPN enriched with branched-chain amino acids may be caused by increased insulin elaboration.[226] Bessey and Lowe induced accelerated skeletal muscle protein catabolism in normal subjects by blocking insulin elaboration during the first day of a 3-day infusion of stress hormones,[98] thereby simulating the typical hormonal profiles of injured patients. When insulin elaboration was allowed to rise unchecked or when exogenous insulin was administered to limit the rise of blood glucose, net muscle protein breakdown did not increase.

Table 8 Factors Affecting Metabolic Response to Critical Illness and Patient Outcome

Factors that *cannot* be directly controlled or influenced at present
  Patient's genetic makeup and premorbid state of health
  Gene transcription and translation
  Expression of hormones, cytokines, and growth factors
  Expression of hormone, cytokine, growth factor, and other specific cell receptors
  Expression of secondary messengers
  Generation of nitric oxide and other reactive oxygen intermediates
  Signal transduction mechanisms
  Intracellular transporters and other regulatory peptides and organelles
  CNS neural pathway traffic and cytokine expression
  Futile cycles
  Enzymes controlling protein synthesis and breakdown
  Bacterial virulence factors
  Expression of adhesion molecules
  Inflammatory and noninflammatory cell proliferation
  Apoptosis
  Wound-healing biology

Factors that *can* be directly controlled or influenced at present
  Whole-body oxygenation
  Whole-body perfusion
  Pain, anxiety
  Body temperature
  Acid-base balance
  ECF electrolyte composition and balance
  Nutrient supply
  Glucose concentration
  Anabolic factors
  Gut mucosal integrity
  Focal infection and bacteremia
  Wound repair and closure

Although some degree of hyperglycemia may facilitate glucose uptake by the inflammatory cells in the wound, excessive elevations—in excess of 10 mmol/L (180 mg/dl)—have been associated with a variety of adverse effects, including impaired phagocytosis and immune function, increased CO_2 production and ventilatory requirements, increased vascular tone and reduction of regional blood flow, and altered collagen formation.[12] Close control of blood glucose concentration (110 to 160 mg/dl) with insulin therapy may not only prevent these effects but also exert a beneficial effect on net protein loss. The insulin resistance in critically ill patients blunts the hypoglycemic effects of insulin, so that it may be administered continuously and regulated safely at the bedside by means of a standardized algorithm (sliding scale).[227]

One of the most effective means of manipulating the metabolic response to critical surgical illness, however, remains excellent surgical care. Such care is directed toward reducing, limiting, preventing, or neutralizing the signals that initiate these debilitating responses. Aggressive and prompt resuscitation, restoration of tissue oxygenation, debridement of necrotic tissue, drainage of pus, and wound repair all should have a high priority in the early management of a critically ill patient. Maintenance of effective cardiopulmonary function and tissue oxygenation, provision of a warm environment, preservation of GI tract integrity, and control of infection are clinical objectives of later management.

Over the course of the past few decades, close attention to these details has resulted in improved outcome for critically ill patients. For example, Pruitt and Mason analyzed a population of over 8,000 burn patients treated at the US Army Burn Unit from 1950 through 1991.[228] Since the mid-1970s, the burn size associated with a 50% mortality steadily rose from 57% of BSA to 77%. Similarly, Milberg and colleagues demonstrated a reduction in ARDS-related mortality from nearly 70% to 30% between 1983 and 1993.[229]

In a 1995 study, Kelleman and colleagues determined the effect of burn size on resting energy expenditure.[230] This study reproduced that of Wilmore done at the same institution almost 20 years before. In the earlier study, the resting metabolic rate increased steadily with burn size and plateaued at about twice the basal level with burns larger than 50% of BSA. Kelleman found that energy expenditure plateaued at only 1.5 times the basal level with burns of about 25% of BSA or more. This dramatic change in the relationship between burn size (injury severity) and metabolic activity (hypermetabolism) probably reflects the combined effects of improvements in all aspects of burn care, including resuscitation, cardiopulmonary and metabolic support, wound care, nursing practice, occupational and physical therapy, and reduced time to excision and grafting and wound closure. Improvements in care have thus reduced the metabolic cost of critical surgical illness.

Conclusion

The physiologic impact of major trauma, burns, intra-abdominal catastrophe, sepsis, or other critical illness reverberates throughout the body and affects all organ systems. Knowledge about the mechanisms that regulate this comprehensive and commanding response is growing at an exponential rate. These mechanisms are intricate, interrelated, and redundant. Where we once looked for a simple, direct answer, we now see dizzying complexity. The critically ill patient is a true example of controlled inflammation, suspended between anabolic and catabolic forces and between inflammatory and anti-inflammatory forces.

Unfortunately, our ability to apply our improved understanding to the care of critically ill patients still lags far behind. When the patient is not progressing well, we lack the ability to make a specific bedside diagnosis that will pinpoint the part of the system that is out of balance. Even if we could make such a diagnosis, however, we still lack the accurately targeted therapies that would allow us to intervene precisely.

Thus, a wide variety of factors and processes, with both beneficial and adverse effects, appear to be involved in the metabolic response to critical illness, but we are unable to affect many of them directly with the means currently available [see Table 8]. We can remove necrotic tissue, repair wounds, and drain pus. We can also usually ensure excellent cardiovascular performance and maintain extracellular electrolyte and nutrient composition and acid-base balance. We can often suppress bacteremia and can treat some infections effectively with antibiotics. We can prevent many additional insults to and stresses on our patients. These measures may seem unsophisticated and clumsy in the light of our contemporary understanding of the biology of convalescence, but they clearly are capable of nudging the metabolic response to critical illness toward a successful outcome. At present, such measures constitute the essentials of excellent comprehensive care of critically ill patients, and they give these patients their best hope for recovery.

References

1. Wilmore DW: Metabolic Management of the Critically Ill. Plenum Press, New York, 1980
2. Patient-controlled analgesia (editorial). Lancet 1:289, 1980
3. Kehlet H: Multimodal approach to control postoperative pathophysiology and rehabilitation. Br J Anaesth 78:606, 1997
4. MacKersie RC, Shackford SR, Hoyt DB, et al: Continuous epidural fentanyl analgesia: ventilatory function improvement with routine use in treatment of blunt chest injury. J Trauma 27:1207, 1987
5. Bone RC, Balk RA, Cerra FB, et al: Definitions for sepsis and organ failure and guidelines for the use of innovative therapies in sepsis. Chest 101:1644, 1992
6. Rangel-Frausto MS, Pittet D, Costigan M, et al: The natural history of the systemic inflammatory response syndrome (SIRS): a prospective study. JAMA 273:117, 1995
7. Civetta JM, Hudson-Civetta J, Bell S: Decreasing catheter-related infection and hospital costs by continuous quality improvement. Crit Care Med 24:1660, 1996
8. Mandal AK, Monturo J, Thadepelli H: Prophylactic antibiotics and no antibiotics compared in penetrating chest trauma. J Trauma 25:639, 1985
9. Stoutenbeek CP, van Saene HKF, Miranda DR, et al: The effect of oropharyngeal decontamination using topical nonabsorbable antibiotics on the incidence of nosocomial respiratory tract infections in multiple trauma patients. J Trauma 27:357, 1987
10. Goldman DA, Weinstein RA, Wenzel RP, et al: Strategies to prevent and control the emergence and spread of antimicrobial-resistant microorganisms in hospitals: a challenge to hospital leadership. JAMA 275:234, 1996
11. Sise MJ, Hollingsworth P, Brimm JC, et al: Complications of the flow-directed pulmonary artery catheter. Crit Care Med 8:272, 1980
12. Bessey PQ, Watters JM: Glucose metabolism following trauma or sepsis. Trauma, Sepsis, and Shock: The Physiological Basis of Therapy. Burke PA, Forse RA, Eds. Marcel Dekker, New York (in press)
13. Cuthbertson DP: Surgical metabolism: historical and evolutionary aspects. Metabolism and the Response to Injury. Wilkinson AW, Cuthbertson DP, Eds. Year Book Medical Publishers, Chicago, 1977, p 1
14. Thomas L: The Lives of a Cell. Viking Press, New York, 1974, p 75
15. Im MJC, Hoopes JE: Energy metabolism in healing skin wounds. J Surg Res 10:459, 1970
16. Ben-Porat M, Sideman S, Bursztein S: Energy metabolism rate equation for fasting and postabsorptive subjects. Am J Physiol 244:R764, 1983
17. Atwater WO, Benedict FG: Experiments on the metabolism of matter and energy in the human body. US Department of Agriculture Office of Experimental Stations Bulletin, publication No. 136, 1903
18. Dubois EF: Basal Metabolism in Health and Disease. Lea & Febiger, Philadelphia, 1936, p 163
19. Wilmore DW, Long JM, Mason AD Jr, et al: Catecholamines: mediator of the hypermetabolic response to thermal injury. Ann Surg 180:653, 1974
20. Wilmore DW: Metabolic Management of the Critically Ill. Plenum Medical, New York, 1977, p 33
21. Shiozaki T, Kishikawa M, Hiraide A, et al: Recovery from postoperative hypothermia predicts survival in extensively burned patients. Am J Surg 165:326, 1993
22. Wilmore DW, Aulick LH, Mason AD, et al: Influence of the burn wound on local and systemic responses to injury. Ann Surg 186:444, 1977
23. Aulick LH, Wilmore DW, Mason AD Jr, et al: Muscle blood flow following thermal injury. Ann Surg 188:778, 1978
24. Wilmore DW, Goodwin CW, Aulick LH, et al: Effect of injury and infection on visceral metabolism and circulation. Ann Surg 192:491, 1980
25. Aulick LH, Goodwin CW Jr, Becker RA, et al: Visceral blood flow following thermal injury. Ann Surg 193:112, 1981
26. Wilmore DW, Aulick LH: Metabolic changes in burned patients. Surg Clin North Am 58:1173, 1978
27. Cuthbertson DP: The disturbance of metabolism produced by bony and non-bony injury, with notes on certain abnormal conditions of bone. Biochem J 24:1244, 1930
28. Monafo WW: Wound care: physiologic concepts. Treatment of Burns: Principles and Practice. Monafo WW, Pappalardo C, Eds. Warren H Green, Inc, St Louis, 1971, p 111
29. Caldwell FT Jr, Osterholm JL, Sower ND, et al: Metabolic response to thermal trauma of normal and thyroprivic rats at three environmental temperatures. Ann Surg 150:976, 1959
30. Barr PO, Birke G, Liljedahl SO, et al: Oxygen consumption and water loss during treatment of burns with warm dry air. Lancet 1:164, 1968
31. Wilmore DW, Mason AD Jr, Johnson DW, et al: Effect of ambient temperature on heat production and heat loss in burn patients. J Appl Physiol 38:593, 1975
32. Wilmore DW, Orcutt TW, Mason AD Jr, et al: Alterations in hypothalamic function following thermal injury. J Trauma 15:697, 1975
33. Howard JE, Parson W, Stein KE, et al: Studies on fracture convalescence: I. Nitrogen metabolism after fracture and skeletal operations in healthy males. Johns Hopkins Hospital Bulletin 75:156, 1944
34. Cuthbertson DP: Observations on disturbance of metabolism produced by injury to the limbs. Q J Med 25:233, 1932
35. Cuthbertson DP, McGirr JL, Robertson JSM: The effect of fracture of bone on the metabolism of the

rat. Quarterly Journal of Experimental Physiology 29:13, 1939
36. Threlfall CJ, Stoner HB, Galasko CSB: Patterns in the excretion of muscle markers after trauma and orthopedic surgery. J Trauma 21:140, 1981
37. Young VR, Munro HN: N^γ-methylhistidine (3-methylhistidine) and muscle protein turnover: an overview. Federal Proceedings 37:2291, 1978
38. Williamson DH, Farrell R, Kerr A, et al: Muscle protein catabolism after injury in man as measured by urinary excretion of 3-methylhistidine. Clin Sci Molec Med 52:527, 1977
39. Bilmazes C, Kien CL, Rohrbaugh DK, et al: Quantitative contribution by skeletal muscle to elevated rates of whole-body protein breakdown in burned children as measured by N^γ-methylhistidine output. Metabolism 27:671, 1978
40. Long CL, Schiller WR, Blakemore WS, et al: Muscle protein catabolism in the septic patient as measured by 3-methylhistidine excretion. Am J Clin Nutr 30:1349, 1977
41. Cuthbertson DP: The physiology of convalescence after injury. Br Med Bull 3:96, 1945
42. Moore FD, Langohr JL, Ingebretsen M, et al: The role of exudate losses in the protein and electrolyte imbalance of burned patients. Ann Surg 132:1, 1950
43. Soroff HS, Pearson E, Artz CP: An estimation of the nitrogen requirements for equilibrium in burned patients. Surg Gynecol Obstet 112:150, 1961
44. Wilmore DW: Nutrition and metabolism following thermal injury. Clin Plast Surg 1:603, 1974
45. Kinney JM: Energy deficits in acute illness and injury. Proceedings of a Conference on Energy Metabolism and Body Fuel Utilization. Morgan AP, Ed. Harvard University Press, Cambridge, Massachusetts, 1966, p 174
46. Picou D, Taylor-Roberts T: The measurement of total protein synthesis and catabolism and nitrogen turnover in infants on different amounts of dietary protein. Clin Sci 36:283, 1969
47. Birkhahn RH, Long CL, Fitkin D, et al: Effects of major skeletal trauma on whole body protein turnover in man measured by L-[1,^{14}C]-leucine. Surgery 88:294, 1980
48. Kien CL, Young VR, Rohrbaugh DK, et al: Increased rates of whole body protein synthesis and breakdown in children recovering from burns. Ann Surg 187:383, 1978
49. Munro HN: Free amino acid pools and their role in regulation. Mammalian Protein Metabolism, Vol 4. Munro HN, Ed. Academic Press, New York, 1970, p 299
50. Bergström J, Fürst P, Noree L-O, et al: Intracellular free amino acid concentration in human muscle tissue. J Appl Physiol 36:693, 1974
51. Askanazi J, Elwyn DH, Kinney JM, et al: Muscle and plasma amino acids after injury: the role of inactivity. Ann Surg 188:797, 1978
52. Vinnars E, Bergström J, Fürst P: Influence of the postoperative state on the intracellular free amino acids in human muscle tissue. Ann Surg 182:665, 1975
53. Fürst P, Bergström J, Chao L, et al: Influence of amino acid supply on nitrogen and amino acid metabolism in severe trauma. Acta Chir Scand 494(suppl):136, 1979
54. Askanazi J, Carpentier YA, Michelson CB, et al: Muscle and plasma amino acids following injury: influence of intercurrent infection. Ann Surg 192:78, 1980
55. Askanazi J, Fürst P, Michelsen CB, et al: Muscle and plasma amino acids after injury: hypocaloric glucose vs. amino acid infusion. Ann Surg 191:465, 1980
56. Wilmore DW, Black PR, Muhlbacher F: Injured man: trauma and sepsis. Nutritional Support of the Seriously Ill Patient. Winters RW, Greene HL, Eds. Academic Press, New York, 1983, p 33
57. Aulick LH, Wilmore DW: Increased peripheral amino acid release following burn injury. Surgery 85:560, 1979
58. Garber AJ, Karl IE, Kipnis DM: Alanine and glutamine synthesis and release from skeletal muscle: I. Glycolysis and amino acid release. J Biol Chem 251:826, 1976
59. Garber AJ, Karl IE, Kipnis DM: Alanine and glutamine synthesis and release from skeletal muscle: II. The precursor role of amino acids in alanine and glutamine synthesis. J Biol Chem 251:836, 1976
60. Close JH: The use of amino acid precursors in nitrogen-accumulation diseases. N Engl J Med 290:663, 1974
61. Johnson DJ, Jiang ZM, Colpoys M, et al: Branched chain amino acid uptake and muscle free amino acid concentrations predict postoperative muscle nitrogen balance. Ann Surg 204:513, 1986
62. Rennie MJ, Hundal HS, Babij P, et al: Characteristics of a glutamine carrier in skeletal muscle have important consequences for nitrogen loss in injury, infection, and chronic disease. Lancet 2:1008, 1986
63. Windmueller HG: Glutamine utilization by the small intestine. Adv Enzymol 53:201, 1982
64. Souba WW, Wilmore DW: Postoperative alteration of arteriovenous exchange of amino acids across the gastrointestinal tract. Surgery 94:342, 1983
65. Long CL, Spencer JL, Kinney JM, et al: Carbohydrate metabolism in man: effect of elective operations and major injury. J Appl Physiol 31:110, 1971
66. Wolfe RR, Durkot MJ, Allsop JR, et al: Glucose metabolism in severely burned patients. Metabolism 28:1031, 1979
67. Wilmore DW, Mason AD, Pruitt BA Jr: Alterations in glucose kinetics following thermal injury. Forum on Fundamental Surgical Problems 26:81, 1975
68. Ruderman MB: Muscle amino acid metabolism and gluconeogenesis. Annu Rev Med 26:245, 1975
69. Wolfe RR, Herndon DN, Jahoor F, et al: Effect of severe burn injury on substrate cycling by glucose and fatty acids. N Engl J Med 317:403, 1987
70. Shaw JHF, Wolfe RR: An integrated analysis of glucose, fat, and protein metabolism in severely traumatized patients: studies in the basal state and the response to total parenteral nutrition. Ann Surg 209:63, 1989
71. Howard JM: Studies of the absorption and metabolism of glucose following injury: the systemic response to injury. Ann Surg 141:311, 1955
72. Allison SP, Hinton P, Chamberlain MJ: Intravenous glucose-tolerance, insulin, and free-fatty-acid levels in burned patients. Lancet 2:1113, 1968
73. Wilmore DW, Mason AD Jr, Pruitt BA Jr: Insulin response to glucose in hypermetabolic burn patients. Ann Surg 183:314, 1978
74. Black PR, Brooks DC, Bessey PQ, et al: Mechanisms of insulin resistance following injury. Ann Surg 196:420, 1982
75. Brooks DC, Bessey PQ, Black PR, et al: Post-traumatic insulin resistance in uninjured forearm tissue. J Surg Res 37:100, 1984
76. Long JM III, Wilmore DW, Mason AD Jr, et al: Effect of carbohydrate and fat intake on nitrogen excretion during total intravenous feeding. Ann Surg 185:417, 1977
77. Wolfe RR, O'Donnell TF Jr, Stone MD, et al: Investigation of factors determining optimal glucose infusion rate in total parenteral nutrition. Metabolism 29:892, 1980
78. Burke JF, Wolfe RR, Mullany CJ, et al: Glucose requirements following burn injury: parameters of optimal glucose infusion and possible hepatic and respiratory abnormalities following excessive glucose intake. Ann Surg 190:274, 1979
79. Askanazi J, Carpentier YA, Elwyn DH, et al: Influence of total parenteral nutrition on fuel utilization in injury and sepsis. Ann Surg 191:40, 1980
80. Goodenough RD, Wolfe RR: Effect of total parenteral nutrition on free fatty acid metabolism in burned patients. JPEN J Parenter Enteral Nutr 8:357, 1984
81. Roth J, LeRoith D, Lesniak MA, et al: Molecules of intercellular communication in vertebrates, invertebrates, and microbes: do they share common origins? Prog Brain Res 68:71, 1986
82. Davies CL, Newman RJ, Molyneux SG, et al: The relationship between plasma catecholamines and severity of injury in man. J Trauma 24:99, 1984
83. Harrison TS, Seaton JF, Feller I: Relationship of increased oxygen consumption to catecholamine excretion in thermal burns. Ann Surg 165:169, 1967
84. Porte D Jr, Robertson RP: Control of insulin secretion by catecholamines, stress, and the sympathetic nervous system. Fed Proc 32:1792, 1973
85. Bessey PQ, Brooks DC, Black PR, et al: Epinephrine acutely mediates skeletal muscle insulin resistance. Surgery 94:172, 1983
86. Garber AJ, Karl JE, Kipnis DM: Alanine and glutamine synthesis and release from skeletal muscle: IV. β-Adrenergic inhibition of amino acid release. J Biol Chem 251:851, 1976
87. Vaughan GM, Becker RA, Allan JP, et al: Cortisol and corticotrophin in burned patients. J Trauma 22:263, 1982
88. Wilmore DW, Lindsey CA, Moylan JA, et al: Hyperglucagonaemia after burns. Lancet 1:73, 1974
89. Baxter JD, Forsham PH: Tissue effects of glucocorticoids. Am J Med 53:573, 1972
90. Owen OE, Cahill GF Jr: Metabolic effects of exogenous glucocorticoids in fasted man. J Clin Invest 52:2596, 1973
91. Felig P, Wahren J, Hendler R: Influence of physiologic hyperglucagonemia on basal and insulin-inhibited splanchnic glucose output in normal man. J Clin Invest 58:761, 1976
92. Ferrannini E, DeFronze RA, Sherwin RS: Transient hepatic response to glucagon in man: role of insulin and hyperglycemia. Am J Physiol 242:E73, 1982
93. Wolfe BM, Culebras JM, Aoki TT, et al: The effects of glucagon on protein metabolism in normal man. Surgery 86:248, 1979
94. Shamoon HM, Hendler R, Sherwin RS: Synergistic interactions among anti-insulin hormones in the pathogenesis of stress hypoglycemia in humans. J Clin Endocrinol Metab 52:1235, 1981
95. Bessey PQ, Watters JM, Aoki TT, et al: Combined hormonal infusion simulates the metabolic response to injury. Ann Surg 200:264, 1984
96. Bessey PQ, Jiang Z-M, Johnson DJ, et al: Post-traumatic skeletal muscle proteolysis: the role of the hormonal environment. World J Surg 13:465, 1989
97. Vilstrup H, Hansen BA, Aldal T: Glucagon enhances hepatic efficacy for urea production. Clinical Nutrition 7(suppl):35, 1988
98. Bessey PQ, Lowe KA: Early hormonal changes affect the catabolic response to trauma. Ann Surg 218:476, 1993
99. Hulton N, Johnson DJ, Smith RJ, et al: Hormonal blockade modifies post-traumatic protein catabolism. J Surg Res 39:310, 1985
100. Brandt MR, Fernandes A, Mordhorst R, et al: Epidural analgesia improves postoperative nitrogen balance. Br Med J 1:1106, 1978
101. Tsuji H, Shirasaka C, Asoh T, et al: Effects of epidural administration of local anaesthetics or morphine on postoperative nitrogen loss and catabolic hormones. Br J Surg 74:421, 1987
102. Heindorff H, Schulze S, Morgensen T, et al: Hormonal and neural blockade prevents the postoperative increase in amino acid clearance and urea synthesis. Surgery 111:543, 1992
103. Hunt TK: Physiology of wound healing. Trauma, Sepsis, and Shock: The Physiological Basis of Therapy. Clowes GHA Jr, Ed. Marcel Dekker, New York, 1988, p 443
104. Dinarello CA: Proinflammatory and anti-inflammatory cytokines as mediators in the pathogenesis of septic shock. Chest 112:321S, 1997

105. Cinat M, Waxman K, Vaziri ND, et al: Soluble cytokine receptors and receptor antagonists are sequentially released after trauma. J Trauma 39:112, 1995
106. Akira S, Hirano T, Taga T, et al: Biology of multifunctional cytokines: IL-6 and related molecules (IL-1 and TNF). FASEB J 4:2860, 1990
107. Jiang JX, Tian KL, Chen HS, et al: Plasma cytokines and endotoxin levels in patients with severe injury and their relationship with organ damage. Injury 28:509, 1997
108. Drosst AC, Burleson DG, Cioffi WG Jr, et al: Plasma cytokines following thermal injury and their relationship with patient mortality, burn size, and time postburn. J Trauma 35:335, 1993
109. Michie HR, Spriggs DR, Manogue KR, et al: Tumor necrosis factor and endotoxin induce similar metabolic responses in human beings. Surgery 104:280, 1988
110. Michie HR, Sherman ML, Spriggs DR, et al: Chronic TNF infusion causes anorexia but not accelerated nitrogen loss. Ann Surg 209:19, 1989
111. Mealy K, van Lanschot JJB, Robinson BG, et al: Are the catabolic effects of tumor necrosis factor mediated by glucocorticoids? Arch Surg 125:42, 1990
112. Hall-Angeras M, Angeras U, Zamir O, et al: Effect of the glucocorticoid receptor antagonist RU 38486 on muscle protein breakdown in sepsis. Surgery 109:468, 1991
113. Dinarello CA: Interleukin-1. Rev Infect Dis 6:51, 1984
114. Dinarello CA: An update on human interleukin-1: from molecular biology to clinical relevance. J Clin Immunol 5:287, 1985
115. Baracos V, Rodemann HP, Dinarello CA, et al: Stimulation of muscle protein degradation and prostaglandin E_2 release by leukocytic pyrogen (interleukin-1): a mechanism for the increased degradation of muscle proteins during fever. N Engl J Med 308:553, 1983
116. Sobrado JL, Moldawer LL, Dinarello CA, et al: Effect of ibuprofen on fever and metabolic changes induced by leukocytic pyrogen (interleukin-1) and endotoxin. Infect Immun 42:997, 1983
117. Moldawer LL, Svaninger G, Gelin J, et al: Interleukin-1 and tumor necrosis factor do not regulate protein balance in skeletal muscle. Am J Physiol 253:C766, 1987
118. Zamir O, Hasselgren P-O, von Allmen D, et al: The effect of interleukin-1 alpha and the glucocorticoid receptor blocker RU 38486 on total and myofibrillar protein breakdown in skeletal muscle. J Surg Res 50:579, 1991
119. Zamir O, Hasselgren P-O, O'Brien WO, et al: Muscle protein breakdown during endotoxemia in rats and after treatment with interleukin-1 receptor antagonist (IL-1ra). Ann Surg 216:381, 1992
120. Watters JM, Bessey PQ, Dinarello CA, et al: The induction of interleukin-1 in humans and its metabolic effects. Surgery 98:298, 1985
121. Watters JM, Bessey PQ, Dinarello CA, et al: Both inflammatory and endocrine mediators stimulate host responses to sepsis. Arch Surg 121:179, 1986
122. Koj A: The role of interleukin-6 as the hepatic stimulating factor in the network of inflammatory cytokines. Ann NY Acad Sci 557:1, 1989
123. Biffl WL, Moore EE, Moore FA, et al: Interleukin-6 in the injured patient: marker of injury or mediator of inflammation? Ann Surg 224:647, 1996
124. Casey LC, Balk RA, Bone RC: Plasma cytokines and endotoxin levels correlate with survival in patients with the sepsis syndrome. Ann Intern Med 119:771, 1993
125. de Beaux AC, Ross JA, Maingay JP, et al: Proinflammatory cytokine release by peripheral blood mononuclear cells from patients with acute pancreatitis. Br J Surg 83:1071, 1996
126. Guillen I, Blaines M, Gomez-Lechon MJ, et al: Cytokine signaling during myocardial infarction: sequential appearance of IL-1β and IL-6. Am J Physiol 269:R229, 1995
127. Mateo RB, Reichner JS, Albina JE: Interleukin-6 activity in wounds. Am J Physiol 266:R1840, 1994
128. Stouthard JM, Romijn JA, van der Poll T, et al: Endocrinologic and metabolic effects of interleukin-6 in humans. Am J Physiol 268:E813, 1995
129. Tsigos C, Papanicolaou DA, Kyrou I, et al: Dose-dependent effects of recombinant human interleukin-6 on glucose regulation. J Clin Endocrinol Metab 82:4167, 1997
130. De Benedetti F, Alonzi T, Moretta A, et al: Interleukin-6 causes growth impairment in transgenic mice through a decrease in insulin-like growth factor-1. J Clin Invest 99:643, 1997
131. Tsujinaka T, Fujita J, Ebisui C, et al: Interleukin-6 receptor antibody inhibits muscle atrophy and modulates proteolytic systems in interleukin-6 transgenic mice. J Clin Invest 97:244, 1996
132. Rutan RL, Herndon DN: Growth delay in postburn pediatric patients. Arch Surg 125:392, 1990
133. Gonzalez-Hernandez JA, Bornstein SR, Ehrhart-Bornstein M, et al: Interleukin-6 messenger ribonucleic acid expression in human adrenal gland in vivo: new clue to a paracrine or autocrine regulation of adrenal function. J Clin Endocrinol Metab 79:1492, 1994
134. Path G, Bornstein SR, Ehrhart-Bornstein M, et al: Interleukin-6 and the interleukin-6 receptor in the human adrenal gland: expression and effects on steroidogenesis. J Clin Endocrinol Metab 82:2343, 1997
135. Bone RC, Fisher CJ, Clemmer TP, et al: A controlled clinical trial of high-dose methylprednisolone in the treatment of severe sepsis and septic shock. N Engl J Med 317:653, 1987
136. Barber AE, Coyle SM, Maranao MA, et al: Glucocorticoid therapy alters hormonal and cytokine responses to endotoxin in man. J Immunol 150:1999, 1993
137. Hasselgren P-O: Protein Metabolism in Sepsis. RG Landes Co, Austin, Texas, 1993, p 82
138. Wing SS, Goldberg AL: Glucocorticoids activate the ATP-ubiquitin–dependent proteolytic system in skeletal muscle during fasting. Am J Physiol 264:E668, 1993
139. Zamir O, Hasselgren P-O, von Allmen D, et al: In vivo administration of interleukin-1α induces muscle proteolysis in normal and adrenalectomized rats. Metabolism 42:204, 1993
140. Hume DM, Egdahl RH: The importance of the brain in the endocrine response to injury. Ann Surg 150:697, 1959
141. Taylor JW, Hander EW, Skreen R, et al: The effect of central nervous system narcosis on the sympathetic response to stress. J Surg Res 20:313, 1976
142. Dempsey DT, Guenter P, Crosby LO, et al: Barbiturate therapy and energy expenditure in head trauma. Presented at the 42nd Annual Meeting of the American Association for the Surgery of Trauma, Colorado Springs, 1982
143. Fried R, Dempsey D, Guenter P: Barbiturates improve nitrogen balance in patients with severe head trauma (abstr). JPEN J Parenter Enteral Nutr 4:86, 1984
144. Wilmore DW, Long JM, Mason AD, et al: Stress in surgical patients as a neurophysiologic reflex response. Surg Gynecol Obstet 142:257, 1976
145. Wilmore DW, Taylor JW, Handler EW, et al: Central nervous system function following thermal injury. Metabolism and the Response to Injury. Wilkinson AW, Cuthbertson DP, Eds. Year Book Medical Publishers, Chicago, 1977, p 274
146. Chrousos GP: The hypothalamic-pituitary-adrenal axis and immune-mediated inflammation. N Engl J Med 332:1351, 1995
147. Turchik JB, Bornstein DL: Role of the central nervous system in acute-phase responses to leukocyte pyrogen. Infect Immun 30:439, 1980
148. Breder CD, Dinarello CA, Saper CB: Interleukin-1 immunoreactive innervation of the human hypothalamus. Science 240:321, 1988
149. Cunningham ET, Wada E, Carter DB, et al: In situ localization of type I interleukin-1 receptor messenger RNA in the central nervous system, pituitary, and adrenal gland of the mouse. J Neurosci 12:1101, 1991
150. Schöbitz R, DeKloet ER, Sutanto W, et al: Cellular localization of interleukin-6 mRNA and interleukin-6 receptor RNA in rat brain. Eur J Neurosci 5:1426, 1993
151. Lieberman AP, Pitha PM, Shin HS, et al: Production of tumor necrosis factor and other cytokines by astrocytes stimulated with lipopolysaccharide or a neurotrophic virus. Proc Natl Acad Sci USA 86:6348, 1989
152. Maeda Y, Matsumoto M, Hori O, et al: Hypoxia/reoxygenation-mediated induction of astrocyte interleukin-6: a paracrine mechanism potentially enhancing neuron survival. J Exp Med 180:2297, 1994
153. Klir JJ, McClellan JL, Kluger MJ: Interleukin-1β causes the increase in anterior hypothalamic interleukin-6 during LPS-induced fever in rats. Am J Physiol 266:R1845, 1994
154. Nakamori T, Morimoto A, Yamaguchi K, et al: Interleukin-1β production in the rabbit brain during endotoxin-induced fever. J Physiol Lond 476:177, 1994
155. Hill AG, Hiegel J, Rounds J, et al: Metabolic responses to interleukin-1: centrally and peripherally mediated. Ann Surg 225:246, 1997
156. Hill AG, Jacobson L, Gonzalez J, et al: Chronic central nervous system exposure to interleukin-1β causes catabolism in the rat. Am J Physiol 271:R1142, 1996
157. Mastorakos G, Chrousos GP, Weber JS: Recombinant interleukin-6 activates the hypothalamic-pituitary-adrenal axis in humans. J Clin Endocrinol Metab 77:1690, 1993
158. Ling PR, Schwartz JH, Jeevanandam M, et al: Metabolic changes in rats during a continuous infusion of recombinant interleukin-1. Am J Physiol 270:E305, 1996
159. Reyes TM, Coe CL: The proinflammatory cytokine network: interactions in the CNS and blood of rhesus monkeys. Am J Physiol 274:R139, 1998
160. Romero LI, Kakucska I, Lechan RM, et al: Interleukin-6 (IL-6) is secreted from the brain after intercerebroventricular injection of IL-1β in rats. Am J Physiol 270:R518, 1996
161. Senba E, Kashiba K: Sensory afferent processing in multi-responsive DRG neurons. Prog Brain Res 113:387, 1996
162. Thompson SW, Priestley JV, Southall A: gp130 cytokines, leukemia inhibitory factor, and interleukin-6 induce neuropeptide expression in intact adult rat sensory neurons in vivo: time-course, specificity, and comparison with sciatic nerve axotomy. Neuroscience 84:1247, 1998
163. Hirota H, Kiyama H, Kishimoto T, et al: Accelerated nerve regeneration in mice by upregulated expression of interleukin (IL) 6 and IL-6 receptor after trauma. J Exp Med 183:2627, 1996
164. Niijima A: The afferent discharges from sensors for interleukin-1β in the hepatoportal system in the anesthetized rat. J Autonom Nerv Sys 61:287, 1996
165. Ravin HA, Rowley D, Jenkins C, et al: On the absorption of bacterial endotoxin from the gastro-intestinal tract of the normal and shocked animal. J Exp Med 112:783, 1960
166. Caridis DT, Reinhold RB, Woodruff PW, et al: Endotoxaemia in man. Lancet 1:1381, 1972
167. Wilmore DW, Smith RJ, O'Dwyer ST, et al: The gut: a central organ after surgical stress. Surgery 104:917, 1988
168. Marin ML, Greenstein AJ, Geller SA, et al: A freeze fracture study of Crohn's disease of the terminal ileum: changes in epithelial tight junction organization. Am J Gastroenterol 78:537, 1983

169. Dobbins WO III: Gut immunophysiology: a gastroenterologist's view with emphasis on pathophysiology. Am J Physiol 242:G1, 1982
170. Deitch EA, Berg R, Specian R: Endotoxin promotes the translocation of bacteria from the gut. Arch Surg 122:185, 1987
171. Wellmann W, Fink PC, Schmidt FW: Whole-gut irrigation as antiendotoxinaemic therapy in inflammatory bowel disease. Hepatogastroenterology 31:91, 1984
172. Schatten WE, Desprez JD, Holden WD: A bacteriologic study of portal-vein blood in man. Arch Surg 71:404, 1955
173. Ambrose NS, Johnson M, Burdon DW, et al: Incidence of pathogenic bacteria from mesenteric lymph nodes and ileal serosa during Crohn's disease surgery. Br J Surg 71:623, 1984
174. Berg RD: Translocation of indigenous bacteria from the intestinal tract. Human Intestinal Microflora in Health and Disease. Hentges DJ, Ed. Academic Press, New York, 1983
175. Deitch EA, Winterton J, Berg R: Thermal injury promotes bacterial translocation from the gastrointestinal tract in mice with impaired T-cell–mediated immunity. Arch Surg 121:97, 1986
176. Baker JW, Deitch EA, Li M, et al: Hemorrhagic shock induces bacterial translocation from the gut. J Trauma 28:896, 1988
177. Deitch EA, Winterton J, Li M, et al: The gut as a portal of entry for bacteremia: role of protein malnutrition. Ann Surg 205:681, 1987
178. Moore FA, Moore EE, Poggetti R, et al: Gut bacterial translocation via the portal vein: a clinical perspective with major torso trauma. J Trauma 31:629, 1991
179. O'Farrely C: Just how inflamed is the normal gut? Gut 42:603, 1998
180. Guy-Grand E, DiSanto JP, Henchoz P, et al: Small bowel enteropathy: role of intraepithelial lymphocytes and of cytokines (IL-12, IFN-γ, TNF) in the induction of epithelial cell death and renewal. Eur J Immunol 28:730, 1998
181. Wyble CW, Desai TR, Clark ET, et al: Physiologic concentrations of TNFα and IL-1β released from reperfused human intestine upregulate E-selectin and ICAM-1. J Surg Res 63:333, 1996
182. Mainous MR, Ertel W, Chaudry IH, et al: The gut: a cytokine-generating organ in systemic inflammation? Shock 4:193, 1995
183. Mochizuki H, Trocki O, Dominioni L: Mechanism of prevention of postburn hypermetabolism and catabolism by early enteral feeding. Ann Surg 200:297, 1984
184. Saito H, Trocki O, Alexander JW: The effect of route of nutrient administration on the nutritional state, catabolic hormone secretion, and gut mucosal integrity after burn injury. JPEN J Parenter Enteral Nutr 11:1, 1987
185. Alexander JW, MacMillan BG, Stinnett JD: Beneficial effects of aggressive protein feeding in severely burned children. Ann Surg 192:505, 1980
186. Border JR, Hassett J, La Duca J: The gut origin septic states in blunt multiple trauma (ISS = 40) in the ICU. Ann Surg 206:427, 1987
187. Ogle CK, Zuo L, Mao JX, et al: Differential expression of intestinal and splenic cytokines after parenteral nutrition. Arch Surg 130:1301, 1995
188. Lyoumi S, Tamion F, Petit J, et al: Induction and modulation of acute-phase response by protein malnutrition in rats: comparative effect of systemic and localized inflammation on interleukin-6 and acute-phase protein synthesis. J Nutr 128:166, 1998
189. Steiner M, Bourges HR, Freedman LS, et al: Effect of starvation on the tissue composition of the small intestine in the rat. Am J Physiol 215:75, 1968
190. Clarke RM: Evidence for both luminal and systemic factors in the control of rat intestinal epithelial replacement. Clin Sci Mol Med 50:139, 1976
191. Gleeson MH, Dowling RH, Peters TJ: Biochemical changes in intestinal mucosa after experimental small bowel by-pass in the rat. Clin Sci 43:743, 1972
192. Johnson LR, Lichtenberger LM, Copeland EM, et al: Action of gastrin on gastrointestinal structure and function. Gastroenterology 68:1184, 1975
193. Sagor GR, Ghatei MA, Al-Mukhtar MYT, et al: Evidence for a humoral mechanism after small intestinal resection: exclusion of gastrin but not enteroglucagon. Gastroenterology 84:902, 1983
194. Hwang TL, O'Dwyer ST, Smith RJ, et al: Preservation of small bowel mucosa using glutamine-enriched parenteral nutrition. Forum on Fundamental Surgical Problems 37:56, 1986
195. Jacobs DO, Evans DA, O'Dwyer ST, et al: Trophic effects of glutamine-enriched parenteral nutrition on colonic mucosa. JPEN J Parenter Enteral Nutr 12(suppl):6S, 1988
196. O'Dwyer ST, Smith RJ, Scott T: Glutamine enriched nutrition decreases intestinal injury and increases nitrogen retention. Br J Surg 74:1162, 1987
197. Young LS, Stevens P, Kaijser B: Gram-negative pathogens in septicaemic infections. Scand J Infect Dis 31(suppl):78, 1982
198. Fish RE, Spitzer JA: Continuous infusion of endotoxin from an osmotic pump in the conscious, unrestrained rat: a unique model of chronic endotoxemia. Circ Shock 12:135, 1984
199. Revhaug A, Michie HR, Manson JM, et al: Inhibition of cyclooxygenase attenuates the metabolic response to endotoxin in humans. Arch Surg 123:162, 1988
200. Michie HR, Manogue KR, Spriggs DR, et al: Detection of circulating tumor necrosis factor after endotoxin administration. N Engl J Med 318:1481, 1988
201. Fong Y, Tracey KJ, Moldawer LL, et al: Antibodies to cachectin/tumor necrosis factor reduce interleukin 1β and interleukin 6 appearance during lethal bacteremia. J Exp Med 170:1627, 1989
202. Riddington DW, Venkatesh B, Boivin CM, et al: Intestinal permeability, gastric intramucosal pH, and systemic endotoxemia in patients undergoing cardiopulmonary bypass. JAMA 275:1007, 1996
203. O'Dwyer ST, Michie HR, Ziegler TR, et al: A single dose of endotoxin increases intestinal permeability in healthy humans. Arch Surg 123:1459, 1988
204. Coleman W, DuBois EF: Calorimetric observations on the metabolism of typhoid patients with and without food. Arch Intern Med 15:887, 1915
205. Beisel WR, Sawyer WD, Ryll ED, et al: Metabolic effects of intracellular infections in man. Ann Intern Med 67:744, 1967
206. Aulick LH, McManus AT, Mason AD Jr, et al: Effects of infection on oxygen consumption and core temperature in experimental thermal injury. Ann Surg 204:48, 1986
207. Guo L, Lim KB, Gunn JS, et al: Regulation of lipid A modifications by *Salmonella typhimurium* virulence genes phoP-phoQ. Science 276:250, 1997
208. Mekalanos JJ: Environmental signals controlling expression of virulence determinants in bacteria. J Bacteriol 174:1, 1992
209. Springer TA: Traffic signals for lymphocyte recirculation and leukocyte emigration: the multistep paradigm. Cell 76:301, 1994
210. Demling RH: Adult respiratory distress syndrome: current concepts. New Horizons 1:388, 1993
211. Biffl WL, Moore EE, Moore FA, et al: Interleukin-6 delays neutrophil apoptosis via a mechanism involving platelet-activating factor. J Trauma 40:575, 1996
212. Herndon DN, Barrow RE, Rutan TC, et al: Effect of propranolol administration on hemodynamic and metabolic responses of burned pediatric patients. Ann Surg 208:484, 1988
213. Schulze A, Sommer P, Bigler D, et al: Effect of combined prednisolone, epidural analgesia, and indomethacin on the systemic response after colonic surgery. Arch Surg 127:325, 1992
214. Vincent J-L: New therapies in sepsis. Chest 112:330S, 1997
215. Hammarqvist F, Wernerman J, Ali R, et al: Addition of glutamine to total parenteral nutrition after elective abdominal surgery spares free glutamine in muscle, counteracts the fall in muscle protein synthesis, and improves nitrogen balance. Ann Surg 209:455, 1989
216. Ziegler TR, Young LS, Benfell K, et al: Clinical and metabolic efficacy of glutamine-supplemented parenteral nutrition after bone marrow transplantation: a randomized, double blind, controlled study. Ann Intern Med 116: 821, 1992
217. Kudsk KA, Minard G, Croce MA, et al: A randomized trial of isonitrogenous enteral diets after severe trauma: an immune-enhancing diet reduces septic complications. Ann Surg 224:531, 1996
218. Manson JM, Wilmore DW: Positive nitrogen balance with human growth hormone and hypocaloric intravenous feeding. Surgery 100:188, 1986
219. Jiang Z-M, He G-Z, Zhang S-Y, et al: Low dose growth hormone and hypocaloric nutrition attenuate the protein-catabolic response following major operation. Ann Surg 210:513, 1989
220. Herndon DN, Barrow RE, Kunkel KR, et al: Effects of recombinant human growth hormone on donor-site healing in severely burned children. Ann Surg 212:424, 1990
221. Knox J, Demling R, Wilmore D, et al: Increased survival after major thermal injury: the effect of growth hormone therapy in adults. J Trauma 39:526, 1995
222. Pharmacia & Upjohn: Safety statement from Pharmacia & Upjohn regarding the use of recombinant somatropin (Genotropin/Genotonorm) for treatment of acute catabolism in critically ill patients. Kalamazoo, Michigan, 1997
223. Demling RH, DeSanti L: Oxandrolone, an anabolic steroid, significantly increases the rate of weight gain in the recovery phase after major burns. J Trauma 43:47, 1997
224. Tishler ME, Leng E, Al-Kanhal M, et al: Metabolic response of muscle to trauma: altered control of protein turnover. Clinical Nutrition and Metabolic Research: Proceedings of the 7th Congress of ESPEN, Munich 1985. Dietze D, Grünert A, Kleinberger G, et al, Eds. S Karger, Basel, 1986, p 40
225. Inculet RI, Finley RI, Duff JH, et al: Insulin decreases muscle protein loss after operative trauma in man. Surgery 99:752, 1986
226. Bower RH, Muggia-Sullam M, Vallgren S, et al: Branched chain amino acid–enriched solutions in the septic patient: a randomized prospective trial. Ann Surg 203:13, 1986
227. Cole M, Lipp J, Bessey PQ: Effective glucose control in the critically ill using a bedside, algorithm controlled insulin infusion (in preparation)
228. Pruitt BA Jr, Mason AD Jr: Epidemiological, demographic and outcome characteristics of burn injury. Total Burn Care. Herndon, DN. WB Saunders Co, London, 1996, p 5
229. Milberg JA, Davis DR, Steinberg KP, et al: Improved survival of patients with acute respiratory distress syndrome (ARDS) 1983–1993. JAMA 273:306, 1995
230. Kelleman JJ 3rd, Cioffi WG Jr, Mason AD Jr, et al: Effect of ambient temperature on metabolic rate after thermal injury. Ann Surg 223:406, 1996
231. Beisel WR: Magnitude of host nutritional responses to infection. Am J Clin Nutr 30:1237, 1977
232. Michie HR, Wilmore DW: Sepsis, signals, and surgical sequelae. Arch Surg 125:531, 1990

Acknowledgments

Figures 1 and 5   Al Miller.

Figure 3   Nancy Lou Makris.

97 NUTRITIONAL SUPPORT

John L. Rombeau, M.D., Rolando H. Rolandelli, M.D., Douglas W. Wilmore, M.D., and John M. Daly, M.D.

Nutritional Management of Hospitalized Patients

Evaluation of the Need for Nutritional Support

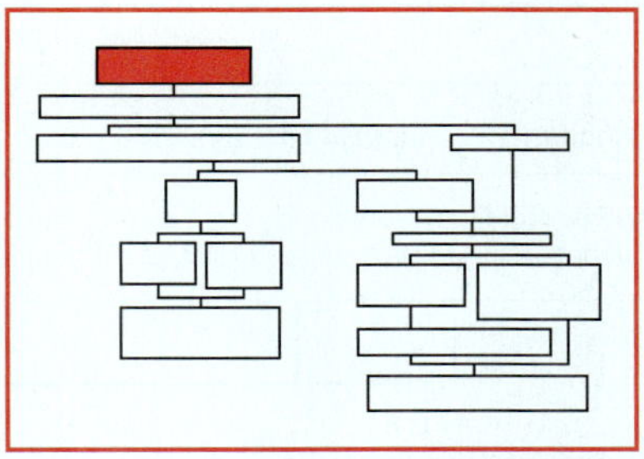

INDICATIONS FOR NUTRITIONAL INTERVENTION

In general, nutritional support should be considered in the following circumstances:

1. The patient has been without nutrition for 5 to 7 days. In a well-nourished individual, body stores are generally adequate to provide nutrients during shorter periods of stress without compromising physiologic functions, altering resistance to infection, or impairing wound healing. Patients who are unable to ingest nutrients orally usually receive intravenous solutions containing 5% dextrose, which provides some energy (approximately 170 kcal/L) and reduces, to varying degrees, protein breakdown. The provision of nutrients becomes more important as body stores become eroded because of inadequate food intake and accelerated catabolism. In general, deficits occur in surgical patients after 7 to 10 days of partial starvation; nutritional intervention should be initiated before this time.

2. The duration of illness is anticipated to be more than 10 days. In patients whose illness is known to have a moderately prolonged course, nutritional support should be considered essential care. Thus, individuals with severe peritonitis or pancreatitis, major injury (injury severity score > 15), or extensive burns (> 20% total body surface area) are candidates for nutritional support because of the known duration of their illness. (The duration of illness in chronically malnourished patients also would be expected to exceed 10 days.)

3. The patient is malnourished (loss of > 15% of usual body weight over 3 months). In general, the degree of weight loss can be used as an index of nutritional deficiency, and recovery may be compromised in patients who do not have adequate body nutrient stores because of an existing nutritional deficit [*see Figure 1*]. The patient should receive nutritional support when the weight loss approaches or exceeds 15% of usual body weight:

$$\% \text{ Weight loss} = \frac{\text{Usual weight} - \text{Present weight}}{\text{Usual weight}} \times 100$$

Patients who do not meet one of these three general indications should be reassessed after 7 days to identify individuals in whom complications develop after admission to the hospital and who require nutritional support. Serum proteins with a short half-life, such as prealbumin, transferrin, or retinol-binding protein, are useful markers for serial assessments.

PRIORITY OF CARDIOPULMONARY FUNCTION

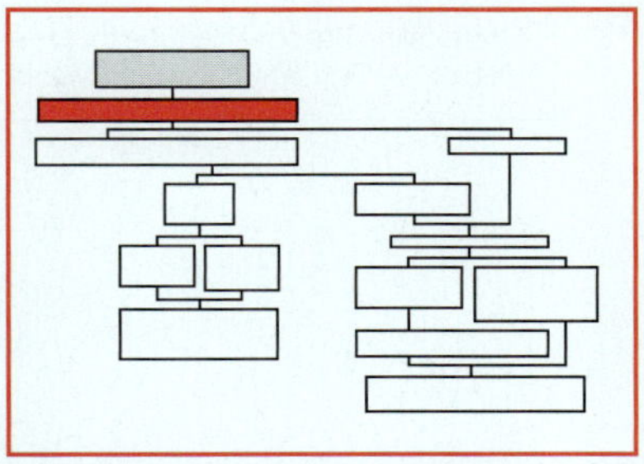

Intensive care unit patients are frequently candidates for nutritional support but often have a number of complex medical and surgical problems that may take precedence. In decreasing order of importance, the priorities are maintenance of airway, breathing, circulation, tissue oxygenation, acid-base neutrality, normal electrolyte concentrations, and adequate nutrition. The six functions that take priority over nutrition are usually impaired by acute and potentially life-threatening disorders that are often correctable over the short term. To optimize nutrient metabolism, circulation and tissue oxygenation must be adequate. In addition, hydrogen ion and electrolyte concentrations should be near normal in the extracellular fluid compartment, as reflected by blood or serum measurements.

If cardiopulmonary function is abnormal, nutrient administration may potentiate the abnormalities and create additional problems. For example, in a patient with respiratory insufficiency, infusion of moderate quantities of carbohydrate could increase carbon dioxide tension (Pco_2) and lower serum potassium concentration. These changes could initiate a life-threatening cardiac

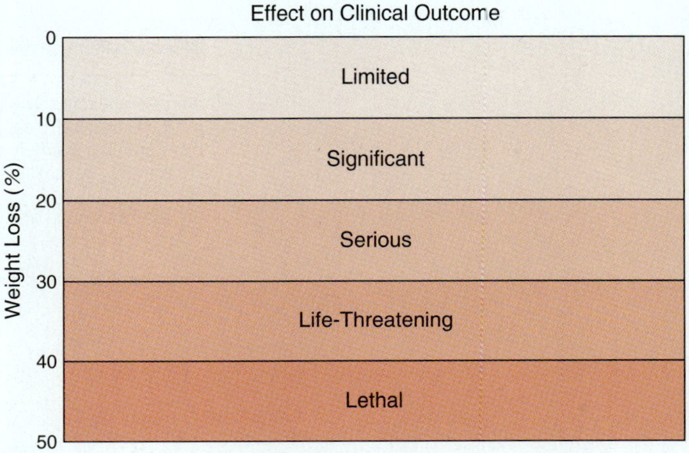

Figure 1 The magnitude of weight loss is a rough predictor of its effect on clinical outcome.

Give nutritional support if any of the following conditions is present:
- Patient has been without nutrition for 7–10 days
- Expected duration of illness > 10 days
- Patient is malnourished (weight loss > 15% of usual weight)

If nutritional intervention is not indicated initially, reassess patient after 5 days.

Initiate nutritional support only if tissue perfusion is adequate and Po_2, Pco_2, electrolyte concentrations, and acid-base balance are near normal

Estimate requirements for fluid, calories, protein, minerals, trace elements, and vitamins according to BMR, disease state, and activity level.

Abdominal distention, diarrhea, massive GI hemorrhage, obstruction, and hemodynamic instability are absent

Use existing nasogastric tube for enteral nutrition. Verify location of NG tube by aspiration of GI contents or by x-ray. Select balanced or disease-specific diet; deliver 30 ml/hr continuously at isotonicity for 24 hr. Elevate head during and after feeding to prevent regurgitation. Assess feeding tolerance.

Enteral feeding is tolerated

Assess risk for aspiration. Risk factors include depressed sensorium, gastroesophageal reflux, and history of aspiration or regurgitation.

Risk for aspiration is low

Give continuous gastric feedings of an isotonic formula at 30 ml/hr. Increase rate daily by 30 ml/hr. Increase tonicity after increasing volume.

Risk for aspiration is high

Pass feeding tube into jejunum; verify tube location by x-ray. Give formulas of 300 mOsm/kg at an initial rate of 30 ml/hr. Increase rate daily by 30 ml/hr. Increase tonicity after volume is fully increased.

Monitor patient; prevent and treat complications as necessary

Irrigate tube routinely with 20–25 ml normal saline or water.
If tube is blocked, clear by injection of a small volume of carbonated beverage.
For persistent diarrhea, give kaolin-pectin, 30 ml q. 3 hr.
To prevent peptic ulcers and bleeding, titrate gastric pH to 4.5–6.5 with antacids if necessary.
If nasoenteric tube dislodgment is recurrent, consider tube enterostomy.
If enterostomy tube leaks persistently, replace with tube of larger diameter.

Nutritional Management of Hospitalized Patients

Abdominal distention, diarrhea, massive GI hemorrhage, obstruction, or hemodynamic instability is present

Enteral feeding not tolerated

Symptoms of intolerance include increased gastric residuum, worsening of diarrhea, emesis, severe abdominal cramping, and abdominal distention.

Administer parenteral nutrition into central or peripheral vein

Initiate central venous infusion

Indications include
- Duration of I.V. feeding > 10 days
- Increased energy needs (≥ 2,200 kcal/day) but normal or limited fluid requirements (< 2.5 L/day)
- Organ failure

Initiate peripheral venous infusion

Indications include
- Duration of I.V. feeding 5–10 days
- Patient is nondepleted, can tolerate 2.5–3.0 L fluid/day, and has near-basal energy requirements
- Central venous catheterization is contraindicated or impossible, or central line is used for other purposes
- Enteral feedings are inadequate and must be supplemented with peripheral infusions

Insert central line (preferably a percutaneously inserted central catheter [PICC]), and order nutrient mix

Use chest x-ray to confirm placement in superior vena cava. Adjust solution for organ failure. Reserve catheter or lumen exclusively for nutrient administration.

Monitor patient

If body weight falls gradually for 2 wk or longer, calculate metabolic rate and increase calorie intake to match.
Give sufficient protein to avoid negative nitrogen balance.
Treat hyperglycemia with insulin; if glucose intolerance is severe, decrease glucose and increase fat emulsion administered.
Ensure catheter asepsis.

Table 1 Alterations in Metabolic Rate

Patient Condition	Basal Metabolic Rate
No postoperative complications Fistula without infection	Normal
Mild peritonitis Long-bone fracture or mild to moderate injury	25% above normal
Severe injury or infection in ICU patient Multiorgan failure	50% above normal
Burn of 40%–100% of TBS	100% above normal

arrhythmia. The need for nutritional support in the ICU patient should always be evaluated with respect to other care problems; acute disorders of cardiorespiratory function, disturbed acid-base status, and altered electrolyte concentrations should generally be corrected before nutritional support is initiated.

NUTRIENT REQUIREMENTS

The energy requirements of an individual are primarily related to body size, age, gender, and energy expenditure of activity (muscular work). In hospitalized patients who are generally inactive, the basal metabolic rate (BMR) accounts for the greatest amount of energy expenditure. The BMR can be calculated according to the Harris-Benedict formulas[1]:

Males: BMR (kcal/day) = 66 + [13.7 × weight (kg)] + [5 × height (cm)] − [6.8 × age (yr)]

Females: BMR (kcal/day) = 665 + [9.6 × weight (kg)] + [1.7 × height (cm)] − [4.7 × age (yr)]

The BMR is influenced by the disease process; hypermetabolism occurs in surgical patients with moderate to severe infection or injury. In these individuals, the magnitude of the increase in the BMR depends on the extent of injury or infection. Patients generally fall into one of four categories according to their metabolic requirements [*see Table 1*].

Estimates that are based on normal basal metabolic requirements and adjusted only for the disease state of the patient should reflect the energy needs of patients requiring mechanical ventilation or those at bed rest. However, further adjustments are necessary for individuals who are out of bed and physically active: they should receive additional calories. To meet the energy needs of physically active patients, who are in a nonbasal state, calculated requirements should be increased an additional 15% to 20%. The metabolic response to stress and critical illness is complex and is mediated by interactions between the neuroendocrine system and circulating cytokines. This interaction produces a metabolic milieu in which the body cannot utilize supranormal amounts of nutritional substrates (i.e., hyperalimentation). In fact, administering excessive nutrients with the purported goal of acutely correcting nutrient deficits is often harmful, leading to an abnormal accumulation of hepatic glycogen, enhancing total energy expenditure, and causing increased urea production and elevation of the blood urea nitrogen (BUN).

Weight gain usually should not be a priority for ICU patients. Complications of nutrient delivery are minimized and nutrient metabolism is generally optimized if the ICU patient receives only the energy necessary for weight maintenance throughout a complex and complicated clinical course. (This quantity of energy rarely exceeds 35 total calories/kg body weight/day in most general surgical patients who are admitted to the ICU for non–trauma-related care.) With resolution of the disease process, the hormonal environment is altered to favor anabolism. In addition, increases in spontaneous activity and in planned exercise stimulate rebuilding of lean body mass.

Table 2 Vitamin Requirements

Vitamin	Units	Recommended Dietary Allowance (RDA) for Daily Oral Intake[134]	Daily Requirement of the Moderately Injured	Daily Requirement of the Severely Injured	Amount Provided by One Vitamin Pill	Daily Amount Provided by Standard Intravenous Preparations[135]
Vitamin A (retinol)	IU	1,760 (females)–3,300 (males)	5,000	5,000	10,000	3,300 (retinal)
Vitamin D (ergocalciferol)	IU	200	400	400	400	200
Vitamin E (tocopherol)	mg TE	8–10	unknown	unknown	15	10 IU*
Vitamin K (phylloquinone)	µg	20–40†	20	20	0	0‡
Vitamin C (ascorbic acid)	mg	60	75	300	100	100
Thiamine (vitamin B_1)	mg	1.0–1.5	2	10	10	3.0
Riboflavin (vitamin B_2)	mg	1.2–1.7	2	10	10	3.6
Niacin	mg	13–19	20	100	100	40
Pyridoxine (vitamin B_6)	mg	2.0–2.2	2	40	5	4.0
Pantothenic acid	mg	4–7 (adults)†	18	40	20	15
Folic acid	mg	0.4	1.5	2.5	0	0.4
Vitamin B_{12}	µg	3.0	2	4	5	5
Biotin	µg	100–200†	unknown	unknown	0	60

*Equivalent to RDA.   †Estimated to be safe and adequate dietary intakes.   ‡Must be supplemented in peripheral venous solutions.

Table 3 Trace Mineral Requirements

Mineral	Recommended Dietary Allowance (RDA) for Daily Oral Intake (mg)	Suggested Daily Intravenous Intake[136] (mg)	Daily Amount Provided by a Commercially Available Mixture (mg)
Zinc	15	2.5–5.0*	5.0
Copper	2–3†	0.5–1.5	1.0
Manganese	2.5–5.0†	0.15–0.8	0.5
Chromium	0.05–0.2†	0.01–0.015	0.1
Iron	10 (males)–18 (females)	3	—

*Burn patients require an additional 2 mg.   †Estimated to be safe and adequate dietary intakes.

Protein

After energy requirements are determined, protein needs are calculated. The protein requirement for most individuals is 0.8 g/kg body weight/day (about 60 to 70 g protein/day). Critically ill patients may need 1.5 to 2.0 g protein/kg/day. Most standard enteral and parenteral feeding mixtures provide this increased quantity of protein if sufficient volume of formula is delivered to meet the increased caloric requirements of these patients. The nitrogen-to-calorie ratio for most feeding formulas prepared for surgical patients is 1:150 (i.e., 1 g of nitrogen for every 150 kcal).

The contraindications to this increased quantity of protein (a daily amount of 100 to 150 g, which is equivalent to the amount of protein in a lean 16 oz steak) are renal failure before dialysis (BUN > 40 mg/dl) and hepatic encephalopathy. Patients with systemic inflammatory response syndrome often require increased quantities of dietary protein [see 95 Multiple Organ Dysfunction Syndrome]. Nutritional support reduces net nitrogen losses in such patients, but positive or even neutral nitrogen balance is generally not achieved because of the disturbance in metabolism and reduced intake of dietary protein.

Vitamins and Minerals

The requirements for vitamins, minerals, and trace elements are usually met when adequate volumes of balanced nutrient formulas are provided [see Tables 2 and 3]. The requirements for most of the major minerals (sodium, potassium, chloride, phosphorus, magnesium, and zinc) are satisfied by monitoring serum concentrations of these elements and adjusting intake to maintain levels within the normal range. Some minerals and electrolytes are restricted in patients with renal failure. Although serum concentrations may not directly reflect total body deficits, sufficient quantities of these nutrients are available to support normal cellular functions if adequate blood concentrations are maintained. Most premixed enteral formulas provide adequate quantities of these substances if caloric needs are met. Vitamins and trace elements must be added to parenteral solutions.

Pharmacologic Recommendations for Stress in Surgical Patients

The doses of vitamins given are often not the recommended dietary allowance (RDA) but rather some multiple of the RDA; for example, stressed patients usually receive three to 10 times the RDA for normal persons.

The prescription of vitamins and minerals for therapeutic use should be based on the patient's nutritional history as well as on estimated requirements for the current disease state. These considerations are particularly important in prescription of the fat-soluble vitamins, which are stored in body fat and thus may become toxic at high levels. Current recommendations stipulate that therapeutic dosages of vitamins not exceed 10 times the recommended dietary allowance.[2] However, it has been suggested that some vitamins may be safe if given at dosages 50 to 100 times the RDA[3] [see Table 4]. Vitamins and minerals are sometimes given in large dosages to exert antioxidant effects. Vitamins A, C, and E and the minerals zinc and selenium can attenuate the tissue-damaging effects of free radicals. Many physicians are giving these vitamins and minerals as supplements to injured and infected patients[4]; supplementation with glutamine should also be considered because of its ability to enhance intracellular glutathione stores, which also play a major antioxidant role [see Discussion, below].

Enteral Nutrition

Enteral nutrition is the provision of liquid-formula diets by mouth or tube into the gastrointestinal tract. The GI tract is the preferred site for feeding the critically ill patient. It cannot be used safely, however, in patients who are hemodynamically unstable or who have abdominal distention, intestinal obstruction, or massive GI bleeding. For patients who are able to receive enteral nutrition, either a balanced or a modified diet is selected on the basis of diagnosis and nutritional requirements. An isotonic (approximately 300 mOsm/kg) diet is given continuously for a trial period of 24 hours. If the patient tolerates this regimen but is at increased risk for aspiration, feeding is delivered into the jejunum rather than into the stomach. A standard protocol is helpful in reducing complications.

SAFE USE OF THE GASTROINTESTINAL TRACT FOR FEEDING

Enteral nutrition should be prescribed only if safety and a low complication rate can be ensured. To determine whether the critically ill patient can be fed safely via the GI tract, a clinical assessment of intestinal function is performed. A good determinant of safe tolerance of enteral nutrition is a GI output of less than 600 ml/24 hr. For the purpose of these guidelines, GI output is defined as the volume of effluent from a nasogastric tube, ostomy, or rectal tube. Examples of conditions in critically ill patients that produce excessively high (> 600 ml/24 hr) GI outputs and therefore preclude the use of enteral nutrition are gastroparesis, intestinal obstruction, paralytic ileus, high-output enteric fistulas, antibiotic-

Table 4 Safety Levels of Vitamins[3]

Safety Level	Vitamin
At least 50 to 100 times RDA	Vitamin B_1 Vitamin B_2 Niacin Vitamin C Vitamin E Biotin Folic acid Pantothenic acid
10 times RDA	Vitamin A Vitamin B_6 Vitamin D Vitamin K

induced colitis, severe idiopathic diarrhea, and the initial phase of short bowel syndrome. Selected patients with enteric losses exceeding 600 ml/24 hr may receive enteral nutrition, however, if carefully monitored by an experienced team.

Another major cause of increased GI output is massive GI bleeding. Conditions that produce bleeding of this magnitude include peptic ulcer disease, esophageal varices, diverticulosis, and angiodysplasia of the colon. Mild bleeding such as that produced by stress gastritis may actually resolve with the delivery of enteral nutrition into the stomach because the liquid diet buffers gastric acid.[5] Enteral nutrition does not exacerbate mild lower intestinal bleeding.

Although commonly used at bedside as indicators of intestinal function, bowel sounds and passage of flatus are nonspecific and are unrelated to the eventual tolerance of enteral nutrition.

In the absence of excessively high GI output, abdominal distention, and massive GI bleeding, a trial of enteral nutrition is warranted to determine if the GI tract can be used safely for feeding.[6] Indications and contraindications for enteral nutrition have been published by the American Society for Parenteral and Enteral Nutrition [see Table 5].[7]

SELECTION OF DIET AND STARTING THE DELIVERY

Before delivery of enteral nutrition, the appropriate diet must be selected on the basis of the patient's nutrient requirements [see Indications for Nutritional Intervention, *above*]. Most liquid-formula diets consist of either a balanced or a modified formula.

Balanced diets contain carbohydrates, proteins, and fats in complex (polymeric) forms in proportions similar to those of a regular Western diet. Frequently, however, the fat content is reduced to 10% to 15% of total calories, and the carbohydrate content is increased. Carbohydrates are present as oligosaccharides, polysaccharides, or maltodextrins; fats consist of medium- or long-chain triglycerides. The nitrogen source is a natural protein, which may be either intact or partially hydrolyzed. In general, balanced diets are isotonic, lactose free, and available in ready-to-use, liquid form. Flavored balanced diets can be used for oral supplementation as well as for enteral tube feeding.

Selection of a balanced diet is based on nutrient and fluid requirements. The caloric density of balanced diets can be 1.0, 1.5, or 2.0 kcal/ml. The largest number of commercially available diets provide 1.0 kcal/ml. The nonprotein caloric content of these diets is derived from either carbohydrates or lipids. Balanced diets formulated with carbohydrates as the main caloric source have higher osmolarity than isocaloric diets containing lipids. These carbohydrate-based diets are well tolerated when adminis-

tered directly into the stomach and may be helpful for patients with steatorrhea. Balanced diets that are fat based may be more appropriate for patients who have diarrhea caused by diet hyperosmolarity, especially when feedings are infused directly into the small intestine. However, fat malabsorption is common in critically ill patients when the fat content of the diet exceeds 30% of total calories. In modified formulas, the proportions and types of nutrients differ from those of a regular Western diet. Manufacturers of enteral diets have introduced these modifications to meet the special nutrient needs of patients with renal failure or short bowel syndrome.

Modified diets are also known as elemental diets or chemically defined diets. These diets contain crystalline amino acids or short peptides in compositions that differ from the reference composition of proteins of high biologic value, such as egg albumin. The fat-to-carbohydrate ratio of these modified diets varies depending on the purpose of the modification. The source of carbohydrate is either dextrose or oligosaccharides; fats are usually in the form of medium-chain triglycerides, essential fatty acids, or both. Because they are not palatable, modified diets are rarely used as oral supplements. Modified diets are further characterized according to the conditions for which they are formulated: stress, immunomodulation, and hepatic, renal, respiratory, or GI dysfunction [see Table 6].

Hepatic formulas are indicated for patients with hepatic failure who are hypercatabolic and encephalopathic. When such patients

Table 5 Indications for Enteral Nutrition (Partial Listing)

Considered Routine Care in the Following:
  Protein-calorie malnutrition with inadequate oral intake of nutrients for the previous 5–7 days
  Normal nutritional status but < 50% of required oral intake of nutrients for the previous 7–10 days
  Severe dysphagia
  Major full-thickness burns
  Low-output enterocutaneous fistulas
  Major trauma

Usually Helpful in the Following:
  Radiation therapy
  Mild chemotherapy
  Liver failure and severe renal dysfunction
  Massive small bowel resection (> 50%) in combination with administration of total parenteral nutrition

Of Limited or Undetermined Value in the Following:
  Intensive chemotherapy
  Immediate postoperative period or poststress period
  Acute enteritis
  > 90% resection of small bowel

Contraindicated in the Following:
  Complete mechanical intestinal obstruction
  Abdominal distention
  Ileus or intestinal hypomotility
  Severe diarrhea
  Severe GI bleeding
  High-output external fistulas
  Severe, acute pancreatitis
  Shock
  Case of aggressive nutritional support not desired by the patient or legal guardian and respect of such wish being in accordance with hospital policy and existing law
  Prognosis not warranting aggressive nutritional support

receive standard protein sources, neurologic symptoms may be aggravated. Hepatic formulas contain increased amounts of branched-chain amino acids (BCAAs) and decreased quantities of aromatic amino acids (i.e., phenylalanine, tyrosine, and tryptophan) and of the sulfur-containing amino acid methionine. These formulas were initially developed for parenteral nutrition to reduce the availability of aromatic amino acids, which are precursors of neurotransmitters synthesized in excess during the development of hepatic encephalopathy.[8]

Renal formulas contain all essential amino acids, including histidine, but lack the nonessential amino acids. These formulas promote the reuse of urea nitrogen associated with hepatic transamination, which is one step in the synthesis of nonessential amino acids.[9,10] Renal diets are indicated for patients with renal failure who do not need dialysis and are not receiving broad-spectrum antibiotics, which reduce urea recycling by colonic bacteria.

The composition of enteral diets can also be altered to reduce carbon dioxide production in ventilator-dependent patients.[11] This reduction is accomplished by increasing the ratio of fat to carbohydrate in the formula. This approach has been shown to be effective when nutrients are given intravenously[12]; however, controlled clinical trials are needed in enterally fed patients.

Diets for patients with GI dysfunction have modified nitrogen and fat composition. Transport of dietary nitrogen across the intestinal mucosa is enhanced when nitrogen is provided in the form of short peptides rather than free amino acids. It is also well documented that the small bowel mucosa utilizes glutamine as the preferred fuel [see Discussion, below]. Consequently, some modified diets contain nitrogen in the form of short peptides, whereas others have an extra amount of glutamine. Medium-chain triglycerides (MCTs) are more easily absorbed and metabolized than long-chain triglycerides (LCTs). Diets modified for improved absorption contain a higher proportion of MCT oil. These diets may be efficacious when used during the transition phase after a period of prolonged bowel rest or when the intestine is inflamed. Controlled trials are necessary to verify their clinical efficacy. Stress formulas are indicated for hypercatabolic patients whose nitrogen balance continues to be negative despite increased intake of a balanced diet. Stress formulas are often enriched with BCAAs (e.g., leucine, valine, and isoleucine) in an attempt to improve nitrogen balance by providing precursors for synthesis of muscle protein.[13] Little evidence supports the use of diets that provide BCAAs in concentrations higher than 20% to 25% of total amino acid content for stressed patients.

The fat sources used for enteral diets are primarily omega-6 fatty acids—the arachidonic acid family. Ongoing research suggests that supplementation with omega-3 fatty acids—the eicosapentaenoic acid family—results in the synthesis of eicosanoids (prostaglandins, leukotrienes, and thromboxanes) that enhance the immune response [see Discussion, below]. The immune response can also be improved by supplemental arginine and glutamine; diets formulated for immunomodulation are enriched with these nutrients. The administration of one of these diets, which also contained RNA, is reported to have reduced postoperative complications and hospital stay after surgery for GI malignancies and trauma.[14]

ASSESSMENT OF FEEDING TOLERANCE

The selected formula is started at isotonicity and delivered continuously at 30 ml/hr for 24 hours. During this initial trial, the formula is delivered via a previously inserted Salem sump or rubber nasogastric (Levin) tube. If a nasogastric tube is not already in place, a soft tube made of either silicone rubber or polyurethane is inserted (see below).

Feeding tolerance is assessed for the first 24 hours. Poor tolerance is indicated by vomiting and severe abdominal cramps, gastric residuum greater than 50% of the volume administered during the previous 4-hour period of feeding, increased abdominal distention (a particularly important factor to assess in comatose patients and individuals being mechanically ventilated), and worsening of diarrhea. If any one of these conditions is present, parenteral nutrition is recommended. If there is no evidence of feeding intolerance, the patient is assessed for the risk for aspiration.

ASSESSMENT OF RISK FOR ASPIRATION

Aspiration is a major complication in patients receiving enteral nutrition.[15] The propensity to aspirate enteral feedings is often related to the patient's primary disease and neurologic status as well as to the site of GI access and the method of delivery.

Important factors in assessing risk for aspiration include depressed sensorium, increased gastroesophageal reflux, and history of previously documented episodes of aspiration. Depressed sensorium in the critical care setting is secondary to organic lesions of the central nervous system, metabolic encephalopathies, or medications. Head trauma, hypoxemia, hepatic and septic encephalopathies, and the use of H_2 receptor blockers are common causes of depressed sensorium in critically ill patients. Increased gastroesophageal reflux may be present in individuals with reduced lower esophageal sphincter pressure and increased intragastric pressure. Many medications used in the ICU, such as theophylline, anticholinergics, calcium channel blocking agents, beta-adrenergic agonists, and alpha-adrenergic antagonists, cause a reduction in lower esophageal sphincter pressure.[16] Finally, a history of aspiration places the patient at increased risk for recurrent episodes.

For most enterally fed patients, safety demands that the head be elevated at feeding time and for some period thereafter to prevent regurgitation. If elevating the patient's head is not possible, an alternative site of nutrient delivery should be considered. Nasogastric intubation, in particular, requires elevation of the head because the tube may render the upper and lower esophageal sphincters incompetent and liable to reflux. Even the presence of a tracheostomy or endotracheal tube does not ensure that regurgitated gastric contents will not be aspirated. Liquid filling the pharynx will inevitably trickle past even an overinflated endotracheal tube cuff and into the lung. Aspiration of liquid formulas can be verified if a bit of food coloring or methylene blue is included in the feeding mixture and subsequently detected in pharyngeal and tracheal secretions.[17]

ACCESS FOR FEEDING

In most general and thoracic surgical patients, access for feeding is most commonly obtained via the stomach or jejunum. Methods of access for intragastric feedings include nasogastric tubes and feeding gastrostomies placed through a laparotomy or percutaneously with the aid of endoscopy, fluoroscopy, or laparoscopy.

To prevent peptic ulcerations and bleeding, gastric acidity is controlled with H_2 receptor blockers in critically ill patients. Although these drugs help control hyperacidity, which is a cause of diarrhea, they also lead to bacterial overgrowth in the intestine.[23] Therefore, the use of H_2 receptor blockers should be avoided in patients who receive feedings into the stomach, because the presence of the liquid formula in the stomach already provides a physiologic means of buffering acid. If necessary, antacids rather than H_2 receptor blockers should be used to titrate gastric pH to 4.5 to 6.5. The amino acid glutamine is also utilized to prevent or treat ulceration of the upper GI tract.

The most common mechanical complications that are related to enteral nutrition are tube dislodgment, clogging of the tube, and leakage of enteric contents around the exit site of the tube onto the skin.[24] Tube dislodgment occurs more frequently in agitated patients and hypoxic patients. Inadvertent removal of the tube is usually prevented by adequate taping of the nasoenteric tube or, in agitated patients, by suturing the tube or using a Velcro abdominal wall binder.

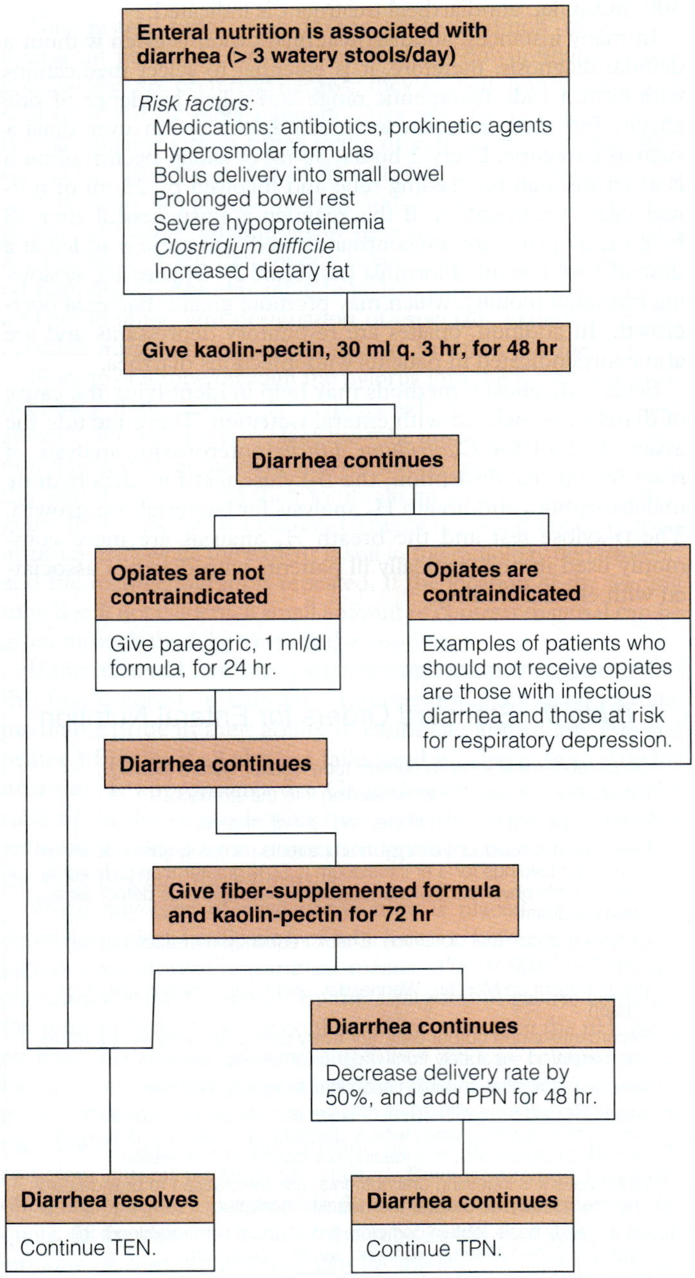

Clogging or plugging of the tube often results from the failure to use saline irrigations after intermittent feedings or the inadvertent delivery of crushed medications through a small-bore tube. This complication is reduced by routine irrigations of 20 to 25 ml of normal saline or water after each intermittent feeding. Liquid medications may also help prevent this complication, although these medications are frequently hyperosmolar and may produce discomfort and diarrhea when delivered rapidly into the jejunum. The injection of a small volume of a carbonated beverage into a plugged tube will often clear the blockage. Occasionally, a guide wire and the help of the interventional radiologist will be needed.

Another mechanical complication is the leakage of enteric contents onto the skin around the exit site of a tube enterostomy. Leakage is often uncomfortable for the patient and may produce a moderate amount of skin irritation. One cause of such leakage is an excessively large incision in the skin at the exit site of the enterostomy tube. Leakage around a tube is prevented by creating the exit site so as to be almost identical in diameter to the tube. A larger tube may also be inserted through the exit site if leakage continues. The enterostomal therapist and the use of products such as karaya gum, zinc oxide, Stomahesive, and locally applied antacid are often helpful. Also problematic is the inappropriate use of urinary catheters for enteral access; these devices were not designed to function as gastrostomy or enterostomy tubes. The catheters currently preferred for these purposes are made of either silicone rubber or polyurethane and include a system to prevent migration of the tube into the stomach.

Parenteral Nutrition

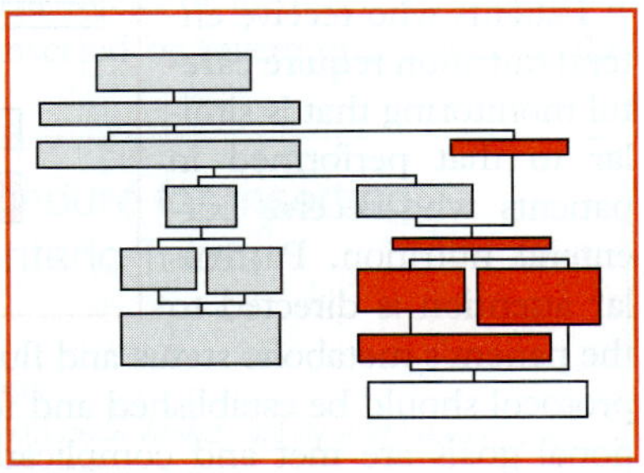

CENTRAL VENOUS VERSUS PERIPHERAL VENOUS INFUSIONS

Central venous infusions are indicated in most critically ill patients who receive parenteral nutrition, because (1) patients in the intensive care unit often require increased quantities of energy and cannot tolerate large fluid volumes and (2) solutions of much greater caloric density and tonicity can be infused into central veins than can be infused into peripheral veins. Nonetheless, peripheral venous infusions may be indicated in certain situations [see Table 10]; peripheral venous infusions will be discussed in detail below.

CENTRAL VENOUS NUTRIENT INFUSION

Hypertonic nutrient solutions are infused into a large-bore central vein. These solutions are rapidly diluted, and the nutrients are delivered throughout the body by the bloodstream. Usually, the hypertonic nutrient solutions contain hypertonic glucose (25%), amino acids (5%), and other essential nutrients. The tonicity of the hypertonic nutrient solutions is so great (> 1,900 mOsm/kg) that administration of the mixture into peripheral veins would cause severe thrombophlebitis and venous sclerosis. If the solution is continuously infused at a constant rate into the superior vena cava, however, the nutrient mixture is rapidly diluted to near-iso-

Figure 2 The decision-making approach for pharmacologic and dietary treatment of diarrhea associated with enteral nutrition is shown.

Table 10 Indications for Central Venous or Peripheral Venous Infusions

Central Venous Infusions
- To provide adequate intravenous nutritional support for 10 days or more
- To satisfy nutrient requirements in patients with increased energy needs and normal or decreased fluid requirements
- To support the patient with single- or multiple-organ failure by infusing modified nutrient solutions in a limited fluid volume

Peripheral Venous Infusions
- To provide initial feeding (< 5 days) before catheter insertion in a patient who will require central venous feedings
- To infuse less concentrated solutions via a multiuse central catheter (i.e., a line for blood drawing, medication, and nutrients) into an individual in whom other venous access cannot be easily or safely obtained
- To supplement enteral feedings that are inadequate because of gastrointestinal dysfunction
- To satisfy energy requirements that are near basal (1,500–1,800 kcal/day) in a nondepleted patient who can tolerate 2.5–3.0 L I.V. solution each day

tonic concentrations, and the nutrients are cleared from the bloodstream by body tissues. The hypertonic nutrient solutions contain at least 1 kcal/ml, and thus, infusion of 2.0 to 2.5 L/day provides 2,000 to 2,500 kcal of energy and all essential nutrients. This calorie load is sufficient to meet energy requirements in more than 90% of surgical patients.

Once positioned, the catheter is used exclusively for administration of the hypertonic nutrient solution. Drawing blood, monitoring central venous pressure, and administering medication through this dedicated lumen are prohibited. Multiple-lumen central venous catheters are now available; manufacturers suggest that at least one port be devoted to the infusion of hypertonic nutrient solutions and additional ports be used for drawing blood, monitoring pressure, and infusing medications. Reports suggest that the rates of catheter sepsis associated with use of these lines are greater than the rates associated with single-lumen feeding catheters.[25,26] In our experience, the infection rate associated with multiple-lumen catheters was similar to that observed with single-lumen catheters (3.3% versus 1.0%, NS), but the multiple-lumen catheters were in place for a shorter period than the single-lumen catheters (7 versus 14 days).[27] Removal of the multiple-lumen catheters was indicated when multiple central access ports were no longer required or when one of the lumens became clotted or malfunctioned. It appears that multiple-lumen catheters can be used in the ICU for central venous nutrient infusions if strict protocols are maintained to ensure that one lumen is dedicated to nutrient infusion, that other lumens are handled safely, and that the catheters are removed when they are no longer required.

Occasionally, a patient may require the infusion of a hypertonic nutrient solution, when percutaneous puncture of central veins is impossible or contraindicated. In these individuals, catheterization of an antecubital vein and insertion of a peripherally inserted central catheter (PICC) with the tip positioned in the superior vena cava should be considered. These catheters are readily inserted by the interventional radiologist, and they eliminate the complications associated with infraclavicular and supraclavicular catheter insertion. The PICC line has become the primary route of central venous access in many institutions.

Newer types of catheters made of Silastic have been safely kept in place for extended periods and provide an additional option for care of patients who require central venous infusions. Catheterization of the femoral vein may provide a route for central venous access in some situations. Because of the high density of skin pathogens in the groin area, these catheters should be replaced every 2 to 3 days. If the catheter tip is positioned in the iliac vein or the inferior vena cava, the concentration of solution infused through the catheter should not exceed 15%. Strict care of the entrance site should be maintained because of the high complication rate associated with lines placed in the groin.[28]

Central Venous Solutions

Central venous solutions are formulated in the hospital pharmacy. These solutions are commonly combinations of 500 ml of 50% dextrose and 500 ml of a 10% amino acid mixture [see Table 11] to which electrolytes, vitamins, and trace elements are added (see below). Each day, 2 L of the solution can be infused. Administration of fat emulsion (500 ml, 20%) 1 day each week meets essential fatty acid requirements. Alternatively, the three major nutrients may be mixed together in a 3 L bag (triple mix or three-in-one) and the entire contents of the single bag infused during the 24-hour period [see Table 11]. Another innovation is the use of an automated mixing device (Auto-mix, Travenol Laboratories) that compounds various proportions of 70% glucose, 10% amino acids, and 20% fat emulsions into 3 L bags. This device allows the hospital pharmacy to manufacture a variety of nutrient combinations with minimal effort. More concentrated solutions can be made, and the computer will generate a label for the bag that allows nurses to verify the order.

Electrolytes and minerals are added to the base formula as required [see Table 12]. Sodium and potassium salts are added as chloride or acetate, depending on the acid-base status of the patient. The solution should usually consist of approximately equal quantities of chloride and acetate. If chloride losses from the body are increased, as in a patient who requires nasogastric decompression, most salts should be administered as chloride. Sodium bicarbonate is incompatible with the nutrient solutions, and acetate is administered when additional base is required (when metabolized, acetate generates bicarbonate). Phosphate is usually given as the potassium salt; sodium phos-

Table 11 Composition of Central Venous Solutions

	Standard Solution	Triple-Mix Solution
Volume		
Amino acids 10% (ml)	500	1,000
Dextrose 50% (ml)	500	1,000
Fat emulsion 20% (ml)	—	250
Total (ml)	1,000	2,250
Contents		
Amino acids (g)	50	100
Dextrose (g)	250 (25%)	500
Total nitrogen (g)	8.4	16.8
Total calories (kcal)	1,050	2,600
Ratio of nitrogen to calories	1:125	1:154
Caloric density (kcal/ml)	1.0	1.15
Osmolarity (mOsm/kg)	≈1,970	≈1,900

phate is used when potassium is contraindicated. Phosphate is also present in fat emulsions.

Commercially available preparations of vitamins, minerals, and trace elements are also added to the nutrient mix for daily administration unless they are contraindicated. A solution containing both fat- and water-soluble vitamins should be added. Vitamin K_1 (phytonadione), 10 mg, is given once a week but is contraindicated in patients receiving warfarin.

Trace elements are given daily. Usual requirements are satisfied by the addition of commercially available mixtures either to 1 L of standard solution or to the triple-mix bag each day. Trace elements are indicated for all patients receiving central venous nutrient solutions, except those with chronic renal failure or severe liver disease. At especially high risk for zinc deficiency are alcoholics and patients with pancreatic insufficiency with malabsorption, massive small bowel resection, renal failure with dialysis, or nephrotic syndrome; at high risk for copper deficiency are patients with short bowel syndrome, jejunoileal bypass, malabsorptive conditions with severe diarrhea, or nephrotic syndrome. Copper and manganese are excreted primarily via the biliary tract. Therefore, in patients with biliary tract obstruction, excess retention of copper and manganese should be avoided by decreasing intake of these ions, monitoring blood levels, or both. Although the main excretory route for zinc and chromium is via the feces, renal excretion will minimize dangers from modest excesses of these elements. In patients with renal insufficiency, however, daily zinc and chromium administration may be contraindicated. ICU patients usually do not require iron. Iron is contraindicated in patients with sepsis because iron supports bacterial growth. Iron may be required to treat iron deficiency anemia, particularly during convalescence from this condition. Rarely does the anemia that is associated with chronic disease and inflammation respond to iron therapy during the active stages of disease.

Like other invasive therapies, total parenteral nutrition (TPN) is associated with potential complications deriving either from central venous access or from the composition of the formula given. Most such complications are preventable with appropriate attention to detail [see Table 13].

PERIPHERAL VENOUS SOLUTIONS

Slightly hypertonic nutrient solutions (approximately 600 to 900 mOsm/kg) can be prepared for peripheral venous infusions from commercially available amino acid mixtures (5%), dextrose solutions (10%), and fat emulsions (20%). These nutrient mixtures have a low caloric density (approximately 0.3 to 0.6 kcal/ml) and thus provide only 1,200 to 2,300 kcal in 2,000 to 3,500 ml of solution. Large volumes of fluid are required.

These dilute nutrient mixtures can be infused through plastic cannulas placed in large-bore peripheral veins. The catheter insertion site and surrounding tissue should be inspected periodically for signs of phlebitis or infiltration, and the infusion site should be rotated every 48 to 72 hours to prevent thrombophlebitis. Only fat emulsion should be administered simultaneously through the same I.V. site as a peripheral venous solution. The nutrient solution should be temporarily stopped if the catheter is used for administration of antibiotics, chemotherapeutic agents, blood, or blood products. The infusion line should then be flushed with saline and infusion of the nutrient solution resumed.

If the fat emulsion is infused in a piggyback manner, administration should be performed during a period of 8 to 12 hours and concluded in the early morning (3:00 A.M.) to allow clearance of the emulsion from the bloodstream. Blood sampling should be avoided during short-term periods of fat infusion because the associated hypertriglyceridemia will interfere with many of the serum measurements. In patients who are receiving peripheral venous solutions by triple mix, hypertriglyceridemia is rare because the rate of infusion has been reduced and infusion extended over a 24-hour period.

Patients receiving peripheral venous feedings should be monitored as suggested for individuals receiving central venous feedings (see below). Mechanical and septic complications are uncommon. Fluid imbalances and alterations in serum electrolyte concentrations are similar to those seen in standard I.V. support, and corrections are made by altering the volume of the infusion or adding or omitting electrolytes. Hyperglycemia and glycosuria are rarely observed unless the patient is diabetic.

MONITORING THE PATIENT: OPTIMIZING NUTRITIONAL SUPPORT, PREVENTING COMPLICATIONS, AND RESOLVING COMMON PROBLEMS

Table 12 Electrolytes Added to Central Venous Solutions

	Usual Electrolyte Concentration	Usual Range of Electrolyte Concentration
Sodium (mEq/L)	30	0–150
Potassium (mEq/L)	30	0–80
Phosphate (mmol/L)	15	0–20
Magnesium (mEq/L)	5	0–15
Calcium* (mEq/L)	4.7	0–10
Chloride (mEq/L)	50	0–150
Acetate (mEq/L)	70	70–220

*As gluconate.

General Measures

Patients receiving central venous feedings should be weighed daily, and accurate intake and output records should be maintained. Urinary glucose should be monitored daily. Persistent glucosuria indicates hyperglycemia and may be associated with a concomitant osmotic diuresis and dehydration. If such glucosuria occurs, a more stringent schedule of monitoring blood glucose should be instituted and specific therapy initiated (see below).

The quantity of energy administered to most ICU patients should maintain lean body mass and adipose tissues. Thus, variations in body weight usually reflect alterations in fluid balance. If sustained weight loss occurs (as characterized by a gradual fall in body weight during a period of 2 weeks or more), caloric intake may be inadequate. Additional calories (500 to 1,000 kcal/day) should be administered to maintain weight. Alternatively, the metabolic rate could be calculated from the volume of oxygen consumed per minute ($\dot{V}O_2$) and calorie intake then matched to equal energy expenditure:

$$\text{Metabolic rate (kcal/hr)} = \dot{V}O_2 \text{ (ml/min)} \times 60 \text{ min/hr} \times 1 \text{ L}/1{,}000 \text{ ml} \times 4.83 \text{ kcal/L}$$

This calculation is required in only 5% of our patients.

Table 13 Diagnosis, Treatment, and Prevention of Potential Mechanical and Metabolic Complications Associated with Total Parenteral Nutrition

	Complications	Diagnosis	Treatment	Prevention
Mechanical	Pneumothorax	Dyspnea, chest x-ray	Tube thoracostomy Observation	Avoid emergency procedures Trendelenburg's position
	Hemothorax	Dyspnea, chest x-ray	Remove catheter Observation	Insert catheter using appropriate technique
	Venous thrombosis	Inability to cannulate	Remove catheter Heparin therapy	Use silicone catheters Add heparin to solution
	Air embolism	Dyspnea, cyanosis, hypotension, tachycardia, precordial murmur	Trendelenburg's position Left lateral decubitus position	Trendelenburg's position Valsalva maneuver Tape intravenous connections
	Catheter embolism	Sheared catheter	Fluoroscopic retrieval	Never withdraw catheter through needle
	Arrhythmias	Catheter tip in right atrium	Withdraw catheter to superior vena cava	Estimate distance to SVC before insertion; confirm position with x-ray
	Subclavian artery injury	Pulsatile red blood	Remove needle Apply pressure Chest x-ray	Review anatomy
	Catheter tip misplacement	Chest x-ray	Redirect with a guide wire	Direct bevel of needle caudally
Metabolic	Hyperglycemic, hyperosmolar, nonketotic coma	Dehydration with osmotic diuresis, disorientation, lethargy, stupor, convulsions, coma, glucose 1,000 mg/dl, osmolarity 350 mOsm/kg	Discontinue TPN; infuse D5 in 0.45% S at 250 ml/hr Insulin 10–20 U/hr Bicarbonate Monitor glucose, potassium, pH	Monitor glucose
	Hypoglycemia	Headache, sweating, thirst, convulsions, disorientation, paresthesias	D50W I.V.	Taper TPN by ½ for 12 hr; then 12 hr of D5W at 100 ml/hr
	CO_2 retention	Ventilator dependence, high respiratory quotient	Taper glucose	Provide 30%–40% of calories with fat
	Azotemia	Dehydration, elevated BUN	Increase nonprotein calories	Monitor fluid balance
	Hyperammonemia	Lethargy, malaise, coma, seizures	Discontinue amino acid infusions Infuse arginine	Avoid casein or fibrin hydrolysate
	Essential fatty acid deficiency	Xerosis, hepatomegaly, impaired healing, bone changes	Fat administration	Provide 25–200 mg/kg/day of essential fatty acids
	Hypophosphatemia	Lethargy, anorexia, weakness	Supplemental phosphate	Treat causative factors: alkalosis, gram-negative sepsis, vomiting, malabsorption Provide 20 mEq/kcal
	Abnormal liver enzymes	Fatty infiltrate in liver	Evaluate for other causes	Provide balanced TPN solution
	Hypomagnesemia	Weakness, nausea, vomiting, tremors, depression, hyporeflexia	Infuse 10% $MgSO_4$	Supply 0.35–0.45 mEq/kg/day
	Hypermagnesemia	Drowsiness, nausea, vomiting, coma, arrhythmia	Dialysis Infuse calcium gluconate	Monitor serum levels

In non–ventilator-dependent patients, oxygen consumption and, in turn, the metabolic rate can be derived from measurements of respiratory gas exchange. Equipment (e.g., the Metabolic Measuring Cart) is commercially available to make these measurements at bedside. In a patient with a Swan-Ganz catheter in place, oxygen consumption can be calculated from cardiac output determinations and simultaneous measurements of mixed venous oxygen content ($C_{mv}O_2$) and arterial oxygen content (C_aO_2):

$$\dot{V}O_2 \text{ (ml/min)} = \text{cardiac output (L/min)} \times (C_aO_2 \text{ [ml/L]} - C_{mv}O_2 \text{ [ml/L]}) \times 1 \text{ L/10 dl}$$

Another objective of nutritional support in the ICU patient is the maintenance of lean body mass, which is reflected by nitrogen equilibration or positive nitrogen balance. Although complete nitrogen balance determination is a complex and sophisticated study, nitrogen equilibration can be estimated by using common analytic procedures. To estimate nitrogen balance, total nitrogen loss is subtracted from total nitrogen intake [see Sidebar Sample Calculation of Nitrogen Balance]. Calculation of total nitrogen loss requires several steps. The urine urea nitrogen (UUN) concentration is multiplied by the total volume of urine output during a given day to yield the 24-hour UUN, that is, the total amount of urea excreted during that period. Because urea accounts for only approximately 80% of the nitrogen excreted in the urine, the value for the 24-hour UUN must be increased by an additional 20%. This quantity and an additional 2 g/day are added to the value for the 24-hour UUN to account for nonurea nitrogen, stool, and integumentary losses:

$$\text{24-hour UUN (g/day)} = \text{UUN (mg/dl)} \times \text{urine output (ml/day)} \times 1\text{ g}/1{,}000\text{ mg} \times 1\text{ dl}/100\text{ ml}$$

$$\text{Total nitrogen loss (g/day)} = \text{24-hour UUN (g/day)} + (0.20 \times \text{24-hour UUN [g/day]}) + 2\text{ g/day}$$

Metabolic Monitoring

A wide variety of metabolic complications may occur during parenteral feeding [*see Table 14*]. They are minimized by frequent monitoring [*see Table 15*] and appropriate adjustment of nutrients in the infusion.

The most common metabolic problems occurring in ICU patients are hyperglycemia and glucosuria. Initially, elevated levels of blood glucose should be treated by the administration of subcutaneous insulin (5.0 units every 4 to 6 hours for glucose 200 to 250 mg/dl; 7.5 units for 250 to 300 mg/dl; 10.0 units for 300 to 350 mg/dl). When the nutritional solution is ordered for the next 24-hour period, half the quantity of insulin administered subcutaneously is added to the bag. At least 10 units of regular insulin per liter of solution should be used as the initial dose, and in some cases, as much as 40 U/L may be required. If larger doses of insulin are needed (> 100 U/day), a separate insulin infusion or drip should be used. Blood glucose levels can be monitored at the bedside by using a small refractometer or other similar devices, and the insulin infusion can be adjusted hourly, if necessary, to control the blood glucose concentration.

In most patients with severe glucose intolerance, the rate of glucose administered should not exceed 5 mg/kg/min (approximately 500 g/day).[29] Additional calories should be administered as fat emulsion. The commercially available fat emulsions are all generally well tolerated by critically ill patients. Triglyceride levels should be monitored, and the rate of administration of the emulsion should be decreased or the emulsion temporarily discontinued if levels exceed 500 mg/dl. Fat emulsion should be used with caution in patients with known hypertriglyceridemia or in those with gram-negative septicemia that is associated with hyperlipidemia.

The infusion of excess glucose or lipid energy may alter pulmonary function and in some patients prevent weaning from a mechanical ventilator. Excessive carbohydrate loads (usually > 500 g/day) increase CO_2 production. If the quantity of CO_2 produced exceeds the ability of the lungs to excrete this oxidative end product, hypercapnia results. CO_2 production can be greatly reduced by diminishing the carbohydrate load; if the patient receives less than 5 mg/kg/min of carbohydrate and cannot be weaned from the ventilator, one approach is to administer only 5% glucose solution overnight and then to attempt weaning the next morning. If the patient can be removed from the ventilator, parenteral feedings may be gradually reinstituted.

Fat emulsion may also interfere with diffusion of gas across the alveolar membranes. This interference is generally related to the concentration of the emulsion in the bloodstream; hence, monitoring triglyceride levels and preventing hypertriglyceridemia will minimize this complication.

Catheter Care and Catheter Sepsis

The most serious problem associated with central venous feedings is catheter sepsis [*see 81 Nosocomial Infection*]. Primary catheter sepsis is defined as the signs and symptoms of infection (usually a febrile episode), with the indwelling catheter being the only anatomic focus of sepsis. After removal of the catheter, the symptoms usually attenuate. Cultures of the catheter tip with semiquantitative techniques yield at least 10^3 organisms.[30] The organisms are the same as those recovered from cultures of blood drawn from a peripheral vein during the initial evaluation of the infection.

Secondary catheter infection, in contrast to primary catheter sepsis, is associated with a second infectious focus that causes bacteremia and thus seeds or contaminates the catheter. The microorganisms cultured from the catheter tip are similar to those cultured from the primary source. The infection clears after specific treatment of the primary infection.

Primary catheter sepsis is prevented or at least greatly reduced by following strict protocols to govern the use and manipulation of the central venous feeding catheter and by employing a systematic method of care and surveillance of the catheter entrance site. Usually, catheter care and its supervision and certification are performed by a nurse with expertise in maintenance of long-term intravenous access (the nurse may be assigned to the nutrition support service or may be experienced in I.V. access or infection control). Every 48 to 72 hours, the dressing that covers the entrance site of the catheter is removed, the site inspected, the area around the entrance site cleaned, a topical antibiotic or antiseptic ointment applied, and the site redressed with a new sterile dressing. This procedure is documented in the clinical record; if drainage or crusting appears at the entrance site, appropriate cultures are taken. In addition, the dressing is changed if it becomes wet or soiled or no longer remains intact. In individuals who have either draining wounds in close proximity to the catheter entrance site or tracheostomies, the entire dressing should be covered with a transparent barrier drape to minimize contamination.

If signs and symptoms of infection develop in a recipient of central venous parenteral nutrition, a history should be taken and a physical examination performed [*see Figure 3*]. Appropriate tests (e.g., complete blood count and urinalysis) and diagnostic studies (including roentgenogram) should also be performed. If blood cultures are needed, they should be drawn from a peripheral vein. If trained nurses have maintained the catheter and no evidence of infection at the exit site has been noted, the catheter dressing should not be removed, and the catheter should not be manipulated. Blood cultures should

---

Sample Calculation of Nitrogen Balance

A 65-year-old man with an infected aortic graft and ileus is receiving 2.2 L triple-mix solution containing 16.8 g nitrogen each day. His UUN is 500 mg/dl, and his urine output is 2,000 ml/day. Is he receiving adequate nitrogen?

24-hour UUN = 500 mg/dl × 2,000 ml/day × 1 g/1,000 mg × 1 dl/100 ml
 = 10 g/day

Nitrogen output
 = 24-hr UUN + (0.20 × 24-hr UUN) + 2 g/day
 = 10 g/day + (0.20 × 10 g/day) + 2 g/day
 = 14 g/day

Nitrogen balance
 = 16.8 g/day (N intake) − 14 g/day (N output)
 = 2.8 g/day

The patient is in positive nitrogen balance, retaining approximately 2 to 3 g nitrogen/day. If positive nitrogen balance had not been achieved, his protein and caloric intake would have had to be increased and the nitrogen balance recalculated.

Table 14 Metabolic Complications of Total Parenteral Nutrition

Problems	Possible Causes	Solutions
Glucose		
Hyperglycemia, glycosuria, osmotic diuresis, hyperosmolar nonketotic dehydration and coma	Excessive total dose or rate of infusion of glucose; inadequate endogenous insulin; increased glucocorticoids; sepsis	Reduce amount of glucose infused; increase insulin; administer a portion of calories as fat emulsion
Ketoacidosis in diabetes mellitus	Inadequate endogenous insulin response; inadequate exogenous insulin therapy	Give insulin; reduce glucose input
Postinfusion (rebound) hypoglycemia	Persistence of endogenous insulin production secondary to prolonged stimulation of islet cells by high-carbohydrate infusion	Administer 5%–10% glucose before infusate is discontinued
Fat		
Pyrogenic reaction	Fat emulsion, other solutions	Exclude other causes of fever
Altered coagulation	Hyperlipidemia	Restudy after fat has cleared bloodstream
Hypertriglyceridemia	Rapid infusion, decreased clearance	Decrease rate of infusion; allow clearance before blood tests
Impaired liver function	May be caused by fat emulsion or by an underlying disease process	Exclude other causes of hepatic dysfunction
Cyanosis	Altered pulmonary diffusion capacity	Discontinue fat infusion
Essential fatty acid deficiency	Inadequate essential fatty acid administration	Administer essential fatty acids in the form of one 500 ml bottle of fat emulsion every 2–3 days
Amino Acids		
Hyperchloremic metabolic acidosis	Excessive chloride and monohydrochloride content of crystalline amino acid solutions	Administer Na^+ and K^+ as acetate salts
Serum amino acid imbalance	Unphysiologic amino acid profile of the nutrient solution; differential amino acid utilization with various disorders	Use experimental solutions if indicated
Hyperammonemia	Excessive ammonia in protein hydrolysate solutions; deficiency of arginine, ornithine, aspartic acid, or glutamic acid, or a combination of these deficiencies in amino acid solutions; primary hepatic disorder	Reduce amino acid intake
Prerenal azotemia	Excessive amino acid infusion with inadequate calorie administration; inadequate free water intake, dehydration	Reduce amino acid intake; increase glucose calories; increase intake of free water
Calcium and Phosphorus		
Hypophosphatemia	Inadequate phosphorus administration; redistribution of serum phosphorus into cells or bones, or both	Administer phosphorous ($\geq$ 20 mEq potassium dihydrogen phosphate/1,000 I.V. calories); evaluate antacid or calcium administration, or both
Hypocalcemia	Inadequate calcium administration; reciprocal response to phosphorus repletion without simultaneous calcium infusion; hypoalbuminemia	Administer calcium
Hypercalcemia	Excessive calcium administration with or without high doses of albumin; excessive vitamin D administration	Decrease calcium or vitamin D
Vitamin D deficiency; hypervitaminosis D	Inadequate or excessive vitamin D	Alter vitamin D administration
Miscellaneous		
Hypokalemia	Potassium intake inadequate relative to increased requirements for protein anabolism; diuresis	Alter nutrient administration
Hyperkalemia	Excessive potassium administration, especially in metabolic acidosis; renal failure	Alter nutrient administration
Hypomagnesemia	Inadequate magnesium administration relative to increased requirements for protein anabolism and glucose metabolism; diuresis; cisplatin administration	Alter nutrient administration
Hypermagnesemia	Excessive magnesium administration; renal failure	Alter nutrient administration
Anemia	Iron deficiency; folic acid deficiency; vitamin B_{12} deficiency; copper deficiency; other deficiencies	Alter nutrient administration
Bleeding	Vitamin K deficiency	Alter nutrient administration
Hypervitaminosis A	Excessive vitamin A administration	Alter nutrient administration
Elevations in AST (formerly SGOT), ALT (formerly SGPT), and serum alkaline phosphatase	Enzyme induction secondary to amino acid imbalance or to excessive deposition of glycogen or fat, or both, in the liver	Reevaluate status of patient

never be taken through the catheter. The one possible exception to this rule is the case in which the initial presentation of infection is characterized by marked hyperpyrexia or hypotension, or both. (In this case, contamination of the catheter is immaterial because the catheter will be removed.) If no other focus of sepsis is identified, the physician may elect to remove all indwelling lines, including the feeding catheter. In addition, either drainage around the catheter or a previous positive culture from the catheter exit site may also indicate immediate removal. If another primary source of the infection is diagnosed, then specific therapy should be instituted, and the parenteral nutrition should be continued. If no source of infection is identified, the catheter should be removed and the catheter tip cultured.

A dilemma arises if another source of infection is identified and if signs and symptoms of infection persist despite what appears to be appropriate therapy. If blood cultures are positive, we favor removal of the catheter to avoid the complications that are associated with a contaminated indwelling catheter (e.g., septic emboli and endocarditis). If, however, peripheral blood cultures are negative, the catheter can be changed over a guide wire and the

Table 15 Variables to Be Monitored during Intravenous Alimentation and Suggested Frequency of Monitoring

Variables	Suggested Monitoring Frequency	
	First Week	Later
Energy Balance		
Weight	Daily	Daily
Metabolic Variables		
Blood measurements		
Plasma electrolytes (Na$^+$, K$^+$, Cl$^-$)	Daily	3 × weekly
Blood urea nitrogen	3 × weekly	2 × weekly
Plasma osmolarity*	Daily	3 × weekly
Plasma total calcium and inorganic phosphorus	3 × weekly	2 × weekly
Blood glucose	Daily	3 × weekly
Plasma transaminases	3 × weekly	2 × weekly
Plasma total protein and fractions	2 × weekly	Weekly
Blood acid-base status	As indicated	As indicated
Hemoglobin	Weekly	Weekly
Ammonia	As indicated	As indicated
Magnesium	2 × weekly	Weekly
Triglycerides	Weekly	Weekly
Urine measurements		
Glucose	Daily	Daily
Specific gravity or osmolarity	Daily	Daily
General measurements		
Volume of infusate	Daily	Daily
Oral intake (if any)	Daily	Daily
Urinary output	Daily	Daily
Prevention and Detection of Infection		
Clinical observations (activity, temperature, symptoms)	Daily	Daily
WBC and differential counts	As indicated	As indicated
Cultures	As indicated	As indicated

*May be predicted from 2 × Na concentration (mEq/L) + [blood glucose (mg/dl) ÷ 18].

catheter tip cultured to confirm that catheter infection does not exist. Central venous feeding can be continued during this interval. If the cultured catheter tip is positive (≥ 10^5 organisms), the catheter should be removed.

Changing the central venous catheter over a guide wire can aid in the diagnosis of primary catheter infection.[31] Because most ICU patients have multiple potential sources for infection, this technique allows culture of the catheter tip but minimizes the risks associated with reinsertion of a new central catheter. Strict aseptic technique is used. The area surrounding the catheter entrance site is sterilized, the I.V. tubing is disconnected from the catheter, a guide wire is passed into the catheter, and the catheter is removed over the guide wire. A new catheter is inserted over the wire and sutured in place. The tip of the old catheter is cut, placed in a transfer vessel, and taken to the microbiology laboratory for semiquantitative culture. With strict care of catheters, the incidence of catheter sepsis should be less than 6%.[32] Septicemia is most commonly caused by growth and invasion of organisms along the catheter tract. Occasionally, bacteria are infused through the catheter because of a breach in sterility during care of the infusion apparatus. The most common bacterial organisms causing catheter sepsis are the skin contaminants *Staphylococcus epidermidis*, *S. aureus*, *Klebsiella pneumoniae*, and *Candida albicans*. In some rare cases, the intravenous solutions may be contaminated.

Moreover, most patients requiring central venous alimentation are immunocompromised hosts; their resistance is lowered further by disease, severe malnutrition, or treatment or by some combination of these factors. Coexisting conditions such as urinary tract infection, abscess, pneumonia, or mucositis secondary to chemotherapy predispose these patients to bacteremia, which may contaminate the central venous catheter.

Immunosuppressed critically ill patients receiving multiple broad-spectrum antibiotics are also at risk for *Candida* septicemia. Blood cultures positive for *C. albicans* in an ICU patient are an indication for catheter removal and treatment with fluconazole. An ophthalmologist should examine the eyegrounds of patients with proven candidemia to exclude the possibility of metastatic *Candida* ophthalmitis [see 85 Fungal Infection].

Home Nutritional Support

Home parenteral nutrition is indicated for patients who are unable to eat and absorb enough nutrients for maintenance.[33] Most of the adult surgical patients who require home parenteral nutrition suffer from short-bowel syndrome caused by (1) extensive Crohn's disease, (2) mesenteric infarction, or (3) severe abdominal trauma. Pseudo-obstruction, radiation enteritis, carcinomatosis, necrotizing enterocolitis, and intestinal fistulas are other indications for home nutritional support. Patients with these conditions cannot receive adequate nutrition enterally, although in some cases compensatory mucosal growth occurs that may either reduce or eventually eliminate the need for continued home parenteral nutrition.

To be eligible for home parenteral nutrition, patients must (1) have an appropriate level of intelligence, (2) be highly motivated, and (3) have adequate support from their families. Patients must receive extensive evaluation, teaching, and training during hospitalization if home parenteral nutrition is to prove successful. These services should be provided by a team consisting of a physician, a nurse, a dietitian, a pharmacist, and a social worker. The team's instructions should be thorough and wide-ranging, covering the basic principles of parenteral nutrition as well as providing mechanical guidelines for catheter care, asepsis, and use of infusion pumps. Patients should be objectively evaluated before being discharged from the hospital to ensure that they have both an adequate understanding of the principles of intravenous nutrition and the technical ability to carry out home parenteral nutrition properly.

A patient who is judged by the nutrition support team to be a candidate for home TPN requires placement of a Silastic catheter designed for more permanent use than the central venous catheter employed during hospitalization.[34] The catheter is typically 90 cm long, with a thin 55 cm intravascular segment that is inserted either by venous cutdown into the internal or external jugular vein or the cephalic vein or directly into the subclavian vein by means of venipuncture. The intravascular portion of the catheter is cut so that its tip will lie at the junction of the superior vena cava and the right atrium. Placement of the catheter is carried out in the operating room by using local anesthesia (1% lidocaine) and adequate sedation. The catheter is tunneled subcutaneously from a small incision lateral to the sternum to the site of venous insertion. The catheter exit site is chosen on the basis of the patient's gender, physique, and hand dominance. In women, lower paraxiphoid or upper abdominal exit sites permit a more natural appearance. If the patient's coagulation status is abnormal, the cephalic vein is isolated in the deltapectoral groove and tied distally, and the catheter is inserted proximally by means of venotomy. Otherwise, a percutaneous approach to the subclavian vein is taken. The pa-

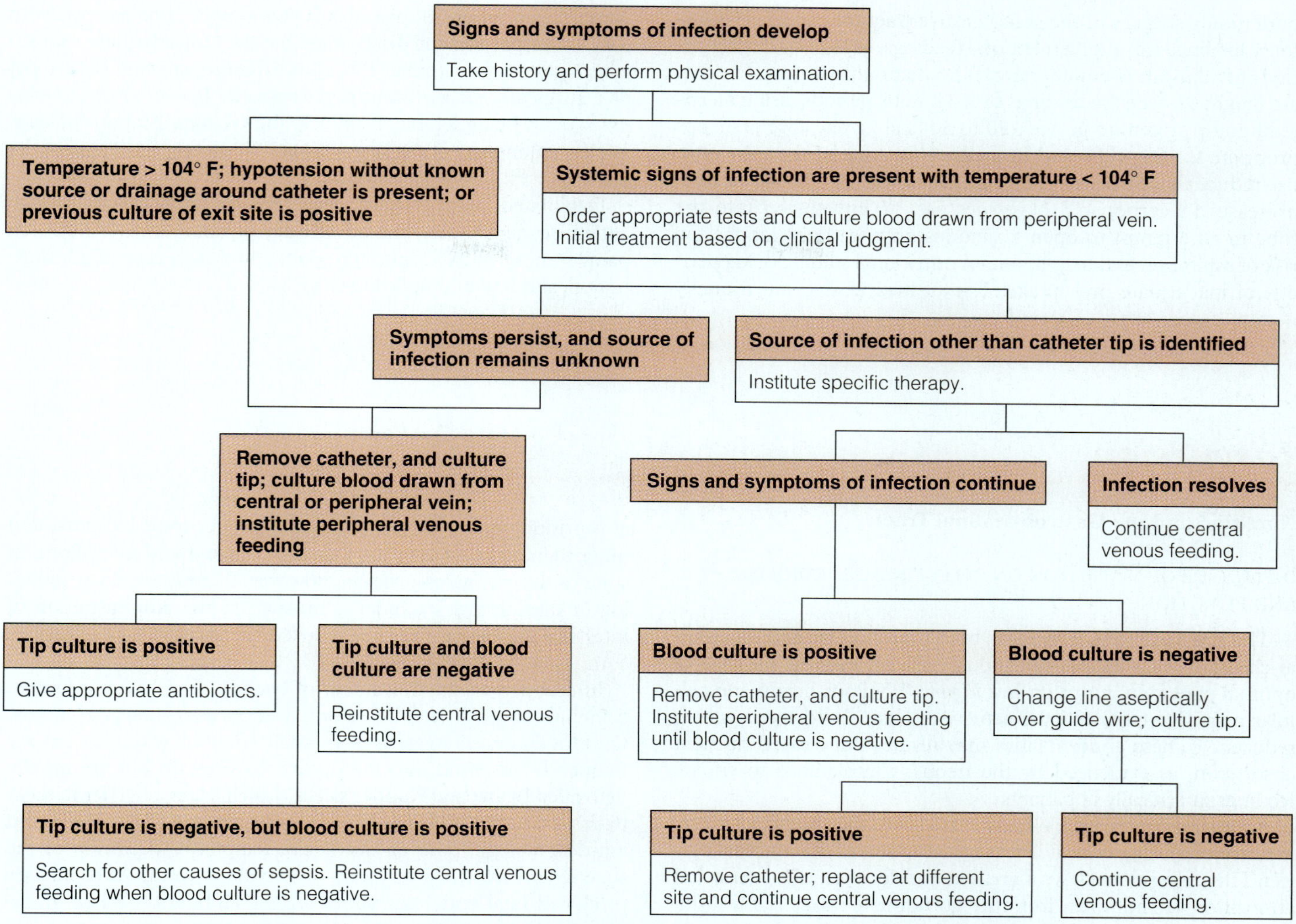

Figure 3 Evaluation of a febrile patient receiving central venous parenteral nutrition is shown.

tient is placed in Trendelenburg's position, and a needle is inserted into the subclavian vein while negative pressure is applied to the attached syringe. Once a flashback of venous blood is obtained, a J-wire is introduced through the needle into the superior vena cava. A large introducer (e.g., a No. 10 tube) that has an internal obturator and an external cannula is then inserted over the guide wire to dilate the tract. After the catheter has been cut to the appropriate length and flushed with heparinized saline, it is inserted into the cannula, which is then peeled away and removed. Proper positioning of the catheter is confirmed by fluoroscopy, and the incisions are closed with absorbable sutures. The catheter is sutured to the skin exit site, and the sutures are left attached for at least 2 weeks while tissue ingrowth into the Dacron velour cuff takes place. After the sutures are placed, sterile dressings are applied.

Calorie, protein, and fluid needs are carefully estimated for each patient, and the administration schedule is arranged so that the total volume may be infused nocturnally over 10 to 12 hours. Electrolytes, micronutrients, and trace minerals are added as indicated. Fat emulsions may be given either separately or admixed with glucose and protein and are used to reduce the requirement for dextrose calories and to prevent essential fatty acid deficiency.

The complications of home TPN are much the same as those of in-hospital TPN. They may be divided into four categories: mechanical, infectious, metabolic, and psychosocial. Mechanical complications, which are generally easy to remedy, include catheter occlusion and dislodgment and damage to the external portion of the catheter. Infectious complications that are superficial to the Dacron cuff usually respond well to antibiotics. Infections of the intravascular catheter may necessitate removal of the catheter after the diagnosis is confirmed by blood cultures obtained through the catheter, but the usual therapeutic approach is to initiate a trial of parenteral antibiotics. Metabolic complications related to individual nutrient deficiencies may be corrected by addition of the appropriate substance to the solution. The role of serum levels of trace minerals and micronutrients in the delineation of nutrient deficiency states remains unclear. In patients receiving insulin, hyperinsulinemia after infusion may be prevented by reducing the rate of administration gradually over the last hour of infusion. Psychosocial complications may vary from slight depression to suicidal tendencies, which must be treated with appropriate counseling.

The costs of a home TPN program may also be divided into four categories: patient training, equipment, supplies, and follow-up. It has been estimated that the average annual cost of home TPN is 70% less than that of in-hospital TPN. The growth of private companies that deliver equipment and supplies to the home, maintain inventory, bill patients, and help with insurance problems has considerably facilitated home care.

Home enteral nutrition is frequently utilized, either as the sole source or as a partial source of nutritional support. It is the preferred method when GI tract function is adequate. In patients undergoing surgery of the aerodigestive tract for cancer, jejunostomy feedings can supplement oral feedings, especially during periods of adjuvant chemotherapy and radiation treatment. Patients are taught to cycle the feedings over 12-hour periods, using an enteral pump system to provide 20 to 30 kcal/kg/day. Use of an appropriate feeding tube and immediate flushing of the tube after use reduce the incidence of clogging at home. If blockage occurs, proteases or carbonated beverages can be introduced into the tube in an attempt to open it. Jejunostomy feedings reduce the risk of aspiration and help maintain nutritional status during periods of inadequate oral intake. Use of inexpensive nutritionally complete commercial formulas is encouraged. For patients who have more permanent disabilities that prevent adequate oral intake, a gastrostomy (either PEG [see 47 Gastrointestinal Endoscopy] or a surgically placed Stamm gastrostomy [see 49 Gastric Procedures]) may be preferable. It reduces the GI complications of feeding by making use of the reservoir and admixing functions of the stomach.

Debilitated patients have been fed for many years through enteral feeding tubes. The advantages of home enteral nutrition parallel those of in-hospital programs: low cost, ease of administration, and fewer complications.

Discussion

Nutrition and the Gastrointestinal Tract

INFLUENCE OF NUTRITION ON INTESTINAL METABOLISM AND FUNCTION

The small intestine undergoes both morphologic and functional changes when enteral nutrition is absent, even in the face of optimal parenteral nutrition [see Figure 4]. Villous height and cellular mass decrease, and the activity of brush border enzymes is reduced.[35] These abnormalities may result in decreased nutrient absorption, as evidenced by the frequent intolerance to enteral feedings in critically ill patients.

Another potential problem associated with the absence of enteral nutrition during critical illness is disruption of the mucosal barrier. This disruption allows increased translocation of bacteria and absorption of endotoxin from the gut lumen.[36] Bacterial translocation is the process of bacterial migration (or invasion) across the mucosal barrier into mesenteric lymph nodes and the portal bloodstream. Factors that are associated with increased bacterial translocation include alterations in the GI microflora, impaired host immunity, and physical disruption of the mucosal barrier.[37]

Bacterial translocation has been studied most extensively in animal models, and it is not known whether much of this information is applicable in humans. For example, the translocation of indigenous enteric bacteria to mesenteric lymph nodes occurred in rats after scald burns of 40% of total body surface area.[38] Because translocation was not associated with increased numbers of bacteria within the intestinal tract, it was thought that the egress of bacteria was caused by a breakdown in the barrier function of the gut associated with the thermal injury. In another model, abscesses were created by intraperitoneal implantation of a fibrin clot contaminated with nonenteric organisms. When cultured at a later time, enteric organisms were present that had presumably translocated from the bowel lumen into the abscess.[39]

More than 40 years ago, intraoperative bacteriologic cultures of the portal venous bloodstream in a heterogeneous group of patients with noninflammatory lesions of the GI tract were performed. Eight of 25 patients had positive portal venous cultures, demonstrating that bacteria pass from the GI tract to the liver via the portal vein.[40] Life-threatening infections from gut-associated bacteria and fungi have been documented in patients with multiorgan failure[36] (now known as multiple organ dysfunction syndrome), in those with cancer who have had chemotherapy[41] or bone marrow transplants,[39] and in those with major burns.[42] These patients are immunocompromised, do not receive adequate enteral nutrition, and are given antibiotics, H_2 receptor blockers, and other therapies that alter the intestinal mucosa and microflora. In spite of this strong association, however, therapy aimed at reducing or diminishing bacterial flora, such as the administration of intestinal antibiotics, has not reduced the incidence of infectious complications in such patients.

In addition to the movement of bacteria from the gut lumen, bacterial endotoxin may be absorbed across abnormal gut mucosa. Current evidence suggests that small amounts of endotoxin are frequently absorbed into the portal bloodstream but are rapidly detoxified by hepatic Kupffer's cells, which act as a barrier to these toxins.[43] Studies were done on rabbits with one of three different injuries: a single dose of endotoxin, temporary occlusion of the superior mesenteric artery, or a 30% scald burn. All three injuries produced fatal endotoxic shock within 12 hours.[44] When gram-negative bacteria were either absent from or present in reduced amounts in the intestinal tract of similar animals, these injuries were not lethal.

Studies in mice reveal that endotoxin given intraperitoneally promotes bacterial translocation from the gut to the mesenteric lymph nodes in a dose-dependent manner.[45] The incidence and magnitude of endotoxin-induced bacterial translocation in endotoxin-resistant mice were similar to those in nonresistant mice, indicating that bacterial translocation was not prevented by genetic resistance to endotoxin. Finally, these same investigators examined the combined effects of malnutrition and endotoxemia on promoting bacterial translocation.[46] This combination was associated with a significantly higher number of translocated bacteria to systemic organs than was seen in normally nourished mice receiving endotoxin.

In clinical studies, circulating endotoxin was found in the blood of individuals with chronic inflammatory bowel disease that progressed despite standard medical treatment.[47] Whole gut lavage with normal saline reduced the levels of endotoxins; as a result, the condition of all patients improved, plasma endotoxin levels dropped rapidly, and abnormal elevations of body temperature were reduced.

The intestinal mucosa is also disrupted in critically ill patients after cardiovascular instability and hypotension. Hypovolemic shock produces sloughing of intestinal mucosal cells and a cessation of mucus production,[48] patchy or diffuse areas of superficial necrosis, openings of tight junctions between epithelial cells, and mucosal edema.[49] These combined effects lead to increased mucosal permeability of the colon and bowel wall edema, process-

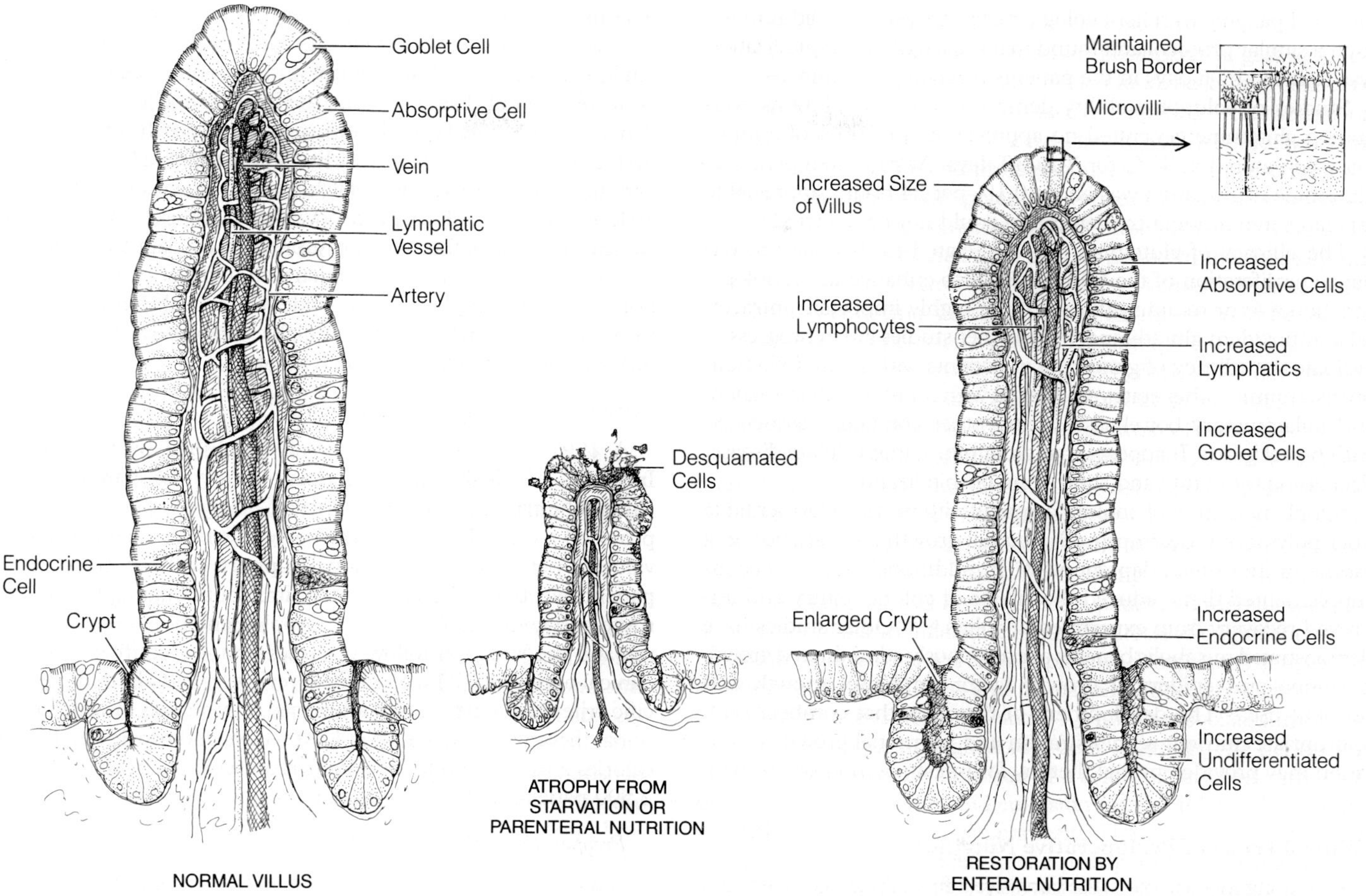

Figure 4 Enteral nutrition maintains and restores intestinal epithelium, whereas starvation or parenteral nutrition causes villous atrophy.

es that have been attenuated by creating a proximal, diverting ileostomy or administering a hydrolyzed chemical diet.[50]

In summary, during critical illness, the GI tract is altered in such a way that the protective barrier function of the gut is lost. This loss allows enteric bacteria to cross the gut wall or accommodates the absorption of endotoxins into the body, or both. Because most patients with critical illness cannot receive enteral feedings and because parenteral nutrition results in gut atrophy, current techniques of nutritional support neither facilitate repair of the intestinal mucosa nor maintain its barrier function.

NUTRITIONAL SUPPORT FOR THE INTESTINAL TRACT

Enteral feedings are the best method of maintaining the integrity of the GI mucosa. The provision of these feedings may have profound effects on the reduction of systemic manifestations of critical illness. For example, early enteral feedings in a 30% burn model not only protected against mucosal atrophy in the GI tract but also decreased the overall elaboration of stress hormones and minimized the catabolic response to this injury.[51]

Glutamine is a nutrient that supports intestinal cell replication and growth and may be useful as specific therapy for the support of the intestinal mucosa. Glutamine is absent from all standard parenteral nutrient solutions unless a specific request is made to provide glutamine-supplemented parenteral nutrition. Glutamine is present in insufficient amounts in most enteral formulas, although there are at least two modified diets that contain adequate glutamine. Glutamine may also be provided as a supplement to standard enteral feedings and is usually given as 0.5 g/kg/day in divided doses. When animals or humans are maintained on parenteral nutrition, atrophy of the intestinal mucosa is observed. When glutamine is added to the parenteral nutrition, this response is greatly attenuated, both in animals[52] and in humans.[53] The effect of this specific bowel nutrient on GI organs has been studied under a variety of conditions in both animals and humans. For example, when rats were treated with the chemotherapeutic agents methotrexate or fluorouracil, growth arrest and GI mucosal atrophy occurred. The addition of glutamine to an enteral diet promoted recovery of the mucosa of the small bowel and colon in animals receiving this diet as compared with animals receiving standard but glutamine-free diets.[54,55] Glutamine solutions also attenuate the pancreatic atrophy and hepatic steatosis associated with standard intravenous formulas. A series of detailed clinical studies have described unique clinical advantages associated with glutamine-supplemented solutions. Glutamine-supplemented solutions were given to postoperative cholecystectomy patients,[56] and parenteral solutions supplemented with the dipeptide of glutamine and alanine were administered to patients after cancer surgery.[57] Glutamine-treated patients in both groups showed improved nitrogen balance as compared with control subjects, who received I.V. feedings. Two randomized, blind, prospective trials have been performed in patients undergoing bone marrow transplantation. In the first study, 45 patients with hematologic malignancies were randomized to receive standard or glutamine-containing I.V. feedings. The patients receiving glutamine feedings had less accumulation of extracellular water,[58] a reduced rate of infection, and a 7-day reduction in the length of hospital stay.[59] The second study, which

were no significant differences in postoperative morbidity between the two groups. It was concluded that early PEG tube feeding (3 hours after tube placement) is as safe as next-day feeding in selected elderly patients.

A 1997 PRCT included 28 patients undergoing esophagectomy or pancreaticoduodenectomy who received either immediate postoperative enteral feeding via jejunostomy (N =13) or no feedings during the first 6 days after operation (N =15).[86] Hand-grip strength, vital capacity, forced expiratory volume in 1 second (FEV_1), and maximal inspiratory pressure were measured before operation and on postoperative days 2, 4, and 6. Postoperative vital capacity ($P < 0.05$) and FEV_1 ($P = 0.07$) were consistently lower in the fed group than in the unfed group, whereas there were no significant differences in grip strength and maximal inspiratory pressure. Postoperative mobility was lower in the fed group, and these patients tended to recover less rapidly. There were no significant differences in fatigue or vigor between the two groups. The investigators concluded that immediate postoperative jejunal feeding is associated with impaired respiratory mechanics and postoperative mobility and does not influence the loss of muscle strength or the increase in fatigue occurring after major surgery; they further concluded that immediate postoperative enteral feeding should not be routine in well-nourished patients who are at low risk for nutrition-related complications. This PRCT is noteworthy not only for its intriguing, unanticipated results but also for its inclusion of an unfed control group, a decision that underscores the importance of such groups in the design of these clinical investigations. Heretofore, many institutional review boards, on ethical grounds, have not permitted investigation of unfed control groups.

Another 1997 PRCT evaluated early enteral feeding after resection of upper GI malignancies.[87] The purpose of the study was to determine whether early postoperative enteral feeding with an immune-enhancing formula could decrease morbidity, mortality, and length of hospital stay. A total of 195 patients with upper GI cancer were randomly selected to receive either the immune-enhancing formula (supplemented with arginine, RNA, and omega-3 fatty acids) via jejunostomy or standard I.V. crystalloid solutions. There were no significant differences between the two groups with respect to the number of minor, major, or infectious wound complications; the length of the hospital stay; or mortality. The two main strengths of this study were (1) its inclusion of an "intent to treat" analysis and (2) the large number of subjects enrolled. It is noteworthy that even though all of the patients had upper GI cancer, the average postoperative weight loss was only 5% to 6%, and serum albumin levels were normal in both groups.

A 1998 report investigated the effects of early postoperative enteral feeding in 43 patients with nontraumatic intestinal perforation and peritonitis.[88] After laparotomy, patients were randomly assigned to either a control group (N = 22) or a study group (N = 21). The study group received a feeding jejunostomy, and enteral feeding was started 12 hours after operation. The mortality rate was high in both groups (18% for the control group versus 19% for the study group). The control group had more septic complications than the study group (22 versus 8, $P < 0.05$).

Complications of Enteral Nutrition

A number of reports have examined the complications of enteral nutrition in different settings. Needle-catheter jejunostomy (NCJ) is the jejunal access method of choice in many centers. Some reports have suggested that this feeding route may be associated with a high rate of complications.[89] In a retrospective review of 2,022 NCJs performed in 1,938 patients, 34 NCJ-related complications occurred in 29 patients (1.5%).[90] The most common complication was premature loss of the catheter from occlusion or dislodgment (N = 15 [0.7%]), and the most serious was bowel necrosis (N = 3 [0.15%]). The investigators concluded that NCJ is associated with low complication rates and that most of the complications that occur can be prevented through greater attention to detail and better monitoring of the physical examination of patients with marginal gut function. Another retrospective review of jejunal feeding was performed in 1,359 patients over a period of 6 years.[91] Small bowel necrosis occurred in 14 patients, and 12 succumbed to this complication. The mechanism of small bowel necrosis was unclear but was thought to be associated with increased intraluminal pressure arising from severe abdominal distention.

As noted, PEG has become the gold standard for the delivery of enteral nutrition into the stomach. Compared with surgical gastrostomy, it is associated with significantly reduced morbidity and cost. Despite the increased use of this technique, however, overall survival remains poor because of the frequent placement of PEGs in patients with terminal disease. A 1997 study reviewed 64 patients consecutively referred for PEGs with the aim of examining possible predictive postoperative variables.[92] Of the 64, 43 survived at least 30 days after tube placement; only one death was directly attributable to tube placement. The 30-day survival correlated directly with the serum albumin concentration and inversely with the serum creatinine concentration. After multivariable logistic regression analysis, only albumin could be identified as an independent predictor of 30-day survival ($P = 0.04$): 83% of patients with a serum albumin level higher than 3.0 g/dl survived for 30 days, compared with 58% of patients with an albumin level lower than 3.0 g/dl. The investigators concluded that serum albumin concentration appeared to be a predictor of early survival in patients undergoing PEG placement.

Conclusions

Parenteral and enteral nutritional support is a valuable adjunctive—and sometimes life-saving—therapy in the management of selective types of surgical patients. It is generally agreed that patients who are unable to ingest adequate nutrients for a prolonged period require nutritional therapy to prevent the adverse effects of malnutrition. It is not entirely clear, however, precisely how "adequate" and "prolonged" should be defined. In practice, the definitions are likely to vary from patient to patient, depending on the amount of body energy stores and lean body mass, the presence or absence of preexisting medical illnesses, the number and severity of postoperative complications, and the nature of the surgical procedure. Summation of the data from the PRCTs suggests that giving nutritional support for 7 days before operation decreases postoperative complications. Severely malnourished patients (defined on the basis of percentage of body weight lost or nutritional risk index score) may derive greater clinical benefit from preoperative nutritional support, but this conclusion is based largely on retrospective analysis of prospective data. In addition, there are subsets of patients who may derive particular benefit from nutritional support, such as patients undergoing hepatic resection for hepatocellular carcinoma and elderly patients with hip fractures. The increased rate of complications in patients given postoperative TPN and the case reports of small bowel necrosis in patients who receive early postoperative enteral nutrition are evidence that nutritional support has risks and should not be given indiscriminately. Future studies are needed for better identification of specific subsets of patients who may benefit from perioperative nutritional therapy, particularly enteral nutrition. Such studies must consider the effect of nutritional therapy on both short-term and long-term outcome.

Nutrition Pharmacotherapy

The role of nutrient administration to surgical patients has evolved from the maintenance of a positive energy and nitrogen balance to the use of nutrients to modulate tissue metabolism and organ system function. This new role is referred to as nutrition pharmacotherapy. Like other forms of adjuvant therapy, nutrition pharmacotherapy is usually a multitargeted therapeutic modality. For instance, one form of nutrition pharmacotherapy, immunonutrition, makes use of combinations of specific amino acids, fatty acids, and, in some enteral formulas, nucleotides. Another form, so-called bowel rehabilitation, uses an amino acid (glutamine) in combination with growth hormone and a modified diet. Inclusion of a specific nutrient as part of a plan of nutrition pharmacotherapy is based either on clinical studies or, more often, on extrapolations from experimental observations.

In what follows, we discuss each of the nutrients used, or proposed for use, in nutrition pharmacotherapy, with emphasis on chemical characteristics, physiologic effects, available forms for exogenous administration, and, if available, clinical data supporting its use for this purpose.

BRANCHED-CHAIN AMINO ACIDS

The BCAAs—leucine, isoleucine, and valine—are unique among amino acids in that they undergo very little, if any, metabolism by the liver. Instead, most absorbed BCAAs remain intact until they reach muscle tissue, where they increase protein synthesis by 50% and decrease protein degradation by 25%.[93] These effects are attributable more to leucine (and its metabolite α-ketoisocaproate) than to isoleucine or valine. These effects reach physiologic significance only during stress or injury, which is why most of the studies that show BCAAs to have beneficial effects have been conducted in animals or patients manifesting the septic response.

In experimental primate models of sepsis, induced by administration of *Salmonella typhimurium* or *Streptococcus pneumoniae*, a positive nitrogen balance can be achieved only by giving high-dose glucose (85 kcal/kg/day) when the nitrogen source is a balanced mixture of amino acids (containing 24% BCAAs). If, however, the formula is enriched to 48% BCAAs, the same amount of nitrogen retention is achieved at a much lower intake of glucose (32 kcal/kg/day). Given the usual glucose intolerance seen in patients with the septic response, this is a highly desirable effect.

In 1986, several clinical studies reported in the late 1970s and early 1980s were reviewed by a panel of experts in a research workshop sponsored by the American Society of Parenteral and Enteral Nutrition.[93] The panel's main conclusion was that whereas some positive parameters of nitrogen metabolism had been noted using BCAA-enriched solutions in the most severely ill patients, a major effect on outcome was not demonstrated.

An entire decade elapsed before a subsequent study attempted to address this issue. In a prospective, randomized, multicenter study conducted in ICUs in Spain, 69 patients with the septic response were randomly selected to receive amino acids in dosages of 1.5 g/kg/day with 23% BCAAs, 1.5 g/kg/day with 45% BCAAs, or 1.1 g/kg/day with 45% BCAAs. Compared with patients who received the standard 23% BCAA solution, patients who received the 45% BCAA solution, at either nitrogen intake, exhibited significantly increased prealbumin and retinol-binding protein levels as well as a lower mortality.[94]

Thus, there are data to support the use of BCAAs in clinical practice, but the indications are very specific. First, the only patients who seem to benefit from BCAA supplementation are those who are in a septic state and critically ill; however, most such patients can be successfully treated either with conventional nutritional therapy or with no nutritional therapy at all. Therefore, a second indication should be a clear need for nutritional therapy, as outlined earlier (see above), coupled with unsuccessful use of conventional amino acid formulations, as demonstrated by persistently low levels of short-lived serum proteins and a negative nitrogen balance.

GLUTAMINE

Glutamine is the most abundant amino acid in the body and appears to be the most versatile. Most free glutamine is synthesized and stored in skeletal muscle, where its concentration is 30 times greater than it is in plasma.[95] Skeletal muscle releases net glutamine for transport to the gut, immune cells, and the kidneys. The cells of the gut and those of the immune system proliferate rapidly, and glutamine acts as the main source of fuel and as a biosynthetic precursor. One of the compounds derived from glutamine is glutathione, a tripeptide (glutamate-cysteineglycine) with potent antioxidant effects. Finally, glutamine participates in acid-base regulation via the release of ammonia, which combines with H^+ to form NH_4^+ and is lost in urine.

Catabolism induced by major injury, surgery, sepsis, or burns results in increased release of glutamine from skeletal muscle.[96] This output of glutamine into the circulation is associated with increased uptake and consumption by the gut, the immune system, the liver, and the kidneys. The net effect is a profound fall in intracellular muscle stores of glutamine. This deficit exceeds all other amino acid deficits and persists even when stores of all other amino acids have already been replenished.[97]

Standard amino acid formulations have always included all of the essential amino acids and most of the nonessential ones. For a long time, glutamine was excluded from parenteral formulations because of its instability in aqueous solutions. In the early formulations, glutamine that had remained in solution for an extended period would undergo spontaneous transformation into a cyclic compound called pyroglutamate, which can cause neurotoxicity. As more knowledge of the potential benefits of glutamine became available, the pharmaceutical industry began to develop ways of keeping glutamine stable in an aqueous solution. For instance, Glamin (Pharmacia & Upjohn, Sweden), an amino acid formulation that is already commercially available in Europe, includes the dipeptide glycyl-L-glutamine, which is readily hydrolyzed to free glutamine in plasma and tissues.

Several clinical studies of supplementation of parenteral formulas with glutamine have been published. The most striking results have been reported in patients undergoing bone marrow transplantation and in patients with short-bowel syndrome. The first randomized, double-blind, controlled study to investigate the effects of glutamine on metabolic parameters and clinical outcome in patients undergoing bone marrow transplantation was published in 1992.[98] A total of 45 adults receiving allogeneic bone marrow transplants for hematologic malignancies were randomly selected to receive L-glutamine, 0.57 g/kg/day, or a standard glutamine-free isonitrogenous formula for an average of 4 weeks after operation. The patients who received the glutamine-supplemented formula had a better nitrogen balance than the control group (−1.4 g/day versus −4.2 g/day); more important, they also had a lower incidence of microbial colonization and clinical infection and a shorter hospital stay. Subsequently, these findings were confirmed by a study performed by a different group of investigators.[99]

One of the most challenging pathologic conditions for surgeons is the short-bowel syndrome that develops after massive small bowel resection. Fortunately, the advent of parenteral nutrition has improved survival for many patients with this condition who previously would have died of dehydration and malnutrition; however, it has also created a dependency on this therapy, which in the long term can have life-threatening complications. For this reason, many surgical scientists have searched for ways of augmenting these patients' intestinal absorption capacity so that their need for parenteral nutrition can be eliminated or at least greatly reduced. Having achieved a better understanding of the roles of glutamine, dietary fiber, short-chain fatty acids, and growth factors in the process of intestinal adaptation, investigators designed clinical trials with the aim of evaluating the effects of supplementation of these substances on patients with short-bowel syndrome.

After a pilot study involving eight patients with short-bowel syndrome, one group of investigators performed a controlled study in which recombinant human growth hormone, 0.14 mg/kg/day; glutamine, 0.45 to 0.63 g/kg/day; and a high-carbohydrate, low-fat diet were given to 31 patients with this syndrome.[100,101] The criteria for inclusion were (1) either the entire colon present with a minimum of 50 cm of small bowel remaining or the colon absent with a minimum of 100 cm of small bowel remaining and (2) previous need for long-term parenteral nutrition. By the end of a 3-week treatment period, there was a significant improvement in nutrient and fluid absorption, and as a result, parenteral nutrition was discontinued in 40% of patients. After an extended follow-up period (6 years) and the inclusion of more patients (87), this bowel rehabilitation regimen led to the discontinuance of parenteral nutrition in 52% of patients and to reduced requirements for parenteral nutrition in an additional 38%.[102] Another group of investigators using a similar protocol found only a modest improvement in electrolyte assimilation and no improvement in gut morphology or nutrient absorption.[103] Although these studies do not settle the issue of how effective the bowel rehabilitation regimen is, they do raise important questions—in particular, how administration of these substances should be timed and whether a multi-institutional study is needed.[104]

All of the studies just cited were conducted according to research protocols that used L-glutamine, which is not practical for I.V. use. As noted, glutamine is now commercially available (in Europe) in a dipeptide form that is stable in an aqueous solution. A 1998 study evaluated the use of the dipeptide glycyl-L-glutamine, 0.3 g/kg/day, in 28 patients who underwent elective abdominal surgery.[105] Over a 5-day period, the mean cumulative nitrogen balance was significantly better with glutamine supplementation than without it (–7 g/day versus –23 g/day). Immune function, as determined by lymphocyte counts and generation of cysteinyl leukotrienes by polymorphonuclear neutrophils, was also improved. In addition, the hospital stay was 6.2 days shorter for the glutamine group. The investigators concluded that glutamine administered as the dipeptide glycyl-L-glutamine appears to be safe and effective.

The precise indications for glutamine supplementation remain to be determined. There is no question regarding the benefits of glutamine administration after bone marrow transplantation. We believe it is safe to assume that glutamine supplementation, when available, is beneficial to stressed surgical patients, particularly those who are immunosuppressed. Further research is needed before its widespread use to augment intestinal absorption can be recommended.

ARGININE

Arginine is a nitrogen-dense amino acid that is considered a semiessential amino acid because it is required for growth.[106] The effect of arginine on growth seems to be mediated by its role in polyamine and nucleic acid synthesis. In addition, arginine is a potent secretagogue of growth hormone, insulin, glucagon, prolactin, and somatostatin.[107-109] When the secretagogue effect of arginine is abolished by hypophysectomy, the stimulatory effect on wound healing is lost.[110] Supplemental dietary arginine has thymotrophic effects and enhances the responsiveness of thymic lymphocytes to mitogens in rats.[111] A similar response occurs in peripheral blood mononuclear cells of healthy human volunteers[112] and postoperative patients,[113] as evidenced by an enhanced response to concanavalin A and phytohemagglutinin.

Arginine enhances cellular immunity, as demonstrated by an increased delayed hypersensitivity response in animals with burns.[51] Dietary supplementation with arginine improves the response to dinitrofluorobenzene (DNFB) and enhances the survival of guinea pigs with 30% body surface burns. However, in a model of acute peritonitis in guinea pigs, supplemental arginine did not improve DNFB response or survival.[114]

Supplemental arginine also has antitumor properties.[115] The inhibition of tumor growth induced by supplemental arginine is associated with increased tumor cyclic adenosine monophosphate levels and decreased ornithine decarboxylase activity.[116] The exact mechanism of action of arginine on tumor growth is not known, but it seems to be twofold: nonspecific immunomodulation and augmentation of the response to immunoregulatory lymphokines. In accordance with this hypothesis, supplemental arginine has been investigated as an immunotherapeutic agent to enhance the effect of interleukin-2 (IL-2).[117] When compared with a glycine-treated group, arginine reduced tumor engraftment and growth and prolonged survival in a model of murine neuroblastoma treated with IL-2.

The experimental evidence currently available demonstrates a physiologic role in growing animals and a therapeutic benefit in posttraumatic states, burns, and cancer. A new enteral formula that includes arginine in combination with fish oil and RNA is now available in the United States (see Fatty Acids, below).

NUCLEOTIDES

Purines and pyrimidines are precursors of DNA and RNA, which are essential for cell proliferation. Purines and pyrimidines are synthesized by the liver de novo from amino acids and reutilized by salvage pathways. Reduction of dietary nucleotides results in suppression of cellular immune responses and prolongation of allograft survival.[118] The mechanism of immunosuppression associated with nucleotide restriction seems to be an inability of T cells to undergo blastogenesis. Dietary supplements containing RNA or uracil (but not adenine) maintain resistance to infection by C. albicans or S. aureus in rodents.[119,120] However, the immune response is not enhanced when compared with a standard control diet.

On the basis of the immunosuppressive effect of dietary restriction of nucleotides, it has been postulated that nucleotide supplementation could provide an immunostimulant effect. This postulate has been tested in studies of the RNA–fish oil–arginine formula now available [see Fatty Acids, below].

FATTY ACIDS

Fatty acids in the systemic circulation can be used in two forms: as fuels to be stored and oxidized as needed by the organism and as precursors for other essential compounds, such as eicosanoids (prostaglandins, leukotrienes, and thromboxanes). The eicosanoids are 20-carbon compounds derived from the essential fatty acids. They function as regulatory compounds in various physiologic processes, such as the immune response. Although organisms can oxidize other compounds to meet caloric needs, fatty acids in minimal amounts are essential as precursors for the synthesis of eicosanoids.

Fatty acids are classified in many different ways. One classification is based on chain length: short (two to five carbons), medium (six to 11 carbons), and long (12 to 26 carbons). Another classification is based on the presence of double bonds in the carbon chain: those with double bonds are called unsaturated and are further classified as either monounsaturated fatty acids or polyunsaturated fatty acids (PUFAs), depending on the number of double bonds. Another classification that has gained popularity is the omega classification, which indicates where the first double bond is located when the carbons are counted from the noncarboxyl end of the chain (e.g., omega-3, omega-6, omega-9).

Humans can synthesize only fatty acids with double bonds at position 7 (counting from the noncarboxyl end toward the carboxyl end). Therefore, fatty acids with double bonds at position 6 or position 3 must be supplied exogenously. Because humans can elongate and desaturate linoleic acid and α-linolenic acid to produce the remaining omega-6 and omega-3 PUFAs, these are considered the essential fatty acids. The requirements for omega-6 PUFAs exceed the requirements for omega-3 PUFAs by a ratio of approximately 5:1.

PUFAs of the omega-6 series are abundant in vegetable oils, such as corn oil and soybean oil, and PUFAs of the omega-3 series are abundant in fish oils, such as menhaden oil. Other oils rich in omega-3 PUFAs are seed oils, such as black currant oil and canola oil (canola oil is derived from rape seeds and genetically modified to optimize the fatty acid composition).

The availability of 20-carbon PUFAs—arachidonic acid in the omega-6 series and eicosapentaenoic acid in the omega-3 series—is the determining factor for the synthesis of eicosanoids [see 100 Eicosanoids in Surgery]. There are two major metabolic pathways for the synthesis of eicosanoids. The cyclooxygenase pathway results in the production of prostanoids. Inasmuch as prostanoids contain two double bonds in the carbon side chain, they are also called di-enoic products, or the two series. These include prostaglandin E_2 (PGE_2), prostaglandin D_2 (PGD_2), prostaglandin F_2 (PGF_2), prostaglandin I_2 (PGI_2, also called prostacyclin), and thromboxane A_2 (TXA_2). The lipoxygenase pathway yields trienoic products (three double bonds in the carbon side chain), such as thromboxane A_3 (TXA_3) and prostaglandin I_3 (PGI_3). All nucleated cells, with the exception of lymphocytes, can synthesize eicosanoids. Platelets are the major sources of thromboxanes, and the leukocytes mainly produce leukotrienes. Prostaglandins have various effects on the tone of blood vessels and the aggregation of platelets. Leukotrienes promote leukocyte migration (chemotaxis) and degranulation, release of lysosomal enzymes, and superoxide production.

Cells obtain arachidonic acid and eicosapentaenoic acid from degradation of phospholipids by phospholipase A_2 and phospholipase C or by elongation and desaturation of linoleic acid and α-linolenic acid. Mature immune cells, such as monocytes, macrophages, lymphocytes, and polymorphonuclear cells, lack δ-6 desaturase, the critical rate-limiting enzyme for transformation of 18-carbon PUFAs into 20-carbon PUFAs.[121] Therefore, the availability of precursors for eicosanoid synthesis in immune cells is largely dependent on their lipid composition. Because lipid intake influences the lipid composition of immune cells, the type of PUFAs ingested can influence the immune response.[122,123] Eicosanoids, especially PGE_2 and the lipoxygenase products leukotriene B_4 (LTB_4), 5-hydroxyeicosatetraenoic acid (5-HETE), and 15-hydroxyeicosatetraenoic acid (15-HETE) are immunomodulatory; when produced in excess (as in posttraumatic states), they are generally immunosuppressive.[124] Dietary supplementation with omega-3 PUFAs has improved survival of endotoxic shock in guinea pigs.[125] The reduced intake of omega-6 PUFAs seems to be as important as the enrichment with omega-3 PUFAs. When animals are made deficient in linoleic acid, they have only a 24% mortality after endotoxin challenge. However, the mortality reaches 100% when arachidonic acid is given 2 days before endotoxin challenge.[126] Similar results have been reported in guinea pigs recovering from flame burns covering 30% of body surface area.[127] When compared with animals fed dietary safflower oil (74% linoleic acid) or linoleic acid alone, animals fed fish oil had less weight loss, better skeletal muscle mass, lower resting metabolic expenditure, better cell-mediated immune responses, better opsonic indices, higher splenic weight, lower adrenal weight, higher serum transferrin levels, and lower serum C3 levels.

In conclusion, high intake of omega-6 PUFAs (e.g., linoleic acid) is associated with increased synthesis of PGE_2, which is immunosuppressive. A reduction in the intake of omega-6 PUFAs appears prudent in patients who are immunocompromised or in posttraumatic states. Dietary supplements with omega-3 PUFAs are associated with incorporation of eicosapentaenoic acid into leukocytes and with concurrent decreases in the incorporation of arachidonic acid. When these cells are challenged, there is a significantly lower production of LTB_4, which exacerbates undesirable immune responses such as those seen in trauma and autoimmune diseases. Formulas for nutritional support should include omega-3 PUFAs, although the exact amount of omega-3 PUFAs and the precise ratio of omega-6 PUFAs to omega-3 PUFAs remain to be determined.

The fat emulsions currently available for I.V. use in the United States are made with long-chain triglycerides derived either from soybean oil alone or from soybean oil and safflower oil. All of the fatty acids in LCTs are in the form of PUFAs, which include the essential fatty acids (i.e., linoleic and linolenic acids). As noted (see above), an excess of omega-6 PUFAs can have an immunosuppressive effect. Intravenously administered LCT emulsions are cleared in part through the reticuloendothelial system (RES).[128] When such emulsions are used as a calorie source, they may impair the ability of the RES to clear bacteria if given too rapidly or in excessively large amounts.

Moreover, the PUFAs in LCT emulsions require carnitine-mediated transport to cross the mitochondrial membrane for oxidation. Carnitine is a quaternary amine derived from two essential amino acids, lysine and methionine. During sepsis, urinary excretion of free carnitine rises significantly, and the plasma acylcarnitine level falls.[129] One way of circumventing these problems is to use emulsions that contain MCTs.

MCT-containing emulsions have long been used in enteral nutrition for their absorptive advantage over LCT-containing emulsions: whereas LCTs are absorbed via lacteals and the lymphatic system, MCTs are absorbed via the portal system. MCTs are obtained from coconut oil and contain saturated fatty acids (with octanoic acids predominating). Because MCTs are smaller than LCTs, they are more water soluble; they are also poorly bound to albumin and diffuse more easily across body compartments.

Several reports on the use of intravenously administered MCT fat emulsions have been published. One study evaluated the effect of a 75% MCT/25% LCT emulsion on RES function as demonstrated by ^{99m}Tc-sulfur colloid (Tc-SC) clearance. Clearance of Tc-SC was significantly higher after 3 days of MCT/LCT administration than after 3 days of LCT administration.[130] Another study investigated the metabolic effects of MCT-containing emulsions on surgical patients.[131] The main finding of this study was the appearance of β-hydroxybutyrate in association with infusion of the MCT emulsion, which was indicative of a ketogenic effect. A tendency toward improved nitrogen balance was also observed, but it was not statistically significant.

Another feature of fat emulsions that is exploited in surgical patients is the salutary effect of omega-3 fatty acids on the immune response. A diet is now commercially available in the United States that contains fish oil in addition to arginine and RNA. This diet was tested in a 1993 study of postoperative patients who underwent surgery for upper GI malignancies.[132] A total of 85 patients were randomly selected to receive either the experimental diet or a standard formula. The patients who received the experimental diet had better nitrogen balance (−2.2 g/day versus −6.6 g/day) and improved in vitro lymphocyte mitogenesis. Infection and wound complication rates were also lower in the experimental group (11% versus 37%), and hospital stay was shorter (15.8 days versus 20.2 days).

This experimental diet was subsequently tested in a randomized, double-blind study in which 325 patients from eight different hospitals were enrolled.[133] The inclusion criteria were (1) admission to the ICU as a result of trauma, operation, or sepsis and (2) an APACHE II score of 10 or higher or a Therapeutic Intervention Scoring System score of 20 or higher. Patients started tube feedings within 48 hours of admission with either the experimental formula (N = 68) or a standard tube-feeding formula (N = 15). Patients receiving the experimental formula had significantly higher plasma levels of arginine, ornithine, eicosapentaenoic acid, and docosahexaenoic acid, with a concomitant decrease in linoleic acid levels. Hospital stay was significantly shorter in several subgroups (including patients who received more than a certain amount of formula and patients in a septic state) in association with a significant reduction in the incidence of acquired infections.

In summary, specific fatty acids have significant potential for use in nutrition pharmacotherapy. Omega-6 fatty acids are potential immunosuppressants, whereas omega-3 fatty acids are potential immunostimulants. In the United States, the only emulsions commercially available for I.V. use at present are made of LCTs containing omega-6 fatty acids. MCTs offer some metabolic advantages over LCTs and obviate the side effects resulting from an excess of omega-6 fatty acids. Enteral diets containing omega-3 fatty acids appear to benefit stressed surgical patients, particularly those who are immunosuppressed as a result of therapy for cancer.

References

1. Wilmore DW: Metabolic Management of the Critically Ill. Plenum Publishing Corp, New York, 1977
2. Vitamin preparations as dietary supplements and as therapeutic agents. Council on Scientific Affairs. JAMA 257:1929, 1987
3. Marks J: The safety of vitamins: an overview. Int J Vitam Nutr Res 30(suppl):12, 1989
4. Demling R, LaLonde C, Saldinger P, et al: Multiple-organ dysfunction in the surgical patient: pathophysiology, prevention, and treatment. Curr Probl Surg 30:345, 1993
5. Pingleton SK, Hadzima SK: Enteral alimentation and gastrointestinal bleeding in mechanically ventilated patients. Crit Care Med 11:13, 1983
6. Koruda MJ, Guenter P, Rombeau JL: Enteral nutrition in the critically ill. Critical Care Clinics 3:133, 1987
7. Guidelines for the use of parenteral and enteral nutrition in adult and pediatric patients. JPEN J Parenter Enteral Nutr 17(4 suppl):1SA, 1993
8. Fischer JE, Rosen HM, Ebeid AM, et al: The effect of normalization of plasma amino acids on hepatic encephalopathy in man. Surgery 80:77, 1976
9. Abel RM: Parenteral nutrition in the treatment of renal failure. Total Parenteral Nutrition. Fischer JE, Ed. Little, Brown & Co, Inc, Boston, 1976, p 143
10. Steffee WP, Anderson CF: Enteral nutrition and renal disease. Clinical Nutrition, Vol 1: Enteral and Tube Feeding. Rombeau JL, Caldwell MD, Eds. WB Saunders Co, Philadelphia, 1984, p 363
11. Heymsfield SB, Head CA, McManus CB III, et al: Respiratory, cardiovascular, and metabolic effects of enteral hyperalimentation: influence of formula dose and composition. Am J Clin Nutr 40:116, 1984
12. Askanazi J, Weissman C, Rosenbaum SH, et al: Nutrition and the respiratory system. Crit Care Med 10:163, 1982
13. Cobb LM, Cartmill AM, Barry M, et al: A tube for enteral nutrition of patients with aphagopraxia and patients with ventilator assistance. Surg Gynecol Obstet 155:81, 1982
14. Daly JM, Lieberman MD, Goldfine J, et al: Enteral nutrition with supplemental arginine, RNA, and omega-3 fatty acids in patients after operation: immunologic, metabolic, and clinical outcome. Surgery 112:56, 1992
15. Winterbauer RH, Durning RB Jr, Barron E, et al: Aspirated nasogastric feeding solution detected by glucose strips. Ann Intern Med 95:67, 1981
16. Rolandelli RH, Rombeau JL: Liquid defined formula diets. Current Therapy in Gastroenterology and Liver Disease. Bayless TM, Ed. BC Decker Inc, Toronto, 1986, p 206
17. Treolar DM, Stechmiller J: Pulmonary aspiration in tube-fed patients with artificial airways. Heart Lung 13:667, 1984
18. McLean GK: Radiologic techniques of gastrointestinal intubation. Clinical Nutrition, Vol 1: Enteral and Tube Feeding. Rombeau JL, Caldwell MD, Eds. WB Saunders Co, Philadelphia, 1984, p 240
19. Rombeau JL, Barot LR, Low DW, et al: Feeding by tube enterostomy. Clinical Nutrition, Vol 1: Enteral and Tube Feeding. Rombeau JL, Caldwell MD, Eds. WB Saunders Co, Philadelphia, 1984, p 275
20. Moss G: Early enteral feeding after abdominal surgery. Nutrition in Clinical Surgery, 2nd ed. Deitel M, Ed. Williams & Wilkins Co, Baltimore, 1985, p 220
21. Ponsky JL, Gauderer MW, Stellato TA, et al: Percutaneous approaches to enteral alimentation. Am J Surg 149:102, 1985
22. Cataldi-Betcher EL, Seltzer MH, Blocum BA, et al: Complications occurring during enteral nutrition support: a prospective study. JPEN J Parenter Enteral Nutr 7:546, 1983
23. Du Moulin GC, Paterson DJ, Hedley-White J, et al: Aspiration of gastric bacteria in antacid-treated patients: a frequent cause of postoperative colonization of the airway. Lancet 1:242, 1982
24. Forlaw L, Chernoff R: Enteral delivery systems. Clinical Nutrition, Vol 1: Enteral and Tube Feeding. Rombeau JL, Caldwell MD, Eds. WB Saunders Co, Philadelphia, 1984, p 228
25. Pemberton LB, Lyman B, Lander V, et al: Sepsis from triple- vs single-lumen catheters during total parenteral nutrition in surgical or critically ill patients. Arch Surg 121:591, 1986
26. Miller JJ, Venus B, Mathru M: Comparison of the sterility of long-term central venous catheterization using single lumen, triple lumen, and pulmonary artery catheters. Crit Care Med 12:634, 1984
27. Belliveau K: Catheter infection rate using multiple lumen catheters. Read before the National Intravenous Therapy Association, New Orleans, April 1986
28. Moncrief JA: Femoral catheters. Ann Surg 147:166, 1958
29. Black PR, Brooks DC, Bessey PQ, et al: Mechanisms of insulin resistance following injury. Ann Surg 196:420, 1982
30. Maki DG, Weise CE, Sarafin HW: A semiquantitative culture method for identifying intravenous-catheter–related infection. N Engl J Med 296:1305, 1977
31. Pettigrew RA, Lang SDR, Haydock DA, et al: Catheter-related sepsis in patients on intravenous nutrition: a prospective study of quantitative catheter cultures and guidewire changes for suspected sepsis. Br J Surg 72:52, 1985
32. Williams WW: Infection control during parenteral nutrition therapy. JPEN J Parenter Enteral Nutr 9:735, 1985
33. Grundfest S, Steiger E: Home parenteral nutrition. JAMA 244:1701, 1980
34. Broviac JW, Scribner BH: Prolonged parenteral nutrition in the home. Surg Gynecol Obstet 139:24, 1974
35. Levine GM, Deren JJ, Steiger E, et al: Role of oral intake in maintenance of gut mass and disaccharidase activity. Gastroenterology 67:975, 1974
36. Border JR: Trauma and sepsis. Principles and Practice of Trauma Care. Worth MH, Ed. Williams & Wilkins Co, Baltimore, 1982, p 330
37. Udall JN, Walker WA: Mucosal defense mechanisms. Immunopathology of the Small Intestine. Marsh MN, Ed. John Wiley & Sons, Inc, New York, 1986, p 3
38. Deitch EA, Maejima K, Berg R: Effect of oral antibiotics and bacterial overgrowth on the translocation of the GI tract microflora in burned rats. J Trauma 25:385, 1985
39. Wells CL, Rotstein OD, Pruett TL, et al: Intestinal bacteria translocate into experimental intraabdominal abscesses. Arch Surg 121:102, 1986
40. Schatten WE, Desprez JD, Holden WD: A bacteriologic study of portal-vein blood in man. Arch Surg 71:404, 1955

41. Bodey GP: Antibiotic prophylaxis in cancer patients: regimens of oral, nonabsorbable antibiotics for prevention of infection during induction of remission. Rev Infect Dis 3(suppl):S259, 1981
42. Jarrett F, Balish L, Moylan JA, et al: Clinical experience with prophylactic antibiotic bowel suppression in burn patients. Surgery 83:523, 1978
43. Keller GA, West MA, Cerra FB, et al: Multiple systems organ failure: modulation of hepatocyte protein synthesis by endotoxin activated Kupffer cells. Ann Surg 201:87, 1985
44. Hammer-Hodges D, Woodruff P, Cuevas P, et al: Role of the intraintestinal gram negative bacterial flora in response to major injury. Surg Gynecol Obstet 138:599, 1974
45. Deitch EA, Berg R, Specian R: Endotoxin promotes the translocation of bacteria from the gut. Arch Surg 122:185, 1987
46. Deitch EA, Winterton J, Li M, et al: The gut as a portal of entry for bacteremia: role of protein malnutrition. Ann Surg 205:681, 1987
47. Wellmann W, Fink PC, Schmidt FW: Whole-gut irrigation as antiendotoxinaemic therapy in inflammatory bowel disease. Hepatogastroenterology 31:91, 1984
48. Bounous G: Acute necrosis of the intestinal mucosa. Gastroenterology 82:1457, 1982
49. Rhodes RS, Depalma RG, Robinson AV: Intestinal barrier function in hemorrhagic shock. J Surg Res 14:305, 1973
50. Bounous G, Cronin RFP, Gurd FN: Dietary prevention of experimental shock lesions. Arch Surg 94:46, 1967
51. Saito H, Trocki O, Alexander JW, et al: The effect of route of nutrient administration on the nutritional state, catabolic hormone secretion, and gut mucosal integrity after burn injury. JPEN J Parenter Enteral Nutr 11:1, 1987
52. Hwang TL, O'Dwyer ST, Smith RJ, et al: Preservation of small-bowel mucosa using glutamine enriched parenteral nutrition. Forum on Fundamental Surgical Problems 37:56, 1986
53. van der Hulst RRWJ, van Kreel BK, von Meyenfeldt MF, et al: Glutamine and the preservation of gut integrity. Lancet 341:1363, 1993
54. Jacobs DO, Evans A, O'Dwyer ST, et al: Disparate effects of 5-fluorouracil on ileum and colon of enterally fed rats with protection by dietary glutamine. Forum on Fundamental Surgical Problems 38:45, 1987
55. Fox AD, Kripke SA, Berman JM, et al: Reduction of the severity of enterocolitis by glutamine-supplemented enteral diets. Forum on Fundamental Surgical Problems 38:43, 1987
56. Hammarqvist F, Wernerman J, Ali R, et al: Addition of glutamine to total parenteral nutrition after elective abdominal surgery spares free glutamine in muscle, counteracts the fall in muscle protein synthesis, and improves nitrogen balance. Ann Surg 209:455, 1989
57. Stehle P, Zander J, Mertes N, et al: Effect of parenteral glutamine peptide supplements on muscle glutamine loss and nitrogen balance after major surgery. Lancet 1:231, 1989
58. Scheltinga MR, Young LS, Benfell K, et al: Glutamine-enriched intravenous feedings attenuate extracellular fluid expansion after a standard stress. Ann Surg 214:385, 1991
59. Ziegler TR, Young LS, Benfell K, et al: Clinical and metabolic efficacy of glutamine-supplemented parenteral nutrition after bone marrow transplantation: a randomized, double-blind, controlled study. Ann Intern Med 116:821, 1992
60. Schloerb PR, Amare M: Total parenteral nutrition with glutamine in bone marrow transplantation and other clinical applications (a randomized, double-blind study). JPEN J Parenter Enteral Nutr 17:407, 1993
61. Hardy G, Bevan SJ, McElroy B, et al: Stability of glutamine in parenteral feeding solutions (letter). Lancet 342:186, 1993
62. Parry-Billings M, Evans J, Calder PC, et al: Does glutamine contribute to immunosuppression after major burns? Lancet 336:523, 1990
63. Jensen GL, Miller RH, Talabiska D, et al: A double-blind prospective randomized study of glutamine-enriched versus standard peptide-based feeding in critically ill. JPEN J Parenter Enteral Nutr 17(suppl):33S, 1993
64. Hong RW, Rounds JD, Helton WS, et al: Glutamine preserves liver glutathione after lethal hepatic injury. Ann Surg 215:114, 1992
65. Welbourne TC, King AB, Horton K: Enteral glutamine supports hepatic glutathione efflux during inflammation. J Nutr Biochem 4:236, 1993
66. Koruda MJ, Rolandelli RH, Settle RG, et al: The effect of a pectin-supplemented elemental diet on intestinal adaptation to massive small-bowel resection. JPEN J Parenter Enteral Nutr 10:343, 1986
67. Koruda MJ, Rolandelli RH, Settle RG, et al: Small bowel disaccharidase activity in the rat as affected by intestinal resection and pectin feeding. Am J Clin Nutr 47:448, 1988
68. Rolandelli RH, Koruda MJ, Settle RG, et al: The effect of enteral feedings supplemented with pectin on the healing of colonic anastomosis in the rat. Surgery 99:703, 1986
69. Rolandelli RH, Saul SH, Settle RG, et al: Comparison of parenteral nutrition and enteral feeding with pectin in experimental colitis in the rat. Am J Clin Nutr 47:715, 1988
70. Jacobs DO, Evans DA, Smith RJ, et al: Combined effects of glutamine and epidermal growth factor on the rat intestine. Surgery 104:358, 1988
71. Klein S, Kinney J, Jeejeebhoy K, et al: Nutrition support in clinical practice: review of published data and recommendations for further research directions. JPEN J Parenter Enteral Nutr 21:133, 1997
72. von Meyenfeldt MF, Meijrink WJHJ, Rouflart MMJ, et al: Perioperative nutritional support: a randomized clinical trial. Clin Nutr 11:180, 1992
73. Shukla HS, Rao RR, Banu N, et al: Enteral hyperalimentation in malnourished surgical patients. Ind J Med Res 80:339, 1984
74. Sagar S, Harland P, Shields R: Early postoperative feeding with elemental diet. Br Med J 1:293, 1979
75. Ryan JA, Page CP, Babcock L: Early postoperative jejunal feeding of elemental diet in gastrointestinal surgery. Am Surg 47:393, 1981
76. Smith RC, Hartemink RJ, Holinshead JW, et al: Fine bore jejunostomy feeding following major abdominal trauma: a controlled randomized clinical trial. Br J Surg 72:458, 1985
77. Tovinelli G, Marsili I, Varrassi G: Nutrition support after total laryngectomy. JPEN J Parenter Enteral Nutr 17:445, 1993
78. Daly JM, Lieberman MD, Goldfine J, et al: Enteral nutrition with supplemental arginine, RNA and omega-3 fatty acids in patients after operation: immunologic, metabolic and clinical outcome. Surgery 112:56, 1992
79. Bastow MD, Rawlings J, Allison S: Benefits of supplementary tube feeding after fractured neck of femur: a randomized controlled trial. Br Med J 187:1589, 1983
80. Delmi M, Rapin CH, Bengoa JM, et al: Dietary supplementation in elderly patients with fractured neck of the femur. Lancet 335:1013, 1990
81. Brennan MF, Pisters PW, Posner M, et al: A prospective randomized trial of total parenteral nutrition after major pancreatic resection for malignancy. Am Surg 220:436, 1994
82. van Berge Henegowen M, Akkermans L, van Gulik T, et al: Prospective, randomized trial on the effect of cyclic versus continuous enteral nutrition on postoperative gastric function after pylorus-preserving pancreatoduodenectomy. Ann Surg 226:677, 1997
83. Fan ST, Lo CM, Lai E, et al: Perioperative nutritional support in patients undergoing hepatectomy for hepatocellular carcinoma. N Engl J Med 331:1547, 1994
84. Bufo A, Feldman S, Daniels G, et al: Early postoperative feeding. Dis Col Rect 37:1260, 1994
85. Choudhry U, Barde C, Markert R, et al: Percutaneous endoscopic gastrostomy: a randomized prospective comparison of early and delayed feeding. Gastrointest Endosc 44:164, 1996
86. Watters JM, Kirkpatrick SM, Norris SB, et al: Immediate postoperative enteral feeding results in impaired respiratory mechanics and decreased mobility. Ann Surg 226:369, 1997
87. Heslin MJ, Latkany L, Leung D, et al: A prospective, randomized trial of early enteral feeding after resection of upper gastrointestinal malignancy. Ann Surg 226:567, 1997
88. Singh G, Ram RP, Khanna SK: Early postoperative enteral feeding in patients with non-traumatic intestinal perforation and peritonitis. J Am Coll Surg 187:142, 1998
89. Smith-Choban P, Max MH: Feeding jejunotomy: a small bowel stress test? Am J Surg 155:112, 1988
90. Myers JG, Page CP, Stewart RM, et al: Complications of needle catheter jejunostomy in 2,022 consecutive applications. Am J Surg 170:547, 1995
91. Schunn CD, Daly JM: Small bowel necrosis associated with postoperative jejunal tube feeding. J Am Coll Surg 180:410, 1995
92. Friedenberg F, Jensen, G, Gujral N, et al: Serum albumin is predictive of 30-day survival after percutaneous endoscopic gastrostomy. JPEN J Parenter Enteral Nutr 21:72, 1997
93. Brennan MF, Cerra F, Daly JM, et al: Report of a research workshop: branched-chain amino acids in stress and injury. JPEN J Parenter Enteral Nutr 10:446, 1986
94. Garcia-de-Lorenzo A, Ortiz-Leyba C, Planas M, et al: Parenteral administration of different amounts of branch-chain amino acids in septic patients: clinical and metabolic aspects. Crit Care Med 25:418, 1997
95. Souba WW, Herskowitz K, Augstgen TR, et al: Glutamine nutrition: theoretical considerations and therapeutic impact. JPEN J Parenter Enteral Nutr 14: 237S, 1990
96. Furst P, Albers S, Stehle P: Stress-induced intracellular glutamine depletion. Contr Infusion Ther Clin Nutr 17:117, 1987
97. Lacey JM, Wilmore DW: Is glutamine a conditionally essential amino acid? Nutr Rev 48:297, 1990
98. Ziegler TR, Young LS, Benfell K, et al: Clinical and metabolic efficacy of glutamine-supplemented parenteral nutrition after bone marrow transplantation. Ann Intern Med 116:821, l992
99. Schloerb PR, Amare M: Total parenteral nutrition with glutamine in bone marrow transplantation and other clinical applications. JPEN J Parenter Enteral Nutr 17:407, 1993
100. Byrne TA, Morrissey T, Naltakom T, et al: Growth hormone, glutamine and a modified diet enhance nutrient absorption in patients with severe short bowel syndrome. JPEN J Parenter Enteral Nutr 19:296, 1995
101. Byrne TA, Persinger RC, Young LS, et al: A new treatment for patients with short bowel syndrome. Ann Surg 222:243, 1995
102. Wilmore DW, Byrne TA, Persinger RL: Short bowel syndrome: new therapeutic approaches. Curr Probl Surg 34:398, 1997
103. Scolapio JS, Camilleri M, Fleming R, et al:

Effect of growth hormone, glutamine, and diet on adaptation in short bowel syndrome: a randomized, controlled study. Gastroenterology 113:1074, 1997
104. Thompson JS: Can the intestine adapt to a changing environment? Gastroenterology 113:1402, 1997
105. Morlion BJ, Stehle P, Wachtler P, et al: Total parenteral nutrition with glutamine dipeptide after major abdominal surgery: a randomized, double blind, controlled study. Ann Surg 227:302, 1998
106. Barbul A: Arginine and immune function. Nutrition 6:53, 1990
107. Rakoff JS, Siler TM, Sinha YN, et al: Prolactin and growth hormone release in response to sequential stimulation by arginine and synthetic TRF. J Clin Endocrinol Metab 37:641, 1973
108. Palmer JP, Walter RM, Ensinck JW: Arginine-stimulated acute phase of insulin and glucagon secretion: I. In normal man. Diabetes 24:735, 1975
109. Utsumi M, Makimura H, Ishihara K, et al: Determination of immunoreactive somatostatin in rat plasma and responses to arginine, glucose and glucagon infusion. Diabetologia 17:319, 1979
110. Barbul A, Rettura G, Levenson SM, et al: Wound healing and thymotropic effects of arginine: a pituitary mechanism of action. Am J Clin Nutr 37:786, 1983
111. Barbul A, Wasserkrug HL, Seifter E, et al: Immunostimulatory effects of arginine in normal and injured rats. J Surg Res 29:228, 1980
112. Barbul A, Sisto DA, Wasserkrug HL, et al: Arginine stimulates lymphocyte immune response in healthy human beings. Surgery 90:244, 1981
113. Daly JM, Reynolds J, Thom A, et al: Immune and metabolic effects of arginine in the surgical patient. Ann Surg 208:512, 1988
114. Gonce SJ, Peck MD, Alexander JW, et al: Arginine supplementation and its effect on established peritonitis in guinea pigs. JPEN J Parenter Enteral Nutr 14:237, 1990
115. Daly JM, Reynolds J, Sigal RK, et al: Effect of dietary protein and amino acids on immune function. Crit Care Med 18(suppl):S86, 1990
116. Cho-Chung YS, Clair T, Bodwin JS, et al: Arrest of mammary tumor growth in vivo by L-arginine: stimulation of NAD-dependent activation of adenylate cyclase. Biochem Biophys Res Commun 95:1306, 1980
117. Lieberman MD, Nishioka K, Redmond HP, et al: Enhancement of interleukin-2 immunotherapy with L-arginine. Ann Surg 215:157, 1992
118. Van Buren CT, Kim E, Kulkarni AD, et al: Nucleotide-free diet and suppression of immune response. Transplant Proc 19:57, 1987
119. Fanslow WC, Kulkarni AD, Van Buren CT, et al: Effect of nucleotide restriction and supplementation on resistance to experimental murine candidiasis. JPEN J Parenter Enteral Nutr 12:49, 1988
120. Kulkarni AD, Fanslow WC, Drath DB, et al: Influence of dietary nucleotide restriction on bacterial sepsis and phagocytic cell function in mice. Arch Surg 121:169, 1986
121. Chapkin RS, Somers SD, Erickson KL: Inability of murine peritoneal macrophages to convert linoleic acid into arachidonic acid. J Immunol 140:2350, 1988
122. Johnston DV, Marshall LA: Dietary fat, prostaglandins and the immune response. Prog Food Nutr Sci 8:3, 1984
123. Meade CJ, Mertin J: Fatty acids and immunity. Adv Lip Res 16:127, 1978
124. Kinsella JE, Lokesh B: Dietary lipids, eicosanoids, and the immune system. Crit Care Med 18(suppl):S94, 1990
125. Mascioli E, Leader L, Flores E, et al: Enhanced survival to endotoxin in guinea pigs fed IV fish oil emulsions. Lipids 23:623, 1988
126. Cook JA, Wise WC, Knapp DR, et al: Essential fatty acid deficient rats: a new model for evaluating arachidonate metabolism in shock. Adv Shock Res 6:93, 1981
127. Alexander JW, Saito H, Trocki O, et al: The importance of lipid type in the diet after burn injury. Ann Surg 204:1, 1986
128. Seidner DL, Mascioli EA, Istfan NW, et al: Effects of long-chain triglyceride emulsions on reticuloendothelial system function in humans. JPEN J Parenter Enteral Nutr 13:614, 1989
129. Nanni C, Pittiruti M, Giovannini I, et al: Plasma carnitine levels and urinary carnitine excretion during sepsis. JPEN J Parenter Enteral Nutr 9:483, 1985
130. Jonsen GL, Mascioli EA, Seidner DL, et al: Parenteral infusion of long- and medium-chain triglycerides and reticuloendothelial system function in man. JPEN J Parenter Enteral Nutr 14:467, 1990
131. Jiang Z, Zhang S, Wang X, et al: A comparison of medium-chain and long-chain triglycerides in surgical patients. Ann Surg 217:175, 1993
132. Daly JM, Lieberman MD, Goldfine J, et al: Enteral nutrition with supplemental arginine, RNA, and omega-3 fatty acids in patients after operation: immunologic, metabolic, and clinical outcome. Surgery 112:56, 1992
133. Bower RH, Cerra FB, Bershadsky B, et al: Early enteral administration of a formula (impact) supplemented with arginine, nucleotides, and fish oil in intensive care unit patients: results of a multicenter, prospective, randomized, clinical trial. Crit Care Med 24:173, 1995
134. Food and Nutrition Board: Recommended Dietary Allowances, 9th ed. National Academy of Sciences, Washington DC, 1980
135. Multivitamin preparations for parenteral use: a statement by the Nutrition Advisory Group, American Medical Association Department of Foods and Nutrition, 1975. JPEN J Parenter Enteral Nutr 3:258, 1979
136. Guidelines for essential trace element preparations for parenteral use: a statement by an expert panel, AMA Department of Foods and Nutrition. JAMA 241: 2951, 1979

Acknowledgments

Figure 2   Talar Agasyan.
Figure 4   Carol Donner.

… 98 FEVER, HYPERPYREXIA, AND HYPOTHERMIA

Douglas W. Wilmore, M.D.

Emergency Management of Life-Threatening Temperature Derangements

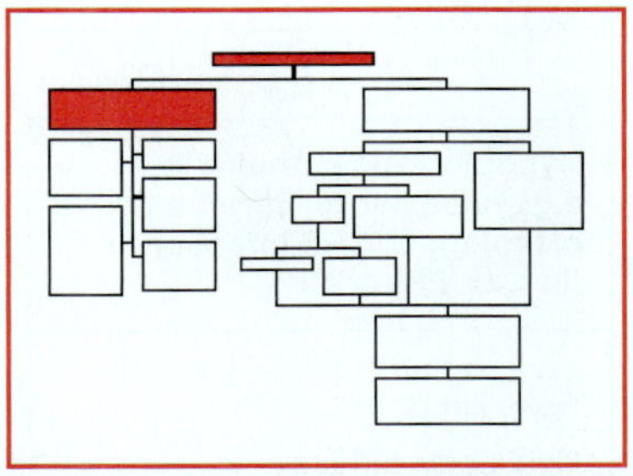

Management of Life-Threatening Fever and Hyperpyrexia

INITIAL CARE

When the physician learns (usually from a member of the nursing staff or an associate) of a dramatic elevation in a patient's temperature, his or her initial response should be to check that the temperature was measured in the rectum, not in the mouth or the axilla. The only situation in which a rectal measurement is unnecessary is when a patient's body temperature must be obtained in the operating room. In this situation, monitoring with an esophageal, nasopharyngeal, or tympanic probe yields acceptable results.

The first step in addressing the problem of life-threatening elevations in body temperature (≥ 40° C [104° F]) [see Figure 1] always is to evaluate the adequacy of the cardiorespiratory system and circulation. If the patient is already intubated and receiving ventilatory support, inspired oxygen should be delivered in generous concentrations; if not, the indications for intubation should be reviewed [see 92 Use of the Mechanical Ventilator]. If ventilatory support is not required, oxygen should be administered by face mask. Finally, if the patient is dehydrated, fluids should be administered intravenously. These measures ensure that sufficient oxygen is delivered to essential organs that have increased metabolic requirements because of the temperature elevation; they also help maintain skin perfusion, which is necessary to offload body heat.

The next step is to institute measures to reduce the patient's temperature. Clothing, bedcovers, and, if possible, operative drapes should be removed to facilitate heat loss from the body surface to the environment. If life-threatening hyperpyrexia is present in an individual who has been exercising and has sustained severe heatstroke, rapid cooling can be achieved by placing the person in an ice bath; this measure, together with rehydration, will lower body temperature dramatically. In extreme situations, uncontrolled malignant hyperthermia in a patient who is undergoing operation may be managed through partial cardiopulmonary bypass with a heat exchanger, an approach that can rapidly offload heat and reduce body temperature [see Treatment of Fever and Hyperpyrexia, Malignant Hyperthermia, below].

Finally, the cause of the temperature elevation should be determined, if it is not already apparent. Because elevation in body temperature is a response to a disease process, returning the temperature to normal can reduce morbidity and potential mortality considerably. However, the underlying disease process that is causing the temperature elevation also requires treatment because in

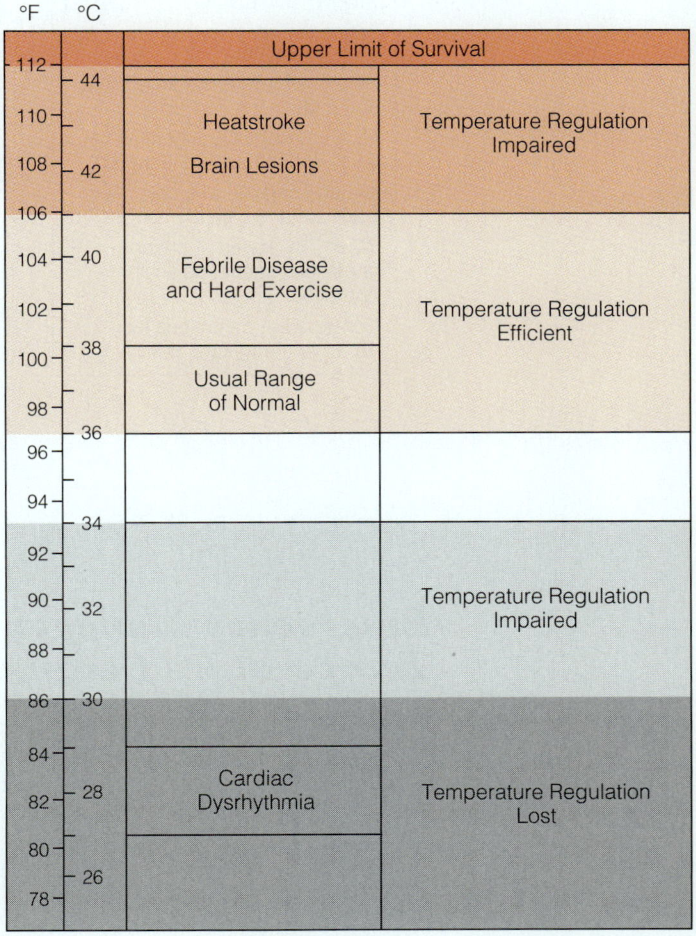

Figure 1 Extreme variations in body temperature are associated with morbidity and mortality.[14]

```
┌─────────────────────────────────────────────────────────────────┐
│ Patient's core T° is outside normal range of 36° to 38° C       │
│ (96.8° to 100.4° F)                                             │
└─────────────────────────────────────────────────────────────────┘
```

Rectal T° ≥ 40° C (104° F); fever or hyperpyrexia is life-threatening

Institute appropriate cardiorespiratory support.
Reduce body T° (e.g., remove clothes, bathe skin with cool H_2O).
Establish diagnosis (may depend to an extent on whether patient is seen in the ER, ICU, or OR), and institute specific therapy.

Infection/inflammation (in ICU, ER, or OR)

Give aspirin or NSAIDs to lower set point.
Cool body surface.
Provide hydration and metabolic support.
Diagnose and treat infection.

Malignant hyperthermia (in OR)

Stop operation.
Stop inhalation anesthesia; give 100% O_2.
Give I.V. $NaHCO_3$ (1–2 mEq/kg) and I.V. dantrolene (2.5 mg/kg).
Reduce body T° with cold solutions and heat exchanger.
When T° is lowered, change anesthetic agent and finish operation.
Continue I.V. dantrolene for 48–72 hr (1 mg/kg q. 6 hr).

Heatstroke (in ER)

Cool the patient.
Rehydrate.

Hypothalamic pathology: e.g., head injury, intracranial bleeding, or CNS infection (in ICU, ER, or OR)

Give aspirin or NSAIDs to lower set point.
Cool body surface.
Treat underlying disease.

Endocrine excess: hyperthyroidism or pheochromocytoma (in OR or ICU)

Cool body surface.
Use appropriate drugs to block end-organ endocrine response.

Emergency Management of Life-Threatening Temperature Derangements

Life-threatening hypothermia: rectal T° ≤ 35° C (95° F) as measured with low-reading thermometer, *not* standard clinical-grade thermometer

Ensure adequate oxygenation and circulation. Establish I.V. access. (Remember: monitoring may be difficult; manipulation may initiate arrhythmias.)

Consider whether hypothermia is primary (caused by exposure to cold or immersion in water) or secondary to concomitant conditions.

Circulatory collapse has not occurred or has been resolved

Patient is breathing spontaneously.

Core T° is ≥ 28° C (82.4° F), and cardiovascular function is stable

Core T° is < 28° C (82.4° F) (patients are usually unconscious at this T°); cardiovascular function is unstable or at risk

Patient is extremely susceptible to arrhythmias. Monitor carefully and prepare for ventricular fibrillation or asystole.

Patient is conscious

Patient is unconscious

Unconsciousness in patients with core T° > 28° C (82.4° F) is rare and suggests underlying disease process.

Circulatory collapse:
- Cold, asystolic, apparently dead patient
- Ventricular fibrillation
- Marked hypotension

Resuscitate; intubate and initiate external cardiac massage.

Rewarm using cardiopulmonary bypass with heat exchanger or peritoneal dialysis.

Use pharmacologic therapy or countershock *only with extreme caution*.

DO NOT TERMINATE resuscitative efforts until T° > 30° C (86° F) but vital signs remain absent.

Distinguish between primary hypothermia and secondary hypothermia (if not already done), and manage accordingly

In secondary hypothermia, initiate evaluation and treatment of life-threatening conditions that may alter consciousness: e.g.,
- Head injury — reduction of intracranial pressure
- Drug overdose — dialysis, naloxone
- Alcohol abuse — dialysis, thiamine
- Hypoglycemia — glucose administration

Rewarm the patient gently

Wrap patient in warm blankets.

Maintain ambient T° at 32° C (89.6° F).

Administer warm fluid (40° C; 104° F) I.V. in conjunction with hot, humidified, O_2-enriched air by face mask.

Consider microwave diathermy to increase body heat.

Table 1 Pathophysiology and Treatment of Common Causes of Elevated Body Temperature

Diagnosis	Pathophysiology	Treatment
Infection and inflammation	Activated macrophages liberate pyrogens (IL-1, TNF, and interferon) to reset the thermoregulatory center in the hypothalamus. This set-point alteration mediates increased heat production and decreased heat loss.	Give drugs that lower the set point: aspirin, acetaminophen, ibuprofen. Cool the body surface and provide general supportive measures. Provide hydration and metabolic support. Diagnose and treat infection or cause of inflammation.
Malignant hyperthermia	Certain inhalation agents or muscle relaxants stimulate abnormal metabolic reactions, particularly in skeletal muscle, that produce increased heat, acidosis, hyperkalemia, skeletal muscle rigidity, alterations in coagulation, and circulatory collapse.	Interrupt the operation. Stop inhalation anesthetics; give 100% O_2. Give I.V. $NaHCO_3$ (1–2 mEq/kg) and I.V. dantrolene (2.5 mg/kg). Reduce body temperature with cold solutions and heat exchanger. When temperature is lowered, change anesthetic agents and complete the operation. Continue dantrolene for 48 to 72 hr (1 mg/kg q. 6 hr).
Heatstroke	Heatstroke usually occurs in healthy individuals exercising on hot days (e.g., runners, football players). Subjects become dehydrated and lose less heat while continuing to produce heat through exercise.	Cool the patient. Rehydrate.
Hypothalamic pathology (head injury, intracranial bleeding, CNS tumors, encephalitis)	Intracerebral pyrogens cause resetting of thermoregulatory set point, or the hypothalamus is directly altered by the disease process.	Give drugs to lower the set point. Cool the body surface and provide general supportive measures. Treat the underlying disease process.
Endocrine excess (pheochromocytoma, hyperthyroidism)	Excess of hormones results in increased heat production.	Cool the body surface and provide general supportive measures. Block the effects of hormones: for pheochromocytoma, use alpha- and beta-adrenergic blockade; for hyperthyroidism, use beta-adrenergic blockade. Consider glucocorticoid administration.

most instances the disease, not the fever, causes mortality. It is essential to diagnose the underlying disease process accurately because each of the many physiologic processes that may be involved requires specific therapy [see Table 1]. The most common cause of fever is infection or inflammation (accounting for the majority of marked temperature elevations in hospitalized adults).[1] Other causes of extreme pyrexia include heatstroke, malignant hyperthermia, hypothalamic pathology, and endocrine excess.

Treatment of Fever and Hyperpyrexia

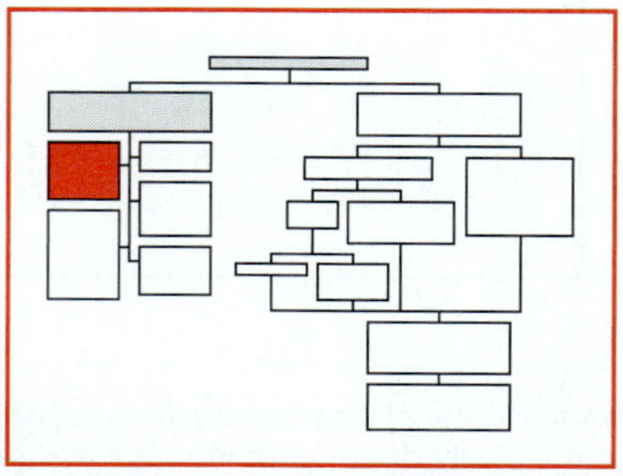

INFECTION AND INFLAMMATION

The inflammatory response activates cytokines that are released locally within the brain or into the bloodstream and act on the hypothalamus. These molecules are pyrogens: they cause an upward resetting of the thermoregulatory apparatus. This shift triggers two physiologic mechanisms for increasing body temperature: vasoconstriction, which limits heat loss from the body, and increased heat production, which is manifested by shivering. These two processes in combination increase body temperature until it reaches the level that is required by the new set point in the hypothalamus [see Figure 2].

The treatment of set-point elevation should begin with administration of a drug that blocks the actions of the pyrogens in the hypothalamus and allows body temperature to return to normal. Aspirin, acetaminophen, and ibuprofen have all been frequently used to reduce fever; they act by blocking the formation of prostaglandins (i.e., PGE_2) in the hypothalamus. Other drugs, including morphine, general anesthetics, chlorpromazine, and certain tranquilizers, have a nonspecific depressive effect on the central nervous system and therefore are capable of decreasing body temperature when used in the ICU or the operating room.

Surface cooling should be started only after administration of the antipyretic because unless the central set point is first pharmacologically reduced, cooling the surface only stimulates additional vasoconstriction and heat production in the form of shivering. Shivering, in turn, increases oxygen consumption dramatically and places additional demands on an already stimulated and possibly overstressed

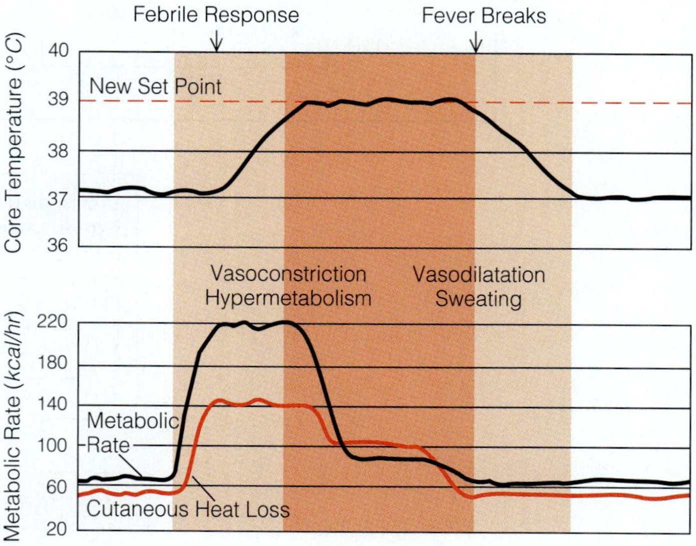

Figure 2 A pyrogenic stimulus to the hypothalamus results in an elevated set point for body temperature. Changes in body temperature reflect the shifting relation between metabolic rate and cutaneous heat loss.[15]

cardiovascular system. Once the antipyretics have been administered and have begun to act, a number of common techniques can be implemented, such as removing bed clothing, lowering the room temperature, sponging the patient with tepid water, increasing airflow over the patient, and applying refrigeration blankets. A 1997 study, however, found that the use of hypothermia blankets was no more effective in reducing core temperature than other cooling methods and was associated with more temperature fluctuations and more episodes of rebound hypothermia.[2] These methods of surface cooling should be used only as long as they do not induce shivering.

Other general measures should also be considered, such as correction of dehydration and electrolyte imbalance and provision of adequate quantities of glucose, a substrate that the body may consume at increased rates when hyperpyrexia is present. A careful physical examination should be performed, and tests should be ordered to diagnose the source of the infection. Antimicrobial therapy should be initiated if indicated, and definitive surgical therapy, such as drainage, extirpation, or debridement, should be considered.

MALIGNANT HYPERTHERMIA

Early diagnosis of malignant hyperthermia is difficult but nevertheless essential for effective therapy [see 41 Perioperative Effects of Anesthesia]. The usual signs are an unexplained tachycardia and an increase in core temperature (i.e., rectal or esophageal temperature), which ordinarily falls in anesthetized patients. Cardiac arrhythmias related to acute acidosis or hyperkalemia, excessive bleeding, a rise in end-tidal carbon dioxide concentration, and marked hyperpyrexia are common developments as the syndrome progresses.[3,4]

If this symptom complex is recognized early in the course of an operation—or if its presence is even suspected—administration of the inhalation agent should be stopped, and 100% oxygen should be given instead. The operation should be halted. To promote heat loss, as many drapes as possible should be removed from the patient without compromising sterility. Sodium bicarbonate, 1 to 2 mEq/kg I.V., should be given to buffer the metabolic acidosis, along with dantrolene sodium, 2.5 mg/kg I.V. Administration of dantrolene should be repeated every 5 to 10 minutes if necessary. Serum electrolytes should be measured. Glucose and insulin therapy may also be required to correct the marked hyperkalemia that may follow. If necessary, body heat can be offloaded by means of partial cardiopulmonary bypass using a heat exchanger.

HEATSTROKE

Acute hyperpyrexia, or heatstroke, often develops in persons who are working or exercising strenuously in a hot, humid environment. Typical victims are marathon runners, members of military units taken on a forced march, and football players practicing and playing in late summer. However, heatstroke may occur without being precipitated by strenuous effort. For instance, elderly persons with circulatory impairment or other chronic diseases often sustain marked increases in body temperature when exposed to high environmental temperatures, such as during a heat wave.[5]

Whatever the cause of the heatstroke, the initial steps in treatment must be to draw heat from the body and to support circulation. The heat overload syndromes, of which heatstroke is the most severe, represent a spectrum of physiologic disturbances that range from mild effects, such as heat cramps, to more severe symptoms, such as headache, vomiting, tachycardia, and hypotension associated with moderate dehydration.[6] The milder manifestations of heat overload generally do not qualify as emergencies; however, heatstroke—diagnosed on the basis of a core temperature greater than 40° C (104° F) coupled with hot, dry skin—can be life-threatening, and thus emergency measures must be taken. Rapid cooling can be achieved by placing the patient in an ice bath, which provides accelerated removal of heat through inductive cooling. The bath also improves venous return and thus enhances cardiac output by initiating venoconstriction in the skin and displacing blood back to the heart to increase ventricular end-diastolic volumes; in addition, it constricts the arterioles and increases the blood pressure. The core temperature of the patient should be reduced at a rate of 0.1 to 0.2° C/min so that it will be below 38° C (100.4° F) within 30 minutes. The patient can then be removed from the ice bath, but core temperature should be monitored frequently to ensure that rebound hyperthermia does not occur.

When treating a previously healthy, exercising person with heatstroke, it is advisable to remove the patient's clothing and to place the patient in a cool room. Further cooling can be achieved by using a fan to circulate air over the body or, if the elevation in body temperature is particularly severe, by packing the patient in ice or even placing him or her in an ice bath. All these techniques accelerate heat removal and minimize damage to vital tissues, particularly those of the central nervous system. Cautious administration of a balanced salt solution replenishes fluid and electrolyte deficits, supports circulation, and enhances blood flow to the skin, thereby further facilitating body heat loss. It is rare that more than 1.5 L of intravenous fluid is required during the first 4 hours.

When treating elderly, nonexercising persons, similar measures—that is, heat unloading and fluid replacement—should be taken; however, because of the relative impairment of physiologic function in the elderly, a more gentle approach to body cooling and fluid resuscitation should be followed.

In all heatstroke patients, inotropic support should be initiated if hypotension persists after volume loading or if heart failure occurs [see 90 Support of the Failing Heart]. Other complications of heatstroke include damage to the CNS, rhabdomyolysis, acute renal failure, disseminated intravascular coagulation, and hepatic and myocardial necrosis. Mannitol administration may be advisable to promote urine output and to prevent acute tubular necrosis in the presence of myoglobinuria. An initial loading dose of 25 g is given, and 12.5 g of mannitol is added to each liter of intravenous fluid. Systemic heparinization is effective for disseminated intravascular coagulation [see 5 Bleeding and Transfusion]. Ventilatory support should be provided if indicated. Appropriate laboratory studies should be performed to evaluate any complications that occur.

Mortality from heatstroke ranges from 10% to 80% and is directly related to the duration and intensity of the hyperthermia, to the length of time that elapses before initiation of therapy, and to the effectiveness of the treatment.

HYPOTHALAMIC PATHOLOGY

A variety of central nervous system disorders can cause fever, including meningitis, brain abscesses, blood present in the subarachnoid space as a consequence of trauma or intracranial hemorrhage, postoperative responses to neurosurgical procedures, and disturbances of the hypothalamus or brain stem, such as those associated with transtentorial (uncal) herniation or localized tumors or those that occur after encephalitic disorders. Although the fever is often mild and indolent, occasionally the temperature may reach a life-threatening level. In the case of more generalized infection of the central nervous system or subarachnoid bleeding, signs of meningismus (e.g., headache, neck guarding, and back pain) accompany the fever; in other disorders, nonspecific or localizing neurologic signs and symptoms may be present. In all cases in which hypothalamic pathology is suspected, a spinal tap should be performed. The fluid should be examined for cells, and the concentrations of protein and glucose should be biochemically determined. Bloody fluid confirms the diagnosis of intracranial hemorrhage, whereas the presence of white cells or frank pus confirms the presence of infection; what specific type of infection is present and which antibiotics should therefore be prescribed are determined on the basis of culture results.

In most patients, general measures aimed at reducing fever should be employed. In patients who have undergone neurosurgery and in those with significant head injuries, the fever may be severe enough to warrant paralysis, ventilation, and heat unloading by means of a cooling blanket. Although the inflammatory response following intracranial injury may be the cause of the elevated temperature, it is still essential to inspect the surgical wounds and to search vigilantly for other sources of infection, particularly in the urinary tract and lungs.

ENDOCRINE EXCESS

Thyrotoxic Crisis

Thyrotoxic crisis, or so-called thyroid storm, is the acute accentuation of thyrotoxicosis. It is an infrequently observed but serious complication of Graves' disease. It may occur after subtotal thyroidectomy or may be precipitated by infection, trauma, a surgical emergency, thyroiditis, or parturition.

The clinical picture is dominated by the signs of acute hyperthyroidism. Fever may be severe and persistent, and sweating may be profuse. A marked tachycardia is frequently associated with congestive heart failure and pulmonary edema. Nausea, vomiting, abdominal pain, delirium, and psychosis may be observed as well.

The goals of treatment are to correct the severe thyrotoxicosis and to provide supportive therapy. The patient should be sedated, cooled, and given oxygen by face mask. Adequate hydration should be maintained with glucose-containing fluids to ensure sufficient exogenous substrate.

The excess thyroid hormone should be counteracted with large doses of an antithyroid agent (propylthiouracil, 200 mg orally every 4 to 6 hours), iodine (five drops of a saturated solution of potassium iodide orally every 6 hours or I.V. infusion of 0.5 g of sodium iodide every 12 hours), and glucocorticoids (dexamethasone, 2 mg orally, or hydrocortisone sodium succinate [Solu-Cortef], 100 mg I.V.). If there is no cardiac insufficiency, an adrenergic blocking drug should be given (propranolol, 40 to 80 mg orally every 6 hours, or up to 2 mg I.V., administered in conjunction with ECG monitoring and repeated when the pulse increases). If heart failure is present, digitalis and diuretics should be administered.

Pheochromocytoma

Occasionally, pheochromocytomas are associated with hyperpyrexia. These endocrine tumors secrete catecholamines that produce a variety of physiologic effects, including an increased metabolic rate. Such an increase is frequently manifested by an increased respiratory rate and weight loss. Tachycardia, hypertension, psychosis, and tremulousness are associated symptoms. Pheochromocytomas should be treated with adrenergic blocking agents such as phentolamine, 1 to 5 mg intravenously, and propranolol, 40 to 80 mg orally every 6 hours or 2 mg I.V. General supportive measures should also be instituted.

Management of Accidental Hypothermia

Life-threatening hypothermia (rectal temperature ≤ 35° C [95° F]) is frequently encountered in the emergency room. In temperate areas, it is most common during the winter, but in regions with cold climates, it is seen throughout the year. Certain patients, such as those who are either very young or very old, those who are mentally ill, those who have a disabling physical illness, and those who are unconscious because of drug overdose or alcohol abuse, appear to be predisposed to hypothermia; lack of adequate housing, homelessness, malnutrition, and low levels of fitness are also contributing factors.[7] Even healthy young persons experience hypothermia after immersion in cold water, after injury and prolonged exposure to cold, or after mild to moderate exertion in a cold environment.

INITIAL CARE

The first step in the treatment of hypothermic patients is to ensure adequate oxygenation and tissue perfusion by following the ABCs of resuscitation [see 1 Initial Emergency Management of Noninjured Patients and 2 Trauma Resuscitation]. Conscious patients may require I.V. fluid resuscitation to counteract fluid losses associated with injury, cold diuresis, or internal fluid shifts. As a rule, the preferred fluid is a 5% solution of dextrose in saline, without added potassium. The fluids can be either warmed before infusion or administered through a blood-warming apparatus. Comatose patients with a detectable heartbeat who are breathing spontaneously, no matter how slowly, should be handled with extreme care. Ventricular fibrillation or asystole may be initiated by intubation, chest compression, insertion of a central line or a Swan-Ganz catheter, or extreme movements (e.g., transferring the patient from a bed to a litter); the reason is that a cold, bradycardic heart is extremely sensitive to potentially arrhythmogenic stimuli [see Figure 1]. If circulatory collapse occurs or is present on admission, resuscitation should be instituted (see below).

If the patient is unconscious but has cardiac activity, measures should be initiated to evaluate and treat conditions that may under-

Table 2 Clinical Manifestations, Treatment, and Outcome of Varying Degrees of Hypothermia

Core Temperature	Clinical Findings	Treatment	Outcome
32°–35° C (90°–95° F)	Cold to touch; confused, disoriented; cardiovascular function stable	Active heating with top and bottom warming blankets	Usually uneventful
28°–32° C (82°–90° F)	Bradycardia, atrial fibrillation, but stable cardiovascular function; muscle rigidity; blood pressure difficult to detect; pupils dilated	Rewarm slowly but actively with blankets, I.V. fluids, heated oxygen, etc.	Depends on underlying disease
< 28° C (< 82° F)	Hypotensive; ventricular fibrillation or cardiac instability; appearing clinically dead (apnea and asystole)	Rewarm with cardiopulmonary bypass or peritoneal dialysis	Mortality high (50%)

lie a life-threatening coma [see 9 *Coma, Seizures, Cognitive Impairment, and Brain Death*]. These conditions include hypoglycemia, which is treated by intravenous administration of glucose; narcotics overdose, which is treated by administration of naloxone; and cardiovascular collapse, which is treated by resolution of the problems associated with airway obstruction, hypovolemia, or severe arrhythmias.

The next step in initial care of a hypothermic patient is to determine the patient's actual temperature. Proper measurement of core temperature is vital because both the choice of treatment and the therapeutic outcome are linked with the extent of the hypothermia [see Table 2]. Because most clinical-grade mercury thermometers read only as low as 34° C (93.2° F), it is possible that when the physician is told that the patient has a low rectal temperature or a temperature of 34° C (93.2° F), the patient's actual temperature is considerably lower. Therefore, in these instances, the physician should remeasure the rectal temperature by using either a low-reading thermometer or a thermistor probe attached to a temperature-monitoring device, such as those that are commonly used in the operating room or the intensive care unit.

The final step, to be taken either during or after initial care, is to make an attempt to diagnose the cause of the hypothermia. The fundamental distinction to be made is between primary hypothermia that occurs in an otherwise healthy person and hypothermia that is secondary to an associated disease that alters heat balance or thermoregulation [see Table 3]. The distinction between primary and secondary hypothermia is an essential one because hypothermia associated with another disease process may necessitate additional therapy or some modification of the approach that is taken for treatment of primary hypothermia, or both.

PATIENTS WITH HYPOTHERMIC CARDIAC ARREST

The most seriously ill hypothermic patients are those who present with circulatory collapse and rectal temperature of less than 28° C (82.4° F). The chances of resuscitating such patients by conventional methods are slight or nonexistent. However, even though young persons suffering from sudden, severe hypothermia because of cold exposure may appear dead, resuscitation should be attempted. Clinical experience demonstrates that such patients often survive with little or no cerebral impairment.[8] (As a rule, a patient should not be pronounced dead until the rectal temperature is greater than 30° C [86° F] but all signs of life remain absent.) The patient should be intubated, intravenous lines should be inserted, and resuscitation should be initiated.

Unfortunately, the cold heart is relatively insensitive to atropine, electrical pacing, countershock, and most antiarrhythmic drugs and pressor agents. Moreover, the hypothermic liver cannot detoxify or conjugate drugs in a normal manner. Pharmacologic therapy must therefore be used with extreme caution in these patients. If ventricular fibrillation is present, it may be appropriate to try countershock once or twice; however, if this measure is unsuccessful, cardiopulmonary resuscitation should be continued until the patient can be placed on cardiopulmonary bypass with a heat exchanger. The core temperature can then be raised to a level above which the arrhythmia can be successfully treated. An alternative but less successful method is to maintain external cardiac massage and to attempt to rewarm the patient using external means and peritoneal dialysis with warm fluid. Thoracotomy and mediastinal lavage with warm fluid should be reserved for persons with persistent ventricular fibrillation or asystole.

HYPOTHERMIC PATIENTS WITH CARDIAC ACTIVITY

Treatment of the hypothermic patient with cardiac activity is determined by the patient's state of consciousness, the clinical findings, and the severity of the hypothermia.

Conscious Patients

Hypothermia in a conscious patient with stable cardiovascular function and rectal temperature of 28° to 30° C (82.4° to 86° F) or higher is relatively easy to manage. The patient's clothing should be removed, and he or she should be dried off and wrapped in warm blankets. The room in which the patient is placed should be warmed to at least 32° C (89.6° F). Warm fluids should be given intravenously, in conjunction with hot, humidified, oxygen-enriched air administered by face mask. Microwave diathermy can also be used to increase body heat.

Table 3 Causes of Hypothermia

Primary hypothermia
Exposure to a cold environment
Immersion in cold water

Secondary hypothermia
Drugs: narcotics, tranquilizers, anesthetics, beta blockers
Metabolic disorders: myxedema, hypopituitarism, hypoadrenalism, diabetes mellitus, hypoglycemia, protein-calorie malnutrition
Impaired thermoregulation as a result of CNS disorders
Impaired muscular activity as a result of paralysis, dementia, or injury
Increased heat loss as a result of burns

Blood tests should be performed to evaluate blood count, electrolyte concentrations, and renal and liver function. Blood culture should also be obtained, and a chest x-ray is imperative. It may also be advisable to screen the blood for toxic substances.

Unconscious Patients

If the patient is unconscious but has stable cardiovascular function and rectal temperature of 28° to 30° C (82.4° to 86° F) or higher, treatment should proceed as outlined above, except that additional measures should be taken to diagnose and treat the altered state of consciousness. Although hypothermia is associated with disorientation and confusion, unconsciousness is rare at body temperatures greater than 28° C (82.4° F); its presence suggests that central nervous system dysfunction may underlie the hypothermia. Because mortality and morbidity are usually linked not with hypothermia but with associated conditions, every effort should be made to diagnose and treat the pathologic state that induced the altered state of consciousness. Drug and alcohol overdose can be treated by dialysis, head injury by operative decompression or standard measures to reduce cerebral edema, and hypoglycemia by glucose administration.

Once a preliminary diagnosis has been reached, it must be confirmed with appropriate tests. Blood test results must be carefully interpreted in hypothermic patients because changes in body temperature have a direct effect on blood chemical values. For example, the initial laboratory findings in a hypothermic patient may include a high hematocrit, an elevated potassium level, a low pH, and altered blood gas tensions. Therefore, the laboratory should correct the blood gas determinations for the altered temperature. When allowances for actual core temperature are made, most hypothermic patients are found to be alkalemic. Blood glucose levels are often elevated, and ketones may be present in blood and urine. However, hypothermic patients are extremely resistant to the hypoglycemic effects of insulin; if the glucose level can be kept below 400 mg/dl, exogenous insulin is seldom indicated.

Every effort should be made to treat hypothermic patients with extreme care. Gradual rewarming will minimize complications. Overhydration and hyperventilation are frequently associated with lethal complications.

A more severe form of hypothermia causes unconsciousness and cardiac instability in patients who retain adequate perfusion but whose rectal temperature is less than 28° C (82.4° F). Such patients are extremely susceptible to cardiac arrhythmias. The cornerstones of management are gentle rewarming, careful monitoring, and preparation for the possibility of ventricular fibrillation or asystole.

Discussion

Thermoregulation in the Hospital Environment

Fever is an upward resetting of the thermoregulatory set point. Hyperpyrexia is an elevation of the core temperature above the body's set point. Patients become febrile as a result of the actions of pyrogens [*see Figure 2*]. When patients are febrile, their central thermoregulatory mechanism works both to minimize heat loss and to accelerate heat production (by adjusting the flow of metabolic substrate) so that body temperature is raised to the level demanded by the new central nervous system set point and is maintained there.

Many of the adaptive mechanisms that respond to alterations in body or environmental temperature are closely linked with behavioral changes. For example, during a febrile episode, a patient may curl up in bed under layers of blankets, as if cold. The reason for this behavior is that the patient's temperature is below the elevated thermoregulatory set point, even though it is above normal. Removing the bedcovers from such patients in an effort to reduce body temperature brings not relief but heightened stress; the preferred approach is to administer an antipyretic at an adequate dosage. The patient will start to sweat and remove the blankets as soon as the set point has been readjusted downward (i.e., as soon as the fever has broken).

Behavioral adaptation allows patients to establish the environmental temperature most comfortable for them. This temperature is called thermal neutrality. Achievement of thermal neutrality can be facilitated by making thermostats available in patients' rooms to allow each person to select the ambient temperature he or she prefers. Studies have demonstrated that certain groups of patients tend to select an ambient temperature that is much warmer than that preferred by the hospital staff.[9] In one study, for example, when burn patients without known infection (but with burn wound colonization) were placed in an environmentally controlled chamber and allowed to regulate the ambient temperature by means of a bedside remote control unit, the mean ambient temperature they selected as most comfortable was significantly higher than the temperature selected by normal individuals [*see Table 4*].[9] Furthermore, when comfortable, the burn patients had significantly higher core and mean skin temperatures than did the normal subjects. These results indicate that in burn patients, the thermoregulatory set point is reset upward because of the pyrogens that are produced during the inflammatory process that is associated with the injury. In these patients, the minimal level of environmental stress is achieved at warmer ambient temperatures (30° to 32° C [86° to 89.6° F]) than in normal subjects, and these conditions are associated with comfort.

Other classes of hospitalized patients also feel cold at temperatures that normal persons consider comfortable: persons with large wounds, peritonitis, pancreatitis, sepsis, and the multiple organ dysfunction syndrome (MODS) all have an elevated central set point. Moreover, very old and very young patients are known to be especially vulnerable to the effects of a cool ambient environment, and the prevailing ambient temperature in a modern air-conditioned hospital may cause them considerable discomfort and additional cold stress. It is clear that ambient temperatures of 23° to 25° C (73.4° to 77° F) are too cold for most patients, particularly those in intensive care areas. In the operating room, temperatures

Table 4 Ambient Temperatures of Comfort[9]

Subjects (N)	Room Comfort Temperature (° C)	Skin Temperature (° C)	Core Temperature (° C)
Control subjects (5)	27.8 ± 0.6	33.4 ± 0.6	36.9 ± 0.1
Burn patients* (9)	30.4 ± 0.7 P < 0.05	35.2 ± 0.4 P < 0.05	38.4 ± 0.3 P < 0.01

Note: mean ± SE.
*Mean burn size was 39% TBS.

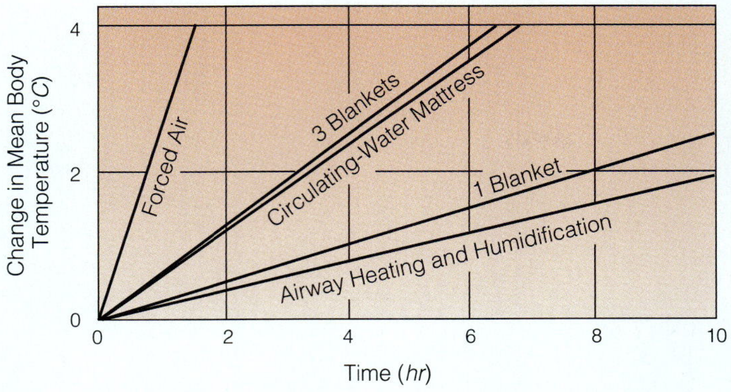

Figure 3 Depicted are the effects of various warming methods on body temperature.[10]

of 21° to 23° C (69.8° to 73.4° F) may induce marked hypothermia in certain critically ill patients: those with burns or sepsis, elderly persons with organ system failure, and infants.

With routine perioperative care, mild hypothermia (a 1° C fall in core temperature) develops in about one half of surgical patients in the OR, and frank hypothermia (a 2° C or greater fall in core temperature) develops in approximately one third. Perioperative cooling occurs because almost all forms of anesthesia impair thermoregulation and because cold ORs accelerate heat loss (open body cavities are exposed to the relatively cold air, and cold I.V. fluids and blood products are frequently administered).

Perioperative hypothermia carries a high morbidity in terms of patient discomfort, shivering, bleeding, nitrogen loss, surgical site infection rate, incidence of morbid cardiac events, and length of hospital stay.[10] A major reason for this morbidity is that even mild hypothermia triggers the dramatic elaboration of catecholamines and other counterregulatory hormones,[11] which is associated with a sequence of cardiovascular events that includes hypertension, systemic vasoconstriction, tachycardia, and cardiac arrhythmias. Accordingly, investigators have recently begun to focus on ways of resolving mild perioperative hypothermia.

One approach is to improve environmental conditions in the OR so as to keep the patient's core temperature at or near normal. Raising the room temperature can achieve this goal, but even an ambient temperature of 25° C (77° F) is uncomfortable for a gowned surgical team. Blankets and heated I.V. solutions appear to be beneficial to an extent [see Figure 3], but in most patients undergoing prolonged procedures (i.e., operations lasting longer than 2 hours), active warming is necessary. Forced-air warming can usually keep the patient's core temperature above 37° C (98.6° F) and seems, on the whole, to be the most effective available method.

Two important studies have examined the use of supplemental warming in the perioperative period. A 1997 study performed at the Johns Hopkins Hospital examined 300 patients undergoing abdominal, thoracic, or vascular surgical procedures who were at high risk for untoward cardiac events.[12] The group was randomized so that one half of the patients received routine thermal care and the other half received supplemental warming via a forced-air warming system. The patients who received standard thermal support had lower core temperatures than those who received supplemental warming; in addition, they experienced many more perioperative morbid cardiac events and showed a higher incidence of postoperative ventricular tachycardia.

Another large study addressed the question of whether perioperative normothermia might reduce the surgical site infection rate.[13] The investigators speculated that perioperative hypothermia, by causing vasoconstriction and reduced tissue oxygen content, could impair host defense and hinder wound healing. A group of 200 patients undergoing colorectal procedures were randomized so that 96 received routine care and 104 received additional warming. As in the Johns Hopkins study, those who received standard care had lower temperatures than those who received additional warming. The hypothermic patients had a higher incidence of surgical site infection than the normothermic patients, as well as a longer average duration of hospitalization.

These two studies demonstrate that the maintenance of near-normothermia in patients during the perioperative period can greatly reduce mortality, morbidity, length of hospital stay, and overall cost. Those who would benefit from supplemental warming include the very young, the very old, those with MODS, burn patients, trauma patients, and all patients undergoing operative procedures that last longer than 2 hours.

Unlike hospitalized critically ill patients, hyperpyrexic heatstroke victims seen in the emergency room feel warm and seek to cool themselves off; they prefer to be in a cool room and drink cold liquids. If adequately hydrated, patients sweat noticeably—a sign that the body temperature is above the set point and that the patients are trying to offload heat. Restoration of blood volume and cessation of exercise lead to markedly increased skin perfusion, which is associated with profuse sweating. Restoration of normal body temperature follows shortly thereafter.

References

1. Sioson PB, Brown RB: Hyperpyrexia among patients in a large community hospital: causes, features, and outcomes. South Med J 86:773, 1993
2. O'Donnell J, Axelrod P, Fisher C, et al: Use and effectiveness of hypothermia blankets for febrile patients in the intensive care unit. Clin Infect Dis 24:1208, 1997
3. Gronert GA: Malignant hyperthermia. Anesthesia. Milla RD, Ed. Churchill Livingstone, New York, 1986, p 1971
4. Meier-Hellman A, Romer M, Hannemann L, et al: Early recognition of malignant hyperthermia using capnometry. Anaesthetist 39:41, 1990
5. Jones TS, Liang AP, Kilbourne EM, et al: Morbidity and mortality associated with the July 1980 heat wave in St. Louis and Kansas City, Mo. JAMA 247:3327, 1982
6. Amundson DE: The spectrum of heat related injury with compartment syndrome. Milit Med 154:450, 1989
7. Hypothermia-related deaths—Suffolk County, New York, January 1999–March 2000, and United States, 1979–1998. MMWR 50:53, 2000
8. Walpoth BH, Walpoth-Aslan BN, Mattle HP, et al: Outcome of survivors of accidental deep hypothermia and circulatory arrest treated with extracorporeal blood warming. N Engl J Med 337:1500, 1997
9. Wilmore DW, Orcutt TW, Mason AD Jr, et al: Alterations in hypothalamic function following thermal injury. J Trauma 15:697, 1975
10. Sessler DI: Mild perioperative hypothermia. N Engl J Med 336:1730, 1997
11. Frank SM, Higgins MS, Breslow MJ, et al: The catecholamine, cortisol, and hemodynamic response to mild perioperative hypothermia. Anesthesiology 82:83, 1995
12. Frank SM, Fleischer LA, Breslow MJ, et al: Perioperative maintenance of normothermia reduces the incidence of morbid cardiac events. JAMA 227:1127, 1997
13. Kurz A, Sessler DI, Lenhardt R, et al: Perioperative normothermia to reduce the incidence of surgical wound infection and shorten hospitalization. N Engl J Med 334:1209, 1996
14. DuBois EF: Fever and the Resolution of Body Temperature. Charles C Thomas, Springfield, Ill., 1948, p 9
15. Wilmore DW: Metabolic Management of the Critically Ill. Plenum Press, New York, 1977, p 70

Acknowledgment

Figures 1 and 2   Albert Miller.

99 REACTIVE OXYGEN METABOLITES

Patrick M. Reilly, M.D., *Susan A. Kelly,* M.D., *Henry J. Schiller,* M.D., *and Gregory B. Bulkley,* M.D.

The ubiquity of molecular oxygen in our environment and the dependence of most organisms on oxygen for metabolic fuel may obscure the fact that oxygen and its metabolites are often quite toxic.[1] This toxicity appears to have influenced the early evolution of metabolic pathways to detoxify oxygen metabolites and make life possible in an aerobic environment.[2] Although aerobic organisms have subsequently evolved to exploit secondarily oxygen's high reactivity and convert this energy into a metabolically useful form [see Table 1], this same reactivity produces a continuous assault on the biochemical integrity of essential structural and functional components of living tissues. Long before the evolution of aerobic energy metabolism, this assault had fostered the development of a number of efficient intracellular biochemical mechanisms of defense against oxidant injury. Nevertheless, whenever the rate of endogenous oxidant generation exceeds these endogenous antioxidant capabilities, tissue injury is sustained.[3,4]

Free radicals and other reactive oxygen metabolites (ROMs) have been implicated in a number of human disease processes [see Table 2]. Postischemic reperfusion injury represents the classic example of free radical–mediated tissue injury. In the cat small intestine, the administration of antioxidants near the end of the ischemic period but before reperfusion largely prevents the microvascular and epithelial injury seen after periods of partial ischemia.[5] The syndromes of ischemic hepatitis,[6] ischemic pancreatitis,[7] and hemorrhagic stress gastritis[8] may all be clinical manifestations of such a free radical–mediated mechanism of injury in the splanchnic bed. The injury seen after myocardial[9] or cerebral[10] ischemia may also be mediated in part by free radicals generated at reperfusion; such injury should be amenable to antioxidant therapy initiated after the ischemic insult has already occurred but before reperfusion has taken place. Extensive research into the precise mechanisms of injury after ischemia and reperfusion and the therapeutic implications of antioxidant therapy in all of these organs is ongoing.

The clinical impact of free radical ablation after ischemia was first demonstrated in the field of renal transplantation. A number of clinical trials have already been completed that demonstrate improvement in postoperative transplant renal function with antioxidant therapy.[11] Moreover, preservation solutions for harvested organs now routinely include antioxidants.[12] More recently, antioxidants have been shown to improve cardiac function in high-risk patients after the global myocardial ischemia of cardiopulmonary bypass.[13,14]

Oxidant injury is a major, often essential, component of the injury process in such apparently disparate diseases as toxin- and radiation-induced carcinogenesis, alcoholic cirrhosis, and Parkinson's disease.[15,16] The injury seen after exposure to pathophysiological levels of oxygen (for example, pulmonary oxygen toxicity or retrolental fibroplasia) is largely oxidant mediated.[17] A number of inflammatory conditions (for example, inflammatory bowel disease and adult respiratory distress syndrome) may also be mediated, at least in part, by toxic oxidants, many of which are produced by the respiratory burst of leukocytes.[18] Moreover, toxic oxidants play important roles in a number of normal physiologic processes, including the phagocytic killing of microorganisms, the generation of prostaglandins and leukotrienes by way of the arachidonic acid cascade, ovulation, and even aging itself.[3,4] Recent data indicate that the high reactivity of these small, highly diffusible molecules has been exploited by natural selection for use in intracellular signaling; the nitric oxide free radical ($NO^\bullet$) is a good example.

The common pathway of tissue injury underlying these varied conditions is the destruction of membranes, proteins, nucleic acids, and components of the intracellular matrix by ROMs. Consequently, the selective pharmacological modification of this pathway by a variety of nontoxic agents may soon become a routine approach to a wide variety of disparate disease processes.

The Biochemistry of Reactive Oxygen Metabolites

The high reactivity of free radicals is explained by their chemical structure. Most stable molecular species contain electrons within their outer orbitals that are arranged so that each electron is paired with another of opposite spin. This arrangement stabilizes (that is, lowers the energy state of) the molecule. A free radical is a molecule that contains one or more unpaired electrons in its outer orbital [see Figure 1]. The presence of such unpaired electrons gives these molecules a higher energy level, rendering them more unstable and therefore quite

Table 1 Roles of Reactive Oxidants in Normal Physiology

Oxidative metabolism of hydrocarbons to generate energy (adenosine triphosphate)
Arachidonic acid cascade
Phagocytic killing of microorganisms
Enzymatic detoxification of xenobiotics
Ovulation
Fertilization
Intracellular signaling

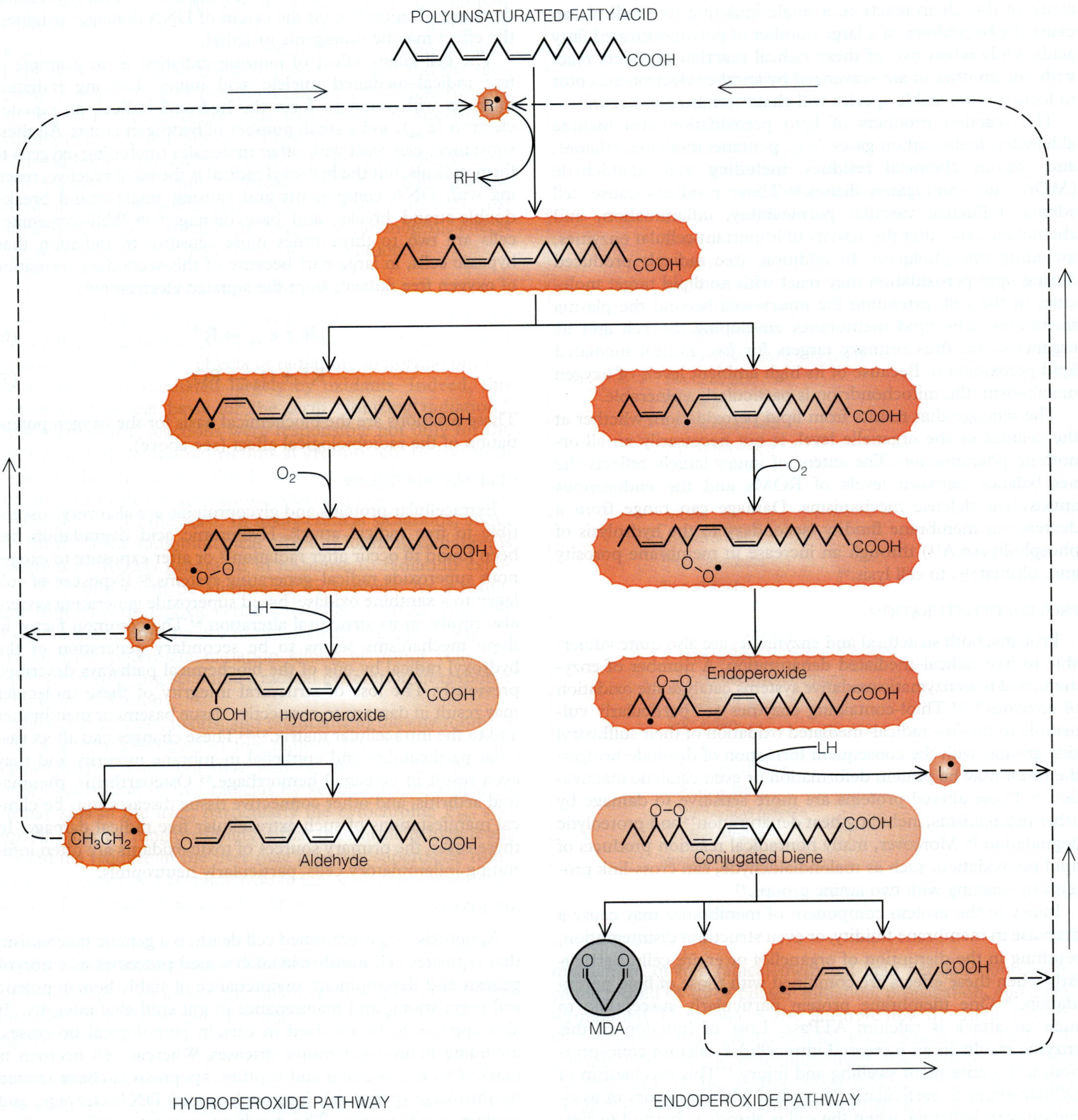

Figure 7 In the presence of oxygen, free radical attack on polyunsaturated fatty acids forms lipid hydroperoxides and endoperoxides. Both of these compounds can subsequently decompose, producing additional radicals. The hydroperoxide pathway generates two radicals from a single radical attack, and the endoperoxide pathway generates three radicals. Each generated radical can itself initiate further lipid peroxidation, a classic chain reaction. The result is extensive peroxidation of many polyunsaturated fatty acid molecules from only a few initiating radicals, leading to membrane damage or even destruction. The detection of these reaction products, especially malondialdehyde (MDA) and ethane, can be used as a marker of free radical–mediated lipid peroxidation in biologic systems.

es apoptosis. Overexpression of bcl-2 can block normal cell death mechanisms,[87] whereas a deficiency in bcl-2 leads to widespread, uncontrolled, pathological apoptosis.[88] This protein appears to be acting after the generation of ROMs to prevent subsequent cellular injury, including lipid peroxidation.[87]

In a recent in vitro model simulating multiple organ dysfunction syndrome (MODS) and its characteristic endothelial injury, intracellular antioxidants such as N-acetylcysteine, dimethyl sulfoxide (DMSO), and o-phenanthroline blocked the induction of apoptosis normally seen in this model.[89] In another model, overexpression of the antioxidant enzyme glutathione peroxidase also protected against apoptotic death.[87] Thus, many diverse stimuli capable of inducing apoptosis all seem to act via a common ROM-mediated pathway.

Antioxidant Defense Mechanisms

ENDOGENOUS ANTIOXIDANTS

A number of endogenous mechanisms enable organisms to prevent or limit damage from ROMs [see Table 5].

Intracellular Compartments

A major defense mechanism is the structural organization of the cell itself, which separates the sites and reactants of free radical reactions from one another, thereby minimizing free radical production and free radical–mediated intracellular injury.[90] This compartmentalization allows scavenging of free radicals at the site of their formation, which is critical in the light of their short radii of reactivity. For example, the respiratory chain in mitochondria prevents most unpaired electrons from escaping to form radicals; however, those radicals that are formed via the univalent leak from this respiratory chain are efficiently scavenged by manganese superoxide dismutase (SOD), a specific form of SOD located almost exclusively within the matrix of the mitochondrion. The lipid-soluble antioxidant vitamins α-tocopherol and β-carotene localize within cellular and organelle membranes, where they are ideally situated to block free radical–mediated lipid peroxidation. Most of the iron in biologic systems is kept inactivated (i.e., in the nonreactive ferric form) by sequestration in proteins such as ferritin, largely preventing the iron-catalyzed generation of hydroxyl (or perferryl) radicals.[91] Similarly, most circulating iron stores are bound to hemoglobin or transferrin, also in a nonreactive state.

Other antioxidants and oxidant scavenging systems are similarly compartmentalized, often at or near the sites of oxidant generation. It is for these reasons that measurements of antioxidant levels from tissue homogenates can be misleading: whereas the total amount of antioxidant may be low, such substances may be present in very high local concentrations at or near sites of ROM generation, thereby acting effectively as physiologic antioxidants.[92]

Enzymatic Antioxidants

The mitochondrial cytochrome oxidase system [see Figure 2] consumes most of the available oxygen within the cell, catalyzing the reduction of 95 to 99 percent of molecular oxygen to water, effectively bypassing the formation of toxic free radical intermediates. In fact, this mechanism, now so important for the generation of energy, appears to have evolved primarily as a mechanism of protection against the toxicity of oxygen.[1,70] The anaerobic blue-green algae, today's most primitive organisms and the organisms most closely resembling those that first evolved in the primordial anaerobic environment, use photosynthesis to synthesize glucose (and generate energy by anaerobic fermentation). A major by-product of photosynthesis is molecular oxygen, which, from the point of view of the anaerobic cell, constitutes not only an unusable but also a highly toxic waste product. As the population of anaerobic organisms increased, they were forced to contend with increasing concentrations of oxygen in both the intracellular and the extracellular environment.[2] Oxygen may react with carbon, hydrogen, and nitrogen in a variety of oxidation reactions, ultimately producing carbon dioxide, water, and nitrous oxide, respectively, but via the generation of highly toxic intermediates by pathways such as the univalent leak. This highly toxic oxidation potential of oxygen would therefore have provided a strong natural selective pressure on these primitive organisms to develop mechanisms for its intracellular detoxification. It seems that some of the first defense mechanisms to appear were the superoxide dismutases and the catalases, which are present in all eukaryotes and even most prokaryotes and are essential for growth in an aerobic environment. For example, SOD-deficient mutants of *Escherichia coli* cannot grow in an aerobic environment.[93] That these enzymes are both basic and essential to life in an aerobic environment is suggested by their ubiquity and by the fact that their amino acid sequences are approximately 90 percent homologous across species, from blue-green algae to humans (i.e., are highly conserved).

The SODs catalyze the conversion (dismutation) of the superoxide anion free radical (O_2^-) to hydrogen peroxide and molecular oxygen at a rate 10,000 times faster than the spontaneous dismutation at physiologic pH[28,94]:

$$O_2^- + 2H^+ \xrightarrow{SOD} H_2O_2 \quad (8)$$

Acceleration of this reaction reduces the quantity of superoxide anion available to reduce ferric salts, thereby decreasing

Table 5 Endogenous Antioxidants

Agent	Comments
Enzymatic antioxidants	
Cytochrome oxidase system	Detoxifies 95%–99% of O_2 in cell
Superoxide dismutase (SOD)	Detoxifies superoxide anion
Catalase	Detoxifies hydrogen peroxide
Glutathione peroxidase	Detoxifies hydrogen peroxide
Nonenzymatic antioxidants	
Lipid phase	
α-Tocopherol	Vitamin E
β-Carotene	Vitamin A precursor
Aqueous phase	
Ascorbic acid	Vitamin C
Urate	Scavenges O_2^-, OH•
Cysteine	Scavenges O_2^-, OH•
Albumin	Scavenges LOOH, HOCl
Bilirubin	Scavenges O_2^-, OH•
Ceruloplasmin	Possible mechanism similar to SOD
Transferrin	Binds circulating iron
Lactoferrin	Binds circulating iron

proteolytic activation of xanthine oxidase during the ischemic period facilitates the generation of ROMs when oxygen is reintroduced at reperfusion.

The Fundamental Mechanism of Reperfusion Injury

This body of work supports the hypothesis of Granger and associates [see Figure 10].[5] Catabolism of ATP during ischemia leads to an increased concentration of the purine metabolites hypoxanthine and xanthine. At the same time, ischemia appears to mediate the conversion of xanthine dehydrogenase to xanthine oxidase. (Although proteolysis is probably involved, the precise mechanism by which ischemia mediates this step is still unclear.[114]) Oxygen, the only substrate lacking for superoxide generation, is reintroduced suddenly, and in excess, at reperfusion. The superoxide generated by xanthine oxidase then triggers a free radical chain reaction that leads to tissue injury. The fact that scavenging the hydroxyl radical, or blocking its secondary generation by iron-catalyzed reactions, has the same protective effect as blockade of the cascade more proximally suggests that some form of the hydroxyl radical, or one of its metabolites, is the final agent of injury.[41,111]

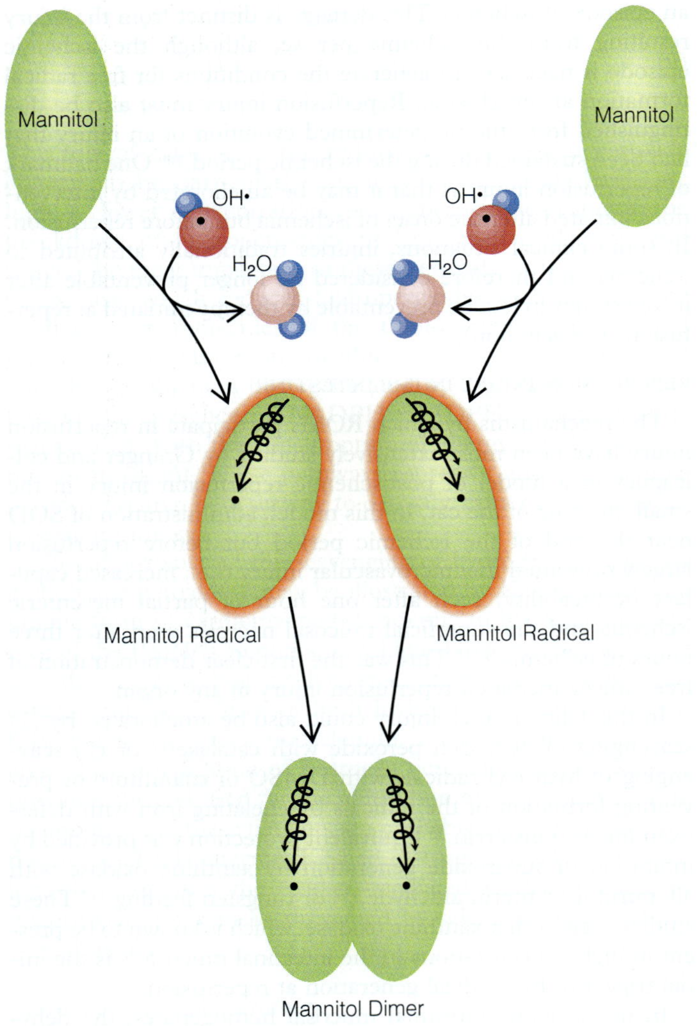

Further studies in this same model suggest that the neutrophil plays an important role in the final mediation of this reperfusion injury. The injury can be largely prevented by treatment of these cats with (1) antineutrophil serum, (2) a monoclonal antibody that blocks neutrophil binding to the endothelial cell,[115] or (3) agents that inhibit platelet-activating factor, which in part mediates neutrophil–endothelial cell interaction.[116] Although this finding might suggest that reperfusion injury is entirely explained by the generation of superoxide by neutrophils, it seems more likely that the neutrophil acts as a necessary amplifier, rather than the initiator, of tissue injury. Superoxide generated endogenously from endothelial cell monolayers exposed to anoxia and reoxygenation, simulating ischemia and reperfusion in vitro, produces cell lysis even in the absence of neutrophils or parenchymal cells.[117] In addition, in some models of organ injury, confirmed neutrophil depletion fails to ameliorate injuries that are blocked with superoxide dismutase and catalase.[118,119] Moreover, neutrophils, which generate superoxide by the NADPH-dependent oxidase system (a process that is not inhibited by allopurinol[120]), also produce a large number of toxic mediators other than oxygen metabolites, including elastase, collagenase, and other proteases.[47] Of crucial importance is the fact that the marked accumulation of neutrophils in the intestinal mucosa of the cat caused by partial ischemia is prevented by inhibition of xanthine oxidase with allopurinol,[121] which also prevents the refusion injury. Other in vivo and in vitro studies suggest that after ischemia, neutrophils accumulate and adhere to the microvascular endothelium in general, and the postcapillary venules in particular [see Figure 11], in response to ROMs generated by a xanthine oxidase–dependent initial event,[115,120] whereas the capillary injury itself is mediated by proteases generated by the accumulated neutrophils [see Figure 12].[115]

REPERFUSION INJURY IN OTHER ORGANS

Splanchnic Organs

After an episode of hypotension or some other form of severe physiologic stress, a mucosal lesion, characterized by hemorrhagic necrosis, is frequently seen in the stomach. Such stress ulcerations can result in hemodynamically significant gastric hemorrhage and even mortality in the critically ill patient. Similar lesions produced by hypotension in animal models of gastric injury can be prevented by either SOD or allopurinol.[8,122] The initiating factor in this injury process is most likely an angiotensin-mediated disproportionate splanchnic vasospasm causing gastric mucosal ischemia,[123] followed by the generation of ROMs at reperfusion. Although loss of mucosal integrity probably appears at this early stage, bleeding usually appears a few days later, concurrent with the return of acid secretion from adjacent, uninjured areas of gastric mucosa.

The liver, which is particularly rich in xanthine oxidase, can also be subjected to postischemic reperfusion injury after shock or preservation for transplantation. In either case, injury may manifest as hepatocellular necrosis in the central portions of the liver lobule, associated with severe impairment of synthetic and catabolic-excretory functions. SOD and catalase, or allopurinol,

Figure 9 Mannitol, an exogenously administered free radical scavenger, reacts with the hydroxyl radical, forming a mannitol radical. Two mannitol radicals subsequently react with one another, resulting in the formation of a more stable, and therefore less reactive, mannitol dimer. Because each electron is now paired in the outer orbital, this dimer is not a toxic oxidant, and the chain reaction is broken. This is an example of chain termination.

Exogenous Antioxidants: The Pharmacological Approach to Injury Mediated by Free Radicals

Enzymatic Scavengers

SUPEROXIDE DISMUTASE

Superoxide dismutase (SOD) catalyzes the dismutation of superoxide anion to hydrogen peroxide.[28,94] SOD alone may be ineffective, particularly in vitro, because it leads to increased production of H_2O_2, which itself is often quite toxic.[117,206] This toxicity can be prevented, especially in vitro, by simultaneous administration of catalase, which catalyzes the reduction of H_2O_2 to water (see below).[95] In many in vivo models, however, especially in intact animals and blood-perfused systems, intravascular administration of SOD alone does effectively block free radical–mediated tissue injury.[5,171] This finding may be explained by the relative abundance of endogenous glutathione peroxidase and catalase, particularly in the erythrocyte, which is accessible to the freely diffusable but less reactive H_2O_2.[25]

Intravenous, intramuscular, or intraperitoneal administration and local instillation are effective routes for administration of SOD.[207,208] Fortunately, both superoxide dismutase and catalase are extremely nontoxic. Recombinant forms of human superoxide dismutase (r-HSOD) have been developed for commercial purposes in response to concern that infusion of a foreign protein might induce an immune response. This is of particular concern in conditions such as arthritis, for which repeated administration might be needed. In most cases, r-HSOD is no more potent than other forms, and in any case, issues of activity and purity are far more important.

Superoxide dismutase is rapidly excreted, unmetabolized, by the kidneys. Its half-life in the circulation is less than 10 minutes[209]; this short half-life potentially limits its therapeutic effectiveness. Accordingly, several approaches have been employed to extend the serum half-life. Through genetic engineering, two human $Cu^{2+}Zn^{2+}$ superoxide dismutase subunits have been linked to the hinge sequence of the human immunoglobulin IgA1.[209] This modification limits glomerular filtration, thereby extending the serum half-life to approximately 145 minutes.

By means of a similar strategy, SOD has been covalently linked to a polyethylene glycol polymer (PEG-SOD).[210-212] PEG-SOD retains its enzymatic activity and has a circulatory half-life of 18 to 40 hours. In addition, PEG-SOD is less immunogenic and is better able to resist proteolysis than the native enzyme. PEG conjugation may also facilitate transmembrane transport of the active enzyme into the cell, where many free radical generation systems are active.[210] Superoxide dismutase has been incorporated into synthetic liposomes,[213] increasing intracellular SOD activity sixfold to 12-fold; moreover, liposome-encapsulated SOD has a circulatory half-life of more than four hours.[190] Nevertheless, an important incremental advantage of PEG-SOD over native SOD has yet to be demonstrated unequivocally.

In addition to the modified forms of superoxide dismutase, several nonprotein compounds may serve as SOD mimics. CuDIPS (copper [II][3,5-diisopropylsalicylic acid]) is a synthetic SOD mimic that is lipophilic and therefore better able to cross cell membranes and act intracellularly.[214] Unfortunately, CuDIPS loses its SOD-mimetic activity in the presence of low levels of albumin, and its clinical utility is thereby limited.[215] Other, more stable copper (II) complexes (e.g., CuφMeTIM, CuTIM, and CuDIM) also mimic SOD but are not as lipid soluble.[214]

Desferal-Mn (DF-Mn), a low-molecular-weight complex of deferoxamine and manganese, also can mimic SOD.[215] DF-Mn can cross the cell membrane to act intracellularly. Unfortunately, it also exhibits a dose-dependent toxicity to cells, probably secondary to the intracellular dissociation of the complex and consequent release of free manganese into the cytoplasm.

Stable cyclic nitroxides derived from oxazolidine have also been employed as free radical scavengers in animal models. These agents have been used extensively as probes in electron spin resonance (ESR) spectroscopy and nuclear magnetic resonance studies. They are extremely stable free radicals of low molecular weight that are membrane permeable, metal independent, and noncytotoxic; they couple rapidly to carbon-centered or oxygen-centered free radicals to produce relatively stable reaction products.[216,217]

CATALASE

Catalase catalyzes the reduction of hydrogen peroxide to water. This enzyme has a half-life of approximately 20 minutes in vivo and is degraded largely by proteolysis unless it is conjugated to polyethylene glycol.[211,218] Because of its high molecular weight, catalase must be modified before it can enter cells. PEG modification and liposomal entrapment have achieved circulatory half-lives of about 18 hours[211] and two and a half hours,[189] respectively, and allow the enzyme to be delivered intracellularly.[190,219]

XANTHINE OXIDASE INHIBITORS

An efficient method of inhibiting superoxide generation by xanthine oxidase is through conventional enzyme inhibition. Allopurinol, a structural analogue of hypoxanthine, competitively inhibits xanthine oxidase–catalyzed urate production, with the subsequent formation of oxypurinol. Oxypurinol forms a stable complex with xanthine oxidase, preventing further enzymatic activity and functioning as a noncompetitive inhibitor. Oxypurinol is therefore sometimes considered to be the "active" form of allopurinol. It is unclear, however, whether administration of oxypurinol offers any practical therapeutic advantage over allopurinol.[220]

Folic acid and pterin aldehyde (a photolytic breakdown product of folic acid) also serve to competitively inhibit xanthine oxidase, although they are structurally dissimilar to allopurinol.[221] These agents bind to the molybdenum at the enzyme active site so that molecular oxygen can no longer be consumed. Some studies suggest that these agents may be as potent as allopurinol.[113,221]

Another method for inhibiting xanthine oxidase activity is dietary administration of tungsten, usually in conjunction with a molybdenum-deficient diet. This acts specifically to prevent the incorporation of molybdenum into the newly synthesized enzyme.[222] The resulting apoenzyme, with tungsten replacing molybdenum, lacks xanthine oxidase activity.

Evidence also suggests that free radical–mediated injury may be ameliorated by preventing irreversible proteolytic conversion of xanthine dehydrogenase to xanthine oxidase (d-to-o conversion).[113,223] Soybean trypsin inhibitor can prevent this conversion and thereby prevent the generation of the superoxide anion in response to reperfusion. A number of other serine proteinase inhibitors are available (e.g., phenylmethylsulfonyl fluoride [PMSF]), but many are too toxic for use in vivo.

Nonenzymatic Scavengers

MANNITOL AND ALBUMIN

Nonenzymatic scavengers of free radicals can also diminish free radical–mediated injury. Mannitol, by virtue of its many hydroxyl groups, can scavenge a hydroxyl radical to form a mannitol free radical. The mannitol free radical then preferentially reacts with another mannitol free radical to form a stable, nonreactive mannitol dimer[38] [see Figure 9] in a classic chain-termination reaction that blocks the destructive oxidant cascade.

Albumin can scavenge lipid hydroperoxides by virtue of its free sulfhydryl groups as well as a separate peroxidaselike activity.[224-226] It has also been shown to prevent the inactivation of α_1-antiproteinase by neutrophil-generated hypochlorous acid.[104] The disadvantage to mannitol and albumin, however, is that they remain extracellular and therefore are probably unable to scavenge free radicals generated intracellularly.

DIMETHYL SULFOXIDE AND DIMETHYLTHIOUREA

Dimethyl sulfoxide (DMSO) is an effective scavenger of the hydroxyl radical. It can freely permeate membranes to act intracellularly at sites of free radical production (e.g., the mitochondria).[227] Dimethylthiourea (DMTU) is also a scavenger of hydroxyl radicals as well as of hydrogen peroxide and hypochlorous acid. Like DMSO, DMTU also crosses lipid membranes easily.[228] Lower tissue levels of DMTU may be adequate for a protective effect, in part because DMTU can scavenge H_2O_2.

(continued)

Exogenous Antioxidants: The Pharmacological Approach (*continued*)

21-AMINOSTEROIDS

The 21-aminosteroids, or lazaroids, represent a new class of steroid virtually without mineralocorticoid or glucocorticoid activity.[229,230] U74006F, the prototype of the series, has been shown to stabilize cellular membranes by inhibiting iron-catalyzed lipid peroxidation; it achieves this inhibition by scavenging lipid hydroperoxides and the superoxide anion.[229] It also serves to block the release of arachidonic acid and attenuates the rise in myocardial depressant factor activity in models of ischemia/reperfusion.[230]

IRON CHELATORS

The extremely high reactivity of the hydroxyl radical causes it to react at diffusion-limited rates; that is, it reacts with the first molecule with which it comes in contact, usually within 1.4 nm and within a period of less than 10^{-6} seconds. Therefore, for a hydroxyl radical scavenger to be effective, it must be present in such a high concentration that it constitutes a significant portion of total molecules. Because hydroxyl radicals are generated by the transition metal–catalyzed Fenton reaction, the prevention of this reaction by chelation of transition metals, particularly iron, represents a more efficient method for preventing hydroxyl radical damage, especially lipid peroxidation.

Deferoxamine, a chelating agent already in clinical use for iron poisoning, strongly binds to Fe^{3+}. Unlike agents such as EDTA, deferoxamine prevents the reduction of Fe^{3+} by ascorbate and superoxide anion and thereby prevents the Fenton reaction.[231] Various models of ischemia/reperfusion have shown a protective effect with this agent.[42,232,233] The conjugation of hydroxyethyl starch or dextran to deferoxamine results in a less toxic agent with a longer circulatory half-life.[234] Although deferoxamine can directly scavenge hydroxide and superoxide radicals, the effect is unlikely to be significant under physiologic conditions.[235]

Agents that possess ferroxidase activity may also sequester iron from the Fenton reaction by maintaining it in the Fe^{3+} form. Ceruloplasmin, a copper-containing protein, has been shown to inhibit hydroxyl ion formation and lipid peroxidation. Although it does have some activity as a superoxide dismutase, ceruloplasmin most likely acts as a ferroxidase.[236] By preventing redox cycling of iron, ceruloplasmin inhibits in vitro lipid peroxidation in some models to a greater extent than either SOD or catalase.

OLTIPRAZ AND EBSELEN

An alternative to the administration of free radical scavengers is the administration of agents that enhance intracellular concentrations of endogenous antioxidants. Oltipraz, a naturally occurring anticarcinogenic dithiolthione found in cabbage, increases hepatic stores of glutathione as well as the hepatic activity of glutathione reductase and glutathione s-transferase. Oltipraz has been shown to decrease the hepatotoxicity of carbon tetrachloride and acetaminophen, both of which exert toxicity by free radical–mediated, cytochrome P_{450}–driven redox cycling mechanisms.[237] Similarly, sulforaphane, another naturally occurring substance with anticarcinogenic properties (found in broccoli and other cruciferous plants), induces enzymes such as glutathione s-transferase and NADPH:quinone reductase (phase II detoxification enzymes).[238]

Ebselen is a selenoorganic compound with anti-inflammatory properties; it mimics glutathione peroxidase in its ability to reduce hydrogen peroxide and lipid hydroperoxides in the presence of glutathione.[239] In addition, ebselen has been found to inhibit the granulocyte oxidative burst by a mechanism independent of its glutathione peroxidase–like activity.[240]

Neutrophil Inhibitors

Free radical–mediated injury may be attenuated if secondary amplification of injury by neutrophils is prevented. This may be accomplished either by depleting neutrophils altogether, by suppressing NADPH oxidase activity, or by hindering neutrophil adhesion.

INHIBITORS OF NADPH OXIDASE

Adenosine, in addition to its well-recognized local vasodilatory effect, inhibits superoxide radical formation by stimulated granulocytes through a receptor-mediated mechanism.[241] Diphenyleneiodonium is another inhibitor to which the NADPH oxidase of neutrophils is extremely sensitive.[242] (This agent inhibits inducible nitric oxide synthase as well.[243]) Other agents that inhibit neutrophil NADPH–dependent oxidase in vitro include local anesthetics, calcium channel blockers, nonsteroidal anti-inflammatory drugs, cetiedil, and CHIP (crude hyphal inhibitory product).[244–248] Unfortunately, many of these agents are nonspecific in action and of such low activity that therapeutically effective concentrations may be difficult to attain in vivo. Mab 1H8.2 is a highly specific monoclonal antibody against NADPH oxidase; it blocks 90 percent of this enzyme's activity.[249]

INHIBITORS OF NEUTROPHIL ADHESION

Monoclonal antibodies have been raised against the CD11/CD18 complex, a neutrophil membrane glycoprotein complex that mediates neutrophil adherence to endothelial cells.[250] These monoclonal antibodies have been shown to inhibit neutrophil chemotaxis and adherence. Platelet-activating factor receptor antagonists (e.g., BN 52021, WEB 2086) also inhibit neutrophil adherence and extravasation.[251] Such agents may offer a highly specific method for minimizing the neutrophil-mediated injury component. GMP 140 is a glycoprotein complex found on endothelial cells that is unrelated to the CD11/CD18 complex but that also mediates adherence of neutrophils to endothelial cells. Administration of GMP 140 has been shown to inhibit neutrophil adherence through competition inhibition.[252]

Polypharmacy Approaches

Just as the endogenous antioxidant system provides several lines of defense, exogenous agents may theoretically be used in combination to prevent free radical–mediated tissue injury. In many studies, however, the benefit of an effective dose of one antioxidant is usually not enhanced by the addition of another agent. The most effective approaches will probably be interventions early in the cascade that prevent initial free radical generation and interventions aimed at those processes in which free radical mechanisms produce a large portion of the injury.

---

have been found to ameliorate this centrilobular necrosis in some studies.[6,124]

The pancreas is susceptible to a form of ischemic injury similar to that seen in the stomach and liver. Ischemic pancreatitis can be seen after shock and after cardiopulmonary bypass.[125] In an ex vivo canine model of ischemic pancreatitis, administration of either allopurinol or superoxide dismutase and catalase at reperfusion provided substantial protection against this injury.[7,126] This does not appear to be a nonspecific antineutrophil effect, because confirmed neutrophil depletion is not protective (see above).[118]

Free radicals appear to play a less important role in other models of pancreatitis, however. Because no currently available experimental model truly mimics the clinical situation, the true role of ROMs as mediators of human pancreatitis will only be defined when the results of ongoing controlled clinical trials of free radical ablation are available.

Heart

Reperfusion injury in the heart may be global, as after cardiac arrest or cardioplegia, or regional, as after transient myocardial ischemia (angina pectoris) or infarction. Several studies in ani-

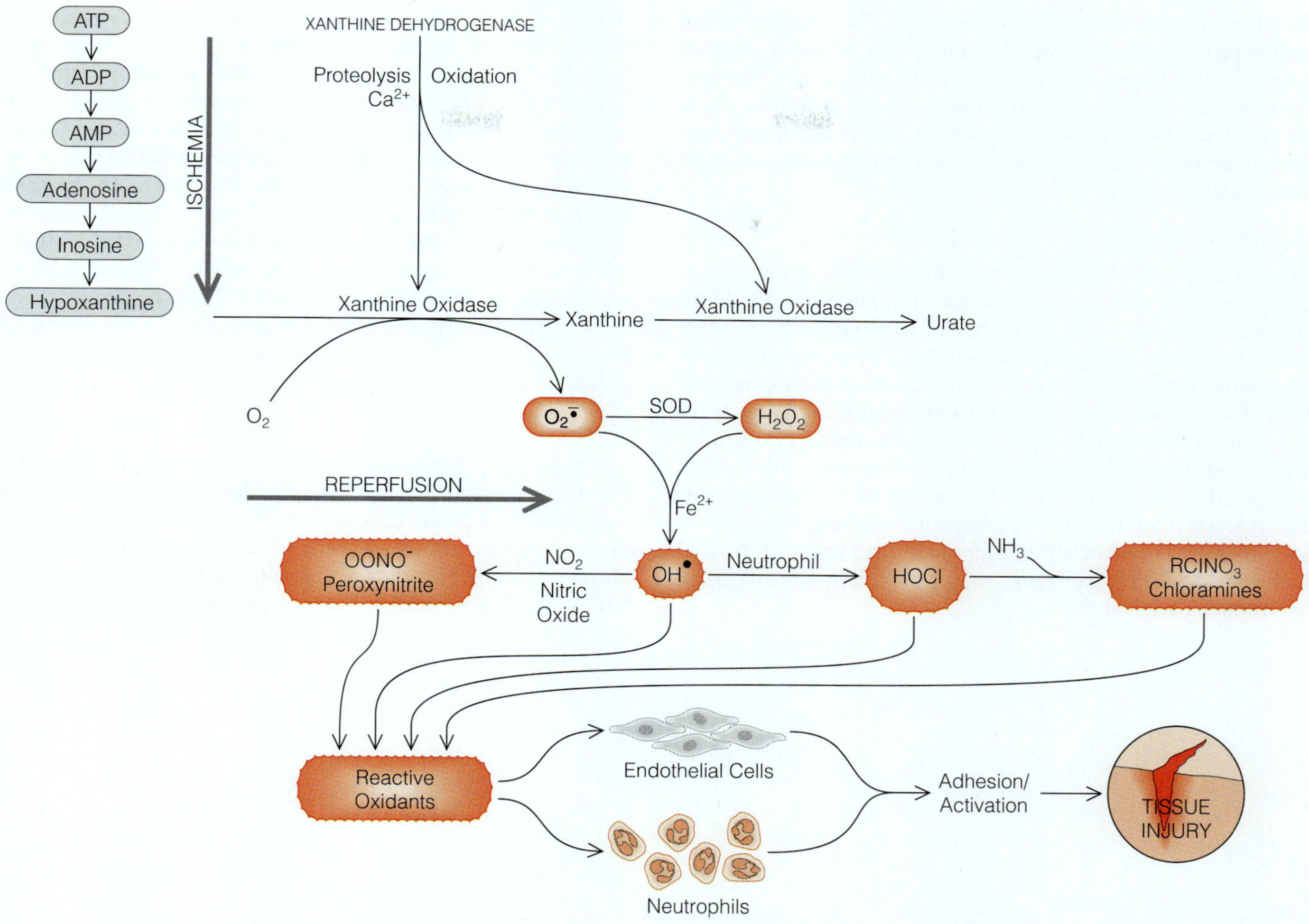

Figure 10 Xanthine oxidase may serve as the initial source of free radical generation in postischemic reperfusion injury. With the onset of ischemia, ATP is degraded to its purine bases (e.g., hypoxanthine), the concentration of which increases. Simultaneously, xanthine dehydrogenase is converted by ischemia to xanthine oxidase. Although the concentrations of substrate and enzyme are high during ischemia, the absence of oxygen prevents purine oxidation until reperfusion. At reperfusion, oxygen becomes available, suddenly and in excess, and the oxidation of hypoxanthine (and xanthine) proceeds rapidly, generating a burst of superoxide radicals as a by-product, probably at or near the endothelial cell surface.

mals have shown that some protection is provided against prolonged global cardiac ischemia by either free radical scavengers or, in some cases, allopurinol.[9,127] In clinical trials, patients given allopurinol showed a significant decrease in the generation of ROMs during and after cardiopulmonary bypass,[14] as well as a significant improvement in cardiac performance, a decreased incidence of postoperative myocardial infarction, and some difference in early mortality after complex coronary bypass surgery.[15,128] At least one phase II multicenter trial of polyethylene glycol–SOD (PEG-SOD) in cardiopulmonary bypass is currently under way.

A major impact of free radical ablation on the postischemic heart appears to be for the ablation of reperfusion arrhythmias. Both SOD[129] and allopurinol[130] have been found to strikingly decrease the incidence of reperfusion-induced arrhythmias after both global and regional ischemia. Although initial studies showed an apparent reduction in infarct size by free radical ablation in models of regional myocardial ischemia,[131] it now appears that the benefit achieved is small to negligible when studies are controlled for anatomic variations in collateral flow and conducted with an appropriate follow-up to determine ultimate infarct size.[132,133] Although xanthine oxidase had not previously been measurable in homogenized preparations of human heart,[134] small, strategically located quantities of this enzyme have now been demonstrated by immunohistochemical studies in the microvascular endothelium of the human heart,[135,136] where it could act as a source of superoxide generation to trigger microvascular reperfusion injury. Other studies suggest an important role for neutrophils and neutrophil-derived oxidants in both global and regional myocardial reperfusion injury in a pattern analogous to that described by Granger and colleagues in the small intestine (see above).[137]

Kidney

Renal ischemia secondary to hypotension frequently results in acute tubular necrosis, with renal microvascular and tubular injury causing acute renal failure. In animals, SOD ameliorates short-term changes in function and morphology after 60 minutes of normothermic renal ischemia.[138] The primary renal lesion is probably a microvascular injury that results in red cell sludging. This lesion is prevented with antioxidant therapy. (These results correspond with analogous microvascular findings in the cat small intestine and rabbit ears[139] and again suggest that the endothelial cell may be the primary source and target of oxidant injury.)

Central Nervous System

The brain has the lowest tolerance for ischemia of any organ. In some models of regional ischemia simulating stroke, SOD improved acute recovery of electrical function (i.e., sensory evoked potentials) after ischemia.[10] In another model of regional ischemia,[140] the combined administration of PEG-conjugated SOD and catalase has been reported to significantly decrease the volume of infarcted brain. In a similar model, both allopurinol and dimethylthiourea (DMTU) decreased the volume of infarcted brain by approximately one third.[141] Although significant levels of endothelial xanthine oxidase have been identified immunohistochemically within the human brain,[136] the role of xanthine oxidase as a primary source of oxygen radicals in the brain remains unclear.[142]

The clinical success of cardiopulmonary resuscitation is severely limited by the susceptibility of the brain to global hypoxia. In a model of global cerebral ischemia caused by cardiac arrest, the combination of 30 seconds of nitrogen ventilation, SOD, and the iron chelator deferoxamine enhanced the recovery of somatosensory evoked potentials.[143] These findings suggest that at least part of the brain damage seen after ischemia is caused by a reperfusion injury, which is potentially treatable after the onset of ischemia but before resuscitation. If this theory proves correct and quantitatively important, it may require that we redefine our concept of brain death.

Free radicals have also been implicated in neural tissue injury after acute spinal cord trauma and may contribute to the failure of injured neurons to recover.[144]

Skin

The construction of skin flaps to cover soft tissue defects may result in a reperfusion injury to the skin. In a rat model, treatment with superoxide dismutase[145] or allopurinol[146] ameliorated the injury caused by seven hours of venous occlusion and reperfusion. Similarly, free radical ablation has been found to protect both island flaps[147] and free skin flaps[148] from similar insults. In

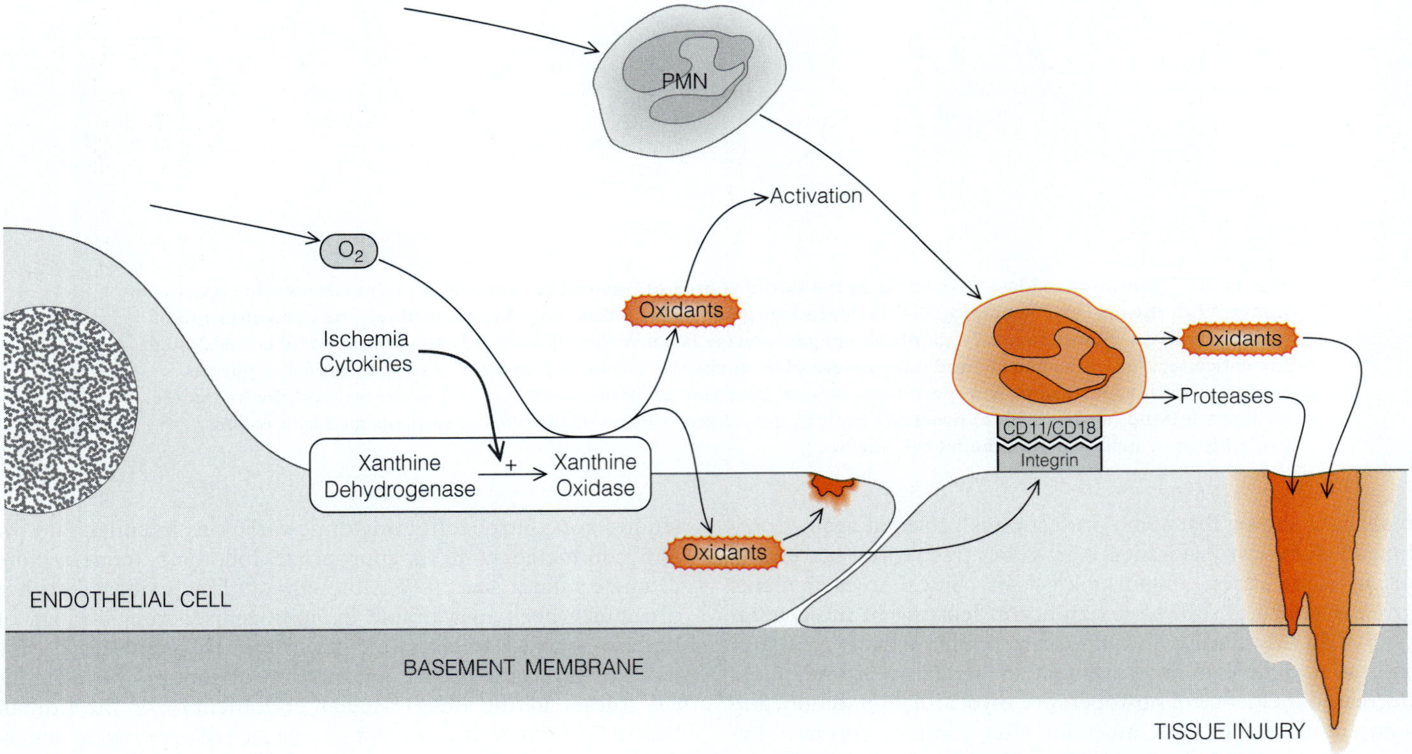

Figure 11 Free radical–mediated reperfusion injury appears to start at the microvascular level, at the interface of the endothelium with the bloodstream. The cascade of events shown in Figure 10 generates the initial oxidants at reperfusion. In some systems, these oxidants alone can produce substantial microvascular injury and consequent parenchymal organ injury. In other organs, however, such as the cat small intestine, these xanthine oxidase–derived oxidants act primarily by stimulating the adhesion of circulating neutrophils to the endothelial cell surface, probably by up-regulation of neutrophil adhesion glycoproteins (e.g., the CD11/CD18 complex) and of the endothelial cellular adhesion molecule (integrin) to which they bind. This process not only arrests the circulating neutrophils but also activates them to produce neutrophil-derived oxidants. In addition, these adherent neutrophils secrete highly toxic proteases, such as elastase. These proteases not only damage tissue directly but also inactivate available enzymatic antioxidants, such as superoxide dismutase and catalase. This serves to amplify the toxic effects of the ambient levels of oxidants, especially within the microenvironment between the endothelium and the adherent neutrophil (not shown).

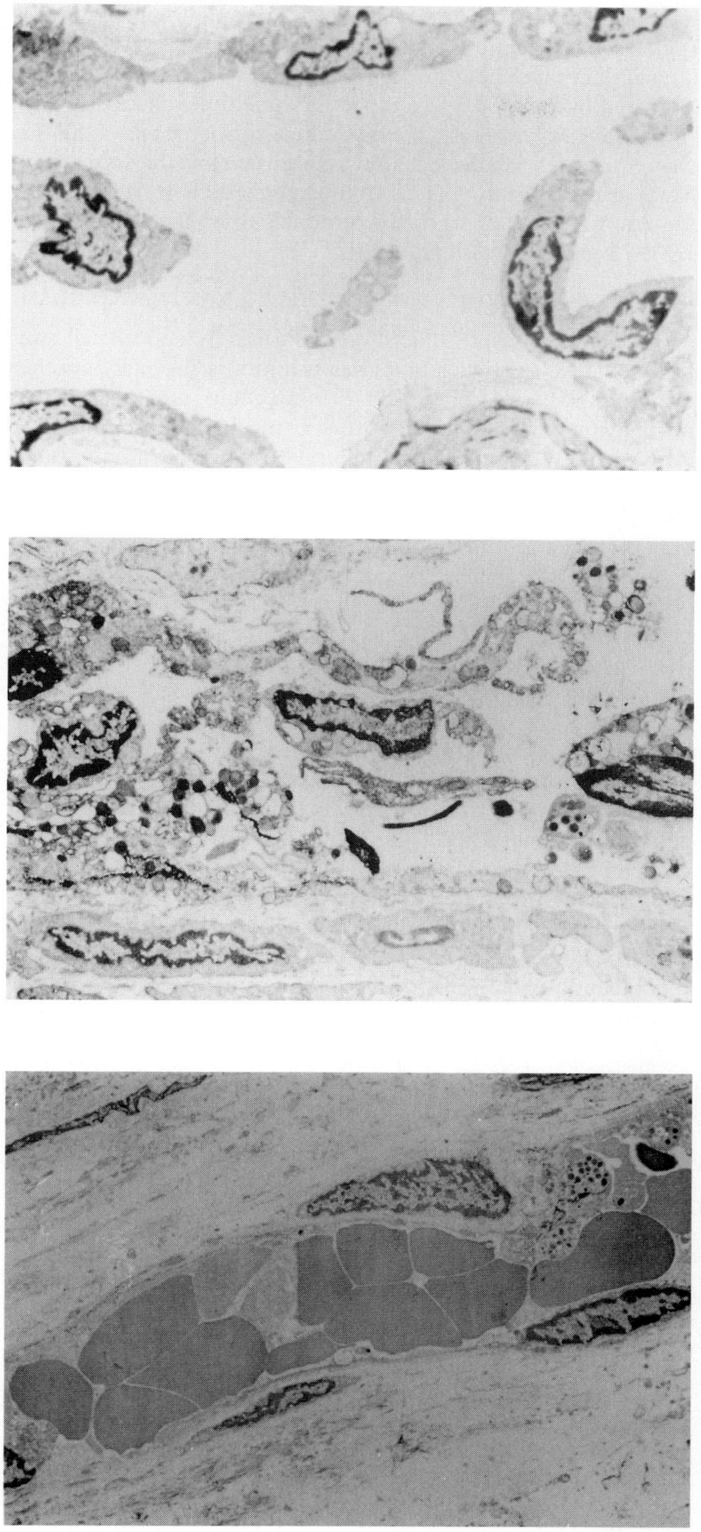

Figure 12 Reperfusion injury is a microvascular phenomenon, with the early loss of endothelial integrity constituting the initial event. In a frostbite model of reperfusion injury, structural damage to the vascular endothelium is seen within 60 seconds of reperfusion (top). Once the endothelial monolayer is injured, neutrophils and platelets accumulate in response to toxic oxidants and more extensive endothelial loss is seen (middle). Eventually, microvascular plugging is seen, with consequent secondary ischemia (bottom).

island flaps, the overall surface area remaining viable after elevation was increased substantially by means of this approach.[147]

Skeletal Muscle

The capillary leak caused by reperfusion injury may result in the compartment syndrome, in which massive swelling and increased hydrostatic pressure in a closed fascial compartment produce secondary ischemia in the tissues within the compartment. Free radical ablation, or leukocyte depletion,[149] has been found to ameliorate the increase in capillary permeability[150] as well as the elevated hydrostatic pressure and consequent muscle ischemia.[151]

Endothelial Cell Trigger Mechanism

Endothelial cells have appropriately received much attention as a possible source of xanthine oxidase–generated superoxide because of the fact that allopurinol can prevent reperfusion injury (even in organs that do not contain measurable quantities of xanthine oxidase within tissue homogenates of their parenchymal cells) and neutrophil accumulation in organs such as the postischemic intestine. Immunohistochemical studies clearly localize xanthine oxidase activity in the microvascular endothelium of a number of organs, including the human heart and brain.[135,136] We have found significant concentrations of xanthine dehydrogenase, which was rapidly converted to the oxidase, in cultured rat pulmonary artery endothelial cells subjected to relatively short periods of anoxia.[117] Moreover, anoxia (simulating ischemia) produced endothelial cell lysis at reoxygenation (simulating reperfusion); cell lysis was prevented by either allopurinol or SOD and catalase, and these agents were equally effective when given at the end of the anoxic period, at the time of reoxygenation. These results indicate that the entire xanthine oxidase–based free radical–generating system is present and operative (i.e., cytotoxic) within the endothelial cell itself, even in the absence of neutrophils and parenchymal cells.

We have proposed that this endothelial cell trigger mechanism is the ubiquitous initiator of free radical–mediated reperfusion injury [*see Figure 10*].[117] In some organs, this endothelial cell injury alone may be sufficient to cause microvascular thrombosis and the ultimate loss of organ function.[152] In other organs (such as the intestine), this injury may only trigger accumulation and activation of neutrophils, which subsequently mediate the major portion of the injury. Neutrophil adherence to endothelial cells is mediated by specific cellular adhesion molecules.[153,154] The adherence of neutrophils to the mesenteric venular endothelium after ischemia and reperfusion can be significantly decreased by scavenging of superoxide with SOD, blockade of its generation from xanthine oxidase with allopurinol, or administration of monoclonal antibodies against the endothelial cell–neutrophil adhesion receptors cited above.[155] The microenvironment created by the adherence of the neutrophil to the endothelial cell plasma membrane seems to be relatively inaccessible to circulating antioxidants and protease inhibitors. As a result, oxidants and proteases are able to initiate and propagate injury. The high concentrations of O_2^- (from both endothelial cells and neutrophils) at this site are sufficient to inactivate SOD, catalase, and some antiproteases as well as to convert endothelium-derived nitric oxide from a protective, vasodilatory agent that helps maintain microvascular integrity to peroxynitrite, a toxic oxidant that may exacerbate microvascular injury.[156] Moreover, the release of endothelial cell mediators such as tumor necrosis factor (TNF) and C'5A, as well as superoxide itself, appears to mediate further conversion of xanthine dehydrogenase to xanthine oxidase, thereby generating positive feedback amplification.[157] Tissue injury occurs as the balance between oxidants and antioxidants (and the balance between proteases and protease inhibitors) is lost. This neutrophil-amplifying system appears to be of variable quantitative importance in different organs, perhaps corresponding to the variable accumulation of neutrophils in different organs subject to ischemia from hemorrhagic shock.[158]

Roles of Reactive Oxygen Metabolites in Intracellular Signaling

The important roles of free radicals in normal cellular function are becoming increasingly evident. In particular, ROMs are now considered to act as intracellular messenger molecules. Among the requisite qualities for such molecules are (1) that they must be small and ubiquitous, (2) that they must be rapidly synthesized and destroyed, (3) that they must be formed as a result of ligand binding at cell membrane receptors, and (4) that they must provide signals to downstream effectors or other intracellular messengers.[159]

NITRIC OXIDE

One example that has already been described in some detail is the nitric oxide free radical. The many functions in which this messenger molecule is involved (in addition to its role in neurotransmission) continue to be elucidated.

ACTIVATION OF NUCLEAR FACTOR κB

Another example of the function of ROMs as messengers is their role in the activation of the transcriptional nuclear factor κB (NFκB). Transcription factors are DNA sequence–specific binding proteins that initiate the synthesis of mRNA from specific target genes. NFκB is found in its inactive form (bound to its inhibitory factor, IκB) in the cytoplasm, where it is activated by diverse stimuli (e.g., cytokines, endotoxin, radiation, and viruses), each of which acts by generating ROMs, primarily H_2O_2. Activation by each of these stimuli is attenuated by antioxidants and also by the overexpression of catalase [see Figure 13].[160,161,162] The activated form of NFκB (dissociated from IκB) translocates to the nucleus, where it initiates the transcription of so-called early response genes—that is, genes encoding cytokines, acute-phase proteins, cellular adhesion molecules, and other immune receptors, all of which help counteract the conditions that caused the cell's activation and thereby help maintain homeostasis.[163]

HEAT SHOCK RESPONSE

The heat shock response is a highly conserved response to certain exogenous stimuli that evolved to protect the cell through the synthesis of a set of specific intracellular stress proteins. These heat shock proteins function in diverse ways: by binding to cytoskeletal proteins (providing tolerance to further injury), by degrading and eliminating damaged cellular proteins, by facilitating the synthesis of proteins to replace those that were damaged, and by facilitating the refolding of proteins to maintain functional tertiary structure.[164,165] In some conditions, activation of the heat shock response preempts other programs of gene expression, such as the acute-phase response.[166] This induction of heat shock proteins has also been found to be triggered by ROMs.[167] In a model of total liver ischemia in pigs, the mRNA expression of the major heat shock protein, HSP-72, was completely abolished after reperfusion by the infusion of SOD at reperfusion.[167] This finding suggests that the superoxide anion is at least partially responsible for the activation of HSP-72 gene expression.

SIGNAL TRANSDUCTION BY ENDOTHELIAL XANTHINE OXIDASE

The generation of O_2^- and other ROMs by endothelial xanthine oxidase to trigger reperfusion injury is probably another example of the role of ROMs as intracellular messengers. It is not obvious why such an intricate mechanism should have evolved: there is no evident natural selective advantage to be derived from reperfusion injury, and this complex system is unlikely to have evolved by chance alone.[109] The explanation may be suggested by the finding that the conversion of form of xanthine dehydrogenase to xanthine oxidase in endothelial cells is effected not only by ischemia but also by proinflammatory cytokines (e.g., TNF-α) and other inflammatory mediators (e.g., lipopolysaccharide [endotoxin] and C'5a).[157] Activating the cascade originally described as the mechanism of reperfusion injury [see Figure 11] then initiates expression of cellular adhesion molecules and consequent neutrophil arrest, trapping, and activation. Thus, endothelial xanthine oxidase–generated O_2^- may trigger an inflammatory response within the microvasculature in general (and the venules in particular) that could cause the trapping and execution of microorganisms in the microvasculature, functionally in the liver and spleen, and perhaps vestigially in other organs. If so, then microvascular endothelial xanthine oxidase could act as the molecular switch of reticuloendothelial function,[34] which would suggest that reperfusion injury is the consequence of the aberrant triggering of this inflammatory signal mechanism by ischemia.

Quantitative Importance of Reperfusion Injury

Although this review has emphasized those studies that have found free radical ablation to ameliorate reperfusion injury, many other studies have failed to find a beneficial effect from this approach.[133,152,168] For example, in the cat small intestine, antioxidants administered at reperfusion clearly prevent the increase in capillary permeability produced after one hour[5] or the necrosis of the villus epithelium seen after three hours of partial ischemia.[110] However, longer periods or more complete degrees of ischemia produce a more severe injury that better corresponds to the clinical syndrome of intestinal ischemia but is largely unaffected by free radical ablation.[31,168,169]

When the quantitative importance of reperfusion injury was formally evaluated in a porcine model of human cadaveric renal transplantation, free radical ablation with either allopurinol or SOD significantly ameliorated acute renal failure after either 24 or 48 hours of cold ischemia preservation, but not after shorter or longer periods of cold ischemia.[170] Regardless of treatment, the kidneys preserved for 18 hours all functioned well, whereas the kidneys preserved for 72 hours all functioned poorly. Thus, there was a defined ischemic period after which ablation of free radical generation at reperfusion provided a measurable and clinically important beneficial effect [see Figure 14].

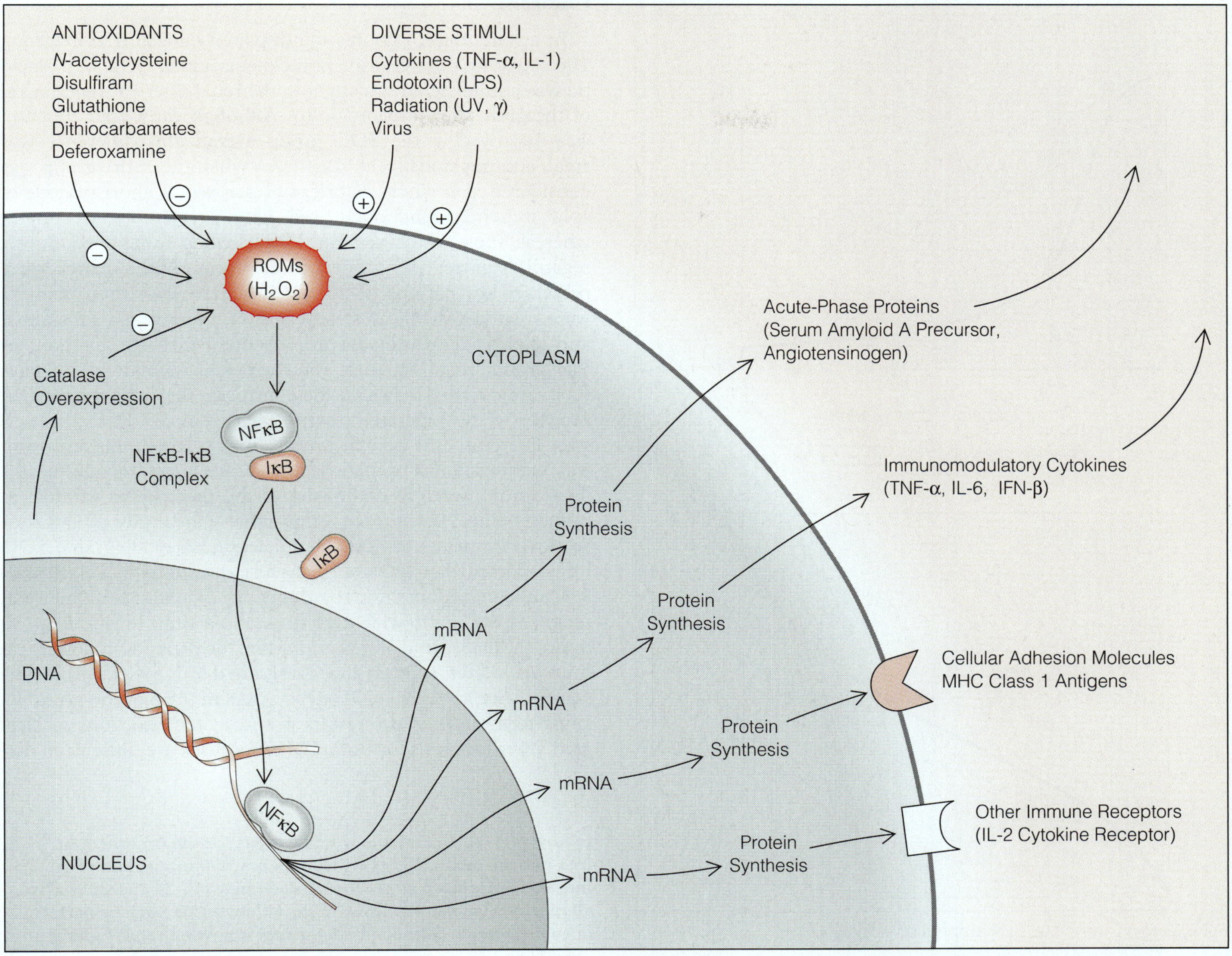

Figure 13 The transcription factor NFκB is activated by its dissociation from an associated inhibitor molecule, IκB, a process that is triggered by a number of disparate agents, including TNF-α, IL-1, and lipopolysaccharide (endotoxin); all of these agents act via the generation of ROMs, most likely H_2O_2. Activation of NFκB is blocked by antioxidants and can be blocked in cells that overexpress catalase. Once activated, NFκB translocates to the nucleus, binds DNA, and activates the transcription of a number of different mRNAs, which, via consequent protein synthesis, increase the expression of cytokines, acute-phase proteins, integrins, and other cell surface immune receptors. In this fashion, ROMs act in a physiologic role as second messengers to trigger gene expression within the cell.

The total injury sustained as a consequence of ischemia reflects the combined effects of ischemia itself and of reperfusion injury. After short periods of ischemia, the degree of injury caused by both ischemia and reperfusion may be so small as to be unmeasurable (and not important clinically); in such cases, ablation of reperfusion injury will have little or no measurable effect. After long ischemic periods, the injury caused by the ischemia itself may be so overwhelming that prevention of the reperfusion injury would have no measurable or clinically meaningful effect. There is, however, a defined period of ischemia after which the major portion of the total injury sustained can be attributed to a preventable reperfusion component rather than to the ischemia itself. This period has been termed the therapeutic window.[171] The clinical relevance of the ablation of reperfusion injury depends fundamentally on the relative size of this therapeutic window. The varying tolerances of different organs to ischemia suggests that the size of this window may be quite variable; this may account for some of the striking discrepancies in the apparent efficacy of free radical ablation reported in the literature. Unfortunately, the size of this window appears to be somewhat organ specific and situation specific and not very amenable to therapeutic manipulation. At present, it places a theoretical upper limit on the efficacy of free radical ablation for the treatment of postischemic injury. This concept is supported by the observation that increasing doses or combinations of different scavengers (all quite nontoxic) have usually failed to further improve outcomes.[171]

Clinical Trials

In a randomized, double-blind, paired clinical trial involving 100 cadaveric renal transplant recipients, either SOD or a placebo was administered directly into the renal artery at reperfusion of the graft after implantation.[11] Although early graft function was improved in the SOD group overall, this difference was small and not statistically significant when the entire group was considered as a whole. Kidneys preserved for short periods of cold ischemia functioned well with or without treatment, whereas those preserved for long periods functioned poorly regardless of treatment. Forty-three percent of the kidneys were preserved for periods of 25 to 28 hours; when these kidneys were treated with SOD at reperfusion, there was a substantial and statistically significant improvement in early function. In this group, renal function returned at a median of six days (compared with 13 days in the control group), and the median number of postoperative dialyses was reduced from three to one. Therefore, the benefit produced by SOD in this subgroup was highly significant statistically, clinically, and economically. This study therefore demonstrates the therapeutic window in human beings. In a subsequent double-blind study of 180 consecutive recipients of human cadaveric kidney allografts, SOD infusion immediately before reperfusion resulted in a statistically significant reduction in the frequency of acute renal failure in recipients of grafts with a cold ischemia time longer than 30 hours.[172] Data from this same group of patients, followed up four years later, showed that the grafted kidneys survived substantially longer in the SOD group than in the placebo group.[173] Long-term graft failure results from chronic rejection, accelerated atherosclerosis, or both; the two causes are difficult to dis-

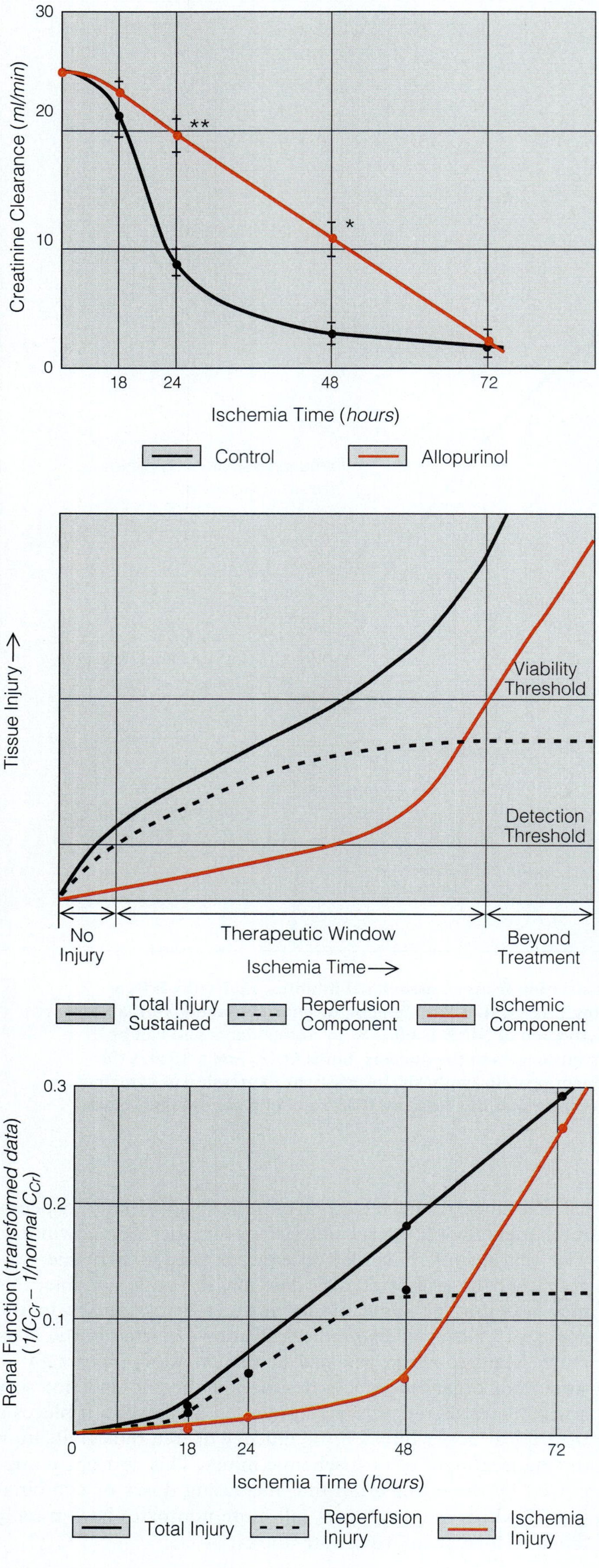

Figure 14 A therapeutic window exists for the treatment of free radical–mediated reperfusion injury. Posttransplant renal function (expressed as creatinine clearance [C_{Cr}]) was studied in allopurinol-treated and control pig kidneys after various periods of cold ischemia. Although allopurinol improved renal function after 24 and 48 hours of cold ischemia (top graph), kidneys subjected to only 18 hours of cold ischemia functioned well, and kidneys subjected to 72 hours of cold ischemia functioned poorly, regardless of therapy (*$P < 0.05$ vs. controls; **$P < 0.01$ vs. controls).

The total injury sustained by an organ during a period of hypoperfusion can be divided into two components: that caused by ischemia and that caused by ROMs generated during reperfusion (middle graph). Each component begins at the onset of ischemia. Initially, neither component is substantial enough to cause measurable injury. As ischemia progresses, the reperfusion component itself appears fixed and may account for as much as two thirds of the total injury sustained. Eventually, however, a point is reached where the ischemic component itself becomes so large that it precludes viability and therefore overwhelms (and renders unmeasurable) the reperfusion component. Only during the therapeutic window will free radical ablation have a substantial beneficial effect on the total postischemic injury.

The actual magnitudes of the two components of postischemic injury can be assessed (bottom graph). Tissue injury has been defined as $1/C_{Cr} - 1/C_{Cr}$ (normal). The data from the top graph have been transformed here. The total injury curve represents the results in the control kidneys. The ischemic injury curve represents the results in the allopurinol-treated kidneys. The reperfusion injury curve was calculated by subtracting ischemic injury from total injury. Note that these empirical data correspond closely to the theoretical curve shown in the middle graph.[170]

tinguish histologically. It is conceivable that SOD, in suppressing endothelial injury at reperfusion, is also inhibiting antigen presentation, thereby reducing graft immunogenicity. If so, such inhibition could explain how a brief period of exposure to an antioxidant at the time of transplantation could result in significant differences in graft survival several years later. Extremely exciting data from a similarly designed and controlled multicenter trial of 400 patients indicate that xanthine oxidase inhibition with allopurinol in the preservation solution substantially and significantly reduced the early incidence both of acute renal failure and of death associated with renal failure.[12]

Other Free Radical–Mediated Human Disease Processes

Although a detailed discussion of all the disease processes in which free radicals have been implicated is beyond the scope of this chapter, some of these processes are particularly representative of free radical–mediated pathology or have particular relevance to circulatory shock.

CENTRAL NERVOUS SYSTEM TOXICITY

Oxidative stress has been implicated in a number of neurodegenerative diseases. Familial amyotrophic lateral sclerosis (ALS, also known as Lou Gehrig's disease), an ultimately lethal degenerative disease of motor neurons in the spinal cord, is associated with several mutations of the gene coding for $Cu^{2+}Zn^{2+}$ SOD.[174] Decreases in SOD activity can result in damage as a result of the action of O_2^- or one of its products (e.g., OH·). Alternatively, increases in SOD activity, which some of these patients manifest, can be cytotoxic by increasing the formation of H_2O_2 or peroxynitrite. Peroxynitrite can react with SOD to form nitrate tyrosine residues. This reaction may be relevant to ALS, in that a number of neurotrophic molecules bind to receptor tyrosine kinases on motor neurons.[175] Moreover, abnormal phosphorylation of neurofilaments by nitrated tyrosine kinases can impair their abnormal assembly and distribution.[176]

Evidence continues to accumulate suggesting that oxidant stress is an important component of Parkinson's disease: increased lipid peroxidation and decreased glutathione reductase activity have been demonstrated in the substantia nigra of affected patients, and decreased activity of NADH-coenzyme Q reductase (complex 1 of the respiratory chain) has been demonstrated in the substantia nigra and platelets of parkinsonian patients.[177] MPTP (1-methyl-4-phenyl-1,2,3,6-tetrahydropyridine), a neurotoxin that induces parkinsonism in humans, is taken up into cells of the dopaminergic nigrostriatal pathway, where it is metabolized to its toxic metabolite, the MPP+ free radical,[177] which may cause toxicity either directly or indirectly through the generation of secondary ROMs via redox cycling. MPP+ also inhibits complex 1 activity in mitochondria, thereby causing increased superoxide generation.[178] Additional evidence for the role of oxidants in Parkinson's disease and MPTP toxicity has been provided by a study involving transgenic mice that overexpress the human *SOD-1* gene and show resistance to MPTP toxicity.[179]

There is also strong evidence linking free radical–mediated injury to Alzheimer's disease. In one study in which brain sections from Alzheimer's patients and control patients were subjected to immunohistochemical staining with anti-SOD and anti-catalase antibodies, staining was observed in 15 to 25 percent of neurofibrillary tangles (cytoskeletal accumulations prominent in Alzheimer's disease) in the Alzheimer's group, in contrast with negligible staining of tangle-free neurons in the Alzheimer's group and in the control group.[164] It is unclear whether oxidative stress precedes or follows the injury seen in Alzheimer's disease; a more precise mechanism for the involvement of ROMs remains to be established. (Given that virtually any cellular injury evokes an inflammatory response, it is not surprising to see evidence for free radical–mediated tissue injury in many pathological conditions. For each condition, it will be important to establish precisely what role or roles ROMs play, whether as causes, consequences, or even epiphenomena.[180])

OXYGEN TOXICITY

Adults can tolerate ventilation with 100 percent oxygen (at 1 atm) for 24 to 48 hours without sustaining lung injury, but extended periods of such exposure have long been known to cause severe pulmonary injury that can lead to death.[18,181,182] Changes in the metabolic activity of pulmonary endothelial cells may precede the earliest detectable morphological changes,[183] which include evidence of endothelial cell injury associated with interstitial edema, followed by the accumulation of platelets and then neutrophils in the pulmonary vasculature.[184] As lung water accumulates, gas exchange is impaired. In some cases, progressive fibrosis subsequently results.

Extensive evidence implicates a pathogenic role for ROMs in this condition. Both the NADH dehydrogenase complex and the ubiquinone–cytochrome b complex of the mitochondrial respiratory chain are responsible for the increased generation of superoxide anions, hydrogen peroxide, and subsequent metabolites as this system is overwhelmed by the excess ambient concentrations of oxygen. Elevated concentrations of these oxidants have been observed in pulmonary cell cytoplasm, nuclear membranes,[185] microsomes, and mitochondria.[186] Attracted, adherent, and diapedetic neutrophils can cause further injury by the generation of both ROMs and proteases. Neutrophil depletion, however, can decrease[187] but not prevent[188] such hyperoxic lung injury.

Immature animals have increased tolerance to increased oxygen concentrations; this greater tolerance is associated with an enhanced ability to induce production of SOD and glutathione peroxidase within 24 hours of exposure to 100 percent oxygen. Moreover, after preliminary exposure to a sublethal concentration (85 percent) of oxygen, rats can subsequently survive pure oxygen; these conditioned animals have been found to have increased levels of superoxide dismutase in their lungs.[18] When SOD and catalase are encapsulated in liposomes to allow passage across cell membranes, they afford protection against oxygen toxicity in experimental models.[189,190] However, no appropriately controlled studies have yet demonstrated convincingly that oxygen radical–scavenging agents can influence the course of human pulmonary oxygen toxicity.

ACUTE RESPIRATORY DISTRESS SYNDROME

Acute respiratory distress syndrome (ARDS) is characterized, at least in part, by pulmonary edema that results from increased vascular permeability. ARDS is often associated with widespread systemic disease and with a high overall mortality. It has been hypothesized that neutrophil recruitment to the lung and the subsequent release of toxic neutrophil products, including ROMs, result in the pathophysiological changes seen in ARDS. In an isolated, perfused lung model,[191] vascular permeability increased when neutrophils and phorbol myristate acetate (a stimulator of the respiratory burst of neutrophils) were infused together into the pulmonary circulation but not when either was infused separately. The increase in vascular permeability was reproduced with enzyme-substrate combinations that produced radicals and was inhibited by free radical scavengers.[192]

Despite these and other studies, the precise role of the neutrophil in ARDS is not clear.[193] ARDS can occur in patients with severe sepsis and neutropenia.[194] Clearly, other factors may also play a role in the pathogenesis of this syndrome, perhaps utilizing neutrophils to amplify, but not initiate, microvasculature endothelial cell injury.[19]

SHOCK

The effect of exogenous agents for free radical ablation after hemorrhagic or septic shock has been studied in animals. Dogs pretreated with allopurinol showed increased survival after hemorrhagic shock, but administration of allopurinol during shock failed to improve survival.[195] Administration of SOD plus catalase early in a 60-minute episode of hemorrhagic shock was found to improve postresuscitation cardiac function.[196] However, administration of these two agents at the end of either one hour or two hours of hemorrhagic shock had no beneficial effect on myocardial function during either the shock or the resuscitation phase of the experiment; these results may reflect a small canine myocardial therapeutic window.[197]

Studies of the role of free radicals in septic shock have also produced mixed results in animal models.[198-201] In many shock studies, free radical ablation improved apparent early organ function without affecting ultimate mortality; this finding has been referred to by Arfors and Rutili as the "cosmetic effect of SOD." In particular, administration of radical inhibitors after the initiation of shock has generally failed to improve survival. Although ROMs undoubtedly play an important role in mortality and morbidity from shock, the relatively simplistic approach of administering a scavenger and recording gross outcome (i.e., death) in experimental models of shock fails to address the precise mechanism of injury. Moreover, until such studies reproducibly vary the degree and duration of the shock state to help define a therapeutic window and look more precisely at specific components of the complex shock state, we can expect to continue to see apparently conflicting reports of positive and negative effects.

MULTIPLE ORGAN DYSFUNCTION SYNDROME

Multiple organ dysfunction syndrome affects a wide variety of critically ill or injured patients, often after initially successful resuscitation from a severe physiologic insult [see 95 Multiple Organ Dysfunction Syndrome]. The inciting agents that subsequently lead to MODS are local injury from trauma, infection, or hypoperfusion, often in combination.[202] A local inflammatory response subsequently occurs, probably as a result of endothelial injury, platelet activation, the release of inflammatory mediators, and activation of the clotting cascade. As a result, the complement, coagulation, and kallikrein systems are all activated, leading to the development of a hyperinflammatory state and a hypermetabolic state, with a marked increase in oxygen consumption and, therefore, demand. While some of this increased oxygen consumption reflects the hypermetabolism itself, some appears to reflect increased superoxide generation as well. The lung is often the first organ to fail, producing ARDS and resulting in prolonged ventilator dependence. Failure of the kidneys, the immune system, the GI tract, and the liver follows, resulting ultimately in sepsis, cardiovascular collapse, and death.

There is increasing evidence that the GI tract plays a central role in the initiation and maintenance of MODS. The breakdown of the gastrointestinal mucosal barrier creates a portal for systemic entry of bacteria (so-called bacterial translocation[193,203]), endotoxin, and other luminal factors that may contribute to a systemic inflammatory response and distant organ injury. Of the proposed triggers for MODS, ischemia and ensuing reperfusion injury to the superficial gut mucosal barrier seems a particularly good candidate. Patients subjected to circulatory shock, hypoxia, sepsis, and other initial forms of severe physiologic stress may sustain a mild, otherwise subclinical level of nonocclusive ischemia of the gut that usually does not progress to frank transmural bowel infarction. Although not recognized clinically as the classic syndrome of intestinal ischemia, this may result in the necrosis of the superficial mucosa, with consequent loss of epithelial barrier function. Indeed, such lesions have long been recognized in critically ill patients at autopsy, but they are often signed out by the pathologist as autolysis and not recognized to be an antemortem change.

Once gut barrier function is lost, the translocation of bacteria—and perhaps of other luminal toxins as well—is facilitated. In rats that have been subjected to hemorrhagic shock and resuscitation, this full sequence of events is seen and is prevented by pretreatment with allopurinol, which suggests that free radicals generated from xanthine oxidase at reperfusion play an important role.[204] Unfortunately, it is not currently known whether it is bacteria, toxins, or digestive enzymes themselves that mediate the systemic injury or whether these agents merely trigger the secondary release of inflammatory mediators (or of xanthine oxidase itself) from the gut, the liver, or elsewhere. In any case, the initial loss of this mucosal epithelial barrier function provides a sound pathophysiological basis for the concept that "the gut is the motor of multiple organ failure."[205]

Summary

The extreme toxicity of free radicals was once thought to make their endogenous generation by living organisms inconsistent with those organisms' evolution and survival. ROMs are now known to be generated continuously by a wide variety of normal metabolic processes throughout the cell and to constitute important components of numerous pathological and even physiologic processes. The ubiquity and importance of free radical toxicity can be inferred from the high concentration and wide distribution of endogenous free radical scavengers and other antioxidants in biologic systems. For example, the enzymes in highest concentration within erythrocytes are SOD, catalase, and glutathione peroxidase. Moreover, the amino acid sequences of endogenous scavengers such as SOD have been highly conserved throughout the evolution of eukaryotic species.[94]

ROMs play a direct role in the tissue damage caused by reperfusion and inflammation. Free radical–mediated processes are among the more important final common pathways of tissue injury in biologic systems, appearing whenever the balance between free radical generation and endogenous scavenging capabilities is disrupted. Although the mechanisms of free radical–mediated injury in some pathophysiological states are still unclear, future investigation will provide a better understanding of the exact role of ROMs in these disease processes. Once the quantitative impact of free radical–mediated injury in a specific pathophysiological state is ascertained with particular cognizance of the therapeutic window, free radical mechanisms may be selectively modified therapeutically to prevent tissue injury at its most basic level. Successful early clinical trials suggest that this remarkable potential for therapeutic benefit has begun to be realized.

References

1. Del Maestro RF: The influence of oxygen derived free radicals on in vitro and in vivo model systems. Acta Univ Upsaliensis 340:32, 1979
2. Gilbert DL: Speculation on the relationship between organic and atmospheric evolution. Perspectives Biol Med 4:58, 1960
3. Babior BM: The respiratory burst of phagocytes. J Clin Invest 73:599, 1984
4. Miyazaki T, Sueoka K, Dharmarajan AM, et al: Effect of inhibition of oxygen free radical on ovulation and progesterone production by the in vitro perfused rabbit ovary. J Reprod Fertil 91:207, 1991
5. Granger DN, Rutili G, McCord JM: Superoxide radicals in feline intestinal ischemia. Gastroenterology 81:22, 1981
6. Adkison D, Hollwarth ME, Benoit JN, et al: Role of free radicals in ischemia-reperfusion injury to the liver. Acta Physiol Scand Suppl 548:101, 1986
7. Sanfey H, Sarr MG, Bulkley GB, et al: Oxygen-derived free radicals and acute pancreatitis: a review. Acta Physiol Scand Suppl 126:109, 1986
8. Perry MA, Wadhwa S, Parks DA, et al: Role of oxygen radicals in ischemia-induced lesions in the cat stomach. Gastroenterology 90:362, 1986
9. Chambers DE, Parks DA, Patterson G, et al: Role of oxygen derived free radicals in myocardial ischemia. Fed Proc 42:1093, 1983
10. Davis RJ, Bulkley GB, Traystman RJ: Role of oxygen free radicals in focal brain ischemia. Fed Proc 46:799, 1987
11. Schneeberger H, Illner WD, Abendroth D, et al: First clinical experiences with superoxide dismutase in kidney transplantation—results of a double-blind randomized study. Transplant Proc 21:1245, 1989
12. Marshall VC, Biguzas M, Jablonski P, et al: UW solution for kidney preservation. Transplant Proc 22:496, 1990
13. England MD, Cavarocchi NC, O'Brien JF, et al: Influence of antioxidants (mannitol and allopurinol) on oxygen free radical generation during and after cardiopulmonary bypass. Circulation 74(suppl III):III-134, 1986
14. Johnson WD, Kayser KL, Brenowitz JB, et al: A randomized controlled trial of allopurinol in coronary bypass surgery. Am Heart J 121:20, 1991
15. Biaglow JE: Oxygen, hydrogen donors and radiation response. Hyperthermia. Bicher HI, Bruley DF, Eds. Plenum Press, New York, 1982, p 147
16. Shaw S, Jayatilleke E: The role of cellular oxidases and catalytic iron in the pathogenesis of ethanol-induced liver injury. Life Sci 50:2045, 1992
17. Crapo JD, Tierney DF: Superoxide dismutase and pulmonary oxygen toxicity. Am J Physiol 226:1401, 1974
18. Swank DW, Moore SB: Role of the neutrophil and other mediators in adult respiratory distress syndrome. Mayo Clin Proc 64:1118, 1989
19. Green MJ, Hill HAD: Chemistry of dioxygen. Methods in Enzymology, Vol 105. Packer L, Ed. Academic Press, Orlando, Florida, 1984, p 3
20. Fee JA, Valentine JS: Chemical and physical properties of superoxide. Superoxide and Superoxide Dismutase. Michelson AM, McCord JM, Fridovich I, Eds. Academic Press, New York, 1977, p 19
21. Michelson AM: Toxic effects of active oxygen. Biochemical and Medical Aspects of Active Oxygen. Hayaishi O, Asada K, Eds. University Park Press, Baltimore, 1977, p 155
22. Anderson JG, Toohey DW, Brune WH: Free radicals within the antarctic vortex: the role of CFCs in antarctic ozone loss. Science 251:39, 1991
23. Boveris A, Chance B: The mitochondrial generation of hydrogen peroxide: general properties and effect of hyperbaric oxygen. Biochem J 134:707, 1973
24. Turrens JF, Boveris A: Generation of superoxide anion by the NADH dehydrogenase of bovine heart mitochondria. Biochem J 191:421, 1980
25. McCord JM, Fridovich I: The reduction of cytochrome c by milk xanthine oxidase. J Biol Chem 243:5753, 1968
26. Rauckman EJ, Rosen GM, Kitchell BB: Superoxide radical as an intermediate in the oxidation of hydroxylamines by mixed function amine oxidases. Mol Pharmacol 15:131, 1979
27. McCord JM, Fridovich I: Superoxide dismutase: an enzymic function for erythrocuprein (hemocuprein). J Biol Chem 244:6049, 1969
28. Waud WR, Rajagopalan KV: Purification and properties of the NAD^+-dependent (type D) and O_2-dependent (type O) forms of rat liver xanthine dehydrogenase. Arch Biochem Biophys 172:354, 1976
29. Parks DA, Granger DN: Xanthine oxidase: biochemistry, distribution, and physiology. Acta Physiol Scand Suppl 548:87, 1986
30. Battelli MG, Della Corte E, Stirpe F: Xanthine oxidase type d (dehydrogenase) in the intestine and other organs of the rat. Biochem J 126:747, 1972
31. McCord JM, Roy RS: The pathophysiology of superoxide: roles in inflammation and ischemia. Can J Physiol Pharmacol 60:1346, 1982
32. Parks DA, Williams TK, Beckman JS: Conversion of xanthine dehydrogenase to oxidase in ischemic rat intestine: a reevaluation. Am J Physiol 254:G768, 1988
33. Bulkley GB: Endothelial xanthine oxidase: a radical transducer of inflammatory signals for reticuloendothelial activation. Br J Surg 80:684, 1993
34. Samuelsson B: Leukotrienes: mediators of immediate hypersensitivity reactions and inflammation. Science 220:568, 1983
35. Kuehl FA, Humes J, Torchiana ML, et al: Oxygen-centered radicals in inflammatory processes. Adv Inflam Res 1:419, 1979
36. Kukreja RC, Kontos HA, Hess ML, et al: PGH synthase and lipoxygenase generate superoxide in the presence of NADH or NADPH. Circ Res 59:612, 1986
37. Freeman BA, Crapo JD: Biology of disease: free radicals and tissue injury. Lab Invest 47:412, 1982
38. Biemond P, van Eijk HG, Swaak AJ, et al: Iron mobilization from ferritin by superoxide derived from stimulated polymorphonuclear leukocytes: possible mechanism in inflammation diseases. J Clin Invest 73:1576, 1984
39. Koppenol WH: The reaction of ferrous EDTA with hydrogen peroxide: evidence against hydroxyl radical formation. J Free Radic Biol Med 1:281, 1985
40. Parks DA, Granger DN: Ischemia-induced vascular changes: role of xanthine oxidase and hydroxyl radicals. Am J Physiol 245:G285, 1983
41. Hernandez LA, Grisham MB, Granger DN: A role for iron in oxidant-mediated ischemic injury to intestinal microvasculature. Am J Physiol 253:G49, 1987
42. Babior BM: Oxygen-dependent microbial killing by phagocytes (pts 1 & 2). N Engl J Med 298:659, 721, 1978
43. Klebanoff SJ: Oxygen metabolism and the toxic properties of phagocytes. Ann Intern Med 93:480, 1980
44. Klebanoff SJ: Phagocytic cells: products of oxygen metabolism. Inflammation: Basic Principles and Clinical Correlates. Gallin JI, Goldstein IM, Snyder R, Eds. Raven Press, New York, 1988, p 391
45. Grisham MB, Jefferson MM, Melton DF, et al: Chlorination of endogenous amines by isolated neutrophils: ammonia-dependent bactericidal, cytotoxic, and cytolytic activities of the chloramines. J Biol Chem 259:10404, 1984
46. Weiss SJ: Tissue destruction by neutrophils. N Engl J Med 320:365, 1989
47. Grisham MB, Jefferson MM, Thomas EL: Role of monochloramine in the oxidation of erythrocyte hemoglobin by stimulated neutrophils. J Biol Chem 259:6757, 1984
48. Tauber AI, Borregaard N, Simons E, et al: Chronic granulomatous disease: a syndrome of phagocyte oxidase deficiencies. Medicine (Baltimore) 62:286, 1983
49. Gross SS, Stuehr DJ, Aisaka K, et al: Macrophage and endothelial cell nitric oxide synthesis: cell type selective inhibition by N^G-aminoarginine, N^G-nitroarginine and N^G-methylarginine. Biochem Biophys Res Commun 170:96, 1990
50. Moncada S, Palmer RM, Higgs EA: Nitric oxide: physiology, pathophysiology and pharmacology. Pharmacol Rev 43:109, 1991
51. Furchgott RF, Zawadzki JV: The obligatory role of endothelial cells in the relaxation of arterial smooth muscle by acetylcholine. Nature 288:373, 1980
52. Katsuki S, Arnold W, Mittal C, et al: Stimulation of guanylate cyclase by sodium nitroprusside, nitroglycerin and nitric oxide in various tissue preparations and comparison to the effects of sodium azide and hydroxylamine. J Cyclic Nucleotide Res 3:23, 1977
53. Vallance P, Collier J, Moncada S: Effects of endothelium-derived nitric oxide on peripheral arteriolar tone in man. Lancet 2:997, 1989
54. Brookes SJH: Neuronal nitric oxide in the gut. J Gastroenterology Hepatology 8:590, 1993
55. Grozdanovic Z, Bruning G, Baumgarten HG: Nitric oxide—a novel autonomic neurotransmitter. Acta Anat 150:16, 1994

56. Ignarro LJ: Biosynthesis and metabolism of endothelium-derived nitric oxide. Annu Rev Pharmacol Toxicol 30:532, 1991
57. Beckman JS, Beckman TW, Chen J, et al: Apparent hydroxyl radical production by peroxynitrite: implications for endothelial injury from nitric oxide and superoxide. Proc Natl Acad Sci USA 87:1620, 1990
58. Li LM, Kilbourn RG, Adams J, et al: Role of nitric oxide in lysis of tumor cells by cytokine-activated endothelial cells. Cancer Res 51:2531, 1991
59. Cohen GM, Doherty M: Free radical mediated cell toxicity by redox cycling chemicals. Br J Cancer 55(suppl VIII):46, 1987
60. Ledwith A: Electron transfer reactions of paraquat. Biochemical Mechanisms of Paraquat Toxicity. Autor AP, Ed. Academic Press, New York, 1977, p 21
61. Powis G: Free radical formation by antitumor quinones. Free Radic Biol Med 6:63, 1989
62. Lyons MJ, Gibson JF, Ingram DJE: Free radicals produced in cigarette smoke. Nature 181:1003, 1958
63. Reynolds ES, Ree HJ: Liver parenchymal cell injury: VII. Membrane denaturation following carbon tetrachloride. Lab Invest 25:269, 1971
64. Hall EJ: Radiobiology for the Radiologist. Harper and Row, Publishers, Hagerstown, Maryland, 1973
65. Southorn PA, Powis G: Free radicals in medicine: II. Involvement in human disease. Mayo Clin Proc 63:390, 1988
66. Oberley LW, Sierra E: Radiation sensitivity testing of cultured eukaryotic cells. CRC Handbook of Methods for Oxygen Radical Research. Greenwald RA, Ed. CRC Press, Boca Raton, Florida, 1985, p 417
67. Fantone JC, Ward PA: Oxygen-Derived Radicals and Their Metabolites: Relationship to Tissue Injury. The Upjohn Company, Kalamazoo, Michigan, 1985
68. Mead JF: Free radical mechanisms of lipid damage and consequences for cellular membranes. Free Radicals in Biology. Pryor WA, Ed. Academic Press, New York, 1976, p 51
69. Southorn PA, Powis G: Free radicals in medicine: I. Chemical nature and biologic reactions. Mayo Clin Proc 63:381, 1988
70. Del Maestro RF: An approach to free radicals in medicine and biology. Acta Physiol Scand Suppl 492:153, 1980
71. Bresnick E, Bailey G, Bonney RJ, et al: Phospholipase activity in skin after application of phorbol esters and 3-methylcholanthrene. Carcinogenesis 2:1119, 1981
72. Fucci L, Oliver CN, Coon MJ, et al: Inactivation of key metabolic enzymes by mixed-function oxidation reactions: possible implication in protein turnover and ageing. Proc Natl Acad Sci USA 80:1521, 1983
73. Kim K, Rhee SG, Stadtman ER: Nonenzymatic cleavage of proteins by reactive oxygen species generated by dithiothreitol and iron. J Biol Chem 260:15394, 1985
74. Chio KS, Tappel AL: Inactivation of ribonuclease and other enzymes by peroxidizing lipids and by malonaldehyde. Biochemistry 8:2827, 1969
75. Oliver CN, Ahn BW, Moerman EJ, et al: Age-related changes in oxidized proteins. J Biol Chem 262:5488, 1987
76. Oliver CN, Fulks R, Levine RL, et al: Oxidative inactivation of key metabolic enzymes during aging. Molecular Basis of Aging. Roy AK, Chatterjee B, Eds. Academic Press, New York, 1984, p 400
77. Tappel AL: Lipid peroxidation damage to cell components. Fed Proc 32:1870, 1973
78. Kunimoto M, Inoue K, Nojima S: Effect of ferrous ion and ascorbate-induced lipid peroxidation on liposomal membranes. Biochem Biophys Acta 646:169, 1981
79. Jones DP, Thor H, Smith MT, et al: Inhibition of ATP-dependent microsomal Ca^{2+} sequestration during oxidative stress and its prevention by glutathione. J Biol Chem 258:6390, 1983
80. Imlay JA, Linn S: DNA damage and oxygen radical toxicity. Science 240:1302, 1988
81. Balazs EA, Davies JV, Phillips GO, et al: Transient intermediates in the radiolysis of hyaluronic acid. Radiat Res 31:243, 1967
82. Del Maestro RF, Arfors KE, Lindblom R: Free radical depolymerization of hyaluronic acid: influence of scavenger substances. 10th Europ Conf Microcirc. Lewis DH, Ed. Karger Press, Basel, Switzerland, 1979, p 132
83. Greenwald RA, Moy WW: Inhibition of collagen gelation by action of the superoxide radical. Arthritis Rheum 22:251, 1979
84. Sundblad L, Balazs EA: Chemical and physical changes of glycosaminoglycans and glycoproteins caused by oxidation-reduction systems and radiation. The Amino Sugars. Balazs EA, Jeanloz RW, Eds. Academic Press, New York, 1966, p 229
85. Bjork J, Del Maestro RF, Arfors KE: Evidence for participation of hydroxyl radical in increased microvascular permeability. AAS 7:208, 1980
86. Wood KA, Youle RJ: Apoptosis and free radicals. Ann NY Acad Sci 738:400, 1994
87. Hockenbery DM, Oltvai ZN, Yin XM, et al: Bcl-2 functions in an antioxidant pathway to prevent apoptosis. Cell 75:241, 1993
88. Veis DJ, Sorenson CM, Shutter JR, et al: Bcl-2-deficient mice demonstrate fulminant lymphoid apoptosis, polycystic kidneys, and hypopigmented hair. Cell 75:229, 1993
89. Abello PA, Fidler SA, Bulkley GB, et al: Antioxidants modulate induction of programmed endothelial cell death (apoptosis) by endotoxin. Arch Surg 129:134, 1994
90. Dormandy TL: Free-radical oxidation and antioxidants. Lancet 1:647, 1978
91. Aust SD, Morehouse LA, Thomas CE: Role of metals in oxygen radical reactions. J Free Radic Biol Med 1:3, 1985
92. Bulkley GB: Evaluating oxidant or antioxidant status: an editorial comment. Shock 1:313, 1994
93. Touati D: Molecular genetics of superoxide dismutases. Free Radic Biol Med 5:393, 1988
94. Fridovich I: The biology of oxygen radicals. Science 201:875, 1978
95. Forman HJ, Fisher AB: Antioxidant defenses. Oxygen and Living Processes: An Interdisciplinary Approach. Gilbert DL, Ed. Springer-Verlag, New York, 1981, p 235
96. Flohe L: Glutathione peroxidase brought into focus. Free Radicals in Biology, Vol IV. Pryor WA, Ed. Academic Press, New York, 1980, p 223
97. Li GS, Wang F, Kang D, et al: Keshan disease: an endemic cardiomyopathy in China. Hum Pathol 16:602, 1985
98. Yang GQ: Selenium-deficiency and endemic Keshan disease in China. Proceedings XIII Int Cong Nutrition 1985. Taylor TG, Jenkins NK, Eds. John Libbey, London, 1986, p 124
99. Witting LA: Vitamin E and lipid antioxidants in free-radical initiated reactions. Free Radicals in Biology, Vol IV. Pryor WA, Ed. Academic Press, New York, 1980, p 295
100. Grisham MB, McCord JM: Chemistry and cytotoxicity of reactive oxygen metabolites. Physiology of Oxygen Radicals. Taylor AE, Matalon S, Ward P, Eds. American Physiological Society, Bethesda, Maryland, 1986, p 1
101. Gaziano JM, Manson JE, Ridker PM, et al: Beta carotene therapy for chronic stable angina. Circulation 82(suppl III):III-201, 1990
102. Packer JE, Slater TF, Willson RL: Direct observation of a free radical interaction between vitamin E and vitamin C. Nature 278:737, 1979
103. Niki E: Antioxidant compounds. Free Radic Biol Med 9(suppl 1):9, 1990
104. Wasil M, Halliwell B, Hutchinson DC, et al: The antioxidant action of human extracellular fluids: effect of human serum and its protein components on the inactivation of alpha 1-antiproteinase by hypochlorous acid and by hydrogen peroxide. Biochem J 243:219, 1987
105. Demple B: Oxidative stress genes and proteins. Free Radic Biol Med 9(suppl):1, 1990
106. Wiese AG, Pacifici RE, Davies KJA: Transient adaptation to oxidative stress in mammalian cells. Arch Biochem Biophys 318:231, 1995
107. Bernstein C, Johns V: Sexual reproduction as a response to H_2O_2 damage in Schizosaccharomyces pombe. J Bacteriol 171:1893, 1989
108. Bernstein H, Hopf FA, Michod RE: The molecular basis of the evolution of sex. Adv Genet 24:323, 1987
109. Bulkley GB: Reactive oxygen metabolites and reperfusion injury: aberrant triggering of reticuloendothelial function. Lancet 344:934, 1994
110. Parks DA, Bulkley GB, Granger DN, et al: Ischemic injury in the cat small intestine: role of superoxide radicals. Gastroenterology 82:9, 1982
111. Granger DN, Hollwarth ME, Parks DA: Ischemia-reperfusion injury: role of oxygen-derived free radicals. Acta Physiol Scand Suppl 548:47, 1986
112. Granger DN: Role of xanthine oxidase and granulocytes in ischemia-reperfusion injury. Am J Physiol 255:H1269, 1988
113. Parks DA, Granger DN, Bulkley GB, et al: Soybean trypsin inhibitor attenuates ischemic injury to the feline small intestine. Gastroenterology 89:6, 1985
114. McKelvey TG, Hollwarth ME, Granger DN, et al: Mechanisms of conversion of xanthine dehydrogenase to xanthine oxidase in ischemic rat liver and kidney. Am J Physiol 254:G753, 1988
115. Hernandez LA, Grisham MB, Twohig B, et al: Role of neutrophils in ischemia-reperfusion-induced microvascular injury. Am J Physiol 253:H699, 1987
116. Kubes P, Ibbotson G, Russell J, et al: Role of platelet-activating factor in ischemia/reperfusion-induced leukocyte adherence. Am J Physiol 259:G300, 1990
117. Ratych RE, Chuknyiska RS, Bulkley GB: The primary localization of free radical generation after anoxia/reoxygenation in isolated endothelial cells. Surgery 102:122, 1987
118. Sarr MG, Bulkley GB, Cameron JL: The role of leukocytes in the production of oxygen-derived free radicals in acute experimental pancreatitis. Surgery 101:292, 1987
119. Toung TJK, Sendak MJ, Rosenfeld BA, et al: Role of leukocytes in the proteolytic enzyme induced lung injury model. Anesthesiology 67:A646, 1987
120. Jones HP, Grisham MB, Bose SK, et al: Effect of allopurinol on neutrophil superoxide production, chemotaxis, or degranulation. Biochem Pharmacol 34:3673, 1985
121. Grisham MB, Hernandez LA, Granger DN: Xanthine oxidase and neutrophil infiltration in intestinal ischemia. Am J Physiol 251:G567, 1986
122. Itoh M, Guth PH: Role of oxygen-derived free radicals in hemorrhagic shock-induced gastric lesions in the rat. Gastroenterology 88:1162, 1985

123. Bailey RW, Bulkley GB, Hamilton SR, et al: The fundamental hemodynamic mechanism underlying gastric "stress ulceration" in cardiogenic shock. Ann Surg 205:597, 1987
124. Nordstrom G, Seeman T, Hasselgren PO: Beneficial effect of allopurinol in liver ischemia. Surgery 97:679, 1985
125. Warshaw AL, O'Hara PJ: Susceptibility of the pancreas to ischemic injury in shock. Ann Surg 188:197, 1978
126. Sanfey H, Bulkley GB, Cameron JL: The pathogenesis of acute pancreatitis: the source and role of oxygen-derived free radicals in three different experimental models. Ann Surg 201:633, 1985
127. Shlafer M, Kane PF, Kirsh MM: Superoxide dismutase plus catalase enhances the efficacy of hypothermic cardioplegia to protect the globally ischemic, reperfused heart. J Thorac Cardiovasc Surg 83:830, 1982
128. Rashid MA, William-Olsson G: Influence of allopurinol on cardiac complications in open heart operations. Ann Thorac Surg 52:127, 1991
129. Woodward B, Zakaria MN: Effect of some free radical scavengers on reperfusion induced arrhythmias in the isolated rat heart. J Mol Cell Cardiol 17:485, 1985
130. Manning AS, Coltart DJ, Hearse DJ: Ischemia and reperfusion-induced arrhythmias in the rat: effects of xanthine oxidase inhibition with allopurinol. Circ Res 55:545, 1984
131. Stewart JR, Crute SL, Loughlin V, et al: Prevention of free radical–induced myocardial reperfusion injury with allopurinol. J Thorac Cardiovasc Surg 90:68, 1985
132. Reimer KA, Jennings RB: Failure of the xanthine oxidase inhibitor allopurinol to limit infarct size after ischemia and reperfusion in dogs. Circulation 71:1069, 1985
133. Miura T, Yellon DM, Kingma J, et al: Protection afforded by allopurinol in the first 24 hours of coronary occlusion is diminished after 48 hours. Free Radic Biol Med 4:25, 1988
134. Eddy LJ, Stewart JR, Jones HP, et al: Free radical–producing enzyme, xanthine oxidase, is undetectable in human hearts. Am J Physiol 253:H709, 1987
135. Jarasch ED, Bruder G, Heid HW: Significance of xanthine oxidase in capillary endothelial cells. Acta Physiol Scand Suppl 548:39, 1986
136. Vickers S, Hildreth J, Kuhajda F, et al: Immunohistoaffinity localization of xanthine oxidase in the microvascular endothelial cells of porcine and human organs (abstr). Circ Shock 31:87, 1990
137. Lucchesi BR: Role of neutrophils in ischemic heart disease: pathophysiologic role in myocardial ischemia and coronary artery reperfusion. Cardiovasc Clin 18:35, 1987
138. Paller MS, Hoidal JR, Ferris TF: Oxygen free radicals in ischemic acute renal failure in the rat. J Clin Invest 74:1156, 1984
139. Marzella L, Jesudass RR, Manson PN, et al: Morphologic characterization of acute injury to vascular endothelium of skin after frostbite. Plast Reconstr Surg 83:67, 1989
140. Liu TH, Beckman JS, Freeman BA, et al: Polyethylene glycol-conjugated superoxide dismutase and catalase reduce ischemic brain injury. Am J Physiol 256:H589, 1989
141. Martz D, Rayos G, Schielke GP, et al: Allopurinol and dimethylthiourea reduce brain infarction following middle cerebral artery occlusion in rats. Stroke 20:488, 1989
142. Lindsay S, Liu TH, Xu J, et al: Role of xanthine dehydrogenase and oxidase in focal cerebral ischemic injury to rat. Am J Physiol 261:H2051, 1991
143. Cerchiari EL, Hoel TM, Safar P, et al: Protective effects of combined superoxide dismutase and deferoxamine on recovery of cerebral blood flow and function after cardiac arrest in dogs. Stroke 18:869, 1987
144. Hall ED: Free radicals and CNS injury. Crit Care Clin 5:793, 1989
145. Manson PN, Anthenelli RM, Im MJ, et al: The role of oxygen-free radicals in ischemic tissue injury in island skin flaps. Ann Surg 198:87, 1983
146. Im MJ, Shem WH, Pak CJ, et al: Effect of allopurinol on the survival of hyperemic island skin flaps. J Plast Reconstr Surg 73:276, 1984
147. Im MJ, Manson PN, Bulkley GB, et al: Effects of superoxide dismutase and allopurinol on the survival of acute island skin flaps. Ann Surg 201:357, 1985
148. Manson PN, Narayan KK, Im MJ, et al: Improved survival in free skin flap transfers in rats. Surgery 99:211, 1986
149. Korthuis RJ, Grisham MB, Granger DN: Leukocyte depletion attenuates vascular injury in postischemic skeletal muscle. Am J Physiol 254:H823, 1988
150. Korthuis RJ, Granger DN, Townsley MI, et al: The role of oxygen derived free radicals in ischemia-induced increases in canine skeletal muscle vascular permeability. Circ Res 57:599, 1985
151. Perler BA, Tohmeh AC, Bulkley GB: Inhibition of the compartment syndrome in post-ischemic skeletal muscle by free radical ablation at reperfusion. FASEB J 2:A1875, 1988
152. Marzella L, Jesudass RR, Manson PN, et al: Functional and structural evaluation of the vasculature of skin flaps after ischemia and reperfusion. Plast Reconstr Surg 81:742, 1988
153. Rice GE, Munro JM, Bevilacqua MP: Inducible cell adhesion molecule 110 (INCAM-110) is an endothelial receptor for lymphocytes: a CD11/CD18-independent adhesion mechanism. J Exp Med 171:1369, 1990
154. Granger DN, Kubes P: The microcirculation and inflammation: modulation of leukocyte–endothelial cell adhesion. J Leukoc Biol 55:662,1994
155. Suzuki M, Grisham MB, Granger DN: Superoxide plays a role in reperfusion-induced leukocyte adherence to microvascular endothelium. Gastroenterology 96:A497, 1989
156. Wennmalm A, Lanne B, Petersson AS: Detection of endothelial-derived relaxing factor in human plasma in the basal state and following ischemia using electron paramagnetic resonance spectrometry. Anal Biochem 187:359, 1990
157. Friedl HP, Till GO, Ryan US, et al: Mediator-induced activation of xanthine oxidase in endothelial cells. FASEB J 3:2512, 1989
158. Grisham MB, Granger DN: Free radicals: reactive metabolites of oxygen as mediators of postischemic reperfusion injury. Splanchnic Ischemia and Multiple Organ Failure. Marston A, Bulkley GB, Fiddian-Green RG, et al, Eds. Edward Arnold, London, 1989, p 135
159. Schreck R, Baeuerle PA: A role for oxygen radicals as second messengers. Trends in Cell Biology 1:39, 1991
160. Schreck R, Albermann K, Baeuerle PA: Nuclear factor κB: an oxidative stress-responsive transcription factor of eukaryotic cells (a review). Free Rad Res Commun 17:221, 1992
161. Schreck R, Rieber P, Baeuerle PA: Reactive oxygen intermediates as apparently widely used messengers in the activation of the NF-κB transcription factor and HIV-1. EMBO J 10:2247, 1991
162. Schmidt KN, Amstad P, Cerutti P, et al: The roles of hydrogen peroxide and superoxide as messengers in the activation of transcription factor NF-κB. Chemistry and Biology 2:13, 1995
163. Baeuerle PA: The inducible transcription activator NF-κB: regulation by distinct protein subunits. Biochim Biophys Acta 1072:63, 1991
164. Pappolla MA, Omar RA, Kim KS, et al: Immunohistochemical evidence of antioxidant stress in Alzheimer's disease. Am J Pathol 140:621, 1992
165. Minowada G, Welch WJ: Clinical implications of the stress response. J Clin Invest 95:3, 1995
166. Schoeniger LO, Reilly PM, Bulkley GB, et al: Heat shock gene expression excludes hepatic acute phase gene expression following resuscitation from hemorrhagic shock. Surgery 112:355, 1992
167. Schoeniger LO, Andreoni KA, Ott GR, et al: Induction of heat shock gene expression in the post-ischemic liver is dependent upon superoxide generation at reperfusion. Gastroenterology 106:177, 1994
168. Haglund U, Bulkley GB, Granger DN: On the pathophysiology of intestinal ischemia. Acta Chir Scand 153:321, 1987
169. Parks DA, Granger DN, Bulkley GB: Superoxide radicals and mucosal lesions of the ischemic small intestine. Fed Proc 41:1742, 1982
170. Hoshino T, Maley WR, Bulkley GB, et al: Ablation of free radical-mediated reperfusion injury for the salvage of kidneys taken from non-heart-beating donors: a quantitative evaluation of the proportion of injury caused by reperfusion following periods of warm, cold, and combined warm and cold ischemia. Transplantation 45:284, 1988
171. Koyama A, Bulkley GB, Williams GM, et al: The role of oxygen free radicals in mediating the reperfusion injury of cold-preserved ischemic kidneys. Transplantation 40:590, 1985
172. Schneeberger H, Schleibner S, Schilling M, et al: Prevention of acute renal failure after kidney transplantation by treatment with rh-SOD: interim analysis of a double-blind placebo-controlled trial. Transpl Proc 22:2224, 1990
173. Land W, Schneeberger H, Schleibner S, et al: The beneficial effect of human recombinant superoxide dismutase on acute and chronic rejection events in recipients of cadaveric renal transplants. Transplantation 57:211, 1994
174. Rosen DR, Siddique T, Patterson D, et al: Mutations in Cu/Zn superoxide dismutase gene are associated with familial amyotrophic lateral sclerosis. Nature 362:59, 1993
175. Olanow CW: A radical hypothesis for neurodegeneration. TINS 16:439, 1993
176. Beckman JS, Carson M, Smith CD, et al: ALS, SOD and peroxynitrite. Nature 364:584, 1993
177. Fahn S, Cohen G: The oxidant stress hypothesis in Parkinson's disease: evidence supporting it. Ann Neurol 32:804, 1992
178. Hasegawa E, Takeshige K, Oishi T, et al: 1-Methyl-4-phenylpyridinium (MPP+) induces NADH-dependent superoxide formation and enhances NADH-dependent lipid peroxidation in bovine heart submitochondrial particles. Biochem Biophys Res Commun 170:1049, 1990
179. Przedborski S, Kostic V, Jackson-Lewis V, et al: Transgenic mice with increased Cu/Zn-superoxide dismutase activity are resistant to N-methyl-4-phenyl-1,2,3,6-tetrahydropyridine-induced neurotoxicity. J Neurosci 12:1658, 1992
180. Harris ML, Schiller HJ, Reilly PM, et al: Free radicals and other reactive oxygen metabolites in inflammatory bowel disease. Pharmacol Ther 53:375, 1992

181. Smith JL: The pathologic effects due to increase of oxygen tension in the air breathed. J Physiol 24:19, 1899
182. Jackson RM: Pulmonary oxygen toxicity. Chest 88:900, 1985
183. Dobuler KJ, Catravas JD, Gillis CN: Early detection of oxygen-induced injury in conscious rabbits: reduced in vivo activity of angiotensin converting enzyme and removal of 5-hydroxytryptamine. Am Rev Respir Dis 126:534, 1982
184. Crapo JD: Morphologic changes in pulmonary oxygen toxicity. Annu Rev Physiol 48:721, 1986
185. Freeman BA, Crapo JD: Hyperoxia increases oxygen radical production in rat lungs and lung mitochondria. J Biol Chem 256:10986, 1981
186. Turrens JF, Freeman BA, Crapo JD: Hyperoxia increases H_2O_2 release by lung mitochondria and microsomes. Arch Biochem Biophys 217:411, 1982
187. Shasby DM, Fox RB, Harada RN, et al: Reduction of the edema of acute hyperoxic lung injury by granulocyte depletion. J Appl Physiol 52:1237, 1982
188. Raj JU, Hazinski TA, Bland RD: Oxygen-induced lung microvascular injury in neutropenic rabbits and lambs. J Appl Physiol 58:921, 1985
189. Turrens JF, Crapo JD, Freeman BA: Protection against oxygen toxicity by intravenous injection of liposome-entrapped catalase and superoxide dismutase. J Clin Invest 73:87, 1984
190. Padmanabhan RV, Gudapaty R, Liener IE, et al: Protection against pulmonary oxygen toxicity in rats by the intratracheal administration of liposome-encapsulated superoxide dismutase or catalase. Am Rev Respir Dis 132:164, 1985
191. Shasby DM, Van Benthuysen KM, Tate RM, et al: Granulocytes mediate acute edematous lung injury in rabbits and in isolated rabbit lungs perfused with phorbol myristate acetate: role of oxygen radicals. Am Rev Respir Dis 125:443, 1982
192. Tate RM, Van Benthuysen KM, Shasby DM, et al: Oxygen-radical-mediated permeability edema and vasoconstriction in isolated perfused rabbit lungs. Am Rev Respir Dis 126:802, 1982
193. Glauser FL, Fairman RP: The uncertain role of the neutrophil in increased permeability pulmonary edema. Chest 88:601, 1985
194. Ognibene FP, Martin SE, Parker MM, et al: Adult respiratory distress syndrome in patients with severe neutropenia. N Engl J Med 315:547, 1986
195. Crowell JW, Jones CE, Smith EE: Effect of allopurinol on hemorrhagic shock. Am J Physiol 216:744, 1969
196. Prasad K, Kalra J, Buchko G: Acute hemorrhage and oxygen free radicals. Angiology 39:1005, 1988
197. Horton JW, Borman KR: Possible role of oxygen-derived, free radicals in cardiocirculatory shock. Surg Gynecol Obstet 165:293, 1987
198. McKechnie K, Furman BL, Parratt JR: Modification by oxygen free radical scavengers of the metabolic and cardiovascular effects of endotoxin infusion in conscious rats. Circ Shock 19:429, 1986
199. Arvidsson S, Falt K, Marklund S, et al: Role of free oxygen radicals in the development of gastrointestinal mucosal damage in *Escherichia coli* sepsis. Circ Shock 16:383, 1985
200. Morgan RA, Manning PB, Coran AG, et al: Oxygen free radical activity during liver E. coli septic shock in the dog. Circ Shock 25:319, 1988
201. Shatney CH, Toledo-Pereyra LH, Lillehei RC: Experiences with allopurinol in canine endotoxin shock. Advances in Shock Research, Vol 4. Schumer W, Spitzer JJ, Marshall BE, Eds. Alan R. Liss, New York, 1980, p 119
202. Cerra FB: The hypermetabolism organ failure complex. World J Surg 11:173, 1987
203. Scheinburg FB, Seligman AM, Fine J: Transmural migration of intestinal bacteria. N Engl J Med 242:747, 1950
204. Deitch EA, Bridges W, Baker J, et al: Hemorrhagic shock-induced bacterial translocation is reduced by xanthine oxidase inhibition or inactivation. Surgery 104:191, 1988
205. Meakins JL, Marshall JC: The gut as the motor of multiple system organ failure. Splanchnic Ischemia and Multiple Organ Failure. Marston A, Bulkley GB, Fiddian-Green RG, Eds. Edward Arnold, London, 1989, p 339
206. Heffner JE, Repine JE: Pulmonary strategies of antioxidant defense. Am Rev Respir Dis 140:531, 1989
207. Flohe L: Superoxide dismutase for therapeutic use: clinical experience, dead ends and hopes. Mol Cell Biochem 84:123, 1988
208. Greenwald RA: Superoxide dismutase and catalase as therapeutic agents for human diseases: a critical review. Free Radic Biol Med 8:201, 1990
209. Hallewell RA, Laria I, Tabrizi A, et al: Genetically engineered polymers of human CuZn superoxide dismutase: biochemistry and serum half-lives. J Biol Chem 264:5260, 1989
210. Beckman JS, Minor RL Jr, White CW, et al: Superoxide dismutase and catalase conjugated to polyethylene glycol increases endothelial enzyme activity and oxidant resistance. J Biol Chem 263:6884, 1988
211. White CW, Jackson JH, Abuchowski A, et al: Polyethylene glycol–attached antioxidant enzymes decrease pulmonary oxygen toxicity in rats. J Appl Physiol 66:584, 1989
212. Pyatak PS, Abuchowski A, Davis FF: Preparation of a polyethylene glycol: superoxide dismutase adduct, and an examination of its blood circulation life and anti-inflammatory activity. Res Commun Chem Pathol Pharmacol 29:113, 1980
213. Freeman BA, Young SL, Crapo JD: Liposome-mediated augmentation of superoxide dismutase in endothelial cells prevents oxygen injury. J Biol Chem 258:12534, 1983
214. Harrison JR, Rillema DP, Ham JH 4th, et al: Inhibition of phorbol ester stimulated interleukin 2 production by copper (II) complexes. Cancer Res 46:5571, 1986
215. Darr DJ, Yanni S, Pinnell SR: Protection of Chinese hamster ovary cells from paraquat-mediated cytotoxicity by a low molecular weight mimic of superoxide dismutase (DF-Mn). Free Radic Biol Med 4:357, 1988
216. Mitchell JB, Samuni A, Krishna MC, et al: Biologically active metal-independent superoxide dismutase mimics. Biochemistry 29:2802, 1990
217. Hearse DJ, Tosaki A: Reperfusion-induced arrhythmias and free radicals: studies in the rat heart with DMPO. J Cardiovasc Pharmacol 9:641, 1987
218. Jones GL, Masters CJ: On the turnover and proteolysis of catalase in tissues of the guinea pig and acatalasemic mice. Arch Biochem Biophys 173:463, 1976
219. Tanswell AK, Freeman BA: Liposome-entrapped antioxidant enzymes prevent lethal O_2 toxicity in the newborn rat. J Appl Physiol 63:347, 1987
220. Spector T, Hall WW, Krenitsky TA: Human and bovine xanthine oxidases: inhibition studies with oxipurinol. Biochem Pharmacol 35:3109, 1986
221. Granger DN, McCord JM, Parks DA, et al: Xanthine oxidase inhibitors attenuate ischemia-induced vascular permeability changes in the cat intestine. Gastroenterology 90:80, 1986
222. Topham RW, Walker MC, Calisch MP: Liver xanthine dehydrogenase and iron mobilization. Biochem Biophys Res Commun 109:1240, 1982
223. Roy RS, McCord JM: Superoxide and ischemia: conversion of xanthine dehydrogenase to xanthine oxidase. Proceedings of the Third International Conference on Superoxides and Superoxide Dismutase. Greenwald R, Cohen G, Eds. Elsevier/North Holland Biomedical Press, New York, 1983, p 145
224. Anbar M, Meyerstein D, Neta P: Reactivity of aliphatic compounds towards hydroxyl radicals. J Chem Soc (B):742, 1966
225. Emerson TE: Unique features of albumin: a brief review. Crit Care Med 17:690, 1989
226. Pirisino R, Di Simplicio P, Ignesti G, et al: Sulfhydryl groups and peroxidase-like activity of albumin as scavenger of organic peroxides. Pharmacol Res Commun 20:545, 1988
227. Jacob SW, Herschler R: Pharmacology of DMSO. Cryobiology 23:14, 1986
228. Portz SJ, Lesnefsky EJ, Van Benthuysen KM, et al: Dimethylthiourea, but not dimethylsulfoxide, reduces canine myocardial infarct size. Free Radic Biol Med 7:53, 1989
229. Hall ED, Braughler JM, McCall JM: New pharmacological treatment of acute spinal cord trauma. J Neurotrauma 5:81, 1988
230. Johnson G 3rd, Lefer AM: Protective effects of a novel 21-aminosteroid during splanchnic artery occlusion shock. Circ Shock 30:155, 1990
231. Halliwell B, Gutteridge JMC: Role of iron in oxygen radical reactions. Methods Enzymol 105:47, 1984
232. Aust SD, White BC: Iron chelation prevents tissue injury following ischemia. Adv Free Radic Biol Med 1(A):1, 1985
233. Illes RW, Silverman NA, Krukenkamp IB, et al: Amelioration of postischemic stunning by deferoxamine-blood cardioplegia. Circulation 80:III-30, 1989
234. Hallaway PE, Eaton JW, Panter SS, et al: Modulation of deferoxamine toxicity and clearance by covalent attachment to biocompatible polymers. Proc Natl Acad Sci USA 86:10108, 1989
235. Halliwell B: Use of desferrioxamine as a 'probe' for iron-dependent formation of hydroxyl radicals: evidence for a direct reaction between desferal and the superoxide radical. Biochem Pharmacol 34:229, 1985
236. Gutteridge JM, Richmond R, Halliwell B: Oxygen free-radicals and lipid peroxidation: inhibition by the protein caeruloplasmin. FEBS Lett 112:269, 1980
237. Stohs SJ, Lawson TA, Anderson L, et al: Effects of oltipraz, BHA, ADT and cabbage on glutathione metabolism, DNA damage and lipid peroxidation in old mice. Mech Ageing Dev 37:137, 1986
238. Zhang Y, Kensler TW, Cho CG, et al: Anticarcinogenic activities of sulforaphane and structurally related synthetic norbornyl isothiocyanates. Proc Natl Acad Sci USA 91:3147, 1994
239. Parnham MJ, Graf E: Seleno-organic compounds and the therapy of hydroperoxide-linked pathological conditions. Biochem Pharmacol 36:3095, 1987
240. Cotgreave IA, Duddy SK, Kass GEN, et al: Studies on the anti-inflammatory activity of ebselen: ebselen interferes with granulocyte oxidative burst by dual inhibition of NADPH oxidase and protein kinase C? Biochem Pharmacol 38:649, 1989
241. Cronstein BN, Rosenstein ED, Kramer SB, et al: Adenosine: a physiologic modulator of superoxide anion generation by human neutrophils: adenosine acts via an A2 receptor on human neutrophils. J Immunol 135:1366, 1985
242. Cross AR, Jones TG: The effect of the inhibitor diphenylene iodinium on the superoxide gener-

ation system of neutrophils: specific labelling of a component polypeptide of the oxidase. Biochem J 237:111, 1986

243. Stuehr DJ, Fasehun OA, Kwon NS, et al: Inhibition of macrophage and endothelial cell nitric oxide synthase by diphenyleneiodonium and its analogs. FASEB J 5:98, 1991

244. Irita K, Fujita I, Takeshige K, et al: Cinchocaine and amethocaine inhibit activation and activity of superoxide production in human neutrophils. Br J Anaesth 58:639, 1986

245. Irita K, Fujita I, Takeshige K, et al: Calcium channel antagonist induced inhibition of superoxide production in human neutrophils: mechanisms independent of antagonizing calcium influx. Biochem Pharmacol 35:3465, 1986

246. Biemond P, Swaak AJG, Penders JMA, et al: Superoxide production by polymorphonuclear leucocytes in rheumatoid arthritis and osteoarthritis: in vivo inhibition by the antirheumatic drug piroxicam due to interference with the activation of the NADPH-oxidase. Ann Rheum Dis 45:249, 1986

247. Chiba T, Asakura T, Kakinuma K: Effect of cetiedil on the superoxide-generating system of porcine neutrophils. J Biochem 98:355, 1985

248. Smail EH, Melnick DA, Ruggeri R, et al: A novel natural inhibitor from *Candida albicans* hyphae causing dissociation of the neutrophil respiratory burst response to chemotactic peptides from other post-activation events. J Immunol 140:3893, 1988

249. Berton G, Dusi S, Serra MC, et al: Studies on the NADPH oxidase of phagocytes: production of a monoclonal antibody which blocks the enzymatic activity of pig neutrophil NADPH oxidase. J Biol Chem 264:5564, 1989

250. Arfors KE, Lundberg C, Lindbom L, et al: A monoclonal antibody to the membrane glycoprotein complex CD18 inhibits polymorphonuclear leucocyte accumulation and plasma leakage in vivo. Blood 69:338, 1987

251. Kubes P, Suzuki M, Granger DN: Platelet-activating factor-induced microvascular dysfunction: role of adherent leukocytes. Am J Physiol 258: G158, 1990

252. Gamble JR, Skinner MP, Berndt MC, et al: Prevention of activated neutrophil adhesion to endothelium by soluble adhesion protein GMP140. Science 249:414, 1990

Acknowledgments

Figures 1 through 3, 5, and 9 Dana Burns.

Figures 4, 6 through 8, 10, 11, and 13 Tom Moore.

Figure 14 Gae Xavier.

100 EICOSANOIDS IN SURGERY

Martin R. Weiser, M.D., James Hill, M.B., Ch.B., Thomas Lindsay, M.D., and Herbert B. Hechtman, M.D.

Prostaglandins, thromboxanes, and leukotrienes all are metabolites of arachidonic acid and belong to a family of biologically active compounds known as the eicosanoids. Eicosanoids are not stored but are rapidly synthesized intracellularly in response to stimuli (e.g., hypoxia, ischemia, or vasoactive agents such as angiotensin, bradykinin, and cytokines); their extracellular release may then influence the activity of other cells in the immediate area. Their plasma half-lives are short—largely as a result of spontaneous hydrolysis or active enzymatic conversion to inactive metabolites—and consequently, they seldom act as circulating hormones.

Prostaglandins were discovered by von Euler in the 1930s when a substance in human semen was found to induce contractions in the myometrium. The active agent, an acidic lipid, was originally thought to be a product of the prostate gland (hence the name prostaglandin). The next major observation was the description of the slow-reacting substance of anaphylaxis (SRS-A) in the early 1940s. It was not until 1980 that SRS-A was identified chemically as the combination of three substances, the so-called cysteinyl leukotrienes—leukotriene C_4 (LTC_4), leukotriene D_4 (LTD_4), and leukotriene E_4 (LTE_4). Thromboxanes were discovered in 1975[1] and leukotrienes in 1979.[2]

Biochemistry of Eicosanoids

Arachidonic acid (eicosatetraenoic acid), the main precursor required for eicosanoid synthesis, is a polyunsaturated fatty acid that is incorporated into the phospholipids of mammalian cell membranes. It is also present in plasma, but it is tightly bound to plasma proteins and thus has little biologic activity. Liberation of arachidonic acid starts when an agonist binds to a receptor on the cell membrane [see Figure 1]. This activates phospholipase C, a membrane component, which then hydrolyzes phosphatidylinositol 4,5-bisphosphate (PIP_2) to the intracellular second messengers inositol 1,4,5-trisphosphate (IP_3) and 1,2-diacylglycerol (DG). IP_3 and DG generate free arachidonic acid by two mechanisms. First, IP_3 increases intracellular calcium ion concentration, thereby activating phospholipase A_2, which then liberates arachidonic acid from the cell membrane phospholipids. Second, DG is degraded by diacylglycerol and monoacylglycerol lipases, and this process generates free arachidonic acid. Phospholipase activation is a crucial aspect of the generation of free arachidonic acid and serves as the rate-limiting step in the production of all the eicosanoids. It would therefore seem likely that agents capable of inhibiting phospholipase activation might be able to reduce inflammation. The antiflammins, a relatively new class of peptides that inhibit phospholipase A_2, have shown promising ability to modify inflammation in arachidonic acid–dependent animal models.[3]

Similarly, steroids have been shown to reduce inflammation by inducing synthesis of lipocortins, which are natural in vivo inhibitors of phospholipase A_2. These phospholipase A_2 antagonists do not, however, inhibit all eicosanoid production: arachidonic acid may still be generated from DG.

Arachidonic acid is metabolized via two enzyme pathways. The cyclooxygenase pathway (mainly in platelets, macrophages, and synovial lining cells) produces prostaglandins and thromboxanes. The lipoxygenase pathway (mainly in neutrophils) produces leukotrienes [see Figures 2 and 3 and Sidebar Dietary Fatty Acids].

CYCLOOXYGENASE PATHWAY

All cells except nonnucleated erythrocytes are capable of generating cyclooxygenase products. In the cytosol, cyclooxygenase (which is also known as prostaglandin endoperoxidase) converts free arachidonic acid into an endoperoxide, prostaglandin G_2 (PGG_2) [see Figure 2], which in turn is converted to prostaglandin H_2 (PGH_2). Cyclooxygenase is fully active in cells; only the presence of arachidonic acid is required for biosynthesis to proceed. PGH_2 is then converted into prostaglandins or thromboxanes by specific enzymes. Cells typically synthesize one of two specific cyclooxygenase products, depending on which enzymes are available. In the vascular system, for instance, platelets produce thromboxane A_2 (TXA_2) through the action of thromboxane synthetase, whereas endothelial cells primarily produce prostaglandin I_2 (PGI_2), or prostacyclin, through the action of prostacyclin synthetase. Some loss of specificity may occur when precursor endoperoxide is lost from cells. For example, endoperoxide synthesized in platelets may escape from these cells by diffusion and then be taken up by endothelial cells for use as a substrate for the synthesis of PGI_2 [see Figure 4]. Drugs that block the action of platelet thromboxane synthetase (e.g., hydralazine) lead to a buildup of precursor endoperoxides in the platelets and increased diffusion from the cells.

Inhibition of Cyclooxygenase by Nonsteroidal Anti-inflammatory Drugs

Nonsteroidal anti-inflammatory drugs (NSAIDs) act primarily by inhibiting cyclooxygenase, thereby decreasing synthesis of all prostaglandins and thromboxanes. NSAIDs may also redirect arachidonic acid metabolism into the lipoxygenase pathway. Thus, aspirin-associated asthma has been hypothesized to be caused by increased synthesis of bronchoconstricting leukotrienes; in addition, the bronchoconstriction is unopposed as a result of reduced synthesis of bronchodilating prostaglandins. A number of side effects are associated with the use of NSAIDs [see Table 1].

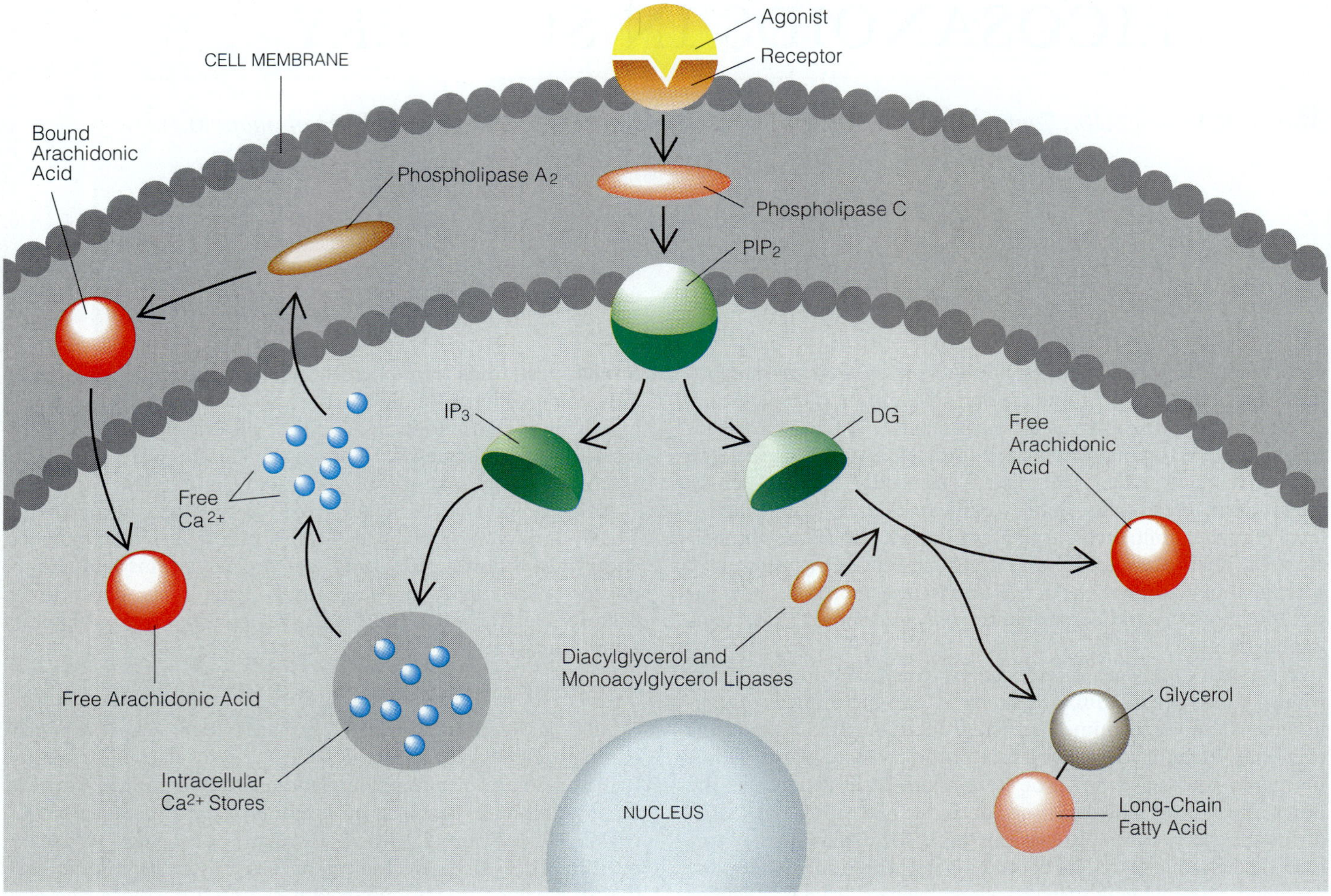

Figure 1 Shown is the production of free arachidonic acid in the cytosol. The binding of an agonist to a receptor activates phospholipase C, which hydrolyzes phosphatidylinositol 4,5-bisphosphate (PIP_2) to inositol 1,4,5-trisphosphate (IP_3) and diacylglycerol (DG). From this point, free arachidonic acid can be generated in two ways. First, IP_3, by increasing the intracellular calcium ion concentration, activates phospholipase A_2, which then liberates arachidonic acid from the cell membrane. Second, DG is broken down enzymatically into several products, one of which is arachidonic acid.

The activity of NSAIDs is determined by the following factors:

1. Dosage and absorption. NSAIDs are rapidly absorbed by passive diffusion in the upper gastrointestinal tract. Concomitant administration of antacids delays but does not reduce absorption. Rectal administration is advantageous when oral therapy is not possible, but peptic side effects, including gastritis and ulcers, still occur because of systemic inhibition of cyclooxygenase.
2. Unbound drug concentration. NSAIDs are extensively bound to human serum albumin, and only free drug is active.
3. Metabolism and catabolism. Some NSAIDs must be metabolically altered to an active form after ingestion. Aspirin, for example, is altered by esterases in gastric mucosa and plasma to salicylate, the active product. Catabolism is limited by hepatic enzymes.

The clinical importance of these considerations is that a reduction in albumin levels will increase the unbound plasma concentration of an NSAID. This increase enhances the action of the drug and may lead to significant alterations in pharmacokinetics in the setting of impaired liver metabolism [*see 107 Pharmacokinetics in Surgical Practice*]. In the presence of hypoalbuminemia combined with hepatic dysfunction, NSAIDs should be avoided or used with care.

LIPOXYGENASE PATHWAY

There are several differences between the lipoxygenase pathway and the cyclooxygenase pathway. Unlike cyclooxygenase, which is ubiquitous, lipoxygenase is present only in myeloid cells (i.e., neutrophils, lymphocytes, monocytes, and macrophages). Moreover, whereas cyclooxygenase is fully active in cells and requires only the presence of arachidonic acid to generate endoperoxides, lipoxygenase is normally quiescent in cells and must be activated before leukotriene synthesis can proceed. Activating stimuli include granulocyte-macrophage colony-stimulating factor, complement component C5a, and *N*-formyl-methionyl-leucyl-phenylalanine.

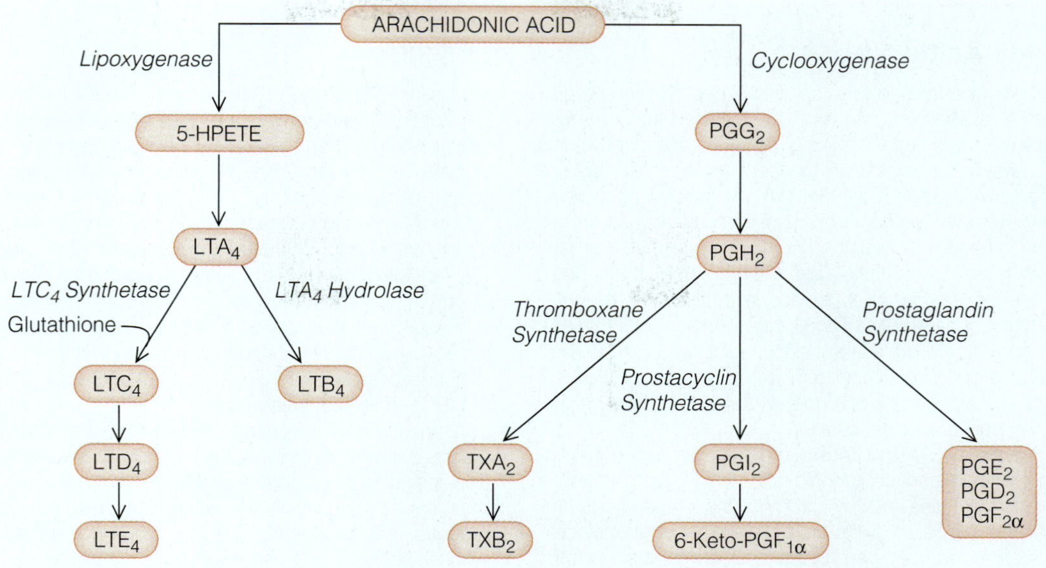

Figure 2 Arachidonic acid is metabolized by two different enzymes, cyclooxygenase and lipoxygenase. The products of cyclooxygenase metabolism are the prostaglandins and the thromboxanes; the products of lipoxygenase metabolism are the leukotrienes.

In the lipoxygenase pathway, arachidonic acid released from myeloid cell membranes via the action of phospholipase A_2 is converted by lipoxygenase to 5-hydroperoxyeicosatetraenoic acid (5-HPETE). The same enzyme then converts 5-HPETE to

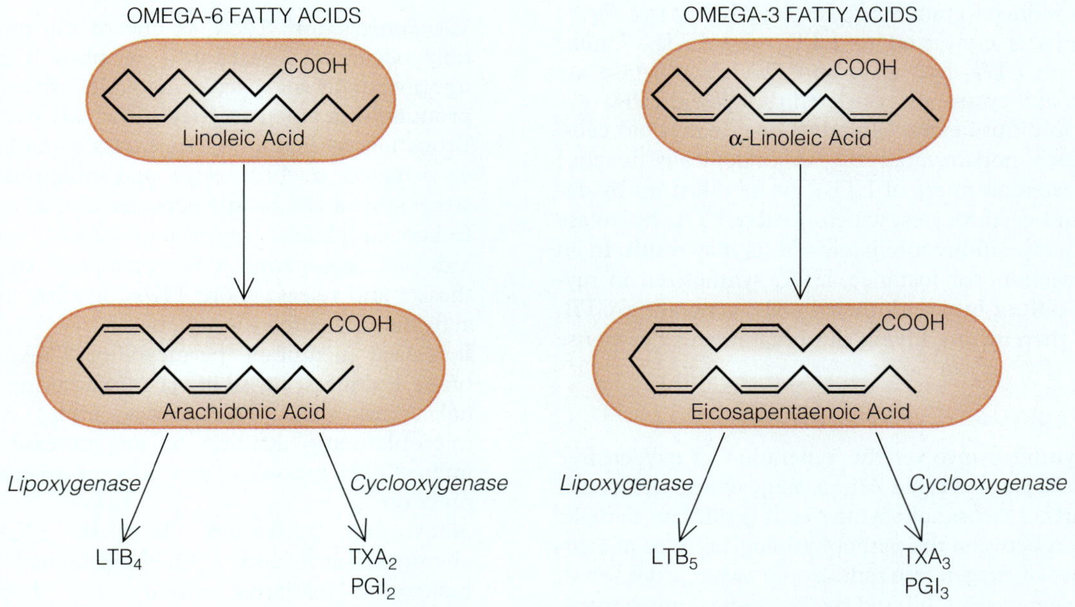

Figure 3 Linoleic acid is the source of arachidonic acid, the main eicosanoid precursor. Both substances belong to a family known as the omega-6 fatty acids (so called because their last double bond is six carbon atoms from the methyl end of the chain). Eicosanoids can also be synthesized from other precursors, such as eicosapentaenoic acid. Eicosapentaenoic acid and its precursor, α-linoleic acid, are omega-3 fatty acids (i.e., the last double bond is only three carbon atoms from the methyl end of the chain). Cyclooxygenase and lipoxygenase act on both arachidonic acid and eicosapentaenoic acid; however, different eicosanoids, with different levels of biologic activity, are produced.

Dietary Fatty Acids

The long-chain polyunsaturated fatty acids that are eicosanoid precursors cannot be synthesized and must be obtained from the diet; consequently, alterations of dietary intake of polyunsaturated fatty acids have important effects on eicosanoid biochemistry and biology. The main source of arachidonic acid in the Western diet is linoleic acid, which is found predominantly in vegetable oils. Linoleic acid and its derivatives are termed omega-6 fatty acids because the last of their four double bonds ends six carbon atoms from the methyl end of the chain [see Figure 3]. In marine fish and, to a lesser extent, in green vegetables, there is a high concentration of two other eicosanoid precursors, eicosapentaenoic acid and docosahexaenoic acid, which are derived from α-linoleic acid. α-Linoleic acid and its derivatives are termed omega-3 fatty acids because the last double bond ends three carbon atoms from the methyl end of the chain.

The relative prevalence of the various precursors has important clinical implications. When eicosapentaenoic acid is the substrate and is processed by cyclooxygenase and then thromboxane synthetase, thromboxane A_3 (TXA_3) is produced, which is biologically inactive; eicosapentaenoic acid also competitively binds cyclooxygenase, thereby reducing TXA_2 synthesis. However, prostaglandin I_3 (PGI_3), the prostacyclin synthesized from omega-3 fatty acids, is fully active. The effects of reducing thromboxane activity while maintaining prostacyclin activity are increased platelet survival, reduced platelet aggregation, and increased bleeding time.

Interest in the clinical effects of dietary omega-3 fatty acids came from the observation that Greenland Eskimos had a low incidence of myocardial infarction despite eating a high-fat diet.[25] Their plasma and platelet lipids were found to contain high concentrations of omega-3 polyunsaturated fatty acids. Furthermore, they had hypoaggregable platelets and increased bleeding times; the same effects were then noted in other populations who were fed dietary supplements of omega-3 fatty acids. Fish and vegetable oils were also found to reduce serum cholesterol and triglycerides by a mechanism that was independent of their effects on eicosanoid synthesis (probably involving suppression of very low density lipoproteins). The potential long-term benefits of increased omega-3 fatty acid intake were suggested by epidemiological studies in the Netherlands and Japan that showed a reduced incidence of coronary artery disease in men whose diet contained large amounts of fish supplements.[26,27]

In animal studies, dietary supplementation with fish oils high in omega-3 fatty acids reduced the severity of experimental vascular occlusion, including myocardial and cerebral infarction. Although the precise mechanisms underlying the protection have not been determined, reduced TXA_2 production is likely to be important. Altered leukotriene biochemistry may play a role as well: the main leukotriene synthesized from omega-3 fatty acids is leukotriene B_5 (LTB_5), which is physiologically less active than LTB_4. Reduced synthesis of LTB_4 by neutrophils may also underlie the observation that fish oil supplements reduce the severity of symptoms in patients with rheumatoid arthritis.[28] Whether increasing intake of omega-3 fatty acids in the Western diet will lower the incidence of degenerative vascular disease or reduce the severity of some chronic inflammatory diseases awaits further determination.

leukotriene A_4 (LTA_4). LTA_4 is either metabolized to leukotriene B_4 (LTB_4) by LTA_4 hydrolase or conjugated via LTC_4 synthetase with reduced glutathione to form LTC_4 [see Figure 2], which in turn is converted to LTD_4 and LTE_4. Unlike lipoxygenase, both LTA_4 hydrolase and LTC_4 synthetase are widely distributed; they are not restricted to myeloid cells.

LTA_4 may also diffuse extracellularly. Outside myeloid cells, it can decompose nonenzymatically to biologically inactive compounds (diastereoisomers of LTB_4) or be taken up by endothelial cells and erythrocytes, which possess LTA_4 hydrolase and LTC_4 synthetase. Indirect biologic effects may result. In an inflammatory reaction, for instance, LTA_4 synthesized in myeloid cells may diffuse into endothelial cells, generating LTB_4 and LTC_4 and thereby amplifying the inflammatory response [see Figure 4].

OXYGEN FREE RADICALS

Eicosanoid synthesis involves the generation of oxygen free radicals [see 99 Reactive Oxygen Metabolites], which can themselves induce further eicosanoid synthesis. It is difficult to make a clear distinction between the pathophysiological roles of eicosanoids and those of oxygen free radicals, for two reasons. First, both classes of agents are inhibited by free radical antagonists. Second, eicosanoid inhibitors are usually redox agents that will also limit free radical synthesis.

Biologic Effects of Eicosanoids

THROMBOXANES

TXA_2, originally called rabbit aortic contracting substance, was identified in 1975 as a substance that contracted vascular smooth muscle and caused platelet aggregation.[1] In picogram amounts, it exerts five major biologic effects:

1. Vasoconstriction. TXA_2 is one of the most potent naturally occurring constrictors of smooth muscle and acts upon virtually all vascular beds. Its effects are particularly prominent in small arteries and arterioles.
2. Bronchoconstriction. TXA_2 exerts a marked spastic effect on isolated tracheal rings and pulmonary parenchymal strips and causes bronchoconstriction in intact animals.
3. Enhanced platelet aggregation. TXA_2 activates platelets, inducing aggregation with subsequent stimulation to synthesize and release more TXA_2, leading to further platelet activation by autocrine action.
4. Increased membrane permeability. TXA_2 increases membrane leakiness, possibly via restructuring of the endothelial cytoskeleton. TXA_2 disassembles endothelial actin microfilaments, leading to an increase in the size of intercellular junctions and loss of microvascular barrier function.
5. Neutrophil activation. Because TXA_2 is both a chemoactivator and a chemoattractant of neutrophils, neutrophil oxidative activity and diapedesis are increased. Specific thromboxane receptors have been identified on platelets and on vascular smooth muscle.

Without stimulation, TXA_2 is synthesized at low levels, but increased synthesis and release by platelets or white blood cells can be rapidly triggered by specific factors. Thrombin or contact with collagen can stimulate release of TXA_2 by platelets. Cytokines, complement fragments, and platelet-activating factor can directly stimulate synthesis of TXA_2 by white blood cells. Thus, clinical settings associated with increased TXA_2 production include vascular injury; arteriosclerosis with endothelial denudation; conditions associated with complement activation, such as sepsis, dialysis, or ischemia; and free radical and cytokine production.

TXA_2 has a plasma half-life of about 30 seconds. It is metabolized by nonenzymatic conversion to thromboxane B_2 (TXB_2), a relatively stable hydrolysis product that is found in plasma. TXB_2 has a plasma half-life of about six minutes. Although it was initially thought to be without any biologic effect, it does in fact have a modest degree of bioactivity; however, TXB_2 is at least 10 times less potent than TXA_2. TXB_2 also enhances endothelial permeability, activates neutrophils, and promotes the diapedesis of neutrophils. Assaying plasma levels of TXB_2 is one method of studying TXA_2 production in vivo. An alternative method is measuring the levels of 2,3-dinor TXB_2, a metabolite that is excreted in urine. The latter method has the advantage of not necessitating blood sampling, which means that platelet activation does not occur and artifactually high TXB_2 levels can be avoided.

PROSTAGLANDINS

Prostacyclin

Prostacyclin (PGI_2) promotes blood flow; its biologic effects are antagonistic to those of TXA_2 [see Table 2]. PGI_2 causes vasodilatation, inhibits platelet aggregation,[4] and is thought to control the release of tissue plasminogen activator (t-PA). The effects of PGI_2 are local; it does not modify systemic vascular resistance or pressure. (Thus, aspirin inhibits PGI_2 production but has no effect on normal blood pressure.) PGI_2 is also cytoprotective.

Prostacyclin is synthesized in response to stimulation of the endothelial cell membrane by agents such as bradykinin, thrombin, serotonin, platelet-derived growth factor (PDGF), and interleukin-1 (IL-1). Its effects are mediated by stimulation of the plasma membrane–bound enzyme adenylate cyclase, which leads to an increase in cyclic adenosine monophosphate (cAMP) in platelets and smooth muscle.

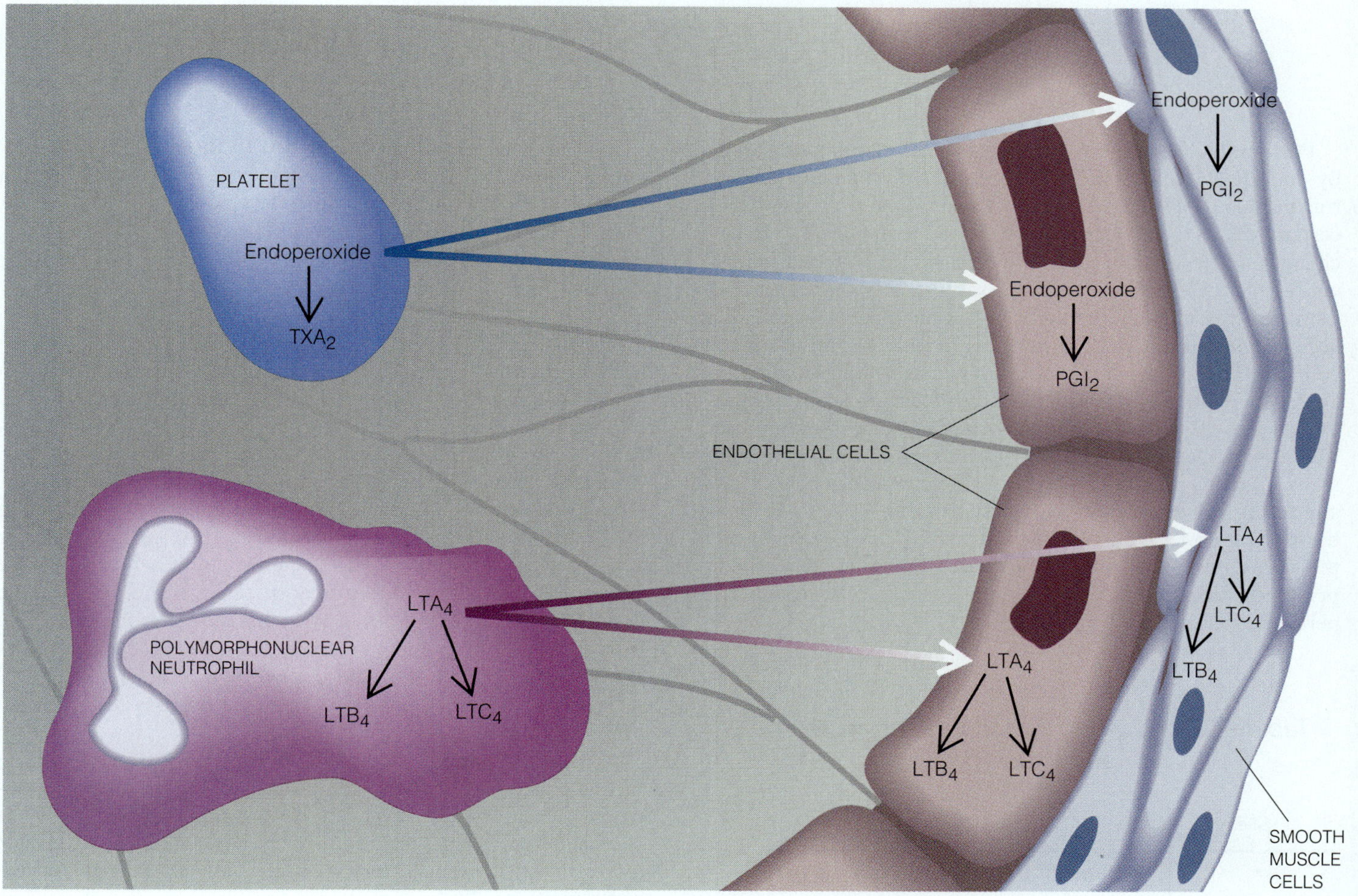

Figure 4 Cellular synthesis of eicosanoids from precursor compounds is generally quite specific, depending on the enzymes present in the cell containing the precursor. When the precursor diffuses out of the cell, however, some specificity is lost. For example, platelets produce TXA_2 from precursor endoperoxide, but if the endoperoxide diffuses extracellularly and is taken up by endothelial cells and smooth muscle cells, PGI_2 is produced instead. LTA_4, the precursor for all the other leukotrienes, may diffuse extracellularly as well. Although LTA_4 is formed only in myeloid cells, it can be metabolized in a variety of cell types. In an inflammatory setting, diffusion of LTA_4 out of myeloid cells and into endothelial cells and smooth muscle cells, with the consequent increased production of LTB_4 and LTC_4, may amplify the inflammatory response.

Table 1 Important Side Effects of NSAIDs

Site	Effect	Comments
Kidney	Renal insufficiency	Caused by inhibition of vasodilating prostaglandins and loss of autoregulation; occurs only in the setting of reduced renal blood flow
	Water and electrolyte retention	Diuretic and natriuretic effects of endogenous prostaglandins lost; antihypertensive medications may be antagonized
	Interstitial nephritis	Uncommon and idiosyncratic; often associated with underlying renal disease
	Papillary necrosis	Rare; associated with high aspirin doses and underlying renal disease, independent of cyclooxygenase inhibition
Gastroduodenal mucosa	Direct mucosal damage with oral intake	Cytoprotection provided by prostaglandins is lost; acid secretion is increased
	Increased complication rate for preexisting peptic ulcers	
Coagulation system	Increased bleeding time	Synergism with warfarin
Liver	Hepatotoxicity in children	—
	Reye's syndrome	
Lungs	Asthma	—

PGI_2 and TXA_2 are the predominant eicosanoids synthesized by endothelial cells and platelets. In healthy persons, the contrasting biologic effects of TXA_2 and PGI_2 are in balance, but certain disease states may disturb the equilibrium. Relative changes in the levels of these two eicosanoids will alter platelet–endothelial cell interactions. For example, PGI_2 synthesized by damaged vascular endothelium will limit platelet aggregation, although it will not prevent platelets from adhering to exposed collagen. The net result is to prevent excess intraluminal platelet aggregation while permitting the local repair process to progress. PGI_2 is also thought to inhibit growth of vascular smooth muscle. This is important in the setting of hypoxic pulmonary hypertension. In acute pulmonary hypoxia, increased PGI_2 production attenuates the vasoconstrictor response. In chronic hypoxia, however, it appears that even though PGI_2 levels remain high, the adenylate cyclase response to PGI_2 is attenuated, leading to persistent vasoconstriction, smooth muscle cell growth, and persistent pulmonary hypertension.

Table 2 Contrasting Actions of Thromboxane A_2 and Prostacyclin

Site	TXA_2	PGI_2
Platelet	Aggregation	Disaggregation
Neutrophil	Chemotaxis and chemoactivation	Nil
Endothelial cell	Disassembly of actin microfilaments, increasing endothelial permeability	Stabilization of actin microfilaments
Vascular smooth muscle	Constriction	Dilation

PGI_2 has a plasma half-life of two to three minutes. Under neutral or acidic conditions, it is converted to 6-keto-$PGF_{1\alpha}$, a stable metabolite that is 100 times less potent as a vasodilator than PGI_2 and is a weak platelet antiaggregator. 6-Keto-$PGF_{1\alpha}$ can be assayed in either plasma or urine. Unlike other prostaglandins, PGI_2 is not inactivated in the lungs.

Prostaglandin E_2

Prostaglandin E_2 (PGE_2) acts directly on smooth muscle in blood vessels and airways [*see Table 3*]. It is an important local regulator of blood flow, particularly in patients with renal insufficiency, in whom it modulates both renal blood flow and glomerular filtration rate. PGE_2 causes local vasodilatation in the kidney and, at the same time, induces systemic vasoconstriction by stimulating the release of renin from the juxtaglomerular apparatus. In addition to its effects on smooth muscle in the kidney, PGE_2 inhibits sodium reabsorption in the distal tubule and limits the action of antidiuretic hormone on the collecting tubule, thereby inducing natriuresis and diuresis. PGE_2 also has a protective effect on the gastric mucosa: it inhibits gastric acid secretion and increases the ability of the mucosa to withstand injury from gastric acid.

Another prominent effect of PGE_2 is hyperalgesia. Prevention of this effect is the most common reason for the use of cyclooxygenase inhibitors. PGE_2 increases pain sensitivity to other chemical and mechanical stimulators. The effects are additive, increasing with both concentration and time of exposure. At high concentrations, PGE_2 stimulates nerve endings directly; at low concentrations, it increases their sensitivity to other chemical and mechanical agents. In humans, intradermal injections of PGE_2 at physiologic concentrations cause erythema and hyperalgesia. Bradykinin and histamine (substances present in the inflammatory milieu) cause intense pain when added, either alone or in combination, to the physiologic concentrations of PGE_2 and injected. Injection of high doses of PGE_2 (one to two orders of magnitude higher than physiologic doses) causes intense pain for as long as two hours.

PGE_2 is unique among the eicosanoids with regard to its thermoregulatory action in the central nervous system. In humans, the thermoregulatory center is situated in the anterior hypothalamus. This center responds to IL-1 (also known as endogenous pyrogen), which is synthesized by phagocytic leukocytes in response to viruses, bacteria, fungi, endotoxins, and antigen-antibody complexes. IL-1 induces synthesis of PGE_2 in the hypothalamus, which functions as a central transmitter in the initiation of fever. When applied in minute amounts to the thermoregulatory center, PGE_2 induces fever by activating heat-gain mechanisms and inhibiting heat-loss mechanisms. During fever, PGE_2 levels in cerebrospinal fluid are elevated. PGE_2 does not moderate normal body temperature.

Both fever and prostaglandin production in the CNS are reduced after administration of cyclooxygenase inhibitors. The antipyretic effect of NSAIDs is well recognized and is known to be mediated centrally via inhibition of prostaglandin synthesis; NSAIDs do not affect IL-1 production. For the most part, one cyclooxygenase inhibitor is about as effective as another in counteracting fever. In children, however, drugs other than aspirin should be used because of aspirin's association with Reye's syndrome.

At physiologic concentrations, PGE_2 has an important immunomodulatory function in lymphocytes and macrophages: it inhibits T cell mitogenesis, clonal proliferation, migration, IL-2 production, natural killer cell activity, and synthesis of immunoglobulin B cells. Release of lysosomal enzymes and production of IL-1 by macrophages are also inhibited. The inhibitory effects of PGE_2 on macrophages are counterbalanced by interferon gamma.

PGE_2 also has potent effects on the uterus and the cervix. Its levels increase in amniotic fluid during labor, and it is an important modulator of uterine contraction during delivery. The physiologic effects of PGE_2 are so potent that it is often used to initiate labor or terminate pregnancy.

Other Prostaglandins

The other endogenous prostaglandins are prostaglandin D_2 (PGD_2) and prostaglandin $F_{2\alpha}$ ($PGF_{2\alpha}$). A number of PGE_2 analogues have been synthesized whose biologic effects are similar to those of PGE_2. Like PGE_2, PGD_2 is a vasodilator and plays a role in regulating renal blood flow; unlike PGE_2, it causes pulmonary artery constriction and bronchoconstriction. $PGF_{2\alpha}$ shares the pulmonary actions of PGD_2 and has the same effects on the uterus and the cervix that PGE_2 does.

Numerous enzymes are involved in the catabolism of PGE_2, $PGF_{2\alpha}$, and PGD_2. In the liver and the lung, oxidation is the typical mechanism for clearance. The lungs have been characterized as metabolic filters, removing 90 percent of PGE_2 and $PGF_{2\alpha}$ in a single pass and ensuring that PGE_2 and $PGF_{2\alpha}$ act as local hormones at the site of synthesis or on the lungs themselves. Pulmonary metabolism of PGE_2 and $PGF_{2\alpha}$ is an important control mechanism that prevents prostaglandin effects; however, the mechanism of pulmonary metabolism is saturable, which means that excess intravenous administration of either prostaglandin may result in spillover into the systemic circulation, leading to systemic effects. Alternatively, lung injury may reduce pulmonary metabolic capacity and allow prostaglandin spillover. A metabolite of PGE_2 can be measured in both blood and urine and is a reliable indicator of in vivo production.

LEUKOTRIENES

The biologic effects of the leukotrienes occur at the level of the microvasculature, particularly at the postcapillary venule; the most important of these effects relate to the role of leukotrienes in allergic and inflammatory diseases [see Table 4]. LTB_4 is a leukocyte chemoactivator. Its effects include increased neutrophil oxidative activity, release of granular enzymes, and enhanced expression of integrins, surface adhesion receptors that increase the adhesiveness of leukocytes to endothelium. In addition, LTB_4 is a potent chemotactic factor for neutrophils and is weakly chemotactic for eosinophils. Specific LTB_4 receptors have been identified on neutrophil cell membranes. LTB_4 also stimulates myelopoiesis and mediates cytokine synthesis [see Table 4].

The cysteinyl leukotrienes, LTC_4, LTD_4, and LTE_4, all increase the permeability of venules; they accomplish this by modifying the state of actin filaments so that the endothelial cell junctions are widened. LTC_4 may be produced at an inflammatory site by adherent neutrophils, eosinophils, basophils, monocytes, or tissue mast cells. Although endothelial cells do not contain lipoxygenase, they are able to generate LTC_4 and LTB_4 from diffusing LTA_4 provided by polymorphonuclear leukocytes. Together, LTC_4 and LTB_4 attract and activate neutrophils, induce their subsequent diapedesis, and increase capillary permeability.

Pulmonary synthesis of leukotrienes has important effects on the airways. In anaphylaxis, IgE-dependent stimulation of mast

Table 3 Biologic Effects of PGE_2

- Vasodilation
- Bronchodilation
- Diuresis and natriuresis
- Inhibition of gastric acid secretion
- Gastric mucosal protection
- Hyperalgesia
- Pyrexia
- Immunomodulation
- Uterine contraction

Table 4 Biologic Effects of Leukotrienes

LTB_4
- Activation of neutrophil superoxide synthesis and elastase release
- Activation of neutrophil integrins, leading to endothelial adhesion
- Induction of neutrophil chemotaxis
- Stimulation of myelopoiesis
- Stimulation of IL-1 production

Cysteinyl leukotrienes
- Alteration of endothelial cell actin filaments and enhancement of microvascular permeability
- Vasoconstriction
- Bronchoconstriction
- Augmentation of bronchial mucus secretion

cells and basophils elicits the generation and release of LTC_4. Human basophils also release LTC_4 when stimulated by IL-3 or C5a. Pulmonary mast cells strategically located adjacent to tracheobronchial mucosa are important generators of leukotrienes in response to airway stimuli. As a consequence of the release of LTC_4 and LTD_4 from mast cells, there is a potent and prolonged contraction of bronchial and small-airway smooth muscle. These leukotrienes also stimulate the secretion of mucus. Consequently, they are thought to be important in the pathophysiology of reversible obstructive airway disease.

LTB_4 is metabolized by LTB_4-20-hydroxylase, an enzyme located exclusively in the microsomes of neutrophils, to 20-hydroxyleukotriene B_4, which retains some biologic activity. This substance is further oxidized to 20-carboxyleukotriene B_4, which is biologically inactive. The key agent necessary for the oxidation is hypochlorous acid, which is generated by activated neutrophils and eosinophils and is present in the extracellular environment of an inflammatory focus. This indicates that activated neutrophils have an increased capacity both to produce and to degrade LTB_4.

LTC_4 is catabolized to LTD_4, with loss of glutamic acid, by γ–glutamyl transpeptidase. Another peptidase catalyzes the conversion of LTD_4 to LTE_4, with the release of glycine. LTD_4 and LTE_4 retain biologic activity; their final inactivation occurs in one pass through the pulmonary circulation, where they are oxidized to diastereoisomers. The leukotrienes can be measured in biologic fluids, but because of inhibitors present in plasma, extraction procedures are necessary before analysis is possible.

Physiologic Roles of Eicosanoids and Therapeutic Implications

REGULATION OF BLOOD FLOW

The eicosanoids may modulate organ and tissue blood flow by adjusting the balance between local production of vasodilating components and local production of vasoconstricting components. Reduction of eicosanoid synthesis—as when age, diabetes, or atherosclerosis decreases the capacity of the endothelium to synthesize PGI_2—may impair normal regulatory mechanisms. In addition to direct eicosanoid effects on vasomotion, altered platelet aggregation can regulate blood flow indirectly. For example, in occlusive vascular disease, acute ischemia might bring about elevated levels of TXA_2 by stimulating synthesis of TXA_2 by platelets and neutrophils, and this increased synthesis and the resulting vasoconstriction may in turn exacerbate the ischemia.

The role of eicosanoids in the control of blood flow is perhaps most apparent with respect to the kidney and the ductus arteriosus.

Kidney

The principal eicosanoids elaborated by the kidney are PGE_2, PGI_2, and TXA_2. These substances play an important role in regulating renal hemodynamics and glomerular filtration rate, particularly in disease states. PGE_2, the major vasodilating prostaglandin, is synthesized primarily in the renal medulla; PGI_2 is synthesized mainly in endothelial cells; and TXA_2 is synthesized mainly in the cortex. Renal eicosanoid synthesis is increased by ureteral obstruction and release of angiotensin, catecholamines, or vasopressin. These vasoconstrictive stimuli are in part reversed by PGE_2 and PGI_2, which reduce the severity of renal ischemia. Experimentally, vasodilating prostaglandins moderate renal damage induced by vasoconstricting agents such as norepinephrine.

Renal blood flow may be reduced in both prerenal and intrarenal disease. In patients with shock, cirrhosis, or congestive heart failure, there is a compensatory increase in renal PGE_2 production. Administration of NSAIDs to these patients reduces prostaglandin production and is frequently associated with impairment of renal function. NSAIDs cause about 20 percent of cases of drug-induced acute renal failure. This failure is not associated with structural damage to the kidney and is usually readily reversible when the drugs are withdrawn. In normal individuals, NSAIDs cause no change in renal plasma flow or glomerular filtration rate.

Ductus Arteriosus

Fetuses have high circulating levels of PGE_2, which decrease after birth in a fashion temporally associated with ductus arteriosus closure. In the 1970s, experiments done on the ductus arteriosus in fetal lambs showed that both PGE_2 and the synthetic agent PGE_1 prevented ductus closure by virtue of their vasodilatory effects, whereas the cyclooxygenase inhibitor indomethacin led to closure. The control that prostaglandins exert over the ductus arteriosus has led to the development of therapies to modulate its patency. Maintenance of a patent ductus arteriosus is necessary in two patient groups: (1) newborns whose systemic blood flow depends on shunting from the pulmonary artery to the aorta (as in the setting of an interrupted aortic arch) and (2) newborns whose pulmonary blood flow depends on shunting from the aorta to the pulmonary artery (as in pulmonary valve atresia). PGE_1 has been highly beneficial for both groups, enabling resuscitation and stabilization even in the face of major respiratory and electrolyte disturbances. Side effects of PGE_1 therapy include pyrexia, bradycardia, hypotension, cutaneous flushing, and diarrhea; less common problems include gastric mucosal hyperplasia with outlet obstruction, CNS irritability, cardiac arrhythmias, anuria, and disseminated intravascular coagulation. PGE_1 is rapidly metabolized: as much as 80 percent of each dose is cleared in one pass through the lungs. Thus, its effects dissipate quickly on withdrawal.

The value of cyclooxygenase inhibition in low-birth-weight infants with persistent patent ductus arteriosus was established in 1983 by a large multicenter clinical trial that demonstrated that indomethacin was safe and effective.[5] Side effects are uncommon with indomethacin therapy. Transient renal dysfunction, bleeding tendency, pneumothorax, and retinopathy have been noted; the last two are mediated by unknown mechanisms. Indomethacin is employed when usual medical therapy, including fluid restriction and diuretics, has failed. In as many as 30 percent of those receiving indomethacin, the ductus arteriosus may not be permanently closed.

Aspirin and other NSAIDs may also be effective in closing a patent ductus arteriosus; however, only indomethacin has been approved for parenteral administration.

ISCHEMIC INJURY

Ischemia stimulates thromboxane synthesis and release: all organs studied to date (including the myocardium, the cerebrum, the kidneys, the liver, the bowel, and skeletal muscle) have been shown to synthesize TXA_2 on reperfusion. Although PGI_2

levels may also be increased, the ratio of TXA_2 to PGI_2 is typically elevated during reperfusion, suggesting that the biologic equilibrium has shifted so as to favor vasoconstriction and reduced flow. In the setting of atheromatous narrowing of arteries in the myocardial and cerebral circulation, the vasoconstrictive and platelet-aggregating effects of TXA_2 could, in theory, exacerbate ischemia. Because of these putative adverse effects of TXA_2, attempts have been made to alleviate myocardial and cerebrovascular ischemia by infusing PGI_2 or its analogues. A number of clinical trials have been performed, but no clinical benefit has been documented. On the other hand, TXA_2 inhibitors have proved beneficial in trials involving experimental myocardial, renal, and skeletal muscle ischemia; however, these agents have not been studied in humans, because none of them has yet been approved.

TXA_2 levels are considerably elevated in patients with rest pain of the legs and in those undergoing aortic clamping for repair of an abdominal aortic aneurysm. There is evidence that high circulating levels of TXA_2 may induce not only local injury but also injury remote from the ischemic organ. Thus, during abdominal aortic aneurysmectomy, TXA_2 release causes constriction of the pulmonary artery and increases mean pulmonary arterial pressure. The effects are transient because of the short half-life of TXA_2. In addition, TXA_2, along with lipoxygenase products that are also released in response to ischemia, activates circulating neutrophils, which become sequestered in the ischemic organ and the lungs. In the lungs, these circulating neutrophils release proteases and reactive oxygen species, thereby producing an increase in microvascular permeability that results in increased transvascular fluid filtration and pulmonary edema. The raised systemic TXA_2 levels, the pulmonary hypertension, and the pulmonary edema that follow abdominal aortic aneurysm repair can be inhibited by mannitol.[6]

Other mediators are also involved in ischemic injury [see 99 Reactive Oxygen Metabolites]. Eicosanoid synthesis appears early and soon leads to cytokine, complement, neutrophil, and free radical activity.

HEMOSTASIS AND COAGULATION

The first step in normal hemostasis is formation of a primary platelet plug. Exposed collagen and thrombin activate platelet adhesion receptors known as the P-selectins. When platelets adhere to injured endothelium, they change shape, and a number of substances, including serotonin, adenosine diphosphate (ADP), α-granule contents (fibrinogen, platelet-derived growth factor, and β-thromboglobulin), and TXA_2, are released. TXA_2 contributes to hemostasis by (1) causing vasoconstriction and (2) activating other platelets to release TXA_2 and to express their adhesion receptors, which leads to further platelet aggregation. NSAIDs, which decrease TXA_2 synthesis by inhibiting cyclooxygenase, reduce platelet function and bring about a rise in measured bleeding time and, in some patients, a bleeding tendency. Salicylates, but not other NSAIDs, cause irreversible acetylation of platelet cyclooxygenase; because platelets have no nucleus, TXA_2 synthesis is inhibited for the life span of the cells. The ability of circulating platelets to produce TXA_2 is restored only when new platelets from the bone marrow pool appear in the circulation. About 10 percent of circulating platelets are replaced every day. Aspirin has an additional effect on bleeding tendency in that it is capable of enhancing fibrinolysis by reducing prothrombin activity.

NSAIDs also displace warfarin from its binding sites on plasma proteins, thereby increasing its anticoagulant effect. The synergism of NSAIDs and warfarin should limit their combined use.

Aspirin Treatment

A single aspirin dose as small as 75 mg can cause a greater than 95 percent inhibition of platelet TXA_2 production for two to three days.[7] Synthesis then slowly returns to normal in eight to 10 days. After aspirin treatment, nucleated cells are able to synthesize more cyclooxygenase within a few hours, so that PGI_2 production by endothelial cells is inhibited for a much shorter period than TXA_2 production by platelets. In addition, the active metabolite of aspirin, salicylate, is absorbed into the portal circulation, where it antagonizes circulating platelets. The salicylate is then largely metabolized by the liver, and systemic cyclooxygenase inhibition is minimized as a result.

It has been found that alternate-day aspirin therapy achieves relatively selective inhibition of TXA_2 while preserving prostaglandin synthesis. The rationale for such treatment would be to inhibit platelet aggregation and thereby to prevent complete occlusion of narrowed and atheromatous arteries in the cerebral and myocardial circulation. Whether this therapy can alter the progress of the underlying arteriosclerotic disease is unknown.

Aspirin has in fact been shown to benefit patients with coronary artery disease.[8] A recent review of six trials (involving a total of 11,136 patients observed for an average of 24 months) that tested the ability of aspirin as an antithrombotic agent found that aspirin led to a 31 percent reduction in subsequent cardiac ischemic events when compared with placebo.[9] A review of four randomized, double-blind studies (involving a total of 3,168 patients with unstable angina) found that aspirin, either alone or in combination with heparin, reduced the risk of myocardial infarction and cardiac death by 50 to 70 percent.[10] Aspirin has also been shown to be effective after invasive treatment for coronary artery disease. When the administration of aspirin was begun within 48 hours of coronary artery bypass surgery, the incidence of saphenous vein bypass graft closure in the six months following the procedure was significantly reduced.[11,12] Similar findings were noted with respect to coronary artery reocclusion after percutaneous angioplasty.[10]

There is some controversy concerning the use of aspirin as primary prevention in individuals who have not yet experienced a thrombotic event, given the small but significant risk of cerebrovascular hemorrhage. The Physicians' Health Study, a randomized, double-blind, placebo-controlled trial of low-dose aspirin (325 mg every other day) in 22,071 participants, found that treatment resulted in a 44 percent reduction in the risk of nonfatal myocardial infarction.[13] The risk of peptic ulcer was slightly greater in the treatment group, and there was a significant increase in reported bleeding problems. Despite the large number of participants, there were still too few patients with the end points of fatal myocardial infarction or fatal stroke to permit definite conclusions regarding the effect of aspirin on the incidence of these events. Surprisingly, a European trial of a significantly higher aspirin dosage (500 mg/day) in 5,000 male British doctors reported that treatment had no beneficial effect on the incidence of nonfatal stroke or nonfatal myocardial infarction.[14] Disparities in study results notwithstanding, the evidence available to date overwhelmingly favors the preventive use of aspirin; there is no question that aspirin can significantly reduce cardiovascular mortality and morbidity in patients who have previously suffered a myocardial infarction.[8] Current recommendations are to give 80 to 160 mg daily as primary prevention in patients with risk factors for atherosclerosis, such as diabetes, smoking, hypertension, and hyperlipidemia.[10]

Studies have shown that aspirin is effective in preventing new or recurrent cerebrovascular accidents and death after transient ischemic attacks and minor strokes; however, there are insufficient data on the use of aspirin in treating patients with evolving or completed major strokes.[10] A study of 20,000 patients is currently under way whose aim is to examine the immediate effects of heparin, aspirin, or both in the setting of major acute ischemic strokes.[15]

Aspirin is also used to treat patients with carotid stenosis. A 1993 study examined the efficacy of surgical treatment of asymptomatic carotid stenosis and employed aspirin in all treatment groups[16]; however, the conclusion of this study and of many others was that surgery is the optimal treatment for both symptomatic[17,18] and asymptomatic carotid stenosis.[16] Aspirin remains an important adjuvant therapy.

The benefits of antiplatelet therapy with cyclooxygenase inhibitors (i.e., NSAIDs) must be weighed against the potential side effects of these drugs [see Table 1]. A 1991 study showed that aspirin was as effective at a dosage of 30 mg/day as at a dosage of 325 mg every other day, with the lower dosage causing fewer adverse consequences.[7] None of the other cyclooxygenase inhibitors has been studied with a view to prophylaxis of cardiac or cerebral thrombotic disease. Aspirin will probably remain the drug of choice for these indications because of its ability to acetylate platelet cyclooxygenase irreversibly. In theory, the ideal therapeutic approach would be to inhibit thromboxane synthetase so that the endoperoxide precursors are redirected into the part of the cyclooxygenase pathway that produces the vasodilating prostaglandins. To date, however, no thromboxane synthetase inhibitors have been approved for use in humans.

Despite the increased bleeding time associated with use of aspirin, cardiovascular surgery and peripheral vascular surgery are routinely conducted without any untoward effects. Indeed, in a randomized trial of aspirin versus placebo in humans, blood loss after abdominal aortic aneurysm surgery in the treatment group was not measurably different from that in the placebo group.[19]

MEDIATION OF INFLAMMATION

Histologically, acute inflammation is characterized by vasodilatation, edema, and early neutrophil accumulation. Eicosanoids are synthesized at the inflammatory site by damaged tissues as well as by invading neutrophils. Production of PGI_2 and PGE_2 leads to vasodilatation. TXA_2, the leukotrienes, and histamine increase vascular permeability both directly, by reorganizing the cytoskeleton and widening the endothelial cell junctions, and indirectly, by promoting entry of neutrophils into tissue, where these cells release oxidative products and proteases. Neutrophil chemoattraction and chemoactivation are largely caused by LTB_4 and TXA_2, as well as by complement fragments. In addition, LTB_4 is a potent stimulus for the production of IL-1 and tumor necrosis factor, cytokines that play key roles in mediating inflammation. Finally, PGE_2, in combination with histamine and bradykinin, produces the symptom complex of inflammation (redness, pain, and warmth). Inhibition of cyclooxygenase reduces pain and yields clinical and microscopic evidence of alleviation of the inflammatory process.

There are several inflammatory conditions in which a mediating role for the cysteinyl leukotrienes is strongly suggested. One study, for example, found elevated levels of LTC_4 and LTD_4 in bronchoalveolar lavage fluid from asthmatic patients.[20] In another trial, a specific LTD_4-receptor antagonist delivered by aerosol inhibited allergic bronchoconstriction in asthmatics.[21] The orally administered lipoxygenase inhibitor zileuton (Abbott-64077) has been shown to reduce symptoms in patients with moderately severe asthma, aspirin-induced asthma, and allergic rhinitis.[9] Animal studies have provided good evidence that leukotriene antagonists can be effective in other acute inflammatory conditions as well. For example, topically applied lipoxygenase inhibitors reduce scaling and erythema in patients with psoriasis; however, oral lipoxygenase inhibitors have no effect on the disease symptoms.[9]

The role of eicosanoids in the production of a pathological inflammatory process can be illustrated by considering rheumatoid arthritis. In this setting, there is a complex interrelationship between the eicosanoids, complement, neutrophils, macrophages, and the interleukins. That eicosanoids play an important part is shown by the fact that inhibition of cyclooxygenase limits the hyperalgesic effects of the arthritis. Unfortunately, the components of the inflammatory process that cause joint destruction are not influenced by NSAIDs.

Several investigators have demonstrated that eicosanoid production by the intestinal mucosa is increased in ulcerative colitis and Crohn's disease. It is unlikely, however, that increased prostaglandin production causes inflammatory bowel disease; indeed, the cyclooxygenase inhibitor flurbiprofen is less effective against active ulcerative colitis than conventionally used drugs. Whether lipoxygenase and its products might mediate inflammatory bowel disease has not yet been resolved.

Selective LTB_4 antagonists and lipoxygenase inhibitors have been reported to reduce acute mucosal inflammation in animals with experimental colitis. Phase II studies in patients with moderately severe ulcerative colitis have shown that treatment with zileuton leads to a significant decrease in symptoms and an improved appearance of the intestinal mucosa at sigmoidoscopy, though it apparently has no effect on intestinal histology.[9]

PROTECTION OF GASTRODUODENAL MUCOSA

Endogenous prostaglandins exert two main homeostatic effects with respect to the gastroduodenal mucosa. The first is cytoprotection, which is thought to result from increases in mucus production, bicarbonate secretion, and mucosal blood flow; the relative importance of the individual factors is not known. The second is modulation of gastric acid release: PGE_2 and its analogues inhibit basal and stimulated production both in normal subjects and in patients with duodenal ulcers.

It is well known that NSAIDs cause damage to the mucosa of the stomach and duodenum and increase the complication rate of preexisting peptic ulcers. They cause mucosal damage by two mechanisms, one local (direct injury to the mucosa) and the other systemic (indicated by the fact that delayed-release and enteric-coated NSAID preparations still cause mucosal injury and predispose to peptic ulcer formation). The first observation that NSAIDs directly damage gastric mucosa was made in 1938, when aspirin therapy was found to be associated with the development of gastritis.[22] All NSAIDs have the potential to cause gastritis: five to 10 percent of NSAID-treated patients complain of epigastric distress, and the risk is increased if there is a history of gastroduodenal pathology. Epigastric pain is the most frequent symptom of gastritis, but in 10 percent of patients with NSAID-induced hemorrhage, there are no warning symptoms. In patients with an NSAID-induced gastric ulcer, coexisting gastritis is almost universal.

Epidemiological studies have shown that NSAIDs are more commonly associated with gastric ulcer than with duodenal ulcer but that their administration increases the risk of hemorrhage and perforation from either type of peptic ulcer. The antiplatelet effect of NSAIDs adds to the problem in that it increases the likelihood of ulcer bleeding. The risk of serious complications secondary to NSAID administration has been estimated to be one per 5,500 prescriptions of an average duration of one month.[23] Even though the incidence of serious complications is low, large numbers of patients are affected each year owing to the huge quantities of NSAIDs consumed. One of the dangers of NSAID-associated peptic ulceration is that many patients with this complication have no symptoms until a life-threatening ulcer problem has developed. It has been suggested that the analgesic effects of NSAIDs mask ulcer symptoms,[24] but the evidence for this view is not convincing. Although the general risk factors for peptic ulcer are known, it is not possible to identify individual patients who are especially sensitive to NSAID effects, aside from those with a history of gastritis or ulcer.

Oral therapy with synthetic analogues of PGE_2 (e.g., PGE_1) has been shown to be effective in healing both gastric and duodenal ulcers, but it is less beneficial than use of H_2 antagonists. Although the prostaglandins have no serious side effects, they do cause annoying diarrhea in about 10 percent of patients. There is evidence that prostaglandins can prevent NSAID-induced gastric and duodenal ulcer, at least in the short term, and their administration does not appear to impair the efficacy of the NSAID. However, patients who are treated on occasion with NSAIDs in moderate doses and who have no history of ulcer usually need not receive prophylactic prostaglandin treatment or H_2-antagonist therapy. Patients with a history of ulcer should receive antacid or H_2-antagonist therapy and should be closely monitored for gastrointestinal bleeding.

INDUCEMENT OF UTERINE FUNCTION

The prostaglandins that are used to induce a uterine response (PGE_2 and $PGF_{2\alpha}$) may be administered intravenously, vaginally, or by an intrauterine route; the vaginal route is preferred because it is effective and carries the lowest risk of side effects. When these prostaglandins are given by the vaginal route to induce labor at term, they have no adverse effects on the fetus even though they cross the fetoplacental barrier. Prostaglandins have been employed to induce second-trimester abortions. They have also been shown to be safe and effective in inducing first-trimester abortions; their ability to soften the cervix during suction termination reduces the likelihood of injury and of subsequent cervical incompetence.

The side effects of PGE_2 and $PGF_{2\alpha}$ include nausea, vomiting, and diarrhea. As noted (see Biologic Effects of Eicosanoids, Prostaglandins, above), $PGF_{2\alpha}$ has pronounced pulmonary effects and thus should be used with caution in patients with asthma.

Dysmenorrhea is associated with increased eicosanoid synthesis. Eicosanoids can be responsible for painful myometrial contractions; in 80 percent of patients, NSAIDs help reduce menstrual discomfort.

Conclusion

Although eicosanoids are both potent and ubiquitous, there are surprisingly few applications for their clinical use. To date, advances in the understanding of the therapeutic benefits of eicosanoid inhibition have been hampered by the lack of specific antagonists.

References

1. Hamberg M, Svensson J, Samuelsson B: Thromboxanes: a new group of biologically active compounds derived from prostaglandin endoperoxides. Proc Natl Acad Sci USA 72:2994, 1975
2. Borgeat P, Samuelsson B: Transformation of arachidonic acid by rabbit polymorphonuclear leukocytes: formation of a novel dihydroxy-eicosatetraenoic acid. J Biol Chem 254:2643, 1979
3. Mukherjee AB, Cordells-Miele E, Miele L: Regulation of extracellular phospholipase A_2 activity: implications for inflammatory diseases. DNA Cell Biol 11:233, 1992
4. Moncada S, Gryglewski R, Bunting S, et al: An enzyme isolated from arteries transforms prostaglandin endoperoxides to an unstable substance that inhibits platelet aggregation. Nature 263:663, 1976
5. Gersony WM, Peckham GJ, Ellison RC, et al: Effects of indomethacin in premature infants with patent ductus arteriosus: results of a national collaborative study. J Pediatr 102:895, 1983
6. Paterson IS, Klausner JM, Goldman G, et al: Pulmonary edema after aneurysm surgery is modified by mannitol. Ann Surg 210:796, 1989
7. Clarke RJ, Mayo G, Price P, et al: Suppression of thromboxane A_2 but not of systemic prostacyclin by controlled-release aspirin. N Engl J Med 325:1137, 1991
8. Aspirin after myocardial infarction (editorial). Lancet 1:1172, 1980
9. Henderson WR Jr: The role of leukotrienes in inflammation. Ann Intern Med 121:684, 1994
10. Roth GJ, Calverley DC: Aspirin, platelets, and thrombosis: theory and practice. Blood 83:885, 1994
11. Chesebro JH, Clements IP, Fuster V, et al: A platelet-inhibitor-drug trial in coronary-artery bypass operations: benefit of perioperative dipyridamole and aspirin therapy on early postoperative vein-graft patency. N Engl J Med 307:73, 1982
12. Lorenz RL, Schacky CV, Weber M, et al: Improved aortocoronary bypass patency by low-dose aspirin (100 mg daily): effects on platelet aggregation and thromboxane formation. Lancet 1:1261, 1984
13. Steering Committee of the Physicians' Health Study Research Group: Final report on the aspirin component of the ongoing Physicians' Health Study. N Engl J Med 321:129, 1989
14. Peto R, Gray R, Collins R, et al: Randomised trial of prophylactic daily aspirin in British male doctors. Br Med J (Clin Res Ed) 296:313, 1988
15. Patrono C: Aspirin as an antiplatelet drug. N Engl J Med 330:1287, 1994
16. Hobson RW 2nd, Weiss DG, Fields WS, et al: Efficacy of carotid endarterectomy for asymptomatic carotid stenosis. The Veterans Affairs Cooperative Study Group. N Engl J Med 328:221, 1993
17. North American Symptomatic Carotid Endarterectomy Trial collaborators: Beneficial effect of carotid endarterectomy in symptomatic patients with high-grade carotid stenosis. N Engl J Med 325:445, 1991
18. European Carotid Surgery Trialists' Collaborative Group: MRC European Carotid Surgery Trial:

interim results for symptomatic patients with severe (70–99%) or with mild (0–29%) carotid stenosis. Lancet 337:1235, 1991
19. Krausz MM, Utsunomiya T, McIrvine AJ, et al: Modulation of cardiovascular function and platelet survival by endogenous prostacyclin released during surgery. Surgery 93:554, 1983
20. Okubo T, Takahashi H, Sumitomo M, et al: Plasma levels of leukotrienes C_4 and D_4 during wheezing attack in asthmatic patients. Int Arch Allergy Appl Immunol 84:149, 1987
21. Dahlen SE, Dahlen B, Eliasson E, et al: Inhibition of allergic bronchoconstriction in asthmatics by the leukotriene-antagonist ICI-204,219. Prostaglandin Thromboxane Leukotriene Res 21A:461, 1991
22. Douthwaite AH, Lintott GAM: Gastroscopic observation of the effect of aspirin and certain other substances on the stomach. Lancet 2:1222, 1938
23. Langman MJ: Epidemiologic evidence on the association between peptic ulceration and anti-inflammatory drug use. Gastroenterology 96:640, 1989
24. Armstrong CP, Blower AL: Non-steroidal anti-inflammatory drugs and life threatening complications of peptic ulceration. Gut 28:527, 1987
25. Bang HO, Dyerberg J, Sinclair HM: The composition of the Eskimo food in north western Greenland. Am J Clin Nutr 33:2657, 1980
26. Kromhout D, Bosschieter EB, de-Lezenne-Coulander C: The inverse relation between fish consumption and 20-year mortality from coronary heart disease. N Engl J Med 312:1205, 1985
27. Kagawa Y, Nishizawa M, Suzuki M, et al: Eicosapolyenoic acids of serum lipids of Japanese islanders with low incidence of cardiovascular diseases. J Nutr Sci Vitaminol (Tokyo) 28:441, 1982
28. Kremer JM, Michalek AV, Bigauoette J, et al: Effects of manipulation of dietary fatty acids on clinical manifestations of rheumatoid arthritis. Lancet 1:184, 1985

Acknowledgments

Figure 1   Andy Christie. Adapted from a drawing by Dana Burns Pizer.

Figures 2 and 4   Tom Moore.

Figure 3   Andy Christie.

101 CYTOKINES AND THE CELLULAR RESPONSE TO INJURY AND INFECTION

Yuman Fong, M.D., and Stephen F. Lowry, M.D.

Patients with injuries or infections exhibit hemodynamic, metabolic, and immune responses orchestrated by endogenous mediators. Some of the best known humoral mediators of the response to injury and infection (e.g., catecholamines and glucocorticoids) are produced by specialized tissues and exert their influence largely through endocrine mechanisms. Recent evidence suggests, however, that certain protein mediators produced both at the site of injury and by diverse immune cells throughout the body are also critical determinants of the response to injury and infection. These small proteins are collectively termed cytokines and include tumor necrosis factor (TNF), interleukins, interferons, and colony-stimulating factors.

Originally, it was thought that the cytokines' primary influence was on immunologic homeostasis, and indeed, cytokines exert significant influences on immune cell production and immune cell function. Recently, cytokines have also been identified as important determinants of other responses to injury, including the cardiovascular and metabolic alterations seen in infection. There is increasing evidence that cytokines broadly influence tissue metabolic pathways. Cytokines potentiate the release of other cytokines and mediators in a convoluted cascade; this cascade appears to amplify the injury response by directing immunologic and metabolic processes both acutely and for an extended period after the initial insult.

Cytokines differ from classic endocrine hormones in their production by many cell types and in their capacity to elicit significant tissue responses at very low concentrations. Cytokines can influence tissue responses locally via direct cell-to-cell interaction, or when produced in excess, they may spill into the circulation and produce systemic responses via endocrine mechanisms. At present, instability and fever associated with cytokine release are the most clinically evident manifestations of cytokine-mediated injury in patients.

The patterns of cytokine release in response to injury, the precise biologic role for each individual protein, and the potential for synergistic action between these mediators remain to be fully defined. It is likely, however, that their activity is indispensable in the immunologic response necessary to eradicate invading organisms and promote wound healing. On the other hand, it is also likely that acute exaggerated production of some cytokines may produce the hemodynamic manifestations of septic shock and that excessive chronic production may be responsible for the debilitating tissue wasting of cachexia.

The potential toxicities of cytokines have led investigators to postulate that there are natural inhibitors that protect the host against aberrant or excessive production of these proteins. A number of such natural inhibitors have recently been identified, including adrenocorticosteroids, interleukin-1 receptor antagonist (IL-1ra), and tumor necrosis factor soluble receptors. It is likely that a complete network of such endogenous inhibitors exists.

Improved understanding of cytokines' biologic influences will allow them to be used more rationally in immunologic and metabolic response modification. Highly selective antibodies against many cytokines are available; these may find a clinical role in the treatment of injured patients. In addition, understanding the actions of natural inhibitors of cytokines may not only increase our understanding of cytokine biology but also lead to other methods for modulating cytokines' potentially deleterious effects after injury.

The number of recognized cytokines is large and increasing rapidly [see Table 1]. This chapter will concentrate on the five cytokines whose roles in the response to injury have been most extensively studied. Specifically, these cytokines are TNF-α, IL-1, IL-2, IL-6, and interferon gamma [see Table 2].

Biologic Activities

TUMOR NECROSIS FACTOR

Immunologic Activities

Tumor necrosis factor influences all myelogenous cell lines, including neutrophils, monocytes, lymphocytes, and eosinophils. TNF elicits the release of neutrophils from the bone marrow and also initiates neutrophil margination, transendothelial passage,[1] and neutrophil activation.[2] TNF also promotes differentiation of bone marrow precursors to monocytes, and it activates mature monocytes against viral and parasitic organisms. Additionally, TNF has been shown to enhance the activities of eosinophils against parasites.

Effects on Wound Healing

Tumor necrosis factor may play important roles in wound formation and remodeling. It increases procoagulant activity on the endothelial cell surface and increases vascular permeability. In addition, because TNF is a growth factor, it has the capacity to stimulate microvascular angiogenesis[3] and fibroblast

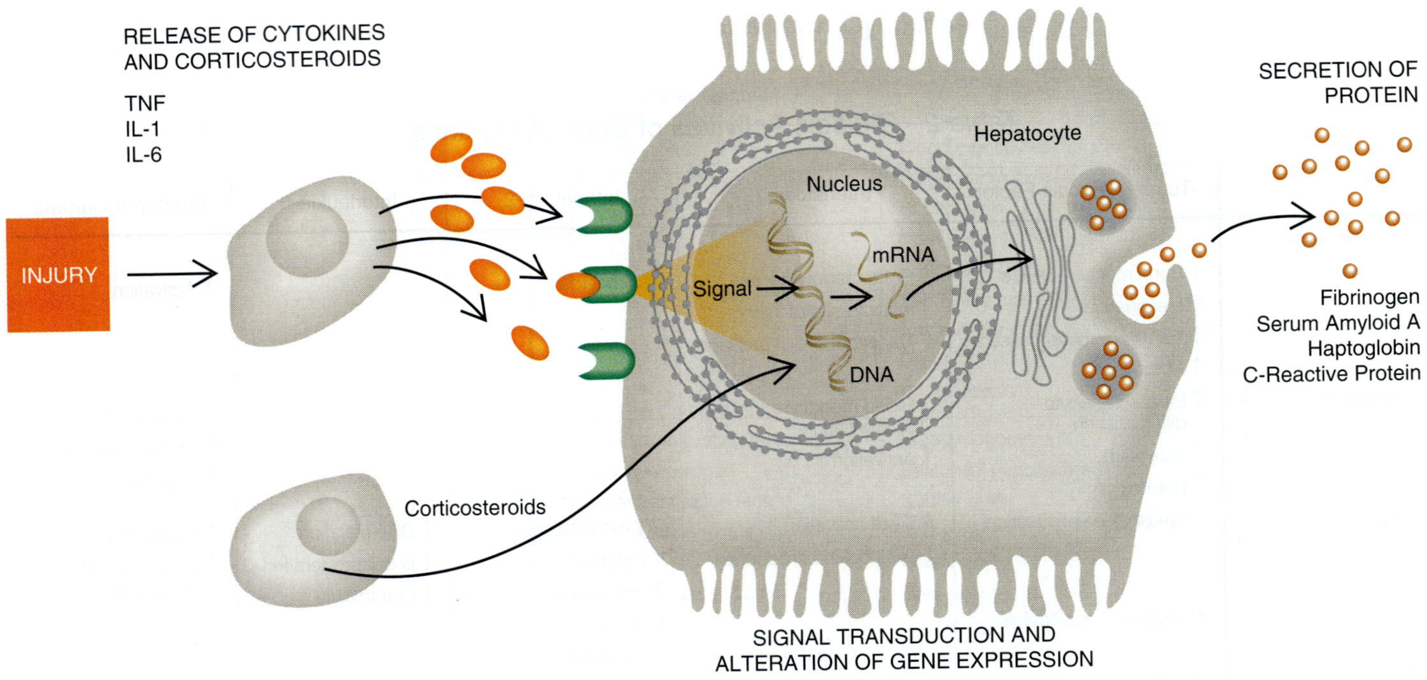

Figure 1 Cytokines released from a variety of cells in response to injury appear to regulate the acute-phase response. (Shown here are circulating cytokines; not shown is the cell-associated form.) Within hours, the cytokines influence gene expression in hepatocytes; corticosteroids released by the adrenal cortex act as cofactors. This so-called reprogramming of hepatocytes is responsible for alterations in plasma levels of numerous proteins after injury and inflammation.[195]

proliferation. A role has also been shown for tumor necrosis factor in bone remodeling.

Metabolic Effects

TNF has potent effects on metabolic homeostasis. In concert, these effects may be acutely beneficial for the host because they promote mobilization of nitrogenous and carbonaceous substrates from peripheral muscle and lipid stores for transport to splanchnic tissue, the site of synthesis of hepatic proteins with important roles as protease inhibitors, local immune modulators, and scavengers for trace minerals and free radicals.

In myocytes, TNF increases cell membrane influx of glucose, depletion of cell glycogen, and cellular efflux of lactate.[4] Secretion of TNF may thus represent an important signal for the induction of anaerobic glycolysis in somatic tissues.

TNF also has profound influences on body protein metabolism. Specifically, it induces a peripheral wasting,[5-7] with a release of amino acids from skeletal muscle.[8] Simultaneously, it promotes increased uptake of these nitrogenous substrates by the liver,[9] contributes to the preservation of liver mass, and enhances hepatic protein synthesis (in particular, of hepatic acute-phase proteins) [see Figure 1].[10]

Finally, TNF elicits changes in fat metabolism that are similar to the changes observed in infection. In some species, TNF promotes loss of triglycerides from adipocytes; it does so by decreasing the clearance of extracellular lipids,[11,12] inhibiting fatty acid synthesis,[13] and increasing cellular lipolysis. Furthermore, TNF stimulates increased hepatic lipogenesis in vivo.[14]

The role of TNF in cachexia It is thought that chronic excessive production of TNF may lead to the clinical syndrome of cachexia, which is characterized by severe losses of peripheral lean tissue, anorexia, and anemia (hence this cytokine's other name, cachectin). Indeed, chronic administration of sublethal doses of TNF in experimental models reproduces many of the physiologic findings observed in cachexia. In rodents, administration of TNF decreases food intake,[6,7,10] increases nitrogen loss,[13] and produces body lipid depletion[7] and weight loss. Tumors secreting human TNF produce a similar syndrome of cachexia with severe weight loss.[15] Additionally, TNF administration produces a reduction in body red blood cell mass[7] by decreasing both red cell synthesis and the red cells' life span.[16]

The role of TNF in sepsis Acute, exaggerated secretion of TNF may be responsible, in part, for the cardiovascular collapse, shock, and death associated with severe infection. High-dose TNF administration in rodents[17] and canines[18] precipitates a syndrome of hypotension, lactic acidosis, and death similar to that seen in human septic shock. Tissue findings are similar to those seen after septic shock, including adrenal necrosis, pulmonary congestion (possibly related to excessive margination of activated neutrophils into pulmonary epithelium), cecal necrosis, and ischemia of other regions of the bowel.[17] Furthermore, blockade of TNF before endotoxin infusions improved the survival rate in mice,[19] rabbits,[20] and primates.[21]

INTERLEUKIN-1

Immunologic Activities

IL-1 acts on a variety of immunologic cells. This cytokine has potent myelopoietic effects, including (1) the ability to increase the numbers of myeloid precursors in the bone mar-

adherence of macrophages; and induces rounding of the monocytes.[103] In addition to having effects on cytokine production, IL-10 inhibits T cell proliferation in response to antigen-presenting monocytes.[104,105] These anti-inflammatory properties of IL-10 have made it an attractive potential candidate for the treatment of injury and the septic response.

The biology of natural antagonists against cytokines is only beginning to unfold. Inhibitory activity against TNF or IL-1 has been observed in patients' sera during a variety of injury states, including infection, trauma, and cancer.[82] Such inhibitory activity can also be elicited in humans by administration of endotoxin.[88,94,106] Study of the actions of antagonists and their interactions with cytokines will provide important insights into the host response to injury. In addition, manipulation of antagonists (i.e., either enhancement of natural production or administration of exogenous antagonists) may evolve into strategies for the treatment of injury and sepsis.

Tissue Levels of Cytokines

Cells of both myeloid and nonmyeloid origin can produce cytokines. TNF, for example, is readily produced in vitro by pulmonary macrophages, Kupffer cells,[107] peritoneal macrophages, and endothelial cells. IL-1 is synthesized not only by blood monocytes and tissue macrophages but also by other cell types, including endothelial cells, keratinocytes, blood neutrophils, and B cells.[108] IL-6 is produced by fibroblasts, monocytes, macrophages, keratinocytes, and endothelial cells in vitro.[109] In rodents, TNF gene transcription is increased at many sites after endotoxin injection,[110] including the liver, kidney, lung, and spleen. In animals, IL-1 gene transcription is also increased at many tissue sites after injury.[111] Furthermore, in humans, endotoxin elicits production of cytokines not only by circulating monocytes but also by splanchnic tissues.[55]

The fact that diverse tissues can produce cytokines in vivo is an important characteristic distinguishing cytokine mediators from classic hormones. Because tissue-fixed macrophages exist near important effector cells in numerous organs, cytokines derived from such tissue macrophages may exert important local paracrine influences. Local tissue levels of the various cytokines in the lung or in hepatic tissues, for example, may be of greater importance than circulating levels in influencing the development of pulmonary failure or hepatic metabolic activities. The existence of cell-associated forms of TNF[112,113] and IL-1α indicates that the forms of cytokines produced in fixed tissues may be different from those that circulate. These tissue-specific forms may be important in localized biologic effects of cytokines through cell-cell interactions. The presence of a cell-associated form of IL-1 can explain the capacity of activated macrophages to induce natural killer cell cytotoxicity, T cell proliferation, and other functions by cell contact in the absence of any releasable IL-1.[114,115]

There is also evidence that cytokine production may be particularly increased at tissue sites near sites of injury. Intratracheal administration of endotoxin to rodents is associated with particularly significant increases in TNF levels in the bronchoalveolar lavage fluid even while TNF remains undetectable in the circulation [see Figure 4].[116] In humans with meningitis, levels of TNF,[117] IL-6,[61] and interferon gamma[65] are decidedly higher in the cerebrospinal fluid than in the systemic circulation. In rodents, IL-1 and IL-6 can be detected locally in healing wounds.[118] Interferon gamma can be detected in injured tissues, such as in the vesicular fluid of herpes simplex, in the lesions of psoriasis, in the lungs of patients with sarcoidosis, and in the synovial fluid of patients with rheumatoid arthritis. Recently, the proximity of an organ to tumor has also been shown to affect tissue cytokine production. In an experimental transplantable tumor model, implantation of tumor in the liver elicited significantly higher local levels of TNF, even in liver tissue remote

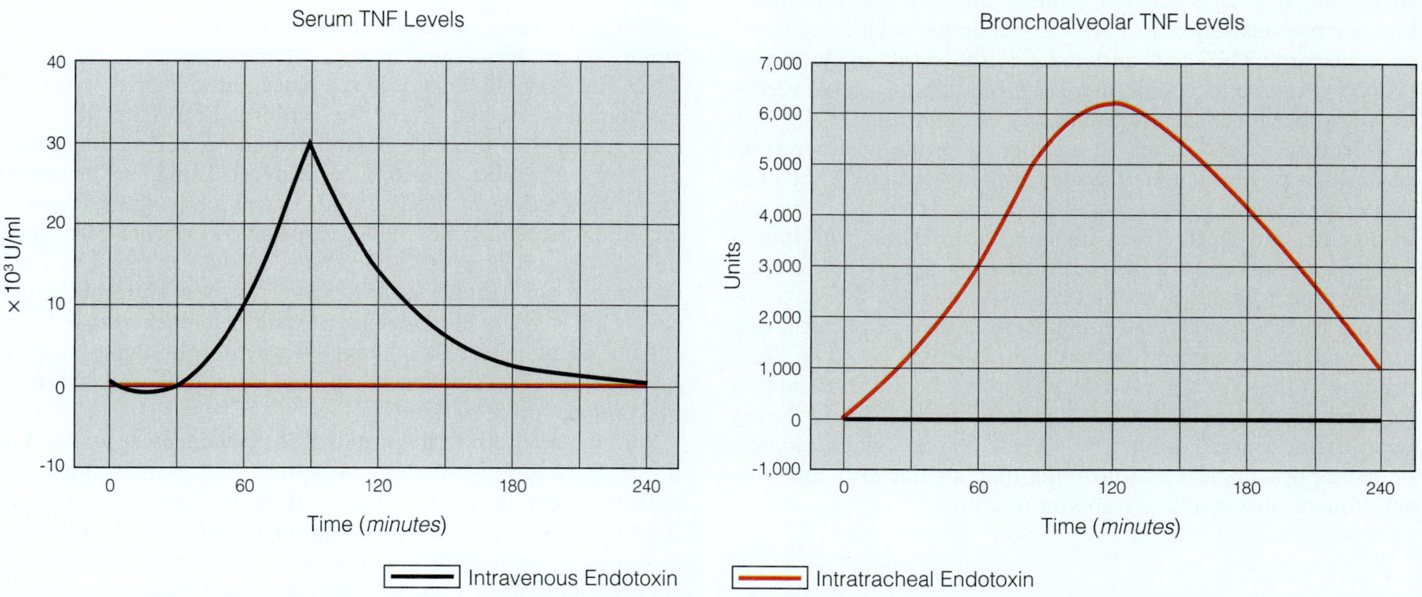

Figure 4 Cytokine production may be increased at tissue sites near sites of injury. Shown here are serum and bronchoalveolar TNF levels after intravenous and intratracheal administration of endotoxin. Intratracheal administration of endotoxin is associated with significantly higher bronchoalveolar TNF levels.[116]

from the tumor, when compared with liver tissue from animals with subcutaneous tumors.[119]

Thus, even though the majority of clinical studies involving cytokines in clinical illness have sought to detect cytokines in the circulation, tissue concentrations of these proteins are more likely to be biologically relevant than those in the circulation.

Role of Cytokines in Endotoxin Tolerance

Even though cytokine appearance is more frequent during clinical injury, absolute cytokine levels have generally correlated poorly with clinical outcome. One explanation for this is that tissue concentrations may be more biologically important than circulating levels. Tolerance may be another explanation: repeated exposure to injurious stimuli may alter host cytokine production and consequently the expression of host responses to injury. This is supported by data from studies on endotoxin tolerance.

Repeated exposure to endotoxin induces a state of tolerance. When rodents, rabbits, or even primates are injected with sublethal doses of endotoxin, many physiologic responses are attenuated, including fever, anorexia, weight loss, and acute-phase responses.[120,121] Experimental models have shown that an endotoxin-tolerant state is protective against oxygen toxicity or against massive infection and burn injury.[122] Two particular alterations in cytokine biology associated with repeated exposure to endotoxin contribute to this tolerance phenomenon. First, repeated exposure to endotoxin appears to blunt cellular production of cytokines.[121,122] LPS administered as a single injection, a short course of repeated injections of the same dose, or a continuous infusion produces an attenuated secretion of the cytokines TNF[121,122] and IL-6.[122] Second, tolerance to endotoxin may be partly related to decreased end-organ responses to cytokines. In a study examining the response of LPS-tolerant rats to exogenous TNF, rats were made tolerant to LPS by repeated injections of endotoxin and then challenged with an LD_{50} dose of TNF.[123] All LPS-tolerant rats survived, suggesting that LPS-tolerant animals also have a diminished biologic responsiveness to TNF.[123,124] Whether such cross-tolerance between TNF and endotoxin is the result of decreased cellular cytokine receptors, increased binding to soluble receptors, or other mechanisms remains to be determined.

Tolerance to endotoxin, in addition to being an interesting physiologic phenomenon, may also have important clinical consequences. Many patient populations are prone to recurrent bacteremia and sepsis. These include burn patients with infected open wounds and surgical patients with undrained or incompletely drained sources of infection. Additionally, the gastrointestinal tract is a potentially significant source of bacteria that may produce recurrent bacteremia. Normal bacterial flora residing in the GI tract can very well cross the intestinal mucosal barrier and appear systemically after injury[125,126] and during poor oral nutritional intake.[127,128] These episodes of physiologic or pathophysiological endotoxemia may significantly alter the subsequent host cytokine response to injury.

Mediator Interactions

The interactions of cytokines with one another and with classic hormones are the subject of increasing interest and active investigation. These mediator interactions can be classified into two primary areas: (1) cytokine interactions that influence the subsequent production of other mediators and (2) influences exerted by cytokines that have a synergistic effect on the actions of other mediators.

PROPAGATION OF MEDIATOR CASCADE

It appears that the release of host cytokines may involve a definitive, but convoluted, cascade. Cytokines are potent stimuli for the release of other mediators [see Figure 5]. Tumor necrosis factor, for example, elicits the release of the counterregulatory hormones glucagon, cortisol, and epinephrine[18] as well as of PGE_2, interleukin-1, granulocyte-macrophage colony-stimulating factor,[129] and tumor necrosis factor itself.[130] Interleukin-1 elicits the release of pituitary neurohormones, including adrenocorticotropic hormone (ACTH), thyroid-stimulating hormone, and somatostatin.[131-133] Interleukin-1 also directly elicits the release of corticosterone, insulin, and glucagon[134,135] and is a strong inducer of the release of GM-CSF, macrophage colony-stimulating factor (M-CSF), and colony-stimulating factor–1.[136] Interleukin-6 can elicit the production of interleukin-2 in vitro,[31] and interleukin-2 in turn can activate transcription of tumor necrosis factor mRNA in alveolar macrophages,[137] leading to increased production of TNF by human monocytes in vitro.

There is evidence that these convoluted positive feedback relations are organized in the fashion of a cytokine cascade during injury. In a primate model of bacteremia, administration of antibodies specific for TNF can block the release of classic hormones, such as cortisol and epinephrine, as well as the release of the cytokines IL-1β and IL-6 [see Figure 6].[21,58] Tumor necrosis factor blockade has also resulted in significantly diminished end-organ responses to bacteremia. Release of an early mediator, such as TNF, thus apparently triggers the release of the complete complement of cytokines that combine to elicit the host responses.

SYNERGISM

Once released, cytokine mediators also exhibit synergy among themselves as well as with other endogenous mediators. TNF, for example, enhances the glucagon-mediated uptake of amino acids by the liver.[9] In rabbits, TNF and IL-1 act synergistically to produce hemodynamic instability, alterations in energy expenditure, and hypertriglyceridemia.[138] The synergistic interaction of TNF and IL-1 in many tissue types—including pituitary cells, bone, vascular endothelial cells, skin, fibroblasts, and islets of Langerhans—is well described.[108] TNF and interferon gamma are synergistic in their antiproliferative effects on certain human and murine cell lines and in their enhancement of fungal killing by polymorphonuclear leukocytes. TNF is also synergistic with colony-stimulating factors in macrophage proliferation.[139]

An increase both in the number of cytokine receptors and in the binding affinity of those receptors is one mechanism for such synergism among cytokines. IL-6, for example, increases the expression of IL-2 receptors on thymocytes.[43] GM-CSF increases the expression of receptors for interferon gamma.[140] Interferon gamma, in turn, increases surface expression of IL-2 receptors on human monocytes.[141] The binding of TNF to adipocytes and fibroblasts is known to be enhanced by preexposure of the cells to interferon gamma.

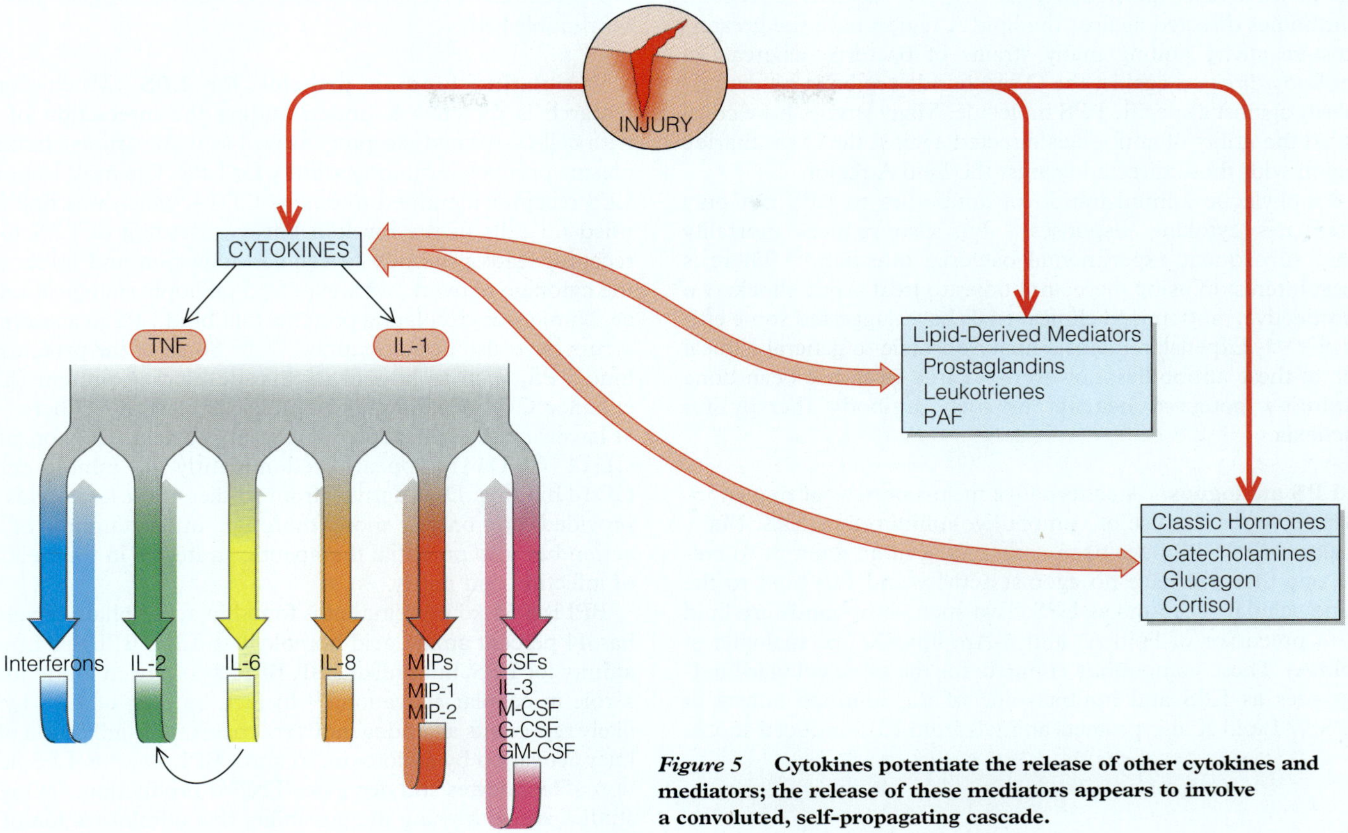

Figure 5 Cytokines potentiate the release of other cytokines and mediators; the release of these mediators appears to involve a convoluted, self-propagating cascade.

Clinical Therapy

Progress in understanding cytokine biology offers increasing potential for the beneficial modulation of host responses to injury. There is potential not only to block the detrimental effects that are triggered by excessive release of various cytokines [see Figure 7] but also to harness the beneficial qualities of many cytokines [see Sidebar Physical Properties of Cytokines and Natural Antagonists to Cytokines].

MODULATION OF ENDOGENOUS CYTOKINE RESPONSE

Certain cytokines, particularly TNF, IL-1, and interferon gamma, play essential roles in detrimental responses to injury, including septic shock and cachexia of disease, and extensive research has been directed at blocking these detrimental effects. Research efforts have focused on five strategies: (1) preventing injurious stimuli from reaching cell sources of cytokine production, (2) decreasing host tissue production of cytokines despite stimulation by injurious stimuli, (3) neutralizing cytokines that are produced, (4) increasing cytokine clearance, and (5) modulating the responses of effector cells to cytokines. Preclinical and clinical studies of many of these strategies are already under way, although it is likely that clinical utility will ultimately result from a combination of approaches.

Preventing Injurious Stimuli from Reaching Cell Sources of Cytokine Production

Paramount in the treatment of injury is eradication of injurious stimuli. Traditional treatments (e.g., excision and allograft coverage of burn wounds, excision of tumors, or surgical drainage and antibiotic treatment of infections) abolish noxious stimuli that can elicit or propagate a host cytokine response. Terminating the injurious stimulus reverses many of the metabolic alterations associated with injury (e.g., the hypermetabolism associated with burn injury or the altered glucose metabolism associated with cancer-bearing states).

In clinical infections, however, even with administration of appropriate antibiotics and surgical therapy, toxins released by killed bacteria may yet elicit host cytokine production sufficient to cause detrimental biologic responses, including shock. Furthermore, incompletely eradicated infections can lead to ongoing toxin release and cachexia. Lipopolysaccharide, one of the most potent bacterial toxins, is an important trigger of the cytokine cascade.[55,58] In the early 1980s, clinical studies were begun to neutralize LPS before it could trigger host mediator production. Initially, the neutralizing agent was polyvalent IgG antibodies from blood donors. In septic patients, administration of such polyvalent IgG reduced the appearance of TNF in the circulation but also reduced the mortality from sepsis.[142]

LPS antibodies The utility of targeting monoclonal antibodies at specific epitopes of the LPS molecule has been examined. LPS has three main regions: the inner core, or lipid A region; the intermediate region; and the outer region, or O saccharide region [see 88 Immunomodulation]. Monoclonal antibodies directed at each of these regions have been produced.[143-146] Directing antibodies against each region has distinct advantages. LPS molecules from different gram-negative bacteria differ in structure, particularly at the O saccharide region. Antibodies directed against the lipid A region have the greatest cross-reactivity among many strains of bacteria, whereas an antibody directed against the O saccharide region is potent primarily against a specific LPS molecule. Many studies have compared the utility of antibodies directed against the O saccharide region with those directed against the lipid A region.

Prophylactic administration of antibodies to LPS not only attenuates cytokine responses[143] but also reduces mortality from subsequent experimental bacterial infection.[144] There is great interest in using these antibodies to treat septic shock; two prospective, randomized clinical trials have suggested some efficacy.[145,147] Expense remains a major obstacle to general clinical use of these antibodies, however.[148] Little work has been done exploring potential benefits of such antibody therapy for cachexia.

LPS analogues An alternative means of neutralizing endotoxin involves the use of competitive inhibitors of LPS. Many analogues of LPS have been constructed in an attempt to create one that will have no agonist activity and will bind to the same cellular receptors as LPS. Two such compounds are lipid X (a precursor of lipid A) and 3-Aza-lipid X (an analogue of lipid A). These compounds compete for the same cellular binding sites as LPS and inhibit some of the immune effects of LPS.[149] Lipid X also protects animals from LPS-induced shock.

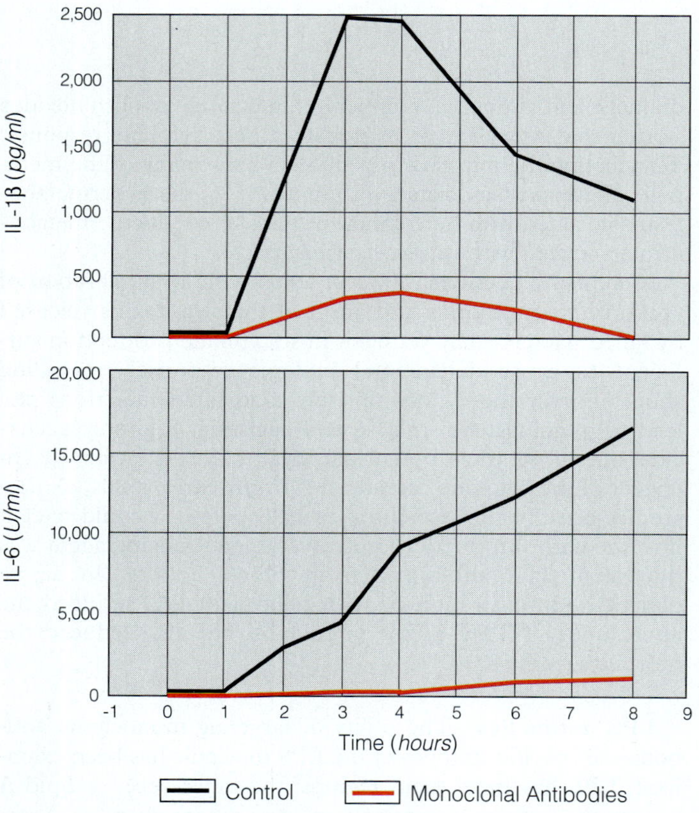

No preclinical or clinical studies of such analogues have yet been published.

Circulating binding proteins for LPS Much current research is directed at understanding the interaction of LPS with cell-associated receptors as well as with various circulating plasma proteins exhibiting affinity for LPS. The most important LPS receptor identified to date is CD14, which was first identified on cells of the myeloid lineage. Binding of LPS to this receptor leads promptly to cellular activation and initiation of the cytokine network, with expected pathophysiological sequelae. Numerous circulating proteins that bind LPS in acute-phase serum have also been identified.[150-153] Some of the proteins that bind LPS, such as lipopolysaccharide-binding protein (LBP), enhance CD14 binding and cellular activation. Others, such as bactericidal/permeability–increasing protein (BPI) or soluble CD14 (sCD14), appear predominantly to inhibit cellular CD14 binding. Data derived from studies of these proteins have provided not only a more thorough understanding of LPS action but also potential therapeutic strategies in the treatment of infection and injury.

BPI is a 55 kd protein that is found in acute-phase serum and has 44 percent amino acid homology to LBP. BPI also has high affinity for LPS, but unlike LBP, BPI has not been found to have a role in cellular activation.[152] In fact, binding of LPS by BPI likely represents an endogenous mechanism for inhibition of cellular activation by endotoxin. In vitro, BPI prevents LPS activation of leukocytes and decreases TNF-α production.[154] Ongoing studies are addressing the possibility that administration of BPI may be useful in diminishing the pathophysiological changes seen in sepsis.[155] Modified forms of BPI are also being tested, including a 23 kd NH_2-terminal fragment of BPI (BPI_{23}).[156,157] Administration of BPI has proved effective in preventing cytokine activation and the resultant physiologic changes from endotoxemia in rodents and other animal models.[156-158]

The cell surface receptor CD14 was originally used as a myeloid marker.[159] CD14 is a 55 kd protein anchored to the cell surface by a glycerophosphorylinositol (GPI) tail. Under normal conditions, CD14 is also found as a soluble protein circulating freely in the plasma at levels of 2 to 6 µg/ml.[153] Administration of LPS increases expression of CD14 by tissue-fixed macrophages, such as liver Kupffer cells.[160] Binding of cell surface CD14 is instrumental in the elaboration not only of cytokines[161] but also of cytokine antagonists such as soluble TNF receptors.[162] Soluble CD14 is released by the actions of phospholipases on the GPI anchor or by protein digestion.[163] Strategies at neutralizing LPS activation of cytokines and the resultant cellular responses have included administration of anti-CD14 antibodies[164] as well as sCD14 as a competitive binder for LPS.[165] No clinical data are yet available.

Decreasing Host Tissue Production of Cytokines

Nutritional manipulation of host tissues As discussed previously, the responsiveness of host macrophages to injury appears to be influenced by previous exposure to noxious stimuli as well as by the prevailing cytokine milieu. Additionally, host macrophage cytokine production appears to be related to nutritional factors. In particular, the lipid composition of a patient's diet and the route of nutrient intake have been shown experimentally to have significant influences on host mediator

Figure 6 Monoclonal antibodies to TNF were administered to baboons two hours before an *E. coli* infusion. As illustrated here, the monoclonal antibodies to TNF attenuated the appearance of IL-1β and IL-6 during bacteremia.[58]

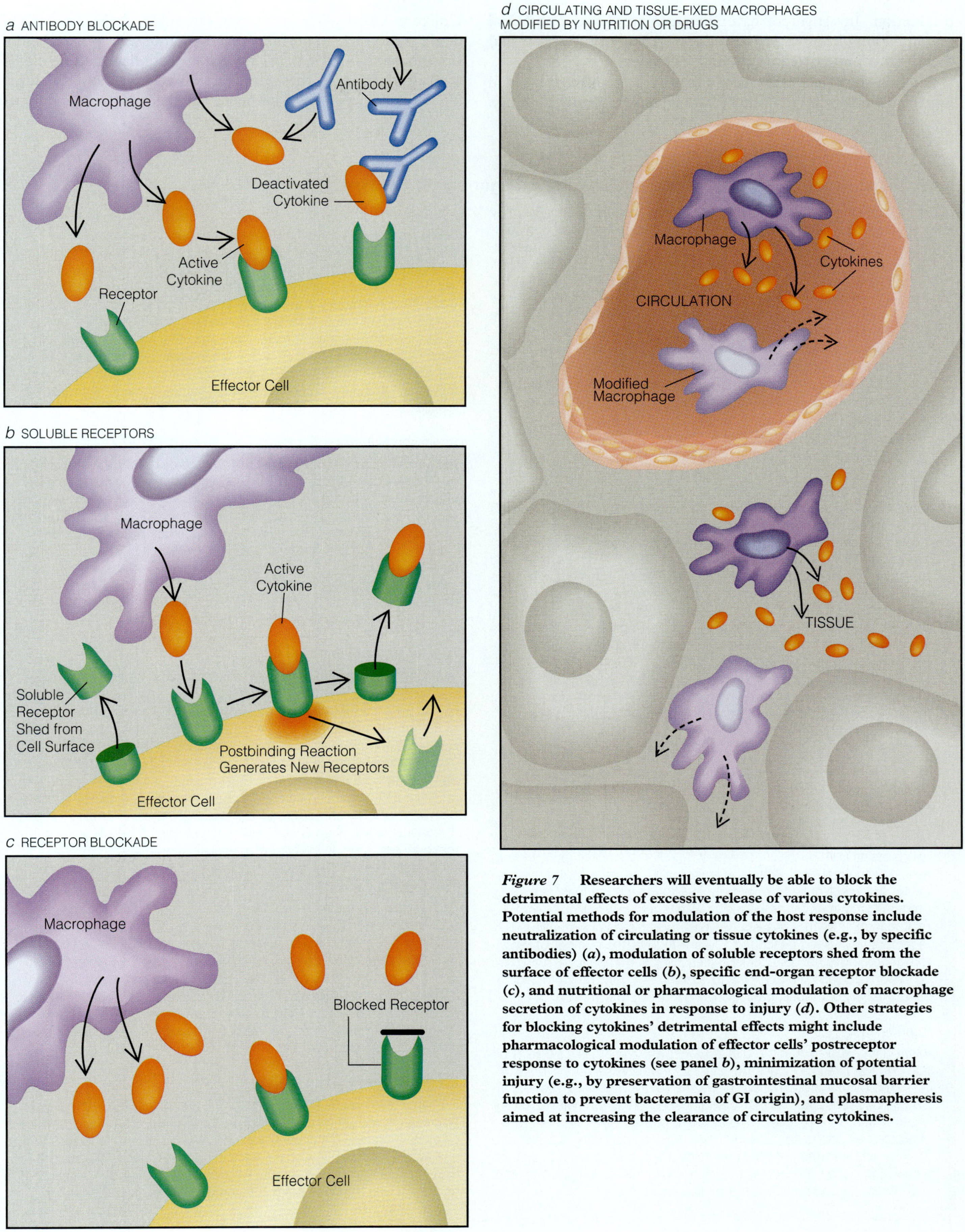

101 CYTOKINES, INJURY, AND INFECTION — 1615

a ANTIBODY BLOCKADE

b SOLUBLE RECEPTORS

c RECEPTOR BLOCKADE

d CIRCULATING AND TISSUE-FIXED MACROPHAGES MODIFIED BY NUTRITION OR DRUGS

Figure 7 Researchers will eventually be able to block the detrimental effects of excessive release of various cytokines. Potential methods for modulation of the host response include neutralization of circulating or tissue cytokines (e.g., by specific antibodies) (*a*), modulation of soluble receptors shed from the surface of effector cells (*b*), specific end-organ receptor blockade (*c*), and nutritional or pharmacological modulation of macrophage secretion of cytokines in response to injury (*d*). Other strategies for blocking cytokines' detrimental effects might include pharmacological modulation of effector cells' postreceptor response to cytokines (see panel *b*), minimization of potential injury (e.g., by preservation of gastrointestinal mucosal barrier function to prevent bacteremia of GI origin), and plasmapheresis aimed at increasing the clearance of circulating cytokines.

production. Investigators have therefore employed nutritional manipulations in attempts to reduce cytokine production and thereby moderate deleterious clinical changes.

Altering the relative amounts of n-6 versus n-3 unsaturated fatty acids in the diet may alter host cytokine response to injury.

Unlike n-3 fatty acids, n-6 unsaturated fatty acids (e.g., arachidonic acid) are important precursors of the prostaglandin, thromboxane, and leukotriene classes of inflammatory mediators. Production of these arachidonic acid metabolites during infection has a positive influence on the release of cytokines.

Physical Properties of Cytokines and Natural Antagonists of Cytokines

Many names exist for some of these protein mediators because they were isolated independently for different properties and named accordingly [see Table 1]. As a group, cytokines are of roughly similar molecular weight, with nonmodified forms between 10 and 30 kilodaltons (kd). They may undergo variable posttranscription modification, including the formation of dimers and trimers (in the case of tumor necrosis factor [TNF]) or glycosylation (in the case of interleukin-6 [IL-6]). Thus, multiple forms of each protein may exist simultaneously in vivo. Cytokines generally have very short circulating half-lives, on the order of minutes, and are generally sensitive to heating and freezing, with significant biologic activity lost with each process. The physical properties of these cytokines have been summarized [see Table 3].

Tumor Necrosis Factor

The circulating form of tumor necrosis factor is a polypeptide with a molecular weight of 17 kd and an isoelectric point (pI) of approximately 5.3. It is translated as a precursor with 233 amino acids; it then undergoes proteolytic cleavages to generate the secreted protein of 157 amino acids.[181] This mature protein contains one intrachain disulfide bond and exists as a dimer, a trimer, or a pentamer in solution.[182] Bioactive, cell-associated forms with molecular weights of 24 to 31 kd have also been identified.[112,113] The synthesis of TNF is elicited by numerous infections or inflammatory stimuli, including bacteria or their cell wall–derived lipopolysaccharide (i.e., endotoxin), bacterial exotoxins, protozoans, fungi, and viral particles. Stimulation induces both increased transcription and increased translation of the protein, leading to the release of mature protein within minutes. The half-life of circulating TNF is brief, approximately 14 minutes in rabbits and approximately 14 to 18 minutes in humans.[183] Injected radiolabeled TNF is degraded in many organ systems, including the liver, the skin, the gastrointestinal tract, and the kidneys.[11]

Interleukin-1

The name interleukin-1 (IL-1) is shared by two distinct proteins; only 30 percent of the amino acids of these proteins are homologous. Both are synthesized as high-molecular-weight precursors of approximately 33 kd, with mature forms of approximately 17 kd. The two bind with equal affinity to the IL-1 receptors. Three physical properties distinguish these two proteins from each other, however: (1) IL-1α is acidic (pI 5), whereas IL-1β is neutral (pI 7); (2) the precursor of IL-1α has bioactivity, whereas the precursor of IL-1β does not; and (3) the mature form of IL-1α is predominantly membrane bound, whereas a significant portion of the mature form of IL-1β is released. At least two classes of high-affinity IL-1 receptors have been described.[184] As with TNF, the number of receptors per cell does not correlate with bioactivity. IL-1α and IL-1β both have very short circulating half-lives (six to 10 minutes)[185] and are both degraded in a variety of tissues, particularly the kidneys, the liver, and the skin.

Interleukin-2

Interleukin-2 (IL-2) is translated as a 15 kd protein and has a single disulfide bond between residues 58 and 105 that is essential for bioactivity.[186] The natural protein undergoes variable glycosylation. The recombinant nonglycosylated molecule also has a short serum half-life, on the order of six to 10 minutes. The IL-2 receptor complex has been well characterized and is composed of two unlinked peptides of 55 kd and 75 kd. Lymphocytes are the predominant cell source of IL-2; antigen stimulation in the lymphocytes triggers rapid increases in transcription of both the IL-2 gene and the gene for IL-2 receptors.

Interleukin-6

Interleukin-6 exists as variably modified phosphoglycoproteins.[187,188] As secreted by human monocytes or fibroblasts in vitro, IL-6 has molecular weights ranging from 23 to 30 kd,[187] although the prevailing circulating form in humans after endotoxin challenge appears to be a 45 kd species.[57] Endotoxins and viruses, as well as other cytokines (e.g., TNF and IL-1), are potent inducers for transcription and production of IL-6 by fibroblasts, monocytes, macrophages, keratinocytes, and endothelial cells in vitro.[109] Transcription of mRNA for this protein by fibroblasts can be detected within 30 minutes after endotoxin stimulation and is sustained for at least 20 hours. A specific receptor for this cytokine has also been identified.[189]

Interferon Gamma

Recombinant nonglycosylated interferon gamma has a molecular weight of 17 kd and a circulating half-life of approximately 30 minutes. The natural proteins of 40 kd and 70 kd exist as polymeric glycoproteins that can be resolved to three mononumeric proteins of 25 kd, 20 kd, and 15.5 kd. Interferon gamma is readily produced by lymphocytes, particularly human helper T cells, in response to microbial antigens[190,191] or cytokines such as IL-2. Increased transcription of interferon gamma T cells occurs within six hours of stimulation,[192] with peak release of this protein at approximately 48 to 72 hours.[190] Alveolar macrophages also appear to be capable of producing interferon gamma.

IL-1 Receptor Antagonist

Interleukin-1 receptor antagonist is a glycosylated protein with a molecular weight of 22 kd. This protein has been isolated as three different forms, varying in the amount of glycosylation.[92] The recombinant form of the protein has a molecular weight of 17 kd.[96] This cytokine shares significant homology to interleukin-1β. It binds to the IL-1 receptor with a kd of 150 pM, which is similar in affinity to IL-1α or IL-1β[193] but appears to have no agonist activity. The protein that has been cloned and recombinantly produced has specific affinity for the interleukin-1 receptor type 1, which is on T cells and fibroblasts, but does not bind to the type 2 receptor, which is on B cells and macrophages.[93] This protein therefore appears to be an inhibitor of interleukin activity.

TNF Binding Proteins

Two distinct proteins have been isolated and cloned, each occurring naturally and each possessing inhibitory activity for TNF bioactivity. The first is a protein with a molecular weight of approximately 30 kd and appears to be the extracellular domain of TNF receptor type I, whereas the second is a protein with a molecular weight of approximately 40 kd and appears to be the extracellular domain of TNF receptor type II.[80–86] These proteins are shed from the cell surface in response to a variety of inflammatory stimuli.[87] Human studies demonstrate that these proteins appear rapidly in response to endotoxemia.[88]

Interleukin-10

Human interleukin-10 (IL-10) is an 18 kd nonglycosylated polypeptide. Sources of the human protein include T cells, macrophages, keratinocytes, and B cells. The DNA sequence is well conserved among various species; homology between human IL-10 and rat IL-10 is 73 percent.[194] One interesting finding is that IL-10 shares great DNA and amino acid homology with the open reading frame of the Epstein-Barr virus.

Replacement of dietary n-6 fatty acids with n-3 fatty acids can theoretically alter host cytokine production [see 100 Eicosanoids in Surgery]. In experimental rodent studies, eicosanoid production—as well as production of TNF and IL-1 by liver tissue macrophages—was significantly reduced after the animals were fed a diet high in fish oils, which are rich in n-3 fatty acids.[166] In other studies, monocytes isolated from human subjects who had been pretreated with fish oils rich in n-3 fatty acids exhibited a diminished TNF and IL-1β response when stimulated with LPS in vitro.[167] Animal studies have demonstrated the efficacy of n-3 fatty acids in attenuating injury in a model of granulomatous colitis.[168] Some clinical evidence suggests that diets rich in n-3 fatty acids reduce the severity of inflammatory and immune conditions, such as rheumatoid arthritis,[169] psoriasis,[170] and systemic lupus erythematosus. Although no data are yet available to demonstrate the efficacy of such a diet in attenuating detrimental responses during sepsis, the results of these experiments certainly encourage studies of long-term administration of fish oils to patients at high risk for infection and sepsis as a method of modulating host responses to injury.

The route of feeding also may influence the production of cytokines during injury. Hormonal and metabolic responses to an endotoxin challenge were compared in two groups of healthy volunteers; during the week before the endotoxin challenge, one group had received 100 percent of feedings by vein, and the other group had received feedings by mouth. The subjects who received only intravenous feedings had twice the TNF response to the same endotoxin challenge as the subjects who had received oral feedings[171] [see Figure 8]. The degree of peripheral nitrogen loss and the acute-phase protein response were also attenuated by previous oral feedings. The cellular mechanisms underlying these altered responses to endotoxemia are as yet unknown. It has long been thought that patients receiving parenteral feedings have compromised clinical responses to injury. The findings of this study suggest that alterations in cytokine production may be responsible and that early enteral feedings may be a method for modulating the responses to injury.

Manipulation with interleukin-10 IL-10 appears to modulate the detrimental host responses to injury by attenuating cytokine release in response to noxious stimuli. Studies in rodents have demonstrated that administration of IL-10 not only dampens the circulating cytokine response to endotoxin but also protects against the consequent pathophysiological effects.[105,172] In mice that were injected with an otherwise lethal dose of endotoxin, IL-10 in doses of 1.0 μg or 0.5 μg administered within 30 minutes of LPS injection protected against lethality.[105] To date, however, only preclinical data exist.

Pharmacological manipulation As stated above, experimental data have firmly documented a role for glucocorticoids in inhibiting production of cytokines such as TNF[67,68] and IL-6.[69] It has also been confirmed by human in vivo studies that cortisol inhibits the production of tumor necrosis factor in response to injury.[71,72] Clinical trials of glucocorticoids for septic shock, however, have produced mixed results,[73,74] which underscores our lack of understanding of the complex relations between cytokines and their natural inhibitors [see Natural Antagonists to Cytokines, above]. At present, it is unclear what role, if any,

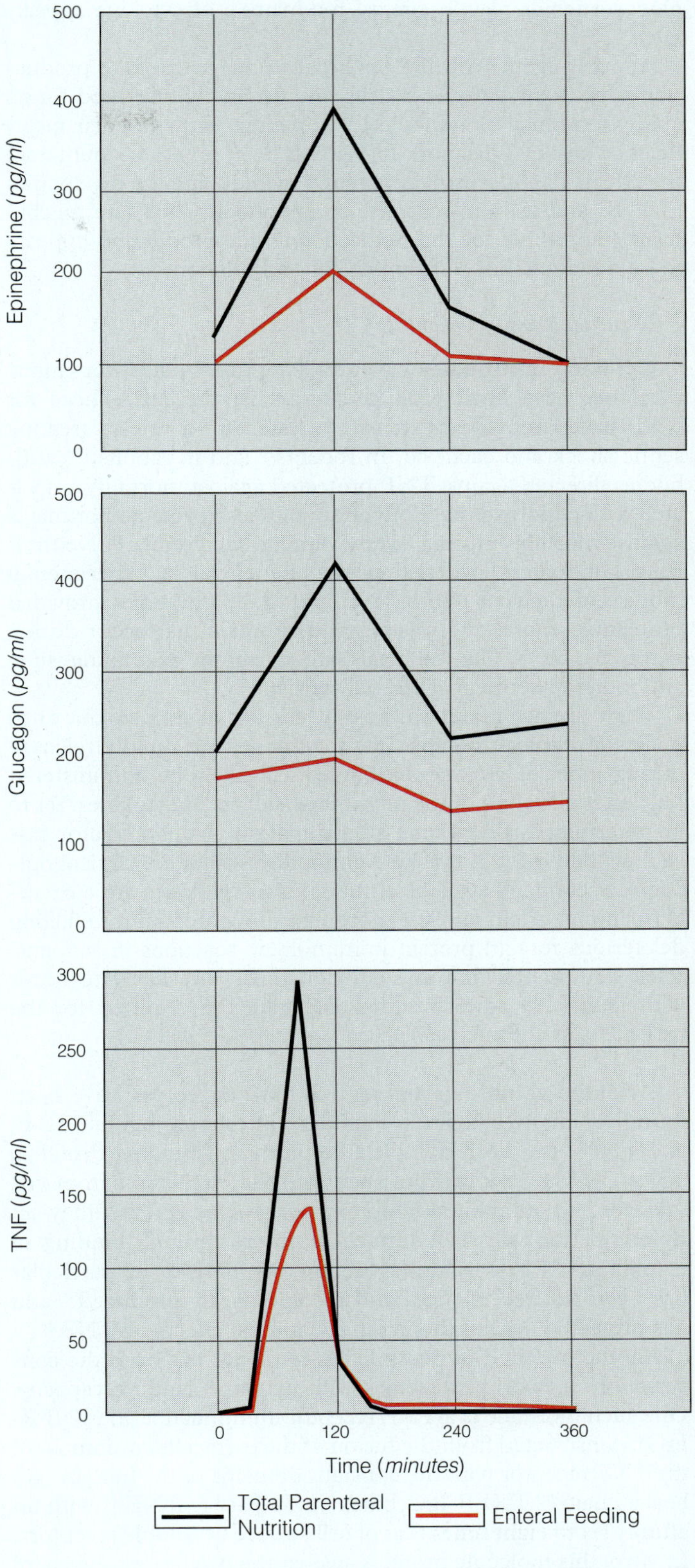

Figure 8 Illustrated is the effect of the route of feedings on the endocrine responses to endotoxin. Circulating levels of epinephrine, glucagon, and tumor necrosis factor in response to an injection of endotoxin are compared in subjects who received only intravenous feedings for one week and subjects who received only enteral feedings. The subjects who received intravenous feedings and gut rest had a markedly exaggerated response to injury.[171]

glucocorticoids play in clinical modulation of cytokine appearance.

Another agent with the potential to affect cytokine production is pentoxifylline. This drug was originally marketed for its ability to reduce blood viscosity in patients with vascular insufficiency and claudication. It has also been noted to counteract the effects of endotoxin, apparently by reducing the production of TNF and IL-6 in response to endotoxin.[173,174] The mechanism responsible for the reduced cytokine production appears to be a reduction in TNF mRNA accumulation.[70]

Neutralization of Cytokines

Cytokine antibodies Neutralizing antibodies for many cytokines have been produced and characterized. Those for TNF have been most extensively tested for a role in treating septic shock and cachexia. In rodents[19] and in rabbits,[175] antibodies directed against TNF protected against mortality associated with endotoxemia. TNF antibodies also protected primates against mortality during overwhelming bacteremia.[21] Neutralizing antibodies have also proved beneficial in experimental models of cachexia. Both TNF and IL-1 antibodies provided protection against the wasting and anorexia that occur during chronic injury.[6] Clinical trials are currently examining such antibodies in settings of clinical sepsis.

There are two major obstacles to the use of anticytokine antibodies as clinical therapy. First, cytokines are rapidly released during injury. Cytokine antibodies will likely be administered only after initiation of the physiologic effects of cytokines. Yet to be determined is how long after initiation of the mediator cascade will delivery of cytokine antibodies still affect clinical outcome. Second, all available antibodies to cytokines are currently of animal origin and therefore have the potential for eliciting deleterious foreign protein immunologic reactions in humans. Such detrimental immune reactions are more likely to occur with long-term administration, as might be required for the treatment of chronic cachexia.

Cytokine soluble receptors Soluble receptors have been found for many cytokines, including interferon gamma, IL-6, and TNF[75] [see TNF Soluble Receptors and Binding Proteins, *above*]. These receptors are shed into the circulation from cell surfaces and are natural inhibitors of cytokine activity; they act by competing with cell surface receptors through binding of cytokines.[46,86] The soluble receptor for TNF-α in particular has been isolated, cloned, and recombinantly produced[86] and has protected against the in vitro cytotoxic effects of TNF.[46]

Another method of neutralizing cytokines has been the construction of hybrid molecules with cytokine binding capacity. One such molecule is a TNF receptor immunoadhesin (TNFR-IgG), constructed from the fusion of the extracellular domain of the TNF receptor with the constant domains of the human IgG heavy chain.[90] TNFR-IgG binds to TNF-α or TNF-β with an affinity six to eight times that of cell surface or soluble receptors. In vitro, this molecule protects against the deleterious effects of TNF.[90] Whether such agents will be important clinically for neutralization of harmful effects of cytokines is an intensive research area. Such hybrid soluble receptors would have an advantage over antibodies; as human proteins, they will not elicit a foreign-protein response.

Increasing Cytokine Clearance

Another strategy for modulating detrimental cytokine responses involves increasing the clearance of cytokines during infection and injury. Attempts are under way to design filters that specifically remove endotoxin or cytokines from the circulation.[176] Activated charcoal and other resins are being tested for their ability to bind TNF, IL-1, IL-6, interferon alfa, and interferon gamma.[176] Although studies are still preclinical, they offer the potential of producing an anticytokine therapy that will not involve injection of foreign protein into patients.

Natural clearance of cytokines occurs through many routes, including the kidney and liver. An interesting question is whether increased renal blood flow or even plasmapheresis during infection would affect circulating cytokine levels and clinical outcome. Hepatic failure has been associated with higher levels of circulating cytokines. No data are available to relate renal failure to circulating levels of cytokines. Important answers to both biologic and clinical questions may be provided by trials of aggressive dialysis for patients with renal failure and trials of extracorporeal filtration of cytokines in renal or liver failure patients at high risk for infection and sepsis.

Modulation of Effector Cells

Receptor antagonists Another option for modulating the biologic effects of cytokines is blockade at the effector cell by specific receptor antagonists. As discussed above, considerable effort has been expended to produce an IL-1 receptor antagonist by recombinant means and to characterize its biologic activities. This receptor antagonist is useful both in experimental models of shock and in models of cachexia. In rabbits, IL-1ra decreased mortality from endotoxemic shock.[101,102] In a model of inflammation and cachexia, IL-1ra protected against anorexia, weight loss, and acute-phase response during injury.[98]

For each cytokine, a number of distinct receptors may exist. Expression of the various receptors may be a characteristic of the tissue involved. For example, in the case of IL-1, at least two types of receptors exist: one expressed mainly by fibroblasts, endothelial cells, hepatocytes, and T cells, and the other found mainly on neutrophils, macrophages, and B cells.[177] Antibodies specific for each receptor may block detrimental end-organ responses while selectively preserving potentially beneficial effects of cytokines.

Pharmacological manipulation Many of the end-organ responses elicited by cytokines appear to be produced by release of secondary mediators at the effector sites. These secondary mediators may include not only other cytokines but also members of other mediator classes (e.g., eicosanoids, platelet-activating factor [PAF], and nitric oxide [NO·]). Cyclooxygenase inhibitors, such as ibuprofen, which inhibit production of eicosanoids, also block physiologic responses to cytokines, such as the febrile response associated with infusions of TNF, IL-1, or IL-6. A competitive inhibitor of NO·—namely, N^G-methyl-L-arginine—has displayed protection against the hypotensive effects of TNF in a canine model,[178] suggesting that the effects of TNF on hemodynamic stability may also be mediated through NO·. Many other antagonists to eicosanoids, PAF, and NO· have been developed and may represent other ways of attenuating the end-organ response to cytokines.

ADMINISTRATION OF EXOGENOUS CYTOKINES

Cytokines also have potent immunostimulatory effects. A number of cytokines are thought to principally influence immune function. Colony-stimulating factors, for example, may have predominantly myeloproliferative effects. IL-2 is thought to affect mainly lymphocyte proliferation, differentiation, and function. Interferon gamma has immunopotentiating effects on lymphocyte function as well as antiviral effects. It is hoped that exogenous administrations of these and other cytokines may be beneficial in times of injury.

Some preliminary studies on the effects of endogenous administration have been encouraging. Administration of IL-2 to immunocompromised rodents confers survival benefit during subsequent infection.[59] Infusion of interferon gamma in patients enhances the oxidative activities of blood monocytes.[39,40] Infusions of human GM-CSF in primates produce leukocytosis that involves neutrophils, lymphocytes, monocytes, and eosinophils. Infusions in neutropenic AIDS patients produce increases in the white blood cell count.[179] Interferon gamma has proved efficacious in the treatment of patients with refractory leishmaniasis.[180] Although these results are preliminary, they encourage further investigations into potential roles for select cytokines as immunoadjuvants during sepsis, particularly in the immunocompromised host.

Conclusion

Cytokines are clearly important mediators of the host responses to infection and injury. These protein mediators are redundant in actions and are released in a convoluted but characteristic cascade. Increasingly clear is the importance of cytokines produced in fixed tissues, particularly at sites of injury. A complex system of natural inhibitors to cytokines exists to protect the host against potential detrimental effects of these proteins. It is hoped that increased understanding of these host mediators and their natural antagonists will lead to improved treatment of the injured patient.

References

1. Moser R, Schleiffenbaum B, Groscurth P, et al: Interleukin 1 and tumor necrosis factor stimulate human vascular endothelial cells to promote transendothelial neutrophil passage. J Clin Invest 83:444, 1989
2. Ulich TR, del Castillo J, Keys M, et al: Kinetics and mechanisms of recombinant human interleukin 1 and tumor necrosis factor-alpha-induced changes in circulating numbers of neutrophils and lymphocytes. J Immunol 139:3406, 1987
3. Frater-Schroder M, Risau W, Hallman R, et al: Tumour necrosis factor type alpha, a potent inhibitor of endothelial cell growth in vitro, is angiogenic in vivo. Proc Natl Acad Sci USA 84:5277, 1987
4. Lee MD, Zentella A, Vine W, et al: Effect of endotoxin-induced monokines on glucose metabolism in the muscle cell line L6. Proc Natl Acad Sci USA 84:2590, 1987
5. Flores EA, Bistrian BR, Pomposelli JJ, et al: Infusion of tumor necrosis factor/cachectin promotes muscle catabolism in the rat: a synergistic effect with interleukin 1. J Clin Invest 83:1614, 1989
6. Fong YM, Moldawer LL, Marano MA, et al: Cachectin/TNF or IL-1 alpha induces cachexia with redistribution of body proteins. Am J Physiol 256:R659, 1989
7. Tracey KJ, Wei H, Manogue KR, et al: Cachectin/tumor necrosis factor induces cachexia, anemia, and inflammation. J Exp Med 167:1211, 1988
8. Warren RS, Starnes HF, Gabrilove JL, et al: The acute metabolic effects of tumor necrosis factor administration. Arch Surg 122:1396, 1987
9. Warren RS, Donner DB, Starnes HF, et al: Modulation of endogenous hormone action by recombinant human tumor necrosis factor. Proc Natl Acad Sci USA 84:8619, 1987
10. Moldawer LL, Anderson C, Gelin J, et al: Regulation of food intake and hepatic protein synthesis by recombinant-derived cytokines. Am J Physiol 254:G450, 1988
11. Beutler B, Mahoney J, Le Trang N, et al: Purification of cachectin, a lipoprotein lipase-suppressing hormone secreted by endotoxin-induced RAW 264.7 cells. J Exp Med 161:984, 1985
12. Zechner R, Newman TC, Sherry B, et al: Recombinant human cachectin/tumor necrosis factor but not interleukin-1 alpha downregulates lipoprotein lipase gene expression at the transcriptional level in mouse 3T3-L1 adipocytes. Mol Cell Biol 8:2394, 1988
13. Fong Y, Lowry SF: Tumor necrosis factor in the pathophysiology of infection and sepsis. Immunol Immunopathol 55:157, 1990
14. Feingold KR, Grunfeld C: Tumor necrosis factor-alpha stimulates hepatic lipogenesis in the rat in vivo. J Clin Invest 80:184, 1987
15. Oliff A, Defeo-Jones D, Boyer M, et al: Tumors secreting human TNF/cachectin induce cachexia in mice. Cell 50:555, 1987
16. Moldawer LL, Marano MA, Wei H, et al: Cachectin/tumor necrosis factor-alpha alters red blood cell kinetics and induces anemia in vivo. FASEB J 3:1637, 1989
17. Tracey KJ, Beutler B, Lowry SF, et al: Shock and tissue injury induced by recombinant human cachectin. Science 234:470, 1986
18. Tracey KJ, Lowry SF, Fahey TJ, et al; Cachectin/tumor necrosis factor induces lethal shock and stress hormone responses in the dog. Surg Gynecol Obstet 164:415, 1987
19. Beutler B, Milsark IW, Cerami AC: Passive immunization against cachectin/tumor necrosis factor protects mice from lethal effect of endotoxin. Science 229:869, 1985
20. Mathison JC, Wolfson E, Ulevitch RJ: Participation of tumor necrosis factor in the mediation of gram negative bacterial lipopolysaccharide-induced injury in rabbits. J Clin Invest 81:1925, 1988
21. Tracey KJ, Fong Y, Hesse DG, et al: Anti-cachectin/TNF monoclonal antibodies prevent septic shock during lethal bacteraemia. Nature 330:662, 1987
22. Chen L, Novick D, Rubinstein M, et al: Recombinant interferon-beta 2 (interleukin-6) induces myeloid differentiation. FEBS Lett 239:299, 1988
23. Watson ML, Lewis GP, Westwick J: Increased vascular permeability and polymorphonuclear leucocyte accumulation in vivo in response to recombinant cytokines and supernatant from cultures of human synovial cells treated with interleukin 1. Br J Exp Pathol 70:93, 1989
24. Baumann H, Isseroff H, Latimer JJ, et al: Phorbol ester modulates interleukin 6- and interleukin 1-regulated expression of acute phase plasma proteins in hepatoma cells. J Biol Chem 263:17390, 1988
25. Moldawer LL, Georgieff M, Lundholm K: Interleukin 1, tumour necrosis factor-alpha (cachectin) and the pathogenesis of cancer cachexia. Clin Physiol 7:263, 1987
26. Nawroth PP, Handley DA, Esmon CT, et al: Interleukin 1 induces endothelial cell procoagulant while suppressing cell-surface anticoagulant activity. Proc Natl Acad Sci USA 83:3460, 1986
27. Miller LC, Dinarello CA: Biologic activities of interleukin-1 relevant to rheumatic diseases. Pathol Immunopathol Res 6:22, 1987
28. Goronzy J, Weyand C, Quan J, et al: Enhanced cell-mediated protection against fatal *Escherichia coli* septicemia induced by treatment with recombinant IL-2. J Immunol 142:1134, 1989
29. Anderson TD, Hayes TJ: Toxicity of human recombinant interleukin-2 in rats. Pathologic changes are characterized by marked lymphocytic and eosinophilic proliferation and multisystem involvement. Lab Invest 60:331, 1989
30. Michie HR, Eberlein TJ, Spriggs DR, et al: Interleukin-2 initiates metabolic responses associated with critical illness in humans. Ann Surg 208:493, 1988
31. Garman RD, Jacobs KA, Clark SC, et al: B-cell-stimulatory factor 2 (β_2 interferon) functions as a second signal for interleukin 2 production by mature murine T cells. Proc Natl Acad Sci USA 84:7629, 1987
32. Kishimoto T: Factors affecting B-cell growth and differentiation. Annu Rev Immunol 3:133, 1985
33. Tosato G, Seamon KB, Goldman ND, et al: Monocyte-derived human B-cell growth factor identified as interferon-β_2 (BSF-2, IL-6). Science 239:502, 1988
34. Ritchie DG, Fuller GM: Hepatocyte-stimulating factor: a monocyte-derived acute-phase regulatory protein. Ann NY Acad Sci 408:490, 1983
35. Castell JV, Gomez-Lechon MJ, David M, et al: Interleukin-6 is the major regulator of acute phase protein synthesis in adult human hepatocytes. FEBS Lett 242:237, 1989

36. Nijsten MW, de Groot ER, ten Duis HJ, et al: Serum levels of interleukin-6 and acute phase responses. Lancet 2:921, 1987
37. Helfgott DC, Fong Y, Moldawer LL, et al: Human interleukin-6 is an endogenous pyrogen. Clin Res 37:564A, 1989
38. Nathan CF, Murray HW, Wiebe ME, et al: Identification of interferon-gamma as the lymphokine that activates human macrophage oxidative metabolism and antimicrobial activity. J Exp Med 158:670, 1983
39. Nathan CF, Horowitz CR, de la Harpe J, et al: Administration of recombinant interferon gamma to cancer patients enhances monocyte secretion of hydrogen peroxide. Proc Natl Acad Sci USA 82:8686, 1985
40. Nathan CF, Kaplan G, Levis WR, et al: Local and systemic effects of intradermal recombinant interferon-gamma in patients with lepromatous leprosy. N Engl J Med 315:6, 1986
41. Kurzrock R, Quesada JR, Talpaz M, et al: Subcutaneous recombinant gamma interferon in cancer patients: toxicity, pharmacokinetics, and immunomodulatory effects. Cancer Immunol Immunother 25:47, 1987
42. Lotz M, Jirik F, Kabouridis P, et al: B cell stimulating factor 2/interleukin 6 is a costimulant for human thymocytes and T lymphocytes. J Exp Med 167:1253, 1988
43. Le JM, Fredrickson G, Reis LF, et al: Interleukin 2-dependent and interleukin 2-independent pathways of regulation of thymocyte function by interleukin 6. Proc Natl Acad Sci USA 85:8643, 1988
44. Marano MA, Fong Y, Moldawer LL, et al: Serum cachectin/TNF in critically ill burn patients correlates with infection and mortality. Surg Gynecol Obstet 170:32, 1990
45. Eastgate JA, Symons JA, Wood NC, et al: Correlation of plasma interleukin 1 levels with disease activity in rheumatoid arthritis. Lancet 2:706, 1988
46. Waage A, Halstensen A, Espevik T: Association between tumour necrosis factor in serum and fatal outcome in patients with meningococcal disease. Lancet 1:355, 1987
47. Scuderi P, Sterling KE, Lam KS, et al: Raised serum levels of tumour necrosis factor in parasitic infections. Lancet 2:1364, 1986
48. Girardin E, Grau GE, Dayer JM, et al: Tumor necrosis factor and interleukin-1 in the serum of children with severe infectious purpura. N Engl J Med 319:397, 1988
49. Balkwill F, Osborne R, Burke F, et al: Evidence for tumour necrosis factor/cachectin production in cancer. Lancet 1:1229, 1987
50. Maury CP, Teppo AM: Raised serum levels of cachectin/tumor necrosis factor alpha in renal allograft rejection. J Exp Med 166:1132, 1987
51. Muto Y, Nouri-Aria KT, Meager A, et al: Enhanced tumour necrosis factor and interleukin-1 in fulminant hepatic failure. Lancet 2:72, 1988
52. Waage A, Brandtzaeg P, Halstensen A, et al: The complex pattern of cytokines in serum from patients with meningococcal septic shock: association between interleukin 6, interleukin 1, and fatal outcome. J Exp Med 169:333, 1989
53. Prieur AM, Kaufmann MT, Griscelli C, et al: Specific interleukin-1 inhibitor in serum and urine of children with systemic juvenile chronic arthritis. Lancet 2:1240, 1987
54. Maury CP, Salo E, Pelkonen P: Circulating interleukin-1β in patients with Kawasaki disease. N Engl J Med 319:1670, 1988
55. Fong Y, Marano MA, Moldawer LL, et al: The acute splanchnic and peripheral tissue metabolic response to endotoxin in humans. J Clin Invest 85:1896, 1990
56. Michie HR, Manogue KR, Spriggs DR, et al: Detection of circulating tumor necrosis factor after endotoxin administration. N Engl J Med 318:1481, 1988
57. Fong Y, Moldawer LL, Marano M, et al: Endotoxemia elicits increased circulating beta 2-IFN/IL-6 in man. J Immunol 142:2321, 1989
58. Fong Y, Tracey KJ, Moldawer LL, et al: Antibodies to cachectin/tumor necrosis factor reduce interleukin 1β and interleukin 6 appearance during lethal bacteremia. J Exp Med 170:1627, 1989
59. Moss NM, Gough DB, Jordan AL, et al: Temporal correlation of impaired immune response after thermal injury with susceptibility to infection in a murine model. Surgery 104:882, 1988
60. Kikuchi Y, Kita T, Oomori K, et al: Interleukin 2 activity in peripheral blood mononuclear cells of patients with gynecologic malignancies. Med Oncol Tumor Pharmacother 5:85, 1988
61. Helfgott DC, Tatter SB, Santhanam U, et al: Multiple forms of IFN-beta 2/IL-6 in serum and body fluids during acute bacterial infection. J Immunol 142:948, 1989
62. Gelin J, Moldawer LL, Lonnroth C, et al: Appearance of hybridoma growth factor/interleukin-6 in the serum of mice bearing a methylcholanthrene-induced sarcoma. Biochem Biophys Res Commun 157:575, 1988
63. Shenkin A, Fraser WD, Series J, et al: The serum interleukin 6 response to elective surgery. Lymphokine Res 8:123, 1989
64. Van Oers MH, Van der Heyden AA, Aarden LA: Interleukin 6 (IL-6) in serum and urine of renal transplant recipients. Clin Exp Immunol 71:314, 1988
65. Abbott RJ, Bolderson I, Gruer PJ, et al: Immunoreactive IFN-gamma in CSF in neurological disorders. J Neurol Neurosurg Psychiatry 50:882, 1987
66. Hesse DG, Tracey KJ, Fong Y, et al: Cytokine appearance in human endotoxemia and primate bacteremia. Surg Gynecol Obstet 166:147, 1988
67. Zuckerman SH, Shellhaas J, Butler LD: Differential regulation of lipopolysaccharide-induced interleukin-1 and tumor necrosis factor synthesis: effects of endogenous glucocorticoids and the role of the pituitary-adrenal axis. Eur J Immunol 19:301, 1989
68. Luedke CE, Cerami A: Interferon-gamma overcomes glucocorticoid suppression of cachectin/tumor necrosis factor biosynthesis by murine macrophages. J Clin Invest 86:1234, 1990
69. Ray A, LaForge KS, Sehgal PB: On the mechanism for efficient repression of the interleukin-6 promoter by glucocorticoids: enhancer, TATA box, and RNA start site (Inr motif) occlusion. Mol Cell Biol 10:5736, 1990
70. Han J, Thompson P, Beutler B: Dexamethasone and pentoxifylline inhibit endotoxin-induced cachectin/tumor necrosis factor synthesis at separate points in the signaling pathway. J Exp Med 172:391, 1990
71. Barber AE, Coyle SM, Fong Y, et al: Impact of hypercortisolemia on the metabolic and hormonal responses to endotoxin in humans. Surg Forum 41:74, 1990
72. Van Zee KJ, Fischer E, Hawes AS, et al: Effects of intravenous IL-8 administration in nonhuman primates. J Immunol 148:1746, 1992
73. Bone RC, Fisher CJ, Clemmer TP, et al: A controlled clinical trial of high-dose methylprednisolone in the treatment of severe sepsis and septic shock. N Engl J Med 317:653, 1987
74. Luce JM, Montgomery AB, Marks JD, et al: Ineffectiveness of high-dose methylprednisolone in preventing parenchymal lung injury and improving mortality in patients with septic shock. Am Rev Respir Dis 138:62, 1988
75. Novick D, Engelmann H, Wallach D, et al: Soluble cytokine receptors are present in normal human urine. J Exp Med 170:1409, 1989
76. Seckinger P, Isaaz S, Dayer JM: A human inhibitor of tumor necrosis factor α. J Exp Med 167:1511, 1988
77. Lantz M, Gullberg U, Nilsson E, et al: Characterization in vitro of a human tumor necrosis factor-binding protein: a soluble form of a tumor necrosis factor receptor. J Clin Invest 86:1396, 1990
78. Peetre C, Thysell H, Grubb A, et al: A tumor necrosis factor binding protein is present in human biological fluids. Eur J Haematol 41:414, 1988
79. Engelmann H, Aderka D, Rubinstein M, et al: A tumor necrosis factor-binding protein purified to homogeneity from human urine protects cells from tumor necrosis factor toxicity. J Biol Chem 264:11974, 1989
80. Kohno T, Brewer MT, Baker SL, et al: A second tumor necrosis factor receptor gene product can shed a naturally occurring tumor necrosis factor inhibitor. Proc Natl Acad Sci USA 87:8331, 1990
81. Loetscher H, Pan YC, Lahm HW, et al: Molecular cloning and expression of the human 55 kd tumor necrosis factor receptor. Cell 61:351, 1990
82. Schall TJ, Lewis M, Koller KJ, et al: Molecular cloning and expression of a receptor for human tumor necrosis factor. Cell 61:361, 1990
83. Seckinger P, Lowenthal JW, Williamson K, et al: A urine inhibitor of interleukin 1 activity that blocks ligand binding. J Immunol 139:1546, 1987
84. Gray PW, Barrett K, Chantry D, et al: Cloning of human tumor necrosis factor (TNF) receptor cDNA and expression of recombinant soluble TNF-binding protein. Proc Natl Acad Sci USA 87:7380, 1990
85. Seckinger P, Zhang JH, Hauptmann B, et al: Characterization of a tumor necrosis factor α (TNF-α) inhibitor: evidence of immunological cross-reactivity with the TNF receptor. Proc Natl Acad Sci USA 87:5188, 1990
86. Himmler A, Maurer Fogy I, Kronke M, et al: Molecular cloning and expression of human and rat tumor necrosis factor receptor chain (p60) and its soluble derivative, tumor necrosis factor-binding protein. DNA Cell Biol 9:705, 1990
87. Porteu F, Nathan C: Shedding of tumor necrosis factor receptors by activated human neutrophils. J Exp Med 172:599, 1990
88. Van Zee KJ, Kohno T, Fischer E, et al: Tumor necrosis factor soluble receptors circulate during experimental and clinical inflammation and can protect against excessive tumor necrosis factor a in vitro and in vivo. Proc Natl Acad Sci USA 89:4845, 1992
89. Aderka D, Engelmann H, Maor Y, et al: Stabilization of the bioactivity of tumor necrosis factor by its soluble receptors. J Exp Med 175:323, 1992
90. Ashkenazi A, Marsters SA, Capon DJ, et al: Protection against endotoxic shock by a tumor necrosis factor receptor immunoadhesin. Proc Natl Acad Sci USA 88:10535, 1991
91. Lesslauer W, Tabuchi H, Gentz R, et al: Recombinant soluble tumor necrosis factor receptor proteins protect mice from lipopolysaccharide-induced lethality. Eur J Immunol 21:2883, 1991
92. Hannum CH, Wilcox CJ, Arend WP, et al: Interleukin-1 receptor antagonist activity of a human

interleukin-1 inhibitor. Nature 343:336, 1990
93. McIntyre KW, Stepan GJ, Kolinsky KD, et al: Inhibition of interleukin 1 (IL-1) binding and bioactivity in vitro and modulation of acute inflammation in vivo by IL-1 receptor antagonist and anti-IL-1 receptor monoclonal antibody. J Exp Med 173:931, 1991
94. Fischer E, Van Zee KJ, Marano MA, et al: Interleukin-1 receptor antagonist circulates in experimental inflammation and in human disease. Blood 79:2196, 1992
95. Turner M, Chantry D, Katsikis P, et al: Induction of the interleukin 1 receptor antagonist protein by transforming growth factor-beta. Eur J Immunol 21:1635, 1991
96. Arend WP, Welgus HG, Thompson RC, et al: Biological properties of recombinant human monocyte-derived interleukin 1 receptor antagonist. J Clin Invest 85:1694, 1990
97. Fischer E, Marano MA, Van Zee KJ, et al: Interleukin-1 receptor blockade improves survival and hemodynamic performance in *Escherichia coli* septic shock, but fails to alter host responses to sublethal endotoxemia. J Clin Invest 89:1551, 1992
98. Gershenwald JE, Fong YM, Fahey TJ III, et al: Interleukin 1 receptor blockade attenuates the host inflammatory response. Proc Natl Acad Sci USA 87:4966, 1990
99. Henricken BE, Neta R, Vogel SN: An interleukin-1 receptor antagonist blocks lipopolysaccharide-induced colony-stimulating factor production and early endotoxin tolerance. Infect Immun 59:1188, 1991
100. Opp MR, Krueger JM: Interleukin 1-receptor antagonist blocks interleukin 1-induced sleep and fever. Am J Physiol 260:R453, 1991
101. Ohlsson K, Björk P, Bergenfeldt M, et al: Interleukin-1 receptor antagonist reduces mortality from endotoxin shock. Nature 348:550, 1990
102. Wakabayashi G, Gelfand JA, Burke JF, et al: A specific receptor antagonist for interleukin 1 prevents *Escherichia coli*-induced shock in rabbits. Faseb J 5:338, 1991
103. Moore KW, O'Garra A, de Waal Malefyt R, et al: Interleukin-10. Annu Rev Immunol 11:165, 1993
104. Taga K, Mostowski H, Tosato G: Human interleukin-10 can directly inhibit T-cell growth. Blood 81:2964, 1993
105. Howard M, Muchamuel T, Andrade S, et al: Interleukin 10 protects mice from lethal endotoxemia. J Exp Med 177:1205, 1993
106. Spinas GA, Bloesch D, Kaufmann MT, et al: Induction of plasma inhibitors of interleukin 1 and TNF-α activity by endotoxin administration to normal humans. Am J Physiol 259:R993, 1990
107. Hesse DG, Davatelis G, Felsen D, et al: Cachectin/tumor necrosis factor gene expression in Kupffer cells. J Leukoc Biol 42:422, 1987
108. Dinarello CA: Biology of interleukin 1. FASEB J 2:108, 1988
109. Helfgott DC, May LT, Sthoeger Z, et al: Bacterial lipopolysaccharide (endotoxin) enhances expression and secretion of beta 2 interferon by human fibroblasts. J Exp Med 166:1300, 1987
110. Ulich TR, Guo K, del Castillo J: Endotoxin-induced cytokine gene expression in vivo: I. Expression of tumor necrosis factor mRNA in visceral organs under physiologic conditions and during endotoxemia. Am J Pathol 134:11, 1989
111. Takacs L, Kovacs EJ, Smith MR, et al: Detection of IL-1α and IL-1β gene expression by in situ hybridization. J Immunol 141:3081, 1988
112. Kriegler M, Perez C, DeFay K, et al: A novel form of TNF/cachectin is a cell surface cytotoxic transmembrane protein: ramifications for the complex physiology of TNF. Cell 53:45, 1988
113. Keogh C, Fong Y, Marano MA, et al: Identification of a novel tumor necrosis factor alpha/cachectin from the livers of burned and infected rats. Arch Surg 125:79, 1989
114. Okubo A, Sone S, Tanaka M, et al: Membrane-associated interleukin 1α as a mediator of tumor cell killing by human blood monocytes fixed with paraformaldehyde. Cancer Res 49:265, 1989
115. Beuscher HU, Fallon RJ, Colten HR: Macrophage membrane interleukin 1 regulates the expression of acute phase proteins in human hepatoma Hep 3B cells. J Immunol 139:1896, 1987
116. Nelson S, Bagby GJ, Bainton BG, et al: Compartmentalization of intraalveolar and systemic lipopolysaccharide-induced tumor necrosis factor and the pulmonary inflammatory response. J Infect Dis 159:189, 1989
117. Leist TP, Frei K, Kam-Hansen S, et al: Tumor necrosis factor α in cerebrospinal fluid during bacterial, but not viral, meningitis: evaluation in murine model infections and in patients. J Exp Med 167:1743, 1988
118. Ford HR, Hoffman RA, Wing EJ, et al: Characterization of wound cytokines in the sponge matrix model. Arch Surg 124:1422, 1989
119. Fong Y, Moldawer LL, He W, et al: Tumor location influences local cytokine production and host metabolism. Surg Oncol 1:65, 1992
120. Greisman SE, Woodward WE: Mechanisms of endotoxin tolerance: III. The refractory state during continuous intravenous infusions of endotoxin. J Exp Med 121:911, 1965
121. Sanchez-Cantu L, Rode HN, Christou NV: Endotoxin tolerance is associated with reduced secretion of tumor necrosis factor. Arch Surg 124:1432, 1989
122. He W, Fong Y, Marano MA, et al: Tolerance to endotoxin prevents mortality in infected thermal injury: association with attenuated cytokine responses. J Infect Dis 165:859, 1992
123. Fraker DL, Stovroff MC, Merino MJ, et al: Tolerance to tumor necrosis factor in rats and the relationship to endotoxin tolerance and toxicity. J Exp Med 168:95, 1988
124. Smith EF III: Thromboxane A2 in cardiovascular and renal disorders: is there a defined role for thromboxane receptor antagonists or thromboxane synthase inhibitors? Eicosanoids 2:199, 1989
125. Deitch EA: The management of burns. N Engl J Med 323:1249, 1990
126. Jones WG II, Minei JP, Richardson RP, et al: Pathophysiologic glucocorticoid elevations promote bacterial translocation after thermal injury. Infect Immun 58:3257, 1990
127. Spaeth G, Berg RD, Specian RD, et al: Food without fiber promotes bacterial translocation from the gut. Surgery 108:240, 1990
128. Alverdy JC, Aoys E, Moss GS: Total parenteral nutrition promotes bacterial translocation from the gut. Surgery 104:185, 1988
129. Kaushansky K, Broudy VC, Harlan JM, et al: Tumor necrosis factor-α and tumor necrosis factor-β (lymphotoxin) stimulate the production of granulocyte-macrophage colony-stimulating factor, macrophage colony-stimulating factor, and IL-1 in vivo. J Immunol 141:3410, 1988
130. Le J, Vilcek J: Tumor necrosis factor and interleukin 1: cytokines with multiple overlapping biological activities. Lab Invest 56:234, 1987
131. Uehara A, Gottschall PE, Dahl RR, et al: Interleukin-1 stimulates ACTH release by an indirect action which requires endogenous corticotropin releasing factor. Endocrinology 121:1580, 1987
132. Beach JE, Smallridge RC, Kinzer CA, et al: Rapid release of multiple hormones from rat pituitaries perfused with recombinant interleukin-1. Life Sci 44:1, 1989
133. Scarborough DE, Lee SL, Dinarello CA, et al: Interleukin-1 beta stimulates somatostatin biosynthesis in primary cultures of fetal rat brain. Endocrinology 124:549, 1989
134. Sandler S, Bendtzen K, Borg LA, et al: Studies on the mechanisms causing inhibition of insulin secretion in rat pancreatic islets exposed to human interleukin-1β indicate a perturbation in the mitochondrial function. Endocrinology 124:1492, 1989
135. Roh MS, Drazenovich KA, Barbose JJ, et al: Direct stimulation of the adrenal cortex by interleukin-1. Surgery 102:140, 1987
136. Bagby GC Jr, Dinarello CA, Wallace P, et al: Interleukin 1 stimulates granulocyte macrophage colony-stimulating activity release by vascular endothelial cells. J Clin Invest 78:1316, 1986
137. Strieter RM, Remick DG, Lynch JP III, et al: Interleukin-2-induced tumor necrosis factor-alpha (TNF-α) gene expression in human alveolar macrophages and blood monocytes. Am Rev Respir Dis 139:335, 1989
138. Tredget EE, Yu YM, Zhong S, et al: Role of interleukin 1 and tumor necrosis factor on energy metabolism in rabbits. Am J Physiol 255:E760, 1988
139. Branch DR, Turner AR, Guilbert LJ: Synergistic stimulation of macrophage proliferation by the monokines tumor necrosis factor-alpha and colony-stimulating factor 1. Blood 73:307, 1989
140. Zuckerman SH, Schreiber RD: Up-regulation of gamma interferon receptors on the human monocytic cell line U937 by 1,25-dihydroxyvitamin D3 and granulocyte macrophage colony stimulating factor. J Leukoc Biol 44:187, 1988
141. Rambaldi A, Young DC, Herrmann F, et al: Interferon-gamma induces expression of the interleukin 2 receptor gene in human monocytes. Eur J Immunol 17:153, 1987
142. Fomsgaard A, Baek L, Fomsgaard JS, et al: Preliminary study on treatment of septic shock patients with antilipopolysaccharide IgG from blood donors. Scand J Infect Dis 21:697, 1989
143. Mayoral JL, Schweich CJ, Dunn DL: Decreased tumor necrosis factor production during the initial stages of infection correlates with survival during murine gram-negative sepsis. Arch Surg 125:24, 1990
144. Priest BP, Brinson DN, Schroeder DA, et al: Treatment of experimental gram-negative bacterial sepsis with murine monoclonal antibodies directed against lipopolysaccharide. Surgery 106:147, 1989
145. Ziegler EJ, Fisher CJ Jr, Sprung CL, et al: Treatment of gram-negative bacteremia and septic shock with HA-1A human monoclonal antibody against endotoxin: a randomized, double-blind, placebo-controlled trial. N Engl J Med 324:429, 1991
146. Harkonen S, Scannon P, Mischak RP, et al: Phase I study of a murine monoclonal anti-lipid A antibody in bacteremic and nonbacteremic patients. Antimicrob Agents Chemother 32:710, 1988
147. Greenman RL, Schein RM, Martin MA, et al: A controlled clinical trial of E5 murine monoclonal IgM antibody to endotoxin in the treatment of gram-negative sepsis. JAMA 266:1097, 1991
148. Schulman KA, Glick HA, Rubin H, et al: Cost-effectiveness of HA-1A monoclonal antibody for

gram-negative sepsis: economic assessment of a new therapeutic agent. JAMA 266:3466, 1991
149. Danner RL, Joiner KA, Parrillo JE: Inhibition of endotoxin-induced priming of human neutrophils by lipid X and 3-Aza-lipid X. J Clin Invest 80:605, 1987
150. Tobias PS, Ulevitch RJ: Lipopolysaccharide binding protein and CD14 in LPS dependent macrophage activation. Immunobiology 187:227, 1993
151. Tobias PS, Soldau K, Hatlen LE, et al: Lipopolysaccharide binding protein. J Cell Biochem 16C:151, 1992
152. Ooi CE, Weiss J, Doerfler ME, et al: Endotoxin-neutralizing properties of the 25 kD N-terminal fragment and a newly isolated 30 kD C-terminal fragment of the 55-60 kD bactericidal/permeability-increasing protein of human neutrophils. J Exp Med 174:649, 1991
153. Bazil V, Strominger JL: Shedding as a mechanism of down-modulation of CD14 on stimulated human monocytes. J Immunol 147:1567, 1991
154. Marra MN, Wilde CG, Griffith JE, et al: Bactericidal/permeability-increasing protein has endotoxin neutralizing activity. J Immunol 148:662, 1992
155. Rogy MA, Oldenburg HSA, Calvano SE, et al: The role of bactericidal/permeability-increasing protein in the treatment of primate bacteremia and septic shock. J Clin Immunol 14:120, 1994
156. Evans TJ, Carpenter A, Moyes D, et al: Protective effects of a recombinant amino-terminal fragment of human bactericidal/permeability-increasing protein in an animal model of gram-negative sepsis. J Infect Dis 171:153, 1995
157. Kohn FR, Ammon S, Horwitz A, et al: Protective effect of a recombinant amino-terminal fragment of bactericidal/permeability-increasing protein in experimental endotoxemia. J Infect Dis 168:1307, 1993
158. Vandermeer TJ, Menconi MJ, O'Sullivan BP, et al: Bactericidal/permeability-increasing protein ameliorates acute lung injury in porcine endotoxemia. Am J Physiol 76:2006, 1994
159. Goyert SM, Ferrero EM, Seremetis SV, et al: Biochemistry and expression of myelomonocytic antigens. J Immunol 137:3909, 1986
160. Matsuura K, Ishida T, Setoguchi M, et al: Upregulation of mouse CD14 expression in Kupffer cells by lipopolysaccharide. J Exp Med 179:1671, 1994
161. Haziot A, Rong GW, Bazil V, et al: Recombinant soluble CD14 inhibits LPS-induced tumor necrosis factor-α production by cells in whole blood. J Immunol 152:5868, 1994
162. Leewenberg FM, Dentener MA, Buurman WA: Lipopolysaccharide LPS-mediated soluble TNF receptor release and TNF receptor expression by monocytes. J Immunol 152:5070, 1994
163. Ziegler-Heitbrock HWL, Ulevitch RJ: CD14: cell surface receptor and differentiation marker. Immunol Today 14:121, 1993
164. Yasul K, Komiyama A, Molski TFP, et al: Pentoxifylline and CD14 antibody additively inhibit priming of polymorphonuclear leukocytes for enhanced release of superoxide by lipopolysaccharide: possible mechanism of these actions. Infect Immun 62:922, 1994
165. Schutt C, Schilling T, Grunwald U, et al: Endotoxin-neutralizing capacity of soluble CD14. Res Immunol 143:71, 1992
166. Billiar TR, Bankey PE, Svingen BA, et al: Fatty acid intake and Kupffer cell function: fish oil alters eicosanoid and monokine production to endotoxin stimulation. Surgery 104:343, 1988
167. Endres S, Ghorbani R, Kelley VE, et al: The effect of dietary supplementation with n-3 polyunsaturated fatty acids on the synthesis of interleukin-1 and tumor necrosis factor by mononuclear cells. N Engl J Med 320:265, 1989
168. Vilaseca J, Salas A, Guarner F, et al: Dietary fish oil reduces progression of chronic inflammatory lesions in a rat model of granulomatous colitis. Gut 31:539, 1990
169. Sperling RI, Weinblatt M, Robin JL, et al: Effects of dietary supplementation with marine fish oil on leukocyte lipid mediator generation and function in rheumatoid arthritis. Arthritis Rheum 30:988, 1987
170. Bittiner SB, Tucker WF, Cartwright I, et al: A double-blind, randomized, placebo-controlled trial of fish oil in psoriasis. Lancet 1:378, 1988
171. Fong YM, Marano MA, Barber A, et al: Total parenteral nutrition and bowel rest modify the metabolic response to endotoxin in humans. Ann Surg 210:449, 1989
172. Gerard C, Bruyns C, Marchant A, et al: Interleukin 10 reduces the release of tumor necrosis factor and prevents lethality in experimental endotoxemia. J Exp Med 177:547, 1993
173. Zabel P, Wolter DT, Schonharting MM, et al: Oxpentifylline in endotoxemia. Lancet 2:1474, 1989
174. Martich GD, Danner RL, Ceska M, et al: Detection of interleukin 8 and tumor necrosis factor in normal humans after intravenous endotoxin: the effect of antiinflammatory agents. J Exp Med 173:1021, 1991
175. Feuerstein G, Hallenbeck JM: Prostaglandins, leukotrienes, and platelet activating factor in shock. Ann Rev Pharmacol Toxicol 27:301, 1987
176. Nagaki M, Hughes RD, Lau JY, et al: Removal of endotoxin and cytokines by adsorbents and the effect of plasma protein binding. Int J Artif Organs 14:43, 1991
177. Chizzonite R, Truitt T, Kilian PL, et al: Two high affinity interleukin-1 receptors represent separate gene products. Proc Natl Acad Sci USA 86:8029, 1989
178. Kilbourn RG, Gross SS, Jubran A, et al: NG-methyl-L-arginine inhibits tumor necrosis factor-induced hypotension: implications for the involvement of nitric oxide. Proc Natl Acad Sci USA 87:3629, 1990
179. Groopman JE, Mitsuyasu RT, DeLeo MJ, et al: Effect of recombinant human granulocyte-macrophage colony-stimulating factor on myelopoiesis in the acquired immunodeficiency syndrome. N Engl J Med 317:593, 1987
180. Badaro R, Falcoff E, Badaro FS, et al: Treatment of visceral leishmaniasis with pentavalent antimony and interferon gamma. N Engl J Med 322:16, 1990
181. Beutler B, Cerami A: Cachectin: more than a tumor necrosis factor. N Engl J Med 316:379, 1987
182. Beutler B, Cerami A: Cachectin and tumour necrosis factor as two sides of the same biologic coin. Nature 320:584, 1986
183. Blick M, Sherwin SA, Rosenblum M, et al: Phase I study of recombinant tumor necrosis factor in cancer patients. Cancer Res 47:2986, 1987
184. Dinarello CA, Savage N: Interleukin-1 and its receptor. CRC Crit Rev Immunol 9:1, 1989
185. Newton RC, Uhl J, Covington M, et al: The distribution and clearance of radiolabeled human interleukin-1 beta in mice. Lymphokine Res 7:207, 1988
186. Yamada T, Fujishima A, Kawahara K, et al: Importance of disulfide linkage for constructing the biologically active human interleukin-2. Arch Biochem Biophys 257:194, 1987
187. May LT, Ghrayeb J, Santhanam U, et al: Synthesis and secretion of multiple forms of beta 2-interferon/B-cell differentiation factor 2/hepatocyte-stimulating factor by human fibroblasts and monocytes. J Biol Chem 263:7760, 1988
188. May LT, Santhanam U, Tatter SB, et al: Phosphorylation of secreted forms of human beta 2-interferon/hepatocyte stimulating factor/interleukin-6. Biochem Biophys Res Commun 152:1144, 1988
189. Yamasaki K, Taga T, Hirata Y, et al: Cloning and expression of the human interleukin-6 (BSF-2/IFN beta 2) receptor. Science 241:825, 1988
190. Kelly CD, Welte K, Murray HW: Antigen-induced human interferon-gamma production: differential dependence on interleukin 2 and its receptor. J Immunol 139:2325, 1987
191. Cunningham AL, Merigan TC: Leu-3+ T cells produce gamma-interferon in patients with recurrent herpes labialis. J Immunol 132:197, 1984
192. Rigby WF, Denome S, Fanger MW: Regulation of lymphokine production and human T lymphocyte activation by 1,25-dihydroxyvitamin D3: specific inhibition at the level of messenger RNA. J Clin Invest 79:1659, 1987
193. Dripps DJ, Brandhuber BJ, Thompson RC, et al: Interleukin-1 (IL-1) receptor antagonist binds to the 80-kDa IL-1 receptor but does not initiate IL-1 signal transduction. J Biol Chem 266:10331, 1991
194. Feng L, Tang WW, Chang JC, et al: Molecular cloning of rat cytokine synthesis inhibitory factor (IL-10) cDNA and expression in spleen and macrophages. Biochem Biophys Res Commun 192:452, 1993
195. Rusher I: C-reactive protein and the acute-phase response. Hosp Pract 25(3A):13, 1990

Acknowledgments

Figures 1 and 7   Dana Burns-Pizer.

Figures 2, 3, and 5   Tom Moore.

Figures 4, 6, and 8   Gae Xavier.

VIII POSTOPERATIVE MANAGEMENT

102 POSTOPERATIVE MANAGEMENT

Samir M. Fakhry, M.D., Edmund J. Rutherford, M.D., and George F. Sheldon, M.D.

Postoperative care is an integral part of the complete surgical care of a patient. Appropriate and compassionate postoperative care, in combination with proper preoperative preparation, can result in superior clinical outcomes and provide the patient with a favorable perioperative experience.

Ongoing changes in health care have affected both preoperative and postoperative care. An increasing number of patients undergo outpatient surgery and are discharged home after their procedure. At least 50% of patients undergoing surgery are discharged 24 hours or less after operation and consequently require outpatient care for problems such as pain, nausea, and bleeding. Advances in surgical knowledge and technological innovations (e.g., minimally invasive surgery) have shortened the hospital stay and resulted in changes in the delivery of postoperative care. Despite these changes, postoperative care remains an important part of a surgeon's responsibility. Though this responsibility can be shared with other physicians and specialists (as in a critical care unit[1,2]) and with other health professionals (as in outpatient surgery supplemented by home nursing), the surgeon's role remains central, since he or she has a singular knowledge of the indications for the procedure, the operative findings, and the potential complications that might arise in the postoperative course.

The complications that follow operation are, in general, directly related to the operative procedure. Appropriate postoperative care, however, can decrease the incidence of complications and enhance the patient's overall recovery. Advances in medical knowledge and technology have brought about a steady decrease in postoperative complications. Aggressive monitoring techniques are now employed more frequently during the postoperative period. In particular, use of the intensive care unit, ventilatory support, and invasive monitoring has increased significantly. These measures have proved extremely valuable in the management of patients with serious surgical illness. However, it is important to use these measures judiciously and to be alert for their potential complications [*see 89 Cardiopulmonary Monitoring*]. The importance of a caring physician who employs good surgical judgment and interacts frequently with the patient and the patient's family members cannot be overemphasized.

Postoperative Orders

The physician communicates the specifics of postoperative management to the nurse and other members of the health care team via the postoperative orders [*see Sidebar Sample Postoperative Orders*]. The postoperative orders should include an admission diagnosis, the operative procedure performed, a request to bring the old chart to the floor (if this has not already been done), and a statement of the patient's condition and known allergies. The postoperative orders should be accurate, legible, reasonable, effective, applicable, and uniform. The physician should be aware of the limits of the particular nursing unit in which the patient is placed and should avoid making unreasonable requests. Similarly, the effectiveness and cost of each order should be considered—for example, studies have now documented that a number of formerly standard respiratory treatments, such as intermittent positive-pressure ventilation (IPPB), ultrasonic nebulization, and room humidifiers, are of little or no value. The use of prophylactic measures against gastritis (especially intravenous H_2 receptor antagonists) in the setting of elective surgery has gained widespread application but is probably unwarranted in the case of most patients who have no history of ulcer diathesis or coagulopathy or who are not in a critical care unit and do not require mechanical ventilation.[3] Some uniformity in the postoperative orders is valuable because it allows a decrease in the floor stock of medications and increases the nursing staff's experience with specific medications and procedures. Physicians should become acquainted with the costs of the various treatments and medications at their institution. Choices made on the basis of both efficacy and expense will become increasingly common as hospital systems adapt to the changing health care environment.

Postoperative Pain Relief

Pain relief is often inadequate after operation.[4,5] This is a major issue because pain can cause serious physiologic and psychological sequelae. For example, unrelieved postoperative pain decreases respiratory function and increases the frequency of splinting and atelectasis. Gastrointestinal complications associated with postoperative pain include ileus, nausea, and vomiting. Pain causes ureteral and bladder hypomotility, which interferes with normal urination, and can prolong immobilization, thereby increasing the risk of deep vein thrombosis and thromboembolic complications. The release of catecholamines with pain results in vasoconstriction, hypovolemia, increased blood viscosity, and increased activation of clotting and platelet aggregation. Catecholamines increase cardiac work, which is particularly undesirable in patients with significant ischemic heart disease.

Treatment of postoperative pain actually begins before the procedure, as the health care team educates the patient about the events that will occur before, during, and after the procedure. Classic studies demonstrated that such an educational approach reduced patients' requirements for analgesics and diminished their perception of pain.[6] Subsequent studies in which patients were instructed in the use of relaxation techniques[7] or methods of hypnosis[8] after operation found that such instruction substantially reduced pain perception and length of convalescence.

Preemptive anesthesia reduces the sensation of pain before the creation of the incision, thereby significantly decreasing pain perception in the postoperative period. Techniques utilizing epidural anesthesia[9] or major field block[10] achieve a greater reduction in perceived pain than general anesthesia does, and

> **Sample Postoperative Orders**
>
> An otherwise healthy 50-year-old, 70 kg man was recently diagnosed with a cecal carcinoma. He has type 2 (adult-onset) diabetes, for which he takes an oral hypoglycemic. He has arrived in the postanesthesia care unit (PACU) in stable condition after an uneventful right hemicolectomy and primary reanastomosis of 2 hours' duration under general anesthesia. Intraoperative blood loss is estimated at 100 ml, fluid replacement was 2,500 ml of lactated Ringer solution, and urine output totaled 250 ml.
>
> [Date and Time]
>
> 1. Admit to PACU; Service: surgery H; Attending: Sheldon; Resident: Fakhry
> 2. Diagnosis: colon cancer; status: post right hemicolectomy
> 3. Condition: stable
> 4. Vital signs per PACU routine, then every 4 hours on ward × 24 hours, then every shift
> 5. Activity: out of bed to chair three times a day, beginning this evening; walk hall three times a day
> 6. Diet: nothing by mouth, but may have sips of ice chips and hard candy
> 7. Allergies: no known drug allergies
> 8. [Daily weight]
> 9. Accurate intake and output
> 10. Foley catheter to gravity
> 11. Fluids: 5% dextrose in lactated Ringer solution at 125 ml/hr
> 12. Antithrombosis prophylaxis
> 13. Medications:
>   patient-controlled analgesia (if indicated): morphine sulfate, 1 to 2 mg I.V. every 10 minutes on demand
>   other medications as indicated (e.g., pain medication, acetaminophen, preoperative medications)
> 14. Insulin sliding scale (for diabetic patients): finger-stick glucose every 6 hours and cover as follows:
>   < 60 ------------------ call physician
>   60–180 ------------- no coverage
>   180–240 ----------- 5 units subcutaneous regular insulin
>   240–300 ----------- 10 units subcutaneous regular insulin
>   > 300 --------------- 15 units subcutaneous regular insulin, and call physician
> 15. Morning laboratory tests: complete blood count and electrolyte panel (if indicated)
> 16. Call physician for
>   systolic blood pressure > 180 mm Hg or < 90 mm Hg
>   diastolic blood pressure > 100 mm Hg
>   heart rate > 120 or < 60 a minute
>   respirations > 32 or < 12 a minute
>   temperature > 38.5° C (101.3° F)
>   urine output < 200 ml every 4 hours

they greatly reduce the need for postoperative analgesics while enhancing postdischarge activity. Epidural anesthesia and other regional techniques are now being applied more frequently as multiple trials demonstrate their superiority to general anesthesia. In the case of epidural anesthesia, the catheter can be used to provide sustained pain relief for several days after operation. This approach is particularly useful in patients who have undergone operations on the lower abdomen or the lower extremities: it can lead to earlier mobilization and return of bowel function after operation, thereby shortening hospital stay.[11]

In a study of 174 patients treated with either systemic or epidural morphine, postoperative pain was less intense and of shorter duration in patients who received epidural morphine.[12] In this and other studies, the patients treated with epidural morphine also required less secondary analgesia and reported an increased feeling of well-being.[13,14] Numerous studies have compared narcotic and regional analgesia with regard to their effects on the restoration of respiratory function. In one such study, systemic narcotics improved respiratory function by about 20%, whereas epidural analgesia effectively restored vital capacity and peak expiratory flow rates to 70% of normal and functional residual capacity to normal[15]; consequently, postoperative hypoxemia was virtually eliminated in the epidural analgesia group. In a study of patients with multiple rib fractures, epidural administration of fentanyl, compared with an I.V. regimen, afforded excellent pain relief and brought about greater improvements in blood gas values and ventilation.[16] In a study of cardiac surgery patients, epidural administration of morphine led to effective pain relief and lower levels of stress hormones, including cortisol and β-endorphin.[17] Field block using long-acting local anesthetic agents extends the period of anesthesia for 12 hours longer, thereby enhancing recovery. In some centers, mastectomy is now being performed as day surgery by using paraspinal anesthesia.[18]

Systemic medications used for postoperative pain relief include opioids, nonsteroidal anti-inflammatory drugs (NSAIDs), and other nonnarcotic agents [see Table 1]. Surgeons are currently moving away from systemic opioids: in addition to their well-recognized capacity for inducing respiratory depression, opioids prolong ileus and increase nausea and vomiting. Regional anesthesia coupled with NSAID administration appears to yield better results in terms of patient recovery.[11]

On occasion, however, systemically administered narcotics are still the best available choice. Studies on postoperative pain have shown that most cases of severe pain are not uniformly relieved by the current practice of narcotic prescription. According to one study of 102 medical residents, physicians prescribe inadequate doses of narcotic analgesics for patients with moderate or severe pain, and nurses give only 40% to 50% of the amount prescribed.[19] In this study, the effective dose of narcotic required for pain relief was underestimated, the fear of respiratory depression was high, the duration of action was overestimated, and the danger of addiction was exaggerated. (Addiction usually does not develop unless narcotics are prescribed regularly for more than 2 weeks).

NSAIDs, though safer than narcotics, have side effects of their own. In particular, they inhibit prostaglandin synthesis, thereby decreasing inflammation. This prostaglandin inhibition may exacerbate renal insufficiency; for this reason, NSAIDs should be used with caution in patients with preexisting renal dysfunction. Other side effects include GI bleeding, inhibition of platelet aggregation, and prolonged bleeding time.

Patient-controlled analgesia (PCA) represents an important advance in pain management [see 104 Postoperative Pain].[20-22] This modality has gained widespread acceptance because it provides improved pain control and greater patient satisfaction,

Table 1 Suggested Dosing of Opioid and Nonopioid Analgesics

Class	Drug	Oral Dosage	Parenteral Dosage	Comments
Opioid agonists	Morphine	10–30 mg q. 4 hr	0.05–0.1 mg/kg I.V. (maximum, 15 mg), followed by 4–6 mg/hr I.V. 5–20 mg I.M. q. 4 hr	—
	Heroin	—	—	Not available in United States
	Fentanyl	—	1–2 µg/kg I.V., followed by 1–2 µg/kg/hr I.V.	Transdermal patches available in 25, 50, 75, and 100 µg/hr release
	Sufentanil	—	0.2–0.6 µg/kg I.V., followed by 0.01–0.05 µg/kg/min I.V.	—
	Alfentanil	—	10–25 µg/kg I.V., followed by 0.5–3.0 µg/kg/min I.V.	Safe in renal insufficiency
	Remifentanil	—	0.0125–0.025 µg/kg/min I.V.	—
	Hydromorphone	2–4 mg q. 4–6 hr	0.5–2 mg I.V. q. 1–2 hr	—
	Oxymorphone	—	1–1.5 mg S.C. or I.M. q. 4–6 hr 0.5 mg I.V.	—
	Levorphanol	2–3 mg q. 4 hr	2–3 mg S.C. q. 4–6 hr	Optimal I.V. dose has not been established
	Methadone	5–20 mg q. 3–4 hr	2.5–10.0 mg S.C., I.M., or I.V. q. 3–4 hr	Excellent I.V.-to-oral bioavailability, 1:2 mg
	Meperidine	50–150 mg q. 3–4 hr	25–100 mg I.V. q. 3–4 hr	Generally not recommended, because of oral effectiveness and active metabolites; increased bioavailability in liver failure exacerbates action of the normeperidine metabolite
	Oxycodone	5–10 mg q. 4–6 hr	—	Certain preparations contain acetaminophen
	Hydrocodone	5–10 mg q. 4–6 hr	—	—
	Acetaminophen with codeine	15–60 mg q. 3–6 hr	15–60 mg S.C., I.M., or I.V. q. 4 hr	—
	Propoxyphene	32–65 mg q. 4 hr	—	—
Opioid agonist antagonists	Buprenorphine	—	0.3 mg I.M. or I.V. q. 6 hr	—
	Pentazocine	25 mg t.i.d.–q.i.d.	30 mg S.C., I.M., or I.V. q. 3–4 hr	—
	Nalbuphine	—	10 mg S.C., I.M., or I.V. q. 3–6 hr	Often used with epidural narcotics to decrease side-effect profile of itching and hypotension
	Butorphanol	—	1 mg I.V. q. 3–4 hr 2 mg I.M. q. 3–4 hr	—
	Dezocine	—	5–20 mg I.M. q. 3–6 hr 2.5–10.0 mg I.V. q. 2–4 hr	—
	Tramadol	50–100 mg q. 4–6 hr	—	—

COX—cyclooxygenase   OA—osteoarthritis   PDA—patent ductus arteriosus   RA—rheumatoid arthritis

which are attributable both to more expedient administration of the drug and to more consistent plasma levels. PCA generally takes the form of intermittent drug doses administered on demand, with a minimal required interval between doses (the lockout interval). A constant background infusion (basal dosage) may be given to supplement the intermittent dose, but it should be used cautiously so as not to induce respiratory depression. The narcotics most commonly used for PCA are morphine, meperidine, and fentanyl. Methadone is rarely given in this setting because of its slow onset and long duration of action [see Table 2]. Nalbuphine, though possessing narcotic analgesic properties of its own, is generally used for its antagonist properties, which act against side effects such as pruritus. Other side effects seen with patient-controlled analgesia are nausea, vomiting, sweating, and the aforementioned respiratory depression.

Physical Signs

A variety of physical signs are important to note in the postoperative period. These include respiratory distress, central nervous system depression, agitation, disorientation, complaints of severe pain that are inappropriate for the operative procedure, development of a hematoma or bleeding from the wound, irregular heart rate, and pale, cool, or clammy extremities (indicating decreased perfusion). Other important physical signs may be pres-

Table 1 Suggested Dosing of Opioid and Nonopioid Analgesics (*continued*)

Class	Drug	Oral Dosage	Parenteral Dosage	Comments
Nonopioid analgesics	Acetaminophen	325–650 mg q. 4 hr	—	Maximum, 4 g/day
	Acetylated salicylate Aspirin	325–650 mg q. 4 hr	—	—
	Nonacetylated salicylates Diflunisal	Loading dose, 1,000 mg, then 500–1,000 mg/day	—	FDA indications: pain, OA, and RA
	Salsalate	1,500 mg b.i.d.	—	FDA indications: RA and OA
	Choline magnesium trisalicylate	1,000–2,000 mg b.i.d.	—	FDA indications: OA, RA, and acute painful shoulder
	Propionic acids Ibuprofen	400–800 mg t.i.d.–q.i.d.	—	FDA indications: RA, OA, pain, and dysmenorrhea
	Fenoprofen	200 mg q. 4–6 hr	—	FDA indications: RA, OA, and pain
	Ketoprofen	50–75 mg t.i.d. or q.i.d.	—	FDA indications: RA, OA, pain, and dysmenorrhea
	Naproxen	500 mg, followed by 250 mg q. 6 hr	—	FDA indications: pain, RA, OA, dysmenorrhea, juvenile arthritis, ankylosing spondylitis, tendinitis, bursitis, and gout
	Flurbiprofen	50–100 mg b.i.d. or t.i.d.	—	FDA indications: RA and OA
	Oxaprozin	1,200 mg q. day	—	FDA indications: OA and RA
	Acetic acids Indomethacin	25 mg b.i.d. or t.i.d.	I.V. used to close PDA	FDA indications: RA, OA, ankylosing spondylitis, acute painful shoulder, and gout
	Sulindac	200 mg b.i.d.	—	FDA indications: OA, RA, ankylosing spondylitis, acute painful shoulder, and gout
	Tolmetin	400 mg t.i.d.	—	FDA indications: RA and OA
	Diclofenac	50 mg t.i.d.	—	FDA indications: RA, OA, and ankylosing spondylitis
	Etodolac	200–400 mg q. 6–8 hr, to maximum of 1,200 mg/day	—	FDA indications: OA and pain
	Nabumetone	1,000 mg/day	—	FDA indications: OA and RA
	Ketorolac	10 mg q. 4 hr	30 mg I.V., followed by 15–30 mg I.V. q. 6 hr 60 mg deep I.M., followed by 30 mg I.V. q. 6 hr	Maximum, 120 mg/day
	Oxicam Piroxicam	20 mg/day	—	FDA indications: OA and RA
	Fenamates Meclofenamate	50 mg q. 4 hr	—	FDA indications: pain, dysmenorrhea, RA, and OA
	Mefenamic acid	500 mg, followed by 250 mg q. 6 hr	—	FDA indications: pain and dysmenorrhea
	COX-2 inhibitors Rofecoxib	12.5–25.0 mg/day	—	FDA indications: OA, pain, and dysmenorrhea
	Celecoxib	100–200 mg q. 12–24 hr	—	FDA indications: OA, RA, and familial adenomatous polyposis

ent after specific operative procedures—for example, changes in pulse after vascular procedures or neurologic changes after neurosurgical procedures. The postoperative orders should alert the nursing staff to the importance of such signs so that they may notify the physician when such signs are present.

Laboratory Tests

A variety of laboratory tests can be obtained postoperatively. Although such tests can be valuable, they are used infrequently. Laboratory tests should not be used as a substitute for careful physical examination of the patient.

Table 2 Guidelines for I.V. Patient-Controlled Analgesia

Drug (Concentration)	Basal Dosage	Demand Dosage	Lockout Interval
Morphine (1–2 mg/ml)	0–0.5 mg/hr	0.5–3.0 mg	5–12 min
Meperidine (10 mg/ml)	0–5 mg/hr	5–30 mg	5–12 min
Fentanyl (10–20 µg/ml)	0–5 µg/hr	10–20 µg	5–10 min
Hydromorphone (0.2–0.5 mg/ml)	0–0.1 mg/hr	0.1–0.5 mg	5–10 min
Oxymorphone (0.25 mg/ml)	—	0.2–0.4 mg	8–10 min
Methadone (1 mg/ml)	0–0.5 mg/hr	0.5–2.5 mg	8–20 min
Nalbuphine (1 mg/ml)	—	1–5 mg	5–10 min

Finger-stick blood glucose measurements are indicated in insulin-resistant patients and should be obtained every 6 hours (see below). Hematocrits should be obtained postoperatively only if serious bleeding is suspected. The white blood cell count routinely increases after the stress of operation and is therefore of little diagnostic value during the first few days after operation. Thrombocytopenia routinely accompanies major trauma, massive transfusion, and major operative procedures (e.g., cardiac bypass operation); platelet counts are necessary only if the patient shows evidence of bleeding. In healthy individuals with normal renal function, serum electrolyte levels are usually well maintained despite major stress. In these patients, infrequent measurements of serum electrolytes are appropriate (every 2 or 3 days). By contrast, in patients with an underlying chronic disease, such as renal or hepatic disease or an illness that routinely results in electrolyte derangement, frequent measurements of electrolytes are indicated. The electrolyte abnormalities that are the most serious and potentially the most immediately life threatening are hypokalemia and hyperkalemia. These abnormalities must be corrected rapidly; multiple potassium measurements to confirm this correction are required. Abnormal levels of sodium and chloride should be corrected over a period of days.

Serum calcium measurements reflect total serum calcium. Only the ionized fraction of serum calcium is active, however, and thus, total serum calcium levels are not reliable indicators of the need for calcium administration.[23] However, after parathyroid operation, measurements of calcium levels are valuable because the other factors that affect the level of ionized calcium are usually unchanged.

Coagulation studies are overused preoperatively and are unnecessary postoperatively, except to monitor anticoagulation therapy or to evaluate the bleeding patient. Arterial blood gas measurements are useful in ventilated or hypoxic patients but should be used judiciously.

Postoperative Monitoring and Triage

In the postoperative period, many patients return to the same room they occupied preoperatively. Some, however, require more advanced monitoring and care and will require admission to a monitored telemetry bed, an intermediate care unit, or a surgical critical care unit.

The selection of postoperative monitoring is guided by a thorough understanding of the patient's preoperative status and medical history, the diagnosis that led to operation, the operation performed, and the circumstances of the operative procedure. The vital signs that are commonly monitored on a surgical ward include temperature, pulse rate, blood pressure, respiratory rate, urine output (hourly or at some other interval), weight (daily), and fluid intake and output. These can generally be obtained at intervals of 2 to 4 hours. Patients requiring more frequent monitoring or nursing care (e.g., frequent suctioning) may be better suited for admission to an intermediate care unit. On a telemetry ward, continuous cardiac monitoring can be provided for patients who have significant cardiopulmonary disease or for those at risk for perioperative myocardial infarction or dysrhythmia. In the critical care setting, additional monitoring is provided,[24,25] including both noninvasive and invasive monitoring with arterial lines, continuous monitoring of central venous pressure (CVP) and right-sided pulmonary arterial pressures via Swan-Ganz catheterization, continuous monitoring of arterial oxygen saturation via pulse oximetry, measurement of end-tidal carbon dioxide tension, and electrocardiographic monitoring [see 89 Cardiopulmonary Monitoring]. Recommended criteria for ICU admission and discharge have been formulated.[26] When resources are limited, such guidelines may be useful in resolving triage difficulties, but each institution and each unit will have to develop its own approach to this sometimes thorny problem.

Controversy continues regarding what level of monitoring is most appropriate for each patient. In many hospitals, requests for ICU beds exceed the number of available critical care beds, and triage of patients is necessary. This sometimes means moving patients from the ICU before their primary physician feels they are ready for transfer, canceling or delaying operative procedures, and providing less than the requested level of postoperative monitoring for some patients. The increased use of intermediate or step-down units has provided some relief in these difficult situations, but appropriate allocation of resources continues to be a major issue in postoperative bed selection. Wiedemann stated, "In some clinical circumstances, our ability to monitor disease may have outpaced our ability to intervene therapeutically."[27] A consensus conference sponsored by the National Institutes of Health in 1983 concluded that although the care provided in ICUs appears beneficial, the only area in which improved outcome could be documented was coronary care.[28] Acceptable indications for admission to critical care units and invasive monitoring with arterial lines and pulmonary arterial catheters have been proposed; they include myocardial infarction, shock, drug overdose, major cardiovascular surgery, acute respiratory distress syndrome (ARDS), and other forms of respiratory failure that require mechanical ventilation[29] [see 89 Cardiopulmonary Monitoring].

Management of Fluid Imbalance, Electrolyte Abnormalities, and Acid-Base-Balance Disorders

Postoperative fluid therapy is guided by the patient's overall preoperative condition, the preoperative diagnosis, and the circumstances of the operative procedure. The presence of cardiac, pulmonary, renal, or hepatic disease will affect the type and rate of fluid required postoperatively. Similarly, peritonitis, the septic response, or other conditions that affect the patient's volume status and peripheral capillary permeability will influence the approach to fluid therapy. In an adequately hydrated patient who has undergone a minor procedure with minimal blood loss and for whom the postoperative recovery period is expected to be short, maintenance fluid alone will be adequate. Maintenance requirements for a 70 kg patient are normally about 100 ml/hr of 5% dextrose in one-half normal saline, with approximately 20 mEq/L of potassium added. By contrast, in a patient with bowel obstruction, small bowel infarction, and bowel perforation, administration of maintenance fluid alone would be inadequate. In these patients, reequilibration and fluid loss from the intravascular space will continue for many hours after operation. Consequently, resuscitation must be continued postoperatively, possibly requiring administration of 7 to 10 L of crystalloid over 24 hours to maintain adequate perfusion.

In patients who require continued postoperative volume resuscitation, hypotonic fluids, even at an increased rate, are not appropriate. Isotonic fluid is required to maintain adequate intravascular volume. Administration of 5% dextrose in lactated Ringer solution at the rate of 150 ml/hr provides about six times as much intravascular volume resuscitation as the maintenance regimen mentioned earlier. Adjustments in volume should be guided by careful monitoring of urine output, pulse rate, and blood pressure. A common error in postoperative fluid therapy is ordering of hypotonic fluids at an increased rate of administration (i.e., 150 ml/hr of 5% dextrose in one-half normal saline) after determining, on the basis of physical examination findings (i.e., tachycardia, decreased blood pressure, and decreased urine output in the appropriate clinical situation), that a patient is relatively hypovolemic. Since fluid losses into the interstitium are isotonic, isotonic fluid replacement is indicated.

In addition, the use of isotonic fluids is important because of the presence of elevated levels of antidiuretic hormone (ADH) and other counterregulatory hormones. In a normal, unstressed person, free-water loading (e.g., the drinking of several glasses of water) results in a fall in ADH levels and excretion of very dilute urine by the kidney, thus allowing the serum sodium and osmolality to return to normal. Various stressful stimuli, including operative procedures, result in an inability to lower ADH levels and an inability to excrete free water.[30-32] The administration of hypotonic fluid, with its free-water content, can lead to hyponatremia in postoperative patients and others with elevated levels of counterregulatory stress hormones. The resultant hyponatremia may cause significant morbidity and mortality.[33,34]

The use of isotonic fluid prevents this problem. In uncomplicated elective procedures of brief duration (e.g., hernia repair, cholecystectomy, uncomplicated bowel surgery), the stress response is short-lived and the patient can be switched to maintenance fluids 24 hours after operation. Patients who undergo operation under local anesthesia do not experience a stress response and generally need little, if any, fluid.

Once recovery from a major insult has begun, the capillary leak will close, and fluid will be mobilized from the periphery into the vascular space. At this point, the fluid orders should be changed to maintenance rates or lower and from isotonic resuscitation fluid to hypotonic saline. An important sign that the capillary leak has reversed is the return of a brisk urine output. Such spontaneous diuresis is a significant marker of the patient's recovery. It is associated with a fall in levels of ADH, aldosterone, steroids, catecholamines, and other counterregulatory hormones and with a rise in atrial natriuretic factor.[35,36] The use of diuretics in an attempt to "diurese off" excess fluid will mask this physiologic response. Diuretics should therefore be reserved for use in patients who have inadequate renal or cardiac function and should be administered only after the capillary leak has reversed, to avoid causing intravascular volume depletion.

Several I.V. fluids are commonly employed for maintenance and resuscitation [see Table 3]. Crystalloids are the fluids of choice for perioperative fluid replacement. Controversy continues regarding the use of colloid solutions instead of or together with crystalloids. The use of colloid solutions offers no clear advantages in perioperative care, and their very high cost makes it difficult to justify their use in the majority of surgical patients.[37-39]

In the first 24 hours after operation, potassium supplementation is unnecessary in most patients. Potassium levels in I.V. fluids should be adjusted according to serum potassium levels. Unfortunately, the serum potassium level provides an extremely inaccurate estimate of total body potassium. A profound depletion may exist despite serum potassium levels in the low to normal range.

Table 3 Commonly Used I.V. Fluids

Solution	Plasma Osmolality (mOsm/L)	pH	Na$^+$ (mEq/L)	Cl$^-$ (mEq/L)	K$^+$ (mEq/L)	Ca^{2+} (mEq/L)	Other Components	Cost* ($)	Comments
D5LR (1,000 ml)	525	5	130	109	4	3	Lactate 28 mEq/L, 50 g dextrose	6	Fluid of choice for initial resuscitation and post-operative replacement
D5NS (1,000 ml)	560	4	154	154	0	0	50 g dextrose	6	Alternative to D5LR, but large amounts may cause metabolic acidosis
D5½NS (1,000 ml)	406	4	77	77	0	0	50 g dextrose	6	Hypotonic maintenance fluid
D5¼NS (1,000 ml)	321	4	34	34	0	0	50 g dextrose	6	Hypotonic maintenance fluid
D5W (1,000 ml)	321	4.5	0	0	0	0	50 g dextrose	6	Free-water source, no role in resuscitation
25% Albumin (100 ml)	Equal to plasma	Equal to plasma	145	0	0	0	25 g albumin	67	Colloid, expensive
5% Plasma protein fraction (250 ml)	Equal to plasma	Equal to plasma	145	0	< 2	0	12.5 g protein	33	Colloid, expensive
6% Hetastarch in 0.9% NaCl (500 ml)	310	3.5–7.0	154	154	0	0	30 g hydroxyethyl starch	42	Use limited volume (500–1,000 ml); coagulation abnormalities with larger volumes

*Reflects sample cost to pharmacy at the University of North Carolina at Chapel Hill School of Medicine. Actual cost to the patient is likely to be significantly higher.
D5LR—5% dextrose in lactated Ringer solution   D5NS—5% dextrose in normal saline solution   D5½NS—5% dextrose in one-half normal saline solution   D5¼NS—5% dextrose in one-quarter saline solution   D5W—5% dextrose in water

The long-term use of diuretics such as furosemide and the thiazides is commonly associated with low body stores of potassium. Patients undergoing nutritional repletion will also tend to have low serum potassium levels. If the patient has questionable renal function, potassium should be withheld until a serum level is available. If renal function is normal and urine output is not compromised, we add 20 mEq/L of potassium to the I.V. fluids after the first 24 postoperative hours.

FLUID IMBALANCE

Patients who undergo uncomplicated elective procedures will usually experience relatively inconsequential abnormalities of their intravascular volume. However, patients who undergo lengthy or complicated procedures or have abnormalities of intravascular volume preoperatively are more likely to develop abnormalities of circulating volume and should be evaluated carefully in the postoperative period to assess their intravascular volume status and tissue perfusion.

Hypovolemia

Hypovolemia is a decrease in the effective intravascular volume, caused by losses incurred either externally (e.g., hemorrhage or loss of transcellular fluid) or internally (e.g., transcapillary leakage of fluid into traumatized tissue). Oxygen delivery and tissue perfusion are dependent on the ability to generate an adequate cardiac output in the presence of hemoglobin that is sufficiently saturated (arterial oxygen saturation [S_aO_2] more than 90%, arterial oxygen tension [P_aO_2] more than 60 mm Hg). An inadequate intravascular volume can lead to poor perfusion either because of a lowered preload that results in a depressed cardiac output or because of a low hemoglobin concentration (e.g., bleeding). Younger patients will usually tolerate a lowered hemoglobin concentration by increasing cardiac output, provided intravascular volume is adequate. Older patients with coronary artery disease will be more likely to suffer deleterious effects if their intravascular volume, hemoglobin concentration, or both are low, because such patients have a limited ability to augment cardiac output under these circumstances.

Standard monitoring of volume status includes vital signs, mental status, and urine output. Because of the effects of general anesthesia, patients may develop unrecognized intravascular volume depletion. If a Foley catheter has been inserted, a decrease in the urine output can be an early sign of such depletion. Hypovolemia with depletion of the intravascular compartment should not be confused with changes in total body water, which may or may not occur in hypovolemia. If body weight is used to assess total body water content, it is possible to assume that a patient is "fluid overloaded" because of an elevated body weight, though in fact the intravascular volume has been depleted and the patient is underperfused and hypovolemic. This is a common scenario in patients who have sustained significant losses of intravascular volume and blood with resulting shock, capillary leakage, and fluid accumulation in the interstitium and the intracellular compartment.[40]

It has been demonstrated that the volume status of an individual patient, especially if he or she has unstable vital signs or is critically ill in the ICU, cannot be easily estimated by clinical assessment alone.[41,42] The use of invasive monitoring is therefore important in determining the status of the intravascular compartment and the ability of the body to maintain tissue perfusion. The use of a pulmonary arterial catheter to determine cardiac filling pressures and cardiac output usually allows a more accurate assessment of the patient's intravascular volume status. In patients who are relatively stable hemodynamically but manifest signs of a contracted intravascular volume (e.g., low urine output, increased heart rate, low or borderline blood pressure, depressed mental status, poor capillary refill), an isotonic fluid challenge should be administered. Between 500 and 1,000 ml of lactated Ringer solution or normal saline solution can be given over 20 to 30 minutes and the patient's response evaluated. If the vital signs normalize and the urine output rises, the patient is assumed to be responding to volume loading. Further observation will determine whether the patient requires more isotonic fluid administration. If the patient does not respond to the initial bolus of fluid or if the patient has significant renal or cardiopulmonary dysfunction, it is generally more prudent to employ invasive monitoring with a pulmonary arterial catheter to determine the status of the intravascular compartment. The use of diuretics in this setting should be limited to patients who have known severe cardiopulmonary dysfunction or advanced renal disease with a known dependency on diuretics. The administration of a diuretic to a patient with intravascular volume depletion can result in further depletion of the intravascular volume despite the production of urine.

Other techniques useful in the assessment of a patient's volume status include measurement of sodium in the urine sediment, cardiac echocardiography, and the determination of serum lactate levels. None of these techniques is entirely accurate or practical. The response to a fluid bolus remains a practical means of assessing the status of the intravascular compartment. Failure to respond to one or more fluid boluses should prompt further evaluation, including invasive monitoring if indicated.

Fluid Overload

Fluid overload in the postoperative surgical patient is reported to occur with varying frequency and has been associated with inferior outcomes.[43] The degree to which a patient may become "overloaded" with fluid is determined by the patient's preoperative status, age, and existing cardiopulmonary, renal, or hepatic disorders; the length of the operative procedure; the fluids administered; and the presence or absence of infection and inflammatory mediators. Although it is generally accepted that patients who require large amounts of fluid and gain weight in the postoperative period are likely to have a less favorable outcome, it is difficult to separate the effect of large-volume resuscitation from the circumstances that prompt such therapy, most commonly shock, a septic response, or both. The judicious use of fluids in the perioperative period and the application of the principles of invasive monitoring outlined above will generally allow appropriate volume resuscitation without precipitating pulmonary edema or congestive heart failure. It should be recognized, however, that patients who sustain shock or manifest a septic response (with or without bacterial infection) will leak fluid from their intravascular compartments and develop total body anasarca. The resultant increase in body weight associated with an increased requirement for fluid infusion will give the impression that the patient is receiving excessive amounts of fluid. Although this may be the case, it is generally difficult in the more seriously ill patients to determine the status of the intravascular volume by simple observation alone.[41,42] The value of invasive monitoring in the ICU should again be emphasized. Patients suspected of being "fluid overloaded" should be carefully evaluated by an experienced clinician, and if they do not respond to preliminary

ELECTROLYTE ABNORMALITIES

Disorders of Sodium Concentration

Hyponatremia Hyponatremia is caused by excess free water in the intravascular space [see 6 Life-Threatening Electrolyte Abnormalities]. The serum sodium concentration is not an accurate measure of total body sodium but rather reflects the concentration of sodium relative to the amount of free water in the intravascular compartment. The serum sodium concentration is not related to the volume state of the intravascular compartment. Patients may be normovolemic, hypovolemic, or hypervolemic in the presence of hyponatremia.

In the postoperative setting, hyponatremia usually results from an excess of free water. This occurs when hypotonic fluid is administered to patients whose ADH levels cannot fall because of the stress of operation or injury. In these patients, the free water administered as hypotonic fluid cannot be eliminated through the kidney, and hyponatremia results. In most cases, the stress subsides in 24 to 48 hours and the ADH levels fall, which allows the kidney to correct the free-water excess. Patients who continue to be ill or under stress and those who have poor renal function may experience difficulty in correcting the free-water excess. Significant morbidity and mortality can occur if the serum sodium concentration falls below 120 mEq/L.[33,34] Hyponatremia in the postoperative setting is best avoided by means of appropriate I.V. fluid management, including the use of isotonic fluid in the immediate postoperative period.

The treatment of hyponatremia depends on the serum sodium concentration and how long it took serum sodium to reach that level. Intravascular volume deficits, if any, should be corrected first. Patients who have chronically depressed serum sodium concentrations will tolerate slow correction with small amounts of relatively hypertonic fluid (e.g., lactated Ringer solution or normal saline solution). Patients who experience an acute, rapid falloff of their serum sodium concentration or those who are symptomatic require correction with hypertonic (3%) saline over 24 to 48 hours.

Hypernatremia Hypernatremia reflects a relative deficiency of free water compared with sodium. Under normal circumstances, hypernatremia stimulates thirst, and the intake of free water returns the serum sodium concentration to normal. Hypernatremia may develop in patients who are unable to regulate their fluid intake (e.g., obtunded patients) or do not have their fluids replaced appropriately. This is especially likely in patients with large free-water losses such as sweat and insensible losses. Patients with diabetes insipidus (e.g., as a result of head injury) develop hypernatremia because of large (>10 L/day) losses of very dilute urine.

Treatment of hypernatremia consists of providing adequate volumes of free water to correct the deficit. Serum sodium concentration is a good indicator of the adequacy of replacement. In the case of diabetes insipidus, treatment with vasopressin or desmopressin acetate, either parenterally or by the nasal route, in concert with careful fluid management will generally alleviate the hypernatremia.

Disorders of Potassium Concentration

Hypokalemia Hypokalemia may have a number of causes in the postoperative patient. Chronic use of diuretics, poor nutrition with total body potassium depletion, and GI losses are all associated with varying degrees of hypokalemia. Among the most common causes is alkalosis, which brings about a shift of potassium into the intracellular compartment.

Since the serum potassium level does not accurately reflect the total body potassium pool, hypokalemia at levels of 3 mEq/L or less is associated with severe total body potassium depletion (usually in excess of 100 mEq). Such patients may require ECG monitoring and should receive I.V. potassium and have levels measured frequently to monitor their progress. Correction of the underlying cause of the problem is important. Potassium should be given only if there is reliable urine flow, however, as dangerously high potassium levels may result in anuric patients. Our practice is to deliver three doses of 10 mEq of potassium chloride in 50 to 100 ml of saline solution and then check serum levels.

Hyperkalemia Hyperkalemia is among the most dangerous of electrolyte abnormalities. It is especially likely to occur in patients with renal dysfunction but can also result from crush injury, hemolysis, myonecrosis, and acidosis. Hyperkalemia can also occur in malignant hyperthermia and after the administration of succinylcholine to patients with spinal cord injury, burns, or neurologic disorders secondary to severe muscle contractions.

The most serious manifestations of hyperkalemia are cardiac in nature and include high-peaked T waves, absent P waves, widened QRS complexes, ventricular arrhythmias, and cardiac arrest (in diastole). Heart block can also occur. Cardiac effects begin at serum potassium levels of around 6.5 mEq/L; serious risk of death is associated with levels exceeding 8 mEq/L. Patients with serum levels above 6.5 mEq/L should be strongly considered for cardiac monitoring until their serum potassium level is under control.

Treatment consists of discontinuance of any exogenous potassium. If acidosis is present, sodium bicarbonate (50 mEq/L I.V.) should be administered. This dose can be repeated after 10 to 15 minutes. Since sodium bicarbonate is hypertonic saline, caution should be exercised in its use if hypernatremia or fluid overload is present. Infusion of glucose and insulin will lower the serum potassium level by driving potassium into the cell. An ampule (50 ml) of 50% dextrose is administered intravenously along with 10 units of regular insulin. Calcium gluconate can also be used to antagonize the effect of potassium on the myocardium. Administration of furosemide with or without a bolus of saline in patients with reasonable kidney function will also decrease potassium levels. The administration of cation-exchange resins (e.g., sodium polystyrene sulfonate) either orally or by enema will decrease potassium levels more slowly by binding to ions in the GI tract. If other measures fail, dialysis is highly effective in reducing potassium levels.

ACID-BASE-BALANCE DISORDERS

Respiratory Acidosis

Homeostatic mechanisms maintain arterial carbon dioxide tension (P_aCO_2) and serum pH within the normal range through the central regulation of minute ventilation (tidal volume × respiratory rate). Respiratory acidosis results when the ability to eliminate the produced CO_2 is exceeded [see 7 Life-Threatening Acid-Base Disorders]. A variety of causes of respiratory acidosis have been identified. They include central causes (e.g., excess sedation and neuromuscular disorders) as well as disorders of ventilation associated with respiratory failure and ventilatory malfunction. Patients with acute respiratory acidosis characteristically have an elevation in their P_aCO_2 associated with a decreased pH. Acute compensation is relatively limited; it is not until the respiratory acidosis has persisted for at least 12 to 24 hours that renal compensatory mechanisms are activated. Serum bicarbonate gradually rises over a period of several days and drives the pH back (but not completely) toward normal. It is thus possible to differentiate between patients with acute respiratory acidosis and those with chronic respiratory acidosis by the assessment of their serum bicarbonate level and pH. Patients should be assessed for potentially reversible factors. Those on mechanical ventilation should have an immediate increase in minute ventilation. If respiratory acidosis fails to resolve in a spontaneously breathing patient and respiratory distress develops, intubation and mechanical ventilation are necessary.

Respiratory Alkalosis

Respiratory alkalosis occurs when CO_2 elimination exceeds CO_2 production. This is usually caused by an increase in minute ventilation with a decrease in P_aCO_2 and an elevation of pH. Only small changes in the serum bicarbonate level occur in the acute form. If respiratory alkalosis persists, renal compensation will lead to a lowering of the serum bicarbonate level and a return of serum pH almost to normal. Patients with respiratory alkalosis generally have mild hypokalemia and hyperchloremia. The hypokalemia is related to the exchange of potassium for hydrogen ions between the intracellular and extracellular compartments in compensation for the alkalemia. In addition, potassium wasting occurs in the kidney. Hyperchloremia results from the renal retention of chloride to offset the gradually falling levels of serum bicarbonate.

The compensation that occurs in the first week of respiratory alkalosis is generally insufficient to return the pH to normal. More chronic forms of alkalosis will ultimately result in a normalization of the serum pH.

Metabolic Acidosis

Metabolic acidosis in the postoperative surgical patient is always worrisome. It occurs when there is either an increase in the production of H^+ or a significant loss of bicarbonate. Increased production of hydrogen ions is generally associated with underperfusion of tissues and the development of lactic acidosis. Although other conditions can result in metabolic acidosis, hypovolemia and poor tissue perfusion must be ruled out in the postoperative patient.

The initial compensatory response to metabolic acidosis in the spontaneously breathing patient is an increase in minute ventilation. Lactic acidosis exhibits a greater increase in minute ventilation than that seen in other forms of metabolic acidosis. If a patient is sedated or mechanically ventilated, this compensation may not occur, in which case the patient will continue to manifest a low serum pH. A pH of 7.2 or greater has not been associated with significant detrimental effects. Once the patient is known to have metabolic acidosis, assessment of the intravascular volume status should be undertaken immediately. If the metabolic acidosis does not resolve with preliminary maneuvers such as fluid bolus therapy, then invasive monitoring should be undertaken to establish the status of the intravascular circulation and the cardiopulmonary system. Persistent acidosis may signal myocardial ischemia, ischemic bowel, sepsis syndrome, or inadequate volume resuscitation in an injured or critically ill patient.

The administration of I.V. bicarbonate generally does not materially affect the outcome of patients who have metabolic acidosis related to inadequate tissue perfusion; the net effect of this measure is a temporary elevation of serum pH associated with an increase of CO_2 production. Bicarbonate combines with hydrogen ions to form carbonic acid and, subsequently, water and CO_2. It should be noted that this increased CO_2 production can result in a worsening of intracellular acidosis if minute ventilation is not increased to allow elimination of the excess CO_2.

Determination of the anion gap and the serum lactate level can be helpful in determining the cause of the metabolic acidosis. Besides poor tissue perfusion, causes may include renal failure, ketoacidosis, lactic acidosis, and poisoning (all associated with an increased anion gap) as well as renal tubular acidosis, diarrhea, ureteral diversion, and a variety of other conditions (all associated with a normal anion gap).

Metabolic Alkalosis

Metabolic alkalosis is most often caused by a loss of hydrogen ions from the GI tract (e.g., through vomiting or nasogastric suction) or in the urine (e.g., as a result of diuretic therapy). The loss of hydrogen ions is associated with the liberation of bicarbonate, as shown in the following equation:

$$CO_2 + H_2O \rightarrow H_2CO_3 = \rightarrow H^+ + HCO_3^-$$

Hypokalemia can result in metabolic alkalosis by causing a shift of hydrogen ions into the cell in exchange for potassium. Although perceived as extracellular metabolic alkalosis, this is in fact an intracellular metabolic acidosis because of the hydrogen ion shift. Prompt repletion of potassium in the hypokalemic patient can minimize the effect of these changes. Metabolic alkalosis can also result from contraction of the extracellular volume. This contraction alkalosis occurs when the lost fluid contains chloride but little or no bicarbonate, as occurs with diuretic therapy.

Of particular significance in the postoperative period is the development of hypokalemic, hypochloremic metabolic alkalosis associated with the loss of significant amounts of gastric secretions. This can occur either through nasogastric suction or with repeated vomiting. Patients develop intravascular volume contraction in addition to alkalosis and hypochloremia as they lose volume and HCl. This is associated with an increase in sodium and water retention in the kidney, mediated by ADH and aldosterone. The volume deficit, hypochloremia, and hypokalemia all result in increased bicarbonate absorption by the kidney. Paradoxical aciduria will result as bicarbonate reabsorption, together with sodium and potassium retention, leads to an increased hydrogen ion concentration in the urine. Treatment of hypokalemic, hypochloremic metabolic alkalosis is directed at decreasing the fluid losses, if possible, and providing significant amounts of volume, potassium, and chloride.

Chloride repletion is important because chloride is the only reabsorbable anion in this setting. If adequate chloride is not given, electroneutrality in the distal nephron can be maintained only by the excretion of hydrogen ions. Since the patient is volume contracted, no excess sodium ions are available for excretion, and hypokalemia precludes the excretion of potassium ions. Bicarbonate is being reabsorbed avidly at this time. Thus, as sodium is reabsorbed in the hypovolemic state, hydrogen ions will of necessity be excreted in the urine. If chloride is provided in adequate amounts, it will be reabsorbed with sodium, thus obviating excretion of hydrogen ion (or potassium ions if they are available) to maintain electroneutrality.

Metabolic alkalosis can be divided into two varieties: saline responsive and saline resistant. Saline-responsive metabolic alkalosis is generally caused by GI losses or by diuresis, whereas saline-resistant metabolic alkalosis is usually a consequence of either severe hypokalemia or an edematous state such as cirrhosis. Patients with the saline-responsive variety generally respond well to volume expansion with sodium chloride.

Management of Tubes and Drains

Guidelines for the perioperative use of tubes and drains should be developed on the basis of scientific data. For the most part, current practices in this regard are not rigorously formulated and tested but are simply passed on to surgical trainees on little basis other than surgical tradition. With the development of evidence-based medicine, these approaches are being evaluated and challenged. As a result, this aspect of surgical care is evolving.

NASOGASTRIC TUBES

Nasogastric tubes have been routinely utilized in patients undergoing GI surgery. Of late, however, this routine practice has come under scrutiny, and a number of randomized trials have been performed to evaluate its utility. A 1995 meta-analysis of 26 trials including 3,964 patients concluded that nasogastric tubes are unnecessary in elective surgical patients and may even add to debility[44] [see Table 4]. Nasogastric decompression is appropriate on a selective basis for any patient in whom severe nausea, vomiting, or gastric distention develops [see Figure 1]. Moreover, it is known to be helpful in patients with intestinal obstruction.

FINE, PLIABLE FEEDING TUBES

The introduction of the Dobbhoff tube by Dobbie and Hoffmeister[45] allowed routine intubation past the pylorus for feeding. The Dobbhoff tube is a highly flexible No. 8 polyurethane tube with two distal side holes and a mercury-weighted tip. A steel wire is used to stent the tube during placement and is removed after the tube is positioned. The Dobbhoff tube and the Entriflex tube (a similar tube with a thin, elongated distal segment, made by the same manufacturer) are placed in a manner similar to that of a nasogastric tube [see Figure 1]. Once in the stomach, the tube can be advanced under fluoroscopic guidance into the duodenum. Alternatively, the tube can be allowed to pass spontaneously through the pylorus by placing the patient in the right lateral decubitus position and allowing enough slack externally. The use of metoclopramide can sometimes facilitate passage into the duodenum. A radiograph should always be obtained before the initiation of feedings through a nasoenteric small-bore catheter [see Figure 2]. These tubes can pass easily into the trachea even in intubated patients and can cause a pneumothorax or a pneumonic process if feedings are given without radiographic confirmation that the location of the tip is correct.[46-50]

LONG INTESTINAL TUBES

Long intestinal tubes (e.g., the Cantor tube and the Miller-Abbott tube) are occasionally used in patients with partial small-bowel obstruction early after operation, although mechanical bowel obstruction usually requires early operation. Use of long intestinal tubes should be reserved for selected patients who are not candidates for early reoperation. Because movement distally is dependent on peristalsis, these tubes are of little value in patients with paralytic ileus. The Cantor tube is made of silicone-coated polyvinyl chloride and has a small balloon tip. The tip is filled with mercury, passed through the nose, and allowed to advance into the small intestine either passively or with fluoroscopy-guided assistance; there, it will aspirate fluid and gas. Removal of the tube is accomplished by pulling approximately 1 ft of tube out of the nose every 1 or 2 hours and either taping or clamping it to prevent slippage.

BILIARY DRAINAGE CATHETERS

Biliary tract drains include cholecystostomy tubes, percutaneous drains of the biliary tract placed under fluoroscopic control, T tubes, and endoscopically placed nasobiliary tubes. Cholecystostomy tubes may be placed under local anesthesia in patients with advanced medical problems who cannot tolerate general anesthesia and formal cholecystectomy. Patients in whom dissection would be technically difficult and associated with a high risk of complications can also be treated by cholecystostomy tube placement. Ultrasound-guided percutaneous cholecystostomy tube placement has gained acceptance for patients who are not considered good candidates for operation.

The use of T tubes is generally limited to operative exploration or repair of the common bile duct (CBD). In most cases, the CBD is explored for the presence of stones. The duct is then closed around the T-shaped end of the tube to stent the duct. The long end of the T tube is then brought out of an incision, sutured to the skin, and attached to a drainage bag. The exit site should be chosen to allow direct percutaneous access into the distal CBD should this become necessary for later stone extraction or duct manipulation. A T tube will usually drain most of the bile produced (600 to 700 ml daily) initially. A decrease in the volume of bile drained indicates patency of the distal duct and free flow into the duodenum. At 7 to 10 days after surgery, a cholangiogram is obtained to assess the patency of the CBD and look for stones. I.V. antibiotics should be administered during the cholangiogram. A normal cholangiogram will show no stones; a patent, nondilated CBD without leakage; and free flow of contrast medium into the duodenum. The tube can be removed by gentle withdrawal; alternatively, the tube is clamped, and if the patient continues to do well, it is removed on an outpatient basis after 1 to 2 weeks. If the cholangiogram is abnormal, the T tube should be left to drain and the problem addressed either through the tract of the T tube or by means of endoscopic retrograde cholangiopancreatography.

Nasobiliary tubes are placed at the time of endoscopic evaluation of the biliary tree, usually to alleviate CBD obstruction. These tubes are left to drain by gravity and can otherwise be managed like nasoenteric tubes in general.

Table 4 Meta-analysis of 26 Clinical Trials of Selective versus Routine Nasogastric Decompression

	Selective Decompression	Routine Decompression	P
Total no. of patients	1,986	1,978	—
Patients with complications	833	1,084	< 0.03
Patients with pneumonia	53	119	< 0.0001
Patients with atelectasis	44	94	0.001
Patients with fever	108	212	0.02
Time to oral feeding (days)	3.53	4.59	0.04

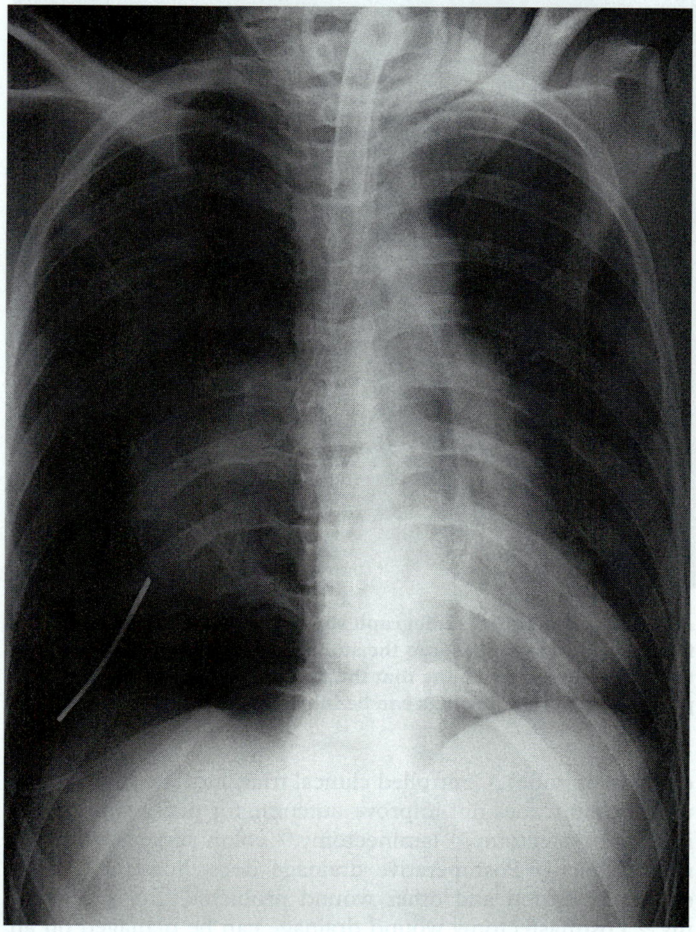

Figure 1 (*a*) The nasogastric tube (generally a No. 18 sump catheter) is passed through the nose to the posterior pharynx, at which point it must make a nearly 90° turn into the esophagus—a maneuver that should be executed gently and with extreme caution. Ideally, the patient should be in a sitting position with head forward and should be sipping liquids, which will help ease the progress of the tube into the stomach. The position of the tube is confirmed by rapid injection of 10 to 20 ml of air into the tube and auscultation over the gastric area of the abdomen. The exterior portion of the tube is gently secured with adhesive tape, preferably to the upper lip or to the nose, without tension or deviation of the alae or septum. If intubation does not drain fluid regularly, the tube may have to be irrigated or repositioned. If the position of the tube is in doubt, a radiograph should be taken (*b*) before feeding is initiated. Examples of inappropriate positioning include passage into the prevertebral fascia, which can cause mediastinitis, or into the lung, which can lead to pneumothorax (*c*) or pneumonia after feeding. At removal, the nasogastric tube is disconnected from the suction tubing and the adhesive tape removed. The patient is instructed to hold his or her breath, and the tube is then withdrawn gently but quickly. After removal, the tube is discarded.

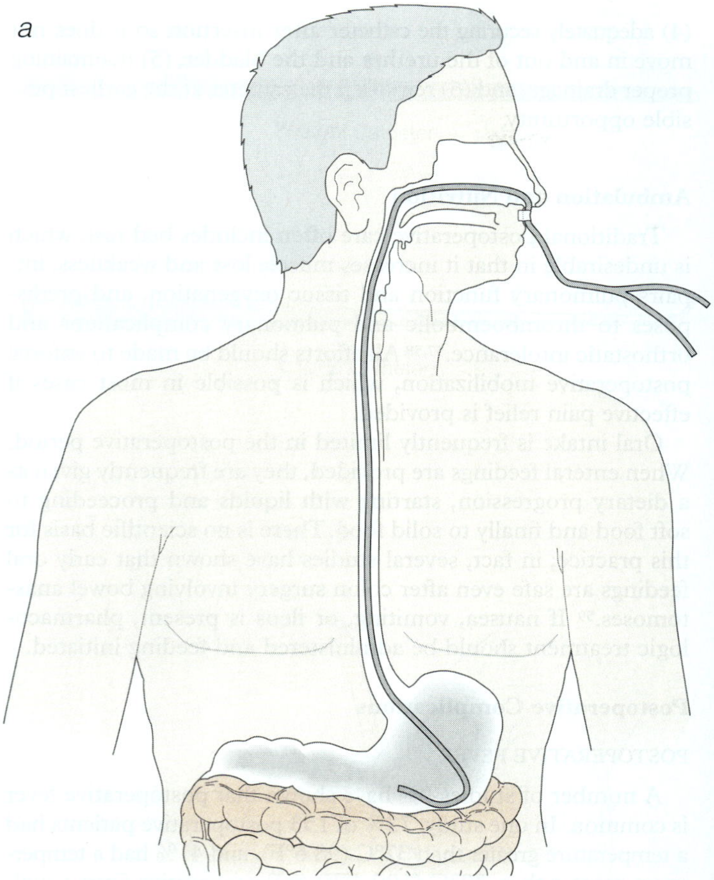

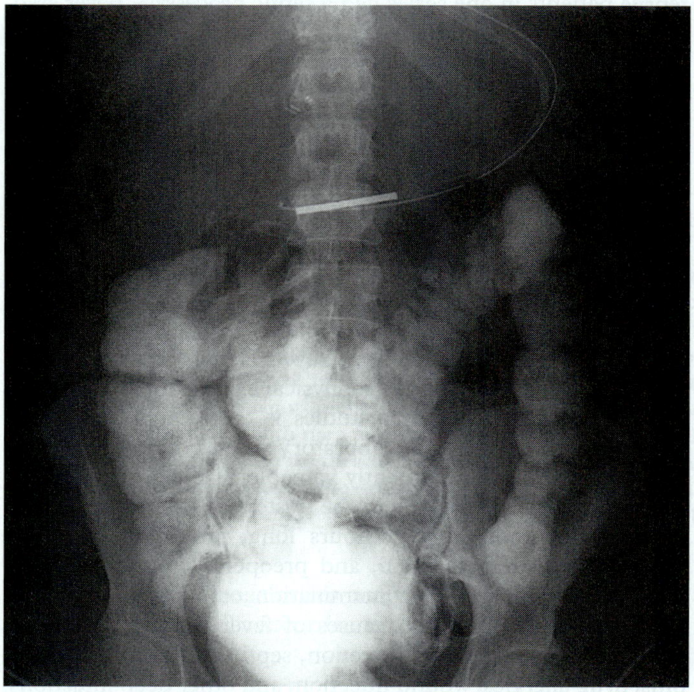

Long intestinal tubes, most commonly a Cantor or Miller-Abbott tube, are passed through the nose and into the stomach in a manner similar to that of a nasogastric tube. Weighted by a balloon tip filled with 5 to 8 ml of mercury, the tube continues on through the stomach and into the small intestine either passively or with assistance under fluoroscopy. Once in the small intestine, it will aspirate fluid and gas as it proceeds. Removal of a long intestinal tube is accomplished gradually; approximately 1 ft of tubing is pulled out through the nose once every 1 or 2 hours and then taped or clamped to prevent slippage.

DRAINS

Various tubes and associated devices have been used to drain purulent materials, blood, or serum from body cavities. These include Penrose drains (very soft rubber tubes with a gauze wick), closed suction drains (commercially available as Jackson-Pratt or Hemovac drains), and sump drains (multiple-lumen tubes that draw air into one interior lumen and fluid from a

myocardial infarction, ventricular failure, and hypertension.[69-72] As the average age of patients undergoing general surgical procedures has increased, so too has the incidence of significant heart disease in this population. Ideally, selective management to prevent significant cardiovascular complications is initiated preoperatively and is continued both intraoperatively and postoperatively.

Table 5 Drugs Used in Urgent and Emergency Treatment of Hypertension[112]

Drug	Administration	Onset of Action	Mechanism of Action	Side Effects	Indications/Contraindications
Sodium nitroprusside	Prepare 50–100 mg/500 ml 5% dextrose in water; administer at rate of 25–50 µg/min and titrate (solution is light sensitive and should be covered with aluminum foil) Patient needs constant monitoring	Immediate	Vasodilatation	Nausea, restlessness, disorientation, severe hypotension, thiocyanate toxicity (check blood levels every 48 hr; discontinue if levels exceed 10 mg/dl), hypothyroidism or methemoglobinemia (rare), ↓ platelet adhesiveness, intracranial hypertension	Especially useful in patients with ischemic heart disease, aortic dissection (combined with a beta blocker), or intracranial hemorrhage
Trimethaphan	Prepare 500 mg/500 ml 5% dextrose in water; administer 1 mg/min initially and titrate Patient needs constant monitoring	Immediate	Ganglionic blockade	Severe hypotension, tachyphylaxis, orthostatic effect, sympathetic blockade (urinary retention, constipation, ileus, pupillary dilatation), respiratory arrest (> 5 mg/min)	Second-choice agent in patients with aortic dissection, intracranial hemorrhage, or ischemic heart disease when sodium nitroprusside cannot be used
Nifedipine	Administer 10–20 mg sublingually or orally as a broken or chewed capsule	5–30 min	Calcium channel blocker	Hypotension, tachycardia, flushing	Drug of choice for hypertensive emergencies when invasive monitoring is not required; contraindicated in patients with aortic dissection
Labetalol	Administer 20–80 mg I.V. at 10-min intervals (maximum cumulative dose 300 mg)	Immediate	Nonselective beta blocker and alpha$_1$ blocker	Pressor response after previous beta-blocker treatment, nausea, paresthesia, headache, hypotension, bradycardia, bronchospasm, urinary retention, ? congestive heart failure	Experience limited; contraindicated for patients with asthma, heart failure, heart block greater than first degree, or bradycardia
Diazoxide	Give 150–300 mg rapid I.V. push or 50–150 mg I.V. every 5 min; to minimize overshoot hypotension, use 7.5–30 mg/min constant I.V. infusion instead Each dose after the first 300 mg should be preceded by furosemide, 40 mg I.V.	Immediate	Vasodilatation	↑ CO, ↑ HR, ↑ blood glucose, ↑ uric acid, Na$^+$ retention; may precipitate angina and cardiac ischemia, nausea, postural hypotension, painful extravasation	Hypertensive encephalopathy, accelerated hypertension, eclampsia; not to be given to patients with ischemic heart disease, intracranial hemorrhage, or aortic dissection
Nicardipine	Administer 5 mg/hr by I.V. infusion and increase by 1–2 mg/hr every 15 min up to 15 mg/hr	1–5 min	Calcium channel blocker	Hypotension, headache, tachycardia, nausea, and vomiting	Similar to other calcium channel blockers; preferential vasodilatory effects; useful in patients who require careful detrition for the control of hypertension
Phentolamine mesylate	Administer 5–20 mg by I.V. bolus or 10–20 mg by I.M. injection	Immediate	Alpha blocker	Hypotension, tachycardia, vomiting, angina, nausea	Drug of choice in patients with pheochromocytoma and monoamine oxidase inhibitor–tyramine interaction; also useful for patients in whom severe hypertension develops after discontinuance of clonidine; short duration of action may require repeated boluses; can precipitate angina and myocardial ischemia in patients at risk
Hydralazine	Administer 5–10 mg I.V. or I.M.	15–30 min	Direct arteriolar vasodilatation	Tachycardia, flushing, angina	Associated with undesirable reflex tachycardia, which may be especially worrisome in patients with coronary artery disease; current usage restricted mostly to patients with renal insufficiency and toxemia
Clonidine	Initial dose 0.2 mg, then 0.1 mg every hr to a maximum of 0.7 mg	30–60 min	Central alpha-adrenergic agonist	Hypotension, sedation, dry mouth; blood pressure should be monitored for 4 hr after last dose	Especially useful in patients with severe hypertension (especially diastolic) without end-organ damage; useful in the emergency department and on the ward

CO—cardiac output   HR—heart rate

Specific measures should be taken to control congestive heart failure; such measures may include aggressive management with careful volume management as well as appropriate use of diuretics, digoxin, afterload reduction therapy, and oxygen therapy. The surgeon should be alert for the presence of angina, cardiac valve disease, and arrhythmias, including heart block, ventricular arrhythmias, and supraventricular tachycardia.[73,74]

Hypertension in the postoperative period frequently occurs secondary to pain or hypoxia. Initial treatment, therefore, consists of administering adequate analgesia to control pain and ensuring adequate oxygenation. Once pain is alleviated and hypoxia corrected, drug treatment may be considered. A variety of agents are available for the treatment of hypertension[75-77] [see Table 5]. The physician should generally become familiar with one or two medications and use them with confidence rather than try to master a large number of them.

RESPIRATORY COMPLICATIONS

Pulmonary complications are common after operative procedures. In one study, dependent atelectasis (3.4% of lung volume) developed in 100% of patients 5 to 10 minutes after administration of anesthesia[78]; 1 hour later, atelectasis was present in 90% of the patients, and 24 hours after operation, it was present in 50%. Up to 40% of obese patients show evidence of basal pulmonary atelectasis on initial postoperative x-ray.[79]

Postoperative respiratory complications include atelectasis, aspiration pneumonia, and other pneumonias. A variety of factors contribute to the development of these complications, and various approaches have been used to prevent and treat them. For example, abdominal incisions cause pain, which limits the patient's activity and shifts predominantly abdominal breathing to chest wall breathing. Fluoroscopy of the diaphragm after operation has demonstrated reduced diaphragmatic movement, with a shift from abdominal to rib cage breathing.[80] This shift begins to reverse after 24 hours. However, the placement of the incision can influence the risk of postoperative respiratory compromise. For example, lower abdominal and transverse incisions are associated with a lower rate of complications and a lower rate of respiratory compromise than longitudinal or midline incisions.[81] Other factors that increase the risk of postoperative pulmonary complications include age, underlying disease, malnutrition, and chronic obstructive pulmonary disease with subsequent colonization.

A variety of preoperative, intraoperative, and postoperative respiratory treatments are available that may be valuable in preventing serious postoperative pulmonary complications. Preoperative treatment with incentive spirometry and chest physical therapy has been studied and appears to be of some value in improving patients' overall pulmonary status in preparation for operation.[82] Underlying pulmonary infection such as bronchitis or pneumonia should always be treated and operation delayed if possible because the ciliary paralysis that occurs with the use of anesthetics has the potential for causing a severe pneumonia after operation.

Routine respiratory therapy is frequently used postoperatively to prevent pulmonary complications. Routine therapeutic measures include administration of bronchodilator aerosol or ultrasonic mist aerosol, IPPB, incentive spirometry, and oxygen therapy. However, some studies have questioned the value of many of these respiratory treatments.[83,84] One study demonstrated that a hospital-wide effort to reduce the use of specific respiratory therapy services did not adversely affect patient outcome.[85] For example, administration of beta agonists was successfully switched from air-driven aerosols to handheld nebulizers. The use of IPPB was nearly completely eliminated, and treatment by incentive spirometry was reduced by 55%. The decrease in the use of incentive spirometry occurred in the late postoperative period, when, studies suggest, it is no longer of value. In patients at high risk, such as those undergoing upper abdominal operation, respiratory therapy is most beneficial when performed in the immediate postoperative period. Patients treated with incentive spirometry return more rapidly to preoperative pulmonary lung volumes than do untreated patients.[82] In this study, use of ultrasonic nebulization was also decreased markedly, whereas oxygen therapy was retained at about the same level.[85] Aerosol ultrasonic nebulization and mist aerosol are of little or no value.

Early mobilization after operation is believed to improve the patient's overall respiratory status. In several studies, early mobilization appeared to be as effective in improving overall respiratory status as chest physical therapy.[86-88] Early mobilization (i.e., turning every 2 hours) in coronary artery bypass patients was shown to decrease the incidence of atelectasis and pneumonia significantly. In high-risk patients, routine postoperative prophylactic chest physical therapy has been shown to decrease the frequency of pulmonary infection significantly.[89] However, in a study of children undergoing cardiac procedures, chest physical therapy had no effect on the development of pulmonary atelectasis.[90]

Atelectasis indicates pulmonary dysfunction and may also presage pneumonia. Postoperative pneumonia is an extremely serious complication and is a major cause of mortality on surgical services [see 103 Early Postoperative Pneumonia]. Factors that increase the risk of postoperative pneumonia include advanced age, gram-negative bacterial infection, emergency operation, use of a ventilator, and postoperative peritonitis.

THROMBOEMBOLISM

Pulmonary Embolism

Pulmonary embolism is the most common acute pulmonary disorder in hospitalized patients [see 70 Thromboembolic Problems]. In the United States, pulmonary embolism occurs in more than 250,00 patients each year[91]; mortality ranges from 8% to 23%.[92] Approximately one third of deaths occur in the first hour after embolism; however, up to 90% of patients survive long enough to be evaluated and for therapeutic intervention to be considered. Aggressive early anticoagulation therapy is associated with 90% survival. Up to 95% of pulmonary emboli originate in the deep veins of the leg; a small percentage originate in pelvic veins and at other sites. There have been reports of pulmonary emboli originating in veins of the upper extremities, but such cases are exceedingly uncommon.

Dyspnea is the most common symptom of pulmonary embolism and is usually of sudden onset. Dyspnea can be transient. The most common physical finding is tachypnea. Rales are present in 50% of cases. Circulatory collapse characterized by shock or syncope occurs in 20% of patients with pulmonary embolism and correlates with larger emboli. Although most patients with pulmonary embolism are hypoxemic, a P_{aO_2} greater than 80 mm Hg was found in 10% of patients in the urokinase-streptokinase pulmonary embolus trial. The chest x-ray, although it may be abnormal, is commonly nondiagnostic. The most common abnormalities evident on the electrocardiogram are T wave inversion, nonspecific ST segment elevation or depression, and sinus tachycardia. Ventilation-perfusion scans are frequently valuable in ruling out pulmonary embolism in a patient with a clear chest x-ray, but recent data cast doubt on the utility of a ventilation-perfusion scan result of low or intermediate probability.[92,93] If the lung scan is equivocal, pulmonary angiography should be performed. Pulmonary arterial pressures are routinely elevated in patients with significant pulmonary embolism.

Treatment of pulmonary embolism is supportive and includes administration of oxygen, adequate maintenance of fluid resuscitation, and rapid I.V. heparinization to increase the partial thromboplastin time to two times the normal value. Patients who cannot receive heparin[94] or who exhibit continued or recurrent signs and symptoms of pulmonary embolus should be considered strongly for vena caval filter placement.[95] Some patients may benefit from thrombolytic therapy administered early, but this option is generally not available for postoperative patients.[96]

Deep Vein Thrombosis

Some degree of deep vein thrombosis develops in approximately 30% of patients after abdominal or thoracic procedures and in up to 80% of patients after hip procedures [see *70 Thromboembolic Problems*]. Some reviews suggest that routine prophylaxis is justified in all surgical patients who are at high risk for deep vein thrombosis (e.g., those older than 40 years, obese patients, patients with malignant disease, patients with prior deep vein thrombosis or pulmonary embolism, or patients undergoing long, complicated operative procedures). Low-dose heparin (5,000 units subcutaneously every 12 hours) should be given until the patient is ambulatory.[97] Increasing the frequency of administration does not decrease the incidence of emboli but does increase the risk of hemorrhagic complications. The addition of dihydroergotamine to heparin may improve efficacy, but the risk associated with its vasoconstrictor effects may outweigh its potential benefits. Dextran in an initial dose of 10 ml/kg appears to be equally effective in decreasing the risk of pulmonary embolism but is more expensive. Dextran 70 and dextran 40 appear to be equally efficacious. External pneumatic compression and gradient elastic stockings can also be employed to prevent deep vein thrombosis.

Findings from several reviews suggest that mortality from pulmonary embolism is decreasing and that effective prophylaxis with either subcutaneous heparin or pneumatic compression devices can decrease the risk of deep vein thrombosis and pulmonary embolism.[98-100] To achieve optimal results, prophylaxis must be started before the operative procedure begins.

CENTRAL VENOUS CATHETER COMPLICATIONS

Central venous catheters, arterial catheters, and triple-lumen catheters may be associated with such complications as perforation of the vascular system, thrombi, and infection.[97,101] In one study, complications related to initial catheter placement occurred in 5.7% of patients, sepsis occurred in 6.5%, and mechanical complications occurred in 9%.[102,103] Complications of catheter placement are hemorrhage and pneumothorax. The most common late mechanical complications are major venous thrombosis and nursing mishaps. Central venous thrombophlebitis and sepsis usually require immediate removal of the central venous catheter and antibiotic therapy. In some patients with Silastic catheters, treatment with I.V. antibiotics and anticoagulants and careful monitoring for potential exploration and drainage of perivascular infection or vein excision may be indicated.[102] Other studies have shown that administration of antibiotics through the indwelling catheter is effective. In one study of catheter-associated infections, 18 patients (86%) were cured without removal of the catheter. Absolute indications for catheter removal are lack of defervescence and continued positive blood cultures despite antibiotic therapy.[103] An effective method of assessing catheter contamination in patients with central lines in place is routine catheter exchange and culture [see *81 Nosocomial Infection*]. Studies have shown a direct link between catheter infection and contamination of the site. To avoid mechanical complications, an x-ray should be obtained after insertion of any central line to document its position. The catheter should be evaluated every 2 to 7 days to ensure that it has not migrated or been displaced.

UPPER GASTROINTESTINAL BLEEDING

Before the advent of routine administration of antacids, life-threatening upper GI bleeding was a common problem in patients undergoing major stress, particularly in those with head injury, burns, or multiple trauma. The protocol for bleeding prophylaxis is 30 to 60 ml of antacids by nasogastric tube every 1 to 2 hours to maintain gastric pH above 4. With adequate prophylaxis, the incidence of massive upper GI bleeding is essentially zero. According to one study, sucralfate may also be effective for bleeding prophylaxis.[104] By comparison, H_2 receptor antagonists have not proved to be more effective than antacids in preventing major upper gastrointestinal bleeding.[105-108]

POSTOPERATIVE TRANSFUSION AND ANEMIA

A decreased hematocrit and relative anemia occur very commonly after major operative procedures. In patients with these conditions, blood transfusion is often considered. It is important, however, to avoid unnecessary transfusions because of the potential for transfusion-associated complications, which include hemolytic transfusion reactions, nonhemolytic transfusion reactions, and transmission of infection (e.g., hepatitis, AIDS, cytome-galovirus, and herpesvirus). In addition, blood transfusion itself may be a significant immunodepressant. Many surgeons consider it reasonable to order a blood transfusion when the hematocrit measures 30% or less. However, there are many situations in which this practice should not be followed. For example, in a young healthy patient who has no other disease and is expected to continue to improve, hematocrits in the low to middle 20s are acceptable. In addition, patients with a variety of other chronic diseases that lead to persistently low hematocrits (e.g., chronic renal insufficiency) have been safely observed at relatively low hematocrit levels without transfusion.

DIABETES MELLITUS

The diabetic patient presents a series of management problems in the postoperative period [see *68 Diabetes Mellitus*]. Careful management of blood glucose levels is necessary to avoid hypoglycemia or hyperglycemia with associated complications such as diabetic ketoacidosis and dehydration secondary to glycosuria. Diabetes has a significant negative impact on wound healing. For patients whose disease is managed by diet alone, additional measures are usually unnecessary. In the postoperative period, careful monitoring, including finger-stick glucose measurements every 6 hours, is appropriate, with a sliding scale of regular insulin administered as needed. In patients who are receiving oral hypoglycemic agents, the medication should be discontinued on the day before operation, and insulin should be given as needed for hyperglycemia. Patients who require insulin should be given a dextrose infusion and one half of the total daily dose of insulin as regular insulin the morning of the operation. Glucose is administered throughout the operation, as guided by measured glucose levels. In patients who require major operations and massive fluid administration, blood glucose should be measured frequently during operation, and insulin should be given I.V. as needed. Postoperatively, glucose levels in some patients will be well controlled by administration of insulin on a sliding scale based on finger-stick glucose monitoring.

Shock, major trauma, or extremely prolonged operations can lead to hypoperfusion of the skin and subcutaneous tissue. In these patients, subcutaneous administration of insulin is inappropriate and dangerous. Instead, monitoring in the ICU, with frequent glucose measurements, and treatment with I.V. insulin should be undertaken. Dextrose should be included in postoperative administration of fluids.

OTHER ENDOCRINE COMPLICATIONS

Another postoperative endocrine complication is hypothyroidism, which usually occurs in the elderly. Hypothyroidism is frequently associated with (1) a low temperature and (2) a low blood pressure that does not respond to fluid management or pressors. The elderly are also at risk for hyponatremia, hypoventilation, and hypoglycemia. In these cases, thyroid levels should be measured and intravenous thyroxine (200 to 500 μg) given. This dose should provide adequate thyroid levels for several days.

Postoperative hypoadrenocorticism occurs in patients who have been receiving oral or parenteral steroids. The stress of operation necessitates replacement with hydrocortisone (300 to 400 mg/day) or its equivalent. The suggested regimen is 100 mg I.V. every 8 hours on postoperative day 1 or 2, which should be rapidly tapered if the level of stress and the length of preoperative therapy allow it. In patients who are treated with steroids, the wound healing process is slowed. This deleterious effect can be reversed by administration of vitamin A (25,000 units orally or by nasogastric tube).

Discharge from Hospital and Follow-up Care

Discharge from the hospital is an important milestone in the postoperative care of a patient. For many patients who return home after their hospitalization, discharge represents a marker of major improvement. For other patients who have more complex problems and require significant care after hospital discharge, it is the beginning of a long and often difficult journey through a rehabilitation system or a skilled nursing facility.

The vast majority of patients admitted for elective surgery and most patients admitted for emergency surgery are discharged from the hospital back to their preoperative domicile. Patients with complex injuries (especially head injury), advanced malignancy, or significant disabilities or elderly patients may require placement in a facility rather than being sent home. In some cases, support from agencies in their community, such as home health care groups, may obviate placement in a nursing facility.

Table 6 Care Services

In-home services	Community services
Telephone reassurance	Congregate meals
Emergency response systems	Senior centers
Home-delivered meals	Day care
Respite care	Retirement communities
Housekeeping/shopping services	**Institutional services**
Congregate housing	Family care home
Home health care	Rest home
Hospice care	Nursing home
	Intermediate care facility
	Skilled nursing facility

Sample Discharge Orders

[Date and Time]
1. Discharge patient home.
2. Return to clinic in 1 wk to see Dr. Smith. Patient may call 919-555-4343 for questions or problems.
3. Prescriptions for discharge medications on the chart.
4. Instructions regarding wound care or care of drains: as indicated.
5. Activity: ambulatory.
6. Patient may bathe or shower.
7. Diet: regular as tolerated.
8. Work status: to be determined at follow-up appointment.
9. Discharge summary dictated.

[Physician's signature and ID number]

Recent data suggest that well-developed family networks contribute significantly to a decreased risk of institutionalization.[109] A continuum of care services exists but may vary from one community to another [see Table 6]. A qualified medical social worker or discharge planner is invaluable in providing access to the various available options in each particular locale.

Most patients are discharged once the physician determines that they have met certain criteria: they must be medically stable and afebrile, tolerant of oral intake, ambulatory, and reasonably comfortable, and they must have wounds or drains that require only minimal care. The physician should then write discharge orders in the hospital chart to notify the nursing staff and the hospital administration [see Sidebar Sample Discharge Orders]. The discharge summary, written or dictated by the physician, should include information from the patient's history; data from physical examinations, laboratory tests, and radiographs; details of the hospital course; and full discharge plans. A copy of the discharge summary may be sent to the referring or family physician, or a personal letter can be forwarded to inform the physician of the patient's progress and plans for follow-up.

Certain patients, however, require significantly more sophisticated discharge planning. These include patients with severe multiple injuries (especially head injury), elderly patients with limited ability to care for themselves, patients with significant disabilities and functional impairment, patients with advanced malignancy, and patients with one or more significant socioeconomic difficulties, including homelessness, history of substance abuse, or AIDS. Such patients will require either significant levels of support at home or placement in a care facility [see Table 7]. Discharge planning for these patients should begin as soon as possible after admission. Once such a patient is identified, the physician should notify a medical social worker or other hospital employee with experience in discharge planning and placement. Such early notification will permit planning for discharge and placement to proceed more efficiently. This is especially relevant for patients with complex needs, such as those requiring placement into a rehabilitation facility or those who have no insurance and who can perhaps be enrolled in Medicaid to provide them with financial support for placement.

DISCHARGE PLANNING

With today's emphasis on decreasing the length of hospitalizations, discharge planning has become a crucial part of the management of patient care in the inpatient setting. Even for the most complicated patient, the issue of a patient's disposition can be addressed from the moment of admission. Comprehensive discharge planning can reduce readmissions, lengthen the interval between discharge and readmission, and decrease the cost of providing health care.[110]

Early in a patient's admission, discharge planning primarily takes the form of assessment. All health care workers involved in the patient's care may provide input based on their interactions with patient and family. How a patient and family cope initially in a crisis and throughout the course of recovery can indicate the strength or weakness of the existing support system. Once a patient progresses beyond the initial crisis, more concrete information pertaining to the patient's financial resources, living situation, physical and emotional supports, and family dynamics is essential. This information is most often obtained by a social worker or trained discharge planner. Once the complete picture of the numerous facets of a patient's life outside of the hospital comes into focus, it can be compared with the new limitations and needs that may have resulted from the illness or injury that necessitated the hospitalization. One should always remember that functioning well in the hospital setting and being independent at home, work, or school can be dramatically different.

A number of options are available for acute care placement for those patients who have special care needs after discharge [see Table 7]. They fall into two categories: in-home care and extended care facilities.

In-Home Care

In-home care consists of home health services, private duty nurses, and community resources such as Meals on Wheels and transportation services. For patients who can be discharged home but require assistance or support, home health services represent an excellent alternative to continued hospitalization. Home health agencies can provide skilled nursing care, assistance in the home (homemakers or aides), physical therapy services, speech therapy services, occupational therapy services, and medical social worker support [see Table 8]. These patients must be otherwise independent, as home health agencies do not provide long periods of custodial care. Patients who require greater assistance must therefore either hire private duty nurses or consider an extended care facility as an alternative after discharge.

Home health agencies charge per service per visit. Charges for skilled therapies, such as skilled nursing, occupational therapy, and physical therapy, may cost up to $100 a visit or an hour. These fees are comparable to those charged in acute care facilities. Charges for nonskilled assistance range from a few dollars an hour to as high as $15 an hour. Services offered through home health providers are time limited under Medicare and Medicaid rules.

The use of home health services has increased dramatically over the past decade. Medicare data indicate that $2.1 billion was spent in 1988, compared with $15 billion in 1999. It has been estimated that this figure may reach $17 billion by 2002. Between 1980 and 1997, home health care costs increased from $842/recipient to $6,595/recipient.[111]

Extended Care Facilities

Extended care facilities, such as rest homes, nursing homes, and rehabilitation centers, are often very successful in maximizing a patient's potential for independence. They offer more intensive skilled therapies than are offered by home health agencies and provide supervision and assistance with activities of daily living that can be difficult for working family members to provide. Rehabilitation facilities are distinguished from skilled nursing facilities primarily by the amount of activity an individual patient can endure. The standard amount of activity for a rehabilitation center is 3 to 4 hours a day, though this need not be constant activity. Physical therapists, occupational therapists,

Table 7 Options for Acute Care after Hospital Discharge

Facility	Approximate Daily Cost ($)	Insurance Coverage	Services Offered
Rest home	40–60*	Medicaid Private payment plans	Convalescent care
Intermediate care facility	85–135*	Medicaid Private payment plans Medicare will cover skilled services but not room and board	Skilled nursing, 4 hr a day Other skilled services (e.g., physical and occupational therapy) only on contractual basis
Skilled nursing facility	100–150*	Medicaid Medicare (for 100 days) Some insurance plans Private payment plans	Skilled nursing, 24 hr a day Other skilled services (e.g., physical and occupational therapy) only on contractual basis; some provide in-house physical therapy
Subacute care facility	400–600	Medicare (for 100 days) Medicaid Some insurance plans Private payment plans	Skilled nursing, 24 hr a day Other skilled services often provided in-house Specialize in complex wound care and ventilator-dependent patients
Rehabilitation facility	800–1,000	Medicare Medicaid Some insurance plans Private payment plans	All skilled services (physical, occupational, and speech therapy) provided in-house Intensive therapy provided 3–5 hr a day
Acute care facility	1,000+	All current payor sources	Therapies provided on less frequent basis and for shorter duration than at rehabilitation facilities

*Includes only room and board; additional fees required for therapies and medications.
Prices reflect average cost in 1998 based on semiprivate room rates.

> **Table 8 Services Offered by Home Health Professionals**
>
> **Skilled nursing**
>   Injections
>   Ostomy care
>   Dressing changes
>   Catheter care
>   Observation
>   Instruction in medication/disease process
>   In-home management training
>   Hospice care
>   Respiratory care
>   Tracheotomy
>   Post–cataract surgery care
>   Instruction in diabetes care and monitoring
>
> **Home health aide/homemaker**
>   Bathing
>   Meal assistance
>   Personal grooming
>   Ambulation assistance
>
> **Physical therapy**
>   Muscle strengthening
>   Gait or prosthesis training
>   Training in ambulation and transfer techniques (e.g., bed to wheelchair)
>   Pulmonary exercises
>   Ultrasound treatments
>
> **Speech therapy**
>   Retraining speech and language function
>   Developing alternative communication skills
>   Swallowing therapy
>
> **Occupational therapy**
>   Preparation for independence in activities of daily living
>   Motor coordination improvement
>   Increase in upper extremity function
>
> **Medical social services**
>   Disability assistance
>   Coordination of community resources

and speech therapists can assist in making judgments about a patient's endurance, potential, and goals for independence.

Patients who require assistance with convalescence that cannot be provided in their home setting are most often referred to a rest home facility. This is a relatively cost-effective alternative and is generally an intermediate step before the patient returns to a home setting.

Patients who require a higher level of care than that provided in either a rest home or through home health care require admission to a nursing home. A nursing home is either an intermediate care facility or a skilled nursing facility. At an intermediate care facility, registered nurses or licensed practical nurses are on duty for at least 4 hours a day to tend to patients' special medical needs; additional care is provided full time by trained staff who are not registered or practical nurses. Patients who require round-the-clock care from either a registered nurse or a licensed practical nurse must be admitted to a skilled nursing facility. Such patients include those who are potentially unstable or who may have a special need such as I.V. fluid administration or oxygen therapy. In addition, such patients may require advanced comprehensive support services such as physical and occupational therapy. Although physical and occupational therapy and related services can be provided at an intermediate care facility, a skilled nursing facility provides a more comprehensive approach to such needs. Both intermediate care and skilled nursing facilities require physician involvement for admission evaluation and supervision of subsequent care. Payment arrangements may vary among different settings, and such information should be obtained with the assistance of a social worker or other discharge planner. In general, Medicare will cover nursing home costs for a period of up to 100 days.

Rehabilitation facilities are ideally suited for patients who have complex problems that require comprehensive care and graded rehabilitation. They offer nursing services as well as physical, occupational, and speech therapy. They can also provide complex care services in addition to general rehabilitation, and many specialize in areas such as head injury, spinal cord injury, respiratory rehabilitation, stroke, burns, or advanced neurologic disorders. The goal of such centers is to allow patients to attain their maximum level of independence and reintegration into society. An interdisciplinary team provides care in a structured, graded fashion. Most rehabilitation centers will send a member of their team to assess a patient while the patient is still in the hospital to determine whether he or she is a candidate for admission. In general, for admission to a rehabilitation facility, the following criteria must be met:

1. Patients must be medically stable.
2. Patients must require an intensive rehabilitation program as offered by the multidisciplinary team. An intensive rehabilitation program is one in which the patient has a demonstrated need for round-the-clock nursing care and is capable of receiving 3 to 4 hours of physical, occupational, or speech therapy.
3. Patients must be able to participate actively in the rehabilitation process and should be able to follow at least simple commands, except in cases of severe brain injury or stroke.
4. The patient must have the potential for attaining significant functional improvement, with the expectation that he or she will return to an acceptable level of functional recovery.

Current trends in posthospital care focus on providing patient care at home and on shortening the length of acute hospital stays. Some skilled nursing facilities are able to provide complex care without the high cost associated with a stay in an acute care hospital. Services provided include ventilator support, I.V. drug therapy, care of advanced decubitus ulcers, total parenteral nutrition, tracheostomy care, and dialysis. These advanced care facilities are often referred to as subacute facilities. If a patient has relatively complex needs, such as ongoing wound care or a need for mechanical ventilation, then admission to a subacute facility would be required. Medicare will cover up to 100 days at such a facility, as will some insurance companies. Because of the generally sophisticated level of care, these facilities tend to have long waiting lists, as do many nursing homes. It is therefore crucial to begin seeking placement for such patients as early as possible in their hospital course to ensure bed availability.

Other Options

Hospice programs provide care for patients who are no longer seeking a cure but rather require care near the end of life. The majority of patients admitted to hospices have terminal illnesses as a result of disseminated malignancy. Hospice care provides the opportunity for patients to gain greater control over decisions regarding their care and allows the family to become more closely involved with the day-to-day progress of the patient. Hospices offer such specialized services as pain management and grief counseling. They are designed to allow patients in the last phase of an incurable illness to live at home or in equally comfortable surroundings for as long as possible. The program strives to keep patients as active as possible and provides them outlets for expressing their feelings in a supportive environment. The hospice team includes members of the family, nurses, social workers, physicians, clergy, and volunteers. Help is available to the patient on a continuous basis. Many of the services provided through the hospice system are covered under Medicare as long as the patient's physician and the hospice medical director certify that the patient is terminally ill, with a life expectancy of less than 6 months, and the hospice providing care is certified by Medicare. Physician services unrelated to hospice care continue to be provided for under standard Medicare Part B coverage.

Some pharmaceutical companies and home health agencies combine skills and efforts to provide I.V. drug therapies at home for patients who are otherwise independent and have adequate family support and assistance. For patients who require more aggressive physical therapy than can be provided at home, outpatient physical therapy at a local hospital or clinic may be a good option to enable the patient to live at home. This option, however, requires extensive family support to provide transportation to therapy and care in the home.

Services for Indigent Patients

Patients without insurance and with no available financial resources can present a difficult problem for discharge planners. Most home health agencies are mandated to set aside funds for indigent clients, but the services provided tend to be the bare minimum. Nursing homes and rehabilitation facilities have no such mandate, however. They set aside a limited number of beds for Medicare and Medicaid patients, but these tend to be in high demand and may represent a resource drain for these facilities. Patients who are not eligible for Medicare can sometimes be enrolled in Medicaid programs. Patients who are not eligible for Medicaid assistance will have to spend their private funds until they qualify for Medicaid. In general, adults are eligible for Medicaid if they are disabled, have dependent children, or have inadequate financial resources.

References

1. Fakhry SM, Buehrer JL, Sheldon GF, et al: A comparison of intensive care unit care of surgical patients in teaching and nonteaching hospitals. Ann Surg 213:19, 1991
2. Trask AL, Faber DR: The intensive care unit—who's in charge? The private practice view. Arch Surg 125:1105, 1990
3. Cook DJ, Fuller HD, Guyatt GH, et al: Risk factors for gastrointestinal bleeding in critically ill patients. N Engl J Med 330:377, 1994
4. Carr BD, Goudas LC: Acute pain. Lancet 353:2051, 1999
5. Warfield CA, Kahn CH: Acute pain management: programs in US hospitals and experiences and attitudes among US adults. Anesthesiology 83:1090, 1995
6. Egbert LD, Battit GE, Welch CE, et al: Reduction of postoperative pain by encouragement and instruction of patients: a study of doctor-patient rapport. N Engl J Med 270:825, 1964
7. Daltory LH, Morlino CL, Eaton HM, et al: Preoperative education for total hip and knee replacement patients. Arthritis Care Res 11:469, 1989
8. Lebovits AH, Twersky R, McEwan B: Intraoperative therapeutic suggestions in day-case surgery: are there benefits for postoperative outcome? Br J Anaesth 82:861, 1999
9. Gottschalk A, Smith DS, Jobes DR, et al: Preemptive epidural analgesia and recovery from radical prostatectomy: a randomized controlled trial. JAMA 279:1076, 1998
10. Kato J, Ogawa S, Katz J, et al: Effects of presurgical local infiltration of bupivacaine in the surgical field on postsurgical wound pain in laparoscopic gynecologic examinations: a possible preemptive analgesic effect. Clin J Pain 16:12, 2000
11. Kehlet H: Acute pain control and accelerated postoperative surgical recovery. Surg Clin Nutr Am 79:431, 1999
12. Lanz E, Theiss D, Riess W, et al: Epidural morphine for postoperative analgesia: a double-blind study. Anesth Analg 61:236, 1982
13. Bromage PR: Epidural Analgesia. WB Saunders Co, Philadelphia, 1978
14. Mackersie RC, Karagianes TG, Hoyt DB, et al: Prospective evaluation of epidural and intravenous administration of fentanyl for pain control and restoration of ventilatory function following multiple rib fractures. J Trauma 31:443, 1991
15. Holland AJ, Srikantha SK, Tracey JA: Epidural morphine and post-operative pain relief. Can Anaesth Soc J 28:453, 1981
16. Zenz M, Piepenbrock S, Otten B, et al: [Epidural morphine analgesia]. Anaesthesist 30:77, 1981
17. El-Baz N, Goldin M: Continuous epidural infusion of morphine for pain relief after cardiac operations. J Thorac Cardiovasc Surg 93:878, 1987
18. Weltz CR, Greengrass RA, Lyerly HK: Ambulatory and surgical management of breast carcinoma using paravertebral block. Ann Surg 222:19, 1995
19. Marks RM, Sachar EJ: Undertreatment of medical inpatients with narcotic analgesics. Ann Intern Med 78:173, 1973
20. Bollish SJ, Collins CL, Kirking DM, et al: Efficacy of patient-controlled versus conventional analgesia for postoperative pain. Clin Pharm 4:48, 1985
21. Graves DA, Foster TS, Batenhorst RL, et al: Patient controlled analgesia. Ann Intern Med 99:360, 1983
22. Bennett RL, Batenhorst RL, Bivins BA, et al: Patient-controlled analgesia: a new concept of postoperative pain relief. Ann Surg 195:700, 1982
23. Burchard KW, Gann DS, Colliton J, et al: Ionized calcium, parathormone, and mortality in critically ill surgical patients. Ann Surg 212:543, 1990
24. Fakhry SM, Meyer AA: Critical care: recent advances. Adv Trauma 4:43, 1989
25. Goldenheim PD, Kazemi H: Cardiopulmonary monitoring of critically ill patients. N Engl J Med 311:717, 1984
26. Recommendations for intensive care unit admission and discharge criteria. Task Force on Guidelines, Society of Critical Care Medicine. Crit Care Med 16:807, 1988
27. Wiedemann HP, Matthay MA, Matthay RA: Cardiovascular-pulmonary monitoring in the intensive care unit (pt 1). Chest 85:537, 1984
28. Critical care medicine. NIH Consensus Conference. JAMA 250:798, 1983
29. Wiedemann HP, Matthay MA, Matthay RA: Cardiovascular-pulmonary monitoring in the intensive care unit (pt 2). Chest 85:656, 1984
30. Moore FD: Common patterns of water and electrolyte change in injury, surgery and disease. N Engl J Med 258:277, 1958
31. Moran WH Jr, Miltenberger FW, Shuayb WA, et al: Relationship of antidiuretic hormone secretion to surgical stress. Surgery 56:99, 1964
32. Ukai M, Moran WH Jr, Zimmerman B: The role of visceral afferent pathways on vasopressin secretion and urinary excretory patterns during surgical stress. Ann Surg 168:16, 1968
33. Ayus JC, Krothapalli RK, Arieff AI: Treatment of symptomatic hyponatremia and its relation to brain damage. N Engl J Med 317:1190, 1987
34. Arieff AI: Hyponatremia, convulsions, respiratory arrest, and permanent brain damage after elective surgery in healthy women. N Engl J Med 314:1529, 1986
35. Needleman P, Greenwald JE: Atriopeptin: a cardiac hormone intimately involved in fluid, electrolyte, and blood-pressure homeostasis. N Engl J Med 314:828, 1986
36. Putensen C, Mutz N, Pomaroli A, et al: Atrial natriuretic factor release during hypovolemia and after volume replacement. Crit Care Med 20:984, 1992
37. Virgilio RW, Rice CL, Smith DE, et al: Crystalloid vs. colloid resuscitation: is one better? Surgery 85:129, 1979
38. Foley EF, Borlase BC, Dzik WH, et al: Albumin supplementation in the critically ill. Arch Surg 125:739, 1990
39. Golub R, Sorrento JJ Jr, Cantu R Jr, et al: Efficacy of albumin supplementation in the surgical intensive care unit: a prospective, randomized study. Crit Care Med 22:613, 1994
40. Shires GT, Canizaro PC: Fluid resuscitation in the severely injured. Surg Clin North Am 53:1341, 1973
41. Eisenberg PR, Jaffe AS, Schuster DP: Clinical evaluation compared to pulmonary artery catheterization in the hemodynamic assessment of critically ill patients. Crit Care Med 12:549, 1984
42. Connors AF, McCaffree DR, Gray BA: Evaluation of right-heart catheterization in the critically ill patient without acute myocardial infarction. N Engl J Med 308:263, 1983
43. Lowell JA, Schifferdecker C, Driscoll DF, et al: Postoperative fluid overload: not a benign problem. Crit Care Med 18:728, 1990
44. Cheatham ML, Chapman WC, Key SP, et al: A meta-analysis of selective versus routine nasogastric decompression after elective laparotomy. Ann Surg 221:469, 1995
45. Dobbie RP, Hoffmeister JA: Continuous pump-tube enteric hyperalimentation. Surg Gynecol Obstet 143:273, 1976
46. Roubenoff R, Ravich WJ: Pneumothorax due to

nasogastric feeding tubes: report of four cases, review of the literature, and recommendations for prevention. Arch Intern Med 149:184, 1989
47. McWey RE, Curry NS, Schabel SI, et al: Complications of nasoenteric feeding tubes. Am J Surg 155:253, 1988
48. Ghahremani GG, Gould RJ: Nasoenteric feeding tubes: radiographic detection of complications. Dig Dis Sci 31:574, 1986
49. Harris MR, Huseby JS: Pulmonary complications from nasoenteral feeding tube insertion in an intensive care unit: incidence and prevention. Crit Care Med 17:917, 1989
50. Lipman TO: Nasopulmonary intubation with feeding tubes: therapeutic misadventure or accepted complication? (editorial). Nutrition in Clinical Practice 2:45, 1987
51. Trowbridge PE: A randomized study of cholecystectomy with and without drainage. Surg Gynecol Obstet 155:171, 1982
52. Payne DH, Fishchgrund JS, Herkowitz HN, et al: Efficacy of closed wound suction drainage after single-level lumbar laminectomy. J Spinal Disord 9:401, 1996
53. Urbach DR, Kennedy ED, Cohen MM: Colon and rectal anastomosis do not require rectal drainage: a systematic review and meta-analysis. Ann Surg 229:174, 1999
54. Wihlborg O, Bergljung L, Martensson H: To drain or not to drain in thyroid surgery: a controlled clinical study. Arch Surg 123:40, 1988
55. Somers RG, Jablon LK, Kaplan MJ, et al: The use of closed suction drainage after lumpectomy and axillary node dissection for breast cancer: a prospective randomized trial. Ann Surg 215:146, 1992
56. Sobel JD, Kaye D: Urinary tract infections. Principles and Practice of Infectious Diseases, 2nd ed. Mandell GL, Douglas RG Jr, Bennett JE, Eds. John Wiley & Sons, New York, 1985
57. Kovacevich GJ, Gaich SA, Lavin JP, et al: The prevalence of thromboembolic events among women with extended bed rest prescribed as part of the treatment for premature labor or preterm premature rupture of membranes. Am J Obstet Gynecol 182:1089, 2000
58. Convertino VA, Goldwater DJ, Sandler H: Effects of orthostatic stress on exercise performance after bedrest. Aviat Space Environ Med 53:652, 1982
59. Kehlet H, Mogensen T: Hospital stay of 2 days after open sigmoidectomy with a multimodal program. Br J Surg 86:227, 1999
60. Yeung RS, Buck JR, Filler RM: The significance of fever following operations in children. J Pediatr Surg 17:347, 1982
61. Galicier C, Richet H: A prospective study of postoperative fever in a general surgery department. Infect Control 6:487, 1985
62. Drago JJ, Jacobs AM, Oloff LM: Elevated temperature in the postoperative patient. J Foot Surg 21:269, 1982
63. Locker D, Norwood SH, Torma MJ, et al: A prospective randomized study of drained and undrained cholecystectomies. Am Surg 49:528, 1983
64. Trowbridge PE: A randomized study of cholecystectomy with and without drainage. Surg Gynecol Obstet 155:171, 1982
65. Lewis RT, Allan CM, Godall RG, et al: The conduct of cholecystectomy: incision, drainage, bacteriology, and postoperative complications. Can J Surg 25:304, 1982
66. Soper DE: Delayed hemolytic transfusion reaction: a cause of late postoperative fever. Am J Obstet Gynecol 153:227, 1985
67. Lewis JH, Zimmerman HJ, Ishak KG, et al: Enflurane hepatotoxicity: a clinicopathologic study of 24 cases. Ann Intern Med 98:984, 1983
68. Siegman-Igra Y: Late postoperative fever—viral infection following multiple blood transfusion. Isr J Med Sci 19:267, 1983
69. Goldman L: Cardiac risks and complications of noncardiac surgery. Ann Surg 198:780, 1983
70. O'Kelly B, Browner WS, Massie B, et al: Ventricular arrhythmias in patients undergoing noncardiac surgery. JAMA 268:217, 1992
71. Lappas DG, Powell WMJ Jr, Daggett WM: Cardiac dysfunction in the perioperative period: pathophysiology, diagnosis, and treatment. Anesthesiology 47:117, 1977
72. Charlson ME, MacKenzie CR, Ales K, et al: Surveillance for postoperative myocardial infarction after noncardiac operations. Surg Gynecol Obstet 167:407, 1988
73. Pritchett ELC: Management of atrial fibrillation. N Engl J Med 326:1264, 1992
74. Salerno DM, Anderson B, Sharkey P, et al: Intravenous verapamil for treatment of multifocal atrial tachycardia with and without calcium pretreatment. Ann Intern Med 107:623, 1987
75. Calhoun DA, Oparil S: Treatment of hypertensive crisis. N Engl J Med 323:1177, 1990
76. McRae RP Jr, Liebson PR: Hypertensive crisis. Med Clin North Am 70:749, 1986
77. Halpern NA, Goldberg M, Neely C, et al: Postoperative hypertension: a multicenter, prospective, randomized comparison between intravenous nicardipine and sodium nitroprusside. Crit Care Med 20:1637, 1992
78. Strandberg A, Tokics L, Brismar B, et al: Atelectasis during anaesthesia and in the postoperative period. Acta Anaesthesiol Scand 30:154, 1986
79. Ramsey-Stewart G: The perioperative management of morbidly obese patients (a surgeon's perspective). Anaesth Intensive Care 13:399, 1985
80. Ford GT, Whitelaw WA, Rosenal TW, et al: Diaphragm function after upper abdominal surgery in humans. Am Rev Respir Dis 127:431, 1983
81. Becquemin JP, Piquet J, Becquemin MH, et al: Pulmonary function after transverse or midline incision in patients with obstructive pulmonary disease. Intensive Care Med 11:247, 1985
82. Minschaert M, Vincent JL, Ros AM, et al: Influence of incentive spirometry on pulmonary volumes after laparotomy. Acta Anaesthesiol Belg 33:203, 1982
83. O'Donohue WJ Jr: National survey of the usage of lung expansion modalities for the prevention and treatment of postoperative atelectasis following abdominal and thoracic surgery. Chest 87:76, 1985
84. Pontoppidan H: Mechanical aids to lung expansion in non-intubated surgical patients. Am Rev Respir Dis 122:109, 1980
85. Zibrak JD, Rossetti P, Wood E: Effect of reductions in respiratory therapy on patient outcome. N Engl J Med 315:292, 1986
86. Kigin CM: Chest physical therapy for the postoperative or traumatic injury patient. Phys Ther 61:1724, 1981
87. Morran CG, Finlay IG, Mathieson M, et al: Randomized controlled trial of physiotherapy for postoperative pulmonary complications. Br J Anaesth 55:1113, 1983
88. Castillo R, Haas A: Chest physical therapy: comparative efficacy of preoperative and postoperative in the elderly. Arch Phys Med Rehabil 66:376, 1985
89. Connors AF Jr, Hammon WE, Martin RJ, et al: Chest physical therapy: the immediate effect on oxygenation in acutely ill patients. Chest 78:559, 1980
90. Reines HD, Sade RM, Bradford BF, et al: Chest physiotherapy fails to prevent postoperative atelectasis in children after cardiac surgery. Ann Surg 195:451, 1982
91. Goldhaber SZ: Pulmonary embolism. N Engl J Med 339:93, 1998
92. Douketis JD, Kearon C, Bates S, et al: Risk of fatal pulmonary embolism in patients with treated venous thromboembolism. JAMA 279:458, 1998
93. Bone RC: Ventilation/perfusion scan in pulmonary embolism: "the emperor is incompletely attired" (editorial). JAMA 263:2794, 1990
94. Laster J, Cikrit D, Walker N, et al: The heparin-induced thrombocytopenia syndrome: an update. Surgery 102:763, 1987
95. Greenfield LJ, Peyton R, Crute S, et al: Greenfield vena caval filter experience. Arch Surg 116:1451, 1981
96. Molina JE, Hunter DW, Yedlicka JW, et al: Thrombolytic therapy for postoperative pulmonary embolism. Am J Surg 163:375, 1992
97. Ducatman BS, McMichan JC, Edwards WD: Catheter-induced lesions of the right side of the heart: a one-year prospective study of 141 autopsies. JAMA 253:791, 1985
98. Collins R, Scrimgeour A, Yusuf S, et al: Reduction in fatal pulmonary embolism and venous thrombosis by perioperative administration of subcutaneous heparin. N Engl J Med 318:1162, 1988
99. Clagett GP, Reisch JS: Prevention of venous thromboembolism in general surgical patients: a meta-analysis. Ann Surg 208:227, 1988
100. Conti S, Daschbach M: Venous thromboembolism prophylaxis: a survey of its use in the United States. Arch Surg 117:1036, 1982
101. Wolfe BM, Ryder MA, Nishikawa RA, et al: Complications of parenteral nutrition. Am J Surg 152:93, 1986
102. Wang EE, Prober CG, Ford-Jones L, et al: The management of central intravenous catheter infections. Pediatr Infect Dis 3:110, 1984
103. Verghese A, Widrich WC, Arbeit RD: Central venous septic thrombophlebitis—the role of medical therapy. Medicine (Baltimore) 64:394, 1985
104. Borrero E, Ciervo J, Chang JB: Antacid vs sucralfate in preventing acute gastrointestinal tract bleeding in abdominal aortic surgery: a randomized trial in 50 patients. Arch Surg 121:810, 1986
105. Poleski MH, Spanier AH: Cimetidine versus antacids in the prevention of stress erosions in critically ill patients. Am J Gastroenterol 81:107, 1986
106. Priebe HJ, Skillman JJ, Bushnell LS, et al: Antacid versus cimetidine in preventing acute gastrointestinal bleeding. N Engl J Med 302:426, 1980
107. Shuman RB, Schuster DP, Zuckerman GR: Prophylactic therapy for stress ulcer bleeding: a reappraisal. Ann Intern Med 106:562, 1987
108. Cheung LY: Pathogenesis, prophylaxis, and treatment of stress gastritis. Am J Surg 156:437, 1988
109. Freedman VA, Berkman LF, Rapp SR, et al: Family networks: predictors of nursing home entry. Am J Public Health 84:843, 1994
110. Naylor MD, Brooten D, Campbell R, et al: Comprehensive discharge planning and home follow-up of hospitalized elders: a randomized clinical trial. JAMA 281:613, 1999
111. Social Security Bulletin. Annual statistical supplement, 1997. Annu Stat Suppl Soc Secur Bull, Dec 1997, p 1
112. Oparil S, Calhoun DA: High blood pressure. Scientific American Medicine, Section 1, Subsection III. Dale DC, Federman DD, Eds. WebMD Corp, New York, 2000

Acknowledgments

Figures 1 and 3   Tom Moore.

Figures 1b, 1c, and 2   Courtesy Samir M. Fakhry, M.D.

The authors wish to thank Ms. Eva Powell, M.S.W., for her invaluable contributions to the section on hospital discharge planning.

103 EARLY POSTOPERATIVE PNEUMONIA

David W. Chang, M.D., and Robert H. Demling, M.D.

Diagnosis and Management of Nosocomial Pneumonia

Treatment of nosocomial pneumonia should focus first on making a rapid and accurate diagnosis. Diagnosis is often difficult in the critically ill patient because of the frequent presence of pulmonary infiltrates, some of which are not the result of infectious processes. Moreover, pharyngeal bacterial colonization makes it difficult to determine the source of the bacteria simply from their appearance in sputum.[1,2]

It is essential to maintain optimal pulmonary support as well as systemic tissue perfusion for maintenance of both local lung and systemic immune defenses. Measures must be initiated to prevent a recurrent or progressive pneumonic process from developing. These preventive measures are based on an understanding of the pathophysiology of the disease process [see Figure 1 and Discussion, below]. Initial antibiotic management is usually empirical: the regimen is selected according to which organisms are most likely to have caused the particular case of nosocomial pneumonia; this determination is made on the basis of Gram's stain, patient history, and clinical experience. A more specific antibiotic approach is initiated once culture and sensitivity results are available (see below).

Diagnosis of Nosocomial Pneumonia

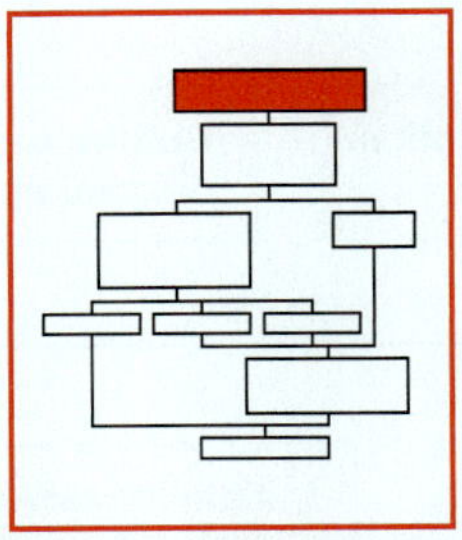

ASSESSMENT OF CLINICAL AND X-RAY FINDINGS

Characteristic signs and symptoms of pneumonia include fever, cough, dyspnea, chest pain, and increased sputum production. Expiratory rales in one or more lobes are often noted. The presence or absence of clinical symptoms depends in large part on the extent of the pneumonic process. For example, bronchopneumonia is often preceded by bronchitis or bronchiolitis. Small airway obstruction by mucus and the resultant local consolidation block diffusion of oxygenated blood through involved areas of lung, with subsequent hypoxemia. Reactive hypoxic pulmonary vasoconstriction, which normally limits the blood flow through nonventilated areas, is hampered by pneumonia, probably as a result of the local release of inflammatory mediators that cause vasodilatation. Carbon dioxide removal is usually adequately maintained as a result of compensatory hyperventilation of uninvolved areas of lung. Additional ventilation-perfusion abnormalities caused by hypovolemia or by chest wall splinting that occurs with pain will magnify the impairment in gas exchange.

The usual criteria for diagnosing pneumonia are fever, leukocytosis, purulent sputum, new or increasing infiltrates on x-ray, and pathogens growing from the sputum[3] [see Table 1]. However, these criteria are of much less value in diagnosing pneumonia in the surgical intensive care unit or postoperative patient than in the non-ICU or preoperative patient. For example, the upper airways of approximately 75 percent of ICU patients are colonized, usually with gram-negative organisms, and purulent sputum in these patients may simply consist of aspirated pharyngeal secretions that have not as yet caused distal lung infection. Pulmonary infiltrates are also a common finding in the postoperative or ICU patient. Approximately 30 percent of new infiltrates in the surgical ICU patient prove not to be pneumonia. Thus, clinical findings alone are not sufficient for a precise diagnosis; however, if they are assessed in the context of chest x-ray findings, they can be very useful in helping to distinguish pneumonia from a noninfectious process or from nonpulmonary infection [see Table 1]. The x-ray picture of pneumonia is one of focal areas of consolidation that include inflammation and airway collapse causing focal atelectasis. (Air bronchograms that indicate a patent airway and surrounding consolidation are common in pulmonary processes, such as acute respiratory distress syndrome [ARDS], that do not start as airway obstruction.)

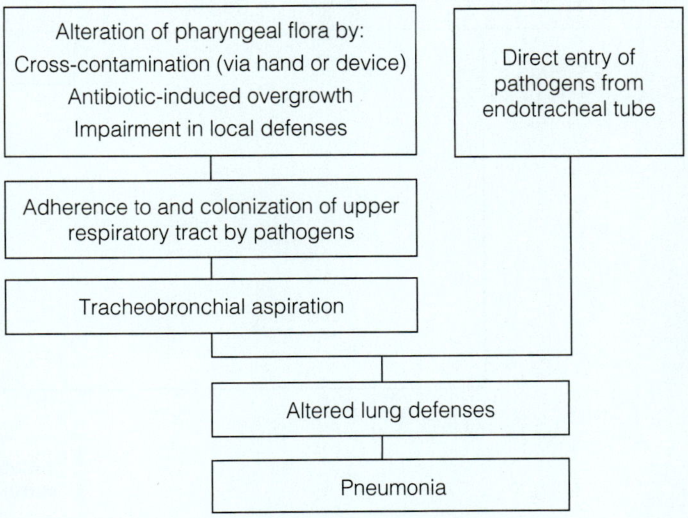

Figure 1 Prevention of nosocomial pneumonia is based on an understanding of the pathogenesis.

Diagnosis and Management of Nosocomial Pneumonia

Pneumonia is suggested by positive physical findings:
- ↑ WBC
- ↑ Temperature
- Purulent sputum
- Lung infiltrate

Findings are not diagnostic but indicate need for further workup.

Proceed to noninvasive testing

Collect sputum sample from tracheobronchial tree; submit sample for immediate plating and culture. Rule out gross oropharyngeal contamination by microscopic inspection of sputum. Obtain good-quality Gram's stain of smear. Obtain blood culture.

Initiate empirical antibiotic therapy based on results of Gram's stain

Give cefazolin plus an aminoglycoside *or* oxacillin plus an aminoglycoside.
- If *Pseudomonas* is suspected, add an antipseudomonal agent or a third-generation cephalosporin.
- If methicillin-resistant *Staphylococcus aureus* is suspected, add vancomycin.
- If *Hemophilus influenzae* is suspected, add ampicillin.

Results of Gram's stain are inconclusive, or there is a significant risk with standard empirical therapy

Response to empirical antibiotics is good

Response to empirical antibiotics is poor

Culture results indicate that original specimen was inadequte

Initiate invasive diagnostic testing

Perform fiberoptic bronchoscopy by using protected specimen brush/plugged telescoping catheter technique. Transtracheal needle aspiration is another option (easier but less reliable). Lung biopsy is usually performed in an immunosuppressed patient, who is at risk for a nonbacterial process.

Initiate specific antibiotic therapy when culture and sensitivity results are available

> **Table 1 Clinical Diagnosis of Pneumonia**
>
> Clinical signs
> - Rales, rhonchi
> - Fever, leukocytosis, impaired lung function
> - New pulmonary infiltrate
> - New onset of purulent sputum
>
> Differential diagnosis
> - Noninfectious pulmonary process (e.g., congestive heart failure, pulmonary embolism, or pulmonary infarction)
> - Nonpulmonary infection, tissue trauma, inflammation
> - Aspiration, lung contusion, postoperative atelectasis
> - Oropharyngeal colonization

In general, reliance on clinical signs results in overdiagnosis of pneumonia. The exception is patients with ARDS, in whom as many as 40 percent of pneumonias are missed because of the difficulty of assessing changes in the x-rays and in the clinical findings. In the absence of any new clinical findings or further lung deterioration, however, routine chest x-rays no longer appear to be indicated; in such cases, the yield of major new findings (including pneumonia) from x-ray is less than 10 percent.[3] The exception, of course, is the case in which x-ray is necessary to assess the effect of a procedure (e.g., positioning an endotracheal tube or a central venous catheter).

Types of Pulmonary Infection

Ventilator-associated pneumonia is an infection of the lung parenchyma that develops in patients who have been on a mechanical ventilator for more than 48 hours. It is characterized by a remarkably consistent spectrum of pathogenic bacteria—primarily aerobic gram-negative bacilli and to a lesser extent *Staphylococcus aureus*—which suggests unique host-bacterial interactions. This pneumonia results from repeated aspiration of secretions harboring these pathogenic organisms, which appear to be endogenously acquired.

S. aureus (coagulase-positive) lung infection is often characterized by migration of the process from one portion of the lung to another; that is, the infection tends to have a multifocal appearance. Infiltrates tend to be patchy, with rounded densities that clear as new ones appear in other lung segments. Formation of abscesses and pneumatoceles (i.e., thin-walled, spherical cysts containing air) reflects the necrotizing nature of staphylococcal pneumonia. Involvement of the pleural cavity with development of pleural effusions and empyema is also common. Copious, purulent sputum production along with evidence of a septic response is usually present; however, sputum is usually not bloody.

Klebsiella pneumoniae infection is characterized by very severe lung inflammation; clinical signs include severe systemic toxicity, pleural pain, cough, and blood-tinged sputum that has a currant-jelly appearance. Chest x-ray reveals moderately discrete areas of homogeneously increased density that may involve several lobes. Upper lobes tend to be involved more than in most other types of pneumonia, and there is a strong tendency toward abscess formation as well as development of pleural effusion and empyema.

Pseudomonas aeruginosa pneumonia does not have distinctive clinical features, although the presence of green-tinged sputum may be a helpful diagnostic clue. The process is quite variable and may involve both upper and lower lobes. The pneumonic process, as in *K. pneumoniae* infection and *S. aureus* infection, is necrotizing. The mortality associated with *P. aeruginosa* pneumonia may be as high as 85 percent. There is a high incidence of recurrent infections, defined as the development of a new infiltrate at least 48 hours after resolution of the initial pneumonia.[4]

Hemophilus influenzae pneumonia produces irregular, homogeneous densities without abscess formation, usually in the lower lobes. The organism is commonly seen with aspiration of oral secretions.

Other types of bacterial pneumonias in general have no specific characteristics and are evidenced on clinical examination and x-ray by localized infiltrates with areas of consolidation but without extensive necrosis.

Viral pneumonias are characterized by minimal physical findings and the frequent absence of large amounts of purulent sputum. Radiographic findings vary from air-space to interstitial disease, depending on the causative organism, and include patterns ranging from widespread, fine, patchy infiltrates, which are often bilateral, to peribronchial and perihilar or reticulonodular infiltrates, to frank consolidation. Confluence of the infiltrate or abscess formation is not seen unless a superinfection develops. Diagnosis is made by testing for antibody titers.

Pneumocystis carinii pneumonia is characterized by severe respiratory dysfunction but an insidious course, with a dry cough and slight or no fever. On radiography, pneumonia that is caused by *Pneumocystis* has the appearance of bilateral bronchopneumonia with the presence of interstitial edema. The infiltrate spreads from the hilum to the peripheral lung in a fanlike fashion, which can be confused with the appearance of pulmonary edema.

EXAMINATION OF SPUTUM

Although microscopic examination of expectorated sputum is not particularly accurate or reliable, it remains the most common method of detecting a respiratory tract infection. The sputum must be obtained by means of a deep cough, with or without the aid of aerosol provocation, or by suctioning well beyond the distal end of the endotracheal or tracheostomy tube [see Table 2]. A process of active infection is reflected in the presence of numerous neutrophils and mac-

> **Table 2 Guidelines for Sputum Analysis**
>
> Criteria for an adequate sputum sample
> - Sample consists of sputum expectorated after deep cough (if necessary, use aerosol provocation) or suctioned from beyond distal endotracheal or tracheostomy tube
> - Presence in sample of more than 25 leukocytes per low-power field
> - Presence in sample of only occasional squamous cells
> - Presence in sample of alveolar macrophages
>
> Causes of errors in sputum analysis
> - Collection of saliva rather than sputum
> - Delay in plating sputum sample
> - Colonization of oropharynx
> - Use of antibiotics before sample was obtained

rophages along with large numbers of organisms, especially of those present in the cytoplasm of phagocytes. Usually, a dominant organism, such as a gram-positive coccus or a gram-negative rod, is present. Cultures should then be obtained from the sputum sample. This approach is reliable in approximately 50 percent of patients. In the other 50 percent, there is a discrepancy between the data from cultures of expectorated sputum and the data from cultures obtained from the lower respiratory tract via more invasive techniques [see Table 2]. The major reason for this discrepancy is contamination of sputum by organisms colonizing the oropharynx and upper airways. This contamination is most evident in ICU patients, especially those with endotracheal tubes in place. Another reason for the discrepancy relates to the handling of specimens. Some organisms, such as *Streptococcus pneumoniae* (pneumococcus) and *H. influenzae*, multiply rapidly and will overgrow a mixed culture, especially if there is a delay in plating. If the patient is receiving antibiotics, growth of the etiologic pathogen may be suppressed in culture. In addition, antibiotics will lead to altered pharyngeal colonization and specimen contamination. The presence of large numbers of squamous cells, for example, indicates that the source of the sample is more likely to be the oropharynx than the lung parenchyma.

There remains considerable interest in and controversy regarding the best method of detecting the pathogens responsible for a pneumonia. A number of methods, all involving bronchoscopy, have been studied (see below), but the ideal method has yet to be agreed upon. It is generally agreed, however, that standard expectorated sputum analysis is not the appropriate method.

EXAMINATION OF TRANSTRACHEAL, TRANSBRONCHIAL, OR BRONCHOSCOPIC ASPIRATES

If sputum analysis has not proved diagnostic, transtracheal aspiration can be done: a small catheter is passed into the lungs through the thyroid membrane in an attempt to obtain lung secretions not contaminated by oral flora. The technique is more reliable in diagnosing true lung pathogens than is standard sputum analysis; however, it cannot be used in the intubated patient. Complications of this method, such as bleeding, are usually minor, but severe complications have been reported; hence, the method cannot be considered to be innocuous.

Bronchoscopic sampling is a more precise diagnostic method used to bypass contamination by upper airway flora.[1,5,6] However, some contamination is inevitable from passage of the bronchoscope through the upper airway. A technique of much greater sensitivity is the tube-within-a-tube technique, in which contamination of the protected specimen brush (PSB) is prevented by a distal biodegradable plug that is not ejected until the catheter reaches the deep area of the lung to be sampled. The brush is then advanced beyond the distal orifice of the scope, the sample taken, and the brush retracted back into its protective tube. This technique, known as plugged telescoping catheter (PTC), has substantially improved the sensitivity and specificity of results obtained for both sputum smear and bacteriologic evaluation. Other techniques in use include direct needle aspiration of lung secretions via a catheter passed through the endotracheal tube and sampling of bronchoalveolar lavage fluid.

Bronchoscopy, however, is not without risk. Hypoxemia and bronchospasm can occur if proper precautions are not taken. Another important consideration is the significant potential false negative rate. In several series, no pathogens could be identified in as many as 20 percent of samples obtained via PSB, PTC, and needle aspiration from patients likely to have pneumonia.[1,5,6] On the whole, however, the false positive rate is significantly lower with these techniques than with standard sputum analysis.

BLOOD CULTURES

If other sources of infection can be ruled out, a positive blood culture in the presence of pneumonic infiltrate can provide information as to the etiologic organism. The organism isolated from the blood in this case can be considered the organism producing the pneumonia. Bacteremia occurring in association with pneumonia, however, is not common. The incidence of bacteremia in patients with pneumonia is five to 15 percent, depending on the type of bacteria involved; with *Klebsiella* pneumonia, the incidence of associated bacteremia is about 15 percent.

LUNG BIOPSY

Open lung biopsy is usually not indicated to diagnose bacterial nosocomial pneumonia. It is used to detect etiologic agents that are difficult or impractical to culture, such as fungi, cytomegalovirus, or protozoa; it is generally considered the technique most likely to provide enough material for an accurate histologic and microbiological diagnosis. It is used most commonly in immunocompromised patients in whom the suspected microorganisms—that is, viruses or protozoa—cannot be readily cultured but can be diagnosed by histology. Transthoracic aspiration and transbronchial biopsy have been used to avoid upper airway contamination. Although contamination is minimized with these techniques, a high rate of complications, especially pneumothoraces, has been reported. The amount of lung material obtained by these methods is small, compared with that obtained by open lung biopsy.

OTHER DIAGNOSTIC TECHNIQUES

The finding of elastin fibers on Gram's stain is indicative of a tissue injury compatible with invasive infection.[7] Immunologic methods are commonly employed to diagnose suspected viral infection. Rising antibody titers support the diagnosis, but consecutive plasma samples are required, and the time frame necessary to observe a titer increase makes the method less practical. Advances have made possible the measurement of specific microbial antigens. Antigenemia (defined as the presence of minute amounts of circulating bacterial antigen) has been found in up to 40 percent of patients with pneumococcal pneumonias. In addition, the presence of antibody-coated bacteria in sputum is considered an indication of a reliable sputum specimen.[8]

Management

Pulmonary toilet is optimized by a strong cough and by frequent patient position changes to allow the secretions from the involved lung to drain from the distal to more proximal airways. Chest physiotherapy, with percussion and vibration followed by coughing, will greatly improve clearance of secretions. Aerosols to assist in mobilization of secretions can be given just before the chest therapy. Bronchodilator agents such as isoetharine hydrochloride (Bronkosol) and metaproterenol sulfate (Alupent) are used commonly, especially when the

Table 3 Empirical Antibiotic Regimens for Nosocomial Pneumonia

Risk Factors	Likely Causative Organisms	Therapeutic Options
Hospitalization	Core organisms: *Staphylococcus aureus*, *Escherichia coli*, *Klebsiella*, *Enterobacter*, *Proteus*, *Serratia marcescens*, *Hemophilus influenzae*	Core antibiotics: cefazolin, gentamicin, second-generation cephalosporins (e.g., cefuroxime), nonantipseudomonal third-generation cephalosporins (e.g., cefotaxime, ceftriaxone), β-lactam–β-lactamase inhibitor combination (e.g., ampicillin-sulbactam)
Gross aspiration, thoracoabdominal surgery	Core organisms and anaerobes	Core antibiotics plus clindamycin or metronidazole A β-lactam–β-lactamase inhibitor combination (e.g., ampicillin-sulbactam, ticarcillin-clavulanate)
Diabetes, coma, head injury, renal failure, previous antibiotic therapy (with possible methicillin-resistant organisms)	Core organisms and, possibly, methicillin-resistant *S. aureus*	Core antibiotics plus vancomycin (if a methicillin-resistant organism is likely)
High-dose corticosteroid therapy, cytotoxic chemotherapy (but no previous antibiotic therapy or alterations of consciousness)	Core organisms and *Legionella*	Core antibiotics plus a macrolide (e.g., erythromycin)
Multiple risk factors, including more than one of the following: previous antibiotic therapy, ICU stay, prolonged hospitalization, malnutrition, prolonged mechanical ventilation, tracheostomy, immunosuppression	Core organisms and *Pseudomonas aeruginosa*, with or without *Candida*	Combination therapy including two of the following: an antipseudomonal penicillin (e.g., piperacillin, azlocillin, mezlocillin), ceftazidime or cefoperazone, aztreonam, imipenem-cilastatin, ticarcillin-clavulanate, ciprofloxacin, an aminoglycoside; fluconazole may be added if needed

pneumonia is accompanied by an element of bronchospasm, which further impairs secretion clearance. The beta-adrenergic activity of these agents gives rise to their side effects: tachycardia, hypertension, and central nervous system irritability. There is increasing interest in early tracheostomy to improve pulmonary toilet in patients with severe lung dysfunction, especially when complicating factors, such as other infections or traumatic injuries, are present.[9] In such patients, early tracheostomy has resulted in improved pulmonary toilet, improved nursing care, and decreased sinusitis, with minimal complications. Side-to-side rotating beds have been shown to decrease the incidence of pneumonia in selected patient populations (especially neurologically impaired patients) by improving postural drainage and secretion clearance.

ANTIBIOTICS

Empirical Therapy

Because there is generally a lag of several days before the specific causative organism can be identified, empirical therapy is usually initiated on the basis of clinical impressions and the findings from Gram's stain [*see Table 3*]. A combination of two or more antibiotics is the standard recommendation for a gram-negative pneumonia, but there is increasing interest in single-drug therapy.[10] Randomized clinical trials using a variety of single agents—in particular, imipenem-cilastatin, ciprofloxacin, aztreonam, and cefoperazone—have reported these agents to be as effective as or more effective than two-drug regimens; however, subset analysis suggests that patients with risk factors for *Pseudomonas* pneumonia may benefit from a combination of antipseudomonal drugs.

Correct dosing of these agents depends on a solid understanding of antibiotic pharmacokinetics [*see 107 Pharmacokinetics in Surgical Practice*]. The biologic elimination half-life and the volume of distribution for antibiotics are determined by studying healthy volunteers or minimally ill patients. Because the data obtained are used to establish dosing schedules for each antibiotic, physicians must be aware that in many circumstances—more commonly encountered by surgeons than by medical specialists—therapeutic antibiotic concentrations may be delayed or may not be achieved at all, with poor clinical outcomes, the emergence of resistant bacteria, or both as the consequences.

Such circumstances include postoperative stress, severe infection, burns, and trauma. The septic response to injury or infection causes increased cardiac output, altered vascular permeability, increased vascular capacitance, and increased extracellular and interstitial water volume. Metabolic changes, such as hypermetabolism, protein catabolism, accelerated gluconeogenesis, and protein-mediated down-regulation of hepatic albumin synthesis, result in reduced plasma oncotic pressure, and this reduced pressure causes fluid shifts that dramatically increase the volume of distribution. A given dose of antibiotic will therefore be distributed within a much

Table 4 Common Antibiotics Used for Specific Nosocomial Pneumonias

Organism	Antibiotics	Dosage*
Staphylococcus aureus	Methicillin Oxacillin Cefazolin Vancomycin	1 g q. 4 hr 1 g q. 4–6 hr 1 g q. 6–8 hr 1 g q. 12 hr
Hemophilus influenzae	Ampicillin Cefuroxime	1–2 g q. 6 hr 2–3 g q. 8 hr
Klebsiella pneumoniae	Cefotaxime Gentamicin Tobramycin Imipenem Aztreonam	1–2 g q. 8 hr 3–5 mg/kg/day 3–5 mg/kg/day 1 g q. 8 hr 1–2 g q. 6–12 hr
Pseudomonas aeruginosa	Gentamicin Tobramycin Ceftazidime Imipenem Ciprofloxacin	3–5 mg/kg/day 3–5 mg/kg/day 1 g q. 8 hr 1 g q. 8 hr 0.5 g q. 12 hr
Escherichia coli	Gentamicin Ampicillin Ceftazidime	3–5 mg/kg/day 1–2 g q. 6 hr 1 g q. 8 hr

*Dosages are for adults with normal renal and hepatic function.

larger volume, and peak concentrations of the drug will necessarily be lower. In one study, the volume of distribution for aminoglycosides in ICU patients increased 36 to 70 percent in comparison with non-ICU patients, necessitating daily doses of 1.4 to 15.5 mg/kg rather than the recommended 3 to 5 mg/kg.[11] Other studies show similar variability in volume of distribution in the critical care setting, with the result that a number of antibiotics, including various cephalosporins, vancomycin, metronidazole, and penicillin, are often given in inadequate dosages.

An important associated concept is the compartmental volume of distribution, which determines the amount of antibiotic present at the target organ. Aminoglycosides penetrate bronchial secretions poorly: the level of the drug in these secretions is usually only 30 to 40 percent of their serum level. Moreover, because aminoglycosides are less effective in acidic environments, they are not optimal for treatment of pneumonia associated with a low endobronchial pH. Their only undisputed advantage is their synergy with β-lactam antibiotics for the treatment of *P. aeruginosa* pneumonia. Most β-lactam antibiotics achieve pulmonary concentrations that are less than 50 percent of serum concentrations[12]; however, the fluoroquinolones achieve pulmonary concentrations that are equal to or greater than serum concentrations.

Drug metabolism and excretion may affect the half-life. For example, the major enzyme system for biotransformation in the liver, cytochrome P-450, may be induced by various agents (most notably phenobarbital), and metabolism may thereby be accelerated. In other situations, biotransformation is necessary for the drug to exert its effect (e.g., clindamycin), or a metabolite of an antibiotic may have antimicrobial activity or even synergy with the parent compound (e.g., cefotaxime). These interactions are affected when competing drugs that use the same system of enzymes are being administered. Renal and hepatic clearance rates of antimicrobial agents may also be increased during hyperdynamic cardiac states.

Specific Therapy

When the specific organisms responsible for pneumonia and the sensitivities of these organisms are known, antibiotic therapy should be tailored appropriately [*see Table 4*]. Monotherapy is acceptable for severe nonpseudomonal nosocomial pneumonia, but a second agent should be added if isolates of *P. aeruginosa* or *Enterobacter* are obtained. *P. aeruginosa* becomes resistant to ciprofloxacin 33 percent of the time and to imipenem 53 percent of the time.[12] Given that resistance does not emerge until after at least 72 hours of treatment, single-agent therapy remains viable if serial respiratory cultures and sensitivity patterns are obtained to detect these and other, less common pathogens.

Once appropriate antibiotic therapy is initiated, a specific duration of therapy should be chosen in accordance with the clinical setting. Excessive length of treatment appears to be the most common form of inappropriate antibiotic administration in current surgical practice.[13] Continuing treatment until the temperature and the white blood cell count are normal is not warranted. Fever and leukocytosis at the end of an antibiotic course often represent a sterile cytokine-mediated inflammatory response. Excessive treatment time prevents the restoration of the protective native oropharyngeal and gastrointestinal flora, increasing the risk of recurrent infection, and predisposes to the emergence of resistant pathogens. This is also true of too-lengthy surgical prophylaxis, which can lead to a higher incidence of nosocomial pneumonia.

In sum, giving antibiotics in higher dosages for shorter periods is generally preferable to giving them in lower dosages for longer periods; however, a persistent inflammatory response is an indication that one should look for other organisms and sources of infection.

MAINTENANCE OF HOST DEFENSES

The main conditions that lead to impairment of host pulmonary defenses are well known [*see Table 5*]. Nutrition is important for preservation of both local lung defenses and systemic immune function.

PREVENTION

The best way of managing nosocomial pneumonia is to prevent both incipient and recurrent infection. In addition to appropriate antibiotic selection and duration of therapy, attention must be paid to hand washing, evaluation of the patient's swallowing mechanism, removal of nasogastric and endotracheal tubes, elevation of the head of the bed, maintenance of gastric acidity, and implementation of preoperative and postoperative respiratory care.

Table 5 Causes of Impaired Lung Defenses

Impairment of nasopharyngeal filter system because of bypass by endotracheal tube, use of nasal tube, rhinitis, or sinusitis

Impairment of cough reflex because of decrease in state of consciousness (from anesthesia, drugs, or head injury) *or* decrease in necessary full inspiration followed by rapid expiration (from chest trauma, pain, muscle weakness, or use of endotracheal tube)

Impairment of mucociliary clearance because of direct mucosal damage with ciliary destruction (from inhalation of smoke, heat, or chemicals) *or* endobronchial obstruction (by thick mucus, tumor, or foreign body)

Impairment of alveolar macrophage function because of inhalation of smoke, hypoxia, hyperoxia, alcohol, or malnutrition

Impairment of containment process because of deficiency in cellular defenses, humoral defenses, or both (from decrease in neutrophil function, impairment of cytokine release, decrease in opsonins, decrease in antibodies), *or* spread of infectious focus by increase in bronchoalveolar fluid, pulmonary congestion, or high- and low-pressure edema

---

Discussion

Pathophysiology of Nosocomial Pneumonia

Pneumonia is defined as inflammation of the lung parenchyma—that is, of the alveoli and terminal bronchioles. The severity of the pneumonia depends not only on the cause of the infection but also on the host immune response and other predisposing pulmonary conditions, if any.

With the exception of the early stages of an aspiration pneumonia [*see 91 Pulmonary Dysfunction*], nearly all pneumonias in surgical patients are caused by microorganisms, the majority of which are bacteria [*see Table 6*]. Several routes for contamination of the lung parenchyma are possible [*see Table 7*]. The most common route is by aspiration of bacterial organisms colonizing the pharynx. A

Table 6 Distribution of Causative Organisms of Nosocomial Pneumonia

Organism	Percent of Total
Pseudomonas aeruginosa	10–15
Proteus mirabilis	5–7
Serratia marcescens	4–6
Escherichia coli	5–8
Klebsiella pneumoniae	10–15
Staphylococcus aureus	10–15
Streptococcus pneumoniae	5–6
Enterobacter species	10
Hemophilus influenzae	8–10
Other gram-negative aerobes	5–8
Gram-negative anaerobes	1–2
Fungi	1

number of organisms can be found in the pharynx of a healthy adult, including *S. pneumoniae, H. influenzae, S. aureus*, and a large number of anaerobic organisms. Coliforms, which are uncommon in healthy adults, are present in seriously ill patients, especially ICU patients who have an endotracheal tube or tracheostomy in place, or in patients who are being treated with broad-spectrum antibiotics.

A major component of bacterial colonization appears to be an increase in the organisms' ability to adhere to the airway epithelium. This increased adherence is probably the result of a decreased secretion of immunoglobulin A (IgA), which normally inhibits the attachment of organisms (particularly gram-negative organisms) to the epithelium[7]; it may also be the result of denaturing proteases released from local inflammatory cells. In addition, any mechanical injury to the mucosa (e.g., from acid aspiration or intubation) will enhance bacterial binding through specific binding glycoproteins. Sucralfate has been reported to help decrease bacterial binding; the mechanism is currently unknown.[14]

The most significant form of pneumonia the surgeon encounters is that which develops after admission to the hospital, in a patient who had no evidence of lung infection on admission. Although other forms of nosocomial infection, such as wound and urinary tract infections, are more common, the mortality for pneumonia is much higher. Patients admitted to the ICU have the greatest risk of acquiring pneumonia; the incidence in patients admitted to the surgical ICU is 12 to 22 percent. The high incidence in this group is caused not only by the presence of virulent organisms in the ICU environment but also by the magnitude of the illness that necessitated hospital admission. Incidence of pneumonia in ARDS patients, who by definition have an acutely injured lung, exceeds

Table 7 Routes of Lung Contamination

Aspiration from naso-oropharynx
Inhalation of contaminated air
Hematogenous spread from distant focus
Direct spread from local infection

50 percent. Mortality in ICU patients in whom pneumonia develops is about 50 percent, compared with a mortality of about five percent in ICU patients without pneumonia. Mortality in patients with ARDS and pneumonia is 70 percent.[1,2]

The high mortality of pneumonia, despite the availability of potent, normally effective antimicrobial agents, reflects two problems: (1) impairment of host defenses, which are affected by a number of factors, including age, the degree of underlying systemic or pulmonary disease, nutritional status, smoking, alcohol, and the adequacy of perfusion, and (2) the difficulty of making the correct diagnosis [*see* Diagnosis of Nosocomial Pneumonia, *above*]. The sequence of major events occurring in the majority of nosocomial lung infections is as follows:

1. Colonization of pathogenic microorganisms in the pharynx and the proximal airways.
2. Aspiration of the tracheobronchial secretions, which are now infected.
3. Impairment of local lung defenses, particularly the ability to clear secretions, which allows the infected aspirated material to develop into a deep lung infection. (Chronic lung disease is one process that markedly impairs local defenses.)
4. Impairment of systemic immune defenses by the septic response, organ dysfunction, and malnutrition, which further increases the risk of infection. (Chronic systemic diseases such as diabetes will result in an increased risk of any infection.)

There is a very close association between the incidence of pneumonia and the duration of endotracheal intubation [*see Table 8*]: the duration of intubation reflects the degree of both lung and systemic diseases. The endotracheal tube also provides a potential conduit for organisms from the ICU environment to the tracheobronchial tree.

AIRWAY COLONIZATION WITH PATHOGENS

The main source of organisms that cause nosocomial pneumonia is the patient's upper respiratory tract—in particular, the oropharynx. Microorganisms are most likely to reach the lower air passages and alveoli by aspiration of pharyngeal secretions. This process occurs in up to 70 percent of sick patients with depressed consciousness and up to 25 percent of healthy individuals during sleep. The concentration of bacteria in the oropharynx frequently exceeds 10^8/ml, with anaerobes outnumbering aerobes by a factor of 10 to 1; hence, a significant bacterial inoculum may result from only 1 ml or less of aspirate.[15] This aspiration of secretions is further facilitated by the presence of an endotracheal tube.

Colonization or bacterial overgrowth of the pharynx with potential pathogens [*see Figure 2*], such as enteric bacteria, occurs in up to eight percent of healthy patients and about 50 percent of critically ill patients in the surgical ICU. Colonization of the oropharynx with pathogens occurs in nearly 100 percent of ICU patients with a major respiratory problem. The chance that a pneumonia will develop in a colonized patient is 75 percent, compared with a three percent chance if colonization is not present. In more than 80 percent of patients in whom nosocomial pneumonia eventually develops, evidence of colonization precedes the pneumonia. The colonization not only provides a source of infection but also makes the diagnosis of pneumonia more difficult: determining the pathogens of the pneumonia in sputum that contains oral contaminants can be very difficult. The marked increase in colonization of sick versus healthy individuals indicates an alteration in local host defenses. In healthy individuals, pathogens are rapidly cleared from

Table 8 Cumulative Incidence of Pneumonia versus Days Intubated

Number of Days Intubated	Patients Who Acquire Pneumonia (%)
1–3	8
7	21
14	32
> 14	45

the oropharynx, whereas in ill or immunocompromised patients, there is increased adherence of organisms to pharyngeal epithelium. Pathogenic colonization most commonly derives from proximate oropharyngeal sources, such as gingival and periodontal spaces, dental plaque, sinuses, or the upper GI tract. The expansion of organisms from their characteristic niche is facilitated by antibiotic therapy and altered host defenses. Prolonged prophylaxis with first-generation cephalosporins eliminates the gram-positive organisms in the normal oral flora and creates ecological pressures that encourage migration of endogenous gram-negative organisms. Fibronectin, found in secretions of the upper and lower respiratory tracts, is an integral component of host defense.[16] This protein mediates binding of the lipoteichoic acid–protein complex on gram-positive bacteria to buccal epithelial cells and inhibits the adherence of gram-negative bacteria. In stress states, increases in salivary protease levels lead to degradation of fibronectin, and trauma from endotracheal or nasogastric tubes denudes fibronectin-lined epithelial cells; both of these changes facilitate adherence of gram-negative bacteria. Bacterial binding to buccal mucosa is also potentiated by smoking. Moreover, the lysozyme in pulmonary secretions cleaves the peptidoglycan in bacterial cell walls, and lactoferrin deprives certain pathogens of iron, thereby killing them. Inadequate perioperative resuscitation may hinder the delivery of all these protective secretions and must therefore be avoided.

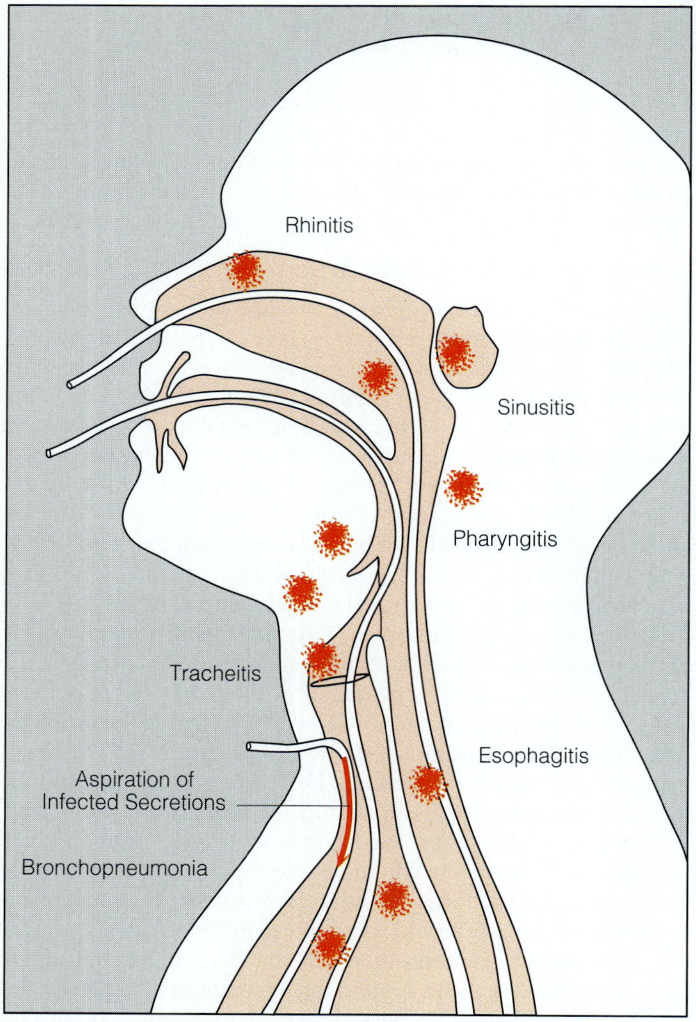

Colonization also occurs by a number of other routes [see Table 9]. Transmission of pathogens on the hands of hospital personnel to patients is a major cause. Up to 50 percent of personnel have been shown to carry either gram-negative bacilli or *S. aureus* on their hands. Frequent hand washing markedly decreases the incidence of transmission by this route. Another important route is from the patient's intestinal tract to the oropharynx—from the hand to the mouth or by retrograde movement of organisms from the stomach to the oropharynx, for example. The routine iatrogenic neutralization of gastric acidity increases the pathogen content of the stomach. This process can lead to colonization of the upper GI tract with pathogens. The presence of a nasogastric tube can contribute to the transmission of these pathogens from the stomach to the oropharynx. The need to control gastric acidity and avoid gastrointestinal distention in these patients makes this route of transmission more difficult to eliminate. However, alternative approaches to antacids and H_2-receptor blockers, such as the use of sucralfate, appear to decrease the risk of upper GI bacterial overgrowth and reduce the incidence of pneumonias in the ICU.

Another approach to decreasing airway colonization, and thereby reducing the incidence of nosocomial pneumonia, is selective gut decontamination.[17] Several combinations of agents have been used. One consists of tobramycin, polymyxin E, and amphotericin B applied to the oropharynx as a paste and administered as a suspension via a nasogastric tube. Another consists of oral gentamicin, vancomycin, and nystatin; polymyxin B is added to neutralize endotoxin. This approach has decreased the incidence of nosocomial pneumonia by more than 50 percent in a number of clinical trials. Overall mortality was not reduced in these studies, however, which indicates that the underlying disease necessitating intensive care is the primary determinant of survival.

The intensive care unit environment contains many other reservoirs of pathogenic organisms, which eventually come in contact

Figure 2 Interventions associated with intensive care and impairment of normal defense mechanisms in surgical patients contribute to the development of infectious complications.

Table 9 Causes of Colonization

Hand-to-mouth transmission of pathogens by patient and hospital personnel

Migration of GI pathogens to oropharynx potentiated by decreased acidity and nasogastric tubes

Direct contamination by aerosols, ventilators, and humidifiers

Alteration of normal flora by antibiotics

Alteration in local defenses that causes increase in bacterial adherence with the airways. Aerosol nebulizers and ventilator tubes, for example, provide moist environments for bacterial growth and are potential sources of infection. The introduction of more disposable equipment and unit-dose packaging of aerosols has decreased the incidence of contamination by these routes.

ASPIRATION OF INFECTED SECRETIONS

Aspiration of infected secretions is the next step in the development of pneumonia following pharyngeal colonization. Aspiration is potentiated by sedation or any process that impairs normal clearance of oral secretions [see Table 10], such as use of a nasogastric tube. The potential for aspiration of secretions is also markedly increased by use of an endotracheal or tracheostomy tube because the tube prevents the glottis and the cords from closing effectively, and secretions can therefore track down both inside and outside the tube. Pooled contaminated secretions present above the cuff of an endotracheal tube can readily be aspirated into the tracheobronchial tree. In one study, a radioisotopic tracer was placed in the stomachs of patients with nasogastric and endotracheal tubes; there was substantial accumulation of the tracer in the lungs within six hours when the patients were supine.[16] Endotracheal tubes provide a surface for colonizing bacteria and do not prevent gastric aspiration. Careful attention should therefore be paid to minimizing supine positioning of intubated patients.

Furthermore, the design of the endotracheal tubes currently in use encourages aspiration. The tube lumen allows the development of a biofilm containing pathogenic organisms, which are expelled centimeters beyond the endotracheal tube with each breath on positive pressure ventilation.[18] Low-pressure, high-volume cuffs cause folds in the balloon along the trachea, which facilitate translocation of secretions with respiratory motion. Nevertheless, every attempt should be made to avoid gross aspiration by suctioning the oropharynx before cuff deflation or extubation.

Other causes of bacterial inoculation include contaminated suction catheters, contaminated lavage fluid, or anything else passed through the tube during management of the patient in the operating room or during the postoperative period.

IMPAIRMENT OF HOST DEFENSES

Even with the introduction of microorganisms, the healthy host should be able to clear bacteria from the lung via normal pulmonary defenses. However, in surgical patients, the normal defense mechanisms are often impaired [see Table 5].

Impairment of the Nasopharyngeal Filter System

In the surgical patient, the nasopharyngeal filter system is frequently bypassed by means of nasogastric tubes and endotracheal tubes. Microorganisms and particulate debris that are normally filtered and trapped in the nasal passages can thereby enter the oropharynx and can then, in turn, enter the tracheobronchial tree.

Impairment of the Cough Reflex

The cough reflex, commonly impaired in the surgical patient, is normally one of the principal means by which airways are cleared of foreign material, excess secretions, and irritating stimuli (e.g., microorganisms). The larynx, the major bronchi, and the terminal bronchioles are especially sensitive to local irritation. Coughing is a reflex response initiated by means of a four-stage process that results in clearance of the irritant. First, as a reflex, the individual takes a large inspiration, usually in excess of 2 L in an adult. Second, the epiglottis closes, and the vocal cords become tightly apposed. Third, internal intercostal and abdominal muscles forcefully contract, pushing the diaphragm up and generating an intrathoracic pressure that usually exceeds 100 mm Hg. Fourth, the epiglottis and cords suddenly open, generating a significant force of expulsion. The rapidly moving air carries with it secretions and any other foreign material.

In the patient receiving anesthetics or postoperative narcotic analgesics, decreased consciousness markedly suppresses both the initiation of the cough reflex and the quality of the cough. Chest pain and abdominal pain, as well as residual muscle weakness if muscle paralysis was employed in general anesthesia, impair the ability to take a large inspiration, which is necessary for the cough mechanism. Pain and the instability of the chest wall mechanism in patients with chest trauma hamper the ability to generate sufficient transpulmonary pressure. The presence of an endotracheal tube decreases the ability to generate a significant propulsive force during forced expiration. The bacteria in any aspirated infected oral secretions will have the opportunity to proliferate if they are not effectively cleared.

Impairment of Mucociliary Action

In healthy individuals, airways are lined by a mucus-coated epithelium with cilia that beat toward the pharynx to assist in the continued clearance of particles and microorganisms. This mechanism for clearance is particularly useful in the smaller airways, which are less effectively cleared by coughing. Ciliary action is directly impeded by inhalation of smoke (including cigarette smoke) or of chemicals such as those found in general inhalation-type anesthetics.

A high oxygen tension also impairs mucociliary function. In a canine model,[16] tracheal mucus velocity was not affected by intubation for up to 30 hours; however, it was reduced by 84 percent at six hours in patients on 100 percent inspired oxygen and by 51 percent at 30 hours in patients on 50 percent inspired oxygen.[15]

Impairment of the cough reflex directly impinges on clearance by mucociliary action. Secretions normally coughed up eventually plug airways, thereby preventing mucociliary clearance. Obstruction by tumor and foreign bodies also impedes this clearance mechanism.

Impairment of Alveolar Macrophage Function

Bacteria and other foreign particles deposited in the alveoli are rapidly phagocytized by alveolar macrophages and either destroyed by direct killing via release of oxygen free radicals or cleared via the mucociliary system. Microorganism-laden macrophages may also migrate through the interstitium and be cleared by the lymphatics into regional lymph nodes and the systemic circulation. A large or continued exposure to organisms initiates an inflammatory response that is mediated by chemoattractants released by the macrophages. The neutrophils that are thereby attracted will later assist

Table 10 Causes of Tracheobronchial Aspiration

Pharmacological impairment of clearance of secretions by sedation, anesthesia, or paralysis

Anatomic impairment of clearance of secretions by oropharyngeal edema, trauma, nasogastric tube, endotracheal tube, or oral airway

Direct contamination of lower airways by catheters, lavage, or deflation of cuff on endotracheal tube

in the containment process. However, a number of factors hamper alveolar macrophage function in the surgical patient, thereby increasing the risk of lung infection. These factors include use of inhalation anesthetics, smoke exposure (acute and chronic), malnutrition, anemia, and hypoxia.

Impairment of Cellular Immunity

Immunosuppressed persons, such as those with human immunodeficiency virus (HIV) infection or cancer, are particularly vulnerable to pneumonia. In HIV infection, depletion and functional impairment of helper (CD4) T cells results in infection with *P. carinii* or intracellular pathogens, such as mycobacteria, cryptococci, and herpesviruses.[15] Antibody responses and vaccination are also suppressed because of disordered T cell regulation and depletion of antigen-presenting cells as well as because of direct effects on B cells. This suppression gives rise to an increased incidence of pneumococcal and *H. influenzae* infections. Coinfection with cytomegalovirus or Epstein-Barr virus may also contribute to immunosuppression.

Impairment of the Containment Process

In healthy individuals, the inflammatory process initiated by macrophages attracts other inflammatory cells to the focus of infection to assist in the process of containment. Containment refers to the process whereby a focus of infection is isolated and prevented from spreading to other portions of the lung. Immunoglobulins constitute part of this defensive process. IgA, which is normally present in the upper respiratory tract, provides protection against viral infection. IgA also decreases the ability of bacteria to attach to mucosal surfaces, thereby rendering them more easily phagocytized. IgG, which enters the lung inflammatory focus via local increases in capillary permeability, both opsonizes bacteria and activates complement, thereby promoting further neutrophil attraction. Activation of the clotting cascade results in local fibrin deposition, which further assists in the infection localization process. Neutrophil migration is assisted by chemoattractant factors released from macrophages and by opsonins and globulins released as part of the humoral system. Any impairment in these humoral and cellular defenses impairs the ability of the host to contain the infection.

The containment process is also impaired by increased amounts of lung water. Movement of edema fluid carries bacteria to uninvolved areas of lung. Edema also allows spread of infection by impairing sequestration.

Types of Pneumonia

ALVEOLAR (LOBAR) PNEUMONIA

In alveolar pneumonia, the pneumonic process involves a large portion of a lobe of a lung or an entire lobe. This process is currently much less common than in the past because of more aggressive pulmonary care. Alveolar pneumonia occurs in all age groups.

Only a few types of organisms cause most cases of lobar pneumonia. The most common type is pneumococcus. Other causative organisms are *Klebsiella, Staphylococcus, Streptococcus, H. influenzae, Pseudomonas,* and *Proteus.*

Pathology

The most common portal of entry of the bacteria that cause lobar pneumonia is the air passages, although the airways themselves remain relatively uninvolved. The causative organism, usually pneumococcus, produces an extensive exudative process that spreads among alveoli via the interconnecting pores of Kohn. The extent of the process depends on host defenses and on bacterial virulence. Segmented boundaries are not preserved, because the process can extend to the boundaries of the lobe.

The extensive suppurative consolidation of alveolar pneumonia evolves and resolves in four classic stages: (1) congestion, (2) red hepatization, (3) gray hepatization, and (4) resolution. Congestion is the initial response to infection, characterized by vascular congestion and increased alveolar fluid in the involved area. The red hepatization that follows is characterized by an intra-alveolar inflammatory exudative process during which the involved area appears airless, red, and firm. Extravasation of red blood cells causes the red color of the lung tissue. White blood cells actively engulf the invading bacteria. Gray hepatization follows, with increasing fibrin deposition and progressive lysis and removal of red blood cells producing the characteristic gray color. A more pronounced pleural reaction and, in some cases, development of empyema are evident during this period. Resolution usually begins about one week after the onset of the pneumonic process. The exudate undergoes progressive enzymatic digestion into semifluid debris, some of which is resorbed by macrophages and some coughed up as sputum.

Clinical Presentation and Course

The pneumococcal variety of alveolar pneumonia can be seen in otherwise healthy adults, whereas the gram-negative bacilli–induced process is seen in immunocompromised hosts—that is, individuals who are elderly, diabetic, alcoholic, or critically ill. The onset of lobar pneumonia is usually sudden, with fever, tachycardia, and lethargy. The cough initially produces a watery sputum indicative of the first stage, which is followed by the rusty, purulent sputum of the red hepatization stage. Chills, indicative of bacteremia, are common. Impairment of gas exchange is usually manifested by hypoxemia caused by passage of blood through nonventilated alveoli. Splinting, which occurs at the onset of any pleuritic reaction, further magnifies ventilation-perfusion mismatch.

Initial physical findings of high-pitched, end-inspiratory crackles reflect the early filling of alveoli with fluid. After two to three days, evidence of consolidation is noted, with fewer rales and dullness to percussion. During resolution, rales return, and the signs of consolidation resolve. Radiographic findings include clear evidence of consolidation, and air bronchograms indicate air-filled airways surrounded by inflammatory infiltrate. The magnitude of physical findings does not always correlate with the x-ray findings. Frequently, the patient is improving clinically before x-ray evidence of resolution. Most lobar pneumonias resolve completely, and mortality is less than 10 percent. However, septicemia can result, as can lung abscess formation. In addition, portions of the damaged lung can be replaced by fibrous tissue.

BRONCHOPNEUMONIA (LOBULAR PNEUMONIA)

The primary characteristic of bronchopneumonia is a patchy consolidation of the lung. The infection frequently represents an extension of a preexisting bronchitis or bronchiolitis caused by, for example, aspiration or smoke inhalation. Impairment of lung defenses allows the pneumonic process to progress. Patient populations that are vulnerable to development of lobular pneumonia include the very young, the very old, and the critically ill, all of whom are immunocompromised.

Any pathogen is capable of causing bronchopneumonia. The most common agents, however, are *Staphylococcus, Streptococcus,* pneumococcus, *H. influenzae, P. aeruginosa,* coliforms, and fungi (in a severely immunocompromised host).

Pathology

In bronchopneumonia, consolidated foci of suppurative inflammation extend down and around involved airways in a segmental distribution that is frequently multilobar. The involved airways become filled with purulent exudate, with subsequent extension into the alveoli. The basal portions are usually more involved as a result of gravitational migration. Confluence of multiple foci can give the appearance of lobar consolidation. Multiple abscess formation is characteristic when the causative organism is *Staphylococcus*. Frequently, bacteria are not visualized in the inflammatory focus, because they have been removed by the white blood cells. If the process resolves, a fibrous scar may persist, or there may be complete restoration of normal lung architecture.

Clinical Presentation and Course

The signs and symptoms of bronchopneumonia depend on the virulence of the invading microorganism and the extent of lung involvement. Increased temperature, productive cough, and expiratory rales are characteristic. Distribution is often patchy, and thus, there is not as much evidence of consolidation as there is with lobar pneumonia. X-rays demonstrate focal areas of consolidation with airway collapse followed by distal atelectasis and an exudative process. Air bronchograms are not characteristic, because the involved airway is usually occluded. Mortality is dependent on the status of the host, who is often elderly and immunosuppressed. When the pneumonic process is caused by organisms that are sensitive to antibiotics, infection is usually readily controlled in the absence of severe underlying systemic or pulmonary disease. Complications of bronchopneumonia include formation of abscesses, spread of infection to the chest cavity with development of empyema, and development of bacteremia.

BACTEREMIC (HEMATOGENOUS) PNEUMONIA

In bacteremic pneumonia, the pneumonic process is initiated by a bacteremia from another source. The process therefore begins in the periphery of the lung rather than in the airway. The x-ray picture is often one of a multifocal process. Abscess formation is common.

In surgical patients, the most common causative organism of bacteremic, or hematogenous, pneumonia is *S. aureus*. Increased sputum production is not an early sign of this condition in view of the lack of large airway involvement. Increased sputum is more evident with extension of the process or during resolution. The clinical signs and symptoms and the mortality are determined primarily by the underlying health of the patient and the initiating focus.

INTERSTITIAL PNEUMONIA

Interstitial pneumonia refers to an acute respiratory infection characterized by inflammatory changes in the lung, largely confined to alveolar septa and pulmonary interstitium. The process is caused by viruses such as respiratory syncytial virus, rhinoviruses, echoviruses, or coxsackieviruses. *Mycoplasma pneumoniae* is also a common cause. In the immunocompromised host, both cytomegalovirus and *P. carinii* are common causes of interstitial pneumonia. Cytomegalovirus is often detected in the lungs of transplant patients in the absence of any lung pathology; identification of cytomegalovirus is not in itself an indication for treatment.

Pathology

The pneumonic involvement may be patchy or may involve entire lobes unilaterally or bilaterally. There is no obvious consolidation. The inflammatory response is localized in the lung interstitium; mononuclear cells are the predominant cell infiltrate. The alveoli may be free of exudate or may be filled with a proteinaceous material with hyaline membranes very similar to that seen in ARDS. In fact, this process is sometimes considered a cause of ARDS.

Clinical Presentation and Course

The presentation is often subtle, with few clinical findings of lung disease except for a dry, nonproductive cough and, in extreme cases, abnormalities in gas exchange. Symptoms are quite varied. A superimposed bacterial pneumonia, usually involving *S. aureus*, is often found in the immunocompromised host, particularly the elderly patient, because local lung immune defenses are impaired by the inflammatory process. Mortality for a viral pneumonia in a relatively healthy host is less than one percent. Mortality in the compromised host is considerably higher and is dependent primarily on the immune status of the host and also on the presence of a superimposed bacterial pneumonia.

References

1. Potgieter PD, Hammond JM: Etiology and diagnosis of pneumonia requiring ICU admission. Chest 101:199, 1992
2. Scheld WM, Mandell GL: Nosocomial pneumonia: pathogenesis and recent advances in diagnosis and therapy. Rev Infect Dis 13(suppl 9):S743, 1991
3. Hall JB, White SR, Karrison T: Efficacy of daily routine chest radiographs in intubated, mechanically ventilated patients. Crit Care Med 19:689, 1991
4. Silver DR, Cohen IL, Winberg PF: Recurrent Pseudomonas aeruginosa pneumonia in an intensive care unit. Chest 101:194, 1992
5. Rodriguez deCastro F, Sole-Violan J, Lafarga-Capuz B, et al: Reliability of the bronchoscopic protected catheter brush in the diagnosis of pneumonia in mechanically ventilated patients. Crit Care Med 19:171, 1991
6. Fagon JY, Chastre J, Domart Y, et al: Nosocomial pneumonia in patients receiving continuous mechanical ventilation: prospective analysis of 52 episodes with use of a protected specimen brush and quantitative culture techniques. Am Rev Respir Dis 139:877, 1989
7. Niederman MS, Merrill WW, Polomski LM, et al: Influence of sputum IgA and elastase on tracheal cell bacterial adherence. Am Rev Respir Dis 133:255, 1986
8. Wunderink RG, Russell GB, Mezger E, et al: The diagnostic utility of the antibody-coated bacteria test in intubated patients. Chest 99:84, 1991
9. Rodriguez JL, Steinberg SM, Luchetti FA, et al: Early tracheostomy for primary airway management in the surgical critical care setting. Surgery 108:655, 1990
10. Aoun M, Klastersky J: Drug treatment of pneumonia in the hospital: what are the choices? Drugs 42:962, 1991
11. Fry DE: The importance of antibiotic pharmacokinetics in critical illness. Am J Surg 172(6A):20S, 1996
12. Niederman MS: An approach to empiric therapy of nosocomial pneumonia. Med Clin North Am 78:1123, 1994
13. Dietmar HW, Schein M: Let us shorten antibiotic prophylaxis and therapy in surgery. Am J Surg 172(6A):26S, 1996
14. Driks MR, Craven DE, Celli BR, et al: Nosocomial pneumonia in intubated patients given sucralfate as compared with antacids or histamine type 2 blockers: the role of gastric colonization. N Engl J Med 317:1376, 1987
15. Skerrett S: Host defenses against respiratory infection. Med Clin North Am 78:941, 1994
16. Estes RJ, Meduri GU: The pathogenesis of ventilator-associated pneumonia: I. Mechanisms of bacterial transcolonization and airway inoculation. Intensive Care Med 21:365, 1995
17. Stoutenbeek CP, van Saene HK, Miranda DR, et al: The effect of selective decontamination of the digestive tract on colonisation and infection rate in multiple trauma patients. Intensive Care Med 10:185, 1984
18. Koerner RJ: Contribution of endotracheal tubes to the pathogenesis of ventilator-associated pneumonia. J Hosp Infect 35:83, 1997

Acknowledgment

Figure 2 Dana Burns-Pizer.

104 POSTOPERATIVE PAIN

Henrik Kehlet, Prof. M.D., Ph.D., and F. Michael Ferrante, M.D.

Approach to the Patient with Postoperative Pain

Pain may usefully be classified into two varieties: acute and chronic. As a rule, postoperative pain is considered a form of acute pain, although it may become chronic if it is not effectively treated.

Postoperative pain consists of a constellation of unpleasant sensory, emotional, and mental experiences associated with autonomic, psychological, and behavioral responses precipitated by the surgical injury. Despite the considerable progress that has been made in medicine during the past few decades, the apparently simple problem of how to provide total or near total relief of postoperative pain remains largely unsolved. Pain management does not occupy an important place in academic surgery. However, government agencies have recently attempted to foster improved postoperative pain relief.[1,2]

Postoperative pain relief has two practical aims. The first is provision of subjective comfort, which is desirable for humanitarian reasons. The second is inhibition of trauma-induced nociceptive impulses to blunt autonomic and somatic reflex responses to pain and to enhance subsequent restoration of function by allowing the patient to breathe, cough, and move more easily. Because these effects reduce pulmonary, cardiovascular, thromboembolic, and other complications, they may lead secondarily to improved postoperative outcome.

Inadequate Treatment of Pain

A common misconception is that pain, no matter how severe, can always be effectively relieved by opioid analgesics. It has repeatedly been demonstrated, however, that in a high proportion of postoperative patients, pain is inadequately treated. This discrepancy between what is possible and what is practiced can be attributed to a variety of causes [*see Table 1*], which to some extent can be ameliorated by increased teaching efforts. In general, however, the scientific approach to postoperative pain relief has not been a great help to surgical patients in the general ward, where intensive surveillance facilities are not available.

Guidelines for Postoperative Pain Treatment

The recommendations provided below are aimed at surgeons working on the general surgical ward; superior regimens have been constructed by specialized groups interested in postoperative pain research, but these regimens are not currently applicable to the general surgical population, unless an acute pain service is available. Consideration is given to the efficiency of each analgesic technique, its safety versus its side effects, and the cost-efficiency problems arising from the need for intensive surveillance. For many of the recommendations, there are not sufficient data in the literature to form a valid scientific data base; accordingly, these recommendations are made on empirical grounds only.

THORACIC PROCEDURES

Pain after thoracotomy is severe, and pain therapy should therefore include a combination regimen, preferably of epidural local anesthetics and opioids plus systemic nonsteroidal anti-inflammatory drugs (NSAIDs). If the epidural regimen is not available, NSAIDs and systemic opioids should be given to obtain the documented synergistic-additive effect. Finally, cryoanalgesia is recommended because it is moderately effective, easy, and without side effects or considerable cost.

Pain after cardiac operation with sternotomy is less severe, and systemic opioids plus NSAIDs are recommended. The combined regimen of epidural local anesthetics and opioids is recommended when more effective pain relief is necessary.

ABDOMINAL PROCEDURES

Pain after major and upper abdominal operations is severe, and a combined regimen of epidural local anesthetics and opioids plus systemic NSAIDs is recommended because it has proved to be very effective and to have few and acceptable side effects. Furthermore, the epidural regimen will reduce postoperative pulmonary complications, as compared with treatment

Table 1 Contributing Causes of Inadequate Pain Treatment

- Insufficient knowledge of drug pharmacology among surgeons and nurses
- Uniform (p.r.n.) prescriptions
- Lack of concern for optimal pain relief
- Failure to give prescribed analgesics
- Fear of side effects
- Fear of addiction

Approach to the Patient with Postoperative Pain

Combine psychological preparation with pharmacological and other interventions to treat postoperative pain

Consider recommended combination regimens.

Thoracic

Cardiac
Give systematic opioids with NSAID.
Consider epidural local anesthetics or epidural opioids, or both.

Noncardiac
Give NSAID with epidural local anesthetics or epidural opioids, or both.
or
Give NSAID with systemic opioids.
Consider cryoanalgesia.

Abdominal

Major
Give epidural local anesthetics or epidural opioids with NSAID, or both.
or
Give systemic opioids with NSAID.

Pelvic

Gynecologic
Give systemic opioids with NSAID.
Consider epidural local anesthetics or epidural opioids, or both.

Prostatectomy
Open: Give epidural local anesthetics or systemic opioids.
Transurethral resection: Give systemic opioids.

Make final choice of treatment modality on the basis of:
- Efficiency of analgesic techniques
- Side effects and additive effects
- Availability of surveillance, if required

Peripheral

Vascular

Give epidural local anesthetics with NSAID.
or
Give systemic opioids with NSAID.

Superficial

Give systemic opioids with NSAID.

Consider incisional local anesthetic.

Major joint procedures (e.g., hip replacement, amputation)

Give epidural local anesthetics or epidural opioids, or both, with NSAID.
or
Give systemic opioids with NSAID.

with systemic opioids. Intrapleural local anesthetics may have some analgesic effect in unilateral procedures, but the combined epidural local anesthetic–opioid regimens are more effective.

After gynecologic operations, systemic opioids with NSAIDs are recommended except in patients in whom more effective pain relief is desirable. In such patients, the combined regimen of epidural local anesthetics and opioids is preferable, possibly in combination with systemic NSAIDs.

Pain following prostatectomy is usually not severe and may be treated with systemic opioids. However, blood loss and thromboembolic complications are reduced when epidural local anesthetics are administered. This method is therefore recommended intraoperatively and continued for pain relief after open prostatectomy and in selected high-risk patients undergoing transurethral resection. In other transurethral resection patients, systemic opioids, NSAIDs, or both provide postoperative pain alleviation.

PERIPHERAL PROCEDURES

After vascular procedures, postoperative pain control is probably best achieved with epidural local anesthetic–opioid mixtures, possibly combined with systemic NSAIDs. This regimen will be effective, and the increase in peripheral blood flow that is documented to occur with epidural local anesthetics may lower the risk of graft thrombosis.

Pain relief after major joint procedures (e.g., hip and knee operations) should also involve an epidural regimen because of the documented reduction in thromboembolic complications and in intraoperative blood loss. The severe pain after knee replacement is probably best treated with epidural local anesthetics combined with opioids. If epidural regimens are not available, combined treatment with systemic opioids and NSAIDs may provide moderately effective pain relief. After arthroscopic joint procedures, instillation of a local anesthetic and an opioid analgesic (e.g., morphine) provides effective early postoperative pain relief.

During superficial procedures, the use of systemic opioids combined with NSAIDs is sufficient. Transcutaneous electrical nerve stimulation (TENS) may have an additional effect during soft tissue procedures but cannot alone alleviate pain very effectively.

Treatment Modalities

PSYCHOLOGICAL INTERVENTIONS

Individuals differ considerably in how they respond to noxious stimuli; much of this variance is accounted for by psychological factors. Cognitive, behavioral, or social interventions should be used in combination with pharmacological therapies to prevent or control acute pain, with the goal of such interventions being to guide the patient toward partial or complete self-control of pain.[3,4] Sophisticated psychological techniques, such as biofeedback and hypnosis therapy, are not applicable to a busy surgical unit, but simple psychological techniques are a valuable part of good medical practice.

Psychological preparation in patients with postoperative pain has been demonstrated to shorten hospital stay and to reduce postoperative narcotic use [see Table 2].[5] Psychological techniques should be combined with pharmacological or other interventions, but care must be taken to ensure that the pharmacological treatment does not compromise the mental function necessary for the success of the planned psychological intervention.

Table 2 **Psychological Preparation of Surgical Patients**

Procedural information   Give a careful and relevant description of what will take place

Sensory information   Describe the sensations that will be experienced either during or after the operation

Pain treatment information   Outline the plan for administering sedative and analgesic medication, and encourage patients to communicate concerns and discomforts

Instructional information   Teach patients postoperative exercises, such as leg exercises, and show them how to turn in bed or move so that pain is minimal

Reassurance   Reassure those who are mentally, emotionally, or physically unable to cooperate that they are not expected to take an active role in coping with pain and will still receive sufficient analgesic treatment

SYSTEMIC OPIOIDS

The terminology associated with the pharmacology of the opioids is confusing, to say the least. Opiate is an appropriate term for any alkaloid derived from the juice of the poppy plant (i.e., from opium). The proper term for the class of agents, whether exogenous, endogenous, natural, or synthetic, is opioid.

Mechanisms of Action

When administered for pain relief, opioids produce analgesia and other physiologic effects by binding to specific receptors in the central nervous system. These receptors normally bind a number of endogenous substances called opioid peptides. These receptor-binding interactions mediate a wide array of physiologic effects [see Table 3]. Five types of opioid receptors and their subtypes have been discovered: mu, delta, kappa, epsilon, and sigma receptors [see Table 3]. Most commonly used opioids bind to mu receptors. The mu_1 receptor is responsible for the production of opioid-induced analgesia, whereas the mu_2 receptor is responsible for the production of respiratory depression, cardiovascular effects, and the inhibition of the gastrointestinal motility commonly seen with the opioids.

The relation between receptor binding and the intensity of the resultant physiologic effect is known as the intrinsic activity of an opioid. Most of the commonly used opioid analgesics are agonists. An agonist produces a maximal biologic response by binding to its receptor. Other opioids, such as naloxone, are termed antagonists because they compete with agonists for opioid receptor binding sites. Still other opioids are partial agonists because they produce a submaximal response after binding to the receptor. (An excellent example of a submaximal response produced by partial agonists is buprenorphine's action at the mu receptor.)

Drugs such as nalbuphine, butorphanol, and pentazocine are known as agonist-antagonists or mixed agonist-antagonists.[6] These opioids simultaneously act at different receptor

Table 3 Opioid Receptor Types and Physiologic Actions

Receptor Type	Prototypical Ligand		Physiologic Actions
	Endogenous	Exogenous	
Mu$_1$	β-Endorphin	Morphine	Supraspinal analgesia
Mu$_2$	β-Endorphin	Morphine	Respiratory depression
Delta	Enkephalin	—	Spinal analgesia
Kappa	Dynorphin	Ketocyclazocine	Spinal analgesia, sedation
Epsilon	β-Endorphin	—	Hormone?
Sigma	—	N-Allylnormetazocine	Psychotomimetic effect, dysphoria

sites; their action is agonistic at one receptor and antagonistic at another [see Table 4]. The agonist-antagonists have certain pharmacological properties that are distinct from those of the more common mu agonists: (1) they exhibit a ceiling effect and cause only submaximal analgesia as compared with mu agonists and (2) administration of an agonist-antagonist and a complete agonist may cause a reduction in the effect of the complete agonist.[6]

Morphine

Morphine is the opioid with which the most clinical experience has been gained, although scientific data, especially pharmacokinetic and pharmacodynamic data, are still scarce. Use of this agent is recommended; it may be given orally, intravenously, or intramuscularly [see Table 5].

Meperidine

Detailed and sufficient pharmacokinetic and pharmacodynamic data are available. Meperidine is less suitable than morphine as an analgesic because of its active metabolite, normeperidine. Normeperidine can accumulate, even in patients with normal renal clearance. This accumulation can result in CNS excitation and seizures.[7] It is recommended that other agents be used before meperidine is considered.[2] Like morphine, meperidine can be given orally, intravenously, or intramuscularly [see Table 5].

Table 4 Intrinsic Activity of Opioids

Opioid	Receptor Type			
	Mu	Kappa	Delta	Sigma
Agonists				
Morphine	Agonist	—	—	—
Meperidine (Demerol)	Agonist	—	—	—
Hydromorphone (Dilaudid)	Agonist	—	—	—
Oxymorphone (Numorphan)	Agonist	—	—	—
Levorphanol (Levo-Dromoran)	Agonist	—	—	—
Fentanyl (Duragesic)	Agonist	—	—	—
Sufentanil (Sufenta)	Agonist	—	—	—
Alfentanil (Alfenta)	Agonist	—	—	—
Methadone (Dolophine)	Agonist	—	—	—
Agonist-Antagonists				
Buprenorphine (Buprenex)	Partial agonist	—	—	—
Butorphanol (Stadol)	Antagonist	Agonist	Agonist	—
Nalbuphine (Nubain)	Antagonist	Partial agonist	Agonist	—
Pentazocine (Talwin)	Antagonist	Agonist	Agonist	—
Dezocine (Dalgan)	Partial agonist	—	—	Agonist
Antagonists				
Naloxone (Narcan)	Antagonist	Antagonist	Antagonist	Antagonist

Table 5 Suggested Regimens for Systemic Opioid Administration

	\multicolumn{4}{c}{Intermittent Administration (Suggested Initial Dose)*}
	p.o.	I.M.	I.V.	Duration (hr)
Morphine	30–50 mg	10 mg	5–10 mg	3–4
Meperidine	300 mg	75–100 mg	25–50 mg	2–4
Buprenorphine	0.4 mg (sublingual)	0.3 mg	0.3 mg	6–8

	Continuous I.V. Infusion†
Morphine	≈ 3 mg/hr (loading dose: 5–10 mg)
Meperidine	≈ 25 mg/hr (loading dose: ≈ 25–50 mg)

*Number of doses to be given is calculated with the following formula:

$$\frac{24 \text{ hr}}{\text{actual duration of single effective dose (hr)}}$$

Single doses should be given at calculated fixed intervals approximately 30 min before expected recurrence of pain. Single dose should be readjusted daily. Elderly patients may be more susceptible to opioids.

†Dose should be adjusted according to effect and side effects.

Methadone

Methadone has a half-life of about 35 hours, and it relieves pain for a comparably long period. Because one dose is effective for so long, there is an increased risk of accumulation if further doses are given. This risk notwithstanding, a single 20 mg dose of methadone may be useful after relatively minor procedures that result in fairly short periods of postoperative pain.[8]

Buprenorphine

Buprenorphine is a mixed agonist-antagonist analgesic with a longer duration of action than morphine.[9] Unlike morphine, it is only partially antagonized by naloxone; however, doxapram, 1.0 to 1.5 mg/kg I.V., is effective. Sublingual and injectable preparations are available [see Table 5].[10] Buprenorphine may lead to respiratory depression with repetitive dosing.

Side Effects

By depressing or stimulating the CNS, opioids cause a number of physiologic effects in addition to analgesia. The depressant effects of opioids include analgesia and altered respiration and mood. The excitatory effects of opioids include nausea, vomiting, and miosis.

All mu agonists produce a dose-dependent decrease in the responsiveness of brain stem respiratory centers to increased carbon dioxide tension (PCO_2).[11] This is clinically manifested as an increase in resting PCO_2 and a shift in the CO_2 response curve. Agonist-antagonist opioids have a limited effect on the brain stem and appear to elicit a ceiling effect on increases in PCO_2.[6,12]

Opioids also have effects on the gastrointestinal tract. Nausea and vomiting are caused by stimulation of the chemoreceptor trigger zone of the medulla. Opioids enhance sphincteric tone and reduce peristaltic contraction. Delayed gastric emptying is caused by decreased motility, increased antral tone, and increased tone in the first part of the duodenum. Delay in passage of intestinal contents because of decreased peristalsis and increased sphincteric tone leads to greater absorption of water, increased viscosity, and desiccation of bowel contents, which cause constipation. Opioids also increase biliary tract pressure.[12,13]

EPIDURAL AND SUBARACHNOID OPIOIDS

Opioids were first used in the epidural and subarachnoid space in 1979. Since that time, they have become the mainstay of postoperative pain management. Epidural opioids may be administered in a single bolus or in continuous infusions. They are usually combined with local anesthetic in a continuous epidural infusion.

Mechanisms of Action

Opioids injected into the epidural or subarachnoid space cause segmental (i.e., selective, spinally mediated) analgesia by binding to opioid receptors in the dorsal horn of the spinal cord. The lipid solubility of an opioid, described by its partition coefficient, predicts its behavior when administered to the epidural or subarachnoid space. Opioids with low lipid solubility (i.e., hydrophilic opioids) have a slow onset of action and a long duration of action. Opioids with high lipid solubility (i.e., lipophilic opioids) have a quick onset of action but a short duration of action [see Table 6]. Thus, the lipid solubility of an opioid determines its access to the dorsal horn via (1) diffusion through the arachnoid granulations and (2) diffusion into spinal radicular artery blood flow.[14-16]

Subarachnoid opioids should be used when the required duration of analgesia after surgery is relatively short. When protracted analgesia is required, epidural administration is preferred; repeated injections may be given through epidural catheters, or continuous infusions may be used. Smaller doses of subarachnoid opioids are generally required to produce analgesia. Ordinarily, no more than 0.25 to 0.50 mg of morphine should be used. This range provides reliable pain relief with few side effects. These doses are about one tenth to one fifth that of effective epidural morphine doses. Fentanyl has also been extensively used in the subarachnoid space in a dose range of 6.25 to 50 μg. Pain relief after administration of subarachnoid fentanyl is as potent but not as prolonged as analgesia after administration of morphine.[15]

Regimens for Acute Pain Relief

Most studies agree that at least 2 mg of epidural morphine is needed to achieve a significant analgesic response [see Table 6], but the criteria used to assess this response have varied greatly in reported studies, and no firm conclusion can be derived from them.[16,17] Epidural opioids are less efficient in the earliest stages of the acute pain state than on subsequent days; moreover, they appear to be more successful at alleviating pain after procedures in the lower half of the body than at alleviating upper abdominal and thoracic pain.[16] In general, 2 to 4 mg of morphine epidurally is sufficient after minor procedures, whereas about 4 mg is needed after vascular and gynecologic procedures and about 4 to 6 mg after major upper abdominal and thoracic procedures.[17-19] On the first postoperative day, however, such a regimen, even when repeated as many as three times, relieves pain completely in fewer than 50 percent of patients in contrast to an increased success rate on subsequent days. Its efficiency will be lowest after major procedures.

Information now suggests that use of continuous epidural morphine in low dosages (0.1 to 0.3 mg/hr) may lower the risk of late respiratory depression and may be more efficient than intermittent higher dosages of morphine.[20-22] It is therefore recommended.

Side Effects

The chief side effects associated with epidural and subarachnoid opioids are respiratory depression, nausea and vomiting, pruritus, and urinary retention.[14-16,23,24] The poor lipid solubility of morphine is responsible for its protracted duration of action but also allows morphine to undergo cephalad migration in the cerebrospinal fluid. This migration can cause delayed respiratory depression with a peak incidence three to 10 hours after an injection.[16,23,24] The high lipid solubility of lipophilic opioids such as fentanyl allows them to be absorbed into lipids close to the site of administration. Consequently, the lipophilic opioids do not migrate rostrally in the CSF and cannot cause delayed respiratory depression. Of course, the high lipid solubility of lipophilic opioids allows them to be absorbed into blood vessels, which may cause early respiratory depression, as is commonly seen with systemic administration of opioids.[14-16]

Naloxone reverses the depressive respiratory effects of spinal opioids. In an apneic patient, 0.4 mg administered intravenously will usually restore ventilation. If a patient has a depressed respiratory rate but is still breathing (i.e., one to four breaths a minute), small aliquots of naloxone (0.04 mg) can be given until the respiratory rate returns to normal. Because naloxone has a short half-life, it is best to start a continuous infusion of naloxone at a rate of 5 mg/kg/hr to prevent respiratory depression from recurring.[15]

Nausea and vomiting are caused by transport of opioids to the vomiting center and the chemoreceptor trigger zone in the medulla via CSF flow or systemic circulation.[15] Nausea can usually be treated with antiemetics, naloxone (small increments of 0.04 to 0.10 mg followed by infusion of 1 mg/kg/hr I.V.), and agonist-antagonist opioids (e.g., butorphanol, 0.25 to 0.50 mg, or nalbuphine 2.5 to 5.0 mg).[15]

Pruritus is probably the most common side effect of the spinal opioids. Histamine is released by certain opioids, but this mechanism probably plays a negligible role in the genesis of itching. The production of spinal opioid-induced pruritus is probably caused by changes in the electrophysiology of neurons of the dorsal horn.[23] The treatment of pruritus is similar to that of nausea.

The mechanism of spinal opioid-induced urinary retention involves inhibition of volume-induced bladder contractions and blockade of the vesical reflex.[24] Naloxone administration is the treatment of choice, though bladder catheterization is sometimes required.

EPIDURAL LOCAL ANESTHETICS AND OTHER REGIONAL BLOCKS

Local anesthetics have gained increasing popularity because of the growing familiarity with the techniques of both epidural catheterization and regional nerve blocks.[17,25] In addition, there is a great deal of experimental evidence that documents the benefits of blocking noxious impulses.[26,27] Local anesthetic neural blockade is unique among available analgesic techniques in that it may offer complete afferent neural blockade, resulting in relief of pain; inhibition of the stress response; reduction in the cardiorespiratory effects of severe pain; avoidance of sedation, respiratory depression, and nausea; and, finally, efferent sympathetic blockade resulting in increased blood flow to the region

Table 6 Dosage Regimens for Epidural Opioids

Drug	Lipid Solubility*	Bolus Dose	Onset (min)	Duration (hr)	Comments
Morphine	1	2–5 mg	30–60	6–24	Because of spread in CSF, preferred when incisions are extensive and injection site is distant from source of pain
Diamorphine	10	4–6 mg	5	10–12	
Meperidine (Demerol)	30	35–50 mg	5–10	6–8	
Methadone (Dolophine)	100	1–10 mg	10	6–10	May accumulate in blood with repeated dosing
Fentanyl (Duragesic)	800	50–100 μg	5	4–6	Not recommended when incision is extensive or injection site is distant from source of pain
Sufentanil (Sufenta)	1,500	10–60 μg	5	2–4	Higher doses may produce excessive sedation or ventilatory depression, presumably because of vascular uptake

*Octanol/pH 7.4 buffer partition coefficient relative to morphine.

of neural blockade.[25-27] Despite the considerable scientific data documenting these beneficial effects, the place of epidural local anesthesia as a method of pain relief remains somewhat controversial in comparison with that of other analgesic techniques; side effects, such as hypotension, urinary retention, and motor blockade, combined with the need for trained staff for surveillance, argue against its use. However, the risk of these side effects can be reduced by use of combination regimens (see below).

Mechanism of Action

Local anesthetic neural blockade is a nondepolarizing block that reduces the permeability of cell membranes to sodium ions.[28] Whether different local anesthetics have different effects on different nerve fibers is debatable.

Choice of Drug

For optimal management of postoperative pain, the anesthetic agent should provide excellent analgesia of rapid onset and long duration without inducing motor blockade. The various local anesthetic agents all meet one or more of these criteria, but it is bupivacaine that comes closest to meeting all of them. This should not preclude the use of other agents, because their efficacy has also been demonstrated.

Continuous Epidural Analgesia

No regimen has been found that provides complete analgesia in all patients all of the time, and it is unlikely that one ever will be found. As a rule, the block should be limited to the area in which pain is felt. Care should be taken to avoid motor blockade and to spare autonomic function to the urinary bladder, as well as to formulate a regimen that requires only minimal attention from staff members and carries no significant toxicity. Given these requirements, continuous infusion is more effective and reliable than intermittent injection [see Table 7]. Whether low hourly volume and high concentration approaches are preferable to high hourly volume and low concentration approaches remains to be determined. The weaker solutions may produce less motor blockade while continuing to block smaller C and A-delta pain fibers and are recommended in lumbar epidural analgesia as a means of reducing the risk of orthostatic hypotension and lower extremity motor blockade.[25]

Specific indications for continuous epidural analgesia that are supported by data from controlled morbidity studies include (1) pain relief and reduction of deep venous thrombosis and of pulmonary embolism and hypoxemia after total hip replacement and prostatectomy; (2) pain relief, facilitation of coughing, and reduction of chest infections after thoracic, abdominal, and orthopedic procedures; (3) pain relief, control of hypertension, and enhancement of graft flow after major vascular operations; and (4) pain relief and reduction of paralytic ileus after abdominal procedures.[27,29]

Side Effects

The main side effects of epidural local anesthesia are hypotension caused by sympathetic blockade, vagal overactivity, and decreased cardiac function (during a high thoracic block). Under no circumstances should epidural local anesthetics be used before a preexisting hypovolemic condition is treated. Hypotension may be treated with ephedrine, 10 to 15 mg I.V., and fluids, with the patient tilted in a head-down position. Atropine, 0.5 to 1.0 mg I.V., may be effective during vagal overactivity.

Urinary retention occurs in 20 to 100 percent of patients. Fortunately, urinary catheterization for only 24 hours in the course of a high-dose regimen probably has no important side effects, and many patients for whom epidural analgesia is indicated need an indwelling catheter for other reasons in any case. The incidence of urinary retention is below 10 percent when epidural local anesthetics are used in weak solutions [see Table 8]. Motor blockade may delay mobilization; however, its incidence can be reduced by using the weakest concentration of local anesthetic that is compatible with adequate sensory blockade. Cerebral and cardiovascular toxicity are seldom encountered, and epidural hematoma

---

Table 8 Procedures for Maintenance of Epidural Anesthesia for Longer Than 24 Hours

1. Administer appropriate drug in appropriate dosage at selected infusion rate as determined by physician.
2. Nurse evaluates vital signs and intake and output as required for a postoperative patient.
3. Nurse checks infusion pump hourly to ensure that it is functioning properly, that infusion rate is proper, and that alarm is on.
4. Nurse also assesses
   - Bladder—for distention, if patient is not catheterized
   - Lower extremities—for status of motor function
   - CNS—for signs of toxicity or respiratory depression
   - Relief of pain (drug dosage may require modification)
   - Skin integrity on back (breakdown may occur if motor function is not present)
   - Tubing and dressing (disconnection of tubing or dislodgment of catheter may occur)
5. Every 48 hr, the catheter dressing should be removed, the catheter entrance site cleaned, and topical antibiotic applied (much as in care of a central venous catheter).

Table 7 Regimen for Pain Relief with Continuous Epidural Bupivacaine during the Initial 24 Postoperative Hours

Type of Operation	Interspace for Catheter Insertion	Concentration (%)	Volume (ml/hr)
Thoracic procedures	T4–6	0.250–0.125	5–10
Upper laparotomy	T7–8	0.250–0.125	4–12
Gynecologic laparotomy	T10–12	0.250–0.125	4–10
Hip procedures	L2	0.125–0.0625	4–8
Vascular procedures	T10–12	0.250–0.125	4–10

Note: indications for postoperative epidural bupivacaine may be strengthened if this method is also indicated for intraoperative analgesia. Dosage requirements may vary and should be assessed 3 hr after the start of treatment, every 6 hr thereafter on the first day, and then every 12 hr (more often if pain occurs). The duration of treatment is 1–4 days, depending on the intensity of the pain. The concentration of bupivacaine employed should be the lowest possible and should be decreased with time postoperatively. Some patients, especially those who have undergone major upper abdominal operation, require 0.5 percent bupivacaine initially.

and abscess are extremely rare. Epidural analgesia should not be employed in patients already receiving anticoagulant therapy, but it may be started with catheter insertion before vascular or other procedures in which controlled heparin therapy is used. Epidural analgesia has been used in patients receiving thromboembolic prophylaxis with low-dose heparin or low-molecular-weight heparin without significantly increased risk.[30,31] The complications associated with the epidural catheter are minimal when proper nursing protocols are followed [see Table 8]. The decision to employ epidural local anesthetics in such patients should be made only after the risks are carefully compared with the documented advantages of such anesthetics.[25-27]

Other Nerve Blocks

The popularity of single-dose intercostal block and intrapleural regional analgesia has decreased in comparison with that of continuous epidural treatment. Intermittent or continuous administration of bupivacaine through a catheter inserted into the intercostal space seems to be a promising approach to providing anesthesia after abdominal procedures, but further data are needed.[32] Intravenous and intraperitoneal administration of local anesthetics cannot be recommended, because they are not efficacious. Intraincisional administration of bupivacaine, which has negligible side effects and demands little or no surveillance, is recommended in shorter procedures[33] but should receive additional study. More detailed information on special blocks can be found in the anesthesiology literature.

In general, despite its disadvantages, neural blockade with local anesthetics is recommended for relief of postoperative pain because of the advantageous physiologic effects it exerts and the reduction in postoperative morbidity it brings about.

NONSTEROIDAL ANTI-INFLAMMATORY DRUGS

NSAIDs are minor analgesics that, because of their anti-inflammatory effect, may be suitable for management of postoperative pain associated with a significant degree of inflammation, such as bone or soft tissue damage. However, they may also have central analgesic effects and may therefore have analgesic efficacy after all kinds of operations. Only a few of them may be given parenterally. The data now available on the use of NSAIDs for postoperative pain are insufficient to allow definitive recommendation of any agent or agents over the others, and selection may therefore depend on convenience of delivery, duration, and cost.[34,35] It is clear, however, that they may play a valuable role as adjuvants to other analgesics—in particular because of their ability to reduce platelet adhesion. All the NSAIDs, except acetaminophen, have a potentially serious side effect: gastrointestinal hemorrhage. Fortunately, this effect is probably of minor importance during short-term postoperative treatment,[35] and it may be further minimized by intravenous, intramuscular, or rectal administration.

The NSAIDs exert their anti-inflammatory effect by inhibiting prostaglandin synthesis at the wound site (and probably also in the CNS), thereby decreasing the release of local inflammatory agents. Because prostaglandins are important for regulation of water and mineral homeostasis by the kidneys[36] in the dehydrated patient, perioperative treatment with NSAIDs may lead to postoperative renal failure. Although little systematic evaluation has been done, extensive clinical experience with these drugs suggests that this risk is not substantial.[34,35] Nonetheless, NSAIDs should be used with caution in patients who have preexisting renal dysfunction.

Although NSAIDs may also prolong bleeding time and inhibit platelet aggregation, increased bleeding does not seem to be a clinically significant risk.[34,35] However, in procedures where strict hemostasis is critical (e.g., cosmetic surgery and eye surgery), these drugs should be given with caution.

Despite the gaps in our current understanding of the workings of NSAIDs, what is known is sufficiently encouraging to suggest that NSAIDs probably should be recommended for baseline analgesic treatment after most operative procedures, except in the earliest part of the postoperative period immediately after heparinization during cardiovascular procedures [see Table 9]. NSAIDs are a valuable component of multimodal pain treatment (see below) and may be of special value in patients undergoing short operations (e.g., laparoscopic procedures) in whom opioid-sparing effects may reduce postoperative nausea and vomiting. Until further data can be obtained on safety and efficacy, four of the available NSAIDs are recommended: acetylsalicylic acid, acetaminophen, indomethacin, and ibuprofen.

CRYOANALGESIA

Cryoanalgesia is the application of low temperatures (–20° to –29° C) to peripheral nerves with the goal of producing axonal degeneration and thus analgesia [see Figure 1].[37] Axonal regeneration takes place at a rate of 1 to 3 mm/day, which means that analgesia after intercostal blocks lasts about 30 days. Cryoanalgesia has no cardiac, respiratory, or cerebral side effects, and local side effects (e.g., neuroma formation) are extremely rare. However, it can be used only on sensory nerves or on nerves supplying muscles of no clinical importance. At present, no information is available on the use of cryoanalgesia in operative procedures other than thoracotomy and herniotomy. Whereas the significance of the data on inguinal nerve cryoanalgesia after herniotomy is debatable, the data on postthoracotomy cryoanalgesia indicate improved pain alleviation and a concomitant reduction in the need for narcotics.[38-41] Furthermore, combining cryoanalgesia with administration of indomethacin may yield an additive analgesic effect after thoracotomy.[42]

The positive results after thoracotomy, together with the simplicity and low cost of the modality and the absence of side effects, present a strong argument for more extensive use of cryoanalgesia.

TRANSCUTANEOUS ELECTRICAL NERVE STIMULATION

Transcutaneous electrical nerve stimulation is the application of a mild electrical current through the skin surface to a specific area, such as a surgical wound, to achieve pain relief; the exact mechanism whereby it achieves this effect is yet to

Table 9 Recommended Dosages of Nonsteroidal Anti-inflammatory Drugs (NSAIDs) for Relief of Postoperative Pain

NSAID	Dosage
Acetylsalicylic acid	500–1,000 mg q. 4–6 hr
Acetaminophen	500–1,000 mg q. 4–6 hr
Indomethacin	50–100 mg q. 6–8 hr
Ibuprofen	200–400 mg q. 4–6 hr
Ketorolac	30 mg q. 4–6 hr

be explained. Many TENS devices are available for clinical use, but the specific value and the proper use of the various stimulation frequencies, waveforms, and current intensities have not been determined; however, most would agree that a high-frequency (50 to 100 Hz), low-intensity (12 to 20 mA at 1,000 Ω) current with an asymmetric biphasic waveform is the most effective current.[43] Whereas TENS has been shown to be effective in reducing postoperative pain and narcotic requirements after knee, hip, and low-back operations,[43] results after abdominal, herniotomy, and thoracic procedures are inconclusive. The effect of TENS on acute pain is too small to warrant a recommendation for routine use.

PATIENT-CONTROLLED ANALGESIA

Patient-controlled administration of opioids has experienced a dramatic increase in use. This increased use may be attributed to (1) awareness of the inadequacy of traditional I.M. opioid regimens, (2) the development of effective and safe biotechnology, and (3) the widespread patient satisfaction with patient-controlled analgesia (PCA).[44-46]

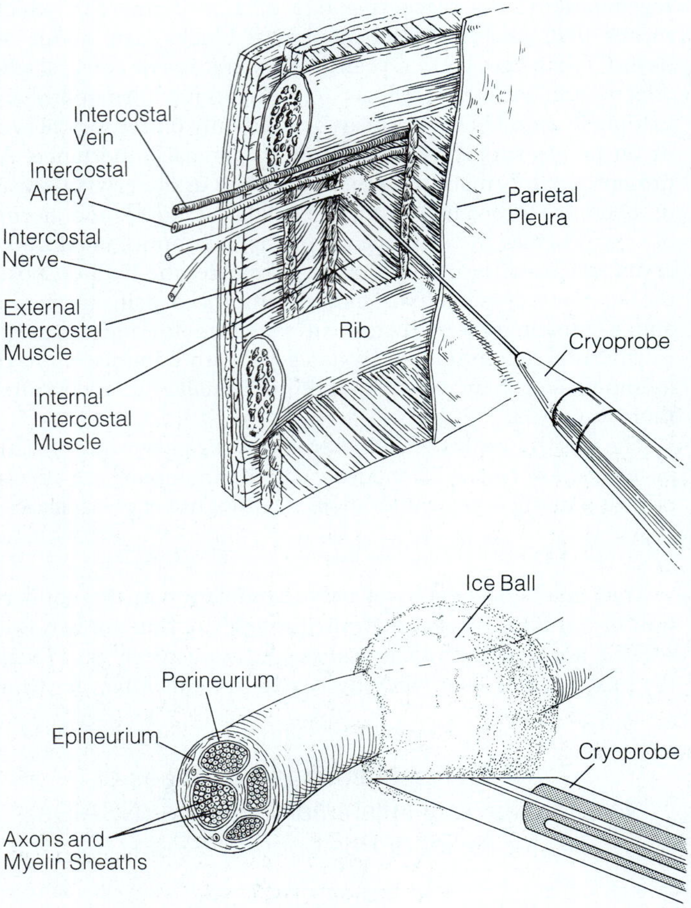

Table 10 Prescription Guidelines for Intravenous Patient-Controlled Analgesia

Drug (Concentration)	Demand Dose	Lockout Interval (min)
Morphine (1 mg/ml)	0.5–3.0 mg	5–12
Meperdine (10mg/ml)	5–30 mg	5–12
Fentanyl (10 μg/ml)	10–20 μg	5–10
Hydromorphone (0.2 mg/ml)	0.1–0.5 mg	5–10
Oxymorphone (0.25 mg/ml)	0.2–0.4 mg	8–10
Methadone (1 mg/ml)	0.5–2.5 mg	8–20
Nalbuphine (1 mg/ml)	1–5 mg	5–10

Mechanism of Action

Traditional I.M. dosing of opioids does not result in consistent blood levels,[47,48] because opioids are absorbed at a variable rate from the vascular bed of muscle. Moreover, administration of traditional I.M. regimens results in opioid concentrations that exceed the concentrations required to produce analgesia only 35 percent of the time during any four-hour dosing interval. PCA avoids these pitfalls by allowing repeated dosing on demand. PCA provides more constant and consistent plasma opioid levels and therefore better analgesia.[47,48]

Modes of Administration and Dosing Parameters

Several modes can be used to administer opioids under patient control. Intermittent delivery of a fixed dose is known as demand dosing. Background infusions may be used to supplement patient-administered doses, but this increases the risk of respiratory depression.[49]

There are several basic prescription parameters for PCA: loading dose, demand dose, lockout interval, background infusion rate, and four-hour limits [see Table 10].[49] When PCA is used for postoperative care, it is usually instituted in the recovery room. The patient is made comfortable by administration of as much opioid as needed (i.e., loading dose). When the patient is sufficiently recovered from the anesthetic, he or she may begin to use the infuser.

Side Effects

Minor side effects associated with PCA include nausea, vomiting, sweating, and pruritus. Clinically significant respiratory depression with PCA is rare. There is no evidence to suggest that PCA is associated with a higher incidence of side effects than are other routes of systemic administration of opioids.[50] Side effects are the result of the pharmacological properties of opioids, not the method of administration.[44,45] One fatality has been reported with PCA.[46]

COMBINATION REGIMENS

Because no single pain treatment modality is optimal, combination regimens (e.g., balanced analgesia or multimodal treat-

Figure 1 Illustrated is the procedure for performing cryoanalgesia in a thoracotomy. The intercostal nerve in the thoracotomy space is isolated, together with the two intercostal nerves above the space and the two below it, and the cryoprobe is applied to the nerves for 45 seconds. The probe is then defrosted and reapplied to the nerves for 45 seconds. The analgesia obtained lasts about 30 days.

ment) offer major advantages over single-modality regimens, whether by maintaining or improving analgesia, by reducing side effects, or by doing both. Combinations of epidural local anesthetics and morphine[51,52] and of NSAIDs and opioids[34,35,52] or cryoanalgesia[43] have been reported to have additive effects, but detailed recommendations must await the results of further studies.

Discussion

Physiologic Mechanisms of Acute Pain

The basic mechanisms of acute pain are (1) afferent transmission of nociceptive stimuli through the peripheral nervous system after tissue damage, (2) modulation of these injury signals by control systems in the dorsal horn, and (3) modulation of the ascending transmission of pain stimuli by a descending control system originating in the brain [see Figure 2].[53-56]

PERIPHERAL PAIN RECEPTORS AND NEURAL TRANSMISSION TO THE SPINAL CORD

Peripheral pain receptors (nociceptors) can be identified by function but cannot be distinguished anatomically. The responsiveness of peripheral pain receptors may be enhanced by endogenous analgesic substances (e.g., prostaglandins, serotonin, bradykinin, and histamine) as well as by increased efferent sympathetic activity.[55] Antidromic release of substance P may amplify the inflammatory response and thereby increase pain transmission. The peripheral mechanisms of visceral pain still are not well understood[57]—for example, no one has yet explained why cutting or burning may provoke pain in the skin but not in visceral organs. Peripheral opioid receptors have been demonstrated to appear in inflammation on the peripheral nerve terminals.[58] Preliminary clinical studies have demonstrated analgesic effects from peripheral opioid administration during arthroscopic knee surgery.[59]

Somatic nociceptive input is transmitted to the CNS through A-delta and C fibers, which are small in diameter and either unmyelinated or thinly myelinated. Visceral pain is transmitted through afferent sympathetic pathways; the evidence that afferent parasympathetic pathways play a role in visceral nociception is inconclusive.[60]

DORSAL HORN CONTROL SYSTEMS AND MODULATION OF INCOMING SIGNALS

All incoming nociceptive traffic synapses in the gray matter of the dorsal horn (Rexed's laminae I to VI). Several substances may be involved in primary afferent transmission of nociceptive stimuli in the dorsal horn: substance P, enkephalins, somatostatin, neurotensin, γ-aminobutyric acid (GABA), glutamic acid, angiotensin II, vasoactive intestinal polypeptide (VIP), and cholecystokinin octapeptide (CCK-8).[54-56] From the dorsal horn, nociceptive information is transmitted through the spinothalamic tracts to the hypothalamus, through spinoreticular systems to the brain stem and reticular formation, and finally to the cerebral cortex.

DESCENDING PAIN CONTROL SYSTEM

A descending control system for sensory input exists that originates in the brain stem and reticular formation and in certain higher brain areas. The main neurotransmitters in this system are norepinephrine, serotonin, and enkephalins. Epidural-intrathecal administration of alpha-adrenergic agonists (e.g., clonidine) may therefore provide pain relief.[58]

SPINAL REFLEXES

Nociperception may be enhanced by spinal reflexes that affect the environment of the nociceptive nerve endings. Thus, tissue damage may provoke an afferent reflex that causes muscle spasm in the vicinity of the injury, thereby increasing nociperception. Similarly, sympathetic reflexes may cause decreased microcirculation in injured tissue, thereby generating smooth muscle spasm, which amplifies the sensation of pain.

POSTINJURY CHANGES IN PERIPHERAL AND CENTRAL NERVOUS SYSTEMS

After an injury, the afferent nociceptive pathways undergo physiologic, anatomic, and chemical changes.[53,55,61] These changes include increased sensitivity on the part of peripheral nociceptors as well as the growth of sprouts from damaged nerve fibers that become sensitive to mechanical and alpha-adrenergic stimuli and eventually begin to fire spontaneously. Moreover, excitability may be increased in the spinal cord, which leads to expansion of receptive fields in dorsal horn cells. Such changes may lower pain thresholds, may increase afferent barrage in the late postinjury state, and, if normal regression does not occur during convalescence, may contribute to a chronic pain state.

In experimental studies, acute pain behavior or hyperexcitability of dorsal horn neurons may be eliminated or reduced if the afferent barrage is prevented from reaching the CNS. Preinjury neural block with local anesthetics or administration of opioids can suppress excitability of the CNS; this is called preemptive analgesia.[53,55] Because similar antinociceptive procedures were less effective in experimental studies when applied after injury, timing of analgesia seems to be important in the treatment of postoperative pain. However, a critical analysis of controlled clinical studies that compared the efficacy of analgesic regimens administered preoperatively with the efficacy of the same regimens administered postoperatively concluded that preemptive analgesia is of no major clinical importance.[62,63] Thus, as long as the afferent input from the surgical wound continues, continuous treatment with multimodal or balanced analgesia may be the most effective method of treating postoperative pain.

Effects of Pain Relief

METABOLIC RESPONSE TO OPERATION

It has not been generally appreciated that acute pain in the postoperative period or after hospitalization for accidental injury not only serves no useful function but also may actually exert harmful physiologic and psychological effects. Therefore,

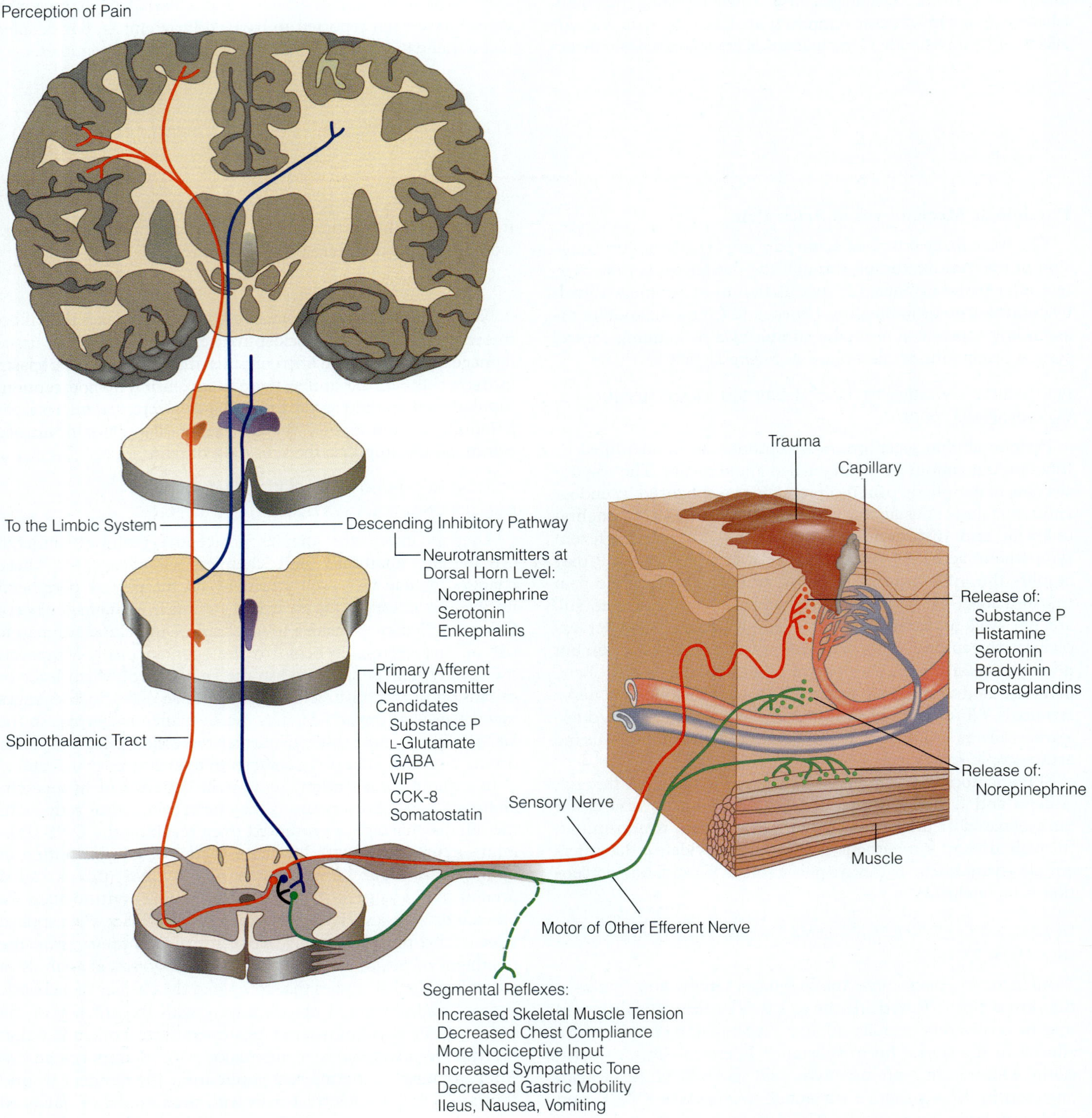

Figure 2 Shown are the major neural pathways involved in nociperception. Nociceptive input is transmitted from the periphery to the dorsal horn via A-delta and C fibers (for somatic pain) or via afferent sympathetic pathways (for visceral pain). It is then modulated by control systems in the dorsal horn and sent via the spinothalamic tracts and spinoreticular systems to the hypothalamus, to the brain stem and reticular formation, and eventually to the cerebral cortex. Ascending transmission of nociceptive input is also modulated by descending inhibitory pathways originating in the brain and terminating in the dorsal horn. Nociception may be enhanced by reflex responses that affect the environment of the nociceptors, such as smooth muscle spasm.

except in the initial stage in acutely injured hypovolemic patients for whom increased sympathetic activity may provide cardiovascular support, the pain-induced reflex responses that may adversely affect respiratory function, increase cardiac demands, decrease intestinal motility, and initiate skeletal muscle spasm (thereby impairing mobilization) should be counteracted by all available means.

The traditional view of the physiologic role of the stress response to surgical injury is that it is a homeostatic defense mechanism that helps the body heal tissue and adapt to injury. However, the necessity for the stress response in modern anesthesiology and surgery has been questioned.[26] Thus, concern about the detrimental effects of operative procedures, such as myocardial infarction, pulmonary complications, and thromboembolism—which cannot be attributed solely to imperfections in surgical technique—has led to the hypothesis that the injury response may instead be a maladaptive response that erodes body mass and physiologic reserve.[26,27] Because neural stimuli play an important role in releasing the stress response to surgical injury, pain relief may modify this response, but this modulation is dependent on the mechanism of action of the pain treatment modality employed.[26,27,63]

Alleviation of pain by antagonism of peripheral pain mediators (i.e., through use of NSAIDs) has no important modifying effect on the response to operation.[34] The effects of blockade of afferent and efferent transmission of pain stimuli by means of regional anesthesia have been studied in detail.[26,27] Spinal or epidural analgesia with local anesthetics prevents the greater part of the classic endocrine metabolic response to operative procedures in the lower region of the body (e.g., gynecologic and urologic procedures and orthopedic procedures in the lower limbs). However, this effect is considerably weaker in major abdominal and thoracic procedures, probably because of insufficient afferent neural blockade. The modifying effect of epidural analgesia on the stress response is most pronounced if the neural blockade takes effect before the surgical insult. The optimal duration of neural blockade for attenuating the hypermetabolic response has not been established, but it probably should include the initial 24 to 48 hours.

Alleviation of postoperative pain by administration of epidural-intrathecal opioids has a smaller modifying effect on the surgical stress response, in comparison with the degree of pain relief it provides[26,27]; furthermore, it does not provide efferent sympathetic blockade. Systemic administration of opioids, either according to a fixed administration regimen or according to a demand-based regimen, has no important modifying effect on the stress response.[26,27] The effects of pain relief by cryoanalgesia or TENS on the stress response are not known.

POSTOPERATIVE MORBIDITY

The effects of nociceptive blockade and pain relief on postoperative morbidity have not been adequately studied, except with respect to epidural local anesthetics, about which the following conclusions can be made[26,27,29,64,65]:

1. Intraoperative blood loss is reduced by about 30 percent after hip replacement, prostatectomy, and other lower body procedures.
2. Thromboembolic complications are reduced by about 30 to 50 percent after hip replacement, knee replacement, and prostatectomy.
3. Pulmonary infectious complications appear to be reduced by about 40 percent, but as yet, too few patients have been studied to permit a firm conclusion.
4. The duration of postoperative ileus after colonic operation is reduced.

At present, it is impossible to determine whether a short-term neural blockade that lasts throughout the operation and shortly thereafter has a more beneficial effect on postoperative morbidity than a prolonged continuous epidural blockade that lasts several days postoperatively.

Controlled studies on the effect of epidural morphine or epidural morphine–bupivacaine combinations on morbidity after abdominal or thoracic operation have yielded inconclusive results,[66-70] although ambulation, cardiovascular and pulmonary complications, and hospital stay were improved in some studies.[67,69,70]

Controlled studies comparing the improved pain relief obtained by patient-controlled opioid analgesia with conventional intermittent opioid treatment have not demonstrated clinically important advantages in outcome.[71-74] The most plausible explanation for the lack of improvement in outcome associated with improved postoperative analgesia is that general postoperative care has not adapted to make optimum use of the postoperative pain-free state. Thus, recent observations suggest that a combination of improved pain relief, enhanced early mobilization, oral feeding, and reinforced psychological preparation of the patient may lead to major improvements in postoperative morbidity, including reduction in fatigue and hospital stay. This level of care is probably best implemented in a postoperative rehabilitation unit.

TOLERANCE, PHYSICAL DEPENDENCE, AND ADDICTION

Continued exposure of an opioid receptor to high concentrations of opioid will cause tolerance. Tolerance is the progressive decline in potency of an opioid with continued use; higher and higher concentrations of the drug are required to cause the same analgesic effect. Physical dependence refers to the production of an abstinence syndrome when an opioid is withdrawn. It is defined by the World Health Organization as follows:

> A state, psychic or sometimes also physical, resulting from interactions between a living organism and a drug, characterized by behavioral and other responses that always include a compulsion to take the drug on a continuous or periodic basis in order to experience its psychic effects, and sometimes to avoid discomfort from its absence.[75]

This definition is very close to the popular conception of addiction. However, it is important to distinguish addiction (implying compulsive behavior and psychological dependence) from tolerance (a pharmacological property) and from physical dependence (a characteristic physiologic effect of a group of drugs). Physical dependence does not imply addiction. Moreover, tolerance can occur without physical dependence; the converse does not appear to be true.

The possibility that the medical administration of opioids could result in a patient's becoming addicted has generated much debate about the use of opioids. In a prospective study of 12,000 hospitalized patients receiving at least one strong opioid for a protracted period of time, there were only four reasonably well documented cases of subsequent addiction.[76] (None of these patients had a prior history of substance abuse.) Thus, the iatrogenic production of opioid addiction may be very rare.

Conclusion

The choice of therapeutic intervention for acute postoperative pain is determined largely by the nature of the patient's problem, the resources available, the efficacy of the various treatment techniques, the risks attendant on the procedures under consideration, and the cost to the patient. It appears that whereas trauma has been the subject of intensive research, the mechanisms of pain associated with trauma and surgical injury and the optimal methods of relieving such pain have received comparatively little attention. The exciting new data on basic pain mechanisms and therapy now being collected, combined with promising data supporting the idea that adequate inhibition of surgically induced nociceptive stimuli may reduce postoperative morbidity, will probably stimulate surgeons to turn their attention to this area. Effective control of postoperative pain, combined with a high degree of surgical expertise and judicious use of other perioperative therapeutic interventions, is certain to improve surgical outcome.

References

1. Report of a working party of the commission on the provision of surgical services. Pain after Surgery. The Royal College of Surgeons of England and the College of Anaesthetists, London, 1990
2. Agency for Health Care Policy and Research: Acute Pain Management and Trauma: Operative or Medical Procedures. Publication No 92-0032. U.S. Department of Health and Human Services, Rockville, Maryland, 1992
3. Chapman CR: Psychological factors in postoperative pain. Acute Pain. Smith G, Covino BG, Eds. Butterworth Publishers, Stoneham, Massachusetts, 1985, p 22
4. Peck CL: Psychological factors in acute pain management. Acute Pain Management. Cousins MJ, Phillips GD, Eds. Churchill Livingstone, Inc, New York, 1986, p 251
5. Egbert LD, Battit GE, Welch CE, et al: Reduction of postoperative pain by encouragement and instruction of patients: a study of doctor-patient rapport. N Engl J Med 270:825, 1964
6. Freye E: Opioid Agonists Antagonists and Mixed Narcotic Analgesics: Theoretical Background and Considerations for Practical Use. Springer-Verlag, Berlin, 1987
7. Kaiko RF, Foley KM, Grabinski PY, et al: Central nervous system excitatory effects of meperidine in cancer patients. Ann Neurol 13:180, 1983
8. Gourlay GK, Cousins MJ: Strong analgesics in severe pain. Drugs 28:79, 1984
9. Rosow CE: Newer synthetic opioid analgesics. Acute Pain. Smith G, Covino BG, Eds. Butterworth Publishers, Stoneham, Massachusetts, 1985, p 68
10. Shah MV, Jones DI, Rosen M: "Patient demand" postoperative analgesia with buprenorphine: comparison between sublingual and I.M. administration. Br J Anaesth 58:508, 1986
11. Bellville JW, Seed JC: The effect of drugs on the respiratory response to carbon dioxide. Anesthesiology 21:727, 1960
12. Ferrante FM: Opioids. Postoperative Pain Management. Ferrante FM, VadeBoncouer TR, Eds. Churchill Livingstone, Inc, New York, 1993, p 145
13. McCammon RL, Stoelting RK, Madura JA: Effects of butorphanol, nalbuphine, and fentanyl on intrabiliary tract dynamics. Anesth Analg 63:139, 1984
14. Cousins MJ, Cherry DA, Gourlay GK: Acute and chronic pain: use of spinal opioids. Neural Blockade in Clinical Anesthesia and Management of Pain, 2nd ed. Cousins MJ, Bridenbaugh PO, Eds. JB Lippincott Co, Philadelphia, 1988, p 955
15. VadeBoncouer TR, Ferrante FM: Epidural and subarachnoid opioids. Postoperative Pain Management. Ferrante FM, VadeBoncouer TR, Eds. Churchill Livingstone, Inc, New York, 1993, p 279
16. Cousins MJ, Mather LE: Intrathecal and epidural administration of opioids. Anesthesiology 61:276, 1984
17. Staren ED, Cullen ML: Epidural catheter analgesia for the management of postoperative pain. Surg Gynecol Obstet 162:389, 1986
18. Allen PD, Walman T, Concepcion M, et al: Epidural morphine provides postoperative pain relief in peripheral vascular and orthopedic surgical patients. Anesth Analg 65:165, 1986
19. Rawal N, Sjöstrand UH, Dahlström B, et al: Epidural morphine for postoperative pain relief: a comparative study with intramuscular narcotic and intercostal nerve block. Anesth Analg 61:93, 1982
20. El-Baz NMI, Faber LP, Jensik RJ: Continuous epidural infusion of morphine for treatment of pain after thoracic surgery: a new technique. Anesth Analg 63:757, 1984
21. Cullen ML, Staren ED, El-Ganzouri A, et al: Continuous epidural infusion for analgesia after major abdominal operations: a randomized, prospective, double-blind study. Surgery 98:718, 1985
22. Chrubasik J, Wiemers K: Continuous-plus-on-demand epidural infusion of morphine for postoperative pain relief by means of a small, externally worn infusion device. Anesthesiology 62:263, 1985
23. Ballantyne JC, Loach AB, Carr DB: Itching after epidural and spinal opiates. Pain 33:149, 1988
24. Durant PA, Yaksh TL: Drug effects on urinary bladder tone during spinal morphine-induced inhibition of the micturition reflex in unanesthetized rats. Anesthesiology 68:325, 1988
25. Bowler GMR, Wildsmith JA, Scott DB: Epidural administration of local anesthetics. Acute Pain Management. Cousins MJ, Phillips GD, Eds. Churchill Livingstone, Inc, New York, 1986, p 187
26. Kehlet H: Modification of responses to surgery and anesthesia by neural blockade. Neural Blockade in Clinical Anesthesia and Management of Pain. Cousins MJ, Bridenbaugh PO, Eds. JB Lippincott Co, Philadelphia, 1987, p 145
27. Kehlet H: General vs. regional anesthesia. Principles and Practice of Anesthesiology, Vol 2. Rogers MC, Tinker JH, Covino BG, et al, Eds. Mosby-Year Book, St. Louis, 1993, p 1218
28. Butterworth JF IV, Strichartz GR: Molecular mechanisms of local anesthesia: a review. Anesthesiology 72:711, 1990
29. Scott NB, Kehlet H: Regional anaesthesia reduces surgical morbidity. Br J Surg 75:299, 1988
30. Wille-Jørgensen P, Jørgensen LN, Rasmussen LS: Lumbar regional anaesthesia and prophylactic anticoagulant therapy: is the combination safe? Anaesthesia 46:623, 1991
31. Bergqvist D, Lindblad B, Mätzsch T: Low molecular weight heparin for thromboprophylaxis and epidural/spinal anaesthesia—is there a risk? Acta Anaesthesiol Scand 36:605, 1992
32. Murphy DF: Continuous intercostal nerve blockade: an anatomical study to elucidate its mode of action. Br J Anaesth 56:627, 1984
33. Dahl JB, Møniche S, Kehlet H: Wound infiltration with local anaesthetics for postoperative pain relief. Acta Anaesthesiol Scand 38:7, 1993
34. Dahl JB, Kehlet H: Non-steroidal anti-inflammatory drugs: rationale for use in severe postoperative pain. Br J Anaesth 66:703, 1991
35. Kehlet H, Mather LE, Eds: The value of NSAIDs in the management of postoperative pain. Drugs 44(suppl 5):1, 1992
36. Harris K: The role of prostaglandins in the control of renal function (editorial). Br J Anaesth 69:233, 1992
37. Cryoanalgesia (editorial). Lancet 1:779, 1982
38. Orr IA, Keenan DJM, Dundee JW: Improved pain relief after thoracotomy: use of cryoprobe and morphine infusion. Br Med J 283:945, 1981
39. Joucken K, Michel L, Schoevaerdts JC, et al: Cryoanalgesia for post-thoracotomy pain. Acta Anaesthesiol Belg 38:179, 1987
40. Roberts D, Pizzarelli G, Lepore V, et al: Reduction of post-thoracotomy pain by cryotherapy of intercostal nerves. Scand J Thor Cardiovasc Surg 22:127, 1988
41. Gough JD, Williams AB, Vaughan RS: The control of post-thoracotomy pain: a comparative evaluation of thoracic epidural fentanyl infusions and cryo-analgesia. Anaesthesia 43:780, 1988
42. Keenan DJM, Cave K, Langdon L, et al: Comparative trial of rectal indomethacin and cryoanalgesia for control of early postthoracotomy pain. Br Med J 287:1335, 1983
43. Tyler E, Caldwell C, Ghia JN: Transcutaneous electrical nerve stimulation: an alternative approach to the management of postoperative pain. Anesth Analg 61:449, 1982
44. Bahar M, Rosen M, Vickers MD: Self-administered nalbuphine, morphine and pethidine: comparison, by intravenous route, following cholecystectomy. Anaesthesia 40:529, 1985
45. Bollish SJ, Collins CL, Kirking DM, et al: Efficacy of patient-controlled versus conventional analgesia for postoperative pain. Clin Pharm 4:48, 1985
46. Grey TC, Sweeney ES: Patient-controlled analgesia (letter). JAMA 259:2240, 1988

47. Austin KL, Stapleton JV, Mather LE: Multiple intramuscular injections: a major source of variability in analgesic response to meperidine. Pain 8:47, 1980
48. Austin KL, Stapleton JV, Mather LE: Relationship between blood meperidine concentrations and analgesic response: a preliminary report. Anesthesiology 53:460, 1980
49. Ferrante FM: Patient-controlled analgesia: a conceptual framework for analgesic administration. Postoperative Pain Management. Ferrante FM, VadeBoncouer TR, Eds. Churchill Livingstone, Inc, New York, 1993, p 255
50. Mather LE, Owen H: The pharmacology of patient-administered opioids. Patient-Controlled Analgesia. Ferrante FM, Ostheimer GW, Covino BG, Eds. Blackwell Scientific Publications, Boston, 1990, p 27
51. Dahl JB, Rosenberg J, Hansen BL, et al: Differential analgesic effects of low-dose epidural morphine and morphine-bupivacaine at rest and during mobilization after major abdominal surgery. Anesth Analg 74:362, 1992
52. Kehlet H, Dahl JB: The value of "multi-modal" or "balanced analgesia" in postoperative pain treatment. Anesth Analg 77:1048, 1993
53. Woolf CJ: Central mechanisms of acute pain. Proceedings of the VIth World Congress on Pain. Bond MR, Charlton JE, Woolf CJ, Eds. Elsevier Science Publishers, Amsterdam, 1991, p 25
54. Raja SN, Meyer RA, Campbell JN: Peripheral mechanisms of somatic pain. Anesthesiology 68:571, 1988
55. Hyperalgesia and Allodynia. Willis WD Jr, Ed. The Bristol-Myers Squibb Symposium on Pain Research. Raven Press, New York, 1992
56. Fields HL, Heinricher MM, Mason P: Neurotransmitters in nociceptive modulatory circuits. Annu Rev Neurosci 14:219, 1991
57. Ness TJ, Gebhart GF: Visceral pain: a review of experimental studies. Pain 41:167, 1990
58. Maze M, Tranquilli W: Alpha-2 adrenoceptor agonists: defining the role in clinical anesthesia. Anesthesiology 74:581, 1991
59. Stein C: Peripheral mechanisms of opioid analgesia. Anesth Analg 76:182, 1993
60. Randich A, Gebhart GF: Vagal afferent modulation of nociception. Brain Res Rev 17:77, 1992
61. Treede R-D, Meyer RA, Raja SN, et al: Peripheral and central mechanisms of cutaneous hyperalgesia. Prog Neurobiol 38:397, 1992
62. McQuay HJ: Pre-emptive analgesia (editorial). Br J Anaesth 69:1, 1992
63. Dahl JB, Kehlet H: The value of pre-emptive analgesia in the treatment of postoperative pain. Br J Anaesth 70:434, 1993
64. Kehlet H: Surgical stress: the role of pain and analgesia. Br J Anaesth 63:189, 1989
65. Sorenson RM, Pace NL: Anesthetic techniques during surgical repair of femoral neck fractures: a meta-analysis. Anesthesiology 77:1095, 1992
66. Rawal N, Sjöstrand U, Christoffersson E, et al: Comparison of intramuscular and epidural morphine for postoperative analgesia in the grossly obese: influence on postoperative ambulation and pulmonary function. Anesth Analg 63:583, 1984
67. Hjortsø N-C, Neumann P, Frøsig F, et al: A controlled study on the effect of epidural analgesia with local anaesthetics and morphine on morbidity after abdominal surgery. Acta Anaesthesiol Scand 29:790, 1985
68. Yeager MP, Glass DD, Neff RK, et al: Epidural anesthesia and analgesia in high-risk surgical patients. Anesthesiology 66:729, 1987
69. Tuman KJ, McCarthy RJ, March RJ, et al: Effects of epidural anesthesia and analgesia on coagulation and outcome after major vascular surgery. Anesth Analg 73:696, 1991
70. Seeling W, Bruckmooser K-P, Hüfner C, et al: No reduction in postoperative complications by the use of catheterized epidural analgesia following major abdominal surgery. Anaesthesist 39:33, 1990
71. Jackson D: A study of pain management: patient controlled analgesia versus intramuscular analgesia. Journal of Intravenous Nursing 12:42, 1989
72. Wasylak TJ, Abbott FV, English MJM, et al: Reduction of post-operative morbidity following patient-controlled morphine. Can J Anaesth 37:726, 1990
73. Egbert AM, Parks LH, Short LM, et al: Randomized trial of postoperative patient-controlled analgesia vs intramuscular narcotics in frail elderly men. Arch Intern Med 150:1897, 1990
74. Kenady DE, Wilson JF, Schwartz RW, et al: A randomized comparison of patient-controlled versus standard analgesic requirements in patients undergoing cholecystectomy. Surg Gynecol Obstet 174:216, 1992
75. World Health Organization: Expert committee on drug dependence, 16th report. Technical Report Series No 407. World Health Organization, Geneva, 1969
76. Porter J, Jick H: Addiction rare in patients treated with narcotics (letter). N Engl J Med 302:123, 1980

Acknowledgments

Figure 1 Carol Donner.
Figure 2 Dana Burns Pizer.

105 STOMAL CARE

M. Joyce Rosenthal, R.N., M.S., C.E.T.N., and Daniel Rosenthal, M.D.

Approach to Perioperative Stomal Care

Preoperative Counseling

Once a surgeon decides that the creation of a stoma is essential to the cure or alleviation of a patient's disease, the next task is to convince the patient that the cure is not worse than the disease. It must be emphasized to the patient that although the stoma will be an inconvenience, the chances are excellent that he or she will go on to live a fruitful life after recovery from operation. Elderly patients or patients with an advanced stage of cancer may not be as receptive to these words of comfort as a younger or healthier patient would be. In such instances, strong emotional support from the entire health care team and from the patient's family is crucial.

Certain specific topics should always be discussed with the patient preoperatively:

1. The procedure itself. The normal intestinal anatomy, the patient's specific disease process, and the planned rerouting of the bowel should be outlined with the help of simple sketches or preprinted diagrams. Common complications associated with the intended operation should be candidly reviewed. Whether the stoma will be temporary or permanent and whether a pouch will have to be worn at all times should also be discussed. Finally, there should be a brief discussion addressing how long the operation is likely to take; what the postoperative recovery room routine will be; when the patient is likely to be able to return to the hospital room; how the nasogastric tube and the urinary catheter are used and how long they are likely to be needed; how soon after the operation the family will be able to visit the patient; and how soon after the operation the patient will be able to eat. These points have no bearing on the actual procedure, but addressing them instills in the patient and the family some sense of participation in the event and provides some answers they can use when questioned by relatives or friends. Such discussion may seem trivial to the surgeon, but it is of great importance for bolstering patient and family morale.
2. Stoma appliances. The stoma appliances currently available should be described to the patient, with special emphasis placed on their inconspicuousness and ability to contain odor completely. An easy-to-use pouch (probably a one-piece appliance) should be selected and shown to the patient and the family, who should be told that in the postoperative period they will receive detailed instruction in its use. The patient should also be made aware that at some future date, whether because of a change in body habitus or out of a desire to try another type of appliance more suitable to a particular lifestyle, he or she may switch to another pouch system. If time permits, the pouch may be worn before the procedure to yield a better idea of the suitability of the stoma site.
3. Bathing and showering. Soap and water do not hurt a stoma: ostomates can bathe or shower, with or without their pouch, as often as they wish. If circumstances permit and the patient is physically able, he or she should take a shower in the hospital after the operation with the pouch off, then reapply the pouch just as would be the routine at home. In so doing, the patient gains confidence in his or her ability to return to normal daily activities. Good hygiene is crucial to the care of the peristomal skin. Soaps with creams or oils may prevent the pouch from adhering properly and thus should not be used in the peristomal area. Often, patients want to use strong lye-based or antimicrobial soaps to sterilize the peristomal skin. This practice should be discouraged because such soaps may cause local irritation and alter the normal skin flora. The use of alcohol to clean the peristomal skin should also be discouraged.
4. Employment and physical activities. Once patients have recovered from their operation, they can generally go back to their former occupations with few or no physical limitations; however, heavy lifting or straining should be avoided because the presence of a stoma predisposes to the development of a peristomal hernia.
5. Diet. After the operation, the patient should be fed in the same manner as any other patient who has undergone a major GI operation (whether conventionally or laparoscopically performed), progressing from sips of water to clear liquids to full liquids and then to a soft, low-roughage, low-fat diet. Moving directly to a regular diet after a full-liquid diet often results in premature exposure to high-fat, gas-forming, high-roughage items. Very often, new ostomates cannot tolerate such a diet and may start vomiting or experience ileus.

In our practice, the Dietary Department is involved in coordinating the foods offered after the patient has shown the ability to tolerate a fluid diet. An "ostomy diet" order on the chart alerts the dietitian to the presence of a newly created stoma, which necessitates adjustments to the patient's diet. An ostomy diet should include three small meals supplemented by between-meal snacks. A soft or regular diet should be changed to a low-residue, low-fat, and low-lactose diet for about 2 days. Snacks should be offered at midmorning, midafternoon, and bedtime. Provided that the hospital course has been uneventful, a sample menu for postoperative day 1 might be as follows:

- Breakfast: orange juice, cream of wheat, scrambled egg, white toast, and coffee, tea, or water.

Approach to Perioperative Stomal Care

Stoma with external pouch

In operating room

Mature the stoma and apply disposable pouch, allowing for 3 mm postoperative swelling. If necessary, trim adhesive area to avoid drains or retention sutures. Support loop colostomy with bridge (e.g., segment of No. 16 rubber catheter with ends folded) inside stoma pouch. If opening of digestive stoma is delayed, cover exteriorized bowel segment with petrolatum gauze and sterile dressing.

First postoperative day

Do not change pouch if it is not leaking and stoma color is good. If stoma color cannot be determined, remove pouch, gently wipe off stoma with wet gauze, and inspect. If stoma appears healthy, apply new disposable pouch.

Start involving patient's family in care. If patient is alert, begin teaching process.

Subsequent days

48 hr after operation: Remove entire pouch system, and clean peristomal skin. Select and apply long-term pouch system. Demonstrate working of clamp or spigot, and gradually increase patient involvement.

- Digestive stoma: During next 48 to 72 hr, whenever pouch is one half to two thirds full, remove clamp, empty pouch, and rinse, using water-filled bulb syringe.
- Urinary stoma: Once a day, rinse pouch through spigot with 20 to 30 ml vinegar; reconnect to drainage.

Change pouch system every other day (unless leakage occurs): carefully detach portion adhering to abdomen with help of moist gauze or washcloth, and gently wipe stoma and peristomal skin clean.

Teach patient to fit adhesive wafer snugly around stoma, connect wafer and pouch, and position appliance over stoma and to recognize potential local skin problems.

Consider use of nonadhesive reusable pouch system (VPI).

In preparation for discharge from hospital

If necessary, ensure assistance of relative, friend, or social worker. Advise patient and caretaker of available social and medical support systems.

Patient or caretaker should be familiar with one type of pouch system, including the following:
- Emptying pouch and cleansing closure tail
- Detaching adhesive portion of pouch
- Caring for peristomal skin
- Measuring stoma and cutting hole of correct size in adhesive portion of pouch
- Applying pouch
- Recognizing, preventing, and correcting peristomal skin problems

Early postoperative skin problems include allergic contact dermatitis, folliculitis, and irritant dermatitis; problems that may arise later include radiation reactions, parastomal abscesses and ulcers, pseudoepithelial hyperplasia, and pyoderma gangrenosum.

Do not change pouch as long as wafer is securely fixed to and protecting peristomal skin. Wearing time generally ranges from 3 to 6 days; if patient has problems, consult enterostomal therapist and consider changing systems.

Counsel patient and family preoperatively

Discuss:
- Procedure itself
- Stoma appliances
- Bathing and showering
- Employment and physical activities
- Diet
- Sports and travel
- Sexual activity
- Reproduction and pregnancy
- Availability of home health care and financial support
- Importance of family support system
- Ostomate Bill of Rights

Enlist services of enterostomal therapist and trained ostomy visitor.
For emergency procedures, explain briefly and clearly what a stoma is and why its creation may be unavoidable.

Select and mark stoma site

Site must be visible to the patient and surrounded by a radius of 5 cm of flat, unencumbered skin; flexing thigh, standing, sitting, or lying should not interfere. Avoid iliac crest, costal margins, umbilicus, symphysis pubis, and folds, grooves, or scars in skin.
Proper sites tend to fall in right or left lower quadrant, below beltline, over body of rectus muscle, and 5 cm lateral to and below umbilicus.

Special considerations in site selection:
- Transverse colostomy or continent stoma
- Multiple stomas
- Abdominal shape in obese patient, newborn, or infant; unusual lower abdominal skin folds; abdominal scars
- Handicaps and prostheses
- Anticipated need for or history of radiation therapy
- Laparoscopic creation of a stoma

To mark stoma site, the preferred technique is intradermal injection of methylene blue. Superficial scratch marks are sometimes used.

Continent stoma (Kock pouch)

Intubate with No. 30 Silastic catheter.
Mark correct position of tube with silk tie at stomal level. Affix tube securely to skin. Leave in place for 10 days, and allow intestinal pouch to empty by gravity.
Irrigate tube with 30 ml normal saline q. 6 hr.

10 days after operation: Teach patient to extubate and intubate intestinal pouch. Do not keep tube out of pouch for > 30 min at a time.

4 wk after operation: Have patient extubate and reintubate stoma at gradually increasing intervals.

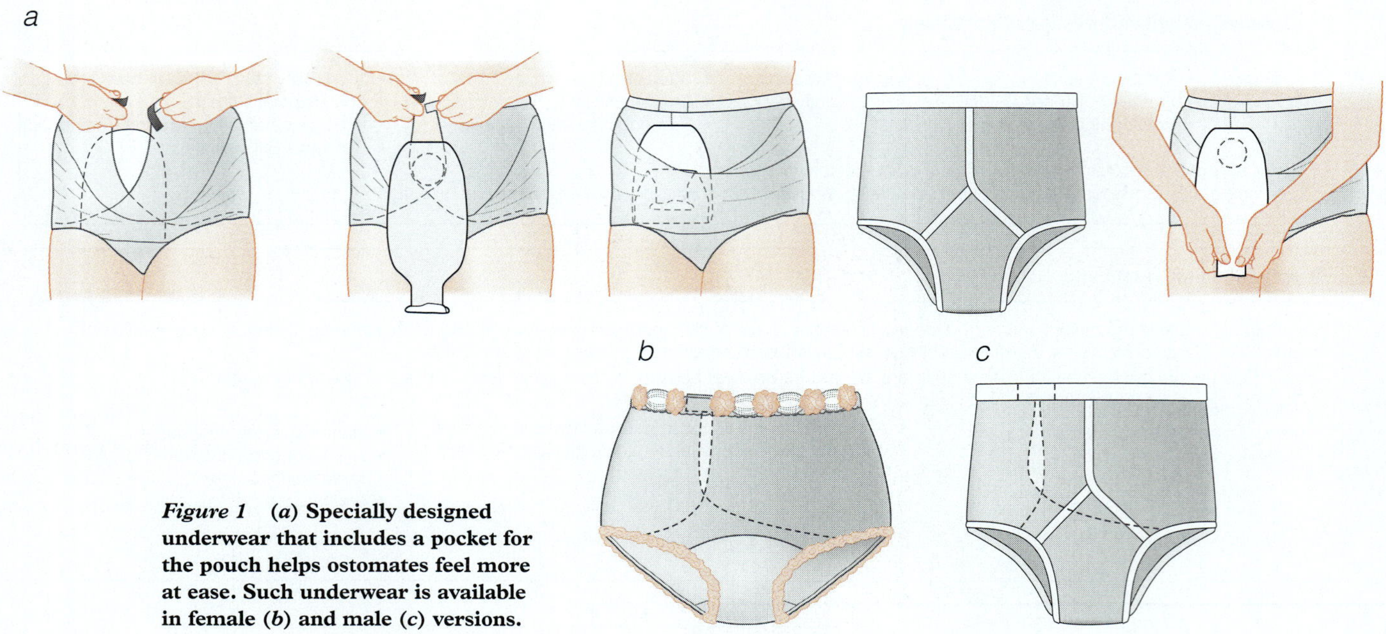

Figure 1 (*a*) Specially designed underwear that includes a pocket for the pouch helps ostomates feel more at ease. Such underwear is available in female (*b*) and male (*c*) versions.

- Lunch: baked chicken, mashed potatoes, boiled carrots, roll, and coffee, tea, or water.
- Dinner: turkey, cup of soup, canned fruit, and coffee, tea, or water.
- Snacks: midmorning, crackers and canned fruit; midafternoon, vanilla wafers with juice; and bedtime, low-fat flavored yogurt with tea or coffee.

Specific instructions are needed for the first week or two at home as more roughage and fats are introduced into the diet. Any lactose-intolerance problems should also be taken into account as milk products are slowly reintroduced into the diet. Patients with an ileostomy should have more fluids in their diet to make up for increased stomal water loss. Patients with cardiac or renal disease should be closely monitored by their physicians so that fluid overload may be prevented.

A sample menu plan for week 1 at home might be as follows:

- Breakfast: orange juice, cream of wheat, toast with jam, and milk, coffee, or tea.
- Lunch: pureed soup, turkey sandwich with reduced mayonnaise, canned fruit, and milk, coffee, or tea.
- Dinner: tomato juice; boneless, skinless chicken breast; white rice; cooked carrots; roll with margarine; and coffee or tea.
- Snacks: midmorning, half a banana and four or five graham crackers with water or juice; midafternoon, applesauce and three or four vanilla wafers with water or juice; and bedtime, low-fat flavored yogurt with milk, coffee, or tea.

Beyond the postoperative period, the diet of an ostomate, except for whatever individual modifications are necessary, can be relatively unrestricted. Overall, there is no specific ostomy diet. Any dietary restrictions adhered to are generally voluntary, and their main purpose is the prevention and relief of gas, diarrhea, constipation, or unusual odor. If any of these problems persist for more than 24 hours, the patient should notify a physician. Most difficulties can be averted if patients follow a few simple instructions, which should be emphasized to the patient before discharge:

- Avoid foods that were troublesome preoperatively. (Often, patients know which foods do not agree with them.)
- Chew foods well to break down bulk and fiber. (Failure to chew adequately may lead to stomal obstruction.)
- Eat slowly to minimize swallowing of air. (Eating fast may also result in stomal obstruction.)
- For the first few weeks after operation, avoid high-residue foods, such as fresh fruits and vegetables and whole-grain breads and cereals.
- About 6 weeks after operation, reintroduce high-residue foods into the diet, one at a time. If any food causes problems, try it again at a later date.
- If you have diarrhea, do not restrict fluid intake; instead, drink beverages that contain salt, such as Gatorade or bouillon.
- Keep well hydrated: drink four to six extra glasses of fluid a day.
- If you wish to drink alcoholic beverages, practice moderation.

Some patients with ileostomies tend to pass enteric-coated tablets or time-release capsules before the medication can be absorbed. In such cases, these products should be avoided. If a liquid form of the medication is available, it should be given instead; alternatively, a similar product that is available as a liquid may be substituted.

6. Sports and travel. Contact sports may injure the stoma and should therefore be avoided. Otherwise, ostomates may enjoy a wide range of sports activities, including swimming, as their general state of health allows. They need not avoid Jacuzzis or hot tubs, and they pose no health threat to themselves or to others if they use community pools. Any fears of possible pouch leakage may be allayed by "picture-framing" the stoma appliance with waterproof tape (i.e., placing tape on all four sides of the wafer).

Ostomates should feel free to travel, although they should be careful not to place all of their stoma supplies in their checked luggage when traveling by air. In areas where it is not safe to drink the water, they should use bottled water to irrigate their colostomies.

7. Sexual activity. Sexual activity will be a paramount consideration to some future ostomates, although probably not to all.

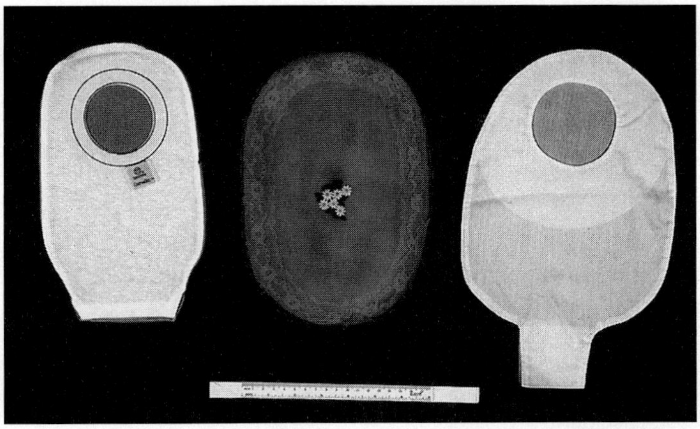

Figure 2 Shown are three different pouch covers: a commercially available cover (ConvaTec), a lace cover, and a plain handmade cover.

This matter is of such importance that it should be candidly discussed not only in the preoperative period but during follow-up visits as well. The surgeon should not hesitate to offer any patient the opportunity to voice his or her concerns about this matter. Male patients should be made aware that the amount of erectile or ejaculatory dysfunction that occurs after pelvic surgery or the removal of the rectum is related to the extent of the pelvic dissection necessary to eradicate the disease as well as to the degree of sexual vigor present before operation. Those male patients who are interested in having children may be advised to bank their sperm for future use; a certain number of patients will have permanent ejaculatory dysfunction in spite of the most careful pelvic surgery.[1] Female patients should be told that loss of the rectum and the presence of a stoma do not preclude sexual activity, even though dyspareunia, increased vaginal discharge, and altered orgasmic response are common complications of total rectal excision in women.[2-4] The use of specially designed underwear [see Figure 1] or pouch covers [see Figure 2] may help patients feel more at ease with their sexuality by enhancing the feeling of normality during intimacy.

8. Reproduction and pregnancy. Women in their reproductive years should be reassured that a stoma is not incompatible with pregnancy and that many female ostomates do in fact become pregnant and undergo normal vaginal delivery. For pregnant women who have an ileal pouch after a proctocolectomy for inflammatory bowel disease, cesarean section may be preferable to vaginal delivery at term, given that anal sphincter damage would be catastrophic in their case. Pregnant women undergoing stoma surgery for Crohn disease should be made aware that recurrent disease and some of the medications required to treat such recurrence may be detrimental to the fetus.[5] As a rule, a pregnant woman undergoing an ostomy procedure should be managed exactly as a nonpregnant woman would be. Major reconstructive procedures, however, should probably be deferred until after delivery. Closer to term, uterine enlargement may preclude even a conventional proctectomy, in which case a staged operation that spares the rectum is appropriate.[6] In our practice, we have seen 11 cases in which pregnant ostomates came to term with normal babies. A few were followed for the entire 9 months of gestation, whereas others were seen only during the last month or two for support and reassurance. We have seen both vaginal deliveries and cesarean sections in patients with ileostomies, colostomies, or ileal conduits; however, we have not been involved in the care of any pregnant patients with Kock or J ileal pouches. One women who had undergone a total colectomy and an ileostomy for Crohn disease and who had a vaginal fistula became pregnant and gave birth to a normal baby girl via cesarean section. These women are some of the best ostomy visitors we know of—living proof that life goes on despite a stoma.

9. Home health care needs. After an ostomy, some patients may require additional nursing care at home or a period of recuperation in a convalescent center.

10. Financial support. The expense of stoma equipment, along with that of home health care needs, may place a heavy financial burden on patients and their families. Surgeons should anticipate such problems preoperatively and should not hesitate to inquire into patients' insurance coverage. Patients who are 65 years of age or older should be made aware that Medicare covers, to some extent, posthospital nursing care facilities, home health care, and stoma appliance expenses. Because Medicare and Medicaid benefits and deductible expenses tend to vary annually, medical personnel may wish to update their knowledge by obtaining new schedules of Medicare and Medicaid benefits. Handbooks listing Medicare Part B benefits are reviewed annually and are available at Medicare state headquarters; their locations can be obtained by calling 800-442-2620. Pamphlets describing Medicaid benefits can be obtained by calling the individual state's department of human services. The help of a hospital social worker familiar with these problems is frequently invaluable. Retired military personnel and military dependents who are not eligible for Medicare or Medicaid should consult an adviser from the Civilian Help and Medical Program of the Uniformed Services (CHAMPUS) to determine the extent of the benefits available to them.

11. Family support system. It is vital that the surgeon keep a relative or friend of the patient informed of the upcoming operation and its consequences. Well-informed relatives who are involved in the patient's care and demonstrate by words and deeds that they will continue to offer love and concern, regardless of the outcome of the procedure, can exert a positive influence on the patient's recovery.

12. The Ostomate Bill of Rights. According to this manifesto, developed by the United Ostomy Association (UOA), the ostomate shall have the following:

- Preoperative counseling.
- An appropriately positioned stoma site.
- A well-constructed stoma.
- Skilled postoperative nursing care.
- Emotional support.
- Individual instruction.
- Information on the availability of supplies.
- Information on community resources.
- Posthospital follow-up and lifelong supervision.
- Team efforts of health care professionals.

The process of counseling can be greatly aided by the publications for patients available from the UOA [see Table 1], 19772 MacArthur Boulevard, Suite 200, Irvine, CA 92612-2405 (800-826-0826; http://www.uoa.org; e-mail uoa@deltanet.com); Crohn's and Colitis Foundation of America, Inc., 386 Park Avenue South, New York, NY 10016-8804 (800-932-2423; http://www.ccfa.org; e-mail info@ccfa.org); and the Wound, Ostomy and Continence Nurses Society, 1550 South Coast Highway, Suite 201, Laguna Beach, CA 92651 (888-224-WOCN [9626]; http://www.wocn.org; e-mail maria@wocn.org).

Table 1 Selected Publications for Patients, Available from the United Ostomy Association

The Ostomy Handbook
Colostomies: A Guide
Transverse Colostomies: A Guide
Ileostomy: A Guide
The Continent Ileostomy
Urostomy: A Guide
My Child Has an Ostomy
All about Jimmy and His Friend
Sex and the Female Ostomate
Sex and the Male Ostomate
Sex, Courtship, and the Single Ostomate
Pregnancy and the Woman with an Ostomy
Employment of the Ostomate
Handicapped Ostomate

CONSULTING AN ENTEROSTOMAL THERAPIST

Before operation, the surgeon may wish to consult an enterostomal therapy (ET) nurse. (In the United States, most enterostomal therapists are registered nurses; however, there are a few very able ones who are not.) By training and experience, ET nurses are ideally suited to the physical and emotional preparation of ostomy candidates for surgery. Reassurance aimed at dispelling any lingering apprehensions about the upcoming operation often allows the ET nurse to establish a good rapport with the patient and his or her family. To alleviate the patient's fears further, the ET nurse may display a sample pouch, which can even be worn by the candidate if desired. The ET nurse can also explain how one cares for the pouch and how one lives comfortably wearing it, provided that the patient is able and willing to assimilate this information. The patient should be assured that he or she will be taught how to take care of the stoma before leaving the hospital. This point should be reinforced by telling the patient that the ET nurse will be caring for the patient's stoma and the peristomal skin after the operation and will be slowly teaching the patient and any other personal care provider how to provide this care.

If the patient is not opposed, the ET nurse may bring in a well-adjusted ostomate of the same gender as the patient, preferably a trained ostomy visitor. This approach can reassure the patient considerably, especially if the visitor appears self-confident, is well dressed, and is about the same age as the patient. It is helpful, but not necessary, for the visitor to have the same type of stoma as the patient. Ostomy visitors are usually quite eager to help; they can generally be contacted through the local chapters of the UOA or the American Cancer Society. Local telephone directories list numbers for both agencies. In communities where no local chapters are present, the location of the nearest facility can be obtained by calling the national headquarters of either organization. The headquarters of the American Cancer Society is located at 1599 Clifton Road N.E., Atlanta, GA 30329 (800-ACS[227]-2345; http://www.cancer.org).

EMERGENCY COUNSELING

When creation of an intestinal stoma is being planned or considered under emergency conditions, the time available for counseling may be short. This time is best used in briefly but clearly explaining to the patient and the family what a stoma is and why its creation may be unavoidable in this case. Emergency stomas must be constructed according to the same basic principles of stoma construction that govern nonemergency stomas.

Preoperative Selection and Marking of the Stoma Site

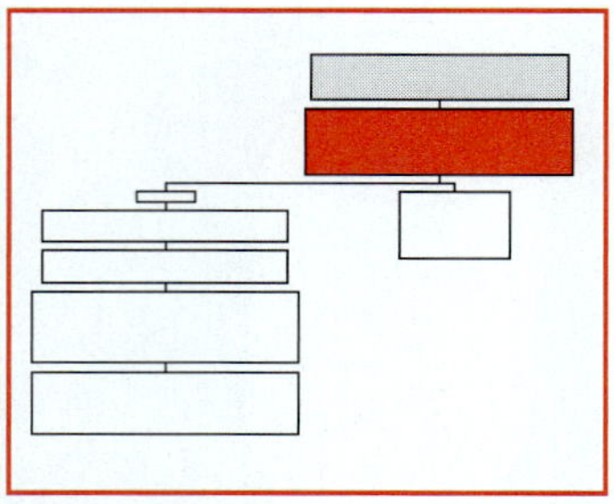

The selection and marking of the stoma site directly affect the likelihood of complications associated with the creation of the stoma.[7,8] Proper location of a stoma can mean the difference between an active, independent life and one of social isolation. Poorly placed stomas are hard to pouch and tend to leak. Accidental pouch leaks are a nuisance and a source of considerable embarrassment to ostomates. Many, in fact, avoid social contacts out of fear of such accidents.

GENERAL CONSIDERATIONS FOR SITE SELECTION

There are several general considerations for site selection that the surgeon must take into account. Proper placement of the stoma may prevent parastomal hernia, prolapse, and leakage (which can lead to skin problems and consequent patient anxiety). Stomas should be placed away from the iliac crest, the costal margins, the umbilicus, the symphysis pubis, and any folds, grooves, or scars in the skin [*see Figure 3*]. There must be a radius of about 5 cm of flat, unencumbered skin around the stoma site if an appliance is to fit well. Flexing the ipsilateral thigh should not interfere with the wearing of the appliance. The stoma site should also be visible to the patient and, ideally, should not interfere with the beltline. If the stoma site is to be placed above the beltline, care should be taken to ensure that pendulous breasts are not hanging over it. In this situation, not only would the patient find it difficult to see the stoma, but the weight of the breast would apply pressure on the appliance wafer, causing it to loosen and thus resulting in leakage.

Because the shape of the abdomen tends to change as an individual stands, sits, or lies down, it is imperative that the stoma site selected be suitable for the wearing of an appliance in all three positions—

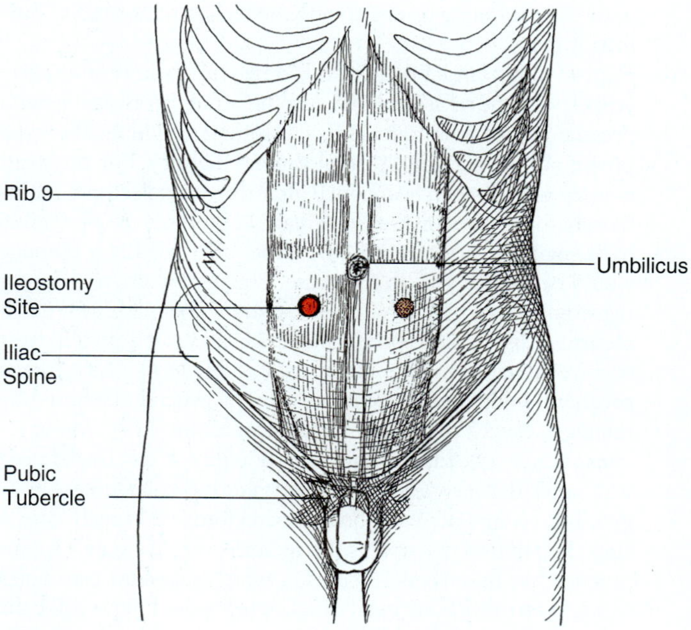

Figure 3 Shown is a stoma site selected for a conventional ileostomy. A site located in the same spot on the left side of the abdomen would be ideally suited for a sigmoid colostomy.

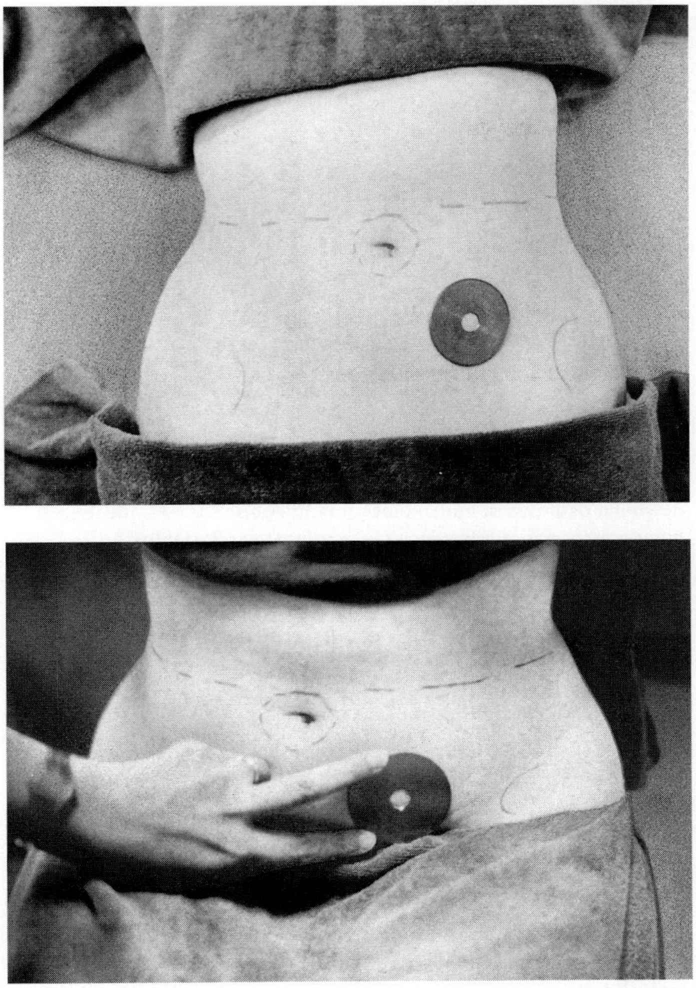

Figure 4 A 5 cm marking disk is used to select the proper stoma site with the patient lying down (*above*) and sitting up (*below*).

especially the sitting position, because it is sitting that brings about the greatest changes in abdominal contours. Often, a lower stoma site is selected so that the patient can wear the beltline low; however, a low site may lead to kinks in the appliance when the patient sits, which could result in overfilling of the upper part of the appliance. The use of a skin barrier wafer or a marking disk [*see Figure 4*] is invaluable for determining the adequacy of the stoma site selection.

The right and left lower quadrants of the abdomen are still the most common locations for digestive and urinary stomas. Properly selected stoma sites in these areas tend to fall below the beltline, over the body of the rectus muscle, about 5 cm lateral to and below the umbilicus. In our experience, creation of the stoma through the rectus sheath and muscle is associated with a lower incidence of peristomal hernia.

SPECIAL CONSIDERATIONS FOR SITE SELECTION

Besides these general considerations, the surgeon must also take into account five special considerations: (1) the type of stoma to be created, (2) whether more than one stoma is to be constructed, (3) the shape of the patient's abdomen, (4) whether the patient is handicapped or wears special prosthetic equipment, and (5) whether future radiation therapy to the abdomen is likely to be necessary.

Type of Stoma

In transverse colostomies, the stoma is generally placed in the right or left upper quadrant of the abdomen, away from the costal margins and the umbilicus. It should also be brought through the rectus sheath and muscle [*see Figure 5*] to minimize the chances of peristomal herniation. Transverse loop colostomies have a tendency to prolapse, particularly if they are created close to the hepatic flexure.

Because with a continent stoma (e.g., Kock pouch or reservoir) there is no need to wear an external pouch, the stoma can be created below the bikini line, in an inconspicuous yet accessible and visible area of the abdomen. A location about 2.5 cm above the pubic hairline over the right rectus sheath area is generally a suitable site.

Multiple Stomas

Unless there is no alternative, two functioning stomas should not be placed on the same side of the abdomen. To do so would greatly reduce the area of peristomal skin available for affixing the appliances and would complicate the emptying of the individual pouches. In addition, the weight of each pouch impinges on the other and makes the wearing of a belt very difficult for the patient. If both a urinary stoma and a digestive stoma are to be created, the stoma that is more likely to necessitate the use of a belt (i.e., the urinary stoma) should be placed somewhat higher than the other. If both stomas were placed at the same level, a belt would interfere with the second one.

Abdominal Shape

A patient must be able to see a stoma to be able to care for it [*see Figure 6*]. As a rule, therefore, a stoma cannot be placed over the lower abdomen in obese patients or patients with unusual lower abdominal skin folds [*see Figure 7*]. The deep skin creases associated with obesity also render the lower abdomen unsuitable for the placement of an appliance. In such patients, the stoma should be placed higher on the abdomen (generally above the belt line), brought through the rectus muscle, and located where it is visible and can easily be pouched [*see Figure 8*]. In a patient with a distended abdomen, the stoma site chosen should be where the stoma is to sit once the abdomen has regained its normal contour.

The general principles of stoma site selection on the abdomen apply to newborns and infants. Because their abdominal walls are more rounded and their hips are usually flexed, however, their abdominal stomas should be placed somewhat higher than is usual in adults. A diaper should not be used instead of a pouch to contain bowel efflux or urine. Many companies make stoma pouches specif-

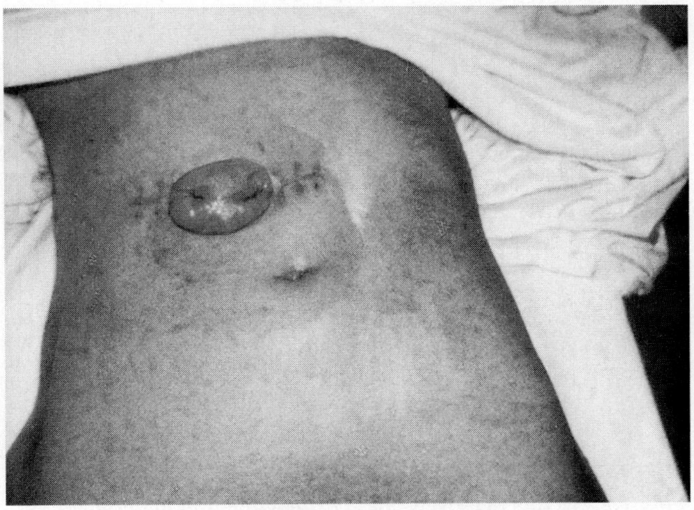

Figure 5 Shown is a properly placed loop colostomy in the right upper quadrant.

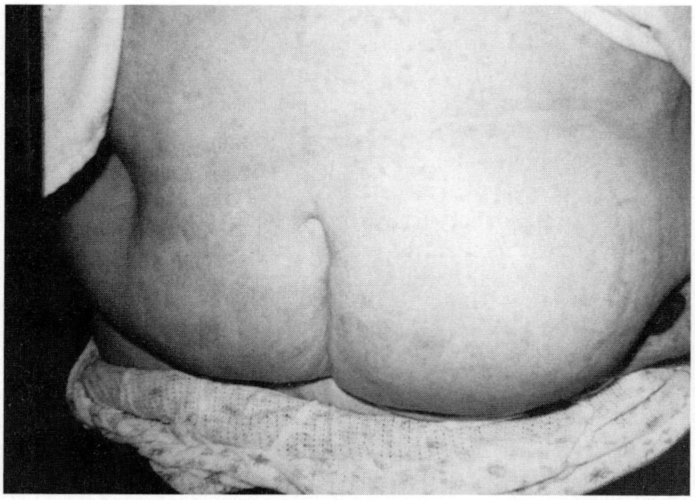

Figure 6 This poorly placed stoma is in a deep skin fold, on top of the iliac crest; it is invisible to the patient.

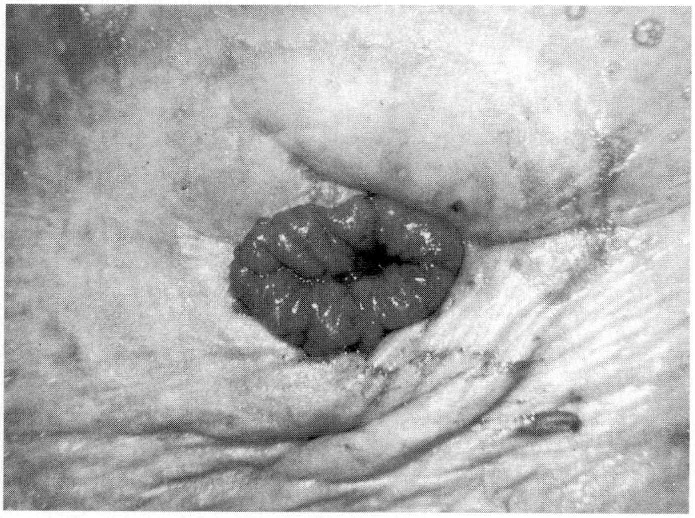

Figure 7 These multiple skin folds make the use of a leakproof pouch system very difficult.

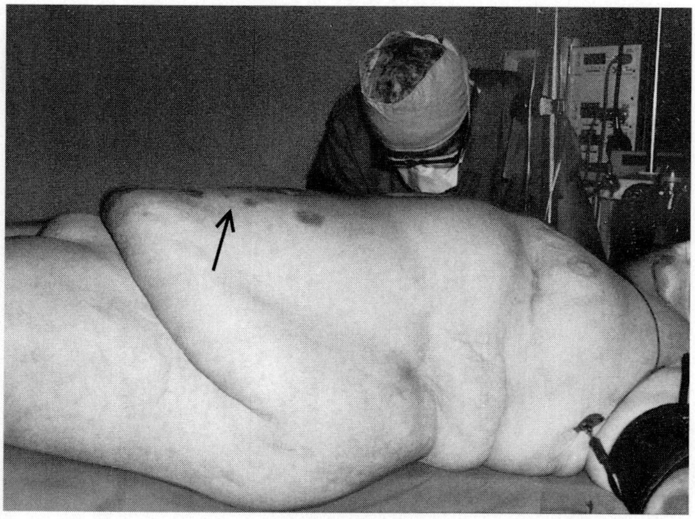

Figure 8 In this massively obese patient about to undergo an abdominoperineal proctectomy, the colostomy site selected (black dot) is above the belt line. The arrow points to the umbilicus.

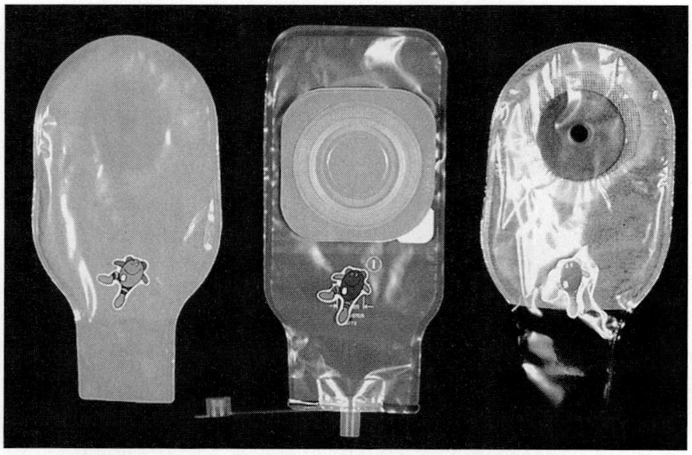

Figure 9 Shown are three pouches that are suitable for infant and newborn ostomates: a one-piece opaque pouch, a two-piece urinary pouch, and a one-piece clear infant pouch (Hollister).

ically for infants and newborns. These pouches not only are smaller but also have skin barriers that are gentler to and safer for newborns' skin [*see Figure 9*].

If the creation of a stoma in the vicinity of a scar is unavoidable, use of easily molded paste or wafers made of pectin, gelatin, and cellulose (e.g., Stomahesive or Hollihesive) can minimize, to some extent, the fitting problems such skin irregularities present.

Stomas for Handicapped Patients

In patients who wear orthopedic braces, are confined to wheelchairs, or are restricted by other handicaps, the stoma may have to be placed in an unconventional location. A surgeon must select a stoma site for such a patient with particular care, taking into consideration both the patient's infirmity and the position in which the patient plans to be when caring for the stoma. Accordingly, it may be advisable to choose the stoma site with the patient sitting in a wheelchair or wearing braces.

Often, with bedridden patients, the surgeon does not select a specific stoma site preoperatively. This is a mistake: when the patient is repositioned, especially into a sitting position, an appliance covering a stoma that was placed in a skin fold or a deep crease, too close to a scar, under a sagging breast, or too close to a feeding tube will tend to loosen and spill its contents. To minimize such problems, the surgeon need only spend a few minutes looking at the patient lying in bed in the usual position and then examine the abdomen for scars, deep folds, feeding tube sites, and other physical features that might impinge on the stoma. This simple step will save the surgeon many calls asking for a revision or a relocation of the stoma.

Stomas and Radiation Therapy

When it is anticipated that radiation therapy through lower abdominal portals will be necessary after operation, the stoma site should be located outside the radiation field, if possible.

When a patient has already undergone irradiation, the stoma should be placed outside the treated area to prevent skin breakdown and delayed healing.

MARKING THE STOMA SITE

It is essential that skin marks placed at the selected stoma site not fade away when the patient showers preoperatively or when his or her abdomen is washed in the operating room. Because truly indelible skin markers are unavailable, the preferred technique for identifying the selected stoma site is intradermal injection of methylene blue. Placement of superficial scratch marks, unless done immediately before operation, can cause local cellulitis that may contribute to postoperative problems with the stoma.

THE LAPAROSCOPICALLY CREATED STOMA

Because the only major difference between laparoscopic and conventional surgery is the access to the operative site,[9] stomal care is, for the most part, the same in patients who have undergone laparoscopic procedures as in those who have undergone open procedures. Creating a stoma laparoscopically involves pulling a segment of intestine through a trocar site and then enlarging the site to deliver the bowel onto the abdomen. Too often, either by necessity or by lack of foresight, the trocar site is not where the stoma site ideally should be. Additional thought must be given to trocar placement when one plans to create a stoma; a good site for the stoma must be selected and marked, even if this means inserting an additional port devoted exclusively to pulling out the stoma. The common practice of enlarging the trocar site by simply incising the adjacent skin is not to be recommended: it causes the stoma to be slit-shaped, with poor projection and a tendency to retract. Instead, the trocar orifice should be enlarged by excising a circular button of skin around the trocar site.

Postoperative Care

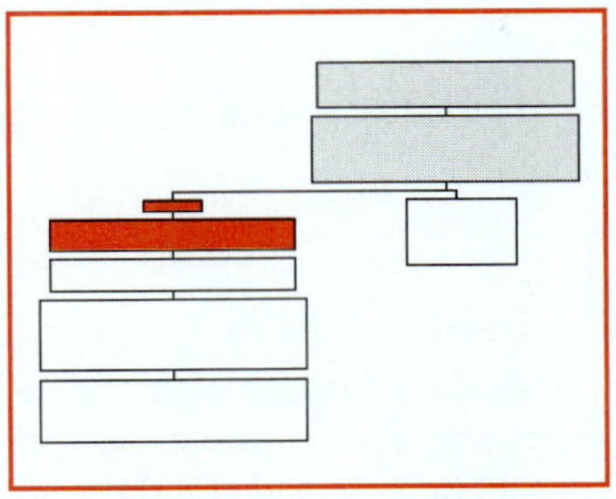

The following discussion is on general principles of stomal care. We do not address care of the various types of stoma separately, because the basic principles governing care are essentially the same for all types, except for some details that will be noted. Care of a continent pouch will be described separately.

IN THE OPERATING ROOM

Provided that the general principles of stoma construction are clearly followed (i.e., that the bowel is brought through the abdominal wall to the skin without tension, is brought through the rectus muscle with a good blood supply, and is everted and sutured primarily to the skin away from the incision, drains, and retention sutures), all electively created stomas, with very few exceptions, are matured and are ready for pouching at the end of the operation. Stomas created under emergency conditions should also be matured. The advantages of maturing the stoma (i.e., the immediate decompression of the bowel and the ease of caring for a matured stoma) far outweigh the disadvantages (i.e., the additional operating time needed to mature the stoma and the theoretical possibility of contaminating the peritoneal cavity with bowel contents). When a surgeon decides to delay the opening of a digestive stoma, the exteriorized bowel segment can simply be covered with a piece of petrolatum gauze and a sterile dressing. The gaseous distention, serositis, and bowel wall edema that eventually develop in such cases often make pouching and caring for these stomas after their opening a challenge.

The pouch used in the operating room should be transparent, drainable, disposable, and of one- or two-piece construction [see Figure 10]. A pouch system is available for digestive stomas that is simple and inexpensive yet fully adequate for the purpose. Before applying the pouch, the surgeon should cut a hole in the adhesive backing about 3 mm larger than the stoma to allow for postoperative swelling. Whereas digestive stoma pouches are closed by means of a clamp, urinary stoma pouches are connected to a drainage system.

Once a segment of bowel (i.e., the future stoma) has been exteriorized, the surgeon should exert his or her utmost efforts to avoid impinging on the peristomal skin necessary for securing the appliance. All too often, one sees retention sutures, drains, and feeding catheters placed carelessly in close proximity to a stoma. Such carelessness makes pouching difficult at best and frequently leads to leaks and the attendant skin problems. The problem of insufficient peristomal skin area can be circumvented to some degree by cutting and reshaping the adhesive area; however, this loss of adhesive surface may reduce the stability of the appliance.

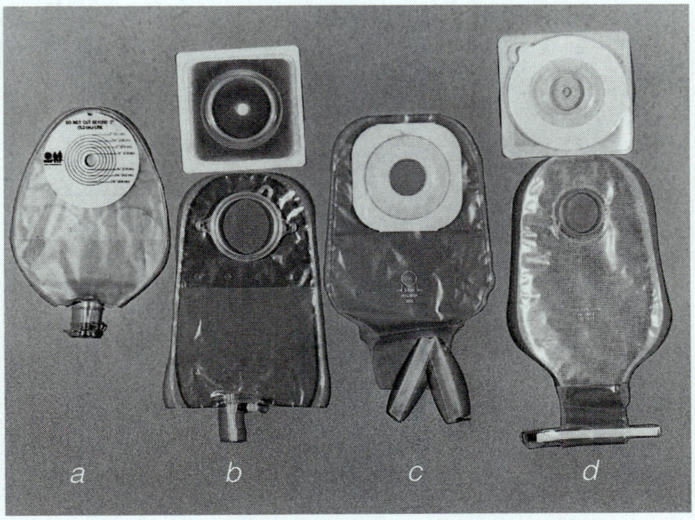

Rigid bridges of various designs are available for support of loop colostomies [see Figure 11]. These bridges should fit inside the stoma pouch; however, many do not. In addition, if these rigid bridges are sewn to the skin, the pouch opening will not fit adequately around the stoma. The peristomal skin will be bathed by stomal efflux, and the stitch holes create an avenue by which urine or stool can infect the skin. We recommend using a segment of No. 16 rubber catheter with its ends folded [see Figure 12]; this will serve the same purpose and can easily be inserted completely into the pouch. If a supporting bridge cannot be accommodated within the pouch, it is difficult

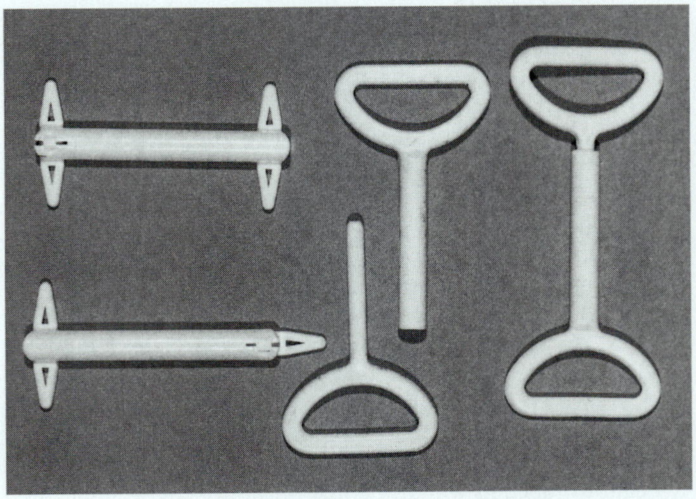

Figure 10 Four different types of pouch are shown: a one-piece urinary system (United) (*a*), a two-piece urinary system (ConvaTec) (*b*), a one-piece digestive pouch system (Hollister) (*c*), and a two-piece digestive pouch system (Coloplast) (*d*).

Figure 11 Rigid colostomy bridges that can fit inside a pouch system are used to support loop colostomies. They come in one- and two-piece forms.

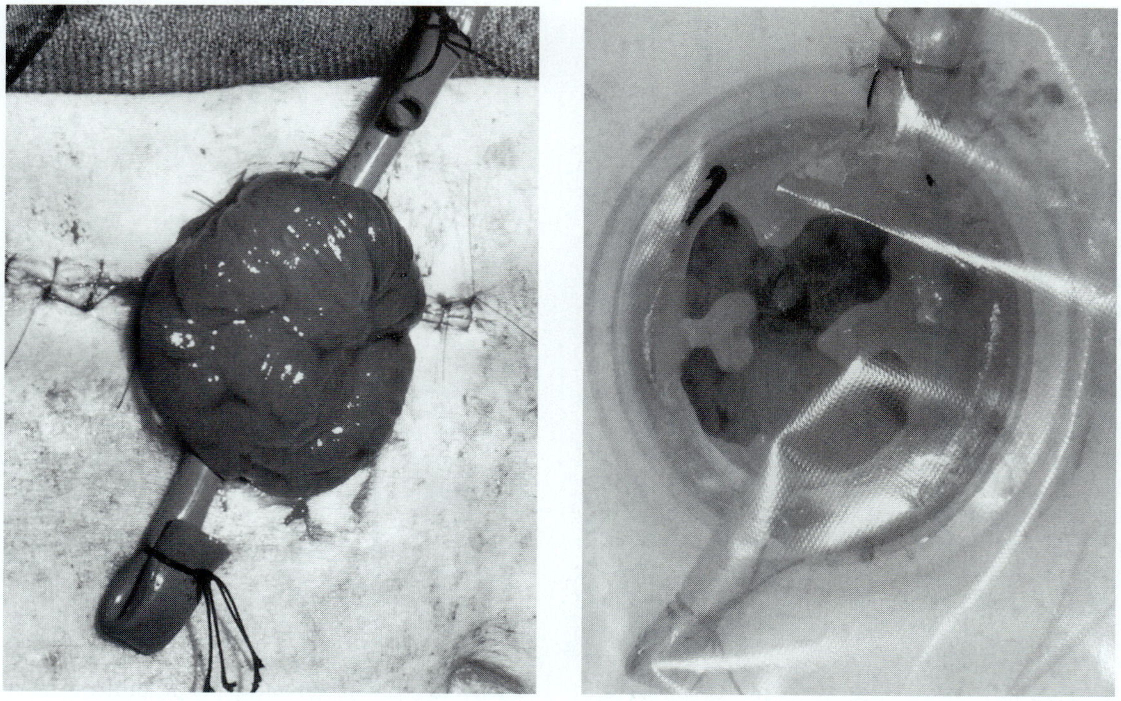

Figure 12 Use of a segment of No. 16 catheter is an easy and practical way to support a loop colostomy (*left*). The rubber bridge shown at left fits into the pouch (*right*).

to make the pouch system leakproof, unless some adhesive paste is used to fill the gap created by the rod between the skin and the adhesive wafer. The bulky plastic rods with rubber tubing that are traditionally used to hold a loop colostomy are out of place in modern stomal care.

FIRST POSTOPERATIVE DAY

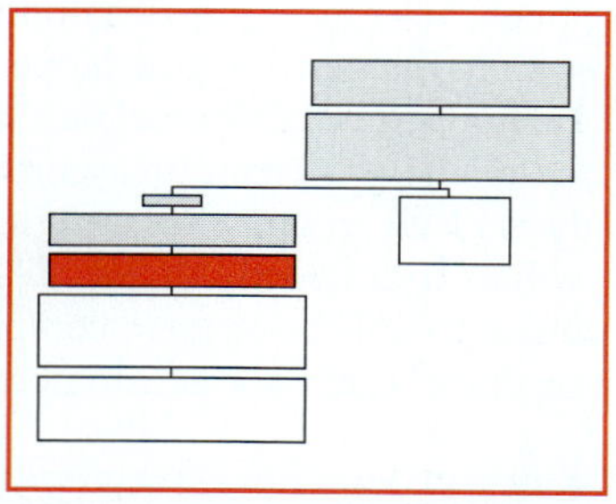

If the pouch is not leaking and the stoma color is good, there is little to be gained by changing the pouch. If a stoma is smeared with stool or its color cannot be determined, the pouch should be removed and the stoma gently wiped off with wet gauze and inspected. If the stoma appears to be healthy, a new disposable pouch should be applied; if not, the surgeon should be notified. The patient should be reassured and told that in the next few days he or she will be thoroughly instructed in the care of the stoma. Given the pressure for accelerated discharges imposed by managed care, it is necessary to begin involving the family in the care of the patient on the day after the operation, even if the patient is still somewhat obtunded. If the patient is alert at this time, the ET nurse or the staff nurse can start the postoperative education process by showing the patient how the pouch is changed and doing it for him or her. On the next day, the ET nurse or the staff nurse helps the patient change the pouch, and by the third day (or at least the third teaching session), the patient should be able to change the pouch unassisted under the guidance of the ET nurse or the staff nurse.

Whereas urinary stomas drain immediately, ileostomies generally begin to function within the first 48 postoperative hours, and colostomies take about twice that long. Stomas created under emergency conditions to relieve bowel obstruction may start to discharge promptly.

SUBSEQUENT DAYS

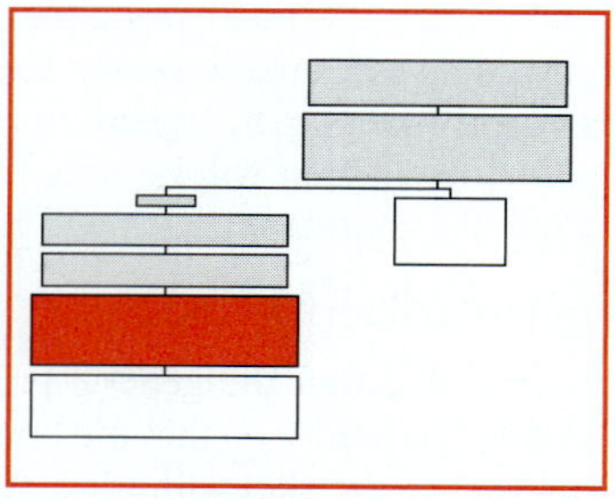

About 48 hours after operation, the entire pouch system should be removed and the peristomal skin cleaned. If any discoloration, retraction, or mucocutaneous separation is noted or, in a urinary stoma, if any of the stents seem displaced, these problems should be promptly reported to the surgeon. Mucocutaneous separation at the base of the stoma may be caused either by the breaking or untying of the sutures uniting the intestine to the skin or by the sutures having cut through the tissues. If such a separation is noted, one must apply a minimum of pressure at the base of the stoma when pouching to prevent further separation. If the separation is superficial, the area can be covered with a coating of Stomahesive powder. If the separation is wider and deeper, it should be filled with Stomahesive paste to protect the area, keep it moist, and promote granulation. The pouch wafer should cover the filled site to protect the subcutaneous tissue from the stoma efflux.

The pouch system with which the patient is to become familiar is then selected. The patient should be shown how the clamp or the spigot at the bottom of the pouch works. If the system is a two-piece one, the pouch and adhesive wafer are connected and then applied over the stoma as a unit, with care taken not to put pressure on the newly created stoma and the sutures fixing it to the skin. The patient should then be invited to place and close the clamp or to connect the spigot to drainage on the newly applied pouch; in this way, he or she is coaxed into looking at the stoma and touching the pouch. Further involvement of the patient in the care of the stoma should progress gradually, under the gentle and patient supervision of a member of the health care team.

During the next 48 to 72 hours, whenever the pouch of a diges-

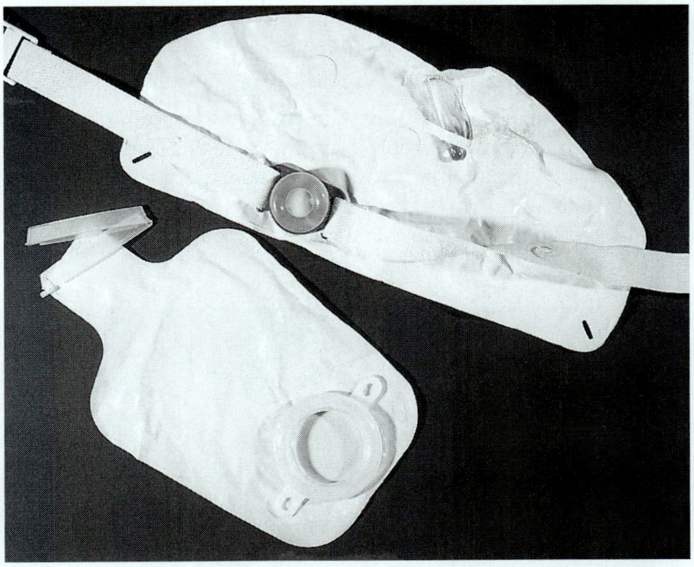

Figure 13 Shown is the VPI nonadhesive pouch system for intestinal and urinary stomas. The urinary appliance is the larger of the two.

tive stoma is one half to two thirds full, the pouch clamp should be removed and the pouch emptied and rinsed out rather than replaced. Rinsing is easily accomplished by means of a bulb syringe filled with tap water. The pouch should not be allowed to fill to the point where its sheer weight pulls it away from the patient's skin.

Once a day, the pouch of a urinary stoma should be rinsed through its spigot with 20 to 30 ml of vinegar to break up mucous plugs and to acidify the pouch wall so as to prevent bacterial proliferation and the formation of uric acid crystals. The pouch should then be reconnected to drainage.

At this stage, the pouch system should be changed every other day, unless leakage occurs. This schedule allows the staff to teach the patient how to care for the stoma. When the patient's appliance is changed, the portion adhering to the patient's abdomen should be carefully detached with the help of a cloth (either a piece of gauze or a washcloth) moistened with tap water; it should never be pulled off. The stoma and the peristomal skin should then be gently wiped clean with a moist cloth. We do not use permanent appliances that are cemented to the skin in the postoperative period. If such appliances are used, it must be remembered that skin cement solvent rather than water is needed to detach them from the skin. Currently, with the large assortment of disposable pouch systems available, the use of cement and rigid faceplates is seldom, if ever, indicated.

A reusable pouch system (the VPI system) [*see Figure 13*] has been developed that uses no adhesive and consists of a Silastic ring held in place with a belt. This system is favored by patients who have problems with adhesive pouch systems or who wish to change their pouch frequently. In particular, it is attractive to active people and to persons in wheelchairs, who appreciate the large capacity of the pouch and the fact that they can easily and atraumatically change their pouch system frequently. All of the components of the system—the belt, the Silastic ring, and the large-capacity pouch—are reusable and easy to clean and care for.

The patient should learn to measure the stoma with a measuring guide [*see Figure 14*] and cut out a properly sized hole in the appliance wafer so that the edge of the wafer is approximately $1/8$ in. away from the stomal mucosa; this allows for expansion. The wafer and the pouch should be connected and the appliance positioned as one piece over the stoma. The importance of a well-fitting stoma appliance to protect the peristomal skin cannot be overemphasized. The patient should be told about some of the potential local skin problems associated with the type of stoma selected and taught how to recognize them. The instructor must stress that most of these skin problems can be prevented by (1) proper fitting of the pouch system, (2) using the least irritating products at the stoma site, and (3) avoiding physical trauma to the skin in the region around the stoma. When a stoma is being pouched, additional support for the appliance can be provided by use of a belt or by framing the adhesive wafer with adhesive tape. Waterproof Perma Type tape can be used by patients planning to swim.

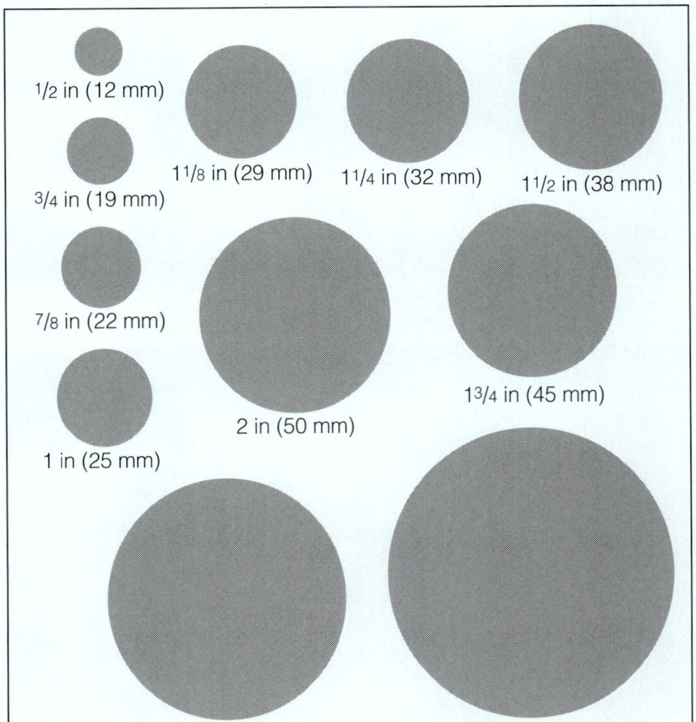

DISCHARGE OBJECTIVES

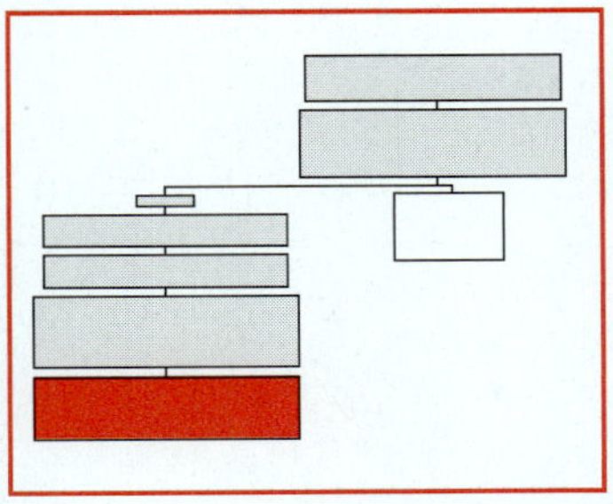

The psychosocial aspects of care discussed earlier [*see Preoperative Counseling, above*] should be reemphasized and elaborated on throughout the postoperative period. If the patient did not see or refused to see an ostomy visitor preoperatively, it may be appropriate to ask if he or she wants to see one at this time. If the patient is willing, a relative may learn to help him or her look after the stoma. If infirmity or age prevents a patient from attending to the stoma, a relative or friend must be called in. If relatives and friends are unavailable or are unable or unwilling to help, the services of a social worker must be obtained as soon as possible. In fact, this need for postdischarge assistance should have been anticipated preoperatively, and steps should have been taken to provide the patient with adequate support. Patients and caretakers should be made aware of the social and medical support systems available to them [*see Table 2*]. Either the surgeon or

Figure 14 Patients must learn to measure their stomas with the help of measuring guides, such as this one, provided by the manufacturers of stoma appliances.

Table 2 Social and Medical Support Systems Available to Ostomates and Caretakers

Social Resources
Hospital social worker
Medicare or CHAMPUS advisers
Local chapter of the United Ostomy Association
United Ostomy Association ostomy visitor
American Cancer Society

Medical Resources
Surgeon
Enterostomal therapy (ET) nurse
Family physician
Psychologist
Dietitian

the ET nurse should provide the patient with written instructions, supplies, and lists of suppliers (including phone numbers).

Before discharge, a patient or caretaker should be familiar with one type of pouch system. He or she should be able to (1) empty the pouch and cleanse the closure tail [see Figure 15], (2) detach the adhesive portion of the pouch system properly, (3) care for the peristomal skin, (4) measure the stoma and cut a hole of the correct size in the adhesive portion of the system, (5) apply the pouch system properly, and (6) be aware of the telltale signs of peristomal skin problems and know how to prevent and correct them.

Peristomal Skin Care

As noted, many skin problems can be prevented by taking a few simple precautions. Fungal infections (most commonly caused by *Candida*) often occur under a wafer because of body heat. These infections respond rapidly to topical antifungal powders such as Mycostatin. Fungal overgrowth can also occur where the warm plastic appliance presses over the abdomen. This problem can often be prevented by using a pouch cover, wearing bikini underpants under the pouch, or wearing specially designed underwear [see Figure 1] to keep the plastic away from the skin.

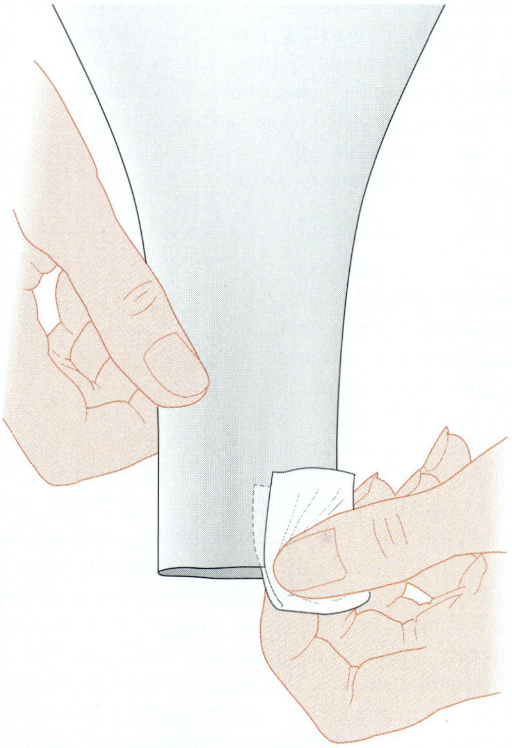

Figure 15 Once an open-end pouch is emptied, the closure tail must be cleansed.

The following three conditions can arise soon after surgery and demand immediate attention if they do:

1. Allergic contact dermatitis. The skin appears erythematous, weepy, or eroded in a pattern exactly corresponding to the shape of the offending product (e.g., tape or a skin barrier). Before a change is made to another skin barrier, a skin-barrier wipe or a transparent dressing should be used on the damaged skin in the interim so that a pouch can be secured. Patch test-

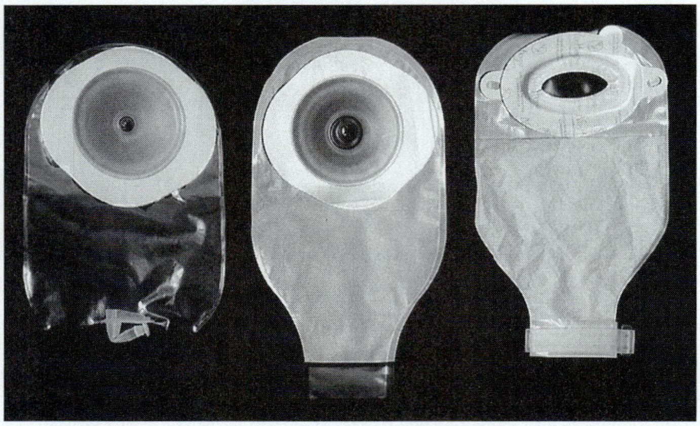

Figure 16 Shown are three convex pouches: a one-piece precut urostomy pouch (ConvaTec), an open-end bowel pouch (ConvaTec), and a one-piece bowel stoma pouch (NuHope).

a

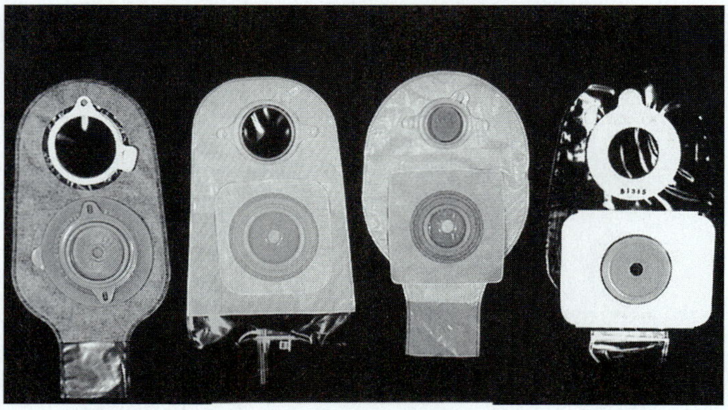

b

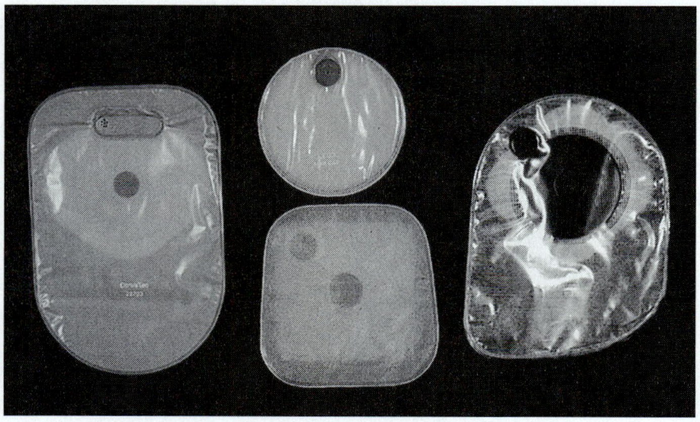

Figure 17 Shown are selected (*a*) two-piece pouches (Coloplast open-end, ConvaTec urinary, and Cymed open-end) and (*b*) closed-end pouches (ConvaTec, Dansac, United, and Hollister).

Table 3 Selected Manufacturers of Ostomy Products

Coloplast Corporation, 1955 W. Oak Circle, Marietta, GA 30062 (800-533-0464; www.us.coloplast.com)

ConvaTec, P.O. Box 5242, Princeton, NJ 08543-5254 (800-422-8811; www.convatec.com)

Cook Wound, 1100 W. Morgan Street, P.O. Box 266, Spencer, IN 47460 (800-843-4851)

Cymed, 1336A Channing Way, Berkeley, CA 94702 (800-582-0707; www.cymed-ostomy.com)

Dansac Ostomy Products, 307-A S. Westgate Drive, Greensboro, NC 27407 (800-538-0890; www.dansac.com)

Hollister, Inc., 2000 Hollister Drive, Libertyville, IL 60048 (800-323-4060; www.hollister.com)

Smith & Nephew United, Inc., 11775 Starkey Road, P.O. Box 1970, Largo, FL 33779 (800-876-1261; www.snwmd.com)

ing of another pouch system can be done by cutting a small piece of the new barrier wafer and tape and placing them on the opposite side of the patient's abdomen, forearm, or back for 24 hours and checking for any reaction.

2. Folliculitis (i.e., inflammation or infection of hair follicles). This condition usually arises when the abdominal hairs have grown back in the peristomal area and are forcibly pulled out with each pouch change. The patient should be instructed to remove the pouch using a wet piece of gauze or washcloth in a push-pull motion. When the folliculitis has healed, the patient should use an electric razor to shave the area and apply a skin sealant to protect the skin during pouch removal. Safety razors may cause small skin cuts that lead to skin infections. Application of an antimicrobial powder after the skin has been cleaned and dried is also helpful.

3. Irritant dermatitis. Either efflux from the stoma or the use of harsh cleansers may cause chemical burns. The skin appears erythematous, weepy, and painful, and the irritation may be restricted to a specific area of leakage. Treatment consists of (1) gently cleansing all of the peristomal skin, (2) dusting with Stomahesive powder, and (3) correcting any pouching problems that may have caused the leak.

Besides these three conditions, all of which may appear in the early postoperative period, there are a number of complications that may arise later, such as radiation reactions, parastomal abscesses, caput medusae, pseudoepithelial hyperplasia, pyoderma gangrenosum, and parastomal ulcers.

The patient should be seen for stomal and pouch evaluation 3 months after the operation and subsequently on an annual basis or as necessary for management of complications. Either weight gain or weight loss may necessitate changing the pouch system. In either event, the use of convex pouches may prove helpful [*see Figure 16*].

The patient must be aware that as long as the wafer is protecting the peristomal skin and is securely fixed to it, there is no compelling reason to change it. Wearing time generally ranges from 3 to 6 days and depends on both the individual and the pouch system used. If a patient has problems with the appliance, he or she should consult the surgeon or an ET nurse, who may recommend a change in the pouching steps or, if necessary, a change of pouch systems. Improvements are constantly being made in the design and manufacture of stoma equipment; some of the newer systems may fit or be worn more comfortably. There are several makers of high-quality equipment whose products [*see Figure 17*] we use regularly [*see Table 3*].

Written Patient Information

Most ostomy patients are under such intense stress after the op-

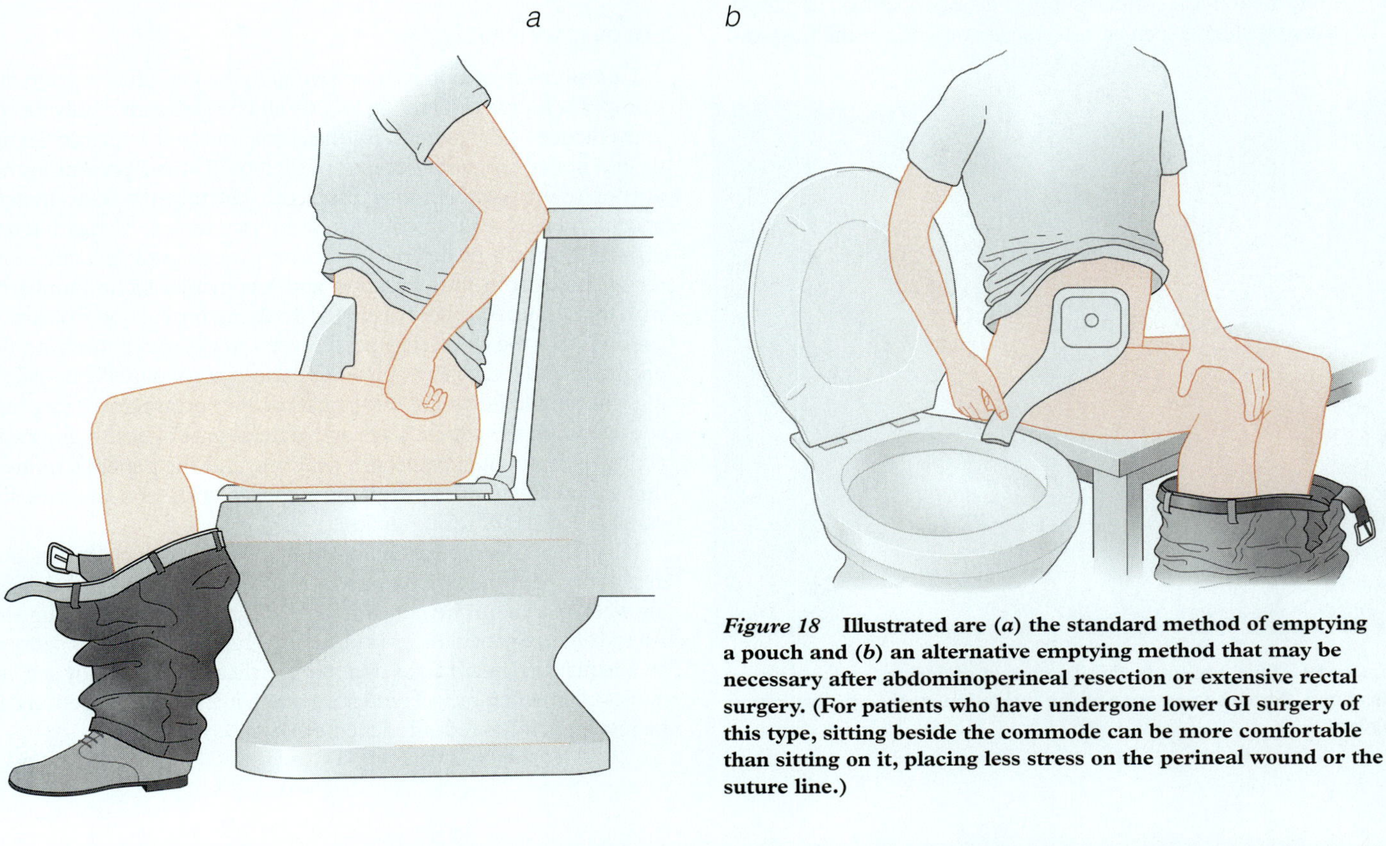

Figure 18 Illustrated are (*a*) the standard method of emptying a pouch and (*b*) an alternative emptying method that may be necessary after abdominoperineal resection or extensive rectal surgery. (For patients who have undergone lower GI surgery of this type, sitting beside the commode can be more comfortable than sitting on it, placing less stress on the perineal wound or the suture line.)

Table 4 Selected Companies Selling Stoma Appliances through Mail-Order Catalogues

AOS—American Ostomy Supply Guide, P.O. Box 13396, Milwaukee, WI 53213-9906; 800-858-5858

Edgepark Surgical, Inc., 1810 Summit Commerce Park, Twinsburg, OH 44087-9931; 800-321-0591

MED EXPRESS, P.O. Box 49850, Minneapolis, MN 55449-9908; 877-409-1234

Parthenon Co., 3311 W. 2400 Street, Salt Lake City, UT 84119; 800-453-8898

eration and the creation of the stoma that they cannot absorb all the oral instructions they receive. For this reason, it is important to give them some written information, preferably in a folder; they may or may not read this material while in the hospital, but they will have it at home to use as a reference after discharge. The patient information folder should contain the following components:

1. General stomal care instructions [see Figure 18].
2. Specific instructions on caring for their particular type of stoma.
3. Specific directions for applying and caring for their particular pouch system.
4. A list of the steps involved in changing the pouch.
5. Some general dietary instructions, along with explanations of what a stoma blockage is, how to prevent it, and what to do before calling the physician.
6. A guide to recognizing signs of urinary infection (for patients with ileal conduits).
7. A number where the ET can be reached for answers to questions and for discussion of any stoma or pouch problems that may arise, along with the date of the 3-month return visit to the ET for evaluation of the stoma and the pouch system.
8. A referral to local ostomy support group meetings. Ideally, the patient will have seen an ostomy visitor while in the hospital.
9. Information on where and how to obtain stoma appliances and a reminder to check with the insurance company to see whether supplies must be purchased from a specific vendor. A list of local pharmacies or medical suppliers should be included, along with, if needed or desired, a mail-order catalogue [see Table 4].

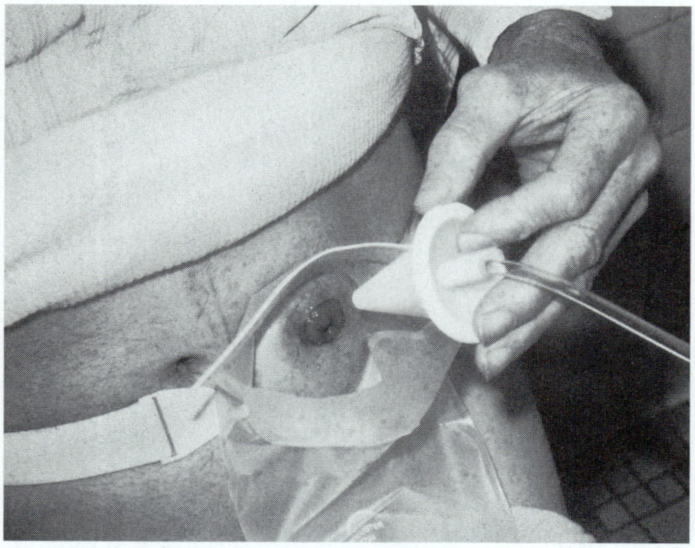

POSTOPERATIVE CARE OF PATIENTS WITH CONTINENT STOMAS

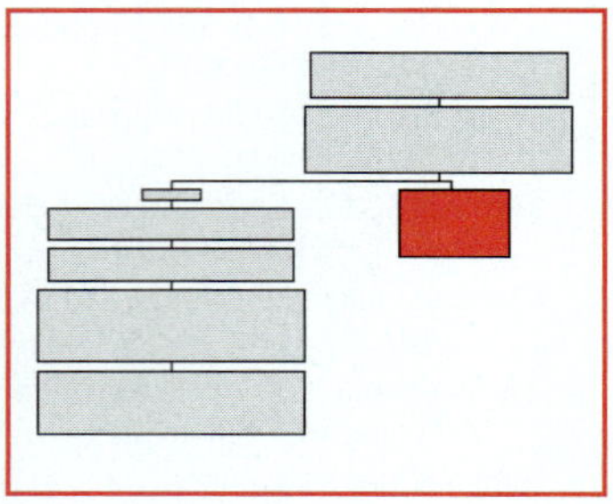

A patient with a continent stoma does not use an external pouch, and hence, certain aspects of his or her care are different. Nevertheless, a patient with a continent stoma also requires the expert planning, counseling, and care that other ostomates require.

After the construction of a continent ileostomy, the surgeon intubates the intestinal pouch with a No. 30 Silastic catheter. A silk tie is placed around the catheter at the level of the stoma to mark the correct position of the tube. The tube is then affixed securely to the skin. It is left in place for about 10 days, and the intestinal pouch is allowed to empty by gravity. The tube must be irrigated with 30 ml of normal saline solution every 6 hours or so to ensure that it remains patent. As soon as the patient expresses interest, he or she may participate in the irrigation of the intestinal pouch and in the washing of the stoma and the surrounding skin. About 10 days after operation, the patient should be taught how to extubate and intubate the intestinal pouch. At this point, the tube should not be kept out of the pouch for more than 30 minutes at a time. Drainage through the catheter is facilitated by saline irrigations.

About 4 weeks after the operation, the patient will extubate and reintubate the stoma at preset times separated by gradually longer intervals, which allows the intestinal pouch to distend progressively.

A similar postoperative approach is required after the creation of a urinary continent pouch, such as the so-called Indiana pouch.[10]

COLOSTOMY IRRIGATION

Colostomy irrigation is not essential to the good functioning of a stoma.[11] It is time consuming and should be performed only for the convenience of the patient. Stomas proximal to the splenic flexure should not be irrigated because of the liquid stools present in that portion of the bowel. In most cases, the teaching of colostomy self-irrigation [see Sidebar Recommended Procedures for Irrigation and Figure 19] should be deferred for several weeks, until the patient has recuperated from the operation and has gained some familiarity with the stoma. Another reason for deferring instruction in self-irrigation is that the colon may need several weeks to recover from the operation and return to its previous pattern of motility. When deciding who should be taught self-irrigation, the surgeon must take into consideration the patient's age and general state of health, the availability of reasonable bathroom facilities, and the patient's motivation and ability to put up with the inconvenience (and, at times, the variable results) of self-irrigation.

If a patient is to receive chemotherapy postoperatively, instruction in self-irrigation should be postponed. If the patient is already irrigating when placed on chemotherapy, irrigation should be discontinued. All too often, a patient receiving chemotherapy is too tired to perform an adequate irrigation; moreover, the diarrhea that frequently accompanies chemotherapy will render irrigation ineffectual. Irrigation can be resumed, if desired, after chemotherapy is completed.

Figure 19 This patient is about to insert an irrigating cone into his stoma. Note the presence of the irrigation sleeve and the retaining belt.

Recommended Procedures for Irrigation

If irrigation is to be performed, the following instructions for the patient are recommended.

Supplies
Irrigation bag with long tube and cone; sleeve with belt.

Water
Tepid tap water, 1,000–1,500 ml.

Procedure

1. Fill the irrigation bag with tepid water, remove air in the tube by allowing water to run through it and into the sink, close the clamp, hang up the irrigation bag at a height that will allow the bottom of the bag to be at the level of your shoulder when you are seated.
2. Sit on the toilet or a chair beside the toilet (if the perineum is still sore).
3. Remove the colostomy appliance.
4. Center the opening of the irrigation sleeve over the stoma, and place the end of the sleeve in the toilet bowl. To avoid splashing, the sleeve need only be long enough to touch the water. If it is too long, it may be cut. Tighten the irrigation sleeve belt to prevent leakage.
5. Lubricate the end of the cone with water or a water-soluble lubricant. Insert the cone tip gently through the top of the open sleeve and into the stoma, and rotate the cone until the water flows in freely. (If the water does not flow in freely, do not push the cone in further; instead, pull the cone back and rotate it because usually the cause of the limited water flow is that the opening of the cone is against the bowel wall.)
6. Press the cone firmly and gently against the stoma to prevent leakage.
7. The water must flow in slowly. It takes about 5 minutes to instill a quart. Stop the flow of water if you become uncomfortable or experience cramps, but do not remove the cone, because removal would allow the water to return too soon.
8. When all the water has been emptied from the irrigation bag and tube, remove the cone from the stoma. Close the top of the irrigation sleeve with clips or ties.
9. Allow about 15 to 20 minutes for the bowel to empty, with the sleeve end remaining in the toilet.
10. Rinse the sleeve with water, and clamp the end closed. You may leave the bathroom and do what you wish for the next 30 to 45 minutes. During this time, additional water and stool may be expelled.
11. Return to the bathroom, unclamp the sleeve, empty any effluence, and rinse the sleeve. With time, you will know when evacuation is completed. Unsnap the belt, and remove the sleeve.
12. Wash the peristomal skin with warm water, rinse well, pat dry, and replace your appliance.
13. Clean the sleeve with detergent and water, rinse it well, and allow it to air-dry. Let any remaining fluid in the irrigation bag and tubing drain out. Wash, rinse, and dry off the cone.

The entire procedure should take about 1 hour.

General Pointers

1. For the first irrigations you perform, write down the amount of water used, the amount of time for the procedure, and the amount and character of the water and stool expelled. If you record this information for the first few irrigations, you will learn how long to wait for a total evacuation, how much fluid to use, and how often you need to irrigate.
2. Good results are obtained by performing the procedure at about the same time each day. Some individuals need to irrigate only every other day.
3. Because you do not eat the same type or amount of food daily, the amount of elimination will vary from day to day. Persons who are dehydrated may at times need extra irrigation fluid because some of that fluid will be quickly absorbed by the colon.
4. Try to relax when performing irrigation. If you are nervous or upset, often this method will not work for you. If you are ill or experiencing diarrhea, you should temporarily discontinue irrigation.
5. Remember: to irrigate or not to irrigate is your choice.

References

1. Rothman CP: Sperm banking. Common Problems in Infertility and Impotence. Rajfer J, Ed. Year Book Medical Publishers, Chicago, 1990, p 200
2. Metcalf AM, Dozois RR, Kelly KA: Sexual function in women after proctocolectomy. Ann Surg 204:624, 1986
3. Emblem R, Stray Pedersen S, Bergan A, et al: Female complaints after proctocolectomy. Proceedings of the Seventh Biennial Congress of the World Council of Enterostomal Therapists. Palex International SA, 1990, p 20
4. Gloeckner MR, Starling JR: Providing sexual information to ostomy patients. Dis Colon Rectum 25:575, 1982
5. Physician's Desk Reference, 51st ed. Medical Economics, Montvale, New Jersey, 1997, pp 1103, 1677, 2588
6. Fazio VW, Erwin-Toth P: Enterostomal therapy. Colon and Rectal Surgery, 4th ed. Corman ML, Ed. Lippincott-Raven, Philadelphia, 1998
7. Ohmura Y: Evaluation of preoperative stoma site marking. Proceedings of the Seventh Biennial Congress of the World Council of Enterostomal Therapists. Palex International SA, 1990, p 27
8. Bass EM, Pino AD, Tan A, et al: Does preoperative stoma marking and education by the enterostomal therapist affect outcome? Dis Colon Rectum 40:440, 1997
9. Milsom JW, Bohm B: Laparoscopic Colorectal Surgery. Springer, New York, 1995
10. Rowland RG, Mitchell ME, Bihrie R, et al: Indiana continent urinary reservoir. J Urol 137:1136, 1986
11. Laucks SS 2nd, Mazier WP, Milsom JW, et al: An assessment of colostomy irrigation. Dis Colon Rectum 31:279, 1988

Reviews

Broadwell DC, Jackson BS: Principles of Ostomy Care. CV Mosby Co, St. Louis, 1982

Celestin LR: Color Atlas of the Surgery and Management of Intestinal Stomas. Year Book Medical Publishers, Chicago, 1987

Dozois R: Alternatives to Conventional Ileostomy. Year Book Medical Publishers, Chicago, 1985

Goldstein BG, Jackson BS: Principles of Ostomy Care. CV Mosby Co, St. Louis, 1982

Gordon PH, Nivatvong S: Colon, Rectum, and Anus. Quality Medical Publishers, St. Louis, 1999

Jeter K: These Special Children: The Ostomy Book for Parents of Children with Colostomies, Ileostomies, and Urostomies. Bull Publishing Co, Palo Alto, 1982

McDougal WS: Use of intestinal segments and urinary diversions. Campbell's Urology, vol 3. Walsh PC, Retik AB, Vaughan ED, et al, Eds. WB Saunders Co, Philadelphia, 1998, p 3121

Smith DB, Johnson DE: Ostomy Care and the Cancer Patient: Surgical and Clinical Considerations. Grune & Stratton, Orlando, Florida, 1986

Acknowledgments

Figures 1, 15, and 18   Tom Moore.

Figure 3 and Sidebar illustrations   Carol Donner.

106 REHABILITATION OF THE BURN PATIENT

Robert H. Demling, M.D.

Return to Normal Function after a Burn

Rehabilitation is the return to normal function. This process is particularly difficult in burn patients because healing is a long-term process and burn scars are permanent.

Rehabilitation begins on the day of admission, with the objectives of restoring cardiopulmonary stability and minimizing musculoskeletal dysfunction. Long-term objectives are the maintenance or restoration of function in affected areas, the control of scarring and wound contractures, the restoration of the whole patient to functional activity, and the adjustment to cosmetic and functional abnormalities. Rehabilitation efforts include the following six components aimed at minimizing disability: early wound closure; exercise, positioning, and splinting; skin care; thermoregulation; psychological support; and restoration of function. Each component requires special expertise, making an integrated team approach essential.

Components of Rehabilitation

EARLY WOUND CLOSURE

Early wound excision can minimize functional loss by removing the nonpliable eschar and eliminating wound pain [*see 33 Burn Care in the Early Postresuscitation Period*]. Even with deep burns, pain develops after eschar separation, which begins approximately 1 week after the burn. A split-thickness skin graft, although more elastic than eschar, does not have normal elasticity, and wound stiffness has to be counterbalanced with aggressive therapy and splinting.

Early grafting can hamper general function in two ways. First, pain at the sites of donor skin can limit the range of motion, often interfering with ambulation. The use of skin substitutes can decrease pain at donor sites and improve mobility. Second, grafted areas must be immobilized to permit neovascularization. From 3 to 5 days of immobilization is usually adequate if the grafts are placed on residual dermis or fascia, but grafts on fatty tissue take 5 to 7 days to revascularize. The use of temporary skin substitutes on superficial second-degree burns and donor sites improves function by decreasing pain and increasing flexibility.

EXERCISE

As soon as feasible, the burn areas should be evaluated for estimates of current and future limitations of motion. This evaluation should be made in the first 24 hours after a small to moderate burn and during the first 24 to 48 hours after a large burn. Supervised motion of burned areas should begin as soon as possible. The goals of exercise are to maintain normal joint range, maintain strength and endurance, and promote functional independence. Although functional independence is the long-range goal, progressive independence is needed throughout rehabilitation. Proper positioning and splinting must be used to maintain the positive effects of exercise.

The selection of exercise techniques depends on the extent of injury and the patient's progress in recovery. In active exercises, the patient achieves a greater range of motion, resistance is increased as the patient progresses, and eventually the patient exercises independently. In active assistive exercise, the patient receives assistance from weights, pulleys, and other devices that permit stretching that exceeds the patient's strength. Passive exercises are used in critically ill patients, often with anesthesia, to increase the range of motion. Passive resistive exercise relies on weights and other mechanical means to increase strength and endurance. Stretching, which can be a component of either active or passive exercise, gradually increases force to increase the range of motion and restore position; stretching is used in conjunction with splints. Any of these active and passive techniques can be used in combination with a stationary bicycle or other means of developing endurance. Ambulation improves the patient's range of motion, strength, endurance, and independence.

Active and passive motion are assisted by the use of hydrotherapy, which relaxes the patient as well as affected muscles. A daily hydrotherapy session is ideal to begin movement in previously immobilized joints. A 3- to 5-minute period of muscle activity every few hours helps maintain joint motion; longer periods of muscle activity (25 to 30 minutes twice daily) help improve muscle strength. With increased muscle action, tissue edema resolves more rapidly, the appetite is stimulated, and the patient's self-image improves with evidence of progress. Between 2 and 3 weeks after injury, weight lifting and isometric exercise can be added to standard exercises to extend the range of motion.

Early exercise for the hand should emphasize finger range of motion, particularly flexion of the metacarpophalangeal joints, extension of the interphalangeal joints, and thumb abduction and opposition. Wrist exercises should emphasize extension and ulnar deviation because flexion and radial deviation are the most common abnormalities. Forearm supination and pronation are performed with the elbow close to the side to keep the shoulder from assuming the motion of the forearm. Elbow extension, shoulder abduction, and external rotation should be emphasized. Riding a stationary bicycle is an excellent means of strengthening the lower extremities while improving cardiopulmonary reserve. Consistent activity is an essential component of care, even in patients with massive burns. The success of the activity program depends on control of pain and anxiety and on motivation. Premedication before exercise is important, and biofeedback techniques are benefi-

Table 1 Positioning of Burn Areas during Rest

Area	Position
Neck	Extended by pillow or rolled towel placed under neck
Arm	Shoulder abducted 80° to 90°, elbow fully extended, wrists extended 30° to 40° by use of pillows and bedside tables
Hand	Elevated, with metacarpophalangeal joint in 90° flexion; fingers separated, with interphalangeal joints in midflexion; and thumb in midabduction
Trunk/hip	Hip abducted 20°, with knee extended; for short periods, prone position promotes hip extension
Foot	Neutral ankle position, with padding for heel

cial, although difficult to learn. A successful exercise program requires a team effort, with the involvement of all care providers.

The criteria of pulse, blood pressure, respiration, fatigue, pain, and electrocardiography are used to monitor exercise tolerance. Pain is probably the most difficult criterion to monitor because it is the most subjective. All components of the exercise plan are essential and must be integrated into other daily activities, especially burn care, sleep, and nutrition. Exercise and nutrition can be combined, for example, by fabricating simple devices that allow the patient to feed himself or herself. This approach increases independence and improves the patient's self-image. Evidence of progress maintains the patient's cooperation and enthusiasm. Simple techniques, such as marking the floor where the last attempt at ambulation stopped or the wall at the height of the last stretch, show progress and establish new goals.

Careful supervision is required if a joint has been immobilized for a long period or muscle atrophy has eliminated joint protection by muscle tone. Heterotopic calcification is particularly difficult to treat because movement is extremely painful and forced movement may exaggerate the local inflammatory process. Early mobilization of injured areas and early ambulation can prevent heterotopic calcification.

POSITIONING AND SPLINTING

Although exercise is effective in preventing loss of function, patients invariably resume the position of comfort between exercise sessions. This position then leads to contractures. For this reason, exercise, positioning [see Table 1], and splinting are closely linked, all being essential to rehabilitation. Splints maintain position in areas not amenable to positioning techniques or, after grafting, allow revascularization. Splints and positioning are often needed for burns of the neck, especially at night or when fatigue develops. Splints are often needed for elbows [see Figure 1], but the area most likely to require splinting is the burned wrist and hand. Wrist flexion is a common abnormality, affecting hand and finger function. If the wrist requires a splint, it should be placed over the wound dressing, from the proximal forearm to the palmar crease, extending the wrist 20° to 40°. The burned hand requires a splint that maintains wrist extension and keeps the metacarpophalangeal joint at 80° to 90° flexion and the interphalangeal joint fully extended. The thumb should be abducted and opposed. Splints may be needed to maintain the foot in neutral, overcoming the powerful pull of the extensors.

Thermoplastic materials used in many splints become pliable in hot water (at 160° to 170° F) and cool rapidly at room temperature, making it possible to mold and readjust them as edema resolves or other gains are made. Splints should be worn at night and during other periods of extended inactivity. Dynamic splinting, with the addition of a pull, adds a component of exercise. Such splinting techniques require a well-trained therapist because improper splints can result in serious complications.

PRESSURE GARMENTS AND SKIN CARE

Constant pressure of 25 to 30 mm Hg on the hypertrophic scar reduces its size and hyperemia. The initial reduction reflects decreased edema and blood flow in the wound. The long-term reduction appears to be caused by decreases in collagen and ground substance deposition, also reflecting decreased blood flow and a decrease in available tissue oxygen. After several weeks of pressure for 22 to 23 hours daily, there is a measurable reduction in wound chondroitin sulfate and myofibroblasts. Pressure garments also improve venous return, which is particularly important if the venous system was compromised by a deep burn or excision to fascia. Because of their contours, areas such as the eyes, nose, mouth, and anterior chest usually do not receive adequate pressure. For these areas, a mold of the contour can be fitted and a garment placed over the mold, providing pressure [see Figure 2]. Custom-made pressure inserts can fit any area. Once the wound is closed, garments are used; at first, they are worn for only a few hours a day, but gradually, the period of use is increased to about 22 hours daily. The pressure has to be applied until the scar matures, as is evident from lack of hyperemia, a process taking 12 to 18 months. Problems can occur if the fitting is not perfect or if rapid weight gain makes the fit too tight. Wound erosions can develop, necessitating removal of the garments until the wounds heal.

The skin must also be constantly lubricated to prevent drying and cracking. Skin moisturizers, usually lanolin based, need to be applied several times a day [see Table 2]. Patients who wear pressure garments need to use a special lubricant that does not harm the fabric. Prolonged exposure to direct sunlight should be avoided until the scar has matured or the skin has thickened. Temperature and humidity extremes must be avoided, especially by patients with large burns. If sweat glands have been destroyed, increased humidity is poorly tolerated in the summer, often requiring the use of an air conditioner and dehumidifier in the home or at work. In cold weather, the dry air often leads to rapid drying of skin, necessitating use of a humidifier in the home. Many of these early problems resolve in 12 to 24 months.

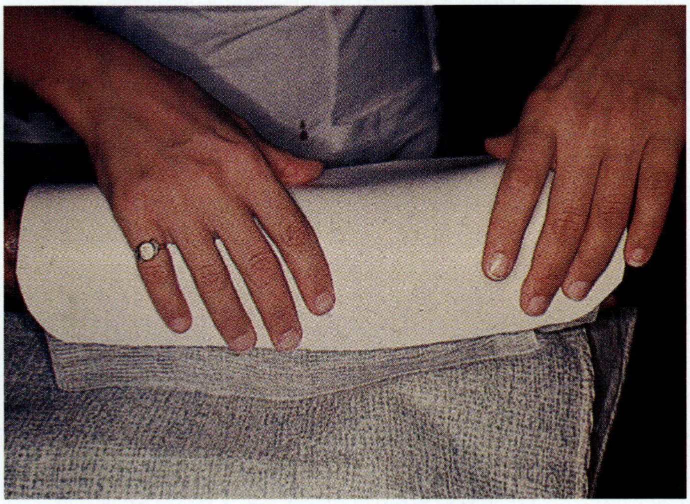

Figure 1 Shown is an elbow splint being molded to hold the joint in the proper position.

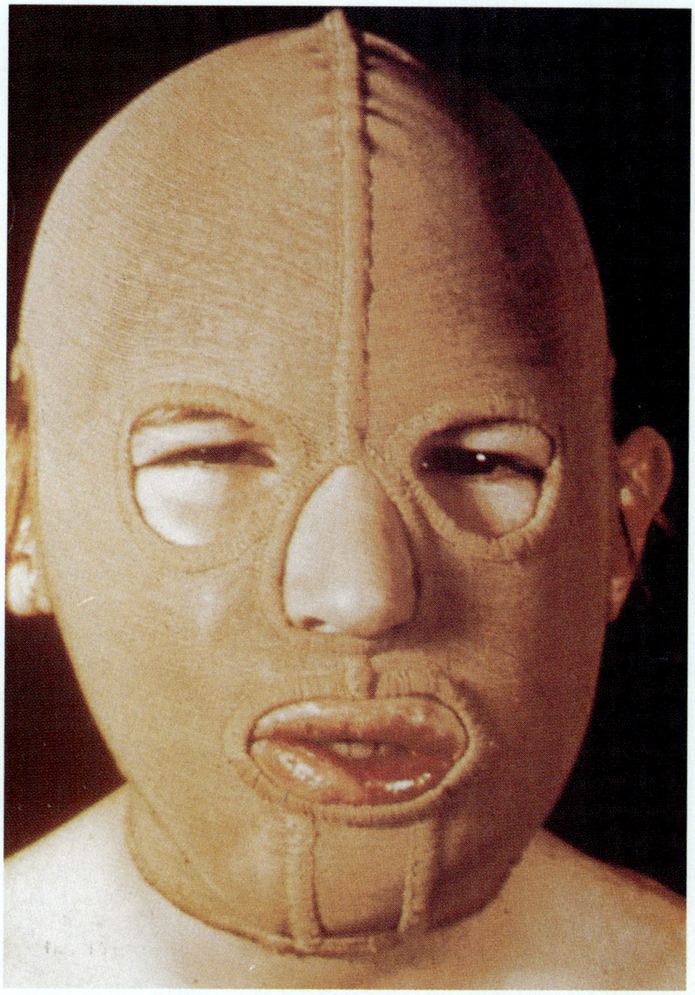

Figure 2 Shown is a compression garment applied to a healed or grafted burn to decrease scar formation.

come dependent, they must be strongly encouraged, if not required, to be as independent as possible. Patients' independence must be maintained by their families as well. A key to this independence is a structured plan for daily activities, allowing each patient a measure of control.

Thus, psychosocial support requires independence, good communication, avoidance of unnecessary anxiety (caused by fear of the unknown), adequate sedation and analgesia, an organized daily plan, adequate sleep, and psychosocial assistance for patients, their families, and staff.

Patients should have some input in the scheduling of daily activities. Initially, staff members may need to establish goals. Because of the close interaction of patients and staff over a long period of time, it is often difficult for staff to remain objective. In addition, patients' family members suffer stress because of the magnitude of injury as well as the time required for healing. A psychiatrist or psychologist and a social worker are key members of the burn team. They must become involved early in the course of treatment and not be called in only when serious difficulties arise, because preventive measures may be much more effective than treatment of psychological problems.

Table 2 Skin Care in Burn Rehabilitation

Problem	Treatment
Skin surface blistering and breakdown	Avoid poorly fitted compression garments, splints, and clothing Use lubricating lotions Use nonadherent dressings Use mild soaps
Pigmentation	Wear pressure garments Avoid direct sunlight until scar matures and skin is thickened
Itching	Consider using antihistamines or hydrocortisone cream Use nonirritating skin lubricants Avoid temperature extremes that induce sweating
Impaired thermoregulation	Avoid temperature extremes Wear loose-fitting clothing appropriate for the season

PSYCHOSOCIAL SUPPORT

Members of the treatment team must be aware of potential problems and be able to recognize them if they occur. Some emotional problems can be prevented or minimized if the staff communicates adequately with patients, preparing them for procedures and discussing their likely outcome. Because patients may regress and be-

Discussion

Pathophysiology

BURN EDEMA AND ESCHAR RIGIDITY

The massive edema that develops beneath the eschar and the nonpliable nature of the eschar seriously impair muscle and joint motion. The edema-induced stiffness lasts 7 to 10 days, long enough for a contracture to develop if the correct position is not maintained. Compared with normal skin, the burn eschar is extremely noncompliant, shrunken by the loss of water and cell substances. Muscle and joint motion depends on the stretching of contiguous nonburned or more superficially burned skin. The eschar may remain in place for extended periods, depending on the approach to grafting and the availability of donor sites. It is important to recognize functional limitations, such as joint stiffness and muscle atrophy.

FUNCTIONAL IMPAIRMENT

Stretching of a burn wound is painful, the comfortable position being the one that minimizes stretch. Continued flexion or adduction at large joints, as well as hyperextension of the metacarpophalangeal joints, often develops. A particularly disabling process with a third-degree hand burn is pressure necrosis of the central slip of the digital extensor tendon at the proximal interphalangeal joint. This is caused by exaggerated flexion when the metacarpophalangeal joint is hyperextended. The most common position abnormalities are adduction of shoulders; flexion at the elbows, wrists, neck, or interphalangeal joints; and hyperextension of the feet.

The patient's motion is limited not only by pain but also by monitoring devices, ventilator tubing, and other equipment. The forced immobility may be necessary if the patient is in a life-threatening situation with cardiopulmonary instability. More often, however, the lack of motion is for the convenience of both patient and medical care providers. In nonburned patients, inactivity is often well tolerated with few, if any, permanent sequelae; in burn patients, immobility may mean losing the battle against the contracting wound. What begins as voluntary immobility rapidly evolves into an intrinsic defect. Another form of restraint occurs after early skin grafting (and later reconstructive procedures). Although it would be ideal to immobilize the graft for 7 to 10 days, as in a nonburned patient, the result in a burn patient would be significant tissue rigidity and muscle atrophy, seriously restricting motion.

Three pathophysiologic processes—contracture and hypertrophic scar formation, muscle loss, and heterotopic calcification and ossification—are potentiated by lack of motion.

CONTRACTURE AND HYPERTROPHIC SCAR FORMATION

The natural course of a wound that remains open for more than 3 weeks is the deposition of dense scar. Complete epithelialization before 3 weeks usually leads to only minimal scarring, but some patients produce incredible amounts of scar despite relatively superficial injuries. Wound contraction is produced by contractile myofibroblasts and the deposition of ground substance and collagen. A shortened noncompliant wound at a joint results in a contracture, the most common contractures being identical to the most common position abnormalities (resulting from inadequate motion). These are flexion contractures (of the elbows, wrists, neck, and interphalangeal joints), adduction contractures of the shoulders, and extension contractures of the feet and metacarpophalangeal joints.

Hypertrophic scarring occurs after continued scar deposition in the reepithelialized wound. The scar is a raised, hyperemic, pruritic wound—a serious physical blemish as well as a cause of rigidity and pain, impairing function. Pain associated with movement limits activity, and continued itching leads to scratching, skin breakdown, and the risk of superficial infection. Exercise may cause the scar to split, especially if the scar becomes dry, increasing pain and the risk of infection. Keloid formation is the exaggerated form of this process, which is more likely to occur if there is any delay in wound closure. Wounds requiring more than 4 weeks to heal, such as deep dermal burns that heal spontaneously, are most likely to produce hypertrophic scars. Grafted wounds produce much less hypertrophic scarring. Both contracture and hypertrophic scarring peak from 3 to 6 months after injury and partially resolve at 12 to 18 months.

Care providers must recognize the delayed onset of hypertrophic scarring so that precautionary measures can be taken. As the inflammatory process diminishes and the rate of collagen lysis exceeds the rate of collagen deposition, the hypertrophic scar decreases in size. Between 12 and 18 months, the scar becomes softer and flatter and less hyperemic. Any hyperemia indicates active scar turnover, but the lack of hyperemia is a good sign that the scar is mature. Although the scar may relax, the underlying tissues can become permanently foreshortened, resulting in joint ankylosis.

MUSCLE LOSS

Inactivity of muscle leads to rapid atrophy, as is evident after a fracture is placed in a cast or, on a more general level, after head or spinal cord injury. The muscle catabolism in burn patients accentuates muscle loss caused by inactivity. The first muscles to decrease in size and strength are the proximal thigh muscles, which are essential for ambulation. Restoration of muscle mass, requiring a continuing increase in work load, is seriously hampered by any contractures or hypertrophic scarring. It is clearly more efficient to maintain muscle mass than to attempt to rebuild muscle, especially in elderly patients who lack the cardiopulmonary reserve needed for an increased work load.

HETEROTOPIC CALCIFICATION AND OSSIFICATION

The earliest sign of calcification, usually appearing 3 to 6 months after injury, is loss of range of motion or increased pain on attempted motion. X-ray evidence of calcium deposition usually postdates initial symptoms by at least 1 week. Calcium and phosphate may be deposited in soft tissue (heterotopic calcification) in 1% to 3% of burn patients, generally patients with major burns involving a joint. Calcium and phosphate deposits may produce bone (ossification), a process that can occur in the ligaments and capsule around a joint or in tissues distant from the joint. The joint most often involved is the elbow, followed by the shoulder. Bone scanning is the most reliable method for monitoring ossification.

Immobility appears to correlate directly with the amount of calcium deposited, although there are usually no measurable changes in serum levels of calcium, phosphorus, or alkaline phosphatase. The mechanism remains unknown, but immobility and hypermetabolism, with rapid tissue turnover, are clearly involved. Both *Staphylococcus aureus* and β-hemolytic streptococci are often found in the wound, but infection does not appear to be a prerequisite. With forceful range-of-motion exercise, there may be bleeding into the joint.

TEMPERATURE REGULATION

Compared with normal skin, thin grafted or healed skin is more prone to heat loss for years after injury. The loss is greatest when there is increased blood flow to the wound. As the scar matures, blood flow to the wound decreases, as does the potential for heat loss. Autoregulation of the microcirculation is impaired, especially for the first few months after injury, limiting the ability to vasoconstrict and vasodilate in response to changes in environmental temperature. Large, deep burns also destroy sweat glands, impairing an important mechanism for eliminating heat generated by pyrogens or exercise. Sensitivity to temperature extremes is a long-term problem in patients who have had burns over large areas of the body.

Recommended Reading

Abdullah A, Herndon D, Robson M: Visible scars and self esteem in pediatric patients with burns. J Burn Care Rehabil 15:164, 1994

Bernstein N, O'Connell K, Chedekel D: Patterns of burn adjustment. J Burn Care Rehabil 13:4, 1992

Evans E: Prevention and correction of deformity after severe burns. Surg Clin North Am 50:1361, 1970

Hallock G: A systematic approach to flap selection for the axillary burn contracture. J Burn Care Rehabil 14:343, 1993

Kealy G, Jensen K, Laubenthal K: Prospective randomized comparison of two types of pressure therapy garments. J Burn Care Rehabil 11:334, 1990

Leivis W, San K: Hypertrophic scar: a genetic hypothesis. Burns 16:176, 1990

Long R, Cope O: Emotional problems of burned children. N Engl J Med 264:1121, 1961

Mann R, Yeong EK, Moore M, et al: Do custom-fitted pressure garments provide adequate pressure? J Burn Care Rehabil 18:247, 1997

Powers P, Crase W: Post traumatic stress disorder in patients with burns. J Burn Care Rehabil 15:147, 1994

Richard R, Staley M, Miller S, et al: To splint or not to splint—past philosophy and practice: part III. J Burn Care Rehabil 18:251, 1997

Robison MC: Prevention and treatment of post burn scars and contracture. World J Surg 16:87, 1992

Rosenberg D, Nelson M: Rehabilitation concerns in electrical burn patients. J Trauma 28:808, 1988

IX MISCELLANEOUS CONCERNS

107 PHARMACOKINETICS IN SURGICAL PRACTICE

C. Edward Hartford, M.D., and G. Patrick Kealey, M.D., M.S.

Drugs are dangerous. The incidence of drug-related adverse reactions in hospitalized patients is about 30 percent, and it has been estimated that the risk of such reactions is about five percent for each course of drug therapy.[1] Risks notwithstanding, drugs can be of tremendous benefit when properly used, and their use to modify the course of illness is an integral part of surgical practice. Application of pharmacokinetic principles enables the surgeon to select dosages and dosing schedules that enhance the efficacy of the drug while minimizing the likelihood of drug-related toxicity. Pharmacokinetics is the study of the interactions that occur between a drug and the body in terms of the drug's absorption, distribution, biotransformation (metabolism), and excretion. These four variables are often described by using mathematical models.

Pharmacokinetic Variables

To be effective, a drug must reach the systemic circulation and be delivered to its site of action. Between the site of administration and the site of action, absorption, distribution, biotransformation, and elimination interplay to determine the amount of drug available. The clinical response to a drug (including both therapeutic and toxic effects) is a function of the concentration of the drug at its site of action. It is assumed, however, that the drug's pharmacological activity correlates with its plasma concentration.[2] The plasma concentration of most drugs can be measured, whereas the concentration at the site of action often cannot.

ABSORPTION

Factors Governing Absorption

Absorption usually refers to the movement of a drug from its site of administration into the systemic circulation; however, the term can also be applied to the movement of a drug across any membrane or barrier (e.g., a cell membrane). Absorption is governed by three variables: ionization, molecular size, and blood flow.

Ionization The ability of a drug to traverse a cell membrane (i.e., to be absorbed) is a function of its lipid solubility, which depends on its state of ionization. Most drugs are weak acids or weak bases that exist in solution in both nonionized and ionized species. In the nonionized state, drugs are nonpolar, have enhanced lipid solubility, and readily traverse cell membranes. In the ionized state, they are polar, are not lipid soluble, and do not readily traverse cell membranes.

Ionization is a function of the pK_a of the drug and the pH of the solution [see Figure 1]. The ratio of nonionized drug to ionized drug can be calculated using the Henderson-Hasselbalch equation:

$$pH = pK_a + \log \frac{[\text{base form}]}{[\text{acid form}]}$$

If, for example, a weakly acidic drug with a pK_a of 3.4 is dissolved in a solution with a pH of 1.4, the nonionized species predominates:

$$1.4 = 3.4 + \log \frac{[A^-]}{[HA]}$$

$$-2 = \log \frac{[A^-]}{[HA]}$$

$$[100] \; HA \rightleftharpoons H^+ + A^- \; [1]$$

where HA (the acid form) represents the nonionized species and A^- (the base form) represents the ionized species. Conversely, if the same drug is dissolved in a solution with a pH of 7.4, the ionized species predominates:

$$7.4 = 3.4 + \log \frac{[A^-]}{[HA]}$$

$$4 = \log \frac{[A^-]}{[HA]}$$

$$[1] \; HA \rightleftharpoons H^+ + A^- \; [10{,}000]$$

When the concentration of the ionized fraction equals that of the nonionized fraction, the ratio equals 1. The log of 1 equals 0. Therefore, the pK_a of a drug is the pH at which 50 percent of the drug is ionized and 50 percent is nonionized.

In most regions of the body, the pores between endothelial cells permit transcapillary movement of most drugs. The limiting factors to movement into the interstitial space are blood flow and molecular size, not pH-dependent lipid solubility. Therefore, that fraction of a drug that is ionized at systemic pH is distributed into the extracellular fluid compartment. (Because the ionized species does not readily traverse lipid cell membranes, it is trapped in the compartment in which it is contained.) In several regions, however, lipid solubility is required for a drug to traverse the capillary wall, because tight apposition of capillary endothelial cells prevents transcapillary movement of ionized moieties. The most notable of these regions is the central nervous system, where the impediment to drug movement is known as the blood-brain barrier.

The role of ionization in renal tubular reabsorption (and hence in elimination) is discussed in more detail elsewhere [see Elimination, Routes of Excretion, *below*].

Molecular size Diffusion through a barrier diminishes exponentially as the drug's molecular weight increases.

Blood flow Absorption of a drug into the systemic circulation is enhanced by increased local blood flow. Many critically ill patients have diminished regional blood flow to nonvital

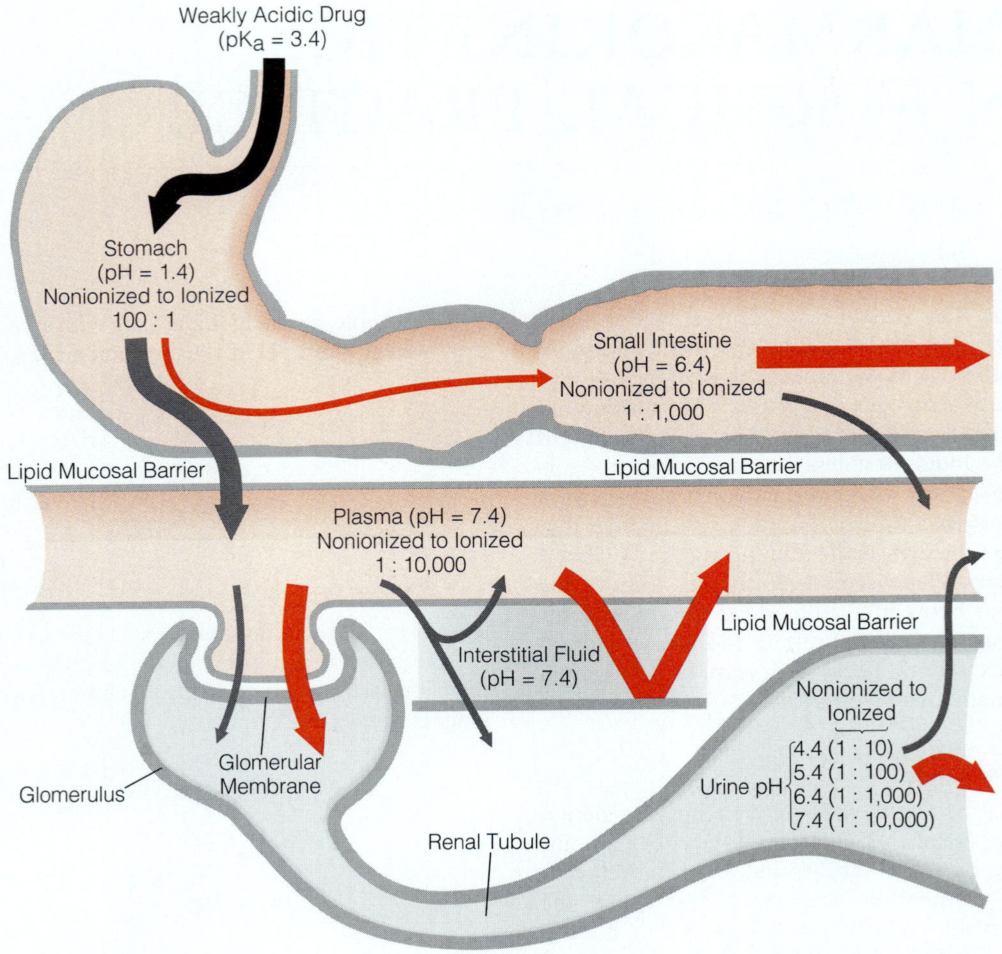

Figure 1 Absorption is governed by ionization, molecular size, and blood flow. The extent to which a drug is ionized depends on its pK_a and on the pH of the solution in which it is dissolved. To illustrate this point, shown here are the ratios of the concentration of nonionized drug to that of ionized drug for a weak acid (pK_a = 3.4) in various regions of the body.

In the stomach, where the pH is 1.4, the large concentration of free hydrogen ions prevents ionization, so that the ratio of nonionized drug to ionized drug is 100:1. The nonionized, lipid-soluble fraction (gray arrows) is readily absorbed across the lipid mucosal barrier of the stomach into the plasma by passive diffusion; the ionized, non–lipid-soluble fraction (red arrows) is not absorbed and passes into the small intestine. There, where the pH is 6.4, a high proportion of the drug will remain in the ionized state: the ratio of nonionized drug to ionized drug is 1:1,000. This favors retention of the drug within the intestinal tract and excretion in stool.

In the plasma, where the pH is 7.4, ionization of the drug is favored: the ratio of nonionized drug to ionized drug is 1:10,000. Because of the pores that exist between endothelial cells throughout most of the vasculature, both ionized and nonionized species of drugs of relatively low molecular weight generally move freely between plasma and interstitial fluid. However, the predominance of the ionized, lipid-insoluble species means that most of the drug cannot pass through lipid cellular membranes. The drug is therefore said to be trapped in the extracellular compartment.

Because of the porosity of the glomerular membrane, both ionized and nonionized species readily pass into the urine. The nonionized fraction in the glomerular filtrate, being lipid soluble, is readily reabsorbed through the renal tubular cell back into the plasma, whereas the ionized fraction is excreted in the urine. As urinary pH rises, the ratio of ionized drug to nonionized drug rises as well. Therefore, elimination of weak acids can be enhanced by alkalinizing the urine.

structures, large pools of inactive sequestered fluid, or both; as a result, absorption is erratic and unpredictable.

Area under the Curve

Total area under the plasma concentration-time curve, commonly referred to as area under the curve (AUC), is the term used by the pharmaceutical industry to indicate the total amount of drug that reaches the systemic circulation after a single test dose. It appears in numerous reference sources, such as drug package inserts and pharmacological publications. Although the concept of AUC has no clinical value, it is used to calculate bioavailability, which has great clinical relevance.

Bioavailability

Bioavailability (F) is that fraction of a drug dose that reaches the systemic circulation. When a drug is given intravenously, its bioavailability is 100 percent (i.e., F = 1); when it is given by any other route, its bioavailability may be less (i.e., F < 1). Information on bioavailability is especially important when the margin between therapeutic efficacy and toxicity is narrow.

Bioavailability is determined by administering equal doses of a drug to a person, first by the intravenous route and then by a test route (e.g., per os). The amount of drug reaching the systemic circulation by the test route is divided by the amount of drug reaching the systemic circulation by the intravenous route to yield the value for F.

First-pass effect Drugs given enterally pass through the liver before they reach the systemic circulation. In the liver, a drug may be eliminated by excretion or inactivated by biotransformation (see below). Loss of pharmacologically active drug by this mechanism is known as the first-pass effect. The result is a decrease in bioavailability. Several clinically useful drugs (e.g., nitroglycerin and naloxone[3]) are so efficiently removed by the liver that they are not given by the enteral route. On the other hand, some drugs that are subject to the first-pass effect in the liver—such as morphine, which has a low bioavailability (F = 0.24 ± 0.12) when given enterally—can still be administered by this route with satisfactory therapeutic results if the oral dose is adjusted upward.

The first-pass effect may occur at sites other than the liver. Many tissues contain the same biotransforming enzymes that the liver does, though usually in lower concentrations. The intestinal mucosa, the lung, and the skin all may contribute to the first-pass effect for drugs administered enterally, by inhalation, and topically, respectively.

In the intensive care setting, most drugs should be delivered intravenously to ensure optimal bioavailability.

DISTRIBUTION

Volume of Distribution

The hypothetical volume into which a drug is distributed after complete equilibration is known as the apparent volume of distribution (V). This quantity is used clinically to estimate the dose needed to achieve a target plasma concentration:

$$A = V \times C$$

where A is the amount of drug needed and C is the target plasma concentration. The most important clinical use of V is in the determination of the loading dose of a drug [*see* Administration of Drugs, Loading Dose, *below*].

V rarely corresponds to a real volume, such as the plasma volume, the extracellular fluid volume, or the volume of total body water. If all of the drug were contained in the plasma, then the plasma volume would represent the volume of distribution. Virtually all drugs, however, are distributed beyond the plasma volume, and most bind at least partially to tissue and plasma proteins (see below), which affects V [*see Table 1*]. Volume of distribution is commonly expressed in liters per kilogram of body weight. For reference purposes, the volume of distribution is 0.05 L/kg for plasma, 0.2 L/kg for extracellular fluid, and 0.6 L/kg for total body water.

Diseases alter the volume of distribution of many drugs. In fact, at the inception of therapy, the actual volume of distribution of a given drug in a given patient is not known. Therefore, the referenced volume of distribution serves only as a guide, and the known alterations in V caused by disease must be taken into consideration before a dosing regimen can be developed. If the plasma concentration of a drug can be measured, V can be calculated:

$$V = \frac{A}{C}$$

where A is the amount of drug in the body and C is the measured plasma concentration. In most instances, the calculation should use a plasma concentration value obtained after a steady state has been achieved.

Multiple compartments The two previous equations are valid for the one-compartment model, which defines the body as a single homogeneous compartment and assumes that drugs are distributed instantaneously and uniformly into the entire compartment. For the majority of drugs, however, this assumption does not hold. Distribution of drugs into tissues beyond the central vascular compartment occurs at varying rates and depends on factors such as blood flow, molecular size, ionization, and affinity for tissues. Consequently, there are usually at least two compartments, and often more; these compartments do not correspond to defined physiologic spaces. To determine V in multiple-compartment models, more complex mathematical formulas are necessary.

Protein Binding

Many drugs bind to plasma and tissue proteins. For example, acidic and neutral drugs bind to albumin, and basic drugs bind to α_1-acid glycoprotein and lipoproteins. In addition, specific drugs may bind to specific proteins. Drugs that are bound are pharmacologically inactive, cannot move through membranes, and are not available for elimination.

Binding is a reversible state. The bound fraction and the unbound fraction of a drug are in dynamic equilibrium. The degree of binding varies greatly among drugs and is expressed as a ratio between the bound fraction and the unbound fraction. The binding ratio ranges from 0 to 1: drugs with a binding ratio higher than 0.9 are regarded as highly bound, those with a binding ratio of 0.2 to 0.9 are regarded as having intermediate binding, and those with a binding ratio of less than 0.2 are regarded as having little binding. The amount of drug bound is a function of the affinity of the protein for the drug, the amount of protein available, and the availability of drug binding sites on the protein. When binding sites are full—whether because more of the drug is available, because less of the protein is available, or because other drugs that compete for the same binding sites are present—the amount of free drug increases. When a drug is mea-

Table 1 Volume of Distribution of Selected Commonly Used Drugs

Drug	V (L/kg)
Amikacin	0.27 ± 0.06
Amphotericin B	0.76 ± 0.52
Ceftazidime	0.23 ± 0.02
Ciprofloxacin	1.8 ± 0.4
Digitoxin	0.54 ± 0.14
Digoxin	10.0 ± 3.0
Dobutamine	0.20 ± 0.08
Furosemide	0.11 ± 0.02
Gentamicin	0.31 ± 0.10
Heparin	0.058 ± 0.011
Lidocaine	1.1 ± 0.4
Metronidazole	0.74 ± 0.10
Morphine	3.3 ± 0.9
Nitroglycerin	3.3 ± 1.2
Phenobarbital	0.54 ± 0.03
Phenytoin	0.64 ± 0.04
Procainamide	1.9 ± 0.3
Propranolol	4.3 ± 0.6
Theophylline	0.50 ± 0.16
Vancomycin	0.39 ± 0.06
Verapamil	5.0 ± 2.1

sured in the plasma, both bound and unbound fractions are measured.

Protein binding influences V. The more extensively a drug is bound to tissue proteins, the greater the apparent volume of distribution. This point can be illustrated by dissolving 10 mg of a drug into 1 L of water. The concentration of the drug would then be 10 mg/L, and V would be 1 L (V = A/C). If, however, an absorbent, such as charcoal, is added in a dose sufficient to bind 9 mg of the drug, the concentration of the drug in solution would then become 1 mg/L, and V would be 10 L.

Binding to plasma proteins influences V differently. The more extensively a drug is bound to plasma proteins, the less available it is to diffuse into tissues, and the apparent volume of distribution of the drug is limited as a result. For example, warfarin is 99 percent bound to albumin. Its volume of distribution is 0.14 L/kg, which is identical to the V for albumin.[4]

Protein binding also plays an important role in the elimination of drugs, irrespective of the mechanism or the site of elimination; only unbound drug can be eliminated. In general, high binding affinity results in low rates of clearance, and low affinity results in enhanced clearance.

BIOTRANSFORMATION (METABOLISM)

Biotransformation comprises the processes by which drugs are enzymatically altered.[5] These processes generally make drugs more water soluble and ionized, reducing their lipid solubility and enhancing their elimination: whereas nonionized lipid-soluble drugs and nonionized biotransformed metabolites filtered through the glomerular membrane into the urine are likely to be reabsorbed into the plasma, ionized species are more readily excreted with the urine. Drugs excreted in the bile that remain in a nonpolar state while in the gastrointestinal tract tend to be reabsorbed.

The biotransforming processes are oxidation, reduction, hydrolysis, and conjugation. The reactions associated with the first three are known as phase 1 reactions, and those associated with conjugation are known as phase 2 reactions [see Table 2]. Many phase 1 reactions are driven by a large family of microsomal enzymes known as cytochrome P-450 mixed-function oxidative isoenzymes. To date, 31 human genes have been identified for various cytochrome P-450 enzymes.[6] The cytochrome P-450 3A subfamily is the most abundant enzyme, representing approximately 30 percent of the total hepatic cytochrome P-450.[7] The major site of drug biotransformation is the smooth endoplasmic reticulum of the hepatocyte. However, the enzymes that drive these processes are also found in the plasma and cells of other body tissues, although in lesser amounts. Biotransformation in the gastrointestinal tract may contribute to the first-pass effect.

Drugs are usually metabolized in a single reaction; however, there may be a series of reactions with intermediate metabolites. Although biotransformed metabolites are usually pharmacologically inactive, this is not always the case. Sometimes, the metabolite is active but less so than the parent compound. Occasionally, the biotransformed moiety is more active: for instance, enalapril is hydrolyzed by a plasma esterase to the active form of the drug, enalaprilat.[8]

Genetic, environmental, and physiologic factors can modify biotransformation of drugs. Additionally, biotransformation can be either induced or inhibited by a variety of substances.

Induction Induction is the process by which enzymes are stimulated to greater metabolic activity and therefore a greater rate

Table 2 Biotransforming Reactions

	Type of Reaction	Example of Drugs Affected
Phase 1	Oxidation	
	P-450 mixed-function oxidation	
	Aliphatic hydroxylation	Phenobarbital
	Aromatic hydroxylation	Phenytoin
	Epoxidation	Carbamazepine
	N-dealkylation	Imipramine
	O-dealkylation	Phenacetin
	N-oxidation	Acetaminophen
	Desulfuration	Thiopental
	Nonmicrosomal oxidation	
	Alcohol dehydrogenase activity	Ethanol
	Aldehyde dehydrogenase activity	Aldehydes
	Monoamine oxidase activity	Catecholamines
	Reduction	
	Nitro reduction	Clonazepam
	Azo reduction	Prontosil
	Carbonyl reduction	Warfarin
	Sulfoxide	Sulindac
	Hydrolysis	
	Esterase activity	Aspirin
	Amidase activity	Lidocaine
	Epoxide hydrolase activity	Carbamazepine epoxide
Phase 2	Conjugation	
	Glucuronide conjugation	
	Aliphatic hydroxyl group	Propranolol
	Aromatic hydroxyl group	Morphine
	COOH group	Fenoprofen
	Sulfate conjugation	
	Aromatic hydroxyl group	Terbutaline
	Glycine conjugation	Salicylic acid
	Acetylation	Procainamide
	Methylation	Norepinephrine

of drug biotransformation. It may be specific for a single enzyme or involve multiple enzymes. Many of the numerous agents that can cause induction resemble phenobarbital or are polycyclic aromatic hydrocarbons.[9] For example, phenobarbital enhances the clearance of cimetidine, digitoxin, oral anticoagulants, and theophylline.[10] Phenytoin increases the rate of biotransformation of cyclosporine, diazepam, digitoxin, glucocorticoids, oral anticoagulants, and theophylline.[10] Various drugs used for nonmedical purposes (e.g., certain opioids,[11] ethanol,[9] and tobacco[9]) are also potent inducers of microsomal enzymes. For instance, cigarette smokers clear theophylline more rapidly than nonsmokers,[12] and recreational opioid users have increased narcotic requirements.[11] Enzyme induction begins and ends slowly, occurring over a period of days to weeks. Dosage adjustment and clinical monitoring are as important at the end of induction as at the beginning.

The metabolism of drugs biotransformed by the same enzyme system may be competitively inhibited. Most of these interactions occur in the liver. Unlike induction, inhibition begins and ends rapidly, and the effect may be seen with a single dose. The most outstanding example is cimetidine's inhibition of the metabolism of many drugs (e.g., theophylline, lidocaine, and warfarin), presumably by competitive inhibition of hepatic cytochrome P-450 mixed-function oxidases.[13]

Of special note are the varied effects of alcohol on hepatic biotransformation of drugs. Whereas the acute ingestion of alcohol competitively inhibits metabolism of many drugs, chronic use encourages induction of enzymes.[14]

ELIMINATION

Elimination is the irreversible loss of drug either through removal from the body or through inactivation by biotransformation. The rate at which a drug is eliminated is the most important pharmacokinetic variable to consider in any attempt to develop a rational regimen for long-term administration (i.e., more than one dose) of a drug.

Clearance

In pharmacological terms, clearance (CL) is defined as the volume of serum, plasma, or blood that loses all the drug it contains in a specified period. A serum creatinine clearance of 100 ml/min, for example, means that each minute, all of the creatinine in 100 ml of serum is removed. Clearance is therefore a measure of the rate at which a drug is removed from serum, plasma, or blood, not of the amount of drug removed. It is a function of volume of distribution and half-life:

$$CL = 0.693 \frac{V}{t^{1/2}}$$

where 0.693 is the natural logarithm of 2 and $t^{1/2}$ is half-life.

Organ clearance measures the rate at which an organ (e.g., the kidney or the liver) removes a drug from perfusing blood and is calculated as follows:

$$CL = E \times Q$$

where E is the extraction ratio and Q is total blood flow through the organ. Total body clearance is the sum of all organ clearances.

Clearance of a drug is usually a linear function of its concentration in the plasma—that is, a first-order kinetic process in which a constant percentage of drug is eliminated in a given period [see Principles of Kinetics, *below*]. If the pathways for elimination become saturated, however, zero-order kinetics come into play, and a constant amount of drug is eliminated in a given period; unless the dosing regimen is modified, the risk of toxicity will be enhanced.

Half-life

The half-life (also referred to as the elimination half-life) of a drug is the time required for the plasma concentration to decrease by one half of its initial value. After a single dose of a drug, 50 percent is eliminated and 50 percent remains at the end of one half-life. During the second half-life, 50 percent of the remaining amount is eliminated, which means that only 25 percent of the original amount is still present. After three half-lives, 12.5 percent of the original amount remains; after four, 6.25 percent remains; after five, 3.125 percent remains; and after 10, only 0.1 percent remains. For practical purposes, virtually all of the drug (96.9 percent) has been eliminated after five half-lives. Theoretically, however, a minuscule fraction would remain even after an infinite number of half-lives.

Half-life varies dramatically from one drug to another, ranging from minutes to days [see Table 3]. Knowledge of a drug's half-life allows the clinician to estimate the dosing interval that will achieve the desired steady-state plasma concentration most reliably and safely. A drug with a short half-life must be administered more frequently than a drug with a long half-life.

It is important to be aware of the factors that can alter a drug's half-life in an individual patient. As noted, half-life and clearance are related; this relation can be expressed as follows:

$$t^{1/2} = 0.693 \frac{V}{CL}$$

Accordingly, half-life is greatly influenced by blood flow and by the functional status of the liver and the kidneys. These organs are important pathways of biotransformation and elimination. Factors that diminish volume of distribution and enhance clearance tend to shorten half-life, whereas slow metabolism, poor excretion, and extensive binding to plasma proteins tend to lengthen half-life.

Routes of Excretion

The major routes of drug removal from the body are renal excretion of unchanged drug, hepatic biotransformation with renal excretion, hepatic biotransformation with enteral excretion, biliary-enteral excretion of unchanged drug, and excretion through the lung.

Most drugs are excreted in the urine. Three processes are involved: glomerular filtration, passive tubular reabsorption, and active tubular secretion. Drugs that are not bound to plasma proteins and that have a low molecular mass (< 500 daltons) are readily filtered through the glomerulus into the urine. Both ionized and nonionized fractions cross the glomerular membrane. The ionized fraction is excreted with the urine; the nonionized (and therefore lipid-soluble) fraction is reabsorbed through the tubule by passive diffusion along a concentration gradient. Most drugs that are reabsorbed in an unaltered state are eventually biotransformed in the liver to ionized metabolites, which are then excreted in urine.

For many drugs, renal tubular reabsorption is a pH-dependent phenomenon. For instance, if the drug is a weak acid (e.g., aspirin or phenobarbital), a more acidic urine leads to reduced ionization and increased reabsorption (i.e., reduced excretion), whereas a more alkaline urine leads to increased ionization and reduced reabsorption (increased excretion). If, however, the drug is a weak base (e.g., ephedrine), a more acidic urine results in increased ionization and reduced reabsorption, whereas a more alkaline urine results in reduced ionization and increased reabsorption. This is the rationale for clinical use of urinary pH alteration to enhance elimination of some drugs. Alteration of urinary flow rate may also have a significant effect on elimination by altering the urinary concentration of those drugs that are subject to reabsorption via the concentration gradient–dependent passive diffusion mechanism.

Active tubular secretion takes place, for the most part, in the pars recta of the proximal renal tubule. Organic anions and cations are transported by separate systems. Transport is not selective: there may be competition for transport between various drugs or between drugs and endogenously produced substances. Therefore, when competing drugs are administered or when levels of certain endogenous organic substances are elevated, as is the case in renal failure, the half-lives of drugs are prolonged and

Table 3 Half-Lives of Selected Drugs

Drug	Half-life
Nitroglycerin	2.3 min
Furosemide	1.5 hr
Gentamicin	2.5 hr
Theophylline	9 hr
Digoxin	36 hr
Phenobarbital	4 days
Digitoxin	9 days

dosing regimens must be modified. Other clinically important sites of active drug transport exist. Digoxin, for example, is secreted in the distal nephron, and spironolactone, quinidine, and verapamil all compete for tubular secretion at this site as well.[15]

Some drugs or their biotransformed metabolites are excreted in bile and either eliminated in the feces or, more frequently, reabsorbed through the GI tract and eventually eliminated by the kidneys. Volatile anesthetics are eliminated through the lung. Other routes of excretion, such as skin, tears, saliva, breast milk, and wounds, are clinically much less important.

Principles of Kinetics

Kinetics is the term used to define the rate at which a drug moves across a barrier. It usually refers to the rate at which a drug is absorbed or eliminated; however, it may also refer to the rate at which a drug moves from one compartment in the body to another (e.g., across the blood-brain barrier or across a cell membrane).

FIRST-ORDER KINETICS

In first-order kinetics (also known as linear or monoexponential kinetics), the rate at which a drug moves across a barrier is proportional to the amount of drug present—that is, over a specified unit of time, the percentage of the drug that traverses the barrier remains constant. If the amount or concentration of the drug increases or decreases, the amount of drug that traverses the barrier increases or decreases proportionately. The unit of time for first-order kinetics is the half-life of the drug [see Pharmacokinetic Variables, Elimination, above], which remains constant.

When a first-order process is displayed as a Cartesian plot, the line defined by the change in the concentration of the drug over time is a parabolic curve [see Figure 2]. When the process is plotted semilogarithmically, however, the line defined is straight [see Figure 3]. A semilogarithmic plot is clinically useful because from the slope of the line one can calculate the first-order rate constant (k) at which the drug moves across the barrier. From this constant, in turn, one can calculate the half-life:

$$t^{1/2} = \frac{0.693}{k}$$

Distribution and Elimination Phases

The preceding description of first-order kinetics is accurate for the one-compartment model of distribution described earlier [see Pharmacokinetic Variables, Distribution, above]. In practice, however, the description would generally require modification. Typically, elimination is preceded by a brief distribution phase, during which the drug diffuses throughout the central vascular compartment. This phenomenon is readily illustrated on a semilogarithmic plot. If a drug that follows first-order kinetics is administered in an I.V. bolus, the line defined by the change in concentration over time generally will have two distinct components, corresponding to the distribution phase and the elimination phase [see Figure 4]. Because the rate of distribution is different from the rate of elimination, the lines representing the two phases have different slopes. The curve that connects these two lines represents the interaction between the end of the distribution phase (which is still incomplete when elimination begins) and the beginning of the elimination phase.

ZERO-ORDER KINETICS

In zero-order kinetics (also known as nonlinear, Michaelis-Menten, or saturation kinetics), the rate at which a drug moves across a barrier is constant. The pathway for movement or elimination of the drug is enzymatically driven; when the system becomes saturated, the amount of drug that moves per unit of time cannot be increased. Consequently, in each unit of time, the same amount of drug traverses the barrier, regardless of the amount that remains to be moved. The proportion of remaining drug that moves increases progressively, whereas the half-life of the drug decreases progressively; thus, a zero-order kinetic process plotted with Cartesian coordinates yields a straight line [see Figure 5].

Although most drugs follow first-order kinetics at clinically useful doses, some follow zero-order kinetics (e.g., salicylic acid, ethanol, phenytoin, mezlocillin, heparin, quinidine, and tetracycline. A given drug may follow both first-order and zero-order

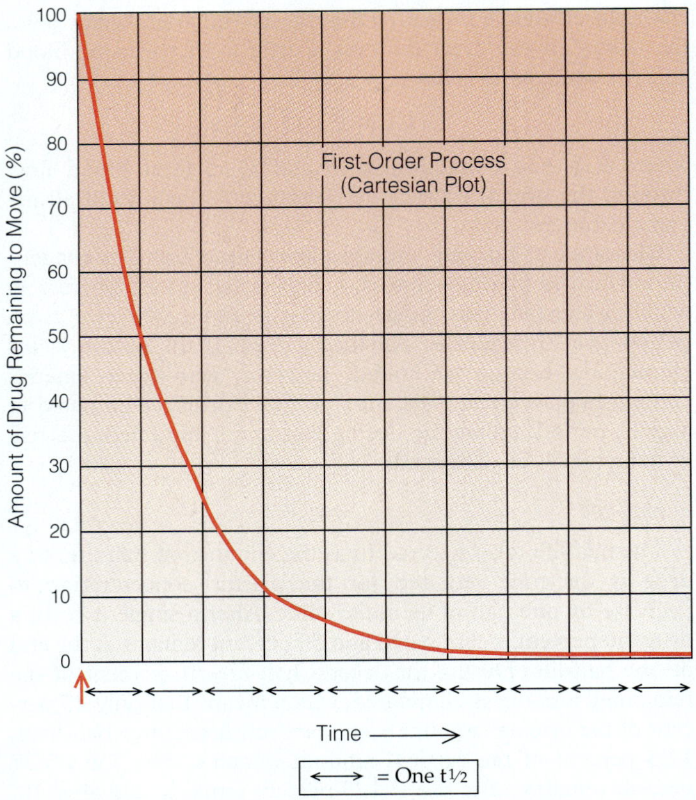

Figure 2 In first-order kinetics, the percentage of a drug dose that moves across a barrier over a given unit of time (i.e., $t^{1/2}$) remains constant. When this process is plotted onto Cartesian coordinates, the change in the plasma concentration of the drug follows a parabolic curve.

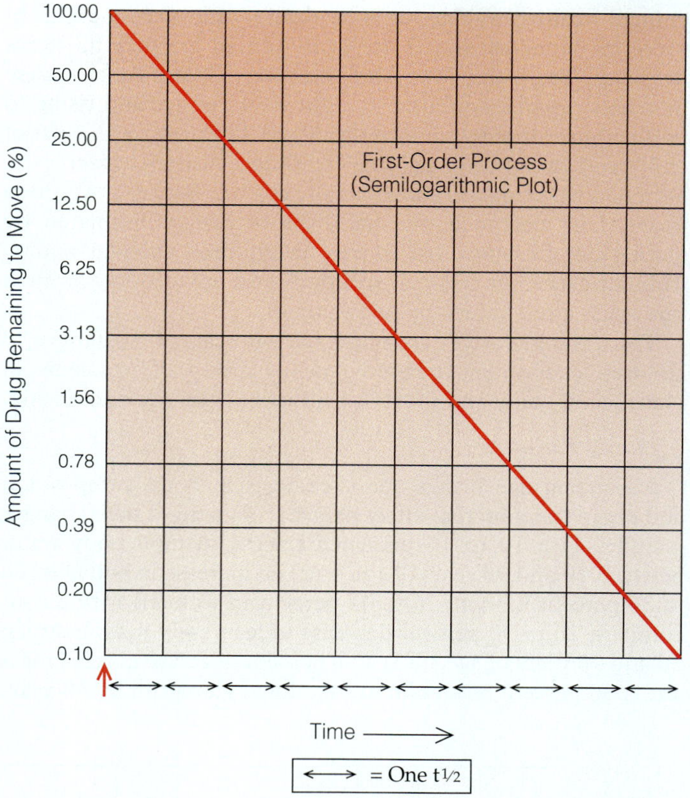

Figure 3 A first-order process plotted semilogarithmically yields a straight line. The slope of this line can be used to determine the first-order rate constant.

kinetics in the same patient, but not at the same time. When the plasma concentration of the drug is relatively low, protein binding, biotransformation, and clearance may proceed according to first-order kinetics. When the plasma concentration increases, however, one or more of the pathways for these processes may be saturated, in which case the drug will display zero-order kinetics. Under these circumstances, the drug may accumulate rapidly, with the result that half-life lengthens (rather than decreases) and the possibility of toxicity increases [see Figure 6]. A small increase in the dose thus may lead to a large increase in serum concentration. Therefore, to prevent toxicity, the dose, the dosing interval, or both must be changed.

Factors That Modify Pharmacokinetics

Most of the pharmacokinetic data in current reference sources are derived from disease-free young adult volunteers. The dosing regimens generally cited in these sources are those that have been found through clinical testing to be safe and effective in most patients. However, these dosing regimens are often unsatisfactory in actual treatment situations. Consequently, it is crucial to incorporate pharmacokinetic concepts into critical care and to take into account factors that may modify pharmacokinetics (e.g., age, nutritional status, burns, and kidney, liver, heart, or lung disease).

AGE

Fetus, Neonate, and Child

As a person grows to adulthood, changes in body composition, metabolic pathways, and organ function occur. These changes affect pharmacokinetic variables and must be considered whenever pharmacotherapy is planned.[16]

Before birth, drugs are mostly biotransformed and excreted by the mother. Enzyme systems in the placenta may defend the fetus against drug-mediated toxicity.

At birth, total body water is 78 percent of body weight. This value decreases by three to five percent by the fifth day of life, then falls more slowly, reaching adult levels (60 to 65 percent of body weight) by one and one-half years of age. Extracellular water, which is 45 percent of body weight at birth, decreases to 40 percent by the fifth day of life, to 33 percent by two months of age, and to adult levels (20 to 25 percent of body weight) by three years of age. These changes alter the volume of distribution of drugs.

Gastric emptying is prolonged in neonates, not reaching the adult rate until six months of age. The neonatal stomach is initially devoid of acid, and it does not attain adult levels of pH until two to three years after birth. Binding of drugs to plasma proteins is reduced in both preterm and full-term neonates because there are lower levels of total protein and albumin and lower levels of plasma globulin. In addition, some proteins, such as fetal albumin, are qualitatively different.[17] Plasma concentrations of proteins reach normal adult levels by one year of age.

Although very young persons have relatively more liver tissue than do adults, their livers are less able to biotransform

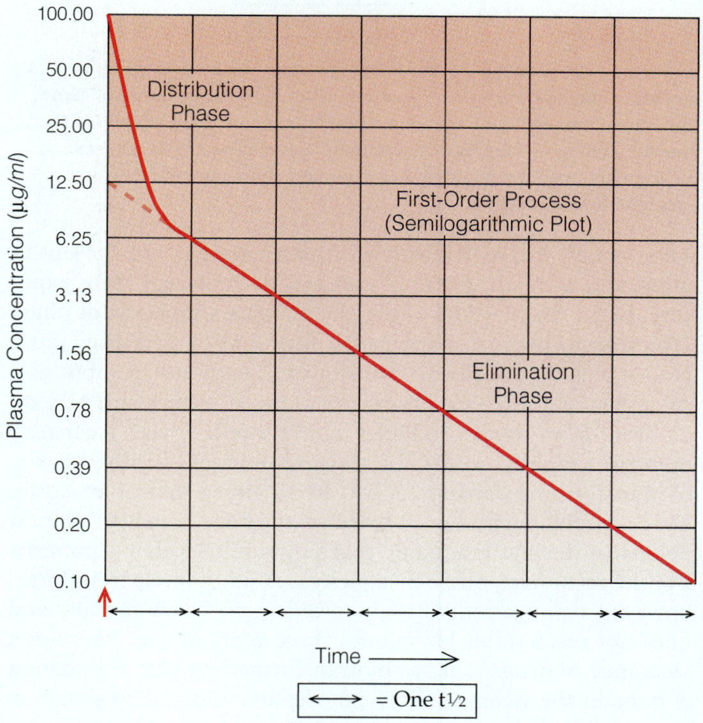

Figure 4 A drug that follows first-order kinetics (according to a one-compartmental model) is administered in an I.V. bolus at time 0. When the change in plasma concentration over time is plotted semilogarithmically, it becomes apparent that the decay curve has two distinct components. The initial steep curve represents the distribution phase, during which the drug diffuses rapidly throughout the central vascular compartment. This phase is not a kinetic process. The straight terminal segment represents the elimination phase (also known as the log-linear phase). The broken line represents the extrapolation of the line for the elimination phase back to time 0. (The value for $t^{1/2}$ is determined by the slope of the line for the elimination phase.)

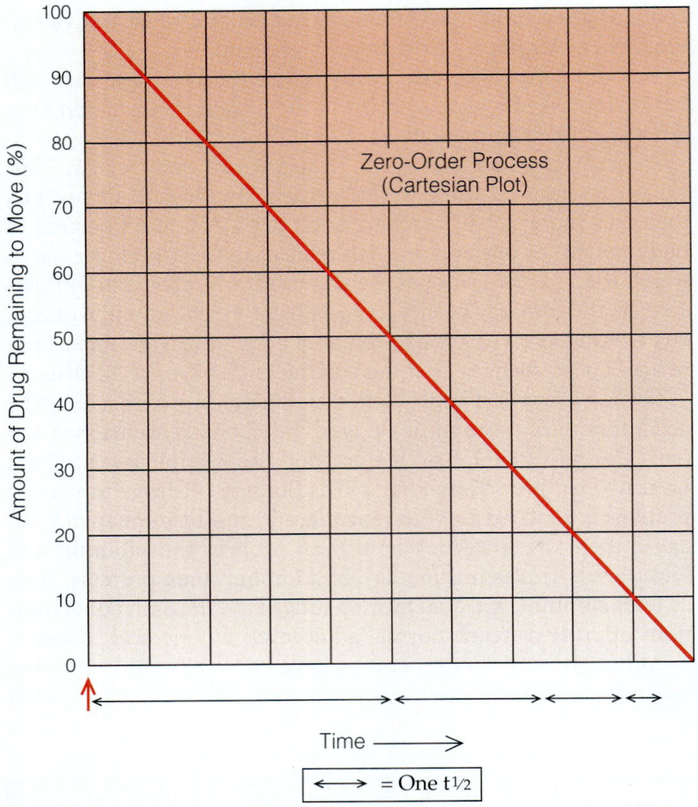

Figure 5 In zero-order kinetics, the rate at which a drug moves across a barrier remains constant; that is, for each unit of time, the same amount (not the same percentage) of drug traverses the barrier. Thus, as plasma concentrate decreases, $t^{1/2}$ decreases. When this process is plotted using Cartesian coordinates, a straight line is defined.

some drugs. Phase 1 biotransforming enzymes are present in utero and at birth, possibly induced by maternal drug exposure. In the first 15 days of life, the neonate's capacity for phase 1 biotransformation is about one fifth that of a healthy adult. Not only is biotransformation slower in early infancy, but as a rule, the metabolic end products produced in early infancy, are different from those produced in adulthood. Phase 1 capacity then rises rapidly, so that by three months of age, the hepatic biotransforming capacity is two to six times that of an adult. This capacity persists until three years of age, at which point it begins to decline gradually, reaching adult levels by puberty. For the most part, phase 2 capacity is at adult levels from birth; however, conjugation with glucuronic acid is low initially and does not reach adult levels until three years of age. Therefore, clearance of drugs that are biotransformed by glucuronidation is poor in the neonate. This exposes the neonate to potential toxicity (e.g., the gray syndrome, caused by chloramphenicol[18]). Narcotics, benzodiazepines, barbiturates, anticonvulsants, antibiotics, and local anesthetics have all been shown to have age- and maturation-dependent variations in metabolic clearance, V, and $t^{1/2}$.[16,19,20]

Drugs that are cleared through the kidney, such as aminoglycosides, penicillins, cephalosporins, and digitalis, also have age- and maturation-dependent changes in V, clearance, and $t^{1/2}$. The glomerular filtration rate (GFR), which is assessed by measuring creatinine clearance, is low in the neonatal kidney: whereas creatinine clearance is greater than 100 ml/min in young, healthy adults, it is typically only 0.8 ml/min in preterm neonates and 2 to 4 ml/min in normal full-term neonates. From this low value, however, creatinine clearance increases rapidly, doubling by eight weeks of age and rising to twice adult values by six months of age. Throughout the rest of childhood, weight-normalized creatinine clearance decreases, although it remains above adult values. Because of these changes in clearance, the half-lives of drugs eliminated by glomerular filtration are shorter in children than in adults. Tubular excretion and reabsorption rates are also low at birth but reach adult values by two years of age.

Thus, the intensive care physician who cares for infants and children encounters a heterogeneous group of problems in pharmacotherapy and must individualize drug use and dosing.

Elderly Patient

Advancing age brings about changes in body composition and organ function that affect pharmacokinetics. These changes include (1) a 10 to 15 percent decrease in total body water between 20 and 90 years of age,[21] (2) an increase in body fat (18 to 36 percent in men, 30 to 45 percent in women) with a concomitant 20 to 30 percent decrease in lean body mass between 20 and 90 years of age,[21] (3) a 20 percent decrease in renal mass and a 30 percent reduction in functional glomeruli by 80 years

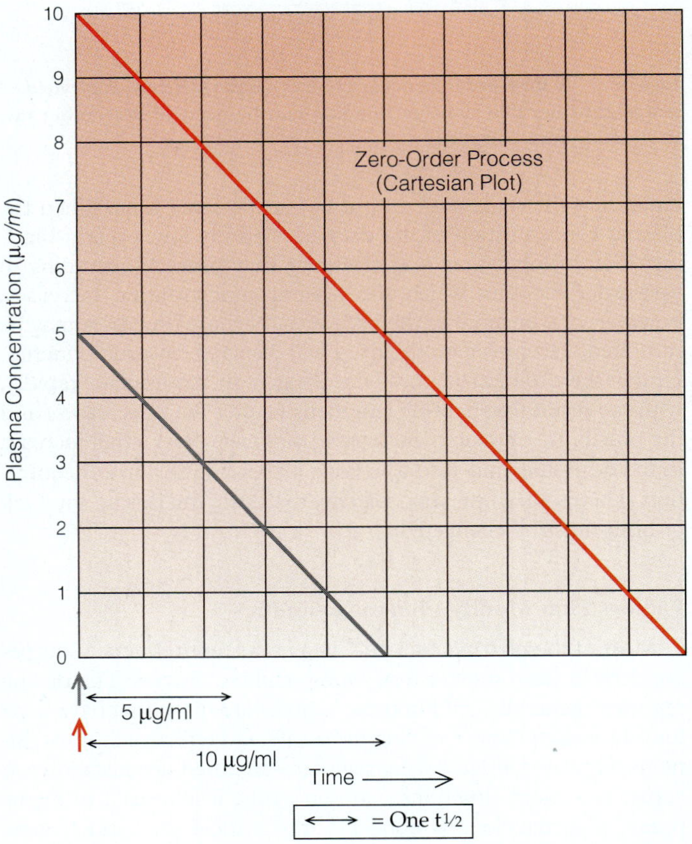

Figure 6 In zero-order kinetics, the same amount of drug moves for a given unit of time, regardless of the amount that remains to be moved. Consequently, if the plasma concentration of a drug that follows zero-order kinetics is increased (e.g., by increasing the dose without extending the dosing interval), the half-life is lengthened; because of the resulting higher plasma concentration of drug, the possibility of toxicity increases.

of age,[22,23] (4) a decrease in hepatic mass and hepatic blood flow,[24] and (5) a one percent yearly decrease in cardiac output as a result of coronary artery disease.[21,25]

The changes in body composition caused by aging modify volume of distribution. For instance, digoxin[21] and alcohol[26] have a decreased volume of distribution.[21] Lipid-soluble drugs, such as benzodiazepines, tend to accumulate in the increasing amounts of fat as the body ages.[21]

Deterioration of renal function with advancing age results in diminished clearance of drugs eliminated by the kidney.[22]

The biotransforming functions of the liver—that is, the activity of phase 1 and phase 2 enzymes and even enzyme induction—are largely unaffected by aging.[27] Therefore, age-associated decreases in clearance of drugs are more likely to be caused by age-related decreases in renal function, hepatic blood flow,[24] and volume of distribution than by a decline in hepatic enzyme activity.[26]

Aging may have a profound effect on the pharmacokinetics of commonly used drugs. For instance, aminoglycosides have a narrow margin of safety, and the diminished renal clearance of these drugs that occurs with aging increases the risk of toxicity.[21] Also, the effects of morphine, given by any route, may be both enhanced and prolonged in the elderly, as compared with young adults, because the rate of morphine clearance is 35 percent lower in the elderly.[28]

NUTRITIONAL STATUS

Malnutrition

Malnourished states are characterized by a rise in total body water associated with a rise in extracellular fluid volume.[29,30] These changes serve to increase V and extend $t_{1/2}$. Malnutrition is also associated with reductions in cardiac output, renal plasma flow, and GFR.[29]

Severely malnourished patients have decreased hepatic clearance of drugs.[29] In general, phase 1 reactions are more adversely affected than phase 2 reactions.[31] For instance, in protein malnutrition, clearance of drugs, many of which are metabolized by oxidation (phase 1), may be decreased by 20 to 40 percent. First-pass clearance is affected, which increases the bioavailability of many drugs.[32] In sum, malnutrition results in increased plasma levels of drug and delayed clearance, which increase the risk of toxicity.

The affinity of plasma proteins for drugs is not altered in malnourished states, but the circulating plasma protein mass may be reduced.[33] This change, coupled with diminished glomerular filtration, tends to increase the unbound fraction of some drugs. For example, the elimination of parenterally administered penicillin is decreased by a factor of 2 in patients with severe malnutrition and anasarca.[30]

It has been demonstrated both in healthy adult volunteers and in children with severe malnutrition that hepatic and renal metabolic function, and thereby the clearance of drugs, can be normalized by means of nutritional support.[29]

Obesity

The most important pharmacokinetic consideration in obesity is the distribution of drugs into the excess body fat. To assess these effects, it is preferable to use total body weight (TBW) and an estimated ideal (lean) body weight (IBW) rather than other variables that have been used to define the extent of obesity, such as the body mass index (BMI = the ratio of the TBW in kilograms to height in meters squared) or skin-fold thickness.[34]

Ideal body weight can be calculated as follows:

Men: 50 kg + 2.3 kg for each inch of height over 5 ft
Women: 45.5 kg + 2.3 kg for each inch of height over 5 ft
For both sexes: Subtract 2.3 kg for each inch below 5 ft

Note that obese persons have a larger absolute amount of lean body mass than do persons of normal weight of the same age, height, and sex.

In obese persons, the normal pathways of absorption, metabolism, and elimination of drugs are intact.[35] Because of the proportionately larger fat mass, however, the potential exists for sequestration of lipophilic drugs into excess adipose tissue. Therefore, the volume of distribution, clearance, and half-life of drugs in a wide variety of therapeutic classes are affected, and dose adjustment, especially for those drugs with a narrow therapeutic index, is often needed.

The extent of a drug's distribution into fat depends on its lipid solubility. Lipophilic drugs are drugs with high lipid solubility; that is, they are not ionized, are therefore nonpolar, and are distributed disproportionately into excess adipose tissue. For example, the lipophilic anesthetics, such as halothane and enflurane, are partitioned extensively into fat and therefore have a great increase in the volume of distribution.[36,37] On the other hand, hydrophilic drugs, which are ionized and polar, have a low lipid solubility and are distributed mainly into lean body mass. Thus, augmentation of the volume of distribution does not occur in obese persons given hydrophilic drugs, such as digitoxin,[38] H_2-receptor blockers,[39] and neuromuscular blockers,[40] so dosing of these drugs is based on ideal body weight.

There are significant discrepancies regarding generalizations about distribution of drugs in obese persons. For example, among the highly lipophilic drugs, such as verapamil,[41] sufentanil,[42] and the benzodiazepines (including diazepam, midazolam, lorazepam, oxazepam, alprazolam, and nitrazepam), there is clear evidence for augmentation of the volume of distribution and half-life in obese persons, as compared with nonobese persons.[43] However, for cyclosporine, which is also lipophilic, there is no difference in the volume of distribution and half-life between obese and nonobese persons.[44,45]

Although beta-adrenergic receptor blockers all have differing lipophilicity, in obese persons the volume of distribution is reduced or similar to that found in lean persons.[34] It has been suggested that because these drugs can induce a vasoconstrictive effect, the blood flow into adipose tissue can be altered, thereby limiting diffusion.

Ciprofloxacin, which is considered hydrophilic, is widely distributed in the body,[46] but it is distributed less in fat than in other tissues. Because of this partial distribution into fat, the dose of ciprofloxacin that will be effective in the obese should be calculated on the basis of ideal body weight plus 45 percent of the excess body weight [IBW + 0.45(TBW − IBW)].[47]

The volumes of distribution of aminoglycosides, all polar at normal blood pH, are larger in obese persons than in nonobese persons. This is thought to result from the diffusion of the aminoglycoside into the extracellular fluid contained in adipose tissue.[48] It has been recommended that the initial dose of aminoglycoside be based on the ideal weight plus 40 percent (1.4 IBW).[34] Subsequent dosing should be calculated on the basis of data derived from therapeutic drug monitoring.

RENAL FAILURE

Because of the kidney's role in excretory function and regulation of fluid and electrolytes, renal disease may have a profound effect on pharmacokinetic variables.

Uremia may impair the enteral absorption of drugs. For instance, the internal urea-ammonia cycle enhances alkalinization of gastric juice, impairing the absorption of drugs whose nonionized state is dependent on an acidic environment in the stomach.[49] Bioavailability may be enhanced as a result of a reduction in the first-pass effect (attributable to altered hepatic metabolism, which is common in renal disease).

Edema increases the apparent volume of distribution of drugs that are water soluble and highly protein bound. Renal disease often leads to diminished plasma protein binding, an effect that is clinically relevant for drugs that are highly protein bound. Reduced binding is a function of a decrease in serum albumin, a reduction in binding affinity, and an accumulation of endogenous substances that compete for protein binding sites. Acidic drugs tend to be more affected than basic drugs. The varied clinical manifestations of diminished protein binding include an enhanced risk of toxicity, an increase in apparent volume of distribution, and, because of the increased availability of unbound drug for metabolism and excretion (and the resulting lower plasma concentration), a reduced half-life.[50]

Renal failure has varying effects on biotransformation. Whereas oxidation, glucuronidation, and sulfate conjugation are unaffected, the rates of reduction and hydrolysis reactions are generally decreased.[51] The biotransformed metabolites, many of which are active or toxic, tend to accumulate.[52]

The excretion of drugs cleared by glomerular filtration and tubular secretion is also impaired in patients with renal failure. The simplest way of estimating the glomerular filtration rate is to estimate creatinine clearance:

$$\text{GFR} = \frac{(140 - \text{age [yr]}) \times \text{ideal body weight (kg)}}{72 \times \text{serum creatinine (mg/dl)}}$$

The formula yields the approximate value for men; to obtain the value for women, multiply the result by 0.85. For this formula to yield accurate results, the serum creatinine level and renal function must be stable.[22] If, however, renal function is not stable, as is often the case in patients who are critically ill, it is preferable to measure creatinine clearance rather than estimate it; a timed urine collection and a midpoint determination of the serum creatinine level are necessary. This measurement is especially important when the patient is receiving drugs whose pharmacokinetics are altered by renal disease and whose margin between efficacy and toxicity is small. For practical purposes, in the presence of oliguria the creatinine clearance is assumed to be less than 10 ml/min.

As renal function worsens, tubular excretion decreases. Consequently, the half-lives of drugs whose elimination depends on active organic ion transport by the renal tubule (i.e., tubular excretion) may be prolonged. Furthermore, endogenously produced substances compete with the drugs for transport. This enzyme-driven transport system often becomes saturated, and the problems associated with zero-order kinetics come into play [see Principles of Kinetics, Zero-Order Kinetics, above].

Dosing Regimens

Variables that should be considered in the planning of drug therapy for patients with renal failure are the patient's state of hydration (which affects V), the patient's estimated renal functional status, and whether a loading dose should be used. Giving a loading dose increases the likelihood of attaining a timely therapeutic plasma concentration. This is especially important when a drug with a long half-life is employed.

It is usually safe to give a dose of a drug once. After the initial dose, the subsequent dosing rate may have to be modified in accordance with the patient's renal functional status. The frequently updated monograph by Bennet and colleagues, "Drug prescribing in renal failure: dosing guidelines for adults,"[53] is an especially good resource. At first, estimation of creatinine clearance (and thus of GFR) is a sufficient indicator of renal function. Subsequently, however, creatinine clearance should be measured, particularly when drugs with a narrow margin of safety are used. Therapeutic drug monitoring is also helpful in enhancing the efficiency of drug therapy in patients with renal failure.

HEPATIC FAILURE

Because of the liver's unique anatomic position between the gut and the systemic circulation and its pivotal role in the disposition of drugs, diseases of the liver can dramatically affect pharmacokinetics. Whereas in renal failure there are functional indices (e.g., creatinine clearance) that can be used to guide drug dosing, no such indices exist in liver dysfunction. There are several reasons for this. First, the changes associated with liver injury can range from the imperceptibly slight (as in mild fatty infiltration) to the severe (as in end-stage liver disease). Second, the liver usually needs only a fraction of its functional capacity to carry out each of its metabolic functions. For instance, liver function must fall below 20 percent of normal before glucose maintenance is impaired, and bilirubin elimination must fall below 10 percent of normal before jaundice develops. Third, disposition of drugs does not correlate with either the histologic changes or the biochemical abnormalities that accompany liver disorders.[54] Fourth, the renal clearance of many drugs is impaired as a result of kidney dysfunction related to liver disease. Although this effect is obvious in the hepatorenal syndrome,[55] even moderate degrees of liver dysfunction impair the renal clearance of drugs.[56] Furthermore, because of a reduction in muscle mass that occurs in patients with liver failure, reduced hepatic conversion of creatine to creatinine,[57] and increased fractional tubular secretion of creatinine as GFR deteriorates,[58] assessments of renal function made on the basis of serum creatinine levels or measurements of creatinine clearance overestimate renal capability for clearance of drugs. Fifth, use of alcohol and other recreational drugs can induce or inhibit drug metabolism, as can concurrent administration of other medications.[9-11,14] Sixth, patients with hepatic disorders often receive multiple drugs, and polypharmacy enhances the risk of adverse drug reactions.[59] The situation is complicated because most information on pharmacokinetics in liver disease is derived from patients with chronic alcoholic cirrhosis. In addition, the clearance of drugs in a variety of liver diseases is not significantly altered unless cirrhosis is also present.

In patients with liver disease, there are three factors that modify pharmacokinetics: (1) hepatic blood flow, (2) protein binding, and (3) hepatic enzyme–driven metabolism.[60] It is clinically useful to distinguish between drugs on the basis of the third factor—specifically, the efficiency with which they are irreversibly removed or extracted as they pass through the normal liver [see Table 4]. If a drug's hepatic extraction ratio is greater than 0.6—that is, if more than 60 percent of it is irreversibly removed as it passes through the liver—it is considered highly extracted. Drugs whose hepatic extraction ratio is less than 0.2 are considered poorly extracted.

Because the elimination of highly extracted drugs is so efficient, the rate at which these drugs are removed is dependent upon the rate at which they are delivered (i.e., on hepatic blood flow); changes in intrahepatic metabolic processes or protein binding do not affect their clearance. When a significant amount of blood bypasses the liver, as occurs in cirrhosis or in surgically created portosystemic shunts, less of the drug is delivered to the liver, which means that bioavailability of an enterally administered drug would increase and clearance of a parenterally delivered drug would decrease. Moreover, the diminished blood flow associated with congestive hepatomegaly, beta-adrenergic blockade, and hypotensive states is capable of decreasing the clearance of highly extracted drugs.[60] For instance, the clearance of highly extracted drugs in diseased livers has been observed to be five to 65 percent lower than the clearance in healthy livers.[61,62] Such changes may have a substantial impact on bioavailability: if, for instance, the hepatic extraction ratio of a drug decreases from 0.95 to 0.90, the bioavailability of that drug doubles, from 0.5 to 1.0.

For most highly extracted drugs, liver disease does not have an appreciable effect on V.[54] Therefore, unless factors that significantly alter bioavailability are present, the amount of drug required to achieve a desired plasma concentration in a patient with liver disease should be much the same as that required in someone with normal liver function. However, because of reduced hepatic blood flow (and, therefore, reduced clearance), the half-life of highly extracted drugs is prolonged.[62] For example, when given a constant infusion of lidocaine, patients with chronic liver disease take 24 hours to attain a steady-state plasma concentration, whereas those with a normal liver attain a steady state in 10 hours.[63] Consequently, the rate of drug administration should be reduced. Most available data suggest that for patients with chronic liver disease, the dosage of highly extracted drugs should be reduced by 50 percent.

Clearance of poorly extracted drugs, unlike that of highly extracted drugs, is not influenced by hepatic blood flow but is influenced by intrahepatic metabolic processes.[60,62] Clearance of those poorly extracted drugs that are also more than 85 percent bound to plasma proteins (e.g., diazepam, phenytoin, and warfarin) can be affected by factors that alter plasma protein binding as well as by factors that alter enzymatic biotransformation. Among the factors that reduce protein binding are (1) a decrease in serum albumin, (2) production of defective or altered plasma proteins, and (3) displacement of drugs from plasma protein binding sites, either by endogenously produced substances (e.g., bilirubin, which has a strong binding affinity for albumin) or by drugs with a stronger competitive affinity.[64] When binding is decreased, more drug is available to distribute to tissues, and both V and $t^{1/2}$ are increased. More drug also becomes available for elimination. When biotransforming enzyme capability is diminished, however, active drug accumulates, and the risk of toxicity increases. Clearance of those poorly extracted drugs that have low binding ratios is not significantly affected by factors that alter plasma protein binding.

Clearance of drugs that have intermediate hepatic extraction ratios is potentially sensitive to altered hepatic blood flow, altered hepatic enzyme clearance, altered protein binding, or any combination thereof.

Table 4 Hepatic Extraction Ratios for Selected Drugs

Drug	Extraction Ratio
Highly extracted	
Labetalol	0.85
Lidocaine	0.60
Morphine	0.75
Propranolol	0.65
Verapamil	0.80
Poorly extracted	
Chlordiazepoxide	0.02
Diazepam	0.02
Diphenylhydantoin	0.03
Theophylline	0.05
Warfarin	0.005

In chronic diseases of the liver, phase 1 biotransforming processes are more affected than phase 2 processes. For example, elimination of the benzodiazepines lorazepam and oxazepam, which are metabolized through glucuronidation, a phase 2 reaction, is not significantly altered, whereas clearance of diazepam and chlordiazepoxide, which are metabolized through phase 1 reactions, is reduced.

In advanced liver disease, altered pharmacodynamic responses may occur independently of altered pharmacokinetic variables, especially in patients at risk for encephalopathy, who have a tendency toward an altered mental state when analgesics, anxiolytics, or hypnotics are used.

Dosing Regimens

The lack of indices of liver function to guide drug dosing and the difficulty of predicting drug disposition in the presence of liver disease make it difficult to define precisely how drug regimens should be modified in patients with hepatic dysfunction. Generally, in patients who have liver disease but not cirrhosis, hepatic elimination of drugs is not significantly impaired. A good background knowledge of the hepatic disorders capable of modifying pharmacokinetic variables, coupled with informed guesswork as to the magnitude of the change in drug dosing needed, can improve the safety of drug administration in patients with liver disease. Whatever drugs are given, the clinician should exercise an extra degree of caution, paying close attention to plasma drug levels (if they are available) and remaining alert for evidence of toxicity. Comprehensive guidelines for dosing in patients with liver dysfunction have been published.[54]

CARDIAC FAILURE

Cardiac failure is associated with changes in systemic, regional and organ blood flow that affect the absorption, distribution, and clearance of many drugs.[65] Because the hemodynamic response to cardiac failure is not uniform, it may not be possible to predict how pharmacokinetics will be modified. In general, however, the principal pharmacokinetic consequences of cardiac failure stem from congestion and hypoperfusion.

In congestive heart failure, congestion of the gut and impaired gastric emptying may reduce enteral absorption of drugs.[65] Absorption of loop diuretics and the angiotensin-converting enzyme inhibitor lisinopril is affected. However, the enteral absorption of digoxin is unchanged in heart failure.[66,67] Hypoperfusion can decrease the rate of absorption of drugs administered subcutaneously, intramuscularly, or cutaneously. Problems of drug absorption can be circumvented in patients with cardiac failure by using the intravenous route.

Because of the increase in total body water in congestive heart failure, the volume of distribution of highly water soluble drugs is increased.[65] On the other hand, the volume of distribution of several antidysrhythmic drugs, such as lidocaine and quinidine, is substantially reduced.[63,65] The reasons for these empirical observations are not clear. The important point, however, is that the usual doses of these drugs may evoke a toxic reaction in the patient with a failing heart. Therefore, when such a patient is given a drug whose volume of distribution is known to be decreased by congestive heart failure, the loading dose should be reduced. It is important to note that the volume of distribution of digoxin, which is huge because of extensive binding to tissues, is unchanged in congestive heart failure.[65]

Congestive heart failure and acute myocardial infarction decrease both hepatic and renal clearance of many drugs secondary to diminished perfusion of these organs as a result of decreased cardiac output.[65] In addition, passive congestion of the liver enhances the potential for diminished hepatic clearance.[63] In congestive heart failure, hepatic blood flow and hepatic enzyme activity are decreased to a greater extent than renal function is.[63] Therefore, toxicity is more likely with drugs metabolized in the liver than with those excreted primarily by the kidney.

Hepatic clearance of drugs with high or intermediate hepatic extraction ratios (e.g., lidocaine) is reduced, and their half-lives are thereby lengthened.[63,65] Infusion of drugs that increase hepatic blood flow (e.g., isoproterenol) may enhance elimination of these drugs; infusion of alpha-adrenergic agonists (e.g., norepinephrine) or beta-adrenergic blockers (e.g., propranolol) may have the opposite effect.[65] Renal blood flow may decrease out of proportion to the reduction in cardiac output, leading to a diminished GFR and, potentially, to diminished tubular excretion and reabsorption of drugs.[65] For instance, excessive diuresis with furosemide can reduce renal clearance of digoxin. On the other hand, afterload reduction with hydralazine or nitroglycerin increases renal blood flow and renal clearance of drugs in patients with cardiac failure.[65]

Because myocardial function (and, therefore, organ blood flow) changes constantly during treatment of heart failure, drug therapy must be continually reassessed. When the drug given has a narrow margin between therapeutic and toxic levels, therapeutic drug monitoring [see Monitoring Drug Therapy, Measurement of Plasma Drug Concentration (Therapeutic Drug Monitoring), below] can be a valuable aid.

CARDIOPULMONARY BYPASS

In cardiopulmonary bypass, there are four factors that alter pharmacokinetics: (1) nonpulsatile blood flow leads to a redistribution of blood flow from nonvital organs as well as from the liver, (2) the pump oxygenator is primed with 1.5 to 2.0 L of balanced electrolyte solution, which causes hemodilution, (3) the patient is heparinized, and (4) hypothermia is induced.[68]

The only blood flow to the lung during a cardiopulmonary bypass procedure is via the bronchial circulation. Therefore, drugs that normally accumulate in the lung (e.g., lidocaine) are unable to do so and exhibit a decreased volume of distribution.[69] After circulation is restored, these drugs, if present in the systemic circulation, accumulate in the lung, and their plasma concentration is abruptly decreased. In addition, any drugs present in the lung before the bypass are washed out.

Concurrent with the hemodilution associated with asanguineous priming of the pump oxygenator, there is an immediate and proportional reduction in plasma drug concentration. This has been documented for a number of drugs, including benzodiazepines, cephalosporins, cardiac glycosides, opiates, and lidocaine.[68] Hemodilution also affects serum protein binding: for highly bound drugs, hemodilution of serum albumin leads to a rise in the unbound fraction, which favors redistribution to tissues and elimination and thus results in decreased plasma drug concentrations.

Heparin may also decrease protein binding of drugs.[70] After cardiopulmonary bypass, the binding of basic drugs is altered because of the substantial rise in α_1-acid glycoprotein.[68]

Hypothermia, by decreasing metabolic activity, reduces the intrinsic biotransforming activity.

RESPIRATORY DISORDERS

The pathophysiological changes induced by respiratory disorders or the treatment of these disorders with mechanical ventilation can potentially alter the pharmacokinetics of drugs.[71,72] Sequelae of respiratory diseases (e.g., pulmonary hypertension) that are known to alter the disposition of drugs include hypoxemia; altered ventilation, resulting in either respiratory alkalosis or acidosis; right ventricular dysfunction from pulmonary hypertension, leading to congestive hepatomegaly; and decreased regional blood flow, especially to the liver and kidney.[71]

The changes in drug absorption and bioavailability associated with pulmonary disorders are predominantly the result of secondary alterations in perfusion and congestive hepatomegaly rather than primary effects of the pulmonary condition. For instance, the increased bioavailability of drugs with high hepatic extraction can result from a decrease in the first-pass effect, which is associated with impaired liver function, secondary to the hemodynamic alterations caused by pulmonary hypertension.

In chronic obstructive lung disease, inflammatory conditions of the lung, respiratory tract infection, and bronchogenic carcinoma, a twofold to threefold increase in circulating α_1-acid glycoprotein occurs.[73] Thus, in these diseases, the protein binding capacity of neutral and basic drugs is vastly enhanced.[73] The best-studied example involves patients with chronic obstructive lung disease who were treated with propranolol. Substantially less unbound propranolol—that is, active drug—was found in these patients than in healthy volunteers.[74]

Theoretically, the tissue distribution of drugs with pK_a values close to the pH of plasma should be significantly altered by small changes in the plasma pH. For instance, if the pH change from a change in minute ventilation results in an increase in the nonionized fraction of a drug, there should be an increase in tissue distribution of that drug, increasing its apparent V. To date, there are no confirmatory studies of this phenomenon in humans, however.[71]

Elimination of drugs is affected by both pulmonary disorders and mechanical ventilation, which are often interrelated. For instance, the pathological sequelae of pulmonary hypertension are exacerbated by positive pressure mechanical ventilation, especially when positive end-expiratory pressure (PEEP) is added.[72]

The decrease in hepatic blood flow can be associated with diminished clearance of drugs that have high hepatic extraction ratios.[75] In one study, for example, healthy persons with normal hepatic function who were given lidocaine either received or did not receive mechanical ventilation. The clearance of lidocaine was found to be 22 percent lower in those who received mechanical ventilation than in those who did not receive mechanical ventilation.[75] Impaired clearance can also be expected with other drugs that have high hepatic extraction ratios, including labetalol, meperidine, metoprolol, propranolol, and verapamil. Interventions that enhance cardiac output and maintain organ perfusion, such as blood volume expansion and inotropic support, and changes in mechanical ventilation that decrease mean airway pressure should reduce the risk of adverse reactions from these drugs.

Data on the renal elimination of drugs in patients with pulmonary disease and in patients who require mechanical ventilation are not available.[71] However, with the known systemic effects of cor pulmonale and mechanical ventilation on renal blood flow, changes in the renal excretion of drugs can be expected.[72] The elimination of those drugs whose clearance depends on GFR (e.g., β-lactam antibiotics, vancomycin, aminoglycosides, and digitoxin) should decrease. The elimination of those drugs whose clearance depends on tubular secretion (e.g., digoxin, furosemide, procainamide, and several penicillins) should also decrease because of the decrease in renal blood flow. Additionally, as urine volume decreases, the gradient for resorption increases, which decreases the elimination of drugs in the glomerular filtrate concentrate (e.g., aminoglycosides and phenobarbital).

The efficacy of an antibiotic against pulmonary infections is related to its sputum concentration rather than its plasma concentration.[72] The higher the ratio of the bronchiolar concentration of an antibiotic to the minimum inhibitory concentration (MIC) of that antibiotic against the infecting organism, the better the therapeutic effect. To be effective, an antibiotic must diffuse through the pulmonary capillary into the bronchiolar alveolar lumen. Because this process involves passive diffusion, it is enhanced by the elevated concentration gradient that results from a higher serum concentration, and it proceeds more freely if the drug is nonionized and lipid soluble at plasma pH. Inflammation may increase the penetration of some drugs.

Administration of Drugs

SELECTION

In selecting drugs, the clinician must consider the diagnosis, the stage of the disease, any coexisting illnesses, and any drugs being used concurrently. He or she must also establish goals of therapy and acceptable limits of toxicity. (For instance, dysarthria associated with administration of lidocaine for emergent control of ventricular tachycardia might be considered inconsequential, whereas sleep disturbances associated with long-term use of propranolol for mild essential hypertension might be unacceptable.) In addition, the physician must be aware of the variability in drug response among people.

Because of the risk of toxicity, only those drugs that are absolutely necessary should be used. ICU patients receive an average of seven to 17 drugs.[76] Critical review shows not only that some of these drugs are unnecessary but also that duplication—such as simultaneously administering an antacid and an H_2-receptor blocker—is common. Physicians should consider using only one or two drugs in each therapeutic class and should be thoroughly familiar with each agent's pharmacological and toxic properties. New drugs are inherently more risky. When a new drug is employed, it is essential to understand the indications for its use and to know how to monitor its effects.

Routine or standard preprinted medication orders should be avoided. For reasons of convenience, many surgeons write such orders for a variety of potential clinical problems. This practice is intrinsically risky. If the patient's clinical state changes, the physician should be notified and the problem investigated before a drug is administered.

Fixed-dose drug combinations do not have a role in the treatment of hospitalized surgical patients whose pathophysiological condition is changing.

ROUTE OF ADMINISTRATION

Because enteral, intramuscular, and subcutaneous absorption of drugs is often impaired in critical illness, the intravenous route is preferable in ICU patients, especially those who are hemodynamically unstable. Continuous intravenous infusion is a convenient and effective method of attaining and sustaining a steady-state plasma concentration of a drug. Often, intravenously administered drugs are given in a bolus. It is important to remember that when a drug is administered intravenously, the entire amount reaches the systemic circulation immediately, yielding complete bioavailability (F = 1). When this route is used, it is essential that the physician remain aware of the margin between therapeutic and toxic plasma concentrations.

INITIAL DOSE

Whether a given drug regimen is therapeutically efficacious or provokes toxic reactions depends on the dosage. If the therapeutic margin is narrow or the effect of the drug is difficult to assess, the drug should be administered at a rate slow enough to prevent toxicity while the drug is being distributed; in general, smaller doses are safer. However, when such a cautious approach is taken, the goals of therapy may not always be met. (Control of seizures, for example, calls for aggressive drug therapy. Inadequate control of infection, especially pneumonia, as a result of underdosing of antibiotics is also frequent.[77,78]) There-

---

Therapeutic Index and Standard Margin of Safety

All drugs are potentially lethal. The therapeutic index and the standard margin of safety are two measures employed by the pharmaceutical industry to quantitate potential lethality. The therapeutic index is the factor by which the dose that is therapeutically effective in 50 percent of the population (ED_{50}) must be increased to cause death in 50 percent of the population (LD_{50}):

$$\text{Therapeutic index} = \frac{LD_{50}}{ED_{50}}$$

This measure of safety is satisfactory when the range of therapeutically effective doses does not overlap with the lowest lethal dose. When these doses overlap, the standard margin of safety is a better index of safety. The standard margin of safety is the factor by which the dose that is effective in 99 percent of the population (ED_{99}) must be increased to cause death in one percent of the population (LD_1):

$$\text{Standard margin of safety} = \frac{LD_1}{ED_{99}}$$

fore, therapy must be aimed at achieving a target plasma concentration. Therapeutic plasma concentrations have been published for a number of drugs whose therapeutic and toxic ranges are separated by a narrow margin[3] (e.g., 10 to 20 µg/ml for theophylline, 1.5 to 6.0 µg/ml for lidocaine, and 0.5 to 2.0 ng/ml for digoxin). If the margin of safety is wide, as with the penicillins, large doses, which ensure therapeutic efficacy and extend the dosing interval, may be given.

Therapy usually starts with an average dose that is known to be effective and safe in most patients. In any individual patient, however, the ultimate plasma concentration of a drug is affected by the patient's age, genetic makeup, weight, and diseases, as well as by any other drugs he or she may be taking. Often, several doses of a drug must be administered before a therapeutically effective plasma concentration is achieved. In critical care situations, this delay is not desirable. To avoid this delay, a loading dose can be given.

LOADING DOSE

When a loading dose is administered, the target plasma concentration is achieved immediately. The loading dose can be calculated from the target plasma concentration, the volume of distribution, and the bioavailability of the drug[3]:

$$\text{Loading dose} = \frac{V \times C}{F}$$

In emergencies, the loading dose is usually given intravenously, and therefore, $F = 1$. The alterations of V associated with many disease states will necessarily affect the size of the loading dose.

If the drug has a narrow margin of safety, the loading dose may be infused over a long period to avoid toxicity, as is done with lidocaine and the aminoglycosides. Alternatively, the total loading dose may be divided, as is done with cardiac glycosides such as digoxin. Digoxin has a half-life of 1.5 days; without loading, it would take about a week to reach an effective plasma concentration and a steady state. To achieve a therapeutic plasma concentration in a more timely fashion without toxic effects, the loading dose is divided into several doses and given over the first day or two of therapy.

From practical clinical experience, an effective plasma concentration can usually be achieved by administering a dose equal to twice the usual maintenance dose and then maintained by repeating the maintenance dose at intervals equal to the elimination half-life of the drug.

MAINTENANCE DOSING

Steady-State Plasma Concentration

The purpose of repetitive dosing is to achieve a steady-state plasma concentration within the drug's therapeutic range. In pharmacological terms, a steady-state plasma concentration is attained when the amount of drug administered is equal to the amount eliminated. It is dependent on the dose, the dosing interval, bioavailability, and clearance:

$$\overline{C}_{ss} = \frac{F \times D}{CL \times \tau}$$

where $\overline{C}_{ss}$ is the mean steady-state plasma concentration, D is the dose, and τ is the dosing interval.

When a drug is given by any route at regular intervals, a steady state is approached in five half-lives [see Figure 7]. Even though the drug continues to accumulate, it does so at an ever-decreasing rate [see Table 5]. Eventually, the rate at which the drug is cleared is equal to the rate at which it is delivered, at which point a true steady state is achieved. During each dosing interval, the plasma concentration rises and falls, exhibiting so-called peak and trough values; however, both the $\overline{C}_{ss}$ and the fluctuation in concentration within the dosing interval remain constant.

If the dose is too small, the dosing interval is too long, bioavailability is limited, or clearance is too rapid, the $\overline{C}_{ss}$ may be too low to be therapeutically efficacious; conversely, if the dose is too large, the dosing interval is too short, bioavailability is high, or clearance is slow, the $\overline{C}_{ss}$ may be higher than desirable and potentially in the toxic range. Any change in one or more of these four factors will eventually lead to a new steady-state plasma concentration, but only after an additional five half-lives have elapsed.

Dosing Adjustments

Regardless of how a pharmacodynamic effect or a steady-state plasma concentration is achieved, to maintain this effect, it is necessary to adjust the dosage (expressed as dose over dosing interval, or D/τ) so that the rate of drug input equals the rate of elimination. The dosage may be determined by restating the equation for $\overline{C}_{ss}$ as follows:

$$\frac{D}{\tau} = \overline{C}_{ss} \times \frac{CL}{F}$$

The most efficient dosing interval for maintaining a mean steady state is one half-life of the drug. When the risk of toxicity is low and clearance is rapid, as with penicillin, the dose can be large and the dosing interval long. When the margin of safety is narrow, however, to maintain an effective mean steady state and avoid toxicity, the dosing interval must match the half-life more closely. Therefore, to design a rational plan, the clinician needs to know a drug's bioavailability, clearance, volume of distribution, half-life, therapeutic margin of safety, and potential for variability among people, as well as the patient's disease. If one can measure the plasma concentration of a drug, one can estimate bioavailability, clearance, and volume of distribution; this allows more precise dosing. Plasma concentration measurements become exceedingly important in the complex milieu of critical care, where numerous drugs with narrow margins of safety are employed.

Monitoring Drug Therapy

Therapeutic efficacy without toxicity is the goal of drug therapy. Efficacy is evaluated in three ways: (1) by assessing the clinical response (subjective or objective), (2) by monitoring a drug-related variable, and (3) by measuring the drug concentration in a biologic fluid (e.g., plasma), a process also known as therapeutic drug monitoring. Because response to drugs varies considerably from one patient to another and sometimes even in a single patient during a single course of therapy, monitoring drug therapy is a dynamic process.

ASSESSMENT OF CLINICAL RESPONSE

For certain classes of drugs, efficacy is most effectively evaluated by subjective or objective measurement of clinical response. The effects of analgesics, nonsteroidal anti-inflammatory drugs, and sedatives are assessed on the basis of subjective response; the effects of other drugs, such as antipyretics and antihypertensive agents, are assessed by objective measurement (i.e., body temperature and blood pressure).

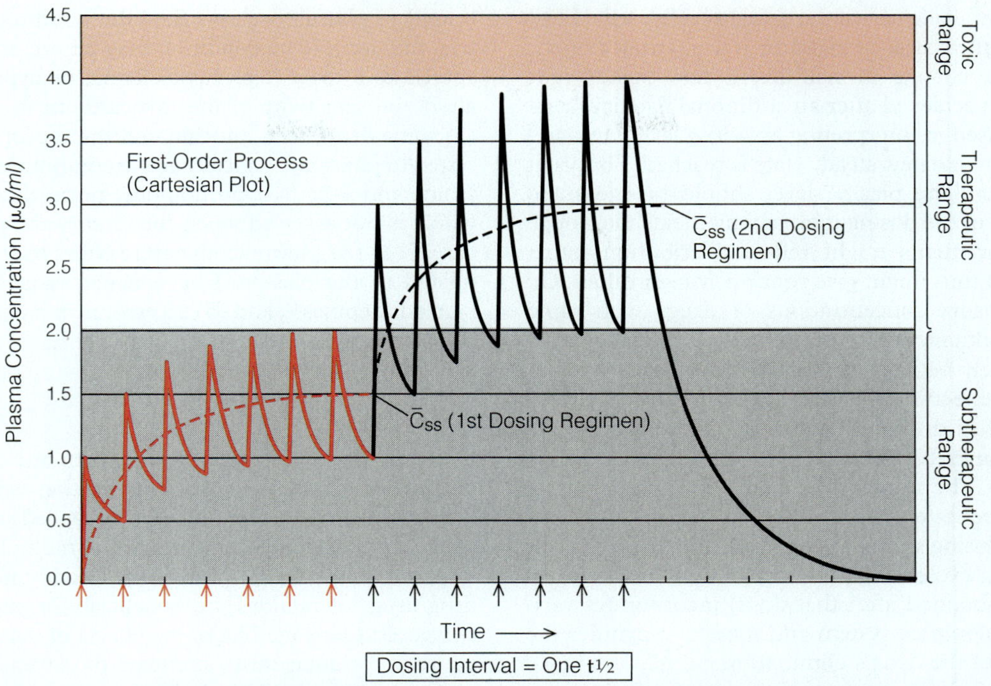

Figure 7 A drug that follows first-order kinetics is given intravenously in a dose that yields a plasma concentration of 1.0 μg/ml. Subsequently, identical doses are given at dosing intervals equal to the half-life of the drug (↑). At the end of each half-life, half the amount of drug present at the beginning of the dosing interval remains. The solid red line reflects the rising and falling of the plasma concentration after each dose; the broken red line represents the mean plasma concentration. The mean plasma concentration rises rapidly through five half-lives, at which point it has reached a virtual steady state ($\overline{C}_{ss}$). In this instance, the $\overline{C}_{ss}$ is in the subtherapeutic range. Accordingly, the dose is doubled after the seventh half-life. Both peak and trough plasma levels rise (solid black line). The mean plasma concentration at the new dose (broken black line) rises to a new $\overline{C}_{ss}$ in an additional five half-lives. The last dose is given at the end of the 13th half-life. By the end of the 18th half-life, 96.9 percent of the drug has been eliminated.

In this illustration, only the dose changed. However, a change in any other variable (e.g., bioavailability, dosing interval, or clearance) would also result in a new $\overline{C}_{ss}$ but, again, only after an additional five half-lives.

When the efficacy of an agent with a narrow margin of safety (e.g., lidocaine, digoxin, or theophylline) is being assessed on the basis of clinical response, it is prudent to monitor plasma levels as well.

MONITORING OF A DRUG-RELATED VARIABLE

Laboratory tests are often used to assess the effects of drug therapy indirectly. Laboratory assessment is especially important when drugs with a narrow margin of safety are used prophylactically. For example, the prothrombin time and international normalized ratio (INR), the partial thromboplastin time, the platelet count, and the bleeding time are used to monitor anticoagulation [see 70 Thromboembolic Problems]. Urine and blood glucose levels guide the use of hypoglycemic agents. Laboratory tests are also used to screen for toxic effects. For instance, the results of hearing tests and serum creatinine measurements may suggest the presence of aminoglycoside toxicity. Acidemia may suggest—and an elevated thiocyanate level may prove—the presence of nitroprusside toxicity.

MEASUREMENT OF PLASMA DRUG CONCENTRATION (THERAPEUTIC DRUG MONITORING)

It is useful to measure the plasma concentration of the following drugs: antidysrhythmics, cardiac glycosides, anticonvulsants, aminoglycosides, tricyclic antidepressants, lithium, vancomycin, and theophylline.[79] With all of these agents, the margin between therapeutic concentrations and toxic concentrations is narrow.

It must be remembered that the published therapeutic ranges of many drugs are not absolute values and must be interpreted in the light of the clinical response. In general, at the lower end of the referenced therapeutic plasma concentration, the desired therapeutic effect will be achieved about half the time. The ceiling of the therapeutic range is determined by toxicity: at the upper end of this range, five to 10 percent of patients will experience toxic reactions.[15] A useful example is digoxin. At plasma concentrations of 0.5 to 2.0 ng/ml, the drug is effective in most patients, and toxic effects are infrequent. However, at plasma concentrations of 1.7, 2.5, and 3.3 ng/ml, the probability of a digoxin-induced dysrhythmia is 10 percent, 50 percent, and 90 percent, respectively.[3]

Obtaining of Samples

To enhance interpretation of plasma drug levels, samples must be obtained at the proper time in the dosing cycle. If the drug is being administered by continuous intravenous infusion, sampling is best done after a steady-state concentration has been achieved (i.e., after five half-lives of the drug have elapsed). If the dose or the dosing interval is changed or if a pharmacokinetic variable produces a change in half-life, a new steady-state concentration will be achieved after an additional five half-lives. Caution should be used in interpreting any drug level measurements obtained before the new steady state is reached. For drugs with slow elimination, the plasma level should be measured during the latter half of the dosing interval; this yields the trough level. Earlier measurements might reflect distribution rather than elimination and thus might give spuriously high values. On the other hand, plasma concentrations of drugs with rapid elimination (e.g., gentamicin,[80] procainamide,[81] and theophylline[82]) fluctuate widely between doses. Therefore, two samples are obtained: one, reflecting the peak concentration, is drawn 30 to 60 minutes after drug administration is completed; the other, reflecting trough concentration, is drawn immediately before the next dose. The slope of the drug's elimination curve is calculated most accurately using peak and trough blood levels from the same dosing cycle. Using peak and trough levels from different dosing cycles (e.g., the trough obtained before a dose and the peak obtained after that dose) incorporates variations inherent in a complex system and thereby magnifies the error in calculation of the drug's elimination curve.

In general, the peak drug concentration is used to assess toxicity, whereas the trough concentration is used to assess therapeutic efficacy. This is true for time-dependent bactericidal antibiotics—that is, all β-lactams and glycopeptides (the most important of which is vancomycin)—for which the bactericidal effect is a function of the length of time the serum concentration of the antibiotic is above the MIC of the target organism.[83] However, among the antibiotics that display concentration-dependent bacterial killing, particularly the aminoglycosides, the peak level assesses efficacy—that is, the higher the concentration, the greater the killing power—and the trough level assesses the risk of nephrotoxicity.[84]

Interpretation of Measurements

The following confounding factors must be taken into account in the interpretation of measurements of plasma concentration: (1) the measured plasma drug level includes not only the unbound, or biologically active, fraction but also the amount bound to plasma proteins (i.e., the bound, or biologically inactive, fraction); (2) a condition may be present that alters the response to a drug (e.g., hypokalemia or hypercalcemia typically alters the sensitivity of the myocardium to cardiac glycosides); (3) some drugs (e.g., procainamide and propranolol) are metabolized to pharmacologically active compounds (N-acetylprocainamide and 4-hydroxypropranolol, respectively), the presence of which is not assessed when the level of the parent drug is measured; (4) the pharmacodynamic effect may not be consistently related to the plasma drug concentration, as is the case with benzodiazepines[84]; and (5) an error may have been made in sampling or assay.

Drug-Drug Interactions

A drug-drug interaction occurs when one drug alters the effect of another. The potential for interaction exists whenever more than one drug is given, and it is enhanced in critical care units, where simultaneous administration of multiple drugs is common. The true scope of the problem is clearly underestimated. Some drug-drug interactions are beneficial: for example, the narcotic antagonist naloxone blocks the effects of narcotics, beta-adrenergic receptor antagonists attenuate the effects of catecholamines, probenecid blocks the tubular secretion of penicillin, and protamine reverses the effects of heparin. Of much greater concern to the clinician are those interactions that either diminish the efficacy of a drug or produce an unforeseen response. Such undesirable interactions are known to affect each pharmacokinetic variable.

ALTERED ABSORPTION

As noted [see Administration of Drugs, Route of Administration, *above*], in critically ill patients, most drugs should be delivered intravenously. I.V. administration avoids the large number of interactions that could occur when multiple agents are given simultaneously by the enteral route. Still, when drugs are coadministered intravenously, the possibility of drug inactivation must be considered. Certain combinations can neither be mixed in the same bottle nor be administered simultaneously through the same intravenous line. These incompatibilities are documented.[85] In addition, most clinical pharmacists have resources that identify potential drug-drug interactions.

Table 5 Accumulation of Drug over Time When Dosing Interval Equals Half-life

		Amount of Drug in Body (mg)	
$t_{1/2}$	Dose (mg)	At Start of $t_{1/2}$	At End of $t_{1/2}$
First	100	100	50
Second	100	150	75
Third	100	175	87.5
Fourth	100	187.5	93.8
Fifth	100	193.8	96.9
Sixth	100	196.9	98.4
Seventh	100	198.4	99.2
Eighth	100	199.2	99.6
Ninth	100	199.6	99.8
Tenth	100	199.8	99.9
Eleventh	100	199.9	99.95

ALTERED DISTRIBUTION

Many drugs compete for the same protein binding sites and may competitively displace each other. As a result, the unbound fraction of the displaced drug is increased. When the routes of biotransformation and elimination are intact and not saturated, there are usually no adverse consequences. When these pathways are impaired or saturated, however, the potential exists for a significant increase in the unbound fraction. From a clinical perspective, the most important recognized interactions involving protein binding displacement occur with the coumarin group of anticoagulants. Drugs that compete with these anticoagulants for protein binding sites include chloral hydrate, ethacrynic acid, phenytoin, salicylates, and many antibiotics.[4] A decrease in the protein binding of coumarin from 99 percent to 96 percent might be considered an inconsequential change, but it represents a quadrupling of the active fraction of drug.

ALTERED BIOTRANSFORMATION

The metabolic pathways by which drugs are biotransformed are the site of a large number of drug-drug interactions. The vast majority of these interactions occur with enzyme induction or inhibition, usually of the P-450 family of mixed-function oxidases. For instance, cigarette smoking, phenobarbital, phenytoin, and rifampin induce the enzymes that increase the rate of biotransformation of theophylline; chronic ethanol use, phenobarbital, phenytoin, and rifampin accelerate the metabolism of oral anticoagulants.[10] Because induction both begins and ends slowly [see Pharmacokinetic Variables, Biotransformation (Metabolism), above], there must be an extended period of drug monitoring when enzyme induction is a possibility. Drugs that are metabolized by the same enzyme may competitively inhibit the biotransformation of each other. For instance, recent alcohol ingestion impedes the metabolism of chloral hydrate, benzodiazepines, propranolol, and phenytoin.[49]

Other drug-drug interactions result from altered regional blood flow. For instance, beta-adrenergic blocking agents decrease hepatic blood flow.[65] Therefore, the biotransformation of drugs with a high hepatic extraction rate, such as lidocaine, will be reduced.[63]

ALTERED ELIMINATION

Many drugs are eliminated through glomerular filtration or renal tubular secretion. Drugs that alter the GFR (such as low-dose dopamine, which increases it,[86] or furosemide, which decreases it[87]) will alter the clearance of other drugs (such as the aminoglycosides and digoxin).

A large number of drugs are eliminated by proximal tubular secretion. There are two active transport pathways: one for organic acids and one for organic bases. These pathways are not drug specific; drugs of the same class compete with each other for transport. A long list of clinically useful organic acids, including many diuretics, nonsteroidal anti-inflammatory drugs, penicillins, and cephalosporins, all compete for the same excretory transport system.[10] Endogenous acids compete for transport as well, which explains the frequently observed need for an increase in the dose of furosemide to obtain a satisfactory clinical effect in the presence of uremia.[88] Tubular secretion of organic bases has been less extensively studied. It is recognized, however, that when cimetidine or ranitidine is given simultaneously with procainamide, competition between these organic bases provokes an increase in the concentration of procainamide.[89,90]

Drugs that increase urine flow provide less time for reabsorption and therefore enhance excretion. Drugs that alter urine pH may coincidentally influence tubular reabsorption.

Additional Resources

To make timely and rational therapeutic decisions, surgeons involved in critical care will inevitably require more resources than are available in this chapter. Drug-drug interactions, pharmacokinetic predictions, and dosing schedules can become highly complex in patients who are receiving multiple drugs (as ICU patients generally are). Hospital-based clinical pharmacists can be of considerable assistance with these problems and should be integrated into the ICU team. There are several good reference sources that can be used to facilitate pharmacokinetic decision making.[53,54] In addition, an increasing number of computerized drug-drug interaction software programs are becoming available. In many institutions, these programs are used by the hospital-based pharmacist. There are also computerized pharmacokinetic programs that can be used to make initial projections and to refine drug dosage schedules in the clinical setting. These software services are routinely updated and can be of great value.

References

1. Jick H: Adverse drug reactions: the magnitude of the problem. J Allergy Clin Immunol 74:555, 1984
2. Benet LZ, Mitchell JR, Sheiner LB: Pharmacokinetics: the dynamics of drug absorption, distribution, and elimination. Goodman and Gilman's The Pharmacological Basis of Therapeutics, 8th ed. Gilman AF, Rall TW, Nies AS, et al, Eds. Pergamon Press, New York, 1990, p 3
3. Benet LZ, Williams RL: Appendix II: Design and optimization of dosage regimens: pharmacokinetic data. Goodman and Gilman's The Pharmacological Basis of Therapeutics, 8th ed. Gilman AF, Rall TW, Nies AS, et al, Eds. Pergamon Press, New York, 1990, p 1650
4. Majerus PW, Broze GJ Jr, Miletich JP, et al: Anticoagulant, thrombolytic, and antiplatelet drugs. Goodman and Gilman's The Pharmacological Basis of Therapeutics, 8th ed. Gilman AR, Rall TW, Nies AS, et al, Eds. Pergamon Press, New York, 1990, p 1311
5. Biological Basis of Detoxication. Caldwell J, Jakoby WB, Eds. Academic Press, New York, 1983
6. Nelson DR, Kamataki T, Waxman DJ, et al: The P_{450} superfamily: update on new sequences, gene mapping, accession numbers, early trivial names of enzymes, and nomenclature. DNA Cell Biol 12:1, 1993
7. Shimada F, Yamazaki H, Mimura M, et al: Individual variations in human liver cytochrome P_{450} enzymes involved in the oxidation of drugs, carcinogens, and toxic chemicals: studies with liver microsomes of 30 Japanese and 30 Caucasians. J Pharmacol Exp Ther 270:414, 1994
8. Garrison JC, Peach MJ: Renin and angiotensin. Goodman and Gilman's The Pharmacologic Basis of Therapeutics, 8th ed. Gilman AR, Rall TW, Nies AS, et al, Eds. Pergamon Press, New York, 1990, p 749
9. Goldstein JA: Mechanism of induction of hepatic drug metabolizing enzymes: recent advances. Trends Pharmacol Sci, July 1984, p 290
10. Vasko MR, Brater DC: Drug interactions. The Pharmacologic Approach to the Critically Ill Patient, 2nd ed. Chernow B, Ed. Williams & Wilkins, Baltimore, 1988, p 21
11. Jaffe JH: Drug addiction and drug abuse. Goodman and Gilman's The Pharmacological Basis of Therapeutics, 8th ed. Gilman AF, Rall TW, Nies AS, et al, Eds. Pergamon Press, New York, 1990, p 522
12. Bierman CW, Williams PV: Therapeutic monitoring of theophylline: rationale and current status. Clin Pharmacokinet 17:377, 1989

13. Sedman AJ: Cimetidine-drug interactions. Am J Med 76:109, 1984
14. Rall TW: Hypnotics and sedatives; ethanol. Goodman and Gilman's The Pharmacological Basis of Therapeutics, 8th ed. Gilman AF, Rall TW, Nies AS, et al, Eds. Pergamon Press, New York, 1990, p 345
15. Hoffman BH, Bigger JT Jr: Digitalis and allied cardiac glycosides. Goodman and Gilman's The Pharmacological Basis of Therapeutics, 8th ed. Gilman AF, Rall TW, Nies AS, et al, Eds. Pergamon Press, New York, 1990, p 814
16. Boréus LO: Principles of Pediatric Pharmacology. Churchill Livingstone, New York, 1982, pp 107, 115
17. Kearns GL, Reed MD: Clinical pharmacokinetics in infants and children: a reappraisal. Clin Pharmacokinet 17(suppl 1):29, 1989
18. Evans LS, Kleinman MB: Acidosis as a presenting feature of chloramphenicol toxicity. J Pediatr 108:475, 1986
19. Bhat R, Chari G, Gulati A, et al: Pharmacokinetics of a single dose of morphine in preterm infants during the first week of life. J Pediatr 117:477, 1990
20. Jacqz-Aigrain E, Wood C, Robieux I: Pharmacokinetics of midazolam in critically ill neonates. Eur J Clin Pharmacol 39:191, 1990
21. Wilkinson GR: Drug distribution and renal excretion in the elderly. J Chron Dis 36:91, 1983
22. Cockcroft DW, Gault MH: Prediction of creatinine clearance from serum creatinine. Nephron 16:31, 1976
23. Cherry KE, Morton MR: Drug sensitivity in older adults: the role of physiologic and pharmacokinetic factors. Int J Aging Hum Dev 28:159, 1989
24. Wynne HA, Cope LH, Mutch E, et al: The effect of age upon liver volume and apparent liver blood flow in healthy man. Hepatology 9:297, 1989
25. Abernethy DR, Azrnoff DL: Pharmacokinetic investigations in elderly patients: clinical and ethical considerations. Clin Pharmacokinet 19:89, 1990
26. Ozdemir V, Fourie J, Busto U, et al: Pharmacokinetic changes in the elderly: do they contribute to drug abuse and dependence? Clin Pharmacokinet 31:272, 1966
27. Woodhouse KW, James OFW: Hepatic drug metabolism and aging. Br Med Bull 46:22, 1990
28. Baillie SP, Bateman DN, Coates PE, et al: Age and pharmacokinetics of morphine. Age Ageing 18:252, 1989
29. Mehta S: Drug disposition in children with protein energy malnutrition. J Pediatr Gastroenterol Nutr 2:407, 1983
30. Buchanan N, Robinson R, Koornhof HJ, et al: Penicillin pharmacokinetics in kwashiorkor. Am J Clin Nutr 32:2233, 1979
31. Walter-Sack I, Klotz U: Influence of diet and nutritional status on drug metabolism. Clin Pharmacokinet 31:47, 1996
32. Basu TK, Dickerson JWT: Inter-relationships of nutrition and the metabolism of drugs. Chem Biol Interact 8:193, 1974
33. Buchanan N: Drug-protein binding and protein energy malnutrition. S Afr Med J 52:733, 1977
34. Cheymol G: Clinical pharmacokinetics of drugs in obesity: an update. Clin Pharmacokinet 25:103, 1993
35. Abernethy DR, Greenblatt DJ: Pharmacokinetics of drugs in obesity. Clin Pharmacokinet 7:108, 1982
36. Saraiva RA, Lunn JN, Mapleson WW, et al: Adiposity and the pharmacokinetics of halothane. Anaesthesia 32:240, 1977
37. Miller MS, Gandolfi AJ, Vaughan RW, et al: Disposition of enflurane in obese patients. J Pharmacol Exp Ther 215:292, 1980
38. Ewy GA, Groves BM, Ball MF, et al: Digoxin metabolism in obesity. Circulation 44:810, 1971
39. Bauer LA, Waring-Tran C, Drew Edwards WA, et al: Cimetidine clearance in the obese. Clin Pharmacol Ther 37:425, 1985
40. Varin F, Ducharme J, Theoret Y, et al: Influence of extreme obesity on the disposition and neuromuscular blocking effect of atracurium. Clin Pharmacol Ther 48:12, 1990
41. Abernethy DR, Schwartz JB: Verapamil pharmacodynamics and disposition in obese hypertensive patients. J Cardiovasc Pharmacol 11:209, 1988
42. Schwartz AE, Matteo RS, Ornstein E, et al: Pharmacokinetics of sufentanil in obese patients. Anesth Analg 73:790, 1991
43. Abernethy DR, Greenblatt DJ: Drug disposition in obese humans: an update. Clin Pharmacokinet 11:199, 1986
44. Yee GC, McGuire TR, Gmur DJ, et al: Blood cyclosporin pharmacokinetics in patients undergoing marrow transplantation: influence of age, obesity, and hematocrit. Transplantation 43:399, 1988
45. Flechner SM, Kolbeinson ME, Tam J, et al: The impact of body weight on pharmacokinetics in renal transplant recipients. Transplantation 47:806, 1989
46. Bergan T: Extravascular penetration of ciprofloxacin. Diagn Microbial Infect Dis 13:103, 1990
47. Allard S, Kinzig M, Boivin G, et al: Intravenous ciprofloxacin disposition in obesity. Clin Pharmacol Ther 54:368, 1993
48. Bauer LA, Drew Edwards WA, Dellinger P, et al: Influence of weight on aminoglycoside pharmacokinetics in normal weight and morbidly obese patients. Eur J Clin Pharmacol 24:643, 1983
49. Anderson RJ, Gambertoglio JW, Schrier RW: Clinical Use of Drugs in Renal Failure. Charles C Thomas, Publisher, Springfield, Illinois, 1976, p 8
50. Reidenberg MM: The binding of drugs to plasma proteins and the interpretation of measurements of plasma concentrations of drugs in patients with poor renal function. Am J Med 62:466, 1977
51. Reidenberg MM: The biotransformation of drugs in renal failure. Am J Med 62:482, 1977
52. Verbeeck RK, Branch RA, Wilkinson GR: Drug metabolites in renal failure: pharmacokinetic and clinical implications. Clin Pharmacokinet 6:329, 1981
53. Bennett WM, Aronoff GR, Golper TA, et al: Drug prescribing in renal failure: dosing guidelines for adults. American College of Physicians, Philadelphia, 1994
54. Bass NM, Williams RL: Guide to drug dosage in hepatic disease. Clin Pharmacokinet 15:396, 1988
55. Shear L, Kleinerman J, Gabuzda GJ: Renal failure in patients with cirrhosis of the liver. Am J Med 39:184, 1965
56. McLean AJ, Morgan DJ: Clinical pharmacokinetics in patients with liver disease. Clin Pharmacokinet 21:42, 1991
57. Morgan DJ, McLean AJ: Clinical pharmacokinetic and pharmacodynamic considerations in patients with liver disease. Clin Pharmacokinet 29:370, 1995
58. Caregaro L, Menon F, Angeli P, et al: Limitations of serum creatinine level and creatinine clearance as filtration markers in cirrhosis. Arch Intern Med 154:201, 1994
59. Naranjo CA, Busto U, Janecek E, et al: An intensive drug monitoring study suggesting possible clinical irrelevance of impaired drug disposition in liver disease. Br J Clin Pharmacol 15:451, 1983
60. Arns PA, Wedlund PJ, Branch RA: Adjustment of medications in liver failure. The Pharmacologic Approach to the Critically Ill Patient, 2nd ed. Chernow B, Ed. Williams & Wilkins, Baltimore, 1988, p 85
61. Blaschke TF, Rubin PC: Hepatic first-pass metabolism in liver disease. Clin Pharmacokinet 4:423, 1979
62. Williams RL: Drug administration in hepatic disease. N Engl J Med 309:1616, 1983
63. Thomson PD, Melmon KL, Richardson JA, et al: Lidocaine pharmacokinetics in advanced heart failure, liver disease, and renal failure in humans. Ann Intern Med 78:499, 1973
64. Blaschke TF: Protein binding and kinetics of drugs in liver disease. Clin Pharmacokinet 2:32, 1977
65. Benowitz NL: Effects of cardiac disease on pharmacokinetics: pathophysiologic considerations. Pharmacokinetic Basis for Drug Treatment. Benet LZ, Massoud N, Gambertoglio JG, et al, Eds. Raven Press, New York, 1984, p 89
66. Ohnhaus EE, Vozeh S, Nuesch E: Absorption of digoxin in severe right heart failure. Eur J Clin Pharmacol 15:115, 1979
67. Meister W, Benowitz NL, Benet LZ: Unchanged absorption of digoxin tablets in patients with cardiac failure. Pharmacology 28:90, 1984
68. Buylaert WA, Herregods LL, Mortier EP, et al: Cardiopulmonary bypass and the pharmacokinetics of drugs: an update. Clin Pharmacokinet 17:10, 1989
69. Roth RA, Wiersma DA: Role of the lung in total body clearance of circulating drugs. Clin Pharmacokinet 4:355, 1979
70. Giacomini KM, Swezey SE, Giacomini JC, et al: Administration of heparin causes in vitro release of non-esterified fatty acids in human plasma. Life Sci 27:771, 1980
71. Taburet A-M, Tollier C, Richard C: The effect of respiratory disorders on clinical pharmacokinetic variables. Clin Pharmacokinet 19:462, 1990
72. Perkins MW, Dasta JF, DeHaven B: Physiologic implications of mechanical ventilation on pharmacokinetics. Drug Intell Clin Pharm 23:316, 1989
73. Kremer JMH, Wilting J, Janssen LHM: Drug binding to human alpha-1-acid glycoprotein in health and disease. Pharmacol Rev 40:1, 1988
74. Paxton JW, Briant RH: Alpha-1-acid glycoprotein concentrations and propranolol binding in elderly patients with acute illness. Br J Clin Pharmacol 18:806, 1984
75. Richard C, Berdeaux A, Delion F, et al: Effect of mechanical ventilation on hepatic drug pharmacokinetics. Chest 90:837, 1986
76. Campos RA, Valle Herraez FX, Marcos RJ, et al: Drug use in an intensive care unit and its relation to survival. Intensive Care Med 6:163, 1980
77. Zaske DE, Bootman JL, Solem LB, et al: Increased burn patient survival with individualized dosages of gentamicin. Surgery 91:142, 1982
78. Moore RD, Smith CR, Lietman PS: The association of aminoglycoside plasma levels with mortality in patients with gram-negative bacteremia. J Infect Dis 149:443, 1984
79. Koch-Weser J: Serum drug concentrations in clinical perspective. Ther Drug Monit 3:3, 1981
80. Barza M, Lauermann M: Why monitor serum levels of gentamicin? Clin Pharmacokinet 3:202, 1978
81. Koch-Weser J: Serum procainamide levels as therapeutic guides. Clin Pharmacokinet 2:389, 1977
82. Hendeles L, Weinberger M, Johnson G: Monitoring serum theophylline levels. Clin Pharmacokinet 3:294, 1978
83. Rotschafer JC, Zabinski RA, Walker KJ: Pharmacodynamic factors of antibiotic efficacy. Pharmacotherapy 12 (suppl):65S, 1992
84. Rickels K: Psychopharmacological approaches to treatment of anxiety. Phenomenology and Treatment of Anxiety. Fann WE, Karacan I, Porkorny AD, et al, Eds. Spectrum Publishers, New York, 1979, p 325
85. Trissel LA: Handbook on Injectable Drugs, 6th ed. American Society of Hospital Pharmacists, Bethesda, Maryland, 1990
86. Kirby MG, Dasta JF, Armstrong DK, et al: Effect of low-dose dopamine on the pharmacokinetics of tobramycin in dogs. Antimicrob Agents Chemother 29:168, 1986

87. Tilstone WJ, Semple PF, Lawson DH, et al: Effects of furosemide on glomerular filtration rate and clearance of practolol, digoxin, cephaloridine, and gentamicin. Clin Pharmacol Ther 22:389, 1977
88. Brater DC: Resistance to loop diuretics: why it happens and what to do about it. Drugs 30:427, 1985
89. Christian CD Jr, Meredith CG, Speeg KV Jr: Cimetidine inhibits renal procainamide clearance. Clin Pharmacol Ther 36:221, 1984
90. Somogyi A, Bochner F: Dose and concentration dependent effect of ranitidine on procainamide disposition and renal clearance in man. Br J Clin Pharmacol 18:175, 1984

Reviews

Ritschel WA: Handbook of Basic Pharmacokinetics: Including Clinical Applications, 3rd ed. Drug Intelligence Publications, Hamilton, Illinois, 1986

Vožeh S, Schmidlin O, Taeschner W: Pharmacokinetic drug data. Clin Pharmacokinet 15:254, 1988

Goodman and Gilman's The Pharmacological Basis of Therapeutics, 8th ed. Gilman AF, Rall TW, Nies AS, et al, Eds. Pergamon Press, New York, 1990

Drug Interactions and Updates. Hanston PD, Horn JR, Eds. Applied Therapeutics, Vancouver, Washington (published quarterly)

AHFS Drug Information 97. McEvoy GK, Ed. American Society of Hospital Pharmacists, Bethesda, Maryland, 1997

Boreus LO: Principles of Pediatric Pharmacology. Churchill Livingstone, New York, 1982

Acknowledgments

Figure 1   Tom Moore.
Figures 2 through 7   Marcia Kammerer.

108 INFECTION CONTROL IN SURGICAL PRACTICE

A. Peter McLean, M.D., and Catherine M. Dixon, R.N., B.A.

Surgical procedures, by their very nature, interfere with the normal protective skin barrier and expose the patient to microorganisms from both endogenous and exogenous sources. The response to infection may not be limited to the surgical site but may produce widespread systemic effects. Prevention of surgical site infections (SSIs) is therefore of primary concern to surgeons and must be addressed in the planning of any operation. Standards of control have been developed for every step of a surgical procedure to help reduce the impact of exposure to microorganisms.[1-3] Traditional control measures include sterilization of surgical equipment, disinfection of the skin, use of prophylactic antibiotics, and expeditious operation.

The Study on the Efficacy of Nosocomial Infection Control (SENIC), conducted in United States hospitals between 1976 and 1986, showed that surgical patients were at increased risk for all types of infection. The nosocomial, or hospital-acquired, infection rate at that time was estimated to be 5.7 cases out of every 100 hospital admissions.[4] These infections included SSIs as well as bloodstream, urinary, and respiratory infections. Today, the increased use of minimally invasive surgical procedures and early discharge from the hospital necessitates postdischarge surveillance[5] in addition to in-hospital surveillance for the tracking of nosocomial infections. With the reorganization of health care delivery programs, nosocomial infections will appear more frequently in the community and should therefore be considered a part of any patient care assessment plan.

Care assessment programs designed to help minimize the risk of nosocomial infections were first introduced in 1951 by the Joint Commission on Accreditation of Healthcare Organizations (JCAHO). Since then, as medical technology has changed, JCAHO has redesigned the survey process. In its latest plan for infection control programs, JCAHO strongly recommends that the survey, documentation, and reporting of infections be made mandatory for the purpose of hospital accreditation.[6]

Effective infection control and prevention requires an organized, hospital-wide program aimed at achieving specific objectives. The program's purpose should be to obtain relevant information on the occurrence of nosocomial infections both in patients and in employees. The data should be documented, analyzed, and communicated with a plan for corrective measures. Such surveillance activities, combined with education, form the basis of an infection control program.

Data relating to host factors are an integral part of infection data analysis. Documentation of host factors has made for a better appreciation of the associated risks and has allowed for comparative evaluation of infection rates. In this century, new surgical equipment and technological advances have influenced the impact of certain risk factors, such as lengthy operation and prolonged hospital stay. Clinical investigations have helped improve the understanding of host factors and have influenced other aspects of surgical practice.[7-12] New problems have arisen as a result of the overuse of and reliance on antibiotics—for example, the emergence of drug-resistant microorganisms, such as methicillin-resistant *Staphylococcus aureus* (MRSA), multidrug-resistant *Mycobacterium tuberculosis*, and multidrug-resistant *Enterococcus* strains.[13-16] Such complications reemphasize the need to focus on infection control as an essential component of preventive medicine.

Apart from the impact of morbidity and mortality on the patient is the cost of treating nosocomial infections—a matter of concern for surgeons, hospital administrators, insurance companies, and government planners alike. Efforts to reduce the occurrence of nosocomial infections are now a part of hospital cost-control management programs.[17,18] The current challenge to clinicians is how to reduce cost while maintaining control over and preventing spread of infection.

The Surgical Wound and Infection Control

Nosocomial infections typically develop in the institution. The incubation period may be 48 to 72 hours after admission. Usually, an apparent infection on the day of admission is considered to be community acquired unless it is epidemiologically linked to a previous admission or to an operative procedure at the time of admission.

IDENTIFICATION OF RISK FACTORS

The risk for development of an SSI depends on host factors, perioperative wound hygiene, and the duration of the surgical procedure. The risk for development of other nosocomial infections depends on these and other factors, including length of the hospital stay and appropriate management of the hospital environment [*see* Activities of an Infection Control Program, *below*]. Identification of host and operative risk factors can help determine the potential for infection and point toward measures that might be necessary for prevention and control.

Host Risk Factors

Under current guidelines,[19] host susceptibility to infection can be estimated according to the following variables: older age, severity of disease, classification of physical status (see below), the presence of infections at other sites, prolonged preoperative hospitalization, morbid obesity, malnutrition, and immunosuppressive therapy.

A scale dividing patients into five classes according to their physical status was introduced by the American Society of Anesthesiologists (ASA) in 1974 and tested for precision in 1978.[20] The test results showed that the ASA scale is a workable system, though it lacks scientific definition [see Table 1].

Significant differences in infection rates have been shown among patients with different illnesses. In one prospective study, the severity of underlying disease (rated as fatal, ultimately fatal, or nonfatal) was shown to have predictive value for endemic nosocomial infections: the nosocomial infection rate in patients with fatal diseases was 23.6 percent, compared with 2.1 percent in patients with nonfatal diseases.[21] Various preexisting medical conditions (e.g., diabetes mellitus, malnutrition, morbid obesity, and cancer) and older age may also increase a patient's susceptibility to infection.[22]

Operative Risk Factors

In addition to host factors, several circumstances related to the operative procedure may be used as indicators for increased risk for development of an SSI, including the following: (1) nonuse of prophylactic antibiotics, (2) use of a razor for hair removal at the surgical site, (3) lower abdominal operation, (4) prolonged duration of the surgical procedure, and (5) wound classification.[19]

Cruse and Foord found that antibiotic prophylaxis was important but only when used appropriately.[8] The influence of hair removal methods has been tested by many investigators[7,9]: one study showed lower infection rates with the use of a depilatory,[7] and another reported a significant reduction in clean wound infection rates with the use of electric clippers.[9]

Operative wounds are susceptible to varying levels of bacterial contamination, by which they are classified as clean, clean-contaminated, contaminated, or dirty[23] [see 39 Prevention of Postoperative Infection]. In most institutions, the responsibility for classifying the incision site is assigned to the operating room circulating nurse; a recent assessment suggests that the accuracy of decisions made by this group is as high as 88 percent.[24]

Composite Risk Indices

Two infection control study groups—SENIC and the National Nosocomial Infections Study (NNIS) conducted by the Centers for Disease Control and Prevention (CDC)—have developed composite indices designed to predict the risk of wound infection.

SENIC risk index Using a multivariate logistic regression analysis of 10 potential risk factors, the SENIC project developed a simple index to predict the risk of wound infection in the immediate postoperative phase. This analysis resulted in the identification of four risk factors to make up the SENIC risk index: (1) abdominal operation, (2) operation lasting longer than two hours, (3) operative wounds classified as contaminated or dirty/infected, and (4) a patient who has three or more diagnoses at discharge from the hospital. The SENIC risk index was shown to be a better predictor of risk of acquiring an SSI than the univariate traditional wound classification system alone.[25]

NNIS risk index Another composite risk index was developed by the NNIS control group of the CDC.[26] Reporting on data collected from 44 United States hospitals between 1987 and 1990, NNIS showed that a risk index using the wound classification system combined with the ASA physical-status scale and the duration of operation is a significantly better predictor of SSI risk than the traditional wound classification system alone.[27,28] An evaluation of the data illustrated significant wound infection risks associated with contaminated or dirty wounds, surgery of over two hours' duration, and ASA perioperative classification scores of 3, 4, or 5. Out of this evaluation was developed the NNIS risk index, which correlates with a surgical patient's risk of acquiring an SSI. The NNIS risk index is scored as 0, 1, 2, or 3 by counting the number of risk factors present from among the following:

- No risk factor identified (0).
- A patient with an ASA preoperative assessment score of 3, 4, or 5.
- A surgical wound that is classified as contaminated or dirty/infected.
- An operation lasting over T hours (T depending on the operative procedure being performed—the 75th percentile of distribution of the duration of each operation rounded to the nearest whole number of hours).

PREVENTIVE MEASURES

In any surgical practice, policies and procedures should be in place pertaining to the making of a surgical incision and the prevention of infection. These policies and procedures should govern the following: (1) skin disinfection and hand-washing practices of the operating team, (2) preoperative preparation of the patient's skin (e.g., hair removal and use of antiseptics), (3) the use of prophylactic antibiotics, (4) techniques for preparation of the operative site, (5) management of the postoperative site if drains, dressings, or both are in place, (6) standards of behavior and practice for the operating team (e.g., the use of gown, mask, and gloves), and (7) special training of the operating team.

Table 1 American Society of Anesthesiologists Physical-Status Scale

Class 1	A normally healthy individual
Class 2	A patient with mild systemic disease
Class 3	A patient with severe systemic disease that is not incapacitating
Class 4	A patient with incapacitating systemic disease that is a constant threat to life
Class 5	A moribund patient who is not expected to survive 24 hr with or without operation
E	Added for emergency procedures

Disinfectants

A disinfectant is a germicide that inactivates virtually all recognized pathogenic microorganisms on inanimate objects. Chemical disinfectants are classified by the CDC according to the level of disinfection achievable (i.e., complete sterilization or high-level, intermediate-level, or low-level disinfection).[29] The rationale for their use should be related to the potential risks for infection in a given patient and for a given procedure. Proper cleaning of the object is essential because mucus, dried secretions, and blood prevent disinfection.

Spaulding proposed in 1972 that the level of disinfection for surgical and other instruments be determined by classifying the instruments into three categories—critical, semicritical, and noncritical—according to the degree of infection risk involved in their use.[30] Objects or instruments that enter directly into the vascular system or sterile areas of the body are categorized as critical and should be sterilized. Semicritical items are those that come into contact with mucous membranes or skin that is not intact (e.g., bronchoscopes and gastroscopes). Although scopes are noninvasive, they have the potential to cause infection if they are improperly cleaned and disinfected. Transmission of infection has been documented after endoscopic investigations, including infection with *Salmonella typhi*[31] and *Helicobacter pylori*[32]—which should emphasize the need for sterilization of the endoscopic biopsy forceps. Given the risks associated with endoscopes, it is recommended that a 20- to 45-minute soak in a two percent solution of alkaline glutaraldehyde disinfectant be performed (i.e., high-level disinfection).[33,34] Noncritical items are those that come in contact with intact skin (e.g., blood pressure cuffs); they require only washing or scrubbing with a detergent and warm water or disinfection with an intermediate- or low-level germicide for 10 minutes.

The reuse of disposable items has become a topic of interest because of the implied cost saving. However, the central concerns must remain the effectiveness of sterilization or disinfection according to category of use as well as the essential mechanical features and the function of the item to be reused.

Hand Hygiene

Although hand washing is considered the single most important measure for preventing nosocomial infections, poor compliance is frequent. Role modeling is important in positively influencing this behavior. One study showed that a hand-washing educational program contributed to a reduction in the rate of nosocomial infections.[35] Good hand-washing habits can be encouraged by making facilities (with sink, soap, and towel) visible and easily accessible in patient care areas. Plain or nonantimicrobial soap cleansers in any form (e.g., bar, liquid, leaflet, or powder) are acceptable for the physical removal of dirt and transient bacteria [see 39 Prevention of Postoperative Infection].

Antiseptics

An antiseptic is a chemical germicide formulated for use on skin or tissue and should be used only to degerm animate subjects. Views differ over whether to use antiseptics or liquid soaps for hand washing. In one study, liquid soap was compared with four percent chlorhexidine gluconate in four percent alcohol, used both on bare hands and on gloves during a *Clostridium difficile* epidemic. No difference between the use of soap and the use of chlorhexidine was shown. At the same time, however, the impact of hand washing was clearly demonstrated; numbers of *C. difficile* were reduced by an estimated 10,000 to 100,000 bacteria after a 20-second hand wash using either agent.[36] Another study showed that a mild, low-iodine soap was more effective for hand washing than natural liquid soap in controlling an outbreak of MRSA.[37] Hand washing with an antiseptic (e.g., chlorhexidine in alcohol) was shown to have a residual degerming effect[38] [see 39 Prevention of Postoperative Infection].

Hair Removal

An infection control program should have a hair-removal policy for preoperative skin preparation [see 39 Prevention of Postoperative Infection].

Interventions

Protocols for the introduction of intravascular catheters should be followed to prevent nosocomial bloodstream infections. The complications associated with indwelling vascular catheters are well known and result from a variety of risk factors, including poor aseptic technique.[39] Raad and colleagues in 1994 studied the use of aseptic techniques for introducing central venous catheters and showed that maximal draping was needed to prevent site contamination. The rate of catheter-related sepsis was 6.3 times higher when small drapes were used.[40] In one random trial, cutaneous disinfection before insertion of vascular catheters was evaluated, comparing the efficacy of chlorhexidine (two percent aqueous solution), povidone-iodine (10 percent solution), and alcohol (70 percent solution). Use of chlorhexidine was associated with the lowest rate (0.5 percent) of catheter-related infections, compared with 2.6 percent for povidone-iodine and 2.3 percent for alcohol.[41]

Patient Care Assessment

The primary need for patient care assessment is determined according to the patient's health status and the operation planned. A multidisciplinary approach may sometimes be needed to evaluate risks to the patient, to employees, to other patients, and to the environment. If the patient has an underlying infection—for example, from human immunodeficiency virus (HIV), hepatitis B virus (HBV), *M. tuberculosis*, or varicella-zoster virus—a collaborative plan that involves infectious disease personnel and infection control personnel should be considered.

Methods for patient care assessment have evolved to include a wider range of patient care activities. Some programs advocate a continuous quality-improvement system in which other services and departments collaborate to create a more comprehensive model for patient care.[42] Whatever the plan, the collection of surveillance data is useful for making changes and preventing the spread of infection and disease.

HEALTH STATUS OF THE HEALTH CARE TEAM

The health care team has a primary role in the prevention of infection. Continued education and reindoctrination of policies are essential: the team must be kept well informed and up to date on concepts of infection control. Inadvertently, team members may also be the source of, or the vector in, transmission of infection. Nosocomial infection outbreaks with MRSA have been repeatedly traced to MRSA carriers among health care workers.[43,44] Screening of personnel to identify carriers is undertaken only when an outbreak of nosocomial infection with specific resistance patterns occurs.

Protecting the health care team from infection is a constant concern. Today, it is widely believed that preventive measures, such as immunizations and preemployment medical examinations, should be undertaken at an employee health care center staffed by knowledgeable personnel. Preventable infectious diseases, such as chicken pox and rubella, should be tightly controlled in hospitals that serve immunocompromised and obstetric patients. It is highly recommended that a record be maintained of an employee's immunizations. Knowledge of the employee's health status on entry to the hospital helps ensure appropriate placement and good preventive care. Many programs have eliminated practices now considered useless, such as stool culture for *Salmonella* in food handlers.

When exposure to contagious infections is unavoidable, susceptible personnel should be located, screened, and given prophylactic treatment. Infection control personnel should define the problem, establish a definition of contact, and take measures to help reduce panic.

Contact with Blood and Body Fluids

The risk of transmission of HIV and hepatitis B virus from patient to surgeon or from surgeon to patient has resulted in a series of recommendations governing contact with blood and body fluids. In 1987, Lynch and Jackson introduced the concept of blood and body substance isolation (BSI), which requires wearing gloves for handling all types of body secretions during any patient care activity.[45] The CDC's recommendation, universal precautions, is similar in principle, requiring the use of gloves when coming in contact with blood, semen, vaginal secretions, and other body fluids with visible blood[46] [see 86 *Viral Infection*]. Another series of recommendations, termed blood and body substance precautions (BSP), was initiated by a Canadian group, the Community Hospital Infection Control Program (CHICA), and differs from BSI in that hand washing is required after glove removal.[47,48] BSP has replaced the traditional disease-specific isolation recommendations except for protective isolation and those involving airborne pathogens.

Protection of the face and hands during operation has become important. A study of 8,502 operations found that the rate of direct blood exposure was 12.4 percent, whereas the rate of parenteral exposure via puncture wounds and cuts was 2.2 percent. Parenteral blood contacts were two times as likely to occur among surgeons as among other operating room personnel.[49] These findings support the need for operating room practice policies and the thoughtful choice of protective garments for the operating room staff. Operating room practice policy should give particular attention to the use of sharp instruments: sharp instruments should be passed in a metal dish, cautery should be used, and great care should be taken in wound closures. It is important that masks protect the operating team from aerosolized fluids. Researchers have shown that for ideal protection, a mask should be fluid-capture efficient and air resistant.[50]

Since the introduction of BSI, gloves have been carefully studied. For invasive surgical procedures, double gloving has become routine. However, there are recognized differences among the gloves available. An important issue is the allergic reaction to latex; nonallergenic alternatives are available for those who are allergic.[51]

Hepatitis B virus For active surgeons and other members of the health care team, HBV infection continues to pose a major risk. Hepatitis B vaccination has proved safe and protective and is highly recommended for all high-risk employees; it should be made available through the employee health care center.

Despite the efficacy of the vaccine, many surgeons and other personnel remain unimmunized and are at high risk for HBV infection.[52] HBV is far more easily transmitted than HIV and continues to have a greater impact on the morbidity and mortality of health care personnel. An estimated 8,700 new cases of hepatitis B are acquired occupationally by health care workers each year; 200 to 250 of these cases result in death.[53] It is important, therefore, that patients infected with HBV be identified to the personnel who care for them.

With HBV infection, as with HIV (see below), the approach to prevention and control is a two-way street—that is, protection should be afforded patients as well as health care personnel. In addition to universal precautions, the CDC has developed recommendations for health care workers that are

---

Table 2 CDC Recommendations for Prevention of HIV and HBV Transmission during Invasive Procedures[52]

Health care workers with exudative lesions or weeping dermatitis should cover any unprotected skin, or they should not provide patient care until the damaged skin has healed.

Hands should be washed after every patient contact.

Health care workers should wear gloves when contact with blood or body substances is anticipated; double gloves should be used during operative procedures; hands should be washed after gloves are removed.

Gowns, plastic aprons, or both should be worn when soiling of clothing is anticipated.

Mask and protective eyewear or face shield should be worn if aerosolization or splattering of blood or body substances is expected.

Resuscitation devices should be used to minimize the need for mouth-to-mouth resuscitation.

Disposable containers should be used to dispose of needles and sharp instruments.

Avoid accidents and self-wounding with sharp instruments by following these measures:
- Do not recap needles.
- Use needleless systems when possible.
- Use cautery and stapling devices when possible.
- Pass sharp instruments in metal tray during operative procedures.

In the case of an accidental spill of blood or body substance on skin or mucous membranes, do the following:
- Rinse the site immediately and thoroughly under water.
- Wash the site with soap and water.
- Document the incident (i.e., report to Occupational Safety and Health Administration or to the Infection Control Service).

Blood specimens from all patients should be considered hazardous at all times.

Prompt attention should be given to spills of blood or body substances, which should be cleaned with an appropriate disinfectant.

designed to prevent transmission of HBV and HIV from health care worker to patient or from patient to health care worker during exposure-prone invasive procedures [see Table 2]. Cognizant of the CDC recommendations, the American College of Surgeons has issued additional recommendations regarding the surgeon's role in the prevention of HBV transmission[53] [see Sidebar ACS Recommendations for Preventing Transmission of HBV].

Human immunodeficiency virus Exposure to blood and body substances of patients who have acquired immunodeficiency syndrome (AIDS) or who are seropositive for HIV constitutes a health hazard to hospital employees. The magnitude of the risk depends on the degree and method of exposure [see 87 Acquired Immunodeficiency Syndrome].

The presence of HIV infection in a patient is not always known. Because the HIV prevalence in the North American patient population is less than one percent (range, 0.09 to 0.89 percent), and as the care giver's risk of seroconversion after needle-stick injury is likewise less than one percent, the CDC recommends utilizing universal precautions [see 86 Viral Infection] and following in all patients the same guidelines for invasive procedures that one would use in cases of known HBV-infected patients [see Table 2].[52] Infection control personnel have introduced realistic control measures and educational programs to help alleviate fears that health care workers might have about coming in contact with patients infected with HIV.

Isolation Procedures

The traditional practice of separating infected patients has undergone change in recent years. New CDC guidelines[54] identify universal precautions as the standard precautions for the traditional disease-specific isolation categories (e.g., wound infection, urinary infection, respiratory infection, and enteric infection); strict isolation measures are now dictated by the mode of disease transmission, whether by air, droplet, or contact. Overall, emphasis has been placed on individualizing the precautionary measures to suit the particular disease. One drawback is the need for a diagnosis to indicate the category of isolation.

An example of the change in isolation procedures is seen in the policy for tuberculosis patients.[55,56] It calls for isolating the patient in a single room with anteroom, ventilated under negative pressure with six air exchanges an hour. Consideration may be given to portable as well as fixed negative pressure ventilation systems with controlled air evacuation using a high-efficiency particulate air (HEPA) filter. All employees must wear a respirator mask before entering the room, and the door must be kept closed at all times. It has been shown that droplets containing tubercle bacilli may aerosolize to form droplet nuclei 1 to 5 μm in diameter, and these can remain airborne and viable for several days.[57] Most hospitals are not physically structured for this change in policy, and the expense of restructuring to accommodate tuberculosis patients should depend on the frequency of admission and exposure. In a very low risk facility (e.g., a nursing or convalescent home with fewer than 50 beds), patients with active tuberculosis are not admitted to inpatient areas but may receive initial assessment and diagnostic outpatient evaluation or management.[55]

ACS Recommendations for Preventing Transmission of HBV[53]

1. Surgeons should continue to utilize the highest standards of infection control, involving the most effective known sterile barriers, universal precautions, and scientifically accepted infection control practices. This practice should extend to all sites where surgical care is rendered.

2. Surgeons have the same ethical obligations to render care to hepatitis B virus (HBV)–infected patients as they have to care for other patients.

3. Surgeons with natural or acquired antibodies to HBV are protected from acquiring HBV from patients. All surgeons (and other members of the operating room team) without natural immunity should be vaccinated against HBV as early as possible in their careers.

4. Surgeons who perform invasive procedures without evidence of immunity to HBV should know their hepatitis B surface antigen (HB_sAg) status and, if that is positive, should also know their hepatitis B e antigen (HB_eAg) status.

5. Surgeons who are infected with HBV (and are HB_eAg positive) should seek counsel from an unbiased expert review panel structured to maintain practitioner confidentiality.

A study of 14 pulmonary physician training programs—where activities such as bronchoscopy, endotracheal intubation, and mechanical ventilation were in use—found that 11 percent of the resident fellows at these centers had positive tuberculin conversion on purified protein derivative testing.[58]

The current CDC recommendation for tuberculosis prevention places emphasis on a hierarchy of control measures, including administrative engineering controls and personal respiratory protection. The following measures should be considered:

1. The use of risk assessments and development of a written tuberculosis control protocol.
2. Early identification and management of persons who have tuberculosis.
3. Tuberculosis screening programs for health care workers.
4. Training and education.
5. Evaluation of tuberculosis infection control programs.[55]

Antibiotics

The arguments for and against MRSA control continue, and different approaches have been suggested. The frequency of outbreaks, however, points to the need for organized control and prevention in surgical units. A recent report suggests that when MRSA is endemic in an institution, there is a risk of transmission to employees.[59] Transmission rates of two to six percent have been reported in point prevalence surveys.[59] Surveillance culture of nares only was shown to be 93 percent sensitive for MRSA.[60]

Antibiotic-resistant bacteria such as MRSA and *Enterococcus* have created a need for the control of antibiotic use, and it has been recommended that antibiogram (i.e., the resistance and sensitivity of a microorganism to antibiotics) become the marker by which SSIs are monitored.

The prophylactic use of antibiotics has clearly been of benefit, particularly in the case of operation for clean-contaminated wounds. A reduction in the wound infection rate is evident in contaminated colonic operations after mechanical cleansing and administration of antibiotics.[10] However, overmanipulation of the colonic environment with antibiotics may contribute to the risk of other infections (e.g., resistant *Pseudomonas* and *C. difficile*). The general consensus is that the use of antibiotics should be controlled, but this step requires the development of better definitions with an outline of the therapeutic options. The Hospital Infection Control Practices Advisory Committee has issued recommendations for preventing the spread of vancomycin-resistant infection.[61]

Activities of an Infection Control Program

SURVEILLANCE

The cornerstone of an infection control program is surveillance. This process depends on the verification, classification, analysis, reporting, and investigation of infection occurrences, with the intent of generating or correcting policies and procedures. Six surveillance methods can be applied[62]:

1. Site-specific surveillance, which focuses on particular types of infection.
2. Unit-directed surveillance, which focuses on infection occurrences in specific areas of the hospital.
3. Rotating surveillance, which includes intensive surveillance of infections and patient care practices by unit or by service at different times of the year.
4. Outbreak surveillance, which deals with the identification and control of outbreaks of infection.
5. Total, or hospital-wide, surveillance, which looks at all types of infection and aims to correct problems as they arise.
6. Surveillance by objective, in which a specific goal is set for reducing certain types of infection. This concept is priority directed and can be further subdivided into two distinct activities:
    a. The setting of outcome objectives, in which the objectives for the month or year would be established and all efforts would be applied to achieve a desired rate of infection. Like the hospital-wide approach, a short-term plan would be made to monitor, record, and measure results and provide feedback on the data.
    b. The setting of process objectives, which incorporates the patient care practices of doctors and nurses as they relate to outcome (e.g., wound infections and their control).

Surveillance techniques include the practice of direct patient observation[7] and indirect observation by review of microbiology reports, nursing Kardex, or the medical record to obtain data on nosocomial infections. The sensitivity of case finding by microbiology reports was found to be 33 to 65 percent; by Kardex, 85 percent; and by total chart review, 90 percent.[19] These methods may be used either separately or in combination to obtain data on clinical outcomes.

One of the uses of surveillance data is to generate information for individual surgeons, service chiefs, and nursing personnel as a reminder of their progress in keeping infections and diseases under control. This technique was used by Cruse in 1980 to show a progressive decrease in infection rates of clean surgical wounds to less than one percent over 10 years.[8] A cluster outbreak of wound infections caused by *Legionella* was detected in post–cardiac surgery patients,[63] and in other settings, endemic rates of bloodstream, respiratory, and urinary tract infections were corrected and reduced by routine monitoring and reporting to medical and nursing staff.[21]

The increasing practice of same-day or short-stay surgical procedures has led to the need for postdischarge surveillance. This may be done by direct observation in a follow-up clinic, by surveying patients through the mail or over the telephone, by reviewing medical records, or by mailing questionnaires directly to surgeons. The original CDC recommendation of 30 days for follow-up was used by one hospital to randomly screen post–joint arthroplasty patients by telephone. This screening identified an infection rate of 7.5 percent, compared with two percent for hospitalized orthopedic patients.[64] New evidence suggests that 90 percent of cases would be captured in a 21-day postoperative follow-up program.[5] Infections that occur after discharge are more likely in clean operations, operations of short duration, and operations in obese patients and in nonalcoholic patients. The use of prosthetic materials for implants requires extending the follow-up period to one year.

Certain clinical markers help establish the presence of a wound infection.

Definition of Surgical Site Infections

The CDC defines an incisional SSI as an infection that occurs at the incision site within 30 days after surgery or within one year if a prosthetic implant is in place. Infection is characterized by redness, swelling, or heat with tenderness, pain, or dehiscence at the incision site and by purulent drainage. Other indicators of infection include fever, deliberate opening of the wound, culture-positive drainage, and a physician's diagnosis of infection with prescription of antibiotics. To encourage a uniform approach among data collectors, the CDC has suggested three categories of SSIs, with definitions for each category [*see Table 3*].[65] The category of organ or space SSI was included to cover any part of the anatomy (i.e., organs or spaces) other than the incision that might have been opened or manipulated during the operative procedure. This category would include, for example, arterial and venous infections, endometritis, disk space infections, and mediastinitis.[65]

Table 8 Surgical Site Infections (SSIs)[65]

Superficial SSIs
  Skin
Deep incisional SSIs
  Fascia
  Muscle layers
Organ or space SSIs
  Body organs
  Body spaces

There should be collaboration between the physician or nurse and the infection control practitioner to establish the presence of a surgical site infection. The practitioner should complete the surveillance with a chart review and document the incident in a computer database program for later analysis. The data must be systematically recorded; many commercial computer programs are available for this purpose. One group reported that their experience with the Health Evaluation through Logically Processing system was useful for identifying patients at high risk for nosocomial infections.[66]

Verification of Infection

A complete assessment should include clinical evaluation of commonly recognized sites (e.g., wound, respiratory system, urinary tract, and intravenous access sites) for evidence of infection, especially when no obvious infection is seen at the surgical site. Microbiological evaluation should identify the microorganism. Such evaluation, however, depends on an adequate specimen for a Gram's stain and culture. For epidemiological reasons, sensitivity and specificity (so-called fingerprinting, through identification of bacteriophage and plasmid and chromosomal DNA restriction endonuclease analysis) may be required, especially when multiresistant microorganisms, such as MRSA, are identified.

A system of internal auditing should alert the infection control service to multiresistant microorganisms—for example, to the presence of MRSA in a patient. Differentiation between infection and colonization is important for the decision of how to treat. In either case, verification of MRSA would generate a discussion on control measures.

Data Interpretation

The predictive value of data is deemed more useful when it is applied to specific situations. According to CDC experts, the scoring for infections depends on specified, related denominators to interpret the data, especially when there is to be interhospital comparison.[27]

Data Analysis

The original practice of presenting overall hospital-wide crude rates provided little means for adjustment of variables (e.g., risk related to the patient or to the operation). The following formulas, however, are said to offer more precision than traditional methods[27]:

$$\frac{\text{Number of nosocomial infections}}{\text{Service operations}} \times 100 \quad (1)$$

$$\frac{\text{Number of site-specific nosocomial infections}}{\text{Specific operations (e.g., number of inguinal hernias)}} \times 100 \quad (2)$$

$$\frac{\text{Number of nosocomial infections}}{\text{Hospital admissions (patient-days)}} \times 1{,}000 \quad (3)$$

Data on infections of the urinary tract, respiratory system, and circulatory system resulting from exposure to devices such as Foley catheters, ventilators, and intravascular lines can be illustrated as device-associated risks according to site, as follows:

$$\frac{\text{Number of device-associated infections of a site}}{\text{Number of device days}} \times 1{,}000 \quad (4)$$

Reporting

Infection notification to surgeons has been shown by Cruse and Foord to have a positive influence on clean-wound infection rates.[7,8] In a medical setting, Britt and colleagues also reported a reduction in endemic nosocomial infection rates for urinary tract infections, from 3.7 to 1.3 percent ($P < .001$), and for respiratory tract infections, from 4.0 to 1.6 percent ($P < .001$), simply by keeping medical personnel aware of the rates.[21]

Investigation

The identification of the microorganism should be verified with the laboratory (e.g., if MRSA is truly MRSA), and the pattern of antibiotic resistance should be determined. The microbiological characteristics (i.e., phage type and plasmid) should be determined for so-called fingerprinting.

On identification of an infectious organism, preliminary control measures should be established. Surveillance data should be reviewed to define whether an outbreak has occurred. The time of an outbreak would start from when the first case occurred to when the others were found, including the current case or cases under investigation. Any outbreak situation requires data from the preepidemic phase (retrospective from six months to one year) to calculate an attack rate for comparison purposes.[67]

$$\text{Attack rate} = \frac{\text{Number of infections}}{\text{Number of operations performed}}$$

For comparative analysis, the Fisher exact test or the chi-squared (χ^2) test should be used to determine whether the P value is less than 0.05 and the significance of change.

The epidemic curve should be described in time (e.g., date, weeks, or months) on the X axis and the number of cases plotted on the Y axis to show the exact time of exposure. The exposed population may be of different groups (e.g., age, sex, ward, surgeons). All the risk factors associated with exposure (e.g., admission time, room, bed number, preinfection tests, and devices used) should be listed in a line.

The data may or may not demonstrate clues; however, if the clues are relevant, the investigation plan should be continued to find the reservoir and the mode of transmission.

It may be necessary at this point to consult with an epidemiologist to receive expert advice if an associated high-risk factor is found and a case-control study is to be the course of action.

For a case-control study, control subjects should be selected from an uninfected surgical population who were hospitalized at the same time as those identified during the epidemic period and matched (e.g., two control subjects for each case) for age, sex, service operation, operation date, time (duration), and health status (by ASA scale). If the P value is large (> 0.05), the problem may not be statistically significant, but a common factor, such as the same person involved with suturing of wounds within the time frame, may be important. At this time, screening of employees may be significant.[67]

Other important features may include a computer search for information on similar outbreaks and keeping surgeons, nurses, and administrators informed and updated as events change. The incident should be reported to the infection control committee, and at the completion of the investigation, a report should be submitted. Communication should be initiated with nursing homes to obtain their agreement in regard to discharge for convalescent care. Finally, the efficacy of the control measures should be reviewed, and any necessary changes should be made to the existing policies and procedures.

ENVIRONMENTAL CONTROL

Control of the microbial reservoir of the patient's immediate environment in the hospital is the goal of an infection control program. Environmental control begins with design of the hospital's physical plant. The design must meet the functional standards for patient care and must be integrated into the architecture to provide traffic accessibility and control. Since the 1960s, the practice of centralizing seriously ill patients in intensive care, dialysis, and transplant units has accentuated the need for more careful analysis and planning of space. The primary standards for these special care units and operating rooms require planning of floor space, physical surfaces, lighting, ventilation, water, and sanitation to accommodate easy cleaning and disinfecting of surfaces, sterilization of instruments, proper food handling, and garbage disposal. These activities should then be governed by workable policies that are understandable to the staff.

Surveillance of the environment by routine culturing of operating room floors and walls was discontinued in the late 1970s. Autoclaves and sterilization systems should, however, be continuously monitored with routine testing for efficiency and performance. The results should be documented and records maintained.

Investigations of the physical plant should be reserved for specific outbreaks, depending on the organism and its potential for causing infection. This was demonstrated by the incident of a cluster outbreak of sternal wound *Legionella* infections in post–cardiovascular surgery patients after they were exposed to tap water during bathing.[63] Because outbreaks of nosocomial respiratory infections caused by *L. pneumophila* continue to be a problem,[68] the CDC has now included precautionary measures for this disease in its pneumonia prevention guidelines.[69] In addition, several water-treatment measures are available to help eradicate or clear the water of these bacteria.[70]

Hospital-acquired aspergillosis is caused by another ubiquitous type of microorganism that is often a contaminant of ambient air during construction. The patients most at risk are usually immunosuppressed (i.e., neutropenic). It is recommended that preventive measures be organized for these patients when construction is being planned.[71] The provision of clean (i.e., HEPA-filtered) air in positive pressure–ventilated rooms, with up to six air exchanges an hour, is the basic requirement for these patients.

EDUCATION

A strategy for routine training of the health care team is necessary at every professional level. The process may vary from institution to institution, but some form of communication should be established for the transmittal of information about the following:

1. Endemic infection rates.
2. Endemic bacterial trends.
3. Updates on infection prevention measures (especially during and after an outbreak).
4. Updates on preventive policies pertaining to intravenous line management, hand washing, isolation, and other areas of concern.

Although members of the infection control team are the responsible resource persons in the hospital system, each member of the health care team also has a responsibility to help prevent infection in hospitalized patients. Under the JCAHO guidelines,[6] education of patients and their families should become a part of teaching plans as well—for example, in such areas as understanding HIV infection and testing and the proper care of an indwelling catheter or line in a home care program.

RESEARCH

Infection control policies are constantly being evaluated and remodeled because most traditional preventive measures are not scientifically proved but based on clinical experience. Although infection data are useful, research in infection control requires microbiological support to conduct realistic studies. Very few infection control programs have the personnel and resources for these activities.

PUBLIC HEALTH AND COMMUNITY HEALTH SERVICE

According to existing public health acts, certain infectious diseases must be reported by law. Differences exist between the reporting systems of one country and those of another, but on the whole, diseases such as tuberculosis and meningococcal meningitis are reported for community follow-up.

Open communication with community hospitals and other health care facilities provides for better management of patients with infections, allowing for notification and planning for additional hospitalization or convalescence as the patient moves to and from the community and hospital.

Discussion

The establishment of an infection control program can greatly benefit a hospital. An infection control program supports patient care activities and is a means for continuous quality improvement in the care that is given, in addition to being an accreditation requirement. In Canada and the United States, the governing agents—the Canadian Council on Hospital Accreditation, JCAHO, the American Hospital Association (AHA), the Canadian Hospital Association, the Association for Practitioners in Infection Control (APIC)–Society of Hospital Epidemiologists of America (SHEA) Joint Commission Task Force, and CHICA—all support the need for infection control programs. The program requires a committee of multidisciplinary members and an infection control practitioner, who may be a nurse or a technician. In the original concept, Infection Control Officer was the title given to the person in charge of the program. As the practice has expanded into research and more sophisticated data analysis, physicians and nurses have had to update their epidemiological skills, and some hospitals have acquired the services of an epidemiologist. The historical development of infection control programs in hospitals dates to the late 1970s. The SENIC project endorsed the use of nurses[72] because of their patient care expertise; the literature contains many examples of collaboration between infection control officers and nurse practitioners.

Controlling and preventing the spread of infections in health care facilities has taken many forms:

1. Prevention of cross-infection between patients.
2. Monitoring environmental systems (e.g., plumbing, ventilation).
3. Procedures for sterilization of equipment and instruments.
4. Policies and procedures for the implementation of sterile technique for surgical and other invasive procedures.
5. Procedures for nursing care activities for the postoperative patient.
6. Policies and procedures for dietary, housekeeping, and other ancillary services.
7. Policies for regulating visitor traffic.
8. Policies for the control of antibiotics.
9. Policies and procedures for occupational health prevention.
10. Educational strategies for the implementation of precautionary measures.

Today's infection control practices have developed into a sophisticated network that does not allow for hospital-wide surveillance as it was once practiced. However, the use of surveillance by objective and the use of indicators to monitor select groups of patients or select situations provide information that will benefit the entire hospital. For example, monitoring blood-borne infections in an intensive care setting will provide data to support an intravenous care plan for general use. Accomplishing a high-quality infection control program requires organization and the dedicated service of all health care employees.

Organization of an Infection Control Program

INFECTION CONTROL COMMITTEE

The chair of the infection control committee should have an ongoing interest in the prevention and control of infection. Members should represent microbiology, nursing, the operating room, central supply, medicine, surgery, pharmacy, and housekeeping. This multidisciplinary group becomes the advocate for the entire hospital. They work with the infection control service to make decisions in the following areas: (1) hygienic control of the hospital environment and (2) assessing the effectiveness and pertinence of policies and protocols in establishing and maintaining hygienic control.

INFECTION CONTROL SERVICE

The collection of surveillance data on nosocomial infections is the benchmark of the infection control service. In the traditional sense, the service provides information on all types of endemic infections (e.g., wound, urinary tract, and bloodstream) to the benefit of the health care system. The cost-effectiveness of data collection was demonstrated by the SENIC study.[4] Since then, other studies have shown that there are benefits in reducing nosocomial infection.[17,18,49] Cruse and Foord presented data to show that clean wound rates could be influenced to fall below 0.8 percent.[8] A recent estimate on the extra costs of treating bloodstream infections in an intensive care setting was shown to be $40,000 per survivor.[73] The global impact of cost saving through infection control programs is presented in *Prevention and Control of Nosocomial Infections*, edited by R. P. Wenzel.[74]

INFECTION CONTROL PRACTITIONERS

The reshaping of hospitals because of cost constraints will have an effect on the work of infection control practitioners. Already, some institutions have regrouped responsibilities and changed the role of these professionals. Given the accreditation mandate, the need to continue an active program may be reviewed. Many training programs are available to assist with professional and organizational development (see below), and the APIC certification program supports continuous professional improvement. A viable and useful program for surveillance and collection of data requires a computer database program networked to microbiology, the operating room, and nursing units. Methods for collecting, editing, storing, and sharing data should be based on the CDC's NNIS system,[26] which promotes the use of high-quality indicators for future monitoring and comparison among health care institutions.

Available training programs for infection control practitioners include the following:

SHEA-CDC-AHA Training Course in Hospital Epidemiology
Contact: SHEA Meetings Department
    875 Kings Highway, Suite 200
    Woodbury, NJ 08096
    Telephone (609-845-1720); Fax (609-853-0411)

The APIC Certification Examination Preparation Study Guide
Contact: APIC
1016 Sixteenth Street NW
Sixth Floor
Washington, DC 20036
Telephone (202-296-2742)
Fax (202-296-5645)

CHICA–Canada Education Program
Contact: Joanna Bernstein, Education Committee
School of Applied Arts and Health Sciences
Centennial College
P.O. Box 631, Station A
Scarborough, Ontario M1P 5E9 CANADA
Telephone (416-694-3241, extension 3391 or 3351)

References

1. Preparation of the operating team and supporting personnel. Manual on Control of Infection in Surgical Patients, 2nd ed. Altemeier WA, Burke JF, Pruitt BA, et al, Eds. JB Lippincott Co, Philadelphia, 1986, p 91
2. LaForce FM: The control of infections in hospitals, 1750 to 1950. Prevention and Control of Nosocomial Infections, 2nd ed. Wenzel RP, Ed. Williams & Wilkins, Baltimore, 1993, p 1
3. US Public Health Service: Disinfection and sterilization: cleaning, disinfection, and sterilization of hospital equipment. US Dept of Health and Human Services (HHS Publication No. [CDC] 3N84-19281). Centers for Disease Control, Atlanta, 1981
4. Haley RW, Culver DH, White JW, et al: The nationwide nosocomial infection rate: a new need for vital statistics. Am J Epidemiol 121:159, 1985
5. Weigelt JA, Dwyer D, Haley RW: The necessity and efficiency of wound surveillance after discharge. Arch Surg 127:77, 1992
6. APIC–SHEA Joint Commission Task Force: Review of 1995 Accreditation Manual for Hospitals [Insert]. APIC News 14(January/February):1, 1995
7. Cruse PJE, Foord R: A five-year prospective study of 23,649 surgical wounds. Arch Surg 107:206, 1973
8. Cruse PJE, Foord R: The epidemiology of wound infection: A 10-year study of 62,939 wounds. Surg Clin North Am 60:27, 1980
9. Alexander W, Fischer JE, Boyajian M, et al: The influence of hair-removal methods on wound infections. Arch Surg 118:347, 1983
10. Clarke JS, Condon RE, Bartlett JG, et al: Preoperative oral antibiotics reduce septic complications of colon operations. Ann Surg 186:251, 1977
11. Farnell MB, Worthington-Self S, Mucha P, et al: Closure of abdominal incisions with subcutaneous catheters: a prospective randomized trial. Arch Surg 121:641, 1986
12. Miles AA, Miles EM, Burke J: The value and duration of defence reactions of the skin to the primary lodgement of bacteria. Br J Exp Pathol 38:79, 1957
13. Rao N, Jacobs S, Joyce L: Cost-effective eradication of an outbreak of methicillin-resistant *Staphylococcus aureus* in a community teaching hospital. Infect Control Hosp Epidemiol 9:255, 1988
14. DiPerri G, Cadeo G, Castelli F, et al: Transmission of HIV-associated tuberculosis to healthcare workers. Infect Control Hosp Epidemiol 14:67, 1993
15. Sepkowitz KA: AIDS, tuberculosis, and the health care worker. Clin Infect Dis 20:232, 1995
16. Nosocomial enterococci resistant to vancomycin—United States, 1989–1993. MMWR 42:597, 1993
17. Miller PJ, Farr BM, Gwaltney JM: Economic benefits of an effective infection control program: case study and proposal. Rev Infect Dis 11:284, 1989
18. Haley RW: Measuring the costs of nosocomial infections: methods for estimating economic burden on the hospital. Am J Med 91(suppl 3B):32S, 1991
19. Consensus paper on the surveillance of surgical wound infections. The Society for Hospital Epidemiology of America, the Association for Practitioners in Infection Control, the Centers for Disease Control, the Surgical Infection Society. Infect Control Hosp Epidemiol 13:599, 1992
20. Owens WD, Felts JA, Spitznagel EL: ASA physical status classifications: a study of consistency of ratings. Anesthesiology 49:239, 1978
21. Britt MR, Schleupner CJ, Matsumiya S: Severity of underlying disease as a predictor of nosocomial infection: utility in the control of nosocomial infection. JAMA 239:1047, 1978
22. Hooton TM, Haley RW, Culver DH, et al: The joint association of multiple risk factors with the occurrence of nosocomial infections. Am J Med 70:960, 1981
23. Manual on Control of Infection in Surgical Patients, 2nd ed. Altemeier WA, Burke JF, Pruitt BA, et al, Eds. JB Lippincott Co, Philadelphia, 1986, p 29
24. Cardo DM, Falk PS, Mayhall CG: Validation of surgical wound classification in the operating room. Infect Control Hosp Epidemiol 14:255, 1993
25. Haley RW, Culver DH, Morgan WM, et al: Identifying patients at high risk of surgical wound infections: a simple multivariate index of patient susceptibility and wound contamination. Am J Epidemiol 121:206, 1985
26. Emori GT, Culver DH, Horan TC, et al: National nosocomial infections system (NNIS): description of surveillance methods. Am J Infect Control 19:19, 1991
27. Nosocomial infection rates for interhospital comparison: limitations and possible solutions. Infect Control Hosp Epidemiol 12:609, 1991
28. Culver DH, Horan TC, Gaynes RP, et al: Surgical wound infection rates by wound class, operative procedure, and patient risk index. Am J Med 91(suppl 3B):152S, 1991
29. Garner JS, Favero MS: Guideline for handwashing and hospital environmental control, 1985. US Dept of Health and Human Services (HHS Publication No. [CDC] PB85-923404). Centers for Disease Control, Atlanta, 1985
30. Favero MS, Bond WW: Chemical disinfection of medical and surgical materials. Disinfection, Sterilization, and Preservation. Lawrence CA, Block SS, Eds. Lea & Febiger, Philadelphia, 1991, p 618
31. Dean AG: Transmission of *Salmonella typhi* by fiberoptic endoscopy. Lancet 2:134, 1977
32. Langenberg W, Rauws EAJ, Oudbier JH, et al: Patient-to-patient transmission of *Campylobacter pylori* infection by fiberoptic gastroduodenoscopy and biopsy. J Infect Dis 161:507, 1990
33. Rutala WA: APIC guideline for selection and use of disinfectants. Am J Infect Control 18:19, 1990
34. Martin MA, Reicheiderfer M: Draft APIC guideline for infection prevention and control in flexible endoscopy. Am J Infect Control 21:1, 1993
35. Conly JM, Hill S, Ross J, et al: Handwashing practices in an intensive care unit: the effects of an educational program and its relationship to infection rates. Am J Infect Control 17:330, 1989
36. Bettin K, Clabots C, Mathie P, et al: Effectiveness of liquid soap vs chlorhexidine gluconate for the removal of *Clostridium difficile* from bare hands and gloved hands. Infect Control Hosp Epidemiol 15:697, 1994
37. Onesko KM, Wienke EC: The analysis of the impact of a mild, low-iodine lotion soap on the reduction of nosocomial methicillin-resistant *Staphylococcus aureus*: a new opportunity for surveillance by objectives. Infect Control 8:284, 1987
38. Ayliffe GAJ: Surgical scrub and skin disinfection. Infect Control 5:23, 1984
39. Moro ML, Vigano EF, Lepri AA: Risk factors for central venous catheter–related infections in surgical and intensive care units. Infect Control Hosp Epidemiol 15:253, 1994
40. Raad II, Hohn DC, Gilbreath J, et al: Prevention of central venous catheter–related infections by using maximal sterile barrier precautions during insertion. Infect Control Hosp Epidemiol 15:231, 1994
41. Maki DG, Ringer M, Alvarado CJ: Prospective randomised trial of povidone-iodine, alcohol, and chlorhexidine for prevention of infection associated with central venous and arterial catheters. Lancet 338:339, 1991
42. Scheckler WE: Continuous quality improvement in a hospital system: implications for hospital epidemiology. Infect Control Hosp Epidemiol 13:288, 1992
43. Bartzokas CA, Paton JH, Gibson MF, et al: Control and eradication of methicillin-resistant *Staphylococcus aureus* on a surgical unit. N Engl J Med 311:1422, 1984
44. Management of methicillin-resistant *Staphylococcus aureus* (MRSA) in health care facilities: 1991 guidelines. Education Committee, Michigan Society for Infection Control. Michigan Society for Infection Control, Detroit, 1991
45. Lynch P, Jackson MM, Cummings MJ, et al: Rethinking the role of isolation practices in the prevention of nosocomial infections. Ann Intern Med 107:243, 1987
46. Recommendations for prevention of HIV transmission in health-care settings. MMWR 36(suppl 2S):3S, 1987
47. Statement on the management of blood and body fluids. CHICA–Canada. Infection Control Canada May–June:18, 1989
48. Duncan IB, Batchelor C: Assessment of the effectiveness of body substance precautions as the infection control system of a large teaching hospital. Am J Infect Control 21:302, 1993
49. White MC, Lynch P: Blood contact and exposure among operating room personnel: a multicenter study. Am J Infect Control 21:243, 1993
50. Chen CC, Willeke K: Aerosol penetration through surgical masks. Am J Infect Control 20:177, 1992
51. Rich P, Belozer ML, Norris P, et al: Allergic contact dermatitis to two antioxidants in latex gloves: 4,4'-thiobis(6-tert-butyl-meta-cresol) (Lowinox 44S36) and butylhydroxyanisole. J Am Acad Dermatol 24:37, 1991
52. Recommendations for preventing transmission of human immunodeficiency virus and hepatitis B virus to patients during exposure-prone invasive procedures. MMWR 40(RR-8):1, 1991

53. Statement on the surgeon and hepatitis B infection. American College of Surgeons. Bulletin of the American College of Surgeons 80(5):33, 1995
54. Draft guideline for isolation precautions in hospitals: notice. Centers for Disease Control and Prevention. Federal Register 59:55552, 1994
55. Guidelines for preventing the transmission of *Mycobacterium tuberculosis* in health-care facilities, 1994. Centers for Disease Control and Prevention. Federal Register 59:54242, 1994
56. OSHA enforcement policy and procedures for occupational exposure to tuberculosis. Infect Control Hosp Epidemiol 14:694, 1993
57. Menzies D, Fanning A, Yuan L, et al: Tuberculosis among health care workers. N Engl J Med 332:92, 1995
58. Malasky C, Jordon T, Potulski F, et al: Occupational tuberculosis infections among pulmonary physicians in training. Am Rev Respir Dis 142:505, 1990
59. Muder RR, Brennen C, Goetz AM: Infection with methicillin-resistant *Staphylococcus aureus* among hospital employees. Infect Control Hosp Epidemiol 14:576, 1993
60. Sanford MD, Widmer AF, Bale MJ, et al: Efficient detection and long-term persistence of the carriage of methicillin-resistant *Staphylococcus aureus*. Clin Infect Dis 19:1123, 1994
61. Recommendations for preventing the spread of vancomycin resistance. Hospital Infection Control Practices Advisory Committee (HICPAC). Infect Control Hosp Epidemiol 16:105, 1995
62. Haley RW: Surveillance by objective: a new priority-directed approach to the control of nosocomial infections. Am J Infect Control 13:78, 1985
63. Lowry PW, Blankenship RJ, Gridley W, et al: A cluster of *Legionella* sternal-wound infections due to postoperative topical exposure to contaminated tap water. N Engl J Med 324:109, 1991
64. Taylor S, McKenzie M, Taylor G, et al: Wound infection in total joint arthroplasty: effect of extended wound surveillance on infection rates (abstr). CHICA–Canada '93 Conference. Can J Infect Control 8:71, 1993
65. Horan TC, Gaynes RP, Martone WJ: CDC definitions of nosocomial surgical site infections, 1992: a modification of CDC definitions of surgical wound infections. Infect Control Hosp Epidemiol 13:271, 1992
66. Evans RS, Burke JP, Classen DC, et al: Computerized identification of patients at high risk for hospital-acquired infection. Am J Infect Control 20:4, 1992
67. Doebbeling BN: Epidemics: identification and management. Prevention and Control of Nosocomial Infections, 2nd ed. Wenzel RP, Ed. Williams & Wilkins, Baltimore, 1993, p 177
68. Arnow PM, Chou T, Weil D, et al: Nosocomial legionnaires' disease caused by aerosolized tap water from respiratory devices. J Infect Dis 146:460, 1982
69. Draft guidelines for prevention of nosocomial pneumonia: notice of comment period. Centers for Disease Control and Prevention. Federal Register 59:4980, 1994
70. Muraca PW, Yu VL, Goetz A: Disinfection of water distribution systems for *Legionella*: a review of application procedures and methodologies. Infect Control Hosp Epidemiol 11:79, 1990
71. Walsh TJ, Dixon DM: Nosocomial aspergillosis: environmental microbiology, hospital epidemiology, diagnosis, and treatment. Eur J Epidemiol 5:131, 1989
72. Haley RW, Gaynes RP, Aber RC, et al: Surveillance of nosocomial infections. Hospital infections, 3rd ed. Bennett JV, Brachman PS, Eds. Little, Brown & Co, Boston, 1992, p 79
73. Pittet D, Tarara D, Wenzel RP: Nosocomial bloodstream infection in critically ill patients: excess length of stay, extra costs, and attributable mortality (abstr). 32nd Interscience Conference on Antimicrobial Agents and Chemotherapy, Anaheim, California, 1992
74. Nettleman MD: The global impact of infection. Prevention and Control of Nosocomial Infections, 2nd ed. Wenzel RP, Ed. Williams & Wilkins, Baltimore, 1993, p 13

109 THE IMPAIRED PHYSICIAN

David B. Hoyt, M.D., Martha C. Martell, M.S., and Peter Rosen, M.D.

Approach to Physician Impairment

There are many causes of physician impairment, but we will concentrate on three of the most important: aging, dysfunctional character traits, and substance abuse. We will not consider the ethical or medical problems of surgeons infected with hepatitis B or human immunodeficiency virus (HIV), nor will we discuss issues related to other major illnesses.

Age-related impairment is the mental and physical deterioration or decline that occurs with advancing age or that may be part of a specific neurologic syndrome, such as Alzheimer's disease.

Character impairment is not a specific psychiatric or psychological disorder but rather a state in which normative error results in suboptimal quality of care. A normative error is an error in behavior, morality, or ethics that is counter to accepted standard practices,[1,2] such as refusing to answer a page or trying to cover up a technical error. A normative error is distinct from a technical error, such as the improper placement of a central line, and also from a judgmental error, such as choosing the wrong surgical procedure.

Substance or chemical abuse is the deliberate use of a substance by any route of administration to produce an alteration of normal consciousness. Cases in which consciousness is altered because a harmful substance was consumed unknowingly or mistaken for a less harmful substance are toxicologic conditions rather than instances of deliberate substance abuse. Chemical dependence is a more severe form of substance abuse that also involves withdrawal effects.[3] Diagnosis of alcohol or drug dependence will not be addressed here; the focus of the discussion will be on identifying the possible abuse of chemicals in a colleague or a medical student for the purpose of making an appropriate referral.

The Age-Impaired Physician

DETECTION

The signs of age-related physical and mental impairment are often subtle and, in general, are similar to those of chemical abuse and addiction [see Table 1].[4-6] Virtually all of the signs may be unnoticed by colleagues or, if noticed, dismissed as insignificant. They are most likely to be noticed by people who have not been working regularly with the aging physician, such as a new nurse or house officer, and who are unlikely to have a means of criticism because of youth, inexperience, or junior hierarchic status.

One clue to the presence of impairment and, perhaps, to a need for retirement is prolonged or repeated absence from work for medical reasons. This may be manifested by last-minute changes in call schedule or sudden cancellations of scheduled operations, clinics, or committee work. Physicians are often reluctant to take care of themselves when ill, and as they age, they are increasingly subject to minor aches and pains. The aging physician may also have more substantive disease processes and greater difficulty with recovery from illness and rehabilitation.

Another clue is a deterioration of language skills. Whereas changes in conversational language skills may be hardly noticeable, decay of written language skills is readily apparent, not only in handwriting but also in language structure and content. Such decay is often first noticed in medical charts and should not be dismissed as simple inattentiveness.

Decision-making skill deficits are more difficult to detect but should be considered when the physician appears uncharacteristically slow to make a decision for an emergency operation or seems to be increasingly noncurrent in his or her practice. Often, inappropriate decisions are hidden because the only witnesses are junior house officers or other personnel who cannot critically appraise the decisions. For example, during an operation for a ruptured sigmoid diverticulitis, a decision not to perform a colostomy may be uncharacteristic for a particular surgeon, but it is unlikely to be perceived as such by a scrub nurse or an assisting first-year resident.

Another indicator of impairment is reluctance to respond to emergency needs of patients. This reluctance may be observed first by night nurses who have trouble obtaining help for patients experiencing deteriorations during the night shift. The aging physician may also be reluctant to operate in the middle of the night, often citing experience or conservatism as a reason. The consequences may be serious for a patient who would have benefited from nighttime relief of a bowel obstruction or who might not have developed perforated appendicitis if timely emergency surgery had been done. Such bad decisions may not reach a point where they can be detected by quality assurance (QA)

Table 1 Signs of Age-Related Impairment

Increasing sick days
Language decay in charting
Decision-making errors
Reluctance to answer emergency calls
Increasing technical errors
Uncharacteristic forgetfulness
Uncharacteristic slovenliness

mechanisms; they may be observed only by the night teams, who have no easy way to report their observations.

An increasing number of technical errors is a common signal of age-related impairment. Not every technical error is of major import, however. Often, it is the performance of minor tasks, such as starting an intravenous line or placing a nasogastric tube, that most clearly reveals failing technical ability. The major procedures may be the last to be performed poorly, because as a rule, more attention is paid to more difficult tasks. In many senior surgeons, errors in performance of minor tasks are rarely observed because such tasks are often delegated to others. Errors in the performance of major tasks may be manifested only by slower performance. Some technical errors can be avoided by recognizing age-related deterioration and attempting to compensate for it (e.g., using magnifying loupes).

Many physicians are absentminded even when young, but if an aging physician with a reasonably good memory starts forgetting important appointments or tasks, there is cause for concern. Absentmindedness during surgery can have severe medical consequences.

Individual physicians place varying degrees of importance on personal appearance. Uncharacteristic slovenliness or omission of ordinary acts of privacy (e.g., failure to zip a fly after urination) may be a sign of impairment. Although anyone is capable of an occasional act of forgetfulness, it may nevertheless be an important clue to failing cognitive awareness.

MANAGEMENT

Physicians generally retire before their skills have been significantly eroded by ordinary aging. Often, institutional rules mandate retirement at a specified age. However, legal challenge to forced retirement regulations has sometimes been successful,[7] and given that there is no mandatory retirement for Supreme Court justices, it can safely be predicted that this trend will continue. The major concern in the management of age-related impairment is the physician who either is unaware of his or her failing capacities or is financially or psychologically incapable of accepting the need for retirement and who is working within a structure that does not mandate retirement at a given age.[8]

Formal review is a key component of management. All members of a department or group should be reviewed regularly, either as part of the credentialing cycle or through a special review called by the department chair. The review should be performed every three to five years; some departments may prefer shorter intervals. The department chair should be reviewed by the dean, the chief of staff, or another designated reviewer. If technical task review is outside the expertise of the chief of staff, a vice-chair of the department or an outside consultant may be called on. The consultant should be chosen by the dean, the chief of staff, or the executive committee from a list submitted by the executive committee and the department chair.

The QA program may identify a need for a special review, but a single red flag from the QA program should not be considered a sufficient reason for removing titles or privileges. Another red flag might be a significant increase in patient morbidity or mortality above what is expected for a particular individual or procedure. It would be unfair, however, to penalize a surgeon solely because of greater than normal cost or length of stay; he or she may be treating especially ill patients referred from other institutions or may have expertise in unusual disease states that are likely to produce statistical outliers.

Besides the regular review process, there should be an established system for the identification and management of the impaired physician. If, between reviews, a physician appears to exhibit age-related impairment, the executive committee should confront him or her with well-documented evidence of impaired performance; this should be done in the presence of a witness who is an ally of, or at least friendly to, the physician. The team confronting the physician should have experience in the management of physician impairment and should include someone who is skilled at evaluating suicide potential. It is commonly feared that confrontation may provoke a suicide attempt, but often, the physician is in fact relieved to be able to bring the problem into the open at last.

In addition, efforts should be made to search for significant coexisting medical conditions that might be causing or contributing to the problems, and a period of reevaluation of the age-related problems should also be instituted. If there is reason to believe that medical disease may be playing a role, it should be department policy to request an emergency consultation from an appropriate specialist. The management team should have access to appropriate treatment facilities and should be ready to place the impaired physician in such a facility immediately if necessary. Immediate hospitalization is advisable in many cases but by no means in all.

If the evaluation identifies significant deficits, the physician may be forced to retire. Forced retirement is never easy, but it is easier to implement in an institution with a formalized personnel system. Fortunately, there are often alternatives to forced retirement, such as removal from direct patient care. A physician who is no longer able to handle active surgical clinical practice might still be able to serve well in an administrative function. If the physician is in private practice, the associated hospital may have to take action to remove his or her clinical privileges. Unless policies and procedures exist for routinely evaluating a physician's competence before noticeable problems arise, removal of privileges is often a battle that becomes mired in the legal system.

Some may take the position that surgeons simply should not operate after a given age. Although mandatory retirement is undoubtedly somewhat unjust, it may in fact be the fairest way to ensure that physicians do not practice past the age of competence. We surgeons must face the reality that surgery is a youthful profession and acknowledge that at some point we must turn the responsibilities over to the next generation. It is up to us to address the issue of retirement before it is forced on us, to provide for financial security at retirement age, and to be willing to adjust our egos to a life without the rewards of an active surgical career.

The Normative Error Maker

DETECTION

Perhaps the fundamental characteristic of normative error makers is a supreme unawareness of their effect on other people, frequently accompanied by hypersensitivity to the way they are treated by others. Normative error makers are arrogant, condescending, irritating, and often intellectually dishonest; however, they are commonly well liked by their superiors because they never display such behavior toward those above them. It is difficult to detect character impairment, especially when, as is often the case, the normative error maker possesses true talent and even a measure of charm (when he or she chooses to exercise it).

One of the clues to the presence of character impairment [see Table 2] is multiple complaints from the staff. The departmental chief is often the last to know: every chief has had the experience of dismissing a physician for unacceptable normative errors that are deemed recent, only to be told by an astonishing number of personnel that they are glad that something has finally been done about the "troublemaker." Ancillary personnel, nurses, and technicians are frequently abused by the normative error maker, but they have no easy way of registering a complaint. Naturally, not every complaint is based on reality, and anyone can have personality conflicts. The existence of complaints, by itself, is less significant than the kind of complaints made and the frequency with which they are reported. Often, character-impaired individuals appear on the surface to have an element of right on their side. Many nurses are driven past ordinary patience by a normative error maker, and when they finally respond, their reactions frequently appear excessive and inappropriate. It is important to have a means of documenting the incidents as they occur because they often seem to be trivial or unrelated until the sheer weight of their number is felt.

Another signal of possible character impairment is unexpected technical errors. Any such errors should be investigated by the supervisor because normative errors can cause technical errors.[2] For example, a normative error maker who is technically skilled may fail to routinely follow up on a deftly performed technical procedure and consequently may miss an important complication that should ordinarily have been recognized. For instance, the normative error maker may fail to obtain a chest x-ray after inserting an endotracheal tube because he or she *knows* that the intubation was done correctly; the tube may be in the mainstem bronchus and remain undiscovered.

Frequently, normative error makers are incapable of fair play in creating a schedule or in sharing scut work. They may relish their power over junior personnel. Unless a legitimate mechanism is put in place that allows junior personnel to score the performance of the physicians in charge of their education and supervision, this problem is unlikely to be corrected. In addition, normative error makers are often reluctant to credit junior faculty with much skill and experience and so may deem it unnecessary to follow their instructions. Sometimes, normative error makers will not even bother to mask their disdain for the recommendations made to them by junior faculty. This attitude is often unnoticed by senior physicians until the error maker undergoes formal review.

The normative error maker frequently complains of impolite or disrespectful treatment from the other staff members. These complaints are more than a grim irony of projection (i.e., a referral of one's own attitudes or behavior to others): they reveal him or her as a person whose only perceptions of the world are based on input without feedback.

Character-impaired physicians tend to make excuses for their errors by blaming a consultant, the referring service, or the nurses caring for the patients. It is easy to overlook their contribution to the problem because their side of the issue is often the only one immediately available when a problem is recognized. This kind of insidious dishonesty leads to frequent turnover among support staff.

MANAGEMENT

Normative error makers may be more difficult to manage than age-impaired or chemically impaired physicians. All too often, the director is reluctant to punish a normative error maker because of the time and energy invested in the physician's education[9]; only after repeated betrayals of trust is dismissal considered. By then, the normative error maker usually is close to the end of training or has passed the barrier to partner selection. The path of least inconvenience is often chosen: residents are allowed to finish their training or junior attending physicians are passed off to someone else without any detailed analysis of their errors. Given the difficulty of proving error to a point of dismissal and given the problems created by dismissing a more senior resident, it is no surprise that normative error making is not punished effectively.[10] Technical and judgmental errors are more likely causes of dismissal than normative errors because they are much easier to document and are more acceptable as reasons for termination. This is unfortunate because technical error and judgmental error often disappear over time with education, practice, and experience, whereas normative error generally does not. In fact, character impairment tends to worsen with age, as the physician becomes more indifferent to the profession and to people in general. When a pattern of errors is first identified, it is imperative to create a detailed paper trail of the problems encountered. The personnel regulations and practices of the institution must be studied carefully, followed closely, and documented thoroughly. The normative error maker is precisely the type of person who will demand and expect a degree of documentation that is difficult to achieve and who may well file a countercomplaint in retaliation.

The normative error maker should be confronted by the department chair and a vice-chair in the presence of a friendly witness. It is wise to avoid having attorneys present at the initial confrontation; the departmental representatives should explain that the meeting's purpose is to communicate a problem, not to initiate legal proceedings. The physician should not be prevented from consulting an attorney, however. The normative error maker should be given specific details, in writing, of the behavioral problems to be resolved. He or she will often respond with excuses or descriptions of extenuating circumstances. The department chair must communicate directly, specifically, and in writing the behavioral changes that are expected and must explicitly establish rules for monitoring these changes. Disciplinary measures are a last resort, to be taken only if the physician denies the problem and refuses to change his or her behavior. At this point, a variety of attorneys may become involved.

The character-impaired physician is unlikely to resign because of criticism or pressure. If the physician does respond to criticism with rage and threatens to resign, it might be prudent to accept the resignation. The resignation should be taken in writ-

---

Table 2 Signs of Character Impairment

Multiple complaints from nurses, technicians, or ancillary personnel
Errors that seem out of character for the known level of talent
Intense dislike from peers, junior residents, or students
Complaints of ineducability from junior faculty
Frequent complaints from the physician about other services, nurses, or ancillary personnel
Unwillingness to accept responsibility for technical or judgmental errors
High turnover in support staff

ing. A cool-down period, with 60 to 90 days of leave, might be considered before the resignation (or dismissal) becomes final.

The Substance-Abusing Physician

DETECTION

It is hard to believe that impairment of a surgeon by drug or alcohol abuse would not immediately be detected by colleagues and coworkers. The reality, however, is that denial, the need to protect the professional image, and our own unwillingness to consider the possibility of substance abuse in those we know, respect, and love all combine to protect the impaired physician from discovery.

Most institutions have protocols for screening employees, but many do not have protocols for screening staff physicians who are not employees. If no screening protocols are in place, it may help to sound out other staff members, such as the OR crew or an ICU nurse who knows the physician. Nurses in particular are quite sensitive to physician impairment: they often spot the clues long before physician colleagues.

Even after a physician has been identified as impaired by substance abuse, it is difficult to pinpoint when the problem began. Chemical dependency is difficult to diagnose in the early stages; the effects of alcohol or drug abuse on major areas of life are the key to diagnosis [see Table 3].[11-14] Patient care is usually the last part of a physician's life to be affected by substance abuse.

Although the impaired physician may attempt (often successfully) to deny and conceal the problem, we must be as alert to the signs and symptoms of substance abuse as we would be to other disease manifestations in a colleague. (Many substance abusers are, of course, well aware that they consume forbidden substances, but part of the disease is the chronic inability to accept that they have a drug or alcohol problem; gaining the ability to face the problem is the true first step in therapy.)

A sign that may be difficult to recognize is the sudden onset of illness in a healthy person. Surgeons, like most physicians, are slow to accept their own human frailty and often will work with a degree of illness that would lead to mandatory hospital admission for any nonphysician. Therefore, when a colleague suddenly has a run of ill health, especially if the problems appear unrelated, chemical abuse should be considered. It may be that the physician has become immunologically suppressed, is sustaining traumatic injuries from falls while under the influence of drugs or alcohol, is experiencing the ravaging effects of substance abuse on general health, or is chronically too intoxicated or hung over to come to work.

Another clue is drug-seeking behavior. A British study of physicians hospitalized for drug dependence over a 20-year period found that the subjects obtained their drugs mainly through self-prescribing.[15] Some authors argue that chemical dependence is an occupational hazard for physicians because of their unlimited access to drugs.[15,16] In particular, opiate addicts frequently request narcotic prescriptions either for themselves or for family members to treat a variety of acutely painful problems, such as dental pain, rib pain, contusions, bruises, or unusual fractures (e.g., rib, humerus, or clavicle fractures). Often, addicts are clever enough to go to several different colleagues so that no single physician will receive a suspiciously high number of narcotic requests. Not until the prescriptions reach a central clearing site (e.g., the pharmacy) or until one physician overhears the addict repeat a request to another physician does it become clear that the impaired physician is engaging in drug-seeking behavior. Uncharacteristic or bizarre behavior, such as spending excessive time in the bathroom or emerging unexpectedly from a closet, should arouse suspicion of surreptitious drug taking. Sudden extreme interest in the analgesic medications of patients who are in the area, a sudden change in the timing of postoperative rounds, the need to see patients at odd hours, and unwillingness to leave the hospital are also behaviors characteristic of opiate addicts.

Table 3 Signs of Substance Abuse–Related Impairment[60]

- Frequent illnesses in a normally healthy person
- Frequent episodes of "flu," especially after weekends or holidays
- Requests for prescriptions for self or family members, especially for narcotics; excessive concern with the ordering of analgesic prescriptions; unwillingness to leave the institution
- Drinking or self-prescribing drugs to relax or sleep
- Inappropriate consumption of alcohol
- Drinking while on call
- Bizarre behavior that might be caused by surreptitious drug taking
- Frequent mood swings with inappropriate irritability or temper tantrums
- Physical confrontations over trivial quarrels
- Poor judgment and inappropriate decision making; hyperdefensiveness to criticism
- Excessive denial of any problem
- Unexplained absences or last-minute changes in schedules
- Failure to meet deadlines or produce reliable work
- Automobile accidents, especially while intoxicated
- Sudden disintegration of marriage or long-standing friendships
- Frequent geographic changes in location
- Lack of concern for grooming and personal habits
- Tendency to be easily distracted
- Increased isolation from others
- Impaired memory
- Depression
- Trembling
- Weight loss
- Deterioration in performance

Obviously, there are grounds for concern when a colleague begins to consume alcohol at a greater than customary rate, in inappropriate places, at odd times of the day, or in a volume that appears to cause anxiety in a spouse or friend. When such signs are combined with recurrent illnesses that are probably hangovers or injuries from traumatic incidents and with episodes of childish anger and confrontations, substance abuse must be strongly suspected. These clues most likely indicate alcoholism, but they may also be associated with chemical dependence of any kind. (In older physicians, however, some of these signs may also be manifestations of incipient Alzheimer's disease.)

Stimulants such as cocaine and amphetamines tend to make the user jumpy and irritable, especially when the user is in a state of withdrawal. When a colleague who has previously been even-tempered begins to act sleep-deprived and irritable, to make normative errors, or to become involved in physical confrontations, the possibility of dependence on a stimulant should be considered.

Similarly, when a talented physician begins to make clinical decisions that seem totally inexplicable, the possibility of drug abuse should be taken into account. Cocaine abuse often causes bizarre thought processes that seem reasonable to the addict. Altered thought processes accompanied by a defensive attitude, especially in a person who has previously been intellectually honest, strongly suggest substance abuse. Another red flag is excessive denial that there is any problem.

Most practicing physicians are well organized. This is especially true of surgeons. Sudden inexplicable unreliability, forgetfulness, and deterioration in the quality of a physician's work are also symptoms of substance abuse.

Sudden breakups of long-standing relationships are another warning sign. Although neither a long-standing marriage nor a long-standing professional partnership is ever absolutely secure, sudden instability and chaos are grounds for serious concern and may well reflect substance abuse.

Numerous geographic moves over a short period signal the possibility of chemical dependence or other impairment. No matter how excellent the reputation and references, candid interviews with former colleagues should be obtained before a surgeon with a recent history of frequent relocation is hired.[17]

Disorderliness and unkempt clothing, especially when they represent a major change in personal appearance, signal possible drug impairment. Other signs of substance abuse include increased isolation, memory impairment, depression, trembling, and weight loss.[11-13]

Each of these warning signs, by itself, could be an innocuous or episodic incident that is unrelated to impairment; it is the context that determines whether they are signals of a problem. When more than one of these signs occur in the same person within a limited time frame, substance abuse must always be considered.

MANAGEMENT

What to do about a probable case of substance abuse can be a difficult question. In addition to the normal reluctance to become involved in another's problems, there is a natural hesitancy to create trouble for a colleague. Although physicians have been called unethical for remaining silent about other physicians' drug abuse,[18] the usual reason for their silence is not so much a conspiracy to cover up the problem as a desire to do no harm; denial, inability to detect the impairment before it has produced harm, and awareness of the financial effects of dismissal play a role as well. Despite the many barriers to taking action, attempts must be made to manage and treat substance abuse: the health and safety of surgeons and their patients are of vastly greater importance than any discomfort, inconvenience, or embarrassment that may result.

In some circumstances, impaired physicians may be reported anonymously. This goes against the idea of fair play, but sometimes, it is the only reasonable step. For example, if the reporting physician is in economic competition with the substance abuser, it is very unlikely that the addict will interpret the competitor's motives as pure and disinterested.

Every state now has developed an impaired-physician program.[19] Many institutions have also developed their own so-called health and well-being committees, designed to identify, evaluate, advise, support, assist, and treat impaired physicians within their institutions. Such committees usually are confidential and nonpunitive and provide education as well as resources. They are also able to monitor physicians for compliance during recovery; such monitoring may include drug testing and behavioral observation.[20,21]

Chemical dependence is a progressive disease that leads to death,[22] not a moral issue. As knowledge of the treatment of chemical dependence has grown, concerns for physician welfare have begun to supplant punitive attitudes toward substance-abusing physicians.[21] In many states, however, it is still necessary to report a chemically dependent physician to the state medical board, though in others, the physician can be granted immunity if he or she enters treatment.[14] In most cases, impaired physicians may receive treatment and return to work without loss of position, as long as they comply with the treatment requirements.[4,23]

Often, the only motivation that will push the physician past denial and into treatment is the threat of serious repercussions (e.g., loss of job or license, impending divorce, or increasing physical deterioration) if treatment is refused.[22] The most effective method of persuading a chemically impaired physician to enter treatment is to hold a formal team intervention,[22] which is a meeting led by a trained facilitator that brings the impaired individual together with significant others and concerned colleagues. The substance abuser is brought into the meeting unexpectedly, at a time when he or she is sober, and asked simply to listen to each person, not responding until all have finished speaking. Each witness recounts one or more situations in which the physician's substance abuse has affected the witness personally, without being judgmental, and then expresses concern for the person and recommends treatment. In the great majority of cases, this team approach is successful.[22] As a rule, it is far more successful than an individual confrontation because the addict is extremely adept at manipulation, denial, and rationalization. When an addict is confronted by a group of concerned people who are united in their recommendation to seek treatment, it is usually possible to penetrate his or her defensiveness and denial. Guidance and leadership for the team intervention can come from the state program, the institution's health and well-being committee, or any community treatment center. The intervention must be well rehearsed, supported by ample evidence, nonjudgmental but firm, and resistant to denial. The group must also have the clout to follow through with the consequences if the physician refuses treatment.[14]

In many states, a substance-abusing physician who voluntarily cooperates with diagnosis and therapy will not lose his or her medical license outright; the license is forfeit only if the physician fails to enter treatment or to follow through with the treatment regimen or relapses while undergoing drug screening.[23-25] Full involvement in and compliance with the aftercare plan are also required.

After assessment by a chemical-dependence specialist, treatment may range from inpatient detoxification and extended hospital treatment to outpatient counseling and attendance at meetings of support groups. No particular effort to conceal the problem from others should be made, but patient confidentiality should be respected. Part of the treatment for addiction is sharing the existence of the problem with others, but the patient should be allowed to choose the timing of this disclosure. After treatment, the key to continuing recovery is the prevention of relapse. The 12-step programs, such as Alcoholics Anonymous, are effective in managing relapse; however, they involve principles that some physicians may find difficult to accept (e.g., admitting powerlessness over the drug and relying on a higher power). If physicians are able to accept the tenets, these programs can be the single most potent element in recovery—more potent than counseling from professional addiction therapists or the support of family members.[13,21]

In some cases, the impaired physician continues to deny the problem and to refuse treatment. It may then be necessary to use the mandatory disciplinary functions of the state licensing agencies. This is especially difficult with long-standing colleagues or friends, but ethics demand such action, for the sake of both patients and physician.

The recovery rate for impaired physicians who enter treatment has been reported to be 85 percent[26] or higher,[19] which is much better than the recovery rates for many other diseases. Furthermore, the recovery rate for chemically dependent physicians who enter treatment is higher than for members of the general population who do so.[12,14,27] Treated physicians probably pose no greater (or perhaps even less) risk to their patients than other physicians do, and treatment-related improvements appear to carry over into practice-related behaviors.[28] This fact should encourage referral. Addicts are known to have a high rate of recidivism.[29] Relapse may well be part of recovery, with periods of special vulnerability occurring three months, six months, 12 months, and 24 months after treatment.[30] Thus, recovery is an ongoing process. Without treatment, the inevitable outcome is premature death.[31]

Discussion

It is estimated that at least 10 to 15 percent of practicing physicians are impaired[19]; however, the true incidence of impairment may be much higher if impairment resulting from abuse of alcohol and other drugs is included.[18,32] Never before in the history of medicine has there been such intense scrutiny of the performance of the physician.[4] Whether this development reflects a change in societal attitudes toward professional authority figures or a change in the ethical behavior expected of physicians, it is clear that the forces that regulate and supervise medicine are less tolerant than ever of physician impairment of any kind.

Although more and more patients are making use of so-called alternative practitioners, there is still a strong societal emphasis on the credentials, competence, and quality of practice of surgeons.[33] Of course, to note that surgeons are held to a high standard is not to argue that this standard is unfair.

The true incidence of the problem is not known. The rate at which sanctions are imposed and treatment mandated by state licensing boards ranges from one to three percent.[34] In 1992, the prevalence of substance abuse was estimated to be 7.9 percent (4.2 percent alcohol only, 1.9 percent drugs only, and 1.8 percent both), with 4.7 percent receiving treatment.[35] It is difficult to say what percentages must be added for character impairment, age-related deterioration of skills, or even transient indiscretions that do not represent true chemical addiction.

In all honesty, it would be easy for any surgeon to think of at least one episode that prevented the performance of duties at an ideal level of competence—for instance, an unexpected visit from an out-of-town colleague that led to overindulgence during a night on the town, or an occasion when the surgeon was distracted by an impending vacation or out-of-town meeting and did not pay sufficient attention to detail. Such episodes produce a kind of transient impairment that, although virtually impossible to measure, can easily result in suboptimal outcome. This kind of impairment is not the focus of our discussion; we mention it in the hope of encouraging better understanding of the problems of the age-impaired, character-impaired, or chemically impaired physician.

Age Impairment

MANIFESTATIONS

Inevitably, skills decay over time. When decay is accompanied by major physical disease, it may manifest itself quickly and be acted on; when it occurs gradually, it may be unnoticed by the practitioner and observed only by persons who are not in a position to take action or make recommendations.

Unfortunately, there are no good objective tests of technical skills for physicians. In many surgical procedures, outcome is not affected by anything less than a major technical error, and in any case, senior surgeons are rarely scrutinized by departmental chairs or hospital administrators. Furthermore, even though technical skills are at their height in the early years after residency, it is often not until years later that a practice builds to the point of maximum activity—by which time it may be only a short while before skills begin to decay. Physicians commonly become busier as they develop a reputation through years of experience, consultation, and consistently good outcomes, and as a result, they become increasingly important contributors to the income of a group, service, or hospital. It is therefore unlikely that anyone will recommend diminished activity for senior physicians, especially if the decay in skills is mild or episodic.

The techniques and wisdom acquired with experience do afford some protection against skills decay. Judgment improves, and decisions are typically less aggressive and more careful and appropriate. Consequently, the experienced physician can often avoid being in a position where maximum technical performance is necessary. For example, after gastrectomy, an experienced surgeon may well choose to perform a gastrojejunostomy to avoid having to wrestle with the deformed duodenal stump.

Physical endurance suffers as well. Coping with long nights of emergency procedures followed by a full elective day schedule becomes increasingly difficult. There are no studies on the ability of older physicians to cope with the physical stress imposed by long hours, which create problems even for young physicians. When this stress is combined with some of the age-related diseases, both judgment and the ability to perform the correct procedures may be impaired.

There is also a variable level of mental decay. Mental decay, however, is often mitigated by the practice environment; it is difficult to teach residents without being taught by them. Some physicians feel a loss of interest in the practice of the profession that may aggravate the natural loss of cognitive ability, and they may become inattentive, lazy, and unmotivated as a result. In such cases, the impairment is likely to be detected because there is generally a higher incidence of complications and often major problems in outcome.

Frequently, the impaired physician recognizes the skills decay and tries to compensate for it (e.g., by voluntarily cutting back on clinical hours and relinquishing some responsibility). On the other hand, the physician may be induced by pride and the impairment itself to deny the problem.

MONITORING AND EVALUATION OF THE AGING PHYSICIAN

To prevent potentially disastrous consequences, it may be prudent to strengthen the requirements for recertification, which should include an independent review of motor and cognitive skills. Many states (perhaps most) require annual driving tests to renew a motor vehicle license after 65 years of age, but apparently no state has special requirements for medical licensure after 65 years of age. Unfortunately, the normal rate of decay in intellect is unknown, as are the normal measures that should be taken to compensate for this decay. The fairest process for curtailing or withdrawing privileges on the grounds of age incompetence has not been identified.

In most programs, hospitals, and universities, there are few or inadequate means of evaluating senior physician performance. Recertification procedures have mostly been aimed at younger physicians, and the promotional criteria are most stringent for unpromoted physicians. There are QA reviews and quality control activities in every medical department, but the kind of deterioration that occurs with aging may not show up on any review until major skills have been lost. Even in universities that have routine performance reviews at regular intervals, it is very difficult to identify nonacademic errors in performance that are attributable to aging.

Even though a university can restrict length of service for departmental chair activities, it is still virtually impossible to remove a physician from a faculty position without mandatory retirement regulations. Most departments do in fact rely on a mandatory retirement age and encourage early retirement[7] because incoming members receive lower salaries and are capable of and interested in performing more activities. In academic departments, there is a natural evolution toward more of the administrative tasks being performed by seasoned physicians, with more of the clinical tasks being given to the younger members of the faculty. Unfortunately, senior faculty members rarely make major contributions to the teaching activities to which their greater experience and wisdom would seem to suit them: often, house-staff education is supervised by a junior faculty member who not only is trying to build a clinical reputation and practice but also must be concerned with maintaining a level of academic productivity that will lead to promotion.

In private groups, it is often the senior surgeon who has the greatest number of patients, the largest clinical responsibility, and the least time for or inclination toward maintenance of skills and knowledge. The bylaws of a private group partnership may require mandatory retirement at a given age. In a solo practice, however, there is usually no method of detecting impairment unless someone complains about the physician.

Clearly, it is imperative to have a system for evaluation in place before there is a problem. The system should evaluate all staff members, and the chairman or director of the service should be evaluated either by the chief of staff or by an independent outside evaluator. Some institutions bring in independent consultants chosen from a list of names submitted by the director. It would be wise to have every staff surgeon undergo something more than a paper application for renewal of staff privileges every few years. The chief of service should personally review the performance of subordinate physicians; however, this may be difficult to accomplish without peer review committees because of the confounding issues that result from economic competition among staff physicians. Efforts to remove staff physicians because of incompetence have frequently foundered in legal suits claiming unfair competition or lack of other objective appraisal.

Individual surgeons should be evaluated with respect to both technical and cognitive performance. If there is a recertification examination available within the specialty, the departmental bylaws should require maintenance of current and active certification. No department should permit the practice of a specialty without certification. Long before age becomes a problem, many surgeons use board eligibility as a cover without attempting or completing board certification. Where there is no board or no certificate of special competence to achieve or maintain, the task of evaluation becomes somewhat more difficult. If evaluation by a chairman or section director involves too many conflicts of interest, the department should retain an outside consultant.

Anyone who works with an attending physician should be able to request a performance review without fear of recrimination, and specified processes and procedures should be formulated for this purpose. Some institutions have forms on which junior personnel can request a review of a problem without identifying themselves as complainants; however, these are rarely effective. Anonymous complaints, besides being inherently unjust, are frequently used to express passive-aggressive responses to personality disputes. On the other hand, it is often junior physicians and staff members who are most likely to make an early identification of age impairment. The optimal approach to monitoring the aging physician must be individualized; however, the establishment of structures and systems for reporting problems without the risk of retribution should be encouraged because it will allow many problems to be identified in a timely fashion. For example, there should be a senior advisor within the department to whom house officers can report without fear of jeopardizing both present and future positions. Similarly, there should be an administrative nurse to whom a section nurse can report and who will then be able to communicate the problem to the chief of service.

Neuropsychological testing can be used to measure intellectual competence. Although it should probably be thought of as an extreme method, to which few physicians will submit on a routine basis, it may be requested when specific problems have been identified.

Clearly, any of the problems described will be exacerbated, and their progression accelerated, if substance abuse is also present. Alcohol, in particular, is a dangerous exacerbating factor. Unfortunately, older physicians are likely to lead a lifestyle that encourages the use of alcohol. Furthermore, age-impaired physicians may attempt to compensate for dimly or subconsciously recognized loss of talents and capabilities with overconsumption of alcohol. They can then blame something other than aging for their failing ability.

Character Impairment

In many ways, character impairment is the saddest of the impairments. Many character-impaired physicians have a great deal of talent, considerable technical skill, and sound judgment when they choose to exercise it. Unfortunately, they are unable to relate well to others, an inability that seems to be based on an assumption of superiority. It is important to distinguish such physicians from those who are simply lazy by nature and unwilling to be compulsive and attentive to detail, especially if fatigued.

Some normative errors are produced by fatigue. There are many people who cannot easily cope with changes in their normal sleep-wake cycles. Because of the sleep deprivation and the long shifts experienced in a surgical residency, such individuals make many normative errors that they would not normally make if they were well rested.

An important means for correcting normative error, however, is the training program. The unfortunate reality is that many training programs do not look for normative error, attempt to correct it, or provide the kind of role models for young physicians that will prevent or alter it.[32,33] Many programs appear to reinforce the very traits that ultimately lead to impairment, rewarding residents for being aggressive, for being intemperate with younger house officers or students, and for being sarcastic on ward rounds or at morbidity and mortality conferences. Many surgical faculty members believe that hazing house staff or junior faculty members is an important part of their education; they feel that this so-called stress teaching will help younger surgeons cope with the ordinary stresses of their subsequent practice. Moreover, there are no mechanisms built into residency training to make allowances for slower development. As a result, slow learners are labeled by their superiors as clumsy, stupid, or inept, and they often react by becoming defensive or by treating their juniors the same way.

Character is formed long before graduation from medical school. It is unlikely that major changes in ethics or temperament will occur during training, and it is equally unlikely that normative error making begins during residency. It is possible to insist on the appropriate behavior during training, but it is unlikely that someone who is forced to work in harmony with others during residency will internalize such behavior. Accordingly, efforts should be directed at detecting character impairment as early in the educational process as possible.

EARLY RECOGNITION OF THE NORMATIVE ERROR MAKER

Unfortunately, although the character impairment is usually present by the time a normative error maker reaches medical school, it is often difficult to identify among medical students.[36] Faculty members rarely witness peer interactions, and students are usually not in a position to quarrel with nurses or ancillary personnel. Nevertheless, it is possible to recognize a character-impaired student, and there should be greater opportunity for the identification of dysfunctional personality traits. All too often, the student's dysfunctional interaction is not noticed on a busy surgical service and does not become an identifiable problem until it deviates drastically from the norm. A model for the early detection of normative error is needed[10] because early identification could lead to appropriate treatment. If a student refuses to change his or her behavior after efforts have been made to intervene, that student could be prevented from becoming a physician.

Residency program coordinators should have open lines of communication with the off-service faculty, nurses, technicians, and ancillary personnel. There must be careful scrutiny of both the quality and the quantity of any complaints that surface: temper tantrums, instrument throwing, personal and sexual innuendo, and biting sarcasm are frequently mentioned. Inappropriate remarks to patients or their relatives are another major type of normative error; they can have disastrous effects on physician-patient relationships, future referrals, and malpractice risk. The director should not pass these off as mere irritabilities induced by overwork or personality conflict but should consider the possibility that a series of complaints is merely the tip of the iceberg.

If there are three or more complaints about the resident that are definable as normative error, the physician's performance should be subjected to a careful and detailed investigation. The resident director must be meticulous in documenting the behavioral errors and should demand that the resident change his or her behavior or face serious penalties. Too few residents are punished or removed because of failure to respond to appropriate warnings. The director must also examine the behavior of the faculty in the department. If faculty members are also normative error makers, it is likely that they will reinforce the resident's deviant behavior and will have their own set of related problems as well. It is crucial that faculty members model ethical behavior for the student's benefit.[33]

New attending physicians are often least guilty of true normative error making, but they may be defensive and lack self-confidence. It is important to distinguish the desire to perform well under extreme pressure from deliberate and characteristic normative error making. The distinction may be partially based on the physician's behavior: normative errors are more likely to be manifested by laziness and inattention, and defensive behavior by hypercompulsivity and perfectionism.

It is wise to institute a probation period before the acceptance of a new member to the group. It is surprising how often a decompensation of character can be observed when new levels of authority are attained. Thus, even someone who performed well as a resident should be watched carefully during his or her transition to new responsibility.

Letters of recommendation should be interpreted in the light of partial disclosure. Even when speaking directly with a reference about a future employee or colleague, it is difficult to obtain complete disclosure. A useful question is "Would you hire this person in your own group, and if not, why not?"

Substance Abuse and Chemical Dependence

Physicians are as much at risk for substance abuse and chemical dependence as any other members of society, and perhaps even more so. Medicine may in fact attract certain addiction-prone personality types, characterized by inadequate coping mechanisms, dissatisfaction with life, and increased physical and psychiatric illness.[37] The risk of substance abuse among physicians does decrease with age.[38] Unfortunately, when faced with such problems, physicians often do not seek treatment. Frequently, they neglect their own principles of care and resort to self-medication and treatment of family members, which increases opportunities for abuse in high-risk situations. Certainly, medical school curricula should teach students about the dangers of self-medication.[39,40]

There are no limits to the substances that physicians may abuse. Recent evidence suggests that impaired physicians are often addicted to more than one drug.[41] The choice of substances may depend on access or may reflect individual taste or societal norms. It is well known that the major drug of choice in all age groups and at all socioeconomic levels is alcohol.[3,42]

No attempt will be made here to describe the toxicology of substance abuse or to outline the diagnosis of chemical dependence. What follows is a brief description of several major categories of drugs commonly abused by physicians.

COMMONLY ABUSED DRUGS

Alcohol

Alcohol is the most widely used and abused drug in the United States.[42,43] It is both socially sanctioned and widely available; these factors, coupled with social pressure to use it, lead many onto the path to addiction. Whereas some people are able to control their drinking behavior, others cannot, and for the latter there is no such thing as a social drink.

The American Medical Association classifies alcoholism as a primary, chronic disease with genetic, psychosocial, and environmental factors influencing its development and manifestations; the disease is often progressive and fatal if not treated.[12,14] In many cases, the progression of the disease is very gradual; there may be 15 to 20 years of alcohol abuse before the chronic stage is reached.[44]

It has been known for many years that alcoholism runs in families.[43] A survey of research studies has demonstrated that approximately one third of all alcoholics have at least one parent who is alcoholic.[3,43] There is a genetic predisposition to alcoholism in the children of alcoholics. Studies on twins reared apart have shown that sons of alcoholics are at least three times more likely to become dependent on alcohol than sons of non-alcoholics, regardless of familial environment.[45-47] There is also evidence of a similarly increased risk of alcohol dependence in daughters of alcoholic mothers.[48]

The disease is usually well advanced by the time the symptoms are noticed in the workplace. Heavy drinking generally goes undetected in medical school, and alcohol abusers often outperform their social-drinking or nondrinking classmates.[49,50] Perhaps youth protects hard-drinking students for a time from the debilitating physiologic effects of chronic alcohol abuse, but performance will inevitably be affected if the pattern of abuse continues.[48] Substance abuse patterns in medical school may be predictive of drinking and drug-taking behavior later in life.[11] As many as half of all chemically dependent physicians first have trouble with substance abuse in medical school.[13] Accordingly, medical schools should establish support programs to deal with abuse of drug and alcohol before it becomes serious.[13]

It should be no surprise that some medical students drink heavily. The prevalence of alcohol use among senior medical students is 87.5 percent. Alcohol is used more often by this group than by other age-related groups, whereas other substances (e.g., marijuana, cocaine, and amphetamines) are used less often.[51] Many colleges introduce students to a lifestyle that revolves around partying (i.e., alcohol and drug consumption). Fortunately, this trend is beginning to be reversed at many college campuses thanks to increased educational efforts beginning in the primary grades.

During residency training, drinking usually becomes more sporadic; the resident spends long hours at work, rarely leaves the hospital to socialize, and frequently is fatigued enough to prefer sleep to parties. Nevertheless, the high degree of stress places residents at high risk for substance abuse. A recent study of surgery residents revealed that 73.5 percent use alcohol regularly and 9.1 percent use it more than 10 times a month.[52] In comparison with residents in other medical specialties, surgery residents have lower rates of abuse for all substances other than alcohol.[53] By the time physicians begin practice, however, any differences between specialties are insignificant.[54]

House officers who are addicted continue to abuse alcohol during residency. They do not do this openly within the institution, because most hospitals in the United States do not serve alcohol in the cafeteria, and many prohibit its consumption completely. It is not a tradition to drink in the hospital, and it is quite likely that being drunk during duty hours will be severely punished. Frequently, the alcoholic resident engages in clandestine consumption of alcohol at work to avoid withdrawal symptoms. On the other hand, off-duty alcohol abuse, even if it has led to a major problem, is not uncommon and may be passed off as a peccadillo. Most training programs do not offer the education on chemical abuse and treatment needed to prevent abuse or to intervene in the progression of abuse to addiction, nor do they provide for the identification and referral of problem drinkers. Since the early 1980s, however, efforts have been made to develop such programs for residents.[32] Like medical school, residency training involves close supervision and thus offers numerous opportunities to notice subtle clues to early chemical impairment.[11]

Once residency is completed, alcohol abuse and dependence are easier to hide. Again, alcohol consumption on duty is unlikely, but there may be times when a physician responds to an emergency call with alcohol on his or her breath. Alcohol use is particularly difficult to hide, which may be why fewer surgeons are drunk in the hospital than outside it. Young surgeons, however, find it almost impossible to avoid situations where they are pressured to drink while on call.

Progression of alcohol abuse to addiction is typically signaled by episodes of intoxication at inappropriate times, such as medical staff dinners or faculty receptions. Such episodes may finally lead the physician's peers to consider the possibility of chemical dependence.

Denial is a primary symptom of alcoholism,[14] and rationalization of associated problems is also part of the syndrome.[44] Alcoholic physicians attempt to hide the problem and to enlist the assistance of everyone around them to hide it through cajolery, promises, and manipulation. Anyone who helps an addict to hide the problem is considered a codependent.[55] The codependent may have the best of intentions but is in effect facilitating progression of the disease. Alcoholic physicians must receive treatment for the disease both for their own sake and for the sake of their patients. The medical community has a moral, legal, and ethical responsibility to ensure that physicians are able to perform their duties competently.[12]

Sedatives

Physicians are known to abuse other sedatives besides alcohol. The many pressures surgeons face—stress, worry, long hours, and tiring shifts—lead to disruption of biologic rhythms, which causes sleep disturbances. Loss of sleep, coupled with the knowledge that in a short time they will again be deprived of sleep, induces some residents to consume sedatives or hypnotics in an attempt to modulate their sleep-wake cycle.

Abuse of sedatives begins in medical school, where sedatives are the only drugs (other than alcohol) that are more frequently used than they were in high school or college.[51] During residency, sedatives are the third most commonly used drugs, after alcohol and marijuana; overall, they account for three to nine percent of substance abuse.[52,56,57] Obviously, long-term use of sedatives and hypnotics leads to impairment. The impairment may not be evident for a number of years, but eventually, judgment is adversely affected, and the diminished capability is noticed in the workplace.

Stimulants

Many residents consume amphetamines during periods of sleep deprivation, some in combination with sedatives in an attempt to control the sleep-wake cycle. Use of amphetamines may have declined since these agents were withdrawn from the market as drugs prescribed for weight control. The street amphetamines are less likely to be used by house officers and graduate physicians; cocaine is now the stimulant of choice.

Cocaine is a powerfully addictive drug that produces impairment and leads to other illnesses. Initially, cocaine is probably used for its euphoric effects. However innocent its initial use may have been, many young physicians have become dependent on cocaine, to the detriment of their lives and careers. We will never know how much heart disease cocaine has caused, nor can we estimate its contribution to sudden deaths of young surgeons that were ascribed to acute myocardial infarction. Its effect on the incidence of the acquired immunodeficiency syndrome among physicians is also unknown.

Opiates

The dictates of fashion have a great deal to do with the form that drug addiction takes. At present, opiates are not fashionable among young physicians for any purposes other than anesthesia. Nevertheless, codeine and its congeners are amply represented in professional drug treatment programs.

Opiates tend to be used more by nonsurgeons than by surgeons,[41] possibly because surgeons do not seek the so-called downer effect that opiates induce. Moreover, needle tracks are harder to hide under the short sleeves of a scrub suit than under a lab coat. Prolonged off-duty use of opiates may go unnoticed for some time, especially if the opiates are taken orally rather than intravenously. Nevertheless, impairment eventually results.

Prevention of Impairment

In the prevention of physician impairment, probably our greatest needs are better education in substance abuse and dependence and a clearer awareness that these represent occupational hazards. Efforts to prevent substance abuse and dependence can be classified as primary, secondary, or tertiary prevention.[11] Primary prevention includes educating physicians on substance abuse, limiting access to prescriptions, discouraging self-prescribing, and seeking to change attitudes about alcohol and drug use. Secondary prevention includes making efforts to detect substance abuse and to impede the progression to addiction through confidential counseling and in-depth seminars on chemical dependency.[13,15] Tertiary prevention includes the development of departmental and institutional policies and procedures to assist chemically impaired physicians.[11]

Better education about addiction is essential[58]: generally, physicians are not trained to develop the attitudes, knowledge, and skills required to prevent, detect, and manage substance abuse.[15,59] Although 93 percent of medical schools and 50 percent of residency programs have some formal instruction in chemical abuse and dependence, it is usually an isolated part of the curriculum and is not integrated into the entire educational process.[59] In what we hope signals a positive trend, the American Boards of Family Practice, Internal Medicine, Obstetrics and Gynecology, and Pediatrics have committed to requiring all residents to be trained in the skills needed (1) to prevent, screen for, and diagnose chemical abuse and dependency, (2) to provide initial therapeutic intervention, (3) to refer patients to appropriate care, and (4) to deliver follow-up care.[59] Medicine in general, and surgery in particular, cannot afford to hide from the problem and buy into denial.

We must address our own lifestyles, and we must squarely face our responsibility for providing a role model that will assist our students and colleagues in avoiding this disease. We must encourage alcohol-free parties and learn to temper our own approach to socializing.

We must learn how to provide appropriate support for our colleagues who suffer from impairment as well as how to prevent and recognize it in ourselves and in our students; this includes appropriate referrals for help, made with the anticipation of good response to treatment.

We must search our own souls for the courage to give up our professional identities and accept the loss of income, prestige, and rewards at the appropriate time so that we do not attempt to practice while senile or otherwise impaired.

We must accept our humanity and its attendant frailties and learn how to care for ourselves as well as for our patients.

References

1. Bosk C: Forgive and Remember. Managing Medical Failure. University of Chicago Press, Chicago, 1979
2. Rosen P, Markovchick V, Dracon D: Normative and technical error in the emergency department. J Emerg Med 1:155, 1983
3. Facts on Teenage Drinking. National Council on Alcoholism, New York, 1982
4. The sick physician: impairment by psychiatric disorders, including alcoholism and drug dependence. JAMA 223:684, 1973
5. Mason SC 3rd: Organic mental disorders and the issue of retirement. Mich Med 87:329, 1988
6. Madden DJ: Cognitive impairment in physicians. Md Med J 37:201, 1988
7. Butler RN: Physicians not exempt from "forced retirement." Geriatrics 44:19, 1989
8. Green W: When is it time to quit? Can Med Assoc J 139:1187, 1988
9. Conner SL: Comparison of impaired physician programs nationwide. Md Med J 37:213, 1988
10. Lohr KM, Engbring NH: Institution-wide program for impaired residents at a major teaching hospital. J Med Educ 63:182, 1988
11. Blondell RD: Impaired physicians. Primary Care 20:209, 1993
12. Arshem EE: Dealing with substance abuse in the medical workplace. Medical Group Management Journal March/April:46 1993
13. Jones D: One in 10 MDs has an addiction problem, physicians warned. Can Med Assoc J 149:77, 1993
14. Bohigian GM, Croughan JL, Sanders K: Substance abuse and dependence in physicians: an overview of the effects of alcohol and drug abuse. Mo Med 91:233, 1994
15. Brooke D, Edward G, Taylor C: Addiction as an occupational hazard: 144 doctors with drug and alcohol problems. Br J Addict 86:1011, 1991
16. Ward RD: Impaired physicians: new law stresses "treatment rather than punishment." Mich Med, 92:41, 1993
17. Brenner LH: Corporate responsibility for physician impairment. Quality Review Bulletin 14:123, 1988
18. Haynes TL: The physician and chemical dependence. Mich Med 87:326, 1988
19. Soter JJ, Dilts SL: The Colorado Physician Health Program. Quality Review Bulletin 14:105, 1988
20. University of California, San Diego, Medical Center Guidelines for Medical Staff Committee on Physician Well-Being. October 1994
21. Carlson HB, Dilts SL, Radcliff S: Physicians with substance abuse problems and their recovery environment: a survey. J Subst Abuse Treat 11:113, 1994
22. Johnson VE: Intervention: How to Help Someone Who Doesn't Want Help. Johnson Institute Books, Minneapolis, 1986
23. Casper E, Dilts SL, Soter JJ, et al: Establishment of the Colorado Physician Health Program with a legislative initiative. JAMA 260:671, 1988
24. Talbott GD, Gallegos KV: The Pilot Impaired Physicians Epidemiologic Surveillance System. Quality Review Bulletin 14:133, 1988
25. Angres DH, Busch KA: The chemically dependent physician: clinical and legal considerations. Legal Im-

plications of Hospital Policies and Practices. Miller RD, Ed. Jossey-Bass, San Francisco, 1989, p 21

26. Martindale JL: Doctors and dependency. J Arkansas Med Soc 85:129, 1988
27. Lloyd G: Alcoholic doctors can recover. BMJ 300:728, 1990
28. Femino J, Nirenberg TD: Treatment outcome studies on physician impairment: a review of the literature. RI Med J 77:345, 1994
29. Alcoholism: A Treatable Disease, rev ed. Johnson Institute, Minneapolis, 1987
30. Gorski TT: Relapse prevention planning: a new recovery tool. Alcohol, Health and Research World Fall: 7, 63, 1986
31. Trent B: Drunk doctors: in Nova Scotia, they're tackling the problem head on. Can Med Assoc J 141:52, 1989
32. Lippert FG 3rd, Farmer J, Schafer MF: Professional behavior in the orthopedic resident: a method for evaluation and development. Clin Orthop 174:188, 1983
33. Organ CH Jr: Reflections concerning resident surgical training. Am Surg 50:6, 1984
34. Centrella M: Physician addiction and impairment—current thinking: a review. J Addictive Dis 13:91, 1994
35. Hughes PH, Brandenburg N, Baldwin DC, et al: Prevalence of substance use among US physicians. JAMA 267:2333, 1992
36. Irby DM, Fantel JI, Milam SD, et al: Legal guidelines for evaluating and dismissing medical students. N Engl J Med 304:180, 1981
37. Serry N, Bloch S, Ball R, et al: Drug and alcohol abuse by doctors. Med J Aust 160:402, 1994
38. Brooke D, Edwards G, Andrews T: Doctors and substance misuse: types of doctors, types of problems. Addiction 88:655, 1993
39. Allibone A: Who treats the doctor? Practitioner 234:984, 1990
40. Wright C: Physician addiction to pharmaceuticals: personal history, practice setting, access to drugs, and recovery. Md Med J 39:1021, 1990
41. Gallegos KV, Browne CH, Veit FW, et al: Addiction in anesthesiologists: drug access and patterns of substance abuse. Quality Review Bulletin 14:116, 1988
42. National Household Survey on Drug Abuse: Population Estimates. National Institute on Drug Abuse, Washington, DC, 1985
43. US Department of Health and Human Services: Fifth Special Report to the US Congress on Alcohol and Health, from the Secretary of Health and Human Services. Alcohol, Drug Abuse, and Mental Health Administration, National Institute on Alcohol Abuse and Alcoholism, Rockville, Maryland, 1984
44. Peterson RL: Reaching the impaired practitioner: the peer assistance network. Journal of the Michigan Dental Association 70:265, 1988
45. Bohman M: Some genetic aspects of alcoholism and criminality: a population of adoptees. Arch Gen Psychiatry 35:269, 1978
46. Goodwin DW, Schulsinger F, Hermansen L, et al: Alcohol problems in adoptees raised apart from alcoholic biological parents. Arch Gen Psychiatry 28:238, 1973
47. Schuckit MA, Goodwin DA, Winokur G: A study of alcoholism in half siblings. Am J Psychiatry 128:1132, 1972
48. Bohman M, Sigvardsson S, Cloninger CR: Maternal inheritance of alcohol abuse: cross-fostering analysis of adopted women. Arch Gen Psychiatry 38:965, 1981
49. Bissell L, Jones RW: The alcoholic physician: a survey. Am J Psychiatry 133:1142, 1976
50. Clark DC: Alcohol and drug use and mood disorders among medical students: implications for physician impairment. Quality Review Bulletin 14:50, 1988
51. Baldwin DC, Hughes PH, Conrad SE, et al: Substance use among senior medical students, a survey of 23 medical schools. JAMA 265:2074, 1991
52. Hyde GL, Wolf J: Alcohol and drug use by surgery residents. J Am Coll Surg 181:1, 1995
53. Hughes PH, Baldwin DC, Sheehan DV, et al: Resident physician substance use, by specialty. Am J Psychiatry 149:1348, 1992
54. Lutsky I, Hopwood M, Abram SE, et al: Use of psychoactive substances in three medical specialties: anaesthesia, medicine and surgery. Can J Anaesth 41:561, 1994
55. Black C: It Will Never Happen to Me. MAC Printing and Publications, Denver, 1982
56. Hughes PH, Conrad SE, Baldwin DC, et al: Resident physician substance use in the United States. JAMA 265:2069, 1991
57. Flaherty JA, Richman A: Substance use and addiction among medical students, residents, and physicians. Psychiatr Clin North Am 16:189, 1993
58. Lloyd G: Supporting the addicted doctor. Practitioner 234:989, 1990
59. Lewis DC: Training about alcohol and substance abuse for all primary care physicians. Report of the Josiah Macy Jr Foundation, New York, July 1, 1994, to June 30, 1995
60. Rosen P, Barkin RM, Sternbach GL: Essentials of Emergency Medicine. CV Mosby, St. Louis, 1991

Bibliography

Adams TL: A new approach to impaired physicians. Wis Med J 87(August):3, 1988

Carden ET: Whither the impaired physician? The politics of impairment. Md Med J 37:206, 1988

Conrad SE, Hughes P, Baldwin D, et al: Substance use and the resident physician: a national study. Proc Annu Conf Res Med Educ 27:256, 1988

Cooper CL, Rout U, Faragher B: Mental health, job satisfaction, and job stress among practitioners. Br Med J 298:366, 1989

The Diagnosis and Treatment of Alcoholism. Mendelson JH, Mello NK, Eds. McGraw-Hill, New York, 1979

Fluharty DG Jr: Portrait of an impaired physician. Va Med 116:266, 1989

Galanter M, Talbott D, Gallegos K, et al: Combined Alcoholics Anonymous and professional care for addicted physicians. Am J Psychiatry 147:64, 1990

Juntunen J, Asp S, Olkinuora M, et al: Doctors' drinking habits and consumption of alcohol. BMJ 297:951, 1988

Kline J: The denial dilemma in fighting substance abuse. Drug Prevention Resources April:79, 1988

Kluge EH: Do you have an ethical obligation to report this impaired colleague? Can Med Assoc J 141:973, 1989

Lewy R: Alcoholism in house staff physicians: an occupational hazard. J Occup Med 28:79, 1986

Marchand WR: The effect of an educational program on the desire for treatment among impaired medical students. J Nerv Ment Dis 176:372, 1988

Marlatt GA, Gordon JR: Relapse Prevention: Maintenance Strategies in the Treatment of Addictive Behaviors. The Guilford Press, New York, 1985

Moffitt EM: MSMA Impaired Physicians Program: an overview. J Miss State Med Assoc 29:377, 1988

Nurse blows whistle on impaired physician. The Regan Report on Nursing Law 29:1, 1989

Scott CD: Coping with stress. JAMA 262:2466, 1989

Smith R: Dealing with sickness and incompetence: success and failure. BMJ 298:1695, 1989

Talbott GD: The impaired physician movement. Md Med J 37:216, 1988

Thomas CB, Santora P, Shaffer JW: Health of physicians in midlife in relation to use of alcohol: a prospective study of a cohort of former medical students. Johns Hopkins Medical Journal 146:1, 1980

Wallot H, Lambert J: Characteristics of physician addicts. Am J Drug Alcohol Abuse 10:53, 1984

INDEX

A

Aaron sign, 236t
Abdomen, great vessels of, traumatic injury to, 437-447
  AAST injury scale for, 437, 438t
  aortic compression device for, 439, 440f
  celiac axis in, 440
  complications of, 447
  damage-control laparotomy in, 446-447
  iliac artery in, 444-445, 445f
  iliac vein in, 441t, 445
  inferior vena cava in, 442-443, 443f
  inframesocolic, 442-443
  infrarenal aorta in, 440t, 442, 442f
  intra-abdominal hematoma in, 437, 437f-438f
  left medial visceral rotation for, 437-438, 439f
  perirenal hematoma in, 443, 443f-444f
  porta hepatis in, 445-446
  proximal renal artery in, 441
  PTFE prosthetic graft for, 439-440, 440f
  renal artery in, 440t, 443-444, 444f
  renal vein in, 441t, 444
  retrohepatic area in, 446
  superior mesenteric artery in, 440-441, 440f-441f, 441t
  superior mesenteric vein in, 441-442, 441t
  supramesocolic, 437-442
  survival rate after, 440, 440t
  zone 1, 437-443
  zone 2, 443-444
  zone 3, 444-445
Abdominal compartment syndrome
  in acute renal failure, 1444, 1446
  in peritonitis, persistent or tertiary, 1256
Abdominal defect(s), flaps for, 980
Abdominal infection. *See* Acute abdominal pain; Intra-abdominal infection; Upper abdominal infection
Abdominal injury, 405-411
  blunt, nonoperative management of, 421-422
  bowel in, damaged or devascularized, 409-410
  closure in, 410-411
    general technique for, 410
    open fascial closure in, 410-411, 411f
    "quick cuts" and damage control in, 411, 411f
    skin closure in, 410
  contamination in, control of, 408
  hemorrhage control in, 408, 409f
  incision in, 405
  initial exploration in, 405-406
  management of, priorities in, 408-410
  operative exposure in, 406-408
    for aorta, 406, 407f
    for biliary tract, 408
    for duodenum, 408
    for pancreas, 408
    for vena cava, 406-408, 407f, 409f
  patient preparation in, 405
  retroperitoneal hematoma in, 406, 406f
  retroperitoneal injury repair in, 410
  vascular repair in, 408-409
Abdominal mass, 241-250
  angiography in, 246
  barium studies, 246
  biopsy in, 248-249
    image-guided percutaneous, 248-249, 248f
    laparoscopic, 249
  clinical history in, 241-244
  computed tomography in, 247, 247f
  differential diagnosis in, 244
  evaluation of, **Algorithm**, 242-243
  excretory urography in, 246
  exploratory laparotomy in, 249
  investigative studies in, 245-249
  laboratory studies in, 245
  magnetic resonance imaging in, 246
  physical examination in, 244-245
  plain abdominal radiography in, 246
  radiographic studies in, 245-247, 246f-247f
  radionucleotide scan in, 246
  ultrasonography in, 246-247
  working diagnosis in, 245
Abdominal pain
  acute. *See* Acute abdominal pain
  in children, 1127
  in elderly patient, 1092-1093
  in pregnancy. *See* Pregnancy
  upper. *See* Upper abdominal infection
Abdominal procedure(s), antibiotic prophylaxis for, 572, 573
Abdominal radiography
  in abdominal mass, 246
  in intestinal obstruction, 267-268, 268f-271f
Abdominal wall hernia(s). *See also under* Femoral hernia(s); Inguinal hernia(s)
  open repair of, 857-875
Abdominoperineal resection, 835-836
  complications of, 836
  operative resection in, 835
  operative technique in, 835-836, 835f
  outcome in, 836
Abortion, prostaglandins for, 1601
Abrasion, in extremity trauma, 476
Abscess
  anal. *See* Anal abscess
  breast, 214
  cerebral, coma in, 151
    treatment of, 156-157
  cutaneous
    confined, 313
    pathogens in, 324
  hepatic, 1271-1272
  intra-abdominal. *See* Intra-abdominal abscess
  pericholecystic, surgical options for, 1244t
  rectal, in neutropenia, 1078
  renal, candidal, 1299
  retroperitoneal, 1248
  splenic, 1273-1275, 1275f
Accident(s). *See also* Trauma
  motorcycle, acute wound management after, 124
  motor vehicle, elderly patient and, 1093
Acetabular fracture, 470-471
Acetaminophen. *See also* Nonsteroidal anti-inflammatory drug(s) (NSAIDs)
  in pregnancy, 1155
  suggested dosing for, 1628t
  toxicity, in acute hepatic failure, 1458
Acetaminophen with codeine, suggested dosing for, 1627t
Acetic acid, contraindicated in acute wound care, 128
Acetylsalicylic acid. *See* Aspirin; Nonsteroidal anti-inflammatory

1741

drug(s) (NSAIDs)
Acid(s), causing chemical burns, 52t
Acid aspiration. *See* Aspiration, acid
Acid-base disorder(s)
  arterial blood samples for temperature correction for, 107
    venous *vs.*, 107
  bicarbonate concentration in, measured *vs.* calculated, 107
  in cardiac arrest, sodium bicarbonate and, 22
  definitions and measurement issues in, 107
  discussion of, 119-120
  evaluation of, *Algorithm*, 108-109
  in infants and neonates, 1127-1128
  life-threatening, 107-120
  mixed, 117-118
    classification of, 117t
    computers in analysis of, 118
    pH in, 117, 118f
    primary *vs.*, 107-110
  postoperative, 1632-1634
  primary. *See also* Metabolic acidosis; Metabolic alkalosis; Respiratory acidosis; Respiratory alkalosis
    expected compensation for, 110, 110t
  in trauma patient, sodium bicarbonate and, 45
Acid-base homeostasis, in elderly patients, 1107-1108
Acidosis. *See* Acid-base disorder(s)
  lactic. *See* Lactic acidosis
  metabolic. *See* Metabolic acidosis
  respiratory. *See* Respiratory acidosis
Acinetobacter infection, antimicrobial agents for, 1198t
Acquired immunodeficiency syndrome (AIDS), 1333-1346. *See also* Human immunodeficiency virus (HIV) infection
  central venous catheterization in, 1338-1339
  choledochoenteric bypass in, 1338
  common infections in, protection from, 1339
  epidemiology of, 1341
  lymph node biopsy in, 1336, 1337f
  major risk groups for, 1335, 1336f
  peritonitis in, 1246
  splenectomy in, 1338
  sterilization of surgical equipment in, 1339
  surgical interventions in, 1338-1339
ACTH stimulation test, 1067, 1067t, 1088
Actinomyces israelii infection, antimicrobial agents for, 1199t
Action potential(s), Purkinje (ventricular muscle), 24-25, 25f
Activated charcoal, for emergency management of substance abuse, 173
Activities of daily living (ADL), during hospitalization, for elderly patient, 1102, 1102t, 1104
Activity, physical. *See* Physical activity
Acute abdominal pain, 225-240
  abdominal pain chart for, 236, 236t-237t

  age as factor in, 232, 235t
  Algorithm, 226-227
  basic investigational studies in, 235-236
  in children, 232, 235t
  clinical history in, 225-231
    associated gastrointestinal symptoms in, 229, 231
    character of pain in, 229
    continuous pain in, 229
    fever in, 231
    intensity of pain in, 229
    intermittent pain in, 229
    location of pain in, 229, 230f
    mode of onset in, 229
    questioning patient in, 229
    referred pain in, 229, 231f
    structured data sheets for, 225-229, 228f
    vomiting in, 229
  differential diagnosis in, tentative, 231-233
  in elderly patients, 232, 235t
  extraperitoneal causes of, 233t
  frequency of specific diagnoses in, 232, 234t
  hospitalization and active observation for
    in surgical abdomen, 238
    in uncertain diagnosis, 239
  indications for laparotomy in
    early or elective, 239
    immediate, 237
    urgent, 237-238
  intraperitoneal causes of, 232t
  laboratory studies in, 235
  nonspecific, 232
  outpatient evaluation in, 239
  physical examination in, 233-235
    auscultation in, 234
    inspection in, 234
    palpation in, 234-235
    percussion in, 234
    rectal, genital, and pelvic, 235
    specific signs in, 235, 236t-237t
  radiologic studies in, 235-236
  suspected nonsurgical abdomen with, 239-240
  suspected surgical abdomen with, 237-239
  uncertain diagnosis in, 239
  working diagnosis in, 236-237
Acute-phase response. *See also* Hypermetabolism; Metabolic response to critical illness; Sepsis
  IL-1 in, 1510, 1606f, 1607
  IL-6 in, 1510-1511
  in multiple organ dysfunction syndrome, 1477
  tumor necrosis factor in, 1606, 1606f
Acyclovir, for herpesvirus infections, 1328
Addison disease (adrenocortical insufficiency), metabolic acidosis in, 114
Adenitis, cervical, 189
Adenopathy, cervical, in Hodgkin and non-Hodgkin lymphoma, 192
Adenosine
  for acute dysrhythmias, after resuscitation, 15-18
  classification of, 23
Admission day surgery, home environment and discharge in,

611
Adrenal crisis, 1063-1066, 1067t
Adrenal hemorrhage, heparin-induced, 1025
Adrenal insufficiency, 1063-1069
  adrenal crisis in, 1063-1066, 1067t
  after surgical correction of endogenous hypercortisolism, 1067-1068
  clinical manifestations of, 1087t, 1088
  discussion of, 1068-1069
  known or suspected, 1066-1067
  management of, 1063-1068
  perioperative
    clinical manifestations of, 1087t, 1088
    management of, 1088, 1087t-1088t
  primary, 1063, 1066, 1088
  recognition and classification of, 1063, 1066
  recognition and management of, *Algorithm*, 1064-1065
  secondary, 1063, 1066, 1088
  tests for, 1088
Adrenergic agonist(s). *See also* Alpha agonist(s); Beta agonist(s)
  cardiovascular effects of, 1393t
  receptor types stimulated by, 1394t
Adrenergic receptor(s). *See* Alpha receptor(s); Beta receptor(s)
Adrenocortical insufficiency (Addison disease). *See also* Adrenal insufficiency
  metabolic acidosis in, 114
Adult respiratory distress syndrome (ARDS), 1405-1407. *See also* Pulmonary insufficiency
  in burn patient, 494
  causes of, 1405-1406, 1406t
  clinical presentation in, 1406, 1407t
  free radicals in, 1583-1584
  in multiple organ dysfunction syndrome, 1478
  neutrophils causing, 1407
  phases of, 1406
  positive-pressure ventilation for, 1407
  radiographic manifestations of, 1405t
  treatment of, 1407
Aerodigestive tract cancers, upper, 192
Aeromonas hydrophilia, antimicrobial agents for, 1198t
Age
  as factor in acute abdominal pain, 232, 235t
  as factor in cardiopulmonary monitoring, 1389
  as factor in immunodeficiency, 1084
  as factor in perioperative outcome, 552
  as factor in selection for outpatient surgery, 541
  as factor in wound healing, 137
Aging patient. *See* Elderly patient
Aging physician. *See* Physician, impaired, due to age
Agitation
  management of, 162-163
  in substance abuse, emergency

management of, 171
AIDS. *See* Acquired immunodeficiency syndrome (AIDS); Human immunodeficiency virus (HIV) infection
Air embolism. *See* Embolism, air
Airway
 in burn care
  in early postresuscitation period, 479
  in immediate resuscitation period, 49-54
 in cervical spine trauma
  discussion on, 42
  precautions, 31-34, 34f
 in coma management, 143
 in CPR, 3-7, 6f-8f
 establishment of. *See also* Endotracheal intubation
  parameters for, 9
 major, traumatic disruption of, 399
 in maxillofacial injury, 369-371
 in neck injury, 379-381
 obstruction of
  alveolar hypoventilation in, 1419
  respiratory acidosis in, 114-115
  in shock, 68
 opening of
  chin lift for, 6-7, 6f
  head tilt for, 6, 6f
  jaw thrust for, 7, 7f
  manual maneuvers for, 6-7, 6f-7f
 patency of, verification of, 6
 in trauma resuscitation, 31-35, 34f-35f
 in unconscious patient, 3-6, 6f
Alanine, in metabolic response to critical illness, 1506
Albumin, as free radical scavenger, 1575
Alcohol(s), isopropyl
 contraindicated in acute wound care, 128
 ingestion of, 177, 178
Alcohol abuse
 as factor in selection for outpatient surgery, 542
 by physician, 1736-1737
Alcoholic liver disease. *See* Cirrhosis
Alcohol intoxication. *See also* Substance abuse
 acute, 176-178
  clinical findings in, 176-177
  laboratory studies in, 177
  management of, 177-178
 chronic, 178
  clinical findings in, 178
  differential diagnosis of, 177
  disulfiram-ethanol reaction in, 177
  hypoglycemia in, 177
  laboratory studies in, 178
  management of, 178
  wound healing and, 137
 coma in, treatment of, 155-156
 emergency management of, 176-180
 nonethanol, 177
 withdrawal in, 178-180
  clinical findings in, 178-179
  delirium tremens in, 179
  hallucinosis in, 178, 180
  ketoacidosis in, 112, 179, 180
  laboratory studies in, 179
  management of, 179-180

minor, 178
 seizures in, 178
Aldosteronism, primary, metabolic alkalosis in, 116
Alfentanil
 for induction of anesthesia, 607t
 preoperative, 544t
 suggested dosing for, 1627t
Alkalies, causing chemical burns, 52t
Alkalosis
 metabolic. *See* Metabolic alkalosis
 respiratory. *See* Respiratory alkalosis
Allen test, for systemic arterial catheterization, 1370
Allergy, to anesthesia, 546-547, 547t
Alpha$_1$ agonist(s), 1394t
Alpha agonist(s), for CPR, 21
Alpha$_1$ receptor(s), cardiovascular effects of, 1393t
Alveolar hypoventilation, 1419
 causes of, 1419, 1419t
 in chest wall instability, 1419
 in impaired respiratory muscle function, 1419
 primary idiopathic, acute respiratory acidosis in, 115
 in stiff lung, 1419, 1420t
 in upper airway obstruction, 1419
Alveolar macrophage(s), in nosocomial pneumonia, 1655-1656
Alveolus(i)
 open, maintenance of, 1415
 recruitment *vs.* distention of, in positive-pressure ventilation, 1431-1432, 1431f
Alzheimer disease, free radicals in, 1583
Amaurosis fugax, 195
Ambulation, postoperative, 1636
American Society of Anesthesiologists physical status classification, 538, 539t
Amikacin, 1210
 for bacterial infections, 1202t-1203t
Amino acid(s), in critical illness, 1501
Amino acid metabolism, in critical illness, 1506-1507
Aminoglycoside(s), 1208-1211
 adverse effects of, 1208t, 1210
 nephrotoxicity of, 1450
 for nosocomial gram-negative bacteremia, 1180t
 for peritonitis, 1252-1253
 pharmacokinetics of, 1210-1211
 in vivo drug interactions with, 1193t
Aminopenicillin(s), 1196
Aminophylline, for asystole, 11
21-Aminosteroid(s), as free radical scavenger, 1576
Amiodarone, for acute dysrhythmias, after resuscitation, 18
Ammonium chloride solution, electrolyte content of, 103t
Amoxicillin, 1196
 for bacterial infections, 1202t-1203t
Amoxicillin-clavulanate, 1214
 for bacterial infections, 1202t-1203t
Amphetamine(s), abuse of, emergency management of, 175
 in acute exposure, 175

in chronic use, 175
 in withdrawal, 175
Amphotericin B, 1300, 1301t
 for candidiasis, 1294-1296, 1295t
 renal tubular acidosis due to, 114
Ampicillin, 1196
 for bacterial infections, 1202t-1203t
Amputation
 ankle, guillotine, 953-954, 954f
 lower-extremity, 949-958
  above-the-knee, 956-957, 956f-957f
  below-the-knee, 954-956, 954f-955f
  general preoperative planning for, 949
  toe, 949-951, 949f-951f
  transmetatarsal, 951-953, 953f
Amrinone, for heart failure, 1395
Amyotrophic lateral sclerosis, familial (Lou Gehrig disease), free radical effects on, 1583
Anaerobic bacteremia, 1180-1181. *See also specific organisms, e.g., Bacteroides fragilis*
Anal abscess, cryptoglandular, 848, 849f
 in Crohn disease, 851, 852f, 853
 in hidradenitis suppurativa, 851-852, 853, 853f
 horseshoe, 851, 852f
 operative management of, 848-853
 operative planning in, 849
 operative technique in, 849-850, 849f-855f
 complications of, 853
 special problems in, 850-851, 852f
 troubleshooting in, 853
Anal fissure
 diagnosis and treatment of, 854
 operative management for
  complications of, 855-856
  outcome evaluation in, 856
  planning in, 854-855
  technique in, 855
  troubleshooting in, 855
Anal fistula, 848, 849f
 in Crohn disease, 851, 852f, 853
 in hidradenitis suppurativa, 851-852, 853, 853f
 operative management of, 848-853
 operative planning in, 849
 operative technique in, 849-850, 849f-855f
 complications of, 853
 special problems in, 850-851, 852f
 troubleshooting in, 853
Analgesia. *See also* Anesthesia
 for burn patient, 488, 488t
 epidural
  for acute pain, 1498
  continuous, 1666, 1666t
  in elderly patients, 1100
  for postoperative pain, 1664-1665, 1665t
 narcotic, preoperative, 606
 patient-controlled. *See* Patient-controlled analgesia (PCA)
 postoperative, in pulmonary insufficiency, 1043
 in pregnancy, 1155
Anal procedures, 843-856
 for hemorrhoids, 843-848. *See also* Hemorrhoid(s), operative

Anal stricture, after hemorrhoid surgery, 848
Anal symptom(s), hemorrhoids vs., 843, 844t
Anal ulcer
  diagnosis and treatment of, 854
  operative management for, 854-856
    complications of, 855-856
    outcome evaluation in, 856
    planning in, 854-855
    technique in, 855
    troubleshooting in, 855
Anaphylaxis, pulseless electrical activity in, 12t
Anastomosis
  biliary, technical issues in, 736-738, 737f-738f
  coloanal, in low anterior resection with coloproctostomy, 834. *See also* Coloproctostomy, low anterior resection with
  colorectal, in low anterior resection with coloproctostomy, 834. *See also* Coloproctostomy, low anterior resection with
  ileoanal, in restorative proctocolectomy with ileoanal pouch, 831-832. *See also* Proctocolectomy, restorative, with ileoanal pouch
  ileorectal, with total colectomy, 827, 828f. *See also* Colectomy, total, with ileorectal anastomosis
  intestinal, 803-813. *See also* Intestinal anastomosis
Anemia
  blood substitutes for, 84, 84t
  in burn patients, in early postresuscitation period, 482
  lowering metabolic rate in, 84
  observation in, 84
  postoperative, 1640
  in renal failure, 1058-1059, 1059f
    blood loss in, 1058
    decreased red cell production in, 1058, 1059f
  transfusion in, 83-84, 83f, 84t
    in active bleeding, 83
    in significant coronary artery disease, 83
    in symptomatic anemia, 83
Anesthesia. *See also* Analgesia
  in burn patients, after first postburn week, 502
  for carotid artery procedures, 922
  in diabetes mellitus, 997
  in elderly patients, 1099-1100
  emergency management of substance abuse and, 173
  epidural, 612-613, 612t
    choice of drug for, 1666
    in elderly patients, 1100
    mechanism of action of, 1666
    nursing protocols for, 1667, 1666t
    for postoperative pain, 615, 1665-1667
    side effects of, 1666-1667
  general, 606-611
    in elderly patients, 1099, 1099f
    emergence from, 610-611, 611t
    induction of, 606-608
      drugs for, 606, 607t
    endotracheal intubation in, 606-608, 608t. *See also* Endotracheal intubation
      neuromuscular-blocking drugs for, 607, 608t
    maintenance of, 608-610
      dysrhythmias in, 609
      hypothermia in, 610
      inhalation anesthesia for, 608, 609t
      positioning of patient in, 609
      recall of intraoperative events in, 610
    immunodeficiency in, 1086
    intrathecal, for postoperative pain, 615
  local
    drugs for, 611, 611t
    in hemorrhoid surgery, 844, 845f
    with sedation, 611
    for wound closure, 127
  malignant hyperthermia in. *See* Malignant hyperthermia
  in maxillofacial injury, 373
  for nonemergency surgery, 545-547
    adjunctive, 546
    local and regional, 545-546, 545t
    nausea and vomiting and, 547
    nonsteroidal anti-inflammatory drugs and, 546
    toxicity and allergy to, 546-547, 547t
  nonemergency surgical care and, 538, 539t-540t
  outpatient, 613-614
  perioperative effects of, 605-617
  as perioperative risk factor, 550
  plexus block, 613
  in pregnancy, 1155-1156
  premedication for, 605-606
    analgesia as, 606
    anxiety and, 605-606
    gastric secretions and, 606
    hemodynamic stability and, 606
    oral secretions and, 606
    preoperative assessment for, 605
  in pulmonary insufficiency, 1042
  recovery issues in, 614-615
    hypertension, 615
    nausea and vomiting, 614, 614t
    pain. *See* Pain, postoperative
    respiratory insufficiency, 615
  regional, 611-613, 612t
    complications of, 613
      hypotension, 613
      post-dural puncture headache, 613
    in elderly patients, 1100
    inadequate, 613
    physiologic effects of, 609t, 611
  in renal failure, 1056
  in respiratory insufficiency, in obesity, 1005
  subarachnoid (spinal), 611-612, 612t
Anesthetic gas(es), hazards of, 597-598
Aneurysm
  aortic. *See* Aortic aneurysm
  false, in chest trauma, 403
Angina pectoris
  in preoperative workup, 561
  unstable, 561
  variant (Prinzmetal), 561
Angiodysplastic lesion(s), of colon, colonoscopy for, 296f, 297
Angiogenesis, in wound healing, 132, 133t
Angiographic embolization, for distal vertebral artery injury, 392
Angiography
  in abdominal mass, 246
  carotid, for asymptomatic carotid bruit, 200-201
  coronary, in preoperative assessment, 562
  in lower gastrointestinal bleeding, 298-299, 299f
  pulmonary, for pulmonary embolism, 1019-1020, 1020f
Angiotensin-converting enzyme (ACE) inhibitor(s), for heart failure, 1393
Angiotensin II, pulmonary metabolism of, 1417
Angle classification, of malocclusion, in maxillofacial injury, 369
Animal bite(s). *See* Bite(s), animal
Ankle, amputation of, guillotine, 953-954, 954f
Anogenital carcinoma(s), in transplant recipients, 1087
Anorectal bleeding. *See* Lower gastrointestinal bleeding
Antacids, preoperative, 545
Antibiotic(s), 1191-1220. *See also specific drugs*
  for acute cholangitis, 1269
  for acute wound, 976
  bactericidal, 1195t
  bacteriostatic, 1195t
  for burn care, 484-485
  complications of, 1216-1217
  for infants and neonates, 1122, 1124t, 1129
  for infected wound, 126
  intestinal microflora and. *See also* Colitis, antibiotic-associated
  for intra-abdominal abscess, 1243t, 1249
  for intra-abdominal infection, 1251-1253
  in multiple organ dysfunction syndrome, 1477-1478
  for nosocomial infections, 1484
  for pancreatic abscess, 1273
  for peritoneal dialysis, 1247
  for peritonitis, 1242-1243, 1243t, 1251-1253
  in peritoneal dialysis, 1247
  in pregnancy, 1195t
  in surgical patients, 1191-1192
    empirical, 1191
    for infection, 1192, 1197t-1200t, 1202t-1205t. *See also specific drugs*
    laboratory tests for, 1192
    variables influencing treatment in, 1191-1192, 1193t-1195t
  topical
    for acute wound, 976
    for burn care, 60-61, 60t
  in vitro susceptibility tests for, 1192
    agar dilution, 1192
    broth dilution, 1192
    disk diffusion, 1192
    serum bactericidal test, 1192, 1195t
Antibiotic prophylaxis
  for acute wounds, 121-124

for burn care, 60, 60t
for endocarditis, 573, 575t
for prosthetic inguinal
herniooplasty, 864
for surgical site infections, 572-573, 574t
Anticholinergic agent(s),
preoperative, 544, 606
Anticoagulant(s), 1022-1028. *See also* Heparin; Warfarin
oral. *See* Warfarin
in renal failure, preoperative, 1058
for thromboembolic prophylaxis, 1034
Anticytokine antibody(ies), 1618
Antidepressant(s), tricyclic,
complications of, 12
Antidiarrheal agent(s), for diarrhea
due to enteric nutrition, 1529, 1530f
Antidiuretic hormone. *See*
Vasopressin (antidiuretic hormone)
Antidysrhythmic agent(s),
classification of, 23
Antiembolic stocking(s), 1034
Antiemetic agent(s), 614t
Antiendotoxin antibody, 1353-1356
biochemical structure of endotoxin and, 1354, 1354f
clinical trials for, 1355-1356, 1355t
experimental data on, 1354-1355
for septic response, 1187
Antiflammin(s), 1591
Antifungal agent(s), systemic, 1300-1302, 1301t-1302t
Antilymphocyte antibody(ies),
immunodeficiency due to, 1086
Antioxidant(s), 1571-1573
for burn patients, 499, 499t
endogenous, 1571-1573, 1571t
enzymatic, 1571-1572, 1572f, 1575
exogenous, 1573, 1574f, 1575-1576
neutrophil inhibitors, 1576
nonenzymatic, 1572-1573, 1575-1576
polypharmacy approach to, 1576
Antipyretic(s), for fever and
hyperpyrexia, in infection, 1552
Antiseptic(s)
for handwashing, 1719
topical, for acute wound, 976
Antithrombin III deficiency, 1030
in nephrotic syndrome, 1058
Anti-TNF antibody, 1357-1358
Antrectomy. *See* Gastric resection,
distal subtotal (antrectomy)
Anuria. *See also* Urine output
in acute renal failure, 1441
Anxiety
in burn patient, 488
in surgical patient, premedication for, 606
Aorta. *See also* Great vessel(s)
cross-clamping of, in trauma
resuscitation, 44
infrarenal, traumatic injury to, 442, 442f, 440t
operative exposure of, in
abdominal injury, 406, 407f
thoracic, traumatic injury to, 398-399, 398f-399f
Aortic aneurysm, abdominal
anatomic variants in, 944
concurrent disease processes in, 944

diagnosis confirmation in, 937-938
elective or urgent repair of,
patient classification in, 938
endovascular repair of, 941-944
device implantation in, 943-944, 946f
procedure-specific preoperative preparation in, 942-943
horseshoe kidney and, 944
inflammatory, 944
infrarenal, repair of, 937-947
open repair of, 939-941
creation of distal anastomosis in, 939-940, 943f-944f
initial incision and choice of approach in, 939, 940f
opening of aneurysm and creation of proximal anastomosis in, 939, 942f
retroperitoneal approach in, 939
transperitoneal approach in, 939, 940f-941f
troubleshooting in, 940-941, 945f
operative planning in, 938
operative technique in, 939-944
outcome evaluation in, 945-947
preoperative evaluation of, 937-938
pulseless electrical activity in, 12t
risk factor identification in, 937
ruptured, 944-945
size determination in, 937-938, 938f-939f
ultrasonography for, 663, 664f
venous anomalies in, 944
Aortic root, pulmonary arterial end-systolic pressure-volume relations and, 1388
Aortoenteric fistula, management of bleeding in, 290
APACHE II scoring system, for peritonitis, 1255
Apneusis, in coma, 148
Apoptosis, *bcl-2* in, 1569-1571
Appendectomy, 815-823
in appendiceal neoplasm, 821
in histologically normal appendix, 820-821
history of, 815
laparoscopic
advantages of, 1244t
open *vs.*, 815, 816t
operative technique in, 817-820, 820f-822f
open
laparoscopic *vs.*, 815, 816t
operative technique in, 815-817, 817f-819f
Appendicitis
in children, 1127
ectopic pregnancy *vs.*, 1150
in elderly patient, 1092-1093
ovarian cyst *vs.*, 822
ovarian torsion *vs.*, 822, 1150
in pregnancy, 1149-1150
diagnosis of, 1149-1150
differential diagnosis of, 1150
management of, 1150
pyelonephritis *vs.*, 1150
surgical options for, 1244t
treatment options in, 815, 817f
Appendix
adenocarcinoma of, 821
adenoma of, 821
carcinoid of, 821
cystadenoma of, 821

in gynecologic conditions, 822
in inflammatory bowel disease, 822
neoplasms of, 821, 822f
Arachidonic acid
free, production of, 1591, 1592f
metabolism of, 1591-1594, 1592f-1595f
cyclooxygenase pathway in, 1591-1592, 1593f
effect of NSAIDS on, 1591-1592
lipoxygenase pathway in, 1592-1594, 1593f
ARDS. *See* Adult respiratory distress syndrome (ARDS)
Arginine
supplemental, for elderly patient, 1109
in supplemental nutritional support, 1544
Argon beam coagulator, for video-assisted thoracic surgery, 676
Arm. *See under* Extremity(ies)
Arrhythmia(s). *See* Cardiac dysrhythmia(s)
Arterial blood gas(es). *See also*
Carbon dioxide; Oxygen; Systemic arterial catheterization
in burn patients, in immediate resuscitation period, 54, 57
in cardiac arrest, 22
in infants and neonates, 1122
measurement of, 1371-1374
in preoperative evaluation, 1041
Arterial blood pH
in cardiac arrest, 22
measurement of, 1374
in mixed acid-base disorders, 117, 118f
Arterial blood sample(s)
measurements obtained by, 1371-1374. *See also* Arterial blood gas(es); Arterial blood pH
temperature correction for, 1374
for acid-base disorders, 107-110
Arterial catheter(s)
pulmonary. *See* Pulmonary arterial (Swan-Ganz) catheterization
systemic. *See* Systemic arterial catheterization
Arterial embolism, 1021-1022
arterial thrombosis *vs.*, 1021, 1021t
cardiac origin of, 1021, 1023f
extremity, 1022, 1024f
fascial compartment swelling in, 1033
incidence of, 1033
irreversible, 1032, 1033f
mesenteric, 1021-1022
outcome in, 1033
pathophysiology of, 1032-1033
prophylaxis for, 1034
renal, 1022
reperfusion injury in, 1033
sites of, 1021, 1022f-1023f
visceral, 1021-1022
management of, 1024f
Arterial injury(ies), of
extremities, 465-466, 465f-466f
Arterial pressure
pulmonary. *See* Pulmonary arterial pressure; Pulmonary arterial wedge pressure
systemic. *See* Systemic arterial pressure
Arterial thrombosis, arterial
embolism *vs.*, 1021, 1021t

Arteriovenous fistula
  in chest trauma, 403
  vascular access for. See Vascular access
Arteriovenous malformation, upper GI bleeding in, 290
Arthritis
  candidal, 1297
  septic, of hand, 1285
Ascites
  in cirrhosis, 1245, 1246
  in portal hypertension, 1463-1465, 1464t
Ascorbic acid. See Vitamin C
Aspergillosis, 1299
  clinical presentation and diagnosis of, 1293t
  hospital-acquired, 1724
  pulmonary, 1299
Aspergillus infection, antimicrobial agents for, 1199t
Aspiration
  acid, 1410-1411
    causes of, 1410, 1410t
    clinical presentation in, 1410-1411, 1410t
    treatment of, 1411
  fine-needle
    of breast, 629-630
    of neck mass, 189
  of gastric contents
    diagnostic, in intestinal obstruction, 267
    in endotracheal intubation, 607-608
    in enteral nutrition, 1527
    in general anesthesia, 609
    metabolic alkalosis due to, 116
    in substance abuse, 169
    in upper GI bleeding, 286
  pneumonitis in, septic response in, 1184
  tracheobronchial, in nosocomial pneumonia, 1655, 1655t
Aspirin. See also Nonsteroidal anti-inflammatory drug(s) (NSAIDs)
  antiplatelet effects of, 80, 1599-1600
  in coronary artery disease, 1599
  in myocardial infarction, 1599-1600
  in pregnancy, 1155
  in stroke, 1599-1600
  suggested dosing for, 1628t
  in transient ischemic attacks, 1600
Asthma
  eicosanoids and, 1600
  postoperative pulmonary insufficiency in, 1043
  respiratory acidosis in, 115
Asystole, management of
  in CPR, 11
  electrical defibrillation in, 11
  epinephrine for, 21
  pacemaker therapy in, 11
  pharmacologic, 11
Atactic breathing, in coma, 148
Atelectasis, 1407-1408
  in nosocomial infection, 1221
  postoperative, 1407-1408, 1639-1640
    pulmonary insufficiency in, 1043
    treatment of, 1044-1045, 1045f
  pulmonary mechanics in, 1430, 1430f
  treatment of, 1408

types and causes of, 1407-1408, 1408t
Atlantoaxial dislocation, 361
Atlanto-occipital dislocation, 361
Atlas (Jefferson) fracture, 361
Atracurium besylate, for induction of anesthesia, 608t
Atropine
  for asystole, 11
  preoperative, 606
Auscultation
  in acute abdominal pain, 234
  in intestinal obstruction, 267
Autonomic neuropathy
  cardiac, diabetic, 997, 995
  in diabetes mellitus, 995
Axillary dissection, for breast cancer, 634-636
  lymph node levels in, 634-635, 635f
  operative technique in, 635-636
  structures to be preserved in, 635, 636f
Axillary lymph node(s), 634-635, 635f
Axis fracture, 361
Azithromycin, 1211-1212
Azlocillin, 1196, 1200
  for bacterial infections, 1202t-1203t
Aztreonam, 1214
  for bacterial infections, 1202t-1203t

B

Bacillus anthracis infection, antimicrobial agents for, 1197t
Bacillus cereus infection, antimicrobial agents for, 1197t
Bacillus subtilis infection, antimicrobial agents for, 1197t
Bacitracin, for burn care, 60t, 61
Back defect(s), flaps for, 979
Bacteremia. See also Blood culture(s)
  in immunosuppressed patient, prevention of, 1076t
  in neutropenia, 1078
Bacterial counts, in acute wound, 976
Bacterial infection. See also *specific organisms*
  in metabolic response to critical illness, 1514-1515
Bacterial overgrowth, of gastrointestinal tract. See Gastrointestinal tract, bacterial overgrowth of
Bacterial translocation, gastrointestinal. See Gastrointestinal tract, bacterial translocation from
Bactericidal/permeability increasing protein (BPI), 1356
Bactericidal/permeability-increasing protein (BPI), lipopolysaccharides and, 1614
Bacteroides fragilis bacteremia, 1180-1181
  antimicrobial therapy for, 1180-1181
  sources of, 1180
Bacteroides infection, antimicrobial agents for, 1197t
Ballance sign, 236t

Barbiturate(s). See also Substance abuse
  for elevated intracranial pressure, 358
Barium enema, contraindicated in lower gastrointestinal bleeding, 299
Barium studies, in abdominal mass, 246
Bartonella henselae infection, antimicrobial agents for, 1198t
Basal cell carcinoma, 303-304, 303f
  of neck, 193
  nodular, 303, 303f
  sclerosing (morpheaform), 303, 303f
  ulceration and pigmentation in, 303, 303f
Basal metabolic rate. See Metabolic rate
Bassini hernioplasty, 859-862, 860f-861f
Bassler sign, 236t
Battered child syndrome, 1141
B cell deficiency, 1083, 1083t
B cell function, in surgical patients, 1074
bcl-2, in apoptosis, 1569-1571
Bed rest. See Immobilization
Beevor sign, 236t
Beta$_1$ agonist(s), 1394t
Beta$_2$ agonist(s), 1394t
Betamethasone, glucocorticoid and mineralocorticoid activities of, 1066t
Beta$_1$ receptor(s), cardiovascular effects of, 1393t
Beta$_2$ receptor(s), cardiovascular effects of, 1393t
Bicarbonate. See also Sodium bicarbonate
  concentration
    calculation of, 1389, 1389t
    Henderson-Hasselbalch equation for, 107
  loss, metabolic acidosis in, 113-114
Bile, normal volume and composition of, 103t
Bile duct
  common. See Common bile duct
  resection of, for tumor, 746-751
    assessment of resectability in, 747-748, 748f
    basic principles of, 746-747
    closure and postoperative care in, 751
    complications of, 751
    division of common bile duct in, 748, 748f
    location of tumor in, 746, 746f
    operative technique in, 747-751, 748f-751f
    proximal dissection in, 748-749, 748f-751f
    reconstruction in, 749, 751
  trauma to, 419-420
Biliary anastomosis, technical issues in, 736-738, 737f-738f
Biliary colic, abdominal pain and fever in, 1263-1266, 1263f, 1266t
Biliary drainage catheter(s), postoperative management of, 1634
Biliary stricture, malignant, ERCP for, 693, 694f

Biliary tract
  infection of, enterococcal
      bacteremia due to, 1179
  obstruction of, management of,
      prior to biliary tract
      procedures, 735
  operative exposure of, in
      abdominal injury, 408
  procedures for, 735-752. *See also*
      specific procedures, e.g.,
      Cholecystectomy
    anastomosis for, 736-738, 737f-
        738f
    exposure of subhepatic field
        for, 736
    positioning for, 735
    postoperative care in, 738
    preoperative preparation for,
        735
    Roux loop for, 738
Biliary tract disease. *See*
    Cholangitis; Cholecystitis
Bilirubin, unconjugated, 251. *See
    also* Jaundice
Billroth I reconstruction, 713-714,
    713f
Billroth II reconstruction, 714,
    714f
Biologic response modifier(s), 1351-
    1353, 1351t
Biopsy. *See also* Laboratory
    method(s)
  of abdominal mass
    image-guided percutaneous, 248-
        249, 248f
    laparoscopic, 249
  of breast, 212, 629-633. *See also*
      Breast, biopsy of
  of burn wound, technique for, 485
  of lung, for nosocomial pneumonia,
      1650
  of lymph node. *See also* Lymphatic
      mapping and sentinel node
      biopsy
    in HIV infection, 1336, 1337f
  of neck mass, 189
  of skin, 301
    in melanoma, 308-309
Biotin, requirements for, in ICU
    patient, 1524t
Birth trauma, 1141
Bite(s)
  animal
    acute wound care for, 126
    antibiotic regimens for, 1280
    of hand, 1283-1285, 1285f
    infection after, 321-322
    rabies prophylaxis for, 126,
        322, 331
    viral infections from, 1330
  black widow spider, 127
  brown recluse spider, 127
  cat
    acute wound care for, 126
    of hand, 1283-1285, 1285f
  coral snake, 126-127
  dog
    acute wound care for, 126
    of hand, 1283-1285, 1285f
    hand infection in, 1283-1285,
        1285f
  human
    acute wound care for, 126
    antibiotic regimens for, 1280
    of hand, 1283-1285, 1285f
    infection after, 322
    viral infections from, 1330

pit viper, 126-127
Black widow spider bite(s), 127
Bladder. *See also entries under*
    Urinary
  exstrophy of, in infants and
      neonates, emergency surgery
      in, 1129
  infection. *See* Urinary tract
      infection
  trauma to, 454-456
    initial evaluation of, 454-455,
        455f
    pelvis fracture and, 454
Blastomyces dermatitidis infection,
    antimicrobial agents for, 1199t
Blastomycosis, clinical presentation
    and diagnosis of, 1293t
Bleeding disorder(s). *See*
    Coagulation disorder(s)
Bleeding (hemorrhage), 77-90. *See
    also* Coagulation disorder(s);
    Hemostasis
  in abdominal injury, 408, 409f
  in acute wound, timing of closure
      for, 124
  adrenal, heparin-induced, 1025
  after hemorrhoid surgery, 847
  Algorithm, 78-79
  anemia in, 83-84, 83f, 84t
  approach to patient with, 77-84
    coagulation parameters in, 80-83
    exclusion of technical bleeding
        in, 77
    increased INR
      normal aPTT and, 81, 82t
      prolonged aPTT and, 82-83, 82t
    normal INR
      normal aPTT and, 80
      prolonged aPTT and, 80, 81t
  in chest trauma, 402
  in chronic hepatic disease, 1467-
      1468
  esophageal variceal. *See*
      Esophageal varices
  gastrointestinal. *See*
      Gastrointestinal bleeding;
      Lower gastrointestinal
      bleeding; Upper
      gastrointestinal bleeding
  laboratory assessment of, 88-89,
      88f, 89t
  maxillofacial, 371
  shock in, 69
  transfusion in, 83
Bleomycin, reactive oxygen
    metabolites created by, 1568
Blood
  arterial. *See under* Arterial blood
  fecal occult. *See* Fecal
      examination
  substitutes for, 84, 84t
  venous. *See under* Venous blood
Blood and body fluid(s), precautions
    for contact with, 1720
Blood and body substance isolation
    (BSI), 1720
Blood and body substance precautions
    (BSP), 1720
Blood culture(s), 1175-1189. *See
    also* Bacteremia
  Algorithm, 1176
  for candidiasis, 1292-1293
  negative, with infection, 1183-
      1184
  evaluation and management of,
      1183-1184, 1183t
  reasons for, 1183

  for nosocomial pneumonia, 1650
  positive
    with infection, 1175-1181, 1177f
      anaerobes in, 1180-1181
      fungi in, 1181, 1182t
      gram-negative
          Enterobacteriaceae in,
          1179-1180, 1180t
      gram-positive cocci in, 1175-
          1179
      staphylococci in, 1175-1178,
          1178t, 1178f
      streptococci in, 1178-1179
    without infection, 1181-1183
      gut barrier function and, 1182
      microbial translocation and,
          1182-1183
Blood donor(s), acceptance policy
    for, 1319, 1320t
Blood flow. *See also* Circulation
  eicosanoids in, 1598
Blood gas(es)
  arterial. *See* Arterial blood
      gas(es)
  venous. *See* Venous blood gas(es)
Blood pressure. *See also*
    Hypertension; Hypotension;
    Pulmonary arterial pressure;
    Systemic arterial pressure
  cuff method for, 1386-1387
  Doppler devices for, 1387
  in infants and neonates, 1121,
      1121t
  noninvasive monitoring of, 1386-
      1387
  in obese patients, 1387
Blood transfusion. *See* Transfusion
    therapy
Blood type and crossmatch, in
    preoperative evaluation, 538
Blood urea nitrogen (BUN)
  in burn patient, 57
  preoperative evaluation of, 537
  unreliable in renal failure, 1051
Blumberg sign, 236t
Body composition, of elderly
    patients, 1110-1111, 1111f
Body fluid(s), precautions for
    contact with, 1720
Body stuffing or packing, in
    substance abuse, 173
Body temperature. *See* Fever and
    hyperpyrexia; Temperature
Body water
  in hyperdynamic state of critical
      illness, 1501
  total, 101
    body weight for, 1631
    in infants and neonates, 1124,
        1126f
Body water compartment(s), 101
  infants and neonates, 1122, 1124,
      1126f
Body weight. *See* Weight, body
Bone demineralization, in uremic
    syndrome, 1059-1060
Bone infection, quinolone for, 1216
Borrelia burgdorferi infection,
    antimicrobial agents for, 1199t
Borrelia recurrentis infection,
    antimicrobial agents for, 1199t
Bowel
  large. *See* Colon
  small. *See* Small bowel
Bowel irrigation, whole, for
    emergency management, of
    substance abuse, 172-173

Bowel preparation, 570, 576t, 577-578, 579t-580t, 584-585
Bowel resections, intestinal anastomosis for, 808-809
Bowen disease, 305
Brachial artery, for systemic arterial catheterization, 1370
Brachial plexus injury, in birth trauma, 1141
Bradycardia
 maintenance anesthesia causing, 609
 in shock, 67
Bradykinin, pulmonary metabolism of, 1417
Brain death, 163-164
 in children, 164
 clinical criteria for, 959
 confirmatory tests for, 164
 guidelines for determination of, 162f, 163-164, 163t
Brain herniation syndromes, 164-165
 central (axial), 165
 lateral (uncal), 164-165
 posterior (tectal), 165
 subfalcial (cingulate), 164
 tonsillar, 165
Brain injury. *See* Head injury
Brain protection, in head injury. *See* Intracranial pressure, reduction of
Branchial cleft cyst, 190
Breast(s)
 abscess of, 214
 biopsy of, 212, 629-633
  core-needle, 630
   image-guided, 631-632
   stereotactic, 631
   ultrasound-guided, 631
  fine-needle aspiration for, 629-630
  in nonpalpable mass, 630-633
   open, 630, 631f
   with needle localization, 632-633, 632f-633f
  in palpable mass, 629-630
  terminal duct excision for, 633-634, 633f-634f
Breast cancer, 214-221
 axillary dissection for, 634-636
  lymph node levels in, 634-635, 635f
  operative technique in, 635-636
  structures to be preserved in, 635, 636f
 drug and hormonal therapy for, 217
 ductal carcinoma in situ, treatment of, 217-218, 218f
 high-risk for, screening in, 214
 incidence of, 643
 invasive, treatment of, 218-220
  early-stage, 218-219, 219f
  locally advanced, 219-220, 220f
  stage IV, 220, 220f
 lobular carcinoma in situ, treatment of, 218
 lumpectomy for, 634
  mastectomy *vs.*, 215-216, 215t
 mastectomy for, 636-639. *See also* Mastectomy
 multidisciplinary care for, 221
 noninvasive, treatment of, 217-218
 in pregnancy, 1157
 radiation therapy for, 216-217
 risk factors for, 207, 210t
 staging of, 214-215, 215t
  lymphatic mapping and sentinel node biopsy for, 650-655. *See also* Lymphatic mapping and sentinel node biopsy
 surgical options for, 634
 TNM classification of, 215t
 treatment of, 215-221
  follow-up after, 220-221
  future directions for, 221
Breast complaints, 207-223
 Algorithm, 208-209
 common presenting symptoms of, 207, 210t
 history in, 207-210
 imaging studies in, 210-211
 infection or inflammation, 214
 magnetic resonance imaging in, 210-211
 mammography in, 210
  abnormal, with normal physical findings, 212-213
 nipple discharge in, 213
  terminal duct excision for, 633-634, 633f-634f
 pain in, 213-214
 palpable mass in, 211
  cystic, 211
  solid, 211
 patient workup in, 207-211
 phyllodes tumor in, 211
 physical examination in, 210
 ultrasonography in, 210, 661-662, 668f-669f, 669
 vague thickening or nodularity in, 213
Breast procedure(s), 629-642. *See also* Breast(s), biopsy of; Breast reconstruction; Mastectomy
Breast reconstruction, 216, 638f, 639-642
 autologous tissue for, 640f-641f, 641-642
  latissimus dorsi myocutaneous flap, 641-642, 641f
  TRAM flap, 640f, 641-642
 implants for, 640-641
 operative technique in, 640-642
 skin-sparing mastectomy incision in, 639f, 640
 steps in, 638f
Breathing. *See also* Mechanical ventilation; Respiration; Ventilation
 atactic, in coma, 148
 cluster, in coma, 148
 in coma management, 143-146
 mouth-to-mouth
  for CPR, 7-8, 8f
  gastric insufflation and, 7
 stimulus for, 1415
 in trauma resuscitation, 31-34
 work of, 1416
Breathing exercises
 postoperative, in pulmonary insufficiency, 1042
 for weaning from mechanical ventilation, 1429, 1429t
Bretylium
 classification of, 23
 for ventricular fibrillation, 10
Bronchitis
 chronic, postoperative pulmonary insufficiency in, 1043
 nosocomial, 1221-1224
Bronchodilator(s), for burn patients, in immediate resuscitation period, 54
Bronchopneumonia
 bacterial, 1412
 nosocomial, 1656-1657
Bronchopulmonary disease, as factor in selection for outpatient surgery, 542
Bronchoscopy
 in mechanical ventilation, 1437
 for nosocomial pneumonia, 1650
Bronchospasm
 in endotracheal intubation, 607
 postoperative pulmonary insufficiency in, 1043
Broviac catheter. *See* Central venous catheterization
Brown recluse spider bite(s), 127
Brucella infection, antimicrobial agents for, 1198t
Brudzinski sign, in coma, 148
Bullet wound(s), acute wound management after, 125
BUN. *See* Blood urea nitrogen (BUN)
Bupivacaine
 comparative pharmacology of, 612t
 for nonemergency surgery, 545t
Buprenorphine
 suggested dosing for, 1627t
 systemic, for postoperative pain, 1664, 1664t
Burn(s)
 chemical, 49, 52t
  agents causing, 52t
  neutralization of, 49
 classification of severity of, 59, 60t
 in elderly patient, 1093-1094
 electrical. *See* Electrical injury
 estimation of size of (Rule of Nines), 54, 54f
 first-degree, 58
 immunodeficiency in, 1085
 physical characteristics of, 58t
 in pregnancy, 1157-1158, 1158t
 second-degree, 58-59, 59f
 third-degree, 59, 59f
Burn care after first postburn week, 491-503
 adult respiratory distress syndrome in, 494
 Algorithm, 492-493
 lung function in, 491-494
 hemodynamic stability in, 494-499
 hydration in, 494
 hypermetabolism-induced respiratory fatigue in, 494
 nosocomial pneumonia in, 494
 nutrition in, 499-501
  administration of, 501
  energy requirements for, 500, 500t, 500f
  nutrient requirements for, 500-501
  stress factors for, 500, 500t
  trace element requirements for, 501
  vitamin requirements for, 501
 perfusion in, 495-496
  hyperdynamic state and, 495, 495t
  multiple organ dysfunction syndrome and, 496
  restoring and maintaining, 495-496
  systemic stress response in, 496-499. *See also* Stress response, in burn patients
Burn care in early postresuscitation period, 479-489. *See also* Burn

wound care
Algorithm, 480-481
blood volume in, 482
endotracheal intubation in, 479
fluid and electrolyte balance in, 482-483, 483t
hemodynamic stability in, 482-483
from hypometabolism to hypermetabolism in, 483
physical therapy and splinting in, 489
pulmonary function in, 479-482
pulmonary injury in, 479-482
diagnosis of, 482
treatment of, 482
stress control in, 488-489
analgesia and sedation in, 488, 488t
gastric pH in, 489
heat loss and, 488
hyperthermia and, 488
nutritional support for, 489
ventilation in, 479
Burn care in immediate resuscitation period, 49-61. *See also* Burn wound care
aggressive pulmonary support in, 54
airway and ventilation in, 49-54
Algorithm, 50-51
arterial blood gas values in, 54, 57
blood glucose level in, 57
blood lactate concentration in, 57
body weight and temperature in, 57
BUN in, 57
carbon monoxide toxicity in, 49, 53t
cardiac output in, 56-57
chest wall escharotomy in, 54, 54f
cyanide toxicity in, 49-52
diuretics in, 58
ECG in, 57
electrolyte status in, 57
hematocrit and hemoglobin in, 57
hemodynamic parameters in, 56-57
hemodynamic stability in, 54-58
inhalation injury in, 52-53, 53f
inotropic support in, 57-58
intake and output in, 57
intravenous access in, 54
intubation for, 53
mean arterial pressure in, 56
mixed venous oxygen tension in, 56-57
neutralization of source in, 49
chemical burns and, 49, 52t
clothing and, 49
PEEP for, 53
perfusion-related parameters in, 56-57
plasma protein and myoglobin level in, 57
prothrombin time, partial thromboplastin time, platelet count in, 57
pulmonary arterial wedge pressure in, 56
pulse rate in, 56
resuscitation fluids for, 55-56, 55t
blood transfusion, 56
colloid, 55-56
crystalloid, 55, 55t
infusion rate for, 56
in young patient without inhalation injury, 55t
serum creatinine in, 57
transfer to specialized facility for, 61
urine output in, 57
white blood cell count in, 57
Burn patient(s)
blood glucose concentrations in, 1502t
hypermetabolism in, 1504
ambient temperature and, 1505, 1505t
insulin concentrations in, 1502t
rehabilitation for, 1691-1694
burn edema and, 1693
contracture and, 1694
early wound closure for, 1691
eschar rigidity and, 1693
exercise for, 1691-1692
functional impairment and, 1693-1694
heterotopic calcification and ossification and, 1694
hypertrophic scar formation and, 1694
muscle loss and, 1694
positioning and splinting for, 1692, 1692t, 1692f
pressure garments for, 1692, 1693f
psychosocial support for, 1693
skin care for, 1692-1693, 1693t
temperature regulation and, 1694
Burn wound care
after first postburn week, 501-502
alterations in care in, 501-502
changes in, 501
hypertrophic scarring, 502-503
infection in, 501
skin lubrication, 503
surgical management in, 502
closure in, 125, 485-488
early, 1691
early excision in, 480, 485-488
excision to fascia, 486-487, 486t
tangential (sequential), 486, 486t, 487f
general principles of, 485-486
grafting in, 480, 487-488
excision to fascia in, 488
tangential excision in, 487-488, 488f
risk assessment in, 485, 485t
for electrical burns, 507
infection control in, 483-485
bedside care for, 484
colonization *vs.* invasive infection in, 484t
daily care for, 483-485
etiology of invasive infection in, 484t
hydrotherapy in, 484
organisms recovered in, 483t
systemic antibiotics for, 484-485
topical antibiotics for, 484
wound biopsy in, 485
initial, 58-61
antibiotic prophylaxis in, 60, 60t
assessment of depth in, 58-59, 58f-59f, 58t
cooling for, 58
for extremities, subeschar edema and, 61
pain medication in, 59
removal of foreign bodies and nonviable tissue in, 59-60
temporary skin substitutes for, 61
tetanus prophylaxis in, 60
topical antibiotics for, 60-61, 60t
morbidity in, factors affecting, 485t
Bursitis, uremic, 1059
Butorphanol, suggested dosing for, 1627t
Butyrate, in colonic metabolism, 1514

C

Cachectin. *See* Tumor necrosis factor
Cachexia, tumor necrosis factor in, 1606
Calcification, heterotopic, in burn patient, 1694
Calcitonin, for hypercalcemia, 97-98
Calcium. *See also* Hypercalcemia; Hypocalcemia
for CPR, 21-22
for heart failure, 1395
in myocardial contractility, 1398-1399, 1398f
serum
measurement of, 96
postoperative evaluation of, 1629
total body, 94t
Calcium metabolism, 105-106, 105t
Calcium sensitizer(s), for heart failure, 1395
Caloric expenditure, in various age groups, 1110f
Caloric requirement(s)
for hyperdynamic state of critical illness, 1501
for infants and neonates, 1131, 1131t
Caloric test, for coma, 148
Calymmatobacterium granulomatis infection, antimicrobial agents for, 1198t
Campylobacter fetus infection, antimicrobial agents for, 1197t
Campylobacter jejuni infection, antimicrobial agents for, 1197t
Cancer. *See* Malignancy; *specific anatomic sites, e.g.,* Breast cancer
Candida albicans, in burn wound, 483t, 484t
Candida endophthalmitis
in hematogenous candidiasis, 1294
management of, 1297
pathologic findings in, 1304, 1304f
Candida infection, antimicrobial agents for, 1199t
Candida species
drug-resistance in, 1303
microbiologic characteristics of, 1302-1303, 1303f
changing microbiologic spectra of, 1302-1303
virulence factors in, 1302
Candidemia
catheter-associated, definition of, 1292
definition of, 1289-1292
management of, 1294-1296, 1295t
in surgical patients, 1181, 1182t

causes of, 1181
therapy for, 1181
Candidiasis, 1289-1299
  arthritis due to, 1297
  cystitis in, 1299
  in immunosuppressed patient, 1082
  deep, 1298-1299
  disseminated
    acute, definition of, 1292
    chronic, definition of, 1292
    in immunosuppression, 1304
    management of, 1294-1296, 1295t
    pathologic findings in, 1304
  endocarditis due to, 1297
  esophageal, 1298, 1298f
    in immunosuppressed patient, 1076t, 1081, 1082
  fungus ball of ureter in, 1299
  gastrointestinal, 1298, 1298f
  genital, 1299
  hematogenous
    antibody detection for, 1293
    antifungal prophylaxis in, 1296
    antigen detection and PCR for, 1293-1294
    Candida endophthalmitis in, 1294
    candiduria in, 1294
    clinical diagnosis of, 1294
    cultures for, 1292-1293
    cytokine therapy for opportunistic infection in, 1296
    histologic analysis for, 1294
    laboratory and clinical assessment in, 1292-1294
    management of, 1294-1297, 1295t
    metabolite detection for, 1294
    pathologic findings in, 1304
    suppurative thrombophlebitis in, 1294, 1297
    surgical patients at risk for, 1292
  incidence of, 1289
  in intra-abdominal abscess, 1298
  meningitis due to, 1297
  nonhematogenous, 1297-1299
  oral (thrush), 1297-1298
  osteomyelitis due to, 1297
  pericarditis due to, 1297
  in peritonitis, antimicrobial agents for, 1252-1253
  peritonitis in, 1298
  pyelitis in, 1299
  in renal abscess, 1299
  septicemia due to, in central venous catheter sepsis, 1536
  superficial, 1297-1298
  in surgical patient
    colonization of gut in, 1303
    pathogenesis of, 1303-1304
    physical disruption of intestinal mucosal barrier in, 1299-1300
  in urinary tract, 1299
  vulvovaginal, 1299
  in wound infection, 1298-1299
Candiduria, 1299
  in hematogenous candidiasis, 1294
Canthus(i), examination of, in maxillofacial injury, 372
Cantor tube(s), postoperative management of, 1634, 1635f
Carbapenem(s), 1213-1214
  for Enterobacteriaceae bacteremia, 1180t
Carbenicillin, 1196

for bacterial infections, 1202t-1203t
Carbenicillin indanyl sodium, for bacterial infections, 1202t-1203t
Carbicarb, for lactic acidosis, 119
Carbohydrate(s), requirements for, in burn patients, 500-501
Carbohydrate metabolism
  in critical illness, 1507-1508
  in pregnancy, 1154
Carbon dioxide
  end-tidal, as monitor of CPR efficacy, 22
  partial pressure of. *See* Carbon dioxide tension (PCO_2)
Carbon dioxide content (CCO_2), measurement of, 1374
Carbon dioxide production (VCO_2)
  definition of, 1413
  in hyperdynamic state of critical illness, 1501
Carbon dioxide removal
  alveolar ventilation in, 1419
  physiology of, 1414-1415
Carbon dioxide tension (PCO_2). *See also* Hypercapnia
  alveolar (P_ACO_2), 1415
  arterial (P_aCO_2), 1415
  in mechanical ventilation. *See* Mechanical ventilation
  preoperative, 1041
  in elderly patient, 1095
  end-expiratory, continuous measurement of, 1386
  measurement of, 1374
Carbonic anhydrase inhibitor(s), renal tubular acidosis due to, 114
Carbon monoxide toxicity
  in burn patient, 49, 53t
  treatment of, 12
Carboxypenicillin(s), 1196
Carcinoid tumor, of appendix, 821
Carcinoma. *See* Malignancy; specific anatomic sites, e.g., Breast cancer
Cardiac arrest
  acid-base disorders in, sodium bicarbonate and, 22
  in electrical injury, 508
  hypothermic, 1555
  in-hospital, prevention of, 13
  management of. *See also* Cardiopulmonary resuscitation (CPR)
    Algorithm, 4-5
  pH in, arterial *vs.* venous, 22
  in trauma, management of, 3
  traumatic, 337-339, 339f-340f
    blunt, 339-340, 340f
    penetrating, 339, 339f
    verification of, 3
Cardiac assessment
  in immunosuppressive therapy, 1080-1081
  preoperative, 536. *See also* Cardiac risk, preoperative assessment of
    in angina pectoris, 561
    in valvular lesions, 559
Cardiac autonomic neuropathy, diabetic, 995, 997
Cardiac bypass, emergency, 18
Cardiac catheterization, in preoperative assessment, 562
Cardiac dysfunction, postoperative, 1637-1639

Cardiac dysrhythmia(s). *See also specific dysrhythmias*
  after resuscitation, 13-18, 15f
    in hemodynamic instability, 13
      cardioversion for, 13
    in hemodynamic stability, 13-18
      adenosine in, 15-18
      amiodarone in, 18
      ECG in, 13-15, 18f
      with fast ventricular rate, 13-18
      magnesium in, 18
      with slow ventricular rate, 13
      verapamil in, 15
    with antidysrhythmic drugs, 19
  automatic, 25-26, 26f
    in digitalis toxicity, 26, 26f
    in elevated catecholamine levels, 26
    in hypercalcemia, 25-26
    in hypokalemia, 25
    in local myocardial hypoxia, 25
  in burn patient, 57
  in elderly patients, 1095
  maintenance anesthesia causing, 609
  pathophysiology of, 25-28
    in automatic dysrhythmias, 25-26, 26f
    in reentrant dysrhythmias, 26-27, 26f-27f
    in slow afterdepolarizations, 28, 28f
  during pregnancy, 19
  preoperative assessment of, 561
  reentrant, 26-27, 26f-27f
  reperfusion, 1577
  in shock, 68
Cardiac failure, pharmacokinetics in, 1707-1708
Cardiac function, in infants and neonates, 1121-1122
Cardiac glycoside(s), for heart failure, 1396
Cardiac index
  in burn patient, 56-57
  definition of, 1413
  in heart failure, 1391
Cardiac massage, open-chest, in trauma resuscitation, 37
Cardiac morbidity and mortality, perioperative, 550-551, 564-565
  cardiac risk index system (CRIS) for, 564, 564t
  risk factors for, 563t, 564
  studies of, 564-565, 565t
Cardiac output
  body surface area in calculation of, 1387
  in burn patient, 56-57
  high
    in hyperdynamic state of critical illness, 1500
  measurement of, 1383, 1384f
    indicator dilution technique for, 1383, 1384f
    noninvasive, 1383
  monitoring of, in cardiac resuscitation, 22-23
  pulmonary arterial catheterization for, 1387
Cardiac risk, 559-566
  preoperative assessment of
    Algorithm, 560
    ambulatory ECG in, 561
    cardiac catheterization in, 562
    coronary angiography in, 562

diagnostic testing in, 561-562
exercise ECG in, 561-562
for high-risk patient, 562-564
  invasive monitoring in, 562-563
  medication in, 563-564
  pacemakers in, 564
history and physical examination in, 559-561
radioisotope imaging in, 562
resting ECG in, 561
Cardiopulmonary arrest. *See* Cardiac arrest
Cardiopulmonary bypass, pharmacokinetics in, 1708
Cardiopulmonary monitoring, 1365-1390
for blood pressure, noninvasive, 1386-1387
central venous. *See* Central venous catheterization; Central venous pressure
continuous, 1386
for arterial oxygen saturation, 1386
for end-expiratory carbon dioxide tension, 1386
for high-risk patients, 562-563
for mixed venous oxygen saturation, 1385, 1385f
for skin temperature, 1386
for tissue oxygen tension, 1386
derived values in, 1387-1390
  aortic root and pulmonary arterial end-systolic pressure-volume relations, 1388
  bicarbonate concentration, 1389, 1389t
  cardiac output, 1387
  influence of age and other variables on, 1389-1390
  left ventricular and right ventricular end-diastolic volume, 1387
  left ventricular and right ventricular end-systolic pressure, 1387-1388
  left ventricular and right ventricular end-systolic pressure-volume relations, 1388
  left ventricular and right ventricular end-systolic unstressed volume, 1387
  left ventricular and right ventricular end-systolic volume, 1387
  oxygen consumption, 1389
  oxygen return, 1389
  oxygen transport, 1388
  power, 1388
  stroke volume, 1387
  thermal stress and, 1389-1390
  vascular resistances, 1388
indications for and uses of, *Algorithm,* 1366-1367
normal values obtained from, 1368t-1369t
pulmonary arterial. *See* Pulmonary arterial (Swan-Ganz) catheterization; Pulmonary arterial wedge pressure
systemic arterial. *See* Systemic arterial catheterization; Systemic arterial pressure
Cardiopulmonary resuscitation (CPR), 3-30
ABCs of, 3
  exceptions to, 3
active compression-decompression (ACD-CPR), 20
acute dysrhythmia after, 13-18. *See also* Cardiac dysrhythmia, after resuscitation
advanced life support in, 8-10
  assisted ventilation in, 8-9
  bag-valve-mask ventilation for, 8-9, 10f
  tracheal intubation in, 9-10
asystole in, 11
basic life support in, 3-8
  airway in, 3-7, 6f-8f. *See also under* Airway
  breathing in, 7-8, 8f
  chin lift for, 6-7, 6f
  circulation in, 8
  external chest compression for, 8, 9f
  head tilt for, 6, 6f
  initial steps in, 3
  jaw thrust for, 7, 7f
  nasopharyngeal airway for, 7, 8f
  oropharyngeal airway for, 7, 7f
  verify pulselessness in, 8
circulation in
  cardiac pump in, 19
  cerebral, 20
  coronary artery, 20
  limited vital organ perfusion and, 20
  physiology of, 19-21
  thoracic pump in, 20
current-based defibrillation in, 20
discussion in, 19-28
drug therapy in, 21-23
  alpha agonists for, 21
  calcium for, 21-22
  central, 23
  end-tidal CO_2 monitoring and, 22
  epinephrine for, 21
  methoxamine in, 21
  peripheral, 23
  pH and, 22-23
  phenylephrine in, 21
  sodium bicarbonate for, 22
  tracheal, 23
effective, measures of, 20
interposed abdominal compression (IAC-CPR), 20
new techniques for, 20
pulseless electrical activity in, 12-13, 12t
survival statistics in, 19
ventricular fibrillation in, 10-11
volume loading in, 20
Cardiovascular assessment. *See* Cardiac assessment
Cardiovascular dysfunction
in obesity, 1003, 1009, 1009f
in toxic epidermal necrolysis, 513
in uremic syndrome, 1057
Cardiovascular failure. *See* Cardiac failure
Cardiovascular infection, in immunosuppression, 1076
Cardiovascular injury
in electrical injury, 508
in lightning strike, 510
Cardioversion (defibrillation)
for acute dysrhythmia, after resuscitation, 13
for asystole, 11
current-based, 20-21
intracardiac cardioverter defibrillator for, 15
technique for, 10, 11f
Carnett test, 235, 236t
Carotid angiography, for asymptomatic carotid bruit, 200-201
Carotid artery, internal
coiling or kinking of, 933-934, 933f-934f
fibromuscular dysplasia of, 932-933, 932f-933f
Carotid artery procedures, 921-935
alternatives to, 935
anesthesia for, 922
endarterectomy, 928-930, 929f-930f
  arteriotomy in, 928, 929f
  for asymptomatic carotid bruit, 201
  prophylactic, 199, 200t
  closure of arteriotomy in, 929-930
  eversion, 930-931, 931f
  irrigation and clearing of debris in, 929
  plaque removal in, 928-929, 930f
follow-up after, 935
imaging for, 921-922
in injury, 384-385
  repair *vs.* ligation, 392
in neck trauma, 382-384, 383f-384f
operative planning for, 922-923, 922f
operative technique in, 923-935
  cerebral circulatory support in, 926-928, 926f-928f
  shunting options in, 926-927, 926f-927f
  shunt placement technique in, 927-928, 928f
  closure in, 935
  in coiling or kinking of internal carotid, 933-934, 933f-934f
  completion imaging in, 934-935
  eversion endarterectomy in, 930-931, 931f
  exposure of carotid artery in, 923-926, 923f-925f
  in fibromuscular dysplasia of internal carotid, 932-933, 932f-933f
  initial incision in, 922f-923f, 923
  open endarterectomy in, 928-930, 929f-930f
  reconstruction for proximal lesions in, 931-932
  reconstruction for recurrent stenosis in, 932
  reconstruction options in, 928-934
patient positioning for, 922-923, 922f
patient selection for
  in asymptomatic critical stenosis, 921
  in prior stroke, 921
  in symptomatic hemodynamically significant stenosis, 921
  in transient ischemic attacks, 921
postoperative management for, 935
preoperative evaluation in, 921-922
Carotid body tumor (chemodectoma), of neck, 191-192

Carotid bruit, asymptomatic, 195-206
  Algorithm, 196-197
  carotid angiography for, 200-201
  carotid endarterectomy and, 199, 200t
  carotid endarterectomy for, 201
  center specific variations and risk-to-benefit ratio in, 204
  clinical assessment of, 195-200
  diagnosis of, 200-201
  duplex ultrasonography for, 200
  economic considerations in, 202
  epidemiology in, 202
  high-risk factors in
    asymptomatic cerebral infarction as, 203
    contralateral disease as, 203
    degree of stenosis as, 202-203, 203t
    plaque ulceration and structure as, 203
    sex as, 202
    subgroup analyses of, 202-203
  indications for surgical intervention in, 198-199, 199t
  other cervical sounds *vs.*, 195
  patient education in, 201
  in preoperative assessment for coronary artery bypass grafting, 203-204
  restenosis or previous carotid surgery and, 203
  risk of carotid stenosis in, 199, 201t, 201f
  screening issues in, 202
  stroke in, 199-200, 202t
  surgical intervention for, patient preference in, 200
  symptomatic *vs.*, 195-198, 195t
  vascular risk assessment in, 198
Carotid stenosis
  asymptomatic, carotid arterial procedures for, 921
  in asymptomatic carotid bruit, 199, 201t, 201f
  lower-grade, patient follow-up in, 202
  prevalence of, 198t, 199
Case cart system, 595
Catabolism. *See also* Hypermetabolism
Catalase, as free radical scavenger, 1575
Cat bite(s)
  acute wound care for, 126
  of hand, 1283-1285, 1285f
Catecholamine(s)
  automatic dysrhythmias and, 26
  in heart failure, 1393-1395, 1393t-1394t
Catheterization. *See also* Intravascular device(s)
  cardiac, in preoperative assessment, 562
  central venous. *See* Central venous catheterization
  Foley. *See* Foley catheterization
  intravenous. *See* Intravenous catheterization
  pulmonary arterial. *See* Pulmonary arterial (Swan-Ganz) catheterization
  sepsis in. *See under* Intravascular device(s)
Catheter whip, in systemic arterial pressure measurement, 1370, 1373f
Causalgia, in chest trauma, 404

CD14, lipopolysaccharides and, 1614
Cecal volvulus
  abdominal radiography in, 268, 271f
  operative therapy in, 273-274
Cecum, angiodysplastic lesions of, colonoscopy for, 296f, 297
Cefaclor, for bacterial infections, 1202t-1203t
Cefadroxil, for bacterial infections, 1202t-1203t
Cefamandole, for bacterial infections, 1202t-1203t
Cefazolin, for bacterial infections, 1202t-1203t
Cefonicid, for bacterial infections, 1202t-1203t
Cefoperazone, for bacterial infections, 1202t-1203t
Ceforanide, for bacterial infections, 1202t-1203t
Cefotaxime, for bacterial infections, 1202t-1203t
Cefotetan, for bacterial infections, 1202t-1203t
Cefoxitin, for bacterial infections, 1202t-1203t
Ceftazidime, for bacterial infections, 1202t-1203t
Ceftizoxime, for bacterial infections, 1202t-1203t
Ceftriaxone, for bacterial infections, 1202t-1203t
Cefuroxime, for bacterial infections, 1202t-1203t
Celecoxib, suggested dosing for, 1628t
Celiac axis, traumatic injury of, 440
Cellular electrophysiology, 24-25
  action potential in, 24-25
  membrane potential in, 24
  Nernst equation in, 24
Cellulitis
  clostridial, 319
  in hand infection, 1281
  necrotizing, Gram-negative synergistic, 329, 329f-330f
  nonoperative, 320-321, 320f-322f
  antibiotics in, 324
  lymphangitis in, 319, 320f
  pathogens in, 324
Central nervous system
  free radical effects on, 1583
  in hepatic failure. *See* Hepatic encephalopathy
  in metabolic response to critical illness, 1511-1513
  reperfusion injury in, 1578
  in stress response, in burn patients, 498
Central nervous system infection, in immunosuppression, 1076
Central nervous system trauma, 355-366. *See also* Head injury; Spinal cord injury
  in lightning strike, 510
Central venous catheterization, 1374-1377
  in AIDS, 1338-1339
  in burn patients, 54
  complications of, 1375-1376
  in high-risk patient, 562
  indications for, 1374-1375
  in infants and neonates, 1122
  infection (sepsis) in, 1534-1536, 1537f

  candidal, 1296
  exit site, 1226
  incidence of, 1232
  prevention of, 1227-1228
  recommendations for changing catheter in, 1227
  septic thrombosis in, 1227
  tunnel, 1226
  insertion of, 1375, 1376f
  sterile technique for, 1227
  postoperative complications of, 1640
Central venous pressure (CVP)
  in heart failure, 1391
  measurement of, 1375f, 1376-1377
    at end-expiratory pressure, 1375t, 1376-1377
  pulmonary arterial catheterization for, 1381
Cephalexin, for bacterial infections, 1202t-1203t
Cephalosporin(s), 1200-1208
  adverse effects of, 1208, 1208t
  antimicrobial spectra of, 1201-1206
  biochemistry of, 1200
  clinical utility of, 1206-1207
  for Enterobacteriaceae bacteremia, 1180t
  first-generation, 1200-1201
  for intra-abdominal infections, 1207
  pharmacokinetics of, 1206
  properties of, 1209t
  for respiratory tract infections, 1206-1207
  second-generation, 1201
  third-generation, 1201
  for urinary tract infections, 1207
  in vivo drug interactions with, 1193t
Cephalothin, for bacterial infections, 1202t-1203t
Cephapirin, for bacterial infections, 1202t-1203t
Cephradine, for bacterial infections, 1202t-1203t
Cerebral abscess, coma in, 151
  radiographic diagnosis of, 153, 154f
  treatment of, 156-157
Cerebral circulation, in CPR, 20
Cerebral edema. *See also* Intracranial pressure
  in hepatic failure, 1460
Cerebral ischemia, reperfusion injury in, 1578
Cerebral perfusion pressure, in head injury, 357-358
Cerebral tumor, coma in, 150
  radiographic diagnosis of, 152, 152f
  treatment of, 156
Cerebrospinal fluid examination, in hypothalamic pathology, 1554
Cerebrospinal fluid leakage, nosocomial meningitis in, 1225
Cervical adenitis, 189
Cervical adenopathy, in Hodgkin and non-Hodgkin lymphoma, 192
Cervical lymph node(s)
  classification of, 186t, 187f
  enlarged, 186, 186t, 187f
Cervical spine fracture, 361-362
  atlantoaxial dislocation in, 361
  atlanto-occipital dislocation in, 361

INDEX — 1753

atlas (Jefferson) fracture in, 361
axis fracture in, 361
extension and compression injury of, 362
flexion and compression injury of, 361-362
flexion and distraction injury of, 361
lower, 361-362
Cervical spine injury, 355. *See also* Spinal cord injury
airway in
discussion on, 42
precautions, 31-34, 34f
in blunt trauma, 350, 352
emergency department management of, 31-34, 34f, 38
Chandelier sign, 236t
Charcoal, activated, for emergency management, of substance abuse, 173
Charcot sign, 236t
Chaussier sign, 236t
Chemical burn(s), 49, 52t
agents causing, 52t
neutralization of, 49
Chemodectoma(s) (carotid body tumor), of neck, 191-192
Chemotherapy
neutropenia in, 1078
reactive oxygen metabolites created by, 1567-1568
wound healing and, 137
Chest
alveolar hypoventilation in, 1419
in chest trauma, 1411
Chest compression, external, for CPR, 8, 9f
Chest defect(s), flaps for, 979
Chest trauma, 395-404
aortic injury in, 398-399, 398f-399f
bleeding in, 402
cardiac complications of, 403
cardiac trauma in, 396-398, 396f-397f
chest tube output in, 402
chest wall complications of, 404
chest wall injury in, 401
damage control tactics for, 402
diaphragmatic complications of, 403-404
esophageal complications of, 403-404
esophageal injuries in, 401, 401f
great vessel complications of, 403
hypothermia in, 402
incision choices in, 395
lung contusion due to, 1411-1412
major airway disruption in, 399
missed injury in, 402-403
oxygenation in, 402
penetrating, emergency management of, 341-342, 342f-343f
in stable patient, 342, 343f
in unstable patient, 341, 342f
postoperative problems in, 402-404
pulmonary complications of, 403
pulmonary lacerations in, 399-401, 400f
reoperation in, 403
resuscitative thoracotomy in, 395
special operative considerations in, 401-402
thoracic outlet injury in, 399
thoracoabdominal, 402
tracheal complications of, 403-404

transmediastinal, 401-402
treatment of, 1411-1412
Chest wall
escharotomy for, in burn patients, 54, 54f
traumatic injury to, 401
complications of, 404
Cheyne-Stokes respiration, in coma, 148
Chilblain (pernio), 511
Child abuse, 1141
Children, 1121-1143. *See also* Infants and neonates
abdominal pain in, 1127
acute, 232, 235t
appendicitis in, 1127
brain death in, 164
inguinal hernioplasty in, 863
mechanical ventilation for, 1437
orotracheal intubation in, tube size for, 34
peritoneal access in, 917
peritonitis in, 1245, 1246
pharmacokinetics in, 1703-1704
trauma in, 1137-1141
abdominal, 1139-1141, 1140f-1141f
blunt, 1138
emergency management of, 1138-1139
general principles of care in, 1137-1138
pediatric trauma score for, 1138, 1139t
Chin lift, for airway patency, 6-7, 6f
Chlamydia pneumoniae infection, antimicrobial agents for, 1199t
Chlamydia psittaci infection, antimicrobial agents for, 1199t
Chlamydia trachomatis infection, antimicrobial agents for, 1199t
Chloramphenicol, 1212
adverse effects of, 1208t
for bacterial infections, 1204t-1205t
in vivo drug interactions with, 1193t
Chlorhexidine, contraindicated in acute wound care, 128
Chloride, for hypokalemic, hypochloremic metabolic alkalosis, 1633
Chloroprocaine, comparative pharmacology of, 612t
Cholangiography
intraoperative, 765, 766f
in jaundice, 254-255
due to malignant obstruction, 258
Cholangiohepatitis, oriental, 1269
Cholangiojejunostomy, intrahepatic, 751-752
operative technique in, 752
Cholangiopancreatography
endoscopic retrograde. *See* Endoscopic retrograde cholangiopancreatography (ERCP)
magnetic resonance (MRCP), in jaundice, 256, 256f
Cholangitis
acute
abdominal pain and fever in, 1263-1266
in AIDS, 1338
antibiotics for, 1269

bacteriology of, 1275-1276
choledochoduodenostomy for, 1270
DIC in, 1269
endoscopic sphincterotomy for, 1270, 1270f
jaundice in, 256
fever and, 1269-1270
nonobstructive, acute cholecystitis in, 1269
pathophysiology of, 1275
percutaneous transhepatic biliary drainage for, 1270
treatment of, 1269-1270
prior to biliary tract procedures, 735
T-tube drainage for, 1270
primary sclerosing, 1269
Cholecystectomy
for acute cholecystitis, 1268-1269. *See also* Cholecystectomy
for gallstone pancreatitis, 1266-1267
for immunosuppressed patient, 1081
laparoscopic, 753-771
acute cholecystitis and, 769
advantages of, 1244t
background of, 753
bleeding complications of, 767
abdominal wall, 767
cystic artery branch, 767
liver bed, 767
mesenteric adhesions, 767
omental adhesions, 767
in common bile duct stones, 769-770
contraindications in, 755
conversion to laparotomy in, 768-769
deep vein thrombosis prophylaxis in, 755
equipment for, 756-758, 757t
hemostatic devices, 758
insufflator, 757
optical system, 756-757
surgical instruments, 757t, 758
trocars, 757-758
in hernia, 755
history and physical examination in, 753
imaging studies in, 753-754, 754f
intraoperative cholangiography in, 765, 766f
intraoperative complications of, 766-767
bleeding, 767
trocar injury, 767
Veress needle injury, 766-767
jaundice after, 260, 260f
laboratory tests for, 754
operative planning for, 755-758
operative technique, 758-766
accessory port placement, 760, 761f
cystic duct and cystic artery, 764-765
dissection of adhesions, 761-762, 762f
dissection of gallbladder, 765-766
exposure of Calot triangle, 762-763, 762f-763f
extraction of gallbladder, 766
perforation of gallbladder, 766
stripping of peritoneum, 763-764, 763f-764f

trocar placement, 758-760, 759f
outpatient, 754
patient positioning for, 755-756, 756f
patient selection for, 754-755
postoperative complications in, 767-768, 768f
  bile leakage, 768
  fever, 768
  fluid collection, 768
  liver function abnormalities, 768, 768f
predictors of choledocholithiasis and, 755-756, 755f
in pregnancy, 755
preoperative evaluation in, 753-755
prophylactic antibiotics for, 755
special problems in, 768-770
ultrasonography in, 765
open, 739-740
  complications of, 740
  operative technique in, 739, 739f
  troubleshooting in, 739-740, 740f
Cholecystitis
acute
  abdominal pain and fever in, 1263-1266, 1266t
  acalculous, 1268, 1268f
  acute nonobstructive cholangitis in, 1269
  in AIDS, 1338
  cholecystectomy for, 1268-1269
  diabetes mellitus and, 1267-1268
  emphysematous cholecystitis vs., 1267, 1268t
  gangrene and perforation of gallbladder in, 1267-1268
  in immunosuppressed patient, 1076t
  laparoscopic cholecystectomy in, 769
  in pregnancy, 1151-1152
  treatment of, 1267-1269
emphysematous, 1267, 1268t, 1268f
  acute cholecystitis vs., 1267, 1268t
perforation in, surgical options for, 1244t
Cholecystojejunostomy
  complications of, 743
  operative technique in, 742-743
Cholecystostomy tube(s), postoperative management of, 1634
Choledochal cyst, resection of, 744-746
  complications of, 746
  operative technique in, 745-746, 745f
  Todani classification of, 744, 744f
  troubleshooting in, 746
Choledochoduodenostomy
  for acute cholangitis, 1270
  complications of, 742
  operative technique in, 742
Choledochoenteric bypass, in AIDS, 1338
Choledochojejunostomy
  complications of, 743
  operative technique in, 743

troubleshooting in, 743
Choledocholithiasis
  in elderly patient, 1092-1093
  ERCP for, 693, 693f
  imaging for, 753-754, 754f
  laparoscopic cholecystectomy for, 769-770
    accessing biliary tree in, 769-770
    diagnostic and therapeutic options in, 769
    endoscopic transcystic bile duct exploration in, 770
    fluoroscopic wire basket transcystic bile duct exploration in, 770
    identification of patients at risk for, 769
    laparoscopic common bile duct exploration in, 770
  in obesity, 1007
  predictors of, 754-755, 755f
  without cholangitis, jaundice in, 256-257
Cholestatic syndrome, 254
Choline magnesium trisalicylate, suggested dosing for, 1628t
Chondritis, costal, in chest trauma, 404
Chromium
  in central venous nutritional support, 1532
  requirements for, in ICU patient, 1525t
Chronic obstructive pulmonary disease (COPD)
  pharmacokinetics in, 1710
  respiratory acidosis in, 115
Chylothorax, in chest trauma, 404
Cigarette smoking
  postoperative pulmonary insufficiency in, 1043
  wound healing and, 136
Ciprofloxacin, for bacterial infections, 1204t-1205t
Circulation
  in coma management, 146
  in CPR, 8
  in trauma resuscitation, 34-35, 36f
Cirrhosis. See also Hepatic disease
  ascites in, peritonitis in, 1245, 1246
  coagulopathy in, 81
Citrobacter infection, antimicrobial agents for, 1197t
Clarithromycin, 1211-1212
Clavicle fracture, in birth trauma, 1141
Clavulanate, 1214-1215
Claybrook sign, 236t
Clean air systems, in operating room, 570-571
Clindamycin, 1212
  adverse effects of, 1208t
  for bacterial infections, 1204t-1205t
  in vivo drug interactions with, 1193t
Clonidine
  for hypertension, 1638t
  preoperative, for hemodynamic stability, 606
Clostridial bacteremia, 1181
Clostridial infection
  cellulitis, 319
  of hand, 1285-1286

myonecrosis, 319
  gas in, 329-330, 330f-331f
  necrotizing, 318-319, 319f
  pathogenesis of, 325
  in surgical wound, 1224
Clostridium difficile
  antimicrobial agents for, 1197t
  in pseudomembranous colitis, 1229, 1229f
Clostridium perfringens, antimicrobial agents for, 1197t
Clostridium tetani, antimicrobial agents for, 1197t
Clotrimazole, 1301t
Clotting. See Coagulation; Thrombosis
Cloxacillin, 1196
  for bacterial infections, 1202t-1203t
Cluster breathing, in coma, 148
Coagulation. See also Factor(s); Hemostasis
  disseminated intravascular (DIC). See Disseminated intravascular coagulation (DIC)
  eicosanoids in, 1599-1600
Coagulation disorder(s). See also Bleeding (hemorrhage); Hemostasis
  acquired, 87-88
  in chronic hepatic disease, 1467-1468
  dilutional, 82, 87
  inherited, 86-87. See also specific types, e.g., Hemophilia
  laboratory assessment of, 88-89, 88f, 89t
  management of, prior to biliary tract procedures, 735
  thrombotic. See entries beginning Thrombo-
  in trauma patient, 44-45, 44f
  in uremic syndrome, 1058
Coagulation factor(s). See Factor(s)
Coagulation test(s), in preoperative evaluation, 537-538
Cocaine. See also Substance abuse
  abuse of, emergency management of, 174-175
  in acute exposure, 174-175
  in chronic use, 175
  in withdrawal, 175
Coccidioides immitis infection, antimicrobial agents for, 1199t
Coccidioidomycosis, 1293t
Codeine, in pregnancy, 1155
Cognitive and sensory defect(s), 158-163. See also Coma; Delirium; Dementia
  agitation in, management of, 162-163
  delirium in, 159-160, 159t-160t
  dementia in, 160-161, 160t-161t
  depression in, 161, 161t
  diagnosis and management of, 159-160
  due to pharmacologic therapy, 162
  head injury in, 161-162, 162t
  perioperative, care in, 158-159, 158t
  postoperative intervention for, in elderly patients, 1104
Cold injury, 510-511. See also Heat loss; Hypothermia
  chilblain (pernio), 511
  frostbite, 510-511, 510t-511t

immersion foot, 511
ophthalmic, 511
treatment of, 511f
trench foot, 511
Colectomy
  laparoscopic, 837-842
    complications of, 841
    indications for, 837
    for left hemicolectomy and sigmoid resection, 839, 840f
    operative planning in, 837
    operative techniques in, 837-839, 838f-840f
    outcome evaluation in, 841
    postoperative care in, 840
    for right hemicolectomy, 837-838, 838f-839f
    troubleshooting in, 840-841
  total, with ileorectal anastomosis, 825-828
    anastomosis technique in, 827, 828f
    completion of, 827
    complications of, 827
    indications for, 825
    mobilization and removal of colon for, 825-827, 826f-827f
    operative planning for, 825
    operative technique in, 825-827
    outcome in, 827-828
    positioning and incision for, 825
Colforsin, for heart failure, 1395
Colistimethate, for bacterial infections, 1204t-1205t
Colitis
  antibiotic-associated, 1229-1230
    clinical and laboratory diagnosis of, 1171
    Clostridium difficile in, 1229
    incidence of, 1233-1234
    diagnosis of, 1229
    drugs implicated in, 1229-1230
    pseudomembranes in, 1229, 1229f
    treatment of, 1230
  pseudomembranous. *See* Colitis, antibiotic-associated
  ulcerative
    appendix in, 822
    eicosanoids and, 1600
    in pregnancy, 1152-1153
    zileuton for, 1600
Collagen
  in intestinal structure, 803
  in wound healing, 133-134
Colloid oncotic pressure, 102
Colloid solution(s). *See also* Fluid resuscitation
  for burn patients, 55-56
Coloanal anastomosis
  double-stapled end-to-end, 810-811
  in low anterior resection with coloproctostomy, 834. *See also* Coloproctostomy, low anterior resection with
Colon
  anastomosis for, 808
  angiodysplastic lesions of, colonoscopy for, 296f, 297
  bleeding in. *See* Lower gastrointestinal bleeding
  diverticulitis of, intestinal obstruction in, 276
  elective resection of, preoperative preparation for, 576t, 577

emergency operation of, preoperative preparation for, 578
metabolism of, nutrients in, 1514
obstruction of
  abdominal radiography in, 268, 269f-271f
  causes of, 267t
  complete, 272
  partial, 277
  in pregnancy, 1151
perforation of, surgical options for, 1244t
pseudo-obstruction of
  abdominal radiography in, 268, 269f
  chronic, 279
  management of, 278-279, 279f
  in pregnancy, 1151
sigmoid. *See under* Sigmoid
trauma to, 432-434
  colostomy for, 433-434
  closure of, 434
  gradation of injury in, 426t
  repair of, 409-410
  treatment algorithm for, 432f
Colonoscopy, 693-696
  for angiodysplastic lesions, 296f, 297
  for colonic bleeding, 695f, 696
  diagnostic, 693-695
  emergency, for lower gastrointestinal bleeding, 296f, 297
  for polyps, 695-696, 695f
  for stricture, 696
  therapeutic indications for, 695-696
Colony-stimulating factor(s)
  as biologic response modifiers, 1351
  granulocyte
    physical properties of, 1610t
    synonyms and cell sources of, 1604t
  granulocyte-macrophage
    physical properties of, 1610t
    synonyms and cell sources of, 1604t
  physical properties of, 1610t
  synonyms and cell sources of, 1604t
Coloproctostomy, low anterior resection with, 833-835
  coloanal anastomosis in, 834
  colorectal anastomosis in, 834
  complications of, 834
  operative planning for, 833
  operative technique in, 833-834, 834f
  outcome in, 834-835
  tumor assessment in, 833
Colorectal anastomosis, in low anterior resection with coloproctostomy, 834. *See also* Coloproctostomy, low anterior resection with
Colorectal procedure(s), 825-836. *See also individual procedures*
  abdominoperineal resection, 835-836
  low anterior resection with coloproctostomy, 833-835
  restorative proctocolectomy with ileoanal pouch, 830-833
  total colectomy with ileorectal anastomosis, 825-828

  total proctocolectomy with conventional ileostomy, 828-830
Colostomy
  for colon trauma, 433-434
  closure of, 434
  irrigation of, 1688, 1688f, 1689
  loop. *See also* Stoma(s)
    rigid bridges for, 1683, 1683f
    support for, 1683-1684, 1684f
Coma, 143-157. *See also* Head injury
  in aneurysmal subarachnoid hemorrhage, 150-151, 150t
    radiographic diagnosis of, 153, 153t, 153f
    treatment of, 156
  in cerebral abscess, 151
    radiographic diagnosis of, 153, 154f
    treatment of, 156-157
  in cerebral tumor, 150
    radiographic diagnosis of, 152, 152f
    treatment of, 156
  in diabetic ketoacidosis, 149
    treatment of, 156
  in electrolyte disturbances, 149
  emergency management of
    Algorithm, 144-145
  in substance abuse, 169-171
  in head injury, radiographic diagnosis of, 153-154, 154f-155f, 155t
  in hepatic encephalopathy, 149
  in hyperglycemia, uncontrolled, 149
  hyperglycemic hyperosmolar nonketotic, treatment of, 156
  hypoglycemic, 149
    treatment of, 156
  in hypothermia, 151
    treatment of, 157
  initial management of, 143-146
    airway in, 143
    breathing in, 143-146
    circulation in, 146
    glucose administration in, 146
    laboratory screening in, 146
  in intoxication, treatment of, 155-156
  in locked-in syndrome, 151
  in meningoencephalitis, 151
    radiologic diagnosis in, 153
    treatment of, 156-157
  metabolic, treatment of, 155-156
  pathophysiology of, 164-165, 165f
  in persistent vegetative state, 151
  physical and neurologic examination of, 146-148
    brain-stem reflexes in, 147-148
    caloric test for, 148
    corneal reflex in, 148
    doll's eye maneuver for, 147
    elevated intracranial pressure in, 148
    eye movements in, 147
    gag reflex in, 148
    level of consciousness in, 146, 147t
    localizing or lateralizing signs in, 146-147
    meningism in, 148
    pupillary size and response in, 147
    respiration in, 148
  prognosis in, 165

psychogenic, 151
radiographic diagnosis of
  CT in, 151-152
  MRI in, 151-152
radiologic diagnosis of, 151-154
  plain skull, 151, 152t
in stroke, 150
  radiographic diagnosis of, 152-153
  treatment of, 156
structural, 149-151, 149t
  treatment of, 156-157
toxic metabolic, 148-149, 149t
  treatment of, 155-157
in uremic encephalopathy, 149
Common bile duct
open exploration of, 740-742
  operative technique in, 740-741, 741f
  troubleshooting in, 741-742
stone(s). *See* Choledocholithiasis
stricture of, ERCP for, 693, 694f
trauma to, 419
Compartment syndrome, 474-476
causes and mechanism of, 475
definition of, 474-475
diagnosis of, 475
operative treatment of, 475-476, 475f-476f
Competency assessment, for elderly patient, 1097-1098
Complement system
defect in, 1083t
in host defense, 1347
tests for, 1074
Complete blood count (CBC)
in pregnancy, 1154
preoperative, 537
Computed tomography (CT)
in abdominal aortic aneurysm, 937-938, 938f-939f
in abdominal mass, 247, 247f
in abdominal trauma, in children, 1139-1141, 1140f-1141f
in coma, 151-152
in intestinal obstruction, 270-271, 273f-274f
in intra-abdominal abscess, 1248-1249, 1257, 1257f
in jaundice, 256
  due to malignant obstruction, 257
in maxillofacial injury, 373
in neck mass, 189
in pancreatitis, 1274f
in splenic abscess, 1274, 1275f
Confusion. *See also* Cognitive and sensory defect(s)
in infection, 1166
Congestive heart failure. *See also* Heart failure
in acute renal failure, fluid therapy precautions for, 1444
in elderly patients, 1095
as factor in selection for outpatient surgery, 542
pharmacokinetics in, 1707-1708
postoperative pulmonary insufficiency in, 1043
preoperative assessment of, 559-561
Consciousness, loss of, in blunt trauma, 349
Constipation, in pregnancy, 1158, 1159t
Contrast agent(s). *See* Radiographic contrast agent(s)

Contusion
in extremity trauma, 476
lung, in chest trauma, 1411-1412
myocardial, emergency management of, 37
Convalescence, postoperative, for elderly patient, 1097
COPD. *See* Chronic obstructive pulmonary disease (COPD)
Copper
in central venous nutritional support, 1532
requirements for, in ICU patient, 1525t
Copperhead bite(s), 126-127
Coral snake bite(s), 126-127
Corneal reflex, in coma, 148
Coronary air embolism, 397-398
Coronary angiography, in preoperative assessment, 562
Coronary artery bypass graft, preoperative assessment for, carotid bruit in, 203-204
Coronary artery circulation, in CPR, 20
Coronary artery disease
aspirin and, 1599
in elderly patients, 1094, 1094f
in obesity, 1003
radioisotope imaging in, 562
transfusion in, 83
Coronary care unit (CCU). *See* Intensive care unit (ICU)
Corticosteroid(s), 1066t
aerosolized, for burn patients, in immediate resuscitation period, 54
deficiency. *See* Adrenal insufficiency
as factor in selection for outpatient surgery, 542
fungal infections due to, clinical presentation and diagnosis of, 1293t
immunodeficiency due to, 1085-1086
properties of, 1088t
therapeutic, perioperative glucocorticoid management and, 1066-1067, 1068, 1087-1088
wound healing and, 137
Cortisol
in metabolic response to critical illness, 1509, 1509t
properties of, 1088t
in stress response, in burn patients, 498
Cortisone
glucocorticoid and mineralocorticoid activities of, 1066t
properties of, 1088t
Corynebacterium, JK group, antimicrobial agents for, 1197t
Corynebacterium diphtheriae infection, antimicrobial agents for, 1197t
Costal chondritis, in chest trauma, 404
Cost-effective nonemergency surgical care, 519-533
assessment of outcomes and, 521-522, 522t
challenges for academic health centers and, 529
determination of cost-effectiveness in, 528-529, 529t-530t

economics of surgical care in, 527-528
ethical and legal issues in, 529
evidence-based decision making and, 522-524
  critical literature analysis in, 523-524, 525t
  statistical analysis in, 522-523, 522f
  technology assessment in, 524, 526t
the future of, 530
performance assessment and, 525-527
preventive approaches and process measures in, 524-525
  coordination of care and disease management and, 524
  critical pathways and, 524-525
quality care and, 519-521, 520t, 521f
U.S. health care expenditures and, 519, 519t
Cough, in nosocomial pneumonia, 1655
Courvoisier sign, 236t
CPR. *See* Cardiopulmonary resuscitation (CPR)
Crack. *See* Cocaine; Substance abuse
Creatinine, serum, 1448
in acute renal failure, 1441
in burn patient, 57
in elderly patients, 1096, 1096f
Creatinine clearance, 1448
in renal failure, 1051
Cricothyrotomy
advantages and disadvantages of, 1404t
conversion to tracheotomy of, 392-393
in maxillofacial injury, 369
in neck injury, 379
technique for, 35f
in trauma resuscitation, 34, 35f
Critical care unit(s) (CCU). *See also* Intensive care unit (ICU)
Critical illness
gastrointestinal mucosa in, 1538-1539
metabolic response to. *See* Metabolic response to critical illness
multiorgan failure in. *See* Multiple organ dysfunction syndrome (MODS)
polyneuropathy of, in multiple organ dysfunction syndrome, 1480
Crohn disease
anal and perineal infections in, 848, 851, 852f, 853
appendix in, 822
eicosanoids and, 1600
in pregnancy, 1152-1153
resection in, anastomotic breakdown in, 803
strictureplasty for, 809
Crush injury, acute wound management for, 125
Cruveilhier sign, 236t
Cryoanalgesia, for postoperative pain relief, 1667, 1668f
Cryptococcosis, clinical presentation and diagnosis of, 1293t
Cryptococcus neoformans infection, antimicrobial agents for, 1199t
Crystalloid solution(s). *See also*

Fluid resuscitation
  for acute renal failure, 1444
  for burn patients, 55, 55t
  for trauma resuscitation, 43
CT. See Computed tomography (CT)
Cullen sign, 236t
Curling ulcer, gastric pH and, 489
Cushing syndrome
  adrenal insufficiency after surgical correction of, 1067-1068
  metabolic alkalosis in, 116
Cyanide toxicity
  in burn patient, 49-52
  nitroprusside causing, 112
  treatment of, 12
Cyanoacrylate tissue adhesive, for acute wound closure, 128
Cyst(s)
  branchial cleft, 190
  choledochal, resection of, 744-746
  ovarian, appendicitis vs., 822
  sebaceous, of neck, 191
  thyroglossal duct, 190
Cystic hygroma, 190
Cystitis, candidal, 1299
  in immunosuppressed patient, 1082
Cystostomy, suprapubic, for urethral trauma, 456-457
Cytokine(s), 1603-1622. See also specific cytokines, e.g., Tumor necrosis factor
  circulating levels of, 1607-1608
    after experimental infusion, 1608
    in infection, 1608
  clinical therapy with, 1613-1619, 1615f-1617f
  in different infectious states, 1511f
  in endotoxin administration, 1348
  in endotoxin tolerance, 1612
  exogenous administration of, 1619
  in host defense, 1348-1350
  as immunostimulants, 1352
  listing of, 1604t
  mediator interactions of, 1612, 1613f-1614f
  propagation of mediator cascade, 1612, 1613f-1614f
  synergism, 1612
  in metabolic response to critical illness, 1510-1511, 1511f
  modulation of responses to, 1613-1618, 1615f-1617f
    decreasing host tissue production, 1614-1618, 1617f
    nutritional methods for, 1614-1617, 1617f
    pharmacologic methods for, 1617-1618
    effector cell modulation, 1618
      pharmacologic methods for, 1618
      receptor antagonists as, 1357-1359, 1357t, 1618
      increasing clearance, 1618
      neutralization, 1618
        antibodies for, 1618
        soluble receptors for, 1618
      preventing injurious stimuli from reaching cell sources, 1613-1614
  names of, 134
  natural antagonists to, 1608-1611, 1616
    glucocorticoids as, 1608-1609

  in peritoneal infection, 1250, 1251
  physical properties of, 1616
  in stress response, in burn patients, 497
  tissue levels of, 1611-1612, 1611f
  in wound healing, 134-135, 133t
Cytomegalovirus immunoglobulin, for immunorepletion, 1356-1357
Cytomegalovirus infection, 1325-1327
  agents effective against, 1329t
  antimicrobial agents for, 1199t
  in immunosuppressed patient, prevention of, 1076t
  in transfusion, 1325-1326
    prevention and treatment of, 1326-1327
  in transplantation, 1326
    prevention and treatment of, 1326-1327

D

Dakin solution, contraindicated in acute wound care, 128
Dance sign, 236t
Danforth sign, 236t
Dantrolene, for malignant hyperthermia, 616-617
Dead space
  increased, causes of, 1418, 1418t
  physiologic (V_D), definition of, 1415
Dead space to tidal volume ratio (V_D/V_T), 1423
  definition of, 1415
Death, brain. See Brain death
Debridement
  of acute wound, 973
  of burn wound. See Burn wound care
  of necrotic tissue, in acute wound management, 125
Deep vein thrombosis. See Thrombosis, deep vein
Defibrillation. See Cardioversion (defibrillation)
Delayed-type hypersensitivity
  for evaluation of operative risk, 553-554, 554t-555t
  in surgical patients, 1074
Delirium, 159-160, 159t-160t
Delirium tremens, in alcohol withdrawal, 179
Demeclocycline, for bacterial infections, 1202t-1203t
Dementia, 160-161, 160t-161t
Depression, cognitive impairment in, 161, 161t
Dermopathy, diabetic, 995
Dexamethasone
  glucocorticoid and mineralocorticoid activities of, 1066t
  properties of, 1088t
Dextran
  for burn patients, 55-56
  for thromboembolic prophylaxis, 1034
Dextrose, intravenous, for altered mental state in substance abuse, 169-171
Dezocine, suggested dosing for, 1627t
Diabetes mellitus, 993-1002
  acute cholecystitis and, 1267-1268
  autonomic neuropathy in, 995

  cardiac autonomic neuropathy in, 995, 997
  criteria for diagnosis of, 993, 995t
  dermopathy in, 995
  diabetic foot in, 999
  evaluation in, 995-996
  as factor in selection for outpatient surgery, 542
  fungal infections in, clinical presentation and diagnosis of, 1293t
  gestational, diagnostic criteria for, 995t
  history in, 995
  immunodeficiency in, 1085
  insulin-dependent, 993
    prevention of, 1000
  insulin pumps for, 1000-1001
    benefits of, 1001
    complications of, 1001
    initiating therapy with, 1000-1001
  intraoperative management of, 997-998
    for elective major procedures, 997, 998t
    for emergency procedures, 998
    insulin and glucose administration in, 997-998, 998t
    metabolic effects of operation and anesthesia and, 997
    for minor procedures, 998, 998t
  laboratory tests in, 996
  lipodystrophy in, 996
  macular edema in, 995
  necrobiosis lipoidica diabeticorum in, 996
  nephropathy in, 995
  nomenclature in, 993
  non-insulin-dependent, 993
  in obesity, 1006-1007
  pancreas and islet cell transplantation in, 1001
  perioperative management of, Algorithm, 994
  peripheral neuropathy in, 995
  peripheral polyneuropathy in, 996
  physical examination in, 995-996
  postoperative complications of, 1640-1641
  postoperative management of, 999, 999t
    cardiovascular assessment in, 999
    infection and, 999
    insulin and glucose administration in, 999
    renal assessment in, 999
  preoperative management of, 996-997, 996t
    cardiovascular assessment in, 996-997
    metabolic monitoring in, 996
    renal assessment in, 996-997
  radiculopathy in, 996
  radiographic contrast studies in, 998
  renal dysfunction in, prevention of, 998
  retinopathy in, 995
  type I, 993
  type II, 993
  wound healing and, 137
Diabetic ketoacidosis. See Ketoacidosis, diabetic

Dialysis. *See* Hemodialysis;
  Peritoneal dialysis
Dialysis dementia, 1060
Dialysis disequilibrium syndrome,
  1060
Diamorphine, epidural, for
  postoperative pain relief, 1665t
Diaphragmatic hernia
  in infants and neonates, 1126
  emergency surgery in, 1129
  posttraumatic, 404
Diaphragmatic rupture, shock in, 68
Diaphragmatic trauma, 420-421
  complications of, 403-404
Diarrhea
  antibiotic-associated, 1229. *See
    also* Colitis, antibiotic-
    associated
  in enteric nutrition, 1529, 1530f
  quinolone for, 1215
Diazepam, preoperative, 544t
Diazoxide, for hypertension, 1638t
DIC. *See* Disseminated intravascular
  coagulation (DIC)
Dichloroacetate (DCA), for lactic
  acidosis, 119-120
Diclofenac, suggested dosing for,
  1628t
Dicloxacillin, 1196
  for bacterial infections, 1202t-
    1203t
Diet. *See also under* Nutrition
  ostomates and, 1679-1680
Dieulafoy lesion, management of
  bleeding in, 290
Digestive tract, selective
  decontamination of, 1477
Digitalis
  classification of, 23
  toxicity, automatic dysrhythmias
    and, 26, 26f
Dimethyl sulfoxide, as free radical
  scavenger, 1575-1576
Dimethylthiourea, as free radical
  scavenger, 1575-1576
Discharge planning, 1641-1644
  for acute care, 1641, 1642t
  care services for, 1641, 1641t
  discharge orders for, 1641
  discharge summary for, 1641
  extended care facilities and, 1642-
    1643
  hospice facilities and, 1643-1644
  for indigent patients, 1644
  in-home care and, 1642, 1643t
Disinfection
  of endoscopes, 1719
  of surgical instruments, 1719
Dislocation
  extremity, in blunt trauma, 352
  hip, 470-471
  knee, popliteal artery injury in,
    466, 466f
Disopyramide, classification of, 23
Disseminated intravascular
  coagulation (DIC), 82-83, 82t,
  87-88
  in acute cholangitis, 1269
  in chronic hepatic disease, 1468
Disulfiram-ethanol reaction, in
  chronic alcohol intoxication,
  177, 178
Diuretic(s)
  in burn patient, 58
  metabolic alkalosis due to, 116
  in renal failure, acute, 1451
Diverticulitis, colonic, intestinal
    obstruction in, 276
Diverticulum(a)
  duodenal, management of upper GI
    bleeding in, 290
  jejunal, management of upper GI
    bleeding in, 290
Dobbhoff tube, 1634
Dobutamine
  for heart failure, 1394
  for pulmonary edema, 1405
  receptor types stimulated by,
    1394t
Dog bite(s)
  acute wound care for, 126
  of hand, 1283-1285, 1285f
Doll's eye maneuver, for coma, 147
Dopamine
  for heart failure, 1394
  for hypovolemic shock, in infants,
    1122
  for multiple organ dysfunction
    syndrome, 1483
  for pulmonary edema, 1405
  receptor types stimulated by,
    1394t
Dopamine agonist(s), 1394t
Dopamine receptor(s), cardiovascular
  effects of, 1393t
Dopexamine
  for heart failure, 1394
  receptor types stimulated by,
    1394t
Doppler effect, 660
Dorsalis pedis artery, for systemic
  arterial catheterization, 1370
Doxorubicin, reactive oxygen
  metabolites created by, 1568
Doxycycline, for bacterial
  infections, 1202t-1203t
Drain(s)
  for acute wound closure, 129
  suction, postoperative management
    of, 1635
  surgical site infection and, 574
Drapes, impermeable, 571
Draping, for infection control in
  operating room, 601
Dressing(s)
  for acute wounds, 130-131
  scab as, 131
  for skin graft donor sites, 130
  for sutured wounds, 130-131
  wet-to-dry, 130
    for acute wound, 976
  wet-to-wet, 130
    for acute wound, 976
Droperidol
  as antiemetic, 614t
  preoperative, 544t
Drug administration, 1709-1710. *See
  also* Pharmacokinetics
  endotracheal, in CPR, 23
  initial dose in, 1709-1710
  loading dose in, 1710
  maintenance dose in, 1710
  route of, 1709
  selection in, 1709
  standard margin of safety for,
    1709
  steady-state plasma concentration
    in, 1710, 1711f, 1712t
  therapeutic index for, 1709
Drug-drug interaction(s), 1712-1713
  absorption in, 1712
  biotransformation in, 1713
  distribution in, 1713
  elimination in, 1713
Drug history, in evaluation of
  operative risk, 536
Drug intoxication. *See also*
  Substance abuse
  coma in, treatment of, 155-156
Drug therapy. *See also*
  Pharmacokinetics; *specific drugs*
  in acute renal failure,
    adjustments for, 1447
  acute renal failure due to, 1445,
    1446, 1450
  immunodeficiency due to, 1085-1086
  monitoring of, 1710-1712
    clinical response in, 1710-1711
    drug-related variables in, 1711
    plasma drug concentration in,
      1711-1712
  in pregnancy, 1155, 1156t
  preoperative
    as factor in selection for
      outpatient surgery, 541-542
    in high-risk patient, 563-564
Ductus arteriosus closure,
  eicosanoids in, 1598
Duodenal diverticulum(a), management
  of upper GI bleeding in, 290
Duodenal exclusion, with
  gastrojejunostomy, 426, 428f
Duodenal ulcer(s)
  chronic, upper GI bleeding in, 286-
    287, 287f
  perforated
    in pregnancy, 1151
    surgical options for, 1244t
Duodenopancreatic crunch, 426
Duodenum
  diverticulization of, 426, 427f
  injuries to, 425-426, 426t, 427f
  operative exposure of, in
    abdominal injury, 408
Duplex, ultrasonography for,
  asymptomatic carotid bruit, 200
Dural puncture, headache after, 613
Dynamic compliance (C_{dyn}),
  definition of, 1416
Dysfibrinogenemia, congenital, 1028-
  1029
Dysfibrinolysis, congenital, 1029-
  1030
Dyspnea. *See* Pulmonary insufficiency
Dysrhythmia(s). *See* Cardiac
  dysrhythmia(s)

E

Ear(s)
  examination of, in maxillofacial
    injury, 372
  external, injuries of, 374
Ebselen, as free radical scavenger,
  1576
Edema
  cerebral. *See also* Intracranial
    pressure
    in hepatic failure, 1460
  macular, diabetic, 995
  pulmonary. *See* Pulmonary edema
  subeschar
    of extremities, 61
    rehabilitation and, 1693
Education, for health care team, for
  infection control, 1724
Effusion
  pericardial
    in chest trauma, 403
    uremic, 1057

pleural, in chest trauma, 403
Eicosanoid(s), 1591-1602. *See also*
    Leukotriene; Prostaglandin;
    Thromboxane
  biochemistry of, 1591-1594
  biologic effects of, 1593-1598
  in ductus arteriosus closure, 1598
  in hemostasis and coagulation,
    1599-1600
  in ischemic injury, 1598-1599
  in mediation of inflammation, 1600
  physiologic roles of, 1598-1601
  precursors of, fatty acids as,
    1593f, 1594
  in protection of gastroduodenal
    mucosa, 1600-1601
  in regulation of blood flow, 1598
  renal blood flow and, 1598
  in stress response, in burn
    patients, 498
  synthesis of
    arachidonic acid metabolism in,
      1591-1593, 1592f-1593f
    oxygen free radicals and, 1594
  in uterine function, 1601
Eikenella corrodens
  antimicrobial agents for, 1198t
  in human bite wound, 126
Elderly patient, 1091-1120
  acute abdominal pain in, 232, 235t
  body composition of, 1110-1111,
    1111f
  burns in, 1093-1094
  clinical presentation in,
    alterations in, 1092-1094
  establishing rapport with, 1097
  functional assessment tools for,
    1092
  heatstroke in, 1553
  hemorrhoid management for, 843
  hospital milieu for, geriatrically
    adapted, 1105-1106
  immune function in, 1114
  intraoperative management of, 1099-
    1101
    anesthesia in, 1099-1100
      general, 1099, 1099f
      regional, 1100
    hypothermia in, 1100-1101
    monitoring in, 1100
    positioning in, 1099
  optimal functional level for,
    achievement of, 1092
  organ systems of, age-related
    changes in, 1111-1114
  oxygen delivery and consumption
    in, 1111-1113, 1112f-1113f
  pain threshold in, 1092-1093
  perioperative management of, 1106-
    1110
    clinical pharmacology in, 1106-
      1107, 1106t
    fluid, electrolyte, acid-base
      homeostasis in, 1107-1108
    nutritional support in, 1108-
      1110, 1108f-1111f
    pharmacokinetics in, 1106-1107,
      1106t, 1704-1705
  postoperative management of, 1101-
    1104
    activities of daily living and,
      1104
    cardiovascular monitoring in,
      1101-1102
    cognition and, 1104
    continence and, 1103-1104
    mechanical ventilation in, 1101

mobility and, 1102-1103, 1103t
    optimizing functional level in,
      1102-1104, 1102t
    pain management in, 1102
    respiratory care in, 1101
  preoperative management of, 1094-
    1098
    cardiovascular assessment in,
      1094-1095, 1094f
    congestive heart failure and,
      1095
    coronary artery disease and,
      1094, 1094f
    dysrhythmias and, 1095
    hypertension and, 1095
    informed consent and competency
      assessment in, 1097-1098
    myocardial infarction and, 1095
    planning for convalescence in,
      1097
    psychological preparation in,
      1096
    pulmonary function assessment
      in, 1095-1096
    renal assessment in, 1096, 1096f
    serum creatinine in, 1096, 1096f
  surgical care for
    factors for best outcome in,
      1091
    principles of, 1091-1094
  surgical risk assessment in, 1114-
    1115
    causes of postoperative
      mortality and, 1115
    medical and physiologic status
      and, 1115
    nature of surgical procedure
      and, 1114-1115
    studies on, 1114
  thermoregulation in, 1113
  trauma in, 1093-1094, 1093t
  wound healing in, 1113-1114
Elective surgery
  remote infection and, 570
  renal failure and, preoperative
    considerations in, 1055-1056
Electrical injury, 505-510
  high-voltage, 505-508
    cardiovascular injury in, 508
    diagnosis of, 505, 506f-507f
    escharotomy in, 507
    fasciotomy in, 507
    fluid management in, 506-507
    infection control in, 507
    managing entrance and exit sites
      in, 507-508
    monitoring in, 505-506
    muscle necrosis in, 505
    neurologic injury in, 508
    ocular injury in, 508
    orthopedic injury in, 508
    otic injury in, 508
    pulmonary injury in, 508
    renal injury in, 508
    wound management in, 507
  lightning, 509-510
    cardiovascular injury in, 510
    central nervous system injury
      in, 510
    diagnosis of, 510
    musculoskeletal injury in, 510
    ocular injury in, 510
    otic injury in, 510
    properties and effects of, 509-
      510
    skin injury in, 510
  low-voltage, 508-509, 509f

oral burns in, 508-509, 509f,
      509t
    terminology in, 514-515, 514t
    pathway of current, 514
    resistance, 514
    type and duration of current,
      515
    voltage and amperage, 514
  treatment of, 506f
Electrocardiography (ECG)
  in acute abdominal pain, 235
  in acute dysrhythmia, after
    resuscitation, 13-15, 18f
  in burn patient, 57
  in high-risk patient, 562-563
  in preoperative evaluation, 537,
    561-562
    ambulatory, 561
    exercise, 561-562
    resting, 561
Electrolyte(s)
  for central venous nutritional
    support, 1531, 1532t
  in parenteral fluids, 103t
  requirement for, in elderly
    patients, 1107
  serum
    postoperative evaluation of,
      1629
    preoperative evaluation of, 537
  total body, 94t
Electrolyte abnormality(ies)
  coma in, 149
  hypercalcemia. *See* Hypercalcemia
  hyperkalemia. *See* Hyperkalemia
  hypermagnesemia. *See*
    Hypermagnesemia
  hypernatremia. *See* Hypernatremia
  hypocalcemia. *See* Hypocalcemia
  hypokalemia. *See* Hypokalemia
  hypomagnesemia. *See* Hypomagnesemia
  hyponatremia. *See* Hyponatremia
  life-threatening, 91-106
    Algorithm, 92-93
    calcium status in, 96-100
    magnesium status in, 100-101
    potassium status in, 95-96
    sodium status in, 94-95
    volume status in, 91
  postoperative assessment of, 1632
Electrolyte status, in burn patient
  in early postresuscitation period,
    483
  in immediate resuscitation period,
    57
Electromechanical dissociation. *See*
    Pulseless electrical activity
    (PEA)
Electrosurgical devices, hazards of,
    594
Embolism
  air
    in chest trauma, 403
    coronary, 397-398
    emergency management of, 37-38
    shock in, 68-69
  arterial. *See* Arterial embolism
  missile, to heart, 397
  pulmonary. *See* Pulmonary embolism
Embolization, angiographic, for
    distal vertebral artery injury,
    392
Emergency management
  of head injury, 355-357
  of multiple injury, 337-353. *See*
    also Trauma, multiple
  of substance abuse, 169-180. *See*

also Substance abuse
Emergency operation
  in diabetes mellitus, 998
  in infants and neonates, 1129
  renal failure and, preoperative considerations in, 1056
Emesis. *See* Nausea and vomiting
EMLA, for anesthesia in wound closure, 127
Emphysema, postoperative pulmonary insufficiency in, 1043
Empyema
  of gallbladder, diagnosis of, 1269
  nosocomial, 1225
  pleural, in chest trauma, 403
Encephalopathy
  hepatic
    in chronic hepatic disease, 1465-1466, 1465t
    coma in, 149
    mechanisms of, 1469
  uremic, 1060
    coma in, 149
  Wernicke. *See* Wernicke-Korsakoff syndrome
Endoanal ultrasonography, 662
Endocarditis
  alpha-hemolytic streptococcal infection in, 1179
  antibiotic prophylaxis for, 573, 575t
  candidal, 1297
Endocrine dysfunction, in uremic syndrome, 1058
Endocrine evaluation
  in immunosuppression therapy, 1081
  preoperative, 536
Endophthalmitis, *Candida*
  in hematogenous candidiasis, 1294
  management of, 1297
  pathologic findings in, 1304, 1304f
Endorectal ultrasonography, 662, 662f
Endoscope(s), disinfection of, 1719
Endoscopic retrograde cholangiopancreatography (ERCP)
  for cholangitis, acute, 1270, 1270f
  for choledocholithiasis, 693, 693f
  for common bile duct stricture, 693, 694f
  diagnostic, 692, 692f-693f
  for gallstone pancreatitis, 1267, 1267f
  for jaundice, 254-255, 256f
  for malignant biliary obstruction, 693, 694f
  therapeutic, 693, 693f-694f
Endothelial xanthine oxidase, in intracellular signaling, 1580
Endothelium-derived relaxing factor. *See* Nitric oxide (endothelium-derived relaxing factor)
Endotoxin
  absorbed from gastrointestinal tract, 1347
  in absence of enteral nutrition, 1538
  in burn patients, 499
  cytokine response to, 1348
  gram-negative bacterial, biochemical structure of, 1354, 1354f
  host tolerance to, 1351-1352
  in metabolic response to critical illness, 1514-1515

  neutralization of, cytokine response modulation for, 1357-1359, 1357t, 1613-1614
  in stress response, in burn patients, 497
  TNF response to, 1511f
  tolerance to, cytokines in, 1357-1358, 1612
Endotracheal drug administration, in CPR, 23
Endotracheal extubation, timing of, 610
Endotracheal intubation, 1401-1404. *See also* Nasotracheal intubation; Orotracheal intubation
  in burn patients
    in early postresuscitation period, 479
    extubation guidelines in, 479
    in immediate resuscitation period, 53
  choice of route for, 1401-1404, 1404t
  complications of, 607-608
    aspiration, 607-608
    bronchospasm, 607
    hypertension, 608
    hypotension, 608
    laryngospasm, 607
    physical limitations, 607
  in CPR, 9
  indications for, 1401
  in induction of anesthesia, 606-607
  neuromuscular-blocking agents for, 607, 608t
  in infants and neonates, 1130, 1130t
  in maxillofacial injury, 369
  nosocomial pneumonia and, 1653-1654, 1654f
  obstruction in, shock in, 68
  postoperative, in pulmonary insufficiency, 1042
Enema, barium, contraindicated in lower gastrointestinal bleeding, 299
Enflurane, for maintenance anesthesia, 609t
Enoxacin, for bacterial infections, 1204t-1205t
Enoximone, for heart failure, 1395
Enterobacteriaceae bacteremia, 1179-1180. *See also specific organisms, e.g., Escherichia coli*
  antibiotic therapy in, 1180, 1180t
  identification of primary focus in, 1179-1180
Enterobacter infection, antimicrobial agents for, 1197t
Enteroclysis, in intestinal obstruction, 271
Enterococcal bacteremia, 1179
Enterococcal infection
  antimicrobial agents for, 1197t
  in peritonitis, 1252-1253
  vancomycin-resistant, 1179
Enterocolitis
  antibiotic-associated. *See* Colitis, antibiotic-associated
  necrotizing, in infants and neonates, 1128
  neutropenic, 1079
Enterocolostomy, double-layered sutured end-to-side, 810, 811f

Enteroenterostomy, single-layer sutured extramucosal side-to-side, 809-810, 810f
Enterostomal therapist(s), 1680
Entriflex tube, 1634
Epidermal growth factor, in experimental wound healing, 135
Epidural analgesia. *See* Analgesia, epidural
Epidural anesthesia. *See* Anesthesia, epidural
Epidural hematoma, emergency management of, 357
Epigastric hernia(s), 871
Epilepsy, classification of, 157, 157t
Epinephrine
  for asystole, 11, 21
  for CPR, 21
  discontinuance of, in lactic acidosis, 112
  for heart failure, 1394
  for pulseless electrical activity, 12-13, 11t
  receptor types stimulated by, 1394t
  for ventricular fibrillation, 10, 11t, 21
  for wound closure, 127
Epithelialization, in wound healing, 132-133
Epstein-Barr virus infection, 1327-1328
  transfusion-related, 1327
  in transplantation, 1327-1328
Erb-Duchenne paralysis, 1141
ERCP. *See* Endoscopic retrograde cholangiopancreatography (ERCP)
Erythromycin, 1211
  adverse effects of, 1208t, 1211
  for bacterial infections, 1204t-1205t
  in vivo drug interactions with, 1193t
Erythromycin estolate, for bacterial infections, 1204t-1205t
Erythropoietin
  recombinant, for uremic syndrome, 1058
  in red cell production, 1058, 1059f
Eschar, rigidity of, rehabilitation and, 1693
Escharotomy
  for chest wall, 54, 54f
  for electrical burns, 507
  for extremities, 61
Escherichia coli, antimicrobial agents for, 1197t
Esophageal atresia, in neonates, 1125
  emergency surgery in, 1129
Esophageal injury
  in chest trauma, 401, 401f
  complications of, 403-404
Esophageal manometry
  for left thoracoscopic myotomy, 702
  for Nissen fundoplication, 697
Esophageal procedure(s), minimally invasive, 697-706
Esophageal rupture, in pregnancy, 1149
Esophageal stricture(s), esophagogastroduodenoscopy for, 689-690, 689f
Esophageal tumors,

esophagogastroduodenoscopy for, 690, 690f
Esophageal varices
  esophagogastroduodenoscopy for, 688-689, 688f
  management of upper GI bleeding in, 287-289, 288f
  in portal hypertension, 1463, 1464t
Esophagectomy, video-assisted thoracic surgery for, 681-682, 682f
Esophagitis
  candidal, 1298, 1298f
  in immunosuppressed patient, 1076t, 1081, 1082
  in immunosuppression, 1078
Esophagogastroduodenoscopy, 687-692
  diagnostic, 687-688
    complications of, 688
    technique in, 687-688, 687f
  for esophageal stricture, 689-690, 689f
  for esophageal tumors, 690, 690f
  for foreign body retrieval, 690-691
  for nonvariceal hemorrhage, 689
  therapeutic, 688-692
  in upper GI bleeding, 286
  for variceal hemorrhage, 688-689, 688f
Esophagojejunostomy, Roux-en-Y, in total gastrectomy, 715-717, 716f
Esophagus
  exposure of, in neck trauma, 384
  Mallory-Weiss tears of, management of upper GI bleeding in, 289
Estrogen level(s), in pregnancy, 1153
Ethanol abuse. See Alcohol intoxication
Ethylene glycol ingestion, 177, 178
  metabolic acidosis in, 113
Ethylene oxide sterilization, hazards of, 598
Etidocaine, comparative pharmacology of, 612t
Etodolac, suggested dosing for, 1628t
Etomidate
  for elevated intracranial pressure, 358
  for induction of anesthesia, 607t
Euthyroid syndrome, sick, in multiple organ dysfunction syndrome, 1480
Exercise. See also Physical activity
  for burn rehabilitation, 1691-1692
Exercise tolerance test, in preoperative evaluation, 550
Extended care facility(ies), 1642-1643
Extracorporeal life support (ECLS), in acute respiratory failure, 1439
Extracorporeal membrane oxygenation (ECMO), in acute respiratory failure, 1438-1439
Extremity(ies)
  arterial embolism of, 1022, 1024f
  burns of, initial wound management for, 61
  lower
    amputation of, 949-958. See also Amputation
    above-the-knee, 956-957, 956f-957f
    below-the-knee, 954-956, 954f-955f
    flaps for defects of, 981
    fracture of, 470-474
    prosthesis for, below-the-knee amputation and, 955
    pulseless, in blunt trauma, 349-350
  upper
    flaps for defects of, 979-980
    fracture of, 470
Extremity trauma, 463-477. See also Fracture(s)
  Algorithm, 464
  blood vessel injury in, 465-466, 465f-466f
    in blunt trauma, 465-466, 466f
    in penetrating trauma, 465
  dislocation, in blunt trauma, 352
  fracture of, in blunt trauma, 352
  initial assessment in, 463-465
  mangled extremity in, 477
  nerve injury in, 466-467, 467t
    classification of, 466-467, 467t
    treatment of, 467
  penetrating, emergency management of, 344-345, 346f
  Roberts Jones dressing for, 465
  secondary evaluation in, 463-465
  soft tissue injury in, 476-477
  splinting for, 463-465
  temporizing of fracture-dislocation in, 463-465
Eye(s), trauma to. See Ocular injury
Eyebrow(s), injuries of, 374
Eyelid(s), injuries of, 374
Eye movement(s), in coma, 147

F

Facial defect(s), flaps for, 979, 981f
Facial examination, in maxillofacial injury, 371-372, 371f-372f
Facial nerve injury
  in birth trauma, 1141
  in maxillofacial trauma, 373
Facial trauma. See Maxillofacial injury
Factor(s). See also under Coagulation
  in coagulopathy, 87
Famciclovir, for herpesvirus infections, 1328
Family, preoperative conference with, for nonemergency surgery, 543
Family support
  for ostomates, 1679
  postoperative, for elderly patients, 1104
Fascial compartment syndrome, in arterial embolism, 1033
Fasciitis, necrotizing. See Necrotizing fasciitis
Fasciotomy
  for crush injury, 125
  for electrical burns, 507
Fatty acid(s)
  as eicosanoid precursors, 1594, 1593f
  omega-3
    in degenerative vascular disease, 1594
    in eicosanoid synthesis, 1593f
    in supplemental nutritional support, 1545-1546
  omega-6, 1594
    in eicosanoid synthesis, 1593f
    in supplemental nutritional support, 1545-1546
  in supplemental nutritional support, 1544-1545
Fatty liver of pregnancy, acute, 1458
Fecal examination, for blood, in preoperative evaluation, 538
Fecal impaction, intestinal obstruction in, 274
Fecal incontinence, postoperative, in elderly patients, 1103-1104
Feet. See Foot
Felon, 1282, 1282f
Femoral artery, for systemic arterial catheterization, 1370
Femoral head fracture, 471, 471f
Femoral hernia, classification of, 857, 858f
Femoral hernioplasty, classic, 862-863, 862f
Femoral neck fracture, 471-472, 471f
Femoral shaft fracture, 472-473, 473f
Fenoldopam, receptor types stimulated by, 1394t
Fenoprofen, suggested dosing for, 1628t
Fentanyl
  epidural, for postoperative pain relief, 1665t
  in induction of anesthesia, 607t
  in patient-controlled analgesia, 1668t
  preoperative, 544t
  suggested dosing for, 1627t
Fetal monitoring, 1156-1157
Fetus. See also Pregnancy
  pharmacokinetics in, 1703-1704
Fever and hyperpyrexia, 1549-1557. See also Heatstroke; Malignant hyperthermia; Temperature
  acute abdominal pain and, 231
  emergency management of, *Algorithm*, 1550-1551
  in endocrine excess, 1554
  in hypothalamic pathology, 1554
  hypothalamic set-point elevation in, 1552, 1552f
  in infection and inflammation, 1166, 1552-1553, 1552t
  life-threatening
    causes of, 1549-1552
    management of, 1549-1552
  morbidity and mortality in, 1549f
  oxygen consumption in, 1420
  in pheochromocytoma, 1554
  postoperative, 1166, 1636-1637. See also Sepsis, in absence of infection
    incidence of, 1231
    infectious cause of vs., 1166, 1498
  in laparoscopic cholecystectomy, 768
  in nosocomial infection, 1221
  prostaglandin E_2 in, 1597
  in thyrotoxic crisis, 1554
  treatment of, 1498-1499, 1552-1554, 1552t
  in upper abdominal infection. See Upper abdominal infection
Fibrillation, ventricular. See Ventricular fibrillation

Fibrin glue, for acute wound closure, 128-129
Fibroblast growth factor, basic, in experimental wound healing, 135
Fibromuscular dysplasia, of internal carotid artery, 932-933, 932f-933f
Fibular fracture, 474
Financial support, ostomates and, 1679
Fine-needle aspiration biopsy
  of breast, 629-630
  of neck mass, 189
Finger(s). See also under Hand(s)
  defects of, flaps for, 980
Fistula
  anal. See Anal fistula
  aortoenteric, management of bleeding in, 290
  arteriovenous, in chest trauma, 403
Flail chest
  alveolar hypoventilation in, 1419
  in chest trauma, 1411
Flap(s), 986-989. See also Skin graft(s)
  for abdomen, 980
  for acute wound care, 130
  for arm, forearm, 979-980
  axial, 130
  blood supply for, 986-989, 987f-988f
  for chest, back, 979
  for foot, 982
  free, 977-979, 977f, 978t
    no-reflow concept, 989
    postoperative care of, 985
  for gluteal area, perineum, 981
  for hand, 980
  for head, neck, 979, 981f
  for knee, proximal leg, mid-leg, 981
  latissimus dorsi myocutaneous, for breast reconstruction, 641-642, 641f
  local, 977-979, 977f, 978t, 979f
    postoperative care of, 984
  for mastectomy, 637
  nomenclature for, 986
  for plastic surgical reconstruction, 977-982, 978t
  random, 130
  resistance to infection of, 989
  for thigh, 981
  TRAM, for breast reconstruction, 640f, 641-642
Flexor tenosynovitis, suppurative, of hand, 1282-1283, 1283f-1284f
Flora. See Microflora
Flubiprofen, suggested dosing for, 1628t
Fluconazole, 1301, 1301t-1302t
  for candidiasis, 1295, 1295t
Flucytosine, 1300-1301, 1301t
Fludrocortisone, glucocorticoid and mineralocorticoid activities of, 1066t
Fluid(s)
  body, total, 101
  extracellular, 101, 102f
    age as factor in, 1124, 1126f
    electrolyte content of, 103t
    in hyperdynamic state of critical illness, 1501
    osmotic pressure and, 102
  intracellular, 101, 102f
    age as factor in, 1124, 1126f

osmotic pressure and, 102
  mixed volume and concentration changes, 104-105
  parenteral, electrolyte content of, 103t
  pathophysiologic changes in, 102-106
    calcium metabolism and, 105-106. See also Hypercalcemia; Hypocalcemia
    magnesium metabolism and, 106. See also Hypermagnesemia; Hypomagnesemia
    potassium concentration and, 105. See also Hyperkalemia; Hypokalemia
    sodium concentration and, 104-105. See also Hypernatremia; Hyponatremia
    volume disturbances as, 103
  plasma, 101, 102f
  requirement for, in elderly patients, 1107
Fluid challenge, for intravascular volume status, 1631
Fluid loss. See also Fluid volume deficit
  evaporative, in burn patients, 482, 483f
  insensible
    in hyperdynamic state of critical illness, 1501
    in infants and neonates, 1126
Fluid management. See Fluid resuscitation
Fluid overload. See Fluid volume excess
Fluid resuscitation
  for burn patients. See also under Burn care, in immediate resuscitation period
    in early postresuscitation period, 482-483
    in immediate resuscitation period, 55-56, 55t
  for electrical burns, 506-507
  for infants and neonates, 1122-1128
  in multiple organ dysfunction syndrome, 1476, 1483
  in peritonitis, 1242
  postoperative, 1629-1634, 1630t
    isotonic vs. hypotonic, 1630
    maintenance, 1629-1630, 1630t
Fluid therapy. See Fluid resuscitation
Fluid volume deficit
  bolus of crystalloid for expansion in, 1444
  calculation of, 95
  extracellular, 103
    evaluation and treatment of, 91
    hyponatremia and, 104
  intravascular, in acute renal failure, 1441-1444
  postoperative, 1631
  postoperative pulmonary insufficiency in, 1043
Fluid volume excess
  in cardiogenic pulmonary edema, 1405
  extracellular, 103
    evaluation and treatment of, 91
    hypernatremia and, 104
    hyponatremia and, 104
  postoperative, 1631-1632
Flumazenil, for altered mental

state, in substance abuse, 171
Fluosol-DA, for trauma resuscitation, 44
Foley catheterization
  in high-risk patient, 562
  postoperative management of, 1636, 1637f
  urinary tract infection due to, 1636
Folic acid, requirements for, in ICU patient, 1524t
Foot
  amputation of, transmetatarsal, 951-953, 953f
  defects of, flaps for, 982
  diabetic, 999
  immersion, 511
  trench, 511
Forced expiratory volume (FEV), preoperative, 1039
  in elderly patient, 1095-1096
Forced vital capacity (FVC), preoperative, 1039
Forearm defect(s), flaps for, 979-980
Foreign body(ies)
  in acute wound, timing of closure for, 124-125
  esophagogastroduodenoscopy for, 690-691
  immunodeficiency due to, 1085
  in immunosuppressed patient, 1082
  removal of, in initial burn care, 59-60
Formula(s), infant, 1132t
Foscarnet, for herpesvirus infections, 1329-1330
Fothergill sign, 236t
Fournier gangrene, of scrotum, 329, 329f
Fractional extraction of sodium (FENa), in acute renal failure, 1053, 1445, 1445t
Fracture(s). See also under anatomic location; Extremity trauma
  acetabular, 470-471
  clavicle, in birth trauma, 1141
  closed, 470-474
  extremity
    in blunt trauma, 352
    lower, 470-474
    upper, 470
  femoral head, 471, 471f
  femoral neck, 471-472, 471f
  femoral shaft, 472-473, 473f
  fibular, 474
  frontal sinus, 375
  hip, 471-472, 471f
  intertrochanteric and subtrochanteric, 471f-472f, 472
  knee, intra-articular, 473
  Le Fort, 375f-376f, 376
  mandibular, 372f, 376-377, 376f
  maxillary, 375f-376f, 376
  nasal, 371f, 375
  naso-orbito-ethmoidal, 375
  open, 467-470
    classification of, 468, 468t
    evaluation of, 468
    stabilization of, 469-470
    treatment of, 468, 469f
    wound care in, 468-469, 469f
  orbital, 375
  patellar, 473
  pelvic. See Pelvic fracture
  pilon, 474

rib, alveolar hypoventilation in, 1419
tibial, 473-474
zygoma, 371f, 375
Francisella tularensis infection, antimicrobial agents for, 1198t
Frank-Starling relation, 1399
Free radical(s), 1561t. *See also* Oxygen metabolite(s), reactive
in Alzheimer disease, 1583
in ARDS, 1583-1584
biochemistry of, 1559-1560
in central nervous system toxicity, 1583
in disease processes, 1583-1584
in familial amyotrophic lateral sclerosis, 1583
in multiple organ dysfunction syndrome, 1584
in oxygen toxicity, 1583
in Parkinson disease, 1583
in reperfusion injury, 1573-1583. *See also* Reperfusion injury
in shock, 1584
Frontal sinus fracture, 375
Frostbite, 510-511, 510t-511t
Functional assessment tools, for elderly patient, 1092
Functional residual capacity (FRC)
definition of, 1416
in general anesthesia, 609
preoperative, 1041
Fundoplication
Nissen. *See* Nissen fundoplication, laparoscopic
partial (Guarner), 702
Fungal infection, 1289-1307. *See also specific pathogens, e.g., Candida*
Algorithm, 1290-1291
clinical presentation and diagnosis of, 1293t
emerging, 1300
in surgical patient, magnitude of problem, 1289
systemic antifungal agents for, 1300-1302, 1301t-1302t
Fungal translocation, gastrointestinal, in candidiasis, 1303-1304
Fungemia, in surgical patients, 1181
Furosemide, for acute renal failure, 1451
Fusobacterium infection, antimicrobial agents for, 1198t

G

Gag reflex, in coma, 148
Galactorrhea, 213
Gallamine, in renal failure, contraindicated, 1056
Gallbladder
empyema of, diagnosis of, 1269
gangrene of, in acute cholecystitis, 1267-1268
trauma to, 419-420
Gallium nitrate, for hypercalcemia, 98
Gallstone(s). *See* Choledocholithiasis
Gallstone pancreatitis. *See* Pancreatitis, gallstone
Ganciclovir, for herpesvirus infections, 1329
Ganglionic blocking agent(s), for heart failure, 1393
Gangrene. *See also* Necrotizing infection
of gallbladder, in acute cholecystitis, 1267-1268
of hand, 1285-1286
postoperative progressive bacterial, Meleney, 317, 316f-317f
of scrotum
Fournier, 329, 329f
idiopathic, 329
streptococcal, 325, 326t
Gardnerella vaginalis infection, antimicrobial agents for, 1198t
Gasoline, causing chemical burns, 52t
Gastrectomy
subtotal, for cancer, 717
total, for cancer, 715-717, 716f
Gastric acid
aspiration of. *See* Aspiration, acid
neutralization of, in multiple organ dysfunction syndrome, complications of, 1482
Gastric aspirate. *See* Aspiration, of gastric contents
Gastric banding, laparoscopic adjustable
complications of, 723f, 724
for morbid obesity, 722-724, 722f-723f
operative technique for, 723, 723f
outcome evaluation in, 724
troubleshooting for, 723-724
Gastric bypass
laparoscopic
complications of, 732
hand-assisted, 730-731
for morbid obesity, 727-732, 728f-731f
postoperative care after, 731-732
total intracorporeal, 728-730, 728f
anastomosis in, 730
closure in, 730, 731f
gastrojejunostomy (circular stapling) in, 730
gastrojejunostomy (linear stapling) in, 730
initial access and trocar placement in, 728, 728f
linear stapling in, 729
Roux limb and jejunojejunostomy in, 729-730
stapling in gastric pouch in, 728-729
stomach dissection and gastric pouch in, 728, 728f
proximal
assessment of anastomosis in, 726-727
closure in, 727
complications in, 727
division of mesentery and stomach dissection in, 725, 725f
gastric stapling and gastrojejunostomy in, 726
initial incision and abdominal exploration in, 724-725
mobilization of esophagus in, 725
for morbid obesity, 724-727, 724f-726f
operative technique for, 724-727, 725f-726f
outcome evaluation in, 727
roux limb and jejunojejunostomy in, 725-726
Gastric colonization. *See* Gastrointestinal tract, bacterial overgrowth of
Gastric content(s), aspiration of. *See under* Aspiration
Gastric distention, in gastric bypass for obesity, 1006
Gastric insufflation, in assisted ventilation, 7, 8f
Gastric juice, normal volume and composition of, 103t
Gastric lavage, for emergency management, of substance abuse, 173
Gastric outlet obstruction, abdominal radiography in, 268
Gastric pH
Curling ulcer and, 489
preoperative H_2-receptor blockers for, 606
Gastric procedure(s), 707-719. *See also individual types, e.g., Vagotomy*
Gastric resection, distal subtotal (antrectomy), 712-715
Billroth I reconstruction after, 713-714, 713f
Billroth II reconstruction after, 714, 714f
difficult duodenal stump in, 714-715
procedure for, 712, 712f
Roux-en-Y jejunal limb in, 715
Gastric ulcer(s)
chronic, upper GI bleeding in, 287, 287f
drug-induced, NSAIDs causing, 1600-1601
perforated, surgical options for, 1244t
Gastric varices
management of upper GI bleeding in, 288f, 289
in portal hypertension, 1463, 1464t
Gastritis
acute hemorrhagic, management of, 289
NSAIDs causing, 1600-1601
Gastrointestinal bleeding
enteral nutrition in, 1526
lower. *See* Lower gastrointestinal bleeding
in occult infection, 1167
postoperative, 1640
pulseless electrical activity in, 12t
upper. *See* Upper gastrointestinal bleeding
Gastrointestinal dysfunction
in dialysis patients, 1057-1058
enteral nutrition in, nutritional formula for, 1527
in uremic syndrome, 1057-1058
Gastrointestinal endoscopy, 687-696
ultrasonography in, 662, 662f
upper. *See also* Esophagogastroduodenoscopy
for upper GI bleeding, 286
Gastrointestinal malignancy, management of bleeding in, 289

Gastrointestinal neoplasm(s),
  benign, management of bleeding
    in, 289
Gastrointestinal secretion(s),
  normal volume and composition
    of, 103t
Gastrointestinal tract. See also
    under Gut
  bacterial translocation from, 1347
    in absence of enteral nutrition,
      1538
    in burn patients, 499
    in critical illness, 1513
    in multiple organ dysfunction
      syndrome, 1488
    recognition and management of,
      1182-1183
  barrier function of
    compromise of, 1182
    critical illness and, 1513, 1538-
      1539
    mechanisms of, 1182
  candidiasis of, 1298, 1298f
  endotoxin absorbed from, 1347
    in absence of enteral nutrition,
      1538
    in burn patients, 499
    in metabolic response to critical
      illness, 1503, 1513-1514
  microbial flora of. See Alimentary
    tract microflora
  nutrition and, enteral, 1513-1514,
      1538, 1539f
    bacterial translocation and,
      1538
    endotoxin absorption and, 1538
    glutamine in, 1539-1540
    pectin in, 1540
    supportive, 1539-1540
  ultrasonography of, 662, 662f
Gastrojejunostomy, duodenal
  exclusion with, 426, 428f
Gastroplasty, vertical banded, for
  morbid obesity, 721-722, 722f
Gastroschisis, in infants and
  neonates, emergency surgery in,
    1129
Gastrostomy
  for enteral nutrition, 1528-1529
  percutaneous endoscopic, 691-692,
    691f
  Stamm, 717-718, 718f
Gated blood-pool scanning, in
  preoperative evaluation, 550
Genital examination, in acute
  abdominal pain, 235
Genitourinary tract evaluation, in
  immunosuppression therapy, 1081
Genitourinary tract infection, in
  immunosuppression, 1078
Gentamicin, 1210
  for bacterial infections, 1202t-
    1203t
Gentamicin sulfate, for burn care,
  60t, 61
Geriatric patient. See Elderly
  patient
Gestational diabetes, diagnostic
  criteria for, 995t
Glasgow Coma Scale, 146, 147t
  in head injury, 355, 356t
Glomerular filtration rate (GFR),
  1448
  in renal failure, 1051
Glomerulonephritis, acute renal
  failure in, 1053
Glove(s)

double, 1720
  for infection control in operating
    room, 601-602
Glucagon
  in metabolic response to critical
    illness, 1509, 1509t
  in stress response, in burn
    patients, 498
Glucocorticoid(s)
  as cytokine antagonists, 1608-1609
  perioperative, for patients
    treated with steroids, 1066-
    1067, 1068, 1087-1088, 1087t
Glucocorticoid response, to injury,
  intestinal anastomotic healing
  and, 803-804
Glucose
  blood
    in burn patients, 57, 1502t
    preoperative evaluation of, 537
  in diabetes mellitus
    intraoperative, 997-998, 998t
    postoperative, 999, 999t
  hepatic synthesis of, 1507
    in critical illness, 1503, 1507
  insulin response to, age-related
    responses to, 1109, 1111f
  intravenous
    for coma management, 146
    thiamine deficiency and, 146
  plasma, in normal vs. trauma
    patients, 1507, 1507t
Glucose tolerance, impaired. See
    also Diabetes mellitus,
    Hyperglycemia
  in critical illness, 1502, 1502t,
    1507
  diagnostic criteria for, 995t
Glutamine, in critical illness, 1506-
  1507
Glutamine-supplemented nutritional
  support, 1543-1544
  for burn patients, 499
  for critical illness, 1515-1516
  intestinal mucosal effects of,
    1514, 1539-1540
Gluteal area defect(s), flaps for,
  981
Goiter(s), nodular, 191
Gowns, impermeable, 571
Graft(s), skin. See Skin graft(s)
Gram-negative infection. See also
    under specific organisms, e.g.,
    Escherichia coli
  antiendotoxin therapy for, 1353-
    1356
Gram-positive cocci. See under
    Staphylococcal; Streptococcal
Granulocytopenia, management of,
  1079
Great vessel(s). See also Aorta
  of abdomen, traumatic injury to,
    437-447
  traumatic injury to, complications
    of, 403
Grey Turner sign, 237t
Groin, superficial and radical
  dissection of, in melanoma, 309-
    311, 309f-310f
Groshong catheter. See Central
  venous catheterization
Growth hormone
  for burn therapy, 499
  for metabolic response to critical
    illness, 1516
  in stress response, in burn
    patients, 498

Guarner (partial) fundoplication,
  702
Gunpowder explosion, acute wound
  management after, 124
Gut. See also Gastrointestinal tract
Gut barrier function. See
    Gastrointestinal tract, barrier
    function of
Gut decontamination, selective, as
  immunostimulation, 1353
Gut metabolism, in response to
  critical illness, 1503, 1513-
    1514
Gynecologic procedure(s)
  antibiotic prophylaxis for, 572
  pain relief after, 1662

H

H_2-receptor blocker(s)
  in enteral nutrition,
    contraindicated, 1530
  preoperative, 545
  to increase gastric pH, 606
Hallucinogen(s). See LSD; PCP
Hallucinosis, in alcohol withdrawal,
  178, 180
Halothane
  for maintenance anesthesia, 609t
  in renal failure, 1056
Hand(s), anatomy of, 1279-1280,
  1279f
Hand defect(s), flaps for, 980
Hand infection, 1279-1287
  bite wound, 1283-1285, 1285f
  cellulitis in, 1281
  felon, 1282, 1282f
  fungal, 1286
  gas-forming, 1285-1286
  general principles of treatment
    of, 1281
  herpetic whitlow, 1285f, 1286
  history and physical examination
    in, 1280
  lymphangitis in, 1281
  midpalmar space, 1283, 1284f
  mycobacterial, 1286
  necrotizing soft tissue, 1285
  osteomyelitis, 1285
  paronychia, 1281-1282, 1281f-1282f
  pathogens in, 1279, 1280t
  septic arthritis, 1285
  splinting in, hand position for,
    1281, 1281f
  sporotrichosis, 1286
  suppurative flexor tenosynovitis,
    1282-1283, 1283f-1284f
  thenar space, 1283, 1284f
  Trichophyton rubrum, 1286
  viral, 1285f, 1286
  web space, 1283, 1284f
Handwashing
  antiseptics for, 1719
  encouraging, 1719
Headache, post-dural puncture, 613
Head and neck procedure(s),
  antibiotic prophylaxis for, 572
Head defect(s), flaps for, 979, 981f
Head injury, 355-358. See also Coma
  blood flow regulation in, 363
    CO_2 reactivity and, 363
    metabolic autoregulation and,
      363
    pressure autoregulation and, 363
    viscosity autoregulation and,
      363

INDEX — 1765

cerebral circulation and
  metabolism after, 363-365
 altered cerebral metabolism and,
   365
 arterial hypoxia and hypotension
   and, 363-364
 cerebral blood volume,
   intracranial pressure,
   cerebral blood flow and, 364
 cerebral ischemia and, 364-365,
   365t
 raised intracranial pressure
   and, 364
 vessel diameter, cerebral blood
   volume, intracranial
   pressure and, 364
cerebral metabolism in, 363
cognitive impairment in, 161-162,
  162t
coma in, radiographic diagnosis
  of, 153-154, 154f-155f, 155t
emergency department management
  of, 355-357
Glasgow Coma Scale in, 355, 356t
ICU management of, 357-358
 brain protection in, 358
 cerebral perfusion pressure in,
   357-358
 hemoglobin, hematocrit, blood
   viscosity in, 358
 intracranial pressure management
   in, 358
 intracranial pressure monitoring
   in, 357
 jugular bulb oximetry in, 357,
   357t
 monitoring in, 357
incidence of, 355
initial management of, 355-356,
  356t, 356f
intracranial hypertension in, 356
operative management of, 356-357
orotracheal intubation in, 355
Head tilt, for airway patency, 6, 6f
Health care personnel
 abortion in, anesthesia exposure
   causing, 600
 education for, for infection
   control, 1724
 health status of, 1719-1722
 hepatitis in, 1323-1324, 1324t-
   1325t, 1340
 hepatitis precautions for, 1340,
   1720-1721, 1720t
 HIV precautions for, 1309-1312,
   1339-1340, 1720t, 1721
 immunizations for, 1344, 1720
 isolation procedures and, 1721
 tuberculosis precautions for, 1721
Heart
 as donor organ, 961
  technique for, 963-964, 964f
 herniation of, in chest trauma,
   403
 missile emboli to, 397
 reperfusion injury in, 1576-1577
 traumatic injury to, 396-398, 396f-
   397f
  complex, 396
  complications of, 403
  simple, 396
  special considerations in, 397-
    398
Heartburn, in pregnancy, 1158, 1159t
Heart disease
 as factor in selection for
   outpatient surgery, 542

 ischemic. *See* Coronary artery
   disease
 valvular, in preoperative
   evaluation, 559
Heart failure, 1391-1400
 afterload-reducing agents for,
   1391-1393
 approach to, **Algorithm,** 1392
 cardiac index in, 1391
 central venous pressure in, 1391
 inotropic agents for, 1393-1396
 intra-aortic balloon
   counterpulsation for, 1396
 pulmonary arterial occlusion
   pressure in, 1391
Heart-lung, as donor organ, 961
Heart rate, in infection, 1166
Heat loss. *See also* Cold injury;
  Hypothermia
 in burn patient, control of, 488
 evaporative, metabolic rate and,
   1505, 1505t
Heat overload syndrome(s), 1553
Heat shock response, in
  intracellular signaling, 1580
Heatstroke, 1553
 complications of, 1553
 in elderly patients, 1553
 in healthy, exercising patients,
   1553
 thermoregulation in, patient
   control of, 1557
 treatment of, 1553
Helicobacter pylori infection,
  antimicrobial agents for, 1197t
Hemangioma, in differential
  diagnosis of neck mass, 190-191
Hemarthrosis, in extremity trauma,
  477
Hematocrit
 in acute abdominal pain, 235
 in burn patient, 57
 in head injury, 358
Hematologic dysfunction. *See also*
  specific disorders, e.g., Anemia
 in uremic syndrome, 1058-1059,
   1059f
Hematologic evaluation
 in immunosuppression therapy, 1082
 preoperative, 536
Hematoma(s)
 epidural, emergency management of,
   357
 posterior fossa, emergency
   management of, 357
 retroperitoneal, 406, 406f
Hematuria
 in blunt trauma, 352
 in renal trauma, 449
Hemicolectomy
 left, laparoscopic, 839, 840f
 right, laparoscopic, 837-838, 838f-
   839f
Hemobilia, management of bleeding
  in, 290
Hemoccult testing, in preoperative
  evaluation, 538
Hemodialysis. *See also* Peritoneal
  dialysis
 for acute renal failure, 1447
 continuous arteriovenous, for
   multiple organ dysfunction
   syndrome, 1483
 continuous venovenous, for
   multiple organ dysfunction
   syndrome, 1483
 dialysis dementia in, 1060

 dialysis disequilibrium syndrome
   in, 1060
 gastrointestinal dysfunction in,
   1057-1058
 for prevention of uremic bleeding,
   1058-1059
 vascular access for. *See* Vascular
   access
Hemodynamic management
 for burn patients
  after first postburn week, 494-
    499
  in early postresuscitation
    period, 482-483
  in immediate resuscitation
    period, 54-58
 in multiple organ dysfunction
   syndrome, 1473-1477
 preoperative, clonidine for, 606
Hemodynamic monitoring. *See also*
  Cardiopulmonary monitoring
 central venous. *See* Central venous
   catheterization; Central
   venous pressure
 pulmonary arterial. *See* Pulmonary
   arterial pressure; Pulmonary
   arterial (Swan-Ganz)
   catheterization
 systemic arterial. *See* Systemic
   arterial catheterization;
   Systemic arterial pressure
Hemoglobin level
 in burn patient, 57
 in head injury, 358
 oxygen delivery and, decreased,
   1420
 P_{50}, 1414
Hemoperitoneum, in birth trauma,
  1141
Hemophilia, 80, 81t
 directed therapy in, 81t
 HIV seropositivity in, incidence
   of, 1333
Hemophilia A, 86
Hemophilia B (Christmas disease), 86
Hemophilus ducreyi infection,
  antimicrobial agents for, 1198t
Hemophilus influenzae infection
 antimicrobial agents for, 1198t
 in cellulitis, 321, 321f
Hemophilus influenzae pneumonia,
  nosocomial, 1649
Hemophilus species, in human bite
  wound, 126
Hemorrhage. *See* Bleeding
  (hemorrhage)
Hemorrhoid(s)
 anal symptoms *vs.*, 843, 844t
 external, 843, 843f, 845-846, 846f
 internal, 843, 843f, 844-845, 845f
 operative management of, 843-848
  bleeding after, 847
  complete hemorrhoidectomy for,
    846, 847f
  complications of, 847-848
  elastic ligation for, 844-845,
    845f
  elderly patients and, 843
  infection after, 847
  intravenous sedation and local
    anesthesia for, 844, 845f
  outcome of, 848
  planning in, 843-844, 843f
  positioning for, 844, 844f
  sphincterotomy for, 844
  stricture after, 848
  technique in, 844-847, 844f-847f

troubleshooting in, 847
urinary retention after, 848
young patients and, 843
in pregnancy, 1158-1159, 1159t
Hemorrhoidectomy, complete, 846, 847f
Hemostasis, 84-86. *See also* Bleeding (hemorrhage); Coagulation disorder(s)
  cellular components of, 84-85
  eicosanoids in, 1599-1600
  endothelium in, 84-85
  erythrocytes and leukocytes in, 85
  plasma components in, 85-86, 86f
    fibrin(ogen)olysis, 85
    procoagulants, 85, 86f
    regulatory factors, 85-86
  platelets in, 85
Hemosuccus pancreaticus, management of bleeding in, 290
Hemothorax
  retained, clotted, 403
  shock in, 68
Henderson-Hasselbalch equation, for bicarbonate concentration, 107
Heparin, 1022-1025
  coagulopathy due to, 87
  complications of, 1025
    adrenal hemorrhage, 1025
  dosage
    high, 1023-1025
    low, 1022-1023
    moderate, 1023
    rationale for varying, 1034-1035
  reversal of, 80, 1025
  for thromboembolic prophylaxis, 1034
Hepatic abscess, 1271-1272
  amebic, 1271-1272
    treatment of, 1272
  pyogenic, 1271-1272
    treatment of, 1271-1272
Hepatic disease. *See also* Cirrhosis
  chronic, 1462-1469
    acute tubular necrosis in, 1466-1467, 1466t
    coagulopathy and nonvariceal bleeding in, 1467-1468
    DIC in, 1468
    etiology of, 1462, 1463t
    hepatic encephalopathy in, 1465-1466, 1465t
    liver transplantation for, 1468-1469, 1468t
    malnutrition in, 1467
    portal hypertension in, 1463-1465, 1463t-1464t
    renal failure in, 1466-1467, 1466t
    treatment of complications of, 1462-1468
  immunodeficiency in, 1085
  laparoscopic cholecystectomy and, 768, 768f
Hepatic duct(s), trauma to, 419
Hepatic encephalopathy
  in chronic hepatic disease, 1465-1466, 1465t
  coma in, 149
  mechanisms of, 1469
Hepatic failure, 1455-1472
  acute, 1458-1462
    acute fatty liver of pregnancy and, 1458
    assessment of prognosis in, 1458-1459, 1459t-1460t
    cerebral edema in, 1460
    coagulopathy and bleeding in, 1461
    drug toxicity in, 1458
    etiology of, 1458, 1459t
    fluid, electrolyte, nutritional abnormalities in, 1461
    infectious complications in, 1461
    liver transplantation for, 1462
    medical therapy for, outcome of, 1461-1462
    pulmonary complications in, 1461
    renal failure in, 1461
    toxic liver syndrome in, 1462
    toxin-induced, 1458
    treatment of complications of, 1460-1461
    viral hepatitis in, 1458
    Wilson disease and, 1458
  Algorithm, 1456-1457
  fulminant, 1458
  in occult infection, 1167
  patient evaluation in, 1455
  pharmacokinetics in, 1706-1707, 1707t
  primary *vs.* secondary, 1455
  risk factors and workup in, 1455
  subfulminant, 1458
  wound healing and, 137-138
Hepatic formula, for enteral nutrition, 1526-1527, 1528t
Hepatic metabolism, in response to critical illness, 1503, 1507
Hepatic rupture, in pregnancy, 1149
Hepatic trauma, 413-419
  AAST liver injury scale for, 413, 413t, 414f
  assessment in, 413, 413t, 414f-415f
  in children, 1140, 1140f
  management of, 413-419
    control of hemorrhage in, 413-416, 415f-416f
      atriocaval shunt for, 415, 416f
      hepatic vascular isolation for, 415
      manual compression for, 414, 415f
      Moore-Pilcher balloon for, 415-416
      perihepatic packing for, 414, 416f
      Pringle maneuver for, 414-415, 415f
      tourniquet for liver clamp for, 415
      venovenous bypass for, 416
    definitive, 416-418
      fibrin glue for, 416
      hepatic arterial ligation for, 417-418
      hepatic resection for, 418
      hepatic transplantation for, 418
      hepatotomy with selective ligation for, 417, 417f
      intrahepatic balloon for, 418, 418f
      manual compression for, 416-417
      omentum for large defects in, 417
      parenchymal suturing for, 417
      perihepatic packing for, 418
      resectional debridement for, 418
      wrapping injured lobe for, 418
    mortality and complications in, 419
    nonoperative treatment of, 421-422
    perihepatic drainage for, 419
    Pringle maneuver in, 413, 414-415, 415f
    subcapsular hematoma in, 418-419
Hepatitis, 1320-1325
  in hospital personnel, 1323-1324, 1324t-1325t
  in immunosuppression, 1078
  of indeterminate etiology, in acute hepatic failure, 1458
  ischemic (shock liver), in multiple organ dysfunction syndrome, 1479-1480
Hepatitis A, 1320-1321
  in acute hepatic failure, 1458
Hepatitis B, 1321
  acute, 1321, 1323f
  in acute hepatic failure, 1458
  antigens in, 1321
  antimicrobial agents for, 1199t
  chronic
    hepatocellular carcinoma and, 1324
    long-term effects of, 1324-1325
  clinical course of, 1321, 1322f
  in immunosuppressed patient, prevention of, 1076t
  management of exposure to, 1314-1315, 1314t
    active immunoprophylaxis for, 1315, 1315t
    after blood exposure, 1315
    passive immunoprophylaxis for, 1314-1315
  persistent, 1321, 1322f
  prevention of transmission of, 1309-1313
    from health care workers to patients, 1312-1313, 1340
    from patients to health care workers, 1309-1312, 1720-1721, 1720t
    risks to surgeons, 1343t, 1343f-1344f, 1344
  serology of, 1321, 1323f, 1323t-1324t
  in transfusion, 1230
    epidemiology of, 1324
Hepatitis B vaccination, 1314-1315, 1315t, 1344
Hepatitis C, 1322-1323
  in acute hepatic failure, 1458
  antimicrobial agents for, 1199t
  chronic, long-term effects of, 1324-1325
  chronic active, 1323
  clinical manifestations of, 1322-1323
  management of exposure to, 1316
  prevention of transmission of, 1309-1313
    from health care workers to patients, 1312-1313
    from patients to health care workers, 1309-1312
  in transfusion, 1230
  transfusion-related, 1322
    epidemiology of, 1324
  transmission of, 1322
Hepatitis D, 1321-1322
  in acute hepatic failure, 1458
  prevention of transmission of, risks to surgeons, 1344
  transfusion-related, epidemiology of, 1324
Hepatitis E, 1322

Hepatocellular carcinoma, chronic hepatitis B and, 1324
Hepato-iminodiacetic acid (HIDA) scan, in jaundice, 255
Hepatorenal syndrome, 1466-1467
  acute renal failure in, 1446
  acute tubular necrosis vs., 1466t
Hernia
  abdominal wall. See also under Femoral hernia; Inguinal hernia
    open repair of, 857-875
  diaphragmatic
    in infants and neonates, 1126
      emergency surgery in, 1129
    posttraumatic, 404
  epigastric, 871
  femoral. See Femoral hernia
  groin. See also under Femoral hernia; Inguinal hernia
    classification of, 857, 858f
    hernioplasty for, 857, 859f
  hiatal, management of bleeding in, 289-290
  incarcerated
    intestinal obstruction in, 272-273
    ultrasonography in, 663, 663f
  incisional, 873-874, 891-893, 892f-893f. See also Incisional hernia
  inguinal. See Inguinal hernia
  internal, in gastric bypass for obesity, 1006
  laparoscopic cholecystectomy in, 755
  laparoscopic repair of, 877-895. See also Incisional hernia repair; Inguinal hernia repair
  lumbar, 872
  parastomal, 872-873
  pelvic, 872
  Spigelian, 871-872
  strangulated, intestinal obstruction in, 272-273
  umbilical, 871
Herniation, of heart, in chest trauma, 403
Heroin, suggested dosing for, 1627t
Herpes simplex virus infection
  agents effective against, 1329t
  antimicrobial agents for, 1199t
  of hand, 1285f, 1286
  in renal transplantation, 1328
Herpesvirus, 1325-1330. See also specific viruses, e.g., Cytomegalovirus infection
  agents effective against, 1328-1330, 1329t
Herpetic whitlow, 1286, 1285f
Hetastarch, for burn patients, in immediate resuscitation period, 56
Hexachlorophene, contraindicated in acute wound care, 127-128
Hiatal hernia, management of bleeding in, 289-290
Hickman catheter. See Central venous catheterization
Hidradenitis suppurativa, anal and perineal infections in, 848, 851-852, 853, 853f
Hip
  dislocation of, 470-471
  fracture of, 471-472, 471f
Histiocytoma(s), malignant fibrous, of neck, 192

Histoplasma capsulatum infection, antimicrobial agents for, 1199t
Histoplasmosis, clinical presentation and diagnosis of, 1293t
HIV infection. See AIDS; Human immunodeficiency virus (HIV) infection
Hodgkin lymphoma, cervical adenopathy in, 192
Home discharge, same day surgery and, 611
Home health care, 1642, 1643t
Horseshoe kidney, abdominal aortic aneurysm and, 944
Hospice care, 1643-1644
Hospital
  geriatrically adapted, 1105-1106
  infection control in, 1724. See also Infection control; Nosocomial infection(s)
  thermoregulation in
    fever in critical illness and, 1498-1499
    patient control of, 1556-1557, 1556t
Host defense(s), 1347-1350. See also entries beginning Immun-
  barriers as, 1347, 1348f
  cell-mediated immunity as, 1347-1348, 1349f
  cytokines in. See Cytokine(s)
  humoral immunity as, 1347
  in immunosuppression, 1071-1074. See also Immunosuppression, evaluation of host defenses in
  modulation of, 1350-1351
    immunotherapy for. See Immunoabrogation; Immunorepletion; Immunostimulation; Immunosuppressive therapy
    surgical, 1350
  in nosocomial pneumonia, 1655-1656
  in surgical patients, depression of, 1347
Human bite(s). See Bite(s), human
Human chorionic gonadotropin level(s), in pregnancy, 1154
Human immunodeficiency virus (HIV) infection. See also Acquired immunodeficiency syndrome (AIDS)
  AIDS in, statistics on, 1333, 1333f
  antimicrobial agents for, 1199t
  CDC classification of, 1333-1339
  Algorithm, 1334
    group I: acute syndrome, 1333-1335
    group II: asymptomatic carrier, 1335
    group III: generalized lymphadenopathy, 1335-1337, 1337f
    group IV: other HIV diseases, 1338
      constitutional disease, 1338
      neurologic disease, 1338
      other conditions in, 1338
      secondary cancers, 1338
      secondary infectious disease, 1338
  ELISA testing for, 1335
  latency period of, 1342
  lymph node biopsy in, 1336, 1337f
  major risk groups for, 1335, 1336f
  management of exposure to, 1313-1314
  pathogenesis of, 1341-1342
  prevention of transmission of, 1309-1313, 1339-1341
    from health care workers to patients, 1312-1313, 1339-1340
    from patients to health care workers, 1309-1312, 1339-1340, 1720t, 1721
    precautions for invasive procedures in, 1309, 1312t
    risks to health care workers and, 1340-1341, 1340t
    risks to patients and, 1339-1340
    risks to surgeons, 1342-1344, 1342t, 1343f
    transfusions and, 1339
    transplantation and, 1339
    universal precautions for, 1309, 1312t, 1340-1341
  seropositivity in, incidence of, 1333
  in transfusion, 1230-1231, 1335
  transmission of, 1319-1320
    to health care workers, 1320
    organ transplantation in, 1320
    transfusion in, 1319-1320
  Western blot assay for, 1335
Humidification, for mechanical ventilators, 1434
Hutchinson freckle (lentigo melanoma), 306, 307f
Hyaline membrane(s), in ARDS, 1407
Hydralazine, for hypertension, 1638t
Hydrocodone, suggested dosing for, 1627t
Hydrocortisone
  glucocorticoid and mineralocorticoid activities of, 1066t
  properties of, 1088t
Hydrogen ion concentration, conversion of pH to, 1389, 1389t
Hydrogen peroxide, contraindicated in acute wound care, 128
Hydromorphone
  for patient-controlled analgesia, 1668t
  suggested dosing for, 1627t
Hydrotherapy, for burn wound care, 484, 1691
Hygroma, cystic, 190
Hyperbilirubinemia. See also Jaundice
  direct vs. indirect, 251, 254t
Hypercalcemia
  automatic dysrhythmias and, 25-26
  causes of, 96t
  differential diagnosis of, 98t
  evaluation and treatment of, 96-99, 97f
  in hyperparathyroidism, 96-98, 98t, 106
  in malignancy, 96-98, 98t, 106
Hypercapnia. See also Carbon dioxide tension (PCO_2)
  definition of, 1418
  permissive, in acute respiratory failure, 1438
Hypercoagulable state. See Thrombotic syndrome(s)
Hyperdynamic state of critical illness, 1500-1501, 1501f
Hyperglycemia. See also Diabetes mellitus
  in central venous nutritional

support, 1534
coma in, 149
in elderly patients, 1109
as metabolic response to critical illness, 1502, 1502t, 1507
in occult infection, 1167
perioperative, 993
Hyperkalemia, 105
causes of, 105
emergency management of, *Algorithm*, 93
evaluation and treatment of, 95-96
postoperative, 1632
pulseless electrical activity in, 12t
Hypermagnesemia, evaluation and treatment of, 101
Hypermetabolism. *See also* Metabolic response to critical illness
in burn patient, 1504
ambient temperature and, 1505, 1505t
in early postresuscitation period, 483
respiratory fatigue due to, 494
in critical illness, 1503-1505, 1504f-1505f
oxygen consumption in, 1505
physiologic reserves and, 1504-1505, 1505f
temperature regulation in, altered, 1505, 1505t
Hypernatremia, 104
emergency management of, *Algorithm*, 92
evaluation and treatment of, 94-95
in extracellular fluid volume deficit, 103
in extracellular fluid volume excess, 104
postoperative assessment of, 1632
Hyperparathyroidism
hypercalcemia in, 96-98, 98t, 106
secondary, in uremic syndrome, 1058
Hyperpigmentation, in uremic syndrome, 1060
Hyperpyrexia. *See* Fever and hyperpyrexia
Hypersensitivity, delayed-type. *See* Delayed-type hypersensitivity
Hypertension. *See also* Blood pressure
in elderly patients, 1095
in endotracheal intubation, 608
as factor in selection for outpatient surgery, 542
intracranial. *See* Intracranial pressure
portal, 1463-1465, 1463t-1464t
postoperative, 1638t, 1639
anesthesia-related, 615
pulmonary. *See* Pulmonary hypertension
urgent and emergent, drug therapy for, 1638t
Hyperthermia. *See also* Fever and hyperpyrexia
in burn patient, 57
malignant. *See* Malignant hyperthermia
Hyperventilation, central neurogenic, in coma, 148
Hypervolemia. *See* Fluid volume excess
Hypoadrenocorticism. *See also* Adrenal insufficiency

postoperative, 1641
Hypoaldosteronism, metabolic acidosis in, 114
Hypocalcemia
blood transfusion causing, 45
causes of, 99, 100t
evaluation and treatment of, 99f, 99-100
Hypoglycemia
in chronic alcohol intoxication, 177
coma in, 149
treatment of, 156
Hypokalemia, 105
automatic dysrhythmias and, 25
causes of, 105
emergency management of, *Algorithm*, 93
evaluation and treatment of, 95
management of, 105
postoperative, 1632
respiratory muscle weakness in, 115
Hypomagnesemia, evaluation and treatment of, 100-101, 100f
Hypometabolism, in burn patient, in early postresuscitation period, 483
Hyponatremia, 104
calculation and replacement in, 94
emergency management of, *Algorithm*, 92
evaluation and treatment of, 94
in extracellular fluid volume deficit, 91, 103, 104
in extracellular fluid volume excess, 104
postoperative assessment of, 1632
in SIADH, 104
in water intoxication, 104
Hypoparathyroidism, hypocalcemia in, 100
Hypopharynx, in differential diagnosis of neck mass, 188
Hypophosphatemia, respiratory muscle weakness in, 115
Hypotension. *See also* Blood pressure
in endotracheal intubation, 608
intermittent, in occult infection, 1167
in regional anesthesia, 613
in shock, 63
in trauma, blunt, 348
Hypothalamic pathology, fever in, 1554
Hypothalamic-pituitary-adrenal axis, 1067, 1067f
Hypothalamic set-point, in fever and hyperpyrexia, 1552, 1552f
Hypothermia. *See also* Cold injury; Heat loss
accidental, 1554-1556
cardiac activity in, 1555-1556
in conscious patients, 1555-1556
in unconscious patients, 1556
cardiac arrest in, 1555
causes of, 1555, 1555t
initial care in, 1549f, 1554-1555
temperature measurement in, 1555, 1555t
varying degrees of, 1555t
blood transfusion causing, 45
in burn patients, 57
in wound excision and grafting, 487

in chest trauma, 402
coma in, 151
treatment of, 157
for elevated intracranial pressure, 358
emergency management of, *Algorithm*, 1550-1551
in general anesthesia, 610
intraoperative, in elderly patients, 1100-1101
morbidity and mortality in, 1549f
postoperative, 1637
Hypothyroidism, postoperative, 1641
Hypoventilation
alveolar. *See* Alveolar hypoventilation
in obesity, 1005, 1008-1009
Hypovolemia. *See* Fluid volume deficit
Hypovolemic shock. *See* Shock, hypovolemic
Hypoxemia
definition of, 1418
in shock, 67
Hypoxia
definition of, 1418
wound healing and, 136

I

Ibopamine, receptor types stimulated by, 1394t
Ibuprofen. *See also* Nonsteroidal anti-inflammatory drug(s) (NSAIDs)
suggested dosing for, 1628t
Ice bath, for heatstroke, 1553
ICU. *See* Intensive care unit (ICU)
ICU patient(s). *See* Critical illness
Idoxuridine, for herpesvirus infections, 1329
Ileoanal anastomosis, in restorative proctocolectomy with ileoanal pouch, 831-832. *See also* Proctocolectomy, restorative, with ileoanal pouch
Ileorectal anastomosis, with total colectomy, 827, 828f. *See also* Colectomy, total, with ileorectal anastomosis
Ileostomy, conventional, with total proctocolectomy, 828-830. *See also* Proctocolectomy, total, with conventional ileostomy
Ileus, 277-278
causes of, 266t
in infants and neonates, in intestinal obstruction, 1124
in infection, 1166
management of, 277, 278f
postoperative, 277
gastric distention in, 268, 269f
mechanical obstruction *vs.*, 277-278
radiographic contrast agent for, 278
Iliac artery, traumatic injury to, 444-445, 445f
Iliac vein, traumatic injury to, 441t, 445
Illness, critical. *See* Critical illness
metabolic response to. *See* Metabolic response to critical illness
Imipenem, in vivo drug interactions

with, 1193t
Imipenem-cilastatin, 1213-1214
  for bacterial infections, 1202t-1203t
Immersion foot, 511
Immobilization
  consequences of, in elderly patient, 1103
  in metabolic response to critical illness, 1500
Immune dysfunction, in uremic syndrome, 1059
Immune evaluation, in immunosuppression therapy, 1082
Immune function, in elderly patients, 1114
Immune response. *See* Host defense(s)
Immunity
  cell-mediated, 1347-1348, 1349f
    tests for, 1074
  humoral, 1347
    tests for, 1074
Immunization(s). *See* Vaccination
Immunoabrogation, 1350, 1350t, 1357-1359
  cytokine antagonism in, 1357-1359
  inhibition of PGE_2 synthesis in, 1359
  leukocyte receptor antagonism in, 1359
  platelet-activating factor antagonism in, 1359
Immunocompromise. *See* Immunodeficiency; Immunosuppression
  infection in. *See under* Infection, in immunocompromise
Immunodeficiency
  acquired, 1083-1086. *See* Acquired immunodeficiency syndrome (AIDS); Human immunodeficiency virus (HIV) infection
  age as factor in, 1084
  in anesthesia, 1086
  anoperineal infection in, 848
  B cell, 1083, 1083t
  in blood transfusion, 1086
  in diabetes mellitus, 1085
  in drug therapy, 1085-1086
  in foreign body implantation, 1085
  in infants and neonates, 1128
  in liver disease, 1085
  in malignancy, 1085
  in malnutrition, 1084
  in obesity, 1084
  in operation, 1086
  primary, 1083, 1083t
  in protein-losing disease, 1085
  in radiation therapy, 1086
  in renal failure, 1085
  in septic response, 1085
  in splenectomy, 1086
  T cell, 1083, 1083t
  in thermal injury, 1085
  in trauma, 1086
Immunoglobulin(s)
  in host defense, 1347
  in infants and neonates, 1128
Immunomodulation, 1347-1362. *See also* Immunoabrogation; Immunorepletion; Immunostimulation; Immunosuppressive therapy
  in multiple organ dysfunction syndrome, 1478
  nutrients for. *See* Nutritional support, in immune modulation

Immunorepletion, 1350, 1350t, 1353-1357
  antiendotoxin antibody for, 1353-1356, 1354f, 1355t
  bactericidal/permeability increasing protein (BPI) for, 1356
  CMV immunoglobulin for, 1356-1357
  other agents for, 1356-1357
Immunostimulation, 1350, 1350t, 1351-1353
  biologic response modifiers for, 1351-1352, 1351t
  cytokines for. *See* Cytokine(s)
  endotoxin and derivatives for, 1351-1352
  nutritional support for. *See* Nutritional support, in immune modulation
  selective gut decontamination for, 1353
  vaccination for. *See* Vaccination
Immunosuppression, 1071-1090. *See also* disorders causing, e.g., Acquired immunodeficiency syndrome (AIDS)
  Algorithm, 1072
  central venous catheterization in, *Candida* septicemia in, 1536
  diagnostic evaluation of, 1073f
  evaluation of, 1074
  evaluation of host defenses in, 1071-1074
    cell-mediated immunity and, 1074
    complement and, 1074
    humoral immunity and, 1074
    local, 1071
    neutrophil function and, 1074
    systemic, 1071, 1074
  infection in, 1075-1078, 1167
    candidiasis in, 1304
    cardiovascular infection in, 1076
    central nervous system infection in, 1076
    genitourinary tract infection in, 1078
    hepatitis in, 1078
    intra-abdominal infection in, 1078
    pneumonia in, 1076
    signs and symptoms of, 1075
    sinusitis in, 1078
    skin infection in, 1076
    workup in, 1075, 1077t
    wound infection in, 1076
  neutropenia in, 1078-1079
  therapy for, 1074-1079
    bacterial infection and, 1075
    microenvironmental conditions and, 1074-1075
    nutritional status and, 1075
    vaccination and, 1075
Immunosuppressive therapy
  complications in
    malignancy as, 1087
    prevention of, 1075, 1076t
  evaluation prior to, 1079-1082
    cardiovascular system in, 1080-1081
    dermal system in, 1081
    digestive system in, 1081
    endocrine system in, 1081
    foreign bodies in, 1082
    genitourinary system in, 1081
    hematologic system in, 1082
    immune system in, 1082

    infectious diseases in, 1082
    musculoskeletal system in, 1081
    nervous system in, 1080
    nutritional state in, 1082
    psychological, social, and financial assessment in, 1082
    respiratory system in, 1081
    workup in, 1079, 1080t
  wound healing and, 137
Immunotherapy. *See* Immunoabrogation; Immunomodulation; Immunorepletion; Immunostimulation; Immunosuppressive therapy
Impaired physician, 1729-1739. *See also* Physician, impaired
Incisional hernia, 873-874
  pathophysiology of, 873
Incisional hernia repair, 871f-872f, 873-874
  laparoscopic, 891-893, 892f-893f
    operative planning in, 891-892
    operative technique in, 892-893, 893f
    outcome evaluation in, 893
    postoperative care in, 893
  Rives-Stoppa incisional hernioplasty for, 871f, 874
Indicator dilution technique, for cardiac output, 1383, 1384f
Indomethacin, suggested dosing for, 1628t
Infant formula, 1132t
Infants and neonates, 1121-1143. *See also* Children
  acid-base status in, 1127-1128
  antibiotics for, 1122, 1124t, 1129
  arterial blood gases in, 1122
  bladder exstrophy in, emergency surgery in, 1129
  body fluid compartment changes in, 1122, 1124, 1126f
  body weight in, 1121
  cardiac function in, 1121-1122
  cystic lung disease in, 1126
  diaphragmatic hernia in, 1126
    emergency surgery in, 1129
  emergency surgical problems in, 1129
  endotracheal intubation in, 1130, 1130t
  enteral nutrition in, 1132, 1132t-1133t
  esophageal atresia in, 1125
    emergency surgery in, 1129
  fluid and electrolytes in, 1122, 1124, 1126-1128
  gastrointestinal water loss in, 1127
  gastroschisis in, emergency surgery in, 1129
  immune function in, 1128
  infection in, 1128-1129
  inguinal hernioplasty in, 863
  insensible water loss in, 1126
  intestinal obstruction in, 1123-1124
  mechanical ventilation for, 1130, 1437
    CPAP, 1130
    CPPV, 1130
    IMV, 1130
  meningocele in, emergency surgery in, 1129
  metabolic response to surgery in, 1131

monitoring in, 1121-1122, 1121t
necrotizing enterocolitis in, 1128
nutritional assessment in, 1131-1132
nutritional requirements of, 1131, 1131t
nutritional support for, 1130-1137
omphalocele in, emergency surgery in, 1129
oxygenation in, 1122
pharmacokinetics in, 1703-1704
postoperative feeding in, 1132, 1134t
potassium requirements in, 1127
pulse oximetry in, 1122
renal function in, 1124, 1126
renal water requirements in, 1126-1127
respiratory distress in, 1125-1126
respiratory failure in, 1129-1130
sepsis in, 1128-1129
shock in, 1122
 antibiotics for, 1122, 1124t
 dopamine for, 1122
 hypovolemic, 1122
 septic, 1122
short-bowel syndrome in, 1137
sodium requirements in, 1127
temperature in, 1121
total parenteral nutrition for, 1132-1137
 administration of, 1134-1135, 1135f
 central vein, 1134, 1134t
 complications of, 1136-1137, 1137t
  liver function, 1136
  metabolic, 1136-1137, 1137t
  sepsis, 1136
 indications for, 1133-1134
 monitoring in, 1135-1136, 1136t
 peripheral vein, 1134, 1135t
 solutions for, 1134, 1134t
urine output in, 1121
ventilatory support in, 1129-1130, 1130t
vital signs in, 1121, 1121t
Infarction
 myocardial. See Myocardial infarction
 pulmonary, pulmonary embolism vs., 1018
 small bowel, surgical options for, 1244t
Infection. See also Sepsis; Shock, inflammatory; Shock, septic; specific infections
 in absence of sepsis, 1184
 blood tests in, 1168
 clinical and laboratory diagnosis of, 1163-1173
  Algorithm, 1164-1165
  general approach to, 1163-1166, 1166t
 evaluation for, 1168-1169
  in immunosuppression therapy, 1082-1083
  in evaluation of operative risk, 536
 fever and hyperpyrexia in, 1166-1167
  management of, 1552-1553, 1552t
 history and physical examination in, 1168
 in immunocompromise, 1167
  clinical signs and symptoms of, 1167
 laboratory signs of, 1167-1168
 normal patient vs., 1163
 in infants and neonates, 1128-1129
 in metabolic response to critical illness, 1499-1500, 1499f
 microbiological studies in, 1168
 in normal patient, 1166-1167
  cardinal signs of inflammation in, 1166
  fever in, 1166
  immunocompromise vs., 1163
  infectious syndrome in, 1167
  miscellaneous signs in, 1166
 nosocomial. See Nosocomial infection(s)
 occult. See Infection, in immunocompromise
 postoperative, prevention of, 567-589. See also Surgical site infection
 radiologic studies in, 1168-1169
 remote, elective surgery and, 570
 sepsis vs., 1163
 soft tissue. See Soft tissue infection
 therapy for, 1169-1170
  in mild to moderate sepsis, 1169
  in septic response without infection, 1169, 1170
  in severe sepsis and septic shock, 1169. See also Sepsis; Shock, septic
 wound. See Wound infection
 wound healing and, 135-136
Infection control, 1717-1727. See also under Nosocomial infection(s)
 health status of health care team and, 1719-1722. See also Health care personnel
 surgical wound and, 1717-1722. See also Wound infection, nosocomial
Infection control committee, 1725
Infection control practitioner(s), 1725
Infection control program(s), 1722-1724
 data interpretation and analysis in, 1723
 discussion on, 1725-1726
 education in, 1724
 environmental control in, 1724
 investigation in, 1723-1724
 organization of, 1725
 public health and community health service in, 1724
 research in, 1724
 surveillance in, 1722-1724
 verification of infection in, 1723
Infection control service, 1725
Infectious hazard(s), in operating room, protection against, 598-599, 599t
Infectious syndrome, 1167
Inflammation
 metabolic response to, 1514-1515
 in metabolic response to critical illness, 1498-1499, 1499t
Inflammatory bowel disease
 appendix in, 822
 eicosanoids and, 1600
 in pregnancy, 1152-1153
Influenza, in immunosuppressed patient, prevention of, 1076t
Influenza A, antimicrobial agents for, 1199t
Informed consent
 for elderly patient, 1097-1098
 for nonemergency surgery, 543-544
Infratentorial tumor, coma in, 149-150
Inguinal anatomy, laparoscopic, 877-881, 878f-880f
 peritoneal intact, 877-879, 878f-879f
  external iliac vessels in, 879
  inferior epigastric vessels in, 878
  obliterated umbilical artery in, 878
  spermatic vessels in, 877-878, 879f
 peritoneal removed, 879-881, 879f-880f
  Cooper's ligament in, 880
  femoral canal in, 881
  genitofemoral nerve in, 881
  ilioinguinal and iliohypogastric nerves in, 881
  iliopubic tract in, 879-880
  internal inguinal ring in, 879
  lateral cutaneous nerve of thigh in, 881
  trapezoid of disaster in, 880f, 881
Inguinal hernia, classification of, 857, 858f
Inguinal hernia repair
 classic, 859-862
  Bassini repair, 859-862, 860f-861f
  in bilateral hernia, 862
  Cooper ligament repair (McVay-Lotheissen hernioplasty), 859-862, 860f-861f
  critique of, 863
  dissection in, 859, 859f, 861
  Marcy repair (simple ring closure), 859-862, 860f-861f
  repair in, 860f-861f, 861-862
  Shouldice-Bassini repair, 860f-861f, 861-862
  special considerations in, 862-863
  surgical technique for, 859f-861f, 859-862
 complications of, 867-871
  neuralgia, 868-871
  testicular atrophy, 867-868
 essentials of, 857, 859f
 in infants and children, 863
 laparoscopic, 877-891
  complications of, 887-889
   dissection and, 887-888
   groin and thigh pain as, 889
   mesh and, 888
   miscellaneous, 889
   peritoneal cavity access as, 887
   urinary, 888-889
   vas deferens and testicular, 889
  disadvantages of, 887
  history and physical examination in, 881
  open mesh repair vs., 888t, 890-891
   bilateral hernias and, 890
   convalescence time and, 890
   hernia recurrence and, 890-891
   postoperative pain and, 890
   quality of life and, 890
  operative planning in, 881-882,

882f
operative technique in, 882-887, 883f-886f
outcome evaluation in, 889-891
patient selection in, 881
postoperative care in, 887-889
preoperative evaluation in, 881
totally extraperitoneal repair in, 885-887, 886f
closure in, 887
creation of preperitoneal space in, 885-886, 886f
dissection of hernial sac, 886-887
mesh placement in, 887
transabdominal preperitoneal repair, 882-885
anatomic landmarks in, 883
closure of fascia and skin in, 885
hernial sac dissection in, 884
mesh placement in, 884-885, 885f
peritoneal closure in, 885, 885f
peritoneal flap in, 883-884, 884f
reidentification of landmarks in, 884, 885f
trocar placement in, 882-883, 883f
transabdominal preperitoneal repair *vs.* extraperitoneal repair in, 891
prosthetic, 863-867
anterior, 864-866
Gilbert sutureless hernioplasty for, 865-866, 866f
infection in, 863-864
management of, 864
prophylaxis in, 864
Lichtenstein tension-free hernioplasty for, 864-865, 865f-866f
posterior (properitoneal), 866-867, 867f
Stoppa giant prosthetic reinforcement of visceral sac for, 866-867, 868f-870f
surgical technique for, 864-867
synthetic prosthesis for, 863
tissue response to, 863
Inhalation injury
in burn patient, in immediate resuscitation period, 52-53, 53f
chemical, 53
mucosal edema in, 52, 53f
thermal, 53
Injection injury, acute wound management after, 125
Injury. *See* Trauma
Inotropic agent(s). *See also* specific drugs, e.g., Dopamine
in burn patient, 57-58
after first postburn week, 495-496
in heart failure, 1393-1395
mechanism of action of, 1399
in multiple organ dysfunction syndrome, 1476
Inspiratory force (IF), definition of, 1415
Instrument(s). *See* Surgical instrument(s)
Insulin
blood, in burn patients, 1502t

in critical illness, resistance to, 1502, 1502t, 1507
in diabetes mellitus
intraoperative, 997-998, 998t
postoperative, 999, 999t
in diabetic ketoacidosis, 112
glucose loading and, age-related responses to, 1109, 1111f
in hyperglycemia of critical illness, 1502, 1502t, 1507
resistance to. *See also* Diabetes mellitus; Hyperglycemia
in occult infection, 1167
serum, in normal *vs.* trauma patients, 1507, 1507t
in stress response, in burn patients, 498
Insulin pump(s), 1000-1001
benefits of, 1001
complications of, 1001
initiating therapy with, 1000-1001
Intensive care unit (ICU). *See also* Critical illness
head injury management in, 357-358
jaundice in, in multiple organ dysfunction syndrome, 1480
monitoring in. *See also* Cardiopulmonary monitoring
indications for and uses of, **Algorithm,** 1366-1367
multiorgan failure in. *See* Multiple organ dysfunction syndrome (MODS)
nosocomial infection and, 1478
in multiple organ dysfunction syndrome, 1483-1484
postoperative admission to, 1627-1628
shock management in. *See also* Shock, ICU management of
sleep deprivation in, 1500
surgical, ultrasonography in, 664, 664f
Intercostobrachial nerve, in axillary dissection, for breast cancer, 635
Interferon gamma, 1607
biologic activities of, 1605t
detection of, in infection, 1608
as immunostimulant, 1352
physical properties of, 1610t, 1616
in sepsis, 1350
synonyms and cell sources of, 1604t
Interleukin-1, 1606-1607
in acute phase response, 1510, 1606f, 1607
biologic activities of, 1605t
blockade of, in vivo protective effects of, 1358-1359
detection of
after experimental infusion, 1608
in infection, 1608
effects on wound healing of, 1607
immunologic activities of, 1606-1607
as immunostimulant, 1352
metabolic effects of, 1606f, 1607
in metabolic response to critical illness, 1510
physical properties of, 1610t, 1616
in propagation of mediator cascade, 1612, 1613f-1614f
in sepsis, 1349

synergism of, 1612
synonyms and cell sources of, 1604t
tissue levels of, 1611-1612
Interleukin-2, 1607
biologic activities of, 1605t
detection of, in infection, 1608
as immunostimulant, 1352
for melanoma, 308
physical properties of, 1610t, 1616
synonyms and cell sources of, 1604t
Interleukin-6, 1607
in acute phase response, 1510-1511
biologic activities of, 1605t
detection of
after experimental infusion, 1608, 1609f
in infection, 1608
in endotoxin tolerance, 1612
glucocorticoids as antagonists of, 1608
physical properties of, 1610t, 1616
in propagation of mediator cascade, 1612, 1613f-1614f
in sepsis, 1349-1350
synergism of, 1612
synonyms and cell sources of, 1604t
tissue levels of, 1611-1612
Interleukin-10, 1610-1611, 1616, 1617
Interleukin-8, in sepsis, 1349-1350
Interleukin-3, physical properties of, 1610t
Interleukin-1*alpha*
physical properties of, 1610t
synonyms and cell sources of, 1604t
Interleukin-1*beta*
physical properties of, 1610t
synonyms and cell sources of, 1604t
Interleukin-1ra, 1609-1610
clinical uses of, 1618
physical properties of, 1616
Internet, health care sites on, 525t
Intertrochanteric fracture, 471f-472f, 472
Intestinal anastomosis, 803-813
for bowel resections, 808-809
breakdown of, 803-806
associated diseases and systemic factors in, 803-804
controversial areas in, 806
hand-sewn *vs.* stapled anastomosis and, 805-806
patient preparation and, 804-805
type and location of anastomosis and, 805-806
unusual anastomosis techniques and, 806
for colon, 808
double-layered sutured end-to-side enterocolostomy, 810, 811f
double-stapled end-to-end coloanal anastomosis, 810-811
handsewn, 806-807
continuous sutures *vs.* interrupted sutures for, 807
single-layer anastomosis *vs.* double-layer anastomosis in, 807
suture material for, 806
healing in, 803, 805f

historical perspective on, 804
for rectum, 808
single-layer sutured extramucosal side-to-side enteroenterostomy, 809-810, 810f
for small bowel, 808
stapled, 807-808
 choice of stapler for, 807, 809f
 single-stapled vs. double-stapled, 808
 staple height for, 808
for strictureplasty, 809
successful, principles of, 804t
Intestinal obstruction, 263-281
abdominal radiography in, 267-268, 268f-271f
in adhesive partial small bowel obstruction, 275-276
adjunctive tests in, 270-271
assessment of, **Algorithm,** 264-265
auscultation in, 267
classification of, 263, 269-271
closed-loop, 272, 274f
colon. *See* Colon, obstruction of
contrast studies in, 271
cost considerations in, 279-280
CT scan in, 270-271, 273f-274f
determination of need for operation in, 269-271
early postoperative, 276
early postoperative technical complications in, 274-275
enteroclysis in, 271
in fecal impaction, 274
gastric aspirate in, 267
history and clinical setting in, 263-267
ileus in. *See* Ileus
imaging studies in, 267-268, 268f-274f
in incarcerated or strangulated hernias, 272-273
in infants and neonates, 1123-1124
in inflammatory conditions, 276
investigative studies in, 267-269
laboratory studies in, 268-269
mechanical, 271-277
 complete, 272
 elective operation for, 276-277
 immediate operation for, 272-274
 no operation in, 275-276
 postoperative ileus vs., 277-278
 in terminal illness, 271-272
 urgent operation in, 274-275
nonmechanical, 277-279
nonoperative therapy in, lack of response to, 274
in nonsigmoid volvulus, 273-274
operative and nonoperative therapy in, guidelines for, 272t
physical examination in, 267
in pregnancy, 1150-1151
pseudo-obstruction, 278-279, 279f
resuscitation in, 267
sigmoidoscopy in, 270
in sigmoid volvulus, 270f-271f, 273-274
small bowel. *See* Small bowel, obstruction of
strangulation, 272, 274f
ultrasonography in, 270-271
Intestinal tube(s), long, postoperative management of, 1634, 1635f
Intestine, reperfusion injury in, 1573-1574

Intoxication
alcohol. *See* Alcohol intoxication
drug. *See* Drug intoxication; Substance abuse
Intra-abdominal abscess, 1248-1250. *See also* Intra-abdominal infection(s); Peritonitis
Algorithm, 1240-1241
antibiotics in, 1243t, 1249
candidal, 1298
clinical presentation and diagnosis of, 1248-1249
CT for, 1257, 1257f
drainage in, 1249-1250, 1249f
 percutaneous, 1258, 1258t
general patient care in, 1249
magnetic resonance imaging for, 1258
management of, 1249-1250
postoperative, incidence of, 1248, 1248f
radiologic evaluation of, 1248-1249, 1256-1258, 1256f-1257f
radionuclide studies for, 1257-1258
ultrasonography for, 1256-1257, 1256f
Intra-abdominal fluid collection(s), in immunosuppression, 1078
Intra-abdominal infection(s). *See also* Intra-abdominal abscess; Peritonitis; Upper abdominal infection
antibiotics for, 1251-1253
cephalosporins for, 1207
nosocomial, 1225
Intra-abdominal procedure(s), pain relief after, 1659-1662
Intra-aortic balloon counterpulsation, for heart failure, 1396
Intracardiac cardioverter defibrillator (AICD), 15
Intracellular signaling
activation of nuclear factor *kappa*B in, 1580, 1581f
endothelial xanthine oxidase in, 1580
heat shock response in, 1580
nitric oxide in, 1580
reactive oxygen metabolites in, 1580
Intracranial hypertension. *See* Intracranial pressure
Intracranial pressure. *See also* Coma; Head injury
in coma, 148
in head injury, 356
in hepatic failure, 1460
monitoring of, in head injury, 357
pressure-volume index of, 364
reduction of, 358
 barbiturates for, 358
 etomidate for, 358
 in head injury, 358
 hypothermia for, 358
 propofol for, 358
Intravascular device(s)
bacteremia due to, 1178t
candidemia due to, 1292, 1296
central venous. *See* Central venous catheterization
enterococcal bacteremia due to, 1179
infection in, 1226-1228
 catheter-site, 1226
 clinical and laboratory

diagnosis of, 1170-1171
culture technique for, 1226, 1226f-1227f
exit-site, 1226
incidence of, 1232
in infants and neonates, 1136
long-term catheterization and, 1228
with multiple internal lumina, 1228
nasal carriage of *Staphylococcus aureus* in, 1247-1248
studies on prevention of, 1719
treatment of, 1226-1227
tunnel, 1226
warfarin and, 1228
intravenous. *See* Intravenous catheterization
nursing care for, 1228
septicemia with, 1226
septic thrombophlebitis in, 1013, 1175, 1227
staphylococcal bacteremia due to, 1175, 1178t, 1178f
Swan-Ganz. *See* Pulmonary arterial (Swan-Ganz) catheterization
systemic arterial. *See* Systemic arterial catheterization
Intravascular fluid volume
in acute renal failure, 1441-1444
postoperative, 1631-1632
Intravenous access, in emergency management, of substance abuse, 169
Intravenous catheterization, for burn patients, in immediate resuscitation period, 54
Intravenous line(s), replacement of, 1500
Intubation
gastric. *See* Nasoenteric intubation; Nasogastric intubation
tracheal. *See* Endotracheal intubation; Nasotracheal intubation; Orotracheal intubation
Iron
in central venous nutritional support, 1532
requirements for, in ICU patient, 1525t
Iron chelator(s), as free radical scavenger, 1576
Irrigation
for acute wounds, 127, 973-976
whole bowel, for emergency management, of substance abuse, 172-173
Ischemia
cerebral, reperfusion injury in, 1578
eicosanoids in, 1598-1599
myocardial, in shock, 67
Ischemic heart disease. *See* Coronary artery disease
Ischemic hepatitis (shock liver), in multiple organ dysfunction syndrome, 1479-1480
Islet cell transplantation, in diabetes mellitus, 1001
Isoflurane, for maintenance anesthesia, 609t
Isolation procedures, 1721
Isopropyl alcohol
contraindicated in acute wound care, 128

ingestion of, 177, 178
Isoproterenol
  for heart failure, 1395
  receptor types stimulated by, 1394t
Itraconazole, 1301, 1301t-1302t
  for candidiasis, 1296

J

Jaundice, 251-262
  Algorithm, 252-253
  in cholangitis, 256
  in choledocholithiasis, without cholangitis, 256-257
  in cholestatic syndromes, 254
  clinical assessment of, 251-254
  hepatic, 255
    causes of, 255t
    Child-Pugh classification of, 255
    posthepatic *vs.*, 254
  hyperbilirubinemia in, direct *vs.* indirect, 251-254, 254t
  ICU, in multiple organ dysfunction syndrome, 1480
  imaging in, 254-256, 256f
  in lesions other than choledocholithiasis, 257-260
  in malignant obstruction, 257-260
    cholangiography and decompression for, 258
    diagnosis and assessment of resectability in, 257-258
    nonoperative management of, 258
    operative management of, 258-260
      in lower-third obstruction, 260
      in middle-third obstruction, 259-260
      in upper-third obstruction, 259
    palliation in, 258
  posthepatic
    causes of, 257, 257t
    hepatic *vs.*, 254
    workup and management of, 256-260
  postoperative, 260-261, 260f
  wound healing and, 137-138
Jaw thrust, for airway patency, 7, 7f
Jefferson (atlas) fracture, 361
Jejunal diverticulum(a), management of upper GI bleeding in, 290
Jejunal limb, Roux-en-Y
  in distal subtotal gastric resection, 715
  drainage of pancreatic pseudocyst into, 781-782, 781f-782f
Jejunal ulcer(s), management of upper GI bleeding in, 290
Jejunum, tissue layers of, 805f
Joint Commission on Accreditation of Healthcare Organizations (JCAHO), 1717
Joint contracture, burn wound rehabilitation and, 1694
Joint infection, quinolone for, 1216
Joint procedure(s), pain relief after, 1662
Jugular bulb oximetry, in head injury, 357, 357t
Jugular vein
  external, for central venous catheterization, 1375

injury to, 385
internal, for central venous catheterization, 1375, 1376f

K

Kanamycin, 1210
  for bacterial infections, 1202t-1203t
Kaolin-pectin, for diarrhea in enteric nutrition, 1529, 1530f
Katz index of basic ADL, 1092
Kehr sign, 235, 237t
Keloid(s), 138
Kernig sign, in coma, 148
Ketamine, for induction of anesthesia, 607t
Ketoacidosis
  alcoholic, 112, 179, 180
  diabetic, 112
    coma in, 149
    treatment of, 156
    metabolic acidosis in, 112
    nitroprusside test for, 112
    therapy for, 112
Ketoconazole, 1301-1302, 1301t-1302t
Ketoprofen, suggested dosing for, 1628t
Ketorolac, suggested dosing for, 1628t
Kidney
  as donor organ, 959
    technique for, 965-966, 966f
  horseshoe, abdominal aortic aneurysm and, 944
Klebsiella pneumoniae infection, antimicrobial agents for, 1197t
Klebsiella pneumoniae pneumonia, nosocomial, 1649
Klumpke paralysis, 1141
Knee
  dislocation, popliteal artery injury in, 466, 466f
  fracture of, intra-articular, 473
Knee defect(s), flaps for, 981
Korsakoff syndrome. *See* Wernicke-Korsakoff syndrome
Kussmaul respiration, in coma, 148
Kustner sign, 237t

L

Labetalol, for hypertension, 1638t
Laboratory method(s), collection and transport of specimen. *See also specific specimens*
Laceration, in extremity trauma, 476-477
Lacrimal duct injury, 373
beta-Lactamase inhibitor(s), 1214-1215
Lactate
  blood, in burn patient, 57
  serum, for lactic acidosis, 1374
Lactated Ringer solution. *See also* Fluid resuscitation
  for burn patients, 55
  electrolyte content of, 103t
Lactation, breast abscess in, 214
Lactic acidosis, 111-112
  biochemical basis of, 121
  classification of, 119, 119t
  pathophysiology of, 111, 111f
  serum lactate for, 1374

severe, 112
therapy for, 119-120
  alkalinizing agents in, 119
  dichloroacetate in, 119-120
Laparoscopic ultrasonography, 663, 765
Laparoscopy
  for cholecystectomy, 753-771. *See also* Cholecystectomy, laparoscopic
  for colectomy, 837-842. *See also* Colectomy, laparoscopic
  for inguinal hernia repair, 877-891. *See also* Inguinal hernia repair, laparoscopic
  for Nissen fundoplication, 697-702. *See also* Nissen fundoplication, laparoscopic
  in peritonitis, 1242
    secondary, 1243-1244
  for splenectomy, 787-801. *See also* Splenectomy, laparoscopic
  for vagotomy, 711-712
Laparotomy
  in abdominal mass, 249
  in acute abdominal pain, 237
  for multiple organ dysfunction syndrome, 1484
  in traumatic injury to great vessels of abdomen, 446-447
Laryngospasm, in endotracheal intubation, 607
Laryngotracheal injury, isolated, 381
Larynx
  in differential diagnosis of neck mass, 188
  tumors of, 192
Laser(s)
  safety requirements for, 594
  for video-assisted thoracic surgery, 676, 676f
Latissimus dorsi myocutaneous flap, for breast reconstruction, 641-642, 641f
Lavage
  gastric. *See* Gastric lavage
  peritoneal. *See* Peritoneal lavage
Laxative use, occult, hyperchloremic metabolic acidosis in, 113
Le Fort fracture, 375f-376f, 376
Left atrial pressure (LAP), pulmonary arterial wedge pressure for, 1381, 1382f
Left ventricular end-diastolic volume
  measurement of, 1387
  pulmonary arterial wedge pressure and, 1383
Left ventricular end-systolic pressure, calculation of, 1387-1388
Left ventricular end-systolic pressure-volume relation(s), 1388
Left ventricular end-systolic volume
  calculation of, 1387
  unstressed, calculation of, 1387
Leg. *See under* Extremity(ies)
Legionella infection(s), hospital environment and, 1724
Legionella micdadei infection, antimicrobial agents for, 1198t
Legionella pneumophila infection, antimicrobial agents for, 1198t
Leptospira infection, antimicrobial agents for, 1199t

Leukocyte receptor antagonist(s), 1359
Leukotriene, 1597-1598
  biologic effects of, 1597t
Leukotriene antagonist(s), for inflammatory conditions, 1600
Levorphanol, suggested dosing for, 1627t
Lichtenstein tension-free hernioplasty, 864-865, 865f-866f
Lidocaine
  for anesthesia in wound closure, 127
  classification of, 23
  comparative pharmacology of, 612t
  for nonemergency surgery, 545t
  for ventricular fibrillation, 10-11
Life support. *See also* Cardiopulmonary resuscitation (CPR)
  advanced, 8-10
  basic, 3-8
  in multiple organ dysfunction syndrome, withdrawal of, 1486
Lightning injury, 509-510. *See also under* Electrical injury, lightning
Lincomycin, for bacterial infections, 1204t-1205t
Linoleic acid, in eicosanoid synthesis, 1593f
Lip(s)
  defects of, flaps for, 979, 981f
  electrical burns of, 508-509, 509f, 509t
  injuries of, 374-375
Lipid metabolism, in critical illness, 1508
Lipocortin(s), as phospholipase A_2 antagonists, 1591
Lipodystrophy, diabetic, 996
Lipoma(s), of neck, 191
Lipopolysaccharide, circulating binding proteins for, 1614
Lipopolysaccharide analogue(s), 1614
Lipopolysaccharide antibody(ies), 1613-1614
Lipoxygenase inhibitor(s), for inflammatory conditions, 1600
Listeria monocytogenes infection, antimicrobial agents for, 1197t
Liver. *See also under* Hepatic
  as donor organ, 961
    technique for, 964-965, 964f-965f
  glucose production in, 1507
  injury to. *See* Hepatic trauma
  reperfusion injury in, 1574-1576
  shock (ischemic hepatitis), in multiple organ dysfunction syndrome, 1479-1480
  trauma to. *See* Hepatic trauma
Liver failure. *See* Hepatic failure
Liver support system, bioartificial, 1469-1470, 1469t-1470t
Liver transplantation
  for chronic hepatic disease, 1468-1469, 1468t
  for hepatic failure, 1462
  for hepatic trauma, 418
Lobectomy, video-assisted thoracic surgery for, 680
Locked-in syndrome, 151
Lou Gehrig disease (familial amyotrophic lateral sclerosis), free radical effects on, 1583

Lower extremity. *See under* Extremity(ies)
Lower gastrointestinal bleeding, 293-300. *See also* Upper gastrointestinal bleeding
  angiography for, 298-299, 299f
  assessment and management of, Algorithm, 294-295
  barium enema contraindicated in, 299
  colonoscopy for, emergency, 296f, 297
  investigation and management of, 293-300
  in minor bleeding, 300
  in stable patients, 296-300
    with bleeding that stops, 299-300
    with continued bleeding, 296-299
  in unstable bleeding patients, 293-296
  physical examination in, 296
  presentation and initial assessment in, 293
  radionuclide scanning for, 297-298, 297f-298f
  resuscitation in, 293
  sigmoidoscopy in, 296
  therapy in, 299
LSD, abuse of, emergency management of, 175-176
Lumbar hernia(s), 872
Lumbar spine injury, 355
Lumpectomy, for breast cancer, 634
  mastectomy *vs.*, 215-216, 215t
Lung(s)
  injury to, in mechanical ventilation, 1427, 1427t
  movement of, 1415-1416
  stiff, alveolar hypoventilation in, 1419
  traumatic lacerations of, 399-401, 400f
    complications of, 403
Lung biopsy, for nosocomial pneumonia, 1650
Lung compliance, definition of, 1416
Lung contusion, in chest trauma, 1411-1412
Lung scan(s), for pulmonary embolism, 1019
Lyell disease. *See* Toxic epidermal necrolysis
Lymphangitis
  in cellulitis, 320, 320f
  in hand infection, 1281
Lymphatic mapping and sentinel node biopsy, 643-658
  for breast cancer, 650-655
    complications of, 654
    intraoperative mapping and node identification in, 652-653, 652f
    nodal staging for, 650-651
    pathologic examination of sentinel node in, 653-654, 653f-654f
    patient selection for, 651
    preoperative lymphoscintigraphy in, 651-652, 651f
    rationale for, 650-651
    reported results of, 654-655, 655t
    sentinel node removal in, 653
    technique for, 651-654
    upstaging in, 653t, 654

  cost considerations in, 657
  for melanoma, 643-650
    clinical implications of, 650
    complications of, 648
    development of, 644-645
    intraoperative mapping and sentinel node identification in, 647-648
    mapping in, 645, 645f
    pathologic examination of sentinel node in, 648
    patient selection for, 645-646
    patterns of failure after negative findings in, 650
    preoperative lymphoscintigraphy in, 646-647, 647f
    radiocolloid and blue dye for, 644
    rationale, 643-645
    reported results of, 648-650
    sentinel node removal in, 648
    technique for, 646-648
    unusual or ambiguous drainage patterns in, 645, 645f
  national protocols for, 656-657
  radiation exposure guidelines and, 657
  training and credentialing in, 655-656
Lymph node(s)
  axillary, 634-635, 635f
  biopsy of, in HIV infection, 1336, 1337f
  cervical
    classification of, 186t, 187f
    enlarged, 186, 186t, 187f
  sentinel. *See* Lymphatic mapping and sentinel node biopsy
Lymphoma(s)
  cervical adenopathy in, 192
  in transplant recipients, 1087
Lytic therapy. *See* Thrombolytic therapy

M

Macrolide(s), 1211-1212. *See also specific drugs, e.g.,* Erythromycin
Macrophage(s)
  alveolar, in nosocomial pneumonia, 1655-1656
  in host defense, 1348, 1349f
Macrophage colony-stimulating factor
  physical properties of, 1610t
  synonyms and cell sources of, 1604t
Macrophage inflammatory protein
  physical properties of, 1610t
  synonyms and cell sources of, 1604t
Macular edema, diabetic, 995
Mafenide, for burn care, 60-61, 60t
Magnesium. *See also* Hypermagnesemia; Hypomagnesemia
  for acute dysrhythmias, after resuscitation, 18
  total body, 94t
Magnesium metabolism, 106
Magnetic resonance cholangiopancreatography (MRCP), in jaundice, 256, 256f
Magnetic resonance imaging (MRI)
  in abdominal mass, 246
  in breast complaints, 210-211
  in coma, 151-152

in intra-abdominal abscess, 1258
in jaundice due to malignant
  obstruction, 257
in spinal cord injury, 359
Malaria, transfusion therapy
  causing, 1230
Malignancy
  as complication of
    immunosuppressive therapy,
    1087
  fungal infections in, clinical
    presentation and diagnosis of,
    1293t
  hypercalcemia in, 96-98, 98t, 106
  immunodeficiency in, 1085
  wound healing and, 136-137
Malignant hyperthermia, 615-617,
  1553
  biochemical basis of, 616
  clinical manifestations of, 616
  clinical signs of, 1553
  diagnosis and treatment of, 616-
    617
    acute-phase, 616
    post-acute-phase, 616
  management of, 1553
  risk factors for, 615-616
Malignant melanoma. See Melanoma
Mallory-Weiss tear(s), management of
  upper GI bleeding in, 289
Malnutrition. See also under
  Nutrition
  in chronic hepatic disease, 1467
  immunodeficiency in, 1084
  in immunosuppressed patient, 1082
  pharmacokinetics in, 1705
  wound healing and, 136
Mammography, 210
Mandible
  examination of, in maxillofacial
    injury, 372
  fracture of, 372f, 376-377, 376f
Manganese
  in central venous nutritional
    support, 1532
  requirements for, in ICU patient,
    1525t
Mangled extremity, 477
Mannitol
  for elevated intracranial
    pressure, 356
  as free radical scavenger, 1574t,
    1575
  for heatstroke, 1553
Mannkopf sign, 237t
Marcy hernioplasty, 859-862, 860f-
  861f
Marjolin ulcer, squamous cell
  carcinoma in, 305
Mask(s), for infection control in
  operating room, 602
Mastectomy, 636-639
  breast reconstruction after, 638f,
    639-642. See also Breast
    reconstruction
  goal of, 637-638
  limited surgery (lumpectomy) vs.,
    215-216, 215t
  operative technique in, 637-639
    borders of dissection in, 637,
      639
    flaps in, 637
    incision in, 637, 637f
    modified radical, 639
    simple, 639
  skin-sparing, incision placement
    for, 639f, 640

Maxilla
  examination of, in maxillofacial
    injury, 372
  fracture of, 375f-376f, 376
Maxillofacial fracture, 375-377
  frontal sinus fracture in, 375
  mandibular fracture in, 376-377,
    376f
  maxillary fracture in, 375f-376f,
    376
  nasal and naso-orbito-ethmoidal
    fracture in, 375
  orbital fracture in, 375
  zygomatic fracture in, 375
Maxillofacial injury, 369-378
  airway assessment in, 369-371
  Angle's classification of
    malocclusion in, 369
  assessment and management of,
    Algorithm, 370
  bleeding in, 371
  computed tomography in, 373
  definitive evaluation in, 371-373
  discussion of, 377
  examination in, 371-372, 371f-372f
  external ear injury in, 374
  eyebrow injury in, 374
  eyelid injury in, 374
  facial nerve injury in, 373
  facial x-rays in, 372-373
  initial survey in, 369-371
  lacrimal duct injury in, 373
  lip injury in, 374-375
  nasal injury in, 374
  parotid duct injury in, 373
  scalp injury in, 373-374
  soft tissue injuries in
    anesthesia for, 373
    treatment of, 373-375
Maximum voluntary ventilation (MVV),
  preoperative, 1039-1041
McClintock sign, 237t
McVay-Lotheissen hernioplasty, 859-
  862, 860f-861f
Mechanical ventilation, 1423-1440
  Algorithm, 1424-1425
  assist-controlled, 1434-1435
  auto-PEEP, 1437
  basic, 1423-1426
  bronchoscopy in, 1437
  in burn care
    in early postresuscitation
      period, 479
    in first postburn week, 491
    in immediate resuscitation
      period, 53
  cardiac effects of, 1404, 1404t
  central venous pressure
    measurement in, 1375f, 1377
  for children, 1437
  continuous positive airway
    pressure (CPAP), 1435, 1435f
    for infants and neonates, 1130
    in pulmonary insufficiency, 1042
  continuous positive pressure
    (CPPV), for infants and
    neonates, 1130
  controlled (CMV), 1434
  defining, 1404
  enteral nutrition in, nutritional
    formula for, 1527
  fighting ventilator in, 1436-1437
  in improving respiratory status,
    1427-1428
  for infants and neonates, 1130,
    1437
  intermittent mandatory (IMV), 1435

central venous pressure
  measurement in, 1375f, 1377
for infants and neonates, 1130
intermittent positive pressure
  (IPP), 1437
  in pulmonary insufficiency, 1042
malfunctioning, shock in, 68
modes of, 1434-1435, 1434f-1435f
in multiple organ dysfunction
  syndrome, 1482-1483
nonpulmonary side effects of,
  1404, 1404t
oxygenation in, 1423-1426, 1426f
oxygen kinetics in, 1432, 1432f
pharmacokinetics in, 1708-1709
positive end-expiratory pressure
  (PEEP), 1404
  alveolar recruitment vs.
    distention in, 1431-1432,
    1431f
  for ARDS, 1407
  for burn patients, 53
  for infants and children, 1130
  in suspected shock, 68
  V/Q ratio in, 1418
postoperative
  in elderly patient, 1101
  in pulmonary insufficiency, 1042
postventilation prophylaxis in,
  1429-1430
pressure support, 1435
pulmonary arterial pressure and,
  1378, 1378f-1379f
pulmonary mechanics and, 1430-
  1432, 1430f-1431f
pulmonary physiology and, 1430-
  1433
renal effects of, 1404, 1404t
in severe respiratory failure,
  1438-1439
  extracorporeal life support and,
    1438-1439
  high-frequency ventilation for,
    1438
  nonventilatory treatment and,
    1438
  permissive hypercapnia in, 1438
  pressure-controlled inverse-
    ratio ventilation for, 1438
  pressure-limitation ventilation
    for, 1438
  tracheal insufflation for, 1438
sigh mode, 1435
supine vs. sitting position for,
  1431-1432
synchronized intermittent
  mandatory (SIMV), 1435
ventilation in, 1423
ventilation-perfusion matching in,
  1433
weaning from, 1428-1429, 1429f,
  1429t
  breathing exercises for, 1429,
    1429t
  difficult, 1428-1429, 1429t
  nutrition and metabolism in,
    1429
  oxygenation in, 1429
  parameters for, 1428
  technique for, 1428, 1429f
  ventilation in, 1428-1429, 1429t
in worsening respiratory status,
  1426-1427, 1426f, 1427t
  lung injury in, 1427, 1427t
  oxygenation in, 1426-1427, 1426f
  PEEP level in, 1426, 1426f
  ventilation in, 1426

writing orders for, 1436, 1437t
Mechanical ventilator(s), 1433-1434
  controls and monitors for, 1433, 1433t
  humidification for, 1434
  inspiratory flow rate control for, 1433
  inspiratory flow wave pattern control for, 1434
  inspiratory hold control for, 1434
  learning to use, 1436, 1436t
  monitors and alarms for, 1435-1436
  pressure-controlled, 1433
  pressure-cycled, 1404
  volume-controlled, 1433, 1433t
  volume-cycled, 1404
Meclofenamate, suggested dosing for, 1628t
Mediastinal infection, nosocomial, 1225
Mediastinal mass, video-assisted thoracic surgery for, 683, 683f
Mediastinal node dissection, video-assisted thoracic surgery for, 680-681
Mediastinal trauma, in chest injury, 401-402
Mediastinum, wide, in blunt trauma, 349
Mefenamic acid, suggested dosing for, 1628t
Megaspleen, laparoscopic splenectomy for, 800
Melanoma, 305-311
  benign nevi *vs.*, 305-306, 305f-306f
  incidence of, 305, 643
  lentigo (Hutchinson's freckle), 306, 307f
  lymphatic mapping and sentinel node biopsy for, 643-650
  metastatic to neck, 194
  of neck, 193
  nodular, 306, 307f
  prognostic markers in, 305
  staging of, 306-308, 307f
    Breslow, 308
    Clark, 306-308, 307f
    elective lymph node dissection for, 643-644
    lymphatic mapping and sentinel node biopsy for. *See also* Lymphatic mapping and sentinel node biopsy
  superficial spreading, 306, 307f
  treatment of, 308-311
    excisional biopsy, 308-309
    IL-2, 308
    superficial and radical groin dissection, 309-311, 309f-310f
    surgical, 308-311
    tumor vaccine, 308
Meningism, in coma, 148
Meningitis
  candidal, 1297
  posttraumatic, nosocomial, 1225
Meningoencephalitis, coma in, 151
  radiographic diagnosis of, 153
  treatment of, 156-157
Mental status
  altered. *See* Cognitive and sensory defect(s); Coma; Delirium; Dementia
  depressed, in emergency management, of substance abuse, 169

in shock, 67
Meperidine
  epidural, for postoperative pain relief, 1665t
  for patient-controlled analgesia, 1668t
  precautions for use in elderly patients, 1102
  in pregnancy, 1155
  preoperative, 544t
  suggested dosing for, 1627t
  systemic, for postoperative pain, 1663, 1664t
Mephentermine, for heart failure, 1395
Mepivacaine
  comparative pharmacology of, 612t
  for nonemergency surgery, 545t
Meropenem, 1214
  for bacterial infections, 1202t-1203t
Mesenteric artery
  embolism of, 1021-1022
  superior, traumatic injury of, 440-441, 440f-441f, 441t
Mesenteric vein, superior, traumatic injury to, 441-442, 441t
Metabolic acidosis, 110-116
  in cardiac arrest, sodium bicarbonate and, 22
  evaluation of, **Algorithm,** 108
  expected compensation for, 110t
  increased anion gap, 111-113
    in acute and chronic renal failure, 112
    in alcoholic ketoacidosis, 112
    in diabetic ketoacidosis. *See* Ketoacidosis, diabetic
    in ethylene glycol ingestion, 113
    laboratory tests for, 111
    in lactic acidosis. *See* Lactic acidosis
    in methanol ingestion, 113
    in paraldehyde intoxication, 113
    in rhabdomyolysis, 113
    in salicylate intoxication, 112-113
    in toxin ingestion, 112-113
  in infants and neonates, 1128
  normal anion gap, 113-114
    in Addison disease, 114
    in excessive acid administration, 114
    in excessive bicarbonate loss, 113-114
    in hypoaldosteronism, 114
    in occult laxative use, 113
    in renal tubular acidosis, 113-114
    in ureterosigmoidoscopy, 113
    urinary anion gap and urinary pH in, 114, 114t
  oxyhemoglobin dissociation curve in, 110, 110f
  postoperative, 1633
  in shock, 67
  sodium bicarbonate for, 110
  in surgical patient, 110-111
Metabolic alkalosis, 116-117
  complications of, 116
  evaluation of, **Algorithm,** 109
  expected compensation for, 110t
  hypokalemic, hypochloremic, postoperative, 1633
  in infants and neonates, 1127-1128
  pathophysiology of, 116

  postoperative, 1633-1634
  saline-responsive, 116
    in gastric aspiration or vomiting, 116
    postoperative, 1633-1634
    thiazide or loop diuretics causing, 116
  saline-unresponsive, 116-117
    in Cushing syndrome, 116
    in primary aldosteronism, 116
Metabolic rate
  ambient temperature and, 1505, 1505t
  basal
    for humans of various ages, 500
    for nutrient requirement, 1524, 1524t
  calculation of, 1503
  in central venous nutritional support, 1532
  in critical illness, 1504, 1504f-1505f
Metabolic response to critical illness, 1495-1520. *See also* Hypermetabolism
  Algorithm, 1496-1497
  amino acid metabolism in, 1506-1507
  bacteria in, 1514-1515
  bacterial translocation in, 1513
  bed rest in, 1500
  carbohydrate metabolism in, 1507-1508
  central nervous system in, 1511-1513
  cytokines in, 1510-1511, 1511f
  discussion of, 1502-1517
  endotoxin in, 1514-1515
  food deprivation in, 1500
  fuel metabolism in, 1508
  glucose intolerance in, 1502, 1502t, 1507
  glucose production in, accelerated, 1507
  gut in, 1503, 1513-1514
  hormones in, 1508-1510, 1509t
  hyperdynamic state in, 1500-1501, 1501f
  hypermetabolism in, 1503-1505, 1505f
  iatrogenic factors in, 1500
  IL-1 in, 1510
  infection in, 1499-1500
  inflammation in, 1498-1499, 1499t
  integration of, 1503, 1504f
  invasive devices in, 1500
  kidneys in, 1503
  lipid metabolism in, 1508
  liver in, 1503, 1507
  manipulation of, 1515-1517, 1516t
    adrenergic blockade for, 1515
    growth hormone for, 1516
    humoral blockade for, 1515
    nutritional support for, 1515
  muscle wasting in, 1501-1502, 1501f
  nitrogen loss in, 1506
  nutritional support and, 1508
  pain in, 1498
  phases of, 1495
  protein metabolism in, 1505-1507, 1506t
  sleep deprivation in, 1500
  systemic mediators of, 1508-1511
  temperature regulation in, altered, 1505, 1505t
  tumor necrosis factor in, 1510

wound in, 1495-1498, 1503, 1504f
Metaraminol, for heart failure, 1395
Methadone
  epidural, for postoperative pain relief, 1665t
  for patient-controlled analgesia, 1668t
  suggested dosing for, 1627t
  systemic, for postoperative pain, 1664
Methanol ingestion, 177, 178
  metabolic acidosis in, 113
Methicillin, 1195
  for bacterial infections, 1202t-1203t
Methicillin-resistant *Staphylococcus aureus* (MRSA), 1717, 1721-1722
Methoxamine, for CPR, 21
Methylprednisolone
  glucocorticoid and mineralocorticoid activities of, 1066t
  properties of, 1088t
  for spinal cord injury, 360, 361
Metoclopramide, as antiemetic, 614t
Metronidazole
  for bacterial infections, 1204t-1205t
  in vivo drug interactions with, 1193t
Mezlocillin, 1196, 1200
  for bacterial infections, 1202t-1203t
Microbial translocation. *See* Gastrointestinal tract, bacterial translocation from
Microbiology. *See also* Laboratory method(s); Microflora
Microflora. *See also specific sites*
  resident, as barrier to microbial invasion, 1347
Midazolam, for induction of anesthesia, 607t
Midpalmar space infection, 1283, 1284f
Miller-Abbott tube(s), postoperative management of, 1634, 1635f
Milrinone, for heart failure, 1395
Mineral(s)
  requirements for, in ICU patient, 1525, 1525t
  for stress, in surgical patients, 1525, 1525t
Minocycline, for bacterial infections, 1204t-1205t
Mirizzi syndrome, 1269
Missile emboli, to heart, 397
Mivacurium, for induction of anesthesia, 608t
Mobility, postoperative, for elderly patient, 1102-1103
Monobactam(s), 1214
  for nosocomial gram-negative bacteremia, 1180t
Moore-Pilcher balloon, for hepatic trauma, 415-416
Moraxella catarrhalis infection, antimicrobial agents for, 1197t
Morbid obesity. *See* Obesity, morbid
Morganella morganii infection, antimicrobial agents for, 1197t
Morphine
  for elderly patients, 1102
  epidural, for postoperative pain relief, 1665t
  for patient-controlled analgesia, 1668t

in pregnancy, 1155
  suggested dosing for, 1627t
  systemic, for postoperative pain, 1663, 1664t
Motorcycle accident(s). *See also* Trauma
  acute wound management after, 124
Motor vehicle accident(s), elderly patient and, 1093
Mouth, trench, antimicrobial agents for, 1198t
M protein(s), Streptococcal, in streptococcal toxic-shock syndrome, 328
MRI. *See* Magnetic resonance imaging (MRI)
Mucormycosis (zygomycosis), 1299-1300
Multiorgan failure. *See* Multiple organ dysfunction syndrome (MODS)
Multiple injury(ies), emergency management of, 337-353. *See also* Trauma, multiple
Multiple organ dysfunction syndrome (MODS), 1171, 1473-1494
  Algorithm, 1474-1475
  in burn patients, 496
  cardiovascular dysfunction in, 1480
  cardiovascular support in, 1483
  definitions of, 1478-1481
  endocrine dysfunction in, 1480
  evaluation in, 1481-1482
    in multiple-organ disease, 1481-1482
    iatrogenic, 1482
    occult, 1481-1482
    in single-organ disease, 1481
  evolution of, 1486
  fluid replacement in, 1476, 1483
  free radicals in, 1584
  gastrointestinal dysfunction in, 1480
  gastrointestinal support in, 1483
  gut hypothesis in, 1488
  hematologic dysfunction in, 1480
  hematologic support, 1483
  hemodynamic support in, 1473-1477
  hepatic dysfunction in, 1479-1480
  hepatic support in, 1483
  host septic response in, 1487
    bacterial translocation in, 1488
    cellular, 1487
    humoral, 1487
    neutrophils in, 1487
  ICU-acquired infection and, 1483-1484
  immunologic dysfunction in, 1480
  immunologic support in, 1477-1478
  laparotomy for, 1484
  life support in, withdrawal of, 1486
  metabolic support in, 1477
  microvascular injury in, 1487-1488
  neurologic dysfunction in, 1480
  nutritional support in, 1477
  pathogenesis of, 1487-1488
  patient support in, 1482-1484
  peritonitis and, persistent, 1255-1256
  preparation for operation in, 1484-1485
    in ICU, 1485
    optimization of patient, 1484
    tracheostomy in, 1485
    transport to operating room, 1484-1485
  prevention of, 1473-1478
  prognosis in, 1485-1486, 1485f, 1485t
  recognition and assessment of, 1478, 1479t
  renal dysfunction in, 1478-1479. *See also* Renal failure, acute
  renal support in, 1483
  reperfusion injury in, 1488
  respiratory dysfunction in, 1478. *See also* Adult respiratory distress syndrome (ARDS)
  respiratory support in, 1482-1483
  risk factors in, 1473, 1476t
  selective decontamination of digestive tract in, 1477
  stress ulcer prophylaxis in, 1477
  susceptible patient in, 1473
  temporal sequence of, 1481, 1481t
  terminology for, 1486-1487
  therapy for
    critical decisions in, 1484
    experimental, 1488-1489, 1488t
    manipulation of inflammatory mediators, 1488-1489
  two-hit theory of, 496-497, 497f, 1488
  wound healing abnormalities in, 1481
Murphy sign, 235, 237t
Muscle(s), necrosis of, in electrical injury, 505
Muscle mass, in elderly patients, 1108, 1108f
Muscle wasting
  in burn patient, 1694
  in disuse, 1502
  as metabolic response to critical illness, 1501-1502, 1503, 1505-1506
Musculoskeletal evaluation, in immunosuppression therapy, 1081
Musculoskeletal injury, in lightning strike, 510
Mushroom poisoning, acute hepatic failure due to, 1458
Mycobacterial infection(s)
  evaluation for, in immunosuppression therapy, 1082
  of hand, 1286
  superficial atypical, 316-317, 316f
Mycobacterium avium complex, antimicrobial agents for, 1198t
Mycobacterium fortuitum, antimicrobial agents for, 1198t
Mycobacterium kansasii, antimicrobial agents for, 1198t
Mycobacterium leprae, antimicrobial agents for, 1198t
Mycobacterium marinum, antimicrobial agents for, 1198t
Mycobacterium tuberculosis, antimicrobial agents for, 1198t
Mycoplasma pneumoniae infection, antimicrobial agents for, 1199t
Myocardial afterload, physiology of contraction and, 1399
Myocardial afterload-reducing agent(s), 1391-1393
Myocardial contractility (inotropism), physiology of, 1397-1399
  afterload and, 1399
  calcium in, 1398-1399, 1398f

inotropic agents and, 1399
preload and, 1399
sarcomeric thick and thin filaments in, 1396f-1397f, 1397-1398
sodium in, 1398f, 1399
Myocardial contusion, emergency management of, 37
Myocardial dysfunction
in acute renal failure, 1444
fluid volume infusion for, 1444
in uremic syndrome, 1057
Myocardial hypoxia, automatic dysrhythmias and, 25
Myocardial infarction
aspirin and, 1599-1600
in elderly patients, 1095
pulmonary arterial catheterization in, 1377
recent, in evaluation of operative risk, 536, 550
Myocardial ischemia, in shock, 67
Myocardial preload, physiology of contraction and, 1399
Myoglobin level, in burn patient, 57
Myoglobinuria, renal failure in, 1450
Myonecrosis, clostridial, 319
gas in, 329-330, 330f-331f
Myopathy, in uremic syndrome, 1059
Myositis, streptococcal, 328-329, 328f
Myotomy
left thoracoscopic, 702-705
operative planning in, 702-703
operative technique in, 703-704, 703f-704f
outcome evaluation in, 705t
postoperative complications in, 704-705
preoperative evaluation in, 702
right thoracoscopic, 705

N

Nabumetone, suggested dosing for, 1628t
NADPH oxidase inhibitor(s), as free radical scavenger, 1576
Nafcillin, 1195-1196
for bacterial infections, 1202t-1203t
Nalbuphine
for patient-controlled analgesia, 1668t
suggested dosing for, 1627t
Nalidixic acid, for bacterial infections, 1204t-1205t
Naloxone
for altered mental state, in substance abuse, 171
for narcotic-induced respiratory depression, 615
Naproxen, suggested dosing for, 1628t
Narcotics. *See also* Opioid(s)
abuse of. *See also* Substance abuse
emergency management of, 173-174
in acute exposure, 173-174
in chronic use, 174
in withdrawal, 174
preoperative, 544-545, 544t
Nasal. *See also* Nose
Nasal carriage, of *Staphylococcus aureus*, catheter-related infection and, 1247-1248

Nasal cavity, in differential diagnosis of neck mass, 188
Nasobiliary intubation, postoperative management of, 1634
Nasoenteric intubation. *See also* Nutritional support, enteral
for enteric nutrition, 1528
procedure for, 1528t
verification of location in, 1528
Nasogastric aspiration. *See* Aspiration, of gastric contents
Nasogastric intubation
confirming position of, 1634, 1635f
postoperative, 1634, 1634t, 1635f
Naso-orbito-ethmoidal fracture, 375
Nasopharyngeal airway, for CPR, 7, 8f
Nasopharynx
in differential diagnosis of neck mass, 188
nosocomial infection of, 1224
Nasotracheal intubation
advantages and disadvantages of, 1404t
in maxillofacial injury, 369
in trauma resuscitation, 34
Nausea and vomiting
acute abdominal pain and, 229
after anesthesia, 547, 614
antiemetic drugs for, 614, 614t
metabolic alkalosis in, 116
Neck defect(s), flaps for, 979
Neck injury, 379-393
airway compromise in, 379-381
cricothyrotomy for, 379
tracheotomy for, 379-381
assessment and management of, Algorithm, 380
at base of neck, 386-387, 387f-388f
incisions for, 395
carotid artery injury in, 384-385
jugular vein injury in, 385
laryngotracheal injury in, 381
management algorithm for carotid artery, jugular vein, pharynx, and esophagus injury in, 382f
penetrating, 379
emergency management of, 340-341, 341f
pharyngoesophageal injury in, 385-386
sternocleidomastoid incision in, 381-384
advantages of, 381
arteries and veins in, 382-384, 383f-384f
exploration and exposure in, 382-384, 383f-384f
operative technique in, 381-382, 382f-384f
pharynx and esophagus in, 384
superficial wounds in, 391
vertebral artery injury in, 387-391
Neck mass, 183-194
assessment of, Algorithm, 184-185
benign neoplasms as, 191-192
biopsy in, 189
cervical lymph nodes in, 186, 186t, 187f
congenital cystic lesions as, 190-191
dissection in, 193
etiology of, 183t

history in, 183
imaging studies in, 189
in inflammatory and infectious disorders, 189-190
initial diagnostic impression in, 188
investigative studies in, 188-189
larynx and hypopharynx in, 188
metastatic tumors as, 193-194
adenocarcinoma, 193-194
melanoma, 194
squamous cell carcinoma, 193
from unknown primary, 194
oral cavity and oropharynx in, 187-188
physical examination in, 183-188
primary malignant neoplasms as, 192-193
salivary glands in, 186-187
thyroid gland in, 186
Necrobiosis lipoidica diabeticorum, 996
Necrotic tissue, in acute wound, identification and debridement of, 125
Necrotizing cellulitis, Gram-negative synergistic, 329, 329f-330f
Necrotizing enterocolitis, in infants and neonates, 1128
Necrotizing fasciitis, 325-328
bacteriologic types in, 326
pathogenesis of, bacterial synergy in, 326
phycomycotic, 326
streptococcal gangrene *vs.*, 325, 326t
with streptococcal toxic-shock syndrome, 326-328, 326t, 327f
characteristics of, 326t
pathogenesis of, 326-328, 327f
streptococcal M proteins in, 328
superantigen theory in, 327-328, 327f
Vibrio, 326
Necrotizing infection, 317-320. *See also* Gangrene
clostridial, 318-319, 319f
pathogenesis of, 325
diffuse
antibiotics in, 324
classification of, 323, 323t
gas in wound in, 329-330, 330f-331f
nonclostridial, 318f, 320
pathogenesis of, 325-329
pathogenesis of, 325-329
requiring operation, 317-320, 323-324
diagnosis of, 317-318, 318f-319f
histologic criteria for, 318
x-ray examination in, 318, 319f
Neisseria gonorrhoeae infection, antimicrobial agents for, 1197t
Neisseria meningitidis infection, antimicrobial agents for, 1197t
Neomycin, 1210
for bacterial infections, 1202t-1203t
Neonate(s). *See* Infants and neonates
Nephron, juxtamedullary, anatomy of, 1448, 1449f
Nephropathy, diabetic, 995
Nephrotic syndrome
coagulopathy in, 82
hypercoagulable state in, 1058
Nephrotoxic agent(s), acute renal

failure due to, 1445, 1446, 1450
Nernst equation, 24
Nerve block(s), local, for postoperative pain, 1667
Netilmycin, 1210
  for bacterial infections, 1202t-1203t
Neurilemmoma(s), of neck, 192
Neurofibroma(s), of neck, 192
Neurogenic shock. See Shock, neurogenic
Neurologic evaluation
  in immunosuppressive therapy, 1080
  in spinal cord injury, 359, 360f
Neurologic injury
  in electrical injury, 508
  in extremity trauma, 466-467, 467t
    classification of, 466-467, 467t
    treatment of, 467
Neuromuscular-blocking agent(s). See also specific drugs, e.g., Succinylcholine
  for endotracheal intubation, 607, 608t
  incomplete reversal of, 615
  in renal failure, contraindicated, 1056
  respiratory muscle weakness due to, 115
Neuromuscular function, impaired, pulmonary dysfunction in, 1412
Neuropathy
  autonomic
    cardiac, diabetic, 995, 997
    in diabetes mellitus, 995
  peripheral, in diabetes mellitus, 995
  uremic, 1060
Neutropenia
  management of, 1078-1079
  prevention of, 1078
Neutropenic enterocolitis, 1079
Neutrophil(s)
  in ARDS, 1407
  defect in, 1083t
  function of, tests for, 1074
  in host defense, 1348
  in multiple organ dysfunction syndrome, 1487
  in reperfusion injury, 1574, 1578f-1579f
Neutrophil adhesion inhibitor(s), as free radical scavenger, 1576
Nevus(i)
  benign, melanoma vs., 305-306, 305f-306f
  compound, 306
  dermal, 306
  dysplastic, 306
  familial dysplastic nevus syndrome, 306
  junctional, 306
Niacin, requirements for, in ICU patient, 1524t
Nicardipine, for hypertension, 1638t
Nifedipine, for hypertension, 1638t
Nimodipine, for spinal cord injury, 360
Nipple disorder(s). See Breast complaints
Nissen fundoplication, laparoscopic, 697-702
  instrumentation for, 698, 698t
  operating table for, 697, 698f
  operative planning in, 697-698
  operative technique for, 698-701, 699f
    crural closure, 700
    esophageal bougie insertion, 700
    final inspection, 701
    gastric fundus window, 700
    gastrohepatic ligament division, 699
    peritoneum and phrenoesophageal membrane division, 699-700
    short gastric vessel division, 700
    trocar insertion, 698-699, 699f
    wrapping of gastric fundus, 700-701
  outcome evaluation in, 702
  postoperative complications, 701-702
  preoperative evaluation in, 697
Nitric oxide (endothelium-derived relaxing factor), for multiple organ dysfunction syndrome, 1483
Nitrogen balance, in central venous nutritional support, 1533-1534
Nitrogen loss, in metabolic response to critical illness, 1506
Nitroglycerin, for heart failure, 1393
Nitroprusside
  cyanide toxicity due to, 112
  discontinuance of, in lactic acidosis, 112
Nitroprusside test, for diabetic ketoacidosis, 112
Nitrous oxide, for maintenance anesthesia, 609t
Nocardia infection, antimicrobial agents for, 1199t
Nociperception. See also Pain, acute
  neural pathways in, 1670f
  physiologic mechanisms of, 1669
Nodule(s)
  pulmonary, video-assisted thoracic surgery for, 678-679, 678f
  thyroid, benign, 191
Non-AIDS immunosuppression. See Immunosuppression
Nonemergency surgical care, 535-557
  anesthesia and, 538, 539t-540t
    American Society of Anesthesiologists physical status classification and, 538, 539t
    surgical categories in, 538, 540t
  anesthesia in, 545-547
    adjunctive use of local, 546
    local and regional, 545-546, 545t
    nausea and vomiting in, 547
    nonsteroidal anti-inflammatory drugs and, 546
    toxicity and allergy of, 546-547, 547t
  consultation for, 538
  cost-effective, 519-533. See also Cost-effective nonemergency surgical care
  discharge after, 548-549, 549t
  history in, 535-536
    current medication, 536
    social, 536
  informed consent for, 543-544
  outpatient, growth of, 554-555
  outpatient vs. inpatient, 538, 541t
  perioperative monitoring in, 547-548
  perioperative risk assessment after, 550-552
    age in, 552
    anesthesia and, 550
    cardiac risk in, 550-551
    pulmonary assessment in, 551-552
  physical examination in, 535-536
    cardiovascular system in, 536
    endocrine system in, 536
    existing infection and, 536
    hematologic system in, 536
    nutritional status in, 536
    respiratory system in, 536
  postoperative care after, immediate, 548
  postoperative pain control after, 549
  postoperative risk assessment after, 552-554, 554t-555t
    delayed-type hypersensitivity skin test for, 553-554, 554t-555t
    statistical data on, 552-554
  premedication for, 544-545, 544t-545t
    antacids in, 545
    anticholinergic drugs in, 544
    histamine antagonists in, 545
    narcotics in, 544-545
    sedatives in, 545
  preoperative conference in, 543
  preoperative tests for, 536-538. See also Preoperative testing
  selection of appropriate site for procedure in, 542-543
  selection of inpatient or outpatient procedures for, 538-539
  selection of patients for inpatient or outpatient procedures for, 539-542, 541t
    adrenocortical steroid therapy and, 542
    age and, 541
    alcohol and drug abuse and, 542
    bronchopulmonary disease and, 542
    congestive heart failure and, 542
    diabetes mellitus and, 542
    heart disease and, 542
    hypertension and, 542
    obesity and, 542
    preoperative drug therapy and, 541-542
    psychiatric illness and, 542
    psychotropic drug therapy and, 542
  risk factors in, 540-542
Nonsteroidal anti-inflammatory drug(s) (NSAIDs)
  anesthesia and, 546
  in burn patients, 499
  complications of, 1667
  cyclooxygenase inhibition by, 1591-1592
  gastric mucosal damage due to, 1600-1601
  mechanism of action of, 1667
  for postoperative pain, 615, 1626, 1667, 1667t
  renal complications of, in elderly patients, 1096
  side effects of, 1596t
Norepinephrine
  in heart failure, 1394-1395
  receptor types stimulated by, 1394t
Norfloxacin, in bacterial infections, 1204t-1205t
Nose. See also under Nasal

examination of, in maxillofacial injury, 372
fracture of, 371f, 375
soft tissue injury of, 374
Nosocomial infection(s), 1221-1238. *See also under* Infection control
Algorithm, 1222-1223
atelectasis in, 1221
broad-spectrum antibiotics for, empirical, 1484
bronchitis, 1221-1224
cost of, 1234
empyema, 1225
enteric, 1229-1230. *See also* Colitis, antibiotic-associated
gram-negative
  aminoglycosides for, 1180t
  penicillins for, 1180t
hospital environment and, 1724
ICU and, 1478
  in multiple organ dysfunction syndrome, 1483-1484
incidence of, 1231-1232
intra-abdominal, 1225
with intravascular devices. *See* Intravascular device(s)
magnitude and significance of, 1231-1234
mediastinal, 1225
meningitis, posttraumatic, 1225
nasopharyngeal, 1224
osteomyelitis, 1225
paranasal sinusitis, 1224
pathogens in, 1232-1233, 1233f, 1233t
peritonitis in, 1221
pneumonia, 1221
  in burn patient, 494
  cephalosporins for, 1206-1207
postoperative fever and, 1221
pulmonary, 1171
respiratory tract, 1221-1224
risk of, 1234
sternal, 1225
surgical site. *See* Wound infection, nosocomial
tracheitis, 1221-1224
transfusion-associated. *See* Transfusion therapy, complications of
urinary tract, 1228-1229
wound infection. *See* Wound infection, nosocomial
NSAID. *See* Nonsteroidal anti-inflammatory drug(s)
Nuclear factor *kappa*B, in intracellular signaling, 1580, 1581f
Nucleotide(s), in supplemental nutritional support, 1544
Nursing home facility(ies), 1643
Nutrient requirement(s), 1524-1525
basal metabolic rate for, 1524, 1524t
in burn patients, 500-501
mineral, 1525, 1525t
protein, 1525
vitamin, 1524t, 1525
Nutrition
for elderly patient, 1108
enteral
  for burn patient, 489
  effect on gastrointestinal tract of, 1513-1514, 1538-1539, 1539f
  for elderly patient, 1109
  for infants and neonates, 1132, 1132t-1133t
  for intestinal tract support, 1539-1540
    glutamine in, 1539-1540
    pectin in, 1540
  for multiple organ dysfunction syndrome, 1483
  perioperative
    clinical trials of, 1540-1542
    cancer patients and, 1541
    complications of enteral nutrition and, 1542
    early postoperative enteral nutrition and, 1541-1542
    hip fractures and, 1541
    perioperative enteral nutrition and, 1540-1541
    postoperative TPN and, 1540
    preoperative TPN and, 1540
    indications for, 1540
  pharmacokinetics and, 1705
  pharmacotherapeutic, 1543-1546
    arginine in, 1544
    branched-chain amino acids in, 1543
    fatty acids in, 1544-1546
    glutamine in, 1543-1544
    nucleotides in, 1544
postoperative, 1636
total parenteral. *See* Nutritional support, parenteral
Nutritional assessment, in infants and neonates, 1131-1132
Nutritional requirement(s), of infants and neonates, 1131, 1131t
Nutritional support, 1521-1548
Algorithm, 1522-1523
in burn patients. *See* Burn care after first postburn week, nutrition in
cardiopulmonary function and, prioritizing, 1521-1524
in critical illness, 1515
metabolic responses to, 1508
in elderly patients, 1108-1110, 1108f-1111f
enteral, 1525-1530
  access for feeding in, 1527-1529, 1528t
  assessment of aspiration risk in, 1527
  assessment of feeding tolerance in, 1527
  balanced diet, 1526
  complications of, 1529-1530
    diarrhea, 1529, 1530f
    leakage of enteric contents, 1530
    peptic ulceration, 1530
    tube clogging, 1530
    tube dislodgement, 1530
  contraindicated in high gastrointestinal output, 1525-1526
  feeding regimens for, 1529, 1529t
  in gastrointestinal bleeding, 1526
  in gastrointestinal dysfunction, 1527
  hepatic formula, 1526-1527, 1528t
  indications for, 1526t
  intragastric, 1529, 1529t
  intrajejunal, 1529, 1529t
  modified (elemental) diet, 1526, 1528t
  monitoring in, 1529-1530, 1529t
  nasoenteric intubation for, 1528t, 1530-1531. *See also* Nasoenteric intubation
  renal formula, 1527, 1528t
  safe use of gastrointestinal tract for, 1525-1526, 1526t
  selection of diet for, 1526-1527, 1528t
  standard orders for, 1529, 1529t
  stress formula, 1527, 1528t
  in ventilator-dependent patients, 1527
evaluation of need for, 1521-1525
home, 1536-1538
  candidates for, 1536
  catheters for, 1536-1537
  complications of, 1537
  costs of, 1537
in hyperdynamic state of critical illness, 1501
in immune modulation, 1352-1353
in surgical patients, 1075
indications for, 1521
in infants and neonates, 1130-1137
in intra-abdominal abscess, 1249
in multiple organ dysfunction syndrome, 1477
in pancreatic abscess, 1273
parenteral, 1530-1536
  central venous, 1530-1532
  catheter care and sepsis in, 1534-1536, 1537f
  electrolytes for, 1531, 1532t
  general measures for, 1532-1534
  hyperglycemia in, 1534
  indications for, 1531t
  infection in, 1534-1536, 1537f
  metabolic monitoring in, 1534, 1535t-1536t
  metabolic rate in, 1532
  multiple-lumen catheters for, 1531
  nitrogen balance in, 1533-1534
  oxygen consumption in, 1533
  peripherally inserted central catheter for, 1531
  peripheral venous *vs.*, 1530
  solutions for, 1531-1532, 1531t-1533t
  trace elements for, 1532
for elderly patient, 1109
glutamine-supplemented
  for burn patients, 499
  for critical illness, 1515-1516
  intestinal mucosal effects of, 1514, 1539-1540
  metabolic complications of, 1534, 1535t
peripheral venous, 1532
  central venous *vs.*, 1530
  indications for, 1531t
preoperative
  nasoenteral. *See also* Nasoenteric intubation; Nutritional support, enteral
  total parenteral. *See also* Nutritional support, total parenteral
total parenteral
  for infants and neonates, 1132-1137. *See also under* Infants and neonates
  in multiple organ dysfunction

syndrome, complications of, 1482
in toxic epidermal necrolysis, 513
in weaning from mechanical ventilation, 1429

O

Obesity, 1003-1011
as abdominal mass, 244
Algorithm, 1004
blood pressure measurement in, 1387
cardiac dysfunction in, 1003, 1009, 1009f
central fat deposition in, morbidity of, 1007-1008
deep venous thrombosis in, 1005
degenerative osteoarthritis in, 1007
diabetes mellitus in, 1006-1007
as factor in selection for outpatient surgery, 542
gallstones in, 1007
gastric bypass for
  acute gastric distention in, 1006
  internal hernia in, 1006
  peritonitis in, 1006
gastric surgery for, 1006
  abdominal catastrophe in, 1006
immunodeficiency in, 1084
morbid
  gastric bypass *vs.* gastric resection for, 721
  gastric procedures for, 721-733. *See also individual procedures*
    failed weight loss and regain after, 732
    postoperative management after, 732
  laparoscopic adjustable gastric banding for, 722-724, 722f-723f
  laparoscopic gastric bypass for, 727-732, 728f-731f
  preparation for operation in, 721
  proximal gastric bypass for, 724-727, 724f-726f
  vertical banded gastroplasty for, 721-722, 722f
operative risks of, 1003
pharmacokinetics in, 1705
pseudotumor cerebri in, 1007
pulmonary embolism in, 1009-1010
respiratory insufficiency in, 1003-1005, 1008-1009, 1008f-1009f
  anesthesia in, 1005
  postoperative management of, 1005
sleep apnea syndrome in, 1003-1005, 1008-1009
thrombophlebitis in, 1009-1010
venous stasis ulcers in, 1009-1010, 1010f
wound care in, 1007
Obesity hypoventilation syndrome, 1005, 1008-1009
Obturator sign, 235, 237t
Octylcyanoacrylate tissue adhesive, for acute wound closure, 128
Ocular injury
  in cold exposure, 511
  in electrical injury, 508
  in lightning strike, 510
Oculocephalic reflex, doll's eye maneuver for, 147
Oculovestibular reflex, caloric test for, 148
Ofloxacin, for bacterial infections, 1204t-1205t
Ogilvie syndrome, in pregnancy, 1151
OKT3, immunodeficiency due to, 1086
Older Americans Retirement Survey (OARS), 1092
Oliguria. *See also* Urine output
  acute, in acute renal failure, 1441
  definition of, 1441
  in shock, 67
Oltipraz, as free radical scavenger, 1576
Omphalocele, in infants and neonates, emergency surgery in, 1129
Ondansetron, as antiemetic, 614t
Operating room
  additional devices in, 595
  air handling in, 592
  asepsis in, 600-602
    drapes for, 601
    gowns for, 601
    hand washing for, 601
    masks for, 602
    scrub suits for, 601
    skin preparation for, 601
    surgical attire and drapes, 601-602
  case carts in, 595
  communication equipment in, 595
  design and construction of, 591
  electrosurgical units in, 594
  equipment in, 593-595, 593t
    basic concerns with, 593
    life-support, anesthetic delivery, monitoring devices and, 593
    occupational injury and, 593
    OR devices and, 593-595, 593t
    patient safety and, 593
    surgical team efficiency and, 593
  heating and insulating devices in, 594
  housekeeping procedures for, 595-596
    dirty cases and, 596
    floor and walls and, 595-596, 596t
    machines from "outside" and, 596
    OR cleaning schedules and, 596t
  instrument tables in, 595
  lasers in, 594
  lighting in, 592-593
  OSHA standards for, 599
  physical aspects of, 591-593
  powered devices in, 594
  preparation of, 591-604
  protecting patient, 596-597
  protecting surgeon and staff, 597-600
    anesthetic gases and, 597-598
    environmental hazards and, 597-598
    ethylene oxide and, 598
    hazards during pregnancy and, 600
    infectious hazards and, 598-599, 599t
  radiologic devices in, 594
  SSI surveillance for, 602
  temperature and humidity in, 592
  traffic flow in, 591
  ultrasonic devices in, 594
  viewing and imaging devices in, 594-595
Operative site, preoperative decontamination of, 576-578
Opioid(s). *See also* Narcotics; *specific drugs*
  abuse of, by physician, 1738
  for acute pain, 1498
  addiction to, 1671-1672
  agonist, 1662
  agonist-antagonist, 1662-1663
  analgesic, preoperative, 606
  antagonist, 1662
    naloxone as, 615
  epidural and subarachnoid, 1664-1665
    mechanism of action of, 1664-1665
    for postoperative pain, 615, 1665, 1665t
    side effects of, 1665
  intrinsic activity of, 1662-1663, 1663t
  oral and parenteral, for postoperative pain, 1627t-1628t
  partial agonist, 1662
  physical dependence on, 1671
  receptor types for, 1662, 1663t
  systemic
    mechanism of action of, 1662-1663, 1663t
    for postoperative pain, 614-615
    regimens for, 1664t
    side effects of, 615, 1664
  tolerance of, 1671
Oral cavity, in differential diagnosis of neck mass, 187-188
Oral injury, in electrical burns, 508-509, 509f, 509t
Oral secretion(s), anticholinergic agents for, preoperative, 606
Orbit
  examination of, in maxillofacial injury, 372
  fracture of, 375
Organ dysfunction, multiple. *See* Multiple organ dysfunction syndrome (MODS)
Organ procurement, 959-971. *See also* Transplantation
  Algorithm, 960
  brain death and, 959
  coordination of donor and recipient activities in, 961-962
  donor for
    basic care for, 961
    evaluation and management in, 959-961
    operation for, 962-967, 962f-968f
  heart
    criteria for, 961
    technique for, 963-964, 964f
  heart-lung, criteria for, 961
  kidney
    criteria for, 959
    technique for, 965-966, 966f
  liver
    criteria for, 961
    technique for, 964-965, 964f-965f
  medical, ethical, and legal

considerations in, 969-970
pancreas, technique for, 967, 967f-968f
preliminary steps for, 959
preservation in, principles and limitations of, 968-969
vascular graft, technique for, 967
Oriental cholangiohepatitis, 1269
Oropharyngeal airway, for CPR, 7, 7f
Oropharynx, in differential diagnosis of neck mass, 187-188
Orotracheal intubation
advantages and disadvantages of, 1404t
in children, tube size for, 34
in CPR, 9-10
intubation technique for, 9-10
patient position for, 9
preparation for, 9
in head injury, 355
in maxillofacial injury, 369
in trauma resuscitation, 34
Orthopedic injury, in electrical injury, 508
Osmotic pressure, 102
Ossification, in burn patient, 1694
Osteoarthritis, degenerative, in obesity, 1007
Osteodystrophy, renal, 1060
Osteomyelitis
candidal, 1297
of hand, 1285
nosocomial, 1225
Ostomy. *See* Colostomy; Stoma(s)
Otic injury
in electrical injury, 508
in lightning strike, 510
Otorrhea, CSF, nosocomial meningitis in, 1225
Outcomes assessment, cost-effective nonemergency surgical care and, 521-522, 521t
Outpatient surgery. *See also* Nonemergency surgical care
anesthesia for, 613-614
growth of, 554-555
Ovary(ies)
cysts of, appendicitis *vs.*, 822
torsion of, appendicitis *vs.*, 822, 1150
trauma to, 458-459, 458f
Overwhelming postsplenectomy infection (OPSI), 420
Oxacillin, 1195-1196
for bacterial infections, 1202t-1203t
Oxaprozin, suggested dosing for, 1628t
Oxidant(s). *See also* Antioxidant(s); Oxygen metabolite(s), reactive
in normal physiology, 1559, 1559t
in pathophysiology, 1559, 1560t
Oxycodone, suggested dosing for, 1627t
Oxygen, partial pressure of. *See* Oxygen tension (PO_2)
Oxygenation
in chest trauma, 402
tissue
in burn patients, 491
physiology of, 1413, 1413t
ventilation *vs.*, 1423
in wound healing, 1495
Oxygen consumption (VO_2)
calculation of, 1389, 1396
in central venous nutritional support, 1533

definition of, 1413
in elderly patients, 1111-1113, 1112f-1113f
in fever, 1420
in hyperdynamic state of critical illness, 1500
in hypermetabolism, 1505
Oxygen content (CO_2)
arterial (C_aO_2), 1413
calculation of, 1413
definition of, 1413
measurement of, 1374
mixed venous ($C_{mv}O_2$), 1413
Oxygen delivery (DO_2)
decreased, causes of, 1419-1420
definition of, 1413
in elderly patients, 1111-1113, 1112f-1113f
Oxygen diffusion, pulmonary, impaired, 1418
Oxygen exchange, physiology of, 1413-1414, 1414t
Oxygen extraction ($C_{a-v}O_2$), definition of, 1413
Oxygen extraction ratio (O_2ER), myocardial effects of, 1397
Oxygen free radical(s). *See* Oxygen metabolite(s), reactive
Oxygen gradient, alveolar-arterial ($A-aDO_2$), definition of, 1414
Oxygen kinetics, in mechanical ventilation, 1432, 1432f
Oxygen metabolite(s), reactive, 1559-1589. *See also* Antioxidant; Free radical(s)
biochemical mechanisms of, 1568-1569
apoptosis as, 1569-1571
cell matrix injury as, 1569
lipid peroxidation as, 1568
nucleic acid denaturation as, 1569
protein denaturation as, 1569
biochemistry, 1559-1560, 1561f
eicosanoid synthesis and, 1594
in intracellular signaling, 1580
endothelial xanthine oxidase in, 1580
heat shock response in, 1580
nitric oxide in, 1580
nuclear factor *kappa*B in, 1580, 1581f
listing of, 1561t
sources of, 1561-1568
arachidonic acid cascade as, 1563, 1565f
chemical toxins as, 1568
chemotherapeutic agents as, 1567-1568
endogenous, 1561-1566
enzymatic oxidases as, 1561, 1563, 1564f
exogenous, 1566-1568, 1568t
ionizing radiation as, 1568
iron-catalyzed reactions as, 1563
NADPH-dependent oxidase as, 1563-1564, 1566f
oxidized metabolites of nitrogen as, 1565-1566
redox cycling of xenobiotics as, 1566-1567
univalent leak from oxidative metabolism as, 1561, 1562f
in stress response, in burn patients, 497-498, 497t
Oxygen return, calculation of, 1389

Oxygen saturation (SO_2)
arterial (S_aO_2)
in burn patients, 491
oxygen content and, 1413
pulse oximetry for, 1386
definition of, 1413
measurement of, 1371
mixed venous ($S_{mv}O_2$)
oxygen content and, 1413
pulmonary arterial catheterization for, 1385, 1385f
Oxygen tension (PO_2)
alveolar (P_AO_2), definition of, 1414
arterial (P_aO_2)
in burn patient, 57
definition of, 1414
in mechanical ventilation. *See* Mechanical ventilation
oxygen content and, 1413
preoperative, 1041
as stimulus to breath, 1415
for ventilation-perfusion matching, 1423
conjunctival, measurement of, continuous, 1386
measurement of, 1371
mixed venous ($P_{mv}O_2$)
in burn patient, 56-57
oxygen content and, 1413
tissue, measurement of, continuous, 1386
transcutaneous ($P_{tc}O_2$), measurement of, continuous, 1386
Oxygen therapy
for burn patients, in immediate resuscitation period, 54
in multiple organ dysfunction syndrome, complications of, 1482
postoperative, in pulmonary insufficiency, 1042
Oxygen toxicity, free radicals in, 1583
Oxygen transport, calculation of, 1388
Oxyhemoglobin dissociation curve, in metabolic acidosis, 110, 110f
Oxymorphone
for patient-controlled analgesia, 1668t
suggested dosing for, 1627t
Oxytetracycline, for bacterial infections, 1204t-1205t

P

Pacemaker(s)
for asystole, 11
preoperative assessment of, 564
troubleshooting for, 16-17
ventricular capture and, 17
ventricular sensing and, 17
Pain
abdominal
acute. *See* Acute abdominal pain
in elderly patient, 1092-1093
in pregnancy. *See* Pregnancy
upper. *See* Upper abdominal infection
acute
descending pain control system in, 1669
dorsal horn control systems and

modulation of incoming
signals in, 1669
epidural analgesia for, 1498
narcotic analgesics for, 1498
patient-controlled analgesia
for, 1498
peripheral receptors and neural
transmission to spinal cord
in, 1669
physiologic mechanisms of, 1669,
1670f
postinjury changes in peripheral
and central nervous systems
in, 1669
spinal reflexes in, 1669
breast, 213-214
burn, 488, 488t
drug therapy for, 59
in infection, 1166
in metabolic response to critical
illness, 1498
phantom, after below-the-knee
amputation, 955-956
postoperative, 1625-1627, 1627t-
1629t, 1659-1673
in abdominal procedures, 1659-
1662
Algorithm, 1660-1661
combination regimens for, 1668-
1669
control of, 549
cryoanalgesia for, 1667, 1668f
in elderly patient, 1102
epidural anesthetics for, 1625-
1626, 1665-1667, 1666t
epidural opioids for, 615, 1664-
1665, 1665t
guidelines for, 1659-1662
inadequate treatment of, 1659,
1659t
intrathecal opioids for, 615
manifestations of, 614
nerve blocks for, 1667
nonsteroidal anti-inflammatory
drugs for, 615, 1667, 1667t
opioids for, 614-615
systemic, 1626, 1627t-1628t,
1662-1664, 1663t-1664t
patient-controlled analgesia
for, 614-615, 1626-1627,
1629t, 1668, 1668t
in peripheral procedures, 1662
psychological interventions for,
1662, 1662t
subarachnoid opioids for, 1664-
1665
in thoracic procedures, 1659
transcutaneous electrical nerve
stimulation for, 1667-1668
treatment of, 1625-1627, 1627t-
1629t, 1662-1669. *See also
under specific drugs and
procedures*
Pain relief
effects of, 1669-1672
on metabolic response to
operation, 1669, 1671
on postoperative morbidity, 1671
postoperative. *See* Pain,
postoperative
Pain threshold, in elderly patient,
1092-1093
Pancreas
as donor organ, technique for,
967, 967f-968f
injuries to, 426t, 427-429, 428f-
431f

grade 1, 427, 429f
grade 2, 427-428
grade 3, 428, 430f
grade 4, 428-429, 431f
grade 5, 429
operative exposure of, in
abdominal injury, 408
reperfusion injury in, 1576
Pancreas transplantation, in
diabetes mellitus, 1001
Pancreatectomy, distal
for chronic pancreatitis, 776-778,
777f
ninety-five percent, 778-780, 778f-
779f
Pancreatic abscess, 1272-1273
treatment of, 1273
antibiotics for, 1273
drainage for, 1273
nutritional support for, 1273
Pancreatic carcinoma
jaundice in, 257. *See also*
Jaundice, in malignant
obstruction
unresectable, palliative bypass
for, 784-786, 784f-786f
Pancreatic juice, normal volume and
composition of, 103t
Pancreatic necrosis, infected, 1272-
1273
Pancreaticoduodenectomy (Whipple
procedure), pylorus-preserving,
773-776, 773f-776f
Pancreaticojejunostomy, longitudinal
(Puestow procedure), 780-781,
780f
Pancreatic procedure(s), 773-786
distal pancreatectomy for chronic
pancreatitis, 776-778, 777f
drainage of pancreatic pseudocyst
into Roux-en-Y jejunal loop,
781-782, 781f-782f
drainage of pancreatic pseudocyst
into stomach, 782-784, 783f
longitudinal
pancreaticojejunostomy
(Puestow procedure), 780-781,
780f
ninety-five percent distal
pancreatectomy, 778-780, 778f-
779f
palliative bypass for unresectable
pancreatic cancer, 784-786,
784f-786f
pylorus-preserving
pancreaticoduodenectomy
(Whipple procedure), 773-776,
773f-776f
Pancreatic pseudocyst
drainage of
into Roux-en-Y jejunal loop, 781-
782, 781f-782f
into stomach, 782-784, 783f
infected, 1272-1273
Pancreatitis
acute
abdominal pain and fever in,
1263-1266, 1266t
septic response in, 1184
chronic, distal pancreatectomy
for, 776-778, 777f
clinical criteria for severity of,
1272, 1272t
gallstone
cholecystectomy for, 1266-1267
ERCP sphincterotomy for, 1267,
1267f

Ranson clinical prognostic index
in, 1266, 1266t, 1274f
treatment of, 1266-1267, 1266t,
1267f
ischemic, 1576
in pregnancy, 1152
Ranson clinical prognostic index
in, 1266, 1266t, 1274f
Pancuronium, for induction of
anesthesia, 608t
p24 antigen testing, for blood
donations, for HIV screening,
1335
Pantothenic acid, requirements for,
in ICU patient, 1524t
Paraldehyde intoxication, metabolic
acidosis in, 113
Paramedic(s), in prehospital trauma
resuscitation, 41-42
Paranasal sinusitis, nosocomial,
1224
Paraplegia, in chest trauma, 403
Parastomal hernia(s), 872-873
Parathyroidectomy, 626-627
complications in, 627
hypocalcemia after, 100
operative planning in, 626
operative technique in, 626-627
outcome evaluation in, 627
Parkinson disease, free radicals in,
1583
Paronychia, 1281-1282, 1281f-1282f
Parotid duct injury, 373
Parotitis, clinical and laboratory
diagnosis of, 1171
Partial thromboplastin time (PTT),
in burn patient, 57
Pasteurella multocida
in animal-bite wound, 126, 322
antimicrobial agents for, 1198t
Patellar fracture, 473
Patient, preoperative conference
with, for nonemergency surgery,
543
Patient-controlled analgesia (PCA)
for acute pain, 1498
mechanism of action of, 1668
modes of administration and dosing
parameters for, 1668, 1668t
for postoperative pain, 614-615,
1626-1627, 1629t, 1668, 1668t
in elderly patient, 1102
side effects of, 1668
PCP, abuse of, emergency management
of, 176
in acute exposure, 176
in chronic use, 176
in withdrawal, 176
Pectin, enteral, intestinal mucosal
effects of, 1540
Pediatric surgical patient, 1121-
1143. *See also* Children; Infants
and neonates
Pediatric trauma score, 1138, 1139t
Pelvic examination, in acute
abdominal pain, 235
Pelvic fracture
in children, 1140
emergency department management
of, 40, 42f
Pelvic hernia(s), 872
Pelvis fracture, bladder rupture in,
454
Penciclovir, for herpesvirus
infections, 1328
Penicillin(s), 1192, 1194-1196, 1200
adverse effects of, 1208t

for Enterobacteriaceae bacteremia, 1180t
for nosocomial gram-negative bacteremia, 1180t
penicillinase-resistant, 1195-1196
semisynthetic, 1207f
in vivo drug interactions with, 1194t
Penicillin G
  aqueous crystalline, 1194-1195
  for bacterial infections, 1202t-1203t
  benzathine, 1195
    for bacterial infections, 1202t-1203t
  procaine, 1195
    for bacterial infections, 1202t-1203t
Penicillin V, 1195
  for bacterial infections, 1202t-1203t
Penrose drain(s), postoperative management of, 1635-1636
Pentazocine, suggested dosing for, 1627t
Pentoxifylline, for cytokine response modulation, 1618
Peptic ulcer
  in enteral nutrition, prevention of, 1530
  in immunosuppressed patient, 1076t, 1081
  NSAIDs causing, 1600-1601
  in pregnancy, 1152
Peptide(s), pulmonary metabolism of, 1417
Peptococcal bacteremia, 1181
Peptostreptococcal bacteremia, 1181
Peptostreptococcal infection, antimicrobial agents for, 1197t
Perfloxacin, for bacterial infections, 1204t-1205t
Perianal ulceration, in immunosuppressed patient, prevention of, 1076t
Pericardial effusion
  in chest trauma, 403
  uremic, 1057
Pericardial tamponade
  pulseless electrical activity in, 12t
  shock in, 68
  traumatic, emergency management of, 36-37, 38f-39f
Pericardial window, video-assisted thoracic surgery for, 682-683, 683f
Pericardiocentesis, for traumatic pericardial tamponade, 37, 38f
Pericarditis
  candidal, 1297
  uremic, 1057
Pericholecystic abscess, surgical options for, 1244t
Perineum, defects of, flaps for, 981
Peripheral nervous system evaluation, in immunosuppressive therapy, 1080
Peripheral neuropathy, in diabetes mellitus, 995
Peripheral polyneuropathy, in diabetes mellitus, 996
Peripheral vascular resistance, in sepsis, 1185
Peripheral venous catheterization, for burn patients, 54
Peritoneal access

alternative technology in, 917
catheter type in, 914, 915f
in children, 917
complications of, 917
operative planning in, 914
operative technique in, 914-917, 916f
  catheter insertion, 915
  catheter maintenance, 917
  catheter removal, 917
  catheter tunneling, 915
outcome evaluation in, 917-918
patient assessment in, 914
Peritoneal cavity, bacterial contamination of, 1250-1251. See also Peritonitis
  local response to, 1250-1251
    cytokines in, 1250, 1251
    mechanical clearance as, 1250
    phagocytosis as, 1250
    sequestration in, 1250
  systemic response to, 1251
Peritoneal dialysis. See also Peritoneal access
  antibiotics for, 1247
  catheters for, infection of, 1247-1248
  peritonitis in, 1247-1248
    antimicrobial agents for, 1247
    clinical presentation and diagnosis of, 1247
    management of, 1247-1248
Peritoneal lavage
  continuous postoperative, in peritonitis, 1253
  diagnostic, 39, 41f
  in multiple organ dysfunction syndrome, 1484
  in peritonitis, 1242, 1245, 1253
  technique for, 41f
  in trauma resuscitation, 39-40, 41f
Peritonitis, 1239-1248. See also Intra-abdominal infection(s); Peritoneal cavity, bacterial contamination of
  in AIDS, 1246
  Algorithm, 1240-1241
  candidal, 1298
  in cirrhotic ascites, 1245, 1246
  common causes of, surgical options for, 1244t
  hypovolemic shock in, 1251
  in infants and neonates, in intestinal obstruction, 1124
  laparoscopic diagnosis of, 1242
  in multiple organ dysfunction syndrome, 1484
  in nosocomial infection, 1221
  in obesity, 1006
  in peritoneal dialysis, 1247-1248
    antimicrobial agents for, 1247
    clinical presentation and diagnosis of, 1247
    management of, 1247-1248
    peritoneal lavage in, 1242, 1245, 1253
    continuous postoperative, 1253
  persistent or tertiary, 1255-1256
    abdominal compartment syndrome in, 1256
    multiorgan failure and, 1255-1256
  postoperative, surgical options for, 1244t
  primary, 1245-1247
    in children, 1245, 1246

clinical presentation and diagnosis of, 1246
management of, 1246
microorganisms in, 1245-1246
prognosis in, 1246-1247
secondary, 1239-1245
  adjuvant surgical techniques for, 1253-1255, 1254f
  antibiotic therapy for, 1242-1243, 1243t, 1251-1253
    aminoglycoside, 1252-1253
    combination, 1251-1252
    enterococci and Candida and, 1252-1253
    monotherapy for, 1252
    peritoneal culture and, 1253
  bacteria causing, 1243, 1243t
  causes of, 1239, 1242t
  clinical presentation and diagnosis in, 1239-1242
  fluid resuscitation in, 1242
  laparoscopic management of, 1243-1244
  management of, 1242-1245, 1251-1255
  operative management of, 1243-1245
  planned relaparotomy for, 1254-1255, 1254f
  preoperative preparation in, 1242-1243
  prognosis in, 1255
    APACHE II score in, 1255
  ultrasonography in diagnosis of, 1242
spontaneous bacterial, in ascites, 1464, 1464t
Pernio (chilblain), 511
Persistent vegetative state, 151
pH
  arterial. See Arterial blood pH
  conversion hydrogen ion concentration to, 1389, 1389t
  gastric. See Gastric pH
  monitoring of, in cardiac resuscitation, 22-23
  as stimulus to breath, 1415
  24-hour
    for left thoracoscopic myotomy, 702
    for Nissen fundoplication, 697
  venous blood, in cardiac arrest, 22
Phantom pain, after below-the-knee amputation, 955-956
Phantom sensation, after below-the-knee amputation, 955-956
Pharmacokinetics, 1697-1715. See also Drug administration; Drug therapy
  absorption in, 1697-1699, 1698f
  area under curve in, 1698
  bioavailability in, 1698
  blood flow in, 1697-1698, 1698f
  first-pass effect in, 1699
  ionization in, 1697, 1698f
  molecular size in, 1697, 1698f
  age of patient and, 1703-1705
  biotransformation in, 1700-1701, 1700t
    induction in, 1700-1701
  in cardiac failure, 1707-1708
  in cardiopulmonary bypass, 1708
  in child, 1703-1704
  in chronic obstructive lung disease, 1708
  distribution in, 1699-1700

protein binding in, 1699-1700
volume of, 1699, 1699t
in elderly patient, 1106-1107, 1106t, 1704-1705
elimination in, 1701-1702
clearance in, 1701
half-life in, 1701, 1702t
routes of excretion in, 1701-1702
factors modifying, 1703-1705
in fetus, 1703-1704
first-order, 1702, 1702f-1703f
in hepatic failure, 1706-1707, 1707t
in infant, 1703-1704
in malnutrition, 1705
nutritional status and, 1705
in obesity, 1705
principles of, 1702-1703
in renal failure, 1706
in respiratory disorders, 1708-1709
variables in, 1697-1702
zero-order, 1702-1703, 1704f
Pharyngoesophageal injury, 385-386
Pharynx, exposure of, in neck trauma, 384
Phenol, causing chemical burns, 52t
Phentolamine mesylate, for hypertension, 1638t
Phenylephrine
for CPR, 21
for heart failure, 1395
Pheochromocytoma, fever and hyperpyrexia in, 1554
Phlebothrombosis. *See* Thrombophlebitis
Phlegmasia cerulea dolens, 1017
Phosphate replacement, in diabetic ketoacidosis, 112
Phosphodiesterase inhibitor(s), for heart failure, 1395
Phospholipase A_2 antagonists, lipocortins as, 1591
Phycomycetes infection, antimicrobial agents for, 1199t
Phyllodes tumor, of breast, 211
Physical activity
elderly patients and, body composition effects of, 1110-1111
long-term effects of, 1110
ostomates and, 1678
postoperative, for elderly patient, 1102-1103
Physical status classification, American Society of Anesthesiologists, 538, 539t
Physical status scale, American Society of Anesthesiologists, 1718t
Physical therapy, for burn patient, 489
Physician, impaired, 1729-1739
discussion of, 1734-1738
due to age, 1729-1730, 1729t
detection of, 1729-1730
management of, 1730
manifestations of, 1734
monitoring and evaluation in, 1735
due to normative error (character impairment), 1730-1732, 1735-1736
detection of, 1730-1731, 1731t
early recognition of, 1736
management of, 1731-1732

due to substance abuse, 1732-1734, 1736-1738
alcohol in, 1736-1737
common drugs in, 1736-1738
detection of, 1732-1733, 1732t
management of, 1733-1734
opiates in, 1738
sedatives in, 1737
stimulants in, 1737-1738
prevention of, 1738
Physiologic dead space (V_D), 1415
Pickwickian syndrome, 1003, 1008-1009
obesity hypoventilation syndrome in, 1008-1009
sleep apnea syndrome in, 1008-1009
Pilon fracture, 474
Pipecuronium, for induction of anesthesia, 608t
Piperacillin, 1196, 1200
for bacterial infections, 1202t-1203t
Piperacillin-clavulanate, 1214
Piperacillin-tazobactam, 1214
Piroxicam, suggested dosing for, 1628t
Pit viper bite(s), 126-127
Plasma, fluid composition of, 101, 102f
Plastic surgical reconstruction, 973-990
acute, 973-982
antibiotics for, 976
antiseptics for, 976
bacterial counts in, 976
coverage procedure for, 976-982
debridement in, 973
evaluation and initial treatment in, 973-976
flaps for, 977-982, 978t. *See also* Flap(s)
high-pressure irrigation for, 973-976
skin grafts for, 977, 977f. *See also* Skin graft(s)
wet dressings for, 976
Algorithm, 974-975
postoperative care of, 984-985
of flaps, 984-985
patient positioning in, 985
of skin grafts, 984
secondary, 982-984
in complex defects, 983-984, 983f
in composite defects, 983-984, 983f
in contour deformity, 984
in functional defects, 984
in shortage of skin and subcutaneous tissue, 982-983
in small localized scar, 982, 982f
tissue expanders for, 982-983, 989
in unstable tissue coverage, 984
Platelet(s). *See also entries beginning* Thrombo-
in coagulopathy, 87, 88f, 89t
effect of aspirin on, 1599-1600
function of, tests of, 89t
in hemostasis, 85
Platelet-activating factor (PAF), antagonists of, 1359
Platelet count, in burn patient, 57
Platelet-derived growth factor, in experimental wound healing, 135
Platelet dysfunction, in uremic

syndrome, 1058
Pleural disease, video-assisted thoracic surgery for, 676-678
Pleural effusion, in chest trauma, 403
Pleural empyema, in chest trauma, 403
Plicamycin, for hypercalcemia, 98
Pneumatic antishock garment (PASG), for prehospital trauma resuscitation, 31, 42
Pneumatic compression, intermittent, for thromboembolic prophylaxis, 1034
Pneumocystis carinii pneumonia
in immunosuppressed patient, prevention of, 1076t
nosocomial, 1649
Pneumonectomy, video-assisted thoracic surgery for, 680
Pneumonia
alveolar (lobar), nosocomial, 1656
bacteremic (hematogenous), nosocomial, 1657
bacterial, 1412
interstitial, nosocomial, 1657
lobar, 1412
developmental stages of, 1412
lobular (bronchopneumonia), nosocomial, 1656-1657
nosocomial, 1221, 1639, 1647-1657
Algorithm, 1648
antibiotics for, 1651t
aspirates in, transtracheal, transbronchial, or bronchoscopic, 1650
blood cultures for, 1650
in burn patients, 494
causative organisms in, distribution of, 1652, 1653t
clinical and x-ray findings in, 1647-1649
diagnosis of, 1647-1650, 1649t
endotracheal intubation and, 1653-1654, 1654f
gram-negative bacillary, cephalosporins for, 1206-1207
Hemophilus influenzae, 1649
in ICU patients, incidence and mortality, 1653
impaired lung defenses in, 1652t
Klebsiella pneumoniae, 1649
lung biopsy for, 1650
lung contamination in, routes of, 1652, 1653t
management of, 1650-1651
pathophysiology of, 1652-1656
airway colonization in, 1653-1655, 1654f, 1654t
alveolar macrophage function in, 1655-1656
aspiration of secretions in, 1655, 1655t
cough reflex in, 1655
host defenses in, 1655-1656
impairment of cellular immunity in, 1656
impairment of containment process in, 1656
mucociliary action in, 1655
nasopharyngeal filter system in, 1655
Pneumocystis carinii, 1649
prevention of, 1647, 1647f
Pseudomonas aeruginosa, 1649
sputum in, 1649-1650, 1649t

Staphylococcus aureus, 1649
  types of, 1649, 1656-1657
  ventilator-associated, 1649
  viral, 1649
  opportunistic, in immunosuppression, 1076
  postoperative. *See* Pneumonia, nosocomial
Pneumonitis
  aspiration, septic response in, 1184
  uremic, 1057
Pneumothorax
  spontaneous, video-assisted thoracic surgery for, 679-680
  tension
    emergency management of, 36-37, 38f
    pulseless electrical activity in, 12t
    in shock, 68
Poisoning, mushroom, acute hepatic failure due to, 1458
Polymorphonuclear leukocyte(s). *See* Neutrophil(s)
Polymyxin(s), in vivo drug interactions with, 1194t
Polymyxin B, for bacterial infections, 1204t-1205t
Polyneuropathy
  critical illness, in multiple organ dysfunction syndrome, 1480
  peripheral, in diabetes mellitus, 996
Popliteal artery injury, in knee dislocation, 466, 466f
Porta hepatis, traumatic injury to, 445-446
Portal hypertension, 1463-1465, 1463t-1464t
  ascites in, 1463-1465, 1464t
    evaluation of, 1463-1464
    medical management of, 1464-1465
    spontaneous bacterial peritonitis and, 1464, 1464t
    surgical management of, 1465
  complications of, 1463, 1464t
  etiology of, 1463, 1463t
  variceal bleeding in, 1463, 1464t
Positioning of patient for operation, 596-597
  anesthetic considerations in, 609
  elderly patient and, 1099
  lateral position and, 597
  organ systems and, 596-597
  prone position and, 597
  sitting position and, 597
Postdural puncture headache, 613
Posterior fossa hematoma, emergency management of, 357
Postischemic injury, cerebral. *See* Reperfusion injury
Postoperative complication(s), 1636-1641
  anemia, 1640
  atelectasis, 1408, 1639
  cardiac, 1637-1639
  central venous catheterization, 1640
  deep vein thrombosis, 1640
  diabetes mellitus, 1640-1641
  fever. *See* Fever and hyperpyrexia, postoperative
  hypertension, 1638t, 1639
  hypoadrenocorticism, 1641
  hypothermia, 1637
  hypothyroidism, 1641
  pain. *See* Pain, postoperative
  peritonitis, surgical options for, 1244t
  pneumonia. *See* Pneumonia, nosocomial
  pulmonary embolism, 1639-1640
  respiratory, 1639
  thromboembolism, 1639-1640
  transfusion therapy, 1640
  upper gastrointestinal bleeding, 1640
  wound infection. *See* Wound infection
Postoperative infection. *See also* Nosocomial infection(s); Wound infection
  prevention of, 567-589. *See also* Surgical site infection
Postoperative management, 1625-1645
  of acid-base disorders, 1632-1634
  of anesthesia emergence, 610-611, 611t
  of biliary drainage catheters, 1634
  of closed suction drains, 1635
  of complications. *See* Postoperative complication(s)
  discharge from hospital and follow-up care, 1641-1644. *See also* Discharge planning
  of electrolyte abnormalities, 1632
  of fluid imbalance, 1631-1632
  of fluid overload, 1631-1632
  of fluid therapy, 1629-1634, 1630t
  of Foley catheters, 1636, 1637f
  of hyperkalemia, 1632
  of hypernatremia, 1632
  of hypokalemia, 1632
  of hyponatremia, 1632
  of hypovolemia, 1631
  of laboratory tests, 1628-1629
  of long intestinal tubes, 1634, 1635f
  of metabolic acidosis, 1633
  of metabolic alkalosis, 1633-1634
  monitoring in, 1629
  of nasogastric tubes, 1634, 1634t, 1635f
  of pain relief. *See* Pain, postoperative
  of Penrose drains, 1635-1636
  of physical signs, 1627-1628
  of renal failure, 1056-1057
  of respiratory acidosis, 1632-1633
  of respiratory alkalosis, 1633
  of sump drains, 1635
  triage in, 1629
  of tubes and drains, 1634-1636
Postoperative order(s), 1625, 1626
Postoperative pain. *See* Pain, postoperative
Postsplenectomy sepsis, in immunosuppressed patient, prevention of, 1076t
Potassium. *See also* Hyperkalemia; Hypokalemia
  balance, regulation of, 105
  in infants and neonates, 1127
  serum, 104f, 105
  postoperative, 1630-1631
  total body, 94t, 104f, 105
Potassium concentration, postoperative, 1632
Potassium replacement, in diabetic ketoacidosis, 112
Povidone-iodine
  for burn care, 60t, 61
  contraindicated in acute wound care, 127-128
Power calculation(s), cardiovascular, 1388
Power of attorney, elderly patients and, 1098
Prednisolone
  glucocorticoid and mineralocorticoid activities of, 1066t
  properties of, 1088t
Prednisone
  glucocorticoid and mineralocorticoid activities of, 1066t
  properties of, 1088t
Pregnancy, 1145-1161
  abdominal pain in
    Algorithm, 1146-1147
    initial management in, 1145
  acute cholecystitis in, 1151-1152
  acute fatty liver of, 1458
  analgesia in, 1155
  anesthesia in, 1155-1156
  antibiotics in, 1195t
  appendicitis in, 1149-1150
    diagnosis of, 1149-1150
    differential diagnosis of, 1150
    management of, 1150
  breast cancer in, 1157
  burns in, 1157-1158, 1158t
  cardiac dysrhythmia during, 19
  constipation in, 1158, 1159t
  deep vein thrombosis in, 1159, 1159t
  drug safety in, 1155, 1156t
  duodenal ulcer in, perforated, 1151
  ectopic, appendicitis *vs.,* 1150
  esophageal rupture in, 1149
  fetal and maternal monitoring in, 1156-1157
  heartburn in, 1158, 1159t
  hemodynamic values in, 1158t
  hemorrhoids in, 1158-1159, 1159t
  hepatic rupture in, 1149
  inflammatory bowel disease in, 1152-1153
  intestinal obstruction in, 1150-1151
  laboratory tests in, 1155
  laparoscopic cholecystectomy in, 755
  minor surgical problems of, 1158-1160, 1159t
  operative considerations in, 1155-1157
  ostomates and, 1679
  pancreatitis in, 1152
  peptic ulcer disease in, 1152
  physiologic alterations in, 1153-1155, 1153t
    chemical, 1153t, 1154-1155
    hematologic, 1153t, 1154-1155
    hormonal, 1154-1155
    mechanical, 1153, 1154f
  postoperative considerations in, 1157
  radiologic investigations in, 1155
  renal rupture in, 1149
  round ligament pain in, 1159t, 1160
  splenic rupture in, 1149
  trauma in, 1145-1149
    altered maternal physiology and, 1145-1148

cesarean section in, 1148-1149
diagnostic procedures in, 1148
management of, 1148-1149
uterine, 459-461, 460f
varicose veins in, 1159, 1159t
visceral rupture in, 1149
Pregnant operating room worker(s), hazards to, 600
Premature ventricular contraction(s) (PVCs)
electrophysiology of, 25
in preoperative workup, 561
Preoperative drug therapy, as factor in selection for outpatient surgery, 541-542
Preoperative shave, 570
Preoperative (surgical) scrub, 580, 583-584, 584t, 601
Preoperative testing, 536-538
blood glucose in, 537
blood urea nitrogen in, 537
cardiac assessment in. See Cardiac insufficiency, preoperative assessment of
chest x-ray in, 537
clotting profile in, 537-538
complete blood count in, 537
electrocardiography, 561-562
electrocardiography in, 537
serum electrolytes in, 537
stool exam for blood in, 538
type and crossmatch in, 538
urinalysis in, 537
Pressure garments, for burn wound rehabilitation, 1692, 1693f
Prilocaine, comparative pharmacology of, 612t
Pringle maneuver, in hepatic trauma, 413, 415f
Prinzmetal angina, 561
Procainamide
classification of, 23
complications of, 12
Procaine
comparative pharmacology of, 612t
for nonemergency surgery, 545t
Prochlorperazine, as antiemetic, 614t
Proctocolectomy
restorative, with ileoanal pouch, 830-833
colectomy and preparation of ileal mesentery in, 831
complications of, 832-833
construction of ileal pouch in, 831, 832f
diverting ileostomy in, 832
ileoanal anastomosis in, 831-832
indications for, 830
operative planning in, 830-831
operative technique in, 831-832, 832f
outcome in, 833
positioning for, 831
proctectomy in, 831
transanal purse-string suture in, 832
total, with conventional ileostomy, 828-830
complications of, 830
indications for, 828
operative planning in, 828
operative technique in, 828-830, 829f-830f
outcome of, 830
Progesterone level(s), in pregnancy, 1153-1154

Promethazine, as antiemetic, 614t
Prophylaxis, antibiotic. See Antibiotic prophylaxis
Propionibacterium infection, antimicrobial agents for, 1197t
Propofol
for elevated intracranial pressure, 358
for induction of anesthesia, 607t
Propoxyphene, suggested dosing for, 1627t
Propranolol, classification of, 23
Propylbutyldopamine, receptor types stimulated by, 1394t
Prostacyclin (PGI$_2$), 1595-1596
biologic effects of, 1595-1596
TXA$_2$ vs., 1595-1596, 1597t
Prostaglandin, 1595-1597
Prostaglandin D$_2$, 1597
Prostaglandin E$_2$
biologic effects of, 1596-1597, 1597t
immunomodulatory functions of, 1597
inhibition of, 1359
in NSAID-induced peptic ulceration, 1600-1601
side effects of, 1601
in thermoregulation, 1597
uterine effects of, 1601
Prostaglandin F$_{2alpha}$, 1597
side effects of, 1601
uterine effects of, 1601
Prostatectomy, pain relief after, 1662
Prostatitis, clinical and laboratory diagnosis, 1171
Prosthesis, leg, below-the-knee amputation and, 955
Prosthetic device infection(s), staphylococcal bacteremia due to, 1175-1177
Protein(s)
acute-phase, in stress response, in burn patients, 498
metabolism of, in critical illness, 1505-1507, 1506t
plasma, in burn patient, 57
requirements for
in burn patients, 501
in critical illness, 1501
in ICU patient, 1525
in infants and neonates, 1131, 1131t
Protein C
activated, resistance to, 1030
deficiency of, 1030-1031
Protein-calorie malnutrition. See Malnutrition; Nutritional support
Protein S deficiency, 1030-1031
Proteus mirabilis infection, antimicrobial agents for, 1197t
Proteus stuartii infection, antimicrobial agents for, 1198t
Proteus vulgaris infection, antimicrobial agents for, 1197t
Prothrombin time (PT), in burn patient, 57
Providencia rettgeri infection, antimicrobial agents for, 1197t
Pruritus, in uremic syndrome, 1060
Pseudomembranous colitis. See Colitis, antibiotic-associated
Pseudomonas aeruginosa
antimicrobial agents for, 1198t
in burn wound, 483t, 484t

Pseudomonas aeruginosa pneumonia, nosocomial, 1649
Pseudomonas cepacia infection, antimicrobial agents for, 1198t
Pseudotumor cerebri, in obesity, 1007, 1010, 1010f
Psoas sign, 235, 237t
Psychiatric illness, as factor in selection for outpatient surgery, 542
Psychogenic coma, 151
Psychological preparation, of surgical patients, 1662, 1662t
elderly, 1096
Psychosocial support, in burn wound rehabilitation, 1693
Psychotropic drug therapy, as factor in selection for outpatient surgery, 542
PT. See Prothrombin time (PT)
PTT. See Partial thromboplastin time (PTT)
Puddle sign, 237t
Puestow procedure (longitudinal pancreaticojejunostomy), 780-781, 780f
Pulmonary abnormalities in surgical patient(s), 1417-1421
alveolar hypoventilation in, 1419, 1419t
in chest wall instability, 1419
in impaired respiratory muscle function, 1419
in physical impairment, 1419
in stiff lung, 1419, 1420t
in upper airway obstruction, 1419
decreased hypoxic pulmonary vasoconstriction in, 1420-1421, 1420t
decreased oxygen delivery in, 1419-1420
impaired diffusion in, 1418
increased shunt in, 1419
pulmonary hypertension in, 1420, 1420t
ventilation-perfusion mismatch in, 1418-1419, 1418t
Pulmonary air leak, in chest trauma, 403
Pulmonary angiography, for pulmonary embolism, 1019-1020, 1020f
Pulmonary arterial end-systolic pressure-volume relation(s), aortic root and, 1388
Pulmonary arterial occlusive pressure (PAOP). See Pulmonary arterial wedge pressure (PAWP)
Pulmonary arterial pressure, 1416-1417
diastolic, wedge pressure vs., 1381
increased, causes of, 1416-1417
mechanical ventilation and, 1378, 1378f-1379f
pulmonary arterial catheterization for, 1381
Pulmonary arterial (Swan-Ganz) catheterization, 1377-1386
in bundle branch block, 1380
in cardiac output, 1383, 1384f
catheter position in, chest x-ray for, 1382f, 1383
in central venous pressure, 1381
complications of, 1378-1381, 1378f-1380f
catheter migration, 1381

dysrhythmias, 1379
  infectious, 1232
  intra-atrial curling, 1378, 1379t
  intracardiac knotting, 1381
  lodging in ventricular trabeculae, 1378, 1380, 1380f
  pulmonary artery perforation and rupture, 1381
  right ventricular puncture, 1380
  valvular damage, 1380-1381
  distance between insertion site and right atrium in, 1379t
  in high-risk patient, 562
  indications for insertion, 1377-1378
  in infants and neonates, 1122
  insertion of, 1378, 1378f
  in intravascular volume status, 1631
  in mixed venous gases, 1384-1386, 1385f
    continuous monitoring of, 1385
    technique for, 1385f
  in pulmonary arterial pressure, 1381
  recommendations for changing catheter, 1227
  in right atrial pressure, 1381
Pulmonary arterial wedge pressure (PAWP), 1381
  in burn patient, 56
  catheter position for, chest x-ray for, 1382f, 1383
  diastolic pressure *vs.*, 1381
  in heart failure, 1391
  high, pulmonary microvascular pressure and, 1381-1382
  in infants and neonates, 1122
  in left atrial pressure, 1381, 1382f
  left ventricular end-diastolic volume and, 1383
  measurement of, 1381-1383, 1382f
  ventricular compliance and, 1383
Pulmonary artery(ies), perforation of, in pulmonary arterial catheterization, 1381
Pulmonary aspergillosis, 1299
Pulmonary assessment. *See* Pulmonary function testing; Respiratory status
Pulmonary blood flow, physiology of, 1416
Pulmonary circulation, 1416-1417
  blood volume and surface area in, 1416
  pulmonary blood flow in, 1416
  vascular permeability in, 1417
  vascular pressure and resistance in, 1416-1417
Pulmonary defense mechanisms, 1417
Pulmonary disease, cystic, in infants and neonates, 1126
Pulmonary dysfunction, 1401-1421. *See also* specific disorders, e.g., Chronic obstructive pulmonary disease (COPD)
  in burn patients, in first postburn week, 494
  clinical recognition of, 1404-1412
  in impaired neuromuscular function, 1412
  management of
    Algorithm, 1402-1403
    endotracheal intubation in. *See*
Endotracheal intubation
    postoperative, 1639
    in uremic syndrome, 1057
Pulmonary edema
  cardiogenic, 1404-1405
    identifying characteristics of, 1406t
    pathophysiology of, 1405
    radiographic manifestations of, 1405, 1405t
    treatment of, 1405
  high-pressure. *See* Pulmonary edema, cardiogenic
  low-pressure
    identifying characteristics of, 1406t
    radiographic manifestations of, 1405t
  postoperative
    effects of lung water in, 1045, 1045f
    pathogenesis of, 1047-1048
    pulmonary insufficiency in, 1043
    treatment of, 1045-1046, 1046f
    pulmonary arterial catheterization in, 1377
Pulmonary embolism, 1018-1021, 1408-1409
  catastrophic, 1020-1021
  classification of, 1408
  clinical findings in, 1018, 1018t, 1409, 1409t
  diagnosis of, 1409
  differential diagnosis of, 1018, 1018t
  incidence of, 1032
  laboratory and radiographic findings in, 1409t
  management of, 1019f
  minor, 1018-1020
    differential diagnosis of, 1018
    laboratory studies for, 1018
    lung scans for, 1019
    pulmonary angiography for, 1019-1020, 1020f
  moderate, 1020, 1409
  in obesity, 1009-1010
  postoperative, 1639-1640
    in pulmonary insufficiency, 1043
  prophylaxis for, 1034
  pulmonary infarction *vs.*, 1018
  pulseless electrical activity in, 12t
  risk factors for, 1018, 1019t
  shock in, 68-69
  treatment of, 1409
  very large, 1409
Pulmonary function testing, preoperative, 1039-1041
  in elderly patients, 1095-1096
Pulmonary hypertension, 1420
  acute, 1420
  in ARDS, 1406
  causes of, 1420, 1420t
  chronic, 1420
Pulmonary infarction, pulmonary embolism *vs.*, 1018
Pulmonary infection, nosocomial, 1171
Pulmonary injury, in electrical injury, 508
Pulmonary insufficiency, 1039-1049. *See also* Adult respiratory distress syndrome (ARDS)
  Algorithm, 1040
  anesthesia-related, 615
  anesthetic choices for, 1042
  intraoperative, prevention of, 1041-1042
  postoperative
    clinical presentation in, 1043-1044, 1044t
    edema and pulmonary interstitium in, 1047-1048
    pathogenesis of, 1047-1048
    in preexisting lung disease, 1043
    prevention of, 1039, 1042-1043
    treatment of, 1044-1046, 1045f-1046f
    ventilation and pulmonary mechanics in, 1047, 1048f
  preoperative assessment of, 1039-1041
    correction of abnormalities and, 1041
Pulmonary interstitial fibrosis, in ARDS, 1406
Pulmonary mechanics
  in acute respiratory failure, 1430, 1430f
  effect of abdominal viscera on, 1431-1432
  in mechanical ventilation, 1430-1432, 1430f-1431f
  in normal lung *vs.* atelectasis, 1430, 1430f
Pulmonary metabolic function, 1417
Pulmonary nodule(s), video-assisted thoracic surgery for, 678-679, 678f
Pulmonary physiology, 1413-1417
  carbon dioxide removal, 1414-1415
  in mechanical ventilation, 1430-1433
    oxygen kinetics in, 1432, 1432f
    pulmonary mechanics and, 1430-1432, 1430f-1431f
    ventilation-perfusion matching in, 1433
  oxygen exchange, 1413-1414, 1414t
  pulmonary circulatory function, 1416-1417
  pulmonary defense mechanism, 1417
  pulmonary metabolic function, 1417
  tissue oxygenation, 1413, 1413t
  ventilation, 1415-1416
Pulmonary shunt fraction (Q_S/Q_T)
  calculation of, 1414
  definition of, 1414
Pulmonary support, for burn patients
  after first postburn week, 491-494
  in immediate resuscitation period, 54
Pulmonary toilet, for burn care, in first postburn week, 491
Pulmonary vascular permeability, 1417
Pulmonary vascular resistance, 1417
  measurement of, 1388
Pulmonary vasoconstriction, hypoxic, 1419
  decreased, 1420-1421, 1420t
Pulmonary wedge section, video-assisted thoracic surgery for, 678-679, 678f
Pulseless electrical activity (PEA), 12-13, 12t
  definition of, 12
  due to drug overdose and toxins, 12
  refractory, 11t, 12-13
  reversible causes of, 12t
  treatment of, 12-13

volume loading in CPR for, 20
Pulse oximetry
  for arterial oxygen saturation, 1386
  in infants and neonates, 1122
Pulse rate, in burn patient, 56
Puncture wound(s), timing of closure for, 124
Pupillary light reflex, in coma, 147
Purkinje (ventricular muscle) action potential, 24-25, 25f
Purpura fulminans, 323
  pathogenesis of, 331
Pyelitis, candidal, 1299
Pyelonephritis
  appendicitis vs., 1150
  nosocomial, 1229
Pyloroplasty, 718-719, 718f
  Weinberg, 718-719, 718f
Pyoderma gangrenosum, 313-316
  clinical signs of, 313-316, 313f
  diagnosis of, 316
  pathogens in, 324
  treatment of, 316
Pyridoxine, requirements for, in ICU patient, 1524t

Q

Quality of care, cost and, 519-521, 520t, 521f
Quinidine
  classification of, 23
  complications of, 12
Quinolone(s), 1215-1216
  adverse effects of, 1216
  clinical utility of, 1215-1216
  in diarrheal disease, 1215
  in intra-abdominal infection, 1216
  in joint and bone infection, 1216
  pharmacokinetics of, 1215
  in respiratory infection, 1216
  in sexually transmitted disease, 1215
  in skin and skin structure infection, 1215
  in urinary tract infection, 1215
  in vivo drug interactions with, 1194t

R

Rabies, 1330
  management of exposure to, 1316-1317, 1316t
Rabies prophylaxis, 1316t
  for animal bites, 126, 322, 331
Radial artery, for systemic arterial catheterization, 1370
Radiation therapy
  for breast cancer, 216-217
  immunodeficiency due to, 1086
  stomal site selection and, 1682
  wound healing and, 136
Radicular pain, in chest trauma, 404
Radiculopathy, diabetic, 996
Radiograph(s)
  abdominal
    in abdominal mass, 246
    in intestinal obstruction, 267-268, 268f-271f
  cervical spine, cross-table lateral, in trauma, 34, 34f, 38

chest
  in atelectasis, 1408
  in preoperative evaluation, 537
  in pulmonary arterial catheter position, 1382f, 1383
  facial, in maxillofacial injury, 372-373
Radiographic contrast agent(s)
  for adhesive obstruction of small bowel, 275-276
  nephrotoxicity of, 1450
  for postoperative ileus, 278
  renal failure and, in diabetes mellitus, 998
Radiologic evaluation
  in abdominal mass, 245-247, 246f-247f
  in acute abdominal pain, 235-236
  in coma, 151-152, 152t
  in emphysematous cholecystitis, 1267, 1268f
  in intra-abdominal abscess, 1248-1249, 1256-1258, 1256f-1257f
  in necrotizing infection, 318, 319f
  in nosocomial pneumonia, 1647-1649
  in pregnancy, 1155
  in pulmonary edema, 1405, 1405t
  safety requirements for, 594
  in spinal cord injury, 359
Radionuclide imaging
  in abdominal mass, 246
  in coronary artery disease, 562
  in intra-abdominal abscess, 1257-1258
  in lower gastrointestinal bleeding, 297-298, 297f-298f
Ransohoff sign, 237t
Rattlesnake bite(s), 126-127
Recall of intraoperative events, in general anesthesia, 610
Receptor(s), adrenergic. See Alpha receptor(s); Beta receptor(s)
Rectal abscess, in neutropenia, 1078
Rectal bleeding. See Lower gastrointestinal bleeding
Rectal examination, in acute abdominal pain, 235
Rectosigmoid trauma, 426t, 432f, 434-435
Rectum
  anastomosis for, 808
  trauma to, 426t, 432f, 434-435
Red cell(s)
  in hemostasis, 85
  production of, erythropoietin in, 1058, 1059f
Rehabilitation facility(ies), 1642
Relaparotomy, planned, for secondary peritonitis, 1254-1255, 1254f
Remifentanil, suggested dosing for, 1627t
Renal abscess, candidal, 1299
Renal artery
  proximal, traumatic injury to, 441
  traumatic injury to, 440t, 443-444, 444f
Renal artery embolism, 1022
Renal artery injury, acute, in acute renal failure, 1444
Renal blood flow
  eicosanoids in, 1598
  physiology of, 1448
  in prerenal renal failure, 1449-1450
Renal cortical necrosis, acute renal failure in, 1053

Renal dysfunction. See Renal failure
Renal failure, 1051-1062. See also Uremic syndrome
  acute, 1053, 1441-1453
    acute oliguria in, 1441
    Algorithm, 1442-1443
    anuria in, 1441
    biliary tract procedures and, 735
    causes of, 1441, 1444t
    chronic vs., 1053, 1055t
    classification of, 1054t
    differential diagnosis of, 1451
    evaluation of, 1444-1446, 1445t
    fractional excretion of sodium in, 1053
    increased serum creatinine, 1441
    intrarenal, 1053, 1054t
    maintenance of intravascular volume in, 1444
    maintenance of urine volume in, 1444
    management of, 1446-1447
    medications and nephrotoxic agents causing, 1445, 1446, 1450
    metabolic acidosis in, 112
    mortality in, 1447, 1448
    in multiple organ dysfunction syndrome, 1478
    parenchymal, 1444t, 1445
      inflammatory and vasculitic, 1450
      ischemic, 1450
      management of, 1446
      pathophysiology of, 1450
      toxic, 1450
    pathophysiology of, 1449-1450
    perfusion status in, 1441-1444
    postrenal, 1053, 1054t, 1444t, 1445
      management of, 1447
    preoperative anticoagulation in, 1058
    prerenal, 1053, 1054t, 1444t, 1445
      management of, 1446
      pathophysiology of, 1449-1450
    renal failure index in, 1451
    prerenal and parenchymal (mixed), management of, 1446-1447
    prevention of, 1448
    prevention of further injury in, 1054-1055
    progressive, 1447
      dialysis for, 1447
      drug dosages in, 1447
      renal replacement therapy in, 1447
    recognition of, 1441
    return to normal function after, 1447
    at risk groups for, 1448
    treatment of, 1450-1451
    urinary tract in, 1441-1444
    urine output in, 1441
      maintenance of, 1444, 1451
  anemia in, 1058-1059, 1059f
    blood loss in, 1058
    decreased red cell production in, 1058, 1059f
  anesthetic considerations in, 1056
  BUN and, 1051
  chronic, 1053-1054
    acute vs., 1053, 1055t
    metabolic acidosis in, 112

in chronic hepatic disease, 1466-1467, 1466t
creatinine clearance for, 1051
definition of, 1051
elective surgery in, preoperative considerations in, 1055-1056
in electrical injury, 508
emergency surgery in, preoperative considerations in, 1056
end-stage, vascular access for. *See* Vascular access
GFR for, 1051
in hepatic failure, 1461
immunodeficiency in, 1085
in occult infection, 1167
pathophysiology of, 1057-1060
disease progression and, 1057
perioperative complications of, 1055-1057
perioperative management of, **Algorithm**, 1052
pharmacokinetics in, 1706
postoperative considerations in, 1056-1057
progression of, extent and rate of, 1051-1053
radiographic contrast agent–associated, in diabetes mellitus, 998
Renal failure index, 1451
Renal formula, for enteral nutrition, 1527, 1528t
Renal function
in immunosuppression therapy, 1081
in infants and neonates, 1124, 1126
Renal injury, reperfusion, 1578-1579
Renal ischemia, acute tubular necrosis in, 1577-1578
Renal metabolism, in response to critical illness, 1503
Renal osteodystrophy, 1060
Renal papillary necrosis, acute renal failure in, 1053
Renal physiology, 1448-1449, 1449f
Renal rupture, in pregnancy, 1149
Renal transplantation
cytomegalovirus immunoglobulin for, 1356-1357
cytomegalovirus infection, 1326
herpes simplex virus infection in, 1328
Renal trauma, 449-452
blunt, 449, 451f
classification of, 449, 450f
hematuria in, 449
initial evaluation in, 449, 451f
operative management of, 449-451, 451f
penetrating, 449, 451f
postoperative care in, 451-452
Renal tubular acidosis
amphotericin B causing, 114
carbonic anhydrase inhibitors causing, 114
distal, hypoaldosteronism in, 114
metabolic acidosis in, 113-114, 114t
urinary anion gap in, 114, 114t
Renal tubular injury, limiting, 1451
Renal tubular necrosis, acute, 1053, 1450
in chronic hepatic disease, 1466-1467, 1466t
hepatorenal syndrome *vs.*, 1466t
in renal ischemia, 1577-1578
Renal tubule(s), functions of, 1448-1449
Renal vein, traumatic injury to, 441t, 444
Renin-angiotensin system, 1448, 1449f
Reperfusion injury
in arterial embolism, 1033
in brain, 1578
in central nervous system, 1578
clinical trials in, 1582-1583
definition of, 1573
endothelial cell trigger mechanism for, 1579-1580
free radical–mediated, 1573-1583
fundamental mechanism of, 1574, 1577f
in heart, 1576-1577
in intestine, 1573-1574
in kidney, 1577-1578
in liver, 1574-1576
in multiple organ dysfunction syndrome, 1488
neutrophil in, 1574, 1578f-1579f
in pancreas, 1576
quantitative importance of, 1580-1581, 1582f
in skeletal muscle, 1579
in skin, 1578-1579
in splanchnic organs, 1574-1576
in stomach, 1574
Respiration. *See also* Breathing; Mechanical ventilation; Ventilation
Cheyne-Stokes, in coma, 148
in coma, 148
Kussmaul, in coma, 148
Respiratory acidosis, 114-116
acute, 114-115
in airway obstruction, 114-115
in asthma, 115
in chronic obstructive pulmonary disease, 115
in depressed respiratory drive, 115
life-threatening, 114
pathophysiology of, 114
in pulmonary disease, 115
in respiratory muscle weakness, 115
treatment of, 114
in cardiac arrest, sodium bicarbonate and, 22
chronic, 115-116
pathophysiology of, 115
treatment of, 115-116
evaluation of, **Algorithm**, 108
expected compensation for, 110t
postoperative, 1632-1633
in salicylate intoxication, 113
Respiratory alkalosis, 117
evaluation of, **Algorithm**, 109
expected compensation for, 110t
postoperative, 1633
Respiratory disease
as factor in perioperative outcome, 551-552
pharmacokinetics in, 1708-1709
Respiratory distress, in infants and neonates, 1125-1126
Respiratory distress syndrome, adult. *See* Adult respiratory distress syndrome (ARDS)
Respiratory drive, depressed, respiratory acidosis in, 115
Respiratory dysfunction. *See* Pulmonary dysfunction
Respiratory failure
acute
diagnostic criteria for, 1401, 1401t
extracorporeal life support in, 1438
mechanical ventilation in. *See under* Mechanical ventilation
nonventilatory treatment in, 1438
permissive hypercapnia in, 1438
postoperative pulmonary insufficiency in, 1043
pulmonary mechanics in, 1430, 1430f
in infants and neonates, 1129-1130
in occult infection, 1167
Respiratory fatigue, hypermetabolism-induced, in burn patients, 494
Respiratory insufficiency. *See* Pulmonary insufficiency
in obesity. *See* Obesity, respiratory insufficiency in
Respiratory muscle impairment
alveolar hypoventilation in, 1419
respiratory acidosis in, 115
Respiratory status. *See also* Pulmonary function testing
in evaluation of operative risk, 536
in immunosuppressive therapy, 1081
preoperative assessment of, 551-552, 1039
for elderly patients, 1095-1096
Respiratory syncytial virus infection, antimicrobial agents for, 1199t
Respiratory therapy, postoperative, 1639
Respiratory tract infection(s). *See also specific infections, e.g.* Pneumonia
cephalosporins for, 1206-1207
nosocomial, 1221-1224
quinolone for, 1216
Rest home facility(ies), 1643
Restless legs syndrome, in uremia, 1060
Resuscitation
cardiopulmonary. *See* Cardiopulmonary resuscitation (CPR)
emergency management of, in substance abuse, 169
fluid. *See* Fluid resuscitation
in lower gastrointestinal bleeding, 293
trauma. *See* Trauma resuscitation
Retinopathy, diabetic, 995
proliferative, 995
Retrohepatic area, traumatic injury to, 446
Retroperitoneal abscess, 1248
Retroperitoneal hematoma, 406, 406f
Retroperitoneal injury, repair of, 410
Retrovirus(es), HIV as, 1341-1342
Rhabdomyolysis, metabolic acidosis in, 113
Rhabdomyosarcoma, of neck, 192-193
Rheumatoid arthritis, eicosanoids and, 1600
Rhinorrhea, CSF, nosocomial meningitis in, 1225
Rib fracture(s), alveolar hypoventilation in, 1419
Riboflavin, requirements for, in ICU patient, 1524t

Rickettsial infection, antimicrobial agents for, 1199t
Right atrial pressure, pulmonary arterial catheterization for, 1381
Right ventricle, puncture of, in pulmonary arterial catheterization, 1380
Right ventricular end-diastolic volume, measurement of, 1383-1384, 1387
Right ventricular end-systolic pressure, calculation of, 1387-1388
Right ventricular end-systolic pressure-volume relation(s), 1388
Right ventricular end-systolic volume
 calculation of, 1387
 unstressed, calculation of, 1387
Ringer solution, lactated. See Lactated Ringer solution
Ritter disease. See Toxic epidermal necrolysis
Rives-Stoppa incisional hernioplasty, 871f, 874
Rofecoxib, suggested dosing for, 1628t
Round ligament pain, in pregnancy, 1159t, 1160
Roux-en-Y esophagojejunostomy, in total gastrectomy, 715-717, 716f
Roux-en-Y jejunal limb, in distal subtotal gastric resection, 715
Rovsing sign, 235, 237t

S

Salicylate intoxication
 metabolic acidosis in, 112-113
 respiratory acidosis in, 113
Saline, hypertonic
 for acute renal failure, 1444
 for burn patients, in immediate resuscitation period, 55
Saliva, normal volume and composition of, 103t
Salivary gland(s)
 benign tumors of, 191
 in differential diagnosis of neck mass, 186-187
Salmonella typhi infection, antimicrobial agents for, 1198t
Salsalate, suggested dosing for, 1628t
Same day surgery. See Surgery, admission day
Saphenous vein cutdown, in trauma resuscitation, 35, 36f
Sarcoma(s), soft tissue, of neck, 192-193
Scab, as wound dressing, 131
Scalp injury, 373-374
Scar(s)
 hypertrophic, 138
 in burn patient, 502-503
 plastic surgical reconstruction of, 982, 982f
Scintigraphy. See Radionuclide imaging
Scopolamine
 as antiemetic, 614t
 preoperative, 606
Scrotum
 gangrene of

Fournier, 329, 329f
 idiopathic, 329
 trauma to, 461-462, 461f
Scrub, preoperative (surgical), 580, 583-584, 584t, 601
Scrub suit, for infection control in operating room, 601
Sebaceous cyst(s), of neck, 191
Sedation
 for burn patient, 488, 488t
 for hemorrhoid surgery, 844, 845f
 preoperative, 545
Sedative abuse, by physician, 1737
Seizure(s), 157-158, 157t. See also Status epilepticus
 in alcohol withdrawal, 179
 causes of, 157
 emergency management of, **Algorithm,** 144-145
 focal, 157, 157t
 generalized, 157, 157t
 in substance abuse, emergency management of, 171
 tonic-clonic, 157
Sellick maneuver, for assisted ventilation, 7, 8f
Sensory defect(s). See Cognitive and sensory defect(s)
Sepsis. See also Infection(s); Shock, inflammatory; Shock, septic
 in absence of infection, 1169, 1184. See also Fever and hyperpyrexia, postoperative
 in acute pancreatitis, 1184
 in aspiration pneumonitis, 1184
 clinical triggers of, 1184
 discussion of, 1184-1185
 therapy in, 1170
 blood cultures in, 1175-1189. See also Blood culture(s)
 catheter. See under Intravascular device(s)
 definition of, 1163
 immunodeficiency in, 1084
 in immunosuppression. See Immunosuppression, infection in
 infection vs., 1163
 inflammatory activation in, 1184-1185
 management of, 1187-1188
 metabolic features of, 1185
 natural history of, 1185-1186, 1185f
 neonatal, 1128-1129
 pathophysiology of, 1186-1187
  local events in, 1186
  systemic events in, 1187, 1187f
 physiologic elements of, 1185
 pulmonary arterial catheterization in, 1377
 reduced peripheral vascular resistance in, 1185
 severe
  definition of, 1163
  therapy in, 1169
 therapy in, 1169
  antibiotic, 1169
  drainage, 1169
 tumor necrosis factor in, 1606
 upper abdominal. See Upper abdominal infection
Septic response. See Sepsis; Shock, inflammatory; Shock, septic
Septic shock. See Shock, inflammatory; Shock, septic

Serotonin, pulmonary metabolism of, 1417
Serratia infection, antimicrobial agents for, 1198t
Serum chemistry(ies), in pregnancy, 1155
Sexual activity, ostomates and, 1678-1679, 1678f-1679f
Sexually transmitted disease, quinolone for, 1215
Shave, preoperative, 570
Shigella infection, antimicrobial agents for, 1198t
Shivering, in fever and hyperpyrexia, 1552-1553
Shock, 63-76
 cardiogenic, 63, 66t
  left-sided, 66t
  traumatic, 37
  treatment of, 72
 classification of, 63, 66t
 cutaneous hypoperfusion in, 67
 extracardiac
  compressive/obstructive, 63, 66t
  treatment of, 69
 hemorrhagic, free radicals in, 1584
 hypotension in, 63
 hypovolemic, 63, 66t
  in infants and neonates, 1122
  in peritonitis, 1251
  pulmonary arterial catheterization in, 1377
  treatment of, 69-71
   acidemia in, 71
   coagulopathy in, 71
   fluid administration in, 70-71
   hypothermia in, 71
   pain in, 71
   underlying cause and, 69
   vascular access and, 69-70
 hypoxemia in, 67
 ICU management of. See also Ventricular contraction
 inflammatory, 63, 66t
  treatment of, 71
 life-threatening conditions in, 67-69
  acute medical conditions as, 69
  bleeding as, 69
  compression or obstruction of heart or great vessels as, 68-69
  dysrhythmias as, 68
  loss of airway or inadequate ventilation as, 68
 mental abnormalities in, 67
 metabolic acidemia in, 67
 myocardial ischemia, 67
 neurogenic, 63, 66t
  treatment of, 71
 oliguria in, 67
 persistent
  invasive monitoring in, 72
  resuscitation in, 72-74, 73t
  treatment of, 72-75
   when heart is priority, 75
   when periphery and heart are equal priorities, 75
   when periphery is priority, 74-75
    fluid administration for, 74-75
    inotropes for, 75
    vasoconstrictors for, 75
 recognition of, 63-67, 67t

septic. *See also* Infection(s); Sepsis
  definition of, 1163
  free radicals in, 1584
  in infants and neonates, 1122
  in intestinal obstruction, 1124
  in occult infection, 1167
  therapy in, 1169
  surgical site infection and, 576, 581f
  tachycardia or bradycardia in, 67
  tachypnea in, 67
  thermodynamic concepts in, 73
  treatment of
    Algorithm, 64-65
    based on physiologic abnormality, 69-72
Shock liver (ischemic hepatitis), in multiple organ dysfunction syndrome, 1479-1480
Shoe cover(s), for infection control in operating room, 602
Short-bowel syndrome, in infants and neonates, 1137
Shouldice-Bassini hernioplasty, 861-862, 860f-861f
Sick euthyroid syndrome, in multiple organ dysfunction syndrome, 1480
Sigmoid colon, resection of, laparoscopic, 839, 840f
Sigmoidoscopy
  in intestinal obstruction, 270
  rigid, in lower gastrointestinal bleeding, 296
Sigmoid volvulus
  abdominal radiography in, 268, 270f
  operative therapy in
    elective, 276-277
    immediate, 273-274
  in pregnancy, 1151
Silver sulfadiazine
  for burn care, 60, 60t
  for infected wound, 126
  for wound dressing, 130
Sinus, frontal, fracture of, 375
Sinusitis
  clinical and laboratory diagnosis, 1171
  in immunosuppression, 1078
  paranasal, nosocomial, 1224
Sisomicin, 1210
Skeletal muscle, reperfusion injury in, 1579
Skilled nursing home facility(ies), 1643
Skin. *See also entries under* Cutaneous
  biopsy of, 301
  evaluation of, in immunosuppression therapy, 1081
  hypoperfusion of, in shock, 67
  microflora of. *See* Cutaneous microflora
  preoperative decontamination of, 576, 583-584
  reperfusion injury in, 1578-1579
Skin carcinoma
  basal cell. *See* Basal cell carcinoma
  in immunosuppressed patient, prevention of, 1076t
  melanoma. *See* Melanoma
  squamous cell, 304-305, 304f
    metastatic to neck, 193

of neck, 193
  in transplant recipients, 1087
Skin care, in burn wound rehabilitation, 1692-1693, 1693t
Skin graft(s), 986. *See also* Flap(s)
  for acute wound care, 129
  for burn wound. *See* Burn wound care, closure in
  donor site for, 129
  dressings for, 130
  healing of, 986
  postoperative care of, 984
  healing, physiology of, 135
  meshed, 129
  for plastic surgical reconstruction, 977, 977f
  postoperative care of, 984-985
  revascularization of, 986
  survival of, 986
Skin infection
  in immunosuppression, 1076
  quinolone for, 1215
Skin injury, in lightning strike, 510
Skin integrity, nursing care for, 1500
Skin lesion(s), 301-312
  Algorithm, 302
  nonsuspicious, 301
  suspicious, 301
    biopsy of, 301
    clinical staging of malignancy in, 301
Skin preparation, for operative site, 601
Skin substitute(s), temporary, for burn care, 49
Skin testing, delayed-type hypersensitivity. *See* Delayed-type hypersensitivity
Sleep apnea syndrome, in obesity, 1003-1005, 1008-1009
Sleep deprivation, in metabolic response to critical illness, 1500
Small bowel
  anastomosis for, 808
  infarction of, surgical options for, 1244t
  obstruction of
    abdominal radiography in, 268, 268f-269f
    adhesive partial, 275-276, 277
    causes of, 266t
    complete, 272
    partial, without previous abdominal operation, 277
    in pregnancy, 1150-1151
  perforation of, surgical options for, 1244t
  trauma to, 426t, 429-432, 431f
  repair of, 409
  volvulus of, operative therapy in, 273-274
Smoking, cigarette
  postoperative pulmonary insufficiency in, 1043
  wound healing and, 136
Snake bite(s), 126-127
Snap test, for catheter-tubing-transducer, in systemic arterial pressure measurement, 1370, 1372f
Social history, in evaluation of operative risk, 536
Sociobiological function, during hospitalization, for elderly

patient, 1102t
Sodium. *See also* Hypernatremia; Hyponatremia
  assessment of, 94
  fractional extraction of (FENa), in acute renal failure, 1053, 1445, 1445t
  in infants and neonates, 1127
  in myocardial contractility, 1398f, 1399
  postoperative assessment of, 1632
  total body, 94t
  urine level of, in acute renal failure, 1445, 1445t
Sodium bicarbonate. *See also* Bicarbonate
  for CPR, 22
  for lactic acidosis, 119
  for metabolic acidosis, 110
  for trauma patient, 45
Sodium chloride solution, electrolyte content of, 103t
Sodium lactate solution, electrolyte content of, 103t
Sodium nitroprusside
  for heart failure, 1391-1393
  for hypertension, 1638t
Soft tissue infection, 313-333. *See also specific types*
  Algorithm, 314-315
  animal bite, 321-322, 330-331
  antibiotics and pathogens in, 324-325
  cellulitis, nonoperative, 320-321
  classification of, 323, 323t
  cutaneous abscess, 313
  diffuse, 317-321
  focal, 313-317
    confined, 313
    spreading, 313-317
  gangrene, postoperative progressive bacterial, 317, 317f
  gas in, 329-330
  human bite, 322, 330-331
  mycobacterial, superficial atypical, 316-317
  necrotizing. *See also* Necrotizing infection
    operation in, 317-320
    pathogenesis of, 325-329
  operation in, 323-324
  purpura fulminans, 323, 331
  pyoderma gangrenosum, 313-316
  recognition of, 323
Soft tissue injury, in extremity trauma, 476-477
Soft tissue sarcoma(s), of neck, 192-193
Somatostatin, for adhesive obstruction of small bowel, 275
Spectinomycin, for bacterial infections, 1204t-1205t
Sphincteroplasty, transduodenal, 743-744, 744f
  operative technique in, 743-744, 744f
  troubleshooting in, 744
Spider bite(s), 127
Spigelian hernia(s), 871-872
Spinal cord injury, 358-362
  cervical. *See* Cervical spine fracture; Cervical spine injury
  complete, 365
  costs of, 355
  diagnosis and initial management of, 358-360, 359f-360f

incidence of, 355
neurological exam in, 359, 360f
radiography in, 359
thoracolumbar spine in, 362, 362f, 362t
treatment of, 360-361
  pharmacologic, 360-361
  surgical, 361
  traction in, 360
Spinal shock, in spinal cord injury, 359
Spinal tap. See Cerebrospinal fluid examination
Spirometry. See Pulmonary function testing
Splenectomy
  in AIDS, 1338
  immunodeficiency in, 1086
  laparoscopic, 787-801
    anatomic considerations in, 788-791, 788f-790f
      branches of splenic artery, 789-790, 788f-789f
      collaterals, 790, 788f
      splenic artery, 788-789, 788f
      suspensory ligaments, 790-791, 790f
    complications of, 799
    for extraction of specimens, 799-800
    in massive splenomegaly, 800
    in megaspleen, 800
    operative planning in, 787-791
    operative technique, 791-799
      anterior approach, 794-797
        lower pole and blood supply, 795, 788f
        splenic extraction, 795-797
        trocar placement, 795, 797f
      lateral approach, 791-794
        accessory spleens and, 792, 793f
        phrenicocolic ligament, 792-793
        splenic extraction, 794, 796f
        splenic hilum, 793-794, 795f-796f
        "splenic tent," 792-793, 793f
        trocar placement, 791-792, 791f-792f
        vessels at lower pole, 792-793, 793f
    in partial splenectomy, 797-798, 798f
    preoperative splenic artery embolization, 798-799
    outcome evaluation in, 800-801, 800t
    postoperative care in, 799
    preoperative evaluation in, 787, 787t
Splenic abscess, 1273-1275, 1275f
  diagnosis of, 1273-1274, 1275f
  treatment of, 1274-1275
Splenic artery, embolization of, preoperative, 798-799
Splenic rupture, in pregnancy, 1149
Splenic trauma, 420, 420t, 421f
  in children, 1139-1140, 1141f
  nonoperative treatment of, 421-422
Splenomegaly, massive, laparoscopic splenectomy for, 800
Splinting
  for burn wound rehabilitation, 1692, 1692f
  for extremity trauma, 463-465
Sporothrix schenckii infection, antimicrobial agents for, 1199t
Sporotrichosis, in hand infection, 1286
Sprain, in extremity trauma, 477
Spray gun injury, acute wound management after, 125
Sputum, in nosocomial pneumonia, 1649-1650, 1649t
Squamous cell carcinoma, 304-305, 304f
  metastatic to neck, 193
  of neck, 193
SSI surveillance program, 602
Staphylococcal bacteremia, 1175-1178
  intravascular devices causing, 1175, 1178t, 1178f
  methicillin-resistant, 1178
  prosthetic materials causing, 1175-1177
Staphylococcal scalded skin syndrome. See Toxic epidermal necrolysis
Staphylococcus aureus
  antimicrobial agents for, 1197t
  in bite wounds, 126
  in burn wound, 483t, 484t
  methicillin-resistant (MRSA), 1717, 1721-1722
  nasal carriage of, catheter-related infection and, 1247-1248
  in toxic-shock syndrome, 1178
Staphylococcus aureus pneumonia, nosocomial, 1649
Staphylococcus epidermidis
  antimicrobial agents for, 1197t
  in surgical infections, 1177
Staple(s)
  for acute wound closure, 128
  for intestinal anastomosis. See Intestinal anastomosis, stapled
Starvation, in metabolic response to critical illness, 1500
Static compliance (C_{stat}), definition of, 1416
Status epilepticus, 157-158
  cellular, metabolic, systemic effects of, 165-166
  management of, 158
  pharmacotherapy for, 158
  prognosis in, 166
Sterilization, of surgical equipment, for AIDS patients, 1339
Sternal infection, nosocomial, 1225
Sternocleidomastoid incision, in neck injury, 381-384. See also under Neck injury
Sternotomy, pain relief after, 1659
Steroid(s). See Corticosteroid(s)
Stevens-Johnson syndrome. See Toxic epidermal necrolysis
Stimulant abuse, by physician, 1737-1738
Stocking(s), antiembolic, 1034
Stoma(s), 1675-1690
  Algorithm, 1676-1677
  continent, postoperative care of, 1688
  discharge objectives for, 1685-1688
  peristomal skin care and, 1686-1687, 1686f, 1687t
  written patient information for, 1687-1688, 1688t
  emergency counseling for, 1680
  enterostomal therapist and, 1680
  manufacturers of products for, 1687t, 1687
  measurement of, 1685, 1685f
  postoperative care for, 1683-1688
    first postoperative day, 1684
    in operating room, 1683-1684, 1683f-1684f
    subsequent days, 1684-1685, 1685f
  pouches for, 1683, 1683f
  preoperative counseling for, 1675-1680
  publications for patients, 1680t
  rigid bridges for, 1683, 1683f
  site selection for, 1680-1683
    abdominal shape and, 1681-1682, 1682f
    general considerations for, 1680-1681, 1680f-1681f
    handicapped patients and, 1682
    marking site, 1682-1683
    multiple stomas and, 1681
    radiation therapy and, 1682
    special considerations for, 1681-1682
    type of stoma and, 1681, 1681f
  social and medical support systems for, 1685, 1686t
Stomach
  injuries to, 425, 425f, 426t
  reperfusion injury in, 1574
Stool. See Fecal
Stoppa giant prosthetic reinforcement of visceral sac, 866-867, 868f-870f
Strain, in extremity trauma, 477
Strength, muscle, in elderly patients, 1108, 1108f-1109f
Streptobacillus moniliformis infection, antimicrobial agents for, 1198t
Streptococcal bacteremia, 1178-1179
  anaerobic, 1181
Streptococcal gangrene, 325, 326t
Streptococcal infection
  alpha-hemolytic
    in bite wounds, 126
    in endocarditis, 1179
    in cellulitis, 320
  group(s) A, C, and G, antimicrobial agents for, 1197t
  group A, in necrotizing soft tissue infection, 1178
  group B, antimicrobial agents for, 1197t
Streptococcal M protein(s), in streptococcal toxic-shock syndrome, 328
Streptococcal myositis, 328-329, 328f
Streptococcal toxic-shock syndrome, necrotizing fasciitis with, 326-328, 326t, 327f
  characteristics of, 326t
  pathogenesis of, 326-328, 327f
  streptococcal M proteins in, 328
  superantigen theory in, 327-328, 327f
Streptococcus bovis infection, antimicrobial agents for, 1197t
Streptococcus pneumoniae infection, antimicrobial agents for, 1197t
Streptococcus viridans, antimicrobial agents for, 1197t
Streptokinase, 1027

Streptomycin, 1209-1210
  for bacterial infections, 1202t-1203t
Stress formula, for enteral nutrition, 1527, 1528t
Stress hormone(s)
  in burn patients, 498-499
  in metabolic response to critical illness, 1508-1509, 1509t
Stress response
  in burn patients, 496-499, 496f
    acute-phase proteins in, 498
    afferent arc: inflammatory response, 496-498
    CNS modulation in, 498
    control methods for, 498-499
      decrease gut leakage, 499
      exogenous inflammatory inhibitors for, 499, 499t
      glutamine for, 499
      modulate stress hormone activity, 499
      modulate stress hormone release, 498-499
      prevent second insult, 499
      remove inflammatory focus, 498
    cytokines in, 497
    efferent arc: stress hormone response, 498
    eicosanoids in, 498
    endotoxin in, 497
    metabolic alterations in, 498, 498t
    reactive oxygen metabolites in, 497-498, 497t
    two-hit theory of, 496-497, 497f
  in wound excision and grafting, 488-489
  effect of pain relief on, 1671
  physiologic role of, 1671
  postoperative, fluid therapy and, 1630
  in surgical patients, vitamin and mineral therapy for, 1525, 1526t
Stress ulcer(s)
  in ischemia, 1574
  prophylaxis against, in multiple organ dysfunction syndrome, 1477
Stricture, anal, after hemorrhoid surgery, 848
Strictureplasty, intestinal anastomosis for, 809
Stroke
  aspirin and, 1599-1600
  coma in, 150
    radiographic diagnosis of, 152-153
    treatment of, 156
  prior, carotid arterial procedures for, 921
  risk of
    annual, in carotid bruit, 198t, 199
    high, in carotid bruit, 199-200, 202t
Stroke volume, calculation of, 1387
Study on the Efficacy of Nosocomial Infection Control (SENIC), 1717
Stupor. *See* Coma
Subarachnoid hemorrhage, coma in, 150-151, 150t
  radiographic diagnosis of, 153, 153t, 153f
  treatment of, 156
Substance abuse. *See also specific drugs*
  alcohol. *See* Alcohol intoxication
  amphetamine. *See* Amphetamine(s)
  barbiturate. *See* Barbiturate(s)
  body packing in, 173
  body stuffing in, 173
  cocaine. *See* Cocaine
  emergency management of, 169-180
    Algorithm, 170
    anesthesia and, 173
    coma and altered mental state in, 169-171
      antidotes for, 169-171
      dextrose for, 169-171
      flumazenil for, 171
      naloxone for, 171
      thiamine for, 171
    enhancing drug elimination in, 173
    laboratory studies in, 172
    patient evaluation in, 171-172
    patient history in, 171-172
    perioperative considerations in, 173
    physical examination in, 172
    preventing drug absorption in, 172-173
    resuscitation in, 169
    seizure in, 171
    severe agitation in, 171
    urgent syndromes in, 169-171
  as factor in selection for outpatient surgery, 542
  hallucinogen. *See* LSD; PCP
  narcotic. *See* Narcotics; Opioid(s)
  by physician. *See* Physician, impaired, due to substance abuse
  stimulant, 174-175. *See also* Cocaine
Subtrochanteric fracture, 471f, 472
Succinylcholine, for induction of anesthesia, 608t
Succus entericus, normal volume and composition of, 103t
Suction drain(s), postoperative management of, 1635
Sufentanil
  epidural, for postoperative pain relief, 1665t
  for induction of anesthesia, 607t
  preoperative, 544t
  suggested dosing for, 1627t
Sulbactam, 1214-1215
Sulfadiazine, for bacterial infections, 1204t-1205t
Sulfisoxazole, for bacterial infections, 1204t-1205t
Sulfonamide(s), in vivo drug interactions with, 1194t
Sulindac, suggested dosing for, 1628t
Summer sign, 237t
Sump drain(s), postoperative management of, 1635
Superantigen(s), streptococcal toxic-shock syndrome, 327-328, 327f
Superoxide dismutase, as free radical scavenger, 1575
Suprapubic cystostomy, for urethral trauma, 456-457
Supratentorial tumor, coma in, 150
Supraventricular tachycardia, in preoperative workup, 561
Surfactant, in maintenance of open alveoli, 1415
Surgery
  admission day, home environment and discharge in, 611
  elective
    remote infection and, 570
    renal failure and, 1055-1056
  emergency. *See* Emergency operation
  nonemergency. *See also* Nonemergency surgical care
  outpatient, anesthesia for, 613-614
Surgical care, cost-effective nonemergency, 519-533. *See also* Cost-effective nonemergency surgical care
Surgical equipment, sterilization of, for AIDS patients, 1339
Surgical instrument(s)
  disinfection of, 1719
  powered, safety requirements for, 594
Surgical procedure(s). *See also* Wound(s); Wound care; Wound infection
  clean, 571t, 596
    antibiotic prophylaxis for, 572
  clean-contaminated, 571t, 596
    antibiotic prophylaxis for, 572
  contaminated, 571t, 596
    antibiotic prophylaxis for, 573
  dirty or infected, 571t, 596
    antibiotic prophylaxis for, 573
  operating room cleanup rituals for, 596
Surgical site infection, 1722-1723, 1722t. *See also* Infection control; Wound infection
  antibiotic prophylaxis of, 572-573, 578-583
    antibiotic selection and administration for, 581-582
    complications of, 583
    current issues with, 583
    patient selection for, 580-581, 582t
    pioneer study on, 580, 582f
    trauma patients and, 582
  bacteria in, 570-573, 574t
    antibiotic-resistant, 572
    control of sources of, 570-571
    inoculum size of, 570, 571f
    probability of contamination and, 571, 571t
    properties of, 571-572
    surgeons and, 572-573, 580f
  bowel barrier function and, 574
  deep incisional, 567, 570f
  definition of, 567, 570f
  determinants of, 567, 567f
  drains and, 574
  duration of operation and, 574
  electrocautery and, 574
  environment: local factors in, 570f-571f, 573-574, 581f
  epidemiology of, 567-578
    Algorithm, 568-569
  host defense mechanisms in, 575-578
    patient factors in, 575-578
    surgeon-related factors in, 575
  integration of determinants of, 578, 581t
  integration of determinants of infection in, 585-586, 586t
  local blood flow and, 574, 581f
  organ/space, 567, 570f
  patient age and, 574
  patient factors in, 574, 581f

shock and, 576, 581f
superficial incisional, 567, 570f
surgeon's influence on, 571f, 573-574
Suture(s), for acute wound closure, 128
Swan-Ganz catheterization. *See* Pulmonary arterial (Swan-Ganz) catheterization
Sympathectomy, video-assisted thoracic surgery for, 683-684
Syndrome of inappropriate antidiuretic hormone secretion (SIADH)
　acute renal failure in, 1446
　diagnosis and treatment of, 1450
　hyponatremia in, 104
Systemic arterial catheterization, 1365-1374
　complications of, 1365
　　heparin flush for, 1365
　　sepsis, 1232, 1365
　　thrombosis, 1365
　in high-risk patient, 562-563
　indications for insertion of, 1365
　insertion technique for, 1370
　measurements obtained by, 1371-1374. *See also* Arterial blood gas(es); Arterial blood pH
　for systemic arterial pressure, 1365-1370, 1371f-1372f, 1373f-1374f
Systemic arterial pressure, 1365-1370, 1371f-1372f, 1373f-1374f
　in burn patient, 56
　catheter-tubing-transducer system for, snap test for, 1370, 1372f
　catheter whip and, 1370, 1373f
　mean pressure for, 1365, 1371f
　pressure differences at varying distances from heart in, 1370, 1374f
Systemic inflammatory response syndrome (SIRS), 1171-1173, 1184, 1487
Systemic vascular resistance, measurement of, 1388

T

TAC, for anesthesia in wound closure, 127
Tachycardia
　in burn patient, 56
　in shock, 67
　supraventricular, in preoperative workup, 561
　ventricular, management of, in CPR, 10-11
Tachydysrhythmia(s), maintenance anesthesia causing, 609
Tachypnea
　in infection, 1166
　in shock, 67
Tamponade
　cardiac. *See* Pericardial tamponade
　pericardial. *See* Pericardial tamponade
Tape, for acute wound closure, 128
Tar, causing chemical burns, 52t
Tazobactam, 1214-1215
T cell(s), in host defense, 1348
T cell deficiency, 1083, 1083t
T cell function, in surgical patients, 1074

Teeth, precautions for, in endotracheal intubation, 607
Temperature. *See also* Fever and hyperpyrexia; Hypothermia
　ambient
　　fever in critical illness and, 1498-1499
　　in hyperdynamic state of critical illness, 1501, 1505, 1505t
　metabolic rate and, 1505, 1505t
　patient control of, 1556-1557, 1556t
　in burn patient, 57
　extreme variations in, morbidity and mortality in, 1549f
　in hypothermia, varying degrees of, 1555t
　in infants and neonates, 1121
　measurement of, in hypothermia, 1555, 1555t
　regulation
　　in burn patient, 1694
　　in elderly patients, 1113
　　in hypermetabolism, 1505, 1505t
　room, in operating room, 592
　skin, continuous measurement of, 1386
Ten horn sign, 237t
Tenosynovitis, suppurative flexor, of hand, 1282-1283, 1283f-1284f
Tension pneumothorax. *See* Pneumothorax, tension
Tetanus prophylaxis
　for acute wounds, 121, 124t
　in burn care, 60
Tetracaine, comparative pharmacology of, 612t
Tetracycline(s), 1211
　adverse effects of, 1208t
　for bacterial infections, 1204t-1205t
　in vivo drug interactions with, 1194t
Thallium scan. *See* Radionuclide imaging
THAM, for lactic acidosis, 119
Thenar space infection, 1283, 1284f
Thermal injury, 505-515. *See also* Cold injury; Electrical Injury; Toxic epidermal necrolysis
Thiamine
　for altered mental state, in substance abuse, 171
　deficiency of. *See also* Wernicke-Korsakoff syndrome
　　glucose administration and, 146
　requirements for, in ICU patient, 1524t
Thiazide, metabolic alkalosis due to, 116
Thigh defect(s), flaps for, 981
Thiopental, for induction of anesthesia, 607t
Thoracic outlet injury, 399
　incisions for, 395
Thoracic spine injury, 355
Thoracic surgery
　pain relief after, 1659
　video-assisted. *See* Video-assisted thoracic surgery (VATS)
Thoracic trauma. *See* Chest trauma
Thoracoabdominal trauma, penetrating, 402
　emergency management of, 342, 344, 344f
Thoracolumbar spine fracture, 362,

362f, 362t. *See also* Spinal cord injury
Thoracoscopy, 673-686
　historical, 673
　for myotomy, 702-705. *See also under* Myotomy
　video-assisted. *See* Video-assisted thoracic surgery (VATS)
Thoracostomy, tube, for tension pneumothorax, 36-37, 38f
Thoracotomy
　in chest injury, 395
　　choices for, 395
　　resuscitative, 395
　emergency, 38, 39f, 44
　　for blunt chest trauma, 346
　　for penetrating chest trauma, 341, 342
　pain relief after, 1659
Thrombocytopenia
　in multiple organ dysfunction syndrome, 1480
　in occult infection, 1167
Thromboembolism, 1013-1037
　postoperative, 1639-1640
　shock in, 68
Thrombolytic therapy, 1026-1028. *See also* Streptokinase; Urokinase
　administration of, 1027
　complications of, 1027-1028
　indications and contraindications for, 1026-1027
　monitoring effects of, 1027
Thrombophlebitis
　deep, 1013-1017
　　clinical manifestations of, 1013-1014
　　incidence of, 1032
　　management of, 1015f-1016f
　　nonocclusive, 1014-1015
　　　phlebography for, 1015, 1017f
　　　risk factors for, 1015t
　　　treatment of, 1015
　　occlusive, 1015-1017
　　　arm, 1016-1017, 1017t
　　　leg, 1015-1016
　in obesity, 1009-1010
　septic, intravascular devices causing, 1013, 1175, 1227
　superficial, 1013
　　clinical manifestations of, 1013
　　management of, 1013, 1014f
　　septic, 1013
　　sterile, 1013
　suppurative, in hematogenous candidiasis, 1294, 1297
Thrombosis
　arterial, arterial embolism *vs.*, 1021, 1021t
　deep vein
　　in obesity, 1005
　　postoperative, 1640
　　in pulmonary insufficiency, 1043
　　in pregnancy, 1159, 1159t
　　prophylaxis for, in laparoscopic cholecystectomy, 755
　septic, in central venous catheterization, 1227
　systemic arterial catheters causing, 1365
　venous
　　as complication of percutaneous catheterization, 913
　　pathophysiology of, 1031-1032
　　prophylaxis for, 1034
Thrombotic syndrome(s), 1028-1032

acquired, 1028, 1029f, 1030t
activated protein C resistance as, 1030
antithrombin III deficiency as, 1030
congenital, 1028-1031, 1029f, 1030t
dysfibrinogenemia as, 1028-1029
dysfibrinolysis as, 1029-1030
initial laboratory assessment in, 1028
in nephrotic syndrome, 1058
protein C deficiency as, 1030-1031
protein S deficiency as, 1030-1031
screening for, 1028-1031, 1029f
treatment of, 1031
Thromboxane, 1593-1595
TXA_2, 1593-1595
PGI_2 vs., 1595-1596, 1597t
TXB_2, 1593-1595
Thrush, 1297-1298
Thyroglossal duct cyst, 190
Thyroid cancer, 192
Thyroidectomy, 621-626
complications of, 625-626
hypocalcemia after, 100
operative planning in, 621
operative technique in, 621-625, 621f-625f
closure in, 624-625
general troubleshooting, 621
identification of recurrent laryngeal nerves, 623-624, 624f
incision, 621-622, 621f
isthmus division, 622
midline dissection, 622, 622f
mobilization of pyramidal lobe, 624, 625f
thyroid mobilization, 622-623, 623f
thyroid resection, 624
outcome evaluation in, 626
special concerns in, 625
invasion of trachea or esophagus, 625
median sternotomy, 625
neck dissection for nodal metastasis, 625
Thyroid gland
in differential diagnosis of neck mass, 186
nodules of, benign, 191
Thyrotoxic crisis
fever and hyperpyrexia in, 1554
treatment of, 1554
Tibial fracture, 473-474
Ticarcillin, 1196
for bacterial infections, 1202t-1203t
Ticarcillin-clavulanate, 1214
for bacterial infections, 1202t-1203t
Tidal volume (V_T), definition of, 1415
Tissue expander(s), 989
Tissue oxygenation. See Oxygenation, tissue
Tissue plasminogen activator, 1027
TNF. See Tumor necrosis factor
Tobramycin, 1210
for bacterial infections, 1202t-1203t
Toe, amputation of, 949-951, 949f-951f
complications and outcome of, 951
operative planning in, 950

operative technique in, 950-951, 949f-951f
ray, 950-951, 951f-952f
transphalangeal, 949f, 950
Tolmetin, suggested dosing for, 1628t
Toma sign, 237t
Torticollis, in birth trauma, 1141
Total parenteral nutrition. See Nutritional support, parenteral; Nutritional support, total parenteral
Toxic epidermal necrolysis, 511-513
clinical manifestations of, 512-513
treatment of, 512f, 513
cardiopulmonary stability in, 513
nutrition in, 513
wound management and infection control in, 513, 513t
Toxic liver syndrome, 1462
Toxic-shock syndrome
staphylococcal, 1178
streptococcal, necrotizing fasciitis with, 326-328, 326t, 327f
characteristics of, 326t
pathogenesis of, 326-328, 327f
streptococcal M proteins in, 328
superantigen theory in, 327-328, 327f
Trace element(s)
for central venous nutritional support, 1532
for elderly patient, 1108
requirements for, in burn patients, 501
Tracheal injury
complications of, 403-404
isolated, 381
Tracheal insufflation, in acute respiratory failure, 1438
Tracheal intubation. See Endotracheal intubation; Nasotracheal intubation; Orotracheal intubation
Tracheitis, nosocomial, 1221-1224
Tracheobronchial aspiration, in nosocomial pneumonia, 1655, 1655t
Tracheostomy
for burn patients
contraindicated, 53
in early postresuscitation period, 479
in first postburn week, 494
in multiple organ dysfunction syndrome, in ICU vs. operating room, 1485
Tracheotomy
advantages and disadvantages of, 1404t
conversion to cricothyrotomy of, 392-393
in maxillofacial injury, 369
in neck injury, 379-381
Tramadol, suggested dosing for, 1627t
TRAM flap, for breast reconstruction, 640f, 641-642
Transbronchial aspiration, for nosocomial pneumonia, 1650
Transcutaneous electrical nerve stimulation (TENS), for postoperative pain relief, 1667-1668

Transduodenal sphincteroplasty, 743-744, 744f
operative technique in, 743-744, 744f
troubleshooting in, 744
Transforming growth factor-*beta*, in experimental wound healing, 135
Transfusion therapy
in anemia, 83-84, 83f, 84t
autologous, for trauma resuscitation, 44
blood substitutes for, 84, 84t
for burn patients
after first postburn week, 496
in immediate resuscitation period, 56
complications of, 45
cytomegalovirus infection, 1325-1327
Epstein-Barr virus infection, 1327
hepatitis B, 1230, 1324
hepatitis C, 1230, 1322, 1324
hepatitis D, 1324
HIV infection, 1230-1231, 1319-1320, 1335
hypocalcemia, 45
hypothermia, 45
infectious, 1230-1231
malaria, 1230
donors for, acceptance policy for, 1319, 1320t
immunodeficiency in, 1086
massive, complications of, 45
in multiple organ dysfunction syndrome, complications of, 1482
O-negative blood for, for trauma resuscitation, 43
red cell
for burn patients, in early postresuscitation period, 482
postoperative, 1640
for trauma resuscitation, 36, 43-44
autotransfusion for, 44
complications of, 45
crystalloid for, 43
discussion of, 43-44
type O-negative blood for, 43
Transhepatic biliary drainage, percutaneous, for acute cholangitis, 1270
Transient ischemic attack(s) (TIAs)
aspirin and, 1600
carotid arterial procedures for, 921
carotid bruit and, 195
Transmetatarsal, amputation, 951-953, 953f
complications and outcome in, 953
operative planning in, 951
operative technique in, 951-953, 953f
Transplantation
cytomegalovirus infection in, 1326
donor organs for. See Organ procurement
Epstein-Barr virus infection in, 1327-1328
HIV infection in, 1320
immunosuppressive therapy in,
malignancy in, 1087
islet cell, in diabetes mellitus, 1001
kidney

cytomegalovirus immunoglobulin for, 1356-1357
cytomegalovirus infection, 1326
herpes simplex virus infection in, 1328
liver
 for chronic hepatic disease, 1468-1469, 1468t
 for hepatic failure, 1462
 for hepatic trauma, 418
pancreas, in diabetes mellitus, 1001
varicella-zoster virus infection in, 1328
Transport, to operating room, in multiple organ dysfunction syndrome, 1484-1485
Transtracheal aspiration, for nosocomial pneumonia, 1650
Trauma. See also under specific anatomic locations
 abdominal. See Abdominal injury
 acute wound care after. See Wound care, acute
 antibiotic prophylaxis for, 573, 582
 aortic, thoracic, 398-399, 398f-399f
 bile duct, 419-420
 birth, 1141
 bladder, 454-456
 cardiac arrest in, management of, 3
 chest. See Chest trauma
 in children, 1137-1141. See also Children, trauma in
 colon, 432-434
 diaphragmatic, 420-421
  complications of, 403-404
 duodenal, 425-426, 426t, 427f
 in elderly patient, 1093-1094, 1093t
 extremity, 463-477
 gallbladder, 419-420
 gastric, 425, 425f, 426t
 great vessels of abdomen, 437-447
 head. See Head injury
 heart, 396-398, 396f-397f
 hepatic, 413-419
 in children, 1140, 1140f
 immunodeficiency in, 1086
 kidney, 449-452
 multiple
  blunt, 346-352
   cervical spine injury in, 350, 352
   extremity fracture or dislocation in, 352
   hematuria in, 352
   hemodynamic stability in, 351f
   loss of consciousness in, 349
   pulseless extremity in, 349-350
   stable patient in, 348-349, 348f
   unstable patient in, 346-348, 347f
   wide mediastinum in, 349
  cardiopulmonary arrest in, 337-339, 339f-340f
  emergency management of, 337-353
   Algorithm, 338
  penetrating, 337-345
   of chest, 341-342, 342f-343f
   of extremities, 344-345, 346f
   of neck, 340-341, 341f
   of thoracoabdominal region, 342-344, 344f-345f
 ovarian, 458-459, 458f
 in pregnancy, 1145-1149
  uterine, 459-461, 460f
 rectal, 426t, 432f, 434-435
 rectosigmoid, 426t, 432f, 434-435
 scrotal, 461-462, 461f
 small bowel, 426t, 429-432, 431f
 spinal. See Spinal cord injury
 splenic, 420, 420t, 421f
  nonoperative treatment of, 421-422
 ureter, 452-454
 urethra, 456-458
 urogenital tract, 449-462
 uterine, 458-459, 458f
  gravid, 459-461, 460f
 vaginal, 458-459, 458f
Trauma resuscitation, 31-47
 Algorithm, 32-33
 emergency department management in, 31-40
 air embolism in, 37-38
 airway, breathing, circulation in, 42
 airway/breathing in, 31-35, 34f-35f
 aortic cross-clamping in, 44
 bicarbonate in, 45
 blood transfusion in, 36, 43-44. See also Transfusion therapy, for trauma resuscitation
 cardiac massage in, 38
 cardiogenic shock in, 36
 cervical spine trauma in, 31-34, 34f
  airway management in, 31-34, 34f, 42
 circulation in, 34-35, 36f
 coagulopathy and, 44-45, 44f
 cricothyrotomy in, 34, 35f
 discussion on, 43-45
 evaluation and continued resuscitation in, 35-38
 hypothermia in, 38, 45
 monitoring in, 44
 myocardial contusion in, 37
 nasotracheal intubation in, 34
 orotracheal intubation in, 34
 pelvic fracture assessment in, 40, 42f
 pericardial tamponade in, 36-37, 36-37, 38f-39f
 pericardiocentesis in, 37, 38f
 peritoneal lavage in, 39-40, 41f
 primary survey and initial resuscitation in, 31-35
 saphenous vein cutdown in, 35, 36f
 secondary survey and definitive diagnosis in, 38-40
 tension pneumothorax in, 36-37, 37f-38f
 thoracostomy in, tube, 36-37, 37f
 venous access in, 35, 36f
 prehospital care in, 31
 basic trauma life support for, 31
 discussion on, 41-42
 paramedics and, 41-42
 pneumatic antishock garment (PASG) for, 31, 42
Trauma Score, Pediatric, 1138, 1139t
Trench foot, 511
Trench mouth, antimicrobial agents for, 1198t
Treponema pallidum infection, antimicrobial agents for, 1199t
Triage, postoperative, 1629
Triamcinolone, glucocorticoid and mineralocorticoid activities of, 1066t
Trichophyton rubrum infection, of hand, 1286
Trimethaphan
 for heart failure, 1393
 for hypertension, 1638t
Trimethoprim
 for bacterial infections, 1204t-1205t
 in vivo drug interactions with, 1194t
Trimethoprim-sulfamethoxazole
 for bacterial infections, 1204t-1205t
 in vivo drug interactions with, 1194t
T tube(s), biliary, postoperative management of, 1634
Tuberculosis, precautions for, health care personnel and, 1721
Tubocurarine, for induction of anesthesia, 608t
Tubular necrosis, renal. See Renal tubular necrosis
Tumor necrosis factor, 1603, 1606
 in acute phase response, 1606, 1606f
 antibodies to, 1618
 biologic activities of, 1605t
 in cachexia, 1606
 detection of
  after experimental infusion, 1608, 1609f
  in infection, 1608
  in different infectious states, 1511f
 effects on wound healing, 1603, 1606
 in endotoxin tolerance, 1357-1358, 1612
 glucocorticoids as antagonists of, 1608-1609
 immunologic activities of, 1603
 metabolic effects of, 1606, 1606f
 in metabolic response to critical illness, 1510
 physical properties of, 1610t, 1616
 in propagation of mediator cascade, 1612, 1613f-1614f
 in sepsis, 1606
 soluble TNF receptors as inhibitors of, 1609, 1610f, 1618
 in stress response, in burn patients, 497
 synergism of, 1612
 synonyms and cell sources of, 1604t
 tissue levels of, 1611-1612, 1611f
Tumor necrosis factor-*alpha*, 1348-1349
 host tolerance to, 1351-1352
Tumor necrosis factor binding protein, physical properties of, 1616
Tumor necrosis factor receptor immunoadhesin (TNFR-IgG), 1618
Tumor vaccine, for melanoma, 308

U

Ulcer(s)
  anal, 854-856. *See also* Anal ulcer
  Curling, gastric pH and, 489
  duodenal. *See* Duodenal ulcer(s)
  gastric. *See* Gastric ulcer(s)
  jejunal, management of upper GI bleeding in, 290
  peptic. *See* Peptic ulcer
  stress. *See* Stress ulcer(s)
  venous stasis, in obesity, 1009-1010, 1010f
Ulcerative colitis
  appendix in, 822
  eicosanoids and, 1600
  in pregnancy, 1152-1153
  zileuton for, 1600
Ultrasonography
  in abdominal aortic aneurysm, 937, 938f
  in abdominal mass, 246-247
  in acute conditions, 663, 663f
    nontraumatic, 663, 663f-664f
    traumatic, 663
  in breast complaints, 210, 661-662, 668f-669f, 669
  in carotid bruit, asymptomatic, 200
  continuous performance improvement in, 665
  documentation for, 664-665
  endoanal, 662
  endorectal, 662, 662f
  endoscopic, 662
  essential principles of, 661t
  FAST in, 663, 665f-668f, 667-669
  of gastrointestinal tract, 662, 662f
  historical, 659-660
  instrumentation for, 664
  in intestinal obstruction, 270-271
  in intra-abdominal abscess, 1256-1257, 1256f
  intraoperative, 663
  in jaundice, 255, 256
    due to malignant obstruction, 257-258
  laparoscopic, 663, 765
  in laparoscopic cholecystectomy, 753
  in neck mass, 189
  patient positioning for, 664, 665f
  in peritonitis, secondary, 1242
  physics and instrumentation in, 659-661, 661t-662t, 662f
  scanning modes for, 661
  surgical applications of, 659-671
  in surgical ICU, 664, 664f
  technical tips in, 665-667
  terminology in assessment of, 661t
  transducer for, 659-660, 662f
  transducer frequencies in, 660, 662t
  of vascular system, 663-664
Umbilical hernia(s), 871
Universal precaution(s), 1720
  for HIV infection, 1309, 1312t, 1340-1341
Upper abdominal infection, 1263-1278
  Algorithm, 1264-1265
  fever and abdominal mass in, 1271-1275
    epigastric or left upper quadrant, 1272-1275
    right upper quadrant, 1271-1272
  fever and jaundice in, 1269-1270
    diagnosis of, 1269
    treatment of, 1269-1270
  pain and fever in, 1263-1269
    diagnosis of, 1263-1266, 1263f, 1266t
    treatment of, 1266-1269
Upper extremity. *See under* Extremity(ies)
Upper gastrointestinal bleeding, 283-291. *See also* Lower gastrointestinal bleeding
  in acute hemorrhagic gastritis, 289
  in aortoenteric fistula, 290
  in arteriovenous malformation, 290
  assessment and management of, *Algorithm,* 284-285
  in chronic duodenal ulcer, 286-287, 287f
  in chronic gastric ulcer, 287, 287f
  in Dieulafoy lesion, 290
  in duodenal diverticula, 290
  in esophageal hiatal hernia, 289-290
  in esophageal varices, 287-289, 288f
  in gastric varices, 288f, 289
  in hemobilia, 290
  in hemosuccus pancreaticus, 290
  history in, 283
  initial assessment and management of, 283
  in jejunal diverticula, 290
  in jejunal ulcer, 290
  in Mallory-Weiss tears, 289
  nasogastric aspiration in, 286
  in neoplasms, 289
  other tests in, 286
  physical examination in, 286
  resuscitation in, 283
  upper GI endoscopy in, 286
  workup in, 283-286
Ureaplasma urealyticum infection, antimicrobial agents for, 1199t
Ureidopenicillin(s), 1196, 1200
Uremic encephalopathy, 1060
  coma in, 149
Uremic syndrome, 1057-1060. *See also* Renal failure
  cardiovascular system in, 1057
  dermal system in, 1060
  endocrine system in, 1058
  gastrointestinal system in, 1057-1058
  hematologic system in, 1058-1059, 1059f
  immune system in, 1059
  major organ systems in, 1057-1060
  musculoskeletal system in, 1059-1060
  nervous system in, 1060
  pulmonary system in, 1057
  wound healing and, 137
Ureter(s)
  fungus ball of, candidal, 1299
  trauma to, 452-454
    initial evaluation in, 452-453, 453f
    operative management in, 453-454, 454f
    postoperative care in, 454
Ureterosigmoidoscopy, hyperchloremic metabolic acidosis in, 113
Urethra
  female, trauma to, 456
  male, trauma to, 456-458
    initial evaluation of, 456
    operative management of, 455f, 456-458
    suprapubic cystostomy for, 456-457
Urinalysis, 235
  in pregnancy, 1154-1155
  in preoperative evaluation, 537
Urinary anion gap, in metabolic acidosis, 114, 114t
Urinary incontinence, postoperative, in elderly patients, 1103
Urinary retention, after hemorrhoid surgery, 848
Urinary tract, Foley catheterization of. *See* Foley catheterization
Urinary tract infection
  bladder *vs.* renal, 1229
  catheter-associated, 1228
    incidence of, 1231-1232
  cephalosporins for, 1207
  clinical and laboratory diagnosis of, 1170
  condom catheter and, 1228
  in Foley catheterization, 1636
  in immunosuppressed patient, prevention of, 1076t
  nosocomial, 1228-1229, 1231-1232
  quinolone for, 1215
Urinary tract obstruction, in acute renal failure, 1444, 1447
Urine
  pH, in metabolic acidosis, 114, 114t
  retention of, local epidural anesthesia causing, 1666
  sodium level, in acute renal failure, 1445, 1445t
Urine output. *See also* Oliguria
  in acute renal failure, 1444, 1451
  in burn patient, 57
  in infants and neonates, 1121
Urogenital tract, trauma to, 449-462
Urography, excretory, in abdominal mass, 246
Urokinase, 1027
Urologic procedure(s), antibiotic prophylaxis for, 572
Uterus, trauma to, 458-459, 458f
  in pregnancy, 459-461, 460f

V

Vaccination, 1353
  for health care personnel, 1344, 1720
  hepatitis B, 1314-1315, 1315t, 1344
  for immunocompromise, in surgical patients, 1075
  tumor, for melanoma, 308
Vagina
  preoperative decontamination of, 576
  trauma to, 458-459, 458f
Vagotomy, 707-712
  highly selective (proximal gastric), 709-711, 711f
  for chronic duodenal ulcer, 287
  complications of, 711
  with patch closure for perforation, 711
  laparoscopic, 711-712
  transthoracic (subdiaphragmatic), 707, 709, 709f
  truncal, 707-709, 708f

types of, 707
Valacyclovir, for herpesvirus infections, 1328
Valvular heart disease, in preoperative evaluation, 559
Vancomycin, 1212-1213
  adverse effects of, 1208t
  for bacterial infections, 1204t-1205t
Vancomycin-resistant enterococcal infection, 1179
Varicella-zoster virus infection, 1328
  agents effective against, 1329t
  antimicrobial agents for, 1199t
Varices
  esophageal. *See* Esophageal varices
  gastric
    management of upper GI bleeding in, 288f, 289
    in portal hypertension, 1463, 1464t
Varicose veins, in pregnancy, 1159, 1159t
Vascular access, 897-919
  arteriovenous fistula for, 897-908
    autogenous
      arterial inflow in, 902
      AV anastomosis in, 902-903
      infection in, 907-908
      late thrombosis in, 905
      operative technique for, 898-901
      troubleshooting for, 902-903
      types of, 898
      venous outflow in, 902
    brachiobasilic, operative technique for, 900-901, 902f
    brachiocephalic, 898
      operative technique for, 899-900, 901f-902f
    choice of type of, 898
    complications of, 904-908
      arterial stenosis as, 905
      central venous stenosis as, 904-905
      early thrombosis as, 905
      inadequate maturation of vein as, 907
      infection as, 907-908
      late thrombosis as, 905-906
      pseudoaneurysm as, 907
      steal syndrome as, 906, 906f
      true aneurysm as, 907
      venous stenosis as, 904-905
    follow-up for, 904
    graft
      arterial anastomosis in, 904
      infection in, 908
      late thrombosis in, 905-906
      operative technique for, 901, 903f
      skin incisions in, 903
      troubleshooting for, 903-904
      tunneling in, 903-904, 904f
      type of, 904
      types of, 898
      venous anastomosis in, 904
    noninvasive preoperative assessment in, 897-898, 898t
    operative planning in, 897-898
    operative technique for, 898-901
    outcome evaluation in, 908
    prosthetic, 898
    radiocephalic, 898
      operative technique for, 898-899, 899f-900f
    troubleshooting for, 902-904
    vein transposition in forearm, 898
      operative technique for, 899, 900f
    venous system assessment in, 897
  percutaneous catheter for, 908-914
    catheter types for, 909
      cuffed, 909
      noncuffed, 909
    complications in, 912-914
      catheter infection as, 913-914
      catheter malfunction as, 913
      central venous thrombosis as, 913
      early, 912-913
      late, 913-914
    femoral vein approach for, 912
    insertion site for, 909-910
    operative planning in, 908-910
    operative technique for, 910-912
    outcome evaluation in, 914
    patient assessment in, 908-909
    right internal jugular approach for, 910-912
      cannulation of right IJ vein in, 910-911, 910f
      evaluation in, 912
      insertion of cuffed catheter in, 911-912, 912f
      insertion of noncuffed catheter in, 911, 911f
    patient preparation for, 910
    subclavian vein approach for, 912
Vascular graft, procurement technique for, 967
Vascular injury, of extremities, 465-466, 465f-466f
Vascular malformation, in differential diagnosis of neck mass, 190-191
Vascular procedure(s), pain relief after, 1662
Vascular repair, in abdominal injury, 408-409
Vascular resistance, measurement of, 1388
Vascular system
  risk assessment for, 198
  ultrasonography of, 663-664
Vasoactive agent(s), for multiple organ dysfunction syndrome, 1476
Vasoconstriction, hypoxic pulmonary, 1419
  decreased, 1420-1421, 1420t
Vasopressin (antidiuretic hormone), elevated, postoperative fluid therapy and, 1630
VATS. *See* Video-assisted thoracic surgery (VATS)
Vecuronium, for induction of anesthesia, 608t
Vegetative state, persistent, 151
Vena cava
  inferior, traumatic injury to, 442-443, 443f
  operative exposure of, in abdominal injury, 406-408, 407f, 409f
Venom, coagulopathy due to, 87
Venous access, in trauma resuscitation, 35, 36f
Venous blood gas(es)
  in cardiac arrest, 22
  mixed
    in cardiac arrest, 22
    continuous monitoring of, 1385
    pulmonary arterial catheterization for, 1384-1386, 1385f
Venous blood pH, in cardiac arrest, 22
Venous catheter(s), central. *See* Central venous catheterization
Venous injury(ies), of extremities, 466
Venous pressure, central. *See* Central venous pressure
Venous stasis ulcers, in obesity, 1009-1010, 1010f
Venous thrombosis. *See under* Thrombophlebitis; Thrombosis
Ventilation. *See also* Breathing; Respiration
  absence of, verification of, 3
  alveolar minute (V_A), 1415
  assisted
    bag-valve-mask, 8-9, 10f
    gastric insufflation due to, 7, 8f
    mouth-to-mouth, 7-8, 8f
      gastric insufflation and, 7
    Sellick maneuver for, 7, 8f
  in burn care
    in early postresuscitation period, 479
    in immediate resuscitation period, 49-54
  insufficient, shock in, 68
  mechanical. *See* Mechanical ventilation
  mechanics of, 1415-1416
    lung movement and, 1415-1416
    maintenance of open alveoli and, 1415
  postoperative, 1047
  stimulus to breath and, 1415
  minute (V_E), 1415, 1423
    in burn patients, 491
  oxygenation *vs.*, 1423
  parameters of, 1415-1416, 1416t
Ventilation-perfusion (V/Q) ratio
  average, 1418
  mismatched, 1418-1419, 1418t
  P_aO_2 for, 1423
  in positive pressure ventilation, 1418
Ventilator(s), mechanical. *See* Mechanical ventilator(s)
Ventilator-associated nosocomial pneumonia, 1649
Ventilatory compliance, decreased, causes of, 1419, 1420t
Ventricle
  left. *See under* Left ventricular
  right. *See under* Right ventricular
Ventricular compliance, pulmonary arterial wedge pressure and, 1383
Ventricular contraction. *See also* Shock, ICU management of
Ventricular dysrhythmia(s), in pulmonary arterial catheterization, 1379
Ventricular fibrillation
  management of, 10-11
    antiarrhythmic drugs for, 10-11
    antifibrillatory agents for, 11
    in CPR, 10-11
    electrical defibrillation for, 10, 11f
    epinephrine for, 21
    in monitored setting, 3

in refractory fibrillation, 11
median-frequency analysis of, 22-23
Ventricular muscle (Purkinje) action potential, 24-25, 25f
Ventricular tachycardia, management of, in CPR, 10-11
Verapamil
  for acute dysrhythmias, after resuscitation, 15
  classification of, 23
Vertebral artery injury, 387-391
  distal, angiographic embolization of, 392
  exposure and exploration in, 388-389, 389f-390f
  management of, 389f
  treatment of, 389-391, 390f-391f
Vibrio cholerae infection, antimicrobial agents for, 1198t
Vibrio infection, in necrotizing fasciitis, 326
Vibrio vulnificus infection, antimicrobial agents for, 1198t
Vidarabine, for herpesvirus infections, 1328-1329
Video-assisted thoracic surgery (VATS), 673-686
  argon beam coagulator for, 676
  for bullous disease, 679-680
  cost of, 684
  dissecting clamps for, 676, 676f
  endoscopes for, 674, 674f
  for esophagectomy, 681-682, 682f
  forceps for, 675-676, 676f
  incisions with, 676, 677f
  indications and contraindications for, 673t
  instrumentation for, 674-676
  lasers for, 676, 676f
  for lobectomy and pneumonectomy, 680
  lung clamps for, 675, 675f
  for mediastinal mass, 683, 683f
  for mediastinal node dissection, 680-681
  miscellaneous uses for, 684
  operative technique for, 676-684
  patient preparation and intraoperative care for, 673-674
  for pericardial window, 682-683, 683f
  for pleural disease, 676-678
  for pulmonary wedge section, 678-679, 678f
  retractors for, 675, 675f
  scissors for, 676, 676f
  for spontaneous pneumothorax, 679-680
  staplers for, 674-675, 675f
  for sympathectomy, 683-684
  training and certification in, 684-685
  trocars for accessing pleural space, 674, 675f
  video equipment for, 674
Vincent stomatitis, antimicrobial agents for, 1198t
Viral infection, 1309-1332. See also specific infections, e.g., Hepatitis
  Algorithm, 1310-1311
  prevention of transmission of, 1309-1313
  from health care workers to patients, 1312-1313

from patients to health care workers, 1309-1312
of surgical interest, epidemiology of, 1319
Virus(es)
  classification of, 1317
  identification of, 1317-1319
    antigen detection for, 1319
    electron microscopy for, 1319
    histologic examination for, 1319, 1319f
    isolation for, 1318, 1318f
    serologic tests for, 1317-1318
    viral nucleic acid detection for, 1319
  size and structure of, 1317, 1318f
Vital capacity (V_C), definition of, 1415-1416
Vital sign(s), in infants and neonates, 1121, 1121t
Vitamin(s)
  for elderly patient, 1108
  requirements for
    in burn patients, 501
    in ICU patient, 1525, 1524t
    safety levels for, 1525, 1526t
  for stress, in surgical patients, 1524t, 1525
Vitamin A
  requirements for, in ICU patient, 1524t
  wound healing and, 136
Vitamin B_{12}, requirements for, in ICU patient, 1524t
Vitamin C
  requirements for, in ICU patient, 1524t
  wound healing and, 136
Vitamin D
  requirements for, in ICU patient, 1524t
  wound healing and, 136
Vitamin E
  requirements for, in ICU patient, 1524t
  wound healing and, 136
Vitamin K, requirements for, in ICU patient, 1524t
Volvulus
  cecal
    abdominal radiography in, 268, 271f
    operative therapy in, 273-274
  sigmoid
    abdominal radiography in, 268, 270f
    operative therapy in
      elective, 276-277
      immediate, 273-274
    in pregnancy, 1151
  small bowel, operative therapy in, 273-274
Vomiting. See Nausea and vomiting
von Willebrand disease, 80, 86
Vulvovaginal candidiasis, 1299

W

Warfarin, 1025-1026
  coagulopathy due to, 81, 87
  complications of, 1026
  dosage for, 1025
  drug interactions with, 1026, 1026t
  recommendations for use of, 1025t
  for thromboembolic prophylaxis,

1034
Water. See also under Fluid
  body. See Body water
Water intoxication, hyponatremia in, 104
Water moccasin bite(s), 126-127
Web space infection, of hand, 1283, 1284f
Weight, body
  in burn patient, 57
  as indication for nutritional support, 1521, 1521f
  of infants and neonates, 1121
  for total body water content, 1631
Weight loss, after gastric procedures for morbid obesity, 732
Weinberg pyloroplasty, 718-719, 718f
Wernicke encephalopathy. See Wernicke-Korsakoff syndrome
Wernicke-Korsakoff syndrome, in glucose load, 146
Whipple procedure (pancreaticoduodenectomy), pylorus-preserving, 773-776, 773f-776f
White blood cell count
  in acute abdominal pain, 235
  in burn patient, 57
White cell(s), in hemostasis, 85
Wilson disease, acute hepatic failure in, 1458
Wound(s)
  bite. See Bite(s)
  bullet. See Bullet wound(s)
  contracture of, burn wound rehabilitation and, 1694
  dehiscence of, ultrasonography in, 663, 663f
  dirty and infected. See also Wound infection
  in metabolic response to critical illness, 1495-1498, 1503, 1504f
  non-tetanus-prone, 121, 121t, 124t
  tetanus-prone, 121, 121t, 124t
Wound care
  acute, 121-141. See also Trauma
    Algorithm, 122-123
    antibiotic prophylaxis in, 121-124
    dressings for, 130-131
    method of closure for, 127-130
      direct approximation as, 127-128
      flaps for, 130
      materials for, 128-129
      skin grafts for, 129. See also Skin graft(s)
    tetanus prophylaxis in, 121, 124t
    timing of closure for, 124-127
      in animal bites, 126-127
      in bacterial contamination, 125-126
      in excessive bleeding, 124
      in foreign-body presence, 124-125
      in necrosis, 125
      in noncontaminated wounds, 124
      in puncture wounds, 124
      in small or superficial wounds, 124
  in burns. See Burn wound care
  in complicated wound, infection. See Wound infection
  in infected wound. See Wound

infection
  in obesity, 1007
  in toxic epidermal necrolysis, 513, 513t
Wound healing, 131-138, 985-986
  angiogenesis in, 132, 133t
  cytokines in, 133t, 134-135
  disturbances of, 135-138
    aging as, 137
    alcoholism as, 137
    cancer as, 136-137
    chemotherapy use as, 137
    diabetes mellitus as, 137
    hypertrophic scars as, 138
    hypoxia as, 136
    immunosuppressant use as, 137
    infection as, 135-136
    irradiation as, 136
    jaundice as, 137-138
    keloids as, 138
    liver failure as, 137-138
    local factors as, 135-136, 135t
    malnutrition as, 136
    smoking as, 136
    steroid use as, 137
    systemic factors as, 135t, 136-138
    uremia as, 137
  in elderly patients, 1113-1114
  epithelialization in, 132-133
  hemostasis in, 131
  inflammation in, 131, 132f
  late phase: scar remodeling in, 132f, 134, 134f
  metabolic responses to, 1503, 1504f
  migratory phase of, 132-133, 132f, 133t
  in multiple organ dysfunction syndrome, 1481
  in occult infection, 1167
  oxygenation in, 1495
  proliferative phase: collagen synthesis in, 132f, 133-134
  in renal failure, 1056
  tissue perfusion in, 1495
  tumor necrosis factor effects on, 1603, 1606
  wound contraction in, 134
Wound infection. *See also* Surgical site infection
  candidal, 1298-1299
  clinical and laboratory diagnosis of, 1170
  definition of, 125
  in diabetes mellitus, 999
  in immunosuppressed transplant recipients, 1076
  in infants and neonates, 1128
  nosocomial, 1221, 1224
    clostridial, 1224
    composite risk indices for, 1718
    host risk factors for, 1718, 1718t
    invasive and necrotizing, 1224
    NNIS risk index for, 1718
    operative risk factors for, 1718
    preventive measures for, 1718-1719
      antiseptics, 1719
      disinfectants, 1719
      hair removal, 1719
      hand hygiene, 1719. *See also* Handwashing
      interventional procedures and, 1719
      patient care assessment in, 1719
    risk factors for, 1717-1718
    SENIC risk index for, 1718
    treatment of, 1224

X

Xanthine oxidase, endothelial, in intracellular signaling, 1580
Xanthomonas maltophilia, antimicrobial agents for, 1198t
X-ray. *See* Radiograph(s)

Y

Yersinia enterocolitica infection, antimicrobial agents for, 1198t
Yersinia pestis infection, antimicrobial agents for, 1198t

Z

Zileuton
  for inflammatory conditions, 1600
  for ulcerative colitis, 1600
Zinc
  in central venous nutritional support, 1532
  deficiency, in elderly patient, 1108
  requirements for, in ICU patient, 1525t
  wound healing and, 136
Zygoma, fracture of, 371f, 375
Zygomycosis (mucormycosis), 1299-1300